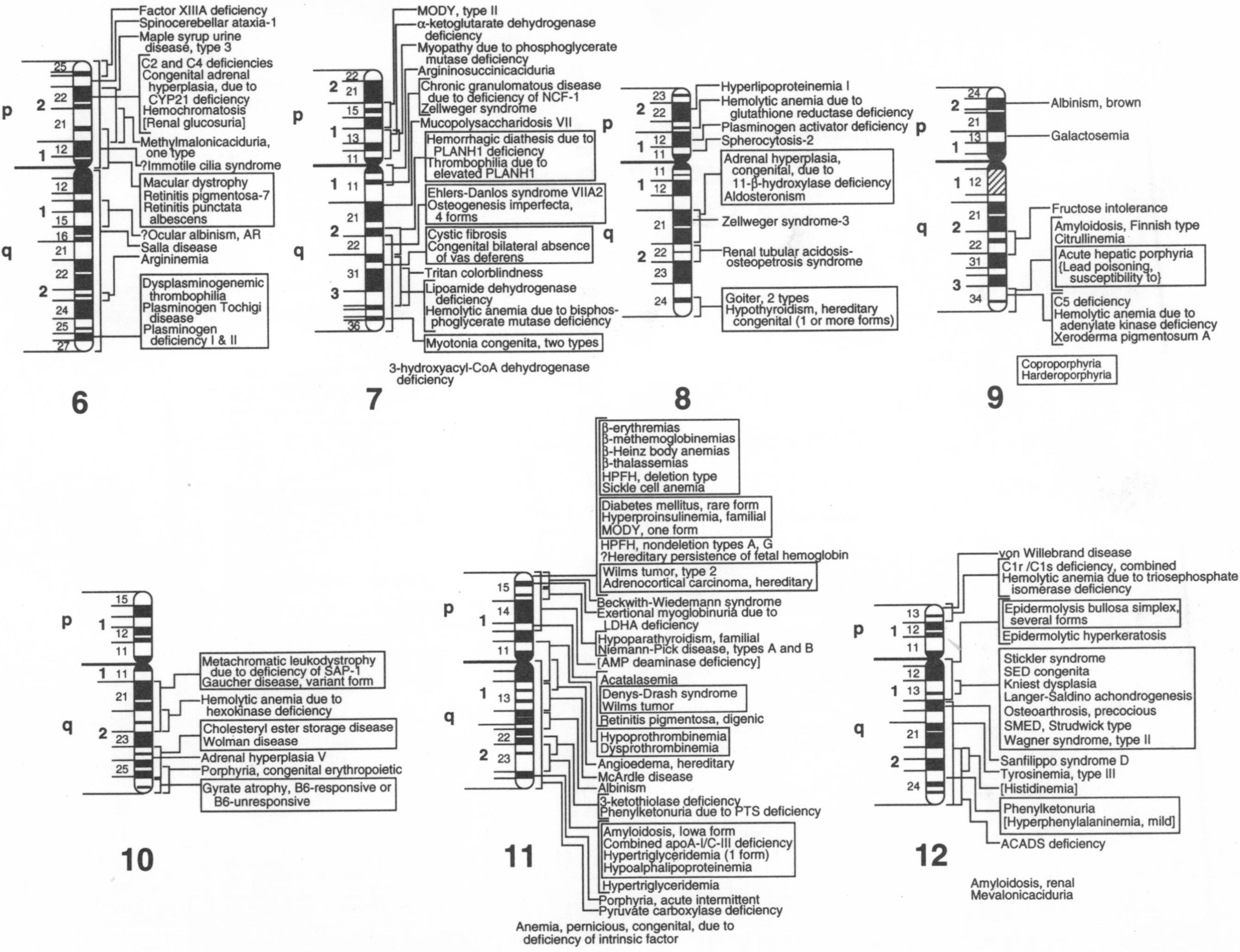

Factor XIIIA deficiency
Spinocerebellar ataxia-1
Maple syrup urine disease, type 3
C2 and C4 deficiencies
Congenital adrenal hyperplasia, due to CYP21 deficiency
Hemochromatosis
[Renal glucosuria]
Methylmalonicaciduria, one type
?Immotile cilia syndrome
Macular dystrophy
Retinitis pigmentosa-7
Retinitis punctata albescens
?Ocular albinism, AR
Salla disease
Argininemia
Dysplasminogenemic thrombophilia
Plasminogen Tochigi disease
Plasminogen deficiency I & II
6
MODY, type II
α-ketoglutarate dehydrogenase deficiency
Myopathy due to phosphoglycerate mutase deficiency
Argininosuccinicaciduria
Chronic granulomatous disease due to deficiency of NCF-1
Zellweger syndrome
Mucopolysaccharidosis VII
Hemorrhagic diathesis due to PLANH1 deficiency
Thrombophilia due to elevated PLANH1
Ehlers-Danlos syndrome VIIA2
Osteogenesis imperfecta, 4 forms
Cystic fibrosis
Congenital bilateral absence of vas deferens
Tritan colorblindness
Lipoamide dehydrogenase deficiency
Hemolytic anemia due to bisphosphoglycerate mutase deficiency
Myotonia congenita, two types
3-hydroxyacyl-CoA dehydrogenase deficiency
7
Hyperlipoproteinemia I
Hemolytic anemia due to glutathione reductase deficiency
Plasminogen activator deficiency
Spherocytosis-2
Adrenal hyperplasia, congenital, due to 11-β-hydroxylase deficiency
Aldosteronism
Zellweger syndrome-3
Renal tubular acidosis-osteopetrosis syndrome
Goiter, 2 types
Hypothyroidism, hereditary congenital (1 or more forms)
8
Albinism, brown
Galactosemia
Fructose intolerance
Amyloidosis, Finnish type
Citrullinemia
Acute hepatic porphyria
{Lead poisoning, susceptibility to}
C5 deficiency
Hemolytic anemia due to adenylate kinase deficiency
Xeroderma pigmentosum A
Coproporphyria
Harderoporphyria
9
Metachromatic leukodystrophy due to deficiency of SAP-1
Gaucher disease, variant form
Hemolytic anemia due to hexokinase deficiency
Cholesteryl ester storage disease
Wolman disease
Adrenal hyperplasia V
Porphyria, congenital erythropoietic
Gyrate atrophy, B6-responsive or B6-unresponsive
10
β-erythremias
β-methemoglobinemias
β-Heinz body anemias
β-thalassemias
HPFH, deletion type
Sickle cell anemia
Diabetes mellitus, rare form
Hyperproinsulinemia, familial
MODY, one form
HPFH, nondeletion types A, G
?Hereditary persistence of fetal hemoglobin
Wilms tumor, type 2
Adrenocortical carcinoma, hereditary
Beckwith-Wiedemann syndrome
Exertional myoglobinuria due to LDHA deficiency
Hypoparathyroidism, familial
Niemann-Pick disease, types A and B
[AMP deaminase deficiency]
Acatalasemia
Denys-Drash syndrome
Wilms tumor
Retinitis pigmentosa, digenic
Hypoprothrombinemia
Dysprothrombinemia
Angioedema, hereditary
McArdle disease
Albinism
3-ketothiolase deficiency
Phenylketonuria due to PTS deficiency
Amyloidosis, Iowa form
Combined apoA-I/C-III deficiency
Hypertriglyceridemia (1 form)
Hypoalphalipoproteinemia
Hypertriglyceridemia
Porphyria, acute intermittent
Pyruvate carboxylase deficiency
Anemia, pernicious, congenital, due to deficiency of intrinsic factor
11
von Willebrand disease
C1r /C1s deficiency, combined
Hemolytic anemia due to triosephosphate isomerase deficiency
Epidermolysis bullosa simplex, several forms
Epidermolytic hyperkeratosis
Stickler syndrome
SED congenita
Kniest dysplasia
Langer-Saldino achondrogenesis
Osteoarthrosis, precocious
SMED, Strudwick type
Wagner syndrome, type II
Sanfilippo syndrome D
Tyrosinemia, type III
[Histidinemia]
Phenylketonuria
[Hyperphenylalaninemia, mild]
ACADS deficiency
Amyloidosis, renal
Mevalonicaciduria
12

(Continued)

SEVENTH EDITION

THE METABOLIC AND MOLECULAR BASES OF INHERITED DISEASE

EDITORS

Charles R. Scriver, M.D.C.M.

Alva Professor of Human Genetics and Professor of Biology and Pediatrics, McGill University, Montreal, Quebec, Canada

Arthur L. Beaudet, M.D.

Investigator, Howard Hughes Medical Institute; Professor, Departments of Molecular and Human Genetics, Pediatrics, and Cell Biology, Baylor College of Medicine, Houston, Texas

William S. Sly, M.D.

Alice A. Doisy Professor of Biochemistry and Molecular Biology and Professor of Pediatrics; Chair, Edward A. Doisy Department of Biochemistry and Molecular Biology, St. Louis University School of Medicine, St. Louis, Missouri

David Valle, M.D.

Investigator, Howard Hughes Medical Institute; Professor of Pediatrics, Medicine, Ophthalmology, and Molecular Biology and Genetics, The Johns Hopkins University School of Medicine, Baltimore, Maryland

CONSULTING EDITORS

John B. Stanbury, M.D.

James B. Wyngaarden, M.D.

Donald S. Fredrickson, M.D.

SEVENTH EDITION

THE METABOLIC AND MOLECULAR BASES OF INHERITED DISEASE

VOLUME III

EDITORS

Charles R. Scriver, M.D.C.M.
Arthur L. Beaudet, M.D.
William S. Sly, M.D.
David Valle, M.D.

CONSULTING EDITORS

John B. Stanbury, M.D.
James B. Wyngaarden, M.D.
Donald S. Fredrickson, M.D.

McGraw-Hill, Inc.
Health Professions Division

New York St. Louis San Francisco Auckland Bogotá Caracas Lisbon London Madrid Mexico City Milan Montreal New Delhi San Juan Singapore Sydney Tokyo Toronto

THE METABOLIC AND MOLECULAR BASES OF INHERITED DISEASE, 7/e

1234567890 KGPKGP 987654

ISBN 0-07-909826-6 (set)
0-07-060729-X (vol. 1)
0-07-060730-3 (vol. 2)
0-07-060731-1 (vol. 3)
This book was set in Times Roman by Monotype Composition Company, Inc.
The editors were J. Dereck Jeffers, Gail Gavert, Mariapaz Ramos Englis, and Peter McCurdy;
the production supervisor was Richard Ruzycka; Barbara Littlewood prepared the index;
the designer was José R. Fonfrias.
Quebecor Printing/Kingsport, Inc. was printer and binder.
This book is printed on acid-free paper.

Library of Congress Cataloging-in-Publication Data

The metabolic and molecular bases of inherited disease / editors,
Charles R. Scriver . . . [et al.] ; consulting editors, John B.
Stanbury, James B. Wyngaarden, Donald S. Fredrickson.—7th ed.
p. cm.
Rev. ed. of: The metabolic basis of inherited disease. 6th ed.
c 1989.
Includes bibliographical references.
ISBN 0-07-909826-6
1. Metabolism, Inborne errors of. 2. Medical genetics.
3. Pathology, Molecular. I. Scriver, Charles R. II. Title:
Metabolic basis of inherited disease.
[DNLM: 1. Hereditary Diseases. 2. Metabolic Diseases.
3. Metabolism, Inborn Errors. WD 200 M5865 1995]
RC627.8.M47 1995
616.3′9042—dc20
DNLM/DLC
for Library of Congress 94-29426

NOTICE

Medicine is an ever-changing science. As new research and clinical experience broaden our knowledge, changes in treatment and drug therapy are required. The editors and the publisher of this work have checked with sources believed to be reliable in their efforts to provide information that is complete and generally in accord with the standards accepted at the time of publication. However, in view of the possibility of human error or changes in medical sciences, neither the editors nor the publisher nor any other party who has been involved in the preparation or publication of this work warrants that the information contained herein is in every respect accurate or complete, and they are not responsible for any errors or omissions or for the results obtained from use of such information. Readers are encouraged to confirm the information contained herein with other sources. For example and in particular, readers are advised to check the product information sheet included in the package of each drug they plan to administer to be certain that the information contained in this book is accurate and that changes have not been made in the recommended dose or in the contraindications for administration. This recommendation is of particular importance in connection with new or infrequently used drugs.

CONTENTS

PART 2
Cancer and Genetics

PART 3
Chromosomes and Autosomes

PART 4

Carbohydrates

PART 5

Amino Acids

PART 6

Organic Acids

VOLUME II

PART 7
Purines and Pyrimidines

PART 8

Lipoprotein and Lipid Metabolism Disorders

PART 9

Porphyrins and Heme

PART 13

Hormones: Synthesis and Action

PART 19

Muscle

PART 20

Eye

PART 21
Skin

PART 22
Intestine

PART 23
Neurogenetics

PART 24
Significant Developments in Progress

CONTRIBUTORS

Milton B. Adesnik, Ph.D. [8]*
Professor, Department of Cell Biology, New York University School of Medicine, New York, New York

Björn A. Afzelius, Ph.D. [131]
Professor, Wenner-Gren Institute, Stockholm University, Stockholm, Sweden

Robert J. Alpern, M.D. [121]
Professor of Medicine; Chief, Division of Nephrology, University of Texas Southwestern Medical Center, Dallas, Texas

Joanna S. Amberger, B.A. [1]
Research Coordinator II, Center for Medical Genetics, The Johns Hopkins University School of Medicine, Baltimore, Maryland

Donald C. Anderson, M.D. [132]
Professor of Pediatrics and Cell Biology, Baylor College of Medicine, Houston, Texas; Executive Director, Discovery Research, Upjohn Laboratories, Kalamazoo, Michigan

Thomas E. Andreoli, M.D. [98]
Professor and Chair, Department of Internal Medicine, University of Arkansas for Medical Sciences, Little Rock, Arkansas

Generoso Andria, M.D. [91]
Professor of Pediatrics, Department of Pediatrics, University of Naples, Naples, Italy

Stylianos E. Antonarakis, M.D. [3, 106]
Director, Division of Medical Genetics, University of Geneva School of Medicine, Geneva, Switzerland; Professor, Center for Medical Genetics, The Johns Hopkins University School of Medicine, Baltimore, Maryland

Irwin M. Arias, M.D. [67]
Professor and Chair, Department of Physiology; Professor of Medicine, Tufts University Medical School, Boston, Massachusetts

Gerd Assmann, M.D. [60, 64, 82]
Director, Institute for Clinical Chemistry and Laboratory Medicine, Central Laboratory; Director, Institute for Arteriosclerosis Research, Westphalian-Wilhelms University, Münster, Germany

*The numbers in brackets following each contributor's name refer to chapters written or co-written by that contributor.

Pertti P. Aula, M.D. [126]
Associate Professor of Medical Genetics, University of Turku, Turku, Finland

Salvatore Auricchio, M.D. [151]
Professor and Chair of Pediatrics, Department of Pediatrics and Faculty of Medicine, University of Naples, Naples, Italy

Andrea Ballabio, M.D. [20, 96, 154]
Associate Professor, Department of Molecular and Human Genetics, Baylor College of Medicine, Houston, Texas

Douglas J. Barrett, M.D. [128]
Professor of Pediatrics, Immunology and Pathology; Chair, Department of Pediatrics, College of Medicine, University of Florida, Gainesville, Florida

Arthur L. Beaudet, M.D. [1, 81, 127, 154]
Investigator, Howard Hughes Medical Institute; Professor, Departments of Molecular and Human Genetics, Pediatrics, and Cell Biology, Baylor College of Medicine, Houston, Texas

Michael A. Becker, M.D. [49]
Professor of Medicine and Chief, Rheumatology Section, Department of Medicine, University of Chicago, Chicago, Illinois

Pamela S. Becker, M.D., Ph.D. [115]
Assistant Professor of Medicine and Cell Biology, Division of Hematology-Oncology, University of Massachusetts Medical Center, Worcester, Massachusetts

David M. O. Becroft, M.D. [55]
Department of Obstetrics and Gynaecology, University of Auckland School of Medicine, Auckland, New Zealand

Merrill D. Benson, M.D. [139]
Professor of Medicine, Medical and Molecular Genetics, Indiana University School of Medicine, Indianapolis, Indiana

Michel Bergeron, M.D. [122]
Professeur titulaire, Département de physiologie, Faculté de médecine, Université de Montréal, Montréal, Québec, Canada

Gerard T. Berry, M.D. [25]
Associate Professor, Department of Pediatrics, University of Pennsylvania School of Medicine; Division of Biochemical Development and Molecular Diseases, The Children's Hospital of Philadelphia, Philadelphia, Pennsylvania

Ernest Beutler, M.D. [86]
Chair, Department of Molecular and Experimental Medicine, The Scripps Research Institute; Clinical Professor of Medicine, University of California, La Jolla, California

Ingemar Björkhem, M.D., Ph.D. [65]
Professor, Department of Clinical Chemistry, Karolinska Institutet, Huddinge University Hospital, Huddinge, Sweden

R. Michael Blaese, M.D. [129]
Chief, Clinical Gene Therapy Branch, National Center for Human Genome Research, National Institutes of Health, Bethesda, Maryland

Thomas F. Boat, M.D. [127]
Professor and Chair, Department of Pediatrics, University of Cincinnati College of Medicine; Director, Children's Hospital Research Foundation, Children's Hospital Medical Center, Cincinnati, Ohio

Kirsten Muri Boberg, M.D., Ph.D. [65]
Department of Clinical Chemistry, University of Oslo, Rikshospitalet, Oslo, Norway

Thomas H. Bothwell, M.D. [69]
Dean and Emeritus Professor of Medicine, Faculty of Medicine, University of the Witwatersrand Medical School, Johannesburg, South Africa

Jan L. Breslow, M.D. [63]
Frederick Henry Leonhardt Professor; Director, Laboratory of Biochemical Genetics and Metabolism, The Rockefeller University, New York, New York

H. Bryan Brewer, Jr., M.D. [64]
Chief, Molecular Disease Branch, National Heart, Lung, and Blood Institute, Bethesda, Maryland

Garrett M. Brodeur, M.D. [15]
Professor of Pediatrics, University of Pennsylvania; Director, Basic Oncology Research, The Children's Hospital of Philadelphia, Philadelphia, Pennsylvania

Michael H. Brooke, M.B., B.Ch. [140]
Director, Division of Neurology, University of Alberta, Edmonton, Alberta, Canada

Michael S. Brown, M.D. [62]
Paul J. Thomas Professor of Genetics and Director, Center for Genetic Diseases; Department of Molecular Genetics, University of Texas Southwestern Medical Center, Dallas, Texas

John D. Brunzell, M.D. [59]
Professor of Medicine, Division of Metabolism, Endocrinology and Nutrition, University of Washington, Seattle, Washington

Saul W. Brusilow, M.D. [32]
Professor of Pediatrics, The Johns Hopkins University School of Medicine, Baltimore, Maryland

Ann Burchell, Ph.D. [24]
Reader and Lister Institute Research Fellow, Ninewells Hospital and Medical School, University of Dundee, Dundee, Scotland

Joseph L. Butler, M.D. [128]
Private Practice, Allergy and Clinical Immunology, Birmingham, Alabama

Peter H. Byers, M.D. [134]
Professor, Departments of Pathology and Medicine (Medical Genetics), University of Washington, Seattle, Washington

C. Thomas Caskey, M.D. [50]
Investigator, Howard Hughes Medical Institute; Professor and Chair, Department of Molecular and Human Genetics, Baylor College of Medicine, Houston, Texas

Webster K. Cavenee, Ph.D. [11]
Director, Ludwig Institute for Cancer Research–San Diego Branch; Professor, Department of Medicine, University of California-San Diego School of Medicine, La Jolla, California

Shu Jin Chan, Ph.D. [22]
Senior Research Associate, Howard Hughes Medical Institute, University of Chicago, Chicago, Illinois

Robert W. Charlton, M.D. [69]
Vice-Chancellor and Principal, University of the Witwatersrand, Johannesburg, South Africa

Lawrence R. Charnas, M.D., Ph.D. [123]
Senior Staff Fellow, Human Genetics Branch, National Institute of Child Health and Human Development, Bethesda, Maryland

Christiane Charpentier, Ph.D. [5]
Assistant Researcher, Department of Biochemistry, Hôpital Necker Enfants Malades, Paris, France

Yuan-Tsong Chen, M.D., Ph.D. [24]
Professor of Pediatrics; Chief, Division of Medical Genetics, Duke University Medical Center, Durham, North Carolina

Russell W. Chesney, M.D. [120]
Le Bonheur Professor and Chair, Department of Pediatrics, University of Tennessee, Memphis, Tennessee

Barton Childs, M.D. [2]
Emeritus Professor of Pediatrics, The Johns Hopkins University School of Medicine, Baltimore, Maryland

David T. Chuang, Ph.D. [34]
Associate Professor, Department of Biochemistry, University of Texas Southwestern Medical Center, Dallas, Texas

Dominic W. Chung, Ph.D. [105]
Research Associate Professor, Department of Biochemistry, University of Washington, Seattle, Washington

Joe T. R. Clarke, M.D., Ph.D. [92]
Professor, Department of Genetics, The Hospital for Sick Children, Toronto, Ontario, Canada

James E. Cleaver, Ph.D. [148]
Professor of Radiology; Associate Director, Laboratory of Radiobiology and Environmental Health, University of California, San Francisco, California

John B. Clegg, M.A., Ph.D. [113]
Reader in Molecular Haematology, M.R.C. Molecular Haematology Unit, Institute of Molecular Medicine, University of Oxford, John Radcliffe Hospital, Oxford, England

Paul M. Coates, Ph.D. [45]
Research Professor, Department of Pediatrics, University of Pennsylvania School of Medicine, Philadelphia, Pennsylvania

Francis S. Collins, M.D., Ph.D. [14]
Director, National Center for Human Genome Research, National Institutes of Health, Bethesda, Maryland

Harvey R. Colten, M.D. [130]
Harriet B. Spoehrer Professor and Chair, Department of Pediatrics, Washington University School of Medicine, St. Louis, Missouri

David N. Cooper, B.Sc., Ph.D. [3]
Senior Lecturer in Molecular Genetics, Charter Molecular Genetics Laboratory, Thrombosis Research Institute, London, England

Max D. Cooper, M.D. [128]
Investigator, Howard Hughes Medical Institute; Professor of Medicine, Pediatrics and Microbiology, Division of Developmental and Clinical Immunology, Departments of Medicine and Pediatrics, University of Alabama at Birmingham, Birmingham, Alabama

David R. Cox, M.D., Ph.D. [6]
Professor, Departments of Genetics and Pediatrics, Stanford University School of Medicine, Stanford, California

Diane Wilson Cox, Ph.D. [138]
Professor, Departments of Paediatrics and of Molecular and Medical Genetics, University of Toronto; Senior Scientist, Research Institute, The Hospital for Sick Children, Toronto, Ontario, Canada

Rody P. Cox, M.D. [33]
Professor of Internal Medicine, University of Texas Southwestern Medical Center at Dallas, Dallas, Texas

Donnell J. Creel, Ph.D. [147]
Research Professor, Departments of Ophthalmology and Anatomy, University of Utah; Research Career Scientist, Veterans' Administration Medical Center, Salt Lake City, Utah

Frans P.M. Cremers, Ph.D. [145]
Assistant Professor, Department of Human Genetics, University Hospital Nijmegen, Nijmegen, The Netherlands

John T. Curnutte, M.D., Ph.D. [133]
Director, Immunology Department, Genentech, Inc., South San Francisco, California

Joseph Dancis, M.D. [33]
Professor, Department of Pediatrics, New York University School of Medicine, New York, New York

David M. Danks, M.D. [68]
Director, Murdoch Institute for Research into Birth Defects, Royal Children's Hospital; Professor of Paediatric Research, University of Melbourne, Melbourne, Australia

Christopher J. Danpure, Ph.D. [75]
Head, M.R.C. Protein Translocation Group, Department of Biology, University College London, London, England

Earl W. Davie, Ph.D. [104]
Professor of Biochemistry, University of Washington, Seattle, Washington

Alessandra d'Azzo, Ph.D. [91]
Associate Member, Department of Genetics, St. Jude Children's Research Hospital, Memphis, Tennessee

Samir S. Deeb, Ph.D. [143]
Research Professor of Medicine, Adjunct Professor of Genetics, University of Washington, Seattle, Washington

Jehan-François Desjeux, M.D. [116]
Professor, Conservatoire National des Arts et Métiers; Director, Research Unit on Intestinal Functions, Metabolism and Nutrition, Institut National de la Santé et de la Recherche Médicale, Paris, France

Robert J. Desnick, Ph.D., M.D. [80, 84, 89]
Arthur J. and Nellie Z. Cohen Professor of Pediatrics and Human Genetics; Chair, Department of Human Genetics, Mount Sinai School of Medicine, New York, New York

Patricia A. Donohoue, M.D. [94]
Associate Professor of Pediatrics, University of Iowa College of Medicine, Iowa City, Iowa

Thaddeus P. Dryja, M.D. [144]
Professor of Ophthalmology, Harvard Medical School, Massachusetts Eye and Ear Infirmary, Boston, Massachusetts

Thomas D. DuBose, Jr., M.D. [121]
Professor of Medicine, Physiology and Cell Biology; Director, Division of Nephrology, University of Texas Medical School at Houston, Houston, Texas

Jacques E. Dumont, M.D., Ph.D. [93]
Professor of Biochemistry; Head, Institut de Recherche Interdisciplinaire, Faculté de Médecine, Université Libre de Bruxelles, Brussels, Belgium

John W. Eaton, Ph.D. [74]
Director, Division of Experimental Pathology; Professor of Pathology and Laboratory Medicine and of Biochemistry and Molecular Biology; Albany Medical College, Albany, New York

Randy C. Eisensmith, Ph.D. [27]
Research Assistant Professor, Department of Cell Biology, Baylor College of Medicine, Houston, Texas

Christine M. Eng, M.D. [89]
Assistant Professor, Departments of Human Genetics and Pediatrics, Mount Sinai School of Medicine, New York, New York

Charles J. Epstein, M.D. [18]
Professor of Pediatrics, University of California, San Francisco, California

Wayne A. Fenton, Ph.D. [41, 102]
Research Scientist, Department of Genetics, Yale University School of Medicine, New Haven, Connecticut

Malcolm A. Ferguson-Smith, M.B., Ch.B., D.Sc. [17]
Professor, Department of Pathology, University of Cambridge, Cambridge, England

Gebhard Flatz, M.D. [150]
Professor Emeritus of Human Genetics, Medizinische Hochschule, Hanover, Germany

Arvan L. Fluharty, Ph.D. [88]
Professor, Department of Psychiatry and Behavioral Sciences, Mental Retardation Research Center, University of California School of Medicine, Los Angeles, California

John R. Forehand, M.D. [133]
Director, Southern Appalachian Center for Pulmonary Studies, Richlands, Virginia

Frank E. Frerman, Ph.D. [42, 47]
Professor of Pediatrics, University of Colorado School of Medicine, Denver, Colorado

Elaine Fuchs, Ph.D. [149]
Investigator, Howard Hughes Medical Institute; Amgen Professor of Basic Sciences, Department of Molecular Genetics and Cell Biology, University of Chicago, Chicago, Illinois

Lars Fugger, M.D., Ph.D. [9]
Postdoctoral Fellow, Department of Microbiology and Immunology, Stanford University School of Medicine, Stanford, California

Werner Fürst, Ph.D. [76]
Boehringer Mannheim GmbH, Penzberg, Germany

William A. Gahl, M.D., Ph.D. [126]
Chief, Human Genetics Branch, National Institute of Child Health and Human Development, National Institutes of Health, Bethesda, Maryland

Richard A. Galbraith, M.D., Ph.D. [66]
Associate Professor, Medical Director and Physician, The Rockefeller University, New York, New York

Hans Galjaard, M.D., Ph.D. [91]
Professor of Cell Biology, Erasmus University; Chair, Department of Clinical Genetics, University Hospital, Rotterdam, The Netherlands

K. Michael Gibson, Ph.D. [38]
Associate Professor of Biomedical Studies; Senior Research Scientist, Kimberly H. Courtwright and Joseph W. Summers Metabolic Disease Center and Baylor Research Institute, Baylor University Medical Center, Dallas, Texas

Richard Gitzelmann, M.D. [23]
Professor, Division of Metabolism, Department of Pediatrics, University of Zurich, Kinderspital Zurich, Zurich, Switzerland

Egil Gjone, M.D. [60]
Professor of Internal Medicine, University of Oslo, Rikshospitalet, Oslo, Norway

John A. Glomset, M.D. [60]
Investigator, Howard Hughes Medical Institute; Professor of Medicine and Biochemistry, University of Washington, Seattle, Washington

Maurice Godfrey, Ph.D. [135]
Assistant Professor of Pediatrics, University of Nebraska Medical Center, Omaha, Nebraska

Joseph L. Goldstein, M.D. [62]
Paul J. Thomas Professor of Genetics and Chair, Department of Molecular Genetics, University of Texas Southwestern Medical Center, Dallas, Texas

Peter N. Goodfellow, B.Sc., D.Phil. [17]
Professor, Department of Genetics, University of Cambridge, Cambridge, England

Stephen I. Goodman, M.D. [42, 47]
Professor of Pediatrics, University of Colorado School of Medicine, Denver, Colorado

André Gougoux, M.D. [122]
Professeur titulaire, Départements de médecine et de physiologie, Université de Montréal, Montréal, Québec, Canada

Gregory A. Grabowski, M.D. [86]
Professor, Departments of Pediatrics, and Molecular Genetics, Biochemistry and Microbiology, University of Cincinnati College of Medicine; Director, Division of Human Genetics, Children's Hospital Medical Center, Cincinnati, Ohio

Denis M. Grant, Ph.D. [4]
Assistant Professor, Departments of Pediatrics and Pharmacology and Faculty of Pharmacy, University of Toronto; Scientist, Division of Clinical Pharmacology and Toxicology Research Institute, The Hospital for Sick Children, Toronto, Ontario, Canada

Roy A. Gravel, Ph.D. [92]
Professor, Departments of Pediatrics and Human Genetics; Scientific Director, McGill University-Montreal Children's Hospital Research Institute, Montreal, Quebec, Canada

Eric D. Green, M.D., Ph.D. [6]
Assistant Professor, Departments of Pathology, Genetics, and Medicine, Washington University School of Medicine, St. Louis, Missouri

James E. Griffin, M.D. [95]
Professor of Internal Medicine, University of Texas Southwestern Medical Center at Dallas, Dallas, Texas

John H. Griffin, Ph.D. [108]
Associate Member, Department of Molecular and Experimental Medicine and of Vascular Biology, The Scripps Research Institute, La Jolla, California

David H. Gutmann, M.D., Ph.D. [14]
Assistant Professor, Departments of Neurology and of Pediatrics and Genetics; Washington University School of Medicine; Co-Director, Neurofibromatosis Program, St. Louis Children's Hospital, St. Louis, Missouri

Daniel A. Haber, M.D., Ph.D. [13]
Assistant Professor of Medicine, Massachusetts General Hospital Cancer Center, Harvard Medical School, Charlestown, Massachusetts

Theodora Hadjistilianou, M.D. [11]
Assistant Professor, Institute of Ophthalmological Sciences, University of Sienna, Sienna, Italy

Judith G. Hall, M.D. [7]
Professor and Chair, Department of Pediatrics, University of British Columbia, British Columbia's Children's Hospital, Vancouver, British Columbia, Canada

Ada Hamosh, M.D., M.P.H. [37]
Assistant Professor of Pediatrics, Center for Medical Genetics, The Johns Hopkins University School of Medicine, Baltimore, Maryland

Peter S. Harper, M.D. [141]
Professor and Consultant in Medical Genetics, Institute of Medical Genetics, University of Wales College of Medicine, Cardiff, Wales

Klaus Harzer, M.D. [76]
Professor, Institut für Hirnforschung der Universität Tübingen, Tübingen, Germany

Richard J. Havel, M.D. [56, 57]
Professor of Medicine, Cardiovascular Research Institute, University of California School of Medicine, San Francisco, California

Michael R. Hayden, M.B., Ch.B., D.Ch., Ph.D. [152]
Professor, Department of Medical Genetics, University of British Columbia, Vancouver, British Columbia, Canada

Vincent J. Hearing, Ph.D. [147]
Senior Investigator, Laboratory of Cell Biology, National Cancer Institute, National Institutes of Health, Bethesda, Maryland

J. Fielding Hejtmancik, M.D., Ph.D. [146]
Medical Officer, Laboratory of Mechanisms of Ocular Diseases, National Eye Institute, National Institutes of Health, Bethesda, Maryland

Michael S. Hershfield, M.D. [52]
Professor of Medicine, Duke University Medical Center, Durham, North Carolina

Howard H. Hiatt, M.D. [26]
Professor of Medicine, Harvard Medical School; Senior Physician, Brigham and Women's Hospital, Boston, Massachusetts

Douglas R. Higgs, M.B., B.S. [113]
Honorary Consultant in Haematology, M.R.C. Molecular Haematology Unit, Institute of Molecular Medicine, University of Oxford, John Radcliffe Hospital, Oxford, England

Rochelle Hirschhorn, M.D. [77]
Professor of Medicine; Chief, Division of Medical Genetics, New York University School of Medicine, New York, New York

Helen H. Hobbs, M.D. [62]
Associate Professor, Departments of Molecular Genetics and Internal Medicine; Head, Division of Medical Genetics, University of Texas Southwestern Medical Center, Dallas, Texas

Edward W. Holmes, M.D. [53]
Professor and Chair, Department of Medicine, University of Pennsylvania Medical Center, Philadelphia, Pennsylvania

Arthur L. Horwich, M.D. [32]
Associate Investigator, Howard Hughes Medical Institute; Associate Professor of Human Genetics and Pediatrics, Yale University School of Medicine, New Haven, Connecticut

David E. Housman, Ph.D. [13]
Professor of Biology, Center for Cancer Research, Massachusetts Institute of Technology, Cambridge, Massachusetts

Peiyi Y. Hu, M.D. [137]
Postdoctoral Fellow, Edward A. Doisy Department of Biochemistry and Molecular Biology, St. Louis University School of Medicine, St. Louis, Missouri

Donald E. Hultquist, Ph.D. [112]
Professor of Biological Chemistry, University of Michigan Medical School, Ann Arbor, Michigan

Akitada Ichinose, M.D., Ph.D. [105]
Professor, Department of Molecular Patho-Biology, Yamagata University, Iida-Nishi, Yamagata, Japan

Yiannis A. Ioannou, Ph.D. [89]
Assistant Professor, Department of Human Genetics, Mount Sinai School of Medicine, New York, New York

Ernst R. Jaffé, M.D. [112]
Distinguished University Professor of Medicine Emeritus, Albert Einstein College of Medicine, Bronx, New York

Jean L. Johnson, Ph.D. [70]
Assistant Research Professor, Department of Biochemistry, Duke University Medical Center, Durham, North Carolina

Michael V. Johnston, M.D. [37]
Professor of Neurology and Pediatrics, The Johns Hopkins University School of Medicine and the Kennedy Krieger Institute, Baltimore, Maryland

Richard B. Johnston, Jr., M.D. [133]
Adjunct Professor of Pediatrics, Yale University School of Medicine, New Haven, Connecticut; Senior Vice President for Programs and Medical Director, March of Dimes Foundation, White Plains, New York

Michael M. Kaback, M.D. [92]
Professor, Departments of Pediatrics and Reproductive Medicine, University of California at San Diego, San Diego, California

Muriel I. Kaiser, M.D. [146]
Chief, Ophthalmic Genetics and Clinical Services Branch, National Eye Institute, National Institutes of Health, Bethesda, Maryland

Werner Kalow, M.D. [4]
Professor Emeritus, Department of Pharmacology, University of Toronto, Toronto, Ontario, Canada

John P. Kane, M.D., Ph.D. [56, 57]
Professor of Medicine; Professor of Biochemistry and Biophysics, University of California School of Medicine, San Francisco, California

Attallah Kappas, M.D. [66]
Sherman Fairchild Professor, Physician-in-Chief Emeritus, The Rockefeller University, New York, New York

Seymour Kaufman, Ph.D. [27]
Chief, Laboratory of Neurochemistry, National Institute of Mental Health, Bethesda, Maryland

Haig H. Kazazian, Jr., M.D. [106]
Seymour Gray Professor of Molecular Medicine in Genetics, Chair, Department of Genetics, University of Pennsylvania School of Medicine, Philadelphia, Pennsylvania

Richard A. King, M.D., Ph.D. [147]
Director, Division of Genetics and Metabolism; Professor, Departments of Medicine and Pediatrics and Institute of Human Genetics, University of Minnesota, Minneapolis, Minnesota

Kenneth W. Kinzler, Ph.D. [12]
Assistant Professor of Oncology, The Johns Hopkins Oncology Center, Baltimore, Maryland

Takashi Kei Kishimoto, Ph.D. [132]
Principal Scientist, Cellular Adhesion-Immunology, Boehringer-Ingelheim Pharmaceuticals, Inc., Ridgefield, Connecticut

Edwin H. Kolodny, M.D. [88]
Bernard A. and Charlotte Marden Professor and Chair, Department of Neurology, New York University School of Medicine, New York, New York

Stuart Kornfeld, M.D. [79]
Professor of Medicine and Biochemistry; Co-Director, Division of Hematology, Department of Medicine, Washington University School of Medicine, St. Louis, Missouri

Kenneth H. Kraemer, M.D. [148]
Research Scientist, Laboratory of Molecular Carcinogenesis, National Cancer Institute, National Institutes of Health, Bethesda, Maryland

Michael Krawczak, Dip.Math., Dr.Rer.Nat. [3]
Research Scientist, Abteilung Humangenetik, Medizinische Hochschule, Hanover, Germany

Berry Kremer, M.D., Ph.D. [152]
Neurologist, Department of Neurology, Academic Hospital-St. Radboud, Nijmegen, The Netherlands

Bert N. La Du, Jr., M.D., Ph.D. [39]
Emeritus Professor, Department of Pharmacology, University of Michigan Medical School, Ann Arbor, Michigan

Marie Lambert, M.D. [28]
Professeur adjoint de clinique, Département de pédiatrie, Université de Montréal; Service de génétique médicale, Hôpital Ste-Justine, Montréal, Québec, Canada

Agne Larsson, M.D. [43]
Professor, Department of Pediatrics at Huddinge Hospital, Karolinska Institutet, Stockholm, Sweden

Paul B. Lazarow, Ph.D. [71]
Professor and Chair, Department of Cell Biology and Anatomy, Mount Sinai School of Medicine, New York, New York

David H. Ledbetter, Ph.D. [19, 20]
Chief, Diagnostic Development Branch, National Center for Human Genome Research, National Institutes of Health, Bethesda, Maryland

Brendan Lee, Ph.D. [135]
Research Assistant Professor of Microbiology and Immunology, Health Science Center at Brooklyn, Brooklyn, New York

Harvey L. Levy, M.D. [29, 35, 119]
Senior Associate in Medicine and Genetics, Children's Hospital; Chief of Biochemical Genetics, State Laboratory Institute, Boston, Massachusetts

Roland Libau, M.D. [9]
Postdoctoral Fellow, Department of Microbiology and Immunology, Stanford University School of Medicine, Stanford, California

Samuel E. Lux, M.D. [115]
Professor of Pediatrics, Harvard Medical School; Chief, Division of Hematology-Oncology, Children's Hospital, Boston, Massachusetts

Lucio Luzzatto, M.D. [111]
Professor of Haematology, Royal Postgraduate Medical School; Consultant Haematologist, Hammersmith Hospital, University of London, London, England

Muchou Ma, M.D., Ph.D. [74]
Division of Experimental Pathology, Albany Medical College, Albany, New York

Robert W. Mahley, M.D., Ph.D. [61]
Director, Gladstone Institute of Cardiovascular Disease, Cardiovascular Research Institute, Departments of Pathology and Medicine, University of California, San Francisco, California

Don Mahuran, Ph.D. [92]
Associate Professor, Department of Clinical Biochemistry, University of Toronto; Senior Scientist, The Hospital for Sick Children, Toronto, Ontario, Canada

Stephen J. Marx, M.D. [100]
Chief, Genetics and Endocrinology Section, National Institute of Diabetes and Digestive and Kidney Diseases, National Institutes of Health, Bethesda, Maryland

Edward R. B. McCabe, M.D., Ph.D. [48]
Professor and Vice Chair for Research, Department of Pediatrics; Professor and Vice Chair, Department of Molecular and Human Genetics, Baylor College of Medicine, Houston, Texas

Hugh O. McDevitt, M.D. [9]
Burt and Marion Avery Professor in Immunology, Department of Microbiology and Immunology, Stanford University School of Medicine, Stanford, California

Roderick R. McInnes, M.D., Ph.D. [29]
Professor of Pediatrics and of Molecular and Medical Genetics, University of Toronto; The Hospital for Sick Children, Toronto, Ontario, Canada

William J. McKenna, M.D. [142]
Professor of Cardiac Medicine, Department of Cardiological Sciences, St. George's Hospital Medical School, University of London, London, England

Victor A. McKusick, M.D. [1]
University Professor of Medical Genetics, The Johns Hopkins University School of Medicine; Physician, Johns Hopkins Hospital, Baltimore, Maryland

Michael J. McPhaul, M.D. [95]
Associate Professor of Internal Medicine, University of Texas Southwestern Medical Center at Dallas, Dallas, Texas

Atul Mehta, M.D. [111]
Consultant Haematologist, Department of Haematology, Royal Free Hospital, University of London, London, England

Alton Meister, M.D. [43]
Professor and Chair, Department of Biochemistry, Cornell University Medical College, New York, New York

Claude J. Migeon, M.D. [94]
Professor of Pediatrics, Division of Pediatric Endocrinology, The Johns Hopkins University School of Medicine, Baltimore, Maryland

Beverly S. Mitchell, M.D. [52]
Professor of Medicine, University of North Carolina School of Medicine, Chapel Hill, North Carolina

Grant A. Mitchell, M.D. [28]
Professeur adjoint, Départements de pédiatrie et de biochimie, Université de Montréal; Service de génétique médicale, Hôpital Ste-Justine, Montréal, Québec, Canada

Ann B. Moser, B.A. [72]
Kennedy Krieger Institute; Research Associate, Department of Neurology, The Johns Hopkins University School of Medicine, Baltimore, Maryland

Hugo W. Moser, M.D. [71, 72, 83]
Kennedy Krieger Institute; University Professor of Neurology and Pediatrics, The Johns Hopkins University School of Medicine, Baltimore, Maryland

Björn Mossberg, M.D. [131]
Associate Professor, Department of Respiratory Medicine and Allergology, Stockholm Söder Hospital, Stockholm, Sweden

Arno G. Motulsky, M.D., D.Sc. [69, 143]
Professor of Medicine and Genetics, University of Washington, Seattle, Washington

S. Harvey Mudd, M.D. [35]
Guest Scientist, Laboratory of General and Comparative Biochemistry, National Institute of Mental Health, Bethesda, Maryland

Joseph Muenzer, M.D., Ph.D. [78]
Associate Professor, Department of Pediatrics, Division of Genetics and Metabolism, University of North Carolina, Chapel Hill, North Carolina

Richard M. Myers, Ph.D. [6]
Associate Professor, Department of Genetics, Stanford University School of Medicine, Stanford, California

Kishio Nanjo, M.D. [22]
Professor, Department of Medicine, Wakayama University of Medical Science, Wakayama, Japan

William M. Nauseef, M.D. [133]
Professor, Department of Internal Medicine, Division of Infectious Diseases, University of Iowa College of Medicine; Veterans Administration Medical Center, Iowa City, Iowa

Elizabeth F. Neufeld, Ph.D. [78]
Professor and Chair, Department of Biological Chemistry, University of California Los Angeles School of Medicine, Los Angeles, California

Peter J. Newman, Ph.D. [110]
Senior Investigator, Platelet Molecular Biology Laboratory, Blood Research Institute, The Blood Center of Southeastern Wisconsin, Milwaukee, Wisconsin

Irene F. Newsham, Ph.D. [11]
Section Head, Ludwig Institute for Cancer Research-San Diego Branch; Assistant Professor, Department of Medicine, University of California-San Diego School of Medicine, La Jolla, California

Takeshi Nishino, M.D., Ph.D. [54]
Associate Professor, Department of Biochemistry, Nippon Medical School, Tokyo, Japan

Yves Nordmann, M.D. [66]
Professor and Chief, French Center of Porphyria, Hôpital Louis Mourier, Colombes, France

Kaare R. Norum, M.D. [60]
Professor, Institute for Nutrition Research, School of Medicine, University of Oslo, Oslo, Norway

Robert L. Nussbaum, M.D. [19, 123]
Chief, Laboratory of Genetic Disease Research, National Center for Human Genome Research, National Institutes of Health, Bethesda, Maryland

William S. Oetting, Ph.D. [147]
Research Associate, Department of Medicine, University of Minnesota, Minneapolis, Minnesota

Akihiro Oshima, M.D. [90]
Senior Investigator, Department of Clinical Genetics, The Tokyo Metropolitan Institute of Medical Science, Tokyo, Japan

Donald E. Paglia, M.D. [114]
Professor of Pathology and Laboratory Medicine, University of California School of Medicine, Los Angeles, California

Morag Park, Ph.D. [10]
Molecular Oncology Group, Royal Victoria Hospital, Departments of Oncology and Medicine, McGill University, Montreal, Quebec, Canada

Keith Parker, M.D., Ph.D. [94]
Assistant Investigator, Howard Hughes Medical Institute; Associate Professor of Medicine and Biochemistry, Duke University Medical Center, Durham, North Carolina

Marc C. Patterson, M.B., B.S. [85]
Assistant Professor, Mayo Medical School; Senior Associate Consultant, Department of Neurology, Section of Child and Adolescent Neurology, Mayo Clinic and Foundation, Rochester, Minnesota

Peter G. Pentchev, Ph.D. [85]
Chief, Cellular and Molecular Pathophysiology Section, Developmental and Metabolic Neurology Branch, National Institute of Neurological Disorders and Stroke, National Institutes of Health, Bethesda, Maryland

James M. Phang, M.D. [30]
Chief, Laboratory of Nutritional and Molecular Regulation, Division of Cancer Prevention and Control, National Cancer Institute, National Institutes of Health, Frederick, Maryland

John A. Phillips III, M.D. [97]
Professor of Pediatrics and Biochemistry; Director, Division of Genetics, Vanderbilt University School of Medicine, Nashville, Tennessee

Joram Piatigorsky, Ph.D. [146]
Chief, Laboratory of Molecular and Development Biology, National Eye Institute, National Institutes of Health, Bethesda, Maryland

Mortimer Poncz, M.D. [110]
Associate Professor, Hematology Division, The Children's Hospital of Philadelphia, Philadelphia, Pennsylvania

Stanley B. Prusiner, M.D. [153]
Professor of Neurology and Biochemistry, Departments of Neurology and of Biochemistry and Biophysics, University of California, San Francisco, California

P. Edward Purdue, Ph.D. [75]
Department of Cell Biology and Anatomy, Mount Sinai School of Medicine, New York, New York

Stanley C. Rall, Jr., Ph.D. [61]
Associate Director, Gladstone Institute of Cardiovascular Disease, Cardiovascular Research Institute, University of California, San Francisco, California

Francesco Ramirez, Ph.D. [135]
Professor of Molecular Biology, Mount Sinai School of Medicine, New York, New York

Howard Rasmussen, M.D., Ph.D. [124]
Professor of Medicine; Director, Institute for Molecular Medicine and Genetics, Medical College of Georgia, Augusta, Georgia

W. Brian Reeves, M.D. [98]
Assistant Professor, Department of Internal Medicine, Division of Nephrology, University of Arkansas for Medical Sciences, Little Rock, Arkansas

Samuel Refetoff, M.D. [93]
Professor of Medicine and Pediatrics, University of Chicago, Chicago, Illinois

Alexander P. Reiner, M.D. [104]
Senior Fellow and Instructor, Department of Medicine, University of Washington, Seattle, Washington

Sebastian Reiter, M.D. [54]
Privatdozent, III-Medizinische Klinik, Klinikum Mannheim, Universität Heidelberg, Heidelberg, Germany

Brian H. Robinson, Ph.D. [44]
Professor, Departments of Biochemistry and Pediatrics, University of Toronto; Research Institute, The Hospital for Sick Children, Toronto, Ontario, Canada

Charles R. Roe, M.D. [45]
Professor, Department of Pediatrics, Duke University School of Medicine, Durham, North Carolina

Blake J. Roessler, M.D. [49]
Assistant Professor of Internal Medicine, Department of Internal Medicine, University of Michigan, Ann Arbor, Michigan

Hans-Hilger Ropers, M.D. [145]
Professor, Department of Human Genetics, University Hospital Nijmegen, Nijmegen, The Netherlands

Leon E. Rosenberg, M.D. [41, 102]
President, Bristol-Myers Squibb Pharmaceutical Research Institute, Princeton, New Jersey

David S. Rosenblatt, M.D. [101]
Director, Divisions of Medical Genetics, Royal Victoria Hospital and Montreal General Hospital; Professor of Medicine, Human Genetics and Pediatrics, McGill University, Montreal, Quebec, Canada

Belinda J.F. Rossiter, Ph.D. [50]
Instructor, Department of Molecular and Human Genetics and Human Genome Center, Baylor College of Medicine, Houston, Texas

Jayanta Roy Chowdhury, M.D. [67]
Professor of Medicine, Marion Bessin Liver Research Center, Albert Einstein College of Medicine, New York, New York

Namita Roy Chowdhury, Ph.D. [67]
Associate Professor of Medicine, Marion Bessin Liver Research Center, Albert Einstein College of Medicine, New York, New York

Arthur H. Rubenstein, M.D. [22]
Professor and Chair, Department of Medicine, University of Chicago, Chicago, Illinois

David W. Russell, Ph.D. [95]
Eugene McDermott Distinguished Professor of Molecular Genetics, University of Texas Southwestern Medical Center at Dallas, Dallas, Texas

David D. Sabatini, M.D., Ph.D. [8]
Frederick L. Ehrman Professor and Chairman, Department of Cell Biology, New York University School of Medicine, New York, New York

Richard L. Sabina, Ph.D. [53]
Associate Professor, Department of Biochemistry, Medical College of Wisconsin, Milwaukee, Wisconsin

J. Evan Sadler, M.D., Ph.D. [107]
Associate Investigator, Howard Hughes Medical Institute; Professor, Departments of Medicine, Biochemistry and Molecular Biophysics, Washington University School of Medicine, St. Louis, Missouri

Amrik S. Sahota, Ph.D. [51]
Associate Scientist; Associate Director, DNA Diagnostic Laboratory, Department of Medical Genetics, Indiana University Medical Center, Indianapolis, Indiana

Hitoshi Sakuraba, M.D. [90]
Chief, Department of Clinical Genetics, The Tokyo Metropolitan Institute of Medical Science, Tokyo, Japan

Konrad Sandhoff, Ph.D. [76, 92]
Professor and Director, Institut für Organische Chemie und Biochemie, Rheinische Friedrich-Wilhelms-Universität, Bonn, Germany

Carmen Sapienza, Ph.D. [7]
Professor of Pathology and Laboratory Medicine, The Fels Institute for Cancer Research and Molecular Biology, Temple University School of Medicine, Philadelphia, Pennsylvania

Shigeru Sassa, M.D., Ph.D. [66]
Associate Professor and Physician, Laboratory of Biochemical Hematology, The Rockefeller University, New York, New York

Jean-Marie Saudubray, M.D., Prof. [5]
Director, Clinique de Génétique Médicale, Department of Pediatrics, Hôpital Necker Enfants Malades, Paris, France

Jerry A. Schneider, M.D. [126]
Bernard L. Maas Professor of Inherited Metabolic Disease, Professor of Pediatrics, University of California, San Diego, La Jolla, California

Edward H. Schuchman, Ph.D. [84]
Associate Professor, Department of Human Genetics, Mount Sinai School of Medicine, New York, New York

C. Ronald Scott, M.D. [36]
Professor, Department of Pediatrics, University of Washington School of Medicine, Seattle, Washington

Charles R. Scriver, M.D.C.M. [1, 27, 30, 38]
Alva Professor of Human Genetics and Professor of Biology and Pediatrics, McGill University, Montreal, Quebec, Canada

Udo Seedorf, Ph.D. [82]
Senior Scientist, Laboratory for Cellular Lipid Metabolism, Institute for Arteriosclerosis Research, Westphalian-Wilhelms University, Münster, Germany

Stanton Segal, M.D. [25, 117]
Professor of Pediatrics and Medicine, University of Pennsylvania School of Medicine; Director, Division of Biochemical Development and Molecular Diseases, The Children's Hospital of Philadelphia, Philadelphia, Pennsylvania

Uri Seligsohn, M.D. [108]
Professor and Chair of Hematology, Sackler School of Medicine, Tel-Aviv University; Director, Institute of Thrombosis and Hemostasis, Chaim Sheba Medical Center, Tel Hashomer, Israel

Giorgio Semenza, M.D. [151]
Professor and Chair of Biochemistry, Swiss Federal Institute of Technology, ETH-Zentrum, Zurich, Switzerland

Larry J. Shapiro, M.D. [96]
Professor and Chair, Department of Pediatrics, University of California, San Francisco, California

Vivian E. Shih, M.D. [34]
Associate Professor of Neurology, Harvard Medical School; Director, Amino Acid Disorder Laboratory, Massachusetts General Hospital, Boston, Massachusetts

John M. Shoffner, M.D. [46]
Assistant Professor, Departments of Genetics and Molecular Medicine and of Neurology, Emory University School of Medicine, Atlanta, Georgia

Olli Simell, M.D. [31, 118]
Professor and Chair, Department of Pediatrics, University of Turku, Turku, Finland

H. Anne Simmonds, Ph.D. [51, 54]
Director, Purine Research Laboratory, United Medical and Dental Schools of Guy's and St. Thomas's Hospitals, London, England

Flemming Skovby, M.D. [35]
Associate Professor, Department of Pediatrics, Clinical Genetics Section, Rigshospitalet, University of Copenhagen, Copenhagen, Denmark

William S. Sly, M.D. [1, 79, 137]
Alice A. Doisy Professor of Biochemistry and Molecular Biology and Professor of Pediatrics; Chair, Edward A. Doisy Department of Biochemistry and Molecular Biology, St. Louis University School of Medicine, St. Louis, Missouri

C. Wayne Smith, M.D. [132]
Professor, Departments of Pediatrics and Microbiology and Cell Biology; Head, Section of Leukocyte Biology, Baylor College of Medicine, Houston, Texas

Kirby D. Smith, Ph.D. [72]
Kennedy Krieger Institute; Associate Professor of Pediatrics, The Johns Hopkins University School of Medicine, Baltimore, Maryland

Oded Sperling, Ph.D. [125]
Dean and Professor of Chemical Pathology, Sackler School of Medicine, Tel-Aviv University; Scientific Director, Felsenstein Medical Research Center; Director of Clinical Biochemistry, Beilinson Medical Center, Petah-Tikva, Israel

Allen M. Spiegel, M.D. [99]
Chief, Metabolic Diseases Branch, National Institute of Diabetes and Digestive and Kidney Diseases, National Institutes of Health, Bethesda, Maryland

Daniel Steinberg, M.D., Ph.D. [73]
Professor, Department of Medicine; Director, Specialized Center of Research on Arteriosclerosis, University of California-San Diego School of Medicine, La Jolla, California

Donald F. Steiner, M.D. [22]
Senior Investigator, Howard Hughes Medical Institute, University of Chicago, Chicago, Illinois

Beat Steinmann, M.D. [23]
Professor, Division of Metabolism, Department of Pediatrics, University of Zurich, Kinderspital Zurich, Zurich, Switzerland

Pietro Strisciuglio, M.D. [91]
Associate Professor of Pediatrics, Department of Pediatrics, University of Reggio Calabria, Catanzaro, Italy

Kathleen E. Sullivan, M.D., Ph.D. [130]
Assistant Professor of Pediatrics, Division of Allergy, Immunology and Infectious Diseases, The Children's Hospital of Philadelphia, Philadelphia, Pennsylvania

D. Parker Suttle, Ph.D. [55]
Associate Member, Department of Molecular Pharmacology, St. Jude Children's Research Hospital, Memphis, Tennessee

Kinuko Suzuki, M.D. [85, 87, 92]
Professor, Department of Pathology, University of North Carolina School of Medicine, Chapel Hill, North Carolina

Kunihiko Suzuki, M.D. [87]
Professor of Neurology and Psychiatry; Director, Brain and Development Research Center, University of North Carolina School of Medicine, Chapel Hill, North Carolina

Yoshiyuki Suzuki, M.D. [87, 90]
Vice-Director, The Tokyo Metropolitan Institute of Medical Science, Tokyo, Japan

Lawrence Sweetman, Ph.D. [40]
Professor of Pediatrics and Pathology, University of Southern California School of Medicine; Director, Biochemical Genetics Laboratory, Children's Hospital, Los Angeles, California

Howard S. Tager, Ph.D. [22]
Professor, Department of Biochemistry and Molecular Biology, University of Chicago, Chicago, Illinois

Kouichi R. Tanaka, M.D. [114]
Professor of Medicine; Chief, Division of Hematology, University of California School of Medicine, Los Angeles, California; Harbor-UCLA Medical Center, Torrance, California

Robert M. Tanguay, Ph.D. [28]
Professeur titulaire, Département de médecine; Laboratoire de génétique cellulaire développementale, Université Laval, Sainte-Foy, Québec, Canada

Simeon I. Taylor, M.D., Ph.D. [21]
Chief, Diabetes Branch, National Institute of Diabetes and Digestive and Kidney Diseases, National Institutes of Health, Bethesda, Maryland

Robin G. Taylor, Ph.D. [29]
Department of Molecular and Medical Genetics, University of Toronto; The Hospital for Sick Children, Toronto, Ontario, Canada

Harriet S. Tenenhouse, Ph.D. [124]
Professor of Pediatrics and Human Genetics, Auxiliary Professor of Biology, McGill University, Montreal, Quebec, Canada

Samuel O. Thier, M.D. [117]
President and Chief Operating Officer, Massachusetts General Hospital, Boston, Massachusetts

George H. Thomas, Ph.D. [81]
Professor of Pediatrics, The Johns Hopkins University School of Medicine; Director, Kennedy Krieger Institute Genetics Laboratory, Baltimore, Maryland

Roland Tisch, Ph.D. [9]
Postdoctoral Fellow, Department of Microbiology and Immunology, Stanford University School of Medicine, Stanford, California

Douglas M. Tollefsen, M.D., Ph.D. [109]
Professor of Medicine, Division of Hematology-Oncology, Washington University Medical School, St. Louis, Missouri

Petros Tsipouras, M.D. [135]
Professor of Pediatrics, University of Connecticut Health Center, Farmington, Connecticut

Lap-Chee Tsui, Ph.D. [127]
Professor, Department of Molecular and Medical Genetics, University of Toronto; Senior Scientist, Department of Genetics, The Hospital for Sick Children, Toronto, Ontario, Canada

Edward G. D. Tuddenham, M.D. [106]
Director, Clinical Research Center, Haemostasis Research Group, Harrow, England

Eric Turk, Ph.D. [116]
Research Physiologist, Department of Physiology, University of California School of Medicine, Los Angeles, California

Gerd M. Utermann, M.D. [58]
Professor and Chair, Institute for Medical Biology and Human Genetics, Leopold Franzens University of Innsbruck, Innsbruck, Austria

David Valle, M.D. [1, 31, 37]
Investigator, Howard Hughes Medical Institute; Professor of Pediatrics, Medicine, Ophthalmology, and Molecular Biology and Genetics, The Johns Hopkins University School of Medicine, Baltimore, Maryland

Karel J. Van Acker, M.D., Ph.D. [51]
Professor, Department of Pediatrics, University of Antwerp, Antwerp, Belgium

Georges Van den Berghe, M.D. [23]
Research Director, Laboratory of Physiological Chemistry, International Institute of Cellular and Molecular Pathology, Brussels; Consultant Physician, Department of Pediatrics, University of Leuven, Leuven, Belgium

Peter van Endert, M.D. [9]
Postdoctoral Fellow, Department of Microbiology and Immunology, Stanford University School of Medicine, Stanford, California

Marie T. Vanier, M.D., Ph.D. [85]
Directeur de Recherche, Institut National de la Santé et de la Recherche Médicale, Unité 189, Département de Biochimie, Faculté de Médecine Lyons-Sud, Lyons, France

Gilbert Vassart, M.D., Ph.D. [93]
Professor of Medical Genetics, Sérvice de Génétique Médicale et Institut de Recherche Interdisciplinaire, Faculté de Médecine, Université Libre de Bruxelles, Brussels, Belgium

Patrick Vinay, M.D. [122]
Professeur titulaire, Départements de médecine et de physiologie, Université de Montréal, Montréal, Québec, Canada

Bert Vogelstein, M.D. [12]
Professor of Oncology, The Johns Hopkins Oncology Center, Baltimore, Maryland

Arnold von Eckardstein, M.D. [64]
Senior Scientist, Institute for Clinical Chemistry and Laboratory Medicine, Central Laboratory; Westphalian-Wilhelms University, Münster, Germany

Sybe K. Wadman, Ph.D. [70]
Professor of Biochemistry of Inherited Metabolic Disease, University Children's Hospital, Het Wilhelmina Kinderziekenhuis, Utrecht, The Netherlands

Douglas C. Wallace, Ph.D. [46]
Robert Woodruff Professor of Medical Genetics, Chair, Department of Genetics and Molecular Medicine, Emory University School of Medicine, Atlanta, Georgia

Anne M. Wang, Ph.D. [80]
Postdoctoral Fellow, Department of Human Genetics, Mount Sinai School of Medicine, New York, New York

Hugh C. Watkins, M.B., B.S. [142]
Lecturer, Department of Cardiological Sciences, St. George's Hospital Medical School, University of London, London, England

Sir David Weatherall, M.D. [113]
Regius Professor of Medicine, University of Oxford, Institute of Molecular Medicine, John Radcliffe Hospital, Oxford, England

Dianne R. Webster, Ph.D. [55]
Director, National Testing Centre, Auckland, New Zealand

Lee S. Weinstein [99]
Senior Staff Fellow, Metabolic Diseases Branch, National Institute of Diabetes and Digestive and Kidney Diseases, National Institutes of Health, Bethesda, Maryland

Michael J. Welsh, M.D. [127]
Investigator, Howard Hughes Medical Institute; Professor, Departments of Internal Medicine and Physiology and Biophysics, University of Iowa College of Medicine, Iowa City, Iowa

Michael P. Whyte, M.D. [136]
Professor of Medicine and Pediatrics, Divisions of Bone and Mineral Diseases and Endocrinology and Metabolism, Washington University School of Medicine; Medical Director, Metabolic Research Unit, Shriners Hospital for Crippled Children, St. Louis, Missouri

Huntington F. Willard, Ph.D. [16]
Henry Willson Payne Professor and Chair, Department of Genetics, Case Western Reserve University School of Medicine; Director, Center for Human Genetics, University Hospitals of Cleveland, Cleveland, Ohio

Julian C. Williams, M.D., Ph.D. [40]
Associate Professor of Pediatrics, University of Southern California School of Medicine; Head, Division of Medical Genetics, Children's Hospital, Los Angeles, California

Jean D. Wilson, M.D. [95]
Charles Cameron Sprague Distinguished Chair in Biomedical Science, Professor of Internal Medicine, University of Texas Southwestern Medical Center at Dallas, Dallas, Texas

Jerry A. Winkelstein, M.D. [130]
Eudowood Professor of Pediatrics; Director, Division of Allergy and Immunology, Department of Pediatrics, The Johns Hopkins University School of Medicine, Baltimore, Maryland

Barry Wolf, M.D., Ph.D. [103]
Professor, Departments of Human Genetics and Pediatrics, Medical College of Virginia, Virginia Commonwealth University, Richmond, Virginia

Allan W. Wolkoff, M.D. [67]
Professor of Medicine, Marion Bessin Liver Research Center, Albert Einstein College of Medicine, New York, New York

Savio L. C. Woo, Ph.D. [27]
Investigator, Howard Hughes Medical Institute; Professor of Cell Biology and Molecular Genetics; Director, Center for Gene Therapy, Baylor College of Medicine, Houston, Texas

William G. Wood, Ph.D. [113]
Senior Scientist, M.R.C. Molecular Haematology Unit, Institute of Molecular Medicine, University of Oxford, John Radcliffe Hospital, Oxford, England

Ronald G. Worton, Ph.D. [140]
Professor, Department of Molecular and Medical Genetics, University of Toronto; Geneticist-in-Chief, The Hospital for Sick Children, Toronto, Ontario, Canada

Ernest Wright, D.Sc., Ph.D. [116]
Professor and Chair, Department of Physiology, University of California School of Medicine, Los Angeles, California

Grace Chao Yeh, Ph.D. [30]
Senior Investigator, Laboratory of Nutritional and Molecular Regulation, Division of Cancer Prevention and Control, National Cancer Institute, National Institutes of Health, Frederick, Maryland

Huda Y. Zoghbi, M.D. [154]
Associate Professor, Departments of Pediatrics, Molecular and Human Genetics, and Neurology, Baylor College of Medicine, Houston, Texas

PREFACE

The sixth edition of *The Metabolic Basis of Inherited Disease* experienced "transition, transformation, and challenge." Transition continues in the seventh edition with the arrival of many new authors. Challenge remains, like the mountain whose peak is never in view while the climb proceeds. And there is transformation again, not least with the title: *The Metabolic and* Molecular *Bases of Inherited Disease*. The new word is significant.

A reviewer of the sixth edition reminds us of the original plan for the book: to present "the pertinent clinical, biochemical, and genetic information concerning those metabolic anomalies grouped under Garrod's engaging term 'inborn errors of metabolism.' "[1] The term *molecular* is a belated but natural homecoming for Garrod. During his lifetime, Garrod's views grew to encompass inherited susceptibility to any disease originating in our chemical individuality. These ideas emerged fully developed, for their time, in Garrod's second book, *The Inborn Factors in Disease*. That we have been slow to perceive the reach of his thinking is a theme of his recent biographer.[2] To accept it and put it to use requires the means to test its validity. Molecular analysis of the genetic variation causing or predisposing to disease provides the opportunity. The inborn errors of metabolism are simply our most obvious illustrations of the genetic variation that affects health and the molecular underpinnings of that variation. A corresponding analysis of multifactorial diseases is the obvious next step in the understanding of disease.[3] Need we say that MMBID-7 is nothing less than a textbook of molecular medicine, encompassing the diseases about which we know most? We predict that the "classic" textbooks of medicine in the future will look more and more like MMBID.

Change in the title of MBID did something else: it solved a problem the editors created for themselves in MBID-6, again commented on by the above-mentioned reviewer.[1] When we included topics not overtly "metabolic" in the sixth edition, for example, Down and fragile X syndromes, primary ciliary dyskinesia, collagen disorders and the muscular dystrophies, we moved well beyond the canonical theme of inborn errors of *metabolism*. The nonmetabolic topics are further expanded in this edition because they conform to *a logic of disease*, as it is called by Barton Childs in Chapter 2. The manifestations of any "genetic" disease are explained by a process (pathogenesis) that originates in part or in full from an intrinsic cause (mutation); and, since genotype is one of the determinants of the phenotype (disease), it follows that diagnosis, treatment, and counseling should be motivated from the genetic point of view because the disease involves both the patient and his or her family.

If there is an identifiable molecular explanation for the disease—and it affects a dynamic phenotype, metabolic or otherwise—then it is a candidate for inclusion in the seventh edition. The expansion of topics here is selective and obviously not inclusive of all possibilities. If this were the case, the table of contents would resemble the McKusick catalog, *Mendelian Inheritance in Man!* Nevertheless, yet a further 32 chapters are new to this edition of MBID while 31 others were introduced in the sixth edition; new ideas appear again and again in virtually all "old" chapters. Will it be three volumes—or more—for the eighth edition? (A CD-ROM format is under serious consideration for the next edition.) The Summary Table, immediately preceding Chapter 1, surveys the information in MMBID-7.

In the first section of the book, the following major new themes appear:

- A logic of disease based on genetic and evolutionary concepts that challenges conventional medical thinking (Chapter 2)
- Mutational mechanisms, including dynamic mutations (elastic or unstable DNA) (Chapter 3) and the methods to detect them (Chapter 1)
- Pharmacogenetics (Chapter 4) as a classical illustration of multifactorial disease (with ultimate and proximate causes) and of the "idiosyncratic reaction to drugs"—to recall Garrod's felicitous phrase
- Diagnostic algorithms for the patient with an inborn error of metabolism (Chapter 5)
- Mapping of genes (genomics) (Chapter 6), along with an increased awareness that mutant gene expression may involve more than conventional Mendelian inheritance; for example, imprinting and mosaicism (Chapter 7)
- How cellular organelles, protein targeting and posttranslational modification, and the HLA complex affect expression of "genetic" disease (the subjects of Chapters 8 and 9, respectively).
- Cancer appears as a major theme for the first time in this edition (Chapters 10 to 15). Cancers are products of genetic damage. Modified events in pathways release cells from the normal controls of replication and growth. The cascades of events controlled by proto-oncogenes are counterparts of Garrod's pathways of metabolism. Because cancers can involve constitutional mutations, somatic mutations, or both, they further expand the conceptual boundaries of the book.
- Processes of inactivation harbored on the X chromosome (Chapter 16) and knowledge about the testis-determining factor and primary sex reversal (Chapter 17) are topics new to the section on chromosomes, itself an innovation of the sixth edition.

An awesome expansion of information continues in old and new chapters. The new chapters include, for example, insulin gene defects (Chapter 22); a completely new look at nonketotic hyperglycinemia (Chapter 37); diseases of the mitochondrial genome (Chapter 46); the apolipoprotein (a) molecule and its association with heart disease (Chapter 58); oxalosis as a peroxisomal disorder (Chapter 75); lysosomal enzyme activator proteins (Chapter 76); Pompe disease as a disease of lysosome function (Chapter 77) rather than a disease of carbohydrate metabolism; Lowe syndrome, separated from the Fanconi syndrome, following positional cloning of the gene (Chapter 123); Marfan syndrome, a disease of fibrillin dysfunction (Chapter 135); the muscular dystrophies (Chapters 140 and 141), and hypertrophic cardiomyopathy (Chapter 142). All is not new; in recognition of tradition, the spelling of *alcaptonuria* has reverted to *alkaptonuria* (Chapter 39).

A new section on diseases of the eye (Chapters 143 to 146) includes retinitis pigmentosa, choroideremia, and disorders of color vision and crystallins. Discussions of epidermolysis bullosa (Chapter 149), Huntington disease (Chapter 152), and prion-related diseases (Chapter 153) reflect emerging molecular information on diseases of skin and brain. Chapter 154, the last in the book, catches recent developments involving half a dozen diseases.

The authors of chapters about particular diseases were asked to remember the needs of physicians and families, and they provide up-to-date information on diagnosis, treatment, and counseling. (These aspects are dealt with in even greater depth in a book that functions as our companion—the excellent *Inborn Metabolic Diseases: Diagnosis and Treatment,* edited by J. Fernandes, J-M. Saudubray, and K. Tada.)

Some 200 authors wrote for MBID-6; 302 have written for MMBID-7; they have achieved the continuing transformation of this text. While so much seems to change overnight in molecular biology and genetics, stability can be found in the life of this book: Gail Gavert, Mariapaz Ramos-Englis, J. Dereck Jeffers, Peter McCurdy, and their colleagues have translated formidable stacks of typescript into a book agreeable to the publisher. The editors are still working with the same colleagues: Lynne Prevost and Huguette Rizziero (C.R.S.), Grace Watson (A.B.), Elizabeth Torno (W.S.), and Sandy Muscelli (D.V.). Loy Denis was again our editorial coordinator until the last stages of this edition; her successor is Catherine Watson. The process of reading manuscripts and proofs was lightened by the tolerant support of our families and by colleagues at the places of business.

As this edition went to press, Harry Harris died. A giant in our field, his imprint is apparent everywhere in the book.

REFERENCES

1. Childs B: Book Review: *The Metabolic Basis of Inherited Disease,* 6th ed. *Am J Hum Genet* **46:**848, 1990.
2. Bearn AG: *Archibald Garrod and the Individuality of Man.* New York, Oxford University Press, 1993, 227 pp.
3. King RA, Rutter JI, Motulsky AG: *The Genetic Basis of Common Diseases.* New York, Oxford University Press, 1993, 978 pp.

SEVENTH EDITION

THE METABOLIC AND MOLECULAR BASES OF INHERITED DISEASE

Part 15

BLOOD AND BLOOD FORMING TISSUE

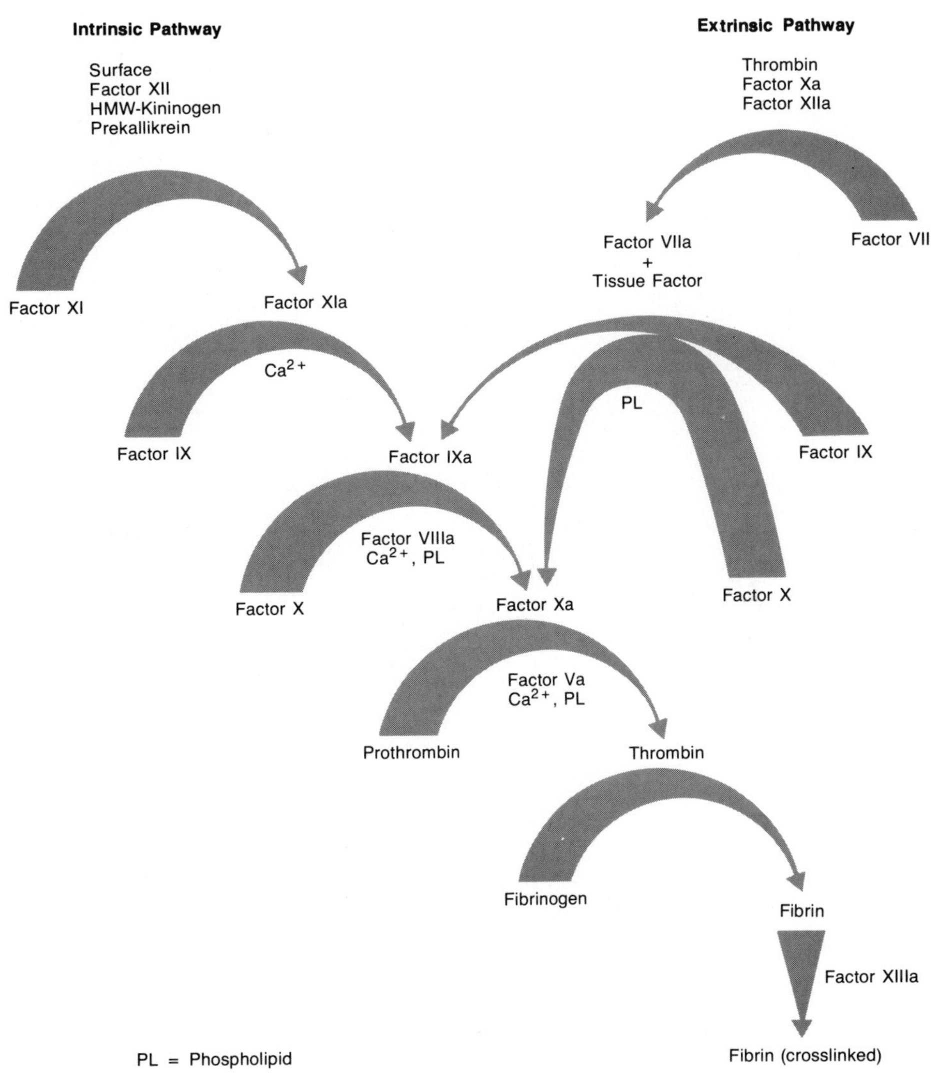

Intrinsic Pathway
Surface
Factor XII
HMW-Kininogen
Prekallikrein
Extrinsic Pathway
Thrombin
Factor Xa
Factor XIIa
Factor VIIa
+
Tissue Factor
Factor VII
Factor XI
Factor XIa
Ca^{2+}
PL
Factor IX
Factor IXa
Factor IX
Factor VIIIa
Ca^{2+}, PL
Factor X
Factor Xa
Factor X
Factor Va
Ca^{2+}, PL
Prothrombin
Thrombin
Fibrinogen
Fibrin
Factor XIIIa
PL = Phospholipid
Fibrin (crosslinked)

CHAPTER 104

Introduction to Hemostasis and the Vitamin K–Dependent Coagulation Factors

Alexander P. Reiner ▪ Earl W. Davie

1. **Six plasma proteins, including prothrombin, factor VII, factor IX, factor X, protein C, and protein S, require vitamin K for their biosynthesis in the liver. Each contains 9 to 12 γ-carboxyglutamic acid residues in the N-terminal portion of their molecule, and these residues are formed by vitamin K–dependent carboxylation of specific glutamic acid residues. The γ-carboxyglutamic acid residues are required for the calcium-dependent binding of the vitamin K–dependent proteins to phospholipid surfaces.**

2. **Prothrombin, factor VII, factor IX, factor X, and protein C circulate in blood as precursor molecules to serine proteases. When the blood coagulation cascade is initiated by exposure to tissue factor, prothrombin, factor VII, factor IX, and factor X are converted to serine proteases by minor proteolysis. Each protease in turn then cleaves a specific protein substrate(s). These reactions eventually lead to the generation of thrombin and fibrin at the site of vascular injury. Protein C is also converted to a serine protease by minor proteolysis during the coagulation cascade. This enzyme, however, plays a regulatory role in blood coagulation in that it inactivates factor Va and factor VIIIa in the presence of protein S. This helps to bring the coagulation cascade to a halt.**

3. **Reduced levels of prothrombin, factor VII, factor IX, and factor X result in bleeding complications in patients with these deficiencies. Reduced levels of protein C or protein S, however, may be associated with thrombotic risk, since the regulation of the coagulation pathway is impaired. Congenital factor IX deficiency, or hemophilia B, is approximately one fourth as common as factor VIII deficiency, also known as hemophilia A. Both are X-linked disorders and are clinically indistinguishable. Clinical manifestations include joint and muscle bleeding, the frequency and severity of which are related to the patient's residual factor IX clotting activity (FIX:C). Patients can be classified as having severe (FIX:C <1%), moderate (FIX:C = 1–5%), or mild (FIXC: = 6–30%) factor IX deficiency. Most severely affected patients have undetectable factor IX antigen levels (CRM$^-$), while moderate-to-mildly affected individuals may have relatively normal (CRM$^+$) or reduced (CRM^R) factor IX antigen levels. At the molecular level, a variety of factor IX mutations, ranging from complete gene deletions to single nucleotide substitutions, have been identified in hemophilia B patients. The identification of molecular defects, as well as the presence of several intragenic factor IX polymorphisms, has led to accurate methods for hemophilia B carrier testing and prenatal diagnosis. Treatment of bleeding episodes in hemophilia B currently consists of replacement therapy using purified plasma-derived factor IX concentrates. Preclinical studies of recombinant factor IX, as well as factor IX gene transfer therapy, are currently in progress.**

4. **The genes for prothrombin, factor VII, factor IX, protein C, and protein S have been well characterized and their chromosomal locations established. Abnormalities in the genes for the vitamin K–dependent proteins have been identified; they range from partial gene deletions to single nucleotide changes or deletions. These abnormalities have been observed in the exons coding for the mature protein and the leader sequence as well as in the intron–exon boundaries and regulatory regions of the genes for these proteins.**

A list of standard abbreviations is located immediately preceding the index in each volume. Additional abbreviations used in this chapter include: APT = activated partial thromboplastin time; DIC = disseminated intravascular coagulation; Gla = γ-carboxyglutamic acid; HCV = hepatitis C virus; PT = prothrombin time; RVV = Russell's viper venom.

GENERAL INTRODUCTION TO HEMOSTASIS

Hemostasis in humans involves a number of plasma proteins and platelets and their interaction with the vascular endothelium. Initially, a platelet plug is formed followed by a fibrin clot at the site of vascular injury. Platelet plug formation requires von Willebrand factor—a plasma protein that forms a bridge between the activated platelet and the subendothelium. This reaction, which is called "platelet adhesion," involves a specific platelet membrane receptor (glycoprotein Ib) that binds to von Willebrand factor. Platelet adhesion is immediately followed by platelet aggregation. In this reaction, fibrinogen forms a bridge between platelets by binding one activated platelet to another. Another platelet membrane receptor, called "glycoprotein IIb/IIIa," is involved in this reaction. During platelet plug formation, phospholipid is made available and the blood coagulation cascade is initiated.

Table 104-1 Nomenclature and Chapter Assignment for the Blood Coagulation Factors, Associated Proteins, and Platelets

Roman Numeral Designation	Common Name	Chapter
Factor I	Fibrinogen	105
Factor II	Prothrombin	104
Factor III	Tissue factor	104
Factor IV	Calcium ions	—
Factor V	Proaccelerin	106
Factor VII	Proconvertin	104
Factor VIII	Antihemophilic factor	106
Factor IX	Christmas factor	104
Factor X	Stuart factor	104
Factor XI	Plasma thromboplastin antecedent	108
Factor XII	Hageman factor	108
Factor XIII	Fibrin-stabilizing factor	105
—	Prekallikrein (Fletcher factor)	108
—	HMW kininogen (high-molecular weight-kininogen)	108
—	Protein C	104
—	Protein S	104
—	Antithrombin III	109
—	Heparin cofactor II	109
—	von Willebrand factor	107
—	Platelets	110

The precise events that trigger the coagulation cascade are not known, but it appears that tissue factor, a subendothelial cell-surface glycoprotein, plays an important role in the process.

The plasma proteins that participate in the coagulation cascade circulate in blood in precursor or inactive forms. When blood coagulation is initiated, these proteins are converted to active enzymes or cofactors that eventually lead to the generation of thrombin and fibrin. The plasma and cellular proteins and their cofactors have been assigned Roman numerals and are listed in Table 104-1, along with their common names. The terms *fibrinogen, prothrombin, tissue factor,* and *calcium* are employed by most investigators working in the field, while the remaining proteins (factors V through XIII) are usually referred to by their Roman numerals alone. No protein has been assigned as factor VI.

In recent years, the amino acid sequences for all the proteins shown in Table 104-1 have been established by a combination of protein sequence analysis and cDNA cloning. Furthermore, the chromosomal location, gene organization, and DNA sequence have also been determined for most of these proteins. These data have shown that the plasma proteins involved in fibrin formation and its regulation often share considerable amino acid sequence homology, physiological function, and mechanism of action. For instance, the vitamin K–dependent proteins (prothrombin; factors VII, IX, and X; protein C; and protein S) all share common domains, and all but protein S are converted to serine proteases by minor proteolysis. Likewise, factors V and VIII are large single-chain glycoproteins with considerable sequence homology. These two proteins also participate in the coagulation cascade as cofactors in the presence of calcium and phospholipid following their activation by minor proteolysis. Similarly, factor XI and plasma prekallikrein are highly homologous molecules that share common domains and are converted to serine proteases by minor proteolysis.

In Chaps. 104 to 110, the plasma proteins and the platelet surface glycoproteins that are involved in hemostasis are discussed and their gene structures are described.

INTRODUCTION TO VITAMIN K–DEPENDENT COAGULATION PROTEINS

The vitamin K–dependent proteins that participate in blood coagulation and its regulation include prothrombin, factor VII, factor IX, factor X, protein C, and protein S. These glycoproteins are synthesized in the liver and secreted into the blood. They circulate in the blood as trace proteins with plasma concentrations that range from 0.47 μg/ml for factor VII to 80 to 90 μg/ml for prothrombin (Table 104-2). Their half-lives in blood also vary considerably, with those for factor VII and protein C being the shortest. Prothrombin, factor VII, factor IX, factor X, and protein C circulate in blood as precursor or zymogen molecules and are converted to active serine proteases during the coagulation cascade (Fig. 104-1). Protein S, however, participates as a cofactor to activated protein C, and these two proteins are involved in the regulation of the coagulation pathway by the inactivation of factor Va and factor VIIIa in the presence of phospholipid (Fig. 104-2).

Each of the six human vitamin K–dependent coagulation factors consists of a series of homologous structural domains. The N-terminal region of each of the vitamin K–dependent coagulation proteins contains from 9 to 12 γ-carboxyglutamic acid (Gla) residues. These residues are formed by carboxylation of glutamic acid residues located within the first 40 to 45 amino acids in the N-terminal region of each protein.[1–3] The γ-carboxyglutamic acid residues constitute the Gla domains in each of the vitamin K–dependent proteins and are required for the calcium-dependent binding of these proteins to phospholipid surfaces.[4] Based on three-dimensional x-ray crystallographic analysis of the N-terminal region of prothrombin, in the presence of calcium ions, the Gla domain maintains a highly ordered structure with nine Gla residues interacting with seven calcium ions.[5] This

Table 104-2 Properties of the Vitamin K–Dependent Proteins

Protein	Molecular Weight	Number of Chains	Number of Gla Residues	Plasma Conc., μg/ml	Plasma Half-Life
Prothrombin	71,600	One	10	80–90	2–5 days
Factor VII	50,000	One	10	0.47	2–5 h
Factor IX	56,800	One	12	4	20–24 h
Factor X	58,800	Two	11	6.4	32–48 h
Protein C	62,000	Two	9	3.9–5.9	6–8 h
Protein S	70,700	One	11	25–35	—

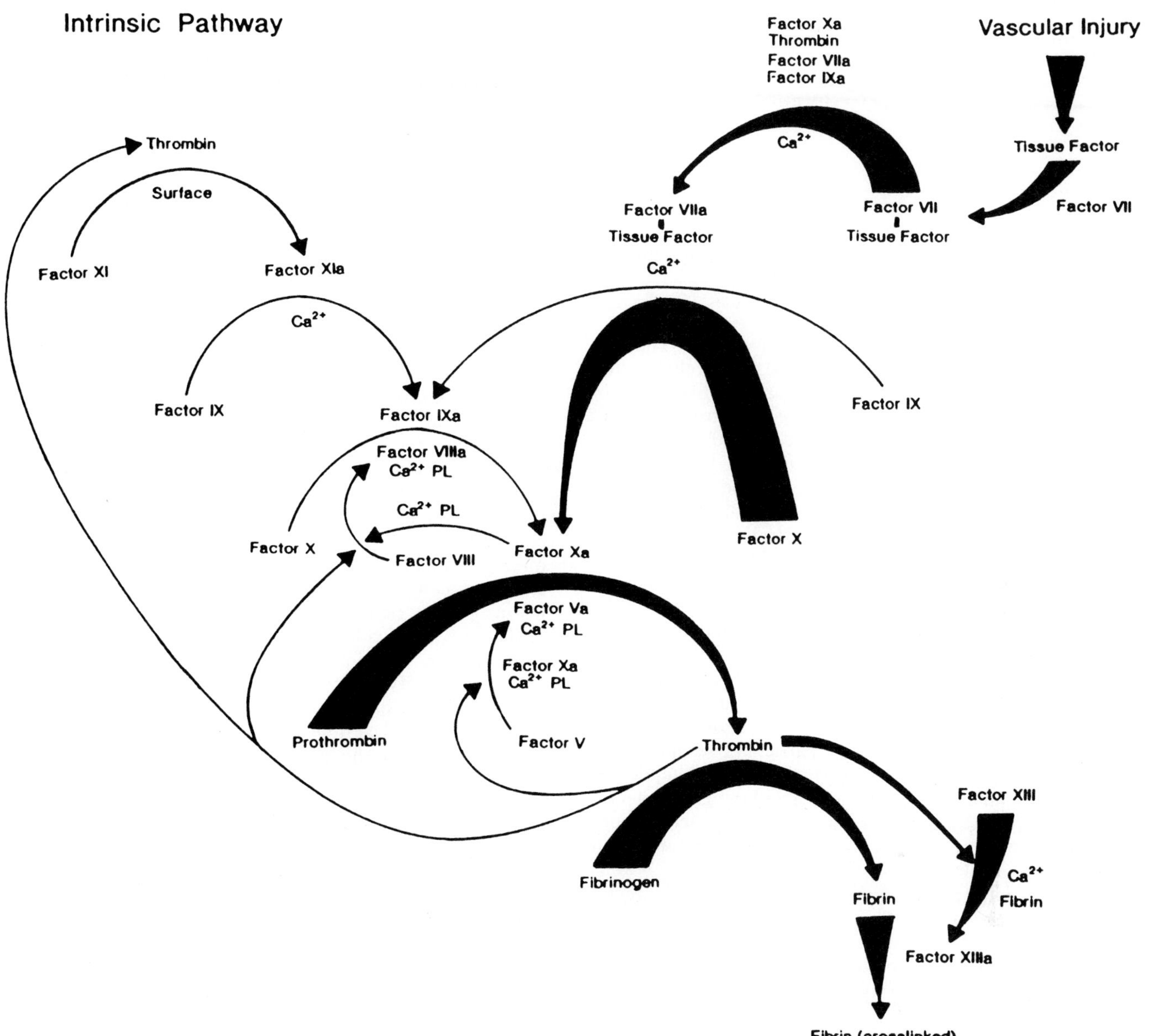

FIG. 104-1 **Coagulation cascade and fibrin formation by the intrinsic and extrinsic pathways. The initiation of the coagulation cascade occurs following vascular injury and the exposure of tissue factor to the blood. This triggers the extrinsic pathway (right side), shown by heavy arrows. The intrinsic pathway (left side) can be triggered when thrombin is generated, leading to the activation of factor XI. The two pathways converge by the formation of factor Xa. The activated clotting factors (except thrombin) are designated by lowercase a, i.e., IXa, Xa, XIa, etc. PL = phospholipid. The phospholipid bound to tissue factor is not shown.** ***(From Davie et al.*[112] *Used by permission.)***

creates an environment in which some of the positively charged calcium ions presumably form an electrostatic bridge between the negatively charged Gla residues and the negatively charged phospholipid of a membrane surface. This binding localizes the vitamin K–dependent coagulation factors at the site of vascular injury where platelet plug formation has occurred and an active phospholipid surface has been made available.

The Gla domain in prothrombin is followed by two kringle domains.[6] These kringle domains are composed of approximately 80 amino acids with disulfide bonds linking the six Cys residues in a pattern of $1 \rightarrow 6$, $2 \rightarrow 4$, and $3 \rightarrow 5$. Kringle structures are also present in factor XII,[7] plasminogen,[8] tissue plasminogen activator,[9] and urokinase.[10] In factor VII,[11] factor IX,[12–14] factor X,[15–17] and protein C,[18,19] the kringle domains are replaced by two growth factor domains. These domains are composed of 40 to 50 amino acids with disulfide bonds linking the six Cys residues in a characteristic pattern of $1 \rightarrow 3$, $2 \rightarrow 4$, and $5 \rightarrow 6$ (Fig. 104-3). These domains show considerable structural similarity to EGF and EGF precursor.[20–22] Protein S contains four growth factor domains present as tandem repeats following the N-terminal Gla domain.[23,24] Homologous growth factor structures are also present in several other hemostatic proteins

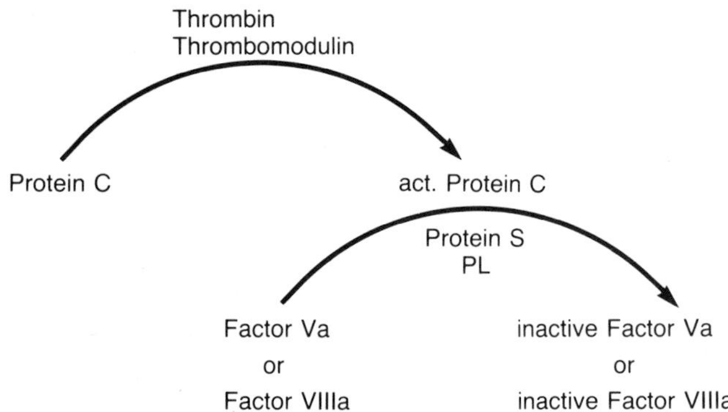

FIG. 104-2 Activation of protein C and the inactivation of factors Va and VIIIa. PL = phospholipid.

(factor XII, urokinase, tissue plasminogen activator) as well as a number of functionally unrelated extracellular and membrane-bound proteins.[25,26] A comparison of two-dimensional NMR spectroscopic studies of the growth factor domains of human,[27,28] mouse,[29] and rat[30] EGF; human transforming growth factor-α (TGF-α)[28,31-33]; human factor IX[34,35]; and bovine factor X[36,37] indicates considerable similarity in overall secondary structure. The structure of these growth factor domains is highly constrained by the three conserved disulfide loops and consists of one major and one minor β-sheet and five β-turns (see Fig. 104-3). In contrast to EGF and TGF-α, however, the N-terminal portion of the growth factor domains of the vitamin K–dependent proteins does not form a third strand of the major β-sheet. Instead, these N-terminal residues apparently constitute Gla-independent high-affinity calcium-binding sites[38-41] that have been demonstrated in factor IX,[42] factor X,[43] protein C,[44] and protein S.[45] In factors IX and X in particular, residues 47 to 50 and 64 and 65 (factor IX numbering) have been implicated in calcium binding.[34,46,47] Both the Gla and the growth factor domains have been implicated in the specific interactions and assembly of the vitamin K–dependent factors and their cofactors on membrane surfaces.[48-64]

The C-terminal region of prothrombin, factor VII, factor IX, factor X, and protein C contains the catalytic or serine protease domain that includes the active site residues Asp, His, and Ser. The amino acid sequence in this domain shows considerable sequence and structural similarity to pancreatic trypsin and chymotrypsin and is responsible for hydrolysis of specific Arg-containing peptide bonds. The serine proteases generated during blood coagulation have a high degree of substrate specificity and cleave only one or two peptide bonds in the protein substrates. Thus, they are far more substrate-specific than the pancreatic serine proteases involved in protein digestion. Based on computer modeling[65] and x-ray crystallographic comparisons[66] with the pancreatic enzymes, several unique insertion loop structures surrounding the active site center are responsible for the substrate specificity of the coagulation serine proteases.

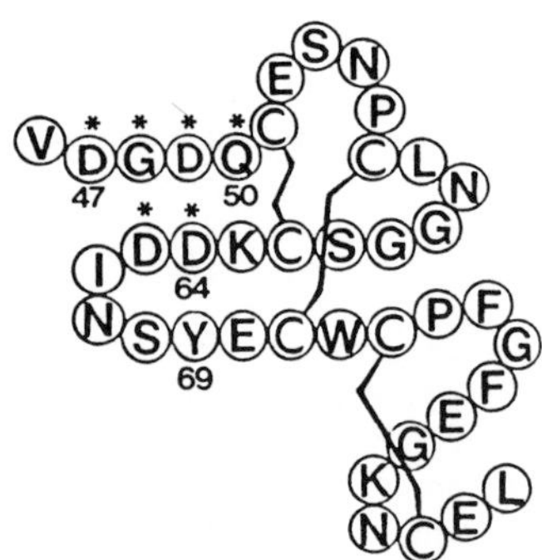

FIG. 104-3 First growth factor domain of human factor IX (residues 46 to 84) based on the NMR structure of human EGF.[27] Single-letter amino acid code is used. Asp 64 is β-hydroxylated. The structure consists of three disulfide loops and two β-sheets (see text). The amino acids denoted by an asterisk indicate residues that have been implicated in a Gla-independent calcium-binding site.[34,46,47] *(Modified from Handford et al.[46])*

BIOSYNTHESIS OF THE VITAMIN K–DEPENDENT COAGULATION PROTEINS

A number of steps are required for the biosynthesis of the vitamin K–dependent proteins in liver. Initially, large mRNA are synthesized in the nucleus of the hepatocyte for each of these proteins and processed by a capping reaction at the 5′ end, removal of the RNA corresponding to the introns and polyadenylation at the 3′ end of the mRNA. This results in a mature mRNA that is transported from the nucleus into the cytoplasm of the cell. Translation of the mature mRNA on the ribosomal machinery results in an immature polypeptide chain that contains a prepro leader sequence of approximately 40 amino acids (Fig. 104-4). Removal of the prepro leader sequence by proteolytic processing gives rise to the mature protein that circulates in plasma.

The prepro leader sequences of the human vitamin K–dependent proteins show considerable amino acid sequence similarity[11,12,16-19,23,24,67,68] (see Fig. 104-4). Each contains an initiator methionine followed by a very hydrophobic region of 13 to 17 residues that is required for transport of these proteins into the lumen of the RER during polypeptide elongation. The pre or signal peptides are 28, 23, and 18 amino acids in factor IX,[68] factor X,[69] and protein C,[70] respectively. The length of the signal peptides for prothrombin, factor VII, and protein S have not been established.

The signal peptide sequence in the vitamin K–dependent proteins is followed by a propeptide ranging from 17 to 24 residues in length. This region is important for the carboxylation of the vitamin K–dependent proteins and serves as a recognition site for the carboxylase complex.[68,70-73] The carboxylation reaction is carried out posttranslationally[74,75] by a membrane-bound enzyme[76,77] in a reaction requiring CO_2, O_2, polypeptide substrate, NADH, and vitamin K.[78,79] The carboxylation of the vitamin K–dependent proteins is inhibited by vitamin K antagonists such as dicumarol or warfarin.[80,81]

The carboxyl end of the propeptide contains highly conserved basic residues and serves as a recognition site for a processing protease(s) that preferentially cleaves peptide bonds, which generally follow an –Arg–X–Lys/Arg–Arg– motif (see Fig. 104-4). Cleavage of the propeptide gives rise to an N-terminal Ala in the mature polypeptide chain of prothrombin, factor VII, factor X, protein C, and protein S and to a Tyr in factor IX. Failure of factor IX propeptide cleavage due to naturally occurring point mutations of the conserved basic residues at either the −1, −2, or −4 positions results in a circulating factor IX molecule devoid of clotting activity.[82-86] The enzyme(s) responsible for propeptide processing of the vitamin K–dependent proteins are unknown, but several candidate proteases have been identified.[87,88]

In addition to γ-carboxylation, several of the vitamin

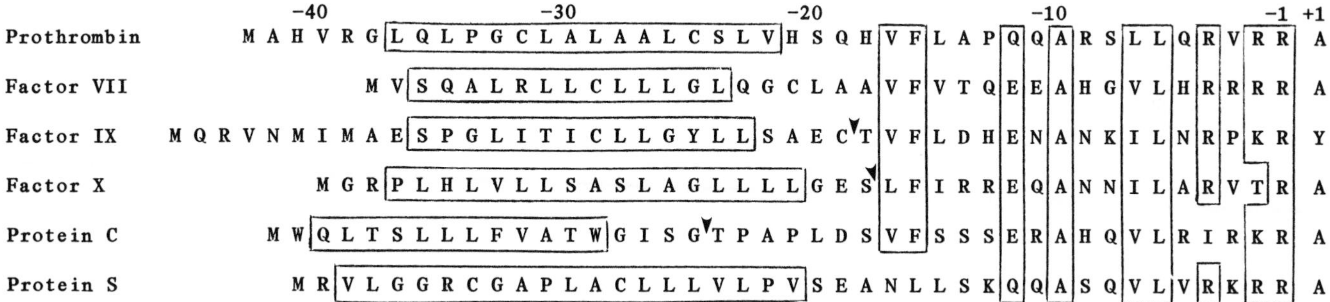

FIG. 104-4 Prepro leader sequences of the vitamin K–dependent proteins present in human plasma. The apparent hydrophobic core of each signal or pre sequence is boxed. The known signal peptidase cleavage sites are indicated by arrowheads. Identical or homologous amino acid residues within the propeptide regions of each protein are also boxed. Numbering of the residues is relative to the N-terminus of the mature proteins circulating in plasma. *(Modified from Foster et al.*[70]*)*

K–dependent coagulation proteins undergo a second type of enzymatic modification of certain amino acid residues during synthesis. A specific aspartic acid residue within the first growth factor domains of factor IX, factor X, protein C, and protein S and a specific Asn residue in the last three growth factor domains of protein S undergo β-hydroxylation to form β-erythro-hydroxyasparatic acid and β-erythro-hydroxyasparagine, respectively.[89–93] Interestingly, hydroxylated aspartic acid or asparagine residues have also been identified in other proteins containing growth factor domains, such as thrombomodulin, uromodulin, the LDL receptor, transforming growth factor-β1, and the complement proteins C1r and C1s.[26] The β-hydroxylation reaction occurs independently of γ-carboxylation and does not require vitamin K.[71,81] The enzyme responsible for β-hydroxylation has been characterized as an α-ketoglutarate-dependent dioxygenase that requires Fe^{2+} for activity.[94,95] The β-hydroxylase is functionally similar to, but structurally distinct from the collagen prolyl- and lysyl-hydroxylases.[96] The β-hydroxylase modifies specific Asp or Asn residues within an eight-residue epidermal growth factor consensus sequence.[93,95] Other sequence or structural requirements for β-hydroxylation must exist, however, since the first growth factor domain of factor VII conforms to this sequence, but does not undergo hydroxylation.[97] Furthermore, in contrast to factor X and protein C, human factor IX and protein S are only partially hydroxylated.[93,98] The functional significance of the β-hydroxyaspartic acid and β-hydroxyasparagine residues within the vitamin K–dependent proteins has yet to be determined.

Like many other synthesized proteins, the vitamin K–dependent protein precursors are modified by the addition of carbohydrate chains to certain Asn (*N*-linked) and Ser or Thr (*O*-linked) residues. Cotranslational glycosylation of specific Asn residues within the consensus sequence -Asn-X-Ser/Thr- occurs in the ER and is catalyzed by the enzyme oligosaccharyltransferase. Subsequently, the *N*-linked oligosaccharides undergo further processing by various glycosidases and glycosyltransferases within the ER and Golgi apparatus to generate complex carbohydrate structures that often terminate in sialic acid residues. Each vitamin K–dependent coagulation protein contains two to four potentially glycosylated Asn residues per molecule. These *N*-linked carbohydrate structures may be important for efficient secretion, proteolytic processing, and proper functioning of the newly synthesized proteins.[75,99]

In addition to *N*-linked carbohydrate, two unique *O*-linked carbohydrate moieties have been identified within the first growth factor domain of several of the vitamin K–dependent proteins. Specifically, Xyl-Glc or Xyl-Xyl-Glc structures are attached to a conserved serine residue in factor VII (Ser 52) and factor IX (Ser 53), as well as to the homologous serine residue within the first growth factor domains of vitamin K–dependent protein Z.[100,101] Secondly, *O*-linked fucose is attached to Ser 60 or Ser 61 in factor VII[102] and factor IX,[103] respectively, as well as to homologous serine or threonine residues in the growth factor domains of prourokinase,[104] tissue plasminogen activator,[105] and factor XII.[106] The function of these unusual *O*-linked sugar chains has yet to be determined, but thus far they have been identified only within proteins containing growth factor domains.

Prothrombin, factor VII, factor IX, and protein S circulate in plasma as single polypeptide chains, while factor X and protein C undergo proteolysis of an internal arginyl bond and circulate in plasma as mature two-chain proteins. Analogous to propeptide processing, this internal cleavage occurs following basic residues, i.e., the dibasic sequence -Lys-Arg- in protein C and the tetrabasic sequence -Arg-Arg-Lys-Arg- in factor X. Proteolytic processing at these internal basic sequences is a calcium-dependent event that occurs late in the secretion pathway.[75,107] While secreted factor X is fully processed to the two-chain form, approximately 10 to 15 percent of plasma protein C exists in the unprocessed single-chain form.[108] Interestingly, the efficiency of proteolytic processing of recombinant protein C to the two-chain form can be increased either by introducing a basic residue at the −4 position[109] or by coexpression of a yeast-processing protease (Kex2) that is capable of cleaving the peptide bond following dibasic sequences.[110] Thus, an enzyme(s) recognizing basic sequences identical or similar to that responsible for propeptide processing of the vitamin K–dependent proteins may also cleave factor X and protein C to their mature forms.

The two-chain forms of factor X and protein C, as well as the activated forms of factor VII, factor IX, and prothrombin, are linked by interchain disulfide bonds between cysteine residues of the N-terminal light chain and the C-terminal heavy chain containing the catalytic domain. In addition, each vitamin K–dependent protein contains several intrachain disulfide bonds in highly conserved positions throughout the molecule. Disulfide bond formation is catalyzed within the ER lumen during protein synthesis by the enzyme protein disulfide isomerase.[111]

PROTHROMBIN

Prothrombin participates in the final stages of the blood coagulation cascade,[112] where it is converted to thrombin in

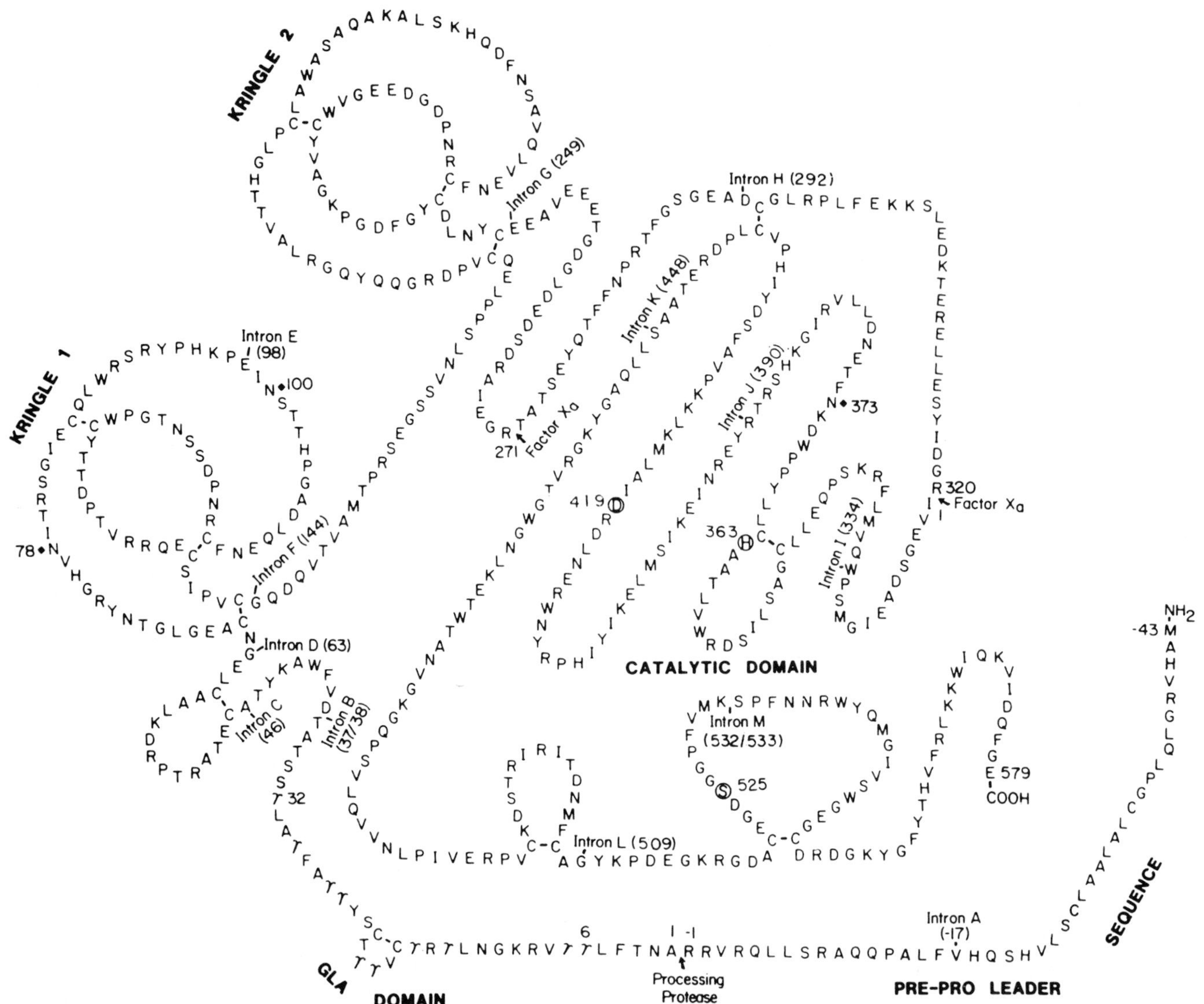

FIG. 104-5 Amino acid sequence and tentative structure of human prepro prothrombin. The locations of the 13 introns (A to M) are shown in the various regions of the protein. The prepro leader sequence is cleaved during protein biosynthesis to give rise to mature protein with an N-terminal sequence of A-N-T-F-. The two peptide bonds cleaved by factor Xa during the activation reaction are shown with small arrows. The three amino acids in the catalytic domain (H 363, D 419, S 525) that participate in catalysis are circled, while the three carbohydrate attachment sites are shown with solid diamonds. The amino acids are numbered as follows, starting with the N-terminal end of the protein: −43 to −1, prepro leader sequence; +1 to 271, prothrombin fragment 1.2; 272 to 320, light chain of thrombin; and 321 to 579, catalytic chain of thrombin. The single letter code for amino acids is as follows: A = Ala; R = Arg; N = Asn; D = Asp; C = Cys; Q = Gln; E = Glu; G = Gly; H = His; I = Ile; L = Leu; K = Lys; M = Met; F = Phe; P = Pro; S = Ser; T = Thr; W = Trp; Y = Tyr; V = Val; γ = γ-carboxyglutamic acid. *(From Degen et al.*[67,129]*)*

the presence of factor Xa, factor Va, calcium ions, and phospholipid (see Fig. 104-1). Thrombin then cleaves fibrinopeptides A and B from the N-terminal end of the two α and two β chains of fibrinogen leading to the formation of the fibrin clot. Thrombin also activates factor V,[113,114] factor VIII,[115–118] factor XIII,[119,120] and protein C[121–123] by limited proteolysis (see Fig. 104-2). In addition, thrombin is capable of factor XI activation in the presence of a negatively charged surface such as sulfatide, heparin, or dextran sulfate.[124,125] Finally, thrombin is capable of a number of cellular interactions.[126] Of particular importance among these, thrombin binds to and cleaves a specific platelet membrane receptor,[127] resulting in platelet activation, aggregation, and release of intracellular granule contents.

Prothrombin is a single-chain glycoprotein with a molecular weight of 71,600 and an N-terminal sequence of Ala-Asn-Thr-Phe-Leu[128] (Fig. 104-5). The mature protein circulating in plasma contains 579 amino acids, including 10 residues of γ-carboxyglutamic acid that constitute the Gla domain.[129] The two kringle structures in prothrombin are located between the Gla domain and the serine protease portion of the molecule. Prothrombin also contains 8.2 percent carbohydrate, which is apparently attached to asparagine residues 78 and 100 located in kringle 1 and Asn 373 in the catalytic domain of the molecule. The catalytic domain also contains the three active site residues that include His 363, Asp 419, and Ser 525.

The activation of human prothrombin involves the cleavage of internal Arg 271-Thr and Arg 320-Ile peptide bonds by factor Xa[130] (Figs. 104-5 and 104-6). The reaction requires calcium ions and is accelerated about 20,000 times by the addition of phospholipid and factor Va.[131,132] The principal

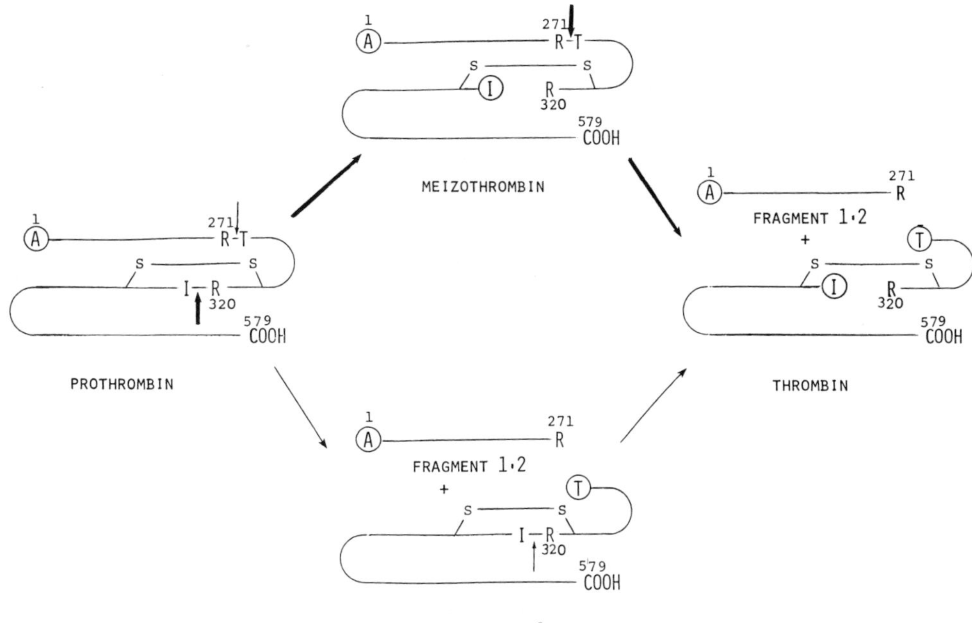

FIG.104-6 Activation scheme for human prothrombin. In the presence of factor Va, the initial cleavage by factor Xa occurs at R_{320}-I_{321} (heavy vertical arrow) generating thrombin and fragment 1.2. In the absence of factor Va, the initial cleavage by factor Xa occurs at R_{271}-T_{272} (thin vertical arrow), generating prethrombin 2 and fragment 1.2. The second cleavage then occurs at R_{320}-I_{321} (thin vertical arrow) generating thrombin. N-terminal amino acids are circled. I = Ile; R = Arg; T = Thr.

effect of the phospholipid is to decrease the K_m for the substrate about 150 times, while factor Va, in a complex with factor Xa at a molar ratio of 1:1, increases the V_{max} of the reaction approximately 1000 times. In the presence of factor Va, the activation of human prothrombin proceeds by the initial cleavage of the Arg 320-Ile bond generating a meizothrombin intermediate.[133] Meizothrombin has peptidase activity toward small synthetic substrates and incorporates di*i*sopropylfluoridate into its active site serine. It is unable, however, to convert fibrinogen to fibrin. A second cleavage occurs in meizothrombin at the Arg 271-Thr bond. This cleavage generates thrombin by the liberation of fragment 1.2, which contains amino acids 1 to 271, including the Gla and kringle domains. The thrombin generated is composed of a light chain of 49 amino acids and a heavy chain of 259 amino acids. These two chains are held together by a disulfide bond. This molecule undergoes further cleavage at Arg 284-Thr in the light chain to form a thrombin molecule with a light chain of 36 amino acids. These reactions reduce the molecular weight of the precursor from 71,600 to about 34,500.

In the absence of factor Va, the activation of prothrombin proceeds by a prethrombin-2 intermediate generated by the initial cleavage at the Arg 271-Thr bond[133] (see Fig. 104-6). In whole plasma, the cleavage in prothrombin occurs primarily at Arg 284-Thr in the light chain as well as the Arg 320-Ile bond.[134] This latter pathway generates a thrombin molecule with an initial light chain of 36 amino acids rather than 49 amino acids and a Gla-kringle fragment of 284 amino acids (fragment 1.2.3). This latter pathway may well represent a major avenue for thrombin generation under physiological conditions.

Activation of prothrombin occurs on phospholipid surfaces, where the protein substrate is concentrated.[135] It appears that factor Va enhances the binding of factor Xa to membrane surfaces[136] and that this association modulates the orientation and conformation of the bound factor Xa and prothrombin.[137,138] The calcium-dependent binding of prothrombin to the phospholipid surfaces involves the Gla region[4,139] and possibly the first kringle structure.[140] In vivo, the phospholipid component of the reaction may be provided by platelets,[141,142] endothelial cells,[143] or leukocytes.[142] When the newly generated thrombin is formed, it is released from the phospholipid surface and is then free to interact with its various substrates, such as fibrinogen and factor XIII.

Prothrombin Gene

The gene for human prothrombin is located on chromosome 11 at p11-q12.[144] It contains about 21 kb of DNA, and its complete sequence has been established.[67] The gene is composed of 14 exons separated by 13 introns. The introns range in size from 84 to 9447 nucleotides, while the exons range in size from 25 to 315 nucleotides (Table 104-3). The intron–exon splice junction sequences follow the GT-AG rule[145] and the typical splice junction consensus,[146] except for the splice site at the 5′ end of intron L (Table 104-4). The exons in the gene for prothombin code for 579 amino acids comprising the mature protein that circulates in plasma, in addition to a prepro leader sequence of 43 amino acids. The first intron (intron A) is located in the prepro leader sequence (Val −17), while the second intron is located just after the Gla domain (between Thr 37 and Asp 38). The third intron occurs nine residues later (Ala 46), while the fourth intron occurs just prior to the first kringle (Gly 63). The fifth intron is located within the first kringle (Glu 98), and the sixth intron is located between kringles 1 and 2 (Gly 144). The second kringle in prothrombin, in contrast to the first kringle, is coded by a single exon. Accordingly, the seventh intron is present immediately following kringle 2 (Glu 249). The remaining introns in the gene for prothrombin occur throughout the molecule, including five within the catalytic domain (see Fig. 104-5).

The gene for human prothrombin contains 30 copies of *Alu* repetitive DNA and two copies of partial *Kpn*I repeats. These repeats comprise approximately 40 percent of the human gene for prothrombin. The *Alu* sequences occur in clusters, with 20 present in the 12th intron (intron L). The human haploid genome contains about 300,000 copies of *Alu* repetitive sequences that are about 300 nucleotides in length and show about 80 percent sequence homology.[147,148] This is equivalent to about one *Alu* repetitive sequence in every 6

Table 104-3 Location and Size of Exons and Introns in the Gene for Human Prothrombin

Exon	Nucleotide Positions	Length, bp	Amino Acids	Intervening Sequence	Nucleotide Positions	Length, bp	Number of *Alu* Repeats
I	+ 1–79	79 + *	− 43 to − 17	A	80–465	386	
II	466–626	161	− 17 to 37	B	627–1285	659	
III	1286–1310	25	38–46	C	1311–1552	242	
IV	1553–1603	51	46–63	D	1604–3929	2326	4
V	3930–4035	106	63–98	E	4036–4131	96	
VI	4132–4268	137	98–144	F	4269–6606	2338	3
VII	6607–6921	315	144–249	G	6922–7245	324	
VIII	7246–7374	129	249–292	H	7375–7458	84	
IX	7459–7585	127	292–334	I	7586–8742	1157	2
X	8743–8910	168	334–390	J	8911–9407	497	
XI	9408–9581	174	390–448	K	9582–10123	542	1
XII	10124–10305	182	448–509	L	10306–19752	9447	20†
XIII	19753–19823	71	509–532	M	19824–19969	146	
XIV	19970–20210	241	533–polyA site				

*The length of the 5′ noncoding region of the mRNA for human prothrombin is unknown; therefore, the length of exon I is measured from the initiator methionine.
†This intervening sequence also has two copies of partial "*Kpn*" repeats.
SOURCE: Degen and Davie.[67]

kb of human DNA. Thus, the prothrombin gene has an unusually high concentration of these repetitive sequences, whose function is presently unknown.

The 5′ region of the prothrombin gene lacks a typical TATA or CCAAT sequence, but appears to have a weak promoter immediately upstream from a heterogeneous transcription initiation site.[149,150] In addition, a bidirectional liver-specific enhancer element is located between nucleotides −940 and −860.[150] The prothrombin enhancer region contains a putative HNF-1 binding site flanked by an inverted CCTCCC sequence that is present in other HNF-1 liver-specific promoters such as the fibrinogen β chain and α_1-antitrypsin promoters.

Three common polymorphisms have been identified within the prothrombin gene. An 800-bp insertion resulting in a *Pst*I RFLP occurs in intron D with a frequency of about 30 percent in Caucasians.[151,152] In Japanese individuals, two common polymorphisms occur within 71 bp: an *Nco*I RFLP due to a T-to-C substitution in exon VI resulting in a Thr–Met polymorphism at residue 122,[153] and a *Mbo*II RFLP in intron E due to a C–G polymorphism at nucleotide 4125.[154]

Prothrombin Deficiency

Prothrombin deficiency is a very rare abnormality, with about 50 reported cases. Patients with this deficiency have been placed in two broad categories: those with normal plasma levels of an abnormal protein that has decreased biologic activity (dysprothrombinemia) and those with decreased biosynthesis and reduced plasma levels (hypoprothrombinemia). Hypoprothrombinemia has been described as an autosomal recessive disorder, and most reported cases

Table 104-4 Intron–Exon Splice Junction Sequences in the Gene for Human Prothrombin

		Splice Junction Sequences			
Intron	Exon	5′	Intron	3′	Exon
A	ATG	GTAAGG	— — — —	CCACCGCCTTTACAG	T
B	ACG	GTGAGC	— — — —	GCCCTTGTTTTTCAG	G
C	CAG	GTGAGC	— — — —	CTGGGTCTTTTCCAG	C
D	AAG	GTGAGC	— — — —	GTGGGGTCTCCGCAG	G
E	TGA	GTGAGT	— — — —	AATTTCCTCTTCCAG	A
F	GTG	GTAGGC	— — — —	CCCCTCACCCACCAG	G
G	GTG	GTGAGC	— — — —	CCTGGGTCCCAACAG	A
H	CAG	GTGAGG	— — — —	TGGCTTGCTCTGCAG	A
I	TTG	GTGTGT	— — — —	TGCTGCCCCTCCCAG	G
J	AAG	GTACAG	— — — —	TTGGGGTCTCTGCAG	G
K	CAG	GTGGGC	— — — —	CTTCCTTCCCCAAAG	C
L	CTG	GCAAGT	— — — —	CTGTTCTCTTTCAAG	G
M	AAG	GTAAGC	— — — —	ATCTTTCTTCTTCAG	A
Consensus sequence*	$^{C}_{A}$AG	GT$^{A}_{G}$AGT	— — — —	$^{T}_{C}$$^{T}_{C}$$^{T}_{C}$$^{T}_{C}$$^{T}_{C}$$^{T}_{C}$$^{T}_{C}$$^{T}_{C}$$^{T}_{C}$$^{T}_{C}$$^{T}_{C}N^{T}_{C}$AG	G

*From Mount.[146]
SOURCE: Degen and Davie.[67]

have been in individuals of Mediterranean descent.[155,156] Patients who are homozygous have bleeding complications, and their prothrombin coagulant activity ranges from 2 to 25 percent of normal. Bleeding complications include bruising easily, epistaxis, gingival hemorrhage, menorrhagia, and postoperative hemorrhage; spontaneous hemarthrosis is rare. Individuals who are heterozygous have prothrombin activity levels of 50 percent or greater and are asymptomatic.

Congenital dysprothrombinemia is also inherited in an autosomal recessive manner and bleeding manifestations are similar to those of congenital hypoprothrombinemia.[157] The severity of bleeding, however, does not necessarily correlate with residual prothrombin clotting activity. Thus far, more than 20 abnormal prothrombins have been reported. Ten have been isolated and characterized, but specific molecular abnormalities have been identified in only six of these. Of the six different molecular abnormalities in prothrombin identified to date, four are the result of C-to-T transitions within codons containing CGX. This type of nucleotide transition occurs fairly commonly, since CG is a major site of methylation in genomic DNA and the deamination of methyl cytosine to thymidine would give rise to this mutation.

Prothrombin$_{\text{BARCELONA}}$[158] and prothrombin$_{\text{MADRID}}$[159] have both been shown to be due to the replacement of an Arg by a Cys residue at position 271.* The Arg 271-Thr bond is one of two peptide bonds that must be cleaved by factor Xa during the conversion of prothrombin to thrombin, and the replacement of an Arg by a Cys residue prevents this cleavage. The Cys residue in prothrombin$_{\text{BARCELONA}}$ and prothrombin$_{\text{MADRID}}$ apparently results from a base change of C to T in the triplet of CGT originally coding for arginine in the gene for human prothrombin. Mutations at the analogous arginine activation sites in factor IX and factor X have also been described in patients with these respective deficiencies (see below).

Prothrombin$_{\text{TOKUSHIMA}}$ is an abnormal protein that is readily converted to thrombin by factor Xa in the presence of factor Va, phospholipid, and calcium ions.[161] The newly generated thrombin, however, shows only 21 percent clotting activity relative to normal thrombin. The abnormal thrombin also exhibits reduced platelet aggregating activity. Amino acid sequence analysis indicates that the reduced clotting activity in this protein is due to the replacement of Arg 418 by Trp in the catalytic region of the abnormal molecule. This mutation can be explained by a single base change of C to T in the triplet of CGG coding for arginine in the normal molecule.[162] The reduced fibrinogen clotting activity for thrombin$_{\text{TOKUSHIMA}}$ also suggests that Arg 418, located adjacent to the essential Asp 419 (see Fig. 104-5), is important for the binding of fibrinogen to the enzyme and is consistent with the increased K_m and decreased catalytic rate constant for the abnormal enzyme.

Prothrombin$_{\text{QUICK}}$ has been separated into two components designated "thrombin$_{\text{QUICK I}}$" and "thrombin$_{\text{QUICK II}}$."[163] In thrombin$_{\text{QUICK I}}$, a mutation of Arg 382 to Cys (presumably due to a mutation of CGC to TGC) in the putative fibrinogen binding site results in decreased thrombin clotting activity, normal amidolytic activity toward chromogenic substrates, decreased platelet aggregating activity, and markedly reduced platelet binding affinity.[164,165] Thrombin$_{\text{QUICK II}}$, on the other hand, is characterized by a mutation of Gly 558 to Val (corresponding to a mutation of GGC to GTC) in the primary substrate binding pocket that completely abolishes both clotting and amidolytic activity as well as platelet aggregation, but has less effect on high-affinity platelet binding.[165,166]

Prothrombin$_{\text{SALAKTA}}$ was isolated from an asymptomatic individual with 17 percent clotting activity and reduced substrate binding affinity.[167] The molecular abnormality has been identified as a substitution of Glu (GAG) to Ala (GCG) at residue 466 of the thrombin heavy chain. Presumably, this substitution affects the conformation of a surface loop surrounding Trp 468 that is thought to be necessary for specific substrate binding.[168]

Although the precise molecular abnormalities involved have not been confirmed, prothrombin$_{\text{CARDEZA}}$[156] and prothrombin$_{\text{CLAMART}}$[169] appear to be due to defects similar to prothrombins$_{\text{BARCELONA}}$ and $_{\text{MADRID}}$ in that the zymogen is not converted to thrombin by factor Xa. In contrast, prothrombin$_{\text{HIMI}}$,[170] prothrombin$_{\text{METZ}}$,[171] and prothrombin$_{\text{MOLISE}}$[172] apparently have abnormalities in the thrombin portion of the molecule, while prothrombin$_{\text{SAN JUAN I}}$[156] shows an abnormality in the calcium binding domain.

Treatment of bleeding episodes in patients with congenital prothrombin deficiency consists of plasma transfusions to maintain plasma prothrombin levels above 30 percent of normal (30 U/dl). Fresh frozen plasma contains 1 unit per milliliter of prothrombin, which has a circulating half-life of ≈3 days. For major bleeding episodes or surgical procedures, prothrombin complex concentrates can be used, but these products carry an increased risk of viral transmission and thromboembolic complications.

COMBINED DEFICIENCY OF THE VITAMIN K–DEPENDENT COAGULATION FACTORS

Combined deficiency of the vitamin K–dependent coagulation factors usually occurs because of vitamin K deficiency. It is commonly found in newborns, and in the settings of liver disease and of malabsorption. A few patients, however, have been described with congenital deficiency of prothrombin as well as factor VII, factor IX, and factor X.[173–179] In some instances, levels of protein C and protein S were also reduced, but generally not as greatly as the procoagulant proteins. Clinical severity has varied in that some patients presented with severe bleeding episodes from early childhood,[173,174,177,179] while others were diagnosed later in life, following postsurgical or mucocutaneous bleeding.[175,176,178] The lack of γ-carboxylation of the vitamin K–dependent proteins[174,176,178,179] and the response to parenteral vitamin K[174,176,177,179] suggest an abnormality in vitamin K–dependent γ-carboxylation in these patients. One patient had associated skeletal abnormalities and was found to have a congenital deficiency of vitamin K epoxide reductase.[178] An abnormality of the liver carboxylase enzyme has been proposed in other patients.[179]

FACTOR VII

Factor VII participates in the extrinsic pathway of blood coagulation,[112] where it is converted to factor VIIa by a trace amount of a circulating protease (e.g., thrombin, factor

*This residue was originally assigned to position 273 according to the early protein sequence analysis of prothrombin.[160] In these studies, a Glu–Glu peptide was reported at positions 266 and 267. Subsequent amino acid sequence analysis and sequence analysis of the cDNA and the gene coding for human prothrombin indicated the absence of this peptide in the normal molecule.

IXa, factor Xa, factor XIIa, factor VIIa) or by some as yet unidentified plasma or cellular enzyme (see Fig. 104-1).[180-186] Factor VIIa in turn converts factor IX to factor IXa[187] and/or factor X to factor Xa. These reactions require a cofactor called "tissue factor."[188] Tissue factor is an integral membrane protein that is present in the vascular subendothelium as well as other extravascular sites.[189-191] It binds circulating factor VII at sites of vascular injury.[192-194] The binding of exposed tissue factor to factor VII or to factor VIIa greatly increases the catalytic efficiency of these reactions,[195-197] apparently by causing a conformational change in the catalytic site of factor VIIa.[198,199] Tissue factor is not accessible to factor VII without prior tissue damage. Thus, generation of the factor VII–tissue factor complex is critical for initiating the blood coagulation cascade leading to fibrin formation. Once the factor VIIa–tissue factor complex is formed and factor Xa is generated, the extrinsic pathway is rapidly inactivated by a lipoprotein-associated inhibitor that forms a quaternary complex with factor VIIa–tissue factor–factor Xa.[200,201]

Human factor VII is a single-chain glycoprotein with a molecular weight of 50,000 and an N-terminal sequence of Ala-Asn-Ala-Phe-Leu[11,202] (Fig. 104-7). The protein is initially synthesized with a prepro leader sequence of 38 amino acids. This prepropeptide is removed by signal peptidase and a processing protease, resulting in a mature protein of 406 amino acids. The Gla-containing region contains 10 γ-carboxyglutamic acid residues and is followed by two growth factor

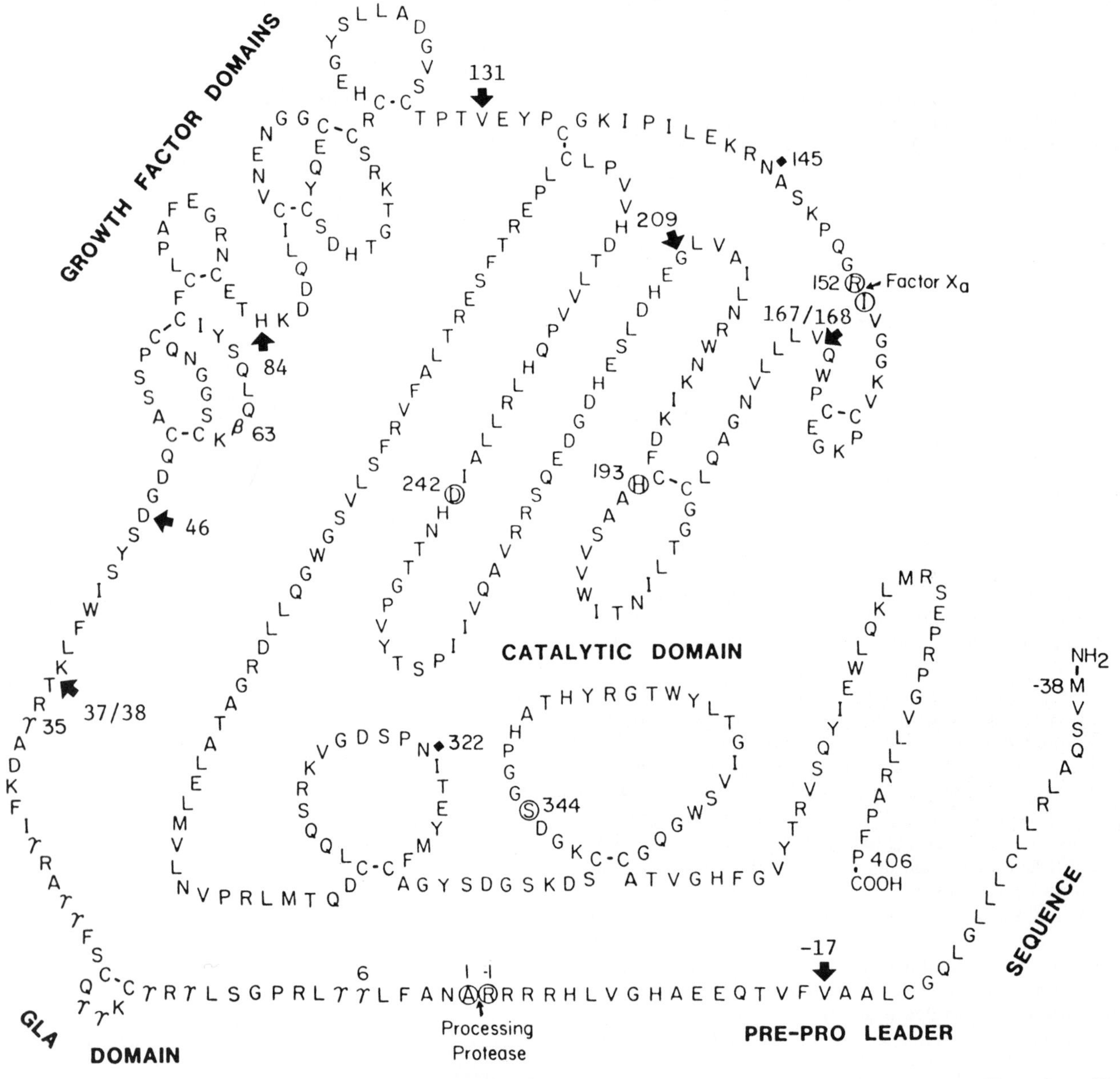

FIG. 104-7 Amino acid sequence and tentative structure of human prepro factor VII. The locations of the seven introns are shown by heavy arrows. The prepro leader sequence is cleaved during protein biosynthesis to give rise to the mature protein with an N-terminal sequence of A-N-A-F-. The single peptide bond cleaved by factor Xa during the activation reaction is shown with a small arrow. The three amino acids in the catalytic domain (H_{193}, D_{242}, S_{344}) that participate in catalysis are circled, while the tentative carbohydrate attachment sites are shown with solid diamonds. The amino acids are numbered as follows, starting with the N-terminal end of the protein: −38 to −1 = prepro leader sequence; +1 to 152 = light chain of factor VIIa; 153 to 406 = catalytic chain of factor VIIa. The single letter codes for amino acids are given in the legend to Fig. 104-5. β = β-hydroxyaspartic acid. *(Modified from Hagen et al.[11] and O'Hara et al.[218])*

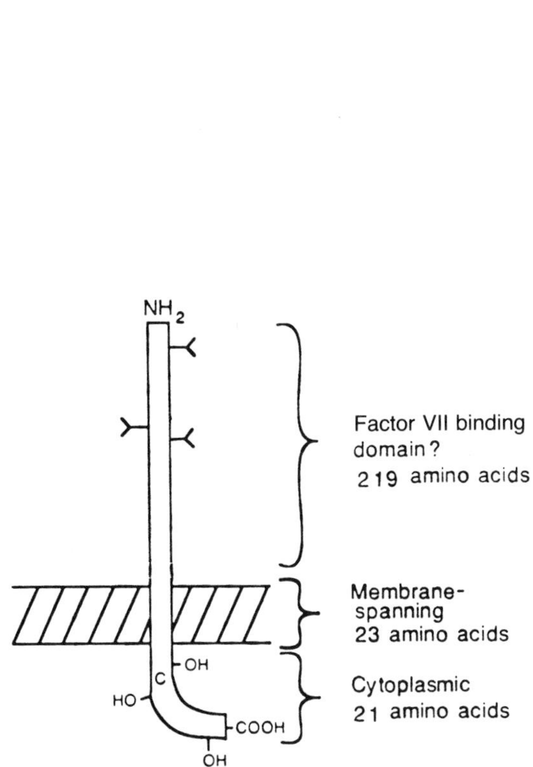

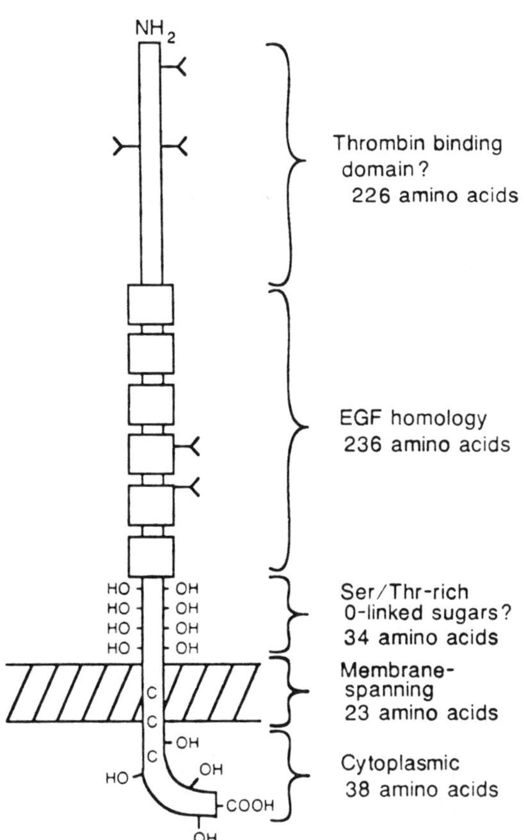

FIG. 104-8 **Structural domains of human tissue factor** ***(left panel)*** **and human thrombomodulin** ***(right panel).*** **The extracellular N-terminal region of each portion is shown above the membrane (diagonal bar) and the cytoplasmic C-terminal region is shown below the membrane. Epidermal growth factor domains (EGF) are shown by open squares. Potential N-glycosylation sites are indicated by Y, while the hydroxy amino acids in the Ser–Thr-rich region and the cytoplasmic region are indicated by —OH. Cysteine residues in the transmembrane region and cytoplasmic regions are also indicated by C.** ***(Modified from Scarpati et al.,[206] Spicer et al.,[207] Morrissey et al.,[208] Fisher et al.,[209] and Wen et al.[484])***

domains. Factor VII also contains carbohydrate, a portion of which is attached to Asn 145 in the light chain and Asn 322 in the heavy chain of the activated molecule.[97] In addition, factor VII contains two unique *O*-linked carbohydrate chains, glucose-(xylose)$_2$ at Ser 52 and fucose at Ser 60.[101,102] The functional importance of these carbohydrate moieties is unknown.

The activation of human factor VII involves the cleavage of an internal Arg 152-Ile peptide bond (see Fig. 104-7). This generates factor VIIa, which is composed of a light chain of 152 amino acids and a heavy chain of 254 amino acids. These two chains are held together by a single disulfide bond. The heavy chain of the molecule contains the catalytic domain, including the active site residues of His 193, Asp 242, and Ser 344. No activation peptide is liberated during the activation reaction; thus, factor VII and factor VIIa have essentially the same molecular weight.

The binding of factor VII/VIIa to tissue factor is calcium-dependent. It appears that several discrete regions within both the light chain (Gla and growth factor domains) and heavy chain (catalytic domain) are required for this specific interaction.[48–52,203–205]

Human tissue factor ($Mr \approx 44{,}000$) is a single-chain glycoprotein composed of 263 amino acids.[206–209] It is initially synthesized with a signal peptide of 32 amino acids cleaved from the growing polypeptide chain by signal peptidase. This generates the mature membrane-bound glycoprotein with an N-terminal sequence of Ser-Gly-Thr-Thr (Fig. 104-8). The extracellular domain at the N-terminal end of the protein is 219 residues in length and contains the potential factor VII or factor VIIa binding sites[197,210] as well as a possible recognition site for factor X.[211] This region is followed by a membrane-spanning region of 23 hydrophobic residues and a cytoplasmic region of 21 residues at the carboxyl end of the molecule. The membrane-spanning region, in addition to the extracellular domain, appears to be required for full cofactor activity.[212–214]

Factor VII and Tissue Factor Genes

The gene for factor VII is located on chromosome 13 in the region q34-qter, which is very close to the gene for factor X.[215–217] The complete sequence for the gene for factor VII has been determined and found to span about 12.8 kb of DNA.[218] The mRNA for factor VII can undergo alternative splicing, forming a major transcript from eight exons and a very minor transcript utilizing nine exons. The additional exon located in the 5′ end of the gene results in a prepro leader sequence of 60 amino acids rather than the usual 38 amino acids. The smallest exon in the gene for factor VII codes for nine amino acids (residues 38 to 46 in the light chain), while the largest exon codes for 198 amino acids (residues 57 to 254 in the heavy chain). The introns range in size from 68 nucleotides (intron C) to 2574 nucleotides (intron A). All the intron–exon splice junctions follow the GT-AG rule.[145] The gene for factor VII is free of *Alu* repetitive sequences. However, it does contain five regions of tandem repeats that are also similar to hypervariable minisatellite DNA.[218,219] A prevalent polymorphism due to the presence or absence of a 37-bp monomer element is present in intron G and is readily detected by PCR.[220,221] In addition, an *Msp*I RFLP in exon VIII is present in ≈10 percent of Caucasian factor VII alleles[222]; this G/A dimorphism results in substitution for Gln for Arg 353.

Five of the seven introns in the gene for factor VII are located in the regions coding for the N-terminal half of the protein (see Fig. 104-6). The first intron occurs in the prepro leader sequence (Val −17), while the second follows the Gla domain (between Thr 37 and Lys 38). The third intron is located just prior to the first growth factor domain (Asp 46). The fourth intron is located between the two growth factor domains (His 84), while the fifth intron is found just after the second growth factor domain (Val 131). The last two introns are present within the catalytic domain (between Gln 167 and Val 168 and at Gly 209). The remaining portion of the protein (from Gly 209 to Pro 406) is coded by a single exon. These seven introns in the gene for factor VII are located in the same position as the seven introns in factor IX, factor X, and protein C and in the same position as the first three introns in prothrombin relative to the amino acid sequence of each of these proteins[13,17,67,218,223,224] (Table 104-5). However, the introns in the genes of this family of vitamin K–dependent proteins differ greatly in their size and DNA sequence, with the exception of intron C in factor VII and protein C. The similarity of the amino acid sequence and the organization of the genes in this family of proteins has led to the proposal that the vitamin K–dependent proteins have evolved from a common ancestor through gene duplication and exon shuffling.[225]

The gene for tissue factor is located on region p21-p22 of chromosome 1[226,227] and includes 12.4 kb.[228] It contains six exons separated by five introns with typical consensus intron–exon boundaries. The first exon encodes the 32-residue signal peptide, while the second through fifth exons encode the N-terminal extracellular domain. The sixth exon contains 1278 bp and includes the transmembrane and cytoplasmic domains as well as a long 3′ untranslated region. The gene for tissue factor also contains three full-length and one partial *Alu* repeat and a single major transcription initiation site 26 bp downstream of a TATA box. Transcription of the tissue factor gene in activated monocytes results in a 2.2-kb mRNA encoding the tissue factor protein and a 3.1-kb mRNA due to an alternative splice site in intron 1 that terminates in a premature stop codon.[229]

Tissue factor is expressed constitutively in a differentiation-dependent manner in extravascular cells and tumor cells and is inducible in fibroblasts, monocytes, and endothelial cells in response to a variety of cytokines and inflammatory mediators.[189,230] Regulation of cell-surface tissue factor expression is complex and probably occurs at both the transcriptional and posttranscriptional levels.[230] The tissue factor promoter region can be divided into two functional regions: a downstream minimal promoter region responsible for maintaining low base-line levels of expression that contains the TATA box and an Spl binding site and an upstream modulator/enhancer region that amplifies transcription to high levels in response to lipopolysaccharide and which contains AP-1 and NF-κB binding sites.

Table 104-5 Comparison of the Location, Splice Junction Type, and Size of the Introns in the Genes for Human Factors VII, IX, and X, Protein C, and Prothrombin

Intron	Protein	Location* (Amino Acid)	Splice Junction Type	Size, bp
A	Factor VII	−17	I	2574
	Factor IX	−17	I	6206
	Factor X	−17	I	≈5000
	Protein C	−19	I	1263
	Prothrombin	−17	I	386
B	Factor VII	37/38	0	1919
	Factor IX	38/39	0	188
	Factor X	37/38	0	≈7400
	Protein C	37/38	0	1462
	Prothrombin	37/38	0	659
C	Factor VII	46	I	68
	Factor IX	47	I	3689
	Factor X	46	I	≈ 950
	Protein C	46	I	92
	Prothrombin	46	I	242
D	Factor VII	84	I	1908
	Factor IX	85	I	7163
	Factor X	84	I	≈1800
	Protein C	92	I	102
E	Factor VII	131	I	971
	Factor IX	128	I	2565
	Factor X	128	I	≈2900
	Protein C	137	I	2668
F	Factor VII	15/16	0	595
	Factor IX	15/16	0	9473
	Factor X	15/16	0	≈3400
	Protein C	15/16	0	873
G	Factor VII	57	I	816
	Factor IX	54	I	668
	Factor X	55	I	≈1700
	Protein C	55	I	1129

NOTE: Type 0 splice junctions have introns between the triplets coding for two amino acids; type I splice junctions have introns between the first and second nucleotides of the triplet coding for one amino acid.
*Numbering for introns A through E refers to light chain and for introns F and G refers to heavy chain.

Clinical Aspects of Factor VII

Elevated levels of factor VII have been associated with a number of clinical conditions. Levels of factor VII rise during pregnancy, delivery, and puerperium, most likely occurring in a complex of factor VII and phospholipid.[231] Elevated levels of factor VII have also been associated with increasing age,[232] hyperglycemia,[233] dietary fat intake,[234] and hyperlipidemia,[233,235,236] particularly large triglyceride-rich lipoproteins such as VLDL and chylomicrons. The effect of lipids on factor VII coagulant activity (factor VII:C) levels may be due to the contact surface activation of factor XII by negatively charged plasma lipid particles, with the subsequent activation of factor VII.[237,238] Finally, raised plasma factor VII:C activity has been associated both retrospectively and prospectively with an increased risk of ischemic heart disease.[239–241] Interestingly, the Gln 353 allele of the *Msp*I RFLP in exon VIII correlates strongly with lower plasma factor VII:C levels.[222]

Congenital factor VII deficiency is a very rare condition. It is inherited as an autosomal recessive disorder with variable expression and high penetrance.[242–244] There is no absolute correlation between a decreased plasma level of factor VII and bleeding symptoms. Cerebral hemorrhage has been reported to occur in 16 percent of factor VII–deficient patients.[245] Other common bleeding manifestations include easy bruising, epistaxis, gingival hemorrhage, and menorrhagia. Hemarthroses generally occur only in severely affected individuals. Paradoxically, some patients with factor VII deficiency have been reported to suffer from thromboembolism.[246–248]

Factor VII deficiency is usually characterized by an isolated prolonged prothrombin time (PT) and normal activated partial thromboplastin time (APTT). Several molecular variants of factor VII have been described that show variable patterns with regard to the level of factor VII:C and factor VII antigen (factor VII:Ag).[249,250] Furthermore, the factor VII activity may vary depending on the thromboplastin used in the coagulation assay.[251]

Several factor VII variants have been characterized at the molecular level. A symptomatic patient with severe factor VII deficiency (factor VII:C <1 percent, factor VII:Ag normal) was found to be homozygous for a G → A mutation resulting in the substitution of Gln for Arg 79 within the first growth factor domain. This patient was also heterozygous for a second mutation of G → A, resulting in the substitution of Gln for Arg 152 at the factor VII activation site.[252] Secondly, an asymptomatic individual was found to have an Arg (CCG) to Gln (CAG) mutation at codon 304 within the catalytic domain.[253] This individual had a factor VII:C level that was undetectable using rabbit tissue factor, but was 30 percent of normal using human tissue factor. The factor VII:Ag level in this patient was normal. A homozygous Cys 310 to Phe mutation (TGC to TTC) was found in an Italian patient with 4 percent factor VII:C activity and a mild bleeding disorder.[221] Finally, a severely affected patient (factor VII:C and factor VII:Ag = 1 percent) was a compound heterozygote for two different single base deletions at codons 260/261 and 289/290, respectively.[254]

When bleeding episodes occur, factor VII–deficient patients may be treated with plasma or a prothrombin complex concentrate that contains significant amounts of all the vitamin K–dependent plasma proteins, including factor VII. Concentrates of purified factor VII have also been prepared for this purpose, but are less readily available.

Recombinant human factor VIIa has been successfully used to treat patients with hemophilia A who have antibodies against factor VIII.[255] The administered recombinant factor VIIa presumably forms a complex with exposed tissue factor at the site of injury that directly activates factor X (see Fig. 104-1) independently of the presence of factors VIII and IX.

FACTOR IX

As is true of most coagulation factors, factor IX was first recognized as a special entity by the revelation that hemophilia could be caused by a deficiency of two different plasma proteins. In 1947, Pavlovsky found that the prolonged coagulation time of plasma from one hemophilia patient normalized the clotting time of another hemophilic plasma. Further studies[256,257] clearly showed two types of hemophilia, both of which were inherited as X-linked recessive disorders that were clinically indistinguishable from each other. One was called "hemophilia A" and was caused by a deficiency of factor VIII. The other was designated "hemophilia B" and was defined as a deficiency of factor IX (Christmas factor, plasma thromboplastin component, β-prothromboplastin).

Factor IX participates in the middle stages of the blood coagulation cascade[112] and is converted to factor IXa in the presence either of factor XIa and calcium ions[258] or of factor VIIa, tissue factor, and calcium ions[187] (see Fig. 104-1). Factor IXa then activates factor X in the presence of factor VIIIa, calcium ions, and phospholipid.

Human factor IX is a single-chain glycoprotein with a molecular weight of 56,800 and an N-terminal sequence of Tyr-Asn-Ser-Gly-Lys[259] (Fig. 104-9). The mature protein circulating in plasma contains 415 amino acids, including 12 residues of γ-carboxyglutamic acid.[12] The human protein also contains 0.3 equivalent of β-hydroxyaspartic acid at position 64 in the first of the two growth factor domains.[91,92] The function of β-hydroxyaspartic acid in factor IX has not been established. Equilibrium dialysis experiments have shown that it does not participate in the high affinity calcium binding sites present in factor IX.[260] In addition, nonhydroxylated recombinant factor IX retains full procoagulant activity.[261] Factor IX also contains 17 percent carbohydrate, a portion of which is attached to asparagine residues 157 and 167 in the activation peptide. Like factor VII, human factor IX also contains two unique *O*-linked carbohydrate structures including Xyl-Glc at Ser 53 within the first growth factor domain[100,101] and a tetrasaccharide at Ser 61, which is *O*-linked through a fucose residue.[103]

Human factor IX is converted to a serine protease during the coagulation process by the cleavage of two internal peptide bonds[258] (Figs. 104-9 and 104-10). Cleavage occurs initially at the Arg 145-Ala bond with the formation of factor IXα followed by cleavage of the Arg 180-Val bond leading to the generation of factor IXaβ. The second cleavage releases an activation glycopeptide of 35 amino acids. The light chain of factor IXaβ contains the Gla domain and the two growth factor domains, while the heavy chain contains the catalytic domain that includes the active site residues of His 221, Asp 269, and Ser 365. The light chain and the heavy chain of factor IXaβ are linked together by a single disulfide bond involving Cys 132 in the light chain and Cys 289 in the heavy chain (See Fig. 104-9). The cleavage of the two internal arginine peptide bonds is catalyzed either by factor XIa in the presence of calcium ions, or by factor VIIa in the presence of tissue factor, phospholipid, and calcium ions. Cleavage of only the Arg 180-Val bond gives rise to factor IXaα, an enzyme with markedly reduced biologic activity. This activation reaction occurs in the presence of a protease from Russell's viper venom (RVV-X).[262]

The binding of calcium ions to the Gla domain is required for the interaction of factor IX with phospholipid membrane surfaces.[263,264] Factor IX contains two additional calcium binding sites located within the first growth factor domain[39,42,46,260] and within the N-terminal portion of the catalytic domain.[265] In addition to binding calcium and phospholipid, the Gla and growth factor domains of the factor IX/IXa light chain have been implicated in the binding of the protein to specific receptors on platelets[60] and endothelial cells.[53,54,58,59] In contrast, interaction of factor IXa with its cofactor (factor VIIIa) and substrate (factor X) appears to require determinants within both the light and heavy chains of factor IXa.[55–57,266]

Factor IX Gene

The genes for human factor IX and factor VIII are located close to each other on the tip of the long arm of the X chromosome at Xq26-Xq27.[267,268] The gene for factor IX is about 34 kb in size, and its complete nucleotide sequence has been established.[13] The gene contains seven introns and eight exons within the coding and 3′ noncoding regions of the gene (Table 104-6). The eight exons code for 415 amino acids comprising the mature protein that circulates in plasma. The first two exons also code for a prepro leader sequence of 46 amino acids (see Figs. 104-4 and 104-9), and the intron–

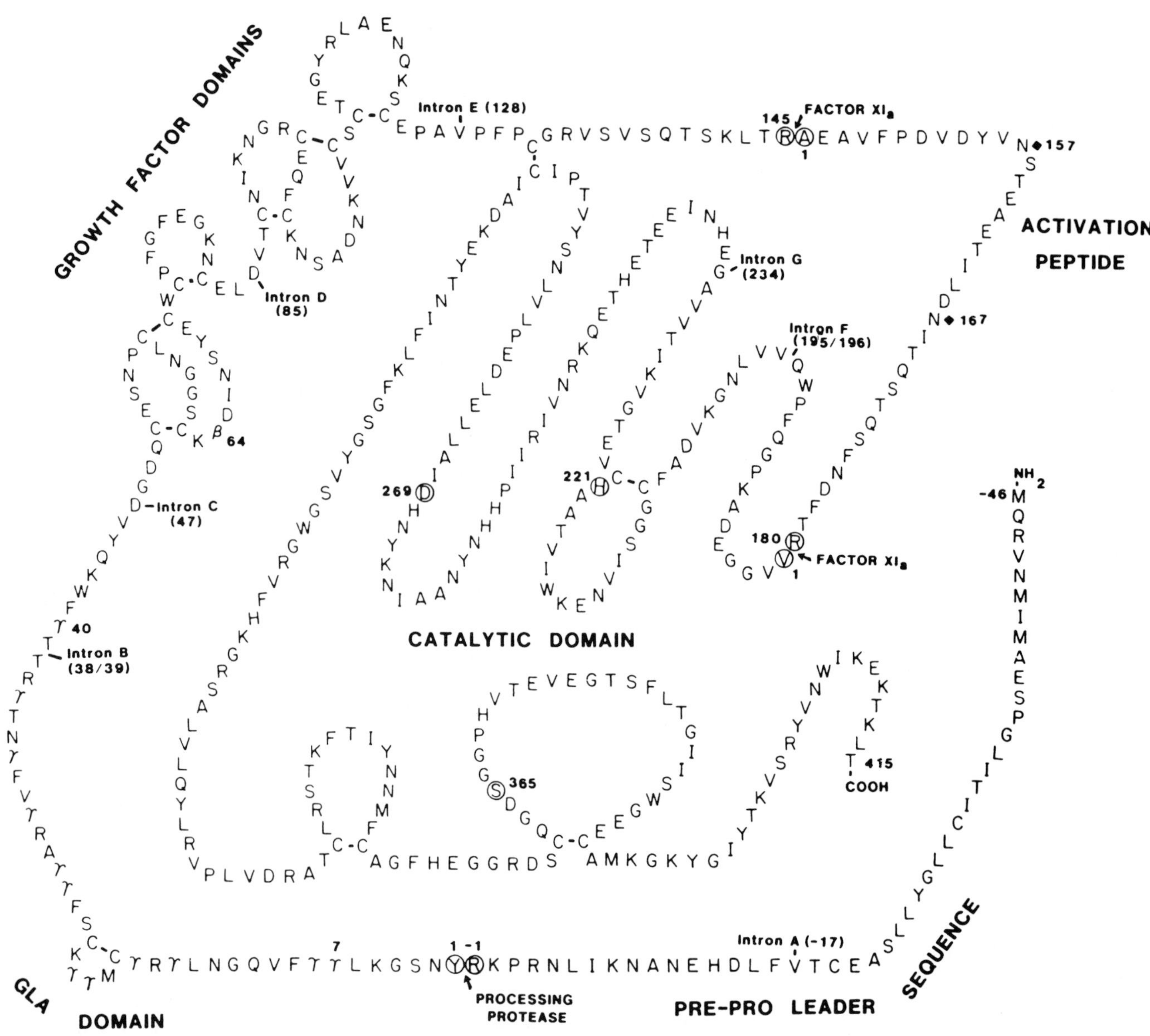

FIG. 104-9 Amino acid sequence and tentative structure for human prepro factor IX. The locations of the seven introns (A to G) are shown in the various regions of the protein. The prepro leader sequence is cleaved during protein biosynthesis to give rise to the mature protein with an N-terminal sequence of Y-N-S-G-. The two peptide bonds cleaved by factor XIa (or factor VIIa) during the activation reaction are shown with small arrows. The three amino acids in the catalytic domain (H 221, D 349, S 365) that participate in the catalysis are circled, while the two potential N-linked carbohydrate attachment sites in the activation peptide are shown with solid diamonds. The amino acids are numbered as follows starting with the N-terminal end of the protein: −46 to −1 = prepro leader sequence; +1 to 145 = light chain of factor IXa; 146 to 180 = activation peptide; 181 to 415 = catalytic chain of factor IXa. The single-letter codes for amino acids are given in the legend to Fig. 104-5. β = β-hydroxyaspartic acid. *(Modified from Yoshitake et al.*[13]*)*

exon splice junction sequences follow the GT-AG rule.[145] The introns contain four *Alu* repetitive sequences and range in size from 188 nucleotides (intron B) to 9473 nucleotides (intron F).

Although the factor IX promoter region contains no obvious TATA- or CCAAT-like sequences, several *cis-* and *trans-*acting regulatory elements have been identified within the 5′ untranslated region of the factor IX gene: a promoter between nucleotides −28 and −17 binds the liver-specific factor LF-A1/HNF-4[269,270]; an enhancer element spanning nucleotides +1 to +18 binds the CCAAT enhancer binding protein (C/EBP)[271]; and another regulatory element within the region −99 to −76 binds nuclear factor liver-1.[271] In addition, an androgen-responsive region may overlap the HNF-4 binding site.[269,270]

Normal Variants of Factor IX

To date, several RFLP have been identified within the gene for human factor IX.[272,273] These include a *Bam*HI site in the 5′ untranslated region, a *Dde*I/*Hin*fI site in intron A, an *Xmn*I site in intron C, a *Taq*I site in intron D, an *Msp*I site also in intron D, an *Mnl*I site in exon VI, and an *Hha*I site in the 3′ untranslated region. The allelic frequencies of these seven RFLP vary considerably among different ethnic groups. The *Bam*HI and *Msp*I sites are more polymorphic in African-Americans, while the *Dde*I/*Hin*fI, *Xmn*I, *Taq*I, and *Mnl*I sites are more polymorphic in Caucasians. The only polymorphic site in Asians is the *Hha*I site in the 3′ flanking region. Most of the known factor IX polymorphisms are in some degree of linkage disequilibrium with one

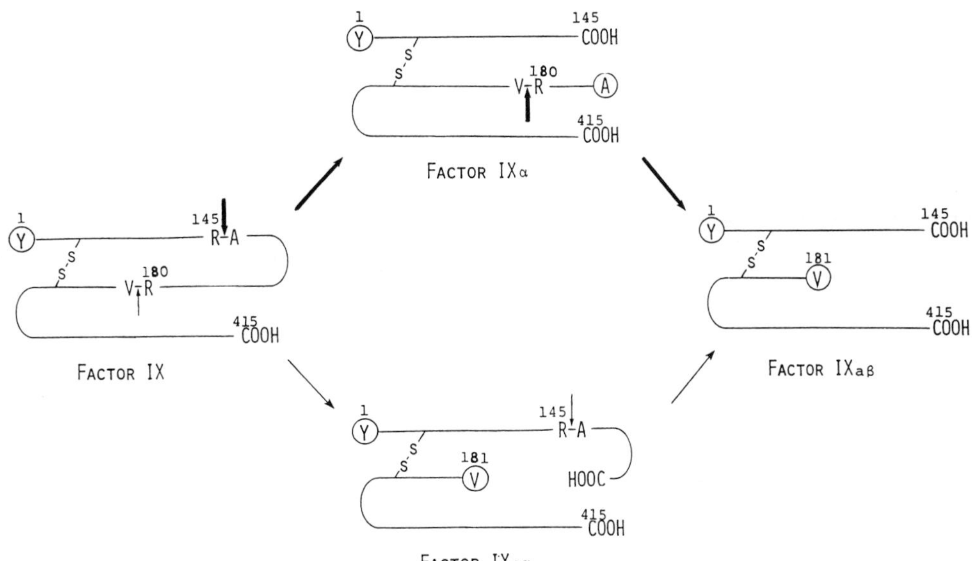

FIG. 104-10 **Activation scheme for human factor IX. In the presence of factor XIa or factor VIIa, the principal cleavage occurs initially at R 145-A 146 (heavy vertical arrow) generating the factor IXα intermediate. The second cleavage then occurs at R 180-V 181 (heavy vertical arrow) generating factor IXaβ and an activation peptide. Factor IX can also be cleaved initially at R 180-V 181 (thin vertical arrow) by factor XIa generating factor IXaα. The second cleavage then occurs at R 145-A 146 (thin vertical arrow) generating factor IXaβ and an activation peptide. N-terminal amino acids are circled.**

another. The exon VI *MnlI* polymorphism results in an amino acid polymorphism of Thr/Ala at residue 148 within the factor IX activation peptide that has no effect on biologic activity,[274] but can be detected by an immunoassay using a monoclonal antibody that recognizes only the more common threonine allele.[275,276]

Abnormal Variants of Factor IX

All patients with hemophilia B have a prolonged coagulation time and decreased factor IX clotting activity (factor IX:C) in their plasma. In 1956, however, two distinct phenotypes of hemophilia B were described. In one case, barium sulfate–absorbed plasma from one patient's blood blocked a specific inhibitor against factor IX in the assay plasma, whereas, in a second case, a similar fraction from another patient had no effect.[277] Later it was shown that approximately 10 percent of all factor IX–deficient patients have factor IX antigenic material (factor IX:Ag) or cross-reacting material (CRM^+) in their plasma.[278] The remaining 90 percent of patients deficient in factor IX either lack cross-reacting material (CRM^-) or have reduced amounts (CRM^R). Patients with severe factor IX deficiency (factor IX:C <1 percent) have lower factor IX:Ag levels, while those with milder defects fall within the low, intermediate, or normal range.[279]

The phenotypic heterogeneity of factor IX deficiency has been reflected by the identification of a large number of molecular abnormalities in hemophilia B patients. As of 1992, ≈300 unique factor IX mutations had been identified in nearly 600 hemophilia B pedigrees worldwide.[272,280] Of the mutations identified, 12 percent are gross gene alterations (complete or partial gene deletions, insertions, or rearrangements), 3 percent are short nucleotide deletions or insertions, and 85 percent are single base substitutions (point mutations). Of the point mutations, over 75 percent are missense mutations and the remainder are nonsense mutations. Molecular abnormalities responsible for factor IX deficiency have been identified in the 5′ noncoding region,

Table 104-6 **Location and Size of Exons and Introns in the Gene for Human Factor IX**

Exon	Nucleotide Positions*	Nucleotide Length*	Amino Acids†	Intron	Nucleotide Position	Nucleotide Length
I	1–117	117	−46 to −17	A	118–6325	6206‡
II	6326–6489	164	−17 to 37	B	6490–6677	188
III	6678–6702	25	38–47	C	6703–10391	3689
IV	10392–10505	114	47–85	D	10506–17668	7163
V	17669–17797	129	85–128	E	17798–20362	2565
VI	20363–20565	203	128–195	F	20566–30038	9473
VII	30039–30153	115	196–234	G	30154–30821	668
VIII	30822–32757	1935	234–415			

*Includes 30 nucleotides at the 5′ end and 1390 nucleotides at the 3′ end that are not translated.
†Amino acids coded for by each exon; negative numbers refer to amino acids in the prepro leader sequence.
‡Includes 50 extra nucleotides present in some polymorphic forms of the gene.
SOURCE: Yoshitake et al.[13]

at intron–exon splice junctions, and in all eight exons of the coding sequence. Over half the identified point mutations, however, are located in exon VII or VIII (i.e., the catalytic domain).

Gross transcriptional abnormalities, such as complete or partial factor IX gene deletions, insertions, frameshift mutations, and nonsense mutations, are almost invariably associated with severe hemophilia B (factor IX:C <1 percent) and levels of circulating factor IX antigen that are markedly reduced or undetectable. In addition, severely affected patients in whom factor IX inhibitors develop usually have one of these gross gene abnormalities. Also associated with CRM^- factor IX deficiency are single base substitutions (missense mutations) that cause mRNA or protein instability or degradation.

Hemophilia B_{LEYDEN} is a particularly interesting CRM^- variant characterized by moderate to severe factor IX deficiency during childhood followed by clinical improvement and near-normalization of factor IX clotting and antigen levels with the onset of puberty.[281] This phenotype has been associated with point mutations within a region of approximately 40 bp (−20 bp to +13) surrounding the putative transcription initiation site of the factor IX gene. Reporter gene analysis shows that several of these mutations (at nucleotides −20, −6, and +13) interfere with gene expression and that androgen stimulates transcription of both the normal and mutant sequences.[271,282] The +13 mutation specifically interferes with binding of the putative factor IX enhancer, C/EBP,[271] while a −20 T-to-A mutation inhibits binding of HNF4/LF-A1 to the factor IX promoter region.[269,270] Furthermore, a −26 G-to-C mutation (hemophilia $B_{BRANDENBURG}$) disrupts not only the LF-A1/HNF-4 binding site, but also a putative overlapping androgen-responsive site; this may explain the absence of clinical improvement following puberty in this phenotype.[269]

Of the many CRM^+ and CRM^R variants of factor IX described, several provide means for understanding the relationship between the factor IX amino acid sequence, protein structure, and coagulant function. Several patients have severe CRM^+ to CRM^R hemophilia B (factor IX:C usually <1 percent) caused by a mutation of one of several highly conserved basic amino acids within the carboxyl end of the −18-residue propeptide.[280] These include mutations of Arg −4 to Gln (factor $IX_{OXFORD\ 3}$,[82] factor $IX_{SAN\ DIMAS}$,[84] and factor $IX_{KAWACHINAGANO}$[85]), Arg −1 to Ser (factor $IX_{CAMBRIDGE}$),[83] and Lys −2 to Asn.[86] These mutations prevent removal of the propeptide prior to secretion from the hepatocyte and result in a circulating dysfunctional factor IX molecule with an 18 amino acid N-terminal extension.

Several CRM^+ variants are caused by mutations within the Gla or first growth factor domains and are characterized by reduced factor IX procoagulant activity; this is presumably due to abnormal calcium binding. Mutations of glutamic acid residues that are normally γ-carboxylated include Gla_7 to Ala (factor $IX_{OXFORD\ B2}$),[283] Gla 21 to Lys (factor $IX_{NAGOYA\ 4}$)[284] and Gla 27 to Lys (factor $IX_{SEATTLE\ 3}$)[285] or to Val (factor $IX_{CHONGQUING}$).[286] The two Gla 27 variants are characterized by severe factor IX deficiency (factor IX:C <1 percent) and reduced factor IX:Ag levels, especially when measured using a calcium-dependent antibody. In addition, site-directed mutagenesis of the equivalent Gla 21 and Gla 27 residues in protein C completely abolishes protein C calcium-dependent anticoagulant activity.[287] These conserved Gla residues are thus important for the calcium-dependent interaction of the vitamin K–dependent proteins with phospholipid membrane surfaces. Several residues within the N-terminal region of the first growth factor domain of factor IX also are involved in calcium binding and factor IX function.[34,46] Factor $IX_{ALABAMA}$ was isolated from a patient with moderately severe CRM^+ hemophilia B (factor IX:C = 10 percent).[288] The mutation was later identified as Asp 47 to Gly, which results in reduced factor IX clotting activity, most notably in the presence of calcium and factor VIIIa.[289] Factor $IX_{NEW\ LONDON}$, described in a severely affected patient (factor IX:C <1 percent; normal factor IX:Ag), is due to a substitution of Gln 50 by Pro, which results in markedly reduced activation of factor IX by factor XIa.[290] Mutation of the normally β-hydroxylated Asp 64 to Gly (factor $IX_{LONDON\ 6}$)[291] or to Asn (factor $IX_{OXFORD\ DL}$)[283] results in moderately severe CRM^+ hemophilia B; the latter variant demonstrated impaired calcium binding affinity.

Factor IX variants caused by mutations at either of the two activation sites have been described. Factor $IX_{CHAPEL\ HILL}$ (IX_{CH}) was first reported in a patient with a mild bleeding disorder (factor IX:Ag = 100 percent, factor IX:C = 20 percent).[292] The molecular defect was later shown to be a substitution of a His for Arg 145, the first or α cleavage site necessary for factor IX conversion to factor IXa[293] (see Fig. 104-8). Factor IX_{CH} is cleaved by factor XIa, however, only at the second or β cleavage site (Arg 180-Val), giving rise to factor IXaα.[294] In this molecule, the activation peptide remains attached to the light chain. Factor $IXa\alpha_{CH}$ has only about 20 percent of the clotting activity of normal factor IXaβ, but is essentially the same as normal factor IXaα. This indicates that both activation cleavages are required for normal factor IXa activity. In factor $IX_{ALBUQUERQUE}$ (factor IX:C = 1 percent, factor IX:Ag = 30 percent), the Arg 145 is replaced by Cys, which similarly results in reduced factor IX activation.[295] A number of mutations involving the β activation site (Arg 180-Val) have also been reported. As opposed to the Arg 145 mutations, the Arg 180-Val mutations are manifested by severe CRM^+ hemophilia B (factor IX:C <1 percent), indicating that the β cleavage is essential for factor IX procoagulant activity. Examples include Arg 180 to Trp (factor $IX_{DEVENTER/NAGOYA}$),[296,297] to Gln (factor $IX_{HILO/NOVARA}$),[296,298] or to Gly (factor IX_{MADRID})[299] and Val 181 to Phe (factor IX_{MILANO}).[296]

As mentioned previously, over half of the identified point mutations associated with factor IX deficiency are located within the catalytic domain or factor IXa heavy chain. Mutations in the catalytic domain characterized by a circulating dysfunctional factor IX protein can interfere with factor IX catalytic activity by several different mechanisms. Once factor IX is activated, the new N-terminus formed at Val 181 of the factor IXa heavy chain forms an ion pair with Asp 364 adjacent to the active center Ser 365 (see Fig. 104-9). By analogy with chymotrypsin, formation of the ion pair results in a conformational change in the active site required for catalysis. Thus, a substitution of Asp 364 with Val[300] or His (factor $IX_{MECHTAL}$)[301] results in severe factor IX deficiency (factor IX:C <1 percent) with normal levels of a circulating dysfunctional protein caused by the lack of ion pair formation. Likewise, mutations at two highly conserved glycine residues, Gly 309 to Val and Gly 311 to Glu (factor $IX_{AMAGASAKI}$), both result in undetectable factor IX clotting activity, but normal factor IX:Ag levels. Computer modeling of the catalytic domain has predicted that both mutations disrupt the active site conformational change accompanying ion pair formation.[302,303]

Several mutations directly affect the catalytic site. Mutations of the active site serine itself (Ser 365 to Gly,[301] to Ile,[301] or to Arg[304]) result in a severely dysfunctional factor

IX molecule (factor IX:C < 1 percent) incapable of catalytic activity. Replacement of Gly 363 with Val (factor $IX_{EAGLE\ ROCK}$) is associated with a moderately severe bleeding disorder (factor IX:C = 1 to 5 percent, factor IX:Ag = 100 percent), because the highly conserved glycine residue is required for stabilization of the factor IXa active site and substrate binding during catalysis.[305]

Another set of CRM+ variants interfere with the extended or secondary substrate binding site(s) within the factor IXa heavy chain. In factor IX_{ANGERS}, substitution of Arg for the highly conserved Gly 396 results in severe hemophilia (factor IX:C <1 percent, factor IX:Ag = 100 percent). It is presumed this is caused by the positively charged arginine amino group binding to the negatively charged side chain of Asp 359 at the base of the substrate binding pocket, thus forming a "self-inhibited" enzyme.[306,307] Similarly, mutation of Ile 397 to Thr (factor $IX_{VANCOUVER}$,[307] factor $IX_{LONG\ BEACH}$,[308] factor $IX_{LOS\ ANGELES}$[309]) causes moderately severe to severe hemophilia (factor IX:C = 1 to 5 percent, factor IX:Ag = 50 to 100 percent). Computer modeling predicts that the new side chain hydroxyl group of Thr 397 forms a hydrogen bond with the carbonyl oxygen of Trp 385, thus disrupting the factor X–binding site.[310,311] Another moderately severe CRM+ variant, factor $IX_{LAKE\ ELSINORE/NIIGATA}$[312,313] results from an Ala 390 to Val substitution, which also may inhibit macromolecular substrate binding.

Hemophilia B_M, a phenotypic variant of CRM+ factor IX deficiency, was initially described by Hougie and Twomey,[314] who found that the one-stage ox brain prothrombin time was prolonged in some patients. Patients with hemophilia B_M synthesize a factor IX devoid of clotting activity (factor IX:C usually <1 percent), but which is capable of inhibiting the activation of factor X catalyzed by factor VIIa and bovine tissue factor.[296,315] At the molecular level, two groups of abnormalities have been found in patients with the B_M phenotype. The first group involves the β activation site (Arg 180-Val) and includes Arg 180 to Trp (factor IX $B_{M\ DEVENTER/NAGOYA}$),[296,297] to Gly (factor IX_{MADRID}),[299] or to Gln (factor $IX_{HILO/NOVARA}$)[296,298]; Val 181 to Phe (factor IX_{MILANO})[296]; and Val 182 to Phe (factor $IX_{KASHIHARA}$)[316] or to Leu (factor $IX_{CARDIFF\ 2}$).[317] The second group of B_M mutations are located near the catalytic center or substrate binding site. These include Gly 311 to Glu (factor $IX_{AMAGASAKI}$),[303] Pro 368 to Thr (factor $IX_{BERGAMO}$),[297] Ala 390 to Val (factor $IX_{LAKE\ ELSINORE/NIIGATA}$),[312,313] Gly 396 to Arg (factor IX_{ANGERS}),[306,307] and Ile 397 to Thr (factor $IX_{VANCOUVER}$).[307]

Overall, about 40 percent of the point mutations identified in patients with hemophilia B are located within CG dinucleotides,[272,280,300] where deamination of methylcytosine results in a transition of C̲G to T̲G or CG̲ to CA̲ depending on whether the mutation occurs in the DNA coding strand or complementary strand, respectively. Thus, CG type transitions account for most of the mutations that recur in more than one pedigree.[318] The remaining "recurrent" mutations identified in multiple hemophilic families appear to represent a "founder effect"—that is, they result from a distant common ancestor. These include factor $IX_{VANCOUVER}$ (Ile 397 to Thr),[319,320] as well as mutations of Thr 296 to Met[86,321] and Gly 60 to Ser[86,322] that are associated with moderately severe (factor IX:C ≈5 percent) and mild (factor IX:C = 10 to 15 percent) hemophilia, respectively.

Genetic Counseling For Hemophilia B

Developments in the molecular biology of factor IX as well as advances in the field of molecular genetics have greatly facilitated genetic counseling of families with hemophilia B. Detection of female carriers and prenatal diagnosis of affected males can now be accomplished in the vast majority of families either indirectly by linkage analysis using RFLP or by direct identification of the causative mutation in the particular hemophilia B pedigree.[323] Linkage analysis is based on the cosegregation of an intragenic factor IX RFLP (see above) with the hemophilic mutation; this approach requires female heterozygosity for the particular RFLP as well as the availability and cooperation of key family members for testing. Most of the known factor IX RFLP were initially detected by Southern blotting.[267,324–327] This technique employs a radiolabeled DNA fragment or probe prepared from factor IX cDNA or genomic DNA. More recently, PCR has simplified detection of previously known factor IX RFLP and also has enabled the identification of new RFLP.[328,329] RFLP linkage analysis by PCR requires only minute amounts of DNA, is nonradioactive, and can be performed much more rapidly than Southern blotting. Taking into account the ethnic frequencies (see above) and degree of linkage equilibrium of the various factor IX RFLP, carrier detection by linkage analysis should be successful in about 90 percent, 80 percent, and 50 percent of African-American, Caucasian, and Asian families, respectively.

Because linkage analysis by RFLP testing is not successful in every family, identification of the actual hemophilic mutation is the ultimate goal for genetic counseling. Furthermore, for the relatively high proportion of families with "sporadic" hemophilia due to a recent or *de novo* mutation (30 to 50 percent), direct detection of the hemophilic mutation is required for accurate assignment of carrier status. The identification of causative factor IX mutations, however, is complicated by the genetic heterogeneity of hemophilia B (see above). Nevertheless, relatively rapid and efficient screening procedures using PCR-based techniques have been applied to detection of hemophilic mutations.[330] These include denaturing gel gradient electrophoresis (DGGE),[307] chemical cleavage of mismatches,[331] single strand conformation polymorphism (SSCP),[332] and direct sequencing of PCR-amplified genomic DNA fragments[291,300] or transcripts.[304] Once the particular mutation in an affected individual is identified by DNA sequencing, family members can be rapidly tested by analysis of the appropriate PCR-amplified DNA fragment.[86,333,334]

Clinical Aspects

Hemophilia B (Christmas disease) like hemophilia A occurs in a severe, moderate, or mild form according to the level of factor IX activity in plasma. Clinical symptoms reflect the factor IX:C level in plasma regardless of the level of factor IX:Ag. Severe factor IX deficiency (factor IX:C <0.01 U/ml) is characterized by spontaneous bleeding, especially in the joints. A unit (U) of factor IX is defined as the amount of coagulant activity in 1 ml of normal pooled plasma. The disease is usually diagnosed when the affected male infant starts crawling or walking. A typical symptom at this stage is the development of large hematomas on the forehead. The hematomas may become the size of a golf ball and cause a dangerous strain on the skin. These hematomas must be watched carefully to avoid skin necrosis or any trauma to the skin. A typical feature for the superficial, subcutaneous hematomas that are often seen in hemophilia patients is the easily palpable subcutaneous infiltrate. These characteristics are otherwise found only in very severely thrombocytopenic patients and never occur in normal individuals.

When the afflicted youngster begins to stand and walk, recurrent joint bleeding is the most obvious clinical manifestation, appearing as swollen, very painful joint regions. The joints most often affected are the large joints, such as knees and ankles. Muscle bleeding may occur both spontaneously and after trauma in severely affected patients.[335,336] Large flexor muscle groups (i.e., ileopsoas, calf, and forearm) are most commonly affected. Large volumes of blood may be extravasated in the muscle tissue, resulting in compression of blood vessels and nerves. Muscle necrosis occurs rapidly due to ischemia. Bleeding into the ileopsoas muscle is rather common and presents with pain in the groin associated with local swelling. The patient is unable to stretch the hip joint. Retroperitoneal bleeding is also rather common and may be difficult to diagnose. Ultrasound, CT, and MRI are of great help in these situations. Muscle and tissue hematomas should never be aspirated or treated surgically. A serious sequela to deep tissue bleeding is the development of pseudotumors (hemophilic blood cysts).[337] The incidence of such cysts has been reported as ≈1 percent. Further bleeding will occur with gradual increase in size, resulting in pressure on surrounding structures. These formations may assume enormous dimensions and erode bone and even destroy adjacent joints and muscles. Finally, they may perforate into the abdomen or intestines. Infections may then supervene. Treatment should be aimed at prevention, and all deep hematomas should be treated vigorously with plasma factor IX concentrates. Established pseudotumors may require surgical removal under the protection of adequate substitution therapy.[338] Gastrointestinal bleeding and bleeding from the urinary tract are also rather common. With the development of better plasma concentrates, surgical intervention in the case of peptic ulcers has often been recommended. Central nervous system hemorrhage can occur in severe hemophilia following relatively minor trauma, and until recently, was the major cause of death in hemophiliacs.[339] Thus, any patient with severe hemophilia with neurologic symptoms should receive replacement therapy and be observed closely until a head CT scan is obtained.

It should be kept in mind that bleeding may imitate any disease in hemophiliacs. Thus, a hematoma in the wall of the bowel mimicked acute appendicitis in a patient, and similar bleeding caused acute hepatic stasis in another patient.[340] A rule of thumb is to regard any symptom in a hemophiliac as caused by bleeding, and substitution therapy should be started immediately as the diagnostic work proceeds.

Patients with moderate hemophilia B (factor IX:C = 0.01 to 0.05 U/ml) most often have less severe bleeding, and massive joint bleeding occurs less frequently. Patients with a factor IX:C level of 0.01 to 0.03 U/ml, however, require substitution treatment to almost the same extent as severe hemophiliacs.

Mild hemophiliacs (factor IX:C = 0.05 to 0.30 U/ml) usually do not have spontaneous joint bleeding. However, they present some special problems. Mild hemophilia often is not diagnosed until adulthood and is then detected at times of surgery or trauma. Such patients may be difficult to treat since they might have unexpected heavy bleeding, and mild hemophilia should be kept in mind as a diagnostic possibility. It should be stressed that gastrointestinal bleeding and hematuria are almost as common in mild hemophilia as in the severe form. After trauma, life-threatening bleeding such as intracranial and muscle bleeding may develop in patients with mild hemophilia. Both the patients and their physicians may tend to underestimate the risk, resulting in an unnecessary delay in starting treatment.

Joint Disease. Typical joint disease is seen mainly in severely affected hemophiliacs. Its clinical pattern is the same in hemophilia A and B. In adults, acute hemarthrosis is most frequent in the knee joints, followed by the elbow, ankle, and wrist.[335,336] The hip is most often spared, probably because it is protected by the large muscle cuff.[341] Repeated joint bleeding leads to long-term changes of hyperplasia and hyperemia of the synovium, which makes the joint more susceptible to recurrent bleeding. This stresses the need for adequate substitution treatment for each joint bleed to minimize the development of chronic synovitis.

Chronic Arthritis. The chronic degenerative lesions of the joints in hemophilia are characterized by the presence of gross deformity with fixed flexion contractures. The muscle cuffs around the joint are often severely atrophied. Often there are also chronic effusions and pain. Microscopically, the synovium is greatly hypertrophied and heavily infiltrated with inflammatory cells and deposits of iron. Extensive fibrosis and bone cysts are seen. The radiologic findings have been described in detail.[342] Osteoporosis is invariable. Loss of cartilage results in loss of joint space, and underlying bone is resorbed with formation of subchondral cysts. Later, osteophytic outgrowth may be marked. Resorption of bone occurs especially in the knee joint with production of an enlarged intercondylar fossa, which may lead to differential overgrowth of one of the femoral condyles. Such deformity may result in posterior subluxation of the tibia and lateral shift of the tibia on the femur.

Treatment

Care of the patient with hemophilia B includes treatment of acute bleeding episodes, rehabilitation and management of the chronic musculoskeletal complications, and prophylaxis. Since hemophilia care involves many special requirements, centralization to hemophilia centers has been recommended.[343] Such centers should be capable of taking care of the psychological and social problems of the family of the patient with hemophilia and should provide orthopedic, dental, and surgical treatment. The centers also should provide the laboratory facilities for diagnosis and for monitoring replacement therapy.

Management of Acute Bleeding Episodes and Surgery. The goal for management of acute bleeding episodes is to normalize the hemostatic function by replacement of the missing coagulation protein, factor IX. Factor IX is relatively stable and the in vivo half-life of ≈24 h[344,345] makes it possible to administer factor IX at longer intervals than those used in hemophilia A. Most often, infusion one to two times daily is enough. The in vivo yield, however, is lower than that of factor VIII and is only 20 to 40 percent of the factor IX activity administered as plasma or factor IX concentrate.[344,345] This has been ascribed to the fact that factor IX is distributed both intravascularly and extravascularly and binds to cellular surfaces.

To achieve hemostasis, the patient's plasma level of factor IX should be increased to 0.6 to 1.0 U/ml (60 U/kg body weight). In minor bleeding situations, it may be enough to reach a plasma level of 0.2 to 0.4 U/ml. Minor bleeding is often managed by treatment for 1 to 3 days. Major hemorrhages, including muscle hematomas, most often require treatment for 7 to 14 days (50 to 60 U/kg the first day, followed by 20 to 30 U/kg on days 2 through 4, and 10 to 20 U/kg for another 4 to 10 days). At major surgery, a plasma level of 0.6 to 1.0 U/ml is desirable during the operation and for the first 1 to 4 days postoperatively, depending on the specific operation. This corresponds to a dose of about 60 U/kg body weight. The dose is then slowly decreased to 30 to 40 U/kg for postoperative days 2 to 4 (a plasma level of 0.3 to 0.4 U/ml) and later to 10 to 20 U/kg (plasma level of 0.1 to 0.2 U/ml) for another 10 to 15 days.[346]

Management of Chronic Musculoskeletal Complications. Surgical correction of chronic musculoskeletal defects in hemophiliacs has become possible with the availability of plasma factor concentrates. Successful total arthroplasty of the knee and hip joints has been performed in hemophiliacs.[347–349] Chronic synovitis has increasingly been treated with synovectomy.[350] Although there has been some uncertainty regarding joint function deterioration after surgical synovectomy, good long-term results have been reported.[351,352] Arthroscopic synovectomy may reduce the postoperative complication rate.[353,354] Chemical synovectomy, using radioisotopes like colloidal ^{198}Au,[355] ^{90}Y,[356] and ^{32}P,[357] has also been reported to be valuable. In chronic hemophilia, physiotherapy for the arthritis is of major importance.

Prophylaxis. Prophylaxis has been applied in cases of severe hemophilia since the 1960s.[358] The principle involves prevention of the development of heavy bleeding in patients with severe hemophilia by raising the concentration of factor IX in plasma to a level ($\approx$0.04 U/ml) at which spontaneous joint bleeding is rare. This approach was based on earlier observations in which substantially less severe musculoskeletal complications were noted in patients with moderate or mild hemophilia. The prophylactic treatment generally consists of regular doses of factor IX concentrate (25 to 30 U/kg) administered about twice per week. Such treatment has decreased the chronic musculoskeletal complications substantially. Similar long-term results have been reported in patients treated only at times of bleeding.[359] The most important point is an increase in the frequency of treatment, whether given regularly without regard to ongoing bleeding or immediately when symptoms are first noted.[360,361]

Home treatment of hemophilia is now widely accepted. The patients receive greater personal freedom, and the delay in receiving treatment is clearly reduced. Also, financial costs are lowered.[362]

Factor IX Concentrates. Factor IX is rather stable and retains about 80 percent of its activity in plasma stored at 4°C for up to 3 months. Therefore, plasma can be used in replacement therapy of mild hemophilia B, but this method does not permit normalization of the plasma level of factor IX in patients with severe hemophilia B.

Crude concentrates of factor IX are prepared by absorption of the vitamin K–dependent coagulation factors (prothrombin and factors VII, IX, and X) on tricalcium phosphate,[363] DEAE-cellulose,[364] or DEAE-Sephadex.[365] The absorbed vitamin K–dependent factors are eluted with phosphate or citrate buffers and the final product is lyophilized. Such concentrates thus contain approximately equal amounts of prothrombin, factor IX, and factor X. The content of factor VII varies substantially in different preparations. The clinical experience of such factor IX concentrates has been documented.[346]

Side Effects of Factor IX Concentrates

Thrombosis. Venous and arterial thrombotic complications as well as disseminated intravascular coagulation (DIC) have been described following the administration of crude concentrates of factor IX.[366,367] The thrombogenic potential varies between different preparations[368] and has been ascribed to contamination of the concentrates by activated coagulation factors (e.g., factors VIIa, IXa, and Xa),[369,370] to the administration of large quantities of the nonactivated vitamin K–dependent factors,[371] and/or to the presence of platelet-derived phospholipid.[372] Patients who are most likely to have thromboembolic complications or DIC are those with concomitant liver disease and those receiving large doses of factor IX concentrate for support during surgery or as treatment to arrest bleeding in patients with a factor VIII inhibitor.

Several more highly purified factor IX concentrates have been developed.[373,374] These products undergo additional purification steps during the manufacturing process, such as pseudoaffinity chromatography on sulfated proteoglycans (e.g., heparin-Sepharose), or monoclonal antibody affinity chromatography. Thus these newer factor IX concentrates are virtually free of the other, contaminating, vitamin K–dependent clotting factors. Preliminary in vivo studies of these more highly purified concentrates indicate reduced thrombogenicity but similar efficacy compared to the older, crude concentrates.[375–380] Some of these newer, highly purified factor IX concentrates have been made available for clinical use and should ultimately replace the crude concentrates for treatment of hemophilia B.

Viral Transmission. Concentrates of factor IX are prepared from plasma pooled from several thousand donors. The risk of transmitting bloodborne viral diseases, such as hepatitis and AIDS, via pooled plasma products increases substantially with the number of plasma donors involved. In the early to mid-1980s, HIV infection was recognized as one of the most serious hazards of blood transfusion, particularly in recipients of coagulation factor concentrates. Compared to hemophilia A, the HIV seropositivity rate for hemophilia B has been somewhat lower (76 vs. 42 percent for severely affected patients).[381] More recently, the introduction of several measures has virtually eliminated HIV from currently available blood products. Since the HIV virus is heat labile and is surrounded by a lipid envelope, the introduction of viral inactivation methods such as heat treatment and solvent–detergent treatment has successfully eliminated HIV from commercial clotting factor concentrates. Furthermore, screening plasma donors for HIV antibody has virtually eliminated infectious individuals from the donor pool.

The transmission of hepatitis viruses is currently the most significant risk associated with the use of plasma products. Although the current risk of hepatitis B infection is negligible due to the introduction of donor screening assays in the late 1970s and the development of a hepatitis vaccine in the mid-1980s, the risk of transmission of hepatitis C virus (HCV; formerly, non A, non B hepatitis) remains. The isolation of the hepatitis C virus[382] has led to the development of a specific immunoassay using recombinant viral antigens.[383] Retrospective serologic studies indicate a prevalence of hepatitis C infection of $\approx$70 percent for both hemophilia A and B,[373] although the actual prevalence is even higher when more sensitive assays are used.[384,385] Furthermore, a significant percentage of hemophiliacs infected with HCV have chronic progressive liver disease, including cirrhosis.[386,387] Screening blood and plasma donors for anti-HCV should reduce the frequency of hepatitis C transmission via blood products.[388] In addition, several procedures have been developed to inactivate viruses present in clotting factor concentrates. These include heat treatment either in the dry state, in solution (i.e., pasteurization), or in the presence of steam or an organic solvent or combined treatment with an organic solvent together with a detergent to destroy the viral envelope. The most effective methods for inactivation of hepatitis C virus appear to be dry heat treatment at 80°C for 72 h,[389,390] pasteurization,[391] and solvent–detergent treatment.[392] Dry heat treatment using lower temperatures (60°C) and shorter durations (<24 h) and heat treatment in the presence of an organic solvent are less effective.[393,394] The crude factor IX concentrates that are currently available have been heated either in the dry state or in the presence of n-heptane. Most of the newer, more highly purified factor IX concentrates, however, have been treated by the solvent–detergent method.

Chronic liver disease secondary to hepatitis C infection is a serious complication of factor IX replacement therapy. Preliminary studies indicate that interferon may be useful in the treatment of hemophiliacs with chronic liver disease.[395,396] Additionally, liver transplantation has been successful in a few selected patients[397]; an additional salutary effect of this procedure is the cure of the patient's hemophilia.

Symptomatic infection with parvovirus B19 has been reported in patients with hemophilia.[398,399] This virus is resistant to current virucidal procedures since it lacks a lipid envelope.

Factor IX Inhibitors. Antibodies against factor IX develop in about 10 percent of patients with severe hemophilia B. In these cases, infused factor IX is rapidly neutralized and does not induce hemostasis until the patient's total amount of anti–factor IX has been neutralized. Furthermore, an anamnestic response follows administration of any product containing factor IX. Hemophilia patients with a substantial anamnestic response following infusion of factor IX are called "high responders." In other patients, the stimulating effect on the antibody formation is not as striking. These patients are called "low responders." Most patients with inhibitors are high responders, and the antibody develops at an early age.

Treatment of patients with factor IX inhibitors includes treatment of acute bleeding episodes as well as attempts to induce tolerance. An acute bleeding episode can be managed by administering factor IX concentrate in amounts high enough to neutralize the inhibitor and also to give a hemostatic effect. This is possible, provided the antibody titer is not too high in relation to the activity of factor IX in the available concentrates. Concomitantly, immunosuppressive treatment can be given to diminish the anamnestic response. Such treatment has been used successfully in a substantial number of patients.[400] In patients with extremely high antibody titers, the inhibitor can be removed by extracorporeal adsorption on protein A-Sepharose[401,402] or by specific immunoadsorption[403] before the administration of factor IX. Recombinant factor VIIa has been used successfully to control bleeding in a factor IX–deficient patient with inhibitor.[404]

It has been claimed that tolerance in patients with hemophilia A will develop after long-term administration of high amounts of coagulation factor concentrates. Repeated treatments using the combination of high amounts of factor IX and cyclophosphamide in hemophilia B patients seemed to result in a similar conversion of high responders to low responders.[405] Another hemophilia B patient became a low responder after two instances of treatment, including extracorporeal adsorption of his anti–factor IX:C on protein A-Sepharose followed by the administration of factor IX, cyclophosphamide, and IV IgG.[406] This led to the Malmo treatment protocol comprised of factor IX, cyclophosphamide, and IV IgG, that has been successful in inducing immune tolerance in several hemophilia B inhibitor patients.[407]

Future Directions

The ability to produce recombinant factor IX on a commercial scale for the treatment of hemophilia B would presumably alleviate the complications of viral transmission and thrombogenicity associated with currently available concentrates of plasma-derived factor IX. To date, a variety of mammalian cell types have been transfected with factor IX cDNA, but secretion of mature, functional factor IX protein has been limited by the γ-carboxylation and propeptide processing activities of the transfected cells.[408,409] These technical problems, combined with the lower economic incentive (hemophilia B is only one-fourth as common as hemophilia A), have limited progress in the development of recombinant factor IX as compared with recombinant factor VIII for the treatment of hemophilia. The identification of cDNAs coding for intracellular enzymes capable of γ-carboxylation[76] and propeptide processing,[87] however, should facilitate the development of commercially produced recombinant factor IX.

A more "curative" approach to the treatment of inherited metabolic disorders such as hemophilia is the concept of gene transfer therapy.[410] Gene transfer involves the transfection of a target cell with a retroviral vector containing a promoter element, the cDNA for the missing protein, and a selectivity marker. The cells containing the missing cDNA are grown in culture and then transplanted into the deficient host, in whom, ideally, the missing protein is now able to circulate. This approach has been approved for clinical trials in patients with adenosine deaminase deficiency. In the area of hemophilia, preclinical research has progressed more rapidly for hemophilia B than for hemophilia A[411,412] because the factor IX cDNA and protein are significantly smaller than those of factor VIII. In addition, because of its extravascular distribution, factor IX should not require direct intravascular secretion to achieve adequate circulating levels. Thus far, several mammalian target cell types (skin fibroblasts, hepatocytes, and endothelial cells) have been transfected with a variety of retroviral vectors containing human factor IX cDNA, and in vitro expression of significant levels of human factor IX (up to 4.6 μg/ml/10^6 cells/24 h for rat fibroblasts)[413] have been achieved. Once the cultured fibroblasts were transplanted into rodents, the expressed human factor IX was detected in rodent plasma, but circulating levels were much lower than predicted in vitro and were maintained for only up to 1 month. The use of alternative types of retroviral vectors and promoters[414,415] and target cell types (e.g., myoblasts)[416] are currently under investigation.

FACTOR X

Factor X (M_r = 59,000) participates in the middle stage of blood coagulation[112] in which it is converted to factor Xa in the intrinsic pathway by the "tenase" complex (factor IXa in the presence of factor VIIIa, phospholipid, and calcium ions) or in the extrinsic pathway by factor VIIa in the presence of tissue factor and calcium ions (see Fig. 104-1). Human factor X is a glycoprotein that circulates in blood as a two-chain molecule.[259,417] It contains a light chain (M_r = 16,900) and a heavy chain (M_r = 42,100), and these two chains are held together by a disulfide bond. The light chain contains 11 residues of γ-carboxyglutamic acid and two growth factor domains[15–17] (Fig. 104-11). It also contains β-hydroxyaspartic acid at position 63 in the first epidermal growth factor domain.[90–92] Calcium binding occurs through both the Gla and first growth factor domains, and the former is responsible for factor X interaction with membrane surfaces.[40,43,47,61] The total length of the light chain is 139 residues, while the heavy chain is composed of 306 residues. The heavy chain also includes the catalytic domain and the active site serine. Human factor X contains 15 percent carbohydrate that includes *N*-linked chains attached to Asn 39 and Asn 49 in the activation peptide.

The activation of human factor X by factor IXa results from the cleavage of an Arg 52-Ile bond in the N-terminal end of the heavy chain[417] (see Fig. 104-11). This releases an activation peptide of 52 amino acids and generates factor

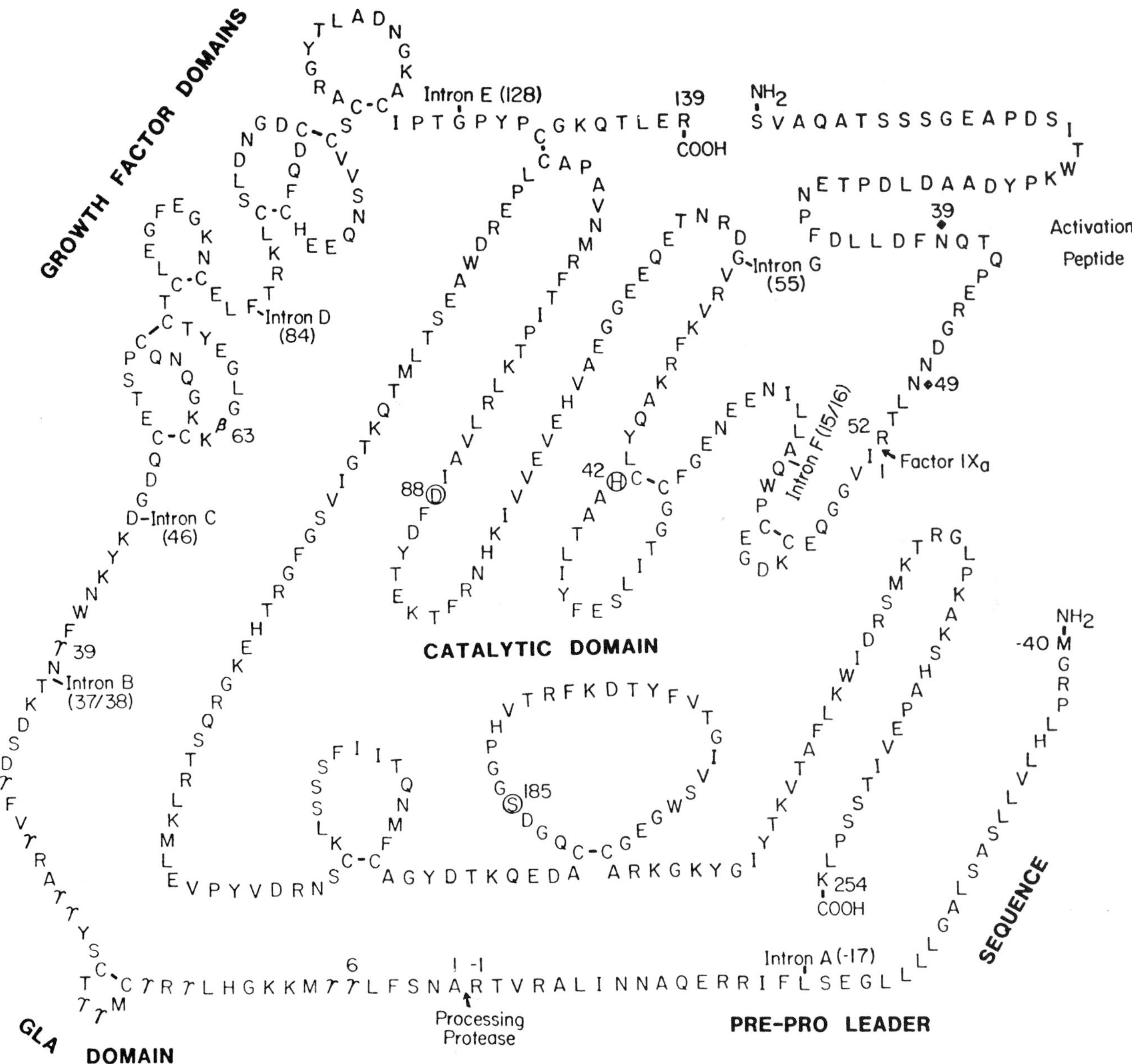

FIG. 104-11 **Amino acid sequence and tentative structure of human prepro factor X. The locations of the seven introns (A to G) are shown in the various regions of the protein. The prepro leader sequence (−40 to −1) is cleaved during protein biosynthesis to give rise to the mature protein with an N-terminal sequence of A-N-S-F- for the light chain. The Arg-Lys-Arg tripeptide that connects the light and heavy chains during biosynthesis is not shown. The peptide bond cleaved by factor IXa during the activation reaction is shown with a small arrow. The three amino acids in the catalytic domain (H_{42}, D_{88}, S_{185}) that participate in catalysis are circled, while the two potential carbohydrate attachment sites in the activation peptide are shown with solid diamonds. The amino acids are numbered as follows, starting with the N-terminal end of the protein: −40 to −1 = prepro leader sequence; +1 to 139 = light chain; 1 to 52 = activation peptide; 1 to 254 = catalytic chain. The single-letter code for amino acids is shown in the legend to Fig. 104-5. β = β-hydroxyaspartic acid.** ***(From Leytus et al.[7] Used by permission.)***

Xa, a serine protease. The V_{max} for the activation reaction is accelerated approximately 200,000 times by the addition of factor VIIIa, while the phospholipid decreases the K_m of the reaction about 3000 times.[418] The participation of factor VIII as a cofactor in the reaction requires its prior activation by thrombin or factor Xa.[115–118] Current evidence suggests that factor VIIIa forms a complex with the enzyme factor IXa in the presence of phospholipid and calcium ions, and this complex functions as the activator of factor X.[135,419] This is analogous to the complex formed by factor Xa, factor Va, phospholipid, and calcium ions that carries out the activation of prothrombin. The activation of factor X by factor IXa/factor VIIIa can occur on the membrane surface of platelets,[419] endothelial cells,[143] or monocytes.[420]

Factor X Gene

The gene for human factor X is located on chromosome 13 in the region of q34-qter.[215–217] It contains approximately 25 kb of DNA and includes seven introns and eight exons.[17] As previously mentioned, the seven introns in the gene for factor X interrupt the coding sequence at essentially identical locations in the amino acid sequence as do the introns in the genes for human factor VII, factor IX, and protein C.

Analysis of the 5′ flanking sequence of the gene for factor X has resulted in the identification of a region upstream of the initiation Met codon ≈20 bp in length that contains multiple transcription initiation sites[421] and a region spanning nucleotides −457 to −1 that contains three distinct elements involved in the regulation of factor X.[422] The first of these, a tissue-specific promoter in the region −63 to −42 (FXP1), is essential for liver-specific transcription and is homologous to the known liver-specific transcription factor recognition sequences for LF-A1 or HNF-4. Two additional regulatory sequences encompassing nucleotides −215 to −149 (FXP2) and −457 to −351 (FXP3) are also present. Like FXP1, FXP3 is liver-specific, while FXP2 is homologous to an Sp-1 binding site.

Several polymorphisms have been identified within the gene for factor X. A *Taq*I site with a frequency of 20 percent, as well as less prevalent *Eco*RI, *Hin*dIII, and *Pst*I RFLP (frequencies of less common alleles = 5 to 10 percent) have been identified by Southern blotting.[423–425] In addition, a highly polymorphic extragenic *Pvu*II site is present ≈3 kb downstream of exon VIII.[425] An *Nla*IV polymorphism in exon VII, due to a C/T dimorphism at codon 817, has been detected by PCR. This polymorphism is silent at the amino acid level and has a frequency of ≈25 percent in Caucasians and 50 percent in African-Americans.[426] Since the genes for factor VII and factor X are separated by only 2.8 kb on chromosome 13,[422] these factor X polymorphisms may be useful in studies of families with either congenital factor X or factor VII deficiency.

Factor X Deficiency

In 1955, Duckert and coworkers reported the presence of a serum factor, called "factor X," that was depressed by coumarin anticoagulants.[427] Inherited deficiencies were identified shortly thereafter, and the plasma protein was called Prower factor[428] and Stuart factor[429] after the families affected by this disorder. Thus far, more than 50 families have been reported with factor X deficiency. The complete deficiency is inherited as an autosomal recessive disorder, although a subtle bleeding tendency occurs in heterozygotes.[430,431] Clinically, severe factor X deficiency can mimic severe hemophilia A or B, but chronic arthropathy is usually not as prominent. Patients whose levels of factor X clotting activity (factor X:C) are above ≈15 percent of normal exhibit abnormal bleeding episodes only in connection with major surgery or trauma.

Factor X deficiency is a heterogeneous disorder at both the phenotypic and genotypic levels. The original Stuart plasma demonstrates equally reduced factor X:C levels using PT, aPTT, or RVV-based clotting assays. Other variants of factor X, on the other hand, demonstrate different levels of factor X:C, depending on whether factor X activation occurs via the extrinsic system, the intrinsic system, or RVV.[432,433] For example, factor X_{PADUA}[434] and factor $X_{VORARLBERG}$[435] show lower clotting activity as determined by extrinsic activation, whereas factor $X_{MELBOURNE}$[436] and factor X_{ROMA}[437] demonstrate selectively reduced intrinsic activation. Measurement of factor X antigen indicates further heterogeneity, as levels may be normal (CRM^+), absent (CRM^-), or reduced (CRM^R).[432]

Several abnormal variants of factor X have been characterized at the molecular level; these have ranged from gross gene deletions to single base substitutions. A patient with severe CRM^- factor X deficiency was found to be heterozygous for two different deletions: a complete gene deletion for which the mother demonstrated germ-line mosaicism, and a partial gene deletion of paternal origin, which included exons VII and VIII.[438] A partial deletion encompassing exon VII and the 5′ portion of exon VIII was described in another patient with severe factor X deficiency, who is presumably a compound heterozygote for an as yet unidentified second mutation.[439]

Seven point mutations have been identified in patients with factor X deficiency, and five of these are transitions within CG dinucleotides. Factor $X_{SANTO\ DOMINGO}$ is characterized by a severe CRM^- bleeding disorder due to a homozygous mutation of G to A in exon I. This mutation causes the substitution of Gly with Arg at residue −20 within the signal peptide and prevents factor X secretion from the liver, presumably by disrupting signal peptidase cleavage of the leader sequence.[69] The molecular defect in the original Stuart pedigree[429] is a homozygous mutation of G to A that results in the substitution of Val 104 with Met and also appears to impair secretion of the mutant factor X protein from the hepatocyte.[440] Factor $X_{VORARLBERG}$ is associated with a clinically mild bleeding tendency, preferentially affecting extrinsic factor X activation. This disorder is characterized by diminished calcium affinity caused by a mutation in exon II of Gal 14 (GAA) to Lys (AAA).[435] A second transition of G to A in exon V, which changes Glu 102 to Lys, was detected in this pedigree, but does not correlate with the factor $X_{VORARLBERG}$ phenotype. Two other mildly affected variants have been preliminarily described: factor X_{OCKERO} is due to a homozygous mutation of Gly 114 to Arg within the second growth factor domain,[441] while an individual with factor $X_{WENATCHEE}$ is heterozygous for a substitution of Arg 142 with Cys at the site that is normally cleaved intracellularly to form two-chain factor X.[442] This mutation is analogous to the α activation site mutations in factor $IX_{CHAPEL\ HILL}$ and $prothrombins_{BARCELONA}$ and $_{MADRID}$. Factor X_{FRIULI} is a variant found in Northern Italian individuals and is characterized by a moderate bleeding tendency in homozygotes with ≈5 percent factor X:C levels as measured by PT and aPTT, though RVV clotting times and factor X:Ag levels remain normal.[432,443,444] The mutation responsible for factor X_{FRIULI} is a substitution of Pro 343 (CCC) with Ser (TCC) within a conserved region of the catalytic domain.[445] Factor X_{SAN}

ANTONIO is a mild CRM^R variant characterized by compound heterozygosity for two mutations within the catalytic domain. The first of these mutations is a single nucleotide deletion at codon 272 in exon VII, which results in the premature termination of translation. The second mutation is a transition of C for T at codon 366 in exon VIII, which results in the substitution of Arg with Cys.[446]

An acquired deficiency of factor X associated with amyloidosis has also been described.[447] Bleeding manifestations in this disorder most commonly involve the skin and gastrointestinal tract.[448] Nine of the 10 patients described by Fair and Edgington had factor X antigen levels ranging from 15 to 73 percent of normal, while the factor X activity was consistently below normal.[432]

Bleeding episodes in patients with congenital factor X deficiency are generally treated with plasma transfusions to maintain plasma factor X levels above 15 to 20 percent.[449] For major bleeding associated with trauma or surgery, crude factor IX concentrates can be used, since these products contain approximately one unit of factor X per unit of factor IX. More highly purified concentrates of factor X are not currently available, though recombinant factor X recently has been expressed in mammalian cells.[450]

PROTEIN C, PROTEIN S, AND THROMBOMODULIN

Protein C is a vitamin K–dependent protein that was described in 1976[451] and was later identified as an important regulator of the coagulation cascade. Protein C is converted to activated protein C, a serine protease, by thrombin[452,453] in a reaction enhanced by an endothelial cell cofactor[121] (see Fig. 104-2). This cofactor, called "thrombomodulin," forms a complex with thrombin resulting in a potent activator of protein C and a marked decrease in the procoagulant function of the enzyme.[454,455] The activated protein C then inhibits the coagulation pathway by inactivating factor Va and factor VIIIa in the presence of phospholipid.[118,453,456–460] The anticoagulant activity of activated protein C requires the presence of protein S,[461,462] another vitamin K–dependent coagulation factor,[259,463] which enhances the activity of activated protein C about 14 times.[464] Protein S functions as a cofactor in the binding of activated protein C to phospholipid and increases the affinity of activated protein C to membrane surfaces.[465,466] The complex of activated protein C and protein S is also readily formed on the endothelial cell surface.[467] Furthermore, the presence of activated protein C decreases the internalization and degradation of protein S by endothelial cells.[468] In addition to its anticoagulant activity, protein C also has a profibrinolytic effect,[469] which may involve in part the inactivation of plasminogen activator inhibitor-1 (PAI-1), a major inhibitor of tissue plasminogen activator.[470,471] This inactivation is also dependent on the presence of protein S.[471,472] Activated protein C is regulated by a specific plasma protein inhibitor that binds to activated protein C to form a 1:1 stoichiometric complex that is promoted by heparin.[473] Additionally, α_1-antitrypsin is the major heparin-independent inhibitor of activated protein C.[474,475]

Human protein C (M_r = 62,000) is a glycoprotein that circulates in blood as a two-chain molecule held together by a single disulfide bond[452,453,476] (Fig. 104-12). The light chain ($M_r \approx$ 22,000) is composed of 155 amino acids and contains nine residues of γ-carboxyglutamic acid and one residue of β-hydroxyaspartic acid at position 71.[89,91,92] The heavy chain ($M_r \approx$ 40,000) is composed of 262 amino acids and contains the catalytic domain. Human protein C also contains 23 percent carbohydrate including *N*-linked chains that are probably attached to Asn 97 in the light chain and Asn 79, Asn 144, and Asn 160 in the heavy chain of the activated protein.

The activation of human protein C by thrombin is due to the cleavage of an Arg 12-Ile bond in the N-terminal region of the heavy chain. This releases an activation peptide of 12 amino acids and gives rise to an active serine protease. The rate of activation of protein C by thrombin is accelerated approximately 1000 times by the presence of thrombomodulin, an endothelial cell surface glycoprotein.[122] The formation of the 1:1 molecular complex of thrombin and thrombomodulin changes the activity of the enzyme from a procoagulant in the coagulation cascade to an anticoagulant involved in the regulation of the coagulation cascade.[454] Apparently, the binding of thrombomodulin to thrombin directly inhibits the interaction of thrombin with its procoagulant substrates.[477,478] Thus, the thrombin bound to thrombomodulin no longer converts fibrinogen to fibrin or factor V to factor Va,[479] nor does it activate platelets,[480] but instead it becomes a specific activator of protein C.

The light chain of protein C contains two calcium binding sites, one within the Gla domain and the other within the growth factor domains, which are required for protein C anticoagulant activity.[38,44,81,287,481] In addition, the Gla and growth factor domains of protein C appear to be involved in the cell-surface interaction with thrombin and thrombomodulin.[63,64] The heavy chain of protein C, on the other hand, probably interacts with the substrates factor Va and factor VIIIa.[482]

Thrombomodulin ($M_r \approx$ 75,000 to 100,000) is a single-chain cell surface glycoprotein containing 557 amino acids[483–485] (see Fig. 104-8). The N-terminal portion of the molecule contains a lectinlike extracellular region (226 amino acids) followed by six growth factor domains present in tandem repeats (236 amino acids), a potential carbohydrate-rich region (34 amino acids including 8 serine and threonine residues), a transmembrane domain (23 residues), and an intracellular domain (38 amino acids) located at the C-terminal end of the protein. The fourth through sixth growth factor domains along with the Ser–Thr-rich region are required for cofactor activity.[486,487] The fifth and sixth growth factor domains are involved in binding to thrombin,[478,488–491] whereas a calcium-dependent binding site for protein C is located within the fourth growth factor domain.[489,491]

Thrombomodulin is synthesized in endothelial cells and is found in arteries, veins, and lymphatics.[492] It is not present in the endothelium of the human brain and hepatic sinusoids.[492,493] Thrombomodulin has also been identified in platelets[494] and the syncytiotrophoblast of human placenta.[492] A soluble, truncated form of thrombomodulin has been isolated from human plasma and urine,[495] but its significance is unknown. Thrombomodulin activity is decreased by endotoxin,[496] interleukin-1,[497] and tumor necrosis factor.[498]

Human protein S ($M_r \approx$ 70,000) is a single-chain glycoprotein containing 11 γ-carboxyglutamic acid residues[259,463] (Fig. 104-13). It also contains three residues of β-hydroxyaspartic acid and one β-hydroxyasparagine,[93,98] but the function of these residues is at present unknown. Protein S is synthesized mainly in the liver,[499] but it is also present in endothelial cells,[500] platelets,[501] and osteoblasts.[502] Approximately 60 percent of plasma protein S circulates as a complex with complement C4 binding protein.[503–505] The binding to C4 binding protein significantly reduces the stimulating effect of protein S on activated protein C.[506] Human protein S is

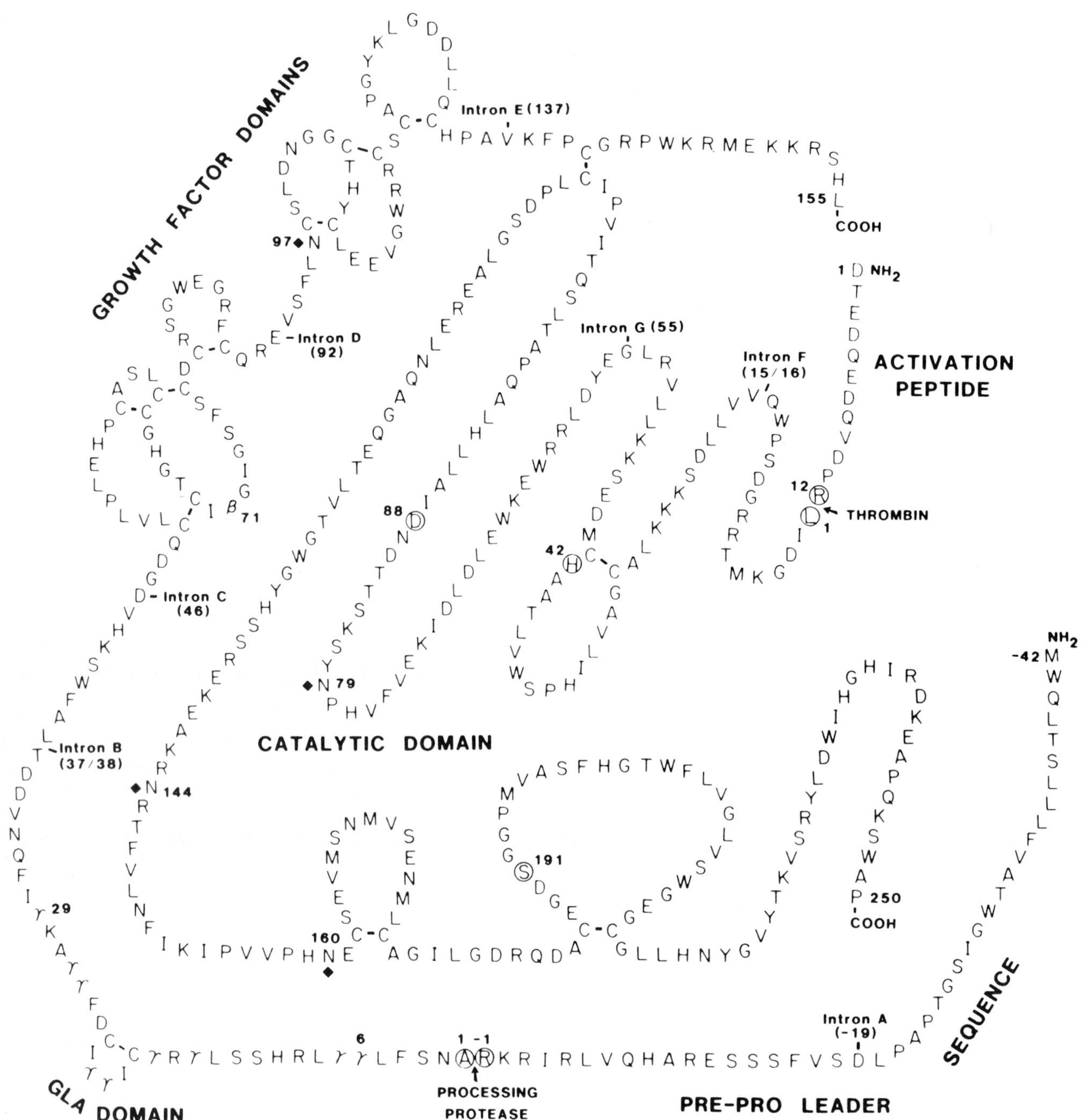

FIG. 104-12 Amino acid sequence and tentative structure for human prepro protein C. The locations of the seven introns (A to G) are shown in the various regions of the protein. An eighth intron located in the 5′ noncoding region of the gene is not shown. The prepro leader sequence (−42 to −1) is cleaved during protein biosynthesis to give rise to the mature protein with an N-terminal sequence of A-N-S-F- for the light chain. The Lys-Arg dipeptide that connects the light and heavy chains during biosynthesis is not shown. The peptide bond cleaved by the thrombin–thrombomodulin complex during the activation reaction is shown with a small arrow. The three amino acids in the catalytic domain (H_{42}, D_{88}, S_{191}) that participate in catalysis are circled, while the four potential carbohydrate attachment sites are shown with solid diamonds. The amino acids are numbered as follows starting with the N-terminal end of the protein: −42 to −1 = prepro leader sequence; +1 to 155 = light chain; 1 to 12 = activation peptide; 1 to 250 = catalytic chain. The single-letter code for amino acids is shown in the legend to Fig. 104-5. β = β-hydroxyaspartic acid. *(From Foster et al.*[223] *and Plutzky et al.*[224] *Used by permission.)*

composed of 635 amino acids, including four growth factor domains following the Gla domain.[23,24] Between the Gla and growth factor domains is a disulfide loop that contains a thrombin-sensitive site.[507] The C-terminal region in protein S, in contrast to the C-terminal regions in the other vitamin K–dependent proteins, does not resemble a serine protease; instead this portion of the molecule contains sequences that are similar to steroid-binding proteins.[508] A segment of the C-terminal portion of protein S has been implicated in the interaction with C4 binding protein.[509,510] Human protein S also contains ≈7.8 percent carbohydrate with potential *N*-linked attachment sites at Asn residues 458, 468, and 489.

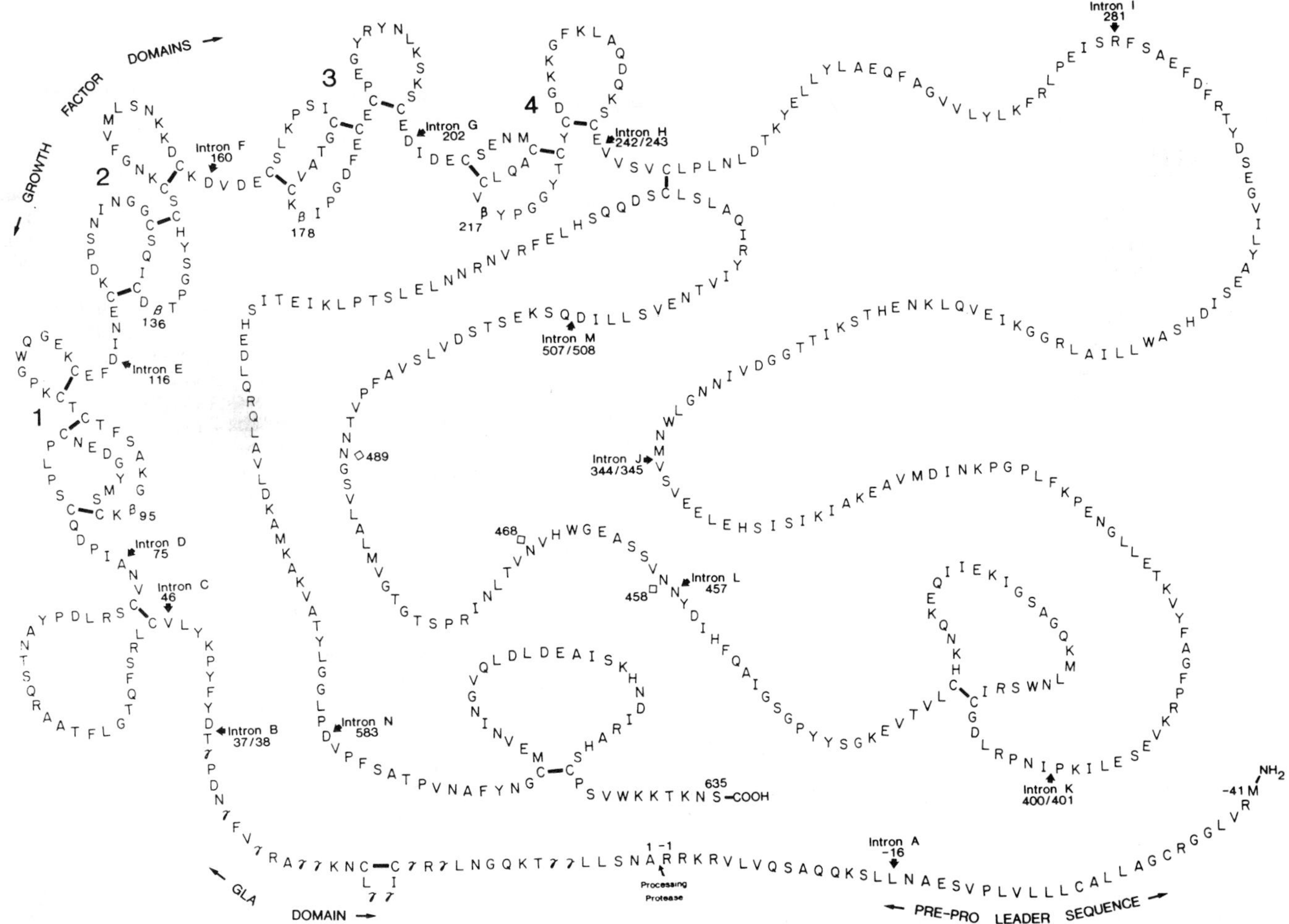

FIG. 104-13 Amino acid sequence and tentative structure of human prepro protein S. The locations of the 14 introns (A to N) are shown in the various regions of the protein. The prepro leader sequence (−41 to −1) is cleaved during protein biosynthesis to give rise to the mature protein with an N-terminal sequence of A-N-S-L-. The three potential N-linked carbohydrate attachment sites are shown with open diamonds. The amino acids are numbered as follows starting with the N-terminal end of the protein: −41 to −1 = preproleader sequence; +1 to 41 = Gla domain; 42 to 75 = thrombin-sensitive region; 76 to 242 = four growth factor domains; 243 to 635 = region homologous to steroid-binding proteins. The single-letter code for amino acids is shown in the legend to Fig. 104-5. β = β-hydroxyaspartic acid (EGF-1 domain) or β-hydroxyasparagine (EGF-2-4 domains). *(From Lundwall et al.,[23] Hoskins et al.,[24] Edenbrandt et al.,[520] Schmidel et al.,[521] and Ploos van Amstel et al.[522])*

Genetic Aspects

The gene for protein C is located in the q13-q14 region of chromosome 2[511,512] and contains approximately 11 kb of DNA.[223,224] It is composed of nine exons and eight introns. As mentioned previously, the seven introns in the gene for protein C that are located within the coding region are present in essentially the same positions in the amino acid sequence as the seven introns in the genes for human factor VII, factor IX, and factor X. The gene for protein C also contains two *Alu* sequences and two homologous repeats of about 160 nucleotides that are located in intron E. Common intragenic protein C polymorphisms include a T/A dimorphism at nucleotide −1476 within the untranslated exon I, and silent substitutions of the third base in five codons: CG<u>C</u>/CG<u>T</u> at Arg 87, TC<u>T</u>/TC<u>G</u> at Ser 99, AA<u>A</u>/AA<u>G</u> at Lys 156, GA<u>T</u>/GA<u>C</u> at Asp 214, and GA<u>T</u>/GA<u>C</u> at Asp 215.[513–516]

Two copies of the gene for protein S (PSα and PSβ) are located near the centromere of chromosome 3,[517–519] but only PSα appears to be transcriptionally active. The PSα gene is ≈ 80 kb long and contains 15 exons, 14 introns, and 6 *Alu* repetitive sequences.[520–522] The first eight exons encode protein segments homologous to factors VII, IX, and X and protein C, whereas the remaining seven exons encode the C-terminal region homologous to sex hormone binding globulin. The coding sequence for the PSβ gene is 97 percent identical to that of the PSα gene, but contains several nonsense and frameshift mutations. It also lacks exon I containing the initiation Met codon, which suggests the PSβ gene is indeed a pseudogene.[520–522]

The gene for human thrombomodulin is located on chromosome 20.[484] Surprisingly, it contains no introns.[485,523] Accordingly, it represents an unusual example of a gene containing growth factor domains that are not separated by introns, as is the case in the genes for factor VII, factor X, protein C, and protein S.

Protein C Deficiency

Plasma protein C levels are determined either immunochemically or functionally.[524] In the functional assays, protein C partially isolated from plasma is activated by thrombin, thrombin–thrombomodulin complex, or a specific snake venom activator; enzymatic activity is then determined either by amidolysis of a chromogenic substrate or by prolongation of a clotting assay.

Normal plasma protein C concentration is about 4 μg/ml (see Table 104-2) and varies between 0.7 and 1.3 U/ml, where 1 U is the amount of protein C found in 1 ml of normal pooled plasma. No significant difference is seen with various ages or between males and females. Like the other vitamin K–dependent coagulation factors, the levels of protein C in infants is low. This probably reflects decreased synthesis relative to that in an older child or an adult.[525,526] Transient severe protein C deficiency (<0.01 U/ml) occurs not infrequently in preterm infants and high-risk term infants, and it may increase the risk of thrombosis.[527] Levels of protein C are also reduced in a number of acquired conditions, such as liver disease,[528–532] DIC,[528,529,533] L-asparaginase therapy,[534] plasma exchange,[535] and following surgery.[528,536] In thrombotic thrombocytopenic purpura (TTP), decreased fibrinolytic activity has been attributed to impaired protein C function.[537] Elevated levels of protein C, on the other hand, have been found in patients with diabetes and ischemic heart disease[538] and the nephrotic syndrome,[539] as well as during late pregnancy[540] and in some women taking oral contraceptives.[541] The attenuated androgens stanazolol[542] and danazol[543] also increase plasma protein C levels.

During anticoagulant treatment with coumarin drugs, the level of γ-carboxylation of each of the vitamin K–dependent coagulation factors is reduced, and nonfunctional proteins are produced. Depending on their different half-lives, the activity of these proteins in plasma decreases with time, with protein C and factor VII showing an activity of only 10 to 20 percent of normal after 1 to 2 days. Factor X, prothrombin, and factor IX, however, have a much longer half-life and require 5 to 6 days to decrease to the same level.[531] It has been proposed that the rapid decrease in protein C levels in patients following administration of oral anticoagulants causes a transient hypercoagulable state (see below). In patients receiving warfarin, activity levels of protein C are generally reduced relative to levels of protein C antigen, particularly when a clotting-based assay is used.

Congenital protein C deficiency is associated with an increased risk of venous thromboembolic disease.[544] Heterozygous protein C deficiency (plasma protein C level ≈40 to 50 percent of normal) is associated with the development of recurrent episodes of deep venous thrombosis, pulmonary embolism, and superficial phlebitis at an early age (under 40 years). The prevalence of heterozygous protein C deficiency in young patients with idiopathic venous thrombosis is approximately 5 percent.[545,546] Intraabdominal venous thrombosis has been reported in a few patients with congenital protein C deficiency.[547,548] Hereditary protein C deficiency should also be considered in young patients with acute or subacute neurologic symptoms associated with cerebral thrombosis or with myocardial infarction.[549–551] Skin necrosis developing soon after the initiation of warfarin therapy also has been associated with heterozygous protein C deficiency.[552,553] It has been proposed that the relatively short half-life of protein C compared to most of the other vitamin K–dependent factors results in a transient hypercoagulable state that leads to the formation of thrombi within the small skin vessels.

Hereditary protein C deficiency is inherited in an autosomal dominant manner, but the clinical expression of heterozygous protein C deficiency is quite variable. Although laboratory evidence of heterozygous protein C deficiency is present in one in every 200 to 300 healthy blood donors without any personal or family history of thrombotic disease,[554] the frequency of clinically apparent heterozygous protein C deficiency has been estimated to be only about 1 in every 16,000 individuals.[544] Furthermore, even within the same affected family, the clinical severity of protein C deficiency may vary among heterozygous individuals.[555] Finally, unrelated individuals with the same molecular abnormality can have different clinical phenotypes.[513,556] Thus, other as yet undefined factor(s) must influence the clinical expression of hereditary protein C deficiency.

Two phenotypes of heterozygous protein C deficiency have been described based on the results of antigenic and functional protein C assays.[544] Type I is characterized by a concomitant decrease in levels of protein C antigen and activity. Type II is marked by a functionally abnormal protein C molecule (i.e., normal antigen but reduced activity). Type I accounts for most described cases of protein C deficiency.

Homozygous protein C deficiency is a rare disorder with an estimated frequency of 1 in every 500,000 to 750,000 births. Protein C levels are usually undetectable (less than 1 percent of normal). The homozygous form of protein C deficiency can be manifested by massive venous thrombosis in the neonatal period or by DIC and purpura fulminans in newborns.[557,558] The clinical spectrum of homozygous protein C deficiency, however, includes moderately affected and even asymptomatic individuals.[559–561]

Patients with heterozygous protein C deficiency who experience recurrent thromboembolic events generally require long-term anticoagulation with warfarin. Infants with homozygous protein C deficiency born with purpura fulminans or DIC are initially treated with frequent plasma infusions for 1 to 2 months until all lesions have healed, followed by long-term oral anticoagulant therapy.[557] Purified protein C concentrates have become available for replacement therapy of homozygous protein C deficiency[562] as well as for heterozygous individuals during periods of increased thrombotic risk.[563]

Molecular abnormalities have been identified in a number of individuals with heterozygous and homozygous protein C deficiency.[564] A variety of defects have been found in type I patients, including deletions, frameshift mutations, splice-junction alterations, promoter region mutations, nonsense mutations, and missense mutations. Some of the mutations have been described in more than one pedigree, and most of these recurrent mutations involve CG dinucleotides. An exception is a recurrent Arg 306 to stop mutation in several Dutch pedigrees that is invariably associated with a rare *Msp*I haplotype; it thus appears to have descended from a common distant ancestor.[513] At the molecular level, patients with severe, "homozygous" protein C deficiency are either true homozygotes or compound heterozygotes.[565,566]

Several missense mutations have been identified in patients with the less common type II deficiency.[564] These are of particular interest from a protein C structure/function standpoint. For example, a homozygous Arg 169 to Trp mutation disrupts the thrombin–thrombomodulin activation site[567] (see Fig. 104-11). A compound heterozygous abnormality, protein $C_{VERMONT}$, is characterized by normal protein C antigen and amidolytic activity but markedly reduced anticoagulant activity due to two mutations within the Gla domain: Glu 20 to Ala and Val 34 to Met.[568] The former amino acid substitution eliminates a site that is normally γ-carboxylated, and thus may disrupt calcium binding.[287]

Protein S Deficiency

Congenital protein S deficiency is also an autosomal disorder associated with a thrombotic tendency.[569–571] Like patients with protein C deficiency, clinically affected individuals usually have venous thromboembolic disease at a young age,[572] and heterozygous protein S deficiency accounts for ≈3 to 5 percent of such cases of recurrent venous thrombosis.[545,546] Arterial thrombosis[573,574] and warfarin-induced skin necrosis[575,576] have also been reported in patients with protein S deficiency. Purpura fulminans has been described in a neonate with homozygous protein S deficiency.[577]

The normal plasma concentration of protein S is about 25 μg/ml,[578] (see Table 104-2) and total protein S levels in normal individuals range from 70 to 125 percent of normal.[505] Levels are somewhat lower for women than for men.[579,580] About 60 percent of plasma protein S forms a 1:1 complex with C4 binding protein,[503–505] and this bound form of protein S is functionally inactive.[506] Total plasma protein S (free plus C4 binding protein–bound) is measured immunologically.[505,570] By adding polyethylene glycol to plasma, the C4 binding protein–bound protein S is precipitated and the free protein S concentration can then be determined.[504,580] Functional assays based on the cofactor ability of protein S to enhance the activated protein C–induced prolongation of clotting times have been described,[569] but these are not yet routinely available.

Most patients with inherited protein S deficiency have little or no free protein S, but a normal (or near-normal) amount of protein S in a complex with C4 binding protein (type I).[504] Individuals with little or no protein S, either free or bound (type II),[504,569,581] appear to be homozygotes (or compound heterozygotes). A patient with low normal free and total protein S levels, but reduced protein S activity, has also been described.[582]

Acquired protein S deficiency has been described in several clinical settings. Total protein S levels decrease during pregnancy and during the postpartum period; a concomitant reduction in free functional protein S also occurs due to redistribution into a complex with C4 binding protein.[583] Furthermore, oral contraceptives have been found to lower levels of both total and free protein S.[579,584] Levels of protein S are also reduced in liver disease, DIC, diabetes, and during warfarin anticoagulation.[585–587] A transient redistribution of free protein S to the complexed form can occur in patients with acute venous thrombosis.[585] The reduced free protein S levels in some patients with the lupus anticoagulant–antiphospholipid antibody syndrome has been implicated in the associated thrombotic diathesis.[588–591] Acquired protein S deficiency has been reported in some patients with AIDS.[592,593]

Abnormalities of C4 binding protein can also affect levels of free protein S. Two patients with a history of venous thrombosis and reduced levels of free protein S presumed secondary to increased binding to C4 binding protein have been described.[594,595] Conversely, a family with hereditary C4 binding protein deficiency had elevated levels of free protein S but no increased risk of bleeding.[596]

In general, molecular genetic analysis of protein S–deficient individuals has been hindered to a large degree by the presence of the protein S pseudogene. To date, two molecular defects responsible for protein S deficiency have been identified: a partial deletion of the middle portion of the PSα gene,[597] and a 5.3-kb partial gene deletion encompassing exon XIII and introns L and M.[598] A common dimorphism of Ser/Pro at residue 460 is due to a T-to-C transition in exon XIII of the PSα gene and can be readily detected by immunoassay.[599] This amino acid substitution disrupts an *N*-linked glycosylation site, but does not correlate with thrombotic risk. The site may be useful, however, as a marker in linkage analysis of protein S–deficient families.

REFERENCES

1. Stenflo J, Fernlund P, Egan W, Roepstorff P: Vitamin K dependent modifications of glutamic acid residues in prothrombin. *Proc Natl Acad Sci USA* **71**:2730, 1974.
2. Nelsestuen GL, Zytkovicz TH, Howard JB: The mode of action of vitamin K isolation of a peptide containing the vitamin K–dependent portion of prothrombin. *J Biol Chem* **249**:6347, 1974.
3. Magnusson S, Sottrup-Jensen L, Petersen TE, Morris HR, Dell A: Primary structure of the vitamin K–dependent part of prothrombin. *FEBS Lett* **44**:189, 1974.
4. Esmon CT, Suttie JW, Jackson CM: The functional significance of vitamin K action: Differences in phospholipid binding between normal and abnormal prothrombin. *J Biol Chem* **250**:4095, 1975.
5. Soriano-Garcia M, Padmanabhan K, de Vos AM, Tulinsky A: The Ca^{+} ion and membrane binding structure of the Gla domain of Ca-prothrombin fragment 1. *Biochemistry* **31**:2554, 1992.
6. Magnusson S, Petersen TE, Sottrup-Jensen L, Claeys H: Complete primary structure of prothrombin: Isolation, structure and reactivity of ten carboxylated glutamic acid residues and regulation of prothrombin activation by thrombin, in Reich E, Rifkin DB, Shaw E (eds): *Proteases and Biological Control*. Cold Spring Harbor, NY, Cold Spring Harbor Laboratory, 1975, p 123.
7. McMullen BA, Fujikawa K: Amino acid sequence of the heavy chain of human a-factor XIIa. *J Biol Chem* **260**:5328, 1985.
8. Sottrup-Jensen L, Claeys H, Zajdel M, Petersen TE, Magnusson S: The primary structure of human plasminogen: Isolation of two lysine-binding fragments and one "mini"-plasminogen (MW, 38,000) by elastase-catalyzed-specific limited proteolysis, in Davidson JF, Rowan RM, Samama MM, Desnoyers PC (eds): *Progress in Chemical Fibrinolysis and Thrombolysis*. New York, Raven, 1978, vol 3, p 191.
9. Pennica D, Holmes WE, Kohr WJ, Harkins RN, Vehar GA, Ward CA, Bennett WF, Yelverton E, Seeburg PH, Heyneker HL, Goeddel DV: Cloning and expression of human tissue-type plasminogen activator cDNA in E. coli. *Nature* **301**:214, 1983.
10. Gunzler WA, Steffens GJ, Otting F, Kim S-MA, Frankus E, Flohe L: The primary structure of high molecular mass urokinase from human urine: The complete amino acid sequence of the A chain. *Hoppe Seyler Z Physiol Chem* **363**:1155, 1982.
11. Hagen FS, Gray CL, O'Hara P, Grant FJ, Saari GC, Woodbury RG, Hart CE, Insley M, Kisiel W, Kurachi K, Davie EW: Characterization of a cDNA coding for human factor VII. *Proc Natl Acad Sci USA* **83**:2412, 1986.
12. Kurachi K, Davie EW: Isolation and characterization of a cDNA coding for human factor IX. *Proc Natl Acad Sci USA* **79**:6461, 1982.
13. Yoshitake S, Schach BG, Foster DC, Davie EW, Kurachi K: Nucleotide sequence of the gene for human factor IX (antihemophilic factor B). *Biochemistry* **24**:3736, 1985.
14. Anson DS, Choo KH, Rees DJG, Giannelli F, Gould K, Huddleston JA, Brownlee GG: The gene structure of human anti-haemophilic factor IX. *EMBO J* **3**:1053, 1984.
15. Leytus SP, Chung DW, Kisiel W, Kurachi K, Davie EW: Characterization of a cDNA coding for human factor X. *Proc Natl Acad Sci USA* **81**:3699, 1984.
16. Fung MR, Hay CS, MacGillivray RTA: Characterization of an almost full-length cDNA coding for human blood coagulation factor X. *Proc Natl Acad Sci USA* **82**:3591, 1985.

17. Leytus SP, Foster DC, Kurachi K, Davie EW: Gene for human factor X, a blood coagulation factor whose gene organization is essentially identical to that of factor IX and protein C. *Biochemistry* **25:**5098, 1986.
18. Foster D, Davie EW: Characterization of a cDNA coding for human protein C. *Proc Natl Acad Sci USA* **81:**4766, 1984.
19. Beckmann RJ, Schmidt RJ, Santerre RF, Plutzky J, Crabtree GR, Long GL: The structure and evolution of a 461 amino acid human protein C precursor and its messenger RNA, based upon the DNA sequence of cloned human liver cDNAs. *Nucleic Acids Res* **13:**5233, 1985.
20. Gray A, Dull TJ, Ullrich A: Nucleotide sequence of epidermal growth factor cDNA predicts a 128,000-molecular weight protein precursor. *Nature* **303:**722, 1983.
21. Doolittle RF, Feng DF, Johnson MS: Computer-based characterization of epidermal growth factor precursor. *Nature* **307:**558, 1984.
22. Carpenter G, Zendegui JG: Epidermal growth factor, its receptor, and related proteins. *Exp Cell Res* **164:**1, 1986.
23. Lundwall A, Dackowski W, Cohen E, Shaffer M, Mahr A, Dahlback B, Stenflo J, Wydro R: Isolation and sequence of the cDNA for human protein S, a regulator of blood coagulation. *Proc Natl Acad Sci USA* **83:**6716, 1986.
24. Hoskins J, Norman DK, Beckmann RJ, Long GL: Cloning and characterization of human liver cDNA encoding a protein S precursor. *Proc Natl Acad Sci USA* **84:**349, 1987.
25. Appella E, Weber IT, Blasi F: Structure and function of epidermal growth factor-like regions in proteins. *FEBS Lett* **231:**1, 1988.
26. Stenflo J: Structure-function relationships of epidermal growth factor modules in vitamin K-dependent clotting factors. *Blood* **78:**1637, 1991.
27. Cooke RM, Wilkinson AJ, Baron M, Pastore A, Tappin MJ, Campbell ID, Gregory H, Sheard B: The solution structure of human epidermal growth factor. *Nature* **327:**339, 1987.
28. Campbell ID, Cooke RM, Baron M, Harvey TS, Tappin MJ: The solution structures of epidermal growth factor and transforming growth factor alpha. *Prog Growth Factor Res* **1:**13, 1989.
29. Montelione GT, Wuthrich K, Nice EC, Burgess AW, Scheraga HA: Solution structure of murine epidermal growth factor: Determination of the polypeptide backbone chain-fold by nuclear magnetic resonance and distance geometry. *Proc Natl Acad Sci USA* **84:**5226, 1987.
30. Mayo KH, Cavalli RC, Peters AR, Boelens R, Kaptein R: Sequence-specific ^{1}H-n.m.r. assignments and peptide backbone conformation in rat epidermal growth factor. *Biochem J* **257:**197, 1989.
31. Montelione GT, Winkler ME, Burton LE, Rinderknecht E, Sporn MB, Wagner G: Sequence-specific ^{1}H-NMR assignments and identification of two small antiparallel β-sheets in the solution structure of recombinant human transforming growth factor α. *Proc Natl Acad Sci USA* **86:**1519, 1989.
32. Kohda D, Shimada I, Miyake T, Fuwa T, Inagaki F: Polypeptide chain fold of human transforming growth factor α analogous to those of mouse and human epidermal growth factors as studied by two-dimensional ^{1}H NMR. *Biochemistry* **28:**953, 1989.
33. Kline TP, Brown FK, Brown SC, Jeffs PW, Kopple KD, Mueller L: Solution structures of human transforming growth factor α derived from ^{1}H NMR data. *Biochemistry* **29:**7805, 1990.
34. Huang LH, Cheng H, Pardi A, Tam JP, Sweeney WV: Sequence-specific 1H NMR assignments, secondary structure, and location of the calcium binding site in the first epidermal growth factor like domain of blood coagulation factor IX. *Biochemistry* **30:**7402, 1991.
35. Baron M, Norman DG, Harvey TS, Handford PA, Mayhew M, Tse AGD, Brownlee GG, Campbell ID: The three-dimensional structure of the first EGF-like module of human factor IX: Comparison with EGF and TGF-α. *Protein Sci* **1:**81, 1992.
36. Selander M, Persson E, Stenflo J, Drakenberg T: ^{1}H NMR assignment and secondary structure of the Ca^{2+}-free form of the amino-terminal epidermal growth factor like domain in coagulation factor X. *Biochemistry* **29:**8111, 1990.
37. Ullner M, Selander M, Persson E, Stenflo J, Drakenberg T, Teleman O: Three-dimensional structure of the Apo form of the N-terminal EGF-like module of blood coagulation factor X as determined by NMR spectroscopy and simulated folding. *Biochemistry* **31:**5974, 1992.
38. Esmon NL, DeBault LE, Esmon CT: Proteolytic formation and properties of γ-carboxyglutamic acid-domainless protein C. *J Biol Chem* **258:**5548, 1983.
39. Morita T, Isaacs BS, Esmon CT, Johnson AE: Derivatives of blood coagulation factor IX contain a high affinity Ca^{2+}-binding site that lacks γ-carboxyglutamic acid. *J Biol Chem* **259:**5698, 1984.
40. Sugo T, Bjork I, Holmgren A, Stenflo J: Calcium-binding properties of bovine factor X lacking the γ-carboxyglutamic acid-containing region. *J Biol Chem* **259:**5705, 1984.
41. Sugo T, Dahlback B, Holmgren A, Stenflo J: Calcium binding of bovine protein S: Effect of thrombin cleavage and removal of the γ-carboxyglutamic acid-containing region. *J Biol Chem* **261:**5116, 1986.
42. Handford PA, Baron M, Mayhew M, Willis A, Beesley T, Brownlee GG, Campbell ID: The first EGF-like domain from human factor IX contains a high-affinity calcium binding site. *EMBO J* **9:**475, 1990.
43. Persson E, Selander M, Linse S, Drakenberg T, Ohlin A-K, Stenflo J: Calcium binding to the isolated β-hydroxyaspartic acid-containing epidermal growth factor-like domain of bovine factor X. *J Biol Chem* **264:**16897, 1989.
44. Ohlin A-K, Linse S, Stenflo J: Calcium binding to the epidermal growth factor homology region of bovine protein C. *J Biol Chem* **263:**7411, 1988.
45. Dahlback B, Hildebrand B, Linse S: Novel type of very high affinity calcium-binding sites in β-hydroxyasparagine-containing epidermal growth factor-like domains in vitamin K-dependent protein S. *J Biol Chem* **265:**18481, 1990.
46. Handford PA, Mayhew M, Baron M, Winship PR, Campbell ID, Brownlee GG: Key residues involved in calcium-binding motifs in EGF-like domains. *Nature* **351:**164, 1991.
47. Selander-Sunnerhagen M, Ullner M, Persson E, Teleman O, Stenflo J, Drakenberg T: How an epidermal growth factor (EGF)-like domain binds calcium: High resolution NMR structure of the calcium form of the NH_2-terminal EGF-like domain in coagulation factor X. *J Biol Chem* **267:**19642, 1992.
48. Sakai T, Lund-Hansen T, Thim L, Kisiel W: The γ-carboxyglutamic acid domain of human factor VIIa is essential for its interaction with cell surface tissue factor. *J Biol Chem* **265:**1890, 1990.
49. Ruf W, Kalnik MW, Lund-Hansen T, Edgington TS: Characterization of factor VII association with tissue factor in solution: High and low affinity calcium binding sites in factor VII contribute to functionally distinct interactions. *J Biol Chem* **266:**15719, 1991.
50. Toomey JR, Smith KJ, Stafford DW: Localization of human tissue factor recognition determinant of human factor VIIa. *J Biol Chem* **266:**19198, 1991.
51. Clarke BJ, Ofosu FA, Sridhara S, Bona RD, Rickles FR, Blajchman MA: The first epidermal growth factor domain of human coagulation factor VII is essential for binding with tissue factor. *FEBS Lett* **298:**206, 1992.
52. Wildgoose P, Jorgensen T, Komiyama Y, Nakagaki T, Pedersen A, Kisiel W: The role of phospholipids and the factor VII Gla-domain in the interaction of factor VII with tissue factor. *Thromb Haemost* **67:**679, 1992.
53. Ryan J, Wolitzky B, Heimer E, Lambrose T, Felix A, Tam JP, Huang LH, Nawroth P, Wilner G, Kisiel W, Nelsestuen GL, Stern DM: Structural determinants of the factor IX molecule mediating interaction with the endothelial cell binding site are distinct from those involved in phospholipid binding. *J Biol Chem* **264:**20283, 1989.
54. Astermark J, Stenflo J: The epidermal growth factor-like domains of factor IX: Effect on blood clotting and endothelial cell binding of a fragment containing the epidermal growth factor-like domains linked to the γ-carboxyglutamic acid region. *J Biol Chem* **266:**2438, 1991.
55. Rees DJG, Jones IM, Handford PA, Walter SJ, Esnouf MP, Smith KJ, Brownlee GG: The role of β-hydroxyaspar-

tate and adjacent carboxylate residues in the first EGF domain of human factor IX. *EMBO J* **7**:2053, 1988.
56. Lin S-W, Smith KJ, Welsch D, Stafford DW: Expression and characterization of human factor IX and factor IX-factor X chimeras in mouse C127 cells. *J Biol Chem* **265**:144, 1990.
57. Astermark J, Hogg PJ, Bjork I, Stenflo J: Effects of γ-carboxyglutamic acid and epidermal growth factor-like modules of factor IX on factor X activation: Studies using proteolytic fragments of bovine factor IX. *J Biol Chem* **267**:3249, 1992.
58. Cheung W-F, Hamaguchi N, Smith KJ, Stafford D: The binding of human factor IX to endothelial cells is mediated by residues 3-11. *J Biol Chem* **267**:20529, 1992.
59. Toomey JR, Smith KJ, Roberts HR, Stafford DW: The endothelial cell binding determinant of human factor IX resides in the γ-carboxyglutamic acid domain. *Biochemistry* **31**:1806, 1992.
60. Rawala-Sheikh R, Ahmad SS, Monroe DM, Roberts HR, Walsh PN: Role of γ-carboxyglutamic acid residues in the binding of factor IXa to platelets and in factor-X activation. *Blood* **79**:398, 1992.
61. Persson E, Valcarce C, Stenflo J: The γ-carboxyglutamic acid and epidermal growth factor-like domains of factor X: Effect of isolated domains on prothrombin activation and endothelial cell binding of factor X. *J Biol Chem* **266**:2453, 1992.
62. Hertzberg MS, Ben-Tal O, Furie B, Furie BC: Construction, expression, and characterization of a chimera of factor IX and factor X: The role of the second epidermal growth factor domain and serine protease domain in factor Va binding. *J Biol Chem* **267**:14759, 1992.
63. Hogg PJ, Ohlin A-K, Stenflo J: Identification of structural domains in protein C involved in its interaction with thrombin-thrombomodulin on the surface of endothelial cells. *J Biol Chem* **267**:703, 1992.
64. Olsen PH, Esmon NL, Esmon CT, Laue TM: Ca^{2+} dependence of the interactions between protein C, thrombin, and the elastase fragment of thrombomodulin. Analysis by ultracentrifugation. *Biochemistry* **31**:746, 1992.
65. Furie B, Bing DH, Feldmann RJ, Robison DJ, Burnier JP, Furie BC: Computer-generated models of blood coagulation factor Xa, factor IXa, and thrombin based upon structural homology with other serine proteases. *J Biol Chem* **257**:3875, 1982.
66. Bode W, Mayr I, Baumann U, Huber R, Stone SR, Hofsteenge J: The refined 1.9 A crystal structure of human α-thrombin: Interaction with D-Phe-Pro-Arg chloromethylketone and significance of the Tyr-Pro-Pro-Trp insertion segment. *EMBO J* **8**:3467, 1989.
67. Degen SJF, Davie EW: Nucleotide sequence of the gene for human prothrombin. *Biochemistry* **26**:6165, 1987.
68. Jorgensen MJ, Cantor AB, Furie BC, Brown CL, Shoemaker CB, Furie B: Recognition site directing vitamin K-dependent γ-carboxylation residues on the propeptide of factor IX. *Cell* **48**:185, 1987.
69. Watzke HH, Wallmark A, Hamaguchi N, Giardina P, Stafford DW, High KA: Factor $X_{SANTO\ DOMINGO}$: Evidence that the severe clinical phenotype arises from a mutation blocking secretion. *J Clin Invest* **88**:1685, 1991.
70. Foster DC, Rudinski MS, Schach BG, Berkner KL, Kumar AA, Hagen FS, Sprecher CA, Insley MY, Davie EW: Propeptide of human protein C is necessary for γ-carboxylation. *Biochemistry* **26**:7003, 1987.
71. Rabiet M-J, Jorgensen MJ, Furie B, Furie BC: Effect of propeptide mutations on post-translational processing of factor IX: Evidence that β-hydroxylation and γ-carboxylation are independent events. *J Biol Chem* **262**:14895, 1987.
72. Ulrich MMW, Furie B, Jacobs MR, Vermeer C, Furie BC: Vitamin K-dependent carboxylation: A synthetic peptide based upon the γ-carboxylation recognition site sequence of the prothrombin propeptide is an active substrate for the carboxylase *in vitro*. *J Biol Chem* **263**:9697, 1988.
73. Huber P, Schmitz T, Griffin J, Jacobs M, Walsh C, Furie B, Furie BC: Identification of amino acids in the γ-carboxylation recognition site on the propeptide of prothrombin. *J Biol Chem* **265**:12467, 1990.
74. Stanton C, Taylor R, Wallin R: Processing of prothrombin in the secretory pathway. *Biochem J* **277**:59, 1991.
75. McClure DB, Walls JD, Grinnell BW: Post-translational processing events in the secretion pathway of human protein C, a complex vitamin K-dependent antithrombotic factor. *J Biol Chem* **267**:19710, 1992.
76. Wu S-M, Cheung W-F, Frazier D, Stafford DW: Cloning and expression of the cDNA for human γ-glutamyl carboxylase. *Science* **254**:1634, 1991.
77. Berkner KL, Harbeck M, Lingenfelter S, Bailey C, Sanders-Hinck CM, Suttie JW: Purification and identification of bovine liver γ-carboxylase. *Proc Natl Acad Sci USA* **89**:6242, 1992.
78. Suttie JW: Vitamin K-dependent carboxylase. *Annu Rev Biochem* **54**:459, 1985.
79. Furie B, Furie BC: Molecular basis of vitamin K-dependent γ-carboxylation. *Blood* **75**:1753, 1990.
80. Friedman PA, Griep AE: In vitro inhibition of vitamin K-dependent carboxylation by tetrachloropyridinol and the imidazopyridines. *Biochemistry* **19**:3381, 1980.
81. Sugo T, Persson U, Stenflo J: Protein C in bovine plasma after warfarin treatment: Purification, partial characterization, and β-hydroxyaspartic acid content. *J Biol Chem* **260**:10453, 1985.
82. Bentley AK, Rees DJG, Rizza C, Brownlee GG: Defective propeptide processing of blood clotting factor IX caused by mutation of arginine to glutamine at position −4. *Cell* **45**:343, 1986.
83. Diuguid DL, Rabiet MJ, Furie BC, Liebman HA, Furie B: Molecular basis of hemophilia B: A defective enzyme due to an unprocessed propeptide is caused by a point mutation in the factor IX precursor. *Proc Natl Acad Sci USA* **83**:5803, 1986.
84. Ware J, Diuguid DL, Liebman HA, Rabiet M-J, Kasper CK, Furie BC, Furie B, Stafford DW: Factor IX San Dimas: Substitution of glutamine for Arg^{-4} in the propeptide leads to incomplete γ-carboxylation and altered phospholipid binding properties. *J Biol Chem* **264**:11401, 1989.
85. Sugimoto M, Miyata T, Kawabata S, Yoshioka A, Fukui H, Iwanaga S: Factor IX Kawachinagano: Impaired function of the Gla-domain caused by attached propeptide region due to substitution of arginine by glutamine at position −4. *Br J Haematol* **72**:216, 1989.
86. Thompson AR, Schoof JM, Weinmann AF, Chen S-H: Factor IX mutations: Rapid, direct screening methods for 20 new families with hemophilia B. *Thromb Res* **65**:289, 1992.
87. Barr PJ: Mammalian subtilisins: The long-sought dibasic processing endoproteases. *Cell* **66**:1, 1991.
88. Kawabata S-i, Davie EW: A microsomal endopeptidase from liver with substrate specificity for processing proproteins such as the vitamin K-dependent proteins of plasma. *J Biol Chem* **267**:10331, 1992.
89. Drakenberg T, Fernlund P, Roepstorff P, Stenflo J: β-Hydroxyaspartic acid in vitamin K-dependent proteins. *Proc Natl Acad Sci USA* **80**:1802, 1983.
90. McMullen BA, Fujikawa K, Kisiel W, Sasagawa T, Howald WN, Kwa EY, Weinstein B: Complete amino acid sequence of the light chain of human blood coagulation factor X: Evidence for identification of residue 63 as β-hydroxyaspartic acid. *Biochemistry* **22**:2875, 1983.
91. McMullen BA, Fujikawa K, Kisiel W: The occurrence of β-hydroxyaspartic acid in the vitamin K-dependent blood coagulation zymogens. *Biochem Biophys Res Commun* **115**:8, 1983.
92. Fernlund P, Stenflo J: β-Hydroxyaspartic acid in vitamin K-dependent proteins. *J Biol Chem* **258**:12509, 1983.
93. Stenflo J, Lundwall A, Dahlback B: β-Hydroxyasparagine in domains homologous to the epidermal growth factor precursor in vitamin K-dependent protein S. *Proc Natl Acad Sci USA* **84**:368, 1987.
94. Gronke RS, VanDusen WJ, Garsky VM, Jacobs JW, Sardana MK, Stern AM, Friedman PA: Aspartyl β-hydroxylase: In vitro hydroxylation of a synthetic peptide based on the structure of the first growth factor-like domain of human factor IX. *Proc Natl Acad Sci USA* **86**:3609, 1989.
95. Stenflo J, Holme E, Lindstedt S, Chandramouli N, Tsai Huang LH, Tam JP, Merrifield RB: Hydroxylation of

aspartic acid in domains homologous to the epidermal growth factor precursor is catalyzed by a 2-oxoglutarate-dependent dioxygenase. *Proc Natl Acad Sci USA* **86**:444, 1989.

96. Jia S, VanDusen WJ, Diehl RE, Kohl NE, Dixon RAF, Elliston KO, Stern AM, Friedman PA: cDNA cloning and expression of bovine aspartyl (asparaginyl) β-hydroxylase. *J Biol Chem* **267**:14322, 1992.
97. Thim L, Bjoern S, Christensen M, Nicolaisen EM, Lund-Hansen T, Pedersen AH, Hedner U: Amino acid sequence and posttranslational modifications of human factor VII_a from plasma and transfected baby hamster kidney cells. *Biochemistry* **27**:7785, 1988.
98. Nelson RM, VanDusen WJ, Friedman PA, Long GL: β-Hydroxyaspartic acid and β-hydroxyasparagine residues in recombinant human protein S are not required for anticoagulant cofactor activity or for binding to C4b-binding protein. *J Biol Chem* **266**:20586, 1991.
99. Grinnell BW, Walls JD, Gerlitz B: Glycosylation of human protein C affects its secretion, processing, functional activities, and activation by thrombin. *J Biol Chem* **266**:9778, 1991.
100. Hase S, Kawabata S-i, Nishimura H, Takeya H, Sueyoshi T, Miyata T, Iwanaga S, Takao T, Shimonishi Y, Ikenaka T: A new trisaccharide sugar chain linked to a serine residue in bovine blood coagulation factors VII and IX. *J Biochem* **104**:867, 1988.
101. Nishimura H, Kawabata S, Kisiel W, Hase S, Ikenaka T, Takao T, Shimonishi Y, Iwanaga S: Identification of a disaccharide (Xyl-Glc) and a trisaccharide (Xyl_2-Glc) *O*-glycosidically linked to a serine residue in the first epidermal growth factor-like domain of human factors VII and IX and protein Z and bovine protein Z. *J Biol Chem* **264**:20320, 1989.
102. Bjoern S, Foster DC, Thim L, Wiberg FC, Christensen M, Komiyama Y, Pedersen AH, Kisiel W: Human plasma and recombinant factor VII: Characterization of O-glycosylations at serine residues 52 and 60 and effects of site-directed metagenesis of serine 52 to alanine. *J Biol Chem* **266**:11051, 1991.
103. Nishimura H, Takao T, Hase S, Shimonishi Y, Iwanaga S: Human factor IX has a tetrasaccharide *O*-glycosidically linked to serine 61 through the fucose residue. *J Biol Chem* **267**:17520, 1992.
104. Kentzer EJ, Buko A, Menon G, Sarin VK: Carbohydrate composition and presence of a fucose-protein linkage in recombinant human pro-urokinase. *Biochem Biophys Res Commun* **171**:401, 1990.
105. Harris RJ, Leonard CK, Guzzetta AW, Spellman MW: Tissue plasminogen activator has an *O*-linked fucose attached to threonine-61 in the epidermal growth factor domain. *Biochemistry* **30**:2311, 1991.
106. Harris RJ, Ling VT, Spellman MW: *O*-linked fucose is present in the first epidermal growth factor domain of factor XII but not protein C. *J Biol Chem* **267**:5102, 1992.
107. Stanton C, Wallin R: Processing and trafficking of clotting factor X in the secretory pathway. Effects of warfarin. *Biochem J* **284**:25, 1992.
108. Miletich JP, Leykam JF, Broze GJ Jr: Detection of single chain protein C in human plasma. *Blood (suppl 1)* **62**:306a, 1983.
109. Foster DC, Sprecher CA, Holly RD, Gambee JE, Walker KM, Kumar AA: Endoproteolytic processing of the dibasic cleavage site in the human protein C precursor in transfected mammalian cells: Effects of sequence alterations on efficiency of cleavage. *Biochemistry* **29**:347, 1990.
110. Foster DC, Holly RD, Sprecher CA, Walker KM, Kumar AA: Endoproteolytic processing of the human protein C precursor by the yeast Kex2 endopeptidase coexpressed in mammalian cells. *Biochemistry* **30**:367, 1991.
111. Freedman RB: Protein disulfide isomerase: Multiple roles in the modification of nascent secretory proteins. *Cell* **57**:1069, 1989.
112. Davie EW, Fujikawa K, Kisiel W: The coagulation cascade: Initiation, maintenance, and regulation. *Biochemistry* **30**:10363, 1991.
113. Suzuki K, Kahlback B, Stenflo J: Thrombin-catalyzed activation of human coagulation factor V. *J Biol Chem* **257**:6556, 1982.
114. Nesheim ME, Foster WB, Mann KG: Characterization of factor V intermediates. *J Biol Chem* **259**:3187, 1984.
115. Vehar GA, Davie EW: Preparation and properties of bovine factor VIII antihemophilic factor. *Biochemistry* **19**:401, 1980.
116. Fulcher CA, Roberts JR, Zimmerman TS: Thrombin proteolysis of purified factor VIII procoagulant protein: Correlation of activation with generation of specific polypeptide. *Blood* **61**:807, 1983.
117. Fay PJ, Anderson MT, Chavin SI, Marder VJ: The size of human factor VIII heterodimers and the effects produced by thrombin. *Biochim Biophys Acta* **871**:268, 1986.
118. Eaton D, Rodriquez H, Vehar GA: Proteolytic processing of human factor VIII. Correlation of specific cleavages by thrombin, factor Xa and activated protein C with activation and inactivation of factor VIII coagulant activity. *Biochemistry* **25**:505, 1986.
119. Schwartz ML, Pizzo SV, Hill RL, McKee PA: Human factor XIII from plasma and platelets. Molecular weights, subunit structures, proteolytic activation, and cross-linking of fibrinogen and fibrin. *J Biol Chem* **248**:1395, 1973.
120. Takagi T, Doolittle RF: Amino acid sequence studies on factor XIII and the peptide released during its activation by thrombin. *Biochemistry* **13**:750, 1974.
121. Esmon CT, Owen WG: Identification of an endothelial cell cofactor for thrombin-catalyzed activation of protein C. *Proc Natl Acad Sci USA* **78**:2249, 1981.
122. Owen WG, Esmon CT: Functional properties of an endothelial cell cofactor for thrombin-catalyzed activation of protein C. *J Biol Chem* **256**:5532, 1981.
123. Esmon NL, Owen WG, Esmon CT: Isolation of a membrane-bound cofactor for thrombin-catalyzed activation of protein C. *J Biol Chem* **257**:859, 1982.
124. Gailani D, Broze GJ Jr: Factor XI activation in a revised model of blood coagulation. *Science* **253**:909, 1991.
125. Naito K, Fujikawa K: Activation of human blood coagulation factor XI independent of factor XII. *J Biol Chem* **266**:7353, 1991.
126. Shuman MA: Thrombin-cellular interactions. *Ann NY Acad Sci* **485**:228, 1986.
127. Vu T-KH, Hung DT, Wheaton VI, Coughlin SR: Molecular cloning of a functional thrombin receptor reveals a novel proteolytic mechanism of receptor activation. *Cell* **64**:1057, 1991.
128. Suttie JW, Jackson CM: Prothrombin structure, activation and biosynthesis. *Physiol Rev* **57**:1, 1977.
129. Degen SJF, MacGillivray RTA, Davie EW: Characterization of the cDNA and gene coding for human prothrombin. *Biochemistry* **22**:2087, 1983.
130. Downing MR, Butkowski RJ, Clark MM, Mann KG: Human prothrombin activation. *J Biol Chem* **250**:8897, 1975.
131. Rosing J, Tans G, Grovers-Riemslag JWP, Zwaal RFA, Hemker HC: The role of phospholipids and factor V_a in the prothrombinase complex. *J Biol Chem* **255**:274, 1980.
132. Nesheim ME, Taswell JB, Mann KG: The contribution of bovine factor V and factor Va to the activity of prothrombinase. *J Biol Chem* **254**:10952, 1979.
133. Krishnaswamy S, Church WR, Nesheim ME, Mann KG: Activation of human prothrombin by human prothrombinase. *J Biol Chem* **262**:3291, 1987.
134. Rabiet MJ, Blashill A, Furie B, Furie BC: Prothrombin fragment 1.2.3, a major product of prothrombin activation in human plasma. *J Biol Chem* **261**:13210, 1986.
135. Mann KG, Nesheim ME, Church WR, Haley P, Krishnaswamy S: Surface-dependent reactions of the vitamin K-dependent enzyme complexes. *Blood* **76**:1, 1990.
136. Krishnaswamy S: Prothrombinase complex assembly. Contributions of protein-protein and protein-membrane interactions toward complex formation. *J Biol Chem* **265**:3708, 1990.
137. Husten EJ, Esmon CT, Johnson AE: The active site of blood coagulation factor Xa. Its distance from the phospholipid surface and its conformational sensitivity to components of the prothrombinase complex. *J Biol Chem* **262**:12953, 1987.
138. Armstrong SA, Husten EJ, Esmon CT, Johnson AE: The active site of membrane-bound meizothrombin. A fluorescence determination of its distance from the phospholipid surface and its conformational sensitivity to calcium and factor Va. *J Biol Chem* **265**:6210, 1990.

139. Pollock JS, Shepard AJ, Weber DJ, Olson DL, Klapper DG, Pedersen LG, Hiskey RG: Phospholipid binding properties of bovine prothrombin peptide residues 1-45. *J Biol Chem* **263:**14216, 1988.
140. Berkowitz P, Huh N-W, Brostrom KE, Panek MG, Weber DJ, Tulinsky A, Pedersen LG, Hiskey RG: A metal ion-binding site in the kringle region of bovine prothrombin fragment 1. *J Biol Chem* **267:**4570, 1992.
141. Rosing J, van Rijn JLML, Bevers EM, van Dieijen G, Comfurius P, Zwaal FA: The role of activated human platelets in prothrombin and factor X activation. *Blood* **65:**319, 1985.
142. Tracy PB, Eide LL, Mann KG: Human prothrombinase complex assembly and function on isolated peripheral blood cell population. *J Biol Chem* **260:**2119, 1985.
143. Stern D, Nawroth P, Handley D, Kisiel W: An endothelial cell-dependent pathway of coagulation. *Proc Natl Acad Sci USA* **82:**2523, 1985.
144. Royle NJ, Irwin DM, Koschinsky ML, MacGillivray RTA, Hamerton JL: Human genes encoding prothrombin and ceruloplasmin map to 11p11-q12 and 3q21-24, respectively. *Somat Cell Mol Genet* **13:**285, 1987.
145. Breathnach R, Benoist C, O'Hare K, Gannon F, Chambon P: Ovalbumin gene: Evidence for a leader sequence in mRNA and DNA sequences at the exon-intron boundaries. *Proc Natl Acad Sci USA* **75:**4853, 1978.
146. Mount SM: A catalogue of splice junction sequences. *Nucleic Acids Res* **10:**459, 1982.
147. Rinehart FP, Ritch TG, Deininger PL, Schmid CW: Renaturation rate studies of a single family of interspersed repeated sequences in human deoxyribonucleic acid. *Biochemistry* **20:**3003, 1981.
148. Schmid CW, Jelinek WR: Tha alu family of dispersed repetitive sequences. *Science* **216:**1065, 1982.
149. Bancroft JD, Schaefer LA, Degen SJF: Characterization of the *Alu*-rich 5'-flanking region of the human prothrombin-encoding gene: Identification of a positive *cis*-acting element that regulates liver-specific expression. *Gene* **95:**253, 1990.
150. Chow BK-C, Ting V, Tufaro F, MacGillivray RTA: Characterization of a novel liver-specific enhancer in the human prothrombin gene. *J Biol Chem* **266:**18927, 1991.
151. de Vetten M, van Amstel HKP, Reitsma PH: RFLP for the human prothrombin (F2) gene. *Nucleic Acids Res* **18:**5917, 1990.
152. McAlpine PJ, Dickson M, Guy C, Wiens A, Irwin DM, MacGillivray RTA: Polymorphism detected by multiple RENS in the human coagulation factor II (F2) gene. *Nucleic Acids Res* **19:**193, 1991.
153. Iwahana H, Yoshimoto K, Itakura M: NcoI RFLP in the human prothrombin (F2) gene. *Nucleic Acids Res* **19:**4309, 1991.
154. Iwahana H, Yoshimoto K, Itakura M: Highly polymorphic region of the human prothrombin (F2) gene. *Hum Genet* **78:**123, 1992.
155. Kattlove HE, Shapiro SS, Spivack M: Hereditary prothrombin deficiency. *N Engl J Med* **282:**57, 1970.
156. Shapiro SS, McCord IS: Prothrombin, in Spaet TH (ed): *Hemostasis and Thrombosis*. New York, Grune & Stratton, 1978, vol 4, p 177.
157. Guillin M-C, Bezeaud A, Rabiet M-J, Elion J: Congenitally abnormal prothrombin and thrombin. *Ann NY Acad Sci* **485:**56, 1986.
158. Rabiet M-J, Furie BC, Furie B: Molecular defect of prothrombin Barcelona. *J Biol Chem* **261:**15045, 1986.
159. Diuguid DL, Rabiet M-J, Furie BC, Furie B: Molecular defects of factor IX Chicago-2 (Arg 145→His) and prothrombin Madrid (Arg 271→Cys): Arginine mutations that preclude zymogen activation. *Blood* **74:**193, 1989.
160. Walz DA, Hewett-Emmett D, Seegers WH: Amino acid sequence of human prothrombin fragments 1 and 2. *Proc Natl Acad Sci USA* **74:**1969, 1977.
161. Miyata T, Morita T, Inomoto T, Kawuchi S, Shirakami A, Iwanaga S: Prothrombin Tokushima, a replacement of arginine-418 by tryptophan that impairs the fibrinogen clotting activity of derived thrombin Tokushima. *Biochemistry* **26:**1117, 1987.
162. Iwahana H, Yoshimoto K, Shigekiyo T, Shirakami A, Saito S, Itakura M: Detection of a single base substitution of the gene for prothrombin Tokushima. The application of PCR-SSCP for the genetic and molecular analysis of dysprothrombinemia. *Int J Hematol* **55:**93, 1992.
163. Henriksen RA, Owen WG: Characterization of the catalytic defect in the dysthrombin, thrombin Quick. *J Biol Chem* **262:**4664, 1987.
164. Henriksen RA, Mann KG: Identification of the primary structural defect in the dysthrombin thrombin Quick I: Substitution of cysteine for arginine-382. *Biochemistry* **27:**9160, 1988.
165. Leong L, Henriksen RA, Kermode JC, Rittenhouse SE, Tracy PB: The thrombin high-affinity binding site on platelets is a negative regulator of thrombin-induced platelet activation. Structure-function studies using two mutant thrombins, Quick I and Quick II. *Biochemistry* **31:**2567, 1992.
166. Henriksen RA, Mann KG: Substitution of valine for glycine-558 in the congenital dysthrombin thrombin Quick II alters primary substrate specificity. *Biochemistry* **28:**2078, 1989.
167. Bezeaud A, Elion J, Guillin M-C: Functional characterization of thrombin Salakta: An abnormal thrombin derived from a human prothrombin variant. *Blood* **71:**556, 1988.
168. Miyata T, Aruga R, Umeyama H, Bezeaud A, Guillin M-C, Iwanaga S: Prothrombin Salakta: Substitution of glutamic acid-466 by alanine reduces the fibrinogen clotting activity and the esterase activity. *Biochemistry* **31:**7457, 1992.
169. Huisse MG, Dreyfus M, Guillin M-C: Prothrombin Clamart: Prothrombin variant with defective Arg 320-Ile cleavage by factor X_a. *Thromb Res* **44:**11, 1986.
170. Morishita E, Saito M, Asakura H, Jokaji H, Uotani C, Kumabashiri I, Yamazaki M, Hachiya H, Okamura M, Matsuda T: Prothrombin Himi: An abnormal prothrombin characterized by a defective thrombin activity. *Thromb Res* **62:**697, 1991.
171. Rabiet MJ, Jandrot-Perrus M, Boissel JP, Elion J, Josso F: Thrombin Metz: Characterization of the dysfunctional thrombin derived from a variant of human prothrombin. *Blood* **63:**927, 1984.
172. Girolami A, Coccheri S, Palareti G, Poggi M, Burul A, Cappellato G: Prothrombin Molise: A "new" congenital dysprothrombinemia, double heterozygosis with an abnormal prothrombin and true prothrombin deficiency. *Blood* **52:**115, 1978.
173. McMillan CW, Roberts HR: Congenital combined deficiency of coagulation factors II, VII, IX, and X. *N Engl J Med* **274:**1313, 1966.
174. Chung K-S, Bezeaud A, Goldsmith JC, McMillan CW, Menache D, Roberts HR: Congenital deficiency of blood clotting factors II, VII, IX and X. *Blood* **53:**776, 1979.
175. Johnson CA, Chung KS, McGrath KM, Bean PE, Roberts HR: Characterization of a variant prothrombin in a patient congenitally deficient in factors II, VII, IX and X. *Br J Haematol* **44:**461, 1980.
176. Goldsmith GH, Pence RE, Ratnoff OD, Adelstein DJ, Furie B: Studies on a family with combined functional deficiencies of vitamin K dependent coagulation factor. *J Clin Invest* **69:**1253, 1982.
177. Vicente V, Maia R, Alberca I, Tamagnini GPT, Lopez Borrasca A: Congenital deficiency of vitamin K-dependent coagulation factors and protein C. *Thromb Haemost* **51:**343, 1984.
178. Pauli RM, Lian JB, Mosher DF, Suttie JW: Association of congenital deficiency of multiple vitamin K-dependent coagulation factors and the phenotype of the warfarin embriopathy: Clues to the mechanism of teratogenecity of coumarin derivatives. *Am J Hum Genet* **41:**566, 1987.
179. Brenner B, Tavori S, Zivelin A, Keller CB, Suttie JW, Tatarsky I, Seligsohn U: Hereditary deficiency of all vitamin K-dependent procoagulants and anticoagulants. *Br J Haematol* **75:**537, 1990.
180. Radcliffe R, Nemerson Y: Activation and control of factor VII by activated factor X and thrombin. Isolation and characterization of a single chain form of factor VII. *J Biol Chem* **250:**388, 1975.
181. Kisiel W, Fujikawa K, Davie EW: Activation of bovine factor VII (proconvertin) by factor XII_a (activated Hageman factor). *Biochemistry* **16:**4189, 1977.
182. Seligsohn U, Osterud B, Brown SF, Griffin JH, Rapa-

port SI: Activation of human factor VII in plasma and in purified systems: Roles of activated factor IX, kallikrein, and activated factor XII. *J Clin Invest* **64:**1056, 1979.
183. Broze GJ Jr, Majerus PW: Purification and properties of human coagulation factor VII. *J Biol Chem* **255:**1242, 1980.
184. Masys DR, Bajaj SP, Rapaport SI: Activation of human factor VII by activated factors IX and X. *Blood* **60:**1143, 1982.
185. Wildgoose P, Kisiel W: Activation of human factor VII by factors IXa and Xa on human bladder carcinoma cells. *Blood* **73:**1888, 1989.
186. Nakagaki T, Foster DC, Berkner KL, Kisiel W: Initiation of the extrinsic pathway of blood coagulation: Evidence for the tissue factor dependent autoactivation of human coagulation factor VII. *Biochemistry* **30:**10819, 1991.
187. Osterud B, Rapaport SI: Activation of factor IX by the reaction product of tissue factor and factor VII: Additional pathway for initiating blood coagulation. *Proc Natl Acad Sci USA* **74:**5260, 1977.
188. Nemerson Y: Tissue factor and hemostasis. *Blood* **71:**1, 1988.
189. Drake TA, Morrissey JH, Edgington TS: Selective cellular expression of tissue factor in human tissues. *Am J Pathol* **134:**1087, 1989.
190. Wilcox JN, Smith KM, Schwartz SM, Gordon D: Localization of tissue factor in the normal vessel wall and in the atherosclerotic plaque. *Proc Natl Acad Sci USA* **86:**2839, 1989.
191. Weiss HJ, Turitto VT, Baumgartner HR, Nemerson Y, Hoffmann T: Evidence for the presence of tissue factor activity of subendothelium. *Blood* **73:**968, 1989.
192. Fair DS, MacDonald MJ: Cooperative interaction between factor VII and cell surface-expressed tissue factor. *J Biol Chem* **262:**11692, 1987.
193. Sakai T, Lund-Hansen T, Paborsky L, Pedersen AH, Kisiel W: Binding of human factors VII and VIIa to a human bladder carcinoma cell line (J82). Implications for the initiation of the extrinsic pathway of blood coagulation. *J Biol Chem* **264:**9980, 1989.
194. Le DT, Rapaport SI, Rao LVM: Relations between factor VIIa binding and expression of factor VII/tissue factor catalytic activity on cell surfaces. *J Biol Chem* **267:**15447, 1992.
195. Bom VJJ, Bertina RM: The contributions of Ca^{2+}, phospholipids and tissue-factor apoprotein to the activation of human blood-coagulation factor X by activated factor VII. *Biochem J* **265:**327, 1990.
196. Komiyama Y, Pedersen AH, Kisiel W: Proteolytic activation of human factors IX and X by recombinant human factor VIIa: Effects of calcium, phospholipids, and tissue factor. *Biochemistry* **29:**9418, 1990.
197. Ruf W, Rehemtulla A, Edgington TS: Phospholipid-independent and -dependent interactions required for tissue factor receptor and cofactor function. *J Biol Chem* **266:**2158, 1991.
198. Nemerson Y, Gentry R: An ordered addition, essential activation model of the tissue factor pathway of coagulation: Evidence for a conformational cage. *Biochemistry* **25:**4020, 1986.
199. Lawson JH, Butenas S, Mann KG: The evaluation of complex-dependent alterations in human factor VIIa. *J Biol Chem* **267:**4834, 1992.
200. Rapaport SI: Inhibition of factor VIIa/tissue factor-induced blood coagulation: With particular emphasis upon a factor Xa-dependent inhibitory mechanism. *Blood* **73:**359, 1989.
201. Broze GJ Jr, Girard TJ, Novotny WF: Regulation of coagulation by a multivalent Kunitz-type inhibitor. *Biochemistry* **29:**7539, 1990.
202. Kisiel W, McMullen BA: Isolation and characterization of human factor VIIa. *Thromb Res* **22:**375, 1981.
203. Wildgoose P, Kazim AL, Kisiel W: The importance of residues 195-206 of human blood clotting factor VII in the interaction of factor VII with tissue factor. *Proc Natl Acad Sci USA* **87:**7290, 1990.
204. Kumar A, Blumenthal DK, Fair DS: Identification of molecular sites on factor VII which mediate its assembly and function in the extrinsic pathway activation complex. *J Biol Chem* **266:**915, 1991.
205. Higashi S, Nishimura H, Fujii S, Takada K, Iwanaga S: Tissue factor potentiates the factor VIIa-catalyzed hydrolysis of an ester substrate. *J Biol Chem* **267:**17990, 1992.
206. Scarpati EM, Wen D, Broze GJ Jr, Miletich JP, Flandermeyer RR, Siegel NR, Sadler JE: Human tissue factor: cDNA sequence and chromosome localization of the gene. *Biochemistry* **26:**5234, 1987.
207. Spicer EK, Horton R, Bloem L, Bach R, Williams KR, Guha A, Kraus J, Lin T-C, Nemerson Y, Konigsberg WH: Isolation of cDNA clones coding for human tissue factor: Primary structure of the protein and cDNA. *Proc Natl Acad Sci USA* **84:**5148, 1987.
208. Morrissey JH, Fakhrai H, Edgington TS: Molecular cloning of the cDNA for tissue factor, the cellular receptor for the initiation of the coagulation protease cascade. *Cell* **50:**129, 1987.
209. Fisher KL, Gorman CM, Vehar GA, O'Brien DP, Lawn RM: Cloning and expression of human tissue factor cDNA. *Thromb Res* **48:**89, 1987.
210. Rehemtulla A, Ruf W, Edgington TS: The integrity of the cysteine 186-cysteine 209 bond of the second disulfide loop of tissue factor is required for binding of factor VII. *J Biol Chem* **266:**10294, 1991.
211. Ruf W, Miles DJ, Rehemtulla A, Edgington TS: Cofactor residues lysine 165 and 166 are critical for protein substrate recognition by the tissue-factor VIIa protease complex. *J Biol Chem* **267:**6375, 1992.
212. Waxman E, Ross JBA, Lane TM, Guha A, Thiruvikraman SV, Lin TC, Konigsberg WH, Nemerson Y: Tissue factor and its extracellular soluble domain: The relationship between intermolecular association with factor VIIa and enzymatic activity of the complex. *Biochemistry* **31:**3998, 1992.
213. Yamamoto M, Nakagaki T, Kisiel W: Tissue factor-dependent autoactivation of human blood coagulation factor VII. *J Biol Chem* **267:**19089, 1992.
214. Neuenschwander PF, Morrissey JH: Deletion of the membrane anchoring region of tissue factor abolishes autoactivation of factor VII but not cofactor function. Analysis of a mutant with a selective deficiency in activity. *J Biol Chem* **267:**14477, 1992.
215. de Grouchy J, Dautzenberg MD, Turleau C, Beguin S, Chavin-Colin F: Regional mapping of clotting factors VII and X to 13q34. Expression of factor VII through chromosome 8. *Hum Genet* **66:**230, 1984.
216. Ott R, Pfeiffer RA: Evidence that activities of coagulation factors VII and X are linked to chromosome 13 (q34). *Hum Hered* **34:**123, 1984.
217. Gilgenkrantz S, Briquel ME, Andre E, Alexandre P, Jalbert P, Le Marec B, Pouzol P, Pommereuil M: Structural genes of coagulation factors VII and X located on 13q34. *Ann Genet* **29:**32, 1986.
218. O'Hara PJ, Grant FJ, Haldeman BA, Gray CL, Insley MY, Hagen FS, Murray MJ: Nucleotide sequence of the gene coding for human factor VII, a vitamin K-dependent protein participating in blood coagulation. *Proc Natl Acad Sci USA* **84:**5158, 1987.
219. O'Hara PJ, Grant FJ: The human factor VII gene is polymorphic due to variation in repeat copy number in a minisatellite. *Gene* **66:**147, 1988.
220. Marchetti G, Gemmati D, Patracchini P, Pinotti M, Bernardi F: PCR detection of a repeat polymorphism within the F7 gene. *Nucleic Acids Res* **19:**4570, 1991.
221. Marchetti G, Patracchini P, Gemmati D, DeRosa V, Pinotti M, Rodorigo G, Casonato A, Girolami A, Bernardi F: Detection of two missense mutations and characterization of a repeat polymorphism in the factor VII gene (F7). *Hum Genet* **89:**497, 1992.
222. Green F, Kelleher C, Wilkes H, Temple A, Meade T, Humphries S: A common genetic polymorphism associated with lower coagulation factor VII levels in healthy individuals. *Arterioscler Thromb* **11:**540, 1991.
223. Foster DC, Yoshitake S, Davie EW: The nucleotide sequence of the gene for human protein C. *Proc Natl Acad Sci USA* **82:**4673, 1985.
224. Plutzky J, Hoskins JA, Long GL, Crabtree GR: Evolution and organization of the human protein C gene. *Proc Natl Acad Sci USA* **83:**546, 1986.
225. Patthy L: Evolutionary assembly of blood coagulation proteins. *Semin Thromb Hemost* **16:**245, 1990.

226. Carson SD, Henry WM, Shows TB: Tissue factor gene localized to human chromosome 1 (1ptr→1p21). *Science* **229**:991, 1985.
227. Kao F-T, Hartz J, Horton R, Nemerson Y, Carson SD: Regional assignment of human tissue factor gene (F3) to chromosome 1p21-p22. *Somat Cell Mol Genet* **14**:407, 1988.
228. Mackman N, Morrissey JH, Fowler B, Edgington TS: Complete sequence of the human tissue factor gene, a highly regulated cellular receptor that initiates the coagulation protease cascade. *Biochemistry* **28**:1755, 1989.
229. van der Logt CPE, Reitsma PH, Bertina RM: Alternative splicing is responsible for the presence of two tissue factor mRNA species in LPS stimulated human monocytes. *Thromb Haemost* **67**:272, 1992.
230. Edgington TS, Mackman N, Brand K, Ruf W: The structural biology of expression and function of tissue factor. *Thromb Haemost* **66**:67, 1991.
231. Dalaker K: Clotting factor VII during pregnancy, delivery and puerperium. *Br J Obstet Gynaecol* **93**:17, 1986.
232. Balleisen L, Bailey J, Epping P-H, Schulte H, van de Loo J: Epidemiological study on factor VII, factor VIII and fibrinogen in an industrial population: I. Baseline data on the relation to age, gender, body-weight, smoking, alcohol, pill-using, and menopause. *Thromb Haemost* **54**:475, 1985.
233. Balleisen L, Assmann G, Bailey J, Epping P-H, Schulte H, van de Loo J: Epidemiological study on factor VII, factor VIII and fibrinogen in an industrial population: II. Baseline data on the relation to blood pressure, blood glucose, uric acid, and lipid fractions. *Thromb Haemost* **54**:721, 1985.
234. Miller GJ, Cruickshank JK, Ellis LJ, Thompson RL, Wilkes HC, Stirling Y, Mitropoulos KA, Allison JV, Fox TE, Walker AO: Fat consumption and factor VII coagulant activity in middle-aged men. *Atherosclerosis* **78**:19, 1989.
235. Miller GJ, Walter SJ, Stirling Y, Thompson SG, Esnouf MP: Assay of factor VII activity by two techniques: Evidence for increased conversion of VII to αVII_a in hyperlipidaemia, with possible implications for ischaemic heart disease. *Br J Haematol* **59**:249, 1985.
236. Mitropoulos KA, Miller GJ, Reeves BEA, Wilkes HC, Cruickshank JK: Factor VII coagulant activity is strongly associated with the plasma concentration of large lipoprotein particles in middle-aged men. *Atherosclerosis* **76**:203, 1989.
237. Mitropoulos KA, Martin JC, Reeves BEA, Esnouf MP: The activation of the contact phase of coagulation by physiologic surfaces in plasma: The effect of large negatively charged liposomal vesicles. *Blood* **73**:1525, 1989.
238. Mitropoulos KA, Miller GJ, Watts GF, Durrington PN: Lipolysis of triglyceride-rich lipoproteins activates coagulant factor XII: A study in familial lipoprotein-lipase deficiency. *Atherosclerosis* **95**:119, 1992.
239. Meade TW, Mellows S, Brozovic M, Miller GJ, Chakrabarti RR, North WR, Haines AP, Stirling Y, Imeson JD, Thompson SG: Haemostatic function and ischaemic heart disease: Principal results of the Northwick Park heart study. *Lancet* **2**:533, 1986.
240. Dalaker K, Smith P, Arnesen H, Prydz H: Factor VII-phospholipid complex in male survivors of acute myocardial infarction. *Acta Med Scand* **222**:111, 1987.
241. Broadhurst P, Kelleher C, Hughes L, Imeson JD, Raftery EB: Fibrinogen, factor VII clotting activity and coronary artery disease severity. *Atherosclerosis* **85**:169, 1990.
242. Hall CA, Rapaport SI, Ames SB, DeGroot JA: A clinical and family study of hereditary proconvertin (Factor VII deficiency). *Am J Med* **37**:172, 1964.
243. Dische FE, Benfield V: Congenital factor VII deficiency: Haematological and genetic aspects. *Acta Haematol (Basel)* **21**:257, 1959.
244. Kupfer HG, Hanna BL, Kinne DR: Congenital factor VII deficiency with normal Stuart activity: Clinical, genetic and experimental observations. *Blood* **15**:146, 1960.
245. Ragni MV, Lewis JH, Spero JA, Hasiba U: Factor VII deficiency. *Am J Hematol* **10**:79, 1981.
246. Gershwin ME, Gude JK: Deep vein thrombosis and pulmonary embolism in congenital factor VII deficiency. *N Engl J Med* **288**:141, 1973.
247. Shifter T, Machtey I, Creter D: Thromboembolism in congenital factor VII deficiency. *Acta Haematol (Basel)* **71**:60, 1984.
248. Godal HC, Madsen K, Nissen-Meyer R: Thromboembolism in a patient with total proconvertin (factor VII) deficiency. *Acta Med Scand* **171**:325, 1962.
249. Mariani G, Mazzucconi MG, Hermans J, Ciavarella N, Faiella A, Hassan HJ, Mannucci PM, Nenci GG, Orlando M, Romoli D, Mandelli F: Factor VII deficiency: Immunological characterization of genetic variants and detection of carriers. *Br J Haematol* **48**:7, 1981.
250. Triplett DA, Brandt JT, McGann Batard MA, Schaeffer Dixon JL, Fair DA: Hereditary factor VII deficiency. Heterogeneity defined by combined functional and immunochemical analysis. *Blood* **66**:1284, 1985.
251. Girolami A, Fabris F, Zanon RDB, Ghiotto G, Burul A: Factor VII Padua: A congenital coagulation disorder due to an abnormal factor VII with a peculiar activation pattern. *J Lab Clin Med* **91**:387, 1978.
252. Chaing SH, High KA: Severe factor VII deficiency associated with two missense mutations in the factor VII gene. *Thromb Haemost* **65**:1262, 1991.
253. O'Brien DP, Gale KM, Anderson JS, McVey JH, Miller GJ, Meade TW, Tuddenham EGD: Purification and characterization of factor VII 304-Gln: A variant molecule with reduced activity isolated from a clinically unaffected male. *Blood* **78**:132, 1991.
254. Millar DS, Cooper DN, Kakkar VV, Schwartz M, Scheibel E: Prenatal exclusion of severe factor VII deficiency by DNA sequencing. *Lancet* **339**:1359, 1992.
255. Hedner U: Experiences with recombinant factor VIIa in haemophiliacs. *Curr Stud Hematol Blood Transfus* **58**:63, 1991.
256. Aggeler PM, White SG, Glendening MG, Page EW, Leake TB, Bates G: Plasma thromboplastin component (PTC) deficiency: A new disease resembling hemophilia. *Proc Soc Exp Biol Med* **79**:692, 1952.
257. Biggs R, Douglas AS, MacFarlane RG, Dacie JV, Pitney WR, Merskey C, O'Brien JR: Christmas disease: A condition previously mistaken for haemophilia. *Br Med J* **2**:1378, 1952.
258. DiScipio RG, Kurachi K, Davie EW: Activation of human factor IX (Christmas factor). *J Clin Invest* **61**:1528, 1978.
259. DiScipio RG, Hermodson MA, Yates SG, Davie EW: A comparison of human prothrombin, factor IX (Christmas factor), factor X (Stuart factor), and protein S. *Biochemistry* **16**:698, 1977.
260. Morita T, Kisiel W: Calcium binding to a human factor IXa derivative lacking γ-carboxyglutamic acid: Evidence for two high-affinity sites that do not involve β-hydroxyaspartic acid. *Biochem Biophys Res Commun* **130**:841, 1985.
261. Derian CK, VanDusen W, Przysiecki CT, Walsh PN, Berkner KL, Kaufman RJ, Friedman PA: Inhibitors of 2-ketoglutarate-dependent dioxygenases block aspartyl β-hydroxylation of recombinant human factor IX in several mammalian expression systems. *J Biol Chem* **264**:6615, 1989.
262. Lindquist PA, Fujikawa K, Davie EW: The activation of bovine factor IX (Christmas factor) by factor XI_a (activated plasma thromboplastin antecedent) and a protease from Russell's viper venom. *J Biol Chem* **253**:1902, 1978.
263. Jones ME, Griffith MJ, Monroe DM, Roberts HR, Lentz BR: Comparison of lipid binding and kinetic properties of normal, variant, and γ-carboxyglutamic acid modified human factor IX and factor IX_a. *Biochemistry* **24**:8064, 1985.
264. Schwalbe RA, Ryan J, Stern DM, Kisiel W, Dahlback B, Nelsestuen GL: Protein structural requirements and properties of membrane binding by γ-carboxyglutamic acid-containing plasma proteins and peptides. *J Biol Chem* **264**:20288, 1989.
265. Bajaj SP, Sabharwal AK, Gorka J, Birktoft JJ: Antibody-probed conformational transitions in the protease domain of human factor IX upon calcium binding and zymogen activation: Putative high-affinity Ca^2-binding site in the protease domain. *Proc Natl Acad Sci USA* **89**:152, 1992.
266. Bajaj SP, Rapaport SI, Maki SL: A monoclonal antibody to factor IX that inhibits the factor VIII:C potentiation of factor X activation. *J Biol Chem* **260**:11573, 1985.

267. Camerino G, Grzeschik KH, Jaye M, de la Salle H, Tolstoshev P, Lecocq JP, Heilig R, Mandel JL: Regional localization on the human X chromosome and polymorphism of the coagulation factor IX gene (hemophilia B locus). *Proc Natl Acad Sci USA* **81**:498, 1984.
268. Chance PF, Dyer KA, Kurachi K, Yoshitake S, Ropers H, Wieacker P, Gartler SM: Regional localization of human factor IX gene by molecular hybridization. *Hum Genet* **65**:207, 1983.
269. Crossley M, Ludwig M, Stowell KM, De Vos P, Olek K, Brownlee GG: Recovery from hemophilia B Leyden: An androgen-responsive element in the factor IX promoter. *Science* **257**:377, 1992.
270. Reijnen MJ, Sladek FM, Bertina RM, Reitsma PH: Disruption of a binding site for hepatocyte nuclear factor 4 results in hemophilia B Leyden. *Proc Natl Acad Sci USA* **89**:6300, 1992.
271. Crossley M, Brownlee GG: Disruption of a C/EBP binding site in the factor IX promoter is associated with haemophilia B. *Nature* **345**:444, 1990.
272. Thompson AR: Molecular biology of the hemophilias. *Prog Hemost Thromb* **10**:175, 1991.
273. Peake I: Registry of DNA polymorphisms within or close to the human factor VIII and factor IX genes. *Thromb Haemost* **67**:277, 1992.
274. McGraw RA, Davis LM, Noyes CM, Lundblad RL, Roberts HR, Graham JB, Stafford DW: Evidence for a prevalent dimorphism in the activation peptide of human coagulation factor IX. *Proc Natl Acad Sci USA* **82**:2847, 1985.
275. Wallmark A, Ljung R, Nilsson IM, Holmberg L, Hedner U, Lindvall M, Sjögren H-O: Polymorphism of normal factor IX detected by mouse monoclonal antibodies. *Proc Natl Acad Sci USA* **82**:3839, 1985.
276. Smith KJ, Thompson AR, McMullen BA, Frazier D, Lin SW, Stafford D, Kisiel W, Thibodeau SN, Chen S-H, Smith LF: Carrier testing in hemophilia B with an immunoassay that distinguishes a prevalent factor IX dimorphism. *Blood* **70**:1006, 1987.
277. Fantl P, Sawers RJ, Marr AG: Investigation of a haemorrhagic disease due to beta-prothromboplastin deficiency complicated by a specific inhibitor of thromboplastin formation. *Aust Ann Med* **5**:163, 1956.
278. Roberts HR, Grizzle JE, McLester WD, Penick GO: Genetic variants of hemophilia B. Detection by means of a specific PTC inhibitor. *J Clin Invest* **47**:360, 1968.
279. Thompson AR: Factor IX antigen by radioimmunoassay. Abnormal factor IX protein in patients on warfarin therapy and with hemophilia B. *J Clin Invest* **59**:900, 1977.
280. Giannelli F, Green PM, High KA, Sommer S, Lillicrap DP, Ludwig M, Olek K, Reitsma PH, Goossens M, Yoshioka A, Brownlee GG: Haemophilia B: Database of point mutations and short additions and deletions—Third edition, 1992. *Nucleic Acids Res (suppl)* **20**:2027, 1992.
281. Briët E, Bertina RM, Van Tilburg NH, Veltkamp JJ: Hemophilia B Leyden. A sex-linked hereditary disorder that improves after puberty. *N Engl J Med* **306**:788, 1982.
282. Hirosawa S, Fahner JB, Salier J-P, Wu C-T, Lovrien EW, Kurachi K: Structural and functional basis of the developmental regulation of human coagulation factor IX gene: Factor IX Leyden. *Proc Natl Acad Sci USA* **87**:4421, 1990.
283. Winship PR, Dragon AC: Identification of haemophilia B patients with mutations in the two calcium binding domains of factor IX: Importance of a β-OH Asp 64-Asn change. *Br J Haematol* **77**:102, 1991.
284. Hamaguchi M, Matsushita T, Tanimoto M, Takahashi I, Yamamoto K, Sugiura I, Takamatsu J, Ogata K, Kamiya T, Saito H: Three distinct point mutations in the factor IX gene of three Japanese CRM$^+$ hemophilia B patients (factor IX B_M Nagoya 2, factor IX Nagoya 3 and 4). *Thromb Haemost* **65**:514, 1991.
285. Chen S-H, Thompson AR, Zhang M, Scott CR: Three point mutations in the factor IX genes of five hemophilia B patients: Identification strategy using localization by altered epitopes in their hemophilic proteins. *J Clin Invest* **84**:113, 1989.
286. Wang NS, Thompson AR, Chen S-H: Factor $IX^{Chongqing}$: A new mutation in the calcium-binding domain of factor IX resulting in severe hemophilia B. *Thromb Haemost* **63**:24, 1990.
287. Zhang L, Jhingan A, Castellino FJ: Role of individual γ-carboxyglutamic acid residues of activated human protein C in defining its in vitro anticoagulant activity. *Blood* **80**:942, 1992.
288. Davis LM, McGraw RA, Ware JL, Roberts HR, Stafford DW: Factor $IX_{ALABAMA}$: A point mutation in a clotting protein results in hemophilia B. *Blood* **69**:140, 1987.
289. McCord DM, Monroe DM, Smith KJ, Roberts HR: Characterization of the functional defect in factor IX Alabama. *J Biol Chem* **265**:10250, 1990.
290. Lozier JN, Monroe DM, Stanfield-Oakley S, Lin S-W, Smith KJ, Roberts HR, High KA: Factor IX New London: Substitution of proline for glutamine at position 50 causes severe hemophilia B. *Blood* **75**:1097, 1990.
291. Green PM, Bentley DR, Mibashan RS, Nilsson IM, Giannelli F: Molecular pathology of haemophilia B. *EMBO J* **8**:1067, 1989.
292. Chung K-S, Madar DA, Goldsmith JC, Kingdon HS, Roberts HR: Purification and characterization of an abnormal factor IX (Christmas factor) molecule. *J Clin Invest* **62**:1078, 1978.
293. Noyes CM, Griffith MJ, Roberts HR, Lundblad RL: Identification of the molecular defect in factor $IX_{CHAPEL\ HILL}$: Substitution of histidine for arginine at position 145. *Proc Natl Acad Sci USA* **80**:4200, 1983.
294. Griffith MJ, Breitkreutz L, Trapp H, Briët E, Noyes CM, Lundblad RL, Roberts HR: Characterization of the clotting activities of structurally different forms of activated factor IX. Enzymatic properties of normal human factor IXaα, factor IXaβ, and activated factor $IX_{CHAPEL\ HILL}$. *J Clin Invest* **75**:4, 1985.
295. Toomey JR, Stafford D, Smith K: Factor IX Albuquerque (arginine 145 to cysteine) is cleaved slowly by factor XIa and has reduced coagulant activity. *Blood (suppl 1)* **72**:312, 1988.
296. Bertina RM, van der Linden IK, Mannucci PM, Reinalda-Poot HH, Cupers R, Poort SR, Reitsma PH: Mutations in hemophilia B_m occur at the Arg^{180}-Val activation site or in the catalytic domain of factor IX. *J Biol Chem* **265**:10876, 1990.
297. Suehiro K, Kawabata S-I, Miyata T, Takeya H, Takamatsu J, Ogata K, Kamiya T, Saito H, Niho Y, Iwanaga S: Blood clotting factor IX B_M Nagoya: Substitution of arginine 180 by tryptophan and its activation by α-chymotrypsin and rat mast cell chymase. *J Biol Chem* **264**:21257, 1989.
298. Monroe DM, McCord DM, Huang M-N, High KA, Lundblad RL: Functional consequences of an $arginine^{180}$ to glutamine mutation in factor IX Hilo. *Blood* **73**:1540, 1989.
299. Solera J, Magallón M, Martin-Villar J, Coloma A: Identification of a new haemophilia B_M case produced by a mutation located at the carboxy terminal cleavage site of activation peptide. *Br J Haematol* **78**:385, 1991.
300. Chen S-H, Zhang M, Lovrien EW, Scott CR, Thompson AR: CG dinucleotide transitions in the factor IX gene account for about half of the point mutations in hemophilia B patients: A Seattle series. *Hum Genet* **87**:177, 1991.
301. Ludwig M, Sabharwal AK, Brackmann HH, Olek K, Smith KJ, Birktoft JJ, Bajaj SP: Hemophilia B caused by five different nondeletion mutations in the protease domain of factor IX. *Blood* **79**:1225, 1992.
302. Thompson AR, Chen S-H, Brayer GD: Severe hemophilia B due to a G to T transversion changing GLY 309 to VAL and inhibiting active protease conformation by preventing ion pair formation. *Blood* **74**:134, 1989.
303. Miyata T, Sakai T, Sugimoto M, Naka H, Yamamoto K, Yoshioka A, Fukui H, Mitsui K, Kamiya K, Umeyama H, Iwanaga S: Factor IX Amagasaki: A new mutation in the catalytic domain resulting in the loss of both coagulant and esterase activities. *Biochemistry* **30**:11286, 1991.
304. Koeberl DD, Bottema CDK, Ketterling RP, Bridge PJ, Lillicrap DP, Sommer SS: Mutations causing hemophilia B: Direct estimate of the underlying rates of spontaneous germ-line transitions, transversions, and deletions in a human gene. *Am J Hum Genet* **47**:202, 1990.
305. Bajaj SP, Spitzer SG, Welsh WJ, Warn-Cramer BJ, Kasper CK, Birktoft JJ: Experimental and theoretical evi-

dence supporting the role of Gly[363] in blood coagulation factor IXa (Gly[193] in chymotrypsin) for proper activation of the proenzyme. *J Biol Chem* **265:**2956, 1990.

306. Vidaud M, Attree O, Schaad O, Vidaud D, Edelstein S, Goossens M: Self-inhibition of factor IX by a Gly to Arg mutation at the substrate binding pocket is linked to severe hemophilia B. *Blood (suppl 1)* **72:**313, 1988.
307. Attree O, Vidaud D, Vidaud M, Amselem S, Lavergene J-M, Goossens M: Mutations in the catalytic domain of human coagulation factor IX: Rapid characterization by direct genomic sequencing of DNA fragments displaying an altered melting behavior. *Genomics* **4:**266, 1989.
308. Ware J, Davis L, Frazier D, Bajaj SP, Stafford DW: Genetic defect responsible for the dysfunctional protein: Factor $IX_{LONG\ BEACH}$. *Blood* **72:**820, 1988.
309. Spitzer SG, Warn-Cramer BJ, Kasper CK, Bajaj SP: Replacement of isoleucine-397 by threonine in the clotting proteinase factor IXa (Los Angeles and Long Beach variants) affects macromolecular catalysis but not L-tosylarginine methyl ester hydrolysis. *Biochem J* **265:**219, 1990.
310. Geddes VA, Le Bonniec BF, Louie GV, Brayer GD, Thompson AR, MacGillivray RTA: A moderate form of hemophilia B is caused by a novel mutation in the protease domain of factor $IX_{VANCOUVER}$. *J Biol Chem* **264:**4689, 1989.
311. Hamaguchi N, Charifson PS, Pedersen LG, Brayer GD, Smith KJ, Stafford DW: Expression and characterization of human factor IX: Factor $IX_{thr-397}$ and factor $IX_{val-397}$. *J Biol Chem* **266:**15213, 1991.
312. Spitzer SG, Pendurthi UR, Kasper CK, Bajaj SP: Molecular defect in factor IX Bm Lake Elsinore: Substitution of Ala[390] by Val in the catalytic domain. *J Biol Chem* **263:**10545, 1988.
313. Sugimoto M, Miyata T, Kawabata S, Yoshioka A, Fukui H, Takahashi H, Iwanaga S: Blood clotting factor IX Niigata: Substitution of alanine-390 by valine in the catalytic domain. *J Biochem* **104:**878, 1988.
314. Hougie C, Twomey JJ: Haemophilia B_M: A new type of factor-IX deficiency. *Lancet* **1:**698, 1967.
315. Osterud B, Kasper CK, Lavine KK, Prodanos C, Rapaport SI: Purification and properties of an abnormal coagulation factor IX (factor IX BM sub): Kinetics of its inhibition of factor X activation by factor VII and bovine tissue factor. *Thromb Haemost* **45:**55, 1981.
316. Sakai T, Yoshioka A, Yamamoto K, Niinomi K, Fujimura Y, Fukui H, Miyata T, Iwanaga S: Blood clotting factor IX Kashihara: Amino acid substitution of valine-182 by phenylalanine. *J Biochem* **105:**756, 1989.
317. Taylor SAM, Liddell MB, Peake IR, Bloom AL, Lillicrap DP: A mutation adjacent to the beta cleavage site of factor IX (valine 182 to leucine) results in mild haemophilia B_M. *Br J Haematol* **75:**217, 1990.
318. Green PM, Montandon AJ, Ljung R, Nilsson IM, Giannelli F: Haplotype analysis of identical factor IX mutants using PCR. *Thromb Haemost* **67:**66, 1992.
319. Thompson AR, Bajaj SP, Chen S-H, MacGillivray RTA: Founder effect in different families with haemophilia B mutation. *Lancet* **335:**418, 1990.
320. Bottema CDK, Koeberl DD, Ketterling RP, Bowie EJW, Taylor SAM, Lillicrap D, Shapiro A, Gilchrist G, Sommer SS: A past mutation at Isoleucine[397] is now a common cause of moderate/mild haemophilia B. *Br J Haematol* **75:**212, 1990.
321. Ketterling RP, Bottema CDK, Koeberl DD, Ii S, Sommer SS: T[296]-M, a common mutation causing mild hemophilia B in the Amish and others: Founder effect, variability in factor IX activity assays, and rapid carrier detection. *Hum Genet* **87:**333, 1991.
322. Ketterling RP, Bottema CDK, Phillips JA III, Sommer SS: Evidence that descendants of three founders constitute about 25% of hemophilia B in the United States. *Genomics* **10:**1093, 1991.
323. Brocker-Vriends AHJT, Bakker E, Kanhai HHH, van Ommen GJB, Reitsma PH, van de Kamp JJP, Briet E: The contribution of DNA analysis to carrier detection and prenatal diagnosis of hemophilia A and B. *Ann Hematol* **64:**2, 1992.
324. Giannelli F, Choo KH, Winship PR, Rizza CR, Anson DS, Rees DJG, Ferrari N, Brownlee GG: Characterization and use of an intragenic polymorphic marker for detection of carriers of haemophilia B (factor IX deficiency). *Lancet* **1:**239, 1984.
325. Winship PR, Anson DS, Rizza CR, Brownlee GG: Carrier detection in haemophilia B using two further intragenic restriction fragment length polymorphisms. *Nucleic Acids Res* **12:**8861, 1984.
326. Camerino G, Oberlé I, Drayna D, Mandel JL: A new Mspl restriction fragment length polymorphism in the hemophilia B locus. *Hum Genet* **71:**79, 1985.
327. Hay CW, Robertson KA, Yong S-L, Thompson AR, Growe GH, MacGillivray RTA: Use of a *Bam*HI polymorphism in the factor IX gene for the determination of hemophilia B carrier status. *Blood* **67:**1508, 1986.
328. Tsang TC, Bentley DR, Nilsson IM, Giannelli F: The use of DNA amplification for genetic counseling related diagnosis in haemophilia B. *Thromb Haemost* **61:**343, 1989.
329. Winship PR, Rees DJG, Alkan M: Detection of polymorphisms at cytosine phosphoguanadine dinucleotides and diagnosis of haemophilia B carriers. *Lancet* **1:**631, 1989.
330. Thompson AR, Chen S-H: Characterization of factor IX defects in hemophilia B patients, in Lorand L, Mann KG (eds): *Proteolytic Enzymes in Coagulation, Fibrinolysis and Complement Fixation*. Orlando, FL, Academic, vol. 222, 1993, pp 143–169.
331. Green PM, Montandon AJ, Ljung R, Bentley DR, Nilsson IM, Kling S, Giannelli F: Haemophilia B mutations in a complete Swedish population sample: A test of new strategy for the genetic counselling of diseases with high mutational heterogeneity. *Br J Haematol* **78:**390, 1991.
332. Fraser BM, Poon M-C, Hoar DI: Identification of factor IX mutations in haemophilia B: Application of polymerase chain reaction and single strand conformation analysis. *Hum Genet* **88:**426, 1992.
333. Chan V, Yip B, Tong TMF, Chang TPT, Lau K, Yam I, Chan TK: Molecular defects in haemophilia B: Detection by direct restriction enzyme analysis. *Br J Haematol* **79:**63, 1991.
334. Matsushita T, Tanimoto M, Yamamoto K, Sugiura I, Takamatsu J, Kamiya T, Saito H: Direct carrier detection in hemophilia B kindreds: Use of modified primers (mutagenic primers) for enzymatic amplification of the factor IX gene. *Thromb Res* **63:**355, 1991.
335. Forbes CD: Clinical aspects of the hemophilias and their treatment, in Ratnoff OD, Forbes CD (eds): *Disorders of Hemostasis*. Orlando, FL, Grune & Stratton, 1984, p 177.
336. Duthie RB, Matthews JM, Rizza CR, Steel WM, Woods CG: *The Management of Musculo-skeletal Problems in the Haemophiliacs*. Oxford, Blackwell, 1972.
337. De Valderrama JAF, Matthews JM: The haemophilic pseudotumour of haemophilic subperiosteal haematoma. *J Bone Joint Surg [Br]* **47:**256, 1965.
338. Gilbert MS: The hemophilic pseudotumor. *Prog Clin Biol Res* **324:**257, 1990.
339. Larsson SA, Wiechel B: Deaths in Swedish hemophiliacs, 1957-1980. *Acta Med Scand* **214:**199, 1983.
340. Forbes CD, Prentice CRM: Mortality in haemophilia-A United Kingdom survey, in Fratantoni JC, Aronson DL (eds): *Unsolved Therapeutic Problems in Hemophilia*. Washington, DC, 1977, DHEW Publication No (NIH) 77-10899, p 15.
341. Duthie RB, Rizza CR: Rheumatological manifestations of the haemophiliacs. *Clin Rheum Dis* **1:**53, 1975.
342. Petersson H, Ahlberg A, Nilsson IM: A radiologic classification of hemophilic arthropathy. *Clin Orthop* **149:**153, 1980.
343. Kasper CK, Dietrich SL: Comprehensive management of haemophilia, in Ruggeri ZM (ed): *Clinics in Hematology Coagulation Disorders*. London, Saunders, 1985, vol 14/no 2, p 489.
344. Zauber NP, Levin J: Factor IX levels in patients with hemophilia B (Christmas disease) following transfusion with concentrates of factor IX or fresh frozen plasma. *Medicine (Baltimore)* **56:**213, 1977.
345. Smith KJ, Thompson AR: Labeled factor IX kinetics in patients with hemophilia-B. *Blood* **58:**625, 1981.
346. Nilsson IM, Ahlberg A, Bjorlin G: Clinical experience

with a Swedish factor IX concentrate. *Acta Med Scand* **19:**257, 1974.

347. Goldberg VM, Heiple KG, Ratnoff OD, Kurczynski E, Arvan G: Total knee arthroplasty in classic hemophilia. *J Bone Joint Surg [Am]* **63:**695, 1981.
348. Lachiewicz PF, Inglis AE, Insall JN, Sculco TP, Hilgartner MW, Bussel JB: Total knee arthroplasty in hemophilia. *J Bone Joint Surg [Am]* **67:**1361, 1985.
349. Nelson IW, Sivamurugan S, Latham PD, Matthews J, Bulstrode CJK: Total hip arthroplasty for hemophilic arthropathy. *Clin Orthop* **276:**210, 1992.
350. Storti E, Ascri E: Surgical and chemical synovectomy. *Ann NY Acad Sci* **240:**316, 1975.
351. Storti E, Ascari E, Gamba G: Postoperative complications and joint function after knee synovectomy in haemophiliacs. *Br J Haematol* **50:**544, 1982.
352. Scarponi R, Silvello L, Landonio G, Baudo F, De Cataldo F: Long-term evaluation of knee-joint function after synovectomy in haemophilia. *Br J Haematol* **52:**337, 1982.
353. Klein K, Aland C, Kim H, Eisele J, Saidi P: Long-term follow-up of arthroscopic synovectomy for chronic hemophilic synovitis. *Arthroscopy* **3:**231, 1987.
354. Wiedel JD: Arthroscopy of the knee in hemophilia. *Prog Clin Biol Res* **324:**231, 1990.
355. Lofqvist T, Pettersson C: Experience with colloid ^{198}Au synoviorthesis in hemophiliacs. *Ric Clin Lab* **16:**97, 1986.
356. Espinosa C, Caballero O, Aznar JA, Querol F: Synoviorthesis with ^{90}Y in hemophilic chronic synovitis. *Ric Clin Lab* **16:**97, 1986.
357. Rivard GE: Synoviorthesis with radioactive colloids in hemophiliacs. *Prog Clin Biol Res* **324:**215, 1990.
358. Nilsson IM, Berntorp E, Lofqvist T, Pettersson H: Twenty-five years' experience of prophylactic treatment in severe haemophilia A and B. *J Intern Med* **232:**25, 1992.
359. Brettler DB, Forsberg AD, O'Connell FD, Cederbaum AI, Chaitman AK, Levine PH: A long-term study of hemophilic arthropathy of the knee joint on a program of factor VIII replacement given at time of each hemoarthrosis. *Am J Hematol* **18:**13, 1985.
360. Steven MM, Yogarajah S, Madhok R, Forbes CD, Sturrock RD: Haemophilic arthritis. *Q J Med* **226:**181, 1986.
361. Guenthner EE, Hilgartner MW, Miller CH, Vienne G: Hemophilic arthropathy: Effect of home care on treatment patterns and joint disease. *J Pediatr* **97:**378, 1980.
362. Ingram GIC, Dykes SR, Creese AL, Mellor P, Swan AV, Karufert J, Rizza CR, Spooner RJD, Biggs R: Home treatment in haemophilia: Clinical, social and economic advantages. *Clin Lab Haematol* **1:**13, 1979.
363. Soulier JP, Blatrix C, Steinbach M: Fractions "coagulants" contenant les facteurs de coagulation absorbables par le phosphate tricalcique. *Presse Med* **72:**1223, 1964.
364. Bidwell E, Booth JM, Dike GWR: The preparation for therapeutic use of a concentrate of factor IX containing also factors II, VII, and X. *Br J Haematol* **13:**568, 1967.
365. Tullis JL, Melin M, Jurgian P: Clinical use of human prothrombin complexes. *N Engl J Med* **273:**667, 1965.
366. Kasper CK: Clinical use of prothrombin complex concentrates: Report on thromboembolic complications. *Thromb Diath Haemorrh* **33:**640, 1975.
367. Lusher JM: Thrombogenicity associated with factor IX complex concentrate. *Semin Hematol (suppl 6)* **28:**3, 1991.
368. Hedner U, Nilsson IM, Bergentz SE: Various prothrombin complex concentrates and their effect on coagulation and fibrinolysis *in vivo*. *Thromb Haemost* **35:**386, 1979.
369. White GC II, Roberts HR, Kingdon HS, Lundblad RL: Prothrombin complex concentrates: Potentially thrombogenic materials and clues to the mechanism of thrombosis in vivo. *Blood* **49:**159, 1977.
370. Hultin MB: Activated clotting factors in prothrombin complex concentrates. *Blood* **54:**1028, 1979.
371. Aronson DL, Menache D: Thrombogenicity of factor IX complex: In vivo investigation. *Dev Biol Stand* **67:**149, 1987.
372. Giles AR, Nesheim ME, Hoogendoorn H, Tracy PB, Mann KG: The coagulant-active phospholipid content is a major determinant of *in vivo* thrombogenicity of prothrombin complex (factor IX) concentrates in rabbits. *Blood* **59:**401, 1982.
373. Smith KJ: Factor IX concentrates: The new products and their properties. *Transfus Med Rev* **6:**124, 1992.
374. Thompson AR: Clinical factor IX concentrates. *Semin Thromb Hemost* **19:**25, 1993.
375. Menache D, Behre HE, Orthner CL, Nunez H, Anderson HD, Triantaphyllopoulos DC, Kosow DP: Coagulation factor IX concentrate: Method of preparation and assessment of potential in vivo thrombogenicity in animal models. *Blood* **64:**1220, 1984.
376. Mannucci PM, Bauer KA, Gringeri A, Barzegar S, Bottasso B, Simoni L, Rosenberg RD: Thrombin generation is not increased in the blood of hemophilia B patients after the infusion of a purified factor IX concentrate. *Blood* **76:**2540, 1990.
377. Bardin JM, Sultan Y: Factor IX concentrate versus prothrombin complex concentrate for the treatment of hemophilia B during surgery. *Transfusion* **30:**441, 1990.
378. MacGregor IR, Ferguson JM, McLaughlin LF, Burnouf T, Prowse CV: Comparison of high purity factor IX concentrates and a prothrombin complex concentrate in a canine model of thrombogenicity. *Thromb Haemost* **66:**609, 1991.
379. Kim HC, McMillan CW, White GC, Bergman GE, Horton MW, Saidi P: Purified factor IX using monoclonal immunoaffinity technique: Clinical trials in hemophilia B and comparison to prothrombin complex concentrates. *Blood* **79:**568, 1992.
380. Goldsmith JC, Kasper CK, Blatt PM, Gomperts ED, Kessler CM, Thompson AR, Herring SW, Novak PL: Coagulation factor IX: Successful surgical experience with a purified factor IX concentrate. *Am J Hematol* **40:**210, 1992.
381. Goedert JJ, Kessler CM, Aledort LM, Biggar RJ, Andes WA, White GC, Drummond JE, Vaidya K, Mann DL, Eyster ME, Ragni MV, Lederman MM, Cohen AR, Gray GL, Rosenberg PS, Friedman RM, Hilgartner MR, Blattner WA, Kroner B, Gail MH: A prospective study of human immunodeficiency virus type 1 infection and the development of AIDS in subjects with hemophilia. *N Engl J Med* **321:**1141, 1989.
382. Choo QL, Kuo G, Weiner AJ: Isolation of a cDNA clone derived from blood borne non A, non B viral hepatitis genome. *Science* **244:**359, 1989.
383. Kuo G, Choo Q-L, Alter HJ, Gitnick GL, Redeker AG, Purcell RH, Miyamura T, Dienstag JL, Alter MJ, Stevens CE, Tegtmeier GE, Bonino F, Colombo M, Lee W-S, Kuo C, Berger K, Shuster JR, Overby LR, Bradley DW, Houghton M: An assay for circulating antibodies to a major etiologic virus of human non-A, non-B hepatitis. *Science* **244:**362, 1989.
384. Allain J-P, Dailey SH, Laurian Y, Vallari DS, Rafowicz A, Desai SM, Devare SG: Evidence for persistent hepatitis C virus (HCV) infection in hemophiliacs. *J Clin Invest* **88:**1672, 1991.
385. Watson HG, Ludlam CA, Rebus S, Zhang LQ, Peutherer JF, Simmonds P: Use of several second generation serologic assays to determine the true prevalence of hepatitis C virus infection in haemophiliacs treated with non-virus inactivated factor VIII and IX concentrates. *Br J Haematol* **80:**514, 1992.
386. Hay CRM, Preston FE, Triger DR: Progressive liver disease in haemophiliacs: An understated problem? *Lancet* **1:**1495, 1985.
387. Makris M, Preston FE, Triger DR, Underwood JCE, Choo Q-L, Kuo G, Moughton M: Hepatitis C antibody and chronic liver disease in haemophilia. *Lancet* **355:**1117, 1990.
388. Esteban JI, Gonzalez G, Hernandez JM, Viladomiu L, Sanchez C, Lopez-Talevera JC, Luccea D, Martin-Vega C, Vidal X, Esteban R, Guardia J: Evaluation of antibodies to hepatitis C virus in a study of transfusion-associated hepatitis. *N Engl J Med* **323:**1107, 1990.
389. Colvin BT, Rizza CR, Hill FGH, Kernoff PBA, Bateman CJT, Bolton-Maggs P, Daly HM, Kenny MW, Taylor PC, Mitchell VE, Wensley RT, Whitmore DN, Lane RS, Smith JK: Effect of dry-heating of coagulation factor concentrates at 80°C for 72 hours on transmission of non-A, non-B hepatitis. *Lancet* **2:**814, 1988.
390. Skidmore SJ, Pasi KJ, Mawson SJ, Williams MD, Hill

FGH: Serological evidence that dry heating of clotting factor concentrates prevents transmission of non-A, non-B hepatitis. *J Med Virol* **30**:50, 1990.

391. Kreuz W, Auerswald G, Bruckmann C, Zieger B, Linde R, Funk M, Auberger K, Sutor AH, Rasshofer R, Roggendorf M: Prevention of hepatitis C virus infection in children with haemophilia A and B and von Willebrand's disease. *Thromb Haemost* **67**:184, 1992.
392. Horowitz MS, Rooks C, Horowitz B, Hilgartner MW: Virus safety of solvent/detergent-treated antihaemophilic factor concentrate. *Lancet* **2**:186, 1988.
393. Blanchette VS, Vorstman E, Shore A, Wang E, Petric M, Jett BW, Alter HJ: Hepatitis C infection in children with hemophilia A and B. *Blood* **78**:285, 1991.
394. Carnelli V, Gomperts ED, Friedman A, Aledort L, Hilgartner M, Dietrich S, Fedor EJ: Assessment for evidence of non A-non B hepatitis in patients given n-heptane-suspended heat-treated clotting factor concentrates. *Thromb Res* **47**:827, 1987.
395. Lee CA, Kernoff PBA, Karayiannis P, Thomas HC: Interferon therapy for chronic non-A non-B and chronic delta disease in haemophilia. *Br J Haematol* **72**:235, 1989.
396. Makris M, Preston FE, Triger DR, Adelman MI, Underwood JCE: A prospective randomized controlled liver biopsy study of recombinant alpha interferon in chronic non-A non-B hepatitis in haemophilia. *Br J Haematol (suppl 1)* **71**:19, 1989.
397. Bontempo FA, Lewis JH, Corenc TJ, Spero JA, Ragni MV, Scott JP, Starzl TE: Liver transplantation in hemophilia A. *Blood* **69**:1721, 1987.
398. Lyon DJ, Chapman CS, Martin C, Brown KE, Clewley JP, Flower AJE, Mitchell VE: Symptomatic parvovirus B19 infection and heat-treated factor IX concentrate. *Lancet* **1**:1085, 1989.
399. Morfini M, Longo G, Rossi Ferrini P, Azzi A, Zakrewska C, Ciappi S, Kolumban P: Hypoplastic anemia in a hemophiliac first infused with a solvent/detergent treated factor VIII concentrate: The role of human B19 parvovirus. *Am J Hematol* **39**:149, 1992.
400. Hedner U, Sundqvist SB, Nilsson IM: Immunosuppressive treatment in haemophiliacs with inhibitors, in *The State of Art of Managing Hemophilia with FVIII Inhibitors, Proceedings of the International Meeting on Activated Prothrombin Complex Concentrates*. New York, Praeger, 1982.
401. Nilsson IM, Jonsson S, Sundqvist S-B, Ahlberg A, Bergentz S-E: A procedure for removing high titer antibodies by extracorporeal protein-A-Sepharose adsorption in hemophilia: Substitution therapy and surgery in a patient with hemophilia B and antibodies. *Blood* **58**:38, 1981.
402. Uehlinger J, Button GR, McCarthy J, Forster A, Watt R, Aledort LM: Immunoadsorption for coagulation factor inhibitors. *Transfusion* **31**:265, 1991.
403. Theodorsson B, Hedner U, Nilsson IM, Kisiel W: A technique for specific removal of factor IX alloantibodies from human plasma: Partial characterization of the alloantibodies. *Blood* **61**:973, 1983.
404. Schmidt ML, Smith HE, Gamerman S, DiMichele D, Glazer S, Scott JP: Prolonged recombinant activated factor VII (rFVIIa) treatment for severe bleeding in a factor-IX-deficient patient with an inhibitor. *Br J Haematol* **78**:460, 1991.
405. Hedner U, Nilsson IM: Induced tolerance in hemophilia patients with antibodies against IX:C. *Acta Med Scand* **214**:191, 1983.
406. Nilsson IM, Sundqvist S-B, Ljung R, Holmberg L, Freiburghaus C, Bjorlin G: Suppression of secondary antibody response by intravenous immunoglobulin in a patient with haemophilia B and antibodies. *Scand J Haematol* **30**:458, 1983.
407. Nilsson IM, Berntorp E, Zettervall O: Induction of split tolerance and clinical cure in high-responding hemophiliacs with factor IX antibodies. *Proc Natl Acad Sci USA* **83**:9169, 1986.
408. Kaufman RJ, Wasley LC, Furie BC, Furie B, Shoemaker CB: Expression, purification, and characterization of recombinant γ-carboxylated factor IX synthesized in Chinese hamster ovary cells. *J Biol Chem* **261**:9622, 1986.
409. Balland A, Faure T, Carvallo D, Cordier P, Ulrich P, Fournet B, de la Salle H, Lecocq J-P: Characterization of two differently processed forms of human recombinant factor IX synthesized in CHO cells transformed with a polycistronic vector. *Eur J Biochem* **172**:565, 1988.
410. Miller AD: Progress toward human gene therapy. *Blood* **76**:271, 1990.
411. Thompson AR: Status of gene transfer for hemophilia A and B. *Thromb Haemost* **66**:119, 1991.
412. Brinkhous KM: Gene transfer in the hemophilias: Retrospect and prospect. *Thromb Res* **67**:329, 1992.
413. Palmer TD, Thompson AR, Miller AD: Production of human factor IX in animals by genetically modified skin fibroblasts: Potential therapy for hemophilia B. *Blood* **73**:438, 1989.
414. Palmer TD, Rosman GJ, Osborne WRA, Miller AD: Genetically modified skin fibroblasts persist long after transplantation but gradually inactivate introduced genes. *Proc Natl Acad Sci USA* **88**:1330, 1991.
415. Scharfmann R, Axelrod JH, Verma IM: Long-term *in vivo* expression of retrovirus-mediated gene transfer in mouse fibroblast implants. *Proc Natl Acad Sci USA* **88**:4626, 1991.
416. Dai Y, Roman M, Naviaux RK, Verma IM: Gene therapy via primary myoblasts: Long-term expression of factor IX protein following transplantation *in vivo*. *Proc Natl Acad Sci USA* **89**:10892, 1992.
417. DiScipio RG, Hermondson MA, Davie EW: Activation of human factor X (Stuart factor) by a protease from Russell's viper venom. *Biochemistry* **16**:5253, 1977.
418. van Dieijen G, Tans G, Rosing J, Hemker HC: The role of phospholipid and factor VIII_a in the activation of bovine factor X. *J Biol Chem* **256**:3433, 1981.
419. Ahmad SS, Rawala-Sheikh R, Walsh PN: Components and assembly of the factor X activating complex. *Semin Thromb Hemost* **18**:311, 1992.
420. McGee MP, Li LC: Functional difference between intrinsic and extrinsic coagulation pathways. Kinetics of factor X activation on human monocytes and alveolar macrophages. *J Biol Chem* **266**:8079, 1991.
421. Huang M-N, Hung H-L, Stanfield-Oakley SA, High KA: Characterization of the human blood coagulation factor X promoter. *J Biol Chem* **267**:15440, 1992.
422. Miao CH, Leytus SP, Chung DW, Davie EW: Liver-specific expression of the gene coding for human factor X, a blood coagulation factor. *J Biol Chem* **267**:7395, 1992.
423. Jaye M, Ricca G, Kaplan R, Howk R, Mudd R, Ngo KY, Fair DS, Drohan W: Polymorphism associated with the human coagulation factor X (F10) gene. *Nucleic Acids Res* **13**:8286, 1985.
424. Hay CW, Robertson KA, Fung MR, MacGillivray RTA: RFLPs for PstI and EcoRI in the human blood clotting factor X gene. *Nucleic Acids Res* **14**:5118, 1986.
425. Hassan HJ, Guerriero R, Chelucci C, Leonardi A, Mattia G, Leone G, Mariani G, Mannucci PM, Peschle C: Multiple polymorphic sites in factor X locus. *Blood* **71**:1353, 1988.
426. Wallmark A, Rose VL, Ho C, High KA: A NlaIV polymorphism within the human factor X gene. *Nucleic Acids Res* **19**:426, 1991.
427. Duckert F, Fluckiger P, Matter M, Koller F: Clotting factor X: Physiologic and physico-chemical properties. *Proc Soc Exp Biol Med* **90**:17, 1955.
428. Telfer TP, Denson KW, Wright DR: A "new" coagulation defect. *Br J Haematol* **2**:308, 1956.
429. Hougie C, Barrow EM, Graham JB: Stuart clotting defect. I. Segregation of an hereditary hemorrhagic state from the heterogeneous group heretofore called "stable factor" (SPCA, proconvertin, factor VII) deficiency. *J Clin Invest* **36**:485, 1957.
430. Graham JB, Barrow EM, Hougie C: Stuart clotting defect II: Genetic aspects of a "new" hemorrhagic state. *J Clin Invest* **36**:497, 1957.
431. Lechler E, Webster WP, Roberts HR, Penick GD: The inheritance of Stuart disease: Investigation of a family with factor X deficiency. *Am J Med Sci* **249**:191, 1965.
432. Fair DS, Edgington TS: Heterogeneity of hereditary and acquired factor X deficiencies by combined immunochemical and functional analyses. *Br J Haematol* **59**:235, 1985.

433. Girolami A: Tentative and updated classification of factor X variants. *Acta Haematol* **75**:58, 1986.
434. Girolami A, Vicarioto M, Ruzza G, Cappellato G, Vergolani A: Factor X Padua: A 'new' congenital factor X abnormality with a defect only in the extrinsic system. *Acta Haematol* **73**:31, 1985.
435. Watzke HH, Lechner K, Roberts HR, Reddy SV, Welsch DJ, Friedman P, Mahr G, Jagadeeswaran P, Monroe DM, High KA: Molecular defect ($Gla^{+14}\rightarrow Lys$) and its functional consequences in a hereditary factor X deficiency (factor X "Vorarlberg"). *J Biol Chem* **265**:11982, 1990.
436. Parkin JD, Madares F, Sweet B, Castaldi PA: A further inherited variant of coagulation factor X. *Aust N Z J Med* **4**:561, 1974.
437. De Stefano V, Leone G, Ferrelli R, Hassa HJ, Macioce G, Bizzi B: Factor X Roma: A congenital factor X variant defective at different degrees in the intrinsic and the extrinsic activation. *Br J Haematol* **69**:387, 1988.
438. Wieland K, Millar DS, Grundy CB, Mibashan RS, Kakker VV, Cooper DN: Molecular genetic analysis of factor X deficiency: Gene deletion and germline mosaicism. *Hum Genet* **86**:273, 1991.
439. Bernardi F, Marchetti G, Patracchini P, Volinia S, Gemmati D, Simioni P, Girolami A: Partial gene deletion in a family with factor X deficiency. *Blood* **73**:2123, 1989.
440. Asakai R, Davie EW: Unpublished.
441. Wallmark A, Ho C, Monroe DM, Tengborn L, High KA: Molecular defect in F.X 'Ockero,' a mild congenital F.X deficiency. *Thromb Haemost* **65**:1263, 1991.
442. James HL, Kumar A, Thompson AR, Fair DS: A point mutation destroys a processing site between the light and heavy chains of factor $X_{WENATCHEE}$. *FASEB J* **5**:A1661, 1991.
443. Girolami A, Molaro G, Lazzarin M, Scarpa R, Brunetti A: A new congenital hemorrhagic condition due to the presence of an abnormal factor X (factor X Friuli): Study of a large kindred. *Br J Haematol* **19**:179, 1970.
444. Fair DS, Revak DJ, Hubbard JG, Girolami A: Isolation and characterization of the factor X Friuli variant. *Blood* **73**:2108, 1989.
445. James HL, Girolami A, Fair DS: Molecular defect in coagulation factor X_{FRIULI} results from a substitution of serine for proline at position 343. *Blood* **77**:317, 1991.
446. Reddy SV, Zhou Z-Q, Rao KJ, Scott JP, Watzke H, High KA, Jagadeeswaran P: Molecular characterization of human factor $X_{SAN\ ANTONIO}$. *Blood* **74**:1486, 1989.
447. Korsan-Bengsten L, Hjort PF, Ygge J: Acquired factor X deficiency in a patient with amyloidosis. *Thromb Diath Haemorrh* **7**:558, 1962.
448. Greipp PR, Kyle RA, Bowie EJW: Factor-X deficiency in amyloidosis: A critical review. *Am J Hematol* **11**:443, 1981.
449. Knight RD, Barr CF, Alving BM: Replacement therapy for congenital factor X deficiency. *Transfusion* **25**:78, 1985.
450. Messier TL, Pittman DD, Long GL, Kaufman RJ, Church WR: Cloning and expression in COS-1 cells of a full-length cDNA encoding human coagulation factor X. *Gene* **99**:291, 1991.
451. Stenflo J: A new vitamin K dependent protein: Purification from bovine plasma and preliminary characterization. *J Biol Chem* **251**:355, 1976.
452. Kisiel W: Human plasma protein C: Isolation, characterization and mechanism of activation by α-thrombin. *J Clin Invest* **64**:761, 1979.
453. Marlar RA, Kleiss AJ, Griffin JH: Mechanism of action of human activated protein C, a thrombin dependent anticoagulant enzyme. *Blood* **59**:1067, 1982.
454. Esmon CT: The roles of protein C and thrombomodulin in the regulation of blood coagulation. *J Biol Chem* **264**:4743, 1989.
455. Dittman WA, Majerus PW: Structure and function of thrombomodulin: A natural anticoagulant. *Blood* **5**:329, 1990.
456. Walker FJ, Sexton PW, Esmon CT: The inhibition of blood coagulation by activated protein C through the selective inactivation of activated factor V. *Biochim Biophys Acta* **571**:333, 1979.
457. Suzuki K, Stenflo J, Dahlback B, Theodorsson B: Inactivation of human coagulation factor V by activated protein C. *J Biol Chem* **258**:1914, 1983.
458. Fulcher CA, Gardiner JE, Griffin JH, Zimmerman TS: Proteolytic inactivation of human factor VIII procoagulant protein by activated human protein C and its analogy with factor V. *Blood* **63**:486, 1984.
459. Odegaard B, Mann K: Proteolysis of factor Va and activated protein C. *J Biol Chem* **262**:11233, 1987.
460. Fay PJ, Smudzin TM, Walker FJ: Activated protein C-catalyzed inactivation of human factor VIII and factor VIII_a. Identification of cleavage sites and correlation of proteolysis with cofactor activity. *J Biol Chem* **266**:20139, 1991.
461. Walker FJ: Regulation of activated protein C by a new protein: A possible function for bovine protein S. *J Biol Chem* **255**:5221, 1980.
462. Walker FJ: Regulation of activated protein C by protein S: The role of phospholipid in factor Va inactivation. *J Biol Chem* **256**:1128, 1981.
463. DiScipio RG, Davie EW: Characterization of protein S, a γ-carboxyglutamic acid containing protein from bovine and human plasma. *Biochemistry* **18**:899, 1979.
464. Mitchell CA, Hau L, Salem HH: Control of thrombin-mediated cleavage of protein S. *Thromb Haemost* **56**:151, 1986.
465. Walker FJ: Protein S and the regulation of activated protein C. *Semin Thromb Hemost* **10**:131, 1984.
466. Harris K, Esmon C: Protein S is required for platelets to support activated protein C binding and activity. *J Biol Chem* **260**:2007, 1985.
467. Nawroth PP, Handley D, Stern DM: The multiple levels of endothelial cell-coagulation factor interactions, in Chesterman CN (ed): *Clinics in Haematology. Thrombosis and the Vessel Wall.* London, Saunders, 1986, vol 15/no 2, p 293.
468. Stern DM, Nawroth PP, Harris K: Activated protein C regulates cellular processing of protein S. *Thromb Haemost* **54**:707, 1985.
469. Comp PC, Esmon CT: Generation of fibrinolytic activity by infusion of activated protein C into dogs. *J Clin Invest* **68**:1221, 1981.
470. Sakata Y, Curriden S, Lawrence D, Griffin JH, Loskutoff DJ: Activated protein C stimulates the fibrinolytic activity of cultured endothelial cells and decreases antiactivator activity. *Proc Natl Acad Sci USA* **82**:1121, 1985.
471. van Hinsbergh VWM, Bertina RM, van Wijngaarden A, van Tilburg NH, Emeis JJ, Haverkate F: Activated protein C decreases plasminogen activator inhibitor activity in endothelial cell conditioned medium. *Blood* **65**:444, 1985.
472. D'Angelo A, Lockhart MS, D'Angelo SV, Taylor FB: Protein S is a cofactor for activated protein C neutralization of an inhibitor of plasminogen activation released from platelets. *Blood* **69**:231, 1987.
473. Suzuki K, Deyashiki Y, Nishioka J, Toma K: Protein C inhibitor: Structure and function. *Thromb Haemost* **61**:337, 1989.
474. Heeb MJ, Griffin JH: Physiologic inhibition of human activated protein C by α_1-antitrypsin. *J Biol Chem* **263**:11613, 1988.
475. van der Meer FJM, van Tilburg NH, van Wijngaarden A, van der Linden IK, Briët E, Bertina RM: A second plasma inhibitor of activated protein C: α_1-antitrypsin. *Thromb Haemost* **62**:756, 1989.
476. Kisiel W, Davie EW: Protein C. *Methods Enzymol* **80**:320, 1981.
477. Suzuki K, Nishioka J: A thrombin-based peptide corresponding to the sequence of the thrombomodulin-binding site blocks the procoagulant activities of thrombin. *J Biol Chem* **266**:18498, 1991.
478. Ye J, Liu L-W, Esmon CT, Johnson AE: The fifth and sixth growth factor-like domains of thrombomodulin bind to the anion-binding exosite of thrombin and alter its specificity. *J Biol Chem* **267**:11023, 1992.
479. Esmon CT, Esmon NL, Harris KW: Complex formation between thrombin and thrombomodulin inhibits both thrombin catalyzed fibrin formation and factor V activation. *J Biol Chem* **257**:7944, 1982.
480. Esmon NL, Carroll RC, Esmon CT: Thrombomodulin blocks the ability of thrombin to activate platelets. *J Biol Chem* **258**:12238, 1983.
481. Öhlin A-K, Björk I, Stenflo J: Proteolytic formation and properties of a fragment of protein C containing the γ-carboxy-

glutamic acid rich domain and the EGF-like region. *Biochemistry* **29**:644, 1990.

482. Mesters RM, Houghten RA, Griffin JH: Identification of a sequence of human activated protein C (residues 390-404) essential for its anticoagulant activity. *J Biol Chem* **266**:24514, 1991.
483. Suzuki K, Kusumoto H, Deyashiki Y, Nishioka J, Maruyama I, Zushi M, Kawahara S, Honda G, Yamamoto S, Horiguchi S: Structure and expression of human thrombomodulin, a thrombin receptor on endothelium acting as a cofactor for protein C activation. *EMBO J* **6**:1891, 1987.
484. Wen D, Dittman WA, Ye RD, Deaven LL, Majerus PW, Sadler JE: Human thrombomodulin: Complete cDNA sequence and chromosome location of the gene. *Biochemistry* **26**:4350, 1987.
485. Jackman RW, Beeler DL, Fritze L, Soff G, Rosenberg RD: Human thrombomodulin gene is intron depleted: Nucleic acid sequences of the cDNA and gene predict protein structure and suggest sites of regulatory control. *Proc Natl Acad Sci USA* **84**:6425, 1987.
486. Zushi M, Gomi K, Yamamoto S, Maruyama I, Hayashi T, Suzuki K: The last three consecutive epidermal growth factor-like structures of human thrombomodulin comprise the minimum functional domain for protein C-activating cofactor activity and anticoagulant activity. *J Biol Chem* **264**:10351, 1989.
487. Tsiang M, Lentz SR, Sadler JE: Functional domains of membrane-bound human thrombomodulin. EGF-like domains four to six and the serine/threonine-rich domain are required for cofactor activity. *J Biol Chem* **267**:6164, 1992.
488. Stearns DJ, Kurosawa S, Esmon CT: Microthrombomodulin. Residues 310-486 from the epidermal growth factor precursor homology domain of thrombomodulin will accelerate protein C activation. *J Biol Chem* **264**:3352, 1989.
489. Hayashi T, Zuahi M, Yamamoto S, Suzuki K: Further localization of binding sites for thrombin and protein C in human thrombomodulin. *J Biol Chem* **265**:20156, 1990.
490. Parkinson JF, Nagashima M, Kuhn I, Leonard J, Morser J: Structure-function studies of the epidermal growth factor domains of human thrombomodulin. *Biochem Biophys Res Commun* **185**:567, 1992.
491. Zushi M, Gomi K, Honda G, Kondo S, Yamamoto S, Hayashi T, Suzuki K: Aspartic acid 349 in the fourth epidermal growth factor-like structure of human thrombomodulin plays a role in its Ca^{2+}-mediated binding to protein C. *J Biol Chem* **266**:19886, 1991.
492. Maruyama I, Bell CE, Majerus PW: Thrombomodulin is found on endothelium of arteries, veins, capillaries, and lymphatics, and on syncytiotrophoblast of human placenta. *J Cell Biol* **101**:363, 1985.
493. Ishii H, Salem HH, Bell CE, Laposata EA, Majerus PW: Thrombomodulin, an endothelial anticoagulant protein, is absent from the human brain. *Blood* **67**:362, 1986.
494. Suzuki K, Nichioka J, Hayaoni T, Kosaka Y: Functionally active thrombomodulin is present in human platelets. *J Biochem* **104**:628, 1988.
495. Ishii H, Majerus PW: Thrombomodulin is present in human plasma and urine. *J Clin Invest* **76**:178, 1985.
496. Moore KL, Andreoli SP, Esmon NL, Esmon CT, Bang NU: Endotoxin enhances tissue factor and suppresses thrombomodulin expression of human vascular endothelium in vitro. *J Clin Invest* **79**:124, 1987.
497. Nawroth PP, Handley DA, Esmon CT, Stern DM: Interleukin 1 induces endothelial cell procoagulant while suppressing cell-surface anticoagulant activity. *Proc Natl Acad Sci USA* **83**:3460, 1986.
498. Naworth PP, Stern DM: Modulation of endothelial cell hemostatic properties by tumor necrosis factor. *J Exp Med* **163**:740, 1986.
499. Fair DS, Marlar RA: Biosynthesis and secretion of factor VII, protein C, protein S and the protein C inhibitor by a human hepatoma cell line. *Blood* **67**:64, 1986.
500. Fair DS, Marlar RA, Levin EG: Human endothelial cells synthesize protein S. *Blood* **67**:1168, 1986.
501. Schwartz HP, Heeb MJ, Wencel-Drake JD, Griffin JH: Identification and quantitation of protein S in human platelets. *Blood* **66**:1452, 1985.
502. Maillard C, Berruyer M, Serre CM, Dechavanne M, Delmas PD: Protein-S, a vitamin K-dependent protein, is a bone matrix component synthesized and secreted by osteoblasts. *Endocrinology* **130**:1599, 1992.
503. Dahlback B, Stenflo J: High molecular weight complex in human plasma between vitamin K-dependent protein S and complement component C4b-binding protein. *Proc Natl Acad Sci USA* **78**:2512, 1981.
504. Comp PC, Doray D, Patton D, Esmon CT: An abnormal plasma distribution of protein S occurs in functional protein S deficiency. *Blood* **67**:504, 1986.
505. Bertina RM, van Wijngaarden A, Reinalda-Poot J, Poort SR, Bom VJJ: Determination of plasma protein S—The protein cofactor of activated protein C. *Thromb Haemost* **53**:268, 1985.
506. Dahlback B: Inhibition of protein Ca cofactor function of human and bovine protein S by C4b-binding protein. *J Biol Chem* **261**:12022, 1986.
507. Dahlback B, Lundwall A, Stenflo J: Localization of thrombin cleavage sites in the amino-terminal region of bovine protein S. *J Biol Chem* **261**:5111, 1986.
508. Baker ME, French FS, Joseph DR: Vitamin K-dependent protein S is similar to rat androgen-binding protein. *Biochem J* **243**:293, 1987.
509. Walker FJ: Characterization of a synthetic peptide that inhibits the interaction between protein S and C4b-binding protein. *J Biol Chem* **264**:17645, 1989.
510. Nelson RM, Long GL: Binding of protein S to C4b-binding protein. Mutagenesis of protein S. *J Biol Chem* **267**:8140, 1992.
511. Kato A, Miura O, Sumi Y, Aoki N: Assignment of the human protein C gene (PROC) to chromosome region 2q14-q21 by in situ hybridization. *Cytogenet Cell Genet* **47**:46, 1988.
512. Patracchini P, Aiello V, Palazzi P, Calzolari E, Bernardi F: Sublocalization of the human protein C gene on chromosome 2q13-q14. *Hum Genet* **81**:191, 1989.
513. Reitsma PH, Poort SR, Allaart CF, Briët E, Bertina RM: The spectrum of genetic defects in a panel of 40 Dutch families with symptomatic protein C deficiency type I: Heterogeneity and founder effects. *Blood* **78**:890, 1991.
514. Yamamoto K, Tanimoto M, Matsushita T, Kagami K, Sugiura I, Hamaguchi M, Takamatsu J, Saito H: Genotype establishments for protein C deficiency by use of a DNA polymorphism in the gene. *Blood* **77**:2633, 1991.
515. Yamamoto K, Takamatsu J, Saito H: Two novel sequence polymorphisms of the human protein C gene. *Nucleic Acids Res* **19**:6973, 1991.
516. Gandrille S, Alach M: Polymorphism in the protein C gene detected by denaturing gradient gel electrophoresis. *Nucleic Acids Res* **19**:6982, 1991.
517. Ploos van Amstel JK, van der Zanden AL, Bakker E, Reitsma PH, Bertina RM: Two genes homologous with human protein S cDNA are located on chromosome 3. *Thromb Haemost* **58**:982, 1987.
518. Long GL, Marshall A, Gardner JC, Naylor SL: Genes for human vitamin K-dependent plasma proteins C and S are located on chromosomes 2 and 3, respectively. *Somat Cell Mol Genet* **14**:93, 1988.
519. Watkins PC, Eddy R, Fukushima Y, Byers MG, Cohen EH, Dackowski WR, Wydro RM, Shows TB: The gene for protein S maps near the centromere of human chromosome 3. *Blood* **71**:238, 1988.
520. Edenbrandt C-M, Lundwall Å, Wydro R, Stenflo J: Molecular analysis of the gene for vitamin K dependent protein S and its pseudogene. Cloning and partial gene organization. *Biochemistry* **29**:7861, 1990.
521. Schmidel DK, Tatro AV, Phelps LG, Tomczak JA, Long GL: Organization of the human protein S genes. *Biochemistry* **29**:7845, 1990.
522. Ploos van Amstel HK, Reitsma PH, van der Logt CPE, Bertina RM: Intron-exon organization of the active human protein S gene PSα and its pseudogene PSβ: Duplication and silencing during primate evolution. *Biochemistry* **29**:7853, 1990.
523. Shira T, Shiojiri S, Ito H, Yamamoto S, Kusumoto H, Deyashiki Y, Maruyama I, Suzuki K: Gene structure of human thrombomodulin, a cofactor for thrombin catalyzed activation of protein C. *J Biochem* **103**:281, 1988.
524. Marlar RA, Adcock DM: Clinical evaluation of protein C:

A comparative review of antigenic and functional assays. *Hum Pathol* **20:**1040, 1989.
525. Andrew M, Paes B, Milner R, Johnston M, Mitchell L, Tollefsen DM, Powers P: Development of the human coagulation system in the full-term infant. *Blood* **70:**165, 1987.
526. Ankola P, Nardi M, Karpatkin M: Functional activity of protein C in newborn infants. A report of a study and a review of the literature. *Am J Pediatr Hematol Oncol* **14:**140, 1992.
527. Manco-Johnson MJ, Abshire TC, Jacobson LJ, Marlar RA: Severe neonatal protein C deficiency: Prevalence and thrombotic risk. *J Pediatr* **119:**793, 1991.
528. Mannucci PM, Viganò S: Deficiencies of protein C, an inhibitor of blood coagulation. *Lancet* **2:**463, 1982.
529. Griffin JH, Mosher DF, Zimmerman TS, Kleiss AJ: Protein C, an antithrombotic protein is reduced in hospitalized patients with intravascular coagulation. *Blood* **60:**261, 1982.
530. Viganò S, Mannucci PM, Rumi MG, Viganò P, Delninno E, Colombo M, Podda M: The significance of protein C antigen in acute and chronic liver and biliary disease. *Am J Clin Pathol* **89:**454, 1985.
531. D'Angelo SV, Comp PC, Esmon CT, D'Angelo A: Relationship between protein C antigen and anticoagulant activity during oral anticoagulation and in selected disease states. *J Clin Invest* **77:**416, 1986.
532. Bell H, Ødegaard OR, Andersson T, Raknerud N: Protein C in patients with alcoholic cirrhosis and other liver diseases. *J Hepatol* **14:**163, 1992.
533. Marlar RA, Endres-Brooks J, Miller C: Serial studies of protein C and its plasma inhibitor in patients with disseminated intravascular coagulation. *Blood* **66:**59, 1985.
534. Barbui T, Finazzi G, Viganò S, Mannucci PM: L-asparaginase lowers protein C antigen. *Thromb Haemost* **52:**216, 1984.
535. Mannucci PM, D'Angelo A, Viganò S, Lewis JH, Spero JA, Baicchi U, Gremignai G, Rao AK, Walsh PN: Decrease and rapid recovery of protein C after plasma exchange. *Transfusion* **26:**156, 1986.
536. Blamey SL, Lowe GDO, Bertina RM, Kluft C, Sue-Ling HM, Davies JD, Forbes DC: Protein C antigen levels in major abdominal surgery: Relationship to deep vein thrombosis, malignancy and treatment with stanozolol. *Thromb Haemost* **54:**622, 1985.
537. Glas-Greenwalt P, Hall JM, Panke TW, Kant KS, Allen CM, Pollak VE: Fibrinolysis in health and disease: Abnormal levels of plasminogen activator inhibitor, and protein C in thrombotic thrombocytopenic purpura. *J Lab Clin Med* **108:**415, 1986.
538. Viganò S, Mannucci PM, D'Angelo A, Gelfi C, Gensini GF, Rostangno C, Neri Serneri GG: Protein C antigen is not an acute phase reactant and is often high in ischemic heart disease and diabetes. *Thromb Haemost* **52:**263, 1984.
539. Pabinger-Fasching I, Lechner K, Niessner H, Schmidt P, Balzar E: High levels of plasma protein C in nephrotic syndrome. *Thromb Haemost* **53:**5, 1985.
540. Mannucci PM, Viganò S, Bottasso B, Candotti G, Bozzetti P, Rossi E, Pardi G: Protein C antigen during pregnancy, delivery and puerperium. *Thromb Haemost* **52:**217, 1984.
541. Meade TW, Stirling Y, Wilkes H, Mannucci PM: Effects of oral contraceptives and obesity on protein C antigen. *Thromb Haemost* **53:**198, 1985.
542. Kluft C, Bertina RM, Preston FE, Malia RG, Blamey SL, Lowe GDO, Forbes CF: Protein C, an anticoagulant protein, is increased in healthy volunteers and surgical patients after treatment with stanozolol. *Thromb Res* **33:**297, 1984.
543. Thorisdottir H, Evans JA, Schwartz HJ, Comp P, Haluschak J, Ratnoff OD: Some clotting factors in plasma during danazol therapy: Free and total protein S, but not C4b-binding protein, are elevated by danazol therapy. *J Lab Clin Med* **119:**698, 1992.
544. Marlar RA: Protein C in thromboembolic disease. *Semin Thromb Hemost* **11:**387, 1985.
545. Gladson CL, Scharrer I, Hach V, Beck KH, Griffin JH: The frequency of type I heterozygous protein S and protein C deficiency in 141 unrelated young patients with venous thrombosis. *Thromb Haemost* **59:**18, 1988.
546. Ben-Tal O, Zivelin A, Seligsohn U: The relative frequency of hereditary thrombotic disorders among 107 patients with thrombophilia in Israel. *Thromb Haemost* **61:**50, 1989.
547. Green D, Ganger DR, Blei AT: Protein C deficiency in splanchnic venous thrombosis. *Am J Med* **82:**1171, 1987.
548. Orozco H, Guraieb E, Takahashi T, Garcia-Tsao G, Hurtado R, Anaya R, Ruiz-Arguelles G, Hernandez-Ortiz J, Casillas MA, Guevara L: Deficiency of protein C in patients with portal vein thrombosis. *Hepatology* **8:**1110, 1988.
549. Wintzen AR, Broekmans AW, Bertina RM, Briët PE, Zecha A, Vielvoye GJ, Bots STAM: Cerebral hemorrhagic infarction in young patients with hereditary protein C deficiency: Evidence for "spontaneous" cerebral venous thrombosis. *Br Med J* **290:**350, 1985.
550. Camerlingo M, Finazzi G, Casto L, Laffranchi C, Barbui T, Mamoli A: Inherited protein C deficiency and nonhemorrhagic arterial stroke in young adults. *Neurology* **41:**1371, 1991.
551. De Stefano V, Leone G, Micalizzi P, Teofili L, Falappa PG, Pollari G, Bizzi B: Arterial thrombosis as clinical manifestation of congenital protein C deficiency. *Ann Hematol* **62:**180, 1991.
552. Broekmans AW, Bertina RM, Loeliger EA, Hofmann V, Klingemann HG: Protein C and the development of skin necrosis during anticoagulant therapy. *Thromb Haemost* **49:**251, 1983.
553. McGehee WG, Klotz TA, Epstein DJ, Rapaport SI: Coumarin necrosis associated with hereditary protein C deficiency. *Ann Intern Med* **101:**59, 1984.
554. Miletich J, Sherman L, Broze G Jr: Absence of thrombosis in subjects with heterozygous protein C deficiency. *N Engl J Med* **317:**991, 1987.
555. Bovill EG, Bauer KA, Dickerman JD, Callas P, West B: The clinical spectrum of heterozygous protein C deficiency in a large New England kindred. *Blood* **73:**712, 1989.
556. Bernardi F, Patracchini P, Gemmati D, Boninsegna S, Guerra S, Legnani C, Ballerini G, Marchetti G: Rapid detection of a protein C gene mutation present in the asymptomatic and not in the thrombosis-prone lineage. *Br J Haematol* **81:**277, 1992.
557. Marlar RA, Montgomery RR, Broekmans AW, the Working Party: Diagnosis and treatment of homozygous protein C deficiency. Report of the Working Party on Homozygous Protein C Deficiency of the Subcommittee on Protein C and Protein S, International Committee on Thrombosis and Haemostasis. *J Pediatr* **114:**528, 1989.
558. Marlar RA, Neumann A: Neonatal purpura fulminans due to homozygous protein C or protein S deficiencies. *Semin Thromb Hemost* **16:**299, 1990.
559. Sharon C, Tirindelli MC, Mannucci PM, Tripodi A, Mariani G: Homozygous protein C deficiency with moderately severe clinical symptoms. *Thromb Res* **41:**483, 1986.
560. Melissar E, Kakkar VV: Congenital severe protein C deficiency in adults. *Br J Haematol* **72:**222, 1989.
561. Tripodi A, Franchi F, Krachmalnicoff A, Mannucci PM: Asymptomatic homozygous protein C deficiency. *Acta Haematol* **82:**152, 1990.
562. Dreyfus M, Magny JF, Bridey F, Schwarz HP, Planché C, Dehan M, Tchernia G: Treatment of homozygous protein C deficiency and neonatal purpura fulminans with a purified protein C concentrate. *N Engl J Med* **325:**1565, 1991.
563. Manco-Johnson M, Nuss R: Protein C concentrate prevents peripartum thrombosis. *Am J Hematol* **40:**69, 1992.
564. Thompson AR: Molecular genetics of hemostatic proteins, in Colman RW, Hirsh J, Marder VJ, Salzman EW (eds): *Hemostasis and Thrombosis: Basic Principles and Clinical Practice*, 3d ed. Philadelphia, Lippincott, 1994, chap 3, pp 55–80.
565. Yamamoto K, Matsushita T, Sugiura I, Takamatsu J, Iwasaki E, Wada H, Deguchi K, Shirakawa S, Saito H: Homozygous protein C deficiency: Identification of a novel missense mutation that causes impaired secretion of the mutant protein C. *J Lab Clin Med* **119:**682, 1992.
566. Sugahara Y, Miura O, Yuen P, Aoki N: Protein C deficiency Hong Kong 1 and 2: Hereditary protein C deficiency caused by two mutant alleles, a 5-nucleotide deletion and a missense mutation. *Blood* **80:**126, 1992.

567. Matsuda M, Sugo T, Sakata Y, Murayama H, Mimuro J, Tanabe S, Yoshitake S: A thrombotic state due to an abnormal protein C. *N Engl J Med* **319:**1265, 1988.
568. Bovill EG, Tomczak JA, Grant B, Bhushan F, Pillemer E, Rainville IR, Long GL: Protein $C_{VERMONT}$: Symptomatic type II protein C deficiency associated with two GLA domain mutations. *Blood* **79:**1456, 1992.
569. Comp P, Esmon CT: Recurrent venous thromboembolism in patients with a partial deficiency of protein S. *N Engl J Med* **311:**1525, 1984.
570. Schwarz HP, Fisher M, Hopmeier P, Batard MA, Griffin JH: Plasma protein S deficiency in familial thrombotic disease. *Blood* **64:**1297, 1984.
571. Szatkowski NS, Miller CM, Endres-Brooks JL, Madden RM, Marlar RA: Clinical studies of human protein S and identification of a patient with protein S deficiency and thrombotic complication. *Circulation* **70(II):**204, 1984.
572. Engesser L, Broekmans AW, Briët E, Brommer EJP, Bertina RM: Hereditary protein S deficiency: Clinical manifestation. *Ann Intern Med* **106:**677, 1987.
573. Girolami A, Simioni P, Lazzaro AR, Cordiano I: Severe arterial cerebral thrombosis in a patient with protein S deficiency (moderately reduced total and markedly reduced free protein S): A family study. *Thromb Haemost* **61:**144, 1989.
574. Sié P, Boneu B, Biermé R, Wiesel ML, Grunebaum L, Cazenave JP: Arterial thrombosis and protein S deficiency. *Thromb Haemost* **62:**1040, 1989.
575. Friedman KD, Marlar RA, Houston JG, Montgomery RR: Warfarin-induced skin necrosis in a patient with protein S deficiency. *Blood* **68:**333a, 1986.
576. Grimaudo V, Gueissaz F, Hauert J, Sarraj A, Kruithof EKO, Bachmann F: Necrosis of skin induced by coumarin in a patient deficient in protein S. *Br Med J* **298:**233, 1989.
577. Mahasandana C, Suvatte V, Marlar RA, Manco-Johnson M, Jacobson L, Hathaway HE: Neonatal purpura fulminans associated with homozygous protein S deficiency. *Lancet* **335:**61, 1990.
578. Dahlback B: Purification of human vitamin K-dependent protein S and its limited proteolysis by thrombin. *Biochem J* **209:**837, 1983.
579. Boerger LM, Morris PC, Thurnau GR, Esmon CT, Comp PC: Oral contraceptives and gender affect protein S status. *Blood* **69:**692, 1987.
580. Edson JR, Vogt JM, Huesman DA: Laboratory diagnosis of inherited protein S deficiency. *Am J Clin Pathol* **94:**176, 1990.
581. Chafa O, Fischer AM, Meriane F, Chellali F, Rahal S, Sternberg C, Benabadji M: A new case of 'type II' inherited protein S deficiency. *Br J Haematol* **73:**501, 1989.
582. Mannucci PM, Valsecchi C, Krachmalnicoff A, Faioni EM, Tripodi A: Familial dysfunction of protein S. *Thromb Haemost* **62:**763, 1989.
583. Comp PC, Thurnau GR, Welsh J, Esom CT: Function and immunologic protein S levels are decreased during pregnancy. *Blood* **68:**881, 1986.
584. Malm J, Laurell M, Dahlback B: Changes in the plasma levels of vitamin K-dependent proteins C and S and of C4b-binding protein during pregnancy and oral contraception. *Br J Haematol* **68:**437, 1988.
585. D'Angelo A, Vigano-D'Angelo S, Esmon CT, Comp PC: Acquired deficiencies of protein S: Protein S activity during oral anticoagulation, in liver disease and in disseminated intravascular coagulation. *J Clin Invest* **81:**1445, 1988.
586. Schwarz HP, Schernthaner G, Griffin JH: Decreased plasma levels of protein S in well-controlled type I diabetes mellitus (letter). *Thromb Haemost* **57:**240, 1987.
587. Heeb MJ, Mosher D, Griffin JH: Activation and complexation of protein C and cleavage and decrease of protein S in plasma of patients with intravascular coagulation. *Blood* **73:**455, 1989.
588. Friedman KD, Marlar RA, Gill JC, Endres-Brooks J, Montgomery RR: Protein S deficiency in patients with lupus anticoagulant. *Blood (suppl)* **68:**333a, 1986.
589. Greaves M, Malia RG, Cooper P, Preston FE: Reduced free protein S in patients with lupus anticoagulant. *Br J Haematol* **69:**81, 1988.
590. Moreb J, Kitchens CS: Acquired functional protein S deficiency, cerebral venous thrombosis, and coumarin skin necrosis in association with antiphospholipid syndrome: Report of two cases. *Am J Med* **87:**207, 1989.
591. Parke JL, Weinstein RE, Bona RD, Maier DB, Walker FJ: The thrombotic diathesis associated with the presence of phospholipid antibodies may be due to low levels of free protein S. *Am J Med* **93:**49, 1992.
592. Bissuel F, Berruyer M, Causse X, Dechavanne M, Trepo C: Acquired protein S deficiency: Correlation with advanced disease in HIV-1-infected patients. *J Acquir Immune Defic Syndr* **5:**484, 1992.
593. Culpepper RM, Carr ME: Case Report: A novel form of free protein S deficiency in an HIV-positive patient on hemodialysis. *Am J Med Sci* **303:**403, 1992.
594. Bona RD, Weinstein RE, Walker FJ: Pseudo protein S deficiency due to a defect in C4BP. *Blood* **76:**500a, 1990.
595. Stankiewicz AJ, Steiner M, Lally EV, Kaplan SR: Abnormally high level of C4b binding protein and deficiency of free fraction of protein S in a patient with systemic lupus erythematosus and recurrent thromboses. *J Rheumatol* **18:**82, 1991.
596. Comp PC, Forristall J, West CD, Trapp RG: Free protein S levels are elevated in familial C4b-binding protein deficiency. *Blood* **76:**2527, 1990.
597. Ploos van Amstel HK, Huisman MV, Reitsma PH, Wouter ten Cate J, Bertina RM: Partial protein S gene deletion in a family with hereditary thrombophilia. *Blood* **73:**479, 1989.
598. Schmidel DK, Nelson RM, Broxson EH Jr, Comp PC, Marlar RA, Long GL: A 5.3-kb deletion including exon XIII of the protein S alpha gene occurs in two protein S-deficient families. *Blood* **77:**551, 1991.
599. Bertina RM, Ploos van Amstel HK, van Wijngaarden A, Coenen J, Leemhuis MP, Deutz-Terlouw PP, van der Linden IK, Reitsma PH: Heerlen polymorphism of protein S, an immunologic polymorphism due to dimorphism of residue 460. *Blood* **76:**538, 1990.

CHAPTER 105

Hereditary Disorders of Fibrinogen and Factor XIII

Dominic W. Chung ▪ Akitada Ichinose

1. Fibrinogen is a dimeric protein consisting of six polypeptide chains ($\alpha_2\beta_2\gamma_2$) held together by disulfide bonds and folded in a trinodular structure in which the globular nodules are connected by triple-stranded α helixes. Fibrinogen is converted to fibrin by thrombin, which removes fibrinopeptides from the α and β chains. Fibrin monomers polymerize into protofibrils through reciprocal half-staggered interactions. Protofibrils form macroscopic fibers through lateral aggregation and branch point formation. Fibrinogen binds to the integrin glycoprotein IIb-IIIa on activated platelets and is essential for platelet aggregation. The genes for the constituent chains of fibrinogen are linked and are located on chromosome 4. Fibrinogen genes are regulated by glucocorticoids and interleukin 6. High circulating levels of fibrinogen are associated with an increased risk of myocardial infarction and stroke.

2. Genetic abnormalities of fibrinogen are rare and include afibrinogenemia, hypofibrinogenemia, and dysfibrinogenemia, which refer to the complete absence of fibrinogen, reduced amounts of plasma fibrinogen, or the presence of dysfunctional fibrinogen molecules, respectively. Afibrinogenemia is characterized by neonatal umbilical cord hemorrhage, ecchymoses, mucosal hemorrhage, internal hemorrhage, recurrent abortion, and autosomal recessive inheritance. Hypofibrinogenemia is characterized by fibrinogen levels below 100 mg per deciliter of plasma (normal 250 to 350 mg/dl) and can be inherited or acquired. The symptoms in hypofibrinogenemia are similar but milder than for afibrinogenemia. Dysfibrinogenemia is highly heterogeneous and may affect any one of the functional properties of fibrinogen leading to various manifestations that include hemorrhage, spontaneous abortion, and thromboembolism. Most cases of dysfibrinogenemia are heterozygous for amino acid substitutions; homozygous occurrence is rare but known.

3. Factor XIII is a proenzyme for a plasma transglutaminase. It is converted to the active form, factor XIIIa, by thrombin in the presence of calcium ions. It catalyzes the formation of γ-glutamyl–ε-lysine bonds between fibrin monomers and between fibrin and α-$_2$-plasmin inhibitor. Factor XIII in plasma is a tetramer (a_2b_2) held together by noncovalent bonds. The a subunit contains the active site and the b subunit is thought to stabilize the a subunit. The sequence around the active site is identical among all members of the transglutaminase family. The b subunit contains 10 tandem repeats, which have been designated as Sushi domains or GP-I structures. Homologous Sushi domains have been found in 25 other proteins/genes. The a subunit of plasma factor XIII is synthesized at least in part by hemopoietic cells, whereas the a subunit is also present in many tissues. The site of synthesis for the b subunit is the liver.

4. The genes for the a and b subunits of factor XIII are localized at 6p24-p25 and 1q32-q32.1, respectively. Thus, factor XIII deficiency is inherited as an autosomal recessive trait and is caused by the absence of either subunit. Genetic defects have been identified at the DNA level in several patients with either a or b subunit deficiency. This disease is characterized by delayed bleeding, although primary hemostasis is normal. Manifestations include neonatal bleeding from the umbilical cord after birth, intracranial hemorrhage, and soft-tissue hematomas. In addition, abnormal wound healing and recurrent spontaneous abortion are not uncommon. Infusion of factor XIII concentrates has been successful both for treatment of acute bleeding and for prophylaxis.

FIBRINOGEN

Fibrinogen participates in two crucial events in hemostasis. It is an adhesive protein essential for platelet aggregation and platelet plug formation that reduces or temporarily stops the loss of blood at the site of vascular damage. On the surface of the activated platelets, a series of zymogen activations are triggered that culminates in the formation of thrombin. Thrombin catalyzes the conversion of soluble circulating fibrinogen to fibrin, resulting in an insoluble fibrin clot. The fibrin clot is further crosslinked by factor XIIIa (fibrin-stabilizing factor), which introduces a small number of covalent bonds between adjacent fibrin monomers, giving rise to a tough, insoluble clot. Congenital fibrinogen deficiency, which results in the complete absence of fibrinogen in the circulation (afibrinogenemia), is rare and is usually fatal. Individuals with reduced circulating levels (hypofibrinogenemia) may exhibit a predisposition to bleeding. Individuals with inherited structural defects in the fibrinogen molecule (dysfibrinogenemia) may be asymptomatic or exhibit hemorrhagic tendency, abnormal wound healing, or even thrombosis.

A list of standard abbreviations is located immediately preceding the index in each volume. Additional abbreviations used in this chapter include: DIC = disseminated intravascular coagulation; and tPA = tissue plasminogen activator.

Structure of Fibrinogen

Fibrinogen is a plasma glycoprotein of 340 kDa.[1,2] It is a dimeric protein composed of three pairs of nonidentical but homologous polypeptide chains held together by disulfide bonds. The polypeptide chains, designated as the α, β, and γ chains, are 63, 56, and 47 kDa, and fibrinogen can be represented by the formula $(\alpha\beta\gamma)_2$. At the final stage of blood coagulation, thrombin proteolytically removes fibrinopeptides A and B from the N-termini of the α and β chains.[3] The resultant molecule, a fibrin monomer, possesses new N-termini on the α and β chains, while the γ chains remain unchanged. The removal of the fibrinopeptides exposes polymerization sites that make it possible for the monomers to polymerize into insoluble fibrin composed of networks of fibers.

Fibrinogen exhibits properties of both globular and fibrous proteins; it contains globular domains as well as triple-stranded α helixes or "coiled coils."[4,5] These structural features are preserved in the molecule after conversion of fibrinogen to fibrin.

The amino acid sequences of the three chains of fibrinogen have been determined.[6–8] The sequences, although nonidentical, are homologous and are derived from a common ancestor. The α chain is composed of 610 amino acids and does not contain carbohydrate. The N-terminal 16 residues (1 to 16), fibrinopeptide A, are removed by thrombin during the conversion of fibrinogen to fibrin. Gly17 thus becomes the new N-terminal residue in the α chain of fibrin. The region from residue Cys45 to Cys165 forms part of the coiled coil and the associated flanking disulfide bonds with the β and γ chains. The sequence between residues 195 and 239 has a high proline content, suggesting that this region is folded into an exposed and vulnerable conformation, accessible to many proteases, including plasmin.[9,10] The region from residues 240 to 424 is exceptionally rich in glycine, serine, threonine, proline, and tryptophan residues and consists of eight tandem repeats, each 13 residues in length. These tandem repeat sequences and the remaining C-terminal sequence is hydrophilic and varies greatly among species.[11–14] Two Arg-Gly-Asp (RGD) sequences are present in the α chain. The proximal RGD sequence (95 to 97) occurs in the middle of the coiled-coil region, and the distal RGD sequence (572 to 574) is present in the C-terminal region and is not conserved among species.

The β chain of human fibrinogen contains 461 amino acids. The N-terminal 14 amino acids (1 to 14), fibrinopeptide B, is removed by thrombin during clotting, and Gly15 becomes the new N-terminus of the β chain of fibrin. The first 75 residues at the N-terminus show 15 percent identity to the corresponding region of the α chain. The region from Cys76 to Cys201 participates in disulfide-ring and coiled-coil formation. The remaining sequence (202 to 461) apparently folds into a globular domain. Asn364 is the only site for *N*-linked carbohydrate attachment on the β chain.

The γ chain is 411 amino acids in length. It does not contain sequences removed by thrombin during clotting. The N-terminal region (1 to 18) preceding the coiled-coil region and the flanking disulfide rings (19 to 139) is significantly shorter than that of the α and β chains. A single *N*-linked carbohydrate attachment site has been identified in the middle of the coiled-coil region at Asn52. The C-terminal half (140 to 411) of the γ chain is 35 percent identical to the corresponding region of the β chain and apparently folds into a globular structure. The γ chain appears to have gained a C-terminal extension of 18 amino acids that participates in intermolecular crosslinking. The β chain is devoid of such sequences and does not participate in the crosslinking process.

A naturally occurring variant of the γ chain, referred to as γ′ or γ_B, has a higher molecular weight than γ. Amino acid sequencing shows that in the γ′ form, the C-terminal four amino acids are replaced by a sequence of 20 amino acids.[15,16] Hence, the γ′ form is not a precursor to the γ form. Studies of the cDNA and gene structure show that the two forms arise by alternative processing of the γ-chain transcript. Use of an alternative polyadenylation site in the ninth intron removes the 3′ acceptor site of this intron and the following tenth exon that encodes the last four amino acids (408 to 411) of the γ chain. This infrequent polyadenylation event enables the immediate 5′ end of the ninth intron to serve as an extension of the ninth exon. Translation of this mRNA leads to the replacement of residues 408 to 411 by a peptide of 20 amino acids (γ′ 408 to 427).[17,18] In humans, the γ′ form amounts to ~10 percent of the total γ-chain population.[19] In rats, the γ′ form constitutes ~30 percent of the total γ chain.[20] Both polypeptides are assembled into the dimeric fibrinogen molecule and function normally in fibrin polymerization and in γ-chain crosslinking.

Electron microscopic studies[21] provide evidence that fibrinogen is folded into a trinodular structure connected by coiled coils (Fig. 105-1). The central globular nodule (E domain or fragment E) is approximately 50 Å in diameter and is comprised of the N-termini of all six polypeptide chains.[22] The two outer globular nodules (D domains or fragment D) are approximately 60 Å in diameter and are made up of the C-terminal two thirds of the β and γ chains.[23,24] The three domains are linked by triple-stranded α helixes or coiled coils, formed by the folding of stretches of 111 or 112 amino acids from each of the three polypeptide chains.[25] The coiled coils are flanked on both sides by a characteristic arrangement of disulfide bonds called the "disulfide rings" that hold the three strands in alignment for the formation of triple-stranded helixes. The amino acid sequences of the coiled-coil region from each chain consist of alternating polar and nonpolar clusters and are extremely low in proline content. This composition favors the formation of helixes. The coiled-coil region is briefly interrupted in the middle by a short region of nonhelical structure, which has been implicated as a region sensitive to proteolytic cleavages. The coiled coils are approximately 150 to 160 Å in length.

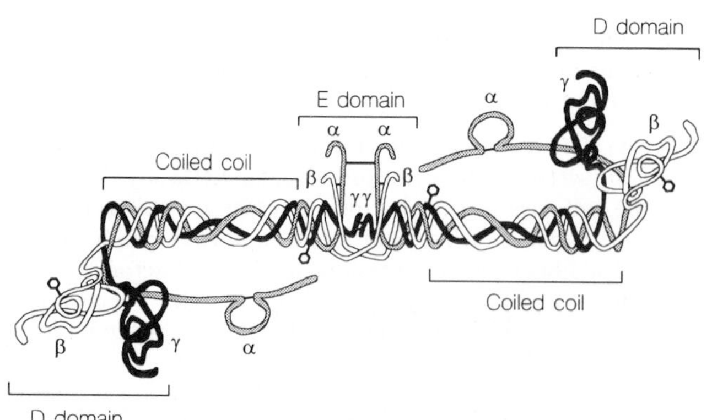

FIG. 105-1 **Schematic representation of fibrinogen. The molecule is depicted in a trinodular structure containing a central nodule, the E domain, connected to two outer nodules, the D domains, by triple-stranded α helixes designated as coiled coils. *N*-linked carbohydrate chains are represented by open hexagons.**

The overall length of the trinodular structure is approximately 450 Å. The disulfide rings and the coiled coils impart rigidity and mechanical strength to the molecule. The C-terminal half of the α chain folds into an extended domain around the coiled coils.

Fibrinogen isolated from plasma is heterogeneous; the heterogeneity is attributed to the varying extent of proteolysis in the C-terminus of the α chain.[26] Fibrinogen II, a fraction of 305 kDa, has been isolated and analyzed in detail. The level of this species increases in patients with progressive liver diseases and occlusive vascular diseases. This species is composed of two types of α chains: a normal homogeneous intact α-chain population and a second population (α′) that has been proteolytically cleaved to terminate predominantly at Asn269, Gly297, or Pro309.[27] These cleavage-site sequences bear no resemblance to plasmin-specific cleavage sites. The identity of the proteases responsible for these cleavages remains to be determined.

The structure of carbohydrate attached to β Asn364 and γ Asn52 has been studied by proton-NMR techniques in conjunction with sequential exoglycosidase digestions.[28] The carbohydrate chains on each polypeptide are identical in structure and contain a core pentasaccharide with biantennary oligosaccharide branch points. Approximately 20 percent of the carbohydrate chains are desialylated. Increased sialic acid content in fibrinogen preparations from patients with inherited dysfibrinogenemia or chronic liver disease[29] usually causes delayed polymerization. Deglycosylation in vitro accelerates polymerization and increases lateral aggregation of fibrin fibers.[30]

Removal of Fibrinopeptides

The conversion of fibrinogen to fibrin can be divided into several stages. The process is initiated by thrombin, which specifically cleaves at Arg-Gly bonds close to the N-termini of the α and β chains to release two molecules of fibrinopeptide A (α1 to α16) and two molecules of fibrinopeptide B (β1 to β14) per molecule of fibrinogen. The release of fibrinopeptide A proceeeds more rapidly than that of fibrinopeptide B,[31] but the release of fibrinopeptide A is not a prerequisite for the removal of fibrinopeptide B. Removal of fibrinopeptide A exposes a new N-terminal sequence, Gly-Pro-Arg, on the α chain and is sufficient to initiate polymerization. Assembly into a polymeric form induces conformational changes in the molecule that enhance the rate of fibrinopeptide B release.[32] In addition to thrombin, several snake venom enzymes have been shown to remove fibrinopeptides from fibrinogen. Batroxobin (reptilase), isolated from the venom of *Bothrops atrox* and ancrod (arvin), from *Agkistrodon rhodostoma*, exclusively remove fibrinopeptide A from fibrinogen.[33,34] A different enzyme from the venom of *Agkistrodon contortrix contortrix* preferentially releases fibrinopeptide B but also releases fibrinopeptide A slowly.[35,36]

Protofibril Assembly

The removal of fibrinopeptide A exposes new N-termini on the α chains with the sequence of Gly-Pro-Arg, and these termini interact with complementary sites on the D domain of a second fibrin monomer. The N-terminus of the α chain of the second molecule binds in a reciprocal manner to the D domain of the first molecule (Fig. 105-2). This reciprocal binding positions the two molecules in a half-staggered overlap structure.[37] The addition of a third molecule and

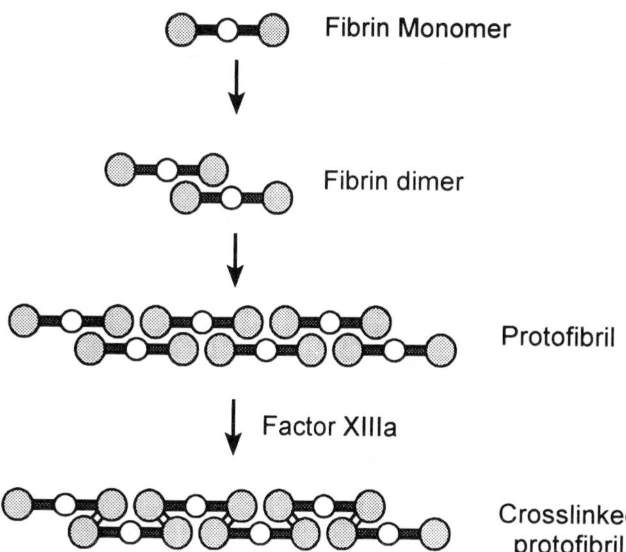

FIG. 105-2 **Polymerization and crosslinking of fibrin. Fibrin monomers polymerize into fibrin protofibrils by half-staggered interactions. Covalent crosslinks between γ chains of adjacent fibrin molecules are introduced by factor XIIIa.**

subsequent linear elongation align the D domains of adjacent fibrin monomers next to each other, and bring together "end-to-end" contacts between adjacent fibrin monomers. The two-stranded linear polymer structure composed of two rows of end-to-end monomers is called a "protofibril," and is an obligatory intermediate in fibrin assembly under physiological conditions.[38,39] A tripeptide with a sequence identical to the N-terminus of the fibrin α chain (Gly-Pro-Arg) can bind to the γ chain in the D domains of fibrinogen and fibrin and is an effective inhibitor of protofibril elongation and fibrin polymerization.[40] The polymerization sites in the D domain are composed of the C-terminal globular domain of the γ chain. Photoaffinity labeling shows the primary fibrin polymerization site involves Tyr363 of the γ chain. Analysis of dysfunctional fibrinogens defective in polymerization also shows involvement of amino acids between Arg275 and Asp330. These results imply that the C-terminal region of the γ chain is essential in forming a polymerization pocket for the Gly-Pro-Arg sequence. Removal of fibrinopeptide B promotes branch point formation in protofibrils and allows protofibrils to associate laterally into thick fibrin strands.[37–40] The process of lateral aggregation is not well defined and is thought to include lateral D–D domain and D–E domain interactions.[41] A tripeptide with sequence identical to the N-terminus of the β chain (Gly-His-Pro) binds to the D domain but does not completely inhibit fibrin polymerization.[40,42] Selective removal of β-chain N-terminal residues 1 to 42 by protease III from the venom of *Crotalus atrox* results in a fibrinogen derivative without a removable fibrinopeptide B.[43] This species can be clotted by thrombin subsequent to the release of fibrinopeptide A. However, lateral aggregation of protofibrils and thickening of fiber bundles are severely impaired. Kinetic modeling and electron microscopic studies show that protofibrils must reach a minimum length of 10 to 20 monomers before lateral aggregation can occur, which is indicative of a process involving nucleation polymerization. This requirement indicates lateral aggregation needs the cumulative or cooperative effect of many weak interactions along the protofibrils of a minimum length. To simulate fiber diameters observed experimentally, it is also necessary to postulate that the addition of protofibrils to existing fibers is kinetically favored over initiation of new fibers. Similarly, addition of fibrin monomers to protofibrils leading to growth is favored over initiation of protofibrils.[44]

Crosslinking

Because the interactions among the individual fibrin monomers are noncovalent, a fibrin gel can be resolubilized by chemical agents such as 6 *M* urea. The fibrin clot is stabilized by the introduction of covalent bonds that crosslink individual fibrin molecules. The crosslinking reaction is catalyzed by a plasma transglutaminase, factor XIIIa. These covalent linkages, in the form of isopeptide bonds between glutamine and lysine residues, impart mechanical strength to the clot. The crosslinking reaction initially involves adjacent γ chains, where Lys406 of the γ chain from one fibrin molecule is crosslinked to the Gln398 or Gln399 of the γ chain of a second adjacent fibrin molecule and the Lys406 of the second molecule is reciprocally crosslinked to Gln398 or Gln399 of the first molecule.[45,46] This crosslinking leads to the formation of covalent γ-chain dimers. In a considerably slower process, multiple crosslinks among α chains involving Gln328, Gln366, Lys508, Lys556, and Lys562 are also introduced.[47–49] The presence of multiple acceptor and donor sites on each α chain leads to the formation of α-chain multimers that act as a "wraparound" of the coiled-coil regions and protect these regions from proteolytic attack.[50] In addition to these two major types of crosslinks, the presence of crosslinked γ trimers and tetramers supports the proposal that these crosslinked molecules occur at protofibril branch points and interfibrillar junctions.[51] Other plasma proteins, α_2-plasmin inhibitor and fibronectin, are also crosslinked to the α chain.

Degradation of Fibrin

After a fibrin clot is formed at the site of vascular injury, tissue remodeling and regeneration eventually lead to repair of the damaged vessels. The fibrin clot is then removed by plasmin. The folding of fibrinogen and fibrin into an extended trinodular structure predisposes the molecule to proteolytic attack in the exposed coiled-coil regions. Initially, the multiple crosslinked α chains are removed, exposing the connecting coiled-coil regions betwen D and E domains. Further cleavage in the coiled-coil region between the D and E domains ultimately releases DD-E (D dimer E) complexes that consist of crosslinked D domains and a noncovalently bound E domain.[52,116]

Platelet Aggregation

Platelet aggregation is mediated by the binding of fibrinogen to the platelet surface receptor glycoprotein IIb-IIIa (GPIIb-IIIa), which is a member of the integrin family of receptors.[52] This binding can be competitively inhibited by RGD-containing peptides and a peptide containing the C-terminal 12 amino acids of the γ chain (γ400 to γ411, HHLGGAK-QAGDV).[53,54] These findings suggest that the platelet binding site on fibrinogen is either located at the C-terminus of the γ chain or at the two RGD sequences in the α chain (α95 to α97 and α572 to α574). Studies on recombinant fibrinogens containing an RGD to RGE mutation at either position α97 or α574, and a variant fibrinogen containing two γ′ chains show that the homodimeric γ′ variant is markedly defective in platelet aggregation despite the presence of intact RGD sites in the α chain.[55] Fibrinogens with RGE mutations in the α chain are functionally indistinguishable from normal fibrinogen in platelet aggregation. These results support the proposal that the C-terminal region of the γ chain is essential for platelet aggregation. Effective competition by RGD-containing peptides probably reflects a similarity in conformation of RGD peptides and the γ C-terminus sequence. Although the two RGD sequences in fibrinogen are not essential for binding to GPIIb-IIIa, they may be important in binding to other receptors of the integrin family. Consistent with the γ-chain terminal sequence as the primary site for platelet binding, electron micrographs show that GPIIb-IIIa binds to fibrinogen at the two outer nodules or D domains in which the C-termini of the γ chains are located.[56]

Interaction with Other Molecules

Fibrinogen contains three calcium-binding sites. Two of these sites are localized in the D domain and involve γ-chain residues 311 to 336, which bear sequence resemblance to the calcium-binding regions of calmodulin.[57] A third binding site is located within the E domain.[58] Calcium binding enhances lateral association of protofibrils and renders the γ chain resistant to proteolysis by plasmin.[59] Substitution of γ chain Arg375 by Gly in fibrinogen Osaka V[60] and deletion of γ-chain residues 319 to 320 in fibrinogen Vlissingen[61] show defective calcium binding and delayed fibrin polymerization.

In addition to the removal of fibrinopeptides from fibrinogen, thrombin specifically binds to fibrin at a nonsubstrate site in the E domain composed of sequences from α17 to α51, β51 to β118 and γ1 to γ53.[62] There is apparently less than one (0.4) binding site per molecule of fibrin. Bound thrombin retains enzymatic activity and is protected from inactivation by circulating inhibitors and is released in an active form following fibrinolysis.[63] This nonsubstrate binding is physiologically important in limiting the diffusion of thrombin from the site of fibrin clot formation. A dysfunctional fibrinogen with a β-chain deletion of amino acids 9 to 72, fibrinogen New York I, fails to bind thrombin and is associated with recurrent thromboembolism.[64]

Fibrinogen circulates as a complex with factor XIII; this interaction involves regions of the α and β chains in the D domain.[65] Activation of factor XIII to factor XIIIa by thrombin and dissociation of b subunits is enhanced by polymerized fibrin. However, crosslinked fibrin does not promote factor XIIIa activation.

The α_2-plasmin inhibitor is a major inhibitor of plasmin and tissue plasminogen activator (tPA). A small but significant amount (20 percent of α_2-plasmin inhibitor is crosslinked to Lys303 of the α chain of fibrinogen or fibrin by factor XIIIa.[66] The α_2-plasmin inhibitor bound to fibrin prevents and delays the initiation of fibrinolysis. Congenital α_2-plasmin inhibitor deficiency results in a severe hemorrhagic disorder characterized by reduced resistance of fibrin clots to lysis.[67]

Fibrin binds to tPA and enhances the rate of tPA-catalyzed plasminogen activation. This cofactor effect is unmasked only when fibrinogen is converted to fibrin. Two regions of the molecule, accessible to monoclonal antibodies only after conversion of fibrin, are responsible for high-affinity binding to tPA. These two sites are localized to α148 to α160 and γ311 to γ379; the disulfide bond between γ Cys326 and γ Cys339 is essential for tPA binding and cofactor activity.[68]

Plasminogen binds weakly to fibrinogen ($K_d \sim 1 \times 10^{-3}$ M),[69] but binds fibrin with high affinity ($K_d \sim 1 \times 10^{-6}$ M). After fibrinolysis is initiated, plasmin progressively cleaves fibrin and generates peptide segments with C-terminal lysines that serve as additional binding sites for plasminogen. Recruitment of additional plasminogen to partially degraded fibrin further promotes clot lysis.[70]

Fibrinogen binds to and coprecipitates with fibronectin as a complex in the cold (cold-insoluble globulin). This binding is mediated through sites on the α chain.[71] Under physiological conditions, fibronectin is incorporated into the fibrin clot and is crosslinked to lysine residues in the α chain of fibrin by factor XIIIa.[72] Crosslinking of fibronectin to fibrin greatly enhances the attachment and spreading of cells on a fibrin-coated surface and may be important for the adhesion and migration of fibroblasts, endothelial cells, and monocytes at the site of a fibrin clot.

Fibrinogen is mitogenic for hemopoietic cells such as early bone marrow progenitor cells or lymphoma-derived cell lines such as Raji or JM cells. This mitogenic effect is mediated by a low-affinity receptor on these cells that is distinctly different from GPIIb-IIIa. Affinity chromatography and chemical crosslinking studies show this receptor is 94 kDa, and its binding to fibrinogen is not inhibited by RGD-containing peptides or by a monoclonal antibody against the γ chain C-terminus. Binding is apparently mediated by other regions of the D domain.[73,74]

Biosynthesis of Fibrinogen

Gene Structure. Fibrinogen is synthesized in the liver by hepatic parenchymal cells and is secreted into the circulation and maintained at a level of ~250 to 350 mg/dl.[75] The amount of fibrinogen synthesized ranges from 1.7 to 5 g/day, and the half-life in plasma is approximately 3 to 5 days.[76,77] The three chains of fibrinogen are encoded by three single-copy genes that are linked in a cluster located at chromosome 4q23-q32.[78,79] The three genes extend over approximately 45 kb and are arranged in the order of γ-α-β, with the genes for the γ and α chains transcribed in the same direction and the gene for the β chain transcribed in the opposite direction.[79]

Similarity in sequence and conservation in exon organization provide evidence that the three genes are derived from a common ancestor.[80] Studies of a rare α-chain transcript show the presence of an additional 3′ exon (exon 6) with high sequence identity of the γ chain.[81] These results support the proposal that in the evolution of the α-chain gene an insertion was introduced that was subsequently recruited to become an exon. This insertion displaces the original exon sequences that bear high sequence identity to the γ chain further in the 3′ direction. This additional exon is expressed at a low frequency in liver as an extended α chain of 100 kDa. The function of this extended α-chain variant is unclear.

Assembly. Analysis of isotope uptake in whole animals and in cultured hepatocytes[82,83] shows the presence of an existing pool of α and γ chains in the cell. The sequence of fibrinogen chain assembly was studied in HepG2 cells and in baby hamster kidney cells transfected with combinations of human fibrinogen cDNAs.[84] Assembly apparently begins with a γ chain combining with either a β or an α chain to form heterodimeric αγ, or βγ intermediates. Subsequently, a third β or α chain is added to these intermediates to form half molecules consisting of one α, one β, and one γ chain (αβγ). Half molecules dimerize in the last step to yield fully assembled fibrinogen molecules, which are then secreted into circulation. Dimerization of two half molecules involves the formation of five disulfide bonds in the E domain. These include the two reciprocal disulfide bonds between γ Cys8 in one half molecule with γ Cys9 in the complementary half molecule, one disulfide bond between α Cys28 in one half and the corresponding α Cys28 in the second half, and two reciprocal disulfide bonds between α Cys36 in one half molecule to β Cys65 in the complementary half molecule.[85] Partially assembled fibrinogen intermediates accumulate intracellularly and are not secreted, except the αγ complex, which is secreted at a low level both by HepG2 cells and transfected baby hamster kidney cells.

Platelet Fibrinogen. Fibrinogen is present in the α granules of platelets in which it constitutes ~15 percent of the protein content.[86] Platelet fibrinogen lacks the γ′ variant form,[87] and its origin is controversial. Some evidence has shown that megakaryocytes and platelets can directly endocytose and incorporate plasma fibrinogen into α granules.[88,89] Although the mechanism is unclear, uptake may involve a receptor on megakaryocytes and unstimulated platelets. In Glanzmann thrombasthenia patients who have a deficiency of GPIIb-IIIa, an unexplained deficiency of platelet fibrinogen was also observed.[90] Uptake of fibrinogen into α granules from plasma was readily demonstrated in an afibrinogenemic patient within 24 h after cryoprecipitate infusion.[91] The sensitive technique, RT-PCR, fails to detect transcripts for any of the three chains of fibrinogen in megakaryocytes,[92] suggesting that platelet fibrinogen is not synthesized in megakaryocytes. Furthermore, rat platelets matured under a defibrinated state maintained by injection of ancrod contain only trace amounts of fibrinogen in the α granules.[93]

Regulation. Fibrinogen synthesis is liver-specific and occurs constitutively. Extrahepatic transcription of the γ chain has been detected in bone marrow, lung, and brain.[94] However, in the absence of α- and β-chain transcripts, no functional fibrinogen is derived from these tissues. It is unclear if the γ-chain transcript is translated or if this polypeptide is incorporated into other protein complexes. The gene for the γ chain contains a 12 bp sequence in the 5′ flanking region that shows high affinity for a ubiquitous transcription factor, the major late transcription factor (MLTF). This sequence may be responsible for nonhepatic transcription.[95] Liver-specific transcription of the genes for the α and β chains is attributed to the presence of the regulatory sequence ATTAAC that interacts with the liver-specific transcription factor hepatocyte nuclear factor 1 (HNF1).[96]

As an acute-phase protein, the level of fibrinogen in circulation rises in response to trauma and inflammation. Massive defibrination and exposure to fibrinogen degradation products, fragments D and E, lead to a fourfold to sevenfold increase in fibrinogen synthesis in the liver.[97] Exposure of peripheral blood leukocytes (including monocytes and macrophages) to fibrinogen degradation product fragment D causes these cells to release the cytokine interleukin 6 (IL-6), which in turn stimulates fibrinogen synthesis in hepatocytes. The response of hepatocytes to IL-6 is mediated through the IL-6 receptor,[98] which is composed of two functionally different transmembrane subunits, a ligand-binding subunit (IL-6R) and a signal-transducing subunit (gp130). IL-6 binding to the receptor triggers tyrosine phosphorylation of gp130, and through unidentified intermediary steps, leads to serine phosphorylation and activation of transcription factor NF-IL.[99] Okadaic acid, a specific inhibitor of protein phosphatases 1 and 2A can overcome the effects of IL-6 induction, suggesting that activation of phosphatase 1 or 2A is also involved in signal transduction.[100] The effect of IL-6 on hepatocytes is dependent on the presence of glucocorticoids, which not only directly stimulate transcription, but also up-regulate the level of IL-6 receptors on the hepatocyte membrane.[101, 102] Reporter gene analysis of the 5′ flanking region of the β-chain gene identified a distal regulatory sequence (−1500 to −2900 bp from the transcription initiation site) involved in dexamethasone response. A separate IL-6 responsive sequence has also been identified at −82 to −150 bp in the β-chain gene.[101]

CLINICAL ABNORMALITIES OF FIBRINOGEN

Cardiovascular Risk Factor

As a consequence of the acute-phase response or through other unidentified mechanisms, elevated plasma fibrinogen levels have been observed in patients with coronary arterial disease, peripheral arterial disease, diabetes, hypertension, hyperlipoproteinemia, and hypertriglyceridemia. Oral contraceptives, pregnancy, menopause, smoking, and high plasma cholesterol levels also increase plasma fibrinogen levels. Clinical studies show that about half the patients who have ischemic heart disease have high plasma fibrinogen levels (>320 mg/dl). These observations also suggest that the atherogenic effects of smoking may be attributed to the fact that smoking raises fibrinogen levels.[103] It is possible that smoking stimulates macrophages in the lung to release IL-6 and chronically stimulates fibrinogen synthesis. These studies conclude that fibrinogen level is an independent risk factor for myocardial infarction and for stroke in men. Although not completely understood, elevated fibrinogen levels may contribute to these disease processes by promoting a state of platelet hyperaggregation, thrombosis, and atherogenesis.

Variations in plasma fibrinogen levels have been, in part, attributed to a nucleotide polymorphism in the 5′ flanking region of the gene for the β chain.[104] An *Hae*III restriction-length polymorphism (designation as H2 allele) located at −453 bp from the transcription initiation site of the β-chain gene shows a significant association with elevated levels of plasma fibrinogen. The effects of genotype and smoking on fibrinogen level are independent and additive. The association suggests the polymorphic base change may be involved, directly or through linkage disequilibrium, in transcription of the β chain gene.

Genetic Disorders of Fibrinogen

Congenital abnormalities of fibrinogen are rare and include afibrinogenemia, hypofibrinogenemia, and dysfibrinogenemia characterized, respectively, by the complete absence of fibrinogen, reduced amounts of fibrinogen, or the presence of dysfunctional fibrinogen molecules in circulation. A nomenclature similar to that for abnormal hemoglobins has been adopted, and dysfunctional fibrinogens are designated according to the city of origin of the patient, for example, fibrinogen Detroit, fibrinogen Paris I, fibrinogen Bethesda II, etc.

Afibrinogenemia. Afibrinogenemia was first reported in 1920, when the existence of other coagulation factors had not been discovered. The patient was anemic and suffered from repeated epistaxis and gingival bleeding.[105] Subsequent studies showed that afibrinogenemia corresponds to the homozygous state of an autosomal recessive disorder with phenotypic heterogeneity and is distinctly different from the hemophilias, which are X-linked disorders. To date, over 160 cases have been reported. The cardinal symptom is umbilical cord bleeding at birth followed by a lifelong predisposition to easy bruising, mucosal hemorrhage (especially epistaxis), prolonged bleeding from acute wounds and trauma, delayed wound healing, and sudden gastrointestinal bleeding. Uncontrollable internal bleeding, especially intracranial bleeding, is usually a fatal complication. Laboratory findings show that afibrinogenemic blood has an indefinitely prolonged clotting time while the levels of all other coagulation factors are within the normal range. Afibrinogenemia is usually accompanied by mild thrombocytopenia,[106] and platelets from afibrinogenemic patients show normal adhesion and spreading properties but defective aggregation. Because of the early onset and severity of the hemorrhages, few affected individuals survive beyond the age of 20. Therapy has mainly been focused on management of acute bleeding by infusion of fibrinogen-containing preparations, for example, whole blood, fresh frozen plasma, fibrinogen concentrate, or cryoprecipitate, aimed to bring the circulating fibrinogen level to 100 mg/dl. Afibrinogenemic children, especially those 1 to 3 years of age, have an increased incidence of bleeding following trauma and minor injuries and an increased risk of intracranial bleeding. In one report, prophylactic infusion of cryoprecipitate was effective.[107] In this report, weekly cryoprecipitate infusion was initiated at 12 months to achieve a circulating level of 150 mg/dl. At 24 months, infusions were reduced to once every 10 days. Infusion was discontinued at age 3 and was used only to control acute bleeding. Afibrinogenemic women present special complications of recurrent spontaneous abortions and postpartum hemorrhage. Without intervention, only one of eight pregnancies is successful. Successful pregnancies have been achieved by prophylactic infusion of fibrinogen to establish a stable level of 100 mg/dl through term.[108] Maintenance of fibrinogen at 40 and 50 mg/dl was not adequate to prevent miscarriage. These observations are consistent with the hypothesis that minute placental separations and hemorrhages occur in a normal pregnancy and are controlled by prompt conversion of maternal fibrinogen to fibrin.[109] In an afibrinogenemic patient, this normal function may be lacking.

Hypofibrinogenemia. Hypofibrinogenemia is a rare and heterogeneous disorder. It may be inherited as the heterozygous state of afibrinogenemia. Hypofibrinogenemia can roughly be categorized into two groups: fibrinogen levels below 50 mg/dl of plasma and levels between 50 and 100 mg/dl of plasma. Patients with fibrinogen levels below 50 mg/dl of plasma exhibit hemorrhagic symptoms resembling those of afibrinogenemia but occurring less frequently and with less severity. Umbilical cord bleeding occurs frequently (15 percent), and hemorrhage (especially cerebral hemorrhage) is a major cause of death.[110] Recurrent spontaneous abortion, placenta separation, and postpartum hemorrhage are frequent obstetric complications. In patients with fibrinogen levels between 50 and 100 mg/dl of plasma, symptoms are much milder. These patients are usually undiagnosed until routine preoperative hemostatic screening. Acute bleeding is treated by replacement therapy.

Dysfibrinogenemia. Several hundred cases of dysfunctional fibrinogen caused by mutations in one or more of the amino acids in the fibrinogen polypeptide chains have been described.[111] Depending on the locations of the amino acid changes, any one of the many functional properties of fibrinogen may be affected. Defective fibrinopeptide release, delayed polymerization, defective crosslinking, decreased thrombin binding, and defective secretion from hepatocytes have been described. The nature of the dysfunction causes varied manifestations, including hemorrhage, spontaneous abortion, thromboembolism, and thrombosis. Most reported cases of dysfibrinogenemia are heterozygous, with the mutations affecting approximately half of a polypeptide population. Since each fibrinogen molecule contains two of each chain, approximately 25 percent of the fibrinogen molecules are normal, 50 percent contain one defective and one normal chain, and 25 percent contain two defective chains. This distribution accounts for the usually mild and undetected symptoms in most cases of heterozygous dysfibrinogenemia. Elucidation of the precise amino acid changes have been useful in studying the structure and function relationships in fibrinogen. Frequently observed amino acid substitutions at and around the cleavage site of the α chain (e.g., α Arg16 → His, Asp7 → Asn, Gly12 → Val, Arg19 → Asn) abolish or delay fibrinopeptide A release.[112] Removal of amino acids 9 to 72 of the β chain (exon 2) abolishes fibrinopeptide B release and removes a putative thrombin-binding site in fibrin, resulting in recurrent thromboembolism.[64] Numerous mutations at the C-terminus of the γ chain (amino acids 275 to 375) affect fibrin polymerization and calcium binding. Attachment of an additional carbohydrate chain in this region of the γ chain caused by a mutation that creates a new N-linked attachment site[113] also impairs fibrin polymerization. Enhanced fibrin polymerization and enhanced binding to stimulated platelets are associated with a change in the β chain of fibrinogen Oslo I, although the precise amino acid substitution has not been identified.[114] Fibrinogen Paris I is characterized by delayed fibrin polymerization and defective γ chain crosslinking. The abnormal γ chain is longer than the normal γ chain and apparently contains inserted sequences at or around the crosslinking site.[115]

Acquired Abnormalities. Acquired fibrinogen abnormalities are usually associated with liver diseases, for example, cirrhosis, hepatitis, and hepatocarcinoma. The most common functional abnormality is delayed polymerization caused by an increase in carbohydrate content, particularly sialic acid. The additional carbohydrate probably occurs through additional branch points in the existing carbohydrate side chains on the β and γ chains. Treatment with neuraminidase in vitro restores the rate of polymerization to normal.

Hypofibrinogenemia may be acquired as a consequence of disseminated intravascular coagulation (DIC) in which fibrinogen, platelets, and other coagulation factors are being consumed in abnormal coagulation. Injury to the vascular endothelium—for example, infections and endotoxemia and tissue injury with the release of tissue factor—are major causes of DIC.[119] Snake bite and envenomation of proteases that directly activate or degrade fibrinogen can cause hypofibrinogenemia. Some venom proteases activate prothrombin and cause fibrinogen consumption indirectly. Similarly, thrombolytic therapy may cause systemic fibrinogenolysis leading to transient reductions in circulating fibrinogen levels.

Patients with multiple myeloma or Waldenström macroglobulinemia may show hemostatic abnormalities attributed to monoclonal plasma paraprotein inhibitors. The most commonly described paraprotein inhibitors are directed against fibrin, and these paraproteins inhibit fibrin polymerization, resulting in a clot with reduced opacity and poor clot retraction.[117, 118]

Fetal fibrinogen isolated from cord blood shows delayed fibrin aggregation and is different from adult plasma fibrinogen. The functional difference of fetal fibrinogen resembles fibrinogen associated with liver diseases and has been attributed, in part, to a high phosphate and sialic acid content. Delayed polymerization has also been attributed to the presence of trace amounts of fibrinogen degradation product in fetal fibrinogen preparations.[120]

FACTOR XIII

Factor XIII (fibrin stabilizing factor or fibrinoligase) is a plasma glycoprotein that plays an important role in the final stage of blood coagulation, in the regulation of fibrinolysis, and in tissue repair

Thrombin generated during blood coagulation converts the proenzyme (factor XIII) to an active enzyme (factor XIIIa) in the presence of calcium ions. Factor XIIIa is a transglutaminase that catalyzes the crosslinking of fibrin monomers and the crosslinking of fibrin and α_2-plasmin inhibitor through the formation of intermolecular γ-glutamyl-ϵ-lysine bonds. These reactions result in a fibrin with considerable physical strength and increased resistance to proteolytic degradation by plasmin. Crosslinking of fibronectin to fibrin or to collagen is also catalyzed by factor XIIIa, and this reaction appears to be related to wound healing.

Deficiency of factor XIII results in a severe lifelong bleeding tendency and defective wound healing in affected individuals, and habitual spontaneous abortion in affected females. Congenital deficiency is due to the absence of either the a or the b subunit of factor XIII. This disorder is inherited in an autosomal recessive manner. The genes coding for the a and b subunits exist on chromosomes 6 and 1, respectively. Disease-causative defects of these two genes have been identified in patients with factor XIII deficiency.

Structure of Factor XIII

Physical Properties. Factor XIII circulates in blood as a tetramer (Fig. 105-3), a_2b_2 (about 320 kDa), consisting of two a subunits (75 kDa each) and two b subunits (80 kDa each).[121,122] The molecular complex of four polypeptide chains is held together by noncovalent bonds.[121] The carbohydrate content has been reported to be 1.5 percent and 8.5 percent for the a and b subunits, respectively.[123,124] The a subunit

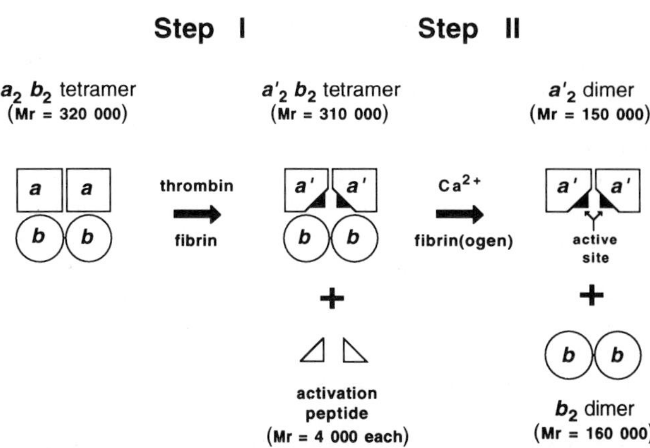

FIG. 105-3 Subunit structure and activation of factor XIII. The a subunits are indicated by squares, and the b subunits by circles. Active sites are shown by solid triangles. Fibrin acts as a cofactor for thrombin-catalyzed cleavage of the activation peptide (step I). Fibrin(ogen) promotes calcium-dependent dissociation of a'_2 and b_2 dimers and exposure of the active sites (step II).

has six free sulfhydryl groups, while the b subunit has no free sulfhydryl groups.[122] Factor XIII in plasma is in a complex with fibrinogen.[125,126] Both native factor XIII (a_2b_2) and factor XIIIa′ (a'_2b_2) potentiated by thrombin (see "Metabolism of Factor XIII" below) bind similarly to calcium ions,[127] although the native factor XIII remains as a heterotetramer.[122,128] Thus, plasma factor XIII (a_2b_2) circulates in blood in a complex with both fibrinogen and calcium ions.

The three-dimensional structure of factor XIII has been demonstrated by an electron microscopic study. The a subunit and the b subunit appear to be a globular particle and a filamentous strand, respectively.[129] The a subunits of platelet[123] and placenta[130,131] and recombinant proteins[131,132] have also been crystallized, and the unit cell dimensions determined by x-ray analysis are fairly consistent.

Primary Structure. The a subunit of factor XIII consists of 731 amino acid residues.[133,134] Accordingly, the molecular weight of the polypeptide portion of the molecule was calculated to be 83,150. The addition of 1.5 percent carbohydrate[123] gives a molecular weight of approximately 84,400 for each of the a subunits. The b subunit is synthesized with a signal peptide of 20 amino acids,[135] which is removed by signal peptidase(s) later. The mature b subunit is composed of 641 amino acid residues,[136] with a calculated molecular weight of 73,183. The addition of 8.5 percent carbohydrate[124] gives a molecular weight of about 79,700 for each of the b subunits of human factor XIII. These molecular weights are in agreement with those estimated by SDS-PAGE.[121,122]

The N-terminus of the a subunit is acetylated,[137] while that of the b subunit is a free Glu residue.[136,137] The a subunit contains several functional regions, including an activation peptide (37 amino acids), an active site, putative calcium-binding sites, and a thrombin inactivation site. The amino acid sequence around the active site (Tyr-Gly-Gln-Cys-Trp) is identical to those of other transglutaminases.[138–140]

The a subunit of factor XIII is also present in other tissues, such as platelets, megakaryocytes, placenta, uterus, and monocytes/macrophages, etc. (see "Synthesis of Factor XIII" below). The amino acid sequences of the corresponding regions of the a subunits from plasma,[133,137] platelet,[137] and placenta[133,134,141] are indistinguishable. The purified a subunit from human placenta is reported to contain various molecules, which differ in length at the C-termini.[141]

The a subunit of factor XIII is highly homologous to other human transglutaminases (Titani, Zenita, Ando, and Kannagi; shown in refs. 139, 140, and 142). The degree of identity ranges from 40 to 45 percent. The middle portion of these proteins contains most of the identical sequences, while their N- and C-terminal regions are more diverse. A transglutaminase has been isolated from horseshoe crab hemocytes, and its primary structure was found to be homologous to the a subunit of factor XIII (37 percent amino acid identity).[143] This provides strong evidence to support the idea that these transglutaminases ultimately derive from a common ancestor. The amino acid sequence of human erythrocyte membrane band 4.2 protein is also similar to those of the transglutaminases[144,145]; however, it lacks enzymatic activity because of the substitution of the active site Cys by Ala.

The b subunit contains 10 tandem repeats. These repeats each consist of about 60 amino acids, two disulfide bonds, and highly conserved Pro, Gly, Tyr, and Trp residues.[136] They have been called "Sushi domains" because of their shape[142,146] or "GP-I structures"[147] because the disulfide bond pairing was partly established in human β_2-glycoprotein I between the first and third, and the second and fourth Cys residues in each repeat.[148] This pattern is true in the bovine counterpart[146] and in the α chain of human C4-binding protein.[149] Therefore, it is likely that a similar pairing occurs with the disulfide bonds in the Sushi domains present in other homologous proteins, including the b subunit of factor XIII. At least 25 other proteins/genes are found to contain similar Sushi domains.[142] Nearly half of these 26 proteins are involved in the complement system and the others in diverse systems such as blood coagulation and lymphocyte regulation. Sushi domains are found even in proteins of invertebrates and virus, suggesting that the genes for these proteins might have evolved from a common ancestor through gene duplication and exon shuffling.

In the middle of the last Sushi domain of the b subunit of factor XIII there is an Arg-Gly-Asp (RGD) sequence that is reported to be responsible for the cell attachment of various adhesive proteins.[150] It remains to be determined, however, whether this RGD sequence of the b subunit is related to its function.

Function of Factor XIII

The a subunit of factor XIII contains the catalytic site,[122,151] while the b subunit is thought to protect or stabilize the a subunit[152–154] or regulate the activation of the zymogen.[122,151]

Factor XIIIa catalyzes a γ-glutamyl-ϵ-lysine crosslinking reaction between several proteins. Fibrin acts as both an amino donor and acceptor,[46] while α_2-plasmin inhibitor and fibronectin preferentially serve as amino acceptors.[155,156]

Crosslinking of Fibrin Monomers. The crosslinking reaction catalyzed by factor XIIIa leads to dimerization of the γ chains of fibrin followed by polymerization of the α chains of fibrin.[121] The crosslinking sites between the γ chains are Gln398 and Lys406[46] near the C-terminal end of the polypeptide chain. Gln328 and Gln366[47] and Lys508[49] are involved in the α-chain polymerization. The γ-dimerization and α-polymerization reactions result in a fibrin with considerable mechanical strength and elasticity[157–159]; thus, these polymerization reactions aid in primary hemostasis.

A formation of γ-trimer, γ-tetramer, and $\alpha\gamma_2$-triad has been demonstrated following the γ-dimerization of both fibrin and fibrinogen.[51,160] These reactions may be important for the introduction of branching points into the growing fibrin network.

Crosslinking of α_2-Plasmin Inhibitor. The crosslinking reaction of α_2-plasmin inhibitor to the α chain of fibrin[161] or fibrinogen[162] by factor XIIIa occurs at a faster rate than with other proteins. Accordingly, in plasma, α_2-plasmin inhibitor and fibrin are considered to be the best substrates of factor XIIIa.[163] The crosslinking site in each substrate has been identified as Gln2 in α_2-plasmin inhibitor[156,164] and Lys303 in the α chain of fibrinogen.[66]

The crosslinking of α_2-plasmin inhibitor to fibrin renders the fibrin clot resistant to digestion by plasmin[165,166] Consequently, the crosslinked α_2-plasmin inhibitor protects the hemostatic fibrin clot from premature lysis by plasmin.

Crosslinking of Fibronectin. Factor XIIIa catalyzes the crosslinking of fibronectin to the α chain of fibrin[161,167] and to collagen.[168] The crosslinking site of fibronectin is Gln 3 at its N-terminus.[155]

The crosslinking between fibronectin and fibrin may result in the anchorage of fibrin clots to cells or the structural matrix in vessel walls at the site of vascular injury. In a cell culture system, fibronectin is crosslinked by factor XIIIa and accumulates in fibroblast cell layers. This reaction may be important for a particular assembly process to organize and stabilize the growing extracellular matrix.[169,170] Factor XIII is also reported to enhance fibroblast proliferation[171] and to generate a monocyte chemotactic factor derived from complement component 5.[172] These reactions appear to be related to wound healing.[173–175]

Other Protein Substrates. The contractile proteins actin and myosin have also been shown to be substrates of factor XIIIa.[176–178] Since these proteins exist in platelets, they might be involved in the crosslinking of structural proteins under certain conditions.[178]

Several other plasma proteins such as von Willebrand factor,[179,180] thrombospondin,[181] factor V,[182] and apolipoprotein(a)[183] have been reported to be crosslinked to themselves or to other substrates by factor XIIIa; however, the precise functions of these reactions have not been established.

Synthesis of Factor XIII

Concentrations of the a and b subunits of factor XIII in normal plasma have been determined by an ELISA to be 11 μg/ml and 21 μg/ml, respectively.[184] Since all of the a subunit in plasma is in the form of an equimolar complex with the b subunit, about half of the b subunit (10 μg/ml) exists as a "free" form in plasma.[153,185,186] The "free" b subunit may act as a reserve for binding and stabilization of the a subunit immediately after its release from cells into circulation.

Site of Synthesis for Factor XIII. The liver has long been thought to be a major site of synthesis for both the a and b subunits of plasma factor XIII.[187,188] In addition, biosynthesis and secretion of both subunits by a human hepatoma cell line, HepG2, have been reported[189]; however, no cDNA clone for the a subunit was obtained from liver libraries despite extensive trials for screening[133], (and Ichinose A: unpublished data). Northern blotting analyses of mRNA samples of normal liver, HepG2 cells, and fibroblasts also showed little or no detectable hybridization signal, while a single mRNA species (about 4.0 kb) for the a subunit was obtained from mRNA samples of placenta, macrophages, and osteosarcoma U-2 cells[134,190,191] (and Ichinose A, Sakariassen KS, unpublished data). These results suggest that placenta and macrophages synthesize the a subunit, but liver does not.

The a subunit free from the b subunit is also present in a number of organs, tissues, and cells, such as placenta, uterus, prostate, platelets, megakaryocytes, and monocytes/macrophages.[192–197] The a subunit in these cells, however, is found to be localized in cytoplasm by immunohistochemical and immunobiochemical methods. Platelets in particular contain an equal amount of the a subunit as does plasma,[198,199] but the a subunit of platelets is present in cytoplasm[197,199] and is not secreted.[198,199] An acetylated N-terminus, and the absence of glycosylation and disulfide bonds are also consistent with the fact that the a subunit is a typical cytoplasmic protein. At present, the function of the intracellular form of the a subunit is not known, although other cytosolic transglutaminases are thought to be related to apoptosis (programmed cell death).[200,201]

Cells peculiar to the dermis, called "dendrocytes," have been found to contain the a subunit of factor XIII.[202] Since dendrocytes share several common epitopes with monocytes/macrophages, they are also considered to be derived from bone marrow and to become perivascular resident macrophages. Accordingly, most of the a subunit–containing cells are of hemopoietic lineage.

After bone marrow transplantation, the phenotype of the a subunit in plasma of the donors was seen to replace that of the recipients, while the phenotype of the b subunit was unchanged.[203] In addition, complete or partial conversion of the phenotype of the a subunit in monocytes and platelets as well as plasma has been detected in patients after bone marrow transplantation.[204] Therefore, the a subunit of plasma factor XIII is produced at least in part by hemopoietic cells.

It has been suggested that the b subunit of factor XIII is synthesized in liver.[187,188] HepG2 and PLC/PRF/5 hepatoma cells secrete the b subunit,[189] and cDNA clones coding for the b subunit have been obtained from a normal human liver library.[136,205] In addition, the phenotype of the b subunit of the recipients changed to the donors' phenotype after liver transplantation, while that of the a subunit remained unchanged.[203] Therefore, it is clear that liver is the major site of synthesis for the b subunit.

Mechanism for Release of the a Subunit of Factor XIII. Like those of other transglutaminases, the 5′ end of the cDNA for the placental a subunit does not encode a typical hydrophobic leader sequence for secretion.[133,134] The search for a possible prepro-leader sequence or an internal signal inside the mature protein portion has been unsuccessful, although the corresponding regions of its genomic clones were examined extensively.[205,206] Because the a subunit of factor XIII remains in cytoplasm of placenta,[192] macrophages,[195,196] megakaryocytes,[194] and platelets,[197,199] it is very likely that the Met at position −1 functions as the initiator for biosynthesis. The removal of the Met by an aminopeptidase(s) would then be followed by acetylation of the N-terminal for Ser residue.[137]

If any of the cells or tissues listed above is the major source of the a subunit of "plasma" factor XIII, there should be a unique mechanism(s) for its release into circulation, where the free b subunit readily binds the released a subunit and forms an a_2b_2 tetramer. The results of an expression study of recombinant a and/or b subunits in a mammalian cell system suggest that the recombinant a subunit is not secreted through the conventional secretory pathway but is released from transfected cells by cell damage.[205] There are several proteins that lack a typical hydrophobic leader sequence and a distinct internal hydrophobic signal but are present and function in extracellular spaces.[207–211] In the case of interleukin-1β, two different mechanisms—a novel pathway and apoptosis—are proposed for its release from cells.[212,213]

The 5′ end of the cDNA and the corresponding exon of the gene for the b subunit code for a typical hydrophobic leader sequence that aids in secretion of the b subunit from hepatocytes into circulation.[135,153] This is supported by the fact that HepG2 and PLC/PRF/5 hepatoma cells secrete the b subunit[189] and that the recombinant b subunit is secreted through the conventional secretory pathway in the mammalian cell system.[205]

Regulation of Concentration of the b Subunit. Patients with congenital factor XIII deficiency lack an immunologically detectable a subunit (less than 1 percent of normal), and have a reduced amount (about 50 percent of normal) of the b subunit.[153,214] Heterozygotes have about 50 percent and 80 percent of the a and b subunits, respectively.[215] Furthermore, administration of the a subunit obtained from placenta increased not only the a subunit level in plasma but also the level of the b subunit, which reached a maximum after several days and remained increased for a time.[188,216] An ELISA study revealed that the plasma concentration of the complex form of the b subunit is decreased to almost 0 percent of normal in homozygotes of a subunit deficiency and to about 50 percent in heterozygotes, while that of the free b subunit is essentially the same among normal individuals, homozygotes, and heterozygotes.[184] Therefore, it is likely that the concentration of the complex form of the b subunit (a_2b_2) is dependent on the amount of the a subunit in plasma and that the concentration of the free b subunit is controlled to be constant. An increase in the level of the a subunit by infusion of exogenous a subunit may induce synthesis of the b subunit as a response to the increase of the a subunit or the decrease of the free b subunit. This response is absent in a patient whose complete b subunit deficiency is genetic in origin.[217]

Metabolism of Factor XIII

The half-life for the a subunit of factor XIII has been reported to be about 10 days.[175,188,218,219] It is of interest that the half-life of placental factor XIII concentrate (a_2 alone) in the patient with complete b subunit deficiency was shorter than that in patients with a subunit deficiency.[217] The placental a_2 dimer may be stabilized through immediate formation of an a_2b_2 tetramer with the free b_2 dimer in plasma of the patients with a subunit deficiency. This complex formation does not occur in the plasma of b subunit deficiency because of the absence of the b subunit.

Factor XIIIa (the activated form) is removed from circulation faster than native factor XIII (the zymogen form) probably through the reticuloendothelial system in liver.[187] The uptake of factor XIIIa into fibrin clots[220] could be an additional mechanism for its clearance from plasma.

Activation of the Zymogen. During the final stage of blood coagulation, thrombin converts the proenzyme (factor XIII) to a potentiated form (factor XIIIa′) by releasing an activation peptide (4 kDa) from the N-terminus of each of the a subunits.[121,137] The site of cleavage by thrombin is between Arg37 and Gly38). This reaction is stimulated by fibrin monomers.[221] The cofactor activity of fibrin I (polymerized des-A fibrinogen) has been attributed to formation of a fibrin I—factor XIII complex (K_d = 65 nM), which is potentiated by α-thrombin 80 times more efficiently than free factor XIII.[222] In contrast, fibrin crosslinked by factor XIIIa in the presence of calcium ions loses this accelerating capability as γ-dimers appear.[221] Thus, crosslinking of fibrin may function as a negative-feedback mechanism to prevent wasteful continued generation of factor XIIIa.

In the presence of calcium ions, the potentiated a'_2 dimer dissociates from the b_2 dimer[122,123,151,152] and binds to fibrin more tightly,[223] while the b_2 dimer remains in a liquid phase.[220] Calcium ions bind to the a′ subunit and also unmask its active site.[127,151,152,224] Fibrin(ogen) lowers the calcium concentration, required both for the dissociation of the a'_2 and b_2 dimers and for the exposure of the active site, to the physiological level (1.5 mM).[225,225]

Several other enzymes, including trypsin, factor Xa, elastase, and cathepsin C, are reported to activate (potentiate) factor XIII.[121,195,226–228] Some of these thrombin-independent reactions may actually play an important role in the activation of intracellular factor XIII (a_2 alone), since thrombin does not exist in cytoplasm.

Degradation of the Enzyme. The loss of biologic activity of factor XIIIa during prolonged incubation with thrombin occurs parallel to the generation of fragments of 56 and 24 kDa from the a subunit, while the molecular weight of the b subunit remains unchanged.[121,229] It has been reported, however, that the loss of activity is not correlated with the appearance of the small peptides,[230] An expression study of mutant a subunits suggested that the removal of its C-terminal portion makes the molecule unstable.[205] Degradation of factor XIII or factor XIIIa has also been reported to occur by digestion with elastase and trypsin.[121,227]

Acquired deficiencies in factor XIII and its elevated plasma levels are seen in various disease states (see refs. 175 and 231).

Chromosomal Localization and Gene Structures

The gene for the a subunit of factor XIII is located on chromosome 6p24-p25,[232] while that encoding keratinocyte (epidermal) transglutaminase is located on chromosome 14q11.2-q13.[233,234] Gene loci for the other transglutaminases have not yet been reported. The gene for the b subunit is located on chromosome 1q32-q32.1.[235] It is noteworthy that the genes for other proteins containing multiple Sushi domains, such as factor H, the α and β chains of C4b binding protein, complement receptors type I and type II, membrane cofactor protein, and decay accelerating factor, are also clustered in the same region.[236,237] Because of the existence of many genes homologous to either the a or b subunit, the chromosomal localization of the genes for both subunits has been reexamined and confirmed by in vitro amplification of genomic DNAs from human–hamster hybrid cell lines employing gene-specific primers.[205]

The genes for both the a and b subunits of human factor XIII have been characterized.[135,206] The gene for the a subunit spans more than 160 kb (Fig. 105-4). It consists of 15 exons interrupted by 14 introns, and each functional region is encoded by a separate exon. The genomic structures of keratinocyte transglutaminase and erythrocyte membrane band 4.2 protein are nearly identical to the structure of the a subunit, while these genes are much smaller in size.[238,239]

The gene for the b subunit is about 28 kb in length (Fig. 105-5). It is composed of 12 exons interrupted by 11 introns. Each of the 10 Sushi domains is encoded by a single exon. This is also true of the genes for other Sushi domain–containing proteins.

Genetic Polymorphism. Using agarose gel electrophoresis, several different allelic forms of the a subunit of factor XIII have been identified in normal populations.[240,241] The heterogeneity in the a subunit has been confirmed by both amino acid and DNA sequencing.[133,134,141,206] All of these amino acid substitutions can be explained by point mutations. It is also shown by restriction-fragment length polymorphism that DNA polymorphism exists at the a subunit locus[206,241,242] (and Ichinose A: unpublished data).

Microheterogeneity of the b subunit[224] was also classified into several alleles.[243] However, differences in the amino acid sequence of the b subunit have not been identified,[135,136] while several nucleotide substitutions were found in noncoding parts of its gene (Hashiguchi T, Ichinose A: unpublished data).

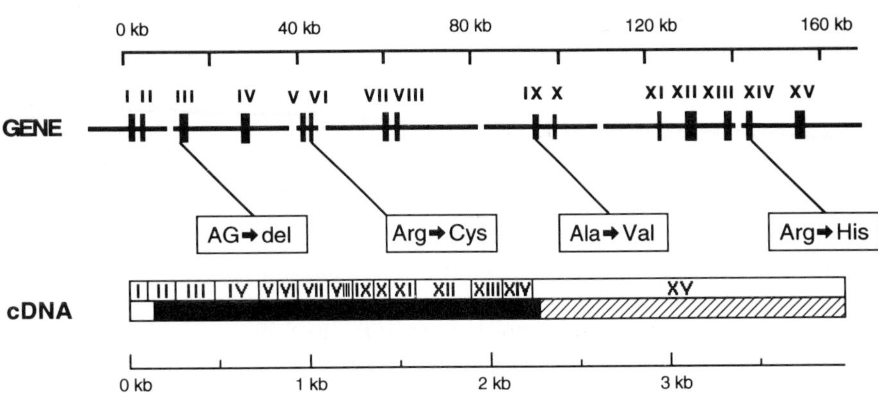

FIG. 105-4 Structure of gene and cDNA for the a subunit of factor XIII. Exons are indicated by wide vertical bars and Roman numerals. The 5′-noncoding, coding, and 3′-noncoding regions of the cDNA are shown by open, closed, and hatched boxes, respectively. A deletion of a dinucleotide, AG, at the 5′ end of exon III and amino acid substitutions of Arg by Cys in exon VI, Ala by Val in exon IX, and Arg by His in exon XIV depicted in the middle have been identified in patients with a subunit deficiency.

HEREDITARY DISORDERS OF FACTOR XIII

Congenital Deficiency and Molecular Abnormality

The incidence of congenital factor XIII deficiency (with less than 1 percent of the normal level of factor XIII activity) is reported to be in the range of 1 in 5 million in the United Kingdom[175] and in Japan.[244] Most patients appear to be deficient in the a subunit in plasma. The mode of inheritance is autosomal recessive,[175,215] which is consistent with the a subunit locus on chromosome 6.

In affected individuals, the first manifestation of bleeding is usually from the umbilical cord after birth, and this occurs in approximately 90 percent of the cases.[173] Intracranial hemorrhage occurs in one fourth of the patients and is the leading cause of death. Superficial bruising and hematomas in subcutaneous tissue and muscle are common, and bleeding at these sites may recur if not treated. Patients may bleed around joints after trauma, but have much less spontaneous hemarthrosis than do hemophiliacs.

Deficiency of either factor XIII[174,175] or α_2-plasmin inhibitor[67] results in "delayed bleeding" after trauma, while primary hemostasis in individuals with these traits is normal. The delayed bleeding is caused by premature lysis of hemostatic clots because of the absence of crosslinking between α_2-plasmin inhibitor and fibrin, which results in decreased resistance of the clots to proteolytic degradation by plasmin.[165,166]

In addition to a lifelong bleeding tendency, abnormal wound healing in affected individuals and habitual spontaneous abortion in affected females are not uncommon.[174,175] It is noteworthy that recurrent abortion has also been described in patients with congenital hypofibrinogenemia or afibrinogenemia.[245,246] Moreover, abnormal wound healing and repetitive abortion are reported in patients with congenital dysfibrinogenemia (for review, see ref. 247). These facts suggest the real functions of factor XIII and fibrin and their importance in vivo.

Mutations in the gene for the a subunit have been detected by in vitro amplification of DNA samples obtained from patients with a subunit deficiency; however, effects of these mutations on the a subunit biosynthesis are not confirmed. A deletion of a dinucleotide at the intron B–exon III boundary may lead to premature termination.[248] Amino acid substitutions of Arg260 by Cys and Ala394 by Val may result in instability of the a subunit molecule.[205] A point mutation at the end of exon XIV that causes an amino acid change of Arg681 to His may also lead to abnormal splicing of the pre-mRNA for the a subunit.[249]

A case with complete deficiency of the b subunit of factor XIII has been found in Japan and characterized.[217] The patient, who manifested a mild bleeding tendency, had no b subunit and a significantly reduced level of the a subunit in plasma. The half-life of an infused placental concentrate (a_2) in the patient was shorter than that in the plasma of patients

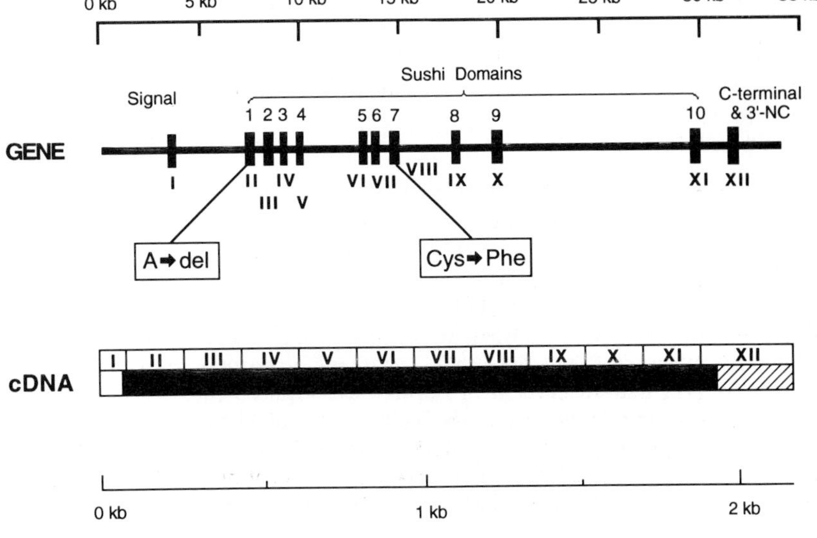

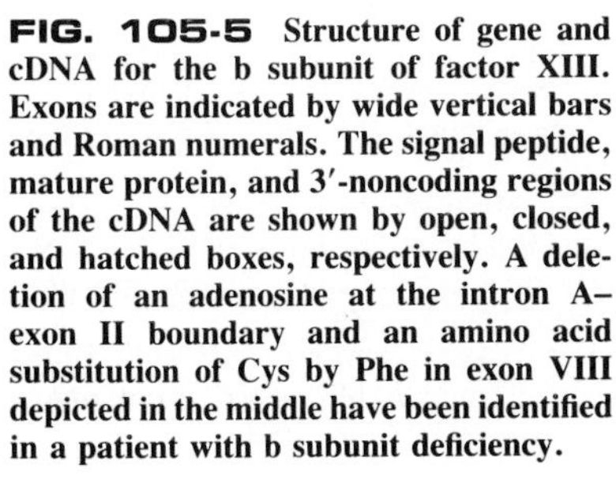
FIG. 105-5 Structure of gene and cDNA for the b subunit of factor XIII. Exons are indicated by wide vertical bars and Roman numerals. The signal peptide, mature protein, and 3′-noncoding regions of the cDNA are shown by open, closed, and hatched boxes, respectively. A deletion of an adenosine at the intron A–exon II boundary and an amino acid substitution of Cys by Phe in exon VIII depicted in the middle have been identified in a patient with b subunit deficiency.

with a subunit deficiency; therefore, the lack of the b subunit most likely causes instability of the a subunit. Nucleotide sequencing analysis of the DNA sample of this patient has revealed that the patient is a genetic compound heterozygote for two separate defects in the b subunit gene. The deletion of an adenosine at the splicing acceptor junction of the intron A–exon II boundary and the nucleotide substitution of a guanosine in exon VIII by thymidine will result in abnormal splicing of pre-mRNA and breakup of a disulfide bond in the seventh Sushi domain, respectively (Hashiguchi T, Ichinose A: unpublished data). At least two more patients seem to be deficient in the b subunit, although the half-life of the infused placental a subunit was not shortened.[219]

A rare case of congenital deficiency of factor XIII was also reported, which could be caused by the presence of "unstable" a subunits.[250] If the a subunit of this patient is intact, the b subunit may be defective in stabilization of the a subunit.

Diagnosis for Factor XIII Deficiency and Factor XIII Assay

The diagnosis for a homozygote with congenital deficiency is based on the pattern of inheritance, clinical symptoms, and laboratory tests. In addition to the typical umbilical cord bleeding after birth, the characteristic delayed bleeding after trauma strongly suggests this disorder. Deficiencies and molecular abnormalities of α_2-plasmin inhibitor and fibrinogen should be excluded since these disorders show similar symptoms, as described above.

The screening tests for factor XIII deficiency are based on the transglutaminase activity. These are thromboelastography and, more specifically, the solubility test of the recalcified plasma clot in 5 *M* urea or 1 percent monochloroacetic acid. Visualization of a γ-dimer or α-polymers of fibrin by SDS-PAGE is useful to estimate roughly the functional level of factor XIII in plasma. The transglutaminase activity of factor XIII is quantitatively measured by amine incorporation assays.[251, 252]

Immunologic quantitation of the a and b subunits in plasma is essential to determine which subunit is primarily deficient, although the incidence of b subunit deficiency appears to be rare. Concentration of the a and b subunits are measured by the Laurell rocket electrophoresis method,[153,214] or more precisely, by an ELISA.[184] Other laboratory coagulation tests are within normal range.

The diagnosis for a heterozygote, who usually lacks symptoms of factor XIII deficiency, can be made only by the specific quantitative measurements of both the a and b subunits. Genetic diagnosis at the DNA level will help both in prenatal detection of affected patients and in determination of carrier states.

Therapy for Factor XIII Deficiency

Both congenital and acquired factor XIII deficiencies have been treated successfully with fresh frozen plasma, cryoprecipitate, and crude factor XIII concentrates from placenta.[253,254] Maintaining the level of plasma factor XIII at 10 to 20 percent of normal is sufficient, since bleeding occurs frequently in patients with less than 1 percent of normal, and levels of 1 and 10 percent of normal are required for the in vitro γ-dimerization and α-polymerization of fibrin, respectively. The long half-life of factor XIII in plasma and its minimum requirement for hemostasis are beneficial both for the treatment of acute bleeding and for prophylaxis. Prophylactic therapy by factor XIII concentrates would be desirable for patients with severe cases, who may otherwise bleed frequently. Although development of inhibitors to factor XIII following multiple infusions is rare, it must be considered when bleeding is uncontrollable by a therapeutic dosage of factor XIII. In such a case, immunosuppressive therapy may be required as well.

The cloning of human factor XIII[133,134] made it possible to prepare recombinant a subunit as a therapeutic material that is free of viral contamination. The recombinant a subunit is confirmed to be comparable to the native a subunit protein in the structural and functional properties[255]; thus, it will substitute for the current placental factor XIII concentrates in transfusion therapy. It will be included also as an essential component in "tissue glue," which is in use widely for all types of surgery and for the treatment of trauma.

REFERENCES

1. Scheraga HA, Laskowski M Jr: The fibrinogen-fibrin conversion. *Adv Protein Chem* **12**:1, 1957.
2. Doolittle RF: Structural aspects of the fibrinogen-fibrin conversion. *Adv Protein Chem* **27**:1, 1973.
3. McKee PA, Rogers LA, Marler E, Hill RL: The subunit polypeptides of human fibrinogen. *Arch Biochem Biophys* **116**:271, 1966.
4. Bailey K, Astbury WT, Rudall KM: Fibrinogen and fibrin as members of the keratin-myosin group. *Nature* **151**:716, 1943.
5. Hall CE, Slayter HS: The fibrinogen molecule: Its size, shape and mode of polymerization. *J Biophys Biochem Cytol* **5**:11, 1959.
6. Doolittle RF, Watt KWK, Cottrell BA, Strong DD, Riley M: The amino acid sequence of the α-chain of human fibrinogen. *Nature* **280**:464, 1979.
7. Henschen A, Lottspeich F: Amino acid sequence of human fibrin. Preliminary note on the completion of the β chain sequence. *Hoppe Seyler Z Physiol Chem* **358**:1643, 1977.
8. Henschen A, Lottspeich F: Amino acid sequence of human fibrin: Preliminary note on the γ chain sequence. *Hoppe Seyler Z Physiol Chem* **358**:935, 1977.
9. Tagaki T, Doolittle RF: Amino acid sequence studies on the α chain of human fibrinogen. Location of four plasmin attack points and a covalent cross-linking site. *Biochemistry* **14**:5149, 1975.
10. Takagi T, Doolittle RF: The amino acid sequences of those portions of human fibrinogen Fragment E which are not included in the amino-terminal disulfide knot. *Thromb Res* **7**:813, 1975.
11. Chung DW, Rixon MW, Davie EW: The biosynthesis of fibrinogen and the cloning of its cDNA, in Bradshaw RA, Hill RL, Tang J, Liang CC, Tsao TC, Tsou CL (eds): *Proteins in Biology and Medicine*. New York, Academic, 1982, p 309.
12. Crabtree GR, Comeau CM, Fowlkes DM, Fornace AJ, Malley JD, Kant JA: Evolution and structure of the fibrinogen genes. Random insertion of introns or selective loss? *J Mol Biol* **185**:1, 1985.
13. Weissbach L, Grieninger G: Bipartite mRNA for chicken alpha-fibrinogen potentially encodes an amino acid sequence homologous to beta- and gamma-fibrinogens. *Proc Natl Acad Sci USA* **87**:5198, 1990.
14. Pan Y, Doolittle RF: cDNA sequence of a second fibrinogen alpha chain in lamprey: An archetypal version alignable with full-length beta and gamma chains. *Proc Natl Acad Sci USA* **89**:2066, 1992.
15. Wolfenstein-Todel C, Mosesson MW: Human plasma fibrinogen heterogeneity: Evidence for an extended carboxyl-terminal sequence in a normal gamma chain variant (gamma'). *Proc Natl Acad Sci USA* **77**:5069, 1980.
16. Wolfenstein-Todel C, Mosesson MW: Carboxyl-terminal amino acid sequence of a human fibrinogen gamma-chain variant (gamma'). *Biochemistry* **20**:6146, 1981.

17. Chung DW, Davie EW: γ and γ' chains of human fibrinogen are produced by alternative mRNA processing. *Biochemistry* **23**:4232, 1984.
18. Fornace AJ, Cummings D, Comeau CM, Kant JA, Crabtree GR: The γ_B chain of human fibrinogen is produced by alternate splice patterns of mRNA from a single gene. *J Biol Chem* **259**:12826, 1984.
19. Mosesson MW, Finlayson JS, Umfleet RA: Human fibrinogen heterogeneities. III. Identification of chain variants. *J Biol Chem* **247**:5223, 1972.
20. Legrele CD, Wolfenstein-Todel C, Hurbourg Y, Mosesson MW: Evidence for two classes of rat plasma fibrinogen gamma chains differing by their COOH-terminal amino acid sequences. *Biochem Biophys Res Commun* **105**:521, 1982.
21. Hall CE, Slayter HS: The fibrinogen molecule: Its size, shape and mode of polymerization. *J Biophys Biochem Cytol* **5**:11, 1959.
22. Blomback B: *Symp Zool Soc Lond* **27**:167, 1970.
23. Weisel JW, Stauffacher CV, Bullit E, Cohen C: A model for fibrinogen: Domains and sequence. *Science* **230**:1388, 1985.
24. Medved LV, Litvinovich SV, Privalov PL: Domain organization of the terminal parts in the fibrinogen molecule. *FEBS Lett* **202**:298, 1986.
25. Doolittle RF, Goldbaum DM, Doolittle LR: Designation of sequences involved in the "coiled coil" interdomainal connector in fibrinogen: Construction of an atomic scale model. *J Mol Biol* **120**:311, 1978.
26. Mosesson MW: Fibrinogen heterogeneity. *Ann NY Acad Sci* **408**:97, 1983.
27. Nakashima A, Sasaki S, Miyazaki K, Miyata T, Iwanaga S: Human fibrinogen heterogeneity: The COOH-terminal residues of defective Aα chains of fibrinogen II. *Blood Coagul Fibrinolysis* **3**:361, 1992.
28. Townsend RR, Hilliker E, Li YT, Laine RA, Bell WR, Lee YC: Carbohydrate structure of human fibrinogen: Use of 300 MHz 1H-NMR to characterize glycosidase-treated glycopeptides. *J Biol Chem* **257**:9704, 1982.
29. Martinez J, Palascak JE, Dwasniak D: Abnormal sialic acid content of the dysfibrinogenemia associated with liver disease. *J Clin Invest* **61**:535, 1978.
30. Langer BG, Weisel JW, Dinauer PA, Nagaswami C, Bell WR: Deglycosylation of fibrinogen accelerates polymerization and increases lateral aggregation of fibrin fibers. *J Biol Chem* **263**:15056, 1988.
31. Blomback B, Vestermark A: Isolation of fibrinopeptides by chromatography. *Ark Kemi* **12**:173, 1958.
32. Lewis SD, Shields PP, Shafer JA: Characterization of the kinetic pathway for liberation of fibrinopeptides during assembly of fibrin. *J Biol Chem* **260**:10192, 1985.
33. Bilezikian SB, Nossel HL, Butler VP Jr, Canfield RE: Radioimmunoassay of human fibrinopeptide B and kinetics of fibrinopeptide cleavage by different enzymes. *J Clin Invest* **56**:438, 1975.
34. Stocker K, Fischer H, Meier J: Thrombin-like snake venom proteinases. *Toxicon* **20**:265, 1982.
35. Shainoff JR, Dardik BN: Fibrinopeptide B and aggregation of fibrinogen. *Science* **204**:200, 1979.
36. Dyr JE, Blomback B, Kornalik F: The fibrinogenolytic and procoagulant activity of southern copperhead venom enzymes. *Thromb Res* **30**:185, 1983.
37. Fowler WE, Hantgan RR, Hermans J, Erickson HP: Structure of the fibrin protofibril. *Proc Natl Acad Sci USA* **78**:4872, 1981.
38. Hantgan RR, Hermans J: Assembly of fibrin: A light scattering study. *J Biol Chem* **254**:11272, 1979.
39. Hantgan RR, Fowler RW. Erickson HP, Hermans J: Fibrin assembly: A comparison of electron microscopic and light scattering results. *Thromb Haemost* **44**:119, 1980.
40. Laudano AP, Doolittle RF: Studies on synthetic peptides that bind to fibrinogen and prevent fibrin polymerization. *Proc Natl Acad Sci USA* **75**:3085, 1978.
41. Yamazumi K, Doolittle RF: Photoaffinity labeling of the primary fibrin polymerization site: Localization of the label to gamma-chain Tyr-363. *Proc Natl Acad Sci USA* **89**:2893, 1992.
42. Laudano AP, Doolittle RF: Studies on synthetic peptides that bind to fibrinogen and prevent fibrin polymerization. Structural requirements, number of binding sites, and species differences. *Biochemistry* **19**:1013, 1980.
43. Mosesson MW, Siebenlist KR, DiOrio JP, Budzynski AZ: Studies on the conversion of des Bbetal-42 fibrin, in Matsuda M (ed): *Fibrinogen*. Amsterdam, Elsevier, 1989, Vol 4.
44. Weisel JW, Nagaswami C: Computer modeling of fibrin polymerization kinetics correlated with electron microscope and turbidity observations: Clot structure and assembly are kinetically controlled. *Biophys J* **63**:111, 1992.
45. Chen R, Doolittle RF: Identification of the polypeptide chains involved in the cross-linking of fibrin. *Proc Natl Acad Sci USA* **63**:420, 1969.
46. Chen R, Doolittle RF: γ-γ cross-linking sites in human and bovine fibrin. *Biochemistry* **10**:4486, 1971.
47. Cottrell BA, Strong DD, Watt KWK, Doolittle RF: Amino acid sequence studies on the α chain of human fibrinogen. Exact location of cross-linking acceptor sites. *Biochemistry* **18**:5405, 1979.
48. Fretto LJ, Ferguson EW, Steinman HM, McKee PA: Localization of the α-chain cross-link acceptor sites of human fibrin. *J Biol Chem* **253**:2184, 1978.
49. Corcoran DH, Ferguson EW, Fretto LJ, McKee PA: Localization of a cross-link donor site in the alpha-chain of human fibrin. *Thromb Res* **19**:883, 1980.
50. Gaffney PJ, Whitaker AN: Fibrin crosslinks and lysis rates. *Thromb Res* **14**:85, 1979.
51. Mosesson MW, Siebenlist KR, Amrani DL, DiOrio JP: Identification of covalently linked trimeric and tetrameric D domains in crosslinked fibrin. *Proc Natl Acad Sci USA* **86**:1113, 1989.
52. Bennett JS: Integrin structure and function in hemostasis and thrombosis. *Ann NY Acad Sci* **614**:214, 1991.
53. Kloczewiak M, Timmons S, Hawiger J: Recognition site for the platelet receptor is present on the 15-residue carboxy-terminal fragment of the gamma chain of human fibrinogen and is not involved in the fibrin polymerization reaction. *Thromb Res* **29**:249, 1983.
54. Kloczewiak M, Timmons S, Lukas TJ, Hawiger J: Platelet receptor recognition site on human fibrinogen. Synthesis and structure-function relationship of peptides corresponding to the carboxy-terminal segment of the γ chain. *Biochemistry* **23**:1767, 1984.
55. Farrell DH, Thiagarajan P, Chung DW, Davie EW: Role of fibrinogen α and γ chain sites in platelet aggregation. *Proc Natl Acad Sci USA* **89**:10729, 1992.
56. Weisel JW, Nagaswami C, Vilaire G, Bennett JS: Examination of the platelet membrane glycoprotein IIb-IIIa complex and its interaction with fibrinogen and other ligands by electron microscopy. *J Biol Chem* **267**:16637, 1992.
57. Dang CV, Ebert RF, Bell WR: Localization of a fibrinogen calcium binding site between γ subunit positions 311 and 336 by terbium fluorescence. *J Biol Chem* **260**:9713, 1985.
58. Nieuwenhuizen W, Haverkate F: Calcium binding regions in fibrinogen. *Ann NY Acad Sci* **408**:92, 1983.
59. Hardy JJ, Carrell NA, McDonagh J: Calcium ion functions in fibrinogen conversion to fibrin. *Ann NY Acad Sci* **408**:279, 1983.
60. Yoshida N, Hirata H, Morigami Y, Imaoka S, Matsuda M, Yamazumi K, Asakura S: Characterization of an abnormal fibrinogen Osaka V with the replacement of γ-arginine 375 by glycine. The lack of high affinity calcium binding to D-domains and the lack of protective effect of calcium on fibrinolysis. *J Biol Chem* **267**:2753, 1992.
61. Koopman J, Haverkate F, Brieet E, Lord ST: A congenitally abnormal fibrinogen (Vlissingen) with a 6-base deletion in the gamma-chain gene, causing defective calcium binding and impaired fibrin polymerization. *J Biol Chem* **266**:13456, 1991.
62. Vali Z, Scheraga HA: Localization of the binding site on fibrin for the secondary binding site of thrombin. *Biochemistry* **27**:1956, 1988.
63. Francis CW, Markham RE Jr, Barlow GH, Florak TM, Dobrzynski DM, Marder VJ: Thrombin activity of fibrin thrombi and soluble plasmic derivatives. *J Lab Clin Med* **102**:220, 1983.
64. Liu CY, Koehn, JA, Morgan FJ: Characterization of

fibrinogen New York 1. A dysfunctional fibrinogen with a deletion of Bβ(9-72) corresponding exactly to exon 2 of the gene. *J Biol Chem* **260**:4390, 1985.

65. Mary A, Achyuthan KE, Greenberg CS: Factor XIII binds to the A alpha- and B beta-chains in the D domain of fibrinogen: An immunoblotting study. *Biochem Biophys Res Commun* **147**:608, 1987.
66. Kimura S, Aoki N: Cross-linking site in fibrinogen for α_2-plasmin inhibitor. *J Biol Chem* **261**:15591, 1986.
67. Aoki N, Saito H, Kamiya T, Koie K, Dakata Y, Kobokura M: Congenital deficiency of α_2-plasmin inhibitor associated with severe hemorrhagic tendency. *J Clin Invest* **63**:877, 1979.
68. Yonekawa O, Voskuilen M, Nieuwenhuizen W: Localization in the fibrinogen γ chain of a new site that is involved in the acceleration of the tissue-type plasminogen activator-catalysed activation of plasminogen. *Biochem J* **283**:187, 1992.
69. Lucas MA, Fretto LJ, McKee PA: The binding of human plasminogen to fibrin and fibrinogen. *J Biol Chem* **258**:4249, 1983.
70. Tran-Thang C, Kruitkof EKO, Atkinson J, Bachmann F: High affinity binding sites for glu-plasminogen unveiled by limited plasmic degradation of human fibrin. *Eur J Biochem* **160**:599, 1986.
71. Mosesson MW, Umfleet RA: The cold-insoluble globulin of human plasma. I. Purification, primary characterization, and relationship to fibrinogen and other cold-insoluble fraction components. *J Biol Chem* **245**:5728, 1970.
72. Stathakis NE, Mosesson MW, Chen AB, Galanakis DK: Cryoprecipitation of fibrin-fibrinogen complexes induced by the cold-insoluble globulin of plasma. *Blood* **51**:1211, 1978.
73. Levesque JP, Hatzfeld A, Hatzfeld J: Fibrinogen mitogenic effect on hemopoietic cell lines: Control via receptor modulation. *Proc Natl Acad Sci USA* **83**:6494, 1986.
74. Levesque JP, Hatzfeld J, Hatzfeld A: A mitogenic fibrinogen receptor that differs from glycoprotein IIb-IIIa. Identification by affinity chromatography and by covalent cross-linking. *J Biol Chem* **265**:328, 1990.
75. Straub PW: A study of fibrinogen production by human liver slices in vitro by immunoprecipitin method. *J Clin Invest* **42**:130, 1963.
76. Collen D, Tygat GN, Claeys H, Piessens R: Metabolism and distribution of fibrinogen. I. Fibrinogen turnover in physiological conditions in humans. *Br J Haematol* **22**:681, 1972.
77. Rausen AA, Cruchaud A, McMillan CW, Gitlin D: A study of fibrinogen turnover in classical hemophilia and congenital afibrinogenemia. *Blood* **18**:710, 1961.
78. Henry I, Uzan G, Weil D, Nicolas H, Kaplan JC, Marguerie C, Kahn A, Junien C: The genes coding for A alpha-, B beta-, and gamma-chains of fibrinogen map to 4q2. *Am J Hum Genet* **36**:760, 1984.
79. Kant JA, Fornace AJ Jr, Saxe D, Simon ML, McBride OW, Crabtree GR: Organization and evolution of the human fibrinogen locus on chromosome four. *Proc Natl Acad Sci USA* **82**:2344, 1985.
80. Chung DW, Harris JE, Davie EW: Nucleotide sequences of the three genes coding for human fibrinogen. *Adv Exp Med Biol* **281**:39, 1990.
81. Fu Y, Weissbach L, Plant PW, Oddoux C, Cao Y, Liang J, Roy SN, Redman CM, Grieninger G: Carboxy-terminal-extended variant of the human fibrinogen α subunit: A novel exon conferring marked homology to β and γ subunits. *Biochemistry* **31**:11968, 1992.
82. Alving BM, Chung SI, Murano G, Tang DB, Finlayson JS: Rabbit fibrinogen: Time course of constituent chain production in vivo. *Arch Biochem Biophys* **217**:1, 1982.
83. Yu S, Sher B, Kudryk B, Redman CM: Intracellular assembly of human fibrinogen. *J Biol Chem* **258**:13407, 1983.
84. Huang S, Mulvihill ER, Farrell DH, Chung DW, Davie EW: Biosynthesis of human fibrinogen: Subunit interactions and potential intermediates in the assembly. *J Biol Chem* **268**:8919, 1993.
85. Huang S, Cao Z, Davie EW: The role of amino-terminal disulfide bonds in the structure and assembly of human fibrinogen. *Biochem Biophys Res Commun* **190**:488, 1993.
86. Castaldi PA, Caen J: Platelet fibrinogen. *J Clin Pathol* **18**:579, 1965.
87. Mosesson MW, Homandberg GA, Amrani DL: Human platelet fibrinogen gamma chain structure. *Blood* **63**:990, 1984.
88. Hadagama PJ, George JN, Shuman MA, McEver RP, Bainton DF: Incorporation of a circulating protein into megakaryocyte and platelet granules. *Proc Natl Acad Sci USA* **84**:861, 1987.
89. Hadagama PJ, Shuman MA, Bainton DF: Incorporation of intraveneously injected albumin, immunoglobulin G, and fibrinogen in guinea pig megakaryocyte granules. *J Clin Invest* **84**:73, 1989.
90. George JN, Nurden AT, Phillips DR: Molecular defects in interactions of platelets with the vessel wall. *N Engl J Med* **311**:1084, 1984.
91. Harrison P, Wilbourn B, Debili N, Vainchenker W, Breton-Gorius J, Lawrie AS, Masse JM, Savidge GF, Cramer EM: Uptake of plasma fibrinogen into the alpha granules of human megakaryocytes and platelets. *J Clin Invest* **84**:1320, 1989.
92. Louache F, Debili N, Cramer E, Breton-Gorius J, Vainchenker W: Fibrinogen is not synthesized by human megakaryocytes. *Blood* **77**:311, 1991.
93. Hadagama PJ, Shuman MA, Bainton DF: In vivo defibrination results in markedly decreased amounts of fibrinogen in rat megakaryocytes and platelets. *Am J Pathol* **137**:1393, 1990.
94. Haidaris PJ, Courtney MA: Tissue-specific and ubiquitous expression of fibrinogen gamma-chain mRNA. *Blood Coagul Fibrinolysis* **1**:433, 1990.
95. Chodish LA, Carthew RW, Morgan JG, Crabtree GR, Sharp PA: The adenovirus major late transcription factor activates the rat γ-fibrinogen promoter. *Science* **238**:684, 1987.
96. Courtois G, Morgan JG, Campbell LA, Fourel G, Crabtree GR: Interaction of a liver-specific nuclear factor with the fibrinogen and α1-antitrypsin promoter. *Science* **238**:688, 1987.
97. Ritchie DG, Fuller GM: Hepatocyte-stimulating factor: A monocyte-derived acute-phase regulatory protein. *Ann NY Acad Sci* **408**:490, 1983.
98. Kishimoto T, Akira S, Taga T: Il-6 receptor and mechanism of signal transduction. *Int J Immunopharmacol* **14**:431, 1992.
99. Akira S, Isshiki H, Sugita T, Tanabe O, Kinoshita S, Nishio Y, Nakajima T, Hirano T, Kishimoto T: A nuclear factor for Il-6 expression (NF-IL6) is a member of a C/EBP family. *EMBO J* **9**:1897, 1990.
100. Ganapathi MK: Okadaic acid, an inhibitor of protein phosphatases 1 and 2A, inhibits induction of acute-phase proteins by interleukin-6 alone or in combination with interleukin-1 in human hepatoma cell lines. *Biochem J* **284**:645, 1992.
101. Huber P, Laurent M, Dalmon J: Human β-fibrinogen gene expression. *J Biol Chem* **265**:5695, 1990.
102. Rose-John S, Schooltink H, Lenz D, Hipp E, Dufhues G, Schmitz H, Schiel X, Hirano T, Kishimoto T, Heinrich PC: Studies on the structure and regulation of the human hepatic interleukin-6 receptor. *Eur J Biochem* **190**:79, 1990.
103. Kannel WB, D'Agostino RB, Belanger AJ: Fibrinogen, cigarette smoking, and risk of cardiovascular disease: Insights from the Framingham Study. *Am Heart J* **113**:1006, 1987.
104. Thomas AE, Green FR, Kelleher CH, Wilkes HC, Brennan PJ, Meade TW, Humphries SE: Variation in the promoter region of the β fibrinogen gene is associated with plasma fibrinogen levels in smokers and non-smokers. *Thromb Haemost* **65**:487, 1991.
105. Rabe F, Salomon E: Ueber Faserstiffmangel im Blut bei einem Fallen con Hamophilie. *Dtsch Arch Klin Med* **132**:240, 1920.
106. Flute PT: Disorders of plasma fibrinogen synthesis. *Br Med Bull* **33**:253, 1977.
107. Rodriguez RC, Buchanan GR, Clanton MS: Prophylactic cryoprecipitate in congenital afibrinogenemia. *Clin Pediatr (Phila)* **27**:543, 1988.
108. Grech H, Majumdar G, Lawrie AS, Savidge GF: Pregnancy in congenital afibrinogenaemia: Report of a successful case and review of the literature. *Br J Haematol* **78**:571, 1991.
109. Pritchard JA: Chronic hypofibrinogenaemia and pregnant placental abruption. *Obstet Gynecol* **18**:146, 1961.

110. Fried K, Kaufman S: Congenital afibrinogenemia in 10 offspring of uncle-niece marriages. *Clin Genet* **17**:223, 1980.
111. Ebert RF: Index of variant human fibrinogens. Boca Raton, FL, CRC, 1991.
112. Henschen A, Lottspeich F, Kehl M, Southan C: Covalent structure of fibrinogen. *Ann NY Acad Sci* **408**:28, 1983.
113. Yamazumi K, Shimura K, Terukina S, Takahashi N, Matsuda M: A gamma methionine-310 to threonine substitution and consequent N-glycosylation at gamma asparagine-308 identified in a congenital dysfibrinogenemia associated with posttraumatic bleeding, fibrinogen Asahi. *J Clin Invest* **83**:1590, 1989.
114. Thorsen LI, Brosstad F, Solum NO, Stormorken H: Increased binding to ADP-stimulated platelets and aggregation effect of the dysfibrinogen Oslo I as compared with normal fibrinogen. *Scand J Haematol* **36**:203, 1986.
115. Denninger MH, Jandrot-Perrus M, Elion J, Bertrand O, Homandberg GA, Mosesson MW, Guillin MC: ADP-induced platelet aggregation depends on the conformation or availability of the terminal gamma chain sequence on fibrinogen. Study of the reactivity of fibrinogen Paris 1. *Blood* **70**:558, 1987.
116. Francis CW, Marder VJ, Barlow GH: Plasmic degradation of crosslinked fibrin. Characterization of new macromolecular soluble complexes and a model of their structure. *J Clin Invest* **66**:1033, 1980.
117. Coleman M, Bigliano EM, Weksler ME, Nachman RL: Inhibition of fibrin monomer polymerization by lambda myeloma globulins. *Blood* **9**:210, 1972.
118. Davey F: Immunoglobulin inhibition of fibrin clot formation. *Ann Clin Lab Sci* **6**:72, 1976.
119. Marder VJ, Martin SE, Francis CW, Colman RW: Consumptive thrombohemorrhagic disorders, in Colman RW, Hirsh J, Marder VJ, Salzman EW (eds): *Hemostasis and Thrombosis, Basic Principles and Clinical Practices*. Philadelphia, Lippincott, 1987, p 975.
120. Hamulyak K, Nieuwenhuizen W, Devilee PP, Hemker HC: Reevaluation of some properties of fibrinogen, purified from cord blood of normal newborns. *Thromb Res* **32**:301, 1983.
121. Schwartz ML, Pizzo SV, Hill RL, McKee PA: Human factor XIII from plasma and platelets. *J Biol Chem* **248**:1395, 1973.
122. Chung SI, Lewis MS, Folk JE: Relationships of the catalytic properties of human plasma and platelet transglutaminases (activated blood coagulation factor XIII) to their subunit structures. *J Biol Chem* **249**:940, 1974.
123. Bohn H: Isolierung und Charakterisierung des fibrinstabilisierenden Faktors aus menschlichen Thrombozyten. *Thromb Diath Haemorrh* **23**:455, 1970.
124. Bohn H, Haupt H, Kranz T: Die molekulare Struktur der fibrinstabilisierenden Faktoren des Menschen. *Blut* **25**:235, 1972.
125. Loewy AG, Dahlberg A, Dunathan K, Kriel R, Wolfinger HL: Fibrinase: Some physical properties. *J Biol Chem* **236**:2634, 1961.
126. Greenberg CS, Shuman MA: The zymogen forms of blood coagulation factor XIII bind specifically to fibrinogen. *J Biol Chem* **257**:6096, 1982.
127. Lewis BA, Freyssinet J-M, Holbrook JJ: An equilibrium study of metal ion binding to human plasma coagulation factor XIII. *Biochem J* **169**:397, 1978.
128. Freyssinet J-M, Lewis BA, Holbrook JJ, Shore JD: Protein-protein interaction in blood clotting. *Biochem J* **169**:403, 1978.
129. Carrell NA, Erickson HP, McDonagh J: Electron microscopy and hydrodynamic properties of factor XIII subunits. *J Biol Chem* **264**:551, 1989.
130. Bohn H, Schwick HG: Isolation and characterization of a fibrin-stabilizing factor from human placentas. *Arzneimittelforschung* **21**:1432, 1971.
131. Hilgenfeld R, Liesam A, Storm R, Metzner HJ, Karges HE: Crystallization of blood coagulation factor XIII by an automated procedure. *FEBS Lett* **265**:110, 1990.
132. Bishop PD, Teller DC, Smith RA, Lasser GW, Gilbert T, Seale RL: Expression, purification, and characterization of human factor XIII in *Saccharomyces cerevisiae*. *Bichemistry* **29**:1861, 1990.
133. Ichinose A, Hendrickson LE, Fujikawa K, Davie EW: Amino acid sequence of the a subunit of human factor XIII. *Biochemistry* **25**:6900, 1986.
134. Grundmann U, Amann E, Zettlmeissl G, Kupper HA: Characterization of cDNA coding for human factor XIIIa. *Proc Natl Acad Sci USA* **83**:8024, 1986.
135. Bottenus RE, Ichinose A, Davie EW: Nucleotide sequence of the gene for the b subunit of human factor XIII. *Biochemistry* **29**:11195, 1990.
136. Ichinose A, McMullen BA, Fujikawa K, Davie EW: Amino acid sequence of the b subunit of human factor XIII, a protein composed of ten repetitive segments. *Biochemistry* **25**:4633, 1986.
137. Takagi T, Doolittle RF: Amino acid sequence studies on factor XIII and the peptide released during its activation by thrombin. *Biochemistry* **13**:750, 1974.
138. Connellan JM, Chung SI, Whetzel NK, Bradley LM, Folk JE: Structural properties of guinea pig liver transglutaminase. *J Biol Chem* **246**:1093, 1971.
139. Phillips MA, Stewart BE, Qin Q, Chakravarty R, Floyd EE, Jetten AM, Rice RH: Primary structure of keratinocyte transglutaminase. *Proc Natl Acad Sci USA* **87**:9333, 1990.
140. Gentile V, Saydak M, Chiocca EA, Akande O, Birckbichler PJ, Lee KN, Stein JP, Davies PJA: Isolation and characterization of cDNA clones to mouse macrophage and human endothelial cell tissue transglutaminases. *J Biol Chem* **266**:478, 1991.
141. Takahashi N, Takahashi Y, Putnam FW: Primary structure of blood coagulation factor XIIIa (fibrinoligase, transglutaminase) from human placenta. *Proc Natl Acad Sci USA* **83**:8019, 1986.
142. Ichinose A, Bottenus RE, Davie EW: Structure of transglutaminase. *J Biol Chem* **265**:13411, 1990.
143. Tokunaga F, Muta T, Iwanaga S, Ichinose A, Davie EW, Kuma K, Miyata T: Limulus hemocyte transglutaminase: cDNA cloning, amino acid sequence, and tissue localization. *J Biol Chem* **268**:262, 1993.
144. Sung LA, Chien S, Chang L-S, Lambert K, Bliss SA, Bouhassira EE, Nagel RL, Shwartz RS, Rybicki AC: Molecular cloning of human protein 4.2: A major component of the erythrocyte membrane. *Proc Natl Acad Sci USA* **87**:955, 1990.
145. Korsgren C, Lawler J, Lambert S, Speicher D, Cohen CM: Complete amino acid sequence and homologies of human erythrocyte membrane protein band 4.2. *Proc Natl Acad Sci USA* **87**:613, 1990.
146. Kato H, Enjoji K: Amino acid sequence and location of the disulfide bonds in bovine β_2 glycoprotein I: The presence of five Sushi domains. *Biochemistry* **30**:11687, 1992.
147. Davie EW, Ichinose A, Leytus S: Structural features of the proteins participating in blood coagulation and fibrinolysis. *Cold Spring Harb Symp Quant Biol* **51**:509, 1986.
148. Lozier J, Takahashi N, Putnam FW: Complete amino acid sequence of human plasma β_2-glycoprotein I. *Proc Natl Acad Sci USA* **81**:3640, 1984.
149. Janatova J, Reid KBM, Willis AC: Disulfide bonds are localized within the short consensus repeat units of complement regulatory proteins: C4b-binding protein. *Biochemistry* **28**:4754, 1989.
150. Pierschbacher MD, Ruoslahti E: Cell attachment activity of fibronectin can be duplicated by small synthetic fragments of the molecule. *Nature* **309**:30, 1984.
151. Lorand L, Gray AJ, Brown K, Credo RB, Curtis CG, Domanik RA, Sternberg P: Dissociation of the subunit structure of fibrin stabilizing factor during activation of the zymogen. *Biochem Biophys Res Commun* **56**:914, 1974.
152. Cooke RD: Calcium-induced dissociation of human plasma factor XIII and the appearance of catalytic activity. *Biochem J* **141**:683, 1974.
153. Bohn H, Becker W, Trobisch H: Die molekulare Struktur der fibrinstabilisierenden Faktoren des Menschen. *Blut* **26**:303, 1973.
154. Lorand L: Activation of blood coagulation factor XIII. *Ann NY Acad Sci* **485**:144, 1986.

155. McDonagh RP, McDonagh J, Petersen TE, Thorgersen HC, Skorstengaard K, Sottrup-Jensen L, Magnusson S: Amino acid sequence of the factor XIIIa acceptor site in bovine plasma fibronectin. *FEBS Lett* **127**:174, 1981.
156. Tamaki T, Aoki N: Cross-linking of α_2-plasmin inhibitor to fibrin catalyzed by activated fibrin-stabilizing factor. *J Biol Chem* **257**:14767, 1982.
157. Lorand L: Fibrinoligase: The fibrin-stabilizing factor system of blood plasma. *Ann NY Acad Sci* **202**:6, 1972.
158. Shen LL, Hermans J, McDonagh J, McDonagh RP, Carr M: Effects of calcium ion and covalent crosslinking on formation and elasticity of fibrin gels. *Thromb Res* **6**:255, 1975.
159. Shen L, Lorand L: Contribution of fibrin stabilization to clot strength. *J Clin Invest* **71**:1336, 1983.
160. Shainoff JR, Urbanic DA, Dibello PM: Immunoelectrophoretic characterization of the cross-linking of fribrinogen and fibrin by factor XIIIa and tissue transglutaminase. *J Biol Chem* **266**:6429, 1991.
161. Tamaki T, Aoki N: Cross-linking of α_2-plasmin inhibitor and fibronectin to fibrin by fibrin-stabilizing factor. *Biochim Biophys Acta* **661**:280, 1981.
162. Ichinose A, Aoki N: Reversible cross-linking of α_2-plasmin inhibitor to fibrinogen by fibrin-stabilizing factor. *Biochim Biophys Acta* **706**:158, 1982.
163. Carmassi F, Chung SI: Regulation of fibrinolysis by factor XIII. *Prog Fibronolysis* **6**:281, 1983.
164. Ichinose A, Tamaki T, Aoki N: Factor XIII-mediated cross-linking of NH_2-terminal peptide of α_2-plasmin inhibitor to fibrin. *FEBS Lett* **153**:369, 1983.
165. Sakata Y, Aoki N: Cross-linking of α_2-plasmin inhibitor to fibrin by fibrin-stabilizing factor. *J Clin Invest* **65**:290, 1980.
166. Sakata Y, Aoki N: Significance of cross-linking of α_2-plasmin inhibitor to fibrin in inhibition of fibrinolysis and in hemostasis. *J Clin Invest* **69**:536, 1982.
167. Mosher D: Cross-linking of cold-insoluble globulin by fibrin-stabilizing factor. *J Biol Chem* **250**:6614, 1975.
168. Mosher DF, Schad PE, Kleinman HK: Cross-linking of fibronectin to collagen by blood coagulation factor XIIIa. *J Clin Invest* **64**:781, 1979.
169. Barry ELR, Mosher DF: Factor XIII cross-linking of fibronectin at cellular matrix assembly sites. *J Biol Chem* **263**:10464, 1988.
170. Barry ELR, Mosher DF: Factor XIIIa-mediated cross-linking of fibronectin in fibroblast cell layers. *J Biol Chem* **264**:4179, 1989.
171. Grinnell F, Feld M, Minter D: Fibroblast adhesion to fibrinogen and fibrin substrate: Requirement for cold-insoluble globulin (plasma fibronectin). *Cell* **19**:517, 1980.
172. Okamoto M, Yamamoto T, Matsubara S, Kukita I, Takeya M, Miyauchi Y, Kambara T: Factor XIII-dependent generation of 5th complement component (C5)-derived monocyte chemotactic factor coinciding with plasma clotting. *Biochim Biophys Acta* **1138**:53, 1992.
173. Duckert F: Documentation of the plasma factor XIII deficiency in man. *Ann NY Acad Sci* **202**:190, 1972.
174. Folk JE, Finlayson JS: The ϵ-(γ-glutamyl)lysine crosslink and the catalytic role of transglutaminases. *Adv Protein Chem* **31**:1, 1977.
175. Lorand L, Losowsky MS, Miloszewski KJM: Human factor XIII: Fibrin-stabilizing factor. *Prog Hemost Thromb* **5**:245, 1980.
176. Mui PTK, Ganguly P: Cross-linking of actin and fibrin by fibrin-stabilizing factor. *Am J Physiol* **233**:H346, 1977.
177. Cohen I, Young-Bandala L, Blankenberg TA, Siefring GE, Bruner-Lorand J: Fibrinoligase-catalyzed cross-linking of myosin from platelet and skeletal muscle. *Arch Biochem Biophys* **192**:100, 1979.
178. Cohen I, Glaser T, Veis A, Bruner-Lorand J: Ca^{2+}-dependent cross-linking processes in human platelets. *Biochim Biophys Acta* **676**:137, 1981.
179. Hada M, Kaminski M, Bockenstedt P, McDonagh J: Covalent crosslinking of von Willebrand factor to fibrin. *Blood* **68**:95, 1986.
180. Bockenstedt P, McDonagh J, Handin RI: Binding and covalent cross-linking of purified von Willebrand factor to native monomeric collagen. *J Clin Invest* **78**:551, 1986.
181. Bale MD, Mosher DF: Thrombospondin is a substrate for blood coagulation factor XIIIa. *Biochemistry* **25**:5667, 1986.
182. Francis RT, McDonagh J, Mann KG: Factor V is a substrate for the transamidase factor XIIIa. *J Biol Chem* **261**:9787, 1986.
183. Borth W, Chang V, Bishop P, Harpel PC: Lipoprotein(a) is a substrate for factor XIIIa and tissue transglutaminase. *J Biol Chem* **266**:18149, 1991.
184. Yorifuji H, Anderson K, Lynch GW, van de Water L, McDonagh J: B protein of factor XIII: Differentiation between free B and complexed B. *Blood* **72**:1645, 1988.
185. Cooke RD, Holbrook JJ: The calcium-induced dissociation of human plasma clotting factor XIII. *Biochem J* **141**:79, 1974.
186. Bannerjee D, Mosesson MW: Characterization of platelet protransglutaminase (factor XIII)-binding activity in human plasma. *Thromb Res* **7**:323, 1975.
187. Lee SY, Chung SI: Biosynthesis and degradation of plasma protransglutaminase (factor XIII). *Fed Proc* **35**:1486, 1976.
188. Ikematsu S: An approach to the metabolism of factor XIII. *Acta Haematol Jpn* **44**:1499, 1981.
189. Nagy JA, Henriksson P, McDonagh J: Biosynthesis of factor XIII b subunit by human hepatoma cell lines. *Blood* **68**:1272, 1986.
190. Weisberg LJ, Shiu DT, Greenberg CS, Kan YW, Shuman MA: Localization of the gene for coagulation factor XIII a-chain to chromosome 6 and identification of sites of synthesis. *J Clin Invest* **79**:649, 1987.
191. Weisberg LJ, Shiu DT, Conkling PR, Shuman MA: Identification of normal human peripheral blood monocytes and liver as sites of synthesis of coagulation factor XIII a-chain. *Blood* **70**:579, 1987.
192. Fear JD, Jackson P, Gray C, Miloszewski KJA, Losowsky MS: Localization of factor XIII in human tissues using an immunoperoxidase technique. *J Clin Pathol* **37**:560, 1984.
193. Chung SI: Comparative studies on tissue transglutaminase and factor XIII. *Ann NY Acad Sci* **202**:240, 1972.
194. Kiesselbach TH, Wagner RH: Demonstration of factor XIII in human megakaryocytes by a fluorescent antibody technique. *Ann NY Acad Sci* **202**:318, 1972.
195. Henriksson P, Becker S, Lynch G, McDonagh J: Identification of intracellular factor XIII in human monocytes and macrophages. *J Clin Invest* **76**:528, 1985.
196. Muszbek L, Adany R, Szegedi G, Plogar J, Kavai M: Factor XIII of blood coagulation in human monocytes. *Thromb Res* **37**:401, 1985.
197. Sixma JJ, Van Den Berg A, Schiphorst M, Gueze HJ, McDonagh J: Immunocytochemical localization of albumin and factor XIII in thin cryo sections of human blood platelets. *Thromb Haemost* **51**:388, 1984.
198. McDonagh J, McDonagh RP, Delage JM, Wagner RH: Factor XIII in human plasma and platelets. *J Clin Invest* **48**:940, 1969.
199. Lopaciuk S, Lovette KM, McDonagh J, Chuang HYK, McDonagh RP: Subcellular distribution of fibrinogen and factor XIII in human blood platelets. *Thromb Res* **8**:453, 1976.
200. Fesus L. Thomazy V, Autuori F, Ceru MP, Tarcsa E, Piacentini M: Apoptotic hepatocytes become insoluble in detergents and chaotropic agents as a result of transglutaminase action. *FEBS Lett* **245**:150, 1989.
201. Knight CRL, Rees RC, Griffin M: Apoptosis: A potential role for cytosolic transglutaminase and its importance in tumour progression. *Biochim Biophys Acta* **1096**:312, 1991.
202. Cerio R, Griffiths CEM, Cooper KD, Nickoloff BJ, Headington JT: Characterization of factor XIIIa positive dermal dendritic cells in normal and inflamed skin. *Br J Dermatol* **121**:421, 1989.
203. Wolpl A, Lattke H, Board PG, Arnold R, Schmeiser T, Kubanek B, Robin-Winn M, Pichelmayr R, Goldmann SF: Coagulation factor XIII a and b subunits in bone marrow and liver transplantation. *Transplantation* **43**:151, 1987.
204. Poon M-C, Russell JA, Low S, Sinclair GD, Jones AR, Blahey W, Ruether BA, Hoar DI: Hemopoietic origin of factor XIII A subunits in platelets, monocytes, and plasma. *J Clin Invest* **84**:787, 1989.
205. Ichinose A, Kaetsu H: Molecular approach to the structure-

function relationship of human coagulation factor XIII. *Methods Enzymol* **222**:36, 1993.

206. Ichinose A, Davie EW: Characterization of the gene for the a subunit of human factor XIII (plasma transglutaminase), a blood coagulation factor. *Proc Natl Acad Sci USA* **85**:5829, 1988.
207. Auron PE, Webb AC, Rosenwasser LJ, Mucci SF, Rich A, Wolff SM, Dinarello CA: Nucleotide sequence of human monocyte interleukin 1 precursor cDNA. *Proc Natl Acad Sci USA* **81**:7907, 1984.
208. Wallner BP, Mattaliano RJ, Hession C, Cate RL, Tizard Pepinsky RB: Cloning and expression of human lipocortin, a phospholipase A_2 inhibitor with potential anti-inflammatory activity. *Nature* **320**:77, 1986.
209. Jaye M, Howk R, Burgess W, Ricca GA, Chiu IM, Ravera MW, O'Brien SJ, Modi WS, Maciag T, Drohan WN: Human endothelial cell growth factor: Cloning, nucleotide sequence, and chromosome localization. *Science* **233**:541, 1986.
210. Kurokawa T, Sasada R, Iwane M, Igarashi K: Cloning and expression of cDNA encoding human basic fibroblast growth factor. *FEBS Lett* **213**:189, 1987.
211. Ye RD, Wun TC, Sadler JE: cDNA cloning and expression in Escherichia coli of a plasminogen activator inhibitor from human placenta. *J Biol Chem* **262**:3718, 1987.
212. Hogquist KA, Nett MA, Unanue ER, Chaplin DD: Interleukin 1 is processed and released during apoptosis. *Proc Natl Acad Sci USA* **88**:8485, 1991.
213. Rubartelli A, Cozzolino F, Talio M, Sitia R: A novel secretory pathway for interleukin-1b, a protein lacking a signal sequence. *EMBO J* **9**:1503, 1990.
214. Barbui T, Cartei G, Chisesi T, Dini E: Electroimmunoassay of plasma subunits-A and -S in a case of congenital fibrin stabilizing factor deficiency. *Thromb Diath Haemorrh* **32**:124, 1974.
215. Barbui T, Rodeghiero F, Dini E, Mariani G, Papa ML, De Biasi R, Murillo RC, Umana CM: Subunits A and S inheritance in four families with congenital factor XIII deficiency. *Br J Haematol* **38**:267, 1978.
216. Rodeghiero F, Morbin M, Barbui T: Subunit a of factor XIII regulates subunit b plasma concentration. *Thromb Haemost* **46**:621, 1981.
217. Saito M, Asakura H, Yoshida T, Ito K, Okafuji K, Yoshida T, Matsuda T: A familial factor XIII subunit b deficiency. *Br J Haematol* **74**:290, 1990.
218. Fear JD, Miloszewski KJA, Losowsky MS: The half life of factor XIII in the management of inherited deficiency. *Thromb Haemost* **49**:102, 1983.
219. Rodeghiero F, Tosetto A, Bona ED, Castaman G: Clinical pharmacokinetics of a placenta-derived factor XIII concentrate in type I and type II factor XIII deficiency. *Am J Hematol* **36**:30, 1991.
220. Folk JE, Chung SI: Blood coagulation factor XIII: Relationship of some biological properties to subunit structure, in Reich E, Rifkin DB, Show E (eds): *Proteases and Biological Control*. Cold Spring Harbor, NY, Cold Spring Harbor Laboratory, 1975, p 157.
221. Lewis SD, Janus TJ, Lorand L, Shafer JA: Regulation and formation of factor XIIIa by its fibrin substrates. *Biochemistry* **24**:6772, 1985.
222. Naski MC, Lorand L, Shafer JA: Characterization of the kinetic pathway for fibrin promotion of α-thrombin-catalyzed activation of plasma factor XIII. *Biochemistry* **30**:934, 1991.
223. Hornyak TJ, Shafer JA: Role of calcium ion in the generation of factor XIII activity. *Biochemistry* **30**:6175, 1991.
224. Curtis CG, Brown KL, Credo RB, Domanik RA, Gray A, Stenberg P, Lorand L: Calcium-dependent unmasking of active center cysteine during activation of fibrin stabilizing factor. *Biochemistry* **13**:3774, 1974.
225. Credo RB, Curtis CG, Lorand L: α-chain domain of fibrinogen controls generation of fibrinoligase (coagulation factor XIIIa). *Biochemistry* **20**:3770, 1981.
226. McDonagh J, McDonagh RP: Alternative pathways for the activation of factor XIII. *Br J Haematol* **30**:465, 1975.
227. Henriksson P, Nilsson IM, Ohlsson K, Stenberg P: Granulocyte elastase activation and degradation of factor XIII. *Thromb Res* **18**:343, 1980.
228. Lynch GW, Pfueller SL: Thrombin-independent activation of platelet factor XIII by endogenous platelet acid protease. *Thromb Haemost* **59**:372, 1988.
229. Schrode J, Chung SI, Folk JE: Thrombin cleavage products of human placental transglutaminase. *Fed Proc* **35**:1487, 1976.
230. Hornyak TJ, Bishop PD, Shafer JA: α-Thrombin-catalyzed activation of human platelet factor XIII: Relationship between proteolysis and factor XIIIa activity. *Biochemistry* **28**:7326, 1989.
231. Chung D, Ichinose A: Hereditary disorders related to fibrinogen and factor XIII, in Scriver CR, Beaudet AL, Sly WS, Valle D (eds): *The Metabolic Basis of Inherited Disease*, 6th ed. New York: McGraw-Hill, 1989, vol 2, p 2135.
232. Board PG, Webb GC, McKee J, Ichinose A: Localization of the coagulation factor XIII A subunit gene (F13A) to chromosome bands 6p24-p25. *Cytogenet Cell Genet* **48**:25, 1988.
233. Polakowska RR, Eddy RL, Shows TB, Goldsmith LA: Epidermal type I transglutaminase (TGM1) is assigned to human chromosome 14. *Cytogenet Cell Genet* **56**:105, 1991.
234. Kim I-G, McBride OW, Wang M, Kim S-Y, Idler WW, Steinert PM: Structure and organization of the human transglutaminase 1 gene. *J Biol Chem* **267**:7710, 1992.
235. Webb GC, Coggan M, Ichinose A, Board PG: Localization of the coagulation factor XIII B subunit gene (F13B) to chromosome bands 1q31-32.1. *Hum Genet* **81**:157, 1989.
236. de Cordoba SR, Rey-Campos J, Dykes DD, McAlpine PJ, Wong P, Rubinstein P: Coagulation factor XIII B subunit is encoded by a gene linked to the regulator of complement activation (RCA) gene cluster in man. *Immunogenetics* **28**:452, 1988.
237. Pardo-Manuel F, Rey-Campos J, Hillarp A, Dahlback B, de Cordoba SR: Human genes for the a and b chains of complement C4b-binding protein are closely linked in a head-to-tail arrangement. *Proc Natl Acad Sci USA* **87**:4529, 1990.
238. Korsgren C, Cohen CM: Organization of the gene for human erythrocyte membrane protein 4.2: Structural similarities with the gene for the a subunit of factor XIII. *Proc Natl Acad Sci USA* **88**:4840, 1991.
239. Phillips MA, Stewart BE, Rice RH: Genomic structure of keratinocyte transglutaminase. *J Biol Chem* **267**:2282, 1992.
240. Board PG: Genetic polymorphism of the a subunit of human coagulation factor XIII. *Am J Hum Genet* **31**:116, 1979.
241. Castle SL, Board PG: An extended survey of the genetic polymorphism of the coagulation factor XIII: A subunit structural locus. *Hum Hered* **35**:101, 1985.
242. Zoghbi HY, Daiger SP, McCall A, O'Brien WE, Beaudet AL: Extensive DNA polymorphism at the factor XIIIa (F13A) locus and linkage to HLA. *Am J Genet* **42**:877, 1988.
243. Board PG: Genetic polymorphism of the b subunit of human coagulation factor XIII. *Am J Hum Genet* **32**:348, 1980.
244. Fukui H: Hemophilia and the related diseases. *Nihon Rinsho* **41**:704, 1983.
245. Hahn L, Lundberg PA, Teger-Nilsson AC: Congenital hypofibrinogenemia and recurrent abortion. *Br J Obstet Gynaecol* **85**:790, 1978.
246. Evron S, Anteby SO, Brzezinsky A, Samueloff A, Eldor A: Congenital afibrinogenemia and recurrent early abortion: A case report. *Eur J Obstet Gynecol Reprod Biol* **19**:307, 1985.
247. McDonagh J, Carrell N: Disorders of fibrinogen structure and function, in Colman RW, Hirsh J, Marder VJ, Salzman EW (eds): *Hemostasis and Thrombosis, Basic Principles and Clinical Practice*. Philadelphia, Lippincott, 1987, p 301.
248. Kamura T, Okamura T, Murakawa M, Tsuda H, Teshima T, Shibuya T, Harada M, Niho Y: Deficiency of coagulation factor XIII A subunit caused by the dinucleotide deletion at the 5′ end of exon III. *J Clin Invest* **90**:315, 1992.
249. Board P, Coggan M, Miloszewski K: Identification of a point mutation in factor XIII A subunit deficiency. *Blood* **80**:937, 1992.
250. Castle SL, Board PG, Anderson RAM: Genetic heterogeneity of factor XIII deficiency: First description of unstable a subunits. *Br J Haematol* **48**:337, 1981.

251. Lorand L, Campbell-Wilkes LK, Cooperstein L: A filter paper assay for transamidating enzymes using radioactive amine substrates. *Anal Biochem* **50:**623, 1972.
252. Nishida Y, Ikematsu S, Fukutake K, Fujimaki M, Fukutake K, Kakishita E: A new rapid and simple assay for factor XIII activity using dancylcadaverine incorporation and gel filtration. *Thromb Res* **36:**123, 1984.
253. Trobisch H, Egbring R: Substitution treatment of factor XIII deficiency with a new factor XIII concentrate. *Dtsch Med Wochenschr* **97:**499, 1972.
254. Kuratsuji T, Oikawa T, Fukumoto T, Shimizu S, Iwasaki Y, Tomita Y, Meguro T, Yamada K: Factor XIII deficiency in antibiotic-associated pseudomembranous colitis and its treatment with factor XIII concentrate. *Haemostasis* **11:**229, 1982.
255. Bishop PD, Teller DC, Smith RA, Lasser GW, Gilbert T, Seale RL: Expression, purification, and characterization of human factor XIII in *Saccharomyces cerevisiae*. *Biochemistry* **29:**1861, 1990.

CHAPTER **106**

Hemophilia A and Parahemophilia: Deficiencies of Coagulation Factors VIII and V

Haig H. Kazazian, Jr. ▪ Edward G. D. Tuddenham
Stylianos E. Antonarakis

1. Hemophilia A (classic hemophilia) is an X-linked bleeding disorder characterized by a deficiency in the activity of factor VIII, a key component of the coagulation cascade. Roughly 1 in 5,000 to 10,000 males are affected in all populations.

2. Affected individuals suffer joint and muscle hemorrhage, easy bruising, and prolonged bleeding from wounds. Because platelet function is not affected, blood loss from minor cuts and abrasions is not excessive. Of hemophilia A patients, 50 to 70 percent of patients have severe hemophilia with factor VIII activity <1 percent, while the remainder have mild to moderate disease with factor VIII levels of 1 to 20 percent. Nearly all patients with severe disease have no factor VIII protein in their plasma (CRM−), but a small proportion of these patients (about 5 percent) have inactive factor VIII protein circulating in their plasma (CRM+).

3. Factor VIII functions as a cofactor in the activation of factor X to factor Xa in a reaction catalyzed by factor IXa on a phospholipid surface. Factor VIII is activated by specific proteolytic cleavage by thrombin and factor Xa, which results in an effective amplification of the signal through this step of the cascade. Factor VIII is inactivated by limited proteolysis by factor Xa or by activated protein C.

4. Hemophilia A arises from a variety of mutations within the factor VIII gene, which is located near the telomere of the long arm of the X chromosome. The gene comprises 26 exons and spans 186 kb. The cDNA sequence reveals that factor VIII is synthesized as a large precursor molecule (2332 amino acids). The amino acid sequence of the protein has considerable sequence similarity to that of ceruloplasmin and coagulation factor V.

5. About 95 percent of patients with hemophilia A in whom mutations have been characterized have point mutations in the gene. Although the functional consequences of some of the 150-odd point mutations producing the disease are known (for example, some alter a thrombin cleavage site or a von Willebrand factor binding site), the structure–function relationships of most mutations remain unknown. An unusual inversion accounts for about 25 percent of the total mutations producing the disease.

6. Treatment of hemophilia A is accomplished by infusions of factor VIII concentrates prepared either from human plasma or by recombinant DNA technology. The in vivo half-life of such preparations is approximately 12 h. While such therapy is effective in most cases, approximately 15 percent of affected individuals eventually develop neutralizing antibodies (inhibitors) that complicate further therapy.

A list of standard abbreviations is located immediately preceding the index in each volume. Additional abbreviations used in this chapter include: AHG = antihemophilic globulin; APC = activated protein C; DDAVP = 1-desamino-8-D-arginine vasopressin; FVIII = factor VIII; vWF = von Willebrand factor.

HISTORICAL PERSPECTIVE

Sex-linked hemophilia, of which factor VIII deficiency is the leading cause, was first recognized by Rabbi Simon ben Gamaliel in the 2nd century A.D. He gave dispensation from circumcision to an infant whose three maternal cousins had died after the operation (Babylonian Talmud,[1,2]). The first reference to a male-specific bleeding disorder in the medical literature appeared eight centuries later. Khalif ibn Abbas, a great surgical writer of the Moorish period in Spain, wrote of a certain village where there were men who, when wounded, suffered uncontrollable hemorrhage that caused death.[3] In the modern medical literature, the first report of hemophilia was by John Otto (ref 4, reprinted in ref 5). He noted the pattern of transmission: "It is a surprising circumstance that the males only are subject to this strange affection and that all of them are not liable to it. Although the females are exempt, they are still capable of transmitting it to their children." Severe bleeding from trivial injury was the major clinical feature noted.

In 1813, an account was published of another North American family of bleeders—the Appleton-Swain kindred.[6] The founder of this kindred was a certain Oliver Appleton who came to Massachusetts from England in the 18th century. He was himself a bleeder and had three daughters (Fig. 106-1). Both of the daughters who married had "bleeder" sons who themselves had daughters who bore bleeder sons—the great-great-grandsons of Oliver Appleton. This family was later studied by Osler.[7]

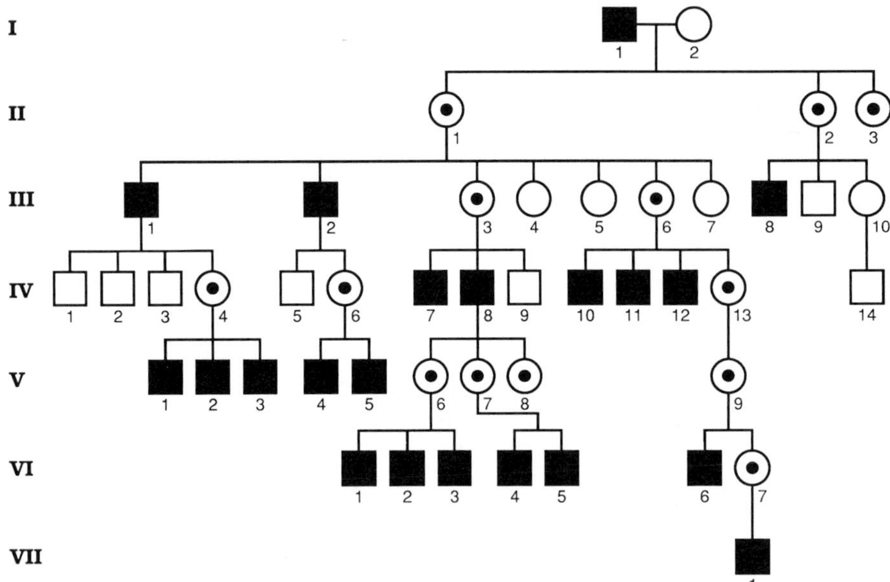

FIG. 106-1 Appleton–Swain kindred, the first kindred published in 1813 showing all the characteristics of a sex-linked bleeding disorder.[6] Solid squares = bleeder males; open squares = normal males; circles with dot = obligatory carrier females.

The first recorded usage of the term *hemophilia* was by Hopff at the University of Würzburg in 1828.[8] The cases referred to were four brothers who bled to death either from a trivial injury or, in one case, from a ruptured tumor of the thigh. From the clinical description, the latter was probably a hemophilic pseudotumor.

In a monumental compilation in 1911, Bulloch and Fildes critically reviewed almost 1000 publications on hemophilia and related conditions, extracting from them 224 pedigrees.[1] Almost all of the clinical features of untreated hemophilia that we recognize today were well described in 1911. A satisfactory theory of the genetics of sex-linked disorders had just become available. Bateson's 1909 book *Mendel's Principles of Heredity* contains an account of sex-linked recessive color blindness.[9] He made the correct interpretation that female carriers are heterozygous, therefore unaffected. Bateson realized the importance of the normality of affected men's sons and the carrier status of their daughters and rightly concluded that this implied dimorphism of spermatozoa (X or Y). It was soon realized that hemophilia, as classically defined, fit perfectly the prediction of an X-linked recessive disorder. The occurrence of homozygous affected females was also predicted and correctly explained by Bateson.[9]

The most famous hemophilic kindred is that descended from Queen Victoria (Fig. 106-2). None of Victoria's ancestors suffered from a bleeding tendency, but she was clearly a carrier of X-linked hemophilia since one of her sons (Leopold) was affected and two of her daughters (Alice and Beatrice) were carriers, transmitting the disease to their descendants.[10] Through dynastic marriage and intermarriage, the gene was passed to three other royal families in Europe, with particularly tragic consequences for the Russian royal family. Among the affected males in this kindred, only Leopold lived to have children, and he died at the age of 31. All the other hemophilic males had died of bleeding without issue by 1945, demonstrating the short life expectancy and low reproductive fitness of hemophiliacs before replacement therapy. Since their death predated the discovery that X-linked hemophilia can be due to either factor VIII or factor IX deficiency, we do not know to which type the royal hemophilia belonged. A plausible origin for the royal hemophilia gene is the gamete supplied by Victoria's father, Edward, Duke of Kent, who was 54 at the time of Victoria's birth.

Research into the defect in the blood of hemophiliacs began in the late 19th century. Almroth Wright[11] showed that whereas normal blood clotted in a capillary tube in 6 min, blood from a boy with typical clinical features of severe hemophilia took over 10 min to clot. Thomas Addis[12,13] showed that the prolonged clotting time of hemophilic blood could be corrected by a fraction from normal blood. He also demonstrated a delay in the conversion of prothrombin to thrombin and concluded that this was sufficient to completely explain the hemostatic failure. The fraction of plasma that Addis used to study prothrombin content was a euglobulin fraction that contains both prothrombin and factor VIII among many other proteins. Therefore, Addis concluded that hemophilia is due to prothrombin deficiency, an inescapable conclusion in terms of the theory of blood coagulation proposed by Morawitz,[14] which prevailed then and for 30 years after. Based on this theory, the coagulation defect of hemophilia could *only* be due to a deficiency of prothrombin, calcium, thrombokinase, or fibrinogen. The last option was excluded by the finding that hemophilic blood could form a firm clot if "thrombokinase" or tissue extract was added to it.[11] Although Addis' experiment pointed to a prothrombin defect, Govaerts and Gratia[15] demonstrated that the correcting fraction in normal plasma was not absorbed by tricalcium phosphate and therefore could not be prothrombin. Furthermore, prothrombin was later shown to be normal in hemophilic blood by Quick[16] using his newly devised prothrombin time. Addis had shown that hemophilic blood clotted more slowly than normal in response to diluted tissue extract, but the explanation for this correct observation has only recently come to light.[17]

Morawitz and Lossen had studied the blood of a hemophilic boy in 1908 and concluded there was a deficiency of thrombokinase production by the corpuscles.[18] Sahli drew the similar conclusion that the tissues were deficient in thrombokinase.[19] Neither hypothesis was supported by later experiments. Thus, an intellectual impasse was reached which could only be surmounted by a new attack on theory. This came in 1937, when Patek and Taylor re-examined a plasma fraction similar to Addis' and confirmed that it would correct the prolonged clotting time of hemophilic blood.[20]

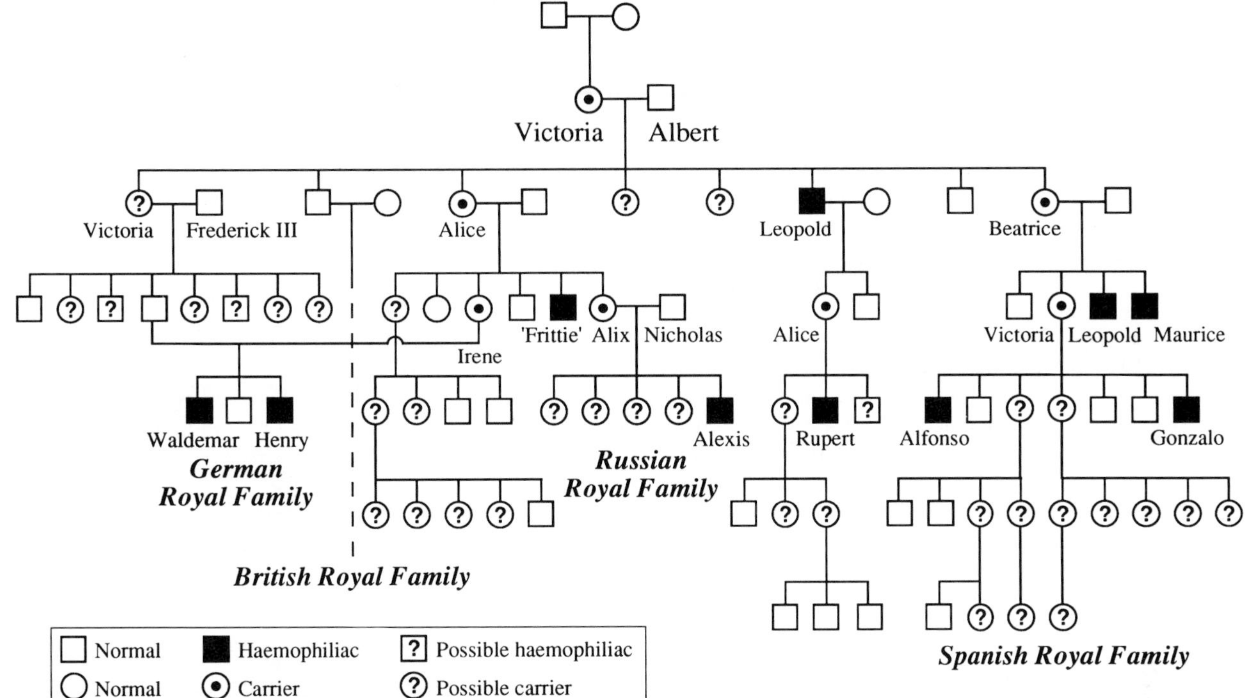

FIG. 106-2 The royal hemophilia pedigree of Queen Victoria's descendants, emphasizing the lines affected by bleeding. The present British royal family is unaffected, being descended through a normal male. The defective gene almost certainly died out with Leopold's daughter Alice in 1980.

They called this fraction "globulin" and, later, "antihemophilic globulin" (AHG).[21]

A further advance came when quantitative assays were devised for measuring the correcting fraction.[22,23] Hemophilia became defined as the condition that results from a deficiency of AHG and is inherited in a sex-linked recessive fashion, with sporadic cases due to new mutation. In 1952, three groups[24–26] simultaneously reported that one hemophiliac's blood could cross-correct that of other clinically identical cases, and that hemophilia, therefore, can be caused by deficiency of more than one factor. The new factor was factor IX, and its deficiency is responsible for about one-sixth of the cases of X-linked hemophilia. By international convention, AHG was assigned the Roman number VIII.[27] The two disorders are now called hemophilia A and B (factor VIII and factor IX deficiency, respectively). Attempts to purify factor VIII began in the 1950s as soon as an assay became available. In retrospect, it is easy to see that the early work failed for the following reasons: (1) factor VIII copurifies with its carrier protein, von Willebrand factor (vWF) and (2) factor VIII is unstable and is present in a very low concentration in blood. In 1972, Owen and Wagner used gel filtration[28] to establish that 0.25 M $CaCl_2$ was highly effective at lowering the molecular weight of factor VIII. Furthermore, a high molecular weight for factor VIII was restored by dialyzing off the $CaCl_2$.

In 1971 Zimmerman and colleagues showed that an antigen detected by antisera raised in rabbits against partially purified factor VIII was at reduced concentration in the blood of patients with von Willebrand disease[29] (see Chap. 107) but present in normal quantities in the blood of hemophilia A patients. This antigen was first called by its discoverers factor VIII-related antigen (VIIIR:Ag), but is now designated von Willebrand antigen (vW:Ag).

In 1973, Zimmerman and Edgington used immobilized antibodies to obtain differential absorption of VIII:C and vWF.[30] They concluded that "Factor VIII coagulant activity resides on a molecule distinct from that expressing the von Willebrand's antigen."

In 1979, it was shown that factor VIII could be completely separated from von Willebrand factor by immunoaffinity purification.[31] In 1982, Fass and colleagues succeeded in isolating porcine factor VIII using a monoclonal antibody.[32] These techniques were used by several groups to isolate sufficient factor VIII for partial sequence determination, and the availability of a partial protein sequence made possible the cloning of factor VIII cDNA and its gene.[33–35] In this chapter, we describe the clinical features of hemophilia A, the structure and physiology of factor VIII in blood coagulation, the molecular pathology of the disease and the general biological lessons learned from studies of its mutational basis, carrier and antenatal diagnosis of hemophilia A, and treatment of the disease.

CLINICAL FEATURES OF HEMOPHILIA A

Incidence

The frequency of this disorder is often stated to be 1 in 10,000 male births. This is certainly an underestimate, because countries that compile central records (e.g., the U.K. and Sweden) have a much higher frequency in the general population. Currently, the U.K. has 5,000 cases of hemophilia A known to the Haemophilia Centre Directors, which, in a population of about 58,000,000, approaches 1:5,000 male births (allowing for a shorter than normal life expectancy), or 1:10,000 in the general population.[36] A possible cause of the lower estimates could be underreporting of moderate and mild hemophilia A; these forms of the disease account for up to half of all cases and present later in life than severe hemophilia.

Clinical Features

Almost all patients are male (see "Hemophilia A in Females" below). The severity and frequency of bleeding in X-linked factor VIII deficiency is inversely correlated with the residual factor VIII level. Table 106-1 summarizes this relationship and gives the relative frequencies of categories, based on U.K. national data.[36] The joints most affected are the main load- or strain-bearing articulations—ankles, knees, hips, and elbows—but any joint can be the site of bleeding. If untreated, this intracapsular bleeding causes severe swelling, pain, stiffness, and inflammation, which gradually resolve over days or weeks (for a vivid account of a classical case, see *Journey* by Robert and Anne Massie[37]). Blood is highly irritating to the synovium and causes synovial overgrowth, with a tendency to rebleed from friable vascular tissue, thus setting up a vicious cycle. Probably through accumulation of iron in chondrocytes, a rapid degenerative arthritis occurs, leading to irregularity of the articular contour, then to thinning of the cartilage and bony overgrowth, and finally to ankylosis (Figs. 106-3 to 106-5). A particular joint or joints tend to be the target for this destructive process in a given patient, while other joints may be relatively spared.

Muscle bleeding can be seen in any anatomical site but most often presents in the large, load-bearing groups of the thigh, calf, posterior abdominal wall, and buttocks. Local pressure effects often cause entrapment neuropathy, particularly of the femoral nerve with iliopsoas bleeding. The latter causes a common symptom triad of groin pain, hip flexure, and cutaneous sensory loss over the femoral nerve distribution. Bleeding into the calf, forearm, or peroneal muscles can lead to ischemic necrosis and contracture (Fig. 106-6).

Hematuria is less common than joint or muscle bleeding in hemophiliacs, but most severely affected patients have one or two episodes per decade. These may be painless and resolve spontaneously, but, if bleeding is heavy, they can produce severe pain owing to obstruction by a large blood clot. Usually, no anatomical abnormality is found on radiological investigation to account for the hematuria.

Central nervous system bleeding is uncommon, but can occur after slight head injury and was formerly the most common cause of death in hemophilia A. Intestinal tract bleeding usually presents as obstruction due to intramural hemorrhage, but hematemesis and melena occur occasionally and should be routinely investigated since they may be due to peptic ulcer or malignancy.

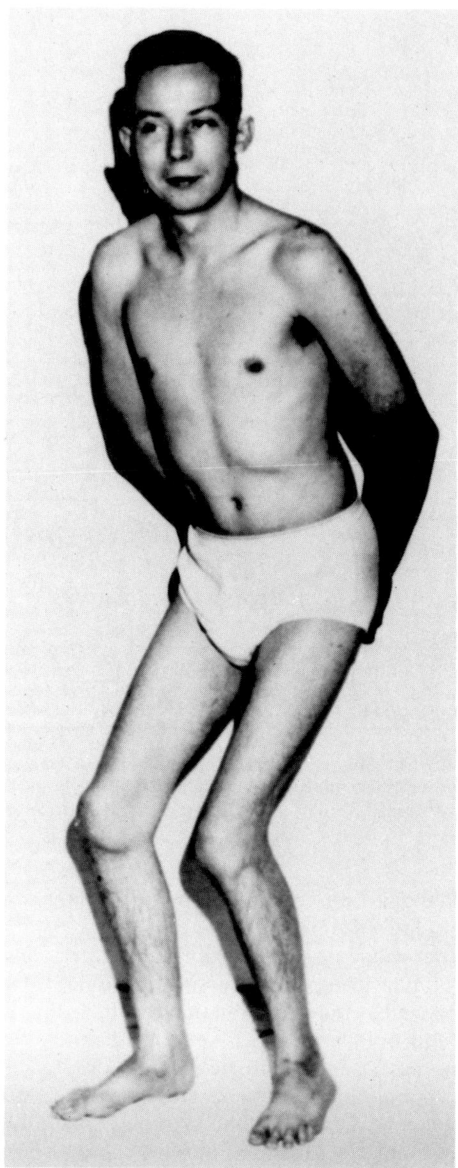

FIG. 106-3 Patient with hemophilia A who grew to maturity before the availability of factor VIII concentrate. He has fixed flexion deformities of both knees and both elbows owing to hemarthroses.

Table 106-1 Relationship of Factor VIII Activity to Severity of Hemophilia A

Factor VIII (U/dl)	Bleeding Tendency	Relative Incidence of Cases (percent)
<2	Severe; frequent spontaneous* bleeding into joints, muscles, and internal organs	50
2–10	Moderately severe; some spontaneous bleeds; bleeding after minor trauma	30
>10–30	Mild; bleeding only after significant trauma or surgery	20

*"Spontaneous bleeding" refers to episodes where no obvious precipitating event precedes the bleed. Presumably, minor tissue damage caused by everyday activities actually initiates bleeding.

Oropharyngeal bleeding, although uncommon, is clinically dangerous since extension through the soft tissue of the floor of the mouth can lead to respiratory obstruction (Fig. 106-7). Bleeding from the tongue after laceration can be very persistent and troublesome because of the fibrinolytic substances in saliva and the impossibility of immobilizing the part.

Surgery and open trauma invariably lead to dangerous hemorrhage in the untreated hemophiliac. The most impressive feature is not the rate of hemorrhage but its persistence, often after an initial short-lived period of hemostasis. Clots, if formed, are bulky and friable and break off, with renewed hemorrhage occurring intermittently over days and weeks. Occasionally, a hemorrhage into a large muscle such as the gluteus fails to resolve, instead becoming encysted and enlarging slowly as a result of repeated bleeding, thus forming

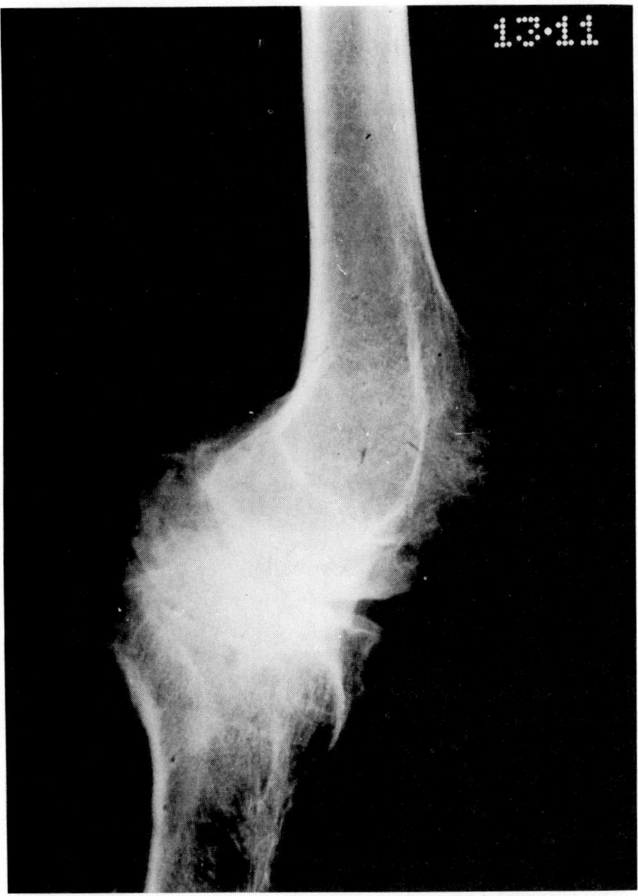

FIG. 106-4 X-ray of the right knee of a hemophiliac showing end-stage hemophilic osteoarthropathy. Note loss of cartilage, osteoporosis, cysts in bone near joint surface, anterior subluxation, deformity, and ankylosis.

a hemophilic pseudotumor (Fig. 106-8). This development is only seen today in patients who are resistant to conventional replacement therapy owing to the presence of inhibitors (see below) or who live where little treatment is available—that is to say, in most developing countries.

Bruising is a feature of hemophilia A, but usually is of only cosmetic significance since it remains superficial and

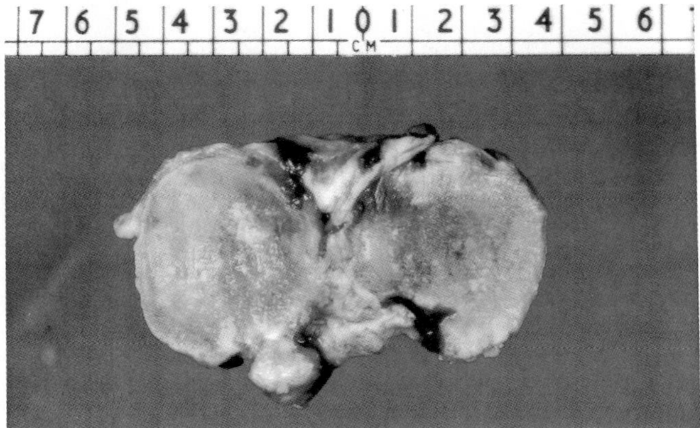

FIG. 106-5 Tibial condyles removed from the knee of a hemophiliac undergoing total knee replacement for advanced arthropathy. Note severe roughening of joint surface with aberrant vascular tissue in the normally avascular area and brown hemosiderin deposition in synovial tissues, the residue of repeated bleeding episodes.

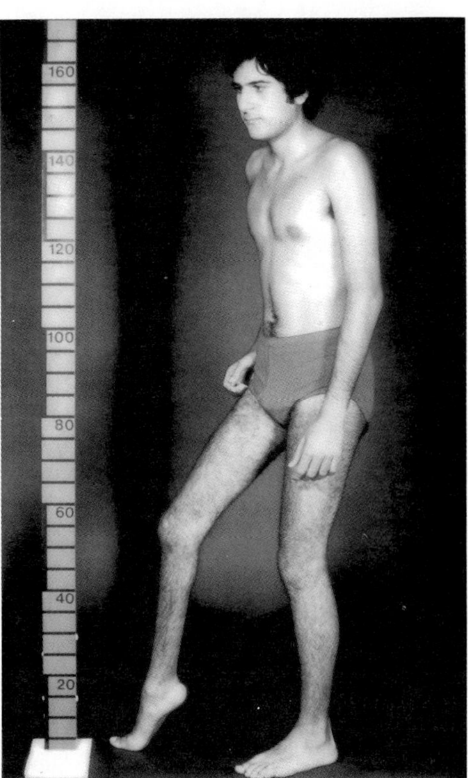

FIG. 106-6 Joint contractures in a patient with hemophilia A. Talipes equinovarus of right foot secondary to untreated bleeding into the calf muscles with ischemic necrosis, followed by contraction and fibrosis causing fixed extension of the ankle. The patient's right elbow is held in fixed flexion owing to hemarthrosis leading to osteoarthropathy.

self-limiting. Large, extending ecchymoses may occasionally require treatment.

When a woman is known to be a carrier or at high risk, a cord blood factor VIII level will establish the diagnosis in her infant. One-third of cases are sporadic, however, and in these the hemophilic condition may come to light in the neonatal period as a result of cephalohematoma or prolonged bleeding from the cord. In cultures where early circumcision is the rule, it will cause prolonged hemorrhage, as was noted in the Babylonian Talmud.[1] Quite often the diagnosis is not made until the infant is noticed to have many large bruises caused by the pressure of being lifted or by minor bumps on the crib (Fig. 106-9). These sometimes cause diagnostic confusion and the erroneous label of "battered baby syndrome," with needless psychological trauma to the parents. As soon as the infant starts to crawl actively, joint bleeding will begin to appear. In other children, excessive bleeding from eruption of primary dentition or from lacerations leads to the performance of diagnostic tests. Patients with mild disease present in later life when severe trauma or surgery provoke unusual bleeding.

Pathophysiology

All the clinical features of hemophilia A are due directly or indirectly to lack of clotting factor VIII. Sufferers are unable to produce normal levels of factor VIII because of various mutations (see below) at the factor VIII locus. Lack of the cofactor drastically slows the rate of generation of factor Xa, even though all other coagulation factors and platelets

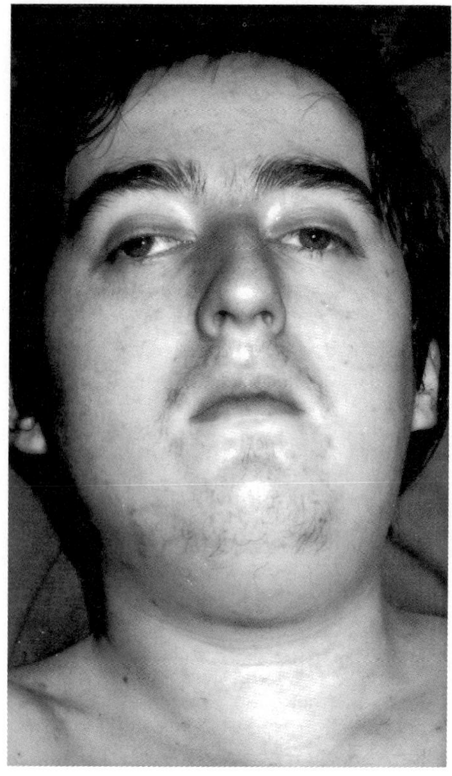

A

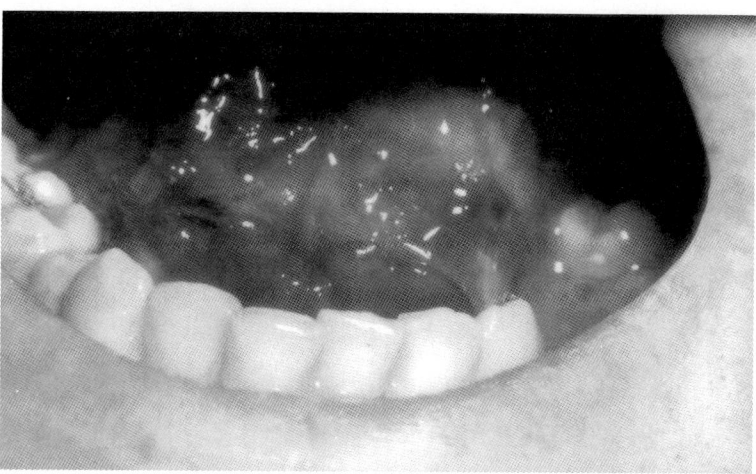

B

FIG. 106-7 Hemophilia A patient with a factor VIII inhibitor. *A*. Sublingual bleeding with extension to oropharyngeal region. The patient developed respiratory distress before the bleeding could be controlled by porcine factor VIII. *B*. Infralingual soft tissues distended with blood.

are present in normal amounts. Conversely, replacement of factor VIII by intravenous infusion completely normalizes the hemophiliac's hemostatic mechanism for as long as the infused factor remains in the circulation at physiological concentration (see "Treatment of Hemophilia A" below).

Laboratory Diagnosis

Screening tests show a prolonged partial thromboplastin time (PTT), normal prothrombin time (PT), normal thrombin clotting time (TCT), normal bleeding time, and normal platelet count. Specific assays show factor VIII clotting activity below 35 U/dl with all other factors normal, including vWF antigen and ristocetin cofactor. A test for antibodies to factor VIII should also be performed.

A normal bleeding time and ristocetin cofactor assay help to distinguish mild hemophilia A from von Willebrand disease, the only condition with which it is likely to be confused on laboratory test results. Quite recently, a number

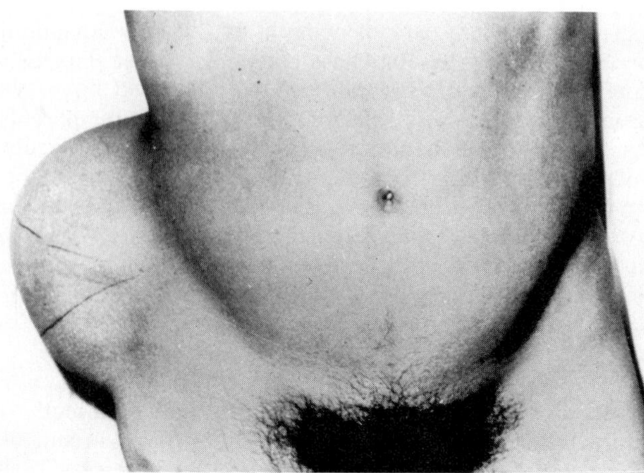

FIG. 106-8 Hemophilic pseudotumour arising in the gluteus muscle. Surgical excision of the entire pseudotumor is mandatory, since rupture and infection of such lesions is invariably fatal.

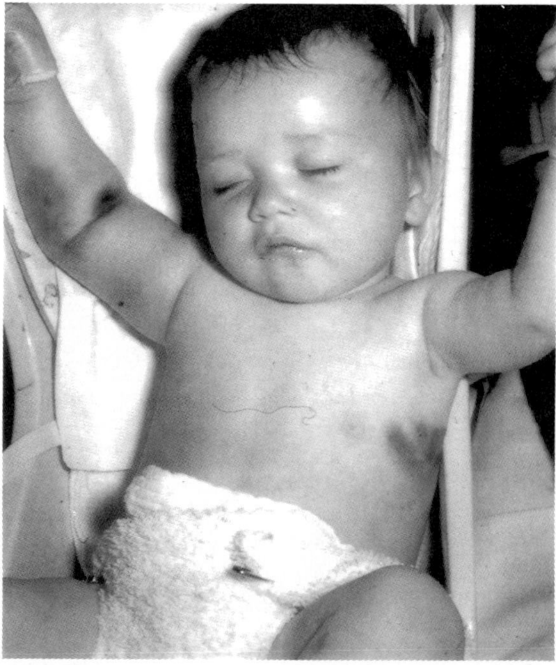

FIG. 106-9 Hemophilia A presentation in infancy with bruising on left chest wall. This led to unsuccessful attempts to obtain a blood sample via the right antecubital fossa, resulting in further bruising.

of individuals have been described with apparently autosomal recessive hemophilia A due to defects in the region of vWF involved in binding to factor VIII.[38] Specific assays for the interaction of vWF with factor VIII are required to identify these rare cases.

THE STRUCTURE AND PHYSIOLOGY OF FACTOR VIII

The Factor VIII Gene and Its Deduced Protein Structure

The gene for factor VIII was first cloned in 1984.[33–35,39] The cloning was accomplished by screening bacteriophage λ genomic libraries with oligonucleotide probes synthesized to correspond to sequenced tryptic peptides from purified human[39] or porcine factor VIII.[35]

Factor VIII genomic DNA is 186-kb long (approximately 0.1 percent of the DNA of the X chromosome) and contains 26 exons and 25 introns. The nucleotide sequence of the exons, intron–exon boundaries, and 5′ flanking region has been determined.[33–35,39] The exon length varies from 69 to 262 bp except for exon 14, which is 3106-bp long, and the last exon (exon 26), which is 1958-bp long (Fig. 106-10). Some of the intervening sequences are quite large; intron 22 is 32 kb, and introns 1, 6, 13, 14, and 25 are 14 to 23 kb.

The normal factor VIII mRNA consists of approximately 9 kb, of which the coding sequence is 7053 nucleotides. There is a CpG island in intron 22, which is associated with two additional transcripts. One transcript of 1.8 kb is produced abundantly in a wide variety of cells. The orientation of this transcript is opposite to that of factor VIII and contains no intervening sequence.[40] This 1739-nucleotide-long cDNA has been termed "factor VIII-associated gene A" (F8A) and is conserved in the mouse.[41] The second transcript, of 2.5 kb, is transcribed in the same direction as factor VIII. After a short exon that may code for eight amino acids, it uses exons 23 to 26 of the factor VIII gene.[42] This gene has been termed "factor VIII-associated gene B" (F8B). The two transcripts, F8A and F8B, originate within 122 bases of each other. The function of these transcripts and their potential protein products are unknown.

Factor VIII is expressed in the liver, spleen, lymph nodes, and a variety of other human tissues but not in bone marrow, peripheral blood lymphocytes, or endothelial cells.[43] In the liver, the hepatocyte is the predominant cell that synthesizes factor VIII mRNA.[43,44]

The gene for factor VIII encodes a precursor protein of 2351 amino acid residues (Fig. 106-11). The first 19 amino acids constitute the leader peptide.[33] This peptide contains 10 hydrophobic amino acids flanked by two charged residues, a structure that is observed in the leader sequences of most proteins. The mature protein contains 2332 amino acids with a calculated molecular weight of 264,763. There are 25 potential asparagine-linked glycosylation sites and 23 cysteine residues.

Factor VIII has several domains with internal homology. The first three are the A1 (amino acid residues 1 to 329), A2

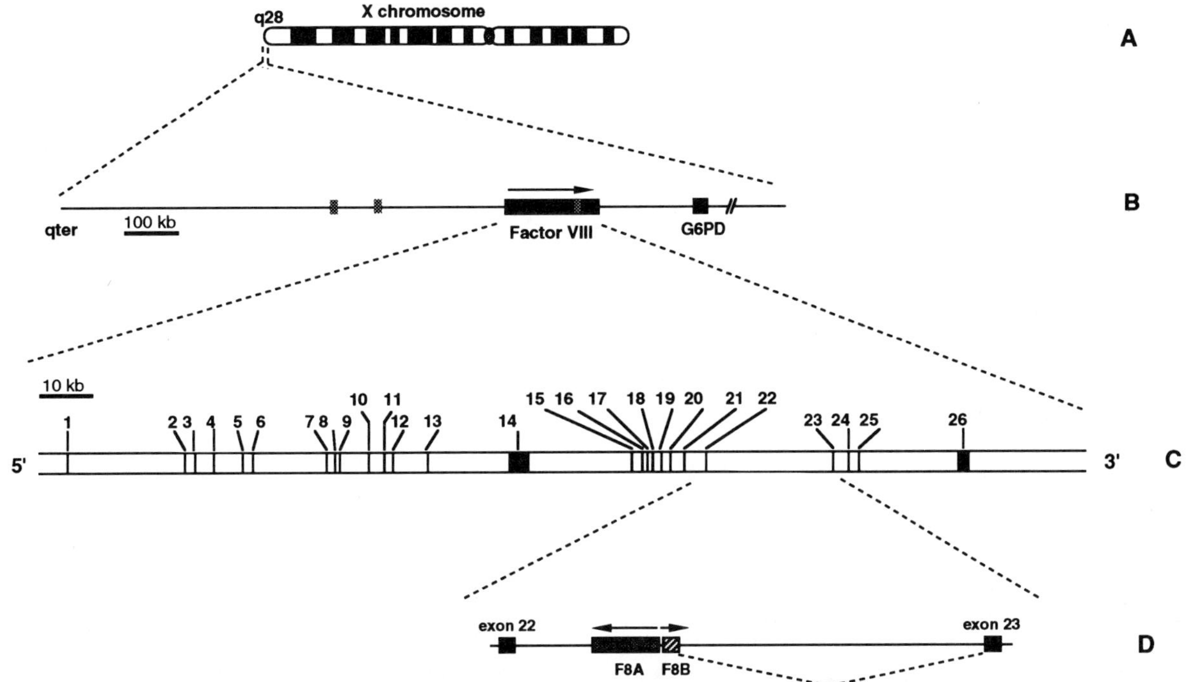

FIG. 106-10 Chromosomal location and structure of the factor VIII genes. *A*. The 186 kb gene is located near the tip of Xq. It contains 26 exons and an unusual bifunctional promoter in intron 22. *B*. Enlargement. The G-6-PD rectangle represents the G-6-PD gene, and the two small rectangles to the right of the factor VIII gene are copies of the F8A gene, which is seen in *C* . in intron 22. *D*. Within intron 22 are the two non–factor-VIII coding sequences, F8A and F8B, which can be transcribed from the bifunctional promoter mentioned above in opposite directions, as shown by the arrows.

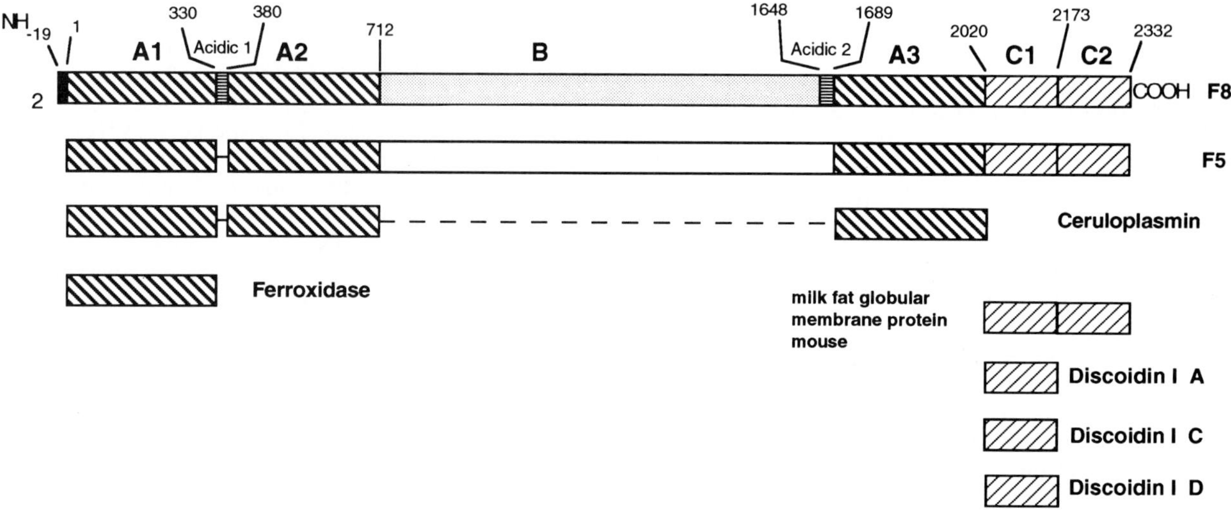

FIG. 106-11 Amino acid homologies of factor VIII domains. The A and C domains have significant homology with factor V. All three A domains have homology with ceruloplasmin and ferroxidase. The C domains also have homology with the milk fat globule membrane protein of mouse and the discoidins of *Dictyostelium*.

(residues 380 to 711) and A3 (residues 1649 to 2019) domains. These domains have an amino acid sequence homology of approximately 30 percent. The A1 domain is encoded by exons 1 through 8, A2 by exons 9 through 13 and a small region of exon 14, and A3 by the 3′ end of exon 14 and exons 15 through 18. These A domains are homologous to similar A domains of ferroxidase, ceruloplasmin, and factor V.[33,45,46] The A2 and A3 domains are separated by a region of 983 amino acids, the B domain, which contains 19 of the 25 potential *N*-glycosylation sites. The B domain has no known function; it is encoded by nearly all of the large exon 14, and it is not conserved between factor VIII and factor V.[47] The B domain is discussed further in "The Mystery of the B Domain" below.

At the C-terminus of the mature factor VIII protein, there are two homologous domains, C1 and C2. These domains are also homologous to the A, C, and D chains of discoidin I; the C domains of factor V, and mouse milk fat globule protein.[33,48,48a] Domain C1 is encoded by exons 20 to 23 and includes amino acid residues 2020 to 2172; domain C2 includes amino acids 2173 to 2332 and is encoded by exons 24 to 26 of the factor VIII gene. The order of the six domains described above from the N-terminus to the C-terminus is A1-A2-B-A3-C1-C2 (Fig. 106-11).

In addition, there are two acidic regions in the factor VIII protein. One lies between the A1 and A2 domains, includes amino acid residues 331 to 379, and contains 15 aspartic acid and glutamic acid residues. The second consists of amino acid residues 1649 to 1689 and also contains 15 aspartic acid and glutamic acid residues. Of the 23 cysteine residues in factor VIII, 14 are conserved between factors V and VIII, suggesting that these proteins may be folded in a similar manner. The murine factor VIII cDNA was recently cloned and sequenced.[49] The mouse cDNA encodes a protein of 2319 amino acids with an overall identity of 74 percent with the human sequence. The amino acid identity in the A and C domains is 84 to 93 percent, whereas the B domain and the two acidic regions are more divergent, with identities of 42 to 70 percent. All thrombin cleavage sites and sulfated tyrosine residues are conserved. Five of six potential *N*-glycosylation sites in the non-B domain regions of factor VIII are conserved. The B domain of the murine deduced protein sequence contains 19 potential *N*-glycosylation sites in positions different from the human sequence. The human sequence contains the same number of potential *N*-glycosylation sites, suggesting that glycosylation of the B domain is important for the biosynthesis of factor VIII.

Genomic Mapping of Factor VIII. The factor VIII gene is located on the long arm of the X chromosome, in the most distal band Xq28. Haldane and Smith[50] reported linkage of hemophilia A with color blindness, and Boyer and Graham[51] demonstrated close linkage of hemophilia A with polymorphisms at the G-6-PD locus. Additional studies confirmed the close linkage of factor VIII with G-6-PD.[52] Patterson et al.[53] showed that the G-6-PD and factor VIII genes lie within 500 kb of each other. Pulsed field gel electrophoresis and physical mapping of Xq28 using yeast artificial chromosomes suggested that the factor VIII gene maps distal to G-6-PD.[54,55] The order of these loci and the direction of transcription is Xcen-G-6-PD-3′F8-5′F8-Xqter.[55,56] The distance from the factor VIII gene to the Xq telomere is approximately 1 Mb.

Biosynthesis and Activation of Factor VIII

Several excellent reviews describe the biosynthesis, proteolytic cleavages, activation, and inactivation of factor VIII.[57,58]

Activated factor VIII is a critical participant in the intrinsic pathway of blood coagulation (see Chap 104 for an overview of hemostasis). It is essential for the activation of factor X by factor IXa. Factor IXa is a serine protease; in the presence of active factor VIII, negatively charged phospholipids, and calcium ions, it cleaves an approximately

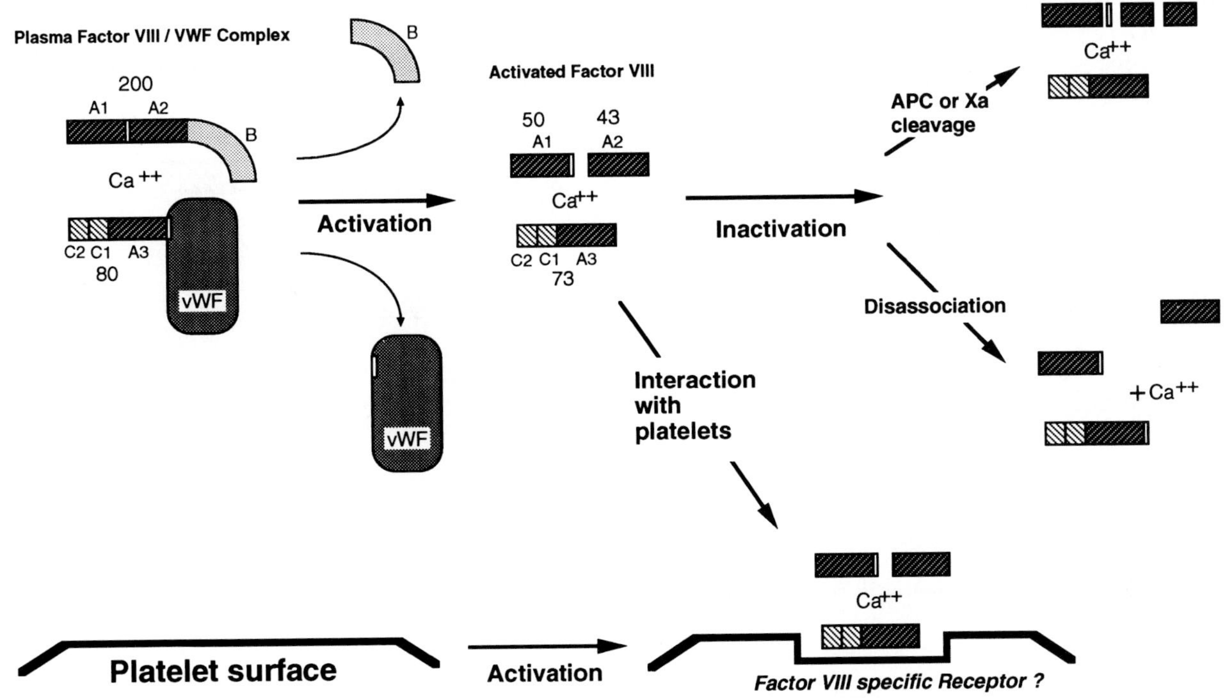

FIG. 106-12 A model for activation and inactivation of factor VIII. Activation involves protease cleavages and interaction with Ca^{2+} ions and platelet surfaces. Inactivation requires proteolysis or dissociation of the subunits. (*Modified from Kaufman.*[58] *Used with permission.*)

11-kDa N-terminal activation peptide from factor X to produce factor Xa. The catalytic activity of factor IXa is increased by approximately 10^4 when factor VIIIa is added to IXa, Ca^{2+}, and phospholipids.[59] This increased activity is believed to result from a direct association of factor VIIIa with factor IXa on the phospholipid surface.

In plasma, factor VIII exists as a heavy chain of 90 to 200 kDa (multiple partially processed polypeptides) in a metal-ion association with a light chain of 80 kDa[33,35] (Fig. 106-12). The complex is stabilized by association with vWF.[60,61] The concentration of factor VIII in plasma is about 100 to 200 ng/μl,[62] and the protein is extremely sensitive to proteolysis. The cloning of factor VIII and its heterologous expression in mammalian cells have made possible the analysis of some aspects of its biosynthesis, processing, and function. Liver transplantation and in situ hybridization of factor VIII mRNA suggest that the liver is the site of its synthesis[63,64]; however, factor VIII mRNA has been detected in many other tissues.[43] There are no known natural cell lines that synthesize factor VIII. The experiments of Kaufman using factor VIII cDNA cloned in expression vectors and introduced into mammalian cells (either Chinese hamster ovary cells or COS-1 monkey kidney cells) showed that factor VIII is synthesized as a single polypeptide chain precursor of 2351 amino acid residues, from which the 19-amino-acid signal peptide is cleaved on translocation into the endoplasmic reticulum (ER).[60] In the ER, high-mannose oligosaccharide is added to asparagine residues. A significant portion of factor VIII in the ER is bound to a protein called GRP78 (glucose-regulated protein 78 kDa or BiP).[64,65] It is not known if the GRP78-associated factor VIII is secreted or degraded. The factor VIII to be secreted moves to the Golgi apparatus, where it is cleaved at sites R1313/A1314 and R1648/E1649 in the B domain to generate the 90- to 200-kDa N-terminal heavy chain(s) and the 80-kDa C-terminal light chain[60] (Fig. 106-13). Within the Golgi apparatus, factor VIII is modified by addition of carbohydrate to serine and threonine residues, modification of asparagine-linked high-mannose oligosaccharides, and sulfation of six specific tyrosine residues in the heavy and light chains.[60,66] In cultured cells, factor VIII synthesized without vWF in the medium is secreted as separate chains and degraded. Addition of vWF results in stable association of the two chains.[60,67]

Proteolytic Activation of Factor VIII. Factor VIII is activated by proteolytic cleavages by proteases such as thrombin (factor IIa) or factor Xa in the presence of phospholipid surfaces. The following cleavages by thrombin occur in factor VIII after secretion (Figs. 106-12 and 106-13).[68,69] Cleavage of the heavy chain at R740/S741 generates a 90-kDa polypeptide, which is subsequently cleaved at R372/S373 to generate polypeptides of 50 kDa and 43 kDa. The light chain is cleaved at R1689/S1690 to produce a 73-kDa polypeptide. Factor Xa cleaves at the same sites and at R1721/A1722. Transfection of COS-1 cells with factor VIII cDNA mutated to alter the Arg residues at these cleavage sites to Ile or Leu suggests that the cleavages at R740 or R1721 have no effect on coagulation activity.[70,71] However, the cleavages at R372 or R1689 are important for the procoagulant activity of factor VIII. The cleavage at R1689 releases factor VIII from vWF and permits factor VIII to interact with phospholipids and platelets.[71,72] The Arg resi-

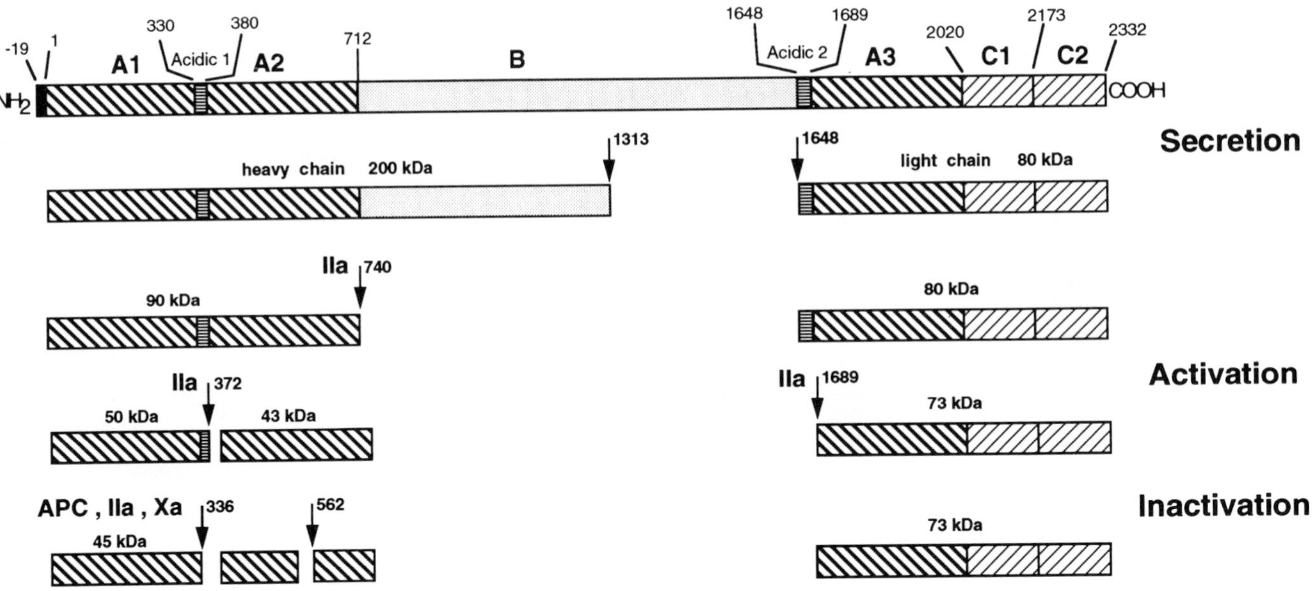

FIG. 106-13 Relationship of proteolytic cleavages of factor VIII to its secretion, activation, and inactivation. (*Modified from Kaufman.*[58] *Used by permission.*)

dues at positions 372, 740, 1689, and 1721 are conserved in murine and porcine factor VIII.[49]

Missense mutations have been described in factor VIII at R372 and R1689 residues in patients with hemophilia A. The mutations R372C and R372H at the first cleavage site, and R1689C and R1689H at the second site, have been found in more than a dozen unrelated patients.[73–80] All of these patients have CRM+ hemophilia A with normal levels of circulating factor VIII protein but very low activity (1 to 7 percent). The circulating dysfunctional plasma factor VIII from these patients, isolated by immunopurification, cannot be cleaved in vitro by thrombin at the site of the amino acid substitution.[78–80a]

After cleavage with thrombin and activation, factor VIII exists as a heterotrimer consisting of the 50-kDa A1 subunit, 43-kDa A2 subunit, and 73-kDa A3-C1-C2 subunit.[66,81,82] Dissociation or deletion of the A2 subunit results in loss of activity, and addition of the A2 domain restores the procoagulant activity.[81–85] It is therefore clear that the A2 domain is required for the activity of factor VIII; however, its function is not yet known. A total of 25 missense mutations have been identified in the A2 domain in patients with hemophilia A, underscoring the importance of the A2 domain (in the A1 and A3 domains, 20 and 19 missense mutations have been identified, respectively).

The Mystery of the B Domain. The B domain (amino acid residues 740 to 1648) is cleaved during proteolytic activation.[60] Deletions of the B domain by mutagenesis (amino acid residues 797 to 1652) in one experiment[86] and 759 to 1639 in another[87] resulted in normal cofactor activity. In addition, plasma factor VIII was activated by thrombin to the same extent as native factor VIII. Furthermore, the derived factor VIII interacted normally with vWF with a half-life of about 13 h, similar to that of factor VIII encoded by the full-length cDNA. The function of the B domain is unknown. It is possible that it may regulate the intracellular processing and/or secretion of factor VIII, since B-domain-deleted molecules are expressed at 5- to 10-fold higher levels than non-B-deleted factor VIII and have decreased association with GRP78 in the ER.[64,87] Surprisingly, the B domain is not well conserved during evolution. The murine B domain of factor VIII is only 55 percent identical to the human domain in amino acid sequence[49] (the other domains have identities of 84 to 93 percent between the two species). The murine B domain contains 19 potential *N*-glycosylation sites, most in positions different from the 19 potential *N*-glycosylation sites in the human B domain.[49] Thus, the number of *N*-glycosylation sites may be of functional importance. The B domains of human and bovine factor V contain 26 and 18 potential *N*-glycosylation sites, respectively, and otherwise have no similarity with the human factor VIII B domain.[47,88,89] Finally, the B domain may have coagulant, anticoagulant, vasoactive, or other properties at present unknown and unsuspected. Only two natural missense mutations have been described in this region in patients with hemophilia A. The L1462P mutation probably has no functional significance, since expression of this variant in COS-1 cells results in factor VIII indistinguishable from normal (SEA, HHK, and R. Kaufman, unpublished observations). The functional significance of a E1038K mutation in a patient with moderate hemophilia A with 2.4 percent factor VIII activity is not known.[90]

Inactivation of Factor VIII

Physiological inactivation of factor VIII activity may not require a proteolytic event,[68] nor is it known if the dissociation of the A2 subunit is necessary. On the other hand, activated protein C (APC) cleaves and inactivates factor VIII.[91–93] Two APC cleavage sites, at R336/M337 and R562/G563, have been identified in factor VIII.[64,87] The cleavage at R562 correlates most significantly with inactivation.[94] R^{336} is not conserved in the murine factor VIII sequence[49]; however, site-directed mutagenesis of R[336] to I resulted in a factor VIII molecule with increased activity, possibly because of resistance to proteolytic inactivation.[70] Factor Xa and thrombin also cleave at R336.[68,70] Factor IXa has been shown to inactivate factor VIII by specific cleavages at R336/M337 and R1719/N1720.[94a] No natural missense mutations have been identified in the inactivation cleavage sites. Recently, an inherited increased ability to form blood clots, called "hereditary thrombophilia," which is due to resistance of factor VIII to APC, has been reported.[95] The molecular defect behind this condition remains unknown.

Interactions of Factor VIII with Other Molecules

Binding to von Willebrand Factor. Von Willebrand factor is required for normal stability of factor VIII in plasma and is encoded by a gene on chromosome 12p. It is synthesized by endothelial cells and megakaryocytes[96,97] and binds to factor VIII in the extracellular fluid.[60] Infused factor VIII–vWF complex in hemophilia A patients has a half-life of 12 h.[98,99] Infused factor VIII is cleared at a rate similar to the factor VIII–vWF complex, probably because factor VIII binds immediately to vWF. However, infused factor VIII in patients with vWF disease or in vWF-deficient dogs has a half-life of only 2.4 h.[99,100] Infusion of vWF in patients with vWF deficiency also elevates factor VIII levels.[98,99] vWF plays an important role in the regulation of factor VIII activity in a number of other ways: (1) In addition to its stabilizing effect, it promotes the association of light and heavy chains of factor VIII[67,101]; (2) it protects factor VIII from inactivation by activated protein C[93,102]; (3) it facilitates cleavage of the light chain of factor VIII by thrombin[103] and does not interfere with the other thrombin cleavages[104]; and (4) it inhibits the binding of factor VIII to phospholipids and activated platelets.[105–107]

Several investigators have localized the portion of vWF protein that interacts with factor VIII to the first 272 amino acids of the secreted vWF.[108–110] In fact, missense mutations such as T28M,[111] R53W, and R91Q[112,113] in this portion of vWF result in defective binding to factor VIII and a clinical phenotype that mimics hemophilia A (autosomal recessive hemophilia).[114]

The N-terminus of the light chain of factor VIII has also been shown to interact with vWF.[104,115] After thrombin cleavage at residue R1689 of the factor VIII light chain, vWF no longer binds to factor VIII, suggesting that the peptide from E1649 to R1689 contains the vWF binding capacity of factor VIII.[116] This region, E1649 to R1689, corresponds to the second acidic region, which contains 15 aspartic and glutamic acid residues. The use of monoclonal antibodies against specific residues of factor VIII further localized the vWF binding site of factor VIII to amino acids K1673 to E1684.[116,117]

Deletion of the acidic region of the light chain results in a factor VIII molecule that does not bind vWF but has normal specific activity when compared to normal factor VIII.[118] In addition, the second acidic region contains two tyrosine residues, Y1664 and Y1680, which are sulfated.[66] Site-directed mutagenesis of Y1680 to F, which cannot be sulfated, results in a molecule that lacks high-affinity binding to vWF.[119] Patients with the naturally occurring Y1680F mutation[76] have moderately severe, CRM-reduced hemophilia (10 percent factor VIII activity and about 20 percent factor VIII antigen). Therefore, the sulfation of Y1680 is an important posttranslational modification required for proper binding of factor VIII to vWF.

Binding to Phospholipids. The C1 and C2 domains of factor VIII are thought to interact with phospholipids. These domains have amino acid homology with discoidins, which are *Dictyostelium* lectins that are capable of binding negatively charged phospholipid.[120] Phospholipids are important components in the activation of factor X by activated factor IX and the factor-VIII co-factor activity.[59,121] The light chain of factor VIII contains a phospholipid binding site,[122,123] which is not abolished after thrombin cleavage and elimination of the vWF binding domain.[106]

A subset of human factor VIII inhibitor antibodies that have epitopes contained in the C2 domain inhibit the binding of factor VIII to immobilized phosphatidylserine.[124] Furthermore, a study of the ability of synthetic peptides to inhibit the binding of purified factor VIII to immobilized phosphatidylserine indicated that the region between residues T2303 and Y2332—i.e., the C-terminal portion of the C2 domain—is an important phospholipid-binding domain of factor VIII.[125]

The surface of thrombin-activated platelets binds factor VIII, and vWF inhibits this binding.[107] Activated platelets have more phosphatidylserine in their membrane surface,[126] and factor VIII has specific affinity to this phospholipid.[127] Alternatively, factor VIII may bind to a specific, unidentified receptor that appears in the platelet membrane after activation. There are approximately 400 factor VIII sites per activated platelet.[128,129] Although factor V has a C2 domain similar to that of factor VIII, it cannot compete with factor VIII for platelet binding.

Several natural mutations have been identified in the last 30 amino acid residues of factor VIII in patients with hemophilia A. These include R2304C, R2307Q, and R2307L, which result in both mild and severe forms of the disease. However, the role of these residues in phospholipid binding is not known.[130–133] Endothelial cells are important components of the coagulation mechanism; however, it is not known if these cells have specific binding sites for factor VIII.

Tyrosine Sulfation. Using ^{35}S metabolic labeling in cultured Chinese hamster ovary cells expressing human recombinant factor VIII, Pittman and Kaufman[66] identified six sulfated tyrosine residues. Of these residues, Y346, Y718, Y719, and Y723 are in the heavy chain, and Y1664 and Y1680 are in the light chain.

Tyrosine sulfation is a posttranslational modification that occurs on a number of secretory proteins as they traverse the Golgi apparatus,[134] and it is required for full factor VIII activity. It may also affect the interaction of factor VIII with other components of the coagulation cascade. However, inhibition of tyrosine sulfation does not alter the synthesis or secretion of factor VIII. The sulfated tyrosine residues of human factor VIII are conserved in murine and porcine factor VIII.[49] Y1680 has been shown to be important for interaction with vWF,[117,119] and, as mentioned earlier, site-directed mutagenesis of Y1680 to F resulted in a factor VIII molecule with defective binding to vWF.[71,119]

Binding to Factors IXa and X. The contact sites of factor VIII with the protease factor IXa and its substrate factor X, have not yet been established. The analogous interaction of factor V with the protease factor Xa and substrate prothrombin can be used as a model. In this latter system, factor Va binds to prothrombin via the heavy chain and to factor Xa via the light chain with a contribution by the heavy chain.[89,135–137]

There is indirect evidence that the heavy chain of factor VIII binds factor IXa, because the latter factor protects factor VIII from inactivation by APC, which cleaves only the heavy chain.[138–140] Recently, Leuting et al.[141] demonstrated that the isolated light chain of factor VIII contains a high-affinity binding site for factor IXa that does not require the presence of phospholipids or the factor VIII heavy chain. The use of monoclonal antibodies has suggested that the binding occurs in the region N1770 to D1840 of factor VIII. A number of natural missense mutations have been identified in this region, including M1772T, R1781H, R1781C, S1784Y, L1789F, M1823I, P1825S, T1826P, and A1834V, most of which result in mild to moderate hemophilia A (see next section). It is not known if these mutations affect binding of factor VIII to factor IXa.

MOLECULAR PATHOLOGY OF HEMOPHILIA A

Until recent times, hemophilia A was a lethal genetic disease, and affected males had little chance of reproduction. Therefore, the observed gene frequency for the disorder indicates that a large fraction of cases must arise by new mutation. In fact, in the 1930s, Haldane predicted that one-third of all isolated cases would arise by new mutation in noncarrier females, and that another one-third of the remaining cases would have arisen by new mutation in the grandparent generation.[142] This prediction has now been verified in studies of the molecular basis of the disease.[143] A corollary of the Haldane hypothesis is that if a number of potential molecular defects can give rise to hemophilia A, multiple new mutations will be significantly heterogenous. One might even predict that, in the absence of "mutation hotspots" in the factor VIII gene, nearly every unrelated hemophilic male would carry a different mutation in the factor VIII gene. As it turns out, a large number of mutations can produce the disease, and over 50 percent of unrelated patients have a different mutation. A database of nucleotide substitutions, deletions, insertions, and rearrangements of the factor VIII gene in hemophilia A was compiled in late 1991.[144] From November 1991 to May 1993, 19 new mutations were described, and a mutation hotspot has been discovered.[145–149e] The total number of different point mutations described to date is 148.

Deletions in the Factor VIII Gene

Nearly 95 percent of the factor VIII mutations characterized by scanning the entire coding region of the gene are point mutations consisting of nucleotide substitutions, deletions, and insertions of a small number of nucleotides in a coding region. Deletions account for most of the remaining characterized mutations (about 5 percent), while large insertions (see "L1 Retrotransposition" below) account for under 1 percent of factor VIII alleles.[144] Deletions usually produce severe hemophilia A with no factor VIII activity. An exception is a deletion that eliminates only the 156-bp exon 22 from the coding region of the gene. This deletion is associated with moderate disease, probably because of in-frame splicing of exon 21 to exon 23.[150] Large deletions are often associated with inhibitor formation (see "Etiology of Inhibitors in Hemophilia A" below), and they show no particular predilection for one or another region of the factor VIII gene. They nearly all result from nonhomologous loss of a region of the gene[151]—that is, they generally are not caused by mispairing of homologous DNA, such as *Alu* sequences, followed by unequal crossing over. They also demonstrate no common nucleotide sequences at their breakpoints.

Point Mutations in the Factor VIII Gene

The observed nucleotide substitutions, which usually produce amino acid substitutions, are spread throughout the factor VIII gene (Table 106-2). However, there are regions, such as the A2 domain, where they concentrate.[90,145] For most of the missense mutations, the antigen level is commensurate

Table 106-2 Missense Mutations in the Factor VIII Gene Producing Hemophilia A

Mutation*	Domain	CRM Status	Severity†	Remarks	Reference
E11V	A1		Mi		227
G73V	A1		Mi		227
V85D	A1		Mi		227
K89T	A1		Mi		133
M91V	A1		Mo		133
G111R	A1		S		226
G145V	A1		Mi		227
P146S	A1		S		226
V162M	A1		Mi-Mo		227
K166T	A1		Mi		90
S170L	A1	CRM red	Mo		228
G205W	A1		Mo		90
V266G	A1		Mi		133
E272G	A1		Mo		229
E272K	A1		—		239
R282H	A1	CRM red	S		133
S289L	A1	CRM+	Mo		145
F293S	A1		Mo		133
T295A	A1		Mi		90
V326L	A1		Mo-S		230
C329R	A1		S		230
R372H	Acidic 1	CRM+	Mi-Mo	Thrombin cleavage site	78
R372C	Acidic 1	CRM+	Mo	Thrombin cleavage site	73
S373L	Acidic 1		Mi	?? thromin cleavage	231
L386S	A2		S		226
L412F	A2		Mi		90
K425R	A2	CRM red	S		133
Y473H	A2		Mi		133
Y473C	A2		Mo		90
G479R	A2		Mo		148
R527W	A2	CRM+	Mi		90
R531C	A2		Mi		90
R531G	A2		Mi		90
S535G	A2		—		240
D542G	A2	CRM red	S		133
S558F	A2	CRM+	Mi		145
Q565K	A2		Mi-Mo		90
I566T	A2	CRM+	S	New *N*-glycosyl (NQI-NQT)	153
S577P	A2		S		240
S584I	A2		—	Loss of *N*-glycosyl?	240
W585C	A2		S		226
R593C	A2		Mi		133

Table 106-2 Missense Mutations in the Factor VIII Gene Producing Hemophilia A (Continued)

Mutation*	Domain	CRM Status	Severity†	Remarks	Reference
N612S	A2		—		240
V634A	A2	CRM +	Mi		145
V634M	A2	CRM +	S		145
A644V	A2	CRM red	Mi		90
F652del	A2	CRM red	S		145
R698W	A2		Mi		227
A704T	A2		Mi		133
E1038K	B	CRM red	Mo	? B domain mutation	90
Y1680F	Acidic 2	CRM red	Mi	vWF binding site	76
R1689C	A3	CRM +	Mo-S	Thrombin cleavage site	74
R1689H	A3	CRM +	Mi	Thrombin cleavage site	232
R1696G	A3		—		144
E1704K	A3		S		233
Y1709C	A3		Mo		152
G1760E	A3		S		226
M1772T	A3	CRM +	S	New *N*-glycosyl (NIM-NIT)	153
R1781H	A3		Mo		133
R1781C	A3		Mi		146
S1784Y	A3		S		133
L1789F	A3		Mi		227
M1823I	A3		Mo		226
P1825S	A3		Mi		90
T1826P	A3		Mi		234
A1834V	A3		Mi		226
H1848R	A3		Mo		90
E1885K	A3		S		226
N1922D	A3		Mo-S		152
N1922S	A3		S		133
R1941Q	A3	CRM red	Mi-Mo		235
R1941L	A3		Mo		147
R1997W	A3		Mo		90
W2046R	C1		Mo		227
F2101L	C1		Mi		90
Y2105C	C1		Mi		148
R2116P	C1		S		236
S2119Y	C1		Mi		90
R2150H	C1		Mi-Mo		90
T2154I	C1		Mi		146
R2159C	C1	CRM red	Mi		90
R2163H	C1		Mo		240
L2166S	C1		S		235
A2192P	C2		Mo		226
P2205del	C2		S		234
R2209Q	C2	CRM red	Mo-S		229
R2209L	C2		Mo		237
V2223M	C2		—	Poly-morphism?	90
W2229C	C2		Mo		238
P2300L	C2		Mi		90
P2300S	C2		Mi		233
P2304C	C2		S		133
R2307Q	C2		Mi-Mo		131
R2307L	C2		Mo-S		130

*Most mutations listed in this table are also discussed in review ref. 144.
†S, severe; Mo, moderate; Mi, mild.

with the factor VIII activity, that is, very low. Indeed, for most of these mutations, the mechanism that produces reduced factor VIII in plasma is unknown and is very difficult to study. Only for eight of the point mutations are the structure–function relationships known. Mutations at the thrombin cleavage sites—arginine residues 372 and 1689—are known to block activation of factor VIII by thrombin, producing CRM+ hemophilia in which FVIII:Ag levels are normal[73–80a] (Fig. 106-14). The mutation Y1680F produces a mild CRM-reduced phenotype owing to a block in tyrosine sulfation and concomitant vWF binding to factor VIII.[76,133] A nearby tyrosine substitution, Y1709C, causes a severe hemophilia A.[152]

Two other CRM+ mutations produce severe hemophilia A phenotypes by creating new *N*-glycosylation sites in the protein.[153] The consensus amino acid sequence for *N*-glycosylation is Asn-X-Ser/Thr. One of these newly created sites is in the A2 domain of the heavy chain at position 566, producing a glycosylation site at N564 (Asn-X-Ile to Asn-X-Thr). The second new site is in the A3 domain of the light chain at residue 1772, creating a glycosylation site at N1770 (Asn-X-Met to Asn-X-Thr). In both cases, factor VIII is present at normal levels in the plasma but is completely inactive. In either case, deglycosylation of the plasma restores factor VIII activity to a significant degree.[153] Whether the abnormal glycosylation of these proteins prevents binding of one or more key proteins to factor VIII remains to be shown.

Other CRM+ mutations that greatly reduce factor VIII activity while leaving factor VIII antigen levels intact or only modestly reduced should provide clues to important sites of interaction of factor VIII with other molecules, such as factor IXa, factor Xa, APC, phospholipid surfaces, and calcium ions. Sites of CRM+ mutations include S289, R527, and S558, defects of which produce mild factor VIII deficiency, and V634.[145,133] A V634A substitution produces moderate hemophilia A, while a V634M substitution leads to severe hemophilia A.[145] An R282H substitution in domain A1 leads to a severe hemophilia with 18 percent of normal antigen.[90] An E1038K mutation in a moderately affected patient with 10 to 20 percent of normal factor VIII antigen is of interest because it occurs in the B region of the protein, which is thought not to participate in factor VIII function.[90] Although this substitution was the only one found in the patient's DNA after scanning all the factor VIII exons for mutation, functional studies are needed to confirm whether it causes the CRM-reduced hemophilia A in the patient.

In general, studies of the small numbers of CRM+ and CRM-reduced patients point to potentially important residues in the protein. Since about 50 percent of the known CRM+ mutations (11 of 26) occur in the A2 domain, which consists of 228 amino acids, or about 10 percent of the coding region of factor VIII, this region must be important in procoagulant activity.[145] The great majority of mutations are CRM−, and these probably affect protein folding and stability. Since these mutations result in an absence of secreted factor VIII, and in vitro functional studies depend on analysis of the protein produced in eukaryotic cells after transfection with factor VIII cDNA, the mechanisms of action of these mutations are difficult to elucidate.

General Lessons from the Study of Factor VIII Mutations

The factor VIII gene was one of the first genes studied at the molecular level that was large and, because of its high

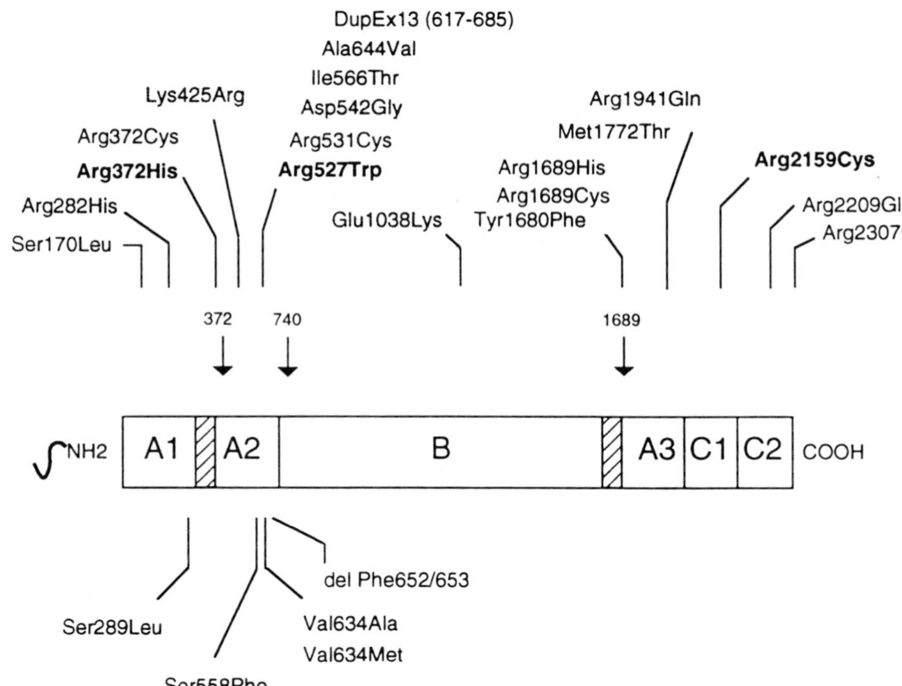

FIG. 106-14 Mutations in the human factor VIII gene responsible for CRM-reduced and CRM-positive hemophilia A. The domain structure of factor VIII is shown, and arrows show the thrombin cleavage sites. The cross-hatched areas depict the two highly acidic regions.

rate of new mutations, contained a broad spectrum of mutations. Thus, a few general lessons concerning human mutation were learned from the factor VIII gene. These are described below.

CpG Dinucleotide Hypermutability. A general mutation hotspot exists in human genomic DNA at CpG dinucleotides in which the canonical mutation is a CG-to-TG, or, if the C-T substitution occurs in the antisense strand, a CG-to-CA substitution.[154–156] These CG dinucleotides are the only general hotspot known, and the mutations occur because cytosine residues 5′ to guanine are the only methylation site in mammalian DNA. These cytosines are methylated by a methyltransferase to produce 5-methylcytosine. When 5-methylcytosine is spontaneously deaminated in a nonenzymatic reaction, thymine is produced. Canonical CG-to-TG or -CA substitutions account for about 35 percent of the mutations observed in the factor VIII gene after scanning the exons for mutations in patients,[90,133] and they account for 25 to 40 percent of the mutations observed in a wide variety of other human genes (see ref. 156a and Chap 3).

L1 Retrotransposition. The first insertions of a transposable element in humans were observed in the factor VIII gene in 1987. Although transposable elements are present in a large variety of organisms, including yeast, maize, *Drosophila*, and mouse, they had not been seen in humans until hemophilia A—a disorder with a wide spectrum of mutations—was studied. Two patients were found with truncated L1 elements inserted into exon 14 of the factor VIII gene.[157]

L1 elements make up about 5 percent of the human genome and are present in about 100,000 copies, most of which are defective. About 3000 copies are full length and are potential transposable elements.[158] A few of these elements are retrotransposable, in that they produce a new insertion through an RNA intermediate; they are transcribed into RNA and then reverse transcribed into DNA, and the double-stranded DNA is then reinserted into another genomic site. Thus, they are "copy and paste" mobile elements.[159] In the case of the de novo L1 insertions into exon 14 of the factor VIII gene, one insertion that contained the 3′ two-thirds of an L1 element was shown to result from retrotransposition of an active element located on chromosome 22.[160] The number of active L1 elements is not known, but, as of May 1993, a total of seven new insertions of different L1 elements into the factor VIII gene,[157] the adenomatosis polyposis coli gene,[161] and the dystrophin gene[162–164] were known. In addition, four insertions of *Alu* elements have been reported.[165–168]

Exon Skipping Owing to Nonsense Mutations. An important observation concerning the pathophysiology of nonsense codon mutations has recently been made in the factor VIII gene.[148] This observation, independently made in the fibrillin and ornithine aminotransferase genes,[169] indicates that a nonsense mutation can on occasion lead to aberrant RNA processing whereby the exon harboring the mutation is skipped. The mechanism for this unusual RNA processing is unknown. At least two instances of the skipping of an exon containing a nonsense codon have been discovered in the factor VIII gene.[148] The fraction of factor VIII mRNA missing the exon of interest was nearly 100 percent in one case and about 50 percent in the other, and in both cases the skipping of an in-frame exon would lead to an otherwise normal factor VIII protein missing the amino acids encoded by the skipped exon. In both cases the phenomenon explains the lack of inhibitor formation by the patient (see "Etiology of Inhibitors in Hemophilia A" below.) Presumably, a small amount of near-normal protein protects the patient from producing factor VIII antibodies.

Exon skipping in factor VIII gene mutants was demonstrated by taking advantage of the low level of factor VIII transcripts, so-called illegitimate transcripts, present in lymphocytes.[170] As mentioned earlier, the major site of factor VIII transcription is the liver, but transcript levels of about one factor VIII mRNA per 10 cells can be detected in lymphocytes using reverse transcriptase followed by PCR. In a number of gene systems, these transcripts have been shown to accurately reflect the transcription and splicing of the gene of interest at its major site of expression. Thus, illegitimate transcripts can be used to characterize mutations in genomic DNA.[171]

A Mutation "Hotspot" in Intron 22 and Common Inversions Involving the Factor VIII Gene

After scanning all the exons of the factor VIII gene using denaturing gradient gel electrophoresis (DGGE), Higuchi et al. found the causative mutation in about 90 percent of patients with mild to moderate hemophilia A.[90] However, when severely affected patients were similarly extensively studied, the causative mutation was found in only about 60 percent of patients.[133]

The difficulty of characterizing mutations in severe hemophilia A was a mystery, even leading to speculation that another site of mutations outside the factor VIII gene might be responsible for many cases of severe disease. Naylor et al. used a study of illegitimate transcription of the factor VIII gene to debunk this speculation and provide the beginnings of an answer to the mystery.[149] They found that RNA transcripts were interrupted between exons 22 and 23 in 40 percent of patients with severe hemophilia A. These patients must all have one or more different mutations at a hotspot in the large intron 22. Since other unusual duplicated genes lie in this intron (see Fig. 106-10), along with a promoter that can result in a transcript containing eight codons from the intron-22 sequence connected to exons 23 through 26, this region has interesting possibilities for an unusual mutation hotspot. Thus, 25 percent of all hemophilia A patients (40 percent of those with severe disease) may turn out to have a single type of easily detectable mutation, thereby making direct detection of the mutation for prenatal and carrier diagnosis feasible in this subset of patients.

Recently, Gitschier and colleagues suggested a model to account for these observations.[172] They propose that the region encompassing gene A in intron 22 inappropriately pairs with one of the two homologous regions upstream of the factor VIII gene on the same X chromosome (Figs. 106-10 and 106-15). This unusual pairing is sometimes followed by homologous recombination, resulting in one of two potential large inversions that disrupt the factor VIII gene (Fig. 106-15). This inversion places exons 1 to 22 some 400 kb upstream of exons 23 to 26 and oriented in the opposite direction. Experimental results from affected patients are consistent with this model: (1) Two of the three fragments containing gene A are altered; (2) one of the two altered fragments always contains gene A of intron 22; (3) no DNA appears to be lost or gained; and (4) the altered factor VIII transcript includes sequences from the vicinity of an upstream gene A.

CARRIER AND ANTENATAL DIAGNOSIS

At present, the two inversions mentioned above are easily detectable by Southern blotting and account for up to 40 percent of factor VIII mutations in families seeking genetic counseling. Thus, this observation is greatly altering our ability to provide exact counseling for a sizable fraction of families that have only one case of hemophilia A. Previously, the high incidence of new mutations meant that DNA diagnosis was not available for many families to whom accurate carrier diagnosis would be very valuable. This has

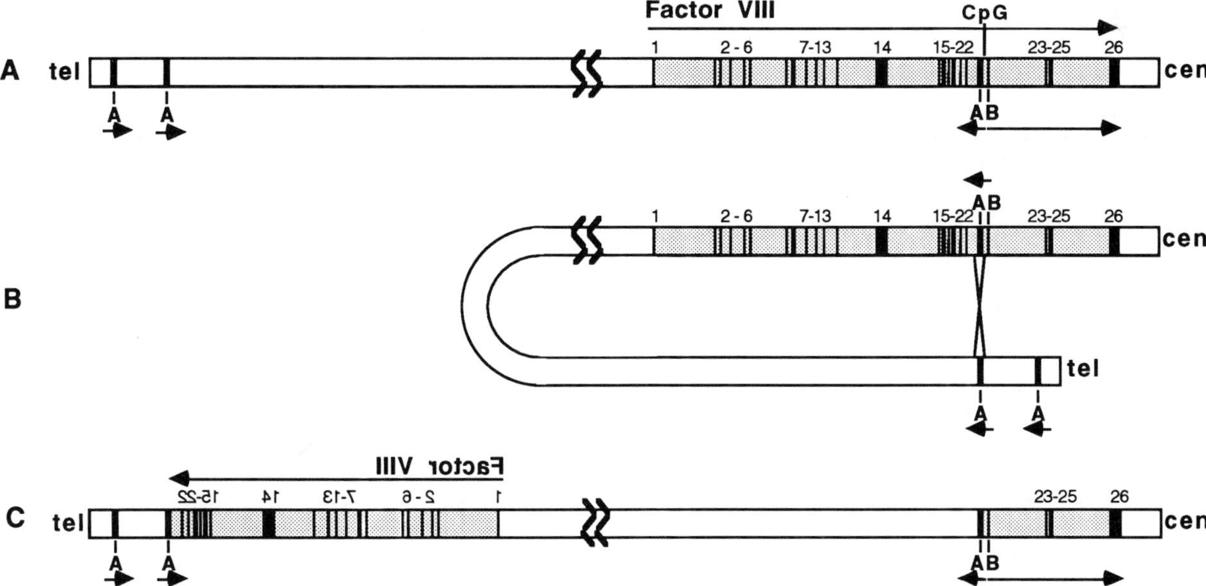

FIG. 106-15 Inversions involving the factor VIII gene. *A*. The region of Xq28 that includes the factor VIII gene, oriented with the telomere at the left. Three copies of gene A are indicated, two lying upstream of factor VIII and one inside intron 22 of factor VIII. The location of the B transcript is also shown. The arrows indicate the direction of transcription of the factor VIII and internal A and B genes. The direction of the upstream A genes is hypothesized to be as shown. *B*. The proposed homologous recombination between the intron-22 copy of gene A and one of the two upstream copies. A crossover between these two identical regions, oriented in the manner illustrated, would result in an inversion of sequence between the two recombined A genes, as shown in *C*. A recombination could involve either of the upstream A genes, but only one is presented. The crossover could occur anywhere in the region of homology that includes the A genes.

now changed for those families whose affected member carries an inversion involving the factor VIII gene.

However, because of the enormous variety of other mutations producing the disease, in the remaining 60 percent of cases, carrier and antenatal diagnosis by DNA analysis is carried out by indirect detection using linked DNA polymorphisms. The affected factor VIII gene is tracked in these families using DNA polymorphisms both within the gene (*Bcl*I, *Xba*I, *Bgl*I restriction site polymorphisms)[172–174] and outside the gene.[175,176] Simple sequence repeats (CA_n repeats) have been found in two introns of the factor VIII gene and are also valuable in this process.[177,178] Nearly all families are informative with one or more DNA polymorphism, but 20 to 30 percent of families are informative for extragenic polymorphisms only. In these families, the chance of error in the diagnosis is 2 to 3 percent in some and 4 to 6 percent in others, depending on the number of meioses in question. When an intragenic polymorphism is used for the diagnosis of carrier or affected status, the chance of an error is under 1 percent.

In families with only one affected male who does not carry an inversion, however, there is often further uncertainty in determining carrier status by linkage analysis, and one must often rely heavily on biochemical determinations of factor VIII levels for determination of carrier status. Carriers of defective factor VIII genes have, on average, 50 percent of the normal mean level of factor VIII in their plasma. However, owing to random X-inactivation (lyonization) and several other physiological influences, including age, blood group, acute-phase response, and hormonal status, there is a large overlap between the factor VIII levels in carriers and normal individuals. Improved separation of the two groups can be obtained by measuring the ratio of factor VIII coagulant activity to vWF antigen. The "odds favoring carriership" can then be calculated by applying statistical analysis to the data and taking account of age and blood group. The odds are then combined with the probability of carriership derived from pedigree analysis to reach a final probability of carriership.[178] Activity-to-antigen ratios of 0.6 or less suggest carriership for hemophilia A, while ratios of 0.9 or above are generally noncarrier results. The test is accurate when it produces a clear-cut result (either carrier-female or normal-female). When it produces a test result in the inconclusive range (ratios of 0.6 to 0.9), it is of little value.

In current genetic counseling practice, biochemical analysis for carrier detection in hemophilia A kindreds is only resorted to when an inversion is not detected in the proband and linkage analysis fails owing to family structure, as mentioned above. However, it remains a valuable adjunct to DNA analysis.

As of 1993, hundreds of families have undergone carrier and antenatal diagnosis for factor VIII deficiency by DNA analysis, with generally satisfactory results and a minimum of error. Although exact numbers of pregnancy terminations for affected fetuses are hard to obtain, a sizable percentage of couples (perhaps 40 percent) who have undergone antenatal diagnosis and been informed that their fetus was affected decided to carry the pregnancy to term.

It was the hope of many in this field that by 1993, mutation detection would improve to the point where family members of an affected child could be offered a 100 percent accurate diagnosis of their status through the determination of the causative mutation in the child and analysis for that mutation in each family member. This would be an important service for families at risk. Now that the hotspot mutation in intron 22 has been delineated, this hope has been partially realized. Indeed, if the study of illegitimate transcripts and their analysis using the chemical cleavage method, as presently used by Naylor et al.,[148] can be carried out in a number of laboratories after the factor VIII gene of a patient has been found to be free of an inversion, it could take as little as 1 to 2 weeks to scan the factor VIII gene for mutations and to detect the causative mutation in nearly all the remaining affected individuals. This leads one to the optimistic forecast that further technical improvements along with new knowledge should make rapid mutation analysis in carriers and antenatal diagnosis an available service within the next 5 years. The ability to analyze each family member for the pertinent mutation causing hemophilia A in his or her family will have a major effect on the genetic counseling for this important condition.

TREATMENT OF HEMOPHILIA A

The mainstay of treatment is replacement therapy by means of intravenous infusion with factor VIII. Until two years ago, all factor VIII used was blood-derived (Table 106-3). Now two recombinant products have been licensed. Ideally, all severely affected patients would be maintained on long-term prophylaxis with daily or alternate-day infusions to keep spontaneous hemorrhages to a minimum. This has been impossible for most patients owing to limitations of supply and finance. Since the half-life of factor VIII is 8 to 12 h, twice-daily infusions are needed to maintain a normal level at all times. However, for prophylactic purposes a fairly wide fluctuation is still very effective. In practice, most patients are treated on demand, which means that they receive an infusion of factor at the first symptom of bleeding. Patients become skilled at recognizing very early joint bleeding and, provided that an infusion of factor VIII is given within a few minutes to 1 h of onset, the bleeding can be halted before a significant amount of blood has leaked into a joint. Normal activities can then be resumed almost immediately.

It was realized in the 1960s that such prompt treatment could only be achieved if the patient or his relatives gave the injection. Therefore, home therapy programs were instituted, leading to a dramatic fall in time lost from school or work and a marked reduction in the onset of new joint damage and the progression of old joint damage. In contrast to older patients or patients from developing countries, who nearly all have severe damage in several joints, which increases relentlessly with age and number of bleeds, severely affected patients who have grown up under this regimen are now reaching their twenties with little arthritis. However, it is becoming clear that to completely prevent joint damage a high-dose prophylactic regimen is necessary (L. Aledort, personal communication).

The dosage of factor VIII is adjusted to obtain a desired level in the circulation (Table 106-4). Formulas based on plasma volume and expected recovery give a rough guide to dosage, but where the level is critical, as for surgery or in case of serious bleeding, it should always be checked by assay after infusion. On average, factor VIII infusion produces a plasma increment of 2 U/dl per unit infused per kilogram body weight. From this a simple formula can be derived:

$$\text{Dose to be infused (Units)} = \frac{\text{weight (kg)} \times \text{increment needed (U/dl)}}{2.0}$$

Table 106-3 Therapeutic Materials for Treatment of Hemophilia A

Material	Factor VIII (U/ml)	vWF (U/ml)	Donors per Unit	Advantages	Disadvantages
Cryo-precipitate	5–10	5–10	1	Low infection hazard (unless many units used); simple to prepare	Storage at −20°C. Allergic reactions. Not virus-inactivated. Potency not assayed.
Heat or solvent detergent treated factor VIII concentrate	20–50	20–50	3,000–15,000	Assayed higher potency, HIV and hepatitis B and C infectivity. Store at 4°C. Few allergic reactions	Heavy load of non-factor-VIII proteins, including B_2-microglobulin iso-anti-A, anti-B, β_2-microglobulin, fibrinogen, etc. Falling CD4 count in HIV-positive patients.
DDAVP	—	—	0	No infection risk as totally synthetic	Only effective in mild cases
High-purity plasma-derived factor VIII	~5000U/mg*	0	3,000–15,000	Convenience. Preserves CD4 count in HIV-positive cases	High cost; ? increased incidence of inhibitors
Recom-binant factor VIII	~5000U/mg*	0	0	No infectious risk. Totally pure	High cost; ? increased incidence of inhibitors

*Before addition of albumen carrier.

Assessing the period of treatment required is a matter of clinical judgment with respect to the individual episode or lesion. An early joint bleed will often resolve with a single infusion. For surgery other than very minor procedures, treatment needs to be continued at full dosage twice daily, adjusted according to pre- and posttreatment assays, for a week or more, followed by a period of treatment at reduced dosage during convalescence.

Detailed discussion of the orthopedic management of hemophilic arthropathy is beyond the scope of this chapter, and the reader is referred to the texts on comprehensive care.[179–181] Suffice it to say that large numbers of patients have had total hip or knee joint replacements with good results and that arthrodesis of the knee or ankle can provide pain relief and improved locomotor function where arthroplasty is impractical.

Physical therapy plays a very important role in maintaining and improving the function of joints and muscles damaged or weakened by bleeding and enforced periods of immobilization.

Table 106-4 Plasma Levels of Factor VIII required for Hemostasis

Clinical Indication	Plasma Factor VIII (U/dl)	Dosage (U/kg)
Early hemarthrosis or muscle bleeding	15–20	8–10
More severe bleeding, minor trauma	30–50	15–25
Surgery, major trauma, head injury	80–120	40–60

Factor VIII concentrate, with its advantages of storage, convenience, and assayed potency, is the material of choice in severe hemophilia and in the treatment of major bleeding where it is essential to maintain high levels. The realization that it carries a risk of infection (see "Complications of Therapy" below) has given rise to intensive and by now successful efforts to (1) inactive viruses in concentrate, (2) use recombinant factor VIII, and (3) use a non-blood-derived alternative—DDAVP (desamino-D-arginine vasopressin). This synthetic analogue of vasopressin was noted to cause a rise in factor VIII and vWF levels without pressor effects. DDAVP retains the antidiuretic action of natural vasopressin and also stimulates the release of vascular plasminogen activator. In practice, these effects can be used to elevate the plasma factor VIII level two- to fourfold above baseline, presumably by inducing release from a storage site(s).

Given together with a fibrinolytic inhibitor such as tranexamic acid (to neutralize the fibrinolytic stimulus), DDAVP can correct the hemostatic defect in mild hemophilia A or von Willebrand disease well enough to cover minor surgery or treat a minor bleeding episode. A typical regimen would be to give 0.3 μg per kilogram body weight by slow intravenous infusion over 20 min together with 1 g of tranexamic acid. The effect reaches a maximum at 1 h, at which point, for example, the factor VIII level in a mild hemophiliac may have risen from 10 to 40 U/dl. The half-life of the endogenously released factor VIII is about 8 h, and repeat doses can be given, but with progressively diminishing response. The maximum useful number of doses is three in 24 h, after which a rest period is needed to allow stores to reaccumulate. Fibrinolytic inhibition is also useful for management of oral and intestinal tract bleeding. It must be strictly avoided when there is upper urinary tract bleeding, since it can cause obstructive nephropathy and acute renal failure owing to mechanical outflow occlusion by blood clots.

Complications of Therapy

Inhibitors. Development of antibodies to factor VIII (often termed *inhibitors*) after exposure to factor VIII occurs in about 5 percent of all patients with hemophilia A but in 10 to 25 percent of severely affected individuals.[182] The time of appearance of such antibodies is unpredictable but is usually after the first or first few exposures. Routine testing for factor VIII antibodies is therefore always performed before elective surgery and regularly at follow-up in severe cases. Laboratory tests for antibody rely on neutralization of clotting activity in mixtures of normal and patient plasma. Since the plasma concentration of factor VIII is very low (200 ng/ml, or 0.5 n*M*), it is necessary to prolong the incubation of the mixture to attain equilibrium binding of antibody to antigen. This test is standardized to Bethesda units,[183] 1 unit being the amount of antibody that neutralizes 50 percent of the factor VIII in 1 ml of normal plasma after 2 h incubation at 37°C. Three aspects of an individual patient's antibody are of clinical importance: the level in units at the time of treatment, the type of immune response to infusion of factor VIII (low or high), and whether there is cross-reaction with porcine factor VIII. When the antibody titer is low (Table 106-5), treatment can consist of an increased dose of factor, so that enough factor will remain after the circulating inhibitor has been neutralized to give a hemostatic level. In some patients, the level of antibody remains low to moderate (low responders), but, in others, treatment with factor VIII elicits a sharp "anamnestic" response (high responders). The low responders can be treated repeatedly with human or porcine factor VIII, but high responders become refractory, so that alternative therapies have been developed. Most often, the antibody is species-specific to human factor VIII and has little or no cross-reactivity with porcine factor VIII.

A concentrate from pig plasma (Hyate C, Table 106-5) is available that has much better clinical characteristics than earlier animal factor VIII preparations. This material is effective on many occasions when the titer against human factor VIII is too high to be neutralized. About half of the patients treated with Hyate C have become resistant owing to development of an alloantibody, but the remainder can be treated repeatedly with good response. When the factor VIII inhibitor titer rises sharply to hundreds or even thousands of units per milliliter, factor VIII therapy is ineffective. In this situation, an alternative strategy is to attempt to bypass factor VIII with partly activated mixtures of the vitamin K-dependent factors. Conventional factor IX concentrate contains activated species (and is, in fact, liable to produce thrombosis, particularly in patients with liver damage). Controlled trials have shown it to be more effective than albumin solution in hastening recovery from a hemarthrosis. More effective are the deliberately activated coagulation factor mixtures FEIBA and AUTOPLEX. It is not clear what the active principle in these products consists of, nor how to monitor the response by blood tests. Empirical dosage regimens have been established, and the fact remains that these products have been strikingly effective on some occasions but have failed to control bleeding on others. Elective surgical procedures should not be attempted on the basis of treatment with these products. Recently, recombinant factor VIIa has been used for these patients, with excellent results in most cases and a few failures. Doses are high, and there is a risk of inducing generalized coagulation activation in the presence of infection.[184]

Induction of immune tolerance has been attempted on many occasions. Immunosuppressive agents, such as glucocorticoids and alkylating agents, are of no benefit (although probably valuable for treatment of spontaneous acquired autoantibodies to factor VIII). Brackman[185] demonstrated that a megadose regimen of factor VIII infusion continued over many months is effective in abolishing inhibitory antibodies in over 90 percent of cases. In the long term, a medium intermittent dose regimen is also fairly effective in blunting or abolishing immune response to factor VIII.[186] Various schemes have been proposed for inducing specific immune tolerance, but, to date, no consistently successful protocol has been reported. Infusion of intravenous gamma globulin has been successful in temporarily lowering inhibitor titers,[187] presumably through the action of anti-idiotypic antibodies.

The multiplicity of therapies proposed and the space devoted to this topic reflects the lack of any universally successful regimen and the large amount of time, expense, and effort required for the management of these unfortunate

Table 106-5 Guidelines for Treatment of Patients with Factor VIII Inhibitors

Inhibitor Level (BU/ml)*			
Anti-human	Anti-orcine	Type of Therapeutic Responder	Strategies
1–5	1–5	Low	Human factor VIII at increased dosage
		High	1. Institute immune-tolerance-inducing regimen 2. Human factor VIII at high dose first, then as below
5–13	1–5	Low	Porcine factor VIII for all bleeds
		High, developing antiporcine antibodies	1. Factor VIIa or activated factor complex for minor bleeds; reserve Hyate C for major bleeds 2. Attempt to induce tolerance
>13	>13	High	1. Treat bleeds with factor VIIa or activated factor complex 2. Plasmapheresis with extracorporeal antibody binding column for severe bleeds, then high-dose human or porcine factor VIII 3. Attempt to induce tolerance

*BU = Bethesda units.

patients. For further details, the reviews of Kasper[188] and Bloom[189] should be consulted.

Etiology of Inhibitors in Hemophilia A. Inhibitors occur predominantly but not exclusively in severely affected patients (factor VIII:C and factor VIII:Ag undetectable) after treatment with factor VIII. The phenomenon is a fairly typical immune response to foreign protein, in that several doses are required to produce a maximum response. Most such antibodies are IgG subtype 4.[189] Epitope mapping has shown that specificities against the heavy chain or light chain or both can be detected in different patients.[190] Other than neutralization of infused factor VIII, no additional immune-complex-type pathology occurs. A relationship to HLA subtype BFF, C4A4, and C4B2 was detected in one survey.[191] More recently, Lippert and colleagues[192] found a highly significant association between inhibitor formation and HLA class II genes but no association with HLA-DR. Likewise, Aly et al.[193] found a strong association between HLA-Cw5 ad inhibitors (16 out of 16) in their survey of 44 patients, but no linkage to HLA-DR. Conversely, Simmoney et al.[194] detected an association between inhibitors and HLA-DR4. All these surveys involved rather small numbers of patients, but an association with the HLA class II locus seems well established.

Familial incidence of antibodies was noted before the recent molecular genetic analysis of hemophilia A. From the published database of mutations,[144] it is now possible to draw some inferences about mutational associations with inhibitor development. Mild hemophilia A is almost always associated with missense mutations and a very low incidence of inhibitors (only two cases have been reported). Perhaps the missense mutations in these cases (R2209Q and W2229C) create local structural variations such that the wild-type sequence presents an immunogenic epitope.

All other reported patients with inhibitors have nonsense mutations or deletions in their factor VIII gene. The incidence varies for different sites; R336X is associated with inhibitors in none of six cases, R1941X in five of seven, R2147X in three of four, and R2209X in three of five. The low incidence for R336X may be explained by exon skipping, which has been observed specifically in the mutant processed mRNA,[148] giving rise to synthesis of factor VIII del exon 8 in sufficient quantity to induce tolerance to most of the factor VIII sequence (see above).

Patients with gross deletions (>2 kb) in the factor VIII gene have five times the incidence of inhibitors as patients without deletions detectable by Southern blotting.[195] Of 49 deletion patients in the database, 18 have inhibitors, but that is a biased estimate since many patients were selected for screening who had antibodies. Evaluation of the total contribution of genotype to inhibitor development must await nonselective molecular genetic analysis of a large group of patients with and without inhibitors, including those with the intron 22 defect mentioned earlier.[149]

Recently, intensive observation of previously untreated patients after exposure to new, high-purity (recombinant or plasma-derived) factor VIII has revealed a worryingly high incidence of inhibitors (up to 30 percent).[183] The implications of this observation are debatable, since exactly comparable historical controls treated with low-purity concentrate are not available. Thus, it is unclear whether the high incidence of inhibitors reflects increased surveillance or a higher immunogenicity of high-purity factor VIII. No consensus has yet emerged on this issue. It is highly desirable to identify the genotypes most at risk and subject these patients to preemptive regimens to induce tolerance, since development of high-titer inhibitors is now the only important complication of factor VIII therapy.

Viruses Transmitted by Factor VIII Concentrates. Multiple-donor concentrates were introduced in the late 1960s. Very soon thereafter, it was noted that a high incidence of hepatitis occurred in patients treated with them, and that the newly discovered Australia antigen was present in most attacks. Most older patients now test positive for hepatitis B antibody or are chronically antigen-positive. During the 1970s, despite screening of blood for hepatitis B antigen, both acute and chronic hepatitis continued to appear in hemophiliacs, and it was realized that this was mainly due to another virus, now known to be hepatitis C. Up to half of hemophiliacs have chronically or intermittently elevated liver enzymes[197] that developed after a first attack of hepatitis C: this disease may cause a very severe acute episode before converting to chronicity. Liver biopsies show characteristic histologic features[198] and chronic active or chronic persistent hepatitis in a high proportion of cases.[197] The long-term effect of this process is eventual liver failure.[198] Prevention of hepatitis B is now assured by vaccinating all nonimmune patients. The management of chronic viral hepatitis, especially when there is coexisting delta agent, includes interferon, which is effective in suppressing biochemical signs of hepatitis in about 25 percent of cases. Whether this treatment will prevent eventual liver failure or hepatocarcinoma remains to be seen.

The first hemophilic patient to develop AIDS was reported from the United States in 1983. Retrospective surveys of stored blood serum of hemophiliacs in the U.K. and United States show that seroconversion to HIV-antibody-positive began in 1978. Currently, all factor concentrates are from HIV-antibody-negative plasma and are treated with heat or solvent detergent, which successfully prevents transmission. Tragically, 30 to 90 percent of hemophiliacs (the rate varies in different countries) were infected by HIV before the cause of AIDS and the means of avoiding it were discovered. The conversion rate of HIV-antibody-positive patients to clinical AIDS is similar for hemophiliacs and other high risk groups (70 percent conversion rate at 11 years).[199]

AIDS has now become the most common cause of death in hemophilia A. The only clinical point of difference between AIDS in hemophiliacs and in other high-risk groups is that Kaposi's sarcoma is very uncommon in hemophiliacs. Surveys of the families of HIV-antibody-positive hemophiliacs show that up to 5 percent of wives and sexual partners test positive but that no other household contacts do. Several wives of hemophiliacs have died of AIDS. This devastating situation has thrown a great strain on patients, their families, and those who care for them. Intensive counseling and treatment of the condition, once it develops, with AZT and appropriate antimicrobials for infections are all that can be offered at present. Patients have been strongly advised to use barrier contraception if they test positive.

Prospects for Gene Therapy

Hemophilia A is considered a suitable condition for gene therapy for several reasons. Since the action of the protein is in the circulation, any convenient tissue or site can be targeted for expression, provided the protein is exported to plasma. In vitro studies show that a wide variety of cell types will make functional factor VIII, including fibroblasts, endothelial cells, hepatocytes, and kidney-derived cell lines.

Tight control of the expression level is not essential, and a partial correction, for example, from 0 to 10 percent, would make a very large difference to the clinical bleeding tendency. The present treatments, though effective, are inconvenient to administer and expensive. Several animal models of hemophilia are available for experimental correction. Liver transplantation (for end-stage liver failure) cures hemophilia A.[63]

The argument against gene therapy for hemophilia A is that the disease is not usually a lethal condition and that replacement therapy is effective, with a long history of success. Therefore, gene therapy of any type would need to be completely free of harmful side effects, a stricture that few therapies of any kind can meet.

The most worrisome aspects of current approaches to gene therapy based on retroviral vectors are the potentials for insertional mutagenesis and for reversion of the virus to replication competence. Many workers would now consider retrovirus vectors contraindicated in hemophilia A gene therapy for those reasons. Furthermore, studies in mice, where retroviral vectors have been used to transfer a factor VIII cDNA to fibroblasts and to hematopoietic progenitor cells, have shown either no expression or short-lived expression of factor VIII.[200] Recent work suggests that this is particularly associated with sequences in the A2 and A3 domains (Dusty Miller, personal communication). However, gene therapy is an extremely active research field, with new strategies being devised almost weekly. Therefore, animal trials with effective vectors are likely to be reported within the next 5 to 10 years. When or indeed whether all reasonable safety issues can be met well enough to allow human clinical trials, time alone can tell.

HEMOPHILIA A IN FEMALES

Hemophilia A is very rare in females; yet a number of biologic bases exist for the observation. If the frequency of affected males in the population is 1 in 5000, and one-third of affected males result from new mutations occurring in females who are not carriers of the disease, then about 1 in 7000 males inherit the disease from a carrier female. Since carrier females have a 1 in 2 chance of having an affected male with each pregnancy, the incidence of carrier females should be roughly 1 in 3500. A true homozygous female will result from matings of affected males and carrier females, with an incidence of 1 in every 2 female offspring. Thus, the general population frequency of homozygous affected females should be roughly ($^1/_{7000}$) × ($^1/_{3500}$) × ($^1/_2$), or about 1 in 50 million females. Such cases have been described.[201-203]

Another cause of hemophilia in a phenotypic female is a defective factor VIII gene in an XO, or Turner syndrome, female.[204] In such females, Turner syndrome should be suspected on the basis of the typical dysmorphic features, including short stature, webbed neck, and shield chest.

A potentially more frequent cause of hemophilia A in a female is inappropriate lyonization such that by chance, the X chromosome bearing the mutant factor VIII gene in a female heterozygote is the active X chromosome in the vast majority of factor VIII-producing cells in the liver.

A fourth cause of hemophilia A in a female is an X–autosome translocation involving a breakpoint within the factor VIII gene.[56] Since cells with one or three copies of autosomal genes are at a survival disadvantage to those with two copies of all autosomal genes, the normal X chromosome is the inactive X in all cells in females carrying such an X–autosome translocation. Since the factor VIII gene is very close to the telomere of the long arm of the X chromosome, translocations involving the factor VIII gene and the tip of an autosomal arm would by cryptic and impossible to detect by conventional cytogenetic analysis. This type of translocation, though rarely reported to date, could be a significant contributor to the incidence of females with hemophilia A.

A fifth possible cause of hemophilia A in a female is uniparental isodisomy, the inheritance of two copies of one chromosomal homologue of a pair from one parent and no copies of that chromosome from the other parent. In this instance, uniparental isodisomy would require inheritance in an affected female of two copies of the X chromosome bearing a factor VIII mutation from her carrier mother. Such a female, who is homozygous for all genes on the X chromosome, may not be viable. Isodisomy has been observed in one case of male-to-male transmission of hemophilia A, in which an affected male passed both his X chromosome and his Y chromosome to his affected son, who received no sex chromosome from his mother.[205]

COMBINED FACTOR V AND FACTOR VIII DEFICIENCY

About 30 families with this surprising combined defect, inherited as an autosomal recessive, have been described worldwide (for a review, see Soff and Lein[206])

Parental consanguinity is common in these patients, and homozygotes have factor V and factor VIII levels generally below 20 U/dl. Patients have excessive blood loss after dental extraction or other surgery, epistaxes, and large bruises. A few cases have had hemarthroses or muscle hematomas. Treatment with fresh frozen plasma is effective. Factor VIII concentrates contain insufficient factor V to be effective.

The pathophysiology of this disorder remains mysterious. The level of factor VIII antigen is reduced to about the same extent as the coagulant activity,[207] but the level of factor V antigen was normal in one study[108] and reduced in another.[209] A chance association of the two isolated deficiencies [parahemophilia (factor V deficiency) and hemophilia A] is ruled out by the autosomal inheritance pattern and the improbability of a chance combination of the two diseases. Although it was originally claimed that the plasma level of a protein C inhibitor also was reduced in these patients,[210] subsequent studies proved that the protein C inhibitor is labile and is present in normal amounts in fresh plasma samples from combined-deficiency patients.[211-213] Excessive inactivation of factor V and factor VIII by activated protein C remains a possible cause of this disorder.

Factor V

Protein Structure

Factor V is a cofactor in the activation of prothrombin by activated factor X. Indeed, it has both functional and structural similarities to factor VIII. Both are cofactors required for optimal coagulant activity as a result of their interaction with vitamin K-dependent serine proteases. Both proteins are activated by thrombin and factor Xa and are inactivated by activated protein C. Both proteins are initially synthesized as proteins of M_r greater than 300,000 (see refs.

214 to 219 for factor V). For both proteins, proteolytic activation occurs in the N-terminal heavy chain and the C-terminal light chain, producing the active form of these cofactors. In the primary sequence, the two functional subunits are separated by a large and highly glycosylated peptide, the B domain. Both proteins are also posttranslationally modified by sulfation of tyrosine residues.[66,220] Amino acid[221] and nucleic acid sequence[222] analysis has demonstrated a high degree of homology between these factors. Thus, both their structure and their function indicate that factors V and VIII are closely related.

Gene Structure

The gene for factor V spans about 80 kb, has 25 exons, and is generally quite similar to the factor VIII gene.[222a] The size difference between the factor V and factor VIII genes is due to the smaller size of six of the factor V introns relative to their factor VIII counterparts. Of 24 intron–exon boundaries, 21 are at identical locations in the two genes. Although the B domains of factor V and factor VIII are unrelated in sequence, both are encoded within a single large exon, possibly owing to the insertion of a processed mRNA into the evolutionary precursor of the two genes.

Factor V Deficiency

Factor V deficiency is a rare autosomal recessive bleeding disorder (less than one per million) first described by Owen,[223] who gave it the name *parahemophilia*. A curious feature of the condition is that the plasma factor V levels do not correlate with the bleeding tendency.[224] However, it has been shown that the platelet surface-associated factor V levels are the critical determinants of the bleeding tendency.[225] Thus, patients may have no detectable plasma factor V but little bleeding. These patients have normal or slightly reduced platelet factor Xa-binding capacity, a measure of platelet surface-associated factor V. Other cases have no platelet or plasma factor V, and these patients bleed readily, especially after trauma or surgery. Many such individuals have a prolonged bleeding time, emphasizing the close relationship between factor V and platelet function. Some patients are reported to have nonfunctional factor V antigen in their plasma, but there is no further information on the underlying genotype.

Laboratory diagnosis shows prolonged prothrombin and partial thromboplastin times, since factor V functions in both the intrinsic and extrinsic pathways.

None of the commercially available plasma concentrates have sufficient factor V to be useful in treating a hemorrhagic episode. However, treatment with fresh frozen plasma is effective, and hemostasis may be normal at plasma levels of 20 U/dl or 20 percent of normal levels.

ADDENDUM

The parental origin of the inversion mutations[141a,241] that account for over 25% of hemophilia A has importance for genetic counselling. One may hypothesize that pairing of the long arm of the X chromosome with its homolog inhibits the inversion process, and that, therefore, the event would originate predominantly in male germ cells. In one study, 20 of 20 informative cases in which the inversion originated in a maternal grandparent occurred in a male meiosis. In addition, all but one of 50 mothers of sporadic cases due to an inversion were carriers.[242] The data support the hypothesis that an unpaired Xq is much more likely to be involved in an intrachromosomal inversion and indicate that factor VIII gene inversions leading to severe hemophilia A occur almost exclusively in male germ cells. This means that nearly every mother of a sporadic, severely affected patient with an inversion is a carrier. The carrier frequency in all mothers of sporadic, severe cases is therefore much greater than 2/3, and it approaches 5/6.

REFERENCES

1. Bulloch W, Fildes P: Haemophilia. in *Treasury of Human Inheritance* Parts V and VI, *Eugenics Laboratory Memoirs* Vol 12. Dulau, London, p. 173, 1911.
2. Rosner F: Hemophilia in the Talmud and Rabbinic writings. *Ann Intern Med* **70**:833.
3. Alsaharavius: *Liber Theoricae Necnon Practicae Alsaharavii . . . qui Vulgo caravius Dicitur; Jam. . . . Depromptus in Lucem*. tractatus XXXI, sectio II, capitulum XV, folio CXLV. Augsburg, published by S. Grim and M. Vuirsung, 1519. Translated from the original Arabic into Latin by Paul Ricius.
4. Otto JC: An account of an haemorrhagic disposition existing in certain families. The Medical Repository, New York. vol. 6, no. 1, p.1, 1803.
5. Major M: *Classic Descriptions of Disease* 3rd ed. Springfield, IL, Charles C Thomas, p. 521, 1945. (Reproduction of J. C. Otto's classic paper, with a short biographical note on Otto.)
6. Hay J: An account of a remarkable haemorrhagic disposition existing in many individuals of the same family. *N Engl J Med Surg Boston* **2**:221, 1813.
7. Osler W: Haemophilia, in *Pepper's System of Medicine*, vol. 3. London, p. 933, 1885.
8. Hopff F: *Ueber die Haemophilie oder die erbliche Anlage zu tödtlichen Blutungen*. Germany, Würzburg University, 1828. Inaugural Dissertation.
9. Bateson W: *Mendel's Principles of Heredity*. Cambridge, Cambridge University Press, p. 222, 1909.
10. McKusick VA: The Royal Hemophilia. *Sci Am* **213**:88, 1965.
11. Wright AE: On a method of determining the condition of blood coagulability for clinical and experimental purposes and on the effect of the administration of calcium salts in haemophilia and actual or threatened haemorrhage. *Br Med J* **2**:223, 1893.
12. Addis T: Hereditary haemophilia: Deficiency in the coagulability of the blood the only immediate cause of the condition. *Q J Med* **4**:14, 1910.
13. Addis T: The pathogenesis of hereditary haemophilia. *J Pathol Bacteriol* **15**:427, 1911.
14. Morawitz P: Die Chemie der Blutgerinnung. *Ergebnisse der Physiologie biologischen Chemie und experimental Pharmackologie* **4**:307, 1905.
15. Govaerts P, Gratia A: Contribution à l'étude de l'hémophilie. *Rev Belg Sci Med* **3**:689, 1931.
16. Quick AJ, Stanley-Brown M, Bancroft FW: A study of the coagulation defect in hemophilia and in jaundice. *Am J Med Sci* **190**:501, 1935.
17. Repke K, Gemmell CH, Guha A, Turitto VT, Broze GJ, Nemerson Y: Hemophilia as a defect of the tissue factor pathway of blood coagulation. Effect of factors VIII and IX on factor X activation in a continuous flow reactor. *Proc Natl Acad Sci USA* **87**:7623, 1990.
18. Morawitz P, Lossen J: Ueber Hämophilie. *Deutsch Arch Klin Med*. Leipzig. Bd. XCIV, S.110, 1908.
19. Sahli H: Ueber das Wesen der Häemophilie. *Z Klin Med Berlin*. Bd. LVI, S.264, 1904.
20. Patek AJJ, Taylor FHL: Hemophilia II. Some properties of a substance obtained from normal human plasma effective in accelerating the coagulation of hemophilic blood. *J Clin Invest* **16**:113, 1937.
21. Lewis JH, Tagnon HJ, Davidson CS, Minot GR, Taylor FHL: The relation of certain fractions of the plasma globulins to the coagulation defect in hemophilia. *Blood* **1**:166, 1946.

22. Merskey C: The laboratory diagnosis of haemophilia. *J Clin Pathol* **3**:301, 1950.
23. Merskey C, MacFarlane RG: The female carrier of haemophilia: A clinical and laboratory study. *Lancet* **1**:487, 1951.
24. Aggeler PM, White SG, Glendening MB, Page EW, Leake TB, Bates B: Plasma thromboplastin component (PTC) deficiency: A new disease resembling haemophilia. *Proc Soc Exp Biol Med* **79**:692, 1952.
25. Biggs R, Douglas AS, Macfarlane RG, Dacie JV, Pitney WR, Merskey C, O'Brien JR: Christmas disease: A condition previously mistaken for haemophilia. *Br Med J* **2**:1378, 1952.
26. Schulman I, Smith CH: Hemorrhagic disease in an infant due to deficiency of a previously undescribed clotting factor. *Blood* **7**:794, 1952.
27. Wright IS: The nomenclature of blood clotting factors. *Thromb Diath Haemorrh* **7**:381, 1962.
28. Owen WG, Wagner RH: Antihemophilic factor: Separation of an active fragment following dissociation by salts or detergents. *Thromb Diath Haemorrh* **27**:502, 1972.
29. Zimmerman TS, Ratnoff OD, Powell AE: Immunologic differentiation of classic haemophilia (factor VIII deficiency) and von Willebrand's disease. *J Clin Invest* **50**:244, 1971.
30. Zimmerman TS, Edgington TS: Factor VIII coagulant activity and factor VIII like antigen: Independent molecular entities. *J Exp Med* **138**:1015, 1973.
31. Tuddenham EGD, Trabold NS, Collins JA, Hoyer LW: The properties of factor VIII coagulant activity prepared by immunoadsorbent chromatography. *J Lab Clin Med* **93**:40, 1979.
32. Fass DN, Knutson GJ, Katzmann JA: Monoclonal antibodies to porcine factor VIII coagulant and their use in the isolation of active coagulant protein. *Blood* **59**:594, 1982.
33. Vehar GA, Keyt B, Eaton D, Rodriguez H, O'Brien DP, Rotblat F, Oppermann H, Keck R, Wood WI, Harkins RN, Tuddenham EGD, Lawn RM, Capon DJ: Structure of human factor VIII. *Nature* **312**:337, 1984.
34. Wood WI, Capon DJ, Simonsen CC, Eaton DL, Gitschier J, Keyt B, Seeburg PH, Smith DL, Hollingshead P, Wion KL, Delwart E, Tuddenham EGD, Vehar GA, Lawn RM: Expression of active human factor VIII from recombinant DNA clones. *Nature* **312**:330, 1984.
35. Toole JJ, Knopf JL, Wozney JM, Sultzman LA, Buecker JL, Pittman DD, Kaufman RJ, Brown E, Shoemaker C, Orr EC, Amphlett GW, Foster WB, Coe ML, Knutson GJ, Fass DN, Hewick RM: Molecular cloning of a cDNA encoding human antihaemophilic factor. *Nature* **312**:342, 1984.
36. Rizza CR, Spooner RJD: Treatment of haemophilia and related disorders in Britain and Northern Ireland during 1976–80: Report on behalf of the Directors of Haemophilia Centres in the United Kingdom. *Br Med J* **286**:929, 1983.
37. Massie R, Massie S: *Journey*. New York, Knopf, 1973.
38. Mazurier C: von Willebrand's disease masquerading as haemophilia A. *Thromb Haemost* **67**:391, 1992.
39. Gitschier J, Wood WI, Goralka TM, Wion KL, Chen EY, Eaton DE, Vehar GA, Capon DJ, Lawn RM: Characterization of the human factor VIII gene. *Nature* **312**:326, 1984.
40. Levinson B, Kenwrick S, Lakich D, Hammonds G, Gitschier J: A transcribed gene in an intron of the human factor VIII gene. *Genomics* **7**:1, 1990.
41. Levinson B, Bermingham JR, Metzenberg A, Kenwrick S, Chapman V, Gitschier J: Sequence of the human factor VIII-associated gene is conserved in mouse. *Genomics* **13**:862, 1992.
42. Levinson B, Kenwrick S, Gamel P, Fisher K, Gitschier J: Evidence for a third transcript from the human factor VIII gene. *Genomics* **14**:585, 1992.
43. Wion KL, Kelly D, Summerfield JA, Tuddenham EGD, Lawn RM: Distribution of factor VIII mRNA and antigen in human liver and other tissues. *Nature* **317**:726, 1985.
44. Zelechowska MG, van Mourik JA, Brodniewicz-Proba T: Ultrastructural localization of factor VIII procoagulant antigen in human liver hepatocytes. *Nature* **317**:729, 1985.
45. Koschinsky ML, Funk WD, van Ooar BA, MacGillivray TRA: Complete cDNA sequence of human preceruloplasmin. *Proc Natl Acad Sci USA* **83**:5086, 1986.
46. Kane WH, Davie EW: Cloning of a cDNA coding for human factor V, a blood coagulation factor homologous to factor VIII and ceruloplasmin. *Proc Natl Acad Sci USA* **83**:800, 1986.
47. Kane WH, Ichinose A, Hagen FS, Davie EW: Cloning of cDNAs coding for the heavy chain region and connecting region of human factor V, a blood coagulation factor with four types of repeats. *Biochemistry* **26**:6508, 1987.
48. Stubbs JD, Lekutis C, Singer KL, Bui A, Yuzuki D, Srinivasan U, Parry G: cDNA cloning of a mouse mammary epithelial cell surface protein reveals the existence of epidermal growth factor-like sequences. *Proc Natl Acad Sci USA* **87**:8417, 1990.
48a. Larocca D, Paterson JA, Urrea R, Kuniyoshi J, Bistrain AM, Ceriono RL: A M_r 46,000 human milk globule protein that is highly expressed in human breast tumours contains factor VIII-like domains. *Cancer Res* **51**:4994, 1991.
49. Elder B, Lakich D, Gitschier J: Sequence of the murine Factor VIII cDNA. *Genomics* **16**:374, 1993.
50. Haldane JBS, Smith CAB: A new estimate of the linkage between the genes for colour-blindness and haemophilia in man. *Ann Eugen* **14**:10, 1947.
51. Boyer SH, Graham JB: Linkage between the X chromosome loci for G6PD electrophoretic variation and hemophilia A. *Am J Hum Genet* **17**:320, 1965.
52. Filippi G, Mannucci PM, Coppola R, Farris A, Rinaldi A, Siniscalco M: Studies on hemophilia A in Sardinia bearing on the problems of multiple allelism, carrier detection and differential mutation rate in the two sexes. *Am J Hum Genet* **36**:44, 1984.
53. Patterson M, Schwartz C, Bell M, Sauer S, Hofker M, Trask B, van den Engh G, Davies KE: Physical mapping studies on the human X chromosome in the region Xq27-Xqter. *Genomics* **1**:297, 1987.
54. Poustka A, Detrich A, Langenstein G, Toniolo D, Warren ST, Lehrach H: Physical map of Xq27-Xqter: Localizing the region of the fragile X mutation. *Proc Natl Acad Sci USA* **88**:8302, 1991.
55. Freije D, Schlessinger D: A 1.6 mb contig of yeast artificial chromosomes around the human factor VIII gene reveals three regions homologous to probes for the DXS115 locus and two for the DXYS64 locus. *Am J Hum Genet* **51**:66, 1992.
56. Migeon BR, McGinnis MJ, Antonarakis SE, Axelman J, Stasiowski B, Youssoufian H, Keams WG, Chung A, Pearson PL, Kazazian HH Jr, Muneer RS: Severe hemophilia A in a female by cryptic translocation: Order and orientation of factor VIII within Xq28. *Genomics* **16**:20, 1993.
57. Kaufman RJ: Structure and biology of factor VIII in Hoffman R, Benz EJ, Shattil SJ, Furie B, Cohen HJ (eds): *Hematology: Basic Principles and Practice*. New York: Churchill Livingstone, 1276, 1991.
58. Kaufman RJ: Biological regulation of Factor VIII activity. *Annu Rev Med* **43**:325, 1992.
59. van Dieijen G, Tans G, Rosing J, Hemker HC: The role of phospholipid and factor VIIIa in the activation of bovine factor X. *J Biol Chem* **256**:3433, 1981.
60. Kaufman RJ, Wasley LC, Dorner AJ: Synthesis, processing and secretion of recombinant human factor VIII expressed in mammalian cells. *J Biol Chem* **263**:6352, 1988.
61. Weiss HJ, Sussman I, Hoyer LW: Stabilization of factor VIII in plasma by the von Willebrand factor. Studies on posttransfusion and dissociated factor VIII and in patients with von Willebrand disease. *J Clin Invest* **60**:390, 1977.
62. Fulcher CA, Zimmerman TS: Characterization of the human factor VIII procoagulant protein with a heterologous precipitating antibody. *Proc Natl Acad Sci USA* **79**:1648, 1982.
63. Bontempo FA, Lewis JH, Gorenc TJ, Spero JA, Ragni MV, Scott JP, Starzl TE: Liver transplantation in hemophilia A. *Blood* **68**:1721, 1986.
64. Dorner AJ, Bole DG, Kaufman RJ: The relationship of N-linked glycosylation and heavy chain binding protein association with the secretion of glycoproteins. *J Cell Biol* **105**:2665, 1987.
65. Munro S, Pelham HRB: An Hsp70-like protein in the ER: Identity with the 78 kD glucose-regulated protein and immunoglobulin heavy chain binding protein. *Cell* **46**:291, 1986.

66. Pittman DD, Wang JH, Kaufman RJ: Identification and functional importance of tyrosine sulfate residues within recombinant factor VIII. *Biochemistry* **31**:3315, 1992.
67. Wise RJ, Dorner AJ, Krane M, Pittman DD, Kaufman RJ: The role of von Willebrand factor multimers and propeptide cleavage in binding and stabilization of factor VIII. *J Biol Chem* **266**:21948, 1991.
68. Eaton D, Rodriguez H, Vehar GA: Proteolytic processing of human factor VIII. Correlation of specific cleavages by thrombin, factor Xa, and activated protein C with activation and inactivation of factor VIII coagulant activity. *Biochemistry* **25**:505, 1986.
69. Fulcher CA, Roberts JR, Zimmerman TS: Thrombin proteolysis of purified factor VIII. Correlation of activation with generation of a specific polypeptide. *Blood* **61**:807, 1983.
70. Pittman DD, Kaufman RJ: Proteolytic requirements for thrombin activation of antihemophilic factor (factor VIII). *Proc Natl Acad Sci USA* **85**:2429, 1988.
71. Pittman DD, Kaufman RJ: Structure-function relationships of factor VIII elucidated through recombinant DNA technology. *Thromb Haemost* **61**:161, 1989.
72. Hill-Eubanks DC, Parker CG, Lollar P: Differential proteolytic activation of factor VIII-von Willebrand factor complex by thrombin. *Proc Natl Acad Sci USA* **86**:6508, 1989.
73. Shima M, Ware J, Yoshioka A, Fukui H, Fulcher CA: An arginine to cysteine amino acid substitution at a critical thrombin cleavage site in a dysfunctional factor VIII molecule. *Blood* **74**:1612, 1989.
74. Gitschier J, Kogan S, Levinson B, Tuddenham EGD: Mutations of factor VIII cleavage sites in hemophilia A. *Blood* **72**:1022, 1988.
75. Pattinson J, Millar DS, McVey J, Grundy CB, Wieland K, Mibashsan RS, Martinowitz U, Tan-Un K, Vidaud M, Goossens M, Sampietro M, Manucci PM, Krawczak M, Reiss J, Zoll B, Whitmore D, Bowcock S, Wensley R, Ajani A, Mitchell V, Rizza C, Maia R, Winter P, Mayne EE, Schwartz M, Green PJ, Kakker VV, Tuddenham EGD, Cooper DN: The molecular genetic analysis of hemophilia A: A directed search strategy for the detection of point mutations in the human factor VIII gene. *Blood* **76**:2242, 1990.
76. Higuchi M, Wong C, Kochhan L, Olek K, Aronis S, Kasper CK, Kazazian HH, Antonarakis SE: Characterization of mutations in the factor VIII gene by direct sequencing of amplified genomic DNA. *Genomics* **6**:65, 1990.
77. Schwaab R, Ludwig M, Kochhan L, Oldenburg J, McVey JH, Egli H, Brackmann HH, Olek K: Detection and characterisation of two missense mutations at a cleavage site in the factor VIII light chain. *Thromb Res* **61**:225, 1991.
78. Arai M, Inaa H, Higuchi M, Antonarakis SE, Kazazian HH, Fujimaki M, Hoyer LW: Detection of a mutation altering a thrombin cleavage site (arginine-372-histidine) *Proc Natl Acad Sci USA* **86**:4277, 1989.
79. O'Brien D, Pattinson JK, Tuddenham EGD: Purification and characterization of factor VIII 372-cys: A hypofunctional cofactor from a patient with moderately severe hemophilia A. *Blood* **75**:1664, 1990.
80. Arai M, Higuchi M, Antonarakis SE, Kazazian HH, Phillips JA, Janco RL, Hoyer LW: Characterization of a thrombin cleavage site mutation (arg 1689 to cys) in the factor VIII gene of two unrelated patients with cross-reacting material positive hemophilia A. *Blood* **75**:384, 1990.
80a. O'Brien DP, Tuddenham EGD: Purification and characterization of factor VIII 1689Cys: A non-functional cofactor occurring in a patient with severe haemophilia A. *Blood* **73**:2117, 1989.
81. Lollar C, Parker CG: Subunit structure of thrombin-activated porcine factor VIII. *Biochemistry* **28**:666, 1989.
82. Fay PJ, Haidaris PJ, Smudzin TM: Human factor VIIIa subunit structure: Reconstitituion of factor VIIIa from the isolated A1/A3-C1-C2 dimer and A2 subunit. *J Biol Chem* **266**:8957, 1991.
83. Lollar P, Parker CG: pH-dependent denaturation of thrombin-activated porcine factor VIII. *J Biol Chem* **265**:1688, 1990.
84. Lollar P, Parker ET: Structural basis for the decreased procoagulant activity of human factor VIII compared to the porcine homolog. *J Biol Chem* **266**:12481, 1991.
85. Pittman DD, Millenson M, Marquette K, Bauer K, Kaufman RJ: The A2 domain of human recombinant derived factor VIII is required for procoagulant activity but not for thrombin cleavage. *Blood*. In press.
86. Eaton DL, Wood WI, Eaton D, Hass PE, Hollingshead P, Wion K, Mather J, Lawn RM, Vehar GA, Gorman C.: Construction and characterization of an active factor VIII variant lacking the central one-third of the molecule. *Biochemistry* **25**:8343, 1987.
87. Toole JJ, Pittman DD, Orr EC, Murtha P, Wasley LC, Kaufman RJ: A large region (= 95 kDa) of human factor VIII is dispensable for *in vitro* procoagulant activity. *Proc Natl Acad Sci USA* **83**:5939, 1986.
88. Jenny RJ, Pittman DD, Toole JJ, Kriz RW, Aldape RA, Hewick RM, Kaufman RJ, Mann KG: Complete cDNA and amino acid sequence of human factor V. *Proc Natl Acad Sci USA* **84**:4846, 1986.
89. Guinto ER, Esmon CT: Loss of prothrombin and of factor Xa-factor Va interactions upon inactivation of factor Va by activated protein C. *J Biol Chem* **259**:13986, 1983.
90. Higuchi M, Antonarakis SE, Kasch L, Oldenburg J, Economou-Petersen E, Olek K, Inaba H, Kazazian HH: Towards a complete characterization of mild to moderate hemophilia A: Detection of the molecular defect in 25 of 29 patients by denaturing gradient gel electrophoresis. *Proc Natl Aca Sci USA* **88**:8307, 1991.
91. Walker FJ, Scandella D, Fay PJ: Identification of the binding site for activated protein C on the light chain of factors V and VIII. *J Biol Chem* **265**:1484, 1990.
92. Fulcher CA, Gardiner JE, Griffin JH, Zimmerman TS: Proteolytic inactivation of human factor VIII procoagulant protein by activated protein C and its analogy with factor V. *Blood* **63**:486, 1984.
93. Fay PJ, Walker FJ: Inactivation of human factor VIII by inactivated protein C: Evidence that the factor VIII light chain contains the activated protein C binding site. *Biochim Biophys Acta* **994**:142, 1989.
94. Fay PJ, Smudzin TM, Walker FJ: Activated protein C-catalyzed inactivation of human factor VIII and factor VIIIa. Identification of cleavage sites and correlation of proteolysis with cofactor activity. *J Biol Chem* **266**:20139, 1991.
94a. O'Brien DP, Johnson D, Byfield P, Tuddenham EGD: Inactivation of factor VIII by factor IXa. *Biochemistry* **31**:2805, 1992.
95. Dahlback B, Carlsson M: Factor VIII defect associated with familial thrombophilia. *Thromb Haemost* **65**:658, 1991. Abstract 39.
96. Bonthron DT, Hardin R, Kaufman RJ, Wasley LC, Orr EC, Mitsork LM, Ewenstein B, Loscalzo J, Ginsburg D, Orkin SH: Structure of pre-pro-von Willebrand factor and its expression in heterologous cells. *Nature* **324**:270, 1986.
97. Marcuso DJ, Tuley EA, Westfield LA, Worval NK, Shelton-Inloes BB, Sorace JM, Alevy YG, Sadler JE: Structure of the gene for human von Willebrand factor. *J Biol Chem* **264**:19514, 1989.
98. Pver K. Sixma JJ, Bruine MH, Trieschnigg AM, Vlooswijk RA, Beeser-Visser NH, Bonnon B: Survival of ^{125}iodine-labeled factor VIII in normals and patients with classic hemophilia. Observations on the heterogeneity of human factor VIII. *J Clin Invest* **62**:233, 1978.
99. Tuddenham EGD, Lane RS, Rotblat F, Johnson AJ, Snapp TJ, Middleton S, Kernoff PB: Response to infusions of polyelectrolyte fractionated human factor VIII concentrate in human hemophilia A and von Willebrand's disease. *Br J Haematol* **52**:259, 1982.
100. Brinkhous KM, Sandberg H, Garris JB, Mattsson C, Palm M, Griggs T, Read MS: Purified human factor VIII procoagulant protein: Comparative hemostasis response after infusions into hemophilic and von Willebrand disease dogs. *Proc Natl Acad Sci USA* **82**:8752, 1985.
101. Fay PJ, Coumans J-V, Walker FJ: Von Willebrand factor mediates protection of factor VIII from activated protein C-catalyzed inactivation. *J Biol Chem* **266**:2172, 1991.
102. Koedam JAS, Meijers JCM, Sixma JJ, Bouma BN: Inactivation of human factor VIII by activated protein C cofactor activity of protein S and protective effect of von Willebrand factor. *J Clin Invest* **82**:12336, 1988.

103. Hill-Eubanks DC, Lollar P: Von Willebrand factor is a cofactor for thrombin-catalyzed cleavage of the factor VIII light chain. *J Biol Chem* **265:**17854, 1990.
104. Hamer RJ, Koedam JA, Beeser-Visser NH, Bertina RM, van Mourik JA, Sixma JJ: Factor VIII binds to von Willebrand factor via its M_r-80,000 light chain. *Eur J Biochem* **166:**37, 1987.
105. Andersson L-O, Brown JE: Interaction of factor VIII-von Willebrand factor with phospholipid vesicles. *Biochem J* **200:**161, 1981.
106. Lajmonovich A, Hudry-Clergeon G, Freyssinet JM, Marguerie G: Human factor VIII procoagulant activity and phospholipid interaction. *Biochim Biophys Acta* **678:**123, 1991.
107. Nesheim M, Pittman DD, Giles AR, Fass DN, Wang JH, Slonosky D, Kaufman RJ: The effect of von Willebrand factor on the binding of factor VIII to thrombin activated platelets. *J Biol Chem* **266:**17815, 1991.
108. Foster PA, Fulcher CA, Marti T, Titani K, Zimmerman TS: A major factor VIII binding domain resides within the amino-terminal 272 amino acid residues of von Willebrand factor. *J Biol Chem* **262:**8443, 1987.
109. Takahashi Y, Kalafatis M, Girma J-P, Sewerin K, Andersson L-O, Meyer D: Localization of factor VIII binding domain on a 34 kilodalton fragment of the N-terminal portion of von Willebrand factor. *Blood* **70:**1679, 1987.
110. Bahou WF, Ginsburg D, Sikkink R, Litwiller R, Fass DN: A monoclonal antibody to von Willebrand factor (vWF) inhibits factor VIII binding. *J Clin Invest* **84:**56, 1989.
111. Tuley EA, Gaucher C, Jorieux S, Worrall NK, Sadler JE, Mazurier C: Expression of von Willebrand factor "Normandy": An autosomal mutation that mimics hemophilia A. *Proc Natl Acad Sci USA* **88:**6377, 1991.
112. Gaucher C, Mercier B, Jorieux S, Oufkir D, Mazurier C: Identification of two point mutations in the von Willebrand factor gene of three families with the "Normandy" variant of van Willebrand disease. *Br J Haematol* **78:**506, 1991.
113. Cacheris PM, Nichols WC, Ginsburg D: Molecular characterization of a unique von Willebrand disease variant. *J Biol Chem* **266:**13499, 1991.
114. Nishino M, Girma J-P, Rothschild C, Fressinaud E, Meyer D: New variant of von Willebrand disease with defective binding to factor VIII. *Blood* **74:**1591, 1989.
115. Leyte A, Verbeet MP, Brodniewicz-Proba T, Van Mourik JA, Mertens K: The interaction between human blood-coagulation factor VIII and von Willebrand factor: Characterization of a high-affinity binding site on factor VIII. *Biochem J* **257:**679, 1989.
116. Lollar P, Hill-Eubanks DC, Parker CG: Association of the factor VIII light chain with von Willebrand factor. *J Biol Chem* **263:**10451, 1988.
117. Foster PA, Fulcher CA, Houghten RA, Zimmerman TS: An immunogenic region within amino acid residues Val^{1670}-Glu^{1684} of the factor VIII chain induces antibodies which inhibit binding of factor VIII to von Willebrand factor. *J Biol Chem* **264:**5230, 1988.
118. Pittman DD, Kaufman RJ: Internal deletions of factor VIII identify potentially important peptide sequences for binding to von Willebrand factor. *Blood* **70:**392, 1987.
119. Leyte A, van Schijndel HB, Niehrs C, Huttner WB, Verbeet M Ph et al: Sulfation of Tyr^{1680} of human blood coagulation factor VIII is essential for the interaction of factor VIII with von Willebrand factor. *J Biol Chem* **266:**17572, 1991.
120. Poole S, Firtel RA, Lamar E, Rowekamp W: Structure and expression of the discoidin I gene family in *Dictyostelium discoideum*. *J Mol Biol* **153:**273, 1981.
121. Brown JE, Baugh RF, Hougie C: Effect of exercise on the factor VIII complex: A correlation of the von Willebrand antigen and factor VIII coagulant antigen increase. *Thromb Res* **15:**61, 1979.
122. Bloom JW: The interaction of rDNA, factor VIII, factor $VIII_{des\text{-}797\text{-}1562}$ and factor $VIII_{des\text{-}797\text{-}1562}$-derived peptides with phospholipid. *Thromb Res* **48:**439, 1987.
123. Kemball-Cook G, Edwards SJ, Sewerin K, Andersson L-O, Barrowcliffe TW: The phospholipid-binding site of factor VIII is located on the 80 kD light chain. *Thromb Haemost* **58:**222, 1987.
124. Arai M, Scandella D, Hoyer LW: Molecular basis of factor VIII inhibition by human antibodies. *J Clin Invest* **83:**1978, 1989.
125. Foster PA, Fulcher CA, Houghten RA, Zimmerman TS: Synthetic factor VIII peptides with amino acid sequences contained within the C2 domain of factor VIII inhibit factor VIII binding to phosphatidylserine. *Blood* **75:**1999, 1990.
126. Bevers EM, Comfurius P, Zwaal RF: Changes in membrane phospholipid distribution during platelet activation. *Biochim Biophys Acta* **736:**57, 1983.
127. Gilbert GE, Furie BC, Furie B: Binding of human factor VIII to phospholipid. *J Biol Chem* **265:**815, 1990.
128. Nesheim ME, Pittman DD, Wang JH, Slonosky D, Giles AR, Kaufman RJ: The binding of ^{35}S-labeled recombinant factor VIII to activated and unactivated human platelets. *J Biol Chem* **263:**16467, 1988.
129. Muntean W, Leschnik B, Haas J: Factor VIII coagulant moiety binds to platelets by binding to phospholipids of the platelet membrane. *Thromb Res* **45:**345, 1987.
130. Inaba H, Fujimaki M, Kazazian HH, Antonarakis SE: Mild hemophilia A resulting from Arg to Leu substitution in exon 26 of the factor VIII gene. *Hum Genet* **81:**335, 1989.
131. Gitschier J, Wood WI, Shuman MA, Lawn RM: Identification of a missense mutation in the factor VIII gene of a mild hemophiliac. *Science* **232:**1415, 1986.
132. Casula L, Murru S, Pecorara M, Ristaldi MS, Restagno G, Mancuso G, Morfini M, DeBiasi R, Baudo F, Carbonara A, Mori PG, Cao A, Pirastu M: Recurrent mutations and three novel deletions in the factor VIII gene of hemophilia A patients of Italian descent. *Blood* **75:**662, 1990.
133. Higuchi M, Kazazian HH, Kasch L, Warren TC, McGinniss MJ, Phillips JA, Kasper C, Janco R, Antonarakis SE: Molecular characterization of severe hemophilia A suggests that about half the mutations are not within the coding region and splice junctions of the factor VIII gene. *Proc Natl Acad Sci USA* **88:**7405, 1991.
134. Baeuerle PA, Huttner WB: Tyrosine sulfation is a trans-Golgi-specific protein modification. *Mol Cell Biol* **6:**97, 1988.
135. Tucker MM, Foster WB, Katzmann JA, Mann KG: A monoclonal antibody which inhibits the factor Xa interaction. *J Biol Chem* **258:**1210, 1983.
136. Tracy PB, Mann KG: Prothrombinase complex assembly on the platelet surface is mediated through 74,000-dalton component of factor Va. *Proc Natl Acad Sci USA* **80:**2380, 1983.
137. Annamalai AE, Ran AK, Chin HC, Wang D, Dutta-Roy AK, Walsh PN, Colman RW: Epitope mapping of functional domains of human factor Va with human and murine monoclonal antibodies. Evidence for the interaction of heavy chain with factor Xa and calcium. *Blood* **70:**139, 1987.
138. Bertina RM, Cupers R, van Wijngaarden A: Factor IXa protects activated factor VIII against inactivation by activated protein C. *Biochem Biophys Res Commun* **125:**177, 1984.
139. Walker FJ, Chavin SI, Fay PJ: Inactivation of factor VIII by activated protein C and protein S. *Arch Biochem Biophys* *252:*322, 1987.
140. Rick MF, Kriezek DM, Esmon NL: Factor IXa modifies the degradation of factor VIII by activated protein C. *Clin Res* **36:**4127, 1988.
141. Leuting PJ, Donath MJSH, van Mourik JA, Mertens K: Identification of a high affinity binding site for factor IXa on the factor VIII light chain. 14th Congress of the International Society for Thrombosis and Hemostasis, New York, NY, 1993. Abstract.
142. Haldane JBS: The rate of spontaneous mutation of a human gene. *J Genet* **31:**317, 1935.
143. Antonarakis SE, Kazazian HH Jr: The molecular basis of hemophilia A in man. *Trends Genet* **4:**233, 1988.
144. Tuddenham EGD, Cooper DN, Gitschier J, Higuchi M, Hoyer L, Yoshioka A, Peake I, Schwaab R, Olek K, Kazazian H, Lavergne J-M, Giannelli F, Antonarakis S: Haemophilia A: Database of nucleotide substitutions, deletions, insertions and rearrangements of the factor VIII gene. *Nucleic Acids Res* **19:**4821, 1991.
145. McGinniss MJ, Kazazian HH Jr, Hoyer LW, Bi L, Inaba H, Antonarakis SE: Spectrum of mutations in CRM-positive and CRM-reduced hemophilia A. *Genomics* **15:**392, 1993.

146. Jonsdottir S, Diamond C, Levinson B, Magnusson S, Jensson O, Gitschier J: Missense mutations causing mild hemophilia A in Iceland detected by denaturing gradient gel electrophoresis. *Hum Mutation* **1**:506, 1992.
147. Kafa K, Baudis M, Deburgrave N, Bardin JM, Sultan Y, Kaplan JC, Delpech M: A novel mutation (Arg→Leu in exon 18) in factor VIII gene responsible for moderate hemophilia A. *Hum Mutation* **1**:1,77, 1992.
148. Naylor JA, Green PM, Rizza CR, Ginnelli F: Analysis of factor VIII mRNA reveals defects in every one of 28 haemophilia A patients. *Hum Mol Genet* **2**:11, 1993.
149. Naylor JA, Green PM, Rizza CR, Giannelli F: Factor VIII gene explains all cases of haemophilia A. *Lancet* **340**:1066, 1992.
149a. Lavergne JM, Bahnak BR, Vidaud M, Laurian Y, Meyer D: A directed search for mutations in hemophilia A using restriction enzyme and analysis and denaturing gradient gel electrophoresis. A study of seven exons in the factor VIII gene of 170 cases. *Nouv Rev Fr Hematol* **34**:85, 1992.
149b. Reiner AP, Thompson AR: Screening for nonsense mutations in patients with severe hemophilia A can provide rapid, direct carrier detection. *Hum Genet* **89**:88, 1992.
149c. Lin SW, Lin SR, Shen MC: Characterization of genetic defects of hemophilia A in patients of Chinese origin. *Genomics* **18**:496, 1993.
149d. Economou EP, Kazazian HH Jr, Antonarakis SE: Detection of mutations in the factor VIII gene using single-stranded conformational polymorphism (SSCP). *Genomics* **13**:909, 1992.
149e. Paynton C, Sancar G, Sommer SS: Identification of mutations in two families with sporadic hemophilia A. *Hum Genet* **87**:397, 1991.
150. Youssoufian H, Antonarakis SE, Aronis S, Triftis G, Phillips DG, Kazazian HH Jr: Characterization of five partial deletions of the factor VIII gene. *Proc Natl Acad Sci USA* **84**:3772, 1987.
151. Woods Samuels P, Kazazian HH Jr, Antonarakis SE: Nonhomologous recombination in the human genome: Deletions in the human factor VIII gene. *Genomics* **10**:94, 1991.
152. Traystman MD, Higuchi M, Antonarakis SE, Kazazian HH Jr: Use of denaturing gradient gel electrophoresis to detect point mutations in the factor VIII gene. *Genomics* **6**:293, 1990.
153. Aly AM, Higuchi M, Kasper CK, Kazazian HH Jr, Antonarakis SE, Hoyer LW: Hemophilia A due to mutations that create new N-glycosylation sites. *Proc Natl Acad Sci USA* **89**:4933, 1992.
154. Barker D, Schafer M, White R: Restriction sites containing CpG show a higher frequency of polymorphism in human DNA. *Cell* **36**:343, 1984.
155. Gitschier J, Wood WI, Tuddenham EGD, Shuman MA, Goralka TM, Chen EY, Lawn RM: Detection and sequence of mutations in the factor VIII gene of haemophiliacs. *Nature* **315**:427, 1985.
156. Youssoufian H, Kazazian HH Jr, Phillips DG, Aronis S, Tsiftis G, Brown VA, Antonarakis SE: Recurrent mutations in haemophilia A give evidence for CpG mutations hotspots. *Nature* **324**:380, 1986.
156a. Sommer S: Assessing the underlying pattern of human germline mutations: Lessons from the factor IX gene. *FASEB J* **6**:2767, 1992.
157. Kazazian HH Jr, Wong C, Youssoufian HG, Scott AF, Phillips D, Antonarakis SE: A novel mechanism of mutation in man: Hemophilia A due to de novo insertion of L1 sequences. *Nature* **332**:164, 1988.
158. Fanning TG, Singer MF: LINE-1: A mammalian transposable element. *Biochem Biophys Acta* **910**:203, 1987.
159. Kazazian HH Jr, Scott AF: "Copy and paste" transposable elements in the human genome. *J Clin Invest* **91**:1859, 1993.
160. Dombroski BA, Mathias SL, Nanthakumar E, Scott AF, Kazazian HH Jr: Isolation of a human transposable element. *Science* **254**:1808, 1991.
161. Miki Y, Nishisho I, Horii A, Miyoshi Y, Utsunomiya J, Kinzler KW, Vogelstein B, Nakamura Y: Disruption of the APC gene by a retrotransposal insertion of L1 sequence in a colon cancer. *Cancer Res* **52**:643, 1992.
162. Narita N, Nishio H, Kitoh Y, Ishikawa Y, Ishikawa Y, Minami R, Nakamura H, Matsuo M: Insertion of a 5′ truncated L1 element into the 3′ end of exon 44 of the dystrophin gene resulted in skipping of the exon during splicing in a case of Duchenne muscular dystrophy. *J Clin Invest* **91**:1862, 1993.
163. Bakker E, van Omenn G, personal communication.
164. Dombroski BA, Holmes SH, Boehm CD, Krebs C, Kazazian HH Jr: Unusual insertion of an L1 element with its unique 3′ flanking sequence into an exon of the dystophin gene. *Am J Hum Genet*, 1993. Abstract.
165. Wallace MR, Andersen LB, Saulino AM, Gregory TW, Collins FS: A de novo Alu insertion results in neurofibromatosis type 1. *Nature* **353**:864, 1991.
166. Muratani K, Hada T, Yamamoto Y, Kaneko T, Shigeto Y, Ohue T, Furuyama J, Higashino K: Inactivation of the cholinesterase gene by Alu insertion: Possible mechanism for human gene transposition. *Proc Natl Acad Sci USA* **88**:11315, 1991.
167. Vidaud D, Vidaud M, Bahnak BR, Siguret V, Sanchez SG, Laurian Y, Meyer D, Goossens M, Lavergne JM: Haemophilia B due to a de novo insertion of a human-specific Alu subfamily member within the coding region of the factor IX gene. *Eur J Hum Genet* **1**:30, 1993.
168. Goldberg YP, Rommens JM, Andrew SE, Hutchinson GB, Lin B, Theilmann J, Graham R, Glaves ML, Starr E, McDonald H, Nasir J, Schappert K, Kalchman MA, Clarke LA, Hayden MR: Identification of an Alu retrotransposition event in close proximity to a strong candidate gene for Huntington's disease. *Nature* **362**:370, 1993.
169. Dietz HC, Valle D, Francomano CA, Kendzior RJ Jr, Pyeritz RE, Cutting GR: The skipping of constitutive exons in vivo induced by nonsense mutations. *Science* **259**:680, 1993.
170. Naylor JA, Green PM, Montandon AJ, Rizza CR, Giannelli F: Detection of three novel mutations in two haemophilia A patients by rapid screening of whole essential region of factor VIII gene. *Lancet* **337**:635, 1991.
171. Kaplan J-C, Kahn A, Chelly J: Illegitimate transcription: Its use in the study of inherited disease. *Hum Mutation* **1**:357, 1992.
171a. Lakich D, Kazazian HH Jr, Antonarakis SE, Gitschier J: Inversions disrupting the factor VIII gene as a common cause of severe hemophilia A. *Nat Genet* **5**:236, 1993.
172. Gitschier J, Drayne D, Tuddenham EGD, White RL, Lawn RM: Genetic mapping and diagnosis of haemophilia A achieved through a *Bcl*I polymorphism in the factor VIII gene. *Nature* **314**:738, 1985.
173. Wion KL, Tuddenham EGD, Lawn RM: A new polymorphism in the factor VIII gene for prenatal diagnosis of hemophilia A. *Nucleic Acids Res* **14**:4535, 1986.
174. Antonarakis SE, Waber PG, Kittur SD, Patel AS, Kazazian HH Jr, Mellis MA, Stamatoyannopoulos G, Counts RB, Bowie EJW, Fass DN, Pittman DD, Wozney JM, Toole JJ: Hemophilia A: Molecular defects and carrier detection by DNA analysis. *N Engl J Med* **313**:843, 1985.
175. Harper K, Winter RM, Pembrey ME, Hartley D, Davies KE, Tuddenham EGD: A clinically useful DNA probe linked to haemophilia A. *Lancet* **2**:6, 1984.
176. Oberle I, Camerino G, Heilig R, Grunebaum L, Cazenave J-P, Crapanzano C, Manucci P, Mandel JL: Genetic screening for hemophilia A (classic hemophilia) with a polymorphic DNA probe. *N Engl J Med* **312**:682, 1985.
177. Lalloz MR, McVey JH, Pattinson JK, Tuddenham EGD: Haemophilia A diagnosis by analysis of a hypervariable dinucleotide repeat within the factor VIII gene. *Lancet* **338**:207, 1991.
178. Peake IR, Lillicrap DP, Boulyjenkov V, Briët E, Chan V, Ginter EK, Kraus EM, Ljung R, Mannucci PM, Nicolaides K, Tuddenham EGD: Report of a joint WHO/WFH meeting on the control of haemophilia: Carrier detection and prenatal diagnosis. *Blood Coagul Fibrinolysis* **4**:313, 1993.
179. Biggs R: *The Treatment of Haemophilia A and B and von Willebrand's Disease*. Oxford, Blackwell, 1978.
180. Boone DC: *Comprehensive Management of Haemophilia*. Philadelphia, FA Davis, 1976.
181. Gilbert MS, Aledort L: Comprehensive Care in Hemophilia: A team approach. *Mount Sinai Med*. **44**:3, 1977.
182. Lusher JM, Arkin S, Abildgaard CF, Schwartz RS and the Kogenate Previously Untreated Patient Study

Group: Recombinant factor VIII for the treatment of previously untreated patients with hemophilia A. *N Engl J Med* **328**:453, 1993.
183. Kasper CK, Aledort LM, Counts RB, Edson JR, Fratantoni J, Green D, Hampton JW, Hilgartner MW, Lazerson J, Levine PH, McMillan CW, Pool JG, Shapiro SS, Shulman NR, van Eys J: A more uniform measurement of factor VIII inhibitors. *Thromb Diath Haemorrh* **34**:869, 1975.
184. Hedner U, Glazer S, Pingel K, Alberta KA, Blombaeck M, Schulman S, Johnson M: Successful use of recombinant factor VIIa in patient with severe haemophilia A during synovectomy. *Lancet* **2**:1193, 1988.
185. Brackman HH: The treatment of inhibitor against factor VIII by continuous treatment with factor VIII and activated prothrombin complex concentrate, in Mariani G, Russo MA, Mandelli F (eds): *Activated Prothrombin Complex Concentrates*. New York, Praeger Publishers, 1982.
186. Rizza CR, Mathews JM: Effect of frequent factor VIII replacement on the level of factor VIII antibodies in haemophiliacs. *Br J Haematol* **52**:13, 1982.
187. Sultan U, Maisonneuve D, Kazatchkine MD, Nydegger UE: Anti-idiotypic suppression of autoantibodies to factor VIII (antihaemophilic factor) by high dose intravenous gammaglobulin. *Lancet* **2**:765, 1984.
188. Kasper CK: Treatment of factor VIII inhibitors. *Progr Hemost Thromb* **9**:57, 1989.
189. Bloom AL: The treatment of factor VIII inhibitors, in Verstraete M, Vermylen J, Lijnene R, Arnout J (eds): *Thrombosis and Haemostasis 1987*. Leuven University Press, p. 447, 1987.
190. Fulcher CA, de Graaf S, Mahoney S, Zimmerman TS: FVIII inhibitor IgG subclass and FVIII polypeptide specificity determined by immunoblotting. *Blood* **69**:1475, 1987.
191. Alper CA, Raum DD, Awdeh ZL, Sahpiro SS, Yunis EJ: Major histocompatibility complex (MHC)-linked complement alleles as markers for the development of anti-factor VIII in hemophiliacs, in Hyouer L (ed): *Factor VIII Inhibitors*. New York, Alan R. Liss, p. 141, 1984.
192. Lippert LE, Fisher LM, Schook LB: Relationship of major histocompatibility complex class II genes to inhibitor antibody formation in hemophilia A. *Thromb Haemost* **64**:564, 1990.
193. Aly AM, Aledort LM, Lee TD, Hoyer LW: Histocompatibility antigen patterns in patients with factor VIII antibodies. *Br J Haematol* **76**:238, 1990.
194. Simmoney N, DeBosch N, Argueyo A, Garcia E. Layrise Z: HLA antigens in hemophiliacs A with or without factor VIII antibodies in a Venezuelan Mestizo population. *Tissue Antigens* **25**:216, 1985.
195. Millar DS, Steinbrecher RA, Wieland K, Grundy CB, Martinowitz U, Krawczak M, Zoll B, Whitmore D, Stephenson J, Mibashan RS, Kakkar VV, Cooper DN: The molecular genetic analysis of haemophilia A; characterization of six partial deletions in the factor VIII gene. *Hum Genetics* **86**:219, 1990.
196. Preston FE, Underwood JCE, Mitchell VE: Percutaneous liver biopsy and chronic liver disease in haemophiliacs. *Lancet* **2**:292, 1978.
197. Aledort LM, Levine PH, Hilgartner M, Blatt P, Spero JA, Goldberg JD, Bianchi L, Desmet V, Scheuer P, Popper H, Berk PD: A study of liver biopsies and liver disease among haemophiliacs. *Blood* **66**:367, 1985.
198. Triger DR, Preston FE: Chronic liver disease in haemophiliacs. *Br Med J* **74**:241, 1990. Annotation.
199. Lee CA, Phillips AN, Elford J, Janossy G, Griffiths P, Kernoff PBA: Progression of HIV disease in a haemophiliac cohort followed for 11 years and the effect of treatment. *Br Med J* **303**:1093, 1991.
200. Hoeben RC, Einerhand MPW, Briet E, Von Ormondt H, Valerio D, Vander Erb AJ: Towards gene therapy in haemophilia A: Retrovirus-mediated transfer of a factor VIII gene into murine haematopoietic progenitor cells. *Thromb Haemost* **67**:341, 1992.
201. Merskey C: The occurrence of haemophilia in the human female. *Q J Med* **3**:301, 1951.
202. Lusher JM, Zuelaer WW, Evans RK: Hemophilia A in chromosomal female subjects. *J Pediatr* **74**:265, 1969.
203. Morita H: The occurrence of homozygous hemophilia in the female. *Acta Haematol* **45**:112, 1971.
204. Panarello C, Acquila M, Caprino D, Gimelli G, Pecorara M, Mori PG: Concomitant Turner syndrome and hemophilia A in a female with an idic (X) (p11) heterozygous at locus DXS52. *Cytogenet Cell Genet* **59**:241, 1992.
205. Vidaud D, Vidaud M, Plassa F, Gazengel C, Noel B, Goossens M: Father-to-son transmission of hemophilia A due to uniparental disomy. *Am J Hum Genet* **45**:A226, 1989.
206. Soff GA, Lein J: Familial multiple coagulation factor deficiencies. *Semin Thromb Hemost* **7**:112, 1981.
207. Seligsohn V, Zivelin A, Zwang E: Decreased factor VIII clotting antigen levels in the combined factor V and VIII deficiency. *Thromb Res* **33**:95, 1983.
208. Giddings JC, Sugrue A, Bloom AL: Quantitation of coagulant antigens and inhibition of activated protein C in combined factor V and VIII deficiency. *Br J Haematol* **52**:495, 1982.
209. Tracy PB, Eide LL, Bowie EJW, Mann KG: Radioimmunoassay of factor V in human plasma and platelet. *Blood* **60**:59, 1982.
210. Marlar RA, Griffin JH: Deficiency of protein C inhibitor in combined factor V/VIII deficiency disease. *J Clin Invest* **66**:1186, 1980.
211. Canfield WM, Kisiel W: Evidence of normal functional levels of activated protein C inhibitor in combined factor V/VIII deficiency disease. *J Clin Invest* **70**:1260, 1982.
212. Gardiner JE, Griffin JH: Studies on human protein C inhibitor in normal and factor V/VIII deficient plasmas. *Thromb Res* **36**:197, 1984.
213. Suzuki K, Nishioka J, Hashimoto S, Kamiya T, Saito H: Normal titer of functional and immunoreactive protein C-inhibitor in plasma of patients with congenital combined deficiency of factor V and factor VIII. *Blood* **62**:1266, 1983.
214. Esmon CT: The subunit structure of thrombin-activated factor V. Isolation of activated factor V, separation of subunits, and reconstruction of biological activity. *J Biol Chem* **254**:964, 1979.
215. Nesheim ME, Mann K: Thrombin-catalyzed activation of single chain bovine factor V. *J Biol Chem* **254**:1326, 1979.
216. Nesheim ME, Myrmel KH, Hibbard L, Mann KG: Isolation and characterization of human coagulation factor V. *J Biol Chem* **254**:508, 1979.
217. Kane WH, Majerus PW: Purification and characterization of human coagulation factor V. *J Biol Chem* **256**:1002, 1981.
218. Katzman JA, Nesheim ME, Hibbard LS, Mann KG: Isolation of functional human coagulation factor V by using a hybridoma antibody. *Proc Natl Acad Sci USA* **78**:162, 1981.
219. Suzuki K, Dahlback B, Stenflo J: Thrombin-catalyzed activation of human coagulation factor V. *J Biol Chem* **257**:6556, 1982.
220. Hortin GL: Sulfation of tyrosine residues in coagulation factor V. *Blood* **76**:946, 1990.
221. Church WR, Jernigan RL, Toole J, Hewick RM, Knopf J, Knutson GJ, Nesheim ME, Mann KG, Fass DN: Coagulation factors V and VIII and ceruloplasmin constitute a family of structurally related proteins. *Proc Natl Acad Sci USA* **81**:6934, 1984.
222. Kane WH, Davie EW: Cloning of a cDNA coding for human factor V, a blood coagulation factor homologous to factor VIII and ceruloplasmin. *Proc Natl Acad Sci USA* **83**:6800, 1986.
223. Owren PA: Parahemophilia, hemorrhagic diathesis due to the absence of a previously unknown clotting factor. *Lancet* **1**:446, 1947.
224. Seeler RA: Parahemophilia factor V deficiency. *Med Clin North Am* **56**:119, 1972.
225. Tracy PB, Eide LL, Bowie EJW, Mann KG: Radioimmunoassay of factor V in human plasma. *Blood* **60**:59, 1982.
226. Lin S-W, Lin S-R, Shen M-C: Characterization of genetic defects of hemophilia A patients of Chinese origin. *Genomics* **18**:496, 1993.
227. Diamond D, Kogan S, Levinson B, Gitschier J: Amino acid substitutions in conserved domains of factor VIII and related proteins: Study of patients with mild and moderately severe hemophilia A. *Hum Mutation* **1**:248, 1992.
228. Chan V, Chan TK, Tong TMF, Todd D: A novel missense mutation in exon 4 of the factor VIII gene resulting in moderately severe hemophilia A. *Blood* **74**:2688, 1989.

229. Youssoufian H, Antonarakis SE, Bell W, Griffin AM, Kazazian HH Jr: Nonsense and missense mutations in hemophilia A: Estimate of the relative mutation rate at CpG dinucleotides. *Am J Hum Genet* **42**:718, 1988.
230. Kogan S, Gitschier J: Mutations and a polymorphism in the factor VIII gene discovered by denaturing gradient gel electrophoresis. *Proc Natl Acad Sci USA* **87**:2092, 1990.
231. Acquila M, Caprino D, Pecorara M, Baudo F, Morfini M, Mori PG: Two novel mutations at codon 373 of FVIII gene detected by DGGE. *Thromb Haemost* **69**:225, 1991.
232. Schwaab R, Ludwig M, Kochhan L, Oldenburg J, McVey JH, Egli H, Brackmann HH, Olek K: Detection and characterization of two missense mutations at a cleavage site in the factor VIII light chain. *Thromb Res* **6**:225, 1991.
233. Paynton C, Sarkar G, Sommer SS: Identification of mutations in two families with sporadic hemophilia A. *Hum Genet* **87**:397, 1991.
234. Economou EP, Kazazian HH, Antonarakis SE: Detection of mutations in the factor VIII gene using single stranded conformational analysis. *Genomics* **13**:909, 1992.
235. Levinson B, Lejesjoki AE, de la Chapelle A, Gitschier J: Molecular analysis of hemophilia A mutations in the Finnish population. *Am J Hum Genet* **46**:53, 1990.
236. Levinson B, Janco R, Phillips JA, Gitschier J: A novel missense mutation in the factor VIII gene identified by analysis of amplified hemophilia DNA sequences. *Nucleic Acids Res* **15**:9797, 1987.
237. Millar DS, Zoll B, Martinowitz U, Kakkar VV, Cooper DN: The molecular genetics of haemophilia A: Screening for point mutations in the factor VIII gene using the restriction enzyme *Taq*I. *Hum Genet* **87**:607, 1991.
238. Naylor JA, Green PM, Montandon JA, Rizza CR, Giannelli F: Detection of three novel mutations in two hemophilia A patients by rapid screening of whole essential region of factor VIII gene. *Lancet* **337**:635, 1991.
239. Krepelova A, Vorlava Z, Acquila M, Mori P: GAA (Glu) 272 to AAA (Lys) and CGA (Arg) 1941 to CAA (Gln) in the factor VIII gene in two haemophilia A patients of Czech origin. *Br J Haematol* **81**:458, 1992.
240. Antonarakis SE, Kazazian HH Jr, unpublished data.
241. Naylor J, Brinke A, Hassock S, Green PM, Giannelli F: Characteristic mRNA abnormality found in half the patients with severe haemophilia A is due to large DNA inversions. *Hum Molec Genet* **2**:1773, 1993.
242. Rossiter JP, Young M, Kimberland ML, Hutter P, Ketterling RP, Gitschier J, Horst J, Morris MA, Schaid DJ, de Moerloose P, Sommer SS, Kazazian HH, Jr., Antonarakis SE: Factor VIII gene inversions causing severe hemophilia A originate almost exclusively in male germ cells. *Hum Molec Genet*, in press.

CHAPTER 107

von Willebrand Disease

J. Evan Sadler

1. von Willebrand factor (vWF) is a complex multimeric glycoprotein that is found in plasma, in platelet α granules, and in subendothelial connective tissue. vWF performs two biologic functions required for normal hemostasis. It binds to specific receptors on the platelet surface and in subendothelial connective tissue to form a bridge between the platelet and areas of vascular damage, and it binds to and stabilizes blood coagulation factor VIII. This interaction between vWF and factor VIII is necessary for normal survival of factor VIII in the circulation. Deficiency of vWF results in defective platelet adhesion and also causes a secondary deficiency of factor VIII. Consequently, deficiency of vWF may cause bleeding that mimics either platelet dysfunction or hemophilia.

2. Inherited deficiency of vWF causes von Willebrand disease (vWD), the most common inherited bleeding disorder of human beings. By sensitive laboratory tests, asymptomatic inherited abnormalities of vWF function can be detected in approximately 8000 people per million. Clinically significant vWD affects approximately 125 people per million, a prevalence approximately twice that of hemophilia A.

3. vWD is a very heterogeneous disorder that has been classified into several major subtypes. The most common form (type 1) is transmitted as an autosomal dominant trait and appears to be due to simple quantitative deficiency of all vWF multimers. A clinically severe variant (type 3) is characterized by recessive inheritance and virtual absence of vWF. Variants that are characterized by a dysfunctional protein are classified as type 2. These usually exhibit a relative deficiency of the larger vWF multimers in plasma. Type 2 vWD is further subdivided according to whether the dysfunctional protein has decreased or paradoxically increased function in certain laboratory tests that reflect binding of vWF to platelets. Additional variants are characterized by other functional defects or by structural abnormalities that are detected on gel electrophoresis of the mutant vWF multimers.

4. Bleeding in severe vWD is treated with blood products containing factor VIII–vWF complex; these include certain factor VIII concentrates and plasma cryoprecipitate. Clinically milder variants can often be treated without exposure to blood products through pharmacologic manipulation of plasma vWF levels. For many patients with vWD, the intravenous or intranasal administration of the vasopressin analogue DDAVP causes a rise in plasma vWF that is sufficient to treat spontaneous and traumatic bleeding, or to sustain normal hemostasis during surgery.

5. Molecular defects have been characterized in many types of vWD. Nonsense mutations and gene deletions are causes of severe vWD (type 3). Gene deletions predispose to the development of alloantibody inhibitors to transfused vWF, a rare complication of therapy. Missense mutations have been characterized that cause specific gain of function and loss of function variants of type 2 vWD. Many polymorphisms have been described for the vWF gene, and these can be used in linkage analysis to augment biochemical testing for genetic counseling and prenatal diagnosis.

HISTORICAL ASPECTS

von Willebrand factor (vWF) and the corresponding inherited deficiency state take their name from Erik von Willebrand, who in 1926 described a bleeding disease that affected several branches of a large family from the Åland Islands in the Gulf of Bothnia, Finland.[1,2] In contrast to classic hemophilia, the mode of inheritance was autosomal dominant rather than X-linked, and the bleeding was usually from mucocutaneous sites rather than joints and deep tissues. The disorder was characterized by a prolonged bleeding time, with normal coagulation time, clot retraction, and platelet count. von Willebrand named the condition *hereditary pseudohemophilia*, distinguishing it from thrombocytopenic purpura and Glanzmann thrombasthenia.

The pathogenesis of von Willebrand disease (vWD) remained controversial for over 30 years. von Willebrand and subsequent investigators thought that the bleeding disorder was caused either by platelet dysfunction or by a lesion of the vasculature.[3,4] In 1953, several reports described patients with prolonged bleeding times who also had decreased plasma factor VIII activity, suggesting that an abnormality of the blood might be responsible for their apparent platelet or vascular dysfunction.[4–6] These patients were not immediately recognized to have vWD, but later studies showed that the original patients described by von Willebrand were indistinguishable and also had reduced factor VIII activity.[7,8]

The concept of a plasma deficiency was confirmed when the prolonged bleeding time and factor VIII deficiency in vWD were shown to be corrected by transfusion of a plasma factor VIII concentrate.[7,8] The same plasma fraction prepared from patients with severe hemophilia A was also effective,[9] indicating that the hemostatic defect in vWD could be corrected by a "von Willebrand factor" that was

A list of standard abbreviations is located immediately preceding the index in each volume. Additional abbreviations used in this chapter include: DDAVP = 1-desamino-8-D-arginine vasopressin; GPIb (GPIIb, GPIIIa) = platelet glycoprotein Ib (IIb, IIIa); GPIIb-IIIa = platelet glycoprotein IIb-IIIa complex; RIPA = ristocetin-induced platelet aggregation; RGD = Arg-Gly-Asp sequences; vWAg = von Willebrand antigen; vWD = von Willebrand disease; vWF = von Willebrand factor.

found in normal or hemophilia A plasma. This vWF clearly was not identical to factor VIII.

Despite this clinical evidence that vWF and factor VIII were different, recognition that they were distinct proteins was obscured by the fact that factor VIII is usually deficient in vWD. Furthermore, the transfusion of vWF into patients with vWD produces a sustained rise in plasma factor VIII levels that cannot be explained by the content of factor VIII transfused. Factor VIII may remain elevated for several days, and it decays with a half-life much longer than that of factor VIII in normal subjects.[9–12]

The relationship between factor VIII and vWF was further confused because early partial purifications of factor VIII activity yielded a protein that by immunochemical assays was clearly deficient in vWD plasma, but was present in normal antigenic amounts in hemophilia A plasma.[13–17] Conversely, the autoantiserums to factor VIII that developed in some patients with hemophilia A did not recognize this "factor VIII–related antigen."[18–20] To reconcile these data, some investigators proposed that vWF was a protein specified by an autosomal gene that served as a precursor to factor VIII, which was produced when a protein specified by an X-linked gene acted on vWF.[21–23] These observations gave rise to one of the most persistent confusions in the study of hemostasis, in which the term *factor VIII* referred either to (antihemophilic) factor VIII or to vWF, depending on the context.

The first evidence that vWF was specifically required for platelet adhesion in vivo was obtained in 1960 by Borchgrevink, who found that patients with vWD had higher platelet counts in blood from capillary lesions than did normal controls.[24] Subsequently, decreased platelet adhesion in vitro was demonstrated by the perfusion of blood from patients with vWD through a column of glass beads.[25,26] Transfusion of either normal plasma, hemophilia A plasma, or factor VIII concentrate was shown to correct both the bleeding time and the in vitro platelet adhesion defect in vWD.[7,8,25,27] This glass bead retention assay was used for the first documented purification of vWF.[15]

A more convenient assay for human vWF was developed in 1971 by Howard and Firkin, who discovered that the antibiotic ristocetin induced platelet aggregation in normal platelet-rich plasma but not in plasma from patients with vWD.[28] The defect was corrected by normal plasma, hemophilia A plasma, or partially purified vWF. A similar defect could be induced in normal plasma by heteroantiserums to vWF.

Factor VIII was known to behave as a very large macromolecule that could apparently be dissociated into a smaller active species by buffers of high ionic strength.[29] This salt-induced transition was shown to resolve factor VIII from the ristocetin-dependent platelet aggregating activity of vWF, which did not decrease in apparent size.[30] Bovine plasma aggregates human platelets in the absence of ristocetin, and similar experiments demonstrated that bovine platelet aggregating activity, or vWF, could also be resolved from factor VIII.[31]

Conclusive proof that factor VIII and vWF were independent proteins was subsequently obtained by protein sequencing and cDNA cloning, as discussed below for vWF and in Chap. 106 for factor VIII. Together, these methods demonstrated that the two proteins have unique primary sequences that are encoded by distinct genes. Furthermore, the product of each gene has the appropriate biologic activity in the absence of the other.

At one time, vWD was thought to be a single entity that was characterized in part by deficiency of both vWF activity and the corresponding protein antigen. In 1972 Holmberg and Nilsson showed that a subgroup of patients with vWD have a normal plasma concentration of vWF antigen.[32] By crossed immunoelectrophoresis, the vWF antigen in these patients was shown to have excessively rapid mobility, consistent with a structural abnormality.[33,34] Subsequent studies have revealed still more evidence of phenotypic heterogeneity in vWD.

BIOCHEMISTRY OF VON WILLEBRAND FACTOR

Knowledge of the biochemistry of vWF provides a necessary framework for organizing and understanding the pathogenesis of the many variants of vWD. vWF has a particularly complex structure that requires a correspondingly complicated biosynthesis. Accordingly, vWF deficiency could result from defects in biosynthetic processing or from the structural alteration of specific functional domains.

Biosynthesis and Localization of von Willebrand Factor

vWF is synthesized by endothelial cells,[35,36] megakaryocytes,[37,38] and perhaps by the syncytiotrophoblast of placenta.[39] The structure of vWF was determined by a combination of protein chemistry methods and cDNA cloning. The ~9-kb mRNA for vWF encodes a primary translation product of 2813 amino acids (Fig. 107-1) that includes a conventional signal peptide of 22 residues, an unusually large propeptide of 741 residues or ~100 kDa, and the mature subunit of 2050 residues or ~270 kDa.[40–47] The pro-vWF contains four distinct

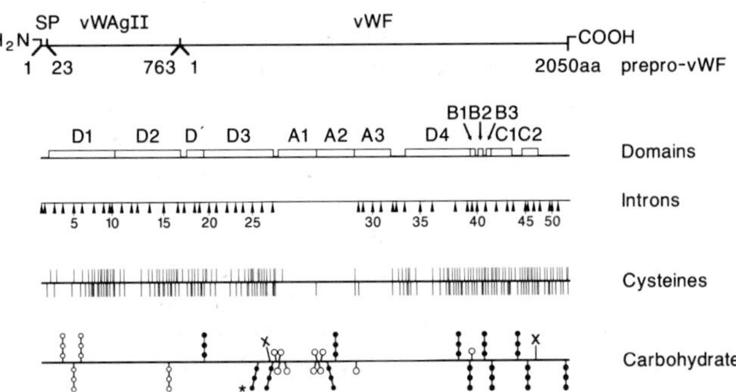

FIG. 107-1 Structural features of the human vWF precursor. Prepro-vWF: The schematic structure of the primary translation product employs separate amino acid (aa) numbering systems for the prepro-peptide (aa 1 to 763) and the mature vWF subunit (aa 1 to 2050). The signal peptide or prepeptide consists of aa 1 to 22, the von Willebrand antigen II (vWAgII) propeptide consists of aa 23 to 763. Domains: The repeated domains are labeled A to D. Introns: The locations within the amino acid sequence of the 51 vWF introns are indicated by arrowheads, and every fifth intron is numbered. Cysteines: The sites of cysteine residues are indicated by vertical marks. In regions with a very high density of cysteine residues one mark may represent several cysteines. Carbohydrate: The sites of potential *N*-linked glycosylation sites are indicated by the open symbols, ○—○—○. The filled symbols, ●—●—●, indicate sites shown to be glycosylated by protein sequencing. The asterisk (*) marks a glycosylated asparagine residue in the unusual sequence Asn-Ser-Cys. The symbol *X* indicates potential *N*-linked glycosylation sites that are not glycosylated in mature vWF. The large open circles (◯) mark sites of *O*-linked glycosylation. (*From Sadler JE.*[291] *Reprinted by permission.*)

types of repeated domains that together make up over 90 percent of the sequence. The A domains contain from 193 to 200 amino acids and are found in three imperfect tandem copies. The triplicated B domains contain 25 to 35 residues, and the duplicated C domains contain 116 to 119 residues. Finally, the D domains contain 351 to 376 residues and are present in four copies. There is also a small D′ fragment that represents the C-terminal fourth of a complete D domain. The propeptide cleavage site lies between the second D domain and the D′ fragment that occurs at the N-terminal end of the third complete D domain.

vWF contains a remarkable amount of cysteine. In fact, cysteine is the most abundant amino acid in the protein, comprising 234 of the total 2813 residues (8.3 percent). The cysteines are clustered at the N-terminal and C-terminal ends of the sequence, and the triplicated A domains correspond to a cysteine-poor region in the middle of the protein.

Shortly after removal of the signal peptide, the ~370 kDa pro-vWF dimerizes by disulfide bond formation between the C-terminal ends of the subunits (Fig. 107-2) to yield the basic repeating unit of vWF.[48–52] The dimers undergo further polymerization by forming disulfide bonds between the N-terminal ends of subunits to yield a series of oligomers. This polymerization appears to occur at about the same time that the pro-vWF dimers arrive in the Golgi apparatus, and is associated with removal of the propeptide from all but ~1 percent of the subunits.[51] The oligomers in plasma range in size from ~500 kDa dimers to species of over 10 million daltons and 20 subunits.[53–56] Subunits that retain the propeptide are found in all of the multimers.[51]

The propeptide of vWF is identical to von Willebrand antigen II (vWAgII),[57] a ~100 kDa protein found in blood plasma and platelet α granules.[58,59] The free vWAgII propeptide spontaneously forms noncovalent dimers.[60] Many deletions or insertions within the propeptide lead to the formation of vWF dimers but not higher multimers,[61–63] although missense mutations that abolish propeptide cleavage are compatible with normal multimer assembly.[62,64] These observations suggest that the propeptide may be needed for vWF multimer assembly; whether it has an independent biologic function is not known.

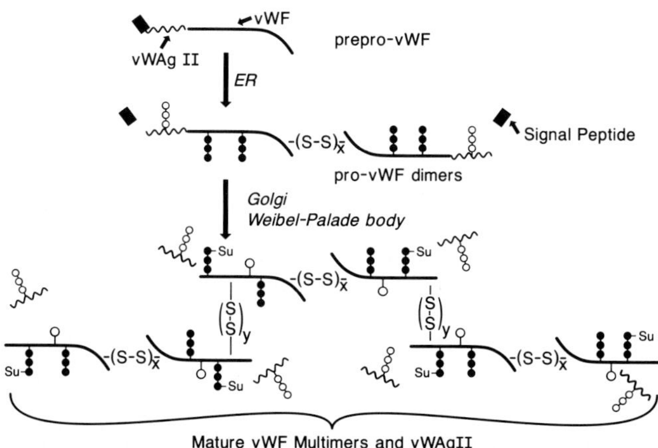

FIG. 107-2 Biosynthesis of vWF. The primary translation product of the mRNA for vWF is translocated into the lumen of the rough endoplasmic reticulum (ER), where the signal peptide is removed and *N*-linked glycosylation begins. The resultant pro-vWF rapidly dimerizes by the formation of a number (*x*) of disulfide bonds in the C-terminal region of the protein sequence. Pro-vWF dimers are transported to the Golgi apparatus and then to Weibel-Palade bodies. In one or both of these locations, *O*-linked and *N*-linked glycosylation is completed, inorganic sulfate (Su) is incorporated into some *N*-linked oligosaccharides, the vWAgII propeptide is cleaved from almost all the subunits, and multimers are created by the formation of a number (*y*) of intersubunit disulfide bonds near the N-terminal end of the subunits. The symbols for *N*-linked and *O*-linked oligosaccharides are as in Fig. 107-1.

In addition to proteolytic processing and disulfide bond formation, vWF is subject to several other posttranslational modifications that may affect its function. There are a total of 17 potential *N*-linked glycosylation sites in prepro-vWF with the sequence Asn-X-Thr/Ser (see Fig. 107-1). Plasma vWF contains ~19 percent carbohydrate by weight,[65] distributed among 12 asparagine-linked and 10 serine/threonine-linked oligosaccharides.[46] All but two of the 13 potential *N*-linked sites in the mature subunit are glycosylated, and one glycosylated asparagine residue occurs in the unusual sequence Asn-Ser-Cys. Additional carbohydrate may be attached to the vWAgII propeptide. The antibiotic tunicamycin inhibits the asparagine-linked glycosylation of nascent vWF. The resultant carbohydrate-deficient pro-vWF monomers do not dimerize and the propeptide is not removed, suggesting that this glycosylation is required for the normal assembly of vWF structure.[66] Also, cultured endothelial cells incorporate sulfate into some *N*-linked oligosaccharides of vWF (see Fig. 107-2). Sulfate has been found in both the 270 kDa and 370 kDa subunits of all vWF multimers except the intracellular pro-vWF dimer.[67]

Mature vWF and vWAgII are both stored in endothelial cells in a unique organelle, the Weibel-Palade body.[68] These are 0.1 × 2- to 0.1 × 3-μm vesicles containing regularly spaced longitudinal tubular structures[69] that may represent closely packed vWF molecules. Whether they participate in the assembly of vWF multimers or are simply storage organelles is not known. vWF is also found at the periphery of the α granules of platelets in tubular structures that resemble those of Weibel-Palade bodies,[70] as well as in subendothelial connective tissue[71,72] and the syncytiotrophoblast of placenta.[39] vWF isolated from plasma, endothelial cells, subendothelium, and platelets displays similar multimeric structure, although the multimers and associated minor "satellite" bands of plasma and platelet vWF appear to have slightly different mobilities in high-resolution gel electrophoresis systems.[73]

Metabolism

The plasma concentration of vWF is ~10 μg/ml, with a wide range of normal concentration from 40 to 200 percent of the mean.[74] Some of this variability may be due to an effect of blood type. Both vWF antigen levels[75,76] and ristocetin-cofactor activity[77] are lower in individuals with blood type O. Plasma vWF levels appear to increase slightly with increasing age.[76,77] Approximately 15 percent of circulating vWF is found in platelets.[78]

The plasma concentration of vWF increases in response to many physiological stimuli, including adrenergic stress, vasopressin, growth hormone, and estrogens (reviewed in Bloom[79]). Adrenergic agents and vasopressin act through independent pathways. The effect of adrenergic agonists is blocked by propranolol and is probably mediated by β-adrenergic receptors. Propranolol has no effect on the response to the vasopressin analogue, 1-desamino-8-D-arginine vasopressin (DDAVP). Neither epinephrine nor vasopressin stimulate the secretion of vWF by cultured vascular endothelial cells.[80,81] In vivo, DDAVP may indirectly induce the secretion of vWF stored in Weibel-Palade bodies.

Estrogen stimulates vWF synthesis in cultured endothelial

cells.[82] This in vitro response may explain the elevated vWF levels that occur during pregnancy and long-term estrogen therapy (reviewed in Bloom[79]).

Certain products of blood coagulation act directly on endothelial cells to stimulate the secretion of vWF. Human α thrombin induces the rapid release of vWF that appears to be complete after 10 min of exposure to thrombin and does not require continued protein synthesis.[83,84] Release requires the presence of extracellular calcium, is associated with depletion of the Weibel-Palade bodies,[84] and requires the thrombin active site.[83] Fibrin also induces the release of vWF, and this effect is not duplicated by fibrinogen, fibrinopeptides A and B, factor XIII, or tissue plasminogen activator. Fibrin prepared by clotting with reptilase is not effective, indicating that a specific fibrin structure is required.[85] Thus, products of thrombosis may have localized effects on the adjacent vascular endothelium to recruit additional vWF to the clot environment. In addition, the vWF secreted by endothelial cells in response to such stimuli appears to contain especially large and biologically potent vWF multimers.[86]

The metabolic fate of vWF is not known in much detail. Clearance from the circulation of ^{125}I-labeled vWF occurs in two phases. In both normal persons and patients with hemophilia A, an initial rapid phase with a half-life of 4.5 h is followed by a slower phase with a half-life of 20 h. The larger multimers seem to be cleared more rapidly than small multimers.[11] The catabolism of vWF probably involves proteolysis within the circulation. Specific proteolytic fragments of the basic subunit are present in plasma vWF.[65,87] These fragments are reduced or absent in the larger vWF multimers that are released into the circulation by the administration of DDAVP, and with time both the multimer pattern and subunit fragmentation pattern return to those present before DDAVP.[88] This proteolysis may contribute to the relatively rapid disappearance of larger multimers from the circulation, whether transfused or endogenous.

Biologic Activities and Structure–Function Relationships of von Willebrand Factor

vWF has two well-characterized biologic functions. It is necessary for the adhesion of platelets to regions of vascular damage, and it is necessary for the normal survival of factor VIII in circulation. These functions have been dissected in vitro into several distinct binding interactions that are dependent on specific domains of the protein sequence as well as higher orders of structure that include organization into multimers (Table 107-1). Abnormalities in any of these interactions might contribute to the phenotype of von Willebrand disease.

Table 107-1 Binding Activities of von Willebrand Factor

Ligand	Biologic Function
Collagens	May mediate platelet adhesion to subendothelium
Other connective-tissue elements	May mediate platelet adhesion to subendothelium
Platelet glycoprotein Ib	Required for platelet adhesion to subendothelium
Platelet glycoprotein IIb-IIIa	May mediate platelet adhesion to subendothelium and vWF-dependent platelet aggregation
Factor VIII	Stabilizes factor VIII in the circulation
Heparin	Unknown
Sulfated glycolipids	Unknown

NOTE: References can be found in the text.

Role of von Willebrand Factor in Platelet Adhesion to Subendothelial Connective Tissue. Several in vitro perfusion systems have been described for the study or vWF function in promoting platelet adhesion to damaged blood vessels and connective-tissue constituents. When whole blood is perfused over everted blood vessel segments, platelets adhere to the surface if the endothelium has been removed.[89] Platelet adherence to the subendothelium is decreased in blood from patients with vWD,[90–92] but can be corrected by the addition of purified vWF.[92,93] Conversely, platelet adherence using blood from patients from hemophilia A is normal,[91,92] and that observed with normal blood is inhibited by antibodies to vWF.[94,95] This dependence on vWF is seen only at the high wall shear rates that may occur in the microcirculation.[91,94] The platelet adhesion observed at low shear rates is not increased by vWF and may depend on other proteins in the blood or subendothelium.

There are three principal sites of vWF localization that might contribute to vWF-dependent platelet adhesion: plasma, platelet α granule, and subendothelial connective tissue. The importance of plasma vWF for platelet adhesion is readily demonstrated in the perfusion systems just discussed and is evident from the successful treatment of bleeding in vWD by transfusion of vWF. An independent contribution by the vWF already localized in the subendothelium is strongly supported by perfusion studies using rabbit[96] and human[97] vessel segments. The activation of platelets induces the release of additional vWF from platelet α granules that could augment vWF-dependent processes. Platelet vWF has been shown to promote adhesion to collagen in perfusates that lack vWF[98] and to correlate inversely with the bleeding time in some patients with vWD type 1.[99] The relative role of vWF in these three pools in normal hemostasis is difficult to assess, but all of them may participate in vWF-mediated platelet adhesion in vivo.

Binding of von Willebrand Factor to Subendothelial Connective Tissue. The substances in subendothelial connective tissue that support vWF-dependent platelet adhesion have not been completely characterized, and more than one may be important. Among connective-tissue constituents, vWF binds to fibrillar collagens, collagen type VI (a nonfibrillar collagen), and heparin; furthermore, vWF mediates platelet adhesion to native collagen types I and III[100,101] but not to denatured collagens.[102–104] vWF binds to extracellular matrix that is depleted of fibrillar collagens with collagenase or α,α′-dipyridyl.[105] Also, a monoclonal anti-vWF antibody that inhibits vWF binding to collagen types I and III does not inhibit binding to extracellular matrix; conversely, another monoclonal antibody that inhibits vWF binding to extracellular matrix does not inhibit binding to the same collagens.[106] These results suggest that interaction of vWF with fibrillar collagens might not be required for platelet adhesion. Collagen type VI consists mostly of large noncollagenous domains (reviewed in Colombatti and Bonaldo[107]) and binds vWF.[108] Since this collagen is abundant in subendothelium[108] and is resistant to both collagenase[109] and α,α′-dipyridyl,[110] collagen type VI may be a physiologically significant vWF binding site in the subendothelium.

The vWF propeptide also has at least one binding site for collagen.[111] The physiological significance of this interaction is not known.

Interaction of von Willebrand Factor with Specific Platelet Receptors. Two distinct receptors for vWF have been identified in the platelet plasma membrane. Platelet glycoprotein Ib (GPIb) appears to be the principal receptor responsible for vWF-dependent platelet adhesion to vascular subendothelium. Patients afflicted with Bernard-Soulier disease, which is characterized by deficiency of platelet membrane glycoprotein Ib,[112, 113] have a severe bleeding disorder associated with defective vWF-dependent platelet adhesion to subendothelium in vitro (see Chap. 110).[91, 114] This phenomenon is mimicked by treatment of normal platelets with antibodies to GPIb.[115] This same receptor also mediates the ristocetin-dependent platelet-aggregating activity of vWF.[116, 117] This interaction does not require platelet activation and can be demonstrated with formalin-fixed normal platelets.[118, 119] Ristocetin-induced binding of vWF to platelets is deficient in Bernard-Soulier disease,[120] and binding to normal platelets is inhibited by monoclonal antibodies to GPIb.[121, 122]

A second receptor for vWF is present on activated platelets. The platelet glycoprotein IIb-IIIa complex (GPIIb-IIIa) does not bind vWF in resting platelets. On activation with thrombin or other agonists, GPIIb-IIIa acquires the ability to bind several plasma proteins, including fibrinogen,[123–125] fibronectin,[126] and vWF.[127] These proteins appear to interact competitively with a common site on GPIIb-IIIa.[128] This may reflect the presence of similar short Arg-Gly-Asp-containing recognition sequences in all three proteins. Additional sequences may contribute to the binding of certain of these proteins to GPIIb-IIIa, particularly the C-terminal 12 amino acids of the γ chain of fibrinogen.[129] Binding of vWF to normal activated platelets is inhibited by antibodies to GPIIb-IIIa,[122] and does not occur at all in Glanzmann thrombasthenia, which is characterized by deficiency of GPIIb-IIIa (see Chap. 110).[130] The binding of vWF to GIIb-IIIa requires calcium ions,[127] in contrast to the ristocetin-induced binding of vWF to GPIb, which is calcium-independent.[131]

The physiological importance of the interaction between vWF and GPIIb-IIIa is not certain. Concentrations of fibrinogen found in plasma are sufficient to prevent the binding of soluble vWF to activated platelets,[132–134] and this suggests that vWF binding to GPIIb-IIIa should not occur, except perhaps in patients with afibrinogenemia.[135] However, vWF immobilized in the vessel wall may bind with higher affinity to activated platelets than does soluble vWF. Resting platelets do not adhere to surfaces coated wtih vWF, but thrombin-activated platelets bind avidly to such surfaces. This interaction with surface-bound vWF is not inhibited by physiological concentrations of fibrinogen.[136] Furthermore, adhesion of platelets to collagen is inhibited either by antibodies[137] or by synthetic peptides[138] that prevent binding of vWF to GPIIb-IIIa, so that this interaction might be significant in vivo.

The GPIb and GPIIb-IIIa sites may interact during vWF-mediated platelet adhesion. Human vWF treated with neuraminidase (asialo-vWF) will bind to normal platelets in the absence of ristocetin.[139–141] This binding is inhibited by antibodies to GPIb, so that asialo-vWF appears to bind to the same site as does the native vWF in the presence of ristocetin.[142] The binding of asialo-vWF to platelets initiates platelet activation, causes platelet granule release and stimulates the subsequent binding of fibrinogen to GPIIb-IIIa to cause platelet aggregation.[142, 143] Similar platelet activation responses are elicited by native vWF in the presence of ristocetin.[144] Thus, vWF bound to GPIb appears to act as a platelet agonist and can induce platelet aggregation through a pathway dependent on GPIIb-IIIa.

Stabilization of Factor VIII by von Willebrand Factor. Factor VIII is noncovalently bound to vWF in the blood, and the two proteins can be resolved by chromatography in buffers of high ionic strength.[29, 30] Activation of factor VIII by thrombin also appears to cause dissociation from vWF.[145] The vWF binding site is on the light chain of factor VIII.[146] Factor VIII is a minor constituent of this factor VIII–vWF complex, comprising only ~1 percent of the mass of circulating vWF. This interaction is necessary for the normal survival of factor VIII in the circulation. Pure factor VIII transfused into patients with hemophilia A or normal volunteers disappears from the circulation with a half-life of about 12 h, and this is similar to the half-life of the factor VIII–vWF complex.[11, 12] In contrast, pure factor VIII transfused into patients with severe vWD has a half-life of only ~2.4 h.[12] As discussed under "Historical Aspects," above, the transfusion of vWF in severe vWD produces a rise in plasma factor VIII that may persist for several days, while the bleeding time and ristocetin cofactor activity are corrected only for several hours.[9, 10, 12] This response to transfusion appears to be adequately explained by a model in which endogenously synthesized factor VIII binds to and is stabilized by the infused vWF. The larger multimers that can correct the bleeding time and ristocetin cofactor levels are more rapidly metabolized,[11] and the remaining smaller multimers continue to protect factor VIII. Thus, severe deficiency of vWF causes a secondary deficiency of factor VIII. Defective interaction between vWF and factor VIII would give rise to a phenotype of apparent autosomal dominant hemophilia A with normal vWF function; as described below, several such patients have been reported.

Other Binding Activities of von Willebrand Factor. Additional binding activities of vWF have been described that have no physiological function known at this time. vWF binds to immobilized heparin,[147] and this interaction was used for the purification of vWF by affinity chromatography on heparin agarose.[148] It is possible that binding to heparin-like glycosaminoglycans contributes to the interaction of vWF with the vascular subendothelium. vWF also binds specifically and with high affinity to certain sulfated glycolipids. This interaction is inhibited only weakly by heparin and may be mediated by an independent binding site.[149, 150] Whether appropriate sulfated glycolipids are accessible to vWF in vivo is not known.

Structure–Function Relationships of von Willebrand Factor. The multimeric structure of vWF is important for its function in promoting platelet adhesion. The larger multimers in plasma adhere selectively to resting platelets in the presence of risotocetin[151] and to collagen,[152] while the small multimers do not. The large multimers in cryoprecipitate support platelet adhesion to subendothelium in perfusion systems, while the small multimers found in cryosupernatant do not.[153] Accordingly, some degree of polymerization may be necessary for optimal vWF function. The apparent relationship between multimer size and function has been invoked to explain the functional defect in subtypes of von Willebrand disease that are characterized by a lack of large multimers. This correlation may instead reflect the greater proportion of degraded subunits in naturally occurring small multimers.[65, 87] If small multimers are made in vitro by partial reduction of large multimers, they retain the ability to support platelet adhesion to subendothelium in perfusion assays, although ristocetin-dependent platelet aggregation is reduced.[153] Thus, the relationship between multimer structure, ristocetin cofactor activity, and hemostatic function of vWF remains poorly understood.

Binding sites for several ligands have been localized to specific segments of the vWF subunit (Fig. 107-3). The site of interaction with platelet glycoprotein Ib has been placed within a 48- to 52-kDa tryptic peptide that contains amino acid residues 448 to 729 of the mature subunit and correlates with repeated domain A1.[154] This same fragment also contains binding sites for collagen[155] and heparin.[156] A second collagen-binding site appears to lie within domain A3.[157] A second heparin-binding site has been reported in the first ~300 amino acids of the mature subunit overlapping with domains D′ and part of D3, although specificity and affinity for heparin were not determined.[158] This same region contains a binding site for factor VIII.[159] The tetrapeptide sequence, Arg-Gly-Asp-Ser, occurs near the C-terminus of domain C1[40] and appears to mediate the binding of vWF to the platelet glycoprotein IIb-IIIa complex of activated platelets.[160–162] Several other adhesive glycoproteins appear to interact with receptors through sites that contain Arg-Gly-Asp sequences (also known as RGD sequences in single letter code), including fibronectin, vitronectin, and fibrinogen (reviewed in Ruoslahti and Pierschbacher[163]). None of these proteins are known to be homologous, and the presence of similar functional binding sites may represent convergent evolution. A second Arg-Gly-Asp sequence occurs in the vWF propeptide[47]; whether it has any function is not known.

The glycosidically bound oligosaccharides of vWF have nonspecific but nevertheless essential functions. The sialic acid and galactose residues appear to protect the native protein from degradation by proteases.[164] The sialic acid residues are necessary to prevent clearance of vWF from the circulation by the liver.[165] They also prevent spontaneous interaction of vWF with platelet GPIb in the absence of ristocetin, as discussed above under "Interaction of von Willebrand Factor with Specific Platelet Receptors."

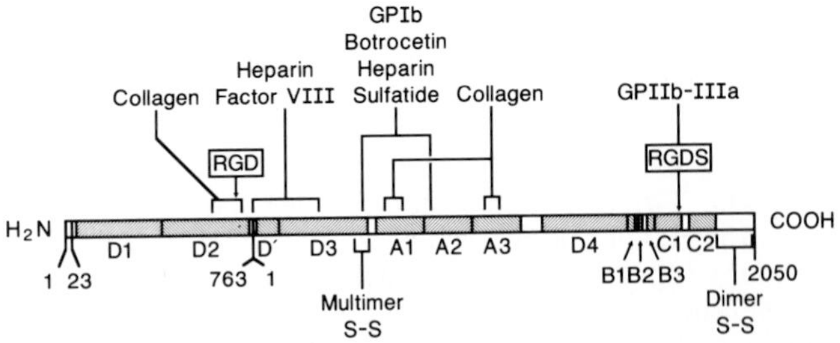

FIG. 107-3 **Structure–function relationships of vWF. The repeated domains are shaded and labeled, and the positions of the signal peptide, vWAgII propeptide, and mature subunit sequences are indicated. The locations of intersubunit disulfide bonds, Arg-Gly-Asp (RGD) sequences, and of various binding sites are shown.** *(From Sadler.[291] Reprinted by permission.)*

MOLECULAR BIOLOGY OF VON WILLEBRAND FACTOR

Chromosome Localization and Structure of the von Willebrand Factor Gene and Pseudogene

The gene for vWF is located near the tip of the short arm of human chromosome 12.[42,43] It spans ~180 kb of DNA and consists of 52 exons.[166–168] There is a rough correlation between the placement of certain intron–exon boundaries and the repeated domains defined by examination of the protein sequence, which lends support to the hypothesis that these domains evolved by gene segment duplication.[166,168]

The vWF locus has been ordered with other loci into a continuous genetic map of chromosome 12 and is the most teleomeric marker yet available on chromosome 12p. vWF lies within a region for which recombination is more frequent in males than in females, in contrast to the rest of chromosome 12 for which recombination is more frequent in females.[169]

A partial, unprocessed vWF pseudogene is located on chromosome 22q11-13.[170,171] The vWF pseudogene spans ~21 to 29 kb of DNA and corresponds to exons 23 through 34 of the vWF gene. These exons encode mainly the triplicated A domains of vWF. The vWF gene and pseudogene have diverged only ~3.1 percent in nucleotide sequence; this is consistent with a relatively recent origin of the pseudogene, perhaps less than 20 to 30 million years ago.[171]

Evolution of von Willebrand Factor and Possible Homology to Other Proteins

The highly repeated structure of vWF indicates that the vWF gene has a complex evolutionary history, including several gene segment duplications. Comparison of the vWF amino acid sequence to other protein sequences further indicates that vWF shares domains with a variety of proteins that otherwise do not appear to be homologous; thus, vWF also is a mosaic protein that has evolved in part by exon shuffling. Homologues of the vWF A domains are present in proteins from at least five other protein "superfamilies" (reviewed in Colombatti and Bonaldo[107]): (1) the complement protease zymogens factor B and component C2; (2) the α-subunits of a subset of heterodimeric cell-surface integrins, the leukocyte adhesion molecules (Mac-1, LFA-1, and p150,95) and collagen receptors (α1β1 and α2β2); (3) cartilage matrix protein; (4) unusual collagens with large noncollagenous domains, including homotrimeric collagen type XII[172] and all three chains of collagen type VI; and (5) undulin, a member of the fibronectin-tenascin family of extracellular matrix proteins.[173] Several of these proteins bind collagen, including the collagen receptor integrins, cartilage matrix protein, and undulin. Because at least two of the vWF A domains appear to bind collagen, the presence of A domains in these other proteins may contribute to their collagen-binding activity.

Portions of the C domains of vWF have some sequence similarity to cysteine-rich segments of thrombospondin,[174] α_1-procollagen types I[175] and III,[176,177] and a *Xenopus laevis* mucin.[178] Most of this sequence similarity is due to the apparent alignment of numerous cysteine residues. The functional significance of these potential homologies is not known.

CLINICAL ASPECTS OF VON WILLEBRAND DISEASE

Diagnosis

von Willebrand disease should be suspected in any patient with mucocutaneous bleeding despite a normal platelet count.

The symptoms may be highly variable with time in a single patient, and all affected members of a given pedigree may not have the same difficulty with bleeding.[74,179–181] Even for severely affected patients with symptoms since birth and a clear family history, the pattern of bleeding is not specific for von Willebrand disease. Thus, final diagnosis depends on laboratory testing and may require repeated examinations of patients and family members.

Detailed reviews of the laboratory assessment of vWD can be found elsewhere.[182,183] Tests commonly applied to the diagnosis of vWD fall into four general categories: (1) *The template bleeding time.* This test assesses the formation of the platelet plug in vivo by determining the time required to stop bleeding from a standard skin laceration. It is difficult to standardize, and consistent results depend strongly on the skill of the tester. A prolonged bleeding time is not at all specific for vWD because connective-tissue and platelet disorders may also exhibit this abnormality. It is a sensitive test, since the bleeding time is prolonged at some time in essentially all patients with symptomatic vWD. Patients with mild vWD may have intermittently normal bleeding times.[74] (2) *Platelet aggregation stimulated by the antibiotic ristocetin.* This test measures vWF binding to platelet glycoprotein Ib. Two variations are used. One (ristocetin-induced platelet aggregation, or RIPA) employs patient platelets suspended in autologous plasma. The second (ristocetin cofactor activity) employs patient plasma with washed and fixed allogeneic platelets. In each assay, platelet aggregation as a function of ristoctein concentration is compared with that of normal controls, and the concentration required to achieve a specific degree or rate of aggregation is noted. The snake venom factor botrocetin has effects similar but not identical to those of ristocetin and can also be used to measure the ability of vWF to bind to resting platelets.[184,185] (3) *Measurement of factor VIII antigen or activity in patient plasma.* Factor VIII binds to plasma vWF, so factor VIII levels usually reflect vWF antigen concentration. Comparison of ristocetin cofactor activity with factor VIII level provides an estimate of the specific activity of the residual vWF protein in patient plasma. This ratio of ristocetin cofactor activity to factor VIII level is expected to be normal for quantitative deficiencies of vWF and reduced for variants of vWD with a qualitatively abnormal protein. (4) *Physical characterization of patient vWF.* Gel electrophoresis and immunochemical assays measure vWF concentration and also multimer distribution. This category of assays includes the quantitative immunoassay of vWF antigen and the qualitative assessment of multimer distribution by counter-immunoelectrophoresis. More precise assessment of multimer distribution is obtained by electrophoresis of plasma on agarose or agarose/acrylamide copolymer gels in the presence of sodium dodecyl sulfate (Fig. 107-4). In such systems, the vWF multimers are separated according to size and can be visualized by reaction with ^{125}I-labeled antihuman vWF antibody and autoradiography[55,56] or by immunoenzymatic methods.

Comparison of platelet and plasma vWF with these assays may be useful in the further characterization of specific variants of vWD.[186,187] In addition, the time course of response of plasma factor VIII, vWF antigen, ristocetin cofactor activity, and vWF multimer structure to a trial infusion of the vasopressin analogue DDAVP can distinguish still more phenotypic heterogeneity.[187–189] Assays of vWF binding to collagen, heparin, or factor VIII have also been described, but have not been applied widely. Finally, the detailed investigation of family members to show inheritance of vWD is useful so that acquired conditions that may mimic vWD may be firmly excluded.

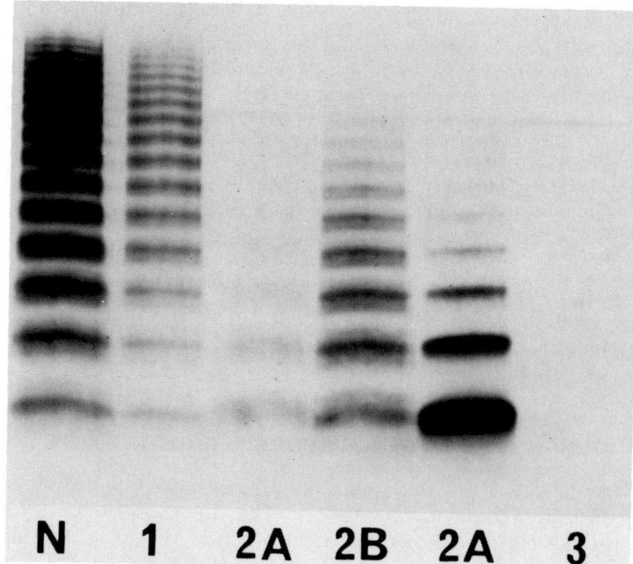

FIG. 107-4 Multimer patterns in variants of von Willebrand disease. Plasma vWF multimers in type 1 vWD have mobility similar to those from normal controls (N). Larger multimers are missing in vWD type 2A (lanes 3 and 5) and type 2B (lane 4). Some type 2A variants exhibit a characteristic absence of so-called satellite bands that usually bracket the intense central multimer species (lane 5). No multimers are visualized in vWD type 3 (lane 6). (*Adapted from Sadler,*[292] *by permission.*)

Prevalence

von Willebrand disease appears to be the most common inherited bleeding disorder of human beings, but the prevalence is difficult to determine precisely because of substantial variation in the severity of disease. If all cases that come to the attention of specialized referral centers are included, the prevalence of symptomatic vWD is approximately 125 per million.[191] However, the screening of an unselected population of school children in Italy has suggested that the prevalence of inherited vWF abnormalities is much higher and closer to ~8000 per million.[77] Severe vWD with essentially no detectable circulating vWF antigen is quite rare and affects 0.5 to 3 per million in western Europe and Scandinavia,[191] and perhaps as many as 5.3 per million among selected Arab populations in the Middle East.[192]

The genetics of vWD illustrate some of the problems in the use of the terms *dominant* and *recessive* to describe human phenotypes (see Chap. 1). In many families, heterozygosity is consistently associated with obvious phenotypic effects, and the dominant description is satisfactory. In other instances, heterozygosity is relatively or totally asymptomatic and may be associated with subtle laboratory abnormalities, thus blurring the separation between dominant and recessive phenotypes. In addition, it is likely that the genotype at other loci and nongenetic factors influence the phenotype, particularly in individuals heterozygous for vWD. Recognizing these limitations, it is still useful to separate phenotypes generally as dominant or recessive disorders.

In most pedigrees, vWD is transmitted as an autosomal dominant trait. By contrast, many patients with severe vWD who appear to be homozygotes or compound heterozygotes for a mutant allele at the vWF locus are born to clinically normal parents. Sensitive testing may disclose mild functional abnormalities in such parents who are obligate heterozygotes, but these families are usually considered to be affected by a recessive disease. Selected pedigrees may exhibit both dominant and recessive patterns of inheritance.[180,181] This variability suggests that some interplay between specific mutant alleles and the genetic background of the host determines whether clinically significant bleeding may occur. Certain variants of type 2 vWD consistently exhibit recessive inheritance, although most are dominant.

One unlinked modifier of plasma vWF levels appears to be related to ABO blood type. Both vWF antigen[75,76] and ristocetin cofactor activity[77] are lower in persons of blood type O as compared with blood types A and B.

Classification and Molecular Defect

The classification of vWD recently was revised based on pathophysiologic mechanism.[192a] The correspondence with previous classifications is straightforward.[192a] vWD is divided into three broad categories based on whether the vWF in blood plasma is qualitatively normal (type 1), abnormal (type 2), or absent (type 3). These categories correlate fairly well with the vWF multimer pattern observed in plasma. In type 1 vWD, all normal multimer species are present but reduced proportionally; assays of vWF antigen and function also are reduced proportionally. This pattern suggests a simple quantitative deficiency of vWF. In type 2 vWD disease, the plasma vWF exhibits defective structure or function, indicating a qualitative abnormality of the protein. In most such variants, the larger vWF multimers are absent (see Fig. 107-4). Further subdivision of type 2 vWD is made based on the response of a patient's vWF to ristocetin, on the details of vWF multimer structure, or on other functional assays. A third category, type 3 vWD, is distinguished by the virtual absence of vWF antigen and activity from plasma and by clinically recessive inheritance.

This scheme has the advantage that the major subdivisions identify patient groups with distinctive biochemical and clinical characteristics. As more sensitive and discriminating tests have been devised, however, additional heterogeneity has been demonstrated in all types of vWD. In particular, certain patients with a normal multimer distribution clearly have structural and functional abnormalities of the vWF subunit. Thus, the distinction between quantitive (type 1) and qualitative (type 2) vWD has become more difficult.

In principle, deficiency of vWF activity could result from lesions within the vWF gene or indirectly as a consequence of mutations that affect biosynthesis or metabolism. No cause of vWD that is not linked to the vWF locus has been described to date.

This chapter will emphasize the properties of vWD types for which molecular defects have been defined (Table 107-2). A more complete database of mutations that cause vWD has been published and will be updated periodically[193]; that database contains comprehensive references for the characterization of specific mutations. A catalogue of virtually all known variants of vWD has been compiled by Zaverio Ruggeri[194]; that review and selected more recent publications[195,196] can be consulted for references to case reports for rare or unclassified variants.

Type 1 von Willebrand Disease. This is the most common form of vWD and is the type originally identified by Erik von Willebrand. It accounts for approximately 70 percent of cases seen in specialized treatment centers.[190,197] Plasma vWF is reduced; ristocetin cofactor activity and factor VIII usually are reduced proportionately, and multimer distribution is normal. This is compatible with a simple quantitative deficiency of vWF with no intrinsic functional abnormality. Inheritance is autosomal dominant.

vWD type 1 is a heterogeneous disorder. Some pedigrees have normal content of platelet vWF, while others have similar deficiencies of both plasma and platelet vWF.[186,187] These distinctions may correlate with the efficacy of therapy with DDAVP.[187]

A normal-appearing multimer distribution does not correlate perfectly with normal function. Because type 1 vWD is

Table 107-2 Classification of von Willebrand Disease

von Willebrand Disease	Genetics	Factor VIII	vWF Antigen	Ristocetin Cofactor Activity	RIPA	Multimer Structure
Type 1	Dominant	Decreased	Decreased	Decreased	Decreased	Normal in plasma and platelets
Type 2A	Dominant (usually)	Decreased or normal	Decreased or normal	Decreased relative to antigen	Decreased relative to antigen	Large and intermediate multimers absent from plasma; variable in platelets
Type 2B	Dominant	Decreased or normal	Decreased or normal	Decreased or normal	Increased	Large multimers usually absent from plasma; normal in platelets
Type 2M	Dominant (usually)	Decreased or normal	Decreased or normal	Decreased relative to antigen	Decreased relative to antigen	Large and intermediate multimers present in plasma and platelets
Type 2N	Recessive	Moderately decreased	Normal	Normal	Normal	Normal in plasma and platelets
Type 3	Recessive	Moderately to markedly decreased	Absent or trace	Absent	Absent	None or trace in plasma or platelets

RIPA = Ristocetin-induced platelet aggregation in platelet-rich plasma.

constrained to include only quantitative disorders, some variants previously designated as type 1 have been reclassified under type 2, mainly as type 2M.

Type 2 von Willebrand Disease. In most forms of type 2 vWD, but not all, the larger multimers are missing from plasma vWF.[56] This structural difference from normal vWF reflects a qualitative abnormality. Additional subdivision of type 2 vWD is made on the basis of ristocetin-dependent assays, analysis of vWF multimer patterns by high-resolution gel electrophoresis (see Fig. 107-4), and other assays.

Type 2A von Willebrand Disease. In type 2A vWD, both ristocetin-induced platelet aggregation and ristocetin cofactor activity are disproportionately decreased relative to vWF antigen, indicating that the residual plasma vWF has reduced function.[56] Large and intermediate plasma vWF multimers are absent, and the smallest multimer may be relatively increased. This subgroup is structurally and immunochemically[206] heterogeneous. The plasma vWF levels may be normal or decreased. The distribution of platelet vWF multimers is variable.[56,186] In some patients, the plasma and platelet multimers exhibit similar decreases in large multimers that suggest a defect in polymerization. In other patients, the platelet multimer distribution appears normal, and increased sensitivity to proteolysis may contribute to the abnormal plasma vWF multimer distribution.[207,208] This heterogeneity is supported by the variable response to DDAVP in vWD type 2A. Some patients show at least a partial correction of both bleeding time and multimer distribution after treatment with DDAVP; others consistently fail to respond.[189,208,209] The mode of inheritance is typically dominant, and this variant accounts for approximately three fourths of all type 2 vWD.

Several missense mutations that cause type 2A vWD have been characterized, most of which are within vWF domain A2 (Fig. 107-5).[193] As was predicted from the phenotypic variability of type 2A vWD, these mutations can be divided into two groups that appear to cause similarly abnormal plasma vWF multimer patterns by distinct mechanisms.[210] One group includes the mutations V844$_m$D, S743$_m$L, and G742$_m$R. (Missense mutations will be designated in single letter code with the normal amino acid followed by the number of the position followed by the mutant amino acid, positions in the prepro-region by subscript p, and those in the mature subunit by subscript m [e.g. V844$_m$D is Val at position 844 in the mature subunit mutated to Asp].) These particular mutations were shown to impair the assembly and secretion of normal vWF multimers, and patients with these mutations have decreased large vWF multimers in both plasma and platelets. The second group includes the mutations R834$_m$W and G742$_m$E, which are compatible with the sythesis and secretion of normal-appearing vWF multimers. Patients with these mutations have normal platelet vWF multimer patterns, and the deficiency of plasma vWF multimers apparently is caused by increased proteolytic degradation in the circulation.[210] For some patients with type 2A vWD, a major site of proteolytic cleavage in the vWF subunit was shown to be the Tyr842$_m$–Met843$_m$ bond[211]; it is not known which protease is responsible.

Many rare type 2 variants have been reclassified as type 2A. In general, these loss-of-function variants were defined initially by unique features of individual multimers on gel electrophoresis. These include the former type IIC[222–226] type IID,[227,228] type IIE,[87,229] type IIF,[230] type IIG,[231] type IIH,[232] and type II-I.[196] The latter four types represent single case reports.

Type 2B von Willebrand Disease. In type 2B vWD there is hyperresponsiveness of platelet-rich plasma to ristocetin,[212] although ristocetin cofactor activity may be decreased or normal. Plasma vWF multimers usually show a decrease in large multimers, but platelets contain a normal multimer distribution.[56] Administration of DDAVP to patients with type 2B vWD causes the release of large multimers into the circulation, but the larger species are rapidly cleared, apparently through spontaneous binding to platelet glycoprotein Ib. This is accompanied by transient thrombocytopenia that can be severe.[213] Thus, the small multimer pattern in this variant is at least partly due to enhanced clearance of

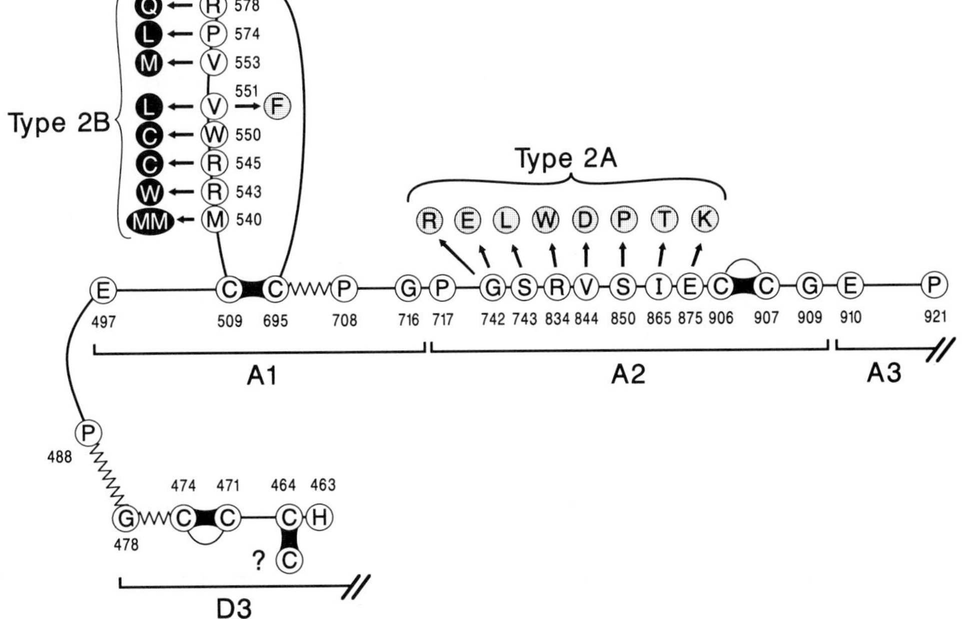

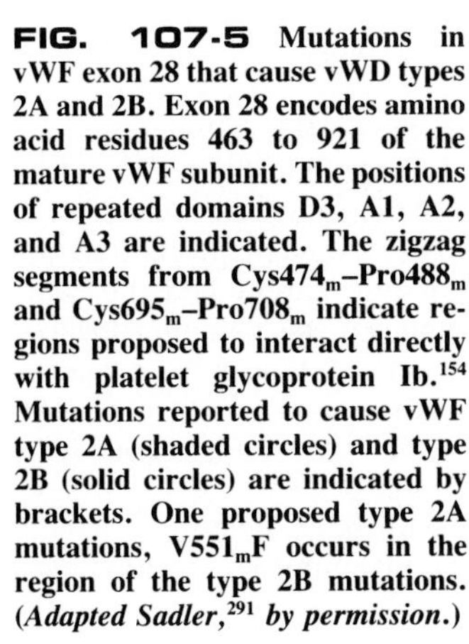
FIG. 107-5 Mutations in vWF exon 28 that cause vWD types 2A and 2B. Exon 28 encodes amino acid residues 463 to 921 of the mature vWF subunit. The positions of repeated domains D3, A1, A2, and A3 are indicated. The zigzag segments from Cys474$_m$–Pro488$_m$ and Cys695$_m$–Pro708$_m$ indicate regions proposed to interact directly with platelet glycoprotein Ib.[154] Mutations reported to cause vWF type 2A (shaded circles) and type 2B (solid circles) are indicated by brackets. One proposed type 2A mutations, V551$_m$F occurs in the region of the type 2B mutations. (*Adapted Sadler,*[291] *by permission.*)

large multimers rather than to a polymerization defect. The increased ristocetin-induced platelet aggregation is due to the presence of large, abnormal, hyperresponsive vWF multimers adsorbed to patient platelets in platelet-rich plasma. The normal or decreased ristocetin cofactor activity is due to the absence of these same multimers from (platelet-poor) patient plasma, so that added allogeneic platelets are not agglutinated by them. Probable variants of this subtype have been reported with chronic thrombocytopenia, circulating platelet aggregates, and spontaneous platelet aggregation in vitro.[214,215] The disorder is transmitted as a dominant trait; a few families with *de novo* mutations have been reported.[193,216,217] The few cases described of normal multimer distribution with hyperresponsiveness to ristocetin[200,201] may represent a mild form of type 2B defect. Type 2B vWD accounts for less than 20 percent of all type 2 vWD.

Mutations that cause vWD type 2B (see Fig. 107-5)[193] cluster within sequences of vWF domain A1 that are proposed to interact with botrocetin, a snake venom protein that binds to vWF and induces binding of vWF to platelet glycoprotein Ib.[218] These mutations may promote a conformational change in vWF that is similar to the effect of botrocetin binding. The gain of function phenotype of vWF type 2B may therefore be due to abnormal regulation of its affinity for platelet glycoprotein Ib.

Type 2M von Willebrand Disease. Type 2M (for "multimer") refers to variants with decreased platelet-dependent function that is not caused by the absence of large vWF multimers.[192a] Despite the normal sized multimers, the presence of a structural or functional defect indicates that the multimers must contain qualitatively abnormal vWF subunits. Type 2M includes variants with normal vWF multimers but decreased ristocetin cofactor activity,[198,199] and variants with subtle differences from normal multimer structure with characteristic abnormalities of "satellite" bands,[198] the presence of large amounts of uncleaved pro-vWF in the multimers,[202] or larger than normal plasma multimers.[203] Such variants often were classified previously as "type I."

One mechanism that causes type 2M vWD is decreased binding affinity for platelet glycoprotein Ib due to mutations in vWF domain A1. For example, two unrelated patients with normal multimer distributions were found to have mutations within the $Cys509_m$-$Cys695_m$ disulfide loop of vWF domain A1. One patient had a deletion of 11 amino acids,[204] and the other had the single amino acid substitution $F606_mI$.[205] Both patients had disproportionately low ristocetin cofactor activity, consistent with qualitative vWF abnormalities. Similarly, the missense mutation $G561_mS$ does not impair multimer assembly but results in an interesting dissociation between ristocetin cofactor activity (absent) and botrocetin cofactor activity (normal).[193,233]

Type 2N von Willebrand Disease. An interesting variant of type 2 vWD is characterized by factor VIII deficiency that is caused indirectly by mutations in vWF.[219,220] The abnormal vWF does not bind to factor VIII and consequently does not stabilize it in the circulation; otherwise it apparently is normal, with normal levels of vWF antigen, normal indexes of platelet-dependent vWF function such as bleeding time and ristocetin cofactor activity, and normal vWF multimer distribution. Thus, this type 2 vWD variant mimics hemophilia A except that the pattern of inheritance is autosomal recessive rather than X-linked recessive. This phenotype was tentatively named vWD "Normandy" after the province in which one proband was born,[220] and currently is designated type 2N.[192a]

In one affected family, a male patient with vWD type 2N was misdiagnosed with hemophilia A, and moderate factor VIII deficiency in a sister was incorrectly attributed to extreme lyonization in a carrier of hemophilia A.[221] The prevalence of vWD type 2N is not known; it probably is rare. Nevertheless, this diagnosis should be considered in patients with congenital factor VIII deficiency in whom the disorder is not clearly X-linked, because correct diagnosis may lead to significant changes in therapy and in genetic counseling.[221]

Patients with the vWD type 2N phenotype have been reported from the United States, France, the Netherlands, and Spain.[193] Several causative mutations were identified within the factor VIII binding domain of vWF: $T28_mM$, $R53_mW$, and $R91_mQ$. In some patients, defects in factor VIII binding were associated with symptomatic decreases in platelet-dependent vWF functions. Such intermediate phenotypes may be due to coinheritance of vWD type 1 and 2N alleles, and suggest that compound heterozygosity can strongly influence the clinical presentation of vWD variants.

Type 3 von Willebrand Disease. Patients with type 3 vWD have essentially no detectable vWF antigen or activity in blood plasma and usually have factor VIII levels of ≤ 1 to 10 percent of normal.[27,234,235] Patients with undetectable factor VIII activity generally have low levels of detectable factor VIII antigen.[19,236] These patients appear to have received two defective vWF alleles, and many such patients have clinically unaffected parents. The traces of vWF detected in the plasma or platelets of some patients with type 3 vWD have exhibited several different structural abnormalities,[235] indicating that this subgroup is heterogeneous.

Because the prevalence of recessive type 3 vWD (q^2) is 0.5 to 3 per million, heterozygotes (2pq) should comprise at least 1400 to 3500 per million persons; however, the prevalence of symptomatic type 1 vWD appears to be at least tenfold lower. Clearly, most heterozygous relatives of patients with type 3 vWD are not symptomatic, and type 3 vWD does not appear to be explained completely as the inheritance of two alleles for type 1 vWD. There is variability in expression among heterozygotes within families that contain patients with type 3 vWD, and deficiencies of vWF antigen and ristocetin cofactor activity can often be detected in clinically normal relatives.[180,181] In type 1 vWD, a similar apparent quantitative vWF deficiency is associated with a dominantly inherited bleeding diathesis. Until the mutations in type 1 and type 3 vWD can be compared, the contrast between the dominant inheritance of type 1 vWD and the recessive inheritance of type 3 vWD will remain unexplained.

Deletions were found in the vWF genes of several patients with type 3 vWD.[193] One patient from each of two unrelated Italian families[170] and four affected siblings from a third Italian family[237] were shown to have total deletions of both vWF alleles. One patient had a heterozygous total deletion of the vWF gene. An asymptomatic parent had the same abnormality by Southern blotting, so the patient appeared to have inherited a second defective allele with a normal hybridization pattern from the other parent.[237] One patient, whose parents were second cousins, was homozygous for a 2.3-kb deletion that contained exon 42.[238]

Among the seven patients with gene deletions in both alleles, in all but one alloantibody inhibitors to transfused vWF had developed.[170,237,238] The one patient without this complication had three affected siblings who did have antibodies to vWF.[238] In contrast, none of the patients reported to date with vWD type 3 and normal Southern-blot patterns has had alloantibodies, which suggests that vWF gene deletions predispose to the development of inhibitors during therapy. A similar but less consistent correlation has been noted for hemophilia B and the factor IX gene[239,240] (see Chap. 104).

Nonsense mutations (designated X in single letter code) in CGA arginine codons were found in several patients with type 3 vWD: In codon 365 of the prepro-region designated $R365_pX$, and in codons 1659 and 2535 of the mature vWF subunit designated $R896_mX$ and $R1772_mX$.[241-243] All of these represent C→T transitions within CpG dinucleotides, which appear to be hotspots for mutation in the human genome.[244]

Clinical Course. For patients with a quantitative deficiency of vWF (vWD types 1 and 3), the severity of disease generally correlates with the degree of vWF functional deficiency, and may vary from clinically insignificant to life-threatening. The severity of the disease in patients with qualitative disorders of vWF (vWD type 2) may exceed what might be expected based on the functional deficiency ascertained by laboratory tests.[223,226,227,230] Symptoms are usually present from childhood and often from birth.[7,8,10,27,180] These commonly include easy bruisability, cutaneous hematomas, epistaxis, bleeding from gums, and prolonged bleeding from cuts. Persistent severe bleeding after minor oral trauma and after dental extraction is common. More than half of affected women have menorrhagia that may require blood transfusion. Bleeding from a ruptured ovarian follicle or corpus luteum may also be severe.[190,226] Gastrointestinal bleeding seems to be relatively rare but may be life-threatening. Patients with vWD type 3 and essentially undetectable vWF can have factor VIII levels low enough to predispose to spontaneous hemarthrosis, joint deformities, and soft-tissue bleeding.[7,8,27,180] Milder forms of vWD are almost never associated with hemarthrosis. The bleeding tendency of vWD has been reported to decrease with advancing age,[7,27,180] although this is not a uniform feature of the disease.

During pregnancy, the plasma vWF levels are increased in normal individuals and in patients with most forms of vWD other than type 3.[245-248] This increase is most marked in the third trimester, and reflects in part the influence of estrogens on vWF levels. If this increase represents functional vWF, then labor and delivery are usually uncomplicated. Plasma vWF levels return to base line within a few days, and patients with vWD should be monitored closely for serious postpartum bleeding during at least the first week after delivery. Patients with dysfunctional vWF (type 2 variants) frequently have severe difficulty with hemorrhage during labor and delivery.[200,223,227]

Type 2B vWD can present special problems during pregnancy. The increased plasma concentration of abnormal vWF that is a consequence of the physiological stimulus of pregnancy can cause severe and prolonged thrombocytopenia, with marked blood loss during delivery.[249] Children born with vWD type 2B may present with congenital thrombocytopenia.[217]

The development of alloantibodies to vWF is distinctly uncommon in vWD (reviewed in Mannucci and Mari[250]). All of the reported cases have occurred in patients with vWD type 3 who produce no immunologically recognizable vWF-like protein. In the type 3 subgroup, the prevalence of alloantibodies to vWF is about 7.5 percent; this is similar to the prevalence of alloantibodies to factor VIII in hemophilia A. Antibodies do not develop in all severely affected patients, and there may be a familial predisposition to this complication of therapy. The apparent association between deletions within the vWF gene and the development of such antibodies was discussed above.

Differential Diagnosis. The symptoms that occur in vWD are not at all specific, and many conditions of quite different pathogenesis may be associated with a similar bleeding diathesis. These include primary platelet disorders such as Bernard-Soulier disease and the ingestion of antiplatelet drugs. In particular, the use of aspirin by patients with hemophilia A can produce a clinical picture quite like severe vWD.[251] In most cases, vWD can be excluded easily by appropriate laboratory testing.

vWD type 2B can cause thrombocytopenia that may be confused with idiopathic thrombocytopenic purpura. Such patients who present during pregnancy have received unnecessary therapy with prednisone[249,252] or intravenous gamma globulin,[253,254] while appropriate therapy with cryoprecipitate and platelet transfusions was withheld. Two men, who were ultimately found to have vWD type 2B, underwent splenectomy for presumed idiopathic thrombocytopenic purpura unresponsive to prednisone.[214,255] This subtype of vWD also is associated with postoperative thrombocytopenia[256] and has presented as congenital thrombocytopenia.[217]

Two conditions are especially difficult to distinguish from vWD because they may cause low vWF levels and even mimic vWD type 2 multimer distributions. These are the acquired von Willebrand syndrome and "platelet-type" or "pseudo" vWD. The *acquired von Willebrand syndrome* refers to a condition of spontaneous bleeding associated with decreased vWF occurring in adults without a prior personal or family history of vWD. More than 60 cases have been reported (reviewed in Mannucci and Mari[250]). Most have been associated with a recognized autoimmune or lymphoproliferative disorder that suggests an immunologic cause. Some patients have lacked such underlying diseases, and fewer than half of afflicted patients were shown to possess autoantibodies to vWF. The multimer distribution in plasma may resemble type 1 or type 2 vWD. In the latter case, discrimination between vWD type 2B and the aquired von Willebrand syndrome may be difficult. Both conditions are characterized by relatively normal platelet vWF structure and concentration and by shortened survival in the circulation of the endogenous vWF released by DDAVP. In contrast to vWD type 2B, the ristocetin sensitivity of platelet vWF is normal in the acquired von Willebrand syndrome, and exogenous vWF administered by transfusion has shortened survival.

Platelet-type or pseudo-vWD is clinically very similar to vWD type 2B, but the abnormality lies with the platelet rather than with the vWF.[257-259] The condition is inherited as an autosomal dominant trait. Symptoms resemble those of moderately severe vWD, and laboratory abnormalities include a prolonged bleeding time, decreased plasma vWF and factor VIII levels, increased ristocetin-induced platelet aggregation, absence of larger multimers from plasma, and presence of all multimers in platelets. The response to DDAVP is like that of vWD type 2B, with transient thrombocytopenia and spontaneous platelet aggregation.[260] In contrast to vWD type 2B, the addition of normal plasma, hemophilic plasma, cryoprecipitate, or purified vWF to platelet-rich plasma in this disorder causes platelet aggregation without the addition of ristocetin.[258,259,261] Candidate mutations within the gene for platelet GPIbα were found in two patients: G233V[262] and M239V.[263]

Therapy. Patients with severe vWD may bleed either because they lack sufficient vWF to support normal platelet function or because they are factor VIII-deficient, and the response to therapy in vWD emphasizes the distinct functions of these molecules in hemostasis. Hemarthroses, soft-tissue hematomas, and postoperative bleeding often respond to elevations of factor VIII, whereas mucocutaneous bleeding responds to infusions of functional vWF.

Factor VIII levels are usually easy to support because even limited amounts of small vWF multimers can stabilize and cause a prolonged elevation of plasma factor VIII level. Correction of the platelet adhesion abnormality is more difficult. Fresh-frozen plasma and cryoprecipitate consistently contain functional vWF multimers. The utility of fresh-frozen plasma is limited by the large volume needed to infuse sufficient vWF. Frozen cryoprecipitate is widely available and will reliably shorten the bleeding time in most forms of vWD, but the possible transmission of disease by cryoprecipitate makes it less than an ideal therapy. Lyophilized cryoprecipitate may not be as effective.[264] Some virucidally treated factor VIII concentrates that are used for the treatment of hemophilia A appear to be ineffective in the treatment of vWD, probably because the larger vWF multimers in these preparations have been denatured or degraded.[265,266] Certain of these concentrates, however, do contain therapeutically effective vWF.[267,268] In preliminary clinical studies, a very-high-purity vWF concentrate that contains little factor VIII was effective in several types of vWD.[269-271] Such preparations are not yet widely available.

Many patients with mild vWD can avoid exposure to blood products through the pharmacological manipulation of plasma vWF levels. In many patients, the vasopressin analogue DDAVP administered intravenously or intranasally causes a threefold to sixfold elevation of vWF and factor VIII levels that is maximal in 30 to 90 min.[272-276] Levels decrease to base-line levels over several hours to several days. Repeated doses often elicit a diminished response,[274] but this is not consistently observed, and the efficacy of repeated doses should be evaluated in individual patients as indicated. For therapy with DDAVP to be effective, the patient must be able to synthesize at least a partially functional vWF. Consequently, DDAVP is expected to be most useful in vWD type 1 with a simple quantitative deficiency of vWF. Patients with vWD type 3 generally do not have a useful response to DDAVP (reviewed in Rodeghiero et al.[275]).

The response to DDAVP in vWD type 2 variants is variable and frequently is unsatisfactory.[188,189,275] However, patients who will respond favorably apparently can be identified with a test infusion, which should be considered for all variants with low ristocetin cofactor activity.[277] In type 2N vWD, DDAVP increases plasma vWF levels but does not significantly increase factor VIII levels; this pattern is consistent with the inability of vWF type 2N to bind and stabilize factor VIII.[278]

In patients with vWD type 2B, DDAVP causes thrombocytopenia and spontaneous platelet aggregation,[213,276] and the bleeding time usually is not shortened.[209,213,277] Concerns over the potential for promoting thrombosis have led to the recommendation that DDAVP should not be used in type 2B vWD.[213,276] Experience with DDAVP in this vWD subtype is very limited and the risk of thrombosis is not known, but no thrombotic complications have been described to date. In a few patients with vWD type 2B, DDAVP was therapeutically effective and did not cause a significant decrease in platelet count.[275,279,280] Thus, DDAVP may be acceptable therapy for a subset of patients with type 2B vWD.

Fibrinolytic inhibitors may be useful adjuncts for the control of nasopharyngeal and oral bleeding. Menorrhagia in women with vWD can be treated successfully with oral contraceptives. Estrogens have also been used to control hemorrhage from other sites and as preparation for surgery in women with vWD type 1.[281,282]

Genetic Counseling. Assessment of the risk of vWD is usually straightforward and requires only the determination of whether a family is affected by a dominant or recessive variant. For families affected with vWD type 3, genetic counseling is the same as for any severe recessive disorder. Prenatal diagnosis has been accomplished for vWD type 3 by assays of factor VIII and vWF in fetal blood samples.[283,284] The vWF multimer distribution in fetal blood may be diagnostic of many type 2 vWD variants even if the levels of antigen are not depressed, provided there is no intercurrent disease that might consume large vWF multimers.[285] The vWF gene is highly polymorphic; at least 32 marker systems are available for genetic studies in vWD.[286] The most informative of these is a tetranucleotide repeat polymorphism in intron 40, with ≥98 alleles,[287] and this system was used for prenatal diagnosis of severe vWD.[288] DNA sequence polymorphisms also have been used to confirm the neonatal diagnosis of vWD.[289,290]

Carriers of the defective allele in mildly affected pedigrees could be identified with greater certainty by combining the currently employed vWF and factor VIII assays with analysis of DNA sequence polymorphisms. Such families should receive counseling, but most families do not choose to alter reproductive plans because of the mild phenotype.

REFERENCES

1. von Willebrand EA: Hereditär pseudohemofili. *Fin Laekaresaellsk Hand* **68**:87, 1926.
2. von Willebrand EA: Über hereditäre pseudohämophilie. *Acta Med Scand* **76**:521, 1931.
3. von Willebrand E, Jürgens R: Über eine neue Bluterkrankheit, die konstitutionelle Thrombopathie. *Klin Wochenschr* **12**:414, 1933.
4. Alexander B, Goldstein B: Dual hemostatic defect in pseudohemophilia. *J Clin Invest* **32**:551, 1953.
5. Larrieu MJ, Soulier JP: Déficit en facteur antihémophilique A chez une fille associé à un trouble saignement. *Rev Hematol* **8**:361, 1953.
6. Quick AJ, Hussey VV: Hemophilic condition in the female. *J Lab Clin Med* **42**:929, 1953.
7. Nilsson IM, Blombäck M, Jorpes E, Blombäck B, Johansson S-A: v. Willebrand's disease and its correction with human plasma fraction 1-0. *Acta Med Scand* **159**:179, 1957.
8. Nilsson IM, Blombäck M, von Francken I: On an inherited autosomal hemorrhagic diathesis with antihemophilic globulin (AHG) deficiency and prolonged bleeding time. *Acta Med Scand* **159**:35, 1957.
9. Nilsson IM, Blombäck M, Blombäck B: von Willebrand's disease in Sweden. Its pathogenesis and treatment. *Acta Med Scand* **164**:263, 1959.
10. Cornu P, Larrieu MJ, Caen J, Bernard J: Transfusion studies in von Willebrand's disease: Effect on bleeding time and factor VIII. *Br J Haematol* **9**:189, 1963.

11. Over J, Sixma JJ, Doucet-de Bruïne MHM, Trieschnigg AMC, Vlooswijk RAA, Beeser-Visser NH, Bouma BN: Survival of [125] iodine-labeled factor VIII in normals and patients with classic hemophilia. *J Clin Invest* **62**:223, 1978.
12. Tuddenham EGD, Lane RS, Rotblat F, Johnson AJ, Snape TJ, Middleton S, Kernoff PBA: Response to infusions of polyelectrolyte fractionated human factor VIII concentrate in human haemophilia A and von Willebrand's disease. *Br J Haematol* **52**:259, 1982.
13. Stites DP, Hershgold EJ, Perlman JD, Fudenberg HH: Factor VIII detection by hemagglutination inhibition: Hemophilia A and von Willebrand's disease. *Science* **171**:196, 1971.
14. Zimmerman TS, Ratnoff OD, Powell AE: Immunologic differentiation of classic hemophilia (factor VIII deficiency) and von Willebrand's disease. *J Clin Invest* **50**:244, 1971.
15. Bouma BN, Wiegerinck Y, Sixma JJ, van Mourik JA, Mochtar IA: Immunological characterization of purified antihaemophilic factor A (factor VIII) which corrects abnormal platelet retention in von Willebrand's disease. *Nature New Biol* **236**:104, 1972.
16. Legaz ME, Schmer G, Counts RB, Davie EW: Isolation and characterization of human factor VIII (antihemophilic factor). *J Biol Chem* **248**:2946, 1973.
17. Shapiro GA, Andersen JC, Pizzo SV, McKee PA: The subunit structure of normal and hemophilic factor VIII. *J Clin Invest* **52**:2198, 1973.
18. Zimmerman TS, Edgington TS: Factor VIII coagulant activity and factor VIII-like antigen: Independent molecular entities. *J Exp Med* **138**:1015, 1973.
19. Lazarchick J, Hoyer LW: Immunoradiometric measurement of the factor VIII procoagulant antigen. *J Clin Invest* **62**:1048, 1978.
20. Peake IR, Bloom AL: Immunoradiometric assay of procoagulant factor VIII antigen in plasma and serum and its reduction in haemophilia. Preliminary studies on adult and fetal blood. *Lancet* **1**:473, 1978.
21. Bennett B, Ratnoff OD, Levin J: Immunologic studies in von Willebrand's disease. Evidence that the antihemophilic factor (AHF) produced after transfusions lacks an antigen associated with normal AHF and the inactive material produced by patients with classic hemophilia. *J Clin Invest* **51**:2597, 1972.
22. Gralnick HR, Coller BS: Molecular defects in haemophilia A and von Willebrand's disease. *Lancet* **1**:837, 1976.
23. Graham JB: Genetic control of factor VIII. *Lancet* **1**:340, 1980.
24. Borchgrevink CF: A method for measuring platelet adhesiveness in vivo. *Acta Med Scand* **162**:361, 1960.
25. Salzman EW: Measurement of platelet adhesiveness: A simple in vitro technique demonstrating an abnormality in von Willebrand's disease. *J Lab Clin Med* **62**:724, 1963.
26. Zucker MB: In vitro abnormality of the blood in von Willebrand's disease correctable by normal plasma. *Nature* **197**:601, 1963.
27. Larrieu MJ, Caen JP, Meyer DO, Vainer H, Sultan Y, Bernard J: Congenital bleeding disorders with long bleeding time and normal platelet count. II. Von Willebrand's disease (report of thirty-seven patients). *Am J Med* **45**:354, 1968.
28. Howard MA, Firkin B: Ristocetin: A new tool in the investigation of platelet aggregation. *Thromb Diath Haemorrh* **26**:362, 1971.
29. Thelin GM, Wagner RH: Sedimentation of plasma antihemophilic factor. *Arch Biochem Biophys* **95**:70, 1961.
30. Weiss HJ, Hoyer LW: Von Willebrand factor: Dissociation from antihemophilic factor procoagulant activity. *Science* **182**:1149, 1973.
31. Griggs TR, Cooper HA, Webster WP, Wagner RH, Brinkhous KM: Plasma aggregating factor (bovine) for human platelets: A marker for study of antihemophilic and von Willebrand factors. *Proc Natl Acad Sci USA* **70**:2814, 1973.
32. Holmberg L, Nilsson IM: Genetic variants of von Willebrand's disease. *Br Med J* **3**:317, 1972.
33. Kernoff PBA, Bruson R, Rizza CR: A variant of factor VIII related antigen. *Br J Haematol* **26**:435, 1974.
34. Peake IR, Bloom AL, Giddings JC: Inherited variants of factor VIII-related protein in von Willebrand's disease. *N Engl J Med* **291**:113, 1974.
35. Jaffe EA, Hoyer LW, Nachman RL: Synthesis of antihemophilic factor antigen by cultured human endothelial cells. *J Clin Invest* **52**:2757, 1973.
36. Jaffe EA, Hoyer LW, Nachman RL: Synthesis of von Willebrand factor by cultured human endothelial cells. *Proc Natl Acad Sci USA* **71**:1906, 1974.
37. Nachman R, Levine R, Jaffe EA: Synthesis of factor VIII antigen by cultured guinea pig megakaryocytes. *J Clin Invest* **60**:914, 1977.
38. Sporn LA, Chavin SI, Marder VJ, Wagner DD: Biosynthesis of von Willebrand protein by human megakaryocytes. *J Clin Invest* **76**:1102, 1985.
39. Maruyama I, Bell CE, Majerus PW: Thrombomodulin is found on endothelium of arteries, veins, capillaries, and lymphatics, and on syncytiotrophoblast of human placenta. *J Cell Biol* **101**:363, 1985.
40. Sadler JE, Shelton-Inloes BB, Sorace JM, Harlan JM, Titani K, Davie EW: Cloning and characterization of two cDNAs coding for human von Willebrand factor. *Proc Natl Acad Sci USA* **82**:6394, 1985.
41. Lynch DC, Zimmerman TS, Collins CJ, Brown M, Morin MJ, Ling EH, Livingston DM: Molecular cloning of cDNA for human von Willebrand factor: Authentication by a new method. *Cell* **41**:49, 1985.
42. Verweij CL, De Vries CJM, Distel B, Van Zonneveld A-J, Van Kessel AG, Van Mourik JA, Pannekoek H: Construction of cDNA coding for human von Willebrand factor using antibody probes for colony-screening and mapping of the chromosomal gene. *Nucleic Acids Res* **13**:4699, 1985.
43. Ginsburg D, Handin RI, Bonthron DT, Donlon TA, Bruns GAP, Latt SA, Orkin SH: Human von Willebrand factor (vWF): Isolation of complementary DNA (cDNA) clones and chromosome localization. *Science* **228**:1401, 1985.
44. Bonthron DT, Orr EC, Mitsock LM, Ginsburg D, Handin RI, Orkin SH: Nucleotide sequence of pre-pro-von Willebrand factor cDNA. *Nucleic Acids Res* **14**:7125, 1986.
45. Shelton-Inloes BB, Titani K, Sadler JE: cDNA sequences for human von Willebrand factor reveal five types of repeated domains and five possible protein sequence polymorphisms. *Biochemistry* **25**:3164, 1986.
46. Titani K, Kumar S, Takio K, Ericsson LH, Wade RD, Ashida K, Walsh KA, Chopek MW, Sadler JE, Fujikawa K: Amino acid sequence of human von Willebrand factor. *Biochemistry* **25**:3171, 1986.
47. Verweij CL, Diergaarde PJ, Hart M, Pannekoek: Full-length von Willebrand factor (vWF) cDNA encodes a highly repetitive protein considerably larger than the mature vWF subunit. *EMBO J* **5**:1839, 1986.
48. Wagner DD, Marder VJ: Biosynthesis of von Willebrand protein by human endothelial cells. Identification of a large precursor polypeptide chain. *J Biol Chem* **258**:2065, 1983.
49. Lynch DC, Williams R, Zimmerman TS, Kirby EP, Livingston DM: Biosynthesis of the subunits of factor VIIIR by bovine aortic endothelial cells. *Proc Natl Acad Sci USA* **80**:2738, 1983.
50. Lynch DC, Zimmerman TS, Kirby EP, Livingston DM: Subunit composition of oligomeric human von Willebrand factor. *J Biol Chem* **258**:12757, 1983.
51. Wagner DD, Marder VJ: Biosynthesis of von Willebrand protein by human endothelial cells: Processing steps and their intracellular localization. *J Cell Biol* **99**:2123, 1984.
52. Wagner DD, Lawrence SO, Ohlsson-Wilhelm BM, Fay PJ, Marder VJ: Topology and order of formation of interchain disulfide bonds in von Willebrand factor. *Blood* **69**:27, 1987.
53. van Mourik JA, Bouma BN, LaBruyère WT, de Graf S, Mochtar IA: Factor VIII, a series of homologous oligomers and a complex of two proteins. *Thromb Res* **4**:155, 1974.
54. Counts RB, Paskell SL, Elgee SK: Disulfide bonds and the quaternary structure of factor VIII/von Willebrand factor. *J Clin Invest* **62**:702, 1978.
55. Hoyer LW, Shainoff JR: Factor VIII-related protein circulates in normal plasma as high molecular weight multimers. *Blood* **55**:1056, 1980.
56. Ruggeri ZM, Zimmerman TS: Variant von Willebrand's disease. Characterization of two subtypes by analysis of multimeric composition of factor VIII/von Willebrand factor in plasma and platelets. *J Clin Invest* **65**:1318, 1980.

57. Fay PJ, Kawai Y, Wagner DD, Ginsburg D, Bonthron D, Ohlsson-Wilhelm BM, Chavin SI, Abraham GN, Handin RI, Orkin SH, Montgomery RR, Marder VJ: Propolypeptide of von Willebrand factor circulates in blood and is identical to von Willebrand antigen II. *Science* **232**:995, 1986.
58. Montgomery RR, Zimmerman TS: von Willebrand's disease antigen II. A new plasma and platelet antigen deficient in severe von Willebrand's disease. *J Clin Invest* **62**:1498, 1978.
59. Scott JP, Montgomery RR: Platelet von Willebrand's antigen II: Active release by aggregating agents and a marker of platelet release reaction in vivo. *Blood* **58**:1075, 1981.
60. Wagner DD, Fay PJ, Sporn LA, Sinha S, Lawrence SO, Marder VJ: Divergent fates of von Willebrand factor and its propolypeptide (von Willebrand antigen II) after secretion from endothelial cells. *Proc Natl Acad Sci USA* **84**:1955, 1987.
61. Verweij CL, Hart M, Pannekoek H: Expression of variant von Willebrand factor (vWF) cDNA in heterologous cells: Requirement of the pro-polypeptide in vWF multimer formation. *EMBO J* **6**:2885, 1987.
62. Wise RJ, Pittman DD, Handin RI, Kaufman RJ, Orkin SH: The propeptide of von Willebrand factor independently mediates the assembly of von Willebrand multimers. *Cell* **52**:229, 1988.
63. Mayadas TN, Wagner DD: Vicinal cysteines in the prosequence play a role in von Willebrand factor multimer assembly. *Proc Natl Acad Sci USA* **89**:3531, 1992.
64. Verweij CL, Hart M, Pannekoek H: Proteolytic cleavage of the precursor of von Willebrand factor is not essential for multimer formation. *J Biol Chem* **263**:7921, 1988.
65. Chopek MW, Girma J-P, Fujikawa K, Davie EW, Titani K: Human von Willebrand factor: A multivalent protein composed of identical subunits. *Biochemistry* **25**:3146, 1986.
66. Wagner DD, Mayadas T, Marder VJ: Initial glycosylation and acidic pH in the Golgi apparatus are required for multimerization of von Willebrand factor. *J Cell Biol* **102**:1320, 1986.
67. Carew JA, Browning PJ, Lynch DC: Sulfation of von Willebrand factor. *Blood* **76**:2530, 1990.
68. Wagner DD, Olmsted JB, Marder VJ: Immunolocalization of von Willebrand protein in Weibel-Palade bodies of human endothelial cells. *J Cell Biol* **95**:355, 1982.
69. Weibel ER, Palade GE: New cytoplasmic components in arterial endothelia. *J Cell Biol* **23**:101, 1964.
70. Cramer EM, Meyer D, Le Menn R, Breton-Gorius J: Eccentric localization of von Willebrand factor in an internal structure of platelet α-granule resembling that of Weibel-Palade bodies. *Blood* **66**:710, 1985.
71. Bloom AL, Giddings JC, Wilks CJ: Factor VIII on the vascular intima: Possible importance in haemostasis and thrombosis. *Nature New Biol* **241**:217, 1973.
72. Hoyer LW, de los Santos RP, Hoyer JR: Antihemophilic factor antigen. Localization in endothelial cells by immunofluorescent microscopy. *J Clin Invest* **52**:2737, 1973.
73. López-Fernández MF, López-Berges C, Nieto J, Martin R, Batlle J: Platelet and plasma von Willebrand factor: Structural differences. *Thromb Res* **44**:125, 1986.
74. Abildgaard CF, Suzuki Z, Harrison J, Jefcoat K, Zimmerman TS: Serial studies in von Willebrand's disease: Variability versus "variants." *Blood* **56**:712, 1980.
75. Wahlberg TB, Blombäck M, Magnusson D: Influence of sex, blood group, secretor character, smoking habits, acetylsalicylic acid, oral contraceptives, fasting and general health state on blood coagulation variables in randomly selected young adults. *Haemostasis* **14**:312, 1984.
76. Gill JC, Endres-Brooks J, Bauer PJ, Marks WJ Jr, Montgomery RR: The effect of ABO blood group on the diagnosis of von Willebrand disease. *Blood* **69**:1691, 1987.
77. Rodeghiero F, Castaman G, Dini E: Epidemiological investigation of the prevalence of von Willebrand's disease. *Blood* **69**:454, 1987.
78. Nachman RL, Jaffe EA: Subcellular platelet factor VIII antigen and von Willebrand factor. *J Exp Med* **141**:1101, 1975.
79. Bloom AL: The biosynthesis of factor VIII. *Clin Haematol* **8**:53, 1979.
80. Shearn SAM, Peake IR, Giddings JC, Humphrys J, Bloom AL: The characterization and synthesis of antigens related to factor VIII in vascular endothelium. *Thromb Res* **11**:43, 1977.
81. Tuddenham EGD, Lazarchick J, Hoyer LW: Synthesis and release of factor VIII by cultured human endothelial cells. *Br J Haematol* **47**:617, 1981.
82. Harrison RL, McKee PA: Estrogen stimulates von Willebrand factor production by cultured endothelial cells. *Blood* **63**:657, 1984.
83. Levine JE, Harlan JM, Harker LA, Joseph ML, Counts RB: Thrombin-mediated release of factor VIII antigen from human umbilical vein endothelial cells in culture. *Blood* **60**:431, 1982.
84. Loesberg C, Gonsalves MD, Zandbergen J, Willems C, van Aken WG, Stel HV, van Mourick JA, de Groot PG: The effect of calcium on the secretion of factor VIII-related antigen by cultured human endothelial cells. *Biochim Biophys Acta* **763**:160, 1983.
85. Ribes JA, Francis CW, Wagner DD: Fibrin induces release of von Willebrand factor from endothelial cells. *J Clin Invest* **79**:117, 1987.
86. Sporn LA, Marder VJ, Wagner DD: Inducible secretion of large, biologically potent von Willebrand factor multimers. *Cell* **46**:185, 1986.
87. Zimmerman TS, Dent JA, Ruggeri ZM, Nannini LH: Subunit composition of plasma von Willebrand factor. Cleavage is present in normal individuals, increased in IIA and IIB von Willebrand disease, but minimal in variants with aberrant structure of individual oligomers (types IIC, IID, and IIE). *J Clin Invest* **77**:947, 1986.
88. Batlle J, Lopez-Fernandez MF, Lopez-Borrasca A, Lopez-Berges C, Dent JA, Berkowitz SD, Ruggeri ZM, Zimmerman TS: Proteolytic degradation of von Willebrand factor after DDAVP administration in normal individuals. *Blood* **70**:173, 1987.
89. Baumgartner HR: The role of blood flow in platelet adhesion, fibrin deposition and formation of mural thrombi. *Microvasc Res* **5**:167, 1973.
90. Tschopp TB, Weiss HJ, Baumgartner HR: Decreased adhesion of platelets to subendothelium in von Willebrand's disease. *J Lab Clin Med* **83**:296, 1974.
91. Weiss HJ, Turitto VT, Baumgartner HR: Effect of shear rate on platelet interaction with subendothelium in citrated and native blood. I. Shear rate-dependent decrease of adhesion in von Willebrand's disease and the Bernard-Soulier syndrome. *J Lab Clin Med* **92**:750, 1978.
92. Sakariassen KS, Bolhuis PA, Sixma JJ: Human blood platelet adhesion to artery subendothelium is mediated by factor VIII-von Willebrand factor bound to the subendothelium. *Nature* **279**:636, 1979.
93. Weiss HJ, Baumgartner HR, Tschopp TB, Turitto VT, Cohen D: Correction by factor VIII of the impaired platelet adhesion to subendothelium in von Willebrand disease. *Blood* **51**:267, 1978.
94. Baumgartner HR, Tschopp TB, Meyer D: Shear rate dependent inhibition of platelet adhesion/aggregation on collagenous surfaces by antibodies to human factor VIII/von Willebrand factor. *Br J Haematol* **44**:127, 1980.
95. Meyer D, Baumgartner HR, Edgington TS: Effect of hybridoma antibodies to human factor VIII/von Willebrand factor on the adhesion of platelets to the subendothelium. *Blood* **58**:237, 1981.
96. Turitto VT, Weiss HJ, Zimmerman TS, Sussman II: Factor VIII/von Willebrand factor in subendothelium mediates platelet adhesion. *Blood* **65**:823, 1985.
97. Stel HV, Sakariassen KS, de Groot PG, van Mourik JA, Sixma JJ: von Willebrand factor in the vessel wall mediates platelet adherence. *Blood* **65**:85, 1985.
98. Fressinaud E, Baruch D, Rothschild C, Baumgartner HR, Meyer D: Platelet von Willebrand factor: Evidence for its involvement in platelet adhesion to collagen. *Blood* **70**:1214, 1987.
99. Gralnick HR, Rick ME, McKeown LP, Williams SB, Parker RI, Maisonneuve P, Jenneau C, Sultan Y: Platelet von Willebrand factor: An important determinant of the bleeding time in type I von Willebrand's disease. *Blood* **68**:58, 1986.
100. Muggli R, Baumgartner HR, Tschopp TB, Keller H: Automated microdensitometry and protein assays as a measure for platelet adhesion and aggregation on collagen-coated slides under controlled flow conditions. *J Lab Clin Med* **95**:195, 1980.

101. Sakariassen KS, Aarts PAMM, de Groot PG, Houdijk WPM, Sixma JJ: A perfusion chamber developed to investigate platelet interaction in flowing blood with human vessel wall cells, their extracellular matrix, and purified components. *J Lab Clin Med* **102:**522, 1983.
102. Santoro SA: Adsorption of von Willebrand factor/factor VIII by the genetically distinct interstitial collagens. *Thromb Res* **21:**689, 1981.
103. Santoro SA, Cowan JF: Adsorption of von Willebrand factor by fibrillar collagen—Implications concerning the adhesion of platelets to collagen. *Coll Relat Res* **2:**31, 1982.
104. Morton LF, Griffin B, Pepper DS, Barnes MJ: The interaction between collagens and factor VIII/von Willebrand factor: Investigation of the structural requirements for interaction. *Thromb Res* **32:**545, 1983.
105. Wagner DD, Urban-Pickering M, Marder VJ: von Willebrand protein binds to extracellular matrices independently of collagen. *Proc Natl Acad Sci USA* **82:**471, 1984.
106. de Groot PG, van Mourik JA, Sixma JJ: Primary binding site of von Willebrand factor in the subendothelium which mediates platelet adhesion is not collagen. *Thromb Haemost* **58:**213, 1987.
107. Colombatti A, Bonaldo P: The superfamily of proteins with von Willebrand factor type A-like domains: One theme common to components of extracellular matrix, hemostasis, cellular adhesion, and defense mechanisms. *Blood* **77:**2305, 1991.
108. Rand JH, Patel ND, Schwartz E, Zhou S-L, Potter BJ: 150-kD von Willebrand factor binding protein extracted from human vascular subendothelium is type VI collagen. *J Clin Invest* **88:**253, 1991.
109. von der Mark H, Aumailley M, Wick G, Fleischmajer R, Timpl R: Immunochemistry, genuine size and tissue localization of collagen VI. *Eur J Biochem* **142:**493, 1984.
110. Colombatti A, Bonaldo P: Biosynthesis of chick type VI collagen. II. Processing and secretion in fibroblasts and smooth muscle cells. *J Biol Chem* **262:**14461, 1987.
111. Takagi J, Fujisawa T, Sekiya F, Saito Y: Collagen-binding domain within bovine propolypeptide of von Willebrand factor. *J Biol Chem* **266:**5575, 1991.
112. Nurden AT, Caen JP: Specific roles for platelet surface glycoproteins in platelet function. *Nature* **255:**720, 1975.
113. Nurden AT, Dupuis D, Kunicki TJ, Caen JP: Analysis of the glycoprotein and protein composition of Bernard-Soulier platelets by single and two-dimensional SDS-polyacrylamide gel electrophoresis. *J Clin Invest* **67:**1431, 1981.
114. Weiss HJ, Tschopp TB, Baumgartner HR, Sussman II, Johnson MM, Egan JJ: Decreased adhesion of giant (Bernard-Soulier) platelets to subendothelium: Further implication on the role of the von Willebrand factor in hemostasis. *Am J Med* **57:**920, 1974.
115. Sakariassen KS, Nievelstein PFEM, Coller BS, Sixma JJ: The role of platelet membrane glycoproteins Ib and IIb-IIIa in platelet adherence to human artery subendothelium. *Br J Haematol* **63:**681, 1986.
116. Caen JP, Nurden AT, Jeanneau C, Michel H, Tobelem G, Levy-Toledano S, Sultan Y, Valensi F, Bernard J: Bernard-Soulier syndrome: A new platelet glycoprotein abnormality. Its relationship with platelet adhesion to subendothelium and with the factor VIII/von Willebrand protein. *J Lab Clin Med* **87:**586, 1976.
117. Jenkins CSP, Phillips DR, Clemetson KJ, Meyer D, Larrieu MJ, Luscher EF: Platelet membrane glycoproteins implicated in ristocetin-induced aggregation. Studies on the proteins on platelets from patients with Bernard-Soulier syndrome and von Willebrand's disease. *J Clin Invest* **57:**112, 1976.
118. MacFarlane DE, Zucker MB: A method for assaying von Willebrand factor (ristocetin cofactor). *Thromb Diath Haemorrh* **34:**306, 1975.
119. Allain JP, Cooper HA, Wagner RM, Brinkhous KM: Platelets fixed with paraformaldehyde: A new reagent for assay of von Willebrand factor and platelet aggregation factor. *J Lab Clin Med* **85:**318, 1975.
120. Moake JL, Olson JD, Troll JH, Tang SS, Funicella T, Peterson DM: Binding of radioiodinated human von Willebrand factor to Bernard-Soulier, thrombasthenic and von Willebrand's disease platelets. *Thromb Res* **19:**21, 1980.
121. Coller BS, Peerschke EI, Scudder LE, Sullivan CA: Studies with a murine monoclonal antibody that abolishes ristocetin-induced binding of von Willebrand factor to platelets: Additional evidence in support of GPIb as a platelet receptor for von Willebrand factor. *Blood* **61:**99, 1983.
122. Ruggeri ZM, De Marco L, Gatti L, Bader R, Montgomery RR: Platelets have more than one binding site for von Willebrand factor. *J Clin Invest* **72:**1, 1983.
123. Marguerie GA, Plow EF, Edgington TS: Human platelets possess an inducible and saturable receptor specific for fibrinogen. *J Biol Chem* **254:**5357, 1979.
124. Coller BS, Peerschke EI, Scudder LE, Sullivan CA: A murine monoclonal antibody that completely blocks the binding of fibrinogen to platelets produces a thrombasthenic-like state in normal platelets and binds to glycoproteins IIb and/or IIIa. *J Clin Invest* **72:**325, 1983.
125. Bennett JS, Hoxie JA, Leitman SF, Vilaire G, Cines DB: Inhibition of fibrinogen binding to stimulated human platelets by a monoclonal antibody. *Proc Natl Acad Sci USA* **80:**2417, 1983.
126. Plow EF, Ginsberg MH: Specific and saturable binding of plasma fibronectin to thrombin-stimulated human platelets. *J Biol Chem* **256:**9477, 1981.
127. Fujimoto T, Ohara S, Hawiger J: Thrombin-induced exposure and prostacyclin inhibition of the receptor for factor VIII/von Willebrand factor on human platelets. *J Clin Invest* **69:**1212, 1982.
128. Plow EF, Srouji AH, Meyer D, Marguerie G, Ginsberg MH: Evidence that three adhesive proteins interact with a common recognition site on activated platelets. *J Biol Chem* **259:**5388, 1984.
129. Kloczewiak M, Timons S, Lukas TJ, Hawiger J: Platelet receptor recognition site on human fibrinogen. Synthesis and structure-function relationship of peptides corresponding to the carboxy-terminal segment of the γ-chain. *Biochemistry* **23**:1767, 1984.
130. Ruggeri ZM, Bader R, De Marco L: Glanzmann thrombasthenia: Deficient binding of von Willebrand factor to thrombin-stimulated platelets. *Proc Natl Acad Sci USA* **79**:6038, 1982.
131. Kao K-J, Pizzo SV, McKee PA: Demonstration and characterization of specific binding sites for factor VIII/von Willebrand factor on human platelets. *J Clin Invest* **63**:656, 1979.
132. Schullek J, Jordan J, Montgomery RR: Interaction of von Willebrand factor with human platelets in the plasma milieu. *J Clin Invest* **73**:421, 1984.
133. Gralnick HR, Williams SB, Coller BS: Fibrinogen competes with von Willebrand factor for binding to the glycoprotein IIb/IIIa complex when platelets are stimulated with thrombin. *Blood* **64**:797, 1984.
134. Piétu G, Cherel G, Marguerie G, Meyer D: Inhibition of von Willebrand factor-platelet interaction by fibrinogen. *Nature* **308**:648, 1984.
135. De Marco L, Girolami A, Zimmerman TS, Ruggeri ZM: von Willebrand factor interaction with the glycoprotein IIb/IIIa complex. Its role in platelet function as demonstrated in patients with congenital afibrinogenemia. *J Clin Invest* **77**:1272, 1986.
136. Santoro SA, Cowan JF: Thrombin enhanced adhesion of platelets to von Willebrand factor substrates. *Thromb Res* **43**:57, 1986.
137. Fressinaud E, Baruch D, Girma J-P, Sakariassen KS, Baumgartner HR, Meyer D: von Willebrand factor-mediated platelet adhesion to collagen involves platelet membrane glycoprotein IIb-IIIa as well as glycoprotein Ib. *J Lab Clin Med* **112**:58, 1988.
138. Fressinaud E, Girma J-P, Sadler JE, Baumgartner HR, Meyer D: Synthetic RGDS-containing peptides of von Willebrand factor inhibit platelet adhesion to collagen. *Thromb Haemost* **64**:589, 1990.
139. Vermylen J, de Gaetano G, Donati MB, Verstraete M: Platelet-aggregating activity in neuraminidase-treated human cryoprecipitates: Its correlation with factor-VIII-related antigen. *Br J Haematol* **26**:645, 1974.
140. Vermylen J, Bottecchia D, Szpilman H: Factor VIII and human platelet aggregation. III. Further studies on aggregation of human platelets by neuraminidase-treated human factor VIII. *Br J Haematol* **34**:321, 1976.

141. De Marco L, Shapiro SS: Properties of human asialo-factor VIII. A ristocetin-independent platelet-aggregating agent. *J Clin Invest* **68**:321, 1981.
142. De Marco L, Girolami A, Russell S, Ruggeri ZM: Interaction of asialo von Willebrand factor with glycoprotein Ib induces fibrinogen binding to the glycoprotein IIb/IIIa complex and mediates platelet aggregation. *J Clin Invest* **75**:1198, 1985.
143. Williams SB, McKeown LP, Gralnick HR: Asialo von Willebrand factor binding to and aggregation of platelets: Effects of inhibitors of platelet metabolism and function. *J Lab Clin Med* **109**:560, 1987.
144. Kroll MH, Harris TS, Moake JL, Handin RI, Schafer AI: von Willebrand factor binding to platelet GpIb initiates signals for platelet activation. *J Clin Invest* **88**:1568, 1991.
145. Cooper HA, Reisner FF, Hall M, Wagner RH: Effects of thrombin treatment on preparations of factor VIII and the Ca^{2+}-dissociated small active fragment. *J Clin Invest* **56**:751, 1975.
146. Hamer RJ, Koedam JA, Beeser-Visser NH, Bertina RM, Van Mourik JA, Sixma JJ: Factor VIII binds to von Willebrand factor via its Mr-80,000 light chain. *Eur J Biochem* **166**:37, 1987.
147. Madaras F, Bell WR, Castaldi PA: Isolation and insolubilisation of human F VIII by affinity chromatography. *Haemostasis* **7**:321, 1978.
148. Fowler WE, Fretto LJ, Hamilton KK, Erickson HP, McKee PA: Substructure of human von Willebrand factor. *J Clin Invest* **76**:1491, 1985.
149. Roberts DD, Williams SB, Gralnick HR, Ginsburg V: von Willebrand factor binds specifically to sulfated glycolipids. *J Biol Chem* **261**:3306, 1986.
150. Christophe O, Obert B, Meyer D, Girma J-P: The binding domain of von Willebrand factor to sulfatides is distinct from those interacting with glycoprotein Ib, heparin, and collagen and resides between amino acid residues Leu 512 and Lys 673. *Blood* **78**:2310, 1991.
151. Martin SE, Marder VJ, Francis CW, Barlow GH: Structural studies on the functional heterogeneity of von Willebrand protein polymers. *Blood* **57**:313, 1981.
152. Aihara M, Kimura A, Chiba Y, Yoshida Y: Plasma collagen cofactor correlates with von Willebrand factor antigen and ristocetin cofactor but not with bleeding time. *Thromb Haemost* **59**:485, 1988.
153. Sixma JJ, Sakariassen KS, Beeser-Visser NH, Ottenhof-Rovers M, Bolhuis PA: Adhesion of platelets to human artery subendothelium: Effect of factor VIII-von Willebrand factor of various multimeric composition. *Blood* **63**:128, 1984.
154. Mohri H, Fujimura Y, Shuima M, Yoshioka A, Houghten RA, Ruggeri ZM, Zimmerman TS: Structure of the von Willebrand factor domain interacting with glycoprotein Ib. *J Biol Chem* **263**:17901, 1988.
155. Pareti FI, Fujimura Y, Dent JA, Holland LZ, Zimmerman TS, Ruggeri ZM: Isolation and characterization of a collagen binding domain in human von Willebrand factor. *J Biol Chem* **261**:15310, 1986.
156. Fujimura Y, Titani K, Holland LZ, Roberts JR, Kostel P, Ruggeri ZM, Zimmerman TS: A heparin-binding domain of human von Willebrand factor. Characterization and localization to a tryptic fragment extending from amino acid residue Val-449 to Lys-728. *J Biol Chem* **262**:1734, 1987.
157. Roth GJ, Titani K, Hoyer LW, Hickey MJ: Localization of binding sites within human von Willebrand factor for monomeric type III collagen. *Biochemistry* **25**:8357, 1986.
158. Fretto LJ, Fowler WE, McCaslin DR, Erickson HP, McKee PA: Substructure of human von Willebrand factor. Proteolysis by V8 and characterization of two functional domains. *J Biol Chem* **261**:15679, 1986.
159. Foster PA, Fulcher CA, Marti T, Titani K, Zimmerman TS: A major factor VIII binding domain resides within the amino-terminal 272 amino acid residues of von Willebrand factor. *J Biol Chem* **262**:8443, 1987.
160. Beacham DA, Wise RJ, Turci SM, Handin RI: Selective inactivation of the Arg-Gly-Asp-Ser (RGDS) binding site in von Willebrand factor by site-directed mutagenesis. *J Biol Chem* **267**:3409, 1992.
161. Berliner S, Niiya K, Roberts JR, Houghten RA, Ruggeri ZM: Generation and characterization of peptide-specific antibodies that inhibit von Willebrand factor binding to glycoprotein IIb-IIIa without interacting with other adhesive molecules. Selectivity is conferred by Pro^{1743} and other amino acid residues adjacent to the sequence Arg^{1744}-Gly^{1745}-Asp^{1746}. *J Biol Chem* **263**:7500, 1988.
162. Plow EF, Pierschbacher MD, Ruoslahti E, Marguerie GA, Ginsberg MH: The effect of Arg-Gly-Asp-containing peptides on fibrinogen and von Willebrand factor binding to platelets. *Proc Natl Acad Sci USA* **82**:8057, 1985.
163. Ruoslahti E, Pierschbacher MD: New perspectives in cell adhesion: RGD and integrins. *Science* **238**:491, 1987.
164. Federici AB, Elder JH, De Marco L, Ruggeri ZM, Zimmerman TS: Carbohydrate moiety of von Willebrand factor is not necessary for maintaining multimeric structure and ristocetin cofactor activity but protects from proteolytic degradation. *J Clin Invest* **74**:2049, 1984.
165. Sodetz JM, Pizzo SV, McKee PA: Relationship of sialic acid to function and in vivo survival of human factor VIII/von Willebrand factor protein. *J Biol Chem* **252**:5538, 1977.
166. Sorace JM, Shelton-Inloes BB, Sadler JE: Isolation and characterization of genomic clones for human von Willebrand factor (vWF). *Fed Proc* **45**:1639, 1986.
167. Collins CJ, Underdahl JP, Levene RB, Ravera CP, Morin MJ, Dombalagian MJ, Ricca G, Livingston DM, Lynch DC: Molecular cloning of the human gene for von Willebrand factor and identification of the transcription initiation site. *Proc Natl Acad Sci USA* **84**:4393, 1987.
168. Mancuso DJ, Tuley EA, Westfield LA, Worrall NK, Shelton-Inloes BB, Sorace JM, Alevy YG, Sadler JE: Structure of the gene for human von Willebrand factor. *J Biol Chem* **264**:19514, 1989.
169. O'Connell P, Lathrop GM, Law M, Leppert M, Nakamura Y, Hoff M, Kumlin E, Thomas W, Elsner T, Ballard L, Goodman P, Azen E, Sadler JE, Lai GY, Lalouel J-M, White R: A primary genetic linkage map for human chromosome 12. *Genomics* **1**:93, 1987.
170. Shelton-Inloes BB, Chehab FF, Mannucci PM, Federici AB, Sadler JE: Gene deletions correlate with the development of alloantibodies in von Willebrand disease. *J Clin Invest* **79**:1459, 1987.
171. Mancuso DJ, Tuley EA, Westfield LA, Lester-Mancuso TL, Le Beau MM, Sorace JM, Sadler JE: Human von Willebrand factor gene and pseudogene: Structural analysis and differentiation by polymerase chain reaction. *Biochemistry* **30**:253, 1991.
172. Yamagata M, Yamada KM, Yamada SS, Shinomura T, Tanaka H, Nishida Y, Obara M, Kimata K: The complete primary structure of type XII collagen shows a chimeric molecular with reiterated fibronectin type III motifs, von Willebrand factor A motifs, a domain homologous to a noncollagenous region of type IX collagen, and short collagenous domains with an Arg-Gly-Asp-site. *J Cell Biol* **115**:209, 1991.
173. Just M, Herbst H, Hummel M, Dürkop H, Tripier D, Stein H, Schuppan D: Undulin is a novel member of the fibronectin-tenascin family of extracellular matrix glycoproteins. *J Biol Chem* **266**:17326, 1991.
174. Lawler J, Hynes RO: The structure of human thrombospondin, an adhesive glycoprotein with multiple calcium-binding sites and homologies with several different proteins. *J Cell Biol* **103**:1635, 1986.
175. Chu M-L, De Wet W, Bernard M, Ding J-F, Morabito M, Meyers J, Williams C, Ramirez F: Human proα1(I) collagen gene structure reveals evolutionary conservation of a pattern of introns and exons. *Nature* **310**:337, 1984.
176. Yamada Y, Liau G, Mudryj M, Obici S, De Crombrugghe B: Conservation of the sizes for one but not another class of exons in two chick collagen genes. *Nature* **310**:333, 1984.
177. Hunt LT, Barker WC: von Willebrand factor shares a distinctive cysteine-rich domain with thrombospondin and procollagen. *Biochem Biophys Res Commun* **144**:876, 1987.
178. Probst JC, Gertzen E-M, Hoffmann W: An integumentary mucin (FIM-B.1) from *Xenopus laevis* homologous with von Willebrand factor. *Biochemistry* **29**:6240, 1990.

179. Silwer J: von Willebrand's disease in Sweden. *Acta Paediatr Scand Suppl.* **238**:5, 1973.
180. Bloom AL, Peake IR: Apparent 'dominant' and 'recessive' inheritance of von Willebrand's disease within the same kindreds. Possible biochemical mechanisms. *Thromb Res* **15**:505, 1979.
181. Miller CH, Graham JB, Goldin LR, Elston RC: Genetics of classic von Willebrand's disease. I. Phenotypic variation within families. *Blood* **54**:117, 1979.
182. Hoyer LW: The assessment of von Willebrand's disease, in Bloom AL (ed): *The Hemophilias*. Edinburgh, Churchill Livingstone, 1982, pp 106–121.
183. Zimmerman TS, Roberts JR, Ruggeri ZM: Factor VIII-related antigen: Characterization by electrophoretic techniques, in Bloom AL (ed): *The Hemophilias*. Edinburgh, Churchill Livingstone, 1982, pp 81–91.
184. Read MS, Shermer RW, Brinkhous KM: Venom coagglutinin: An activator of platelet aggregation dependent on von Willebrand factor. *Proc Natl Acad Sci USA* **75**:4514, 1978.
185. Brinkhous KM, Read MS: Use of venom coagglutinin and lyophilized platelets in testing for platelet-aggregating von Willebrand factor. *Blood* **55**:517, 1980.
186. Weiss HJ, Piétu G, Rabinowitz R, Girma JP, Rogers J, Meyer D: Heterogeneous abnormalities in the multimeric structure, antigenic properties, and plasma-platelet content of factor VIII/von Willebrand factor in subtypes of classic (type I) and variant (type IIA) von Willebrand's disease. *J Lab Clin Med* **101**:411, 1983.
187. Mannucci PM, Lombardi R, Bader R, Vianello L, Federici AB, Solinas S, Mazzucconi MG, Mariani G: Heterogeneity of type I von Willebrand disease: Evidence for a subgroup with an abnormal von Willebrand factor. *Blood* **66**:796, 1985.
188. Hanna WT, Slywka J, Dent J, Ruggeri ZM, Zimmerman TS: Case report: 1-Deamino-8-D-Arginine vasopressin and cryoprecipitate in variant von Willebrand disease. *Am J Hematol* **20**:169, 1985.
189. Gralnick HR, Williams SB, McKeown LP, Rick ME, Maisonneuve P, Jenneau C, Sultan Y: DDAVP in type IIA von Willebrand's disease. *Blood* **67**:465, 1986.
190. Holmberg L, Nilsson IM: von Willebrand disease. *Clin Haematol* **14**:461, 1985.
191. Mannucci PM, Bloom AL, Larrieu MJ, Nilsson IM, West RR: Atherosclerosis and von Willebrand factor. I. Prevalence of severe von Willebrand's disease in western Europe and Israel. *Br J Haematol* **57**:163, 1984.
192. Berliner SA, Seligsohn U, Zivelin A, Zwang E, Sofferman G: A relatively high frequency of severe (type III) von Willebrand's disease in Israel. *Br J Haematol* **62**:535, 1986.
192a. Sadler JE: A revised classification of von Willebrand disease. *Thromb Haemost* **71**:520, 1994.
193. Ginsburg D, Sadler JE: von Willebrand disease: A database of point mutations, insertions, and deletions. *Thromb Haemost* **69**:177, 1993.
194. Ruggeri ZM: Structure and function of von Willebrand factor: Relationship to von Willebrand's disease. *Mayo Clin Proc* **66**:847, 1991.
195. Lopez-Fernandez MF, Gonzalez-Boullosa R, Blanco-Lopez MJ, Batlle J: Abnormal proteolytic degradation of von Willebrand factor after desmopressin infusion in a new subtype of von Willebrand disease (ID). *Am J Hematol* **36**:163, 1991.
196. Castaman G, Rodeghiero F, Lattuada A, Mannucci PM: A new variant of von Willebrand disease (type II I) with a normal degree of proteolytic cleavage of von Willebrand factor. *Thromb Res* **65**:343, 1992.
197. Hoyer LW, Rizza CR, Tuddenham EG, Cara CA, Armitage H, Rotblat F: von Willebrand factor multimer patterns in von Willebrand's disease. *Br J Haematol* **55**:493, 1983.
198. Ciavarella G, Ciavarella N, Antoncecchi S, De Mattia D, Ranieri P, Dent J, Zimmerman TS, Ruggeri ZM: High-resolution analysis of von Willebrand factor multimeric composition defines a new variant of type I von Willebrand disease with aberrant structure but presence of all size multimers (type IC). *Blood* **66**:1423, 1985.
199. Tavori S, Tatarsky I: Additional variant of type I von Willebrand disease. *Am J Hematol* **24**:189, 1987.
200. Weiss HJ, Sussman II: A new von Willebrand variant (Type I, New York): Increased ristocetin-induced platelet aggregation and plasma von Willebrand factor containing the full range of multimers. *Blood* **68**:149, 1986.
201. Holmberg L, Berntorp, Donnér M, Nilsson IM: von Willebrand's disease characterized by increased ristocetin sensitivity and the presence of all von Willebrand factor multimers in plasma. *Blood* **68**:668, 1986.
202. Montgomery RR, Dent J, Schmidt W, Kyrle P, Hiessner H, Ruggeri ZM, Zimmerman TS: Hereditary persistence of circulating pro von Willebrand factor (pro-vWF). *Circulation (suppl II)* **74**:406, 1986.
203. Mannucci PM, Lombardi R, Castman G, Dent JA, Lattuada A, Rodeghiero F, Zimmerman TS: von Willebrand disease "Vicenza" with larger-than-normal (supranormal) von Willebrand factor multimers. *Blood* **71**:65, 1988.
204. Mancuso DJ, Adam PA, Kroner PA, Montgomery RR: The molecular basis of a type I von Willebrand disease variant. *Circulation (suppl II)* **84**:418, 1991.
205. Mancuso DJ, Montgomery RR, Adam P: The identification of a candidate mutation in the von Willebrand factor gene of patients with a variant form of type I von Willebrand disease. *Blood (suppl 1)* **78**:67a, 1991.
206. Girma JP, Piétu G, Lavergne JM, Meyer D, Larrieu MJ: Abnormal antigenic reactivity of factor VIII/von Willebrand factor subunit in variants of von Willebrand's disease. *J Lab Clin Med* **99**:481, 1982.
207. Gralnick HR, Williams SB, McKeown LP, Maisonneuve P, Jenneau C, Sultan Y, Rick ME: In vitro correction of the abnormal multimeric structure of vWF in type IIA vWD. *Proc Natl Acad Sci USA* **82**:5968, 1985.
208. Batlle J, Lopez Fernandez MF, Campos M, Justica B, Berges C, Navarro JL, Diaz Cremades JM, Kasper CK, Dent JA, Ruggeri ZM, Zimmerman TS: The heterogeneity of type IIA von Willebrand's disease: Studies with protease inhibitors. *Blood* **68**:1207, 1986.
209. Ruggeri ZM, Mannucci PM, Lombardi R, Federici AB, Zimmerman TS: Multimeric composition of factor VIII/von Willebrand factor following administration of DDAVP: Implications for pathophysiology and therapy of von Willebrand's disease subtypes. *Blood* **59**:1272, 1982.
210. Lyons SE, Bruck ME, Bowie EJW, Ginsburg D: Impaired intracellular transport produced by a subset of type IIA von Willebrand disease mutations. *J Biol Chem* **267**:4424, 1992.
211. Dent JA, Berkowitz SD, Ware J, Kasper CK, Ruggeri ZM: Identification of a cleavage site directing the immunochemical detection of molecular abnormalities in type IIA von Willebrand factor. *Proc Natl Acad Sci USA* **87**:6306, 1990.
212. Ruggeri ZM, Pareti FI, Mannucci PM, Ciavarella N, Zimmerman TS: Heightened interaction between platelets and factor VIII/von Willebrand factor in a new subtype of von Willebrand's disease. *N Engl J Med* **302**:1047, 1980.
213. Holmberg L, Nilsson IM, Borge L, Bunnarsson M, Sjorin E: Platelet aggregation induced by 1-desamino-8-D-arginine vasopressin (DDAVP) in type IIB von Willebrand's disease. *N Engl J Med* **309**:816, 1983.
214. Saba HI, Saba SR, Dent J, Ruggeri ZM, Zimmerman TS: Type IIB Tampa: A variant of von Willebrand disease with chronic thrombocytopenia, circulating platelet aggregates, and spontaneous platelet aggregation. *Blood* **66**:282, 1985.
215. Gralnick HR, Williams SB, McKeown LP, Rick ME, Maisonneuve P, Jenneau C, Sultan Y: von Willebrand's disease with spontaneous platelet aggregation induced by an abnormal plasma von Willebrand factor. *J Clin Invest* **76**:1522, 1985.
216. Federici AB, Mannucci PM, Bader R, Lombardi R, Lattuada A: Heterogeneity in type IIB von Willebrand disease: Two unrelated cases with no family history and mild abnormalities of ristocetin-induced interaction between von Willebrand factor and platelets. *Am J Hematol* **23**:381, 1986.
217. Donnér M, Holmberg L, Nilsson IM: Type IIB von Willebrand's disease with probable autosomal recessive inheritance and presenting as thrombocytopenia in infancy. *Br J Haematol* **66**:349, 1987.
218. Sugimoto M, Mohri H, McClintock RA, Ruggeri ZM: Identification of discontinuous von Willebrand factor sequences involved in complex formation with botrocetin. A model for

the regulation of von Willebrand factor binding to platelet glycoprotein Ib. *J Biol Chem* **266**:18172, 1991.

219. Nishino M, Girma J-P, Rothschild C, Fressinaud E, Meyer D: New variant of von Willebrand disease with defective binding to factor VIII. *Blood* **74**:1591, 1989.
220. Mazurier C, Dieval J, Jorieux S, Delobel J, Goudemand M: A new von Willebrand factor (vWF) defect in a patient with factor VIII (FVIII) deficiency but with normal levels and multimeric patterns of both plasma and platelet vWF. Characterization of abnormal vWF/FVIII interaction. *Blood* **75**:20, 1990.
221. Mazurier C, Gaucher C, Jorieux S, Parquet-Gernez A, Goudemand M: Evidence for a von Willebrand factor defect in factor VIII binding in three members of a family previously misdiagnosed mild haemophilia A and haemophilia A carriers: Consequences for therapy and genetic counselling. *Br J Haematol* **76**:372, 1990.
222. Ruggeri ZM, Nilsson IM, Lombardi R, Holmberg L, Zimmerman TS: Aberrant multimeric structure of von Willebrand factor in a new variant of von Willebrand's disease (type IIC). *J Clin Invest* **70**:1124, 1982.
223. Mannucci PM, Lombardi R. Pareti FI, Solinas S, Mazzucconi MG, Mariani G: A variant of von Willebrand's disease characterized by recessive inheritance and missing triplet structure of von Willebrand factor multimers. *Blood* **62**:1000, 1983.
224. Batlle J, Lopez Fernandez MF, Lasierra J, Fernandez Villamor A, Lopez Berges C, Lopez Borrasca A, Ruggeri ZM, Zimmerman TS: von Willebrand disease type IIC with different abnormalities of von Willebrand factor in the same sibship. *Am J Hematol* **21**:177, 1986.
225. Batlle J, Lopez Fernandez MF, Fernandez Villamor A, Lopez Berges C, Zimmerman TS: Multimeric pattern discrepancy between platelet and plasma von Willebrand factor in type IIC von Willebrand disease. *Am J Hematol* **22**:87, 1986.
226. Mazurier C, Mannucci PM, Parquet-Gernez A, Goudemand M, Meyer D: Investigation of a case of subtype IIC von Willebrand disease: Characterization of the variability of this subtype. *Am J Hematol* **22**:301, 1986.
227. Kinoshita S, Harrison J, Lazerson J, Abildgaard CF: A new variant of dominant type II von Willebrand's disease with aberrant multimeric pattern of factor VIII-related antigen (type IID). *Blood* **63**:1369, 1984.
228. Hill FGH, Enayat MS, George AJ: Investigation of a kindred with a new autosomal dominantly inherited variant type von Willebrand's disease (possible type IID). *J Clin Pathol* **38**:665, 1985.
229. Triplett D, Musgrave K, Daniels T, Bowie EJW: Identification and further characterization of type IIE von Willebrand disease. *Thromb Haemost* **58**:360, 1987.
230. Mannucci PM, Lombardi R, Federici AB, Dent JA, Zimmerman TS, Ruggeri ZM: A new variant of type II von Willebrand disease with aberrant multimeric structure of plasma but not platelet von Willebrand factor (type IIF). *Blood* **68**:269, 1986.
231. Gralnick HR, Williams SB, McKeown LP, Maisonneuve P, Jenneau C, Sultan Y: A variant of type II von Willebrand disease with an abnormal triplet structure and discordant effects of protease inhibitors on plasma and platelet von Willebrand factor structure. *Am J Hematol* **24**:259, 1987.
232. Mannucci PM, Lombardi R, Lattuada A, Muleo G, Federici AB: High resolution multimeric analysis identifies a new variant of type II von Willebrand's disease (type IIH) inherited in an autosomal recessive manner. *Ric Clin Lab* **62**:237a, 1986.
233. Howard MA, Salem HH, Thomas KB, Hau L, Perkin J, Coghlan M, Firkin BG: Variant von Willebrand's disease type B—Revisited. *Blood* **60**:1420, 1982.
234. Italian Working Group: Spectrum of von Willebrand's disease: A study of 100 cases. *Br J Haematol* **35**:101, 1977.
235. Zimmerman TS, Abildgaard CF, Meyer D: The factor VIII abnormality in severe von Willebrand's disease. *N Engl J Med* **301**:1307, 1979.
236. Peake IR, Bloom AL, Giddings JC, Ludlam CA: An immunoradiometric assay for procoagulant factor VIII antigen: Results in haemophilia, von Willebrand's disease and fetal plasma and serum. *Br J Haematol* **42**:269, 1979.
237. Ngo KY, Glotz T, Koziol JA, Lynch D, Gitscher J, Ranieri P, Ciavarella N, Ruggeri ZM, Zimmerman TS: Homozygous and heterozygous deletions of the von Willebrand factor gene in patients and carriers of severe von Willebrand disease. *Proc Natl Acad Sci USA* **85**:2753, 1988.
238. Peake IR, Liddell MB, Moodie P, Standen G, Mancuso DJ, Tuley EA, Westfield LA, Sorace JM, Sadler JE, Verweij CL, Bloom AL: Severe type III von Willebrand's disease caused by deletion of exon 42 of the von Willebrand factor gene: Family studies that identify carriers of the condition and a compound heterozygous individual. *Blood* **75**:654, 1990.
239. Giannelli F, Choo KH, Rees DJG, Boyd Y, Rizza CR, Brownlee GG: Gene deletions in patients with haemophilia B and anti-factor IX antibodies. *Nature* **303**:181, 1983.
240. Matthews RJ, Anson DS, Peake IR, Bloom AL: Heterogeneity of the factor IX locus in nine hemophilia B inhibitor patients. *J Clin Invest* **79**:746, 1987.
241. Bahnak BR, Lavergne J-M, Rothschild C, Meyer D: A stop codon in a patient with severe type III von Willebrand disease. *Blood* **78**:1148, 1991.
242. Eikenboom JCJ, Briët E, Reitsma PH, Ploos van Amstel HK: Severe type III von Willebrand's disease in the Dutch population is often associated with the absence of von Willebrand factor messenger RNA. *Thromb Haemost* **65**:1127, 1991.
243. Zhang ZP, Falk G, Blombäck M, Egberg N, Anvret M: Identification of a new nonsense mutation in the von Willebrand factor gene in patients with von Willebrand disease type III. *Hum Mol Genet* **1**:61, 1992.
244. Barker D, Schafer M, White R: Restriction sites containing CpG show a higher frequency of polymorphism in human DNA. *Cell* **36**:131, 1984.
245. Straus HS, Diamond LK: Elevation of factor VIII (antihemophilic factor) during pregnancy in normal persons and in a patient with von Willebrand's disease. *N Engl J Med* **269**:1251, 1963.
246. Noller KL, Bowie EJW, Kempers RD, Owen CA: von Willebrand's disease in pregnancy. *Obstet Gynecol* **41**:865, 1973.
247. Bennett B, Oxnard SC, Douglas AS, Ratnoff OD: Studies on antihemophilic factor (AHF, factor VIII) during labor in normal women, in patients with premature separation of the placenta, and in a patient with von Willebrand's disease. *J Lab Clin Med* **84**:851, 1974.
248. Telfer MC, Chediak J: Factor-VIII-related disorders and their relationship to pregnancy. *J Reprod Med* **19**:211, 1977.
249. Rick ME, Williams SB, Sacher RA, McKeown LP: Thrombocytopenia associated with pregnancy in a patient with type IIB von Willebrand's disease. *Blood* **69**:786, 1987.
250. Mannucci PM, Mari D: Antibodies to factor VIII-von Willebrand factor in congenital and acquired von Willebrand's disease, in Hoyer LW (ed): *Factor VIII Inhibitors*. New York, Alan R. Liss, 1984, pp 109–122.
251. Kaneshiro MM, Mielke CH Jr, Kasper CK, Rapaport SI: Bleeding times after aspirin in disorders of intrinsic clotting. *N Engl J Med* **281**:1039, 1969.
252. Giles AR, Hoogendoorn H, Benford K: Type IIb von Willebrand's disease presenting as thrombocytopenia during pregnancy. *Br J Haematol* **67**:349, 1987.
253. Valster FAA, Feijen HLM, Hutten JWM: Severe thrombocytopenia in a pregnant patient with platelet-associated IgM and known von Willebrand's disease; a case report. *Eur J Obstet Gynecol Reprod Biol* **36**:197, 1990.
254. Ieko M, Sakurama S, Sagawa A, Yoshikawa M, Satoh M, Yasukouchi T, Nakagawa S: Effect of a factor VIII concentrate on type IIb von Willebrand's disease-associated thrombocytopenia presenting during pregnancy in identical twin mothers. *Am J Hematol* **35**:26, 1990.
255. Sakariassen KS, Nieuwenhuis HK, Sixma JJ: Differentiation of patients with subtype IIb-like von Willebrand's disease by means of perfusion experiments with reconstituted blood. *Br J Haematol* **59**:459, 1985.
256. Hultin MB, Sussman II: Postoperative thrombocytopenia in type IIB von Willebrand disease. *Am J Hematol* **33**:64, 1990.

257. Takahashi H: Studies on the pathophysiology and treatment of von Willebrand's disease. IV. Mechanism of increased ristocetin-induced platelet aggregation in von Willebrand's disease. *Thromb Res* **19:**857, 1980.
258. Miller JL, Castella A: Platelet-type von Willebrand's disease: Characterization of a new bleeding disorder. *Blood* **60:**790, 1982.
259. Weiss HJ, Meyer D, Rabinowitz R, Piétu G, Girma JP, Vicic WJ, Rogers J: Pseudo-von Willebrand's disease. An intrinsic platelet defect with aggregation by unmodified human factor VIII/von Willebrand factor and enhanced adsorption of its high-molecular-weight multimers. *N Engl J Med* **306:**326, 1982.
260. Takahashi H, Nagayama R, Hattori A, Shibata A: Platelet aggregation induced by DDAVP in platelet-type von Willebrand's disease. *N Engl J Med* **310:**722, 1984.
261. Miller JL, Kupinski JM, Castella A, Ruggeri ZM: von Willebrand factor binds to platelets and induces aggregation in platelet-type but not type IIB von Willebrand disease. *J Clin Invest* **72:**1532, 1983.
262. Miller JL, Cunningham D, Lyle VA, Finch CN: Mutation in the gene encoding the α chain of platelet glycoprotein Ib in platelet-type von Willebrand disease. *Proc Natl Acad Sci USA* **88:**4761, 1991.
263. Russell SD, Roth GJ: A mutation in the platelet glycoprotein (GP) Ib alpha gene associated with pseudo-von Willebrand disease. *Blood (suppl 1)* **78:**281a, 1991.
264. Mannucci PM, Moia M, Rebulla P, Altieri D, Monteagudo J, Castillo R: Correction of the bleeding time in treated patients with severe von Willebrand disease is not solely dependent on the normal multimeric structure of plasma von Willebrand factor. *Am J Hematol* **25:**55, 1987.
265. Blatt PM, Brinkhous KM, Culp HR, Krauss JS, Roberts HR: Antihemophilic factor concentrate therapy in von Willebrand's disease: Dissociation of bleeding time factor and ristocetin-cofactor activities. *JAMA* **236:**2770, 1976.
266. Green D, Potter EV: Failure of AHF concentrate to control bleeding in von Willebrand's disease. *Am J Med* **60:**357, 1976.
267. Berntorp E, Nilsson I-M: Use of a high-purity factor VIII concentrate (Hemate P) in von Willebrand's disease. *Vox Sang* **56:**212, 1989.
268. Cumming AM, Fildes S, Cumming IR, Wensley RT, Redding OM, Burn AM: Clinical and laboratory evaluation of National Health Service factor VIII concentrate (8Y) for the treatment of von Willebrand's disease. *Br J Haematol* **75:**234, 1990.
269. Mazurier C, Jorieux S, de Romeuf C, Samor B, Goudemand M: In vitro evaluation of a very-high purity, solvent/detergent-treated, von Willebrand factor concentrate. *Vox Sang* **61:**1, 1991.
270. Lawrie AS, Goubran HA, Harrison P, Holland LJ, Weston-Smith SG, Savidge GF: Comparison of factor VIII concentrates and vWF:THP for the treatment of von Willebrand's disease. *Thromb Haemost* **65:**1128, 1991.
271. Rothschild C, Fressinaud E, Wolf M, Dreyfus M, Laurian Y, Peynaud-Debayle E, Gazengel C, Meyer D, Larrieu MJ: Unexpected results following treatment of patients with von Willebrand disease with a new highly purified von Willebrand factor concentrate. *Thromb Haemost* **65:**1126, 1991.
272. Mannucci PM, Ruggeri ZM, Pareti FI, Capitano A: DDAVP, a new pharmacological approach to the management of haemophilia and von Willebrand's disease. *Lancet* **1:**869, 1977.
273. Mannucci PM, Canciani MT, Rota L, Donovan BS: Response of factor VIII/von Willebrand factor to DDAVP in healthy subjects and patients with haemophilia A and von Willebrand's disease. *Br J Haematol* **41:**437, 1979.
274. Theiss W, Schmidt G: DDAVP in von Willebrand's disease: Repeated administration and the behaviour of the bleeding time. *Thromb Res* **13:**1119, 1978.
275. Rodeghiero F, Castaman G, Mannucci PM: Clinical indications for desmopressin (DDAVP) in congenital and acquired von Willebrand disease. *Blood Rev* **5:**155, 1991.
276. De La Fuente B, Kasper CK, Rickles FR, Hoyer LW: Response of patients with mild and moderate hemophilia A and von Willebrand's disease to treatment with desmopressin. *Ann Intern Med* **103:**6, 1985.
277. Rodeghiero F, Castaman G, Di Bona E, Ruggeri M: Consistency of responses to DDAVP infusions in patients with von Willebrand's disease and hemophilia A. *Blood* **74:**1997, 1989.
278. López-Fernandez MF, Blanco-López MJ, Castiniera MP, Batlle J: Further evidence for recessive inheritance of von Willebrand disease with abnormal binding of von Willebrand factor to factor VIII. *Am J Hematol* **40:**20, 1993.
279. Fowler WE, Berkowitz LR, Roberts HR: DDAVP for type IIB von Willebrand disease. *Blood* **74:**1859, 1989.
280. Kyrle PA, Niessner H, Dent J, Panzer S, Brenner B, Zimmerman TS, Lechner K: IIB von Willebrand's disease: Pathogenetic and therapeutic studies. *Br J Haematol* **69:**55, 1988.
281. Glueck HI, Flessa HC: Control of hemorrhage in von Willebrand's disease and a hemophiliac carrier with norethynodrelmestranol. *Thromb Res* **1:**253, 1972.
282. Alperin JB: Estrogens and surgery in women with von Willebrand's disease. *Am J Med* **73:**367, 1982.
283. Hoyer LW, Lindsten J, Blombäck M, Hagenfeldt L, Cordesius E, Strömberg P, Gustavii B: Prenatal evaluation of fetus at risk for severe von Willebrand's disease. *Lancet* **2:**191, 1979.
284. Mibashan RS, Millar DS: Fetal haemophilia and allied bleeding disorders. *Br Med Bull* **39:**392, 1983.
285. Montgomery RR, Marlar RA, Gill JC: Newborn haemostasis. *Clin Haematol* **14:**443, 1985.
286. Sadler JE, Ginsburg D: A database of polymorphisms in the von Willebrand factor gene and pseudogene. *Thromb Haemost* **69:**185, 1993.
287. Mercier B, Gaucher C, Mazurier C: Characterization of 98 alleles in 105 unrelated individuals in the F8VWF gene. *Nucleic Acids Res* **19:**4800, 1991.
288. Peake IR, Bowen D, Bignell P, Liddell MB, Sadler JE, Standen G, Bloom AL: Family studies and prenatal diagnosis in severe von Willebrand disease by polymerase chain reaction amplification of a variable number tandem repeat region of the von Willebrand factor gene. *Blood* **76:**555, 1990.
289. Bignell P, Standen GR, Bowen DJ, Peake IR, Bloom AL: Rapid neonatal diagnosis of von Willebrand's disease by use of the polymerase chain reaction. *Lancet* **336:**638, 1990.
290. Mannhalter C, Kyrle PA, Brenner B, Lechner K: Rapid neonatal diagnosis of type IIB von Willebrand disease using the polymerase chain reaction. *Blood* **77:**2538, 1991.
291. Sadler JE: von Willebrand factor. *J Biol Chem* **266:**22777, 1991.
292. Sadler JE: von Willebrand disease, in Bloom AL, Forbes CD, Thomas DP, and Tuddenham EGD (eds): *Haemostasis and Thrombosis*. Edinburgh, Churchill Livingstone, 1994, pp. 843–857.

CHAPTER 108

Contact Activation and Factor XI

Uri Seligsohn ▪ John H. Griffin

1. The contact of blood with a variety of negatively charged surfaces triggers a series of interactions involving factor XII, prekallikrein (PK), high molecular weight kininogen (HK), and factor XI that lead to blood coagulation, fibrinolysis, and kinin generation. This phenomenon is known as contact activation.

2. Factor XI is the only protein among the aforementioned contact activation factors that is physiologically essential since its severe hereditary deficiency confers an injury-related bleeding tendency, whereas a severe hereditary deficiency of HK, PK, or factor XII is not associated with any clinical manifestations. One mechanism, in which factor XI is activated by thrombin, thereby bypassing the contact activation reactions, appears to clarify the variable phenotypic expressions of these coagulation factor deficiencies.

3. Factor XI deficiency is very common in Ashkenazic Jews with a gene frequency of 0.07, and some DNA studies have shown that two point mutations account for most of these cases. Homozygotes for these two mutations present different extents of bleeding manifestations and factor XI activity levels.

4. The amino acid sequences have been established and functional domains have been identified for all four contact factors. Factor XII, factor XI, and PK are zymogens with C-terminal domains that are characteristic of trypsin-like serine proteases and with N-terminal domains that contain functionally important binding sites. These binding sites are responsible for the recognition of factor IX by factor XIa, of factor XI and PK by HK, and of negative surfaces by factor XII. Factor XI is a homodimer with each subunit having extensive structural similarity to PK. Both factor XI and PK circulate as noncovalent complexes with HK, which is a nonenzymatic cofactor. HK is a multidomain protein of 110 kDa that contains bradykinin. HK also has two cysteine protease inhibitor domains, a cell-binding domain, one domain for binding to either factor XI or PK, and one domain for binding to negatively charged surfaces.

5. The contact activation reactions involve the activation of surface-bound factor XII and require the assembly of HK:PK and $(HK)_2$:XI complexes with factor XIIa at the surface. Kallikrein generated from PK by factor XIIa greatly amplifies factor XII activation, releases bradykinin from HK, and converts prourokinase to urokinase. Factor XIa generated from factor XI by factor XIIa activates factor IX to trigger subsequent blood coagulation reactions.

6. The regulation of the contact activation enzymes is accomplished by several plasma protease inhibitors, including C1 inhibitor, α_1-antitrypsin, α_2-macroglobulin, antithrombin III, and protein C inhibitor.

7. The genes for PK, HK, factor XII, and factor XI have been characterized and their chromosomal localizations identified. For hereditary deficiencies of each factor, a number of gene mutations has been described.

The contact of blood or plasma with a wide variety of negatively charged surfaces triggers a series of host defense reactions which involve the plasma proteins, factor XII, prekallikrein (PK), high molecular weight kininogen (HK), and factor XI. These "contact activation reactions," illustrated schematically in Fig. 108-1, lead to the initiation of blood coagulation,[1,2] fibrinolysis,[3] and kinin formation[4,5] through the generation of specific proteases. The recognition of four principal proteins responsible for contact activation followed the identification of patients with inherited deficiencies of each of them.[1,2,6-12]

During the past 20 years, the molecular interactions at the surface have been extensively studied, and considerable progress in defining the contact activation has been made (see Fig. 108-1). The characterization of the amino acid sequences of all four proteins and of their genes combined with the discovery of several inherited mutations in contact factors have provided the foundation for establishing the molecular basis for contact activation reactions. Contrasting with this advance in the description of molecules, genes, and protein–protein interactions is the incomplete understanding of the role of the contact activation reactions in normal physiology and in pathophysiology. Any attempt to assign to the contact activation system an essential in vivo function has so far appeared futile since patients with a severe hereditary deficiency of factor XII, PK, or HK do not present with any clinical manifestations. Conceivably, alternative physiological mechanisms compensate for the deficiency of these proteins. Surprisingly, very few clinical research studies have been carried out in patients deficient in factor XII, PK, and HK regarding more subtle dysfunctions of various physiological mechanisms, for example, the complement system and the prorenin–renin reaction. On the other hand, there is extensive literature implicating the contact factors in a wide variety of pathological conditions, but conclusive evidence for these implications remains to be presented. The liver is the major site of biosynthesis of factor XII, PK, factor XI, and HK. For reviews of the issues

A list of standard abbreviations is located immediately preceding the index in each volume. Additional abbreviations used in this chapter include: APTT = activated partial thromboplastin time; HK = high molecular weight kininogen; LK = low molecular weight kininogen; PAI-1 plasminogen activator inhibitor-1; PK = prekallikrein; PTA = plasma thromboplastin antecedent; proUK = prourokinase; U = units; UK = urokinase.

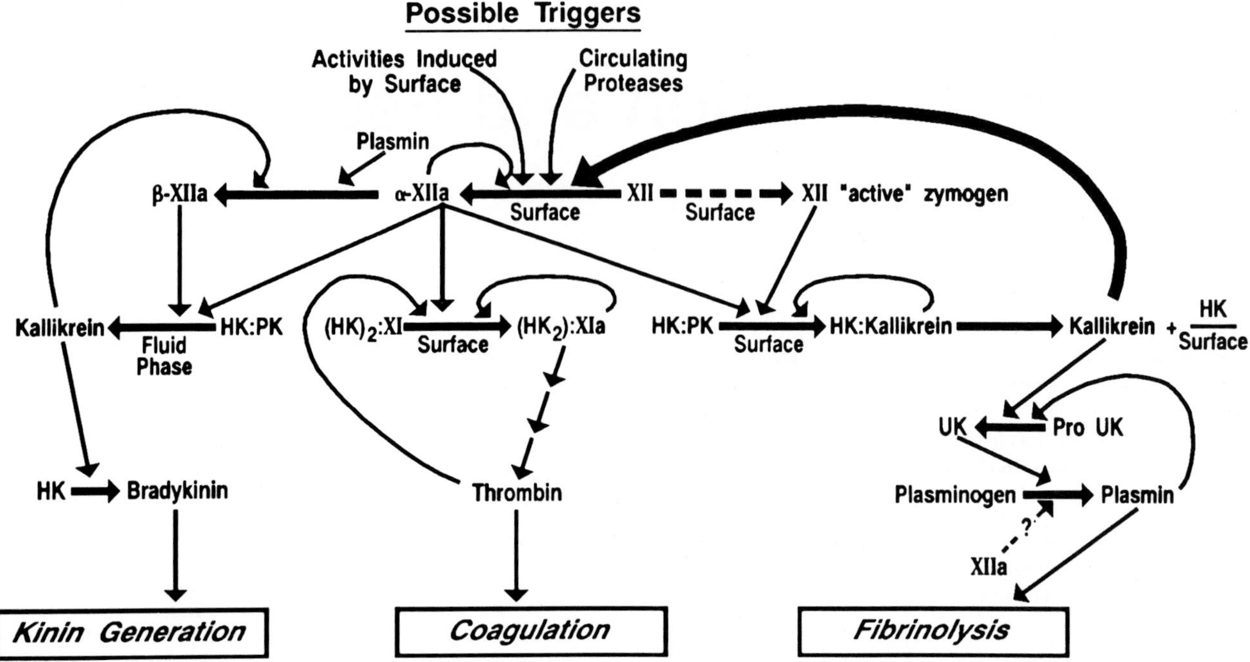

FIG. 108-1 Schematic diagram of the contact activation reactions in which negatively charged surfaces initiate the kinin formation, blood coagulation, and fibrinolytic pathways. A series of proteolytic activations of zymogens is shown; arrows indicate activation by cleavage or the release of bradykinin. Reciprocal proteolytic activation of factor XII by kallikrein and of PK by factor XIIa is a central theme. HK is a nonenzymatic cofactor that associates with PK giving a PK:HK complex and homodimeric factor XI giving XI:HK_2. Autoactivations of factor XII by factor XIIa, of PK by kallikrein, and of factor XI by factor XIa are indicated. Kinin formation is mediated by kallikrein and plasminogen activation by the conversion of proUK to UK. The cluster of consecutive arrows represents the several reactions of the intrinsic coagulation pathway that leads to thrombin generation (Chap. 104). The positive feedback activation of factor XI by thrombin provides a potential mechanism for factor XI activation that bypasses the surface-dependent contact factors, PK, factor XII, and HK. Broken lines represent reactions of questionable significance, that is, the surface-induced activation of factor XII and the activation of plasminogen by factor XIIa. See text for details.

that are not addressed in this chapter, the reader may consult other articles.[13-19]

Factor XI is exceptional among the contact factors. Unlike factor XII, PK, and HK, factor XI is physiologically essential for blood coagulation, as can be inferred from the injury-related bleeding tendency in patients with severe inherited factor XI deficiency, whereas there is no bleeding tendency in patients with severe hereditary deficiencies of factor XII, PK, or HK (see below). This apparent paradox has been possibly resolved by the demonstration of direct activation of factor XI by thrombin,[20,21] thereby bypassing the initial contact reactions which involve factor XII, PK, and HK (see Chap. 104). It remains possible that additional as yet unidentified activators of factor XI may also bypass the contact activation mechanism. Factor XI apparently has no obvious significant role in kinin generation or in the initiation of fibrinolysis.

In this chapter, special emphasis is given to new molecular and clinical data and especially to factor XI because of its clinical and physiological importance. This chapter does not generally cover hereditary deficiencies of contact factors in animals or studies of animal proteins or genes. Because of space limitations we do not cover many excellent biochemical studies of purified bovine contact factors (see Fujikawa and Saito[19]). Previous reviews may be consulted for additional information.[13-19,22-24]

CONTACT ACTIVATION REACTIONS

Exposure of blood or plasma to a variety of negatively charged materials initiates the contact activation reactions[1-5] depicted in Fig. 108-1. Coagulation factor XII is central to a number of surface-dependent reactions. Surface-bound factor XII is a serine protease zymogen that can be activated by limited proteolysis to a two-chain active enzyme designated α factor XIIa of 80 kDa. Enzymes capable of converting factor XII to α factor XIIa include plasma kallikrein, plasmin, trypsin, factor XIa, and possibly other as yet unidentified circulating proteases. The α factor XIIa converts the serine protease zymogens, prekallikrein or factor XI, to the active serine proteases, kallikrein or factor XIa, respectively (see Fig. 108-1). Subsequently, these two enzymes propagate the blood coagulation, kinin formation, and intrinsic fibrinolytic pathways.

Kallikrein is a potent kininogenase that liberates bradykinin from HK.[18,23,25] Kallikrein also converts prourokinase (proUK) to urokinase (UK) and thereby stimulates plasminogen activation.[26-29] Plasmin that is generated by UK is also an activator of proUK and participates in a positive feedback loop that generates intrinsic fibrinolytic activity.[29] Factor XIIa may also convert plasminogen to plasmin, although this reaction has not been shown to be potent.[30-32]

Factor XIa propagates the intrinsic blood coagulation pathway via the activation of factor IX, with subsequent activations of factor X and conversion of prothrombin to thrombin (see Chap. 104). In 1991, investigators at two laboratories demonstrated that thrombin can activate factor XI by limited proteolysis in the presence of negatively charged surfaces,[20,21] thus providing a positive feedback activation of factor XI by thrombin. Notably, the extrinsic coagulation pathway initiated by tissue factor may provide the thrombin which subsequently activates factor XI, thereby bypassing the contact activation mechanism for factor XI activation (see Chap. 104). This direct activation of factor XI by thrombin may be physiologically important, since patients with a severe deficiency of factor XI present with a bleeding tendency whereas those with severe deficiencies of factor XII, prekallikrein, or HK are not subject to a bleeding tendency (see below).

Contact activation reactions require HK as an essential nonenzymatic cofactor[8,9,11,25,33-36] (see Fig. 108-1). HK reversibly associates with PK and factor XI with high affinity, and HK has a strong affinity for negatively charged surfaces.[37-40] Biochemical studies using purified proteins demonstrated that HK is a cofactor for the activation of factor XI by surface-bound α factor XIIa, for the activation of PK by surface-bound α factor XIIa, and for the proteolytic activation of surface-bound factor XII by kallikrein or factor XIa.[34] In exerting these cofactor activities, HK is responsible for the binding of PK or factor XI to negatively charged surfaces, where α factor XIIa activates these zymogens,[39-44] and HK also binds kallikrein to surfaces, thereby facilitating proteolytic activation of factor XII.[41,45-48]

The normal mechanism for contact activation of factor XII involves reciprocal proteolytic activations of factor XII and prekallikrein as first proposed by Cochrane and his colleagues[49] and subsequently updated following the discovery of HK and its cofactor properties.[40,46,50-53] Nonetheless, other less potent mechanisms exist for factor XII activation in plasma since the defective coagulation of PK-deficient plasma undergoes autocorrection on prolonged incubation with contact activators such as kaolin.[54] Several speculations have been advanced for the source of the proteolytic activity that may trigger contact activation reactions through the activation of surface-bound factor XII. Autoactivation of factor XII by α factor XIIa may provide such a mechanism,[55-58] as might activation of surface-bound factor XII by other trace proteases in plasma. Interestingly, both prekallikrein and factor XI exhibit autoactivation on negatively charged surfaces when these purified proteins are incubated with themselves in the presence of a negatively charged surface.[20,21,59] Proteases derived from damaged tissue or cells such as basophils[60] or endothelial cells[61] may function in the capacity of triggering factor XII activation as suggested in Fig. 108-1. Surface-binding of factor XII might possibly convert the molecule to an enzymatically active form,[62] although a number of critical biochemical studies using purified factor XII failed to detect significant enzymatic activity for surface-bound factor XII[63,64] (and Griffin JH: unpublished results). Although surface binding per se does not induce significant amounts of activity in single-chain factor XII, it has been speculated that surface binding might alter factor XII so that it is capable of "substrate-induced activation" by PK or factor XI,[65,66] although this remains to be clearly proven. If either factor XII or PK functions as a weakly "active zymogen" in analogy to trypsinogen or chymotrypsinogen,[52,64,67,68] then proteolytic activation of either factor XII or PK might occur when these two molecules are brought close to each other by binding to a negative surface. Based on enzyme kinetic studies,[69] it must be emphasized that reciprocal proteolytic activation of factor XII by kallikrein and of PK by factor XIIa is orders of magnitude more potent than autoactivation or other hypothesized activation mechanisms for this system.

The contact activation reactions which are initially localized to specific surface sites can be propagated to distant sites through fluid phase reactions in two ways (see Fig. 108-1). First, surface-bound kallikrein can dissociate from HK into the fluid phase and disseminate its activities of liberating bradykinin from HK and of activating surface-bound factor XII.[40,47] Second, α factor XIIa of 80 kDa can be cleaved by kallikrein, trypsin, or plasmin near the C-terminus of its heavy chain and liberate β factor XIIa, a 28-kDa serine protease which does not bind to negatively charged surfaces and which is a potent activator of prekallikrein in the fluid phase.[49,70-75] Importantly, β factor XIIa, in contrast to α factor XIIa, is not a potent activator of factor XI.[75]

The complement system can be activated as a consequence of contact activation. The β factor XIIa can activate the classical pathway via activation of C1,[76,77] while kallikrein can replace complement factor D in the activation of C3 in stimulating the alternative complement pathway.[78] Kallikrein, like plasmin, apparently can inactivate C1.[79]

Plasma kallikrein converts prorenin to renin by limited proteolysis of prorenin.[80-83]

The spectrum of negatively charged materials that initiate contact activation reactions when added to plasma is broad and heterogeneous. No highly specific naturally occurring structures have been identified with certainty as "physiological" activators of contact activation, although the role of many materials as potential activators has been speculated. Crude extracts of human articular cartilage, certain heparin preparations, chondroitin sulfate, sulfatide, cholesterol sulfate (but not cholesterol), a variety of acidic phospholipids, and a variety of proteoglycans have all been shown to stimulate contact activation reactions under particular conditions.[84-91] Bacterial endotoxins stimulate contact activation.[92,93] Sulfatides exhibit a potent stimulatory activity, and because they can be chemically pure and provide a well-defined and homogeneous negatively charged surface, they are useful as a model surface for contact activation studies,[57,87] as is dextran sulfate.[69,94,95]

The regulation of the active proteases, factor XIa, kallikrein, and α and β factors XIIa, is accomplished through the action of plasma protease inhibitors (see subsections for each protease below). The primary serine protease inhibitor (serpin) that neutralizes the contact activation enzymes is C1 inhibitor, and the inherited deficiency of this protein is associated with angioedema (see Chap. 130). The α_1-antitrypsin and antithrombin III proteins also play inhibitory roles (see below) and are reviewed in Chaps. 109 and 139.

Inhibitors of contact activation of plasma include β_2-glycoprotein I, complement component C1q, certain preparations of placental collagen, and certain endothelial-cell culture supernatants.[96-100] These inhibitors are naturally occurring substances and may therefore be of physiological relevance. A number of other nonphysiological inhibitors have been identified, including the synthetic positively charged polymer Polybrene, cytochrome *c*, and basic oligomeric peptides, and such inhibitors are useful for preventing contact activation of plasma. It is often difficult to evaluate whether a reported inhibitor of contact activation is specific in some sense at the molecular level or is trivially due to nonspecific binding to the negatively charged activating surface.

THE PROTEINS AND GENES

Factor XI

Coagulation factor XI complexes noncovalently with HK and is a glycoprotein of 160 kDa present in plasma at 4 μg/ml (Table 108-1).[101-104] Except for von Willebrand factor,

Table 108-1 Characteristics of the Contact Factors and Their Genes

	Factor XI	PK	Factor XII	HK
Protein				
Plasma concentration (μg/ml)	4	50	30	70
Molecular mass (kDa)	160 (homodimer)	85	80	110
Amino acids (AA)	607	619	596	626
Heavy chain (AA)	369	371	353	362
function	HK binding Factor IX binding	HK binding	Surface binding	Cysteine-protease inhibitor and cell binding
Light chain (AA)	238	248	243	255
function	Protease domain	Protease domain	Protease domain	Binding to surface, factor XI, and PK
Activated by	Factor XIIa Thrombin Factor XIa	Factor XIIa Kallikrein	Kallikrein Factor XIIa plasmin Factor XIa	Kallikreins Factor XIIa Factor XIa Elastase Plasmin
Substrates of activated factor	Factor IX Factor XII HK Factor XI	Factor XII HK ProUK PK Prorenin Factor B Plasminogen Factor IX Complement C3	PK Factor XI Factor XII HK Factor VII Complement C1 Plasminogen	None
Other activities of factor or active enzyme	Platelet binding	Chemotaxis Neutrophil aggregation Elastase release from neutrophils	Vascular permeability Mitogenesis	Contact cofactor Stabilization of factor XI and PK Bradykinin: Vasodilatation, increased vascular permeability, bronchospasm, pain Binding to platelets, endothelilal cells, and neutrophils Inhibition of cell spreading Cysteine protease inhibitor
Inhibitors	α_1-Antitrypsin Antithrombin III C1-inhibitor Protein C inhibitor PAI-1* α_2-Antiplasmin	C1-inhibitor α_2-Macroglobulin Antithrombin III Protein C inhibitor	C1-inhibitor Antithrombin III α_2-Macroglobulin α_2-Antiplasmin PAI-1 Protein C inhibitor	
Gene				
kb	23	22	12	27
Exons	15	15	14	11
Introns	14	14	13	—
Chromosomal location	4q34-q35	4q34-q35	5q33	3q26-qter

*PAI-1 = Plasminogen activator inhibitor-1.

human factor XI is the only coagulation factor that circulates in polymeric form, as it is a covalently linked homodimer containing two identical polypeptide chains of 80 kDa[10,102,105]; its primary sequence with disulfide locations is shown in Fig. 108-2.[106,107] Based on cDNA and genomic DNA sequences combined with chemical identification of disulfide bonds, the mature protein is predicted to contain 607 amino acids representing a zymogen of a trypsin-like serine protease with the protease located in the C-terminus and with four tandem repeats of 90 or 91 amino acids, designated "apple domains" (A_1 to A_4), located in the N-terminus.[107] The identical polypeptide chains of factor XI are linked by a single symmetric disulfide bond involving Cys 321.[107] The overall structural motif of factor XI is identical to that of PK, which shares 58 percent identity in amino acid sequence.[106,108]

When factor XI is activated by limited proteolysis by factor XIIa, thrombin, factor XIa, or trypsin, it contains disulfide-linked heavy and light chains of 50 and 33 kDa (see Table 108-1),[20,21,101-103] and each molecule contains two active sites.[102] Activation is due to cleavage at the bond between Arg 369 and Ile 370 (see Fig. 108-2).[106] The expression of

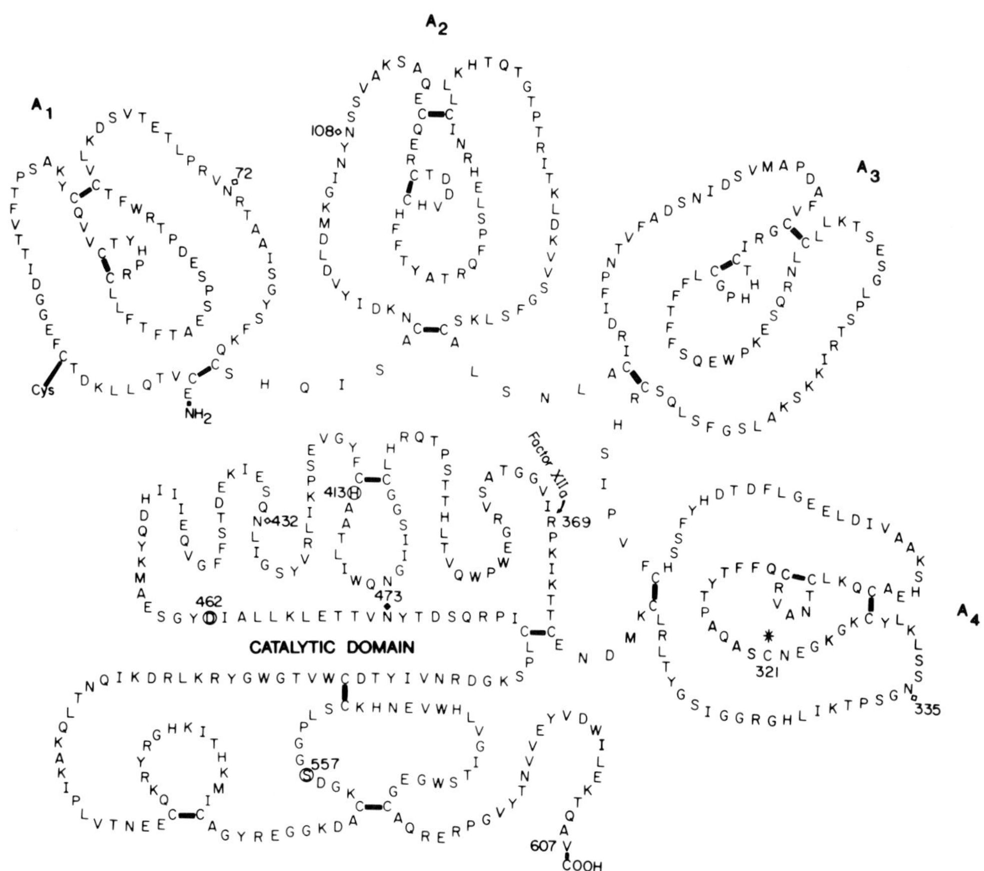

FIG. 108-2 **The amino acid sequence of factor XI monomer with its disulfide bonds. The first apple-shaped domain (A_1) is the site of HK binding[117] and the second apple-shaped domain (A_2) is the site of factor IX binding.[116] The asterisk in the fourth apple-shaped domain (A_4) shows the disulfide bond linking the two identical subunits of factor XI. The arrow marks the site of cleavage by α-factor XIIa, thrombin, or factor XIa. The residues of the catalytic triad are circled, the potential sites for attachment of carbohydrate chains are marked by open diamonds, and the solid diamond at Asn 473 marks an additional identified carbohydrate attachment site.** ***(From McMullen et al.[145] Reprinted by permission.)***

the coagulant activity of factor XIa (see Fig. 108-1) involves the activation of factor IX by limited proteolysis of two peptide bonds in a Ca^{2+}-dependent reaction that is not stimulated by negative surfaces, HK, or phospholipids.[109-112]

In addition to factor IX, factor XIa can cleave and activate factor XII and plasminogen,[31,32,52,113] and it can undergo autoactivation.[20,21] Factor XIa can also cleave HK and liberate bradykinin.[114] The physiological significance of these reactions is not clear.

Studies in which the heavy and light chains of factor XIa were isolated following mild reduction and alkylation showed that the light chain possesses full enzymatic activity and that the heavy chain containing the four apple domains is responsible for binding to HK and for Ca^{2+}-dependent recognition of factor IX.[112] Some work suggested that the HK binding site includes amino acids between residues 56 and 86 in the A_1 domain and that factor IX recognition involves sequences between residues 145 and 176 in the A_2 domain.[115-117]

The inhibition of factor XIa involves principally α_1-antitrypsin and to a much lesser extent might involve antithrombin III, C1 inhibitor, or α_2-antiplasmin.[102,103,118-123] Factor XIa also reacts with plasminogen activator inhibitor-1[124] and protein C inhibitor.[125] Although it was reported that HK protects factor XIa from inhibition by C1 inhibitor and α_1-antitrypsin,[126] no influence of HK on the rate of factor XIa inhibition was found by another laboratory (Bouma BN: unpublished data).

The factor XI gene of 23 kb has been localized to chromosome 4q34-35, and its structure involves 15 exons and 14 introns (see Table 108-1).[127,128]

Factor XI and XIa bind to activated platelets and perturbed endothelial cells in the presence of HK and Zn^{2+} ions.[129-133] Conceivably, HK mediates the localization of factor XI to the surface of these cells similarly to its function at negatively charged surfaces. Since both endothelial cells and platelets also possess binding sites for factor IX,[134] it seems likely that the initiation of coagulation by the contact reactions can take place on the surface of these cells, particularly when platelets are activated or endothelial cells are perturbed.[61,131,135] The localization of HK and factor XIa to the surface of endothelial cells may also exert regulatory functions, as factor XIa was shown to be a potent inactivator of plasminogen activator inhibitor-1 (PAI-I) thereby possibly enhancing fibrinolysis.[124] Platelets not only bind factor XI but contain small amounts of a 230-kDa protein which shows factor XI-like activity and reacts with specific antibodies against factor XI.[22] The roles of this factor XI–related protein and of two inhibitors of factor XIa isolated from platelets remain to be established (see Walsh[22]).

Plasma Prekallikrein

Plasma PK forms a noncovalent complex with HK and is a glycoprotein of 85 kDa present in plasma at 50 μg/ml (see Table 108-1).[37,45,136-143] It should be noted that plasma PK is

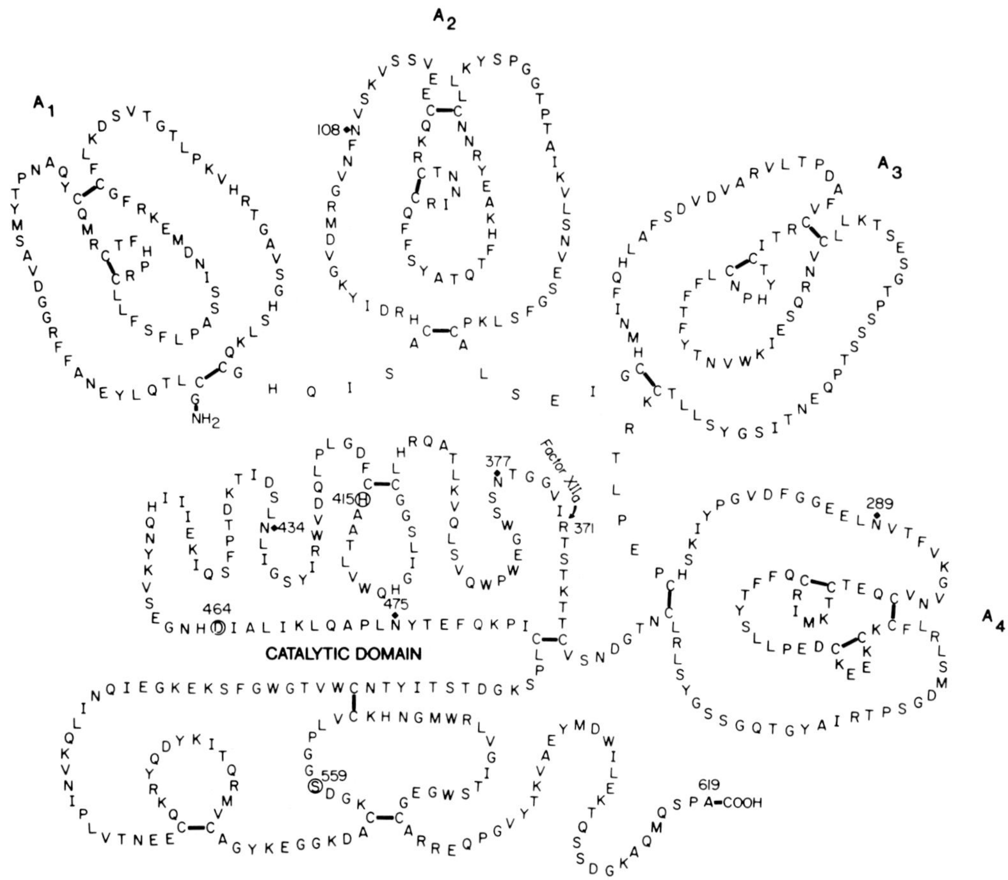

FIG. 108-3 **The amino acid sequence of PK with its disulfide bonds. The arrow at Arg 371 marks the site of cleavage by factor XIIa. Note the striking similarity to the factor XI monomer (Fig. 108-2), including the four apple domains, cleavage site for factor XIIa, and catalytic domain. Asn residues marked by solid diamonds are attachment sites for carbohydrate chains, and circled residues are members of the catalytic triad characteristic of serine proteases.** ***(From McMullen et al.[107] Reprinted by permission.)***

quite distinct from the family of kininogenases known as glandular or tissue-type kallikreins.[23,144] The PK amino acid sequence with disulfide bond locations was determined from cDNA sequencing and chemical analysis and is shown in Fig. 108-3.[108,145] The mature protein is predicted to contain 619 amino acids representing a trypsin-like serine protease zymogen with the protease domain in the C-terminus and with four tandem repeats of 90 or 91 residues, designated "apple domains" (A_1 to A_4), in the N-terminal region.[108,145] PK is highly homologous to factor XI and exhibits 58 percent identity in amino acid sequence.[106,108]

When PK is activated by limited proteolysis by α factor XIIa, β factor XIIa, kallikrein, or trypsin, it contains disulfide-linked heavy and light chains of 50 and 33 kDa (see Table 108-1).[136-138] Activation is due to cleavage at the bond between Arg 371 and Ile 372 (see Fig. 108-3).[108]

Studies in which the heavy and light chains of kallikrein were isolated following mild reduction and alkylation showed that the light chain possesses full enzymatic activity and that the heavy chain containing the four apple domains is responsible for the reversible binding to HK that promotes potent surface-dependent activation of surface-bound factor XII.[45] Some investigators have suggested that the sequence of residues 56 to 86 in the A_1 domain are essential for the binding of factor XI to HK,[115,117] and since factor XI is highly homologous to PK, it may be speculated that the A_1 domain of PK may be responsible at least in part for binding to HK.[146] In the absence of HK, the heavy chain of kallikrein binds to negatively charged surfaces, whereas the light chain does not bind well to negative surfaces.[45,46] Two-chain kallikrein of 85 kDa, sometimes designated α kallikrein, can undergo cleavage in its heavy chain to give β kallikrein of 65 kDa, which has fivefold lower clotting activity than α kallikrein and is not able to stimulate neutrophils.[147,148] The significance of this cleavage of kallikrein is not clear.

The expression of the various activities of kallikrein (see Fig. 108-1) involves limited proteolysis of kininogens to liberate bradykinin,[23,25,149-151] of surface-bound factor XII to generate α factor XIIa and β factor XIIa,[49,50,52] of proUK to form UK,[29] and of plasminogen to generate plasmin.[32,138,152] Kallikrein can activate factor IX to factor IXa in a Ca^{2+}-independent reaction with the same efficiency as factor XIa in the absence of Ca^{2+} ions; interestingly, Ca^{2+} ions stimulate factor XIa action by more than two orders of magnitude but have no effect on kallikrein action.[111] The action of kallikrein on factor IX has been shown to be essential for activation of factor VII during "cold activation" of citrated plasma, that is, when plasma of some individuals is incubated at 4°C.[153,154] During cold activation of plasma, β factor XIIa can directly convert single-chain factor XII to two-chain active factor VIIa.[153,154] Surface-dependent autoactivation of PK by kallikrein can also occur.[59] Kallikrein also activates the renin–angiotensin system by converting prorenin to renin.[80-83]

The inhibition of kallikrein involves neutralization by protease inhibitors, principally by C1 inhibitor and α_2-macroglobulin with a minor contribution by antithrombin III.[155-157] Some investigators have also shown that kallikrein reacts with PAI-1 and protein C inhibitor.[124,125,158] Although it was reported that HK protects kallikrein from inhibition by C1 inhibitor,[159,160] later studies reported no influence of HK on the rate of kallikrein inhibition.[161,162]

The PK gene of 22 kb has been localized to human chromosome 4q34-35 and to mouse chromosome 8, and the rat plasma prekallikrein gene has 15 exons and 14 introns, thus indicating a high homology to the human factor XI gene structure.[163]

Kallikrein exerts strong effects on neutrophils, as it was shown to aggregate neutrophils, express chemotactic activity, and stimulate elastase release (see reviews by Kaplan and Silverberg,[13] Colman,[16] and Gustafson and Colman[164]). These fluid phase reactions are localized at the neutrophil surface, since it was shown that HK in complex with PK binds to neutrophils at high affinity sites in the presence of Zn^{2+} ions.[165] One study reported that α kallikrein does not directly activate neutrophils.[166] The physiological importance of these kallikrein activities remains to be established.

High Molecular Weight Kininogen

Plasma contains two distinct forms of kininogens differing in molecular weight, designated HK and LK (low molecular weight kininogen),[25,167] which release bradykinin or Lys-bradykinin on proteolysis by plasma or glandular kallikreins. Bradykinin is very potent in causing hypotension, smooth muscle contraction, and pain. HK and LK are glycoproteins of 110 and 65 kDa present in plasma at 70 and 160 μg/ml, respectively.[25,139,168-170] HK and LK are also cysteine proteases inhibitors evolutionarily related to cystatins and stefins,[25] and LK is identical to α_2-thiol protease inhibitor.[171-173] HK but not LK is a contact activation cofactor (see above). The amino acid and the cDNA sequences for HK and LK have been reported,[174-177] and HK contains 626 amino acid residues while LK has 409 residues. Both HK and LK are encoded by the same gene, and their messenger RNAs result from alternative RNA splicing and the use of different polyadenylation sites.[25,178,179]

The structures of HK and LK are schematically depicted in Fig. 108-4 and show the identity between HK and LK for residues 1 through 383, which contain four domains designated D1 to D4. These four domains represent three homologous repeats, D1 to D3, characteristic of cysteine protease inhibitors, and domain D4, which contains bradykinin. Two domains, D2 and D3, are functionally active as inhibitors of cystein proteases,[180,181] and domain D3 is also responsible for the binding of HK to cells.[182] Domain D4 releases bradykinin when cleaved by plasma kallikrein at residues Lys 362 and Arg 371 (see Fig. 108-4). Cleavage by glandular kallikrein releases Lys-bradykinin.

The marked structural differences between HK and LK following residue 383 (see Fig. 108-4) explain the marked functional differences, as HK is a contact activation cofactor but LK is not. Following cleavage of HK and LK to release kinins, each molecule contains an N-terminal heavy chain linked by a single disulfide bond to a C-terminal light chain (see Fig. 108-4). Studies in which the heavy and light chains of kinin-free HK were isolated following reduction and alkylation showed that the light chain of HK—domains D5 and D6 comprising residues 384 to 626—expresses the full procoagulant activity of HK.[139,169] Domain D5 of HK contains an unusually long basic sequence in which out of 91 residues, 25 are His, 13 are Lys, 5 are Arg, and 19 are Gly.[174,176,183] This "His-rich region" of domain D5 is responsible for the binding of HK to negatively charged surfaces,[43,184] including a Zn^{2+}-enhanced binding of HK to surfaces.[185] The isolated light chain of HK is responsible for the binding of PK and factor XI with 1:1 stoichiometry represented as PK:HK and XI:HK_2 complexes (see Fig. 108-1).[37-39,104,139,186,187] The binding sites for PK and factor XI in the light chain of HK were identified in domain 6 as residues 565 to 595 and 556 to 613, respectively (see Fig. 108-4).[188-190] These important binding sites for PK and XI in HK were further characterized in other studies.[191,192]

In the proteolytic release of kinin from kininogens, plasma kallikrein is 40 times more active on HK than on LK, whereas glandular kallikrein is equally potent on HK and on LK. Factors XIIa and XIa and plasmin have been reported

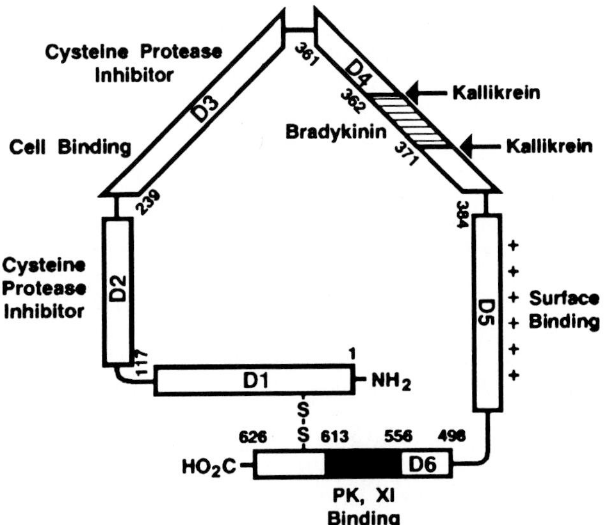

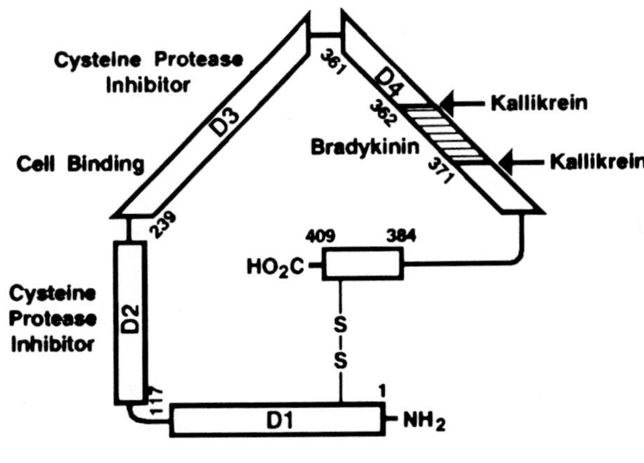

FIG. 108-4 The schematic structures of HK and LK showing their domains and functionally important sites. HK and LK, which are produced from one gene by RNA splicing, are identical between residues 1 and 383, that is, through the first four domains, designated D1 to D4. Cleavage by kallikrein at two sites in domain D4 releases bradykinin. Two domains, D2 and D3, are active as cysteine protease inhibitors, and domain D3 binds to cells. The sequences beyond residue 384 are totally different. HK, but not LK, is a contact activation cofactor. Domain D5, containing an unusual His-rich region, is responsible for binding to negatively charged surfaces, while domain D6 has binding sites for PK or factor XI. See text for further discussion.

to be kininogenases, although the physiological significance of such activity is not clear.[114,193,194] Neutrophil elastase cleaves HK and destroys its contact activation cofactor activity.[195]

The gene for HK and LK of 27 kb contains 11 exons and has been mapped to chromosome 3q26-qter.[196,197] This single gene gives rise to HK and LK by alternative RNA splicing.[179]

Endothelial cells, platelets, and neutrophils not only contain HK[198,199] but also possess high affinity binding sites for HK which require the presence of Zn^{2+} ions.[131,165,200-202] The D3 domain of HK (see Fig. 108-4) has been identified as a platelet and endothelial-cell binding site,[182] while other less well defined sites in HK have been described as important for binding to cells.[203] The presence of such a multifunctional protein as HK on the surface of these cells might play important regulatory roles in blood coagulation, fibrinolysis, and the inflammatory response. For example, HK was found to inhibit platelet activation by thrombin[182] and to displace fibrinogen from platelet and neutrophil surfaces.[204] HK mediates localization of factor XI and XIa on perturbed endothelial cells and platelets and of PK and kallikrein on neutrophils (see above). Moreover, kinin-free HK interferes with platelet spreading on surfaces coated with fibrinogen and vitronectin,[205] and this inhibitory activity of HK may explain the puzzling observation that an HK-deficient individual had an elevated number of inflammatory cells on the "Rebuck skin window" test.[206]

Factor XII

Factor XII is a glycoprotein of 80 kDa present in plasma at 30 μg/ml (see Table 108-1).[72,207,208] The amino acid sequence of factor XII has been elucidated using both protein chemical sequencing and cDNA sequencing methods and is shown in Fig. 108-5, wherein the disulfide bond locations were inferred based on homology to known structures.[209-211] Factor XII contains 596 amino acids with a trypsin-like protease domain in the C-terminus and with a most unusual collection of domains in the N-terminus. The various domains are defined based on homology to known structural motifs and are depicted in Fig. 108-5. Beginning at the N-terminus, factor XII has a fibronectin type II domain, an epiderminal growth factor–like domain, a fibronectin type I domain, another growth factor–like domain, a kringle domain, a novel "proline-rich" domain spanning approximately 55 residues, and a serine protease domain that is responsible for catalytic activity.

When factor XII is proteolytically activated by kallikrein, plasmin, factor XIa, factor XIIa, or trypsin, the bond between Arg 353 and Val 354 is cleaved to generate α factor XIIa[209,210] (see Fig. 108-5). Cleavage at this site occurs 100 to 500 times faster when factor XII is bound to negative surfaces than when it is in solution, presumably because surface-binding induces a conformational change resulting in an increased susceptibility to proteolytic activation.[52] Subsequent cleavages of α factor XIIa can occur at Arg 334 and Arg 343[209,210] (see Fig. 108-5) to generate β factor XIIa of 28 kDa which has remarkably different enzymatic properties than α factor XIIa.[18,49,58,71,72,75,212]

The N-terminal heavy chain of 353 amino acids is responsible for the binding of factor XII or α factor XIIa to negatively charged surfaces.[73] A monoclonal antibody that blocks surface-dependent activation of factor XII was initially suggested to bind near the N-terminus near the fibro-

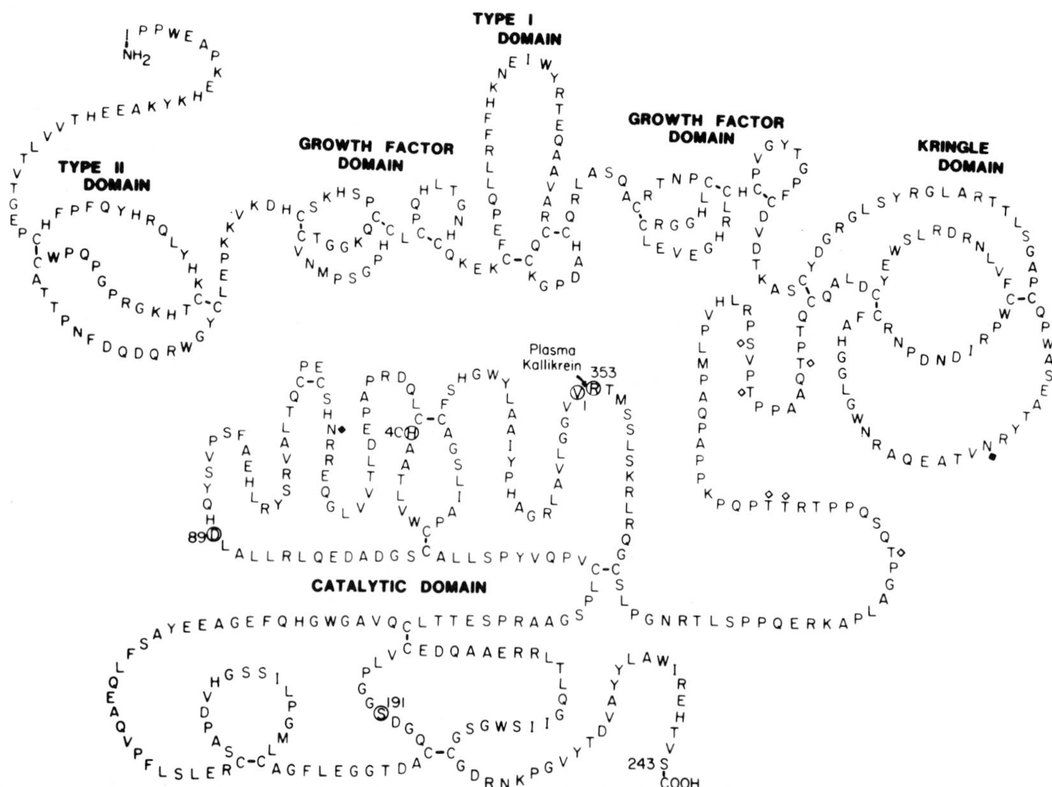

FIG. 108-5 The amino acid sequence of factor XII and its functional domains. The site of proteolytic cleavage by kallikrein that converts factor XII to α-factor XIIa is depicted by an arrow. The residues characteristic of the serine protease catalytic triad are circled. The various domains exhibiting homology to fibronectin types I and II domains, two growth factor–like domains, and a kringle domain are indicated. The closed diamonds denote *N*-glycosylation sites, and the open diamonds depict possible *O*-glycosylation sites. *(From Fujikawa, and based on available sequence data,[209-211] by permission.)*

nectin type I domain[213] and later suggested to bind the N-terminal 15 residues,[214] suggesting that one or both of these regions may mediate surface binding. A recombinant factor XII deletion mutant of 32 kDa has been described that contains the C-terminal protease domain plus only part of the proline-rich domain—residues 320 to 596—and this mutant was reported to exhibit full procoagulant factor XII activity in activated partial thromboplastin time (APTT) assays.[215] If this report is confirmed, it surprisingly suggests that only a small part of the C-terminal region of the heavy chain is essential for the surface-dependent reactions of factor XII that initiate coagulation. Studies of such recombinant deletion mutant factor XII molecules will be very useful to identify the potential functions of the various domains of the heavy chain.

Since the major binding site(s) for negatively charged surfaces resides in the heavy chain of α factor XIIa,[73] β factor XIIa does not bind to negative surfaces, and hence does not exhibit the surface-dependent enhanced activation of factor XI or PK.[75] Nevertheless, β factor XIIa remains a potent activator of PK in the fluid phase, albeit a weak activator of factor XI.[49,58,71,75,212] Contamination of therapeutic plasma protein fraction products by β factor XIIa caused a hypotensive response in patients receiving the products.[216,217] Thus, proteolytic processing of α factor XIIa may modulate the substrate specificity of factor XIIa and thereby regulate the preferential activation of the different factor XII-dependent pathways depicted in Fig. 108-1.

The expression of the various activities of factor XIIa involves limited proteolysis of PK to generate kallikrein,[49,58,71,75,212,218] of factor XI to form factor XIa,[101,102] and of plasminogen to form plasmin.[30,32] Surface-dependent autoactivation of factor XII by factor XIIa can also occur[55-58] and may contribute to the initiation of contact activation in the absence of kallikrein. Divalent metal ions such as Zn^{2+} or Cu^{2+} stimulate this autoactivation reaction[219] as well as contact activation reactions in plasma or in purified reaction mixtures[86,219,220] (and Lämmle B, Griffin JH: unpublished data.) Purified factor XIIa is capable of cleaving HK and liberating bradykinin in reaction mixtures of purified proteins, although the potential for this reaction in plasma is uncertain.[193] Factor XIIa can convert single-chain factor VII to two-chain factor VIIa and thereby enhance the activation of the extrinsic coagulation pathway.[105,153]

The neutralization of factor XIIa activity by plasma protease inhibitors involves principally C1 inhibitor with minor contributions by antithrombin III and possibly α_2-antiplasmin.[123,221-225]

The factor XII gene of 12 kb is located on human chromosome 5q33 and has 14 exons and 13 introns (see Table 108-1).[226,227]

Factor XII and factor XIIa are mitogenic for HepG2 liver cells but not for L cells.[228] It was demonstrated that antisera against mouse epidermal growth factor (EGF) cross-reacted with 80-kDa factor XII, presumably recognizing the EGF-like region in factor XII, and it was suggested that the EGF-like region of factor XII and XIIa was responsible for mitogenic activity.[228]

CLINICAL DISORDERS

Hereditary Factor XI Deficiency

A "new" hemophilia, initially termed *hemophilia C,* was described in 1953 by Rosenthal et al.[1] in two sisters and their maternal uncle. It presented as a mild to moderate bleeding tendency and, unlike X-linked hemophilia A and B, was an autosomal trait. The coagulation factor missing in these patients eventually was designated factor XI, although initially it was called plasma thromboplastin antecedent (PTA). Rosenthal and colleagues[229] erroneously believed that the mode of transmission of factor XI deficiency was autosomal dominant with variable expressivity, but it was later clearly established that the inheritance was autosomal recessive[230] and that most patients were Jewish.[230-232] Several instances of vertical transmission of severe factor XI deficiency in nonconsanguineous Ashkenazic Jewish kindreds (due to homozygote–heterozygote matings) provided the first suggestion that the gene frequency in this population might be extremely high, as was later proven.[233]

Inheritance and Mutations. Factor XI deficiency is an autosomal disorder that presents in homozygotes or compound heterozygotes with severely reduced factor XI levels (less than 15 U/dl) and in heterozygotes with partially deficient or low normal factor XI levels.[230,231,233-235] Unlike the hereditary deficiencies of other blood coagulation factors, such as factors VIII and IX, for which a large number of dysfunctional variants have been described, dysfunctional factor XI deficiency is exceedingly rare. For example, of 121 reported patients of different ethnic backgrounds who had severe factor XI deficiency,[234,236-240] only one patient of German origin had a normal factor XI antigen level with a discordantly low factor XI clotting activity.[239]

DNA mutations responsible for factor XI deficiency have been identified. Three independent point mutations in the factor XI gene were found in Ashkenazic Jews with factor XI deficiency[241] and are summarized in Table 108-2. The first mutation, so far found in only one patient and here designated Ex14+1G→A, is a G→A change at the splice junction boundary of the last intron (intron N) of the factor XI gene. This mutation interrupts the coding region of the mRNA between amino acids Lys 185 and Gly 186 just before the active site Ser 188 of the light chain of factor XIa. The

Table 108-2 Characteristics of Three Mutations in the Factor XI Gene Identified in Ashkenazic Jews

Mutation	Class	Site	Frequency	Factor XI Coagulant Activity Level in Homozygotes (U/dl), Means ±SD*	Number of Injury-Related Bleeding Events in Homozygotes, Means ±SD*	Restriction Enzyme Used for Detection in Amplified DNA Segments
Ex14+1G→A	Splice junction	Intron N	Rare	Unknown	—	*Mae*III
E117X	Nonsense	Exon 5	Common	1.2±0.5 (n = 16)†	1.6±2.4 (n = 16)‡	*Bsm*I
F283L	Missense	Exon 9	Common	9.7±1.6 (n = 13)†	1.0±1.1 (n = 13)‡	*Mbo*I

* Based on Asakai et al.[246]
† $p<0.001$
‡ $p<0.05$

second mutation, designated E117X, involves the introduction of a stop codon for Glu 117 in exon 5 with a change from GAA to TAA, and presumably leads to premature polypeptide termination. The third mutation, designated F283L, is located in exon 9 and consists of a change of TTC, coding for Phe 283, to CTC coding for Leu. This missense mutation at residue 283 is at the fourth apple domain of the molecule and is near the site of a disulfide bond holding together the factor XI dimer. The F283L mutation has been formed in a recombinant mutant factor XI that was expressed in baby hamster kidney cells and was found to cause a diminished secretion of factor XI apparently due to defective intracellular dimerization of factor XI.[242]

Frequency. In 1958 Biggs et al.[243] suggested that factor XI deficiency might be more frequent among Jews than among other populations, thereby accounting for the significantly different proportions of factor XI–deficient patients among all the hemophiliacs observed in series reported from European countries and the United States.[244] Indeed, the subsequently reported series of patients affected by factor XI deficiency were from Los Angeles,[230] Capetown, South Africa, and New York,[232] Israel,[231,233] Philadelphia,[234] and London,[235] where sizable Jewish communities reside. Sporadic cases have also been reported among Italians, Germans, Japanese, Chinese, Koreans, Indians, American blacks, and Arabs.[234,238,244] The vast majority of Jewish patients are of Ashkenazic origin, that is, central and eastern European origin.[233] Two surveys among a total of 1141 Ashkenazic Jews in Israel disclosed a frequency of about 1/190 (q^2) for severe factor XI deficiency.[245] Strikingly, this implies a gene frequency (q) of factor XI deficiency of the square root of 1/190, or 0.0725, and the expected heterozygote frequency (2 pq) was 0.135, or 13.5 percent. Since roughly one half (or 6.7 percent) of such heterozygotes are detectable by a factor XI:C assay,[233] these data agreed with the 8 percent (35:428) partially deficient subjects actually found in one of the surveys.[233] Two molecular genetic studies have shown that the E117X and F283L mutations account for most affected patients in this population and that these two mutations are equally frequent among Ashkenazic Jews.[246,247]

Unlike Tay-Sachs disease,[248] no aggregation of geographic origins of ancestry was found for factor XI deficiency.[233] This may indicate that the mutations which cause factor XI deficiency in Ashkenazic Jews occurred more distantly in time than those responsible for Tay-Sachs disease. Interestingly, four unrelated Iraqi Jewish families with affected members have been reported, and all were found to have the E117X mutation.[249] The Iraqi Jews represent the original "gene pool" of the Jewish people and have stayed in the Middle East for more than 2500 years.[250] If more cases of only the E117X mutation are identified in Iraqi Jews, such a finding might indicate that this mutation in both Ashkenazic and Iraqi Jews stems from a common founder effect, whereas the F283L mutation might have occurred at a later time, for example, after the divergence of the Jews into Ashkenazic, Sephardic (Spanish), and Oriental (Middle Eastern) communities.

The extremely high gene frequency of factor XI deficiency among Ashkenazic Jews probably originates from genetic drifts caused by profound changes in population size, migration, and founder effects,[248,250] rather than selection, since no advantage for carriers of factor XI deficiency has so far been demonstrated or hypothesized.

Bleeding Manifestations. Since the description of the first cases with severe factor XI deficiency,[1] it has been repeatedly shown that most bleeding manifestations in these patients are related to injuries and that spontaneous bleeding manifestations are uncommon.[230,231,233-235,251] Bleeding can be brisk at the time of injury and continue for hours or days unless treated. Alternatively, bleeding can begin several hours after injury and persist as an oozing for many days. Several studies have shown that some patients with severe factor XI deficiency may not bleed at all following trauma[230,252,253] and that sometimes the bleeding tendency may vary in the same patient following hemostatic challenges.[235,246] This apparent enigma has been clarified to some extent by the finding that both the genotype of the patient and the site of surgery may have a marked influence on the bleeding tendency.[246] Thus, patients with genotype F283L/F283L had significantly fewer injury-related bleeding events than patients with genotypes E117X/E117X or E117X/F283L. Conceivably, this relative advantage of homozygotes for the F283L mutation stemmed from their significantly higher factor XI:C level (see Table 108-2). Surgical procedures involving tissues with a high content of plasminogen activators, such as dental extractions, tonsillectomy, urologic surgery, and nasal surgery were found to be frequently associated with excessive bleeding in all patients with severe factor XI deficiency independently of their genotype.[246] In contrast, other surgical procedures, such as appendectomy, orthopedic surgery, cholecystectomy, and hysterectomy were significantly less likely to be accompanied by excessive bleeding. Another explanation for the apparent lack of bleeding manifestations in some patients may be related to a normal content of factor XI–like coagulant activity in their platelets in spite of greatly reduced plasma factor XI levels.[254] However, it is not known whether patients who do bleed indeed have a concomitantly low level of platelet factor XI–like activity; consequently, definitive conclusions cannot be drawn in this regard. An apparent clustering of bleeding manifestations in affected members of certain families[234] may suggest yet another factor contributing to the variability of symptoms in different patients, although this idea has been rejected by others.[230,235,255]

An injury-related bleeding tendency in heterozygotes for factor XI deficiency has been a controversial issue. In one extensive study, heterozygotes had almost no bleeding manifestations following a variety of surgical procedures, including numerous tooth extractions, tonsillectomy, and nasal surgery[230]; and in another study of urologic surgical cases, all heterozygotes did well without plasma replacement except for one patient whose factor XI was the lowest in the group, at 25 U/dl.[256] Two additional studies demonstrated only a gross correlation between factor XI levels and bleeding manifestations,[235,247] whereas other investigators described similar mean factor XI levels in "bleeders" and "nonbleeders."[231,234,255] These discrepancies seem to be related in part to the lack of uniformity of definitions as to what constitutes "excessive bleeding" and to the great variability of injuries and to the different proportions of unchallenged patients in these studies. Conceivably, the variable manifestations are related to different genotypic forms of the heterozygotes or to other as yet unknown causes. We maintain that, although heterozygotes may rarely bleed excessively following trauma when it is inflicted at sites specifically prone to bleeding, patients with severe factor XI deficiency present a substantially greater risk of bleeding at surgery or following trauma.

Diagnosis. Two alternative events usually lead to the diagnosis of factor XI deficiency, either injury-related bleeding or an incidental finding of a prolonged APTT.[233,234,255] Spontaneous bleeding manifestations are rarely the cause for referral of such patients for diagnosis. A history of mild to moderate bleeding, particularly after tooth extractions, urologic surgery, tonsillectomy, or nasal surgery, is helpful for prediction of factor XI deficiency, especially in Ashkenazic Jews.

All patients with severe factor XI deficiency with less than 15 U/dl clotting activity have an APTT that is longer than two standard deviations above the normal mean.[257] Among patients with the E117X or F283L mutations (see Table 108-2), E117X homozygotes have the longest mean APTT values, F283L homozygotes the relatively shortest, and E117X/F283L compound heterozygotes have intermediate mean values.[246] The APTT values of heterozygotes with partial factor XI deficiency substantially overlap the normal range of APTT values,[246,257] and this assay is not a good screening test for identification of heterozygotes.

Factor XI is commonly measured by a clotting assay using a modified APTT system and factor XI–deficient plasma.[230] Unless performed by specialized laboratories, this method was found to have a substantial intra-assay coefficient of variation, and notable interlaboratory differences were reported.[258] Amidolytic assays for factor XI have also been devised[259,260] but are more complicated than clotting assays which provide the preferred activity assay. Factor XI antigen can be assayed by electroimmunoassay[104] or by radioimmunoassay.[238,259]

Factor XI coagulant activity levels in homozygotes or compound heterozygotes are below 15 U/dl and correspond very well with factor XI antigen levels.[238] Significant differences in mean factor XI activity values were described among three genotypically defined groups of patients (see Table 108-2) with severe factor XI deficiency.[246] Patients with F283L homozygosity had the relatively highest mean values (9.7±1.2 U/dl), E117X homozygotes had the lowest values (1.2±0.5 U/dl), and E117X/F283L compound heterozygotes had intermediate values (3.3±1.6 U/dl).[246] Similar differences were obtained in another study.[247] In view of the high and equal frequencies of the E117X and F283L mutations in Ashkenazic Jews and the low frequency among non-Jews, the results of factor XI activity assays in severely deficient patients might be helpful in predicting the genotype of a given patient. For example, an extremely low level (≤1 U/dl) of activity would be consistent with E117X homozygosity and relatively high values (10 to 14 U/dl) with F283L homozygosity, although direct assessment of the genotype is easily performed and is preferable.

Mean factor XI coagulant activity levels in heterozygotes are significantly lower than the normal mean. However, for individual patients there may be a problem in diagnosis since a substantial number of obligatory carriers were shown to have factor XI activity levels within the normal range.[233] Another study described a smaller overlap between the factor XI activity values of heterozygotes and controls and provided an approach for calculating the probability of given patients to be heterozygous or normal.[235] Heterozygotes for the E117X mutation were observed in one study[246] to have a significantly lower mean factor XI activity level than F283L heterozygotes, yet in another study similar values were found in these two genotypes.[247]

Genotypic analysis of patients with factor XI deficiency is possible for the three mutations so far discovered among Ashkenazic Jewish patients. All three mutations can be detected using the polymerase chain reaction method and restriction enzymes.[246] The enzyme *Mae*III is used for the splicing mutation, *Bsm*I for the E117X mutation and *Mbo*I for the F283L mutation. By employing these techniques, one can conclusively differentiate between carriers of factor XI deficiency and normal subjects.

Acquired Inhibitors of Factor XI. Inhibitors with specific neutralizing activity against factor XI have been reported in patients with hereditary factor XI deficiency.[261-267] Twelve of the 13 patients had severe factor XI deficiency prior to the development of the circulating inhibitor, and one patient had a partial deficiency. All but two presented with the inhibitor after they had been infused with plasma. In eight well-studied patients, the inhibitory activity was related to polyclonal IgG antibodies.[262-264,266,267] The antibodies bound to the heavy chain of factor XIa, thereby neutralizing the following: surface binding of factor XI,[262-264] binding to high molecular weight kininogen,[262,266] activation of factor XI by factor XIIa,[262] and cleavage of factor IX by factor XIa.[262,266] Interestingly, only one patient presented with severe spontaneous bleeding, which apparently was related to the very high titer of the inhibitor and to its capacity to neutralize several functions of factor XI—binding to high molecular weight kininogen, cleavage by factor XIIa, and activation of factor IX.[262] In other patients, bleeding manifestations did not seem to be aggravated by the development of these inhibitors, yet correction of the defect became resistant to plasma infusions. This might constitute a problem when such patients have to undergo surgery. However, uneventful surgical procedures have been carried out following the infusion of an activated factor IX concentrate,[262] after plasmapheresis and the use of an antifibrinolytic agent,[265] or following administration of an antifibrinolytic agent only.[268] Specific inhibitors against factor XI have also been described in patients with systemic lupus erythematosus.[269]

Association with Other Disorders. In view of the high frequency of hereditary factor XI deficiency among Ashkenazic Jews, coincidental occurrence of other inherited disorders may not be uncommon. Gaucher disease, also commonly observed in Ashkenazic Jews (see Chap. 86), was described to coexist with hereditary factor XI deficiency but was found to segregate independently.[270] Patients with Noonan syndrome were found to have reduced factor XI levels, for which no explanation has been provided.[255] A variety of other inherited disorders of hemostasis have been described in association with factor XI deficiency, including factor VIII deficiency,[235,271] factor IX deficiency,[272] combined factor VIII and IX deficiency,[272] platelet dysfunction,[273] and von Willebrand disease.[274] In one study of patients with partial factor XI deficiency, a relatively common association with mild von Willebrand disease was described and appeared related to enhanced bleeding manifestations.[275] However, in another related study these findings could not be confirmed.[276] It appears that the coincidental additional defects in hemostasis do not worsen bleeding in patients with factor XI deficiency.[235,255]

Thrombosis. Although factor XI seems to play an important role in hemostasis, a severe deficiency state does not provide protection against venous or arterial thrombosis. Acute myocardial infarction or pulmonary embolism developed in several patients with severe factor XI deficiency.[277] We are aware of three additional patients with severe factor XI deficiency who had an acute myocardial infarction and were successfully treated by recombinant tissue plasminogen activator followed by heparin without experiencing excessive bleeding.

Treatment. Surgical trauma in patients with severe factor XI deficiency, as stated above, can be accompanied by serious and prolonged bleeding.[251,278] Particularly severe bleeding complications are observed after urologic surgery unless treatment is given.[256,278-280] Therefore, careful evaluation of such patients and meticulous planning are indispensable prior to surgery. Some considerations and guidelines are: (1) the surgical procedure should be absolutely indicated; (2) the genotype of the patient should be determined, as it has been shown to be related to the risk of bleeding[246]; (3) ingestion of aspirin or other platelet antiaggregating agents should be avoided for at least a week before surgery; (4) the platelet count and prothrombin time should be normal, and the presence of an inhibitor of factor XI must be excluded; (5) the surgeon should ligate bleeding vessels rather than use cauterization, since at such sites oozing can occur after surgery; (6) for surgical procedures in areas where there is local fibrinolysis, the use of antifibrinolytic agents should be considered; and (7) replacement therapy should be started before surgery and carefully monitored thereafter by APTT or factor XI coagulant activity assays. A policy of "wait and see whether the patient bleeds" is inappropriate, since once bleeding commences, all measures to arrest it are much less effective.[279] For major surgery, replacement should last 10 to 14 days, while 5 days of replacement therapy may suffice for minor surgery.[255,256,280]

Traditionally, fresh-frozen plasma has been used for replacement therapy in patients with factor XI deficiency. This treatment method has the limitations of volume overload, potential transmission of infectious agents, and allergic reactions. More recently, a factor XI concentrate was produced and found to be effective, easy to administer, and safe.[281] With either plasma or factor XI concentrate treatments, the recovery of factor XI following infusion was more than 90 percent,[281,282] and the half-life of factor XI determined in 19 patients was 52±22 h (mean ±SD).[281] This excellent recovery and extended half-life facilitate the treatment of patients by replacement therapy. A controversial issue is the level of factor XI that should be attained at surgery and maintained during the postoperative course. The recommended "hemostatic level of factor XI" has ranged between 20 and 100 U/dl.[230,232,255,256,281] These inconsistencies stem, on the one hand, from observations of some patients who bled excessively following surgery, although they had factor XI levels of 50 to 60 U/dl,[234,235,255] and, on the other hand, from observations of patients who underwent the most risky operation, namely prostatectomy, and did well as long as their factor XI level was 30 to 35 U/dl.[256,280] These reports notwithstanding suggest that for major surgery it seems safe to aim at a nadir factor XI level of 45 U/dl and for minor surgery a nadir of 30 U/dl. These targets can also be used as a guide for planning surgical procedures in patients with partial factor XI deficiency whose initial levels might range between 20 and 60 U/dl. For surgery of the lower urinary tract, adding an antifibrinolytic agent for inhibition of local fibrinolysis might be helpful, but has not so far been studied systematically.

Oral surgery, unless adequately treated, is associated very frequently with hemorrhage in patients with severe factor XI deficiency.[230,251] Plasma infusion with or without antifibrinolytic agents has been successfully used in prevention of this bleeding complication.[282,283] It has been demonstrated that treatment using only tranexamic acid, an antifibrinolytic agent, from 12 h before dental surgery until 7 days after it, prevented bleeding complications in 19 patients with severe factor XI deficiency.[284] For dental surgery, therefore, no plasma infusion or factor XI concentrate administration is necessary.

As already stated, spontaneous bleeding is rare in patients with severe factor XI deficiency, and when it occurs it is usually mild and abates by itself without treatment. Kitchens[255] noted that spontaneous hemorrhage in such patients is sometimes related to aspirin ingestion and hence its discontinuation resolves the problem. For pregnant factor XI–deficient patients, deliveries are infrequently complicated by bleeding[255,285]; thus, preventive plasma infusion for delivery is not advocated.

Hereditary Prekallikrein Deficiency

An incidental finding of a prolonged APTT in four asymptomatic sibs produced by a consanguineous marriage led to the discovery of a "new" clotting factor,[6] which was initially designated Fletcher factor after the surname of the index family. The nature of the clotting factor remained unknown for several years but seemed related to the contact phase of the intrinsic coagulation system. In 1973 Wuepper[7] demonstrated that Fletcher factor was identical to plasma prekallikrein, and thus the name of the disorder was changed to prekallikrein (PK) deficiency. PK deficiency is very rare worldwide. It has so far been diagnosed by a specific PK assay and reported in 47 patients belonging to 35 unrelated families.[6,54,143,286-303]

Inheritance and Heterogeneity. PK deficiency is inherited as an autosomal trait expressed in homozygotes or compound heterozygotes by a markedly low PK level (≤1 U/dl) and in heterozygotes by partially reduced or normal PK levels. Of 27 obligatory carriers of PK deficiency—parents and offspring of patients with a severe deficiency—15 had a PK level less than 2 SD below the normal mean and 12 had levels within the normal range.[54,143,287-289,294-296,300-302]

A dysfunctional PK deficiency is relatively common among patients with severe PK deficiency (Table 108-3). Out of 38 patients with very low PK activity levels belonging to 29 unrelated families, 19 had PK antigen levels of 10 to 54 U/dl, and were thus cross-reacting material positive (CRM$^+$), whereas 19 were cross-reacting material negative (CRM$^-$). Interestingly, 15 of the 18 CRM$^-$ families are Black American, a finding that might be related to a common founder effect. All 11 CRM$^+$ families are Caucasian or Japanese. In two CRM$^+$ families, the characteristics of the variant protein were studied[143,303]; in both instances, the dysfunctional PK was immunologically indistinguishable from normal PK and formed a normal complex with HK. In contrast, both CRM$^+$ variants were cleaved by β-factor XIIa at a much slower rate than normal PK and showed no enzymatic activity. In one of these families, three affected sibs were compound heterozygotes who inherited a CRM$^+$ allele from their mother and a CRM$^-$ allele from their father.[143] No DNA mutation responsible for PK deficiency has been reported.

Clinical Manifestations. Severe PK deficiency is usually not associated with a bleeding tendency. However, several anecdotal cases with bleeding episodes have been described. Of 27 PK-deficient individuals who had documented severe PK deficiency and for whom the bleeding history was described, 23 had no bleeding manifestation in spite of surgical trauma in most of them. One patient had epistaxis, but the authors stated that it was probably unrelated to PK deficiency,[294] and another patient had "easy bruising," but underwent uneventful hysterectomy and tooth extractions.[54]

Table 108-3 Relative Frequency of Prekallikrein Deficiency with No Detectable PK Antigen in Blood (CRM⁻) and Dysfunctional Prekallikrein Deficiency with Circulating Variant Molecules (CRM⁺)

	CRM⁻	CRM⁺	Total
All patients	19	19	38
Families	18	11	29
Black	15	—	15
Caucasian	3	8	11
Japanese	—	3	3

Two patients did bleed excessively following tonsillectomy.[289,300] Thus, in only 2 of 27 patients with severe PK deficiency, excessive bleeding was conceivably related to PK deficiency.

Arterial or venous thrombosis occurred in seven patients with severe PK deficiency at a relatively young age (<45 years). Among these individuals, three patients had thrombotic stroke,[277,296,299] and one of these had diabetes, hypertension and cardiomyopathy[299]; one patient had an acute myocardial infarction[288]; two additional sibs had deep-vein thrombosis but were obese; and one patient had pulmonary infarction related to fatal systemic lupus erythematosus.[304] These data suggest that severe PK deficiency provides no protection against arterial or venous thrombosis, although no conclusions can be drawn regarding a possible association between severe PK deficiency and excessive risk of thrombosis. In order to establish such a linkage, more extensive observations will have to be made as well as rigorous exclusion in affected patients of other risk factors for thrombosis, including associated inherited hypercoagulable states.

A limited number of patients with severe PK deficiency have been challenged by a variety of tests in searches for possible abnormalities in their inflammatory response or fibrinolytic system resulting from their impaired capacity to form kallikrein or bradykinin. The extent of leukocyte migration to a site of skin injury with local stimulation by foreign antigens was normal in one patient[286] but was slightly delayed in two other patients.[206,294] Immediate and delayed hypersensitivity skin reactions were normal in two patients.[286] Elevation of fibrinolytic activity by venous occlusion or DDAVP (1-deamino-8-D-arginine vasopressin) infusion was normal in three patients[286,302] but impaired in another patient.[305] A normal euglobulin lysis time was found for two additional patients, indicating an unimpaired intrinsic fibrinolytic function at least in this particular assay. Consequently, it seems that in spite of the severe PK deficiency, alternative mediators of inflammatory responses and of fibrinolysis that do not require PK can operate effectively in these patients.

Diagnosis. A diagnosis of severe PK deficiency is usually established after an incidental finding of a prolonged APTT in an asymptomatic patient. An isolated finding of a prolonged APTT can result from various clotting factor deficiencies of the intrinsic coagulation system or from the presence of lupus anticoagulant. For the diagnosis of PK deficiency, systematic assays of these factors are unnecessary since, unlike other deficiency states, the abnormal APTT of patients with PK deficiency is correctable by prolonged incubation with strong contact activation reagents such as kaolin.[54]

It should be noted that the diagnosis of severe PK deficiency can be missed if the contact trigger in the APTT assay is ellagic acid, since it usually yields normal values depending on the preincubation time with the contact activation reagent prior to recalcification.[287] Conceivably, many cases remain undiagnosed at present since ellagic acid is commonly used for the APTT tests performed by automated coagulometers. Heterozygotes who have a partial PK deficiency have a normal APTT, since only small amounts of PK (≥2 U/dl) are sufficient to correct the APTT in plasma that is severely deficient in PK.[7] For a definitive diagnosis of severe or partial PK deficiency, a specific modified APTT assay is performed using PK-deficient plasma.[287] Also available are amidolytic assays in which plasma kallikrein generation is measured following contact activation using a chromogenic substrate.[143,260] PK antigen level can be determined by electroimmunoassay[143] or radioimmunoassay[292] using monospecific antibodies.

High Molecular Weight Kininogen Deficiency

In 1974 Schiffman and Lee provided evidence that an unrecognized plasma activity, different from PK, participated in the activation of factor XI by factor XIIa.[306] During the following year three independent groups of investigators described three asymptomatic patients with an inherited deficiency of a clotting factor that indeed was essential for the contact phase of the intrinsic coagulation system.[8-12] The missing factor was initially named after the surnames of these three index families (Fitzgerald, Williams, Flaujac), but once its identity with high molecular weight kininogen (HK) was demonstrated, the terms HK and HK deficiency prevailed.[9]

Reports of HK deficiency are exceedingly rare. It has so far been described in 18 patients belonging to 16 unrelated families of Black American, Caucasian, Japanese, Pakistani, and Aboriginal origins.[8,10-12,33,170,307-316]

Inheritance and Heterogeneity. In spite of the limited number of family studies, there is good evidence that HK deficiency is transmitted as an autosomal recessive disorder. It is expressed in the homozygous state by severe HK deficiency and in the heterozygous state by partially reduced or normal levels of HK. Of 18 homozygotes, 16 had an HK level of less than 1 U/dl, one patient had a level which ranged between 0.7 and 1.7 U/dl,[309] and one patient had a level of 5 U/dl.[315] Of 22 obligatory carriers in 8 families, 15 had an HK level below the lower limit of the normal range, and three had an activity within the normal range.[8,11,12,308,309,313,314,316] No compound heterozygotes have so far been reported.

Heterogeneity of HK deficiency as evidenced by dysfunctional variants or by the presence or absence of LK is typical for this disorder. Thus, of 15 unrelated patients who were tested for dysfunctional HK deficiency, 12 were found to have extremely low HK coagulant and antigen levels

(CRM⁻), whereas three had measurable amounts of HK antigen by radioimmunoassay.[170] In 13 unrelated patients, the levels of both HK and LK were determined. Seven patients had an isolated HK deficiency,[170,310,312] whereas six had a combined HK and LK deficiency.[11,33,311,312] Because the synthesis of both HK and LK is controlled by the same gene with alternative RNA splicing of the primary transcripts yielding mRNAs for HK and LK,[174] the phenotypic variability that was found in these patients indicates that several mutations account for HK deficiency. Two mutations have been found in HK-deficient patients. In one patient who lacks both HK and LK, a homozygous C→T change was located at nucleotide 587, resulting in a TGA (stop) mutation located in exon 5 of the kininogen gene.[317] Since the mutation was localized before the differential splicing of the HK-mRNA and LK-mRNA in exon 10, the data explain the lack of both HK and LK. In another patient who had isolated HK deficiency, restriction analysis by Southern blotting revealed a homozygous deletion in intron 7, which was assumed to account for the abnormality.[312] In four additional patients with combined HK and LK deficiency, Southern-blot analysis did not reveal any gross abnormality of the gene.[312]

Clinical Manifestations. Hypertension has been reported in two patients.[307,318] In one of these patients[318] an excessively increased diastolic blood pressure was observed during an exercise test, which in the investigators' opinion could have resulted from a lack of HK-derived bradykinin known to be a strong vasodilator. In another patient[319] sodium depletion did not induce an increase in renin or angiotensin II levels, a finding that was interpreted to mean that kallikrein, which presumably converts prorenin to renin in such circumstances, was not generated from PK because of the lack of HK. These interesting but very limited observations deserve further investigation.

Neither thrombosis nor spontaneous bleeding manifestations have been described in patients with severe HK deficiency. Eight patients were challenged by surgery or trauma but did not present with excessive bleeding.[10,12,33,309-311,313] Furthermore, no predisposition for infections or other clinical problems have been documented.

The inflammatory response was studied in one patient with severe HK deficiency by the skin window test.[206] Paradoxically, unlike three patients with severe factor XII deficiency who had a substantially impaired response and two patients with severe PK deficiency who had a slightly diminished response, the patient with severe HK deficiency had an exuberant migration of leukocytes to the site of skin abrasion. No explanation for this unusual response was provided, although some work suggests that HK may inhibit cell migration.[205]

While kaolin-activated fibrinolysis was defective in all studied patients with severe HK deficiency, spontaneous fibrinolysis measured by the euglobulin lysis time was normal in one patient,[11] but abnormal in another.[311] A normal elevation of fibrinolytic activity was observed in two patients in the venous occlusion test.[309,310] From these observations and the lack of clinical manifestations in cases with severe HK deficiency, there does not seem to be any in vivo function for which HK is absolutely essential.

Diagnosis. All patients with severe HK deficiency have a very prolonged APTT no matter what contact reagents are used. Thus, a laboratory distinction can be made between severe PK deficiency and HK deficiency by APTT assays performed with ellagic acid, since in HK deficiency clotting times are very prolonged, whereas in PK deficiency they approach normal values. Furthermore, unlike PK-deficient plasma the abnormally prolonged APTT of HK-deficient plasma is not correctable by prolonged incubation with kaolin. A modified APTT clotting assay using severely HK-deficient plasma is the most simple diagnostic test. A bioassay based on kallikrein-induced bradykinin generation is less practical.[170] For determination of HK antigen level, highly specific antibodies have been used in an accurate radioimmunoassay.[170]

Interestingly, a partial PK deficiency is commonly observed in patients with severe HK deficiency. In 13 of 15 patients with severe HK deficiency, the functional PK levels ranged from 10 to 50 U/dl and in 4, for whom studies were performed, a concordantly reduced PK antigen was found.[11,33,310,311] Only two patients have so far been shown to have PK levels within the normal range.[309,315] Interesting, these were the only two patients in whom an HK level of more than 1 U/dl was measured. It was suggested that the reduced PK levels observed in patients with severe HK deficiency stem from excessive catabolism of plasma PK due to its instability when uncomplexed with HK,[308] although no experimental evidence supporting this hypothesis is available at present.

Factor XII Deficiency

In 1955 three patients were described with a remarkably prolonged clotting time not associated with a bleeding tendency.[2] The plasma component missing in these patients seemed to participate in the early phase of blood coagulation and was initially named Hageman factor after the surname of the index case. The striking dissociation between the clinical presentation and the profound in vitro effect in blood coagulation and additional laboratory test abnormalities found later in kinin generation and fibrinolysis, as well as the demise of Mr. Hageman from massive pulmonary embolism,[320] sparked numerous studies, disputes, and speculations. Factor XII deficiency is not as rare as PK or HK deficiencies. It has been reported in many populations, but its true frequency is hard to assess in view of its asymptomatic nature.[17]

Inheritance and Heterogeneity. Factor XII deficiency is an autosomal recessive disorder. Homozygotes and compound heterozygotes have an extremely low factor XII activity, and heterozygotes have a partially reduced or normal factor XII activity.[321-323] In an exceptional nonconsanguineous family, an autosomal dominant mode of inheritance was described, and evidenced by two instances of vertical transmission of severe factor XII deficiency.[324]

Most patients with severe factor XII deficiency have an extremely low activity as well as a similarly reduced antigen level. Among more than 108 patients from different populations who were tested for both activity and antigen,[15,323,325] only five unrelated patients were found to have dysfunctional factor XII deficiency.[15,326-330] Some of the characteristics of these variants, four of which were termed after the city of origin of the patients, are summarized in Table 108-4. All were single-chain polypeptides with a normal 80-kDa molecular weight and immunologic cross-reactivity with normal factor XII, and all adsorbed well to negatively charged surfaces. An apparently normal proteolytic cleavage of the bond between Arg 353 and Val 354, which is essential for the conversion of factor XII to α-factor XIIa, was

Table 108-4 Characteristics of Factor XII Deficiency Variants*

Assigned Name of Variant (Reference)	Factor XII, U/dl		Adsorption to Kaolin	Proteolytic Cleavage of Arg 353–Val 354 Bond	Generation of Factor XIa by Activated Variant	Generation of Kallikrein by Activated Variant
	Activity	Antigen				
Washington[328,331,343]†	<1	39	Normal	Positive by trypsin and kallikrein‡	Negative	Negative‡
Toronto[327,343]†	<1	80	Normal	ND	ND	Negative‡
Bari[326]	<1	30	Normal	Positive by prolonged contact activation	Positive by prolonged contact activation	ND
Bern[329]	<1	11	Normal	Positive by kallikrein	Negative	Negative
Locarno[330]	<1	46	Normal	Negative by kallikrein	Negative	Negative

* ND = not determined.
† Three obligate carriers had factor XII activity between 49 and 51 U/dl and antigen level between 105 and 112 U/dl.
‡ Berrettini M, et al.: unpublished data.

demonstrated in three variants treated with trypsin or kallikrein or following prolonged contact activation.[326,329,331] In contrast, the Locarno variant[330] was proteolytically cleaved by kallikrein only at an alternative site. So far only the Washington variant has been characterized in which the alteration was biochemically identified as a replacement of Cys 571 by Ser.[328]

A *Taq*I polymorphism localized in intron 2 of the factor XII gene was detected in several homozygotes and heterozygotes of five unrelated Italian families, but not in the normal Italian population.[332,333] The gene alteration was suggested to represent either the mutation causing factor XII deficiency or to constitute an RFLP tightly linked to it.

Clinical Manifestations. Patients initially described with severe factor XII deficiency did not have spontaneous bleeding manifestations, nor did they bleed following surgical trauma.[2] Occasionally, patients who experienced excessive bleeding have been reported,[334-336] but other causes for bleeding were not rigorously excluded in all of them, and currently it is widely believed that there is no risk of bleeding associated with factor XII deficiency.

In contrast, thromboembolism has been described more frequently in patients with severe factor XII deficiency[277,323,325,337-340] and even in patients with a partial deficiency.[341] These observations led some investigators to hypothesize that factor XII deficiency might confer a predisposition to thrombosis, possibly stemming from the patient's diminished capacity to generate fibrinolytic activity.[342] However, a critical analysis of the reported data on 23 patients with severe factor XII deficiency who presented with arterial (12 patients) or venous (11 patients) thrombosis reveals that 14 of them had well-known risk factors such as heavy smoking, hypertension, diabetes, hypercholesterolemia, late pregnancy, puerperium, carcinoma, and pelvic fracture. Among the remaining 9 patients, in whom no apparent risk factors were described, 5 patients were over 50 years old and no clinical history was provided for one. In another study of 107 patients with recurrent venous thromboembolism, 11 patients had a partially deficient factor XII level as the only apparent abnormality.[341] The authors of this study suggested that this finding might be considered as a cause of thrombophilia. However, they failed to rule out protein S deficiency or functional protein C deficiency in their patients. Based on the aforementioned clinical data, one cannot conclude that factor XII deficiency is clearly associated with an excessive risk of thrombosis, and caution plus further studies are needed concerning this hypothesis. Nonetheless, the data do clearly indicate that severe factor XII deficiency, similar to several other inherited coagulation factor deficiencies,[277] confers no obvious protection against arterial or venous thromboembolism.

Patients with severe factor XII deficiency have no predisposition to infection.

Diagnosis. An incidental finding of a prolonged APTT in an asymptomatic patient is the common mode of identification of severe factor XII deficiency. The diagnosis can be established by a modified APTT using factor XII–deficient plasma. Factor XII antigen can be determined by electroimmunoassay or radioimmunoassay.[343] Immunoblotting analysis affords an excellent means to study quantitative and qualitative aspects of the deficiency.[344]

ACKNOWLEDGMENT

We are indebted to K. Fujikawa, E.W. Davie, and B.A. McMullen for providing us prints of their published figures displaying the structures of factors XII, XI, and PK. We are also grateful to the following colleagues who shared with us their latest data: P. Bolton-Maggs, G.J. Broze, D. Chung, F. Citarella, R.W. Colman, V.H. Donaldson, A. Fantoni, K. Fujikawa, A.P. Kaplan, B. Lämmle, W. Müller-Esterl, O.D. Ratnoff, H. Saito, J.K. Smith, P.N. Walsh, and W.A. Wuillemin.

REFERENCES

1. Rosenthal RL, Dreskin OH, Rosenthal N: New hemophilia like disease caused by efficiency of a third plasma thromboplastin factor. *Proc Soc Exp Biol Med* **82:**171, 1953.
2. Ratnoff OD, Colopy JE: A familial hemorrhagic trait associated with a deficiency of a clot-promoting fraction of plasma. *J Clin Invest* **34:**602, 1955.
3. Niewiarowski S, Prou-Wartelle O: Role du facteur contact (facteur Hageman) dans la fibrinolyse. *Thromb Diath Haemorrh* **3:**593, 1959.
4. Armstrong D, Keele CA, Jepson JB, Stewart JW: Development of pain-producing substance in human plasma. *Nature* **174:**791, 1954.

5. Margolis J: Activation of plasma by contact with glass: Evidence of a common reaction which releases plasma kinin and initiates coagulation. *J Physiol (Lond)* **144:**1, 1958.
6. Hathaway WE, Belhasen LP, Hathaway HS: Evidence for a new plasma thromboplastin factor. I. Case report, coagulation studies and physiochemical properties. *Blood* **26:**521, 1965.
7. Wuepper KD: Prekallikrein deficiency in man. *J Exp Med* **138:**1345, 1973.
8. Saito H, Ratnoff OD, Waldmann R, Abraham JP: Deficiency of a hitherto unrecognized agent, Fitzgerald factor, participa.ing in surface-mediated reactions of clotting, fibrinolysis, generation of kinins, and the property of diluted plasma enhancing vascular permeability (PF/Dil). *J Clin Invest* **55:**1082, 1975.
9. Wuepper KD, Miller DR, Lacombe MJ: Flaujeac trait. Deficiency of human plasma kininogen. *J Clin Invest* **56:**1663, 1975.
10. Waldmann R, Abraham JP, Rebuck JW, Caldwell J, Saito H, Ratnoff OD: Fitzgerald factor: A hitherto unrecognized coagulation factor. *Lancet* **1:**949, 1975.
11. Colman RW, Bagdasarian A, Talamo RC, Scott CF, Seavey M, Guimaraes JA, Pierce JV, Kaplan AP: Williams trait: Human kininogen deficiency with diminished levels of plasminogen proactivator and prekallikrein associated with abnormalities of the Hageman factor-dependent pathways. *J Clin Invest* **56:**1650, 1975.
12. Lacombe M-J, Varet B, Levy J-P: A hitherto undescribed plasma factor acting at the contact phase of blood coagulation (Flaujeac factor): Case report and coagulation studies. *Blood* **46:**761, 1975.
13. Kaplan AP, Silverberg M: The coagulation-kinin pathway of human plasma. *Blood* **70:**1, 1987.
14. Kaplan AP, Silverberg M: Mediators of inflammation: An overview. *Methods Enzymol* **163:**3, 1988.
15. Saito H: Contact factors in health and disease. *Semin Thromb Hemost* **13:**35, 1987.
16. Colman RW: Contact systems in infectious disease. *Rev Infect Dis (suppl 4)* **11:**S689, 1989.
17. Ratnoff OD, Saito H: Surface-mediated reactions. *Curr Top Hematol* **2:**1, 1979.
18. Cochrane CG, Griffin JH: The biochemistry and pathophysiology of the contact system of plasma. *Adv Immunol* **33:**241, 1982.
19. Fujikawa K, Saito H: Contact activation, in Scriver CR, Beaudet AL, Sly WS, Valle D (eds): *The Metabolic Basis of Inherited Disease,* 6th ed. New York, McGraw-Hill, 1989, vol II, p 2189.
20. Gailani D, Broze GJ Jr: Factor XI activation in a revised model of blood coagulation. *Science* **253:**909, 1991.
21. Naito K, Fukikawa K: Activation of human blood coagulation Factor XI independent of Factor XII. *J Biol Chem* **266:**7353, 1991.
22. Walsh PN: Factor XI: A renaissance. *Semin Hematol* **29:**189, 1992.
23. Movat H: The plasma kallikrein-kinin system and its interrelationship with other components of blood, in Erdos EG (ed): *Bradykinin, Kallidin and Kallikrein.* Berlin, Springer-Verlag, 1979, p 1.
24. Kluft C, Dooijewaard G, Emeis JJ: Role of the contact system in fibrinolysis. *Semin Thromb Hemost* **13:**50, 1987.
25. Muller-Esterl W, Iwanaga S, Nakanishi S: Kininogens revisited. *TIBS* **11:**336, 1986.
26. Miles LA, Rothschild Z, Griffin JH: Dextran sulfate stimulated fibrinolytic activity in whole human plasma. Dependence on the contact activation system and a urokinase-related antigen. *Thromb Haemost* **46:**211, 1981.
27. Kluft C, Wijngaards G, Jie AFH: Intrinsic plasma fibrinolysis: Involvement of urokinase-related activity in the factor XII-independent plasminogen proactivator pathway. *J Lab Clin Med* **103:**408, 1984.
28. Hauert J, Bachmann F: Prourokinase activation in euglobulin fractions. *Thromb Haemost* **54:**122, 1985.
29. Ichinose A, Fujikawa K, Suyama T: The activation of pro-urokinase by plasma kallikrein and its inactivation by thrombin. *J Biol Chem* **261:**3486, 1986.
30. Goldsmith G, Saito H, Ratnoff OD: The activation of plasminogen by Hageman factor (factor XII) and Hageman factor fragments. *J Clin Invest* **12:**54, 1978.
31. Mandle RJ Jr, Kaplan AP: Hageman factor dependent fibrinolysis. Generation of fibrinolytic activity by the interaction of human activated factor XI and plasminogen. *Blood* **54:**850, 1979.
32. Miles LA, Greengard JS, Griffin JH: A comparison of the abilities of plasma kallikrein, β-factor XIIa, factor XIa and urokinase to activate plasminogen. *Thromb Res* **29:**407, 1983.
33. Donaldson VH, Glueck HI, Miller MA, Movat HZ, Habal F: Kininogen deficiency in Fitzgerald trait: Role of high molecular weight kininogen in clotting and fibrinolysis. *J Lab Clin Med* **87:**327, 1976.
34. Griffin JH, Cochrane CG: Mechanisms for the involvement of high molecular weight kininogen in surface-dependent reactions of Hageman factor. *Proc Natl Acad Sci USA* **73:**2554, 1976.
35. Schiffman S, Lee P, Feinstein DI, Pecci R: Relationship of contact activation cofactor procoagulant activity to kininogen. *Blood* **49:**935, 1977.
36. Saito H: Purification of high molecular weight kininogen and the role of this agent in blood coagulation. *J Clin Invest* **60:**584, 1977.
37. Mandle RJ, Colman RW, Kaplan AP: Identification of prekallikrein and high-molecular-weight kininogen as a complex in human plasma. *Proc Natl Acad Sci USA* **73:**4179, 1976.
38. Thompson RE, Mandle R Jr, Kaplan AP: Association of factor XI and high molecular weight kininogen in human plasma. *J Clin Invest* **60:**1376, 1977.
39. Thompson RE, Mandle R Jr, Kaplan AP: Studies of binding of prekallikrein and factor XI to high molecular weight kininogen and its light chain. *Proc Natl Acad Sci USA* **76:**4862, 1979.
40. Wiggins RC, Bouma BN, Cochrane CG, Griffin JH: Role of high-molecular-weight kininogen in surface-binding and activation of coagulation factor XI and prekallikrein. *Proc Natl Acad Sci USA* **74:**4636, 1977.
41. Silverberg M, Nicoll JE, Kaplan AP: The mechanism by which the light chain of cleaved HMW-kininogen augments the activation of prekallikrein, factor XI, and Hageman fctor. *Thromb Res* **70:**173, 1980.
42. Scott CF, Silver LD, Schapira M, Colman RW: Cleavage of human high molecular weight kininogen markedly enhances its coagulant activity: Evidence that this molecule exists as a procofactor. *J Clin Invest* **73:**954, 1984.
43. Sugo T, Ikari N, Kato H, Iwanaga S, Fujii S: Functional sites of bovine high molecular weight kininogen as a cofactor in kaolin-mediated activation of factor XII (Hageman factor). *Biochemistry* **19:**3215, 1980.
44. Sugo T, Kato H, Iwanaga S, Fujii S: The accelerating effect of bovine plasma HMW-kininogen on the surface-mediated activation of factor XII: Generation of a derivative form (active kininogen) with maximal cofactor activity by limited proteolysis. *Thromb Res* **24:**329, 1981.
45. van der Graaf F, Tans G, Bouma BN, Griffin JH: Isolation and functional properties of the heavy and light chains of human plasma kallikrein. *J Biol Chem* **257:**14300, 1982.
46. Rosing J, Tans G, Griffin JH: Surface-dependent activation of human factor XII (Hageman factor) by kallikrein and its light chain. *Eur J Biochem* **151:**531, 1985.
47. Cochrane CG, Revak SD: Dissemination of contact activation in plasma by plasma kallikrein. *J Exp Med* **152:**608, 1980.
48. Espana F, Ratnoff OD: The role of prekallikrein and high molecular weight kininogen in the contact activation of Hageman factor (factor XII) by sulfatides and other agents. *J Lab Clin Med* **102:**487, 1983.
49. Cochrane CG, Revak SD, Wuepper KD: Activation of Hageman factor in solid and fluid phase. *J Exp Med* **138:**1564, 1973.
50. Griffin JH, Cochrane CG: Mechanisms for the involvement of high molecular weight kininogen in surface dependent reactions of Hageman factor. *Proc Natl Acad Sci USA* **73:**2559, 1976.
51. Meier HL, Pierce JV, Colman RW, Kaplan AP: Activation and function of human Hageman factor. The role of high molecular weight kininogen and prekallikrein. *J Clin Invest* **60:**18, 1977.

52. Griffin JH: Role of surface-dependent activation of Hageman factor (blood coagulation factor XII). *Proc Natl Acad Sci USA* **75:**1998, 1978.
53. Tankersley DL, Alving BM, Finlayson JS: Activation of factor XII by dextran sulfate. The basis for an assay of factor XII. *Blood* **62:**448, 1983.
54. Hattersley PG, Hayse D: Fletcher factor deficiency: A report of three unrelated cases. *Br H Haematol* **18:**411, 1970.
55. Wiggins RC, Cochrane CG: The autoactivation of rabbit Hageman factor. *J Exp Med* **150:**1122, 1979.
56. Silverberg M, Dunn JT, Garen L, Kaplan AP: Autoactivation of human Hageman factor: Demonstration utilizing a synthetic substrate. *J Biol Chem* **255:**7281, 1980.
57. Tans G, Rosing J, Griffin JH: Sulfatide-dependent autoactivation of human blood coagulation factor XII (Hageman factor). *J Biol Chem* **258:**8215, 1983.
58. Dunn JT, Silverberg M, Kaplan AP: The cleavage and formation of activated Hageman factor by autodigestion and by kallikrein. *J Biol Chem* **275:**1779, 1982.
59. Tans G, Rosing J, Berrettini M, Lämmle B, Griffin JH: Autoactivation of human plasma prekallikrein. *J Biol Chem* **262:**11308, 1987.
60. Newball H, Revak S, Cochrane CG, Griffin JH, Lichtenstein L: Activation of Hageman factor by a leucocytic protease. *Adv Exp Med Biol* **120A:**139, 1979.
61. Wiggins RC, Loskutoff DJ, Cochrane CG, Griffin JH, Edgington TS: Activation of rabbit Hageman factor by homogenates of cultivated rabbit endothelial cells. *J Clin Invest* **65:**197, 1980.
62. Ratnoff OD, Saito H: Amidolytic properties of single chain activated Hageman factor. *Proc Natl Acad Sci USA* **76:**1411, 1979.
63. Silverberg M, Kaplan AP: Enzymatic activities of activated and zymogen forms of human Hageman factor (factor XII). *Blood* **60:**64, 1982.
64. Griffin JH, Beretta G: Molecular mechanisms of surface-dependent activation of Hageman factor (factor XII). *Adv Exp Med Biol* **120B:**39, 1979.
65. Heimark RL, Kurachi K, Fujikawa K, Davie EW: Surface activation of blood coagulation, fibrinolysis and kinin formation. *Nature* **286:**456, 1980.
66. Kurachi K, Fujikawa K, Davie EW: Mechanism of activation of bovine factor XI by factor XII and factor XII. *Biochemistry* **19:**1330, 1980.
67. Morgan PH, Robinson NC, Walsh KA, Neurath H: Inactivation of bovine trypsinogen and chymotrypsinogen by diisopropyl phosphofluoridate. *Proc Natl Acad Sci USA* **69:**3312, 1972.
68. Bouma BN, Miles LA, Barretta G, Griffin JH: Human plasma prekallikrein. Studies of its activation by activated factor XII and of its inactivation by diisopropyl phosphofluoridate. *Biochemistry* **19:**1151, 1980.
69. Tankersley DL, Finlayson JS: Kinetics of activation and autoactivation of human factor XII. *Biochemistry* **23:**273, 1984.
70. Kaplan AP, Austen KF: A prealbumin activator of prekallikrein. *J Immunol* **105:**802, 1970.
71. Kaplan AP, Austen KF: A prealbumin activator of prekallikrein II. Derivation of activators of prekallikrein from activated Hageman factor with plasmin. *J Exp Med* **133:**672, 1971.
72. Revak SD, Cochrane CG, Griffin JH: Structural changes accompanying enzymatic activation of human Hageman factor. *J Clin Invest* **54:**619, 1974.
73. Revak SD, Cochrane CG: The relationship of structure and function in human Hageman factor. *J Clin Invest* **57:**852, 1976.
74. Revak SD, Cochrane CG, Griffin JH: The binding and cleavage characteristics of human Hageman factor during contact activation. A comparison of normal plasma with plasmas deficient in factor XI, prekallikrein, or high molecular weight kininogen. *J Clin Invest* **59:**1167, 1977.
75. Revak SD, Cochrane CG, Bouma BN, Griffin JH: Surface and fluid phase activities of two forms of activated Hageman factor produced during contact activation of plasma. *J Exp Med* **147:**719, 1978.
76. Ghebrehiwet B, Silverberg M, Kaplan AP: Activation of the classical pathway of complement by Hageman factor fragment. *J Exp Med* **153:**665, 1981.
77. Ghebrehiwet B, Randazzo BP, Dunn JT, Silverberg M, Kaplan AP: Mechanisms of activation of the classical pathway of complement by Hageman factor fragment. *J Clin Invest* **71:**1450, 1983.
78. DiScipio RG: The activation of the alternative pathway C3 convertase by human plasma kallikrein. *Immunology* **45:**587, 1982.
79. Cooper NR, Miles LA, Griffin JH: Effects of plasma kallikrein and plasmin on the first complement component. *J Immunol* **124:**1517, 1980. (abstr.)
80. Sealey JE, Atlas SA, Laragh JH, Silverberg M, Kaplan AP: Initiation of plasma prorenin activation by Hageman factor-dependent conversion of plasma prekallikrein to kallikrein. *Proc Natl Acad Sci USA* **76:**5914, 1979.
81. Derkx FHM, Bouma BN, Schalekamp MPA, Schalekamp MADH: An intrinsic factor XII-prekallikrein-dependent pathway activates the human plasma renin-angiotensin system. *Nature* **280:**315, 1979.
82. Blumberg AL, Sealey JE, Atlas SA, Laragh JH, Dharmgrongartama B, Kaplan AP: Contact activation of human plasma prorenin *in vitro*. *J Lab Clin Med* **97:**771, 1981.
83. Derkx FHM, Schalekamp MPA, Bouma B, Kluft C, Schalekamp MADH: Plasma kallikrein-mediated activation of the renin-angiotensin system does not require prior acidification. *J Clin Endocrinol Metab* **54:**343, 1982.
84. Moskowitz RW, Schwartz HJ, Michel B, Ratnoff OD, Astrup T: Generation of kinin-like agents by chondroitin sulfate, heparin, chitin sulfate, and human articular cartilage: Possible pathophysiologic implications. *J Lab Clin Med* **76:**790, 1970.
85. Hojima Y, Cochrane CG, Wiggins RC, Austen KF, Stevens RL: *In vitro* activation of the contact (Hageman factor) system of plasma by heparin and chondroitin sulfate E. *Blood* **63:**1453, 1984.
86. Shimada T, Kato H, Iwanaga S, Iwamori M, Nagai Y: Activation of factor XII and prekallikrein with cholesterol sulfate. *Thromb Res* **38:**21, 1985.
87. Tans G, Griffin JH: Properties of sulfatides in factor XII-dependent contact activation. *Blood* **59:**69, 1982.
88. Griep MA, Fujikawa K, Nelsestuen GL: Possible basis for the apparent surface selectivity of the contact activation of human blood coagulation factor XII. *Biochemistry* **25:**6688, 1986.
89. Griep MA, Fujikawa K, Nelsestuen GL: Binding and activation properties of human factor XII, prekallikrein, and derived peptides with acidic lipid vesicles. *Biochemistry* **24:**4124, 1985.
90. Kellermeyer RW, Breckenridge RT: The inflammatory process in acute gouty arthritis, I. Activation of Hageman factor by sodium urate crystals. *J Lab Clin Med* **63:**307, 1965.
91. Ginsberg M, Jacques B, Cochrane CG, Griffin JH: Urate crystal-dependent cleavage of Hageman factor in human plasma and synovial fluid. *J Lab Clin Med* **95:**497, 1980.
92. Kimball HR, Melmon KL, Wolff SM: Endotoxin-induced kinin production in man. *Proc Soc Exp Biol Med* **139:**1078, 1972.
93. Morrison DC, Cochrane CG: Direct evidence for Hageman factor (factor XII) activation by bacterial lipopolysaccharides (endotoxins). *J Exp Med* **140:**787, 1974.
94. Kluft C: Determination of prekallikrein in human plasma: Optimal conditions for activating prekallikrein. *J Lab Clin Med* **91:**83, 1978.
95. van der Graaf F, Keus FJA, Vlooswijk RAA, Bouma BN: The contact activation mechanism in human plasma: Activation induced by dextran sulfate. *Blood* **59:**1225, 1982.
96. Schousboe I: β_2-glycoprotein I: A plasma inhibitor of the contact activation of the intrinsic blood coagulation pathway. *Blood* **66:**1086, 1985.
97. Henry ML, Everson B, Ratnoff OD: Inhibition of the activation of Hageman factor (factor XII) by β_2-glycoprotein I. *J Lab Clin Med* **111:**519, 1988.
98. Rehmus EH, Greene BM, Everson BA, Ratnoff OD: Inhibition of the activation of Hageman factor (factor XII) by complement subcomponent C1q. *J Clin Invest* **80:**516, 1987.
99. Koenig JM, Chahine A, Ratnoff OD: Inhibition of the activation of Hageman factor (factor XII) by soluble human placental collagens types III, IV, and V. *J Lab Clin Med* **117:**523, 1991.

100. Ratnoff OD, Everson B, Embury P, Ziats NP, Anderson JM, Emanuelson MM, Malemud CJ: Inhibition of the activation of Hageman factor (factor XII) by human vascular endothelial cell culture supernates. *Proc Natl Acad Sci USA* **88:**10740, 1991.
101. Bouma BN, Griffin JH: Human blood coagulation factor XI. Purification, properties, and mechanism of activation by activated factor XII. *J Biol Chem* **252:**6432, 1977.
102. Kurachi K, Davie EW: Activation of human factor XI (plasma thromboplastin antecedent) by factor XII_a (activated Hageman factor). *Biochemistry* **16:**5831, 1977.
103. Heck LW, Kaplan AP: Substrates of Hageman factor: I. Isolation and characterization of human factor XI (PTA) and inhibition of the activated enzyme by α_1 antitrypsin. *J Exp Med* **140:**1615, 1974.
104. Bouma BN, Vlooswijk RA, Griffin JH: Immunologic studies of human coagulation factor XI and its complex with high molecular weight kininogen. *Blood* **62:**1123, 1983.
105. Kisiel W, Fujikawa K, Davie EW: Activation of bovine factor VII (Proconvertin) by factor XII_a (activated Hageman factor). *Biochemistry* **16:**4189,1977.
106. Fujikawa K, Chung DW, Hendrickson LE, Davie EW: Amino acid sequence of human factor XI, a blood coagulation factor with four tandem repeats that are highly homologous with plasma prekallikrein. *Biochemistry* **25:**2417, 1986.
107. McMullen BA, Fujikawa K, Davie EW: Location of the disulfide bonds in human coagulation factor XI: The presence of tandem apple domains. *Biochemistry* **30:**2056, 1991.
108. Chung DW, Fujikawa K, McMullen Ba, Davie EW: Human plasma prekallikrein, a zymogen to a serine protease that contains four tandem repeats. *Biochemistry* **25:**2410, 1986.
109. Fujikawa K, Legaz ME, Kato H, Davie EW: The mechanism of activation of bovine factor IX (Christmas factor) by bovine factor XI_a (activated plasma thromboplastin antecedent). *Biochemistry* **13:**4508, 1974.
110. DiScipio RG, Kurachi K, Davie EW: Activation of human factor IX (Christmas factor). *J Clin Invest* **61:**1528, 1978.
111. Osterud B, Bouma BN, Griffin JH: Human blood coagulation factor IX. Purification, properties and mechanism of activation by activated factor XI. *J Biol Chem* **253:**5946, 1978.
112. van der Graaf F, Greengard JS, Bouma BN, Kerbiriou DM, Griffin JH: Isolation and functional characterization of the active light chain of activated human blood coagulation factor XI. *J Biol Chem* **258:**9669, 1983.
113. Saito H: The participation of plasma thromboplastin antecedent (Factor XI) in contact-activated fibrinolysis. *Proc Soc Exp Biol Med* **164:**153, 1980.
114. Scott CF, Purdon DA, Silver LD, Colman RW: Cleavage of high molecular weight kininogen (HMWK) by plasma factor XIa. *J Biol Chem* **260:**10856, 1985.
115. Baglia FA, Jameson BA, Walsh PN: Localization of the high molecular weight kininogen binding site in the heavy chain of human factor XI to amino acids Phe-56 through Ser-86. *J Biol Chem* **265:**4149, 1990.
116. Baglia FA, Jameson BA, Walsh PN: Identification and chemical synthesis of a substrate-binding site for factor IX on coagulation factor XIa. *J Biol Chem* **266:**24190, 1991.
117. Baglia FA, Jameson BA, Walsh PN: Fine mapping of the high molecular weight kininogen binding site on blood coagulation factor XI through the use of rationally designed synthetic analogs. *J Biol Chem* **267:**4247, 1992.
118. Forbes CD, Pensky J, Ratnoff OD: Inactivation of activated Hageman factor and activated plasma thromboplastin antecedent by purified serum C1 inactivator. *J Lab Clin Med* **76:**809, 1970.
119. Walsh PN, Sinha D, Kueppers F, Blankstein KB, Seaman FS: Regulation of factor XIa activity by platelets and alpha-1 protease inhibitor. *J Clin Invest* **80:**1578, 1987.
120. Damus PS, Hicks M, Rosenberg RD: Anticoagulant action of heparin. *Nature* **240:**355, 1973.
121. Soons H, Janssen-Claesson T, Tans G, Hemker HC: Inhibition of factor XIa by antithrombin III. *Biochemistry* **26:**4624, 1987.
122. Meijers JC, Vlooswijk RA, Bouma BN: Inhibition of human blood coagulation factor XIa by C-1 inhibitor. *Biochemistry* **27:**959, 1988.
123. Saito H, Goldsmith G, Moroi M, Aoki N: Inhibitory spectrum of α_2-plasmin inhibitor. *Proc Natl Acad Sci USA* **76:**2103, 1979.
124. Berrettini M, Schleef RR, España F, Loskutoff DJ, Griffin JH: Interaction of type 1 plasminogen activator inhibitor with the enzymes of the contact activation system. *J Biol Chem* **264:**11738, 1989.
125. España F, Berrettini M, Griffin JH: Purification and characterization of plasma protein C inhibitor. *Thromb Res* **55:**369, 1989.
126. Scott CF, Schapira M, James HL, Cohen AB, Colman RW: Inactivation of factor XIa by plasma protease inhibitors. Predominant role of alpha 1-protease inhibitor and protective effect of high molecular weight kininogen. *J Clin Invest* **69:**844, 1982.
127. Asakai R, Davie EW, Chung DW: Organization of the gene for human factor XI. *Biochemistry* **26:**7221, 1987.
128. Kato A, Asakai R, Davie EW, Aoki N: Factor XI gene (F11) is located on the distal end of the long arm of human chromosome 4. *Cytogenet Cell Genet* **52:**77, 1989.
129. Greengard JS, Heeb MJ, Ersdal E, Walsh PN, Griffin JH: Binding of coagulation factor XI to washed human platelets. *Biochemistry* **25:**3884, 1986.
130. Greengard JS, Heeb MJ, McGann M, Ersdal E, Griffin JH: Coordinate Zn^{++} and Ca^{++} ion-dependent binding of high MW kininogen and Factor XI to platelets. *Circulation (suppl II)* **70:**1409, 1984.
131. Berrettini M, Schleef RR, Heeb MJ, Hopmeier P, Griffin JH: Assembly and expression of an intrinsic factor IX activator complex on the surface of cultured human endothelial cells. *Thromb Haemost* **65:**693, 1991. (abstr.)
132. Sinha D, Seaman FS, Koshy A, Walsh PN: Blood coagulation factor XIa binds specifically to a site on activated human platelets distinct from that of factor XI. *J Clin Invest* **73:**1559, 1984.
133. Tuszynski GP, Bevacona SJ, Schmaier AH, Colman RW, Walsh PN: Factor XI antigen and activity in human platelets. *Blood* **59:**1148, 1982.
134. Stern DM, Drillings M, Nossel HL, Hurlet-Jensen A, LaGamma KS, Owen J: Binding of factors IX and IX_a to cultured vascular endothelial cells. *Proc Natl Acad Sci USA* **80:**4119, 1983.
135. Walsh PN, Griffin JH: Contributions of human platelets to the proteolytic activation of blood coagulation factors XII and XI. *Blood* **57:**106, 1981.
136. Wuepper KD, Cochrane CG: Plasma prekallikrein: Isolation, characterization and mechanism of activation. *J Exp Med* **135:**1, 1972.
137. Mandle R Jr, Kaplan AP: Hageman factor substrates. Human plasma prekallikrein: Mechanism of activation by Hageman factor and participation in Hageman factor-dependent fibrinolysis. *J Biol Chem* **252:**6097, 1977.
138. Bouma BN, Miles LA, Beretta G, Griffin JH: Human plasma prekallikrein. Studies of its activation by activated factor XII and of its inactivation by diisopropyl phosphofluoridate. *Biochemistry* **19:**1151, 1980.
139. Kerbiriou DM, Bouma BN, Griffin JH: Immunochemical studies of human high molecular weight kininogen and of its complexes with plasma prekallikrein or kallikrein. *J Biol Chem* **255:**3952, 1980.
140. Bock PE, Shore JD, Tans G, Griffin JH: Protein-protein interactions in contact activation of blood coagulation. Binding of high molecular weight kininogen and the 5-(iodoacetamido)fluorescein-labeled kininogen light chain to prekallikrein, kallikrein, and the separated kallikrein heavy and light chains. *J Biol Chem* **260:**12434, 1985.
141. Bouma BN, Keribiriou DM, Vlooswijk RAA, Griffin JH: Immunological studies of prekallikrein, kallikrein, and high molecular weight kininogen in normal and deficient plasmas and in normal plasma after cold-dependent activation. *J Lab Clin Med* **96:**693, 1980.
142. Saito H, Poon M-C, Vicic W, Goldsmith GH, Menitove JE: Human plasma prekallikrein (Fletcher factor) clotting activity and antigen in health and disease. *J Lab Clin Med* **92:**84, 1978.
143. Bouma BN, Kerbiriou DM, Baker J, Griffin JH: Characterization of a variant prekallikrein, prekallikrein Long Beach, from a family with mixed cross-reacting material-positive and

cross-reacting material-negative prekallikrein deficiency. *J Clin Invest* **78**:170, 1986.

144. Drinkwater CC, Evans BA, Richards RI: Kallikreins, kinins and growth factor biosynthesis. *TIBS* **13**:169, 1988.
145. McMullen BA, Fujikawa K, Davie EW: Location of the disulfide bonds in human plasma prekallikrein: The presence of four novel apple domains in the amino-terminal portion of the molecule. *Biochemistry* **30**:2050, 1991.
146. Page JD, Colman RW: Localization of distinct functional domains on prekallikrein for interaction with both high molecular kininogen and activated factor XII in a 28-kDa fragment (Amino Acids 141-371). *J Biol Chem* **266**:8143, 1991.
147. Colman RW, Wachtfogel YT, Kucich U, Weinbaum G, Hahn S, Pixley RA, Scott CF, de Agostini A, Burger D, Schapira M: Effect of cleavage of the heavy chain of human plasma kallikrein on its functional properties. *Blood* **65**:311, 1985.
148. Burger D, Schleuning WD, Schapira M: Human plasma prekallikrein. Immunoaffinity purification and activation to α- and β-kallikrein. *J Biol Chem* **261**:324, 1986.
149. Keribiriou DM, Griffin JH: High molecular weight kininogen. Studies of structure-function relationships and of proteolysis of the molecule occurring during contact activation of plasma. *J Biol Chem* **254**:12020, 1979.
150. Nakayasa T, Nagasawa S: Studies on human kininogen I. Isolation, characterization and cleavage by plasma kallikrein of high molecular weight (HMW) kininogen. *J Biochem* **85**:249, 1979.
151. Mori K, Nagasawa S: Studies on human high moelcular weight (HMW) kininogen II. Structural change of HMW-kininogen by the action of human plasma kallikrein II. *J Biochem* **84**:1465, 1981.
152. Colman RW: Activation of plasminogen by plasma kallikrein. *Biochem Biophys Res Commun* **351**:373, 1969.
153. Seligsohn U, Osterud B, Brown JF, Griffin JH, Rapaport SI: Activation of human factor VII in plasma and in purified systems. *J Clin Invest* **64**:1056, 1979.
154. Seligsohn U, Osterud B, Griffin JH, Rapaport SI: Evidence for the participation of both activated factor XII and activated factor IX in cold-promoted activation of factor VII. *Thromb Res* **13**:1049, 1978.
155. van der Graaf F, Koedam JA, Bouma BN: Inactivation of kallikrein in human plasma. *J Clin Invest* **71**:149, 1983.
156. van der Graaf F, Rietveld A, Keus FJA, Bouma BN: Interaction of human plasma kallikrein and its light chain with α_2-macroglobulin. *Biochemistry* **23**:1760, 1984.
157. Harpel PC, Lewin MF, Kaplan AP: Distribution of plasma kallikrein between C1 inactivator and α_2 macroglobulin in plasma utilizing a new assay for α_2-macroglobulin-kallikrein complexes. *J Biol Chem* **260**:4257, 1985.
158. Meijers JC, Kanters DH, Vlooswijk RA, van Erp HE, Hessing M, Bouma BN: Inactivation of human plasma kallikrein and factor XIa by protein C inhibitor. *Biochemistry* **27**:4231, 1988.
159. Schapira M, Scott CF, Colman RW: Protection of human plasma kallikrein from inactivation by C1 inhibitor and other protease inhibitors. The role of high molecular weight kininogen. *Biochemistry* **20**:2739, 1981.
160. Schapira M, Scott CF, James A, Silver LD, Kueppers F, James HL, Colman RW: High molecular weight kininogen or its light chain protects human plasma kallikrein from inactivation by plasma protease inhibitors. *Biochemistry* **11**:567, 1982.
161. van der Graaf F, Koedam JA, Griffin JH, Bouma BN: Interaction of human plasma kallikrein and its light chain with C1-inhibitor. *Biochemistry* **22**:4860, 1982.
162. Silverberg M, Longo J, Kaplan AP: Study of the effect of high molecular weight kininogen upon the fluid-phase inactivation of kallikrein by C1 INH. *J Biol Chem* **261**:14965, 1986.
163. Beaubien G, Rosinski-Chupin I, Mattei MG, Mbikay M, Chretien M, Seidah NG: Gene structure and chromosomal localization of plasma kallikrein. *Biochemistry* **30**:1628, 1991.
164. Gustafson EJ, Colman RW: Interaction of polymorphonuclear cells with contact activation factors. *Semin Thromb Hemost* **13**:95, 1987.
165. Gustafson EJ, Schmaier AH, Waschtfogel YT, Kaufman N, Kucich U, Colman RW: Human neutrophils contain and bind high molecular weight kininogen. *J Clin Invest* **84**:28, 1989.
166. Burgher D, Maechler P, Schapira M: Studies on the human plasma kallikrein system: α kallikrein does not directly activate blood neutrophils. *Thromb Res* **55**:109, 1989.
167. Habal FM, Movat HZ, Burrowes CE: Isolation of two functionally different kininogens from human plasma-separation from proteolytic inhibitors and interaction with plasma kallikrein. *Biochem Pharmacol* **23**:2291, 1974.
168. Kerbiriou DM, Griffin JH: Human high molecular weight kininogen: Studies of structure-function relationships and of proteolysis of the molecule occurring during contact activation of plasma. *J Biol Chem* **254**:12020, 1979.
169. Thompson RE, Mandle R Jr, Kaplan AP: Characterization of human high molecular weight kininogen. Procoagulant activity assessed with the light chain of kinin-free high molecular weight kininogen. *J Exp Med* **147**:488, 1978.
170. Proud D, Pierce JV, Pisano JJ: Radioimmunoassay of human high molecular weight kininogen in normal and deficient plasma. *J Lab Clin Med* **95**:563, 1980.
171. Ohkubo I, Kurachi K, Takasawa T, Shiokawa H, Sasaki M: Isolation of a human cDNA for α_2-thiol proteinase inhibitor and its identity with low molecular weight kininogen. *Biochemistry* **23**:5691, 1984.
172. Sueyoshi T, Enjyoji K, Shimada T, Kato H, Iwanaga S, Bando Y, Kominami E, Katunuma N: A new function of kininogens as thiol-proteinase inhibitors: Inhibition of papain and cathepsins B, H and L by bovine, rat and human plasma kininogens. *FEBS Lett* **182**:193, 1985.
173. Muller-Esterl W, Fritz H, Machleidt IW, Ritonja A, Brzin J, Kotnik M, Turk V, Kellerman J, Lottspeich F: Human plasma kininogens are identical with α-cysteine protease inhibitors. Evidence from immunological, enzymological, and sequence data. *FEBS Lett* **182**:310, 1985.
174. Takagaki Y, Kitamura N, Nakanishi S: Cloning and sequence analysis of cDNAs for human high molecular weight and low molecular weight prekininogens. *J Biol Chem* **260**:8601, 1985.
175. Kellerman J, Lottspeich F, Henschen A, Muller-Esterl W: Completion of the primary structure of human high-molecular-mass kininogen. The amino acid sequence of the entire heavy chain and evidence for its evolution by gene triplication. *Eur J Biochem* **154**:471, 1986.
176. Lottspeich F, Kellermann J, Henschen A, Rauth G, Muller-Esterl W: Human low-molecular-mass kininogen: Amino-acid sequence of the light chain; homology with other protein sequences. *Eur J Biochem* **142**:227, 1984.
177. Han YN, Kim YM, Iwanaga S, Suzuki T: Studies on the primary structure of bovine high molecular weight kininogen. Amino acid sequence of a fragment ("histidine-rich peptide") released by plasma kallikrein. *J Biochem* **77**:55, 1985.
178. Kitamura N, Kitagawa H, Fukushima D, Takagaki Y, Miyata T, Nakanishi S: Structural organization of the human kininogen gene and a model for its evolution. *J Biol Chem* **260**:8610, 1985.
179: Kitamura N, Takagaki Y, Furuto S, Tanaka T, Nawa H, Nakanishi S: A single gene for bovine high molecular weight and low molecular weight kininogens. *Nature* **305**:545, 1983.
180. Salvesen G, Parker C, Abrahamson M, Grubb A, Barrett AJ: Human low-M_r kininogen contains three copies of a cystatin sequence that are divergent in structure and in inhibitory activity for cysteine proteinases. *Biochem J* **234**:429, 1986.
181. Higashiyama S, Ohkubo I, Ishiguro H, Kunimatsu M, Sawaki K, Sasaki M: Human high molecular weight kininogen as a thiol proteinase inhibitor: Presence of the entire inhibition capacity in the native form of heavy chain. *Biochemistry* **25**:1669, 1986.
182. Jiang Y, Muller-Esterl W, Schmaier AH: Domain 3 of kininogens contains a cell-binding site and a site that modifies thrombin activation of platelets. *J Biol Chem* **267**:3712, 1992.
183. Lottspeich F, Kellermann J, Henschen A, Foertsch B, Müller-Esterl W: The amino acid sequence of the light chain of human high-molecular-mass kininogen. *Eur J Biochem* **152**:307, 1985.
184. Ikari N, Sugo T, Fujii S, Kato H, Iwanaga S: The role of bovine high-molecular-weight (HMW) kininogen in contact-

mediated activation of bovine factor XII: Interaction of HMW kininogen with kaolin and plasma prekallikrein. *J Biochem* **89:**1699, 1981.

185. DeLa Cadena RA, Colman RW: The sequence HGLGHGHEQQHGLGHGH in the light chain of high molecular weight kininogen serves as a primary structural feature for zinc-dependent binding to an anionic surface. *Protein Sci* **1:**151, 1992.
186. Bock PE, Shore JD: Protein-protein interactions in contact activation of blood coagulation. Characterization of fluorescein-labeled human high molecular weight kininogen-light chain as probe. *J Biol Chem* **258:**15079, 1983.
187. Warn-Cramer BJ, Bajaj SP: Stoichiometry of binding of high molecular weight kininogen to factor XI/XIa. *Biochem Biophys Res Commun* **133:**417, 1985.
188. Tait JF, Fujikawa K: Identification of the binding site for plasma prekallikrein in human high-molecular-weight kininogen: A region from residues 185 to 224 of the kininogen light chain retains full binding activity. *J Biol Chem* **261:**15396, 1986.
189. Tait JF, Fujikawa K: Primary-structure requirements for the binding of human high molecular weight kininogen to plasma prekallikrein and factor XI. *J Biol Chem* **262:**11651, 1987.
190. Vogel R, Kaufmann J, Chung DW, Kellermann J, Müller-Esterl W: Mapping of the prekallikrein-binding site of human H-kininogen by ligand screening of λgt11 expression libraries. *J Biol Chem* **265:**12494, 1990.
191. Scarsdale JN, Harris RB: Solution phase conformation studies of the prekallikrein binding domain of high molecular weight kininogen. *J Protein Chem* **5:**647, 1990.
192. You J-L, Scarsdale JN, Harris RB: Calorimetric and spectroscopic examination of the solution phase structures of prekallikrein binding domain peptides of high molecular weight kininogen. *J Protein Chem* **10:**301, 1991.
193. Wiggins RC: Kinin release from high molecular weight kininogen by the action of Hageman factor in the absence of kallikrein. *J Biol Chem* **258:**8963, 1983.
194. Kleniewski J, Donaldson VH: Comparison of human HMW kininogen digestion by plasma kallikrein and by plasmin. A revised method of purification of HMW-kininogen. *J Lab Clin Med* **110:**469, 1987.
195. Kleniewski J, Donaldson V: Granulocyte elastase cleaves human high molecular weight kininogen and destroys its clot-promoting activity. *J Exp Med* **167:**1895, 1988.
196. Fong D, Smith DI, Hsieh W-T: The human kininogen gene (KNG) mapped to chromosome 3q26-qter by analysis of somatic cell hybrids using the polymerase chain reaction. *Hum Genet* **87:**189, 1991.
197. Cheung PP, Cannizzaro LA, Colman RW: Chromosomal mapping of human kininogen gene (KNG) to 3q26→qter. *Cytogenet Cell Genet* **59:**24, 1992.
198. van Iwaarden F, Bouma BN: Role of high molecular weight kininogen in contact activation. *Semin Thromb Hemost* **13:**15, 1987.
199. Figueroa CD, Henderson LM, Kaufmann J, de la Cadena RA, Colman RW, Müller-Esterl W, Bhoola KD: Immunovisualization of high (HK) and low (LK) molecular weight kininogens on isolated human neutrophils. *Blood* **79:**754, 1992.
200. Gustafson EJ, Schutsky D, Knight LC, Schmaier AH: High molecular weight kininogen binds to unstimulated platelets. *J Clin Invest* **78:**310, 1986.
201. Colman RW: Interactions between the contact system, neutrophils and fibrinogen. *Adv Exp Med Biol* **281:**105, 1990.
202. Greengard JS, Griffin JH: Receptors for high molecular weight kininogen on stimulated washed human platelets. *Biochemistry* **23:**6863, 1984.
203. Meloni FJ, Gustafson EJ, Schmaier AH: High molecular weight kininogen binds to platelets by its heavy and light chains and when bound has altered susceptibility to kallikrein cleavage. *Blood* **79:**1233, 1992.
204. Gustafson EJ, Lukasiewicz H, Wachtfogel YT, Norton KJ, Schmaier AH, Neiwiarowski S, Colman RW: High molecular weight kininogen inhibits fibrinogen binding to cytoadhesins of neutrophils and platelets. *J Cell Biol* **109:**377, 1989.
205. Asakura S, Hurley RW, Skorstengaard K, Ohkubo I, Mosher DF: Inhibition of cell adhesion by high molecular weight kininogen. *J Cell Biol* **116:**465, 1992.
206. Rebuck JW: The skin window as a monitor of leukocytic functions in contact activation factor deficiencies in man. *Am J Clin Pathol* **79:**405, 1983.
207. Griffin JH, Cochrane CG: Human factor XII (Hageman factor). *Methods Enzymol* **45:**56, 1976.
208. Fujikawa K, Davie EW: Human factor XII (Hageman factor). *Methods Enzymol* **80:**198, 1981.
209. Fujikawa K, McMullen BA: Amino acid sequence of human β-factor XII_a. *J Biol Chem* **258:**10924, 1983.
210. McMullen BA, Fujikawa K: Amino acid sequence of the heavy chain of human α-factor XIIa (activated Hageman factor). *J Biol Chem* **260:**5328, 1985.
211. Cool DE, Edgell CJS, Louie GV, Zoller MJ, Brayer GD, MacGillivray RTA: Characterization of human blood coagulation factor XII cDNA. *J Biol Chem* **260:**13666, 1985.
212. Dunn JT, Kaplan AP: Formation and structure of human Hageman factor fragments. *J Clin Invest* **70:**627, 1982.
213. Pixley RA, Stumpo LG, Birkmeyer K, Silver L, Colman RW: A monoclonal antibody recognizing an inosapeptide sequence in the heavy chain of human factor XII inhibits surface-catalyzed activation. *J Biol Chem* **262:**10140, 1987.
214. Clarke BJ, Cote HCF, Cool DE, Clark-Lewis I, Saito H, Pixley RA, Colman RW, MacGillivray RTA: Mapping of a putative surface-binding site of human coagulation factor XII. *J Biol Chem* **264:**11497, 1989.
215. Citarella F, La Porta C, Aiuti A, Misiti S, Fantoni A: Recombinant human Factor XII: Activation and substrate specificity are controlled by a proline-rich, 15 amino acid region. *Thromb Haemost* **65:**660, 1991. (abstr.)
216. Alving BH, Hojima Y, Pisano JJ, Mason BL, Buckingham RE Jr, Mozen MM, Finlayson JI: Hypotension associated with prekallikrein activator (Hageman factor fragments) in plasma protein fraction. *N Engl J Med* **229:**66, 1978.
217. Alving BH, Tankersley OL, Mason BL, Rossi F, Aronson DL, Finlayson JS: Contact activation factors: Contaminants of immunoglobulin preparations with coagulant and vasoactive properties. *J Lab Clin Med* **96:**334, 1980.
218. Mandle RJ Jr, Kaplan AP: Hageman factor substrates. II. Human plasma prekallikrein. Mechanism of activation by Hageman factor and participation in Hageman factor-dependent fibrinolysis. *J Biol Chem* **252:**6097, 1977.
219. Shore JD, Day DE, Bock PE, Olson ST: Acceleration of surface-dependent autocatalytic activation of blood coagulation factor XII by divalent metal ions. *Biochemistry* **26:**2250, 1987.
220. Bock PE, Srinivasan KR, Shore JD: Activation of intrinsic blood coagulation by ellagic acid: Insoluble ellagic acid-metal ion complexes are the activating species. *Biochemistry* **20:**7258, 1981.
221. Ratnoff OD, Pensky J, Ogston D, Naff GB: The inhibition of plasmin, plasma kallikrein, plasma permeability factor, and the Clr subcomponent of the first component of complement by serum C1-esterase inhibitor. *J Exp Med* **129:**315, 1969.
222. Schreiber AD, Kaplan AP, Austen KF: Inhibition by C1 INH of Hageman factor fragment activation of coagulation, fibrinolysis, and kinin generation. *J Clin Invest* **52:**1402, 1973.
223. Stead NW, Kaplan AP, Rosenberg RD: The inhibition of human activated Hageman factor (HF) by human antithrombin-heparin cofactor (AT). *J Biol Chem* **251:**6481, 1976.
224. DeAgostini A, Lijnen HR, Pixley RA, Colman RW, Schapira M: Inactivation of factor XII active fragment in normal plasma. Predominant role of C1-inhibitor. *J Clin Invest* **73:**1542, 1984.
225. Pixley RA, Schapira M, Colman RW: The regulation of human factor XIIa by plasma proteinase inhibitors. *J Biol Chem* **260:**1723, 1985.
226. Cool DE, MacGillivray RTA: Characterization of the human blood coagulation factor XII gene. *J Biol Chem* **262:**13662, 1987.
227. Royle NJ, Nigli M, Cool D, MacGillivray RT, Hamerton JL: Structural gene encoding human factor XII is located at 5q33-qtr. *Somat Cell Mol Genet* **14:**217, 1988.
228. Schmeidler-Sapiro KT, Ratnoff OD, Gordon EM: Mitogenic effects of coagulation factor XII and factor XIIa on HepG2 cells. *Proc Natl Acad Sci USA* **88:**4382, 1991.

229. Rosenthal RL, Dreskin H, Rosenthal N: Plasma thromboplastin antecedent (PTA) deficiency: Clinical, coagulation, therapeutic and hereditary aspects of a new hemophilia-like disease. *Blood* **10:**120, 1955.
230. Rapaport SI, Proctor RR, Patch MJ, Yettra M: The mode of inheritance of PTA deficiency: Evidence for the existence of major PTA deficiency and minor PTA deficiency. *Blood* **18:**149, 1961.
231. Leiba H, Ramot B, Many R: Heredity and coagulation studies in ten families with factor XI (plasma thromboplastin antecedent) deficiency. *Br J Haematorl* **11:**654, 1965.
232. Nossel HL, Niemetz J, Mibashan RS, Schulze WG: The measurement of factor XI (plasma thromboplastin antecedent). *Br J Haematol* **12:**133, 1966.
233. Seligsohn U: High gene frequency of factor XI (PTA) deficiency in Ashkenazi Jews. *Blood* **51:**1223, 1978.
234. Ragni MV, Sinha D, Seaman F, Lewis JH, Spero JA, Walsh PW: Comparison of bleeding tendency, factor XI coagulant activity, and factor XI antigen in 25 factor XI-deficient kindreds. *Blood* **65:**719, 1985.
235. Bolton-Maggs PHB, Young-Wan-Yin R, McCraw A, Slack J, Kernoff PBA: Inheritance and bleeding in factor XI deficiency. *Br J Haematol* **69:**521, 1988.
236. Forbes CD, Ratnoff OD: Studies on plasma thromboplastin antecedent (factor XI), PTA deficiency and inhibition of PTA by plasma: Pharmacologic inhibitors and specific antiserum. *J Lab Clin Med* **79:**113, 1972.
237. Rimon A, Schiffman S, Feinstein DI, Rapaport SI: Factor XI activity and factor XI antigen in homozygous and heterozygous factor XI deficiency. *Blood* **48:**165, 1976.
238. Saito H, Ratnoff OD, Bouma BN, Seligsohn U: Failure to detect variant (CRM+) plasma thromboplastin antecedent (PTA, factor XI) molecules in hereditary PTA deficiency: A study of 125 patients of several ethnic backgrounds. *J Lab Clin Med* **106:**718, 1985.
239. Mannhalter C, Hellstern P, Deutsch E: Identification of a defective factor XI cross-reacting material in a factor XI deficient patient. *Blood* **70:**31, 1987.
240. Ohkubo Y, O'Brien DP, Kanehiro T, Fukui H, Tuddenham EGD: Characterization of a panel of monoclonal antibodies to human coagulation factor XI and detection of factor XI in Hep G2 cell conditioned medium. *Thromb Haemost* **63:**417, 1990.
241. Asakai R, Chung DW, Ratnoff OD, Davie EW: Factor XI (plasma thromboplastin antecedent) deficiency in Ashkenazi Jews is a bleeding disorder that can result from three types of point mutations. *Proc Natl Acad Sci USA* **86:**7667, 1989.
242. Meijers JCM, Davie EW, Chung DW: Expression of human blood coagulation factor XI: Characterization of the defect in factor XI type III deficiency. *Blood* **79:**1435, 1992.
243. Biggs R, Sharp AA, Margolis J, Hardisty RM, Stewart J, Davidson WM: Defects in the early stages of blood coagulation: A report of four cases. *Br J Haematol* **4:**177, 1958.
244. Kurtides ES: Plasma thromboplastin antecedent deficiency. Quarterly Bulletin, Northwestern University Medical School **36:**329, 1962.
245. Seligsohn U: Factor XI (PTA) deficiency, in Goodman RM, Motulsky AG (eds): *Genetic Diseases Among Ashkenazi Jews.* New York, Raven, 1979, p 141.
246. Asakai R, Chung DW, Davie E, Seligsohn U: Factor XI deficiency in Ashkenazi Jews in Israel. *N Engl J Med* **325:**153, 1991.
247. Hancock JF, Wieland K, Pugh RE, Martinowitz U, Schulman S, Kakkar VV, Kernoff PBA, Cooper DN: A molecular genetic study of factor XI deficiency. *Blood* **77:**1942, 1991.
248. Meals RA: Paradoxical frequencies of recessive disorders in Ashkenazic Jews. *J Chron Dis* **23:**547, 1971.
249. Seligsohn U, Peretz H, Spielberg O, Eichel R, Asakai R, Davie EW: A nonsense (Type II) mutation accounts for Factor XI deficiency in 4 unrelated Iraqi-Jewish families. *Thromb Haemost* **65:**808, 1991. (abstr.)
250. Goodman RM: A perspective on genetic disease among the Jewish people, in Goodman RM, Motulsky AG (eds): *Genetic Diseases Among Ashkenazi Jews.* New York, Raven, 1979, p 1.
251. Britten AFH, Salzman EW: Surgery in congenital disorders of blood coagulation. *Surg Gynecol Obstet* **123:**1333, 1966.
252. Egeberg O: A family with antihemophilic factor (AHC = plasma thromboplastin antecedent) deficiency without bleeding tendency. *Scand J Clin Lab Invest* **14:**478, 1962.
253. Edson JR, White JG, Krivit W: The enigma of severe factor XI deficiency without hemorrhagic symptoms. *Thromb Diath Haemorrh* **18:**342, 1967.
254. Lipscomb MS, Walsh RN: Human platelets and factor XI. Localization in platelet membranes of factor XI-like activity and its functional distinction from plasma factor XI. *J Clin Invest* **63:**1006, 1979.
255. Kitchens CS: Factor XI: A review of its biochemistry and deficiency. *Semin Thromb Hemost* **17:**55, 1991.
256. Sidi A, Seligsohn U, Jonas P, Many M: Factor XI deficiency: Detection and management during urologic surgery. *J Urol* **119:**528, 1978.
257. Seligsohn U, Modan M: Definition of the population at risk of bleeding due to factor XI deficiency in Ashkenazic Jews and the value of the activated partial thromboplastin time in its detection. *Isr J Med Sci* **17:**413, 1981.
258. Pearson RW, Triplett DA: Factor XI assay results in the CAP survey (1981). *Am J Clin Pathol* 7 (*suppl*) **78:**615, 1982.
259. Scott CF, Sinha D, Seaman FS, Walsh PN, Colman RW: Amidolytic assay of human factor XI in plasma: Comparison with a coagulant assay and a new rapid radioimmunoassay. *Blood* **63:**42, 1984.
260. Retzios AD, Rosenfeld R, Schiffman S: Enzymes of the contact phase of blood coagulation: Kinetics with various chromogenic substrates and a two-substrate assay for the joint estimation of plasma prekallikrein and factor XI. *J Lab Clin Med* **112:**560, 1988.
261. Josephson AM, Lisker R: Demonstration of a circulating anticoagulant in plasma thromboplastin antecedent deficiency. *J Clin Invest* **37:**148, 1958.
262. Stern D, Nossel HL, Owen J: Acquired antibody to factor XI in a patient with congenital factor XI deficiency. *J Clin Invest* **69:**1270, 1982.
263. Morgan K, Schiffman S, Feinstein D: Acquired factor XI inhibitors in two patients with hereditary factor XI deficiency. *Thromb Haemost* **51:**371, 1984.
264. Goldsmith GHJ, Silverman P: Inhibitors of plasma thromboplastin antecedent (factor XI): Studies on mechanism of inhibition. *J Lab Clin Med* **106:**279, 1985.
265. Schnall SF, Duffy TP, Clyne LP: Acquired factor XI inhibitors in congenitally deficient patients. *Am J Hematol* **26:**323, 1987.
266. de la Cadena RA, Baglia FA, Johnson CA, Wenk RE, Amernick R, Walsh PN, Colman RW: Naturally occurring human antibodies against two distinct functional domains in the heavy chain of FXI/FXIa. *Blood* **72:**1748, 1988.
267. Musclow CE, Amato D, Ofosu F, Armstrong AL, Abbott D: Transfusion-induced specific anti-factor XI inhibitor in a patient with previously unrecognized factor XI deficiency. *Am J Clin Pathol* **89:**418, 1988.
268. McKenna R, Cole ER, Jones P: Lack of bleeding after tonsillectomy in a patient with a specific Factor XI inhibitor. *Thromb Haemost* **65:**1167, 1991. (abstr.)
269. Reece EA, Clyne LP, Romero R, Hobbins JC: Spontaneous factor XI inhibitors. Seven additional cases and a review of the literature. *Arch Intern Med* **144:**525, 1984.
270. Seligsohn U, Zitman D, Many A, Klibansky C: Coexistence of factor XI (plasma thromboplastin antecedent) deficiency and Gaucher disease. *Isr J Med Sci* **12:**1448, 1976.
271. Lian ECYI, Deykin D, Harkness DR: Combined deficiencies of factor VIII (AHF) and factor XI (PTA). *Am J Hematol* **1:**319, 1976.
272. Soff GA, Levin J, Bell WR: Familial multiple coagulation factor deficiencies. II. Combined factor VIII, IX and XI deficiency and combined factor IX and XI deficiency: Two previously uncharacterized familial multiple factor deficiency syndromes. *Semin Thromb Hemost* **7:**149, 1981.
273. Winter M, Needham J, Barkhan P: Factor XI deficiency and a platelet defect. *Haemostasis* **13:**83, 1983.
274. Chediak J, Lambert E, Johnson EI, Telfer MC: Combined severe factor XI deficiency and von Willebrand's disease. *Am J Clin Pathol* **74:**108, 1980.

275. Tavori S, Brenner B, Tatarsky I: The effect of combined factor XI deficiency with von Willebrand factor abnormalities on haemorrhagic diathesis. *Thromb Haemost* **63**:36, 1990.
276. Bolton-Maggs PHB, Patterson DA, Hay CRM, Wensley R: Bleeding in factor XI deficiency is not related to abnormalities of the factor VIII complex. *Br J Haematol (suppl 1)* **77**:41, 1991. (abstr.)
277. Goodnough LT, Saito H, Ratnoff OD: Thrombosis or myocardial infarction in congenital clotting factor abnormalities and chronic thrombocytopenias: A report of 21 patients and a review of 50 previously reported cases. *Medicine (Baltimore)* **62**:248, 1983.
278. Bashevkin ML, Nawabi IU: Factor XI deficiency in surgical patients. *NY State J Med* **79**:1360, 1979.
279. Kaufman JM: Prostatectomy in factor XI deficiency. *J Urol* **117**:75, 1977.
280. Jonas P, Sidi AA, Goldwasser B, Many M: Prostatectomy in factor XI (Plasma thromboplastin antecedent) deficiency. *J Urol* **128**:1209, 1982.
281. Bolton-Maggs PHB, Wensley RT, Kernoff PBA, Kasper CK, Winkelman L, Lane RS, Smith JK: Production and therapeutic use of a factor XI concentrate from plasma. *Thromb Haemost* **67**:314, 1992.
282. Nossel HL, Niemetz J, Sawitsky A: Blood PTA (factor XI) levels following plasma infusion. *Proc Soc Exp Biol Med* **115**:896, 1964.
283. Williams JLL: Plasma thromboplastin antecedent deficiency. *Br J Oral Surg* **10**:126, 1972.
284. Berliner S, Horowitz I, Martinowitz U, Brenner B, Seligsohn U: Safe dental surgery in patients with severe factor XI deficiency by administration of tranexamic acid only. *Thromb Haemost* **66**:1263, 1991. (abstr.)
285. Steinberg MH, Saletan S, Funt M, Baker D, Coller BS: Management of factor XI deficiency in gynecologic and obstetric patients. *Obstet Gynecol* **68**:130, 1986.
286. Hathaway WE, Wuepper KD, Weston WL, Humbert JR, Rivers RPA, Genton E, August CS, Montgomery RR, Mass MF: Clinical and physiologic studies of two siblings with prekallikrein (Fletcher factor) deficiency. *Am J Med* **60**:654, 1976.
287. Abildgaard CF, Harrison J: Fletcher factor deficiency: Family study and detection. *Blood* **43**:641, 1974.
288. Currimbhoy Z, Vinciguerra V, Palakavongs P, Kuslansky P, Degnan TJ: Fletcher factor deficiency and myocardial infarction. *Am J Clin Pathol* **65**:970, 1976.
289. Aznar JA, España F, Aznar J, Tascon A, Jimenez C: Fletcher factor deficiency: Report of a new family. *Scand J Haematol* **21**:94, 1978.
290. Ragni MV, Lewis JH, Hasiba U, Spero JA: Prekallikrein (Fletcher factor) deficiency in clinical disease states. *Thromb Res* **18**:45, 1980.
291. Waddell CC, Brown JA, Udden MM: Plasma prekallikrein (Fletcher factor) deficiency in a patient with chronic lymphocytic leukemia. *South Med J* **73**:1653, 1980.
292. Saito H, Goodnough LT, Soria J, Soria C, Aznar J, Espana F: Heterogeneity of human prekallikrein deficiency (Fletcher trait). Evidence that five of 18 cases are positive for cross-reacting material. *N Engl J Med* **305**:910, 1981.
293. Entes K, LaDuca FM, Tourbaf KD: Fletcher factor deficiency, source of variations of the activated partial thromboplastin time test. *Am J Clin Pathol* **75**:626, 1981.
294. Poon MC, Moore MR, Castleberry RP, Lurie A, Huang ST, Lehmeyer J: Combined deficiencies of Fletcher factor (plasma prekallikrein) and Hageman factor (factor XII). Report of a case with observation on *in vivo* and *in vitro* leukocyte chemotaxis. *Am J Hematol* **12**:261, 1982.
295. Kyrle PA, Neissner H, Deutsch E, Lechner K, Korninger C, Mannhalter C: CRM+ severe Fletcher factor deficiency associated with Graves' disease. *Haemostasis* **14**:302, 1984.
296. Harris MG, Exner T, Rickard KA, Kronenberg H: Multiple cerebral thrombosis in Fletcher factor (prekallikrein) deficiency: A case report. *Am J Hematol* **19**:387, 1985.
297. De Stefano V, Leone G, Teofili L, De Marinis L, Micalizzi P, Fiumara C, Bizzi B: Association of Graves' disease and prekallikrein congenital deficiency in a patient belonging to the first CRM+ prekallikrein-deficient Italian family. *Thromb Res* **60**:397, 1990.
298. Joggi J, Stalder M, Knecht H, Hauert J, Bachmann F: Deficience en prekallicreine: À propos de 2 cas. *Schweiz Med Wochenschr* **120**:1942, 1990.
299. Hess DC, Krauss JS, Rardin D: Stroke in a young adult with Fletcher trait. *South Med J* **84**:507, 1991.
300. Raffouxl C, Alexandre P, Perrier P, Briquel ME, Streiff F: HLA typing in a new family with Fletcher factor deficiency. *Hum Genet* **60**:71, 1982.
301. Saade M: Fletcher factor deficiency with mildly prolonged activated PTT. *South Med J* **73**:958, 1980.
302. Castaman G, Ruggeri M, Rodeghiero F: A new Italian family with severe prekallikrein deficiency. Desmopressin-induced fibrinolysis and coagulation changes in homozygous and heterozygous members. *Res Clin Lab* **20**:239, 1990.
303. Wuillemin WA, Furlan M, von Felten A, Lämmle B: Functional characterization of a variant prekallikrein (PK Zurich). *Thromb Haemost* **70**:427, 1993.
304. Hathaway WE: Correspondence. Fletcher factor. *Blood* **46**:817, 1975.
305. Estelles A, Aznar J, España F: The absence of release of the plasminogen activator after venous occlusion in a Fletcher trait patient. *Thromb Haemost* **49**:66, 1983.
306. Schiffman S, Lee P: Preparation, characterization, and activation of a highly purified factor XI. Evidence that a hitherto unrecognized plasma activating factor participates in the interaction of factors XI and XII. *Br J Haematol* **27**:101, 1974.
307. Lutcher CL: A new expression of high molecular weight kininogen (HMW-kininogen) deficiency. *Clin Res* **34**:440, 1979. (abstr.)
308. Donaldson VH, Kleniewski J, Saito H, Sayed JK: Prekallikrein deficiency in a kindred with kininogen deficiency and Fitzgerald trait clotting defect. *J Clin Invest* **60**:571, 1977.
309. Lefrère J-J, Horellou M-H, Gozin D, Conard J, Muller J-Y, Clark M, Soulier J-P, Samama M: A new case of high-molecular-weight kininogen inherited deficiency. *Am J Hematol* **22**:415, 1986.
310. Vicente V, Alberca I, Gonzalez R, Alegre A, Redondo C, Moro J: New congenital deficiency of high molecular kininogen and prekallikrein (Fitzgerald trait). Study of response to DDAVP and venous occlusion. *Haematologic* **19**:41, 1986.
311. Stormorken H, Briseid K, Hellum B, Hoem NO, Johansen HT, Ly B: A new case of total kininogen deficiency. *Thromb Res* **60**:457, 1990.
312. Hayashi H, Ishimaru F, Fujita T, Tsurumi N, Tsuda T, Kimura I: Molecular genetic survey of five Japanese families with high-molecular-weight kininogen deficiency. *Blood* **75**:1296, 1990.
313. Hayashi H, Koya H, Kuroda M, Kitazima K, Kimura I, Katori M, Oh-ishi S: The first cases of Fitzgerald factor deficiency in the orient: Three cases in one family. *Acta Haematol* **63**:107, 1980.
314. Nakamura K, Iijima K, Fukuda C, Kadowaki H, Ikoma H, Oh-ishi S, Uchida Y, Katori M: Tachibana trait: Human high molecular weight kininogen deficiency with diminished levels of prekallikrein and low molecular weight kininogen. *Acta Haematol Jpn* **48**:1473, 1985.
315. Exner T, Barber S, Naujalis J: Fitzgerald factor deficiency in an Australian Aborigine. *Med J Aust* **146**:545, 1987.
316. Hayashi H, Ishimaru F, Fujita T, Takai Y, Tsurumi N, Tsuda T, Fujiwara K, Kimura I: The fifth case of high molecular weight kininogen deficiency in Japan. *Jpn J Clin Hematol* **29**:2358, 1988.
317. Cheung PP, Kunapuli SP, Wachtfogel YT, Scott CF, Colman RW: Total kininogen deficiency (Williams Trait) is due to an arg-stop mutation in exon 5 of the human kininogen gene. *Blood (suppl 1)*: **78**:391a, 1991. (abstr.)
318. James FW, Donaldson VH: Decreased exercise tolerance and hypertension in severe hereditary deficiency of plasma kininogens. *Lancet* **1**:889, 1981.
319. Wong PY, Williams GH, Colman RW: Studies on the renin-angiotensin system in a kininogen-deficient individual. *Clin Sci* **65**:121, 1983.
320. Ratnoff OD, Busse RJ, Sheon RP: The demise of John Hageman. *N Engl J Med* **279**:760, 1968.

321. Veltkamp JJ, Drion EF, Leoliger EA: Detection of the carrier state in hereditary coagulation disorders. *Thromb Diath Haemorrh* **19:**403, 1968.
322. Sano M, Saito H, Sugihara T, Suzuki H, Kojima T, Shirakawa M, Kamiya T, Ohya I: Hereditary hageman factor (factor XII) deficiency: Report of three families and review of the literature published in Japan. *Acta Haematol Jpn* **49:**1275, 1986.
323. Lämmle B, Wuillemin WA, Huber I, Krauskopf M, Zürcher C, Pflugshaupt R, Furlan M: Thromboembolism and bleeding tendency in congenital factor XII deficiency—A study on 74 subjects from 14 Swiss families. *Thromb Haemost* **65:**117, 1991.
324. Bennett B, Ratnoff OD, Holt JB, Roberts HR: Hageman trait (factor XII deficiency): A probable second genotype inherited as an autosomal dominant characteristic. *Blood* **40:**412, 1972.
325. Rodeghiero F, Castaman G, Ruggeri M, Cazzavillan M, Ferracin G, Dini E: Fibrionolytic studies in 13 unrelated families with factor XII deficiency. *Hematologic* **76:**28, 1991.
326. Berrettini M, Lämmle B, Ciavarella G, Ciavarella N: Functional and immunological studies of abnormal factor XII in a cross reacting material positive (CRM+) factor XII deficiency. *Thromb Haemost* **54:**120, 1985. (abstr.)
327. Takahashi I, Saito H: A rapid purification with high recovery of factor XII (Hageman factor) on immunoaffinity column: Application to an abnormal clotting factor XII (factor $XII_{TORONTO}$). *J Biochem* **103:**641, 1988.
328. Miyata T, Kawabata S-I, Iwanaga S, Takahasi I, Alving B, Saito H: Coagulation factor XII (Hageman factor) Washington DC: Inactive factor XIIa results from Cys-571→Ser substitution. *Proc Natl Acad Sci USA* **86:**8319, 1989.
329. Wuillemin WA, Huber I, Furlan M, Lämmle B: Functional characterization of an abnormal factor XII molecule (F XII Bern). *Blood* **78:**997, 1991.
330. Wuillemin WA, Furlan M, Stricker H, Lämmle B: Functional characterization of a variant factor XII (F XII Locarno) in a cross reacting material positive F XII deficient plasma. *Thromb Haemost* **67:**219, 1992.
331. Saito H, Scialla SJ: Isolation and properties of an abnormal Hageman factor (factor XII) molecule in a cross-reacting material-positive Hageman trait plasma. *J Clin Invest* **68:**1028, 1981.
332. Bernardi F, Marchetti G, Patracchini P, del Senno L, Tripodi M,Fantoni A, Bartolai S, Vannini F, Felloni L, Rossi L, Panicucci F, Conconi F: Factor XII gene alteration in Hageman trait detected by *Taq*I restriction enzyme. *Blood* **69:**1421, 1987.
333. Bernardi F, Marchetti G, Volinia S, Patracchini P, Casonato A, Girolami A, Conconi F: A frequent factor XII gene mutation in Hageman trait. *Hum Genet* **80:**149, 1988.
334. Haanen C, Hommes F, Bernraad H, Morselt G: A case of hageman-factor deficiency and a method to purify the factor. *Thromb Diath Haemorrh* **5:**201, 1960.
335. Didisheim P: Hageman factor deficiency (Hageman trait). *Arch Intern Med* **110:**74, 1962.
336. Ikkala E, Myllylä G, Nevanlinna HR: Rare congenital coagulation factor defects in Finland. *Scand J Haematol* **8:**210, 1971.
337. Hellstern P, Köhler M, Schmengler K, Doenecke P, Wenzel E: Arterial and venous thrombosis and normal response to streptokinase treatment in a young patient with severe Hageman factor deficiency. *Acta Haematol* **69:**123, 1983.
338. Lodi S, Isa L, Pollini E, Bravo AF, Scalvini A: Defective intrinsic fibrinolytic activity in a patient with severe factor XII-deficiency and myocardial infarction. *Scand J Haematol* **33:**80, 1984.
339. Londino AV Jr, Luparello FJ: Factor XII deficiency in a man with gout and angioimmunoblastic lymphadenopathy. *Arch Intern Med* **144:**1497, 1984.
340. Kelsey PR, Bottomley J, Grotte GJ, Maciver JE: Congenital factor XII deficiency: Successful open heart surgery and anticoagulation. *Clin Lab Haematol* **7:**379, 1985.
341. Mannhalter C, Fischer M, Hopmeier P, Deutsch E: Factor XII activity and antigen concentrations in patients suffering from recurrent thrombosis. *Fibrinolysis* **1:**259, 1987.
342. Levi M, Hack CE, de Boer JP, Brandjes DPM, Büller HR, ten Cate JW: Reduction of contact activation related fibrinolytic activity in factor XII deficient patients. *J Clin Invest* **88:**1155, 1991.
343. Saito H, Scott JG, Movat HZ, Scialla SJ: Molecular heterogeneity of Hageman trait (factor XII deficiency). Evidence that two of 49 subjects are cross-reacting material positive (CRM+). *J Lab Clin Med* **94:**256, 1979.
344. Lämmle B, Berrettini M, Griffin JH: Immunoblotting studies of coagulation factor XII, plasma prekallikrein, and high molecular weight kininogen. *Semin Thromb Hemost* **13:**106, 1987.

CHAPTER 109

Antithrombin Deficiency

Douglas M. Tollefsen

1. **Antithrombin is a 58-kDa glycoprotein that is present in human plasma at a concentration of ~2.6 μ*M*. It inhibits several activated coagulation factors, including thrombin, factor IXa, and factor Xa. Inhibition occurs by formation of a stable 1:1 complex between antithrombin and the protease.**
2. **Heparin and heparan sulfate increase the rate of the antithrombin-protease reaction at least 1000 times by a catalytic mechanism that requires binding of the glycosaminoglycan chain to antithrombin. The binding site for antithrombin is a specific pentasaccharide sequence that contains an unusual 3-O-sulfated glucosamine residue. This structure occurs in ~30 percent of heparin molecules isolated from mast cells and in 1 to 10 percent of heparan sulfate molecules synthesized by vascular endothelial cells. Current evidence suggests that heparan sulfate proteoglycans anchored in the vessel wall interact with circulating antithrombin to inhibit thrombus formation.**
3. **Antithrombin deficiency is present in ~2 percent of patients with venous thromboembolic disease, in whom it is generally inherited as an autosomal dominant trait. The prevalence of symptomatic antithrombin deficiency has been estimated to range from 1 per 2000 to 1 per 5000 in the general population. Affected heterozygous individuals have ~50 percent of the normal plasma antithrombin activity. Deficiency results from mutations that affect the biosynthesis or stability of antithrombin and hence lower the amount of antithrombin antigen detectable in plasma, or from mutations that affect the protease and/or heparin binding sites and are associated with essentially normal levels of antithrombin antigen. Mutations confined to the heparin binding site appear to be more common than the other types of mutations and are usually asymptomatic unless present in a homozygous state.**
4. **Clinical manifestations of antithrombin deficiency include deep vein thrombosis and pulmonary embolism. Thrombosis may occur spontaneously or in association with pregnancy, trauma, or surgery. Arterial thrombosis is rare. Many patients experience recurrent thromboembolic disease beginning in early adulthood. It has been estimated that by 30 years of age ~60 percent of patients with antithrombin deficiency will have had at least one thrombotic episode. Acute episodes are treated with a 5- to 7-day infusion of heparin followed by oral anticoagulant therapy for an indefinite period of time. Prophylactic therapy of asymptomatic patients remains controversial.**
5. **Heparin cofactor II, which is homologous to antithrombin, inhibits thrombin in the presence of heparin or dermatan sulfate but does not inhibit other coagulation proteases. The concentration of heparin cofactor II in plasma is normal (~1.2 μ*M*) in patients with inherited antithrombin deficiency. Several patients with thrombosis and inherited deficiency of heparin cofactor II have been reported, but a causal relationship between these phenomena has not been established.**

Blood coagulation results from activation of a series of protease zymogens in the presence of nonenzymatic protein cofactors, calcium, and platelets (Fig. 109-1) (reviewed in Davie et al.[1]). The initial event in coagulation is exposure of plasma to tissue factor, a protein expressed on the surface of many cells not normally in contact with the bloodstream, which leads to the generation of factors IXa and Xa by the factor VIIa–tissue factor complex. This triggering mechanism is inactivated rapidly by the tissue factor pathway inhibitor,[2] but additional factor Xa can be generated by the factor IXa–VIIIa complex. Factor Xa in complex with factor Va then converts prothrombin to thrombin, the final protease in the coagulation cascade.

Thrombin is a trypsinlike serine protease that hydrolyzes specific Arg-X peptide bonds. It cleaves fibrinogen near the N-terminal ends of the Aα and Bβ chains to produce fibrin monomers that polymerize to form the clot, and it activates factor XIII, a transglutaminase that covalently crosslinks the polymerized fibrin. Thrombin cleaves the platelet thrombin receptor to generate a peptide ligand that stimulates platelet aggregation and secretion.[3] The aggregated platelets serve as the primary hemostatic plug and provide a surface on which the factor IXa–VIIIa and Xa–Va complexes are localized. Thrombin directly activates factors V and VIII, which serve as the nonenzymatic cofactors in these complexes. In addition, thrombin converts factor XI to XIa, which activates factor IX.[4,5] The reactions of thrombin with platelets and factors V, VIII, and XI provide positive feedback to accelerate thrombin generation at the site of a wound. If thrombin is generated within a normal blood vessel, it binds to the endothelial membrane protein thrombomodulin and activates protein C, which produces a local anticoagulant effect by proteolytically inactivating factors Va and VIIIa.

Thrombin has a number of other activities that are not directly related to coagulation (reviewed in Coughlin et al.[6]). It is mitogenic for lymphocytes and vascular smooth muscle cells, induces chemotaxis in monocytes, promotes adhesion of neutrophils to endothelial cells, and stimulates endothelial cells to produce prostacyclin, platelet-activating factor, plasminogen activator inhibitor-1, and platelet-derived growth factor. These activities may be important in wound healing

A list of standard abbreviations is located immediately preceding the index in each volume.

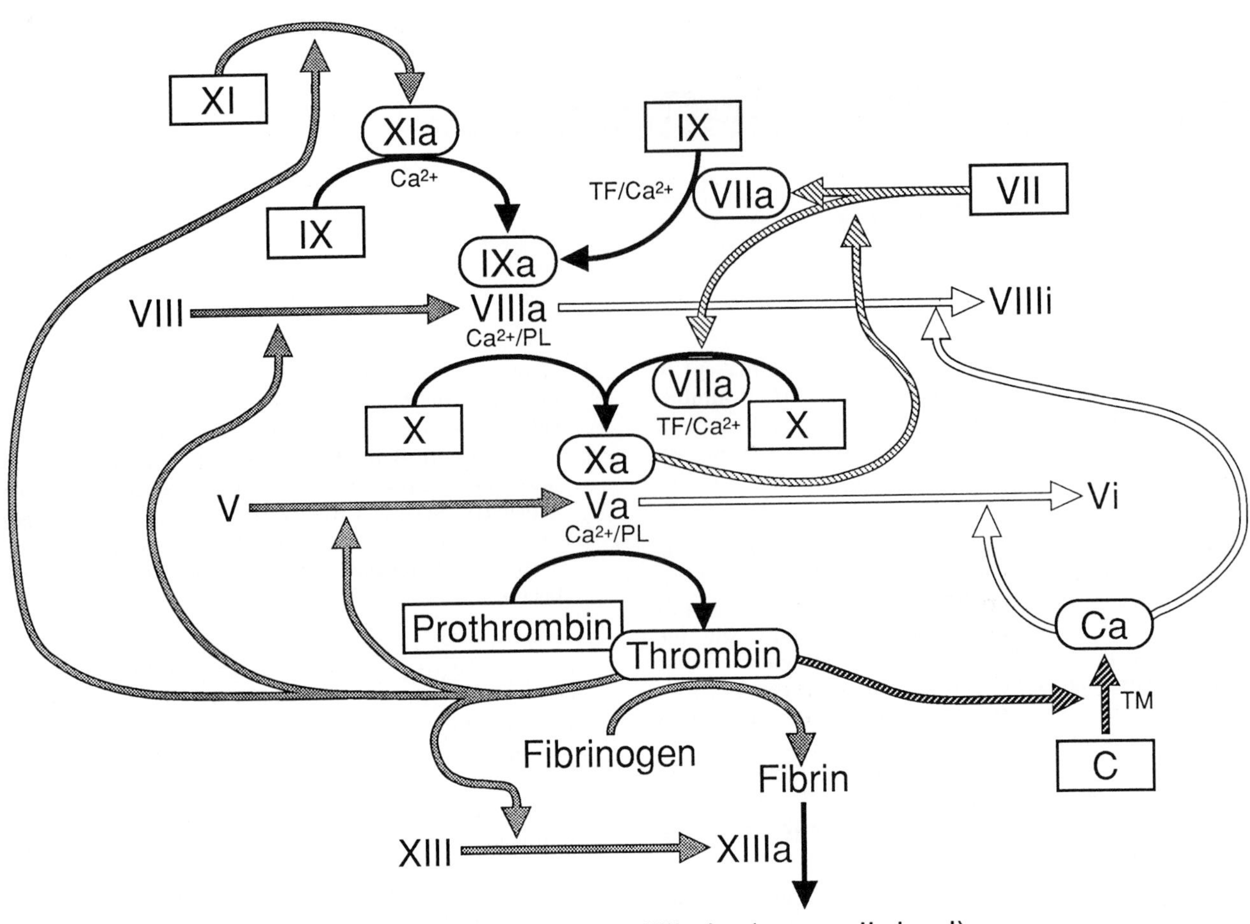

FIG. 109-1 Schematic diagram of coagulation reactions. Protease zymogens are indicated by rectangles and active proteases by ovals. The activated forms of the nonenzymatic protein cofactors V and VIII are designated Va and VIIIa, respectively. The inactive (proteolytically degraded) forms of these cofactors are designated Vi and VIIIi. Other symbols include: TF = tissue factor; TM = thrombomodulin; PL = platelets or negatively charged phospholipids; and Ca^{2+} = calcium ions. The procoagulant activities of thrombin are indicated by the stippled arrows on the left. Activation of protein C by thrombin to produce an anticoagulant effect is indicated by the darkly hatched arrows on the right. Inactivation of factors Va and VIIIa by activated protein C is indicated by the open arrows. Activation of factor VII by factor Xa is indicated by the lightly hatched arrows.

and inflammation. Thrombin also inhibits neurite outgrowth in neuroblastoma cells and sympathetic neurons, a process that may be regulated by glial-derived nexin (protease nexin-I) in the brain.[7]

Thrombin is inhibited by two plasma proteins, antithrombin and heparin cofactor II,* both of which require the presence of a glycosaminoglycan such as heparin for maximal activity.[8,9] The term *heparin* was used by Howell in 1923 to describe an aqueous extract of canine liver that inhibited blood coagulation in vitro.[10] Similar extracts were shown later to consist of mixtures of sulfated polysaccharides containing uronic acid and glucosamine.[11] In 1939, heparin was first used to treat thrombosis and pulmonary embolism,[11,12] and Brinkhous and coworkers discovered that the anticoagulant activity of heparin is mediated by an endogenous plasma component(s) termed "heparin cofactor."[13] Antithrombin was purified from plasma in 1968 by Abildgaard, who showed that this protein has heparin cofactor activity.[14] Rosenberg and Damus later purified a sufficient amount of antithrombin for biochemical characterization.[8]

*Synonyms include "antithrombin III" and "antithrombin/heparin cofactor" for antithrombin and "leuserpin-2" for heparin cofactor II.

Heparin cofactor II, a distinct but less abundant thrombin inhibitor with heparin cofactor activity, was first observed in 1974[15] and was purified subsequently.[9]

The association between antithrombin deficiency and recurrent venous thromboembolism, first reported by Egeberg in 1965,[16] established the idea that antithrombin plays a critical role in the regulation of blood coagulation. The biochemical abnormality in symptomatic individuals most often consists of a reduction of ~50 percent in the activity of antithrombin in plasma.[17] Some patients possess variant forms of the protein in which specific amino acid substitutions have been identified. Some experiments have suggested that heparan sulfate, a heparinlike glycosaminoglycan synthesized by vascular endothelial cells, constitutively activates antithrombin to prevent thrombosis from occurring within normal blood vessels.[18]

BIOCHEMISTRY AND MOLECULAR BIOLOGY OF ANTITHROMBIN

Structure and Biosynthesis

Structure. Antithrombin is a single-chain glycoprotein with a molecular mass of 58 kDa (Fig. 109-2). The cDNA for

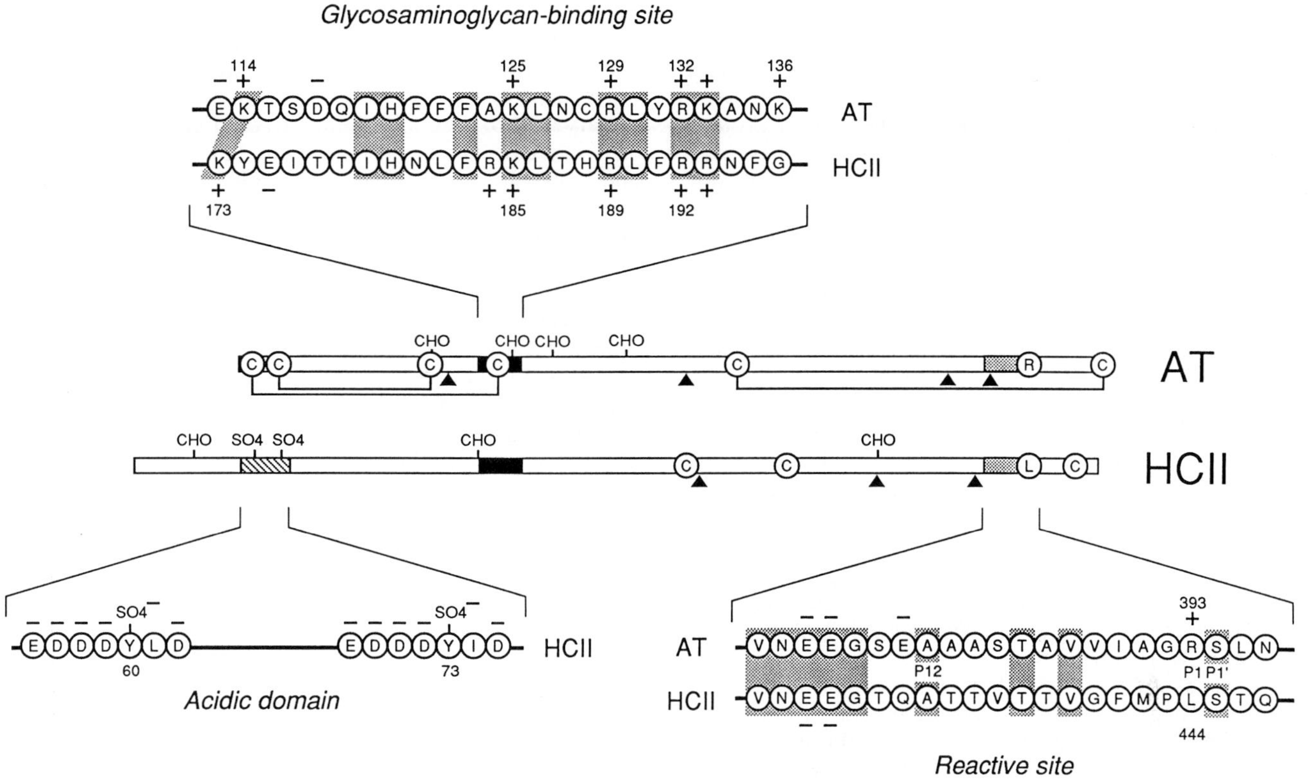

FIG. 109-2 **Structural features of antithrombin and heparin cofactor II. The antithrombin (AT) and heparin cofactor II (HCII) polypeptides are aligned according to amino acid sequence homology in the center of the figure. The positions of cysteine residues (C), P1 leucine (L) and arginine (R) residues, asparagine-linked glycosylation sites (CHO), and sulfate groups (SO4) are indicated. The triangles show the positions of introns in the coding sequence of each gene. The glycosaminoglycan binding sites (solid boxes) and reactive sites (stippled boxes) of both proteins, as well as the N-terminal acidic domain of heparin cofactor II (cross-hatched box), are enlarged to show details of the amino acid sequences. The numbers indicate the positions of residues in the polypeptide chains, and minus or plus symbols indicate ionic charge.**

antithrombin encodes a polypeptide 432 amino acids in length preceded by a 32-residue signal peptide.[19–21] Antithrombin is ~30 percent identical in sequence to members of the serpin superfamily, a group of more than 40 proteins, most of which have serine protease inhibitor activity (e.g., α_1-antitrypsin, α_2-antiplasmin, C_1 inhibitor).[22] Antithrombin contains three disulfide bonds[23,24] and four biantennary asparagine-linked oligosaccharides in its fully glycosylated form.[25]

Two forms of antithrombin that differ in their carbohydrate content have been isolated from normal human plasma by heparin-agarose affinity chromatography.[26] The major form (α-antithrombin), which comprises ~90 percent of the total antithrombin, is eluted from the affinity matrix with 1 *M* NaCl and is fully glycosylated. The minor form (β-antithrombin) is eluted at a higher salt concentration and lacks the oligosaccharide unit linked to Asn 135 near the proposed heparin binding site.[27] Both α- and β-antithrombin inhibit thrombin rapidly in the presence of heparin, but β-antithrombin requires a lower concentration of heparin for maximal activity.

Nonenzymatic glycation of one or two lysine residues of antithrombin occurs in vitro in the presence of high concentrations of glucose. This modification decreases the heparin-dependent thrombin inhibitory activity ~10 to 20 percent.[28]

Gene. The antithrombin gene is present as a single copy per haploid genome[20] and is located on human chromosome 1q23-q25.[29,30] The gene contains seven exons distributed over ~19 kb of DNA.[31–33] The positions of introns in the serpin genes are not strictly conserved (see Fig. 109-2), which suggests the possibility of selective loss of introns during evolution from a common ancestral gene.[34] A number of RFLP have been identified in the antithrombin gene (reviewed in Cooper[35]). In addition, a DNA-length polymorphism of unknown significance has been identified, in which either 32 or 108 bp of DNA have been inserted at the position 345 bp upstream from the translation initiation codon.[36]

The 5′ flanking sequence of the antithrombin gene lacks a TATA-like sequence at the expected location 25 to 30 bp upstream from the transcription initiation site but contains two short sequences (13 and 22 bp) that are similar to an enhancer element found in the immunoglobulin Jκ-Cκ gene.[37,38] Constructs containing the enhancer element ligated to the chloramphenicol acetyltransferase gene give preferential expression of chloramphenicol acetyltransferase in transfected Alexander hepatoma (liver) and COS-1 (kidney) cells, suggesting that the enhancer is involved in tissue-specific expression of the antithrombin gene. The 5′ flanking region of the antithrombin gene also contains a 10-bp sequence that binds Tf-LF1, a *trans*-acting factor that binds to a similar sequence in the transferrin gene.[39]

Biosynthesis. Antithrombin mRNA of ~1500 nucleotides in length is present in the liver, and synthesis of antithrombin has been demonstrated in cultured human hepatoma cells.[40] Alternative splicing of the antithrombin mRNA occurs in the liver.[37] The alternative splicing event introduces a 42-nucleotide segment between codons −19 and −18 of the signal peptide. This segment of mRNA contains an in-frame termination codon such that the protein encoded by the alternatively spliced mRNA would be only 19 amino acids long. Although the alternatively spliced mRNA accounts for 20 to 40 percent of the antithrombin mRNA in human liver, it is not known whether translation of the shorter product occurs. In the adult rat, antithrombin mRNA has been detected in the kidney at a level ~20 percent of that found in the liver.[41] Conflicting data on the biosynthesis of antithrombin in endothelial cells have been reported.[42,43]

Little is known about the regulation of antithrombin biosynthesis. Biosynthesis of antithrombin in isolated rat hepatocytes is unaffected by the presence of protease–antithrombin complexes or by the supernatant medium of macrophages incubated with these complexes.[44] However, antithrombin biosynthesis is stimulated by the supernatant medium of macrophages incubated with endotoxin or fibrinogen fragment D. Under these conditions, fibrinogen and α_1-antitrypsin biosynthesis are stimulated concurrently.

Protease Inhibition by Antithrombin

Specificity. Antithrombin inhibits several of the proteases involved in blood coagulation, including thrombin, factor Xa, factor IXa, and factor XIa,[18] but it has very little activity against factor VIIa[45] or activated protein C.[46] In vitro experiments in which ^{125}I-labeled proteases were incubated with plasma in the absence of heparin suggest that antithrombin is the major inhibitor of factor IXa, factor Xa, and thrombin, although α_1-antitrypsin and α_2-macroglobulin also contribute to inhibition of the latter two proteases.[47–49] In the presence of heparin at concentrations likely to be achieved therapeutically, factor IXa, factor Xa, and thrombin are inhibited almost exclusively by antithrombin. In the presence of higher concentrations of heparin or dermatan sulfate, thrombin is inhibited primarily by heparin cofactor II.[50,51] Factor Xa is also inhibited by tissue factor pathway inhibitor, which is present in plasma bound to lipoproteins at about one-thousandth the concentration of antithrombin,[52] and it is the factor Xa–tissue factor pathway inhibitor complex that inhibits factor VIIa–tissue factor.[53] Factor XIa is inhibited primarily by α_1-antitrypsin in plasma[54] or by protease nexin-II, a form of the amyloid precursor protein released from platelets.[55,56]

Antithrombin may regulate several proteases in addition to those involved in blood coagulation. In the presence of heparin, the streptokinase–plasminogen complex (which has plasminlike activity) is inhibited more rapidly by antithrombin than by α_2-antiplasmin,[57] whereas plasmin itself is inhibited more rapidly by α_2-antiplasmin.[58,59] Antithrombin also inhibits granzyme A (tryptase), a protease from cytotoxic T lymphocytes,[60,61] and one or more of the steps in complement activation.[62]

Mechanism. Antithrombin forms an essentially irreversible, equimolar complex with each of its target proteases.[8] During complex formation, thrombin, factor Xa, or factor IXa attacks a single peptide bond in antithrombin (Arg 393 to Ser 394) termed the "reactive site."*[63] The antithrombin–protease complex resists dissociation in denaturing agents. The denatured complex can be dissociated by treatment with nucleophilic reagents, which release the protease along with a two-chain form of antithrombin cleaved at the reactive site.[64,65] These properties are consistent with the presence of an ester linkage between the active center serine hydroxyl group of thrombin and the α-carbonyl group of Arg 393 in the reactive site of antithrombin. It is debatable whether cleavage of the reactive site peptide bond occurs in the native antithrombin–protease complex or is an artifact of denaturation.

X-ray crystallography of intact ovalbumin (a noninhibitory serpin) suggests that the P1 to P12 residues N-terminal to the cleavage site form an exposed loop on the surface of the protein (Fig. 109-3).[66] This structure is consistent with the observation that the region immediately upstream from the reactive site in many serpins is susceptible to proteolytic cleavage by enzymes other than the target protease, which results in loss of the inhibitory activity of the serpin.[67,68] Antithrombin and other inhibitory serpins undergo a striking conformational change after proteolytic cleavage at the reactive site. In cleaved α_1-antitrypsin, movement of the

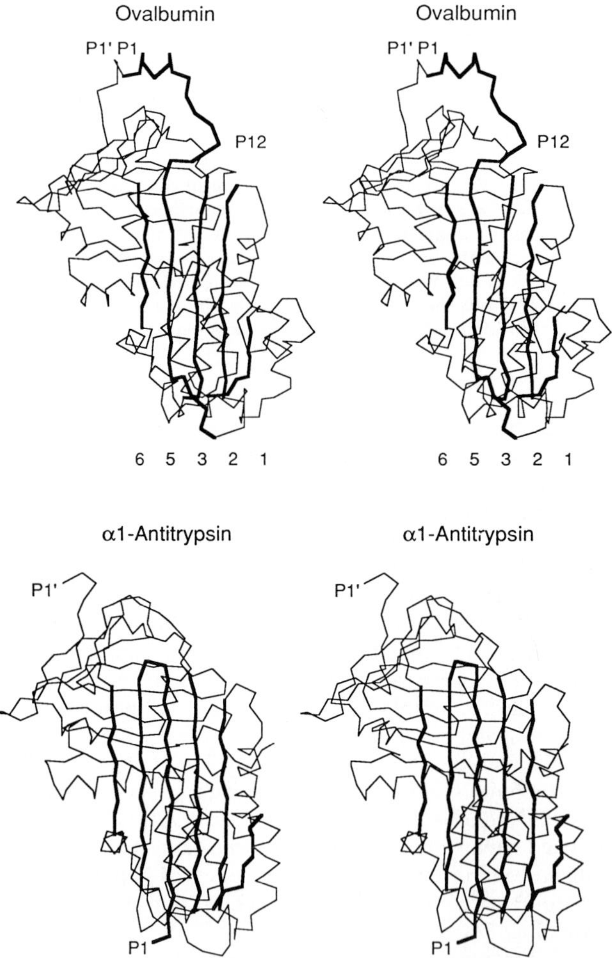

FIG. 109-3 Structures of native and cleaved serpins. The structures of native ovalbumin[66] and cleaved α_1-antitrypsin[69] were determined by x-ray crystallography. The α-carbon tracing of the polypeptide backbone is shown in stereo for each protein. The P1 to P2 residues of ovalbumin form an exposed loop on the surface of the protein that is susceptible to proteolytic attack. After cleavage, the P1 and P1′ amino acid residues of α_1-antitrypsin are separated by 69 Å, and residues P1 to P12 are incorporated into a β-sheet structure (thick lines; strands numbered according to α_1-antitrypsin).

*Residues that extend in the N-terminal direction from the reactive site are numbered P1, P2, P3, . . . beginning with Arg 393, whereas those extending in the C-terminal direction are numbered P1′, P2′, P3′, . . . beginning with Ser 394.

exposed loop about a hinge located near P12 allows residues P1 to P12 to become the fourth strand of a six-membered β-sheet, separating the P1 and P1′ amino acids by 69 Å (see Fig. 109-3).[69] This conformational change results in greater stability of the cleaved ("relaxed") form in comparison to the intact ("stressed") form of the serpin.[68] Mutations of the hinge region of antithrombin (i.e., Ala 384 → Pro at the P10 position or Ala 382 → Thr at the P12 position), which may interfere with insertion of the exposed reactive site loop into the β-sheet, prevent the "stressed" to "relaxed" conformational change and convert antithrombin from an inhibitor to a substrate for thrombin and factor Xa.[70,71] Antithrombin is also converted from an inhibitor to a substrate by a monoclonal antibody that recognizes the sequence Ala-Ala-Ala-Ser-Thr (P8 to P12)[72] and by a synthetic peptide corresponding to P1 to P14.[73,74] These reagents may also prevent insertion of the reactive site loop into the β sheet.

Proteolytic Inactivation. Neutrophil elastase inactivates antithrombin by proteolytic cleavage in the reactive site loop to yield the "relaxed" conformation of the inhibitor.[75] Inactivation by this protease may explain the decreased antithrombin activity observed in patients with sepsis.[76] Other proteases involved in inflammation, including matrix metalloproteinases-1, -2, and -3, inactivate antithrombin very slowly or not at all.[77] Antithrombin is also inactivated by certain snake venom proteases.[78]

Proteolytic inactivation of antithrombin by target proteases such as thrombin and factor Xa occurs in the presence of heparin at low ionic strength.[79,80] For example, the stoichiometry of inhibition of thrombin in the presence of heparin decreases from ~0.9 to ~0.1 mol of thrombin per mole of antithrombin as the ionic strength is lowered from 0.3 to 0.01.[79] The mechanism by which heparin at low ionic strength favors cleavage of the reactive site rather than stable complex formation has not been elucidated.

Stimulation of Antithrombin by Heparin

Kinetics. The concentration of antithrombin in plasma (2 to 3 μM) greatly exceeds that of any of the target proteases generated during coagulation. Under these conditions, protease inhibition follows pseudo-first-order kinetics. In the absence of heparin, thrombin and factor Xa are inhibited by antithrombin in plasma with $t_{1/2}$s of 0.5 to 1.5 min, while factor IXa is inhibited about 10 times more slowly.[81] Addition of heparin to plasma increases the rate of inhibition of all three proteases ~1000 times. As a result, inhibition of thrombin, factor Xa, and factor IXa by antithrombin becomes essentially instantaneous ($t_{1/2}$ = 10 to 60 ms).[81] Heparin also stimulates inhibition of factor XIa and plasmin, but the magnitude of the effect is much less.

The anticoagulant effect produced by an IV infusion of heparin is caused mainly by stimulation of antithrombin-protease reactions, although inhibition of thrombin by heparin cofactor II[50] and factor Xa by tissue factor pathway inhibitor may also contribute.[82] The major effect of heparin is apparently to blunt the positive-feedback reactions of thrombin on activation of factors V and VIII (see Fig. 109-1) and thus to decrease the rate of generation of thrombin.[83–85]

Structure of Heparin and Heparan Sulfate. Heparin occurs in the secretory granules of mast cells. A closely related glycosaminoglycan, heparan sulfate, is found on the surface of most eukaryotic cells and in the extracellular matrix. Heparin and heparan sulfate are synthesized from UDP-sugar precursors as linear polymers of alternating D-glucuronic acid and *N*-acetyl-D-glucosamine.[86,87] Each glycosaminoglycan chain is built on a core structure consisting of one xylose and two galactose residues covalently attached to serine in a polypeptide backbone. About 10 to 15 glycosaminoglycan chains, each containing 200 to 300 monosaccharide units, are attached to a single core protein to yield the heparin proteoglycan, which has a molecular mass of 750 to 1000 kDa. By contrast, heparan sulfate proteoglycans vary considerably in structure. They are generally smaller than the heparin proteoglycan and contain fewer glycosaminoglycan chains linked to a larger core protein. In some cases, the core protein has a hydrophobic domain that anchors the proteoglycan to a cell membrane.

As the glycosaminoglycan chains are being synthesized, they undergo a series of modification reactions that include the following[86,87]: (1) *N*-deacetylation of glucosamine residues, followed by sulfation of the free amino groups to yield *N*-sulfated glucosamine; (2) epimerization at the C-5 position of D-glucuronic acid to yield L-iduronic acid; (3) O-sulfation of iduronic acid residues at the C-2 position; and (4) O-sulfation of glucosamine residues at the C-6 position. In addition, several minor but important reactions occur, including O-sulfation of glucuronic acid at C-2 and C-3 and glucosamine at C-3. The reactions that modify the glycosaminoglycan chain appear to be catalyzed by membrane-bound enzymes in the ER or Golgi apparatus and are completed within minutes of synthesis of the core protein. Many of these reactions are regulated by modifications that have occurred on neighboring sugar residues. Furthermore, all the reactions with the exception of *N*-sulfation are incomplete, yielding heterogeneous oligosaccharide structures within the glycosaminoglycan chain. Heparan sulfate undergoes less polymer modification than heparin and, therefore, contains higher proportions of glucuronic acid and *N*-acetylglucosamine and fewer sulfate groups.

Binding Site in Heparin for Antithrombin. About 30 percent of heparin chains extracted from porcine intestinal mucosa bind to antithrombin with high affinity, and only the high-affinity fraction stimulates protease inhibition by antithrombin.[88–90] The high-affinity antithrombin binding site in heparin is the pentasaccharide shown in Fig. 109-4.[91–93] This structure contains a 3-O-sulfated glucosamine residue that is characteristic of the high-affinity binding site. Several other sulfate groups within the pentasaccharide structure are also essential for binding to antithrombin. A similar pentasaccharide structure can arise during the biosynthesis of heparan sulfate, although usually at a much lower frequency in comparison to mast cell heparin. Other types of glycosaminoglycans (e.g., dermatan sulfate, chondroitin 4-sulfate, and chondroitin 6-sulfate) do not interact with antithrombin.[51]

About 1 to 10 percent of the heparan sulfate chains synthesized by vascular endothelial cells contain antithrombin binding sites and stimulate protease inhibition by antithrombin.[94] The high-affinity heparan sulfate chains appear to be segregated from the low-affinity chains on different subpopulations of endothelial cell core proteins.[95] A variety of other cells, including fibroblasts and melanoma cells, also synthesize high-affinity heparan sulfate chains.[96] Antithrombin binding sites are particularly abundant in heparan sulfate isolated from mouse Reichert's membrane (an extraembryonic uterine basement membrane)[97] and the basement membrane of mouse mammary epithelial cells.[98]

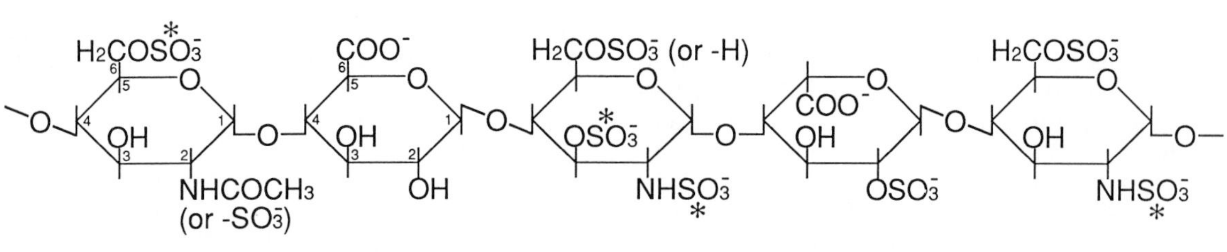

FIG. 109-4 **Structure of the antithrombin binding pentasaccharide of heparin. Sulfate groups marked with asterisks are essential for high-affinity binding to antithrombin. The first residue may be either *N*-sulfated or *N*-acetylated, and the C-6 position of the third residue may or may not be sulfated.**

Binding Site in Antithrombin for Heparin. Antithrombin binds to heparin with a dissociation constant of ~20 n*M*.[99,100] Binding is disrupted at high ionic strength and, therefore, appears to result primarily from electrostatic interactions between sulfate or carboxylate groups in heparin and basic amino acid residues in antithrombin. Several types of evidence suggest that amino acid residues between positions 107 and 145 are involved in binding to heparin: (1) Heparin blocks the chemical modification of Lys 107, Lys 114, Lys 125, Arg 129, Lys 136, and Arg 145, and these modifications decrease the heparin cofactor activity of antithrombin without affecting its ability to inhibit thrombin in the absence of heparin.[101–104] (2) An antibody against residues 124 to 145 blocks heparin binding and partially mimics the ability of heparin to stimulate formation of the thrombin–antithrombin complex.[105] (3) The synthetic peptide corresponding to residues 123 to 139, but not a random peptide of the same composition, competes with antithrombin for binding to heparin.[106] (4) The presence of an oligosaccharide linked to Asn 135 decreases the affinity of α-antithrombin for heparin relative to that of β-antithrombin.[27] (5) The disulfide bond between Cys 8 and Cys 128 is required for the integrity of the heparin binding site.[107]

Other studies suggest that the heparin binding site includes residues in the N-terminal portion of antithrombin. For example, natural mutations of Ile 7, Arg 24, Pro 41, and Arg 47[108–112] as well as chemical modification of Trp 49[113] decrease the affinity of antithrombin for heparin. In addition, proton NMR experiments implicate His 1 and possibly His 65 in heparin binding.[114] An alternative model for the heparin binding site is based on the selective denaturation of an α-helical domain in antithrombin by exposure to low concentrations of guanidine-HCl.[115] This treatment is accompanied by loss of heparin binding activity, while the ability of antithrombin to react with thrombin is retained. The unstable α-helical domain of antithrombin has been identified tentatively as the segment containing Lys 290, Lys 294, and Lys 297 based on secondary structure modeling.

When the sequence of antithrombin is superimposed on the tertiary structure of the cleaved form of α_1-antitrypsin, it appears that Arg 47 and the cluster of basic amino acid residues in the vicinity of Lys 125 occur in close proximity on the surface of the protein (Fig. 109-5).[22] If so, these residues could form a single heparin binding site. Estimates of the number of ion pairs (four or five) that exist in the antithrombin–heparin complex imply that not all of the basic amino acid residues identified in the experiments mentioned above participate directly in heparin binding.[80]

Mechanism of Action of Heparin. Kinetic analyses indicate that heparin binding induces a conformational change in antithrombin that locks the glycosaminoglycan into place on the surface of the protein.[100] Antithrombin with heparin bound to it then reacts rapidly with a target protease. The latter reaction reduces the affinity of antithrombin for heparin, which allows the stable antithrombin–protease complex to dissociate from the heparin molecule.[116] Thus, a single heparin molecule can catalyze the formation of many antithrombin–protease complexes.

Two models have been proposed to explain the catalysis of antithrombin–protease reactions by heparin. In the first model, heparin binding induces a conformational change in the reactive site of antithrombin that allows a target protease to interact more efficiently with this site.[8,81] In the second model, the heparin chain functions as a template that binds antithrombin and the target protease simultaneously, and catalysis occurs mainly by an approximation effect.[117] Current evidence suggests that both mechanisms are valid but differ in their relative importance depending on the target protease.

The balance between the two mechanisms may explain differences in the rate enhancement for inhibition of thrombin and factor Xa produced by heparin chains of varying length (Table 109-1). For example, the synthetic pentasaccharide that contains only the antithrombin binding site of heparin increases the rate of inhibition of factor Xa ~270 times but has relatively little effect on the rate of inhibition of thrombin.[80] Because an oligosaccharide of this size is unlikely to function as a template, induction of a conformational change in antithrombin may be sufficient to catalyze inhibition of factor Xa. Longer heparin chains produce an additional twofold increase in the rate of factor Xa inhibition, which may represent the contribution of the template mechanism. Stimulation of the thrombin–antithrombin reaction requires heparin molecules that contain at least 18 sugar residues, which is the smallest chain able to form a ternary complex with antithrombin and active site-blocked thrombin.[118] The factor IXa–antithrombin reaction has a similar requirement for longer heparin chains. Therefore, inhibition of thrombin and factor IXa may depend primarily on the template mechanism.

Full-length heparin chains and the pentasaccharide bind to antithrombin with similar affinities and induce nearly identical conformational changes in the protein detected by fluorescence, UV absorption, circular dichroism, and proton NMR spectroscopy.[92,119–121] It is not clear whether the small differences observed by some of these techniques represent

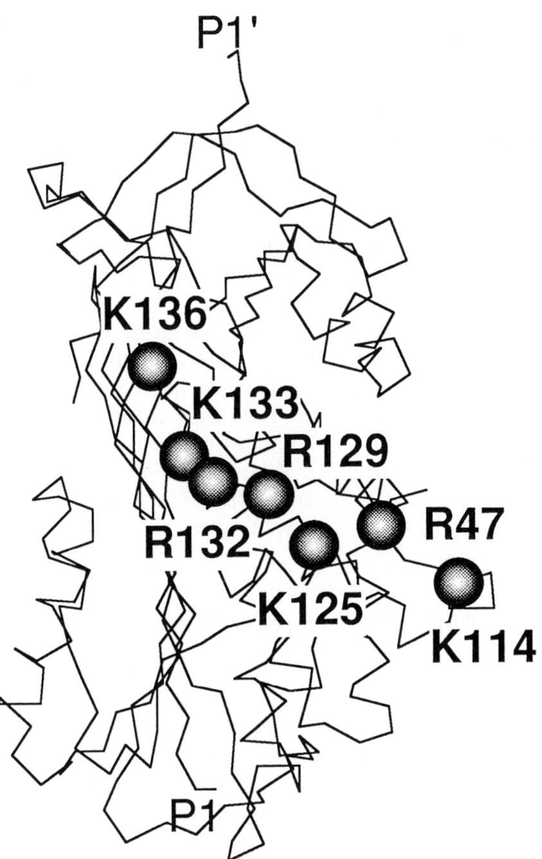

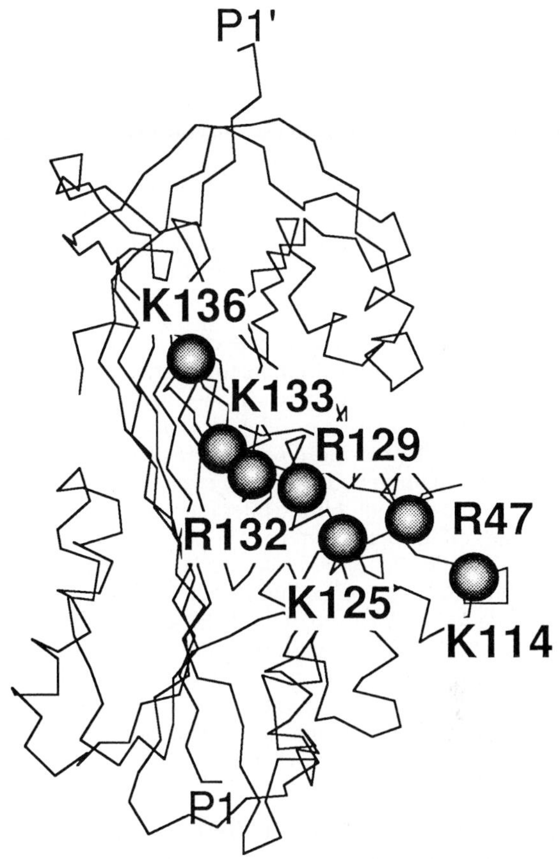

FIG. 109-5 Structure of the proposed heparin binding site of antithrombin. The polypeptide backbone shown in the diagram is that of α_1-antitrypsin. The positions of residues in antithrombin thought to be involved in heparin binding are superimposed on this backbone. In comparison with Fig. 109-3, the projection is rotated approximately 90° about the vertical axis.

nonspecific electrostatic interactions between antithrombin and heparin or a further conformational change induced by full-length heparin that is required for rapid inhibition of thrombin and factor IXa.[80] However, chemical modification of antithrombin in such a way as to diminish the spectroscopic changes induced by heparin does not affect the maximal rate of inhibition of thrombin.[122] These experiments have been interpreted to indicate that the heparin-induced conformational change in antithrombin plays a minor role in the inhibition of thrombin.

Thrombin binds to heparin with a dissociation constant of 6 to 10 μM under physiological conditions.[123] An increase in the NaCl concentration from 0.15 to 0.30 M causes parallel reductions of 20 to 30 times in the affinity of thrombin for heparin and in the rate of inhibition of thrombin by antithrombin in the presence of full-length heparin.[80,117] By contrast, the thrombin–antithrombin reaction in the absence of heparin is much less dependent on the ionic strength. Chemical modifications of thrombin that decrease its affinity for heparin greatly reduce the ability of heparin to stimulate the thrombin–antithrombin reaction.[124] Factor Xa also binds to heparin, but apparently with a much lower affinity in comparison to thrombin. Inhibition of factor Xa by antithrombin in the presence or absence of heparin is essentially unaffected by changes in ionic strength or by chemical modification of factor Xa to reduce its affinity for heparin.[80,125] These observations suggest that binding of thrombin, but not factor Xa, to heparin is required for catalysis of the antithrombin–protease reaction.

At low heparin concentrations, the rate of inhibition of

Table 109-1 Second-Order Rate Constants for Inhibition of Proteases by Antithrombin–Heparin Complexes

	Thrombin	Factor Xa
	$\times 10^6\ M^{-1}s^{-1}$ (increase)	
Antithrombin	0.0087	0.0023
Antithrombin + pentasaccharide	0.0146 (1.7)	0.61 (270)
Antithrombin + full-length heparin*	37 (4300)	1.3 (570)

*24 to 28 monosaccharide units in length. Data from Olson et al.[80]

thrombin or factor Xa is proportional to the concentration of heparin–antithrombin complexes present in the incubation.[81,99] The rate of inhibition plateaus at a concentration of heparin (usually in the micromolar range) that is sufficient to saturate the antithrombin. Higher concentrations of heparin decrease the rate of inhibition of thrombin, presumably by favoring the binding of thrombin and antithrombin to separate heparin chains, but do not decrease the rate of inhibition of factor Xa.[81,99] These observations are consistent with the template mechanism for catalysis of the thrombin–antithrombin reaction.[117]

Modulators of Heparin Catalysis. Several proteins competitively inhibit binding of antithrombin to heparin. They include histidine-rich glycoprotein[126] and vitronectin (complement S protein),[127] both of which are present in plasma at micromolar concentrations. Whether these proteins regulate hemostasis remains to be determined. In this regard, histidine-rich glycoprotein does not inhibit the interaction of antithrombin with heparan sulfate on the surface of cultured aortic endothelial cells.[128] Platelet factor 4 is released from the α granules during platelet aggregation and binds tightly to heparin.[126] It may promote local clot formation at the site of hemostasis by blocking the binding of antithrombin to heparan sulfate. Soluble fibrin monomers decrease the rate of inhibition of thrombin by antithrombin in the presence or absence of heparin,[129] and thrombin bound to a fibrin clot is protected from inhibition by antithrombin in the presence of heparin.[130]

Activity of Antithrombin in Vivo

Protease Inhibition. Radiolabeled thrombin rapidly forms complexes with antithrombin after IV injection in rabbits.[131] Furthermore, low concentrations of thrombin–antithrombin complex (0.02 to 0.10 n*M*) can be detected in plasma from healthy human subjects and may reflect the basal rate of generation of thrombin under normal circumstances.[132] The concentration of the thrombin–antithrombin complex is increased in certain pathological conditions such as disseminated intravascular coagulation.[132,133]

Formation of factor IXa–antithrombin complexes also occurs rapidly in vivo.[47] By contrast, factor Xa mainly forms complexes with α_2-macroglobulin after IV injection in the mouse, although the major inhibitors of factor Xa incubated with murine plasma in vitro are α_1-antitrypsin and antithrombin.[134] Factor Xa is protected from inhibition by antithrombin in vitro when the protease is bound to platelets[135] or to the prothrombinase complex, which contains factor Va, prothrombin, and phospholipids.[136] It is uncertain whether these mechanisms also protect factor Xa from inhibition by antithrombin in vivo.

Clearance of Antithrombin–Protease Complexes. Antithrombin–protease complexes are cleared from the circulation by hepatocytes with a half-life of 2 to 3 min,[47,137] which is considerably more rapid than the rate of clearance of free antithrombin ($t_{1/2} \approx 3$ days).[138] The hepatocyte uptake mechanism is saturable both in vivo and in vitro.[139] Uptake of antithrombin–protease complexes is not inhibited by free antithrombin, α_2-macroglobulin-methylamine, asialoorosomucoid, fucosyl-bovine serum albumin, *N*-acetylglucosaminyl-bovine serum albumin, or mannosyl-bovine serum albumin, and therefore appears to be mediated by a novel hepatocyte receptor.[140] Cross-competition experiments indicate that this receptor also recognizes complexes of proteases with α_1-antitrypsin, α_1-antichymotrypsin, and heparin cofactor II.[141]

An abundant receptor ($\sim 4.5 \times 10^5$ receptors per cell) with high affinity ($K_d \approx 40$ n*M*) for serpin–enzyme complexes has been identified on human HepG2 cells and monocytes.[142] The receptor mediates internalization and degradation of the complexes.[143] Binding of serpin–enzyme complexes to the receptor is blocked by a synthetic peptide (Phe-Val-Phe-Leu-Met) that corresponds to a conserved sequence found in the C-terminal portion of many serpins[144]; this sequence may represent a receptor binding site that becomes exposed on the surface of the serpin after complex formation with a protease.

In human serum, the thrombin–antithrombin complex is associated with vitronectin.[145] Vitronectin mediates binding of the thrombin–antithrombin complex to endothelial cells in vitro,[146] and internalization of the thrombin–antithrombin complex by cultured human umbilical vein endothelial cells has been demonstrated.[43] Whether these processes contribute to the clearance of thrombin–antithrombin complexes from the circulation or serve some other function remains to be determined.

Activation of Antithrombin by Vascular Heparan Sulfate

Because of the dramatic effect of heparin on the activity of antithrombin in vitro, it has been assumed that an endogenous heparinlike substance must stimulate antithrombin in vivo. Under normal circumstances, heparin is not released from mast cells into the circulation and cannot be detected in plasma. However, a small amount of heparin may appear in the circulation of patients with systemic mastocytosis and produce a mild prolongation of the activated partial thromboplastin time.[147] Occasionally, heparan sulfate released into the circulation from damaged tissues causes marked prolongation of the activated partial thromboplastin time and bleeding in a severely ill patient.[148–150] Current evidence suggests that heparan sulfate proteoglycans anchored in the vessel wall interact with circulating antithrombin to produce an antithrombotic effect.

Binding of Antithrombin to Endothelial Cells. Antithrombin binds to cultured bovine aortic endothelial cells ($\sim 6 \times 10^4$ sites per cell) with a dissociation constant of ~ 12 n*M*.[94] Binding is diminished by pretreatment of the cells with heparinase, which hydrolyzes glycosidic linkages following *N*-sulfated glucosamine residues in heparin and heparan sulfate. Similar results have been obtained with intact segments of bovine aorta.[151] However, the binding of antithrombin to intact rabbit aortic endothelium is weak. In this case, antithrombin appears to bind more avidly to heparinase-sensitive components beneath the endothelial cell layer.[152]

Electron microscopic autoradiography of ^{125}I-labeled antithrombin bound to endothelial cells in culture or after perfusion of segments of rat aorta ex vivo indicates that >90 percent of the antithrombin is associated with the extracellular matrix located in the subendothelium.[153] Binding of antithrombin to the subendothelial matrix of the aorta is greatly increased after crush injury, which causes detachment of most of the endothelial cells. It has been suggested that interaction of coagulation proteases with antithrombin bound to subendothelial heparan sulfate proteoglycans may inhibit thrombosis.[153] However, thrombin bound to dermatan sulfate in the extracellular matrix of cultured endothelial cells appears to be protected from inhibition by antithrombin[154] and may be more susceptible to inhibition by heparin cofactor II.

Interleukin-1 and tumor necrosis factor decrease heparan sulfate biosynthesis in cultured endothelial cells and reduce the amount of antithrombin that can be bound per cell by ~50 percent.[155] This mechanism may contribute to the increased thrombogenicity of the endothelium induced by cytokines.

Stimulation of Antithrombin Activity in Vivo. Evidence for the stimulation of antithrombin by vascular heparan sulfate in vivo has been obtained in a rodent hind limb preparation.[156] The hind limb was first perfused with thrombin to saturate thrombin binding sites (e.g., thrombomodulin) present in the microvasculature. When the concentration of thrombin present in the venous effluent had reached a steady state, antithrombin was perfused through the preparation, and the amount of thrombin–antithrombin complex recovered in the effluent was determined. Complex formation occurred fifteenfold to nineteenfold more rapidly within the microvasculature as compared with in vitro incubations in the absence of heparin. The rate enhancement was diminished by prior perfusion of the hind limb preparation with heparinase or by chemical modification of the antithrombin at Trp 49 to decrease the affinity for heparin, suggesting that interaction of antithrombin with microvascular heparan sulfate was responsible for the enhanced rate of inhibition.

Role of Thrombomodulin. When a trace amount of thrombin is injected into the circulation, the thrombin appears to become bound initially to thrombomodulin on the endothelial cell surface.[131] Thrombomodulin mediates internalization of thrombin by endothelial cells in vitro, but the importance of this pathway for the clearance of thrombin in vivo is uncertain.[157] In comparison with free thrombin, thrombin bound to bovine lung thrombomodulin reacts less rapidly with fibrinogen and heparin cofactor II, more rapidly with protein C, and at about the same rate with antithrombin.[158] The net effect of these changes in substrate specificity may be a small increase (approximately threefold) in the rate of the thrombin–antithrombin reaction because of diminished competition from other substrates. According to this hypothesis, only when thrombomodulin becomes saturated with thrombin will the excess thrombin be inhibited rapidly by antithrombin bound to heparan sulfate proteoglycans.

Rabbit lung thrombomodulin is a proteoglycan that bears a single chondroitin sulfate chain.[159] It accelerates the thrombin–antithrombin reaction fourfold to eightfold by a mechanism that depends on the presence of both the protein and glycosaminoglycan components. Expression of recombinant human thrombomodulin in human embryonal kidney cells yields two forms of the protein; the higher-molecular-weight form contains a chondroitin sulfate chain and stimulates the thrombin–antithrombin reaction.[160] By contrast, thrombomodulin purified from human placenta or bovine lung does not have these properties.[158,161] Thus, thrombomodulin may have different effects on the thrombin–antithrombin reaction depending on the tissue or species of origin.

ANTITHROMBIN DEFICIENCY

Antithrombin deficiency was the first inherited abnormality to be associated with a thrombotic tendency.[16] The diagnosis is usually made in a patient who experiences the onset of recurrent thromboembolic disease at an early age or in whom a positive family history of thromboembolic disease is obtained. The diagnosis is established by determination of the antithrombin activity in the patient's plasma.

Assay Methods

The antithrombin concentration in plasma is determined with a functional assay that measures the capacity of a sample to inhibit exogenous thrombin or factor Xa over a short time in the presence of heparin (i.e., heparin cofactor assay). Such assays are conveniently performed with a chromogenic substrate to detect the residual protease activity at the end of the incubation.[162] Heparin cofactor assays that use thrombin as the target protease may overestimate the concentration of antithrombin to a modest degree due to the presence of heparin cofactor II in the sample.[50,163,164] The use of factor Xa should allow greater specificity, since heparin cofactor II does not react with this protease.[165] An assay that measures the inhibition of thrombin over a longer time in the absence of heparin (i.e., progressive antithrombin assay) gives a rough indication of the antithrombin concentration but may also be influenced by α_1-antitrypsin and α_2-macroglobulin.[166] Immunologic assays are used in conjunction with functional assays to detect inactive variants of antithrombin. Crossed immunoelectrophoresis in the presence and absence of heparin is commonly used to detect variants with altered heparin-binding properties.

Normal Levels

The mean concentration of antithrombin in plasma from adults is ~2.6 μM (150 μg/ml).[167] In normal individuals, heparin cofactor activities range from 84 to 166 percent (mean ±2SD) and antithrombin antigen concentrations from 72 to 128 percent (mean ±2SD) of the mean value.[168] Healthy, full-term newborn infants have antithrombin antigen concentrations 39 to 87 percent of the mean adult value.[169] The level gradually increases into the normal adult range by 3 months of age. Levels of antithrombin are approximately the same in men and women until the sixth decade of life, when the level appears to decrease slightly (~ 5 percent) in males and increase slightly in females.[170,171]

Classification of Inherited Deficiencies

Classical (type Ia)* antithrombin deficiency is inherited as an autosomal dominant trait. Affected heterozygous subjects have 25 to 60 percent of the normal plasma levels of both heparin cofactor activity and antithrombin antigen.[168] Total absence of antithrombin has not been reported and may be lethal in utero. Oral anticoagulant therapy may increase the antithrombin level in some deficient patients and make the diagnosis more difficult.[172] Classical antithrombin deficiency has been reported to result from deletion of one of the two antithrombin genes,[173] from a dysfunctional gene,[173,174] or from mutations in the coding sequence that cause a frameshift or a premature stop codon (Table 109-2). The catabolic rate of radiolabeled antithrombin is normal in patients with inherited antithrombin deficiency, which indicates that the decreased plasma concentration is not caused by accelerated clearance of normal antithrombin.[175,176] Patients who have about half of the normal plasma antithrombin activity and antigen, but in whom a small amount of an abnormal

*There is no universally accepted nomenclature for the various types of antithrombin deficiency. The nomenclature used here is that proposed by Lane et al.[274]

Table 109-2 Antithrombin Mutations*

Patient	Antigen (Percent)	Activity (Percent)	Mutation	Amino Acid Change	Comments	Ref.
Type Ia (Classical): Reduced Levels of Normal Antithrombin						
1 family	45	40	+T, codon 48	Frameshift	Stop codon 72	275
1 family	53	47	−T, codon 81	Frameshift	Met 89 → stop	276
1 family	60	63	−T, codon 119	Frameshift	Stop Codon 126	277
6 families	<60	<60	CGA → TGA	Arg 129 → stop		278, 279
1 family	48	47	+A, codon 208	Frameshift	Stop codon 209	275
1 family	<60	<60	+A, codon 228	Frameshift	Glu 232 → stop	280
1 family	54	55	−A, codon 245	Frameshift	Stop codon 251	281
1 family	54	53	2 bp del, codon 245	Frameshift	Stop codon 264	281
1 family	<60	<60	2 bp del, codon 290-1	Frameshift	Asp 309 → stop	280
1 family	<60	<60	4 bp del, codon 308-9	Frameshift	Glu 313 → stop	280
1 family	46	29	−A, codon 370	Frameshift	Stop codon 375	275
1 family	<60	<60	+A, codon 408	Frameshift	Stop codon 432	278
Type Ib: Reduced Levels of Normal Antithrombin and the Presence of a Low Level of Variant						
Unnamed	<60	<60	G to A, intron 4	Frameshift	13 nt 5′ to exon V → new 3′ splice site, stop codon 379	282
Dublin	110	71	GTG → GAG	Val (−3) → Glu	Signal peptidase cleavage after Gly 2	283
Unnamed	60	40	TCC → CCC	Ser 349 → Pro		284
Rosny	70	52	TTC → TGC	Phe 402 → Cys		285
Torino	69	46	TTC → TCC	Phe 402 → Ser		285
Oslo	40	58	GCC → ACC	Ala 404 → Thr		286
Unnamed	70		AAC → AAG	Asn 405 → Lys	Also Val (−3) → Glu	Unpublished
Kyoto	58	57	AGG → ATG	Arg 406 → Met		287
Utah	50	50	CCT → CTT	Pro 407 → Leu		33
Budapest 5	100	70	CCT → ACT	Pro 407 → Thr	Also protein C deficiency	Unpublished
Unnamed	75	52	+G, codon 423-4	Frameshift	Stop codon 432	276
Unnamed			9 bp del, codon 427-9	Frameshift	Stop codon 430; also Arg 47 → His	288
Types IIa and IIb: Defects in the Reactive Site or Both the Reactive Site and Heparin-Binding Site						
Glasgow III	121		AAC → AAA	Asn 187 → Lys		Unpublished
Unnamed	98	55	AAC → GAC	Asn 187 → Asp		Unpublished
Hamilton	100	50	GCA → ACA	Ala 382 → Thr	Transformed into substrate	289, 290
Charleville	100	60	GCA → CCA	Ala 384 → Pro	Transformed into substrate	291, 292
Cambridge II	103	75	GCA → TCA	Ala 384 → Ser		293
Stockholm			GGC → GAC	Gly 392 → Asp		294
Northwick Park	162	65	CGT → TGT	Arg 393 → Cys	Complex with albumin	295, 296
Glasgow	87	43	CGT → CAT	Arg 393 → His	Increased heparin affinity	296
Pescara	100	62	CGT → CCT	Arg 393 → Pro	Increased heparin affinity	297, 298
Denver	92	54	TCG → TTG	Ser 394 → Leu	Increased clearance?	299
Budapest	75	20	CCT → CTT	Pro 429 → Leu	Homozygous	300
Type IIc: Defects Limited to the Heparin-Binding Site						
Rouen III			ATC → AAC	Ile 7 → Asn	Additional carbohydrate	108
Whitechapel	92		ATG → ACG & TAT → TGT	Met 20 → Thr & Trp 166 → Cys	Double mutation	Unpublished
Rouen IV	105	56	CGC → TGC	Arg 24 → Cys		109
Basel	104	60	CCG → CTG	Pro 41 → Leu		110
Toyama	100	26	CGT → TGT	Arg 47 → Cys	Homozygous	111
Rouen I	111	55	CGT → CAT	Arg 47 → His		112
Rouen II	102	64	CGT → AGT	Arg 47 → Ser		301
Budapest 3				Leu 99 → Phe		302
Geneva	100	50	CGA → CAA	Arg 129 → Gln		303
Truro			GAA → AAA	Glu 237 → Lys		Unpublished

*Only variants in which the mutations have been identified are listed. Adapted from Lane et al.[274]

antithrombin is also detectable, are classified as having type Ib deficiency. The mutations found in these patients apparently cause decreased synthesis or accelerated clearance of the abnormal antithrombin.

Patients who have normal concentrations of antithrombin antigen but decreased activity have type II deficiencies. Variants of this type have provided important insights into the mechanism of action of antithrombin and can be grouped into several categories (see Table 109-2): type IIa mutations affect both the reactive site and the heparin-binding site; type IIb mutations are limited to the reactive site; and type IIc mutations are limited to the heparin-binding site. Type II variants appear to have normal rates of synthesis and normal half-lives in the circulation. In most instances, the plasma of an affected heterozygous subject contains approximately equimolar amounts of normal and variant antithrombin. Type IIc deficiency is distinguishable from the other types because the heterozygous carriers are generally asymptomatic, whereas thrombosis occurs in the rare homozygous patients.[111,177,178]

Prevalence

The prevalence of inherited antithrombin deficiency has been estimated to range from 1 per 2000 to 1 per 5000, based on the number of symptomatic patients identified in large referral populations.[179,180] However, one recent study of 4189 healthy blood donors 18 to 65 years of age in Scotland identified 16 unrelated individuals with antithrombin deficiency (1 type I, 2 type IIb, and 13 type IIc), suggesting that the prevalence may be closer to 1 per 250.[181] Only one of the deficient individuals in this series had a history of thrombosis, which is consistent with previous estimates for the prevalence of symptomatic antithrombin deficiency.

The prevalence of antithrombin deficiency in patients with thrombosis has been estimated to range from 2 to 6 percent.[17] In a series of 752 patients with thromboembolic disease, inherited antithrombin deficiency was established in 13 (1.7 percent) by family studies.[182] Only 1 of the 13 deficient patients in this series had a type II abnormality, in contrast to the much more frequent occurrence of type II abnormalities in asymptomatic individuals.[181] The observation that antithrombin deficiency is more common in patients with thromboembolism than in asymptomatic individuals suggests that antithrombin deficiency increases the risk for development of the disease.

Clinical Manifestations

The prevalence of thromboembolic complications in patients with inherited antithrombin deficiency has been estimated from retrospective reviews of published case reports.[17,168,183] Clinical data from 62 families with antithrombin deficiency, excluding 14 families with type IIc deficiency, are summarized in Table 109-3.[184] About half of the 964 individuals studied had low plasma antithrombin activities and were apparently heterozygous. The mean prevalence of venous thromboembolism was 50.8 percent in the deficient subjects in comparison with 1.5 percent in the nondeficient subjects. However, the prevalence of venous thromboembolism in the deficient members of different families ranged from 15 to 100 percent. Thrombosis occurred with approximately equal frequency in male and female patients and included deep vein thrombosis of the lower extremities or pulmonary embolism (89.9 percent), mesenteric vein thrombosis (3.1 percent), and cerebral vein thrombosis (0.9 percent). Arterial occlusion was rare. Risk factors such as pregnancy or surgery were associated with 32 percent of the thrombotic episodes and were absent in 16 percent; however, information about risk factors was not included in the majority of case reports.

Thrombosis has been reported rarely in antithrombin-deficient patients before 15 years of age. It has been suggested that the high levels of α_2-macroglobulin present during childhood (two to three times the adult level) protect antithrombin-deficient children from thrombosis.[185] The incidence of thrombosis in the reported cases was greatest between 15 and 35 years of age and decreased thereafter, presumably because the majority of individuals who became symptomatic were given long-term oral anticoagulant therapy. By 30 years of age, ~60 percent of the antithrombin-deficient subjects had had at least one thromboembolic episode.[184] Despite the high incidence of thrombosis, the mortality of patients with antithrombin deficiency appears to be no different from that of the general population.[186,187]

Most reported cases of antithrombin deficiency have been discovered by laboratory investigation of patients with recurrent thromboembolic disease. The bias of ascertainment inherent in such reports may lead to overestimation of the frequency of complications in patients with antithrombin deficiency. Furthermore, the diagnosis of the thromboembolism was established by objective tests in only 17 percent of the reported episodes (see Table 109-3). Since the clinical manifestations of deep vein thrombosis and pulmonary embolism are nonspecific, thromboembolism has probably been misdiagnosed in at least some individuals with antithrombin deficiency. In a large Canadian family, type IIa antithrombin deficiency was established in 31 of 67 individuals by analysis of genomic DNA.[184] Only 6 episodes of venous thromboembolism, 5 of which were associated with known risk factors, were documented by objective tests in the 31 deficient subjects (mean age, 36 years), whereas none occurred in the 36 nondeficient subjects. This study suggests that idiopathic thrombosis may occur less frequently than previously estimated in antithrombin-deficient patients.

The clinical manifestations of patients with type IIc antithrombin deficiency, in which abnormalities are limited to the heparin-binding site, are distinguishable from those of patients with the other types of deficiencies. Only 3 episodes of thrombosis have been reported among 51 individuals with inherited type IIc antithrombin deficiency[17]; all 3 of these episodes occurred in homozygous patients. For example, one family included a child born to consanguineous parents, both of whom had asymptomatic antithrombin deficiency.[178] The child had undetectable heparin cofactor activity and died at 3 years of age of massive intracardiac thrombosis while receiving oral anticoagulant therapy.

Laboratory Abnormalities

With the exception of decreased plasma antithrombin activity, no laboratory abnormalities are associated consistently with antithrombin deficiency. Immunoassays of plasma for prothrombin activation fragment 1 + 2 and fibrinopeptide A, which are indicative of factor Xa and thrombin activity, respectively, have been used to assess the degree of activation of the coagulation system in vivo. A report that fragment 1 + 2 levels are elevated twofold to threefold in patients with antithrombin deficiency was later found to be incorrect due to an artifact of sample collection.[188,189] A more recent study found a small but statistically significant increase in mean plasma fragment 1 + 2 concentration in deficient adults not

Table 109-3 Summary of Clinical Data from 62 Families with Antithrombin Deficiency

	Number of Subjects	Percent
Prevalence of antithrombin deficiency	449/964	46.6
Prevalence of venous thromboembolism in nondeficient subjects	6/400*	1.5
Prevalence of venous thromboembolism in deficient subjects	228/449	50.8
Site of venous thromboembolism		
Deep vein thrombosis/pulmonary embolism	205	89.9
Mesenteric vein thrombosis	7	3.1
Cerebral vein thrombosis	2	0.9
No information provided	14	6.1
Subtotals	228	100.0
Diagnostic tests		
Venogram	27	11.8
Surgery	3	1.3
Autopsy	3	1.3
Lung scan	2	0.9
Angiogram	2	0.9
CT scan	1	0.4
No information provided	190	83.3
Subtotals	228	100.0
Risk factors		
None identified	36	15.8
Postpartum	22	9.6
Surgery	19	8.3
Pregnancy	18	7.9
Oral contraceptives	5	2.2
Trauma	4	1.8
Immobilization	4	1.8
No information provided	120	52.6
Subtotals	228	100.0

*Includes only studies that provided prevalence of venous thrombosis for nondeficient subjects. Data from Demers et al.[184]

receiving warfarin (0.87±0.26 n*M*) in comparison with nondeficient adults (0.70±0.21 n*M*, $p=0.03$).[190] However, most of the fragment 1+2 values in the deficient adults were within the normal range. No increase in fibrinopeptide A has been found in antithrombin-deficient subjects.[188,190]

Treatment

Anticoagulant therapy is indicated for patients with antithrombin deficiency following acute episodes of deep vein thrombosis or pulmonary embolism. The treatment is similar to that used for patients with normal antithrombin and consists of a 5- to 7-day course of heparin administered by continuous IV infusion followed by oral anticoagulation with warfarin.[191] Warfarin is initiated on the first hospital day to allow time for depletion of the vitamin K–dependent coagulation factors before the heparin is discontinued. Patients with antithrombin deficiency generally respond to standard doses of IV heparin as indicated by an increase in the activated partial thromboplastin time.[192] However, an occasional patient with inherited antithrombin deficiency, as well as patients with severe acquired antithrombin deficiency (<10 percent of normal), may be resistant to heparin.[193] In theory, treatment with a concentrate of purified antithrombin in combination with IV heparin might benefit patients with heparin resistance. Heparin itself can cause a modest (~15 percent) decrease in the circulating antithrombin concentration, but this effect is unlikely to have clinical significance.[194]

The duration of therapy with warfarin remains controversial. Most authorities recommend lifelong treatment of antithrombin-deficient patients after the first thromboembolic episode. Others advocate treatment of asymptomatic family members with documented antithrombin deficiency who have never had a thromboembolic episode. These recommendations are based on anecdotal experience and may not be warranted in view of the morbidity due to hemorrhage associated with long-term anticoagulant therapy.[195] However, patients with recurrent thromboembolism are candidates for indefinite oral anticoagulant therapy. Newer, less intense oral anticoagulant regimens that prevent recurrence of idiopathic deep vein thrombosis may be preferable in patients with antithrombin deficiency because of the lower expected morbidity.[196]

The incidence of thrombotic complications in women with antithrombin deficiency during pregnancy and immediately post partum has been estimated to range from 44 to 70 percent.[197,198] Therefore, it is reasonable to treat asymptomatic patients prophylactically during pregnancy and post partum. Because warfarin is associated with an increase in the incidence of fetal hemorrhage, stillbirth, and developmental abnormalities,[199] subcutaneous heparin regimens have been developed that appear to be effective in preventing thrombosis in these patients.[200] Some physicians have used antithrombin concentrates and a lower dose of heparin in the peripartum period to minimize the risk of bleeding.[201] However, delivery has been managed successfully without the use of antithrombin concentrates in antithrombin-deficient patients.[192,202]

Antithrombin concentrates[203,204] and androgens[205–207] have been used in the treatment of deep vein thrombosis and to prevent thrombosis at the time of surgery. Although these agents increase the plasma concentration of antithrombin in deficient individuals, their clinical efficacy is unproven.

Acquired Deficiencies

Acquired antithrombin deficiency with very low plasma concentrations (10 to 30 percent of normal) can occur in liver disease,[208] in the nephrotic syndrome,[209] and during disseminated intravascular coagulation.[210] Whether antithrombin deficiency contributes to the thrombotic complications associated with these conditions is unclear. Less severe acquired deficiencies have been reported in preeclampsia[211] and diabetes mellitus.[212] Antithrombin is mildly decreased in patients taking estrogens[213] and diethylstilbesterol,[214] and these medications should probably be avoided in patients with inherited antithrombin deficiency. A more profound decrease in antithrombin occurs in patients receiving L-asparaginase.[215] The levels of procoagulant factors such as prothrombin are decreased concomitantly by L-asparaginase, and there is uncertainty about whether a hypercoagulable state attributable to antithrombin deficiency exists in these patients.[216,217]

HEPARIN COFACTOR II

Antithrombin was initially thought to be the only heparin-dependent inhibitor of thrombin in plasma.[8,218] However, experiments that suggested the presence of a second heparin cofactor activity[15,50] were confirmed by the isolation of heparin cofactor II from human plasma.[9] Heparin cofactor II has a more restricted protease specificity than antithrombin and is stimulated by dermatan sulfate as well as heparin.[51,219] These properties suggest that the physiological function of heparin cofactor II is distinct from that of antithrombin.

Structure and Biosynthesis

Heparin cofactor II is a single-chain glycoprotein with a molecular mass of 66 kDa (see Fig. 109-2).[9] The cDNA for heparin cofactor II encodes a polypeptide 480 amino acids in length preceded by a 19 residue signal peptide.[220,221] Heparin cofactor II is ~30 percent identical in sequence to antithrombin and other serpins, the greatest similarity occurring in the C-terminal two thirds of the protein. By contrast, the first 80 amino acid residues at the N-terminal end of heparin cofactor II, which include two tyrosine residues that become O-sulfated during biosynthesis,[222] share no homology with other serpins. Peptides cleaved from this portion of heparin cofactor II by neutrophil proteases have potent chemotactic activity.[223] Heparin cofactor II contains three asparagine-linked glycosylation sites and three cysteine residues that apparently do not form disulfide bonds.[224]

The gene for heparin cofactor II is located on human chromosome 22q11.[225] It contains five exons distributed over ~16 kb of DNA.[225,226] The positions of the introns are shown in Fig. 109-2 in comparison with those of the antithrombin gene. Several RFLP have been identified in the heparin cofactor II gene.[225,227] No TATA or CAAT sequences have been identified in the 5′ flanking region of the heparin cofactor II gene, and transcription may initiate at several positions.[226] Human liver contains a 2200-nucleotide mRNA for heparin cofactor II,[220] and biosynthesis has been demonstrated in cultured human hepatoma cells.[222,228]

Protease Specificity

Heparin cofactor II differs from antithrombin with respect to its protease specificity. Among the proteases involved in coagulation and fibrinolysis, heparin cofactor II inhibits only thrombin.[219] The reactive site peptide bond attacked by thrombin contains a leucine residue in the P1 position, which is atypical of thrombin substrates.[229] In fact, heparin cofactor II inhibits chymotrypsin more rapidly than it inhibits thrombin in the absence of a glycosaminoglycan.[230] Mutation of the P1 leucine to arginine increases the basal rate of inhibition of thrombin in the absence of a glycosaminoglycan ~100 times and eliminates the ability of heparin cofactor II to inhibit chymotrypsin.[231] These results emphasize the importance of the P1 residue as a determinant of the protease specificity and suggest that heparin cofactor II has evolved to be essentially inactive toward thrombin in the absence of a glycosaminoglycan.

Stimulation by Glycosaminoglycans

The rate of inhibition of thrombin by heparin cofactor II is increased ~1000 times by heparin, heparan sulfate, or dermatan sulfate.[51] The affinity of heparin cofactor II for heparin is lower than that of antithrombin, and a tenfold higher concentration of heparin is required to accelerate thrombin inhibition by heparin cofactor II.[9,51] Heparin cofactor II does not require the specific pentasaccharide structure shown in Fig. 109-4 for stimulation by heparin.[232,233] Moreover, heparin cofactor II appears to bind nonspecifically to heparin oligosaccharides that contain ≥4 monosaccharide units regardless of their composition.[234] Heparin chains containing ≥26 monosaccharide units stimulate thrombin inhibition by heparin cofactor II, although shorter oligosaccharides also possess weak activity.[235,236]

Heparin cofactor II is unique with regard to its ability to be stimulated by dermatan sulfate. Dermatan sulfate is a repeating polymer of D-glucuronic or L-iduronic acid and *N*-acetyl-D-galactosamine.[87] O-Sulfation of iduronic acid residues at the C-2 position, and O-sulfation of galactosamine residues at the C-4 and C-6 positions occurs to a variable extent, yielding heterogeneous structures within the polymer. Like heparan sulfate, dermatan sulfate is a component of proteoglycans on the cell surface and in the extracellular matrix. Heparin cofactor II binds preferentially to a minor subpopulation of dermatan sulfate oligosaccharides, in contrast to the nonspecific binding observed with heparin oligosaccharides. The high-affinity binding site for heparin cofactor II in dermatan sulfate is a tandem repeat of three iduronic acid 2-sulfate → *N*-acetylgalactosamine 4-sulfate disaccharide subunits, which appear to be clustered within the polymer.[237] The high-affinity hexasaccharide increases the rate of inhibition of thrombin by heparin cofactor II ~50 times,[237] although dermatan sulfate chains containing ≥14 monosaccharide units are required for maximal stimulation.[238] Addition of dermatan sulfate to plasma in vitro causes prolongation of the thrombin time and the activated partial thromboplastin time,[239] and IV infusion of dermatan sulfate produces an antithrombotic effect in experimental animals[240–243] and humans.[244–246] These effects appear to be mediated primarily by heparin cofactor II.[51,247,248]

Glycosaminoglycan-Binding Site

Analysis of the natural variant heparin cofactor II Oslo (Arg 189 → His) established that heparin and dermatan sulfate interact with different amino acid residues on the surface of the inhibitor.[249,250] This mutation causes a large decrease (~60 times) in the affinity of heparin cofactor II for dermatan sulfate but does not affect the affinity of the inhibitor for heparin. Arg 189 occurs within a cluster of basic amino acid residues that can be aligned with basic residues in the proposed heparin-binding site of antithrombin (see Fig. 109-2) but are poorly conserved in other serpins. Mutations of Lys 173, Arg 184, and Arg 185 in recombinant heparin cofactor II affect heparin binding, whereas mutations of Arg 184, Arg 185, Arg 189, Arg 192, and Arg 193 affect dermatan sulfate binding.[251–254] These results indicate that the binding sites for heparin and dermatan sulfate overlap but are not identical.

Mechanism of Stimulation by Glycosaminoglycans

The stimulatory effect of heparin and dermatan sulfate depends on the presence of an acidic polypeptide domain near the N-terminus of heparin cofactor II.[255] The acidic domain contains a tandem repeat of two nearly identical sequences (see Fig. 109-2), each of which is similar to the C-terminal sequence of hirudin, a potent thrombin inhibitor in the saliva of the medicinal leech. The C-terminal portion of hirudin binds with high affinity to the anion binding exosite (fibrinogen recognition site) of thrombin, while the N-terminal domain of hirudin occupies the catalytic site.[256,257] A synthetic peptide that corresponds to the acidic domain of heparin cofactor II competes with hirudin for binding to thrombin but does not affect the ability of thrombin to hydrolyze a tripeptide *p*-nitroanilide substrate.[258] Furthermore, γ-thrombin, which lacks the anion binding exosite, cannot be inhibited rapidly by heparin cofactor II in the presence of a glycosaminoglycan.[255,259] Thus, binding of the acidic domain of heparin cofactor II to the anion binding exosite of thrombin may facilitate inhibition by bringing the active site of thrombin into approximation with the reactive site of heparin cofactor II.

Experiments with recombinant heparin cofactor II have established the importance of the N-terminal acidic domain.[252,253,255] Although deletion of both acidic repeats does not affect the rate of inhibition of thrombin or chymotrypsin in the absence of a glycosaminoglycan, deletion of the first acidic repeat greatly diminishes the ability of dermatan sulfate or heparin to stimulate the inhibition of thrombin.[255] The deletion mutants bind heparin more tightly, which suggests that the acidic domain occupies the glycosaminoglycan-binding site in native heparin cofactor II. These findings are consistent with a model in which heparin or dermatan sulfate displaces the N-terminal acidic domain from the glycosaminoglycan-binding site of heparin cofactor II, thus enabling the acidic domain to interact with thrombin (Fig. 109-6). The model could explain the ability of dermatan sulfate hexasaccharides to produce a moderate increase in the rate of thrombin inhibition. Dermatan sulfate or heparin

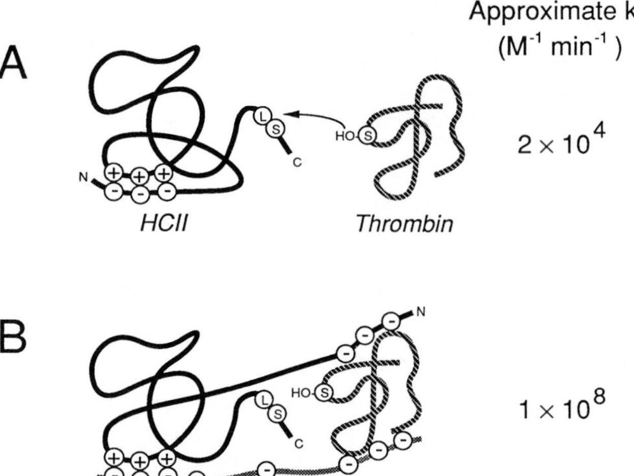

FIG. 109-6 **Model for inhibition of thrombin by heparin cofactor II. *A*. The active site serine (S) hydroxyl group of thrombin attacks the reactive site leucyl-serine (LS) peptide bond of heparin cofactor II to form a covalent complex. In the absence of a glycosaminoglycan, the N-terminal acidic domain of heparin cofactor II (−) forms ionic bonds with the glycosaminoglycan-binding site (+) and is unable to interact with thrombin. *B*. A glycosaminoglycan chain displaces the N-terminal acidic domain of heparin cofactor II from the glycosaminoglycan-binding site. The acidic domain then interacts with anion-binding exosite I of thrombin. Binding of thrombin both to the N-terminal acidic domain of heparin cofactor II and to the glycosaminoglycan template greatly increases the rate of covalent complex formation. Approximate second-order rate constants (k_2) for the thrombin–heparin cofactor II reaction are indicated.[255]**

chains of sufficient length to bind thrombin and heparin cofactor II simultaneously may accelerate the inhibitory reaction further by a template mechanism.

Physiology of Heparin Cofactor II

The function of heparin cofactor II in vivo remains obscure. Heparin cofactor II is present in normal human plasma at a concentration of 1.2±0.4 μ*M* (mean ±2 SD),[260] and several individuals with inherited partial deficiency of heparin cofactor II (~50 percent of normal) have been reported in association with histories of thrombotic disease.[261,262] In one series, however, 4 of 379 apparently healthy individuals had heparin cofactor II levels <60 percent of normal.[263] Thus, heterozygous deficiency of heparin cofactor II may be a coincidental finding in ~1 percent of patients with thrombosis, and it is premature to conclude that heparin cofactor II deficiency is a risk factor for development of the disease.[264] No patients with homozygous heparin cofactor II deficiency have been identified.

The concentration of heparin cofactor II is markedly decreased in some patients with liver disease, disseminated intravascular coagulation, and obstetric complications.[260,265–267] In these situations, the heparin cofactor II and antithrombin levels are usually decreased to a similar degree. A moderately elevated concentration of heparin cofactor II is present in women who are pregnant or use oral contraceptives.[268,269] Normal levels are present in patients taking oral anticoagulants, in the vast majority of patients with venous thromboembolic disease,[264,266,267] and in symptomatic patients with inherited antithrombin deficiency.[265,266,270]

Cultured fibroblasts and vascular smooth muscle cells accelerate inhibition of thrombin by heparin cofactor II, whereas endothelial cells do not.[271] In the case of fibroblasts, a dermatan sulfate proteoglycan was demonstrated to be responsible for the stimulatory effect. These results suggest that heparin cofactor II may inhibit thrombin in the connective tissues rather than within the blood vessels and perhaps modulate wound healing or inflammation. During pregnancy, both the maternal and fetal plasma contain a dermatan sulfate proteoglycan that stimulates inhibition of thrombin by heparin cofactor II approximately twofold.[272] The placenta is rich in dermatan sulfate and may be the source of this proteoglycan.[273] Thus, heparin cofactor II could be activated locally to inhibit coagulation within the placenta.

REFERENCES

1. Davie EW, Fujikawa K, Kisiel W: The coagulation cascade: initiation, maintenance, and regulation. *Biochemistry* **30:**10363, 1991.
2. Broze GJ Jr, Girard TJ, Novotny WF: Regulation of coagulation by a multivalent Kunitz-type inhibitor. *Biochemistry* **29:**7539, 1990.
3. Vu TK, Hung DT, Wheaton VI, Coughlin SR: Molecular cloning of a functional thrombin receptor reveals a novel proteolytic mechanism of receptor activation. *Cell* **64:**1057, 1991.
4. Naito K, Fujikawa K: Activation of human blood coagulation factor XI independent of factor XII. Factor XI is activated by thrombin and factor XIa in the presence of negatively charged surfaces. *J Biol Chem* **266:**7353, 1991.
5. Gailani D, Broze GJ Jr: Factor XI activation in a revised model of blood coagulation. *Science* **253:**909, 1991.
6. Coughlin SR, Vu T-KH, Hung DT, Wheaton VI: Characterization of a functional thrombin receptor. Issues and opportunities. *J Clin Invest* **89:**351, 1992.
7. Gurwitz D, Cunningham DD: Neurite outgrowth activity of protease nexin-1 on neuroblastoma cells requires thrombin inhibition. *J Cell Physiol* **142:**155, 1990.
8. Rosenberg RD, Damus PS: The purification and mechanism of action of human antithrombin-heparin cofactor. *J Biol Chem* **248:**6490, 1973.
9. Tollefsen DM, Majerus DW, Blank MK: Heparin cofactor II. Purification and properties of a heparin-dependent inhibitor of thrombin in human plasma. *J Biol Chem* **257:**2162, 1982.
10. Howell WH: Heparin, an anticoagulant. *Am J Physiol* **63:**434, 1923.
11. Jorpes E: *Heparin: Its Chemistry, Physiology, and Application in Medicine*. London, Oxford University Press, 1939.
12. Murray GDW: Heparin in thrombosis and embolism. *Br J Surg* **27:**567, 1939.
13. Brinkhous KM, Smith HP, Warner ED, Seegers WH: The inhibition of blood clotting: An unidentified substance which acts in conjunction with heparin to prevent the conversion of prothrombin into thrombin. *Am J Physiol* **125:**683, 1939.
14. Abildgaard U: Highly purified antithrombin III with heparin cofactor activity prepared by disc electrophoresis. *Scand J Clin Lab Invest* **21:**89, 1968.
15. Briginshaw GF, Shanberge JN: Identification of two distinct heparin cofactors in human plasma. Separation and partial purification. *Arch Biochem Biophys* **161:**683, 1974.
16. Egeberg O: Inherited antithrombin deficiency causing thrombophilia. *Thromb Diath Haemorrh* **13:**516, 1965.
17. Hirsh J, Piovella F, Pini M: Congenital antithrombin III deficiency. Incidence and clinical features. *Am J Med* **87:**34, 1989.
18. Rosenberg RD: Regulation of the hemostatic mechanism, in Stamatoyannopoulos G, Nienhuis AW, Leder P, Majerus PW (eds): *The Molecular Basis of Blood Diseases*. Philadelphia, Saunders, 1987, p 534.
19. Bock SC, Wion KL, Vehar GA, Lawn RM: Cloning and expression of the cDNA for human antithrombin III. *Nucleic Acids Res* **10:**8113, 1982.
20. Prochownik EV, Markham AF, Orkin SH: Isolation of a cDNA clone for human antithrombin III. *J Biol Chem* **258:**8389, 1983.
21. Stackhouse R, Chandra T, Robson KJ, Woo SL: Purification of antithrombin III mRNA and cloning of its cDNA. *J Biol Chem* **258:**703, 1983.
22. Huber R, Carrell RW: Implications of the three-dimensional structure of α1-antitrypsin for structure and function of serpins. *Biochemistry* **28:**8951, 1989.
23. Petersen TE, Dudek-Wojciechowska G, Sottrup-Jensen L, Magnusson S: Primary structure of antithrombin-III (heparin cofactor). Partial homology between α1-antitrypsin and antithrombin-III, in Collen D, Wiman B, Verstraete M (eds): *The Physiological Inhibitors of Coagulation and Fibrinolysis*. Amsterdam, Elsevier/North Holland, 1979, p 43.
24. Zhou ZR, Smith DL: Location of disulfide bonds in antithrombin III. *Biomed Environ Mass Spectrom* **19:**782, 1990.
25. Franzén L-E, Svensson S, Larm O: Structural studies on the carbohydrate portion of human antithrombin III. *J Biol Chem* **255:**5090, 1980.
26. Peterson CB, Blackburn MN: Isolation and characterization of an antithrombin III variant with reduced carbohydrate content and enhanced heparin binding. *J Biol Chem* **260:**610, 1985.
27. Brennan SO, George PM, Jordan RE: Physiological variant of antithrombin-III lacks carbohydrate sidechain at Asn 135. *FEBS Lett* **219:**431, 1987.
28. Hall PK, Roberts RC: Phosphate promotes glycation of antithrombin III which interferes with heparin binding. *Biochim Biophys Acta* **993:**217, 1989.
29. Kao FT, Morse HG, Law ML, Lidsky A, Chandra T, Woo SL: Genetic mapping of the structural gene for antithrombin III to human chromosome 1. *Hum Genet* **67:**34, 1984.
30. Bock SC, Harris JF, Balazs I, Trent JM: Assignment of the human antithrombin III structural gene to chromosome 1q23-25. *Cytogenet Cell Genet* **39:**67, 1985.
31. Prochownik EV, Bock SC, Orkin SH: Intron structure of the human antithrombin III gene differs from that of other members of the serine protease inhibitor superfamily. *J Biol Chem* **260:**9608, 1985.
32. Jagd S, Vibe-Pedersen K, Magnusson S: Location of two of the introns in the antithrombin-III gene. *FEBS Lett* **193:**213, 1985.
33. Bock SC, Marrinan JA, Radziejewska E: Antithrombin III Utah: Proline 407 to leucine mutation in a highly conserved region near the inhibitor reactive site. *Biochemistry* **27:**6171, 1988.
34. Strandberg L, Lawrence D, Ny T: The organization of the human-plasminogen-activator-inhibitor-1 gene. Implications on the evolution of the serine-protease inhibitor family. *Eur J Biochem* **176:**609, 1988.
35. Cooper DN: The molecular genetics of familial venous thrombosis. *Blood Rev* **5:**55, 1991.
36. Bock SC, Levitan DJ: Characterization of an unusual DNA length polymorphism 5′ to the human antithrombin III gene. *Nucleic Acids Res* **11:**8569, 1983.
37. Prochownik EV, Orkin SH: In vivo transcription of a human antithrombin III "minigene." *J Biol Chem* **259:**15386, 1984.
38. Prochownik EV: Relationship between an enhancer element in the human antithrombin III gene and an immunoglobulin light-chain enhancer. *Nature* **316:**845, 1985.
39. Ochoa A, Brunel F, Mendelzon D, Cohen GN, Zakin MM: Different liver nuclear proteins bind to similar DNA sequences in the 5′ flanking regions of three hepatic genes. *Nucleic Acids Res* **17:**119, 1989.
40. Fair DS, Bahnak BR: Human hepatoma cells secrete single chain factor X, prothrombin, and antithrombin III. *Blood* **64:**194, 1984.
41. D'Souza SE, Mercer JF: Antithrombin III mRNA in adult rat liver and kidney and in rat liver during development. *Biochem Biophys Res Commun* **142:**417, 1987.
42. Chan TK, Chan V: Antithrombin III, the major modulator of intravascular coagulation, is synthesized by human endothelial cells. *Thromb Haemost* **46:**504, 1981.
43. van Iwaarden F, Acton DS, Sixma JJ, Meijers JCM, de Groot PG, Bouma BN: Internalization of antithrombin

III by cultured human endothelial cells and its subcellular localization. *J Lab Clin Med* **113**:717, 1989.

44. Hoffman M, Fuchs HE, Pizzo SV: The macrophage-mediated regulation of hepatocyte synthesis of antithrombin III and α1-proteinase inhibitor. *Thromb Res* **41**:707, 1986.
45. Broze GJ Jr, Majerus PW: Purification and characterization of human coagulation factor VII. *J Biol Chem* **150**:1242, 1980.
46. Suzuki K, Nishioka J, Hashimoto S: Protein C inhibitor: Purification from human plasma and characterization. *J Biol Chem* **258**:163, 1983.
47. Fuchs HE, Trapp HG, Griffith MJ, Roberts HR, Pizzo SV: Regulation of factor IXa in vitro in human and mouse plasma and in vivo in the mouse. Role of the endothelium and the plasma proteinase inhibitors. *J Clin Invest* **73**:1696, 1984.
48. Gitel SN, Medina VM, Wessler S: Inhibition of human activated Factor X by antithrombin III and α1-proteinase inhibitor in human plasma. *J Biol Chem* **259**:6890, 1984.
49. Vogel CN, Kingdon HS, Lundblad RL: Correlation of in vivo and in vitro inhibition of thrombin by plasma inhibitors. *J Lab Clin Med* **93**:661, 1979.
50. Tollefsen DM, Blank MK: Detection of a new heparin-dependent inhibitor of thrombin in human plasma. *J Clin Invest* **68**:589, 1981.
51. Tollefsen DM, Pestka CA, Monafo WJ: Activation of heparin cofactor II by dermatan sulfate. *J Biol Chem* **258**:6713, 1983.
52. Novotny WF, Brown SG, Miletich JP, Rader DJ, Broze GJ Jr: Plasma antigen levels of the lipoprotein-associated coagulation inhibitor in patient samples. *Blood* **78**:387, 1991.
53. Broze GJ Jr, Warren LA, Novotny WF, Higuchi DA, Girard JJ, Miletich JP: The lipoprotein-associated coagulation inhibitor that inhibits the factor VII-tissue factor complex also inhibits factor Xa: Insight into its possible mechanism of action. *Blood* **71**:335, 1988.
54. Scott CF, Colman RW: Factors influencing the acceleration of human factor XIa inactivation by antithrombin III. *Blood* **73**:1873, 1989.
55. Smith RP, Higuchi DA, Broze GJ Jr: Platelet coagulation factor XIa-inhibitor, a form of Alzheimer amyloid precursor protein. *Science* **248**:1126, 1990.
56. Van Nostrand WE, Wagner SL, Farrow JS, Cunningham DD: Immunopurification and protease inhibitory properties of protease nexin-2/amyloid beta-protein precursor. *J Biol Chem* **265**:9591, 1990.
57. Anonick PK, Wolf B, Gonias SL: Regulation of plasmin, miniplasmin, and streptokinase-plasmin complex by α2-antiplasmin, α2-macroglobulin, and antithrombin III in the presence of heparin. *Thromb Res* **59**:449, 1990.
58. Highsmith RF, Rosenberg RD: The inhibition of human plasmin by human antithrombin-heparin cofactor. *J Biol Chem* **249**:4335, 1974.
59. Wiman B, Collen D: On the kinetics of the reaction between human antiplasmin and plasmin. *Eur J Biochem* **84**:573, 1978.
60. Masson D, Tschopp J: Inhibition of lymphocyte protease granzyme A by antithrombin III. *Mol Immunol* **25**:1283, 1988.
61. Poe M, Bennett CD, Biddison WE, Blake JT, Norton GP, Rodkey JA, Sigal NH, Turner RV, Wu JK, Zweerink HJ: Human cytotoxic lymphocyte tryptase. Its purification from granules and the characterization of inhibitor and substrate specificity. *J Biol Chem* **263**:13215, 1988.
62. Weiler JM, Linhardt RJ: Antithrombin III regulates complement activity in vitro. *J Immunol* **146**:3889, 1991.
63. Björk I, Jackson CM, Jörnvall H, Lavine KK, Nordling K, Salsgiver WJ: The active site of antithrombin. Release of the same proteolytically cleaved form of the inhibitor from complexes with factor IXa, factor Xa, and thrombin. *J Biol Chem* **257**:2406, 1982.
64. Owen WG: Evidence for the formation of an ester between thrombin and heparin cofactor. *Biochim Biophys Acta* **405**:380, 1975.
65. Fish WW, Björk I: Release of a two-chain form of antithrombin from the antithrombin-thrombin complex. *Eur J Biochem* **101**:31, 1979.
66. Stein PE, Leslie AGW, Finch JT, Turnell WG, McLaughlin PJ, Carrell RW: Crystal structure of ovalbumin as a model for the reactive centre of serpins. *Nature* **347**:99, 1990.
67. Carrell RW, Owen MC: Plakalbumin, α1-antitrypsin, antithrombin and the mechanism of inflammatory thrombosis. *Nature* **317**:730, 1985.
68. Mast AE, Enghild JJ, Salvesen G: Conformation of the reactive site loop of α1-proteinase inhibitor probed by limited proteolysis. *Biochemistry* **31**:2720, 1992.
69. Loebermann H, Tokuoka R, Deisenhofer J, Huber R: Human α1-proteinase inhibitor. Crystal structure analysis of two crystal modifications, molecular model and preliminary analysis of the implications for function. *J Mol Biol* **177**:531, 1984.
70. Perry DJ, Harper PL, Fairham S, Daly M, Carrell RW: Antithrombin Cambridge, 384 Ala to Pro: A new variant identified using the polymerase chain reaction. *FEBS Lett* **254**:174, 1989.
71. Austin RC, Rachubinski RA, Ofosu FA, Blajchman MA: Antithrombin-III-Hamilton, Ala 382 to Thr: An antithrombin-III variant that acts as a substrate but not an inhibitor of α-thrombin and factor Xa. *Blood* **77**:2185, 1991.
72. Asakura S, Hirata H, Okazaki H, Hashimoto-Gotoh T, Matsuda M: Hydrophobic residues 382-386 of antithrombin III, Ala-Ala-Ala-Ser-Thr, serve as the epitope for an antibody which facilitates hydrolysis of the inhibitor by thrombin. *J Biol Chem* **265**:5135, 1990.
73. Carrell RW, Evans DL, Stein PE: Mobile reactive centre of serpins and the control of thrombosis. *Nature* **353**:576, 1991.
74. Björk I, Ylinenjärvi K, Olson ST, Bock PE: Conversion of antithrombin from an inhibitor of thrombin to a substrate with reduced heparin affinity and enhanced conformational stability by binding of a tetradecapeptide corresponding to the P1 to P14 region of the putative reactive bond loop of the inhibitor. *J Biol Chem* **267**:1976, 1992.
75. Jordan RE, Nelson RM, Kilpatrick J, Newgren JO, Esmon PC, Fournel MA: Inactivation of human antithrombin by neutrophil elastase. Kinetics of the heparin-dependent reaction. *J Biol Chem* **264**:10493, 1989.
76. Duswald K-H, Jochum M, Schramm W, Fritz H: Released granulocytic elastase: An indicator of pathobiochemical alterations in septicemia after abdominal surgery. *Surgery* **98**:892, 1985.
77. Mast AE, Enghild JJ, Nagase H, Suzuki K, Pizzo SV, Salvesen G: Kinetics and physiologic relevance of the inactivation of α1-proteinase inhibitor, α1-antichymotrypsin, and antithrombin III by matrix metalloproteinases-1 (tissue collagenase), -2 (72-kDa gelatinase/type IV collagenase), and -3 (stromelysin). *J Biol Chem* **266**:15810, 1991.
78. Kress LF, Catanese JJ: Identification of the cleavage sites resulting from enzymatic inactivation of human antithrombin III by Crotalus adamanteus proteinase II in the presence and absence of heparin. *Biochemistry* **20**:7432, 1981.
79. Olson ST: Heparin and ionic strength-dependent conversion of antithrombin III from an inhibitor to a substrate of α-thrombin. *J Biol Chem* **260**:10153, 1985.
80. Olson ST, Björk I, Sheffer R, Craig PA, Shore JD, Choay J: Role of the antithrombin-binding pentasaccharide in heparin acceleration of antithrombin-proteinase reactions. Resolution of the antithrombin conformational change contribution to heparin rate enhancement. *J Biol Chem* **267**:12528, 1992.
81. Jordan RE, Oosta GM, Gardner WT, Rosenberg RD: The kinetics of hemostatic enzyme-antithrombin interactions in the presence of low molecular weight heparin. *J Biol Chem* **255**:10081, 1980.
82. Abildgaard U, Lindahl AK, Sandset PM: Heparin requires both antithrombin and extrinsic pathway inhibitor for its anticoagulant effect in human blood. *Haemostasis* **21**:254, 1991.
83. Ofosu FA, Sié P, Modi GJ, Fernandez F, Buchanan MR, Blajchman MA, Boneu B, Hirsh J: The inhibition of thrombin-dependent positive-feedback reactions is critical to the expression of the anticoagulant effect of heparin. *Biochem J* **243**:579, 1987.
84. Béguin S, Lindhout T, Hemker HC: The mode of action of heparin in plasma. *Thromb Haemost* **60**:457, 1988.
85. Ofosu FA, Hirsh J, Esmon CT, Modi GJ, Smith LM, Anvari N, Buchanan MR, Fenton JW II, Blajchman MA: Unfractionated heparin inhibits thrombin-catalysed am-

plification reactions of coagulation more efficiently than those catalysed by factor Xa. *Biochem J* **257:**143, 1989.

86. Lindahl U, Kusche M, Lidholt K, Oscarsson L-G: Biosynthesis of heparin and heparan sulfate. *Ann NY Acad Sci* **556:**36, 1989.
87. Conrad HE: Structure of heparan sulfate and dermatan sulfate. *Ann NY Acad Sci* **556:**18, 1989.
88. Höök M, Björk I, Hopwood J, Lindahl U: Anticoagulant activity of heparin: Separation of high-activity and low-activity species by affinity chromatography on immobilized antithrombin. *FEBS Lett* **66:**90, 1976.
89. Andersson L-O, Barrowcliffe TW, Holmer E, Johnson EA, Sims GEC: Anticoagulant properties of heparin fractionated by affinity chromatography on matrix-bound antithrombin III and by gel filtration. *Thromb Res* **9:**575, 1976.
90. Lam LH, Silbert JE, Rosenberg RD: The separation of active and inactive forms of heparin. *Biochem Biophys Res Commun* **69:**570, 1976.
91. Choay J, Petitou M, Lormeau JC, Sinay P, Casu B, Gatti G: Structure-activity relationship in heparin: A synthetic pentasaccharide with high affinity for antithrombin III and eliciting high anti-factor Xa activity. *Biochem Biophys Res Commun* **116:**492, 1983.
92. Lindahl U, Thunberg L, Bäckström G, Riesenfeld J, Nordling K, Björk I: Extension and structural variability of the antithrombin-binding sequence in heparin. *J Biol Chem* **259:**12368, 1984.
93. Atha DH, Lormeau JC, Petitou M, Rosenberg RD, Choay J: Contribution of monosaccharide residues in heparin binding to antithrombin III. *Biochemistry* **24:**6723, 1985.
94. Marcum JA, Atha DH, Fritze LM, Nawroth P, Stern D, Rosenberg RD: Cloned bovine aortic endothelial cells synthesize anticoagulantly active heparan sulfate proteoglycan. *J Biol Chem* **261:**7507, 1986.
95. Kojima T, Leone CW, Marchildon GA, Marcum JA, Rosenberg RD: Isolation and characterization of heparan sulfate proteoglycans produced by cloned rat microvascular endothelial cells. *J Biol Chem* **267:**4859, 1992.
96. Piepkorn M, Hovingh P, Hentschel WM: Isolation of heparan sulfates with antithrombin III affinity and anticoagulant potency from BALB/c 3T3, B16.F10 melanoma, and cutaneous fibrosarcoma cell lines. *Biochem Biophys Res Commun* **151:**327, 1988.
97. Pejler G, Bäckström G, Lindahl U, Paulsson M, Dziadek M, Fujiwara S, Timpl R: Structure and affinity for antithrombin of heparan sulfate chains derived from basement membrane proteoglycans. *J Biol Chem* **262:**5036, 1987.
98. Pejler G, David G: Basement-membrane heparan sulphate with high affinity for antithrombin synthesized by normal and transformed mouse mammary epithelial cells. *Biochem J* **248:**69, 1987.
99. Jordan R, Beeler D, Rosenberg R: Fractionation of low molecular weight heparin species and their interaction with antithrombin. *J Biol Chem* **254:**2902, 1979.
100. Olson ST, Srinivasan KR, Björk I, Shore JD: Binding of high affinity heparin to antithrombin III. Stopped flow kinetic studies of the binding interaction. *J Biol Chem* **256:**11073, 1981.
101. Pecon JM, Blackburn MN: Pyridoxylation of essential lysines in the heparin-binding site of antithrombin III. *J Biol Chem* **259:**935, 1984.
102. Peterson CB, Noyes CM, Pecon JM, Church FC, Blackburn MN: Identification of a lysyl residue in antithrombin which is essential for heparin binding. *J Biol Chem* **262:**8061, 1987.
103. Chang J-Y: Binding of heparin to human antithrombin III activates selective chemical modification at lysine 236. Lys-107, Lys-125, and Lys-136 are situated within the heparin-binding site of antithrombin III. *J Biol Chem* **264:**3111, 1989.
104. Sun X-J, Chang J-Y: Evidence that arginine-129 and arginine-145 are located within the heparin binding site of human antithrombin III. *Biochemistry* **29:**8957, 1990.
105. Smith JW, Dey N, Knauer DJ: Heparin binding domain of antithrombin III: Characterization using a synthetic peptide directed polyclonal antibody. *Biochemistry* **29:**8950, 1990.
106. Lellouch AC, Lansbury PT Jr: A peptide model for the heparin binding site of antithrombin III. *Biochemistry* **31:**2279, 1992.
107. Sun XJ, Chang JY: Heparin binding domain of human antithrombin III inferred from the sequential reduction of its three disulfide linkages. An efficient method for structural analysis of partially reduced proteins. *J Biol Chem* **264:**11288, 1989.
108. Brennan SO, Borg J-Y, George PM, Soria C, Soria J, Caen J, Carrell RW: New carbohydrate site in mutant antithrombin (7Ile→Asn) with decreased heparin affinity. *FEBS Lett* **237:**118, 1988.
109. Borg JY, Brennan SO, Carrell RW, George P, Perry DJ, Shaw J: Antithrombin Rouen IV 24 Arg to Cys. The amino terminal contribution to heparin binding. *FEBS Lett* **266:**163, 1990.
110. Chang JY, Tran TH: Antithrombin III Basel. Identification of a Pro-Leu substitution in a hereditary abnormal antithrombin with impaired heparin cofactor activity. *J Biol Chem* **261:**1174, 1986.
111. Koide T, Odani S, Takahashi K, Ono T, Sakuragawa N: Antithrombin III Toyama: Replacement of arginine-47 by cysteine in hereditary abnormal antithrombin III that lacks heparin-binding ability. *Proc Natl Acad Sci USA* **81:**289, 1984.
112. Owen MC, Borg JY, Soria C, Soria J, Caen J, Carrell RW: Heparin binding defect in a new antithrombin III variant: Rouen, 47 Arg to His. *Blood* **69:**1275, 1987.
113. Blackburn MN, Smith RL, Carson J, Sibley CC: The heparin-binding site of antithrombin III. Identification of a critical tryptophan in the amino acid sequence. *J Biol Chem* **259:**939, 1984.
114. Gettins P, Wooten EW: On the domain structure of antithrombin III. Tentative localization of the heparin binding region using ^{1}H NMR spectroscopy. *Biochemistry* **26:**4403, 1987.
115. Villanueva GB: Predictions of the secondary structure of antithrombin III and the location of the heparin-binding site. *J Biol Chem* **259:**2531, 1984.
116. Olson ST, Shore JD: Transient kinetics of heparin-catalyzed protease inactivation by antithrombin III. The reaction step limiting heparin turnover in thrombin neutralization. *J Biol Chem* **261:**13151, 1986.
117. Olson ST, Björk I: Predominant contribution of surface approximation to the mechanism of heparin acceleration of the antithrombin-thrombin reaction. Elucidation from salt concentration effects. *J Biol Chem* **266:**6353, 1991.
118. Danielsson Å, Raub E, Lindahl U, Björk I: Role of ternary complexes, in which heparin binds both antithrombin and proteinase, in the acceleration of the reactions between antithrombin and thrombin or factor Xa. *J Biol Chem* **261:**15467, 1986.
119. Stone AL, Beeler D, Oosta G, Rosenberg RD: Circular dichroism spectroscopy of heparin-antithrombin interactions. *Proc Natl Acad Sci USA* **79:**7190, 1982.
120. Gettins P: Antithrombin III and its interaction with heparin. Comparison of the human, bovine, and porcine proteins by ^{1}H NMR spectroscopy. *Biochemistry* **26:**1391, 1987.
121. Gettins P, Choay J: Examination, by ^{1}H-n.m.r. spectroscopy, of the binding of a synthetic, high-affinity heparin pentasaccharide to human antithrombin III. *Carbohydr Res* **185:**69, 1989.
122. Peterson CB, Blackburn MN: Antithrombin conformation and the catalytic role of heparin. II. Is the heparin-induced conformational change in antithrombin required for rapid inactivation of thrombin? *J Biol Chem* **262:**7559, 1987.
123. Olson ST, Halvorson HR, Björk I: Quantitative characterization of the thrombin-heparin interaction. Discrimination between specific and nonspecific binding models. *J Biol Chem* **266:**6342, 1991.
124. Pomerantz MW, Owen WG: A catalytic role for heparin. Evidence for a ternary complex of heparin cofactor, thrombin and heparin. *Biochim Biophys Acta* **535:**66, 1978.
125. Owen BA, Owen WG: Interaction of factor Xa with heparin does not contribute to the inhibition of factor Xa by antithrombin III-heparin. *Biochemistry* **29:**9412, 1990.
126. Lane DA, Pejler G, Flynn AM, Thompson EA, Lindahl U: Neutralization of heparin-related saccharides by histidine-rich glycoprotein and platelet factor 4. *J Biol Chem* **261:**3980, 1986.
127. Preissner KT, Müller-Berghaus G: S protein modulates

the heparin-catalyzed inhibition of thrombin by antithrombin III. Evidence for a direct interaction of S protein with heparin. *Eur J Biochem* **156:**645, 1986.

128. Shimada K, Kawamoto A, Matsubayashi K, Ozawa T: Histidine-rich glycoprotein does not interfere with interactions between antithrombin III and heparin-like compounds on vascular endothelial cells. *Blood* **73:**191, 1989.
129. Hogg PJ, Jackson CM: Fibrin monomer protects thrombin from inactivation by heparin-antithrombin III: Implications for heparin efficacy. *Proc Natl Acad Sci USA* **86:**3619, 1989.
130. Weitz JI, Hudoba M, Massel D, Maraganore J, Hirsh J: Clot-bound thrombin is protected from inhibition by heparin-antithrombin III but is susceptible to inactivation by antithrombin III-independent inhibitors. *J Clin Invest* **86:**385, 1990.
131. Lollar P, Owen WG: Clearance of thrombin from the circulation in rabbits by high-affinity binding sites on the endothelium. Possible role in the inactivation of thrombin by antithrombin III. *J Clin Invest* **66:**1222, 1980.
132. Boisclair MD, Lane DA, Wilde JT, Ireland H, Preston FE, Ofosu FA: A comparative evaluation of assays for markers of activated coagulation and/or fibrinolysis: Thrombin-antithrombin complex, D-dimer and fibrinogen/fibrin fragment E antigen. *Br J Haematol* **74:**471, 1990.
133. Deguchi K, Noguchi M, Yuwasaki E, Endou T, Deguchi A, Wada H, Murashima S, Nishikawa M, Shirakawa S, Tanaka K, Kusagawa M: Dynamic fluctuations in blood of thrombin/antithrombin III complex (TAT). *Am J Hematol* **38:**86, 1991.
134. Fuchs HE, Pizzo SV: Regulation of factor Xa in vitro in human and mouse plasma and in vivo in mouse. Role of the endothelium and plasma proteinase inhibitors. *J Clin Invest* **72:**2041, 1983.
135. Miletich JP, Jackson CM, Majerus PW: Properties of the factor Xa binding site on human platelets. *J Biol Chem* **253:**6908, 1978.
136. Lindhout T, Baruch D, Schoen P, Franssen J, Hemker HC: Thrombin generation and inactivation in the presence of antithrombin III and heparin. *Biochemistry* **25:**5962, 1986.
137. Shifman MA, Pizzo SV: The in vivo metabolism of antithrombin III and antithrombin III complexes. *J Biol Chem* **257:**3243, 1982.
138. Collen D, de Cock F, Verstraete M: Quantitation of thrombin-antithrombin III complexes in human blood. *Eur J Clin Invest* **7:**407, 1977.
139. Fuchs HE, Shifman MA, Michalopoulos G, Pizzo SV: Hepatocyte receptors for antithrombin III-proteinase complexes. *J Cell Biochem* **24:**197, 1984.
140. Fuchs HE, Michalopoulos GK, Pizzo SV: Hepatocyte uptake of α1-proteinase inhibitor-trypsin complexes in vitro: Evidence for a shared uptake mechanism for proteinase complexes of α1-proteinase inhibitor and antithrombin III. *J Cell Biochem* **25:**231, 1984.
141. Pizzo SV, Mast AE, Feldman SR, Salvesen G: In vivo catabolism of α1-antichymotrypsin is mediated by the serpin receptor which binds α1-proteinase inhibitor, antithrombin III and heparin cofactor II. *Biochim Biophys Acta* **967:**158, 1988.
142. Perlmutter DH, Glover GI, Rivetna M, Schasteen CS, Fallon RJ: Identification of a serpin-enzyme complex receptor on human hepatoma cells and human monocytes. *Proc Natl Acad Sci USA* **87:**3753, 1990.
143. Perlmutter DH, Joslin G, Nelson P, Schasteen C, Adams SP, Fallon RJ: Endocytosis and degradation of α1-antitrypsin-protease complexes is mediated by the serpin-enzyme complex (SEC) receptor. *J Biol Chem* **265:**16713, 1990.
144. Joslin G, Fallon RJ, Bullock J, Adams SP, Perlmutter DH: The SEC receptor recognizes a pentapeptide neodomain of α1-antitrypsin-protease complexes. *J Biol Chem* **266:**11282, 1991.
145. Ill CR, Ruoslahti E: Association of thrombin-antithrombin III complex with vitronectin in serum. *J Biol Chem* **260:**15610, 1985.
146. de Boer HC, Preissner KT, Bouma BN, de Groot PG: Binding of vitronectin-thrombin-antithrombin III complex to human endothelial cells is mediated by the heparin binding site of vitronectin. *J Biol Chem* **267:**2264, 1992.
147. Nenci GG, Berrettini M, Parise P, Agnelli G: Persistent spontaneous heparinaemia in systemic mastocytosis. *Folia Haematol (Leipz)* **109:**453, 1982.
148. Khoory MS, Nesheim ME, Bowie EJW, Mann KG: Circulating heparan sulfate proteoglycan anticoagulant from a patient with a plasma cell disorder. *J Clin Invest* **65:**666, 1980.
149. Bussel JB, Steinherz PG, Miller DR, Hilgartner MW: A heparin-like anticoagulant in an 8-month-old boy with acute monoblastic leukemia. *Am J Hematol* **16:**83, 1984.
150. Palmer RN, Rick ME, Rick PD, Zeller JA, Gralnick HR: Circulating heparan sulfate anticoagulant in a patient with a fatal bleeding disorder. *N Engl J Med* **310:**1696, 1984.
151. Stern D, Nawroth P, Marcum J, Handley D, Kisiel W, Rosenberg R, Stern K: Interaction of antithrombin III with bovine aortic segments. Role of heparin in binding and enhanced anticoagulant activity. *J Clin Invest* **75:**272, 1985.
152. Hatton MW, Moar SL, Richardson M: On the interaction of rabbit antithrombin III with the luminal surface of the normal and deendothelialized rabbit thoracic aorta in vitro. *Blood* **67:**878, 1986.
153. de Agostini AI, Watkins SC, Slayter HS, Youssoufian H, Rosenberg RD: Localization of anticoagulantly active heparan sulfate proteoglycans in vascular endothelium: Antithrombin binding on cultured endothelial cells and perfused rat aorta. *J Cell Biol* **111:**1293, 1990.
154. Bar-Shavit R, Eldor A, Vlodavsky I: Binding of thrombin to subendothelial extracellular matrix. Protection and expression of functional properties. *J Clin Invest* **84:**1096, 1989.
155. Kobayashi M, Shimada K, Ozawa T: Human recombinant interleukin-1β-and tumor necrosis factor α-mediated suppression of heparin-like compounds on cultured porcine aortic endothelial cells. *J Cell Physiol* **144:**383, 1990.
156. Marcum JA, McKenney JB, Rosenberg RD: Acceleration of thrombin-antithrombin complex formation in rat hindquarters via heparinlike molecules bound to the endothelium. *J Clin Invest* **74:**341, 1984.
157. Maruyama I, Majerus PW: The turnover of thrombin-thrombomodulin complex in cultured human umbilical vein endothelial cells and A549 lung cancer cells. Endocytosis and degradation of thrombin. *J Biol Chem* **260:**15432, 1985.
158. Jakubowski HV, Kline MD, Owen WG: The effect of bovine thrombomodulin on the specificity of bovine thrombin. *J Biol Chem* **261:**3876, 1986.
159. Bourin M-C, Lundgren-Åkerlund E, Lindahl U: Isolation and characterization of the glycosaminoglycan component of rabbit thrombomodulin proteoglycan. *J Biol Chem* **265:**15424, 1990.
160. Koyama T, Parkinson JF, Sié P, Bang NU, Müller-Berghaus G, Preissner KT: Different glycoforms of human thrombomodulin. Their glycosaminoglycan-dependent modulatory effects on thrombin inactivation by heparin cofactor II and antithrombin III. *Eur J Biochem* **198:**563, 1991.
161. Preissner KT, Koyama T, Müller D, Tschopp J, Müller-Berghaus G: Domain structure of the endothelial cell receptor thrombomodulin as deduced from modulation of its anticoagulant functions. Evidence for a glycosaminoglycan-dependent secondary binding site for thrombin. *J Biol Chem* **265:**4915, 1990.
162. Abildgaard U, Lie M, Ødegård OR: Antithrombin (heparin cofactor) assay with "new" chromogenic substrates (S-2238 and Chromozym TH). *Thromb Res* **11:**549, 1977.
163. Tran TH, Duckert F: Influence of heparin cofactor II (HCII) on the determination of antithrombin III (AT). *Thromb Res* **40:**571, 1985.
164. Conard J, Bara L, Horellou MH, Samama MM: Bovine or human thrombin in amidolytic AT III assays. Influence of heparin cofactor II. *Thromb Res* **41:**873, 1986.
165. Andersson N-E, Menschik M, van Voorthuizen H: New chromogenic ATIII activity kit which is insensitive to heparin cofactor II and designed for use on automated instruments. *Thromb Haemost* **65:**912, 1991. (abstr.)
166. Downing MR, Bloom JW, Mann KG: Comparison of the inhibition of thrombin by three plasma protease inhibitors. *Biochemistry* **17:**2649, 1978.
167. Conard J, Brosstad F, Lie-Larsen M, Samama M, Abildgaard U: Molar antithrombin concentration in normal human plasma. *Haemostasis* **13:**363, 1983.

168. Thaler E, Lechner K: Antithrombin III deficiency and thromboembolism. *Clin Haematol* **10**:369, 1981.
169. Andrew M, Paes B, Milner R, Johnston M, Mitchell L, Tollefsen DM, Powers P: Development of the human coagulation system in the full-term infant. *Blood* **70**:165, 1987.
170. Ødegård OR, Fagerhol MK, Lie M: Heparin cofactor activity and antithrombin III concentration in plasma related to age and sex. *Scand J Haematol* **17**:258, 1976.
171. Tait RC, Walker ID, Davidson JF, Islam SIA, Mitchell R: Antithrombin III activity in healthy blood donors: Age and sex related changes and prevalence of asymptomatic deficiency [letter]. *Br J Haematol* **75**:141, 1990.
172. Marciniak E, Farley CH, DeSimone PA: Familial thrombosis due to antithrombin III deficiency. *Blood* **43**:219, 1974.
173. Prochownik EV, Antonarakis S, Bauer KA, Rosenberg RD, Fearon ER, Orkin SH: Molecular heterogeneity of inherited antithrombin III deficiency. *N Engl J Med* **308**:1549, 1983.
174. Bock SC, Harris JF, Schwartz CE, Ward JH, Hershgold EJ, Skolnick MH: Hereditary thrombosis in a Utah kindred is caused by a dysfunctional antithrombin III gene. *Am J Hum Genet* **37**:32, 1985.
175. Ambruso DR, Leonard BD, Bies RD, Jacobson L, Hathaway WE, Reeve EB: Antithrombin III deficiency: Decreased synthesis of a biochemically normal molecule. *Blood* **60**:78, 1982.
176. Knot EA, de Jong E, ten Cate JW, Iburg AH, Henny CP, Bruin T, Stibbe J: Purified radiolabeled antithrombin III metabolism in three families with hereditary AT III deficiency: Application of a three-compartment model. *Blood* **67**:93, 1986.
177. Fischer AM, Cornu P, Sternberg C, Meriane F, Dautzenberg MD, Chafa O, Beguin S, Desnos M: Antithrombin III Alger: A new homozygous AT III variant. *Thromb Haemost* **55**:218, 1986.
178. Boyer C, Wolf M, Vedrenne J, Meyer D, Larrieu MJ: Homozygous variant of antithrombin III: AT III Fontainebleau. *Thromb Haemost* **56**:18, 1986.
179. Ødegård OR, Abildgaard U: Antithrombin III: Critical review of assay methods. Significance of variations in health and disease. *Haemostasis* **7**:127, 1978.
180. Rosenberg RD: Actions and interactions of antithrombin and heparin. *N Engl J Med* **292**:146, 1975.
181. Tait RC, Walker ID, Perry DJ, Carrell RW, Islam SIA, McCall F, Mitchell R, Davidson JF: Prevalence of antithrombin III deficiency subtypes in 4000 healthy blood donors. *Thromb Haemost* **65**:839, 1991. (abstr.)
182. Vikydal R, Korninger C, Kyrle PA, Niessner H, Pabinger I, Thaler E, Lechner K: The prevalence of hereditary antithrombin-III deficiency in patients with a history of venous thromboembolism. *Thromb Haemost* **54**:744, 1985.
183. Cosgriff TM, Bishop DT, Hershgold EJ, Skolnick MH, Martin BA, Baty BJ, Carlson KS: Familial antithrombin III deficiency: Its natural history, genetics, diagnosis and treatment. *Medicine (Baltimore)* **62**:209, 1983.
184. Demers C, Ginsberg JS, Hirsh J, Henderson P, Blajchman MA: Thrombosis in antithrombin-III-deficient persons. Report of a large kindred and literature review. *Ann Intern Med* **116**:754, 1992.
185. Mitchell L, Piovella F, Ofosu F, Andrew M: α-2-Macroglobulin may provide protection from thromboembolic events in antithrombin III-deficient children. *Blood* **78**:2299, 1991.
186. Rosendaal FR, Heijboer H, Briët E, Büller HR, Brandjes DPM, de Bruin K, Hommes DW, Vandenbroucke JP: Mortality in hereditary antithrombin-III deficiency—1830 to 1989. *Lancet* **337**:260, 1991.
187. Rosendaal FR, Heijboer H: Mortality related to thrombosis in congenital antithrombin III deficiency [letter]. *Lancet* **337**:1545, 1991.
188. Bauer KA, Goodman TL, Kass BL, Rosenberg RD: Elevated factor Xa activity in the blood of asymptomatic patients with congenital antithrombin deficiency. *J Clin Invest* **76**:826, 1985.
189. Bauer KA, Barzegar S, Rosenberg RD: Influence of anticoagulants used for blood collection on plasma prothrombin fragment F1+2 measurements. *Thromb Res* **63**:617, 1991.
190. Demers C, Ginsberg JS, Henderson P, Ofosu FA, Weitz JI, Blajchman MA: Measurement of markers of activated coagulation in antithrombin III deficient subjects. *Thromb Haemost* **67**:542, 1992.
191. Hirsh J: Treatment of pulmonary embolism. *Annu Rev Med* **38**:91, 1987.
192. Leclerc JR, Geerts W, Panju A, Nguyen P, Hirsh J: Management of anti-thrombin III deficiency during pregnancy without administration of anti-thrombin III. *Thromb Res* **41**:567, 1986.
193. Nielsen LE, Bell WR, Borkon AM, Neill CA: Extensive thrombus formation with heparin resistance during extracorporeal circulation. A new presentation of familial antithrombin III deficiency. *Arch Intern Med* **147**:149, 1987.
194. Holm HA, Kalvenes S, Abildgaard U: Changes in plasma antithrombin (heparin cofactor activity) during intravenous heparin therapy: Observations in 198 patients with deep venous thrombosis. *Scand J Haematol* **35**:564, 1985.
195. Petitti DB, Strom BL, Melmon KL: Duration of warfarin anticoagulant therapy and the probabilities of recurrent thromboembolism and hemorrhage. *Am J Med* **81**:255, 1986.
196. Hull R, Hirsh J, Jay R, Carter C, England C, Gent M, Turpie AG, McLoughlin D, Dodd P, Thomas M, Raskob G, Ockelford P: Different intensities of oral anticoagulant therapy in the treatment of proximal-vein thrombosis. *N Engl J Med* **307**:1676, 1982.
197. Conard J, Horellou MH, Van Dreden P, Lecompte T, Samama M: Thrombosis and pregnancy in congenital deficiencies in AT III, protein C or protein S: Study of 78 women. *Thromb Haemost* **63**:319, 1990.
198. Hellgren M, Tengborn L, Abildgaard U: Pregnancy in women with congenital antithrombin III deficiency: Experience of treatment with heparin and antithrombin. *Gynecol Obstet Invest* **14**:127, 1982.
199. Hall JG, Pauli RM, Wilson KM: Maternal and fetal sequellae of anticoagulation during pregnancy. *Am J Med* **68**:122, 1980.
200. Hirsh J, Cade JF, O'Sullivan EF: Clinical experience with anticoagulant therapy during pregnancy. *Br Med J* **1**:270, 1970.
201. Owen J: Antithrombin III replacement therapy in pregnancy. *Semin Hematol* **28**:46, 1991.
202. Blondel-Hill E, Mant MJ: The pregnant antithrombin III deficient patient: Management without antithrombin III concentrate. *Thromb Res* **65**:193, 1992.
203. Menache D, O'Malley JP, Schorr JB, Wagner B, Williams C, Alving BM, Ballard JO, Goodnight SH, Hathaway WE, Hultin MB, Kitchens CS, Lessner HE, Makary AZ, Manco-Johnson M, McGehee WG, Penner JA, Sanders JE: Evaluation of the safety, recovery, half-life, and clinical efficacy of antithrombin III (human) in patients with hereditary antithrombin III deficiency. *Blood* **75**:33, 1990.
204. Menache D: Replacement therapy in patients with hereditary antithrombin III deficiency. *Semin Hematol* **28**:31, 1991.
205. Winter JH, Fenech A, Bennett B, Douglas AS: Prophylactic antithrombotic therapy with stanozolol in patients with familial antithrombin III deficiency. *Br J Haematol* **57**:527, 1984.
206. Fairfax AJ, Ibbotson RM: Effect of danazol on the biochemical abnormality of inherited antithrombin III deficiency. *Thorax* **40**:646, 1985.
207. Eyster ME, Parker ME: Treatment of familial antithrombin-III deficiency with danazol. *Haemostasis* **15**:119, 1985.
208. Knot E, ten Cate JW, Drijfhout HR, Kahle LH, Tytgat GN: Antithrombin III metabolism in patients with liver disease. *J Clin Pathol* **37**:523, 1984.
209. Kauffmann RH, Veltkamp JJ, van Tilburg NH, van Es LA: Acquired antithrombin III deficiency and thrombosis in the nephrotic syndrome. *Am J Med* **65**:607, 1978.
210. Spero JA, Lewis JH, Hasiba U: Disseminated intravascular coagulation. Findings in 346 patients. *Thromb Haemost* **43**:28, 1980.
211. Brenner B: Antithrombin III and preeclampsia [editorial]. *Isr J Med Sci* **26**:121, 1990.
212. Ceriello A, Quatraro A, Marchi E, Barbanti M, Dello Russo P, Lefebvre P, Giugliano D: The role of hyperglycaemia-induced alterations of antithrombin III and factor X

activation in the thrombin hyperactivity of diabetes mellitus. *Diabetic Med* **7**:343, 1990.
213. Fagerhol MK, Abildgaard U, Bergsjø P, Jacobsen JH: Oral contraceptives and low antithrombin III concentration. *Lancet* **1**:1175, 1970.
214. Henny CP, ten Cate H, Dabhoiwala NF, Büller HR, ten Cate JW: The effect of different hormonal approaches in treatment of prostatic cancer on the plasma antithrombin III activity. *Thromb Haemost* **50**:50, 1983. (abstr.)
215. Conard J, Cazenave B, Maury J, Horellou MH, Samama M: L-asparaginase, antithrombin III, and thrombosis. *Lancet* **1**:1091, 1980.
216. Bauer KA, Teitel JM, Rosenberg RD: L-asparaginase induced antithrombin III deficiency: Evidence against the production of a hypercoagulable state. *Thromb Res* **29**:437, 1983.
217. Gugliotta L, D'Angelo A, Mattioli Belmonte M, Viganò-D'Angelo S, Colombo G, Catani L, Gianni L, Lauria F, Tura S: Hypercoagulability during L-asparaginase treatment: The effect of antithrombin III supplementation in vivo. *Br J Haematol* **74**:465, 1990.
218. Holmer E, Soderstrom G, Andersson L-O: Properties of antithrombin III depleted plasma. I. Effect of heparin. *Thromb Res* **17**:113, 1980.
219. Parker KA, Tollefsen DM: The protease specificity of heparin cofactor II. Inhibition of thrombin generated during coagulation. *J Biol Chem* **260**:3501, 1985.
220. Ragg H: A new member of the plasma protease inhibitor gene family. *Nucleic Acids Res* **14**:1073, 1986.
221. Blinder MA, Marasa JC, Reynolds CH, Deaven LL, Tollefsen DM: Heparin cofactor II: cDNA sequence, chromosome localization, restriction fragment length polymorphism, and expression in Escherichia coli. *Biochemistry* **27**:752, 1988.
222. Hortin G, Tollefsen DM, Strauss AW: Identification of two sites of sulfation of human heparin cofactor II. *J Biol Chem* **261**:15827, 1986.
223. Church FC, Pratt CW, Hoffman M: Leukocyte chemoattractant peptides from the serpin heparin cofactor II. *J Biol Chem* **266**:704, 1991.
224. Church FC, Meade JB, Pratt CW: Structure-function relationships in heparin cofactor II: Spectral analysis of aromatic residues and absence of a role for sulfhydryl groups in thrombin inhibition. *Arch Biochem Biophys* **259**:331, 1987.
225. Herzog R, Lutz S, Blin N, Marasa JC, Blinder MA, Tollefsen DM: Complete nucleotide sequence of the gene for human heparin cofactor II and mapping to chromosomal band 22q11. *Biochemistry* **30**:1350, 1991.
226. Ragg H, Preibisch G: Structure and expression of the gene coding for the human serpin hLS2. *J Biol Chem* **263**:12129, 1988.
227. Turner J, Grundy CB, Kakkar VV, Cooper DN: MspI RFLP in the human heparin cofactor II (HCF2) gene. *Nucleic Acids Res* **18**:1664, 1990.
228. Jaffe EA, Armellino D, Tollefsen DM: Biosynthesis of functionally active heparin cofactor II by a human hepatoma-derived cell line. *Biochem Biophys Res Commun* **132**:368, 1985.
229. Griffith MJ, Noyes CM, Tyndall JA, Church FC: Structural evidence for leucine at the reactive site of heparin cofactor II. *Biochemistry* **24**:6777, 1985.
230. Church FC, Noyes CM, Griffith MJ: Inhibition of chymotrypsin by heparin cofactor II. *Proc Natl Acad Sci USA* **82**:6431, 1985.
231. Derechin VM, Blinder MA, Tollefsen DM: Substitution of arginine for Leu444 in the reactive site of heparin cofactor II enhances the rate of thrombin inhibition. *J Biol Chem* **265**:5623, 1990.
232. Hurst RE, Poon M-C, Griffith MJ: Structure-activity relationships of heparin. Independence of heparin charge density and antithrombin-binding domains in thrombin inhibition by antithrombin and heparin cofactor II. *J Clin Invest* **72**:1042, 1983.
233. Maimone MM, Tollefsen DM: Activation of heparin cofactor II by heparin oligosaccharides. *Biochem Biophys Res Commun* **152**:1056, 1988.
234. Maimone MM: Characterization of heparin and dermatan sulfate molecules that bind and activate heparin cofactor II. Ph. D. Thesis. St. Louis, Washington University, 1990.
235. Sié P, Petitou M, Lormeau J-C, Dupouy D, Boneu B, Choay J: Studies on the structural requirements of heparin for the catalysis of thrombin inhibition by heparin cofactor II. *Biochim Biophys Acta* **966**:188, 1988.
236. Bray B, Lane DA, Freyssinet J-M, Pejler G, Lindahl U: Anti-thrombin activities of heparin. Effect of saccharide chain length on thrombin inhibition by heparin cofactor II and by antithrombin. *Biochem J* **262**:225, 1989.
237. Maimone MM, Tollefsen DM: Structure of a dermatan sulfate hexasaccharide that binds to heparin cofactor II with high affinity. *J Biol Chem* **265**:18263, 1990.
238. Tollefsen DM, Peacock ME, Monafo WJ: Molecular size of dermatan sulfate oligosaccharides required to bind and activate heparin cofactor II. *J Biol Chem* **261**:8854, 1986.
239. Teien AN, Abildgaard U, Höök M: The anticoagulant effect of heparan sulfate and dermatan sulfate. *Thromb Res* **8**:859, 1976.
240. Fernandez F, van Ryn J, Ofosu FA, Hirsh J, Buchanan MR: The haemorrhagic and antithrombotic effects of dermatan sulfate. *Br J Haematol* **64**:309, 1986.
241. Maggi A, Abbadini M, Pagella PG, Borowska A, Pangrazzi J, Donati MB: Antithrombotic properties of dermatan sulphate in a rat venous thrombosis model. *Haemostasis* **17**:329, 1987.
242. Merton RE, Thomas DP: Experimental studies on the relative efficacy of dermatan sulphate and heparin as antithrombotic agents. *Thromb Haemost* **58**:839, 1987.
243. Van Ryn-McKenna J, Gray E, Weber E, Ofosu FA, Buchanan MR: Effects of sulfated polysaccharides on inhibition of thrombus formation initiated by different stimuli. *Thromb Haemost* **61**:7, 1989.
244. Agnelli G, Cosmi B, Di Filippo P, Ranucci V, Veschi F, Longetti M, Renga C, Barzi F, Gianese F, Lupattelli L, Rinonapoli E, Nenci GG: A randomised, double-blind, placebo-controlled trial of dermatan sulphate for prevention of deep vein thrombosis in hip fracture. *Thromb Haemost* **67**:203, 1992.
245. Lane DA, Ryan K, Ireland H, Curtis JR, Nurmohamed MT, Krediet RT, Roggekamp MC, Stevens P, ten Cate JW: Dermatan sulphate in haemodialysis. *Lancet* **339**:334, 1992.
246. Cofrancesco E, Boschetti C, Leonardi P, Cortellaro M: Dermatan sulphate in acute leukaemia. *Lancet* **339**:1177, 1992.
247. Ofosu FA, Modi GJ, Smith LM, Cerskus AL, Hirsh J, Blajchman MA: Heparan sulfate and dermatan sulfate inhibit the generation of thrombin activity in plasma by complementary pathways. *Blood* **64**:742, 1984.
248. Sié P, Ofosu F, Fernandez F, Buchanan MR, Petitou M, Boneu B: Respective role of antithrombin III and heparin cofactor II in the in vitro anticoagulant effect of heparin and of various sulphated polysaccharides. *Br J Haematol* **64**:707, 1986.
249. Andersson TR, Larsen ML, Abildgaard U: Low heparin cofactor II associated with abnormal crossed immunoelectrophoresis pattern in two Norwegian families. *Thromb Res* **47**:243, 1987.
250. Blinder MA, Andersson TR, Abildgaard U, Tollefsen DM: Heparin cofactor II Oslo. Mutation of Arg-189 to His decreases the affinity for dermatan sulfate. *J Biol Chem* **264**:5128, 1989.
251. Blinder MA, Tollefsen DM: Site-directed mutagenesis of arginine 103 and lysine 185 in the proposed glycosaminoglycan-binding site of heparin cofactor II. *J Biol Chem* **265**:286, 1990.
252. Ragg H, Ulshöfer T, Gerewitz J: On the activation of human leuserpin-2, a thrombin inhibitor, by glycosaminoglycans. *J Biol Chem* **265**:5211, 1990.
253. Ragg H, Ulshöfer T, Gerewitz J: Glycosaminoglycan-mediated leuserpin-2/thrombin interaction. Structure-function relationships. *J Biol Chem* **265**:22386, 1990.
254. Whinna HC, Blinder MA, Szewczyk M, Tollefsen DM, Church FC: Role of lysine 173 in heparin binding to heparin cofactor II. *J Biol Chem* **266**:8129, 1991.
255. Van Deerlin VMD, Tollefsen DM: The N-terminal acidic

domain of heparin cofactor II mediates the inhibition of α-thrombin in the presence of glycosaminoglycans. *J Biol Chem* **266:**20223, 1991.
256. Grutter MG, Priestle JP, Rahuel J, Grossenbacher H, Bode W, Hofsteenge J, Stone SR: Crystal structure of the thrombin-hirudin complex: A novel mode of serine protease inhibition. *EMBO J* **9:**2361, 1990.
257. Rydel TJ, Ravichandran KG, Tulinsky A, Bode W, Huber R, Roitsch C, Fenton JW II: The structure of a complex of recombinant hirudin and human α-thrombin. *Science* **249:**277, 1990.
258. Hortin GL, Tollefsen DM, Benutto BM: Antithrombin activity of a peptide corresponding to residues 54-75 of heparin cofactor II. *J Biol Chem* **264:**13979, 1989.
259. Rogers SJ, Pratt CW, Whinna HC, Church FC: Role of thrombin exosites in inhibition by heparin cofactor II. *J Biol Chem* **267:**3613, 1992.
260. Tollefsen DM, Pestka CA: Heparin cofactor II activity in patients with disseminated intravascular coagulation and hepatic failure. *Blood* **66:**769, 1985.
261. Sié P, Dupouy D, Pichon J, Boneu B: Constitutional heparin co-factor II deficiency associated with recurrent thrombosis. *Lancet* **2:**414, 1985.
262. Tran TH, Marbet GA, Duckert F: Association of hereditary heparin co-factor II deficiency with thrombosis. *Lancet* **2:**413, 1985.
263. Andersson TR, Larsen ML, Handeland GF, Abildgaard U: Heparin cofactor II activity in plasma: Application of an automated assay method to the study of a normal adult population. *Scand J Haematol* **36:**96, 1986.
264. Bertina RM, van der Linden IK, Engesser L, Muller HP, Brommer EJP: Hereditary heparin cofactor II deficiency and the risk of development of thrombosis. *Thromb Haemost* **57:**196, 1987.
265. Tran TH, Duckert F: Heparin cofactor II determination—levels in normals and patients with hereditary antithrombin III deficiency and disseminated intravascular coagulation. *Thromb Haemost* **52:**112, 1984.
266. Abildgaard U, Larsen ML: Assay of dermatan sulfate cofactor (heparin cofactor II) activity in human plasma. *Thromb Res* **35:**257, 1984.
267. Ezenagu LC, Brandt JT: Laboratory determination of heparin cofactor II. *Arch Pathol Lab Med* **110:**1149, 1986.
268. Massouh M, Jatoi A, Gordon EM, Ratnoff OD: Heparin cofactor II activity in plasma during pregnancy and oral contraceptive use. *J Lab Clin Med* **114:**697, 1989.
269. Toulon P, Bardin JM, Blumenfeld N: Increased heparin cofactor II levels in women taking oral contraceptives. *Thromb Haemost* **64:**365, 1990.
270. Griffith MJ, Carraway T, White GC, Dombrose FA: Heparin cofactor activities in a family with hereditary antithrombin III deficiency: Evidence for a second heparin cofactor in human plasma. *Blood* **61:**111, 1983.
271. McGuire EA, Tollefsen DM: Activation of heparin cofactor II by fibroblasts and vascular smooth muscle cells. *J Biol Chem* **262:**169, 1987.
272. Andrew M, Mitchell L, Berry L, Paes B, Delorme M, Ofosu F, Burrows R, Khambalia B: An anticoagulant dermatan sulfate proteoglycan circulates in the pregnant woman and her fetus. *J Clin Invest* **89:**321, 1992.
273. Brennan MJ, Oldberg A, Pierschbacher MD, Ruoslahti E: Chondroitin/dermatan sulfate proteoglycan in human fetal membranes: Demonstration of an antigenically similar proteoglycan in fibroblasts. *J Biol Chem* **259:**13742, 1984.
274. Lane DA, Ireland H, Olds RJ, Thein SL, Perry DJ, Aiach M: Antithrombin III: A database of mutations. *Thromb Haemost* **66:**657, 1991.
275. Daly M, Perry DJ, Harper PL, Daly HM, Roques AWW, Carrell RW: Insertions/deletions in the antithrombin gene: 3 mutations associated with non-expression. *Thromb Haemost* **67:**521, 1992.
276. Olds RJ, Lane DA, Ireland H, Leone G, De Stefano V, Cazenave JP, Wiesel ML, Thein SL: Novel point mutations leading to type Ia antithrombin deficiency and thrombosis. *Br J Haematol* **78:**408, 1991.
277. Olds RJ, Lane DA, Finazzi G, Barbui T, Thein SL: A frameshift mutation leading to type I antithrombin deficiency and thrombosis. *Blood* **76:**2182, 1990.
278. Gandrille S, Vidaud D, Emmerich J, Clauser E, Sié P, Fiessinger JN, Alhenc-Gelas M, Priollet P, Aiach M: Molecular basis for hereditary antithrombin III quantitative deficiencies: A stop codon in exon IIIa and a frameshift in exon VI. *Br J Haematol* **78:**414, 1991.
279. Olds RJ, Lane DA, Ireland H, Finazzi G, Barbui T, Abildgaard U, Girolami A, Thein SL: A common point mutation producing type Ia antithrombin III deficiency: AT129 *C*GA to *T*GA (Arg to Stop). *Thromb Res* **64:**621, 1991.
280. Vidaud D, Emmerich J, Sirieix ME, Sié P, Alhenc-Gelas M, Aiach M: Molecular basis for antithrombin III type I deficiency: Three novel mutations located in exon IV. *Blood* **78:**2305, 1991.
281. Grundy CB, Thomas F, Millar DS, Krawczak M, Melissari E, Lindo V, Moffat E, Kakkar VV, Cooper DN: Recurrent deletion in the human antithrombin III gene. *Blood* **78:**1027, 1991.
282. Vidaud D, Gandrille S, Emmerich J, Sirieix ME, Alhenc-Gelas M, Fiessinger JN, Sié P, Gouault-Heilman M, Aiach M: Identifications of 6 novel mutations responsible for type I AT III deficiencies. *Thromb Haemost* **65:**991, 1991. (abstr.)
283. Daly M, Bruce D, Perry DJ, Price J, Harper PL, O'Meara A, Carrell RW: Antithrombin Dublin (-3 Val→Glu): An N-terminal variant which has an aberrant signal peptidase cleavage site. *FEBS Lett* **273:**87, 1990.
284. Grundy CB, Holding S, Millar DS, Kakkar VV, Cooper DN: A novel missense mutation in the antithrombin III gene (Ser349→Pro) causing recurrent venous thrombosis. *Hum Genet* **88:**707, 1992.
285. Olds RJ, Thein SL, Ireland H, Lane DA, Boisclair M, Conard J, Horellou MH: Identification of 402 phenylalanine as a functionally important residue in antithrombin. *Thromb Haemost* **65:**670, 1991. (abstr.)
286. Bock SC, Silberman JA, Wikoff W, Abildgaard U, Hultin MB: Identification of a threonine for alanine substitution at residue 404 of antithrombin III Oslo suggests integrity of the 404-407 region is important for maintaining normal inhibitor levels. *Thromb Haemost* **62:**494, 1989. (abstr).
287. Nakagawa M, Tanaka S, Tsuji H, Takada O, Uno M, Hashimoto-Gotoh T, Wagatsuma M: Congenital antithrombin III deficiency (AT-III Kyoto): Identification of a point mutation altering arginine-406 to methionine behind the reactive site. *Thromb Res* **64:**101, 1989.
288. Vidaud D, Sirieix ME, Alhenc-Gelas M, Chadeuf G, Aillaud MF, Juhan-Vague I, Aiach M: A double heterozygosity in 2 brothers with antithrombin (ATIII) deficiency due to the association of an Arg 47 to His mutation with a 9 base pair (bp) deletion in exon VI. *Thromb Haemost* **65:**838, 1991. (abstr.)
289. Devraj-Kizuk R, Chui DHK, Prochownik EV, Carter CJ, Ofosu FA, Blajchman MA: Antithrombin III Hamilton: A gene with a point mutation (guanine to adenine) in codon 382 causing impaired serine protease reactivity. *Blood* **72:**1518, 1988.
290. Ireland H, Lane DA, Thompson E, Walker ID, Blench I, Morris HR, Freyssinet JM, Grunebaum L, Olds R, Thein SL: Antithrombin Glasgow II: Alanine 382 to threonine mutation in the serpin P12 position, resulting in a substrate reaction with thrombin. *Br J Haematol* **79:**70, 1991.
291. Mohlo-Sabatier P, Aiach M, Gaillard I, Fiessinger JN, Fischer AM, Chadeuf G, Clauser E: Molecular characterization of antithrombin III (ATIII) variants using polymerase chain reaction. Identification of the ATIII Charleville as an Ala384 Pro mutation. *J Clin Invest* **84:**1236, 1989.
292. Caso R, Lane DA, Thompson EA, Olds RJ, Thein SL, Panico M, Blench I, Morris H, Freyssinet JM, Aiach M, Rodeghiero F, Finazzi G: Antithrombin Vicenza, Ala 384 to Pro (GCA to CCA) mutation transforming the inhibitor into a substrate. *Br J Haematol* **77:**87, 1990.
293. Perry DJ, Daly M, Harper PL, Tait RC, Price J, Walker ID, Carrell RW: Antithrombin Cambridge II, 384 Ala to Ser. Further evidence of the role of the reactive centre loop in the inhibitory function of the serpins. *FEBS Lett* **285:**248, 1991.

294. Blajchman MA, Fernandez-Rachubinski F, Sheffield WP, Austin RC, Schulman S: Antithrombin-III-Stockholm: A codon 392 (Gly→Asp) mutation with normal heparin binding and impaired serine protease reactivity. *Blood* **79:**1428, 1992.
295. Erdjument H, Lane DA, Ireland H, Panico M, DiMarzo V, Blench I, Morris HR: Formation of a covalent disulfide-linked antithrombin complex by an antithrombin variant, antithrombin Northwick Park. *J Biol Chem* **262:**13381, 1987.
296. Erdjument H, Lane DA, Panico M, DiMarzo V, Morris HR: Single amino acid substitutions in the reactive site of antithrombin leading to thrombosis. Congenital substitution of arginine 393 to cysteine in antithrombin Northwick Park and to histidine in antithrombin Glasgow. *J Biol Chem* **263:**5589, 1988.
297. Lane DA, Erdjument H, Thompson E, Panico M, DiMarzo V, Morris HR, Leone G, De Stefano V, Thein SL: A novel amino acid substitution in the reactive site of a congenital variant antithrombin. Antithrombin Pescara, Arg 393 to Pro, caused by CGT to CCT mutation. *J Biol Chem* **264:**10200, 1989.
298. Owen MC, George PM, Lane DA, Boswell DR: P1 variant antithrombins Glasgow (393 Arg to His) and Pescara (393 Arg to Pro) have increased heparin affinity and are resistant to catalytic cleavage by elastase. Implications for the heparin activation mechanisms. *FEBS Lett* **280:**216, 1991.
299. Stephens AW, Thalley BS, Hirs CHW: Antithrombin-III Denver, a reactive site variant. *J Biol Chem* **262:**1044, 1987.
300. Olds RJ, Lane DA, Caso R, Panico M, Morris HR, Sas G, Dawes J, Thein SL: Antithrombin III Budapest: A single amino acid substitution (429Pro to Leu) in a region highly conserved in the serpin family. *Blood* **79:**1206, 1992.
301. Borg JY, Owen MC, Soria C, Soria J, Caen J, Carrell RW: Arginine 47 is a prime heparin binding site in antithrombin. A new variant Rouen II, 47 Arg to Ser. *J Clin Invest* **81:**1292, 1988.
302. Olds RJ, Lane DA, Boisclair M, Sas G, Bock SC, Thein SL: Antithrombin Budapest 3. An antithrombin variant with reduced heparin affinity resulting from the substitution L99F. *FEBS Lett* **300:**241, 1992.
303. Gandrille S, Aiach M, Lane DA, Vidaud D, Mohlo-Sabatier P, Caso R, de Moerloose P, Fiessinger JN, Clauser E: Important role of Arg 129 in heparin binding site of antithrombin III: Identification of novel mutation Arg 129 to Gln. *J Biol Chem* **265:**18997, 1990.

CHAPTER 110

Inherited Disorders of Platelets

Peter J. Newman ▪ Mortimer Poncz

1. **Human platelets participate in a number of adhesive events that are crucial for repair of the vasculature. Though lacking in protein synthetic capability, platelets come equipped with a variety of plasma membrane receptors and intracellular organelles that make them highly efficient "adhesion machines" for mediating the primary hemostatic process. Adhesion itself is an activating event, and it results in the transmission of signals to the cell interior by virtue of cell-surface receptors that form cytoplasmic connections with intracellular kinases, G proteins, and cytoskeletal components. Platelet activation, in turn, elicits the secretion of several types of intracellular granules, the contents of which serve to embellish further the formation of the platelet plug by providing additional adhesive ligands that can add to the local concentration of intercellular glue molecules.**

2. **The glycoprotein (GP) IIb-IIIa complex (integrin $\alpha_{IIb}\beta_3$) is one of the most abundant receptors on the platelet surface, representing nearly 15 percent of total surface protein. Glanzmann thrombasthenia is a rare, inherited, autosomal recessive bleeding disorder, the hallmark of which is the failure of platelets to bind fibrinogen and aggregate following stimulation by physiological agonists such as ADP, thrombin, epinephrine, or collagen. Underlying this disorder is an abnormality of the genes encoding GPIIb or GPIIIa. Glanzmann thrombasthenia is characterized by often unpredictable mucocutaneous bleeding and is usually noticed at an early age. Though nearly 200 individuals with Glanzmann thrombasthenia have been described in the literature, to date only 12 of these have been solved at the molecular level. As in most genetic disorders, the molecular abnormalities have been found to range from major deletions and inversions easily detectable by Southern blot analysis to single point mutations identified only by nucleotide sequence analysis of platelet mRNA-derived PCR products.**

3. **The GPIb complex is crucial for initial attachment and proper adhesion to the extracellular matrix of a damaged vessel. Bernard-Soulier syndrome represents the second most recognized inherited platelet disorder, and is characterized by a prolonged bleeding time, giant platelets on blood smear, normal platelet aggregation with ADP, collagen, and epinephrine, with delayed response to thrombin, but absent platelet agglutination in the presence of ristocetin. The Bernard-Soulier syndrome is an autosomal recessive disorder in which most patients have a decrease to absence of all four members of the GPIb complex, which is comprised of four subunits: $GPIb_\alpha$, $GPIb_\beta$, GPIX, and GPV. Only a small number of patients have had the responsible defect defined on a molecular level. Defects in the GPIb complex may also be involved in another bleeding disorder—platelet-type (or pseudo-) von Willebrand disease—in which the platelet receptor exhibits increased affinity for von Willebrand factor (vWf).**

4. **In addition to amino acid changes that disrupt function and result in bleeding diatheses, several platelet membrane glycoproteins have naturally occurring allelic forms within the human gene pool. Two clinically recognized immunologic syndromes are attributable to "platelet-specific" polymorphisms. Neonatal alloimmune thrombocytopenia is characterized by thrombocytopenia in neonates due to passively transmitted maternal antibody directed against a fetal platelet antigen inherited from the father and lacking on the mother's platelets. Posttransfusion purpura is quite rare, with less than 200 cases reported to date, and is characterized by acute, usually severe, thrombocytopenia occurring 7 to 10 days after a blood transfusion. As the precise nucleotide sequence polymorphisms associated with the major human platelet alloantigen systems have become defined, it has become possible to develop and apply DNA-based diagnostic tests for the molecular analysis of these clinically important molecular variations.**

5. **Human platelets contain several different types of intracytoplasmic granules that can be distinguished by electron microscopy, including α-granules, dense granules (δ-granules), and lysosomes. These granules play a major role in platelet plug formation following platelet activation. Patients with defects in the platelet-dense granules have a storage pool deficiency. The two most common platelet storage pool disorders are known as Hermansky-Pudlak syndrome and Chediak-Higashi syndrome. A number of patients have been described who have a deficiency in α-granules, a disorder known as the gray platelet syndrome. These platelets are markedly deficient in α-granule-specific proteins such as platelet factor 4, β-thromboglobulin, vWf, factor V, fibronectin, and platelet-derived growth factor.**

6. **Following the binding of an agonist to its platelet receptor, a signal is transferred across the cell membrane into the cell either directly by the membrane receptor or through intervening $G_{\alpha\beta\delta}$ heterotrimeric proteins. Signal transduc-**

A list of standard abbreviations is located immediately preceding the index in each volume. Additional abbreviations used in this chapter include: BSS = Bernard-Soulier syndrome; βTG = β-thromboglobulin; CFU–GEMM = colony-forming unit–granulocyte, erythrocyte, monocyte, megakaryocyte; DMS = demarcation membrane system; GP = glycoprotein; GT = Glanzmann thrombasthenia; LRD = leucine-rich domain; MK-CSA = megakaryocyte colony-stimulating activity; NAT = neonatal autoimmune thrombocytopenia; PTP = posttransfusion purpura; TAR = thrombocytopenia and absent radii syndrome; TPO = thrombopoietin; VNR = vitronectin receptor; vWD = von Willebrand disease; vWf = von Willebrand factor.

tion results in secondary changes within the platelet that include ionic calcium fluxes, cAMP formation, phospholipase A_2 and C activation, changes in arachidonate pathway metabolism, protein kinase C activation, and protein phosphorylation. A small number of patients with inherited disorders of platelet signal transduction have been described.

7. **Activated platelets play a role in accelerating the proteolytic events that take place as part of the coagulation cascade, and this property has been termed "platelet factor 3 activity." The procoagulant properties have been attributed to a number of characteristics unique to the surface of activated platelets, including exposure of phosphatidylserine moieties, redistribution of specific receptors for factors V and X, and development of platelet microvesicles. One of the best-characterized inherited disorders of platelet factor 3 activity is known as Scott syndrome. The defect in this disorder is not limited to platelet membranes, as erythrocytes from patients with Scott syndrome also have decreased microvesiculation and fewer factor Va binding sites than normal following A23187 ionophore stimulation.**
8. **The process by which platelet formation occurs is a fascinating one, which is only now beginning to be understood. Megakaryocytopoiesis begins with the self-renewing hematopoietic stem cell in the bone marrow that becomes progressively committed to the megakaryoblast lineage, eventually resulting in the production of a mature megakaryocyte that "terminally differentiates" by releasing a shower of 10^3 to 10^4 platelets. The size variation and heterogeneity in platelets seen in various disease states may be related to the site and mechanism of formation, and a number of the inherited platelet disorders involve abnormal platelet size, including the macrothrombocytopenic states seen in Bernard-Soulier syndrome and the May-Hegglin anomaly, as well as the microthrombocytopenia seen in Wiskott-Aldrich syndrome. Several of these disorders may result from abnormal hematopoietic-stem-cell commitment to the megakaryocyte lineage, while others may involve defects in the final process of differentiation into mature megakaryocytes and the subsequent shedding of platelets.**

INTRODUCTION: THE ROLE OF PLATELETS IN HEMOSTASIS AND THROMBOSIS

Human platelets are anucleate cellular derivatives of bone marrow megakaryocytes that circulate throughout the bloodstream at a concentration of 150,000 to 400,000/μl. With a life span of only approximately 10 days, resting platelets maintain a disklike shape unless activated, usually by exposure to a damaged vessel wall. Following activation, platelets undergo a rapid metamorphosis from nonadherent plate-shaped cells into highly adherent, pseudopod-containing, ameba-like entities, and participate in the formation of the so-called platelet plug that helps to stop or slow the flow of the other blood components from the site of vascular injury.

Platelet Adhesion and Aggregation

Though lacking in protein synthetic capability, human platelets come equipped with a variety of plasma membrane receptors and intracellular organelles that make them highly efficient "adhesion machines" for mediating the primary hemostatic process. The mechanisms by which platelets become activated are multiple and complex, and have a great deal of built-in redundancy to ensure rapid, efficient sealing of the wound. As illustrated in Fig. 110-1, platelets can be activated by numerous agonists, both soluble and insoluble. Commonly, damage to a vessel wall leads to disruption of the normally present endothelial cell barrier, with subsequent exposure of extracellular matrix components, including fibronectin, collagen, and vWf. Platelets have on their surface specialized receptors for these ligands, and rapidly initiate an adhesive cascade at the site of injury. Membrane glycoprotein (GP) receptor complexes—Ib-V-IX and $\alpha_2\beta_1$—bind vWf and collagen, respectively, and mediate the primary adhesion of an initial layer of platelets that in effect apply a thin bandage to the injury. Nearby platelets become secondarily exposed to extracellular agonists, such as thrombin, epinephrine, ADP, and various thromboxane metabolites that have become generated or liberated as a result of local tissue injury. Platelets in the general vicinity of the wound become activated by one or more of these soluble agonists, and mobilize still another adhesive receptor, the GPIIb–IIIa complex. On activation, this receptor complex undergoes conformational changes that allow it to bind the plasma protein fibrinogen, which, due to its symmetrical structure, serves to crosslink platelets to each other, a process known as "platelet–platelet cohesion" or "platelet aggregation." Thus, the initial attachment of platelets to the exposed subendothelial matrix results in the generation of an adhesive cascade that rapidly seals off the wound by forming the initial platelet plug. The membrane receptors and their ligands that mediate these important adhesive interactions are summarized in Fig. 110-2.

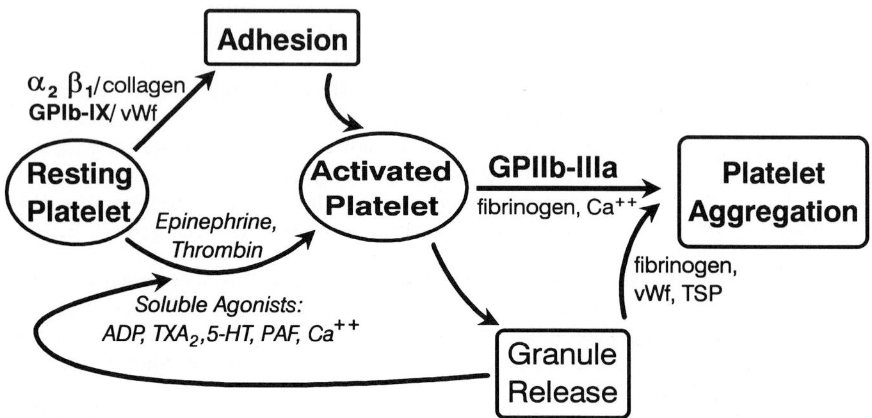

FIG. 110-1 Role of platelets in hemostasis. The transformation of platelets from a resting into an adherent state is depicted, together with several of the known soluble and insoluble agonists that can trigger the event. Adhesion to extracellular matrix components, exposed as a result of endothelial cell damage, is itself an activating event, and leads to granule release and the conversion of cell-surface receptors into an adhesive conformation. Additional soluble agonists, including thrombin, ADP, and epinephrine, generated at the site of the injury, serve to enhance the activation process, and recruit additional platelets into the developing platelet aggregate. TSP = thrombospondin.

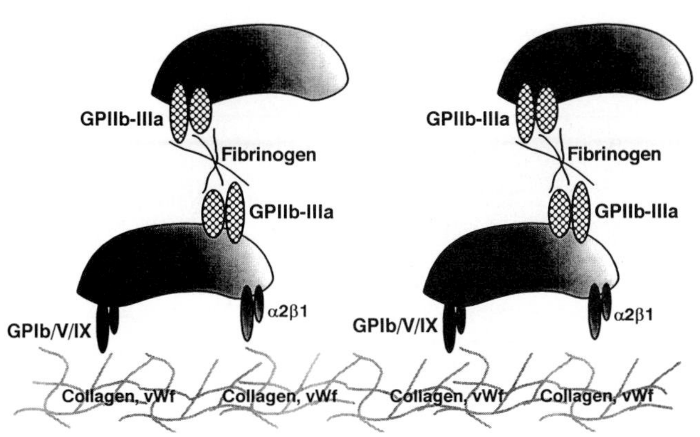

FIG. 110-2 **Platelet adhesive interactions. Platelet receptors involved in platelet–platelet interactions are shown, together with the adhesive ligands with which they interact.**

Platelet Granules

Adhesion itself is an activating event; it causes the secretion of several types of intracellular granules, the contents of which serve to embellish further the formation of the platelet plug by providing additional adhesive ligands that can add to the local concentration of intercellular glue molecules. A number of soluble agonists that aid in recruiting other platelets to the site of injury are also secreted. The three major types of platelet granules, as well as some of their more interesting physiological components, are shown in Table 110-1. α Granules contain a large number of adhesive protein ligands, some of which, on secretion, bind to specific platelet plasma membrane receptors and help to crosslink platelets to each other during the platelet aggregation process. Dense, or δ granules, contain most of the platelet calcium, as well as large storage pools of ADP and serotonin. Though the function of serotonin in platelet function is not well understood, released calcium and ADP play important supportive roles in mediating the subsequent platelet aggregation process. Lysosomal granules, as in other cell types, probably function in degrading various endocytosed plasma constituents, and may also play a role in receptor recycling, though evidence for the latter phenomenon in platelets is just starting to accumulate.

Platelet Adhesion Receptors

Central to the role of platelets in their ability to adhere to both extracellular matrix components (adhesion) and to each other (aggregation) is an abundant supply of cell-surface adhesion molecules that exist in multiple states of activation. These cell adhesion receptors, in turn, are capable of transmitting signals to the cell interior by virtue of their ability to form cytoplasmic connections with intracellular kinases, G proteins, and cytoskeletal components. Through the efforts of many laboratories over the past 10 years, many platelet cell-surface receptors have now been cloned and characterized at the molecular biologic and biochemical level. Fortunately, though more than 50 platelet plasma membrane proteins are recognizable by two-dimensional electrophoretic analysis, many of them, on inspection of their deduced amino acid sequences, have fallen into a limited number of well-recognizable gene families. Four such gene families, the integrins, the leucine-rich glycoproteins, the immunoglobulin gene superfamily, and the selectins, as well as their members that are present in human platelets, are summarized in Table 110-2. A brief description of the major distinguishing characteristics of each gene family follows.

The Leucine-Rich Glycoprotein Family. Platelets contain four members of the leucine-rich glycoprotein family[1,2] and, interestingly enough, all four proteins (GPIbα, GPIbβ, GPV, and GPIX) exist in a complex on the platelet surface,[3,4] and will be referred to for the remainder of this chapter as the GPIb complex. All except GPV have been cloned and sequenced, and are known to derive from distinct genes.[1,5] Each platelet expresses 20,000 to 30,000 copies of the GPIb complex on its surface, and all four components of the complex are missing from the platelet surface in patients with the Bernard-Soulier syndrome, a defect in platelet adhesion to the subendothelium[6] that will be discussed in greater detail below.

The Immunoglobulin Gene Superfamily. The distinguishing feature of the immunoglobulin gene (Ig) superfamily is the presence of one or more immunoglobulin-like homology domains. Structurally, these homology domains resemble antibodies, containing seven β-strands folded into two β-pleated sheets held together by two cysteines spaced approximately 50 residues apart. Ig family members are widely distributed, and members of the Ig superfamily are present on most, if not all, human cell types, where they function in cellular adhesion or cell–cell recognition. Platelets are known to express three members of the Ig superfamily: class I histocompatibility antigens (HLA), FcγRIIA receptors, and the cell adhesion molecule, PECAM-1. Of these, class I HLA molecules are extremely polymorphic, and probably account for the development of the majority of cases of platelet transfusion refractoriness.

The Selectins. Selectins are a relatively recently described gene family, which to date contains only three members, each named for the cell type in which it was first discovered: P-selectin, originally described in human platelets[7,8]; E-selectin, which is present only on endothelium[9,10]; and L-selectin, found on lymphocytes. Selectins share a common

Table 110-1 **Platelet Granules and Their Contents**

Alpha Granules	Dense Granules	Lysosomes
Fibrinogen	Serotonin	β-*N*-acetylglucosaminidase
vWf	Calcium	β-Glucuronidase
Fibronectin	ADP	β-Galactosidase
Thrombospondin	Guanine nucleotides	Other acid hydrolases
Platelet factor 4	ATP, AMP	
Platelet-derived growth factor	Inorganic pyrophosphate	

Table 110-2 Cell Adhesion Molecule Families in Human Platelets

Gene Family	Members on Human Platelets	Functions
Integrins	GPIIb-IIIa (αIIb-β_3), αVβ_3, $\alpha_2\beta_1$, $\alpha_5\beta_1$, $\alpha_6\beta_1$	Cell–cell and cell–matrix interactions
Leucine-rich glycoprotein	GPIbα, GPIbβ, GPV, GPIX	Adhesion to subendothelium
Immunoglobulin gene superfamily	Fc receptor, Class I HLA, PECAM-1	Immunoregulation, adhesion
Selectins	P-selectin (GMP-140, PADGEM)	Platelet–leukocyte interactions

N-terminal lectinlike domain that is capable of interacting with carbohydrate moieties on nearby cellular receptors, and it is this structural motif that gives the family its name.[10] P-selectin, known as GMP-140 or PADGEM before the nomenclature was standardized,[9] is the only platelet selectin, and resides within the membrane of α-granules of resting platelets. On platelet activation, the α-granules fuse with the plasma membrane, exposing 10,000 to 15,000 P-selectin molecules to the platelet surface, where they participate in recruiting monocytes and neutrophils to the site of vascular injury.[11]

The Integrins. Integrins are composed of two-chain $\alpha\beta$ integral membrane protein heterodimer complexes that mediate cell–cell and cell–extracellular matrix adhesive interactions. At least 8 different β subunits and 11 different α-chains have been cloned and sequenced, and it is now recognized that distinct $\alpha\beta$ subunits can pair in different cell types to form distinct functional entities. To date, more than 15 members of this heterodimer family have been identified in species ranging from Drosophila to humans,[12,13] with at least 5 members ($\alpha_2\beta_1$, $\alpha_5\beta_1$, $\alpha_6\beta_1$, $\alpha_{IIb}\beta_3$, and $\alpha_v\beta_3$) expressed on the platelet surface. Of these, the integrin $\alpha_{IIb}\beta_3$, more commonly known as the GPIIb-IIIa complex, is uniquely expressed on platelets, and is by far the most abundant member of the integrin family to be found on the platelet surface, with 40,000 to 50,000 molecules/platelet.[14,15] Other platelet integrins, though not as extensively studied as GPIIb-IIIa, are thought to share similar overall structure due to the presence of multiple highly conserved cysteine residues.[16,17] The integrin most closely related to GPIIb-IIIa is the receptor for vitronectin, $\alpha_v\beta_3$. This integrin shares an identical β_3 subunit, GPIIIa, but forms a complex with the vitronectin receptor (VNR) α-chain that shares 74 percent sequence similarity with GPIIb.[16] Although there are at most 50 to 100 $\alpha_v\beta_3$ molecules per platelet,[18] there are nearly 100,000 VNR per endothelial cell,[19] and they probably play an important adhesive function in this and other cell types. The other three known platelet integrins share a different common β subunit (β_1), which forms a complex with either an α_2, α_5, or α_6 chain to form receptors for collagen, fibronectin, or laminin, respectively.[20–23] $\alpha_2\beta_1$ is most commonly referred to in the platelet literature as the GPIa-IIa complex, whereas $a_5\beta_1$ and $\alpha_6\beta_1$ are known as GPIc-IIa and Ic′-IIa, respectively. Of the β_1 integrin α chain subunits present on the platelet surface, α_2 (GPIa) is unique in that it contains an inserted, or "I," domain of approximately 200 amino acids. The I domain is normally present in α subunits that pair with leukocyte β_2 integrin subunits (LFA-1, p150,95, and MAC-1). Interestingly, of the three β_1 integrin α subunits that are present on platelets, only GPIa (α_2) is known to be naturally polymorphic in humans and will be discussed in that regard below. The major inherited disorder affecting a platelet integrin is known as Glanzmann thrombasthenia, and it will be described in detail below.

DISEASES ASSOCIATED WITH THE GPIIb-IIIa COMPLEX

The GPIIb-IIIa complex ($\alpha_{IIb}\beta_3$) is one of the most abundant receptors on the platelet surface, representing nearly 15 percent of total surface protein. In addition to its role as the major receptor for adhesive ligands such as fibrinogen, vWf, and fibronectin, GPIIb-IIIa is also highly immunogenic and is the target molecule for human auto-, allo-, and drug-dependent antibodies in immune-mediated platelet disorders. Because of its clinical significance in both immunologic, hemostatic, and thrombotic platelet disorders, GPIIb-IIIa is one of the most completely characterized membrane glycoproteins in humans, and an abundant literature exists describing its biochemical, immunologic, and cell and molecular biologic properties (for reviews, see refs. 24 to 26).

Biology of GPIIb-IIIa

The GPIIb and GPIIIa subunits are derived from separate mRNA transcripts,[27,28] though the genes encoding them are closely linked,[29] lying within a 250-kb segment of chromosome 17.[30,31] The amino acid sequences of both these membrane glycoproteins have been determined in full from cloned cDNA, and a schematic diagram of the GPIIb-IIIa complex is shown in Fig. 110-3. GPIIb is a typical integrin α subunit, approximately 145 kDa in size, and it contains 18 cysteine residues arranged into nine disulfide bonds that are rather evenly spaced throughout its length.[32] Like most other integrin α chains, GPIIb contains four calcium-binding domains, similar in sequence to those found in calcium-binding proteins such as troponin C, tropomyosin, and calmodulin.[17,32] Marguerie and coworkers have shown that all four sites must be occupied by divalent cations for proper functioning, and several groups have demonstrated that the ability of GPIIb to associate with GPIIIa depends on the continuous presence of at least micromolar levels of calcium.[33–35] The importance of the four calcium-binding regions for the normal functioning of GPIIb will be further illustrated below by examination of specific mutations that lead to dysfunctional platelet aggregation responses.

Characteristic of other integrin β chains, GPIIIa (integrin β_3) is approximately 90 kDa in molecular mass, and contains 762 amino acid residues in its mature form.[36–38] GPIIIa contains five cysteine-rich regions—one at the N-terminus and four located proximal to the membrane.[37] In total, GPIIIa, like all other known integrin β subunits, contains 56 cysteine residues in locations that are highly conserved

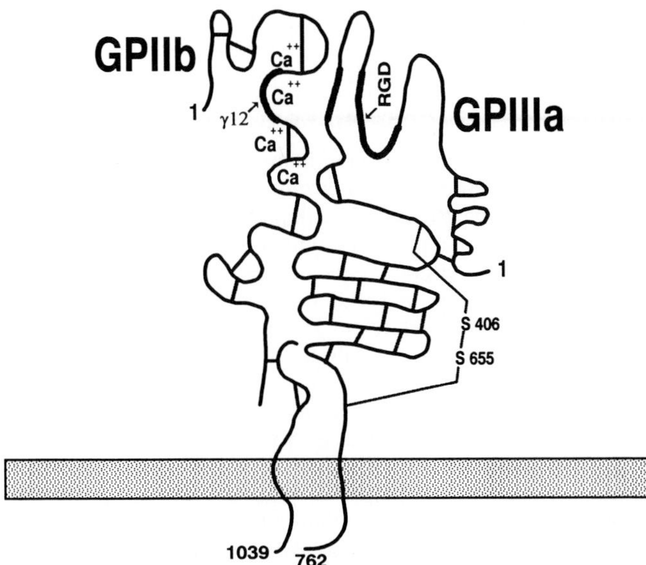

FIG. 110-3 Schematic representation of the major platelet integrin, the GPIIb-IIIa complex ($\alpha_{IIb}\beta_3$). The major features of GPIIIa include the presence of five cysteine-rich regions, including one at the N-terminus, and four cysteine-rich repeats positioned closed to the membrane. Two long-range disulfide bonds (5–435, and 406–655) are depicted, as well as likely sites of interaction with fibrinogen (stippled areas). The four calcium-binding domains of GPIIb are shown, as well as the site on this integrin α subunit that has been shown to bind the γ chain of fibrinogen (H12). RGD = the tripeptide sequence Arg-Gly-Asp.

in both other human integrin β subunits as well as across species. Each cysteine is involved in the formation of disulfide bonds that stabilize the overall three-dimensional structure of the mature glycoprotein complex. Another distinguishing feature of GPIIIa, and presumably other integrin β subunits, is the presence of a large disulfide-bonded loop[39–41] that extends from amino acids Cys_5 to Cys_{435}.[42] At least one critical fibrinogen-binding functional domain of GPIIIa has been localized within this loop[43] (see below). Treatment of intact platelets with the proteolytic enzyme chymotrypsin results in cleavage of GPIIIa at residues 121 and 348,[41] effectively removing approximately half the loop and leaving a nonfunctional 66-kDa fragment associated with the plasma membrane. The 66-kDa remnant is thus composed of two disulfide linked chains—an N-terminal 17-kDa chain containing amino acids 1 to 120 and a larger fragment extending from residues 349 to 762. As will be seen below, immunochemical analyses of such proteolytic fragments have been useful in determining the antigenic epitopes that form the targets of alloimmune antibodies.

In order to understand the molecular nature of inherited disorders associated with GPIIb and GPIIIa, it is necessary first to understand the mechanism by which these two glycoproteins are synthesized, associate to form a complex, and finally are transported through the intercellular organelles of the megakaryocyte before reaching the cell surface. The biosynthetic pathway for the formation of the GPIIb-IIIa complex is illustrated in Fig. 110-4. As shown, both GPIIb and GPIIIa are synthesized in the RER as single-chain precursor molecules that, after a short time, associate to form a pre-GPIIb-IIIa complex. Both proteins are cotranslationally modified with high-mannose carbohydrate moieties, which represent approximately 15 percent of each subunits' molecular mass.[44–46] Following subunit association, the pre-GPIIb-IIIa complex moves to the Golgi apparatus, where a number of posttranslational modifications take place. Pre-GPIIb (1039 amino acids in length) is cleaved at amino acid 859 into a heavy and a light chain[27,47] that remain linked by a disulfide bridge formed by residues Cys_{826} to Cys_{880}.[48] The high-mannose carbohydrate residues of GPIIb, but not GPIIIa, are converted in the Golgi apparatus to complex sugars, as indicated by a change in the susceptibility of GPIIb to endoglycosidase H. There is evidence from endoglycosidase studies that O-linked sugars may be added to the protein backbone of GPIIb as well.[45] Following posttranslational processing, the mature GPIIb-IIIa complex is rapidly transported to the cell surface, where it is maintained in a resting conformation.

There are approximately 60,000 to 80,000 GPIIb-IIIa complexes per platelet.[14,49] Though a substantial proportion (>70 percent) are always present on the platelet surface,[14,50,51] the GPIIb-IIIa complex exists in a resting, nonadhesive state, and as such does not normally interact with its major ligand fibrinogen, despite being bathed in 3 to 4 mg/ml concentrations of this abundant plasma protein. If, however, the platelet becomes activated by thrombin, ADP, thromboxane A_2, or some other agonist, an inside-out signaling event takes place[52–54] that results in the conversion of the complex into an active, adhesive receptor that is now capable of binding its ligand.

It is now recognized that ligands for many integrins contain the tripeptide sequence Arg-Gly-Asp (RGD).[55] Thus, fibrinogen, fibronectin, vWf, and collagen all contain one or more RGD sequences as part of their primary structure.[55–58] Fibrinogen, which is an elongated, cigar-shaped, six-chain molecule composed of two Aα, two Bβ, and two γ chains held together in symmetrical fashion by a centrally located disulfide-dependent knot, contains four such RGD sequences, two on each Aα chain. On conversion of GPIIb-IIIa into the active state, one of the fibrinogen Aα chains binds,[59] presumably through the RGD sequence found at residues 572 to 575.[60] Due to its symmetrical nature, the other fibrinogen Aα chain is free to interact with a GPIIb-IIIa molecule on a nearby platelet, thus serving to bridge the two cells and mediate platelet–platelet cohesion (see Fig. 110-2). Synthetic RGD peptides block fibrinogen binding and platelet aggregation in a competitive fashion,[56,61,62] and

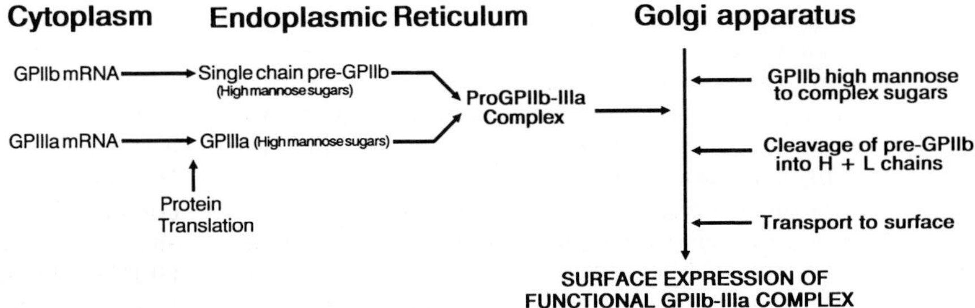

FIG. 110-4 Flow chart of the biosynthetic pathway of the GPIIb-IIIa complex. Each subunit is translated from separate mRNA transcripts into single-chain precursors within the ER of the megakaryocyte, and assembled into a pro-GPIIb-IIIa complex before transport to the golgi. Modification of GPIIb carbohydrate chains and cleavage of GPIIb into heavy and light chains takes place before eventual transport of the now mature complex to the cell surface.

Table 110-3 Sites of Interaction between GPIIb-IIIa and Fibrinogen

Region of the GPIIb-IIIa Complex	Region on Fibrinogen
GPIIIa 109-171	Aα Chain RGD residues 572 to 575
GPIIIa 211-222	Unknown
GPIIb 296-313	γ-Chain residues 400 to 411

photoaffinity-labeled RGD peptides have been shown to interact directly with the GPIIIa subunit at residues 109 to 171,[43] thus defining molecularly at least one mechanism of interaction between the fibrinogen receptor complex and its ligand.

The binding of fibrinogen to GPIIb-IIIa on the platelet surface, however, seems to be multivalent,[59] as fibrinogen is also known to interact with its receptor via a dodecapeptide sequence (labeled γ12 in Fig. 110-3) located at residues 400 to 411 at the C-terminus of its γ chain.[63–65] Like RGD peptides, the γ12 peptide competitively inhibits fibrinogen binding and platelet aggregation,[59,63,66,67] but unlike the RGD sequence, which binds to GPIIIa, the γ12 has been shown to bind to amino acids 296 to 313 of the GPIIb subunit.[68,69] Finally, fibrinogen likely interacts with at least one other region on the GPIIb-IIIa complex, as a small linear synthetic peptide corresponding to GPIIIa amino acids 211 to 222 blocks fibrinogen binding to platelets and the subsequent platelet aggregation response.[70] The three regions on the GPIIb-IIIa complex that interact with fibrinogen that have been defined biochemically, as well as the corresponding site on the fibrinogen molecule, are summarized in Table 110-3.

Molecular Genetic Characterization of Platelet-Specific Defects

Because human platelets are anucleate, they were thought, until 1988, to possess little or no intact mRNA. Consequently, investigators in the field of platelet molecular biology lacked the ability to examine the sequences of platelet-specific mRNA transcripts and identify the molecular origins of clinically and scientifically important inherited platelet disorders. The advent of the PCR in 1985,[71] technical improvements in the PCR reaction in 1987 and 1988,[72,73] and finally the discovery that human platelets contained sufficient levels of intact mRNA that can be enzymatically converted into cDNA and then PCR-amplified,[74] together served to open up the field of platelet molecular biology. As a result, it became possible for the first time to determine rapidly the mRNA sequences of specific platelet membrane glycoproteins from a large number of individuals without the need for cloning or constructing multiple libraries. Using the technique of platelet RNA PCR, a number of laboratories began to determine the cDNA sequences of normal platelet proteins and compare them with those derived from individuals with a wide variety of inherited platelet disorders. In this manner, many of the molecular genetic defects responsible for such diseases as Glanzmann thrombasthenia, Bernard-Soulier syndrome, von Willebrand disease, and the alloimmune thrombocytopenias have been elucidated, and our ability to diagnose these disorders, both prenatally and postnatally, has become a reality in an extremely short time. Much of the remainder of this chapter will describe our current understanding of the molecular biologic basis of inherited platelet defects, and describe lessons learned from these findings.

Glanzmann Thrombasthenia

In 1918, an Swiss pediatrician named Glanzmann described a somewhat heterogeneous group of disorders, which he termed "thrombasthenie" ("weak platelets"), that were characterized by normal platelet counts but abnormal clot retraction.[75] Braunsteiner and Pakesch added to our understanding of what is now termed "Glanzmann thrombasthenia" by noting in 1956 that platelets from these patients failed to spread onto a surface,[76] while the laboratories of Hardisty[77] and Zucker[78] first described the failure of thrombasthenic platelets to stick to each other (aggregate). The disease Glanzmann thrombasthenia is now known to be a rare, inherited, autosomal recessive bleeding disorder, the hallmark of which is the failure of platelets to bind fibrinogen and aggregate following stimulation by physiological agonists such as ADP, thrombin, epinephrine, or collagen. Underlying this disorder is an abnormality of the genes encoding GPIIb or GPIIIa.

Clinical Features. Glanzmann thrombasthenia (GT) is a lifelong disease characterized by often unpredictable mucocutaneous bleeding; it is usually noticed at an early age. Thus, epistaxis, gingival bleeding, and purpura at sites of excessive pressure or minor trauma are the most common features. Menorrhagia is a critical problem in teenage girls and younger women, when bleeding during menstruation is more likely to be severe.[79] Bleeding that normally accompanies pregnancy, surgical procedures, tooth extractions, or physical trauma can be excessive in GT patients, though the severity of hemorrhage is not predictable, even in defined subtypes of the disease (see below). Severe unprovoked intracranial or gastrointestinal hemorrhages, though reported in several GT patients, are rare but sometimes fatal occurrences. Spontaneous joint bleeding or visceral hematomas characteristic of coagulation protein disorders have not been observed in thrombasthenia.[79]

Incidence. Though GT is a rare disorder, there is an unusually high incidence of this disease among certain geographically restricted population clusters in which intermarriage or consanguinity are commonplace. Thus, in spite of its infrequent occurrence worldwide, a high carrier rate for thrombasthenia exists among Iraqi Jews,[80–82] selected Arab populations,[81–83] French gypsies,[84–86] and individuals from southern India.[87] Due to the low frequency of abnormal GPIIb or GPIIIa genes in the overall human gene pool, and the recessive nature of the disease, GT is not often found to occur spontaneously, and a large proportion of the remaining GT patients are the progeny of marriages between first or second cousins.

Classification and Laboratory Diagnosis. Despite several attempts to categorize Glanzmann thrombasthenia into subtypes, it will become apparent from the studies discussed below that there are almost as many molecular biologic etiologies of thrombasthenia as there are patient populations carrying the disease. In 1972, Caen proposed the first classification of this disease based on platelet intracellular fibrinogen content and the ability of platelets to retract a fibrin clot.[88] Type I patients, representing 80 percent of those studied, lacked platelet fibrinogen and had absent clot retraction, whereas type II thrombasthenic platelets contained appreciable levels of platelet fibrinogen and maintained some clot retraction capability. Soon thereafter, the technique of SDS-PAGE became widespread, and Nurden and Caen used this method to detect an abnormal "glycoprotein II" pattern in three cases of GT.[89,90] Phillips and Agin used two-dimensional SDS-PAGE analysis of radiolabeled platelets to show convincingly that both glycoproteins IIb and IIIa were specifically decreased in GT versus normal platelets.[91] Several laboratories made the observation that whereas type I patients lacked detectable levels of GPIIb-IIIa, type II GT platelets expressed moderate (15 to 25 percent) levels of this glycoprotein, as measured using immunochemical[92–94] and electrophoretic[95] techniques. So-called variant forms of thrombasthenia have also been described with increasing frequency, and are characterized by having normal to near-normal levels of a dysfunctional form of GPIIb-IIIa present on the cell surface.[96–99] It is important to note that platelets from these patients are functionally indistinguishable from type I and II platelets in that laboratory diagnosis for all three GT subgroups have in common the complete failure to aggregate in response to physiological agonists such as ADP, thrombin, or epinephrine, as illustrated in Fig. 110-5. Failure to bind fibrinogen,[100] vWf,[101] and other adhesive ligands, normally mediated by the GPIIb-IIIa complex, is responsible for the inability of platelets to cohere.

As the genetic defects underlying the thrombasthenic phenotype have become defined at a molecular level, the rationale for maintaining these three traditional categories of GT becomes less convincing, and alternatively, more complicated classifications based on surface expression or on the fate of GPIIb and GPIIIa subunits as they traffic through the cell to reach the plasma membrane,[102] have been proposed. None of these are entirely satisfying, as biologic exceptions to each seem to appear as readily as classification schemes are devised. Furthermore, no correlation exists between any of the proposed subtypes of GT and the severity of bleeding symptoms in patients.[79] Some patients with absolutely no GPIIb-IIIa have relatively mild clinical symptoms, while others with a full complement of GPIIb-IIIa, albeit dysfunctional, can have frequent bleeding episodes requiring multiple platelet transfusions. Nonetheless, even in the absence of predictive value, it remains instructive for both clinical diagnosis and research purposes to determine the level of GPIIb-IIIa complex surface expression in GT patients soon after clinical laboratory findings allow a diagnosis of thrombasthenia using the criterion of absent platelet aggregation response.

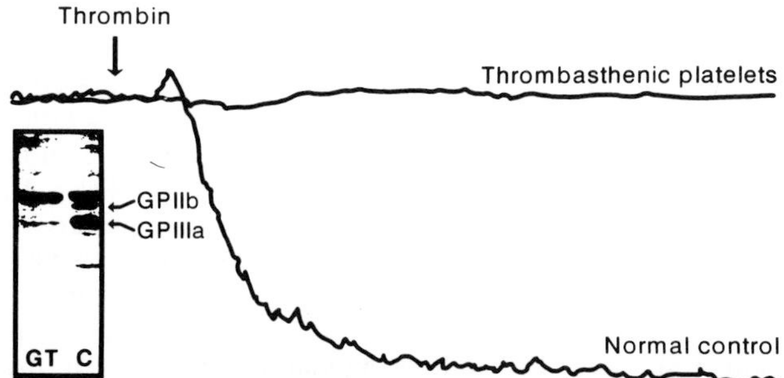

FIG. 110-5 **Typical platelet aggregation profiles of normal versus Glanzmann thrombasthenic (GT) individuals. Whereas normal platelets aggregate readily when exposed to thrombin or other agonists, platelets from a patient with thrombasthenia fail to respond.** ***Inset:*** **Immunoblot of detergent lysates from normal control (C) and GT platelets. Rabbit polyclonal antibodies specific for GPIIb, GPIIIa, and PECAM-1 (top band) were exposed to Immobilon strips containing 100 μg each of a platelet lysate, and developed with an alkaline phosphatase–conjugated second antibody. Platelets from the GT patient shown express less than 5 percent of normal GPIIIa levels, and no GPIIb can be detected, typical of a GPIIb genetic defect.**

Currently, the most common methods used for determining the levels of GPIIb-IIIa on GT patient platelets are flow cytometry[103] and western blot (immunoblot) analysis,[104] each of which offer the advantage of increased sensitivity over previously used crossed immunoelectrophoretic[93,94] or radiolabeled monoclonal antibody binding techniques.[49,105,106] An immunoblot illustrating GPIIb-IIIa content of both a normal control and typical type I GT patient platelet lysate is shown in the inset to Fig. 110-5, and demonstrates the severe deficiency of GPIIb-IIIa in this patient. In patients with less than 5 percent of the normal GPIIb-IIIa content, a trace of even one of the two integrin subunits can be instructive as to the nature of the molecular defect.[107] In the example shown, a trace amount of GPIIIa is apparent, while there is no detectable GPIIb. This patient was later found to have a large deletion in the GPIIb gene (see below), consistent with the immunoblot analysis. Since it is known that GPIIIa does not survive intracellular trafficking in the absence of an integrin α subunit, it is presumed that a small number of GPIIIa molecules expressed on the platelet surface were "rescued" by virtue of their ability for form a complex with the VNR α subunit (see the sections on "The Integrins" and "Biology of GPIIb-IIIa" above). One group has used VNR expression as a reliable indicator of GPIIb versus GPIIIa genetic defects, and has found, somewhat surprisingly, that in the absence of GPIIb synthesis, VNR expression on the platelet surface is actually increased from the normal 50 to 100 molecules up to 150 to 200 VNR molecules.[18] The increase was attributed to the lack of competition among α subunits for β_3 (GPIIIa). Defects in the gene encoding GPIIIa, on the other hand, resulted in lack of expression of both the $\alpha_{IIb}\beta_3$ as well as $\alpha_v\beta_3$, as would be expected of two integrin receptors sharing a common defective subunit.

Molecular Abnormalities of GPIIb and GPIIIa Genes Resulting in Glanzmann Thrombasthenia. Though nearly 200 individuals with GT have been described in the literature, to date only 12 of these have been solved at the molecular level. As in most genetic disorders, the molecular abnormalities have been found to range from major deletions and inversions easily detectable by Southern blot analysis[108,109] to single point mutations identified only by nucleotide sequence analysis of platelet mRNA-derived PCR products.[110–114] The locations of the mutations resulting in the Glanzmann phenotype have shown no preference for either GPIIb or GPIIIa, with seven mutations so far having been localized to the GPIIIa gene and five to GPIIb. In vitro studies have indicated that production of both protein subunits is required for proper surface expression and function,[115] and this concept has been nicely corroborated at the level of human biology through the molecular biologic analysis of GT defects. Not surprisingly, the nature of the molecular defect is often related to the level of GPIIb-IIIa complex surface expression, with a few notable exceptions. Thus, in the two individuals thus far reported with major deletions in either the GPIIb (patient KW[108]) or GPIIIa (patient GT3[109,116]) genes, the corresponding mRNA transcript is altered such that its corresponding subunit is either translated into nascent partial proteins, or not translated at all, resulting in a classical type I phenotype (<5 percent levels of GPIIb-IIIa). Thus, the major abnormalities in these two patients are best categorized as tran-

Table 110-4 Summary of Molecular Abnormalities Causing Glanzmann Thrombasthenia

Patient	Molecular Defect	Biochemical Defect	% Surface Expression	Reference
GT3	GPIIIa gene inversion deletion	Transcriptional	<5	109, 116
I-J	GPIIIa—13-bp deletion/stop codon at AA 654	Truncated, unstable GPIIIa subunit	<5	117
SH	GPIIIa—$Arg_{216} \rightarrow$ Gln	Complex maturation, ligand binding	20–30	Unpublished
Paris 1	GPIIIa—$Ser_{752} \rightarrow$ Pro	Receptor activation	50	53
ET	GPIIIa—$Arg_{214} \rightarrow$ Gln	Ligand binding, complex stability	100	111
Stras 1	GPIIIa—$Arg_{214} \rightarrow$ Trp	Ligand binding, complex stability	100	112
CAM	GPIIIa—Asp_{119}Tyr	Ligand binding	100	110
KW	GPIIb—4-kb gene deletion	Transcriptional	<5	108
Arab	GPIIb—Δ amino acids 106 to 111	Unstable GPIIb subunit	<5	117
FLD	GPIIb—$Gly_{273} \rightarrow$ Asp	Complex maturation, Ca^{2+} binding?	<5	113
LM	GPIIb—$Gly_{418} \rightarrow$ Asp	Complex maturation, Ca^{2+} binding?	<5	114
KJ	GPIIb—$Arg_{327} \rightarrow$ His	Complex maturation	10–20	Unpublished

*Abbreviations explained in text.

scriptional in nature, and are indicated as such in Table 110-4, which summarizes the known molecular abnormalities underlying GT.

Smaller gene deletions characterize the Iraqi-Jewish and Arab thrombasthenia populations living in Israel[117] (referred to as I-J and Arab in Table 110-4), but both result in the translation of unstable integrin subunits and undetectable levels of GPIIb-IIIa expression on the platelet surface. In I-J thrombasthenia, an 11-base deletion in exon 12 of the GPIIIa gene produces a frameshift leading to protein termination at amino acid 654, shortly before the polypeptide chain would enter the lipid bilayer of the plasma membrane. As shown in Fig. 110-3, amino acid Cys_{655}, missing in the I-J GPIIIa molecule, normally participates in the formation of a long-range disulfide bond with Cys_{405},[42] and its absence likely leads to a failure to stabilize this integrin β_3-subunit.

Though many Arab thrombasthenic patients presently live in the same small country as the I-J population, this was not historically true 2000 to 3000 years ago, when the mutational events are thought to have taken place, and Arab thrombasthenia, though clinically indistinguishable, is in fact unrelated in molecular etiology to its I-J counterpart. In three of five kindreds examined, Arab thrombasthenia was found to be caused by a 13-base deletion encompassing the splice acceptor site of exon 4 of the GPIIb gene.[117] This deletion leads to forced alternative splicing to a downstream AG acceptor site, and results in a six amino acid deletion in the GPIIb polypeptide chain, including a single cysteine residue. Again, the loss of a cysteine that normally participates in disulfide-bond formation is thought to be a destabilizing event, and it is likely that complex formation with GPIIIa and subsequent intracellular trafficking are impaired sufficiently to produce the observed severe lack of surface expression of the GPIIb-IIIa complex.

I-J thrombasthenia has a carrier frequency of one in 44 of the approximately 270,000 Iraqi Jews living in Israel (i.e., the gene frequency of the abnormal allele is approximately 2.3 percent in this population).[82] Israeli Arabs also have a high prevalence of this disease, with more than 13 patients from five kindreds thus far identified. Fortunately, elucidation of the molecular genetic defects in each of these relatively large, "at-risk" populations has made possible the development of rapid DNA-based diagnostic assays,[117,118] and opportunities for genetic counseling and family planning are now becoming readily available to suspected carriers of the abnormal GPIIb or GPIIIa genes.

A number of patients with point mutations in either GPIIb or GPIIIa genes leading to defects in the maturation of the GPIIb-IIIa complex have been identified. Depending on the location of the mutation, the blockade can take place at the level of subunit association in the ER (complex formation), sorting to the Golgi apparatus, or trafficking to the cell surface (see Fig. 110-3). In fact, examples for all of these scenarios seem to have been found, and each is characterized by absent to reduced levels of GPIIb-IIIa on the cell surface, though significant intracellular pools of the affected subunit can be recovered in transfection/immunoprecipitation studies of recombinant forms of the mutated subunit. In patients FLD (GPIIb $Gly_{273} \rightarrow$ Asp[113]) and LM (GPIIb $Gly_{418} \rightarrow$ Asp[114]) (see Table 110-4), mutations in the first and fourth calcium-binding domains of GPIIb, respectively, likely lead to improperly folded pre-GPIIb subunits that are stable, but unable to assemble with GPIIIa properly. At least in the case of LM, the abnormal complex has been shown to accumulate within the ER. Thus, LM platelets do not express GPIIb-IIIa on their surface, as illustrated in the representative flow cytometric profiles shown in Fig. 110-6. The defects in patients SH (GPIIIa $Arg_{216} \rightarrow$ Gln) and KJ (GpIIb $Arg_{327} \rightarrow$ His) differ somewhat from LM and FLD in that moderate amounts of their abnormal GPIIb-IIIa complex actually reach the cell surface (see Fig. 110-6). This group of GT patients can best be categorized as having maturational defects in the GPIIb-IIIa complex, as suggested by the decreased to absent levels that reach the cell surface, and by the inability of the residual surface receptor to bind fibrinogen or fibrinogen mimetics. Failure of complex-, but not subunit-specific monoclonal antibodies to bind to residual pools of abnormal subunits that accumulate intracellularly may also be a common feature.

The final group of thrombasthenic defects is characterized

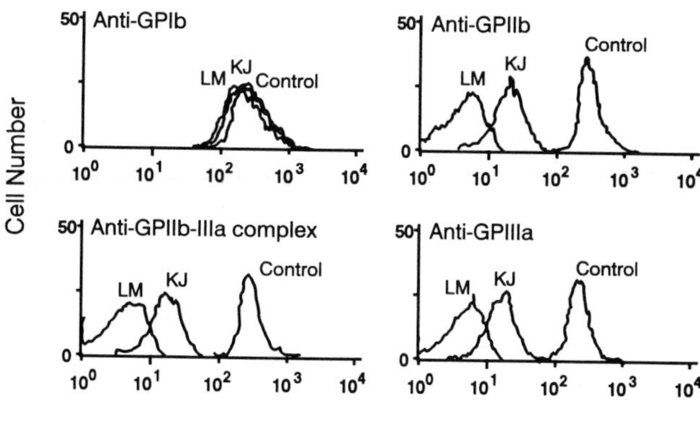

FIG. 110-6 Flow cytometric profile of two patients with GT as compared with a normal control individual. Both patients KJ and LM have mutations that affect the maturation of the GPIIb-IIIa complex, but differ in that the mutation in patient LM is within the calcium-binding domain of GPIIb and perturbs maturation such that no part of the complex is able to traffic to the cell surface. The nature of the mutation in KJ is such that 20 to 30 percent levels of GPIIb-IIIa are expressed, but fail to function normally.

by significant levels of GPIIb-IIIa surface expression, though the complex is not able to interact with fibrinogen or other physiological ligands. In contrast to the platelets of patients having integrin maturational defects, the binding of many GPIIb-IIIa complex-specific antibodies are normal in this group, indicating that subunit association and intracellular trafficking are largely unaffected by the nature of the mutation. That the GPIIb-IIIa complex is not normal is indicated by the fact that divalent-cation dependent regulation of its conformation can be affected (patient CAM, GPIIIa $Asp_{119} \rightarrow Tyr$[110]) and the complex may be easily dissociable by chelation of external calcium ions with EDTA. Examples of thrombasthenic patients with complex stability/ligand binding defects include ET (GPIIIa $Arg_{214} \rightarrow Gln$[111]), patient Stras I (GPIIIa $Arg_{214} \rightarrow Trp$[112]), and patient CM,[98] who has not been characterized at the molecular biologic level. Finally, the Paris I variant of GT (GPIIIa $Ser_{752} \rightarrow Pro$[53,97]) represents a particularly interesting example of an integrin that may be defective in inside-out signal transduction, in that a point mutation within the cytoplasmic tail of GPIIIa prevents the GPIIb-IIIa complex from transforming from an inactive to an active conformation. Classification of Glanzmann thrombasthenia subtypes by the biochemical consequences of their molecular genetic abnormality is shown in Table 110-5.

INHERITED DISORDERS OF THE PLATELET GPIb COMPLEX

Biology of the GPIb Complex

One of the initial events that occurs when circulating platelets come into contact with the arterial subendothelium at a site of injury is adhesion to vWf molecules that have themselves become insolubilized onto the subendothelial matrix.[1,119] This process is especially important in arterioles and in the microcirculation, where high shear rates are present.[1,120–122] Following this initial adhesion event, additional platelets aggregate to the site of injury, forming the platelet plug.[123–125]

Platelet membranes contain two binding sites for vWf.[126] One of these sites requires prior platelet activation, and is located on the platelet membrane GPIIb-IIIa complex.[126] The second binding site involves the GPIb complex, and it is this membrane complex that is crucial for initial attachment and proper adhesion to the extracellular matrix of a damaged vessel wall[127,128] (see Fig. 110-2). The GPIb complex repre-

Table 110-5 Classification of Glanzmann Thrombasthenia Subtypes by Biochemical Consequence of the Molecular Genetic Abnormality

Defect (Examples)	Characteristics	mRNA	Subunit Synthesis	Surface Expression
Transcriptional (KW, GT3)	Major gene deletions, insertions, or rearrangements	−/+	—	—
Subunit stability (I-J, Arab)	Small deletions or insertions leading to a change in the number of amino acids, or substitution to a destabilizing amino acid. Binding of GPIIb-IIIa complex–specific antibodies and at least one subunit-specific antibody, even to intracellular pools are absent.	+	Absent to reduced	—
Complex maturation (LM, FLD, KJ, SH)	Point mutations affecting Ca^{2+}-binding, subunit association, etc. that affect intracellular trafficking and surface expression. Binding of complex-specific antibodies is often affected, though subunit-specific antibodies bind to intracellular forms.	+	Near normal	Absent to reduced
Ligand Binding A. Complex stability (CAM, ET, Stras I) B. Activatability (Paris I)	Normal to somewhat reduced levels of GPIIb-IIIa complex on the platelet surface, though it fails to bind ligands. Often easily dissociable with EDTA. Binding of many subunit- and complex-specific molecular abnormalities and normal.	+	Normal to mildly reduced	Normal to mildly reduced

sents the second most common receptor on the platelet membrane surface, with ~25,000 copies per platelet.[129] As shown in Fig. 110-7, the GPIb complex actually consists of four different proteins. $GPIb_\alpha$ is the largest subunit (143 kDa), and is susceptible to cleavage by trypsin or by the calcium-dependent platelet protease, calpain, giving rise to a water-soluble, heavily glycosylated 135-kDa N-terminal fragment known as "glycocalicin."[130,131] In addition to containing the binding site for vWf, the glycocalicin portion of $GPIb_\alpha$ may also contain a binding site for thrombin.[132–136] The biologic role of the thrombin-binding site is unclear, since enzymatic cleavage of the GPIb complex, while leading to a loss of vWf-mediated platelet agglutination, does not significantly affect the ability of platelets to respond to thrombin.[137,138] These data may be explained by the cloning of a unique seven-membrane-spanning functional thrombin receptor found on several cells of the vasculature, including the platelet surface.[139]

$GPIb_\alpha$ is disulfide-bonded to the 23-kDa $GPIb_\beta$ polypeptide chain,[3,140,141] through a single cysteine residue located in each subunit near the transmembrane domains of $GPIb_\alpha$ and $GPIb_\beta$. These two proteins are, in turn, noncovalently associated with platelet glycoproteins V and IX.[4,140] GPV is a transmembrane protein that is susceptible to digestion by calpain, and in addition is the only known proteolytic substrate for thrombin on the platelet surface, releasing a 69-kDa soluble fragment.[2,142,143] GPIX is the smallest member of the GPIb complex, with a molecular mass of only 17 kDa.[144,145]

The genes encoding the subunits of the GPIb complex are widely dispersed in the human genome. $GPIb_\alpha$ is on the short arm of chromosome 17,[5] while the gene for GPIX is on chromosome 3.[146] The $GPIb_\alpha$ gene has been shown to consist of only two exons, one containing the 5′-untranslated region and the other containing the remainder of the coding region.[5,147] Like the GPIIb gene, this gene also does not have a TATA or CAAT-gene promoter in its 5′-flanking region.[5,147]

The cDNA for $GPIb_\alpha$, $GPIb_\beta$, and GPIX have been characterized, and encode mature proteins of 610, 181, and 160 amino acids, respectively.[144–146,148–150] All three proteins have an N-terminal signal peptide and a hydrophobic transmembrane domain near the C-terminus. The three proteins also share an interesting structural element known as the leucine-rich domain (LRD), which is comprised of a 24 amino acid motif that contains seven conserved leucine positions. There is one such domain in the extracytoplasmic domains of $GPIb_\beta$ and GPIX, and 7 LRD in $GPIb_\alpha$. While the primary structure of GPV is not known in its entirety, it appears to contain at least one LRD motif.[2,151] Other proteins have been described with this leucine-rich repeat, but the biologic significance of this structure is unknown, as the proteins have disparate functions such as a photoreceptor (chaoptin),[152] a hormone receptor (lutropin-choriogonadotropin receptor),[153] and adenylate cyclase.[154] In addition, these repeats have some similarity with the DNA-binding leucine zipper proteins.[155–157]

All four chains of the GPIb complex are glycosylated. $GPIb_\alpha$ has four *N*-glycosylation sites, while $GPIb_\beta$ and GPIX each have a single *N*-glycosylation site. In $GPIb_\alpha$, O-linked carbohydrates are associated with a series of five nine-amino-acid repeats in a region of glycocalicin that is heavily glycosylated.[158] Thus, members of the GPIb complex contain carbohydrate moieties ending with sialic acid residues, contributing significantly to the negative charge of the platelet surface.[132]

In between the LRD and the O-linked glycosylation sites of $GPIb_\alpha$ is a region from amino acid residues 220 to 310 that contains the vWf and thrombin-binding regions. Studies with peptide inhibitors suggest that amino acids 269 to 301 contain two charged domains that represent the major binding site for vWf.[159,160] In vivo, plasma vWf does not bind to the GPIb complex, and it is likely that changes in vWf conformation occur once it has bound to components of the subendothelium that enable it to then interact with its platelet receptor. In vitro, the antibiotic ristocetin is used to mimic this effect, and similarly induces conformational changes in vWf that promote binding to GPIb in stirred platelet-rich plasma.[161]

Studies utilizing proteolytic fragments of vWf have localized the GPIb binding domain to vWf residues 480 to 718.[162,163] Studies of patients with type IIB von Willebrand disease (vWD), in which vWf multimers have increased affinity for nonactivated platelets, have further defined a small disulfide loop in vWf between Cys^{509} and Cys^{695} that is necessary for GPIb binding. Multiple mutations in this loop in patients with type IIB vWD have been defined at the molecular level,

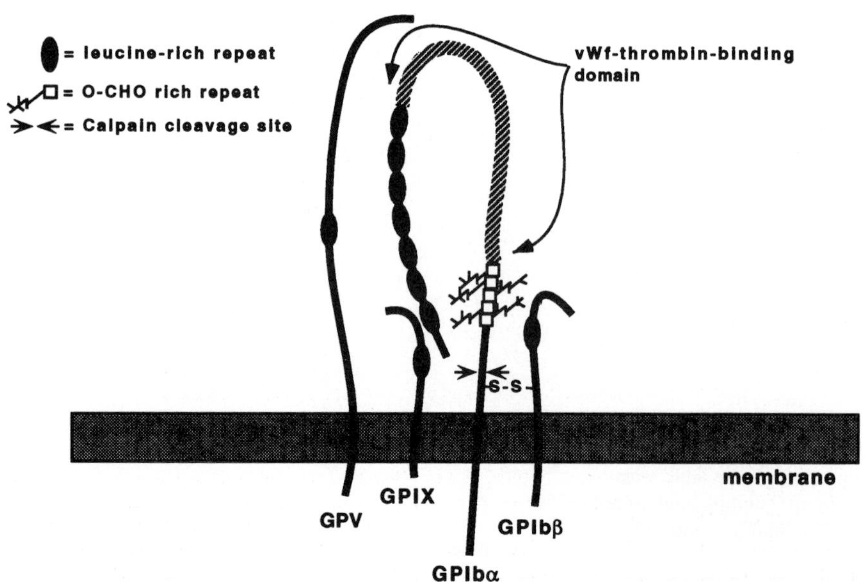

FIG. 110-7 The GPIb complex on platelets consist of four separately encoded proteins: GPIbα, GPIbβ, GPV, and GPIX. Some of the structural features found in this receptor complex are depicted, including the leucine-rich repeats found in each protein, the O-linked carbohydrate-rich region of GPIbα, the calpain cleavage site in GPIbα, the disulfide bond linking GPIbα and GPIbβ, and the thrombin- and vWf-binding domain of GPIbα.

and each appears to be capable of increasing the affinity of vWf for the platelet surface.[163–170] It will become important to distinguish the increased vWf–GPIb interactions seen in this disorder with an inherited disorder of $GPIb_\alpha$, known as platelet-type or pseudo-vWD, which will be discussed below.

Binding of vWf/ristocetin or vWf/collagen to the GPIb complex is itself an activating event (see Fig. 110-1), and operates through an arachidonic acid metabolite–dependent activation of phospholipase C. This signal results in the mobilization of protein kinase C, which together with increases in $(Ca^{2+})_i$ promotes platelet secretion and potentiates platelet aggregation.[171,172] Whether the GPIb complex directly transduces the signal into the platelet or works through an associated coupling protein is unknown. In this regard it is interesting to note that the GPIb complex can become phosphorylated on the cytoplasmic tail of the GPIbβ subunit,[173,174] and the complex exists in its resting state linked to the actin cytoskeleton through a direct linkage to actin binding protein.[175,176] As will be noted below, this linkage to the platelet cytoskeleton may be important for maintaining platelet size and shape.[177]

Bernard-Soulier Syndrome

Bernard-Soulier syndrome (BSS) was first described in 1948 in a 5-month-old infant with a prolonged bleeding time, giant platelets on blood smear, and a sib who had died from hemorrhage at the age of 3 years.[178] Over the following years, additional patients with the combination of mucocutaneous bleeding; enlarged platelets; normal platelet aggregation with ADP, collagen, and epinephrine with a delayed response to thrombin; and absent platelet aggregation with human vWf with ristocetin or with bovine vWf alone were described as having Bernard-Soulier syndrome.[6,179–196] This syndrome represents the second most recognized inherited platelet disorder.

Clinical Features. The bleeding manifestations of these patients are similar to other patients with platelet dysfunctions and center on mucocutaneous bleeding with purpuric skin bleeding epistaxis, gastrointestinal hemmorhage, and menorrhagia.[197] Alloantibodies to components of the GPIb complex can develop following platelet transfusions, and thereby secondary complications from their refractoriness to platelet therapy develop.[198,199] In addition to local forms of therapy such as proper pressure and topical thrombin, platelet transfusion therapy, and hormonal management of menses, there have been several reports that have suggested that the synthetic vasopressin homologue DDAVP (1-deamino-8-D-arginine vasopressin) may be useful in the treatment of a number of inherited bleeding disorders such as BSS.[195,200–202] These studies have demonstrated improved bleeding times in these patients following DDAVP therapy, although the improvement did not correlate with the ability of the DDAVP to increase the levels of circulating vWf.

Incidence. BSS is an autosomal recessive disorder in which most patients have a decrease to absence of all four members of the GPIb complex—$GPIb_\alpha$, $GPIb_\beta$, GPIX, and GPV.[203,204] In 1969, platelets from these patients were shown to have an altered electrophoretic mobility and sialic acid content,[181] and in 1975 membrane protein fractionation of platelets by SDS-PAGE demonstrated a marked decrease in a major 155-kDa glycoprotein, then termed "GPI," in these patients.[90,189] Since that time, further refinements in protein analysis have demonstrated a variable decrease, ranging from the GPIb complex being almost fully present to being virtually absent in homozygous patients.[6,190–194]

Classification and Laboratory Diagnosis. Laboratory evaluation of BSS patients demonstrates a variable degree of thrombocytopenia. Most patients are thrombocytopenic to some degree, but some patients may have platelet counts as low as 20,000/μl.[182,184,185,190] The platelets tend to be increased in size, with a mean diameter ranging from 3 to 20 times normal[190] (Figure 110-8). Other cell types appear normal. As mentioned below in the section on "Platelet Size and Production Disorders," the circulating total platelet mass is more precisely conserved than is platelet count,[205,206] and part of the decrease in platelet count in this disease may well reflect this compensation mechanism. Megakaryocytes in this disorder appear normal in size and appearance by light microscopic examination. However, on electron microscopy, a striking feature in these cells is the variable and intermittent nature of the demarcation system, which is often vacuolar.[207] The relationship between this structural feature in the megakaryocyte and the giant platelet is not understood. It is believed that the absence of interactions between the GPIb complex and the platelet cytoskeleton underlies both the morphologic abnormality seen in the megakaryocyte and the size of the platelets.

Bleeding times are prolonged in these patients, but the distinctive abnormality of BSS platelets is the failure of agglutination in the presence of ristocetin, an abnormality that cannot be corrected by the addition of normal plasma.[184] Aggregation by other agonists such as ADP, collagen, and epinephrine are normal, though the response to low-dose thrombin may be delayed.[184,187,190]

Molecular Abnormalities. Only a small number of patients have had the responsible defect defined on a molecular level. The first described mutation was found within the coding sequence of the $GPIb_\alpha$ gene,[208] in which a TGG → TGA mutation resulted in the conversion of Trp_{343} → stop codon. The resulting $GPIb_\alpha$ chain lacks a portion of the extracellular

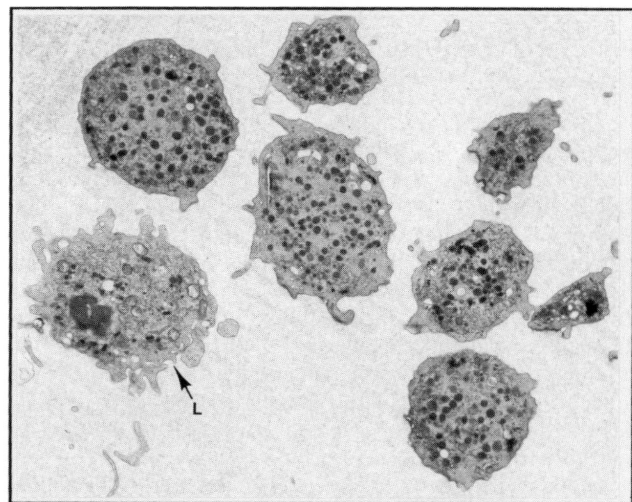

FIG. 110-8 **Thin-section electron micrograph of platelets from a patient with BSS. Whereas normal platelets are 1 to 2 μm in diameter, several of the BSS platelets in this section are the same size as a lymphocyte (L) (8 to 10 μm). Aside from their increased size, the morphology of BSS platelets is comparable to that of normal platelets. Magnification ×5000. (*Electron micrographs generously provided by Dr. James G. White, University of Minnesota.*)**

domain and the entire transmembrane and cytoplasmic domains, providing a likely explanation for the absence of GPIb complex expression on the platelet surface.

Two previously described dominant variants of BSS have been defined in which surface expression of the GPIb complex is approximately 50 percent of normal.[193,209,210] In two cases, point mutations within the leucine-rich repeat region of $GPIb_{\alpha}$ were found to be associated with the defect.[211] In the Balzano variant, an $Ala_{156} \rightarrow$ Val substitution within the leucine-rich repeat domain of $GPIb_{\alpha}$ was identified and was shown to be responsible for the defect in that a recombinant $GPIb_{\alpha}$ protein containing this substitution, when reconstituted into an otherwise normal GPIb complex, was shown to have impaired binding to vWf. In an American variant, a $Leu_{57} \rightarrow$ Phe mutation was found.[210] It is of interest that the American variant mutation occurs in one of the highly conserved leucine residues, whereas the Balzano mutation is positioned within a nonconserved position.[1] Both variants have in common an abnormally small $GPIb_{\alpha}$ protein, and the mutations may lead to increased susceptibility of the N-terminus of the GPIbα chain to cleavage. A monoclonal antibody AS-7, which is directed to the N-terminus of GPIbα, binds to GPIbα of normal platelets but does not bind to the faster-migrating band in the American variant.

Not all BSS patients have defects in $GPIb_{\alpha}$. Transient expression studies of $GPIb_{\alpha}$, GPI_{β}, and GPIX cDNA into Chinese hamster ovary cells have demonstrated that all three of these glycoproteins are necessary to reconstitute a functional binding receptor.[212] In a patient with marked absence of the platelet GPIb complex, restriction polymorphism analysis of one family demonstrated discordance between the inheritance of a $GPIb_{\alpha}$ *Taq*I RFLP and the Bernard-Soulier phenotype.[213] Given the fact that at least $GPIb_{\alpha}$, $GPIb_{\beta}$, GPIX, and perhaps GPV are necessary for complex formation, and that the genes for these proteins are widely dispersed in the human genome, it is not surprising that a classic form of BSS may occur not linked to the $GPIb_{\alpha}$ gene. It is likely that, like the GPIIb-IIIa complex described above, all the subunits comprising the GPIb complex may need to be normally synthesized to achieve complex stability and proper trafficking to the cell surface.[212]

Platelet-Type (Pseudo-) von Willebrand Disease

Platelet-type vWD is an autosomal dominant bleeding disorder often associated with a prolonged bleeding time, mild thrombocytopenia, and decreased circulating levels of high-molecular-weight vWf multimers.[214–217] The patients with this disorder have a mild-to-moderate bleeding diathesis. Platelet-type vWD is very similar to type IIB vWD in that both are characterized by platelet agglutination in the presence of lower than normal concentrations of ristocetin, and by decreased circulating levels of high-molecular-weight vWf. Binding of vWf to the circulating platelet pool results in the reduced levels of circulating levels of vWf seen in these patients, as well as some degree of platelet activation and mild thrombocytopenia.

Unlike type IIB vWD, where mutations in vWf result in increased affinity for normal platelet GPIb, pseudo-vWD is caused by an alteration in the platelet GPIb receptor that leads to increased affinity for normal vWf multimers. Thus, platelet-type vWD can be distinguished with some difficulty from type IIB vWD by addition of normal vWf to patient platelet-rich plasma, which results in spontaneous aggregation of pseudo-vWD, but not type IIB vWD, platelets.[215,216,218] It is important to distinguish patients with platelet-type vWD from other vWD patients, as the standard form of therapy for vWD involves infusion of cryoprecipitate or DDAVP and can lead to severe thrombocytopenia in these patients.[218,219] A patient with mild thrombocytopenia and a prolonged bleeding time should be evaluated for this disorder as described above, and if it is found, treatment should be limited to low-dose cryoprecipitate.[220,221]

The molecular basis of platelet-type vWd has been defined in two patients.[222,223] Both mutations occur in the region of $GPIb_{\alpha}$ that has been previously shown to be important in vWf binding.[159,160] These mutations are a $Gly_{233} \rightarrow$ Val and $Met_{239} \rightarrow$ Val. It is hypothesized that these mutations alter $GPIb_{\alpha}$ such that it is maintained in an adhesive conformation. Further examination of mutations in this region of GPIb may provide important insights on how this receptor becomes activated on exposure to components of the extracellular matrix at sites of vascular injury.

OTHER PLATELET MEMBRANE GLYCOPROTEIN DEFECTS

The integrin $\alpha_2\beta_1$ (platelet GPIa-IIa) is a heterodimer complex that, like GPIIb-IIIa, is held together by noncovalent, divalent cation–dependent interactions.[224] In platelets and other cell types $\alpha_2\beta_1$ serves as a receptor for collagen[20,21,225] and functions in mediating platelet–extracellular matrix interactions as well as cellular activation events, since adherence to fibrillar collagen causes platelets to change their shape rapidly, secrete the contents of their granules, and transform surface receptors into an adhesive phenotype (see Fig. 110-1). The physiological and clinical significance of $\alpha_2\beta_1$ was underscored by the discovery that human platelets from a patient with a long bleeding time, normal platelet count, and normal aggregation response to thrombin, ADP, and epinephrine fail to aggregate in response to collagen, and have a parallel absence of GPIa (α_2) on the platelet surface.[226] A defect in platelet spreading on collagen-coated surfaces has also been associated with α_2 defects.[226,227]

Platelet GPIV, also known as the CD36 differentiation antigen, is an 88-kDa transmembrane glycoprotein found in a wide variety of cells types, including platelets, endothelial cells, erythrocytes, and melanoma cells.[228] GPIV is a multifunctional protein that has been implicated in mediating platelet adherence to collagen[229] and thrombospondin[203] and also serves as a receptor on endothelial cells, monocytes, and platelets for the binding of *Plasmodium falciparum*–infected erythrocytes.[231–233] Several years ago, a population of healthy Japanese individuals, known as Nak^a-negative,[234] was identified, and its members were shown to lack expression of GPIV on their platelets.[235] Interestingly, platelets from these individuals displayed normal platelet function, in that thrombospondin binding and platelet aggregation in response to collagen were normal,[236,237] though platelet adhesion to collagen under conditions of minimal shear flow was mildly diminished.[236] In light of the fact that up to 3 percent of the Japanese population[238] do not express GPIV on the platelet surface and are at the same time free of any overt bleeding abnormality, it would appear that the adhesive functions mediated by this major platelet membrane glycoprotein are adequately compensated for by other adhesive receptors.

ALLOIMMUNE DISORDERS

In addition to amino acid changes that disrupt function and result in bleeding diatheses, several platelet-membrane glycoproteins have naturally occurring allelic forms within the human gene pool. Though the molecular variants of these platelet-surface glycoproteins are thought to function identically, their presence has important clinical consequences not unlike those found in other cellular and organ systems, in that the polymorphisms can be and are recognized as immunologic targets in a transplant setting, broadly defined. Such settings include organ transplantation, blood transfusion, and pregnancy. A detailed understanding of the molecular basis of these naturally occurring variations, therefore, is crucial for our ability to design rational therapeutic and diagnostic approaches for the management of platelet immunologic disorders.

Two clinically recognized immunologic syndromes are attributable to "platelet-specific" polymorphisms. The first such syndrome, posttransfusion purpura, or PTP, is quite rare, with less than 200 cases reported to date.[239] PTP is characterized by acute, usually severe, thrombocytopenia occurring 7 to 10 days following a blood transfusion, and it is thought to be induced by platelets or platelet fragments bearing an incompatible allelic form of one or more platelet membrane glycoproteins, usually GPIIIa. Neonatal alloimmune thrombocytopenia (NAT) is the second immunologically related bleeding disorder due to platelet-antigen incompatibility and is characterized by thrombocytopenia in the neonate due to passively transmitted maternal antibody directed against a fetal platelet antigen inherited from the father and lacking on the mother's platelets. The incidence of NAT is about 1 in 2500 live births,[240] and like PTP, it is usually caused by an alloimmune response to an incompatible allelic form of GPIIIa.

There are currently six known molecular variants of GPIIIa in the human gene pool, and these are shown in Table 110-6. The Pl^{A1} allele of GPIIIa, as defined serologically, is by far the most common, with a gene frequency in Caucasians of about 85 percent, and it is this allelic form of GPIIIa that is most often responsible for inducing the alloimmune response causing both PTP and NAT in individuals that have inherited one of the other, less common, GPIIIa isoforms. With the application of platelet RNA PCR techniques to this field, the molecular basis of the polymorphisms underlying NAT and PTP is now known to involve, almost exclusively, single amino acid substitutions along the length of the polypeptide chain. Thus, a $Leu_{33} \rightarrow$ Pro substitution controls the formation of the Pl^{A1}/Pl^{A2} alloantigen system,[241,242] while an $Arg_{143} \rightarrow$ Gln polymorphism is responsible for the Pen^a/Pen^b alloantigens.[243] Other, rare allelic forms of GPIIIa that can elicit an alloimmune response have also been reported,[244–248] and are summarized in Table 110-6.

In addition to GPIIIa, more than one allele each is known to exist for GPIa, GPIb, and GPIIb, and they too have been defined at the molecular biologic level and shown to be caused by single amino acid substitutions. As shown in Table 110-6, these include a $Gly_{505} \rightarrow$ Lys polymorphism of GPIa associated with the Br^a/Br^b alloantigen system,[249] a $Thr_{145} \rightarrow$ Met substitution in GPIb,[250] and $Ile_{843} \rightarrow Ser_{843}$ allelic forms of GPIIb that control the formation of the Bak^a and Bak^b alloantigens.[242,251] As the precise nucleotide sequence polymorphisms associated with the major human platelet alloantigen systems have become defined, our ability to design novel diagnostic and therapeutic approaches for the treatment of patients with NAT and PTP has improved, and it has now become a routine matter to develop and apply DNA-based diagnostic tests for the molecular analysis of these clinically important molecular variations.[252]

Table 110-6 Naturally Occurring Allelic Forms of Platelet Membrane Glycoproteins That Can Induce Immune Thrombocytopenias

Allelic Form	*Gene Frequency (%)	Serologic Designation
GPIa: Glu_{505}	89	Br^b
GPIa: Lys_{505}	11	Br^a
GPIb: Thr_{145}	93	Ko^b
GPIb: Met_{145}	7	Ko^a
GPIIb: Ile_{843}	61	Bak^a
GPIIb: Ser_{843}	39	Bak^b
GPIIIa: Leu_{33}, Arg_{143}, Pro_{407}, Arg_{489}, Arg_{636}	85	Pl^{A1}
GPIIIa: $\underline{Pro}_{33}$, Arg_{143}, Pro_{407}, Arg_{489}, Arg_{636}	15	Pl^{A2}
GPIIIa: Leu_{33}, $\underline{Gln}_{143}$, Pro_{407}, Arg_{489}, Arg_{636}	$\ll 1$	Pen^b
GPIIIa: Leu_{33}, Arg_{143}, $\underline{Ala}_{407}$, Arg_{489}, Arg_{636}	$\ll 1$	Mo
GPIIIa: Leu_{33}, Arg_{143}, Pro_{407}, $\underline{Gln}_{489}$, Arg_{636}	$\ll 1$	CA
GPIIIa: Leu_{33}, Arg_{143}, Pro_{407}, Arg_{489}, $\underline{Cys}_{636}$	$\ll 1$	Sr

*In the Caucasian population. Gene frequencies in African and Asian populations differ. The amino acid substitutions in allelic forms of GPIIIa are underlined.

PLATELET STORAGE GRANULE DEFECTS

Biology of the Platelet Granules

As mentioned in the introduction, human platelets contain several different types of intracytoplasmic granules that can be distinguished by electron microscopy, including α granules, dense granules (δ granules), and lysosomes[253] (see Table 110-1). These granules play a major role in platelet plug formation following platelet activation. This is especially true for the α and δ granules, which are uniquely designed to participate in the clotting process.

δ Granules are the most rapidly secreted granules following platelet activation; they contain ADP, ATP, serotonin, and calcium.[254] Released ADP serves as a potent agonist for recruiting other platelets,[255] and ATP is an agonist for other cells.[256] Two thirds of platelet adenine nucleotides are stored in these granules, with an ADP:ATP ratio of 3:2, as opposed to the 1:8 ratio in the cytoplasmic pool.[257] Serotonin is a biogenic amine that can influence vascular tone, while secreted calcium ions mediate adhesive interactions and serve in addition as an intracellular second messenger for signal transduction within the activated platelet (discussed below).

Platelet α granules contribute a vast array of proteins uniquely involved in platelet plug formation. Following platelet activation, the α granules move to the center of the platelet and release their contents into the bloodstream via membrane fusion with the open canalicular system.[258,259] Interestingly, not all proteins present in α granules have the same origin. Some, like vWf, thrombospondin, and platelet factor 4 (PF4) are synthesized in and packaged by the megakaryocyte during maturation,[260,261] while others, such as albumin, IgG, and fibrinogen, are acquired by endocytosis of plasma components.[262,263] Secreted α-granule products participate in important ways in hemostasis: fibrinogen, fibronectin, vitronectin, vWf, and thrombospondin serve as adhesive ligands; platelet derived-growth factor (PDGF), β-thromboglobulin (βTG), PF4, tissue-growth factor-β, and thrombospondin modulate cell growth; and factors V and XI, high-molecular-weight kininogen, C1 inhibitor, fibrinogen, plasminogen activator inhibitor-1, and protein S each participate in the coagulation process.[15,260–266] The membrane of the α granule itself also contributes to platelet adhesiveness in that it harbors P-selectin (PADGEM or GMP-140),[267,268] which becomes expressed on the surface of activated platelets and endothelial cells following granule fusion, and mediates the subsequent binding of neutrophils and monocytes during the inflammatory process.[11]

Dense Granule Defects

Storage Pool Diseases. Patients with defects in the platelet dense granules have a storage pool deficiency.[269–273] These patients present with mild-to-moderate bleeding diatheses as well as abnormalities in their platelet aggregation patterns. The second wave of aggregation is absent in response to ADP and epinephrine, and virtually absent in response to collagen. Bleeding times in these patients are often prolonged. In 1969, it was shown that these patients have a deficiency in total platelet ADP,[273] and this deficit was subsequently localized to the ADP pool of the δ granule (known as the nonmetabolic pool).[274,275] Direct measurements of other platelet dense granular components have confirmed their absence as well.[276,277] Platelets from these patients have a defect in their ability to take up serotonin from their environment,[271,278] and electron microscopic examination has revealed an absence of characteristic dense granule.[253] In addition to the δ granule storage pool deficit seen in all of these patients, a subset of individuals have other associated defects. The two most common platelet storage pool disorders are known as Hermansky-Pudlak syndrome[271,279,280] and Chediak-Higashi syndrome,[271,281–285] and will be discussed below.

Hermansky-Pudlak Syndrome. This disorder is characterized by tyrosinase-positive severe oculocutaneous albinism that is associated with photophobia rotatory nystagmus and loss of visual acuity, excessive accumulation of ceroidlike material in reticuloendothelial cells in the bone marrow and other tissues, and a mild-to-moderate hemorrhagic diathesis (see Table 110-7). This disease is inherited as an autosomal recessive disorder, and while it occurs in many populations, it occurs with higher frequency in the Puerto Rican population.[286] Although their platelets completely lack δ granules, these patients often have no significant bleeding diathesis unless complicated by aspirin exposure or by pregnancy.[271,287] However, in one study deaths from bleeding were second only to deaths from pulmonary fibrosis, a complication that probably is secondary to the serotonin released from failure to package the serotonin into δ granules.[253] Hermansky-Pudlak syndrome is also associated with a higher incidence of granulomatous colitis,[288] although the connection of this gastrointestinal disorder and the granule defect is unclear.

Chediak-Higashi Syndrome. Chediak-Higashi syndrome involves only partial albinism, with patients often having a white forelock or ashen hair, secondary to abnormally large melanosomes.[281–285] Platelets from these patients are characterized by the presence of large intracytoplasmic granules (Fig. 110-9*A*). In addition, these patients have an associated immune defect, as characterized by the presence of large intracellular granules in their leukocytes (Fig. 110-10*A*), with a concurrent immune dysfunction involving poor mobilization of the marrow leukocyte pool,[289] defective chemotaxis,[290,291] and decreased bacteriocidal activity[292] (Table 110-7). Many other tissues also contain abnormal granules, including renal tubular cells, pneumocytes, chief and parietal gastric cells, hepatocytes, neuronal cells, and fibroblasts.[293] Chediak-Higashi patients often die in the first two decades of life from either overwhelming infections or lymphoproliferative disorders, especially in what has been

Table 110-7 Inherited Platelet Defects Associated with Morphologic Abnormalities

Category	Disease	Major Feature
δ-Granule defect	Storage pool disease	Absence of dense granules in plates associated with a mild-to-moderate bleeding diathesis. Decrease level of platelet serotonin and decreased ADP:ATP ratio. Absent second wave on platelet aggregation.
	Chediak-Higashi syndrome	Same as storage pool deficiency, but also associated with partial albinism and large cytoplasmic granules in white cells with a mild bleeding diathesis and an immune dysfunction.
	Hermansky-Pudlak syndrome	Same as storage pool deficiency, but also associated with severe albinism and a very mild bleeding diathesis.
α-Granule defect	Gray platelet	Absence of α granules in platelets, associated with a very mild bleeding diathesis and decreased α-granular content.
Large platelets	Bernard-Soulier syndrome	Deficiency of the platelet GPIIb complex associated with a moderate bleeding. Associated with large platelets and often a mild thrombocytopenia.
	May-Hegglin anomaly	Large platelets without a bleeding diathesis, associated with mild thrombocytopenia, no syndrome bleeding diathesis and Dohle body inclusions in white cells.
	Fechtner syndrome	Same as May-Hegglin, but with associated deafness, nephritis and ocular abnormalities.
	Montreal platelet syndrome	Large platelets and a mild bleeding diathesis. Spontaneous platelet aggregation at pH 7.4.
Small platelets	Wiskott-Aldrich syndrome	Presplenectomy has small platelets, severe thrombocytopenia. Has eczema and immune dysfunction ultimately resulting in severe infections, immune complex diseases, and lymphomas/leukemias.

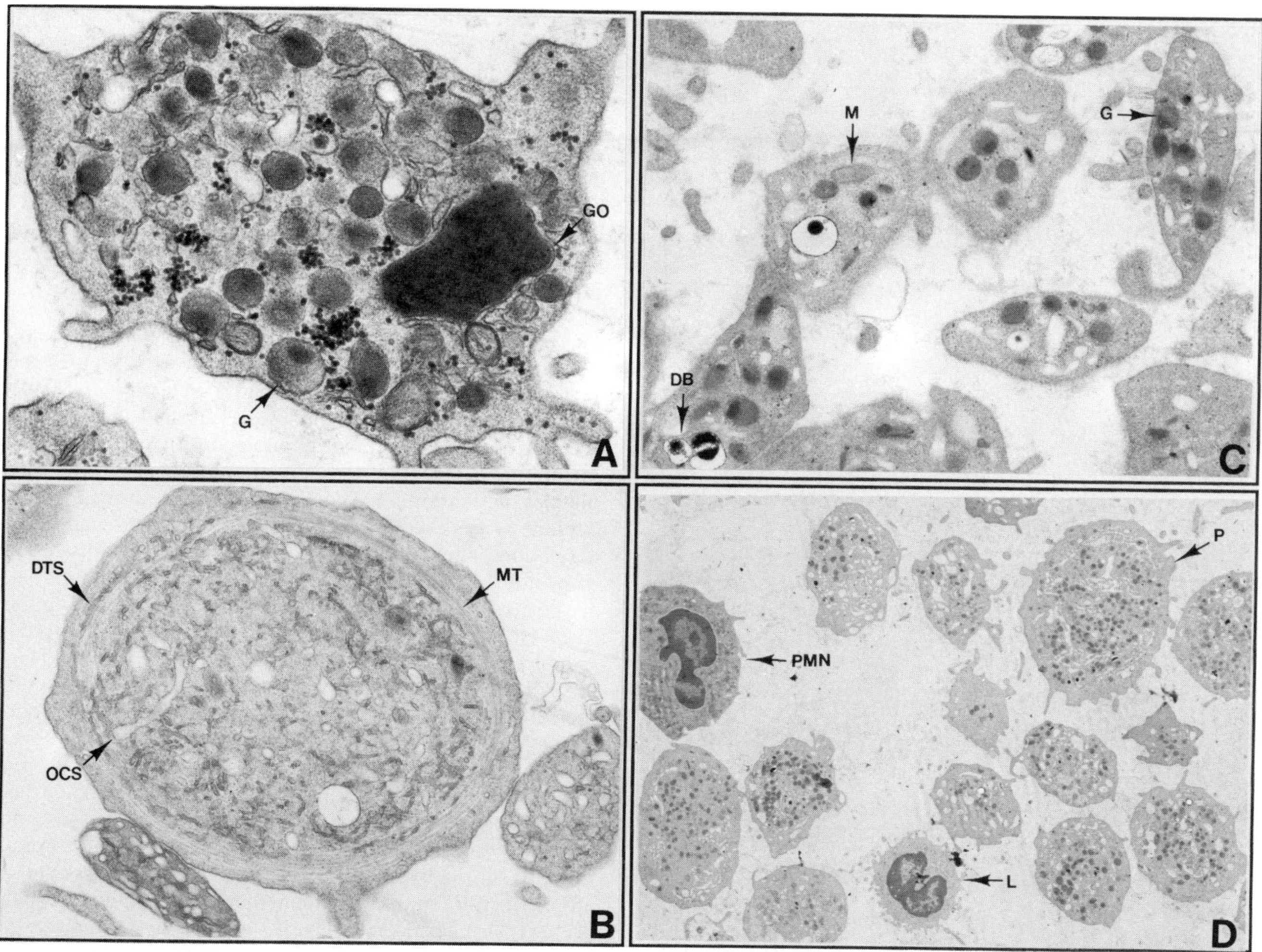

FIG. 110-9 Thin-section electron micrographs of platelets. *A*. Chediak-Higashi platelet demonstrating a giant organelle (GO) present among many normal sized granules (G). Magnification ×32,000. *B*. A platelet from a patient with gray platelet syndrome reveals the presence of the normal circumferential band of microtubules (MT), elements of the open canalicular system (OCS), and dense tubular system (DTS), but lacks other organelles. Magnification ×23,000. *C*. Wiscott-Aldrich platelets are about half normal size, but contain normal-appearing α granules (G), dense bodies (DB), and mitochondria (M), all of which appear large by comparison. Magnification ×22,000. *D*. Platelets from patients with May-Hegglin anomaly are as large as lymphocytes (L), and a few platelets (P) are larger than polymorphonuclear leukocytes (PMN). Occasional large α granules are present, and channels of both the OCS and the DTS are prominent in the cytoplasm. (Magnification ×3500). *(Courtesy of Dr. James G. White, University of Minnesota.)*

termed the "accelerated phase" of the disease.[294] These patients are particularly susceptible to Epstein-Barr infections.[289,295]

The molecular bases of the Hermansky-Pudlak and Chediak-Higashi syndromes are unknown. Certainly, a number of different defects could give the same phenotypic expression, so that sorting out the molecular defect may depend on an improved understanding of how granules are formed and proteins become targeted and processed so that they ultimately become properly localized within the platelet. A 40-kDa δ-granule protein termed "granulophysin" has been characterized and shown to be deficient in Hermansky-Pudlak platelets.[296,297] This protein appears to share immunologic properties with a synaptic vesicle protein called "synaptophysin." Whether absence of this or other granule-specific proteins can account for the Chediak-Higashi syndrome is uncertain. Because the large granules in Chediak-Higashi appear as though they represent the fusion of multiple smaller granules, it has been suggested that there may also be a microtubular defect.[298] Treatment of normal leukocytes with the microtubular assembly inhibitor colchicine mimics these disorders to some extent in that it results in leukocytes with large granules. However, leukocytes isolated from patients with Chediak-Higashi syndrome contain normal numbers of assembled microtubules.[299,300]

A number of animal models have been described for these defects. Examination of animals with pigmen. mutations has defined a large number of associated platelet storage pool deficiencies. Thus, multiple different Hermansky-Pudlak-like mice have been defined involving different genetic loci, suggesting that the observed platelet defect seen in Hermansky-Pudlak syndrome may be secondary to a variety of different defects.[301] For Chediak-Higashi syndrome, animal models have been defined in cows, minks, foxes, cats, and whales[302] Comparison of human Chediak-Higashi characteristics with several animal models indicates a lack of complementation between humans, cats, and mink diseases, suggesting that a single gene is responsible for the illness in all three species.[302] DDAVP has been shown to be effective in the treatment of bleeding manifestations in these syndromes.[303] Platelet transfusions may be necessary to alleviate major bleeding episodes. Bone marrow transplantation has been accomplished in Chediak-Higashi cats, with resolution of the platelet dysfunction and neutrophil migration.[304] How-

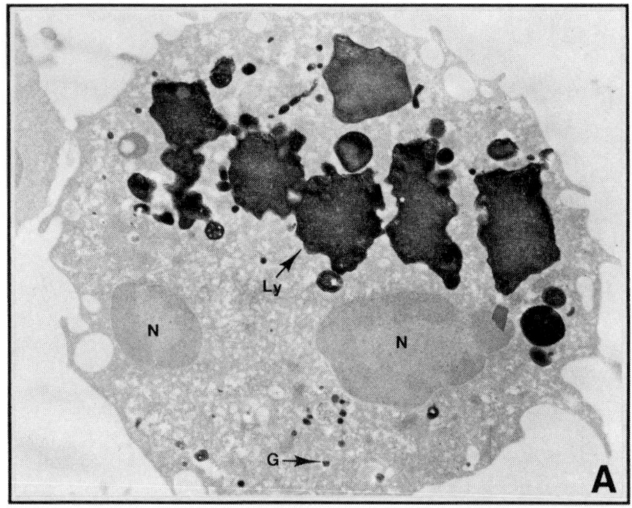

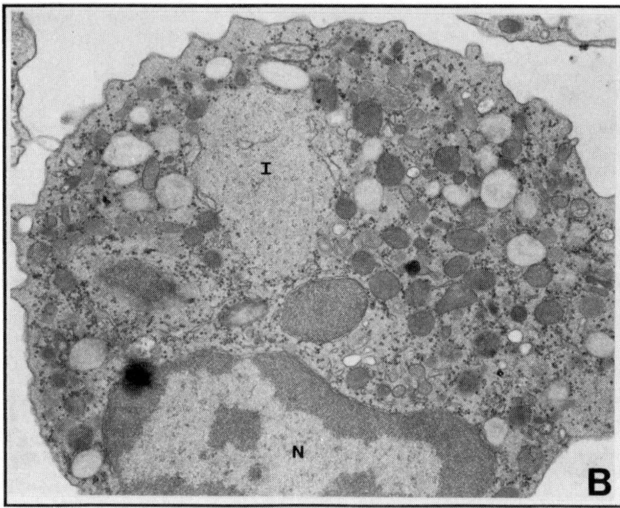

FIG. 110-10 *A*. **Thin-section electron micrographs of a typical neutrophil from a patient with Chediak-Higashi syndrome stained for myeloperoxidase. Osmium black reaction product identifies a few normal size granules (G) and numerous huge lysosomes (Ly) characteristic of this disorder. Nuclear lobes (N) are not stained. Magnification ×14,500.** *B*. **Neutrophil from a patient with May-Hegglin anomaly (MHA), containing a characteristic spindle-shaped inclusion (I) present in nearly all granulocytes from these patients. Fibers resembling intermediate filaments are oriented in the long axis of the inclusions, and are probably responsible for their shape. Clusters of ribosomes are present on the filaments and produce the basophilia of the occlusions on smears stained with Wright-Giemsa. Membrane segments are close by, but do not enclose MHA inclusions. Magnification ×25,000.** ***(Courtesy of Dr. James G. White, University of Minnesota.)***

ever, inclusion bodies seen in the liver and kidney of these animals remained after bone marrow transplantation.

α-Granule Defects: The Gray Platelet Syndrome

A number of patients have been described who have a deficiency in α granules.[305–310] These patients have a bleeding history similar to δ-granule storage pool defective patients, with mild to moderate bleeding, mild thrombocytopenia, and a prolonged bleeding time (see Table 110-7). Because of the initial light microscopic observation of gray platelets in the peripheral blood smear of these patients following Romanovsky stain,[307] this disorder was termed the "gray platelet syndrome." On electron microscopy, these platelets appear somewhat enlarged, but are most notable for the absence or marked reduction of α granules, as shown in Fig. 110-9*B*.[253] These platelets are also markedly deficient in α-granule-specific proteins such as PF4, βTG, vWf, factor V, fibronectin, and PDGF.[305,306,310] Gray platelet aggregation to various agonists, especially to thrombin, appears to be impaired. There have been many mild alterations noted in platelet aggregation, such as a delayed and blunted Ca^{2+} mobilization response in these platelets.[311] The observed platelet aggregation abnormalities may be secondary effects of the absence of any of the many different α-granule components.

The vacuolar structures seen in gray platelets appear to be aborted α granules.[312] Immunocytochemical studies show that these structures contain both P-selection (GMP-140) and GPIIb/IIIa in their membranes, and that these proteins are transferred to and, via granule fusion with the plasma membrane, expressed normally on the cell surface following platelet activation.[309] The vacuolar structures appear to become centralized like normal α granules following platelet activation. They also appear to contain significant amounts of proteins, including immunoglobulin and albumin,[309] that are normally incorporated into α granules by passive endocytosis (see above). Further, endogenously synthesized α-granule-specific proteins such as PDGF, PF4, and βTG do not seem to be retained within the platelet, leaking out of the cell instead.[305,306,313] This latter phenomenon may account for several reports of myelofibrosis and pulmonary fibrosis associated with gray platelet syndrome.[313,314]

The biologic basis of how proteins are processed intracellularly and targeted to particular organelles is just now beginning to be understood.[315] Since multiple α-granule proteins normally synthesized in the megakaryocyte are affected, while granule proteins derived by endocytosis are present at near-normal levels, and since this disease is limited to megakaryocytes and platelets, it appears that a platelet-specific chaperon-like protein necessary to transport proteins to, or retain them in, the α granules may be missing or defective.

Patients with gray platelet syndrome have a mild bleeding diathesis that may be treated by administration of DDAVP or local care of a bleeding site through the use of ϵ-amino caproic acid.[316,317] Platelet transfusions are not often necessary, but may be lifesaving. There is one report of a 68-year-old man in whom the diagnosis of gray platelet syndrome was made while he was being evaluated for thrombocytopenia.[318] Bone marrow analysis demonstrated mild reticular fibrosis that may have resulted from the unregulated secretion of α-granule constituents from megakaryocytes and platelets. The clinical importance of the marrow myelofibrosis in this disorder is as yet unclear.

A variant of the gray platelet syndrome has been described in the Wistar-Furth rat, in which there is thrombocytopenia and platelet size heterogeneity with small α granules and a canalicular system containing α-granular material.[319] The defect in this disorder may be different than in the human disorder and may involve a protein important in the division of the megakaryocyte into platelets as well as in the formation of α granules.

A small number of patients have been described with a combined α/δ-granule deficiency.[277,320] the δ-granule deficiency was often much more severe than the α-granule deficiency. These patients also have mild to moderate bleeding histories, and the laboratory evaluation is similar to that of the δ-granule-deficient patient, with a decreased platelet ADP:ATP ratio in the cells and low levels of serotonin. In one patient with a severe deficiency of both α- and δ-granules, there was a deficiency in total platelet GMP-140,[321] suggesting that, unlike the gray platelet syndrome in which there may be a granule-targeting defect, platelet granule formation itself may underlie this disorder.

Therapeutic treatment of these patients is the same as other storage-pool-deficient patients. Whether there are concomitant, related syndromes such as pulmonary fibrosis, myelofibrosis, or granular defects in other tissues is unknown.

DEFECTS IN SIGNAL TRANSDUCTION

Following the binding of an agonist to its platelet receptor, a signal is transferred across the cell membrane into the cell either directly by the membrane receptor or through intervening $G_{\alpha\beta\delta}$ heterotrimeric proteins.[322] The following G_α proteins have been described in platelets: G_s, $G_{\alpha i1}$, $G_{\alpha i2}$, $G_{\alpha i3}$, G_z, and G_o.[322] These different G proteins have separate roles in the biology of signal transduction and may modulate the response of a particular receptor to a given agonist. Signal transduction results in secondary changes within the platelet that include ionic calcium fluxes, cAMP formation, phospholipase A_2 and C activation, changes in arachidonate pathway metabolism, protein kinase C activation, and protein phosphorylation. These diverse pathways interact with each other in multiple complex ways that are still being defined. For example, phospholipase C releases diacylglycerol,[323,324] which, in turn, activates protein kinase C[325,326] and consequently phosphorylation of numerous intracellular proteins, including cytoskeletal elements.[327,328]

With multiple overlapping pathways of activation, as well as overlapping phenotypes, it has been difficult to define specific defects in patients with inherited disorders of platelet signal transduction. Nonetheless, a small number of patients have been described, many of whom have a mild bleeding diathesis with moderate prolongation of the bleeding time. Most studies have demonstrated abnormal platelet aggregation patterns, with only partial response to certain agonists, which resemble those in patients with storage pool disorders (see above). One such group of patients lack the ability to liberate arachidonic acid.[329,330] This may be due to a phospholipase A_2 deficiency in at least one of the described patients.[329] In others, the failure of phospholipase A_2 to release arachidonic acid may be due to decreased thrombin mobilization of Ca^{2+}.[257]

Other patients have diminished cyclooxygenase enzyme activity that mimics an aspirin-like defect.[331–334] These patients have abnormal platelet aggregation in response to ADP, epinephrine, collagen, and arachidonic acid, while responding normally to prostaglandin G_2, suggesting a defect in cyclooxygenase and subsequent thromboxane A_2 synthesis. In one study, radioimmunoassay using an anticyclooxygenase antibody showed that five of six patients with this disorder had normal antigen levels of an apparently functionally abnormal protein.[335] Additionally, two affected patients have been described who appear to lack thromboxane synthetase that converts prostaglandin H_2 to thromboxane A_2.[336,337] Bassett hound hereditary thrombopathy represents a possible animal model of a signal transduction defect in platelets.[338] Originally thought to be an animal model of Glanzmann thrombasthenia, it appears that fibrinogen binding is normal in these animals, but that there is a delay in platelet activation following fibrinogen binding.[339]

DISORDERS OF PLATELET PROCOAGULANT ACTIVITY

Activated platelets play a role in accelerating the proteolytic events that take place as part of the coagulation cascade, and this property has been termed "platelet factor 3 activity."[340] The procoagulant properties have been attributed to a number of characteristics unique to the surface of activated platelets, including exposure of phosphatidylserine moieties, the redistribution of specific receptors for factors V and X, and the development of platelet microvesicles.

One of the best-characterized inherited disorders of platelet factor 3 activity is known as Scott syndrome.[341,342] In the first case studies of this bleeding disorder, the patient presented with prolonged bleeding after dental extractions, excessive postoperative bleeding, and a spontaneous retroperitoneal hemorrhage.[341] Serum prothrombin time was short, with normal prothrombin and partial thromboplastin times, normal bleeding times, and normal platelet aggregation and secretion. Measurement of prothrombinase activity of the patient's activated platelets demonstrated a 75 percent reduction in factor Xa binding even in the presence of added factor Va, implying a defect in a membrane component necessary for factor Va-Xa assembly. These platelets are ineffective at moderate shear rates in promoting fibrinopeptide A formation and in fibrin deposition on subendothelium.[343] The molecular basis of this decrease in prothrombinase activity is unknown, although it has been shown that these platelets have less phosphatidylserine on their activated platelet surfaces[344] and decreased microvesicle formation.[345] The defect in this disorder is not limited to platelet membranes, as erythrocytes from patients with Scott syndrome also have decreased microvesiculation and fewer factor Va binding sites than normal following A23187 ionophore stimulation.[346]

PLATELET SIZE AND PRODUCTION DISORDERS: THE INHERITED THROMBOCYTOPENIAS

General Comments

The process by which platelet formation occurs is a fascinating one, which is only now beginning to be understood. Megakaryocytopoiesis begins with the self-renewing hematopoietic stem cell in the bone marrow that becomes progressively committed to the megakaryoblast lineage, eventually resulting in the diploid megakaryoblast, a cell that is indistinguishable from other lymphocytic-like cells by routine staining techniques. Over an approximately 4-day period, this precursor cell then undergoes an explosive series of changes, with endoreduplication of the nucleus, an increase in cytoplasmic content to an average volume of ~ 10^3 to 10^4 μm^3, and an accumulation of proteins and morphologic features characteristics of platelets. Eventually, either in the bone marrow or in the pulmonary vascular bed,[347] each megakaryocyte sheds several thousand 7-to-10 μm^3 platelets.

The study of the process of platelet formation is of considerable clinical interest. Regulating this process may be valuable in altering thrombotic tendency and in limiting the incidence of clinically significant thrombocytopenia during chemotherapeutic treatment of tumors. In addition, there are a large number of inherited disorders resulting in decreased platelet production. A number of these are well-defined clinical syndromes such as thrombocytopenia and absent radii (TAR) syndrome, in which skeletal abnormalities occur in association with clinically significant thrombocytopenia[348] (also see below). Interestingly, in most of these patients, the thrombocytopenia disappears with time. Other inherited thrombocytopenic states occur in conjunction with more recognized platelet disorders such as platelet-type vWD (discussed above), the storage pool platelet defects, and May-Hegglin syndrome, in which there are large, often bizarre-shaped platelets associated with the thrombocytopenia and inclusion bodies in the lymphocytes and neutrophils (see below). In many of these states, decreased production may be related to increased platelet size, so that total platelet mass is conserved.

Some of the above described disorders may involve a defect in hematopoietic stem cell commitment to the megakaryocyte lineage, while others may involve defects in the final process of differentiation into mature megakaryocytes and the subsequent shedding of platelets. Below, we discuss the state of knowledge of these two interrelated processes—megakaryocytopoiesis and platelet formation.

Megakaryocytopoiesis

Megakaryocytes are large, polyploid, terminally differentiated hematopoietic cells that release platelets into the peripheral bloodstream.[349] As shown in Fig. 110-11, these cells arise from self-regenerating pluripotent stem cells that also give rise to all other hematopoietic lineages. Megakaryocyte lineage commitment involves a number of precursor stages that are distinguishable by the final differentiated cells to which they can give rise. The earliest precursor after the pluripotent stem cell appears to be the CFU-GEMMK (colony-forming unit—granulocyte, erythrocyte, monocyte, megakaryocyte) that in culture results in a mix of granulocytes, erythrocytes, monocytes, and megakaryocytes. The next apparent stage of commitment appears to be the CFU-EMM that gives rise to mixed colonies of erythrocytes, monocytes, and megakaryocytes. The BFU-MK (burst-forming unit—megakaryocyte) gives rise to a burst of approximately 10 to 20 megakaryocytes after 3 weeks in culture, and the CFU-MK gives rise to a smaller megakaryocyte colony after 10 days in culture.[349–354] This process of differentiation appears to be regulated by extracellular factors including interleukin-1 (IL-1), IL-3, IL-6, granulocyte colony-stimulating factor, granulocyte/macrophage, IL-11, and c-*kit* ligand[349,355–361] that also serve as important regulatory factors for many other hematopoietic lineages. The exact role of these cytokines in the process of commitment into the megakaryocyte lineage is not well understood.

Human marrow is a highly organized tissue containing supportive nutritive accessory cells that may be intimately involved in these processes, so that the immediate microenvironment of a cell may be of critical importance in its differentiation. The development of growth conditions that allow serum-free cultures of well-defined cell populations and long-term bone marrow cultures, together with the isolation, characterization, and recombinant expression of a growing number of cytokines and their receptors, should permit greater insights into these processes. It has become apparent that multiple factors may be required for regulating megakaryocytopoiesis. Some of these cytokines act directly on megakaryocyte precursors, while others may induce helper cells to secrete important cytokines. In addition, cytokines may be stage-specific, and a number of them may

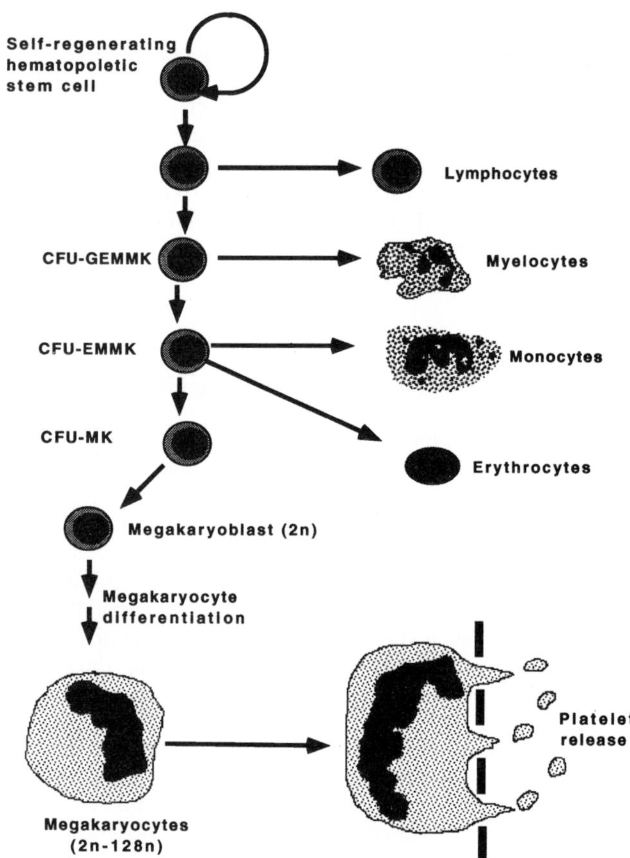

FIG. 110-11 Megakaryocyte development from the pluripotent hematopoietic stem cell involves two steps. In the first, the mononuclear stem cell undergoes increasing commitment toward the megakaryocyte cell lineage. These cells undergo proliferation. In the second, the mononuclear megakaryoblast undergoes nuclear endoreduplication, increases in cell size, and develops special structures and organization. This terminally differentiated cell eventually releases a shower of platelets.

be required to observe megakaryocyte differentiation, as each may play a critical role at different stages of commitment. For example, IL-11 does not stimulate megakaryocytopoiesis by itself.[360] Yet in combination with IL-3, IL-11 increased the number and ploidy of the megakaryocytes that developed from purified primitive hematopoietic stem cells in a serum-free agar culture system. Whether this augmentation commonly seen for a number of the cytokines is due to an increased number of primitive cells differentiating to a more mature form on which the other cytokines are active, or whether the observed phenomenon is due to a cytokine having an effect on an accessory cell (or the megakaryocyte progenitor itself) to secrete an important secondary cytokine needs further study. Certainly, a defect in the ability to produce a cytokine or its receptor may be the basis of the thrombocytopenia seen in an inherited disorder such as the TAR syndrome (see below) or Fanconi's anemia. The relationship between the marrow dysfunction in these disorders and the inherited skeletal abnormality is intriguing.

Intuitively, one would have expected that the production of megakaryocytes would, at least in part, be regulated by a unique cytokine. A number of laboratories have reported such megakaryocyte colony-stimulating activity (MK-CSA) and have partially purified these factors, usually from the urine or serum of patients with a physiological stress that should increase platelet production.[354,362–365] To date none of these materials have been fully purified and characterized, and the assigned molecular weights for this factor have varied enormously.[362,365,366] A number of these MK-CSA factors may turn out to be previously described cytokines, though the possibility exists that a unique megakaryocyte progenitor stimulatory factor remains to be discovered, as studies utilizing neutralizing antibodies (either against MK-CSA or specific cytokine) are consistent with a distinct factor separate from known cytokines.[347,367,368]

Cell and Molecular Biology of Platelet Formation

The end product of this lineage commitment is the megakaryoblast, a small lymphocyte-like cell that undergoes the process of nuclear endoreduplication,[347] cytoplasmic enlargement, and differentiation to form the mature megakaryocyte having a cell volume of approximately 10^4 to 10^5 μm^3 (see Fig. 110-11). Each of these huge cells eventually results in the formation of approximately 10^3 to 10^4 platelets. Since erythrocytes and white cells are directly released from the bone, it has naturally been assumed that platelets are released from there as well. The findings of naked megakaryocyte nuclei[369] in the marrow and the presence of proplatelets in the central venous blood[370] support the hypothesis that platelets are formed in the marrow. It is possible, however, that platelets are, at least in part, released from megakaryocytes that have migrated to the pulmonary bed.[371–374] Studies have demonstrated that there are more circulating megakaryocytes in the pulmonary artery than in the pulmonary venous system and that the opposite is true for platelet numbers.[373,374]

The process by which platelets actually derive from megakaryocytes is not well understood. The mature megakaryocyte contains an extensive membrane system termed the "demarcation membrane system" (DMS) that may represent inverted membranes. Two hypotheses for the mechanism of platelet production have been proposed: that the DMS fuses and the megakaryocyte cytoplasm fractures to release a shower of platelets, or that the DMS represents reserve plasma membrane that allows the formation of projections from the megakaryocyte surface that then break off to form proplatelets and platelets.[375,376] There has been a great deal of effort directed at establishing an in vitro megakaryocyte system that sheds platelets. In some cases, cultured cells have been shown to form spindles, while in others, cellular processes take on a beaded appearance that fragment to form particles with the size and ultrastructural appearance of platelets.[376] This process can be inhibited by agents that disrupt microtubules[377,378] and promoted by actin filaments depolymerizing agents,[378,379] suggesting involvement of the cytoskeleton in this process. The size variation and heterogeneity in platelets seen in various disease states may be related to the site and mechanism of formation, and a number of the inherited platelet disorders to be discussed below appear to involve abnormal platelet size, including the macrothrombocytopenic states seen in Bernard-Soulier syndrome, May-Hegglin anomaly, and the Wistar-Furth rat, and the microthrombocytopenia seen in Wiskott-Aldrich syndrome.

The normal range of platelet counts is 150 to 400 × $10^3/\mu l$.[380] Even more constant than the circulating platelet count, however, is the circulating platelet mass in which the platelet count is multiplied by the mean platelet volume, so that there is an inverse relationship between platelet count and platelet size.[205,206] Certainly, thrombogenic tendency may be related to total platelet mass rather than to platelet count alone.[380] The mechanisms by which the body determines the level of circulating platelets and regulates platelet production are currently unknown. The feedback may involve an MK-CSA factor as described above and/or a factor involved in the maturation of the megakaryoblast to a megakaryocyte with subsequent platelet formation. Such a factor would be similar to erythropoietin, and has been termed "thrombopoietin" (TPO). TPO activity, defined as a lineage-specific promoter of megakaryocyte maturation, has been detected in thrombocytopenic rodent and human plasma.[381–387] Partially purified preparations of TPO are capable of accelerating cytoplasmic maturation of megakaryocytes, promoting nuclear endoreduplication and protein synthesis. However, a specific TPO has not as yet been convincingly isolated, and partially purified TPO has been variously assigned molecular weights of 15,000 to 48,000. While several laboratories have claimed to have purified the factor, there have not been any corroboration or follow-up to these initial reports.[386,387]

Additional factors, including GM-CSF, IL-3, erythropoietin, and IL-6, have been reported to have thrombopoietin-like activity.[355,388–392] Recombinant erythropoietin has been shown to stimulate increased platelet activity in animal models.[388,393] IL-6 appears to behave very much like TPO in that it can increase, in a somewhat specific fashion, nuclear endoreduplication, cytoplasmic size, and the accumulation of megakaryocyte-specific enzymes.[390–392,394,395] In addition, IL-6 stimulation of megakaryocytes results in a positive autocrine effect, with increased production of IL-6 by the megakaryocytes.[395] Animal models show that infusions of IL-6 can stimulate increased circulating platelet counts.[392] As the evidence accumulates for additional multilineage factors having MK-CSA and TPO activities, the strongly held belief that there are additional megakaryocyte-specific as well as more general environmental factors will likely need to be reexamined.

The molecular biology of the above processes is only now beginning to be understood. Two platelet-specific genes, rat PF4 and human GPIIb, have been studied and have provided some interesting information about the 5′-flanking region of these genes. Transgenic mice containing a 1.1-kb segment from the 5′-flanking region of the rat PF4 gene linked to the prokaryote β-galactosidase gene drove expression in a virtually megakaryocyte-specific fashion.[396] Further deletional studies with the 5′-flanking region of the rat PF4 gene and a transient expression assay utilizing rat marrow and a growth hormone expression vector demonstrated the presence of three enhancer regions and one silencer region in the 5′-flanking region.[397] As shown in Fig. 110-12, these regions define the elements that partially control tissue specificity, and include a GATA consensus sequence 31 bp upstream from the transcriptional start site that may contribute to tissue-specific expression.

GATA-binding proteins are nuclear transcription factors that were first defined in erythroid cells.[393] At least one of these proteins, GATA-1, was thought to be restricted in its expression to erythroid tissues.[398,399] More recently, this transcription factor has also been shown to be present in megakaryocytes, megakaryocyte cell lines, and monocytes.[400,401] As these three cell lines share a common progenitor, it is not surprising that there is a common nuclear regulatory factor like GATA-1. The role of GATA-1 in megakaryocyte-specific expression is uncertain, as transgenic mice in which the GATA-1 gene was "knocked out" had a defect limited to

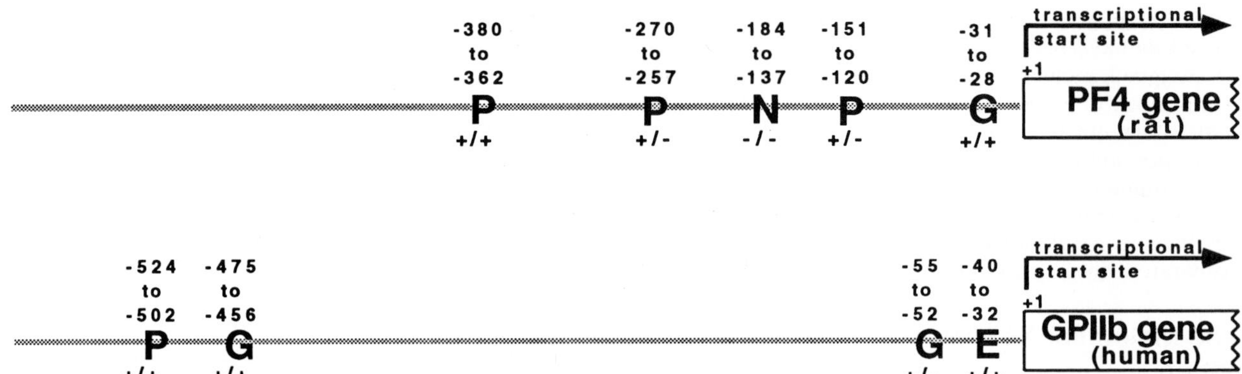

FIG. 110-12 Promoter, enhancer, and silencer elements in the 5′-flanking regions of the rat PF4 and human GPIIb genes that influence megakaryocyte-specific gene expression. Both genes are numbered from the transcriptional start site. P = promoter element; N = silencer element; G = GATA consensus sequence; E = Ets promoter element; The three different P regions do not share significant sequence similarity. The first + or − refers to whether the element enhances or silences transcriptional activity, while the second + or − refers to whether the element is megakaryocyte specific (+) or not (−).

the erythroid lineage.[402] Site-directed mutation of the GATA sequence to TATA increases expression in nonmegakaryocyte cells and makes transcription from this site more dependent on the enhancer sequences for megakaryocyte expression.

A GATA box may also play an important role in the regulation of expression of the human GPIIb gene. DNase I protection sites have been defined within the 5′-flanking region of this gene (see Fig. 110-12),[403] with two of them shown to be megakaryocyte-specific. Transient expression assays using constructs in which these two regions, beginning 456 and 502 bp upstream to the transcriptional start site, have been deleted resulted in a threefold decrease in expression. The −456 bp site contains a GATA consensus sequence, and a second GATA site at −55 has also been defined, and may be an important regulator of megakaryocyte-specific expression.[404]

Defects in Platelet Size and Production

Wiskott-Aldrich Syndrome. A number of inherited disorders involve platelets as part of a much wider syndrome. This can be seen for several of the storage pool disorders discussed above, and is also seen in Wiskott-Aldrich syndrome (see Table 110-7), which was first recognized in two case reports, one in 1973 and one in 1954, as a sex-linked disorder of thrombocytopenia and eczema.[405,406] Platelets are small (Fig. 110-9*C*), usually half-normal volume, and the platelet mass is decreased.[406,407] There appears to be an associated platelet storage pool defect.[406,407] The thrombocytopenia seen is severe, and can be less than 10,000 platelets/μl. It has become apparent that these patients have a severe immune defect, in addition to the platelet disorder and eczema. Many die during the first decade from overwhelming infections or immune-based disorders such as immune thrombocytopenia or hemolytic anemia and from lymphoma-like illnesses during the second decade of life.[408,409] These patients have an impaired ability to form antibodies to carbohydrate antigens[410] and appear to have a defect in both B and T lymphocytes, but primarily in the latter.[411–414] In fact, the defect in T-lymphocyte function has been used clinically to confirm carrier status, since female carriers for this condition have selective inactivation of their X chromosome in their T lymphocytes.[412–414]

Studies have demonstrated that all circulating cells except erythrocytes share a common antigen CD43 (also known as sialophorin, leukosialin, large sialoglycoprotein, or GPII5).[415] The cDNA for CD43 has been cloned and the mature protein is a 381 amino acid transmembrane protein with 50 percent of the extracellular residues as potential O-glycosylation sites.[416] Interestingly, this glycoprotein has been noted to be abnormal in Wiskott-Aldrich patients.[417] Since the gene encoding CD43 is not X-linked, it is probably not directly involved in this syndrome, but may be secondarily involved in the final phenotypic expression of a number of disorders that either directly affect CD43 or enzymes involved in O-glycosylation.[418,419] It has been shown that CD43 binds to the intercellular adhesion molecule, ICAM-1,[420] a member of the immunoglobulin gene superfamily found on neutrophils, lymphocytes, and other lymphoid tissues.[421] In addition to interaction with CD43, ICAM-1 is also the counter-receptor for the integrin receptor LFA-1[422] in an important immunologic intercellular adhesion mechanism. DC43/ICAM-1 interactions are much more limited in scope, but appear to be important in T-cell activation,[423] and the absence of the CD43/ICAM-1 interaction may underlie the severe immunodeficiency seen in this disorder.

Splenectomy, although it increases the risk of opportunistic infection, often alleviates the thrombocytopenia and bleeding diathesis in this disorder[424] and should be undertaken in spite of the increased risk of bleeding. Immune-related complications respond variably to steroids, IV immunoglobulin, vincristine, or plasmapheresis. Bone marrow transplantation has been efficacious in treating this disorder,[425,426] although the success rate with nonrelated marrow donors has been poor.[427]

In addition, there are variations on the classical Wiskott-Aldrich presentation, in which initially the thrombocytopenia is the predominant feature or in which X-linked thrombocytopenia occurs alone.[414,428–431] Linkage analysis studies have shown that both the X-linked thrombocytopenia and Wiskott-Aldrich syndrome are localized to the same pericentric region of the X chromosome.[432,433] In fact, maternal X-chromosome inactivation studies in one of these families demonstrated nonrandom X-inactivation limited to T and B cells and granulocytes, similar to that seen in Wiskott Aldrich syndrome.[430] Whether there is a defect in the CD43 membrane protein in these patients needs to be pursued.

The X-linked scurfy mouse phenotype may be a mouse model of the Wiskott-Aldrich syndrome.[434] This animal has scaliness of its skin and has thrombocytopenia and anemia that may be due to gastrointestinal bleeding. The degree of immunocompromise and the molecular basis of this disorder in the scurfy mouse have not yet been determined.

Several platelet abnormalities have been described associated with large platelets and thrombocytopenia. The most common of these is the May-Hegglin anomaly, in which macrothrombocytes (see Fig. 110-9*D*) are associated with thrombocytopenia and normal coagulation studies.[435,436] In addition, leukocytes appear to contain large spindle-shaped inclusions known as Dohle bodies (Fig. 110-10*B*). A similar disorder, but with inclusions that look different, is Sebastian syndrome.[437] Again, no intrinsic platelet defect has been described. The association of the morphologic finding of May-Hegglin anomaly with sensorineural deafness, nephritis, and ocular abnormalities has been called "Fechtner syndrome."[438] In Montreal platelet syndrome there are macrothrombocytes, a prolonged bleeding time, and spontaneous aggregation of platelets at pH 7.4.[439,440] The molecular bases of these abnormalities are unknown.

Inherited disorders in platelet production alone without defects in other hematopoietic cell lines are rare. The most common ones are the TAR syndrome[348,441,442] and familial thrombocythemia.[433] TAR syndrome was first described in 1951,[441] and is a relatively common disorder involving hypomegakaryocytic thrombocytopenia and bilateral absence of the radii.[348,441,442] These patients are born with a low platelet count in the approximately 10,000/mm^3 range, which improves slowly, reaching normal levels after the first year. During infancy, environmental stress such as viral illness can precipitate episodes of severe thrombocytopenia. Several TAR patients have an associated storage pool defect.[444] In addition, these patients have other hematologic changes, including leukemoid reactions to the 30,000 40,000/mm^3 range and anemia, at least in part due to blood loss.[442] The skeletal manifestations include complete absence of the radii, but presence of functional thumbs. Other orthopedic abnormalities are seen in 50 percent of cases, and the more severe the upper limb deformity, the more likely the patient is to have a lower limb deformity. In about 30 percent of the patients there are cardiac anomalies, including tetralogy of Fallot and atrial septal defects.

The etiology of this disorder is unknown. Megakaryocytes are present in the bone marrow, although there may be some decrease as compared with what one would see in thrombocytopenia secondary to increased peripheral destruction.[445] While measurements of humoral factors involved in megakaryocytopoiesis appear to be normal, bone marrow cultures from TAR patients fail to develop megakaryocyte colonies, while erythroid and myeloid colony formation appears to be intact.[446] In long-term cultures of bone marrow from these patients, megakaryocyte and mixed colonies were decreased in number as compared with normal controls, and rather large, multinucleate cells developed with the characteristic staining of osteoclasts.[447] These latter cells were not seen in normal marrow cultures. The appearance of osteoclast-like cells in the long-term marrow cultures from patients with TAR, a disorder that affects primarily hematopoiesis and bone formation, is intriguing. Certainly other disorders such as Fanconi's anemia and Schwachman syndrome also have a similar relationship in which skeletal abnormalities occur in conjunction with hematopoietic defects.[448,449] Whether a common growth factor or shared environmental factors underlie these disorders remains to be established.

ACKNOWLEDGMENTS

We are grateful to Dr. James G. White (University of Minnesota) for providing the electron micrographs used in this chapter. This research was supported by grants HL-44612 (to P.J.N.) and HL-40387 (to M.P.) from the National Institutes of Health, and by grant 3152 (to M.P.) from the Council for Tobacco Research—U.S.A. P.J.N. is an Established Investigator (92001390) of the American Heart Association.

REFERENCES

1. Roth GJ: Developing relationships: Arterial platelet adhesion, glycoprotein Ib, and leucine-rich glycoproteins. *Blood* **77**:5, 1991.
2. Shimomura T, Fujimura K, Maehama S, Takemoto M, Oda K, Fujimoto T, Oyama R, Suzuki M, Ichihara-Tanaka K, Titani K, Kuramoto A: Rapid purification and characterization of human platelet glycoprotein V: The amino acid sequence contains leucine-rich repetitive modules as in glycoprotein Ib. *Blood* **75**:2349, 1990.
3. DuX, Beutler L, Ruan C, Castaldi PA, Berndt MC: Glycoprotein Ib and glycoprotein IX are fully complexed in the intact platelet membrane. *Blood* **69**:1524, 1987.
4. Modderman PW, Admiraal LG, Sonnenberg A, von dem Borne AEGK: Glycoprotein-V and glycoprotein-Ib-IX form a noncovalent complex in the platelet membrane. *J Biol Chem* **267**:364, 1992.
5. Wenger RH, Wicki AN, Kieffer N, Adolph S, Hameister H, Clemetson KJ: The 5′ flanking region and chromosomal localization of the gene endocing human platelet membrane glycoprotein Ib alpha. *Gene* **85**:517, 1989.
6. Nurden AT, Dupuis D, Kunicki TJ, Caen JP: Analysis of the glycoprotein and protein composition of Bernard-Soulier platelets by single and two dimensional sodium dodecyl sulfate-polyacrylamide gel electrophoresis. *J Clin Invest* **67**:1431, 1981.
7. McEver RP, Martin MN: A monoclonal antibody to a membrane glycoprotein binds only to activated platelets. *J Biol Chem* **259**:9799, 1984.
8. Hsu-Lin S, Berman CL, Furie BC, August D, Furie B: A platelet membrane protein expressed during platelet activation and secretion. Studies using a monoclonal antibody specific for thrombin-activated platelets. *J Biol Chem* **259**:9121, 1984.
9. Bevilacqua M, Butcher E, Furie B, Furie B, Gallatin M, Gimbrone M, Harlan J, Kishimoto K, Lasky L, McEver R, Paulson J, Rosen S, Seed B, Siegelman M, Springer T, Stoolman L, Tedder T, Varki A, Wagner D, Weissman I, Zimmerman G: Selectins: A family of adhesion receptors. *Cell* **67**:233, 1991.
10. McEver RP: Selectins: Novel receptors that mediate leukocyte adhesion during inflammation. *Thromb Haemost* **65**:223, 1991.
11. Larsen E, Celi A, Gilbert GE, Furie BC, Erban JK, Bonfanti R, Wagner DD, Furie B: PADGEM protein: A receptor that mediates the interaction of activated platelets with neutrophils and monocytes. *Cell* **59**:305, 1989.
12. Albelda SM, Buck CA: Integrins and other cell adhesion molecules. *FASEB J* **4**:2868, 1990.
13. Hynes RO: Integrins, a family of cell surface receptors. *Cell* **48**:549, 1987.
14. Pidard D, Montgomery RR, Bennett JS, Kunicki TJ: Interaction of AP-2, a monoclonal antibody specific for the human platelet glycoprotein IIb-IIIa complex, with intact platelets. *J Biol Chem* **258**:12582, 1983.
15. Beckstead JH, Stenberg PE, McEver RP, Shuman MA, Bainton DF: Immunohistochemical localization of membrane and alpha-granule proteins in human megakaryocytes: Application to plastic-embedded bone marrow biopsy specimens. *Blood* **67**:285, 1986.
16. Fitzgerald LA, Poncz M, Steiner B, Rall SC Jr, Bennett

JS, Phillips DR: Comparison of cDNA-derived protein sequences of the human fibronectin and vitronectin receptor alpha-subunits and platelet glycoprotein IIb. *Biochemistry* **26**:8158, 1987.
17. Poncz M, Newman PJ: Analysis of rodent platelet glycoprotein IIb: Evidence for evolutionarily conserved domains and alternative proteolytic processing. *Blood* **75**:1282, 1990.
18. Coller BS, Cheresh DA, Asch E, Seligsohn U: Platelet vitronectin receptor expression differentiates Iraqi-Jewish from Arab patients with Glanzmann thrombasthenia in Israel. *Blood* **77**:75, 1991.
19. Thiagarajan P, Shapiro SS, Levine E, DeMarco L, Yalcin A: A monoclonal antibody to human platelet Glycoprotein IIIa detects a related protein in cultured human endothelial cells. *J Clin Invest* **75**:896, 1985.
20. Santoro SA: Identification of a 160,000 dalton platelet membrane protein that mediates the initial divalent cation-dependent adhesion of platelets to collagen. *Cell* **46**:913, 1986.
21. Kunicki TJ, Nugent DJ, Staats SJ, Orchekowski RP, Wayner EA, Carter WG: The human fibroblast class II extracellular matrix receptor mediates platelet adhesion to collagen and is identical to the platelet glycoprotein Ia-IIa complex. *J Biol Chem* **263**:4516, 1988.
22. Piotrowicz RS, Orchekowski RP, Nugent DJ, Yamada KY, Kunicki TJ: Glycoprotein Ic-IIa functions as an activation-independent fibronectin receptor on human platelets. *J Cell Biol* **106**:1359, 1988.
23. Sonnenberg A, Modderman PW, Hogervorst F: Laminin receptor on platelets in the integrin VLA-6. *Nature* **336**:487, 1988.
24. Phillips DR, Charo IF, Scarborough RM: GPIIb-IIIa: The responsive integrin. *Cell* **65**:459, 1991.
25. Plow EF, Ginsberg MH: Cellular adhesion: GPIIb-IIIa as a prototypic adhesion receptor. *Prog Hemost Thromb* **9**:117, 1989.
26. Newman PJ: Platelet GPIIb-IIIa: Molecular variations and alloantigens. *Thromb Haemost* **66**:111, 1991.
27. Bray PF, Rosa JP, Lingappa VR, Kan YW, McEver RP, Shuman MA: Biogenesis of the platelet receptor for fibrinogen: Evidence for separate precursors for glycoproteins IIb and IIa. *Proc Natl Acad Sci USA* **83**:1480, 1986.
28. Silver SM, McDonough MM, Vilaire G, Bennett JS: The in vitro synthesis of polypeptides for the platelet membrane glycoproteins IIb and IIIa. *Blood* **69**:1031, 1987.
29. Letellier SJ, Hunter JB, Aster RH: Probable genetic linkage between genes coding for platelet-specific antigens of the PlA and Bak systems. *Am J Hematol* **29**:139, 1988.
30. Bray PF, Barsh G, Rosa JP, Luo XY, Magenis E, Shuman MA: Physical linkage of the genes for platelet membrane glycoproteins IIb and IIIa. *Proc Natl Acad Sci USA* **85**:8683, 1988.
31. Bray PF, Rosa JP, Johnston GI, Shiu DT, Cook RG, Lau C, Kan YW, McEver RP, Shuman MA: Platelet glycoprotein IIb. Chromosomal localization and tissue expression. *J Clin Invest* **80**:1812, 1987.
32. Poncz M, Eisman R, Heidenreich R, Silver SM, Vilaire G, Surrey S, Schwartz E, Bennett JS: Structure of the platelet membrane glycoprotein IIb. Homology to the alpha subunits of the vitronectin and fibronectin membrane receptors. *J Biol Chem* **262**:8476, 1987.
33. Brass LF, Shattil SJ, Kunicki TJ, Bennett JS: Effect of calcium on the stability of the platelet membrane glycoprotein IIb-IIIa complex. *J Biol Chem* **260**:7875, 1985.
34. Kunicki TJ, Pidard D, Rosa J-P, Nurden AT: The formation of Ca^{++} – dependent complexes of platelet membrane glycoproteins IIb and IIIa in solution as determined by crossed immunoelectrophoresis. *Blood* **58**:268, 1981.
35. Fitzgerald LA, Phillips DR: Calcium regulation of the platelet membrane glycoprotein IIb-IIIa complex *J Biol Chem* **260**:11366, 1985.
36. Zimrin AB, Eisman R, Vilaire G, Schwartz E, Bennett JS, Poncz M: Structure of platelet glycoprotein IIIa. A common subunit for two different emembrane receptors. *J Clin Invest* **81**:1470, 1988.
37. Fitzgerald LA, Steiner B, Rall SC, Jr, Lo SS, Phillips DR: Protein sequence of endothelial glycoprotein IIIa derived from a cDNA clone. Identity with platelet glycoprotein IIIa and similarity to "integrin." *J Biol Chem* **262**:3936, 1987.
38. Rosa JP, Bray PF, Gayet O, Johnston GI, Cook RG, Jackson KW, Shuman MA, McEver RP: Cloning of glycoprotein IIIa cDNA from human erythroleukemia cells and localization of the gene to chromosome 17. *Blood* **72**:593, 1988.
39. Calvete JJ, Rivas G, Maruri M, Alvarez MV, McGregor JL, Hew CL, Gonzalez-Rodriguez J: Tryptic digestion of human GPIIIa. Isolation and biochemical characterization of the 23 kDa N-terminal glycopeptide carrying the antigenic determinant for a monoclonal antibody (P37) which inhibits platelet aggregation. *Biochem J* **250**:697, 1988.
40. Biewiarowski S, Norton KJ, Echardt A, Lukasiewicz H, Holt JC, Kornecki E: Structural and functional characterization of major platelet membrane components derived by limited proteolysis of glycoprotein IIIa. *Biochim Biophys Acta* **983**:91, 1989.
41. Beer J, Coller BS: Evidence that platelet glycoprotein IIIa has a large disulfide-bonded loop that is susceptible to proteolytic cleavage. *J Biol Chem* **264**:17564, 1989.
42. Calvete JJ, Henschen A, Gonzalez-Rodriguez J: Assignment of disulphide bonds in human platelet GPIIIa. A disulphide pattern for the beta-subunits of the integrin family. *Biochem J* **274**:63, 1991.
43. D'Souza SE, Ginsberg MH, Lam SC, Plow EF: Chemical cross-linking of arginyl-glycyl-aspartic acid peptides to an adhesion receptor on platelets. *J Biol Chem* **263**:3943, 1988.
44. McEver RP, Baenziger JU, Majerus PW: Isolation and structural characterization of the polypeptide subunits of membrane glycoprotein IIb-IIIa from human platelets. *Blood* **59**:80, 1982.
45. Newman PJ, Martin LS, Knipp MA, Kahn RA: Studies on the nature of the human platelet alloantigen, Pl_{A1}: Localization to a 17,000-dalton polypeptide. *Mol Immunol* **22**:719, 1985.
46. Tsuji T, Osawa T: Structures of the carbohydrate chains of membrane glycoproteins IIb and IIIa of human platelets. *Biochem* **100**:1387, 1986.
47. Duperray A, Berthier R, Chagnon E, Ryckewaert JJ, Ginsberg M, Plow E, Marguerie G: Biosynthesis and processing of platelet GPIIb-IIIa in human megakaryocytes. *J Cell Biol* **104**:1665,1987.
48. Calvete JJ, Henschen A, Gonzalez-Rodriguez J: Complete localization of the intrachain disulphide bonds and the N glycosylation points in the alpha-subunit of human platelet glycoprotein IIB. *Biochem J* **261**:561, 1989.
49. Newman PJ, Allen RW, Kahn RA, Kunicki TJ: Quantitation of membrane glycoprotein IIIa on intact human platelets using the monoclonal antibody, AP-3. *Blood* **65**:227, 1985.
50. Woods VL Jr, Wolff LE, Keller DM: Resting platelets contain a substantial centrally located pool of glycoprotein IIb-IIIa complex which may be accessible to some but not other extracellular proteins. *J Biol Chem* **261**:15242, 1986.
51. Wencel-Drake JD, Plow EF, Kunicki TJ, Woods VL, Keller DM, Ginsberg MH: Localization of internal pools of membrane glycoproteins involved in platelet adhesive responses. *Am J Pathol* **124**:324, 1986 – 52.
52. O'Toole TE, Mandelman D, Forsyth J, Shattil SJ, Plow EF, Ginsberg MH: Modulation of the affinity of integrin-alphaIIbbeta3 (GPIIb-IIIa) by the cytoplasmic domain of alphaIIb. *Science* **254**:845, 1991.
53. Chen Y-P, Djaffar I, Pidard D, Steiner B, Cieutat A-M, Caen JP, Rosa J-P: Ser-752 —> Pro mutation in the cytoplasmic domain of integrin β_3 subunit and defective activation of platelet integrin $\alpha_{IIIb}\beta_3$ (glycoprotein IIb-IIIa) in a variant of Glanzmann thrombasthenia. *Proc Natl Acad Sci USA* **89**:10169, 1992.
54. Ginsberg MH, Du X, Plow EF: Inside-out integrin signalling. *Curr Opin Cell Biol* **4**:766, 1992.
55. Pierschbacher MD, Ruoslahti E: Cell attachment activity of fibronectin can be duplicated by small synthetic fragments of the molecule. *Nature* **309**:30, 1984.
56. Haverstick DM, Cowan JF, Yamada KM, Santoro SA: Inhibition of platelet adhesion to fibronectin, fibrinogen, and von Willebrand factor by a synthetic tetrapeptide derived from the cell-binding domain of fibronectin. *Blood* **66**:946, 1985.

57. Pytela R, Pierschbacher MD, Ginsberg MH, Plow EF, Ruoslahti E: Platelet membrane glycoprotein IIb/IIIa: Member of a family of Arg-Gly-Asp-specific adhesion receptors. *Science* **231**:1559, 1986.
58. Ginsberg MH, Pierschbacher MD, Ruoslahti E, Marguerie G, Plow EF: Inhibition of fibronectin binding to platelets by proteolytic fragments and synthetic peptides which support fibroblast adhesion. *J Biol Chem* **260**:3931, 1985.
59. Hawiger J, Timmons S, Kloczewiak M, Strong DD, Doolittle RF: Gamma and alpha chains of human fibrinogen possess sites reactive with human platelet receptors. *Proc Natl Acad Sci USA* **79**:2068, 1982.
60. Amrani DL, Newman PJ, Meh D, Mosesson MW: The role of fibrinogen A alpha chains in ADP-induced platelet aggregation in the presence of fibrinogen molecules containing gamma' chains. *Blood* **72**:919, 1988–61.
61. Gartner TK, Bennett JS: The tetrapeptide analogue of the cell attachment site of fibronectin inhibits platelet aggregation and fibrinogen binding to activated platelets. *J Biol Chem* **260**:11891, 1985.
62. Plow EF, Pierschbacher MD, Ruoslahti E, Marguerie G, Ginsberg MH: The effect of Arg-Gly-Asp-containing peptides on fibrinogen and von Willebrand factor binding to platelets. *Proc Natl Acad Sci USA* **82**:8057, 1985.
63. Kloczewiak M, Timmons S, Lukas TJ, Hawiger J: Platelet receptor recognition site on human fibrinogen. Synthesis and structure-function relationships of peptides corresponding to the carboxy-terminal segment of the gamma chain. *Biochemistry* **23**:1767, 1984.
64. Timmons S, Bednarek MA, Kloczewiak M, Hawiger J: Antiplatelet "hybrid" peptides analogous to receptor recognition domains on gamma and alpha chains of human fibrinogen. *Biochemistry* **28**:2929, 1989.
65. Hawiger J, Timmons S: Binding of fibrinogen and von Willebrand factor to platelet glycoprotein IIb-IIIa complex. *Methods Enzymol* **215**:228, 19982.
66. Plow EF, Strouji AH, Meyer D, Marguerie GA, Ginsberg MH: Evidence that three adhesive proteins interact with a common recognition site on activated platelets. *J Biol Chem* **5388**:5391, 1984.
67. Bennett JS, Shattil SJ, Power JW, Gartner TK: Interaction of fibrinogen with its platelet receptor. Differential effects of alpha and gamma chain fibrinogen peptides on the glycoprotein IIb-IIIa complex. *J Biol Chem* **263**:12948, 1988.
68. D'Souza SE, Ginsberg MH, Burke TA, Plow EF: The ligand binding site of the platelet integrin receptor GPIIb-IIIa is proximal to the second calcium binding domain of its alpha subunit. *J Biol Chem* **265**:2440, 1990.
69. D'Souza SE, Ginsberg MH, Matsueda GR, Plow EF: A discrete sequence in a platelet integrin is involved in ligand recognition. *Nature* **350**:66, 1991.
70. Charo IF, Nannizzi L, Phillips DR, Hsu MA, Scarborough RM: Inhibition of fibrinogen binding to GP IIb-IIIa by a GP IIIa peptide. *J Biol Chem* **266**:1415, 1991.
71. Saiki RK, Scharf S, Faloona F, Mullis KB, Horn GT, Erlich HA, Arnheim N: Enzymatic amplification of β-globin gene sequences and restriction site analysis for diagnosis of sickle cell anemia. *Science* **230**:1350, 1985.
72. Kogan SC, Doherty M, Gitschier J: An improved method for prenatal diagnosis of genetic diseases by analysis of amplified DNA sequences. Application to Hemophilia A. *N Engl J Med* **317**:985, 1987.
73. Saiki RK, Gelfand DH, Stoffel S, Scharf SJ, Higuchi RG, Horn GT, Mullis KB, Erlich HA: Primer-directed enzymatic amplification of DNA with a thermostable DNA polymerase. *Science* **239**:487, 1988.
74. Newman PJ, Gorski J, White GC, Gidwitz S, Cretney CJ, Aster RH: Enzymatic amplification of platelet-specific messenger RNA using the polymerase chain reaction. *J Clin Invest* **82**:739, 1988.
75. Glanzmann E: Hereditare hamorrhagische thrombasthenie: ein beitrag zur pathologie der blut plattchen. *J Kinderkr* **88**:113, 1918.
76. Braunsteiner H, Pakesch F: Thrombocytoasthenia and thrombocytopathia. Old names and new diseases. *Blood* **2**:965, 1956.
77. Hardisty RM, Dormandy KM, Hutton RA: Thrombasthenia: Studies on three cases. *Br J Haematol* **10**:371, 1964.
78. Zucker MB, Pert JH, Hilgartner HR: Platelet function in a patient with thrombasthenia. *Blood* **28**:524, 1966.
79. George JN, Caen JP, Nurden AT: Glanzmann's thrombasthenia: The spectrum of clinical disease. *Blood* **75**:1383, 1990.
80. Reichert N, Seligsohn U, Ramot B: Thrombasthenia in Iraqi Jews, *Isr J Med Sci* **9**:1406, 1973.
81. Reichert N, Seligsohn U, Ramot B: Clinical and genetic aspects of Glanzmann's thrombasthenia in Israel. Report of 22 cases. *Thromb Diath Haemorrh* **34**:806, 1975.
82. Seligsohn U, Rososhansky S: A Glanzmann's thrombasthenia cluster among Iraqi Jews in Israel. *Thromb Haemost* **52**:230, 1984.
83. Awidi AS: Increased incidence of Glanzmann's thrombasthenia in Jordan as compared with Scandinavia. *Scand J Haematol* **30**:218, 1983.
84. Caen JP, Castaldi PA, Leclerc JC, Inceman S, Larrieu M-J, Probst M, Bernard J: Congenital bleeding disorders with long bleeding time and normal platelet count. I. Glanzmann's thrombasthenia (report of fifteen patients). *Am J Med* **41**:4, 1966.
85. Bentegeat J, Verger P, Boisseau M, De Ioigny C, Guiliard JM, Le Menn R: Considerations cliniques, genetiques, biologiques et physiologiques sur la thrombasthenie de Glanzmann (a propos de 5 cas). *Coagulation* **1**:237, 1968.
86. Levy JM, Mayer G, Sacrez R, Ruff R, Francfort JJ, Rodier L: Glanzmann thrombasthenia-Naegeli. Study of a strongly endogamous ethnic group [Fre]. *Semin Hop Paris* **47**:129, 1971.
87. Khanduri U, Pulimood R, Sudarsanam A, Carman RH, Jadhav M, Pereira S: Glanzmann's thrombasthenia. A review and report of 42 cases from South India. *Thromb Haemost* **46**:717, 1981.
88. Caen JP: Glanzmann's thrombasthenia. *Clin Haematol* **1**:383, 1972.
89. Nurden AT, Caen JP: An abnormal platelet glycoprotein pattern in three cases of Glanzmann's thrombasthenia. *Br J Haematol* **28**:253, 1974.
90. Nurden AT, Caen JP: Specific roles for platelet surface glycoproteins in platelet function. *Nature* **255**:720, 1975.
91. Phillips DR, Agin PP: Platelet membrane defects in Glanzmann's thrombasthenia. Evidence for decreased amounts of two major glycoproteins. *J Clin Invest* **60**:535, 1977.
92. Kunicki TJ, Aster RH: Deletion of the platelet-specific alloantigen Pl^{A1} from platelets in Glanzmann's thrombasthenia. *J Clin Invest* **61**:1225, 1978.
93. Hagen I, Nurden AT, Bjerrum OJ, Solum NO, Caen JP: Immunochemical evidence for protein abnormalities in platelets from patients with Glanzmann's thrombasthenia and Bernard Soulier syndrome. *J Clin Invest* **65**:722, 1980.
94. Kunicki TJ, Nurden AT, Pidard D, Russell NR, Caen JP: Characterization of human platelet glycoprotein antigens giving rise to individual immunoprecipitates in crossed-immunoelectrophoresis. *Blood* **58**:1190, 1981.
95. Holahan JR, White GC: Heterogeneity of membrane surface proteins in Glanzmann's thrombasthenia. *Blood* **57**:174, 1981.
96. Ginsberg MH, Lightsey A, Kunicki TJ, Kaufmann A, Marguerie G, Plow EF: Divalent cation regulation of the surface orientation of platelet membrane glycoprotein IIb. Correlation with fibrinogen binding function and definition of a novel variant of Glanzmann's thrombasthenia. *J Clin Invest* **78**:1103, 1986.
97. Caen JP, Rosa JP, Boizard B, Nurden AT: Thrombasthenia Paris I Lariboisiere variant, a model for the study of the platelet glycoprotein (GP) IIb-IIIa complex. *Blood* **62**:951a, 1983. (Abstr.).
98. Nurden AT, Rosa JP, Fournier D, Legrand C, Didry D, Parquet A, Pidard D: A variant of Glanzmann's thrombasthenia with abnormal glycoprotein IIb-IIIa complexes in the platelet membrane. *J Clin Invest* **79**:962, 1987.
99. Fournier DJ, Kabral A, Castaldi PA, Berndt MC: A variant of Glanzmann's thrombasthenia characterized by abnormal glycoprotein IIb/IIIa complex formation. *Thromb Haemost* **62**:977, 1989.
100. Bennett JS, Vilaire G: Exposure of platelet fibrinogen

receptors by ADP and epinephrine. *J Clin Invest* **64**:1393, 1979.

101. Ruggeri ZM, Bader R, De Marco L: Glanzmann thrombasthenia: Deficient binding of von Willebrand factor to thrombin-stimulated platelets. *Proc Natl Acad Sci USA* **79**:6038, 1982.
102. Kato A, Yamamoto K, Aoki N: Classification of Glanzmann's thrombasthenia based on the intracellular transport pathway of GPIIb-IIIa. *Thromb Haemost* **68**:615, 1992.
103. Jennings LK, Ashmun RA, Wang WC, Docker ME: Analysis of human platelet glycoproteins IIb-IIIa and Glanzmann's thrombasthenia in whole blood by flow cytometry. *Blood* **68**:173, 1986.
104. Nurden AT, Didry D, Kieffer N, McEver RP: Residual amounts of glycoproteins IIb and IIIa may be present in the platelets of most patients with Glanzmann's thrombasthenia. *Blood* **65**:1021, 1985.
105. McEver RP, Baenziger NL, Majerus PW: Isolation and quantitation of the platelet membrane glycoprotein deficient in thrombasthenia using a monoclonal hybridoma antibody. *J Clin Invest* **66**:1311, 1980.
106. Montgomery RR, Kunicki TJ, Taves C, Pidard D, Corcoran M: Diagnosis of Bernard-Soulier syndrome and Glanzmann's thrombasthenia with a monoclonal assay on whole blood. *J Clin Invest* **71**:385, 1983.
107. Coller BS, Seligsohn U, Little PA: Type I Glanzmann thrombasthenia patients from the Iraqi-Jewish and Arab populations in Israel can be differentiated by platelet glycoprotein IIIa immunoblot analysis. *Blood* **69**:1696, 1987.
108. Burk CD, Newman PJ, Lyman S, Gill J, Coller BS, Poncz M: A deletion in the gene for glycoprotein IIb associated with Glanzmann's thrombasthenia. *J Clin Invest* **87**:270, 1991.
109. Bray PF, Shuman MA: Identification of an abnormal gene for the GPIIIa subunit of the platelet fibrinogen receptor resulting in Glanzmann's thrombasthenia. *Blood* **75**:881, 1990.
110. Loftus JC, O'Toole TE, Plow EF, Glass A, Frelinger AL, Ginsberg MH: A beta 3 integrin mutation abolishes ligand binding and alters divalent cation-dependent conformation. *Science* **249**:915, 1990.
111. Bajt ML, Ginsberg MH, Frelinger AL, Berndt MC, Loftus JC: A spontaneous mutation of integrin-alphaIIb/beta3 (platelet glycoprotein-IIb-IIIa) helps define a ligand binding site. *J Biol Chem* **267**:3789, 1992.
112. Lanza F, Stierle' A, Fournier D, Morales M, Andre' G, Nurden AT, Cazenave J-P: A new variant of Glanzmann's thrombasthenia (Strasbourg I). Platelets with functionally defective glycoprotein IIb-IIIa complexes and a glycoprotein IIIa ^{214}Arg—>^{214}Trp mutation. *J Clin Invest* **89**:1995, 1992.
113. Rifat S, Coller BS, Newman PJ, Shattil SJ, Parella T, Fortina P, Bennett JS, Poncz M: Glanzmann thrombasthenia secondary to a Gly^{273}—>Asp mutation in the 1st calcium-binding domain of platelet glycoprotein IIb. *Clin Res* **40**:210a, 1992. (abstr.).
114. Wilcox DA, Wautier JL, Pidard D, Newman PJ: An amino acid substitution within the fourth calcium binding domain of GPIIb results in degradation of the integrin GPIIb-IIIa and Type I Glanzmann thrombasthenia. *Circulation* **86**:682a, 1992. (abstr.).
115. O'Toole TE, Loftus JC, Plow EF, Glass AA, Harper JR, Ginsberg MH: Efficient surface expression of platelet GPIIb-IIIa requires both subunits. *Blood* **74**:14, 1989.
116. Li L, Bray PF: Homologous recombination among 3 alu sequences in the GPIIIa gene causes a deletion-inversion in Glanzmann thrombasthenia. *Blood* **80**:164a, 1992.
117. Newman PJ, Seligsohn U, Lyman S, Coller BS: The molecular genetic basis of Glanzmann thrombasthenia in the Iraqi-Jewish and Arab populations in Israel. *Proc Natl Acad Sci USA* **88**:3160, 1991.
118. Peretz H, Seligsohn U, Swang E, Coller BS, Newman PJ: Detection of the Glanzmann thrombasthenia mutations in Arab and Iraqi-Jewish patients by polymerase chain reaction and restriction analysis of blood or urine samples. *Thromb Haemost* **66**:500, 1991.
119. Baumgartner HR, Muggli R: Adhesion and aggregation: Morphological demonstration and quantitation in vivo and in vitro, in Gordon JL (ed): *Platelets in Biology and Pathology. New York*, Elsevier, 1976, p. 23.
120. Baumgartner HR, Tschopp TB, Meyer D: Shear rate dependent inhibition of platelet adhesion and aggregation on collagenous surfaces by antibodies to Factor VIII/von Willebrand factor. *Br J Haematol* **44**:127, 1980.
121. Turritto VT, Weiss HJ, Zimmerman TS, Sussman II: Factor VIII/von Willebrand factor in subendothelium mediates platelets adhesion. *Blood* **65**:823, 1985.
122. Turritto VT, Weiss HJ, Baumgartner HS: Decreased platelet adhesion on vessel segment in von Willebrand's disease: A defect in initial platelet attachment. *J Lab Clin Med* **102**:551, 1983.
123. Jorgensen L, Borchgrevink CF: The hemostatic mechanism in patients with haemorrhagic diseases: A histological study of wounds made for primary and secondary bleeding time tests. *Acta Pathol Microbiol Scand* **60**:55, 1964.
124. Hovig T, Stormorken H: Ultrastructural studies on the platelet plug in bleeding time wounds from normal individuals and patients with von Willebrand's Disease. *Acta Pathol Microbiol Immunol Scand* **248**:105, 1974.
125. Sixma JJ, Wester J: The hemostatic plug. *Semin Hematol* **14**:265, 1977.
126. Ruggeri ZM, De Marco L, Gatti L, Bader R, Montgomery RR: Platelets have more than one binding site for von Willebrand factor. *J Clin Invest* **72**:1, 1983.
127. Sixma JJ, Sakariassen KS, Besser-Visser NH, Ottenhof-Rovers M, Bolhuis PA: Adhesion of platelets to human artery subendothelium: Effect of factor VIII- von Willebrand factor of various multimeric composition. *Blood* **63**:128, 1984.
128. Chopek MW, Gilma J-P, Fujikawa K, Davis EW, Titani K: Human von Willebrand factor: A multivalent protein composed of identical subunits. *Biochemistry* **25**:3146, 1986.
129. Coller BS, Peerschke EL, Scudder IE, Sullivan CA: Studies with a murine monoclonal antibody that abolishes ristocetin-induced bindign of von Willebrand factor to platelets: Additional evidence in support of GPIb as a platelet receptor for von Willebrand factor. *Blood* **61**:99, 1983.
130. Phillips DR, Jakabova M: Ca2+-dependent protease in human platelets. Specific cleavage of platelet polypeptides in the presence of added Ca2+. *J Biol Chem* **252**:5602, 1977.
131. Okumura T, Lombart C, Jamieson GA: Platelet glycocalicin II. Purification and characterization. *J Biol Chem* **251**:5950, 1976.
132. Handa M, Titani K, Holland LZ, Roberts JR, Ruggeri Z: The von Willebrand factor-binding domain of platelet membrane glycoprotein Ib. *J Biol Chem* **261**:12579, 1986.
133. Wicki AN, Clemetson KJ: Structure and function of platelet membrane glycoprotein Ib and V. Effects of leucocyte elastase and other proteases on platelets response to von Willebrand factor and thrombin. *Eur J biochem* **153**:1, 1985.
134. Ganguly P: Binding of thrombin to functionally defective platelets. A hypothesis on the nature of the thrombin receptor. *Br J Haematol* **37**:47, 1977.
135. Okumura T, Hasitz M, Jamieson GA: Platelet glycocalicin: Interaction with thrombin and role as a thrombin receptor on the platelet surface. *J Biol Chem* **253**:435, 1978.
136. Yamamoto K, Yamamoto N, Kitagawa H, Tanoue K, Kosaki G, Yamazaki H: Localization of a thrombin-binding site on human platelet membrane Ib determined by a monoclonal antibody. *Thromb Haemost* **55**:162, 1986.
137. Berndt MC, Gregory C, Dowden G, Castaldi PA: Thrombin interactions with platelet membrane proteins. *Ann NY Acad Sci* **485**:374, 1986.
138. McGowan EB, Detweiler TC: Modified platelet responses to thrombin. Evidence for two types of receptors or coupling mechanisms. *J Biol Chem* **261**:739, 1986.
139. Vu T-KH, Hung DT, Wheaton VI, Coughlin SR: Molecular cloning of a functional thrombin receptor reveals a novel proteolytic mechanism of receptor activation. *Cell* **64**:1057, 1991.
140. Phillips DR, Agin PP: Platelet plasma membrane glycoproteins. Evidence for the presence of nonequivalent disulfide bonds using nonreduced-reduced two-dimensional gel electrophoresis. *J Biol Chem* **252**:2121, 1977.
141. Fox JEB, Aggerbeck LP, Berndt MC: Structure of the glycoprotein Ib-IX complex from platelet membranes. *J Biol Chem* **263**:4882, 1988.
142. Bienz D, Schnippering W, Clemetson KJ: Glycoprotein

V is not the thrombin activation receptor on human blood platelets. *Blood* **68**:720, 1986.
143. Zafar RS, Walz DA: Platelet membrane glycoprotein V: Characterization of the thrombin-sensitive glycoprotein from human platelets. *Thromb Res* **53**:31, 1989.
144. Hickey MJ, Williams SA, Roth GJ: Human platelet glycoprotein IX: An adhesive prototype of leucine-rich glycoproteins with flank-center-flank structures. *Proc Natl Acad Sci USA* **86**:6773, 1989.
145. Roth GJ, Ozols J, Nugent DJ, Williams SA: Isolation and characterization of human platelet glycoprotein IX. *Biochem Biophys Res Commun* **156**:931, 1988.
146. Hickey MJ, Deaven LL, Roth GJ: Human platelet glycoprotein IX. Characterization of cDNA and localization of the gene to chromosome 3. *FEBS LETT* **274**:189, 1990.
147. Wenger RH, Kieffer N, Wicki AN, Clemetson KJ: Structure of the human blood platelet membrane glycoprotein Ib alpha gene. *Biochem Biophys Res Commun* **156**:389, 1988.
148. Lopez JA, Chung DW, Fujikawa K, Hagen FS, Papayannopoulou T, Roth GJ: Cloning of the alpha chain of human platelet glycoprotein Ib: A transmembrane protein with homology to leucine-rich alpha 2-glycoprotein. *Proc Natl Acad Sci USA* **84**:5615, 1987.
149. Lopez JA, Chung DW, Fujikawa K, Hagen FS, Davie EW, Roth GJ: The alpha and beta chains of human platelet glycoprotein Ib are both transmembrane proteins containing a leucine-rich amino acid sequence. *Proc Natl Acad Sci USA* **85**:2135, 1988.
150. Canfield VA, Ozols J, Nugent D, Roth GJ: Isolation and characterization of the alpha and beta chains of human platelet glycoprotein Ib. *Biochem Biophys Res Commun* **147**:526, 1987.
151. Roth GJ, Church TA, McMullen BA, Williams SA: Human platelet glycoprotein V: A surface leucine-rich glycoprotein related to adhesion. *Biochem Biophys Res Commun* **170**:153, 1990.
152. Reinke R, Krantz DE, Yen D, Zipursky SL: Chaoptin, a cell surface glycoprotein required for Drosophila photoreceptor cell morphogenesis, contains a repeat motif found in yeast and human. *Cell* **52**:291, 1988.
153. McFarland KC, Sprengel R, Phillips HS, Kohler M, Rosemblit N, Nikolics K, Segaloff DL, Seeburg PH: Lutropin-choriogonadotropin receptor: An unusual member of the G protein-coupled receptor family. *Science* **245**:494, 1989.
154. Kataoka T, Broek D, Wigler M: DNA sequence and characterization of the S. cerevisae gene encoding adenylate cyclase. *Cell* **43**:493, 1985.
155. Landschultz WH, Johnson OF, McKnight SL: The leucine zipper: A hypothetical structure common to a new class of DNA binding proteins. *Science* **240**:1759, 1990.
156. Bohmann D, Bos TJ, Admon A, Nishimura T, Vogt PK, Tjian R: Human proto-oncogene c-jun encodes a DNA binding protein with structural and functional properties of transcription factor AP-1. *Science* **238**:1386, 1987.
157. Setoyama C, Frunzio R, Liau G, Mudryj M, de Crombrugghe B: Transcription activation encoded by the v-fos gene. *Proc Natl Acad Sci USA* **83**:3213, 1986.
158. Pepper DS, Jamieson GA: Isolation of a macroglycopeptide from human platelets. *Biochemistry* **9**:3706, 1970.
159. Vicente V, Houghten RA, Ruggeri ZM: Identification of a site in the alpha chain of platelet glycoprotein Ib that participates in von Willebrand factor binding. *J Biol Chem* **265**:274, 1990.
160. Handin RI, Peterson E: Production of recombinant glycoprotein Ibalpha fragments and delineation of the von Willebrand factor binding site. *Blood* **74**:4777, 1989.
161. Howard MA, Firkin BG: Ristocetin—a new tool in the investigation of platelet aggregation. *Thromb Diath Haemorrh* **26**:362, 1971.
162. Andrews RK, Gorman JJ, Booth WJ, Corino GL, Castaldi PA, Berndt MC: Cross-linking of a monomeric 39/34-kDa dispase fragment of von Willebrand factor (Leu 480/Val-481-Gly-718) to the N-terminal region of the α-chain of membrane glycoprotein Ib on intact platelets with bis(sulfosuccinimidyl)suberate. *Biochemistry* **28**:8326, 1989.
163. Mohri H, Yoshioka A, Zimmerman TS, Ruggeri ZM: Isolation of the von Willebrand factor domain interacting with platelet glycoprotein Ib, heparin, and collagen and characterization of its three distinct functional sites. *J Biol Chem* **264**:17361, 1989.
164. Randi AM, Rabinowitz I, Mancuso DJ, Mannucci PM, Sadler JE: Molecular basis of von Willebrand disease type IIB. Candidate mutations cluster in one disulfide loop between proposed platelet glycoprotein Ib binding sequences. *J Clin Invest* **87**:1220, 1991.
165. Cooney KA, Nichols WC, Bruck ME, Bahou WF, Shapiro AD, Bowie EJW, Gralnick HR, Ginsberg D: The molecular defect in type IIB von Willebrand disease. *J Clin Invest* **87**:1227, 1991.
166. Ribba AS, Lavergne JM, Bahnak BR, Derion A, Pietu G, Meyer D: Duplication of a methionine within the glycoprotein Ib binding domain of von Willebrand factor detected by denaturing gradient gel electrophoresis in a patient with type IIB von Willebrand disease. *Blood* **78**:1738, 1991.
167. Lillicrap D, Murray EW, Benford K, Blanchette VS, Rivard GE, Wensley R, Giles AR: Recurring mutations at CpG dinucleotides in the region of the von Willebrand factor gene encoding the glycoprotein Ib binding domain, in patients with type IIB von Willebrand's disease. *Br J Haematol* **79**:612, 1991.
168. Holmberg L, Donner M, Dahlback B, Nilsson IB: Apparently recessive IIB von Willebrand disease (vWD) is caused by de novo mutations (Arg543->Trp; Val551->Leu). *Blood* **78**:150, 1991.
169. Randi AM, Tuley EA, Jorieux S, Rabinowitz I, Sadler JE: A missense mutation (R578Q) in von Willebrand disease (vWD) affects von Willebrand factor (vWF) binding to GPIb but not to collagen or heparin: Studies with recombinant vWF. *Blood* **78**:179, 1991.
170. Rabinowitz I, Mancuso DJ, Tuley EA, Randi AM, Firkin BG, Howard MA, Sadler JE: von Willebrand disease (vWd) type B, a variant with absent ristocetin—but normal ristocetin cofactor activity is caused by a missense mutation in the GPIb binding domain of von Willebrand factor (vWf). *Blood* **78**:179, 1991.
171. Weiss HJ, Rodgers J, Brand H: Defective ristocetin-induced platelet aggregation in von Willebrand's disease and its correction by factor VIII. *J Clin Invest* **52**:2697, 1973.
172. Krolls MH, Harris TS, Moake JL, Handin RI, Schafer AI: von Willebrand factor binding to platelet GPIb initiates signals for platelet activation. *J Clin Invest* **88**:1568, 1991.
173. Fox JEB, Reynolds CF, Johnson MM: Identification of glycoprotein Ibβ as oen of the major proteins phosphorylated during exposure of intact platelets to agents that activate cyclic AMP-dependent protein kinase. *J Biol Chem* **12627, 1987.**
174. Krools MH, Schafer AI: Biochemical mechanisms of platelet activation. *Blood* **74**:1181, 1989.
175. Fox JEB: Identification of actin-binding protein as the protein linking the membrane skeleton to glycoproteins on platelet plasma membranes. *J Biol Chem* **260**:11970, 1985.
176. Okita JR, Pidard D, Newman PJ, Montgomery RR, Kunicki TJ: On the association of glycoprotein Ib and actin-binding protein in human platelets. *J Cell Biol* **100**:317, 1985.
177. White JG, Burris SM, Hasegawa D, Johnson M: Micropipette aspiration of human blood platelets. A defect in Bernard-Soulier syndrome. *Blood* **63**:1249, 1984.
178. Bernard J, Soulier JP: Sur une nouvele variete de dystrophie thrombocytaire haemoragipare congenitale. *Semin Hop Paris* **24**:3217, 1948.
179. Kanska B, Niewiarowski S, Ostrowski L, Poplawski A, Prokopowicz J: Macrothrombocytic thrombopathia. Clinical, coagulation and hereditary aspects. *Thromb Diath Haemorrh* **10**:88, 1963.
180. Cullum C, Cooney DP, Schrier SL: Familial thrombocytopenic thrombocytopathy. *Br J Haematol* **13**:147, 1967.
181. Grottum KA, Solum NO: Congenital thrombocytopenia with giant platelets: A defect in the platelet membrane. *Br J Haematol* **16**:277, 1969.
182. Bithell TC, Parekh SJ, Strong RR: Platelet-function studies in the Bernard-Soulier syndrome. *Ann NY Acad Sci* **201**:145, 1972.
183. Jenkins CS, Phillips DR, Clemetson KJ, Meyer D, Larrieu MJ, Luscher EF: Platelet membrane glycoproteins implicated in ristocetin-induced aggregation. Studies of the proteins on platelets from patients with Bernard-Soulier syn-

drome and von Willebrand's disease. *J Clin Invest* **57**:112, 1976.
184. Howard MA, Hutton RA, Hardisty RM: Hereditary giant platelet syndrome: A disorder of a new aspect of platelet function. *Br Med J* **2**:586, 1973.
185. Evensen SA, Solum NO, Grottum KA, Hovig T: Familial bleeding disorder with a moderate thrombocytopenia and giant platelets. *Scand J Haematol* **13**:203, 1974.
186. Maldonado JE, Gilchrist GS, Brigden LP, Bowie EJW: Ultrastructure of platelets in Bernard-Soulier syndrome. *Mayo Clin Proc* **50**:402, 1975.
187. Weiss HJ, Tschopp TB, Baumgartner HR, Sussman II, Johnson MM, Egan JJ: Decreased adhesion of giant (Bernard-Soulier) platelets to subendothelium. Further implications on the role of the von Willebrand factor in hemostasis. *Am J Med* **57**:920, 1974.
188. Walsh PN, Mills DCB, Pareti FI, Stewart GJ, MacFarlane DE, Johnson MM, Egan JJ: Hereditary giant platelet syndrome. Absence of collagen-induced coagulant activity and deficiency of factor-XI binding to platelets. *Br J Haematol* **29**:639, 1975.
189. Caen JP, Nurden AT, Jeanneau C, Michel H, Tobelem G, Levy-Toledano S, Sultan Y, Valensi F, Bernard J: Bernard-Soulier syndrome: A new platelet glycoprotein abnormality. It relationship with platelet adhesion to the subendothelium and with the Factor VIII von Willebrand protein. *J Lab Clin Med* **87**:586, 1976.
190. George JN, Reimann TA, Moake JL, Morgan RK, Cimo PL, Sears DA: Bernard-Soulier disease: A study of four patients and their parents. *Br J Haematol* **48**:459, 1981.
191. Ingerslev J, Stenbjerg S, Taaning E: A case of Bernard-Soulier syndrome: Study of platelet glycoprotein Ib in a kindred. *Eur J Haematol* **39**:182, 1987.
192. Stevens MC, Blanchette VS, Freedman MH, Sparling C, Kunicki TJ: A variant form of Bernard-Soulier syndrome: Mild haemostatic defect associated with partial platelet GPIb deficiency. *Clin Lab Haematol* **10**:443, 1988.
193. De Marco L, Mazzucato M, Fabris F, De Roia D, Coser P, Girolami A, Vicente V, Ruggeri ZM: Variant Bernard-Soulier syndrome type bolzano. A congenital bleeding disorder due to a structural and functional abnormality of the platelet glycoprotein Ib-IX complex. *J Clin Invest* **86**:25, 1990.
194. Poulsen LO, Taaning E: Variation in surface platelet glycoprotein Ib expression in Bernard-Soulier syndrome. *Haemostasis* **20**:155, 1990.
195. Waldenstrom E, Holmberg L, Axelsson U, Winqvist I, Nilsson IM: Bernard-Soulier syndrome in two Swedish families: Effect of DDAVP on bleeding time. *Eur J Haematol* **46**:182, 1991.
196. Arkel YS, Kamiyama M, Chen K, Lynch J, Kunicki J, Schacht N, Soni R: Variant Bernard-Soulier syndrome unassociated with excessive bleeding. *Blood* **78**:148, 1991.
197. Blanchette VS, Sparling C, Turner C: Inherited bleeding disorders. *Baillieres Clin Haematol* **4**:291, 1991.
198. Peng TC, Kickler TS, Bell WR, Haller E: Obstetric complications in a patient with Bernard-Soulier syndrome. *Am J Obstet Gynecol* **165**:425, 1991.
199. Saade G, Homsi R, Seoud M: Bernard-Soulier syndrome in pregnancy: A report of four pregnancies in one patient and review of the literature. *Eur J Obstet Gynecol Reprod Biol* **40**:149, 1991.
200. Cuthbert RJG, Watson HH, Handa SI, Abbott I, Ludlam CA: DDAVP shortens the bleeding time in Bernard-Soulier syndrome. Thromb Res 49:649, 1988.
201. Mant MJ: DDAVP in Bernard-Soulier syndrome. *Thromb Res* **52**:77, 1988.
202. DiMichele DM, Hathaway WE: Use of DDAVP in inherited and acquired platelet dysfunction. *Am J Haematol* **33**:39, 1990.
203. Clemetson KJ, McGregor JL, James E, Dechavanne M, Luscher EF: Characterization of the platelet membrane glycoprotein abnormalities in Bernard-Soulier syndrome and comparison with normal by surface labeling techniques and high resolution two-dimensional electrophoresis. *J Clin Invest* **70**:304, 1982.
204. Bernard J: History of congenital hemorrhagic thrombocytopathic dystrophy. *Blood Cells* **9**:179, 1983.
205. Bessman JD, Williams LJ, Gilmer PR Jr: Mean platelet volume. The inverse relation between platelet size and count in normal subjects and an artifact of other particles. *Am J Clin Pathol* **76**:289, 1981.
206. Odell TT Jr, McDonald TP, Detweiter TC: Stimulation of platelet production by serum of platelet depleted rats. *Proc Soc Exp Biol Med* **108**:428, 1961.
207. Hourdille P, Pico M, Jandrot-Perrus M, Lacaze D, Lozano M, Nurden At: Studies on the megakaryocytes of a patient with the Bernard-Soulier syndrome. *Br J Haematol* **76**:521, 1990.
208. Ware J, Russell SR, Vicente V, Scharf RE, Tomer A, McMillan R, Ruggeri ZM: Nonsense mutation in the glycoprotein Ib alpha coding sequence associated with Bernard-Soulier syndrome. *Proc Natl Acad Sci USA* **87**:2026, 1990.
209. Aakhus AM, Stavem P, Hovig T, Pedersen TM, Solum NO: Studies on a patient with thrombocytopenia, giant platelets and a platelet membrane Ib with reduced sialic acid. *Br J Haematol* **74**:320, 1987.
210. Miller JL, Lyle VA, Cunningham D: Mutation of leucine-57 to phenylanine in a platelet glycoprotein Ibα leucine tandem repeat occurring in patients with an autosomal dominant variant of Bernard-Soulier disease. *Blood* **79**:439, 1992.
211. Ware J, Russell SR, Murata M, Mazzucato M, De Marco L, Ruggeri ZM: Ala156->Val substitution in platelet glycoprotein Ibα impairs von Willebrand factor binding and is the molecular basis of Bernard-Soulier syndrome type Bolzano. *Blood* **78**:278a, 1991. (abstr.)
212. Lopez JA, Leung B, Reynolds CC, Li CQ, Fox JEB: Efficient membrane expression of a functional platelet glycoprotein Ib-IX complex requires the presence of its three subunits. *J Biol Chem* **267**:12851, 1992.
213. Finch CN, Miller JL, Lyle VA, Handin RI: Evidence that an abnormality in the glycoprotein Ib alpha gene is not the cause of abnormal platelet function in a family with classic Bernard-Soulier disease. *Blood* **75**:2357, 1990.
214. Takahashi H: Studies of the pathophysiology and treatment of von Willebrand's disease. IV. Mechanism of increased ristocetin-induced platelet aggregation in von Willebrand's disease. *Trhomb Res* **19**:857, 1980.
215. Weiss HJ, Meyer D, Rabinowitz R, Grima J-P, Vicic WJ, Rogers J: Pseudo-von Willebrand's disease. An intrinsic platelet defect with aggregation by unmodified human factor VIII/von Willebrand factor and enhanced absorption of its high-molecular-weight multimers. *N Engl J Med* **306**:326, 1982.
216. Gralnick HR, Williams SB, Shafer BC, Corash L: Factor VIII/von Willebrand factor for binding to von Willebrand's disease platelets. *Blood* **60**:328, 1982.
217. Miller JL, Castella A: Platelet-type von Willebrand's disease: Characterization of a new bleeding disorder. *Blood* **60**:790, 1982.
218. Miller JL, Kupinski JM, Castella A, Ruggeri ZM: Von Willebrand factor binds to platelets and induces aggregation in platelet-type but not type IIb von Willebrand disease. *J Clin Invest* **72**:1532, 1983.
219. Takahashi H: Replacement therapy in platelet-type von Willebrand disease. *Am J Hematol* **18**:351, 1985.
220. Takahashi H, Handa M, Watanabe K, Ando Y, Nagayama R, Hattori A, Shibata A, Federici A, Ruggeri ZM, Zimmerman TS: Further characterization of platelet-type von Willebrand's disease in Japan. *Blood* **64**:1254, 1984.
221. Miller JL: Platelet-type von Willebrand's disease. *Clin Lab Med* **4**:319, 1984.
222. Miller JL, Cunningham D, Lyle VA, Finch CN: Mutation in the gene encoding the alpha chain of platelet glycoprotein Ib in platelet-type von Willebrand disease. *Proc Natl Acad Sci USA* **88**:4761, 1991.
223. Russell SD, Roth GJ: A mutation in the platelet glycoprotein (GP) Ibα gene associated with pseudo-von Willebrand disease. *Blood* **78**:131a, 1991. (Abstr.).
224. Santoro SA, Rajpara SM, Staatz WD, Woods VL: Isolation and characterization of a platelet surface collagen binding complex related to VLA-2, *Biochem Biophys Res Commun* **153**:217, 1988.
225. Staatz WD, Rajpara SM, Wayner EA, Carter WG, Santoro SA: The membrane glycoprotein Ia-IIa (VLA-2) complex mediates the Mg + + -dependent adhesion of platelets to collagen. *J Cell Biol* **108**:1917, 1989.

226. Nieuwenhuis HK, Akkerman JWN, Houdijk WPM, Sixma JJ: Human blood platelets showing no response to collagen fail to express surface glycoprotein Ia. *Nature* **318**:470, 1985.
227. Kehrel B, Balleisen L, Kokott R, Mesters R, Stenzinger W, Clemetson KJ, van de Loo J: Deficiency of intact thrombospondin and membrane glycoprotein Ia in platelets with defective collagen-induced aggregation and spontaneous loss of disorder. *Blood* **71**:1074, 1988.
228. Greenwalt DE, Lipsky RH, Ockenhouse CF, Ikeda H, Tandon NN, Jamieson GA: Membrane glycoprotein CD36: A review of its roles in adherence, signal transduction, and transfusion medicine. *Blood* **80**:1105, 1992.
229. Tandon NN, Kralisz U, Jamieson GA: Identification of glycoprotein IV (CD36) as a primary receptor for platelet-collagen adhesion. *J Biol Chem* **264**:7576, 1989.
230. Silverstein RL, Asch AS, Nachman RL: Glycoprotein IV mediates thrombospondin-dependent platelet-monocyte and platelet-U937 cell adhesion. *J Clin Invest* **84**:546, 1989.
231. Ockenhouse CF, Tandon NN, Magowan C, Jamieson GA, Chulay JD: Identification of a platelet membrane glycoprotein as a falciparum malaria sequestration receptor [see comments]. *Science* **243**:1469, 1989.
232. Oquendo P, Hundt E, Lawler J, Seed B: CD36 directly mediates cytoadherence of Plasmodium falciparum parasitized erythrocytes. *Cell* **58**:95, 1989.
233. Barnwell JW, Asch AS, Nachman RL, Yamaya M, Aikawa M, Ingravallo P: A human 88-kD membrane glycoprotein (CD36) functions in vitro as a receptor for a cytoadherence ligand on *Plasmodium falciparum*-infected erythrocytes. *J Clin Invest* **84**:765, 1989.
234. Tomiyama Y, Take H, Ikeda H, Mitani T, Furubayashi T, Mizutani H, Yamamoto N, Tandon NN, Sekiguchi S, Jamieson GA, Kurata Y, Yonezawa T, Tarui S: Identification of the platelet-specific alloantigen, Naka, on platelet membrane glycoprotein IV. *Blood* **75**:684, 1990.
235. Yamamoto N, Ikeda H, Tandon NN, Herman J, Tomiyama Y, Mitani T, Sekiguchi S, Lipsky R, Kralisz U, Jamieson GA: A platelet membrane glycoprotein (GP) deficiency in healthy blood donors: Naka- platelets lack detectable GPIV (CD36). *Blood* **76**:1698, 1990.
236. Tandon NN, Ockenhouse CF, Greco NJ, Jamieson GA: Adhesive functions of platelets lacking glycoprotein-IV (CD36). *Blood* **78**:2809, 1991.
237. Yamamoto N, Akamatsu N, Yamazaki H, Tanoue K: Normal aggregations of glycoprotein IV (CD36)-deficient platelets from seven healthy Japanese donors. *Br J Haematol* **81**:86, 1992.
238. Ikeda H, Mitani T, Ohnuma M, Haga H, Ohtzuka S, Kato T, Nakase T, Sekiguchi S: A new platelet-specific antigen, Nak^{a} involved in the refractoriness of HLA-matched platelet transfusions. *Vox Sang* **57**:213, 1989.
239. Aster RH: The immunologic thrombocytopenias, in Kunicki TJ, George JN (eds): *Platelet Immunobiology*. Philadelphia, Lippincott, 1989, p 387.
240. Blanchette VS, Peters MA, Pegg-Feige K: Alloimmune thrombocytopenia: Review from a neonatal intensive care unit. *Curr Stud Hematol Blood Transfus* **52**:87, 1986.
241. Newman PJ, Derbes RS, Aster RH: The human platelet alloantigens, Pl^{A1} and Pl^{A2}, are associated with a leucine$_{33}$/proline$_{33}$ amino acid polymorphism in membrane glycoprotein IIIa, and are distinguishable by DNA typing. *J Clin Invest* **83**:1778, 1989.
242. Goldberger A, Kolodziej M, Poncz M, Bennett JS, Newman PJ: Effect of single amino acid substitutions on the formation of the Pl^{A} and Bak alloantigenic epitopes. *Blood* **78**:681, 1991.
243. Wang R, Furihata K, McFarland JG, Friedman K, Aster RH, Newman PJ: An amino acid polymorphism within the RGD binding domain of platelet membrane glycoprotein IIIa is responsible for the formation of the Pen^{a}/Pen^{b} alloantigen system. *J Clin Invest* **90**:2038, 1992.
244. Kroll H, Kiefel V, Santoso S, Mueller-Eckhardt C: Sra, a private platelet antigen on glycoprotein IIIa associated with neonatal alloimmune thrombocytopenia. *Blood* **76**:2296, 1990.
245. Santoso S, Newman PJ, Kalb R, Kroll H, Walka M, Kiefel V, Mueller-Eckhardt C: An unpaired cysteine residue is involved in epitope formation but has no influence on platelet GPIIIa expression and function. *Blood* **80**:128a, 1992.
246. Kuijpers RWAM, Simsek S, Faber NM, Goldschmeding R, van Wermerkerken RKV, von dem Borne AEGK: Single point mutation in human glycoprotein IIa is associated with a new platelet-specific alloantigen (Mo) involved in neonatal alloimmune thrombocytopenia. *Blood* **81**:70, 1993.
247. McFarland JG, Blanchette V, Collins J, Wang R, Newman PJ, Aster RH: Neonatal alloimmune thrombocytopenia due to a new platelet-specific alloantibody. *Blood* **81**:3318, 1993.
248. Wang R, McFarland JG, Kekomaki R, Newman PJ: Amino acid 489 is a mutational "hot spot" on the β3 integrin chain. The CA/Tu human platelet alloantigen system. *Blood* **82**:3386, 1993.
249. Santoso S, Kalb R, Walka M, Kiefel V, Mueller-Eckhardt C, Newman PJ: The human platelet alloantigens Br^{a} and Br^{b} are associated with a single amino acid polymorphism on glycoprotein Ia (integrin subunit α2). *J Clin Invest* **92**:2427, 1993.
250. Kuijpers RW, Faber NM, Cuypers HT, Ouwehand WH, von dem Borne AE: The N-terminal globular domain of human platelet glycoprotein Ibα has a methionine145/threonine145 amino acid polymorphism which is associated with the HPA-2 (Ko) alloantigens. *J Clin Invest* **89**:381, 1992.
251. Lyman S, Aster RH, Visentin GP, Newman PJ: Polymorphism of human platelet membrane glycoprotein IIb associated with the Bak^{a}/Bak^{b} alloantigen system. *Blood* **75**:2343, 1990.
252. McFarland JG, Aster RH, Bussel JB, Gianopoulos JG, Derbes RS, Newman PJ: Prenatal diagnosis of neonatal alloimmune thrombocytopenia using allele-specific aligonucleotide probes. *Blood* **78**:2276, 1991.
253. White JG: Inherited abnormalities of the platelet membrane and secretory granules. *Hum Pathol* **18**:123, 1987.
254. Ginsberg MH, Taylor L, Painter RG: The mechanism of thrombin-induced platelet factor 4 secretion. *Blood* **55**:661, 1980.
255. Grant JA, Scrutton MC: Positive interaction between agonists in the aggregation response of human blood platelet: Interaction between ADP, adrenaline and vasopressin. *Br J Haematol* **44**:109, 1980.
256. Sung SS, Young JD, Origlio AM, Heiple JM, Kaback HR, Silverstein SC: Extracellular ATP perturbs transmembrane ion fluxes, elevates cytosolic (Ca2+), and inhibits phagocytosis in mouse macrophages. *J Biol Chem* **260**:13442, 1985.
257. Rao AK: Congenital disorders of platelet function. *Hematol Oncol Clin North Am* **4**:65, 1990.
258. White JG, Krumwiede M: Further studies on the secretory pathway in thrombin-stimulated human platelets. *Blood* **69**:1196, 1987.
259. Painter RG, Ginsberg MH: Centripetal myosin redistribution in thrombin-stimulated platelets. Relationship to platelet factor 4 secretion. *Exp Cell Res* **155**:198, 1984.
260. Cramer EM, Debili N, Martin JF, Gladwin A-M, Breton-Gorius J, Harrison P, Savidge GF, Vainchecker W: Uncoordinated expression of fibrinogen compared with thrombospondin and von Willebrand factor in maturing megakaryocytes. *Blood* **73**:1123, 1989.
261. Nachman R, Levine R, Jaffe EA: Synthesis of factor VIII antigen by cultured guinea pig megakaryocytes. *J Clin Invest* **60**:914, 1977.
262. Handagama P, Rappolee DA, Werb Z, Levin J, Bainton DF: Platelet α-granule fibrinogen, albumin and immunoglobulin G are not synthesized by rat and mouse megakaryocytes. *J Clin Invest* **86**:1364, 1990.
263. Handagama PJ, George JN, Shuman MA, McEver RP, Bainton DF: Incorporation of a circulating protein into megakaryocyte and platelet granules. *Proc Natl Acad Sci USA* **84**:861, 1987.
264. Gewirtz AM, Keefer M, Doshi K, Annamalai AE, Chiu HC, Colman RW: Biology of human megakaryocyte Factor V. *Blood* **67**:1639, 1986.
265. Stenberg PE, Beckstead JH, McEver RP, Levin J: Immunohistochemical localization of membrane and alpha-granule proteins in plastic-embedded mouse bone marrow

megakaryocytes and murine megakaryocyte colonies. *Blood* **68**:696, 1986.
266. Ross R: Platelet-derived growth Factor. *Lancet* **1**:1179, 1989.
267. Berman CL, Yeo EL, Wencel-Drake JD, Furie BC, Ginsberg MH, Furie B: A platelet alpha granule membrane protein that is associated with the plasma membrane after activation. *J Clin Invest* **78**:130, 1986.
268. Stenberg PE, McEver RP, Shuman MA, Jacques YV, Bainton DF: A platelet alpha-granule membrane protein (GMP-140) is expressed on the plasma membrane after activation. *J Cell Biol* **101**:880, 1985.
269. Caen JP, Sultan Y, Larrieu M: New familial platelet disease. *lancet* **1**:203, 1967.
270. Oski FA, Naiman JL, Allen DM, Diamond LK: Leukocytic inclusions-Dohle bodies associated with platelet abnormality (the May-Hegglin anomaly). Report of a family and review of the literature. *Blood* **20**:657, 1962.
271. Hardisty RM, Mills DCB, Ketsa-Ard K: The platelet defect associated with albinism. *Br J Haematol* **23**:679, 1972.
272. Sahud MA, Aggeler PM: Platelet dysfunction: Differentiation of a newly-recognized primary type from that produced by aspirin. *N Engl J Med* **280**:453, 1969.
273. Weiss HJ, Chervenick PA, Zalusky R, Factor A: A familial defect in platelet function associated with impaired release of adenosine diphosphate. *N Engl J Med* **281**:1264, 1969.
274. Holmsen H, Weiss HJ: Hereditary defect in the release reaction caused by a deficiency int he storage pool of platelet adenine nucleotides. *Br J Haematol* **19**:643, 1970.
275. Holmsen H, Weiss HJ: Further evidence for a deficient storage pool of adenine nucleotides in platelets from some patients with thrombocytopathia—"storage pool disease." *Blood* **39**:197, 1972.
276. Lages B, Scrutton M, Holmsen H, Day HJ, Weiss HJ: Metal ion content of gel-filtered platelets from patients with storage pool disease. *Blood* **46**:119, 1975.
277. Weiss HJ, Witte LD, Kaplan KL, Lages BA, Chernoff A, Nossel HL, Goodman DS, Baumgartner HR: Heterogeneity in storage pool deficiency: Studies on granule-bound substances in 18 patients including variants deficient in alpha-granules, platelet factor 4, β-thromboglobulin and platelet-derived growth factor. *Blood* **54**:1296, 1979.
278. Weiss HJ, Tschopp TB, Rogers J, Brand H: Studies on platelet 5-hydroxytryptamine (serotonin) in patients with storage-pool disease and albinism. *J Clin Invest* **54**:421, 1974.
279. White JG, Gerrard JM: Ultrastructural features of abnormal blood platelets. *Am J Pathol* **83**:590, 1976.
280. DePinho RA, Kaplan KL: The Hermansky-Pudlak syndrome. Report of three cases and review of the pathophysiology adn management considerations. *Medicine (Baltimore)* **64**:192, 1985.
281. Barak Y, Nir E: Chediak-Higashi syndrome. *Am J Pediatr Hematol Oncol* **9**:42, 1987.
282. Bequez-Cesar A: Neutropenia cronica maligna familiar con granulaciones atipicas de los leucocitos. *Soc Cubana Pediatr Bol* **15**:900, 1943.
283. Steinbrink W: Uber eine neue Granulationsanomalie der keukocyten. *Disch Arciv Klin Med* **193**:577, 1948.
284. Chediak MM: Nouvelle anomalie leucocytaire de caractere constitutionnel et familial. *Rev Hematol* **7**:362, 1952.
285. Higashi O: Congenital gigantism of peroxidase granules. *Tohoku J Exp Med* **59**:315, 1959.
286. Witkop CJ, Almadovar C, Pineeiro B, Nunez-Babcock M: Hermansky-Pudlak syndrome (HPS). An epidemiological study. *Ophthalmic Paediatr Genet* **11**:245, 1990.
287. Witkop CJ Jr, White JG, King RA: Oculocutaneous albinism, in Nyhan WL (ed): *Heritable Disorders of Amino Acid Metabolism. Pattern of Clinical Expression and Genetic Variation*. New York, John Wiley, 1974, p 177.
288. Mahadeo R, Markowitz J, Fisher S, Daum F: Hermansky-Pudlak syndrome with granulomatous colitis in children. *J Pediatr* **118**:904, 1991.
289. Blume RS, Bennet JM, Yankee RA, Wolff SM: Defective granulocyte regulation in the Chediak-Higashi syndrome. *N Engl J Med* **279**:1009, 1969.
290. Clark R, Kimball H: Defective granulocyte chemotaxis in the Chediak-Higashi syndrome. *J Clin Invest* **50**:2645, 1971.
291. Barak Y, Karov Y, Nir E, Wagner Y, Kristal H, Levin S: Chediak-Higashi syndrome: Expression of the cytoplasmic defect by in vitro cultures of bone marrow progenitors. *Am J Pediatr Hematol Oncol* **8**:128, 1981.
292. Root RK, Rosenthal AS, Balestra DJ: Abnormal bactericidal metabolic and lysosomal functions of Chediak-Higashi syndrome. *J Clin Invest* **51**:649, 1979.
293. Spicer SS, Sato A, Vincent R, Eguchhi M, Poon KC: Lysosomal enlargement in the Chediak-Higashi syndrome. *Fed Prod* **40**:1451, 1981.
294. Blume RS, Wolff SM: The Chediak Higashi syndrome: Studies in four patients and a review of the literature. *Medicine (Baltimore)* **51**:247, 1972.
295. Merino F, Henle W, Ramirez-Duque P: Chronic active Epstein-Barr virus infection in patients with Chediak-Higashi syndrome. *J Clin Immunol* **6**:299, 1986.
296. Gerrard JM, Lint D, Sims P, Wiedmer T, Fugate RD, McMillan E, Robertson C, Israels SJ: Identification of a platelet dense granule membrane protein that is deficient in a patient with Hermansky-Pudlak syndrome. *Blood* **77**:101, 1991.
297. Israels SJ, Gerrard JM, Jaques YV, Bainton DF: Human platelet dense granule membranes contain both granulophysin and GMP-140. *Blood* **78**:278, 1991.
298. Oliver JM: Impaired microtubule function correctable by cyclic GMP and cholinergic agonists in the Chediak-Higashi leukocytes. *Am J Pathol* **85**:395, 1976.
299. White JG: Platelet microtubules and giant granules in the chediak-Higashi syndrome. *Am J Med Technol* **44**:273, 1979.
300. Ostlundd RE Jr, Tucker RW, Leung JT, Okun N, Williamson JR: The cytoskeleton in Chediak-Higashi syndrome. *Blood* **56**:806, 1980.
301. Swank RT, Reddington M, Howlett O, Novak EK: Platelet storage deficiency with inherited abnormalities of the inner ear in the mouse pigment mutants Muted and Mocha. *Blood* **78**:2036, 1991.
302. Panner JD *Prieur DJ: Interspecific genetic complementation analysis with fibroblasts from humans and four species of animals with Chediak-Higashi syndrome. Am J Med Genet* **28**:455, 1987.
303. Wijermans PW, Van Dorp DB: Hermansky-Pudlak syndrome: Correction of bleeding time by 1-desamino-8D-arginine vasopressin. *Am J Hematol* **30**:154, 1989.
304. Colgan SP, Hull-Thrall MA, Gasper PW, Gould DH, Rose BJ, Fulton R, Blanquaert AM, Bruyninckx WJ: Restoration of neutrophil and platelet function in feline Chediak-Higashi syndrome by bone marrow transplantation. *Bone Marrow Transplant* **7**:365, 1991.
305. Gerrard JM, Phillips DR, Rao GH, Plow EF, Walz DA, Ross R, Harker LA, White JG: Biochemical studies of two patients with the gray platelet syndrome. Selective deficiency of platelet alpha granules. *J Clin Invest* **66**:102, 1980.
306. Levy-Toledano S, Caen JP, Breton-Gorius J, Rendu F, Cywiner-Golenzer C, Dupuy E, Legrand Y, Maclouf J: Gray platelet syndrome: Alpha-granule deficiency. Its influence on platelet function. *J Lab Clin Med* **98**:831, 1981.
307. Raccuglio G: Grey platelet syndrome: A variety of qualitative platelet disorder. *Am J Med* **51**:818, 1971.
308. White JG: Ultrastructural studies of the gray platelet syndrome. *Am J Pathol* **95**:445, 1979.
309. Rosa JP, George JN, Bainton DF, Nurden AT, Caen JP, McEver RP: Gray platelet syndrome. Demonstration of alpha granule membranes that can fuse with the cell surface. *J Clin Invest* **80**:1138, 1987.
310. Nurden AT, Kunicki TJ, Dupuis D, Soria C, Caen JP: Specific protein and glycoprotein deficiencies in platelets isolated from two patients with the gray platelet syndrome. *Blood* **59**:709, 1982.
311. Srivastava PC, Powling MJ, Nokes TJ, Patrick AD, Dawes J, Hardisty RM: Grey platelet syndrome: Studies on platelet alpha granules, lysosomes and defective response to thrombin. *Br J Haematol* **65**:441, 1987.
312. Breton-Gorius J, Vainchecker W, Nurden A, Levy-Toledano S, Caen J: Defective α-granule production in megakaryocytes from platelet gray syndrome: Ultrastructural studies of bone marrow cells and megakaryocytes growing in culture from blood precursors. *Am J Pathol* **102**:10, 1981.
313. Caen JP, Deschamps JF, Bodevin E, Byckaerrt MC,

Dupuy E, Wasteson A: Megakaryocytes and myelofibrosis in gray platelet syndrome. *Nouv Rev Fr Hematol* **29**:109, 1987.

314. Facon T, Goudemand J, Caron C, Zandecki M, Estienne MH, Fenaux P, Cosson A: Simultaneous occurrence of grey platelet syndrome and idiopathic pulmonary fibrosis: A role for abnormal megakaryocytes in the pathogenesis of pulmonary fibrosis. *Br J Haematol* **74**:542, 1990.
315. Rothman JE, Orci L: Molecular dissection of the secretory pathway. *Nature* **355**:409, 1992.
316. Pfueller SL, Howard MA, White JG, Menon C, Berry EW: Shortening of bleeding time by 1-deamino-8-arginine vasopressin (DDAVP) in the absence of platelet von Willebrand factor in gray platelet syndrome. *Thromb Haemost* **18**:1060, 1987.
317. Kohler M: Treatment of gray platelet syndrome. *Thromb Haemost* **60**:123, 1988.
318. Berrebi A, Klepfish A, Varon D, Shtalrid M, Vorst E, Nir E, Lahav J: Gray platelet syndrome in the elderly. *Am J Hematol* **28**:270, 1988.
319. Jackson CW, Hutson NK, Steward SA, Saito N, Cramer EM: Platelets of the Wistar Furth rat have reduced levels of alpha-granule proteins. An animal model resembling gray platelet syndrome. *J Clin Invest* **87**:1985, 1991.
320. Weiss HJ: Inherited disorders of platelet secretion, in Coleman RW, Hirsch J, Marder VJ, Salzman EW (eds): *Hemostasis and Thrombosis: Basic Principles and Practice*. Philadelphia, Lippincott, 1987, p 741..
321. Lages B, Shattil SJ, Bainton DF, Weiss HJ: Decreased content and surface expression of alpha-granule membrane protein GMP-140 in one of two types of platelet alpha delta storage pool deficiency. *J Clin Invest* **87**:919, 1991.
322. Brass LF: The biochemistry of platelet activation, in Hoffman R, Benz EJ Jr, Shattil SJ, Furie B, Cohen JJ (eds): *Hematology: Basic Principles and Practice*. New York, Churchill Livingstone, 1991, p 1176.
323. Rittenhouse SE, Sasson JP: Mass changes in myoinositoltrisphosphate in human platelet stimulated by thrombin. Inhibitory effects of phorbol esters. *J Biol Chem* **260**:8657, 1985.
324. Lapetina EG: Inositol phospholipids and GTP-binding in signal transduction in stimulated platelets. *Adv Prostaglandin Thromboxane Leukotriene Res* **16**:217, 1986.
325. Irvine RF: Metabolism and function of inositol phosphates: Synthetsis and degradation. *ISI Atlas Sci Biochem* **1**:337, 1988.
326. Majerus PW, Connolly TM, Bansal VS, Inhorn RC, Ross TS, Lips DL: Inositol phosphates: Synthesis and degradation. *J biol Chem* **263**:3051, 1986.
327. Naka M, Nishikawa M, Adelstein RS, Hidaka H: Phorbol ester-induced activation of human platelets in associated with protein kinase C phosphorylation of myosin light chains. *Nature* **306**:490, 1983.
328. Litchfield DW, Ball EH: Phosphorylation of caldesmon 77 by protein kinase C in vitro and in intact platelets. *J Biol Chem* **262**:8056, 1987.
329. Rendu F, Breton-Gorius J, Trugnan G, Malaspina HC, Andrieu JM, Bereziat G, Lebret M, Caen JP: Studies on a new variant of the Hermansky-Pudlak syndrome: Qualitative, ultrastructural, and functional abnormalities of the platelet-dense bodies associated with a phospholipase A defect. *Am J Hematol* **4**:387, 1978.
330. Rao AK, Koike K, Willis J, Daniel JL, Beckett C, Hassel B, Day HJ, Smith JB: Platelet secretion defect associated with impaired liberation of arachidonate metabolism and normal myosin light chain phosphorylation. *Blood* **64**:914, 1984.
331. Malmsten C, Hamberg M, Samuelsson B: Physiological role of an endoperoxide in human platelets: Hemostatic defect due to platelet cyclooxygenase deficiency. *Proc Natl Acad Sci USA* **72**:1446, 1975.
332. Horellou MH, Lecompte T, Lecrubier C, Fouque F, Chignard M, Conard J, Vargaftig BB, Dray F, Samama M: Familial and constitutional bleeding disorder due to platelet cyclo-oxygenase deficiency. *Am J Hematol* **14**:1, 1983.
333. Lagarde M, Byron PA, Vargaftig BB, Dechavanne M: Impairment of platelet thromboxane A2 generation and of the platelet release reaction in two patients with cogenital deficiency of platelet cyclooxygenase. *Br J Haematol* **38**:251, 1978.
334. Pareti FI, Manucci PM, D'Angelo A, Smith JB, Sautebini L, Galli G: Congenital deficiency of thromboxane and prostacyclin. *Lancet* **1**:898, 1980.
335. Roth GJ, Machuga R: Radioimmune assay of human platelet prostaglandin synthetase. *J Lab Clin Med* **99**:187, 1982.
336. Defryn G, Machin SJ, Carreras LO, Dauden M, Chamone AF, Vermylen J: Familial bleeding tendency with partial platelet thromboxane synthetase deficiency: Reorientation of cyclic endoperoxide metabolism. *Br J Haematol* **49**:29, 1981.
337. Mestel F, Oetliker O, Beck E, Felix R, Imbach P, Wagner H-P: Severe bleeding associated with defective thromboxane synthetase. *Lancet* **1**:157, 1980.
338. Bell TG, Leader RW, Olsen PM, Padgett GA, Penner JA, Patterson WR: Basset hound hereditary thrombopathy: An autosomally recessively inherited platelet dysfunction with 11 cases in a kindred of 56 dogs, in Ryder OA, Byrd ML (eds): *One Medicine*. Springer-Verlag, 1984, p 335.
339. Patterson WR, Estry DW, Schwartz KA, Borchert RD, Bell TG: Absent platelet aggregation with normal fibrinogen binding in Basset hound hereditary thrombopathy. *Thromb Haemost* **62**:1011, 1989.
340. Walsh PN, Schmaier AH: Platelet-coagulation protein interactions, in Colman RW, Hirsh J, Marder VJ, Salzman EW (eds): *Hemostasis and Thrombosis: Basic Principles and Clinical Practice*. Philadelphia, Lippincott, 1992, p 689.
341. Weiss HJ, Vicic WJ, Lages BA, Rogers J: Isolated deficiency of platelet procoagulant activity. *Am J Med* **67**:206, 1979.
342. Miletich JP, Kane WH, Hofmann SL, Stanford N, Majerus PW: Deficiency of factor Xa-factor Va binding sites on the platelets of a patient with a bleeding disorder. *Blood* **54**:1015, 1979.
343. Weiss HJ, Turitto VT, Baumgartner HR: Role of shear rate and platelets in promoting fibrin formation on rabbit subendothelium. *J Clin Invest* **78**:1073, 1986.
344. Rosing EM, Bevers P, Comfurius P, Hemker HC, van Diejan G, Weiss HJ, Zwaal RFA: Impaired factor X- and prothrombin activation associated with decreased phospholipid exposure in platelets from a patient with a bleeding disorder. *Blood* **65**:1557, 1985.
345. Sims PJ, Wiedmer T, Esmon CT, Weiss HJ, Shattil SJ: Assembly of the platelet prothrombinase complex is linked to vesiculation of the platelet plasma membrane: Studies in Scott Syndrome: An isolated defect in platelet procoagulant activity. *J Biol Chem* **264**:17049, 1989.
346. Bevers EM, Wiedmer T, Comfurius P, Shattil SJ, Weiss HJ, Zwaal RFA, Sims PJ: Defective Ca2+-induced microvesiculation and deficient expression of procoagulant activity in erythrocytes from a patient with a bleeding disorder: A study of the red blood cells of Scott syndrome. *Blood* **79**:380, 1992.
347. Gewirtz AM, Poncz M: Megakaryocytopoiesis and platelet production, in Hoffman R, Benz EJ Jr, Shattil SJ, Furie B, Cohen HJ (eds): *Hematology: Basic Principles and Practice*. New York, Churchill Livingstone, 1991, p 1148.
348. Hall JG: Thrombocytopenia and absent ra''us (TAR) syndrome. *J Med Genet* **24**:79, 1987.
349. Hoffman R: Regulation of megakaryocytopoiesis. *Blood* **74**:1196, 1989.
350. Metcalf D, MacDonald HR, Odartchenko N, Sordat B: Growth of mouse megakaryocyte colonies in vitro. *Proc Natl Acad Sci USA* **72**:1744, 1975.
351. Nakahata T, Ogawa M: Identification in culture of a new class of hematopoietic colony forming units with extreme capability to self-renew and generate multipotential colonies. *Proc Natl Acad Sci USA* **79**:39, 1982.
352. Geissler DG, Konwalinka G, Peschel CH, Boyd J, Odavic R, Braumsteiner H: Clonal growth of human megakaryocyte progenitor cells in a microagar culture system: Simultaneous proliferation of megakaryocyte, granulocyte, erythroid progenitors (CFU-M, CFU-C, BFU-E) and T lymphocyte colonies (CFU-TL). *Int J Cell Cloning* **1**:377, 1983.
353. Kimura H, Burstein SA, Thorning SA, Powell JS, Harker LA, Fialkow PJ, Adamson JW: Human megakaryocytic progenitors (CFU-M) assaying in methylcellulose: Physi-

cal characteristics and requirements for growth. *J Cell Physiol* **118**:87, 1984.

354. Hoffman R, Mazur EM, Bruno E, Floyd V: Assay of an activity in the serum of patients with disorders of thrombopoiesis that stimulates formation of megakaryocytic colonies. *N Engl J Med* **305**:533, 1981.
355. Burstein SA: Interleukin-3 promotes maturation of murine megakaryocyte in vitro. *Blood Cells* **11**:469, 1986.
356. Teramura M, Katahira J, Hoshino S, Motoji T, Oshimi K, Mizoguchi H: Effect of recombinant hematopoietic growth factors on human megakaryocyte colony formation in serum-free cultures. *Exp Hematol* **17**:1011, 1989.
357. Lu L, Briddell RA, Graham CD, Brandt JE, Bruno E, Hoffman R: Effect of recombinant and purified human hematopoietic growth factors on in vitro colony formation by enriched populations of human megakaryocyte progenitor cells. *Br J Hematol* **70**:149, 1988.
358. Briddell RA, Brandt JE, Straneva JE, Srour EF, Hoffman R: Characterization of the human burst-forming unit-megakaryocyte. *Blood* **74**:145, 1989.
359. Briddell RA, Hoffman R: Cytokine regulation of the human burst-forming unit-megakaryocyte. *Blood* **76**:516, 1989.
360. Teramura M, Kobayashi S, Hoshino S, Oshimi K, Mizoguchi H: Interleukin-11 enhances human megakaryocytopoiesis in vitro. *Blood* **79**:327, 1992.
361. Avraham H, Vannier E, Cowley S, Jiang S, Chi S, Dinarello CA, Zsebo KM, Groopman JE: Effects of the stem cell factor, c-kit ligand, on human megakaryocytic cells. *Blood* **79**:365, 1992.
362. Kawakita M, Enomoto K, Katayama N, Kishimoto S, Miyake T: Thrombopoiesis and megakaryocyte colony stimulating factors in the urine of patients with idiopathic thrombocytopenic purpura. *Br J Haematol* **48**:609, 1981.
363. Kawakita M, Ogawa M, Goldwasser E, Miyake T: Characterization of human megakaryocyte colony stimulating factor in the urinary extracts from patients with aplastic anemia and idiopathic thrombocytopenic purpura. *Blood* **61**:556, 1983.
364. Yamasaki K, Solberg LA, Jamal N, Lockwood G, Tritcher D, Curtis JE, Minden M, Mann KG, Messner HA: Hemopoietic colony growth-promoting activities in the plasma of bone marrow transplant recipients. *J Clin Invest* **82**:255, 1988.
365. Abe T, Fuher P, Bregman MD, Kuramoto A, Murphy MJ Jr: Factors regulating megakaryocytopoiesis and platelet formation, in Tavassoli M, Zanjani ED, Ascensao JL, Abraham NG, Levene A (eds): *Molecular Biology of Hemopoiesis*. New York, Plenum, 1988, p 183.
366. Hoffman R, Yang HH, Bruno E, Staneva JE: Purification and partial characterization of a megakaryocyte colony-stimulating factor from human plasma. *J Clin Invest* **75**:1174, 1985.
367. Stravena JE, Yang HH, Hui SL, Bruno E, Hoffman R: Effects of megakaryocyte colony stimulating factor on terminal cytoplasmic maturation of human megakaryocytes. *Exp Hematol* **15**:657, 1987.
368. Mazur EM, de Alarcon P, South K, Miceli L: Human serum megakaryocyte colony stimulating activity increases in response to intensive cytotoxic chemotherapy. *Exp Hematol* **12**:624, 1984.
369. Radley JM, Haller CJ: Fate of senescent megakaryocytes in the bone marrow. *Br J Haematol* **53**:277, 1983.
370. Tong M, Seth P, Pennington DG: Proplatelets and stress platelets. *Blood* **69**:522, 1987.
371. Kaufman RM, Airo R, Pollack S, Crosby WH: Circulating megakaryocytes and platelet release in the lung. *Blood* **26**:720, 1985.
372. Pederson NT: Occurrence of megakaryocytes in various vessels and their retention in the pulmonary capillaries in man. *Scand J Haematol* **21**:369, 1978.
373. Scheinen TM, Koivuiniemi AP: Megakaryocytes in the pulmonary circulation. *Blood* **22**:82, 1963.
374. Kallinikos-Maniatis A: Megakaryocytes and platelets in central venous and arterial blood. *Acta Haematol (Bosel)* **42**:330, 1969.
375. Radley JM, Haller CJ: The demarcation membrane system of the megakaryocyte: A misnomer? *Blood* **60**:213, 1982.
376. White JG: Interaction of membrane systems in blood platelet. *Am J Pathol* **66**:295, 1972.
377. Handagama PJ, Feldman BF, Jain NC, Farver TB, Kono CS: In vitro platelet release by rat megakaryocytes: Effects of metabolic inhibitors and cytoskeletal disrupting agents. *Am J Vet Res* **48**:1142, 1987.
378. Tablin F, Gastro M, Leven RM: Blood platelet formation in vitro. The role of the cytoskeleton in megakaryocyte fragmentation. *J Cell Sci* **97**:59, 1990.
379. Radley JM, Scurfield G: The mechanism of platelet release. *Blood* **56**:996, 1980.
380. Williams WJ: Clinical evaluation of the patient, in Williams WJ, Beutler E, Erslev AJ, Lichtman MA (eds): *Hematology*. New York, McGraw-Hill, 1983, p 9.
381. Ebbe S, Stohlman F Jr, Donavan J, Overcash J: Megakaryocytic maturation rate in thrombocytopenic rats. *Blood* **32**:787, 1968.
382. Adams WH, Liu YK, Sullivan LW: Humoral regulation of thrombopoiesis in man. *J Lab Clin Med* **91**:141, 1977.
383. Levin J, Levin FC, Pennington DG, Metcalf D: Measurement of ploidy distribution in megakaryocyte colonies obtained from culture with studies of the effect of thrombopoietin. *Blood* **57**:287, 1981.
384. Hill R, Levin J: Partial purification of thrombopoietin using lectin chromatography. *Exp Hematol* **14**:752, 1986.
385. McDonald TP: Thrombopoietin: Its biology, purification and characterization. *Exp Hematol* **16**:201, 1988.
386. Tayrien G, Rosenberg RD: Purification adn properties of a megakaryocyte stimulating factor present both in the serum free conditioned medium of human embryonic kidney cells and in thrombocytopenic plasma. *J Biol Chem* **262**:3262, 1987.
387. McDonald TP, Clift RE, Cottrell MB: A four-step procedure for the purification of thrombopoietin. *Exp Hematol* **17**:865, 1989.
388. Burstein SA, Ishibashi T: Erythropoietin and megakaryocytopoiesis. *Blood Cells* **15**:193, 1988.
389. Ishibashi T, Koziol JA, Burnstein SA: Human recombinant erythropoietin promotes differentiation of murine megakaryocytes in vitro. *J Clin Invest* **79**:286, 1986.
390. Kimura H, Ishibashi T, Uchida T, Maruyama Y, Friese P, Burstein SA: Interleukin 6 is a differentiation factor for human megakaryocytes in vitro. *Eur J Immunol* **20**:1927, 1990.
391. Mei R, Burstein SA: Megakaryocytic maturation in murine long-term bone marrow culture: Role of interleukin-6. *Blood* **78**:1438, 1991.
392. Carrington PA, Hill RJ, Stenberg P, Levin J, Corash L, Schreurs J, Baker G, Levin F: Multiple in vivo effects of interleukin 3 and interleukin 6 on murine megakaryocytopoiesis. *Blood* **77**:34, 1991.
393. Martin DIK, Tsai S-F, Orkin SH: Increased gamma-globin expression in a nondeletional HPFH mediated by an erythroid-specific DNA-binding factor. *Nature* **338**:435, 1989.
394. Hill RJ, Warren MK, Stenberg P, Levin J, Corash L, Crummond R, Baker G, Levin F, Mok Y: Stimulation of megakaryocytopoiesis in mice by human recombinant interleukin-6. *Blood* **77**:42, 1991.
395. Navarro S, Devili N, LeCouedic JP, Klein B, Breton-Gorius J, Doly J, Vainchecker W: Interleukin-6 and its receptor are expressed by human megakaryocytes: In vitro effects on proliferation and endoreduplication. *Blood* **77**:461, 1991.
396. Ravid K, Beeler DL, Rabin MS, Ruley HE, Rosenberg RD: Selective targeting of gene products with the megakaryocyte platelet factor 4 gene. *Proc Natl Acad Sci USA* **88**:1521, 1991.
397. Ravid K, Doi T, Beeler DL, Kuter DJ, Rosenberg RD: Transcriptional regulation of the rat platelet factor 4 gene: Interaction between an enhancer/silencer domain and the GATA site. *Mol Cell Biol* **11**:6116, 1991.
398. Tsai S-F, Martin DIK, Zon L, D'Andrea A, Wong G, Orkin SH: Cloning of the cDNA for the major DNA-binding protein of the erythroid lineage through expression in mammalian cells. *Nature* **339**:446, 1989.
399. Zon LI, Tsai S-F, Burgess S, Matsudaira P, Bruns GAP, Orkin SH: The major human erythroid DNA-binding protein (FG-1;NF-E1; Eryf 1): Primary sequence and localization of the gene to the X chromosome. *Proc Natl Acad Sci USA* **78**:668, 1990.
400. Martin DIK, Zon LI, Mutter G, Orkin SH: Expression

of the erythroid transcription factor in megakaryocytic and mast cell lineages. *Nature* **344**:444, 1990.

401. Romeo P-H, Prandini M-H, Joulin V, Mignotte V, Prenant M, Vainchenker W, Marguerie G, Uzan G: Megakaryocytic and erythrocytic lineages share specific transcription factors. *Nature* **344**:447, 1990.
402. Pevny L, Simon CS, Robertson E, Klein WH, Tsai S-F, D'Agati V, Orkin SH, Constantini F: Erythroid differentiation in chimaeric mice blocked by a targeted mutation in the gene for transcription factor GATA-1. *Nature* **349**:257, 1991.
403. Uzan G, Prenant M, Prandini MH, Martin F, Marguerie G: Tissue-specific expression of the platelet GPIIb gene. *J Biol Chem* **266**:8932, 1991.
404. Lemarchandel V, Ghysdael J, Mignotte V, Rahuel C, Romeo P-H: GATA and Ets cis-acting sequences mediate megakaryocyte-specific expression. *Mol Cell Biol* **13**:668, 1993.
405. Wiskott A: Familiarer angeborener Morbus Werlhofi? Monatsschr Kinderheilkd **68**:212, 1937.
406. Aldrich RA, Steinberg AG, Campbell DC: Pedigree demonstrating a sex-linked recessive condition characterized by draining ears, eczematoid dermatitis and bloody diarrhea. *Pediatrics* **13**:133, 1954.
407. Grottum KA, Hovig T, Holmsen H, Abramsen AF, Jeremic M, Seip M: Wiscott-Aldrich syndrome: Qualitative platelet defects and short platelet survival. *Br J Haematol* **17**:373, 1969.
408. Perry GS, Spector BD, Schuman LM, Mandel JS, Anderson E, McHugh RB, Hanson MR, Fahlstrom SM *Krivitz W, Kersey JH: The Wiskott-Aldrich syndrome in the United States and Canada (1892 – 1979). J Pediatr* **97**:72, 1980.
409. Cotelingam JD, Witebsky FG, Hsu SM, Blaese RM, Jaffe ES: Malignant lymphoma in patients with the Wiskott-Aldrich syndrome. *Cancer Invest* **3**:515, 1985.
410. Cooper MD, Chase HP, Lowman JT, Krivit W, Good RA: Wiskott-Aldrich Syndrome. An immunologic deficiency disease involving the afferent limb of immunity. *Am J Med* **44**:499, 1968.
411. Gahmberg CG, Autero M, Mermonen J: Major O-glycosylated sialoglycoproteins of human hematopoietic cells: Differentiation antigens with poorly understood functions. *J Cell Biochem* **37**:91, 1988.
412. Gealy WJ, Dwyer JM, Harley JB: Allelic exclusion of glucose-6-phosphate dehydrogenase in platelet and T lymphocytes from a Wiskott-Aldrich syndrome carrier. *Lancet* **1**:63, 1980.
413. Prchal JT, Carroll AJ, Prchal JF, Crist WM, Skalka HW, Gealy WJ, Harley J, Malluh A: Wiskott-Aldrich syndrome: Cellular impairments and their implications for carrier detection. *Blood* **56**:1048, 1980.
414. Puck JM, Siminovitch KA, Poncz M, Greenberg CR, Rottem M, Conley ME: Atypical presentation of Wiskott-Aldrich syndrome: Diagnosis in two unrelated males based on studies of maternal T cell X-chromosome inactivation. *Blood* **75**:2369, 1990.
415. Remold-O'Donnell E, Zimmerman C, Kenney D, rosen FS: Expression on blood cells of sialophorin, the surface glycoprotein that is defective in Wiskott-Aldrich syndrome. *Blood* **70**:104, 1987.
416. Shelley CS, Remold-O'Donnell E, Davis A E III, Bruns GA, Rosen FS, Carroll MC, Whitehead AS: Molecular characterization of sialophorin (CD43), the lymphocyte surface sialoglycoprotein defective in Wiskott-Aldrich syndrome. *Proc Natl Acad Sci USA* **86**:2819, 1989.
417. Parkman R, Remold-O'Donnell E, Kenney DM, Perrine S, rosen FS: Surface protein abnormalities in lymphocytes and platelets from patients with Wiskott-Aldrich syndrome. *Lancet* **1**:1387, 1981.
418. Piller F, LeDist F, Weinberg KI, Parkman R, Fukuda M: Altered O-glycan synthesis in lymphocytes from patients wtih Wiskott-Aldrich syndrome. *J Exp Med* **1731501**:1991.
419. Higgins EA, Siminovitch KA, Zhuang DL, Brockhausen I, Dennis JW: Aberrant O-linked oligosaccharide in lymphocytes and platelets from patients with the Wiskott-Aldrich syndrome. *J Biol Chem* **266**:6280, 1991.
420. Rosenstein Y, Park JK, Hahn WC, rosen FS, Bierer BE, Burakoff SJ: CD43, a molecule defective in Wiskott-Aldrich syndrome, binds ICAM-1. *Nature* **354**:233, 1991.
421. Simmons D, Makgoba MW, Seed B: ICAM, an adhesion ligand of LFA-1 is homologous to the neural cell adhesion molecule NCAM. *Nature* **331**:624, 1988.
422. Stauton DE, Marlin SD, Stratowa C, Dustin M, Springer TA: Primary structure of intercellular adhesion molecule 1 (ICAM-1) demonstrates interaction between members of the immunoglobulin and integrin supergene families. *Cell 52*:925, 1988.
423. Park JK, Rosenstein YJ, Remold-O'Donnell E, Bierer BE, Rosen FS, Burakoff SJ: Enhancement of T cell activation by the CD43 molecule whose expression is defective in Wiskott-Aldrich syndrome. *Nature* **350**:706, 1991.
424. Stormoken H, Hellum B, Egeland T, Abrahamsen TG, Hovig T: X-linked thrombocytopenia and thrombocytopathia: Attenuated Wiskott-Aldrich syndrome. Functional and morphological studies of platelet and lymphocytes. *Thromb Haemost* **65**:300, 1991.
425. Brochstein JA, gillio AP, Ruggerio M, Kernan N, Emanuel D, Laver J, Small T, O'Reilly RJ: Marrow transplantation from human leucocyte antigen-identical or haploidentical donors for correction of Wiskott-Aldrich syndrome year follow-up of a patient with Wiskott-Aldrich syndrome. *J Pediatr* **119**:907, 1991.
426. Rimm IJ, rappeport JM: Bone marrow transplantation for the Wiskott-Aldrich syndrome: Long-term follow-up. *Transplantation* **50**:617, 1990.
427. Brochstein JA, Gillio AP, Ruggiero M, Kernan NA, Emanuel M, Small T, O'Reilly RJ: Marrow transplantation from human leukocyte antigen-identical or haploidentical donors for correction of Wiskott-Aldrich syndrome. *J Pediatr* **119**:907, 1991.
428. Ata M, Fisher OF, Holman CA: Inherited thrombocytopenic purpura. *Lancet* **1**:119, 1965.
429. Canales L, Mauer AM: Sex-linked hereditary thrombocytopenia with immunological defects. *N Engl J Med* **277**:899, 1967.
430. Cohn J, Hauge M, Anderson V, Kenningsen K, Nielson LS, Thomsen M, Iversen T: Sex-linked hereditary thrombocytopenia with immunological defects. *Hum Hered* **25**:309, 1975.
431. Notarangelo LD, Parolini O, Faustini R, Porteri V, Albertini A, Ugazio AG: Presentation of Wiskott Aldrich syndrome as isolated thrombocytopenia. *Blood* **77**:1125, 1991.
432. Greer WL, Somani A-K, Wong PC, Peacocke M, Rubin LA, Siminovitch KA: Linkage analysis of the Wiskott-Aldrich syndrome to ten loci in the pericentromeric region of the human X chromosome. *Genomics* **6**:568, 1990.
433. Donner M, Schwartz M, Carlsson KU, Holmberg L: Hereditary X-linked thrombocytopenia maps to the same chromosomal region as the Wiskott-Aldrich syndrome. *Blood* **72**:1849, 1988.
434. Lyon MF, Peters J, Glenister PH, Ball S, Wright E: The scurfy mouse mutant has previously unrecognized hematological abnormalities and resembles Wiskott-Aldrich syndrome. *Proc Natl Acad Sci USA* **87**:2433 1990.
435. Goodwin HA, Ginsberg AD: May-Hegglin anomaly: A defect in megakaryocyte fragmentation? *Br J Haematol* **26**:117, 1975.
436. Coller BS, Zarrabi MH: Platelet membrane studies in the May-Hegglin anomaly. *Blood* **58**:279, 1981.
437. Greinacher A, Mueller-Eckhardt C: Hereditary types of thrombocytopenia with giant platelets and inclusion bodies in the leukocytes. *Blut* **60**:53, 1990.
438. Greinacher A, Nieuwenhuis HK, White JG: Sebastian platelet syndrome: A new variant of hereditary macrothrombocytopenia with leukocyte inclusions. *Blud* **61**:282, 1990.
439. Milton JG, Frojmovic MM: Shape-change agent produce abnormally large platelets in hereditary "giant platelet syndrome (MPS)." *J Lab Clin Med* **93**:154, 1979.
440. Milton JG, Frojmovic MM, Tang SS, White JG: Spontaneous platelet aggregation in a hereditary giant platelet syndrome (MPS). *Am J Pathol* **114**:336, 1984.
441. Bernhardt SG, Gore I, Kelby RA: Congenital leukemia. *Blood* **6**:990, 1951.
442. Hall JG, Levin J, Kuhn JP, Ottenheimer EJ, van Ber-

kum KAP, McKusick VA: Thrombocytopenia with absent radius (TAR). *Medicine (Baltimore)* **48**:411, 1969.

443. Murphy S: Hereditary thrombocytopenia. *Clin Haematol* **1**:358, 1972.
444. Day HJ, Holmsen H: Platelet adenine nucleotide "storage pool deficiency" in thrombocytopenic absent radii syndrome. *JAMA* **221**:1053, 1972.
445. de Alarcon PA, Graeve JA, Levine RF, McDonald TP, Beal DW: Thrombocytopenia and absent radii syndrome: Defective megakaryocytopoiesis-thrombocytopoiesis. *Am J Pediatr Hematol Oncol* **13**:77, 1991.
446. Homans AC, Cohen JL, Mazur EM: Defective megakaryocytopoiesis in the syndrome of thrombocytopenia with absent radii. *Br J Haematol* **70**:205, 1988.
447. Michaelovicz R, Baron S, Burstein Y: Osteoclast-like cells grow in cultures of multipotent hematopoietic progenitors in thrombocytopenia and absent radii. *Isr J Med Sci* **24**:42, 1988.
448. Alter BP: The bone marrow failure syndrome, in Nathan DG, Oski F (eds): *Hematology of Infancy and Childhood.* Philadelphia, Saunders, 1981, p 159.
449. Aggett PJ, Cavanagh NP, Matthew DJ, Pincott JR, Sutcliffe J, Harries JT: Schwachman's syndrome: A review of 21 cases. *Arch Dis Child* **55**:331, 1980.

CHAPTER 111

Glucose 6-Phosphate Dehydrogenase Deficiency

Lucio Luzzatto ▪ Atul Mehta

QUOD ALIIS CIBUS EST,
ALIIS FUAT ACRE VENENUM

What is food to some men
may be fierce poison to others

Lucretius Caro

De Rerum Natura 4: 641, 65 B.C.

1. Glucose-6-phosphate dehydrogenase (G-6-PD) is a cytoplasmic enzyme that is distributed in all cells. G-6-PD catalyzes the first step in the hexose monophosphate pathway, and it produces NADPH, which is required for reactions of various biosynthetic pathways as well as for the stability of catalase and the preservation and regeneration of the reduced form of glutathione (GSH). Since catalase and glutathione (via glutathione peroxidase) are essential for the detoxification of hydrogen peroxide, the defense of cells against this compound depends ultimately and heavily on G-6-PD. This is especially true in red cells, which are exquisitely sensitive to oxidative damage and in which other NADPH-producing enzymes are lacking.
2. G-6-PD in its active enzyme form is made up of either two or four identical subunits, each having a molecular mass of about 59 kDa. The complete primary sequence of 515 amino acids has been determined from the cDNA sequence, and it shows a high degree of homology with the protein sequence obtained from rat liver G-6-PD. The gene encoding G-6-PD maps to the telomeric region of the long arm of the X chromosome (band Xq28), about 400 kb centromeric to the factor VIII gene. Therefore, one of the two G-6-PD alleles is subject to inactivation in females. As determined from overlapping genomic phage clones, the gene spans 18 kb and consists of 13 exons (the first of which is noncoding). The sequence of the DNA region upstream from the major transcription initiation site has features similar to those found in other housekeeping gene promoters.
3. G-6-PD deficiency is the most common known enzymopathy; it is estimated to affect 400 million people worldwide. The highest prevalence rates (with gene frequencies in the range of 5 to 25 percent) are found in tropical Africa, in the Middle East, in tropical and subtropical Asia, in some areas of the Mediterranean, and in Papua New Guinea. The most common clinical manifestations are neonatal jaundice and acute hemolytic anemia. In some cases, the neonatal jaundice is severe enough to cause death or permanent neurologic damage. The acute hemolytic anemia can be triggered by a number of drugs, by infections, or by the ingestion of fava beans. In a proportion of cases these manifestations may be life-threatening, especially favism in children. The detailed mechanism of hemolysis is not fully known, but it undoubtedly results from the inability of G-6-PD-deficient red cells to withstand the oxidative damage produced, directly or indirectly, by the triggering agents mentioned above. Red-cell destruction in these acute hemolytic events is largely intravascular and therefore is associated with hemoglobinuria. Fortunately, apart from these episodes of hemolytic anemia, most G-6-PD-deficient individuals are entirely asymptomatic. A very small proportion of G-6-PD-deficient individuals have instead a chronic hemolytic disorder, which may be quite severe.
4. G-6-PD deficiency is genetically heterogeneous. About 400 different variants have been reported on the basis of diverse biochemical characteristics; this diversity suggests that these variants result from as many allelic mutations in the G-6-PD gene. In addition, several structural mutants without enzyme deficiency have been characterized. Molecular analysis has confirmed that the basis for G-6-PD deficiency is widely heterogeneous. In some cases, variants that had been assigned different names turned out to be identical; conversely, however, some variants that had been thought to be homogeneous have turned out to be heterogeneous on the molecular level. Thus far, some 60 different point mutations have been identified, but only two deletions of one to two codons and no larger deletions have been observed. Different mutants, each one having a polymorphic frequency, underlie G-6-PD deficiency in the various parts of the world where this abnormality is prevalent. Genetic heterogeneity also explains to a large extent the diversity of clinical manifestations. Different mutations are responsible for the less common patients who have chronic hemolytic anemia and for the frequent

A list of standard abbreviations is located immediately preceding the index in each volume. Additional abbreviations used in this chapter include: CNSHA = chronic nonspherocytic hemolytic anemia; GSHPX = glutathione peroxidase; NNJ = neonatal jaundice.

patients who are only at risk of developing episodic hemolysis.

5. **The high prevalence of G-6-PD mutants that have arisen independently suggests a pattern of convergent evolution through balanced polymorphism. Epidemiologic data indicate that G-6-PD deficiency confers relative resistance against *Plasmodium falciparum* malaria, and clinical data indicate that this may be confined to heterozygous females. In vitro culture studies have shown that the growth of malaria parasites is impaired on first passage from normal to G-6-PD-deficient red cells, but that through subsequent passages they can adapt and grow normally, thus explaining clinical protection of heterozygotes but not of deficient hemizygotes. The adaptation phenomenon, and the failure of adaptation in heterozygotes, point to a special type of interaction between the parasite and the host in the context of red-cell mosaicism resulting from X-chromosome inactivation.**

The recognition of human pathology associated with deficiency of glucose 6-phosphate dehydrogenase (G-6-PD) in red blood cells is quite ancient. It has gone through several stages.[1] First came the anecdotal observation by the Greek philosopher and mathematician Pythagoras, who is said to have warned his disciples against the dangers of eating fava beans (*Vicia faba;* broad beans). Second was the clinical picture of favism drawn at the turn of the century by a number of physicians in Southern Italy and Sardinia.[2–4] In contrast to some other inborn errors of metabolism, the mode of inheritance was not easy to establish, because exposure and response to fava beans is erratic; thus both a "toxic theory" and an "allergic theory" of the pathogenesis of favism were popular.[5] However, observant general practitioners had noticed that the condition did "run in families."[2] The third stage was the recognition of hemolytic anemia caused by drugs. It soon became clear that only some individuals were susceptible, and the term "primaquine sensitivity" was appropriately coined.[6] For hematology, this syndrome was important because hemolytic anemia had been traditionally classified as being due to either intracorpuscular or extracorpuscular causes. Here was one that was caused by an exogenous agent, but only in people who presumably already had abnormal red cells.[7] The final stage was the discovery by Carson et al.[8] in Chicago that, indeed, primaquine-sensitive people had a very low level of G-6-PD activity in their red cells. Soon thereafter, similar observations were made in Germany[9] and in Italy on the red cells of people with a past history of favism.[10] The genetic heterogeneity of this abnormality then became quickly apparent,[11,12] and the question arose as to whether G-6-PD deficiency was due mainly to qualitative or to quantitative changes in the enzyme. In other words, it was not clear whether it was more similar to a structural hemoglobinopathy or to a thalassemia-like disorder. Over the last 30 years, the biochemical basis and the clinical implications of G-6-PD deficiency have been largely established, and thus far the only known causes of G-6-PD deficiency are a multitude of different structural allelic mutants. More recently, the molecular structures of the normal gene and of many mutants have been elucidated. Since the previous edition of this book, several reviews dealing with G-6-PD have appeared.[13–17] The hematologic aspects of G-6-PD deficiency have also been covered in textbooks and monographs.[18–21]

STRUCTURE OF G-6-PD

G-6-PD in its active form is either a dimer or a tetramer consisting of identical subunits.[22,23] Both the dimer and the tetramer are active, and the two forms are in a pH-dependent equilibrium with each other, with about equal proportions present at neutral pH.[24,25] There are two molecules of tightly bound NADP per molecule of dimer,[26] but the relationship between this "structural" NADP and substrate NADP is not yet clear.

The primary structure of the single subunit polypeptide chain has been determined from the cDNA sequence (see below). It consists of 515 amino acids (Fig. 111-1), with a molecular weight of 59,265 daltons. The rat liver G-6-PD amino acid sequence, obtained by protein analysis,[27] shows 94 percent homology with the human sequence and provides evidence that the N-terminal amino acid is *N*-acetyl-alanine, which must result from posttranslational cleavage of the N-terminal methionine followed by acetylation. It is likely that the same is true of the human enzyme. The C-terminal peptide predicted by the DNA sequence agrees with that determined by analysis of red-cell G-6-PD[28] despite previous claims that it is different from leukocyte G-6-PD.[29] Sequence information that has become available on the G-6-PD from a variety of organisms, ranging from prokaryotes[30,31] to yeasts[32,33] to *Drosophila*[34] to the human, has now made it possible to outline the evolution of the corresponding gene. A recent analysis[33] has revealed a total of 75 fully conserved amino acid residues. Not surprisingly, these are not randomly distributed. Indeed, one can identify several stretches of conserved residues, which presumably correspond to important functional domains. Thus far, the only domain that has a known function is the one surrounding lysine 205 of the human sequence, which was previously shown to be the

```
MAEQVALSRT  HVCGILREEL  FQGDAFHQSD  THIFIIMGAS  GDLAKKKIYP   50
TIWWLFRDGL  LPENTFIVGY  ARSRLTVADI  RKQSEPFFKA  TPEEKLKLED  100
FFARNSYVAG  QYDDAASYQR  LNSHMNALHL  GSQANRLFYL  ALPPTVYEAV  150
TKNIHESCMS  QIGWNRIIVE  KPFGRDLQSS  DRLSNHISSL  FREDQIYRID  200
HYLGKEMVQN  LMVLRFANRI  FGPIWNRDNI  ACVILTFKEP  FGTEGRGGYF  250
DEFGIIRDVM  QNHLLQMLCL  VAMEKPASTN  SDDVRDEKVK  VLKCISEVQA  300
NNVVLGQYVG  NPDGEGEATK  GYLDDPTVPR  GSTTATFAAV  VLYVENERWD  350
GVPFILRCGK  ALNERKAEVR  LQFHDVAGDI  FHQQCKRNEL  VIRVQPNEAV  400
YTKMMTKKPG  MFFNPEESEL  DLTYGNRYKN  VKLPDAYERL  ILDVFCGSQM  450
HFVRSDELRE  AWRIFTPLLH  QIELEKPKPI  PYIYGSRGPT  EADELMKRVG  500
FQYEGTYKWV  NPHKL
```

FIG. 111-1 **Amino acid sequence of human G-6-PD. The N-terminal methionine is not present in the mature protein, and the N-terminal alanine is acetylated. Highlighted residues are fully conserved in G-6-PD from nine different organisms, ranging from bacteria and yeast to mammals. It is seen that lysine 205 is within the longest highly conserved peptide. This residue is part of the G-6-P-binding site.**

binding site for the substrate glucose 6-phosphate (G6P).[35] There are 11 cysteine residues per subunit, and one or more of them must be important for enzyme activity, since sulfhydryl group inhibitors, such as hydroxymercuribenzoate and *N*-ethylmaleimide, cause marked inhibition.[36]

METABOLIC ROLE OF G-6-PD

G-6-PD is depicted classically in intermediary metabolism as a step in the conversion of glucose 6-phosphate to pentose phosphate. Indeed, it is the first enzyme in the so-called pentose phosphate pathway, also referred to as the oxidative "shunt" (by contrast to the "mainstream" glycolytic Embden-Meyerhof pathway). However, pentose can be produced alternatively by the concerted action of transketolase and transaldolase, thus bypassing G-6-PD. There are limited data on what fraction of pentose is normally produced via G-6-PD as opposed to the transketolase–transaldolase route, and the ratio may vary in different cells and under different circumstances. However, Chinese hamster ovary cells[37] and human fibroblasts[38] with less than 5 percent of normal G-6-PD activity can grow normally, suggesting that G-6-PD does not need to contribute much to the large amount of pentose that is needed for nucleic acid synthesis. On the other hand, G-6-PD produces NADPH, the coenzyme that is the main hydrogen donor for numerous other enzymatic reactions. Some of these reactions are essential steps in biosynthetic pathways; another, catalyzed by glutathione reductase, is essential in protecting cells against oxidative damage (Fig. 111-2). Glutathione converts H_2O_2 to H_2O stoichiometrically via glutathione peroxidase (GSHPX). Thus, the detoxification of each molecule of hydrogen peroxide requires one molecule of NADPH, ultimately provided by G-6-PD. An alternative pathway of H_2O_2 detoxification is via catalase. This route has been regarded as ineffective under normal circumstances,[39] because the affinity of catalase for H_2O_2 is much lower than that of GSHPX. In addition, the rare genetic defect acatalasemia is not associated with hemolytic anemia.[40] However, Kirkman and Gaetani[41,42] have discovered that catalase has four moles of tightly bound NADPH per mole of enzyme dimer, thereby bringing to light a further unexpected link between the G-6-PD coenzyme and H_2O_2 detoxification. From a comparison of normal and catalase-deficient red cells, they further inferred that catalase accounts for more than half of the destruction of H_2O_2 when the latter is generated at a rate comparable to that which leads to hemolysis in G-6-PD-deficient erythrocytes.[43] Thus, we must now regard NADPH as essential for both pathways of H_2O_2 detoxification. Its role is stoichiometric when GSHPX is used, whereas it is catalytic when catalase is used. It has been postulated that when NADPH is in short supply owing to a G-6-PD deficiency, catalase may become much more important in H_2O_2 detoxification.[44]

REGULATION OF G-6-PD ACTIVITY

As for all enzymes, the activity of G-6-PD in a cell could in theory be changed by two general mechanisms. These are discussed below.

Variation in the Number of G-6-PD Molecules

Enzyme activity measured in cell extracts under optimal conditions and with saturating substrate concentrations is assumed to be proportional to the number of molecules present. While G-6-PD is found in all cells, its level varies over a range of about two orders of magnitude in different tissues (Table 111-1) regardless of whether the activity is expressed per cell or per milligram of protein. These tissue-specific differences may result from variations in the rate of transcription, in posttranscriptional processing, in mRNA stability, in the rate of translation, or in posttranslational changes, especially the rate of proteolytic degradation. Each of these possibilities is likely to be important in specific circumstances. For instance, an increase in G-6-PD-specific mRNA has been observed in the liver of rats in which fatty acid synthesis is stimulated by a high-carbohydrate diet after starvation,[45,46] and variation of mRNA is seen in various fetal and adult human organs.[47] Different rates of proteolysis are suggested by the wide difference between the half-life of normal G-6-PD in fibroblasts (about 2 days[48]) and in red cells (about 60 days[49]). Variation in the rate of transcription has not yet been conclusively proven, but its occurrence is suggested by the finding of an empirical correlation between the extent of methylation of cytosine residues in a DNA region located 3′ to the G-6-PD gene and the level of G-6-PD activity in a variety of fetal and adult organs.[47]

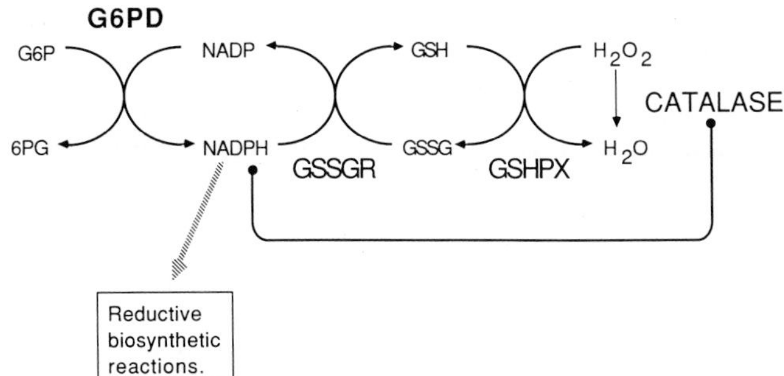

FIG. 111-2 The main metabolic role of G-6-PD in red cells is the defense against oxidizing agents, epitomized by hydrogen peroxide. NADPH, a product of the G-6-PD reaction, is both the hydrogen donor for regeneration of reduced glutathione and a ligand for catalase (see text). GSSGR = glutathione reductase; GSHPX = glutathione peroxidase; G-6-P = glucose-6-phosphate; 6PG = phosphogluconate.

Variation in the Enzyme Activity of Existing G-6-PD Molecules

The actual intracellular activity of G-6-PD, like that of any other enzyme, may be very different from what is measured

Table 111-1 G-6-PD Activity in Selected Tissues

	In normal subjects, milliunits/mg protein*	In G-6-PD-deficient subjects, % of normal⁺
Erythrocytes	8.5	1–50
Granulocytes	851	1–90
Fibroblasts	174	2–90
Muscle	3.3	—
Liver	7.2	15–50
Brain⁺⁺	85	—

*From Battistuzzi et al.[47]
⁺From Luzzatto and Battistuzzi[335] and unpublished results. The range is very wide because the expression of G-6-PD deficiency, defined by assaying erythrocytes, varies widely with different *Gd*⁻ alleles.
⁺⁺Fetal.

under optimal conditions in cell-free extracts. Many effects, including pH,[24,25] divalent cations,[50] inorganic phosphate, phosphorylated intermediates, and other compounds[51,52] have been found to affect G-6-PD activity. Among known metabolites, at least three must be major determinants of the intracellular G-6-PD activity: the two substrates, G-6-P and NADP, and one of the reaction products, NADPH, which is a potent, partially competitive inhibitor of G-6-PD.[53,54] In red cells, the estimated concentration of G-6-P is about 32 μM (well below the K_m of G-6-P of 72 μM) and the concentration of NADP is extremely low (probably less than 1 μM[55]), whereas the concentration of NADPH is high. (Estimating the concentrations of NADP and NADPH is made complicated by the fact that substantial fractions of these compounds are bound to catalase and NADPH diaphorase, respectively[56].) Thus, it can be predicted that the intracellular G-6-PD activity is only a small fraction of the maximum activity that would be available if substrate concentrations were saturating.[52] It is practically impossible to faithfully simulate intracellular conditions, but in the case of G-6-PD the intracellular activity can be measured experimentally by the rate of production of $^{14}CO_2$ from [1-^{14}C]glucose. By using this technique, Kirkman and Gaetani[57] validated the above predictions. They estimated that, in normal red cells, G-6-PD operates at only about 1 to 2 percent of its maximal potential, even under the stimulatory action of methylene blue (which tends to continuously reoxidize the NADPH produced by G-6-PD). This finding quantifies the vast reserve of reductive potential that is available to normal red cells, and which is substantially decreased in G-6-PD-deficient red cells, thus determining their pathophysiological features (see below).

GENETICS

Inheritance of G-6-PD shows a characteristic X-linked pattern, and the much higher incidence of favism in males than in females was recognized even before G-6-PD deficiency was discovered.[58] In contrast to several other X-linked conditions, however, there are many populations in which the frequency of G-6-PD deficiency is so high that homozygous females are not rare (see Luzzatto[59]). In biochemical terms, the inheritance of G-6-PD is typically codominant, as can be seen easily when electrophoretic variants segregate in a pedigree (Fig. 111-3). In terms of clinical expression, G-6-PD deficiency is sometimes classified as X-linked recessive.[60] Although X-linked, it is not truly recessive since heterozygous females can develop hemolytic attacks, even severe ones. This is explained by the coexistence in heterozygotes of two cell populations, G-6-PD(+) and G-6-PD(−), as a result of X-chromosome inactivation (see Fig. 111-7). Beutler et al.[61] first demonstrated this physiological mosaicism in human red cells using G-6-PD as a marker. Soon afterward, Davidson et al.[62] obtained cellular clones expressing different G-6-PD alleles (*Gd^B* and *Gd^A*) from skin fibroblasts of heterozygotes, thus proving conclusively that mosaicism was genetically determined in somatic cells by faithful maintenance of the active state of one or the other X chromosome in each cell and its progeny.

Formal genetic analysis has already established that *Gd* was closely linked to several other X-linked genes,[63,64] including those for hemophilia A, color blindness, and adrenoleukodystrophy. The use of somatic cell hybrids[65] and of *in situ* hybridization with G-6-PD-specific probes[66,67] firmly mapped *Gd* as being distal to the fragile site Xq27.3. Subsequently, physical linkage between *Gd* and the factor VIII gene has been established, within a length of about 400 kb, through analysis by pulsed-field gel electrophoresis of large DNA restriction fragments.[68] Yeast artificial chromosome (YAC) contigs have now fully established the physical relationship between *Gd,* factor VIII, and the color vision genes.[69]

The G-6-PD Gene

Comparison of cDNA clones with genomic clones has revealed that the G-6-PD gene consists of 13 exons and 12 introns[70] (Fig. 111-4). The coding exons vary in size from 38 to 236 bp. All introns are small (less than 1 kb), except for intron II, which is about 11 kb long. The 5′ untranslated portion of the mRNA corresponds to exon I and part of exon II; the initiation codon is in exon II, and the large intron, the significance of which is unknown, interrupts the coding sequence at codon 36. The size of the G-6-PD mRNA expected from the sequence is 2269 nucleotides. This is in good agreement with the size of about 2.4 kb [including the poly(A) tail] measured on northern blots.[71] A sequence previously reported as the 3′ end of the G-6-PD gene[72] turns out to belong to a separate gene, located only 40 kb downstream from the G-6-PD gene itself, referred to provisionally as GdX,[70] that encodes a protein having significant sequence homology to ubiquitin.[73] The relationship of this gene to G-6-PD is not yet known. It appears that a third gene exists between G-6-PD and GdX,[74] and that G-6-PD is embedded in a gene-rich region.[75] It has been claimed that

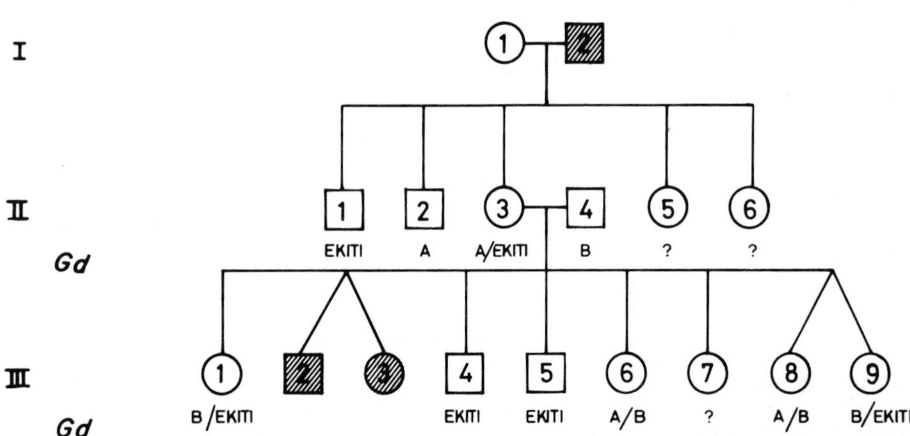

FIG. 111-3 X-linked inheritance of G-6-PD in a family segregating three different alleles (A, B, and EKITI) at the G-6-PD locus, *Gd*. Shaded symbols denote deceased subjects. *(From Usanga et al.,[516] with permission.)*

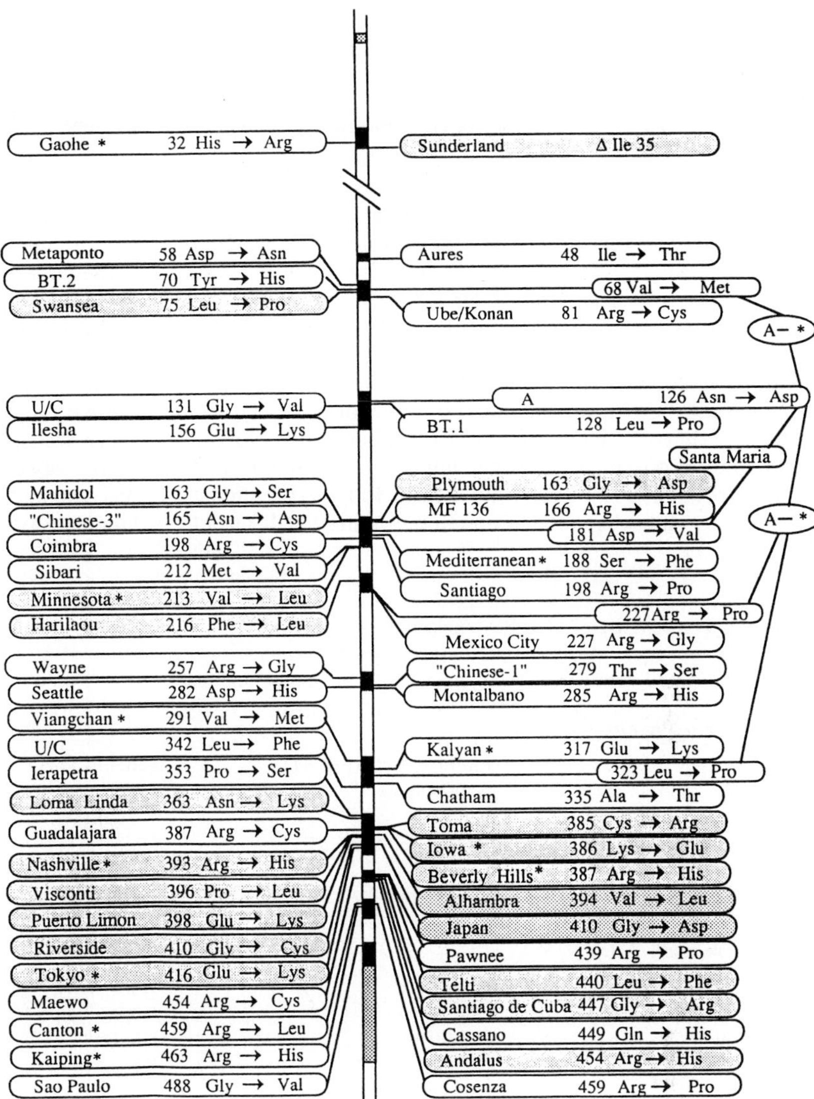

FIG. 111-4 Genomic structure of the human G-6-PD gene. The variants with known mutations are shown individually. The background is white for non-deficient variants (class IV) and for deficient variants associated only with acute hemolytic anemia (classes II and III). The background is gray for the more severe variants associated with chronic non-spherocytic hemolytic anemia (class I).

a portion of the G-6-PD protein is encoded by an autosomal gene mapped to chromosome 6.[76] However, this latter gene turns out to encode instead guanosine monophosphate reductase,[77] and the claim has been now refuted[78,79] and retracted.[80]

The G-6-PD mRNA, like that of most genes, has a relatively short 5′ untranslated region of 69 bp and a longer 3′ untranslated region of 655 bp (Table 111-2). The entire genomic gene has now been sequenced,[81] including about 2 kb of sequence upstream of the transcription initiation site. The mouse genomic gene also has been characterized and has considerable similarity to the human gene, not only in the coding region but also in its overall organization.[82] The G-6-PD promoter[70] is very GC-rich (more than 70 percent), and it contains several SP1-binding elements, GGCGGG and CCGCCC, reminiscent of the 21-bp repeats of the SV40 early promoter.[83] This region contains, therefore, a considerable number of CG dinucleotides, many of which are not methylated. They constitute an island of HTF (*Hpa*II tiny fragments), a feature currently regarded as characteristic of DNA flanking a gene.[84] In this respect, this region is similar to other housekeeping gene promoters.[85,86] It also contains an ATTAAA element at position −30 to −25, which may play the role of a "TATA box" (present in some housekeeping genes but not in others).[70] The size of the G-6-PD "minimal promoter" has been narrowed down to about 160 bp by deletion analysis.[87] However, it remains to be defined what structural element, if any, determines the rate of transcription in different cells, under different physiological conditions (e.g., in response to changes in diet[88] or to hormones[89]), or

Table 111-2 Molecular Numerology of Human G-6-PD

DNA	
Size of gene, kb	18.5
Total number of exons	13
Coding exons	12
mRNA	
Size in nucleotides	2269
5′ untranslated region	69
Coding region	1545
3′ untranslated region	655
Protein	
Amino acids, number	515
Molecular weight	59,265
Subunits per molecule of active enzyme	2 or 4
Molecules of tightly bound NADP per subunit	1

in tissues with markedly increased G-6-PD activity, such as the lactating mammary gland[90] or certain tumors.[91]

Genetic Polymorphism of G-6-PD

It became apparent almost immediately after the discovery of G-6-PD deficiency that the condition was caused not by a single mutation but by a variety of genetic changes. The initial criteria for this inference were the level of residual activity and the electrophoretic mobility. Subsequently, the study of other physicochemical properties (thermostability, chromatographic behavior), and of kinetic properties (K_m for G6P, K_m for NADP, pH dependence, utilization of substrate analogues) revealed that numerous variants must exist even within a set having the same or very similar residual activity and electrophoretic mobility. In 1967, a WHO study group made recommendations on standardized methods of analysis,[92] which have been followed by most investigators and subsequently updated.[93] Some 400 different variants have been reported to date (Tables 111-3A and 111-3B). For taxonomic purposes, it is convenient to classify G-6-PD variants according to the level of enzyme activity and to the clinical manifestations (classes I to V) or according to whether they are sporadic or polymorphic. Not surprisingly, these classification criteria are not unrelated to each other. For instance, variants in class I (chronic nonspherocytic hemolytic anemia, CNSHA) are never polymorphic, presumably because their clinical expression is too severe to become balanced by malaria selection. Among variants in class IV (normal activity), nearly all are electrophoretically different from the wild type (B), because otherwise they would not be detected. A new approach to testing the identity of G-6-PD variants and the relationships among them by multivariate analysis has been proposed.[94] Although there were several reports in the earlier literature of "complete" absence of G-6-PD[95,96] complete G-6-PD deficiency has yet to be identified; all the human mutants are, in the language of classic microbial genetics, "leaky." Therefore,

Table 111-3A List of G-6-PD variants

Class I (Associated with chronic non-spherocytic hemolytic anemia)			
Electrophoretically Fast			
Andalus[c] (ref. 126)	Fukuoka[d] (ref. 413)	Lincoln Park[s]	Puerto Limon (ref. 414)
Barcelona[b]	Gaudalajara[b]	Linda Vista[bd]	San Diego[d]
Baudelocque[bd]	Heian[c]	Nagano[b]	St. Louis
Birmingham[b]	Hotel Dieu[b]	Ohio[cd]	Torrance
Charleston[bd]	Jackson[b]	Pawnee[2bb] (ref. 14)	Varadero
East Harlem[c]	Lawndale[c]	Pea Ridge	Wayne
Electrophoretically Normal			
Aarau[bd]	Dothan[d]	Hong Kong[b]	New York
Akita[b]	Duarte[d]	Iowa City (ref. 14)	Ogikubo[bd]
Albuquerque[cd]	Dublin	Kaluga[b]	Oklahoma[c]
Bangkok[d]	Englewood	Kanazawa	Regensburg[b]
Bat-Yam[bd]	Galveston[b]	Kilgore[b]	Sapporo
Boston[b]	Hamburg[cd]	Kremenchug[b]	Tokushima[d] (ref. 14)
Chinese	Hawaii[bd]	Kyoto[c]	Yokohama
Clinic (ref. 415)	Hayem[b]	Missoula[b]	
**Cornell[d]	Helsinki[b]	Nancy[c]	
Electrophoretically Slow			
Alhambra	Hongkong Pokfulam	Minneapolis[c]	Santiago[d]
Arlington Heights[cd]	Indianapolis[d] (ref. 14)	Moosburg[d] (ref. 418)	Santiago de Cuba (ref. 101)
Ashdod[c]	Iowa[d] (ref. 14)	Panama[b]	Sendagi[b]
Atlanta[d]	Iwate[d] (ref. 417)	Pompton Plains (ref. 14)	Tokyo[d]
Beverly Hills (ref. 14)	Johannesburg[c]	Portici[cd] (ref. 419)	Tripler[bd]
Chicago*[d]	Kobe[cd]	Rennes[c]	Tsukui[d] (ref. 420)
Freiburg[c]	Long Prairie[bd]	Riverside[cd] (ref. 14)	Walter Reed[b]
Genova[c] (ref. 416)	Loma Linda[d] (ref. 14)	Rotterdam[b]	West Town[d]
Grand Prairie[bd]	Manchester	San Francisco[cd]	Worcester[bd]
Huron[bd]	Milwaukee[c]	Santa Barbara[d]	
Class II (Severely deficient, less than 10% residual activity)			
Electrophoretically Fast			
Amboin[b]*	Dhon (ref. 422)	Long Xuyen*[c]	San Jose
Amman I	Ferrara[bd]	Lublin[b]	Taipei Hakka*[b]
Ankara	Ferrara III	Mali*[b]	Taiwan Hakka*[b]
Azerbaijan[b]	Haad Yai*[c]	Markham*[b]	Tehran
Baku	Hualien[bd]	Matam	Union*
Betika*	Hualien Chi[b]	N-Sawan*[bd]	Union-Markham*[b]
Boluo (ref. 421)	Huazhou (ref. 421)	Padrew*[b]	Zaehringen[b]
Castilla-Like*[b]	Huiyang (ref. 421)	Palmi I	

Table 111-3A List of G-6-PD variants *(Continued)*

Class II (Severely deficient, less than 10% residual activity) *Continued*

Electrophoretically Normal

Abrami[b]	Dakar[b]	Hamm[bd]	Petrich[*b]
Baghdad	Dushanba II	Indonesia	Rudosem[b]
Bielefeld[b]	El Fayoum[*b]	Iserlohn[b]	Sassari[*b]
Blida[*b]	Espoo[b]	Kaiping[d] (ref. 421)	Schwaben[b]
Bnei-Brak	Fort Worth[b]	Mediterranean[*b]	Selim[b]
Bodensee	Gaomin[b] (ref. 421)	Moscow[b]	Songhkla[bd] (ref. 423)
Cagliari[*b]	Gifu	N-Pathom[c*]	Strasbourg[c]
Campbell-Pore[*bd]	Goodenough[c]	Nukus[c]	Tarsus
Columbus[*c]	Gotze Delchev[*bd]	Ogori[b]	Viangchan[c] (ref. 424)
Corinth[*b]			

Electrophoretically Slow

Aachen	Dushanba 1[b]	Onoda[b]	Shirin-Bulakh[bd]
Adana[cd] (ref. 425)	Fukushima[b]	Orchomeros[*b]	Stella[d]
Alger[*bd]	Jammu	Palakau	Swit[*b]
Amman II[b]	Kaluan[*cd]	Panay	Titteri[*b]
Angoram[*b]	Kar Kar[*b]	Popondetta[*b]	Toulouse[d]
Asahikawa[c]	Kirovograd[b]	Port Elizabeth[bd]	Wakayama[bd]
Avenches[bd] (ref. 418)	Kurume[bd]	Posillipo[d]	Waterloo[bd] (ref. 14)
Bideiz[bd]	Laos (ref. 14)	Poznan[*b]	West Bengal[*b]
Bogia[A]	Lifta[bd]	Ramat Gan[*bd]	Wewak[*b]
Caltanissetta[b]	Madang[*]	Salata[c]	Wroclaw[d]
Ciudad de la Habana[b]	Mainoki	Samandag[b] (ref. 425)	Yamaguchi[bd]
Chainat	Manus	Santa Maria[b]	Zakataly[b]
Colomiers[b]	Menorca	Shekii[bd]	Zhitomir[b]
Dallas[bd] (ref. 14)	Okhut 1[b]		

Class III (Moderately deficient, 10–60% residual activity)

Electrophoretically Fast

A^{-}[*] (ref. 425)	East Africa[c]	Kephalonia[b]	Puerto Rico[b]
Alabama	Galliera	Konan[*b]	Qing Baijan[b] (ref. 414)
Attica[b]	Gallura[b]	Laghouat[*b]	San Juan[bd]
Canton	Guang Zhou[c] (ref. 421)	Lazere	Selma (ref. 14)
Castilla	Guantanamo[b] (ref. 426)	Matera (ref. 101)	Tahta[*b]
Caujeri (ref. 426)	Hiroshima-1 (ref. 428)	Melissa	Tel-Hashomer[*b]
Central City (ref. 427)	Hiroshima-3 (ref. 428)	Muret	Tepic
Chiapas[b]	Jalisco[b]	Nagasaki-2[b] (ref. 428)	Toronto[b]
Chibuto[b]	Junut[c]	Nagasaki-3 (ref. 428)	Ube[*]
Debrousse[*]	Kabyle[*]	Nanhai[b] (ref. 421)	Velletri[cd]
Djynet[b]			

Electrophoretically Normal

Camaldow	El Morro[b]	Kamiube[*b]	Tashkent[b]
Chatham[d]	Handi (ref. 429)	Mahidol[*b]	Trapani
Columbus	Hillbrow[b]	Nedelino	Villa Clara[b] (ref. 430)
El Kharga[*]	Hofu[b]	Siriraj[*b]	Vin Fu (ref. 429)

Electrophoretically Slow

Agrigento[b]	Gaohe[b] (ref. 421)	Mercury (ref. 14)	Regar[b]
Anant[*b]	Gaozhou	Metaponto	Santa Clara[b] (ret. 430)
Athens[*b]	Great Lakes[d] (ref. 14)	Mexico[b]	Seattle[*b]
Avvocato	Ilesha[c]	Montalbano[b] (ref. 121)	Siwa[*b]
Benevento[b]	Intanon	Musashino (ref. 432)	Tenganan[*b]
Camaldoli	Kalyan[b]	Napoli[b]	Thenia[*]
Camperdown[b]	Kerala[b]	Okhut II[*b]	Trinacria[b]
Carswell[b]	Kobe[cd]	Palepoli[*d]	Tursi[b] (ref. 121)
Ferrara II[b]	Kuanyama[b]	Pallonetto[*d]	Vientiane[b]
Fort Pierce (ref. 14)	Lodi (ref. 431)	Petilia	Washington
Frankfurt	Lizu-Baisha	Pordenone[c]	Yangoru[*b]
Gabrovizza[b]	Los Angeles		

Continued

Table 111-3A List of G-6-PD variants *(Continued)*

Class IV: (Normal activity, 60–150%)

Electrophoretically Fast

A*	King County[c]	Lynn (ref. 14)	S. Dona[c]
Bali*	Kiwa*	Mammola[b]	Singapore (ref. 433)
Barbieri[c]	Lourenco Marquez*	Miseno	S-Sakorn*[c]
Hiroshima-2 (ref. 428)	Levadia[b]	Nagasaki I (ref. 428)	Steilacom
Inhambane*[b]	Luz Saint Sauveur[b]	Pamli II	Titusille (ref. 434)

Electrophoretically Normal

B*
Cuiaba[c]
Huntsville (ref. 435)

Electrophoretically Slow

Abeokuta[c]	Gambia*	Madrona	Port Alegre[b]
Adame[b]	Ibadan-Austin*	Manjacase*[c]	Port Royal[b]
Alessandria[b]	Ijebu-Ode	Minas Gerais[b]	Pozzallo[c]
Alexandra	Ita-Bale[c]	Morelia[b]	Regar (ref. 436)
Ayutthaya*[c]	Kardista[b]	Pinar del Rio[b]	Tacoma*[c]
Baltimore-Austin	Laguna[b]	Pisticci[b] (ref. 121)	Thessaly[b]
Ekiti	Lanlate[b]	Porbander	Western[b]
Capetown[b]			

Class V (Increased Activity)

Electrophoretically Fast

Hektoen*	Verona[c] (ref. 437)

* = polymorphic
b = low K_m G6P
c = high K_m G6P
d = very labile
**Probably identical with Chicago.
References are given only for those variants which were not included in the previous edition which lists all other pertinent references.

we must understand the pathophysiology of G-6-PD deficiency in terms of the quantity and quality of the residual mutant enzyme.

As for any other genetically determined enzymopathy, deficiency of G-6-PD might be due to a quantitative reduction in the number of enzyme molecules, to a qualitative change in the structure of the enzyme molecule, or to both. The findings reviewed in the previous section strongly supported the notion that most subjects with G-6-PD deficiency have a qualitatively abnormal enzyme, and that a wide range of different mutational changes have taken place in human populations. As soon as it became possible to sequence variants, these expectations were in broad outline verified. From an analysis of 59 variants characterized at the molecular level[129] (Table 111-4) a reasonably clear pattern is beginning to emerge for the molecular basis of G-6-PD deficiency. First, in nearly all the G-6-PD variants, we find a single amino acid replacement, caused by a single missense point mutation. In a few cases (the three types of A^- variant, G-6-PD$_{\mathrm{SANTAMARIA}}$ and G-6-PD$_{\mathrm{MOUNT\ SINAI}}$) we find two amino acid replacements, and in all of these one of the replacements is that of G-6-PD A. Since this variant is polymorphic in Africa, the most likely explanation is that a second point mutation has taken place in a Gd^A gene. In one case, three separate amino acid replacements have been reported (G-6-PD$_{\mathrm{VANCOUVER}}$). Although this finding is thus far unique, we note that one of these replacements is the same as the one in G-6-PD$_{\mathrm{COIMBRA}}$, which is polymorphic in the

Table 111-3B Summary of G-6-PD variants

	Polymorphic		Electrophoretic mobility				
Class	**Number**	**%**	**Fast**	**Normal**	**Slow**	**Altered electrophoretic mobility, %**	**Total**
I	1	1	24	34	39	64	97
II	37	30	31	37	54	70	122
III	22	21	41	16	46	84	103
IV	12	23	20	3	29	94	52
V	0		2			100	2
Total	72	19	118	90	168	76	376

Table 111-4 Genetic Variants of G-6-PD Characterized at the Molecular Level

Name	Amino Acid Number	Amino Acid Replacement	Class	Electrophoretic Mobility	K_{mG6P}, μM	Population	References
Gaohe	32	His→Arg	III	96	31	Chinese*	97
Sunderland	35	Δ Ile	I	95		English	98
Aures	48	Ile→Thr	II	100	59	Algerian*	99
Metaponto	58	Asp→Asn	III	90	47	Italian	100, 101
A⁻	68	Val→Met	III	110	60	African*	102, 148
	126	Asn→Asp					
Swansea	75	Leu→Pro	I			Welsh	MacDonald et al., unpublished
Ube	81	Arg→Cys	III	108	52	Japanese*	103
Lagosanto	81	Arg→His	III			Italian	152
Vancouver	106	Ser→Lys	I			Canadian	104
	182	Arg→Trp					
	198	Arg→Cys					
A	126	Asn→Asp	IV	110	60	African*	105
Quing-Yan	131	Gly→Val	III	100	56	Chinese*	106
Ilesha	156	Glu→Lys	III	75	83	Nigerian	107
Mahidol	163	Gly→Ser	II	100	40	Thai/Cambodian*	108
Plymouth	163	Gly→Asp	I	103	48	English	Town et al., unpublished
Chinese-3	165	Asn→Asp	II			Chinese	109
Santamaria	181	Asp→Val	II	98	16	Costa Rican	110
	126	Asn→Asp					
Mediterranean	188	Ser→Phe	II	100	23	Mediterranean/ Indian	101
Coimbra	198	Arg→Cys	II	100	7	Mediterranean*	112
Santiago	198	Arg→-Pro	I			Chilean	113
Sibari	212	Met→Val	III	100	31	Italian*	114
Minnesota	213	Val→Leu	I	95	88	USA–white	115
Harilaou	216	Phe→Leu	I	100		Greek	116
Mexico City	227	Arg→Gln	III	110		Mexican	113
A⁻	227	Arg→Leu	III	110		USA–black	117
	126	Asn→Asp					
Stonybrook	242–243	Δ Gly, Thr	I				Beutler et al., unpublished
Wayne	257	Arg→Gly	I	107	78		118
Chinese-1	279	Thr→Ser	II			Chinese*	119
Seattle	282	Asp→His	III	80	20	European*	120
Montalbano	285	Arg→His	III	93	49	Italian*	121
Viangchan	291	Val→Met	III	100	105	Laotian*	118
Kalyan	317	Glu→Lys	III	75	105	Indian*	122
Nara	Δ319–326	—	I	—	—	Japanese	143
A⁻	323	Leu→Pro	III	110		USA–black/ Spanish*	102
	126	Asn→Asp					
Chatham	335	Ala→Thr	III	100	60	Indian*	101
Chinese-5	342	Leu→Phe	III	91	65	Chinese*	106
Ierapetra	353	Pro→Ser	II			Greek	113
Loma Linda	363	Asn→Lys	I	98	70	USA–Mexican	11
Tomah	385	Cys→Arg	I				123
Iowa	386	Lys→Glu	I	100	65	USA–white	123
Guadalajara	387	Arg→Cys	I	100	36	Mexican	113
Mount Sinai	387	Arg→Cys	I				Vlachos et al., unpublished
	126	Asn→Asp					
Beverly Hills	387	Arg→His	I	95	41	Italian	123
Nashville	393	Arg→His	I	100	87	USA	115
Alhambra	394	Val→Leu	I	96	55	Finnish/Swedish	113
Puerto Limon	398	Glu→Lys	I	98	32	Costa Rican	110
Riverside	410	Gly→Cys	I	100	326	German/English	123
Japan	410	Gly→Asp	I			Japanese	115
Tokyo	416	Glu→Lys	I	90	65	Japanese	124
Atlanta-I	428	Tyr→STOP	I				Beutler et al., unpublished
Pawnee	439	Arg→Pro	I	103	50	USA–N. European	113

Continued

Table 111-4 *(Continued)*

Name	Amino Acid Number	Amino Acid Replacement	Class	Electrophoretic Mobility	K_{mG6P}, μM	Population	References
Telte	440	Leu→Phe	I	100		Italian	Busuttil et al., unpublished
Santiago de Cuba	447	Gly→Arg	I	80	50	Cuban	101
Cassano	449	Gln→His	II	93	14	Italian*	114
Union	454	Arg→Cys	II	105	8	Polynesian/ Filipino*	111
Andalus	454	Arg→His	I	100	14	Spanish	126
Canton	459	Arg→Leu	II	105	28	Chinese*	127
Cosenza	459	Arg→Pro	II	100	27	Italian	114
Kaiping	463	Arg→His	II	100	40	Chinese*	128
Campinas	488	Gly→Val	I			Brazilian	Baronciani et al., unpublished

SOURCE: Modified from ref 129. Used by permission.
*These variants are polymorphic.

Mediterranean area. In one case we find a deletion of a single amino acid (G-6-PD$_{SUNDERLAND}$), and in one case a deletion of two adjacent amino acids (G-6-PD$_{STONYBROOK}$).

Conspicuous by their absence are large deletions or major rearrangements. This is in contrast to what is abundantly documented in this volume with respect to most genes causing human disease. An important functional difference between this majority of genes and G-6-PD is that G-6-PD is a housekeeping gene expressed in all tissues. Hypoxanthine-guanine phosphoribosyltransferase (HPRT) is also regarded as a housekeeping gene, yet deletions have been reported. In order to explain the difference, we may then have to take into account another functional characteristic: namely, some housekeeping genes, although by definition expressed in all cells, may not be indispensable for cell viability. Thus, complete absence of HPRT activity is compatible with life and has no apparent consequence on the function of many types of cells, although unfortunately at the price of serious pathology affecting mainly the central nervous system. By contrast, at least a low level of G-6-PD activity may be indispensable for most cells, and therefore complete inactivation of the gene (e.g., by a large deletion) may be lethal early in embryonic life.

If G-6-PD deletions are not encountered because the gene is indispensable, can we identify any rule as to why certain point mutations are seen in preference to others? In this respect we can only offer some speculations.

1. Sporadic Mutations These are probably the majority (see Table 111-4), and most of them have been detected because they cause clinical manifestations in the form of CNSHA. These mutations must fulfill two requirements. On the one hand, they cannot cause complete loss of G-6-PD activity; otherwise they would fall in the same category as deletions (see above). On the other hand, they must cause sufficient loss of activity in red cells to become limiting for their in vivo survival. This in turn may result, in principle, from two (non-mutually-exclusive) mechanisms. (1) Severe alterations in the interaction with the substrates, particularly G-6-P (see above under regulation). (2) Marked intracellular instability. With both mechanisms, the changes must be relatively subtle, as they seem to affect red cells more than other somatic cells. Although we do not yet know how exactly this is brought about, it is not too difficult to imagine that intracellular stability, for instance, has very different consequences in red cells, which have a long life span after they have lost the ability to synthesize proteins, compared to other somatic cells, which are capable of regenerating continuously effete protein molecules. There is also evidence that protease activity is different in red cells.[48,130] Sporadic variants associated with CNSHA are not likely to spread by genetic drift. Thus, the fact that the same variant may be found repeatedly in people who are almost certainly not ancestrally related is not trivial. We have found, for instance, G-6-PD$_{TOKYO}$ in Dundee, Scotland, and G-6-PD$_{BEVERLY\ HILLS}$ in Genoa, Italy. These observations further corroborate the notion that subtle constraints make it necessary for a sporadic variant to have a distinctly severe clinical expression while remaining compatible with life.

2. Polymorphic Mutations Most known mutations in this category are again associated with G-6-PD deficiency (see Table 111-3B), and there is overwhelming evidence that they have become polymorphic as a result of malaria selection (see "G-6-PD Deficiency and Malaria" below). For these mutations we can visualize more stringent constraints. While they cause deficiency in red cells probably by similar mechanisms, they must not affect the red cells so severely as to outweigh the advantage with respect to malaria. Thus, it is not surprising that nearly all the polymorphic variants fall in classes II or III, and none of them causes CNSHA (class I). There is only one well-characterized variant in class IV, i.e., with normal activity. It is G-6-PD A, which was discovered and is easy to recognize because of its altered electrophoretic mobility. In view of the fact that we know of at least five G-6-PD double mutants that are derivatives of G-6-PD A, we infer that this variant must be quite ancient. Finally, we must remember that, as for other protein polymorphisms, electrophoretically silent, and therefore undetected, G-6-PD variants are likely to exist as well.

Spread of Polymorphic Variants of G-6-PD

The world distribution of G-6-PD deficiency is shown in Fig. 111-5. This figure represents what we could call a "phenotypic map," because it reflects the prevalence of G-6-PD deficiency as a whole, rather than that of individual variants. Ideally, the genetic epidemiology of the G-6-PD polymorphism should tell us both the distribution of a given allele and the set of polymorphic alleles that account for the overall prevalence of G-6-PD deficiency in a given population.

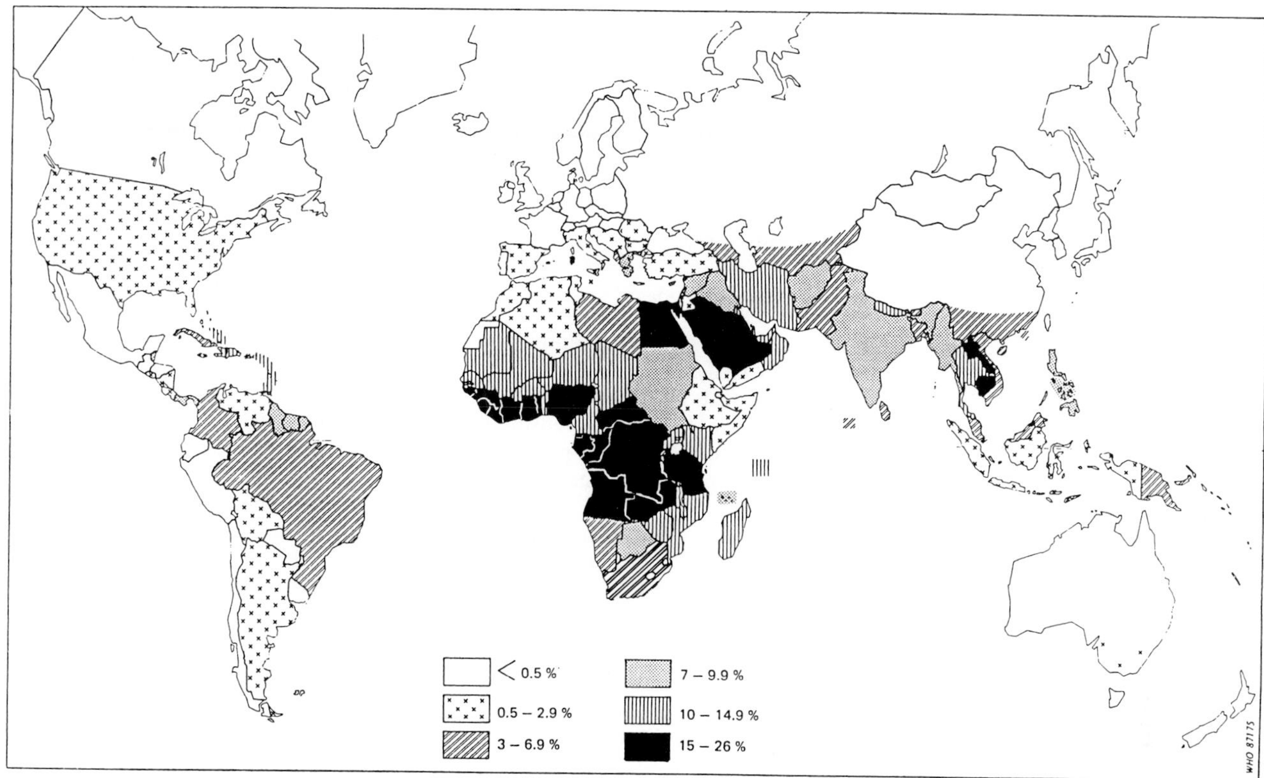

FIG. 111-5 World distribution of G-6-PD deficiency (from ref. 93). The values shown by the different shadings are frequencies in the populations of the various countries of G-6-PD-deficient males (which are also gene frequencies, since the gene is X-linked).

With respect to the distribution of individual alleles, detailed information is not yet available, but we can begin to visualize a pattern in broad strokes. *G-6-PD A*$^-$ is widespread all over Africa, in the West Indies, in the Americas, and wherever there are immigrant populations of African origin. In addition, G-6-PD A$^-$ is present with significant frequency in Southern Europe (for instance in Southern Italy,[101,114] Spain,[117] and Portugal[131]), and in the Arabian peninsula.[132] We have also found G-6-PD A$^-$ in 'white' Brazilians,[133] in a white American from South Carolina, and in Corsica. *G-6-PD*$_{\mathrm{MEDITERRANEAN}}$ turns out to have been named very appropriately, because it is polymorphic in all countries surrounding the Mediterranean sea, including North African countries.[134] But it is also widespread in the Middle East, including the Arab countries and Israel, and it accounts for almost all the G-6-PD deficiency in Kurdish Jews,[135] the population that has the highest known frequency of this trait (estimated gene frequency = 0.65). In addition, G-6-PD$_{\mathrm{MEDITERRANEAN}}$ is one of the most common G-6-PD deficient variants in the Indian subcontinent. *G-6-PD*$_{\mathrm{SEATTLE}}$ was first reported in a subject of Welsh ancestry in the United States.[136] Since then it has been found at polymorphic frequency in Sardinia,[120] Greece,[137] and Southern Italy,[100,114] and we have identified it also in subjects from Algeria, Germany, and Ireland. Thus, although we cannot say where it originated, it is likely to be very ancient, since its origin appears to predate the radiation of European and North African populations. *G-6-PD*$_{\mathrm{MAEWO}}$ had been reported in the Chinese[125] and in Southern Italy,[114] but we have given it this name because we know it is polymorphic in the island Maewo of the Vanuatu archipelago.[138] It has now been called G-6-PD$_{\mathrm{UNION}}$.[111] Unlike the mutations of G-6-PD A$^-$, G-6-PD$_{\mathrm{MEDITERRANEAN}}$, and G-6-PD$_{\mathrm{SEATTLE}}$, the mutation of G-6-PD$_{\mathrm{MAEWO}}$ consists of a C→T replacement in a CpG doublet, and its presence in disparate parts of the globe might result from independent mutational events in a mutational hotspot rather than from the spread of a single mutation. As for nondeficient variants, G-6-PD A is the only one known to be polymorphic, and its distribution is practically the same as that of G-6-PD A$^-$.

With respect to the set of polymorphic alleles that account for the overall prevalence of G-6-PD deficiency in individual populations, it is interesting that in most areas of high prevalence, multiple polymorphic alleles are found. For instance, this is true in the Mediterranean,[100,114,139] the Middle East,[132] India,[122] Southeast Asia,[129,140,141] China,[128,142] and Algeria.[134] The notable exception is tropical Africa, where G-6-PD A$^-$ accounts for at least 90 percent of G-6-PD deficiency,[144] and about 90 percent of G-6-PD A$^-$ is accounted for by the allele with the Val68Met mutation in addition to the Asn126Asp mutation.

Structure-Function Relationships

In the classic example of hemoglobin, the understanding of how individual amino acid replacements cause specific phenotypic changes—for instance, instability or altered oxygen affinity—has been greatly facilitated by the detailed knowledge of the three-dimensional structure of the molecule. Unfortunately we are not so privileged with G-6-PD. The only crystallographic data thus far available have been obtained on the *Leuconostoc mesenteroides* enzyme.[145] Although work on this protein has continued (M. Adams, personal communication), the complete structure has not yet been solved. We and others have obtained crystals of the human enzyme but they have not yielded sufficiently informative diffraction patterns. Thus, we are left for the moment with predictions of secondary structure (α-helix and β-sheet) based on conventional algorithms,[146,147] and perhaps we can glean some information from a reverse approach—namely, by drawing inferences from what is conserved in evolution and from the phenotypes of mutants. It has been noted, for instance, that about one-half of the conserved amino acid stretches correspond to predicted turns in the polypeptide chain, so they may mark the principal folds characteristic of the enzyme's tertiary structure.[33] As far as the human mutants are concerned, we can make only a few general observations, which can be summarized as follows.

1. Mutations causing loss of enzyme activity are scattered throughout the coding sequence. In most cases, loss of activity is due to decreased intracellular stability (which may or may not be reflected by in vitro stability tests). Therefore it appears that amino acid replacements in many different positions can reduce stability, either by affecting the conformation of the G-6-PD molecule or by increasing its susceptibility to proteolytic enzymes.

2. It is more difficult to make a general statement about changes in substrate binding. However, the corresponding mutations appear not to be randomly distributed. Indeed, there is a cluster of low-K_m^{G6P} values in variants with mutations in the neighborhood of lysine 205, the putative G6P binding site. Although it is intriguing that a variety of amino acid replacements increase rather than decrease substrate affinity, that may mean that the normal K_m^{G6P} is optimal for the purposes of erythrocyte physiology. Although it has been suggested that the cluster of class I variants around residue 386 correspond to changes near the NADP binding site, that is still uncertain, because the K_m^{NADP} is more difficult to measure and because we do not yet have hard biochemical evidence as to the location of the NADP binding site.

A special case is that of G-6-PD A$^-$. Because, as stated above, this deficient variant of G-6-PD results from a second mutation in the nondeficient variant G-6-PD A, one might surmise that the second mutation is responsible for loss of enzyme activity. However, when either of the two mutations was introduced into the normal gene by site-directed mutagenesis, and the single mutants were expressed in *E. coli*, the enzyme activity recovered was almost normal. Only the two mutations together caused severe enzyme deficiency.[148] Thus, the two mutations appear to have a synergistic effect on enzyme stability.

G-6-PD Haplotypes

Apart from mutations causing changes in the primary structure of the G-6-PD molecule, one synonymous codon polymorphism[149] and several polymorphic sites in introns[120,150,151,153] have been identified. Not surprisingly, these exhibit marked linkage disequilibrium among themselves and with coding sequence polymorphisms. For instance, in a study of African populations, only 7 out of 128 possible haplotypes have been observed and, as in other systems, they have been used in an attempt to infer the evolutionary history of the G-6-PD gene.[150] In this case it appears that the mutation underlying G-6-PD A$^-$ is the most recent in a sequence of mutational events that have spread in the population. Very recently, linkage disequilibrium has been revealed over a much larger region (about 3 Mb) surrounding the G-6-PD gene and extending from the factor VIII gene to the color vision genes. Again, haplotype analysis in a Southern Italian population indicates that the mutation underlying the deficient variant G-6-PD$_{MEDITERRANEAN}$ is more recent than other polymorphic sites not associated with enzyme deficiency.[154] It can be presumed in both cases that the more ancient mutations spread by genetic drift and migration, whereas the most recent (A$^-$ and Mediterranean) were selected by malaria.

CLINICAL MANIFESTATIONS

The vast majority of individuals with G-6-PD deficiency are asymptomatic and go through life without being aware of their genetic abnormality. The only common clinical manifestation is acute hemolysis, which may be rapidly compensated and often remains undetected. Clinical expression results from an interaction of the molecular properties of each individual G-6-PD variant with exogenous factors and, possibly, with additional genetic factors specific for a certain population. No significant adverse effects of G-6-PD deficiency were discernible on the health and military performance of young, enlisted U.S. black males.[155,156] However, G-6-PD deficiency can cause much human pathology, and the following clinical syndromes are recognized:

Drug-induced hemolysis
Infection-induced hemolysis
Favism
Neonatal jaundice (NNJ)
Chronic nonspherocytic hemolytic anemia (CNSHA)

Hemolysis has also been reported to occur in association with diabetic ketoacidosis[157,158] and hypoglycemia[159]; however, coexistent infection and/or oxidant drug exposure cannot always be excluded.[160] Pregnancy does not, of itself, precipitate hemolysis.[161]

Drug-Induced Hemolytic Anemia

As stated above, G-6-PD deficiency was discovered as a direct consequence of investigations into the development of hemolysis in some individuals, usually blacks, who had received primaquine (30 mg daily), which in other individuals causes no red cell destruction.[162,163] Thus, the acute hemolytic anemia associated with G-6-PD deficiency has become virtually a prototype of hemolytic episodes arising from a unique interaction between genetic and exogenous factors.[6] Clinical hemolysis and jaundice typically begin within 2 to 3 days of starting the drug.[164] The hemolysis is largely intravascular (although to what extent has been recently questioned[165]), and it is characteristically associated with hemoglobinuria. The anemia worsens until the 7th to 8th day. Heinz bodies (Fig. 111-6) are a characteristic finding in the peripheral blood. A reticulocyte response then sets in, and the hemoglobin level begins to recover on the 8th to 10th day. A self-limited course is characteristic with some G-6-PD variants,[162–164] because newly produced red cells, having higher G-6-PD activity, are less susceptible than the older cells, which have been selectively destroyed. However, a high drug dosage or the presence of a severely deficient G-6-PD variant will cause more protracted hemolysis.[166] A critical analysis of the data whereby individual drugs have been implicated in the causation of hemolysis in G-6-PD-deficient subjects has been conducted by Beutler,[167,168] who uncovered a discrepancy between the relatively small list of drugs for which there is strong evidence linking them to hemolytic anemia (Table 111-5) and a much larger list of agents for

Table 111-5 Drugs and Chemicals Associated with Significant Hemolysis in Subjects with G-6-PD Deficiency*

Drugs	Definite association	Possible association†	Doubtful association
Antimalarials	Primaquine Pamaquine Pentaquine	Chloroquine[438–442]	Quinacrine[438] Quinine[443]
Sulfonamides	Sulfanilamide Sulfacetamide Sulfapyridine Sulfamethoxazole	Sulfamethoxypyridazine Sulfadimidine Sulfamerizine	Sulfoxone[445] Sulfadiazine Sulfisoxazole[443]
Sulfones	Thiazolesulfone Dapsone		
Nitrofurans	Nitrofurantoin		
Antipyretic/analgesic	Acetanilid	Aspirin[438,446]	Aminopyrine Acetaminophen[447] Phenacetin[445]
Other drugs	Nalidixic acid Niridazole Methylene blue Phenazopyridine[449]	Ciprofloxacin‡ Norfloxacin‡ Chloramphenicol[169,170] Vitamin K analogues[172] Ascorbic acid[450]	PAS[445] L-DOPA Doxorubicin[448] Probenecid[443] Dimercaprol
Other chemicals	Naphthalene Trinitrotoluene Toluidine blue		

*Based on refs. 18, 167, 168, and 452–455 and on the additional references given in the body of the table.
†These agents will cause significant hemolysis, but only when given in large therapeutic doses, to subjects with severely deficient variants, or to neonates.
‡Personal observations.

which the evidence is less secure. This discrepancy arises for two reasons. First, clinical hemolysis is not always reproducible after administration of a particular drug, presumably because a number of factors influence both its interaction with the erythrocyte and the clinical consequences of the interaction (Table 111-6). Certain drugs are reported to cause oxidative hemolysis (but not necessarily anemia) in some populations but not in others (e.g., chloramphenicol[169,170] and vitamin K[171,172]). Probably for the same reason, the same dose of primaquine given to G-6-PD-deficient subjects of different ethnic origins gives rise to different degrees of hemolysis.[173] Genetic differences in drug metabolism and pharmacokinetics may also affect drug toxicity, while concurrent infection is an important source of additional oxidant stress, particularly in the neonate. Since the oldest red cells have the lowest enzyme activity, the preexisting hemoglobin and reticulocyte count will influence the severity of hemolysis.[144]

Second, clinical and hematologic assessment of hemolysis has notoriously low sensitivity, in that even a two- to threefold increase in red cell destruction may not produce a significant anemia or reticulocytosis. In addition, mere clinical association is not an ideal way of assessing the hemolytic potential of drugs in G-6-PD deficiency, because clinical situations are often complex. For instance, antibiotic, antipy-

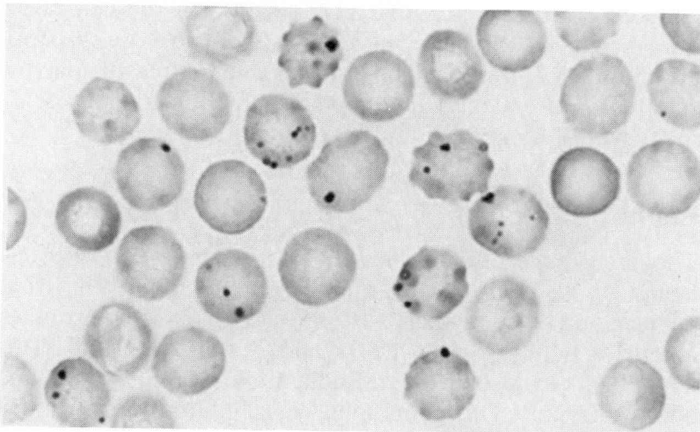

FIG. 111-6 Heinz bodies in erythrocytes from a G-6-PD-deficient person. These particles of denatured protein, adhering to the red cell membrane and staining with basic dyes, are seen in large numbers in the red cells of G-6-PD-deficient individuals after drug exposure. They can also be produced in vitro in both G-6-PD of deficient and normal red cells after incubation with certain oxidant chemicals such as acetylphenylhydrazine.

Table 111-6 Factors Which Influence Individual Susceptibility to, and Severity of, Drug-induced Oxidative Hemolysis

Inherited
Metabolic integrity of the erythrocyte
Precise nature of enzyme defect
Genetic differences in pharmacokinetics
Acquired
Age
Dose, absorption, metabolism, and excretion of drug
Presence of additional oxidative stress, e.g., infection
Effect of drug or metabolite on enzyme activity
Preexisting hemoglobin level
Age distribution of red blood cell population

retic, or analgesic drugs[174] are often administered to patients with infection, which may itself precipitate hemolysis. Similarly, it is unclear whether lead poisoning[167] or dimercaprol therapy[175] causes hemolysis in G-6-PD deficiency. Simultaneous administration of more than one drug makes it particularly difficult to assess the contribution of each. Thus, while the clinical association is very convincing for some agents (e.g., naphthalene,[176] nalidixic acid[177]) it is less so for others (e.g., sodium metasolphan noramidipyrine[178]). The most reliable technique to assess the hemolytic potential of a drug would be to administer it to a normal volunteer who has received a transfusion of ^{51}Cr-labeled G-6-PD-deficient cells and to follow the cells' survival.[179,180] It was always difficult to do this type of experiment in statistically valid numbers of cases, and it would be regarded today as unethical. Because of these difficulties, in vitro tests (Table 111-7) have been developed that aim to predict whether a drug will cause hemolysis in vivo.[181–183] Although these tests have been generally validated by analysis of drugs already known to cause hemolysis in vivo, they have not been widely used, less still made compulsory. In our view, they should be carried out before a new drug is introduced to a population in which G-6-PD deficiency is prevalent.

Infection-Induced Hemolysis

Outside the areas where favism is prevalent, infection is probably the most common cause of hemolysis in subjects with G-6-PD deficiency. One estimate attributed up to a third of these episodes of hemolysis to coincidentally administered drugs,[184] but that was probable an overestimate[185]; the true precipitant is probably usually infection. The severity and clinical consequences of hemolysis are, again, influenced by a number of factors, including concurrent administration of oxidant drugs, the preexisting level of hemoglobin, hepatic function, and age. Numerous bacterial, viral, and rickettsial infections have been reported as precipitants, but particularly important are infectious hepatitis,[184,186,187] pneumonia,[184,188,189] and typhoid fever.[169,170] Viral infections that affect the upper respiratory or gastrointestinal tract are reported[185] to cause more severe hemolysis than bacterial infections in G-6-PD-deficient children. Hemolysis is nearly four times more frequent in children with G-6-PD deficiency who develop viral hepatitis than in normal children,[190] but the degree and duration of jaundice in such children[191] and in adults is frequently out of proportion to the degree of hemolysis,[192] suggesting that the jaundice is in part of hepatocellular origin. Indeed, hepatic dysfunction may contribute to the hyperbilirubinemia seen in G-6-PD deficiency complicated by viral hepatitis[191–193] and pneumonia.[194] On the other hand, erythrocyte G-6-PD activity is reported to be transiently depressed in individuals with normal G-6-PD and typhoid or paratyphoid fever.[195] Renal failure is a well-recognized complication in adults,[184,188,189,196–198] whereas it is rare in children.[199] It may be particularly common after urinary tract infection[189] and in patients with preexisting renal disease,[197] while the concurrent administration of nephrotoxic drugs and pathologic changes in the kidney directly attributable to the underlying infection[200] may contribute to its severity. Acute renal failure is a serious complication in patients with viral hepatitis and G-6-PD deficiency,[186,196,201,202] but it also occurs in subjects with normal G-6-PD.[203] The pathogenesis is likely to be multifactorial, but the pathologic lesion is probably acute tubular necrosis caused by renal ischemia. Tubular obstruction by hemoglobin casts may also be important in pathogenesis.[204] Most patients with infection-induced hemolysis make a complete recovery, even when the course has been complicated by renal failure, provided hemodialysis is instituted promptly when indicated. The mechanism of infection-induced hemolysis is not well understood. Incubation of influenza A virus with normal red cells leads to increased hexose monophosphate shunt activity. In contrast, this increase is not seen upon incubation of the virus with G-6-PD-deficient cells, which, instead, show increased autohemolysis with Heinz body formation.[205] Generation of hydrogen peroxide by activated polymorphonuclear neutrophils in close apposition to G-6-PD-deficient red cells in vitro can lead to a reduction in the reduced form of glutathione (GSH) content and diminished survival of red cells thus treated.[206] The phenomenon of "immune adherence,"[207] whereby opsonized bacteria adhere to red cells in a process mediated by complement, may be important in promoting close apposition of neutrophils to red cells.[208] Hepatic dysfunction may further aggravate the oxidant stress on red cells by permitting accumulation of metabolites capable of oxidizing red-cell SH groups.[201] Activated neutrophils can also mediate lipid peroxidation of red-cell membranes, but G-6-PD-deficient red cells seem no more susceptible than normal red cells.[209] A variable degree of marrow suppression frequently accompanies infection and may delay recovery of the hemoglobin level.

Table 111-7 Techniques Used to Evaluate the Hemolytic Potential of Drugs Administered to G-6-PD-Deficient Subjects

Clinical association
- The occurrence of otherwise unexplained hemolysis in an individual known to be G-6-PD-deficient

Clinical challenge
- Administration of drugs in controlled studies to individuals known to be G-6-PD-deficient[162]
- Administration of drugs to normal volunteers transfused with ^{51}Cr-labelled G-6-PD deficient erythrocytes[443]
- Administration of drugs to animals followed by *in vitro* studies of erythrocytes[439]

In vitro studies
- GSH stability test[440]
- Effect of drug metabolites on mechanical fragility of erythrocytes[454,455]
- Measurement of $^{14}CO_2$ evolution and glucose utilization of normal erythrocytes suspended in homologous serum before and after drug ingestion[331,456]
- Measurement of hydrogen peroxide levels within erythrocytes after incubation with drugs[39]

Favism

The occurrence of acute hemolysis after ingestion of broad beans *(Vicia faba)* has been noted since antiquity.[2,4] It has occurred on an epidemic scale, particularly in Mediterranean countries (Italy,[5] Greece,[210] Spain, Portugal, and Turkey[211,212]), but also in the Middle East, the Far East, and North Africa.[212] This geographic distribution correlates best with the geography of customary consumption of fava beans. Most[18,213,214] but not all[215,216] of the patients reported in North America and the United Kingdom have direct Mediterranean ancestry. Once the similarity between favism and primaquine-induced hemolytic anemia had been noticed,[217] it became clear that all patients with favism are G-6-PD-deficient.[10,218,219] However, not all G-6-PD-deficient subjects are sensitive to fava beans,[220,221] and even those who are show striking variability from one exposure to the next. When ^{51}Cr-labeled G-6-PD-deficient cells from individuals with a clinical history of favism are infused into normal subjects, challenge with primaquine always leads to hemolysis of the deficient cells, whereas challenge with fava beans leads to hemolysis only in some cases.[222,223] One or more factors in addition to G-6-PD deficiency are therefore required for the development of favism,[224] and they help determine the severity of the individual attack.

Clinical favism presents characteristically with sudden onset of acute hemolytic anemia within 24 to 48 h of ingesting the beans. Pallor and hemoglobinuria are the hallmarks. Jaundice is always present, because not all the hemolysis is intravascular,[225] but the bilirubin level is less than in hemolytic attacks triggered by drugs or infection, presumably because the hemoglobinuria is more massive and hemoglobin catabolism within the body is therefore relatively reduced. The anemia is often severe.[210] Acute renal failure may supervene in adults,[226] but it is very rare in children.[199] However, fatalities in children were not uncommon prior to the availability of transfusion therapy.[4] An increase in the proportion of young erythrocytes leads to a decrease in the level of glycosylated hemoglobin (HbA1).[227] The highest incidence is in children aged 2 to 6 years. Boys are affected two to three times more often than girls[228] because of the greater number, in every population, of hemizygous males than heterozygous females. However, it is well documented that heterozygous girls are affected, although the condition is usually milder in these subjects.[216,229] Favism can occur after ingestion of fresh,[228] dried[210] or frozen[228] beans, but fresh beans are by far the most common offender, and, therefore, favism is most common during the spring. Hemolysis in breast-fed babies whose mothers have eaten fava beans is well documented.[210,230,231]

The pathophysiology of hemolysis in favism has recently been authoritatively reviewed.[232] The injury to red cells in favism is likely to consist in oxidant damage due to a chemical agent. On the basis of studies of the effect of fractionated extracts on erythrocyte metabolism, it has been suggested that the toxic components of fava beans are the pyrimidine aglycones divicine and isouramil[233–236] in combination with ascorbic acid. Possible bases for the erratic development of favism might then be variable absorption of toxic compounds from the gut or variability of the concentrations in the beans of the toxic glucosides themselves or of β-glucosidases required for their release. β-glucosidase levels in small intestinal biopsies of subjects with favism do not differ from those in normal and G-6-PD-deficient control subjects.[237] However, important determinants of intrapersonal variability in clinical expression include the amount and form in which the bean is eaten, the season of consumption,[212] and gastric pH.[232] On the other hand, interpersonal variability may have an additional and possibly genetic component (inherited perhaps as an autosomal recessive gene or as part of the genetic heterogeneity of G-6-PD deficiency itself[237–239]). The activity of erythrocyte acid phosphatase has been suggested to be lower in G-6-PD-deficient males sensitive to fava beans than in the general population, owing to a higher frequency of the Pa and Pc alleles of the acid phosphatase gene.[240] Decreased urinary D-glutaric acid and defective hepatic glucuronide formation[241,242] have also been reported in these subjects. A reduction in the number of sheep red-cell rosetting lymphocytes[243] and inversion of the peripheral blood helper T cell (CD4) to suppressor T cell (CD8) ratio owing to a decrease of CD4+ and an increase of CD8+ cells[244] have been described during the hemolytic crisis of favism. These changes may be the consequence of the hemolysis rather than an important pathogenic factor in favism, and similar changes have been reported in hypertransfused subjects with hemoglobinopathies.[245]

Oxidant damage causes crosslinking of erythrocyte membrane proteins, leading to the formation of distorted erythrocytes. It has been suggested that disturbed erythrocyte calcium homeostasis (specifically, reduced activity of the membrane Ca^{2+}-ATPase, leading to increased intraerythrocytic calcium and decreased intraerythrocytic potassium) mediates activation of proteolytic activity in erythrocytes in favic subjects.[246,247] The distorted erythrocytes are rapidly cleared from the circulation,[248] and there is increasing evidence that extravascular mechanisms are important in this process. They include opsonization by immunoglobulins and complement and phagocytosis within the reticuloendothelial system and bone marrow.

The mainstay of prevention is avoidance of fava beans. Experience in Sardinia has demonstrated the value of neonatal screening and health education in reducing the incidence of favism in that community.[249] The mainstay of treatment remains blood transfusion in severe cases.[199] The original observation suggesting arrest of hemolysis by desferrioxamine[250] has been disputed,[251] but a recent, larger study appears to confirm that a single bolus of desferrioxamine may be useful as an adjuvant to red-cell transfusion.[252] The proposed mechanism is that desferrioxamine reduces iron-dependent formation of damaging oxidant radicals (e.g., hydroxyl ions).

It has been widely held that favism is only associated with the more severely deficient variants of G-6-PD (particularly G-6-PDMediterranean); and, specifically, that G-6-PD A$^-$ is not associated with favism. That is not correct, as typical attacks of favism have been well documented in subjects of African origin with the A$^-$ variant.[253] In addition, favism in Spain,[117] Portugal,[131,211] and Algeria[143] has been quite prominent in G-6-PD-deficient individuals who have been shown to be also A$^-$.

Neonatal Jaundice

G-6-PD deficiency is the most common red-cell enzymopathy to cause neonatal hemolysis and jaundice.[254] The earliest reports[255,256] gave the impression that this complication occurred particularly in Greece, Sardinia, and the Far East, but the condition subsequently emerged as a major problem in Africa,[257] and it has been reported in North America.[258] Jaundice usually appears by 1 to 4 days of age, at about the same time as or slightly earlier than so-called physiological jaundice,[254,259] and later than in blood group alloimmunization. There may be a slightly higher threshold for its clinical detection in black infants.[260] The relative contributions of red-cell destruction and impaired hepatic function to the pathogenesis of unconjugated neonatal hyperbilirubinemia are disputed.[18] Reports of abnormal red-cell morphology,[261] mild anemia,[262] and reticulocytosis suggest an element of hemolysis, but impaired hepatic function, similar to that seen in normal neonates, may well be the major cause[263,264] in both premature and full-term[265] G-6-PD-deficient infants. Several distinctive features of neonatal erythrocytes may contribute to the degree of jaundice,[254,261] including elevated levels of ascorbic acid[385] and depressed levels of vitamin E,[266] glutathione reductase,[267] and catalase.[268]

A striking feature of neonatal jaundice (NNJ) in association with G-6-PD deficiency is the wide variation in its

Table 111-8 G-6-PD Deficiency and Neonatal Jaundice (NNJ)

Population	Incidence of G-6-PD Deficiency	Incidence of NNJ Among G-6-PD Deficient Individuals	Incidence of NNJ in Control Groups	Incidence of G-6-PD Deficiency Among NNJ Patients
Africa				
W. Africa[457,459]	21	26	10	31
S. Africa[265,460] (Bantu)	1.3	—	—	3.1 (All) 10 (Full term)
America				
Jamaica[461]	14.7	—	—	20.5
USA[172,462]	7.2 11.2	6	11.6	12.5
Asia				
China/Hong Kong[270,271]	3.6	—	1.2	15–30
Thailand[463,464]	7.5	30	3.0	30–60
Singapore[256,465–467]	1.3	20	25	—
Europe				
Greece[171,468–470]	3	30	9.1	15
Sardinia[282,471]	8.8	20–30	10	8.5

All figures are percentage values *in males only*.

frequency and severity in different populations (Table 111-8). Thus, in West Africa and Southeast Asia, deficiency accounts for a very high proportion (more than 30 percent) of all NNJ and for more than 50 percent of all cases of otherwise unexplained NNJ. Although kernicterus is a rare complication, the most common cause of it in both Africa[269] and Southeast Asia[270,271] is G-6-PD deficiency. In communities with a culturally and genetically heterogeneous population (e.g., Singapore[262] and Israel[272,273]), these differences in incidence seem to be population-specific.

The cause of this variability is incompletely understood, and both genetic and environmental factors are likely to be important. Of the genetic factors, the type of G-6-PD variant that is prevalent in a population is likely to be relevant, and is clearly of importance with respect to unusual or sporadic variants in the USA.[274,275] In Sardinia, where at least three polymorphic variants are associated with NNJ, the severity of NNJ does not correlate with red-cell G-6-PD activity, suggesting that additional variables (e.g., the expression and activity of the G-6-PD-deficient variant in the liver) may be important. Another possible genetic factor is the incidence of superimposed red-cell incompatibility between mother and infant. Ethnic differences in plasma bilirubin levels of full-term neonates may also reflect genetic differences in the activity of liver and red-cell enzymes.

Environmental or cultural factors are likely to be at least as important as genetic factors. G-6-PD deficiency is a less frequent cause of NNJ among individuals of African descent in the USA, and of Greek ancestry in Australia, than in the countries of origin of these populations,[276] although the differences are perhaps less marked than originally thought. Among these environmental factors are maternal exposure to oxidant drugs,[277,278] herbal remedies[262] and naphthalene (mothballs),[279] all of which may precipitate or exacerbate NNJ. Gestational age and maturity is an important consideration, as NNJ is more common, severe, and potentially harmful in premature infants.[261,280] Environmental factors will also affect the incidence of neonatal infection, hypoglycemia, acidosis, and the normal level of neonatal hemoglobin in a population.[144] Cultural factors, including exposure to icterogenic agents, have been identified as important precipitants of NNJ in the G-6-PD-deficient population of Nigeria.[281]

Management of NNJ generally includes avoiding oxidant drugs and promptly treating hypoxia, sepsis, and acidosis in newborns. Specific measures include eliminating the use of mothballs, prophylactic administration of phenobarbital to at-risk infants to improve hepatic conjugation of bilirubin,[282] and exchange transfusion if the bilirubin level is 20 mg/dl or more.[283,284] With respect to phototherapy, although it has been suggested that it could worsen hemolysis by leading to riboflavin deficiency and consequent loss of antioxidant activity,[285,286] several studies have shown conclusively that this treatment is effective in reducing hyperbilirubinemia,[283,287,288] and phototherapy remains in fact a mainstay of the treatment of NNJ whenever the bilirubin level is not so high as to warrant exchange blood transfusion.

Chronic Nonspherocytic Hemolytic Anemia

Although a slight degree of chronic hemolysis invariably accompanies G-6-PD deficiency, the vast majority of individuals with G-6-PD deficiency experience significant hemolysis and anemia only under conditions of oxidant stress. Some G-6-PD variants (class I, Table 111-3A), however, are characterized by overt chronic hemolytic anemia that is further exacerbated by oxidant stress. Such variants have been described (almost invariably in males) in many parts of the world, regardless of whether the common types of G-6-PD deficiency are endemic in the region. For instance, many cases have been reported from Japan.[289] Mostly a single kindred is known for each variant, but sometimes what is apparently the same variant (e.g., G-6-PD$_{CHICAGO}$) has been reported in unrelated individuals in different parts of the world.[290–293] Because the clinical phenotype is similar in affected members of a family and also among unrelated individuals having the same variant, it has been suggested that these variants represent structural and functional changes in the enzyme caused by mutations in the G-6-PD gene.[144] However, additional factors (genetic or environmental) may also operate to influence the clinical picture, and severe-deficiency variants can cause more severe hemolysis in some family members than in others.[294–296] The causative link of a G-6-PD variant with chronic nonspherocytic hemolytic anemia (CNSHA) is usually based on clinical evidence. The degree of enzyme deficiency may be very severe, and detailed biochemical characterization of the residual enzyme is often made even more difficult by its instability. In rare cases with associated granulocyte dysfunction,[297] hemolysis can be made worse by increased susceptibility to infection. Sometimes chronic hemolysis may arise from an association of mild G-6-PD deficiency with an unrelated, genetically transmitted erythrocyte abnormality, such as congenital dyserythropoietic anemia,[298] hereditary spherocytosis,[299,300] pyruvate kinase deficiency,[301,302] or 6-phosphogluconolactonase deficiency.[303]

Since the original descriptions,[304] a large number of detailed clinical observations have been reported. Many patients present with or give a history of neonatal jaundice, often requiring exchange transfusion.[274,305–309] A history of infection or drug-induced hemolysis is also common.[310,311] Gallstones may be a prominent feature.[312] Splenomegaly is usually (but not always) present.[310,313] While occasionally the hemoglobin concentration is normal and the hemolysis well-compensated,[295,305,314] oxidant stress can lead to a dramatic fall in the hemoglobin level.[315] The ^{51}Cr-labeled red-cell half life is shortened to 2 to 17 days, and all patients have a reticulocytosis (4 to 34 percent),[306] which may become extreme after splenectomy. Occasionally, the level of reticulocytosis is inappropriately low (3 percent) in relation to the shortening of the ^{51}Cr-labeled red-cell half life (12 days[316]); the cause is not clear, but folic acid deficiency[294] could be a factor. The increase in red-cell production at puberty can ameliorate the clinical findings. Red cells usually show no abnormal osmotic fragility, whereas a moderate increase in autohemolysis (with partial correction by added glucose) is reported.[307,310,317] Female heterozygotes have been shown to have two populations of cells,[318] one with normal and one with severely deficient G-6-PD; because the severely deficient red cells disappear from the circulation rapidly, these individuals usually have normal G-6-PD levels in peripheral blood cells.

Hemolysis in CNSHA is only partly intravascular (in contrast to the acute hemolysis caused by G-6-PD deficiency), and studies with ^{51}Cr usually indicate increased uptake in both liver and spleen.[310] Splenic sequestration has occasionally been demonstrated,[300] although markedly increased osmotic fragility was also present in that patient, and hereditary spherocytosis cannot be excluded as a coexistent abnormality.[167] Accelerated red cell aging also implies a role for the spleen in steady-state hemolysis. Increased levels of membrane cholesterol and phospholipids are also reported.[319]

There have been claims that high-dose vitamin E, by acting as an antioxidant, may be useful in the management of chronic hemolysis due to G-6-PD deficiency,[320,321] and that oral selenium may have an additive beneficial effect.[322] The reported benefit is only modest (e.g., an increase in red cell half-life from a mean of 15.6 days to 24.3 days, as measured by ^{51}Cr labeling), and such therapy may perhaps be useful in individuals who are deficient in vitamin E. Other studies have failed to show any benefit,[323] and no change in erythrocyte membrane polypeptide aggregates was observed after such treatment.[324] A therapeutic option, especially in severe cases, is splenectomy. On theoretical grounds, one might question its advisability, since selective red-cell destruction in the spleen is seldom documented. In fact, little or no benefit has been reported in some patients,[295,306,314,325–327] but significant improvement has been reported in others.[305–307,309,317] We are personally aware of at least three patients who needed regular blood transfusions before splenectomy but needed few or none over several years after splenectomy (see also Luzzatto[144]).

There is considerable variability in almost every manifestation of CNSHA associated with G-6-PD deficiency. This variability makes it somewhat problematic to give firm guidelines on management. Unlike the G-6-PD variants without CNSHA, many of which are polymorphic, those associated with CNSHA are all sporadic, and most, if not all, result from independent mutations (see Table 111-4). It is therefore not surprising that the red-cell pathophysiology and, ultimately, the clinical manifestations are subtly different in different cases.

MECHANISM OF HEMOLYSIS

The mammalian red cell is notorious for having a very limited biochemical apparatus and therefore an equally limited range of responses to pathologic changes. Typically, the failure of any metabolic pathway will cause the cell as a whole to fail—in other words, to be destroyed prematurely. In essence, G-6-PD deficiency entails failure of the glutathione GSH pathway (Fig. 111-2), and the result is hemolysis. Since a large number of G-6-PD-deficient variants (classes II and III) are not associated with chronic hemolysis, we can infer that a small amount of residual G-6-PD activity is sufficient for the steady state requirements of the red cells. Below that level (class I variants), it is evident that NADPH production has become inadequate, although we do not yet know precisely how this leads to hemolysis. A reasonable model is that the GSH level becomes so low that critical sulfhydryl groups in some key proteins are not maintained in reduced form, and intramolecular or intermolecular disulfides are formed. The most pertinent observation is probably that of membrane-cytoskeletal protein aggregates in red cells from patients with class I variants.[328,329] Such aggregates decrease red cell deformability,[330] and they may alter the cell surface sufficiently to make it recognizable by macrophages as abnormal (much like an aged red cell), thus leading to extravascular hemolysis. With class II and class III variants, hemolysis depends, by definition, on an exogenous trigger. Again, the exact sequence of events is incompletely known, but the following points are well established:

1. Some of the agents that can cause hemolysis stimulate the hexose monophosphate shunt pathway in normal red cells, indicating that in their presence increased NADPH production is required.[331]
2. A fall in GSH is invariably associated with hemolytic events in G-6-PD-deficient individuals.
3. In some cases, particularly in favism, acute hemolysis is associated with massive formation of Heinz bodies (consisting of denatured hemoglobin), which, by their very presence, certainly mediate red cell destruction (Fig. 111-6).
4. Oxygen radicals generated by the auto-oxidation of hemoglobin and in other ways also cause Heinz body formation,[332] intracellular proteolysis, and peroxidation of membrane lipids.[333,334]

These facts, taken together, indicate clearly that acute hemolysis in G-6-PD deficiency results from a failure of the cell, when challenged, to supply enough NADPH for the detoxification of hydrogen peroxide and oxygen radicals, thus justifying the popular phrase "oxidative hemolysis."[19] The question of why some G-6-PD-deficient variants are associated with CNSHA (class I) while others are not (classes II and III) is not yet fully answered. Residual G-6-PD activity is certainly a factor, but the values in classes I and II overlap extensively. Analysis of kinetic data has revealed that variants in class II often have abnormally high substrate affinities for G6P, NADP, or both, whereas variants in class I often have low substrate affinities and decreased affinity for the inhibitor NADPH.[335] For reasons explained more fully elsewhere,[52] we think it is likely that residual enzyme activity and the K_m for G6P may be the most important determinants of whether a particular G-6-PD-deficient variant causes CNSHA or not.

OTHER CLINICAL STUDIES

Occasional patients have been described in whom deficiency of G-6-PD in tissues other than the red cells contributes to

Table 111-9 G-6-PD Deficiency in Non-erythroid Tissues

Tissue	Clinical effects	Refs
Hematologic		
Leukocytes		
Granulocytes	Increased susceptibility to infection	[297,338–340,472]
Lymphocytes	Probably none	[243,244]
Platelets	Probably none	[343,344,474,475]
Nonhematologic		
Lens	Cataracts	[476–479]
Liver	Possible contributory factor in hyperbilirubinemia, e.g., of NNJ	[480,482]
Renal, adrenal,	Probably none	[481]
myocardial, sperm, saliva, muscle		[481–483]

SOURCE: Valentine and Paglia,[484] Luzzatto and Battistuzzi[335] and Marks et al.[485]

Table 111-10 Reported Clinical and Genetic Associations of G-6-PD Deficiency*

	References
Hematologic	
Heterozygosity for sickle-cell anemia, beta-thalassemia, and alpha-thalassemia	[345–350]
Nonhematologic	
Case reports	
Optic atrophy	[95,351]
Malignant hyperthermia	[486]
Xeroderma pigmentosum	[487]
Cystic fibrosis	[488]
Population studies	
Schizophrenia	[489,490]
Abnormal glucose tolerance	[491,492]
Abnormal steroid metabolism	[493]
Pernicious anemia	[494]
Regional enteritis	[495]
Coronary artery disease	[496]
Hypertension	[497]

*We do not regard that a significant effect of G-6-PD deficiency on any of these conditions has been proven.

the clinical picture (Table 111-9). This is to be expected, since the same G-6-PD gene is expressed in all tissues. It is also not surprising that erythroid manifestations predominate, as the red cell is unable to renew its supply of G-6-PD and is also uniquely dependent on the integrity of the hexose monophosphate shunt for its ability to withstand oxidant stress. Other cells can replace G-6-PD molecules (if they are abnormally unstable) and may have alternative means of producing NADPH. Thus, for instance, the shortage of G-6-PD in G-6-PD-deficient leukocytes is much less than in erythrocytes[335] (Table 111-1). A decreased leukocyte G-6-PD level has no clinical consequences in most cases.[336,337] However, it may be important in patients with very rare mutants[297,338–340]; a residual G-6-PD activity less than 5 percent of normal may be associated with defective neutrophil function. The functional defect in these cases is similar to that seen in chronic granulomatous disease, and it arises through disturbance of an NADPH-linked pathway required for killing ingested bacteria. Low levels of leukocyte G-6-PD in chronic granulomatous disease[341,342] are not due to a mutation at the G-6-PD locus, and they probably do not contribute to the neutrophil dysfunction. Low levels of G-6-PD activity in platelets are variably associated with in vitro abnormalities,[343,344] but with no demonstrable clinical consequences. Well-designed population studies have given little or no evidence that any disorders other than hemolytic anemia arise more frequently in G-6-PD-deficient individuals than in nondeficient control subjects.[155] Nevertheless, a number of associations have been reported, some from population studies (Table 111-10). Reported genetic associations may in part arise because an ethnically heterogeneous population (African-Americans) has been studied; in such cases, an apparent association of a disorder with G-6-PD deficiency may simply reflect the presence of more than one gene of African origin in the population. The bulk of evidence from Africa[257,345–347] and from the United States[348–350] suggests that there is no true and independent association of G-6-PD deficiency and sickle-cell anemia. In some cases, the association was proposed based on coinheritance of linked X-chromosome loci (e.g., optic atrophy[94,351]), but in these, as with most other single-case reports, there are no detailed family and molecular studies to support a genuine association. At a phenotypic level, the biochemical changes of G-6-PD deficiency in certain tissues (hematopoietic and nonhematopoietic) may predispose to the development of other conditions. In the presence of another abnormality, G-6-PD deficiency may act in an additive or synergistic way to influence clinical expression. Thus, the coexistence of G-6-PD deficiency with another cause of hemolytic anemia may exacerbate the clinical picture. The clinical effects of deficient G-6-PD levels in nonhematopoietic tissues are largely a topic of speculation, but may, for example, be important in the development of cataracts (Table 111-9).

G-6-PD activity in malignant cells from a variety of human tumors (breast,[352,353] prostate,[354] colon, and stomach[355]) is often higher than in benign cells, and this difference forms the basis for cytochemical tests used in the characterization of these tumors.[355,356] The high G-6-PD activity of tumors, which has been known for 30 years,[91] is presumably related to a high rate of cell division. Perhaps it is this idea that led to studies in which the incidence of G-6-PD deficiency was reported to be lower in cancer patients than in control individuals,[357,358] as though G-6-PD deficiency afforded a degree of protection against cancer. However, a controlled study failed to demonstrate a protective effect of G-6-PD deficiency against the development of hematologic neoplasm.[359]

DIAGNOSIS

The diagnosis of G-6-PD deficiency is easy. However, careful attention must be paid to methodology and to the interpretation of the results. Prenatal diagnosis has been reported.[383] Important considerations include the following.

1. There is very wide geographical distribution of this defect and a high prevalence in developing countries, which makes it important to adopt tests that are simple and inexpensive.
2. The actual enzyme activity of G-6-PD must be measured, rather than the amount of G-6-PD protein.

Table 111-11 Diagnosis of G-6-PD Deficiency

Method	Comments	References
Definitive assay	Spectrophotometer required. Measures 6PGD as well as G6PD (activities can be separated).	[167,498–500] [492]
Screening assays		
Fluorescent spot test	Same principle as definitive assay, but special equipment not required. Cheap, simple, reliable. Stored blood usable. Semiquantitative results available.	[501–505]
Ascorbate cyanide test	Cheap and simple. Fresh blood required.	[506,507]
MTT (tetrazolium) staining test	Highly reliable cytochemical technique for detecting heterozygotes.	[508–511]
Methemoglobin reduction methods	Cheap and simple, but prolonged incubation time required. Fresh blood required. False positives reported. Lends itself to cytochemical modification suitable for heterozygote detection.	[512,513]
Dye decolorization	Cheap, simple, reliable, and extensively used, but prolonged incubation time required. Fresh blood required.	[514,515]

3. The level of activity in young erythrocytes is higher than in older ones. Thus, a reticulocytosis can lead to a false normal result. One way of circumventing this difficulty is to centrifuge the sample to be tested and to assay separately the enzyme activity in erythrocytes from the bottom (older cells) and from the top (younger cells) of the resulting column of cells, as well as the activity of the whole unfractionated sample.[360,361] Alternatively, or additionally, one can determine the ratio of G-6-PD activity to the activity of another age-dependent enzyme, e.g., hexokinase.

4. Because of red-cell mosaicism arising from random X-chromosome inactivation, heterozygotes have a mixture of normal and deficient erythrocytes, and the proportions of the two cell types (maternally and paternally derived) can vary enormously, ranging from completely normal activity to complete deficiency. A cell lysate may therefore not reveal heterozygosity if the proportion of enzyme-deficient cells is small. Microscopic examination of individual cells on a blood film slide is preferable. All the existing methods for measuring G-6-PD activity depend essentially on the production of NADPH. The direct enzyme assay gives an accurate quantitative measurement. A number of other procedures provide convenient screening tests, aiming only to classify subjects as G-6-PD-normal or G-6-PD-deficient. Some of them are semiquantitative (Table 111-11).

ADDITIONAL NOTES ON MANAGEMENT

The vast majority of individuals with G-6-PD deficiency do not need treatment, as they suffer no ill effects in the steady state. Screening of all newborns, except in areas where low-risk populations predominate (e.g., in Northern Europe and among South American Indians), has been proposed,[254,362] and detection of male hemizygotes and most female heterozygotes has been shown to be feasible.[363,364] Such a program would obviously make it possible for susceptible individuals to avoid potentially hemolytic agents (certain drugs and fava beans) or, in the case of necessary drugs, to ensure they are used in subhemolytic doses. These are the most important aspects of management. With respect to neonatal jaundice, there has been recent controversy on treatment policies in relation to the levels of bilirubin.[444] We think at the moment there is not sufficient evidence for NNJ associated with G-6-PD deficiency to be regarded as less dangerous than that associated with classical HDN. Indeed, one might only speculate as to whether the basal nuclei cells from G-6-PD deficient babies may be more vulnerable to hyperbilirubinemia than those of G-6-PD-normal babies. Therefore we definitely recommend phototherapy when the bilirubin concentration exceeds 150 μm/L and exchange transfusion when the bilirubin level exceeds 300 μm/L. Patients with acute and chronic hemolysis may also need blood transfusion.

Because the viability of G-6-PD-deficient erythrocytes after storage may not be as high as that of normal erythrocytes,[365] it has been suggested that blood from G-6-PD-deficient donors should not be used for transfusion purposes.[366,367] There have also been occasional reports of hemolysis of transfused G-6-PD-deficient erythrocytes,[366–368] although it was not proven that hemolysis was the result of this enzyme defect. Indeed, G-6-PD-deficient erythrocytes have been shown to be perfectly satisfactory for transfusion purposes,[369] and refusing to use deficient individuals as blood donors would severely deplete the number of available donors in parts of the world where the deficiency is common.[257] Thus, with the exception of exchange transfusion in severe neonatal jaundice and in the management of severe hemolytic anemia due to favism,[199] G-6-PD-deficient blood should be considered safe for transfusion purposes.

G-6-PD AS A CLONAL MARKER

Somatic cells in females heterozygous for the G-6-PD locus will be of two types, each type expressing only one or the other allele[52] (Fig. 111-7). If a tumor arises by neoplastic transformation of a single cell, all its cells will be expected to express a single G-6-PD allele. The product of this locus can therefore be used as a clonal marker. Since the original studies of uterine tumors using this approach,[370] a large number of other neoplasms have been studied,[370–374] and most have been shown to be of clonal origin. In the case

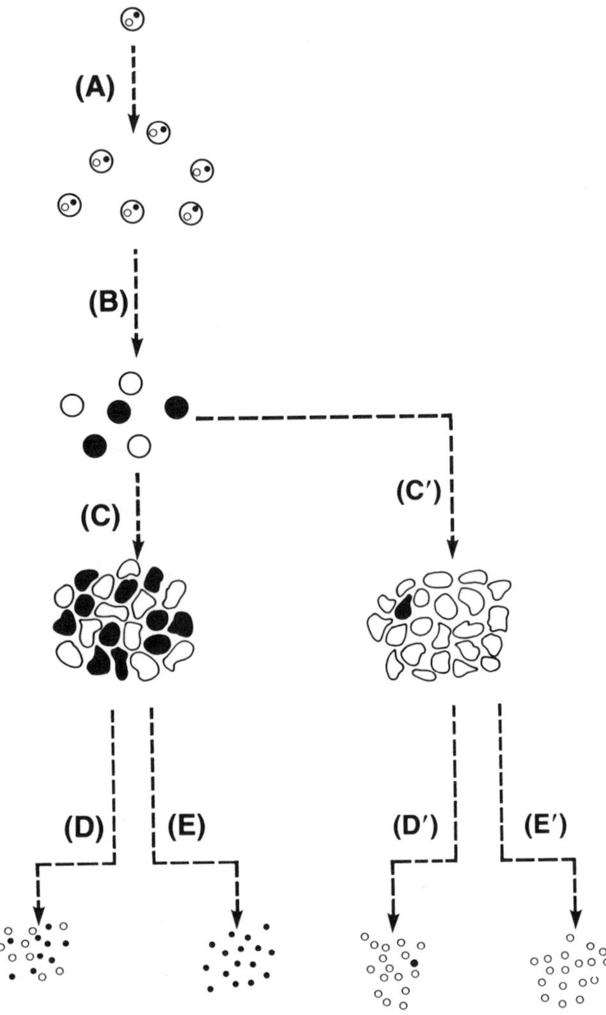

FIG. 111-7 The G-6-PD phenotype in heterozygotes can yield information on clonal proliferation and somatic cell selection. At the top, embryonic cells (A) before x-chromosome inactivation: the two dots represent expression of two different alleles of G-6-PD. B. Inactivation of one x chromosome per cell produces two cell populations (empty and filled circles) distinguishable by their G-6-PD phenotype. C. Proliferation of cells at about even rates produces mosaicism in the adult. C′. Differential growth rate of the two cell types arising from X inactivation (somatic cell selection) may produce in the adult a (nearly) homogeneous population. This could apply to the whole body, or it may occur in one tissue and not in another, because a particular X-linked gene, for which the subject is heterozygous, may confer a growth advantage only in a tissue where the gene is expressed. D. Pathologic tissue (for instance, an inflammatory process or the healing of a wound) will still produce a mosaic. E. Pathologic proliferation arising from a single cell ("monoclonal") of an adult tissue (for instance, a tumor) will produce a homogeneous population. D′ and E′. If pathologic proliferation arises in a tissue that is already homogeneous as a result of C′, the resulting cell population will still be homogeneous, regardless of whether the proliferative process is monoclonal or polyclonal.

of hematologic malignancies,[375,376] it has been shown that neoplastic cells that have differentiated along different pathways (e.g., erythrocytes, granulocytes, and platelets in chronic myeloid leukemia[377,378] and polycythemia rubra vera[379]) nevertheless have a common stem-cell origin. Paroxysmal nocturnal hemoglobinuria is a nonmalignant hematologic disorder that has also been shown to be of clonal origin,[380] and clonal proliferation may be important in the pathogenesis of atheromatous plaques.[381] G-6-PD has been used as a marker in experiments aiming to investigate somatic mutations in intestinal crypts of the mouse.[382] There are several possible sources of error in the interpretation of G-6-PD phenotypes as clonal markers.[335,384] An admixture of normal cells (e.g., in a solid tumor biopsy), which will have both G-6-PD phenotypes, may mask the presence of a single G-6-PD phenotype in the malignant cells. The relative activity of the two phenotypes may vary from one tissue to another and at different sites within the same tissue and, thus, may not be the same in the tissue from which the tumor originated as in other tissues. It is also possible that the tumor arose by clonal proliferation of more than one cell (i.e., is of multicentric origin) but that the original cells were by coincidence of the same G-6-PD phenotype. A further consideration (Fig. 111-7) is somatic cell selection,[107,384,386] whereby X-linked genes other than that for G-6-PD may influence the proliferation of cells after the inactivation process has taken place.

G-6-PD DEFICIENCY AND MALARIA

The now classic notion that G-6-PD deficiency has become widespread as a result of malaria selection[387] can be visualized easily by comparing the geographic distribution of this red-cell phenotype (Fig. 111-5), with an epidemiologic map of *P. falciparum* malaria (see, for instance, ref. 86). Several discrepancies are easy to explain. In Southern Europe, G-6-PD deficiency is common and there is no malaria, but the latter has been eradicated only over the last two generations. In North America there is no malaria, but the prevalence of G-6-PD deficiency in this continent is entirely accounted for by migrations that have taken place in relatively recent times. Geographic correlation alone is of course no proof of the "malaria hypothesis." The body of more compelling evidence has been reviewed elsewhere,[388] and it can be only briefly summarized here.

Micromapping Analysis of relatively narrow geographic areas has consistently shown a good correlation between the frequency of G-6-PD deficiency and the intensity of malaria transmission, for instance, in East Africa,[389] Papua New Guinea,[390] Sardinia,[391] and Greece.[392] In the last two areas, the evidence is strengthened by the fact that the population is genetically relatively homogeneous, and the variance of frequencies of other genes was shown to be significantly lower than that of G-6-PD deficiency.[393]

Genetic Heterogeneity of Polymorphic G-6-PD Variants. If G-6-PD deficiency had spread by genetic drift, the same mutant would be found everywhere. Instead, diverse point mutations (see above) must have arisen independently and then spread centrifugally to establish themselves at polymorphic frequencies—a good example of convergent microevolution in the human species. In this respect the G-6-PD deficiency polymorphism is more reminiscent of the highly heterogeneous thalassemia system than of the unique mutation of hemoglobin S.

Clinical Studies. Studies in the field have yielded ambiguous data when prevalence of malaria or malaria parasitemia was compared between normal and G-6-PD-deficient males or in subjects of both sexes.[394–397] However, in the single study in which girls heterozygous for G-6-PD deficiency (Gd^B/Gd^{A-}) were rigorously classified, a significantly lower *P. falciparum* parasitemia was observed.[398,399] It would be highly desirable that this somewhat laborious test be reproduced independently in malaria-endemic areas in heterozygotes for this and for other G-6-PD-deficient variants.

In Vitro Studies. Once a culture system for the intraerythrocytic cycle of *P. falciparum* was developed by Trager and Jensen,[400] it became possible to test in controlled experiments whether the G-6-PD genotype of red cells affected their ability to host the parasite. Several groups have independently reported that the growth of *P. falciparum* was impaired in G-6-PD-deficient red cells,[401–403] although in some studies the difference was apparent only when the cultures were subjected to oxidative stress.[404] The preferential development of parasites in G-6-PD-normal as opposed to G-6-PD-deficient red cells is in keeping with previous evidence obtained in vivo.[405]

Mechanism of Protection Against Malaria

The findings summarized above leave little doubt that the G-6-PD deficiency polymorphism is balanced by malaria selection. At the same time, the mechanism that effects this is not fully explained. In our own view, the most significant clue is that in vivo protection against malaria is a prerogative of heterozygotes. Therefore, two questions must be answered:

1. How does G-6-PD deficiency hinder the parasite cycle? In vitro culture experiments show clearly that the invasion stage is not affected, but intracellular schizogony is.[403] The most likely explanation is that the G-6-PD-deficient red-cell environment causes oxidative injury to the parasite.[406,407]

2. Why are hemizygous or homozygous G-6-PD-deficient individuals not protected as well or better than heterozygotes? This situation is paradoxical, since hemizygotes and homozygotes have only G-6-PD-deficient red cells in their blood, whereas heterozygotes, who are genetic mosaics, have on the average only 50 percent of them. Recent evidence suggests that it is the very coexistence of two different red cell populations in heterozygotes that may be responsible for their relative resistance to malaria.[408] Parasites that have survived passage through G-6-PD-deficient red cells become adapted to this type of host cell after several cycles,[409] thus explaining why hemizygotes and homozygotes are not protected. On the other hand, this process of adaptation is hindered when parasites cycle through G-6-PD-normal red cells, thus explaining the lower parasitemia in heterozygotes. The mechanism of this adaptation phenomenon is not yet known, but this finding has been a stimulus to characterizing the G-6-PD molecule encoded by *P. falciparum* itself. The parasite enzyme has an unusually large size (about 430 kDa[259,411]), and its sequence has revealed unexpected features.[411,412]

ACKNOWLEDGMENTS

We are immensely indebted to Dr. Ernest Beutler who, having been a pioneer of research in this area, has authoritatively reviewed G-6-PD deficiency in five previous editions of this textbook over a span of 23 years. We are grateful to him and to others, including H. N. Kirkman, G. F. Gaetani, T. Meloni, and P. Arese, for communicating unpublished results; and to G. M. Persico, D. Toniolo, M. D'Urso, G. Battistuzzi, E. A. Usanga, G. Martini, D. Schlessinger, P. M. Mason, T. J. Vulliamy, M. Town, E. O'Brien, B. Kurdi-Haidar, and others for sharing in experimental work and many discussions. Work in the authors' laboratory has been supported by a Programme Grant from the Medical Research Council of Great Britain.

REFERENCES

1. Beutler E: Study of glucose-6-phosphate dehydrogenase: History and molecular biology. *Am J Hematol* **42:**53, 1993.
2. Fermi C, Martinetti P: Studio sul favismo. *Ann Igiene Sper* **15:**76, 1905.
3. Gasbarrini A: Il favismo. *Policlinico Sez Prat* **22:**1505, 1915.
4. Luisada L: Favism: A singular disease affecting chiefly red blood cells. *Medicine* **20:**229, 1941.
5. Sansone G, Piga AM, Segni G: *Il Favismo,* Torino, Italy, Minerva Medica, 1958.
6. Beutler E: The hemolytic effect of primaquine and related compounds. *Blood* **14:**103, 1959.
7. Beutler E: Glucose 6-phosphate dehydrogenase deficiency, in Stanbury JB, Wyngaarden JB, Fredrickson DS (eds): *The Metabolic Basis of Inherited Disease.* New York, McGraw-Hill, 1960.
8. Carson PE, Flanagan CL, Ickes CE, Alving A: Enzymatic deficiency in primaquine-sensitive erythrocytes. *Science* **124:**484, 1956.
9. Waller HD, Löhr GW, Tabatabai M: Hämolyse und Fehlen von Glucose-6-phosphate-dehydrogenase in roten Blutzellen (eine Fermentanomalie der Erythrozyten). *Klin Wochenschr* **35:**1022, 1957.
10. Sansone G, Segni G: Nuovi aspetti dell'alterato biochimismo degli eritrociti dei favici: assenza pressochè completa della glucos-6-P deidrogenasi. *Boll Soc Ital Biol Sper* **34:**327, 1958.
11. Marks PA: Glucose 6-phosphate dehydrogenase, in Bishop C (ed): *The Red Blood Cell.* New York, Academic Press, 1964.
12. Shows TB, Tashian RE, Brewer GJ: Erythrocyte glucose 6-phosphate dehydrogenase in Caucasians: New inherited variant. *Science* **145:**1056, 1964.
13. Beutler E: Glucose-6-phosphate dehydrogenase: New perspectives. *Blood* **73:**1397, 1989.
14. Beutler E: The genetics of glucose-6-phosphate dehydrogenase deficiency. *Semin Hematol* **27:**137, 1990.
15. Beutler E: Glucose 6-phosphate dehydrogenase deficiency. *N Engl J Med* **324:**169, 1991.
16. Vulliamy T, Mason P, Luzzatto L: The molecular basis of glucose 6-phosphate dehydrogenase deficiency. *Trends Genet* **8:**138, 1992.
17. Hirono A, Miwa S: Human glucose-6-phosphate dehydrogenase: Structure and function of normal and variant enzymes. *Hematologia* **25:**85, 1993.
18. Dacie JV: Hereditary enzyme deficiency haemolytic anaemias. III: Deficiency of glucose-6-phosphate dehydrogenase, in: Dacie JV (ed): *Haemolytic Anaemias. The Hereditary Haemolytic Anaemias.* London, Churchill Livingstone, 1985, p 364.
19. Jandl JH: *Blood: Textbook of Hematology,* Boston, Little, Brown, 1987.
20. Lukens JN: Glucose-6-phosphate dehydrogenase deficiency and related deficiencies involving the pentose phosphate pathway and glutathione metabolism, in Lee GR, Bithell TC, Foerster J, Athens JW, Lukens JN (eds): *Wintrobe's Clinical Hematology.* Philadelphia, Lea & Febiger, 1993, p 1006.
21. Luzzatto L: Glucose 6-phosphate dehydrogenase deficiency and hemolytic anemia, in Nathan DG, Oski FA (eds): *Hematology of Infancy and Childhood.* Philadelphia, Saunders, 1993, p 674.
22. Cohen P, Rosemeyer MA: Subunit interactions of human glucose 6-phosphate dehydrogenase from human erythrocytes. *Eur J Biochem* **8:**8, 1969.
23. Bonsignore A, De Flora A: Regulatory properties of G6PD. *Curr Top Cell Regul* **6:**21, 1972.
24. Babalola AOG, Beetlestone JG, Luzzatto L: Genetic variants of human erythrocyte glucose 6-phosphate dehydroge-

nase. Kinetic and thermodynamic parameters of variants A, B, and A⁻ in relation to quaternary structure. *J Biol Chem* **251**:2993, 1976.

25. Bonsignore A, Cancedda R, Nicolini A, Damiani G, De Flora A: Metabolism of human erythrocyte glucose 6-phosphate dehydrogenase. VI. Interconversion of multiple molecular forms. *Arch Biochem Biophys* **147**:493, 1971.
26. DeFlora A, Morelli A, Giuliano F: Human erythrocyte G6PD. Content of bound coenzyme. *Biochem Biophys Res Commun* **59**:406, 1974.
27. Jeffery J, Soderling-Barros J, Murray LA, Wood I, Hansen RJ, Szepesi B, Jornvall H: Glucose 6-phosphate dehydrogenase. Characteristics revealed by the rat liver enzyme. *Eur J Biochem* **186**:551, 1989.
28. Descalzi-Cancedda E, Caruso C, Romano M, di Prisco G, Camardella I: Amino acid sequence of the carboxy-terminal end of human erythrocyte glucose-6-phosphate dehydrogenase. *Biochem Biophys Res Commun* **118**:332, 1984.
29. Khan A, Bertrand O, Cottreau D, Boivin P, Dreyfus JC: Evidence for structural differences between human glucose-6-phosphate dehydrogenase purified from leukocytes and erythrocytes. *Biochem Biophys Res Commun* **77**:65, 1977.
30. Rowley DL, Wolf RE: Molecular characterization of the *Escherichia coli* K12 *zwf* gene encoding glucose 6-phosphate dehydrogenase. *J Bacteriol* **173**:968, 1991.
31. Lee WT, Flynn TG, Lyons C, Levy HR: Cloning and amino acid sequence of glucose 6-phosphate dehydrogenase from *Leuconostoc mesenteroides*. *J Biol Chem* **266**:13028, 1991.
32. Jeffery J, Soderling-Barros J, Murray LA, Hansen RJ, Szepesi B, Jornvall H: Molecular diversity of glucose-6-phosphate dehydrogenase: Rat enzyme structure identifies NH2-terminal segment, shows initiation from sites nonequivalent in different organisms and establishes otherwise extensive sequence conservation. *Proc Natl Acad Sci USA* **85**:7840, 1988.
33. Jeffery J, Persson B, Wood I, Bergman T, Jeffery R, Jörnvall H: Glucose-6-phosphate dehydrogenase. Structure function relationships and the *Pichia jadinii* enzyme structure. *Eur J Biochem* **212**:41, 1993.
34. Fouts D, Ganguly R, Gutierrez AG, Lucchesi JC, Manning JE: Nucleotide sequence of the *Drosophila* glucose-6-phosphate dehydrogenase gene and comparison with the homologous human gene. *Gene* **63**:261, 1988.
35. Camardella L, Caruso C, Rutigliano B, Romano M, diPrisco G, Descalzi-Cancedda F: Human erythrocyte glucose-6-phosphate dehydrogenase. Identification of a reactive lysyl residue labelled with pyridoxal 5′-phosphate. *Eur J Biochem* **171**:485, 1988.
36. Luzzatto L, Afolayan A: Enzymic properties of different types of human erythrocyte glucose-6-phosphate dehydrogenase, with characterization of two new genetic variants. *J Clin Invest* **47**:1833, 1968.
37. Rosenstraus M, Chasin LA: Isolation of mammalian cell mutants deficient in glucose-6-phosphate dehydrogenase activity: Linkage to hypoxanthine phosphoribosyl transferase. *Proc Natl Acad Sci USA* **72**:493, 1975.
38. Town M, Athanasiou Metaxa M, Luzzatto L: Intragenic interspecific complementation of glucose 6-phosphate dehydrogenase in human-hamster cell hybrids. *Somat Cell Mol Genet* **16**:97, 1990.
39. Cohen G, Hochstein P: Generation of hydrogen peroxide in erythrocytes by haemolytic agents. *Biochemistry* **3**:895, 1964.
40. Aebi HE, Wyss SR: Acatalasemia, in Stanbury JB, Wyngaarden JB, Fredrickson DS (eds): *The Metabolic Basis of Inherited Disease*, 4th ed. New York, McGraw-Hill, 1978, p 1792.
41. Kirkman HN, Gaetani GF: Catalase: A tetrameric enzyme with four tightly bound molecules of NADPH. *Proc Natl Acad Sci USA* **81**:4343, 1984.
42. Kirkman HN, Galiano S, Saetani GF: The function of catalase-bound NADPH. *J Biol Chem* **262**:660, 1987.
43. Gaetani GF, Galiano S, Canepa L, Ferraris A-M, Kirkman HN: Catalase and glutathione peroxidase are equally active in detoxification of hydrogen peroxide in human erythrocytes. *Blood* **73**:334, 1989.
44. Gaetani GF, Ferraris AM: Recent developments on Mediterranean G6PD. *Br J Haematol* **68**:1, 1988.
45. Tepperman HM, Tepperman J: On the response of hepatic G6PD activity to changes in diet composition and food intake pattern, in Weber G (ed): *Advances in Enzyme Regulation*. New York, Pergamon, 1963, p 121.
46. Kletzien RF, Fritz RS, Prostko CR, Jones EA, Dreher KL: Hepatic glucose-6-phosphate dehydrogenase: Nutritional and hormonal regulation of mRNA levels, in Yoshida A, Beutler E (eds): *Glucose-6-phosphate Dehydrogenase*. Orlando, FL, Academic, 1986.
47. Battistuzzi G, D'Urso M, Toniolo D, Persico GM, Luzzatto L: Tissue specific levels of G6PD with methylation at the 3′ end of the gene. *Proc Natl Acad Sci USA* **82**:1465, 1985.
48. Persico M, Battistuzzi G, Mareni C, Nobile C, D'Urso M, Toniolo D, Luzzatto L: Genetic variants of human glucose 6-phosphate dehydrogenase (G6PD): Studies of turnover and of G6PD-specific mRNA, in Weatherall DJ, Fiorelli G, Gorini S (eds): *Advances in Red Blood Cell Biology*. New York, Raven, 1982, p 309.
49. Piomelli S, Corash LM, Davenport DD, Miraglia J, Amorosi EL: In vivo lability of glucose-6-phosphate dehydrogenase in Gd A and Gd Mediterranean deficiency. *J Clin Invest* **47**:940, 1968.
50. Bonsignore A, Lorenzoni I, Cancedda R, Consulich ME, De Flora A: Effect of divalent cations on the structure of human erythrocyte G6PD. *Biochem Biophys Res Commun* **42**:159, 1971.
51. Yoshida A: Haemolytic anaemia and G6PD deficiency. *Science* **179**:532, 1973.
52. Luzzatto L, Testa U: Human erythrocyte G6PD: Structure and function in normal and mutant subjects. *Curr Top Hematol* **1**:1, 1978.
53. Luzzatto L: Regulation of the activity of glucose-6-phosphate dehydrogenase by NADP⁺ and NADPH. *Biochim Biophys Acta* **146**:18, 1967.
54. Morelli A, Benatti U, Giuliano F, De Flora A: Human erythrocyte glucose-6-phosphate dehydrogenase. Evidence for competitive binding of NADP and NADPH. *Biochem Biophys Res Commun* **70**:600, 1976.
55. Kirkman HN, Gaetani GD, Clemons EH, Mareni C: Red cell NADP and NADPH in glucose-6-phosphate dehydrogenase deficiency. *J Clin Invest* **55**:875, 1975.
56. Kirkman HN, Gaetani GF, Clemons EH: NADP-binding proteins causing reduced availability and sigmoid release of NADP⁺ in human erythrocytes. *J Biol Chem* **261**:4039, 1986.
57. Gaetani GF, Parker JC, Kirkman HN: Intracellular restraint: A new basis for the limitation in response to oxidation stress in human erythrocytes containing low activity variants of glucose 6-phosphate dehydrogenase. *Proc Natl Acad Sci USA* **71**:3584, 1975.
58. Sartori E: Elementi per la genetica del favismo. *Studi Sassar* **35**:1, 1957.
59. Luzzatto L: Glucose-6-phosphate dehydrogenase deficiency, in Brown MJ (ed): *Advanced Medicine, 21*. London, Churchill Livingstone, 1986, p 398.
60. Nora JJ, Frazer FC: *Medical Genetics*. Philadelphia, Lea & Febiger, 1974.
61. Beutler E, Yeh M, Fairbanks VF: The normal human female as a mosaic of X-chromosome activity: Studies using the gene for G-6-PD deficiency as a marker. *Proc Natl Acad Sci USA* **48**:9, 1962.
62. Davidson RG, Nitowsky HM, Childs B: Demonstration of two populations of cells in the human female heterozygous for glucose-6-phosphate dehydrogenase variants. *Proc Natl Acad Sci USA* **50**:481, 1963.
63. Adam A: Linkage between deficiency of glucose 6-phosphate dehydrogenase and colour-blindness. *Nature* **189**:686, 1961.
64. Keats B: Genetic mapping: X chromosome. *Hum Genet* **64**:28, 1983.
65. Pai GS, Sprenkle JA, Do TT, Mareni CE, Migeon BR: Localization of loci for hypoxanthine phosphoriboxyltransferase and glucose-6-phosphate dehydrogenase and biochemical evidence of non-random X-chromosome expression from studies of a human X-autosome translocation. *Proc Natl Acad Sci USA* **77**:2810, 1980.
66. Szabo P, Purrello M, Rocchi M, Archidiacono N, Alha-

deff B, Filippi G, Toniolo D, Martini G, Luzzatto L, Siniscalco M: Cytological mapping of the human glucose-6-phosphate dehydrogenase gene distal to the fragile-X site suggests a high rate of meiotic recombination across this site. *Proc Natl Acad Sci USA* **81**:7855, 1984.

67. Trask BJ, Massa H, Kenwrick S, Gitschier J: Mapping of human chromosome Xq28 by two-color fluorescence in situ hybridization of DNA sequences to interphase cell nuclei. *Am J Hum Genet* **48**:1, 1991.
68. Patterson M, Schwartz C, Bell M, Sauer S, Hofker M, Trask B, Van den Engh G, Davies KE: Physical mapping studies on the human X chromosome in the region Xq27-Zqter. *Genomics* **1**:297, 1987.
69. Freije D, Schlessinger D: A 1.6-Mb contig of yeast artificial chromosomes around the human factor VIII gene reveals three regions homologous to probes for the DXS115 locus and two for the DXYS64 locus. *Am J Hum Genet* **51**:66, 1992.
70. Martini G, Toniolo D, Vulliamy T, Luzzatto L, Dono R, Viglietto G, Paonessa G, D'Urso M, Persico MG: Structural analysis of the X-linked gene encoding human glucose 6-phosphate dehydrogenase. *EMBO J* **5**:1849, 1986.
71. Persico MG, Viglietto G, Martini G, Toniolo D, Paonessa G, Moscatelli C, Dono R, Vulliamy T, Luzzatto L, D'Urso M: Isolation of human glucose-6-phosphate dehydrogenase (G6PD) cDNA clones: Primary structure of the protein and unusual 5′ non-coding region. *Nucleic Acids Res* **14**:2511, 1986.
72. Persico L, Toniolo D, Nobile C, D'Urso M, Luzzatto L: cDNA sequences of human glucose 6-phosphate dehydrogenase cloned in pBR322. *Nature* **294**:778, 1981.
73. Toniolo D, Persico M, Alcalay M: A "Housekeeping" gene on the X chromosome encodes a protein similar to ubiquitin. *Proc Natl Acad Sci USA* **85**:851, 1988.
74. Toniolo D, Martini G, Migeon BR, Dono R: Expression of the G6PD locus on the human X-chromosome is associated with demethylation of three CpG clusters within 100 kb of DNA. *EMBO J* **7**:401, 1988.
75. Maestrini E, Tamanini F, Kioschis P, Gimbo E, Marinelli P, Tribioli C, D'Urso M, Palmieri G, Poustka A, Toniolo D: An archipelago of CpG islands in Xq28: Identification and fine mapping of 20 new CpG islands of the human X-chromosome. *Hum Mol Genet* **1**:275, 1992.
76. Kanno H, Huang I-Y, Kan YW, Yoshida A: Two structural genes on different chromosomes are required for encoding the major subunit of human red cell glucose-6-phosphate dehydrogenase. *Cell* **58**:595, 1989.
77. Henikoff S, Smith JM: The human mRNA that provides the N-terminus of chimeric G6PD encodes GMP reductase. *Cell* **58**:1021, 1989.
78. Mason PJ, Bautista J, Villiamy TJ, Turner N, Luzzatto L: Human red cell glucose 6-phosphate dehydrogenase is encoded only on the X-chromosome. *Cell* **63**:9, 1990.
79. Beutler E, Gelbart T, Kuhl W: Human red cell glucose-6-phosphate dehydrogenase: All active enzyme has sequence predicted by the X chromosome-encoded cDNA. *Cell* **62**:7, 1990.
80. Yoshida A, Kan YW: Origin of "fused" glucose-6-phosphate dehydrogenase. *Cell* **62**:11, 1990.
81. Chen EY, Cheng A, Lee A, Kuang W-J, Hillier L, Green P, Schlessinger D, Ciccodicola A, D'Urso M: Sequence of human glucose 6-phosphate dehydrogenase cloned in plasmids and a yeast artificial chromosome. *Genomics* **10**:792, 1991.
82. Toniolo D, Filippi M, Dono R, Lettieri R, Martini G: The CpG island in the 5′-region of the G6PD gene of man and mouse. *Gene* **102**:197, 1991.
83. Dynan WS, Tjian R: Control of eukaryotic messenger RNA synthesis by sequence-specific DNA-binding proteins. *Nature* **316**:774, 1985.
84. Bird AP: CpG rich islands and the function of DNA methylation. *Nature* **321**:209, 1986.
85. Reynolds GA, Bam SK, Osborne TF, Chu DJ, Gil G, Brown MS, Goldstein JL, Luskey KL: HMG CoA reductase: A negatively regulated gene with unusual promoter and 5′ untranslated regions. *Cell* **38**:275, 1984.
86. Bruce-Chwatt LJ: *Essential Malariology,* 2d ed. London, Heinemann, 1988.
87. Ursini MV, Scalera L, Martini G: High level of transcription driven by a 400 bp segment of the human G6PD promoter. *Biochem Biophys Res Commun* **170**:1203, 1990.
88. Morikawa N, Nakayawa R, Holtein D: Dietary induction of glucose-6-phosphate dehydrogenase synthesis. *Biochem Biophys Res Commun* **120**:1022, 1984.
89. Manos P, Taylor N, Rudach-Garcia D, Morikawa N, Nakayawa R, Holten D: Signals regulating G6PD levels in rat liver, in Yoshida A, Beutler E (eds): *Glucose-6-phosphate Dehydrogenase*. Orlando, FL, Academic, 1986.
90. Richards AH, Hilf R: Influence of pregnancy, lactation and involution on glucose 6-phosphate dehydrogenase and lactate dehydrogenase isoenzymes in the rat mammary gland. *Endocrinology* **91**:287, 1972.
91. Weber G, Cantero A: Glucose-6-phosphate utilization in hepatoma, regenerating and newborn rat liver, and in the liver of fed and fasted normal rats. *Cancer Res* **17**:995, 1957.
92. Betke K, Brewer GJ, Kirkman HN, Luzzatto L, Motulsky AG, Ramot B, Siniscalco M: Standardization of procedures for the study of glucose-6-phosphate dehydrogenase. *WHO Tech Rep Ser* **366**:53p, 1967.
93. WHO Working Group: Glucose 6-phosphate dehydrogenase deficiency. *Bull WHO* **67**:601, 1989.
94. Vergnes HA, Bonnet LG, Grozdea JD: Genetic variants of human erythrocyte glucose-6-phosphate dehydrogenase: New characterization data obtained by multivariate analysis. *Ann Hum Genet* **49**:1, 1985.
95. Escobar MA, Heller P, Trobaugh FEJ: "Complete" erythrocyte glucose 6-phosphate dehydrogenase deficiency. *Arch Intern Med* **113**:428, 1964.
96. Junien C, Kaplan JC, Heienhofer HC, Malgret P, Sender A: G 6 PD Baudelocque: A new unstable variant characterized in cultured fibroblasts. *Enzyme* **18**:48, 1974.
97. Chao L, Du CS, Louie E, Zuo L, Chen E, Lubin B, Chiu TY: A to G substitution identified in exon 2 of the G6PD gene among G6PD deficient Chinese. *Nucleic Acids Res* **19**:6056, 1991.
98. MacDonald D, Town M, Mason PJ, Vulliamy TJ, Luzzatto L, Goff MC: Deficiency in red blood cells. *Nature* **350**:115, 1991.
99. Nafa K, Reghis A, Osmani N, Baghli N, Benabadji M, Vulliamy T, Luzzatto L: G6PD Aures: A new mutation (48 Ile → Thr) causing mild G6PD deficiency is associated with favism. *Hum Mol Genet* **2**:81, 1993.
100. Calabrò V, Giacobbe A, Vallone D, Montanaro V, Cascone A, Filosa S, Battistuzzi G: Genetic heterogeneity at the glucose 6-phosphate dehydrogenase locus in southern Italy: A study on a population from the Matera district. *Hum Genet* **86**:49, 1990.
101. Vulliamy TJ, D'Urso M, Battistuzzi G, Estrada M, Foulkes NS, Martini G, Calabrò V, Poggi V, Giordano R, Town M, Luzzatto L, Persico MG: Diverse point mutations in the human glucose-6-phosphate dehydrogenase gene cause enzyme deficiency and mild or severe hemolytic anemia. *Proc Natl Acad Sci USA* **85**:5171, 1988.
102. Hirono A, Beutler E: Molecular cloning and nucleotide sequence of cDNA for human glucose-6-phosphate dehydrogenase variant A(−). *Proc Natl Acad Sci USA* **85**:3951, 1988.
103. Hirono A, Fujii H, Miwa S: Molecular abnormality of G6PD Konan and G6PD Ube. *Hum Genet* **91**:507, 1993.
104. Maeda M, Constantoulakis P, Chen CS, Stamatoyannopoulos G, Yoshida A: Molecular abnormalities of a human glucose 6-phosphate dehydrogenase variant associated with undetectable enzyme activity and immunologically cross-reacting material. *Am J Hum Genet* **51**:386, 1992.
105. Takizawa T, Yoneyama Y, Miwa S, Yoshida A: A single nucleotide base transition is the basis of the common human glucose-6-phosphate dehydrogenase variant A(+). *Genomics* **1**:228, 1987.
106. Chiu DTY, Zuo L, Chen E, Louie LT, Lubin BH, Du CS: DNA sequence abnormalities in Chinese glucose 6-phosphate dehydrogenase (G6PD) variants. *Blood* **78(Suppl 1)**:252a, 1991 (abstract).
107. Luzzatto L, Usanga EA, Bienzle U, Esan GJF, Fasuan FA: Imbalance in X-chromosome expression: Evidence for a human X-linked gene affecting growth of haemopoietic cells. *Science* **205**:1418, 1979.

108. Vulliamy TJ, Wanachiwanawin W, Mason PJ, Luzzatto L: G6PD Mahidol, a common deficient variant in South East Asia is caused by a (163)glycine → serine mutation. *Nucleic Acids Res* **17**:5868, 1989.
109. Tang TK, Huamg C-S, Huamg M-J, Tam K-B, Yeh C-H, Tang C-JC: Diverse point mutations result in glucose 6-phosphate dehydrogenase (G6PD) polymorphism in Taiwan. *Blood* **79**:2135, 1992.
110. Beutler E, Kuhl W, Saenz GF, Rodriguez W: Mutation analysis of glucose-6-phosphate dehydrogenase (G6PD) variants in Costa Rica. *Hum Genet* **87**:462, 1991.
111. Rovira A, Vulliamy TJ, Pujades A, Luzzatto L, Vives Corrons J-L: The glucose-6-phosphate dehydrogenase (G6PD) deficient variant G6PD Union (454 Arg → Cys) has a worldwide distribution possibly due to recurrent mutation. *Hum Mol Genet* **3**:833, 1994.
112. Corcoran CM, Calabro V, Tamagnini G, Town M, Haidar B, Vulliamy TJ, Mason P, Luzzatto L: Molecular heterogeneity underlying the G6PD Mediterranean phenotype. *Hum Genet* **88**:688, 1992.
113. Beutler E, Westwood B, Prchal JT, Vaca G, Bartsocas CS, Baronciani L: New glucose 6-phosphate dehydrogenase mutations from various ethnic groups. *Blood* **80**:255, 1992.
114. Calabrò V, Mason PJ, Civitelli D, Cittadella R, Filosa S, Tagarelli A, Martini G, Brancati C, Luzzatto L: Genetic heterogeneity at the glucose 6 phosphate dehydrogenase locus revealed by single-strand conformation and sequence analysis. *Am J Hum Genet* **52**:527, 1993.
115. Beutler E, Kuhl W, Gelbart T, Forman M: DNA sequence abnormalities of human glucose 6-phosphate dehydrogenase variants. *J Biol Chem* **266**:4145, 1991.
116. Poggi V, Town M, Foulkes NS, Luzzatto L: Identification of a single base change in the G6PD gene by PCR amplification of the entire coding region from genomic DNA. *Biochem J* **271**:157, 1990.
117. Beutler E, Kuhl W, Vives-Corrons JL, Prchal JT: Molecular heterogeneity of glucose 6-phosphate dehydrogenase A−. *Blood* **74**:2550, 1989.
118. Beutler E, Prchal JT, Westwood B, Kuhl W: Definition of the mutations of G6PD Wayne, G6PD Viangchan, G6PD Jammu and G6PD "LeJeune." *Acta Haematol* **86**:179, 1991.
119. Beutler E, Westwood B, Kuhl W, Hsia HE: Glucose 6-phosphate dehydrogenase variants in Hawaii. *Hum Hered* **42**:327, 1992.
120. DeVita G, Alcalay M, Sampietro M, Cappellini MD, Fiorelli G, Toniolo D: Two point mutations are responsible for G6PD polymorphism in Sardinia. *Am J Hum Genet* **44**:233, 1989.
121. Viglietto G, Montanaro V, Calabrò V, Vallone D, D'Urso M, Persico MG, Battistuzzi G: Common glucose 6-phosphate dehydrogenase (G6PD) variants from the Italian population: Biochemical and molecular characterization. *Ann Hum Genet* **54**:1, 1990.
122. Ahluwalia A, Corcoran CM, Vulliamy TJ, Ishwad CS, Naidu JM, Argusti A, Stevens DJ, Mason PJ, Luzzatto L: G6PD Kalyan and G6PD Kerala: Two deficient variants in India caused by the same 317Glu→Lys mutation. *Hum Mol Genet* **1**:209, 1992.
123. Hirono A, Kuhl W, Gelbart T, Forman L, Fairbanks VF, Beutler E: Identification of the binding domain for $NADP^+$ of human glucose-6-phosphate dehydrogenase by sequence analysis of mutants. *Proc Natl Acad Sci USA* **86**:10015, 1989.
124. Hirono A, Fujii H, Hirono K, Kanno H, Miwa S: Molecular abnormality of a Japanese glucose 6-phosphate dehydrogenase variant (G6PD Tokyo) associated with hereditary non-spherocytic hemolytic anemia. *Hum Genet* **88**:347, 1992.
125. Perng L, Chiou S-S, Liu TC, Chang JG: A novel C to T substitution at nucleotide 1360 of cDNA which abolishes a natural *Hha*I site accounts for a new G6PD deficiency gene in Chinese. *Hum Mol Genet* **1**:205, 1992.
126. Vives-Corrons J-L, Kuhl W, Pujades MA, Beutler E: Molecular genetics of the glucose-6-phosphate dehydrogenase (G6PD) Mediterranean variant and description of a new G6PD mutant, G6PD Andalus1361A. *Am J Hum Genet* **47**:575, 1990.
127. Stevens DJ, Wanachiwanawin W, Mason PJ, Vulliamy TJ, Luzzatto L: G6PD Canton: A common deficient variant in South East Asia cause by a 459 Arg → Leu mutation. *Nucleic Acids Res* **18**:7190, 1990.
128. Chiu DTY, Zuo L, Chen E, Chao LT, Louie E, Lubin B, Liu TZ, Du CS: Two commonly occurring nucleotide base substitutions in Chinese G6PD variants. *Biochem Biophys Res Commun* **180**:988, 1991.
129. Vulliamy TJ, Beutler E, Luzzatto L: Variants of glucose 6-phosphate dehydrogenase are due to missense mutations spread throughout the coding region of the gene. *Hum Mutat* **2**:159, 1993.
130. Morelli A, Grasso M, Meloni T, Forteleoni G, Zocchi E, De Flora A: Favism: Impairment of proteolytic systems in red blood cells. *Blood* **69**:1753, 1987.
131. Tamagnini G: 1993. (Unpublished.)
132. Daar S: 1993. (Unpublished.)
133. Marquez A: 1993. (Unpublished.)
134. Nafa K, Reghis A, Osmani N, Baghli L, Ait-Abbes H, Benabadji M, Kaplan J-C, Vulliamy T, Luzzatto L: At least five polymorphic mutants account for the prevalence of glucose 6-phosphate dehydrogenase deficiency in Algeria. *Hum Genet* 1994, (in press).
135. Oppenheim A, Jury CL, Rund D, Vulliamy TJ, Luzzatto L: G6PD Mediterranean accounts for the high prevalence of G6PD deficiency in Kurdish Jews. *Hum Genet* **91**:293, 1993.
136. Kirkman HN, Simon ER, Pickard BM: Seattle variant of glucose 6-phosphate dehydrogenase. *J Lab Clin Med* **66**:834, 1965.
137. Rattazzi MC, Lenzerini L, Meera Khan P, Luzzatto L: Characterization of glucose 6-phosphate dehydrogenase variants. II. G6PD Kephalonia, G6PD Attica and G6PD "Seattle-like" found in Greece. *Am J Hum Genet* **21**:154, 1969.
138. Ganczakowski M, Town M: Unpublished results, 1993.
139. Corcoran CM, Calabrò V, Tamagnini G, Town M, Kurdi-Haidar B, Vulliamy TJ, Mason PJ, Luzzatto L: Molecular heterogeneity underlying the G6PD Mediterranean phenotype. *Hum Genet* **88**:688, 1992.
140. Vulliamy TJ, Wanachiwanawin W, Mason PJ, Luzzatto L: G6PD Mahidol, a common deficient variant in South East Asia is caused by a 163 Glycine→Serine mutation. *Nucleic Acids Res* **17**:5868, 1989.
141. Vulliamy TJ, D'Urso M, Battistuzzi G, Estrada M, Foulkes NS, Martini G, Calabro V, Poggi V, Giordano R, Town M, Luzzatto L, Persico MG: Diverse point mutations in the human glucose-6-phosphate dehydrogenase gene cause enzyme deficiency and mild or severe hemolytic anemia. *Proc Natl Acad Sci USA* **85**:5171, 1988.
142. Chiu DTY, Zuo L, Chao L, Chen E, Louie E, Lubin B, Liu TZ, Du CS: Molecular characterization of glucose-6-phosphate dehydrogenase (G6PD) deficiency in patients of Chinese descent and identification of new base substitutions in the human G6PD gene. *Blood* **81**:2150, 1993.
143. Hirono A, Fujii H, Shima M, Miwa S: $G6PD_{NARA}$: A new class I glucose-6-phosphate dehydrogenase variant with an eight amino acid deletion. *Blood* **82**:3250, 1993.
144. Luzzatto L: Inherited haemolytic states: Glucose-6-phosphate dehydrogenase deficiency. *Clin Hematol* **4**:83, 1975.
145. Adams MJ, Levy HR, Moffat K: Crystallization of glucose 6-phosphate dehydrogenase from *Leuconostoc mesenteroides*. *J Biol Chem* **258**:5867, 1983.
146. Eliopoulos E, Geddes AJ, Brett M, Pappin DJC, Findlay JBC: Prediction of secondary strcuture in proteins by a combination of different algorithms. *Int J Biol Macromol* **4**:263, 1982.
147. Sharff A: *Structure Studies on Glucose 6-phosphate Dehydrogenase*. Thesis, Oxford University, Oxford, U.K., 1991.
148. Town M, Bautista JM, Mason PJ, Luzzatto L: Both mutations in G6PD A− are necessary to produce the G6PD deficient phenotype. *Hum Mol Genet* **1**:171, 1992.
149. D'Urso M, Luzzatto L, Perroni L, Ciccodicola A, Gentile G, Peluso I, Persico MG, Pizzella T, Toniolo D, Vulliamy TJ: An extensive search for RFLP in the human glucose-6-phosphate dehydrogenase locus has revealed a silent mutation in the coding sequence. *Am J Hum Genet* **42**:735, 1988.
150. Vulliamy TJ, Othman A, Town M, Nathwani A, Falusi

AG, Mason PJ, Luzzatto L: Polymorphic sites in the African population detected by sequence analysis of the glucose 6-phosphate dehydrogenase gene outline the evolution of the variants A and A−. *Proc Natl Acad Sci USA* **88:**8568, 1991.
151. Yoshida A, Takizawa T, Prchal JT: RFLP of the X chromosome linked glucose 6-phosphate dehydrogenase locus in blacks. *Am J Hum Genet* **42:**872, 1988.
152. Ninfali P, Baronciani L, Ruzzo A, Fortini C, Amadori E, Dallara G, Magnani M, Beutler E: Molecular analysis of G6PD variants in northern Italy: A study on the population from the Ferrara district. *Hum Genet* **92:**139, 1993.
153. Maestrini E, Rivella S, Tribioli C, Rocchi M, Camerino G, Santachiara-Benerecetti S, Paolini O, Notarangelo LD, Toniolo D: Identification of novel RFLPs in the vicinity of CpG islands in Xq28: Application to the analysis of the pattern of X chromosome inactivation. *Am J Hum Genet* **50:**156, 1992.
154. Filosa S, Calabrò V, Lania G, Vulliamy TJ, Brancati C, Tagarelli A, Luzzatto L, Martini G: G6PD haplotypes spanning Xq28 from F8C to red/green color vision. *Genomics* **17:**6, 1993.
155. Heller P, Best WR, Nelsen RB, Becktel J: Clinical implications of sickle cell trait and glucose 6-phosphate dehydrogenase deficiency in hospitalized black male patients. *N Engl J Med* **300:**1001, 1979.
156. Hoiberg A, Ernst J, Uddin DE: Sickle cell trait and glucose-6-phosphate dehydrogenase deficiency. Effects on health and military performance in black naval enlistees. *Arch Intern Med* **141:**1485, 1981.
157. Gant FL, Winks GFJ: Primaquine sensitive hemolytic anaemia complicating diabetic acidosis. *Clin Res* **9:**27, 1961.
158. Gellady A, Greenwood RD: G6PD hemolytic anaemia complicating diabetic ketoacidosis. *J Pediatr* **80:**1037, 1972.
159. Shalev O, Eliakim R, Lugassy GZ, Menczel J: Hypoglycemia-induced hemolysis in glucose-6-phosphate dehydrogenase deficiency. *Acta Haematol* **74:**227, 1985.
160. Shalev O, Wollner A, Menczel J: Diabetic ketoacidosis does not precipitate haemolysis in patients with the Mediterranean variant of glucose-6-phosphate dehydrogenase deficiency. *Br Med J* **288:**179, 1984.
161. Perkins RP: The significance of glucose-6-phosphate dehydrogenase deficiency in pregnancy. *Am J Obstet Gynecol* **125:**215, 1976.
162. Dern RJ, Beutler E, Alving AS: The hemolytic effect of primaquine. II. The natural course of the hemolytic anemia and the mechanism of its self-limiting character. *J Lab Clin Med* **44:**171, 1954.
163. Beutler E, Dern RJ, Alving AS: The hemolytic effect of primaquine. IV. The relationship of cell age to hemolysis. *J Lab Clin Med* **44:**439, 1954.
164. Tarlov AR, Brewer GJ, Carson PE, Alving AS: Primaquine sensitivity—Glucose 6-phosphate dehydrogenase deficiency. *Arch Int Med* **109:**209, 1962.
165. Arese P, Mannuzzo L, Turrini F, Faliano S, Gaetani GE: Etiological aspects of favism, in Yoshida A, Beutler E (eds): *Glucose-6-Phosphate Dehydrogenase*. Orlando, FL, Academic, 1986, p 45.
166. Pannacciulli IM, Tizianello A, Ajmar F, Salvidio E: The causes of experimentally induced haemolytic anaemia in a primaquine sensitive Caucasian. *Blood* **25:**92, 1965.
167. Beutler E: Glucose 6-phosphate dehydrogenase deficiency, in Beutler E (ed): *Hemolytic Anemia in Disorders of Red Cell Metabolism*. New York, Plenum, 1978, p 23.
168. Beutler E: Sensitivity to drug-induced hemolytic anemia in glucose-6-phosphate dehydrogenase deficiency, in *Barnbury Report 16: Genetic Variability in Responses to Chemical Exposure*. Cold Spring Harbor, NY, Cold Spring Harbor Laboratory, 1984, p 205.
169. McCaffrey RP, Halsted CH, Wahab MFA, Robertson RP: Chloramphenicol-induced hemolysis in Caucasian glucose-6-phosphate dehydrogenase deficiency. *Ann Intern Med* **74:**722, 1971.
170. Chan TK, Chesterman CN, McFadzean AJS, Todd D: The survival of glucose-6-phosphate dehydrogenase deficient erythrocytes in patients with typhoid fever on chloramphenicol therapy. *J Lab Clin Med* **77:**177, 1971.
171. Doxiadis SA, Valaes F: The clinical picture of glucose-6-phosphate dehydrogenase deficiency in early infancy. *Arch Dis Child* **39:**545, 1964.
172. Zinkham WH: Peripheral blood and bilirubin values in normal full term primaquine-sensitive negro infants: Effects of vitamin K. *Pediatrics* **31:**983, 1963.
173. George JN, Sears DA, McCurdy PR, Conrad ME: Primaquine sensitivity in Caucasians: Hemolytic reactions induced by primaquine in G6PD deficient subjects. *J Lab Clin Med* **70:**80, 1967.
174. Herman J, Ben-Meir S: Overt hemolysis in patients with glucose-6-phosphate dehydrogenase deficiency. A survey in general practice. *Isr J Med Sci* **11:**340, 1975.
175. Janakiraman N, Seeler RA, Royal JE, Chen ME: Hemolysis during BAL chelation therapy for high blood lead levels in two G6PD deficient children. *Clin Pediatr (Phila)* **17:**485, 1978.
176. Valaes T, Dokiadis S, Fessas PH: Acute hemolysis due to naphthalene inhalation. *J Pediatr* **63:**904, 1963.
177. Mandal BK, Stevenson J: Haemolytic crisis produced by nalidixic acid. *Lancet* **1:**614, 1970.
178. JSansone G, Reali S, Sansone R, Allegranza F: Acute hemolytic anemia induced by a pyrazolonic drug in a child with glucose-6-phosphate dehydrogenase deficiency. *Acta Haematol* **72:**285, 1984.
179. Beutler E, Dern RJ, Alving AS: The hemolytic effect of primaquine. IV. The relationship of cell age to hemolysis. *J Lab Clin Med* **44:**439, 1954.
180. Chan TK, Todd D, Tso SC: Red cell survival studies in glucose-6-phosphate dehydrogenase deficiency. *Bull Hong Kong Med Assoc* **26:**41, 1974.
181. Gaetani GF, Mareni C, Ravazzolo R, Salvidio E: Haemolytic effect of two sulphonamides evaluated by a new method. *Br J Haematol* **32:**183, 1976.
182. Magon AM, Leipzig RM, Zannoni VG, Brewer GJ: Interactions of glucose 6-phosphate dehydrogenase deficiency with drug acetylation and hydroxylation reactions. *J Lab Clin Med* **97:**764, 1981.
183. Luzzatto L: Glucose-6-phosphate dehydrogenase and other genetic factors interacting with drugs. *Prog Clin Biol Res* **214:**385, 1986.
184. Burka ER, Weaver Z, Marks PA: Clinical spectrum of hemolytic anemia associated with glucose-6-phosphate dehydrogenase deficiency. *Ann Intern Med* **64:**817, 1966.
185. Shannon K, Buchanan GR: Severe hemolytic anemia in black children with glucose-6-phosphate dehydrogenase deficiency. *Pediatrics* **70:**364, 1982.
186. Agarwal RK, Moudgil A, Kishore K, Srivastava RN, Tandon RK: Acute viral hepatitis, intravascular haemolysis, severe hyperbilirubinaemia and renal failure in glucose-6-phosphate dehydrogenase deficient patients. *Postgrad Med J* **61:**971, 1985.
187. Clearfield HR, Brody JI, Tumen HJ: Acute viral hepatitis, glucose-6-phosphate dehydrogenase deficiency and hemolytic anemia. *Arch Intern Med* **123:**6879, 1969.
188. Mengel CE, Metz E, Yancey WS: Anemia during acute infections. Role of glucose-6-phosphate dehydrogenase deficiency in Negroes. *Arch Intern Med* **119:**287, 1967.
189. Owusu SK, Addy J, Foli AK, Janosi M, Konotey-Ahulu FID, Larbi EB: Acute reversible renal failure associated with glucose-6-phosphate dehydrogenase deficiency. *Lancet* **1:**1255, 1972.
190. Kattamis CA, Tjortjatou F: The hemolytic process of viral hepatitis in children with normal or deficient glucose 6-phosphate dehydrogenase activity. *J Pediatr* **77:**422, 1970.
191. Choremis C, Kattamis CA, Kyriazakou M, Gavrillidou E: Viral hepatitis in G6PD deficiency. *Lancet* **1:**269, 1966.
192. Morrow RH, Smetana HE, Sai FT, Edgcomb JH: Unusual features of viral hepatitis in Accra, Ghana. *Ann Intern Med* **68:**1250, 1968.
193. Oluboyede L, Francis TI, Esan GJF, Luzzatto L: Genetically determined deficiency of glucose 6-phosphate dehydrogenase (type A$^-$) is expressed in the liver. *J Lab Clin Med* **93:**783, 1979.
194. Tugwell P: Glucose 6-phosphate dehydrogenase deficiency in Nigerians with jaundice associated with lobar pneumonia. *Lancet* **1:**968, 1973.
195. Crowell SB, Crowell EB, Mathew M: Depression of

erythrocyte glucose-6-phosphate dehydrogenase (G6PD) activity in enteric fever. *Trans R Soc Trop Med Hyg* **78:**183, 1984.

196. Phillips SM, Silvers NP: Glucose-6-phosphate dehydrogenase deficiency, infectious hepatitis, acute hemolysis and renal failure. *Ann Intern Med* **70:**99, 1969.
197. Selroos O: Reversible renal failure and G6PD deficiency. *Lancet* **2:**284, 1972.
198. Angle CR: Glucose-6-phosphate dehydrogenase deficiency and acute renal failure. *Lancet* **2:**134, 1972.
199. Luzzatto L, Meloni T: Hemolytic anemia due to glucose 6-phosphate dehydrogenase deficiency, in Brain MC, Carbone PP (eds): *Current Therapy in Hematology-Oncology: 1985–1986*. Toronto, Decker–Mosby, 1985, p 21.
200. Walker DH, Hawkins HK, Hudson P: Fulminant rocky mountain spotted fever. Its pathologic characteristics associated with glucose-6-phosphate dehydrogenase deficiency. *Arch Pathol Lab Med* **107:**121, 1984.
201. Salen G, Goldstein F, Haurani F, Wirts CW: Acute hemolytic anemia complicating viral hepatitis in patients with glucose-6-phosphate dehydrogenase deficiency. *Ann Intern Med* **65:**1210, 1966.
202. Chan TK, Todd D: Haemolysis complicating viral hepatitis with glucose-6-phosphate dehydrogenase deficiency. *Br Med J* **1:**131, 1975.
203. Wilkinson SP, Davis MH, Portman B, Williams R: Renal failure in otherwise uncomplicated viral hepatitis. *Br Med J* **2:**338, 1978.
204. Gulati PD, Rizvi SNA: Acute reversible renal failure in G6PD deficient siblings. *Postgrad Med J* **52:**83, 1976.
205. Necheles TF, Gorshein D: Virus-induced hemolysis in erythrocytes deficient in glucose-6-phosphate dehydrogenase. *Science* **160:**535, 1968.
206. Baehner RL, Nathan DG, Castle WB: Oxidant injury of Caucasian glucose-6-phosphate dehydrogenase deficient red blood cells by phagocytosing leukocytes during infection. *J Clin Invest* **50:**2466, 1971.
207. Nelson RA: The immune adherence phenomenon—An immunologically specific reaction between microorganisms and erythrocytes leading to phagocytosis. *Science* **118:**733, 1953.
208. Kaser ML, Miller WJ, Jacob HS: G6PD deficiency infectious hemolysis: A complement dependent innocent bystander phenomenon. *Br J Haematol* **63:**85, 1986.
209. Claster S, Tsun-Yee Chiu D, Quintanilha A, Lubin B: Neutrophils mediate lipid peroxidation in human red cells. *Blood* **64:**1079, 1984.
210. Kattamis CA, Kyriazakou M, Chaidas S: Favism: Clinical and biochemical data. *J Med Genet* **6:**34, 1969.
211. Kahn A, Marie J, Desbois JC, Boivin P: Favism in a Portuguese family due to a deficient glucose-6-phosphate dehydrogenase variant of Canton or Canton like type 1. *Acta Haematol* **56:**58, 1976.
212. Belsey MA: The epidemiology of favism. *Bull WHO* **48:**1, 1973.
213. Discombe G, Meslitz W: Favism in an English-born child. *Br Med J* **1:**1023, 1956.
214. Holt JM, Sladden RA: Favism in England. Two more cases. *Arch Dis Child* **40:**271, 1965.
215. Davies P: Favism: A family study. *Q J Med* **122:**157, 1962.
216. Stockley R, Dawson A, Slade R: Favism in two British women. *Lancet* **2:**1013, 1985.
217. Crosby WH: Favism in Sardinia (Newsletter). *Blood* **11:**91, 1956.
218. Szeinberg A, Sheba C, Hirschorn N, Bodonyi E: Studies on erythrocytes in cases with past history of favism and drug induced acute hemolytic anemia. *Blood* **12:**603, 1957.
219. Gross AT, Hurwitz RA, Marks PA: An hereditary enzymatic defect in erythrocyte metabolism. Glucose-6-phosphate dehydrogenase deficiency. *J Clin Invest* **37:**1176, 1958.
220. Siniscalco M, Bernini L, Latte B, Motulsky AG: Favism and thalassaemia in Sardinia and their relationship to malaria. *Nature* **190:**1179, 1961.
221. Kattamis CA, Chaidas A, Chaidas S: G6PD deficiency and favism in the island of Rhodes. *J Med Genet* **6:**286, 1969.
222. Vullo C, Panizon F: The mechanism of hemolysis in favism. Transfusion experiments with ^{51}Cr tagged erythrocytes. *Acta Haematol* **26:**337, 1961.
223. Panizon F, Vullo C: The mechanism of hemolysis in favism. Researches on the role of non corpuscular factors. *Acta Haematol* **26:**337, 1961.
224. Sartori E: On the pathogenesis of favism. *J Med Genet* **8:**462, 1971.
225. Arese P, Mannuzzu L, Turrini F: Pathophysiology of favism. *Fol Haematol* **116:**745, 1989.
226. Symvoulidis A, Voudiclaris S, Mountokalakis TH, Pougounias H: Acute renal failure in G6PD deficiency. *Lancet* **2:**819, 1972.
227. Baule GM, Onorato D, Tola G, Forteleoni G, Meloni T: Hemoglobin A1 in subjects with G6PD deficiency during and after hemolytic crisis due to favism. *Acta Haematol* **69:**15, 1983.
228. Meloni T, Forteleoni G, Dore A, Cutillo S: Favism and hemolytic anemia in glucose-6-phosphate dehydrogenase deficiency subjects in North Sardinia. *Acta Haematol* **70:**83, 1983.
229. Ruggo G, Mollica G, Pavone L, Schiliro G: Hemolytic crisis of favism in Sicilian females heterozygous for G6PD deficiency. *Pediatrics* **49:**854, 1972.
230. Schiliro G, Russo A, Curreri R, Marino S, Sciotto A, Russo G: Glucose-6-phosphate dehydrogenase deficiency in Sicily. Incidence, biochemical characteristics, and clinical implications. *Clin Genet* **15:**183, 1979.
231. Kattamis C: Favism in breast-fed infants. *Arch Dis Child* **46:**741, 1971.
232. Arese P, De Flora A: Pathophysiology of hemolysis in glucose 6-phosphate dehydrogenase deficiency. *Semin Hematol* **27:**1, 1990.
233. Chevion M, Navok T, Glaser G, Mager J: The chemistry of favism-inducing compounds. The properties of isouramil and divicine and their reaction with glutathione. *Eur J Biochem* **127:**405, 1982.
234. Arese P: Favism: A natural model for the study of haemolytic mechanisms. *Rev Pur Appl Pharmacol Sci* **3:**1234, 1982.
235. Lin JY, Ling KH: Studies on favism. I. Isolation of an active principle from fava beans *(Vicia faba)*. *J Formosan Med Assoc* **61:**484, 1962.
236. Mager J, Glaser G, Razin A, Izak G, Bien S, Noam M: Metabolic effects of pyrimidines derived from fava bean glycosides on human erythrocytes deficient in glucose-6-phosphate dehydrogenase. *Biochem Biophys Res Commun* **20:**235, 1965.
237. Mareni C, Repetto L, Foreteleoni G, Meloni T, Gaetani GF: Favism: Looking for an autosomal gene associated with glucose-6-phosphate dehydrogenase deficiency. *J Med Genet* **21:**278, 1984.
238. Stamatoyannopoulos G, Fraser GR, Motulsky AG, Fessas PH, Akrivakis A, Papayannopoulou T: On the familial predisposition to favism. *Am J Hum Genet* **18:**253, 1966.
239. Battistuzzi G, Morellini M, Meloni T, Gandini E, Luzzatto L: Genetic factors in favism, in Wetherall DJ, Fiorelli G, Gorino S (eds): *Advances in Red Cell Biology*. New York, Raven, 1982, p 339.
240. Bottini E, Lucarelli P, Agostino R, Palmarino R, Businco L, Antognoni G: Favism: Association with erythrocyte acid phosphatase phenotype. *Science* **171:**409, 1971.
241. Cassimos CHR, Malaka-Zafiriu K, Tsiures J: Urinary D-glucaric acid excretion in normal and G6PD deficient children with favism. *J Pediatr* **84:**871, 1974.
242. Cutillo S, Costa S, Vintuledou MC, Meloni T: Salicylamide glucuronide formation in children with favism and their parents. *Acta Haematol* **55:**296, 1976.
243. Schiliro G, Sciotto A, Russo A, Bottard G, Minniti C, Musumeci S, Russo G: Lymphocyte changes in favism: In vitro evidence of a modifying effect of bilirubin and hemoglobin on T-lymphocyte receptors. *Acta Haematol* **69:**230, 1983. 1983.
244. Schiliro G, Minniti C, Sciotto A, Bellino A, Russo A: T lymphocyte subpopulation changes during haemolysis in glucose-6-phosphate dehydrogenase (G6PD) deficient children. *Am J Hematol* **21:**73, 1986.
245. Kaplan J, Saraik S, Gitlin J, Lusher J: Diminished helper/suppressor ratios and natural killer activity in recipients of repeated blood transfusions. *Blood* **64:**308, 1984.

246. De Flora A, Benatti U, Guida L, Forteleoni G, Meloni T: Favism: Distorted erythrocyte calcium hemostasis. *Blood* **66**:294, 1985.
247. Lorani L, Weissman LB, Epel DL, Bruner-Lorand J: Role of intrinsic transglutaminase in the Ca^{++} mediated crosslinking of erythrocyte proteins. *Proc Natl Acad Sci USA* **73**:4479, 1976.
248. Fischer TM, Pescarmona GP, Bosia A, Maitana A, Turrini F, Arese P: Membrane cross-banding in red cells in favic crisis—A missing link in the mechanism of extravascular haemolysis. *Br J Haematol* **66**:294, 1985.
249. Meloni T, Forteleoni G, Meloni GF: Marked decline of favism after neonatal glucose-6-phosphate dehydrogenase screening and health education: The northern Sardinian experience. *Acta Haematol* **87**:29, 1992.
250. Ekert H, Rawlinson I: Deferoxamine and favism. *N Engl J Med* **312**:1260, 1985.
251. Meloni T, Forteleoni G, Gaetani GF: Desferrioxamine and favism. *Br J Haematol* **63**:394, 1986.
252. Khalifa AS, El-Alfy MS, Mokhtar G: Effect of desferrioxamine B on hemolysis in glucose 6-phosphate dehydrogenase deficiency. *Acta Haematol* **82**:113, 1989.
253. Galiano S, Saetani GF, Barabino A, Cottafava F, Zeitlin H, Town M, Luzzatto L: Favism in the African type of glucose-6-phosphate deficiency (A−). *Br Med J* **300**:236, 1990.
254. Matthay KK, Mentzer WC: Erythrocyte enzymopathies in the newborn. *Clin Haematol* **10**:31, 1981.
255. Smith GD, Vella F: Erythrocyte enzyme deficiency in unexplained kernicterus. *Lancet* **1**:1133, 1960.
256. Panizon F: Erythrocyte enzyme deficiency in unexplained kernicterus. *Lancet* **2**:1093, 1960.
257. Bienzle U: Glucose-6-phosphate dehydrogenase deficiency. Part 1: Tropical Africa. *Clin Haematol* **10**:785, 1981.
258. Karayalcin G, Acs H, Lanzkowsky P: G6PD deficiency and hyperbilirubinaemia in black American full-term infants. *NY State J Med* **79**:22, 1979.
259. Ling IT, Wilson RJM: G6PD activity of the malarial parasite *Plasmodium falciparum*. *Mol Biochen Parasit* **31**:47, 1988.
260. Tarnow-Mordi WO, Pickering D: Missed jaundice in black infants a hazard? *Br Med J* **286**:463, 1983.
261. Lopez R, Cooperman JM: Glucose-6-phosphate dehydrogenase deficiency and hyperbilirubinaemia in the newborn. *Am J Dis Child* **122**:66, 1971.
262. Brown WR, Boon WH: Hyperbilirubinaemia and kernicterus in glucose-6-phosphate dehydrogenase deficient infants in Singapore. *Pediatrics* **41**:1055, 1968.
263. Meloni T, Costa S, Sutillo S: Haptoglobin, hemopexin, hemoglobin and hematocrit in newborns with erythrocyte glucose-6-phosphate dehydrogenase deficiency. *Acta Haematol* **54**:284, 1975.
264. Malaka-Zafiriu K, Tsiures I, Danielides B, Cassimos C: Salicylamide glucuronide formation in newborns with severe jaundice of unknown aetiology and due to glucose-6-phosphate dehydrogenase deficiency in Greece. *Helv Paediatr Acta* **28**:323, 1973.
265. Levin SE, Charlton RW, Freiman I: Glucose-6-phosphate dehydrogenase deficiency and neonatal jaundice in South African Bantu infants. *J Pediatr* **65**:757, 1964.
266. Gross S: Hemolytic anemia in premature infants: Relationship to vitamin E, selenium, glutathione peroxidase and erythrocyte lipids. *Semin Hematol* **3**:187, 1976.
267. Bienzle U, Effiong CE, Aimaku VE, Luzzatto L: Erythrocyte enzymes in neonatal jaundice. *Acta Haematol* **55**:10, 1976.
268. Jones PEH, McCance RA: Enzyme activities in the blood of infants and adults. *Biochem J* **45**:464, 1949.
269. Ifekwunigwe AE, Luzzatto L: Kernicterus in G6PD deficiency. *Lancet* **1**:667, 1966.
270. Lai HC, Lai MPY, Leung KS: Glucose-6-phosphate dehydrogenase deficiency in Chinese. *J Clin Pathol* **21**:44, 1968.
271. Lu T-C, Wei H, Blackwell RQ: Increased incidence of severe hyperbilirubineamia among newborn Chinese infants with G6PD deficiency. *Pediatrics* **37**:994, 1966.
272. Szeinberg A, Oliver M, Schmidt R, Adam A, Sheba C: Glucose-6-phosphate dehydrogenase deficiency and hemolytic disease of the newborn in Israel. *Arch Dis Child* **38**:23, 1963.
273. Milbauer B, Peled N, Svirsky S: Neonatal hyperbilirubineamia and glucose-6-phosphate dehydrogenase deficiency. *Isr J Med Sci* **9**:547, 1973.
274. Beutler E, Grooms AM, Morgan SK, Trinidad F: Chronic severe hemolytic anemia due to G-6-PD Charleston: A new deficient variant. *J Pediatr* **80**:1005, 1972.
275. Feldman R, Gromisch DS, Luhby AL, Beutler E: Congenital nonspherocytic hemolytic anemia due to glucose-6-phosphate dehydrogenase East Harlem: A new deficient variant. *J Pediatr* **90**:89, 1977.
276. Drew JH, Smith MB, Kitchen WH: Glucose-6-phosphate dehydrogenase in immigrant Greek infants. *J Pediatr* **90**:659, 1977.
277. Brown AK, Cevik N: Hemolysis and jaundice in the newborn following maternal treatment with sulfamethoxpyridazine (Kynex). *Pediatrics* **36**:742, 1965.
278. Perkins RP: Hydrops fetalis and stillbirth in a male glucose-6-phosphate dehydrogenase deficient fetus possibly due to maternal ingestion of sulfisoxazole. *Am J Obstet Gynecol* **11**:379, 1971.
279. Valaes T, Doxiadis SA, Fessas PH: Acute hemolysis due to naphthalene inhalation. *J Pediatr* **63**:904, 1963.
280. Eshaghpour E, Oski FA, Williams M: The relationship of erythrocyte glucose-6-phosphate dehydrogenase deficiency to hyperbilirubinemia in Negro premature infants. *J Pediatr* **70**:595, 1967.
281. Owa JA: Relationship between exposure to icterogenic agents, G6PD deficiency and severe neonatal jaundice in Nigeria. *Acta Paediatr Scand* **78**:848, 1989.
282. Meloni T, Cagnazzo G, Dore A, Cutillo S: Phenobarbital for prevention of hyperbilirubinemia in glucose 6-phosphate dehydrogenase-deficient newborn infants. *J Pediatr* **82**:1048, 1973.
283. Luzzatto L, Meloni T: Hemolytic anemia due to glucose-6-phosphate dehydrogenase deficiency, in Brain MC, Carbone PP (eds): *Current Terhapy in Hematology/Oncology 2*. Philadelphia, Marcel Dekker, 1985, p 21.
284. Mallouh AA, Imseeh G, Abu-Osba YK, Hamdan JA: Screening for glucose-6-phosphate dehydrogenase deficiency can prevent severe neonatal jaundice. *Ann Trop Paediatr* **12**:391, 1992.
285. Koperman EY, Ey JL, Lee H: Phototherapy in newborn infants with glucose-6-phosphate dehydrogenase deficiency. *J Pediatr* **93**:497, 1978.
286. Lopez R, Gromisch DS, Cole HS, Cooperman JM: Phototherapy in G6PD deficient infants. *J Pediatr* **102**:326, 1983.
287. Meloni T, Costa S, Dore A, Cutillo S: Phototherapy for neonatal hyperbilirubinemia in mature newborn infants with G6PD deficiency. *J Pediatr* **85**:560, 1974.
288. Meloni T, Corti R, Naitana AF, Arese P: Lack of effect of phototherapy on glucose 6-phosphate dehydrogenase activity in normal and G6PD deficient subjects with neonatal jaundice. *J Pediatr* **100**:972, 1982.
289. Miwa S, Fujii H: Glucose 6-phosphate dehydrogenase variants in Japan, in Yoshida A, Beutler E (eds): *Glucose 6-phosphate Dehydrogenase*. Orlando, FL, Academic, 1986, p 261.
290. Fairbanks VF, Nepo AG, Beutler E, Dickson ER, Honig G: Glucose-6-phosphate dehydrogenase variants: Reexamination of G6PD Chicago and Cornell and a new variant (G6PD Pea Ridge) resembling G6PD Chicago. *Blood* **55**:216, 1980.
291. Kirkman HN, Rosenthal IM, Simon ER, Carson PE, Brinson AG: "Chicago I" variant of glucose-6-phosphate dehydrogenase in congenital hemolytic disease. *J Lab Clin Med* **63**:715, 1964.
292. McCurdy PR, Kamel K, Selim O: Heterogeneity of red cell glucose 6-phosphate dehydrogenase (G6PD) deficiency in Egypt. *J Lab Clin Med* **84**:673, 1974.
293. McCurdy PR, Maldonado N, Dillon DE, Conrad ME: Variants of glucose-6-phosphate dehydrogenase (G-6-PD) associated with G-6-PD deficiency in Puerto Ricans. *J Lab Clin Med* **82**:432, 1973.
294. Karadsheh NS, Awibi AS, Tarawneh MS: Two new glucose-6-phosphate dehydrogenase (G6PD) variants associated with hemolytic anemia. *Am J Hematol* **22**:185, 1986.

295. Beutler E, Mathai CK, Sith JE: Biochemical variants of glucose-6-phosphate giving rise to congenital non-spherocytic hemolytic disease. *Blood* **31:**131, 1968.
296. Ben-Ishay D, Izak G: Chronic hemolysis associated with glucose-6-phosphate dehydrogenase deficiency. *J Lab Clin Med* **63:**1002, 1964.
297. Vives-Corrons JL, Feliu E, Pujades MA, Cardellach F, Rozman C, Carreras A, Jou JM, Vallespi MT, Zuazu FJ: Severe glucose-6-phosphate dehydrogenase (G6PD) deficiency associated with chronic hemolytic anemia, granulocyte dysfunction and increased susceptibility to infections. Description of a new molecular variant ($G6PD_{BARCELONA}$). *Blood* **59:**428, 1982.
298. Ventura A, Panizon F, Soranzo MR, Veneziano G, Sansone G, Testa U, Luzzatto L: Congenital dyserythropoietic anaemia Type II associated with a new type of G6PD deficiency (G6PD Gabrovizza). *Acta Haematol* **71:**227, 1984.
299. Rotoli B: Personal communication, 1992.
300. Ben-Bassat J, Ben-Ishay D: Hereditary hemolytic anemia associated with glucose-6-phosphate dehydrogenase deficiency Mediterranean type. *Isr J Med Sci* **5:**1053, 1969.
301. Mahendra P, Dollery CT, Luzzatto L, Bloom SR: Pyruvate kinase deficiency: Association with G6PD deficiency. *Br Med J* **305:**760, 1992.
302. Zanella A, Colombo M, Mintero R, Perroni L, Meloni T, Sirchia G: Erythrocyte pyruvate kinase deficiency—11 new cases. *Br J Haematol* **69:**399, 1988.
303. Beutler E, Kuhl W, Gilbart T: 6-phosphogluconolactonase deficiency, a hereditary erythrocyte enzyme deficiency: Possible interaction with glucose 6-phosphate dehydrogenase deficiency. *Proc Natl Acad Sci USA* **82:**3876, 1985.
304. Newton WAJ, Frajola WJ: Drug-sensitive chronic hemolytic anemia: Family studies. *Clin Res* **6:**392, 1958.
305. Miller DR, Wollman MR: A new variant of glucose-6-phosphate dehydrogenase deficiency hereditary hemolytic anemia, G6PD Cornell: Erythrocyte, leukocyte, and platelet studies. *Blood* **44:**323, 1974.
306. Rattazzi MC, Corash LM, Van Zanen GE, Jaffe ER, Piomelli S: G6PD deficiency and chronic hemolysis: Four new mutants—Relationships between clinical syndrome and enzyme kinetics. *Blood* **38:**205, 1971.
307. Balinsky D, Gomperts E, Cayanis E, Jenkins T, Bryer D, Bersohn I, Metz J: Glucose-6-phosphate dehydrogenase Johannesburg: A new variant with reduced activity in a patient with congenital non-spherocytic haemolytic anaemia. *Br J Haematol* **25:**385, 1973.
308. Sonnet J, Lievens M, Verpoorten C, Kriekemans J, Eeckels R: Sporadic G6PD deficiency with haemolytic anemia in two children of West European ancestry. *Br J Haematol* **28:**299, 1974.
309. Zinkham WH, Lenhard RE: Metabolic abnormalities of erythrocytes from patients with congenital non-spherocytic hemolytic anemia. *J Pediatr* **55:**319, 1959.
310. Mohler DN, Crockett CLJ: Hereditary hemolytic disease secondary to glucose-6-phosphate dehydrogenase deficiency. Report of 3 cases with special emphasis on ATP metabolism. *Blood* **23:**427, 1964.
311. Kirkman HN, Riley HD: Congenital non-sperocytic hemolytic anemia. Studies on a family with a qualitative defect in glucose-6-phosphate dehydrogenase. *Am J Dis Child* **102:**313, 1961.
312. Engstrom PF, Beutler E: G-6-PD Tripler: A unique variant associated with chronic hemolytic disease. *Blood* **36:**10, 1970.
313. Huskisson EC, Murphy B, West G: Glucose-6-phosphate dehydrogenase deficiency and chronic hemolysis in an English family. *J Clin Pathol* **23:**135, 1970.
314. Vuopio P, Harkonen M, Helske T, Naveri H: Red cell glucose-6-phosphate dehydrogenase deficiency in Finland. Characterisation of a new variant with severe enzyme deficiency. *Scand J Haematol* **15:**145, 1975.
315. Johnson GJ, Kaplan ME, Beutler E: G6PD Long Prairie: A new mutant exhibiting normal sensitivity to inhibition by NADPH and accompanied by non-spherocytic hemolytic anaemia. *Blood* **49:**247, 1977.
316. Ramot B, Ben-Bassat I, Shchory M: New glucose-6-phosphate dehydrogenase variants observed in Israel and their association with congenital nonspherocytic hemolytic disease. *J Lab Clin Med* **74:**895, 1969.
317. Greenberg LH, Tanaka KR: Hereditary hemolytic anemia due to glucose-6-phosphate dehydrogenase deficiency. *Am J Dis Child* **110:**206, 1965.
318. De Mars R: A temperature sensitive glucose-6-phosphate dehydrogenase in mutant cultured human cells. *Proc Natl Acad Sci USA* **61:**562, 1968.
319. Bapat JP, Baxi AJ: Mechanism of hemolysis of G6PD deficient red cells: Changes in membrane lipids and polypeptides. *Blut* **44:**355, 1979.
320. Corash L, Spielberg S, Bartsocas C, Boxer L, Steinhertz R, Sheetz M, Egan M, Schlessleman J, Schulman JD: Reduced chronic haemolysis during high dose vitamin E administration in Mediterranean-type glucose-6-phosphate dehydrogenase deficiency. *N Engl J Med* **303:**416, 1980.
321. Spielberg SP, Boxer LA, Corash LM, Schulman JD: Improved erythrocyte survival with high dose vitamin E in chronic haemolyzing G6PD and glutathione synthetase deficiency. *Ann Intern Med* **90:**53, 1979.
322. Hafez M, Amar ES, Zedan M, Hammad H, Sorour AH, Eldesouky ESA, Gamil N: Improved erythrocyte survival with combined vitamin E and selenium therapy in children with glucose-6-phosphate dehydrogenase deficiency and mild chronic haemolysis. *J Pediatr* **108:**558, 1986.
323. Johnson GJ, Vatassery GR, Finkel B, Allen DW: High dose vitamin E does not decrease the rate of chronic hemolysis in G6PD deficiency. *N Engl J Med* **303:**432, 1983.
324. Newman GJ, Newman TB, Bowie LJ, Mendlesohn J: An examination of the role of vitamin E in G6PD deficiency. *Clin Biochem* **12:**149, 1979.
325. Tanaka KR, Beutler E: Hereditary hemolytic anemia due to glucose-6-phosphate dehydrogenase Torrance: A new variant. *J Lab Clin Med* **73:**657, 1969.
326. Mentzer WCJ, Warner R, Addiego J, Smith B, Walter T: G6PD San Francisco: A new variant glucose-6-phosphate dehydrogenase associated with congenital nonspherocytic hemolytic anemia. *Blood* **55:**1295, 1980.
327. Blackburn EK, Lorber J: Chronic hemolytic anemia due to glucose-6-phosphate dehydrogenase deficiency. *Proc R Soc Med* **56:**505, 1963.
328. Allen DW, Johnson GJ, Cadman S, Kaplan ME: Membrane polypeptide aggregates in glucose-6-phosphate dehydrogenase deficient and in vitro aged red blood cells. *J Lab Clin Med* **91:**321, 1978.
329. Johnson GJ, Allen DW, Cadman S, Fairbanks VF, White JG, Lampkin BC, Kaplan ME: Red cell polypeptide aggregates in glucose-6-phosphate dehydrogenase mutants with chronic hemolytic disease. A clue to the mechanism of hemolysis. *N Engl J Med* **301:**522, 1979.
330. Tillman W, Gahr M, Labitke N, Schroter W: Membrane deformability of erythrocytes with glucose-6-phosphate dehydrogenase Hamburg. *Acta Haematol* **57:**162, 1977.
331. Welt SI, Jackson EH, Kirkman HN, Parker JC: The effects of certain drugs on the hexose monophosphate shunt of human red cells. *Ann NY Acad Sci* **179:**625, 1971.
332. Carrell RW, Winterbourn CC, Rachmilewitz EA: Activated oxygen and haemolysis. *Br J Haematol* **30:**259, 1975.
333. Winterbourn CC: Free radical production and oxidative reactions of hemoglobin. *Environ Health Perspect* **64:**321, 1985.
334. Davies KJ, Goldberg AL: Oxygen radicals stimulate intracellular proteolysis and lipid peroxidation by independent mechanisms in erythrocytes. *J Biol Chem* **262:**8220, 1987.
335. Luzzatto L, Battistuzzi G: Glucose 6-phosphate dehydrogenase. *Adv Hum Genet* **14:**217, 1985.
336. Schiliro G, Russo A, Mauro L, Pizzarelli G, Marino S: Leucocyte function and characterisation of leukocyte glucose-6-phosphate dehydrogenase in Sicilian mutants. *Pediatr Res* **10:**739, 1976.
337. Cowan JM, Ammann AJ: Immunodeficiency syndromes associated with inherited metabolic disorders. *Clin Haematol* **10:**139, 1981.
338. Cooper MR, De Chatelet LR, McCall CE, La Via MF, Spurr CL, Baehner RL: Complete deficiency of leucocyte glucose-6-phosphate dehydrogenase with defective bactericidal activity. *J Clin Invest* **51:**769, 1972.

339. Gray FR, Klebanoff SJ, Stamatoyannopoulos G, Austin T, Naiman SC, Yoshida A, Kilman MR, Robinson GCF: Neutrophil dysfunction, chronic granulomatous disease and non-spherocytic haemolytic anemia caused by complete deficiency of glucose-6-phosphate dehydrogenase. *Lancet* **2**:530, 1973.
340. Baehner RL, Johnston RB, Nathan DG: Comparative study of the metabolic and bactericidal characteristics of severely glucose-6-phosphate dehydrogenase deficient polymorphonuclear leucocytes and leucocytes from children with chronic granulomatous disease. *J Reticuloendothelial Soc* **12**:150, 1972.
341. Bellanti JA, Cantz BE, Schlegel RJ: Accelerated decay of glucose-6-phosphate dehydrogenase activity in chronic granulomatous disease. *Pediatr Res* **4**:405, 1970.
342. Corberand J, De Larrard B, Vergnes H, Carriere JP: Chronic granulomatous disease with leukocyte glucose-6-phosphate dehydrogenase deficiency in a 28 month old girl. *Am J Clin Pathol* **70**:296, 1978.
343. Hoffmann J, Bosia A, Arese P, Losche W, Pescarmona GP, Tazartes O, Till U: Glucose-6-phosphate dehydrogenase deficiency in human platelets and its effect on platelet aggregation. *Acta Biol Med Germanica* **40**:1707, 1981.
344. Schwartz JP, Cooperberg AA, Rosenberg A: Platelet function studies in patients with glucose-6-phosphate dehydrogenase deficiency. *Br J Haematol* **27**:273, 1974.
345. Bienzle U, Sodeinde O, Effiong CE, Luzzatto L: G6PD deficiency and sickle cell anemia: Frequency and features of the association in an African community. *Blood* **46**:591, 1975.
346. Luzzatto L, Allan NC: Relationship between the genes for glucose-6-phosphate dehydrogenase and for haemoglobin in a Nigerian population. *Nature* **219**:1041, 1968.
347. Nhonoli AM, Kujwalile JM, Kigoni EP, Masawe A: Correlation of glucose-6-phosphate dehydrogenase (G6PD) deficiency and sickle cell trait (Hb-AS). *Trop Geogr Med* **30**:99, 1978.
348. Steinberg MH, Dreiling BJ: Glucose-6-phosphate dehydrogenase deficiency in sickle cell anemia. A study in adults. *Ann Intern Med* **80**:217, 1974.
349. Beutler E, Johnson C, Powars D, West C: Prevalence of glucose-6-phosphate dehydrogenase deficiency in sickle cell disease. *N Engl J Med* **280**:826, 1974.
350. Steinberg MH, West MS, Gallagher D, Mentzer W: Cooperative Study of Sickle Cell Disease: Effects of glucose-6-phosphate dehydrogenase deficiency upon sickle cell anemia. *Blood* **71**:748, 1988.
351. Snyder LM, Necheles TF, Reddy WJ: G-6-PD Wocester: A new variant, asssociated with X-linked optic atrophy. *Am J Med* **49**:125, 1970.
352. Petersen OW, Briand P, van Deurs S: Identification of malignant cells in primary monolayer cultures of human breast tumors. *Acta Pathol Microbiol Immunol Scand* **92**:103, 1984.
353. Bezwoda WR, Derman DP, See N, Mansoor N: Relative value of oestogen receptor assay, lactoferrin content and glucose-6-phosphate dehydrogenase activity as prognostic indicators in primary breast cancer. *Oncology* **42**:7, 1985.
354. Zempella EJ, Bradley EL, Pretlow TG: Glucose-6-phosphate dehydrogenase: A possible indicator for prostatic carcinoma. *Cancer* **49**:384, 1982.
355. Ibrahim KS, Husain OAN, Bitensky L, Chayen J: A modified tetrazolium reaction for identifying malignant cells from gastric and colonic cancer. *J Clin Pathol* **36**:133, 1983.
356. Petersen OW, Hoyer PE, van Deurs B: Effect of oxygen on the tetrazolium reaction for glucose-6-phosphate dehydrogenase in cryosections of human breast carcinoma, fibrocystic disease and normal breast tissue. *Virchows Arch (B)* **50**:13, 1985.
357. Naik SN, Anderson DE: G6PD deficiency and cancer. *Lancet* **1**:1060, 1970.
358. Sulis E: G6PD deficiency and cancer. *Lancet* **1**:1185, 1972.
359. Ferraris AM, Broccia G, Meloni T, Forteleoni G, Gaetani GF: Glucose-6-phosphate dehydrogenase deficiency and incidence of haemological malignancy. *Am J Hum Genet* **42**:516, 1988.
360. Herz F, Kaplan E, Scheye ES: Diagnosis of erythrocyte glucose-6-phosphate dehydrogenase deficiency in the Negro male despite hemolytic crisis. *Blood* **35**:90, 1970.
361. Ringelhahn B: A simple laboratory procedure for the recognition of the A− (African type) G6PD deficiency in acute haemolytic crisis. *Clin Chim Acta* **36**:272, 1972.
362. Mallouh AA, Imseeh G, Abu-Osba YK, Hamdan JA: Screening for glucose-6-phosphate dehydrogenase deficiency can prevent severe neonatal jaundice. *Ann Trop Paed* **12**:391, 1992.
363. Solem E: Glucose-6-phosphate dehydrogenase deficiency: An easy and sensitive quantitative assay for the detection of female heterozygotes in red blood cells. *Clin Chim Acta* **142**:153, 1984.
364. Solem E, Pirzer C, Siege M, Kollman F, Romero-Saravia O, Barktsch-Trefs O, Kornhuber B: Mass screening for glucose-6-phosphate dehydrogenase deficiency. Improved fluorescent spot test. *Clin Chim Acta* **152**:135, 1985.
365. Orlina AR, Josephson AM, McDonald BJ: The poststorage viability of glucose-6-phosphate dehydrogenase deficient erythrocytes. *J Lab Clin Med* **75**:930, 1970.
366. van der Saar A, Schouter H, Struyker Boudier AM: Glucose-6-phosphate dehydrogenase deficiency in red cells. Incidence in the Curacao population, its clinical and genetic aspects. *Enzyme* **27**:289, 1964.
367. Mimouni F, Shohat S, Reismer SH: G6PD-deficient donor blood as a cause of haemolysis in two pre-term infants. *Isr J Med Sci* **22**:120, 1986.
368. Shalev D, Manny N, Sharon R: Posttransfusional hemolysis in recipients of glucose-6-phosphate dehydrogenase deficient erythrocytes. *Vox Sang* **64**:94, 1993.
369. McCurdy PR, Morse EE: Glucose-6-phosphate dehydrogenase deficiency and blood transfusion. *Vox Sang* **28**:230, 1975.
370. Linder D, Gartler SM: Glucose 6-phosphate dehydrogenase mosaicism. Utilization as a cell marker in the study of leiomyomas. *Science* **150**:67, 1965.
371. Vogels IMC, Van Noorden CJF, Worf BHM, Saelman DEM, Tromp A, Schutgens RBH, Weening RS: Cytochemical determination of heterozygous glucose-6-phosphate dehydrogenase deficiency in erythrocytes. *Br J Haematol* **63**:402, 1986.
372. Ramot B, Szeinberg A, Adam A, Sheba C, Gafni D: A study of subjects with glucose-6-phosphate dehydrogenase deficiency. I. Investigation of platelet enzyme. *J Clin Invest* **38**:1659, 1959.
373. Beutler E, Collins Z, Irwin LE: Value of genetic variants of glucose-6-phosphate dehydrogenase in tracing the origin of malignant tumours. *N Engl J Med* **176**:389, 1967.
374. Fialkow PJ: Clonal origin of human tumours. *Annu Rev Med* **30**:135, 1979.
375. Povey S, Hopkinson DA: The use of polymorphic enzyme markers of human blood cells in genetics. *Clin Haematol* **10**:161, 1981.
376. Adamson JW: Analysis of hemopoiesis: The use of cell markers and in vitro culture techniques in studies of clonal hemopathies in man. *Clin Haematol* **13**:489, 1984.
377. Fialkow PJ, Gartler SM, Yoshida A: Clonal origin of chronic myelocytic leukaemia in man. *Proc Natl Acad Sci USA* **58**:1468, 1967.
378. Fialkow PJ, Jacobsen RJ, Papyannopoulou T: Chronic myelocytic leukaemia: Clonal origin in a stem cell common to the granulocyte, erythrocyte, platelet and monocyte/macrophage. *Am J Med* **63**:125, 1977.
379. Adamson JW, Fialkow PJ, Murphy S, Prchal JF, Steinman L: Polycythaemia vera stem cell and probable clonal origin of the disease. *N Engl J Med* **295**:913, 1976.
380. Oni SB, Osunkoya BO, Luzzatto L: Paroxysmal nocturnal hemoglobinuria: evidence for monoclonal origin of abnormal red cells. *Blood* **36**:145, 1970.
381. Pearson TA, Dillman J, Hepinstall RH: The clonal characteristics of human aortic intima. Comparison with fatty streaks and normal media. *Am J Pathol* **113**:33, 1983.
382. Griffiths DFR, Davies SJ, Williams D, Williams GT, Williams ED: Demonstration of somatic mutation and colonic crypt clonality by X-linked enzyme histochemistry. *Nature* **333**:461, 1988.
383. Beutler E, Kuhl W, Fox M, Tabsh K, Crandall BF: Prenatal diagnosis of glucose 6-phosphate dehydrogenase deficiency. *Acta Haematol* **87**:103, 1992.

384. Fialkow PJ: Clonal origin of human tumors. *Biochim Biophys Acta* **458:**283, 1976.
385. Hamil BM, Munks B, Moyer EZ, Kaucher M, Williams HH: Vitamin C in the blood and urine of the newborn and in the cord and maternal blood. *Am J Dis Child* **74:**417, 1947.
386. Williams CKO, Esan GJF, Luzzatto L, Town MM, Ogunmola GB: X-linked somatic-cell selection and polycythemia rubra vera. *N Engl J Med* **310:**1265, 1984.
387. Motulsky AG: Metabolic polymorphisms and the role of infectious diseases in human evolution. *Hum Biol* **32:**28, 1960.
388. Luzzatto L: Genetics of red cells and susceptibility to malaria. *Blood* **54:**961, 1979.
389. Allison AC: Glucose 6-phosphate dehydrogenase deficiency in red blood cells of East Africans. *Nature* **186:**531, 1960.
390. Yenchitsomanus P, Summers KM, Board PG, Bhatia KK, Jones GL, Johnston K, Nurse GT: Alpha-thalassemia in Papua New Guinea. *Hum Genet* **74:**432, 1986.
391. Siniscalco M, Bernini L, Filippi G, Latte B, Meera-Khan P, Piomelli S, Rattazzi M: Population genetics of hemoglobin variants, thalassemia and glucose-6-phosphate dehydrogenase deficiency, with particular reference to the malaria hypothesis. *Bull WHO* **34:**379, 1966.
392. Stamatoyannopoulos G, Panayotopoulos A, Motulsky AG: The distribution of glucose-6-phosphate dehydrogenase deficiency in Greece. *Am J Hum Genet* **18:**296, 1966.
393. Piazza A, Mayr WR, Contu L, Amoroso A, Borelli I, Curtoni ES, Marcello C, Moroni A, Olivetti E, Richiardi P, Ceppellini R: Genetic and population structure of four Sardinian villages. *Ann Hum Genet* **49:**47, 1985.
394. Martin SK, Miller LH, Alling D: Severe malaria and glucose 6-phosphate dehydrogenase deficiency: A reappraisal of the malaria/G6PD hypothesis. *Lancet* **1:**524, 1979.
395. Luzzatto L, Bienzle U: The malaria/G6PD hypothesis. *Lancet* **1:**1183, 1979.
396. Segal HE, Noll WW, Thiemanun W: Glucose 6-phosphate dehydrogenase deficiency and falciparum malaria in two Northeast Thai villages. *Proc Helminth Soc Wash* **39:**79, 1972.
397. Gilles HM, Fletcher KA, Hendrickse RG, Lindner R, Reddu S, Allan N: Glucose-6-phosphate dehydrogenase deficiency, sickling, and malaria in African children in Southwestern Nigeria. *Lancet* **1:**138, 1967.
398. Bienzle U, Ayeni O, Lucas AO, Luzzatto L: Glucose-6-phosphate dehydrogenase deficiency and malaria. Greater resistance of females heterozygous for enzyme deficiency and of males with non-deficient variant. *Lancet* **1:**107, 1972.
399. Guggenmoos-Holzmann I, Bienzle U, Luzzatto L: *Plasmodium falciparum* malaria and human red cells. II. Red cell genetic traits and resistance against malaria. *Int J Epidemiol* **10:**16, 1981.
400. Trager W, Jensen JB: Human malaria parasites in continuous culture. *Science* **193:**673, 1976.
401. Luzzatto L: Genetics of human red cells and susceptibility to malaria, in Michal F (ed): *Modern Genetic Concepts and Techniques in the Study of Parasites*. Basel, Schwabe, 1981, p 257.
402. Roth EFJ, Raventos-Suarez C, Rinaldi A, Nagel RL: Glucose-6-phosphate dehydrogenase deficiency inhibits in vitro growth of *Plasmodium falciparum*. *Proc Natl Acad Sci USA* **80:**298, 1983.
403. Miller J, Golenser J, Spira DT, Kosower NS: *Plasmodium falciparum:* Thiol status and growth in normal and glucose-6-phosphate dehydrogenase deficient human erythrocytes. *Exp Parasitol* **57:**239, 1984.
404. Friedman MJ: Oxidant damage mediates variant red cell resistance to malaria. *Nature* **280:**245, 1979.
405. Luzzatto L, Usanga EA, Reddy S: Glucose 6-phosphate dehydrogenase deficient red cells: Resistance to infection by malarial parasites. *Science* **164:**839, 1969.
406. Eckman JR, Eaton JW: Dependence of plasmodial glutathione metabolism on the host cells. *Nature* **278:**754, 1979.
407. Clark IA, Hunt NH: Evidence for reactive oxygen intermediates causing hemolysis and parasite death in malaria. *Infect Immun* **39:**1, 1983.
408. Luzzatto L, O'Brien S, Usanga E, Wanachiwanawin W: Origin of G6PD polymorphism: Malaria and G6PD deficiency, in Yoshida A, Beutler E (eds): *Glucose 6-phosphate Dehydrogenase*. Orlando, FL, Academic, 1986, p 181.
409. Usanga EA, Luzzatto L: Adaptation of *Plasmodium falciparum* to glucose 6-phosphate dehydrogenase deficient host red cells by production of parasite-encoded enzyme. *Nature* **313:**793, 1985.
410. Yoshida A, Roth EF: Glucose-6-phosphate dehydrogenase of malaria parasite *Plasmodium falciparum*. *Blood* **69:**1528, 1987.
411. Kurdi-Haidar B, Luzzatto L: Expression and characterization of glucose 6-phosphate dehydrogenase of *Plasmodium falciparum*. *Mol Biochem Parasit* **41:**83, 1990.
412. O'Brien E, Kurdi-Haidar B, Wanachiwanawin W, Carvajal J-L, Vulliamy TJ, Cappadoro M, Mason PJ, Luzzato L: Cloning of the glucose 6-phosphate dehydrogenase gene from *Plasmodium falciparum*. *Mol Biochem Parasit* **64:**313, 1994.
413. Fujii H, Miwa S, Takegawa S: Gd(-)Gifu and Gd(-) Fukuoka: Two new variants of glucose 6-phosphate dehydrogenase found in Japan. *Hum Genet* **66:**276, 1984.
414. Elizondo J, Saenz GF, Paez CA, Ramon M, Garcia M, Gutierrez A, Estrada M: G6PD-Puerto Limon: a new deficient variant of glucose 6-phosphate dehydrogenase associated with congenital nonspherocytic hemolytic anemia. *Hum Genet* **62:**110, 1982.
415. Vives-Corrons JL, Pujades MA, Petit J, Colomer D, Corbella M, Aguilar y Bascompte JL, Merino A: Chronic nonspherocytic hemolytic anemia (CNSHA) and glucose 6 phosphate dehydrogenase (G6PD) deficiency in a patient with familial amyloidotic polyneuropathy (FAP). *Hum Genet* **81:**161, 1989.
416. Gaetani GF, Galiano S, Melani C, Miglino M, Forni GL, Napoli G, Perrone L, Ferraris AM: A new glucose-6-phosphate dehyrogenase variant with congential nonspherocytic hemolytic anemia (G6PD Genova). Biochemical characterization and mosaicism expression in the heterozygote. *Hum Genet* **84:**337, 1990.
417. Kanno H, Takano T, Fujii H: A new glucose 6-phosphate dehydrogenase variant, G6PD Iwate, associated with CNSHA. *Acta Haematologica Japonica* **51:**715, 1988.
418. Pekrun A, Eber SW, Schroter W: G6PD Avenches and G6PD Moosburg: biochemical and erythrocyte membrane characterization. *Blut* **58:**11, 1989.
419. Filosa S, Calabro V, Vallone D, Poggi V, Mason P, Pagnini D, Alfinito F, Rotoli B, Martini G, Luzzatto L, Battistuzzi G: Molecular basis of chronic non-spherocytic haemolytic anaemia: a new G6PD variant (393Arg→His) with abnormal K_mG6P and marked *in vivo* instability. *Br J Haematol* **80:**111, 1992.
420. Ogura H, Morisaki T, Kanno H, Tsutsumi H, Takahashi K, Miyamori T, Fujii H, Miwa S: A new glucose-6-phosphate dehydrogenase variant (G6PD Tsukui) associated with congenital hemolytic anemia. *Hum Genet* **78:**369, 1988.
421. Du CS, Xu YK, Hua XY, Wu QL, Liu LB: Glucose-6-phosphate dehydrogenase variants and their polymorphic frequency in Guangdong, China. *Hum Genet* **80:**385, 1988.
422. Panich V, Na-Nakorn S, Wasi P: G6PD variants in Chinese in Thailand. *Southeast Asian J Trop Med Public Health* **11:**250, 1980.
423. Panich V, Na-Nakorn S: G6PD variants in Thailand. *J Med Assoc Thai* **63:**537, 1980.
424. Poon MC, Hall K, Scott CW: G6PD Viangchan: a new glucose 6-phosphate dehydrogenase variant from Laos. *Hum Genet* **78:**98, 1988.
425. Aksoy K, Yuregir GT, Dikmen H: Three new G6PD variants: G6PD Adana, G6PD Samandag and G6PD Baleali in Cukorova, Turkey. *Hum Genet* **76:**199, 1987.
426. Gutierrez A, Garcia M, Estrada M: Glucose 6-phosphate dehydrogenase Guantanamo and G6PD Caujeri: two new glucose 6-phosphate dehydrogenase deficient variants found in Cuba. *Biochemical Genetics* **25:**231, 1987.
427. Csepreghy M, Yielding A, Lilly M, Hall K, Scot CW, Prchal JT: Characterization of a new glucose 6-phosphate dehydrogenase variant, G6PD Central City. *Am J Hematol* **28:**61, 1988.
428. Kageoka T, Satoh C, Goriki K: Electrophoretic variants of blood proteins in Japanese. IV. Prevalence and enzymological characteristics of G6PD variants in Hiroshima and Nagasaki. *Hum Genet* **70:**101, 1985.

429. Toncheva D: Variants of glucose-6-phosphate dehydrogenase in a Vietnamese population. *Hum Hered* **36**:348, 1986.
430. Gonzalez OL, Espina AL, Calcines PH: G6P-DH Santa Clara and G6P-DH Villa Clara: two new Cuban variants. *Acta Paediatr Hung* **30**:17, 1990.
431. Ninfali P, Bresolin N, Baronciani L, Fortunato F, Comi G, Magnani M, Scarlato G: Glucose-6-phosphate dehydrogenase Lodi 844 C: a study on its expression in blood cells and muscle. *Enzyme* **45**:180, 1991.
432. Kumakawa T, Suzuki S, Fujii H: Frequency of glucose 6-phosphate dehydrogenase deficiency in Tokyo and a new variant, G6PD Musashino. *Acta Haematologica Japonica* **50**:250, 1987.
433. Saha N, Hong SH, Wong HA, Jeyaseelan K, Tay JSH: Biochemical characteristics of glucose 6-phosphate dehydrogenase variants among the Malays of Singapore with report of a new non-deficient variant (GD Singapore) and three deficient variants. *Jpn J Hum Genet* **36**:307, 1991.
434. Csepreghy M, Hall MK, Berkow RL, Jackson S, Prchal JT: Characterization of a new G6PD variant: G6PD Titusville. *Am J Med Sci* **297**:114, 1989.
435. Hall K, Schreeder MT, Prchal JT: G6PD Huntsville: a new glucose 6-phosphate dehydrogenase variant associated with chronic hemolytic anemia. *Hum Genet* **79**:90, 1988.
436. Ermakov NV, Chernyak NB, Tokarev YN: Properties of a new variant of glucose 6-phosphate dehydrogenase (Regar variant). Glucose metabolism in erythrocytes containing abnormal enzyme. *Biokhimiia* **48**:577, 1983.
437. Perona G, Guidi GC, Tummarello D, Mareni C, Battistuzzi G, Luzzatto L: A new glucose 6-phosphate dehydrogenase variant (G6PD Verona) in a patient with myelodysplastic syndrome. *Scand J Haematol* **30**:407, 1983.
438. Kellermeyer RW, Tarlov AR, Brewer GJ, Carson PE, Alving AS: Hemolytic effect of therapeutic drugs. Clinical considerations of the primaquine-type hemolysis. *JAMA* **180**:388, 1962.
439. Ham TH, Grauel JA, Dunn RF, Murphy JR, White JG, Kellermeyer RW: Physical properties of red cells as related to effects in vivo. IV. Oxidant drugs producing abnormal intracellular concentration of hemoglobin (eccentrocytes) with a rigid-red-cell hemolytic syndrome. *J Lab Clin Med* **82**:898, 1973.
440. Beutler E: The glutathione instability of drug-sensitive red cells. A new method for the in vitro detection of drug sensitivity. *J Lab Clin Med* **49**:84, 1957.
441. Chan TK, Todd D, Tso L: Drug induced haemolysis in glucose-6-phosphate dehydrogenase deficiency. *Br Med J* **ii**:1227, 1976.
442. Sicard D, Kaplan J-C, Labie D: Haemoglobinopathies and G6PD deficiency in Laos. *Lancet* **ii**:571, 1978.
443. Zail SS, Charlton RW, Bothwell TH: The haemolytic effect of certain drugs in Bantu subjects with a deficiency of glucose-6-phosphate dehydrogenase. *S Afr J Med Sci* **27**:95, 1962.
444. Newman TB, Maisels MJ: Evaluation and treatment of jaundice in the term newborn: a kinder, gentler approach. *Pediatrics* **89**:809, 1992.
445. Dern RJ, Beutler E, Alving AS: The haemolytic effect of primaquine V. Primaquine sensitivity as a manifestation of a multiple drug sensitivity. *J Lab Clin Med* **45**:30, 1955.
446. Meloni T, Forteleoni G, Ogana A, Francavilla V: Aspirin-induced acute hemolytic anemia in glucose 6-phosphate dehydrogenase deficient children with systemic arthritis. *Acta Haematol* **81**:208, 1989.
447. Beutler E: Acetaminophen and G6PD deficiency. *Acta Haematol* **72**:211, 1984.
448. Doll DC: Oxidative hemolysis after administration of doxorubicin. *Br Med J* **287**:180, 1983.
449. Mercieca JF, Clarke MF, Phillips ME, Curtis JR: Acute hemolytic anemia due to phenazopyridine hydrochloride in a G6PD deficient subject. *Lancet* **ii**:564, 1982.
450. Mehta JB, Singhal SB, Mehta BC: Ascorbic acid-induced haemolysis in G6PD deficiency. *Lancet* **ii**:930, 1990.
451. Kuby SA, Wu JT, Roy RN: Glucose 6-phosphate dehydrogenase from brewer's yeast (Zwischenferment). Further observations on the ligand-induced macromolecular association phenomenon. *Arch Biochem Biophys* **165**:153, 1974.
452. Gordon-Smith EC: Drug-induced oxidative hemolysis. *Clin Haematol* **9**:557, 1980.
453. Wintrobe MM, Lee GR, Boggs DR, Bithell TC, Foerster J, Athens JW, Lukens JN: *Clinical Haematology*. Philadelphia: Lea & Febiger, 1981.
454. Fraser IM, Vesell ES: Effects of drugs and drug metabolites on erythrocytes from normal and glucose-6-phosphate dehydrogenase deficient individuals. *Ann NY Acad Sci* **151**:777, 1968.
455. Fraser IM, Tilton BE, Vesell ES: Effects of some metabolites of hemolytic drugs on young and old, normal and G6PD deficient human erythrocytes. *Ann NY Acad Sci* **179**:644, 1971.
456. Gaetani GD, Mareni C, Ravazzolo R, Salvidio E: Hemolytic effect of two sulphonamides evaluated by a new method. *Br J Haematol* **32**:183, 1976.
457. Capps FPA, Gilles HM, Jolly H, Worlledge SM: Glucose-6-phosphate dehydrogenase deficiency and neonatal jaundice in Nigeria. Their relation to the prophylactic use of vitamin K. *Lancet* **ii**:379, 1963.
458. Harris R, Gilles HM: Glucose-6-phosphate dehydrogenase deficiency in the people of the Niger Delta. *Ann Hum Genet* **25**:199, 1961.
459. Bienzle U, Effiong CE, Luzzatto L: Erythrocyte glucose 6-phosphate dehydrogenase deficiency (G6PD type A^-) and neonatal jaundice. *Acta Paed Scand* **65**:701, 1976.
460. Bernstein RE: Occurrence and clinical implications of red cell glucose-6-phosphate dehydrogenase deficiency in South African racial groups. *S Afr Med J* **37**:447, 1963.
461. Gibbs WN, Gray R, Lowry M: Glucose 6-phosphate dehydrogenase deficiency and neonatal jaundice in Jamaica. *Br J Haematol* **43**:263, 1979.
462. O'Flynn MED, Hsia DY: Serum bilirubin levels and glucose-6-phosphate dehydrogenase deficiency in newborn American Negros. *J Pediatr* **63**:160, 1963.
463. Flatz G, Sringam S, Premyothin C, Penbharkkul S, Ketusingh R, Chulajata R: Glucose-6-phosphate dehydrogenase deficiency and neonatal jaundice. *Arch Dis Child* **38**:566, 1963.
464. Phornphutkul C, Whitaker JA, Worathumrong N: Severe hyperbilirubinemia in Thai newborns in association with erythrocyte G6PD deficiency. *Clin Pediatr* **8**:275, 1969.
465. Weatherall DJ: Enzyme deficiency in hemolytic disease of the newborn. *Lancet* **ii**:835, 1960.
466. Vella F: The incidence of erythrocyte glucose-6-phosphate dehydrogenase deficiency in Singapore. *Experientia* **17**:181, 1961.
467. Lie-Injo LE, Virjk HK, Lim PW, Lie AK, Ganesan J: Red cell metabolism and severe neonatal jaundice in West Malaysia. *Acta Haematol* **58**:152, 1977.
468. Doxiadis SA, Fessas PH, Valaes T: Erythrocyte enzyme deficiency in unexplained kernicterus. *Lancet* **ii**:44, 1960.
469. Doxiadis SA, Valaes T, Karaklis A, Stavrakakis D: Risk of severe jaundice in glucose 6-phosphate dehydrogenase deficiency of the newborn. Differences in population groups. *Lancet* **ii**:1210, 1964.
470. Fessas PH, Doxiadis SA, Valaes T: Neonatal jaundice in glucose-6-phosphate dehydrogenase deficient infants. *Br Med J* **ii**:1359, 1962.
471. Meloni T, Forteleoni G, Dore A, Cutillo S: Neonatal hyperbilirubinaemia in heterozygous glucose-6-phosphate dehydrogenase deficient females. *Br J Haematol* **53**:241, 1983.
472. Cooper MR, De Chatelet LR, McCall CE, La Via MF, Spurr CL, Baehner RL: Complete deficiency of leukocyte glucose 6-phosphate dehydrogenase with defective bactericidal activity. *J Clin Invest* **51**:769, 1972.
473. Clark M, Root RK: Glucose-6-phosphate dehydrogenase deficiency and infection: A study of hospitalized patients in Iran. *Yale J Biol Med* **52**:169, 1979.
474. Wurzel H, McGeary T, Baker L, Gumerman L: Glucose-6-phosphate dehydrogenase deficiency in plateles. *Blood* **17**:314, 1961.
475. Gray GR, Naiman SC, Fobinson GCF: Platelet function and G6PD deficiency. *Lancet* **i**:997, 1974.
476. Cohn J, Carter N, Warburg M: Glucose-6-phosphate dehydrogenase deficiency in a native Danish family. *Scand J Haematol* **23**:403, 1979.
477. Westring DN, Pisciotta AV: Anemia, cataracts and seizures in a patient with glucose-6-phosphate dehydrogenase deficiency. *Arch Intern Med* **118**:385, 1966.

478. Moro F, Gorgone G, Li-Volti S, Cavallaro N, Faro S, Curreri R, Mollica F: Glucose 6-phosphate dehydrogenase deficiency and incidence of cataract in Sicily. *Ophthalmic Paediatr Genet* **5**:197, 1985.
479. Zinkham WH: A deficiency of glucose-6-phosphate dehydrogenase activity in lens from individuals with primaquine-sensitive erythrocytes. *Johns Hopkins Med J* **109**:206, 1961.
480. Oluboyede OA, Esan GJF, Francis TI, Luzzatto L: Genetically determined deficiency of glucose 6-phosphate dehydrogenase (type A−) is expressed in the liver. *J Lab Clin Med* **93**:783, 1979.
481. Chan TK, Todd D, Wong CC: Tissue enzyme levels in erythrocyte glucose-6-phosphate dehydrogenase deficiency. *J Lab Clin Med* **66**:937, 1965.
482. Sarkar S, Nelson AJ, Jones OW: Glucose-6-phosphate dehydrogenase (G6PD) activity of human sperm. *J Med Genet* **14**:250, 1977.
483. Ramot B, Sheba C, Adam A, Ashkenasi I: Erythrocyte glucose-6-phosphate dehydrogenase deficient subjects: Enzyme-level in saliva. *Nature* **185**:931, 1960.
484. Valentine WN, Paglia DE: Erythrocyte enzymopathies, hemolytic anemia and multi system disease: An annotated review. *Blood* **64**:583, 1984.
485. Marks PA, Gross RT, Hurwitz RE: Gene action in erythrocyte deficiency of glucose-6-phosphate dehydrogenase: Tissue enzyme levels. *Nature* **183**:1266, 1959.
486. Younker D, De Vore M, Hartzage PL: Malignant hyperthermia and glucose-6-phosphate dehydrogenase deficiency. *Anesthesiology* **60**:601, 1984.
487. Harper JI, Coperman PWM: A child with xeroderma pigmentosum and G6PD deficiency. *Clin Exp Dermatol* **7**:213, 1982.
488. Congdon PJ, Littlewood JM, Aggarwal RK, Shapiro H: Glucose-6-phosphate dehydrogenase deficiency and cystic fibrosis. *Postgrad Med J* **57**:453, 1981.
489. Dern RJ, Glynn MF, Brewer GJ: Studies on the correlation of the genetically determined trait, glucose-6-phosphate dehydrogenase deficiency with behavioral manifestations in schizophrenia. *J Lab Clin Med* **62**:319, 1963.
490. Bowman J, Brewer GJ, Frischer H, Carter JL, Eisentein RB, Bayrakci C: A re-evaluation of the relationship between glucose-6-phosphate dehydrogenase deficiency and behavioral manifestations. *J Lab Clin Med* **65**:222, 1965.
491. Chanmugan D, Frumin AM: Abnormal oral glucose tolerance response in erythrocyte glucose-6-phosphate dehydrogenase deficiency. *N Engl J Med* **271**:1202, 1964.
492. Eppes RB, Brewer GJ, De Gowin RL, Mcnamara JV, Flanagan CL, Schrier SL, Tarlov AR, Powell RD, Carson PE: Oral glucose tolerance in Negro men deficient in G6PD. *N Engl J Med* **275**:855, 1966.
493. Borkowski AJ, Marks PA, Katz FH, Lipman MM, Christty NP: An abnormal pathway of steroid metabolism in patient with glucose-6-phosphate dehydrogenase deficiency. *J Clin Invest* **41**:1346, 1962.
494. McCurdy PR: An apparent association between red cell glucose-6-phosphate dehydrogenase deficiency and pernicious anemia in negro males. *Clin Res* **14**:91, 1966.
495. Sheehan RG, Lindeman RJ, Meyer J, Patterson JF, Nechelles TF: The possible association of erythrocyte glucose-6-phosphate dehydrogenase deficiency and regional enteritis. *J Clin Invest* **44**:1098, 1965.
496. Long WK, Wilson SW, Frenkel EP: Associations between red cell glucose-6-phosphate dehydrogenase variants and vascular diseases. *Am J Hum Genet* **19**:35, 1967.
497. Wiesenfeld SL, Petrakis NL, Sams BJ, Collen MF, Cutler JL: Elevated blood pressure, pulse rate and serum creatinine in Negro males deficient in glucose-6-phosphate dehydrogenase. *N Engl J Med* **282**:1001, 1970.
498. Deutsch J: Maleimide as an inhibitor in measurement of erythrocyte glucose-6-phosphate dehydrogenase activity. *Clin Chem* **24**:885, 1978.
499. Catalano EW, Johnson GF, Solomon HM: Measurement of erythrocyte glucose-6-phosphate dehydrogenase activity with a centrifugal analyzer. *Clin Chem* **21**:134, 1975.
500. Ardern JC, Edwards N, Hyde K, Jardine-Wilkinson C, Cintokai KI, Power DN, MacIver JE: A proposal for further standardization of red blood cell glucose 6-phosphate dehydrogenase determinations. *Clin Lab Haematol* **10**:409, 1988.
501. Beutler E: A series of new screening procedures for pyruvate kinase deficiency, glucose-6-phosphate dehydrogenase deficiency. *Blood* **32**:816, 1968.
502. Beutler E, Blume KG, Kaplan JC, Lohr GW, Ramot B, Valentine WN: International Committee for Standardization in Haematology: Recommended screening test for glucose-6-phosphate dehydrogenase (G6PD) deficiency. *Br J Haematol* **43**:465, 1979.
503. Beni A, Fortini G, Salvati AM, Tentori L, Torlontano G: Quantitation of the ultraviolet light test for erythrocyte glucose-6-phosphated dehydrogenase, pyruvate kinase and glutathione reductase. *Clin Chim Acta* **49**:41, 1973.
504. Beutler E, Mitchell M: Special modifications for the fluorescent screening test for glucose 6-phosphate dehydrogenase deficiency. *Blood* **32**:816, 1968.
505. Abdalla SH, Phelan L, Hussain HA: The value of screening tests for glucose 6-phosphate dehydrogenase deficiency. *Clin Lab Haematol* **12**:208, 1989.
506. Jacob H, Jandl HJ: A simple visual screening test for glucose-6-phosphate dehydrogenase deficiency employing ascorbate and cyanide. *N Engl J Med* **274**:1162, 1966.
507. Fairbanks VF, Fernadez MN: The identification of metabolic errors associated with hemolytic anemia. *JAMA* **208**:316, 1969.
508. Fairbanks VF, Lampe LT: A tetrazolium-linked cytochemical method for estimation of glucose 6-phosphate dehydrogenase activity in individual erythrocytes: applications in the study of heterozygotes for glucose 6-phosphate dehydrogenase deficiency. *Blood* **31**:589, 1968.
509. Van Noorden CJF, Vogels IMC, James J, Tas J: A sensitive cytochemical staining method for glucose 6-phosphate dehydrogenase activity in individual erythrocytes. *Histochemistry* **75**:493, 1982.
510. Gordon PA, Stewart J: Red cell cytochemistry in glucose-6-phosphate dehydrogenase deficiency. *Br J Haematol* **27**:358, 1974.
511. Van Noorden CJF, Vogels IMC: A sensitive cytochemical staining method for glucose-6-phosphate dehydrogenase activity in individual erythrocytes. *Br J Haematol* **60**:57, 1985.
512. Brewer GJ, Tarlov AR, Alving AS: The methemoglobin reduction test for primaquine-type sensitivity of erythrocytes. A simplified procedure for detecting a specific hypersusceptibility to drug hemolysis. *JAMA* **180**:386, 1962.
513. Bapat JP, Baxi AJ, Bhatia HM: Is methemoglobin reduction test a true index of G6PD deficiency? *Indian J Med Res* **64**:1687, 1976.
514. Motulsky AG, Campbell-Kraut JM: Population genetics of glucose 6-phosphate dehydrogenase deficiency of the red cell, in: Blumberg BS (ed): *Proceedings of Conference on Genetic Polymorphisms and Geographic Variations in Disease*. New York: Grune & Stratton, 1961, p 159.
515. Bernstein RE: Brilliant cresyl blue screening test for demonstrating glucose-6-phosphate dehydrogenase deficiency in red cells. *Clin Chim Acta* **8**:158, 1963.
516. Usanga EA, Bienzle U, Cancedda R, Fasuan FA, Ajayi O, Luzzatto L: Genetic variants of human erythrocyte glucose 6-phosphate dehydrogenase: new variants in West Africa characterized by column chromatography. *Ann Hum Genet Lond* **40**:279, 1976.
517. Beutler E: Glucose-6-phosphate dehydrogenase deficiency, in: Stanbury JB, Wyngaarden JB, Frederickson DS, Goldstein JL, Brown MS (eds): *The Metabolic Basis of Inherited Disease*, 5th ed. New York: McGraw-Hill, 1983, p 1629.

CHAPTER 112

Cytochrome b_5 Reductase Deficiency and Enzymopenic Hereditary Methemoglobinemia

Ernst R. Jaffé ▪ Donald E. Hultquist

1. **The major pathway for the reduction of methemoglobin to functional hemoglobin in human erythrocytes involves a NADH-dependent methemoglobin reductase system. In addition to NADH, this system requires the presence in the cytosol of both cytochrome b_5 reductase, a 32,000-dalton protein, and cytochrome b_5, a 12,000-dalton protein. These proteins are presumed to arise from larger parent molecules in the erythroid precursors by proteolytic cleavage of their hydrophobic tails.**
2. **Enzymopenic hereditary methemoglobinemia is a rare recessively inherited disorder caused, in most cases, by deficiency of cytochrome b_5 reductase only in erythrocytes (type I). Generalized cytochrome b_5 reductase deficiency, demonstrable in all tissues that have been examined, occurs in 10 to 15 percent of cases and is accompanied by methemoglobinemia and severe, progressive, lethal neurologic disability (type II). Cytochrome b_5 reductase deficiency limited to hematopoietic cells is also manifested by methemoglobinemia, but without neurologic effects (type III). Deficiency of cytochrome b_5 may also lead to methemoglobinemia (type IV).**
3. **The gene regulating the synthesis of cytochrome b_5 reductase has been assigned to chromosome 22. Deficiency of cytochrome b_5 reductase has a worldwide distribution, and electrophoretic variants of the enzyme with normal catalytic properties may have an incidence as high as 1:100. Heterozygotes for cytochrome b_5 reductase deficiency are asymptomatic but have an increased propensity to develop toxic methemoglobinemia induced by drugs or other chemicals.**
4. **The diagnosis of enzymopenic hereditary methemoglobinemia may be made by relatively simple laboratory determinations, but definition of the specific defect requires more sophisticated studies.**
5. **Effective treatment may be provided by the administration of methylene blue, ascorbic acid, or riboflavin but is often not indicated, except for cosmetic reasons. Such therapy, however, has had no demonstrable effect on the neurologic aberrations in the generalized type II disorder.**

A list of standard abbreviations is located immediately preceding the index in each volume. Additional abbreviations used in this chapter include: DPG = 2,3-diphosphoglycerate; DCIP = 2,6-dichlorophenolindophenol.

HISTORY

Hereditary methemoglobinemia, an interesting albeit rare disorder, has a worldwide distribution and has been known for a century and a half. In 1845, François[1] described a patient with long-standing congenital cyanosis without obvious cardiac or pulmonary disease. Although altered hemoglobin pigments and drug-induced cyanosis had been reported frequently, it was 1891 before Dittrich[2] established that the methemoglobinemia that developed in dogs given *Blutgifte,* such as nitroglycerine and acetanilide, eventually disappeared without the occurrence of anemia. He also pointed out that the methemoglobinemic cyanosis that developed in patients receiving certain medicines tended to disappear and suggested that the methemoglobin was reduced to hemoglobin within the circulating erythrocytes. Subsequently, other authors described "enterogenous cyanosis" attributed to the absorption of toxic substances from the gastrointestinal tract.[3] Sulfhemoglobin present in some of these patients' erythrocytes was differentiated from methemoglobin in 1905.[4]

Hitzenberger[5] in 1932 was probably the first to describe a familial incidence of idiopathic cyanosis. He suggested the possibility of congenital, familial methemoglobinemia. Between 1943 and 1945, Gibson[6] and his associates[7] suggested that there was a decreased ability of the erythrocytes to reduce methemoglobin formed continuously at a normal rate in patients with familial, idiopathic methemoglobinemia. The classic investigations of Gibson[8] in 1948 provided substantial experimental evidence for a deficiency of a factor (a methemoglobin reductase) in the erythrocytes of patients with idiopathic methemoglobinemia. In 1959, Scott and Griffith[9] identified an enzyme in normal human erythrocytes that catalyzed the reduction of methemoglobin with NADH and called this enzyme a "diaphorase." The enzyme was subsequently named and assayed as a NADH dehydrogenase, NADH-methemoglobin reductase, NADH-methemoglobin-ferrocyanide reductase, NADH-ferricyanide reductase, and, most recently, NADH-cytochrome b_5 reductase. Scott et al. described a severe deficiency of this enzyme in the erythrocytes of native Alaskans with methemoglobinemia, and intermediate levels of activity in the cells of their acyanotic parents and children.[10,11] To explain the typically recessive pattern of inheritance of idiopathic methemoglobinemia suggested by the family histories of many patients, they proposed that affected individuals inherited one abnormal gene from each parent. These observations have been extended and confirmed by other investigators.[12]

Hultquist and Passon[13] subsequently identified the NADH-dependent enzyme as a cytochrome b_5 reductase and demonstrated that the catalysis of methemoglobin reduction by this reductase involved the participation of a cytochrome b_5 present in normal human erythrocytes. This enzyme system is considered to be the most important one for the conversion of any methemoglobin formed in normal human erythrocytes to functional, oxygen-carrying hemoglobin. The activity of this system is markedly reduced in the erythrocytes of most patients with enzymopenic hereditary methemoglobinemia.

More than 500 cases of hereditary methemoglobinemia have been cited in the literature. Those patients with family histories suggesting dominant inheritance of the methemoglobinemia have usually been proved or presumed to have a hemoglobin M, a hemoglobin that results from a mutation in the hemoglobin gene which makes the hemoglobin more susceptible to oxidation and/or makes the resulting methemoglobin more resistant to reduction (see Chap. 113). More than half of the total reported cases, however, have had family histories or laboratory evidence consistent with inheritance of an autosomal recessive abnormality. With rare exceptions, these latter patients have been presumed or demonstrated to have an abnormality in the methemoglobin reductase activity of their erythrocytes. Their disorder has become known as enzymopenic hereditary methemoglobinemia to differentiate it from the hemoglobin M disorders.

STRUCTURE AND PROPERTIES OF METHEMOGLOBIN

Fully Oxidized Hemoglobin

Methemoglobin is the derivative of hemoglobin obtained by oxidizing the iron of the heme group of deoxyhemoglobin or oxyhemoglobin from the ferrous (Fe^{2+}) state to the ferric (Fe^{3+}) state. For tetrameric hemoglobin, this transformation corresponds to a four-electron loss. Because methemoglobin is incapable of binding molecular oxygen, oxidation of hemoglobin leads to loss of its biologic function and, when carried out to a sufficient extent, leads to pathologic consequences.

Structural and physical studies have established that in methemoglobin, the sixth coordination position of the iron is occupied by a water molecule, whereas this axial position is empty in deoxyhemoglobin and is occupied by O_2 in oxyhemoglobin. The coordinated water molecule of methemoglobin dissociates with a pK of approximately 8 to form a hydroxide ion which remains bound to the iron.[14] Thus, under physiological conditions, methemoglobin is present predominantly as the "aquo" form; the "hydroxy" form becomes more prevalent as the pH is raised.

The differences in valence and axial ligand between ferrous and ferric hemoglobin are the basis for the differences in the chemical, physical, and biologic properties of these forms of the protein. In contrast to ferrous forms of hemoglobin, methemoglobin has a *net* charge of +1 on the iron atom of each heme moiety, with the consequence that ferrous and ferric forms can be readily separated by electrophoretic techniques. Moreover, the net positive charge on the iron of methemoglobin causes it to bind small anionic ligands such as CN^-, N_3^-, F^-, and Cl^-, but methemoglobin has little affinity for the classic hemoglobin ligands O_2 and CO. The valence and ligand changes that accompany oxidation of hemoglobin also explain the dramatic change in color. In contrast to the bright red color of oxyhemoglobin, aquomethemoglobin is chocolate brown and has absorbance maxima at 500 and 631 nm, and hydroxymethemoglobin is dark red with absorbance maxima at 540 and 575 nm. these spectral differences are responsible for the slate-blue skin color of Caucasian individuals with elevated methemoglobin levels.

X-ray diffraction studies carried out by Perutz and coworkers have established that the protein structure of the tetrameric methemoglobin molecule is very similar to that of the "R-state" conformation of oxyhemoglobin but different from the "T-state" conformation of deoxyhemoglobin.[15] Methemoglobin, like deoxyhemoglobin, binds to polyanionic compounds such as 2,3-diphosphoglycerate (DPG), and the accompanying conformational shift has been termed an "R-to-T-state shift."[16] This binding of polyanions results in changes in physical properties which have been interpreted by some as an increase in the spin state of the hemes.

Valence Hybrids of Hemoglobin

The conversion of tetrameric hemoglobin to tetrameric methemoglobin is a four-step oxidation. Both the oxidation of hemoglobin and the reduction of methemoglobin proceed in sequential one-electron steps, and thus there exist valence hybrids in which one, two, or three hemes are in the ferric form. These valence hybrids, rather than fully oxidized hemoglobin, are central participants in methemoglobin homeostasis. Because the hemoglobin molecule comprises two α chains and two β chains and because each of the two αβ dimers is relatively stable, eight different valence hybrids should exist (Fig. 112-1). This number of forms can be detected in a partially oxidized sample of hemoglobin under conditions that minimize the interconversion of hybrid forms.[17] However, under physiological conditions that allow for the dissociation of tetramers to αβ dimers, dimer dissociation, electron exchange, and heme exchange reactions, only two valence hybrids accumulate in appreciable amounts[18,19];

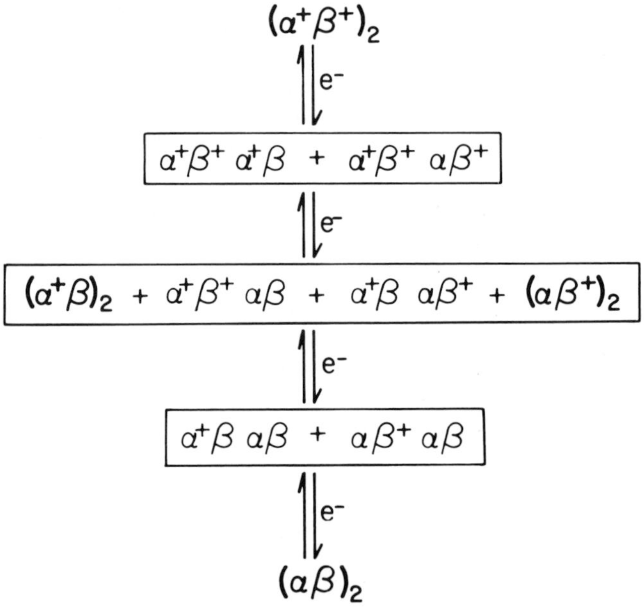

$$(\alpha^+\beta^+)_2$$

$$\rightleftharpoons e^-$$

$$\alpha^+\beta^+\,\alpha^+\beta \;+\; \alpha^+\beta^+\,\alpha\beta^+$$

$$\rightleftharpoons e^-$$

$$(\alpha^+\beta)_2 \;+\; \alpha^+\beta^+\,\alpha\beta \;+\; \alpha^+\beta\,\alpha\beta^+ \;+\; (\alpha\beta^+)_2$$

$$\rightleftharpoons e^-$$

$$\alpha^+\beta\,\alpha\beta \;+\; \alpha\beta^+\,\alpha\beta$$

$$\rightleftharpoons e^-$$

$$(\alpha\beta)_2$$

FIG. 112-1 Valence hybrids of hemoglobin A.

these are the two symmetric forms $(\alpha^+\beta)_2$ and $(\alpha\beta^+)_2$, each of which comprises two identical half-oxidized dimers.

The stepwise *oxidation* of hemoglobin subunits, like the stepwise *oxygenation* of hemoglobin, shows cooperativity, has a Bohr (pH) effect, and is influenced by the binding of polyanions (see reviews in Refs. 20 and 21). Both the standard reduction potential (E'_0) and the degree of cooperativity (n, from a Hill plot) depend on pH. The reduction potential is increased by adding polyanions or lowering the pH. Under physiological conditions, tetrameric hemoglobin A shows an $E'_0 = +0.14$ V. In the tetramer, α chains are slightly stronger reductants than the β chains ($E'_0 = +0.12$ and $+0.16$ V, respectively). Valence hybrids of hemoglobin show a greater affinity for oxygen than does hemoglobin.[20,22] This "left shift" of the oxygen saturation curve by ferric subunits has been interpreted as a shifting of the conformational equilibrium of the tetramer to its high-oxygen-affinity R state by the ferric subunits, which themselves are present in an "R-type" conformation.

Throughout this chapter, *methemoglobin* is used in a general sense to include all forms of hemoglobin in which one or more of the subunits are in the ferric form, and *methemoglobinemia* includes those states in which the valence hybrids are elevated in intact, circulating erythrocytes.

METHEMOGLOBIN HOMEOSTASIS

Observations from the nineteenth century demonstrated that methemoglobin can be generated in red blood cells as a consequence either of hereditary disorders or of the ingestion of toxic compounds and that normal red blood cells possess the capacity to restore methemoglobin to its functional ferrous form. Subsequent studies have demonstrated that methemoglobin is present at low concentrations in normal human erythrocytes and that both generation and reduction of methemoglobin are normal processes for the erythrocyte.[20,23] Moreover, the evidence that hemoglobin is synthesized in reticulocytes as the ferric form suggests that methemoglobin reduction may be a part of the normal biosynthesis of this hemeprotein.[24]

The steady-state level of methemoglobin in normal erythrocytes is low, with most methods of measurement giving values of less than 1 percent of the total hemoglobin. This finding indicates that the capacity to reduce methemoglobin far exceeds the normal rate of hemoglobin oxidation. In isolated, intact erythrocytes, methemoglobin reduction proceeds at a rate of about 5 percent total hemoglobin per hour (1 μmol hemoglobin subunit per hour per milliliter)[8]; the normal rate of hemoglobin oxidation is believed to be 0.02 to 0.12 percent total hemoglobin per hour.

The sustained reduction of methemoglobin in suspensions of intact erythrocytes proceeds only in the presence of a metabolite which can enter the cell and be used in a process that leads to the generation of reduced pyridine nucleotide. Among the substrates that allow for rapid methemoglobin reduction are glucose and a variety of other sugars, lactate, malate, and purine nucleosides such as inosine.[3,23] Studies of the stoichiometry of hemoglobin and pyruvate production in reactions with glucose or lactate as substrate, together with metabolic inhibitor studies, have demonstrated that electrons for methemoglobin reduction are generated primarily by glycolysis and primarily in the form of NADH (Fig. 112-2). However, the rapid methemoglobin reduction that is observed with xylitol and other nonglycolytic substrates[25] suggests that pathways other than glycolysis may be involved with the generation of the NADH used for methemoglobin reduction, at least under conditions where levels of methemoglobin are high.

The steady-state level of methemoglobin is a consequence of all the methemoglobin-reducing reactions (Fig. 112-2) and methemoglobin-generating reactions (Fig. 112-3) in erythrocytes. The major pathway of methemoglobin reduction is catalyzed by erythrocyte cytochrome b_5 reductase and cytochrome b_5; deficiencies of these proteins lead to methemoglobinemia. More difficult to evaluate is the possible role of an erythrocyte NADPH reductase that requires flavin or a redox dye in order to reduce methemoglobin. Likewise, it has been difficult to assess the physiological significance of nonenzymatic reduction reactions, which methemoglobin has been shown to undergo with a number of intracellular compounds. Since methemoglobin reduction proceeds to some extent in red cells severely deficient in cytochrome b_5 reductase activity, the minor pathways, collectively, may be of some importance to the erythrocyte.

A variety of reactions oxidize deoxyhemoglobin and oxyhemoglobin. Among the endogenous compounds that have been identified as reacting with hemoglobin to form methemoglobin are molecular oxygen, hydrogen peroxide (H_2O_2), and a number of free radicals, including superoxide anion ($O_2^{\cdot-}$) and hydroxyl radical ($HO^{\cdot}$). The rate of methemoglobin formation depends on the concentrations of these compounds. The steady-state concentrations of these oxidants, in turn, depend on the rates at which they are generated during metabolism, are consumed by reactions with other cellular components, and are destroyed by protective erythrocyte enzymes such as catalase, superoxide dismutase, and glutathione peroxidase.

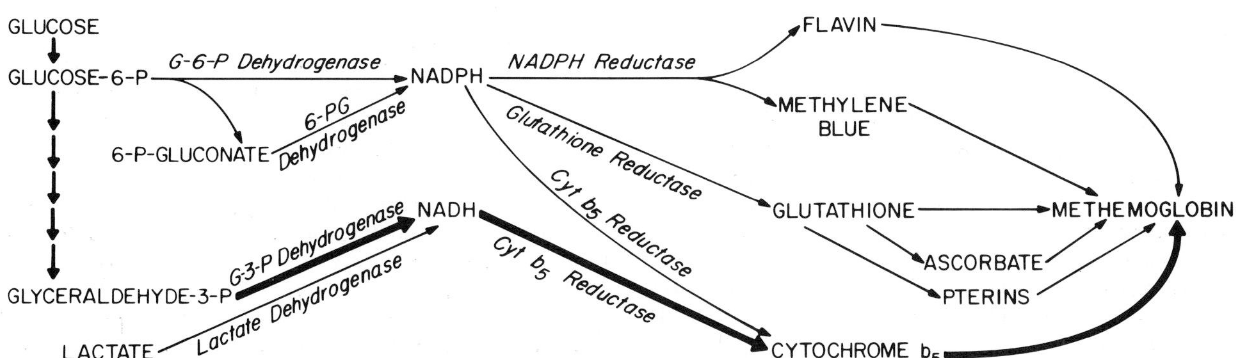

FIG. 112-2 Erythrocyte pathways for the transfer of electrons from metabolites to methemoglobin.

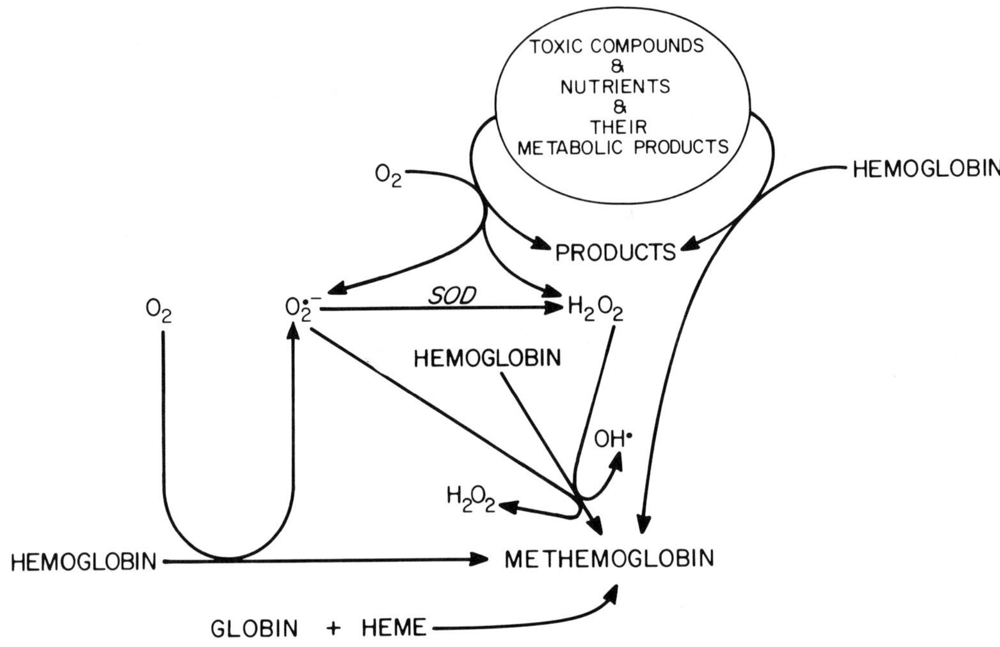

FIG. 112-3 Generation of methemoglobin in erythrocytes.

Elevation of methemoglobin in erythrocytes results either from acceleration of an oxidation reaction or from diminution of a reduction reaction. Such alterations in reaction rates may arise from a hereditary defect or from an environmental stress. The most frequent cause of methemoglobinemia is rapid oxidation arising from ingestion of a toxic compound which either is an oxidant itself or gives rise to oxidants during its metabolism. Methemoglobinemia also arises from rapid autoxidation of a mutant hemoglobin belonging to the hemoglobin M class. Methemoglobinemia due to depressed reduction usually results from deficiency of erythrocyte cytochrome b_5 reductase. A case of methemoglobinemia due to deficiency of cytochrome b_5 has recently been reported.[26] Diminished methemoglobin reduction rates and methemoglobinemia have been observed with hemoglobins $N_{BALTIMORE}$, $I_{TOULOUSE}$, and $M_{MILWAUKEE\text{-}1}$. These mutant hemoglobins presumably fail to interact efficiently with the cytochrome b_5 reductase/cytochrome b_5 system.[27,28] In contrast, methemoglobinemia has not been reported in cases of hereditary hemolytic disorders associated with severe deficiencies of glycolytic enzymes, although an impaired ability to reduce NAD^+ might have been expected to lead to an impaired capacity to reduce methemoglobin, just as inhibition of glycolysis with iodoacetate diminishes methemoglobin reduction.[8]

Methemoglobinemia may also develop if a modest decrease in the ability to reduce methemoglobin is coupled with an environmental stress. The erythrocytes of individuals who are heterozygous for cytochrome b_5 reductase deficiency reduce methemoglobin at approximately 50 percent of the normal rate[29] and are especially susceptible to the methemoglobin-inducing effects of exogenous oxidant agents.[30–32] Similarly, the erythrocytes of newborns have about half the methemoglobin-reducing ability of adults' cells[33,34] and show an increased susceptibility to methemoglobin-producing drugs and chemicals.

OXIDATION OF HEMOGLOBIN

Although the conversion of a ferrous subunit of hemoglobin to the ferric subunit by the removal of an electron can be written as the simplest of chemical reactions, it actually involves a number of complex reactions. In the absence of foreign compounds, much of the oxidation of hemoglobin results from its interaction with O_2 or the partially reduced forms of oxygen, $O_2^{\cdot -}$, H_2O_2, and $HO^{\cdot}$. Following ingestion of foreign compounds, methemoglobin is formed by mechanisms which include direct oxidation by the ingested compound, oxidation by a metabolite derived from the compound, and oxidation by $O_2^{\cdot -}$ and H_2O_2 generated during the metabolism of the compound. The subject of hemoglobin oxidation has been reviewed comprehensively.[21,23,35]

Auto-oxidation of Hemoglobin

Hemoglobin reacts slowly with molecular oxygen to yield methemoglobin and superoxide anion. The reaction corresponds to the transfer of an electron from the iron of the ferrous heme to molecular oxygen. Since oxyhemoglobin apparently exists as a ferric–superoxide anion complex,[36] auto-oxidation may be visualized as the release of the $O_2^{\cdot -}$ from this complex. Whereas auto-oxidation of free ferrous heme in aqueous solution proceeds very rapidly, the auto-oxidation of hemoglobin is slow. The hydrophobic environment provided by the globin is envisioned as hindering the release of the superoxide anion while allowing rapid release of molecular oxygen. This hypothesis is supported by the observation that mutant hemoglobins in which the heme environment is modified show altered rates of autoxidation. Auto-oxidation is accelerated by chloride and other small anions, which may function by displacing the superoxide anion from the oxyhemoglobin. Polyanions and reduced pH also accelerate the reaction. In tetrameric hemoglobin, the

α subunits auto-oxidize more rapidly than the β subunits, with the result that the valence hybrid $(\alpha^+\beta)_2$ is the predominant intermediate in auto-oxidation.[37,38]

The mechanism of auto-oxidation is more complex than the simple release of $O_2^{\cdot-}$ described above. The rate of auto-oxidation increases as the oxygen tension decreases. A maximum rate is achieved when approximately two molecules of oxygen are bound per tetramer.[39] This observation can be interpreted either as evidence that heme is more readily oxidized in deoxyhemoglobin than in oxyhemoglobin or as evidence that $O_2^{\cdot-}$ is more readily released from oxyhemoglobin in the T conformation than in the R conformation. Regardless of the correct mechanism for auto-oxidation, it is clear that the $O_2^{\cdot-}$ generated by auto-oxidation, together with the H_2O_2 and $HO^{\cdot}$ derived from the $O_2^{\cdot-}$, react with hemoglobin to generate additional methemoglobin.

Reactions of Hemoglobin with $O_2^{\cdot-}$ and H_2O_2

$O_2^{\cdot-}$ is generated in erythrocytes not only by the auto-oxidation of hemoglobin but by the auto-oxidation of a number of redox proteins, including cytochrome b_5 and cytochrome b_5 reductase. H_2O_2 is derived from the $O_2^{\cdot-}$ both by a rapid nonenzymatic dismutation reaction and by an even more rapid catalysis of this reaction by superoxide dismutase. H_2O_2 is also an expected end product of oxidase reactions in erythrocytes.

Both $O_2^{\cdot-}$ and H_2O_2 oxidize oxyhemoglobin to methemoglobin. The reaction with $O_2^{\cdot-}$ is a slow one in which the bound molecular oxygen of oxyhemoglobin receives one electron from $O_2^{\cdot-}$ and a second electron from the heme iron:

$$HbFeO_2 + O_2^{\cdot-} + 2H^+ \rightarrow HbFe^+ + H_2O_2 + O_2$$

The overall reaction of H_2O_2 with oxyhemoglobin and deoxyhemoglobin may be written as follows:

$$2HbFeO_2 + H_2O_2 \rightarrow 2HbFe^+ + 2OH^- + 2O_2$$

$$HbFe + H_2O_2 \rightarrow HbFe^+ + OH^- + HO^{\cdot}$$

The highly reactive $HO^{\cdot}$ generated in the latter reaction may react with additional ferrous hemoglobin to form methemoglobin.

The generation of $O_2^{\cdot-}$, H_2O_2, and $HO^{\cdot}$ not only leads to the formation of more methemoglobin but may also promote further oxidation of both the globin and the heme of methemoglobin. One intermediate in this pathway is *hemichrome,* a derivative of methemoglobin in which a functional group of the protein replaces the water molecule bound to the heme. The additional oxidative changes lead to denaturation of the hemoglobin, the formation of intracellular Heinz bodies, and ultimately cell lysis.

The concentrations of $O_2^{\cdot-}$, H_2O_2, and $HO^{\cdot}$ in erythrocytes are normally maintained at low levels by the actions of superoxide dismutase, catalase, and glutathione peroxidase. Superoxide dismutase catalyzes the dismutation of $O_2^{\cdot-}$, catalase the dismutation of H_2O_2, and glutathione peroxidase the reduction of H_2O_2 by reduced glutathione. Because of the relative affinity of catalase and glutathione peroxidase for the substrate H_2O_2, glutathione peroxidase is presumed to be the main agent of the destruction of H_2O_2 under physiological conditions. The ingestion of toxic compounds can lead to rates of $O_2^{\cdot-}$ and H_2O_2 production that overwhelm the protective enzymatic mechanisms.

Oxidation of Hemoglobin by Toxic Compounds

Many drugs, commercial products, other chemical compounds, and metabolic derivatives of such compounds react with hemoglobin to form methemoglobin. If such compounds gain entry into the human circulation, the rate of methemoglobin formation may be several orders of magnitude faster than the rate resulting from the reaction of hemoglobin with oxygen and oxidants generated by normal metabolism. Under such oxidative stress, the erythrocyte methemoglobin reduction systems may be unable to maintain hemoglobin in its functional ferrous form.

The direct reaction of ferrous hemoglobin with various oxidants proceeds with remarkably different reaction rates, reaction mechanisms, preference for α or β chains, and capacity to cause methemoglobinemia. Ferricyanide is an example of an oxidant that accepts one electron from a ferrous heme of hemoglobin. Although this reaction is very rapid, ferricyanide does not lead to methemoglobinemia because it cannot penetrate the red cell membrane. Ferricyanide oxidizes the β subunit somewhat faster than the α subunit, with the result that the $(\alpha\beta^+)_2$ valence hybrid predominates.[40] The reaction of ferricyanide contrasts with that of cupric ion, which exclusively oxidizes the β subunit,[41] and with that of O_2, which favors α-subunit oxidation.

While oxidation of hemoglobin by metal ions results in a valence change of the metal, direct reaction of hemoglobin with organic oxidants yields free radicals. Thus, a variety of oxidant drugs, dyes, and industrial products (including paraquat, menadione, doxorubicin, and methylene blue) react with hemoglobin to form methemoglobin and a free radical; for a quinone, the product is a semiquinone. Many of the free radicals are highly reactive reductants that react with O_2 to form $O_2^{\cdot-}$.

$$R + HbFe \rightarrow HbFe^+ + R^{\cdot-}$$

$$R^{\cdot-} + O_2 \rightarrow R + O_2^{\cdot-}$$

The resulting $O_2^{\cdot-}$ leads to further oxidation of hemoglobin and cell damage. Cell damage may also result from direct reaction with the free radicals.

A number of methemoglobinemia-inducing compounds are reducing rather than oxidizing agents. Nitrites, hydrazines, hydrazides, thiols, phenylenediamines, and aminophenols are among the classes of compounds that oxidize hemoglobin indirectly by reducing O_2 to $O_2^{\cdot-}$, H_2O_2, or $HO^{\cdot}$. With several of these toxic compounds, reduction of O_2 to H_2O_2 proceeds with the bound O_2 of oxyhemoglobin in a reaction analogous to the reaction of oxyhemoglobin with $O_2^{\cdot-}$.

Methemoglobinemia also results from the ingestion of inorganic and organic compounds that are metabolized in vivo to oxidants or reductants that oxidize hemoglobin either directly or indirectly. Nitrate, aniline, and a number of drugs including primaquine, sulfanilamide, dapsone, phenacetin, acetanilide, benzocaine, and phenazopyridine are among the compounds that exert their toxic effects in this manner. Thus, the toxic effect of nitrate in infants arises from its transformation to nitrite in the digestive tract. Likewise, the methemoglobin-forming effect of aniline is dependent on its prior metabolic conversion to phenylhydroxylamine.

REDUCTION OF METHEMOGLOBIN BY MINOR PATHWAYS

Under normal conditions, most of the methemoglobin reduction carried out by the erythrocyte is catalyzed by the cytochrome b_5/cytochrome b_5 reductase system. Only a small fraction of methemoglobin reduction can be attributed to direct reduction of methemoglobin with endogenous reductants in the cell or to catalysis by another methemoglobin reductase system. In individuals with cytochrome b_5 reductase deficiency or in the presence of oxidant stress, these minor pathways may become more important (or even essential) to the cell. These minor pathways also provide the basis for the therapy of methemoglobinemia.

Direct Reaction with Endogenous and Ingested Reductants

Methemoglobin is reduced directly by ascorbic acid, reduced glutathione, reduced flavin, tetrahydropterin, cysteine, cysteamine, and the tryptophan metabolites 3-hydroxyanthranilic acid and 3-hydroxykynurenine.[12,21,23] In order for these endogenous compounds to function in methemoglobin reduction, their reduced forms must be regenerated in the erythrocyte. Indeed, in erythrocytes, reduction of oxidized glutathione is catalyzed by a NADPH-dependent reductase, oxidized ascorbic acid by a glutathione-dependent reductase, and free flavin by a NADPH-dependent reductase, while dihydropterin reacts with reduced glutathione. Under normal conditions, these pathways contribute little to the overall reduction of methemoglobin. The reactions are slow at the concentrations of reductants present in the cell. Methemoglobinemia is not associated with ascorbic acid deficiency (scurvy)[12] or with glutathione deficiency.[42] An increase in the ascorbic acid concentration, however, leads to an increase in the rate of the nonenzymatic reaction between methemoglobin and ascorbic acid both in vitro and in vivo.[6,43] After ingestion of ascorbic acid, the rate of this reaction is sufficiently fast to allow this reductant to be used therapeutically in patients with hereditary methemoglobinemia due to cytochrome b_5 reductase deficiency. Ascorbic acid reduces the β subunit faster than the α subunit, with the result that partial reduction of methemoglobin yields predominantly the $(\alpha^+\beta)_2$ valence hybrid.[44] Polyanions markedly stimulate this reaction.

A number of foreign redox compounds also accelerate the rate of methemoglobin reduction in vitro and in vivo. Methylene blue, Nile blue, and divicine (2,6-diamino-4,5-dihydroxypyrimidine) are among the compounds that are reduced in the erythrocyte and whose reduced forms then reduce methemoglobin directly. Reductions of such foreign redox compounds involve glutathione, cytochrome b_5 reductase, cytochrome b_5, or the NADPH-reductase. The action of many of these reducing agents is complicated by side reactions that alter the amount of H_2O_2 generated.

Role of NADPH-Dependent Reductase of Erythrocytes

A NADPH-dependent reductase present in the cytoplasm of erythrocytes rapidly catalyzes the reduction of methemoglobin, but only in the presence of an electron transfer mediator such as methylene blue or free flavin. By analogy with the erythrocyte NADH-dependent enzyme, this NADPH-dependent enzyme has been variously referred to in the literature as an erythrocyte "dehydrogenase," "reductase," "diaphorase," "methemoglobin reductase," or "ferrihemoglobin reductase." More recently, it has been called "NADPH-flavin reductase." Under normal conditions and in the absence of exogenous redox mediators, the role of this enzyme in methemoglobin reduction is minor, as evidenced by the fact that deficiency of the enzyme does not lead to methemoglobinemia.[45] The extent to which this enzyme catalyzes methemoglobin reduction in cytochrome b_5 reductase deficiency is debatable, but its central role in the treatment of methemoglobinemia is unequivocal.

The studies of Kiese,[23,46] Gibson,[8] and Warburg et al.[47] led to the conclusion that this reductase transferred electrons form NADPH to methylene blue and that the resulting leukomethylene blue then transferred electrons directly to methemoglobin (see Fig. 112-2). Two forms of the NADPH-dependent enzyme with similar properties have been described. Purification procedures have led to increasingly pure enzyme preparations.[23] The enzyme appears to be present in the erythrocyte at nearly 10 μM concentration. The activity does not appear to decline with aging of the cell.

One form of the enzyme has been isolated as a homogeneous protein of 22,000 daltons.[48] The enzyme is unrelated to erythrocyte cytochrome b_5 reductase. Although the isolated protein contains no prosthetic group, it binds FMN or riboflavin and catalyzes either the rapid reduction of these flavins with NADPH as electron donor or a slower reduction with NADH.[49] The resulting reduced form of the flavin rapidly reduces methemoglobin. The β chain is reduced more rapidly than the α chain with the consequence that the $(\alpha^+\beta)_2$ hybrid is an intermediate form.[50] This NADPH-dependent, flavin-mediated pathway (Fig. 112-2) has been presented as a physiological pathway of methemoglobin reduction. The low concentration of flavin in the erythrocyte relative to the K_m values for flavin, however, relegates the pathway to a minor role under normal conditions. When methemoglobin concentration or flavin concentration is high, NADPH-flavin reductase might be expected to play a more significant role.

ERYTHROCYTE CYTOCHROME b_5 REDUCTASE

The early studies of Kiese[46] and Gibson[8] provided the insight that electrons for methemoglobin reduction were transferred from glyceraldehyde-3-phosphate or lactate to NADH by specific dehydrogenases of the glycolytic pathway, and then transferred from NADH to methemoglobin by a reductase (Fig. 112-2). Gibson demonstrated a deficiency of this "methemoglobin reductase" in the red blood cells of two families with idiopathic methemoglobinemia and correctly deduced that this was the basic defect of hereditary methemoglobinemia.

Scott and his colleagues isolated two forms of NADH-dependent reductase from the cytoplasm of normal human erythrocytes and demonstrated that one of these enzymes was absent in an individual with hereditary methemoglobinemia.[51,52] The normal reductase that was deficient in methemoglobinemic individuals rapidly catalyzed the reduction of 2,6-dichlorophenolindophenol (DCIP) and ferricyanide. Further purification of this human erythrocyte reductase has been achieved by Hegesh and Avron,[53] Niethammer and Huennekens,[54] Sugita et al.,[55] Passon and Hultquist,[56] Kuma and Inomata,[57] and Yubisui and Takeshita.[58]

The ability of the enzyme to catalyze the reduction of

DCIP and ferricyanide has been used to detect, quantitate, and study the enzyme. These "diaphorase" activities are much faster with NADH than with NADPH as electron donor. In contrast to the very rapid electron transfer to the artificial acceptors, the reductase catalyzes the direct transfer of electrons from NADH to methemoglobin very slowly; the rate of methemoglobin reduction is approximately 0.01 percent of the rate of DCIP reduction. The catalysis of methemoglobin reduction is greatly facilitated by ferricyanide.[59] Ferricyanide is believed to act by transferring electrons between the reductase and methemoglobin.[60] DPG and other polyanionic effectors of hemoglobin stimulate the ferricyanide-facilitated reduction of methemoglobin,[61] suggesting that the T state of methemoglobin is more readily reduced by ferricyanide than is the R state.

The purified reductase is a flavoprotein with a noncovalently bound FAD prosthetic group.[51,56,57] The flavoprotein shows absorbance maxima at 390 and 462 nm and a shoulder at 488 nm. During isolation or storage, the protein may develop electrophoretic heterogeneity owing either to protein alteration or, in the absence of EDTA, to loss of the FAD prosthetic group.

Human erythrocyte cytochrome b_5 reductase is a 32,000 dalton protein comprising a single peptide chain and one FAD residue. Amino acid sequence analysis[62] has recently established that the structure of the enzyme corresponds to the sequence of 275 residues shown in Fig. 112-4. Notable structural features include four cysteine residues and a high content of proline. Although this slightly acidic protein is water soluble, several regions of its peptide chain are highly hydrophobic.

In normal adult human erythrocytes, cytochrome b_5 reductase is present at approximately a 0.1 μM concentration. The mean, standard deviation, and range of reported values vary considerably from laboratory to laboratory and depending on the method of analysis. The more recent studies have shown a standard deviation from the mean of approximately ± 15 percent. The reductase activity decreases slowly as erythrocytes age in the circulation, with a half-life of 240 days.[63] Modest changes in the kinetic parameters of the enzyme also occur during aging in vivo.[64] The activity in erythrocytes of cord blood and newborns is normally 50 to 60 percent of the activity in the adult, and activity in the premature infant is even lower. Within a few months of birth, the levels have risen to those of an adult. The reductase activity is very low in individuals homozygous for deficiency of erythrocyte cytochrome b_5 reductase. Individuals heterozygous for the deficiency generally have 50 to 60 percent of normal activity.

In addition to cytoplasmic cytochrome b_5 reductase, erythrocytes contain membrane-bound, NADH-dependent reductase activities.[65,66] One of these activities present in erythrocyte ghosts have been shown to be related to the cytoplasmic cytochrome b_5 reductase.[67–70] This membrane-bound reductase is an integral part of the red cell membrane, and detergent is required to extract it. The detergent-solubilized reductase is a flavoprotein with enzymatic properties indistinguishable from the erythrocyte cytoplasmic cytochrome b_5 reductase. The two forms of the enzyme are immunologically cross-reactive. They appear to be encoded by the same gene, since both enzymes have been reported to be deficient in six patients with enzymopenic hereditary methemoglobinemia.[68] The solubilized membrane reductase differs from the cytoplasmic reductase in that it has a measurably larger molecular weight and undergoes aggregation to form high-molecular-weight forms. Proteolytic digestion of erythrocyte ghosts releases the reductase from the membrane in a lower molecular weight form. This proteolyzed form has full enzymatic activity but does not aggregate.

The fraction of erythrocyte cytochrome b_5 reductase present in the membrane-bound form varies markedly among species. This form represents only 2 percent of the activity of rat erythrocytes, but nearly 100 percent of the activity of bird, reptile, and fish erythrocytes. In the erythrocytes of adult humans, 20 to 35 percent of the activity is bound to the membrane. The erythrocytes of human adults and newborns contain the same level of membrane-bound cytochrome b_5 reductase, but this form constitutes a larger fraction of the total activity in the newborn because of the lower levels of cytosolic enzyme in such erythrocytes.[69]

ERYTHROCYTE CYTOCHROME b_5

A hemeprotein with spectral properties of cytochrome b_5 and a flavoprotein that catalyzed the reduction of this hemeprotein were detected in the cytoplasm of human erythrocytes in 1969.[71] Erythrocyte cytochrome b_5 at physiological concentrations markedly enhanced the ability of the cytochrome b_5 reductase to catalyze the transfer of electrons from NADH to methemoglobin.[13,72] One major and two minor forms of human erythrocyte cytochrome b_5 have

```
                    5                        10                       15                       20                       25
Phe-Gln-Arg-Ser-Thr-Pro-Ala-Ile-Thr-Leu-Glu-Ser-Pro-Asp-Ile-Lys-Tyr-Pro-Leu-Arg-Leu-Ile-Asp-Arg-Glu-
                    30                       35                       40                       45                       50
Ile-Ile-Ser-His-Asp-Thr-Arg-Arg-Phe-Arg-Phe-Ala-Leu-Pro-Ser-Pro-Gln-His-Ile-Leu-Gly-Leu-Pro-Val-Gly-
                    55                       60                       65                       70                       75
Gln-His-Ile-Tyr-Leu-Ser-Ala-Arg-Ile-Asp-Gly-Asn-Leu-Val-Val-Arg-Pro-Tyr-Thr-Pro-Ile-Ser-Ser-Asp-Asp-
                    80                       85                       90                       95                      100
Asp-Lys-Gly-Phe-Val-Asp-Leu-Val-Ile-Lys-Val-Tyr-Phe-Lys-Asp-Thr-His-Pro-Lys-Phe-Pro-Ala-Gly-Gly-Lys-
                   105                      110                      115                      120                      125
Met-Ser-Gln-Tyr-Leu-Glu-Ser-Met-Gln-Ile-Gly-Asp-Thr-Ile-Glu-Phe-Arg-Gly-Pro-Ser-Gly-Leu-Leu-Val-Tyr-
                   130                      135                      140                      145                      150
Gln-Gly-Lys-Gly-Lys-Phe-Ala-Ile-Arg-Pro-Asp-Lys-Lys-Ser-Asn-Pro-Ile-Ile-Arg-Thr-Val-Lys-Ser-Val-Gly-
                   155                      160                      165                      170                      175
Met-Ile-Ala-Gly-Gly-Thr-Gly-Ile-Thr-Pro-Met-Leu-Gln-Val-Ile-Arg-Ala-Ile-Met-Lys-Asp-Pro-Asp-Asp-His-
                   180                      185                      190                      195                      200
Thr-Val-Cys-His-Leu-Leu-Phe-Ala-Asn-Gln-Thr-Glu-Lys-Asp-Ile-Leu-Leu-Arg-Pro-Glu-Leu-Glu-Glu-Leu-Arg-
                   205                      210                      215                      220                      225
Asn-Lys-His-Ser-Ala-Arg-Phe-Lys-Leu-Trp-Tyr-Thr-Leu-Asp-Arg-Ala-Pro-Glu-Ala-Trp-Asp-Val-Gly-Gln-Gly-
                   230                      235                      240                      245                      250
Phe-Val-Asn-Glu-Glu-Met-Ile-Arg-Asp-His-Leu-Pro-Pro-Pro-Glu-Glu-Glu-Pro-Leu-Val-Leu-Met-Cys-Gly-Pro-
                   255                      260                      265                      270                      275
Pro-Pro-Met-Ile-Gln-Tyr-Ala-Cys-Leu-Pro-Asn-Leu-Asp-His-Val-Gly-His-Pro-Thr-Glu-Arg-Cys-Phe-Val-Phe
```

FIG. 112-4 Primary structure of humane erythrocyte cytochrome b_5 reductase.

```
                                  10                                      20
Ac-Ala-Glu-Gln-Ser-Asp-Glu-Ala-Val-Lys-Tyr-Tyr-Thr-Leu-Glx-Glu-Ile-Glx-Lys-His-Asn-
                                  30                                      40
His-Ser-Lys-Ser-Thr-Trp-Leu-Ile-Leu-His-His-Lys-Val-Tyr-Asp-Leu-Thr-Lys-Phe-Leu-
                                  50                                      60
Glu-Glu-His-Pro-Gly-Gly-Glu-Glu-Val-Leu-Arg-Glu-Gln-Ala-Gly-Gly-Asp-Ala-Thr-Glu-
                                  70                                      80
Asx-Phe-Glu-Asp-Val-Gly-His-Ser-Thr-Asp-Ala-Arg-Glu-Met-Ser-Lys-Thr-Phe-Ile-Ile-
                                  90
Gly-Glu-Leu-His-Pro-Asp-Asp-Lys-Pro-Arg-Leu-Asn-Lys-Pro-Pro-Glu-Pro
```

FIG. 112-5 **Primary structure of human erythrocyte cytochrome b_5.**

been isolated,[73] and the major form has been purified to homogeneity.[74] Cytochrome b_5 has also been isolated from the cytoplasm of rabbit, mouse, and steer erythrocytes.[73,75–77] Another "*b*-type" cytochrome was isolated from the membrane of human erythrocytes in relatively large amounts, but this "S-protein"[78] did not appear to be structurally or functionally related to erythrocyte cytochrome b_5.

Erythrocyte cytochrome b_5 is a small red protein of approximately 12,000 daltons. It is highly anionic with an isoelectric point of 4.9 and is readily water soluble. It contains a single protoheme IX prosthetic group, present as a low-spin complex that does not bind carbon monoxide. The hemeprotein, isolated in its ferric state, shows a sharp absorbance maximum at 413 nm. The spectrum of the ferrous form shows sharp maxima at 423, 527, and 556 nm, and a prominent shoulder at 560 nm. The standard reduction potential at pH 7.0 is -2 mV.[79] The ferrous form autoxidizes at a moderate rate.

Erythrocyte cytochrome b_5 comprises 97 amino acid residues in a single peptide chain. No carbohydrate or other nonamino acid groups, other than the heme, are bound to the protein. The protein has a blocked N terminus, which recently has been identified as an *N*-acetylalanine residue.[80] Bovine erythrocyte cytochrome b_5 was the first of these proteins for which it was possible to deduce the amino acid sequence.[81] The sequences have now been deduced for the rabbit,[82] human,[80,83] and pig[80] erythrocyte proteins. The structure of human erythrocyte cytochrome b_5 is shown in Fig. 112-5.

Erythrocyte cytochrome b_5 can be quantitated on the basis of its distinct spectral properties or on the basis of its ability to stimulate the cytochrome b_5 reductase-catalyzed reduction of methemoglobin.[73,79,84–86] Mean values for cytochrome b_5 concentration in erythrocytes range from 0.2 to 0.6 μM. The protein is present in higher concentration in reticulocytes than in erythrocytes. Cytochrome b_5 concentrations decrease both during cell aging in the circulation and during cell storage under blood-bank conditions. The apparent half-life in vivo is 44 days.[63]

RELATIONSHIP BETWEEN THE ERYTHROCYTIC AND MICROSOMAL PROTEINS

The erythrocyte cytochrome is named cytochrome b_5 on the basis of its similarity to microsomal cytochrome b_5. They have identical visible spectra, EPR spectra, prosthetic groups, chemical reactivity at the iron atom, and ability to serve as substrate for cytochrome b_5 reductase.[73] The erythrocyte reductase has been identified as a cytochrome b_5 reductase on the basis of its capacity to catalyze the reduction of cytochrome b_5 and its similarity to microsomal cytochrome b_5 reductase in terms of prosthetic group, substrate specificity, and effects of ionic strength, pH, and EDTA on catalytic activity.[56] The erythrocyte and microsomal proteins differ, however, in that the erythrocyte proteins are smaller, are water soluble, and are located in the cytoplasm rather than the endoplasmic reticulum. These comparisons have led to the suggestion that erythrocyte cytochrome b_5 and cytochrome b_5 reductase correspond to the microsomal proteins without their hydrophobic tails.[56] In liver and other tissues, it is the hydrophobic domains of these proteins that are embedded in the endoplasmic reticulum.

Erythrocyte cytochrome b_5 has been shown to be structurally related to the hydrophilic domain of liver microsomal cytochrome b_5. Trypsin degrades *human* cytochrome b_5 from liver and erythrocytes to electrophoretically identical heme peptides.[74] Likewise, trypsin degrades the 97-residue *bovine* erythrocyte cytochrome b_5 and the 133-residue bovine liver cytochrome b_5 to the same 82-residue heme peptide.[76] The amino acid sequence of the bovine erythrocyte protein corresponds precisely to the sequence of 97 residues starting at the blocked N terminus of the liver protein,[87] with the possible exception that an asparagine residue in the liver is present as an aspartate residue in the erythrocyte. Like the bovine erythrocyte protein, *rabbit* erythrocyte cytochrome b_5 is a 97-residue protein with near identity to residues 1 to 97 of the 133-residue rabbit liver protein. Of the 97 residues, only the one at position 97 differs; it is C-terminal proline in rabbit erythrocyte cytochrome b_5 and threonine in the liver protein.[82] Likewise, *pig* and *human* cytochrome b_5 molecules comprise 97-residue erythrocyte proteins and 133-residue liver microsomal proteins in which there is identity between the first 96 residues but a difference at residue 97.[80] In the pig, residue 97 is serine in erythrocytes and threonine in liver. In humans, residue 97 is proline in erythrocytes (Fig. 112-5) and threonine in liver.

Erythrocyte cytochrome b_5 reductase has been shown to be structurally related to microsomal cytochrome b_5 reductase. The two proteins are immunologically cross-reactive.[67,88,89] They are genetically related, as evidenced by the finding that both erythrocyte cytochrome b_5 reductase and the microsomal enzyme of other tissues are defective in the generalized cytochrome b_5 reductase deficiency of humans.[90] The reductases from bovine erythrocytes and liver are degraded by cathepsin D to electrophoretically identical flavopeptides.[91,92] Nucleotide sequencing of cDNA that codes for human liver cytochrome b_5 reductase has recently established that human erythrocyte cytochrome b_5 reductase is a piece of the liver microsomal cytochrome b_5 reductase.[93] These human liver cDNA sequence data, together with amino acid sequence data for bovine liver cytochrome b_5 reductase, establish that the 275-residue sequence of the human erythrocyte protein corresponds precisely to the 275 residues at the C terminus of the human liver protein. The erythrocyte reductase does not possess the membrane-binding, hydrophobic peptide of approximately 25 residues that is present at the N terminus of the liver reductase.

The structural relationship between the erythrocyte and microsomal proteins led to the proposition that erythrocyte cytochrome b_5 and cytochrome b_5 reductase were derived during erythroid maturation from microsomal precursor proteins.[74,94] This postulate was supported by the finding that an immature erythroid cell line contained only the amphipathic forms of cytochrome b_5 and cytochrome b_5 reductase, whereas mature erythrocytes contained the cytoplasmic forms of these proteins.[77] Moreover, a cathepsin D isolated from a membranous fraction of rabbit reticulocytes was shown to catalyze efficiently the proteolytic removal of the hydrophobic tails of microsomal cytochrome b_5 and cytochrome b_5 reductase without causing cleavage in their hydrophilic domains.[91,95,96] With rabbit liver cytochrome b_5 as substrate, the cathepsin removed peptides sequentially from the C terminus and generated a 98-residue limit heme peptide which was one residue longer than rabbit erythrocyte cytochrome b_5; The extra residue was leucine-98.[82] Similarly, an ATP-dependent protease of rabbit reticulocytes released cytochrome b_5 and cytochrome b_5 reductase as water-soluble proteins from rat liver microsomes.[97] The cytoplasmic form of erythrocyte cytochrome b_5 reductase was postulated by Kaplan and coworkers[70,98] to arise from proteolysis of the reductase that was bound to the erythrocyte membrane. Autoincubation of erythrocyte membranes released a solubilized form of the reductase, a process stimulated by calcium ion.

Thus, acidic, ATP-dependent, and calcium-dependent proteases of reticulocytes are potential candidates for the putative enzyme responsible for converting microsomal proteins of immature erythroid cells to the cytoplasmic forms found in mature erythrocytes. If indeed such a proteolytic event occurs, the processing would be responsible for the conversion of amphiphatic, membrane-bound proteins that function in the desaturation of fatty acids to water-soluble proteins that function to reduce methemoglobin. However, the detection of the structural difference between the two forms of cytochrome b_5 at residue 97 brings into question whether such protein processing actually occurs during erythroid maturation. If it does occur, a form of microsomal cytochrome b_5 distinct from liver microsomal cytochrome b_5 (with a proline residue at position 97) must be present in immature erythroid cells.

THE MECHANISM OF METHEMOGLOBIN REDUCTION BY CYTOCHROME b_5 REDUCTASE AND CYTOCHROME b_5

The marked stimulation of the erythrocyte cytochrome b_5 reductase-catalyzed reduction of methemoglobin by physiological concentrations of erythrocyte cytochrome b_5 led to the postulate that methemoglobin is reduced in vivo by the following sequence of electron transfers:

$$\text{NADH} \xrightarrow{e^-} \text{cytochrome } b_5 \text{ reductase} \xrightarrow{e^-} \text{cytochrome } b_5 \xrightarrow{e^-} \text{methemoglobin}$$

These findings had been anticipated in 1959 by Petragnani and coworkers,[99] who demonstrated that solubilized forms of pig liver cytochrome b_5 reductase and cytochrome b_5 together catalyzed the reduction of methemoglobin. Unaware that cytochrome b_5 or cytochrome b_5 reductase was present in erythrocytes, these workers uncannily suggested that ". . . the erythrocyte methemoglobin reductase may be a similar multienzymatic system. . . ."

The mechanism of this major pathway of methemoglobin reduction has been deduced from studies in many laboratories.[13,51,55–57,79,91,100–105] The rate of methemoglobin reduction in intact cells can be reproduced in crude hemolysates or in systems reconstituted from purified NADH, cytochrome b_5 reductase, cytochrome b_5, and methemoglobin, demonstrating that no additional component plays an essential role in this pathway. Under conditions close to physiological, the rate of methemoglobin reduction is first-order with respect to methemoglobin and cytochrome b_5 reductase and second-order with respect to cytochrome b_5. Thus, methemoglobin reduction proceeds more rapidly when the concentration of methemoglobin is elevated and more slowly when either cytochrome b_5 reductase or cytochrome b_5 is present at less than normal concentration.

The results of the mechanistic studies are compatible with the scheme depicted in Fig. 112-6. After NADH binds to the oxidized flavoprotein (step 1), a pair of electrons is transferred from NADH to FAD (step 2). The reduced flavoprotein sequentially binds and reduces first one and then a second molecule of ferric cytochrome b_5, with the resulting formation of ferrous cytochrome b_5 and oxidized flavoprotein (steps 3 and 4). The generation of a complex between cytochrome b_5 reductase and cytochrome b_5 involves ionic interactions between anionic residues of cytochrome b_5 and cationic residues of cytochrome b_5 reductase. These first four steps are presumably identical with the extensively studied reduction of microsomal cytochrome b_5 catalyzed by microsomal cytochrome b_5 reductase.[106,107]

The reduction of methemoglobin is accomplished by the formation of an ionic complex between ferrous cytochrome b_5 and a ferric subunit of a hemoglobin tetramer (step 5) and the subsequent electron transfer in this complex between the hemes of these proteins (step 6). The cytochrome b_5-methemoglobin complex has been detected by isoelectric focusing[108] and by spectral perturbation of the absorbance spectra.[109,110] The formation of the complex and the transfer of electrons between the proteins of this complex have been separated kinetically.[91,101,103] Computer modeling studies by Poulos and Mauk[111] suggest that the complex is stabilized by ionic interactions between carboxylate anions on the face of a cytochrome b_5 molecule from which the heme group protrudes and lysyl cations on the face of methemoglobin subunits from which their heme groups protrude. Optimatization of four such ionic bonds with the α subunit and five ionic bonds with the β subunit places the interacting hemes in a coplanar orientation, which presumably leads to facile electron transfer. Support for the validity of this model is provided by the observations that mutant hemoglobins in which one of these cationic residues is not present have decreased capacities to be reduced by the cytochrome b_5 reductase/cytochrome b_5 system.[27,28]

The overall rate of methemoglobin reduction in vivo depends on the concentration of the ferrous cytochrome b_5–ferric hemoglobin complex. The interaction between these proteins is weak, and under physiological conditions the concentration of the complex depends on the concentrations of ferrous cytochrome b_5 and methemoglobin. The fraction of cytochrome b_5 present in the ferrous form, in turn, is determined by the concentration of cytochrome b_5 reductase. Complex formation between ferric hemoglobin and cytochrome b_5 appears to be inhibited by ferrous hemoglobin. Complexation proceeds more readily with the R state of

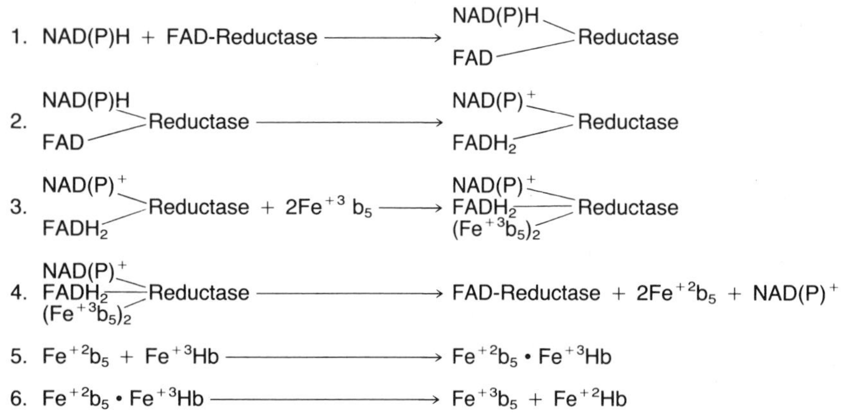

$$1.\quad NAD(P)H + FAD\text{-}Reductase \longrightarrow \begin{matrix}NAD(P)H\\ FAD\end{matrix}\!>\!Reductase$$

$$2.\quad \begin{matrix}NAD(P)H\\ FAD\end{matrix}\!>\!Reductase \longrightarrow \begin{matrix}NAD(P)^+\\ FADH_2\end{matrix}\!>\!Reductase$$

$$3.\quad \begin{matrix}NAD(P)^+\\ FADH_2\end{matrix}\!>\!Reductase + 2Fe^{+3}\,b_5 \longrightarrow \begin{matrix}NAD(P)^+\\ FADH_2\\ (Fe^{+3}b_5)_2\end{matrix}\!>\!Reductase$$

$$4.\quad \begin{matrix}NAD(P)^+\\ FADH_2\\ (Fe^{+3}b_5)_2\end{matrix}\!>\!Reductase \longrightarrow FAD\text{-}Reductase + 2Fe^{+2}b_5 + NAD(P)^+$$

$$5.\quad Fe^{+2}b_5 + Fe^{+3}Hb \longrightarrow Fe^{+2}b_5 \cdot Fe^{+3}Hb$$

$$6.\quad Fe^{+2}b_5 \cdot Fe^{+3}Hb \longrightarrow Fe^{+3}b_5 + Fe^{+2}Hb$$

FIG. 112-6 Scheme for the reduction of methemoglobin by cytochrome b_5 reductase and cytochrome b_5.

methemoglobin than with the T state,[103] and the β subunit of methemoglobin is reduced preferentially in the presence of inositol hexaphosphate.[101] The concentrations of cytochrome b_5 reductase, cytochrome b_5, methemoglobin, and polyanionic effector determine the concentration of the ferrous cytochrome b_5–methemoglobin complex and in this manner determine the rate of methemoglobin reduction in vivo.

The significance of NADPH as an electron donor for this system is debatable. The reduction of cytochrome b_5 reductase (steps 1 and 2) proceeds so much slower in vitro with NADPH than with NADH that the role of NADPH has been assumed to be insignificant. However, the transfer of electrons from reductase to methemoglobin (steps 3 through 6) is rate limiting as a consequence of the very low concentration of cytochrome b_5 in the erythrocyte (far below the K_m of the reductase). In a crude hemolysate or in a system reconstituted from purified cytochrome b_5 reductase and cytochrome b_5, methemoglobin reduction proceeds nearly as rapidly with a saturating level of NADPH as with a saturating level of NADH. Thus, it appears that in vivo steps 1 and 2 are the fast steps in the pathway, even with NADPH as electron donor. This conclusion in not compatible with other studies, which indicate only a minor role for NADPH in methemoglobin reduction.

CLINICAL ASPECTS AND CLASSIFICATION

Subjects with enzymopenic hereditary methemoglobinemia present with persistent slate-gray cyanosis, often dating from birth. A concentration of 1.5 to 2.0 g/dl of methemoglobin (10 to 15 percent of total hemoglobin) produces visible cyanosis, whereas 5 g/dl of deoxygenated hemoglobin is required to produce a comparable degree of cyanosis.[112] In most instances, the patients are really more blue than sick (see, however, type II, below). They lack evidence of cardiac or pulmonary disease. Significant erythrocytosis is observed only occasionally, and the oxygen dissociation curve is normal or shifted only slightly to the left.[3] The absence of manifestations of anoxia may be due to differences in the proportions of valence hybrids in the erythrocytes.[20,22] Hardly any systemic symptoms are reported when the methemoglobin level is 25 percent or less, except for the subjects' odd "cyanotic" appearance. Even with levels up to 40 percent, the only complaints may be headache, easy fatigue, and exertional dyspnea. Life expectancy is normal, and pregnancies are not compromised. The methemoglobinemia is quite well tolerated, and may be readily controlled with appropriate therapy.

Recently, a clinical–biochemical classification of enzymopenic hereditary methemoglobinemia has been proposed on the basis of important differences in the pathophysiology of the disorder.[113]

Type I Enzymopenic Hereditary Methemoglobinemia (Erythrocyte Reductase Deficiency)

Most patients appear to have type I, the classic syndrome with the signs and symptoms described above, that has been extensively studied since the pioneering investigations of Gibson[8] and Scott and Griffith.[9] The subjects have methemoglobinemia alone because the deficiency of cytochrome b_5 reductase is limited to the erythrocytes. Their erythrocytes' metabolic machinery is otherwise intact, so there is no hemolysis.

Type II Enzymopenic Hereditary Methemoglobinemia (Generalized Reductase Deficiency)

A much more severe and lethal disorder occurs in perhaps 10 to 15 percent of patients with enzymopenic hereditary methemoglobinemia; it is referred to as "type II." In addition to methemoglobinemia, signs of a progressive neurologic abnormality become apparent before age 1 year and may be observed even at birth. The association of these two aberrations was described in 1953.[114] The fully expressed syndrome is characterized by severe mental retardation, microcephaly, retarded growth, opisthotonus, attacks of bilateral athetoid movements, strabismus, and generalized hypertonia.[12,29] Death usually supervenes soon. Pathologic examinations of the brains of three sibs with this disorder have revealed only nonspecific alterations, including reduced numbers of nerve elements and retarded myelinization.[29] Not only is the activity of cytochrome b_5 reductase markedly reduced in the patients' erythrocytes, but nearly total deficiency of microsomal cytochrome b_5 reductase is demonstrable in their leukocytes, muscle, liver, fibroblasts, and brain.[90,115,116] Because the microsomal cytochrome b_5/cytochrome b_5 reductase system participates in other tissues in the desaturation of fatty acids, it has been suggested that impairment of fatty acid desaturation, especially in the central nervous system, may account for the generalized systemic manifestations.[90] Lipid analyses of tissues from a child with the type II disorder have revealed decreased cerebroside (48 percent of normal) in the white matter of the brain,[117] decreased linoleic acid and increased palmitic acid in adipose tissue, decreased proportions of unsaturated fatty acids in the ethanolamine phosphoglycerides of the liver, and less than half of normal concentrations of linoleic acid in the ethanolamine phosphoglycerides of the liver, kidney, and spleen.[118] Cholesterol and lipid phosphorus concentrations, however, were normal in the liver, kidney, spleen, muscle, and adrenals. Thus, the effect of the generalized cytochrome b_5 reductase deficiency was unexpectedly slight, but the reduction in cerebroside content might have caused a decrease in myelination, leading to mental retardation.[118] The generalized deficiency of cytochrome b_5 reductase activity in patients with type II, as well as in their fetal amniotic cells, has made antenatal diagnosis feasible.[119]

Type III Enzymopenic Hereditary Methemoglobinemia (Hematopoietic Reductase Deficiency)

In addition to a German family reported only in an abstract,[120] a detailed study of a Japanese family has provided evidence for the occurrence of enzymopenic hereditary methemoglobinemia without neurologic involvement but with cytochrome b_5 reductase deficiency demonstrable in erythrocytes, platelets, lymphocytes, and granulocytes.[121] The enzyme stained normally in the two male sibs' hair root and buccal cells. The only clinical manifestations were their cyanotic appearance with methemoglobin concentrations of about 25 percent. These reports have made it necessary to exercise caution in drawing conclusions from assays of cytochrome b_5 reductase activities in detergent-treated leukocytes, the procedure advocated for making the diagnosis of the generalized type II disorder in infants younger than 1 year old or in newborns.

Type IV Enzymopenic Hereditary Methemoglobinemia (Cytochrome b_5 Deficiency)

The discovery of a patient with long-standing methemoglobinemic cyanosis (methemoglobin concentrations 12 to 19 percent) associated with an erythrocyte cytochrome b_5 concentration about 23 percent of normal has completed the current roster of pathophysiological mechanisms for this disorder.[26] This observation has provided direct evidence for the physiological role of cytochrome b_5 in the reduction of methemoglobin to hemoglobin in vivo in human erythrocytes. The precise nature of this currently unique abnormality remains to be defined.

THE GENETICS OF CYTOCHROME b_5 REDUCTASE

The gene coding for soluble NADH-cytochrome b_5 reductase has been assigned to chromosome 22. This assignment is based on studies of the electrophoretic mobility and isoelectric focusing patterns of soluble enzyme in the cytosol of rodent–human fibroblast hybrids and concurrent cytogenetic analyses.[122–123] The same gene is assumed to code for the full length of the microsomal enzyme polypeptide chain (i.e., polar plus membrane segments).

The diaphorase activity of cytochrome b_5 reductase has been exploited to permit its visualization after electrophoresis of hemolysates or tissue extracts on starch or polyacrylamide gels.[12,124] A survey of 2783 healthy subjects has revealed five electrophoretic phenotypes with normal staining intensity and suggests an incidence of variants of about 1 in 100.[125] Studies of patients with enzymopenic hereditary methemoglobinemia have disclosed at least 14 different phenotypes, based on electrophoretic mobility and/or kinetic aberrations.[12,126] Thus, the mutations causing reductase deficiency are heterogeneous, with several different mutant alleles occurring at the reductase locus. The molecular basis of these mutations is as yet unknown.

An unusually high incidence of enzymopenic hereditary methemoglobinemia is reported among Alaskan Eskimos and Indians, Navajo Indians, Puerto Ricans, people of Mediterranean origins, and natives of the Yakutsk region of Siberia, 1000 miles west of the Bering Sea.[12]

Type I, uncomplicated, benign enzymopenic hereditary methemoglobinemia is attributable to mutations that affect the catalytic activity or stability of the enzyme in the erythrocytes. Clinically affected subjects are homozygous or genetic compounds for cytochrome b_5 reductase deficiency. Exaggerated lability characterizes at least five enzyme variants.[127,128] The role of altered proteolytic processes in erythrocyte precursors in enzymopenic hereditary methemoglobinemia remains to be defined.[129] The asymptomatic heterozygote may have an increased tendency to develop toxic methemoglobinemia on exposure to methemoglobin-inducing drugs or chemicals, such as malaria chemoprophylaxis,[30] phenazopyridine administration,[32] or the "recreational" sniffing of volatile nitrites.[130]

Type II, severe, lethal enzymopenic hereditary methemoglobinemia is a generalized disorder with defective cytochrome b_5 reductase in all tissues. This disorder is presumed to result from mutation(s) that affect the enzyme's activity, thermal stability, or resistance to proteolysis in all tissues.

The apparently rather benign type III disorder may simply be a variant of type II in that the enzyme is altered by selective activity of proteolytic enzymes only in the hematopoietic tissues.[121,129] On the other hand, it may represent a catalytically less significant mutation affecting cytochrome b_5 reductase, analogous to the variants observed in glucose 6-phosphate dehydrogenase deficiency.

The type IV disorder is a deficiency of cytochrome b_5 alone; the activity of cytochrome b_5 reductase is normal.[26] The concentration of cytochrome b_5 is normal in the erythrocytes of the parents and sibs of the only known patient with this form of hereditary methemoglobinemia. The genetics of cytochrome b_5 deficiency, therefore, remain to be determined.

DIAGNOSIS OF CYTOCHROME b_5 REDUCTASE DEFICIENCY

Blood with more than about 10 percent methemoglobin appears unusually dark red or even brown. It does not become bright red upon vigorous shaking with air, and it leaves a dark reddish brown stain on white filter paper or a white laboratory coat. The presence of methemoglobin may be established by the characteristic absorption spectrum of a clear, stroma-free hemolysate with peaks at 500 and 631 nm at an acid pH.[126] The latter peak should disappear promptly after the addition of a neutralized cyanide solution.

If the spectrum in the 600- to 640-nm region is atypical and the peak near 631 nm is shifted toward a lower wavelength and does not change significantly or quickly on the addition of cyanide, hemoglobin M should be suspected. A hemoglobin M should also be suspected if there is a family history of apparent parent-to-child transmission of long-standing, unexplained cyanosis. Electrophoresis of the methemoglobin form and amino acid analysis of the globin are required for the confirmation of the diagnosis of a hemoglobin M.

Congenital cyanosis in sibs, especially with a history of consanguinity, is suggestive of enzymopenic hereditary methemoglobinemia. Presumptive evidence for cytochrome b_5 reductase deficiency may be obtained by comparing the rate of reduction of methemoglobin in a patient's nitrite-treated, washed erythrocytes incubated with glucose or other substrates before and after the addition of methylene blue with the rate observed with cells from a normal subject.[12] Reductase deficiency may be confirmed by direct assay for NADH-diaphorase,[10] NADH-methemoglobin-ferrocyanide reductase,[131] cytochrome b_5 reductase,[56] or NADH-ferricyanide reductase[132] activity in hemolysates of the patient's erythrocytes. Assay of NADH-ferricyanide reductase activity has been advocated as the simplest because of the ready availability of the substrate potassium ferricyanide. A rapid screening spot test for NADH-diaphorase deficiency has also been described.[133]

TREATMENT OF CYTOCHROME b_5 REDUCTASE DEFICIENCY

Because subjects with type I cytochrome b_5 reductase deficiency have only mild symptoms from the methemoglobinemia, therapy is mainly cosmetic. It may be indicated, however, for psychological reasons. A single dose of methylene blue, 1 mg/kg intravenously, will rapidly reduce the methemoglobin concentration to normal, provided that the subject is not glucose 6-phosphate dehydrogenase-deficient, since the methylene blue-stimulated NADPH-methemoglobin reductase system requires the reduction of $NADP^+$. Methylene blue has been reported to cause urinary tract irritation and, of course, makes the urine blue or bright green. Oral ascorbic acid, 500 to 1000 mg daily, can maintain the methemoglobin concentration at acceptable levels, but its prolonged administration may be responsible for hyperoxaluria and renal stone formation. Oral riboflavin, 20 to 60 mg daily, has been reported to be as effective as ascorbic acid in keeping the methemoglobin level at about 5 percent.[134] These therapeutic agents would also be expected to be effective in patients with the type III and type IV disorders. Although methylene blue will control the methemoglobinemia in the type II disorder, it has had no effect on the progressive neurologic dysfunction.

ADDENDUM

Since the appearance of the previous edition of this text, there has been a limited number of publications on the hereditary methemoglobinemias, including a recent concise review.[135] Most of the reports have been on the molecular biology and genetic defects of cytochrome b_5 reductase. What follows is a summary of this recent work.

Clinical

A patient with type I methemoglobinemia, started on methylene blue, 150 mg/day at age 18 years, developed carcinoma *in situ* of the bladder at age 47 (Jaffé, personal communication, 1993). Dusky cyanosis recurred with cessation of therapy. The relationship of the methylene blue therapy to the carcinoma, if any, is uncertain.

Yawata and colleagues reported an interesting case of a Japanese male with type II methemoglobinemia whose clinical phenotype included short stature, deformation of both small and large joints, cyanosis, and mild mental retardation.[136] Partial deficiency of cytochrome b_5 reductase was demonstrated in red cells, platelets, lymphocytes, and cultured skin fibroblasts. The molecular defect(s) was not described.

In an important paper, Nagai et al. re-evaluated the standard classification of hereditary methemoglobinemia phenotypes into types I–III.[137] They pointed out that earlier assays of NADH-reductase activity used artificial electron acceptors such as 2,6-dichloroindophenol, which give high background activity and thus make it difficult to detect mild reductions in b_5 reductase activity in nonerythyroid cells. Recent assays by the authors and others using cytochrome b_5 as the electron acceptor showed a decrease in b_5 reductase activity in platelets and leukocytes as well as in the erythrocytes of patients with type I. This result suggested that the separation of types I and III methemoglobinemia was based on an artifact caused by the way b_5 reductase activity was assayed in the past. Furthermore, Nagai et al. re-evaluated the best-characterized type III patient using a cytochrome b_5 based assay and found lymphocyte and platelet b_5 reductase activities in the range of those of patients with type I methemoglobinemia. The authors conclude that it is now "unnecessary" to have a type III category for the classification of hereditary methemoglobinemia phenotypes.

Biochemistry

Mutagenesis studies of bovine and human cytochrome b_5 reductase have investigated the roles of specific residues in the catalytic function of the enzyme. Lysine-110 appears to be involved in the interactions of the enzyme with NADH,[138] as does the nearby serine-127.[139] The latter residue was investigated when it was found to be involved in a naturally occurring mutation (see below). Cysteine residues at position 273 and 283 also appear to interact with the NADH binding site but are not essential for catalytic function.[140]

NADPH-dependent methemoglobin reductase has been reviewed and compared to NADH-dependent b_5 reductase.[141] Under normal circumstances the former plays no role in methemoglobin reduction but does contribute when the latter is deficient.

Molecular Genetics

Biochemical studies described in this chapter had shown two forms of NADH-cytochrome b_5 reductase: (1) a 34-kDa myristylated, membrane-associated enzyme found in hepatocytes and other cells and involved in the desaturation and elongation of fatty acids; (2) a soluble, 31-kDa, erythrocyte enzyme crucial for methemoglobin reduction. The mechanism by which these two forms of the enzyme are generated was revealed by molecular studies of the b_5 reductase gene.

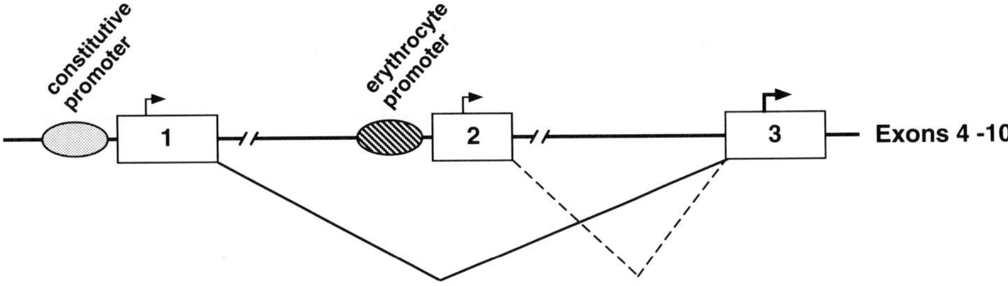

FIG. 112-7 The b_5 reductase gene structure at the 5′ end. The gene has two promoters, one upstream for the ubiquitous (liver) transcript, the other downstream for erythroid cell-specific transcript. The upstream promoter is GC-rich, the downstream promoter has TATAA and GATA boxes. See Addendum text for details.

Human, rat and bovine liver and human placental NADH-cytochrome b_5 reductase cDNAs were cloned[141–144] and alignments described.[143] The human liver cDNA has a 903-bp open reading frame predicting a protein of 301 residues. The N-terminal methionine is followed by a myristylation consensus sequence (G-X-X-X-S/T), and this, together with the observation that the bovine enzyme is myristylated, suggests that the human enzyme also undergoes cotranslational myristylation. As in the bovine enzyme, there is an N-terminal hydrophobic domain of 14 amino acids (residues 11 through 24 of the primary translation product). This domain and the myristyl moiety form an anchor which tethers nonerythrocyte b_5 reductase to the outer mitochondrial and endoplasmic reticulum membranes. The sequence of the C-terminal 275 residues of the protein predicted by the liver cDNA coincides perfectly with the complete sequence of the enzyme purified from erythrocytes,[142] in agreement with the notion that one gene encodes both forms of the enzyme.

The organization of the NADH-cytochrome b_5 reductase gene has been determined in rats[143] and humans.[145] The human gene is about 31 kb long and initially was thought to contain nine exons. The translational start site is in exon 1. Exon 2 contains the junction of the hydrophobic membrane-binding domain with the downstream catalytic portion of the protein. The promoter region resembles that of a constitutively expressed gene in that it lacks a TATAA box, has five GC box elements (GGGCGG) and overall is very GC rich (86 percent).[145] Primer extension experiments indicate multiple transcription start sites. The promoter of the rat gene has a similar organization.[143] In both species, the mature mRNA produced by the b_5 reductase gene is ~2.0 kb long.

To investigate the origin of the erythrocyte form of the enzyme, Pietrini and colleagues compared b_5 reductase cDNAs cloned from rat reticulocyte and liver cDNA libraries.[144] They showed that b_5 reductase cDNAs isolated from reticulocytes (R-cDNA) differed from those isolated from liver (L-cDNA) in the 5′ noncoding and early coding region, where the seven codons specifying the myristylation consensus sequence of the liver protein were replaced by an erythrocyte-specific sequence of 13 noncharged amino acids. This observation lead them to re-examine the gene structure, looking in particular for sequences corresponding to the 5′ end of the R-cDNA. Ultimately, they found that the rat b_5 reductase gene has two promoters: an upstream constitutive GC-rich promoter responsible for the ubiquitous or liver transcript and a downstream, erythroid-specific promoter with TATAA and GATA boxes located in what was previously considered to be intron 1 (Fig. 112-7). The upstream promoter drives expression of a transcript that originates in exon 1, which encodes the N-terminal 25 amino acids including the myristylation consensus sequence, and splices to exon 3. The downstream promoter directs expression of a transcript that originates in the newly recognized exon 2 and encodes two erythrocyte-specific forms of the enzyme, which differ at their N-terminal owing to alternative translation start sites in the erythrocyte-specific message. The quantitatively minor translation product has 307 amino acids and includes a sequence of 13 noncharged N-terminal residues found only in this form of the erythrocyte enzyme. The more abundant erythrocyte translation product starts from an internal methionine (encoded in exon 3) that corresponds to methionine-24 of the liver transcript and methionine-30 of the longer erythrocyte protein (Fig. 112-7). This methionine is two residues upstream of the phenylalanine that is the N-terminal residue of the mature soluble erythrocyte protein. Thus, in rats and presumably in humans, a combination of transcriptional and translational mechanisms produces, from one gene, three forms of NADH-cytochrome b_5 reductase differing at their N terminals. These include a widely expressed membrane-bound protein of 301 residues (processed

Table 112-1 Missense Mutations Described in Patients with Hereditary Methemoglobinemia

Number	Allele*	Phenotype	No Pedigrees	Ethnic Origin	Nucleotide Change†	Comment	Reference
1	S127P	II	1	Japanese	T 382 → C	Unstable	139,147
2	R57Q	I	3	Japanese	G 173 → A	Mutant enzyme has 62% of normal activity but is unstable	146
3	L148P	I	1	Japanese	T 446 → C	Patient previously classified as type III Mutant enzyme has 60% of normal activity but is unstable	137,148
4	V105M	I	1	Italian	G 316 → A	Mutant enzyme has 77% of normal activity but is unstable	146

*By convention, codons are numbered on the basis of the amino acid sequence of the mature membrane-bound constitute or liver enzyme with the initiation methionine removed; i.e. codon 1 refers to the N-terminal glycine of the mature myristylated enzyme. For reference, the N-terminal amino acid of the soluble erythrocyte enzyme is Phe-26.

†The A of the initiation methionine codon equals +1.

to 300 residues in conjunction with myristylation), an erythrocyte-specific, presumptive membrane-associated minor form of 307 residues, and an erythrocyte-specific soluble form of 275 residues. The latter is entirely contained in the C-terminal 275 residues of the former two.

Genetic Defects

Four missense mutations have already been described in the NADH-cytochrome b_5 reductase gene in patients with hereditary methemoglobinemia (see Table 112-1). Thus, allelic heterogeneity is sufficient to account for the phenotypic differences of the various types of the disorder. Mutations that reduce stability and leave catalytic function intact mainly cause a problem in the erythrocyte, because the erythrocyte depends on enzyme synthesized in the reticulocyte persisting for its ~12 day life span.[146] Conversely, mutations that markedly reduce catalytic function cause problems in all cells expressing cytochrome b_5 reductase and result in the so-called type II phenotype. Presumably, the neurologic involvement derives from loss of the fatty acid desaturation and elongation function, while the cyanosis results from inability to reduce methemoglobin to hemoglobin.

Interestingly, consideration of the structure and function of the b_5 reductase gene predicts that mutations that affect the constitutive promoter and/or exon 1 and leave the erythrocyte promoter and downstream exons intact would produce an autosomal recessive neurologic phenotype without accompanying methemoglobinemia. No examples of this putative disorder have been recognized to date.

REFERENCES

1. François: Cas de cyanose congéniale sans cause apparente. *Bull Acad Roy Med Belg* **4**:698, 1845.
2. Dittrich P: Ueber methämoglobinbildende Gifte. *Naunyn-Schmiedeberg's Arch Exp Pathol Pharmacol* **29**:247, 1891.
3. Jaffé ER: Hereditary methemoglobinemias associated with abnormalities in the metabolism of erythrocytes. *Am J Med* **41**:786, 1966.
4. van den Bergh AAH: Enterogene Cyanose. *Dtsch Arch Klin Med* **83**:86, 1905.
5. Hitzenberger K: Autotoxische Zyanose (Intraglobuläre Methämoglobinamie). *Wien Arch Inn Med* **23**:85, 1932.
6. Gibson QH: The reduction of methameoglobin by ascorbic acid. *Biochem J* **37**:615, 1943.
7. Barcroft H, Gibson QH, Harrison DC, McMurray J: Familial idiopathic methaemoglobinaemia and its treatment with ascorbic acid. *Clin Sci* **5**:145, 1945.
8. Gibson QH: The reduction of methaemoglobin in red blood cells and studies on the cause of idiopathic methaemoglobinaemia. *Biochem J* **42**:13, 1948.
9. Scott EM, Griffith IV: The enzymic defect of hereditary methemoglobinemia: Diaphorase. *Biochim Biophys Acta* **34**:584, 1959.
10. Scott EM: The relation of diaphorase of human erythrocytes to inheritance of methemoglobinemia. *J Clin Invest* **39**:1176, 1960.
11. Balsamo P, Hardy WR, Scott EM: Hereditary methemoglobinemia due to diaphorase deficiency in Navajo Indians. *J Pediatr* **65**:928, 1964.
12. Schwartz JM, Reiss AL, Jaffé ER: Hereditary methemoglobinemia with deficiency of NADH cytochrome b_5 reductase, in Stanbury JB, Wyngaarden JB, Fredrickson DS, Goldstein JL, Brown MS (eds): *The Metabolic Basis of Inherited Disease*, 5th ed. New York, McGraw-Hill, 1983, p 1654.
13. Hultquist DE, Passon PG: Catalysis of methaemoglobin reduction by erythrocyte cytochrome b_5 and cytochrome b_5 reductase. *Nature* **229**:252, 1971.
14. Haurowitz F: Zur Chemie des Blutfarbstoffes; zur Kenntnis das Methämoglobins und seiner Derivative. *Z Physiol Chem* **138**:68, 1924.
15. Ladner RC, Heidner EJ, Perutz MF: The structure of horse methaemoglobin at 2.0 Aå resolution. *J Mol Biol* **114**:385, 1977.
16. Perutz MF, Fersht AR, Simon SR, Roberts GCK: Influence of globin structure on the state of the heme. II. Allosteric transitions in methemoglobin. *Biochemistry* **13**:2174, 1974.
17. Perrella M, Cremonesi L, Benazzi L, Rossi-Bernardi L: Isolation of intermediate valence hybrids between ferrous and methemoglobin at subzero temperatures. *J Biol Chem* **256**:11098, 1981.
18. Itano HA, Robinson E: Electrophoretic separation of intermediate compounds in two reactions of ferrihemoglobin. *Biochim Biophys Acta* **29**:545, 1958.
19. Bunn HF, Drysdale JW: The separation of partially oxidized hemoglobins. *Biochim Biophys Acta* **229**:51, 1971.
20. Bodansky O: Methemoglobinemia and methemoglobin-producing compounds. *Pharmacol Rev* **3**:144, 1951.
21. Bunn HF, Forget BG: *Hemoglobin: Molecular, Genetic, and Clinical Aspects*. Philadelphia, Saunders, 1986, p 638.
22. Darling RC, Roughton FJW: The effect of methemoglobin on the equilibrium between oxygen and hemoglobin. *Am J Physiol* **137**:56, 1942.
23. Kiese M: *Methemoglobinemia: A Comprehensive Treatise*. Cleveland, CRC Press, 1974.
24. Schulman HM, Martinez-Medellin J, Sidloi R: The oxidation state of newly synthesized hemoglobin. *Biochem Biophys Res Commun* **56**:220, 1974.
25. Asakura T, Adachi K, Minakami S, Yoshikawa H: Non-glycolytic sugar metabolism in human erythrocytes. I. Xylitol metabolism. *J Biochem (Tokyo)* **62**:184, 1967.
26. Hegesh E, Hegesh J, Kaftory A: Congenital methemoglobinemia with a deficiency of cytochrome b_5. *N Engl J Med* **314**:757, 1986.
27. Nagai M, Yubisui T, Yoneyama Y: Enzymatic reduction of hemoglobins M Milwaukee-1 and M Saskatoon by NADH-cytochrome b_5 reductase and NADPH-flavin reductase purified from human erythrocytes. *J Biol Chem* **255**:4599, 1980.
28. Gacon G, Lostanlen D, Labie D, Kaplan J-C: Interaction between cytochrome b_5 and hemoglobin: Involvement of β66 (E10) and β95 (FG2) lysyl residues of hemoglobin. *Proc Natl Acad Sci USA* **77**:1917, 1980.
29. Jaffé ER, Neumann G, Rothberg H, Wilson FT, Webster RM, Wolff JA: Hereditary methemoglobinemia with and without mental retardation: A study of three families. *Am J Med* **41**:42, 1966.
30. Cohen RJ, Sachs JR, Wicker DJ, Conrad ME: Methemoglobinemia provoked by malarial chemoprophylaxis in Vietnam. *N Engl J Med* **279**:1127, 1968.
31. Horne MK, Waterman MR, Simon LM, Garriott JC, Foerster EH: Methemoglobinemia from sniffing butyl nitrite. *Ann Intern Med* **91**:417, 1979.
32. Daly JS, Hultquist DE, Rucknagel DL: Phenazopyridine induced methaemoglobinaemia associated with decreased activity of erythrocyte cytochrome b_5 reductase. *J Med Genet* **20**:307, 1983.
33. Ross JD: Deficient activity of DPNH-dependent methemoglobin diaphorase in cord blood erythrocytes. *Blood* **21**:51, 1963.
34. Kanazawa Y, Hattori M, Kosaka K, Nakao K: The relationship of NADH-dependent diaphorase activity and methemoglobin reduction in human erythrocytes. *Clin Chim Acta* **19**:524, 1968.
35. Winterbourn CC: Free-radical production and oxidative reactions of hemoglobin. *Environ Health Perspect* **64**:321, 1985.
36. Wittenberg JB, Wittenberg BA, Peisach J, Blumberg WE: On the state of the iron and the nature of the ligand in oxyhemoglobin. *Proc Natl Acad Sci USA* **67**:1846, 1970.
37. Mansouri A, Winterhalter KH: Nonequivalence of chains in haemoglobin oxidation. *Biochemistry* **12**:4946, 1973.
38. Tomoda A, Yoneyama Y, Tsuji A: Changes in intermediate haemoglobins during autoxidation of haemoglobin. *Biochem J* **195**:485, 1981.
39. Brooks J: The oxidation of haemoglobin to methaemoglobin by oxygen. II. The relation between the rate of oxidation and

the partial pressure of oxygen. *Proc R Soc London (B)* **118:**560, 1935.

40. Tomoda A, Yoneyama Y: Analysis of intermediate hemoglobins in solutions of hemoglobin partially oxidized with ferricyanide. *Biochem Biophys Acta* **581:**128, 1979.
41. Winterbourn CC, Carrell RC: Oxidation of human haemoglobin by copper. *Biochem J* **165:**141, 1977.
42. Mohler DN, Majerus PW, Minnich V, Hess CE, Garrick MD: Glutathione synthetase deficiency as a cause of hereditary hemolytic disease. *N Engl J Med* **283:**1253, 1970.
43. Vestling CS: The reduction of methemoglobin by ascorbic acid. *J Biol Chem* **143:**439, 1942.
44. Tomoda A, Tsuji A, Matsukawa S, Takeshita M, Yoneyama Y: Mechanism of methemoglobin reduction by ascorbic acid under anaerobic conditions. *J Biol Chem* **253:**7420, 1978.
45. Sass MD, Caruso CJ, Farhangi M: TPNH-methemoglobin reductase deficiency: A new red-cell enzyme defect. *J Lab Clin Med* **70:**760, 1967.
46. Kiese M: Die Reduktion des Hämiglobins. *Biochem Z* **316:**264, 1944.
47. Warburg O, Kubowitz F, Christian W: Über die katalytische Wirkung von Methylenblau in lebenden Zellen. *Biochem Z* **227:**245, 1930.
48. Yubisui T, Matsuki T, Takeshita M, Yoneyama Y: Characterization of the purified NADPH-flavin reductase of human erythrocytes. *J Biochem (Tokyo)* **85:**719, 1979.
49. Yubisui T, Takeshita M, Yoneyama Y: Reduction of methemoglobin through flavin at the physiological concentration by NADPH-flavin reductase of human erythrocytes. *J Biochem (Tokyo)* **87:**1715, 1980.
50. Tomoda A, Yubisui T, Tsuji A, Yoneyama Y: Changes in intermediate haemoglobins during methaemoblobin reduction by NADPH-flavin reductase. *Biochem J* **179:**227, 1979.
51. Scott EM, McGraw JC: Purification and properties of diphosphopyridine nucleotide diaphorase of human erythrocytes. *J Biol Chem* **237:**249, 1962.
52. Scott EM, Duncan IW, Ekstrand V: The reduced pyridine nucleotide dehydrogenases of human erythrocytes. *J Biol Chem* **240:**481, 1965.
53. Hegesh E, Avron M: The enzymatic reduction of ferrihemoglobin. II. Purification of a ferrihemoglobin reductase from human erythrocytes. *Biochim Biophys Acta* **146:**397, 1967.
54. Niethammer D, Huennekens FM: Electrophoretic separation and characterization of the multiple forms of methemoglobin reductase. *Arch Biochem Biophys* **146:**564, 1971.
55. Sugita Y, Nomura S, Yoneyama Y: Purification of reduced pyridine nucleotide dehydrogenase from human erythrocytes and methemoglobin reduction by the enzyme. *J Biol Chem* **246:**6072, 1971.
56. Passon PG, Hultquist DE: Soluble cytochrome b_5 reductase from humane erythrocytes. *Biochim Biophys Acta* **275:**62, 1972.
57. Kuma F, Inomata H: Studies on methemoglobin reductase. II. The purification and molecular properties of reduced nicotinamide adenine dinucleotide-dependent methemoglobin reductase. *J Biol Chem* **247:**556, 1972.
58. Yubisui T, Takeshita M: Characterization of the purified NADH-cytochrome b_5 reductase of humane erythrocytes as a FAD-containing enzyme. *J Biol Chem* **255:**2454, 1980.
59. Hegesh E, Avron M: The enzymatic reduction of ferrihemoglobin. I. The reduction of ferrihemoglobin in red blood cells and hemolysates. *Biochim Biophys Acta* **146:**91, 1967.
60. Reiss A, Schwartz JS, Patel S: Mechanism of the enzyme-dependent reduction of methemoglobin in the presence of NADH and ferrocyanide. *Blood* 50 *Suppl* **1:**84, 1977.
61. Taketa F, Chen JY: Activation of the NADH-methemoglobin reductase reaction by inositol hexaphosphate. *Biochem Biophys Res Commun* **75:**389, 1977.
62. Yubisui T, Miyata T, Iwanaga S, Tamura M, Takeshita M: Complete amino acid sequence of NADH-cytochrome b_5 reductase purified from human erythrocytes. *J Biochem (Tokyo)* **99:**407, 1986.
63. Takeshita M, Tamura M, Yubisui T, Yoneyama Y: Exponential decay of cytochrome b_5 and cytochrome b_5 reductase during senescence of erythrocytes: relation to the increased methemoglobin content. *J Biochem (Tokyo)* **93:**931, 1983.
64. Yubisui T, Tamura M, Takeshita M: Studies on NADH-cytochrome b_5 reductase activities in hemolysates of human and rabbit red cells by isoelectric focusing. *Biochem Biphys Res Commun* **102:**860, 1981.
65. Zamudio I, Canessa M: Nicotinamide-adenine dinucleotide dehydrogenase activity of human erythrocyte membranes. *Biochim Biophys Acta* **120:**165, 1966.
66. Wang C-S, Alaupovic P: Isolation and partial characterization of human erythrocyte membrane NADH: (acceptor) oxidoreductase. *J Supramol Str* **9:**1, 1978.
67. Goto-Tamura R, Takesue Y, Takesue S: Immunological similarity between NADH-cytochrome b_5 reductase of erythrocytes and liver microsomes. *Biochim Biophys Acta* **423:**293, 1976.
68. Choury D, Leroux A, Kaplan J-C: Membrane-bound cytochrome b_5 reductase (methemoglobin reductase) in human erythrocytes. Study in normal and methemoglobinemic subjects. *J Clin Invest* **67:**149:1981.
69. Kitajima S, Yasukochi Y, Minakami S: Purification and properties of human erythrocyte membrane NADH-cytochrome b_5 reductase. *Arch Biochem Biophys* **210:**330, 1981.
70. Choury D, Reghis A, Pichard A-L, Kaplan J-C: Endogenous proteolysis of membrane-bound red cell cytochrome b_5 reductase in adults and newborns: Its possible relevance to the generation of the soluble "methemoglobin reductase." *Blood* **61:**894, 1983.
71. Hultquist DE, Reed DW, Passon PG: Isolation, characterization, and enzymatic reduction of cytochrome B (556) from human erythrocytes. *Fed Proc* **28:**862, 1969.
72. Passon PG, Hultquist DE: Participation of erythrocyte cytochrome b_5 in methemoglobin reduction and evidence for the occurrence of erythrocyte P-420. *Fed Proc* **29:**732, 1970.
73. Passon PG, Reed DW, Hultquist DE: Soluble cytochrome b_5 from human erythrocytes. *Biochim Biophys Acta* **275:**51, 1972.
74. Hultquist De, Dean RT, Douglas RH: Homogeneous cytochrome b_5 from human erythrocytes. *Biochem Biophys Res Commun* **60:**28, 1974.
75. Capalna S: The erythrocyte cytochrome b_5. *Physiologie* **14:**85, 1977.
76. Douglas RH, Hultquist DE: Evidence that two forms of bovine erythrocyte cytochrome b_5 are identical to segments of microsomal cytochrome b_5. *Proc Natl Acad Sci USA* **75:**3118, 1978.
77. Slaughter SR, Hultquist DE: Membrane-bound redox proteins of the murine Friend virus-induced erythroleukemia cell. *J Cell Biol* **83:**231, 1979.
78. Hultquist DE, Reed DW, Passon PG, Andrews WE: Purification and properties of S-protein (hemoprotein 559) from human erythrocytes. *Biochim Biophys Acta* **229:**33, 1971.
79. Abe K, Sugita Y: Properties of cytochrome b_5 and methemoglobin reduction in human erythrocytes. *Eur J Biochem* **101:**423, 1979.
80. Abe K, Kimura S, Kizawa R, Anan FK, Sugita Y: Amino acid sequences of cytochrome b_5 from human, porcine, and bovine erythrocytes and comparison with liver microsomal cytochrome b_5. *J Biochem (Tokyo)* **97:**1659, 1985.
81. Slaughter SR, Williams CH, Hultquist DE: Demonstration that bovine erythrocyte cytochrome b_5 is the hydrophilic segment of liver microsomal cytochrome b_5. *Biochim Biophys Acta* **705:**228, 1982.
82. Schafer DA, Hultquist DE: Purification and structural studies of rabbit erythrocyte cytochrome b_5. *Biochem Biophys Res Commun* **115:**807, 1983.
83. Imoto M: The purification and primary structure of human erythrocyte cytochrome b_5. *Juzen Igakkai Zasshi* **86:**256, 1977.
84. Hultquist DE, Slaughter SR, Douglas RH, Sannes LJ, Sahagian GG: Erythrocyte cytochrome b_5; Structure, role in methemoglobin reduction, and solubilization from endoplasmic reticulum. *Prog Clin Biol Res* **21:**199, 1978.
85. Takeshita M, Yubisui T, Tanishima K, Yoneyama Y: A simple enzymatic microdetermination of cytochrome b_5 in erythrocytes. *Anal Biochem* **107:**305, 1980.
86. Kaftory A, Hegesh E: Improved determination of cytochrome b_5 in human erythrocytes. *Clin Chem* **30:**1344, 1984.
87. Ozols J, Strittmatter P: Correction of the amino acid sequence of calf liver microsomal cytochrome b_5. J Biol Chem **244:**6617, 1969.

88. Leroux A, Kaplan J-C: Presence of red cell type NADH-methemoglobin reductase (NADH-diaphorase) in human non-erythroid cells. *Biochem Biophys Res Commun* **49**:945, 1972.
89. Kuma F, Prough RA, Masters BSS: Studies on methemoglobin reductase. Immunochemical similarity of soluble methemoglobin reductase and cytochrome b_5 of human erythrocytes with NADH-cytochrome b_5 reductase and cytochrome b_5 of rat liver microsomes. *Arch Biochem Biophys* **172**:600, 1976.
90. Leroux A, Junien C, Kaplan J-C, Bamberger J: Generalised deficiency of cytochrome b_5 reductase in congenital methaemoglobinemia with mental retardation. *Nature* **258**:619, 1975.
91. Hultquist DE, Sannes LJ, Schafer DA: The NADH/NADPH-methemoglobin reduction system of erythrocytes. *Prog Clin Biol Res* **55**:291, 1981.
92. Hultquist DE, Peters CL, Schafer DA: Proteolytic generation of erythrocyte cytochrome b_5 and cytochrome b_5 reductase from endoplasmic reticulum (ER). *Proc XIth Intl Cong Biochem* 490, 1979.
93. Yubisui T, Naitoh Y, Zenno S, Tamura M, Takeshita M, Sakaki Y: Molecular cloning of cDNAs of human liver and placenta NADH-cytochrome b_5 reductase. *Proc Natl Acad Sci USA* **84**:3609, 1987.
94. Hultquist DE, Douglas RH, Dean RT: The methemoglobin reduction system of erythrocytes. *Prog Clin Biol Res* **1**:297, 1975.
95. Schafer DA, Hultquist DE: Isolation of an acid protease from rabbit reticulocytes and evidence for its role in processing redox proteins during erythroid maturation. *Biochem Biophys Res Commun* **100;**1555, 1981.
96. Schafer DA, Hultquist DE: Isolation and characterization of cathepsin D from reticulocyte membranes. *Prog Clin Biol Res* **165**:549, 1984.
97. Raw I, Difini F: The possible role of ATP-dependent proteolysis on the solubilization of methemoglobin reductase during reticulocyte maturation. *Biochem Biophys Res Commun* **116**:357, 1983.
98. Choury D, Wajcman H, Boissel JP, Kaplan J-C: Evidence for endogenous proteolytic solubilization of human red-cell membrane NADH-cytochrome b_5 reductase. *FEBS Lett* **126**:172, 1981.
99. Petragnani N, Nogueira OC, Raw I: Methaemoglobin reduction through cytochrome b_5. *Nature* **184**:1651, 1959.
100. Sannes LJ, Hultquist DE: Effects of hemolysate concentration, ionic strength and cytochrome b_5 concentration on the rate of methemoglobin reduction in hemolysates of human erythrocytes. *Biochem Biophys Acta* **544**:547, 1978.
101. Tomoda A, Yubisui T, Tsuji A, Yoneyama Y: Kinetic studies of methemoglobin reduction by human red cell NADH cytochrome b_5 reductase. *J Biol Chem* **254**:3119, 1979.
102. Kuma F: Properties of methemoglobin reductase and kinetic study of methemoglobin reduction. *J Biol Chem* **256**:5518, 1981.
103. Juckett DA, Hultquist DE: Magnetic circular dichroism studies of hemoglobin. The reduction of ferrihemoglobin by ferrocytochrome b_5 and characterization of the high-spin hydroxy species of mixed-valence hemoglobin. *Biophys Chem* **19**:321, 1984.
104. Hultquist DE, Sannes LJ, Juckett DA: Catalysis of methemoglobin reduction, in DeLuca M, Lardy H, Cross RL (eds): *Current Topics in Cellular Regulation*. New York, Academic, 1984, vol 24, p 287.
105. Lostanlen D, Gacon G, Kaplan J-C: Direct enzyme titration curve of NADH:cytochrome b_5 reductase by combined isoelectric focusing/electrophoresis. *Eur J Biochem* **112**:179, 1980.
106. Strittmatter P: NADH-cytochrome b_5 reductase, in Slater EC (ed): *Flavins and Flavoproteins*. New York, Elsevier, 1966, p 325.
107. Dailey HA, Strittmatter P: Modification and identification of cytochrome b_5 carboxyl groups involved in protein-protein interaction with cytochrome b_5 reductase. *J Biol Chem* **254**:5388, 1979.
108. Righetti PG, Gacon G, Gianazza E, Lostanlen D, Kaplan J-C: Titration curves of interacting cytochrome b_5 and hemoglobin by isoelectric focusing-electrophoresis. *Biochem Biophys Res Commun* **85**:1575, 1978.
109. Mauk MR, Mauk AG: Interaction between cytochrome b_5 and human methemoglobin. *Biochemistry* **21**:4730, 1982.
110. Mauk MR, Reid LS, Mauk AG: Conversion of oxyhaemoglobin into methaemoglobin by ferricytochrome b_5. *Biochem J* **221**:297, 1984.
111. Poulos TL, Mauk AG: Models for the complexes formed between cytochrome b_5 and the subunits of methemoglobin. *J Biol Chem* **258**:7369, 1983.
112. Finch CA: Methemoglobinemia and sulfhemoglobinemia. *N Engl J Med* **239**:470, 1948.
113. Jaffé ER: Enzymopenic hereditary methemoglobinemia: A clinical/biochemical classification. *Blood Cells* **12**:81, 1986.
114. Worster-Drought C, White JC, Sargent F: Familial idiopathic methaemoglobinaemia associated with mental deficiency and neurological abnormalities. *Br Med J* **2**:114, 1953.
115. Kaplan JC, Leroux A, Beauvais P: Formes cliniques et biologiques du déficit en cytochrome b_5 réductase. *CR Seances Soc Biol* **173**:368, 1979.
116. Kaplan JC, Leroux A, Bakouri S, Grangaud JP, Benabadji M: La lésion enzymatique dans la méthémoglobinémie congénitale récessive avec encéphalopathie. *Nouv Rev Fr Hematol* **14**:755, 1974.
117. Hirono H: Lipids of myelin, white matter and gray matter in a case of generalized deficiency of cytochrome b_5 reductase in congenital methemoglobinemia with mental retardation. *Lipids* **15**:272, 1980.
118. Hirono H: Lipids of liver, kidney, spleen and muscle in a case of generalized deficiency of cytochrome b_5 reductase in congenital methemoglobinemia with mental retardation. *Lipids* **19**:60, 1984.
119. Junien C, Leroux A, Lostanlen D, Reghis A, Boue J, Nicolas H, Boue A, Kaplan JC: Prenatal diagnosis of congenital enzymopenic methaemoglobinaemia with mental retardation due to generalized cytochrome b_5 reductase deficiency: First report of two cases. *Prenat Diagn* **1**:17, 1981.
120. Arnold H, Bötcher HW, Hufnagel D, Löhr GW: Hereditary methemoglobinemia due to methemoglobin reductase deficiency in erythrocytes and leukocytes without neurological symptoms. *Abstracts, XVII Congress of the International Society of Hematology, Paris*, 1978, p 752.
121. Tanishima K, Tanimoto K, Tomoda A, Mawatari K, Matsukawa S, Yoneyama Y, Ohkuwa H, Takazakura E: Hereditary methemoglobinemia due to cytochrome b_5 reductase deficiency in blood cells without associated neurologic and mental disorders. *Blood* **66**:1288, 1985.
122. Fisher RA, Povey S, Borrow M, Solomon E, Boyd Y, Carritt B: Assignment of the DIA/1 locus to chromosome 22. *Ann Hum Genet* **41**:151, 1977.
123. Junien C, Vibert M, Weil D, Van-Cong N, Kaplan J-C: Assignment of NADH-cytochrome b_5 reductase (DIA_1 locus) to human chromosome 22. *Hum Genet* **42**:233, 1978.
124. Kaplan J-C, Beutler E: Electorphoresis of red cell NADH- and NADPH-diaphorases in human subjects and patients with congenital methemoglobinemia. *Biochem Biophys Res Commun* **29**:605, 1967.
125. Hopkinson DA, Corney G, Cook PJL, Robson EB, Harris H: Genetically determined electrophoretic variants of human red cell NADH diaphorase. *Ann Hum Genet* **34**:1, 1970.
126. Jaffé ER: Methemoglobinemia in the differential diagnosis of cyanosis. *Hosp Pract* **20**:92, 1985.
127. Schwartz JM, Paress PS, Ross JM, Dipillo F, Rizek R: Unstable variant of NADH methemoglobin reductase in Puerto Ricans with hereditary methemoglobinemia. *J Clin Invest* **51**:1594, 1972.
128. Feig SA, Nathan DG, Gerald PS, Zarkowski HS: Congenital methemoglobinemia: The result of age-dependent decay of methemoglobin reductase. *Blood* **39**:407, 1972.
129. Beutler E: Selectivity of proteases as a basis for tissue distribution of enzymes in hereditary deficiencies. *Proc Natl Acad Sci USA* **80**:3767, 1983.
130. Sharp CW, Stillman RC: Blush not with nitrites. *Ann Intern Med* **92**:700, 1980 (editorial).
131. Hegesh E, Calmanovici N, Avron M: New method for determining ferrihemoglobin reductase (NADH-methemoglobin reductase) in erythrocytes. *J Lab Clin Med* **72**:339, 1968.
132. Board PG: NADH-ferricyanide reductase, a convenient ap-

proach to the evaluation of NADH-methaemoglobin reductase in human erythrocytes. *Clin Chim Acta* **109**:233, 1981.

133. Kaplan J-C, Nicolas AM, Hanzlickova-Leroux A, Beutler E: A simple spot screening test for fast detection of red cell NADH-diaphorase deficiency. *Blood* **36**:330, 1970.

134. Kaplan JC, Chirouze M: Therapy of recessive congenital methaemoglobinaemia by oral riboflavine. *Lancet* **2**:1043, 1978.

135. Mansouri A, Lurie AA: Methemoglobinemia. *Am J Hematol* **42**:7, 1993.

136. Yawata Y, Ding L, Tanishima K, Tomoda A: New variant of cytochrome b_5 reductase deficiency ($b_5R_{Kurashiki}$) in red cells, platelets, lymphocytes and cultured fibroblasts with congenital methemoglobinemia, mental and neurologic retardation and skeletal anomalies. *Am J Hematol* **40**:299, 1992.

137. Nagai T, Shirabe K, Yubisui T, Takeshita M: Analysis of mutant NADH-cytochrome b_5 reductase: Apparent "type III" methemoglobinemia can be explained as type I with an unstable reductase. *Blood* **81**:808, 1993.

138. Strittmatter P, Kittler JM, Coghill JE: Characterization of the role of lysine 110 of NADH-cytochrome b_5 reductase in the binding and oxidation of NADH by site-directed mutagenesis. *J Biol Chem* **267**:20164, 1992.

139. Yubisui T, Shirabe K, Takeshita M, Kobayashi Y, Fukumaki Y, Sakaki Y, Takano T: Structural role of serine 127 in the NADH-binding site of human NADH-cytochrome b_5 reductase. *J Biol Chem* **266**:66, 1991.

140. Shirabe K, Yubisui T, Nishino T, Takeshita M: Role of cysteine residues in human NADH-cytochrome b_5 reductase studied by site-directed mutagenesis. *J Biol Chem* **266**:7531, 1991.

141. Hultquist DE, Xu F, Quandt KS, Shlafer M, Mack CP, Till GO, Seekamp A, Betz AL, Ennis SR: Evidence that NADPH-dependent methemoglobin reductase and administered riboflavin protect tissues from oxidative injury. *Am J Hematol* **42**:13, 1993.

141a. Ozols J, Korza G, Heinemann FS, Hediger MA, Strittmatter P: Complete amino acid sequence of steer liver microsomal NADH-cytochrome b_5 reductase. *J Biol Chem* **260**:11953, 1985.

142. Yubisui T, Naitoh Y, Zenno S, Tamura M, Takeshita M, Sakaki Y: Molecular cloning of cDNAs of human liver and placenta NADH-cytochrome b_5 reductase. *Proc Natl Acad Sci USA* **84**:3609, 1987.

143. Zenno S, Hattori M, Misumi Y, Yubisui T, Sakaki Y: Molecular cloning of a cDNA encoding rat NADH-cytochrome b_5 reductase and the corresponding gene. *J Biochem* **107**:810, 1990.

144. Pietrini G, Carrera P, Borgese N: Two transcripts encode rat cytochrome b_5 reductase. *Proc Natl Acad Sci USA* **85**:7246, 1988.

145. Tomatsu S, Kobayashi Y, Fukumaki Y, Yubisui T, Orii T, Sakaki Y: The organization and the complete nucleotide sequence of the human NADH-cytochrome b_5 reductase gene. *Gene* **80**:353, 1989.

146. Shirabe K, Yubisui T, Borgese N, Tang C, Hultquist DE, Takeshita M: Enzymatic instability of NADH-cytochrome b_5 reductase as a cause of hereditary methemoglobinemia type I (red cell type). *J Biol Chem* **267**:20416, 1992.

147. Kobayashi Y, Fukumaki Y, Yubisui T, Inoue J, Sakaki Y: Serine-proline replacement at residue 127 of NADH-cytochrome b_5 reductase causes hereditary methemoglobinemia, generalized type. *Blood* **75**:1408, 1990.

148. Katsube T, Sakamoto N, Kobayashi Y, Seki R, Hirano M, Tanishima K, Tomoda A, Takazakura E, Yubisui T, Takesha M, Sakaki Y, Fukumaki Y: Exonic point mutations in NADH-cytochrome b_5 reductase genes of homozygotes for hereditary methemoglobinemia, types I and III: Putative mechanisms of tissue-dependent enzyme deficiency. *Am J Hum Genet* **48**:799, 1991.

CHAPTER 113

The Hemoglobinopathies

D. J. Weatherall ▪ J. B. Clegg ▪ D. R. Higgs ▪ W. G. Wood

1. The inherited disorders of hemoglobin fall into three overlapping groups: structural variants; thalassemias, all characterized by a reduced rate of synthesis of one or more of the globin chains of hemoglobin; and conditions in which fetal hemoglobin synthesis persists beyond the neonatal period, known collectively as hereditary persistence of fetal hemoglobin. Taken together, they are the most common single gene disorders in the world population.

2. Because the different hemoglobin disorders coexist at a high frequency in many populations, and individuals may inherit more than one type, they are responsible for an extremely complex series of clinical phenotypes. Their molecular pathology has been elucidated in many cases, and a start has been made in relating primary molecular defects to associated clinical phenotypes.

3. The β thalassemias are divided into β^+ thalassemia, in which some β globin chains are produced, and β^0 thalassemia, in which there is no β chain synthesis. The α thalassemias are similarly divided into α^0 and α^+ thalassemias. Over 100 different mutations have been identified as the cause for β thalassemia, most of which interfere with the transcription of β globin mRNA, or its processing or translation. A few types of β thalassemia result from the production of highly unstable β globin chains. The common forms of α thalassemia result from deletions which involve either both or one of the linked α globin genes. Some less common forms of α thalassemia result from point mutations which interfere with the translation of α1 globin mRNA or transcription of the α globin genes.

4. The development of rapid methods for studying the globin genes has also made it possible to analyze their population genetics and the mechanisms that underlie their high gene frequencies.

5. The carrier states for most of the important hemoglobin disorders are easily identifiable. Their homozygous or compound heterozygous states can be identified in fetal life by fetal blood sampling or analysis of DNA obtained from chorionic villi. Hence the disease can be avoided in an affected family by reproductive counseling and a choice of options.

6. Apart from marrow transplantation there is no definitive treatment, and management is symptomatic.

A list of standard abbreviations is located immediately preceding the index in each volume. Additional nonstandard abbreviations used in this volume include: ATR = α thalassemia mental retardation; CHBA = congenital Heinz body hemolytic anemia; ES = embryonic stem (cell); HPFH = hereditary persistent fetal hemoglobin; HS = hypersensitive site; HVR = hypervariable regions; ISC = irreversibly sickled cells; LCR = locus control region; MGC = minimum gelling concentration; NFE-2 = nuclear factor erythroid 2; PSR = proliferative sickle retinopathy; and RE = reticuloendothelial.

INTRODUCTION

The inherited disorders of hemoglobin are the commonest single gene conditions in humans. The World Health Organization has suggested that, at a conservative estimate, about 5 percent of the world's population are carriers for different inherited disorders of hemoglobin and that about 300,000 severely affected homozygotes or compound heterozygotes are born each year.[1] In the developing countries, in which there is still a very high mortality from infection and malnutrition in the first year of life, many of these conditions go unrecognized. However, as economic conditions improve and infant death rates fall, they pose an increasingly heavy burden on health services.

As the result of mass migrations of populations from high prevalence areas, the hemoglobin disorders are being seen with increasing frequency in parts of the world in which they have not been recognized previously. Because some of them, particularly sickle cell anemia and the more severe forms of thalassemia, can produce life-threatening medical emergencies or chronic ill health, it is important for clinicians in all countries of the world to have a working knowledge of their clinical features, genetic transmission, management, and, in particular, prevention. The other reason why the hemoglobin disorders are of particular current interest is that they were the first diseases to be analyzed by the methods of recombinant DNA technology. More is known about their molecular pathology than any other genetic disease, and it is likely that their study has already given us a relatively complete picture of the repertoire of mutations that underlie single gene disorders.

In this chapter we shall review the main clinical, genetic, and population aspects of these conditions. It will not be possible to provide an all-encompassing picture of the enormous amount of work that has been carried out in this field. Readers who wish to study this subject in greater depth are referred to two extensive monographs on the subject.[2,3]

HISTORICAL BACKGROUND

The fascinating story of the evolution and development of the human hemoglobin field has been the subject of several reviews and monographs that contain extensive bibliographies.[3–6]

In trying to understand why the human hemoglobin field has paved the way for the application of molecular biology to the study of human disease it is helpful to trace three historical threads that finally came together in the 1950s. The first is the story of the discovery of hemoglobin and the elucidation of its structure and function. The second encompasses the early description of sickle cell anemia, the realization that it is an inherited disease, and the characterization of its molecular pathology. And, finally, there is the even more complex saga of the gradual amalgamation of observations from many parts of the world that led to the notion that the thalassemias are also genetic disorders of hemoglobin with many features in common with the structural hemoglobin variants. The final chapter of this biologic defective story, which is not yet complete, is how, given all this diverse information and the new tools of molecular and cell biology, it has been possible in less than 10 years to describe so much of the molecular pathology of hemoglobin that, at the time of writing, it is likely that we already have a very good idea about the repertoire of the molecular defects that underlie single gene disorders.

Following the studies of William Harvey on the circulation of the blood, two English workers, Robert Boyle and the Oxford eccentric Richard Lower, established that the function of the pulmonary circulation is to aerate venous blood. The mechanism of the binding of oxygen to blood was a subject of intense interest during the second half of the 19th century, and in 1862, Hoppe-Seyler first used the term *hemoglobin* to describe the oxygen-carrying pigment. The structure of heme was worked out by Kuster in 1912 but it was not until the mid-1950s, following pioneering work on protein structure by Sanger, that Ingram, Rhinesmith, Schroeder, Pauling, and others established that hemoglobin is a tetramer composed of two pairs of unlike peptide chains, α and β. Using the newly developed techniques of amino acid sequence analysis the primary structures of these chains were rapidly determined. At the same time Perutz and his colleagues, following years of painstaking work, were gradually arriving at a solution for the three-dimensional structure of hemoglobin by x-ray analysis. Thus, by the early 1960s a start could be made in relating the structure of hemoglobin to its functional properties that had been so elegantly described by Bohr and Krogh in Denmark, Barcroft, Haldane, Hill, and Roughton in England, and Henderson in the United States.

This new knowledge, together with the discovery of the abnormal hemoglobins, led to rapid progress toward an understanding of the genetic control of human hemoglobin. But part of the work that laid the basis for this remarkably productive period of hemoglobin research had started half a century before with the discovery of sickle cell anemia.

The first description of sickle cell anemia appeared in 1910 in Herrick's classic paper.[7] The genetic basis of this disease was established by workers in the United States, particularly Neel, and in Africa, notably the Lambotte-Legrands and Beet. The discovery that sickle cell anemia results from a structural change in hemoglobin, following the famous conversation between Castle and Pauling in 1945, was announced by Pauling and his colleagues in 1949,[8] and the amino acid substitution in Hb S was determined by Ingram in 1956.[9] Once it was realized that there are two globin chains, α and β, and that the amino acid substitution in sickle hemoglobin is in the β chain, the one-gene–one-enzyme (or peptide chain) concept, which had been proposed earlier by Beadle and Tatum from their work on Neurospora, was confirmed for higher organisms. More hemoglobin variants were soon discovered by electrophoresis, and by studying families in which genes for both α and β globin variants segregated, the independent genetic control of the α and β chains was established. The different chains of fetal and the adult minor hemoglobin, A_2, were characterized, and by careful analysis of families with different genetic variants, and appropriate linkage studies, a reasonable working model of the order of the α-like and β-like globin genes on their respective chromosomes was obtained.

The third thread in the story starts in 1927 with the first description of thalassemia by Cooley and Lee.[10] Although the carrier state for this condition was probably identified at about the same time in Italy[6] it was more than a quarter of a century before the genetic transmission of thalassemia was fully appreciated. During this period reports of the disease appeared from all over the world, and as soon as hemoglobin analysis became part of the armamentarium of clinicians during the 1950s it was soon realized that thalassemia is not only one of the commonest genetic diseases but is also extremely heterogeneous. Studies of the hemoglobin patterns of patients with different types of thalassemia and structural hemoglobin variants carried out in the late 1950s led to the suggestion by Ingram and Stretton[11] that there might be two main types—α and β thalassemia. The development of a method for studying hemoglobin synthesis in the test tube[12,13] led to the experimental validation of this hypothesis and to the further analysis of thalassemia, so that by the early 1970s it was known that there are many different forms, and it was also possible to make a guess at their underlying defects.

Thus, by the mid-1970s a great deal was known about the genetic control of human hemoglobin, the structural variants, and the biosynthetic defects and remarkable heterogeneity of the thalassemias. The field was ready for the techniques of recombinant DNA. Over the past 15 years these methods have been used successfully to determine the molecular pathology of the globin disorders, thereby paving the way toward an understanding of the molecular basis for many single gene disorders.

STRUCTURE, GENETIC CONTROL, AND SYNTHESIS OF HEMOGLOBIN

Structure

All normal hemoglobins have a tetrameric structure consisting of two pairs of unlike peptide chains (Fig. 113-1). In normal adults the major component, comprising about 97 percent of the total is Hb A ($\alpha_2\beta_2$) with the remainder being Hb A_2 ($\alpha_2\delta_2$). The main hemoglobin in fetal life is Hb F ($\alpha_2\gamma_2$) [although traces of it (~0.5 percent) are found in adults], and this is preceded in the embryo by Hbs Gower 1 ($\zeta_2\epsilon_2$) and 2 ($\alpha_2\epsilon_2$) and hemoglobin Portland ($\zeta_2\gamma_2$). There are also various minor components that are the result of postsynthetic modifications that take place in vivo. The most common of these are Hb A_{1c}, formed by the reaction of glucose with hemoglobin, and Hb F_1, an acetylated form of fetal hemoglobin. The amino acid sequences of all the normal globins are known and they are clearly related to each other, retaining many key features in common. Broadly speaking, they can be regarded as "α-like" (ζ and α, each of 141 amino acids) and "β-like" (ε, γ, δ, and β, 146 amino acids), and it appears that they arose from a single ancestral globin by successive duplications and divergence of the duplicated genes (see below).

The three-dimensional structure of human hemoglobin has been determined by Perutz and colleagues to a resolution

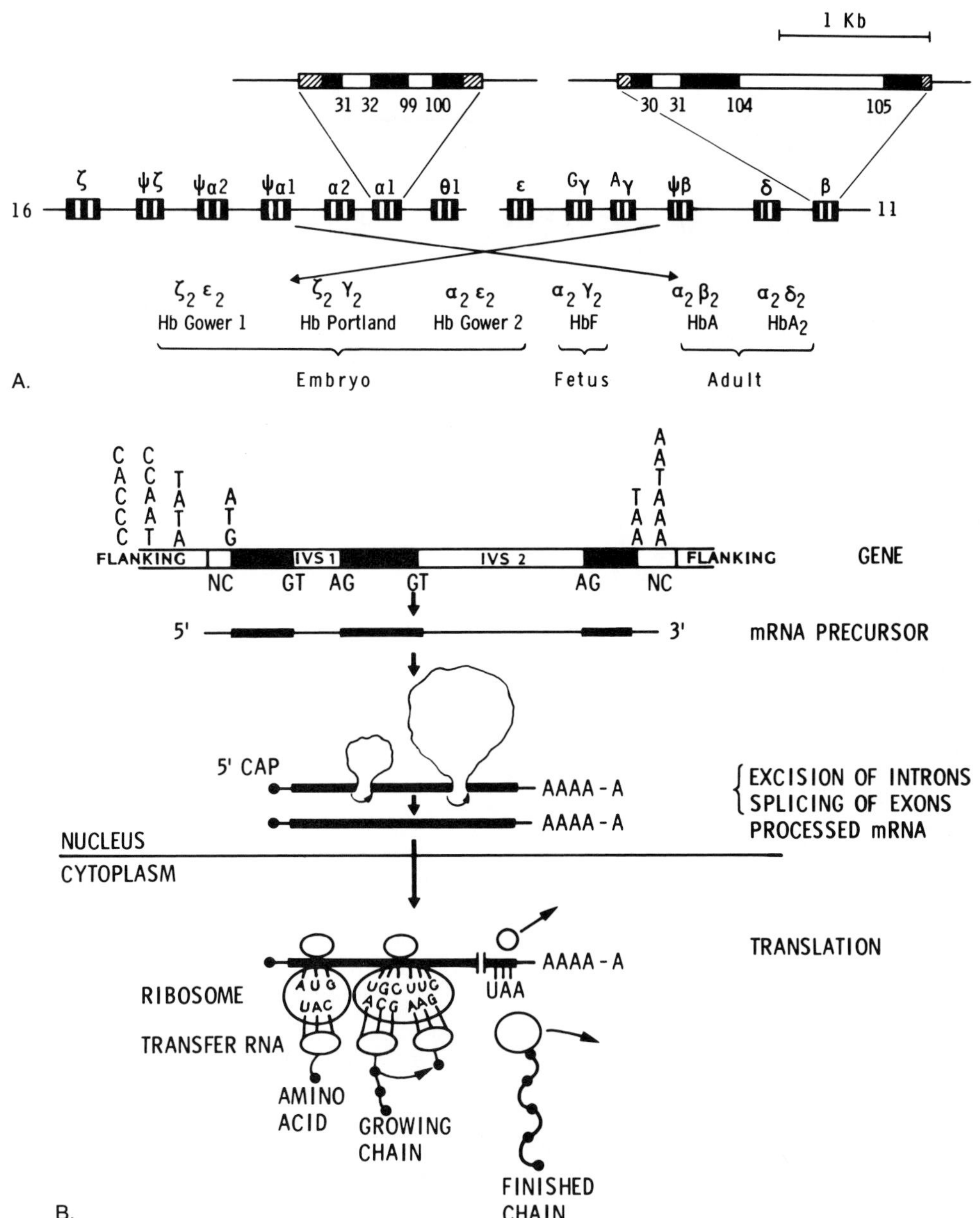

FIG. 113-1 **Genetic control of human hemoglobin. *A*. The human hemoglobins and globin gene clusters. *B*. The mechanism of globin synthesis. The exons are shown in dark shading and the introns (IVS1 and IVS2) unshaded. The positions of the 5′ regulatory boxes and the 5′ and 3′ noncoding (NC) regions are also shown. Further details, including location of RFLPs, VNTRs and *Alu* repeats, are given in refs. 3, 50, 70, 208, 439, and 440.**

better than 2.7Å by x-ray crystallography.[14,15] It consists of an ellipsoid approximately 64×55×50Å in which the subunits are oriented in a unit with a twofold symmetry axis running down a central water-filled cavity. Seventy-five percent of the native hemoglobin molecule is in the form of α-helix. Where the α-helix is interrupted (e.g., by a proline residue) the polypeptide chains can turn corners, thus enabling them to fold and take up the compact shape seen in the tetrameric molecule. Within the tetramer individual polypeptide chains have only a limited contact with each other, and there is relatively little interaction between them compared with the forces that maintain their individual secondary and tertiary structures. The individual subunit chains of hemoglobin have similar three-dimensional structures, with analogous helical segments. Eight helical regions (A–H) are present in the β chain and seven in α, which lacks a region corresponding to the β-chain D helix. Amino acids can thus be identified with specific helical positions.

The interiors of the subunits are made up almost entirely of nonpolar (hydrophobic) residues, which contact neighboring residues by low-energy, short-range (van der Waals) forces. All the side chains that are ionizable under normal physiological conditions are on the surface of the subunits, as are most of the polar (hydrophilic) side groups. The exterior surface of hemoglobin is thus covered with polar groups that generally interact with water rather than other hydrophilic groups.

Oxygen Binding

Binding of oxygen to hemoglobin is mediated by the prosthetic group, heme, a ferroporphyrin molecule in which the iron atom is located at the centre of the porphyrin ring (Fig.

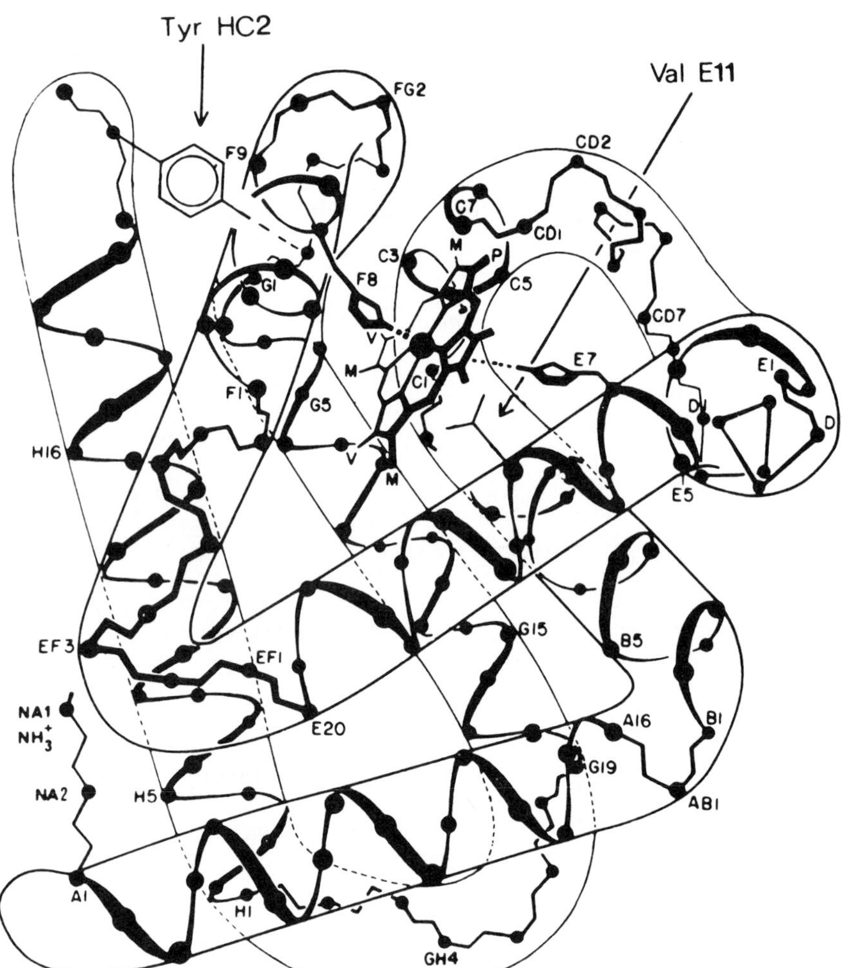

FIG. 113-2 The α-globin subunit showing the structure and relationships of the heme pocket.

113-2). The heme is situated within clefts in the globin subunits that are lined with nonpolar residues and lies between two histidines, one of which (the "proximal histidine") is bonded directly to the heme iron atom through the nitrogen atom of its imidazole group, while the other, or "distal" histidine, lies opposite the oxygen-binding site, but is not directly attached to the heme (see Fig. 113-2). The orientation of the heme within the pocket allows its nonpolar vinyl groups to be buried within the hydrophobic interior while the polar proprionic acid groups reside on the hydrophilic surface of the globin subunit. A large number of interatomic contacts (<4 Å) between the heme and side chains of amino acid residues of the E and F helices stabilize this structure.

The residues that surround the heme group are invariant throughout the animal kingdom, suggesting a highly conservative structure that is essential if it is to function normally as an oxygen carrier. Indeed, hemoglobin variants with mutations in the heme pocket often show profound alterations in their stability or oxygen-binding properties.

There is a marked difference in the three-dimensional structures of the oxy- and deoxy-forms of hemoglobin, implying that the subunit chains change their relative orientation with respect to each other during oxygenation and *vice versa*. In the tetramer each α chain is in contact with the two β chains; the two contacts can thus be defined as $\alpha_1\beta_1$ and $\alpha_1\beta_2$, and the twofold symmetry generates the structurally identical $\alpha_2\beta_1$ and $\alpha_2\beta_2$ contacts (Fig. 113-3). Most of the movement during oxygenation/deoxygenation takes place at the $\alpha_1\beta_2$ ($\alpha_2\beta_1$) interfaces, while the $\alpha_1\beta_1$ ($\alpha_2\beta_2$) interfaces remain relatively immobile, in keeping with the much greater number of contacts, 40, at the latter interface compared with the 17 at the weaker $\alpha_1\beta_2$ interface.[16]

Good contacts between subunits can be made only when key regions of the two αβ dimers are in the same relative orientation, thus favoring the formation of two specific quarternary states, oxy or "relaxed" (R) and deoxy or "tense" (T), without any stable intermediates.[17,18] Owing to the movement that occurs at the $\alpha_1\beta_2$ interface, the nature and number of contacts change during oxygen/deoxygenation. In the deoxy (T) state there are about 40 contacts (which include 19 hydrogen bonds), and this drops by almost half (to 22 and 12, respectively) in the oxy (R) state. Not surprisingly, the $\alpha_1\beta_2$ contact, like the heme pocket, is a highly conserved structure, which has remained unchanged through long periods of evolution. Mutations involving residues in this contact can have drastic functional consequences.

Deoxyhemoglobin has a more stable quaternary structure than oxyhemoglobin because of the increased number of contacts at the $\alpha_1\beta_2$ interface, and because there are additional intersubunit and intrasubunit salt linkages that are absent or much weaker in oxyhemoglobin. Thus, the carboxyl group of the C-terminal arginine of one α chain interacts with the ε-amino group of a lysine residue at position 132 (H10) in the other α chain, and the guanidine group of this same C-terminal arginine interacts with the carboxyl group of the aspartic acid residue at position 131 (H9) of the other

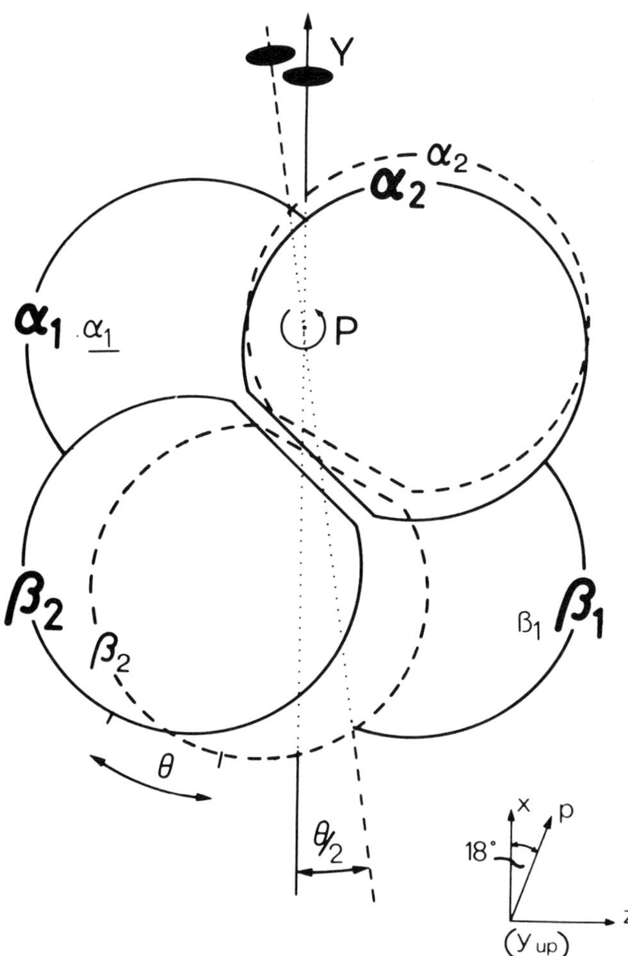

FIG. 113-3 Schematic diagram of quarternary structure of hemoglobin and the relative changes in orientation of the subunits during oxygenation. *Bold*: deoxy; *light*: oxy. *(From Fermi G, Perutz MF:* Haemoglobin and Myoglobin *Oxford University Press. Used by permission.)*

α chain. There is also a chloride ion-mediated link between the C-terminal guanidine group and the opposite α chain's α-NH_2 group. None of these α–α salt linkages can be formed in oxyhemoglobin because of steric hindrance effects.[18] In a similar manner the β chain C-terminal histidines are involved in two interactions—through the imidazole group with the aspartate residue at position 94 (FG1) of the same β chain, and through the carboxyl group with the ε-NH_2 group of lysine α40 (C5) forming a salt bridge that spans the $\alpha_1\beta_2$ interface. In oxyhemoglobin these residues are displaced too far for these interactions to occur, and no salt bridges are formed.

Physiological measurements indicate that there is a free energy change of 10 to 12 kcal per mole of tetramer on the transition of oxy to deoxy states, a figure in accordance with the energy estimated to reside in the salt bridges of 1 to 2 kcal per bond. The salt bridges thus represent a considerable reservoir of stored energy maintaining the deoxyhemoglobin molecule in a high-energy or "tense" (T) state.

Structure–Function Relationships

The role of hemoglobin as oxygen carrier depends on its ability to absorb and release oxygen in response to the relatively small changes in partial pressures encountered under physiological conditions. The function of oxygen bound versus partial pressure is sigmoid, a property that depends crucially on a heterotetrameric structure [it does not occur in monomeric myoglobin or in the homotetrameric hemoglobins H (β_4) and Bart's (γ_4)] and which is achieved by cooperative interactions between the heme groups as the oxygenation at one enhances the subsequent O_2 binding at the others. Hemoglobin thus behaves as an allosteric molecule. In addition, O_2 binding is influenced by the interaction of small molecules such as 2,3-diphosphoglycerate (2,3-DPG) and is sensitive to changes in pH, a phenomenon known as the Bohr effect.

Heme–heme Interaction. The heme–heme interaction that promotes the cooperative binding of oxygen depends on small rearrangements that occur when oxygen is taken up. During oxygenation the β-chain hemes move apart by about 7Å in a process that depends on interactions between the α and β subunits. It is likely that the $\alpha_1\beta_2$ contact is particularly important in these cooperative interactions. The three-dimensional structure indicates that α_1 and β_2 (or α_2 and β_1) subunits can have much more direct interaction than can α_1 and β_1 (or α_2 and β_2). Furthermore, oxygenation of the β_2 subunit causes it to rotate much more with respect to α_1 than does oxygenation of the β_1 subunit. And, as we have seen earlier, the overall structure of the $\alpha_1\beta_2$ contact has remained invariant throughout mammalian evolution. Most hemoglobin variants with abnormalities in heme–heme interactions have mutations in or close to the $\alpha_1\beta_2$ interface.

The molecular origin for the conformational changes that take place in the subunits during oxygenation lies in the heme molecule. When there is no O_2 molecule bound, the atomic diameter of the iron atom is too great to allow it to sit flush in the plane of the porphyrin ring and it is thus displaced 0.6 Å toward the proximal histidine residue. When the heme iron binds oxygen, the resulting changes in the distribution of electrons orbiting the iron atom nucleus lead to an effective reduction in its atomic diameter and it can move into the plane of the porphyrin ring. This movement results in a tilt of the heme into its pocket, and this is amplified as a change in the tertiary structure of the subunit which ultimately pushes the penultimate tyrosine from between the F and H helices, resulting in rupture of the C-terminal salt bridges. The transition of the quaternary structure from the deoxy (T) to oxy (R) conformation occurs abruptly as the salt bridges successively break apart and constraints on the $\alpha_1\beta_2$ interface are relaxed. Since the α subunit hemes are relatively more accessible to oxygen, they are probably oxygenated first. The shift from T to R structure then opens up the clefts of the unliganded β chain hemes, greatly increasing their affinity for oxygen.

Modification of Oxygen-Binding Properties by 2,3-Diphosphoglycerate. Some organic phosphates increase the stability of deoxyhemoglobin. In human erythrocytes the major effector of this type is 2,3-DPG.[19,20] This binds specifically to the β chains of hemoglobin in the T state through electrostatic bonds between the 2,3-DPG phosphate groups and the N-terminal amino and imidazole groups of the β2 and β143 histidine residues and the ε-amino group of β82 lysine.[21] When the structure changes from the T to R state the bound 2,3-DPG molecules are released because the β chain H helices are now too close and the N-terminal amino groups too far apart for the 2,3-DPG to bind. Thus 2,3-DPG and oxygen binding are mutually exclusive, and the overall effect is that 2,3-DPG reduces the oxygen affinity of hemoglobin by stabilizing the deoxy (T) form. The cellular concentration of 2,3-DPG thus has an important influence on oxygen affinity. Differences in oxygen affinity between fetal and adult red cells are largely due to the fact that 2,3-DPG has only a weak affinity for deoxyhemoglobin F.[22,23]

Bohr Effect. The binding of oxygen to hemoglobin is sensitive to changes in pH, a phenomenon that has physiological importance through its effect on the transport of CO_2 in the blood. Carbon dioxide released on respiration is too insoluble to be transported in any quantity in the blood except as bicarbonate ion, produced by reaction with water:

$$CO_2 + H_2O \rightarrow HCO_3^- + H^+$$

The released protons can combine with hemoglobin, forcing the reaction toward bicarbonate formation. Protons stabilize the deoxy (T) state of the hemoglobin molecule, thus favoring oxygen release in the tissues. On oxygen binding (in the lungs) the converse occurs. Protons are released, driving the bicarbonate–CO_2 reaction toward CO_2 formation and thus release from the blood. The Bohr effect therefore mediates a reciprocal CO_2–O_2 exchange.[16,24,25]

Hemoglobin is also responsible for the direct transport of about 10 percent of respired CO_2 through the formation of a carbamate linkage with the N-terminal amino groups. Since CO_2 binds more readily to the deoxy form, this again facilitates the removal of CO_2 from the circulation.

Hemoglobin Genes

Organization and Chromosomal Location. Six different types of globin chain (α, β, γ, δ, ϵ, and ζ) are found in normal human hemoglobins at different stages of development, thus requiring a minimum of six different structural genes.[25] Genetic analyses of families in which abnormal Hb variants were segregating established that the α- and β-globin genes are on separate chromosomes, and that it was likely that the fetal and adult non-α genes were present in a single cluster. The relationships between the amino acid sequences of the ζ and α chains, and ϵ, γ, δ, and β chains suggested that they had arisen by successive duplications and divergences of ancestral genes.

The localization of these groups of genes to specific chromosomes was achieved by the use of hybrid rodent–human somatic cell lines containing one or a few human chromosomes. The α gene cluster was found on chromosome 16, and the β-like genes on chromosome 11[26–28] (see Fig. 113-1). These assignments have been refined by *in situ* hybridization studies and by gene mapping of cell lines containing different translocations and deletions. Such analyses place the β-like cluster distal to band p14 on the short arm of chromosome 11,[29–33] and the α-like cluster in band 16p13.3 at the tip of chromosome 16.[34,35]

Restriction enzyme mapping of genomic DNA coupled with fine structure mapping of cloned DNA from the globin gene complexes on chromosomes 11 and 16 has enabled a very detailed picture to be built up of the precise chromosomal organization of the two complexes. The conclusions that had been reached by conventional genetic and structural analyses of hemoglobin variants have been vindicated by the molecular analyses, and in addition the loci for the embryonic ζ and ϵ genes have been found to be linked to the clusters containing the adult genes (see Fig. 113-1).[36–38]

Unexpectedly, other genes or gene-like structures, unsuspected prior to these molecular analyses, and with considerable structural homology to the "real" genes have been identified within the clusters, one ($\psi\beta$[39,40]) between the $^A\gamma$ and γ genes and no fewer than four ($\psi\zeta1$,[41] $\psi\alpha1$,[38] $\psi\alpha2$,[42] and $\theta1$[43]) in the α cluster (see Fig. 113-1). With the exception of $\theta1$ these (nonfunctional) genes are designated pseudogenes and are thought to be relics of past evolutionary changes within the globin gene clusters. The conserved structure of $\theta1$ and the fact that it contains no inactivating mutations, suggests that it may be functional. However, no protein product has been identified, and protein structural considerations indicate that the predicted protein could not form a viable globin.[44] The role of $\theta1$ is thus at present enigmatic.

Several regions of the α (but not β) cluster contain highly polymorphic tandemly repeated segments of DNA [hypervariable regions (HVR), variable number of tandem repeats (VNTR) varying from a few to hundreds of repeat units. Both α and β clusters contain *Alu*-family elements, some of which are polymorphic at their 3′ ends. References to more detailed descriptions of these structural aspects of the globin genes are given in the caption to Fig. 113-1.

Evolution. By comparing the nucleotide sequences of the genes and using estimates of the average rates of nucleotide substitution derived from species comparisons, it is possible to establish an evolutionary history for the human globin genes. Various estimates put the time of α and β gene divergence from a single ancestral gene at approximately 450 million years (my) ago, during early vertebrate evolution.[5,45] In birds and mammals the α and β gene clusters subsequently became established on different chromosomes. The ζ-α gene split was probably the most ancient of the subsequent duplications,[46] followed by β/γ at 200 my, and γ/ϵ at 100 my.[45] The δ/β divergence appears at 40 my, although this is probably the time of a gene conversion following on from a much more ancient duplication event.[47] Duplication of the α genes, like the ζ-α split appears to have been a relatively early event while the γ duplication is more recent, with the subsequent near-identity of the two α genes and two γ genes being maintained by rounds of gene conversion. From this history it can be inferred that developmental patterns of hemoglobin synthesis have changed considerably during evolution, presumably a reflection in part on the changing physiological and environmental circumstances that hemoglobin has had to respond to.

It can be seen from Fig. 113-1 that the globin genes are arranged in the order in which they are expressed during development and are all in the same transcriptional orientation. The significance of this, which is a feature of many (but not all, chicken and goat are exceptions) animal species, in terms of the changes in gene expression that take place during development is at present unclear.

Individual Variation of Globin Gene Structure. The effort involved in producing very fine structure (down to the nucleotide level) maps of the globin gene clusters has been considerable. Consequently, most of the sequence information available has come from intensive analyses of just one or two chromosomes, and it gives little indication of the variation that might be found if large numbers of individuals were to be studied. The initial indications that sequence variations might be relatively common came from the work of Jeffreys[48] who found two *Hin*dIII polymorphisms in the γ genes of a number of individuals and estimated that perhaps 1 percent of nucleotide sites might be polymorphic. Subsequent studies have shown many such polymorphisms throughout the globin gene clusters. Some of these are common and present in all racial groups while others may have a much more restricted distribution.

Of particular interest and importance is the fact that in general the polymorphisms do not normally occur in association with each other in a random fashion, rather they are present in linked groups called haplotypes[49,50] (Fig. 113-4). Within any given population there are usually a small number of common haplotypes and a larger number of rarer ones, only some of which are clearly related to the more common types, for example, by a difference at a single site. The frequency and types of haplotype present in various populations can provide some interesting insights into racial affinities and evolution.[50–54] At a more practical level, the fact that haplotypes exist at all implies that within the region defined by the restriction enzyme cleavage sites comprising the haplotype, there has been little if any recombination between chromosomes (since, if there had been, the nonrandom association between polymorphic sites would have been destroyed). The knowledge that these chromosome arrangements are relatively stable has thus enabled the polymorphisms comprising the various haplotypes to be used in linkage analysis of hereditary disorders affecting globin genes. For example, establishing the particular haplotype carrying a β thalassemia defect enables the affected chromosome to be followed within a pedigree, and it can also be used for prenatal diagnostic purposes by analysis of DNA from fetuses at risk.[55–57]

Although the features of the α- and β-like gene clusters noted in Fig. 113-1 are the norm, many examples are now known of individuals with various rearrangements within the clusters, most of which have little or no phenotypic effects of clinical significance. Most often seen are the variations in copy number of genes that are usually duplicated (or have an associated, nearly identical, pseudogene such as ζ). Thus, many individuals with triplicated ζ,[58] γ,[59] and α[60] genes have been documented, and even quadruplicate α and γ arrangements are known. Likewise, there are numerous examples of single ζ,[58] that is, lacking ψζ, α,[61,62] and γ[63] gene chromosomes that have probably arisen through unequal crossing-over events. While most of these rearrangements are found at very low frequency in most populations, the single α-gene chromosomes are extremely common in many tropical countries because they appear to be at a selective advantage in malarial environments[64,65] (see below).

Rare cases of homogenization of the $^{G}\gamma$ or $^{A}\gamma$ genes, to form $^{G}\gamma$-$^{G}\gamma$ or $^{A}\gamma$-$^{A}\gamma$ arrangements[66] and of ψζ by ζ to form a ζ-ζ arrangement,[67] are also known, possibly the result of localized gene conversion events.

Structural Features of Globin Genes. Since 1977 it has been apparent that the coding regions of most mammalian genes, and globin genes are no exception, are interrupted by stretches of noncoding DNA, usually referred to as "intervening sequence" or "intron" DNA. All globin genes possess two introns in identical positions relative to the coding sequence but of variable length, the shortest being the first intron (IVS1) of the α genes at 117 bp and the largest of 1264 bp in IVS1 of the ζ gene. The fact that introns are found in identical positions in all globin genes suggests that they were in place before the expansion of the globin gene repertoire from an ancestral gene took place. Molecular sequence analysis of the β-like genes reveals little or no homology among the larger IVS2 introns except in the case of the duplicated $^{G}\gamma$ and $^{A}\gamma$ genes, and variable homology among the small IVS1 introns. Within the α-like genes, the duplicated α1 and α2 genes show considerable homology between IVS1 and IVS2 of those genes, but very little with the linked upstream ζ gene or the ψζ gene.

Comparisons of the sequences of introns from many different genes reveal only a few common features, most notably in the sequences immediately adjacent to and around the coding sequences they interrupt[68] and a sequence 20 to 40 bases from the 3′ end involved in the formation of the branched splicing intermediate. Intron sequences are removed (spliced out) of the initial precursor mRNA transcript in order to form the final mature mRNA product and the necessary signals for correct splicing reside at the 5′ (consensus sequence $^{C}_{A}$AG ↓ GU $^{A}_{G}$AGU) and 3′ (consensus $^{U}_{C}$ X $^{C}_{U}$AG ↓ G) ends of the introns.[69] The importance of these sequences is illustrated by the fact that mutations within them can interfere, or even abolish, correct splicing leading to abnormal processing of globin mRNA precursors, the molecular basis of a number of the thalassemias (see below).

The regions flanking the coding sequences of globin genes contain a number of sequence motifs that are necessary for correct expression[25,70] (see Fig. 113-1*B*). The first of these is the ATA box, which serves to locate accurately the site of transcription initiation at the "cap" site, usually about 30 bases downstream, and which also appears to influence the level of transcription. Natural mutations within the ATA region can reduce transcription quite markedly (see later section). Seventy or eighty base pairs upstream is a second conserved sequence, the CCAAT box (in δ the sequence is CCAAC and the γ genes have a duplicated structure). In

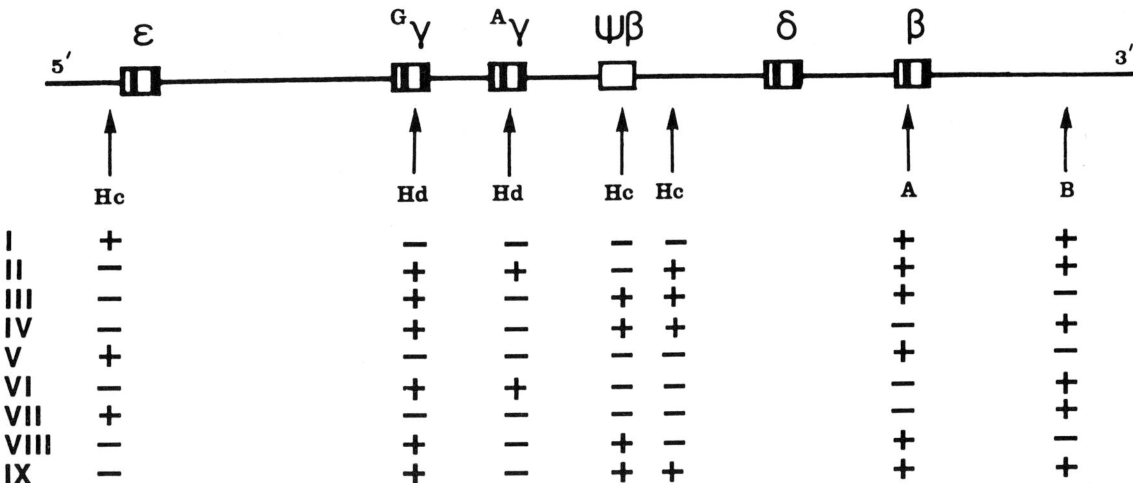

FIG. 113-4 Polymorphic restriction enzyme sites in the human β-globin complex and nine of the common haplotypes derived from them.

model systems, mutations introduced into CCAAT sequences also lead to reductions in the level of transcription.[71] Further 5′, approximately 80 to 100 bp from the cap site is a GC-rich region with general structure GGGG$^{T}_{C}$G or C$^{A}_{G}$CCCC, which can be inverted and/or duplicated. These sequences resemble those required for optimal transcription of the simian virus 40 (SV40) early region, and mutations with this region in β-globin genes adversely affect expression.[72,73]

Other nonglobin mammalian genes contain similar conserved sequences upstream of the mRNA cap sites, each of which has been shown to be necessary for normal gene expression, presumably because they provide binding sites for transcription factors which influence the rate of interaction of transcription by RNA polymerase II. In vitro experiments involving modification or deletion of the sequences are consistent with this, and natural mutations within them may result in decreased expression of the associated gene (see below).

Globin Gene Expression. The mechanism of protein synthesis in eukaryotes has been elucidated in considerable detail (for reviews see references 25, 70, 74, and 75). In this section, only the aspects of globin gene expression that are particularly relevant to the molecular basis of the hemoglobinopathies are considered.[25,70]

Transcription of the globin genes initiates at the cap site, which is ~50 bp upstream of the AUG initiation codon, and which becomes the 5′ end of the mature mRNA after processing. Although mature mRNA terminates 10 to 20 bp downstream of the AATAAA polyadenylation signal, there is evidence from in vitro studies that the initial transcript may extend beyond this site and that the specific cleavage distal to the polyadenylation signal takes place subsequently. Supporting this is evidence from a case of β thalassemia with a mutation in the AATAAA sequence,[76] in which elongated β gene transcripts were observed in RNA isolated from erythroid cells of the affected individual, and in vitro experiments on a similar case of α thalassemia.[77]

The large initial precursor mRNA transcript is rapidly processed after synthesis. The first events, capping the 5′ end and polyadenylation of the 3′ end, probably serve to stabilize the transcript and prevent attack by exonucleases. Capping involves a GTP-mediated modification of the 5′ residue, usually an A or G, to form a 5′ppp5′ linkage, while *polyadenylation*, as the term implies, results in the addition of a long string of A residues (>50) to the 3′ end of the transcript formed by cleavage of the initial precursor 10 to 20 bp downstream of the AATAAA signal.

Subsequent to these steps the intervening sequences are removed from the pre-mRNA in a two-stage process. In the first, pre-mRNA is cut at the 5′ splice site to generate two intermediates, a linear first exon and a branched lariat-type molecule containing the intron and second exon. In the second step, the 3′ splice site is cleaved, the lariat intron released, and the two exons joined.[69] Introns may be removed in a sequential manner until the mature mRNA is produced. This is then transported from the nucleus into the cytoplasm, where ribosomal translation of mRNA into globin can take place. The details of the translational phase of protein synthesis are well known and have been extensively reviewed.[74,75] The synthesis of globin closely follows the pattern of other eukaryotic proteins; indeed many aspects of the general mechanism were elucidated with cell-free systems synthesizing rabbit globins.

Regulation of Globin Gene Expression. Experimental work has begun to dissect the important elements involved in both tissue-specific and developmental-stage-specific regulation of gene expression from the two globin gene complexes. It is clear that this involves critical regulatory sequences around and within the genes themselves as well as at the 5′ end of each gene cluster. These sequences interact with a number of transcriptional factors, some of which have a ubiquitous tissue distribution while others are more or less erythroid-cell restricted. An outline of current understanding of globin gene regulation is given below; more detailed reviews can be found in Evans et al.[78] and Stamatoyannopoulos and Nienhuis.[79]

β-Globin Locus Control Region and α-Globin Hypersensitivity Site 40 kb Upstream of the ζ Globin Gene (Fig. 113-5). Transfection of human α- or β-globin genes into mouse erythroleukemia cells and analysis of their expression in stable cell lines has demonstrated variable, but generally

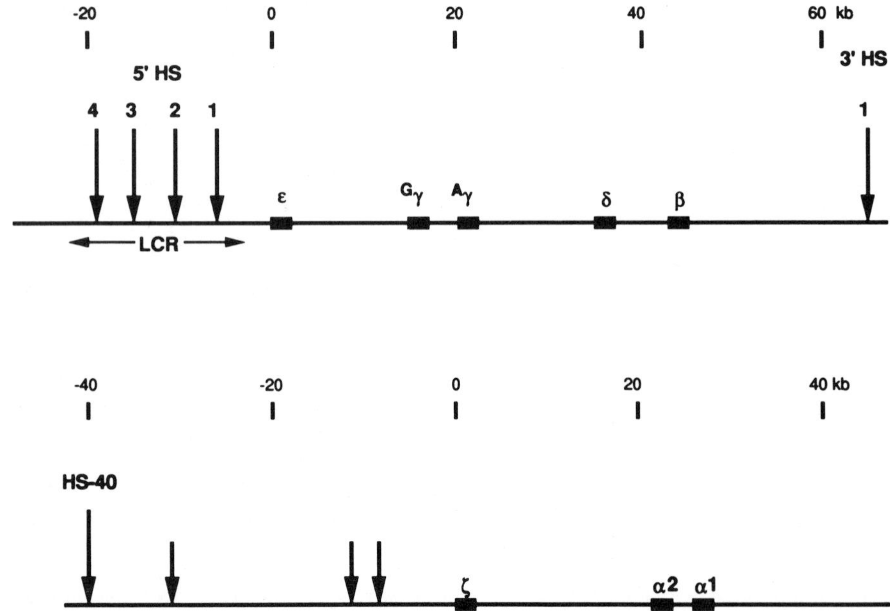

FIG. 113-5 Location of the erythroid-specific DNase I hypersensitive sites in the human α- and β-globin gene complexes. The major regulatory regions, the β locus control region and α hypersensitivity site 40 kb upstream of the ζ globin gene are indicated.

low, levels of expression which appear to depend on the site of their integration into the mouse chromosomes.[80,81] Similar results were obtained when human γ or β genes were injected into fertilized mouse eggs and expression analyzed in the resulting transgenic mice; human globin mRNA was either undetectable or present at low levels.[82,83] In most cases, expression was confined to erythroid cells, suggesting that the sequences around the genes contained elements important in tissue specificity. Furthermore, both the γ and β genes showed developmental-stage specificity, the fetal γ gene being transcribed during the embryonic stage of erythropoiesis in the mouse (which lacks a true fetal hemoglobin), while the adult β gene was expressed only in postembryonic erythroid cells.[84,85] Again, this suggests that information relating to the appropriate time of gene expression is contained within the sequences in and around the genes themselves.

In these experiments high-level expression of human genes was achieved only when they were attached to a 20-kb region immediately upstream of the ε-globin gene.[86] This region, now known as the β-globin locus control region (LCR), is marked by four sites which are hypersensitive (HS) to digestion with DNase I but only in erythroid cells.[87,88] Two of these sites are capable of subsuming much of the LCR function on their own but the whole region is necessary for maximum effect.[89] The LCR confers high-level, tissue-specific expression on attached genes (globin or heterologous) and shows copy-number dependence to some degree. The importance of this region has been confirmed by analysis of patients in whom the LCR is deleted, but the globin genes have been spared; there is no expression from globin genes on chromosomes carrying LCR deletions[90] (see below).

Deletions of a region upstream of the α-globin genes also result in lack of expression from the genes *cis* to the lesion, indicating that there is an equivalent LCR in the α-globin gene cluster.[91,92] Experimental analysis in transfected cell lines and transgenic mice have suggested that the region around a DNase I hypersensitive site 40 kb upstream of the ζ-globin gene (HS-40) is the major regulator of the α-globin gene expression.[93,94] Other erythroid-specific hypersensitive sites, as well as several constitutive sites have been found in this region but as yet have not been shown to affect expression levels, either alone or in combination with HS-40.

Sequence analysis of the hypersensitive sites, combined with binding studies using nuclear protein extracts (in vitro "footprinting"), have demonstrated that each region is rich in sequence motifs which form the recognition sites for the binding of various proteins involved in transcription. The β LCR 5′ HSs 2, 3, and 4, as well as α HS-40 have binding sites for two proteins, GATA-1 and NFE-2, whose tissue distribution is limited largely to erythroid cells, as well as sites for other less well characterized erythroid-restricted proteins. In addition, these regions, which span a few hundred base pairs, contain multiple binding sites for ubiquitously expressed transcription factors. It appears that cooperative activity between the proteins bound at these sites is necessary for full function of the region.

Chromatin Structure In nonerythroid cells, the β-globin cluster exists in a chromatin structure which is insensitive to digestion with DNase I whereas in erythroid cells the whole region is in a more open conformation which is more readily susceptible to DNase I digestion.[95] In addition to the hypersensitive sites which mark the LCR, the promoter regions at the 5′ end of the genes also display hypersensitive sites; in fetal liver these sites are found in front of the $^{G}\gamma$, $^{A}\gamma$, δ and β genes, while in adult bone marrow the γ gene sites are no longer present.[96] The LCR seems to be an essential element in setting up this chromatin structure, since in somatic-erythroid-cell hybrids containing a chromosome 11 with most of the LCR deleted, the whole region around the β-globin gene cluster is DNase I–insensitive and the remaining DNase hypersensitive sites are no longer present.[96] Furthermore, while in hybrids containing a normal chromosome 11 the β-globin cluster replicates in early S phase of the cell cycle, this region becomes late replicating when the LCR is absent, as is the case for the normal chromosome in nonerythroid cells.

There are marked differences in the structures of the α and β complexes. The α gene cluster lies in a GC-rich region, contains several CpG islands and, unlike the β gene complex, has no potential sites for binding to the nuclear matrix.[97] However, like the β gene complex, the α gene region is more sensitive to DNase I digestion in erythroid cells as compared with nonerythroid cells,[98] although the presence of constitutive DNase I hypersensitive sites within the cluster suggest that its chromatin structure may be less tightly compacted in nonerythroid cells than that of the β gene complex. In addition to the upstream DNase hypersensitive sites, the α gene cluster also has hypersensitive sites at the 5′ end of the genes when they are expressed. Interestingly, four other genes have been detected in the region at the 5′ end of the α gene cluster, all of which are expressed in a wide variety of different cell types, and the major regulatory region of the α genes, HS-40, actually lies in the intron of one of these genes. The significance of these observations and their relationship to the concept that the α and β gene clusters might lie in distinct regulatory "domains" has been discussed.[99]

Methylation. The role of DNA methylation, the only known chemical modification of DNA, in the regulation of gene expression, is still unclear. The methylation of cytosine residues in CpG dinucleotides is frequently associated with inactive genes, although whether this relationship is causal or a secondary response to gene repression is unclear. The β-globin gene cluster is extensively methylated in nonerythroid cells, while the pattern of methylation in erythroid cells varies with stages of development.[100] In embryonic erythroblasts, the ε gene is unmethylated while the $^{G}\gamma$,$^{A}\gamma$ and β genes remain methylated. This situation is reversed in fetal liver erythroblasts, where both γ and β genes are active, while in adult bone marrow, the γ genes become remethylated and the β gene remains unmethylated.

In the α-globin gene cluster the expressed genes themselves show little or no methylation in any tissue. This is in keeping with other CpG-rich areas and is also compatible with the concept that the α-globin gene complex has a more open conformation in nonerythroid cells than the β genes.

Trans-acting factors. Protein–DNA interactions are of major importance in the regulation of tissue-specific gene expression and may well be critical in the differential expression of genes within clusters at different developmental stages. Erythroid cells contain general transcription factors common to all cell types but in addition, contain DNA-binding proteins with a very restricted tissue distribution. The best characterized of these is GATA-1,[101–103] found in megakaryocytes and mast cells as well as erythroid cells, and a member of a family of at least three proteins recognizing the consensus sequence (T/A)GATA(A/G). The other members, GATA-2 and GATA-3, are also expressed in erythroid cells, albeit at lower levels than GATA-1, but have a wider tissue distribution.[104] The GATA-1 protein regulates expression of its own gene as well as a wide range of erythroid-specific genes. In mice, it shows higher levels in fetal and adult erythroid cells than in embryonic erythroblasts, and it has also been shown to increase in amount during erythroid differentiation.[105] Its major role in erythroid cell development has been demonstrated in chimeric mice produced by injecting blastocysts with embryonic stem (ES) cells from which the GATA-1 was deleted. Chimeric mice showed variable anemia (leading to fetal death in some cases) and while the ES cells contributed 15 to 50 percent of the cells in most tissues, no detectable erythroid cells were derived from these cells.[106]

Other erythroid-restricted *trans*-acting factors include NFE-2, a protein which binds to sequences similar to those recognized by AP1, the heterodimer product of the *jun* and *fos* oncogenes. Binding sites for NFE-2 are found in the β LCR HS 2 and 4, αHS-40 as well as in the regulatory regions of other erythroid genes. Deletion or mutation of the NFE-2 sites generally leads to significant reduction in gene expression in experimental systems.

It is clear that *trans*-acting factors play a major role in determining tissue-specific gene expression, but their role in developmental gene regulation has yet to be clarified. Several lines of evidence suggest that they play a critical role in the selection of genes for expression. In chicks, a protein which binds to the β-globin gene promoter is found in extracts from adult erythroid nuclei but not in nuclear extracts from embryonic cells, a stage at which the β gene is not expressed.[107] Heterokaryons formed between erythroid and nonerythroid cells or between erythroid cells expressing different globin genes can result in the induction of previously silent globin genes. In the K562 cell line, the β-globin genes are inactive, yet they are fully functional when transferred to other erythroid cell lines by cell fusion.[108] Conversely, normal β genes transferred to K562 are inactive. This suggests that K562 cells either lack an essential *trans*-activating factor or contain a suppressor of β-globin gene expression. Several families have been described who have an X-linked syndrome of mental retardation and α thalassemia (see "α Thalassemia Associated with Mental Retardation" below). Considerable down-regulation of α gene expression is observed from both chromosomes 16, yet they function normally after fusion with mouse erythroleukemia cells.[109] Since the β-globin genes remain unaffected it appears that the X chromosome encodes a gene with a specific role in α-globin gene expression. Finally, a number of genetic disorders involving expression of the β-globin gene cluster have been described which do not segregate with the gene cluster, again suggesting that a gene-specific *trans*-acting factor is involved.

As yet, no developmental stage–specific or gene-specific *trans*-acting factor has been identified in any mammalian globin gene system, and the determination of whether such factors play the major role in developmental selection of gene expression has yet to be established.

Developmental Changes in Globin Gene Expression. The pattern of Hb synthesis changes during development. In the very early embryo Hb synthesis is restricted to the yolk sac and the production of Hbs Gower 1 ($\zeta_2\epsilon_2$) and Gower 2 ($\alpha_2\epsilon_2$) and Portland ($\zeta_2\gamma_2$). Subsequently, at about 8 weeks of gestation, the fetal liver takes over, synthesising predominantly Hb F ($\alpha_2\gamma_2$)and a small amount (<10 percent) of Hb A. Between about 18 weeks and birth, liver is progressively replaced by bone marrow as the major site of red-cell production, and this is accompanied in the later stages of gestation with a reciprocal switch in production of Hbs F and A, which continues, until by the end of the first year Hb F production has dropped to less than 2 percent (Fig. 113-6).

The mechanism by which fetal erythroid cells switch from the production of Hb F to Hb A remains elusive and has been (and still is) the subject of a considerable research effort, not only for its own intrinsic interest, but also because of the important therapeutic implications that would arise from the ability to manipulate the switching process.

In humans, the switch from Hb F to Hb A production seems to be closely related to the gestational age of the fetus and largely independent of environmental factors. Experiments in sheep (which provide a good model system with close developmental parallels to humans) have shown

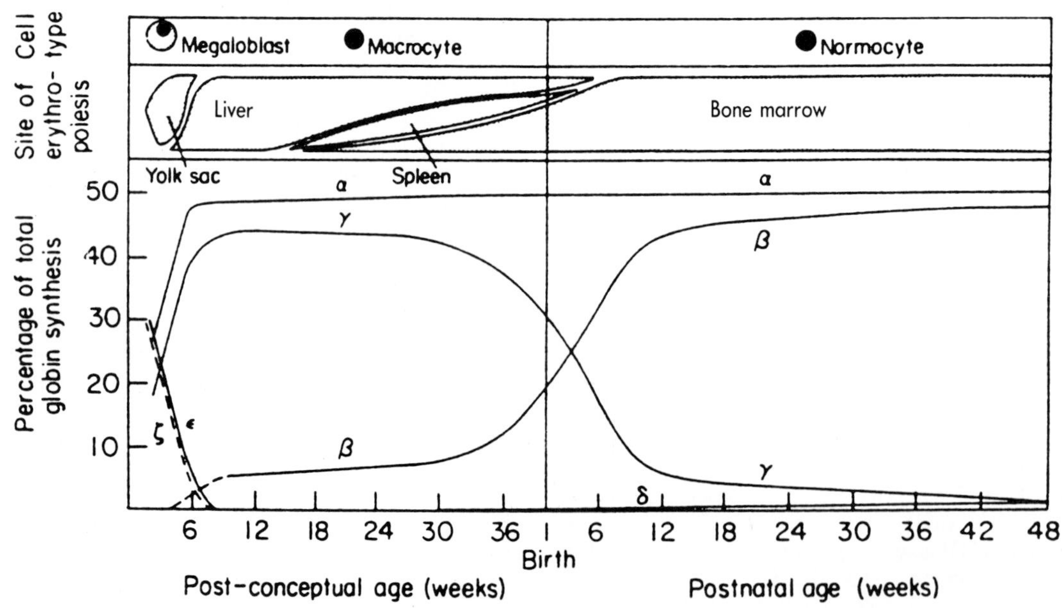

FIG. 113-6 **Globin synthesis at various stages of embryonic and fetal development.**

that while various treatments, such as fetal hypophysectomy in the lamb, may alter the *rate* at which the developmental changes occur, they do not affect the *time* of switching.[110]

Similarly, transplantation experiments involving the introduction of fetal (liver) cells into lethally irradiated adult animals show that the pattern of hemoglobin synthesis in the treated adults is that expected of a fetus of the same age as the donor cells, with switching to the production of adult hemoglobin only at the appropriate time.[111] The reverse experiments, transplanting adult cells into a fetus *in utero*, showed continued production of adult Hb in the fetal environment, until the appropriate time for switching, when the fetus began producing its own adult Hb.[112] These observations provide evidence for preprogrammed globin gene expression that is not appreciably affected by environmental changes. However, it has been found that infants of diabetic mothers show a delayed pattern of hemoglobin switching, possibly due to butyric acid. Injection of butyric acid analogues into fetal sheep *in utero* can delay switching.[113] Thus, environmental factors may play a role in fine tuning the time of switching.

The use of transgenic mouse models has enabled a start to be made in dissecting the processes which govern the developmental regulation of the globin genes. The β LCR and α HS-40 regions are essential for high-level expression of all the genes in their respective complexes, but it is not clear whether they play a determinant role in selective gene expression at different stages of development. The embryonic ζ and ε genes appear to be autonomously regulated; the ε gene alone, or attached to the β LCR is only expressed during the embryonic period of erythropoiesis in transgenic mice.[114] A similar situation appears to apply to γ gene or LCR-γ gene constructs in transgenic mice, at least when they are present in only one to two copies.[115] The adult β gene is developmentally regulated in transgenic mice in the absence of the β LCR but is expressed at all stages of development in the presence of the LCR and in the absence of the other β-like genes. Developmental regulation of the β gene is restored in mice carrying larger LCR-γ-β constructs, suggesting that there may be competition between the γ and β genes which is necessary for down-regulatory β gene transcription during early developmental stages.[116,117] However, there is evidence that the organization of the genes in such constructs, their distance from the LCR, and their order, for example, affects their pattern of expression.[118] Therefore, caution must be exercised in the interpretation of experiments using artificial gene constructs, often present in multiple tandem arrays in these transgenic mice.

In the α gene complex, no expression of the genes has been reported in transgenic mice in the absence of HS-40 except when β LCR elements are substituted for HS-40. Embryonic ζ gene expression is restricted to the embryonic phase of erythropoiesis in β LCR-ζ constructs and also shows a similar pattern of transcription in mice bearing HS-40-ζ-α constructs. Both mouse and human α-globin genes are expressed at the earliest stages of erythropoiesis in these transgenic mice.

At this stage therefore, our understanding of the developmental regulation of globin genes is extremely limited. It is clear that the overall organization of the complexes is important, and it is likely that sequences specifying developmental stage–specific expression lie in the vicinity of the genes, but the role of the upstream regulatory regions, the importance of *trans*-acting factors, and the possible effects of developmentally induced modifications of the complexes have yet to be clarified.

Table 113-1 Genetic Disorders of Hemoglobin

Structural hemoglobin variants
α Chain
β Chain
γ Chain
δ Chain
Fusion chains
δβ
βδ
γβ
Thalassemias
α Thalassemia
β Thalassemia
δβ Thalassemia
γδβ Thalassemia
γ Thalassemia
δ Thalassemia
Hereditary persistence of fetal hemoglobin
Deletion
Nondeletion
Linked to β-globin gene cluster
Unlinked to β-globin gene cluster

CLASSIFICATION OF HEMOGLOBIN DISORDERS

The main groups of hemoglobin disorders are summarized in Table 113-1. They are divided into those in which there is a structural change in a globin chain and those in which there is a reduced rate of production of one or more of the globin chains–the thalassemias. In addition, there is a group of conditions characterized by a defect in the normal switching of fetal to adult hemoglobin production, known collectively as hereditary persistence of fetal hemoglobin. Although the latter are of no clinical significance, they are useful models for studying the regulation of gene switching during development.

Although offering a useful conceptual framework on which to describe the hemoglobin disorders this classification is not entirely satisfactory. In particular, there is an overlap between the structural hemoglobin variants and the thalassemias; some abnormal hemoglobins are produced at a reduced rate and are associated with the clinical phenotype of thalassemia.

It should be remembered that in many populations there is a high incidence of structural hemoglobin variants and different forms of thalassemia. It is not uncommon therefore for an individual to have inherited more than one genetic determinant for a hemoglobin variant and/or different forms of thalassemia. In some countries these interactions produce a bewildering collection of genetic disorders of hemoglobin production with widely varying clinical phenotypes; in Thailand, for example, over 60 different combinations have been observed.[2]

STRUCTURAL HEMOGLOBIN VARIANTS

Extensive population studies using hemoglobin electrophoresis and analyses of the hemoglobin of patients with specific hematologic conditions have led to the discovery of over 400 structural hemoglobin variants. In this section only abnormal hemoglobins associated with clinical disorders will be described in detail. Complete lists of the human hemoglobin variants together with their structural alterations and functional properties are listed in a monograph on the subject.[3]

Nomenclature

When the first hemoglobin variants were described after the discovery of sickle cell hemoglobin in 1949[8] they were designated by letters of the alphabet. By the late 1950s all the letters of the alphabet had been used up and it became customary to name a new hemoglobin by its place of origin. As pointed out by Bunn and Forget[3] there is no consistent usage. Names range from the exotic (Hb_{AIDA}), through the chauvinistic ($Hb_{BRIGHAM}$) or parochial ($Hb_{RIVERDALE\text{-}BRONX}$) to the patriotic ($Hb_{ABRAHAM\ LINCOLN}$); they could also have added the poetic ($Hb_{CONSTANT\ SPRING}$).

Although for many years there have been no formal recommendations for nomenclature of the abnormal hemoglobins, certain conventions are observed in the hemoglobin literature. Heterozygotes for hemoglobin variants are usually described as having the trait–for example, sickle cell trait, Hb C trait. Homozygotes are described as having the "disease," e.g., sickle cell disease, Hb C disease, Hb D disease. In fact, with the exception of the three β-globin variants that occur at polymorphic frequencies in many populations—Hbs S, C, and E—the homozygous states for other β chain variants are extremely rare and have usually been encountered in consanguineous marriages.[3] Individuals who inherit a different β-globin chain variant from each parent, that is compound heterozygotes, are described as having SC, SD, or SE disease, and so on. Similarly, a person who has inherited a β-globin chain variant such as Hb S from one parent and a β thalassemia gene from the other is said to have Hb S β thalassemia. The homozygous state for α chain variants is also extremely uncommon and, because there are two α-globin genes per haploid genome, such individuals also have hemoglobin A.

There are a number of γ and δ chain variants that result from single amino acid substitutions.[3] Abnormal fetal hemoglobins that contain γ chain variants are usually described after their place of origin, Hb F_{MALTA}, Hb F_{POOLE} for example. The first structural δ chain variant was called Hb A_2' or B_2. Subsequently, they were named after their place of discovery, Hb $A_{2CANADA}$, for example.

Since α chains are shared by Hbs F, A, and A_2 it follows that heterozygotes for α chain variants will have both normal Hbs F, A, and A_2 and variant forms composed of abnormal α chains combined with normal γ, β, and δ chains, respectively. These abnormal fetal and adult hemoglobins are usually named after the α chain variant. For example, individuals heterozygous for the α chain variant Hb $G_{PHILADELPHIA}$ have an abnormal fetal hemoglobin variant, Hb GF ($\alpha_2{}^G\gamma_2$), and an abnormal Hb A_2 called Hb G_2 ($\alpha_2{}^G\delta_2$).

The situation becomes even more complex when an individual is heterozygous for both an α chain variant and a β chain variant. Random association of subunits produces four main hemoglobin species. For instance, an individual who has inherited an α globin variant designated X and a β chain variant Y, would have the following hemoglobins: $\alpha_2^A\beta_2^A$, $\alpha_2^X\beta_2^A$, $\alpha_2^A\beta_2^Y$, and $\alpha_2^X\beta_2^Y$. If the β chain variant was Hb S and the α chain variant Hb G, these hemoglobins would become A, G, S, and SG. Of course things are even more complicated because such individuals also have an abnormal form of Hb A_2 and an abnormal fetal hemoglobin due to the association of abnormal α chains with δ and γ chains. Thus, in adult life they would have six hemoglobins; during the switch from fetal to adult hemoglobin there would be eight!

Molecular Pathology

The majority of the 400 or more human hemoglobin variants that have been isolated to date result from single amino acid substitutions in one of the globin chains. In addition, there are a few variants with either elongated or shortened globin chains or chains that are fusion products, part β and part δ or part β and part γ.

Single Base Substitutions. The single amino acid replacements that are found in the structural hemoglobin variants nearly all result from a single base substitution in the corresponding triplet codon of the particular globin gene. A few variants have amino acid replacements at two different sites on the same subunit. Three of them involve the Hb S substitution. It is believed that they arose either by a new mutation on the β^S gene or by crossing over between the β^S gene and a β gene containing another structural variant.[3]

A total of 2583 single base substitutions are possible for the 140 residues of the α chain and the 146 residues of the β chain.[3] Of these, 1690 would result in an amino acid replacement, but only one third of these would cause a change in charge that would allow the identification of the variant by electrophoresis. Remarkably, about 45 percent of these charged variants have already been discovered. The relatively few known hemoglobin variants with neutral mutations have been discovered because the amino acid substitution has altered the stability of the hemoglobin molecule and hence caused a hemolytic anemia.

Elongated Globin Chain Variants. Ten different elongated globin chain variants have been discovered (Table 113-2). They are caused by either single base substitutions in a chain termination codon, frameshift mutations, or by mutations that cause failure of cleavage of the initiator methionine residue.

The chain termination mutants are all α chain variants in which there is a single base substitution in the chain termination codon UAA[119] (see Fig. 113-6). Thus, instead of coding for "termination" an amino acid is inserted into the growing peptide chain. Messenger RNA that is not normally translated is then read through until another in-phase chain termination codon is reached. The result is an elongated α chain. For example, $Hb_{CONSTANT\ SPRING}$ has an α chain with 31 additional amino acid residues at its C-terminal end. The residue at position 142, next to what is normally the C-terminal arginine

Table 113-2 Hemoglobin Variants with Elongated or Shortened Subunits[3,119–128]

Elongated globin chains	
Chain termination mutations	$Hbs_{CONSTANT\ SPRING,\ ICARIA,\ KOYA\ DORA,\ SEAL\ ROCK}$
Frameshift mutations	$Hbs_{WAYNE,\ SAVERNE,\ TAK,\ CRANSTON}$
Reduplication	Hb_{GRADY}
Persistent *N*-terminal Met	$Hbs_{MARSEILLE,\ S.\ FLORIDA,\ LONG\ ISLAND}$
Shortened globin chains	
Deletions	$Hbs_{LEIDEN,\ LYON,\ FREIBURG,\ GUNN\ HILL,\ MCKEES\ ROCKS}$, and others

residue, is glutamine. This is because of a single base change in the chain termination codon UAA to CAA; the latter codes for glutamine. In fact there is a family of α chain termination variants, all of which differ at position 142 but have identical residues in their elongated portions (Fig. 113-7). These variants all reflect different base substitutions in the chain termination codon. Because $Hb_{CONSTANT\ SPRING}$ and its related family of elongated α-chain variants are all associated with the clinical phenotype of α thalassemia[119] they will be considered further in a later section.

Several elongated hemoglobin variants have been found that appear to result from frameshift mutations. Hb_{WAYNE} is an α-chain variant that has five additional amino acid residues at its C-terminal end.[120] This results from the loss of a single base at codons 138 or 139 that throws the reading frame out of phase and hence generates a completely new sequence. Since the α-chain termination codon is also out of phase,

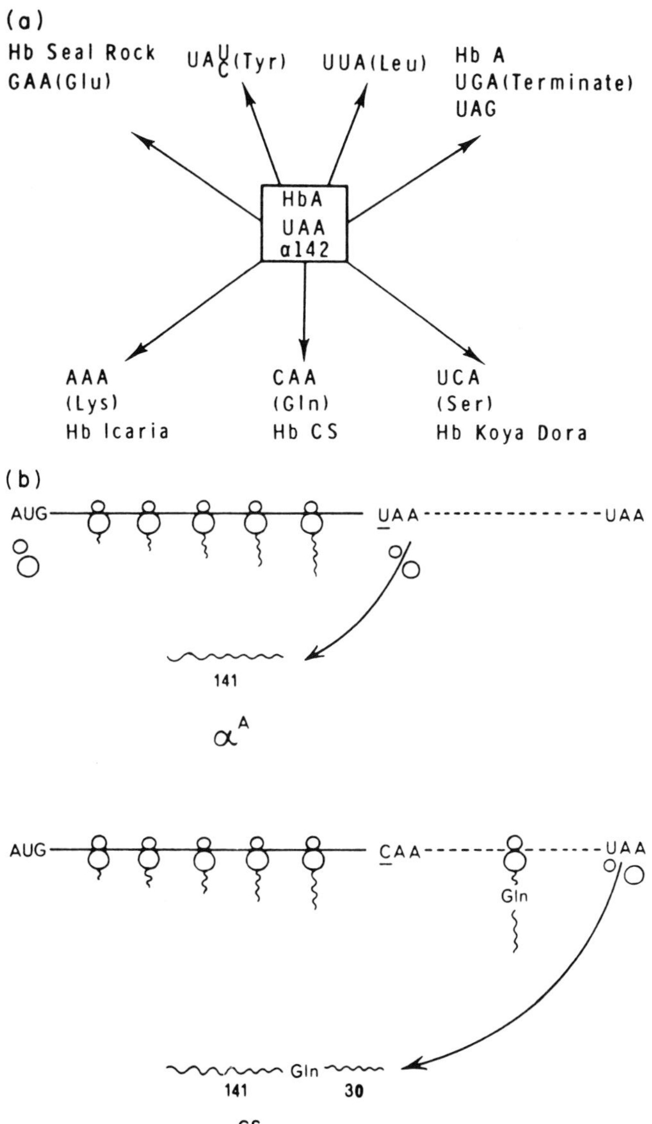

FIG. 113-7 The α-chain termination mutants. *A*. The various replacements in the α-chain termination codon which give rise to the family of termination mutants. *B*. Schematic representation of the synthesis of the elongated α chain of $Hb_{CONSTANT\ SPRING}$ (α^{CS}). *(From Weatherall and Clegg.[2] Used by permission.)*

translation continues until a new in-phase termination codon is reached. The elongated β-globin chain variant Hb_{TAK} also appears to have arisen by a frameshift mutation involving the duplication of two bases—CA, at positions 146/147, or AC, at position 147.[121] Another elongated β-chain variant, $Hb_{CRANSTON}$, has also arisen from a frameshift mutation.[122]

$Hemoglobin_{GRADY}$ has an α chain which is normal in every way except for the insertion of nine bases that result in repetition of the Glu-Phe-Thr sequence at positions 116 to 118.[123] Several mechanisms have been suggested for its generation, including unequal crossing over between allelic α-chain genes or, as seems more likely, the production of a break in a DNA strand, mispairing at an adjacent short repeated dinucleotide sequence, and filling in and repair with the insertion of the additional bases, in this case the in-phase codons for Glu-Phe-Thr.

Several hemoglobin variants with elongated amino terminal ends have been found; in each case there is an additional methionine residue. For example, $Hb_{LONG\ ISLAND}$[124] has two amino acid substitutions in the β chain; an extension of the N-terminus by a methionine residue and a histidine to proline change at the normal second position. Hemoglobin $_{MARSEILLE}$[125] has the same structure, while $Hb_{SOUTH\ FLORIDA}$[126] has an extra N-terminal methionine, and the normal N-terminal valine is replaced by methionine. Methionine is the first residue to be incorporated during translation of globin chains and many other peptide chains. During translation of the nascent peptide chain, the amino terminal methionine is normally cleaved, leaving, in the case of the β-globin chain, valine as the N-terminal residue. It has been suggested that the amino acid substitutions in these variants somehow inhibit the activity of a peptidase that normally cleaves the N-terminal methionine.[124] Thus, they are all single amino acid replacements; the additional N-terminal methionine reflects posttranslational modification.

None of these elongated globin chain variants, with the exception of the α-chain termination mutants, is associated with any major hematologic abnormalities.

Shortened Globin Chains.[3] Several hemoglobin variants with shortened globin chains have been described (see Table 113-2). In each case, one or more adjacent amino acids are missing from the abnormal chains and the remainder of the chain is completely normal. These variants probably involve deletion of one or more intact codons; if an entire codon is lost, the reading frame will remain in-phase and the remainder of the amino acid sequence will not differ from normal. In some cases, $Hb_{GUN\ HILL}$,[127] for example, the deletion results in molecular instability and the clinical picture of an unstable hemoglobin disorder (see "Unstable Hemoglobin Disorders" below). Interestingly, the sequence of globin mRNA in the regions where these deletions have occurred always shows a reiterated nucleotide sequence from two to eight bases in length. These deletion mutants may have arisen by chromosomal mispairing and nonhomologous crossing over in these regions.

One hemoglobin variant with a shortened β chain, $Hb_{MCKEES\ ROCKS}$, may have arisen from a nonsense mutation, that is, a single base change that results in a chain termination codon within the coding region of the β-globin gene.[128] Although, as we shall see later, this is the cause of several forms of β thalassemia, in the case of this variant the premature termination codon is at position 145, thus producing a viable globin chain lacking its two C-terminal residues, tyrosine and histidine.

Fusion Hemoglobins. There are several hemoglobin variants that contain fused or hybrid globin chains. The first to be discovered, Hb_{LEPORE}, contains normal α chains and non–α chains that consist of the first 50 to 80 amino acid residues of the δ chains and the last 60 to 90 residues of the normal C-terminal amino acid sequence of the β chains.[129] Thus the Hb_{LEPORE} non–α chain is a δβ fusion chain. Three different varieties of H_{LEPORE} have been described in which the transition from δ to β sequences occurs at different points.[129–131] $Hemoglobin_{KENYA}$ is analogous except that the abnormal hybrid chain contains γ and β sequences—that is, it is a γβ fusion chain.[132]

The fusion chains have probably arisen by nonhomologous crossing over between part of the δ locus on one chromosome and part of the β locus on the complementary chromosome (Fig. 113-8). This event results from misalignment of chromosome pairing during meiosis so that a δ-chain gene pairs with a β-chain gene instead of its homologous partner. As shown in Fig. 113-8, such a mechanism should give rise to two abnormal chromosomes; the first, the Lepore chromosome, will have no normal δ or β loci but simply a δβ fusion gene. On the opposite of the homologous pairs of chromosomes there should be an anti-Lepore (βδ) fusion gene together with normal δ and β loci. Similarly, in the case of Hb_{KENYA} there should be an anti-Kenya chromosome with intact $^{A}\gamma$, δ, and β loci. A variety of anti-Lepore hemoglobins have been discovered, including Hb_{MIYADA}, $Hb_{P\text{-}CONGO}$, $Hb_{LINCOLN\ PARK}$, and $Hb_{P\text{-}NILOTIC}$.[133–136]

Another variant with fusion chains, $Hb_{PARCHMAN}$, is more complex in that the non–α chain has a δ sequence at the N- and C-terminal ends and a β sequence in the middle. It seems likely that this arose by a double crossover or gene conversion.[137]

The Lepore variants result in the clinical phenotype of β or δβ thalassemia and hence will be considered further in a later section. The anti-Lepore variants and Hb_{KENYA} are not associated with any significant hematologic changes.[2]

Structural Hemoglobin Variants of Clinical Importance

The structural hemoglobin variants that cause clinical disorders are summarized in Table 113-3. The three that reach polymorphic frequencies, and hence cause a major public health problem, are Hbs S, C, and E. The other clinically important variants are much less common. They fall into two major groups. First there are those that alter the oxygen-carrying properties of hemoglobin and result either in hereditary polycythemia or methemoglobinemia. The second group is composed of unstable variants that produce a hemolytic anemia of varying severity. Finally, there are several hemoglobin variants that are ineffectively synthesized and are therefore associated with the clinical phenotype of α or β thalassemia.

Sickling Disorders

Hemoglobin S was the first hemoglobin variant to be discovered[8] and the first to have its amino acid substitution determined.[9] Sickle cell anemia is the cause of considerable mortality and morbidity in Africa, and in every population where there has been migration of individuals of African descent, in parts of the Mediterranean region, and in the Middle East and Indian subcontinent. However, despite the fact that the molecular lesion has been known for over 30

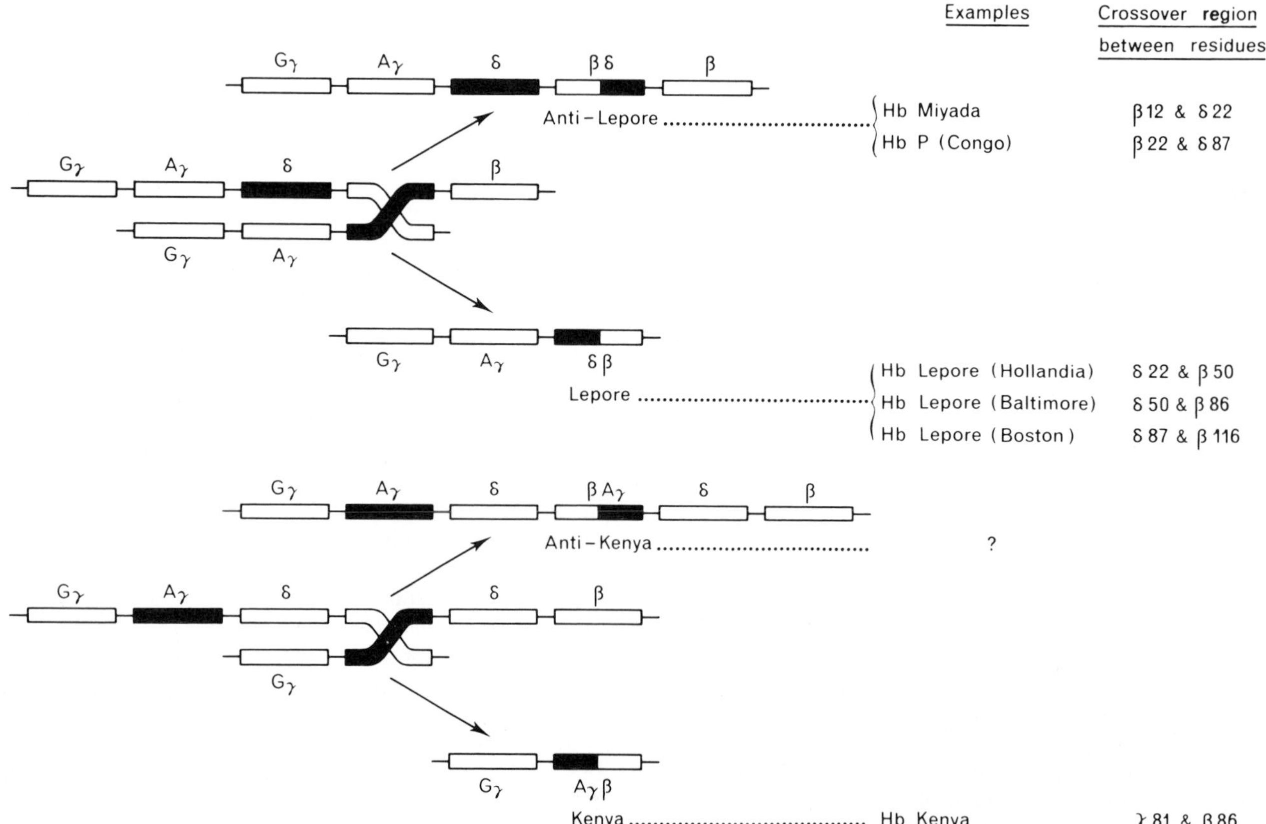

FIG. 113-8 The generation of Hb_{LEPORE} and Hb_{KENYA}. *(From Weatherall and Clegg.[2] Used by permission.)*

Table 113-3 Spectrum of Clinical Disorders Due to Structural Hemoglobin Variants

Hemolytic anemia
  Sickling disorders
  Hb C
  Unstable variants
Abnormal oxygen transport
  High-affinity variants
  Low-affinity variants
Thalassemia phenotypes
  Ineffectively synthesized variants
    Hb E
    $Hb_{KNOSSOS}$
  Chain termination variants
  Fusion variants
  Highly unstable variants
    $Hb_{INDIANAPOLIS}$

years, many questions remain about its pathophysiology, clinical heterogeneity, prognosis, and, above all, its clinical management.

Classification (Table 113-4). The sickling disorders include the heterozygous state [sickle-cell trait (AS)], the homozygous condition [sickle-cell disease (SS)], and the compound heterozygous states for the sickle cell gene in association with other β-globin chain variants such as Hbs C and D (SC and SD disease) or β thalassemia (Hb S β thalassemia). The sickle cell gene is also found in association with α chain variants and different forms of α thalassemia.

Molecular Pathology. Hemoglobin S differs from Hb A by the substitution of valine for glutamic acid at position 6 of the β-globin chain.[9] This reflects an A-to-T substitution in the triplet codon for the sixth residue of the β-globin chain. In concentrated hemoglobin solutions that are partially or fully deoxygenated this amino acid substitution leads to polymerization and the formation of intracellular fibers that cause the sickle cell deformity. The latter results in reduced deformability of the red cell and hence in its defective passage through the microcirculation. This is the basis for the vasoocclusive manifestations of sickle cell disease. In addition, these structural changes of the red cell lead to a shortened survival and a chronic hemolytic anemia.

Despite an enormous amount of work over the past half century, the final story of how sickle cells sickle remains to be told. Early workers in the field observed that sickling is associated with the formation of liquid crystals or tactoids.[138] Electron micrography of sickled erythrocytes shows long thin bundles of Hb S fibers that tend to run parallel to the long axis of the cell and that are probably responsible for its abnormal morphology[139,140] (Fig. 113-9). The precise ultrastructure of these fibers has been the subject of considerable controversy. A number of different models have been proposed in which 6, 8 or, more probably, 14 strands are twisted in a helical configuration to form hollow fibers with an external diameter of 170 to 220 Å.[141,142] The stabilization of these structures depends on interactions between individual globin chains. The precise localization of the contact points and the identification of the amino acid residues involved have been derived from a variety of techniques, particularly x-ray defraction studies. One model based on x-ray data identifies β6 Val, β73 Asp, β121 Glu, and α23 Glu as being among a number of residues that are probably important in generating intermolecular contacts[143]; many others may be implicated (reviewed by Schechter et al.[144]).

Polymer Formation. The way in which Hb S polymerizes to form a high-molecular-weight gel that is in equilibrium with monomeric hemoglobin solution is not fully understood. Monomers are stable in solution at a particular concentration of Hb S, pH, ionic strength, and temperature. However, small alterations in any of these variables lead to a rapid change to the gel form of Hb S. It is probably this sol-to-gel transition that leads to the viscosity changes, abnormalities of cell morphology, and sludging in the microcirculation and organ infarction which are the hallmarks of the sickling disorders.

The sol-to-gel transformations have been studied using many different techniques including light scattering and turbidimetry,[145,146] sedimentation,[147] birefringence optics,[148] calorimetry,[149] and MRI.[150] Although no unifying model has arisen from these studies, several important factors emerge. There appear to be two distinct steps in the transition. The first is a lag phase that corresponds to the construction of a polymer of a critical size. Once this has occurred the reaction proceeds more rapidly and results in the formation of a high-molecular-weight polymer with closely aligned fibers. The delay time varies as the 30th power of the hemoglobin concentration; it has been calculated that by decreasing the intracellular hemoglobin concentration from 35 to 34 g/dl the delay phase is doubled. The sol-to-gel transformation is also extremely sensitive to changes in temperature and pH.

The kinetics of gel formation by Hb S in red cells is probably similar to that in solution. In some models of the pathophysiology of sickling the delay time is thought to have important pathophysiological consequences. Oxygenation and deoxygenation of red cells in the circulation takes approximately the same time as for the sol-to-gel transformation of Hb S in solution.[151] This means that in the pulmonary circulation, at a high oxygen tension, Hb S gels melt in less than half a second. They will remain more or less in this state in the arterial circulation, but in the microcirculation, where oxygen saturation rapidly declines, there will be a concomitant reduction in hemoglobin solubility. The red cell

Table 113-4 Common Sickling Disorders

Disorder	Genotype	Hemoglobins
Homozygous for Hb S		
Sickle cell disease	$\alpha\alpha/\alpha\alpha\ \beta^S\beta^S$	S, F, A_2
With α thalassemia	$-\alpha/-\alpha\ \beta^S\beta^S$	S, F, A_2 ↑
	$-\alpha/\alpha\alpha\ \beta^S\beta^S$	S, F, A_2
Heterozygous for Hb S		
Sickle cell trait	$\alpha\alpha/\alpha\alpha\ \beta^A\beta^S$	A, S, A_2
With α thalassemia	$-\alpha/-\alpha\ \beta^A\beta^S$	A, S↓, A_2
	$-\alpha/\alpha\alpha\ \beta^A\beta^S$	A, S, A_2
With β thalassemia*	$\alpha\alpha/\alpha\alpha\ \beta^0\beta^S$	S, F, A_2 ↑
	$\alpha\alpha/\alpha\alpha\ \beta^+\beta^S$	S, A, F, A_2 ↑
With β-chain variants	$\alpha\alpha/\alpha\alpha\ \beta^S\beta^C$	S, C, A_2
	$\alpha\alpha/\alpha\alpha\ \beta^S\beta^D$	S, D, A_2
	$\alpha\alpha/\alpha\alpha\ \beta^S\beta^O{}_{ARAB}$	S, O_{ARAB}, A_2
	Many others	
With α-chain variants	$\alpha^G\alpha/\alpha\alpha\ \beta^A\beta^S$	A, S, G, A_2, G_2, SG
	Several other interactions	
With HPFH†	$\alpha\alpha/\alpha\alpha\ \beta^S-$	S, F, A_2

*β^0 and β^+ indicate β thalassemia with complete and partial deficiency of β-chain genes.
†Represents a chromosome with a deleted β-chain gene.

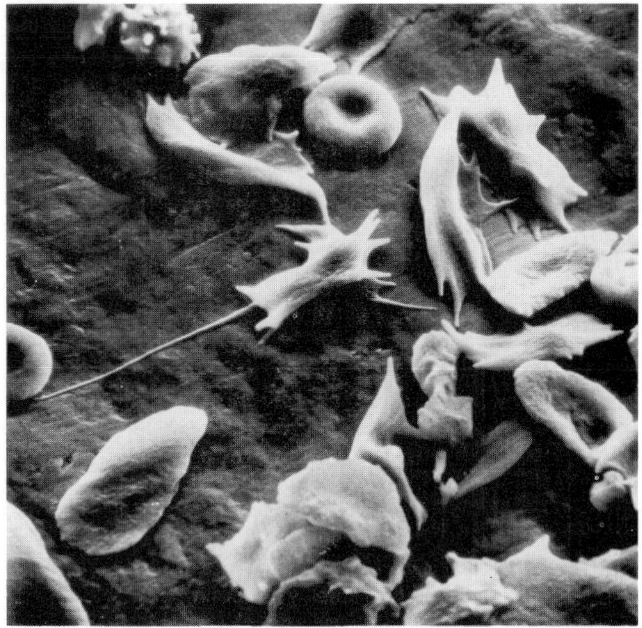

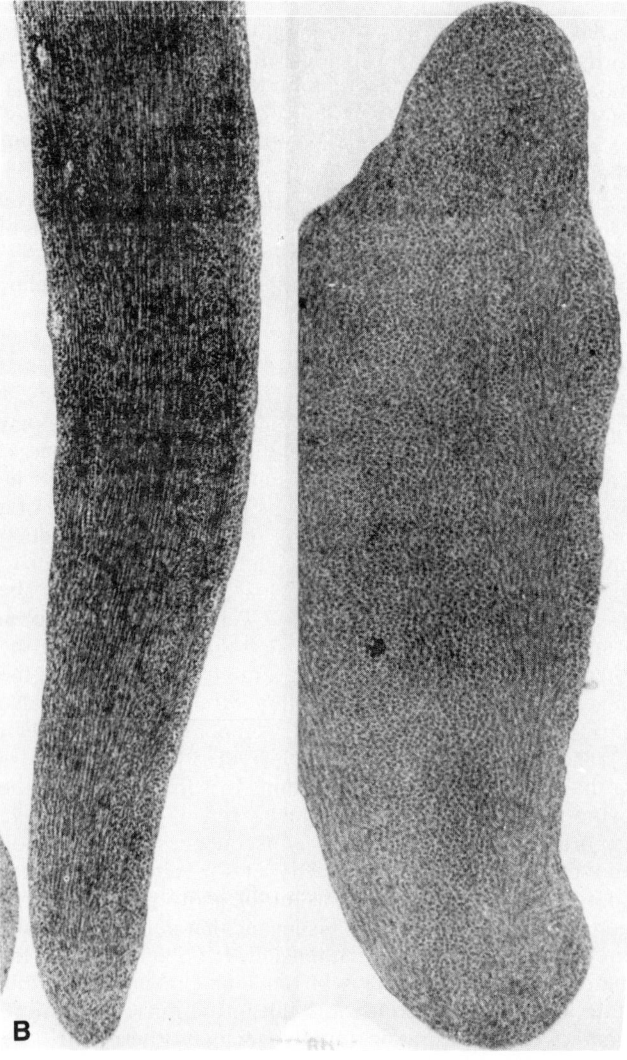

spends approximately 1 s in the capillary circulation; if the delay time is less, cells could sickle and occlude the microcirculation. On the other hand if the delay time is prolonged, sickling should not occur in the capillaries, and hence the microculation will remain patent. In other words, if the transit time is shorter than the delay time occlusion will not occur. The type of environment that red cells may encounter in the renal medulla or spleen—where there may be a low pH, high hemoglobin concentration, and high ionic strength, all of which shorten the delay time—will favor sickling. But although this type of mechanism may be important, other interpretations of the kinetics of sickling, which will be considered later, suggest that the situation may be more complex than this. In particular, the physiological significance of the delay time has been questioned.[144]

Interactions between Sickle and Other Hemoglobins. If known proportions of solutions of purified Hb S and other hemoglobins are mixed under appropriate conditions and are then completely deoxygenated, the degree of interaction of a particular hemoglobin in the sickling process can be assessed by determining the minimum concentration of the final mixture in grams per deciliter at which gelling occurs (MGC).[152] Hence, a low MGC indicates an increased tendency to sickle and a high MGC vice versa. For example, mixtures of Hb S and Hb C have a higher MGC than solutions of Hb S alone, indicating that the substitution of the basic lysine does not cause sickling as efficiently as a hydrophobic valine. Hemoglobins D and O Arab involve substitutions in the β121 region, an area that x-ray data suggest is an important contact region. Gelation studies show that these variants interact with sickle cell hemoglobin and support sickling as efficiently as Hb S. On the other hand, experiments of this type show that Hbs A and F have an inhibitory effect on sickling. Interestingly, x-ray studies that have analyzed contacts between double strands have provided information that is in very good agreement with the location of mutations that affect gelation. The extensive data that have been generated on the various contact points and intermolecular interactions that may be important in the genesis of sickling are all consistent with a 14-strand structure of the sickle cell fiber (reviewed in Bunn and Forget[3] and Schechter et al.[144]).

Cellular Heterogeneity. Films prepared from well-oxygenated blood samples from patients with sickle cell anemia show a number of sickled forms. Such irreversibly sickled cells (ISC) are derived from a relatively young erythrocyte population with a low content of Hb F.[153] They are thought to be the end result of cycles of sickling and unsickling. The ISC is a particularly rigid cell that is partly responsible for the abnormal viscosity of oxygenated whole blood of patients with sickle cell anemia. Their decreased deformability is related directly to the degree of cellular dehydration.

FIG. 113-9 Sickle cells. *A*. Scanning electron microscopy appearances showing deoxygenated sickle cells with bizarre shapes and long filaments, short spicules, and chiseled surfaces. *B*. Electron microscopy (×20,770). The cells are shown in longitudinal section on the left and in cross section on the right. The figures are of deoxygenated irreversibly sickled cells (ISC). In contrast to a more random pattern of filaments on deoxygenated non-ISC there is a distinctive regularity of filament arrangements. *(From Bertles and Dobler.[153] Used by permission.)*

The formation of the ISC is thought to occur in several stages. Cycles of sickling cause damage to the red-cell membrane that becomes abnormally permeable to cations, resulting in a low K^+, high Na^+, high Ca^{2+} concentration. In an effort to restore cation homeostasis ATP-dependent pumps are activated with a consequent decrease in intracellular ATP. At this stage the erythrocyte is calcium-loaded and ATP-depleted and hence may undergo the "Gardos effect," that is, gross dehydration with loss of potassium and water (reviewed by Schechter et al.[144]). There has been considerable progress in defining the roles of the different red-cell cation channels in determining the MCHC of sickle cells.[154,155] It is believed that the dehydrated cell, with its high MCHC, has a decreased delay time and hence tends to remain in the sickled configuration. It seems likely that the low level of Hb F in these cells is a major factor in their termination in the irreversibly sickled state.

Rheology[144] The transition from the sol to the gel state is accompanied by a marked increase in viscosity. Hemoglobin, whether in free solution or in red cells, is a non-Newtonian fluid, meaning its viscosity is critically dependent on shear rate. Above minimum gelling concentration of deoxy Hb S the viscosity increases dramatically; the rheological properties of the gel are probably the most immediate cause of the vasoocclusive manifestations of the sickling disorders.

Oxygen Affinity Although Hb S in dilute solution has a normal oxygen dissociation curve, blood from patients with sickle cell anemia shows a decreased oxygen affinity.[3] There are probably several factors responsible for the shift in the oxygen dissociation curve. Though individuals with sickle cell anemia have higher levels of red cell 2,3-DPG the major cause is intracellular polymerization of Hb S.

Pathophysiology. The sickling disorders are all characterized by two major pathological processes, anemia and vasoocclusion. Over the years, the thinking about the pathophysiology of sickling disorders has changed.[144] Originally it was thought to be the result of a vicious circle, whereby the sickling of cells in the circulation led to stasis, decreased oxygen saturation, further sickling, and hence further stasis. In the 1970s this view was modified to develop a more kinetic concept of what happens in the vasculature of patients with the sickling disorders. It was suggested that the delay time of intracellular polymerization is determined by the intracellular Hb S concentration and by other factors, including temperature, pH, and the circulatory dynamics. Obstruction might be viewed as the end result of the interaction of a number of variables but, overall, to reflect the relationship between delay and transit times. However, it was pointed out that the extremely rapid polymerization time expected to occur in the body, especially if there is preexisting polymer in many cells, makes it unlikely that this delay time is physiologically critical.

An alternate view[144] suggests that the actual sickling of red cells is relatively unimportant and that the major pathological mechanisms in the sickling disorders reflect the rheological effects of continuous variations in intracellular deoxy Hb S polymers. Because of the low mixed arterial saturation in patients with sickle cell anemia due to pulmonary ventilatory abnormalities and shunting, and the right shift in the oxygen dissociation curve caused by sickle hemoglobin, sickle erythrocytes are below 85 to 90 percent oxygen saturated even in the aorta. It is likely, therefore, that many cells will contain polymer while on the arterial side of the microcirculation. This will produce a marked decrease in the flexibility of red cells. Hence, resistance to flow increases in the terminal arterioles, and there is a tendency for stasis leading to local anoxia and tissue damage. In this model hemolysis is visualized as the end result of chronic impedance of relatively inflexible cells as they try to negotiate areas of high resistance.[144]

Whatever the precise pathophysiological mechanisms involved it is necessary to explain both the anemia and vascular occlusion that characterize the sickling disorders. It is likely that similar mechanisms are involved in both processes.

Anemia and Vasoocclusion The anemia of sickle cell disease has an extremely complex pathophysiology. It seems likely that physical trapping of erythrocytes in the microcirculation due to their decreased deformability plays a major role in shortening red-cell survival. It turns out that even when they are fully oxygenated sickle cells exhibit decreased deformability. Both static and dynamic deformability of oxygenated sickle cells decrease with increasing dehydration.[156] Since polymerization of Hb S is highly dependent on hemoglobin concentration, dehydrated sickled red cells show the most marked changes during partial deoxygenation. The decreased deformability is thought to cause trapping of rigid cells in small vessels.

There are other mechanisms that may be of importance in causing vasoocclusion and premature red-cell destruction. Sickle cells have a tendency to adhere to vascular endothelial cells.[157] Furthermore, in vitro studies have shown that these cells are recognized more actively by monocytes and macrophages, suggesting that one component of the anemia of the sickling disorders is accelerated erythrophagocytosis.[158] Some studies (reviewed by Nagel[154]) have demonstrated other novel mechanisms which may be involved in the increased propensity for sickle cells to adhere to the vascular endothelium. It has been found that high multimers of von Willebrand factor greatly increase the adherence of these cells to the lining of small vessels. Furthermore, it has been found that this phenomenon is more marked in young red cells.

It is also possible that autooxidation plays a role in the destruction of sickle cells. Sickle cell membranes have increased amounts of membrane-associated hemichrome that is known to have the property of targeting autooxidative damage to membrane components. Oxidative damage may also be mediated by free heme and iron.[159] Excessive amounts of the biproducts of lipid peroxidation and the modification of membrane constituents by potential cross-linking agents such as malondialdehyde have also been demonstrated.[160] These oxidative mechanisms may render sickle cells susceptible to immunological attack; there is an antibody in normal serums that opsonizes malondialdehyde-modified red cells.[161] Work on oxidant damage to sickle cells has been reviewed in detail by Nagel.[154]

We have already seen how irreversibly sickled cells are dehydrated, have a high calcium and low potassium content, and are extremely rigid. It seems likely therefore that the anemia of the sickling disorders reflects a shortened red-cell survival consequent on decreased deformability, adherence to endothelial cells, erythrophagocytosis, autooxidation, and gross membrane abnormalities. Finally, it has been observed that there may be a suboptimal proliferative response by the bone marrow in this condition, probably because of the low oxygen affinity of Hb S in red cells.[162] Thus, part of the anemia of patients with sickle cell anemia may be a physiological adaptation to the altered oxygen-carrying properties of their blood.

The vasoocclusive manifestations of the sickling disorders probably result from the altered rheological properties of red cells containing a high concentration of Hb S. It is likely that the tendency for sickle cells to adhere to vascular endothelium may also be involved and that plasma constituents may play a role in their interaction with endothelial cells.[163] Adherent cells may retard the flow of other sickle cells, thereby increasing the time available for sickling as cells pass through hypoxic tissues. Ultimately, the mass of adherent red cells and rigid cells free within small vessels may lead to microvascular occlusion and subsequent tissue infarction. To this complicated picture we must add the flow properties and regulation of the diameter of the microcirculation itself. This important topic has not been studied extensively, although the existing evidence suggests that there are important differences in microcirculation flow kinetics in patients with sickle cell anemia as compared with normal individuals (reviewed by Schechter et al.[144] and Nagel[154]).

Although these mechanisms may well contribute to vascular occlusion in sickle cell disease, the triggering mechanisms for the acute occlusive episodes which are the basis for the painful crises of the disease are still not understood. Similarly, we have no information about the factors which cause the curious hypertrophic changes in some of the cerebral vessels which seem to be responsible for the neurological complications of sickle cell anemia (see "Crises" below). There is some epidemiological evidence that cold may be a precipitating factor in the painful crisis,[164] and it seems likely that other factors which alter the dynamics of the microcirculation, either generally or regionally, may be important triggering mechanisms.[144] But all this is speculation and, in effect, virtually nothing is known about the pathogenesis of the painful crisis.

Sickle Cell Trait. The life expectancy of individuals with the sickle cell trait is probably the same as normal persons.[164] Although a number of clinical abnormalities have been reported in individuals with the trait, most of them are anecdotal, and the association may be coincidental. It seems likely that such persons are at risk for splenic infarction when flying at high altitudes under conditions of inadequate cabin pressurization. Except in very unusual circumstances this problem should not be encountered in commercial aircraft. There is no justification for denial of employment or life insurance to individuals with the sickle cell trait who fly in normally pressurized aircraft.

There is some evidence that otherwise unexplained hematuria may be associated with the sickle cell trait, as may the ability to concentrate urine. Other associations based on less firm data include a slightly increased risk of pulmonary embolism, renal papillary necrosis, and avascular necrosis of bone. There have been a few reports of episodes of infarction following the application of a limb tourniquet for orthopedic procedures or following poorly administered anesthesia.

Sickle Cell Anemia. Sickle cell anemia is characterized by a lifelong hemolytic anemia, the occurrence of acute exacerbations called "crises," and a variety of complications resulting from an increased propensity to infection and the deleterious effects of repeated vasoocclusive episodes. Despite so much knowledge about the molecular pathology of the condition the reason the course of the illness is so variable, even within individual sibships let alone between different racial groups, is poorly understood. In this section we shall describe the typical features of sickle cell anemia and then attempt to define what is known about the factors that modify the clinical phenotype.

Clinical and Hematologic Features and Course of the Illness.[144,164] Sickle cell anemia usually presents during the first or second year of life, although in milder cases later presentation is common and some patients may be ascertained as adults only during family studies or by chance. The usual presenting features are failure to thrive, repeated infections in infancy, attacks of painful dactylitis (the hand–foot syndrome; see below) or pallor. At this stage the infant looks pale, there may be slight icterus, the spleen is usually palpable, and the typical hematologic findings of sickle cell anemia are established. The hemoglobin value varies between 7 and 11 g/dl, although higher levels are encountered with unusually mild forms of the illness. There are typical features of hemolysis with a raised reticulocyte count in the 10 to 20 percent range, marked variation in the depth of staining of the red cells, and some sickled erythrocytes on the blood film. The serum bilirubin level is slightly elevated, and the urinary urobilinogen level is increased.

The subsequent course is variable. Overall, patients with this disorder show early retardation of growth; weight is affected more than height. Although the mean height is generally reduced in childhood, data from studies in older children and adolescents are less clear. Usually by the age of 20 years the height curves in males approach those of control groups, and in females they may actually exceed those of normal individuals.[164] Although there has been much controversy, it appears that patients with sickle cell disease have an abnormal body habitus characterized by long limbs and hence a decrease in the upper-to-lower-segment ratio. Other features of abnormal anthropometry include narrow pectoral and pelvic girdles, increased anteroposterior chest diameters, a reduced arm circumference, and thinner skin folds. The onset of puberty is often delayed.

Splenomegaly is usually present in infancy and early childhood; in a large Jamaican study, 77 percent of patients had palpable spleens by the age of 24 months.[164] The organ gradually becomes impalpable in the majority of patients during later childhood; persistent splenomegaly occurs in patients with high levels of Hb F and in those who are homozygous for α^+ thalassemia (see below). The gradual splenic fibrosis and atrophy reflects repeated infarction of the organ. These changes in spleen size are mirrored by the presence of pitted red cells that result from reduced splenic function[165]; the pitted red-cell count in sickle cell anemia correlates with other assessments of splenic function such as the clearance of heat-damaged autologous red cells and the uptake of labeled sulfacolloid.[166]

Because of the right-shifted oxygen dissociation curve, patients with sickle cell anemia tend to compensate well for their anemia, and tolerance for their exercise is good. The main clinical problems encountered early in life are crises (see below) and an increased propensity to infection.

It is clear that children with this condition have an increased susceptibility to infection although many of the published studies lack adequate controls. There is no doubt, however, that they are prone to infections due to *Streptococcus pneumoniae*, Salmonella species, *Escherichia coli*, and

Haemophilus influenzae.[144] The Salmonella infections may be gastrointestinal, but osteomyelitis is also common and probably results from infection of infarcted bone. The pattern of other infections is also variable, but pneumococcal pneumonia and septicemia are particularly important; overwhelming septicemia and shock is a common cause of death, particularly during infancy and childhood.

Undoubtedly a major factor in this proneness to infection is impaired splenic function together with generalized reticuloendothelial blockade; the pattern of infection in childhood is very similar to that of children who have had their spleens removed for other reasons. The precise mechanism whereby splenic hypofunction increases susceptibility to infection is not clear; both antibody production and antigen processing may be involved. There may be other factors, particularly in children with sickle cell anemia, including defective neutrophil function and abnormalities of the alternative pathway of complement activation, although such changes are found in only a small proportion of patients.[164] Infection is a major cause of death at all ages, an observation that suggests that hyposplenism is not the only factor involved in increased susceptibility.

Crises. Acute exacerbations of the illness in patients with sickle cell anemia are called "crises." They can take many clinical forms. Although the subdivision of crises into specific entities is useful for descriptive purposes it should be emphasized that in many sickling crises a number of different pathophysiological mechanisms seem to be involved.

The *painful crisis*[164] is the most common and important manifestation of sickle cell anemia. These episodes are characterized by the rapid onset of pain in the limbs, back, abdomen, or chest. The mechanism is still unknown. There is good epidemiological evidence that cold may be a factor, and in some cases there may be an underlying infection. But in many instances no precipitating factor can be found. There are no consistent changes in blood platelets or coagulation factors. It is clear, however, that these are vasoocclusive episodes; bone marrow biopsy over regions of bone pain invariably shows infarcted marrow. On theoretical grounds a vasoocclusive episode of this type could be caused either by enhancement of intravascular sickling or an alteration in the flow kinetics in the microcirculation. Other factors that may be involved include acidosis, hypoxia, and dehydration, all of which are known to potentiate intracellular polymerization.

The clinical course of the painful crisis is characteristic. The pain follows no particular pattern and tends to be severe for 2 or 3 days, after which it settles spontaneously. It is quite common to observe a mild pyrexia on the second or third day even in patients in whom an extensive search has not demonstrated any source of infection. This is presumably due to bone infarction. In an uncomplicated painful crisis the hematologic findings remain unchanged.

One particularly important form of painful crisis, which occurs early in infancy, is the so-called *hand–foot* syndrome. This is a dactylitis characterized by the sudden onset of painful swelling of the dorsum of the hands and feet. Two pathophysiological mechanisms are involved. First, at this age bones are growing rapidly and may have a limited blood supply. Second, the occlusion of vessels by sickled cells may not be easily compensated by a coaxial blood supply to the bone. Autopsy studies have shown complete necrosis of the marrow and the inner third of the cortex, lesions similar to those that can be produced in experimental animals by interruption of both the metaphyseal and nutrient artery supplies to long bones. In later life almost any bone can be involved in a painful crisis, and local swelling of the bone, that presumably reflects a periosteal reaction over an infarct, is commonly observed. Although painful crises always settle, repeated vasoocclusive episodes may lead to destruction of bone and soft tissue.

While painful crises are usually self-limiting—and therefore not life-threatening—there are other forms of acute exacerbation of the clinical course of sickle cell anemia that are more serious and, together with infection, are the most common causes of death. There are a variety of *sequestration crises*. The commonest type involves the spleen in the first 2 years of life.[164,167] The clinical picture is characterized by a rapid enlargement of the spleen that becomes engorged with sickled erythrocytes. This may progress to a stage at which a large proportion of the circulating blood volume is entrapped in the spleen, leading to profound anemia and death. These episodes may occur more than once, particularly in children with persistent splenomegaly. A similar type of sequestration may occur in the liver in later life; the organ rapidly enlarges, while at the same time there is a dramatic fall in the hematocrit.[168]

Another important type of sequestration crisis is called the *chest syndrome*,[169] recognized increasingly as a cause of morbidity and mortality in patients of all ages. It is characterized by pleuritic pain, fever, cough, and increasing dyspnea. These symptoms reflect widespread blockage of the pulmonary arteries with sickled cells leading to pulmonary infarction. Initially there may be no radiological findings; but as the condition develops, pulmonary infiltrates appear and may progress to an almost complete "white-out" of the lung fields. Blood gas analysis shows increasing hypoxemia. It is often difficult to distinguish between an acute chest syndrome and a chest infection, and it is possible that infection may precipitate the syndrome in some patients. A history of an upper respiratory infection, infected sputum, marked leukocytosis on presentation, and lower lobe disease is more in keeping with a pneumonia, but these features are by no means always present, and the distinction may be extremely difficult. A falling hematocrit and/or platelet count and rapidly deteriorating pO_2 values are useful indicators of an impending chest syndrome.[169]

Attacks of acute abdominal pain resembling a "surgical abdomen" occur frequently in patients with sickle cell anemia and constitute an *abdominal crisis*.[164] The pain is usually widespread and may be associated with tenderness without guarding, distension, and a reduction or absence of bowel sounds. These features may be difficult to distinguish from peritonitis, although in the abdominal crisis, rebound tenderness is absent and the patient's general condition is usually not as poor as in patient's with peritonitis. It is important for this syndrome to be recognized in order to avoid unnecessary surgical exploration.

Another important cause of death in patients with sickle cell anemia of all ages is the *aplastic crisis*. Extensive studies have implicated a human parvovirus-like agent as the commonest cause of this condition.[170] Infection with this agent in normal people causes transient erythroid hypoplasia and a slight drop in the hemoglobin level. In patients with sickle cell anemia, who have a very short red-cell survival, temporary marrow aplasia may lead to profound anemia. This is characterized by a very sudden drop in the hematocrit and the disappearance of reticulocytes from the peripheral blood. The bone marrow shows a marked reduction or absence of erythroid precursors. Recovery occurs in a few days and is heralded by a rising reticulocyte count. Aplastic crises occur in epidemics and often involve more than one family member. This reflects the periodic epidemicity of parvovirus infections in the general population.

Acute neurological episodes or *neurological crises* are a particularly important and distressing accompaniment of sickle cell anemia.[171] The prevalence has ranged in different series from 5.5 to 17 percent.[172] These episodes usually reflect cerebral infarction in younger patients and hemorrhage in older ones. Angiographic studies suggest that these neurological episodes may be the result of occlusion or stenosis of large arteries in the carotid distribution. Histological studies have shown both thrombosis and intimal thickening in the large and small arteries.[173] It has been suggested that these changes result from intimal damage from a combination of high-velocity flow, rigidity of the red cells, and their adherence to the vessel wall—all associated with intravascular sludging. The clinical features of these disorders are similar to those that result from carotid occlusion due to atherosclerotic disease, including premonitory transient ischemic attacks.[174] The work of some investigators has suggested that the regular study of the cerebral vessels using Doppler ultrasonography, possibly with magnetic resonance angiography, is a valuable approach to assessing the likely occurrence of this important complication.[172]

The term *hemolytic crisis* is often used to describe an acute exacerbation of the hemolytic component of sickle cell anemia. In patients with intercurrent infection or painful crises the reticulocyte count may rise, but it is doubtful if the hemolytic crisis is a separate entity. *Priapism* occurs acutely, resulting from occlusion of the outflow vessels from the corpora cavernosa by sickled cells. This is an extremely distressing complication that may last for several days and may lead to permanent deformity of the penis.[164]

Chronic Organ Damage. Repeated vasoocclusive episodes may lead to chronic organ damage resulting from repeated infarction with subsequent healing and fibrosis.

Renal involvement occurs in virtually every patient with sickle cell anemia.[164] In early life there is impairment of renal function that is correctable by blood transfusion. In later life this defect is irreversible. It probably results from derangement of the normal countercurrent distribution in the medullary circulation; blood flow to the glomeruli is maintained, whereas flow to the vasa recta in the medulla is reduced. Injection of kidneys at autopsy has demonstrated decreased filling of these vessels, with dilated capillaries and extravasation of contrast media from ruptured vessels. In addition, there may be a mild form of distal tubular acidosis. Otherwise unexplained hematuria is common and probably results from lesions of the papillae. It appears that chronic progressive renal failure is a common form of death in adults with the sickling disorders.[164]

In early life the concentrating defect of the kidney may be reflected in thirst and polyuria, and it is thought that nocturnal enuresis is common. In addition, there have been a number of reports of a true nephrotic syndrome, although more recent analyses have cast doubt on the true association between the sickling disorders and nephrosis.[164]

Many other organs may be involved in the chronic damage resulting from vascular blockage. Permanent penile deformity has already been mentioned. *Avascular necrosis* of the femoral or humoral heads occurs (Fig. 113-10) although it is not clear whether this is as common in sickle cell disease as in Hb SC disease (see below). Involvement of the

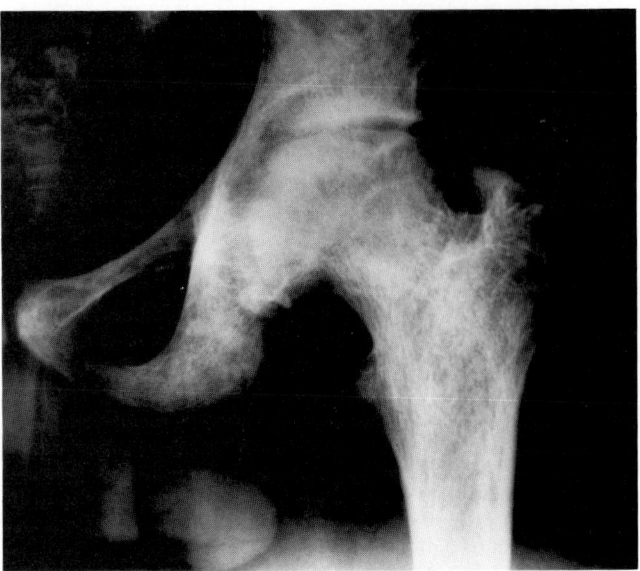

FIG. 113-10 Aseptic necrosis of the head of the left humerus in a patient with HB SC disease. *(From Weatherall and Clegg.[2] Used by permission.)*

mandible, skull, ribs and sternum, and vertebral bodies may all give rise to deformity or chronic bone tenderness. Chronic *leg ulceration* is also very common. The lesions occur just above the medial or lateral malleoli; presumably this reflects the precarious vascularization of the skin of this region. *Proliferative retinopathy* also occurs in sickle cell anemia, although it is commoner in hemoglobin SC disease; it is described in a later section. As mentioned earlier, the *central nervous system* may be involved in a variety of chronic complications following acute vasoocclusive episodes. Stroke is the most important; two thirds of strokes occur in children, and in many cases there are recurrent episodes.[174] Although there may be a remarkable degree of restoration of neurological function, many children are left with permanent defects in cognitive, sensory, and motor function.

Hepatic involvement occurs in a variety of forms. There is invariably iron loading of the Kupffer cells and hepatocytes, and true macronodular cirrhosis has been observed, although the frequency of this condition seems to vary; for example, it is very rare in Jamaica. *Chronic pulmonary involvement* with progressive obliteration of the pulmonary vascular bed and associated pulmonary hypertension and right ventricular hypertrophy is being recognized as shunting, with increasing frequency in adults.[175] Similarly, the *heart* seems to escape infarction. There is nearly always some degree of cardiac enlargement, and a variety of flow murmurs have been described together with all the other manifestations of a hyperdynamic circulation. It is surprising that, although the myocardium extracts more oxygen than any other tissue, vasoocclusive episodes involving the myocardium do not seem to occur, and coronary occlusion is not a recognized complication. This probably reflects the rapidity of blood flow in the myocardium, especially in a hyperdynamic heart. The question of whether there is a specific sickle *cardiomyopathy* remains open, although autopsy series have revealed only minor histological changes in cardiac muscle.[164]

Other Complications There is a large volume of literature on the effects of sickle cell anemia on *pregnancy*. The most recent series estimate a very low maternal mortality, although it should be noted that most of these studies have been carried out in developed Western societies.[164] Such data as are available from Nigeria indicate that there is still a high maternal mortality.[176] Fetal wastage from abortion, stillbirth, and neonatal death is increased in all populations.[164] The anemia is exacerbated, and there appears to be an increased incidence of crises during pregnancy; the acute chest syndrome is particularly important. The association of preeclamptic toxemia remains controversial.

Because of the chronic hemolysis and high turnover of bilirubin, the formation of pigment stones in the gallbladder is extremely common. It seems likely that this complication has been underrecognized in the past, and many patients with sickle cell anemia have attacks of biliary colic and cholecystitis and require cholecystectomy.[164]

Because of the rapid marrow turnover *folate deficiency* may occur, particularly in pregnancy, although this seems to be uncommon in patients maintained on adequate diets. Although *Plasmodium falciparum* malaria may be less severe in sickle cell heterozygotes, there is no doubt that it is a major cause of morbidity and mortality in homozygotes living in endemic areas. Audiometry has revealed *sensorineural hearing loss* in about 12 percent of patients with sickle cell anemia.[164] However, this is usually subclinical; rarely, sudden deafness may occur during a painful crisis.

Factors that Influence Prognosis Surprisingly little is known about the natural history of sickle cell anemia except for the pioneering studies of Serjeant and his colleagues in Jamaica.[164] Until recently it appeared that both in the United States and Jamaica there was a 10 percent mortality in the first few years of life. The most important causes of death were infection and splenic sequestration, with a number of sudden, unexpected deaths of uncertain etiology. With the advent of cord blood screening and the use of prophylactic penicillin, in the United States it appears that this early mortality peak may be diminishing.[177] Studies in Jamaica show a 10-year survival of 84 percent, with the suggestion of a second peak in the mortality curve in the 20-to-24-year age group; data about longevity are extremely sparse.[164] Similarly, little is known about the prognosis for the disease in rural Africa, although such data as are available suggest that few patients survive to adult life. As mentioned earlier, infection remains the commonest cause of death at all ages but, at least in Jamaica, progressive renal failure is being seen with increasing frequency in older age groups.[146]

Unfortunately, knowledge about the factors that modify the course of sickle cell anemia is extremely scanty. In certain populations such as those of eastern Saudi Arabia and Orissa, India, there is a relatively mild form of the disease.[178,179] This is characterized by higher hemoglobin levels, lower reticulocyte counts, and persistence of splenomegaly into adult life. In both these populations the majority of patients have unusually high levels of fetal hemoglobin, in the 15 to 25 percent range, and there is high prevalence of α thalassemia. While, overall, it appears that elevated levels of fetal hemoglobin are protective in sickle cell anemia the relationship is not straightforward.[180] Studies in Saudi Arabia have compared the clinical course in low- versus high-fetal-hemoglobin-producing populations of patients with sickle cell anemia. Although these studies have confirmed that the disease is milder in some respects in patients with the higher levels of fetal hemoglobin, they have also demonstrated that this group may not be protected against certain complications—particularly painful crises and bone disease.[181] The occurrence of severe, destructive aseptic necrosis of the femoral heads was equally common in both groups. Much may depend on the intracellular level and distribution of Hb F. It is only in patients who are compound heterozygotes for the sickle cell and have hereditary persistence of fetal hemoglobin genes that there is a relatively uniform distribution of Hb F among the red cells; this disorder is particularly mild. Even in the populations of Saudi Arabia and Orissa, where there may be fetal hemoglobin levels of similar magnitude, the Hb F is much less uniformly distributed.

While the elevated level of hemoglobin F in patients with sickle cell anemia undoubtedly results from selection of cells containing relatively greater amounts of this hemoglobin in the peripheral circulation, there is no doubt that many different genetic factors are involved in setting the final level of fetal hemoglobin.[154] We shall return to this question in more detail in a later section when we describe the genetic factors responsible for the variable elevation of hemoglobin F in different forms of β thalassemia.

Another factor that modifies the course of sickle cell anemia is the coinheritance of α thalassemia.[154,182] About 2 percent of American black and Jamaican populations are homozygous for the deletion form of α^+ thalassemia. Comparison of such individuals, who also have sickle cell anemia, with those who have sickle cell anemia without α thalassemia shows that the α thalassemia group have higher hemoglobin levels, typical thalassemic red-cell indices, a greater likelihood of splenomegaly after childhood, and fewer episodes of the acute chest syndrome and chronic leg ulceration. They also have lower levels of Hb F. In vitro studies show that the deformability of sickle cells is enhanced if α thalassemia is also present, providing a cellular basis for these observations.[183] Evidence still conflicts about the effect on survival of the coinheritance of α thalassemia.

But if high levels of Hb F and α thalassemia are excluded, the clinical picture of sickle cell anemia still remains remarkably heterogeneous, and the factors that are involved in modifying the course are not understood. As we shall see later, a second mutation in the β-globin gene might account for some of this heterogeneity, but undoubtedly other factors remain to be identified.

Hemoglobin Constitution. In the sickle cell trait there is usually about 30 percent Hb S with a normal Hb A_2 level (Fig. 113-11). The relative amount of Hb S varies. The main factor that seems to be responsible is the number of active α-globin genes. Individuals with the sickle cell trait who are also heterozygous for α^0 thalassemia, or heterozygous or homozygous for α^+ thalassemia have lower levels of Hb S. Those with triplicated α-globin genes have higher levels.[184]

In sickle cell anemia the hemoglobin consists mainly of Hb S with a normal Hb A_2 level and a variable amount of Hb F ranging from 1 or 2 percent up to 30 percent. Hemoglobin S can be distinguished from other variants with a similar electrophoretic migration on standard electrophoresis at alkaline pH by its different properties on agar gel electrophoresis (Fig. 113-12). However, the presence of Hb S should always be confirmed by carrying out a test for sickling. Individuals homozygous for Hb S who also have α thalassemia have slightly raised Hb A_2 levels.

Other Sickling Disorders. The sickle cell gene has been found in association with many structural hemoglobin variants.[3,164,185] However, only a minority of these conditions are common enough to warrant separate description. A new sickling syndrome (Hb $S_{ANTILLES}$, see below) has been de-

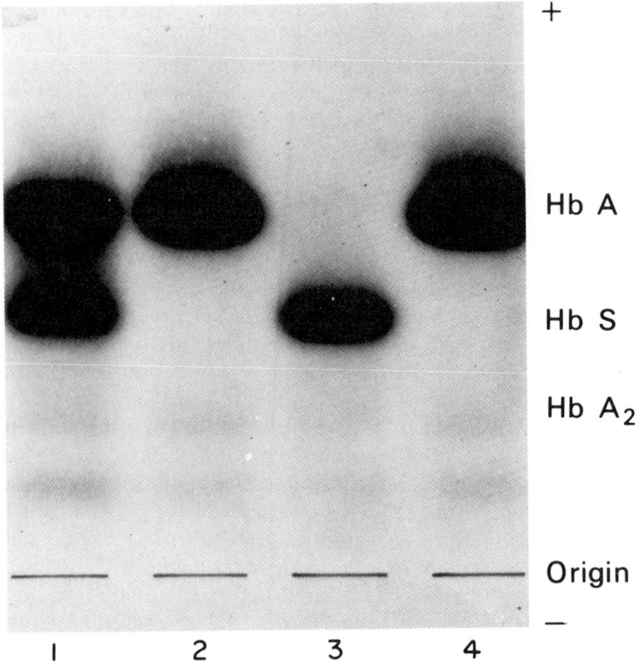

FIG. 113-11 **Hemoglobin electrophoresis (starch gel; protein stain, pH 8.6). The following are shown from left to right: 1 = sickle cell trait; 2 = normal; 3 = sickle cell anemia; 4 = normal.** ***(From Weatherall and Clegg.[2] Used by permission.)***

scribed that is symptomatic in the heterozygous state and that results from the coinheritance of a second mutation in a β-globin gene containing the sickle cell mutation.

Hemoglobin SC Disease Hemoglobin SC disease[3,144,164,185] occurs in individuals of West African origin. It is a milder disorder than sickle cell anemia, although almost all the complications of the latter have been observed. Growth, development, and body habitus are normal; the only abnormal physical sign is splenomegaly, which occurs in about 65 percent of cases. The disease may not present until mid or even late life with one of the complications. The blood picture shows a mild anemia with hemoglobin levels in the 11 to 13 g/dl range and a reticulocytosis of 3 to 5 percent. The peripheral blood film is particularly striking, showing sickled cells, many target cells, and cells that contain linear crystalline structures that tend to lie across their centers.

The main importance of Hb SC disease is that because it is mild it often goes unrecognized until a serious complication occurs. These include otherwise unexplained hematuria, aseptic necrosis of the femoral or humoral heads, and, particularly, ocular manifestations. All these changes reflect the abnormal rheology of red cells that contain both Hbs S and C; the pathophysiology of Hb C is considered in a later section.

The ocular complications are particularly important and are characterized by what is termed a proliferative sickle retinopathy (PSR).[164] The latter seems to develop through successive stages, starting with peripheral arteriolar occlusions, the development of arteriolar–venular anastomoses, neovascularization, and, finally, the development of vitreous hemorrhages and retinal detachment. In a large series studied in Jamaica about one third of patients with hemoglobin SC disease had PSR at varying stages of development, and this complication seems to be more prevalent in patients with higher steady-stage hematocrits.[164]

The other serious complication of Hb SC disease is the development of widespread pulmonary vasoocclusion with the rapid onset of a typical chest syndrome, as described in the section on sickle cell anemia. This complication is particularly common during pregnancy or the puerperium.

Sickle Cell β Thalassemia.[3] The coinheritance of the sickle cell and β thalassemia genes generates a wide spectrum of clinical disorders, the severity of which range from a disorder identical to sickle cell anemia to a completely asymptomatic condition that is identified only by chance. Much of this heterogeneity depends on the type of β thalassemia mutation (see "β and δβ Thalassemias and Hereditary Persistence of Fetal Hemoglobin" below). In those who inherit β^0 thalassemia the clinical disorder is very similar to sickle cell anemia. In those who have a mild β^+ thalassemia mutation there may be as much as 30 percent hemoglobin A in the red cells, and the clinical picture is no more severe than sickle cell or β thalassemia trait.

Other Compound Heterozygous Disorders.[13,164] *Hemoglobin* $S/D_{LOS\ ANGELES}$ is a relatively severe disorder that resembles sickle cell anemia; this reflects the enhanced copolymerization of Hb $D_{LOS\ ANGELES}$ with Hb S due to the β121 substitution at an important contact point in the sickle cell fiber. *Hemoglobin* S/O_{ARAB} is also a severe disorder that is very similar to sickle cell anemia. The various combinations of *Hb S with*

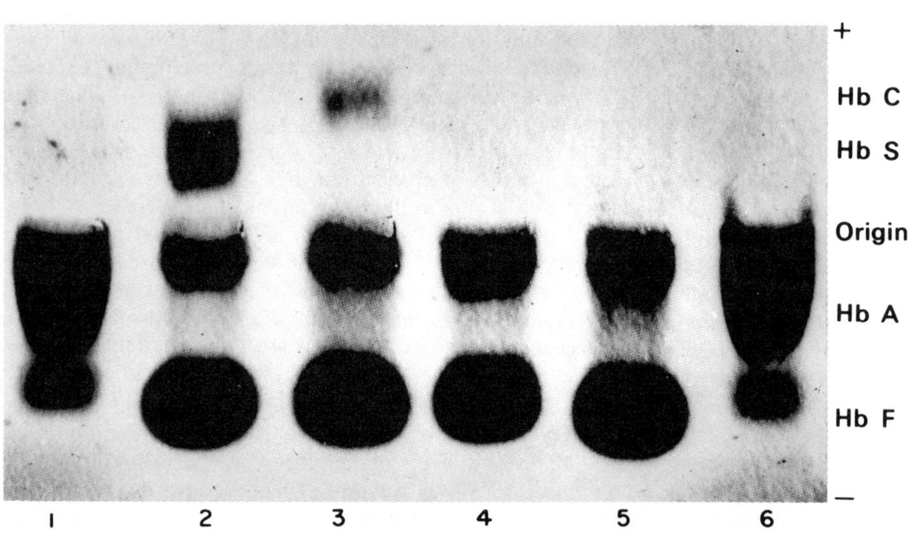

FIG. 113-12 **Hemoglobin electrophoresis (agar gel, pH 6.0). The following are shown from left to right: 1 = normal; 2 = sickle cell trait in newborn period; 3 = Hb C trait in newborn period; 4 and 5 = normal newborns; 6 = normal adult.** ***(From Weatherall and Clegg.[2] Used by permission.)***

hereditary persistence of fetal hemoglobin are all extremely mild. There are numerous other examples of the interaction of α- or β-globin-chain variants with Hb S. In most cases they result in an asymptomatic disorder identical to the sickle cell trait. The effects of α thalassemia on the course of sickle cell anemia were considered in an earlier section.

Sickle Cell Disease in Heterozygotes; HB $S_{ANTILLES}$. This sickling hemoglobin with two substitutions in the β-globin chain, 6 Glu to Val and 23 Val to Ile[186] is of particular phenotypic interest. This variant has the same electrophoretic mobility as Hb S, and the erythrocytes of heterozygotes tend to sickle at partial pressures of oxygen similar to those that induce sickling in Hb SC disease. Heterozygotes have a mild hemolytic anemia, splenomegaly, and, in some cases, painful crises. Thus, the condition resembles Hb SC disease. Nuclear magnetic spin resonance studies suggest that the β23 substitution induces slight structural perturbations throughout the β subunit.

The discovery of this mutation is of particular interest because it raises the possibility that some of the reported heterogeneity of the sickle cell trait and sickle cell anemia might result from substitutions of this type that do not alter the charge of sickle hemoglobin and hence that cannot be identified on routine electrophoresis.

Other Common Hemoglobin Variants

The only other hemoglobin variants that are encountered commonly are Hbs C, D, and E.

Hemoglobin C. Hemoglobin C was the second variant to be identified electrophoretically. It results from the substitution of lysine for glutamic acid at position 6 in the β chain.[187] It is restricted in its distribution to areas of west Africa and countries in which there has been movement of populations from this region. The gene frequency in American blacks, for example, ranges from 0.01 to 0.02.

A number of observations suggest that Hb C is less soluble than Hb A, and hence it tends to crystallize within red cells.[188] This is probably due to intermolecular interactions arising from the β^6 substitution. Interestingly, crystal formation is favored by the oxyhemoglobin configuration, and the crystals tend to melt when red cells undergo deoxygenation in the capillaries.[189] The red cells of Hb C homozygotes contain less water than normal and have an enhanced rate of potassium efflux. It has been suggested that these changes result from the direct interaction of the positively charged Hb C with negatively charged proteins on the cytoplasmic surface of the red-cell membrane.[190] Because of the resulting increased MCHC and the tendency to crystal formation, red cells containing Hb C are less deformable than normal. It seems likely that this is the major mechanism whereby their survival is shortened in the circulation. They also have decreased oxygen affinity.

Hemoglobin C heterozygotes have no hematologic changes except for an increased number of target cells on a stained blood film. The homozygous state for Hb C is characterized by a mild hemolytic anemia with splenomegaly. The blood film shows nearly 100 percent target cells, and there is a slightly elevated reticulocyte count. The peripheral blood film also shows a number of intracellular crystals.

The important interactions of Hb C are with Hb S (see previous section) and with β thalassemia. The compound heterozygous state with β^0 thalassemia produces a clinical picture very similar to Hb C disease.

Hemoglobin D. *Hemoglobin D* is the term used to describe a number of hemoglobin variants that have an identical rate of migration to Hb S on electrophoresis at an alkaline pH. The only common abnormal hemoglobin with these properties is Hb $D_{LOS\ ANGELES}$ (D_{PUNJAB}). This variant occurs frequently in the Punjab region and a number of homozygotes have been reported.[191] Their hemoglobin pattern shows almost all Hb D with normal levels of Hb A_2 and normal or only slightly elevated levels of Hb F. They have normal or only slightly reduced hemoglobin levels, and their red cells are normal except for increased numbers of target forms.

Hemoglobin E. This is probably the most common hemoglobin variant in the world population. It results from the substitution of glutamic acid by lysine at position 26 in the β chain.[192] It occurs mainly in a region stretching east from Bangladesh through Burma and reaches its highest frequency in eastern Thailand and Laos. It occurs in parts of China, and its distribution extends south down into the Indonesian islands. Gene frequencies in these populations are considered in a later section.

The pathophysiology of Hb E is still not fully understood. There seems little doubt that it is synthesized inefficiently as compared with Hb A and hence is associated with the clinical phenotype of a mild form of β thalassemia.[193] One reason for this is that the base substitution responsible for Hb E may activate a cryptic splice site within exon 1, leading to abnormal splicing of β-globin mRNA.[194]

The heterozygous state for Hb E is associated with no clinical disability and with normal hemoglobin levels, although the red cells are slightly microcytic and hypochromic. There is usually about 30 to 35 percent Hb E. Similarly, Hb E homozygotes are asymptomatic and are only slightly anemic, although they have red-cell indices that are very similar to those of heterozygous β thalassemic patients.

The importance of Hb E lies in the different phenotypes that result from its interaction with β thalassemia.[195] Compound heterozygotes for Hb E and β thalassemia have a variable clinical picture ranging from a condition indistinguishable from homozygous β thalassemia to a mild form of β thalassemia intermedia (see "Thalassemia" below). The hemoglobin pattern varies; in Hb E β^0 thalassemia compound heterozygotes there is usually about 50 to 75 percent Hb F, the remainder being Hb E. Compound heterozygotes for Hb E and β^+ thalassemia tend to have a milder disorder and produce variable amounts of Hb A. The reason for the severity of these interactions is not absolutely clear but probably is related to the gross chain imbalance together with the unusual properties of Hb E which make it more sensitive to oxidant stress and render it less stable than normal.[196]

In Southeast Asia there is a family of disorders due to the coinheritance of Hb E with different forms of α thalassemia. Heterozygotes for Hb E who inherit either α^+ or α^0 thalassemia have unusually low levels of Hb E.[195] The heterozygous state for Hb E in association with the genotype that produces Hb H disease (see "α Thalassemia" below) is responsible for a well-defined clinical syndrome characterized by moderate anemia, splenomegaly, and a hemoglobin pattern consisting of Hbs A, E, and Bart's. The reason such patients produce Hb Bart's and no Hb H is not clear, although one factor may be the increased affinity of α chains for normal β chains as compared with β^E chains and the inability of the latter to form stable tetramers. Another complex group of anemias result from the various interactions of α thalassemia with the homozygous state for Hb E.[2,195]

Unstable Hemoglobin Disorders

Over 90 different unstable hemoglobins have been reported.[3] However, the term *unstable hemoglobin disorder* is usually reserved for the clinical phenotype associated with variants, the instability of which is sufficient to cause clinically recognizable hemolysis. The clinical picture associated with such abnormal hemoglobins is also called *congenital Heinz body hemolytic anemia* (CHBA).

Molecular Basis of Hemoglobin Instability.[3,197–199] There are five different classes of mutations that can result in instability of the hemoglobin molecule (Fig. 113-13). The first is comprised of amino acid substitutions in the vicinity of the heme pocket. The binding of heme to globin involves specific interactions with particular nonpolar amino acid residues in the CD, E, F, and FG regions of the globin subunits. Most of these residues are invariant; hence, it is not surprising that their substitution leads to a decrease in the stability of

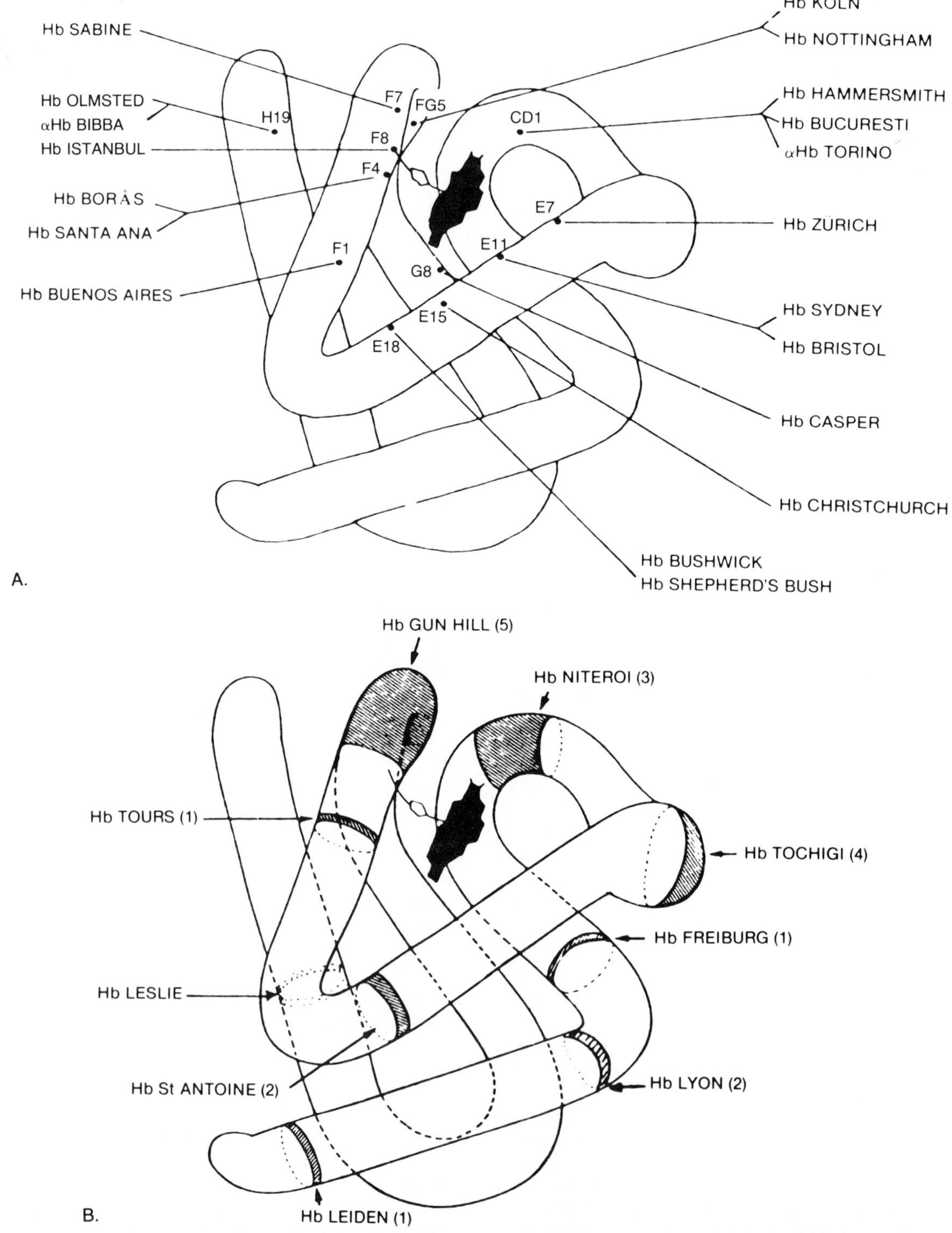

FIG. 113-13 Unstable hemoglobin variants. *A*. Three-dimensional representation of the β chain, showing sites of amino acid substitutions at the heme pocket. *B*. Three-dimensional representation of the β chain, showing sites of amino acid deletions that cause unstable hemoglobins. *(From Milner and Wrightstone.[199] Used by permission.)*

the binding of heme to globin; some examples are summarized in Fig. 113-13. At least three of these variants have amino acid substitutions at the proximal (heme-linked) histidine; two others have substitutions at the distal histidine. Some abnormal hemoglobins of this type are particularly susceptible to drug-induced precipitation and hemolysis. $Hb_{ZÜRICH}$, for example, has a substitution that leaves the heme pocket wide open, thus allowing drugs such as sulfonamides ready access to the heme iron.

A second group of unstable variants result from amino acid substitutions that disrupt the secondary structure of the globin chains. About 75 percent of globin is in the form of α helix, in which proline cannot participate except as part of one of the initial three residues. Eleven unstable hemoglobin variants have been described that result from the substitution of proline for leucine, five that are caused by an alanine to proline change, and three in which proline is substituted by histidine. Another group of variants that cause disruption of the normal configuration of the hemoglobin molecule involve internal substitutions that interfere with its stabilization by hydrophobic interactions. Some of these variants result in alterations in tertiary structure and hence allow access of water to the hydrophobic interior of globin subunits.

Finally, there are two groups of unstable hemoglobins that result from gross structural abnormalities of the globin subunits. At least 11 variants have been found that contain deletions ranging from one to five residues, many of which involve regions at or near interhelical corners. A few unstable variants have elongated globin chains. For example, $Hb_{CRANSTON}$ and $Hb_{SAVERNE}$ are associated with a mild hemolysis that is probably due to the hydrophobic segments attached to the C-terminal ends of their β-globin chains.

Mechanism of Hemoglobin Denaturation.[197-199] The major result of these substitutions is the precipitation of hemoglobin with the formation of rigid Heinz bodies. The latter causes retardation of the passage of red cells through the microcirculation and hence leads to their premature destruction.

Although the precise details of the mechanisms of hemoglobin precipitation in these disorders are unknown, some general conclusions can be drawn. Hemoglobin can autooxidize into methemoglobin with the dissociation of superoxide anion. The latter, and its reduction product hydrogen peroxide, are able to generate more methemoglobin. The unstable hemoglobins show a more rapid rate of autooxidation than normal hemoglobin. Furthermore, methemoglobin can be converted into hemichrome, in which globin undergoes sufficient internal distortion to allow direct bonding of an amino acid side chain to the distal aspect of the heme iron. Initially, this process is reversible, but ultimately irreversible hemichrome formation occurs, and this is followed by precipitation of hemoglobin with the production of a Heinz body. In addition, some unstable variants interact with glutathione to form mixed disulfides. Furthermore, as mentioned above, the formation of methemoglobin favors the dissociation of heme from globin.

A scheme for the denaturation of unstable hemoglobin with the production of Heinz bodies is shown in Fig. 113-14.

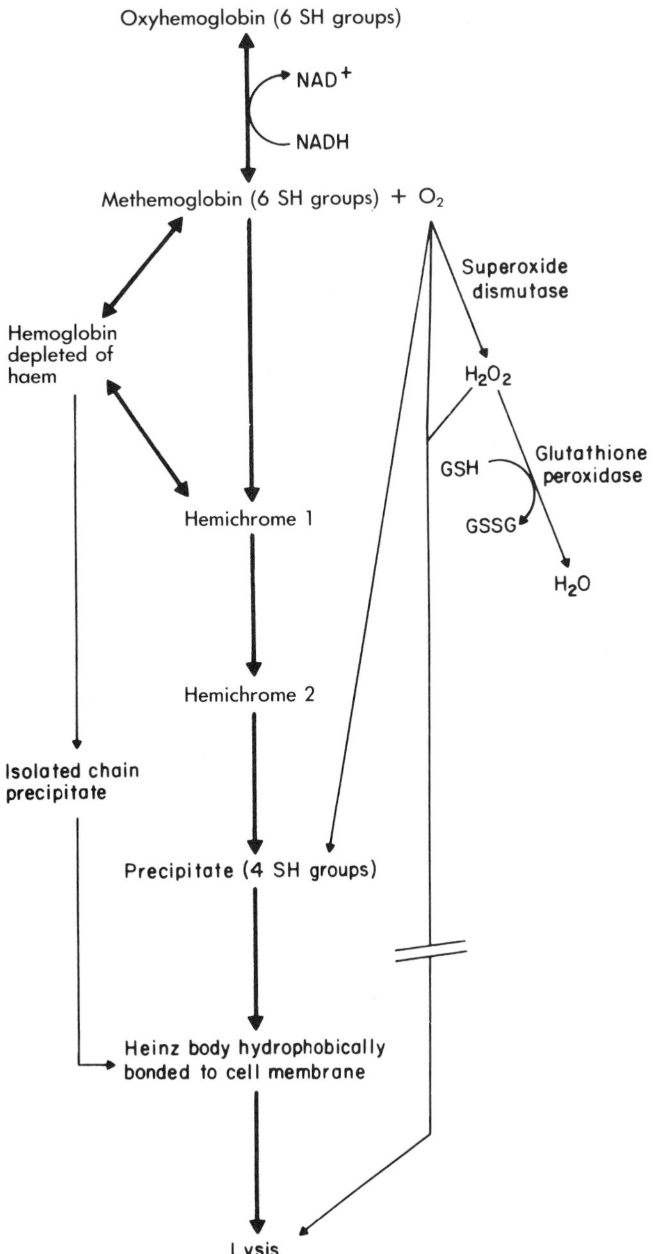

FIG. 113-14 Schematic representation of the mechanism of hemoglobin precipitation in the unstable hemoglobin disorders. *(From Weatherall and Clegg.[2] Used by permission.)*

Mechanism of Hemolysis.[199-201] Red cells that contain Heinz bodies have decreased pliability and hence negotiate the microcirculation with difficulty. These cells are trapped during their transit between the cords and sinuses of the spleen. In this way a Heinz body may be "pulled out" of the cell during its passage through the spleen, after which the remainder of the cell reseals. This process causes membrane damage that also may be mediated by the adherence of Heinz bodies to the inner surface of the red-cell membrane. The red cells of patients with unstable hemoglobin disorders show an increased rate of potassium leak and, in some cases, reduced levels of ATP. Furthermore, because unstable hemoglobins may favor release of reactive oxidants such as hydrogen peroxide, superoxide, and free hydroxyl radical, these toxic side products may also damage the red-cell membrane by causing lipid peroxidation and cross-linking of membrane proteins.

Clinical and Hematologic Findings. Patients with CHBA have varying degrees of hemolysis inherited as autosomal dominants. In several cases no affected relatives have been found, and the hemoglobin variants are thought to be the result of new mutations.[200]

The clinical course is characterized by anemia and splenomegaly and the intermittent passage of dark urine. The latter is not due to hemoglobinuria but to pigmenturia; the pigments have not been identified with certainty but may be related to dipyrrolmethanes of the mesobilifuscin group. Hematologic studies show the features of a hemolytic anemia with a raised reticulocyte count and variation in the shape and size of the red cells. In patients with an intact spleen this may be all that is found. However, after splenectomy many of the red cells contain Heinz bodies.

The hemoglobin variants associated with this condition often have neutral mutations—that is, they cannot be identified by electrophoresis. However, if dilute hemoglobin solutions are incubated in a neutral phosphate buffer at 50°C for 1 to 2 h unstable variants precipitate. A similar effect can be induced by incubation of hemolysates in 17 percent isopropanol at 37°C. Hemoglobin electrophoresis may show no abnormality, but sometimes after the red-cell lysate has been stored for a few days, a variety of bands appear, some of which are heme-depleted and therefore are seen only with a protein stain. The hemoglobin A_2 level may be slightly increased in patients with unstable β-chain variants. The position of the oxygen dissociation curve varies; both high- and low-affinity unstable hemoglobins have been reported.

Course and Prognosis. The majority of patients with CHBA have a mild anemia and are not incapacitated. Because some of these variants are precipitated by oxidant drugs, exacerbations may occur after drug therapy or with intercurrent illnesses, particularly infection. Rarely, there may be progressive splenomegaly with hypersplenism. Sustained thrombocytosis has been observed after splenectomy.

Hemoglobin Variants with Abnormal Oxygen Binding

Several clinical syndromes result from abnormalities of oxygen binding by abnormal hemoglobins (Table 113-5). Both low- and high-oxygen-affinity variants have been encountered. About a third of the unstable variants described in the previous section have increased oxygen affinity, but in these disorders the clinical manifestations are due to accelerated red-cell destruction; the hemoglobin level may be modified by the oxygen affinity of the particular variant. There are, however, over 40 abnormal hemoglobins in which increased oxygen affinity occurs without instability. These variants are sometimes associated with the clinical syndrome of genetic polycythemia. On the other hand, variants characterized by a low oxygen affinity may result in a dominantly inherited form of cyanosis.

Table 113-5 Hemoglobin Variants with Altered Oxygen Affinity

High-oxygen-affinity variants	
Mutations at $\alpha_1\beta_2$ contacts	
$Hb_{CHESAPEAKE}$	α92 Arg → Leu
$Hb_{J\text{-}CAPE\ TOWN}$	α92 Arg → Gln
$Hb_{TARRANT}$	α126 Asp → Asn
$Hb_{LEGNANO}$	α141 Arg → Leu
Mutations at 2,3-DPG binding sites	
Hb_{RAHERE}	β86 Lys → Thr
$Hb_{HELSINKI}$	β82Lys → Met
$Hb_{PROVIDENCE}$	β82Lys → Asn
Heme binding site	
$Hb_{HEATHROW}$	β103 Phe → Leu
Low-oxygen-affinity variants	
Mutations at $\alpha_1\beta_2$ contact	
Hb_{KANSAS}	β102 Asn → Thr
$Hb_{BETH\ ISRAEL}$	β102 Asn → Ser
Mutations at 2,3-DPG binding site	
$Hb_{RALEIGH}$	β1 Val → Acet.Ala

NOTE: A complete list with references is given in Bunn and Forget.[3]

High-Oxygen-Affinity-Variants and Hereditary Polycythemia.[3,202–204] As mentioned earlier, hemoglobin exists in equilibrium between two quaternary conformations, R and T. When it is fully deoxygenated it assumes the T, or tense, state in which it has a low affinity for oxygen and a relatively high affinity for allosteric molecules such as Bohr protons and 2,3-DPG. On the other hand, oxyhemoglobin exists in the R, or relaxed, state in which it has a high affinity for oxygen and a low affinity for allosteric effectors. The transition between these two conformations requires cooperativity between the subunits that is the molecular basis for heme–heme interaction. Most of the high-affinity variants result from mutations that cause amino acid substitutions that affect the equilibrium between the R and T states. Many of them are found at the $\alpha_1\beta_2$ interface, the C-terminal end of the β chain, and at the 2,3-DPG binding sites (see Table 113-5).

The clinical findings vary in patients with high-oxygen affinity hemoglobin variants. There is usually an erythrocytosis with an elevated hemoglobin level but no changes in the white cell or platelet counts, and no splenomegaly, features that distinguish these conditions from polycythemia vera, a myeloproliferative disorder involving hemopoietic stem cells. The whole blood oxygen dissociation curve is shifted to the left with a reduced p50; many of the high-affinity hemoglobins also show a decreased alkaline Bohr effect. In some cases there is reduced interaction with 2,3-DPG. The other physiological properties of these variants have been the subject of a number of extensive reviews.[3,203,204]

The majority of patients with high-oxygen-affinity variants are asymptomatic and are ascertained only because they are found to have a modest erythrocytosis on routine hematologic examination. The diagnosis is made by ruling out other causes of polycythemia and by demonstrating a decreased p50 associated with a hemoglobin variant. It is important to remember that there are other causes of a left-shifted oxygen dissociation curve, methemoglobin, or carboxyhemoglobin, for example, that must be excluded by spectroscopic analysis.

Low-Oxygen-Affinity Variants. There are far fewer hemoglobin variants with low oxygen affinities (see Table 113-5). As mentioned earlier, some unstable variants fall into this group, and some of the M hemoglobins also have decreased oxygen affinity.

The best-studied low-oxygen variant is Hb_{KANSAS}[205] Carriers have normal hemoglobin levels but are cyanosed from birth. The condition is associated with a reduced oxygen saturation of the arterial blood despite a Pa_{O_2} of 100 mmHg. When these individuals breathe 100 percent oxygen the oxygen saturation increases by about 30 percent, suggesting that there is a marked decrease in whole-blood oxygen affinity. $Hemoglobin_{KANSAS}$ has a threonine substitution for asparagine at position 102 in the β chain. Interestingly, this residue is at the $\alpha_1\beta_2$ interface, similar to some of the high-affinity variants described earlier. The low affinity of Hb_{KANSAS} seems to be due in part to a relatively unstable R structure, although the precise mechanism is not understood.

The clinical picture associated with two other low-affinity variants, $Hb_{BETH\ ISRAEL}$ and $_{ST.\ MANDE}$, is similar.

Congenital Cyanosis Due to Hemoglobin Variants. Congenital methemoglobinemia may result either from an inherited structural hemoglobin or from a defect in one of the enzyme systems involved in maintaining a normal level of reduced hemoglobin in the red cells; the latter group of conditions is considered in Chap. 112.

The five structural hemoglobin variants that are associated with methemoglobinemia are all designated *Hb M*; they are further defined by their place of discovery—that is, Hb M_{BOSTON}, Hb $M_{HYDE\ PARK}$, and so on. Their structure–function relationships have been the subject of several detailed reviews.[3,206] As mentioned earlier in this chapter, the iron atom of heme is normally linked to the imidazole group of the proximal histidine residue of the α and β chains. There is another histidine residue on the opposite side, near the sixth coordination position of the heme iron; this, the so-called distal histidine residue, is the normal binding site for oxygen. The imidazole group of the distal histidine does not form a bond with heme iron except, as mentioned earlier, in the pathological conditions in which hemichrome is formed.

Four of the five M hemoglobins result from the substitution of a tyrosine for either the proximal or distal histidine residues in either the α or β chains. It is likely that the phenolic group of the abnormal tyrosine residue forms a covalent link with the heme iron, thus stabilizing the iron atom in the oxidized (Fe^{3+}) configuration. The first three hemoglobin Ms to be discovered were Hb M_{BOSTON} (α58 His→Tyr), Hb $M_{SASKATOON}$ (β63 His→Tyr), and Hb $M_{MILWAUKEE}$ (β67 Val→Glu). Another variant, Hb M_{IWATE} (α87 His→Tyr), was discovered later in Japan, although it subsequently turned up in other populations. A fifth variant, Hb $M_{HYDE\ PARK}$ (β92 His→Tyr) was first encountered in the United Kingdom. A fetal hemoglobin variant associated with methemoglobinemia, Hb FM_{OSAKA} (γ63 His→Tyr) has been found in a Japanese infant.

X-ray crystallographic studies have confirmed that these amino acid substitutions stabilize the heme group of the mutant hemoglobins in the oxidized forms. Once in this form the abnormal subunit is resistant to reduction by both enzymes and reducing agents.

Individuals who are heterozygous for the M hemoglobins are cyanosed from early in life but are otherwise asymptomatic. The condition can often be distinguished from congenital methemoglobinemia because of an enzyme defect in the family history; the pattern of inheritance of Hb M is typically dominant. Furthermore, if the cyanosis is present from birth, it is usually due to an α-chain Hb M methemoglobin variant; alternatively, if cyanosis appears only during the first few months of life, the disorder is likely to be due to a β-chain variant. It is interesting that conjunctival cyanosis is present in children with methemoglobin but not in those in whom the cyanosis is due to defective oxygenation of the blood; the conjunctival sac provides such close apposition of the red cells to air that it acts as a "second lung"; even in cases of severe cyanotic heart disease or pulmonary disease conjunctival cyanosis is usually absent.

The diagnosis of methemoglobinemia is made by demonstrating increased amounts of methemoglobin in the red cells. The M hemoglobins give a characteristic spectral abnormality provided the hemoglobin is completely oxidized to the Fe^{3+} state with ferricyanide. They are not demonstrable by hemoglobin electrophoresis under routine conditions, although some of them separate on agar gel at pH 7.1. They can be demonstrated more effectively if the red-cell lysate is first oxidized with ferricyanide.

No treatment is required for congenital methemoglobinemia due to an M hemoglobin. Affected individuals tolerate major surgery without difficulty; the main task for the clinician is to arrive at an accurate diagnosis and to provide adequate reassurance.

THALASSEMIA

The thalassemias are the commonest single gene disorders in the world population. They have been the subject of several monographs[2,6,207] and reviews.[208–211] In this section, after defining and classifying these conditions we shall describe their pathophysiology as a group; since they are very heterogeneous they have much in common with respect to the mechanisms of disordered erythropoiesis and red-cell destruction. We shall then describe the molecular pathology and clinical and hematologic features of each of the main varieties.

Definition and Classification

The thalassemias are a heterogeneous group of inherited disorders of hemoglobin synthesis, all characterized by the absence or reduced output of one or more of the globin chains of hemoglobin. This leads to the imbalanced globin-chain synthesis that is the hallmark of all the thalassemia syndromes.[3]

The main types of thalassemia are summarized in Table 113-6. The commonest and clinically most important forms are α, β, and δβ thalassemias. Each of these can be classified into disorders in which no chains are produced from the affected chromosomes—α^0, β^0, and $(\delta\beta)^0$ thalassemia—and those in which some chains are synthesized, but at a reduced rate—α^+, β^+, and $(\delta\beta)^+$ thalassemia. The related condition, hereditary persistence of fetal hemoglobin, can be regarded as a particularly mild form of β or δβ thalassemia in

Table 113-6 Thalassemias and Related Disorders

α Thalassemia
α^0
α^+ Deletion, nondeletion
With α-chain Hb variants
With β-chain Hb variants
With β thalassemia
β Thalassemia
β^0
β^+
With β-chain Hb variants
With α-chain Hb variants
With α thalassemia
δβ Thalassemia
$(\delta\beta)^0$ Thalassemia
$(^A\gamma\delta\beta)^0$ Thalassemia
$(\epsilon\gamma\delta\beta)^0$ Thalassemia
δ Thalassemia
γ Thalassemia
Hereditary persistence of fetal hemoglobin
Deletion
$(\delta\beta)^0$ HPFH
Nondeletion
Linked to β-globin gene cluster
Unlinked to β-globin gene cluster

which defective β-chain production is fully compensated by persistent γ-chain synthesis beyond the neonatal period.

In many populations the thalassemias coexist with a variety of different structural hemoglobin variants. Thus, it is quite common to inherit both types of condition. Furthermore, it is equally common for individuals to receive genes for more than one type of thalassemia. These complex interactions give rise to an extremely diverse series of clinical disorders that, taken together, constitute the thalassemia syndromes.[3]

Pathophysiology

One of the most remarkable aspects of the thalassemia field is how it has been feasible to relate the diverse clinical manifestations, that may affect almost any organ system, to primary molecular defects in the α- or β-globin genes. In fact it is possible to trace almost all of the pathophysiological features of these conditions back to a primary imbalance of globin chain synthesis (Fig. 113-15). It is this phenomenon that makes the thalassemias fundamentally different from all the other genetic and acquired disorders of hemoglobin production and, to a large extent, explains their extreme severity in the homozygous or compound heterozygous states.

Imbalanced Globin-Chain Synthesis. Measurements of in vitro globin-chain synthesis in the peripheral blood or bone marrows of patients with different types of thalassemia,[12] together with genetic studies that enable the action of the thalassemia genes to be examined in patients who have also inherited α- or β-globin structural variants, provide a clear picture of the action of the thalassemia determinants.[3] In homozygous β thalassemia, β-globin synthesis may be either absent or markedly reduced. This results in the production of an excess of α-globin chains. Unpaired α-globin chains are incapable of forming a viable hemoglobin tetramer and hence precipitate in red-cell precursors.[212,213] The resulting inclusion bodies can be demonstrated by both light and electron microscopy (Fig. 113-16). In the bone marrow, precipitation can be seen in the earliest hemoglobinized precursors and right through the erythroid maturation pathway. These large inclusions are responsible for the intramedullary destruction of red-cell precursors and hence the ineffective erythropoiesis that characterizes all the β thalassemias. It has been calculated that a large proportion of the developing erythroblasts are destroyed within the bone marrow in severe cases.[3] The red cells that are released are prematurely destroyed by mechanisms considered below.

β-Thalassemia heterozygotes also have imbalanced globin-chain synthesis, but in this case the magnitude of the

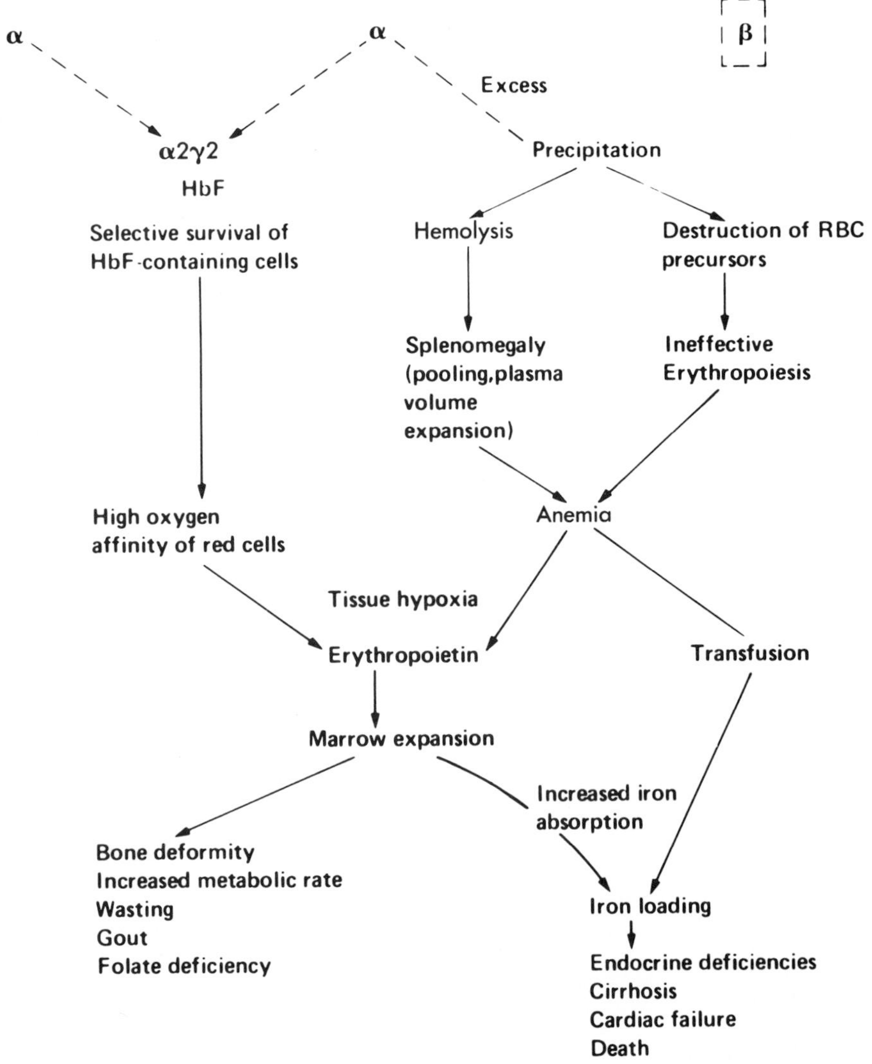

FIG. 113-15 Pathophysiology of β thalassemia.

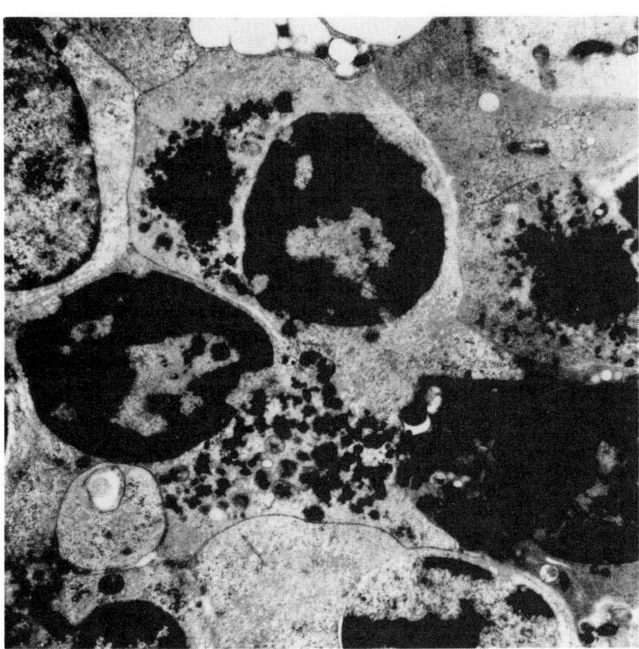

FIG. 113-16 **Inclusion bodies in the red-cell precursors in homozygous β thalassemia (electron microscopy ×9000).** ***(From Weatherall and Clegg.[2] Used by permission; original preparations supplied by Dr. A. Polliack.)***

excess of α chains is much less and presumably can be dealt with successfully by the proteolytic enzymes of the red-cell precursors.[214] Nevertheless, there is a mild degree of ineffective erythropoiesis.

From these considerations it is clear that the anemia of β thalassemia has three major components. First and most important, there is ineffective erythropoiesis with intramedullary destruction of a variable proportion of the developing red-cell precursors. Second, there is a hemolytic component due to destruction of mature red cells containing α-chain inclusions. Finally, because of the overall reduction in hemoglobin synthesis the red cells are hypochromic and microcytic.

Because the primary defect in β thalassemia is in β-chain production, the synthesis of hemoglobins F and A_2 should be unaffected. Fetal hemoglobin production in utero is normal, and it is only when the neonatal switch from γ- to β-chain production occurs that the clinical manifestations of β thalassemia first appear. However, fetal hemoglobin synthesis persists beyond the neonatal period in nearly all forms of β thalassemia; we shall return to the reasons for this in the section on "Persistent Fetal Hemoglobin Production and Cellular Heterogeneity." In β-thalassemia heterozygotes there is an elevated level of Hb A_2. This appears to reflect both a relative decrease in Hb A due to defective β-chain synthesis but also to an absolute increase in the output of δ chains both *cis* and *trans* to the mutant β-globin gene.[3] The question of Hb A_2 production in homozygous β thalassemia is extremely complex and will be discussed in the following section.

The consequences of excess non–α chain production in the α thalassemias are quite different. α Chains are shared by both fetal and adult hemoglobin and therefore defective α-chain production is manifest in both fetal and adult life.[208] In the fetus, a reduced output of α chains leads to excess γ-chain production; similarly, in the adult excess β chains are produced. Excess γ chains combine to form γ_4 homotetramers, or Hb BART'S; excess β chains form β_4 homotetramers or Hb H. It is this ability of γ and β chains to form homotetramers that is the basis of the fundamental difference in the pathophysiology of α and β thalassemia.[208] Because γ_4 and β_4 tetramers are soluble they do not precipitate to any significant degree in the bone marrow; therefore, the α thalassemias are not characterized by a severe degree of ineffective erythropoiesis. However, β_4 tetramers precipitate as red cells age, forming inclusion bodies. Thus, the anemia of the more severe forms of α thalassemia in adults is due mainly to a shortened red-cell survival consequent on their damage in the microvasculature of the spleen due to the presence of the inclusions. In addition, because of the defect in hemoglobin synthesis the cells are hypochromic and microcytic. Hemoglobin BART'S is more stable than Hb H and does not appear to form inclusions.

But there is another factor that exacerbates the tissue hypoxia of the anemia of the α thalassemias. Both Hb BART'S and Hb H show no heme–heme interaction and have almost hyperbolic oxygen dissociation curves with very high oxygen affinities. Thus, they are not able to give up oxygen at physiological tissue tensions and are, in effect, useless as oxygen carriers.[3]

It follows, therefore, that infants with high levels of Hb BART'S have severe intrauterine hypoxia. This is a major component of the clinical picture of homozygous α^0 thalassemia, which results in the stillbirth of hydropic infants late in pregnancy or at term. Severe intrauterine oxygen deprivation is reflected by the grossly hydropic state of the infant, presumably due an increase in capillary permeability consequent on hypoxia, and severe erythroblastosis. Deficient fetal oxygenation is probably responsible for the enormously hypertrophied placentas that occur with the severe forms of intrauterine α thalassemia.[208]

Persistent Fetal Hemoglobin Production and Cellular Heterogeneity. One of the earliest observations on the hemoglobin patterns of children with severe thalassemia was that there is a variable amount of Hb F production that persists into childhood and later.[3] Indeed, in the β thalassemias, except for small amounts of Hb A_2, Hb F is the only hemoglobin produced. Examination of the peripheral blood using staining methods that are specific for Hb F show that it is heterogeneously distributed among the red cells. Persistent Hb F production is not a feature of the more severe forms of α thalassemia, although in some cases persistent γ-chain synthesis is reflected by the presence of Hb Bart's after the first 6 months of life.

There are still many unanswered questions about the mechanisms of persistent γ-chain synthesis in the thalassemias. Normal adults have small quantities of Hb F that are heterogeneously distributed among the red cells; cells with demonstrable Hb F are called "F cells." It is clear that one important mechanism for persistent Hb F production in β thalassemia is cell selection.[3,211] As already mentioned, the major cause of ineffective erythropoiesis and shortened red-cell survival in β thalassemia is the deleterious effects of excess α chains on erythroid maturation and survival of red cells in the blood. It follows therefore that any red-cell precursors that produce significant numbers of γ chains will be at an advantage in an environment in which there are excess α chains; the latter will combine with γ chains to produce Hb F, and therefore the magnitude of α-chain precipitation will be less. Differential centrifugation experiments and in vivo labeling studies have shown that populations of red cells with relatively large amounts of Hb F are more efficiently produced and survive longer in the peripheral blood than those with low levels or no Hb F (reviewed by Weatherall and Clegg[2]). The peripheral blood of homozygous β thalassemia patients shows remarkable cellular heterogeneity with respect to red-cell survival times; there are populations of cells that contain predominantly Hb A that are very rapidly destroyed in the spleen and elsewhere, cells with a much longer survival that contain relatively more Hb F, and populations of intermediate age and hemoglobin constitution.

Whether cell selection of this type is the only mechanism for persistent γ-chain production in β thalassemia is not clear. It is possible that there may be an absolute increase in Hb F production; this is certainly so in some milder forms of homozygous β thalassemia, but in these cases there may be other genetic factors that are responsible for the relatively high level of γ-chain synthesis (see below).

Since there is a reciprocal relationship between γ- and δ-chain synthesis, it follows that the red cells of β-thalassemia homozygotes that contain large amounts of Hb F have relatively low levels of Hb A_2.[2] Thus, the measured percent of Hb A_2 in these individuals is the average of a very heterogeneous cell population. This probably accounts for the extreme variability in the levels of Hb A_2 reported in patients with this disorder.

A further consequence of the persistence of Hb F in β thalassemia is that the red cells have a high oxygen affinity. Thalassemic red cells adapt poorly to anemia, as reflected by inappropriately low levels of 2,3-DPG and a high oxygen affinity.[3]

Consequences of Compensatory Mechanisms for the Anemia of Thalassemia. The profound anemia of homozygous β thalassemia combined with the high oxygen affinity of such blood as is produced combines to produce severe tissue hypoxia. Because of the properties of Hb BART'S and Hb H a similar defect in tissue oxygenation occurs in the more severe forms of α thalassemia. The major response is erythropoietin production and expansion of the dyserythropoietic bone marrow. This in turn leads to deformities of the skull and face and porosity of the long bones.[2] In extreme cases, extramedullary hemopoietic tumors may develop. Apart from the production of severe skeletal deformities, bone marrow expansion may cause pathological fractures, sinus disease, and chronic middle ear infection.

Another effect of the enormous expansion of the marrow mass in severe thalassemia is to divert calories required for normal development to the ineffective red-cell precursor population. Thus, severely affected thalassemic patients show poor development and wasting. The massive turnover of erythroid precursors may result in secondary hyperuricemia and gout and severe folate deficiency.

The effects of gross intrauterine hypoxia in homozygous α^0 thalassemia have already been described. In the symptomatic forms of α thalassemia, such as Hb H disease, that are compatible with survival into adult life, bone changes and other consequences of erythroid expansion are seen, although to a much lesser degree than in β thalassemia.

Splenomegaly; Dilutional Anemia. The constant bombardment of the spleen with abnormal red cells gives rise to the phenomenon of "work hypertrophy." Progressive splenomegaly occurs in both α and β thalassemia and may exacerbate the anemia.[3,207] Large spleens act as a sump for red cells and may sequestrate a considerable proportion of the peripheral red-cell mass. Furthermore, splenomegaly may also cause plasma volume expansion, a complication that may be exacerbated by massive expansion of the erythroid bone marrow. The combination of pooling of the red cells in the spleen together with plasma volume expansion may cause worsening of the anemia in both α and β thalassemia. The same process may occur in an enlarged liver, particularly after splenectomy.

Abnormal Iron Metabolism. In β-thalassemia homozygotes who are anemic there is an increase in intestinal iron absorption that is related to the degree of expansion of the red-cell precursor population; iron absorption is decreased by blood transfusion.[207] Increased absorption causes a steady accumulation of iron, first in the Kupffer cells of the liver and in the reticuloendothelial (RE) cells of the spleen but later in the parenchymal cells of the liver (Fig. 113-17). Most homozygous β thalassemia patients require regular blood transfusions, and thus transfusional siderosis adds to the iron accumulation. Iron accumulates in the endocrine glands, particularly the parathyroids and adrenals, pancreas, skin, and, most important, the liver and the myocardium. The latter leads to death, either by involving the conducting tissues or by causing intractable cardiac failure. Other consequences of iron loading include diabetes, hypoparathyroidism, and hypogonadism, mainly due to end-organ failure.[3,207]

Disordered iron metabolism is less common in the adult forms of α thalassemia. The reason is not clear, but the milder degree of anemia, less marked erythroid expansion of the marrow, and the fact that Hb H may not bind to haptoglobin and may be excreted in the urine, all play a part.

There appears to be an increased susceptibility to bacterial infection in all forms of severe thalassemia.[3,207] The reason is not known. It has been suggested that the relatively high serum iron levels may favor bacterial growth. Another possible mechanism is blockage of the RE system due to the increased rate of destruction of red cells. No consistent defects in white-cell or immune function have been demonstrated, but it remains to be shown unequivocally that high serum iron levels are an important factor.

Disordered Red-Cell Metabolism. As we have seen, the presence of α- or β-chain inclusions in the red cells of thalassemic patients is explanation enough for their shortened survival. However, many abnormalities of red-cell metabolism that might also play a role have been demonstrated.[3,215]

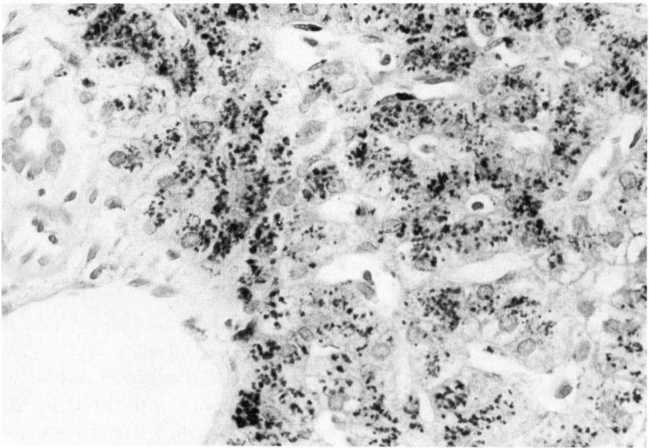

FIG. 113-17 Iron loading of the liver in β thalassemia intermedia (×600, iron stain).

These include oxidant damage to the membrane as a consequence of lipid peroxidation resulting from generation of superoxide and the formation of hemichrome by the precipitated globin chains. The significance of hemichromes was discussed in the section that deals with the unstable hemoglobin disorders. These abnormalities may be enhanced by vitamin E deficiency and excess iron in the red cells. Damage to the red-cell membrane is reflected by a variety of abnormalities of permeability, including an increase in the rate of potassium loss from the cells of both homozygotes and heterozygotes for β thalassemia and of individuals with the more severe forms of α thalassemia. Centrifugation experiments show that these changes are more severe in the fast-turning-over, low-Hb F/high-Hb A population of red cells of β thalassemic patients.

Clinical Heterogeneity. The pathophysiological mechanisms outlined in the previous sections provide a basis for the remarkable clinical diversity of the thalassemia syndromes. It is clear that all the clinical manifestations of β thalassemia can be related to excess α-chain production. It follows that any mechanism that tends to reduce the excess of α chains in β thalassemia should modify the clinical course of the disease. A number of elegant experiments of nature have shown that this is the case. For example, β-thalassemia homozygotes who inherit one or more α-thalassemia genes tend to run a much milder course than those with β thalassemia alone.[216,217] Similarly, the coinheritance of one or more genetic determinants that favor persistent γ-chain synthesis after the neonatal period ameliorates the condition. In other words if α thalassemia is coinherited, the magnitude of excess α chains is less; if there is a higher than usual output of γ chains, some of the excess α chains combine with γ chains to produce Hb F. In either case, the overall excess of α chains is less, and therefore the degree of ineffective erythropoiesis and hemolysis is reduced. These clinical observations have provided strong support for the various pathophysiological concepts outlined in the previous sections.

It is clear that if patients with β thalassemia undergo adequate transfusion, most of the consequences of excess α-chain production can be overcome. The drive to erythroid expansion is diminished, hence the skeletal and growth abnormalities do not develop. Iron absorption from the gastrointestinal tract is reduced, and because endogenous red-cell production is turned off, hepatosplenomegaly does not occur. Thus, adequately transfused thalassemic children grow and develop normally, although if iron is not removed by chelation therapy, they succumb to the effects of iron loading of the tissues in the second or third decade.

α Thalassemia

Classification. Until the late 1970s the various determinants of α thalassemia could be defined only in terms of their effect on the phenotype (MCV, MCH, α/β-globin-chain synthesis ratio) and the way in which they interact to produce the carrier states for α thalassemia (α thalassemia minor), Hb H disease, or the Hb BART'S hydrops fetalis syndrome (Table 113-7).[2] More recently, many of the underlying molecular defects have been identified; therefore it is possible to establish a more comprehensive system for classifying the mutant alleles.[208,211]

α Thalassemias in which no normal α-globin is produced from the α-gene complex are called α^0 thalassemias, and those in which the output is reduced are referred to as α^+ thalassemia. This brings the classification of the α thalassemias in line with that for the β thalassemias. The α^0 and α^+ thalassemias can be further subdivided, according to the precise nature of the underlying molecular defect, into deletion and nondeletion types.

The α-globin haplotype may be written αα, representing the α2 and α1 genes, respectively. Therefore, a normal individual has the genotype αα/αα. A deletion involving one (-α) or both (− −) α genes may be further classified on the basis of its size, written as a superscript thus $-\alpha^{3.7}$ indicates a deletion of 3.7 kb DNA, including one α gene. When the size of a deletion has not yet been established, a superscript

Table 113-7 Genotype/Phenotype Relations in the α Thalassemias

Phenotype	Equivalent Number of Functional α Genes	Level of Hb Bart's at Birth, %*	% HbH (Inclusions)	MCV (fl)†	MCH (pg)†	α/β-Globin Chain Synthesis Ratio	Interacting‡ Haplotypes	Most frequently Encountered Genotypes
Normal	4	0§	0 (None)	90±5	30±2	~1.0	α/α	αα/αα
α Thalassemia¶ minor (mild)	3	0–2	0 (Rare)	81±7	26±2	~0.8	α^+/α	−α/αα
α Thalassemia¶ minor (severe)	2	2–8	0 (Occasional)	69±4	22±2	~0.6	α°/α or α^+/α^+	− −/αα $\alpha^T\alpha/\alpha\alpha$ −α/−α
HbH disease	1	10–40	2–40 (Many)	65±7	19±2	~0.3	α°/α^+ or α^+/α^+	− −/−α $--/\alpha^T\alpha$ $\alpha^T\alpha/\alpha^T\alpha$
Hb BART'S hydrops fetalis	0	~80	Present (Present)	110–120	Reduced	0.0	$\alpha^\circ/\alpha^\circ$	− −/− − $--/\alpha^T\alpha$

*Hb BART'S gradually disappears from peripheral blood in the 3 to 6 months following birth.
†These values vary considerably depending on the age of the patient,[208] and the figures given are a guide to the indices seen in adults with the deletion forms of α thalassemia.[208]
‡α = normal haplotype; α^+ = α^+ thalassemia; α° = α° thalassemia.
§Very small amounts of Hb BART'S have been detected in normal infants at birth.[211]
¶The mild and severe forms of α-thalassemia trait are often referred to as α-thalassemia-2 and α-thalassemia-1, respectively.

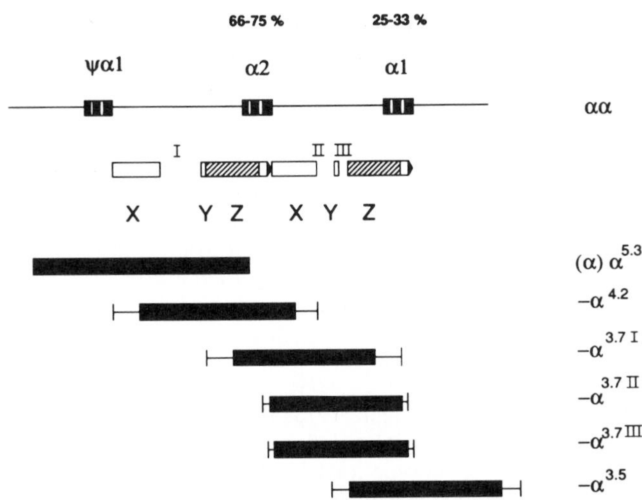

FIG. 113-18 Fine structure around the duplicated α-globin genes (above). The pseudo-α gene (ψα1) and duplicated α genes (α1 and α2) are shown. Above, the relative levels of expression of the α2 and α1 genes are shown. Black boxes indicate exons; white boxes show the size and positions of introns. Below, the X, Y, and Z boxes are shown, marking the positions and extent of the duplication that gave rise to the two α genes. The deletions that involve one or other of the α genes are shown below. Thick black bars indicate the extent of the deletions and thin bars the regions of uncertainty for the breakpoints.

describing the geographical or individual origin of the deletion is used; thus $--^{\text{MED}}$ describes a deletion of both α genes first identified in individuals of Mediterranean origin. In thalassemic haplotypes in which both genes are intact the nomenclature $\alpha^{T}\alpha$ or $\alpha\alpha^{T}$ is given, depending on whether the α2 or α1 gene is affected. When the precise molecular defect is known, as in Hb CONSTANT SPRING,[119] for example, $\alpha^{T}\alpha$ can be replaced by the more informative $\alpha^{CS}\alpha$.

This system provides an accurate shorthand way of describing various interactions. For example the genotype $--^{\text{SEA}}/\alpha^{CS}\alpha$ denotes an interaction of the Hb CONSTANT SPRING mutation with the common Southeast Asian α^{0} defect. The relationship of these genotypes to the commonly observed phenotypes of α thalassemia are outlined in Table 113-7 and discussed in the section on "Interactions of α-Thalassemia Haplotypes," below.

Molecular Pathology. ***α^{+} Thalassemia Due to Deletions.*** The most common molecular defects underlying α thalassemia ($-\alpha^{3.7}$ and $-\alpha^{4.2}$) involve the deletion of one or other of the duplicated α-globin genes[61,62] (Fig. 113-18). One or both of these determinants occur in all populations in which thalassemia is common.

The mechanism by which some of the α^{+} thalassemia deletions occur has now been established, and it is clearly related to the underlying molecular structure of the α-globin complex.[38,218] Each α gene is located within a region of homology approximately 4 kb long, interrupted by small nonhomologous regions (see Fig. 113-18). It is thought that the homologous regions result from an ancient duplication event. Subsequently, during evolution these homologous segments were subdivided, presumably by insertions and deletions, to give three homologous subsegments referred to as X, Y, and Z (see Fig. 113-18). The duplicated Z boxes are 3.7 kb apart, and the X boxes are 4.2 kb apart. Misalignment and reciprocal crossover between these segments at meiosis can give rise to chromosomes with either single $(-\alpha)$[218] or triplicated $(\alpha\alpha\alpha)$[60,219–221] α-globin genes (Fig. 113-19). Such an occurrence between homologous Z boxes deletes 3.7 kb of DNA (referred to as a rightward deletion, $-\alpha^{3.7}$), whereas a similar crossover between the two X blocks deletes 4.2 kb of DNA (referred to as a leftward deletion, $-\alpha^{4.2}$). The corresponding triplicated α gene arrangements are referred to as $\alpha\alpha\alpha^{\text{anti3.7}}$ and $\alpha\alpha\alpha^{\text{anti4.2}}$. Further examples of chromosomes with four α genes ($\alpha\alpha\alpha\alpha^{\text{anti3.7}}$ and $\alpha\alpha\alpha\alpha^{\text{anti4.2}}$) presumably result from similar crossovers involving the $\alpha\alpha\alpha^{\text{anti3.7}}$ and $\alpha\alpha\alpha^{\text{anti4.2}}$ chromosomes, respectively.[222] Crossovers between single $-\alpha$ and duplicated αα chromosomes have also been described.[223] Indeed, several independent lines of evidence suggest that

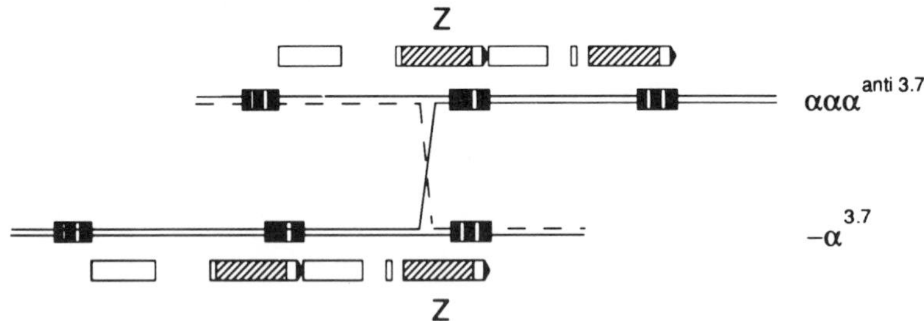

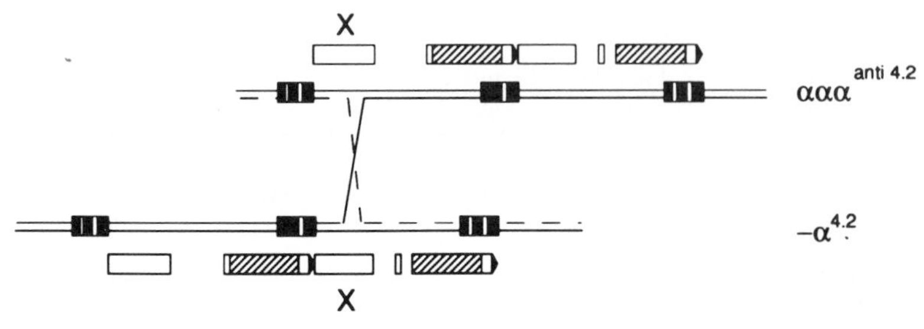

FIG. 113-19 Mechanism of unequal crossover that gives rise to the $-\alpha^{3.7}$ and $-\alpha^{4.2}$ deletions. The rightward crossover occurs when genetic exchange takes place between the misaligned homologous Z boxes, giving rise to chromosomes with either one ($-\alpha^{3.7}$) or three ($\alpha\alpha\alpha^{\text{anti3.7}}$) α-globin genes. The leftward crossover occurs when genetic exchange takes place between the misaligned homologous X boxes, giving rise to chromosomes with either one ($-\alpha^{4.2}$) or three ($\alpha\alpha\alpha^{\text{anti 4.2}}$) α-globin genes.

this type of homologous genetic recombination occurs relatively frequently in globin[224,225] and other[226,227] loci. At present it is not known whether such rearrangements take place between misaligned chromosomes or between chromatids during meiosis.

The mechanism by which two rare deletions that cause α^+ thalassemia (see Fig. 113-19) have arisen are not clear. In one of them, a $(\alpha)^{5.3}$ described in an Italian patient,[228] recombination appears to have taken place by an illegitimate process involving partially homologous sequences (see next section). In the other, $-\alpha^{3.5}$ described in an Asian patient,[229] sequence data across the breakpoint are not available.

From the geographical distribution and relative frequencies of the common $-\alpha$ chromosomes it appears that rearrangements involving the Z box are more frequent than those involving the X or Y regions. It is possible to subdivide the common Z box rearrangements into three types ($-\alpha^{3.7I}$, $-\alpha^{3.7II}$, and $-\alpha^{3.7III}$) depending on exactly where the crossover has taken place with respect to three restriction enzyme sites that differ between the $\alpha 1$ and $\alpha 2$ Z boxes[224] (see Fig. 113-18). In general, it appears that the frequency of each of these subtypes ($-\alpha^{3.7I}$, $-\alpha^{3.7II}$ and $-\alpha^{3.7III}$; Y-box crossovers have not been identified) are simply related to the length of homology within each subsegment. It remains to be seen whether more complex physical constraints also play a role in determining the relative frequency of recombination in this region.

The level of expression of the remaining α gene from these chromosomes (-α) can be assessed by the effect of the deletions on phenotype (see Table 113-7) and more directly by measuring the production of α-specific mRNA from such chromosomes. The level of expression of the $\alpha 2$ gene is two to three times greater than that of the $\alpha 1$ gene, and this appears to be controlled at the level of transcription.[230–233] All six deletions ($-\alpha^{3.7I}$, $-\alpha^{3.7II}$, $-\alpha^{3.7III}$, $-\alpha^{4.2}$, $-\alpha^{3.5}$, and $-\alpha^{5.3}$) reduce α-chain production from the affected chromosome. The similar phenotypes of homozygotes for the $-\alpha^{4.2}$ determinant, in which both $\alpha 2$ genes are removed, and $-\alpha^{3.7III}$ homozygotes, in which, effectively, the $\alpha 1$ genes are deleted, suggests that removal of the $\alpha 2$ gene results in a partial, compensatory increase in the expression of the remaining $\alpha 1$ gene on the $-\alpha^{4.2}$ chromosome[234]; increase in expression of the $\alpha 1$ gene has been clearly demonstrated at the level of mRNA.[235] The mechanism by which this change in gene expression takes place is not understood at present, although clearly this observation may be of importance in understanding the molecular mechanisms that normally maintain the difference in expression of the $\alpha 2$ and $\alpha 1$ genes. At present there are insufficient phenotypic data to compare the relative levels of expression of the less common -α chromosomes.

α° Thalassemia Due to Deletions. To date, 18 deletions have been described that involve both α genes[208,211,236–239] and thereby abolish α-chain production from the affected chromosome (Fig. 113-20); four of them[236–239] extend beyond the current limits of the cloned DNA around the α genes. In general, they are large deletions (5.2 kb to >200 kb). Unlike the $-\alpha^{3.7}$ and $-\alpha^{4.2}$ defects there seem to be several different ways in which they can arise.

Some of these deletions have been analyzed in detail to see if the underlying mechanisms could be established.[240] Several features have emerged; first there appears to be a clustering of breakpoints. Many of the 3′ breakpoints fall within a 6-to-8-kb region at the 3′ end of the α-globin complex, suggesting that this may represent a breakpoint cluster region similar to those observed in the chromosomal translocations associated with certain malignant diseases, or in Duchenne muscular dystrophy, for example. In addition, many of the 5′ breakpoints also appear to cluster. This gives rise to a situation in which the 5′ breakpoints are located approximately the same distance apart and in a similar order along the chromosome as their respective 3′ breakpoints. These findings are consistent with observations on a group of deletions from the β-globin cluster.[241] In both cases it has been proposed that such staggered deletions may result from illegitimate recombination events deleting an integral number of chromatin loops as they pass through their nuclear attachment points during replication.[240,241]

One of the deletions ($--^{MED}$) involves a more complex rearrangement that introduces a new piece of DNA bridging the two breakpoints in the α cluster (see Fig. 113-20). This new DNA originates upstream from the α cluster and appears to have been replicated into the junction in a manner that suggests that the upstream segment of DNA also lies at the base of a replication loop. This region possibly lies close to

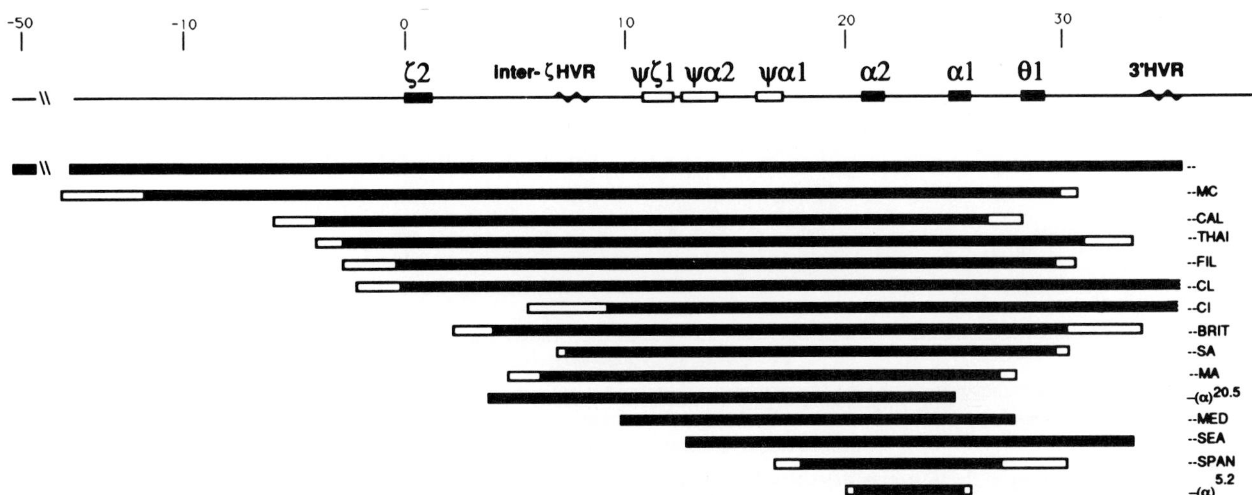

FIG. 113-20 **Map of the human α-globin locus (above) with a summary of currently described α^0 thalassemia deletions below. Coordinate 0 corresponds to the ζ mRNA cap site; the scale is in kilobases. Solid blocks represent the genes, open boxes denote pseudogenes, and zigzag lines denote segments of minisatellite DNA.**

the bases of the proposed replication loops involved in the group of clustered deletions described above.

Sequence analysis has shown that members of the dispersed family of *Alu* repeats[242] are frequently found at or near the breakpoints of these deletions. These repeats may simply provide partially homologous sequences that promote DNA strand exchanges during replication, or possibly a subset of *Alu* sequences may be more actively involved in the process, particularly if they function as origins of replication.[242] It is interesting that similar illegitimate recombination events in the β locus do not seem to involve *Alu* sequences, suggesting that this type of recombination may be to some extent locus-specific.[243]

In contrast to the $-\alpha^{3.7}$ and $-\alpha^{4.2}$ defects, the set of deletions that cause α° thalassemia are of limited geographical distribution[208] and each one probably represents a single example of an uncommon type of genetic mishap. Perhaps the most extreme example of this is the $--^{BRIT}$ mutation, which is predominantly seen in individuals originating from the north of England.[244,245] Nevertheless, this type of molecular defect underlies many common genetic disorders.

Since both α genes are involved in this group of deletions, α-globin synthesis is abolished by these mutants. The similarity of these deletions to deletions of the β cluster that give rise to HPFH, δβ thalassemia and γδβ thalassemia, raises the question of how they affect the expression of neighboring genes. In heterozygotes for the two common α° thalassemia determinants ($--^{SEA}/\alpha\alpha$ and $--^{MED}/\alpha\alpha$) it has been shown, using a sensitive radioimmunoassay, that there is a very small increase in ζ-globin expression.[246,247] In homozygotes for these mutants ($--^{SEA}/--^{SEA}$ and $--^{MED}/--^{MED}$) large amounts (~20 to 30 percent of Hb PORTLAND ($\zeta_2\gamma_2$) are produced. However, it seems more likely that this results from intensive cell selection rather than from specific enhancement of ζ-globin expression. Hence, the change in pattern of gene expression in these deletions may not be comparable to the more dramatic changes in γ expression associated with HPFH. Perhaps it is more relevant to ask why the expression of the embryonic genes, ζ and ε, is not much changed by these deletions of the α- and β-globin cluster, whereas γ-gene expression is markedly altered.

α Thalassemia Due to Deletions of the α-Globin Regulatory Element. It has been shown that expression of the α genes is critically dependent on a segment of DNA that lies 40 kb upstream of the ζ-globin gene.[93] This region is associated with an erythroid-specific DNase I hypersensitive site and is referred to as HS -40. Detailed analysis of HS -40 has shown that this segment of DNA contains multiple binding sites for the erythroid restricted *trans*-acting factors GATA-1 and NF-E2.[94,248]

The first indication that such a remote regulatory sequence might exist came from the observation of a patient with α thalassemia.[249] Analysis of the abnormal chromosome, $(\alpha\alpha)^{RA}$, from this patient demonstrated a 62-kb deletion from upstream of the α complex (Fig. 113-21) which includes HS -40. Although both α genes on this chromosome are intact and entirely normal they appear to be nonfunctional. Since this observation, three more patients with α thalassemia due to a deletion of HS -40 and a variable amount of the flanking DNA have been described[250–252] (see Fig. 113-21). All these mutations give rise to the phenotype associated with α° thalassemia.

The mechanisms by which these mutations have arisen are quite diverse. In the $(\alpha\alpha)^{RA}$ chromosome the deletion resulted from a recombination event between partially homologous *Alu* repeats that are normally 62 kb apart. Another of these mutations $(\alpha\alpha)^{TI}$ involved truncation of the tip of chromosome 16 so that all material between the deletion breakpoint and the end (telomere) of the chromosome has been deleted. This truncated chromosome was healed by the addition of telomere repeat sequence, $(TTAGGG)_n$, to give a stable chromosome.[250] The breakpoints of the other two deletions, $(\alpha\alpha)^{IJ}$ and $(\alpha\alpha)^{MM}$, have not yet been analyzed, but one of them has been shown to be a *de novo* deletion.

α⁺ Thalassemia Due to Nondeletion Defects. The nondeletion α thalassemias are classified in this way because analysis of DNA from patients with these disorders reveals no gross abnormality by Southern blotting. In fact, in most cases they result from single or oligonucleotide mutations at regions of the α-gene sequence that are critical for normal expression. Similar mutations in the β-globin gene are much more common and are discussed in detail in a later section.

Since the expression of the α2 gene is two to three times greater than that of the α1 gene,[230–233] it is not surprising that most of the nondeletion mutants predominantly affect expression of the α2 gene. Clearly, such mutations have a greater effect on phenotype and presumably a greater selective advantage (in the heterozygote). Unlike the deletion of the α2 gene in the $-\alpha^{4.2}$ defect, that results in a compensatory increase in expression of the remaining α1 gene, there appears to be no increase in expression of the α1 gene when the α2 gene is inactivated by a point mutation. Therefore the nondeletion α thalassemias have a greater effect on phenotype than the -α mutants.

The molecular lesions that underlie nondeletion forms of α thalassemia are relatively uncommon when compared with the $-\alpha^{3.7}$ and $-\alpha^{4.2}$ mutants; furthermore, the geographical distribution of each mutant is relatively limited (Table 113-8). As for the β-thalassemia mutants, they may be classified according to the level of gene expression that they affect

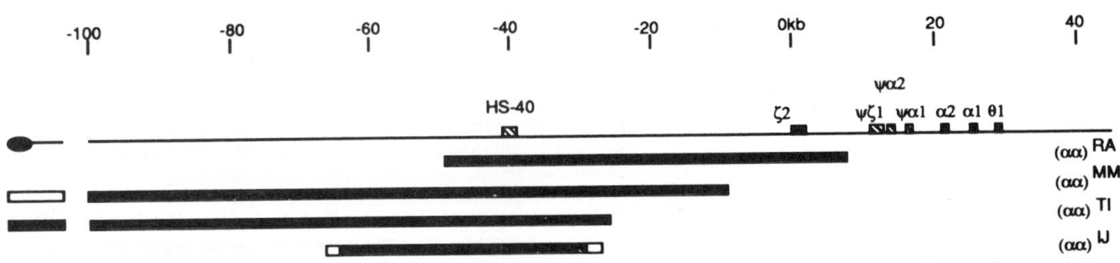

FIG. 113-21 Summary of the upstream deletions that cause α thalassemia. The long-range structure of the α-gene cluster with the telomere is indicated by a black oval. Coordinate 0 indicates the ζ mRNA cap site; the scale is in kilobases. The positions of the globin genes, pseudogenes, and HS -40 are shown. The extent of each deletion is indicated below by a solid black line; white boxes indicate the regions of uncertainty in defining the breakpoints.

Table 113-8 Nondeletion Mutants That Cause α Thalassemia

	Affected Gene	Affected Sequence	Mutation	Geographical Distribution
RNA processing	α2	IVS1 donor site	GAGGTGAGG → GAGG– – – – –	Mediterranean
	α2*	Poly(A) signal	AATAAA → AATAAG	Middle Eastern, Mediterranean
	α2	Poly(A) signal	AATAAA → AATGAA	Mediterranean
RNA translation†	α2	Initiation codon	CCACCATGG → CCACCACGG	Mediterranean
	α1	Initiation codon	CCACCATGG → CCACCGTGG	Mediterranean
	–α	Initiation codon	CCACCATGG → CCACCGTGG	Black
	$-\alpha^{3.7II}$	Initiation codon	CCACCATGG → CC– –CATGG	North African, Mediterranean
	α2	Exon III	α116 GAG → TAG	Black
	α2	Termination codon	α142 TAA → CAA	Southeast Asian
	α2	Termination codon	α142 TAA → AAA	Mediterranean
	α2	Termination codon	α142 TAA → TCA	Indian
	α2	Termination codon	α142 TAA → GAA	Black
	–α	Exon I	α30/31 GAGAGG → GAG– –G	Black
Posttranslational instability	α2	Exon III	α125 Leu → Pro	Southeast Asian
	α2	Exon III	α109 Leu → Arg	Southeast Asian
	α	Exon III	α110 Ala → Asp	Middle Eastern
	–α	Exon I	α14 Trp → Arg	Black
Uncharacterized	α	Unknown	Not determined	Black
	α	Unknown	Not determined	Greek‡

*This mutation has been found in both α2-like genes on an $\alpha\alpha\alpha^{3.7}$ chromosome present in Saudi Arabian individuals.
†The elongated α chains associated with Hb WAYNE, which results from a frameshift (deletion of either C at α138 or A at α139 of the α2-globin gene) and Hb GRADY, which results from a crossover in phase (with insertion of three residues at α118) are not known to be associated with α thalassemia, although the critical interactions that would clearly reveal this have not been described.
‡Its interaction with α^0-thalassemia determinants to produce the Hb BART'S hydrops fetalis syndrome suggests that both α-globin genes may be affected.
NOTE: Full details and references are summarized in Higgs et al.[208]

(see Table 113-8). Three nondeletion mutants that affect processing of the primary mRNA transcript have been identified. The first consists of a pentanucleotide deletion including the 5′ splice site of IVS1 of the α2 globin gene ($\alpha^{Hph}\alpha$). This deletion involves the invariant GT donor splicing sequence (GAGGTGAGG→GAGG), thus abolishing the normal removal of IVS1 during processing.[253,254] The second mutant in this group, $\alpha^{T\ SAUDI}\alpha$, involves the poly(A) addition signal (AATAAA→AATAAG) and down-regulates the α2 gene by interfering with the 3′ end processing[77,255] and possibly with termination of transcription.[256] At present, it is not clear whether a failure to terminate transcription of the α2 gene correctly also down-regulates the linked α1 gene. Whatever the mechanism, it appears that both α2 and α1 genes are affected by this mutation.[255] A second mutation, involving the poly(A) addition site (AATAAA→AATGAA) has been described.[257]

A second group of mutations exert their effect by interfering with the translation of mature mRNA. In one case ($\alpha^{Nco}\alpha$) the initiation codon is completely inactivated by a T-to-C transition (CCATGG→CCACGG),[258] and in another the efficiency of initiation is reduced by a dinucleotide deletion in the consensus sequence around the start signal (CCCACCATG→CC– –CATG).[259] Another results from a single base substitution in the α1 gene initiation codon.[260] Four mutations that affect termination of translation and give rise to elongated α-globin chains have been identified [Hb CONSTANT SPRING ($\alpha^{CS}\alpha$) Hb ICARIA ($\alpha^{I}\alpha$), Hb KOYA DORA ($\alpha^{KD}\alpha$), and Hb SEAL ROCK ($\alpha^{SR}\alpha$)]. Each specifically changes the termination codon (TAA).[119] Another mutation identified in a black patient from Mississippi ($\alpha^{MS}\alpha$),[261] causes premature termination of translation by changing codon 116 in exon III to an in-phase terminator (GAG→UAG).

A group of four structural mutations that cause α thalassemia give rise to highly unstable α-globin chains; these are Hb QUONG SZE ($\alpha^{QS}\alpha$),[262] Hb SUAN DOK ($\alpha\alpha^{SD}$),[263] Hb PETAH TIKVAH ($\alpha\alpha^{PT}$),[264] and Hb EVANSTON.[265]

Many nondeletion α-thalassemia mutations remain to be characterized. Of particular interest are those associated with the Hb Bart's hydrops fetalis syndrome, in which the nondeletion chromosome presumably has a substantially reduced α-chain production.[266,267] Perhaps these will turn out to be similar to the Saudi Arabian type of defect in which both α2 and α1 genes appear to be down-regulated; or possibly, they represent yet more severe defects, for example, mutations involving the α-globin regulatory element HS -40.

Interactions of α-Thalassemia Haplotypes. At present, approximately 50 α haplotypes have been described; thus, there are a large number of potential interactions. Phenotypically, these result in one of four broad categories: a normal phenotype; α thalassemia minor, in which there are mild hematologic changes but no major clinical abnormalities; Hb H disease, and the Hb Bart's hydrops fetalis syndrome. These clinical syndromes and the broad classes of interactions that underlie them are summarized in Table 113-7 and are reviewed in detail in the following sections.

Normal Phenotype. Although the majority of normal individuals have four α-globin genes (αα/αα), between 1 and 2 percent in most populations have five genes (ααα/αα). Furthermore, in populations in which α thalassemia is common, the genotype -α/ααα also occurs.[184] It has been shown that the additional α gene in the ααα haplotype produces a slight excess of α_2 mRNA,[231] although this is not always reflected in the α/β-globin-chain synthesis ratio[60] or at the phenotypic level; individuals with these interactions are often indistinguishable from normal.[60] Rare individuals with $\alpha\alpha\alpha\alpha/\alpha\alpha$ or $\alpha\alpha\alpha/\alpha\alpha\alpha$ may produce excess α globin, but again their phenotype is essentially normal.[222]

It should also be noted that within normal individuals there is a considerable amount of variation in the sequence and structure of the α-globin complex with no apparent effect on the expression of the α-globin genes.[50]

α Thalassemia Minor. α Thalassemia minor most frequently results from the interaction of a normal haplotype ($\alpha\alpha$) with one of the α^+ or α° thalassemia determinants (e.g., $-\alpha^{3.7}/\alpha\alpha$, $-\alpha^{4.2}/\alpha\alpha$, or $\alpha^T\alpha/\alpha\alpha$). In populations in which α thalassemia is common, two α^+ thalassemias can also interact to produce α thalassemia minor, $-\alpha^{3.7}/-\alpha^{3.7}$. Since each α-thalassemia determinant may be associated with a different degree of suppression of α-globin chain synthesis, these interactions produce disorders spanning a clinical and hematologic spectrum from a normal phenotype to Hb H disease (see Table 113-7). The variation in severity of the α^+ and α° mutations is demonstrated by the degree of anemia, MCV, MCH, α/β-globin-chain synthesis ratio, and level of Hb Bart's at birth when different determinants interact with each other or a normal chromosome (see Fig. 113-22).

In general, chromosomes with a single α gene ($-\alpha$) produce the mildest phenotype, with the $-\alpha^{4.2}$ producing a greater reduction in α-globin chain synthesis than $-\alpha^{3.7}$.[234] Nondeletion mutants ($\alpha^T\alpha$) that affect the predominant $\alpha 2$ gene (see Table 113-8) cause a more pronounced reduction in α-chain synthesis and deletion mutants involving both α genes (e.g., $--^{MED}$ and $--^{SEA}$) lead to the most severe phenotype. As shown in Fig. 113-22, it is not possible to predict accurately the genotype from any given phenotype and in some cases ($-\alpha/\alpha\alpha$, for example), it may be impossible to diagnose a carrier of α thalassemia using any of the conventional phenotypic criteria. Therefore, to perform accurate genetic counseling in families with α thalassemia, genotype determination is essential.

Homozygotes for Nondeletion Types of α Thalassemia. The chain termination mutant Hb CONSTANT SPRING causes a severe reduction in $\alpha 2$-globin expression from the affected chromosome. Sufficient homozygotes ($\alpha^{CS}\alpha/\alpha^{CS}\alpha$) have been described to establish that the phenotype is more severe than α thalassemia minor but not as severe as most cases of Hb H disease.[268] The subjects are anemic, with thalassemic red-cell changes and a reticulocytosis. Basophilic stippling of the red cells is often prominent. They have mild jaundice and a variable degree of hepatosplenomegaly and are therefore quite unlike patients with α thalassemia minor. Patients homozygous for the chain termination mutant Koya Dora ($\alpha^{KD}\alpha/\alpha^{KD}\alpha$) have been described, but their phenotype was not given.[269]

The only other homozygotes for mutations affecting the predominant $\alpha 2$ gene are a single Sardinian patient with a very mild form of Hb H disease ($\alpha^{Nco}\alpha/\alpha^{Nco}\alpha$)[258] and Saudi Arabian patients with typical Hb H disease ($\alpha^{T\ SAUDI}\alpha/\alpha^{T\ SAUDI}\alpha$).[77,255] Comparing the phenotype of homozygotes for Hb CS ($\alpha^{CS}\alpha/\alpha^{CS}\alpha$) with the Sardinian patient ($\alpha^{Nco}\alpha/\alpha^{Nco}\alpha$) it appears that these interactions may lie on either side of a critical level of α-chain synthesis below which the syndrome of Hb H disease occurs.

Hb H Disease. Hb H disease most frequently results from the interaction of α^+ and α° thalassemia; therefore, it is

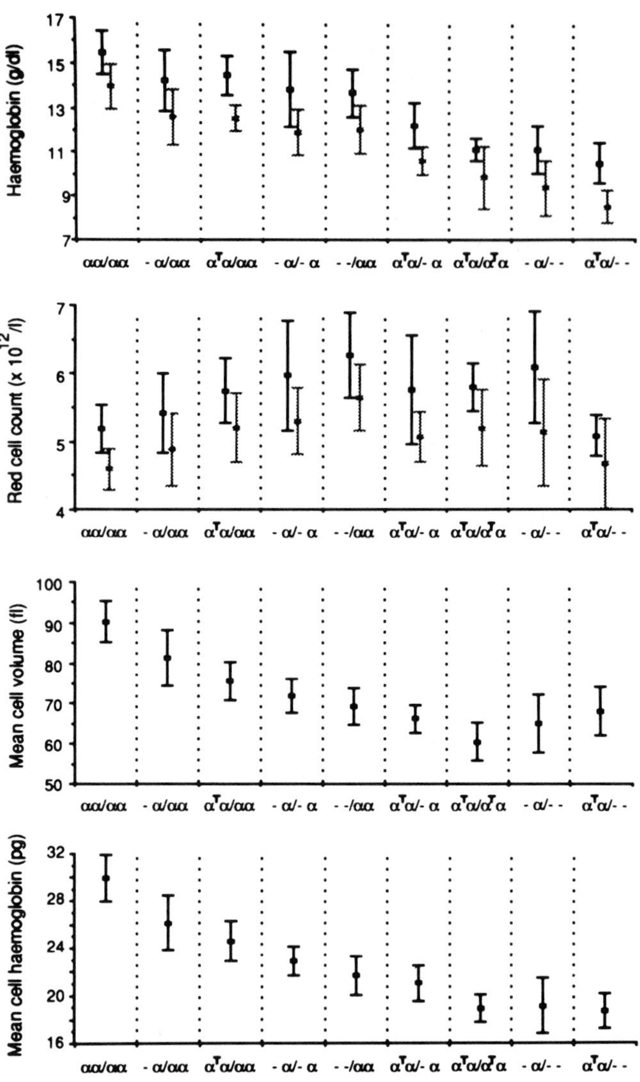

FIG. 113-22 **Mean and standard deviation of the Hb, RBC, MCV, and MCH are plotted for each of nine possible genotypes, arranged in order of increasing severity from $\alpha\alpha/\alpha\alpha$ (left) to $\alpha^T\alpha/--$ (right). For Hb and RBC, results are shown separately for males (black bars) and females (gray bars).** ***(We are grateful to Dr. A.O.M. Wilkie who collated the data presented in this figure.)***

predominantly found in Southeast Asia (commonly, $--^{SEA}/-\alpha^{3.7}$) and the Mediterranean basin (commonly, $--^{MED}/-\alpha^{3.7}$), where both α^+ and α° thalassemia are common. Hb H disease may also result from the interaction of nondeletion mutations affecting the predominant $\alpha 2$-globin gene ($\alpha^{Nco}\alpha/\alpha^{Nco}\alpha$, $\alpha^{T\ SAUDI}\alpha/\alpha^{T\ SAUDI}\alpha$). In Algeria, homozygotes for the $-\alpha^{3.7II\ T}$defect ($-\alpha^{3.7II\ T}/-\alpha^{3.7II\ T}$) (see Table 113-8) have typical Hb H disease.[270]

The genetic basis for Hb H disease is diverse, and as more molecular defects are characterized the underlying interactions will become even more complex. It is not yet clear to what extent this molecular diversity is reflected in the variable clinical and hematologic features of Hb H disease. The clinical picture of hemoglobin H disease is usually thalassemia intermedia, although there is considerable variation in the severity of this condition. The predominant features are a hypochromic, microcytic anemia, with jaundice and hepatosplenomegaly. Since the main mechanism of the anemia is hemolysis rather than dyserythropoiesis only one third of patients have clinical evidence of an

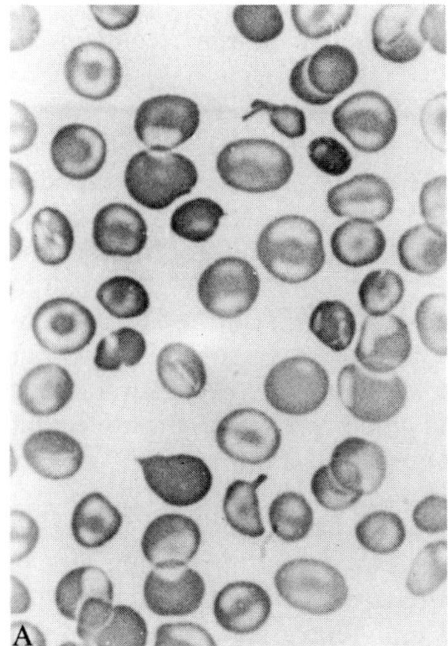

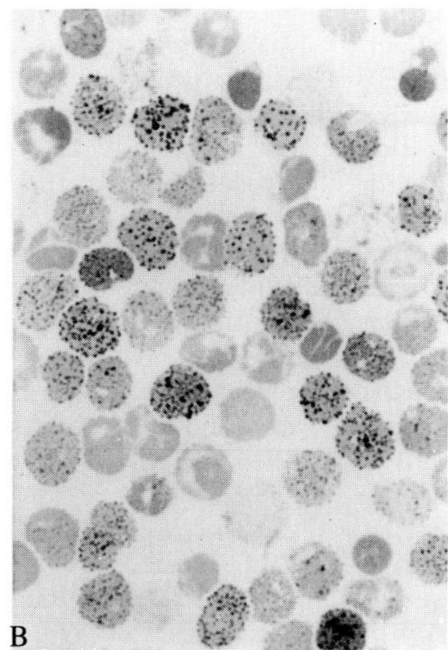

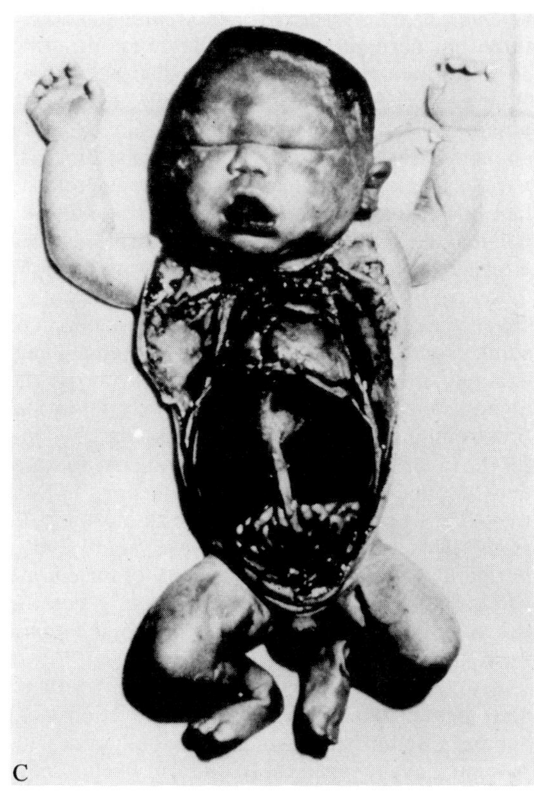

FIG. 113-23 **Clinical manifestations of α thalassemia. *A*. A blood smear of a patient with Hb H disease. *B*. The cells were supravitally stained with brilliant cresyl blue to demonstrate Hb H inclusions. *C*. An infant with the hemoglobin Bart's hydrops fetalis syndrome.**

expanded erythron. The commonest complication is the development of severe splenomegaly with hypersplenism. Other complications include infection, leg ulcers, gallstones, and folic acid deficiency.

The hematologic features of Hb H disease are also quite variable.[2,195] Hemoglobin levels ranging from 2.6 to 12.4 g/dl have been recorded, in association with reticulocytosis and typical thalassemia changes of the red-cell indices. The hemoglobin consists of Hb A with a variable amount of Hb H and sometimes Hb BART'S. The proportion of Hb H varies from 2 to 40 percent. When peripheral blood is incubated with redox dyes this is reflected in the number of cells that contain typical Hb H inclusions (Fig. 113-23).

As yet there have been few systematic attempts to correlate the genotype with the phenotype of Hb H disease. However, in general it appears that, as expected, patients with a nondeletion defect (affecting the predominant $\alpha2$ gene) interacting with an α° thalassemia determinant ($--\alpha^T\alpha$) have higher levels of Hb H (β_4), a greater degree of anemia and, anecdotally, a more severe clinical course than patients with the $--/-\alpha$ genotype.[271-274] At the extreme of this spectrum, a few patients have been described in whom severe Hb H disease was associated with hydrops fetalis.[266]

In Thailand, where there is an abundance of well-documented cases of Hb H disease, it is known that despite the relatively homogeneous nature of the molecular basis ($--^{SEA}/-\alpha^{3.7}$ in 80 percent)[275] the clinical course is quite variable. This suggests that other genetic and environmental factors play an important role in clinical and hematologic variation seen in this syndrome.

Hemoglobin BART'S Hydrops Fetalis Syndrome. Nearly all cases of Hb BART'S hydrops fetalis syndrome are due to the interaction of two α^0-thalassemia determinants. As with Hb H disease, this condition is almost exclusively seen in patients of Southeast Asian (commonly, $--^{SEA}/--^{SEA}$) or Mediterranean (commonly, $--^{MED}/--^{MED}$) origin. Infants with this syndrome either die in utero (at 30 to 40 weeks of gestation) or soon after birth (see Fig. 113-23). However, long-term survival has been recorded: two infants with this syndrome were delivered at 28 and 32 weeks, underwent transfusion, and were intensively nursed.[276,277] Such individuals require lifelong transfusion and iron chelation therapy.

Usually, the clinical picture is that of a pale edematous infant with signs of cardiac failure and prolonged intrauterine hypoxia (see Fig. 113-23). Hepatosplenomegaly is always present, and there are often other congenital abnormalities. The hemoglobin levels range from 3 to 20 g/dl, and the blood film is characterized by anisopoikilocytosis with large hypochromic macrocytes; many nucleated cells are present in the peripheral blood. The hemoglobin consists of ~80 percent Hb BART'S, the remainder being hemoglobins H and Portland. Of these hemoglobins, only Hb PORTLAND is efficient in the transport of oxygen, hence the severe degree of fetal hypoxia. There is a high incidence of maternal complications, including toxemia and postpartum hemorrhage.

Although the Hb BART'S hydrops fetalis syndrome is usually associated with a complete absence of α-globin chain synthesis, there have been a few reports of hydrops fetalis in Greek[267,278] and Southeast Asian infants[266,279] with very low levels of α-chain synthesis. Gene mapping shows that they result from the interaction of common α^0 determinants with nondeletion mutations ($\alpha\alpha^T$), although the latter have not been characterized. The Greek mutation has been called $(\alpha\alpha)^{T\ KARDITSA}$[267,278] (see Table 113-8). It is possible that the nondeletion mutations in these cases are like the $\alpha^{T\ SAUDI}\alpha$ defect in that the output of the two α genes is less than expected for the $\alpha1$ gene alone; thus, α-chain production falls below 12 percent of normal.

A survey of Chinese infants has shown that some hydropic babies have a nondeletion mutation in which there is no α-chain production, thus identifying an entirely new type of disorder.[280] Finally, a stillborn hydropic infant of Iraqi-Kurdish origin has been reported; in this case the infant had thalassemia red-cell changes but only 40 percent Hb BART'S.[281] It is possible that this child was hydropic for other reasons.

α Thalassemia Associated with Mental Retardation. In 1981 three northern European families were described in which severely mentally retarded sons also had Hb H disease.[282] Whereas the common forms of Hb H disease are always inherited in a Mendelian fashion, in these families this appeared not to be so. By 1990, a total of 13 subjects with various forms of α thalassemia and mental retardation (ATR) had been identified, and two distinct syndromes had been delineated.[283,284] One group of patients had large (1- to 2-megabase) deletions of the tip of chromosome 16, including the α-globin gene cluster. The clinical features of this so-called ATR-16 syndrome are rather variable, in part because some patients have additional chromosomal aneuploidy. For example, one child with the ATR-16 syndrome has inherited an unbalanced submicroscopic 16:1 chromosomal translocation from one of his parents.[285] Thus, this child is monosomic for the tip of chromosome 16p—giving rise to α thalassemia—and trisomic for the tip of chromosome 1. Some cases of the ATR-16 syndrome have pure monosomy for the tip of 16p.[286] This suggests that there are other genes, critical for normal development, in the vicinity of the α genes at the tip of chromosome 16. Deletion of these genes together with the α-globin genes may give rise to the combination of mental retardation and α thalassemia.

By contrast, a second group of patients with α thalassemia and mental retardation have no deletions or any other apparent abnormalities of the α-globin gene cluster. These patients have a remarkably uniform phenotype, comprising severe mental retardation, characteristic dysmorphic facies (Fig. 113-24), genital abnormalities, and an unusually mild form of the Hb H disease. A total of 16 cases of this syndrome have been identified.[287] In one remarkable pedigree,[288] including four affected males, it is clear that α thalassemia segregates independently of the α cluster on chromosome 16p.

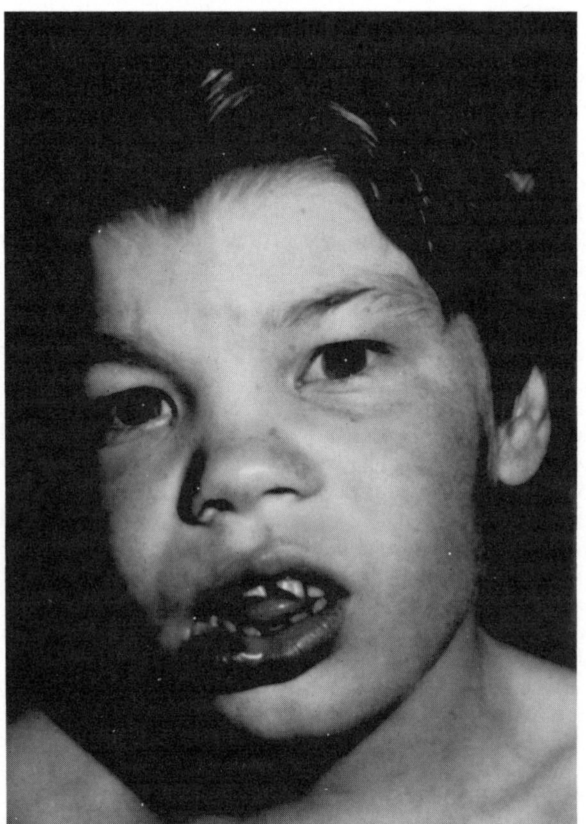

FIG. 113-24 Characteristic facial features of an individual with ATR-X syndrome.

It has now been shown that this disorder maps to the X chromosome[289]; it is referred to as the ATR-X syndrome. Therefore, there appears to be a *trans*-acting factor encoded on the X chromosome which when mutated is capable of down-regulating expression of the α genes (on chromosome 16) in addition to exerting pleiotropic effects throughout development, giving rise to mental retardation and dysmorphism. Elucidation of the molecular basis of this disorder promises to be of great value in advancing our understanding of globin-gene expression and our knowledge of the molecular basis of some forms of mental handicap.

α Thalassemia Associated with Myeloproliferative Disorders. Most cases of Hb H disease result from inheritance of the α-thalassemia determinants described in previous sections. However, several individuals have now been described in whom Hb H disease appears to be an acquired disorder associated with the development of one form or other of myelodysplasia[290]; previous hematologic assessments in these patients were entirely normal. This particular form of α thalassemia seems to be much more frequent in males than in females. The structure of the α-globin complex appears to be normal, but there is a severe reduction in α-specific mRNA and α-globin chain synthesis. The molecular basis for this syndrome thus appears to involve an acquired defect in transcription of the α genes,[290] although the precise mechanism and its relationship to the hematologic malignancy is not yet known.

β and δβ Thalassemias and Hereditary Persistence of Fetal Hemoglobin

The β and δβ thalassemias show considerable heterogeneity, not only in clinical severity but also in the phenotypic characteristics revealed by hematologic measurements and hemoglobin analysis. When the underlying defect is studied at the DNA level, it is clear that the phenotypic diversity hides even further molecular heterogeneity. The equally diverse group of conditions called, collectively, "hereditary persistence of fetal hemoglobin" (HPFH), can be regarded as very mild β or δβ thalassemias in which defective β-chain production is compensated by γ-chain production.

Classification. There are two approaches to subdividing this group of disorders. For clinical purposes they can be described as thalassemia major (transfusion-dependent), thalassemia intermedia (of intermediate severity), and thalassemia minor (asymptomatic). At the biosynthetic level they are categorized by the affected globin chains and whether there is a partial or complete defect in chain production (see Table 113-6).

The β thalassemias are subdivided into β^0 and β^+, representing disorders with complete or partial defects in β-chain production. Similarly, the δβ thalassemias are divided into $(\delta\beta)^+$ and $(\delta\beta)^0$ thalassemia, depending on whether there is any output of δ or β chains from the affected chromosome. The $(\delta\beta)^+$ thalassemias are the result of the production of δβ fusion genes as mentioned in the section "Fusion Hemoglobins" above. The $(\delta\beta)^0$ thalassemias are further divided according to the structure of the Hb F which is produced in the $(\delta\beta)^0$ thalassemias, in which the Hb F contains both ${}^G\gamma$ and ${}^A\gamma$ chains, and $({}^A\gamma\delta\beta)^0$ thalassemia, in which only ${}^G\gamma$ chains are produced.

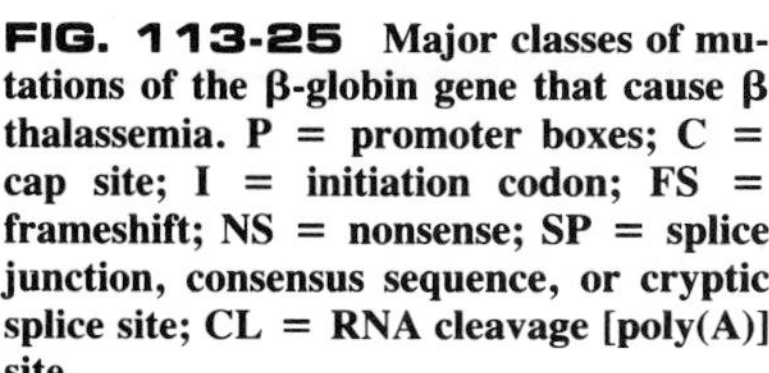

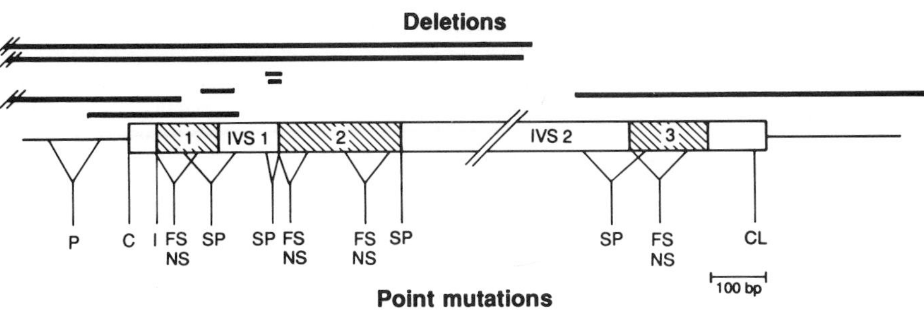

FIG. 113-25 Major classes of mutations of the β-globin gene that cause β thalassemia. P = promoter boxes; C = cap site; I = initiation codon; FS = frameshift; NS = nonsense; SP = splice junction, consensus sequence, or cryptic splice site; CL = RNA cleavage [poly(A)] site.

The different forms of HPFH are classified into three groups according to the underlying defect (see Table 113-6): (1) deletions of the δ and β genes (as well as sequences 3′ to these genes) with continued high level expression of the $^{G}\gamma$ and $^{A}\gamma$ genes (5 to 25 percent Hb F) in adult life ($\delta\beta^0$ HFPH); (2) point mutations in the promoter regions of one or other γ gene resulting in increased expression (2 to 20 percent Hb F) of that gene in adults but with persistent β-gene expression in *cis* ($^{G}\gamma\beta^+$ or $^{A}\gamma\beta^+$ HPFH); and (3) a heterogeneous group of disorders with persistent Hb F in adult life (usually low levels) in which the determinant may segregate independently of the β-globin gene complex. Previous classifications of these disorders have also been based on whether the intercellular distribution of hemoglobin F was pancellular or heterocellular. It now appears that such differences are more likely to be related to the overall hemoglobin F level than to fundamental differences in the underlying molecular pathology.

Molecular Pathology. β *Thalassemia*. The deficiency or absence of β chains that characterizes β thalassemia could potentially arise from defects affecting any of the stages in the complex process by which the β-globin gene is transcribed into RNA, processed into mRNA, and transported to the cytoplasm for translation into polypeptide chains. The molecular basis has been determined in over 100 different β-thalassemia alleles, largely by cloning the abnormal gene and then comparing its sequence with that of the normal β^A gene. The identification of new defects was originally facilitated by the observation that within any population, each mutation is in strong linkage disequilibrium with specific RFLP haplotypes.[73] Some of the mutations characterized to date are listed in Table 113-9, grouped according to the mechanism by which they inactivate β-gene expression, and illustrated in Figs. 113-25 and 113-26.

***Gene Deletions*.** Several different deletions affecting only the β-globin gene have been described[291–297] (see Fig. 113-26). Of these, only the 619-bp deletion at the 3′ end of the β gene is common, and even that is restricted to the Sind populations of India and Pakistan, where it accounts for ~30 percent of the β-thalassemia alleles.[291]

The other deletions are all rare and result in the phenotype of β thalassemia with an unusually high Hb A_2.[292–297] In these cases the 5′ end of the β gene is missing while the δ gene remains intact. It seems that the increased δ-chain production results mainly from increased δ-gene transcription from the gene in *cis* to the deletion.

***Mutations Affecting Transcription*.** A number of β^+ thalassemia genes have a single base substitution in two regions immediately in front of the cap site close to or within the CCAAT and ATA boxes that are known to be important in transcriptional efficiency.[72,298–300] These mutant genes show decreased β mRNA production in transient expression systems ranging from 10 to 25 percent of the output from a normal gene, indicating that these substitutions are responsible for the associated thalassemia phenotype.[298] In general, the level of expression in vitro correlates well with the clinical severity of the condition, in cases in which this is known.

One mutation of this type, C→T at position −101 nt to the β-globin gene appears to cause an extremely mild deficit of β-globin mRNA.[300] This allele is so mild that it is completely silent in carriers but can be identified by its interaction with more severe β thalassemia alleles in compound heterozygotes.

***Splice Site Mutations Involving the Intron–Exon Boundaries*.** The boundaries of exons and introns are marked by almost invariant dinucleotides—GT at the donor (5′) site and AG at the acceptor (3′) site (see "Structural Features of Globin Genes" above). Base substitutions that affect either of those sites totally abolish normal splicing and result in β^0 thalassemia.[73,210,299] Transcription of these genes appears to be normal, but abnormal processing products accumulate at low levels both in erythroid cells in vivo and in in vitro expression systems, as a result of splicing to cryptic splice sites in the surrounding exon or intron.

***Splice Site Consensus Sequence Mutations*.** Although only the GT dinucleotide is invariant at the donor splice site, there is conservation of the surrounding nucleotides, and a consensus sequence of these regions can be derived. Mutations within this sequence can reduce the efficiency of splicing to varying degrees, with alternative splicing occurring at the surrounding cryptic splice sites.[73,210,301–306] Mutations of the G at position 5 of IVS1 to C or T result in moderately severe β^+ thalassemia,[301] whereas the substitution of C for T at position 6 leads to the very mild β^+ thalassemia (Portuguese type) that is fairly common in the Mediterranean.[217,302]

***Mutations in Cryptic Sites in Exons*.** One of the cryptic splice sites used for alternative splicing in mutations affecting the IVS1 donor site covers codons 24 to 27 of exon 1 (Fig. 113-27). This site contains a GT dinucleotide, and substitutions surrounding this dinucleotide that alter the cryptic site so that it more closely resembles the consensus donor splice

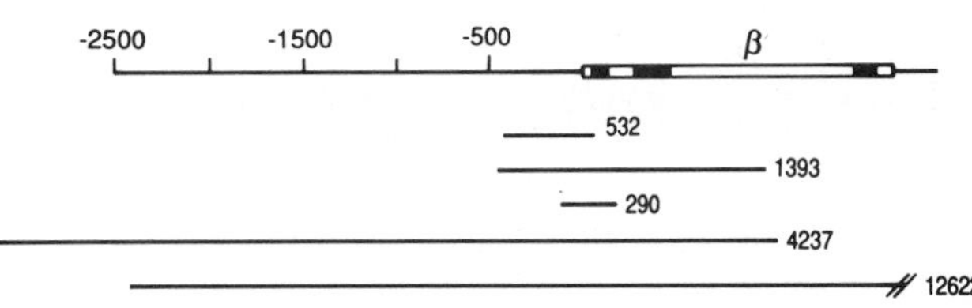

FIG. 113-26 Some of the deletions of the β-globin gene that results in β thalassemia.

Table 113-9 Molecular Pathology of the β Thalassemias

Mutation	β^0 or β^+ Thalassemia	Racial Origin
Nonfunctional mRNA		
Nonsense mutants:		
Codon 17 (A-T)	0	Chinese
Codon 39 (C-T)	0	Mediterranean, European
Codon 15 (G-A)	0	Asian Indian
Codon 121 (A-T)	0	Polish, Swiss
Codon 37 (G-A)	0	Saudi Arabian
Codon 43 (G-T)	0	Chinese
Codon 61 (A-T)	0	Black
Codon 35 (C-A)	0	Thai
Frameshift mutants		
−1 codon 1 (−G)	0	Mediterranean
−2 codon 5 (−CT)	0	Mediterranean
−1 codon 6 (−A)	0	Mediterranean
−2 codon 8 (−AA)	0	Turkish
+1 codons 8/9 (+G)	0	Asian Indian
−1 codon 11 (−T)	0	Mexican
+1 codon 14/15 (+G)	0	Chinese
−1 codon 16 (−C)	0	Asian Indian
+1 codon 27–28 (+C)	0	Chinese
−1 codon 35 (−C)	0	Indonesian
−1 codon 36–37 (−T)	0	Iranian
−1 codon 37 (−G)	0	Kurdish
−7 codon 37–39	0	Turkish
−4 codons 41/42 (−CTTT)	0	Asian Indian, Chinese
−1 codon 44 (−C)	0	Kurdish
+1 codon 47 (+A)	0	Surinamese black
−1 codon 64 (−G)	0	Swiss
+1 codon 71 (+T)	0	Chinese
+1 codons 71/72 (+A)	0	Chinese
−1 codon 76 (−C)	0	Italian
−1 codon 82/83 (−G)	0	Azerbaijani
+2 codon 94 (+TG)	0	Italian
+1 codons 106/107 (+G)	0	American black
−1 codon 109 (−G)	+	Lithuanian
−2, +1 codon 114 (−CT, +G)	+	French
−1 codon 126 (−T)	+	Italian
−4 codons 128–129)		
−11 codons 132–135)	0	Irish
+5 codon 129)		
Initiator codon mutants		
ATG-AGG	0	Chinese
ATG-ACG	0	Yugoslavian
RNA Processing mutants		
Splice junction changes:		
IVS1 position 1 (G-A)	0	Mediterranean
IVS1 position 1 (G-T)	0	Asian Indian, Chinese
IVS2 position 1 (G-A)	0	Mediterranean Tunisian, American black
IVS1 position 2 (T-G)	0	Tunisian
IVS1 position 2 (T-C)	0	Black
IVS1 3′-end −17 bp	0	Kuwaiti
IVS1 3′-end −25 bp	0	Asian Indian
IVS1 3′-end (G-C)	0	Italian
IVS2 3′-end (A-G)	0	American black
IVS2 3′-end (A-C)	0	American black
IVS1 5′-end −44bp	0	Mediterranean
IVS1 3′-end (G-A)	0	Egyptian
Consensus changes		
IVS1 position 5 (G-C)	+	Asian Indian, Chinese, Melanesian
IVS1 position 5 (G-T)	+	Mediterranean, black
IVS1 position 5 (G-A)	+	Algerian
IVS1 position 6 (T-C)	+	Mediterranean

Table 113-9 Molecular Pathology of the β Thalassemias (Continued)

Mutation	β^0 or β^+ Thalassemia	Racial Origin
IVS1 position −1 (G-C) (codon 30)	?	Tunisian, black
IVS1 position −1 (G-A) (codon 30)	?	Bulgarian
IVS1 position −3 (C-T) (codon 29)	?	Lebanese
IVS2 3′-end CAG-AAG	+	Iranian, Egyptian, black
IVS1 3′-end TAG-GAG	+	Saudi Arabian
IVS2 3′-end −8 (T-G)	+	Algerian
Internal IVS changes		
IVS2 position 110 (G-A)	+	Mediterranean
IVS1 position 116 (T-G)	0	Mediterranean
IVS1 position 705 (T-G)	+	Mediterranean
IVS2 position 745 (C-G)	+	Mediterranean
IVS2 position 654 (C-T)	0	Chinese
Coding region substitutions affecting processing		
Codon 26 (G-A)	E	Southeast Asian, European
Codon 24 (T-A)	+	American black
Codon 27 (G-T)	Knossos	Mediterranean
Codon 19 (A-G)	Malay	Malaysian
Transcriptional mutants		
−101 C-T	+	Turkish
−92 C-T	+	Mediterranean
−88 C-T	+	American black, Asian Indian
−88 C-A	+	Kurdish
−87 C-G	+	Mediterranean
−86 C-G	+	Lebanese
−31 A-G	+	Japanese
−30 T-A	+	Turkish
−30 T-C	+	Chinese
−29 A-G	+	American black, Chinese
−28 A-C	+	Kurdish
−28 A-G	+	Chinese
RNA cleavage + polyadenylation mutants		
AATAAA-AACAAA	+	American black
AATAAA-AATAAG	+	Kurdish
AATAAA = A(del.AATAA)	+	Arab
AATAAA-AATGAA	+	Mediterranean
AATAAA-AATAGA	+	Malaysian
Cap site mutants		
+1 A-C	+	Asian Indian

SOURCE: From refs. 209, 210, and 211, which contain references to original descriptions.

site result in some use of this site even though the normal splice site is intact. For example, mutation of codon 24 from GGT to GGA does not alter the amino acid (glycine), but because some splicing occurs at this site instead of the exon–intron boundary, it results in a moderately severe β^+ thalassemia phenotype.[307]

Mutations of codons 19 (A→G), 26 (G→A) and 27 (G→T) result in both reduced production of mRNA and an amino acid substitution when the mRNA which is spliced normally is translated into protein. The abnormal hemoglobins produced are Hb MALAY, E, and Hb KNOSSOS, respectively.[194,308,309] It may be the mild thalassemic nature of the β^E allele that is responsible for its high prevalence in Southeast Asia, rather than an altered property resulting from the amino acid change.

Mutations at Cryptic Sites in Introns. Cryptic splice sites within introns can also undergo mutations that cause them to be used even though the normal site remains intact. The first β-thalassemia mutation characterized was of this type—a base substitution at position 110 in IVS1.[310,311] This region contains a sequence similar to a 3′ acceptor splice site but lacks the invariant AG dinucleotide. Mutation of the G at nt 110 to an A supplies the dinucleotide, and ~90 percent of the RNA transcripts splice to this site and only ~10 percent splice at the normal site, resulting in a phenotype of severe β^+ thalassemia. The result of the abnormal splicing is a nonfunctional mRNA molecule containing an extra 19 nucleotides from IVS1 that can be detected in low amounts in reticulocyte or marrow RNA. This lesion is the most common β^+ thalassemia mutation among Mediterraneans.[73]

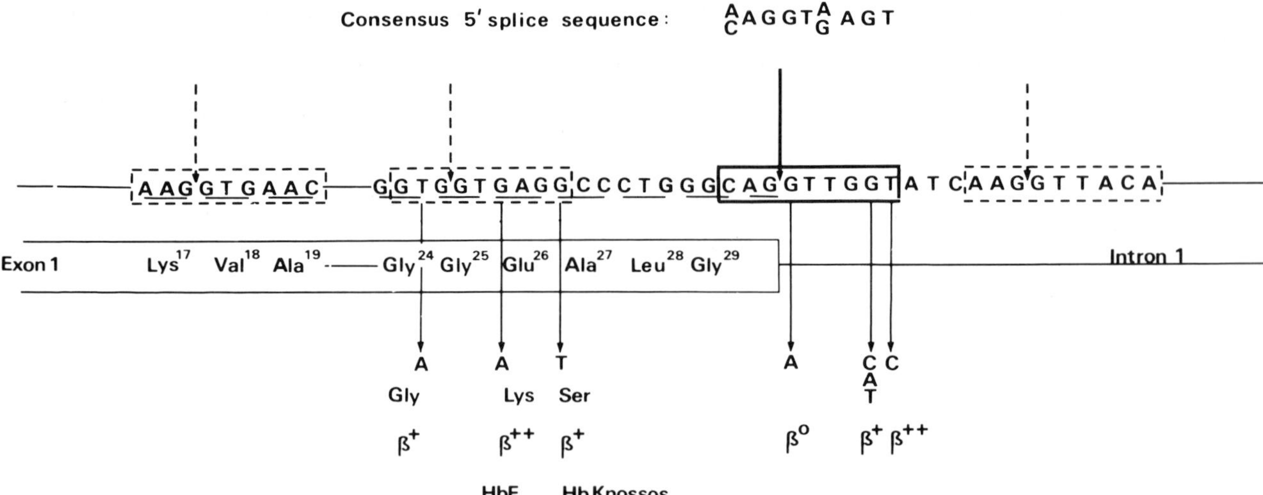

FIG. 113-27 **Normal and abnormal splicing at the boundary of exon 1 and intron 1 of the β-globin gene. Solid box and arrow: normal splice site showing consensus sequence and site of cleavage. dashed boxes and arrows: alternate splice sites used in various β-thalassemia lesions.**

Several β-thalassemia mutations have been described which generate new donor sites within IVS2 of the β-globin gene.[73,303] In each case a cryptic acceptor site within IVS2 following nucleotide 580 is used for processing abnormal transcripts. No normal β-globin mRNA appears to be processed from a gene with an A-to-G substitution at IVS2 position 654; hence the clinical phenotype is β^0 thalassemia. This is a curious finding because the IVS2 donor and acceptor sites are entirely normal. It appears that all stable transcripts are spliced from the normal IVS2 donor to the cryptic acceptor site and from the abnormal new donor site to the normal IVS2 acceptor. The processed β-globin mRNA contains an insertion derived from IVS2. It is not clear why splicing from the normal donor to acceptor sites does not occur.

Cap Site Mutations. One example of a mutation involving the β-globin mRNA cap site has been described.[312] This involves the substitution of the first A residue by C. It is not clear how this change leads to defective β-globin production. It could be mediated by a reduction in the rate of transcription or by slowing down the 5′ capping process which, in turn, might reduce β-globin mRNA stability.

Polyadenylation Signal Mutations. The sequence AAUAAA in the 3′ untranslated region of β-globin mRNA is the signal for cleavage and polyadenylation of the β-gene transcript. Several different mutations of this region have been described.[210,313–315] For example, a T-to-C substitution in the β-globin gene in this sequence leads to only one tenth of the normal amount of β-globin mRNA transcript and hence to a phenotype of severe β^+ thalassemia. A small amount of an extended β-globin mRNA molecule can be found in reticulocytes, presumably polyadenylated at a downstream site.[313]

Mutations to Termination Codons. Base substitutions that change an amino acid codon to a chain termination codon prevent translation of the mRNA and result in β^0 thalassemias. Several mutations of this type have been described, a codon 17 mutation[316] being common in Southeast Asia and the codon 39 mutations[317] occurring at a high frequency in the Mediterranean. The low levels of nuclear and cytoplasmic RNA found in cells with these mutations has yet to be explained.[318]

Frameshift Mutations. The insertion or deletion of one or a few nucleotides in the coding region of the β-globin gene disrupts the normal reading frame and results, on translation of the mRNA, in the addition of anomalous amino acids until a termination codon is reached in the new reading frame.[73,210,315] The abnormal mRNA is found only in very low levels in erythroid cells. This type of mutation leads to β^0 thalassemia, and one, the deletion of four nucleotides in codons 41 and 42, is common in Southeast Asia.

Unstable β-Globin Chain Products. Some studies have shed light on the complex clinical phenotypes which may result from synthesis of unstable β-globin products.[211,319,320] The phenotypic effects of termination codon or frameshift mutations in the β-globin gene seem to depend on their particular position. Mutations that produce truncated β chains up to 72 residues in length are usually associated with a mild phenotype in heterozygotes; presumably the short fragments are degraded and the resulting excess of α chains are removed in the same way. However, many exon-3 mutations produce longer truncated products, and it is likely that the severe heterozygous phenotypes associated with them reflect their heme-binding properties and stability. Truncated products of 120 or more residues should bind heme since only helix H is missing. Furthermore, such heme-containing products should have secondary structure and hence be less susceptible to proteolytic degradation. These mutations are associated with a dominantly inherited form of thalassemia.[321,322] Presumably, the large inclusion bodies seen in the erythroid precursors in the marrow of heterozygotes result from both excess α chains and aggregates of precipitated β-chain products. Some unstable β-globin variants are associated with a milder phenotype similar to heterozygous β thalassemia. A partial list of these mutations is shown in Table 113-10.

Deletions Causing δβ Thalassemia or HPFH. The unequal crossover events that give rise to the Lepore-like hemoglobins and the phenotype of $(\delta\beta)^+$ thalassemia were described earlier in this chapter. The majority of the $(\delta\beta)^0$ and $(^{A}\gamma\delta\beta)^0$

Table 113-10 Molecular Forms of Dominant β Thalassemia and Structural Variants Associated with a β Thalassemia Phenotype

Mutation	Exon	Phenotype	Designation	Race
		Dominant β Thalassemia		
Codons 128 −4 bp, +5 bp, −11 bp. Frameshift terminates codon 154	III	Thalassemia intermedia Inclusion bodies	—	Irish
Codon 121 GAA→TAA*	III	Thalassemia intermedia Inclusion bodies	—	Swiss-French Greek-Polish
Codon 127 CAA → TAA	III	Thalassemia intermedia	—	English
Codon 114 −CT +G Frameshift terminates codon 157	III	Thalassemia intermedia	β Geneva	Swiss-French
Codon 126-T Frameshift terminates codon 157*	III	Thalassemia intermedia Inclusion bodies	β Vercelli	Italian
Codon 94 +TG Frameshift terminates codon 157*	II	Severe thalassemia intermedia Inclusion bodies	β Agnana	Italian
Codon 123 −A Frameshift terminates codon 157	III	Thalassemia intermedia Inclusion bodies	β Makabe	Japanese
Codons 123 to 125 −8 bp β-chain 135 residues	III	Severe thalassemia intermedia with Hb E Inclusion bodies	β Khon Kaen	Thai
Codon 127 Gln → Pro	III	Thalassemia intermedia	β Houston	British
Codons 109 to 110 −G Frameshift terminates codon 157	III	Thalassemia intermedia	β Manhattan	Ashkenazi Jew
Codons 32/34-GGT*	II	Thalassemia intermedia	β Korea	Korean
Codon 106 Leu → Arg†	III	Thalassemia intermedia	β Terre Haute	European
Codon 28 Leu → Arg	I	Thalassemia intermedia Inclusion bodies	β Chesterfield	English
Codon 60 Val → Glu	II	Thalassemia intermedia	β Cagliari	Italian
		Thalassemia Trait		
Codon 110 Leu → Pro	III	β-thalassemia trait	β Showa-Yakushiji	Japanese
Codons 127 and 128 −3 bp β-chain 145 residues	III	β-thalassemia trait	β Gunma	Japanese
β132 Lys → Gln	III	β-thalassemia trait	$\beta^{K\ Woolwich}$	British
β134 Lys → Gln	III	Mild microcytosis S/β thalassemia interaction with Hb S	Hb North Shore-Caracas	

**De novo* mutations.
†Originally reported as $Hb_{INDIANAPOLIS}$.
SOURCE: Original descriptions given in Ref. 211.

thalassemias, as well as different forms of $(\delta\beta)^0$ HPFH (including Hb KENYA) are the result of deletions affecting various parts of the β-globin locus. These disorders have attracted considerable interest, since an understanding of how the deletions result in the γ genes remaining active in adult life may provide valuable insights into the normal developmental regulation of the globin genes. Many deletions have now been characterized, and the breakpoints have been cloned and sequenced; they are summarized in Fig. 113-28 and reviewed in detail by Poncz et al.[323] and Bollekens and Forget.[324] The mechanisms by which they arose are largely unknown. While Hb LEPORE, Hb KENYA, and the γ thalassemias occur as a result of misaligned crossovers between homologous genes, the remaining deletions all involve some type of illegitimate recombination, with little or no sequence homology at the breakpoints.

The *$(\delta\beta)^0$ thalassemia* deletions remove or inactivate only the δ and β genes. They are relatively small and are contained within the β-gene cluster. There is one exception however—the Spanish type, in which the deletion extends much further on the 3′ side, beyond the 3′ end of $(\delta\beta)^0$ HPFH lesions.[325] Phenotypically they are all similar, except that Hb Lepore is associated with a minimal increase in Hb F production.

The *$(^A\gamma\delta\beta)^0$ thalassemia* deletions extend into or beyond the $^A\gamma$ gene on the 5′ side as well as removing the δ and β genes. On the 3′ side, most of them terminate within 20 kb of the β gene. But again, there is one exception—the Chinese type—that extends much further. The Indian form is not a simple linear deletion but a complex rearrangement with two deletions, one affecting the $^A\gamma$ gene and the other the δ and β genes; the intervening region remains but is inverted.[326,327] Again, the phenotypic results of these very different deletions are quite similar. The overall level of Hb F production is similar to that in the $(\delta\beta)^0$ thalassemias but in this case only the $^G\gamma$ gene is active, not both.

The two African forms of $(\delta\beta)^0$ HPFH are both due to extensive deletions, of similar length (>70 kb) but with staggered ends, differing phenotypically only in the proportions of $^G\gamma$ and $^A\gamma$ chains produced.[328] The third type (Indian), although producing a similar amount of Hb F in heterozygotes, has a more severe phenotype than the other two when coinherited with β thalassemia.[329]

Deletions of the β-Globin Locus Control Region; $(\epsilon\gamma\delta\beta)^0$ Thalassemia. This rare group of thalassemias results from several different long deletions which start approximately

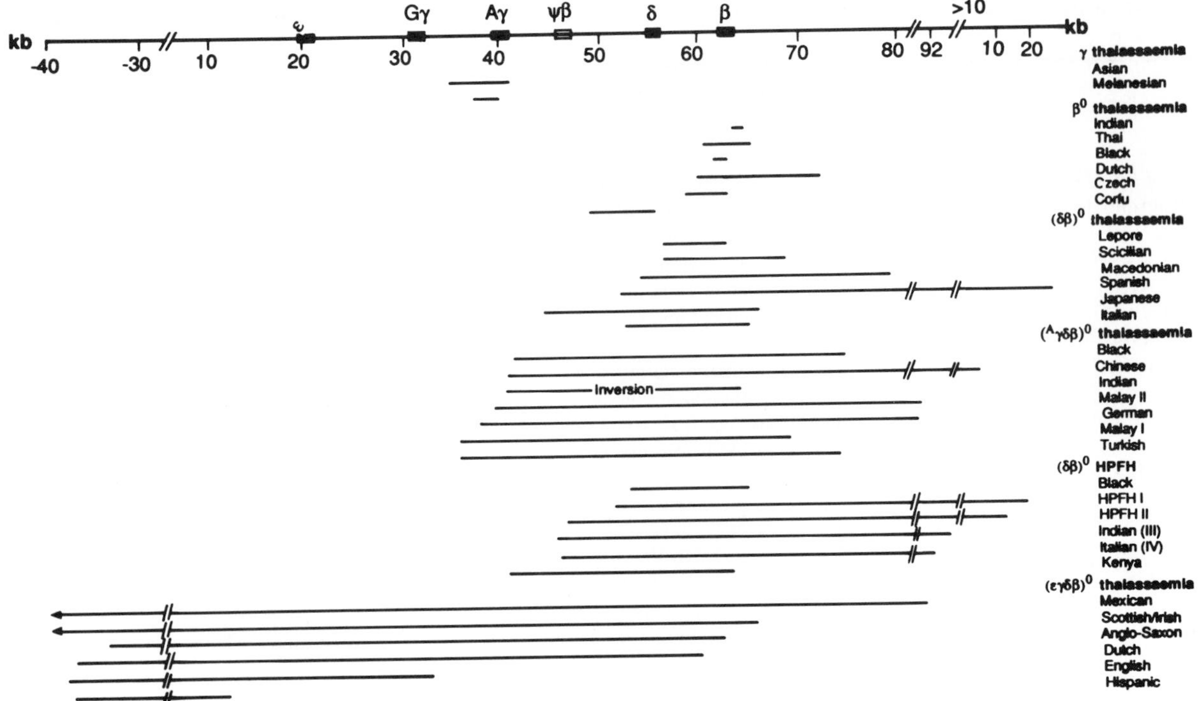

FIG. 113-28 **Deletions affecting the β-globin gene cluster, arranged according to their phenotypic effects. (Note the discontinuities at the 5′ and 3′ ends and the change of scale at the 3′ end.)**

50 to 100 kb upstream from the β-globin gene cluster and extend 3′, where they remove all or part of the cluster.[211,323,324] Even if the β-globin gene is spared it is still inactivated, so they are all $(\epsilon\gamma\delta\beta)^0$ thalassemias. The approximate extent of these deletions is shown in Fig. 113-28. In cases in which the deletion leaves the β-globin gene intact (the Dutch and English forms, for example), no β-chain production occurs, even though the gene is expressed in heterologous systems.[330–332] It is clear, therefore, that any deletion which involves the LCR completely inactivates the downstream globin gene complex. The Hispanic form of this condition[90] results from a deletion which includes most of the LCR, including three of the four DNase I hypersensitive sites. All these lesions appear to shut down the chromatin domain which is usually open in erythroid tissues. They also delay the replication of the β genes in the cell cycle.

Deletion Phenotype Analysis. Analysis of the size and position of deletions of the β-like globin gene cluster are of considerable interest because of their potential for demonstrating critical regulatory regions of this gene complex.[333] Although much remains to be learned about the reasons for their phenotypic effect, certain conclusions can be drawn. First, it is clear that deletions which either completely or partially remove the β-globin LCR inactivate the entire complex. On the other hand, deletions starting within the complex and extending 3′ to it, appear to leave the surviving γ genes active in adult life, when they would normally be repressed. While this could be the result of the newly apposed 3′ sequences, the number of different deletions of this type make it difficult to imagine that each one has a similar effect. Furthermore, two of the deletions [Hb KENYA and Hb INDIAN $(^A\gamma\delta\beta)^0$ thalassemia] leave the 3′ of the β gene and beyond intact.

Comparison of $(\delta\beta)^0$ thalassemia and $(\delta\beta)^0$ HPFH does not identify any single region between the $^A\gamma$ and δ genes that remains intact in the one but is lost in the other, precluding any simple explanation for the difference in γ gene output between these two conditions. $(^A\gamma\delta\beta)^0$ thalassemia appears to act more like $(\delta\beta)^0$ HPFH in terms of output per gene. Furthermore, the internal deletion that results in one form of normal Hb A_2 β thalassemia removes much of the area in which a putative switching sequence might reside, yet causes little or no increase in Hb F in heterozygotes.[334]

Overall, therefore, analysis of the deletions has yet to explain their phenotypic consequences. The phenotypic pattern of the 5′ and 3′ deletions suggests some form of polarity within the globin-gene complex.[335] It is likely, however, that there is more than one mechanism by which deletions within the complex affect the expression of the surviving genes. In fact, one important lesson that can be learned from these conditions is that, within this cluster, the genes are not regulated solely by the sequences immediately surrounding them but are subject to control acting over a considerable distance.

Nondeletion Hereditary Persistence of Fetal Hemoglobin. Analysis of the nondeletion $^G\gamma\beta^+$ and $^A\gamma\beta^+$ forms of HPFH by cloning and sequencing of the overexpressed γ gene has revealed, in each case, a single base substitution in the region immediately upstream from the transcription start site (Table 113-11).[336–340] The clustering of these substitutions and the lack of similar changes in normal γ genes suggests that they are responsible for the persistent Hb F production. This interpretation is strengthened by the observation that when these promoter regions are mutated the amounts of transcription in transfected erythroid cells relative to the normal promoter is increased. It seems likely that these mutations affect the binding of a *trans*-acting protein involved in the normal developmental repression of γ-gene expression, either by decreasing the affinity for an inhibitory factor normally present in adult life or by increasing the affinity for a factor-promoting gene expression. The decrease in β-chain production that accompanies the persistent γ-chain synthesis has yet to be explained, but the fact that it is only the β gene in *cis* that is affected, precludes any simple explanation involving competition for *trans*-acting factors.

As shown in Table 113-11, and discussed in a later section, it is becoming clear that nondeletion HPFH is very heterogeneous. In some cases the genetic determinant is unlinked to the β-globin gene cluster, but so far the genes have not been isolated. Thus, the molecular basis for these conditions remains to be determined.

δβ *Thalassemia-like Disorders Due to Two Mutations in the β-Globin Gene Cluster.* Several disorders with features similar to δβ thalassemia have been described in which more than one mutation in the β-globin gene cluster has been found. For example, in the Sardinian form of δβ thalassemia the β-globin gene has the common Mediterranean codon 39 nonsense mutation which leads to an absence of β-globin synthesis.[341] However, there is a relatively high expression of the $^{A}\gamma$ gene in *cis* which gives this condition the phenotype of $\delta^{+}\beta^{0}$ thalassemia; this is because there is a point mutation at position −196 upstream from the $^{A}\gamma$ gene. Another condition which was originally designated as δβ thalassemia has been described in the Corfu population.[334,342] Again, this results from two different mutations. First, there is a 7201-bp deletion which starts in the δ-globin gene and extends upstream to a 5′ breakpoint located 1719 to 1722 bp 3′ to the ψβ gene termination codon. In addition there is a C-to-A mutation at position 5 in the donor site consensus region of IVS1 of the β-globin gene. The output from this novel chromosome consists of relatively high levels of γ chains in homozygotes and extremely low levels of β chains.

Clinical and Hematologic Characteristics of the β Thalassemias.[2,207] **β *Thalassemia Major.*** This condition may result from the homozygous state for a β-thalassemia mutation or, more commonly, from the compound heterozygous state for two different β thalassemias.

At birth, when Hb F production is still high, β thalassemia homozygotes are asymptomatic, but as Hb F production declines, affected infants present with severe anemia, usually during the first 1 to 2 years of life. Left untreated, they are incapable of maintaining a hemoglobin level above 5 g/dl and show marked growth retardation. The skin shows pallor and icterus, often accompanied by brown pigmentation. Expansion of the bone marrow in response to anemia leads to characteristic skeletal changes, including the development of "thalassemic" facies due to frontal bossing of the skull and protrusion of the jaws and cheekbones. On radiography, the skull has a "hair on end" appearance, while the long bones show considerable thinning and trabeculation and are prone to repeated fractures. The magnitude of the increase in erythropoiesis (estimated to be as much as twentyfold to thirtyfold) may result in extramedullary masses, arising usually from the sternum and ribs. Progressive hepatosplenomegaly is a constant finding, often leading to secondary dilutional anemia, leukopenia, and thrombocytopenia. Gallstones and leg ulcers are common. Intercurrent infections are a frequent complication, and in inadequately transfused patients they are a major cause of morbidity and mortality.

With frequent transfusions to maintain a hemoglobin level above 9 to 11 g/dl, growth and development are relatively normal until early puberty. Splenectomy is often necessary during this period to reduce the transfusion requirements but is associated with an increased incidence of septicemia. By the age of 10 to 11 years, treated patients begin to show signs of progressive hepatic, cardiac, and endocrine disturbances, associated with a reduced or absent pubertal growth spurt and failure of sexual maturation. These changes are due largely to accumulation of iron from transfusion and its deposition in the tissues. Unless iron overload is controlled by chelation therapy, it results in death in the second or third decade, usually from cardiac failure.

The peripheral blood shows grossly abnormal red-cell morphology (see Fig. 113-24). There is marked anisocytosis and poikilocytosis, target cells, and red-cell fragments, all associated with extreme hypochromia. Nucleated red cells are usually present in the blood and often contain inclusion bodies, particularly after splenectomy. White-cell and platelet counts are usually normal or elevated, unless there is hypersplenism.

The bone marrow shows intense erythroid hyperplasia (myeloid:erythroid ratio, ~0.1) with a shift to the less mature basophilic forms. Hypochromia is evident, and inclusion bodies of precipitated α chains can be demonstrated in many of the normoblasts.[212,213] Nuclear and cytoplasmic abnormalities typical of ineffective erythropoiesis, and increased phagocytic activity, are also prominent. This pattern of highly expanded but ineffective erythropoiesis is reflected

Table 113-11 Hereditary Persistence of Fetal Hemoglobin[336–340]

Race and Type	Mutation	Percent Hb F in Heterozygote	γ Chain
Deletion			
Black; Indian $(\delta\beta)^0$	Deletions of δ and β gene	15–25	$^{G}\gamma^{A}\gamma$
Black, Hb KENYA	Deletion, $(^{A}\gamma\beta)$ fusion genes	5–20	$^{G}\gamma$
Nondeletion, involving β-like globin-gene cluster			
Black	$^{G}\gamma$ −202 C → G	15–25	$^{G}\gamma$
Black; Sardinian	$^{G}\gamma$ −175 T → C	17–21	$^{G}\gamma$
Japanese	$^{G}\gamma$ −114 C → T	11–14	$^{G}\gamma$
Italian; Chinese	$^{A}\gamma$ −196 C → T	12–20	$^{A}\gamma$
Black	$^{A}\gamma$ −175 T → C	—	$^{A}\gamma$
Greek (+ others)	$^{A}\gamma$ −117 G → A	10–20	$^{A}\gamma$
Black	$^{A}\gamma$ −114 to −102 deleted	30–32	$^{A}\gamma$
Black	$^{A}\gamma$ −202 C → T	1.5–3.9	$^{A}\gamma$
British	$^{A}\gamma$ −198 T → C	3.5–10	$^{A}\gamma$
Brazilian	$^{A}\gamma$ −195 C → T	4–7	$^{A}\gamma$
Nondeletion segregating independently from β-like globin-gene cluster			
Several types	Unknown		$^{G}\gamma^{A}\gamma$

by the results of ferrokinetic and erythrokinetic studies.[2] Cells that do survive to enter the circulation show a markedly reduced red-cell life span of 7 to 22 days.

Hemoglobin analysis in patients who have not undergone transfusion usually shows a high proportion of Hb F. In patients with no β-chain production there is a corresponding lack of Hb A, and except for a small proportion of Hb A_2 (1 to 3 percent) the remainder is Hb F. In those with reduced β-chain output, a variable amount of Hb A is present, but this rarely exceeds 30 percent. The Hb A_2 level is variable and of no diagnostic help. After transfusion, endogenous erythropoiesis is suppressed and analysis of hemoglobin composition, even immediately prior to transfusion, is unreliable as an indicator of the type of β thalassemia.

More detailed clinical descriptions of severe thalassemia will be found in two monographs.[2,207]

Thalassemia Intermedia. Thalassemia intermedia is an ill-defined clinical term used to describe patients with anemia and splenomegaly but without the full spectrum of clinical severity found in thalassemia major.[2,207,343] Although far less common than thalassemia major, the condition encompasses a much broader clinical spectrum so that it is sometimes further divided into mild or severe thalassemia intermedia. The criteria on which the diagnosis is made are that patients do not present until later in life than those with thalassemia major and that they are capable of maintaining a hemoglobin level about 6 g/dl without undergoing transfusion.

At the severe end of the spectrum, patients present between the ages of 2 and 6 years, and although they are capable of surviving with a hemoglobin level of 5 to 7 g/dl it is clear that they will not develop normally and will show many of the skeletal and facial changes seen in patients with untreated thalassemia major. Thus, they are treated with transfusions, but their blood requirement is not as great as patients with thalassemia major. In general, they are prone to the same complications, though they may occur later in life.

At the other end of the spectrum, patients may not become symptomatic until they reach adult life, and may never undergo transfusion, with hemoglobin levels of 8 to 10 g/dl except during infections. There is usually some degree of hepatosplenomegaly, and the development of hypersplenism may render patients transfusion-dependent; this may be reversed by splenectomy. Sexual development may be normal, and several successful pregnancies have been reported, although the anemia is exacerbated in the later stages.

Even patients who have few transfusions tend to accumulate iron with age, presumably as a result of increased absorption in response to the chronic anemia. Thus, evidence of iron overload may develop in the third and fourth decades, with diabetes mellitus and impairment of other endocrine functions. The chronic hemolysis and ineffective erythropoiesis leads to a high incidence of gallstones. Presumably because of extreme marrow expansion bone and joint disease develop later in life in some patients.

The hematologic picture of thalassemia intermedia, except for the severity of the anemia, is similar to thalassemia major. The hemoglobin composition is extremely variable. Rare cases are homozygous for β^0 thalassemia and hence have only Hbs F and A_2, while in others the level of Hb F may be as low as 5 to 10 percent. This variability reflects the wide genetic heterogeneity that can produce this clinical picture; this is summarized in Table 113-12.

The main causes of a relatively mild phenotype in β

Table 113-12 Causes of β Thalassemia Intermedia

Mild β-chain deficit
Homozygous β^{++} thalassemia*
Compound heterozygous β^{+}/β^{++} thalassemia
Homozygous normal Hb A_2 β thalassemia type I
Compound heterozygous β^{+} or β^{0}/normal Hb A_2 β thalassemia type 1
Severe heterozygous β thalassemia
Interacting α thalassemia
Homozygous β^{+}/β^{+} thalassemia with $\alpha\alpha/-\alpha$
Homozygous β^{0}/β^{0} thalassemia with $-\alpha/-\alpha$
Compound heterozygous β^{0}/β^{+} thalassemia with $-\alpha/-\alpha$
Hb E/β^{0} thalassemia with $-\alpha/-\alpha$
Increased Hb F production
Homozygous $(\delta\beta)^0$ thalassemia
Homozygous $(^{A}\gamma\delta\beta)^0$ thalassemia
Compound heterozygous β^{+} or $\beta^{0}/(\delta\beta)^0$ thalassemia
Homozygous β^{+} or β^{0} thalassemia with high Hb F determinant (allelic or nonallelic)
Homozygous Hb LEPORE, Hb LEPORE/$(\delta\beta)^0$ thalassemia, and Hb LEPORE/β^{0} thalassemia

*β^{++} Thalassemia indicates a particular mild defect in β-chain synthesis.

thalassemia homozygotes or compound heterozygotes are "mild" β thalassemia mutations, the coinheritance of α thalassemia, and various genetic determinants that increase Hb F production (see Table 113-12). The latter interactions are described in a later section. However, there are many cases in which the mild course remains unexplained.

Heterozygous β Thalassemia. The heterozygous state for β thalassemia is asymptomatic and, despite the genetic heterogeneity, remarkably uniform hematologically. The diagnosis is usually straightforward and is based on low MCV and MCH together with an increased proportion of Hb A_2. This is an important consideration for genetic counseling and prenatal diagnosis. The hematologic findings are listed in Table 113-13. The peripheral blood film shows hypochromia and microcytosis with some anisocytosis and poikilocytosis and basophilic stippling. Red-cell survival is normal.

Hemoglobin analysis shows a raised level of Hb A_2, 3.5 to 6.5 percent (mean, ~5 percent), that is only found in this condition and occurs in nearly all cases (see below). It may be accompanied by a slight increase (1 to 3 percent) in Hb F in about half the cases. Although there is globin chain imbalance, with an α-chain excess of about twofold, there is little evidence of ineffective erythropoiesis or of free α chains remaining in the red cell. It appears that the proteolytic mechanisms within the red cell have the capacity to deal with this degree of chain imbalance.

Subtypes of β Thalassemia. The phenotypes of the various forms of β thalassemia detectable by hemoglobin analysis are listed in Table 113-13. Numerically, the β^0 and β^+ forms are by far the most important; the other types shown in Table 113-12, although widespread, do not usually account for more than 10 percent of the β thalassemia alleles within a population.

β^0 Thalassemia genes are found in all affected populations, although they are rare in persons of African origin. In the homozygous state they are detected by the lack of Hb A in patients who have not undergone transfusion, and whose hemoglobin pattern comprises Hb F plus 1 to 3 percent

Table 113-13 Phenotypic Characteristics of the β Thalassemias

Condition	Heterozygotes			Homozygotes		
	MCH, pg	% Hb A_2	% Hb F	% Hb A	% Hb F	Clinical status
β^0 Thalassemia	21±2	3.8–6.5	<4	0	~98	Major
β^+ Thalassemia	22±2	3.8–6.5	<4	5–50	50–90	Major
β^{++} Thalassemia	24±2	3.8–6.5	<2	50–90	10–50	Intermedia
High Hb A_2 β thalassemia	21±2	6.0–10.0	3–10	0	~98	Intermedia
Normal Hb A_2 β thalassemia I	27±2	2.3–3.4	<2	75–90	5–25	Intermedia
Normal Hb A_2 β thalassemia II	23±2	2.8–3.5	<2		—	
Severe heterozygous β thalassemia	21±2	3.5–5.3	1–12		—	

SOURCE: From Weatherall and Clegg.[2] Used by permission.

Hb A_2. The β^0 thalassemia gene can also be identified in compound heterozygotes with a β-chain variant such as Hb S by the absence of Hb A. In populations with both β^0 and β^+ alleles, distinction between β^0/β^+ compound heterozygotes and $\beta^+\beta^+$ homozygotes is not usually possible because of the considerable overlap in the amount of Hb A produced in the two conditions. Heterozygotes for β^0 thalassemia cannot be distinguished from individuals heterozygous for the common β^+ forms of thalassemia.

There are numerous β^+ thalassemia alleles with variable levels of residual β-chain production, and several may be relatively common within the same population. By and large the extent of the β-chain deficit determines the clinical severity, but homozygosity or compound heterozygosity for most of the common alleles causes thalassemia major. The extent of the deficiency in β-chain production dictated by specific β^+ thalassemia alleles can be determined only by the amount of Hb A in compound heterozygotes with β-chain structural variants. Since many alleles have not been observed in such an association, and the molecular defect has not been established in many of those that have, the correlation between the molecular lesion and the extent of β-chain deficit remains to be established in many cases.

In some cases the deficit in β-chain production is so mild that a separate category of β^{++} thalassemia may be warranted. Homozygotes may not come to clinical attention, and compound heterozygotes with β^0 or the more severe β^+ alleles have thalassemia intermedia.

Normal Hb A_2 β Thalassemia. Family studies of β thalassemia patients occasionally reveal a parent without the raised Hb A_2 level characteristic of most heterozygotes. Two forms of this condition have been described[344]—type 1, in which the red-cell indices are almost normal but in which deficient β-chain production is observed when the globin chain synthesis ratio is measured, and type 2, in which only the Hb A_2 level differs from the usual heterozygous β thalassemia picture.

The type 1 form of normal Hb A_2 β thalassemia appears to be heterogeneous at the molecular level. Heterozygotes show no abnormalities; therefore, this condition is sometimes called *silent β thalassemia*. Some cases, as mentioned earlier, seem to result from point mutations upstream from the β-globin gene.[300] One of the commonest varieties is associated with the abnormal β-chain variant, Hb KNOSSOS, which is undetectable on standard hemoglobin electrophoresis, although it can be demonstrated by isoelectric focusing. The Hb KNOSSOS β chain is produced at a slightly reduced rate, resulting in a mild thalassemia phenotype.[309,345] It has been found that the low Hb A_2 level in this condition occurs because in many cases the Hb KNOSSOS mutation occurs on the same chromosome as a form of δ thalassemia.[346]

There is also heterogeneity within type 2 normal Hb A_2β thalassemia, and several different defects have been observed. Many cases are likely to be due to the coinheritance of a defective δ gene (δ thalassemia) which may occur either in *cis* or *trans* to the β thalassemia gene, which itself may be of the β^0 or β^+ type.[346,347] Deletion of the complete complex results in this phenotype,[348,349] as do deletions that remove the ε and $^G\gamma$ or ε, $^G\gamma$, $^A\gamma$, and δ genes but spare the β gene.[330,332,350] These conditions, the εγδβ thalassemias, may result in an unusually severe hemolytic anemia at birth which disappears within the first few months.[351] Heterozygotes for the conditions like the Corfu form of δβ thalassemia, described earlier, also have the clinical phenotype of normal Hb A_2 β thalassemia; the β-globin gene is partially inactivated by a mutation and the δ-globin gene in *cis* is deleted.

Unusually High Hb A_2 Thalassemia. Several β thalassemias have been described in which the proportion of Hb A_2 in heterozygotes is unusually high (>7 percent). This phenotype appears to identify certain specific β^0 thalassemia mutations in which there is a deletion involving at least the 5′ end of the β gene but sparing the δ gene (see "Molecular Pathology. β-Thalassemia" above).

Severe Heterozygous β Thalassemia. Many families have been described in which the inheritance of a mild Thalassemia intermedia phenotype follows a dominant pattern.[321,322] The molecular pathology that underlies these dominantly inherited forms of β thalassemia was described in the section on "Unstable β-Globin Chain Products" (see Table 113-10). Many, but not all of them result from exon 3 mutations of the β-globin gene. There is a spectrum of disorders which range from severe ineffective erythropoiesis and splenomegaly through a moderately severe hypochromic anemia to heterozygous β thalassemia with more severe anemia than usual. This phenotypic variability seems to reflect the properties of the unstable gene products which underlie these conditions.[211]

The coinheritance of the ααα gene arrangement with

heterozygous β thalassemia may also produce this phenotype.[352–354]

Clinical and Hematologic Features of the δβ Thalassemias (Table 113-14). ***Hb LEPORE.*** The structures and molecular mechanisms underlying the Lepore hemoglobins were described in the section "Fusion Hemoglobins."

Homozygotes for Hb LEPORE produce only Hb LEPORE (15 to 20 percent) and Hb F. Clinically, their phenotype is either thalassemia major or thalassemia intermedia; the basis for this variable picture is not understood.[2,355] Although cases have been described from many racial groups it appears to be relatively common only in the Campania region of Italy.

$(\delta\beta)^0$ Thalassemias. $(\delta\beta)^0$ Thalassemias are widely distributed but are relatively rare. Only in the Mediterranean do they constitute a significant proportion of the β thalassemias. They are characterized in the homozygous state by a clinical picture of thalassemia intermedia, while hemoglobin analysis shows 100 percent Hb F containing a mixture of both $^G\gamma$ and $^A\gamma$ chains. Hematologic changes are less marked than in β thalassemia homozygotes.

Heterozygotes are distinguished from β-thalassemia heterozygotes by normal levels of Hb A_2 together with an increased Hb F level of 5 to 20 percent. The Hb F is heterogeneously distributed, with only a proportion of cells positive after acid elution. The red-cell indices of heterozygotes are reduced but not as severely as in β-thalassemia heterozygotes.[356]

In general, the clinical and hematologic findings appear to be very similar in all these disorders, regardless of their underlying defects. However, too few cases have been studied in which the underlying lesions is known to be sure that there are no phenotypic differences.

$(^A\gamma\delta\beta)^0$ Thalassemias. These are also rare but widespread disorders. Clinically and hematologically they are very similar to the $(\delta\beta)^0$ thalassemias, with a similar amount and distribution of Hb F. They can be distinguished only by analysis of the γ-chain composition of the Hb F, which in the $(^A\gamma\delta\beta)^0$ thalassemias consists only of $^G\gamma$ chains. Again, there are few if any phenotypic differences between the various types which have been distinguished by the size and position of the underlying gene deletions.[357]

Hematologic Features of Hereditary Persistence of Fetal Hemoglobin (Table 113-14). HPFH is the term used to describe genetically determined increase in Hb F in adult life, a nomenclature that was introduced before the nature of these varied disorders was understood. As mentioned earlier, there are three major types of lesion that come under this definition, each with distinctive phenotype: (1) deletions similar to those observed in $(\delta\beta)^0$ and $(^A\gamma\delta\beta)^0$ thalassemia,which remove the δ and β genes and differ from δβ thalassemia only in that the resulting level of Hb F is sufficient to make the condition asymptomatic; (2) nondeletion forms, in which fairly high levels of Hb F in heterozygotes (5 to 15 percent) are associated with continued, but reduced, β-chain output from the same chromosome; and (3) a group of conditions, probably heterogeneous, in which much lower levels of Hb F (2 to 5 percent) are found in otherwise normal families. There is evidence that in some of these cases the genetic determinant may not be linked to the β-globin gene cluster.

$(\delta\beta)^0$ Hereditary Persistence of Fetal Hemoglobin. This condition is usually found in individuals of African origin, although cases have been described from India and Southeast Asia. Homozygotes have 100 percent Hb F containing a mixture of both $^G\gamma$ and $^A\gamma$ chains, but they are asymptomatic. Their red cells are microcytic and hypochromic, and globin chain imbalance can be demonstrated (α/γ, ~2.0) but they maintain Hb levels above 15 g/dl, compensating for the increased oxygen affinity associated with having only Hb F. Heterozygotes have normal hematology and 20 to 35 percent Hb F, which has a pancellular but uneven distribution. Three different deletions of the globin gene complex have been found in Africans, affecting the phenotype only in the proportion of $^G\gamma$ chains, (30 percent or 70 percent). A fourth similar deletion underlies the Indian form, giving ~50 percent $^G\gamma$. While the phenotype of the Indian heterozygotes is similar to their African counterparts, the two conditions produce different effects on interaction with β thalassemia. The African compound heterozygotes are similar to β-thalassemia heterozygotes, while Indians with this combination have thalassemia intermedia, similar to that seen in a $(\delta\beta)^0/\beta^0$ thalassemia combination. This underlines the overlap in the clinical and hematologic effects of $(\delta\beta)^0$ thalassemia and $(\delta\beta)^0$ HPFH (see Table 113-14).

HB KENYA. Misaligned crossing over between the $^A\gamma$ and β genes results in a fusion $^A\gamma\beta$ gene which produces the non–α chain of Hb KENYA.[132] This condition has not been observed in the homozygous state, but heterozygotes and compound heterozygotes with Hb S have been found in East Africa.

In the few families studies, the level of Hb KENYA in heterozygotes appears to fall into two groups, comprising 7 to 12 and 20 to 23 percent of the total[358–360]; it is not clear whether this reflects further genetic heterogeneity. This condition is also accompanied by persistent Hb F, with levels of 5 to 10 percent containing only $^G\gamma$ chains. Red-cell morphology is normal, and globin synthesis is balanced.

Table 113-14 Characteristics of the Deletion Forms of δβ Thalassemia and HPFH

	Heterozygotes			Homozygotes		
Condition	**MCH, pg**	**% Hb F**	**% $^G\gamma$**	**% Hb F**	**% $^G\gamma$**	**Clinical Status**
Hb_{LEPORE}	22±2	1–3	20–45	70–90	48–62	Intermedia/major
$(\delta\beta)^0$ Thalassemia	23±2	5–18	25–56	100	47–64	Intermedia
$(^A\gamma\delta\beta)^0$ Thalassemia	24±2	9–18	96–100	100	100	Intermedia
$\delta\beta)^0$ HPFH	27±3	17–35	25–75	100	52–65*	Normal
Hb_{KENYA}	26±3	4–9	100	—	—	—

*African type I 51±4%, type II 32±5%; Indian type 69±4%

SOURCE: From Weatherall and Clegg.[2] Used by permission.

Nondeletion Types of Hereditary Persistence of Fetal Hemoglobin. Compound heterozygotes for HPFH and β-globin chain variants do not usually produce any Hb A, but several conditions have been found in which this is not the case. Family studies have made it clear that these genetic defects are tightly linked to the β-globin locus and that there is β-chain production from the chromosome responsible for the increased γ-chain output. Several types have been described (see Table 113-11); sequencing of the overproduced γ gene has demonstrated various single base substitutions within the promoter region in each of these types (see "Molecular Pathology. Nondeletion Hereditary Persistence of Fetal Hemoglobin" above).

Compound heterozygotes for $^{G}\gamma\beta^{+}$ *HPFH*[361–363] and Hb S or Hb C produce 45 percent of the abnormal hemoglobin, 30 percent Hb A and 20 percent Hb F containing only $^{G}\gamma$ chains. Similar Hb F levels are seen in simple heterozygotes. Globin synthesis is balanced and so the combined output of $^{G}\gamma$ and β^{A} chains from the affected chromosome is equal to the normal β-chain output. This rare condition, which has been found mainly in persons of African origin, is not associated with any hematologic abnormalities.

The most common of the nondeletion types of HPFH, a form of $^{A}\gamma\beta^{+}$ *HPFH*,[364–366] is found most commonly in Greeks. Heterozygotes are hematologically normal, but have 10 to 20 percent Hb F, almost all of the $^{A}\gamma$ type. Homozygotes have about 25 percent Hb F and 0.8 percent Hb A_2.[366] Compound heterozygotes with β thalassemia have a hematologic phenotype slightly more severe than β-thalassemia trait, and the presence of Hb A in compound heterozygotes with β^0 thalassemia confirms that the β gene in *cis* to the HPFH defect is active. Conditions with a similar phenotype have also been described in several other racial groups (see Bollekens and Forget[324]).

In a British family with $^{A}\gamma\beta^{+}$ HPFH it has been possible to study the behavior of the γ genes at birth and during the transition from fetal to adult hemoglobin production.[340,367] Heterozygotes have 3.5 to 10 percent Hb F, consisting mostly of $^{A}\gamma$ chains, and homozygotes, who are hematologically normal, show balanced globin chain synthesis, low normal levels of Hb A_2, and Hb F levels of ~20 percent. The offspring of these homozygotes, obligate heterozygotes, have normal levels of Hb F and normal $^{G}\gamma$:$^{A}\gamma$ ratios at birth, suggesting that the $^{A}\gamma$ gene functions normally during fetal life.[368] After birth, however, there is a markedly delayed decline in Hb F ($^{A}\gamma$) production accompanied by a rapid decline in $^{G}\gamma$-chain production.

Nondeletion Hereditary Persistence of Fetal Hemoglobin with Low Levels of Hb F. The majority of normal adults have less than 1 percent Hb F. However, it has been recognized for many years that slightly elevated levels of Hb F (1 to 3 percent) can be traced through families and hence have a genetic component.[369] Later studies have confirmed this,[370] although neither the pattern of inheritance nor the amount of genetic heterogeneity which might underlie the condition has been elucidated. It has been suggested, for example, that an X-linked determinant may be involved in setting the level of Hb F at these low levels.[371] The importance of this condition (or these conditions) is that its coinheritance with the more severe forms of β thalassemia can lead to a considerable amelioration in clinical severity through the increased ability to produce Hb F.[372,373]

It is clear from family studies of some cases of β thalassemia or Hb S with unusually high Hb F levels that the high level is genetically determined and that the determinant is not linked to the β-globin locus.[373] Other families, however, have been reported in which the high Hb F determinant does appear to be linked to the cluster (reviewed by Bollekens and Forget[324]). In most of these cases, only the nuclear family has been studied, and the small numbers of individuals give limited opportunities for assortment. Given the possibility of genetic heterogeneity of this condition, combining results from several families for genetic analysis may be misleading, and it is not clear to what degree ascertainment bias may have contributed to the published reports.

One further difficulty in genetic studies of such families is whether the determinant shows complete penetrance. In the largest family of this type studied to date,[373] there appeared to be clear-cut examples of impenetrance; this may well be why the genetics of this disorder have not been clarified in Mendelian terms, even within single families. This may be related to the observation that the high Hb F determinant may be expressed to a much greater degree under conditions of erythroid stress. Thus, families in which β-thalassemia heterozygotes coinherit a high Hb F determinant and produce ~5 percent Hb F may contain β-thalassemia homozygotes whose level of Hb F production (10 to 12 g/dl) is sufficient to produce a very mild or asymptomatic condition.

Summary of Genetic Factors Associated with Increased Hemoglobin F Production in β-Chain Globin Disorders. Despite the fact that it has been evident for a long time that genetic factors play a major role in determining the level of Hb F production in sickle cell anemia and β thalassemia, knowledge about their nature remains incomplete. However, from information that is available it appears that they fall into three major groups (reviewed by Weatherall[211]). First, there is growing evidence that the mutations that involve the β-globin genes in some forms of thalassemia may themselves have some effect on the output of Hb F. Second, it appears that certain polymorphisms involving the εγδβ-globin gene cluster may be associated with increased Hb F production in response to defective β-chain production. Finally, as mentioned above, there are genetic determinants unlinked to the cluster which seem to modify the level of Hb F production in adult life, both in normal individuals and in those with β thalassemia or sickle cell anemia. These different mechanisms for modifying Hb F production in the β-globin disorders are summarized in Fig. 113-29.

There is some evidence that individuals who are homozygotes or compound heterozygotes for promoter mutations of the β-globin gene may have a relatively high output of Hb F.[211] It is possible, therefore, that in conditions of relative hemopoietic stress in which γ-chain synthesis is more likely

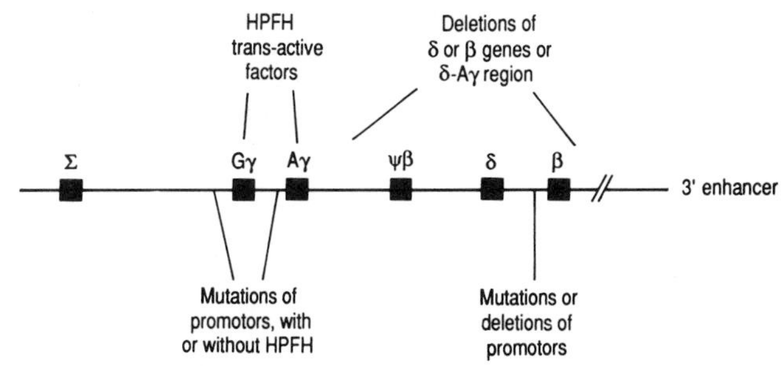

FIG. 113-29 Summary of some of the genetic mechanisms which modify the level of Hb F production in β thalassemia.

to occur, the level of γ-chain production may be modified by competition for transcriptional regulatory sequences between the γ- and β-chain loci; mutations in or near these transcriptional boxes that cause β thalassemia may favor γ-chain production.

Another approach to determining whether *cis*-acting sequences can modify γ-chain production is to determine whether there are any particular β-globin RFLP haplotypes associated with β thalassemia or sickle cell anemia and unusually high levels of Hb F. There has been particular interest in the relationship between Hb F production and a C-to-T polymorphism at position −158 in the $^{G}\gamma$-globin gene.[374] This substitution can be identified with a restriction enzyme *Xmn*I which makes it possible to analyze large populations for its presence or absence. Studies in Asia, the Mediterranean, and the Middle East have shown that this polymorphism is associated predominantly with one β-globin RFLP haplotype.[375–378] Extensive analyses of β thalassemia patients and those of African, Asian, Mediterranean, and Turkish backgrounds who have sickle cell anemia have shown a strong though not absolute correlation between increased γ-chain production and the presence of *Xmn*I polymorphisms.[379–382] It is not clear whether this change at position −158 is responsible for increased γ-chain production in these cases. The whole relationship between this polymorphism and increased γ-chain production remains to be clarified.

Some studies have suggested that other polymorphisms, including those which involve the β-globin LCR may be involved in increased γ-chain production in sickle cell anemia.[383]

Finally, as mentioned earlier, there is clear evidence that the inheritance of some forms of HPFH, the determinants of which are not linked to the β-globin gene cluster, may cause an increased output of Hb F in patients with sickle cell anemia or β thalassemia.

In summary, Hb F response to the β-globin disorders probably reflects a complex series of genetic variables including the nature of the individual globin gene mutations, polymorphisms of the γ-globin gene *cis* to the affected β-globin gene, and the interaction of other genes unlinked to the β-globin gene cluster, all set against a background of variable intramedullary or extramedullary selection of red-cell precursors or red cells with an increased amount of γ chains.

Interaction of β Thalassemia with α-Gene Mutations. The geographical distribution of α and β thalassemias is largely coincident, and relatively high frequencies of both occur in many populations. At least among Mediterraneans, the clinical and hematologic consequences of their coinheritance have been established and the findings are likely to be applicable to other groups (Table 113-15).

Homozygous β Thalassemia and α Thalassemia. In early studies it was established that β-thalassemia homozygotes who also inherited an α-thalassemia allele sometimes had a milder clinical course.[2] Since much of the pathology of β thalassemia is due to the pool of excess α chains, this observation can be readily explained, since the effect of α thalassemia is to reduce α-chain synthesis and hence the degree of excess α chains. However, until gene mapping allowed the ready detection of α thalassemia, it was not clear to what extent α thalassemia played a part in producing the milder forms of the disease.

Extensive data collected from the populations of the Mediterranean and Southeast Asia indicate that the coexistence of α thalassemia may modify the phenotype of homozygotes or compound heterozygotes for different β-thalassemia mutations.[211] The resulting phenotypes are complex and depend on the number of α-globin genes which are inactivated, together with whether the β thalassemia is of the β^0 or β^+ variety.[216,217,384,385] For example, it is clear that the coexistence of the heterozygous state for α^+ thalassemia with homozygous β^0 thalassemia has very little effect on the phenotype of the latter. On the other hand, individuals that are either α^+-thalassemia homozygotes or α^0-thalassemia heterozygotes and who also are homozygous for β^+ thalassemia may have a mild form of β thalassemia intermedia. The same applies even to patients who have the genotype of Hb H disease together with homozygous β^+ thalassemia. These remarkable experiments of nature are the best evidence that we have that the most important factor in determining the phenotype of β thalassemia is the degree of imbalanced globin chain synthesis.

Heterozygous β Thalassemia and α Thalassemia. Studies of β-thalassemia heterozygotes who also have α thalassemia (as determined by gene mapping) have a reduced amount of chain imbalance and fewer hematologic abnormalities.[386,387] Hemoglobin levels, MCV, and MCH all increase across the series −α/αα and −α/−α but decrease again in those with −α/−− (see Table 113-15). These results point to a potential problem in screening for β thalassemia on electronic counters by the reduced MCV, since in β-thalassemia heterozygotes with an −α/−α genotype there is considerable overlap with normal values. However, screening by Hb A_2 levels should not be affected, since the levels remain raised in all these groups. We shall return to this question later when considering population screening.

Table 113-15 Hematologic Findings in Heterozygous β Thalassemia with Normal or Abnormal α-Gene Rearrangements

Condition	n	Hb, g/dl	MCV, fl	MCH, pg	Hb A_2, %	Hb F, %	α:β ratio
αα/αα	53	12.5±1.2	65±4	21±1	4.9±0.7	1.3±1.1	2.2±0.3
αα/−α	36	13.0±1.4	67±4	22±1	5.2±0.7	1.2±0.3	1.4±0.1
−α/−α	11	13.9±1.1	77±3	25±1	5.1±0.6	1.1±0.7	0.8±0.1
−α/−−	6	11.8±0.8	55±3	18±1	4.6±0.2	−	0.5±0.1
αα/ααα*	7	11.7±1.9	65±5	21±2	5.0±0.9	2.3±1.5	2.1±0.4
	11	9.1±0.9	70±8	21±2	4.9±0.6	4.3±2.1	2.9±0.6
ααα/ααα	3	9.3±0.9	65±3	21±1	4.6±0.3	6.8±2.9	4.0±0.4

*Seven cases presenting with phenotype of thalassemia trait, 11 presenting as thalassemia intermedia.

***Homozygous* β *Thalassemia and* ααα.** Given the frequency of the ααα genotype in many populations, it will undoubtedly occur in β-thalassemia homozygotes, and individuals with this interaction and the picture of thalassemia major have been reported. Unexpectedly, four homozygotes with this genotype have been described with the milder pattern of thalassemia intermedia. It is probable that in at least some of these cases, there are nondeletion α-thalassemia mutations affecting genes within the triplicated α-gene arrangement.[388]

***Heterozygous* β *Thalassemia and* ααα.** The clinical and hematologic picture of double heterozygotes for β thalassemia and the triplicated α-gene arrangement (see Table 113-15) may be indistinguishable from simple heterozygotes for β thalassemia in some cases,[338] while others present with thalassemia intermedia.[389,390] The reason for this difference remains unexplained; it does not seem to be due to the nature of the β-thalassemia allele, and in several of the asymptomatic patients all three α genes on the triple α chromosome appeared to be active. Both phenotypes may coexist within the same family.[391]

β-Thalassemia heterozygotes who are homozygous for the ααα arrangement usually have the clinical phenotype of thalassemia intermedia.[392,393]

Interaction of β Thalassemia with Structural Variants.[2,3] The association of β thalassemia with Hbs S, C, and E is described in the section on "Structural Hemoglobin Variants."

Although β thalassemia has been reported in association with several other hemoglobin variants, few result in any clinical disability. Hb D/β thalassemia is not uncommon in parts of India but, apart from a mild anemia which may be exacerbated in pregnancy, it is largely asymptomatic.

Hb O Arab/β^0 thalassemia causes a moderately severe disorder with a hemoglobin level of 6 to 8 g/dl and splenomegaly. Several cases with this combination have been reported from Bulgaria. It is not clear why this interaction is so severe, but homozygotes for Hb O Arab are also anemic.

WORLD DISTRIBUTION AND POPULATION GENETICS

Although our knowledge of the prevalence and distribution of the hemoglobin disorders is still scanty, enough information has been obtained to suggest that they are the commonest single gene disorders. Very conservative data compiled by the World Health Organization indicate that about 5 percent of the world population are carriers for important hemoglobin disorders.[1] Since these data were compiled before anything was known about the distribution of α thalassemia, as assessed by more recently developed gene mapping techniques, it is clear that these figures represent a considerable underestimate of the total problem.

Structural Hemoglobin Variants

The only structural hemoglobin variants to reach polymorphic frequencies are Hbs S, C,and E. The sickle cell gene is most concentrated in west Africa, although its distribution spreads across central Africa, and it is found at lower frequencies in some non-African Mediterranean populations.[3,164] It also occurs patchily throughout the Middle East and central India but, apart from some Indian populations in north Malaya, it has not been observed in Southeast Asia. Hemoglobin C is restricted to parts of West Africa,[3] while Hb E is distributed in a region stretching from the eastern parts of India through Burma to Southeast Asia, where it reaches its highest frequency in parts of Thailand, Laos, and Cambodia. Hemoglobin E is found sporadically in parts of Southern China, and it extends in a line stretching south through Thailand and down the Malay peninsula and into some of the island populations of Indonesia.[3]

The approximate gene frequencies for the structural hemoglobin variants, where known, have been catalogued by several workers.[3,394] In parts of west central Africa, Nigeria, Ghana, Gabon, and Zaire, for example, the gene frequency for Hb S can exceed 0.15; in other words, heterozygotes comprise over 25 percent of the newborn population. Similar frequencies are found in parts of eastern Saudi Arabia, and the condition is almost as common in parts of central India. Hemoglobin C is found exclusively in African populations and reaches its highest frequency in Ghana and Upper Volta, with gene frequencies approaching 0.15. The gene frequency for Hb E in Thailand and Burma is 0.05 to 0.10, although higher values have been recorded in parts of Eastern Thailand near the Vietnamese border—the so-called Hb E triangle. At a minimum estimate there are about 30 million heterozygotes for Hb E and about 1 million homozygotes in Southeast Asia. For more extensive population data, broken down into different racial groups, refer to the catalog of Livingstone.[394]

These remarkably high gene frequencies pose two important questions. How did these variants become distributed among the high-incidence populations, and what are the factors that have maintained these polymorphisms?

Population Distribution. Before it was possible to analyze human DNA directly, a great deal was written about the distribution of the sickle cell gene and other hemoglobin variants under the assumption that population movements could be derived from the distribution of genetic markers of this type. It was believed, reasonably, that the distribution of the β^S gene in the New World is based entirely on emigration from West Africa during the transportation of slaves. But it was also thought that the high prevalence of the sickle cell gene in Saudi Arabia and India may have reflected migration out of East Africa (the transport of slaves from east Africa to the Persian Gulf flourished from 200 to 1500 AD).

More recently, however, it has been possible to analyze the origins of the sickle cell gene and other structural hemoglobin variants by examining the pattern of RFLPs in and around the β-globin gene carrying the sickle mutation. The first study of this type employed a single polymorphism identified by the enzyme *Hpa*I.[395] Nearly all Caucasians and about 97 percent of individuals of African origin with a normal hemoglobin phenotype have a 7.6-kb or, less commonly, a 7.0-kb *Hpa*I fragment that encompasses the entire β-globin gene. Only 3 percent have a 13-kb fragment. In contrast, among American blacks who have Hb S, nearly 70 percent have the 13-kb fragment. Similarly, nearly all blacks with Hb C have the 13-kb fragment. How can this type of linkage disequilibrium be explained? It seems likely that the β^S and β^C mutations both arose on a β gene carrying the 13-kb mutation that may have arisen in a relatively small geographical area corresponding to what is now called Upper Volta and Ghana. Presumably because the β^S and β^C genes offered protection against malaria (see below) their frequency increased, and the linked 13-kb mutation "hitchhiked" along with them. On the other hand, the prevalence of the ancestral 13-kb β^A gene remained low because it lacked a selective advantage. The β^S/13-kb fragment association has also been found in North Africans and Sicilians, although not in individuals from East Africa, Saudi Arabia, or India. These observations suggested an independent origin of the sickle cell gene in West and East Africa.[344]

More recently, extensive RFLP analyses using a variety of single point polymorphisms in the β-globin gene cluster have been carried out in many populations in an attempt to obtain further information about the origins of both the sickle cell and Hb E mutations.[154,396–399] The particular arrangement of RFLPs is referred to as the β-globin gene haplotype. Studies both in Jamaica and West Africa indicate that the β^S mutation can be found in association with a wide variety of haplotypes—SS BENIN, SS BANTU, SS SENEGAL, and SS ARAB INDIA, for example. At first these results suggest that the mutation may have had multiple origins. However, these data must be interpreted with caution because it is possible that a number of gene conversion events could have given rise to at least some of the variability in β^S/haplotype associations. However, the occurrence of a common haplotype associated with a β^S gene in parts of eastern Saudi Arabia and Orissa in central India, and the finding of completely different haplotypes in some African populations, make it more likely that the β^S mutation had at least two origins, one in east Africa and the other in the Middle East or India[399] (see Fig. 113-25).

Similar haplotype data suggests that the β^E mutation may have occurred on more than one occasion.[400] The same reservations apply as in the case of Hb S; gene conversion events might also account for these different haplotype associations.

Maintenance of the Polymorphisms for Structural Hemoglobin Variants. In 1949 J. B. S. Haldane suggested that individuals with red-cell disorders such as thalassemia might be protected against malaria.[401] Early epidemiological studies in Africa suggested that Hb S heterozygotes are protected against *Plasmodium falciparum* malaria.[402] More recent work in Nigeria and The Gambia confirms these studies.[403,403a] For example, the prevalence of the sickle cell trait in Nigerian newborns was 24 percent, as compared with 29 percent over the age of 5 years. Above this age no differences were noted. These data suggest that the Hb S trait confers a relative fitness of about 0.20 as compared with normal individuals in the same population. This figure gives a calculated gene frequency of about 0.15, a value very close to that observed in Nigeria. Furthermore, it can be calculated that it would take about 50 generations (representing 1000 years) to reach the present equilibrium, assuming that the homozygous condition is 100 percent lethal.

If protection against *P. falciparum* malaria is the major mechanism for maintaining the Hb S polymorphism, how is this effect mediated? This problem has been approached by studying the rates of sickling of parasitized and nonparasitized cells under reduced oxygen tension and by examining the patterns of invasion and growth of parasites in red cells containing Hb S using in vitro culture systems. At least three possible protective mechanisms have been demonstrated. First, it has been found that under low oxygen tensions AS cells containing *P. falciparum* sickle more readily than nonparasitized cells. It has been suggested, therefore, that in vivo sickling may provide a mechanism for the rapid clearance of parasitized cells and their subsequent destruction in the RE system. It would follow that the parasite could not complete its life cycle.[404] In vitro culture studies have shown that, under ambient oxygen tensions, parasites invade and grow in sickle cells at the same rate as in normal cells. However, under reduced oxygen conditions, both invasion and growth are inhibited.[405] It has been suggested that this effect may be mediated by the relatively low levels of potassium in AS cells that have undergone sickling.[406]

It is possible that several mechanisms are involved; the major reason the entrapment of sickle cells has been favored is the observation that individuals who are homozygous for the sickle cell gene undergo severe malarial infection, an observation that would be hard to explain if parasites could not survive adequately in cells containing a large concentration of Hb S. On the other hand, even a mild malaria infection might have catastrophic consequences for a child with sickle cell anemia.

In vivo studies of invasion and growth of *P. falciparum* in the cells of Hb E heterozygotes or homozygotes have not provided a clear answer as to why Hb E might be protective against malaria. However, since the Hb E mutation produces a thalassemia phenotype, we shall return to this problem in a later section.

The Thalassemias

The world distribution of the α and β thalassemias is summarized in Figs. 113-30 and 113-31; a more detailed breakdown of published data for the gene frequencies of different forms of thalassemia can be found in several monographs and reviews.[208–210,394]

Adequate gene frequency data for β thalassemia are available for only a small number of populations. It is clear that, with a few exceptions such as Liberia, the condition occurs at only a low frequency throughout tropical Africa, although higher frequencies have been observed in North Africa. The disease is common throughout the Mediterranean region, parts of the Middle East, and India and Burma, although accurate gene frequency data are sparse. It is also common throughout Southeast Asia in a line starting in southern China, stretching through Thailand, Cambodia, and Laos, and down the Malay peninsula into some of the island populations. It is distributed sporadically in Melanesia.

The world distribution of the α thalassemias is summarized in Fig. 113-30. The α^+ thalassemias are extremely common in parts of Africa, the Mediterranean region, the Middle

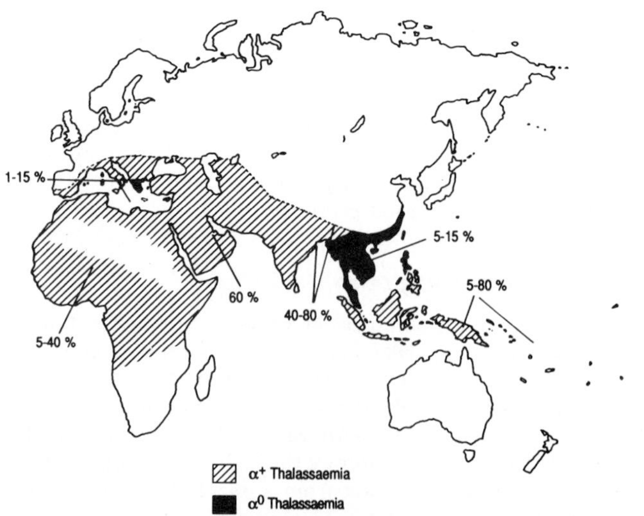

FIG. 113-30 World distribution of α thalassemia.

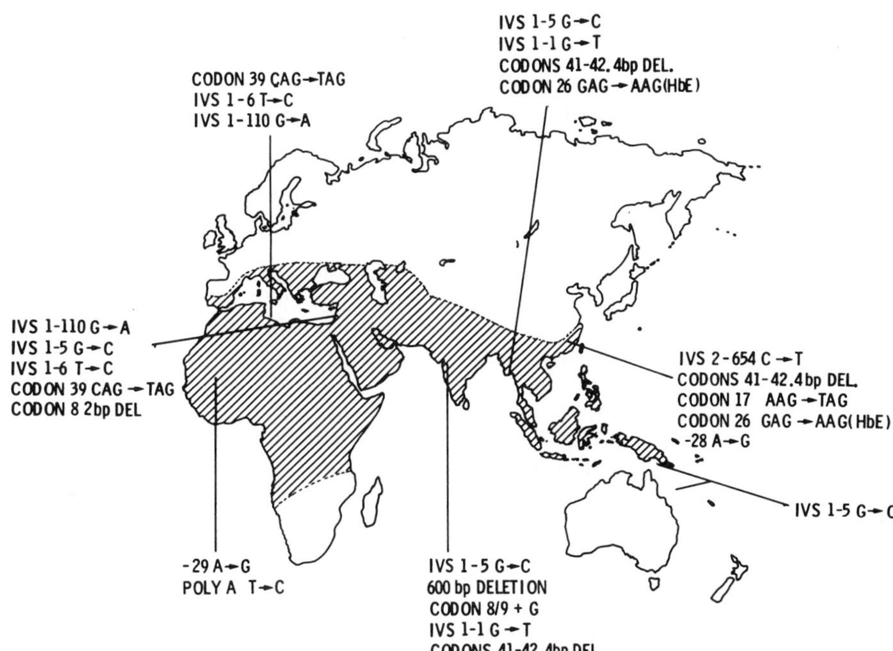

FIG. 113-31 World distribution of β thalassemia.

East, and throughout Southeast Asia and the Pacific island populations. Indeed, α^+ thalassemia appears to be reaching fixation in some regions, notably the coastal regions of Papua New Guinea. On the other hand, α^0 thalassemia is restricted to the Mediterranean region and Southeast Asia.

Population Distribution. As was the case for the sickle cell gene, before the advent of DNA technology and the realization of the remarkable heterogeneity of β thalassemia, much was written about the movement of populations based on the distribution of the β-thalassemia mutations. However, more recent work, in which the precise molecular lesions have been defined and β-globin gene RFLP haplotypes determined, has provided a much clearer picture about the population distribution of the β thalassemias.[73,209,210,407,408]

It is now apparent that in each of the high-frequency areas there are a few common mutations together with varying numbers of rare ones (see Fig. 113-27). Furthermore, in each of these regions the pattern of mutations is different. And even where the same mutation occurs in different populations, it is usually found together with a different β-globin gene RFLP haplotype. It seems likely, therefore, that the β-thalassemia mutations have arisen independently in different populations and then achieved their high frequency by selection. Although there may have been some movement of the β-thalassemia genes between populations, by drift and so on, there is little doubt that the independent mutation and selection provide the overall basis for the world distribution of β thalassemia.

Molecular studies of the α thalassemias lead to similar conclusions.[64,65,208] The deletions that cause α^0 thalassemia in the Mediterranean and Southeast Asia are different.[409] Furthermore, detailed analysis of the RFLP haplotypes in the α-globin gene cluster, together with studies of the crossover events that produce the α^+ thalassemias, have shown that the common form of α^+ thalassemia due to a 3.7-kb deletion ($-\alpha^{3.7I}$), has occurred on many different occasions in different populations.[65] $-\alpha^{3.7III}$ is, on the other hand, confined to parts of Melanesia and Polynesia. Haplotype analysis suggests that the α^+ thalassemias arose *de novo* in Melanesia and reached their high frequencies by selection[65]; haplotypes of the α^+ thalassemias in Southeast Asia are completely different. These studies suggest that, even allowing for a certain amount of drift and founder effect, the different types of α^+ thalassemia have arisen independently in different populations.

Maintenance of the Thalassemia Polymorphism. Haldane's suggestion that thalassemia has been maintained at a high frequency by the protection of heterozygotes against *P. falciparum* malaria was an extremely attractive hypothesis, but it has been very difficult to provide the experimental data with which to validate it.

Studies in Sardinia, which showed that β thalassemia is less common in the mountainous regions where malaria transmission is relatively low, suggested that β thalassemia might have reached its high frequency because of protection against malarial infection.[410] For many years these data remained the only convincing evidence for the protective effect of thalassemia against malaria. However, studies utilizing malaria endemicity data and globin gene mapping have shown a very clear altitude-related effect on the frequency of α thalassemia in Papua New Guinea.[65] Furthermore, a sharp decline in the frequency of α thalassemia has been found in a region stretching north from Papua New Guinea, through the island populations of Melanesia to New Caledonia. A similar gradient in the distribution of malaria has been demonstrated from data on parasites and spleen sizes collected in this region over many years. This relationship might, of course, have resulted from gene drift and founder effect in these island populations. In other words, a population with a high frequency of α thalassemia might have moved through the islands from the north and the gene frequency might have been diluted during the migration southward. This explanation is unlikely, however, because there is a random pattern of the distribution of other DNA polymorphisms throughout these island populations.[65] Thus, the frequency of α^+ thalassemia, but not other DNA polymorphisms, shows an altitude- and latitude-dependent correlation with malarial endemicity throughout Melanesia.

These findings suggest that the α^+ thalassemia determinants found throughout this malaria cline originated in

Melanesia and were amplified to a high frequency by a locally operated selective mechanism rather than being imported by population migrations from outside the region—from Southeast Asia, for example. In a series of control studies, α-thalassemia gene frequencies have been analyzed in areas where malaria has never been recorded.[52,411] These include Iceland and Japan and many of the island archipelagoes of Micronesia and Polynesia as Oceanic controls. There is virtually no α thalassemia in either Iceland or Japan but, surprisingly, gene frequencies as high as 12 percent are seen in parts of Polynesia. However, population studies suggest that the variant has been carried into the eastern Pacific from Melanesia during the migrations of proto-Polynesian colonizers.[411]

The remarkable diversity of the different thalassemia mutations and their widespread distribution, taken together with population data that indicate that heterozygotes are protected against *P. falciparum* malaria, suggests that there may be properties common to the cells of carriers for different forms of thalassemia that make them less attractive to the malarial parasite. Several in vitro studies have shown no major differences between the rates of invasion and growth of *P. falciparum* in α- or β-thalassemic red cells as compared with normal cells.[412] However, it has been found that infected thalassemic cells bind significantly more antibody from the sera of patients with acute *P. falciparum* malaria than do normal red cells.[413] It is not yet clear whether this reflects more efficient exposure of malarial antigens by the thalassemic cells or whether these cells expose red-cell neoantigens related to senescence more effectively than normal cells when invaded by the parasite; changes of this kind have been well documented in parasitized red cells. These observations raise completely new avenues of investigation for the protective effect of thalassemia against *P. falciparum* malaria and suggest that it could be immune-mediated rather than due to the particular properties of the small thalassemic red cell.

DIAGNOSIS, PREVENTION, AND TREATMENT

The practical aspects of the diagnosis, prevention, and management of the hemoglobinopathies are the subject of a number of monographs and reviews,[2,3,207,414–417] and they will only be outlined here.

Diagnosis

The diagnosis of a hemoglobin disorder involves the characterization of the homozygous or compound heterozygous state for a structural hemoglobin variant or one form or other of thalassemia in a patient with an appropriate clinical picture, or the identification of a heterozygote as part of a family study or population screening program. In the routine clinical laboratory, a few relatively simple investigations will suffice in the majority of cases. These include the preparation of a well-stained blood film, analysis of the hemoglobin level and hematocrit together with a determination of the red-cell indices with an electronic cell counter, hemoglobin electrophoresis, estimation of the Hb F level by alkali denaturation, and a quantitative assessment of the Hb A_2 level. To this may be added a heat stability or isopropanol test for unstable hemoglobin. Figure 113-32 shows a flow chart of the order in which these investigations should be carried out to obtain maximum information. In addition, it may be necessary to carry out confirmatory investigations for the sickling disorders such as the metabisulfite or solubility tests and, in cases of suspected high- or low-affinity hemoglobin variants, to determine the p50.

This simple battery of investigations will allow the identification of the important sickling disorders, hemoglobins C and E, the high-oxygen-affinity variants, and the unstable hemoglobins. For unequivocal structural identification it is necessary to "fingerprint" and determine the amino acid substitution, but this is rarely required in clinical practice.

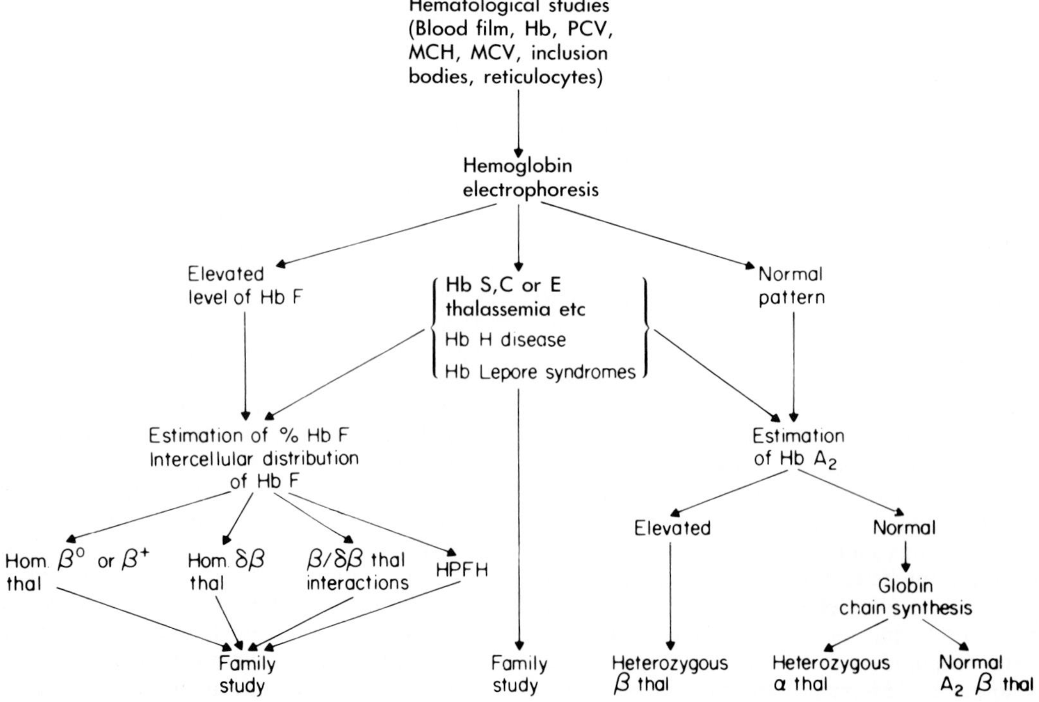

FIG. 113-32 Flow chart showing the approach to the laboratory diagnosis of the hemoglobin disorders. *(From Weatherall and Clegg.[2] Used by permission.)*

The diagnosis of the common sickling disorders is usually straightforward. In sickle cell anemia the Hb A_2 level is normal, and both parents show the sickle cell trait. The other common sickling disorders, such as SC, SD, and S/O ARAB diseases, can be identified provisionally by agar gel electrophoresis or isoelectric focusing. Sickle cell β^0 thalassemia is diagnosed by finding the β thalassemia trait in one parent and a raised Hb A_2 in the patient. It is important to carry out family studies when a raised Hb A_2 is found in an individual who is apparently homozygous for the sickle cell gene, because the coexistence of α thalassemia and homozygous Hb S can also produce a raised Hb A_2 level; in this case, both parents have the sickle cell trait and hematologic evidence of coexistent α thalassemia.

It is usually easy to diagnose the homozygous or compound heterozygous states for the important forms of β and δβ thalassemia by measuring Hb F and Hb A_2 levels and carrying out a family study. The hemoglobin pattern of heterozygotes for these conditions is quite characteristic; β-thalassemia heterozygotes have typical thalassemic indices and a raised Hb A_2, while δβ-thalassemia heterozygotes have a normal Hb A_2 but Hb F levels in the 5 to 15 percent range. In homozygous β-thalassemia patients who have undergone transfusion before referral, it may be necessary to repeat the investigations after an interval or to carry out globin chain synthesis studies on the marrow or blood.

The diagnosis of Hb BART'S hydrops fetalis syndrome and Hb H disease usually presents no difficulties. It should be remembered that the level of Hb H varies considerably in Hb H disease and because Hb H is unstable, it is necessary to examine fresh red-cell lysates. It is also important to carry out hemoglobin electrophoresis on concentrated red-cell lysates, so as not to miss the form of Hb H disease associated with Hb CONSTANT SPRING or one of the other α-chain termination mutants.

The diagnosis of the α-thalassemia carrier states is more difficult. Heterozygous α^0 thalassemia is characterized by typical thalassemic red-cell indices with a normal Hb A_2; a small proportion of the cells may contain Hb H bodies. Heterozygous α^+ thalassemia is extremely difficult to identify, as the red-cell indices may be normal. The heterozygous state for α^0 thalassemia and the homozygous state for α^+ thalassemia produce identical red-cell changes, and the two conditions can be distinguished only in an individual patient by a family study or, better, by α-gene mapping.

Screening. Screening for the hemoglobin variants and thalassemias is required for the prenatal identification of the carrier states for important disorders such as Hb S, β thalassemia, and α^0 thalassemia. It may also be required for identification of the sickling disorders or thalassemia in newborn infants or as part of a population screening program.

Screening for the sickle cell trait in adults can be carried out by hemoglobin electrophoresis or one of the solubility tests for Hb S. Screening for thalassemia is best done by determining the red-cell indices and, if they suggest thalassemia, by carrying out a serum iron or ferritin estimation to exclude iron deficiency. Once thalassemia is suspected, an Hb A_2 estimation should be done. In most cases this will serve to distinguish β-thalassemia trait from α^0 -thalassemia trait. In populations in which β thalassemia with a normal Hb A_2 level is common it is necessary to carry out globin chain synthesis or gene mapping analysis to distinguish this condition from heterozygous α^0 thalassemia. There is one pitfall that may be encountered in populations in which α and β thalassemias are common. Individuals who are heterozygous for both α and β thalassemia may have relatively normal red-cell indices. Thus, in these populations it is wise to use an Hb A_2 estimation as the initial screening procedure because such doubly affected heterozygotes have an elevated Hb A_2.[364] Typical red-cell indices for the different heterozygous forms of thalassemia are summarized in Table 113-14.

Neonatal screening for the sickle cell gene is best carried out using agar gel electrophoresis. Screening for α thalassemia can be carried out by estimating Hb Bart's levels on cord blood, although this will miss many cases of heterozygous α^+ thalassemia. The diagnosis of β thalassemia can be made at birth but only by globin chain synthesis; when heterozygous or homozygous β thalassemia is suspected it is better to delay hemoglobin analysis until after the first 6 months of life, at which time the typical changes are usually well established.

Prevention

Programs for the prevention of the common hemoglobinopathies can be carried out either by population screening of young adults followed by marital advice, or by screening pregnant women and—in cases in which their partners are also carriers—offering prenatal diagnosis followed, when appropriate, by termination of pregnancy. In early studies that were adequately documented, the former approach was not successful,[418] but experience in Montreal suggests that community screening may have a valuable effect in reducing the frequency of β thalassemia.[418a]

Prenatal diagnosis can be carried out in either the second trimester of pregnancy by fetal blood sampling or examination of the DNA of amniotic fluid cells, or by chorionic villus sampling and DNA analysis in the first trimester.[419] Fetal blood sampling followed by globin chain synthesis analysis has been applied widely for the prenatal diagnosis of the hemoglobin disorders.[419] The method is extremely effective for the recognition of the sickling disorders and α and β thalassemias. It carries a 1 to 2 percent risk of fetal loss, and there is about a 1 percent error rate. It has been used widely throughout the Mediterranean region, the Middle East, Britain, and North America. The application of this method has reduced the incidence of homozygous β thalassemia considerably in a number of Mediterranean populations.[420–422]

More recently, fetal DNA analysis following chorionic villus sampling has been developed and is now being widely used for the prenatal diagnosis of all the important hemoglobin disorders.[420,423] It is currently estimated that the fetal loss following this procedure is approximately 2 percent.[419] So far there are no good long-term data on infants who have been born following this procedure; therefore, its safety is still *sub judice*. It is possible to obtain 20 to 100 μg of fetal DNA from chorionic villus material, and if the procedure is carried out correctly, it is usually uncontaminated by maternal cells.

The diagnostic techniques used for fetal DNA analysis have evolved over the past 10 years. The first approach involved Southern blotting of fetal DNA using either RFLP linkage analysis[423,424] or, in cases in which the mutation was known, a restriction enzyme which identifies the base change, or an oligonucleotide probe.[425] The use of RFLP analysis for prenatal detection of genetic disease entails three steps. First, an appropriate RFLP marker is chosen which is either within or closely linked to the disease locus and for which an individual at risk of transmitting the disease is heterozygous.

Second, it is necessary to determine which of the marker alleles is on the chromosome carrying the disease allele; this involves a study of family members—ideally a previously affected or normal child. Finally, using the markers, fetal DNA is examined to see whether the fetus has inherited the chromosomes carrying the genes for the particular form of hemoglobin disorder or its normal allele. The disadvantage of this method is that it is necessary to establish, by a family study, that the appropriate markers are available. Although it has been largely superceded by more direct approaches for identifying thalassemia mutations in fetal DNA it is still a valuable fallback in families at risk for having children with rare forms of thalassemia. α^0 Thalassemia and a few forms of β^0 thalassemia that result from gene deletions can also be identified directly by Southern blotting. There are approximately 30 different β-thalassemic mutations that alter a particular restriction enzyme site and which can therefore be identified directly.[419] Sickle cell anemia and many structural hemoglobin variants can also be diagnosed using this approach.

More recently, following the development of the PCR, the identification of thalassemia mutations and those for structural hemoglobin variants in fetal DNA has been greatly facilitated. For example, PCR can be used for the rapid detection of mutations that alter restriction enzyme cutting sites.[426] The appropriate fragment of the β-globin gene is amplified approximately 30 cycles, after which the DNA fragments are digested with the particular enzyme and separated by electrophoresis. These fragments can be detected by either ethidium bromide or silver staining of DNA bands on gels; radioactive probes are not required.

Now that the mutations are known for so many different forms of α and β thalassemia, most prenatal diagnosis programs are based on the direct detection of these mutations as the first-line approach. The development of PCR, combined with the use of oligonucleotide probes to detect individual mutations, has offered a variety of new approaches for increasing the speed and accuracy of carrier detection and prenatal diagnosis.[427–429] For example, diagnoses can be made using hybridization of specific ^{32}P-end-labeled oligonucleotides to an amplified region of the β-globin gene dotted onto a nylon membrane. A number of variations on this theme have been developed. For example, mutations can be rapidly identified using a modification of PCR called the amplification refractory mutation system (ARMS).[430] This is based on the observation that, in many cases, oligonucleotides for the 3′ mismatched residue will, under appropriate conditions, not function as primers in the PCR. Two primers are prepared. The normal one is refractory to PCR on mutant template DNA; the mutant sequence is refractory to PCR on normal DNA. The difference between normal DNA and that carrying a particular mutation is identified by size differences of the amplified fragments (Fig. 113-33). Other modifications of PCR involve the use of nonradioactively labeled probes. For example, it is possible to use horseradish-peroxidase labeling of the 5′ end of oligonucleotides designed to detect individual mutations.

To develop a comprehensive prenatal diagnosis program for β thalassemia, the first step is to determine the common mutations in the population. Once this has been done, a large proportion of cases can be identified by one of these PCR methods. For those in which the mutation is not known, RFLP linkage analysis can be carried out. For the rare cases in which DNA analysis is unsuccessful, it is still possible to carry out second-trimester diagnosis by fetal blood sampling. Several large series of first-trimester prenatal diagnosis have

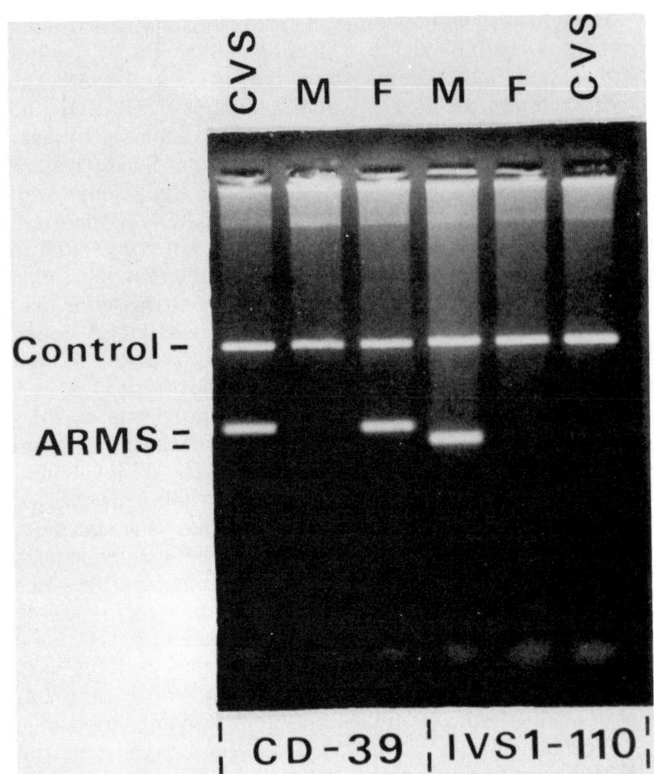

FIG. 113-33 **Rapid prenatal diagnosis of β thalassemia by ARMS, a development for the rapid identification of mutations based on the PCR. One parent has the common Mediterranean codon 39 (CD) mutation, the other the IVS1 110 to G→A mutation. The fetus is heterozygous for the codon 39 mutation. M = mother; F = father; CVS = fetal DNA from chorionic villus sampling.** ***(Kindly prepared by Dr. John Old.)***

now been published, and it is quite clear that the approach is feasible.[421–423] Potential difficulties include plasmid or maternal tissue contamination, crossovers, and nonpaternity. In these series the error rate is about the same as or lower than that for fetal blood sampling followed by globin chain synthesis.

Treatment

Apart from bone marrow transplantation there is no definitive treatment for any of the important hemoglobin disorders, but there has been considerable improvement in their symptomatic management.

The Sickling Disorders.[164,174,416] Individuals with the sickle cell trait require no treatment beyond simple genetic counseling and the avoidance of conditions of extreme oxygen deprivation or dehydration.

Because so many of the serious complications occur in the first 2 years of life, the diagnosis of sickle cell anemia should be made as early as possible. Once established, the parents should be counseled about the dangers of infection during the early years of life. Although there are only limited data there is a good case for the use of prophylactic penicillin in infants and young children. The use of polyvalent pneumococcal vaccines is still under evaluation. The parents and family physician should be advised to seek hospital advice at the onset of any unusual symptoms. Mothers can be counseled about splenic sequestration and taught to assess spleen size. No other treatment is required for sickle cell anemia in the steady state; folic acid supplements are often given but are probably unnecessary if the infant is receiving a good diet.

The management of sickle cell crises usually requires hospital admission and an extremely competent level of clinical care. The painful crisis is managed by bed rest, hydration, and adequate analgesia. Although it may be possible to manage mild painful crises with first-line analgesics such as paracetamol, more powerful agents are often required, at least for a few days; although there is a risk of addiction, patients cannot be left in excruciating pain. A source of infection should be sought, and the hematocrit and reticulocyte count should be monitored twice daily. There is no indication for blood transfusion unless the hematocrit is falling. Splenic or hepatic sequestration crises should be managed by prompt transfusion; if the spleen remains large there is a good case for splenectomy to prevent second episodes. Lung crises should be managed by treatment of any associated infection, adequate oxygenation and hydration, and, if the patient is deteriorating despite these measures, exchange transfusion. Neurological crises should be treated by hypertransfusion or, if the initial hematocrit is relatively high, by exchange transfusion. The management of priapism is difficult. If treated conservatively the condition usually fails to respond, and there may be permanent penile deformity. It has been suggested that the best approach is to use adequate hydration and analgesia for 24 h followed by an exchange transfusion or hypertransfusion for a further 24 h. If the condition does not resolve after these measures a cavernosal–spongiosal shunt should be considered.[164]

Hemoglobin SC disease should be managed in the same way as sickle cell anemia. There is increasing evidence that the retinal complications of this disorder may progress to blindness; therefore, all patients with this condition, and probably sickle cell anemia as well, should have regular ophthalmological surveillance and laser therapy when indicated.

The management of pregnancy in sickle cell anemia is still controversial. Although hypertransfusion regimens have been advocated in the United Kingdom there is no evidence that they are effective. The best compromise is to follow the patient very carefully and transfuse only if there are recurrent crises or a fall in the hematocrit during late pregnancy.

The observation[170] that aplastic crises in sickle cell anemia result from parvovirus infections has important implications. This condition should be suspected in any patient with sickle cell anemia with a falling hematocrit, particularly if the reticulocyte count is also reduced. It requires very careful hospital observation and early transfusion. The possibility of developing a vaccine may make it feasible to prevent this life-threatening complication.

Currently, no antisickling agent has been found to be useful in clinical practice.

Unstable Hemoglobin Variants. The majority of patients require no treatment. If there is severe hemolysis with a large spleen, splenectomy may be helpful. There are, however, insufficient data to evaluate the likely benefit fully.

Thalassemia. No treatment is required for α- or β-thalassemia heterozygotes, although they should be followed carefully during pregnancy because they may become anemic during the second or third trimester. They should receive appropriate genetic counseling.

The clinical management of homozygous β thalassemia is unsatisfactory. It has been the subject of an enormous amount of work,[3,415] and only a few principles can be outlined here. When the condition is suspected in early infancy the patient should be observed carefully to make sure that they are going to fall into the transfusion-dependent category. This usually becomes obvious by the end of the first year of life; the infant fails to thrive, feeding is difficult, and the hemoglobin level falls below 6 to 7 g/dl. It is important not to transfuse before this stage because a child with thalassemia intermedia may be wrongly categorized. Transfusion-dependent homozygous β-thalassemic patients require blood, chelating agents,and, in some cases, splenectomy.

Transfusion-dependent thalassemic children grow and develop best if their hemoglobin levels are maintained as close to normal as possible. This entails regular transfusions to maintain hemoglobin values between 10 and 14 g/dl. They should receive washed or frozen red cells uncontaminated by white cells and plasma proteins. When possible, a program of chelation with deferoxamine should be instituted. The precise age at which this can be started varies, but it should not be delayed much after the second year. The ideal route is subcutaneously into the abdominal wall using an overnight infusion with a clockwork or electric pump. The dose of deferoxamine varies according to age, and in any case it should be monitored by regular measurement of urinary iron excretion. The best response to deferoxamine is obtained in ascorbate-replete patients, although high doses of ascorbate should be avoided. Because of the rare ocular complications of deferoxamine therapy, children treated in this way should have regular ophthalmological surveillance. When it is not possible to use subcutaneous deferoxamine, bolus injections can be given, although they are much less effective. There is increasing evidence that children maintained on an adequate transfusion regimen and subcutaneous deferoxamine will grow and develop normally and that secondary sexual development at puberty may be normal.[415] So far, there are insufficient long-term follow-up data to be absolutely sure about the prognosis for these patients. There is some evidence that children who are already grossly iron-loaded, even if they have cardiac involvement, may be "rescued" at least temporarily by the use of deferoxamine given intravenously in an attempt to remove large amounts of iron.

Hypersplenism is unusual in children who have been adequate transfused. However, in those who have not been so fortunate, or in non-transfusion-dependent patients with β thalassemia intermedia, hypersplenism is common, and the spleen should be removed. The operation should be avoided in the first few years of life, and in any case should be followed up by the use of prophylactic penicillin for an indefinite period. Splenectomy is also indicated occasionally in patients with Hb H disease, although it should be done only if there is severe hypersplenism. There are several reports of migrating thrombophlebitis and more severe thromboembolic disease in splenectomized patients with Hb H disease[3]; the reason this occurs with this condition and not in β-thalassemic patients is not clear.

Good general pediatric care is essential for thalassemic children. If they are inadequately transfused they are prone to infection and to a variety of skeletal complications due to expansion of the bone marrow. When iron loading leads to delayed puberty patients should have a hormone profile carried out and, if indicated, careful replacement therapy instituted. Unfortunately, this is not always successful because sexual underdevelopment is often due to target-organ unresponsiveness due to iron deposition.

Marrow Transplantation. There has been increasing interest in the use of bone marrow transplantation, particularly for β thalassemia but also for selected cases of sickle cell anemia.[431,432] Encouraging results have been obtained, provided that the procedure is carried out early in life, although some experiences have suggested that it is possible to use transplantation in patients up to the age of 20 years or over. Unfortunately, however, successful engraftment requires the availability of a sib or relative with a complete HLA match. Therefore, this form of treatment is available to only a small proportion of children with thalassemia.

Experimental Procedures. Several therapeutic approaches to the hemoglobin disorders are being explored. There are some promising oral chelating agents which are presently under evaluation in clinical trials (reviewed by Piomelli and Lowe[415]). Their precise role and safety remain to be determined. Since it is clear that the production of high levels of fetal hemoglobin have the potential to protect patients with β thalassemia and sickle cell anemia there has been much interest in finding ways to stimulate Hb F production. The methods that are being explored are based on the old observation that there is a transient reversal to fetal hemoglobin synthesis during recovery from marrow suppression after the use of cytotoxic drugs for the treatment of leukemia, or after bone marrow transplantation.[2] It is assumed, therefore, that cytotoxic agents alter the pattern of erythropoiesis in such a way that it favors the expression of the γ-globin genes. Several agents have been used, including the demethylating agent 5-azacytidine, and hydroxyurea. The current status of these studies has been reviewed.[433] While there is no doubt that the use of cytotoxic agents or, under certain circumstances, erythropoietin, can produce a significant rise in the number of Hb F–containing reticulocytes and in the level of Hb F, it is still not certain whether this approach will be of value in the management of the hemoglobinopathies.

The other major area of research in the management of these disorders is somatic gene therapy. The present status of this work has been the subject of several reviews.[434–436] Currently, retroviruses seem to be the most promising vectors for gene transfer. The genes for viral proteins, which comprise nearly 80 percent of the retroviral genome, can be deleted and replaced by DNA sequences encoding the gene to be transferred. Specific packaging lines have been developed, and it has been possible to transfect bone marrow cells from mice, primates, and humans with a reasonable degree of efficiency. Problems are still being encountered in obtaining long-term expression of genes introduced into hemopoietic stem cells. Better results have been obtained by the use of constructs including the LCR, and in this way it has been possible to obtain high-level, tissue-specific expression of the globin genes. However, there are still many difficulties to be overcome. The pluripotent stem cell makes up only a small proportion of bone marrow cells. Furthermore, for successful transfection, these cells must be in cycle. Some improvements have resulted from the addition of hemopoietic growth factors during infection and a variety of approaches to select for transfected cells are being explored. Efforts have also been made to insert globin gene sequences into the human β-globin locus by site-directed homologous recombination. However, although there have been some successes, the major difficulty with this approach is its extremely low efficiency.

Thus, while there are still some formidable obstacles to be overcome in the cell biology of gene therapy, successes in defining the major regulatory loci for the α- and β-globin genes together with the gradual improvement in the efficiency of gene transfer systems suggests that, ultimately, it may be possible to correct some of the hemoglobin disorders in this way.

REFERENCES

1. WHO Working Group: Hereditary anaemias: Genetic basis, clinical features, diagnosis and treatment. *Bull World Health Organ* **60**:643, 1982.
2. Weatherall DJ, Clegg JB: *The Thalassaemia Syndromes*, 3rd ed. Oxford, Blackwell Scientific, 1981.
3. Bunn HF, Forget BG: *Hemoglobin: Molecular, Genetic and Clinical Aspects*. Philadelphia, Saunders, 1986.
4. Conley CL: Sickle-cell anemia—the first molecular disease, in Wintrobe MM (ed): *Blood, Pure and Eloquent*. New York, McGraw-Hill, 1980, p 319.
5. Weatherall DJ: Toward an understanding of the molecular biology of some common inherited anemias: The story of thalassemia, in Wintrobe MM (ed): *Blood, Pure and Eloquent*. New York, McGraw-Hill, 1980, p 373.
6. Bannerman RM: *Thalassemia. A survey of some aspects*. New York, Grune & Stratton, 1961.
7. Herrick JB: Peculiar elongated and sickle-shaped red blood corpuscles in a case of severe anemia. *Arch Intern Med* **6**:517, 1910.
8. Pauling L, Itano HA, Singer SJ, Wells IG: Sickle-cell anemia, a molecular disease. *Science* **110**:543, 1949.
9. Ingram VM: Specific chemical difference between the globins of normal human and sickle-cell anaemia haemoglobin. *Nature* **178**:792, 1956.
10. Cooley TB, Lee P: A series of cases of splenomegaly in children with anemia and peculiar bone changes. *Trans Am Pediatr Soc* **37**:29, 1925.
11. Ingram VM, Stretton AOW: Genetic basis of the thalassemia diseases. *Nature* **184**:1903, 1959.
12. Weatherall DJ, Clegg JB, Naughton MA: Globin synthesis in thalassemia: An *in vitro* study. *Nature* **208**:1061, 1966.
13. Clegg JB, Naughton MA, Weatherall DJ: Abnormal human haemoglobins. Separation and characterisation of the α and β chains by chromatography, and the determination of two new variants Hb Chesapeake and Hb J (Bangkok). *J Mol Biol* **19**:91, 1966.
14. Fermi G, Perutz MF, Shaanan B, Fourme B: The crystal structure of human deoxyhemoglobin at 1.7 A resolution. *J Mol Biol* **175**:159, 1984.
15. Baldwin JM: The structure of human carbonmonoxyhaemoglobin at 2.7 Å resolution. *J Mol Biol* **136**:103, 1980.
16. Perutz MF: Stereochemistry of cooperative effects in haemoglobin. *Nature* **228**:726, 1970.
17. Perutz MF: Stereochemical mechanism of oxygen transport by haemoglobin. *Proc R Soc Lond [Biol]* **208**:135, 1980.
18. Baldwin J: Structure and cooperativity of haemoglobin. *Trends Biol Sci* **5**:224, 1980.
19. Chanutin A, Curnish RR: Effect of organic and inorganic phosphates on the oxygen equilibrium of human erythrocytes. *Arch Biochem Biophys* **121**:96, 1967.
20. Benesch R, Benesch RE: The effect of organic phosphates from the human erythrocyte on the allosteric properties of hemoglobin. *Biochem Biophys Res Commun* **26**:162, 1967.
21. Arnone A: X-ray diffraction study of binding of 2,3 diphosphoglycerate to human deoxyhaemoglobin. *Nature* **237**:146, 1972.
22. Bauer C, Ludwig I, Ludwig M: Different effects of 2,3 diphosphoglycerate and adenosine triphosphate on the oxygen affinity of adult and foetal human haemoglobin. *Life Sci* **7**:1339, 1968.
23. Tyuma I, Shimizu K: Different response to organic phosphates of human fetal and adult hemoglobins. *Arch Biochem Biophys* **129**:404, 1969.
24. Perutz MF: The Bohr effect and combination with organic phosphates. *Nature* **228**:734, 1970.
25. Nienhuis AW, Maniatis T: Structure and expression of globin genes in erythroid cells, in Stamatoyannopoulos G,

Nienhuis AW, Leder P, Majerus PW (eds): *The Molecular Basis of Blood Diseases*. Philadelphia, Saunders, 1987, p 28.

26. Deisseroth A, Velez R, Nienhuis AW: Hemoglobin synthesis in somatic cell hybrids. Independent segregation of the human alpha- and beta-globin genes. *Science* **191**:1262, 1976.
27. Deisseroth A, Nienhuis A, Turner P, Velez R, Anderson WF, Ruddle F, Lawrence J, Creagan R, Kucherlapati R: Localization of the human α-globin structural gene to chromosome 16 in somatic cell hybrids by molecular hybridization assay. *Cell* **12**:205, 1977.
28. Deisseroth A, Nienhuis A, Lawrence J, Giles R, Turner P, Ruddle FH: Chromosomal localization of human β globin gene in human chromosome 11 in somatic cell hybrids. *Proc Natl Acad Sci USA* **75**:1456, 1978.
29. Gusella JF, Varsanyi-Breiner A, Kao FT, Jones C, Puck TT, Keys C, Orkin SH, Houseman D: Precise localization of human β-globin gene complex on chromosome 11. *Proc Natl Acad Sci USA* **76**:5239, 1979.
30. Jeffreys AJ, Craig IW, Francke U: Localisation of the $^{G}\gamma^{A}\gamma\delta$ and β globin genes on the short arm of chromosome 11. *Nature* **281**:606, 1979.
31. Lebo RV, Carrano AV, Burkhardt-Schultz K, Dozy AM, Yu L-C, Kan YW: Assignment of human β-, γ-, and δ-globin genes to the short arm of chromosome 11 by chromosome sorting and DNA restriction analysis. *Proc Natl Acad Sci USA* **76**:5804, 1979.
32. Sanders-Haigh L, Anderson WF, Francke U: The β-globin gene is on the short arm of chromosome 11. *Nature* **283**:683, 1980.
33. Scott AF, Phillips JA, Migeon BR: DNA endonuclease analysis for localisation of human β- and δ-globin genes on chromosome 11. *Proc Natl Acad Sci USA* **76**:4563, 1979.
34. Koeffler HP, Sparkes RS, Stang H, Mohandas T: Regional assignment of genes for human α globin and phosphoglycerate phosphatase to the short arm of chromosome 16. *Proc Natl Acad Sci USA* **78**:7015, 1981.
35. Nicholls RD, Jonasson JA, McGee JO, Patil S, Ionasescu VV, Weatherall DJ, Higgs DR: High resolution mapping of the human α-globin locus. *J Med Genet* **24**:39, 1987.
36. Lawn RM, Fritsch EF, Parker RC, Blake G, Maniatis T: The isolation and characterization of linked δ and β-globin genes from a cloned library of human DNA. *Cell* **15**:1157, 1978.
37. Fritsch EF, Lawn RM, Maniatis T: Molecular cloning and characterization of the human β-like globin gene cluster. *Cell* **19**:959, 1980.
38. Lauer J, Shen C-KJ, Maniatis T: The chromosomal arrangement of human α-like globin genes: Sequence homology and α-globin gene deletions. *Cell* **20**:119, 1980.
39. Jagedeeswaran P, Pan J, Forget BG, Weissman SM: Sequences of human repetitive DNA, non-α-globin genes, and major histocompatibility locus genes. II. Sequences of non-α-globin genes in man. *Cold Spring Harb Symp Quant Biol* **47**:1081, 1983.
40. Chang L-YE, Slightom JL: Isolation and nucleotide sequence analysis of β-type globin pseudogene from human, gorilla and chimpanzee. *J Mol Biol* **180**:767, 1984.
41. Proudfoot NJ, Gill A, Maniatis T: The structure of the human zeta-globin gene and a closely linked, nearly identical pseudogene. *Cell* **31**:553, 1982.
42. Hardison RC, Sawada I, Cheng J-F, Shen C-KJ, Schmid CW: A previously undetected pseudogene in the human alpha globin gene cluster. *Nucleic Acids Res* **14**:1903, 1986.
43. Marks J, Shaw J-P, Shen C-KP: Sequence organization and genomic complexity of primate θ globin gene, a novel α-like gene. *Nature* **321**:785, 1986.
44. Clegg JB: Can the product of θ gene be a real globin? *Nature* **329**:465, 1987.
45. Efstratiadis A, Posakony JW, Maniatis T, Lawn RM, O'Connell C, Spritz RA, DeRiel JK, Forget BG, Weissman SM, Slightom JL, Blechl AE, Smithies O, Baralle FE, Shoulders CC, Proudfoot NJ: The structure and evolution of the human β-globin gene family. *Cell* **21**:653, 1980.
46. Goodman M, Koop BF, Czelusniak J, Weiss ML: The η-globin gene. Its long evolutionary history in the β-globin globin family of mammals. *J Mol Biol* **180**:803, 1984.
47. Hardison RL, Morgot JB: Rabbit-globin pseudogene ψβ2 is a hybrid of δ- and β-globin gene sequences. *Mol Biol Evol* *1*:302, 1984.
48. Jeffreys AJ: DNA sequences in the $^{G}\gamma$-, $^{A}\gamma$-, δ- and β-globin genes of man. *Cell* **18**:1, 1979.
49. Antonarakis SE, Boehm CD, Giardina PVJ, Kazazian HH: Non random association of polymorphic restriction sites in the β-globin gene complex. *Proc Natl Acad Sci USA* **79**:137, 1982.
50. Higgs DR, Wainscoat JS, Flint J, Hill AVS, Thein SL, Nicholls RD, Teal H, Ayyub H, Peto TEA, Jarman A, Clegg JB, Weatherall DJ: Analysis of the human α globin gene cluster reveals a highly informative genetic locus. *Proc Natl Acad Sci USA* **83**:5156, 1986.
51. Wainscoat JS, Hill AVS, Boyce A, Flint J, Hernandez M, Thein SL, Lynch JR, Falusi Y, Weatherall DJ, Clegg JB: Evolutionary relationships of human populations from an analysis of nuclear DNA polymorphisms. *Nature* **319**:491, 1986.
52. O'Shaughnessy DF, Hill AVS, Bowden DK, Weatherall DJ, Clegg JB: Globin genes in Micronesia: Origins and affinities of Pacific Island peoples. *Am J Hum Genet* **46**:144, 1990.
53. Lang JC, Chakravarti A, Boehm CD, Antonarakis S, Kazazian HH: Phylogeny of human β-globin haplotypes and its implication for recent human evolution. *Am J Phys Anthropol* **81**:113, 1992.
54. Chen LZ, Easteal S, Board PG, Kirk RL: Evolution of β-globin haplotypes in human populations. *Mol Biol Evol* **7**:423, 1990.
55. Boehm CD, Antonarakis SE, Phillips JA, Stetten G, Kazazian HH: Prenatal diagnosis using DNA polymorphisms. *N Engl J Med* **308**:1054, 1983.
56. Old JM, Wainscoat JS: A new DNA polymorphism in the β-globin gene cluster can be used for antenatal diagnosis of β thalassaemia. *Br J Haematol* **53**:336, 1983.
57. Old JM: Haemoglobinopathies, in Brock DJH, Rodeck CH, Ferguson-Smith MA (eds): *Prenatal Diagnosis and Screening*. Edinburgh, Churchill Livingstone, 1992, p 425.
58. Winichagoon P, Higgs DR, Goodbourn SEY, Clegg JB, Weatherall DJ: Multiple arrangement of the human embryonic zeta globin genes. *Nucleic Acids Res* **10**:5853, 1982.
59. Trent RJ, Bowden DK, Old JM, Wainscoat JS, Clegg JB, Weatherall DJ: A novel rearrangement of the human β-like globin gene cluster. *Nucleic Acids Res* **9**:6723, 1981.
60. Higgs DR, Old JM, Pressley L, Clegg JB, Weatherall DJ: A novel α-globin gene arrangement in man. *Nature* **284**:632, 1980.
61. Higgs DR, Old JM, Clegg JB, Pressley L, Hunt DM, Weatherall DJ, Serjeant GR: Negro α-thalassaemia is caused by a deletion of a single α-globin gene. *Lancet* **2**:272, 1979.
62. Dozy AM, Kan YW, Embury SH, Mentzer WC, Wang WC, Lubin B, Davis JR, Koenig HM: α-globin gene organisation in blacks precludes the severe form of α-thalassaemia. *Nature* **280**:605, 1979.
63. Sukumaran PK, Nakatsuji T, Gardiner MB, Reese AL, Gilman JG, Huisman THJ: Gamma thalassaemia resulting from the deletion of a γ-globin gene. *Nucleic Acids Res* **11**:4635, 1983.
64. Hill AVS: The population genetics of α thalassemia and the malaria hypothesis. *Cold Spring Harb Symp Quant Biol* **51**:489, 1986.
65. Flint J, Hill AVS, Bowden DK, Oppenheimer SJ, Sill PR, Serjeantson SW, Bana-Koiri J, Bhatia K, Alpers MP, Boyce AJ, Weatherall DJ, Clegg JB: High frequencies of α thalassaemia are the result of natural selection by malaria. *Nature* **321**:744, 1986.
66. Powers PA, Altay C, Huisman THJ, Smithies O: Two novel arrangements of the human fetal globin genes: $^{G}\gamma$-$^{G}\gamma$ and $^{A}\gamma$-$^{A}\gamma$. *Nucleic Acids Res* **12**:7023, 1984.
67. Hill AVS, Nichols RD, Thein SL, Higgs DR: Recombination within the human embryonic ζ-globin locus: A common ζ-ζ chromosome produced by gene conversion of the ψζ gene. *Cell* **42**:809, 1985.
68. Mount SM: A catalogue of splice junction sequences. *Nucleic Acids Res* **10**:459, 1982.

69. Green MR: Pre-mRNA splicing. *Annu Rev Genet* **20**:671, 1986.
70. Collins FS, Weissman SM: The molecular genetics of human hemoglobin, in Cohn WE, Moldave K (eds): *Progress in Nucleic Acids Research and Molecular Biology*. New York, Academic, 1984, p 315.
71. Grosveld GC, DeBoer E, Shewmaker CK, Flavell RA: DNA sequences necessary for transcription of the rabbit β-globin gene *in vitro*. *Nature* **295**:120, 1982.
72. Orkin SH, Antonarakis SE, Kazazian HH: Base substitution at position −88 in a β-thalassemic globin gene: Further evidence for the role of the distal promoter element ACACCC. *J Biol Chem* **259**:8679, 1984.
73. Orkin SH, Kazazian HH, Antonarakis SE, Goff SC, Boehm CD, Sexton JP, Waber PG, Giardina PJV: Linkage of β-thalassaemia mutations and β-globin gene polymorphisms with DNA polymorphisms in human β globin gene cluster. *Nature* **296**:267, 1982.
74. Lewin B: *Genes*, 5th ed. New York, J Wiley, 1994.
75. Alberts B, Bray D, Lewis J, Raff M, Roberts R, Watson JD: *Molecular Biology of the Cell*, 2d ed. New York, Garland, 1989.
76. Orkin SH, Cheng T-C, Antonarakis SE, Kazazian HH: Thalassaemia due to a mutation in the cleavage-polyadenylation signal of the human β-globin gene. *EMBO J* **4**:453, 1985.
77. Higgs DR, Goodbourn SEY, Lamb J, Clegg JB, Weatherall DJ, Proudfoot NJ: α-Thalassaemia caused by a polyadenylation signal mutation. *Nature* **306**:398, 1983.
78. Evans T, Felsenfeld G, Reitman M: Control of globin gene transcription. *Annu Rev Cell Biol* **6**:95, 1990.
79. Stamatoyannopoulos G, Nienhuis AW: Hemoglobin switching, in Stamatoyannopoulos G, Nienhuis AM, Leder P, Majerus PW (eds): *The Molecular Basis of Blood Diseases*. Philadelphia, Saunders, 1987, p 66.
80. Wright S, de Boer E, Grosveld FG, Flavell RA: Regulated expression of the human beta-globin gene family in murine erythroleukaemia cells. *Nature* **305**:333, 1983.
81. Charnay P, Treisman R, Mellon P, Chao M, Axel R, Maniatis T: Differences in human alpha- and beta-globin expression in mouse erythroleukemia cells: The role of intragenic sequences. *Cell* **38**:251, 1984.
82. Costantini F, Radice G, Magram J, Stamatoyannopoulos G, Papayannopoulou T: Developmental regulation of human globin genes in transgenic mice. *Cold Spring Harb Symp Quant Biol* **50**:361, 1985.
83. Townes TM, Lingrel JB, Chen HY, Brinster RL, Palmiter RD: Erythroid-specific expression of human β globin genes in transgenic mice. *EMBO J* **4**:1715, 1985.
84. Chada K, Magram J, Costantini F: An embryonic pattern of expression of a human fetal globin gene in transgenic mice. *Nature* **319**:685, 1986.
85. Kollias G, Hurst J, de Boer E, Grosveld F: Regulated expression of human $^{A}\gamma$-, β- and hybrid γβ-globin genes in transgenic mice: Manipulation of the developmental expression patterns. *Cell* **46**:89, 1986.
86. Grosveld F, Blom van Assendelft G, Greaves DR, Kollias G: Position independent, high level expression of the human β globin gene in transgenic mice. *Cell* **51**:975, 1987.
87. Tuan D, Solomon W, Li Q, London I: The β-like globin gene domain in human erythroid cells. *Proc Natl Acad Sci USA* **82**:6384, 1985.
88. Forrester W, Thompson C, Elder JT, Groudine M: A developmentally stable chromatin structure in the human β-globin gene cluster. *Proc Natl Acad Sci USA* **83**:1359, 1986.
89. Fraser P, Hurst J, Collis P, Grosveld F: DNase 1 hypersensitive sites 1, 2 and 3 of the human β globin dominant control region direct position independent expression. *Nucleic Acids Res* **15**:10159, 1990.
90. Driscoll C, Dobkin CS, Alter BP: γδβ Thalassemia due to a *de novo* mutation deleting the 5′ β-globin locus activating region hypersensitive sites. *Proc Natl Acad Sci USA* **86**:7470, 1989.
91. Hatton CSR, Wilkie AOM, Drysdale HC, Wood WG, Vickers MA, Sharpe JA, Ayyub H, Pretorius I-M, Buckle VJ, Higgs DR: Alpha thalassemia caused by a large (62kb) deletion upstream of the human α globin gene cluster. *Blood* **76**:221, 1990.
92. Wilkie AOM, Lamb J, Harris PC, Finney RD, Higgs DR: A truncated human chromosome 16 associated with α thalassaemia is stabilized by addition of telomeric repeat (TTAGGG)n. *Nature* **346**:868, 1990.
93. Higgs DR, Wood WG, Jarman AP, Sharpe JA, Lida J, Pretorius I-M, Ayyub H: A major positive regulatory region is located far upstream of the human α globin locus. *Genes Dev* **4**:1588, 1990.
94. Jarman AP, Wood WG, Sharpe JA, Gourdon G, Ayyub H, Higgs DR: Characterization of the major regulatory element upstream of the human α globin gene cluster. *Mol Cell Biol* **11**:4679, 1991.
95. Groudine M, Kohwi-Shigematsu T, Gelinas R, Stamatoyannopoulos G, Papayannopoulou T: Human fetal to adult hemoglobin switching: Changes in chromatin structure of the β-globin gene locus. *Proc Natl Acad Sci USA* **80**:7551, 1983.
96. Forrester WC, Epner E, Driscoll CM, Enver T, Brice M, Papayannopoulou T, Groudine M: A deletion of the human β globin locus activation region causes a major alteration in chromatin structure and replication across the entire β-globin locus. *Genes Dev* **4**:1637, 1990.
97. Jarman AP, Higgs DR: Nuclear scaffold attachment sites in the human globin gene complexes. *EMBO J* **7**:3337, 1988.
98. Yagi M, Gelinas R, Elder JT, Peretz M, Papayannopoulou T, Stamatoyannopoulos G, Groudine M: Chromatin structure and developmental expression of the human α globin cluster. *Mol Cell Biol* **6**:1108, 1986.
99. Vyas P, Vickers M, Simmons DL, Ayyub H, Craddock CF, Higgs DR: Cis-acting sequences regulating expression of the human α globin cluster lie within constitutively open chromatin. *Cell* **69**:781, 1992.
100. Mavilio F, Giampaolo A, Care A, Migliaccio G, Calandrini M, Russo G, Pagliardi GL, Mastroberardino G, Marinucci M, Peschle C: Molecular mechanisms of human hemoglobin switching: Selective undermethylation and expression of globin genes in embryonic, fetal and adult erythroblasts. *Proc Natl Acad Sci USA* **80**:6907, 1983.
101. Wall L, de Boer E, Grosveld F: The human beta-globin gene 3′ enhancer contains multiple binding sites for an erythroid specific protein. *Genes Dev* **2**:1089, 1988.
102. Evans T, Felsenfeld G: The erythroid specific transcription factor Eryf1: A new finger protein. *Cell* **58**:877, 1989.
103. Martin DIK, Tsai S-F, Orkin S: Increased γ globin expression in a nondeletion HPFH mediated by an erythroid specific DNA binding factor. *Nature* **338**:435, 1989.
104. Yamamoto M, Ko LJ, Leonard MW, Beng H, Orkin S, Engel JD: Activity and tissue specific expression of the transcription factor NF-E1 mutigene family. *Genes Dev* **4**:1650, 1990.
105. Whitelaw E, Tsai S-F, Hogben P, Orkin SH: Regulated expression of globin chains and the erythroid transcription factor GATA-1 during erythropoiesis in the developing mouse. *Mol Cell Biol* **10**:6596, 1990.
106. Pevny L, Simon MC, Robertson E, Klein W-H, Tsai S-F, D'Agati V, Orkin SH, Costantini F: Erythroid differentiation in chimeric mice blocked by a targeted mutation in the gene for transcription factor GATA-1. *Nature* **349**:257, 1991.
107. Gallarda JL, Foley KP, Yang Z, Engel JD: The β globin stage selector element factor is erythroid-specific promoter-enhancer binding protein NF-E4. *Genes Dev* **3**:1845, 1989.
108. Papayannopoulou T, Lindsley D, Kurachi S, Lewison K, Hemenway T, Melis M, Anagnou NP, Najfeld V: Adult and fetal human globin genes are expressed following chromosomal transfer into MEL cells. *Proc Natl Acad Sci USA* **82**:780, 1985.
109. Gibbons RJ, Wilkie AO, Weatherall DJ, Higgs DR: A newly defined X linked mental retardation syndrome associated with α thalassaemia. *J Med Genet* **28**:729, 1991.
110. Wood WG, Pearce K, Clegg JB, Weatherall DJ, Robinson JS, Thorburn GD, Dawes G: The switch from foetal to adult haemoglobin synthesis in normal and hypophysectomised sheep. *Nature* **264**:799, 1976.
111. Wood WG, Bunch C, Kelly SJ, Gunn Y, Breckon G: Control of haemoglobin switching by a developmental clock? *Nature* **313**:320, 1985.

112. Zanjani ED, Lim G, McGlave PB, Clapp JF, Mann LI, Northwood TH, Stamatoyannopoulos G: Adult haemopoietic cells transplanted to sheep foetuses continue to produce adult globins. *Nature* **295**:244, 1982.
113. Perrine SP, Rudolph A, Faller DV, Roman C, Cohen RA, Shen S-J, Kan YW: Butyrate infusions in the ovine fetus delay the biologic clock for globin gene switching. *Proc Natl Acad Sci USA* **85**:8540, 1988.
114. Raich N, Enver T, Nakamoto B, Josephson B, Papayannopoulou T, Stamatoyannopoulos G: Autonomous developmental control of human embryonic globin gene switching in transgenic mice. *Science* **250**:1147, 1990.
115. Dillon N, Grosveld F: Human γ globin genes silenced independently of other genes in the β-globin locus. *Nature* **350**:252, 1991.
116. Behringer RR, Ryan TM, Palmiter RD, Brinster RL, Townes TM: Human γ- to β-globin gene switching in transgenic mice. *Genes Dev* **4**:376, 1990.
117. Enver T, Raich N, Ebers AJ, Papayannopoulou T, Costantini F, Stamatoyannopoulos G: Developmental regulation of human fetal-to-adult globin gene switching in transgenic mice. *Nature* **344**:309, 1990.
118. Hanscombe O, Whyatt D, Fraser P, Yannoutsos N, Greaves D, Dillon N, Grosveld F: Importance of globin gene order for correct developmental expression. *Genes Dev* **5**:1387, 1991.
119. Weatherall DJ, Clegg JB: The α-chain termination mutants and their relationship to the α-thalassaemias. *Philos Trans R Soc Lond [Biol]* **271**:411, 1975.
120. Seid-Akhaven M, Winter WP, Abramson RK, Rucknagel DL: Hemoglobin Wayne: A frameshift mutation detected in human hemoglobin alpha chains. *Proc Natl Acad Sci USA* **73**:882, 1976.
121. Lehmann H, Casey R, Lang A, Stathopoulou R, Imai K, Tuchinda S, Vinai P, Flatz G: Haemoglobin Tak: A β-chain elongation. *Br J Haematol* **31**:119, 1975.
122. Bunn HF, Schmidt GJ, Haney DN, Dluhy RG: Hemoglobin Cranston, an unstable variant having an elongated β chain due to nonhomologous crossover between two normal β chain genes. *Proc Natl Acad Sci USA* **72**:3609, 1975.
123. Huisman THJ, Wilson JB, Gravely M, Hubbard M: Hemoglobin Grady: The first example of a variant with elongated chains due to an insertion of residues. *Proc Natl Acad Sci USA* **71**:3270, 1974.
124. Prchal JT, Cashman DP, Kan YW: Hemoglobin Long Island is caused by a single mutation (adenine to cytosine) resulting in a failure to cleave amino-terminal methionine. *Proc Natl Acad Sci USA* **83**:24, 1986.
125. Blouquit Y, Lena-Russo D, Delanoe J, Arous N, Bardakjian J, Lancombe C, Orsini A, Rosa J, Galacteros F: Hb Marseille ($\alpha_2\beta_2$ 1(A1) NH→met, 2(A2) His→3(A3) Pro): First variant having an N-terminal elongated β chain. *Blood* **64**:55, 1984.
126. Boissel J-P, Kasper T, Shah S, Malone T, Bunn HF: NH_2-terminal processing of protein: Hb South Florida, a variant with retention of initiation methionine and N^{α}-acetylation. *Proc Natl Acad Sci USA* **82**:8448, 1985.
127. Rieder RF, Bradley TB: Hemoglobin Gun Hill: An unstable protein associated with chronic hemolysis. *Blood* **32**:355, 1968.
128. Winslow RM, Swenberg ML, Gross E, Chervenick P, Buchman RR, Anderson WF: Hemoglobin McKees Rocks ($\alpha_2\beta_2^{145Tyr\text{-}Term}$), a human "nonsense" mutation leading to a shortened β-chain. *Am J Hum Genet* **27**:95, 1975.
129. Baglioni C: The fusion of two peptide chains in hemoglobin Lepore and its interpretation as a genetic deletion. *Proc Natl Acad Sci USA* **48**:1880, 1962.
130. Barnabus J, Muller CJ: Hemoglobin Lepore Hollandia. *Nature* **194**:931, 1962.
131. Ostertag W, Smith EW: Hb Lepore Baltimore, a third type of a δβ crossover (δ^{50}, β^{86}). *Eur J Biochem* **10**:371, 1969.
132. Huisman THJ, Wrightstone RN, Wilson JB, Schroeder WA, Kendall AG: Hemoglobin Kenya, the product of a fusion of γ and β polypeptide chains. *Arch Biochem Biophys* **153**:850, 1972.
133. Ohta Y, Yamaoka K, Sumida I, Fujita S, Fujimura T, Hadana M, Yanase T: Two structural and synthetical variants, Hb Miyada and homozygous δ-thalassaemia, discovered in Japanese, in *XIII International Congress of Haematology*. Munich, Verlag, 1970.
134. Lehmann H, Charlesworth D: Observations on hemoglobin P (Congo type). *Biochem J* **119**:43, 1970.
135. Honig GR, Mason RG, Tremaine LM, Vida LN: Unbalanced globin chain synthesis by Hb Lincoln Park (anti-Lepore) reticulocytes. *Am J Hematol* **5**:335, 1978.
136. Badr FM, Lorkin PA, Lehmann H: Haemoglobin P-Nilotic: Containing β-δ chain. *Nature New Biol* **242**:107, 1973.
137. Adams JG, Morrison WT, Steinberg MH: Double crossover within a single human gene. *Science* **218**:291, 1982.
138. Harris JW: Studies on the destruction of red blood cells. VII. Molecular orientation in sickle cell hemoglobin solutions. *Proc Soc Exp Biol Med* **75**:197, 1950.
139. Edelstein SJ, Telford JN, Crepeau RH: Structure of fibers of sickle cell hemoglobin. *Proc Natl Acad Sci USA* **70**:1104, 1973.
140. Finch JT, Perutz MF, Bertles JF, Dobler J: Structure of sickled erythrocytes and of sickle-cell hemoglobin fibers. *Proc Natl Acad Sci USA* **70**:718, 1973.
141. Garrell RL, Crepeau RH, Edelstein SJ: Cross-sectional views of hemoglobin S fibers by electron microscopy and computer modeling. *Proc Natl Acad Sci USA* **76**:1140, 1979.
142. Dykes G, Crepeau R, Edelstein SJ: Three-dimensional reconstruction of the fibres of sickle cell haemoglobin. *Nature* **272**:506, 1978.
143. Wishner BC, Hanson JC, Ringle WM, Love WE: Crystal structure on sickle cell deoxyhemoglobin, in *Proceedings of the Symposium on Molecular and Cellular Aspects of Sickle Cell Disease. Bethesda, MD, U.S. Department of Health, Education and Welfare, 1976.*
144. Schechter AN, Noguchi CT, Rodgers GP: Sickle cell disease, in Stamatoyannopoulos G, Nienhuis AW, Leder P, Majerus PW (eds): *The Molecular Basis of Blood Diseases.* Philadelphia, Saunders, 1987, p 179.
145. Wilson WW, Luzzana MR, Penniston JT, Johnson CS: Pregelation aggregation of sickle cell hemoglobin. *Proc Natl Acad Sci USA* **71**:1260, 1974.
146. Morrat K, Gibson QH: The rates of polymerization and depolymerization of sickle cell hemoglobin. *Biochem Biophys Res Commun* **61**:237, 1974.
147. Williams RC: Concerted formation of the gel of hemoglobin S. *Proc Natl Acad Sci USA* **70**:1506, 1973.
148. Hofrichter J, Ross PD, Eaton WA: Supersaturation in sickle cell hemoglobin solution. *Proc Natl Acad Sci USA* **73**:3035, 1976.
149. Ross PD, Hofrichter J, Eaton WA: Calorimetric and optical characterization of sickle cell hemoglobin gelation. *J Mol Biol* **96**:239, 1975.
150. Zipp A, James TL, Kuntz ID, Shohet ID: Water proton magnetic resonance studies of normal and sickle erythrocytes. Temperature and volume dependence. *Biochim Biophys Acta* **428**:291, 1976.
151. Eaton WA, Hofrichter J, Ross PD: Delay time in gelation: A possible determinant of clinical severity in sickle cell disease. *Blood* **47**:621, 1976.
152. Singer K, Singer L: Studies on abnormal hemoglobins. VIII. The gelling phenomenon of sickle cell hemoglobin: Its biologic and diagnostic significance. *Blood* **8**:1008, 1953.
153. Bertles JF, Dobler J: Reversible and irreversible sickling; a distinction by electron microscopy. *Blood* **33**:884, 1969.
154. Nagel RL: Severity, pathobiology, epistatic effects, and genetic markers in sickle cell anemia. *Semin Hematol* **28**:180, 1991.
155. Canessa M: Red cell volume-related ion transport systems in hemoglobinopathies. *Hematol Oncol Clin North Am* **5**:495, 1991.
156. Kaul DK, Fabry ME, Windisch P, Baez S, Nagel RL: Erythrocytes in sickle cell anemia are heterogeneous in their rheological and hemodynamic characteristics. *J Clin Invest* **72**:22, 1983.
157. Hebbel RP, Schwartz RS, Mohandas N: The adhesive sickle erythrocyte: Cause and consequence of abnormal interactions with endothelium, monocytes, macrophages and model membranes. *Clin Haematol* **14**:141, 1985.
158. Hebbel RP, Miller WJ: Phagocytosis of sickle erythrocytes:

Immunologic and oxidative determinants of hemolytic anemia. *Blood* **64**:733, 1984.

159. Kuross SA, Hebbel RP: Nonheme iron in sickle erythrocyte membranes: Association with phosphilipids and potential role in lipid peroxidation. *Blood* **72**:1278, 1988.
160. Hebbel RP: Auto-oxidation and a membrane-associated "Fenton Reagent": A possible explanation for development of membrane lesions in sickle erythrocytes. *Clin Haematol* **14**:129, 1985.
161. Kay MMB, Goodman SR, Sorensen K, Whitfield CF, Wong P, Zaki L, Rudloff V: Senescent cell antigen is immunologically related to band 3. *Proc Natl Acad Sci USA* **80**:1631, 1983.
162. Sherwood JB, Goldwasser E, Chilcote E, Carmichael E, Charmichael LD, Nagel RL: Sickle cell anemia patients have low erythropoietin levels for their degree of anemia. *Blood* **67**:46, 1986.
163. Mohandas N, Evans E: Sickle cell adherence to vascular endothelium: Morphologic correlates and the requirement for divalent cations and collagen binding plasma proteins. *J Clin Invest* **76**:1605, 1985.
164. Serjeant GR. *Sickle Cell Disease*. Oxford, Oxford University Press, 1985.
165. Rogers DW, Serjeant BE, Serjeant GR: Early rise in 'pitted' red cell count as a guide to susceptibility to infection in childhood sickle cell anaemia. *Arch Dis Child* **57**:338, 1982.
166. Zago M, Bottura C: Splenic function in sickle-cell diseases. *Clin Sci* **65**:297, 1983.
167. Rogers DW, Clarke JM, Cupidore L, Ramlal AM, Sparke BR, Serjeant GR: Early deaths in Jamaican children with sickle cell disease. *Br Med J* **1**:1515, 1978.
168. Hatton CSR, Bunch C, Weatherall DJ: Hepatic sequestration in sickle cell anaemia. *Br Med J* **290**:744, 1985.
169. Davies SC, Luce PJ, Win AA, Riordan JF, Brozovic M: Acute chest syndrome in sickle-cell disease. *Lancet* **1**:36, 1984.
170. Pattison JR, Jones SE, Hodgson J, Davies LR, White JM, Stroud CE, Murtaza L: Parvovirus infections and hypoplastic crises in sickle-cell anaemia. *Lancet* **1**:664, 1981.
171. Powars D, Wilson B, Imbus C, Pegelow C, Allen J: The natural history of stroke in sickle cell disease. *Am J Med* **65**:461, 1978.
172. Mohr JP: Sickle cell anemia, stroke, and transcranial studies. *N Engl J Med* **326**:637, 1992.
173. Rothman SM, Fulling KH, Nelson JS: Sickle cell anemia and central nervous system infarction: A neuropathological study. *Ann Neurol* **20**:684, 1986.
174. Ohene-Frempong K: Stroke in sickle cell disease: Demographic, clinical, and therapeutic considerations. *Semin Hematol* **28**:213, 1991.
175. Powars D, Weidman JA, Odom-Maryon T, Niland JC, Johnson C: Sickle cell chronic lung disease: Prior morbidity and the risk of pulmonary failure. *Medicine (Baltimore)* **67**:66, 1988.
176. Hendrickse JP, Harrison KA, Watson-Williams EJ, Luzzatto L, Ajabor LN: Pregnancy in homozygous sickle-cell anaemia. *J Obstet Gynaecol Br Commonw* **79**:396, 1972.
177. Leikin SL, Gallagher D, Kinney TR, Sloane D, Klug P, Rida W: Mortality in children and adolescents with sickle cell disease. *Pediatrics* **84**:500, 1989.
178. Perrine RP, Brown MJ, Clegg JB, Weatherall DJ, May A: Benign sickle-cell anaemia. *Lancet* **2**:1163, 1972.
179. Kar BC, Satapathy RK, Kulozik AE, Kulozik M, Sirr S, Serjeant BE, Serjeant GR: Sickle cell disease in Orissa State, India. *Lancet* **2**:1198, 1986.
180. Powars DR, Weiss JN, Chan LS, Schroeder WA: Is there a threshold level of fetal hemoglobin that ameliorates morbidity in sickle cell disease? *Blood* **63**:921, 1988.
181. Padmos MA, Roberts GT, Sackey K, Kulozik A,Bail S, Morris JS, Serjeant BE: Two different forms of homozygous sickle cell disease occur in Saudi Arabia. *Br J Haematol* **79**:93, 1991.
182. Higgs DR, Aldridge BE, Lamb J, Clegg JB, Weatherall DJ, Hayes RJ, Grandison Y, Lowrie Y, Mason KP, Serjeant BE, Serjeant GR: The interaction of alpha-thalassemia and homozygous sickle cell disease. *N Engl J Med* **306**:1441, 1982.
183. Noguchi CT, Dover GJ, Rodgers GP, Serjeant GR, Antonarakis SE, Anagnou NP, Higgs DR, Weatherall DJ, Schechter AN: α Thalassemia changes erythrocyte heterogeneity in sickle cell disease. *J Clin Invest* **75**:1632, 1985.
184. Higgs DR, Clegg JB, Weatherall DJ, Serjeant BE, Serjeant GR: Interaction of the $\alpha\alpha\alpha$ globin gene haplotype and sickle haemoglobin. *Br J Haematol* **58**:671, 1984.
185. Nagel RL, Lawrence C: The distinct pathobiology of sickle cell-hemoglobin C disease. *Hematol Oncol Clin North Am* **5**:433, 1991.
186. Monplaisir N, Merault G, Poyart C, Rhode M-D, Craescu C, Vidaud M, Galacteros F, Blouquit Y, Rosa J: Hemoglobin S Antilles: A variant with lower solubility than hemoglobin S and producing sickle cell disease in heterozygotes. *Proc Natl Acad Sci USA* **83**:9363, 1986.
187. Itano HA, Neel JV: A new inherited abnormality of human hemoglobin. *Proc Natl Acad Sci USA* **36**:613, 1950.
188. Diggs LW, Kraus AO, Morrison DB, Rudnicki RPT: Intra-erythrocyte crystals in a white patient with hemoglobin C in the absence of other types of hemoglobin. *Blood* **9**:1172, 1954.
189. Hirsch RE, Raventos-Suarez C, Olson JA, Nagel RL: Ligand state of intraerythrocyte circulating Hb C crystals in homozygote CC patients. *Blood* **66**:775, 1985.
190. Reiss G, Ranney HM, Shaklai N: The association of hemoglobin C with red cell ghosts. *J Clin Invest* **70**:946, 1982.
191. Vella F, Lehmann H: Haemoglobin D Punjab (D Los Angeles). *J Med Genet* **11**:341, 1974.
192. Hunt JA, Ingram VM: Abnormal human haemoglobins. VI. The chemical difference between haemoglobins A and E. *Biochim Biophys Acta* **49**:520, 1961.
193. Traeger J, Wood WG, Clegg JB, Weatherall DJ, Wasi P: Defective synthesis of Hb E is due to reduced levels of β^E mRNA. *Nature* **288**:497, 1980.
194. Orkin SH, Kazazian HH, Antonarakis SE, Ostrer H, Goff SC, Sexton JP: Abnormal RNA processing due to the exon mutation of β^E-globin gene. *Nature* **300**:768, 1982.
195. Wasi P, Na-Nakorn S, Pootrakul S, Sookanek M, Disthasongchan P, Pornpatkul M, Panich V: Alpha- and beta-thalassemia in Thailand. *Ann NY Acad Sci* **165**:60, 1969.
196. Weatherall DJ, Clegg JB, Na-Nakorn S, Wasi P: The pattern of disordered haemoglobin synthesis in homozygous and heterozygous β-thalassaemia. *Br J Haematol* **16**:251, 1969.
197. Winterbourn CC, Carrell RW: Studies of hemoglobin denaturation and Heinz body formation in the unstable hemoglobins. *J Clin Invest* **54**:678, 1974.
198. Rachmilewitz EA: Denaturation of the normal and abnormal hemoglobin molecule. *Semin Hematol* **11**:441, 1974.
199. Milner PF, Wrightstone RN: The unstable hemoglobins: A review, in Wallach DFH (ed) *The Function of Red Blood Cells: Erythrocyte Pathobiology*. New York, Alan R. Liss, 1981, p 197.
200. Miller DR, Weed RI, Stamatoyannopoulos G, Yoshida A: Hemoglobin Koln disease occurring as a fresh mutation: Erythrocyte metabolism and survival. *Blood* **38**:715, 1971.
201. Flynn TP, Allen DW, Johnson GJ, White JC: Oxidant damage of the lipids and proteins of the erythrocyte membranes in unstable hemoglobin disease. Evidence for the role of lipid peroxidation. *J Clin Invest* **71**:1215, 1983.
202. Charache S, Weatherall DJ, Clegg JB: Polycythemia associated with a hemoglobinopathy. *J Clin Invest* **45**:813, 1966.
203. Charache S: Haemoglobins with altered oxygen affinity. *Clin Haematol* **3**:357, 1974.
204. Adamson JW: Familial polycythemia. *Semin Hematol* **12**:383, 1975.
205. Bonaventura J, Riggs A: Hemoglobin Kansas, a human hemoglobin with a neutral amino acid substitution and an abnormal oxygen equilibrium. *J Biol Chem* **243**:980, 1968.
206. Nagel RL, Bookchin RM: Human hemoglobin variants with abnormal oxygen binding. *Semin Hematol* **11**:385, 1974.
207. Modell CB, Berdoukas VA: *The Clinical Approach to Thalassemia*. New York, Grune & Stratton, 1981.
208. Higgs DR, Vickers MA, Wilkie AOM, Pretorius I-M, Jarman AP, Weatherall DJ: A review of the molecular genetics of the human α-globin gene cluster. *Blood* **73**:1081, 1989.

209. Kazazian HH, Boehm CD: Molecular basis and prenatal diagnosis of β-thalassemia. *Blood* **72**:1107, 1988.
210. Kazazian HH: The thalassemia syndromes: Molecular basis and prenatal diagnosis in 1990. *Semin Hematol* **27**:209, 1990.
211. Weatherall DJ: Thalassemia, in Stamatoyannopoulos G, Nienhuis AW, Leder P, Majerus PW (eds): *The Molecular Basis of Blood Diseases*, 2nd ed. Philadelphia, Saunders, 1994, p. 157.
212. Fessas P: Inclusions of hemoglobin in erythroblasts and erythrocytes of thalassemia. *Blood* **21**:21, 1963.
213. Wickramasinghe SN, Hughes M: Some features of bone marrow macrophages in patients with homozygous β-thalassaemia. *Br J Haematol* **38**:23, 1978.
214. Chalevelakis G, Clegg JB, Weatherall DJ: Imbalanced globin chain synthesis in heterozygous β-thalassemic bone marrow. *Proc Natl Acad Sci USA* **72**:3835, 1975.
215. Shinar E, Rachmilewitz EA: Differences in the pathophysiology of hemolysis of α- and β-thalassemia red blood cells. *Ann NY Acad Sci* **612**:106, 1990.
216. Weatherall DJ, Pressley L, Wood WG, Higgs DR, Clegg JB: The molecular basis for mild forms of homozygous β thalassaemia. *Lancet* **1**:527, 1981.
217. Wainscoat JS, Old JM, Weatherall DJ, Orkin SH: The molecular basis for the clinical diversity of β thalassaemia in Cypriots. *Lancet* **1**:1235, 1983.
218. Embury SH, Miller JA, Dozy AM, Kan YW, Chan V, Todd D: Two different molecular organizations account for the single α-globin gene of the α-thalassemia-2 genotype. *J Clin Invest* **66**:1319, 1980.
219. Goossens M, Dozy AM, Embury SH, Zachariades Z, Hadjiminas MG, Stamatoyannopoulos G, Kan YW: Triplicated α-globin loci in humans *Proc Natl Acad Sci USA* **77**:518, 1980.
220. Trent RJ, Higgs DR, Clegg JB, Weatherall DJ: A new triplicated α-globin gene arrangement in man. *Br J Haematol* **49**:149, 1981.
221. Lie-Injo LE, Herrera AR, Kan YW: Two types of triplicated α globin loci in humans. *Nucleic Acids Res* **9**:3707, 1981.
222. Gu YC, Landman H, Huisman THJ: Two different quadruplicated α globin gene arrangements. *Br J Haematol* **66**:245, 1987.
223. Ramsay M, Jenkins T: The $\alpha\alpha\alpha^{anti3.7}$ globin haplotype with an additional *Bgl* II site mutation ($\alpha\alpha\alpha^{anti\text{-}3.7}$ *Bgl* II(−)). *Hemoglobin* **9**:385, 1985.
224. Higgs DR, Hill AVS, Bowden DK, Weatherall DJ: Independent recombination events between duplicated human α globin genes: Implications for their concerted evolution. *Nucleic Acids Res* **12**:6965, 1984.
225. Powers PA, Smithies O: Short gene conversions in the human fetal globin gene region: A by-product of chromosome pairing during meiosis? *Genetics* **112**:343, 1986.
226. Nathans J, Piantanida TP, Eddy RL, Shows TB, Hogness DS: Molecular genetics of inherited variation in human color vision. *Science* **232**:203, 1986.
227. Taub RA, Hollis GF, Hieter PA, Korsmeyer S, Waldmann TA, Leder P: Variable amplification of immunoglobulin κ light-chain genes in human populations. *Nature* **304**:172, 1983.
228. Lacerra G, Fioretti G, De Angioletti M, Pagano L, Guarino E, De Bonis C, Viola A, Maglione G, Scarollo A, De Rosa L, Carestia C: A novel α^+-thalassemia deletion with the breakpoints in the α2-globin gene and in close proximity to an Alu family repeat between the ψα2- and ψα1-globin genes. *Blood* **78**:2740, 1991.
229. Kulozik A, Kar BC, Serjeant BE, Serjeant GR, Weatherall DJ: The molecular basis of α thalassemia in India; its interaction with the sickle cell gene. *Blood* **71**:467, 1988.
230. Orkin SH, Goff SC: The duplicated human α-globin genes: Their relative expression as measured by RNA analysis. *Cell* **24**:345, 1981.
231. Liebhaber SA, Kan YW: Differentiation of the mRNA transcripts originating from the α1- and α2-globin loci in normals and α-thalassemics. *J Clin Invest* **68**:439, 1981.
232. Shakin SH, Liebhaber SA: Translational profiles of alpha 1-, alpha 2-, and beta-globin messenger ribonucleic acids in human reticulocytes. *J Clin Invest* **78**:1125, 1986.
233. Liebhaber SA, Cash FE, Ballas SK: Human α-globin gene expression. The dominant role of the α2-locus in mRNA and protein synthesis. *J Biol Chem* **261**:15327, 1986.
234. Bowden DK, Hill AVS, Higgs DR, Oppenheimer SJ, Weatherall DJ, Clegg JB: Different hematologic phenotypes are associated with leftward ($-\alpha^{4.2}$) and rightward ($-\alpha^{3.7}$) α^+-thalassemia deletions. *J Clin Invest* **79**:39, 1987.
235. Liebhaber SA, Cash FE, Main DM: Compensatory increase in α1-globin gene expression in individuals heterozygous for the α-thalassemia-2 deletion. *J Clin Invest* **76**:1957, 1985.
236. Fortina P, Dianzani I, Serra A, Gottard E, Saglio G, Farinasso L, Piga A, Gabutti V, Camaschella C: A newly-characterized α-thalassaemia-1 deletion removes the entire α-like globin gene cluster in an Italian family. *Br J Haematol* **78**:529, 1991.
237. Villegas A, Calero F, Vickers MA, Ayyub H, Higgs DR: α Thalassemia in two Spanish families. *Eur J Haematol* **44**:109, 1989.
238. Felice AE, Cleek MP, McKie K, Mckie V, Huisman THJ: The rare α-thalassemia-1 of Blacks is a ζα-thalassemia-1 associated with deletion of all α- and ζ-globin genes. *Blood* **63**:1253, 1984.
239. Waye JS, Eng B, Chui DHK: Identification of an extensive ζ-α globin gene deletion in a Chinese individual. *Br J Haematol* **80**:378, 1992.
240. Nicholls RB, Fischel-Ghodsian N, Higgs DR: Recombination at the human α-globin gene cluster: Sequence features and topological constraints. *Cell* **49**:369, 1987.
241. Vanin EF, Henthorn PS, Kioussis D, Grosveld F, Smithies O: Unexpected relationships between four large deletions in the human β-globin gene cluster. *Cell* **35**:701, 1983.
242. Jelinek WR, Schmid CW: Repetitive sequences in eukaryotic DNA and their expression. *Annu Rev Biochem* **51**:813, 1982.
243. Henthorn PS, Smithies O, Mager DL: Molecular analysis of deletions in the human β-globin gene cluster: Deletion junctions and locations of breakpoints. *Genomics* **6**:226, 1990.
244. Higgs DR, Ayyub H, Clegg JB, Hill AVS, Nicholls RD, Teal H, Wainscoat JS, Weatherall DJ: α-Thalassaemia in British people. *Br Med J* **290**:1303, 1985.
245. Bhavnani M, Wickham M, Ayyub H, Higgs DR: α-thalassaemia in the North West of England. *Clin Lab Haematol* **11**:293, 1989.
246. Chung S-W, Wong SC, Clarke BJ, Patterson M, Walker WHC, Chui DHK: Human embryonic ζ-globin chains in adult patients with α-thalassemias. *Proc Natl Acad Sci USA* **81**:6188, 1984.
247. Chui DHK, Wong SC, Chung S-W, Patterson M, Bhargava S, Poon M-C: Embryonic ζ-globin chains in adults: A marker for α-thalassemia-1 haplotype due to a >17.5 kb deletion. *N Engl J Med* **31**:76, 1986.
248. Strauss EC, Andrews NC, Higgs DR, Orkin SH: *In vivo* footprinting of the human α-globin locus upstream regulatory element by guanine/adenine ligation-mediated PCR. *Mol Cell Biol* **12**:2135, 1992.
249. Hatton CSR, Wilkie AOM, Drysdale HC, Wood WG, Vickers MA, Sharpe JA, Ayyub H, Pretorius I-M, Buckle VJ, Higgs DR: Alpha thalassemia caused by a large (62kb) deletion upstream of the human α globin gene cluster. *Blood* **76**:221, 1990.
250. Wilkie AOM, Lamb J, Harris PC, Finney RD, Higgs DR: A truncated human chromosome 16 associated with α thalassaemia is stabilized by addition of telomeric repeat (TTAGG)n. *Nature* **346**:868, 1990.
251. Romao L, Osorio-Almeida L, Higgs DR, Lavinha J, Liebhaber SA: α-thalassemia resulting from deletion of regulatory sequences far upstream of the α-globin structural genes. *Blood* **78**:1589, 1991.
252. Liebhaber SA, Griese E-U, Cash FE, Ayyub H, Higgs DR, Horst J: Inactivation of human α-globin gene expression by a *de novo* deletion located upstream of the α-globin gene cluster. *Proc Natl Acad Sci USA* **81**:9431, 1990.
253. Orkin SH, Goff SC, Hechtman RL: Mutation in an intervening sequence splice junction in man. *Proc Natl Acad Sci USA* **78**:5041, 1981.
254. Felber BK, Orkin SH, Hamer DH: Abnormal RNA splicing causes one form of α thalassemia. *Cell* **29**:895, 1982.
255. Thein SL, Wallace RB, Pressley L, Clegg JB, Weath-

erall DJ, Higgs DR: Phenotypic expression of the polyadenylation site mutation in the α-globin gene cluster. *Blood* **71**:313, 1988.
256. Whitelaw E, Proudfoot N: α-thalassemia caused by a poly(A) site mutation reveals that transcriptional termination is linked to 3′ end processing in the human α2 globin gene. *EMBO J* **5**:2915, 1986.
257. Yüregir GT, Aksoy K, Cüruk MA, Dikmen N, Fei Y-J, Baysal E, Huisman THJ: Hb H disease in a Turkish family resulting from the interaction of a deletional α-thalassaemia-1 and a newly discovered poly A mutation. *Br J Haematol* **80**:527, 1992.
258. Pirastu M, Saglio G, Chang JC, Cao A, Kan YW: Initiation codon mutation as a cause of α thalassemia. *J Biol Chem* **259**:12315, 1984.
259. Morle F, Lopez B, Henni T, Godet J: α-thalassaemia associated with the deletion of two nucleotides at position -2 and -3 preceding the AUG codon. *EMBO J* **4**:1245, 1985.
260. Moi P, Cash FE, Liebhaber SA, Cao A, Pirastu M: An initiation codon mutation (AUG→GUG) of the human α1-globin gene: Structural characterisation and evidence for a mild thalassemic phenotype. *J Clin Invest* **80**:1416, 1987.
261. Liebhaber SA, Coleman MB, Adams JG III, Cash FE, Steinberg MH: Non-deletion α-thalassemia in a Black kindred resulting from a nonsense mutation (α2 116GAG-UAG). *Blood* **68**:75, 1986.
262. Liebhaber SA, Kan YW: α-thalassemia caused by an unstable α-globin mutant. *J Clin Invest* **71**:461, 1983.
263. Sanguansermsri T, Matragoon S, Changloah L, Fletz G: Hemoglobin Suan-Dok ($\alpha 2^{109(G16)LEU\text{-}ARG}\beta 2$): An unstable variant associated with α thalassemia. *Hemoglobin* **3**:161, 1979.
264. Honig GR, Shamsuddin M, Zaizov R, Steinherz M, Solar I, Kirschman C: Hemoglobin Petah Tikvah (α110 Ala→Asp): A new unstable variant with α-thalassemia-like expression. *Blood* **57**:705, 1981.
265. Honig GR, Shamsuddin M, Vida LN, Mompoint M, Valcourt E, Bowie LJ, Jones EC, Powers PA, Spritz RA, Guis M, Embury SH, Conboy J, Kan YW, Mentzer WC, Weil SC, Hirata RK, Waloch J, O'Riordan JF, Goldstick TK: Hemoglobin Evanston (α14 Trp→Arg): An unstable α-chain variant expressed as α-thalassemia. *J Clin Invest* **73**:1740, 1984.
266. Chan V,Chan TK, Liang ST, Ghosh A, Kan YW, Todd D: Hydrops Fetalis due to an unusual form of Hb H disease. *Blood* **66**:224, 1985.
267. Trent RJ, Wilkinson T, Yakas J, Carter J, Lammi A, Kronenberg H: Molecular defects in 2 examples of severe Hb H disease. *Scand J Haematol* **36**:272, 1986.
268. Lie-Injo LE, Ganesan J, Clegg JB, Weatherall DJ: Homozygous state for Hb Constant Spring (slow-moving Hb X components). *Blood* **43**:251, 1974.
269. De Jong WW, Khan PM, Bernini LF: Hemoglobin Koya Dora: High frequency of a chain termination mutant. *Am J Hum Genet* **27**:81, 1975.
270. Henni T, Morle F, Lopez B, Colonna P, Godet J: α-thalassemia halpotypes in the Algerian population. *Hum Genet* **75**:272, 1987.
271. Kattamis C, Tzotzos S, Kanavakis E, Synodinos J, Metaxatous-Mavromati A: Correlation of clinical phenotype to genotype in haemoglobin H disease. *Lancet* **1**:442, 1988.
272. Galanello R, Pirastu M, Melis MA, Paglietti E, Moi P, Cao A: Phenotype-genotype correlation in haemoglobin H disease in childhood. *J Med Genet* **20**:425, 1983.
273. Fuchareon S, Winichagoon P, Pootrakul P, Piankijagum A, Wasi P: Differences between two types of Hb H disease, α-thalassemia 1/α-thalassemia 2 and α-thalassaemia 1/Hb Constant Spring. *Birth Defects* **23**:309, 1988.
274. George E, Ferguson V, Yakas J, Kornenberg H, Trent RJ: A molecular marker associated with mild hemoglobin H disease. *Pathology* **21**:27, 1989.
275. Winichagoon P, Higgs DR, Goodbourn SEY, Clegg JB, Weatherall DJ, Wasi P: The molecular basis of α thalassaemia in Thailand. *EMBO J* **3**:1813, 1984.
276. Beaudry MA, Ferguson DJ, Pearse K, Yanofsky RA, Rubin EM, Kan YW: Survival of a hydropic infant with homozygous α-thalassemia-1. *J Pediatr* **108**:713, 1986.
277. Bianchi DW, Beyer EC, Stark AR, Saffan D, Sachs BP, Wolfe L: Normal long-term survival with α-thalassemia. *J Pediatr* **108**:716, 1986.
278. Sharma RS, Yu V, Walters WAW: Haemoglobin Bart's hydrops fetalis syndrome in an infant of Greek origin and prenatal diagnosis of alpha-thalassaemia. *Med J Aust* **2**:433, 1979.
279. Ko T-M, Hsieh F-J, Hsu P-M, Lee T-Y: Molecular characterization of severe α-thalassemias causing hydrops fetalis in Taiwan. *Am J Med Genet* **39**:317, 1990.
280. Todd D: Personal communication.
281. Halbrecht I, Shabita F: An unusual case of hemoglobin Bart's hydrops fetalis. *Acta Genet Med Gemellol (Roma)* **24**:97, 1975.
282. Weatherall DJ, Higgs DR, Bunch C, Old JM, Hunt DM, Pressley L, Clegg JB, Bethlenfalvay NC, Sjolin S, Koler RD, Magenic E, Francis JL, Bebbington D: Hemoglobin H disease and mental retardation. A new syndrome or a remarkable coincidence? *N Engl J Med* **305**:607, 1981.
283. Wilkie AOM, Buckle VJ, Harris PC, Lamb J, Barton NJ, Reeders ST, Lindenbaum RH, Nicholls RD, Barrow M, Bethlenfalvay NC, Hutz MH, Tolmie JL, Weatherall DJ, Higgs DR: Clinical features and molecular analysis of the α thalassemia/mental retardation syndromes. I. Cases due to deletions involving chromosome band 16p13.3. *Am J Hum Genet* **46**:1112, 1990.
284. Wilkie AOM, Pembrey ME, Gibbons RJ, Higgs DR, Porteous MEM, Burn J, Winter RM: The non-deletion type of α thalassaemia/mental retardation: A recognisable dysmorphic syndrome with X linked inheritance. *J Med Genet* **28**:724, 1991.
285. Lamb J, Wilkie AOM, Harris PC, Buckle VJ, Lindenbaum RH, Barton NJ, Reeders ST, Weatherall DJ, Higgs DR: Detection of breakpoints in submicroscopic chromosomal translocation, illustrating an important mechanism for genetic disease. *Lancet* **2**:819, 1989.
286. Lamb J, Higgs DR: *De novo* truncation of chromosome 16p and healing with (TTAGGG)n in a case of α-thalassemia/mental retardation. *Am J Hum Genet* **52:**668, 1993.
287. Gibbons RJ, Wilkie AO, Weatherall DJ, Higgs DR: A newly defined X linked mental retardation syndrome associated with α thalassemia. *J Med Genet* **28**:729, 1991.
288. Donnai D, Clayton-Smith J, Gibbons RJ, Higgs DR: The non-deletion α thalassaemia/mental retardation syndrome: Further support for X linkage. *J Med Genet* **28**:742, 1991.
289. Gibbons RJ, Suthers GK, Wikie AOM, Buekle VJ, Higgs DR: X-linked α thalassemia/mental retardation (ATR-X) syndrome: Localisation to Xq12-21.31 by X-inactivation and linkage analysis. *Am J Hum Genet* **51:**1136, 1992.
290. Higgs DR, Wood WG, Barton C, Weatherall DJ: Clinical features and molecular analysis of acquired Hb H disease. *Am J Med* **75**:181, 1983.
291. Thein SL, Old JM, Wainscoat JS, Weatherall DJ: Population and genetic studies suggest a single origin for the Indian deletion β^0 thalassaemia. *Br J Haematol* **57**:271, 1984.
292. Gilman JG, Huisman THJ, Abels J: Dutch β^0-thalassaemia: A 10 kilobase DNA deletion associated with significant γ-chain production. *Br J Haematol* **56**:339, 1984.
293. Padanilam BJ, Felice AE, Huisman THJ: Partial deletion of the 5′ β globin gene region causes β^0 thalassemia in members of an American black family. *Blood* **64**:941, 1984.
294. Popovich BW, Rosenblatt DS, Kendall AG, Nishioka Y: Molecular characterization of an atypical β-thalassemia caused by a large deletion in the 5′ β-globin gene region. *Am J Hum Genet* **39**:797, 1986.
295. Diaz-Chico JC, Yang KG, Kutlar A, Reese AL, Aksoy M, Huisman THJ: A 300 bp deletion involving part of the 5′ β-globin gene region is observed in members of a Turkish family with β-thalassemia. *Blood* **70**:583, 1987.
296. Anand R, Boehm CD, Kazazian HH, Vanin EF: Molecular characterization of a β^0-thalassemia resulting from a 1.4 kb deletion. *Blood* **72**:636, 1988.
297. Aulehla-Scholtz C, Spielberg R, Horst J: A β-thalassemia mutant caused by a 300 bp deletion in the human β-globin gene. *Hum Genet* **81**:298, 1989.
298. Orkin SH, Sexton JP, Cheng TC, Goff SC, Giardina

PJV, Lee JI, Kazazian HH: ATA box transcription mutation in β-thalassemia. *Nucleic Acids Res* **11**:4727, 1983.
299. Antonarakis SE, Orkin SH, Cheng T-C, Scott AF, Sexton JP, Trusko S, Charache S, Kazazian HH: β-thalassemia in American blacks: Novel mutations in the TATA box and IVS-2 acceptor splice site. *Proc Natl Acad Sci USA* **81**:1154, 1984.
300. Gonzalez-Redondo JH, Stoming TA, Kutlar A, Kutlar F, Lanclos KD, Howard EF, Fei YJ, Aksoy M, Altay C, Gurgey A, Basak AN, Efremov GD, Petkov G, Huisman THJ: A C→T substitution at nt −101 in a conserved DNA sequence of the promoter region of the β-globin gene is associated with "silent" β-thalassemia. *Blood* **73**:1705, 1989.
301. Kazazian HH, Orkin SH, Antonarakis SE, Sexton JP, Boehm CD, Goff SC, Waber PG: Molecular characterization of seven β-thalassemia mutations in Asian Indians. *EMBO J* **3**:593, 1984.
302. Tamagnini GP, Lopes MC, Castanheira ME, Wainscoat JS, Wood WG: $β^+$ thalassaemia—Portuguese type: Clinical, haematological and molecular studies of a newly defined form of β thalassaemia. *Br J Haematol* **54**:189, 1983.
303. Cheng T, Orkin SH, Antonarakis SE, Potter MJ, Sexton JP, Markham AF, Giardina PJV, Lia A, Kazazian HH: β-thalassemia in Chinese: Use of *in vivo* RNA analysis and oligonucleotide hybridization in systematic characterization of molecular defects. *Proc Natl Acad Sci USA* **81**:2821, 1984.
304. Gonzalez-Redondo JH, Stoming TA, Lanclos KD, Gu YC, Kutlar A, Kutlar F, Nakasuji T, Deng B, Han IS, McKie VC, Huisman THJ: Clinical and genetic heterogeneity in Black patients with homozygous β-thalassemia from the Southeastern United States. *Blood* **72**:1007, 1988.
305. Hill AVS, Bowden DK, O'Shaughnessy DF, Weatherall DJ, Clegg JB: β-thalassemia in Melanesia: Association with malaria and characterization of a common variant. *Blood* **72**:9, 1988.
306. Lapoumeroulie C, Pagnier J, Bank A, Labie D, Kirshnamoorthy R: β-thalassemia due to a novel mutation in IVS-1 sequence donor site consensus sequence creating a restriction site. *Biochem Biophys Res Commun* **139**:709, 1986.
307. Goldsmith ME, Humphries RK, Bey T, Cline A, Kantor JA, Nienhuis AW: 'Silent' nucleotide substitution in $β^+$ thalassemia globin gene activated splice site in coding sequence RNA. *Proc Natl Acad Sci USA* **88**:2318, 1983.
308. Yang KG, Kutlar F, George E, Wilson JB, Kutlar A, Stoming TA, Gonzalez-Redondo JM, Huisman THJ: Molecular characterization of β-globin gene mutations in Malay patients with Hb E-β-thalassaemia major. *Br J Haematol* **72**:73, 1989.
309. Orkin SH, Antonarakis SE, Loukopoulos D: Abnormal processing of β Knossos RNA. *Blood* **64**:311, 1984.
310. Spritz RA, Jagadeeswaran P, Choudary PV, Biro PA, Elder JT, DeRiel JK, Manley JL, Gefter ML, Forget VG, Weissman SM: Base substitution in an intervening sequence of a $β^+$ thalassemic human globin gene. *Proc Natl Acad Sci USA* **78**:2455, 1981.
311. Busslinger M, Moschanas N, Flavell RA: $β^+$ thalassemia: Aberrant splicing results from a single point mutation in an intron. *Cell* **27**:289, 1981.
312. Wong C, Antonarakis SE, Goff SC, Orkin SH, Boehm CD, Kazazian HH: On the origin and spread of β-thalassemia: Recurrent observation of four mutations in different ethnic groups. *Proc Natl Acad Sci USA* **83**:6529, 1986.
313. Orkin SH, Cheng T-C, Antonarakis SE, Kazazian HH: Thalassaemia due to a mutation in the cleavage-polyadenylation signal of the human β-globin gene. *EMBO J* **4**:453, 1985.
314. Jankovic L, Efremov GD, Petkov G, Kattamis C, George E, Yang K-G, Stoming TA, Huisman THJ: Three novel mutations leading to β-thalassemia. *Blood* **74**:226A, 1989.
315. Rund D, Filon D, Rachmilewitz EA, Cohan T, Dowling C, Kazazian HH, Oppenheim A: Molecular analysis of β-thalassemia in Kurdish Jews: Novel mutations and expression studies. *Blood* **74**:821A, 1989.
316. Chang JC, Kan YW: β-thalassemia: A nonsense mutation in man. *Proc Natl Acad Sci USA* **76**:2886, 1979.
317. Trecartin RF, Liebhaber SA, Chang JC, Lee KY, Kan YW, Furbetta M, Angius A, Cao A: β thalassemia in Sardinia is caused by a nonsense mutation. *J Clin Invest* **68**:1012, 1981.
318. Takeshita K, Forget BG, Scarpa A, Benz EJ: Intranuclear defect in β globin mRNA accumulation to a premature termination codon. *Blood* **64**:13, 1984.
319. Thein SL, Hesketh C, Taylor P, Temperley P, Hutchison RM, Old JM, Wood WG, Clegg JB, Weatherall DJ: Molecular basis for dominantly inherited inclusion body β thalassemia. *Proc Natl Acad Sci USA* **87**:3924, 1990.
320. Kazazian HH, Dowling CE, Hurwitz RL, Coleman M, Adams JG: Thalassemia mutations in exon 3 of the β-globin gene often cause a dominant form of thalassemia and show no predilection for malarial-endemic regions of the world. *Am J Hum Genet* **45**:A242, 1989.
321. Weatherall DJ, Clegg JB, Knox-Macaulay HHM, Bunch C, Hopkins CR, Temperley IJ: A genetically determined disorder with features both of thalassaemia and congenital dyserythropoietic anaemia. *Br J Haematol* **24**:681, 1973.
322. Stamatoyannopoulos G, Woodson R, Papayannopoulou T, Heywood D, Kurachi MS: A form of β thalassemia producing clinical manifestations in simple heterozygotes. *N Engl J Med* **290**:939, 1974.
323. Poncz M, Henthorn P, Stoeckert C, Surrey S: Globin gene expression in hereditary persistence of fetal haemoglobin and $(δβ)^0$-thalassaemia, in Maclean N (ed): *Oxford Surveys on Eukaryotic Genes*. Oxford, Oxford University Press, 1988, p 163.
324. Bollekens JA, Forget BG: δβ thalassemia and hereditary persistence of fetal hemoglobin. *Hematol Oncol Clin North Am* **5**:399, 1991.
325. Ottolenghi S, Giglioni B, Taramelli R, Comi P, Mazza U, Saglio G, Camaschella C, Izzo P, Cao A, Galanello R, Gimferrer E, Baiget M, Gianni AM: Molecular comparison of δβ-thalassemia and hereditary persistence of fetal hemoglobin DNAs: Evidence of a regulatory area. *Proc Natl Acad Sci USA* **79**:2347, 1982.
326. Jones RW, Old JM, Trent RJ, Clegg JB, Weatherall DJ: Major rearrangement in the human β-globin gene cluster. *Nature* **291**:39, 1981.
327. Jennings MW, Jones RW, Wood WG, Weatherall DJ: Analysis of an inversion within the human beta globin gene cluster. *Nucleic Acids Res* **13**:2897, 1985.
328. Kutlar A, Gardiner MB, Headlee MG, Reese AL, Cleek MP, Nagle S, Sukumaran PK, Huisman THJ: Heterogeneity in the molecular basis of three types of hereditary persistence of fetal hemoglobin and the relative synthesis of the $^Gγ$ and $^Aγ$ types of γ chain. *Biochem Genet* **22**:21, 1984.
329. Wainscoat JS, Old JM, Wood WG, Trent RJ, Weatherall DJ: Characterization of an Indian $(δβ)^0$ thalassaemia. *Br J Haematol* **58**:353, 1984.
330. Van Der Ploeg LHT, Konings A, Cort M, Roos D, Bernini L, Flavell RA: γ-β-thalassaemia studies showing that deletion of the γ- and δ-genes influence β-globin gene expression in man. *Nature* **283**:637, 1980.
331. Taramelli R, Kioussis D, Vanin E, Bartram K, Groffen J, Hurst J, Grosveld FG: γδβ-thalassaemia 1 and 2 are the result of a 100 kbp deletion in the human β-globin cluster. *Nucleic Acids Res* **14**:7017, 1986.
332. Curtin P, Pirastu M, Kan YW, Gobert-Jones JA, Stephens AD, Lehmann H: A distant gene deletion affects β-globin gene function in an atypical γδβ-thalassemia. *J Clin Invest* **76**:1554, 1985.
333. Weatherall DJ: The regulation of the differential expression of the human globin genes during development. *J Cell Sci* **4**:319, 1986.
334. Wainscoat JS, Thein SL, Wood WG, Weatherall DJ, Tzotos S, Kanavakis E, Metaxatou-Mavromati A, Kattamis C: A novel deletion in the β globin gene complex. *Ann NY Acad Sci* **445**:20, 1985.
335. Bernards R, Flavell RA: Physical mapping of the globin gene deletion in hereditary persistence of foetal haemoglobin. *Nucleic Acids Res* **8**:1521, 1980.
336. Collins FS, Stoeckert CJ, Serjeant GR, Forget BG, Weissman SM: $^Gγβ^+$ hereditary persistence of fetal hemoglobin: Cosmid cloning and identification of a specific mutation 5′ to the $^Gγ$ gene. *Proc Natl Acad Sci USA* **81**:4894, 1984.
337. Giglioni B, Casini C, Mantovani R, Merli S, Comi P,

Ottolenghi S, Saglio G, Camaschella C, Mazza U: A molecular study of a family with Greek hereditary persistence of fetal hemoglobin and β-thalassemia. *EMBO J* **3**:2641, 1984.

338. Collins FS, Metherall JE, Yamakawa M, Pan J, Weissman SM, Forget BG: A point mutation in the $^A\gamma$-globin gene promoter in Greek hereditary persistence of fetal haemoglobin. *Nature* **313**:325, 1985.
339. Gelinas R, Endlich B, Pfeiffer C, Yagi M, Stamatoyannopoulos G: G to A substitution in the distal CCAAT box of the $^A\gamma$-globin gene in Greek hereditary persistence of fetal haemoglobin. *Nature* **313**:323, 1985.
340. Tate VE, Wood WG, Weatherall DJ: The British form of hereditary persistence of fetal haemoglobin results from a single base mutation adjacent to an S1 hypersensitive site 5′ to the $^A\gamma$ globin gene. *Blood* **68**:1389, 1986.
341. Ottolenghi S, Giglioni B, Pulazzini A, Comi P, Camaschella C, Serra A, Guerrasio A, Saglio G: Sardinian $\delta\beta^0$-thalassemia: A further example of a C to T substitution at position −196 of the $^A\gamma$ globin gene cluster. *Blood* **69**:1058, 1987.
342. Kulozik A, Yarwood N, Jones RW: The Corfu $\delta\beta^0$ thalassemia: A small deletion acts at a distance to selectively abolish β globin gene expression. *Blood* **71**:457, 1988.
343. Wainscoat JS, Thein SL, Weatherall DJ: Thalassaemia intermedia. *Blood Rev* **1**:273, 1987.
344. Kattamis C, Metaxatou-Mavromati A, Wood WG, Nash JR, Weatherall DJ: The heterogeneity of normal Hb A_2-β thalassaemia in Greece. *Br J Haematol* **42**:109, 1979.
345. Fessas P, Loukopoulos D, Loutradi-Anagnostou A, Komes G: 'Silent' β thalassemia caused by a 'silent' β chain mutant: The pathogenesis of a syndrome of thalassemia intermedia. *Br J Haematol* **51**:577, 1982.
346. Olds RJ, Sura T, Jackson B, Wonke B, Hoffbrand AV, Thein SL: A novel δ^0 mutation in *cis* with Hb Knossos: A study of different interactions in three Egyptian families. *Br J Haematol* **78**:430, 1991.
347. Pirastu M, Ristaldi MS, Loudianos G, Murru S, Sciarratta GV, Parodi MI, Leone D, Agosti S, Cao A: Molecular analysis of atypical β-thalassemia heterozygotes. *Ann NY Acad Sci* **612**:90, 1990.
348. Fearon EF, Kazazian HH, Waber PG, Lee JI, Antonarakis E, Orkin SH, Vanin EF, Henthron PA, Grosveld FG, Scott F, Buchanan GR: The entire β-globin gene cluster is deleted in a form of γδβ-thalassemia. *Blood* **61**:1269, 1983.
349. Pirastu M, Kan YW, Lin CC, Baine R, Holbrook CT: Hemolytic disease of the newborn caused by a new deletion of the entire β-globin cluster. *J Clin Invest* **72**:602, 1983.
350. Orkin SH, Goff SC, Nathan DG: Heterogeneity of DNA deletion in γδβ-thalassemia. *J Clin Invest* **67**:878, 1981.
351. Kan YW, Forget BG, Nathan DG: Gamma-beta thalassemia: A cause of hemolytic disease of the newborn. *N Engl J Med* **286**:129, 1972.
352. Sampietro M, Cazzola M, Cappellini MD, Fiorelli G: The triplicated alpha-gene locus and heterozygous beta thalassaemia: A case of thalassaemia intermedia. *Br J Haematol* **55**:709, 1983.
353. Kulozik AE, Thein SL, Wainscoat JS, Gale R, Kaye L, Weatherall DJ, Wood JK, Huenhs ER: Thalassaemia intermedia; interaction of the triple α-globin gene arrangement and heterozygous β-thalassaemia. *Br J Haematol* **66**:109, 1987.
354. Camaschella C, Bertero MT, Serra A, DAII'Acqua M, Gasparini P, Trento M, Vettore L, Perona G, Saglio G, Mazza U: A benign form of thalassaemia intermedia may be determined by the interaction of triplicated α locus and heterozygous β thalassaemia. *Br J Haematol* **66**:103, 1987.
355. Efremov GD: Hemoglobins Lepore and anti-Lepore. *Hemoglobin* **2**:197, 1978.
356. Wood WG, Clegg JB, Weatherall DJ: Hereditary persistence of fetal haemoglobin (HPFH) and δβ-thalassaemia. *Br J Haematol* **43**:509, 1979.
357. Trent RJ, Jones RW, Clegg JB, Weatherall DJ: $(^A\gamma\delta\beta)^0$ thalassaemia: Similarity of phenotype in four different molecular defects, including one newly described. *Br J Haematol* **57**:279, 1984.
358. Kendall AG, Ojwang PJ, Schroeder WA, Huisman THJ: Hemoglobin Kenya, the product of a γ-β fusion gene: Studies of the family. *Am J Hum Genet* **25**:548, 1973.
359. Smith DH, Clegg JB, Weatherall DJ, Gilles HM: Hereditary persistence of foetal haemoglobin associated with a γβ fusion variant, Haemoglobin Kenya. *Nature New Biol* **246**:184, 1973.
360. Nute PE, Wood WG, Stamatoyannopoulos G, Olweny C, Fialkow PJ: The Kenya form of hereditary persistence of fetal haemoglobin; structural studies and evidence for homogeneous distribution of haemoglobin F using fluorescent anti-haemoglobin F antibodies. *Br J Haematol* **32**:55, 1976.
361. Huisman THJ, Miller A, Schroeder WA: $^G\gamma$ type of the hereditary persistence of fetal hemoglobin with β chain production in *cis*. *Am J Hum Genet* **27**:765, 1975.
362. Friedman S, Schwartz E: Hereditary persistence of foetal haemoglobin with β-chain synthesis in *cis* position ($^G\gamma$-β^+-HPFH) in a negro family. *Nature* **259**:138, 1976.
363. Higgs DR, Clegg JB, Wood WG, Weatherall DJ: $^G\gamma\beta^+$ type of hereditary persistence of fetal haemoglobin in association with Hb C. *J Med Genet* **16**:288, 1979.
364. Fessas P, Stamatoyannopoulos G: Hereditary persistence of fetal hemoglobin in Greece. A study and a comparison. *Blood* **24**:223, 1964.
365. Clegg JB, Metaxatou-Mavromati A, Kattamis C, Sofroniadou K, Wood WG, Weatherall DJ: Occurrence of $^G\gamma$ Hb F in Greek HPFH: Analysis of heterozygotes and compound heterozygotes with β thalassaemia. *Br J Haematol* **43**:521, 1979.
366. Camaschella C, Oggiano L, Sampietro M, Gottardi E, Alfarano A, Pistidda P, Dore F, Taramelli R, Ottolenghi S, Longinotti M: The homozygous state of G to A −117 $^A\gamma$ hereditary persistence of fetal hemoglobin. *Blood* **73**:1999, 1989.
367. Weatherall DJ, Cartner R, Clegg JB, Wood WG, Macrae I, Mackenzie A: A form of hereditary persistence of fetal haemoglobin characterised by uneven cellular distribution of haemoglobin F and the production of haemoglobins A and A_2 in homozygotes. *Br J Haematol* **29**:205, 1975.
368. Wood WG, Macrae IA, Darbre PD, Clegg JB, Weatherall DJ: The British type of non-deletion HPFH: Characterisation of developmental changes *in vivo* and erythroid growth *in vitro*. *Br J Haematol* **50**:401, 1982.
369. Marti HR: *Normale und abnormale menschliche Haemoglobine*. Berlin, Springer-Verlag, 1963.
370. Zago MA, Wood WG, Clegg JB, Weatherall DJ, O'Sullivan M, Gunson HH: Genetic control of F-cells in human adults. *Blood* **53**:977, 1979.
371. Miyoshi K, Kaneto Y, Kawai H, Huisman THJ: X-linked dominant control of F-cells in normal adult life. *Blood* **72**:1854, 1988.
372. Cappellini MD, Fiorelli G, Bernini LF: Interaction between homozygous β^0 thalassaemia and the Swiss type of hereditary persistence of fetal haemoglobin. *Br J Haematol* **48**:561, 1981.
373. Jeffreys AJ, Wilson V, Thein SL, Weatherall DJ, Ponder BAJ: DNA "fingerprints" and segregation analysis of multiple markers in human pedigrees. *Am J Hum Genet* **39**:11, 1986.
374. Gilman JG, Huisman THJ: DNA sequence variation associated with elevated fetal $^G\gamma$ globin production. *Blood* **66**:783, 1985.
375. Thein SL, Sampietro M, Old JM, Cappellini MD, Fiorelli G, Modell B, Weatherall DJ: Association of thalassaemia intermedia with a beta-globin gene haplotype. *Br J Haematol* **65**:370, 1987.
376. Thein SL, Hesketh C, Wallace RB, Weatherall DJ: The molecular basis of thalassaemia major and thalassaemia intermedia in Asian Indians: Application to prenatal diagnosis. *Br J Haematol* **70**:225, 1988.
377. Diaz-Chico JC, Yang KG, Stoming TA, Efremov DG, Kutlar A, Kutlar F, Aksoy N, Altay C, Gurgey A, Kilinc Y, Huisman THJ: Mild and severe β-thalassaemia among homozygotes from Turkey: Identification of the types by hybridization of amplified DNA with synthetic probes. *Blood* **71**:248, 1988.
378. Kulozik AE, Wainscoat JS, Serjeant GR, Al-Awamy

B, Essan F, Falusi Y, Haque SK, Hilali AM, Kate S, Sanasinghe WAEP, Weatherall DJ: Geographical survey of β^S-globin gene haplotypes: Evidence for an independent Asian origin of the sickle-cell mutation. *Am J Hum Genet* **39**:239, 1986.

379. Nagel RL, Fabry ME, Pagnier J, Zohoun I, Wajcman H, Baudin V, Labie D: Hematologically and genetically distinct forms of sickle cell anemia in Africa. *N Engl J Med* **312**:880, 1985.
380. Labie D, Dunda-Belkhodja O, Rouabhi F, Pagnier J, Ragusa A, Nagel RL: The − 158 site 5′ to the $^G\gamma$ gene and $^G\gamma$ expression. *Blood* **66**:1463, 1987.
381. Kulozik AE, Kar BC, Satapathy RK, Serjeant BE, Serjeant GR, Weatherall DJ: Fetal hemoglobin levels and β^S globin haplotypes in an Indian population with sickle cell disease. *Blood* **69**:1742, 1987.
382. Kulozik AE, Thein SL, Kar BC, Wainscoat JS, Serjeant GR, Weatherall DJ: Raised HB F levels in sickle cell disease are caused by a determinant linked to the β globin gene cluster, in Stamatoyannopoulos G (ed): *Hemoglobin Switching*. New York, Alan R. Liss, 1987, p 427.
383. Oner C, Dimovski AJ, Altay C, Gurgey A, Gu YC, Huisman THJ, Lanclos KD: Sequence variations in the 5′ hypervariable site-2 of the locus control region of β^S chromosomes are associated with different levels of fetal globin in hemoglobin S homozygotes. *Blood* **79**:813, 1992.
384. Wainscoat JS, Kanavakis E, Wood WG, Letsky EA, Huehns ER, Marsh GW, Higgs DR, Clegg JB, Weatherall DJ: Thalassaemia intermedia in Cyprus—the interaction of α- and β-thalassaemia. *Br J Haematol* **53**:411, 1983.
385. Wainscoat JS, Bell JI, Old JM, Weatherall DJ, Furbetta M, Galanello R, Cao A: Globin gene mapping studies in Sardinian patients homozygous for β^0 thalassaemia. *Mol Biol Med* **1**:1, 1983.
386. Kanavakis E, Wainscoat JS, Wood WG, Weatherall DJ, Cao A, Furbetta M, Galanello R, Georgiou D, Sophocleous T: The interaction of α thalassaemia with heterozygous β thalassaemia. *Br J Haematol* **52**:465, 19982.
387. Rosatelli C, Falchi AM, Scalas MT, Tuveri T, Furbetta M, Cao A: Hematological phenotype of double heterozygous state for alpha and beta thalassemia. *Hemoglobin* **8**:25, 1984.
388. Kanavakis E, Metaxatous-Mavromati A, Kattamis C, Wainscoat JS, Wood WG: The triplicated α gene locus and β thalassaemia. *Br J Haematol* **54**:201, 1983.
389. Sampietro M, Cazzola M, Cappellini MD, Fiorelli G: The triplicated alpha-gene locus and heterozygous beta thalassaemia: A case of thalassaemia intermedia. *Br J Haematol* **55**:709, 1983.
390. Kulozik AE, Thein SL, Wainscoat JS, Gale R, Kaye L, Weatherall DJ, Wood JK, Huenhs ER: Thalassaemia intermedia; interaction of the triple α-globin gene arrangement and heterozygous β-thalassaemia. *Br J Haematol* **66**:109, 1987.
391. Acuto S, Buttice G, Saitta B, Pirrone AM, Gambino R, Costa C, Giambina A, Lo Gioco P, Di Marzo R, Maggio A: $\alpha\alpha\alpha^{anti\ 4.2}$ haplotype and heterozygous β^0 thalassemia in a Sicilian family. *Hum Genet* **70**:31, 1985.
392. Galanello R, Ruggeri R, Paglietti E, Addis M, Melis A, Cao A: A family with segregating triplicated alpha globin loci and beta thalassemia. *Blood* **62**:1035, 1983.
393. Thein SL, Al-Hakin I, Hoffbrand AV: Thalassaemia intermedia—a new molecular basis. *Br J Haematol* **56**:333, 1984.
394. Livingstone FB: *Frequencies of Hemoglobin Variants*. New York, Oxford University Press, 1985.
395. Kan YW, Dozy AM: Evolution of the hemoglobin S and C genes in world populations. *Science* **209**:388, 1980.
396. Mears JG, Lachman HM: Sickle gene: Its origin and diffusion from West Africa. *J Clin Invest* **68**:606, 1981.
397. Antonarakis SE, Boehm CD, Serjeant GR, Theisen CE, Dover GJ, Kazazian HH: Origin of the β^S-globin gene in blacks: The contribution of recurrent mutation or gene conversion or both. *Proc Natl Acad Sci USA* **81**:853, 1984.
398. Wainscoat JS, Bell JI, Thein SL, Higgs DR, Serjeant GR, Peto TEA, Weatherall DJ: Multiple origins of the sickle mutation: Evidence from β^S globin gene cluster polymorphisms. *Mol Biol Med* **1**:191, 1983.
399. Kulozik AE, Wainscoat JS, Serjeant GR, Al-Awamy B, Essan F, Falusi Y, Haque SK, Hilali AM, Kate S, Sanasinghe WAEP, Weatherall DJ: Geographical survey of β^S-globin gene haplotypes: Evidence for an independent Asian origin of the sickle-cell mutation. *Am J Hum Genet* **39**:239, 1986.
400. Kazazian HH, Waber PG, Boehm CD, Lee JI, Antonarakis SE, Fairbank VF: Hemoglobin E in Europeans—further evidence for multiple origins of the beta-E-globin gene. *Am J Hum Genet* **36**:212, 1984.
401. Haldane JBS: The rate of mutation of human genes, in Proceedings of the VIII International Congress of Genetics and Heredity, 1949, p 367.
402. Allison AC: Protection afforded by sickle cell trait against subtertian malarial infection. *Br Med J* **1**:290, 1954.
403. Fleming AF, Storey J, Molineaux L, Iroko EA, Attai EDE: Abnormal haemoglobins in the Sudan savanna of Nigeria. I. Prevalence of haemoglobins and relationships between sickle cell trait, malaria and survival. *Ann Trop Med Parasitol* **73**:161, 1979.

403a. Hill AVS, Allsopp CEM, Kwiatkowski D, Anstey NM, Twumasi P, Rowe PA, Bennett S, Brewster D, McMichael AJ, Greenwood BM: Common west African HLA antigens are associated with protection from severe malaria. *Nature* **352**:595, 1991.

404. Luzzatto L, Nwachuku ES, Reddy S: Increased sickling of parasitized erythrocytes is mechanism of resistance against malaria in the sickle trait. *Lancet* **1**:319, 1970.
405. Pasvol G, Weatherall DJ: A mechanism for the protective effect of haemoglobin S against *P. falciparum* malaria. *Nature* **274**:701, 1978.
406. Friedman MJ, Roth EF, Nagel RL, Trager W: *Plasmodium falciparum:* Physiological interactions with the human sickle cell. *Exp Parasitol* **47**:73, 1979.
407. Orkin SH, Antonarakis SE, Kazazian HH: Polymorphisms and molecular pathology of the human β-globin gene. *Prog Hematol* **13**:49, 1983.
408. Orkin SH, Kazazian HH: The mutation and polymorphism of the human β-globin gene and its surrounding DNA. *Annu Rev Genet* **18**:131, 1984.
409. Pressley L, Higgs DR, Clegg JB, Weatherall DJ: Gene deletions in an α thalassemia prove that the 5′ ζ locus is functional. *Proc Natl Acad Sci USA* **77**:3586, 1980.
410. Siniscalco M, Bernini L, Filippi G, Latte B, Khan M, Piomelli S, Rattazzi M: Population genetics of haemoglobin variants, thalassemia and glucose-6-phosphate dehydrogenase deficiency, with particular reference to malaria hypothesis. *Bull World Health Organ* **34**:379, 1966.
411. Flint J, Hill AVS, Weatherall DJ, Clegg JB, Higgs DR: Alpha globin genotypes in two North European populations. *Br J Haematol* **63**:796, 1986.
412. Pasvol G, Wilson RJM: The interaction of malaria parasites with red blood cells. *Br Med Bull* **38**:133, 1982.
413. Luzzi GA, Merry AH, Newbold CI, Marsh K, Pasvol G, Weatherall DJ: Surface antigen expression on *Plasmodium falciparum*-infected erythrocytes is modified in α- and β-thalassaemia. *J Exp Med* **173**:785, 1991.
414. Weatherall DJ: *Methods in Hematology. The Thalassemias*. Edinburgh, Churchill Livingstone, 1983.
415. Piomelli S, Lowe T: Management of thalassemia major (Cooley's anemia). *Hematol Oncol Clin North Am* **5**:557, 1991.
416. Davies SC, Brozovic M: The presentation, management and prophylaxis of sickle cell disease. *Blood Rev* **3**:29, 1989.
417. Weatherall DJ: Prenatal diagnosis of inherited blood diseases. *Clin Haematol* **14**:747, 1985.
418. Stamatoyannopoulos G: Problems of screening and counselling in the hemoglobinopathies, in Proceedings of the IV International Conference on Birth Defects, Vienna, 1973.

418a. Scriver CR, Bardanis M, Cartier L, Clow CL, Lancaster GA, Ostrowsky JT: β-Thalassemia disease prevention: Genetic medicine applied. *Am J Hum Genet* **36**:1024, 1984.

419. Weatherall DJ: Prenatal diagnosis of haematological disease, in Hann IM, Gibson BES, Letsky EA (eds): *Fetal and Neonatal Haematology*. London, Baillière Tindall, 1991, p 285.
420. Cao A, Rosatelli MC, Battista G, Tuveri T, Scalas MT,

Monni G, Olla G, Galanello R: Antenatal diagnosis of β-thalassemia in Sardinia. *Ann NY Acad Sci* **612**:215, 1990.
421. Loukopoulos D, Hadji A, Papadakis M, Karababa P, Sinopoulou K, Boussiou M, Kollia P, Xenakis M, Antsaklis A, Mesoghitis S, Loutradi A, Fessas P: Prenatal diagnosis of thalassemia and of the sickle cell syndromes in Greece. *Ann NY Acad Sci* **612**:226, 1990.
422. Alter BP: Antenatal diagnosis: Summary of results. *Ann NY Acad Sci* **612**:237, 1990.
423. Old JM, Fitches A, Heath C, Thein SL, Weatherall DJ, Warren R, McKenzie C, Rodeck CH, Modell B, Petrou M, Ward RHT: First trimester fetal diagnosis for haemoglobinopathies: Report on 200 cases. *Lancet* **2**:763, 1986.
424. Kazazian HH, Phillips JAI, Boehm CD, Vik T, Mahoney MJ, Ritchey AK: Prenatal diagnosis of β-thalassemia by amniocentesis: Linkage analysis of multiple polymorphic restriction endonuclease sites. *Blood* **56**:926, 1980.
425. Pirastu M, Kan YW, Cao A, Conner BJ, Teplitz RL, Wallace RB: Prenatal diagnosis of β-thalassemia: Detection of a single nucleotide mutation in DNA. *N Engl J Med* **309**:284, 1983.
426. Chehab F, Doherty M, Cai S, Cooper S, Rubin E: Detection of sickle cell anaemia and thalassaemia. *Nature* **329**:293, 1987.
427. Saiki RK, Chang C-A, Levenson CH, Warren TC, Boehm CD, Kazazian HH, Erlich HA: Diagnosis of sickle cell anemia and β-thalassemia with enzymatically amplified DNA and non-radioactive allele-specific oligonucleotide probes. *N Engl J Med* **319**:537, 1988.
428. Cai SP, Chang CA, Zhang JZ, Saiki RK, Erlich HA, Kan YW: Rapid prenatal diagnosis of β-thalassemia using DNA amplification and nonradioactive probes. *Blood* **73**:372, 1989.
429. Saiki RK, Walsh PS, Levenson CH, Erlich HA: Genetic analysis of amplified DNA with immobilized sequence-specific oligonucleotide probes. *Proc Natl Acad Sci USA* **86**:6230, 1989.
430. Old JM, Varawalla NY, Weatherall DJ: The rapid detection and prenatal diagnosis of β-thalassaemia in the Asian Indian and Cypriot populations in the UK. *Lancet* **336**:834, 1990.
431. Lucarelli G, Galimberti M, Polchi P, Angelucci E, Baronciani D, Durazzi SMT, Giardini C, Nicolini G, Politi P, Albertini F: Bone marrow transplantation in thalassemia. *Hematol Oncol Clin North Am* **5**:549, 1991.
432. Kirkpatrick DV, Barrios NJ, Humbert JH: Bone marrow transplantation for sickle cell anemia. *Semin Hematol* **28**:240, 1991.
433. Ley TJ: The pharmacology of hemoglobin switching: Of mice and men. *Blood* **77**:1146, 1991.
434. Hesdorffer C, Markowitz D, Ward M, Bank A: Somatic gene therapy. *Hematol Oncol Clin north Am* **5**:423, 1991.
435. Weatherall DJ: Gene therapy in perspective. *Nature* **349**:275, 1991.
436. Miller AD: Human gene therapy comes of age. *Nature* **357**:455, 1992.
437. Onita M, Sekiya T, Hayashi K: DNA sequence polymorphisms in Alu repeats. *Genomics* **8**:271, 1990.
438. Economou EP, Bergen AW, Warren AC, Antonarakis SE: The polyadenylate tract of Alu repetitive elements is polymorphic in the human genome. *Proc Natl Acad Sci USA* **87**:2950, 1990.

CHAPTER **114**

Pyruvate Kinase and Other Enzymopathies of the Erythrocyte

Kouichi R. Tanaka ▪ Donald E. Paglia

1. Pyruvate kinase (PK) deficiency is the most common enzymopathy of anaerobic glycolysis resulting in hereditary hemolytic anemia. The disorder occurs worldwide and is characterized clinically by lifelong chronic hemolysis of variable severity. Splenectomy often results in amelioration of the hemolytic process in more severely affected patients, but is less effective, if at all, in milder cases. Defective PK catalysis in affected erythrocytes generally results in elevated concentrations of 2,3-diphosphoglycerate (2,3-DPG) and decreased ATP, relative to cells of comparable age. Changes in the ATP:2,3-DPG ratio aid in the diagnosis, but confirmation depends on quantitative in vitro assays of erythrocyte PK.

2. PK deficiency is inherited as an autosomal recessive disorder. Heterozygous carriers usually display 40 to 60 percent of the PK activity found in normal red cells, but they are devoid of significant hematologic or clinical abnormalities. In the absence of consanguinity, clinically affected individuals are usually compound heterozygotes for two mutant alleles, often resulting in intracellular mixtures of defective PK isoenzymes, which complicates interpretation of biochemical data. Genes encoding the principal natural isoenzymes of human PK have been identified, as have several specific mutations resulting in hemolytic anemia.

3. Severe deficiencies of hexokinase, glucosephosphate isomerase (GPI), phosphofructokinase (PFK), aldolase, triosephosphate isomerase (TPI), phosphoglycerate kinase (PGK), diphosphoglycerate mutase (DPGM), diphosphoglycerate phosphatase, and lactate dehydrogenase (LDH) have also been identified. Partial deficiency of enolase has been reported. All are recessively transmitted except for PGK, which is X-linked, and enolase, which appears to be dominantly inherited. The gene for each enzyme has been cloned, except for GPI, and mutations have been identified for most. Deficiencies of DPGM and diphosphoglycerate phosphatase are associated with mild erythrocytosis secondary to virtual absence of 2,3-DPG. LDH deficiency is also not associated with hemolysis, but in one form there is myopathy. All others are associated with hemolytic anemia of variable severity with partial response to splenectomy, except for PFK deficiency, which usually has a compensated hemolytic process.

4. Hexokinase deficiency is rare, but genetic polymorphism is the rule. GPI deficiency is second to PK deficiency in frequency; all tissues have decreased GPI activity, but clinical manifestations are usually limited to a chronic hemolytic process, though in some instances mental retardation and myopathy may occur. In PFK deficiency (glycogen storage disease type VII), clinical hallmarks are male predominance with early-onset gout, compensated hemolytic process, and prominent myopathy. Severe deficiency of aldolase activity has been documented in only three patients.

5. TPI deficiency is the most severe of the enzymatic defects of the glycolytic pathway; it is characterized by multisystem disease, including progressive neurologic dysfunction, increased susceptibility to infections, cardiomyopathy, and death usually during early childhood. All body tissues investigated are deficient in TPI. PGK deficiency in hemizygous males most frequently is accompanied by hemolytic anemia and a variety of neurologic abnormalities; the phenotypic picture is variable. Heterozygous females may exhibit only hemolytic anemia of variable degree depending on random X inactivation.

6. Enzyme deficiencies involving the pentose phosphate shunt and associated glutathione metabolism are documented. Severe deficiency of 6-phosphogluconate dehydrogenase is rare, is not associated with hemolysis, and is inherited as an autosomal dominant mutation. Partial deficiency of glutathione peroxidase has been reported in association with hemolytic syndromes but requires additional evaluation, since half-normal activity is observed in healthy subjects in certain ethnic groups. Most reported instances of glutathione reductase deficiency have proved to be secondary to inadequate flavin cofactor. A single kindred with severe apoenzyme deficiency demonstrated episodes of hemolysis associated with fava bean ingestion and possible cataracts in affected members.

7. Rare, autosomal recessive deficiency of γ-glutamylcysteine synthetase is manifested by a virtual lack of red-cell glutathione and moderate hemolytic anemia with neurologic features in some cases. Deficiency of the second enzyme of glutathione synthesis, glutathione synthetase, presents as two phenotypes. The first exhibits hemolytic

A list of standard abbreviations is located immediately preceding the index in each volume. Additional abbreviations used in this chapter include: AK-1 = adenylate kinase 1; 2,3-DPG = 2,3-diphosphoglycerate; DPGM = diphosphoglycerate mutase; F-1,6-P_2 = fructose 1,6-diphosphate; GPI = glucosephosphate isomerase; HMP = hexose monophosphate (shunt); PEP = phospho*eno*/pyruvate; PFK = phosphofructokinase; PGK = phosphoglycerate kinase; PK = pyruvate kinase; TPI = triosephosphate isomerase.

anemia alone; the second, presumably due to a generalized deficiency of the enzyme, is characterized by multisystem disease with metabolic acidosis, massive 5-oxoprolinuria and often neurologic dysfunction accompanying a hemolytic syndrome.

8. **Disturbances in erythrocyte nucleotide metabolism that are clearly associated with shortened red-cell life span and hemolytic anemia of variable severity include (1) overproduction of biochemically normal adenosine deaminase and (2) severe deficiency of pyrimidine nucleotidase. Overproduction of adenosine deaminase is a dominantly inherited disorder characterized by decreases in total erythrocyte adenine nucleotides (less than half-normal values), elevations in pyrimidine nucleotidase activity (three- to fourfold), and approximately one-hundred-fold elevations in adenosine deaminase activity. Severe deficiency of pyrimidine nucleotidase is inherited as an autosomal recessive disorder or is acquired secondary to lead toxicity. It is characterized by ineffective clearance of RNA degradation products from maturing reticulocytes with consequent accumulation of diverse pyrimidine conjugates and ribonucleotides, prominent basophilic stippling, two-fold increased concentrations of erythrocyte glutathione, and intermediate (25 percent) reductions in ribose-phosphate pyrophosphokinase activity.**

9. **Adenylate kinase deficiency, previously thought to induce hemolytic anemia, may not do so without certain coexistent abnormalities, since a severe deficiency state (<0.1 percent of normal mean) has been observed with no adverse hematologic effects.**

10. **Erythrocyte enzymopathies may also have hematologic expression other than hemolysis, may have no obvious deleterious consequences, or may be associated with clinical disorders affecting other than hematopoietic tissue.**

The phylogeny of erythrocytes can be traced from hemolymph solutions of primitive respiratory pigments, to discrete globules of hemerythrin circulating within closed vascular systems, culminating finally in the pliable biconcave capsules of hemoglobin that are characteristic of most upper vertebrates and mammals.[1] In humans, the result of this evolutionary process is a plasma membrane enveloping a nearly saturated, highly viscous solution of hemoglobin. These cells are devoid of nuclei and cytoplasmic organelles, simplifying their physiology but simultaneously restricting their metabolic capacities and their ability to adapt to changing environmental conditions.

Unique molecular properties of tetrameric hemoglobin allow it to mediate gas transport and exchange without expending energy. However, maintenance of membrane plasticity depends on an adequate source of high-energy phosphate, specifically ATP, which is also necessary for a number of other essential cell functions. These include maintenance of cation fluxes in opposition to electrochemical gradients, preservation or generation of membrane components and intracellular nucleotides, synthesis of glutathione, and initiation and maintenance of glycolysis itself. In addition, reducing energy is required to preserve the functional valence of hemoglobin iron and to protect enzyme and structural proteins, as well as hemoglobin itself, from irreversible oxidative denaturation.

These energy requirements are fulfilled almost entirely by catabolism of plasma glucose, with the consequent generation and storage of high-energy phosphates, principally ATP, or as reducing equivalents in the form of glutathione (GSH) and pyridine nucleotides (NADH and NADPH).[2-4] Figure 114-1 summarizes these principal metabolic pathways. Glucose is assimilated by facilitated transport and phosphorylated at the 6-carbon position by hexokinase, providing a common substrate for either anaerobic glycolysis through the Embden-Meyerhof pathway or for oxidative glycolysis via the hexose monophosphate (HMP) shunt. Normally, anaerobic glycolysis predominates by a factor of nearly 10, but that ratio can be reversed by oxidant stimulation of HMP shunt activity.

Key features of anaerobic glycolysis that are pertinent to consideration of erythroenzymopathies are discussed below:

Kinase-mediated reactions, principally phosphofructokinase, hexokinase, and pyruvate kinase (PK), are the principal rate limiting steps, and these are sensitive to a multitude of feedback regulators, including substrates, products, cofactors, intermediates, and electrolyte and hydrogen ion concentrations.

Fixation of inorganic phosphate occurs at the glyceraldehyde 3-phosphate dehydrogenase step, allowing generation and subsequent transfer of a high-energy phosphate to ADP. This permits a maximal net gain of two molecules of ATP for every one of catabolized glucose.

The 1,3-phosphodiester can revert to a low-energy state by mutation to 2,3-diphosphoglycerate (2,3-DPG), which comprises half to two-thirds of all organic phosphates in the erythrocyte and has an important regulatory influence on hemoglobin oxygen affinity.[5] Diversion through this pathway (the Rapoport-Luebering shunt)[6] bypasses an ATP-generating step but simultaneously contributes to a large reservoir of potential substrate for PK, thus providing a sensitive regulator to optimize ATP:ADP ratios.

The pyridine nucleotide (NAD^+/NADH) cycled by anaerobic glycolysis is an essential cofactor in methemoglobin reduction via cytochrome b_5 reductase.

Pertinent features of oxidative glycolysis include the following:

HMP shunt activity serves to maintain high concentrations of reduced GSH, a cysteine-containing tripeptide with a very low oxidation potential, allowing it to protect other cellular proteins from oxidant damage by serving as a sacrificial reductant.

$NADP^+$ is the obligate cofactor for each dehydrogenase reaction in the shunt, and the $NADP^+$:NADPH ratio provides the principal regulator of glucose catabolism via this pathway. HMP shunt activity can be stimulated twenty- to thirty-fold or more in response to oxidant challenge.

Glucose is oxidized at the 1-carbon position, generating CO_2 and ribulose 5-phosphate. The latter can be modified and recombined into two intermediates of anaerobic glycolysis by sequential actions of pentose epimerase, isomerase, transketolase, and transaldolase. One of these intermediates, fructose 6-phosphate, can undergo isomerization back to glucose 6-phosphate, providing additional substrate for recycling back through the HMP shunt if the $NADP^+$:NADPH ratio so compels it.

Based on the known physiologic functions of these two major pathways, defective enzymes in either can be expected to interfere with erythrocyte metabolism with predictable consequences. It is generally true that enzymopathies of anaerobic glycolysis result in increased concentrations of glycolytic intermediates proximal to the defective enzyme, impaired production of ATP, and chronic hemolysis with its characteristic clinical sequelae. By contrast, enzymopathies

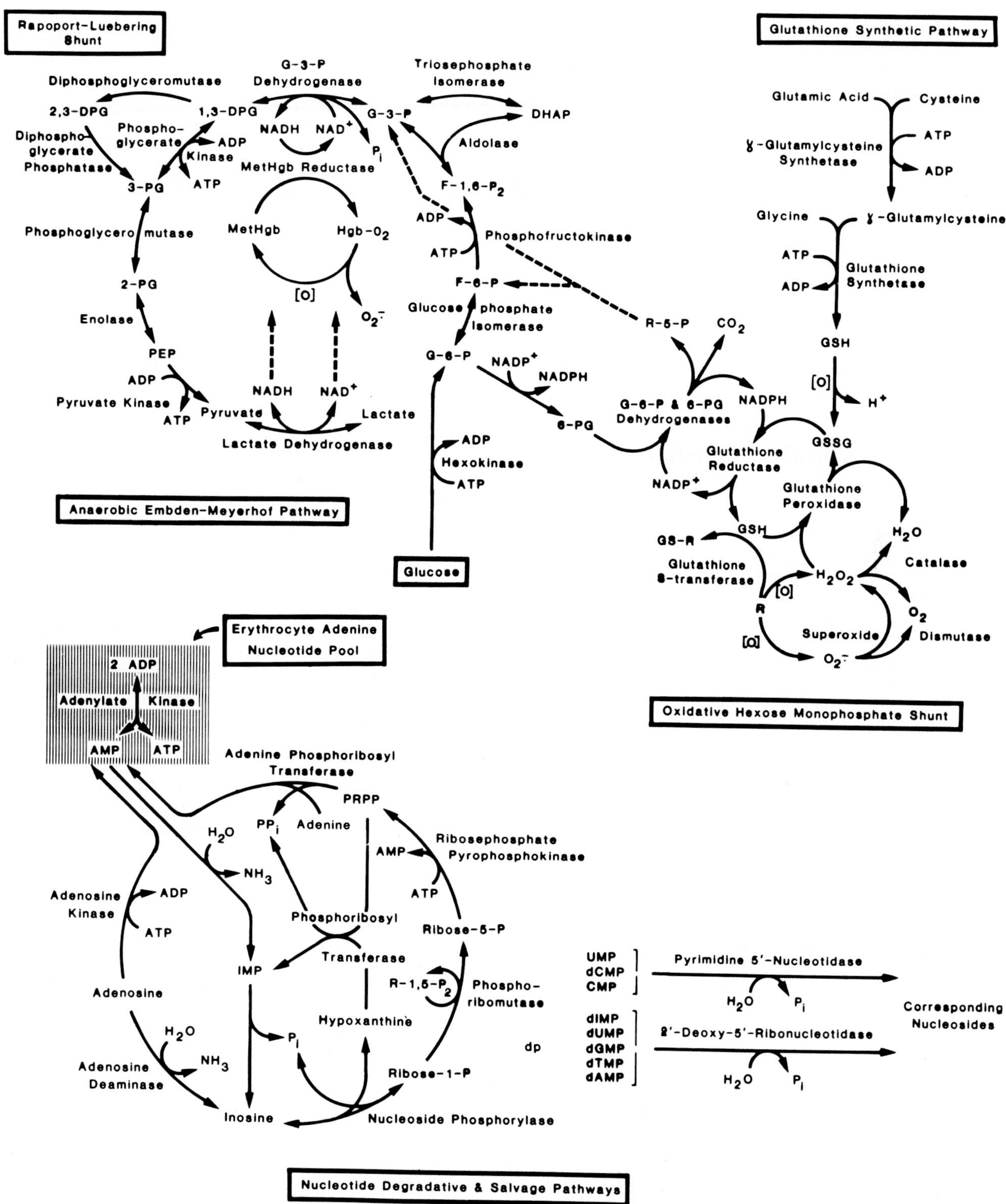

FIG. 114-1 Pathways of energy metabolism in human erythrocytes. Glucose 6-phosphate (G-6-P) may be degraded anaerobically to 2 mol of lactate via the Embden-Meyerhof pathway on the upper left, or oxidatively via the dehydrogenases of the pentose phosphate pathway (hexose monophosphate shunt) on the right. Pentose phosphates. (R-5-P) can reenter anaerobic glycolysis as fructose 6-phosphate (F-6-P) and glyceraldehyde 3-phosphate (G-3-P) after conversion by enzymes of the terminal pentose phosphate pathway or as a product of adenosine or inosine degradation. 2,3-Diphosphoglycerate (2,3-DPG) may be generated instead of ATP by diversion of triose through the Rapoport-Luebering shunt. Glutathione may be directly synthesized from constituent amino acids, and its cycling from oxidized (GSSG) to reduced form (GSH) depends on reduced pyridine cofactor (NADPH) generation. (From Paglia[3], by permission of Churchill Livingstone.)

of the HMP shunt are more often characterized by susceptibility to oxidant stresses, inducing acute episodic hemolysis in otherwise hematologically normal individuals, although chronic hemolytic anemia can also be observed in some severe cases. Glucose 6-phosphate dehydrogenase (G-6-PD) deficiency is the paradigm for the latter group of disorders, as pyruvate kinase deficiency is for the former.

In addition, abnormalities affecting a number of nonglycolytic enzymes have also been observed in association with hemolytic processes. These include deficiencies of glutathione synthesis and of nucleotide clearance and cycling. They also include hyperactivity of an enzyme, ADA, that impairs normal nucleotide salvage via direct phosphorylation of adenosine. Finally, a small group of erythrocyte enzymes can exhibit significant impairment without apparent deleterious effects on cell function or life span. In these instances, erythrocyte enzyme assays provide a simple means of detection and diagnosis of multisystem disorders.[7]

PYRUVATE KINASE DEFICIENCY

Clinical Characteristics

Prevalence. In approximately equal numbers, PK and (class 1) G-6-PD deficiencies comprise the two most common erythrocyte enzymopathies associated with chronic hemolytic anemia.[8–16] By contrast, all the other enzyme defects combined account for less than 20 percent of such cases. Since its original description,[17,18] several hundred patients with various types of PK deficiency have been reported, but many more documented cases remain unreported in the absence of unusual clinical or biochemical features.

PK deficiency exhibits no gender preponderance. It is most commonly observed in kindreds of Northern European ancestry, but it has also been widely reported throughout the United States, Canada, Japan, Western Europe, peri-Mediterranean regions, Southeast Asia, Australia, and New Zealand. Geographic distribution appears to be worldwide, even though its prevalence in many regions remains unknown. PK deficiency has been observed in Mexicans, Filipinos, Arabs, Africans, American Blacks, and in patients with partial American Indian ancestry. An Amish Dutch kindred in Pennsylvania carries a particularly high prevalence of a clinically severe form of this disorder.[19]

PK deficiency is common in Basenji dogs and also occurs in beagles.[20,21]

Clinical Features. PK deficiency is transmitted as an autosomal recessive trait with clinical consequences occurring only in homozygotes or compound heterozygotes. Except in rare instances,[22–24] heterozygotes are hematologically normal. In affected individuals, the primary clinical manifestation is chronic hemolytic anemia varying in severity from asymptomatic and fully compensated to life-threatening cases with heavy lifelong transfusion requirements.[8,9,11,25,26] The latter often present as severe neonatal anemia and jaundice necessitating exchange transfusions.

PK deficiency has no distinguishing or pathognomonic clinical features. Like anemias due to other glycolytic enzymopathies, these cases carry the usual hallmarks of chronic hemolytic processes—variable degrees of jaundice, slight to moderate splenomegaly, and increased incidence of gallstones. In most instances, anemia and/or jaundice are apparent by infancy or early childhood, if not in the neonatal period; but some escape detection until late adulthood.[27,28]

Early onset of symptoms is characteristic of more severe forms of the disorder, just as late onset is typical of milder cases. The latter are often asymptomatic, and diagnoses may emerge only as incidental findings during evaluation of pregnancy[29–31] or acute illnesses. The full spectrum of clinical severity is thus represented, with the severest cases requiring multiple transfusions or even splenectomy in early childhood in order to sustain acceptable hemoglobin levels. Beyond early childhood, or following splenectomy, transfusion requirements often diminish, and hemoglobin concentrations tend to stabilize 1 to 3 g/dl higher. Lower hemoglobin levels may be well tolerated because of decreased oxygen affinity induced by the characteristically elevated concentrations of red-cell 2,3-DPG.[31–34] This organic phosphate also inhibits HMP shunt activity,[35] possibly contributing to increased susceptibility to oxidant stress and consequent acute exacerbations of hemolysis observed in some PK-deficient patients.

Chronic hemolysis may be exacerbated by pregnancy or acute illnesses, particularly viral infections. Parvolike viruses have also been reported in association with aplastic crises in PK deficiency.[36] Depending on the severity of the enzymopathy, pregnancies may be well tolerated, but transfusions have been necessary in some cases in which previous transfusions were rare or nonexistent.[29–31,37–39]

Other clinical effects of PK deficiency include growth retardation and frontal bossing, although general development usually is not impaired.[8,11] Following splenectomy of severely affected children, growth and development may be enhanced. Kernicterus,[19,40,41] hydrops fetalis,[42] chronic leg ulcers,[43–45] acute pancreatitis secondary to biliary tract disease,[46] iron overload,[45,47,48] splenic abscess,[49] spinal cord compression by extramedullary hematopoietic tissue,[50] and migratory phlebitis with arterial thrombosis[51] are rare complications. Cholelithiasis is common and may occur at an early age.[11]

Hematologic Findings. Red-cell morphologic abnormalities are not a prominent feature of PK deficiency.[11] Those that do occur vary among different cases depending on their relative clinical severity. Milder forms may show only minimal macrocytosis and a few smaller, irregularly contracted or spiculated cells or echinocytes. All of these findings are more conspicuous in severe cases, particularly following splenectomy when siderocytes, target cells, and Pappenheimer and Howell-Jolly bodies also become prominent. Such changes, however, are nonspecific, although the presence of many crenated red cells of unusual type (shrunken echinocytes) on a postsplenectomy blood smear is considered to be suggestive of PK deficiency.[52]

As variable as the anemia may be in terms of severity, it is usually normochromic and macrocytic, the latter commensurate with the degree of reticulocytosis rather than any reflection of folate or vitamin B_{12} deficiency.[11] Splenectomy characteristically induces a paradoxical rise in percentage of circulating reticulocytes, sometimes as high as 40 to 70 percent, but again this is not a pathognomonic finding.[11,15,38,52–54] Hemoglobin concentrations generally range from 6 to 12 g/dl, with packed-cell volumes of 17 to 37 percent. Hemoglobin is normal adult type (AA), and hemoglobins F and A_2 are within normal limits. Leukocyte and platelet counts are normal or slightly increased.

Erythrocyte osmotic fragility is usually normal, but slight and variable abnormalities may be apparent following erythrocyte incubation. Antiglobulin (Coombs) and acid serum (Ham) tests are negative, and Donath-Landsteiner antibody and cold agglutinins are absent. Incubated Heinz body formation may be increased.

In most instances, erythrocyte life span is moderately to severely shortened as measured by radiochromium labeling. In some studies, the biphasic nature of ^{51}Cr cell survival curves suggests the existence of two cell populations, one targeted for almost immediate destruction and the other destined for an appreciable, but still shortened, survival.[55,56]

Data derived from ^{51}Cr labeling conflict with regard to splenic sequestration, but many PK-deficient reticulocytes are selectively sequestered and destroyed in the spleen.[28,57] Although reticulocytes possess the advantage of highly efficient ATP generation through mitochondrial oxidative phosphorylation,[53] that process is greatly suppressed in the hypoxic and acidic environment of the spleen, where PK-deficient cells may be detained in the splenic cords because of their decreased deformability.[52,58–60] Splenectomy permits longer survival of these newly formed cells; thus, the reticulocyte count may paradoxically rise after splenectomy even though anemia is less severe.[53] The liver is also a major site of destruction of young PK-deficient red cells according to organ scans with radioiron. Ferrokinetic studies with the latter usually demonstrate rapid red-cell uptake and plasma clearance.

Leukocytes and platelets do not share the enzyme deficiency, so their cell counts are unaffected.

Other Laboratory Findings. PK deficiency is not associated with specific organ dysfunction other than hemolytic anemia, with its expected manifestations and complications. Indirect hyperbilirubinemia and decreased haptoglobin concentrations occur in proportion to severity of the hemolytic process, and fecal urobilinogen excretion is accordingly increased. Because of the relation between hepatic and erythrocytic isoenzymes (see "Natural Isoenzymes" below), the liver generally shares the abnormality but is not impaired sufficiently to alter standard liver-function tests. This is due in part to ongoing enzyme synthesis in hepatocytes, a process that is not available to erythrocytes. Compensatory erythroid hyperplasia may expand the marrow spaces sufficiently to produce radiologic changes characteristic of the more severe forms of chronic hemolytic anemia.[61]

Pathological Findings. Very few cases of PK deficiency have been evaluated by postmortem examination. Such findings have been nonspecific and predictable: normoblastic erythroid hyperplasia of the marrow, extramedullary hematopoiesis, splenic and hepatic hemosiderosis, and congestion, reticuloendothelial hyperplasia, and erythrophagocytosis by cordal macrophages in the spleen.

Diagnosis

Definitive diagnosis of PK deficiency requires laboratory demonstration of specific erythrocyte enzyme abnormalities,[62–64] such as marked decreases in optimal in vitro activities. The latter may range from 5 to 25 percent of normal control activities in clinically affected individuals and 40 to 60 percent in heterozygous carriers, who remain hematologically normal. Other erythrocyte enzyme abnormalities also occur, however, and these may not be apparent by quantitative assays alone, since in vitro measurements utilize substrate and cofactor concentrations far above those that exist in vivo.[65] A number of qualitative abnormalities have now been identified, alone or in combination, many of which may exhibit minimal or only modest decrements in observed in vitro activities.[8,11,66,67]

Methods for biochemical characterization and designation of mutant PK isoenzymes have been established under the auspices of the International Committee for Standardization in Haematology,[64] but these are rapidly being supplanted by molecular biologic techniques that allow identification of specific gene abnormalities and/or amino acid substitutions in the mutant gene products.[68,69] Care must be taken with laboratory assays to be sure that erythrocyte preparations are free of leukocytes, since white cells possess 300 times more PK activity than erythrocytes on a per-cell basis. Reticulocytes and young erythrocytes have disproportionately higher PK activities than older red-cell populations, a fact that must be considered when interpreting in vitro assays. Screening tests commonly used in standard clinical laboratories yield a high proportion of false-negative results because of the many qualitative abnormalities that exist in this heterogeneous disorder. Quantitative assays conducted simultaneously at high and low substrate concentrations, with and without the allosteric activator fructose 1,6-diphosphate (F-1,6-P_2) may be effective in detecting kinetic abnormalities.[63–65]

The metabolic blockade produced by impaired catalysis at the PK step generally results in increased intracellular concentrations of glycolytic intermediates proximal to that point, particularly 2,3-DPG. This has led some to recommend quantitative assays of these intermediates as an effective diagnostic tool.[70] Since ATP concentrations are often decreased in severely affected erythrocytes, the ratio of ATP and 2,3-DPG concentrations becomes a more reliable indicator.

Genetics

PK deficiency is genetically polymorphic, exhibiting a broad range of molecular heterogeneity. As an autosomal recessive disorder, most affected individuals are compound heterozygotes for two differing mutant alleles, with true homozygotes restricted to a small number of consanguineous families.[37,71–76] A few cases have been reported in support of a dominant inheritance pattern[77] or with hematologic effects apparent in some heterozygotes.[22–24,78] Various population surveys to determine gene frequencies have given values ranging from little more than 0.1 percent to about 6 percent for the occurrence of heterozygosity, with most around 1 to 2 percent.[11,79–86]

Biochemistry and Molecular Biology

Natural Isoenzymes. Figure 114-2 summarizes some molecular features of normal human PK that may aid in clarifying the confusing terminology that has evolved to describe PK isoenzymes and their characteristics. These tissue-related isoenzymes are generally homotetramers of 50- to 60-kDa subunits, products of genes located on chromosomes 1 and 15. As natural isoenzymes, they share a number of molecular and biochemical features but differ in their electrophoretic, kinetic, and/or immunologic properties.[87–92]

PK-M_2, determined by a genetic locus at 15q22,[93] could be considered the prototypical natural isoenzyme, since it is the form present in various tissues during early fetal life. With progressive maturation into late fetal or early postnatal periods, other isoenzymes may become dominant in certain tissues, but PK-M_2 persists as the principal form in leukocytes, platelets, lung, kidney, spleen, and adipose tissue and as a minor component in liver. Cases of PK deficiency that have M_2 and other "immature" bands in their mature red

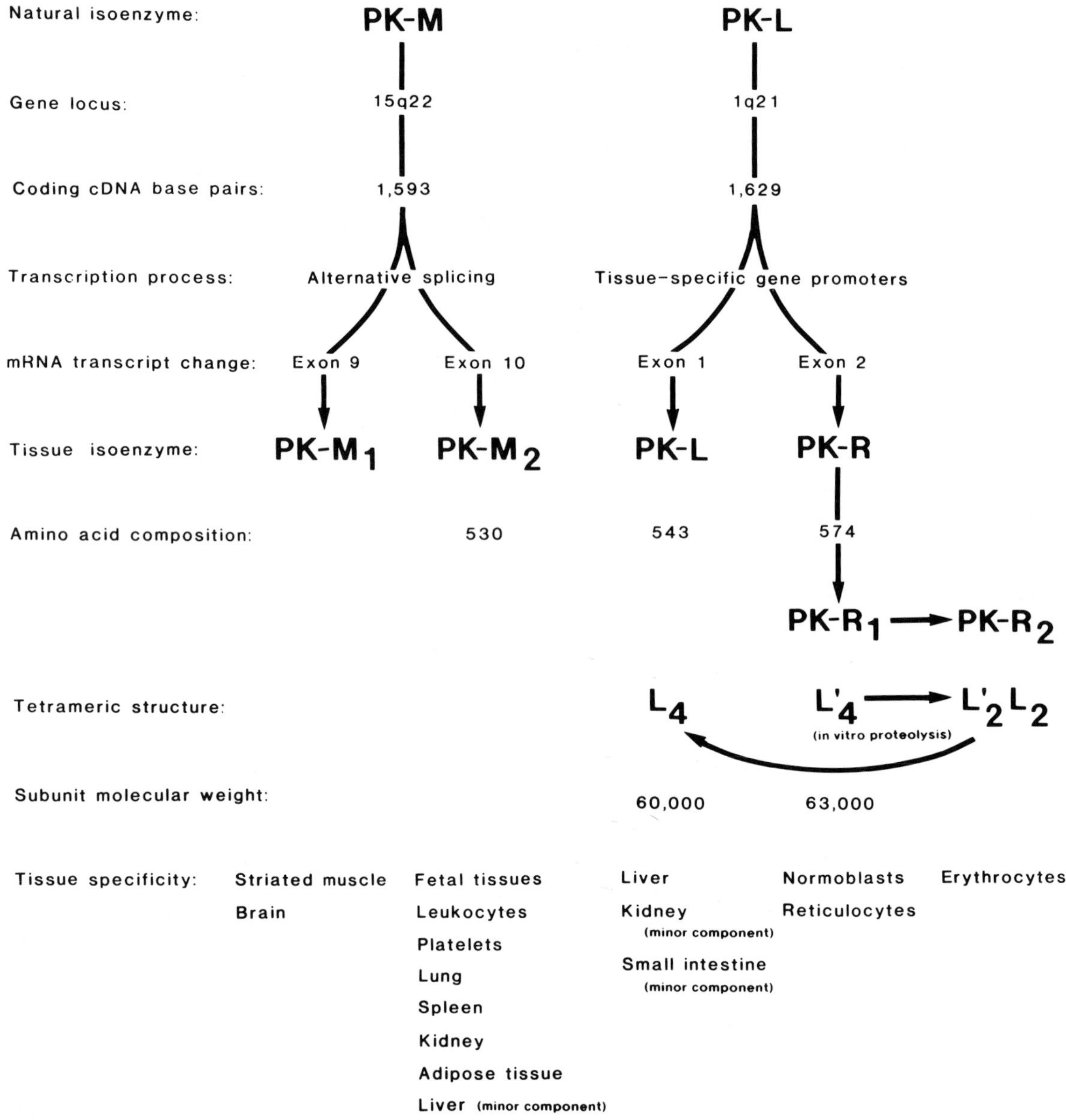

FIG. 114-2 Natural isoenzymes of human pyruvate kinase (PK).

cells have been observed.[72,90,94–97] A similar persistence of PK-M_2 occurs in the PK-deficient Basenji dog.[98]

PK-M_1 is a product of the same genetic locus induced by gene rearrangement or differential splicing,[99–102] and it predominates in mature striated muscle and brain tissue. PK-M_1 is the only natural isoenzyme that is not subject to allosteric modulation by substrate or cofactor.

PK-L, the predominant natural isoenzyme of hepatocytes, is encoded by a gene on chromosome 1q21.[103,104] The third natural isoenzyme, designated PK-R, is unique to mature erythrocytes. PK-R is under control of the same genetic locus as PK-L, but it is a translation product of a distinct mRNA altered at the 5′ terminus by tissue-specific promoters.[102,105] In most instances of erythrocyte PK deficiency, therefore, hepatocytes also exhibit decreased PK activity, but without apparent metabolic or clinical consequences,[106] since the hepatic deficiency is usually only partial[107] and can be compensated by continued or increased enzyme synthesis.

PK-L is a homotetramer of L subunits, each composed of 543 amino acids. As they mature, erythroid precursors begin to produce L subunits, and synthesis of PK-M_2 progressively subsides.[69,108–111] In early erythroid cells, the PK-L subunits have a higher molecular weight than their counterparts in hepatocytes and have been designated L′. L′ subunits can be converted in vitro to L subunits by mild proteolytic conditions, and in vivo proteolysis probably accounts for progressive evolution of the differing erythrocyte isoenzymes as these cells mature.[112–115]

The PK-R of immature erythroid cells is composed predominantly of L′ homotetramers (L'_4) and is designated PK-R_1. Proteolysis converts the L'_4 homotetramer of PK-R_1 into a heterotetramer (L'_2L_2) designated PK-R_2, the major form present in mature erythrocytes. In vitro, the PK-R_2 heterotetramer (L'_2L_2) can be converted into homotetrameric PK-L (L_4) by further proteolysis.

The L and L′ homotetramers and heterotetramers have several differing biochemical characteristics that may be functionally significant.[113,114] PK-R_1 (L'_4) in younger erythroid cells has decreased substrate affinity and stability as compared with PK-R_2 (L'_2L_2) of mature red cells and PK-L, and

PK-R_2 has more effective feedback regulatory properties. This may increase the hemolytic susceptibility of PK-deficient reticulocytes and young erythrocytes, particularly in the relatively static, acidotic, and hypoxic environment of the spleen.

PK-R and PK-L have identical antigenic characteristics but can be separated by electrophoresis.[89,90,116,117] In addition, PK-L is influenced by hormonal and dietary factors, whereas PK-R is not.[87,118]

Biochemical Characteristics. Pyruvate kinase (ATP: Pyruvate 2-*o*-phosphotransferase; EC 2.7.1.40) catalyzes, essentially irreversibly, the conversion of phospho*enol*pyruvate (PEP) to pyruvate with the consequent regeneration of ATP:

$$\begin{array}{ccc} \text{COOH} & & \text{COOH} \\ | & & | \\ \text{C}-\text{O}\sim \textcircled{P} + \text{ADP} & \xrightarrow[\text{Mg}^{2+},\ \text{K}^{+}]{\text{PK}} & \text{C}=\text{O}+\text{ATP} \\ \| & & | \\ \text{CH}_2 & & \text{CH}_3 \\ \text{Phospho}\textit{enol}\text{pyruvate} & & \text{Pyruvic Acid} \end{array}$$

Along with hexokinase and phosphofructokinase, PK serves as a key rate limiting enzyme in anaerobic glycolysis. Magnesium and potassium are necessary for optimal activity, and the latter cation additionally alters affinity for the cofactor nucleotide, ADP. Pyruvic acid is a diffusible product of this reaction, but it also provides a substrate for LDH activity if the intracellular NAD^+:NADH ratio is appropriate. The other product, ATP, exerts a feedback inhibition on the reaction rate.

The natural erythrocyte isoenzyme is highly sensitive to allosteric modulation by F-1,6-P_2.[119–121] Micromolar amounts of this glycolytic intermediate markedly increase affinity for the substrate, PEP, converting a sigmoidal kinetic curve into the classic hyperbola of Michaelis and Menten.

These kinetic properties of PK-R generally follow the $R \Leftrightarrow T$ transformation equilibrium model proposed by Monod et al.,[122] a model that does not adequately account for the properties of some mutants, however.[123,124] In this terminology, R conotes a *relaxed* conformational change in the enzyme molecule, induced by attachment of the substrate, PEP, and the allosteric activator, F-1,6-P_2, both of which cooperatively increase substrate affinity and catalytic activity. The *tight* (T) conformation exhibits a sigmoidal kinetic curve (Hill coefficient $\cong$ 1.5 to 2.0) with decreased substrate avidity and low catalytic activities at physiological concentrations of PEP. In addition, the T conformation is highly sensitive to inhibition by ATP.

These complex regulatory properties reflect a highly ordered, symmetrical tertiary protein structure that is common to all the natural pyruvate kinase isoenzymes and shared by a number of other enzymes possessing helical α-/β-barrel configurations.[125]

Erythrocyte Metabolism in PK Deficiency. Overall glycolytic rates of PK-deficient red cells are perceptibly reduced.[53,126] Ineffective catalysis at the PK step, regardless of the nature of the molecular lesion, generally results in elevated intracellular concentrations of glycolytic intermediates above the blockade, particularly 2,3-DPG and 3-phosphoglycerate. Concentrations of 2,3-DPG often increase two-, three-, or even fourfold, sufficient to shift the oxyhemoglobin dissociation curve significantly to the right in favor of tissue oxygenation, thereby helping to compensate for the anemia and ameliorate symptoms.

Elevated concentrations of 2,3-DPG may also cause deleterious effects by inhibition of other crucial rate limiting enzymes in anaerobic glycolysis, such as hexokinase or phosphofructokinase. Studies have suggested that 2,3-DPG concentration elevations are sufficient to suppress stimulated HMP shunt activity.[35,127] Incubated Heinz body formation is increased[35] and the ascorbate cyanide test has been observed to be positive,[35,128] but red-cell GSH content remains normal.[11,18] Such a suppression may be an additional factor contributing to hemolytic anemia of PK deficiency, particularly during periods of infection or metabolic stress.

NAD^+ and NADH concentrations may be decreased to approximately half-normal levels, impairing the rate of the glyceraldehyde 3-phosphate dehydrogenase reaction in vivo.[129,130] This decrease in diphosphopyridine nucleotides is due in part to impaired NAD synthesis in PK deficiency.[131] PP-ribose-P is an intermediate in the synthesis of adenine nucleotides and NAD. The enzyme responsible for its synthesis (PP-ribose-P synthetase) may be less active in vivo in PK-deficient red cells because of decreased ATP and increased 2,3-DPG concentrations.[132] Impaired PP-ribose-P formation has been documented in intact PK-deficient red cells.[133]

Total adenine nucleotide and ATP concentrations are generally reduced, although this may be masked by the higher concentrations normally present in reticulocytes and young erythrocytes. Reduced ATP alters cation permeability, accelerating potassium and water efflux, thereby contributing to progressive cellular dehydration, crenation, and increasing membrane density and rigidity.[57,134] Impaired ATP generation has traditionally been viewed as the primary metabolic event initiating the sequence of alterations that eventually terminate in premature destruction of PK-deficient erythrocytes in the reticuloendothelial system. The precise pathogenesis, however, remains controversial,[135,136] as does the relative importance of associated phenomena such as impaired antioxidant capacity, translocation of calcium ions, membrane budding without hemoglobin loss, discocyte–echinocyte–spherocyte transformation, and increased susceptibility to phagocytosis.

Molecular Lesions in PK Deficiency. The biochemical heterogeneity of this disorder is well demonstrated by nearly 400 cases documented in the literature, a small proportion of which have been evaluated according to internationally standardized criteria. Interpretation of even these, however, has been complicated by the simultaneous occurrence of multiple isoenzymes in affected cells, since most cases are compound heterozygotes for two dissimilar mutant alleles rather than true homozygotes. A number of the latter have also been reported, and their implications have been discussed in several comprehensive reviews.[8,11,13–16,67–69,92] Additional heterogeneity may occur as a consequence of subunit assembly sequences, possibly resulting in heterotetramers of mutant and normal subunits in various combinations.[137]

Given these complex structural and regulatory features of PK, it is not surprising that mutant gene products might exhibit a variety of biochemical abnormalities depending on the precise site of the molecular lesion and its consequent effects on tertiary structural conformations. This is, indeed, the case with mutant PK isoenzymes. Alterations affecting various regulatory properties, as well as stability or specific activity, occur commonly in this heterogeneous disorder.

These are the phenotypic characteristics documented in reports of cases analyzed according to the criteria of the International Committee for Standardization in Haematology (ICSH).[64] Among the most common alterations are marked enzyme protein instability, decreased affinity for the substrate, PEP, and/or impaired response to the primary allosteric activator of PK, F-1,6-P_2. Other abnormalities, such as increased sensitivity to inhibition by ATP, decreased affinity for the cofactor, ADP, increased substrate affinity, or decreased enzyme protein production, are less commonly encountered. In addition, enzyme protein abnormalities may be reflected by altered electrophoretic migration patterns, isoelectric points, pH optimums, thermal inactivation rates, or optimal cation concentrations. The clinical severity of PK deficiency tends to correlate better with the severity of these qualitative biochemical abnormalities rather than with simple decrements in activity as measured in optimal in vitro assay systems.

Specific Mutations in PK Deficiency. Isolation and nucleotide sequencing of normal human PK-M_2 and PK-L cDNA[93,103,104,138] have provided a basis for similar molecular analyses in cases of PK deficiency. At least six specific point mutations have now been identified in nine unrelated kindreds,[139–144] including a severely hemolytic form present in the Amish deme of Pennsylvania.[144] These are summarized in Table 114-1. The occurrence of identical molecular defects in homozygotes from a Lebanese and two Japanese families, if not fortuitous, suggests that this specific mutation might be evolutionarily ancient.[69] Two other unrelated Japanese families also share an identical point mutation, which results in altered hydrophilic characteristics of the PK-R protein.[141] Comparison of the similarities and differences in biochemical characteristics of these variants provides some insights into the importance of specific regions or domains in the protein matrix relative to substrate, cofactor, and cation binding, and the mechanisms for switching from PK-M_2 to PK-R production during erythroid maturation.[143]

Acquired PK Deficiency. PK deficiency is more often acquired than hereditary, but the clinical significance of acquired changes in PK activity remains uncertain. Reduced PK and pyrimidine 5′-nucleotidase activities are the most frequent combination among multiple enzymatic aberrations of the erythrocyte described in a variety of hematologic malignancies.[8,25,145–149] PK deficiency has been noted particularly in acute myeloblastic leukemia and refractory sideroblastic anemia, but elevated PK activities may occur in myelodysplastic syndromes.[150] Decreased activity of PK is also common following chemotherapy,[151,152] but occurs occasionally prior to treatment of cancer.[151] In most instances of acquired deficiency, PK values are only slightly to moderately reduced, but on occasion they may be markedly decreased. Accumulation of glycolytic intermediates may occur but probably does not result in shortened red-cell survival.[153]

The mechanism of acquired enzyme defects is still unclear, but four types of phenomena have been hypothesized: partial reversion to a fetal form of erythropoiesis, disturbances in gene expression, somatic mutations, and postsynthetic modifications of the enzyme. Arguments exist in favor of each of these hypothetical mechanisms.[8,147] Differentiation between acquired and hereditary PK deficiency (usually the heterozygous state) is occasionally difficult but may be aided by family studies.

PK in High ATP Syndrome. The association of PK hyperactivity (two- to fourfold increase), high ATP (about twice normal), and low 2,3-DPG content in the red cells has been reported in several families.[154–157] In some affected individuals, erythrocytosis developed secondary to a left shift in the oxygen dissociation curve as a result of the low 2,3-DPG content. The mode of inheritance is autosomal dominant. High PK activity may be based either on the presence of PK-M_2 in addition to the L type in erythrocytes,[155,156] or alternatively, on a shift in the R⇔T equilibrium to the relaxed R form (resulting in increased affinity for PEP) together with increased enzyme synthesis or decreased degradation.[157]

Therapy. Nonspecific supportive measures provide the only currently accepted approach to treatment of PK deficiency. Red-cell transfusions may be necessary when hemoglobin levels fall sufficiently, but beyond childhood many patients adapt to a level of compensated hemolysis that may eliminate transfusion needs unless exacerbated by infection, pregnancy, or other conditions.[9,11]

Splenectomy is not curative but is frequently of distinct value, especially in infants and young children with severe disease. Hemoglobin concentrations often increase 1 to 3 g/dl, reducing or even eliminating transfusion requirements. Following splenectomy, growth and development in severely affected children may be accelerated.[11] Splenectomy may be lifesaving in the severely affected Amish patients.[40] On the other hand, anemia in mild cases may be unchanged by the procedure. In contrast to splenectomy in hereditary spherocytosis, hemolysis clearly persists, and aplastic or hemolytic crises may still occur. Erythrocyte survival and

Table 114-1 Specific Molecular Lesions Identified in Pyruvate Kinase Deficiency

Variant PK Isoenzyme	Mutation	Nucleotide Substitution	Nucleotide Position	Amino Acid Substitution	Amino Acid Position	Reference
Beirut	T384M	C→T	1151	Thr→Met	384	139
Tokyo						140
Nagasaki						141
Linz	R163C	C→T	487	Arg→Cys	163	139
Fukushima	Q421K	C→A	1261	Gln→Lys	421	141
Maebashi						141
Sapporo	R426Q	G→A	1277	Arg→Gln	426	142
Osaka	V368F	G→T	1102	Val→Phe	368	143
Amish	R479H	G→A	1436	Arg→His	479	144

sequestration studies utilizing ^{51}Cr-labeled cells are not generally useful in selecting optimal patients for surgery. In any individual case, the beneficial effects remain unpredictable.

Experimental approaches with agents that either modify enzyme activity or circumvent the metabolic aberrations induced by the defective enzyme have been attempted: Administration of AMP, magnesium, riboflavin, methylene blue and ascorbic acid, oral mannose, galactose, and fructose, and infusion of adenine, inosine, and guanosine, mostly in single cases, have produced no convincing clinical improvement and should be considered experimental.[8] Hematopoietic stimulating factors and steroids remain ineffective.[11,158]

OTHER ERYTHROENZYMOPATHIES OF THE GLYCOLYTIC PATHWAY

Hexokinase Deficiency

Hexokinase catalyzes the initial rate limiting step of glycolysis to produce glucose 6-phosphate (see Fig. 114-1). Erythrocyte hexokinase deficiency was described initially as one of multiple abnormalities in Fanconi syndrome.[25,159] Hexokinase deficiency hemolytic anemia was first documented in 1967,[160] and is rare (Table 114-2). About 20 cases have been reported, predominantly in persons of Northern European ancestry, but also in one boy of Chinese ancestry.[8–10,15,25,161–166] The anemia is moderate; it does not require regular transfusion therapy. Splenectomy results in partial benefit, though vigorous hemolysis persists.[25,167] The concentration of 2,3-DPG is low in the red cells, with resultant increased oxygen affinity of the hemoglobin. This may impair exercise tolerance in these subjects.[34] Hexokinase deficiency may involve the platelets and rarely the lymphocytes but without clinical consequences.[161,162,167] The mode of transmission is autosomal recessive. Dominant inheritance has been suggested in some instances,[168,169] but these cases have been atypical, such as the erythrocytes of mother and son demonstrating notable morphologic abnormalities.[169]

Hexokinase, a monomer of 108 kDa, has the lowest catalytic activity of any glycolytic enzyme,[8,170] but it also exhibits the sharpest curve of activity decay with age. The curve is biphasic, with over half the activity loss occurring during the first few days.[171,172] Thus, in severely deficient subjects, hexokinase activity may measure in the normal or modestly subnormal range, but far below the activity expected in reticulocyte-rich red-cell populations.

At least four distinct, tissue-specific isoenzymes of hexokinase are normally identifiable, designated I, II, III, and IV. Red cells possess chiefly type I, which is separable into Ia, Ib, and Ic.[173] Hexokinase Ib predominates in reticulocytes and is presumably responsible for the steep biphasic decay curve observed as reticulocytes mature and erythrocytes age. An isoenzyme specific for the human red blood cell (HK_R) has been proposed.[174] The structural gene for hexoki-

Table 114-2 Summary of Some Features Associated with Glycolytic Enzymopathies

Enzyme	Incidence*	Inheritance	Hemolytic Anemia	Neurologic Abnormalities	Myopathy	Comments
Hexokinase	Rare	Autosomal recessive	Yes			Low 2,3-DPG level; suggestion of poor tolerance of anemia
Glucosephosphate isomerase	Second to pyruvate kinase	Autosomal recessive	Yes	Rarely	Rarely	More than 45 cases reported; decreased activity in leukocytes and platelets
Phosphofructokinase	Rare	Autosomal recessive	Variable		Usually	Hemolysis often fully compensated; predominantly males; early-onset gout
Aldolase	Very rare	Autosomal recessive	Yes			Only three cases; mental retardation and dysmorphic features in one case
Triosephosphate isomerase	Rare	Autosomal recessive	Yes	Usually severe		Generalized, severe disorder; early death, often sudden
Phosphoglycerate kinase	Rare	X-linked recessive	Yes, usually	Usually	Rarely	Neurologic manifestations in males only; generalized enzyme deficiency
Diphosphoglycerate mutase and phosphatase	Very rare	Autosomal recessive	No			Near absence of 2,3-DPG with mild erythrocytosis; both activities reside in same enzyme protein
Enolase	Very rare	Autosomal dominant?	Yes			Partial deficiency with spherocytic phenotype
Pyruvate kinase	Most common	Autosomal recessive	Yes			First described, best studied; nearly 400 cases reported; prototype for group
Lactate dehydrogenase	Very rare	Autosomal recessive	No		M-subunit	No hemolysis with deficiency of H subunit; myopathy with lack of M subunit

*Rare indicates between 15 and 35 cases; very rare fewer than 5 cases reported.

nase I is on chromosome 10 (Table 114-3). The most likely regional assignment appears to be 10p11.2.[175,176] cDNA clones encoding human hexokinase have been isolated from an adult kidney library.[177]

Despite the rarity of severe deficiency, genetic polymorphism is the rule[8,163] and is manifest by differing kinetics for glucose and magnesium-ATP, differing electrophoretic patterns, and variable thermostability. Hexokinase is inhibited by glucose 6-phosphate, by glucose 1,6-diphosphate, and by 2,3-DPG, and is stimulated by P_i. Abnormalities of regulation by inhibitors and insensitivity to P_i have been described.[178,179] The initial step in glycolysis catalyzed by hexokinase is crucial to human erythrocyte metabolism, since mature red cells are almost exclusively dependent on further catabolism of glucose 6-phosphate to generate ATP, reduced glutathione, and pyridine nucleotides, which are the energy sources essential to normal cell survival. In hexokinase-deficient red cells, decreased glucose consumption and reduced content of 2,3-DPG, ATP, and glucose 6-phosphate are usually demonstrable when compared with cells of similar age.[160,161,163] Failure of energy generation is probably the primary cause of premature demise of the red cell is this disorder. An in vitro model utilizing hexokinase-inactivating antibodies has been described.[180]

Glucosephosphate Isomerase Deficiency

More than 45 cases of glucosephosphate isomerase (GPI) deficiency hemolytic anemia have been described worldwide,[8,9,15,25,162,165,166,181] since the initial report in 1968.[182] This disorder ranks second only to that of pyruvate kinase of glycolytic enzymopathies associated with hemolytic syndromes (see Table 114-2). Tissue-specific isoenzymes probably do not exist, and hence in severely deficient subjects not only the red cells but leukocytes, platelets, plasma, fibroblasts, liver, muscle, and presumably other tissues possess decreased GPI activity.[25,183] Despite this, clinical manifestations are usually limited to those accompanying a chronic hemolytic process varying in severity from quite mild to very severe. In some instances, mental retardation, myopathy, and impaired granulocyte function may occur.[184–187] GPI deficiency has been documented as a rare cause of hydrops fetalis[188] and priapism.[189]

Diagnosis depends on detection of the specific deficiency in red cells by quantitative assay for GPI activity. Asymptomatic heterozygotes have about half-normal activity, whereas anemic subjects with homozygosity or compound heterozygosity for GPI deficiency have erythrocytic values approximating 25 percent of the normal mean.[183] Antenatal diagnosis is possible as early as the first trimester of pregnancy by direct enzyme assay of trophoblast cells.[190] Splenectomy in severe cases has been followed by variably positive responses in terms of increased levels of hemoglobin and decreased transfusion requirements.[25,183] Therapeutic attempts to circumvent the partial block at the GPI step have been unsuccessful.[25,183]

Nearly all mutant GPI variants have been manifested chiefly by thermolability in vitro.[162] Erythrocyte GPI activity is normally present in great excess, but this thermal instability presumably results in progressive diminution of activity in vivo, impairment of glycolysis, and hemolysis. Rare, stable mutant enzymes have been identified in association with hemolytic syndromes,[187] as has combined GPI and glucose 6-phosphate dehydrogenase deficiency.[191,192] Red cells deficient in GPI activity are unable to cycle glucose effectively more than once through the pentose phosphate pathway since fructose 6-phosphate, formed through the actions of transketolase and transaldolase, must traverse the GPI step to reenter the shunt (see Fig. 114-1).[183] This limitation of pentose shunt activity on stimulation may account for the increased frequency of hemolytic crises associated with infection in this enzymopathy. The rate of degradation of this enzyme may conceivably be accelerated by the increase of body temperature during febrile episodes.[193]

GPI deficiency is inherited as an autosomal recessive disorder. Extensive heterogeneity exists, with 34 apparently unique mutant forms tabulated.[15] The dimeric enzyme of 134 kDa is encoded by a gene on chromosome 19[194] (see Table 114-3). The gene has been isolated and its 5′ end characterized.[195] An animal model for the human disease occurs in mice.[196]

Phosphofructokinase Deficiency

Phosphofructokinase (PFK) catalyzes the rate limiting reaction in glycolysis, the phosphorylation of fructose 6-phosphate to F-1,6-P_2 (see Fig. 114-1). PFK is a tetrameric protein under the control of three structural loci that code for muscle (M), liver (L), and platelet (P) subunits. Mature granulocytes contain predominantly L subunits, whereas platelets have largely P and some L subunits. Muscle and liver contain the homotetramers M_4 and L_4, respectively. Erythrocytes express both the M and the L subunits, and random tetramerization produces five isoenzymes—M_4, M_3L, M_2L_2, ML_3, and L_4.[197–201]

Severe deficiency of muscle PFK resulting in myopathy

Table 114-3 Molecular Genetics of Glycolytic Enzymopathies

Enzyme	Main Form in Erythrocytes	Chromosome Locus	Gene Cloned	Mutation Identified
Hexokinase	HK I	10p11.2	Yes[177]	No
Glucosephosphate isomerase	Same enzyme*	19cen-q13	No	No
Phosphofructokinase	M, L	1cen→q32;21q22.3	Yes[219-221]	Yes[213,222]
Aldolase	A	16q22-q24	Yes[230,231]	Yes[224]
Triosephosphate isomerase	Same enzyme*	12p13	Yes[258]	Yes[242,260]
Phosphoglycerate kinase	PGK-1	Xq13	Yes[284,285]	Yes[263,271,273,287-290]
Diphosphoglycerate mutase	Only in erythrocytes	7q22-q34	Yes[302,304]	Yes[301]
Enolase	α	1p36.13-pter	Yes[310]	No
Pyruvate kinase	L	1q21	Yes[104]	Yes[139-144]
Lactate dehydrogenase	H	12p12.1-12.2	Yes[318]	Yes[319]

*Same enzyme is present in all cells, including erythrocytes.

was first reported in 1965 by Tarui et al. from Japan[202] and from the United States shortly thereafter.[203] This form of metabolic myopathy has been classified as glycogen storage disease type VII since there is glycogen deposition in muscle.[204] About 35 cases of PFK deficiency have been reported from the United States, Europe, and Japan; most of the patients from the United States are of Ashkenazic Jewish ancestry[15,162,165,198] (see Table 114-2). The clinical hallmarks are a compensated hemolytic process and prominent myopathy manifested by muscle weakness and cramps, exercise intolerance, and myoglobinuria. Hemolysis is clearly demonstrable, but anemia is often absent; in fact, mild erythrocytosis may occur because of the low 2,3-DPG levels, with resultant increased oxygen affinity. Predisposition to hyperuricemia and early-onset gout appears to be secondary to excessive degradation of purines in exercising PFK-deficient muscles. Ammonia, inosine, and hypoxanthine are increased abnormally in venous blood after forearm exercise.[205]

Various clinical phenotypes have been described,[15] but it now appears that most cases of PFK deficiency result from homozygosity for mutant inactive M subunits resulting in hemolysis and myopathy of varying severity. Occasionally individuals with hemolysis but without myopathy may have an L-subunit disorder or possibly an unstable M subunit. Most affected individuals are first detected during adolescence or young adulthood, but the disease may be manifest at birth, with death during infancy[206] or may be so mild as to present in old age.[207] Most patients adjust to their myopathy rather well.[200] Fatigue of active muscles is more rapid after a high-carbohydrate meal.[208]

PFK deficiency should be suspected in an individual with a chronic well-compensated hemolytic process and exercise intolerance or cramps. Muscle biopsies classically reveal virtually absent PFK activity, while activity of the red cell is about half normal.[202,203,209,210] Noninvasive MRI studies of muscle carbohydrate metabolism may also confirm the diagnosis.[211]

Erythrocytes of patients lack the homotetramer M_4 and the hybrid isozymes but still express the homotetramer L_4, and thus have about half-normal PFK activity. This decrease in activity is associated with an accumulation of glycolytic intermediates proximal to the enzyme defect, decreased content of 2,3-DPG, and shortened red-cell survival, although the mechanism of hemolysis is still unclear. Interestingly, the pattern of erythrocyte glycolytic intermediates reflecting the deficiency at the PFK step improves toward normal with exercise, due to large quantities of ammonia, purine nucleosides, and oxypurine released from exercising muscles in these patients.[212]

PFK deficiency is transmitted as an autosomal recessive trait.[213] Obligate heterozygotes with partial deficiency of red-cell PFK activity are normal clinically because sufficient M subunits, which appear to be more critical for adequate glycolytic flux in the erythrocyte, are produced by the unaffected M-subunit allele. Muscle biopsies have not been performed in any parents for direct determination of total PFK activity or analysis of the M subunit.[198] To date there is a strong male predominance. An animal model for PFK deficiency in English springer spaniel dogs manifests chronic hemolytic anemia resulting from total lack of M subunit, but without myopathy, presumably due to both high oxidative potential of the canine muscle and presence of L subunit in the M-deficient muscle.[214]

PFK enzyme is under the control of three structural loci that encode for muscle (M)-, liver (L)-, and platelet (P)-type subunits. These are encoded on chromosome 1cen-q32 for M, chromosome 21q22.3 for L, and chromosome 10 for P (see Table 114-3).[215–218] Both human L- and M-type PFK cDNA have been cloned.[219–221] There is striking structural homology between human-muscle and rabbit-muscle PFK. The first genetic defect described in muscle PFK deficiency was an abnormal splicing of the muscle PFK gene due to a point mutation at the 5′ splice site.[222] Interestingly, another splicing defect, a 5′ splice-junction mutation leading to exon deletion in an Ashkenazic Jewish family with PFK deficiency has been reported.[213] Classification of patients based on the genetic defect may now allow for more definitive grouping of patients with similar symptoms.

Aldolase Deficiency

Aldolase catalyzes the conversion of F-1,6-P_2 to the trioses, dihydroxyacetone phosphate and glyceraldehyde 3-phosphate (see Fig. 114-1). Severe deficiency of erythrocyte aldolase has been reported in only two kindreds[223–225] (see Table 114-2). A severe deficiency of erythrocyte aldolase in association with hemolytic anemia and a galaxy of malformations was first reported in a child of Canadian Jewish parents who were first cousins with normal red-cell aldolase activity.[223] Two boys in a Japanese kindred had mild to moderate hemolytic anemia exacerbated by infections, splenomegaly, and markedly decreased red-cell aldolase activity, but no mental or developmental abnormalities.[225] The enzyme of these cases was thermolabile and had an increased K_m for F-1,6-P_2

Diagnosis of this very rare disorder depends on assay of aldolase activity in erythrocytes. In the Japanese patients, there were greatly increased red-cell concentrations of the substrate for aldolase, F-1,6-P_2, and decreased glucose consumption and lactate formation.[225] In this kindred, transmission was autosomal recessive. Parents of the two patients as well as four other family members had intermediate values for red-cell aldolase activity consistent with heterozygosity and were normal hematologically and clinically.

Aldolase is a tetramer of 158 kDa, and three tissue isoenzymes (A, B, and C) are recognized; A is the principal type found in red cells and muscle.[25,226] The genes for aldolases A and B have been cloned and characterized.[227–232] The aldolase A gene has been localized to chromosome 16q22-q24[233] (see Table 114-3). A cDNA for aldolase A was cloned using RNA isolated from a lymphoblastoid cell line from one of the Japanese patients. Nucleotide sequence analysis revealed an A→G substitution at position 386 in the coding region. This resulted in the replacement of aspartic acid by glycine at codon 128 (D128G) in the mutant enzyme, which was highly thermolabile, suggesting that this mutation causes a functional defect.[224]

Triosephosphate Isomerase Deficiency

Triosephosphate isomerase (TPI), a dimer with two identical subunits containing 248 amino acids and with a calculated subunit mass of 26,750 daltons,[234] catalyzes the reversible isomerization of dihydroxyacetone phosphate and glyceraldehyde 3-phosphate (see Fig. 114-1). The activity of red-cell TPI is the highest of any glycolytic enzyme.

TPI deficiency is the most severe of the enzymatic defects of the glycolytic pathway in its clinical consequences. It is characterized by multisystem disease, including chronic hemolytic anemia, progressive neurologic dysfunction, increased susceptibility to infections, cardiomyopathy, and death, usually during early childhood.[7,165,235–240] About 30 patients have been reported[15] since its original description in 1965[237] (see Table 114-2). The first symptoms relate to a moderately severe hemolytic anemia. The progressive neurologic abnormalities appear at 6 months to 2 years of age, are unrelated to kernicterus, and have been noted in all patients who have survived beyond 1 year, except for one adult man.[241,242] Manifestations include dystonic movements, tremor, pyramidal tract signs, and evidence of spinal motor neuron involvement. Intellect is preserved, sensory impairment is absent, and cerebrospinal fluid has been normal when studied, as have CT brain scans and EEG in two patients.[239] The pathogenesis of the neurologic disease is unclear.

TPI deficiency appears to involve all body tissues.[7,236] While material for study has been limited, TPI activity is reduced greatly in all tissues assayed, including erythrocytes, leukocytes, lymphocytes, platelets, serum, plasma, skeletal muscle, heart, spinal fluid, cultured skin fibroblasts, brain, liver, pancreas, kidney, and intestine.[7,25,236,240,243] There is increased susceptibility to infection, but whether granulocyte function is impaired is controversial.[8,239,240,243,244] TPI-deficient platelets may be functionally impaired.[245]

In the erythrocyte the most striking metabolic abnormality is the twenty- to sixtyfold increase in the concentration of dihydroxyacetone phosphate, the substrate for the enzyme, suggestive of an almost complete metabolic block at this step.[7,235,246] The relationship between high dihydroxyacetone phosphate levels and hemolysis is unclear, since accumulations of this compund also occur in cases of diphosphoglycerate mutase deficiency without hemolysis.[247]

Diagnosis depends on a specific assay for TPI in the erythrocytes. Prenatal identification of heterozygotes has been successful in several instances,[248–250] and diagnosis of affected fetuses should be reliable. Only supportive therapy is available. No significant improvement occurred after splenectomy in one patient.[251]

The mode of inheritance is autosomal recessive.[235,237] Obligate heterozygotes are clinically normal, but their erythrocytes have about half-normal red-cell TPI activity. TPI is encoded by a single structural locus on the short arm of chromosome 12[252] (see Table 114-3). Different electrophoretic forms in normal individuals are due to posttranslational deamination of the parent molecule at asparagines 15 and 71.[253,254] Null alleles (with 50 percent TPI activity and 50 percent of the usual immunologic CRM in heterozygotes) have been found with relatively high frequency in whites (0.37 to 0.48 percent) and especially in American blacks (4.7 percent) in surveys,[255,256] yet clinically identifiable homozygous disease is rare. This discrepancy remains unexplained.[235,256]

The human TPI gene has been isolated and structurally characterized; it spans 3.5 kb and is split into seven exons.[257] The primary structure of TPI has been determined,[234] and the complete amino acid sequence derived.[258] There is clear evidence of heterogeneity among TPI-deficient patients.[242,258,259] A single amino acid substitution, Glu→Asp at position 104 (E104D), was present in a TPI allele from two unrelated patients with severe TPI deficiency and resulted in a thermolabile enzyme.[260] Each DNA-associated sequence exhibited a G→C to C→G transversion in the codon for amino acid 104. The importance of Glu104 to TPI structure and function is suggested by its conservation in TPI of all species thus far characterized.[260] A Hungarian family has been characterized by two mutations, one a Phe (TTC) to Leu (CTC) mutation within codon 240 (F240L), which created a thermolabile protein, and another mutation yet to be localized that reduced TPI mRNA ten to twentyfold.[242]

Phosphoglycerate Kinase Deficiency

Phosphoglycerate kinase (PGK) is a key enzyme for ATP generation in the glycolytic pathway, catalyzing the conversion of 1,3-diphosphoglycerate to 3-phosphoglycerate (see Fig. 114-1). In 1968 PGK was demonstrated to be deficient in a woman whose sole manifestation was hemolytic anemia.[261] Nearly simultaneously, PGK deficiency in erythrocytes and leukocytes in association with hemolytic anemia and neurologic manifestations was documented.[262] Thus far, 14 variants of PGK deficiency have been found in unrelated families.[15,165,166,263] PGK deficiency is the only known X-linked disorder of the Embden-Meyerhof pathway[7,8,262,264,265] (see Table 114-2). Almost all affected males have hemolytic anemia and neurologic manifestations such as behavioral abnormalities, emotional lability, variable mental retardation, movement disorders, hemiplegia, or aphasia. Women heterozygous for PGK deficiency may be normal or have mild hemolytic anemia due to mosaicism associated with random X inactivation; neurologic function has been normal.[7,8,266] Variants with different clinical presentations have been described (Table 114-4).[8,9,162,266–268,271–273]

Specific assay of the erythrocyte enzyme is required for diagnosis of PGK deficiency; values are usually 3 to 20 percent of normal activity in males.[15,271] Variable degrees of expression of the enzyme defect may complicate detection of female carriers of the trait. There is not always a correlation between the degree of PGK deficiency in vitro and clinical severity. Therapy is supportive; red-cell transfusions may be necessary in those most severely affected or during exacerbations usually related to infections. A beneficial response to splenectomy has been noted in three of four patients.[25]

Metabolic abnormalities in erythrocytes consistent with a defect at the PGK step are observed in affected males. Red-cell ATP levels are substantially reduced, and the content of 2,3-DPG may be doubled, favorably shifting the oxygen–hemoglobin equilibrium curve to permit oxygen delivery to most body tissues, including the brain, at better tensions than normal except during a hemolytic crisis.[274] Obligate female heterozygotes may have no or modest increases in 2,3-DPG in their erythrocytes. Leukocytes in hemizygous males in the first studied kindred were found to be deficient in PGK activity, but no increased incidence of infection has been reported.[275]

PGK activity has been demonstrated to be reduced to 5 percent or less of normal activity in lymphocytes, platelets, and muscle of living patients and in brain, cardiac muscle, and liver tissues obtained at autopsy.[276–278] The relationship of PGK deficiency to the neurologic manifestations remains unknown. The selective involvement of muscle, for example, in $PGK_{CRETEIL}$[279] or $PGK_{NEW\ JERSEY}$[280] and, conversely, the lack of myopathy in patients with hemolytic anemia except for $PGK_{SHIZUOKA}$,[273] or the combination of neurologic manifestations and myoglobinuria without hemolytic anemia[272] (see Table 114-4) are not understood.

PGK has two isoenzymes, PGK-1 and PGK-2. PGK-1 is an X-linked gene expressed in all somatic cells, while PGK-2 is an autosomal gene expressed only in spermatozoa.[281] PGK-1 is encoded by a single structural gene at Xq13 in humans[264,282] (see Table 114-3). Rarely, a variant gene may be generated by spontaneous mutation during oogenesis.[263] The complete amino acid sequence, cDNA sequence, and

Table 114-4 Features of Some Phosphoglycerate Kinase Variants

Name of Variant	Clinical Manifestations: Hemolytic Anemia	Neurologic Abnormalities	Muscle Disease	Amino Acid Substitution and Site*	Comments	References
(Classical)	+	+	0		Chinese kindred	265
II (T351N)	0	0	0	Thr→Asn at 351	Electrophoretic variant in Oceania; normal activity	264, 290
Munchen (D267N)	0	0	0	Asp→Asn at 267	20% of normal activity; asymptomatic	268, 288
Uppsala (R205P)	+	+	0	Arg→Pro at 205	Substitution probably affects the ATP and ADP binding site	289
Tokyo (V265M)	+	+	0	Val→Met at 265	Substitution expected to induce conformational change of enzyme	287
Creteil	0	0	+		Rhabdomyolysis	279
New Jersey	0	0	+		Recurrent myoglobinuria; muscle enzyme studied	280
San Francisco	+	0	0		Severe, partially transfusion-dependent anemia; enzyme unusually stable in vitro	267
Hamamatsu	0	+	+		Recurrent convulsions followed by myoglobinuria	272
Matsue (L88P)	+	+	0	Leu→Pro at 88	Rapid in vivo degradation of enzyme	269-271
Shizuoka (G157V)	+	0	+	Gly→Val at 157	First case with both hemolysis and muscle symptoms	273
Michigan (C315R)	+	+	0	Cys→Arg at 315	Variant gene presumably generated by spontaneous mutation during oogenesis	263

*The position of amino acid substitution is counted from the N-terminal Ser.

genomic structure have been elucidated.[283-286] Single amino acid substitutions have been documented in seven variants: PGK II, Munchen, Uppsala, Tokyo, Matsue, Shizuoka, and Michigan[263,271,273,287,289,290] (see Table 114-4).

There is 97 percent homology between the human and horse protein sequences.[284] Structural changes have been related to functional abnormalities of PGK variants by inference from the three-dimensional structure for horse PGK proposed by Banks and colleagues[291] and Yoshida and Tani.[292] For example, the replacement of Arg by Pro in $PGK_{UPPSALA}$ may induce a dislocation at the ATP–ADP binding site, resulting in an inefficient mutant enzyme and hemolytic anemia. The major cause of reduced concentration of PGK_{MATSUE} is most likely a more rapid denaturation and degradation of the variant enzyme originating from the Leu to Pro substitution.[271]

Diphosphoglycerate Mutase (Bisphosphoglycerate Mutase) and Phosphatase Deficiency

Diphosphoglycerate mutase (DPGM) is a trifunctional enzyme whose main function is to synthesize 2,3-DPG (see Fig. 114-1), which profoundly influences the affinity of hemoglobin for oxygen.[5,293] In addition, DPGM displays two other activities, a phosphatase activity that degrades 2,3-DPG and a minor mutase activity identical to that of glycolytic phosphoglycerate mutase.[294,295] In humans, DPGM activity is found only in red blood cells.

DPGM deficiency is very rare. The initial case of a complete deficiency of erythrocyte DPGM was documented in 1978 in a 42-year-old man of French origin who had erythrocytosis.[247] Other findings included a ruddy cyanosis, hemoglobin concentration of 19 g/dl, normal erythrocyte morphology, no evidence of hemolysis, and red-cell 2,3-DPG level below 3 percent of normal values. DPGM activity was undetectable in erythrocytes, as was that of diphosphoglycerate phosphatase, confirming that both activities reside in the same protein. Furthermore, phosphoglycerate mutase activity was reduced to 50 percent of normal. The propositus' three sisters exhibited the same phenotype, while his two children had an intermediate phenotype.[296] In all the deficient subjects, the ATP level was elevated and the pattern of glycolytic intermediates was disturbed, with an increase in fructose 1,6-bisphosphate and triosephosphates. A new minor fraction of glycerylated hemoglobin has been found in these individuals.[297] A marked increase in affinity of hemoglobin for oxygen secondary to the extremely low 2,3-DGP content explains the compensatory erythrocytosis, which requires no therapy.

Complete deficiency of DPGM enzyme activity was shown subsequently to be associated with 30 to 50 percent of an inactive enzyme being detectable by specific antibodies and resulting from a substitution of Arg 89 by Cys (R89C).[298-300] Further studies indicated the presence of two forms of messenger RNA, a major form with the R89C mutation and a minor form with a normal sequence. Sequence studies of the propositus' DNA samples indicated heterozygosity at position 89 and another heterozygosity with the deletion of nucleotide C 205 or C 206. Thus, the total DPGM deficiency results from a genetic compound with one allele coding for an inactive enzyme (mutation $DPGM_{CRETEIL\ I}$) and the other bearing a frameshift mutation ($DPGM_{CRETEIL\ II}$). Both of the children of the propositus were found to have the $DPGM_{CRETEIL\ I}$ mutation.[301]

Molecular cloning and sequencing of human erythrocyte DPGM cDNA have revealed a protein of 258 residues.[302] The DPGM gene has been assigned to region 7q22-q34, and more recently, its organization has been described[303,304] (see Table 114-3).

Enolase Deficiency

Enolase catalyzes the reversible conversion of 2-phosphoglycerate to phospho*enol*pyruvate (see Fig. 114-1). Three classes of isoenzymes exist; each isoenzyme is a homodimeric protein composed of two α, β, or γ subunits. Most tissues contain only αα enolase.[305]

Hemolytic anemia associated with erythrocyte enolase deficiency and exacerbated by nitrofurantoin has been described,[306] but questioned for methodological reasons.[25] A woman who underwent splenectomy for hereditary spherocytosis but who had an incomplete response was found to have 50 percent of normal erythrocyte enolase activity.[307] The propositus' father had died after splenectomy for an undefined hemolytic disorder. Erythrocyte enolase deficiency has been noted in four generations of a Caucasian family.[308] A 13-day-old male infant with hematocrit of 17 percent, reticulocyte count of 11.2 percent, and an elevated bilirubin level had red-cell enolase activity about half that expected for a neonate. The enolase activity of the father, paternal grandmother, and great-grandmother was half normal, strongly suggesting an autosomal dominant mode of transmission. Both the father and a paternal great-uncle had a hematocrit of 40 percent, with 2.5 percent reticulocytes, while the three other enolase-deficient adults had no evidence of anemia or hemolysis. Spherocytes were present on the blood smears of all five affected adults. It appears that partial enolase deficiency has a spherocytic phenotype and a variable clinical expression within this family.

The structural gene for human enolase has been assigned to chromosome 1p36-pter[309] (see Table 114-3). Molecular cloning and nucleotide sequence of a full-length cDNA for human α enolase have been reported.[310]

Lactate Dehydrogenase Deficiency

LDH catalyzes the last step in glycolysis, the conversion of pyruvate to lactate (see Fig. 114-1). LDH is a tetrameric enzyme composed of two subunits, H and M. Complete deficiency of LDH H subunit has been well documented in two adults in unrelated Japanese kindreds.[311-313] Erythrocyte LDH activity was less than 10 percent of normal, but there was no anemia or overt evidence of hemolysis. Pyruvate did not accumulate within the erythrocyte since it is diffusible. However, the concentrations of F-1,6-P_2, dihydroxyacetone phosphate, and glyceraldehyde 3-phosphate were increased markedly, and the concentration of NAD^+ was decreased, owing to the block of LDH-mediated NADH reoxidation. The abnormal pattern for glycolytic intermediates suggests that a metabolic disturbance also exists at the reaction step involving glyceraldehyde 3-phosphate dehydrogenase (see Fig. 114-1). Family studies have demonstrated an autosomal recessive mode of inheritance.

Myopathy without hemolysis and associated with a complete lack of subunit M in muscle, serum, red cells, and leukocytes has been documented in four members of a Japanese family.[314] The mode of inheritance is autosomal recessive.

Somatic-cell hybridization studies have localized the gene locus for LDH-H to chromosome 12[8,315,316] (see Table 114-3) and that for LDH-M to chromosome 11.[317] The gene for LDH has been cloned,[318] and a missense mutation has been reported.[319]

ENZYMOPATHIES INVOLVING THE PENTOSE PHOSPHATE SHUNT AND RELATED GLUTATHIONE METABOLISM

Disorders of glutathione metabolism are discussed in greater detail in Chap. 43.

6-Phosphogluconate Dehydrogenase and 6-Phosphogluconolactonase

Severe deficiency of 6-phosphogluconate dehydrogenase, the second dehydrogenase of the pentose phosphate shunt, while well documented,[320,321] is rare and has never been incriminated in the pathogenesis of a hemolytic syndrome. In fact, subjects with <5 percent of normal activity in erythrocytes have been found in population surveys,[320] but were asymptomatic. Inheritance was thought to be autosomal dominant.[321] Partial deficiency of 6-phosphogluconolactonase coexisting with heterozygous G-6-PD deficiency was found associated with hemolysis in an infant girl with α-thalassemia minor.[322] However, there was no hemolysis in a Hindu boy with combined G-6-PD and 6-phosphogluconate dehydrogenase deficiency.[323]

Glutathione Peroxidase

The enzymatic conversion of harmful peroxides to water and alcohols is catalyzed by the selenoenzyme glutathione peroxidase in a coupled oxidation of reduced glutathione. Partial deficiencies of glutathione peroxidase have been documented in association with otherwise unexplained hemolytic syndromes,[8,10,324] but a cause-and-effect relationship has not been established. About half-normal glutathione peroxidase activity has been demonstrated in the red cells of large numbers of persons of Jewish and Mediterranean origin[325]; certain populations with dietary deficiency of selenium also have decreased enzyme activity.[8] There was no documentation of coexistent hemolysis. Thus, the role of deficient glutathione peroxidase activity in the pathogenesis of a hemolytic syndrome in humans remains unsettled.[325] Glutathione peroxidase is inherited in an autosomal pattern, and the gene has been assigned to chromosome 3.[326]

Glutathione Reductase

A diversity of syndromes, including neurologic disorders, hemolytic anemias, and panmyelopathies, have been reported in association with decreased glutathione reductase activity in erythrocytes.[8,10] Observations that many subjects with such disorders suffered from inadequate synthesis of the cofactor FAD secondary to nutritional riboflavin deficiency or to its defective metabolism did much to resolve this paradox.[8,327] Glutathione reductase deficiency, except when extremely severe, is not associated with hemolysis.[328,329] Virtually complete absence of apoenzyme activity has been documented in three sibs, and partial deficiency was found in their obligate heterozygous parents.[330] This was unaffected by FAD in vitro or riboflavin in vivo, was concomitantly present in leukocytes, and was associated with unstable GSH on incubating red cells with acetylphenylhydrazine. Clinically, this deficiency was manifested by hemolytic crises after eating fava beans in one sib and possibly by cataracts in two sibs. Inheritance of glutathione reductase deficiency is autosomal and the encoding gene resides on chromosome 8.[331]

Enzyme Deficiencies of Glutathione Synthesis: γ-Glutamylcysteine Synthetase and Glutathione Synthetase

The tripeptide GSH is synthesized in two ATP-dependent steps catalyzed respectively by γ-glutamylcysteine and glutathione synthetase.[332,333] The end product, GSH, is present in red cells at the high concentration of 2 m*M* and plays an important role in protecting the cell from oxidative damage.

Virtual absence of GSH results from the rare, autosomal recessive deficiency of γ-glutamylcysteine synthetase, which mediates the first step of glutathione synthesis. The initial probands, brother and sister, were diagnosed in adulthood, had moderate hemolytic anemia, had red-cell GSH only 2 to 3 percent of normal, and had progressive spinocerebellar ataxia.[334,335] Decreased concentrations of GSH in other tissues, such as skeletal muscle (25 percent) and leukocytes (50 percent), were not associated with apparent dysfunction. In contrast to the first kindred studied, another case of severe deficiency with hemolytic anemia demonstrated no neurologic abnormalities.[336]

The second step in glutathione synthesis adds glycine to the dipeptide γ-glutamylcysteine and is mediated by glutathione synthetase. Severe deficiencies of this enzyme are manifested as two phenotypes, one consisting of hemolytic anemia alone and one as multisystem disease with metabolic acidosis, massive 5-oxoprolinuria, and often neurologic dysfunction accompanying a hemolytic syndrome.[8,10] The heterogeneity of glutathione synthetase deficiency may be related to varying effects of unstable mutant enzymes in different tissues, but possibly also to differing tissue distribution of proteases.[337] The loss of feedback inhibition of γ-glutamylcysteine production by glutathione itself allows this dipeptide to accumulate and to affect concentrations of related metabolites. Severe 5-oxoprolinemia and metabolic acidosis requiring bicarbonate therapy are common consequences. In all phenotypes of glutathione synthetase deficiency, obligate heterozygotes have about half-normal enzyme activity, are asymptomatic, and have normal tissue concentrations of GSH. Glutathione synthetase deficiency, when severe, is accompanied by glutathione-*S*-transferase deficiency as well.[338] The latter is not genetically determined but is secondary to increased susceptibility to denaturation when GSH is nearly absent. In addition to chronic hemolysis, subjects with severe deficiencies of either glutathione synthetic enzyme are susceptible to acute episodes of stress-induced hemolysis with Heinz-body production.

DISTURBANCES IN ENZYMES OF NUCLEOTIDE METABOLISM

The metabolic reactions outlined in Fig. 114-1 are delicately balanced to provide optimal concentrations of reducing equivalents and high-energy phosphates. Because many crucial cell functions depend specifically on ATP, perturbations in its generation via glycolysis or its maintenance via salvage pathways often have deleterious effects on erythrocyte function and longevity. Within the adenine nucleotide pool, AMP is in particular jeopardy: AMP deamination, either before or after dephosphorylation, yields IMP or diffusible inosine, and mechanisms do not exist in mature erythrocytes to retrieve the purine moiety from these compounds. This may have special importance in older erythrocytes, where salvage mechanisms probably assume greater relative metabolic roles as glycolytic capacity diminishes with cell age.

Disorders of nucleotide metabolism in erythrocytes include both deficient and hyperactive enzymes.[339] Many of these conditions, (for example, severe deficiencies of ADA, nucleoside phosphorylase, APRT, HPRT, and hyperactive PP-ribose-P synthetase, have no discernible detrimental effects on erythrocytes. A few cases of ribosephosphate pyrophosphokinase and HPRT deficiencies have been associated with megaloblastic changes, but these may have been due to relative folate deficiency rather than to the enzymopathies per se. Megaloblastic features have also been described in cases with severe deficiencies of orotate phosphoribosyltransferase and orotidine 5′-decarboxylase in hereditary orotic aciduria, perhaps reflecting broader disturbances in purine and pyrimidine biosynthesis (see Chap. 55).

Three principal disorders have been reported in association with shortened erythrocyte life span and hemolytic anemia of varying severity—hereditary hyperactivity of ADA, hereditary deficiency of adenylate kinase, and severe hereditary or acquired deficiencies of pyrimidine nucleotidase.

Hemolytic anemia secondary to hyperactive adenosine deaminase (adenosine aminohydrolase, EC 3.5.4.4.) has been identified in three unrelated kindreds in the United States, Japan, and France.[340–344] Affected individuals may be asymptomatic, with well-compensated chronic hemolysis, but they can be identified by moderate reticulocytosis, decrements in erythrocyte ATP to less than half expected concentrations, three- to fourfold increases in pyrimidine nucleotidase activity, and markedly hyperactive adenosine deaminase on the order of one-hundred-fold. The cause and/or effects of elevated pyrimidine nucleotidase activities associated with this disorder remain an enigma. There is no evidence that this nucleotidase is capable of dephosphorylating AMP to cause the observed reductions in ATP.

The ADA molecule itself is normal by all conventional biochemical criteria, including electrophoretic migration, kinetics for various substrates and inhibitors, heat stability, specific activity, pH optimum, immunologic reactivity, amino acid composition, and peptide patterns. The basic abnormality appears to result from overproduction of structurally normal enzyme protein mediated at the level of mRNA translation.[345–348]

The defect is transmitted as a genetic dominant and appears confined to erythroid elements, since granulocytes, lymphocytes, and cultured skin fibroblasts from affected individuals exhibit normal activities. If increased activity were due to altered molecular structure, as in the case of hyperactive ribosephosphate pyrophosphokinase, then specific activity would be increased and other tissues with the same isoenzyme would be expected to share the anomaly. In ADA deficiency associated with immunoincompetence, all tissues exhibit decreased activities. This is consistent with evidence that tissue-specific isoenzymes of ADA share a common protein,[349,350] the production of which is governed by a single genetic locus on chromosome 20.[351] The structure and sequence of this gene have been determined.[352]

Reductions in the adenine nucleotide pool of affected erythrocytes are thought to result from perturbation of the normally delicate balance between ADA and adenosine kinase activities. These two enzymes compete for micromolar amounts of substrate available in the plasma. Under certain conditions adenosine may be preferentially converted to inosine because ADA is normally much more active than the kinase[353,354] and is also in close physical association with the membrane components responsible for facilitated transport of adenosine.[355] At very low adenosine concentrations, however, phosphorylation may predominate because the kinase has a twentyfold lower Michaelis constant as compared with the deaminase.[354]

In the affected cells, adenosine kinase activity is increased almost two orders of magnitude, perhaps even more in subpopulations. This apparently diverts adenosine away from the kinase-mediated pathway, depriving the cells of an effective means to compensate for random nucleotide losses, and low concentrations of adenine nucleotides result. Parenthetically, the converse situation exists in some cases of immunodeficiency disease in which severe impairment of ADA activity is associated with markedly increased concentrations of cellular adenine deoxynucleotides.[356–361] The absence of deaminase activity apparently allows an inordinate amount of adenosine or deoxyadenosine to be phosphorylated to AMP or dAMP, and the nucleotide pool in the cell is consequently expanded. The biochemical abnormalities in these two distinct genetic anomalies strongly suggest that the availability of adenosine, and a balanced competition for it between adenosine kinase and deaminase, are necessary for normal maintenance of the adenine nucleotide pool in mature erythrocytes.

An equally rare disorder, hereditary deficiency of adenylate kinase (myokinase) (ATP:AMP phosphotransferase, EC 2.7.4.3), has been detected in five kindreds, but a causal relation between the deficiency and premature hemolysis remains uncertain. Adenylate kinase activities 10 percent or less of normal were observed in an Israeli Arab[362,363] and a French family[364] and 44 percent of normal in a Japanese child[365] with moderate to severe hemolytic anemia. In one case, anemia was associated with partial G-6-PD deficiency and in another with psychomotor retardation. Parents in each kindred possessed the common adenylate kinase 1 (AK-1) electrophoretic phenotype. Family studies suggested an autosomal recessive (or dominant with variable penetrance) transmission. Nonanemic heterozygotes were identifiable by enzyme activities approximating half-normal mean values.

Studies of a fourth kindred with this disorder, a black American family,[366] cast serious doubt that severe adenylate kinase deficiency alone is capable of inducing shortened erythrocyte survival. Of two children with virtually undetectable adenylate kinase activities, only one had hemolytic anemia, whereas the other was hematologically normal. Erythrocyte concentrations of all adenine nucleotides were only slightly decreased, if at all. The possibility of multiple defects was again raised by the presence of slightly decreased PK activities and increased 2,3-DPG concentrations, but these changes were of comparable degrees in erythrocytes from both children.

AMP, generated from adenine by APRT or from adenosine by adenosine kinase (see Fig. 114-1), cannot be incorporated effectively into ADP and ATP without some minimal amount of kinase activity. Data from this family indicate that less than 0.1 percent of normal activity may be sufficient to maintain normal ATP–ADP concentrations in circulating erythrocytes, despite irreversible losses of the adenine moiety by deamination mediated by ADA or adenylate deaminase. Since severe deficiency of APRT is also not associated with premature hemolysis,[367] this salvage pathway appears less important for maintenance of the ATP–ADP pool than that mediated by adenosine kinase.

Studies of a fifth kindred with this disorder support the concept that adenylate kinase deficiency per se may not be responsible for inducing hemolysis. This proband had undetectable adenylate kinase activity with active hemolysis, but radiolabeled adenine was still incorporated into red-cell nucleotides at half the rates of normal controls, perhaps by an alternative pathway. PK and PP-ribose-P synthetase activities were decreased, and AMP:GTP phosphotransferase was undetectable, suggesting the possibility that the deleterious effects might be a consequence of deficiencies involving multiple phosphotransferases.[368]

The gene encoding AK-1 has been cloned and sequenced and found to be responsible for two species of mRNA.[369] A patient with adenylate kinase deficiency was found to have a CGG → TGG substitution in exon 6 of one allele, causing an Arg to Trp substitution at residue 128 (R128W) of AK-1.

The most common enzyme defect within the category of nucleotide anomalies in red cells is that of pyrimidine nucleotidase deficiency.[370] Nucleotidases (5′-ribonucleotide phosphohydrolase, EC 3.1.3.5), are widely distributed throughout nature as a heterogeneous group of isoenzymes, all of which react with both purine and pyrimidine substrates with variable effectiveness. Catalytic capability of erythrocyte nucleotidase, however, is largely restricted to pyrimidine substrates,[371] an almost mandatory adaptation in erythrocytes, since a nucleotidase also capable of dephosphorylating AMP would impose a constant drain on the adenine nucleotide pool. A second normal isoenzyme of erythrocyte nucleotidase has also been identified, a deoxynucleotidase that acts principally on both purine and pyrimidine deoxyribomononucleotides.[372,373]

Severe hereditary deficiency states of pyrimidine nucleotidase have been identified in a relatively large number of individuals with wide geographic distribution.[370] Those of peri-Mediterranean, Jewish, or African ancestry may be particularly susceptible. The genetic defect is transmitted as an autosomal recessive trait. Heterozygotes exhibit intermediate decrements in nucleotidase activity but are otherwise hematologically and biochemically normal.

Pyrimidine nucleotidase probably functions only during reticulocyte maturation, serving to dephosphorylate the pyrimidine products of RNA degradation without jeopardizing the purine components.[374] Therefore, severe nucleotidase deficiency may result in accumulation of pyrimidines that cannot diffuse from the cells as long as they remain phosphorylated. Impaired degradation of RNA results in aggregates of intact or partially degraded ribosomal nucleoprotein. This provides the most distinctive hematologic finding in this disease, pronounced basophilic stippling on the Wright's stained peripheral smears (Fig. 114-3).

The diagnosis of pyrimidine nucleotidase deficiency is established by demonstration of significantly decreased enzyme activities, generally to about 5 percent of that observed in comparably young cell populations, and/or the identification of an array of intracellular pyrimidine compounds, none of which is normally detectable in erythrocytes. These include conjugates, such as CDP-choline, CDP-ethanolamine, and UDP-glucose as well as pyrimidine monophosphate, diphosphate, and triphosphate. Chromatographic techniques may be required to identify specific pyrimidines,

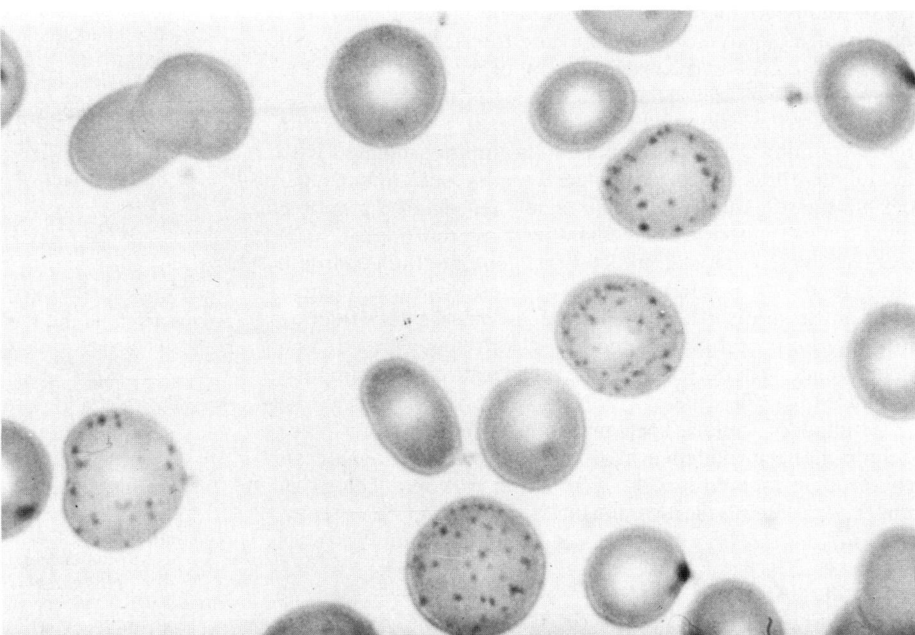

FIG. 114-3 Basophilic stippling in peripheral erythrocytes from a patient with severe hereditary deficiency of pyrimidine nucleotidase (Wright's stain).

but shifts in the UV absorption spectrum of cell extracts can readily detect their presence.[370,374] In subjects with severe hereditary or acquired nucleotidase deficiency, the presence of significant intracellular concentrations of pyrimidine compounds produces spectra with maximal absorption in the region of 265 to 270 nm rather than the usual 257 nm characteristic of adenine compounds. Since the accumulated nucleotides often consist of as much as 80 percent pyrimidine compounds, the adenine nucleotide pool is actually diminished on an absolute scale, and this may be at least partially responsible for premature hemolysis.

Two epiphenomena have been consistently observed in this disorder: Erythrocyte glutathione concentrations are frequently twice normal, and PP-ribose-P synthetase activities are usually reduced to about one-fourth. The etiology of these changes and their pathophysiological significance, if any, remain speculative. Evidence has been presented that pyrimidine nucleotides interfere with the membrane transport system that normally removes oxidized glutathione from the cell.[375] Pyrimidine compounds do not appear to alter the enzymes of glutathione biosynthesis or redox cycling,[376] but they may result in inhibition of HMP shunt activity or response to stimulation.[377,378]

At least six different procedures for partial purification of erythrocyte nucleotidases have been applied in attempts to characterize normal and mutant isoenzymes of erythrocyte nucleotidases. Studies of cases of pyrimidine nucleotidase deficiency have allowed detection and assessment of the biochemical characteristics of residual deoxyribonucleotidase,[372,379–381] but deficiency states for this normal isoenzyme have not yet been observed.

As with other erythrocyte enzymes, the methods of purification and assay strongly influence measurements of maximal activities, kinetic constants, and other biochemical properties, making accurate comparisons untenable.

Pyrimidine nucleotidase and deoxyribonucleotidase may be complementary systems that serve physiologically to clear the cytosol of RNA and DNA degradation products during maturation of erythroid elements by conversion of nucleotide monophosphates to diffusible nucleosides. This implies that erythroid precursors may not lose nuclear material entirely by pitting, but require a deoxynucleotidase system to catabolize residual nucleotides derived from karyolysis or mitochondrial degradation.[372,380]

Deficiencies of pyrimidine nucleotidase may also occur on an acquired basis secondary to lead toxicity. The remarkable sensitivity of this enzyme to inactivation by lead and certain other heavy metals,[371] and the common feature of basophilic stippling, led to elucidation of its role in the pathogenesis of lead-induced hemolytic anemia. Concentrations of lead that totally obliterate pyrimidine nucleotidase activity have minimal effects on most glycolytic and many other erythrocyte enzymes, although they may adversely affect heme biosynthesis. Humans exposed to chronic low-level overburden of industrial lead insufficient to cause anemia or basophilic stippling may still exhibit significant depressions of pyrimidine nucleotidase activity with otherwise normal glycolytic enzyme profiles.[382] When blood lead levels approach 200 μg/dl packed cells, pyrimidine nucleotidase activity is depressed to levels comparable to those found in severe hereditary deficiency states. Basophilic stippling then becomes apparent, and pyrimidine nucleotides begin to accumulate to detectable levels within the erythrocytes.[383–385] Elevated GSH concentrations and decreased PP-ribose-P synthetase activities have also been observed in isolated cases, so it is clear that the lead-induced acquired deficiency is capable of manifesting the full array of changes characteristic of the severe hereditary deficiency state.

A single case of chronic hemolytic anemia with deranged nucleotide metabolism, possibly involving defective choline phosphotransferase, was manifested by selective accumulation of CDP-choline in the range of 15 to 25 times normal erythrocyte concentrations.[386] No other abnormal nucleotides or metabolites were detected.

The three principal conditions reviewed here, hyperactivity of ADA and deficiencies of adenylate kinase and of pyrimidine nucleotidase, have all been reported to occur in association with hemolytic anemias of variable severities. The first two are very rare, and it now seems doubtful that pure adenylate kinase deficiency alone can induce premature hemolysis. The anemia of hyperactive ADA may be subclinical or totally compensated. Life-threatening anemia has been observed in some cases of adenylate kinase deficiency, but these may have been complicated by other defects, since at least one case of severe deficiency has shown no hematologic effects. Pyrimidine nucleotidase deficiency is one of the more common erythroenzymopathies and is associated with hemolytic anemia of intermediate severity, infrequently necessitating transfusions. Acquired deficiencies of pyrimidine nucleotidase activity induced by lead overburden, if sufficiently severe, almost completely recapitulate the syndrome associated with severe hereditary deficiency states. Splenectomy in these disorders has not been consistently effective but may be useful in selected cases with heavy transfusion dependence. Therapy has been largely restricted to supportive measures.

Studies of cellular perturbations resulting from these defects have provided a broader understanding of normal erythrocyte metabolism, as well as the pathophysiology of underlying hemolytic mechanisms.

REFERENCES

1. Bunn HF: Evolution of mammalian hemoglobin function. *Blood* **58**:189, 1981.
2. Brewer GJ, Prasad AS: Biochemistry and function of the erythron, in Bick RL (ed): *Hematology. Clinical and Laboratory Practice*. St. Louis, Mosby, 1990, p 185.
3. Paglia DE: Biochemistry of the red cell, in Hoffman R, Benz EJ Jr, Shattil SJ, Furie B, Cohen HJ (eds): *Hematology: Basic Principles and Practice*, 2d ed. New York, Churchill Livingstone, 1994, in press.
4. Miller DR: Hemolytic anemias: Metabolic defects, in Miller DR, Baehner RL, Miller LP (eds): *Blood Diseases of Infancy and Childhood*. St. Louis, Mosby, 1989, p 294.
5. Benesch R, Benesch RE: Intracellular organic phosphates as regulators of oxygen release by hemoglobin. *Nature* **221**:618, 1969.
6. Rapoport S, Luebering J: The formation of 2,3-diphosphoglycerate in rabbit erythrocytes: The existence of a diphosphoglycerate mutase. *J Biol Chem* **183**:507, 1950.
7. Valentine WN, Paglia DE: Erythrocyte enzymopathies, hemolytic anemia, and multisystem disease. *Blood* **64**:583, 1984.
8. Valentine WN, Tanaka KR, Paglia DE: Pyruvate kinase and other enzyme deficiency disorders of the erythrocyte, in Scriver CR, Beaudet AL, Sly WS, Valle D (eds): *The Metabolic Basis of Inherited Disease*, 6th ed. New York, McGraw-Hill, 1989, p 2341.
9. Valentine WN, Tanaka KR, Paglia DE: Hemolytic anemias and erythrocyte enzymopathies. *Ann Intern Med* **103**:249, 1985.
10. Dacie J: *The Haemolytic Anaemias*, 3rd ed. New York, Churchill Livingstone, 1985, vol 1 (The Hereditary Haemolytic Anaemias), pp 282, 321, 419.
11. Tanaka KR, Paglia DE: Pyruvate kinase deficiency. *Semin Hematol* **8**:367, 1971.
12. Sullivan DW, Glader BE: Erythrocyte enzyme disorders in children. *Pediatr Clin North Am* **27**:449, 1980.
13. Miwa S: Hereditary disorders of red cell enzymes in the Embden-Meyerhof pathway. *Am J Hematol* **14**:381, 1983.
14. Jaffé ER, Valentine WN: Human erythroenzymopathies of the anaerobic Embden-Meyerhof glycolytic and associated pathways, in Nagel R (ed): *Genetically Abnormal Red Cells*. Boca Raton, FL, CRC, 1991, p 105.
15. Mentzer WC Jr: Pyruvate kinase deficiency and disorders of glycolysis, in Nathan DG, Oski FA (eds): *Hematology of Infancy and Childhood*, 4th ed. Philadelphia, Saunders, 1993, p 634.
16. Lukens JN: Hereditary hemolytic anemias associated with abnormalities of erythrocyte anaerobic glycolysis and nucleotide metabolism, in Lee GR, Bithell TC, Foerster J, Athens JW, Lukens JN (eds): *Wintrobe's Clinical Hematology*, 9th ed. Philadelphia, Lea & Febiger, 1993, p 990.
17. Valentine WN, Tanaka KR, Miwa S: A specific erythrocyte glycolytic enzyme defect (pyruvate kinase) in three subjects with congenital nonspherocytic hemolytic anemia. *Trans Assoc Am Physicians* **74**:100, 1961.
18. Tanaka KR, Valentine WN, Miwa S: Pyruvate kinase (PK) deficiency hereditary non-spherocytic hemolytic anemia. *Blood* **19**:267, 1962.
19. Bowman HS, McKusick VA, Dronamraju KR: Pyruvate kinase deficient hemolytic anemia in an Amish isolate. *Am J Hum Genet* **17**:1, 1965.
20. Searcy GP, Miller DR, Tasker JB: Congenital hemolytic anemia in the Basenji dog due to erythrocyte pyruvate kinase deficiency. *Can J Comp Med* **35**:67, 1971.
21. Prasse KW, Crouser D, Beutler E, Walker M, Schall WD: Pyruvate kinase deficiency anemia with terminal myelofibrosis and osteosclerosis in a Beagle. *J Am Vet Med Assoc* **166**:1170, 1975.
22. Sachs JR, Wicker DJ, Gilcher RO: Familial hemolytic anemia resulting from an abnormal red blood cell pyruvate kinase. *J Lab Clin Med* **72**:359, 1968.
23. Bossu M, Dachà M, Fornaini G: Neonatal hemolysis due to a transient severity of inherited pyruvate kinase deficiency. *Acta Haematol (Basel)* **40**:166, 1968.
24. Paglia DE, Valentine WN, Williams KO, Konrad PN: An isozyme of erythrocyte pyruvate kinase (PK-Los Angeles) with impaired kinetics corrected by fructose-1,6-diphosphate. *Am J Clin Pathol* **68**:229, 1977.
25. Beutler E: Hemolytic anemia in disorders of red cell metabolism, in Wintrobe MM (ed): *Topics in Hematology*. New York; Plenum, 1978.
26. Kahn A, Marie J, Vives-Corrons JL, Maigret P, Najman A: Search for a relationship between molecular anomalies of the mutant erythrocyte pyruvate kinase variants and their pathological expression. *Hum Genet* **57**:172, 1981.
27. Schröter W, Tillmann W: Membrane-localized pyruvate kinase of red blood cells in hemolytic anemia associated with pyruvate kinase deficiency. *Klin Wochenschr* **53**:1101, 1975.
28. Nathan DG, Oski FA, Miller DR, Gardner FH: Life-span and organ sequestration of the red cells in pyruvate kinase deficiency. *N Engl J Med* **278**:73, 1968.
29. Levinski U, Fajnholc N, Djaldetti M, De Vries A: Hemolytic anemia in pregnancy associated with erythrocyte pyruvate kinase deficiency. *Clin Sci* **11**:43, 1974.
30. Amankwah KS, Dick BW, Dodge S: Hemolytic anemia and pyruvate kinase deficiency in pregnancy. *Obstet Gynecol* **55**:42S, 1980.
31. Fanning J, Hinkle RS: Pyruvate kinase deficiency hemolytic anemia: Two successful pregnancy outcomes. *Am J Obstet Gynecol* **153**:313, 1985.
32. Van Eys J, Garms P: Pyruvate kinase deficiency hemolytic anemia: A model for correlation of clinical syndrome and biochemical anomalies. *Adv Pediatr* **18**:203, 1971.
33. Delivoria-Papadopoulos M, Oski FA, Gottlieb AJ: Oxygen-hemoglobin dissociation curves: Effect of inherited enzyme defects of the red cell. *Science* **165**:601, 1969.
34. Oski FA, Marshall BE, Cohen PJ, Sugerman HJ, Miller LD: Exercise with anemia. The role of the left-shifted or right-shifted oxygen-hemoglobin equilibrium curve. *Ann Intern Med* **74**:44, 1971.
35. Tomoda A, Lachant NA, Noble NA, Tanaka KR: Inhibition of the pentose phosphate shunt by 2,3-diphosphoglycerate in erythrocyte pyruvate kinase deficiency. *Br J Haematol* **54**:475, 1983.
36. Duncan JR, Potter CG, Cappellini MD, Kurtz JB, Anderson MJ, Weatherall DJ: Aplastic crisis due to parvovirus infection in pyruvate kinase deficiency. *Lancet* **2**:14, 1983.
37. Paglia DE, Valentine WN: Molecular lesion affecting the ADP-combining site in a mutant isozyme of erythrocyte pyruvate kinase. *Proc Natl Acad Sci USA* **78**:5175, 1981.
38. Tanaka KR, Valentine WN: Pyruvate kinase deficiency, in Beutler E (ed): *Hereditary Disorders of Erythrocyte Metabolism*. New York, Grune & Stratton, 1968, p 229.
39. Paglia DE: Enzymopathies, in Hoffman R, Benz EJ Jr, Shattil

SJ, Furie B, Cohen HJ (eds): *Hematology. Basic Principles and Practice*. New York, Churchill Livingstone, 1991, p 504.

40. Bowman HS, Procopio F: Hereditary non-spherocytic hemolytic anemia of the pyruvate-kinase deficient type. *Ann Intern Med* **58**:567, 1963.
41. Gilman PA: Hemolysis in the newborn infant resulting from deficiencies of red blood cell enzymes: Diagnosis and management. *J Pediatr* **84**:625, 1974.
42. Hennekam RCM, Beemer FA, Cats BP, Jansen G, Staal GEJ: Hydrops fetalis associated with red cell pyruvate kinase deficiency. *Genet Couns* **1**:75, 1990.
43. Muller-Soyano A, De Roura ET, Duke PR, De Acquatella GC, Arends T, Guinto E, Beutler E: Pyruvate kinase deficiency and leg ulcers. *Blood* **47**:807, 1976.
44. Curiel Carias D, Velasquez GA, Papa R, Somoza de Martinez R, Linares F, Smith P, Rios de Vielma H, De Acquatella G: Hemolytic anemia and leg ulcers due to pyruvate kinase deficiency. Report of the second Venezuelan family. *Sangre (Barc)* **22**:64, 1977.
45. Vives-Corrons JL, Marie J, Pujades MA, Kahn A: Hereditary erythrocyte pyruvate-kinase (PK) deficiency and chronic hemolytic anemia: Clinical, genetic and molecular studies in six new Spanish patients. *Hum Genet* **53**:401, 1980.
46. Mahour GH, Lynn HB, Hill RW: Acute pancreatitis with biliary disease in erythrocyte pyruvate-kinase deficiency. *Clin Pediatr (Phila)* **8**:608, 1969.
47. Salem HH, Van der Weyden MB, Firkin BJ: Iron overload in congenital erythrocyte pyruvate kinase deficiency. *Med J Aust* **1**:531, 1980.
48. Rowbotham B, Roeser HP: Iron overload associated with congenital pyruvate kinase deficiency and high dose ascorbic acid ingestion. *Aust N Z J Med* **14**:667, 1984.
49. Linos DA, Nagorney DM, McIlrath DC: Splenic abscess—the importance of early diagnosis. *Mayo Clin Proc* **58**:261, 1983.
50. Rutgers MJ, Van der Lugt PJ, Van Turnhout JM: Spinal cord compression by extramedullary hemopoietic tissue in pyruvate-kinase-deficiency-caused hemolytic anemia. *Neurology* **29**:510, 1979.
51. Bertrand P, Feremans WW, Barroy JP, Dereume JP, Goldstein M: Vascular complications in a case of hemolytic anemia due to pyruvate kinase deficiency. *Acta Chir Belg* **82**:533, 1982.
52. Leblond PF, Lyonnais J, Delage JM: Erythrocyte populations in pyruvate kinase deficiency anemia following splenectomy. I. Cell morphology. *Br J Haematol* **39**:55, 1978.
53. Keitt AS: Pyruvate kinase deficiency and related disorders of red cell glycolysis. *Am J Med* **41**:762, 1966.
54. Miwa S, Fujii H, Takegawa S, Nakatsuji T, Yamato K, Ishida Y, Ninomiya N: Seven pyruvate kinase variants characterized by the ICSH recommended methods. *Br J Haematol* **45**:575, 1980.
55. Bowman HS, Oski FA: Laboratory studies of erythrocyte pyruvate kinase deficiency. *Am J Clin Pathol* **70**:259, 1978.
56. Wazewska-Czyzewska M, Guminska M: Cogenital nonspherocytic haemolytic anaemia variants with primary and secondary pyruvate kinase deficiency. I. Erythrokinetic patterns. *Br J Haematol* **41**:115, 1979.
57. Mentzer WC Jr, Baehner RL, Schmidt-Schonbeth H, Robinson SH, Nathan DG: Selective reticulocyte destruction in erythrocyte pyruvate kinase deficiency. *J Clin Invest* **50**:688, 1971.
58. Matsumoto N, Ishihara T, Nakashima K, Miwa S, Uchino F, Kondo M: Sequestration and destruction of reticulocyte in the spleen in pyruvate kinase deficiency hereditary nonspherocytic hemolytic anemia. *Acta Haematol Jpn* **35**:525, 1972.
59. Leblond PF, Lyonnais J, Delage J-M: Erythrocyte populations in pyruvate kinase deficiency anemia following splenectomy II. Cell deformability. *Br J Haematol* **39**:63, 1978.
60. Matsumoto N, Ishihara T, Miwa S, Uchino F: The mechanism of mitochondrial extrusion from reticulocytes in the spleen from patients with erythrocyte pyruvate kinase (PK) deficiency. *Acta Haematol Jpn* **37**:25, 1974.
61. Becker MH, Genieser NB, Piomelli S, Dove D, Mendoza RD: Roentgenographic manifestations of pyruvate kinase deficiency hemolytic anemia. *Am J Roentgenol Radium Ther Nucl Med* **113**:491, 1971.
62. Tanaka KR: Pyruvate kinase, in Yunis JJ (ed): *Biochemical Methods in Red Cell Genetics*. New York; Academic, 1969, p 167.
63. Beutler E: Red cell metabolism. *A Manual of Biochemical Methods*, 3rd ed. Orlando, FL, Grune & Stratton, 1984.
64. Miwa S, Boivin P, Blume KG, Arnold H, Black JA, Kahn A, Staal GEJ, Nakashima K, Tanaka KR, Paglia DE, Valentine WN, Yoshida A, Beutler E: Recommended methods for the characterization of red cell pyruvate kinase variants. International Committee for Standardization in Haematology. *Br J Haematol* **43**:275, 1979.
65. Paglia DE, Valentine WN, Baughan MA, Miller DR, Reed CF, McIntyre OR: An inherited molecular lesion of erythrocyte pyruvate kinase. Identification of a kinetically aberrant isozyme associated with premature hemolysis. *J Clin Invest* **47**:1929, 1968.
66. Miwa S: Hereditary hemolytic anemia due to erythrocyte enzyme deficiency. *Acta Haematol Jpn* **36**:573, 1973.
67. Miwa S: Pyruvate kinase deficiency, in Ogita Z-1, Markert CL (eds): *Isozymes. Structure, Function, and Use in Biology and Medicine*. New York, Wiley-Liss, 1990, p 843.
68. Miwa S, Fujii H: Molecular aspects of erythroenzymopathies associated with hereditary hemolytic anemia. *Am J Hematol* **19**:293, 1985.
69. Miwa S, Kanno H, Fujii H: Pyruvate kinase deficiency: Historical perspective and recent progress in molecular genetics. *Am J Hematol* **42**:31, 1993.
70. Lestas AN, Bellingham AJ: A logical approach to the investigation of red cell enzymopathies. *Blood Rev* **4**:148, 1990.
71. Miwa S, Fujii H, Takegawa S, Nakatsuji T, Yamato K, Ishida Y, Ninomiya N: Seven pyruvate kinase variants characterized by the ICSH recommended methods. *Br J Haematol* **45**:575, 1980.
72. Shinohara K, Tanaka KR: Pyruvate kinase deficiency hemolytic anemia: Enzymatic characterization studies in twelve patients. *Hemoglobin* **4**:611, 1980.
73. Beutler E, Forman L: Coexistence of α-thalassemia and a new pyruvate kinase variant: PK Fukien. *Acta Haematol* **69**:3, 1983.
74. Muir WA, Beutler E, Wasson C: Erythrocyte pyruvate kinase deficiency in the Ohio Amish: Origin and characterization of the mutant enzyme. *Am J Hum Genet* **36**:634, 1984.
75. Tani K, Tsutsumi H, Takahashi K, Ogura H, Kanno H, Hayasaka K, Narisawa K, Nakahata T, Akabane T, Morisaki T, Fujii H, Miwa S: Two homozygous cases of erythrocyte (PK) deficiency in Japan: PK Sendai and PK Shinshu. *Am J Hematol* **38**:186, 1988.
76. Neubauer B, Lakomek H, Winkler H, Parke M, Hofferbert S, Schröter W: Point mutations in the L-type pyruvate kinase gene of two children with hemolytic anemia caused by pyruvate kinase deficiency. *Blood* **77**:1871, 1991.
77. Etiemble J, Picat C, Dhermy D, Buc HA, Morin M, Boivin P: Erythrocytic pyruvate kinase deficiency and hemolytic anemia inherited as a dominant trait. *Am J Hematol* **17**:251, 1984.
78. Kahn A, Marie J, Galand C, Boivin P: Chronic hemolytic anemia in two patients heterozygous for erythrocyte pyruvate kinase deficiency. Electrofocusing and immunological studies of erythrocyte and liver pyruvate kinase. *Scand J Haematol* **16**:250, 1976.
79. Fung RHP, Keung YK, Chung GSH: Screening of pyruvate kinase deficiency and G6PD deficiency in Chinese newborns in Hong Kong. *Arch Dis Child* **44**:373, 1969.
80. Blume KG, Löhr GW, Praetsch O, Rudiger HW: Beitrag zur populationsgenetik der puruvatkinase menschlicher erythrocyten. *Humangenetik* **6**:261, 1968.
81. Garcia SC, Moragon AC, Lopez-Fernandez ME: Frequency of glutathione reductase, pyruvate kinase and glucose-6-phosphate dehydrogenase deficiency in a Spanish population. *Hum Hered* **29**:310, 1979.
82. Satoh C, Neel JV, Yamashita A, Goriki K, Fujita M, Hamilton HB: The frequency among Japanese of heterozygotes for deficiency variants of 11 enzymes. *Am J Hum Genet* **35**:656, 1983.

83. Wu Z-L, Yu W-D, Chen S-C: Frequency of erythrocyte pyruvate kinase deficiency in Chinese infants. *Am J Hematol* **20**:139, 1985.
84. El-Hazmi MAF, Al-Swailem AR, Al-Faleh FZ, Warsy AS: Frequency of glucose-6-phosphate dehydrogenase, pyruvate kinase and hexokinase deficiency in the Saudi population. *Hum Hered* **36**:45, 1986.
85. Mohrenweiser HW: Frequency of enzyme deficiency variants in erythrocytes of newborn infants. *Proc Natl Acad Sci USA* **78**:5046, 1981.
86. Feng C-S, Tsang SS, Mak Y-T: Prevalence of pyruvate kinase deficiency among the Chinese: Determination by the quantitative assay. *Am J Hematol* **43**:271, 1993.
87. Tanaka T, Harano Y, Sue F, Morimura H: Crystallization, characterization and metabolic regulation of two types of pyruvate kinase isolated from rat tissues. *J Biochem (Tokyo)* **62**:71, 1967.
88. Imamura K, Tanaka T: Multimolecular forms of pyruvate kinase from rat and other mammalian tissues. *J Biochem (Tokyo)* **71**:1043, 1972.
89. Imamura K, Taniuchi K, Tanaka T: Multimolecular forms of pyruvate kinase. II. Purification of M_2-type pyruvate kinase from Yoshida ascites hepatoma 130 cells and comparative studies on the enzymological and immunological properties of the three types of pyruvate kinases. L, M_1 and M_2. *J Biochem (Tokyo)* **72**:1001, 1972.
90. Imamura K, Tanaka T, Nishina T, Nakashima K, Miwa S: Studies on pyruvate kinase (PK) deficiency. II. Electrophoretic, kinetic, and immunological studies on pyruvate kinase of erythrocytes and other tissues. *J Biochem (Tokyo)* **74**:1165, 1973.
91. Ibsen KH: Interrelationship and functions of the pyruvate kinase isozymes and their variant forms: A review. *Cancer Res* **37**:341, 1977.
92. Miwa S, Fujii H: Pyruvate kinase deficiency. *Clin Biochem* **23**:155, 1990.
93. Tani K, Yoshida MC, Satoh H, Mitamura K, Noguchi T, Tanaka T: Human M_2-type pyruvate kinase: cDNA cloning, chromosomal assignment and expression in hepatoma. *Gene* **73**:509, 1988.
94. Nakashima K, Miwa S, Oda S, Tanaka T, Imamura K, Nishina T: Electrophoretic and kinetic studies of mutant erythrocyte pyruvate kinases. *Blood* **43**:537, 1974.
95. Miwa S, Nakashima K, Ariyoshi K, Shinohara K, Oda E, Tanaka T: Four new pyruvate kinase (PK) variants and a classical PK deficiency. *Br J Haematol* **29**:157, 1975.
96. Black JA, Rittenberg MB, Bigley RH, Koler RD: Hemolytic anemia due to pyruvate kinase deficiency: Characterization of the enzymatic activity from eight patients. *Am J Hum Genet* **31**:300, 1979.
97. Kahn A, Dreyfus J-C: Molecular basis of the hereditary defects of enzyme activity, in Schewe T, Rapoport S (eds): *Molecular Diseases*. New York, Pergamon, 1979, vol 56, p 1.
98. Black JA, Rittenberg MB, Standerfer RJ, Peterson JS: Hereditary persistence of fetal erythrocyte pyruvate kinase in the Basenji dog, in Brewer GJ (ed): *The Red Cell*. New York, Alan R. Liss, 1978, p 275.
99. Noguchi T, Tanaka T: The M_1 and M_2 subunits of rat pyruvate kinase are encoded by different messenger RNAs. *J Biol Chem* **257**:1110, 1982.
100. Hance AJ, Lee J, Feitelson M: The M_1 and M_2 isozymes of pyruvate kinase are the products of the same gene. *Biochem Biophys Res Commun* **106**:492, 1982.
101. Noguchi T, Inoue H, Tanaka T: The M_1 and M_2-type isozymes of rat pyruvate kinase are produced from the same gene by alternative RNA splicing. *J Biol Chem* **261**:13807, 1986.
102. Noguchi T, Yamada K, Inoue H, Matsuda T, Tanaka T: The L- and R-type isozymes of rat pyruvate kinase are produced from a single gene by use of different promotors. *J Biol Chem* **262**:14366, 1987.
103. Tani K, Fujii H, Tsutsumi H, Sukegawa J, Toyoshima K, Yoshida MC, Noguchi T, Tanaka T, Miwa S: Human liver type pyruvate kinase: cDNA cloning and chromosomal assignment. *Biochem Biophys Res Commun* **143**:431, 1987.
104. Tani K, Fujii H, Nagata S, Miwa S: Human liver type pyruvate kinase: Complete amino acid sequence and the expression in mammalian cells. *Proc Natl Acad Sci USA* **85**:1792, 1988.
105. Tremp GL, Boquet D, Ripoche M-A, Cognet M, Lone Y-C, Jami J, Kahn A, Daegelen D: Expression of the rat L-type pyruvate kinase gene from its dual erythroid- and liver-specific promoter in transgenic mice. *J Biol Chem* **264**:19904, 1989.
106. Nakashima K, Miwa S, Fujii H, Shinohara K, Yamauchi K, Tsuji Y, Yanai M: Characterization of pyruvate kinase from the liver of a patient with aberrant erythrocyte pyruvate kinase, PK Nagasaki. *J Lab Clin Med* **90**:1012, 1977.
107. Bigley RH, Koler RD: Liver pyruvate kinase (PK) isoenzymes in a PK-deficient patient. *Ann Hum Genet* **31**:383, 1968.
108. Takegawa S, Fujii H, Miwa S: Change of pyruvate kinase isozymes from M_2-toL-type during development of the red cell. *Br J Haematol* **54**:467, 1983.
109. Max-Audit I, Testa U, Kechemir D, Titeux M, Vainchenker W, Rosa R: Pattern of pyruvate kinase isozymes in erythroleukemia cell lines and in normal human erythroblasts. *Blood* **64**:930, 1984.
110. Takegawa S, Miwa S: Change of pyruvate kinase (PK) isozymes in classical type PK deficiency and other PK deficiency cases during red cell maturation. *Am J Hematol* **16**:53, 1984.
111. Nijhof W, Wierenga PK, Staal GEJ, Jansen G: Changes in activities and isozyme patterns of glycolytic enzymes during erythroid differentiation in vitro. *Blood* **64**:607, 1984.
112. Marie J, Garreau H, Kahn A: Evidence for a postsynthetic proteolytic transformation of human erythrocyte pyruvate kinase into L-type enzyme. *FEBS Lett* **78**:91, 1977.
113. Kahn A, Marie J, Garreau H, Sprengers ED: The genetic system of the L-type pyruvate kinase forms in man. Subunit structure, interrelation and kinetic characteristics of the pyruvate kinase enzymes from erythrocytes and liver. *Biochim Biophys Acta* **523**:59, 1978.
114. Sprengers ED, Staal GEJ: Functional changes associated with the sequential transformation of L'_4 into L_4 pyruvate kinase. *Biochim Biophys Acta* **570**:259, 1979.
115. Marie J, Simon M-P, Dreyfus J-C, Kahn A: One gene, but two messenger RNAs encode liver L and red cell L′ pyruvate kinase subunits. *Nature* **292**:70, 1981.
116. Marie J, Kahn A, Boivin P: Pyruvate kinase isozymes in man. I. M type isozymes in adult and foetal tissues, electrofocusing and immunological studies. *Humangenetik* **31**:35, 1976.
117. Kahn A, Marie J, Boivin P: Pyruvate kinase in man. II. L-type and erythrocyte-type isozymes. Electrofocusing and immunologic studies. *Hum Genet* **33**:35, 1976.
118. Noguchi T, Inoue H, Chen H-L, Matsubara K, Tanaka T: Molecular cloning of DNA complementary to rat L-type pyruvate kinase mRNA. *J Biol Chem* **258**:15220, 1983.
119. Koler RD, Vanbellinghen P: The mechanism of precursor modulation of human pyruvate kinase I by fructose diphosphate. *Adv Enzyme Regul* **6**:127, 1968.
120. Staal GEJ, Koster JF, Kamp H, van Milligen-Boersma L, Veeger C: Human erythrocyte pyruvate kinase. Its purification and some properties. *Biochim Biophys Acta* **227**:86, 1971.
121. Black JA, Henderson MH: Activation and inhibition of human erythrocyte pyruvate kinase by organic phosphates, amino acids, dipeptides and anions. *Biochim Biophys Acta* **284**:115, 1972.
122. Monod J, Wyman J, Changeux JP: On the nature of allosteric transitions: A plausible model. *J Mol Biol* **12**:88, 1965.
123. Marie J, Vives-Corrons JL, Kahn A: Hereditary erythrocyte pyruvate kinase deficiency: Molecular and functional studies of four mutant PK variants detected in Spain. *Clin Chim Acta* **81**:153, 1977.
124. Paglia DE, Valentine WN, Holbrook CT, Brockway R: Pyruvate kinase isozyme (PK-Greenville) with defective allosteric activation by fructose-1-6-diphosphate: The role of F-1,6-P modulation in normal erythrocyte metabolism. *Blood* **62**:972, 1983.
125. Muirhead H: Triose phosphate isomerase, pyruvate kinase and other α/β-barrel enzymes. *Trends Biochem Sci* **8**:326, 1983.

126. Nathan DG, Oski FA, Sidel VW, Diamond LK: Extreme hemolysis and red cell distortion in erythrocyte pyruvate kinase deficiency. II. Measurements of erythrocyte glucose consumption, potassium flux, and adenosine triphosphate stability. *N Engl J Med* **272**:118, 1965.
127. Glader BE: Salicylate-induced injury of pyruvate-kinase-deficient erythrocytes. *N Engl J Med* **294**:916, 1976.
128. Fairbanks VF, Fernandez MN: The identification of metabolic errors associated with hemolytic anemia. *JAMA* **208**:316, 1969.
129. Grimes AJ, Meisler A, Dacie JV: Hereditary non-spherocytic haemolytic anemia. A study of red-cell carbohydrate metabolism in twelve cases of pyruvate-kinase deficiency. *Br J Haematol* **10**:403, 1964.
130. Loder PB, De Gruchy GC: Red cell enzymes and co-enzymes in non-spherocytic congenital haemolytic anaemias. *Br J Haematol* **11**:21, 1965.
131. Zerez CR, Tanaka KR: Impaired nicotinamide adenine dinucleotide synthesis in pyruvate kinase-deficient human erythrocytes: A mechanism for decreased total NAD content and a possible secondary cause of hemolysis. *Blood* **69**:999, 1987.
132. Zerez CR, Lachant NA, Tanaka KR: Decrease in subunit aggregation of phosphoribosylpyrophosphate synthetase: A mechanism for decreased nucleotide concentrations in pyruvate kinase-deficient human erythrocytes. *Blood* **68**:1024, 1986.
133. Zerez CR, Wong MD, Tanaka KR: Impaired phosphoribosylpyrophosphate (PRPP) formation in intact pyruvate kinase deficient RBC: A mechanism for decreased nucleotide content and hemolysis. *Blood* **68**:59a, 1986.
134. Gardos G, Strau FB: Uber die Rolle der adenosintriphosphor-saure (ATP) in der K-permeabilitat der menschlichen roten Blutkorperchen. *Acta Physiol Acad Sci Hung* **12**:1, 1957.
135. Valentine WN, Paglia DE: The primary cause of hemolysis in enzymopathies of anaerobic glycolysis: A viewpoint. *Blood Cells* **6**:819, 1980.
136. Beutler E: A commentary. *Blood Cells* **6**:827, 1980.
137. Valentine WN, Herring WB, Paglia DE, Steuterman MC, Brockway RA, Nakatani M: Pyruvate kinase Greensboro. A four-generation study of a high $K_{0.5s}$ (phosphoenolpyruvate) variant. *Blood* **72**:1054, 1988.
138. Satoh H, Tani K, Yoshida MC, Sasaki M, Miwa S, Fujii H: The human liver-type pyruvate kinase (PKL) gene is on chromosome 1 at band q21. *Cytogenet Cell Genet* **47**:132, 1988.
139. Neubauer M, Lakomek M, Winkler M, Parke S, Hofferbert S, Schröter W: Point mutations in the L-type pyruvate kinase gene of two children with hemolytic anemia caused by pyruvate kinase deficiency. *Blood* **77**:1871, 1991.
140. Kanno H, Fujii H, Hirono A, Miwa S: cDNA cloning of human R-type pyruvate kinase and identification of a single amino acid substitution ($Thr^{384}\rightarrow$Met) affecting enzymatic stability in pyruvate kinase variant (PK Tokyo) associated with hereditary hemolytic anemia. *Proc Natl Acad Sci USA* **88**:8218, 1991.
141. Kanno H, Fujii H, Hirono A, Omine M, Miwa S: Identical point mutations of the R-type pyruvate kinase (PK) cDNA found in unrelated PK variants associated with hereditary hemolytic anemia. *Blood* **79**:1347, 1992.
142. Kanno H, Fujii H, Miwa S: Low substrate affinity of pyruvate kinase (PK Sapporo) caused by a single amino acid substitution (426 Arg→Gln) associated with hereditary hemolytic anemia. *Blood* **81**:2439, 1993.
143. Kanno H, Fujii H, Tsujino G, Miwa S: Molecular basis of impaired pyruvate kinase isozyme conversion in erythroid cells: A single amino acid substitution near the active site and decreased mRNA content of the R-type PK. *Biochem Biophys Res Commun* **192**:46, 1993.
144. Kanno H, Ballas SK, Miwa S, Fujii H, Bowman HS: Molecular abnormality of erythrocyte pyruvate kinase deficiency in the Amish. *Blood* **88**:2311, 1994.
145. Dharmkrong-At A, Bloom GE: Acquired hemolytic anemia associated with infectious mononucleosis in a patient with congenital pyruvate kinase deficiency. *Clin Pediatr* **12**:119, 1973.
146. Lieberman JE, Gordon-Smith EC: Red cell pyrimidine 5′-nucleotidase and glutathione in myeloproliferative and lymphoproliferative disorders. *Br J Haematol* **44**;425, 1980.
147. Kahn A: Abnormalities of erythrocyte enzymes in dyserythropoiesis and malignancies. *Clin Haematol* **10**:123, 1981.
148. Lintula R: Red cell enzymes in myelodysplastic syndromes: A review. *Scand J Haematol* **36**:56, 1986.
149. Vives-Corrons JL, Pujades MA, Sierra J, Ribera JM: Characteristics of red cell pyruvate kinase (PK) and pyrimidine 5′-nucleotidase (P5N) abnormalities in acute leukemia and chronic lymphoid diseases with leukemic expression. *Br J Haematol* **63**:173, 1987.
150. Tani K, Fujii H, Takahashi K, Kodo H, Asano S, Takaku F, Miwa S: Erythrocyte enzyme activities in myelodysplastic syndromes: Elevated pyruvate kinase activity. *Am J Hematol* **30**:97, 1989.
151. Renoux M, Bernard JF, Torres M, Schlegel N, Amar M, Lopez M, Boivin P: Erythrocyte abnormalities induced by chemotherapy and radiotherapy: Induction of preleukemic states? *Scand J Haematol* **21**:323, 1978.
152. Etiemble J, Bernard JF, Picat CH, Belpomme D, Boivin P: Red blood cell enzyme abnormalities in patients treated with chemotherapy. *Br J Haematol* **42**:391, 1979.
153. Abe S: Secondary red cell pyruvate kinase deficiency. I. Study of 30 subjects of malignant hematological disorders. *Acta Haematol Jpn* **39**:247, 1976.
154. Zurcher C, Loos JA, Prins HK: Hereditary high ATP content of human erythrocytes. *Folia Haematol (Leipz)* **83**:366, 1965.
155. Max-Audit I, Rosa R, Marie J: Pyruvate kinase hyperactivity genetically determined: Metabolic consequences and molecular characterization. *Blood* **56**:902, 1980.
156. Rosa R, Max-Audit I, Izrael V, Beuzard Y, Thillet J, Rosa J: Hereditary pyruvate kinase abnormalities associated with erythrocytes. *Am J Hematol* **10**:47, 1981.
157. Staal GEJ, Jansen G, Roos D: Pyruvate kinase and the "high ATP syndrome." *J Clin Invest* **74**:231, 1984.
158. Tanaka KR: Hemolytic anemia due to abnormalities of enzymes of anaerobic glycolysis and nucleotide metabolism, in Brain MC, Carbone PP (eds): *Current Therapy in Hematology–Oncology*. Philadelphia, B.C. Decker, 1985, p 24.
159. Löhr GW, Waller HD, Anschutz F, Knopp A: Hexokinasemangel in blutzellen bei einer sippe mit familiarer panmyelopathie (Typ Fanconi). *Klin Wochenschr* **43**:870, 1965.
160. Valentine WN, Oski FH, Paglia DE, Baughan MA, Schneider AS, Naiman JL: Hereditary hemolytic anemia with hexokinase deficiency. Role of hexokinase in erythrocyte aging. *N Engl J Med* **276**:1, 1967.
161. Magnani M, Stocchi V, Cucchiarini L, Novelli G, Lodi S, Isa L, Fornaini G: Hereditary nonspherocytic hemolytic anemia due to a new hexokinase variant with reduced stability. *Blood* **66**:690, 1985.
162. Mentzer WC, Glader BE: Disorders of erythrocyte metabolism, in Mentzer WC, Wagner GM (eds): *The Hereditary Hemolytic Anemias*. New York, Churchill Livingstone, 1989, p 267.
163. Paglia DE, Shende A, Lanzkowsky P, Valentine WN: Hexokinase "New Hyde Park": A low activity erythrocyte isozyme in a Chinese kindred. *Am J Hematol* **10**:107, 1981.
164. Magnani M, Stocchi V, Canestrari F, Dacha M, Balestri P, Farnetani MA, Giorgi D, Fois A, Fornaini G: Human erythrocyte hexokinase deficiency: A new variant with abnormal kinetic properties. *Br J Haematol* **61**:41, 1985.
165. Tanaka KR, Zerez CR: Red cell enzymopathies of the glycolytic pathway. *Semin Hematol* **27**:165, 1990.
166. Fujii H, Miwa S: Recent progress in the molecular genetic analysis of erythroenzymopathy. *Am J Hematol* **34**:301, 1990.
167. Rijksen G, Akkerman JWN, van den Wall Bake AWL, Hofstede DP, Staal GEJ: Generalized hexokinase deficiency in the blood cells of a patient with nonspherocytic hemolytic anemia. *Blood* **61**:12, 1983.
168. Necheles TF, Rai US, Cameron D: Congenital nonspherocytic hemolytic anemia associated with an unusual erythrocyte hexokinase abnormality. *J Lab Clin Med* **76**:593, 1970.
169. Newman P, Muir A, Parker AC: Non-spherocytic haemolytic anaemia in mother and son associated with hexokinase deficiency. *Br J Haematol* **46**:537, 1980.
170. Haritos AA, Rosemeyer MA: Purification and physical

properties of hexokinase from human erythrocytes. *Biochim Biophys Acta* **873**:335, 1986.

171. Rogers PA, Fisher RA, Harris H: An examination of the age-related patterns of decay of the hexokinase of human red cells. *Clin Chim Acta* **65**:291, 1975.
172. Zimran A, Torem S, Beutler E: The in vivo ageing of red cell enzymes; direct evidence of biphasic decay from polycythaemic rabbits with reticulocytosis. *Br J Haematol* **69**:67, 1988.
173. Stocchi V, Magnani M, Canestrari F, Dacha M, Fornaini G: Multiple forms of human red blood cell hexokinase. Preparation, characterization, and age dependence. *J Biol Chem* **257**:2357, 1982.
174. Murakami K, Blei F, Tilton W, Seaman C, Piomelli S: An isozyme of hexokinase specific for the human red blood cell (HK_R). *Blood* **75**:770, 1990.
175. Dallapiccola B, Novelli G, Micara G, Delaroche I, Moric-Petrovic S, Magnani M: Regional mapping of hexokinase-I within the short arm of chromosome 10. *Hum Hered* **34**:156, 1984.
176. Danesino C, Lo Curto F, Bonfant G, Cazzadore C, Voltolin G, Bersi S: Deficiency 10p. Report of a case and exclusion mapping of the hexokinase 1 locus to band 10p11.2. *Ann Genet* **27**:162, 1984.
177. Nishi S, Seino S, Bell GI: Human hexokinase: Sequences of amino- and carboxyl-terminal halves are homologous. *Biochem Biophys Res Commun* **157**:937, 1988.
178. Rijksen G, Staal GEJ: Regulation of human erythrocyte hexokinase: The influence of glycolytic intermediates and inorganic phosphate. *Biochim Biophys Acta* **485**:75, 1977.
179. Rijksen G, Staal GEJ: Human erythrocyte hexokinase deficiency. Characterization of a mutant enzyme with abnormal regulatory properties. *J Clin Invest* **62**:294, 1978.
180. Magnani M, Rossi L, Bianchi M, Serafini G, Stocchi V: Human red blood cell loading with hexokinase-inactivating antibodies. An in vitro model for enzyme deficiencies. *Acta Haematol (Basel)* **82**:27, 1989.
181. Arnold H: Inherited glucosephosphate isomerase deficiency. *Blut* **39**:405, 1979.
182. Baughan MA, Valentine WN, Paglia DE, Ways PO, Simon ER, DeMarsh QB: Hereditary hemolytic anemia associated with glucosephosphate isomerase (GPI) deficiency—A new enzyme defect of human erythrocytes. *Blood* **32**:236, 1968.
183. Paglia DE, Valentine WN: Hereditary glucosephosphate isomerase deficiency. A review. *Am J Clin Pathol* **62**:740, 1974.
184. Eber SW, Gahr M, Lakomek M, Prindull G, Schröter W: Clinical symptoms and biochemical properties of three new glucose-phosphate isomerase variants. *Blut* **53**:21, 1986.
185. Schröter W, Eber SW, Bardosi A, Gahr M, Gabriel M, Sitzmann FC: Generalized glucosephosphate isomerase (GPI) deficiency causing haemolytic anaemia, neuromuscular symptoms and impairment of granulocytic function: A new syndrome due to a new stable GPI variant with diminished specific activity (GPI Homburg). *Eur J Pediatr* **144**:301, 1985.
186. Neubauer BA, Eber SW, Lakomek M, Gahr M, Schröter W: Combination of congenital nonspherocytic haemolytic anaemia and impairment of granulocyte function in severe glucosephosphate isomerase deficiency. *Acta Haematol (Basel)* **83**:206, 1990.
187. Zanella A, Izzo C, Rebulla P, Perroni L, Mariani M, Canestri G, Sansone G, Sirchia G: The first stable variant of erythrocyte glucose-phosphate isomerase associated with severe hemolytic anemia. *Am J Hematol* **9**:1, 1980.
188. Ravindranath Y, Paglia DE, Warrier I, Valentine W, Nakatani M, Brockway RA: Glucose phosphate isomerase deficiency as a cause of hydrops fetalis. *N Engl J Med* **316**:258, 1987.
189. Goulding FJ: Priapism caused by glucose phosphate isomerase deficiency. *J Urol* **116**:819, 1976.
190. Dallapiccola B, Novelli G, Ferranti G, Pachi A, Cristiani ML, Magnani M: First trimester monitoring of a pregnancy at risk for glucose phosphate isomerase deficiency. *Prenat Diagn* **6**:101, 1986.
191. Schröter W, Brittinger G, Zimmerschitt E, König E: A new haemolytic syndrome with glucosephosphate isomerase (GPI) and glucose-6-phosphate dehydrogenase (G6PD) deficiency of the erythrocytes: Biochemical studies. *Eur J Clin Invest* **1**:145, 1970.
192. Schröter W, Brittinger G, Zimmerschitt E, König E, Schrader D: Combined glucosephosphate isomerase and glucose-6-phosphate dehydrogenase deficiency of the erythrocytes: A new haemolytic syndrome. *Br J Haematol* **20**:249, 1971.
193. Rijksen G, Jansen G, Manaster J, Ezekiel E, Streichman S, Staal GEJ: Glucose-6-phosphate isomerase deficiency Nahariya: Extreme in vitro and in vivo lability of the mutant enzyme. *Isr J Med Sci* **20**:529, 1984.
194. McMorris FA, Chen TR, Ricciuti F, Tischfield J, Creagan R, Ruddle F: Chromosome assignments in man of the genes for two hexosephosphate isomerases. *Science* **179**:1129, 1973.
195. Walker JIH, Faik P, Morgan MJ: Characterization of the 5′ end of the gene for human glucose phosphate isomerase (GPI). *Genomics* **7**:638, 1990.
196. Merkle S, Pretsch W: Glucose-6-phosphate isomerase deficiency associated with non-spherocytic hemolytic anemia in the mouse: An animal model for the human disease. *Blood* **81**:206, 1993.
197. Kahn A, Meienhofer M-C, Cottreau D, Lagrange J-L, Dreyfus J-C: Phosphofructokinase (PFK) isozymes in man. I. Studies of adult human tissues. *Hum Genet* **48**:93, 1979.
198. Rowland LP, DiMauro S, Layzer RB: Phosphofructokinase deficiency, in Engel AG, Banker BQ (eds): *Myology*. New York, McGraw-Hill, 1986, vol 2, p 1603.
199. Vora S: Isozymes of phosphofructokinase, in Ratazzi MC, Scandalios JG, Whitt GS (eds): *Isozymes: Current Topics in Biological Medical Research*. New York, Alan R. Liss, 1982, vol 4, p 119.
200. Vora S, Davidson M, Seaman C, Miranda A, Noble N, Tanaka K, Frenkel E, DiMauro S: Heterogeneity of the molecular lesions in inherited phosphofructokinase deficiency. *J Clin Invest* **72**:1995, 1983.
201. Vora S, Seaman C, Durham S, Piomelli S: Isozymes of human phosphofructokinase: Identification and subunit structural characterization of a new system. *Proc Natl Acad Sci USA* **77**:62, 1980.
202. Tarui S, Okuno G, Ikura Y, Tanaka T, Suda M, Nishikawa M: Phosphofructokinase deficiency in skeletal muscle. A new type of glycogenosis. *Biochem Biophys Res Commun* **19**:517, 1965.
203. Layzer RB, Rowland LP, Ranney HM: Muscle phosphofructokinase deficiency. *Arch Neurol* **17**:512, 1967.
204. Brown BI, Brown DH: Glycogen storage diseases: Types I, III, IV, V, VII and unclassified glycogenoses, in Dickens F, Randle PJ, Whelan WJ (eds): *Carbohydrate Metabolism and Its Disorders*. New York, Academic, 1968, vol 2, p 123.
205. Mineo I, Kono N, Shimizu T, Hara N, Yamada Y, Sumi S, Nonaka K, Tarui S: Excess purine degradation in exercising muscles of patients with glycogen storage disease Types V and VII. *J Clin Invest* **76**:556, 1985.
206. Servidei S, Bonilla E, Diedrich RG, Kornfeld M, Oates JD, Davidson M, Vora S, DiMauro S: Fatal infantile form of muscle phosphofructokinase deficiency. *Neurology* **36**:1465, 1986.
207. Danon MJ, Servidei S, DiMauro S, Vora S: Late-onset muscle phosphofructokinase deficiency. *Neurology* **38**:956, 1988.
208. Haller RG, Lewis SF: Glucose-induced exertional fatigue in muscle phosphofructokinase deficiency. *N Engl J Med* **324**:364, 1991.
209. Tarui S, Kono N, Nasu T, Nishidawa M: Enzymatic basis for the coexistence of myopathy and hemolytic disease in inherited muscle phosphofructokinase deficiency. *Biochem Biophys Res Commun* **34**:77, 1969.
210. Layzer RB, Rasmussen J: The molecular basis of muscle phosphofructokinase deficiency. *Arch Neurol* **31**:411, 1974.
211. Duboc D, Jehenson P, Dinh ST, Marsac C, Syrota A, Fardeau M: Phosphorus NMR spectroscopy study of muscular enzyme deficiencies involving glycogenolysis and glycolysis. *Neurology* **37**:663, 1987.
212. Shimizu T, Kono N, Kiyokawa H, Yamada Y, Hara N, Mineo I, Kawachi M, Nakajima H, Wang YL, Tarui S:

Erythrocyte glycolysis and its marked alteration by muscular exercise in type VII glycogenosis. *Blood* **71**:1130, 1988.

213. Raben N, Sherman J, Miller F, Mena H, Plotz P: A 5′ splice junction mutation leading to exon deletion in an Ashkenazic Jewish family with phosphofructokinase deficiency (Tarui disease). *J Biol Chem* **268**:4963, 1993.
214. Vora S, Giger V, Turchen S, Harvey JW: Characterization of the enzymatic lesion in inherited phosphofructokinase deficiency in the dog: An animal analogue of human glycogen storage disease Type VII. *Proc Natl Acad Sci USA* **82**:8109, 1985.
215. Van Keuren M, Drabkin H, Hart I, Harker D, Patterson D, Vora S: Regional assignment of human liver-type 6-phosphofructokinase to chromosome 21q22.3 by using somatic cell hybrids and a monoclonal anti-L antibody. *Hum Genet* **74**:34, 1986.
216. Vora S, Durham S, De Martinville B, George DL, Francke U: Assignment of the human gene for muscle-type phosphofructokinase (PFKM) to chromosome 1 (region cen → q32) using somatic cell hybrids and monoclonal anti-M antibody. *Somat Cell Genet* **8**:95, 1982.
217. Vora S, Francke U: Assignment of the human gene for liver-type 6-phosphofructokinase isozyme (PFKL) to chromosome 21 by using somatic cell hybrids and monoclonal anti-L antibody. *Proc Natl Acad Sci USA* **78**:3738, 1981.
218. Vora S, Miranda A, Hernandez E, Francke U: Regional assignment of the human gene for platelet-type phosphofructokinase (PFKP) to chromosome 10p: Novel use of poly-specific rodent antisera to localize human enzyme genes. *Hum Genet* **63**:374, 1983.
219. Levanon D, Danciger E, Dafni N, Groner Y: Construction of a cDNA clone containing the entire coding region of the human liver-type phosphofructokinase. *Biochem Biophys Res Commun* **147**:1182, 1987.
220. Nakajima H, Noguchi T, Yamasaki T, Kono N, Tanaka T, Tarui S: Cloning of human muscle phosphofructokinase cDNA. *FEBS Lett* **223**:113, 1987.
221. Vaisanen PA, Reddy GR, Sharma PM, Kohani R, Johnson JL, Raney AK, Babior BM, McLachlan A: Cloning and characterization of the human muscle phosphofructokinase gene. *DNA Cell Biol* **11**:461, 1992.
222. Nakajima H, Kono N, Yamasaki T, Hotta K, Kawachi M, Kuwajima M, Noguchi T, Tanaka T, Tarui S: Genetic defect in muscle phosphofructokinase deficiency. *J Biol Chem* **265**:9392, 1990.
223. Beutler E, Scott S, Bishop A, Margolis N, Matsumoto F, Kuhl W: Red cell aldolase deficiency and hemolytic anemia: A new syndrome. *Trans Assoc Am Physicians* **86**:154, 1973.
224. Kishi H, Mukai T, Hirono A, Fujii H, Miwa S, Hori K: Human aldolase A deficiency associated with a hemolytic anemia: Thermolabile aldolase due to a single base mutation. *Proc Natl Acad Sci USA* **84**:8623, 1987.
225. Miwa S, Fujii H, Tani K, Takahashi K, Takegawa S, Fujinami N, Sakurai M, Kubo M, Tanimoto Y, Kato T, Matsumoto N: Two cases of red cell aldolase deficiency associated with hereditary hemolytic anemia in a Japanese family. *Am J Hematol* **11**:425, 1981.
226. Penhoet E, Rajkumar T, Rutter WJ: Multiple forms of fructose diphosphate aldolase in mammalian tissues. *Proc Natl Acad Sci USA* **56**:1275, 1966.
227. Izzo P, Costanzo P, Lupo A, Rippa E, Paolella G, Salvatore F: Human aldolase A gene. Structural organization and tissue-specific expression by multiple promoters and alternate mRNA processing. *Eur J Biochem* **174**:569, 1988.
228. Mennecier F, Daegelen D, Schweighoffer F, Levin F, Kahn A: Expression of aldolase A messenger RNAs in human adult and foetal tissues and in hepatoma. *Biochem Biophys Res Commun* **134**:1093, 1986.
229. Rottmann WH, Tolan DR, Penhoet EE: Complete amino acid sequence for human aldolase B derived from cDNA and genomic clones. *Proc Natl Acad Sci USA* **81**:2738, 1984.
230. Sakakibara M, Mukai T, Hori K: Nucleotide sequence of a cDNA clone for human aldolase: A messenger RNA in the liver. *Biochem Biophys Res Commun* **13**:413, 1985.
231. Maire P, Gautron S, Hakim V, Gregori C, Mennecier F, Kahn A: Characterization of three optional promoters in the 5′ region of the human aldolase A gene. *J Mol Biol* **197**:425, 1987.
232. Sakakibara M, Mukai T, Yatsuki H, Hori K: Human aldolase isozyme gene: The structure of multispecies aldolase B mRNAs. *Nucleic Acids Res* **13**:5055, 1985.
233. Kukita A, Yoshida MC, Fukushige S, Sakakibara M, Joh K, Mukai T, Hori K: Molecular gene mapping of human aldolase A (ALDOA) gene to chromosome 16. *Hum Genet* **76**:20, 1987.
234. Lu HS, Yuan PM, Gracy RW: Primary structure of human triosephosphate isomerase. *J Biol Chem* **259**:11958, 1984.
235. Rosa R, Prehu M-O, Calvin M-C, Badoual J, Alix D, Girod R: Hereditary triose phosphate isomerase deficiency: Seven new homozygous cases. *Hum Genet* **71**:235, 1985.
236. Schneider AS, Valentine WN, Baughan MA, Paglia DE, Shore NA, Heins HL: Triosephosphate isomerase deficiency. A. A multi-system inherited enzyme disorder. Clinical and genetic aspects, in Beutler E (ed): *Hereditary Disorders of Erythrocyte Metabolism* Philadelphia, Grune & Stratton, 1968, vol 1, p 265.
237. Schneider AS, Valentine WN, Hattori M, Heins HL: Hereditary hemolytic anemia with triosephosphate isomerase deficiency. *N Engl J Med* **272**:229, 1965.
238. Valentine WN, Schneider AS, Baughan MA, Paglia DE, Heins HL Jr: hereditary hemolytic anemia with triosephosphate isomerase deficiency. Studies in kindreds with coexistent sickle cell trait and erythrocyte glucose-6-phosphate dehydrogenase deficiency. *Am J Med* **41**:27, 1966.
239. Poll-The BW, Aicardi J, Girot R, Rosa R: Neurological findings in triosephosphate isomerase deficiency. *Ann Neurol* **17**:439, 1985.
240. Zanella A, Mariani M, Colombo MB, Borgna-Pignatti C, De Stefano P, Morgese G, Sirchia G: Triosephosphate isomerase deficiency: 2 new cases. *Scand J Haematol* **34**:417, 1985.
241. Hollan S, Miwa S, Fujii H, Natonek K, Hirono A, Hirono K, Kanno H: A unique experiment of nature (a 21 yr old symptom free homozygote for triose phosphate isomerase/TPI/deficiency). *Blood* **76**:35a, 1990.
242. Chang M-L, Artymiuk PJ, Wu X, Hollan S, Lammi A, Maquat LE: Human triosephosphate isomerase deficiency resulting from mutation of Phe-240. *Am J Hum Genet* **52**:1260, 1993.
243. Vives-Corrons J-L, Rubinson-Skala H, Mateo M, Estella J, Feliu E, Dreyfus J-C: Triosephosphate isomerase deficiency with hemolytic anemia and severe neuromuscular disease. Familial and biochemical studies of a case found in Spain. *Hum Genet* **42**:171, 1978.
244. Freycon F, Lauras B, Bovier-Lapierre F, Dorche CL, Goddon R: Anemie hemolytique congenitale par deficit en triosephosphate isomerase. *Pediatrie* **30**:55, 1975.
245. Pogliani EM, Colombi M, Zanella A: Platelet function defect in triosephosphate isomerase deficiency. *Haematologica* **71**:349, 1986.
246. Schneider AS, Dunn I, Ibsen KH, Weinstein IM: Triosephosphate isomerase deficiency. B. Inherited triosephosphate isomerase deficiency. Erythrocyte carbohydrate metabolism and preliminary studies of the erythrocyte enzyme, in Beutler E (ed): *Hereditary Disorders of Erythrocyte Metabolism*. Philadelphia, Grune & Stratton, 1968, vol I, p 273.
247. Rosa R, Prehu M-O, Beuzard Y, Rosa J: The first case of a complete deficiency of diphosphoglycerate mutase in human erythrocytes. *J Clin Invest* **62**:907, 1978.
248. Bellingham AJ, Lestas AN, Williams LHP, Nicolaides KH: Prenatal diagnosis of a red-cell enzymopathy: Triose phosphate isomerase deficiency. *Lancet* **2**:419, 1989.
249. Clark ACL, Szobolotzky MA: Triose phosphate isomerase deficiency: Prenatal diagnosis. *J Pediatr* **106**:417, 1985.
250. Poinsot J, Parent P, Alix D, Toudic L, Castel Y: Un cas d'anemie hemolytique congenitale non spherocytaire, par deficit en triose phosphate isomerase diagnostic prenatal. *J Genet Hum* **34**:431, 1986.
251. Harris SR, Paglia DE, Jaffé ER, Valentine WN, Klein RL: Triosephosphate isomerase deficiency in an adult. *Clin Res* **18**:529, 1970.
252. Jongsma AP, Los WR, Hagemeijer A: Evidence for synteny between the human loci for triose phosphate isomerase,

lactate dehydrogenase-B, and peptidase-B and the regional mapping of these loci on chromosome 12. *Cytogenet Cell Genet* **13**:106, 1974.

253. Decker RS, Mohrenweiser HW: Origin of the triosephosphate isomerase isozyme in humans: Genetic evidence for the expression of a single structural locus. *Am J Hum Genet* **33**:683, 1981.
254. Yuan PM, Talent JM, Gracy RW: Molecular basis for the accumulation of acidic isozymes of triosephosphate isomerase on ageing. *Mech Ageing Dev* **17**:151, 1981.
255. Eber SW, Dunnwald M, Heinemann G, Hofstatter T, Weinmann HM, Belohradsky B: Prevalence of partial deficiency of red cell triosephosphate isomerase in Germany—A study of 3000 people. *Hum Genet* **67**:336, 1984.
256. Mohrenweiser HW, Fielek S: Elevated frequency of carriers for triosephosphate isomerase deficiency in newborn infants. *Pediatr Res* **16**:960, 1982.
257. Brown JR, Daar IO, Krug JR, Maquat LE: Characterization of the functional gene and several processed pseudogenes in the human triosephosphate isomerase gene family. *Mol Cell Biol* **5**:1694, 1985.
258. Maquat LE, Chilcote R, Ryan PM: Human triosephosphate isomerase cDNA and protein structure. Studies of triosephosphate isomerase deficiency in man. *J Biol Chem* **260**:3748, 1985.
259. Kaplan JC, Teeple L, Shore NA, Beutler E: Electrophoretic abnormality in triosephosphate isomerase deficiency. *Biochem Biophys Res Commun* **31**:768, 1968.
260. Daar IQ, Artymiuk PJ, Phillips DC, Maquat LE: Human triosephosphate isomerase deficiency: A single amino acid substitution results in a thermolabile enzyme. *Proc Natl Acad Sci USA* **83**:7903, 1986.
261. Kraus AP, Langston MF, Lynch BL: Red cell phosphoglycerate kinase deficiency. A new cause of non-spherocytic hemolytic anemia. *Biochem Biophys Res Commun* **30**:173, 1968.
262. Valentine WN, Hsieh H-S, Paglia DE, Anderson HM, Baughan MA, Jaffé ER, Garson OM: Hereditary hemolytic anemia: Association with phosphoglycerate kinase deficiency in erythrocytes and leukocytes. *Trans Assoc Am Physicians* **81**:49, 1968.
263. Maeda M, Bawle EV, Kulkarni R, Beutler E, Yoshida A: Molecular abnormalities of a phosphoglycerate kinase variant generated by spontaneous mutation. *Blood* **79**:2759, 1992.
264. Chen S-H, Malcolm LA, Yoshida A, Giblett ER: Phosphoglycerate kinase: An X-linked polymorphism in man. *Am J Hum Genet* **23**:87, 1971.
265. Valentine WN, Hsieh H-S, Paglia DE, Anderson HM, Baughan MA, Jaffé ER, Garson OM: Hereditary hemolytic anemia associated with phosphoglycerate kinase deficiency in erythrocytes and leukocytes. A probable X-chromosome linked syndrome. *N Engl J Med* **280**:528, 1969.
266. Jaffé ER, Valentine WN: Human erythroenzymopathies of the anaerobic Embden-Meyerhof glycolytic and associated pathways, in Nagel RL (ed): *Genetically Abnormal Red Cells*. Boca Raton, FL, CRC, 1988, vol 1, p 105.
267. Guis MS, Karadsheh N, Mentzer WC: Phosphoglycerate kinase San Francisco: A new variant associated with hemolytic anemia but not with neuromuscular manifestations. *Am J Hematol* **25**:175, 1987.
268. Krietsch WKG, Krietsch H, Kaiser W, Dunnwald M, Kuntz GWK, Duhm J, Bucher T: Hereditary phosphoglycerate kinase: A new variant in erythrocytes and leucocytes, not associated with haemolytic anemia. *Eur J Clin Invest* **7**:427, 1977.
269. Miwa S, Nakashima K, Oda S, Ogawa H, Nagafuji H, Arima M, Okuna T, Nakashima T: Phosphoglycerate kinase (PGK) deficiency hereditary nonpherocytic hemolytic anemia: Report of case found in a Japanese family. *Acta Haematol Jpn* **35**:571, 1972.
270. Yoshida A, Miwa S: Characterization of a phosphoglycerate kinase variant associated with hemolytic anemia. *Am J Hum Genet* **26**:378, 1974.
271. Maeda M, Yoshida A: Molecular defect of a phosphoglycerate kinase variant (PGK-Matsue) associated with hemoytic anemia: Leu → Pro substitution caused by T/A → C/G transition in Exon 3. *Blood* **77**:1348, 1991.
272. Sugie H, Sugie Y, Nishida M, Ito M, Tsurui S, Suzuki M, Miyamoto R, Igarashi Y: Recurrent myoglobinuria in a child with mental retardation: Phosphoglycerate kinase deficiency. *J Child Neurol* **4**:95, 1989.
273. Fujii H, Kanno H, Hirono A, Shiomura T, Miwa S: A single amino acid substitution (157 Gly → Val) in a phosphoglycerate kinase variant (PGK Shizuoka) associated with chronic hemolysis and myoglobinuria. *Blood* **79**:1582, 1992.
274. Dodgson SJ, Lee CS, Holland RAB, O'Sullivan WJ, Vowels MR: Erythrocyte phosphoglycerate kinase deficiency: Enzymatic and oxygen binding studies. *Aust N Z J Med* **10**:614, 1980.
275. Strauss RG, McCarthy DJ, Mauer AM: Neutrophil function in congenital phosphoglycerate kinase deficiency. *J Pediatr* **85**:341, 1974.
276. Miwa S, Nakashima K, Oda S, Takahashi K, Morooka K, Nakashima T: Evidence of the decreased muscle enzyme activity in erythrocyte phosphoglycerate kinase deficiency. *Acta Haematol Jpn* **37**:59, 1974.
277. Svirklys LG, O'Sullivan WJ: Tissue levels of glycolytic enzymes in phosphoglycerate kinase deficiency. *Clin Chim Acta* **108**:309, 1980.
278. Tani L, Takizawa T, Yoshida A: Normal mRNA content in a phosphoglycerate kinase variant with severe enzyme deficiency. *Am J Hum Genet* **37**:931, 1985.
279. Rosa R, George C, Fardeau M, Calvin MC, Rapen M, Rosa J: A new case of phosphoglycerate kinase deficiency: PGK Creteil associated with rhabdomyolysis and lacking hemolytic anemia. *Blood* **60**:84, 1982.
280. Bresolin N, Miranda A, Chang HW, Shanske S, DiMauro S: Phosphoglycerate kinase deficiency myopathy: Biochemical and immunological studies of the mutant enzyme. *Muscle Nerve* **7**:542, 1984.
281. McCarrey JR, Thomas K: Human testis specific PGK gene lacks introns and possesses characteristics of a processed gene. *Nature* **326**:501, 1987.
282. Willard HF, Goss SJ, Holmes MT, Munroe DL: Regional localization of the phosphoglycerate kinase gene and pseudogene on the human X chromosome and assignment of a related DNA sequence to chromosome 19. *Hum Genet* **71**:138, 1985.
283. Huang I-Y, Welch CD, Yoshida A: Complete amino acid sequence of human phosphoglycerate kinase. Cyanogen bromide peptides and complete amino acid sequence. *J Biol Chem* **255**:6412, 1980.
284. Michelson AM, Markham AF, Orkin SH: Isolation and DNA sequence of a full length cDNA clone for human X chromosome-encoded phosphoglycerate kinase. *Proc Natl Acad Sci USA* **80**:472, 1983.
285. Singer-Sam J, Simmer RL, Keith DH, Shively L, Teplitz M, Itakura K, Gartler SM, Riggs AD: Isolation of a cDNA clone for human X-linked 3-phosphoglycerate kinase by use of a mixture of synthetic oligodeoxyribonucleotides as a detection probe. *Proc Natl Acad Sci USA* **80**:802, 1983.
286. Michelson AM, Blake CCF, Evans ST, Orkin SH: Structure of the human phosphoglycerate kinase gene and the intron-mediated evolution and dispersal of the nucleotide-binding domain. *Proc Natl Acad Sci USA* **82**:6965, 1985.
287. Fujii H, Chen S-H, Akasuka J, Miwa S, Yoshida A: Use of cultured lymphoblastoid cells for the study of abnormal enzymes: Molecular abnormality of a phosphoglycerate kinase variant associated with hemolytic anemia. *Proc Natl Acad Sci USA* **78**:2587, 1981.
288. Fujii H, Krietsch WKG, Yoshida A: A single amino acid substitution (Asp → Asn) in a phosphoglycerate kinase variant (PGK Munchen) associated with enzyme deficiency. *J Biol Chem* **255**:6421, 1980.
289. Fujii H, Yoshida A: Molecular abnormality of phosphoglycerate kinase-Uppsala associated with chronic non-spherocytic hemolytic anemia. *Proc Natl Acad Sci USA* **77**:5461, 1980.
290. Yoshida A, Watanabe S, Chen S-H, Giblett ER, Malcolm LA: Human phosphoglycerate kinase. II. Structure of a variant enzyme. *J Biol Chem* **247**:446, 1972.
291. Banks RD, Blake CCF, Evans PR, Haser R, Rice DW, Hardy GW, Merrett M, Phillips AW: Sequence, structure,

and activity of phosphoglycerate kinase: A possible hinge-bending enzyme. *Nature* **279**:773, 1979.

292. Yoshida A, Tani K: Phosphoglycerate kinase abnormalities: Functional, structural and genomic aspects. *Biomed Biochim Acta* **42**:S263, 1983.
293. Chanutin A, Curnish RR: Effect of organic and inorganic phosphates on the oxygen equilibrium of human erythrocytes. *Arch Biochem Biophys* **121**:96, 1967.
294. Rosa R, Gaillardon J, Rosa J: Diphosphoglycerate mutase and 2,3-diphosphoglycerate phosphatase activities of red cells: Comparative electrophoretic study. *Biochem Biophys Res Commun* **51**:536, 1973.
295. Sasaki R, Ikura K, Sugimoto E, Chiba H: Purification of bisphosphoglyceromutase, 2,3-bisphosphoglycerate phosphatase and phosphoglyceromutase from human erythrocytes. Three enzyme activities in one protein. *Eur J Biochem* **50**:581, 1975.
296. Galacteros F, Rosa R, Prehu MO, Majean Y, Calvin MC: Deficit en diphosphoglycerate mutase: Nouveaux cas associes a une polyglobulie. *Nouv Rev Fr Hematol* **26**:69, 1984.
297. Blouquit Y, Rhoda M-D, Delanoe-Garin J, Rosa R, Prome J-C, Poyart C, Puzo G, Bernassau JM, Rosa J: Glycerated hemoglobin, $\alpha_2{}^A\beta_2$82 (EF6) N^ϵ-Glyceryllysine. A new post translational modification occurring in erythrocyte bisphosphoglyceromutase deficiency. *J Biol Chem* **261**:6758, 1986.
298. Peterson LL: Red cell diphosphoglycerate mutase. Immunochemical studies in vertebrate red cells, including a human variant lacking 2,3-DPG. *Blood* **52**:953, 1978.
299. Rosa R, Prehu M-O, Albrecht-Ellmer K, Calvin M-C: Partial characterization of the inactive mutant form of human red cell bisphosphoglyceromutase and comparison with an alkylated form. *Biochim Biophys Acta* **742**:243, 1983.
300. Rosa R, Blouquit Y, Calvin M-C, Prome D, Prome J-C, Rosa J: Isolation, characterization, and structure of a mutant 89 Arg → Cys bisphosphoglycerate mutase. Implication of the active site in the mutation. *J Biol Chem* **264**:7837, 1989.
301. Lemarchandel V, Joulin V, Valentin C, Rosa R, Galacteros F, Rosa J, Cohen-Solal M: Compound heterozygosity in a complete erythrocyte bisphosphoglycerate mutase deficiency. *Blood* **80**:2643, 1992.
302. Joulin V, Peduzzi J, Romeo P-H, Rosa R, Valentin C, Dubart A, Lapeyre B, Blouquit Y, Garel M-C, Goossens M, Rosa J, Cohen-Solal M: Molecular cloning and sequencing of the human erythrocyte 2,3-bisphosphoglycerate mutase cDNA: Revised amino acid sequence. *EMBO J* **5**:2275, 1986.
303. Barichard F, Joulin V, Henry I, Garel MC, Valentin C, Rosa R, Cohen-Solal M, Junien C: Chromosomal assignment of the human 2,3-bisphosphoglycerate mutase gene (BPGM) to region 7q34 → 7q22. *Hum Genet* **77**:283, 1987.
304. Joulin V, Garel M-C, LeBoulch PL, Valentin C, Rosa R, Rosa J, Cohen-Solal M: Isolation and characterization of the human 2,3-bisphosphoglycerate mutase gene. *J Biol Chem* **263**:15785, 1988.
305. Zomzely-Neurath CE: Enolase, in Lajtha A (ed): *Handbook of Neurochemistry*, 2 ed. New York, Plenum, 1983, vol 4, p 403.
306. Stefanini M: Chronic hemolytic anemia associated with erythrocyte enolase deficiency exacerbated by ingestion of nitrofurantoin. *Am J Clin Pathol* **58**:408, 1972.
307. Boulard-Heitzmann P, Boulard M, Tallineau C, Boivin P, Tanzer J, Bois M, Barriere M: Decreased red cell enolase activity in a 40-year-old woman with compensated haemolysis. *Scand J Haematol* **33**:401, 1984.
308. Lachant NA, Jennings MA, Tanaka KR: Partial erythrocyte enolase deficiency: A hereditary disorder with variable clinical expression. *Blood* **65**:55a, 1986.
309. D'Ancona GG, Chern CJ, Benn P, Croce CM: Assignment of the human gene for enolase 1 to region pter → p36 of chromosome 1. *Cytogenet Cell Genet* **18**:327, 1977.
310. Giallongo A, Feo S, Moore R, Croce CM, Showe LC: Molecular cloning and nucleotide sequence of a full-length cDNA for human enolase. *Proc Natl Acad Sci USA* **83**:6741, 1986.
311. Kitamura M, Iijima N, Hashimoto F, Hiratsuka A: Hereditary deficiency of subunit H of lactate dehydrogenase. *Clin Chim Acta* **34**:419, 1971.
312. Miwa S, Nishina T, Kakehashi Y, Kitamura M, Hiratsuka A, Shizume K: Studies on erythrocyte metabolism in a case with hereditary deficiency of H-subunit of lactate dehydrogenase. *Acta Haematol Jpn* **34**:228, 1971.
313. Joukyuu R, Mizuno S, Amakawa T, Tsukada T, Nishina T, Kitamura M: Hereditary complete deficiency of lactate dehydrogenase H-subunit. *Clin Chem* **35**:687, 1989.
314. Kanno T, Sudo K, Takeuchi I, Kanda S, Honda N, Nishimura Y, Oyama K: Hereditary deficiency of lactate dehydrogenase M-subunit. *Clin Chim Acta* **108**:267, 1980.
315. Li SS-L, Luedemann M, Sharief FS, Takano T, Deaven LL: Mapping of human lactate dehydrogenase-A, -B, and -C genes and their related sequences: The gene for LDH-C is located with that for LDH-A on chromosome 11. *Cytogenet Cell Genet* **48**:16, 1988.
316. Mayeda K, Weiss L, Lindahl R, Dully M: Localization of the human lactate dehydrogenase B gene on the short arm of chromosome 12. *Am J Hum Genet* **26**:59, 1974.
317. Boone C, Chen T-R, Ruddle FH: Assignment of three human genes to chromosomes (LDH-A to 11, TK to 17, and IDH to 20) and evidence for translocation between human and mouse chromosomes in somatic cell hybrids. *Proc Natl Acad Sci USA* **69**:510, 1972.
318. Sakai I, Sharief FS, Pan Y-CE, Li SS-L: The cDNA and protein sequences of human lactate dehydrogenase B. *Biochem J* **248**:933, 1987.
319. Sudo K, Maekawa M, Ikawa S, Machida K, Kitamura M, Li SS-L: A missense mutation found in human lactate dehydrogenase-B (H) variant gene. *Biochem Biophys Res Commun* **168**:672, 1990.
320. Parr CW, Fitch LI: Inherited quantitative variants of human phosphogluconate dehydrogenase. *Ann Hum Genet* **30**:339, 1967.
321. Brewer GJ, Dern RJ: A new inherited enzymatic deficiency of human erythrocytes: 6-phosphogluconate dehydrogenase deficiency. *Am J Hum Genet* **16**:472, 1964.
322. Beutler E, Kuhl W, Gelbert T: 6-phosphogluconolactonase deficiency, a hereditary erythrocyte enzyme deficiency: Possible interaction with glucose-6-phosphate dehydrogenase deficiency. *Proc Natl Acad Sci USA* **82**:3876, 1985.
323. Dash S, Bhaqwat AG: Combined G-6PD and 6-PGD deficiency in a Hindu boy. *Acta Haematol* **57**:351, 1977.
324. Gondo H, Ideguchi H, Hayashi S. Shibuya T: Acute hemolysis in glutathione peroxidase deficiency. *Int J Hematol* **55**:215, 1992.
325. Beutler E, Matsumoto F: Ethnic variation in red cell glutathione peroxidase activity. *Blood* **46**:103, 1975.
326. Wijnen LMM, Monteba-van Heuvel M, Pearson PL, Khan PM: Assignment of a gene for glutathione peroxidase (GPX_1) to human chromosome 3. *Cytogenet Cell Genet* **22**:232, 1978.
327. Beutler E: Effect of flavin compounds on glutathione reductase activity: In vivo and in vitro studies. *J Clin Invest* **48**:1957, 1969.
328. Beutler E: Red cell enzyme defects as nondiseases and as diseases. *Blood* **54**:1, 1979.
329. Frischer H, Ahmad T: Consequences of erythrocytic glutathione reductase deficiency. *J Lab Clin Med* **109**:583, 1987.
330. Loos H, Roos D, Weening R, Houwerzill J: Familial deficiency of glutathione reductase in human blood cells. *Blood* **48**:53, 1976.
331. Kurcherlapati RS, Nichols EA, Creagan RP, Chen S, Borgaonkar DS, Ruddle FH: Assignment of the gene for glutathione reductase to human chromosome 8 by somatic cell hybridization. *Am J Hum Genet* **26**:51a, 1974.
332. Mooz ED, Meister A: Tripeptide (glutathione) synthetase. Purification, properties, and mechanism of action. *Biochemistry* **6**:1722, 1967.
333. Majerus PW, Brauner MJ, Smith MB, Minnich V: Glutathione synthesis in human erythrocytes. II. Purification and properties of the enzymes of glutathione biosynthesis. *J Clin Invest* **50**:1637, 1971.
334. Konrad PN, Richards F II, Valentine WN, Paglia DE:

γ-Glutamylcysteine synthetase deficiency. A cause of hereditary hemolytic anemia. *N Engl J Med* **286**:557, 1972.

335. Richards F II, Cooper MR, Pearce LA, Cowan RJ, Spurr CL: Familial spinocerebellar degeneration, hemolytic anemia, and glutathione deficiency. *Arch Intern Med* **134**:534, 1974.
336. Beutler E, Moroose R, Kramer L, Gelbart T, Forman L: Gamma-glutamylcysteine synthetase deficiency and hemolytic anemia. *Blood* **75**:271, 1990.
337. Beutler E: Selectivity of proteases as a basis for tissue distribution of enzymes in hereditary deficiencies. *Proc Natl Acad Sci USA* **80**:3767, 1983.
338. Beutler E, Gelbart T, Pegelow C: Erythrocyte glutathione synthetase deficiency leads not only to glutathione but also to glutathione-S-transferase deficiency. *J Clin Invest* **77**:38, 1986.
339. Paglia DE, Valentine WN: Haemolytic anaemia associated with disorders of the purine and pyrimidine salvage pathway. *Clin Haematol* **10**:81, 1981.
340. Valentine WN, Paglia DE, Tartaglia AP, Gilsanz F: Hereditary hemolytic anemia with increased red cell adenosine deaminase (45- to 70-fold) and decreased adenosine triphosphate. *Science* **195**:783, 1977.
341. Paglia DE, Valentine WN, Tartaglia AP, Gilsanz F, Sparkes RS: Control of red blood cell adenine nucleotide metabolism. Studies of adenosine deaminase, in Brewer GJ (ed): *The Red Cell*. New York, Alan R. Liss, 1978, p 319.
342. Miwa S, Fujii H, Matsumoto N, Nakatsuji T, Oda S, Asano H, Asano S, Miura Y: A case of red-cell adenosine deaminase overproduction associated with hereditary hemolytic anemia found in Japan. *Am J Hematol* **5**:107, 1978.
343. Fujii H, Miwa S, Suzuki K: Purification and properties of adenosine deaminase in normal and hereditary hemolytic anemia with increased red cell activity. *Hemoglobin* **4**:693, 1980.
344. Perignon JL, Hamet M, Buc HA, Cartier P, Derycke M: Biochemical study of a case of hemolytic anemia with increased (85-fold) red cell adenosine deaminase. *Clin Chim Acta* **124**:205, 1982.
345. Chottiner EG, Cloft HJ, Tartaglia AP, Mitchell BS: Elevated adenosine deaminase activity and hereditary hemolytic anemia. Evidence for abnormal translational control of protein synthesis. *J Clin Invest* **79**:1001, 1987.
346. Chottiner EG, Ginsburg D, Tartaglia AP, Mitchell BS: Erythrocyte adenosine deaminase overproduction in hereditary hemolytic anemia. *Blood* **74**:448, 1989.
347. Chottiner EG, Ginsburg D, Mitchell BS: Autosomal dominant hemolytic anemia and adenosine deaminase overproduction. *Adv Exp Med Biol* **253A**:493, 1989.
348. Chottiner EG, Gribbin TE, Ginsburg D, Mitchell BS: Erythrocyte-specific overproduction of adenosine deaminase: Molecular genetic studies. *Prog Clin Biol Res* **319**:55, 1989.
349. Hirschhorn R, Levytska V, Pollara B, Meuwissen HJ: Evidence for control of several different tissue-specific isozymes of adenosine deaminase by a single genetic locus. *Nature New Biol* **246**:200, 1973.
350. Hirschhorn R: Conversion of human erythrocyte-adenosine deaminase activity to different tissue-specific isozymes. Evidence for a common catalytic unit. *J Clin Invest* **55**:661, 1975.
351. Tischfield JA, Creagan RP, Nichols EA, Ruddle FH: Assignment of a gene for adenosine deaminase to human chromosome 20. *Hum Hered* 24:1, 1974.
352. Wiginton DA, Kaplan DJ, States JC, Akeson AL, Perme CM, Bilyk IJ, Vaughn AJ, Lattier DL, Hutton JJ: Complete sequence and structure of the gene for human adenosine deaminase. *Biochemistry* **25**:8234, 1986.
353. Parks RE Jr, Brown PR: Incorporation of nucleosides into the nucleotide pools of human erythrocytes. Adenosine and its analogs. *Biochemistry* **12**:3294, 1973.
354. Perrett D, Dean B: The function of adenosine deaminase in the human erythrocyte. *Biochem Biophys Res Commun* **77**:374, 1977.
355. Agarwall RP, Parks RE Jr: A possible association between the nucleoside transport system of human erythrocytes and adenosine deaminase. *Biochem Pharmacol* **24**:547, 1975.
356. Agarwal RP, Crabtree GW, Parks RE Jr, Nelson JR, Keightley R, Parkman R, Rosen FS, Stern RS, Polmar SH: Purine nucleoside metabolism in the erythrocytes of patients with adenosine deaminase deficiency and severe combined immunodeficiency. *J Clin Invest* **57**:1025, 1976.
357. Schmalstieg FC, Goldman AS, Mills GC, Monahan TM, Nelson JA, Goldblum RM: Nucleotide metabolism in adenosine deaminase deficiency. *Pediatr Res* **10**:393, 1976.
358. Cohen A, Hirschhorn R, Horowitz SD, Rubenstein A, Polmar SH, Hong R, Marting DW Jr: Deoxyadenosine triphosphate as a potentially toxic metabolite in adenosine deaminase deficiency. *Proc Natl Acad Sci USA* **75**:472, 1978.
359. Coleman MS, Donofrio J, Hutton JJ, Hahn L, Daoud A, Lampkin B, Dyminski J: Identification and quantitation of adenine deoxynucleotides in erythrocytes of a patient with adenosine deaminase deficiency and severe combined immunodeficiency. *J Biol Chem* **253**:1619, 1978.
360. Nelson JA, Kuttesch JF, Goldblum RN, Goldman AS, Schmalstieg FC: Analysis of adenosine and adenine nucleotides in severe combined immunodeficiency disease, in Baer HP, Drummond GI (eds): *Physiological and Regulatory Functions of Adenosine and Adenine Nucleotides*. New York, Raven, 1979, p 417.
361. Paglia DE, Valentine WN: Genetically induced enzyme anomalies: Insights into normal cellular processes. *Ann NY Acad Sci* **459**:344, 1985.
362. Szeinberg A, Gavendo S, Cahane D: Erythrocyte adenylate-kinase deficiency. *Lancet* **1**:315, 1969.
363. Szeinberg A, Kahana D, Gavendo S, Zaidman J, Ben-Ezzer J: Hereditary deficiency of adenylate kinase in red blood cells. *Acta Haematol* **42**:111, 1969.
364. Boivin P, Galand C, Hakim J, Simony D, Seligman M: Un nouvelle erythroenzymopathie. Anemie hemolytique congenitale non spherocytaire et deficit hereditaire en adenylate-kinase erythrocytaire. *Presse Med* **79**:215, 1971.
365. Miwa S, Fujii H, Tani K, Takahashi K, Takizawa T, Igarashi T: Red cell adenylate kinase deficiency associated with hereditary nonspherocytic hemolytic anemia: Clinical and biochemical studies. *Am J Hematol* **14**:325, 1983.
366. Beutler E, Carson D, Dannawi H, Forman L, Kuhl W, West C, Westwood B: Metabolic compensation for profound erythrocyte adenylate kinase deficiency. A hereditary defect without hemolytic anemia. *J Clin Invest* **72**:648, 1983.
367. Van Acker KJ, Simmonds HA, Potter C, Cameron JS: Complete deficiency of adenine phosphoribosyltransferase. Report of a family. *N Engl J Med* **297**:127, 1977.
368. Lachant NA, Zerez CR, Barredo J, Lee DW, Savely SM, Tanaka KR: Hereditary erythrocyte adenylate kinase deficiency: A defect of multiple phosphotransferases? *Blood* **77**:2774, 1991.
369. Matuura S, Igarashi M, Tanizawa Y, Yamada M, Kishi F, Kajii T, Fujii H, Miwa S, Sakurai M, Nakazawa A: Human adenylate kinase associated with hemolytic anemia. A single base substitution affecting solubility and catalytic activity of the cytosolic adenylate kinase. *J Biol Chem* **264**:10148, 1989.
370. Paglia DE, Valentine WN: Hereditary and acquired defects in the pyrimidine nucleotidase of human erythrocytes. *Curr Top Hematol* **3**:75, 1980.
371. Paglia DE, Valentine WN: Characteristics of a pyrimidine-specific 5′-nucleotidase in human erythrocytes. *J Biol Chem* **250**:7973, 1975.
372. Paglia DE, Valentine WN, Brockway RA: Identification of thymidine nucleotidase and deoxyribonucleotidase activities among normal isozymes of 5′-nucleotidase in human erythrocytes. *Proc Natl Acad Sci USA* **81**:588, 1984.
373. Paglia DE, Valentine WN, Brockway RA, Nakatani M: Substrate specificity and pH sensitivity of deoxyribonucleotidase and pyrimidine nucleotidase activities in human hemolysates. *Exp Hematol* **15**:1041, 1987.
374. Valentine WN, Fink K, Paglia DE, Harris SR, Adams WS: Hereditary hemolytic anemia with human erythrocyte pyrimidine 5′-nucleotidase deficiency. *J Clin Invest* **54**:866, 1974.
375. Kondo T, Dale GL, Beutler E: Glutathione transport by inside-out vesicles from human erythrocytes. *Proc Natl Acad Sci USA* **77**:6359, 1980.
376. Zerez CR, Lachant NA, Tanaka KR: Pyrimidine nucleotides do not affect the enzymes of glutathione biosynthesis. *Enzyme* **34**:94, 1985.
377. David O, Ramenghi U, Camaschella C, Vota MG,

Comino L, Pescarmona GP, Nicolla P: Inhibition of hexose monophosphate shunt in young erythrocytes by pyrimidine nucleotides in hereditary pyrimidine 5′-nucleotidase deficiency. *Eur J Haematol* **47**:48, 1991.

378. Tomoda A, Noble NA, Lachant NA, Tanaka KR: Hemolytic anemia in hereditary pyrimidine 5′-nucleotidase deficiency: Nucleotide inhibition of G6PD and the pentose phosphate shunt. *Blood* **60**:1212, 1982.
379. Swallow DM, Aziz I, Hopkinson DA, Miwa S: Analysis of human erythrocyte 5′-nucleotidases in healthy individuals and a patient deficient in pyrimidine 5′-nucleotidase. *Ann Hum Genet* **47**:19, 1983.
380. Paglia DE, Valentine WN, Keitt AS, Brockway RA, Nakatani M: Pyrimidine nucleotidase deficiency with active dephosphorylation of dTMP: Evidence for existence of thymidine nucleotidase in human erythrocytes. *Blood* **61**:1147, 1983.
381. Hirono A, Fujii H, Natori H, Kurokawa I, Miwa S: Chromatographic analysis of human erythrocyte 5′-nucleotidase from five patients with pyrimidine 5′-nucleotidase deficiency. *Br J Haematol* **65**:35, 1987.
382. Paglia DE, Valentine WN, Dahlgren JG: Effects of low-level lead exposure on pyrimidine 5′-nucleotidase and other erythrocyte enzymes. Possible role of pyrimidine 5′-nucleotidase in the pathogenesis of lead-induced anemia. *J Clin Invest* **56**:1164, 1975.
383. Valentine WN, Paglia DE, Fink K, Madokoro G: Lead poisoning. Association with hemolytic anemia, basophilic stippling, erythrocyte pyrimidine 5′-nucleotidase deficiency, and intraerythrocytic accumulation of pyrimidines. *J Clin Invest* **58**:926, 1976.
384. Paglia DE, Valentine WN, Fink K: Lead poisoning. Further observations on erythrocyte pyrimidine-nucleotidase deficiency and intracellular accumulation of pyrimidine nucleotides. *J Clin Invest* **60**:1362, 1977.
385. Buc HA, Kaplan J-C: Red-cell pyrimidine 5′-nucleotidase and lead poisoning. *Clin Chim Acta* **87**:49, 1978.
386. Paglia DE, Valentine WN, Nakatani M, Rauth BJ: Selective accumulation of cytosol CDP-choline as an isolated erythrocyte defect in chronic hemolysis. *Proc Natl Acad Sci USA* **80**:3081, 1983.

CHAPTER 115

Hereditary Spherocytosis and Hereditary Elliptocytosis

Pamela S. Becker ▪ Samuel E. Lux

1. **The red-blood-cell membrane is composed of a bilayer of lipids and integral membrane proteins laminated to an underlying protein skeleton. The skeleton is a two-dimensional meshwork of spectrin tetramers and oligomers cross-linked by protein 4.1 and short actin filaments. It is attached to the membrane via the binding of spectrin to ankyrin and ankyrin to band 3 (the anion exchanger, designated AE1) and via an interaction between protein 4.1 and glycophorin C. The skeleton is a major determinant of membrane shape, strength, and flexibility and helps to control lipid organization and integral protein mobility and topography.**

2. **Hereditary spherocytosis (HS) is a congenital hemolytic anemia caused by an intrinsic red-cell defect. The progressive loss of membrane surface causes the HS red cell to become increasingly spheroidal and osmotically fragile and rigid and subjects it to detention in the splenic cords, where the metabolically inhospitable environment and the high concentration of macrophages combine, in a still uncertain manner, to accentuate the basic membrane defect and enhance spheroidicity. This process is known as "splenic conditioning." Conditioned red cells appear as microspherocytes in the peripheral circulation and are particularly susceptible to destruction in the spleen. The molecular defects thus far identified include abnormalities in spectrin, ankyrin, pallidin (protein 4.2), and band 3.**

3. **Patients with the common, autosomal dominant form of HS typically have mild to moderate anemia, modest splenomegaly, and intermittent mild jaundice. Individuals with compensated hemolysis and no anemia are common, and occasionally severe, transfusion-dependent anemia occurs. Other complications include neonatal jaundice, gallbladder disease, and intermittent aplastic crises.**

   Although the common form of the disease is inherited as an autosomal dominant trait, in about 25 percent of families neither parent is discernibly abnormal. This apparently recessive form is more severe, on average, than dominant HS. Red-cell conditioning and hemolysis abate following splenectomy, although the basic molecular defect persists.

4. **Hereditary elliptocytosis (HE) is a heterogeneous group of congenital red-cell disorders characterized by elliptically shaped cells and, in its more severe forms, by spherocytes, fragmented red cells, and other bizarre poikilocytes. Three distinct subtypes are discernible: common HE, spherocytic HE, and Southeast Asian ovalocytosis. Common HE is further divided into several different phenotypes: (a) Mild HE, the most common form, is a dominant condition with prominent elliptocytosis. Usually there is little or no hemolysis, but significant red cell destruction can occur in individuals in whom splenomegaly develops in response to exogenous stimuli. (b) Mild HE with poikilocytosis in infancy is clinically similar to mild HE after the first year of life. Neonates with this disorder have moderate hemolytic anemia and marked red-cell fragmentation, which may be due to increased concentrations of unbound 2,3-diphosphoglycerate (2,3-DPG) in fetal red cells. (c) In patients with homozygous mild HE, severe hemolysis is observed. (d) Similar features are observed in hereditary pyropoikilocytosis (HPP), a rare recessive disorder manifested by severe hemolysis, marked poikilocytosis, and a characteristic sensitivity of the red cells to heat-induced fragmentation in vitro. Spherocytic HE clinically resembles HS, with moderate hemolytic anemia and both spherocytosis and elliptocytosis. Southeast Asian ovalocytosis is a variant of HE observed in Indonesian and Melanesian peoples. It is characterized by dominant expression, a unique erythrocyte morphology, a rigid cell membrane, decreased expression of blood group antigens, resistance to malarial parasites, heterozygous deletion of eight amino acids in the anion exchange protein (AE1), and little or no hemolysis. In the forms of HE associated with hemolysis, red-cell destruction is mitigated by splenectomy.**

5. **A number of defects in membrane skeletal proteins have been identified in individuals with HE and HPP. Isolated skeletons retain the elliptocytic or poikilocytic shape of the original red cells. Some of the specific defects thus far identified include diminished spectrin–spectrin interactions due to defects in α or β spectrin, deficiency or dysfunction of protein 4.1, and glycophorin C deficiency. The amount of the mutant α spectrin will vary, depending on the presence of a low expression allele on the other chromosome. Thus, the clinical severity in some types of HE can be affected by the relative expression of the mutant to normal α spectrin alleles.**

A list of standard abbreviations is located immediately preceding the index in each volume. Additional abbreviations used in this chapter include: AE1 = anion exchanger 1; Ank, *Ank*, and *ANK* = ankyrin protein, mouse gene symbol, and human gene symbol, respectively; 2,3-DPG = 2,3-diphosphoglycerate; G-3-PD = glyceraldehyde 3-phosphate dehydrogenase; GP = glycophorin, including GPA, GPB, etc; HE = hereditary elliptocytosis; HPP = hereditary pyropoikilocytosis; HS = hereditary spherocytosis; LELY = low expression Lyon, including LELY allele and α^{LELY}; OF = osmotic fragility; SAO = Southeast Asian ovalocytosis. Missense mutations are indicated in single letter amino acid code, e.g., glycine to cysteine at codon 234 is G234C.

During its 4-month life span, the average human red blood cell travels around the circulation 500,000 times, a distance of several hundred miles. To complete this journey, it must be durable enough to withstand strong circulatory shearing forces and flexible enough to negotiate repetitively the narrow portals connecting the splenic cords and sinuses. The flexibility and durability of the red cell are largely determined by the shape, strength, and pliancy of its membrane, and these properties, in turn, are controlled by a submembranous meshwork of proteins termed the "red-cell membrane skeleton." All the major skeletal proteins have been purified, and many of their interconnections have been defined. Several defects in these proteins have been identified in hereditary disorders. This chapter focuses on the structure of the normal membrane skeleton and on two groups of disorders that are believed to be caused by genetic alterations of this structure: hereditary spherocytosis (HS) and hereditary elliptocytosis (HE).

Reviews are available covering various aspects of normal and abnormal red-cell membrane structure[1-8] and selected specific subjects, including membrane lipids,[9] integral membrane proteins,[10-12] and disorders of red-cell permeability.[13] Red-cell membrane defects also contribute to the pathophysiology of abetalipoproteinemia (Chap. 57), Tangier disease (Chap. 64), lecithin:cholesterol acyltransferase deficiency (Chap. 60), Wilson disease (Chap. 68), some of the porphyrias (Chap. 66), the muscular dystrophies (Chaps. 140 and 141), glucose 6-phosphate dehydrogenase deficiency (Chap. 111), and the hemoglobinopathies (Chap. 113).

STRUCTURE OF THE NORMAL RED-CELL MEMBRANE SKELETON

General Aspects of Membrane Structure

The red-cell membrane contains approximately equal parts of proteins and lipids (Table 115-1). Phospholipids and cholesterol predominate and are present in nearly equal proportions (cholesterol/phospholipid = 0.8). These and the other lipids are organized in an asymmetric planar bilayer. The glycolipids and most of the choline phospholipids (phosphatidylcholine and sphingomyelin) are located in the outer half of the bilayer, while phosphatidylinositols and the aminophospholipids (phosphatidylethanolamine and phosphatidylserine) are concentrated in the inner half[9,14,15] (see Table 115-1). The 10 to 12 major membrane proteins are conventionally separated and classified by SDS-PAGE (Fig. 115-1) and fall into two general classes: integral and peripheral (Table 115-2).

Integral membrane proteins penetrate or traverse the lipid bilayer and interact with the hydrophobic lipid core.[27,28] They characteristically have hydrophobic surfaces exposed at such contact points and tend to aggregate or denature in aqueous solution. Red-cell band 3 (anion exchanger 1, or AE1), which forms the anion exchange channel, and the sialic acid–bearing glycophorins are the major examples of this class (see Table 115-2). These proteins have an external carbohydrate-bearing region, a membrane-spanning hydrophobic portion, and an internal, hydrophilic domain. It is likely that all integral proteins have similar amphipathic properties. Integral membrane proteins form the intramembranous particles seen on freeze-cleave electron microscopy of membranes. In the red cell the 8 to 10 nm intramembranous particles are randomly distributed and are believed to be band 3 dimers and tetramers[29] or a complex of band 3 and glycophorin A molecules.[30,31]

Peripheral proteins are bound to the membrane via interactions with integral proteins or the polar portions of the lipid bilayer. In the red cell, the major peripheral proteins are located on the cytoplasmic membrane surface and include enzymes such as glyceraldehyde 3-phosphate dehydrogenase (G-3-PD, protein 6) and the structural proteins of the membrane skeleton.

Integral Membrane Proteins

The Glycophorins. The glycophorins are a class of red-cell glycoproteins that bear several types of red-cell antigens as well as certain receptors (see refs. 10 and 11 for reviews). There are four types identified by gel electrophoresis, designated glycophorins A, B, C, and D (abbreviated GPA, GPB, GPC, and GPD), and a fifth type (found by molecular cloning studies)—glycophorin E (GPE). GPB and GPE appear to have arisen by gene duplication from GPA, and these types carry the MN and Ss blood group antigens. GPA was the first membrane protein for which the amino acid sequence was ascertained, yet the precise physiological role of GPA and GPB is unclear, since individuals lacking one or both of these genes exhibit no functional erythrocyte abnormalities.[10] Glycophorins C and D carry the Gerbich (Ge) antigens. GPD is a shortened form of GPC, lacking its N-terminal region; GPD arises from the same mRNA by use of an alternative initiation codon.[11] There is a subset of Ge-negative red cells, known as the Leach phenotype, that exhibit elliptocytosis, but without significant hemolysis.[32-34] In patients with homozygous protein 4.1 deficiency and elliptocytosis, there is about 70 percent deficiency of glycophorin C, implying that protein 4.1 in some way regulates the glycophorin C content of the red cell.

Anion Exchange Protein 1 (AE1 or Band 3). Band 3, the major red-cell membrane protein ($\sim 1.2 \times 10^6$ molecules/cell), is a 102-kDa transmembrane glycoprotein that probably exists in the membrane as a noncovalently linked dimer and tetramer. The protein is divided into two structurally and functionally unique domains (see ref. 12 for review). The initial structural information was derived from enzymatic cleavage studies. Cleavage with chymotrypsin cuts at the transmembrane domain and yields 60-kDa N-terminal and 35-kDa C-terminal fragments. The latter is glycosylated, which leads to diffuse mobility and poor staining on SDS-PAGE gels.

The different domains possess distinct functions. The C-terminal region forms the physiologically important anion exchange channel that enables the red cell to exchange Cl^- for HCO_3^- and transport CO_2 from the tissues to the lung. This part of the protein is composed mostly of transmembrane helixes. These presumably cluster together to form the transport channel(s). The sites of covalent binding of the anion transporter, DIDS (4,4′-diisothiocyanostilbene-2,2′-disulfonate), are thought to be at Lys539 and Lys851. A single carbohydrate side chain attached at the outer membrane surface at Asn642 binds concanavalin A and bears the I/i blood group antigens. The glycosylation is heterogeneous, which accounts for the diffuse electrophoretic mobility of the protein on SDS gels.[35,36] The cytoplasmic, N-terminal domain (amino acids 1 to 360) contains the binding sites for a large number of red-cell proteins, including hemoglobin,[37] hemichromes,[38,39] protein 4.1,[40] pallidin (protein 4.2),[41] an-

Table 115-1 Composition of Normal Human Erythrocyte Membranes (Ghosts)

Component	Wt, %	g/Ghost, $\times 10^{13}$	Approximate Number of Molecules/Ghost, $\times 10^{6}$	% in Outer Half of Bilayer*	% in Inner Half of Bilayer*
Proteins and glycoproteins	55	5.7†	5‡		
Lipids					
Phospholipids§	28	3.0	250¶		
Sphingomyelin	6.8	0.73	60	80	20
Phosphatidylcholine	7.0	0.75	63	75	25
Phosphatidylethanolamine	7.4	0.79	65	20	80
Phosphatidylserine	4.3	0.46	40	0	100
Phosphatidylinositols	1.0	0.10	8	0	100
Phosphatidylinositol	0.34	0.036	3		
Phosphatidylinositol-4-P	0.22	0.024	2		
Phosphatidylinositol-4,5-PP	0.39	0.042	3		
Phosphatidic acid	1.0	0.10	8	Unknown	Unknown
Other	0.6	0.06	6	Unknown	Unknown
Cholesterol§	13	1.3	195	~50	~50
Glycolipids**	3	0.3	10	100	100
Free fatty acids††	1	0.1	20	Unknown	Unknown
	100	10.4	480		

*Based on data in refs. 14 to 16.
†An average of three reported values compiled in ref. 17.
‡Calculated from the data in Table 115-2.
§Based on compiled data in ref. 18.
¶Number of phospholipids per ghost based on an average molecular weight of 723 calculated from the average red-cell phospholipid polar head group and fatty acid side chain composition (see ref. 19).
**Based on data in ref. 20.
††An average of two reported values compiled in ref. 21.

kyrin,[42-44] and the glycolytic enzymes G-3-PD,[45,46] phosphofructokinase,[47,48] phosphoglycerate kinase,[49] and aldolase.[48] Hemoglobin, hemichromes, and the glycolytic enzymes bind to a very acidic segment located at the extreme N-terminus.[37] Protein 4.1 also binds within or just beyond this region.[50] The binding sites for ankyrin and pallidin are less well localized. Usually one ankyrin molecule binds avidly (K_d ~10^{-8} *M*) to each band 3 tetramer.[44] With this stoichiometry, approximately 30 to 40 percent of the band 3 molecules will be bound to ankyrin and the membrane skeleton. So far no differences have been detected in the band 3 molecules that are bound and those that are not.[42-44]

As noted earlier, band 3 may also interact with glycophorin A, the other major integral membrane protein.[31] If so, the interaction is weak, since glycophorin and band 3 are not associated when they are extracted (and diluted) in nonionic detergents.

Red-cell band 3 (AE1) is a member of a family of homologous anion transport exchangers designated the AE gene family. AE1 is the erythrocyte form.[12] It is also expressed in the kidney; however, the N-terminal 66 amino acids are not included in the kidney isoform.[51] The 17-kb AE1 gene has been entirely cloned and largely sequenced and predicts a sequence of 911 amino acids.

Components of the Membrane Skeleton

Operationally, the red-cell membrane skeleton is the insoluble proteinaceous residue that remains after extraction of red cells[52] or their ghosts[53] with the nonionic detergent Triton X-100. It comprises 55 to 60 percent of the membrane protein mass and includes all the spectrin, actin, tropomyosin, tropomodulin, adducin, ankyrin, protein 4.1, dematin (protein 4.9), and a portion of band 3, pallidin, and the proteins in the band 7 region on SDS gels (Fig. 115-1). Spectrin, actin, protein 4.1, and dematin form the core of the structure, since the skeleton retains its shape when other components are eluted with hypertonic KCl but disintegrates if spectrin or actin is removed.[52] When the skeleton is isolated in relatively low concentrations of detergent, it contains some residual phospholipid, particularly sphingomyelin,[52,53] but this is not an integral part of the structure since it is absent when higher concentrations of detergent are used.[52] The

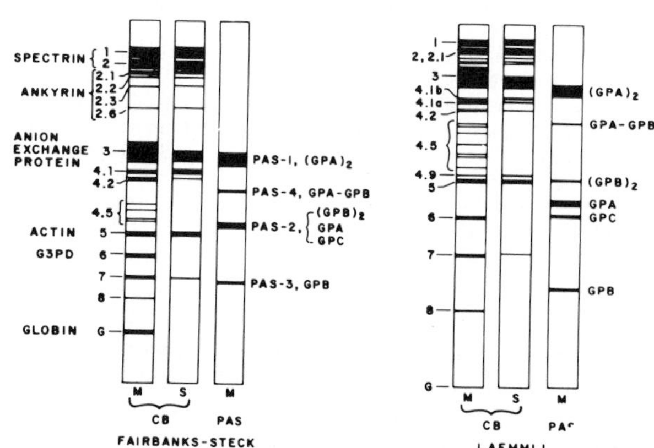

FIG. 115-1 Schematic illustration of the SDS-PAGE patterns of the proteins of red-cell membranes (M) and membrane skeletons (S) stained for proteins with Coomassie blue (CB) and for sialoglycoproteins with PAS. The two gel systems in common use are shown: Fairbands-Steck gels containing 5 percent acrylamide and Laemmli gels containing 11.5 percent acrylamide. GPA, GPB, and GPC refer to glycophorins A, B, and C, respectively. $(GPA)_2$ and $(GPB)_2$ are the dimers and GPA-GPB is the heterodimer of GPA and GPB.

Table 115-2 Major Erythrocyte Membrane Proteins

SDS Gel Band[a]	Protein	Molecular Mass (kDa) Gel	Molecular Mass (kDa) Calc[b]	Monomer Molecules/Cell,[c] Thousands	Oligomeric State	Approximate Proportion,[d] %	Peripheral or Integral	Chromosome Location	Associated Diseases
1	α Spectrin	240	281	242±20	Heterodimer/ tetramer/ oligomer	14	P	1q22-q25	HE,HPP,HS
2	β Spectrin	220	246	242±20		13	P	14q23-q24.2	HE,HPP,HS
2.1[e]	Ankyrin[e]	210	206	124±11[e]	Monomer	6[e]	P	8p11.2	HS
2.9[f]	α Adducin	103	81	~30	Tetramer	<1	P	4p16.3	
	β Adducin	97	80	~30		<1	P	—	—
3	AE1	90–100[g]	102[h]	~1200	Dimer or tetramer	29	I	17q12-q21	HS,SAO,HAc
4.1	Protein 4.1	80+78[i]	66[j]	~200	Monomer	5	P	1p33-p34.2	HE
4.2	Pallidin	72	77	~250	? Dimer or trimer	5	P	15q15-q21	HS[k]
4.9[f]	Dematin[l]	48+52	43+46	~140	Trimer[l]	1	P	—	—
	p55	55	53	~80	? Dimer		P	Xq28	—
5[f]	β Actin	43	42	~500	Oligomer (~14)	6	P	7pter-q22	—
	Tropomodulin	43	41	~30	Monomer		P	9q22	—
6	G3PD	35	36	~500	Tetramer	5[m]	P	12p13	—
7[f]	Stomatin	31	32	—	—	4	I	9q34.1	?HSt[s]
	Tropomyosin	27+29	28[o]	~70	Heterodimer[o]		P	1q31	—
8	Protein 8	23	—	~200	—	1–2	P	—	—
PAS-1[p]	Glycophorin A	36[q]	14[h]	~1000	Dimer	1.6	I	4q31	None
PAS-2[p]	Glycophorin C	32[q]	14[h]	~200[r]	—	0.1	I	2q14-q21	HE
PAS-3[p]	Glycophorin B	20[q]	8[h]	~200	?Dimer	0.2	I	4q31	None
	Glycophorin D	23[q]	11[h]	~200	—	0.02	I	2q14-q21	HE
	Glycophorin E	—[n]	6[h]	—[n]	—[n]	—[n]	I	4q31	—

[a]Numbering system of Fairbanks et al.[17] and Steck.[24] Bands 1 to 8 refer to gels stained with Coomassie blue. PAS-1 to PAS-3 refer to gels stained with PAS.
[b]Calculated from amino acid sequences.
[c]Based on an estimate of 5.7×10^{-13} g protein/ghost[17] and on the approximate proportions of each protein, estimated from densitometry of SDS gels. The data from spectrin and ankyrin were measured directly by radioimmunoassay.[22]
[d]Proteins 1 to 8 were estimated from published data [6,17,23] and from unpublished data (Lux SE, John KM).
[e]Protein 2.1 is full-length anykrin. Other isoforms are evident on SDS gels, including band 2.2 = 195 kDa, band 2.3 = 175 kDa, and band 2.6 = 145 kDa. Band 2.2 is produced by alternate splicing. The origin of the other bands is unknown. The data shown are for ankyrin 2.1 except for the number of copies/cell and approximate proportion (wt %), which includes all isoforms.
[f]The α- and β-adducins lie in the upper part of SDS gel band 3. Band 4.9 contains both dematin and p55; band 5 contains β-actin and tropomodulin; band 7 contains stomatin and tropomyosin.
[g]The protein runs as a broad band on SDS gels because of heterogeneous glycosylation.
[h]The calculated molecular weight does not include the contribution of the carbohydrate chains.
[i]Protein 4.1 is a doublet (4.1a and 4.1b) on SDS gels. Protein 4.1a is derived from 4.1b by slow deamidation.[25] Its proportion is a measure of red-cell age.
[j]Protein 4.1 exists in a very large number of isoforms.[26] The major erythroid isoform is listed here. It is not known why its calculated molecular weight deviates so much from the apparent molecular weight on SDS gels.
[k]Deficiency of pallidin is associated with a variety of morphologies (see text), but spherocytes predominate.[5]
[l]Only the 48-kDa subunit has been cloned. Although dematin is present as a trimer in solution, the 48- and 52-kDa subunits have an apparent stoichiometry of 3:1 on SDS gels.
[m]The amount of G3PD (band 6) associated with the membrane varies from person to person (~3 to 6 wt %).
[n]Glycophorin E mRNA has been identified, but it is not yet certain that the mRNA is translated.
[o]Tropomyosin is a heterodimer of the 27- and 29-kDa subunits. There are about 70,000 copies of each chain per red cell. Data for the calculated molecular weight are for fibroblast tropomyosin. The red-cell isoform has not been sequenced.
[p]The glycophorins (GpA to GpD) are visible only on PAS-stained gels.
[q]Molecular weights, including carbohydrate, estimated from mobilities on SDS gels.[10,11]
[r]Glycophorins C and D are probably synthesized from the same mRNA using different translational start sites[11]. The number of copies is for the total number of glycophorins C and D.
[s]HSt = hereditary stomatocytosis.

chromosomal locations of most of the membrane skeletal proteins are now known and are listed in Table 115-2.

Spectrin. Spectrin is the major skeletal protein and accounts for about 50 to 75 percent of the skeletal mass, depending on the method of preparation.[52,53] It contains two enormous polypeptide chains that are structurally similar but functionally distinct: α chain (protein 1; 281 kDa) and β chain (protein 2; 246 kDa).[54-56] These chains are aligned side by side in an antiparallel arrangement with respect to their N-and C-terminal ends.[57] EM shows spectrin to be a slender, twisted wormlike molecule that extends to a total length of about 100 nm[58,59] (Fig. 115-2). The protein is highly flexible[58,59] and assumes a variety of conformations—an unusual property that may be critical for normal membrane pliancy. The initial model of spectrin structure based on biophysical studies suggested the presence of rigid globular regions containing ionic side chains and α-helical structure joined by hydrophobic, flexible sections of polypeptide chain.[60] Chemical data disclosed a linear arrangement of proteolytically resistant domains joined by protease-sensitive regions[57,61] (Fig. 115-3). There are nine such domains, five on the α chain, designated αI through αV, and four on the β chain, βI through βIV.[61,62] As will be shown, many of the molecular

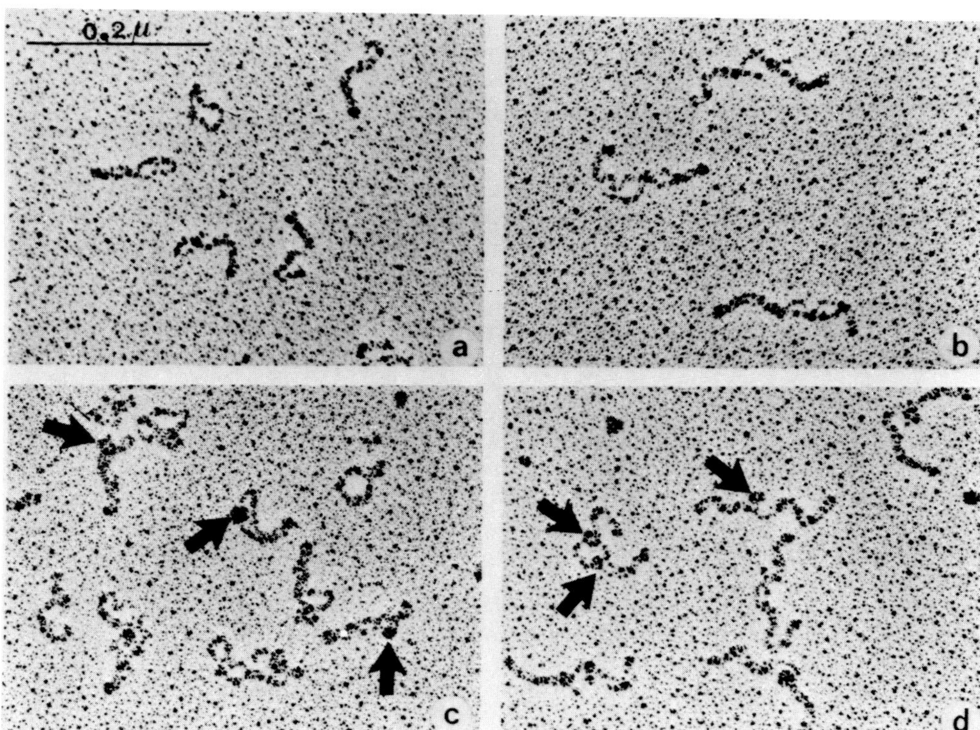

FIG. 115-2 EM of rotary-shadowed specimens of red-cell membrane skeletal proteins: *A*. Spectrin dimers. *B*. Spectrin tetramers. *C*. Spectrin dimers with bound ankyrin (*arrows*). *D*. Spectrin tetramers with bound ankyrin (*arrows*). *(Used by permission of D. Branton,* Cell *24:24, 1981.)*

defects in HE have been identified as abnormalities in spectrin domain maps after proteolytic digestion. Protein sequencing[56] demonstrated the existence of homologous 106 amino acid repeating segments, and this was confirmed by cDNA sequencing.[63,64] There are 22 homologous segments in the α chain, with a nonhomologous tenth segment and a nonhomologous C-terminal region. The latter region appears to contain calcium-binding EF-hand structures. The β chain has 17 repeats, with a nonhomologous N-terminal region that contains the actin and protein 4.1 binding sites, and

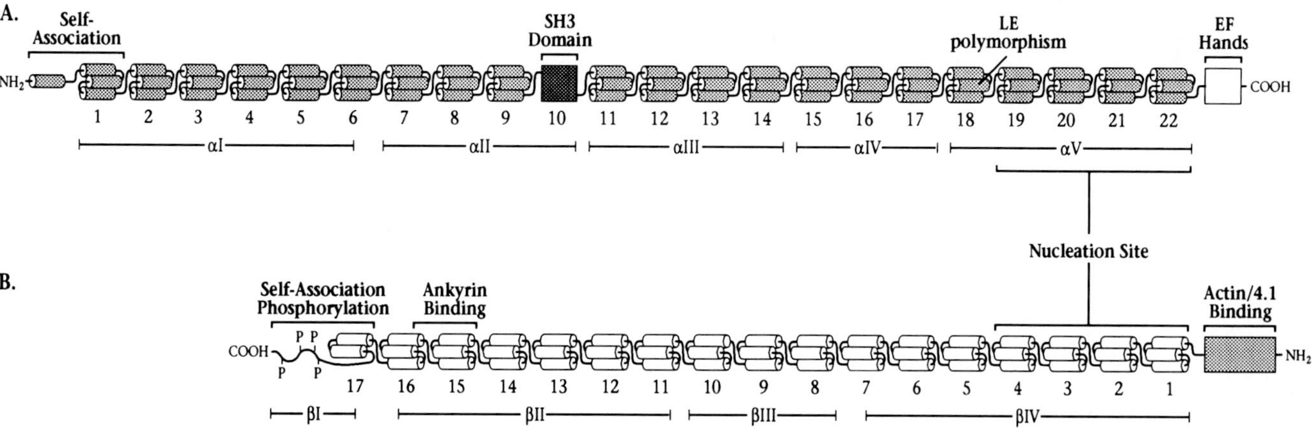

C. Dimer Head-to-Head Self-Association

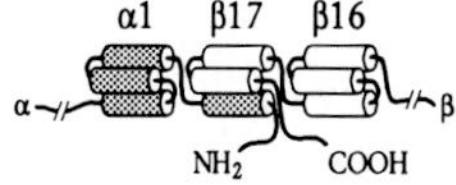

FIG. 115-3 Model of spectrin structure. *A*. The α spectrin molecule is depicted as a series of helical repeating segment. The repeats are designated 1 through 22. The locations of the trypsin-resistant domains are indicated by Roman numerals I through V. The domains are numbered from the proximal "head" of the molecule, the end that contains the spectrin self-association site. The regions of specialized function are indicated, including the N-terminal α-chain self-association site, the atypical segment 10 that contains the SH3 domain, and the C-terminal EF hand structures. *B*. The β spectrin molecule is depicted as a series of triple helical repeating segments. The repeats are designated 1 through 17, beginning from the N-terminus. However, the α and β chains are arranged in antiparallel alignment with respect to their N- and C-terminal ends. The trypsin-resistant domains are indicated below, designated by Roman numerals I through IV. The regions of specialized function are indicated, including actin/protein 4.1 binding on the N-terminal region lacking the repeat structure, ankyrin binding in repeat 15, and the C-terminal phosphorylation site. *C*. The dimer self-association site. The extra helix 3 at the N-terminus of the α chain (α′ repeat segment) associates with the extra helix 2 and helix 3 at the C-terminus of the β chain to form a complete triple helical spectrin repeat. *(Adapted from Winkelmann and Forget,[86] by permission.)*

a short nonhomologous C-terminal segment that contains several casein phosphorylation sites. The repeats contain conserved amino acids at specific positions, such as an invariant tryptophan at position 45 and a leucine at position 26.[56] The 106 amino acid segments are arranged in triple α-helical configurations, with the three helixes arranged in antiparallel alignment and connected by short nonhelical portions[56,65] (see Fig. 115-3). The original repeat segment, based on amino acid sequence data,[56] consisted of the third α-helical region (helix 3) of the following segment and two contiguous α-helical regions (helixes 1 and 2). The newer nomenclature designates a triple helical segment that consists of helixes 1, 2, and 3 (see Figs. 115-2 and 115-3), and the helix 3 at the very beginning of the α chain is designated α′. This latter organization is also known as the conformational repeat and is supported by conformational studies of recombinant spectrin subunits.[66] Thus, helix 3 of repeat 5 (by amino acid sequence designation) is identical to helix 3 of triple helical segment (or conformational repeat) 4. (The designations assigned in Fig. 115-20 and in Table 115-3 refer to the conformational repeats.)

Side-to-side assembly of the α and β spectrin chains occurs in a zipperlike fashion, beginning with a defined nucleation site composed of four repeats from each chain at the end opposite the self-association site, repeats α19 to α22 and β1 to β4.[67] Two of the α repeats and one of the β repeats have an eight-residue insertion in the 106 amino acid repeat unit. The model suggests that after the initial tight association of the complementary nucleation sites, a conformational change is propagated that promotes the pairing of the full remaining length of the two chains.[67] Interestingly, in support of this hypothesis is the finding of a common polymorphism reducing the incorporation of the product of the α spectrin allele into the membrane skeleton. The low expression (LELY, Low Expression Lyon) allele is designated α^{LELY} or $\alpha^{V/41}$, after the peptide that is produced in diminished quantity. Two abnormalities result in the LELY allele: (1) a Leu 1867 to Val mutation, exon 40, repeat α18, helix 2, that causes tryptic cleavage after amino acid 1920, at the αIV-V junction, in the neighboring helix 3; and (2) a linked C-to-T substitution in an acceptor splice site 12 nt before the splice junction that leads to 50 percent inframe skipping of exon 46. This exon is only 18 bp long, and thus the change in the protein is too small to be observed on SDS-PAGE, but the exon lies within the nucleation site for α to β chain association.[68,69] α Spectrin chains lacking exon 46 (i.e., α^{LELY}) probably fail to bind to β spectrin chains and are destroyed. The remaining α chains (~50 percent), which contain the exon, probably function normally. The frequency of the LELY allele is 31 percent in Europeans, 20 percent in Japanese, and 20 percent in African blacks. Expression of this allele can exacerbate the clinical severity of the HE mutations in the trans allele (discussed under "Hereditary Elliptocytosis" below).

Spectrin has the capability to associate to tetramers and higher oligomers.[70-72] This is accomplished by binding in a head-to-head configuration[59,70,71] (see Figs. 115-2 and 3). Both tetramers and oligomers are believed to exist on the intact membrane, but tetramers predominate,[72] probably because the association constant for formation of tetramers is substantially higher than for the larger species.[73] At low ionic strength and physiological temperature (37°C), spectrin dissociates into dimers,[71,73] while physiological ionic strength and lower temperatures (25°C) favor the tetramer and oligomer species. At 4°C the equilibrium is kinetically frozen because of its high activation energy.[70] It is possible to extract spectrin from the membrane at such temperatures and examine its association state directly. Spectrin also binds to other proteins, including ankyrin, protein 4.1, and actin as discussed below.

The tetramer-binding site structure was elucidated by both analysis of mutant spectrin[74] and by proteolytic studies.[75] A triple-stranded conformational unit exists, which comprises a helix 3 derived from the N-terminal α chain, the so-called α′ repeat segment, and modified helixes 1 and 2 from the C-terminal β chain. Specific protease cleavage sites are protected by the formation of the α to β head-to-head complex.[75]

Spectrin is synthesized very early in erythroid development. It is plentiful in pronormoblasts[76] and is detectable in undifferentiated erythroleukemia cells[77] and possibly in immature committed erythroid stem cells, erythroid blast-forming units (BFU-E) and erythroid colony forming units (CFU-E).[78] It is ubiquitous in red cells of both vertebrates[79] and invertebrates,[80-82] and has even been detected in slime molds,[83] sea urchins,[84] and plants.[85] Moreover, a structural and functional analogue of spectrin, fodrin, has been identified in many other cell types (as reviewed elsewhere[86]), and its role in those cells is now being elucidated. Even in the most primitive organisms, regions of spectrin/fodrin are immunochemically (and hence structurally) similar to the human protein.[80-82] This evolutionary conservation suggests that some spectrin function is critical for the survival of the erythrocyte. Spectrin and fodrin are members of a gene superfamily that also includes dystrophin and α actinin. All members contain a series of similar 106 amino acid repeat segments as well as similar N- and C-terminal regions of specialized function.

The α spectrin gene is located on chromosome 1q22-q25,[87] near the Duffy blood group. The β spectrin gene is located on chromosome 14q23-q24.2.[64,88] In chickens, mice, and humans, α spectrin is synthesized in threefold excess relative to β spectrin[89-91] and is degraded by a different, slower pathway.[92] The limited synthesis and more rapid degradation of β spectrin suggests that its association with the membrane is the rate limiting step in spectrin assembly.[92,93]

Actin. Red-cell actin is very similar to other actins, both structurally[94] and functionally.[95] It is the β type,[23] a subtype that is found in a variety of other nonmuscle cells.[96] Unlike the actin in other cells, red-cell actin appears to be organized as short, double helical F-actin filaments ("protofilaments") about 12 to 16 monomers long.[97] It appears that these short filaments are stabilized by their interactions with spectrin, protein 4.1, and tropomyosin (see "Actin-Associated Proteins" below) and by capping of the slow growing or "pointed" end of actin by tropomodulin.[98]

There is also evidence that the state of actin polymerization is functionally important to the red cell, since compounds that inhibit actin polymerization increase membrane flexibility, while compounds that promote its polymerization increase the rigidity of the membrane.[99] Spectrin dimers bind to the side of actin filaments at a site near the tail end of the spectrin molecule[100,101] (Fig. 115-4). A specific peptide in the N-terminal region of β spectrin[102] or an even smaller peptide of 27 amino acids from the analogous region of actin binding protein[103] is capable of binding to actin. Spectrin tetramers are therefore bivalent and can crosslink actin filaments; however, binding is weak ($K_d \sim 10^{-3}$ *M*) and ineffectual in the absence of protein 4.1[104,105]

Protein 4.1. This globular protein (66 kDa, a 5.7-nm sphere)[106] is a core skeletal component and is necessary for normal

Table 115-3 Hereditary Defects of Membrane Skeletal Proteins

Protein Defects*	Clinical Expression: Heterozygote	Clinical Expression: Homozygote or Compound Heterozygote†	Tryptic Cleavage or Other Studies‡	Primary Structural Defect‡/Location	Prevalence and Other Characteristics	Selected References
I. Spectrin (Sp)						
A. Spectrin Deficiency						
Autosomal recessive HS	Silent carrier	Moderate to severe HS	Sp 30–75% of normal	A969D/α9 in many families with severe recessive HS. Probably a linked polymorphism.	Severe forms rare, moderate forms common (−25%); defects in ankyrin and pallidin (see below) may be more common than α-spectrin defects in recessive HS, especially the less severe forms.	237,260,261,263
B. Defects in α-Spectrin that Impair Self-association						
Sp $\alpha^{I/78}$ Sp $_{TUNIS}$	Silent carrier to moderately severe HE	?	78-kDa peptide cleaved at Lys 16	R41W/α′: helix 3 or R45S/α′: helix 3	Especially in North Africa. Single case reports.	506,519,520
Sp $\alpha^{I/74}$	Silent carrier to moderately severe HE	Severe HE to HPP	74-kDa peptide cleaved at Lys 49	R28H/α′: helix 3	Arg 28 mutations are relatively common. Found in whites, blacks, Arabs, and Melanesians.	507,509–511, 521,524
				R28C/α′: helix 3		523
				R28L/α′: helix 3		523,524
				R28S/α′: helix 3		523,524
Sp$_{GENOVA}$			74-kDa peptide cleaved at Arg 45	R34W/α′: helis 3	One report	328
Sp$_{CULOZ}$				G46V/α′: helix 3	One report	522
Sp$_{LYON}$				K48R/α′: helix 3	One report	524
				L49F/α′: helix 3	One report	522
Sp $\alpha^{I/65}$ (Sp $\alpha^{I/68}$)§	Silent carrier to mild HE	Moderate to moderately severe HE	65-kDa peptide cleaved at Arg 137	Dup L154/α1: helix 3	Common in blacks. Homogeneous defect.	328,474,511–513, 515,516,526,545, 587
Sp$_{PONTE\ DE\ SOR}$	Silent carrier	Severe HE		G151D/α1: helix 3	One report	527
Sp $\alpha^{I/61}$	Silent carrier	HPP	61-kDa peptide	?	Single report	514
Sp $\alpha^{I/46}$	Mild HE	HPP	46-kDa peptide cleaved at Lys 258	Deletion of amino acid 178–226 α2 repeat (helix 1–2 link). Exon 5 skipped and ~1-kb insertion in intron 5.	Single report	329
Sp $\alpha^{I/50a}$	Silent carrier to mild HE	HPP	50-kDa peptide cleaved at Arg 256 of Lys 258	L207P/α2: helix 2	Relatively common in blacks	544
				L260P/α2: helix 3		516,545
				S261P/α2: helix 3		516,545
Sp $\alpha^{I/43}$	Mild HE	?	43-kDa peptide	?	Single report	517
Sp $\alpha^{I/36}$ (Sp $_{SFAX}$)	Silent carrier to mild HE	?	36- and 33-kDa peptides cleaved from αI domain	Deletion amino acid 363–371, α3: helix 3, due to cryptic splice site in exon 8.	Single report	518

Continued

Table 115-3 Hereditary Defects of Membrane Skeletal Proteins (Continued)

Protein Defects*	Clinical Expression: Heterozygote	Clinical Expression: Homozygote or Compound Heterozygote†	Tryptic Cleavage or Other Studies‡	Primary Structural Defect‡/Location	Prevalence and Other Characteristics	Selected References
B. Defects in α-Spectrin that Impair Self-association						
Sp $\alpha^{I/50b}$	Mild HE	?	50-kDa peptide cleaved at Arg 468 or Arg 470	H469R/α4: helix 3 E471P/α4: helix 3	Probably rare	546 516,545
Sp ALEXANDRIA	Mild to moderately severe HE			Deletion of H469		547
Sp $\alpha^{II/31}$ (Sp JENDOUBA)	Silent carrier to mild HE	?	Abnormal 31-, 26-, 21-, and 18-kDa peptides; cleavage after Lys 788	D791E/α7: helix 3	Single report, Relatively few, roundish elliptocytes. Only slight defect in Sp self-association.	569
Sp $\alpha^{II/21}$ (Sp ORAN)	Silent carrier	Mild HE	Abnormal 21- and 16-kDa peptides derived from αII domain	Deletion of amino acid 822–862 (exon 18), A → G (−1) in the acceptor splice site (α8: helix 2)	Single report	570
Sp $\alpha^{II/47}$	Silent carrier	HPP	?	?	Single report	543
Truncated α-spectrin	Mild to moderately severe HE	?	235-kDa α′-spectrin band on SDS gels	?	Rare	463,525,528
Decreased amount of α-spectrin	Severe hemolytic HE	?	?	?	Single report	585
C. Defects in β-Spectrin that Impair Self-association						
Sp $\alpha^{I/74}$ Sp CAGLIARI Sp PROVIDENCE	Silent carrier to moderately severe HE	Severe HPP to lethal hydrops fetalis	Increased in the 74-kDa fragment cleaved from the αI domain	A2053P/β17: helix 2 A2018G/β17: helix 1 S2019P/β17: helix 1	Single reports. Mutations in β-Sp that alter cleavage of the neighboring αI domain.	74 542 541
D. Truncated β-Spectrins						
Sp $\beta^{220/218}$ (Sp ROUEN)	Moderate HE	?	218-kDa β′-chain. Reduced phosphorylation.	Truncated, G → T (+3) in donor splice site. Exon Y skipped, premature termination.	Single report. Elliptocytes without poikilocytes; hemolytic crises.	534
Sp $\beta^{220/216}$						
Sp NICE	Moderate HE	?	216-kDa β′-chain. Absent phosphorylation.	Truncated, AG duplication at codons 2045/2046.	Single report. Hemolytic crises.	535
Sp TANDIL	Hemolytic HE	?		Truncated, deletion of 7 bp at codon 2041.	Single report. Rounded elliptocytes.	536

Sp TOKYO	Mild hemolytic HE	?		Truncated, deletion of C in codon 2059.		537
Sp $\beta^{220/214}$						
Sp GÖTTINGEN	Moderately severe HE	?	214-kDa β′-chain. Absent phosphorylation.	Truncated, T → A (+2) in donor splice, exon X skipped.	Single report: Elliptocytes and poikilocytes. Increased OF.	539
Sp LEPUY	Moderate HE	?		Truncated, A → G (+4) in donor splice, exon X skipped.	Single report. Elliptocytes and poikilocytes; OF normal.	538
Sp $\beta^{220/210}$ (Sp YAMAGATA)	?	?		?		540
E. Elongated β-Spectrin						
Sp $\beta^{220/330}$ (Sp DETROIT)	Silent carrier	?	330-kDa β′-chain	?	Single kindred. Giant β′-chain is only 25% of β Sp, probably unstable.	327
F. Defect in β-Spectrin that Impairs Binding of Protein 4.1						
Sp KISSIMMEE	Moderate HS	?	Sp low (80% normal)	W202R. Spontaneous mutation in N-terminal region, between βIV domain and actin binding site. ? Part of 4.1 binding site.	Rare. Some acanthocytes on blood smear. Mutant spectrin unstable, easily oxidized, and binds protein 4.1 very weakly.	277
II. Ankyrin (Ank)						
A. Ankyrin Deficiency						
General case	Mild to moderately severe HS	Moderate to lethal HS	Sp and ankyrin are equally reduced (60–90% of normal) in most patients.	Multiple defects (see below)	Ankyrin defects are a common cause (estimated 30–65%) of dominant HS mutations.	22
B. 5′-Untranslated Region/Promoter Mutations in Ankyrin						
−72/73 mutation	Silent carrier	?Mild AS	Combined Sp-ankyrin deficiency	Deletion of 2 bp (GGTGAG→GGAG) in exon 1, −72/73 bp from translation start site.	2/31 kindreds tested	282
−108 mutation	Silent carrier	?Mild-severe AS	Combined Sp-ankyrin deficiency	T→C exchange (CCTGG→CCCGG) in promoter, −108 bp from translation start site.	4/31 kindreds tested	282
C. Amino Acid Substitutions in Ankyrin						
Ank WALSRODE	Silent carrier	Mild HS	Combined Sp–ankyrin deficiency	V463I, in exon 13 (repeat 14, membrane domain)	1 of 40 HS kindreds tested. Patient (mild HS) is compound heterozygote for clinically silent exon 1 polymorphism.	282

Continued

Table 115-3 Hereditary Defects of Membrane Skeletal Proteins (Continued)

Protein Defects*	Clinical Expression: Heterozygote	Clinical Expression: Homozygote or Compound Heterozygote†	Tryptic Cleavage or Other Studies‡	Primary Structural Defect‡/Location	Prevalence and Other Characteristics	Selected References
D. Truncated Ankyrins						
Ank $_{EINBECK}$	Mild HS	?	Combined Sp–ankyrin deficiency	Extra C in codon 572 (exon 16, repeat 18, membrane domain), 47 extra amino acids and premature termination.	1 of 31 HS kindreds tested	282
Ank $_{MARBURG}$	Moderately severe HS	?	Combined Sp–ankyrin deficiency	4-bp deletion in codons 797–798 (exon 22, end of membrane domain), 6 extra amino acids and premature termination	1 of 31 HS kindreds tested	282
Ank $_{BOVENDEN}$	Moderate HS	?	Combined Sp–ankyrin deficiency	R1436 → Stop (TGA) in exon 36 (regulatory domain), premature termination	1 of 31 HS kindreds tested	282
Ank $_{STUTTGART}$	Moderate HS	?	Combined Sp–ankyrin deficiency	Deletion of GC in codon 329 (exon 10, repeat 10, membrane domain), 25 extra amino acids and premature termination	1 of 31 HS kindreds tested	282
E. Other Ankyrin Defects						
Unstable ankyrin	?	?	Combined Sp–ankyrin deficiency	~50% reduction in ankyrin mRNA. ? Unstable ankyrin.	Single case. Inheritance unclear. Severe HS with unusual poikilocytosis.	270
Ankyrin gene deletions	Severe HS	?	Combined Sp–ankyrin deficiency. Partial lack of pallidin.	Heterozygous interstitial deletions at 8p11-8p22.2. (Ankyrin located at 8p11.2.)	Growth and developmental retardation, hypogonadism. Spontaneous mutations. Six kindreds known.	151
Balanced translocations	HS	?	?	Balanced translocation involving 8p11. (ankyrin gene probably involved but not proven).	Typical HS. Two kindreds known.	151
Ank $_{PRAGUE}$	HS		Deficiency of ankyrin band 2.1. New band at 174 kDa (ankyrin 2.2′).		Single report. Abnormal regulatory domain of ankyrin.	269

III. Protein 4.1						
A. Protein 4.1 Deficiency						
General case	Mild HE	Severe hemolytic HE	Heterozygous: 50% protein 4.1. Homozygous: 0% protein 4.1 and 9% glycophorin C.	Deletion of 318 bp includes downstream (erythroid-type) translation start in one Algerian kindred.	Heterozygous state relatively common, especially North Africa (~33% of HE patients). Most studies on one Algerian kindred.	553,557
Protein 4.1 $_{MADRID}$	Silent carrier	Severe HE		ATG → AGG in the downstream initiation codon.	Single report	558
B. Protein 4.1 Mutations Involving the Sp-actin Binding Region¶						
Protein 4.1$^{68/65}$	Mild HE	?	65- and 68-kDa 4.1 isoforms	Deletion of L407-G486 (2 exons)	Single kindred. Deletion includes exon encoding Sp-actin binding domain. Membranes mechanically unstable.	562,563
Protein 4.1^{95}	Mild HE	?	95-kDa 4.1 isoform	Duplication of L407-Q529 (3 exons)	Single kindred. Duplication at Sp-actin binding domain. Normal membrane stability.	562,563
IV. Pallidin (Protein 4.2)						
A. Pallidin Deficiency						
Pallidin $_{NIPPON}$	Silent carrier	Moderately severe hemolytic anemia	Heterozygous: 50% palladin. Homozygous: <1% pallidin. Faint 74/72-kDa bands on immunoblots.	A142T in alternate spliced segment of pallidin, alters RNA processing.	Rare in Europe, more common in Japan. Morphology may be spherocytic, elliptocytic, stomatocytic, or normal. Normal red cell spectrin.	280
Pallidin $_{TOZEUR}$	Silent carrier	Moderate hemolytic anemia	Trace pallidin, slightly decreased band 3	R310Q	Single report in Tunisian patient. Acanthocytes and poikilocytes	281
Pallidin $_{LISBOA}$	Silent carrier	Moderate hemolytic anemia	Pallidin completely absent	Deletion C in codon 88 or 89, 48 extra amino acids and premature termination	Single Portuguese family. Acanthocytes and poikilocytes	281
V. Glycophorin C (GPC)						
A. GPC Deficiency						
General case	Silent carrier	Mild HE	Heterozygous: 50% GPC	Deletion of exons 3 and 4 in GPC gene.	Rare. Ge^{-} (Leach) blood group.	567,568
			Homozygous: no GPC	Deletion of 2 bp in codons 44–45, frameshift.	One patient	33

Continued

Table 115-3 Hereditary Defects of Membrane Skeletal Proteins (Continued)

Protein Defects*	Clinical Expression: Heterozygote	Clinical Expression: Homozygote or Compound Heterozygote†	Tryptic Cleavage or Other Studies‡	Primary Structural Defect‡/Location	Prevalence and Other Characteristics	Selected References
VI. Band 3 (Anion Exchanger 1)						
A. Band 3 Deficiency						
General case	Mild HS	?	Band 3 = 65–85%	Defect unknown in most cases; presumably multiple.	Probably ~10–15% of dominant HS. Selective loss of band 3 not bound to skeleton, so greatest band 3 deficit in old red cells. Normal or near normal red cell Sp. Some mushroom-shaped red cells on blood smears.	290
Band 3 PRAGUE	HS	?		Duplication of 10 bases after codon 818, involving last predicted transmembrane segment.	Single report	290
Decreased band 3 and protein 4.1	Compensated hemolysis. Normal morphology.	Severe hemolysis. Elliptocytes and poikilocytes.	Band 3 with slightly increased mobility on SDS gels. Protein 4.1 decreased 30%.	?	Single family.	586
B. Defects in Band 3 that Impair Pallidin Binding						
Band 3 TUSCALOOSA	HS	?	Heterozygous; ~70% of normal pallidin.	P327R and linked polymorphism K56E (band 3 MEMPHIS).	Single report. Pallidin binding to inside-out red-cell membranes decreased 30%.	284
Band 3 MONTEFIORE	?	HS	Homozygous: ~12% of normal pallidin. Normal red cell Sp.	E40K	Single patient. Pallidin binding to inside-out red-cell membranes decreased 30%.	283
C. Defects in Band 3 that Reduce Ankyrin Binding						
Hereditary acanthocytosis Band 3 HT (High Transport)	Silent carrier	Acanthocytosis, no hemolysis	Band 3 with slightly increased mobility on SDS gels. Normal amount of band 3.	P868L	Single report. Decreased ankyrin binding (50%) and increased anion transport.	580 580a

D. Defects in Band 3 that Increase Membrane Rigidity

Southeast Asian ovalocytosis (SAO)	Stomatocytic elliptocytosis	Probably lethal	Heterozygous: ~50% SAO band 3	Deletion at A400–A408, linked to Band 3 $_{MEMPHIS}$ polymorphism (K56E). Deletion alters signal sequence in first transmembrane helix, misassembly and inability to transport anions. Deletion at P403 may diminish mobility of cytoplasmic domain.	Very common (up to 25%) in aborigines of Melanesia and Malaysia. Some elliptocytes with characteristic transverse bar. No hemolysis. ? Increased ankyrin binding and decreased protein 3 mobility, very rigid red cells that resist invasion by malaria.	574–576
VII. Some Asymptomatic Membrane Protein Polymorphisms						
A. Spectrin						
Sp $\alpha^{V/41}$ (or α^{LE}) Sp α^{LELY} (or $\alpha^{V/41}$)	Silent carrier	Silent carrier	Enhanced cleavage of α^{IV}–α^{V} junction after K1920, 41-kDa peptide released.	L1867V causes the $\alpha^{V/41}$ cleavage defect. A linked second mutation, C → T (−12), in the acceptor splice site, 60% inframe skipping of exon 46. Exon 46 within nucleation site that initiates side-to-side association of α and β Sp chains.	Very common (~30% of chromosomes in Europeans = 42% heterozygous, 8% homozygous). Clinically silent Sp polymorphism that greatly exacerbates the clinical severity of α-Sp defects in *trans* and mutes the severity of defect in *cis*.	67,68
Sp α^{II}	Silent carrier	Silent carrier	Four polymorphic variants, differ in pI and size.	R701H I809V T853R I: − − − II: + + + III: + + − IV: − + +	Common in blacks	271,504
B. Protein 4.1						
Shortened 4.1 (4.1$_{PRESLES}$)	Silent carrier	Silent carrier	Apparent molecular weight of 73–74 kDa.	Preferential skipping of one exon (34 amino acids) near the beginning of the 22/24-kDa C-terminal domain.	Rare	565
C. Band 3						
Band 3 $_{MEMPHIS}$	Silent carrier	Silent carrier	Band 3 migrates slightly fast on SDS gels.	K56E	Common in blacks, Melanesians.	571,572

*The nomenclature for α spectrin defects includes an abbreviation for spectrin (Sp) followed by a superscript designation of the α-spectrin domain that is altered on tryptic peptide maps (αI to αV) and the size of the largest tryptic peptide that is generated from the mutant domain. Thus Sp α^{V65} indicates that the αI domain is affected and that a 65-kDa peptide is generated by tryptic cleavage instead of the usual 80-kDa peptide. Similarly, the superscript designating β spectrin mutations reflects the size of the abnormal peptide, which is usually a mixture of normal (220 kDa) and abnormal β spectrin. Thus, the 214-kDa Sp LePuy mutation is designated Sp $\beta^{220/214}$. Finally, note that some point mutations of β spectrin cause abnormal tryptic cleavage of the α spectrin chain and are therefore included in the Sp $\alpha^{I/74}$ group—the phenotype of their tryptic cleavage.

†Most HPP patients are compound heterozygotes for an α-spectrin mutant and a second "silent" defect, usually the common low expression α spectrin allele designated α^{LELY} or $\alpha^{V/41}$.

‡The numbering of amino acids and codons of α spectrin is based on the cDNA sequence, which includes six N-terminal amino acids that are not present in the mature protein. In the case of a α-spectrin mutations "located" refers to the repeating segment (α′, α1, α2, etc) and the α helix within the repeating segment (helix 1, 2, or 3) where the primary defect is located.

§The reported differences in molecular weight probably reflect differences in methodology rather than different mutations.

¶The superscript indicates the size (kDa) of the elongated (4.1^{95}) or truncated ($4.1^{68/65}$) protein 4.1 mutants.

skeletal stability.[105] It binds tightly ($K_d \sim 10^{-7}$ M) to spectrin at the tail end of the molecule, very near the actin binding site[101,106] (see Fig. 115-4) on the β chain,[107,108] to actin (K_d 10^{-5} to 10^{-6} M)[109] and greatly amplifies the otherwise weak spectrin–actin interaction.[100,104,105] The resulting ternary complex has an association constant of 10^{12} M^{-2}.[105] In a discontinuous SDS-PAGE system, protein 4.1 appears as a doublet, designated 4.1a and 4.1b. Protein 4.1a arises from 4.1b by deamidation of Asn502 in a time-dependent fashion,[25] resulting in the prominence of 4.1b in younger erythrocytes.[110]

Protein 4.1 also binds to one or more transmembrane proteins. It has been shown to associate with the cytoplasmic portions of both GPA[111] and GPC.[112] The interaction with GPA is regulated by polyphosphoinositides,[113] but the available evidence suggests that binding to GPC predominates in vivo.[114] The protein may also interact with band 3[40] and with phosphatidylserine.[115] Thus, protein 4.1 may provide an alternative site for attachment of the skeleton, through spectrin, to the lipid bilayer.

The protein structure was initially described as a series of proteolytic fragments (30, 15, 10, and 22/24-kDa domains).[116] The sum of these is 77/79 kDa, the apparent molecular weight of protein 4.1 on SDS gels. The actual molecular weight predicted by the cDNA sequence is considerably smaller at 66 kDa. The C-terminal end of the 30-kDa domain is believed to be the region of glycophorin binding, while the 10-kDa region contains the binding site for spectrin and actin,[117] as well as myosin.[118] The 22/24-kDa domain contains the asparagine whose deamidation is responsible for the apparent size difference between 4.1a and 4.1b.[25]

There appear to be multiple protein 4.1 isoforms in erythroid and nonerythroid cells that arise by alternative splicing of pre-mRNA (see ref. 26 for review). There are at least 10 nucleotide sequences ("motifs") that are spliced in or out to produce the various protein 4.1 isoforms. A 63-bp motif contains the region critical for spectrin–actin binding within the 10-kDa domain. A 17-bp motif at the 5′ end of the protein 4.1 gene contains an upstream initiation sequence. In most tissues it is spliced in, and a downstream 80-bp motif is spliced out. This gives rise to an elongated isoform of protein 4.1 containing an additional 209 amino acids attached to the N-terminus of the erythroid form of protein 4.1. Expression of the spectrin–actin binding motif appears to be linked to terminal erythroid differentiation.[119]

Actin-Associated Proteins: Dematin, Adducin, Tropomyosin, and Tropomodulin.

Dematin (Protein 4.9). This 48- and 52-kDa pair of proteins forms a core skeletal component along with spectrin, actin, and protein 4.1.[52] The protein must also attach to a lipid or an integral membrane protein, since it remains associated with the membrane when the other skeletal proteins are extracted; however, this site has not been identified. The native protein is a trimer and is phosphorylated by a cAMP-dependent kinase and protein kinase C.[120-122] It binds to actin and bundles actin filaments into cables.[123] This action is abolished by phosphorylation at the cAMP-dependent site.[124]

Adducin. This protein is a heterotetramer containing α (81-kDa) and β (80 kDa) subunits.[125] There are 30,000 molecules per cell or one per actin protofilament. Adducin is believed to play a role in the early assembly of the spectrin–actin network. The protein binds to actin and, like protein 4.1, increases the binding of spectrin to actin.[125] However, unlike protein 4.1, adducin does not interact directly with spectrin in the absence of actin. The adducin–spectrin–actin complex fosters binding of a second spectrin, a reaction that is blocked by calmodulin.[125] Adducin is phosphorylated by protein kinase C and protein kinase A, but the function of the phosphorylation is unknown.

Tropomyosin. Erythrocyte tropomyosin is a heterodimer of 27- and 29-kDa subunits that run on SDS gels in the region of band 7.[126] The red-cell analogue is similar to other nonmuscle tropomyosins by many criteria.[126] There is one copy for each six to eight actin monomers, which is just enough to cover all of the red-cell actin protofilaments. The length of tropomyosin and the length of the protofilaments also correspond. This suggests a model in which each protofilament bears two tropomyosin molecules, one in each of the two filament grooves. The possible functions include stabilization of the short actin filament and conferring specificity to the site of spectrin interactions along the actin protofilaments.

Tropomodulin. Tropomodulin is a 43-kDa protein that binds to tropomyosin in a 2:1 molar ratio with a K_d of 5×10^{-7} M.[127,128] In erythrocytes, there are 30,000 copies per cell, suggesting that one associates with each actin filament.

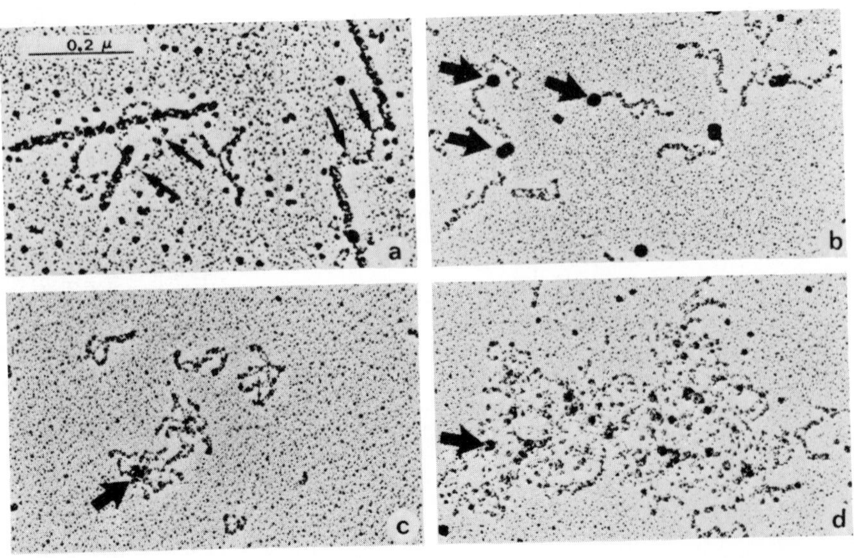

FIG. 115-4 EM of rotary-shadowed specimens of red-cell membrane skeletal proteins: *A*. Spectrin tetramers bound to actin filaments in the presence of protein 4.1. *B*. Ferritin-labeled protein 4.1 (*arrows*) bound to spectrin tetramers. *C*. Complexes of spectrin dimer, actin, and protein 4.1 formed at molar ratios close to those found in the normal red cell (arrow indicates putative actin protofilament); *D*. Complexes formed as in (*C*) except that spectrin tetramer was used instead of dimer, leading to the formation of an extended network (arrow indicates putative actin protofilament). (*Used by permission of D. Branton, Cell 24:24, 1981.*)

Evidence indicates that it associates with the pointed end of the filament and blocks growth at that end.[98] Tropomyosin amplifies this effect. Tropomodulin remains attached to the membrane when spectrin, actin, and tropomyosin are removed. Its binding site has not yet been identified.

Ankyrin (Bands 2.1, 2.2, 2.3, and 2.6). Ankyrin is a large (206 kDa), pyramidal-shaped (8.3×10 nm) protein[106] that serves as the high affinity ($K_d \sim 10^{-7}$ *M*) binding site for the attachment of spectrin to the inner membrane surface.[129-131] Ankyrin binds to spectrin at a site near the end of the molecule involved in dimer–tetramer interactions[106] (see Figs. 115-3 and 115-4). The binding site has been localized to spectrin repeat β15 by functional assay of recombinant spectrin peptides.[132] Judging from its relative abundance (see Table 115-2), each spectrin tetramer probably binds on average only one ankyrin molecule, even though two binding sites are available. Ankyrin is bound with high affinity to the cytoplasmic portion of band 3, the true anchor for the membrane skeleton.[42-44] The ankyrin molecule contains two separate binding domains that can be separated by gentle proteolysis. The spectrin binding site is contained in a 62-kDa fragment.[133-136] A complementary 89-kDa fragment binds to the cytoplasmic domain of band 3.[134,135] Ankyrin also contains a binding site for pallidin (protein 4.2)[41] that has not been localized to a specific domain. Preliminary studies of a patient whose red cells lack pallidin (see "Deficiency of Pallidin" under "Autosomal Dominant HS" below) suggest this protein may modulate ankyrin–band 3 interactions.[41]

Ankyrin is very sensitive to proteolysis and is easily pared from its native size to a number of lower-molecular-weight species. However, the lower-molecular-weight forms also arise by alternative splicing. For example, ankyrin 2.2 (band 2.2) arises by the use of an alternative acceptor site within exon 38 that results in the deletion of 163 highly acidic amino acids.[137] Thus far, at least seven alternatively spliced isoforms of ankyrin have been identified involving differences in the regulatory region.[138] Ankyrin 2.2 binds to more high-affinity band 3 sites than whole ankyrin and has a threefold higher affinity for spectrin. This suggests that the 25-kDa terminal fragment that is missing from the 2.2 isoform is a negative regulator of ankyrin's ability to bind to spectrin or band 3.[139]

There is a family of ankyrin genes (see ref. 4 for review), including the erythroid type, designated *ANK1*, which is also found in muscle, cerebellum, macrophages, and endothelial cells; a neural protein, designated *ANK2* that is localized to neuronal cell bodies and dendrites and to glial cells; and an axonal and epithelial ankyrin called *ANK3*. The latter protein is also found in muscle, megakaryocytes, melanocytes, and hepatocytes. Molecular cloning and nucleotide sequencing of the erythrocyte ankyrin cDNA revealed the presence of three domains, the 62-kDa spectrin binding domain (amino acids 828 to 1382), the 89-kDa band 3 binding domain (amino acids 2 to 827), and the 55-kDa regulatory domain (amino acids 1383 to 1881).[137,140] The 89-kDa domain contains 24 tandem subunits of 33 amino acids. This repeat structure (designated the SWI6/Ank repeat) is found in an enormous variety of proteins in all phyla, including bacteria and viruses.[4] These proteins have little in common except the ability to interact with other proteins. The SWI6/Ank repeat must have been an evolutionarily convenient solution to this recurring need. In ankyrins, the repeat region contains the binding sites for band 3,[42-44] tubulin,[141] the electrogenic and amiloride-sensitive Na^+ channels,[142-144] the cardiac Na^+/Ca^{2+} exchanger,[145] part of the binding site for the Na^+/K^+-ATPase,[146] and a group of neural adhesive proteins related to neurofascin.[147] The 62-kDa domain binds to spectrin and the intermediate filament proteins vimentin and desmin.[148,149] The 55-kDa regulatory domain contains the regions of alternative splicing that result in the formation of ankyrin 2.2 and other isoforms.

Pallidin (Protein 4.2). Pallidin (see ref. 5 for review) is a 77-kDa peripheral membrane protein present in about 500,000 molecules per cell. It can be dissociated from the membrane along with other proteins by extremely alkaline pH (≥11). Pallidin binds to band 3 (AE1) and probably to ankyrin. It certainly binds to ankyrin in solution,[150] but may not bind to ankyrin when ankyrin is attached to band 3 in vitro (i.e., the two proteins would bind to different band 3 molecules).[150] However, in *nb/nb* mice, which lack ankyrin, and in a patient with a deletion of one ankyrin gene, some reduction in pallidin is also observed.[151] This strongly suggests that the two proteins sometimes interact in vivo. Pallidin is also myristylated.[152] The function of this modification is unknown.

The pallidin cDNA has been cloned and sequenced, predicting a protein of 691 amino acids with a calculated molecular weight of 76.9 kDa.[153,154] A slightly larger cDNA (additional 30 bp at 5′ end) is believed to arise by alternative splicing. The sequence demonstrates considerable homology with the sequences of transglutaminase enzymes, although it possesses no such activity itself. The genomic DNA is 20 kb, with 13 exons and 12 introns[155] and has been localized to human chromosome 15q21.[156] In the mouse, it maps to chromosome 2 and is defective in mice with the recessive mutation designated *pallid (pa/pa)*.[157] The phenotype is characterized by hypopigmentation (abnormal melanosomes), prolonged bleeding time (abnormal platelet dense granules), and increased lysosomal enzyme content in the kidneys (defective lysosomes), which suggests a complex defect in granule/organelle formation.[157] Interestingly, *pallid* is 1 of 12 genetically independent mouse mutations that map to unique chromosomal loci but have very similar phenotypes. They resemble the two human platelet storage pool diseases, Hermansky-Pudlak syndrome and Chediak-Higashi disease. In *pallid* mice, mRNA transcripts from affected tissues, such as the skin and kidney, are smaller than normal.[157] Transcripts from erythrocytes and other unaffected tissues are normal.

Organization of the Membrane Skeleton

Complexes of F actin crosslinked by spectrin molecules are visible by high-resolution, negative-stain EM[97,158,159] (Fig. 115-5). Dematin, adducin, and protein 4.1 colocalize with these complexes on immunoelectron microscopy.[1] Most frequently, the complexes are joined by spectrin tetramers and three-legged hexamers.[159] Ankyrin and band 3–containing globular complexes are also noted. These attach to spectrin about 80 nm from its distal end or 20 nm from the site of self-association.[159] The average thickness of the skeletal protein layer has been estimated to be 3 to 6 nm from x-ray diffraction data[160] and 7 to 10 nm from EM.[161] These dimensions suggest that the skeleton is only one or two molecules thick on average, which means it must cover about 25 to 35 percent of the inner membrane surface area.

Models of spectrin and the membrane skeleton based on some of the available evidence are shown in Fig. 115-6. Spectrin dimer is depicted as a twisted, flexible polymer joined head to head to form tetramers and higher-order oligomers. The N-terminal end of the spectrin α chain

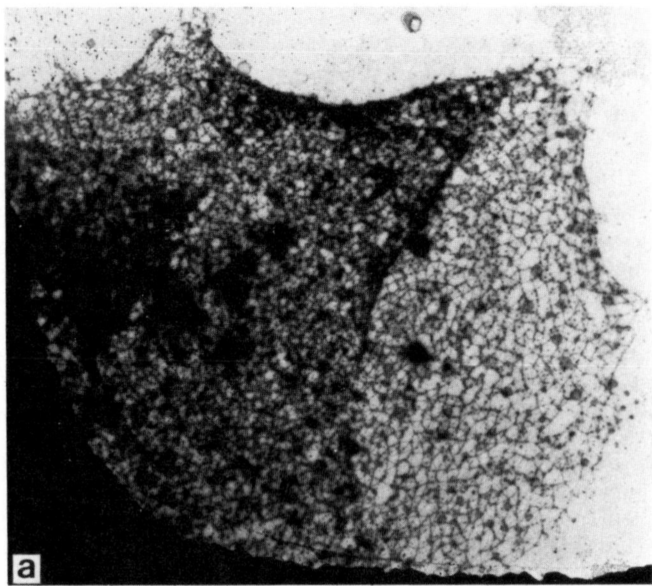

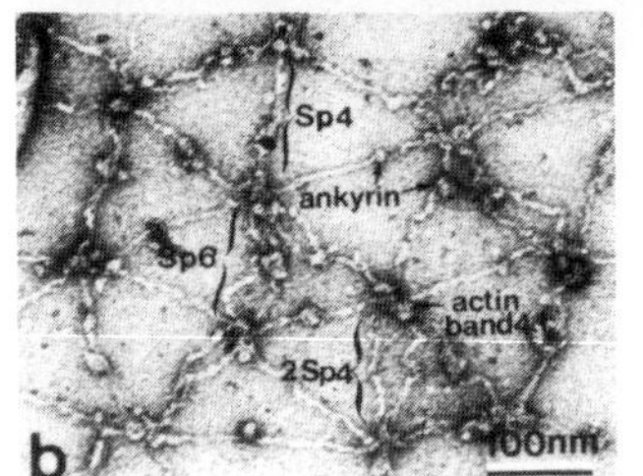

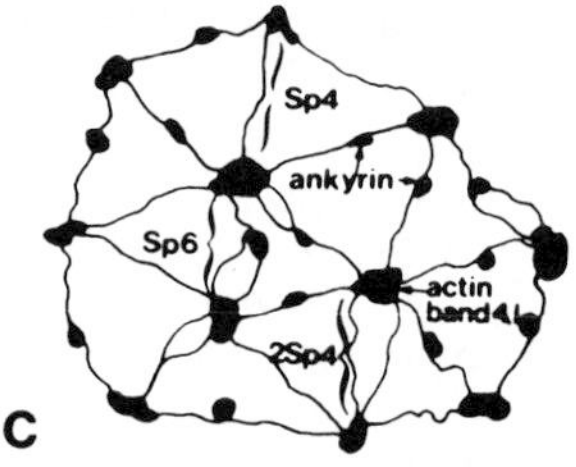

FIG. 115-5 EM of negatively stained erythrocyte membrane skeletons. *A*. Low-power view of spread skeleton. *B*. High-power view, illustrated schematically in *C*, showing a hexagonal lattice of junctional complexes, presumably composed of F-actin protofilaments and protein 4.1 molecules crosslinked by spectrin tetramers (Sp4), three-armed spectrin hexamers (Sp6), and double spectrin filaments (2Sp4). Globular structures of ankyrin or ankyrin-containing complexes are attached to the spectrin molecules at the ankyrin-binding site. *(From Liu, Derick, and Palek.[159] Used by permission of the* Journal of Cell Biology.*)*

and the C-terminal end of the spectrin β chain near the phosphorylated region comprise the self-association site, as described earlier in detail (see "Spectrin" above). Spectrin molecules are linked into a two-dimensional network by interactions with a complex of actin protofilaments, protein 4.1, dematin, adducin, and tropomyosin (see ref. 3 for review). These associations occur at the tail ends of the bifunctional spectrin tetramer. The predicted complexes are morphologically similar to isolated spectrin–actin–protein 4.1 complexes (see Fig. 115-4) and to structures observed *in situ* in normal ghosts (see Fig. 115-5). They appear to serve as a molecular junction or branch point in skeletal construction. Individual spectrin tetramers and oligomers are attached to the overlying lipid bilayer through high affinity interactions with ankyrin and band 3. Current evidence suggests that band 3 is a mixture of dimers and tetramers in the membrane and that the tetramer probably binds only one molecule of anykrin.[44] If so, about 40 percent of the band 3 molecules are involved in anchoring the membrane skeleton. Although the spectrin tetramer contains two ankyrin binding sites, on average only one site can be filled. Interactions between protein 4.1 and either glycophorin C or band 3 provide secondary sites of attachment. In addition, most spectrin molecules probably fold up to about one-third their length and do not extensively overlap or intertwine.[158,159]

Modulation of Membrane Skeletal Structure

Polyanions. Physiological concentrations of organic polyanions such as 2,3-diphosphoglycerate (2,3-DPG) and ATP weaken and dissociate the membrane skeleton[162,163] and increase the lateral mobility of band 3 in ghosts.[164] At the molecular level these compounds dramatically inhibit spectrin–actin interactions, even in the presence of protein 4.1.[165] Whether these or other polyanions (e.g., polyphosphorylated phosphoinositides) are "physiological" mediators in vivo is unknown, as one recent study suggests that even supraphysiological concentrations of 2,3-DPG have little or no effect on *intact* erythrocytes.[166]

Phosphorylation. Almost all of the membrane skeletal proteins are phosphorylated by one or more protein kinases. These include cAMP-independent kinases (spectrin, band 3)[167,168]; cAMP-dependent kinases (ankyrin, protein 4.1, and dematin)[169-171]; tyrosine kinase (band 3)[120-122,172]; and protein kinase C (protein 4.1 and dematin).[120-122] Ankryin phosphorylation abolishes the preference of ankyrin for spectrin tetramer.[173] Phosphorylation of protein 4.1 also diminishes its binding to spectrin[174] and phosphorylation of the distal tyrosine at the N-terminus of band 3 blocks the binding

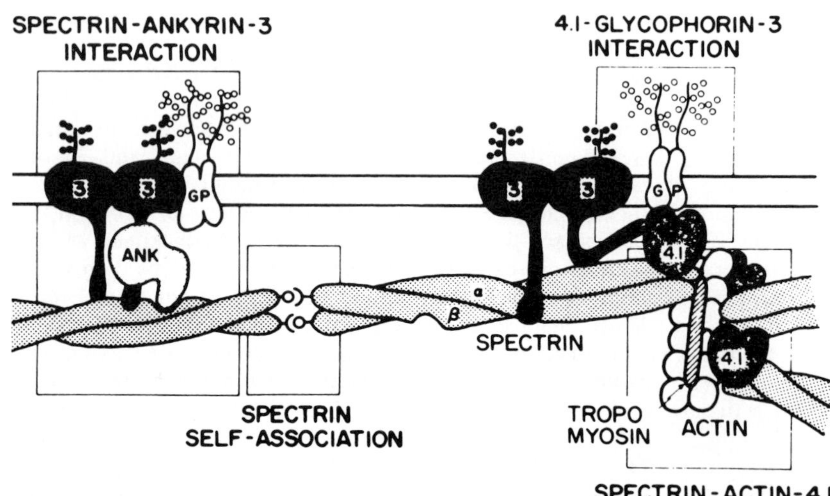

FIG. 115-6 Model (not to scale) of red-cell membrane organization. Ank = ankyrin; GP = glycophorin A and/or C.

of glycolytic enzymes[175] and, presumably, hemoglobin. In contrast, despite extensive study,[176,177] no functional effect of spectrin phosphorylation has yet been identified.

Calmodulin. Calmodulin binds to the spectrin β chain in a Ca^{2+}-dependent manner and inhibits the protein 4.1 stimulated binding of spectrin to actin.[178] However, the affinity of spectrin for calmodulin is not great and it is unclear whether this effect occurs at the concentrations of calmodulin that exist in erythrocytes.

Functions of the Membrane Skeleton

Membrane Flexibility and Durability. Biochemical analyses of the red-cell membrane suggest that its structural properties are determined almost entirely by the membrane skeleton. The best evidence for this hypothesis comes from studies of four mouse mutants with very severe, inherited hemolytic anemias.[90,179,180] The red cells of these mice are spherocytic and fragile and spontaneously vesiculate in the circulation (Fig. 115-7). All the mutants lack spectrin, and the degree of spectrin deficiency correlates with the apparent clinical severity.[180] Red cells from the more deficient mutants lack elasticity, show marked plastic deformation, and mechanically resemble lipid bilayers. Reconstitution of mutant ghosts with normal spectrin restores membrane stability.[181] Numerous other observations attest to the structural importance of the skeleton. In intact red cells, denaturation of spectrin by exposure to heat[182-184] or low pH[183,185,186] destabilizes and rigidifies the membrane and promotes membrane fragmentation and spherocytosis. In isolated membranes vesiculation occurs when spectrin is extracted at low ionic strength[187] or even when spectrin–actin bonds are weakened by 2,3-DPG.[162] Similarly, isolated skeletons become mechanically fragile when spectrin tetramers are converted to dimers by in vitro manipulations of temperature and ionic strength.[188] In contrast, crosslinking of membrane skeletal proteins by a variety of mechanisms increases membrane rigidity.[189-191]

Red-Cell Shape. In general, isolated membrane skeletons retain the shape of the ghosts from which they are derived.[192,193] This and other observations[194,195] confirm the shape-maintaining role of the skeleton. Biomechanical analyses and modeling studies[196] suggest that a membrane formed by a phospholipid bilayer bonded to a membrane skeletal network will assume a biconcave shape spontaneously to minimize mechanical strain. Normally, the red cell rapidly regains this shape if it is temporarily deformed, but if the distortion is maintained for some time, the cell will remain misshaped. This phenomenon, known as "plastic deformation," is probably due to realignment of dynamic skeletal interactions in response to the stress of distortion.[197,198] Diminished skeletal interactions would presumably accelerate this process and foster poikilocytosis. More severe skeletal weakness would permit membrane budding and fragmentation and, in the most extreme cases, lead to the spherical shape characteristic of isolated phospholipid vesicles and spectrin-deficient mouse red cells.[180]

Integral Protein Distribution and Mobility. Perturbations that cause spectrin molecules to precipitate or aggregate on the inner membrane surface immobilize integral proteins in clusters directly over the spectrin aggregates.[199,200] Conversely, congenital absence of spectrin in mice, partial displacement of spectrin from the membrane by a proteolytic fragment of ankyrin, or weakening of spectrin–actin interactions with 2,3-DPG, enhances the lateral diffusion of integral proteins in the bilayer plane.[164,201,202] These experiments clearly show that the membrane skeleton normally restricts the mobility of some integral membrane proteins. The mechanism of this restriction is uncertain. Presumably it is at least partially due to the association between band 3 and the spectrin–ankyrin complex, but because only 30 to 40 percent of the band 3 molecules participate in this interaction,[44] other constituents are probably also involved. Perhaps the cytoplasmic domains of many integral proteins are simply trapped in the skeletal meshwork. Alternatively, poorly described interactions between the skeleton and membrane lipids or between the skeleton and other integral proteins such as the glycophorins may be important. There is some evidence that the distribution of integral membrane proteins influences the interaction of red cells with other cells they encounter in the circulation. The only well-studied example is the abnormal adherence of sickle cells to cultured human umbilical vein endothelial cells.[203,204] This appears to be related to surface charge topography, since it is normalized by desialylation and since negative charges on the sickle-cell surface (presumably sialic acids on glycophorin molecules) are abnormally clustered.[203] It is not known whether the charge clustering in this cell is exacerbated by defects in the membrane skeleton,[205-207] although this is a reasonable possibility.

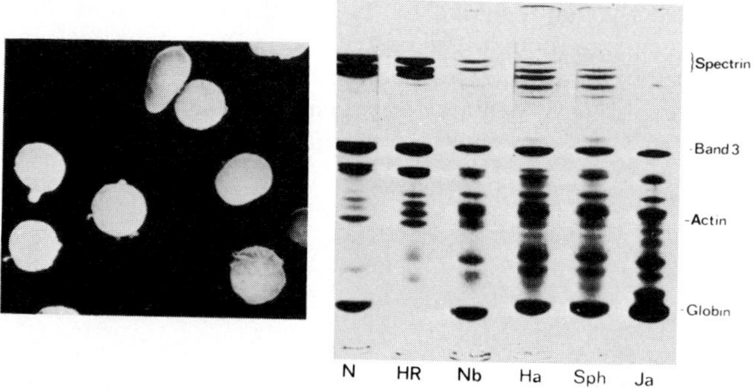

FIG. 115-7 Spectrin-deficient mouse mutants. (*Left*) Scanning EM of red cell from a mouse with the *sph/sph* mutation. Note the intense spherocytosis and membrane budding. Often budding is even more intense, with long strands of linked vesicles dangling from the surface. (*Right*) SDS gels of red-cell membranes from normal (N) and high reticulocyte control (HR) mice, and from mice with the "normoblastosis," *nb/nb* (Nb); "hemolytic anemia," *sph*^{ha}/*sph*^{ha} (Ha); "spherocytosis," *sph/sph* (Sph); and "jaundiced," *ja/ja* (Ja) mutations. (*From Lux.*[180] *Used by permission of* Seminars in Hematology.)

Membrane Endocytosis and Fusion.

In addition to its probable importance in cell–cell interactions, skeletal control of integral protein topography appears to help regulate membrane endocytosis and fusion. Studies have shown that endocytic vacuoles in red cells and ghosts are spectrin-depleted and arise from spectrin-free areas of the membrane, produced by rearrangement of the membrane skeleton.[208,209] Pretreatment of ghosts with alkaline phosphatase blocks endocytosis and spectrin rearrangement, suggesting that phosphorylation of some membrane component is required.[208] The identity of this component has not been established. It appears that a similar process occurs during membrane fusion. Early in the fusion process integral membrane proteins cluster to produce areas of protein-free lipid bilayer.[210] Apparently, fusion results when such bare areas contact each other if the lipids are in the proper configuration.[210] It is known that spectrin is involved in this process.[181,211-213] Antispectrin antibodies inhibit the fusion of red-cell membranes induced by Sendai virus,[211] and crude spectrin extracts prevent Ca^{2+}-induced fusion of phosphatidylserine vesicles.[213] In addition, spectrin-deficient mouse red cells readily fuse with one another in the absence of any inducing agent,[181] a defect that is corrected by reconstituting the cells with normal mouse spectrin.[211] Thus, by immobilizing integral proteins in a diffuse distribution, the membrane skeleton protects the red cell from fusing with the many other cells it encounters in the circulation.

HEREDITARY SPHEROCYTOSIS

Hereditary spherocytosis (HS), is an important, dominantly inherited hemolytic anemia in which defects in spectrin or the proteins that attach spectrin to the membrane (ankyrin, pallidin, band 3) lead to spheroidal, osmotically fragile, often spectrin-deficient cells that are selectively trapped in the spleen and that survive almost normally after splenectomy.

History

HS was first described more than 120 years ago by the Belgian physicians Vanlair and Masius.[214] They reported on a young woman in whom recurrent abdominal pain developed over her enlarged spleen, with associated prostration, vomiting, jaundice, anemia, aphonia, and marked muscular weakness. At the time of this attack (presumably a hemolytic crisis), the authors noted that the majority of the red cells were spherical and much smaller than normal (4 μm diameter). They termed these cells "microcytes" and named the disease "microcythemia." The unstained cells were illustrated in a lithograph drawn and tinted by Vanlair (Fig. 115-8). The drawing clearly shows spherocytosis, although the relatively large number of elliptocytes (19 percent of the evaluable cells) raises the question whether the true diagnosis may not have been spherocytic elliptocytosis. Later, when the patient had improved, her red cells were somewhat larger, but still abnormal, and her spleen remained enlarged. Vanlair and Masius thought the microcytes were senile normal cells ("globules atrophiques") and that the spleen assisted in their aging. They argued that when red cells are sequestered in the pulp of the spleen, they are removed from the active circulation, lose volume, and become dense, spherical, and microcytic. They believed an enlarged spleen produces even more of such cells than a normal spleen and that the liver completes the work of the spleen by destroying the microcytes it receives via the splenic vein. They suggested that the large number of microcytes in their patient was due in part to splenomegaly and in part to atrophy of the liver. Finally, they noted that the patient's older sister had suffered from an identical illness and had died during an apparent crisis. The mother was also subject to jaundice. This remarkable paper must rank among the most prescient in hematology. Not only did the authors describe the first example of hereditary hemolytic anemias well before the microscope was in general use in the analysis of blood diseases, but their deductions concerning the pathophysiology, particularly the role of the spleen, predated Ham and Castle's concept of erythrostasis[215] by more than two-thirds of a century. Their analysis is placed in better perspective when one realizes that 40 to 65 years later HS was ascribed to causes as diverse as hereditary syphilis[216] and splenic hemolysins.[217] Unfortunately, Vanlair and Masius' report and subsequent descriptions of HS by Wilson and Stanley in the 1890s[218,219] went largely unnoticed. The latter authors clearly recognized the hereditary nature of the disease and were the first to describe the pathology of the spleen, which at autopsy was grossly firm and dark and microscopically engorged with red cells. A report by Minkowski in 1900[220] received wide attention, and many additional papers soon appeared,[221,222] including Chauffard's historic definition of osmotic fragility[223] and reticulocytosis[224] as hallmarks of the disease. At about the same time, Widal et al.[225] differentiated an acquired form of "congenital hemolytic jaundice" (now recognizable as Coombs' test-positive immunohemolytic anemia). Because Hayem had previously reported similar cases,[226] the acquired form of the disease soon became the Hayem-Widal type, while the congenital form was given the eponym Minkowski-Chauffard. The use of splenectomy was soon advocated, and in 1911 Micheli[227] removed the spleen from a patient with acquired hemolytic jaundice. The fortunately brilliant result, combined with the subsequent success of splenectomy in the congenital disease,[198,228] soon led to widespread acceptance of the procedure. Actually, the first successful splenectomy for HS was unintentionally performed by Spencer Wells in England in 1887 (three years before Wilson's description of the disease in that country).[229] Operating on a jaundiced woman for a supposed uterine fibroid, he instead encountered and removed an enormous spleen. The patient recovered and the jaundice disappeared. Forty years later Dawson restudied the woman and her son and found the characteristic osmotic fragility.[229] Thus, by the time of Tileston's[230] and Gänsslen's[231] reviews in 1922, almost all the major clinical features of HS were documented, the spleen was thought to be involved in the hemolysis, and splenectomy was known to be curative. Nevertheless, with the exception of Vanlair and Masius' farsighted (and still unrecognized) premonitions, nothing substantive was known

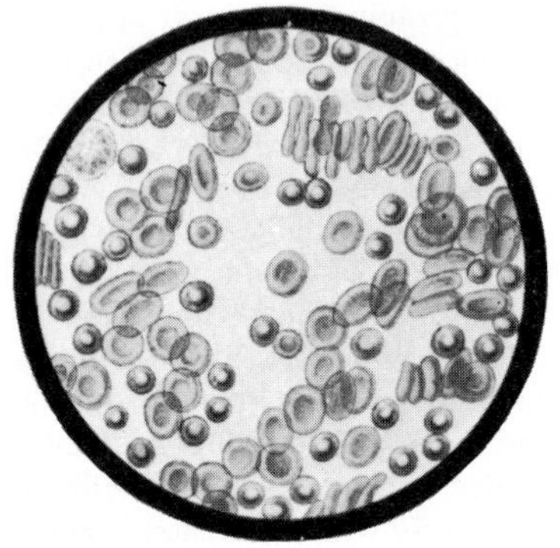

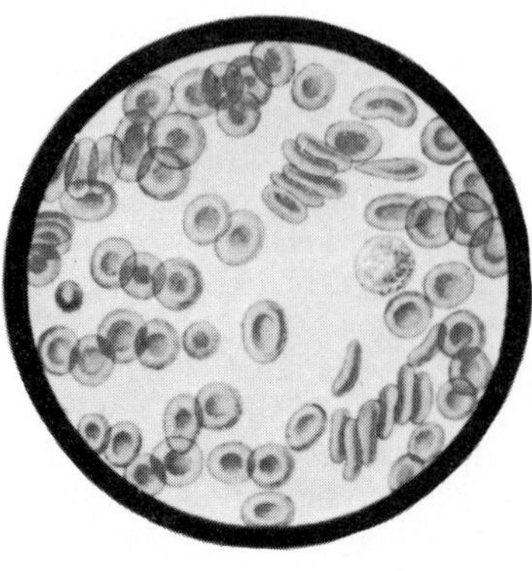

FIG. 115-8 Lithograph of normal red cells (*right*) and cells from a patient (*left*) with "microcythemia" described by Vanlair and Masius in 1871.[214]

about the basic mechanism of the disorder or its pathogenesis. These aspects of the disease will be discussed in the sections that follow. Readers interested in more details of the history of HS should consult the superb chapters by Dacie, Wintrobe, and Crosby in *Blood, Pure and Eloquent,* an account of the history of hematology, edited by Wintrobe.[232]

Prevalence and Genetics

HS is the most common hemolytic anemia in people of Northern European extraction. In this population the prevalence is roughly 1 in 5000,[233] and there is evidence, based on data obtained with sensitive osmotic fragility methods, that very mild forms of the disease may be four or five times more common.[234] The disease occurs, but is less frequent, in other races and ethnic groups. Studies have indicated that there are at least two hereditary forms of HS. Approximately 75 percent of families show the classic autosomal dominant pattern.[233,235] No definite homozygotes for this form of HS have ever been identified, which suggests that homozygosity for the typical dominant disease may be incompatible with life. A family reported by Race[235] supports this supposition. He described a mating between first cousins in which both parents and three children were affected, one child was normal, and two miscarriages had occurred. A French family with 13 successive affected children[236] is sometimes said to be an example of homozygosity, but the mother was normal and the father was not clinically worse than his offspring (as his productivity attests).

Some of the remaining 25 percent are probably examples of an autosomal recessive form of the disease.[237] Others may be examples of dominant HS with reduced penetrance or may be new mutations. It will not be possible to definitively distinguish between these alternatives until specific molecular or genetic markers are identified that can detect heterozygotes.

Etiology

Cross-transfusion experiments clearly show that hereditary spherocytes are intrinsically defective.[238-240] Several precise molecular defects of specific red-cell proteins have been defined. The majority of abnormalities formerly described in HS red cells are believed to be secondary and do not present primary hereditary defects. These include metabolic derangements, alterations in cation transport, abnormal membrane protein phosphorylation, and altered membrane lipid composition. These abnormalities are listed in Table 95-5 of the sixth edition of this book.[241] The discussion here will focus on the membrane skeletal protein defects, since these are likely to be responsible for the disease.

Loss of Membrane Surface. The membrane lesion is expressed as a loss of surface area, but whether this is due to an actual physical loss (i.e., fragmentation) or to contraction of the membrane surface is not completely clear. Most of the evidence favors fragmentation. Careful biomechanical measurements show that the force required to fragment HS membranes is diminished and proportional to the density of spectrin on the membrane.[242,243] Membrane elasticity and bending stiffness are also reduced and proportional to spectrin density.[244,245] In addition, HS red cells lose membrane much more readily than normal when metabolically deprived.[246,247] This has not been shown to occur in metabolically maintained spherocytes, but the surface loss probably occurs slowly under these conditions (~1 to 2 percent per day), and none of the reported studies have been conducted for long periods. The phospholipid and cholesterol contents of isolated spherocytes are decreased by 15 to 20 percent, consistent with the loss of surface area.[246,248-250] Presumably, integral membrane proteins are also lost, but no quantitative measurements have been made. Since budding red cells are only rarely observed in HS blood smears, membrane loss either occurs fairly rapidly (ie., in seconds to minutes) or occurs in bywaters of the circulation such as the reticuloendothelial system. The major evidence that surface loss involves more than simple fragmentation is that the surface deficit exceeds the measured lipid loss. After splenectomy HS red cells are deficient in lipid as compared with splenectomized controls, but their lipid content is similar to that of normal cells from unsplenectomized individuals, despite the fact that they are more spherical and more osmotically fragile.[248] The explanation of this discrepancy is unknown. It is possible that red-cell lipids are more tightly packed in hereditary spherocytes or that the surface is contracted in some other way, but it is not easy to understand how this could occur. Alternatively, integral proteins may be disproportionately lost during fragmentation, or HS red cells may undergo internal as well as external fragmentation. The latter process would decrease surface area without causing a measurable loss of membrane lipid. Thin-section EM do not show cytoplasmic vesicles in hereditary spherocytes,[251] but a careful search has not been reported.

Mouse Mutants with Hereditary Spherocytic Anemia. The structural instability of HS membranes suggests a defect in the membrane skeleton. As noted earlier (see "Functions of the Membrane Skeleton" above), this structure is the major determinant of membrane strength and durability and is defective in certain mutants of the common house mouse, *Mus musculus.* Six types of hereditary hemolytic anemia have been identified. These anemias resemble human hereditary spherocytosis and may share similar genetic defects. They are designated *ja/ja* (jaundice), *sph/sph* (spherocytosis), sph^{ha}/sph^{ha} (hemolytic anemia), sph^{2BC}/sph^{2BC}, sph^{2J}/sph^{2J}, and *nb/nb* (normoblastosis).[252] The nomenclature indicates that anemia is observed only in the homozygous state and that the six mutants represent three loci: *ja, sph,* and *nb.* All of the mutants have severe hemolysis, with reticulocyte counts approaching 100 percent, along with marked spherocytosis, jaundice, bilirubin gallstones, and massive hepatosplenomegaly. The defects are autosomal recessive, and the homozygotes have drastically impaired viability. There is a similar but much milder condition in the deer mouse, *Peromyscus maniculatus,* designated *sp/sp.*[253] Studies of these mouse mutants have revealed various skeletal abnormalities (see Fig. 115-7). The *ja/ja* mutant has no detectable spectrin. The *sph/sph* variants lack spectrin α chains but have small amounts of β spectrin; the *nb/nb* mutant has 50 to 70 percent of the normal quantity of spectrin and no ankyrin.[180] Bone marrow transplantation transfers the phenotypes, confirming their erythroid origin.[252] Studies of spectrin synthesis[253,254] in these mice suggest that *ja* mutants lack the ability to synthesize β chains or synthesize very unstable β chains, and the various *sph* mutants have defects in α spectrin synthesis and/or stability. The *ja* mutation and the mouse β spectrin gene have both been mapped to chromosome 12, and the *sph* mutation and the α spectrin gene have been mapped to chromosome 1[254]—data consistent with these conclusions. The *nb* mutants have normal spectrin synthesis.[253,254] They lack spectrin because their ankyrin is very unstable.[255,256] The *nb* mutation maps to the *Ank-1* locus on mouse chromosome 8[256] and the Ank-1 protein (206 kDa) is markedly reduced in red cells and cerebellar Purkinje cells. Loss of a subset of Purkinje cells in the first 6 months after birth leads to ataxia.[257] Interestingly, fetal *nb/nb* mice have normal reticulocyte counts[258] and no anemia at birth, apparently due to expression of *Ank-1*-related (165 kDa) and *Ank-2*-related (155 kDa) proteins in utero.[259]

Recessively Inherited Spherocytosis in Humans. This disorder was originally described in sibs whose parents were fourth cousins.[237] The clinical condition was characterized by life-threatening anemia, frequent jaundice, and massive splenomegaly. Unlike typical dominant HS, hemolysis improved but was not eliminated by splenectomy. The red cells were microcytic with some acanthocytes and bizarre forms in addition to spherocytes. The red-cell membranes had only 40 to 50 percent of the normal amount of spectrin, as compared to band 3, on SDS gels, and only 26 to 29 percent by radioimmunoassay.[237] The spectrin functioned normally in its ability to self-associate and bind to inside-out vesicles. This severe form of recessive HS is fortunately quite rare; however, less severe variants are common and may affect up to 25 percent of all HS patients.[260] The mechanism of spectrin deficiency in these patients is unknown. The most straightforward explanations are reduced spectrin synthesis, synthesis of an unstable spectrin, or impaired binding of spectrin to the membrane. As noted earlier, in chickens,[89] mice,[90] and humans,[91] α spectrin synthesis exceeds β by a factor of 2 to 3. Thus, heterozygotes for defects in α spectrin synthesis would still make enough normal α spectrin to pair with all or nearly all the β chains produced, so spectrin deficiency would only be evident in the homozygous state. This is exactly what is observed in patients with recessive HS.[237,260] In many, but not all, families with the severe form of recessive HS, a variant α spectrin peptide, designated αIIa, has been identified.[7,261] It bears an amino acid substitution, alanine to asparagine, at position 309 (A309N).[7] Whether this is the cause of the spectrin deficiency or is simply a linked polymorphism is unclear. In addition, one case of hydrops fetalis due to severe HS treated with in utero transfusion has been reported in which there was nearly complete absence of α spectrin synthesis,[262] and molecular studies are now in progress to determine the mechanism.

Autosomal Dominant HS. It is now clear that erythrocyte membranes from almost all HS patients are spectrin-deficient, including both the dominant and recessive forms of the disease, and that the degree of spectrin deficiency correlates closely with the severity of the disease and with the degree of spherocytosis, as measured by the median osmotic fragility of the red cells.[260,263] Moreover, the degree of spectrin deficiency predicts the patient's status postsplenectomy, as judged by reticulocyte count, haptoglobin level, and hematocrit[260] (Fig. 115-9). In general, the dominant forms of HS are milder than the recessive variant(s), although significant overlap is observed.[260] The effect of spectrin deficiency on the hemolytic anemia may be partly explained by the finding that the membrane elastic shear modulus and bending stiffness are directly proportional to the surface density of spectrin.[245] These mechanical membrane properties may relate to the ability of the spectrin-deficient HS red cells to withstand circulatory stresses. Expanding on the reasoning in the previous section, spectrin deficiency in dominant HS might be due to diminished synthesis (or instability) of the relatively scarce spectrin β chains or to a lack of ankyrin molecules, which bind the β chains. Either of these defects should limit the formation of stable, membrane-associated heterodimers and be expressed as a dominant trait. In theory, band 3 might also be a culprit, since ankyrin and spectrin do not bind to the membrane until band 3 is expressed,[264] and there is good evidence that only a fraction of the band 3 molecules are available to bind ankyrin.[44] In fact, defects in all of these proteins, as well as pallidin have been found in hereditary spherocytosis.

***Combined Spectrin–Ankyrin Deficiency*.** The initial clue that an ankyrin defect was related to HS was that two groups had identified families[265,266] with translocations involving chromosome 8 and coexisting HS, suggesting that some protein encoded by chromosome 8 could be responsible. It was later found that the ankyrin gene was on chromosome 8. In addition, Chilcote and his colleagues[267] identified two sisters with moderate to severe splenectomy-responsive anemia, spherocytosis, dysmorphic features, micrognathia, nystagmus, psychomotor retardation, and deletion of a portion of the short arm of chromosome 8 (8p11.1-p21.2). These individuals and another unrelated patient with a similar

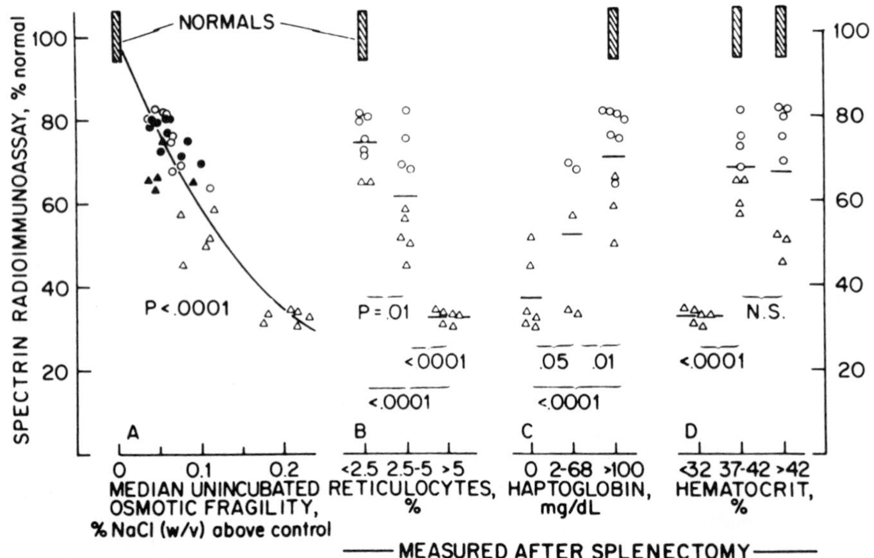

FIG. 115-9 Correlation of red-cell spectrin content with osmotic fragility and measures of hemolysis after splenectomy. The hatched rectangles indicate the normal range for each index. Patients with the nondominant (i.e., probably recessive) form of HS are indicated by triangles, those with the dominant form by circles, and those who have previously undergone splenectomy by open circles or triangles. *(From Agre, Asimos, Casello, and McMillan.[260] Used by permission of the* New England Journal of Medicine.*)*

condition were found to lack the gene encoding ankyrin on chromosome 8.[151] Finally, in one large kindred with typical autosomal dominant HS and no chromosome deletion, linkage could be demonstrated to the ankyrin gene by RFLP analysis, while linkage to the α spectrin, β spectrin, or protein 4.1 genes was excluded.[268] The hypothesis that defective or deficient ankyrin could result in spectrin deficiency was verified by the finding of concomitant spectrin and ankyrin deficiency in 19 of 20 kindreds with HS,[22] with good correlation between the degrees of deficiency of the two proteins. Five distinct molecular defects of ankyrin have been identified in such patients (Table 115-3).

Another kindred with dominant HS was found to have a truncated ankyrin protein (ankyrin$_{PRAGUE}$) due to an incompletely defined abnormality in the regulatory domain.[269]

Coetzer and her colleagues[270] have described two patients with a new, apparently dominantly inherited disease characterized by transfusion-dependent hemolytic anemia, marked spherocytosis, bizarre poikilocytosis, and only a partial response to splenectomy. Red-cell membranes are deficient in both spectrin and ankyrin (about 50 to 60 percent of normal levels). The disease appears to be due to an inability to synthesize ankyrin adequately or to synthesis of an unstable molecule[271] rather than due to a defect in the ankyrin binding capacity of protein 3.[270]

Defective Spectrin–Protein 4.1 Binding. A subset of families with autosomal dominant HS have spectrin that is defective in its capacity to bind protein 4.1. This defect has been observed by two groups in a total of three kindreds.[272-274] The other binding functions of spectrin, such as ankyrin binding and self-association, are preserved.[272-274] Heterozygous individuals have two types of spectrin. The abnormal fraction, approximately 40 percent, lacks the ability to bind protein 4.1 and therefore attaches only weakly to actin.[273,274] Enzymatic digestions with trypsin[272] or chymotrypsin[274] reveal defects toward the tail of the spectrin β chain, near the site where protein 4.1 binds.[101,107,108] The mutant spectrin is unstable and susceptible to thiol oxidation.[274] This oxidation causes or exacerbates the defect in binding to protein 4.1, since chemical reduction almost completely restores normal binding activity.[274] Interestingly, very mild oxidation of normal spectrin[275] or storage of normal cells under aerobic conditions in the blood bank[276] produces similar defects in spectrin–protein 4.1 interactions. Patients with the spectrin–protein 4.1 binding defect are also spectrin-deficient, with spectrin content being only 80 percent of normal.[274] Presumably, the defective spectrin detaches from the membrane more easily than normal and falls prey to proteases that specifically degrade unbound spectrin chains.[69] Loss of the abnormal spectrin explains why the ratio of normal to abnormal spectrin is 60:40 instead of the expected 50:50. A point mutation was identified in β spectrin with a Trp (TGG) to Arg (CGG) mutation at position 202(W202R), in the three affected members of one of these kindreds (Sp$_{KISSIMMEE}$),[277] but not in the other two described kindreds with a similar functional defect. The mutation inserts a positively charged amino acid adjacent to a positive–negative charged pair in a region of largely hydrophobic amino acid sequence, and could thus disrupt a region that is critical for protein 4.1 binding. This sequence is highly conserved among members of the spectrin gene superfamily. The fraction of HS patients with the spectrin–protein 4.1 defect is probably quite small. Clinically, these patients have typical dominant HS with symptoms proportional to the degree of spectrin deficiency. In the family with Sp$_{KISSIMMEE}$, acanthocytes (5 to 15 percent) were present on the peripheral smear in addition to spherocytes,[273] but it is not clear whether this is characteristic of the spectrin–protein 4.1 binding defect.

Deficiency of Pallidin (Protein 4.2). Several patients of Japanese descent, one Portuguese patient, and one Tunisian patient have been described with an apparently recessive disease characterized by moderately severe, splenectomy-responsive hemolytic anemia and complete or nearly complete absence (~99 percent) of pallidin.[41,278,279] The red-cell morphology is different than classic HS[41,278] and varies from normal (in the Tunisian case) to spherocytes, elliptocytes, or ovalostomatocytes.[41,278] In the first Japanese patients,[41] the red cells contained only a trace quantity of a 74/72-kDa pallidin doublet instead of the usual abundant 72-kDa species, because of an Ala142 to Thr mutation (A142T)[280] that affects the processing of pallidin mRNA. Subsequent Japanese patients have the same mutation, which is designated pallidin$_{NIPPON}$. The Portuguese variant (pallidin$_{LISBOA}$) is caused by a single base deletion in codon 88 or 89. No detectable pallidin is synthesized.[281] The Tunisian variant (pallidin$_{TOZEUR}$) is caused by a substitution of Gln for Arg at position 310 (R310Q) and is stable enough to accumulate to low levels in red cells.[282] Finally, red-cell pallidin deficiency has also been associated with mutations in the cytoplasmic domain of band 3 in two patients. One of the mutations lies near the N-terminus of the cytoplasmic domain, Glu40 to Lys (E40K), designated band 3$_{MONTEFIORE}$[283]; the other is near the C-terminal end of the domain, Pro327 to Arg (P327R), designated band 3$_{TUSCALOOSA}$.[284] Presumably, these amino acids form part of the pallidin binding site.

Band 3 Deficiency. Initial estimates suggest that 10 to 15 percent of dominant HS patients have a primary deficiency of band 3. Their red cells contain 20 to 40 percent less band 3 than normal.[285-287] Affected patients have typical HS with mild to moderate hemolysis, except for morphology. In many, but not all cases, a small proportion of "mushroom-shaped" cells are present in addition to the usual spherocytes. The genesis of these unique cells is unknown. Where quantitated, red-cell spectrin is normal in this form of HS. Synthesis of band 3 is also normal,[288] but the molecule is progressively lost as the cells circulate—particularly the "mobile" fraction.[289] This fraction represents band 3 that is not bound to the skeleton, which suggests that the primary defect may affect self-association of band 3 rather than its interactions with various skeletal proteins. In one family, a 10-bp segment of the band 3 gene is duplicated near the C-terminal end of the protein, leading to a shift in the reading frame and an altered C-terminus after amino acid 821 (band 3$_{PRAGUE}$).[290] This mutation affects the last transmembrane helix, and probably alters insertion of band 3 into the membrane and abolishes the transport function.

Inextractable Spectrin. A decreased ability to extract spectrin from the membranes of patients with dominant HS has been observed in a small number of Australian HS patients.[291-293] Inexplicably, the extracted spectrin also resisted reassociation with spectrin-depleted membranes.[292,293] The molecular investigations needed to explain these curious and apparently contradictory findings have not yet been done.

Enolase Deficiency. HS combined with partial enolase deficiency (~50 percent) in four generations of a Caucasian family has been reported.[294] The authors note that the spherocytic red cells resisted lysis in the acidified glycerol lysis test (a characteristic of typical HS) and suggest this indicates that enolase-deficient HS is unique. However, in a previously reported family with enolase deficiency (6 percent of normal) no hemolysis or spherocytosis was evident except during a hemolytic crisis.[295]

Pathophysiology

The major problems of the hereditary spherocyte are the rheologic consequences of its decreased surface:volume ratio. The red-cell membrane is very flexible, but it can expand its surface area only about 3 percent before rupturing.[296] Consequently, as the red cell becomes more and more spherical, it becomes less and less deformable.[297] In the case of HS red cells, this poor deformability is a hindrance only in the spleen, since most hereditary spherocytes survive well after splenectomy.[298,299]

The Spleen. In the spleen most of the arterial blood empties directly into the cords: a narrow, honeycombed maze of passages formed by reticular cells and phagocytes.[300-302] Histologically, this is an "open" circulation, but apparently most of the blood that enters the cords travels in fairly direct (i.e., functionally "closed") pathways.[302,303] If flow through these passages is impeded, red cells are diverted deeper into the labyrinthine portions of the cords, where blood flow is slow and the cells may be detained for minutes to hours. To exit and return to the venous circulation, red cells must squeeze between the endothelial cells that form the walls of the venous sinusoids. Even when maximally distended, these narrow, elliptical fenestrations are much smaller than red cells (Fig. 115-10),[303a] which must undergo considerable contortion during their passage.[301,302,304] It is clear that spherocytic red cells are significantly hindered at this point in the circulation. Isolated hereditary spherocytes are poorly deformable and pass through 3- to 5-μm filters with difficulty,[297,305,306] sometimes bursting in the process.[305] HS red cells are trapped in the cords during in vitro perfusion through spleens removed from patients with idiopathic thrombocytopenic purpura,[307] and ^{51}Cr-labeled spherocytes are selectively sequestered in the spleen in vivo.[308-311] As a consequence, HS spleens characteristically show massively congested cords and relatively empty venous sinuses on light microscopy,[300,312,313] and EM shows relatively few spherocytes traversing the sinus wall,[300,313,314] in contrast to normal spleens, where such cells are easily found.[301] It is also clear that spherocytes are damaged by their detention in the cords. In unsplenectomized HS patients, two populations of spherocytes are detectable—a minor population of hyperchromic "microspherocytes" that form a "tail" of very fragile cells on unincubated osmotic fragility tests and a major population of cells that may be only slightly more spheroidal than normal. Although it was known as early as 1913 that red cells obtained from the splenic vein were more osmotically fragile than those in the peripheral circulation,[315] the significance of this observation was not fully appreciated until the classic studies of Emerson[238] and Young[307] and their colleagues, published in the early 1950s. These investigators clearly showed that osmotically fragile microspherocytes are concentrated in and apparently emanate from the splenic pulp. After splenectomy the tail of hyperfragile cells is no longer evident, although the major population of moderately fragile spherocytes persists.[238,307,316] These and other data led to the conclusion that the spleen detains and conditions circulating HS red cells in a way that increases their spheroidicity and hastens their demise.[238,307] The kinetics of this

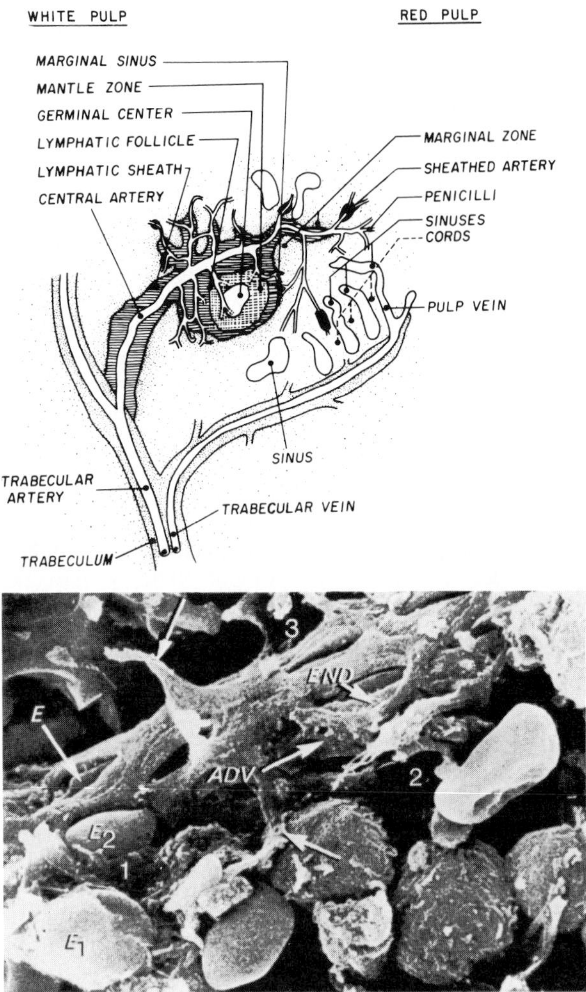

FIG. 115-10 *(Top)* **Schematic illustration of the anatomy of the spleen. Note that blood entering the splenic cords must pass through the walls of the splenic sinuses to reenter the venous circulation.** *(Bottom)* **Scanning EM of a splenic sinus wall viewed from a splenic cord. A portion of the overlying cordal structure has been removed. The narrow transmural slits between the endothelial (END) and adventitial (ADV) cells of the sinus wall are easily seen. It is likely that these cells are normally apposed and that the slits are "potential" structures rather than fixed pores.[300] They are evident here because of a drying artifact. Note that the adjacent erythrocytes (E_1 and E_2) are considerably larger than these slits and must be flexible to pass through them into the splenic sinus.** ***(From Lux and Becker.[582] Used by permission of W. B. Saunders Co.)***

process were beautifully illustrated in vivo by Griggs and his coworkers,[310] who showed that a cohort of ^{59}Fe-labeled HS red cells gradually shifted from the major, less fragile population to the minor, more fragile population during their circulation in vivo. Although most conditioned HS red cells are probably recaptured and destroyed in the spleen, the damage incurred is sufficient to permit their recognition and destruction in extrasplenic sites, since conditioned spherocytes isolated from the spleen at the time of splenectomy and reinfused postoperatively are rapidly destroyed.[310,317] The mechanism of splenic conditioning is less clear. It is difficult to obtain precise information about the cordal environment, but the data that exist suggest that the climate is inhospitable. Arteries supplying the white pulp skim off plasma and dramatically increase congestion in the cords, where the crowded red cells must compete with metabolically voracious phagocytes for limited supplies of glucose.[318] Even if glucose were available, it is questionable whether the HS red cell could use it effectively. Because of the stagnant circulation, lactic acid accumulates[319] and the extracellular pH falls, probably to between 6.5 and 7.0.[238,319] Intracellular pH must also decline, inhibiting hexokinase[320] and phosphofructokinase,[317] the rate limiting enzymes of glycolysis, and retarding glucose utilization. Under these conditions stores of 2,3-DPG will be metabolized to provide energy for the cell. The loss of this polyvalent anion, combined with the decreased anionic charge on hemoglobin that occurs in an acid environment, is compensated by the entry of monovalent chloride ions.[321] The resulting increase in osmolarity causes water to enter the HS red cell and must worsen its already compromising spheroidicity. Thus, the spherocyte, detained in the splenic cords because of its surface deficiency, is severely stressed by erythrostasis in a metabolically threatening environment. Whether this is sufficient to cause its demise is a matter of continuing debate.

Erythrostasis. As Ham and Castle[215] and Dacie[322] first recognized, the HS red cell is particularly vulnerable to erythrostasis. When incubated in the absence of glucose, their physiological substrate, all red cells undergo a series of changes that culminate in autohemolysis. As shown in Fig. 115-11, these changes are accelerated in hereditary spherocytes. HS red cells are initially jeopardized by an increase in the permeability of their membranes to sodium.[323,324] This is normally balanced by increased ATP-dependent sodium pumping and increased glycolysis,[323] a response that is impaired in erythrostasis, during which substrate is limited. Consequently, spherocytes exhaust available glucose and become ATP-depleted more rapidly than normal (Fig. 115-11*A*). As ATP levels fall, cation pumps fail and the cells gain sodium and water and swell (Fig. 115-11*B*). Later, when ATP reaches very low levels, intracellular calcium also rises, owing to failure of the calcium pump. This leads to a selective efflux of red-cell potassium, the so-called Gardós phenomenon.[325,326] The molecular mechanism of this permeability change is not well understood, but its consequences are well defined: As intracellular potassium declines, water exits in response to the change in osmolarity and cells shrink (Fig. 115-11*B*). The sodium gain is accelerated in HS red cells but is insufficient by itself to induce hemolysis in vitro since cation-mediated cell swelling peaks at 12 to 16 h (Fig. 115-11*B*), long before autohemolysis occurs (Fig. 115-11*D*). HS red cells are doubly jeopardized. As noted earlier, they are inherently unstable and fragment excessively during metabolic depletion.[246-248,251] Membrane lipids are lost at more than twice the normal rate (Fig. 115-11*C*).[327] It is not known whether a proportional loss of integral membrane proteins occurs, although this seems likely, particularly in primary band 3 deficiency. At first this surface loss is balanced by cell dehydration (as shown by stabilization of the calculated volume/surface ratio between 20 and 30 h in Fig. 115-11*E*), but eventually membrane loss predominates, the cells exceed their critical hemolytic volume (volume:surface ratio > 100), and autohemolysis ensues (Fig. 115-11*E*).

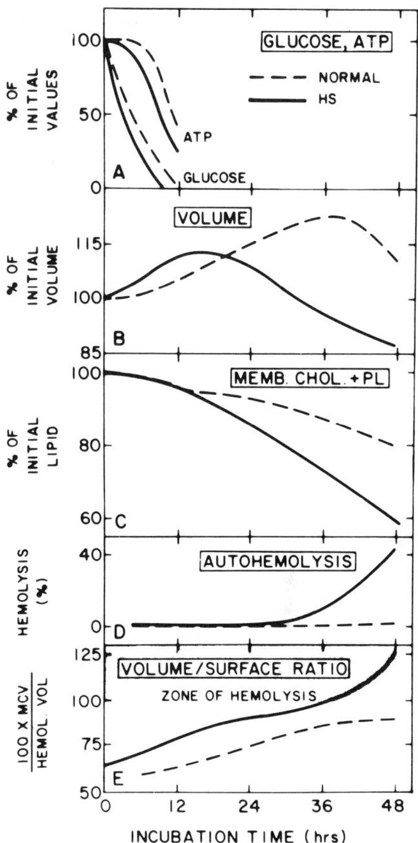

FIG. 115-11 **The effects of erythrostasis on normal (- - -) and HS (—) red cells incubated at 37°C in their own serum at hematocrit values of 25 to 45 percent. Because HS red cells are more permeable to sodium than normal, they require excess ATP for sodium transport and exhaust available serum glucose and red cell ATP more rapidly than normal (*panel A*). This leads to cell swelling, which is followed by cell shrinkage due to calcium accumulation and potassium loss (Gardos phenomenon) (*panel B*). The relatively more rapid loss of membrane fragments (*panel C*) gradually increases the volume/surface ratio (*panel E*) until the critical hemolytic volume is reached (volume:-surface ratio = 100) and autohemolysis ensues (*panel D*). *(From Lux and Glader.[582] Used by permission of W. B. Saunders Co.)***

Dynamics of Splenic Trapping. One of the major unanswered issues about the pathophysiology of HS is whether the events that lead to conditioning and destruction of HS red cells in the spleen are the same as those that lead to increased spheroidicity and autohemolysis during erythrostasis in vitro. In the past, many investigators have assumed this was the case, and the argument focused on the relative importance of membrane leakiness versus membrane fragility in the spherocytes' demise.

In summary, it is clear that HS red cells are selectively detained by the spleen and that this custody is detrimental, leading to a loss of membrane surface that fosters further splenic trapping and eventual destruction (Fig. 115-12). Indeed, studies have shown that the mean splenic transit time correlates inversely ($r = -0.96$) with red-cell survival in HS.[330] It appears likely that splenic trapping is initially promoted by membrane skeletal instability, but the details of how the molecular defect leads to splenic entrapment have yet to be defined. The mechanisms of splenic conditioning and red-cell destruction are also uncertain. Kinetic considerations make it unlikely that red cells are continuously trapped within the cords for the long periods required to induce passive sphering and autohemolysis by metabolic depletion. Repetitious metabolic damage remains a possibility. A special susceptibility of the HS red cell to the acidic environment of the spleen and active intervention of macrophages in the processing of spherocytes damaged

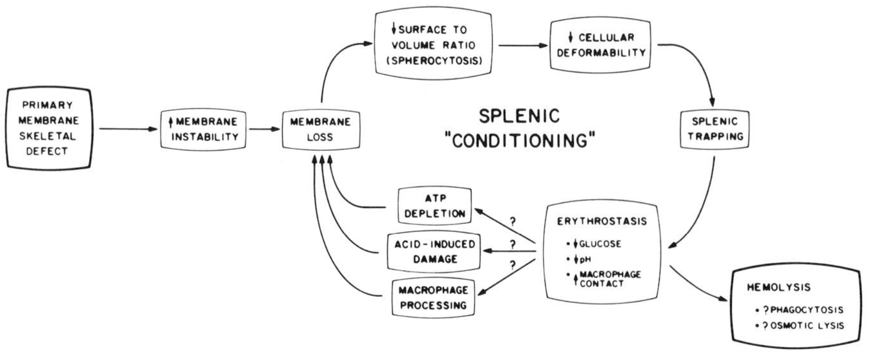

FIG. 115-12 **Pathophysiology of the splenic conditioning and destruction of red cells observed in hereditary spherocytosis.** ***(From Lux and Glader.[582] Used by permission of W. B. Saunders Co.)***

during erythrostasis must also be considered, but direct evidence for these two hypotheses remains to be established.

Clinical Features

The characteristic clinical features of HS are pallor, jaundice, and splenomegaly. The disease typically presents in infancy or childhood, but may present at any age.[331] As noted earlier, in most patients the degree of hemolysis, anemia, and spherocytosis; the need for transfusions (or not); and the response to splenectomy closely parallel the degree of spectrin (and probably ankyrin) deficiency.[260]

Neonatal HS. HS frequently presents as jaundice in the first few days of life.[332,333] The combination of hemolysis and the reduced capacity of the neonatal liver to conjugate bilirubin can cause serum concentrations of unconjugated bilirubin to rise rapidly, and because there is a risk of kernicterus,[333] exchange transfusions are sometimes necessary. Mild anemia is common at this time, but severe anemia is rare. There is no evidence that patients with HS who are symptomatic as neonates have a more severe form of the disease. Indeed most become asymptomatic within the first few weeks of life. However, some infants become progressively more anemic during the first few months of life and require transfusion. In our experience, this usually occurs because the marrow response to anemia is more sluggish than normal. Fortunately, the problem is transient (except in rare patients with severe subtypes of HS) and usually remits after one or two transfusions. Subsequently, the course of the disease depends on the equilibrium established between the rates of red-cell production and destruction.

Mild HS. In a surprisingly large number of patients (~20 to 30 percent), red-cell production and destruction are balanced, and no anemia is present.[334,335] These individuals are said to have "compensated hemolysis." They are often asymptomatic, and in some cases diagnosis may be difficult, since hemolysis, spherocytosis, and splenomegaly are usually mild. Hemolysis may become severe with illnesses that cause the spleen to enlarge, such as infectious mononucleosis.[336] Hemolysis is also exacerbated by pregnancy[337] and by intensive physical effort, to the point at which athletic performance in endurance sports may be impaired, even in patients with mild disease.[338] Many of these patients are diagnosed during family studies or are discovered as adults when splenomegaly or gallstones are detected or when transient episodes of jaundice appear. Although mild HS is usually consistent within families, mild cases may also occur in families with more severely affected members.[334] Presumably this is due to the inheritance of modifying genes, such as those affecting splenic function or, in dominant HS, by genes that affect the expression of the normal or mutant allele.

One of the interesting mysteries about HS is why patients with "compensated hemolysis" continue to have erythroid hyperproduction when their hemoglobin levels are normal. The phenomenon is difficult to reconcile with the generally accepted theory that erythropoiesis is controlled by tissue hypoxia. One possibility is that the concentration of 2,3-DPG, which is low in hereditary spherocytes[339,340] prior to splenectomy, has an effect. Low red-cell 2,3-DPG would increase oxygen affinity and promote erythropoiesis, but this effect is apparently balanced by other factors, since the P_{50} (partial pressure of O_2 at which Hb is half-saturated) of HS blood is normal.[340]

Typical HS. The majority of HS patients (~60 to 75 percent) have incompletely compensated hemolysis and mild to moderate anemia. Intermittent subtle jaundice is common, particularly in children, and is sometimes associated with mild viral infections, presumably due to reticuloendothelial stimulation and an increase in hemolysis. The spleen is palpable in about 50 percent of these patients during infancy and in 75 to 95 percent during late childhood and adult life.[334,341,342] Splenomegaly is usually modest, but it may be massive.[229,230,343,344] There is no published evidence that the size of the spleen correlates with the severity of HS, although such a correlation probably exists, considering the pathophysiology of the disease (see Fig. 115-12).

Severe HS. A small proportion of HS patients (~5 to 10 percent) have severe and sometimes transfusion-dependent anemia. These individuals may present diagnostic difficulties if transfusions are begun before HS is diagnosed, since in the most severe cases the abnormal cells may be destroyed so rapidly that, except for a few spherocytic reticulocytes, only transfused cells are available for testing. In addition to the risks of recurrent transfusion, these patients often suffer from aplastic crises (see "Crises" below), growth retardation,[343,344] and delayed sexual maturation,[343] and frontal bossing or other changes in the facial bones similar to those observed in thalassemia[343] may develop.

Laboratory Features

The major laboratory findings are those common to all hemolytic processes: hyperplasia of erythroid precursors in the bone marrow, an increased concentration of reticulocytes, a slight to moderate rise in unconjugated (indirect) bilirubin in the plasma, and an elevated fecal excretion of urobilinogens.[334,342,345] Plasma hemoglobin is normal,[346] and haptoglobin is only variably reduced,[347] because most of

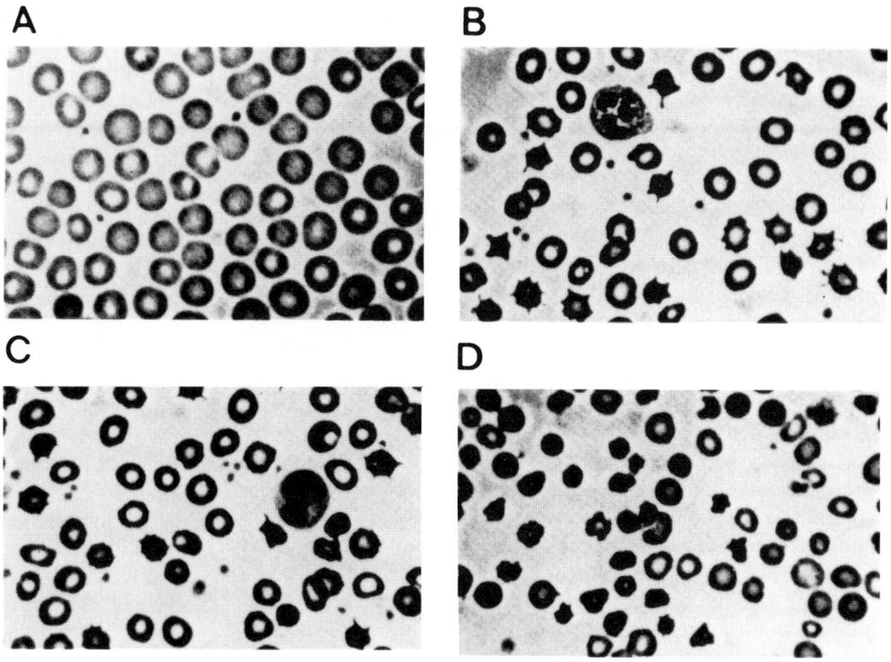

FIG. 115-13 Peripheral blood smears of patients with hereditary spherocytosis. *A*. Typical autosomal dominant HS: spherocytes and cells of normal appearance. *B* and *C*. Autosomal dominant HS with protein 4.1–binding defect of spectrin ($spectrin_{KISSIMMEE}$): acanthocytes, spherocytes, and normal appearing cells. *D*. Autosomal recessive HS with severe spectrin deficiency: microspherocytes, spherocytes, acanthocytes, poikilocytes, and schistocytes. *(From Becker and Lux.[583] Used by permission of* Clinics in Haematology.*)*

the hemoglobin that is released from destroyed hereditary spherocytes is catabolized to bilirubin at the site of destruction (so-called extravascular hemolysis).

Red-Cell Morphology and Indexes. Spherocytosis is the hallmark of HS and, with reticulocytosis, is the most reliable finding. In 20 to 25 percent of patients the typical hyperchromic, conditioned microspherocytes are relatively sparse.[334,342] Peripheral blood smears from these patients may sometimes mistakenly be considered normal, even by relatively experienced observers.[334] Interestingly, although hereditary spherocytes, and particularly the conditioned cells, appear spheroidal in conventional dried smears, most are actually thickened diskocytes or spherostomatocytes when examined on scanning EM.[348] The various types of HS have different morphologic patterns on blood smears, as shown in Fig. 115-13. Patients with classic autosomal dominant HS and most patients with recessive HS have only spherocytes and microspherocytes. Patients with more severe spectrin deficiency have proportionally more misshaped spherocytes, spiculated red cells, and bizarre poikilocytes. In the most severe cases these may dominate the blood smear[237,270] (Fig. 115-13*D*). Spiculated red cells (acanthocytes) are also observed with $Sp_{KISSIMMEE}$[273] and in some other patients whose molecular defects are not known (Fig. 115-13*C*). Oblong spherocytes, combined with elliptocytes, suggest a variant of hereditary elliptocytosis (spherocytic HE). As mentioned previously, a subset of the cells from patients with band 3 deficiency have a mushroom shape. Because the morphologic defect is acquired gradually in the circulation, HS erythroblasts are morphologically and rheologically normal,[349] and circulating reticulocytes are only slightly spheroidal.[350]

The MCHC of HS red cells is increased owing to mild cellular dehydration and exceeds the upper limit of normal (36 percent) in about half of patients.[334] Red-cell sodium concentrations are normal or slightly elevated, but cell potassium and water are low,[351-353] particularly in cells removed from the splenic pulp.[352] MCH and MCV fall within the normal range,[334] but because young red cells normally have a high cell volume, the MCV in HS is actually relatively low, reflecting their dehydration.

Fragility and Autohemolysis Tests. The osmotic fragility (OF) test, particularly its incubated variant, is the most sensitive test generally available for the diagnosis of HS. The unincubated OF provides interesting information on the proportion of conditioned cells in the circulation,[238,316,354] information that is lost in the incubated OF. The test is performed by suspending the cells in aqueous solutions containing various concentrations of sodium chloride.[238] Since there is almost no exchange of cations during the short duration of the test, osmotic equilibrium is achieved almost entirely by the rapid movement of water across the membrane. In hypotonic solutions, red cells swell until they become spheres and then burst. Cells with a decreased surface:volume ratio, such as hereditary spherocytes, can tolerate less swelling than normal and are termed "osmotically fragile." From 20 to 25 percent of HS patients have a normal or near-normal unincubated OF test prior to splenectomy, particularly the mildly affected patients, who are most difficult to diagnose.[341,355] The incubated OF, in contrast, is more often positive[355] since, during the period of preincubation (24 h at 37°C), hereditary spherocytes become metabolically depleted and lose membrane surface more rapidly than normal cells (see Fig. 115-11), which accentuates their spheroidicity and enhances the sensitivity of the test. Occasionally, patients with normal incubated OF have been reported,[356,357] and it seems likely that such patients are even more common than these rare reports suggest, since the OF test detects a secondary property of HS red cells (their loss of membrane surface) rather than the primary molecular defect. A modification of the osmotic fragility test has been described[358] in which the extent of hemolysis in four hypotonic solutions of sodium chloride is assessed. Two parameters are obtained from the logarithmic linearization of the curve, which enable a high level of sensitivity and specificity of the test in diagnosing HS.

The autohemolysis test was first described by Ham and Castle[215] and was carefully standardized by Dacie[322] and

Young[341,359] and their coworkers. The principle of the test is illustrated in Fig. 115-12. Autohemolysis of HS red cells, incubated in their own plasma in the absence of added glucose, is increased at 48 h. In most HS patients much less autohemolysis is observed if supplemental glucose is added.[341,351,359] This is not true in patients with large numbers of conditioned spherocytes,[360] an exception that can lead to considerable diagnostic confusion, since autohemolysis that is unabated in the presence of glucose is a common feature of a number of hemolytic anemias.[359] In general, the autohemolysis test is quite sensitive and is occasionally useful in confirming the diagnosis of HS (e.g., in mild, sporadic cases); however, we do not use it routinely. Other tests for HS are available, including the mechanical fragility test,[238,341] the rate of hemolysis in acidified glycerol,[357,361,362] and the ouabain osmotic fragility test.[363] The former test lacks specificity and has no proven diagnostic benefit, but the latter two procedures appear to be somewhat more sensitive than the standard OF and autohemolysis tests[359,363] (but there is a contradictory view[364] concerning the acidified glycerol lysis test) and may prove diagnostically useful if further studies confirm this increased sensitivity. Lastly, a new method has been described—hypertonic cryohemolysis[365]—that is independent of the surface area:volume ratio of the cells (an advantage over the other diagnostic tests). The hereditary spherocytes appear to be particularly sensitive to cooling at 0°C in hypertonic conditions. The sensitivity was 100 percent, and the specificity 94 percent for healthy controls, and 86 percent for patients with autoimmune hemolytic anemia. One patient with congenital dyserythropoietic anemia type II and one family with spherocytic HE also had positive hypertonic cryohemolysis.

Complications

Crises. Patients with HS, like patients with other hemolytic processes, are subject to various "crises." Mild hemolytic crises are probably most frequent,[334] although this is controversial.[366] They usually occur with common viral syndromes and are characterized by a mild, transient increase in jaundice, splenomegaly, anemia, and reticulocytosis. Severe hemolytic crises are rare but have been reported.[343,367]

Aplastic crises, on the other hand, are less frequent but are often more serious, since severe anemia and even death[229,343] can result. They are mostly[368] caused by infection with human parvovirus B19[369,370] and typically present with fever, vomiting, abdominal pain, arthralgias, headache, pallor, and symptoms of anemia.[366,369-371] A maculopapular rash[372] or even an illness resembling Henoch-Schönlein purpura[368] may also be seen. Sometimes multiple family members or even whole communities are affected simultaneously.[369,373] During the aplastic phase the hematocrit level and reticulocyte count fall, marrow erythroblasts disappear, and unused iron accumulates in the serum.[366] Mild granulocytopenia and thrombocytopenia are common but are not invariably present. Since production of new HS red cells is halted, the cells that remain age, and microspherocytosis and osmotic fragility increase.[374] The bilirubin level declines because of a decrease in the number of abnormal red cells that have to be destroyed. Since the usual aplastic crisis lasts 10 to 14 days[366] (about half the life span of HS red cells), the hemoglobin concentration typically falls to about half its usual value before recovery ensues. It is not uncommon for this severe stress to be the first sign of HS in previously well-compensated patients.[370] The return of marrow function is heralded by a fall in serum iron concentration, a rise in granulocytes and platelets to normal levels, and reticulocytosis.[366]

Megaloblastic crises result when the dietary intake of folic acid is insufficient for the increased needs of the erythroid HS bone marrow. They are usually observed during pregnancy[375,376] when the need for folic acid is particularly high.

Gallbladder Disease. The most common complication of HS from its first reports[218,219] to the present day has been gallbladder disease. Pigment gallstones have been detected in patients as young as 3 years[374] but are most prevalent in adolescents and adults.[377] The available data indicate that 55 to 85 percent of untreated HS patients will eventually acquire stones[341,377,378] and that roughly half these individuals will have symptoms of cholecystitis or, less commonly, biliary obstruction.[229,367,378] However, much more accurate data on the incidence of these complications are needed in patients with bilirubinate gallstones to assess the risk:benefit ratio of cholecystectomy (and splenectomy) in HS accurately.

Other Complications. It is rare for patients with HS to have gout,[230,379] indolent leg ulcers,[380] or a chronic erythematous dermatitis on the legs.[381] Occasionally, patients also have extramedullary masses of hematopoietic tissue, particularly alongside the posterior thoracic or lumbar spine.[229,379,382] These gradually enlarge with time and may be mistaken for neoplasms.[379] Interestingly, Schafer and his colleagues have suggested that untreated HS may predispose patients to a true neoplasm—multiple myeloma.[383] Four patients with HS and myeloma have been reported.[383-385] None was splenectomized, two had gallbladder disease, and one had silicosis. They argue that the association may be due to chronic reticuloendothelial stimulation, since splenic clearance of abnormal red cells induces proliferation of lymphocytes and plasma cells as well as macrophages.[386] HS patients have a mild, polyclonal hypergammaglobulinemia,[383,387] and there is evidence favoring the association of myeloma and chronic gallbladder disease.[383,388] Untreated HS may also exacerbate hemochromatosis in patients who are heterozygous for the hereditary disease,[389-392] and several of the reported patients subsequently died from liver failure or hepatoma.[382,393,394]

Diagnostic Problems

In general, HS is easily diagnosed and differentiated from other causes of spherocytosis, but there are several situations in which diagnosis can be difficult. In the neonatal period it may be hard to differentiate HS from ABO incompatibility since microspherocytosis is prominent in both and the Coombs' test is frequently negative in ABO disease.[395] Fortunately, in most affected infants with ABO incompatibility, anti-A (or anti-B) antibodies can be eluted from the red cells, and free anti-A or anti-B IgG antibodies can be detected in the infant's serum. Occasionally, older patients with immunohemolytic anemias and spherocytosis also have so few antibody molecules attached to their red cells that the Coombs' test is negative and differentiation of the disease from HS is possible only with the use of radioactive antiglobulin reagents.[396]

Diagnostic difficulties also arise in patients who present during an aplastic crisis. Early in the crisis the acute nature of the symptoms may suggest an acquired process, and the absence of reticulocytes may divert the physician from a diagnosis of hemolytic anemia. Later, as marrow function returns, the physician may be misled by the fact that the emerging young HS red cells are initially less spherocytic and osmotically fragile than usual[350] and acquire their typical microspherocytic form only with age and reticuloendothelial conditioning. HS may also be camouflaged by association with disorders that increase the surface:volume ratio of the red cells, such as iron deficiency[397] or obstructive jaundice.[248] Iron deficiency corrects the abnormal shape and fragility of hereditary spherocytes but does not improve their life span,[397] whereas obstructive jaundice improves both shape and survival.[248]

The rare patients with "atypical" HS may also cause diagnostic confusion. Most such patients actually represent combinations of typical HS and diseases affecting other organ systems,[398,399] Coombs-negative immunohemolytic anemias (see above in this section), or very severe HS in which large numbers of very defective spherocytes remain in the circulation owing to saturation of the reticuloendothelial system.[400,401] A few families have been described with unusual forms of hereditary spherocytic hemolytic anemias that resemble HS in some respects but not in others. For example, Boivin and his colleagues have reported a family with a dominantly inherited hemolytic anemia characterized by spherocytosis, decreased spectrin phosphorylation, and failure to improve following splenectomy.[303a] Zail and his coworkers have described a family with a dominantly inherited disorder characterized by spherocytosis and mild compensated hemolysis in which fresh red cells had a normal or decreased osmotic fragility and ^{51}Cr-labeled red cells lacked the characteristic pattern of splenic sequestration that is typical of HS.[403] The relationship of these patients to each other and to typical HS is unclear.

Splenectomy. It is one of the rare absolutes in medicine that patients with true, uncomplicated HS always respond dramatically to splenectomy. The degree of response correlates closely with the degree of spectrin deficiency[260] and is incomplete in the most severely affected patients. The major issues today are who should be splenectomized and how they should be treated postoperatively. The most devastating complication of splenectomy is postsplenectomy sepsis. The data in the literature indicate that overwhelming sepsis occurs in 3.5 percent of patients with HS and that 60 percent of these patients die.[404,405] However, the retrospective studies are seriously flawed[406,407] and the true incidence of fulminant sepsis is undoubtedly much less. The only adequate epidemiologic study suggests an incidence of 0.2 case per 100 person-years for adults, and this rate can presumably be further reduced by use of pneumococcal[408] and other (*Haemophilus influenzae,* meningococcal) bacterial vaccines.

Following splenectomy, spherocytosis persists, but conditioned microspherocytes disappear, and changes typical of the postsplenectomy state—including Howell-Jolly bodies, target cells, acanthocytes, and siderocytes—appear in the peripheral smear.[316,360] Reticulocyte counts fall to normal or near-normal levels, although red-cell life span, if carefully measured, remains slightly shortened (96±13 days).[409] In all cases, anemia and jaundice remit and do not recur except in the rare case of regrowth of a missed accessory spleen. This is the only proven cause of postsplenectomy failure in HS and is sometimes overlooked, since it may not become evident for years[410] or even decades.[411]

HEREDITARY ELLIPTOCYTOSIS

Hereditary elliptocytosis (HE) is a relatively common, clinically and genetically heterogeneous disorder characterized by the presence of a large number of elliptically shaped red cells in the peripheral blood. These cells are sometimes called "ovalocytes," but "elliptocytes" and "elliptocytosis" are the more accurate designations, as the cells are elliptical rather than egg-shaped. In the more severe forms of the disease, spherocytes or bizarre poikilocytes are also present, and sometimes these shapes predominate. Hereditary pyropoikilocytosis (HPP) is an example of the latter situation. Although HPP was previously considered to be a separate entity, emerging biochemical and genetic information clearly indicates it is closely related to HE, and the two disorders will be considered together here.

History

According to Lambrecht,[412] elliptocytosis was first observed by Goltz in Königsburg, Germany, in 1860, but no written report of this observation is known. The disease was first reported in 1904 by Dresbach, a physiologist at Ohio State University, in one of his histology students during a laboratory exercise in which the students were examining their own blood.[413] His brief report elicited some controversy as the student died soon thereafter, leading the prominent American physician Austin Flint to suggest that he had actually had incipient pernicious anemia.[414] Dresbach replied that the student died of acute rheumatic carditis and took his slides to Germany, where famous pathologists such as Ewig, Ehrlich, and Arneth supported his view that the red-cell disorder was primary.[415] This was substantiated during the next two decades by the reports of Bishop,[416] Sydenstricker,[417] and Huck and Bigelow.[418] Hunter's demonstration of elliptocytosis in three generations of one family firmly established the hereditary nature of the disease.[419,420]

In the 1930s and early 1940s there was considerable debate about whether HE was a disease or simply a morphologic curiosity. In retrospect, this is surprising since numerous individuals with hemolytic HE were described during this interval[412,421-425] and some authors had clearly differentiated hemolytic and nonhemolytic forms.[412,421,422] In fact as early as 1928, van den Bergh even reported that anemia and jaundice cleared following splenectomy in one patient.[424] Early on, some confusion also existed in differentiating HE from sickle-cell anemia[426,427] and "hypochromic elliptocytosis" (probably thalassemia)[428] and later in differentiating hemolytic HE from hereditary spherocytosis.[429] These reports illustrate a point that will be emphasized later—namely, that HE, particularly its hemolytic variants, can sometimes be morphologically deceptive.

For the reader interested in the historical and clinical features of the disease, the reports of Wyandt and her coworkers,[429] Wolman and Ozge,[430] Dacie,[431] Josephs and Avery,[432] Weiss,[433] and Cutting and his coworkers[434] are particularly recommended.

Prevalence and Genetics

HE is clearly heterogeneous from a clinical, genetic, or biochemical point of view. This was not appreciated by early investigators. In most papers, all patients with HE were simply lumped together. Accordingly, it is difficult to relate much of the available information to the different clinical forms of the disease.

The prevalence of all forms of HE in the United States is about 250 to 500 per million.[429,435] Elliptocytic red cells have been observed in all racial and ethnic groups, but the distribution of some of the clinical phenotypes is clearly restricted. With the exception of HPP, the disease generally is inherited as an autosomal dominant trait.

Genetic studies show that one of the elliptocytosis genes (El1) is closely linked to the Rh locus on chromosome 1p34-p36.[436-439] This is the location of the protein 4.1 gene.[440] Another gene (El2) is located on the long arm of chromosome 1, near the Duffy blood group locus (1q24),[441] in the region where the spectrin α chain gene is located (1q22-q25).[87] The identification of numerous mutations in both of these proteins in HE confirms the linkage studies.

Clinical Syndromes

Most of the reported cases of HE can be classified into one of three clinical categories: common HE, spherocytic HE, and Southeast Asian ovalocytosis (see Table 115-3). Common HE, the largest group, can be further subdivided on the basis of clinical severity and other characteristic features. It must be emphasized that these appellations denote clinical phenotypes and not specific molecular or genetic etiologies. Several defects in the membrane proteins causing hereditary elliptocytosis have been identified, and the various types of HE can also be classified based on these defects.

Common HE. This the most prevalent form of HE. It can be divided into several subtypes, as discussed below.

Silent Carrier State. This condition has been identified by analyzing asymptomatic members of kindreds with HE or HPP. The affected persons have normal red-cell shape and no evidence of hemolysis, but careful measurements sometimes show a subtle defect in their membrane skeletons, with decreased red-cell thermal stability, decreased mechanical stability of isolated skeletons, abnormal tryptic peptide maps of spectrin, and various combinations of these defects.[442-445] (These tests will be discussed in more detail under "Methods to Define Abnormal Spectrin Structure and Function in HE" below).

More commonly, the "silent carrier" state is associated with an LELY α spectrin allele, $\alpha^{V/41}$ or α^{LELY},[68,69] which has no effect on red-cell properties. This allele (also described in the "Spectrin" and HE "Etiology" sections) decreases the synthesis of the "normal" α spectrin, proportionally increasing spectrin from the HE allele in *trans*. The α^{LELY} locus is clinically silent by itself, even when homozygous, but it greatly augments the effects of the *trans* allele; for example, inheritance of the α^{LELY} allele with a mild HE mutation in *trans* can result in severe hemolytic HE or even pyropoikilocytosis. In addition, the α^{LELY} allele is very common. About 42 percent of Europeans are heterozygous and 9 percent are homozygous. Therefore, it can play a major role in the clinical expression of HE.

Mild HE. The mild form of HE[429,446-450] is typically dominantly inherited and patients have no anemia or splenomegaly (see Table 115-3). Sometimes red-cell survival is normal,[447,451] but more often there is very mild, compensated hemolysis with a slight reticulocytosis and a decreased haptoglobin level.[429,449,450] In these patients HE is little more than a morphologic curiosity. The peripheral blood smear shows prominent elliptocytosis with little red-cell budding or fragmentation and spherocytosis. Elliptocytes almost always exceed 30 percent of the red cells and sometimes approach 100 percent (Fig. 115-14).[429,446,449] Very elongated elliptocytes (rod forms) are common (>10 percent). According to the older literature, normal individuals have less than 15 percent

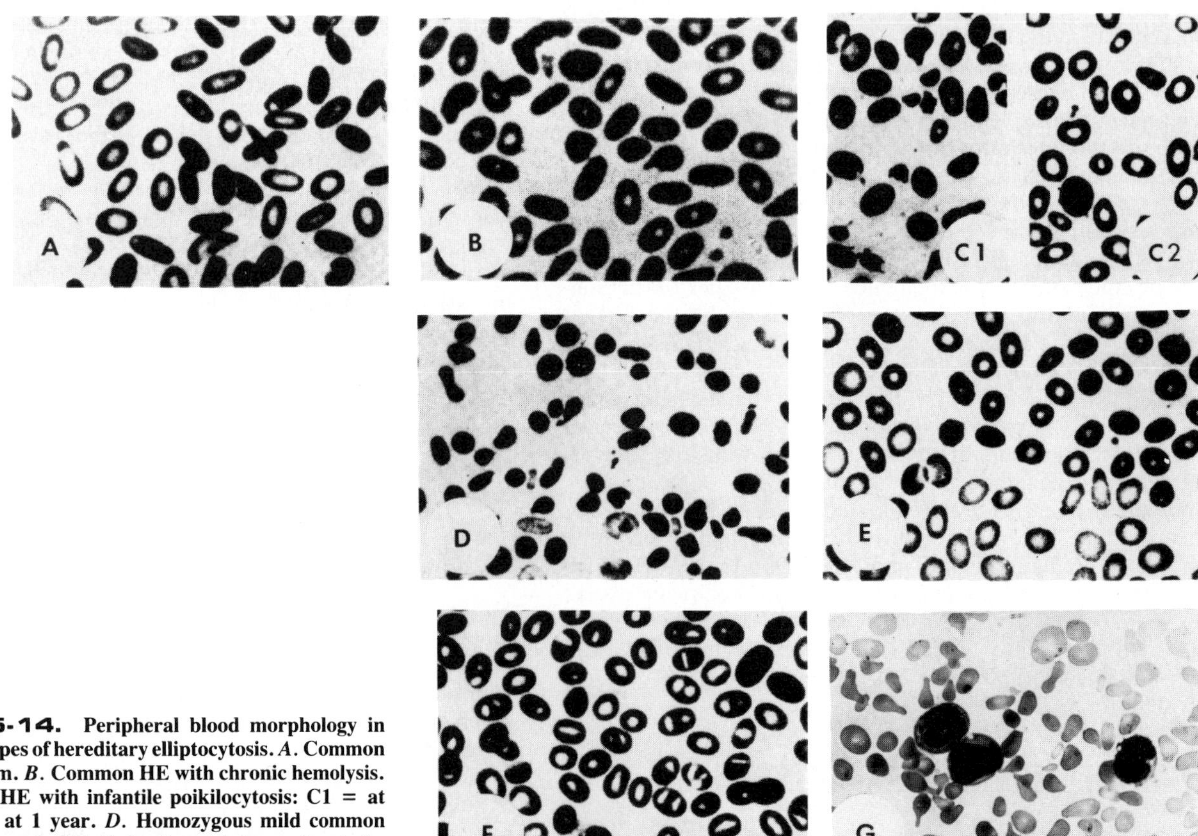

FIG. 115-14. **Peripheral blood morphology in the various types of hereditary elliptocytosis. *A*. Common HE, mild form. *B*. Common HE with chronic hemolysis. *C*. Common HE with infantile poikilocytosis: C1 = at birth, C2 = at 1 year. *D*. Homozygous mild common HE. *E*. Spherocytic HE. *F*. Southeast Asian ovalocytosis. *G*. Hereditary pyropoikilocytosis.**

elliptocytes,[429,446,449] but in our experience this number is too high. We and others[451a,584] find that the upper limit of normal is 2 to 5 percent elliptocytes. Somewhat higher proportions are seen in patients with anemia, particularly megaloblastic and hypochromic–microcytic anemias, but even in these individuals elliptocytes and rod forms do not exceed 35 percent and 15 percent, respectively.[446] Hence, the morphologic diagnosis of mild HE is rarely difficult. This may not be true in the neonatal period. Early investigators noted that elliptocytes are infrequent in the cord blood of infants with mild HE and become more prominent with time.[420,429,452] For example, Wyandt and coworkers detected only 11 percent elliptocytes at birth in one infant, whereas by 4 months of age, 80 percent of the cells were elliptical.[429] These observations, although few, suggest that the disease may be expressed differently in fetal red cells, a point that will be discussed in more detail in the following section. Early workers used a complex system for quantitating ellipticity,[453] but the method is time-consuming and has not proven more useful in diagnosing HE than simple subjective estimation.[446] In addition, it is not prognostically useful since there is no correlation between the proportion of elliptocytes or their ellipticity and the severity of the disease.

Phenotypically identical mild HE is caused by more than one molecular lesion, since in some families mild HE is linked to the Rh gene and in other families it is not.[438,454] The best example of the Rh-linked disease is the large Dutch-American family first described by Hunter[419,420] and van den Bergh[455] and their associates and then restudied by Geerdink et al.[449,454] Moreover, multiple protein defects have been associated with the mild phenotype, including those involving α spectrin, β spectrin, protein 4.1, and glycophorin C (see Table 115-3). These specific defects will be discussed in detail in a later section.

HE with Acute or Chronic Hemolysis. In many large kindreds with typical compensated mild HE, a minority (5 to 20 percent) of the patients have more severe hemolysis and anemia.[456,457] The etiology of this variation is not always clear. In some instances it is a transient acquired state due to hyperplasia of the spleen in response to a variety of stimuli (e.g., cirrhosis,[458] infectious mononucleosis,[450,457] bacterial infections,[450] or malaria).[459,460] For unknown reasons pregnancy may also transiently aggravate the disease,[450] as may transplant rejection and cobalamin (vitamin B_{12}) deficiency.

In other apparently sporadic cases chronic hemolysis exists in the absence of any detectable disease process. Probably many of these individuals coinherit the α^{LELY} allele (see "Silent Carrier State" above). This gene is very common, which could explain how a mother with compensated mild HE bore two children with the uncompensated disease from unrelated fathers.[461]

Except for signs of increased hemolysis and anemia, patients with uncompensated mild HE are similar to their less severely affected relatives. Splenomegaly and morphologic evidence of red-cell destruction (e.g., fragmentation and poikilocytosis) are somewhat more prevalent in this group but are not reliable in differentiating features. It appears that most of these patients respond well to splenectomy, although extensive data are not available.[462-464]

Mild HE with Poikilocytosis in Infancy. Infants with this form of "mild" HE often begin life with moderately severe hemolytic anemia, characterized by marked red-cell budding, fragmentation, and poikilocytosis (see Table 115-3 and Fig. 115-14) and neonatal jaundice.[163,432,465-467] In most cases, sufficient elliptocytes are present to suggest the diagnosis, but sometimes this is not so and the disorder may be mistaken for infantile pyknocytosis, HPP, or a microangiopathic or oxidant-induced hemolytic anemia.[465,466] The correct diagnosis is easily made if the parents' smears are examined, since one will have mild HE. With time, fragmentation and hemolysis decline, and the clinical picture of mild HE emerges. This transition requires from 4 months to 2 years. The change in morphology often occurs somewhat faster than the decline in hemolysis.[467] Subsequently, the disease is clinically indistinguishable from typical mild HE. The prevalence is unknown, but in our experience it is not rare. In particular, it is more common than HPP, with which it is often confused.

The fragmenting neonatal red cells are very sensitive to heat, like hereditary pyropoikilocytes, but unlike pyropoikilocytes this sensitivity lessens as the patients mature.[467] The dense poikilocytic red cells are rich in hemoglobin F,[468] which suggests that the change in the course of the disease is due to the conversion from fetal to adult erythropoiesis. If so, interactions between the genetically defective protein, and other skeletal proteins, must differ in fetal and adult red cells. Mentzer has made the interesting suggestion that 2,3-DPG is the critical agent.[163] Free 2,3-DPG is elevated in fetal red cells since it is not bound by hemoglobin F. The free anion is known to weaken spectrin–actin and protein 4.1–actin bonds[164,165] and to increase the fragility of isolated ghosts at physiological concentrations,[163] although it is controversial whether it does so at physiological concentrations in intact red cells.[166] If so, this would certainly aggravate the underlying defect in spectrin self-association (to be discussed).

Mild HE with Dyserythropoiesis. In a small number of families with otherwise typical mild HE, the sporadic occurrence of hemolysis and anemia is at least partially due to the development of dysplastic and ineffective erythropoiesis. All the reported patients[469] are from central and southern Italy, have somewhat less elongated red cells than is typical for mild HE, and show the characteristic findings of ineffective erythropoiesis (high bilirubin, serum iron, and plasma iron turnover; relatively low reticulocyte count; and low incorporation of iron into circulating erythroid cells).[469] Their bone marrows are hyperplastic, with excessive intermediate erythroblasts, and have some dysplastic features including asynchrony of nuclear-cytoplasmic maturation, binuclearity, and small numbers of ringed sideroblasts. Anemia and presumably erythroid dysplasia usually commence during adolescence or early adult life and advance gradually over a number of years. Because dysplasia persists after splenectomy, response to the operation is incomplete. The available data suggest that dysplasia and elliptocytosis cosegregate, since no individuals with dysplasia have been observed who did not also carry the elliptocytosis gene. If so, these families must represent a unique subtype of mild HE. However, the numbers are small, and it is not clear that the nonelliptocytic members of the reported kindreds have been thoroughly examined.[469]

Homozygous Mild HE. A few patients with homozygous mild HE have been reported.[429,456,470-475] Most have had a very severe or even fatal[472] transfusion-dependent hemolytic anemia (Hb = 2 to 5 g/dl) with marked fragmentation, poikilocytosis, spherocytosis, and elliptocytosis (see Table 115-3 and Fig. 115-14), but in a few patients hemolysis was less rampant (Hb = 7 to 11 g/dl).[429,456] It appears these differences reflect variations in the severity of the many α spectrin mutations that produce mild HE (see Table 115-3). Clinically, the disease is very similar to hereditary pyropoikilocytosis (to be described). All treated patients have responded dramatically to splenectomy.

Hereditary Pyropoikilocytosis. This interesting, rare, recessive disease presents in infancy or early childhood as a severe hemolytic anemia (see Table 115-3) characterized by extreme poikilocytosis with budding red cells, fragments, spherocytes, elliptocytes, triangulocytes, and other bizarre-shaped cells[443,476-478] (see Fig. 115-14). The morphology is similar to that observed in homozygous mild HE and mild HE with poikilocytosis in infancy. Most but not all of the cases have occurred in blacks. Complications of severe anemia including growth retardation,[477] frontal bossing,[477] and early gallbladder disease[477] are reported. Osmotic fragility tests are very abnormal, particularly after incubation,[474-478] and autohemolysis is greatly elevated.[476-478] The MCV is very low (25 to 55 μm^3) because of the large number of fragmented red cells.[477,478]

Another characteristic feature of these cells is their remarkable thermal sensitivity. Hereditary pyropoikilocytes fragment at 45 to 46°C (normal = 49°C) after short periods of heating (10 to 15 min).[476] With prolonged heating (>6 h) they fragment even at body temperatures.[476] Following splenectomy, hemolysis is greatly lessened but not eliminated.[476,477] Typically, the hemoglobin after splenectomy is 7.5 to 10 g/dl with 3 to 7 percent reticulocytes.

Although HPP was initially considered as a separate disease, there is convincing evidence that it is related to HE. First, as noted above, HPP is clinically and morphologically similar to the more severe forms of hemolytic elliptocytosis and shares the characteristic of red-cell heat sensitivity observed in infants with mild HE and poikilocytosis. In addition, in many cases one of the parents or sibs has typical mild HE.[445,476,478] In some of these kindreds an apparently identical functional defect in spectrin (see the following section) is observed in sibs with phenotypically different diseases (i.e., HPP and mild HE). In other families, all the first-degree relatives are phenotypically normal. These findings indicate that HPP is genetically heterogeneous. At present it appears that the HPP phenotype can be produced by homozygosity for certain HE genes, a combination of HE and modifying genes, such as the α^{LELY} allele,[68,89] or compound heterozygosity for two different HE alleles.

Spherocytic HE. This form of HE is a phenotypic hybrid of mild HE and hereditary spherocytosis. It has been reported only in white families of European descent, is not linked to the Rh gene, and appears to be a unique subtype (see Table 115-3).[41,421,433,434,479,480] Its prevalence is unknown, but judging from the number of published reports and our own experience, it is relatively rare, probably accounting for no more than 5 to 10 percent of all HE cases in these populations. Unlike mild HE, almost all the affected patients have some hemolysis. This is usually mild to moderate and is often incompletely compensated. The elliptocytes are less prominent and less elongated than in mild HE, and some spherocytes, microspherocytes, and microelliptocytes are usually present (see Fig. 115-14). Red-cell morphology varies greatly, even within the same family. Some family members may have relatively prominent spherocytes and as few as 10 to 25 percent elliptocytes, while in others elliptocytes predominate and spherocytes are rare.[421,434] This may cause diagnostic confusion initially, particularly if the propositus has few elliptocytes. Family studies will almost always reveal some members with obvious elliptocytosis.

As in HS, the red cells in spherocytic HE are osmotically fragile, particularly after incubation.[433,434,480] Excessive mechanical fragility and increased autohemolysis that responds to glucose are also characteristic.[433,434,479,480] Gallbladder disease is common,[434,480] and aplastic crises are possible. The splenic pathology also mimics HS.[481,482] Splenic sequestration is evident,[434] red cells are conditioned during splenic passage,[479] and hemolysis abates following splenectomy.[41,431,433,434,479-481]

Southeast Asian Ovalocytosis (SAO). This fascinating condition, also known as hereditary ovalocytosis or Melanesian elliptocytosis or stomatocytic elliptocytosis, is inherited in an autosomal dominant pattern.[483-487] It is observed in the aboriginal populations of Melanesia and Indonesia,[484,485,488-490] including portions of the Philippines.[491] The gene is very common in Melanesia, particularly in lowland tribes, in whom malaria is endemic.[483,486,490,492] In these tribes 5 to 25 percent of the natives are affected. In vivo there is evidence that Southeast Asian ovalocytosis provides some protection against malaria, particularly *Plasmodium vivax* and probably *P. falciparum,* but protection is incomplete.[483,486,490,492] In vitro, SAO red cells are very resistant to invasion by all forms of malaria,[490,493,494] apparently because the membrane is much more rigid than normal.[495,496] Other membrane characteristics reflect this property. For example, the cells are usually heat-resistant. They easily withstand heating to 49°C (at which temperature normal red cells disintegrate), they do not undergo endocytosis in response to drugs that produce dramatic endocytosis in normal cells, and they strongly resist crenation,[493,494] even after several days' storage in plasma or buffered salt solutions. This property, combined with the distinctive red-cell morphology (see below), provides a simple means of diagnosing the disease.

The morphology is unique and is characterized by the presence of some elliptical stomatocytes and roundish elliptocytes traversed by one or two transverse bars (elliptical knizocytes) in addition to typical elliptocytes (see Fig. 115-14).[484,488-491] Hemolysis is apparently mild or absent,[484,488,489,491] although extensive hematologic data have not been published. In one well-studied probable patient, red-cell Na^+ and K^+ permeability was increased, glucose consumption was elevated to compensate for increased cation pumping, autohemolysis was increased, and the cells were osmotically resistant.[490] Curiously, many blood group antigens are poorly expressed on the surface of these cells[490]; conceivably, this may occur because the rigid membrane skeleton inhibits their clustering and impedes agglutination, but whatever the explanation, it may prove to be an important property because specific blood group antigens are required for the attachment and invasion of red cells by malarial parasites.[497-499]

Etiology

In all HE patients studied so far, isolated ghosts and membrane skeletons retain the elliptocytic or poikilocytic shape of the parent red cells[193] (Fig. 115-15). The membrane skeletons isolated from individuals with HE are unstable when exposed to mechanical shaking[500] or shear stress[501] (Fig. 115-16). During the past decade a large number of such defects have been defined.

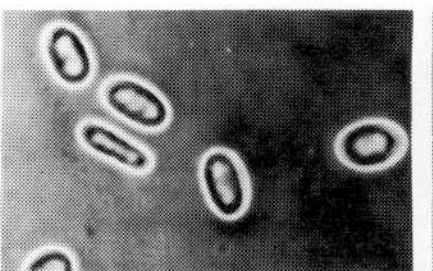
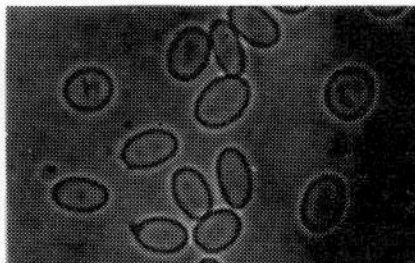
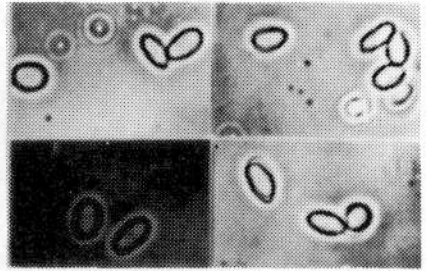

FIG. 115-15. Morphology of HE red cells (*left*), ghosts (*center*), and membrane skeletons (*right*). Essentially all the elliptocytic ghosts form elliptocytic membrane skeletons. *(From Tomaselli, John, and Lux.[193] Used by permission of the* Proceedings of the National Academy of Science of the United States of America.*)*

Methods to Define Abnormal Spectrin Structure and Function in HE. A number of techniques have been utilized to define and analyze the abnormalities of spectrin in HE. These include assays of the thermal sensitivity of spectrin, of spectrin oligomerization, and of mechanical fragility of membranes or membrane skeletons; two-dimensional peptide mapping; and RT-PCR followed by subcloning and nucleic acid sequencing to identify the precise mutations.

Thermal Sensitivity of Spectrin. It has been known for more than 130 years that red cells heated to temperatures approaching 50°C for short periods become unstable and fragment spontaneously.[497] More recent work shows that this phenomenon is probably due to denaturation of spectrin. Normal spectrin denatures at 49°C (10-min exposure),[193,502] and normal red cells fragment at the same temperature.[193]

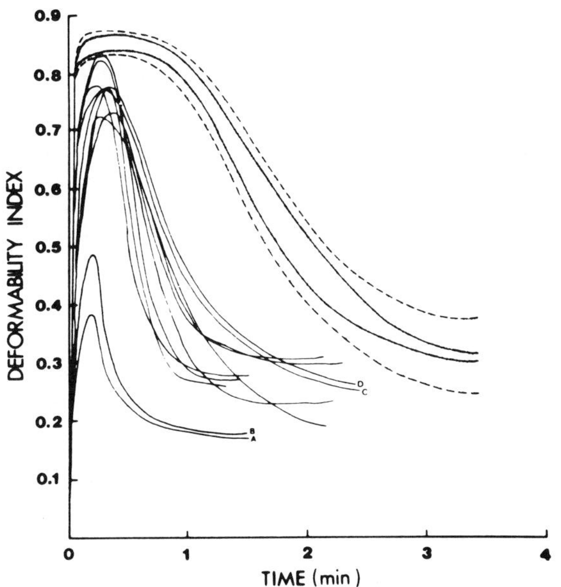

FIG. 115-16. Increased mechanical fragility of red-cell membranes from patients with various elliptocytic disorders. Isolated membranes are resealed and subjected to a constant, high shear stress in a laser diffraction viscometer (ektacytometer). The deformability signal (deformability index) that the instrument provides progressively declines as the deformable cells are sheared into more spheroidal, less deformable fragments. The fragmentation rate for normal cells is shown by the shaded area within the dashed lines. The two curves in this area are from patients with elliptocytosis (60 percent) secondary to myelofibrosis. The curves with intermediate increases in fragmentation are from patients with the typical mild form of common HE due to defects in spectrin self-association (unlabeled curves) or to partial deficiency of protein 4.1 (*C, D*). Two patients with homozygous HE due to absence of protein 4.1 (*A, B*) show the greatest membrane fragility. Patients with hereditary pyropoikilocytosis have very similar curves. *(From Mohandas et al.[59] Used by permission of* Blood.*)*

As noted earlier, all patients with HPP (by definition) and some patients with other forms of HE have thermally sensitive red cells. Hereditary pyropoikilocytes and red cells from infants with mild HE and poikilocytosis fragment after 10 min at 44 to 46°C.[467,476] Red cells from some but not all patients with mild HE fragment at 47 to 48°C.[193] As expected, purified spectrin from these red cells is also heat-sensitive.[193,502] The thermal instability of HE red cells and spectrin is either present or absent in all the affected patients in a kindred.[193,476] This increased thermal sensitivity was the first clue that spectrin was abnormal in many patients with HE and HPP.

Abnormal Spectrin Oligomerization. Thirty percent of patients with HE and all patients thus far tested with HPP have a defect in their ability to associate the dimer form to tetramers and higher-order oligomers (Fig. 115-17). Abnormally high proportions of spectrin dimer are present in 0°C spectrin extracts.[444,503-505] At 0°C the equilibrium between spectrin dimer and tetramer is greatly slowed, virtually frozen.[70] If spectrin is extracted from the membrane at 0°C and carefully protected from warming during separation of dimers, tetramers, and oligomers (usually on nondenaturing polyacrylamide gels), the proportion of each spectrin species reflects its relative proportion on the membrane.[72] As described previously, the head end of the spectrin dimer, consisting of the N-terminus of the α chain and the C-terminus of the β chain, is the functional site for spectrin self-association.[62] The two "extra" helixes (helixes 1 and 2) that extend from the C-terminus of β spectrin engage the "extra" N-terminal helix (helix 3) of the α chain when spectrin associates to tetramers or higher oligomers.[74,75] Abnormalities of α and β spectrin structure have been identified in the kindreds with HE and HPP possessing a defect in spectrin self-association.

Ektacytometry. The ektacytometer, a laser diffraction viscometer, can be used to assess cell deformability as well as membrane fragility in patients with hemolytic disorders.[501]

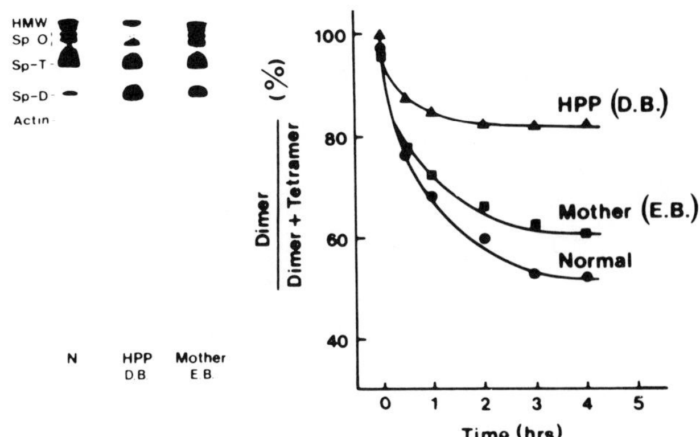

FIG. 115-17. Abnormality in spectrin dimer–tetramer equilibrium in hereditary pyropoikilocytosis. (*Left*) Nondenaturing polyacrylamide gel electrophoresis of spectrin extracts from normal, HPP, and HPP carrier red-cell membranes. The positions of high-molecular-weight spectrin complexes (complex), spectrin tetramers (Sp-T), and spectrin dimers (Sp-D) are indicated. Note the increased proportion of spectrin dimer in the HPP patient (38 percent) and his asymptomatic mother (20 percent) (HPP carrier) compared with normal (5 percent). (*Right*) Kinetics of dimer to tetramer conversion at 30°C of normal, HPP, and HPP carrier spectrin. *(From Liu, Palek, Prchal, and Castlebury.[503] Used by permission of the* Journal of Clinical Investigation.*)*

The cells are subjected to a fixed shear stress, and a deformability index is recorded. The cells are progressively sheared and a curve representing fragment rate is generated. See representative tracings in Fig. 115-16.

Two-Dimensional Domain Maps. Spectrin structure has been analyzed[57,61] by limited tryptic digestion performed at 0°C, then the peptides generated are separated by isoelectric focusing followed by SDS-PAGE in a second dimension. The gels are stained with Coomassie blue and characteristic, reproducible maps are obtained. As described in the section on spectrin, there are five domains on the α chain, designated αI through αV, and four on the β chain, designated βI through βIV. Figure 115-18 shows an example of a normal spectrin domain map. Many defects of spectrin in HE have been identified by this method because of a deficit of a normal peptide, and in most cases, new peptide products were seen. The syndromes are designated by the chain of origin, followed by a superscript consisting of the domain origin and (separated by a slash) the molecular weight of the new peptide produced; for example, $\alpha^{I/74}$ indicates a new or increased amount of the 74-kDa peptide derived from the αI domain. In addition, many defects are now named in the same fashion as the mutant hemoglobins, by the protein followed by the city of residence of the affected proband; for example, $spectrin_{ROUEN}$.

RT-PCR (Reverse Transcription Polymerase Chain Reaction) Subcloning and Sequencing. Reticulocyte mRNA is first isolated from patients with HE. RT-PCR is performed, utilizing specific primers flanking the region suspected to contain the mutation. The cDNA product is subcloned and subjected to nucleic acid sequencing. Several subclones must be obtained and sequenced in the heterozygous patients because on average, only half of the subclones will have the mutant allele. There are many individual variations of this technique that have been used to identify the mutations described in the following sections. In addition, other techniques, such as allele-specific oligonucleotide hybridization, RFLP, direct sequencing of PCR products, and heteroduplex mapping have been utilized in conjunction with these techniques.

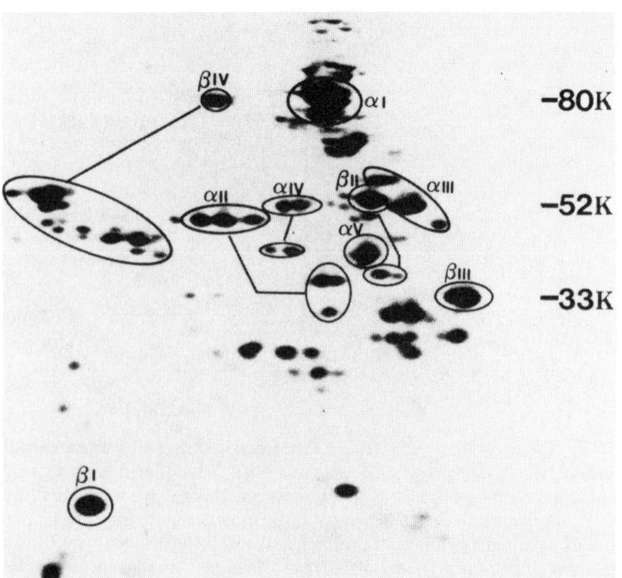

FIG. 115-18 Tryptic domains of spectrin separated by two-dimensional isoelectric focusing, pH 7.2 to 4.5 (*left to right*), followed by SDS gel electrophoresis (*top to bottom*). The major α and β chain domains are labeled. In some cases subdomains derived from further tryptic cleavage of a parent domain are also shown. *(From Marchesi et al.[505] Used by permission of* Blood.)

α Spectrin Defects. Except for the case with $spectrin_{JENDOUBA}$, an elliptocytosis α spectrin variant with normal self-association, all of the other α spectrin mutations with HE result in defective spectrin self-association. The consequence is mechanical instability of the red-cell membrane and disordered structure of the membrane skeleton as assessed by EM. HPP arises from homozygous HE mutations, compound heterozygosity for two different HE mutations, or an HE mutation with a defect in α spectrin synthesis in the other allele (LELY allele). As described in earlier sections, an LELY α spectrin allele arises from skipping of exon 46 and occurs in association with a polymorphism of the $\alpha^{V/41}$ tryptic peptide (exon 40 mutation). Figure 115-19 details how the LELY allele can affect the relative expression of the normal to HE alleles, and thus, the clinical severity. If an HE mutation is on a chromosome bearing the α^{LELY} mutation, a mild defect can be converted into a silent one or a severe one into a mild one. In contrast, a defective HE allele inherited in *trans* (on the opposite chromosome) to the LELY allele results in a more severe clinical condition.

During limited tryptic digestion of normal spectrin, the 80-kDa αI domain, undergoes a second cleavage at Lys45 or Lys48 to produce the 74-kDa domain. When abnormally high quantities of this 74-kDa peptide result in excess of the 80-kDa domain, the $\alpha^{I/74}$ abnormality is identified. This occurs due to a mutation in helix 3 of repeat segment α′. This helix 3 is critical in the head to head α to β contact (see Fig. 115-3). Several point mutations have been identified in repeat segment α′ that give rise to $\alpha^{I/74}$ or $\alpha^{I/78}$. In fact, four different

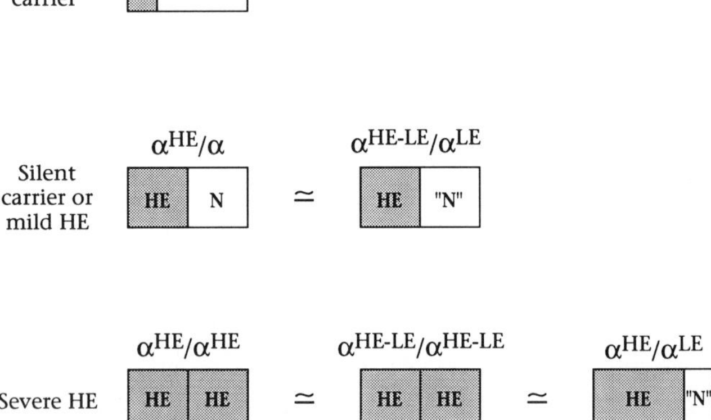

FIG. 115-19 Effect of the α^{LELY} spectrin allele on clinical HE syndromes. The boxes indicate the relative proportions of the products of the normal or mutant α spectrin alleles. The shaded area indicates the HE phenotype and the white area, the normal phenotype. The quotation marks around the N indicate that the allele does not bear a mutation that would cause HE, but does have the LELY polymorphism. A silent carrier state will result if the HE mutation is inherited in *cis* to the LELY allele. Mild HE or a silent carrier state will arise if both the mutant HE allele and the non-HE alleles bear the LELY polymorphism, similar to a heterozygous HE mutation. Severe HE can result from compound heterozygous or homozygous expression of HE mutations, with or without the LELY polymorphisms in *cis* to both alleles, or if the LELY polymorphism is inherited in *trans* to the allele carrying the HE mutation. LELY is indicated as LE in the figure.

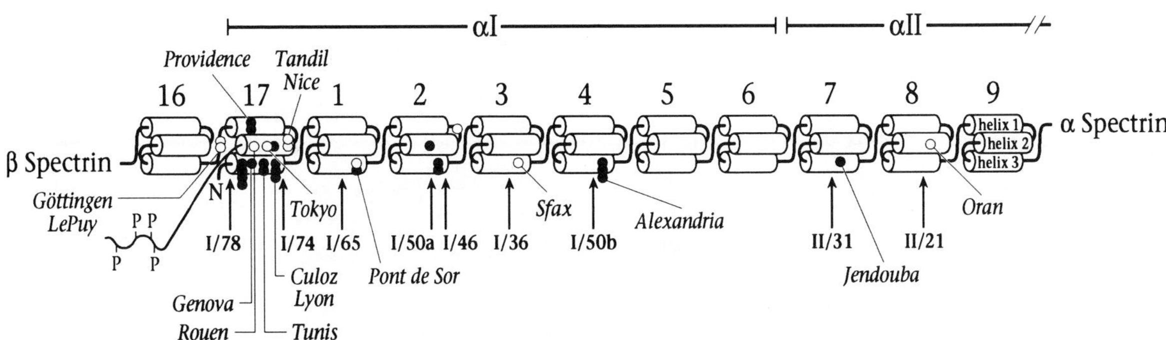

FIG. 115-20 Spectrin mutations causing defective self-association and HE. The diagram illustrates the spectrin α to β contact site (as in Fig. 115-3C) between associating heterodimers. The arrows indicate the areas of mutations giving rise to the types of α spectrin variants designated by the abnormal tryptic peptides. The sites of the named β spectrin mutations are indicated, as are a few of the named α spectrin variants. ***(Adapted from Gallagher PG, Tse WT, Forget BG: Semin Perinatol 14:351, 1992. Used by permission.)***

mutations have been identified at codon 28, evidently a "hot spot" for mutations (see Table 115-3).

The majority of the spectrin mutations are characterized by a decrease in or absence of the normal αI 80-kDa domain and appearance of smaller proteolytic fragments, including: (1) a new 78-kDa peptide ($\alpha^{I/78}$ defect),[506] (2) a new 74-kDa peptide ($\alpha^{I/74}$ defect),[444,507,509-511] (3) a new 65-kDa (or 68-kDa) peptide ($\alpha^{I/65}$ or $\alpha^{I/68}$ respectively),[474,511-513] (4) a new 61-kDa peptide ($\alpha^{I/61}$ defect),[514] (5) two new 46- and 17-kDa (or, in other reports, 50 and 21-kDa) peptides ($\alpha^{I/46}$ or $\alpha^{I/50a}$ defect),[444,505,511,515] (6) another 50-kDa peptide with a more basic isoelectric point ($\alpha^{I/50b}$ defect),[516] (7) a defect with two new peptides ($\alpha^{I/42\text{-}43}$ defect),[517] or (8) a new peptide of 36-kDa ($\alpha^{I/36}$ defect).[518] The precise mutations responsible for hereditary elliptocytosis have been elucidated in the majority of the types of α chain variants. Figure 115-20 indicates the positions of many of these mutations. Of interest, a large number of the mutations occur in the helix 3 segments (see Table 115-3).

The $\alpha^{I/78}$ defect can arise due to changes in codons 41 or 45, CGG to TGG (Arg to Trp, R41W) (spectrin$_{TUNIS}$[519]) or AGG to AGT (Arg to Ser, R45S),[520] respectively. The $\alpha^{I/74}$ defect can arise from four mutations in codon 28 or from changes in codons 46, 48, or 49 (all helix 3 mutations) (see Table 115-3).[521-524] Interestingly, the mutations arising in codon 45 or 48 result in severe HPP, whereas those arising in codons 41, 46, or 49 result in a milder HE condition. The $\alpha^{I/65}$ defect is a mild condition arising from the duplication of Leu154[516,526] or in spectrin$_{PONTE\ DE\ SOR}$ from a Gly151 to Asp (G151D) mutation.[527] The mutation responsible for the $\alpha^{I/61}$ defect has not yet been defined. The $\alpha^{I/50a}$ defect results in changes to proline, an amino acid known to restrict mobility: L207P,[544] L260P[516,545] or S261P.[516,545] The $\alpha^{I/50b}$ defect arises by three mechanisms: H469P,[546] E471P[516,545] or deletion of His 469 (ΔH469) (spectrin$_{ALEXANDRIA}$).[547] The $\alpha^{I/36}$ mutation (spectrin$_{SFAX}$) results from deletion of codons 363 to 371 (helix 3 or repeat α4) due to activation of a cryptic splice site.[518]

Two variants leading to an abnormality in the αII domain have been associated with HE: the $\alpha^{II/31}$ defect (spectrin$_{JENDOUBA}$)[569] and the $\alpha^{II/21}$ defect (spectrin$_{ORAN}$).[570] These are both associated with asymptomatic HE in the heterozygous state. The latter arises due to a deletion of amino acids 822 to 862, from a mutation A → G in the acceptor splice site for exon 18, resulting in skipping of exon 18.[570]

Another abnormality is a short α spectrin chain (234 kDa).[463,528] Although spectrin containing this mutant chain also fails to properly self-associate, studies so far surprisingly suggest the primary defect may lie at the opposite end of the molecule, in the αIV domain.[463]

Several clinical syndromes[529] are associated with these α-chain defects (see Table 115-3). There appears to be an inverse relationship between the distance of a mutation from the self-association site and the clinical severity. In general, the closer to the self-association site, the greater the functional defect, and the more severe the clinical illness. For example, the $\alpha^{I/74}$ defect produces severe disease with a greater proportion of spectrin dimers. In the homozygous state, hemolysis is life-threatening. In contrast, homozygous $\alpha^{I/65}$ spectrin is associated with only mild hemolysis and a lesser defect in spectrin self-association. The $\alpha^{I/46}$ mutation appears to be of intermediate severity.

In addition, HPP patients have also been found to be spectrin-deficient (~30 percent less than the normal quantity),[479] which can be attributed to one of two mechanisms: (1) reduced synthesis of α spectrin or (2) increased degradation of mutant spectrin prior to assembly on the membrane.[530]

β Spectrin Defects. The β spectrin abnormalities include truncations, which delete various amounts of the C-terminus, as well as missense mutations (see Table 115-3). Both groups of mutations alter spectrin self-association. For example, for one of the β spectrin truncated variants, $\beta^{220/216}$, where ~4 kDa is lost from the C-terminus, low-temperature spectrin extracts contain increased spectrin dimer [~50 percent of the dimer–tetramer pool as compared with normal (5 to 10 percent)] and nearly all of the abnormal β^{216} spectrin is found in the dimer fraction (Fig. 115-21),[531-533] indicating that β^{216} is responsible for the functional defect. Seven different defects causing truncated β spectrin chains have thus been identified on a molecular level, named on the basis of the city of origin of the propositus: spectrin$_{ROUEN}$,[534] spectrin$_{NICE}$[535] spectrin$_{TANDIL}$,[536] and spectrin$_{TOKYO}$,[537] due to frameshift mutations; spectrin$_{LEPUY}$[538] or spectrin$_{GÖTTINGEN}$,[539] due to exon skipping; and lastly, spectrin$_{YAMAGATA}$ (a 210-kDa variant for which the mechanism is as yet undefined).[540] The mutations are localized within helix 2 of repeat segment β 17 and can lead to the $\alpha^{I/74}$ abnormality on limited tryptic domain maps. Moreover, missense mutations in this same region of β 17 including A2053P,[74] S2019P (spectrin$_{PROVIDENCE}$)[541] or A2018G (spectrin$_{CAGLIARI}$)[542] can lead to the $\alpha^{I/74}$ abnormality on domain maps and severe HPP in the homozygous state, or in the case of homozygosity for spectrin$_{PROVIDENCE}$, to lethal hydrops fetalis.

Clinically, patients with the β spectrin truncations have mild to moderate hemolysis with rounded elliptocytes and

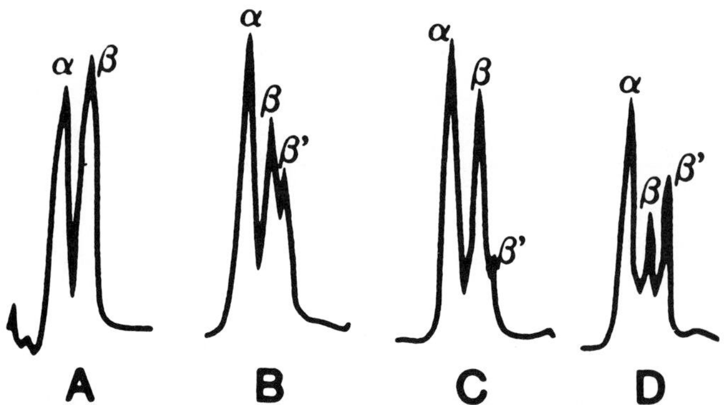

FIG. 115-21 Densitometric tracings of SDS polyacrylamide gels of spectrin from a patient with HE due to deletion of the C-terminal end of the spectrin β chain. *A*. Normal spectrin extract. *B*. Patient's spectrin extract. *C* and *D*. Patient's purified spectrin tetramer and dimer, respectively. Note the presence of an abnormally small (214 kDa) β spectrin component in all of the patient's spectrin preparations, but especially in the spectrin dimer fraction in panel *D*. This suggests that the mutant spectrin cannot participate to a normal extent in spectrin dimer self-assocation. *(From Palek.*[584] *Used by permission of* Clinics in Haematology.*)*

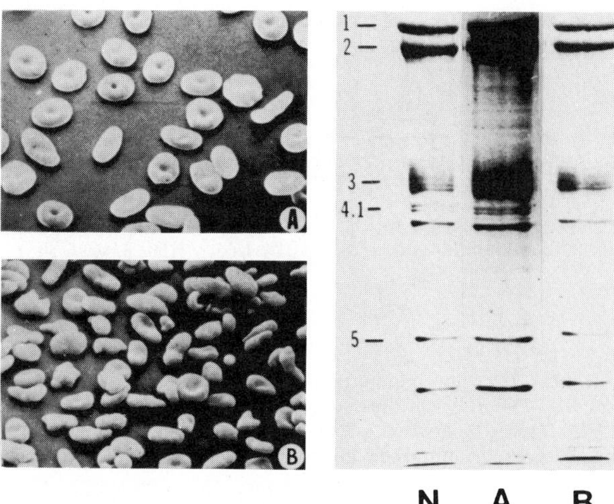

FIG. 115-22 Deficiency of protein 4.1 in HE. (*Right*) SDS polyacrylamide gels (Laemmli system, see Fig. 115-1) of red-cell membranes from a normal individual (N), a heterozygous parent with 50 percent of the normal amount of protein 4.1 (*A*), and a homozygous-deficient daughter (*B*). Note that both components of protein 4.1 (4.1a and 4.1b) are decreased (relative to protein 3) in the parent and missing in the daughter, and that other proteins are present in normal concentrations. (*Left*) Scanning EM of red cells from the parent (*A*) and daughter (*B*). Note that the homozygous-deficient daughter shows marked fragmentation, spherocytosis, elliptocytosis, and bizarre poikilocytosis, while the heterozygous-deficient parent displays only modest elliptocytosis. *(From Tchernia, Mohandas, and Shohet.*[475] *Used by permission of the* Journal of Clinical Investigation.*)*

some fragmented red cells. Where measured, osmotic fragility is increased, suggesting that these disorders should be classified as examples of spherocytic elliptocytosis. Thermal stability is unusual; the red cells become echinocytic at 47°C (normal, 49°C), but do not fragment.

Protein 4.1 Deficiency. In several reported kindreds with HE, protein 4.1 was either partially or fully deficient[548-555] (Fig. 115-22). This variant appears to be more common in patients of French and North African descent.[548-550] Protein 4.1 is decreased about 50 percent in heterozygotes and is absent in homozygotes. Clinically, the heterozygotes have mild HE with prominent elliptocytosis, no red-cell fragmentation, and little or no hemolysis. In contrast, homozygotes have a severe transfusion-dependent hemolytic anemia with marked osmotic fragility, normal thermal stability, bizarre red-cell morphology, and a very good response to splenectomy.[548] The homozygous protein 4.1–deficient membranes are very fragile, but stability can be restored by reconstitution with purified protein 4.1[551] or even by a recombinant peptide containing the region critical for spectrin–actin binding.[556]

Molecular genetic studies in one Algerian kindred show that the disease is caused by a 318-bp deletion that eliminates the initiation codon that gives rise to the 80-kDa erythroid isoform of protein 4.1.[553,557] A second family has an altered downstream initiation codon (ATG to AGG, protein 4.1_{MADRID}),[558] which presumably blocks expression of the erythroid protein 4.1 isoform.

In addition to deficiency in protein 4.1, some of these patients are also missing (partially) other proteins, such as protein 4.9[548] or GPC.[552,555] Patients with complete protein 4.1 deficiency have only 9 percent of the normal amount of glycophorin C. This lends strong support to the theory that protein 4.1 binds to GPC in the membrane.[559]

Structural and Functional Defects of Protein 4.1. Three structural defects of protein 4.1 have been described. One occurred in two generations of a French family with mild HE and moderate chronic hemolysis.[560] The disorder is characterized by prominent elliptocytosis with mechanically fragile membranes. Osmotic and thermal stability and spectrin self-association are normal. SDS gels show a 50 percent decrease in protein 4.1 and two faint new bands, 65 and 68 kDa, that are immunologically related to protein 4.1.[560] Functionally, the protein 4.1 from the patient bound to a crude mixture of normal spectrin and actin only 40 percent as well as normal. A similar variant has been observed in dogs (76/78 kDa).[561] Molecular studies demonstrate that protein $4.1^{68/65}$ is caused by a deletion of 80 amino acids, Lys407 to Gly486,[562,563] which includes the entire spectrin–actin binding domain (Lys407 to Glu427), whereas the canine protein $4.1^{78/76}$ results from a deletion of precisely the 21 amino acid peptide that arises by alternative splicing of a 63-bp exon critical for spectrin–actin binding.[556,564] The second defect has been identified in a single kindred with mild HE. The patients are heterozygous for a large (95 kDa) variant of protein 4.1, designated protein 4.1^{95}, that comigrates with protein 3 and is detected with immunoblots.[562,563] This anomaly results from the internal duplication of a 369-bp segment consisting of three exons that encode Lys407 to Gln529, thus producing two spectrin–actin binding domains. Fortunately, the insertion does not markedly alter spectrin–actin binding, which probably accounts for its relatively mild clinical phenotype.

The third variant, designated $4.1_{PRESLES}$ is a shortened protein 4.1 that migrates as a doublet with apparent sizes of 73 and 74 kDa.[565] This is caused by skipping of one exon that encodes 34 amino acids near the beginning of the C-terminal 22/24-kDa domain.[566] The condition is clinically silent, even in the homozygous state, and so technically is a benign variant of protein 4.1.

Deficiency of GPC. Deficiency of this minor sialoglycoprotein occurs in homozygous protein 4.1 deficiency, as described above, and in patients with the rare Leach phenotype of Gerbich-negative (Ge^-) red cells. The Gerbich antigen system is carried on GPC and GPD. Patients with the Leach subtype of Ge⁻ lack both GPC and GPD.[567,568] These patients, but not other patients with Ge⁻ red cells (who lack the antigen but not GPC and GPD), have mild elliptocytosis[567,568] with increased osmotic fragility (i.e., a form of spherocytic HE). Their red cells contain only 30 percent of the normal amount of protein 4.1,[559] which may account for the elliptocytic phenotype. This and other information, discussed earlier, strongly suggests that GPC is an important binding site for protein 4.1 in normal red cells. In contrast to GPC deficiency, patients lacking GPA, GPB, or both are entirely asymptomatic and have normal red-cell morphology.

Defects of Band 3.

Band $3_{MEMPHIS}$. The band $3_{MEMPHIS}$ polymorphism arises from the point mutation Lys56 to Glu (K56E) (see Table 115-3).[571,572] It results in a change in the electrophoretic mobility such that the variant band 3 migrates more slowly and the N-terminal chymotryptic fragment has an apparent molecular weight on SDS gels of 63,000 instead of 60,000.[573] Six to seven percent of the normal population is heterozygous for this variant, but the polymorphism is entirely silent, even in the homozygous state.

Southeast Asia Ovalocytosis. SAO was described as a clinical entity in the preceding section, where the resistance of the ovalocytes to invasion by *P. falciparum* was highlighted. Patients are heterozygous for a band 3 variant designated band 3_{SAO} which has an electrophoretic migration identical to band $3_{MEMPHIS}$. Molecular genetic analysis has revealed two abnormalities in the SAO allele: the first being the band $3_{MEMPHIS}$ polymorphism, K56E, and the second, the deletion of amino acid residues 400 to 408 at the junction between the cytoplasmic and membrane domains.[574-576] This deletion removes part of the first transmembrane α helix, which is thought to serve as an internal signal sequence, and probably disrupts the structure of the membrane domain.[577] As a consequence, band 3_{SAO} blocks anion transport activity. This may explain why homozygous band 3_{SAO} is not observed (presumably lethal).

As noted earlier, SAO red cells are extraordinarily rigid, the most rigid red cells known. This impedes entry of malarial parasites and accounts for the high frequency of the mutations in the indigenous populations of Southeast Asia. How the 400 to 408 deletion causes this rigidity is less clear. Liu and his colleagues find that band 3_{SAO} binds more ankyrin than normal, perhaps reflecting a tendency for band 3_{SAO} to associate to the ankyrin-binding tetrameric state.[487] Increased ankyrin–band 3 attachments could account for the observed rigidity and for the decreased lateral and rotational mobility of band 3 in SAO red cells[487]; however, the enhanced ankyrin binding of band 3_{SAO} has not been detected by others.[577,578] An alternative hypothesis, advanced by several groups,[575,577,578] is that the SAO deletion may make the flexible section of the cytoplasmic domain just proximal to the membrane more rigid, which would tend to extend the long cytoplasmic domain of band 3 and cause it to become entangled in the spectrin network. In fact, Moriyama and colleagues[577] have observed that band 3 is nonspecifically trapped in isolated skeletons from SAO red cells, which supports this hypothesis. It is reasonable to expect that such entanglement would impede the movement of spectrin chains when the membrane is stretched, leading to membrane rigidity. Remarkably, the rigid SAO red cells negotiate the circulation normally and do not lead to impaired tissue perfusion or hemolysis. Finally, it should be noted that band 3_{SAO} also shows increased phosphorylation of tyrosines in the cytoplasmic domain.[487,579] The cause and consequences of this modification are unknown.

Hereditary Acanthocytosis. One band 3 variant associated with acanthocytosis has been described (Pro868→Leu, P868L) with increased anion transport activity, decreased ankyrin binding sites, and slightly slowed mobility on SDS gels.[580,580a] The effect on ankyrin binding might reflect changes in band 3 oligomerization or indicate previously unrecognized interactions between the C-terminal end of the protein, which lies inside the membrane, and the ankyrin-binding site on the N-terminal, cytoplasmic domain.

Other Considerations

As the previous sections illustrate, HE and HPP are very heterogeneous disorders associated with a large number of molecular defects. In some kindreds, the actual amino acid sequence abnormalities have been identified. However, despite our knowledge of the defective structure and function of the specific membrane proteins, we still do not understand how those abnormalities lead to an elliptical shape.

Any explanation of the various forms of HE must consider the fact that nucleated elliptocytic precursors are round, and elongate or fragment only gradually as they circulate. This process resembles the gradual development of spherocytosis in hereditary spherocytes and aging normal cells, and is consistent with the concept that the change in shape is secondary to the intrinsic structural instability of the skeleton. According to this hypothesis, mild skeletal defects lead to elliptocytosis by increasing membrane plasticity (i.e., plastic deformation). As noted earlier, normal red cells rapidly regain their shape if they are transiently deformed, but they remain misshapen if the distortion is maintained for long periods (minutes to hours).[197,198] Presumably, dynamic skeletal interactions realign in response to stress. In a cell with weakened skeletal interactions, like the hereditary elliptocyte, this process would be accelerated. In vivo, red cells are deformed into a stable elliptical or torpedo shape in very small capillaries and are sometimes detained for short periods. It is easy to imagine how this distortion, repeated thousands of times per day, could cause red cells gradually to elongate and assume their characteristic elliptical shape. Whether this is, in fact, the pathophysiological mechanism remains to be proved.

Red cells with more severe skeletal defects would also tend to elongate, but if skeletal instability were sufficiently compromised, they would be unable to withstand the shear stresses experienced in the normal circulation, and fragmentation or combinations of fragmentation and shape change induced by plastic deformation (i.e., bizarre-shaped poikilocytes) would predominate (see Fig. 115-14G). This process would explain the nearly identical morphology observed in homozygous HE and hereditary pyropoikilocytosis and in neonates with mild HE and poikilocytosis.

In spite of the uncertainties about the molecular mechanisms involved in the different subtypes of HE, the available information suggests that red-cell death in the various hemolytic forms follows a similar pathway. In all cases hemolysis is markedly ameliorated by splenectomy, and where examined, splenic pathology shows cordal congestion essentially identical to that observed in HS.[462,481,482,581] As in HS, the specific pathophysiologic mechanism(s) responsible for splenic sequestration and red-cell destruction remain to be defined.

REFERENCES

1. Liu S-C, Derick LH: Molecular anatomy of the red cell membrane skeleton: Structure-function relationships. *Semin Hematol* **29:**231, 1992.
2. Cohen CM, Gascard P: Regulation and post translational modification of erythrocyte membrane and membrane-skeleton proteins. *Semin Hematol* **29:**244, 1992.
3. Gilligan DM, Bennett V: The junctional complex of the membrane skeleton. *Semin Hematol* **30:**74, 1993.
4. Peters LL, Lux SE: Ankyrins: Structure and function in normal cells and hereditary spherocytes. *Semin Hematol* **30:**85, 1993.
5. Cohen CM, Dotimas E, Korsgren C: Human erythrocyte membrane protein band 4.2 (pallidin). *Semin Hematol* **30:**119, 1993.
6. Palek J, Jarolim P: Clinical expression and laboratory detection of red cell membrane protein mutations. *Semin Hematol* **30:**249, 1993.
7. Gallagher PG, Forget BG: Spectrin genes in health and disease. *Semin Hematol* **30:**4, 1993.
8. Delaunay J, Dhermy D: Mutations involving the spectrin heterodimer contact site: Clinical expression and alterations in specific function. *Semin Hematol* **30:**21, 1993.
9. Schwartz RS, Chiu DT, Lubin B: Plasma membrane phospholipid organization in human erythrocytes. *Curr Top Hematol* **5:**63, 1985.
10. Fukuda M: Molecular genetics of the glycophorin A gene cluster. *Semin Hematol* **30:**138, 1993.
11. Cartron J-P, Le Van Kim C, Colin Y: Glycophorin C and related glycophorins: Structure, function, and regulation. *Semin Hematol* **30:**152, 1993.
12. Tanner MJA: Molecular and cellular biology of the erythrocyte anion exchanger (AE1). *Semin Hematol* **30:**34, 1993.
13. Lande WM, Mentzer WC: Haemolytic anaemia associated with increased cation permeability. *Clin Haematol* **14:**89, 1985.
14. Verkleij AJ, Zwaal RFA, Roelofsen B, Confurius P, Kastelijn D, van Deenen LLM: The asymmetric distribution of phospholipids in the human red cell membrane. A combined study using phospholipase and freeze-etch electron microscopy. *Biochim Biophys Acta* **323:**178, 1973.
15. Low MG, Finean JB: Modification of erythrocyte membranes by a purified phosphatidylinositol-specific phospholipase C (Staphylococcus aureus). *Biochem J* **162:**235, 1972.
16. Blair L, Bittman R: Cholesteol distribution between the two halves of the lipid bilayer of human erythrocyte ghost membranes. *J Biol Chem* **253:**8366, 1978.
17. Fairbanks G, Steck TL, Wallach DFH: Electrophoretic analysis of the major polypeptides of the human erythrocyte membrane. *Biochemistry* **10:**2606, 1971.
18. Ferrel JE Jr, Huestis WH: Phosphoinositide metabolism and the morphology of human erythrocytes. *J Cell Biol* **98:**1992, 1984.
19. Van Deenen LLM, DeGier J: Lipids of the red blood cell membrane, in Surgenor DM (ed): *The Red Blood Cell,* 2d ed. New York, Academic, 1974, p 148.
20. Sweeley CC, Dawson G: Lipids of the erythrocyte, in Jamieson GA, Greenwalt TJ (eds): *Red Cell Membrane Structure and Function*. Philadelphia, Lippincott, 1969, p 172.
21. Cooper RA: Lipids of human red cell membranes: Normal composition and variability in disease. *Semin Hematol* **7:**96, 1970.
22. Savvides P, Shalev O, John KM, Lux SE: Combined spectrin and ankyrin deficiency is common in autosomal dominant hereditary spherocytosis. *Blood* **82:**2953, 1993.
23. Pinder JC, Gratzer WB: Structural and dynamic states of actin in the erythrocyte. *J Cell Biol* **96:**768, 1983.
24. Steck TL: The organization of proteins in the human red cell membrane. *J Cell Biol* **62:**1, 1974.
25. Inaba M, Gupta KC, Kuwabara M, Takahashi T, Benz EJ Jr, Maede Y: Deamidation of human erythrocyte protein 4.1: Possible role in aging. *Blood* **79:**3355, 1992.
26. Conboy JG: Structure, function, and molecular genetics of erythroid membrane skeletal protein 4.1 in normal and abnormal red blood cells. *Semin Hematol* **30:**58, 1993.
27. Bercovich T, Gitler C: 5-[125I]iodonaphthyl azide, a reagent to determine the penetration of proteins into the lipid bilayer of biological membranes. *Biochemistry* **17:**1484, 1978.
28. Kahane I, Gitler C: Red cell membrane glycophorin labelling from within the lipid bilayer. *Science* **201:**351, 1978.
29. Weinstein RS, Khodadad JK, Steck TL: The band 3 protein intramembrane particle of the human red blood cell, in Lassen UV, Ussing HH, Wieth JO (eds): *Membrane Transport in Erythrocytes*. Copenhagen, Munksgaard, 1980, p 35.
30. Gahmberg CG, Tauren G. Virtanen I, Wartiovaara J: Distribution of glycophorin on the surface of human erythrocyte membranes and its association with intramembrane particles: An immunochemical and freeze fracture study of normal and En(a-) erythrocytes, in Lux SE, Marchesi VT, Fox CF (eds): *Normal and Abnormal Red Cell Membranes*. New York, Alan R. Liss, 1979, p 59.
31. Nigg EA, Bron C, Giradet M, Cherry RJ: Band 3-glycophorin A association in erythrocyte membranes demonstrated by combining protein diffusion measurements with antibody-induced cross-linking. *Biochemistry* **19:**1887, 1980.
32. Daniels GL, Shaw M-A, Judson PA, Reid ME, Anstee DJ, Colpitts P, Moore BPL, Cornwall S.: A family demonstrating inheritance of the Leach phenotype, a Gerbich-negative phenotype associated with elliptocytosis. *Vox Sang* **50:**117, 1986.
33. Telen JM, Le Van Kim C, Chung A, Cartron J-P, Colin Y: Molecular basis for elliptocytosis associated with glycophorin C and glycophorin D deficiency in the Leach phenotype. *Blood* **78:**1603, 1991.
34. Sondag D, Alloisio N, Blanchard D, Dueluzeau M-T, Colonna P, Bachir D, Bley C, Cartron J-P: Gerbich reactivity in 4.1 (-) hereditary elliptocytosis and protein 4.1 level in blood group Gerbich deficiency. *Br J Haematol* **65:**43, 1987.
35. Yu J, Steck TL: Isolation and characterization of band 3, the predominant polypeptide of the human erythrocyte membrane. *J Biol Chem* **250:**9170, 1975.
36. Mueller TJ, Li Y-T, Morrison M: Effect of endo-beta-galactosidase on intact human erythrocytes. *J Biol Chem* **254:**8103, 1979.
37. Walder JA, Chatterjee R, Steck TL, Low PS, Musso GF, Kaiser ET, Rogers PH, Arnone A: The interaction of hemoglobin with the cytoplasmic domain of band 3 of the human erythrocyte membrane. *J Biol Chem* **259:**10238, 1984.
38. Waugh SM, Walder JA, Low PS: Partial characterization of the copolymerization reaction of erythrocyte membrane band 3 with hemichromes. *Biochemistry* **26:**1777, 1987.
39. Kannan R, Labotka R, Low PS: Isolation and characterization of the hemichrome-stabilized membrane protein aggregates from sickle erythrocytes. Major site of autologous antibody binding. *J Biol Chem* **263:**13766, 1988.
40. Pasternack GR, Anderson RA, Leto TL, Marchesi VT: Interactions between protein 4.1 and band 3. An alternative binding site for an element of the membrane skeleton. *J Biol Chem* **260:**3676, 1985.
41. Rybicki AC, Heath R, Wolf JL, Lubin B, Schwartz RS: Deficiency of protein 4.2 in erythrocytes from a patient with a Coombs negative hemolytic anemia. Evidence for a role of protein 4.2 in stabilizing ankyrin on the membrane. *J Clin Invest* **81:**893, 1988.
42. Bennett V, Stenbuck PJ: The membrane attachment protein for spectrin is associated with band 3 in human erythrocyte membranes. *Nature* **280,** 468, 1979.
43. Bennett V, Stenbuck PJ: Association between ankyrin and the cytoplasmic domain of band 3 isolated from the human erythrocyte membrane. *J Biol Chem* **255:**6424, 1980.
44. Hargreaves WR, Giedd KN, Verkleij A, Branton D: Reassociation of ankyrin with band 3 in erythrocyte membranes and in lipid vesicles. *J Biol Chem* **255:**11965, 1980.
45. Kliman HJ, Steck TL: Association of glyceraldehyde-3-phosphate dehydrogenase with the human red cell membrane. A kinetic analysis. *J Biol Chem* **255:**6314, 1980.
46. Tsai I-H, Prasanna-Murthy SN, Steck TL: Effect of red cell membrane binding on the catalytic activity of glyceraldehyde-3-phosphate dehydrogenase with the human red cell membrane. *J Biol Chem* **259:**1438, 1982.
47. Higashi T, Richards CS, Uyeda K: The interaction of

phosphofructokinase with erythrocyte membranes. *J Biol Chem* **254:**9542, 1979.

48. Jenkins JD, Madden DP, Steck TL: Association of phosphofructokinase and aldolase with the membrane of the intact erythrocyte. *J Biol Chem* **259:**9374, 1984.
49. De BK, Kirtley ME: Interaction of phosphoglycerate kinase with human erythrocyte membranes. *J Biol Chem* **252:**6715, 1977.
50. Lombardo CR, Willardson BM, Low PS: Localization of the protein 4.1-binding site on the cytoplasmic domain of erythrocyte membrane band 3. *J Biol Chem* **267:**9540, 1992.
51. Brosius FC, Alper SL, Garcia AM, Lodish HF: The major kidney band 3 transcript predicts an aminoterminal truncated band 3 polypeptide. *J Biol Chem* **264:**7784, 1989.
52. Sheetz MP: Integral membrane protein interaction with Triton cytoskeletons of erythrocytes. *Biochim Biophys Acta* **557:**122, 1979.
53. Yu J, Fischman DA, Steck TL: Selective solubilization of proteins and phospholipids of red blood cell membranes by nonionic detergents. *J Supramol Struct* **1:**233, 1973.
54. Dunn MJ, Kemp RB, Maddy AH: The similarity of the two high-molecular weight polypeptides of erythrocyte spectrin. *Biochem J* **173:**197, 1978.
55. Anderson JM: Structural studies on human spectrin. Comparison of subunits and fragmentation of native spectrin. *J Biol Chem* **254:**939, 1979.
56. Speicher DW, Marchesi VT: Erythrocyte spectrin is comprised of many homologous triple helical segments. *Nature* **311:**177, 1984.
57. Speicher DW, Morrow JS, Knowles WJ, Marchesi VT: A structural model of human erythrocyte spectrin: Alignment of chemical and functional domains. *J Biol Chem* **257:**9093, 1982.
58. Elgsaeter A: Human spectrin. I. A classical light scattering study. *Biochim Biophys Acta* **536:**235, 1978.
59. Shotton DM, Burke BE, Branton D: The molecular structure of human erythrocyte spectrin. Biophysical and electron microscopic studies. *J Mol Biol* **131:**303, 1979.
60. Calvert R, Ungewickell E, Gratzer W: A conformational study of human spectrin. *Eur J Biochem* **107:**363, 1980.
61. Speicher DW, Morrow JS, Knowles WJ, Marchesi VT: Identification of proteolytically resistant domains of human erythrocyte spectrin. *Proc Natl Acad Sci USA* **77:**5673, 1980.
62. Morrow JS, Speicher DW, Knowles WJ, Hsu CJ, Marchesi VT: Identification of functional domains of human erythrocyte spectrin. *Proc Natl Acad Sci USA* **77:**6592, 1980.
63. Sahr KE, Laurila P, Kotula L, Scarpa AL, Coupal E, Leto TL, Linnenbach AJ, Winkelmann JC, Speicher DW, Marchesi VT, Curtis PL, Forget BG: The complete cDNA and polypeptide sequences of human erythroid alpha-spectrin. *J Biol Chem* **265:**4434, 1990.
64. Winkelmann JC, Chang J-G, Tse WT, Marchesi VT, Forget BG: Full length sequence of the cDNA for human erythroid beta-spectrin. *J Biol Chem* **265:**11827, 1990.
65. Speicher DW: The present status of erythrocyte spectrin structure: The 106-residue repetitive structure is a basic feature of an entire class of proteins. *J Cell Biochem* **30:**245, 1986.
66. Winograd E, Hume D, Branton D: Phasing the conformational unit of spectrin. *Proc Natl Acad Sci USA* **88:**10788, 1991.
67. Speicher DW, Weglarz L, DeSilva TM: Properties of human red cell spectrin heterodimer (side-to-side) assembly and identification of an essential nucleation site. *J Biol Chem* **267:**14775, 1992.
68. Alloisio N, Morlé L, Maréchal J, Roux A-F, Ducluzeau M-T, Guetarni D, Pothier B, Baklouti F, Ghanem A, Kastally R, Delaunay J: Sp$\alpha^{V/41}$: A common spectrin polymorphism at the α^{IV}-α^{V} domain junction. Relevance to the expression level of hereditary elliptocytosis due to α spectrin variants located in *trans*. *J Clin Invest* **87:**2169, 1991.
69. Wilmotte R, Maréchal J, Morelé L, Baklouti F, Philippe N, Kastally R, Kotula L, Delaunay J, Alloisio N: Low expression allele α^{LELY} of red cell spectrin is associated with mutations in exon 40 ($\alpha^{V/41}$ polymorphism) and intron 45 and with partial skipping of exon 46. *J Clin Invest* **91:**2091, 1993.
70. Ungewickell E, Gratzer W: Self-association of human spectrin. A thermodynamic and kinetic study. *Eur J Biochem* **88:**379, 1978.
71. Morrow JS, Marchesi VT: Self-assembly of spectrin oligomers in vitro: A basis for a dynamic cytoskeleton. *J Cell Biol* **88:**463, 1981.
72. Liu SC, Windisch P, Kim S, Palek J: Oligomeric states of spectrin in normal erythrocyte membranes. Biochemical and electron microscopic studies. *Cell* **37:**587, 1984.
73. Ralston G, Dunbar J, White M: The temperature-dependent dissociation of spectrin. *Biochim Biphys Acta* **491:**345, 1977.
74. Tse WT, Lecomte MC, Costa FF, Garbarz M, Féo C, Boivin P, Dhermy D, Forget BG: Point mutation in the β-spectrin gene associated with $\alpha^{I/74}$ hereditary elliptocytosis. Implications for the mechanism of spectrin dimer self-association. *J Clin Invest* **86:**909, 1990.
75. Speicher DW, DeSilva TM, Speicher KD, Ursitti JA, Hembach P, Weglarz L: Location of the human red cell spectrin tetramer binding site and detection of a related "closed" hairpin loop dimer using proteolytic footprinting. *J Biol Chem* **268:**4227, 1993.
76. Geiduschek JB, Singer SJ: Molecular changes in the membranes of mouse erythroid cells accompanying differentiation. *Cell* **16:**149, 1979.
77. Eisen H, Bach R, Emery R: Induction of spectrin in erythroleukemic cells transformed by Friend virus. *Proc Natl Acad Sci USA* **74:**3898, 1977.
78. Hasthorpe S: Quantification of spectrin-containing erythroid precursor cells in normal and perturbed erythropoiesis. *Exp Hematol* **8:**1001, 1980.
79. Tillack TW, Marchesi SL, Marchesi VT, Steers E Jr: A comparative study of spectrin: A protein isolated from red blood cell membranes. *Biochim Biophys Acta* **200:**125, 1970.
80. Pinder JC, Phethean J, Gratzer WB: Spectrin in primitive erythrocytes. *FEBS Lett* **97:**278, 1978.
81. Dubreuil R, Byers TJ, Branton D, Goldstein CS, Kiehart DP: Drosophila spectrin. I. Characterization of the purified protein. *J Cell Biol* **105:**2095, 1987.
82. Byers TJ, Dubreuil R, Branton D, Kiehart DP, Goldstein LS: Drosophilia spectrin. II. Conserved features of the alpha subunit are revealed by analysis of cDNA clones and fusion proteins. *J Cell Biol* **105:**2103, 1987.
83. Bennett H, Condeelis J: Isolation of an immunoreactive analogue of brain fodrin that is associated with the cell cortex of Dictyostelium amoebae. *Cell Motil Cytoskeleton* **11:**303, 1988.
84. Wessel GM, Chen SW: Molecular identification of spectrin in the sea urchin embryo. *J Cell Biol* **115:**464a, 1991.
85. Michaud D, Guillet GK, Rodgers PA, Charest PM: Identification of a 220 kDa membrane-associated plant cell protein immunologically related to human beta-spectrin. *FEBS Lett* **294:**77, 1991.
86. Winkelmann JC, Forget BG: Erythroid and nonerythroid spectrins. *Blood* **81:**3173, 1993.
87. Huebner K, Palumbo AP, Isobe M, Kozak CA, Monaco S, Rovera G, Croce CM, Curtis PJ: The alpha-spectrin gene is on chromosome 1 in mouse and man. *Proc Natl Acad Sci USA* **82:**3790, 1985.
88. Prchal JT, Morleg BJ, Yoon SH, Coetzer TL, Palek J, Conboy JG, Kan YW: Isolation and characterization of cDNA clones for human erythrocyte beta-spectrin. *Proc Natl Acad Sci USA* **84:**7468, 1987.
89. Moon RT, Lazarides E: Beta-spectrin limits alpha-spectrin assembly on membranes following synthesis in a chicken erythroid cell lysate. *Nature* **305:**62, 1983.
90. Bodine DM, Birkenmeier CS, Barker JE: Spectrin deficient inherited hemolytic anemias in the mouse: Characterization by spectrin synthesis and mRNA activity in reticulocytes. *Cell* **37:**721, 1984.
91. Hanspal M, Yoon S-H, Yu H, Hanspal JS, Lambert S, Palek J, Prchal JT: Molecular basis of spectrin and ankyrin deficiencies in severe hereditary spherocytosis: Evidence implicating a primary defect of ankyrin. *Blood* **77:**165, 1991.
92. Woods CM, Lazarides E: Degradation of unassembled alpha- and beta-spectrin by distinct intracellular pathways: Regulation of spectrin topogenesis by beta-spectrin degradation. *Cell* **40:**959, 1985.
93. Moon RT, Lazarides E: Biogenesis of the avian erythroid

membrane skeleton: Receptor-mediated assembly and stabilization of ankyrin (goblin) and spectrin. *J Cell Biol* **98:**1899, 1984.

94. Puszkin S, Puszkin E, Maimon J, Rouault C, Schook W, Ores C, Kochwa S, Rosenfield R: Alpha-actinin and tropomyosin interaction with a hybrid complex of erythrocyte actin and muscle myosin. *J Biol Chem* **252:**5529, 1977.
95. Tilney LG, Detmers P: Actin in erythrocyte ghosts in its association with spectrin: Evidence for a nonfilamentous form of these two molecules in situ. *J Cell Biol* **66:**508, 1975.
96. Shetevline P: *Mechanisms of Cell Motility. Molecular Aspects of Contractility*. New York, Academic, 1983, p 36.
97. Byers T, Branton D: Visualization of the proteins associations in the erythrocyte membrane skeleton. *Proc Natl Acad Sci USA* **82:**6153, 1985.
98. Fowler VM, Sussmann MA, Miller PG, Flucher BE, Daniels MP: Tropomodulin is associated with the free (pointed) ends of the thin filaments in rat skeletal muscle. *J Cell Biol* **120:**411, 1993.
99. Nakashima K, Beutler E: Comparison of structure and function of human erythrocyte and human muscle actin. *Proc Natl Acad Sci USA* **76:**935, 1979.
100. Ungewickell E, Bennett PM, Calvert R, Ohanian V, Gratzer WB: In vitro formation of a complex between cytoskeletal proteins of the human erythrocyte. *Nature* **280:**811, 1979.
101. Cohen CM, Tyler JM, Branton D: Spectrin-actin associations studied by electron microscopy of shadowed preparations. *Cell* **21:**873, 1980.
102. Karinch AM, Zimmer WE, Goodman SR: The identification and sequence of the actin-binding domain of human red blood cell β spectrin. *J Biol Chem* **265:**11833, 1990.
103. Bresnick AR, Janmey PA, Condeelis J: Evidence that a 27-residue sequence is the actin-binding site of ABP-120. *J Biol Chem* **266:**1991.
104. Cohen CM, Foley SF: The role of band 4.1 in the association of actin with erythrocyte membranes. *Biochem Biophys Acta* **688:**691, 1982.
105. Ohanian V, Wolfe LC, John KM, Pinder JC, Lux SE, Grazer WB: Analysis of the ternary interaction of the red cell membrane skeletal proteins spectrin, actin and protein 4.1. *Biochemistry* **23:**4416, 1984.
106. Tyler JM, Reinhardt BN, Branton D: Associations of erythrocyte membrane proteins. Binding of purified band 2.1 and 4.1 to spectrin. *J Biol Chem* **255:**7034, 1980.
107. Coleman TR, Harris AS, Mische SM, Mooseker MS, Morrow JS: Beta spectrin bestows protein 4.1 sensitivity on spectrin-actin interactions. *J Cell Biol* **104:**519, 1987.
108. Becker PS, Schwartz MA, Morrow JS, Lux SE: Radiolabel-transfer cross-linking demonstrates that the protein 4.1 binds to the N-terminal region of beta spectrin and to actin in binary interactions. *Eur J Biochem* **193:**827, 1990.
109. Morris M, Lux SE: Unpublished observations.
110. Mueller TJ, Jackson CW, Dockler ME, Morrison M: Membrane skeletal alterations during in vivo mouse red cell aging. Increase in the band 4.1a:4.1b ratio. *J Clin Invest* **79:**492, 1987.
111. Anderson RA, Lovrien RE: Glycophorin is linked to band 4.1 protein to the human erythrocyte membrane skeleton. *Nature* **307:**655, 1984.
112. Mueller TJ, Manson M: Glycoconnectin (PAS2), a membrane attachment site for the human erythrocyte cytoskeleton, in Krockeberg W, Eaton J, Greuner G (eds): *Erythrocyte Membranes 2. Clinical and Experimental Advances*. New York, Alan R. Liss, 1981, p 95.
113. Anderson RA, Marchesi VT: Regulation of the association of membrane skeletal protein 4.1 with glycophorin by polyphosphoinositide. *Nature* **318:**295, 1985.
114. Reid M, Takakuwa Y, Conboy JG, Tchernia G, Mohandas N: Glycophorin C content of human erythrocyte membrane is regulated by protein 4.1. *Blood* **75:**2229, 1990.
115. Sato SB, Ohnishi S: Interaction of a peripheral protein of the erythrocyte membrane, band 4.1, with phosphatidylserine containing liposomes and erythrocyte inside-out vesicles. *Eur J Biochem* **130:**19, 1983.
116. Leto TL, Marchesi VT: A structural model of human erythrocyte protein 4.1. *J Biol Chem* **259:**4603, 1984.
117. Correas I, Leto TL, Speicher DW, Marchesi VT: Identification of the functional site of erythrocyte protein 4.1 involved in spectrin-actin associations. *J Biol Chem* **261:**3310, 1986.
118. Pasternack GR, Racusen RH: Erythrocyte protein 4.1 binds and regulates myosin. *Proc Natl Acad Sci USA* **86:**9712, 1989.
119. Chasis JA, Coulombel L, Conboy J, McGee S, Andrews K, Kan YW, Mohandas N: Differentiation-associated switches in protein 4.1 expression. Synthesis of multiple structural isoforms during normal human erythropoiesis. *J Clin Invest* **91:**329, 1993.
120. Horne WC, Leto TL, Marchesi VT: Differential phosphorylation of multiple sites in protein 4.1 and protein 4.9 by phorbol ester-activated and cyclic AMP-dependent protein kinases. *J Biol Chem* **260:**9073, 1985.
121. Palfrey HC, Waseem A: Protein kinase C in the human erythrocyte. Translocation to the plasma membrane and phosphorylation of bands 4.1 and 4.9 and other membrane proteins. *J Biol Chem* **260:**16021, 1985.
122. Faquin WC, Chahwala SB, Cantley LC, Branton D: Protein kinase C of human erythrocytes phosphorylates bands 4.1 and 4.9. *Biochim Biophys Acta* **887:**142, 1986.
123. Siegel DL, Branton D: Partial purification and characterization of an actin-binding protein, band 4.9, from human erythrocytes. *J Cell Biol* **100:**775, 1985.
124. Husain-Chishti A, Levin A, Branton D: Abolition of actin-bundling by phosphorylation of erythrocyte protein 4.9. *Nature* **334:**718, 1988.
125. Gardner K, Bennett V: Modulation of spectrin-actin assembly by erythrocyte adducin. *Nature* **328:**359, 1987.
126. Fowler VM, Bennett V: Tropomyosin: A new component of the erythrocyte membrane skeleton, in Kruckeberg WC, Eaton JW (eds): *Erythrocyte Membrane 3: Recent Clinical and Experimental Advances*. New York, Alan R. Liss, 1984, p 57.
127. Fowler VM: Identification and purification of a novel Mr 43,000 tropomyosin-binding protein from human erythrocyte membranes. *J Biol Chem* **262:**12792, 1987.
128. Fowler VM: Tropomodulin: A cytoskeletal protein that binds to the end of erythrocyte tropomyosin and inhibits tropomyosin binding to actin. *J Cell Biol* **111:**471, 1990.
129. Bennett V, Stenbuck PJ: Identification and partial purification of ankyrin, the high affinity membrane attachment site for human erythrocyte spectrin. *J Biol Chem* **254:**2533, 1979.
130. Luna EJ, Kidd GH, Branton D: Identification by peptide analysis of the spectrin-binding protein in human erythrocytes. *J Biol Chem* **254:**2526, 1979.
131. Yu J, Goodman SR: Syndeins: The spectrin-binding protein(s) of the human erythrocyte membrane. *Proc Natl Acad Sci USA* **76:**2340, 1979.
132. Kennedy SP, Warren SL, Forget BG, Morrow JS: Ankyrin binds to the 15th repetitive unit of erythroid and nonerythroid β spectrin. *J Cell Biol* **115:**267, 1991.
133. Weaver DC, Marchesi VT: The structural basis of ankyrin function. I. Identification of two structural domains. *J Biol Chem* **259:**6165, 1984.
134. Weaver DC, Marchesi VT: The structural basis of ankyrin function II. Identification of two functional domains. *J Biol Chem* **259:**6170, 1984.
135. Wallin R, Culp EN, Coleman DB, Goodman SR: A structural model of human erythrocyte band 2.1: Alignment of chemical and functional domains. *Proc Natl Acad Sci USA* **81:**4095, 1984.
136. Platt OS, Lux SE, Falcone JF: A highly conserved region of human erythrocyte ankyrin contains the capacity to bind spectrin. *J Biol Chem* **268:**24421, 1993.
137. Lux SE, John KM, Bennett V: Analysis of cDNA for human erythrocyte ankyrin indicates a repeated structure with homology to tissue-differentiation and cell-cycle control proteins. *Nature* **344:**36, 1990.
138. Gallagher PG, Tse WT, Scarpa AL, Lux SE, Forget GB: Large number of alternatively spliced isoforms of the regulatory region of human erythrocyte ankyrin. *Trans Assoc Am Physicians* **105:**268, 1992.
139. Davis LH, Davis JQ, Bennett V: Ankyrin regulation: An alternatively spliced segment of the regulatory domain functions as an intramolecular modulator. *J Biol Chem* **267:**18966, 1992.

140. Lambert S, Yu H, Prachal JT, Lawler J, Ruff P, Speicher D, Cheung MC, Kan YW, Palek J: cDNA sequence for human erythrocyte ankyrin. *Proc Natl Acad Sci USA* **87:**1730, 1990.
141. Davis JQ, Bennett V: Brain ankyrin. A membrane-associated protein with binding sites for spectrin, tubulin, and the cytoplasmic domain of the erythrocyte anion channel. *J Biol Chem* **259:**13550, 1984.
142. Srinivasan Y, Elmer L, Davis J, Bennett V, Angelides K: Ankyrin and spectrin associate with voltage-dependent sodium channels in brain. *Nature* **333:**177, 1988.
143. Srinivasan Y, Lewallen M, Angelides KJ: Mapping the site on ankyrin for the voltage-dependent sodium channel from brain. *J Biol Chem* **267:**7483, 1992.
144. Smith P, Saccomani G, Joe E, Angelides K, Benos D: Amiloride-sensitive sodium channel is linked to the cytoskeleton in renal epithelial cells. *Proc Natl Acad Sci USA* **88:**6971, 1991.
145. Li Z, Burke EP, Frank JS, Bennett V, Phillipson KD: The cardiac Na^+-Ca^{2+} exchanger binds to the cytoskeletal protein ankyrin. *J Biol Chem* **268:**11489, 1993.
146. Davis JQ, Bennett V: The anion exchanger and Na^+ K^+-ATPase interact with distinct sites on ankyrin *in vitro* assays. *J Biol Chem* **265:**17252, 1990.
147. Davis JQ, McLaughlin T, Bennett V: Ankyrin-binding proteins related to nervous system cell adhesion molecules: Candidates to provide transmembrane and intercellular connections in adult brain. *J Cell Biol* **121:**121, 1993.
148. Weaver DC, Georgatos SD: Location of the vimentin binding site on erythroid ankyrin. *J Cell Biol* **103:**396a, 1986.
149. Georgatos SD, Weber K, Geisler N, Blobel G: Binding of two desmin derivatives to the plasma membrane and the nuclear envelope of avian erythrocytes: Evidence for the conserved site-specificity in intermediate filament-membrane interactions. *Proc Natl Acad Sci USA* **84:**6780, 1987.
150. Korsgren C, Cohen CM: Associations of human erythrocyte protein 4.2. Binding to ankyrin and to the cytoplasmic domain of band 3. *J Biol Chem* **263:**10212, 1988.
151. Lux SE, Tse WT, Menninger JC, John KM, Harris P, Shalev O, Chilcote RR, Marchesi SL, Watkins PC, Bennett V, McIntosh S, Collins FS, Francke U, Ward DC, Forget BG: Hereditary spherocytosis associated with deletion of the human erythrocyte ankyrin gene on chromosome 8. *Nature* **345:**736, 1990.
152. Risinger M, Dotimas E, Cohen CM: Human erythrocyte protein 4.2, a high copy number membrane protein, is N-myristylated. *J Biol Chem* **267:**5680, 1992.
153. Korsgren C, Lawler J, Lambert S, Speicher D, Cohen CM: Complete amino acid sequence and homologies of human erythrocyte membrane protein band 4.2. *Proc Natl Acad Sci USA* **87:**613, 1990.
154. Sung LA, Chien S, Chang LS, Lambert K, Bliss S, Bouhassira EE, Nagel RL, Schwartz RS, Rybicki AC: Molecular cloning of human protein 4.2: A major component of the erythrocyte membrane. *Proc Natl Acad Sci USA* **87:**955, 1990.
155. Korsgren C, Cohen CM: Organization of the gene for human erythrocyte membrane protein 4.2: Structural similarities with the gene for the subunit of factor XIII. *Proc Natl Acad Sci USA* **88:**4840, 1991.
156. Najfeld V, Ballard SC, Menninger J, Ward DC, Bouhassira EE, Schwartz RS, Nagel RL, Rybicki AC: The gene for human erythrocyte protein 4.2 maps to chromosome 15q15. *Am J Hum Genet* **50:**71, 1992.
157. White RA, Peters LL, Adkinson LR, Korsgren C, Cohen CM, Lux SE: The murine *pallid* mutation is a platelet storage pool disease associated with the protein 4.2 (pallidin) gene. *Nature Genet* **2:**80, 1992.
158. Shen BW, Josephs R, Steck TL: Ultrastructure of the intact skeleton of the human erythrocyte membrane. *J Cell Biol* **102:**997, 1986.
159. Liu S-C, Derick LH, Palek J: Visualization of the hexagonal lattice in the erythrocyte membrane skeleton. *J Cell Biol* **104:**527, 1987.
160. McCaughan L, Krimm S: X-ray and neutron scattering density profiles of the intact human red blood cell membrane. *Science* **207:**1481, 1980.
161. Tsukita S, Tsukita S, Ishikawa H: Cytoskeletal network underlying the human erythrocyte membrane. Thin-section electron microscopy. *J Cell Biol* **85:**567, 1980.
162. Sheetz MP, Casaly J: 2,3-Diphosphoglycerate and ATP dissociate erythrocyte membrane skeletons. *J Biol Chem* **255:**9955, 1980.
163. Mentzer WC Jr, Iarocci TA, Mohandas N, Lane PA, Smith B, Lazerson J, Hayes T: Modulation of erythrocyte membrane mechanical stability by 2,3-diphosphoglycerate in the neonatal poikilocytosis/elliptocytosis syndrome. *J Clin Invest* **79:**943, 1987.
164. Schindler M, Koppel D, Sheetz MP: Modulation of membrane protein lateral mobility by polyphosphates and polyamines. *Proc Natl Acad Sci USA* **77:**1457, 1980.
165. Wolfe LC, Lux SE, Ohanian V: Spectrin-actin binding in vitro; effect of protein 4.1 and polyphosphates. *J Supramol Struct Cell Biochem (suppl)* **5:**123, 1981.
166. Waugh RE: Effects of 2,3-diphosphoglycerate on the mechanical properties of erythrocyte membrane. *Blood* **68:**231, 1986.
167. Avruch J, Fairbanks G: Phosphorylation of endogenous substrates by erythrocyte membrane protein kinases. I. A monovalent cation-stimulated reaction. *Biochemistry* **13:**5507, 1974.
168. Plut DA, Hosey MM, Tao M: Evidence for the participation of cytosolic protein kinases in membrane phosphorylation in intact erythrocytes. *Eur J Biochem* **82:**333, 1978.
169. Fairbanks G, Avruch J: Phosphorylation of endogenous substrates by erythrocyte protein kinases. II. Cyclic adenosine monophosphate-stimulated reactions. *Biochemistry* **13:**5514, 1974.
170. Thomas EL, King LE Jr, Morrison M: The uptake of cyclic AMP by human erythrocytes and its effect on membrane phosphorylation. *Arch Biochem Biophys* **196:**459, 1979.
171. Tao M, Conway R, Cheeta S: Purification and characterization of a membrane-bound protein kinase from human erythrocytes. *J Biol Chem* **255:**2563, 1980.
172. Dekowski SA, Rybicki A, Drickamer K: A tyrosine kinase associated with the red cell membrane phosphorylates band 3. *J Biol Chem* **258:**2750, 1983.
173. Lu PW, Soong C-J, Tao M: Phosphorylation of ankyrin decreases its affinity for spectrin tetramer. *J Biol Chem* **260:**14958, 1985.
174. Eder PS, Soong C-J, Tao M: Phosphorylation reduces the affinity of protein 4.1 for spectrin. *Biochemistry* **25:**1764, 1986.
175. Low PS, Allen DP, Zioncheck TF, Chari P, Willardson BM, Geahlen RL, Hamson ML: Tyrosine phosphorylation of band 3 inhibits peripheral protein binding. *J Biol Chem* **262:**4592, 1987.
176. Harris HW Jr, Levin N, Lux SE: Comparison of the phosphorylation of human erythrocyte spectrin in the intact red cell and in various cell-free systems. *J Biol Chem* **255:**11521, 1980.
177. Anderson JM, Tyler JM: State of spectrin phosphorylation does not affect erythrocyte shape or spectrin binding to erythrocyte membranes. *J Biol Chem* **255:**1259, 1980.
178. Anderson JP, Morrow JS: The interaction of calmodulin with erythrocyte spectrin. Inhibition of protein 4.1-stimulated actin binding. *J Biol Chem* **262:**6365, 1987.
179. Greenquist AC, Shohet SB, Bernstein SE: Marked reduction of spectrin in hereditary spherocytosis in the common house mouse. *Blood* **51:**1149, 1978.
180. Lux SE: Spectrin-actin membrane skeleton of normal and abnormal red blood cells. *Semin Hematol* **16:**21, 1979.
181. Shohet SB: Reconstruction of spectrin-deficient spherocytic mouse erythrocyte membranes. *J Clin Invest* **64:**483, 1979.
182. Mohandas N, Greenquist AC, Shohet SB: Effects of heat and metabolic depletion on erythrocyte deformability, spectrin extractability, and phosphorylation, in Brewer GJ (ed): *The Red Cell.* New York, Alan R. Liss, 1978, p 435.
183. Lux SE, John KM, Ukena TE: Diminished spectrin extraction from ATP-depleted human erythrocytes. Evidence relating spectrin to changes in erythrocyte shape and deformability. *J Clin Invest* **61:**815, 1978.
184. Deeley JDT, Crum LA, Coakley WT: The influence of temperature and incubation time on deformability of human erythrocytes. *Biochim Biophys Acta* **556:**90, 1979.
185. Smith BD, LaCelle PL: Parallel decrease of erythrocyte

membrane deformability and spectrin solubility at low pH. *Blood* **53:**15, 1979.

186. Crandall ED, Critz AM, Osher AS, Keljo DJ, Forster RE: Influence of pH on elastic deformability of the human erythrocyte membrane. *Am J Physiol* **235:**C269, 1978.
187. Marchesi VT, Steers E Jr: Selective solubilization of a protein component of the red cell membrane. *Science* **159:**203, 1968.
188. Liu SC, Palek J: Spectrin tetramer-dimer equilibrium and the stability of erythrocyte membrane skeletons. *Nature* **285:**586, 1980.
189. Nakashima K, Beutler E: Effect of antispectrin antibody and ATP on deformability of resealed erythrocyte membranes. *Proc Natl Acad Sci USA* **75:**3823, 1978.
190. Haest CWM, Fischer TM, Plasa G, Deuticke B: Stabilization of erythrocyte shape by a chemical increase in membrane shear stiffness. *Blood Cells* **6:**539, 1980.
191. Johnson GJ, Allen DW, Flynn TP, Finkel B, White JG: Decreased survival in vivo of diamide-incubated dog erythrocytes. A model of oxidant-induced hemolysis. *J Clin Invest* **66:**955, 1980.
192. Lux SE, John KM, Karnovsky MJ: Irreversible deformation of the spectrin-actin lattice in irreversibly sickled cells. *J Clin Invest* **58:**955, 1976.
193. Tomaselli MB, John KM, Lux SE: Elliptical erythrocyte membrane skeletons and heat-sensitive spectrin in hereditary elliptocytosis. *Proc Natl Acad Sci USA* **78:**1911, 1981.
194. Sheetz MP, Singer SJ: On the mechanism of ATP-induced shape changes in human erythrocyte membranes. I. The role of the spectrin complex. *J Cell Biol* **73:**638, 1977.
195. Johnson RM, Taylor G, Meyer DB: Shape and volume changes in erythrocyte ghosts and spectrin-actin networks. *J Cell Biol* **86:**371, 1980.
196. Elgsaeter A, Stokke BT, Mikkelsen A, Branton D: The molecular basis of erythrocyte shape. *Science* **234:**1217, 1986.
197. Hochmuth RM, Evans EA, Colvard DF: Viscosity of human red cell membranes in plastic flow. *Microvasc Res* **11:**155, 1976.
198. Chien S, Sung K-LP, Skalak R, Usami S, Tozeren A: Theoretical and experimental studies on viscoelastic properties of erythrocyte membranes. *Biophys J* **24:**463, 1978.
199. Nicolson GL, Painter RG: Anionic sites of human erythrocyte membranes. II. Anti-spectrin-induced transmembrane aggregation of the binding sites for positively charged colloidal particles. *J Cell Biol* **59:**395, 1973.
200. Elgsaeter A, Shotton DM, Branton D: Intramembrane particle aggregation in erythrocyte ghosts. II. The influence of spectrin aggregation. *Biochim Biophys Acta* **426:**101, 1976.
201. Fowler V, Bennett V: Association of spectrin with its membrane attachment site restricts lateral mobility of human erythrocyte integral membrane proteins. *J Supramol Struct* **8:**215, 1978.
202. Sheetz MP, Schindler M, Koppel DE: Lateral mobility of integral membrane proteins is increased in spherocytic erythrocytes. *Nature* **285:**510, 1980.
203. Hebbel RP, Yamada O, Moldow CF, Jacob HS, White JG, Eaton JW: Abnormal adherence of sickle erythrocytes to cultured vascular endothelium. Possible mechanism for microvascular occlusion in sickle cell disease. *J Clin Invest* **65:**154, 1980.
204. Mohandas N, Evans E: Adherence of sickle erythrocytes to vascular endothelial cells: Requirement for both cell membrane changes and plasma factors. *Blood* **64:**282, 1984.
205. Platt OS, Falcone JF, Lux SE: Molecular defect in the sickle erythrocyte membrane skeleton: Abnormal spectrin binding to sickle inside-out vesicles. *J Clin Invest* **75:**266, 1985.
206. Schwartz RS, Rybicki AC, Heath RH, Lubin BH: Protein 4.1 in sickle erythrocytes. Evidence for oxidative damage. *J Biol Chem* **262:**15666, 1987.
207. Shinar E, Shalev O, Rachmilewitz EA: Erythrocyte membrane skeleton abnormalities in severe beta-thalassemia. *Blood* **70:**158, 1987.
208. Hardy B, Bensch KG, Schrier SL: Spectrin rearrangement early in erythrocyte ghost endocytosis. *J Cell Biol* **82:**654, 1979.
209. Tokuyasu KT, Schekman R, Singer SJ: Domains of receptor mobility and endocytosis in the membranes of neonatal human erythrocytes and reticulocytes are deficient in spectrin. *J Cell Biol* **80:**481, 1979.
210. Cullis PR, Hope MJ: Effects of fusogenic agents on membrane structure of erythrocyte ghosts and the mechanism of membrane fusion. *Nature* **271:**672, 1978.
211. Sekiguchi K, Asano A: Participation of spectrin in Sendai virus-induced fusion of human erythrocyte ghosts. *Proc Natl Acad Sci USA* **75:**1740, 1978.
212. Lalazar A, Loyter A: Involvement of spectrin in membrane fusion: Induction of fusion in human erythrocyte ghosts by proteolytic enzymes and its inhibition by antispectrin antibody. *Proc Natl Acad Sci USA* **76:**318, 1979.
213. Portis A, Newton C, Pangborn W, Papahadjopoulos D: Studies on the mechanism of membrane fusion: Evidence for an intermembrane Ca^{2+}-phospholipid complex, synergism with Mg^{2+}, and inhibition by spectrin. *Biochemistry* **18:**780, 1979.
214. Vanlair CF, Masius JB: De la microcythémie. *Bull R Acad Med Belg* **5:**515, 1871.
215. Ham TH, Castle WB: Studies on destruction of red blood cells. Relation of increased hypotonic fragility and erythrostasis to the mechanism of hemolysis in certain anemias. *Proc Am Phil Soc* **82:**411, 1940.
216. Chauffard A: Pathogénie de l'ictère hémolytique congénitale. *Ann Med* (Paris) **1:**3, 1914.
217. Dameshek W, Schwartz SO: Hemolysins as the cause of clinical and experimental hemolytic anemias. With particular reference to the nature of spherocytosis and increased fragility. *Am J Med Sci* **196:**769, 1938.
218. Wilson C: Some cases showing hereditary enlargement of the spleen. *Trans Clin Soc (London)* **23:**162, 1890.
219. Wilson C, Stanley D: A sequel to some cases showing hereditary enlargement of the spleen. *Trans Clin Soc (London)* **26:**163, 1893.
220. Minkowski O: Ueber eine hereditare, unter dem Bilde eines chronischen Ikterus mit Urobilinurie, Splenomegalie und Nierensiderosis verlaufende Affection. *Verh Dtsch Kongr Med* **18:**316, 1900.
221. Gilbert A, Castaigne J, Lereboullet P: De l'ictère familial. Contribution à l'étude de la diathèse biliaire. *Bull Mem Soc Med Hop Paris* **17:**948, 1900.
222. Barlow T, Shaw HB: Inheritance of recurrent attacks of jaundice and of abdominal crises with hepatosplenomegaly. *Trans Clin Soc (London)* **35:**155, 1902.
223. Chauffard MA: Pathogènie de l'ictère congénital de l'adulte. *Semin Med (Paris)* **27:**25, 1907.
224. Chauffard MA: Les ictères hemolytique. *Semin Med (Paris)* **28:**49, 1908.
225. Widal F, Abrami P, Brulé M: Differentiation de plusieurs types d'ictères hémolytiques par le procédédes hématies déplasmatisées. *Presse Med* **15:**641, 1907.
226. Hayem G: Sur une variété particulière d'ictère chronique. Ictère infectieux chronique splenomégalique. *Presse Med* **6:**121, 1898.
227. Micheli F: Unmittelbare Effekte der Splenektomie bei einem Fall von erworbenem hämolytischen Splenomegalischen Ikterus Typus-Hayem-Widal (Splenohämolytischer Ikterus). *Wien Klin Wochenschr* **24:**1269, 1911.
228. Giffin HZ: Haemolytic jaundice: A review of 17 cases. *Surg Gynecol Obstet* **25:**152, 1917.
229. Dawson of Penn: The Hume Lectures on haemolytic icterus. *Br Med J* **1:**921 and **1:**1963, 1931.
230. Tileston W: Hemolytic jaundice. *Medicine (Baltimore)* **1:**355, 1922.
231. Gänsslen M: Uber hämolytischen Ikterus. *Dtsch Arch Klin Med* **140:**210, 1922.
232. Wintrobe MM: *Blood, Pure and Eloquent.* New York, McGraw-Hill, 1980.
233. Morton NE, MacKinney AA, Kosower N, Schilling RF, Gray MP: Genetics of spherocytosis. *Am J Hum Genet* **14:**170, 1962.
234. Godal HC, Heist H: High prevalence of increased osmotic fragility of red blood cells among Norwegian donors. *Scand J Haematol* **27:**30, 1981.
235. Race RR: On the inheritance and linkage relations of acholuric jaundice. *Ann Eugenics* **11:**365, 1942.
236. Bernard J, Boiron M, Estager J: Une grande famille

hémolytique. Treize cas de maladie de Minkowski-Chauffard observés dans la même fratrie. *Semin Hop Paris* **28**:3741, 1952.

237. Agre P, Orringer EP, Bennett V: Deficient red-cell spectrin in severe, recessively inherited spherocytosis. *N Engl J Med* **306**:1155, 1982.
238. Emerson CP Jr, Shen SC, Ham TH, Fleming EM, Castle WB: Studies on the destruction of red blood cells. IX. Quantitative methods for determining the osmotic and mechanical fragility of red cells in the peripheral blood and splenic pulp; the mechanism of increased hemolysis in hereditary spherocytosis (congenital hemolytic jaundice) as related to the function of the spleen. *Arch Intern Med* **97**:1, 1956.
239. Dacie JV, Mollison PL: Survival of normal erythrocytes after transfusion to patients with familial haemolytic anaemia (acholuric jaundice). *Lancet* **1**:550, 1943.
240. Wiley JS: Red cell survival in hereditary spherocytosis. *J Clin Invest* **49**:555, 1970.
241. Lux SE, Becker PS: Disorders of the red cell membrane skeleton: Hereditary spherocytosis and hereditary elliptocytosis, in Scriver CR, Beaudet AL, Sly WS, Valle D (eds): *The Metabolic Basis of Inherited Disease,* 6th ed. New York, McGraw-Hill, 1989, vol 2, p 2367.
242. Waugh RE, LaCelle PL: Abnormalities in the membrane material properties of hereditary spherocytes. *J Biomech Eng* **102**:240, 1980.
243. Waugh RE: Effects of abnormal cytoskeletal structure on erythrocyte membrane mechanical properties. *Cell Motil* **3**:609, 1983.
244. Waugh RE: Effects of inherited membrane abnormalities on the viscoeleastic properties of erythrocyte membranes. *Biophys J* **51**:363, 1987.
245. Waugh RE, Agre P: Reductions of erythrocyte membrane viscoelastic coefficients reflect spectrin deficiencies in hereditary spherocytosis. *J Clin Invest* **81**:133, 1988.
246. Reed CF, Swisher SN: Erythrocyte lipid loss in hereditary spherocytosis. *J Clin Invest* **45**:777, 1966.
247. Weed RI, Bowdler AJ: Metabolic dependence of the criticial hemolytic volume of human erythrocytes: Relationship to osmotic fragility and autohemolysis in hereditary spherocytosis and normal red cells. *J Clin Invest* **45**:1137, 1966.
248. Cooper RA, Jandl JH: The role of membrane lipids in the survival of red cells in hereditary spherocytosis. *J Clin Invest* **48**:736, 1969.
249. Langley GR, Felderhof CH: Atypical autohemolysis in hereditary spherocytosis as a reflection of two cell populations: Relationship of cell lipids to conditioning by the spleen. *Blood* **32**:569, 1968.
250. Johnsson R: Red cell membrane proteins and lipids in spherocytosis. *Scand J Haematol* **20**:341, 1978.
251. Schrier SL, Ben-Bassat I, Bensch K, Seeger M, Junga I: Erythrocyte membrane vacuole formation in hereditary spherocytosis. *Br J Haematol* **26**:59, 1974.
251. Bernstein SE: Inherited hemolytic disease in mice: A review and update. *Lab Anim Sci* **30**:197, 1980.
252. Bernstein SE: Inherited hemolytic disease in mice: A review and update. *Lab Anim Sci* **30**:197, 1980.
253. Bodine DM, Birkenmeier CS, Barker JS: Spectrin-deficient inherited hemolytic anemias in the mouse: Characterization by spectrin synthesis and mRNA activity in reticulocytes. *Cell* **37**:721, 1984.
254. Barker JE, Bodine DM, Birkenmeier CS: Synthesis of spectrin and its assembly into the red cell membrane cytoskeleton of normal and mutant mice. *J Cell Biochem (suppl)* **9B**:3, 1985.
255. Falcone JC, Lux SE: Unpublished observations.
256. White RA, Birkenmeier CS, Lux SE, Barker JE: Ankyrin and the hemolytic anemia mutatin, *nb,* map to mouse chromosome 8: Presence of the *nb* allele is associated with a truncated erythrocyte ankyrin. *Proc Natl Acad Sci USA* **87**:3117, 1990.
257. Peters LL, Birkenmeier CS, Bronson RT, White RA, Lux SE, Otto E, Bennett V, Barker JE: Purkinje cell degeneration associated with erythroid ankyrin deficiency in *nb/nb* mice. *J Cell Biol* **114**:1233, 1991.
258. Peters LL, Birkenmeier CS, Barker JE: Fetal compensation of the hemolytic anemia in mice homozygous for the normoblastosis, *nb,* mutation. *Blood* **80**:2122, 1992.
259. Peters LL, Turtzo C, Birkenmeier CS, Barker JE: Distinct fetal *Ank-1* and *Ank-2* related proteins and mRNAs in normal and *nb/nb* mice. *Blood* **81**:2144, 1993.
260. Agre P, Asimos A, Casella JF, McMillan D: Inheritance pattern and clinical response to splenectomy as a reflection of erythrocyte spectrin deficiency in hereditary spherocytosis. *N Engl J Med* **315**:1579, 1986.
261. Marchesi SL, Agre PL, Speicher DW, Tse WT, Forget BG: Mutant spectrin α^{II} domain in recessively inherited spherocytosis. *Blood (suppl 1)* **74**:182a, 1989.
262. Whitfield CF, Follweiler JB, Lopresti-Morrow L, Miller BA: Deficiency of α-spectrin synthesis in burst-forming units-erythroid in lethal hereditary spherocytosis. *Blood* **78**:3043, 1991.
263. Agre P, Casella JF, Zinkham WH, McMillan C, Bennett V: Partial deficiency of erythrocyte spectrin in hereditary spherocytosis. *Nature* **314**:380, 1985.
264. Woods CM, Boyer B, Vogt PK, Lazarides E: Control of erythroid differentiation: Asynchronous expression of the anion transporter and the peripheral components of the membrane skeleton in AEV- and S13-transformed cells. *J Cell Biol* **103**:1789, 1986.
265. Kimberling WJ, Taylor PA, Chapman RG, Lubs HA: Linkage and gene localization of hereditary spherocytosis (HS). *Blood* **52**:859, 1978.
266. Bass EB, Smith SW, Stevenson RE, Rosse WF: Further evidence for location of the spherocytosis gene on chromosome 8. *Ann Intern Med* **99**:192, 1983.
267. Chilcote RR, LeBeau MM, Dampler C, Pergament E, Verlinsky Y, Mohandas N, Frischer H, Rowley JD: Association of red cell spherocytosis with deletion of the short arm of chromosome 8. *Blood* **69**:156, 1987.
268. Costa FF, Agre P, Watkins SM, Winkelmann JC, Tang TK, John KM, Lux SE, Forget BG: Linkage of dominant hereditary spherocytosis to the gene for the erythrocyte membrane-skeleton protein ankyrin. *N Engl J Med* **323**:1046, 1990.
269. Jarolim P, Brabec V, Lambert S, Liu S-C, Zhou Z, Palek J: Ankyrin Prague: A dominantly inherited mutation of the regulatory domain of ankyrin associated with hereditary spherocytosis. *Blood (suppl 1)* **76**:37a, 1990.
270. Coetzer TL, Lawler J, Liu S-C, Prchal J, Gualtieri RJ, Brain MC, Dacie JV, Palek J: Partial ankyrin and spectrin deficiency in severe, atypical hereditary spherocytosis. *N Engl J Med* **318**:230, 1988.
271. Gallagher PG, Kotula L, DiPaulo B, Curtis P, Speicher D, Forget BG: Polymorphisms of the αII domain of α spectrin and of the 3′ untranslated region of α spectrin mRNA. *Blood (suppl 1)* **78**:364a, 1991.
272. Goodman SR, Shiffer KA, Casoria LA, Eyster ME: Identification of the molecular defect in the erythrocyte membrane skeleton of some kindreds with hereditary spherocytosis. *Blood* **60**:772, 1982.
273. Wolfe LC, John KM, Falcone JC, Byrne AM, Lux SE: A genetic defect in the binding of protein 4.1 to spectrin in a kindred with hereditary spherocytosis. *N Engl J Med* **307**:1367, 1982.
274. Becker PS, Morrow JS, Lux SE: Abnormal oxidant sensitivity and beta-chain structure of spectrin in hereditary spherocytosis associated with defective spectrin-protein 4.1 binding. *J Clin Invest* **80**:557, 1987.
275. Becker PS, Cohen CM, Lux SE: The effect of mild diamide oxidation on the structure and function of human erythrocyte spectrin. *J Biol Chem* **261**:4620, 1986.
276. Wolfe LC, Byrne AM, Lux SE: Molecular defect in the membrane skeleton of blood bank-stored red cells. Abnormal spectrin-protein 4.1-actin complex formation. *J Clin Invest* **78**:1681, 1986.
277. Becker PS, Tse WT, Lux SE, Forget BG: β spectrin Kissimmee: A spectrin variant associated with autosomal dominant hereditary spherocytosis and defective binding to protein 4.1. *J Clin Invest* **92**:612, 1993.
278. Nozawa Y, Noguchi T, Iida H, Fukushima T, Sekiya T, Ito Y: Erythrocyte membranes of hereditary spherocytosis: Alteration in surface ultrastructure and membrane proteins, as inferred by scanning electron microscopy and SDS-disc gel electrophoresis. *Clin Chim Acta* **55**:81, 1974.
279. Hayashi S, Koomoto R, Yano A, Ishigami S, Tsujino G, Saeki S, Tanaka T: Abnormality in a specific protein

of the erythrocyte membrane in hereditary spherocytosis. *Biochem Biophys Res Commun* **57**:1038, 1974.

280. Bouhassira EE, Schwartz RS, Yawata Y, Ata K, Kanzaki A, Qiu JJ-H, Nagel RL, Rybicki AC: An alanine-to-threonine substitution in protein 4.2 cDNA is associated with a Japanese form of hereditary hemolytic anemia (protein 4.2_{NIPPON}). *Blood* **79**:1846, 1992.
281. Delaunay J, Hayette S, Cohen C, Korsgren C, Ghanem A, Fattoum S, Dos Santos ME, Dhermy D, Morle L: Hereditary hemolytic anemia associated with the absence of protein 4.2, in *Molecular Biology of Hematopoiesis Symposium Abstracts, 8th Symposium*. Basel, Switzerland, 1993, p 65.
282. Eber SW, Lux ML, Gonzalez JM, Scarpa A, Tse WT, Gallagher PG, Pekrun A, Forget BG, Lux SE: Discovery of 8 ankyrin mutations in hereditary spherocytosis (HS) indicates that ankyrin defects are a major cause of dominant and recessive HS. *Blood (suppl)* **821**:308a, 1993.
283. Rybicki A, Qiu JJH, Musto S, Rosen NL, Nagel RL, Schwartz RS: Human erythrocyte protein 4.2 deficiency associated with hemolytic anemia and a homozygous ^{40}glutamic acid→lysine substitution in the cytoplasmic domain of band 3 (band $3^{Montefiore}$). *Blood* **81**:2155, 1993.
284. Jarolim P, Palek J, Rubin HL, Prchal JT, Korsgren C, Cohen CM: Band 3 Tuscaloosa: Pro^{327}→Arg^{327} substitution in the cytoplasmic domain of erythrocyte band 3 protein associated with spherocytic hemolytic anemia and partial deficiency of protein 4.2 *Blood* **80**:523, 1992.
285. Miraglia del Giudice E, Perrotta S, Pinto L, Cappellini MD, Fiorelli G, Cutillo S, Iolascon A: Hereditary spherocytosis characterized by increased spectrin/band 3 ratio. *Br J Haematol* **80**:133, 1992.
286. Lux S, Bedrosian C, Shalev O, Morris M, Chasis J, Davies K, Savvides P, Telen M: Deficiency of band 3 in dominant hereditary spherocytosis with normal spectrin content. *Clin Res* **38**:300a, 1990.
287. Jarolim P, Ruff P, Coetzer TL, Prchal JT, Ballas SK, Poon M-C, Brabec V, Palek J: A subset of patients with dominantly inherited hereditary spherocytosis has a marked deficiency of the band 3 protein. *Blood (suppl 1)* **76**:37a, 1990.
288. Saad STO, Liu SC, Golan D, et al: Mechanism underlying band 3 deficiency in a subset of patients with hereditary spherocytosis (HS). *Blood* **78**:81a, 1991.
289. Casey JR, Reithmeier AF: Analysis of the oligomeric state of band 3, the anion transport protein of the human erythrocyte membrane, by size exclusion high performance liquid chromatography. Oligomeric stability and origin of heterogeneity. *J Biol Chem* **266**:15726, 1991.
290. Jarolim P, Rubin HL, Liu S-C, Cho MR, Brabec V, Derrick LH, Yi S, Saad STD, Alper S, Brugnara C, Golan DE, Palek J: Duplication of 10 nucleotides in the erythroid band 3 (AEI) gene in a kindred with hereditary spherocytosis and band 3 protein deficiency (Band 3_{PRAGUE}). *J Clin Invest* **93**:121, 1994.
291. Sheehy R, Ralston GB: Abnormal binding of spectrin to the membrane of erythrocytes in some cases of hereditary spherocytosis. *Blut* **36**:145, 1978.
292. Hill JS, Sawyer WH, Howlett GJ, Wiley JS: Hereditary spherocytosis of man: Altered binding of cytoskeletal components to the erythrocyte membrane. *Biochem J* **201**:259, 1981.
293. Sawyer WH, Hill JS, Howlett GH, Wiley JS: Hereditary spherocytosis of man: Detective cytoskeletal interactions in the erythrocyte membrane. *Biochem J* **211**:349, 1983.
294. Lachant NA, Jennings MA, Tanaka KR: Partial erythrocyte enolase deficiency: A hereditary disorder with variable clinical expression. *Blood (suppl 1)* **68**:55a, 1986.
295. Stefanini M: Chronic hemolytic anemia associated with erythrocyte enolase deficiency exacerbated by ingestion of nitrofurantoin. *Am J Clin Pathol* **58**:408, 1972.
296. Evans EA, Waugh R, Melnik C: Elastic area compressibility modulus of red cell membranes. *Biophys J* **16**:585, 1976.
297. Jandl JH, Simmons RL, Castle WB: Red cell filtration and the pathogenesis of certain hemolytic anemias. *Blood* **18**:133, 1961.
298. Chapman RG: Red cell life span after splenectomy in hereditary spherocytosis. *J Clin Invest* **47**:2263, 1968.
299. Baird R, McPherson AS, Richmond J: Red blood cell survival after splenectomy in congenital spherocytosis. *Lancet* **1**:1060, 1971.
300. Barnhart MT, Lusher JM: The human spleen as revealed by scanning electron microscopy. *Am J Hematol* **1**:243, 1976.
301. Chen L-T, Weiss L: Electron microscopy of red pulp of human spleen. *Am J Anat* **134**:425, 1972.
302. Weiss L: A scanning electron microscopic study of the spleen. *Blood* **43**:665, 1974.
303. Knisely MH: Spleen studies. I. Microscopic observations of the circulating system of living unstimulated mammalian spleen. *Anat Rec* **65**:23, 1936.

303a. Boivin P, Delaunay J, Galand C: Altered erythrocyte membrane protein phosphorylation in an unusual case of hereditary spherocytosis. *Scand J Haemoatol* **23**:251, 1979.

304. Chen L-T, Weiss L: The role of the sinus wall in the passage of erythrocytes through the spleen. *Blood* **41**:529, 1973.
305. Johnsson R, Vuopio P: Studies on red cell flexibility in spherocytosis using a polycarbonate membrane filtration method. *Acta Haematol* **60**:329, 1978.
306. Murphy JR: The influence of pH and temperature on some physical properties of normal erythrocytes and erythrocytes from patients with hereditary spherocytosis. *J Lab Clin Med* **69**:758, 1967.
307. Young LE, Platzer RF, Ervin DM, Izzo MJ: Hereditary spherocytosis. II. Observations on the role of the spleen. *Blood* **6**:1099, 1951.
308. Jandl JH, Greenberg MS, Yonemoto R, Castle WB: Clinical determination of the sites of red cell sequestration in hemolytic anemias. *J Clin Invest* **35**:842, 1956.
309. Motulsky AG, Casserd F, Giblett ER, Broun GO Jr, Finch CA: Anemia and the spleen. *N Engl J Med* **259**:1164; **259**:1212, 1958.
310. Griggs RC, Weisman R Jr, Harris JW: Alterations in osmotic and mechanical fragility related to in vivo erythrocyte aging and splenic sequestration in hereditary spherocytosis. *J Clin Invest* **39**:89, 1960.
311. Prankard TAJ: The spleen and anaemia. *BMJ* **2**:517, 1963.
312. Wiland OK, Smith EB: The morphology of the spleen in congenital hemolytic anemia (hereditary spherocytosis). *Am J Clin Pathol* **26**:619, 1956.
313. Molnar Z, Rappaport H: Fine structure of the red pulp of the spleen in hereditary spherocytosis. *Blood* **39**:81, 1972.
314. Fujita T, Kashimura M, Adach K: Scanning electron microscopy (SEM) studies of the spleen-normal and pathological. *Scan Electron Microsc* **Pt 1**:435, 1982.
315. Banti G: Splenomegalie hemolytique au hemopoietique: Le role de la rate dans l'hemolyse. *Semin Med (Paris)* **33**:313, 1913.
316. Dacie JV: Familial haemolytic anaemia (acholuric jaundice), with particular reference to changes in fragility produced by splenectomy. *Q J Med* **12**:101, 1943.
317. Minakami S, Yoshikawa H: Studies on erythrocyte glycolysis. III. The effects of active cation transport, pH and inorganic phosphate concentration on erythrocyte glycolysis. *J Biochem (Tokyo)* **59**:145, 1966.
318. Jandl JH, Aster RH: Increased splenic pooling and the pathogenesis of hypersplenism. *Am J Med Sci* **253**:383, 1967.
319. Murphy JR: The influence of pH and temperature on some physical properties of normal erythrocytes and erythrocytes from patients with hereditary spherocytosis. *J Lab Clin Med* **69**:758, 1967.
320. Rakitzis ET, Mills GC: Relation of red cell hexokinase activity to extracellular pH. *Biochim Biophys Acta* **141**:439, 1967.
321. Parker JC: Ouabain-insensitive effects of metabolism on ion and water content in red blood cells. *Am J Physiol* **221**:338, 1971.
322. Dacie JV: Observations on autohemolysis in familial acholuric jaundice. *J Pathol Bacteriol* **52**:331, 1941.
323. Jacob HS, Jandl JH: Cell membrane permeability in the pathogenesis of hereditary spherocytosis (HS). *J Clin Invest* **43**:1704, 1964.
324. Bertles JE: Sodium transport across the surface of red blood cells in hereditary spherocytosis. *J Clin Invest* **36**:816, 1957.
325. Gárdos G: The function of calcium in the potassium permeability of human erythrocytes. *Acta Physiol Acad Sci Hung* **15**:121, 1959.

326. Sachs JR, Kanuf PA, Dunham PB: Transport through red cell membranes, in Surgenor D, Mac N (eds): *The Red Blood Cell*, 2d ed. New York, Academic Press, 1975, vol 2, p 613.
327. Johnson RM, Rarrhdranath Y, Brohn F, Hussain M: A large erythroid spectrin β-chain variant. *Br J Haematol* **80:**6, 1992.
328. Miraglia del Giudice E, Perrotta S, Sciarratta G, Cutillo L, Pinto L, Iolascon A: $\alpha^{I/72}$ spectrin Geneva: A new elliptocytogenic variant due to Arg→Trp substitution at position 34 of α spectrin. *Blood (suppl)* **80:**2772, 1992.
329. Hassoun H, Coetzer TL, Sahr KE, Saad S, Vassiliadis JN, Palek J: An insertion within the α spectrin gene leading to exon skipping in a family with hereditary elliptocytosis (HE) and pyropoikilocytosis (HPP). *Blood (suppl 1)* **80:**276a, 1992.
330. Ferrant A, Leners N, Michaux JL, Verwilghen RL, Sokal G: The spleen and haemolysis: Evaluation of the intrasplenic transit time. *Br J Haematol* **65:**331, 1987.
331. Mandelbaum H: Congenital hemolytic jaundice: Report of a case on congenital hemolytic jaundice. Initial hemolytic crisis occurring at the age of 75: Splenectomy followed by recovery. *Ann Intern Med* **13:**872, 1939.
332. Trucco JI, Brown AK: Neonatal manifestations of hereditary spherocytosis. *Am J Dis Child* **113:**263, 1967.
333. Burman D: Congenital spherocytosis in infancy. *Arch Dis Child* **33:**335, 1958.
334. MacKinney AA Jr, Morton NE, Kosower NS, Schilling RF: Ascertaining genetic carriers of hereditary spherocytosis by statistical analysis of multiple laboratory tests. *J Clin Invest* **41:**554, 1962.
335. Zanella A, Milani S, Fagnani G, Mariani M, Sirchia G: Diagnostic value of the glycerol lysis test. *J Lab Clin Med* **102:**743, 1983.
336. Gehlbach SH, Cooper BA: Haemolytic anaemia in infectious mononucleosis due to inapparent congenital spherocytosis. *Scand J Haematol* **7:**141, 1970.
337. Ho-Yen DO: Hereditary spherocytosis presenting in pregnancy. *Acta Haematol (Basel)* **72:**29, 1984.
338. Godal HC, Refsum HE: Haemolysis in athletes due to hereditary spherocytosis. *Scand J Haematol* **22:**83, 1954.
339. Palek J, Mircevova L, Brabec V: 2,3-Diphosphoglycerate metabolism in hereditary spherocytosis. *Br J Haematol* **17:**59, 1969.
340. Fernandez LA, Erslev AJ: Oxygen affinity and compensated hemolysis in hereditary spherocytosis. *J Lab Clin Med* **80:**780, 1972.
341. Young LE, Izzo MJ, Platzer RF: Hereditary spherocytosis. I. Clinical, hematologic and genetic features in 28 cases, with particular reference to the osmotic and mechanical fragility of incubated erythrocytes. *Blood* **6:**1073, 1951.
342. Krueger HC, Burgert EO: Hereditary spherocytosis in 100 children. *Mayo Clin Proc* **41:**821, 1966.
343. Debre R, Lamy M, See G, Schrameck G: Congenital and familial hemolytic disease in children. *Am J Dis Child* **56:**1189, 1938.
344. Diamond LK: Indications for splenectomy in childhood. Results in fifty-two operated cases. *Am J Surg (NS)* **39:**400, 1938.
345. Watson CJ: Studies of urobilinogen. III. The per diem excretion of urobilinogen in the common forms of jaundice and disease of the liver. *Arch Intern Med* **59:**206, 1937.
346. Sears DA, Anderson RP, Foy AL, Williams HL, Crosby WH: Urinary iron excretion and renal metabolism of hemoglobin in hemolytic disease. *Blood* **28:**708, 1966.
347. Muller-Eberhard U, Javid J, Liem HH, Hanstein A, Hanna M: Plasma concentrations of hemopexin, haptoglobin and heme in patients with various hemolytic diseases. *Blood* **32:**811, 1968.
348. LeBlond P-F, De Boisfleury A, Bessis M: La forme des érythrocytes dans la sphérocytose héréditaire. Étude au microscope à balayage. Relation avec leur déformabilité. *Nouv Rev Fr Hematol* **13:**873, 1973.
349. LeBlond PF, LaCelle PL, Weed RI: Rhéologie des érythroblastes et des érythrocytes dans la sphérocytose congénitale. *Nouv Rev Fr Hematol* **11:**537, 1971.
350. Paolino W: Variations of the mean diameter in the ripening of the erythrocyte. *Acta Med Scand* **136:**141, 1949.
351. Selwyn JG, Dacie JV: Autohemolysis and other changes resulting from the incubation in vitro of red cells from patients with congenital hemolytic anemia. *Blood* **9:**414, 1954.
352. Mayman D, Zipursky A: Hereditary spherocytosis: The metabolism of erythrocytes in the peripheral blood and in the splenic pulp. *Br J Haematol* **27:**201, 1974.
353. Maizels M: The anion and cation content of normal and anaemic bloods. *Biochem J* **30:**821, 1936.
354. Young LE, Platzer RF, Ervin DM, Izzo MJ: Hereditary spherocytosis II. Observations on the role of the spleen. *Blood* **6:**1099, 1951.
355. Young LE: Observations on inheritance and heterogeneity of chronic spherocytosis. *Trans Assoc Am Physicians* **68:**141, 1955.
356. Jacob HS: Hereditary spherocytosis: A disease of the red cell membrane. *Semin Hematol* **2:**139, 1965.
357. Zanella A, Izzo C, Rebulla P, Zanuso F, Perroni L, Sirchia G: Acidified glycerol lysis test: A screening test for spherocytosis. *Br J Haematol* **45:**481, 1980.
358. Judkiewicz L, Bartosz G, Oplatowska A, Szczepanek A: Modified osmotic fragility test for the laboratory diagnosis of hereditary spherocytosis. *Am J Hematol* **31:**136, 1989.
359. Young LE, Izzo MJ, Altman KI, Swisher SN: Studies on spontaneous in vitro autohemolysis in hemolytic disorders. *Blood* **11:**977, 1956.
360. Langley GR, Felderhof CH: Atypical autohemolysis in hereditary spherocytosis as a reflection of two cell populations: Relationship of cell lipids to conditioning by the spleen. *Blood* **32:**569, 1968.
361. Gottfried EL, Robertson NA: Glycerol lysis time of incubated erythrocytes in the diagnosis of hereditary spherocytosis. *J Lab Clin Med* **84:**746, 1974.
362. Gottfied EL: Acidified glycerol lysis test. *Br J Haematol* **47:**323, 1981.
363. Johnsson R, Salminen S: Effect of ouabain on osmotic resistance and monovalent cation transport of red cells in hereditary spherocytosis. *Scand J Haematol* **29:**323, 1980.
364. Rutherford CJ, Postlewaight BF, Hallowes M: An evaluation of the acidified glycerol lysis test. *Br J Haematol* **63:**119, 1986.
365. Streichman S, Gesheidt Y, Tatarsky I: Hypertonic cryohemolysis: A diagnostic test for hereditary spherocytosis. *Am J Hematol* **35:**104, 1990.
366. Owren PA: Congenital hemolytic jaundice. The pathogenesis of the hemolytic crisis. *Blood* **3:**231, 1948.
367. Barker K, Martin FRR: Splenectomy in congenital microspherocytosis. *Br J Surg* **56:**561, 1969.
368. Lefrere JJ, Courouce AM, Bertrand Y, Soulier JP: Infections a parvovirus B19. *Rev Fr Transfus Immunohematol* **29:**149, 1986.
369. Saarinen UM, Chorba TL, Tattersall P, Young NS, Anderson LJ, Palmer E, Cocela PF: Human parvovirus B19-induced epidemic acute red cell aplasia in patients with hereditary hemolytic anemia. *Blood* **67:**1411, 1986.
370. Lefrere JJ, Courouce MA, Girot R, Bertrand Y, Soulier JP: Six cases of hereditary spherocytosis revealed by human parvovirus infection. *Br J Haematol* **62:**653, 1986.
371. Serjeant GR, Topley JM, Mason K, Serjeant BE, Pattison JR, Jones SE, Mohamed R: Outbreak of aplastic crises in sickle cell anaemia associated with parvovirus-like agent. *Lancet* **2:**595, 1981.
372. Nunove T, Koike T, Koike R, Sanoda M, Tsukoda T, Mortimer PP, Cohen BJ: Infection with human parvovirus infection. *Br J Haematol* **62:**653, 1986.
373. Robins MM: Familial crisis in hereditary spherocytosis. Report of six affected siblings. *Clin Pediatr* **4:**210, 1965.
374. Gairdner D: The association of gall-stones with acholuric jaundice in children. *Arch Dis Child* **14:**109, 1939.
375. Delamore IW, Richmond J, Davies SH: Megaloblastic anaemia in congenital spherocytosis. *BMJ* **1:**543, 1961.
376. Kohler HG, Meynell MJ, Cooke WT: Spherocytic anaemia, complicated by megaloblastic anaemia of pregnancy. *BMJ* **1:**779, 1960.
377. Bates GC, Brown CH: Incidence of gallbladder disease in chronic hemolytic anemia (spherocytosis). *Gastroenterology* **21:**104, 1952.
378. Lawrie GM, Ham JM: The surgical treatment of hereditary spherocytosis. *Surg Gynecol Obstet* **139:**208, 1974.

379. Hanford RB, Schneider GF, MacCarthy JD: Massive thoracic extramedullary hemopoieses. *N Engl J Med* **263:**120, 1960.
380. Taylor ES: Chronic ulcer of the leg associated with congenital jaundice. *JAMA* **112:**1574, 1939.
381. Beinhauer LG, Gruhn JG: Dermatologic aspects of congenital spherocytic anemia. *Arch Dermatol* **75:**642, 1957.
382. Barry M, Scheuer PJ, Sherlock S, Ross CF, Williams R: Hereditary spherocytosis with secondary haemochromatosis. *Lancet* **2:**481, 1968.
383. Schafer AI, Miller JB, Lester EP, Bowers TK, Jacob HS: Monoclonal gammopathy in hereditary spherocytosis: A possible pathogenic relation. *Ann Intern Med* **88:**45, 1978.
384. Lempert KD: Gammopathy and spherocytosis. *Ann Intern Med* **89:**145, 1978.
385. Fukata S, Tamai H, Nogai K, Matsubayashi S, Nagato H, Tashiro T, Yasuda M, Kumagai LF: A patient with hereditary spherocytosis and silicosis who developed an IgA (lambda) monoclonal gammopathy. *Jpn J Med* **26:**81, 1987.
386. Jandl JH, Files NM, Barnett SB, MacDonald RA: Proliferative response of the spleen and liver to hemolysis. *J Exp Med* **122:**299, 1965.
387. Schilling RF: Hereditary spherocytosis; a study of splenectomized persons. *Semin Hematol* **13:**169, 1976.
388. Isobe T, Osserman EF: Pathologic conditions associated with plasma cell dyscrasias: A study of 806 cases. *Ann NY Acad Sci* **190:**507, 1971.
389. Blacklock H, Merkin M: Serum ferritin in patients with hereditary spherocytosis. *Br J Haematol* **49:**117, 1981.
390. Edwards CQ, Skolnick MH, Dadone MM, Kushner JP: Iron overload in hereditary spherocytosis: Association with HLA-linked hemachromatosis. *Am J Hematol* **13:**101, 1982.
391. Fargion S, Cappellini MD, Piperno A, Panajotopoulous N, Ronchi G, Fiorelli G: Assocation of hereditary spherocytosis and idiopathic hemochromatosis. A synergistic effect in determining iron overload. *Am J Clin Pathol* **86:**645, 1986.
392. Mohler DN, Wheby MS: Hemochromatosis heterozygotes may have significant iron overload when they also have hereditary spherocytosis. *Am J Med Sci* **292:**320, 1986.
393. Lawrence RD: Haemochromatosis in three families and in a woman. *Lancet* **1:**736, 1949.
394. Wilson JD, Scott PJ, North JDK: Hemochromatosis in association with hereditary spherocytosis. *Arch Intern Med* **120:**701, 1967.
395. Zipursky A: Isoimmune hemolytic diseases, in Nathan DG, Oski FA (eds): *Hematology of Infancy and Childhood,* 3d ed. Philadelphia, Saunders, 1987, p 44.
396. Gilliland BC, Baxter E, Evans RS: Red cell antibodies in acquired hemolytic anemia with negative antiglobulin serum tests. *N Engl J Med* **285:**252, 1971.
397. Crosby WH, Conrad ME: Hereditary spherocytosis: Observations on hemolytic mechanisms and iron metabolism. *Blood* **15:**662, 1960.
398. McCann SR, Jacob HS: Spinal cord disease in hereditary spherocytosis: Report of two cases with a hypothesized common mechanism for neurologic and red cell abnormalities. *Blood* **48:**259, 1976.
399. Zetterstrom R, Strindberg B: Sporadic congenital spherocytosis associated with congenital hypoplastic thrombocytopenia and malformations. *Acta Paediatr* **47:**14, 1958.
400. Wiley JS, Firkin BG: An unusual variant of hereditary spherocytosis. *Am J Med* **48:**63, 1970.
401. Garwicz S: Atypical spherocytosis, a disease of spleen as well as of red blood cells. *Lancet* **1:**956, 1975.
402. Dunn I, Ibsen KH, Code L, Schneider AS, Weinstein IM: Erythrocyte carbohydrate metabolism in herditary spherocytosis. *J Clin Invest* **42:**1535, 1963.
403. Zail SS, Krawitz P, Viljoen E, Metz J: Atypical hereditary spherocytosis: Biochemical studies and sites of erythrocyte destruction. *Br J Haematol* **13:**323, 1967.
404. Singer DB: Postsplenectomy sepsis, in Rosenberg HS, Bolande RP (eds): *Perspectives in Pediatric Pathology*. Chicago, Year Book, 1973, vol 1, p 285.
405. Krivit W: Overwhelming post-splenectomy infection. *Am J Hematol* **2:**193, 1977.
406. Schwartz PE, Sterioff S, Mucha P, Melton LJ, Offord KP: Postsplenectomy sepsis and mortality in adults. *JAMA* **248:**2279, 1982.
407. Becker PS, Lux SE: Disorders of the red cell membrane, in Nathan DG, Oski FA (eds): *Hematology of Infancy and Childhood,* 4th ed. Philadelphia, Saunders, 1993, p 529.
408. Schwartz JS: Pneumococcal vaccine: Clinical efficacy and effectiveness. *Ann Intern Med* **96:**208, 1982.
409. Chapman RG: Red cell life span after splenectomy in hereditary spherocytosis. *J Clin Invest* **47:**2263, 1968.
410. MacKenzie FAF, Elliot DH, Eastcott HHG, Hughes-Jones NC, Barkhan P, Mollison PL: Relapse in hereditary spherocytosis with proven splenunculus. *Lancet* **1:**1102, 1962.
411. Bart JB, Appel MF: Recurrent hemolytic anemia secondary to accessory spleens. *South Med J* **71:**608, 1978.
412. Lambrecht K: Die Elliptocytose (Ovalocytose) und ihre klinische Bedeutung. *Ergebn Inn Med Kinderheilkd* **55:**295, 1938.
413. Dresbach M: Elliptical human red corpuscles. *Science* **19:**469, 1904.
414. Flint A: Elliptical human erythrocytes. *Science* **19:**796, 1904.
415. Dresbach M: Elliptical human erythrocytes. *Science* **21:**473, 1905.
416. Bishop FW: Elliptical human erythrocytes. *Arch Intern Med* **14:**388, 1914.
417. Sydenstricker VP: Elliptic human erythrocytes. *JAMA* **81:**113, 1923.
418. Huck JG, Bigelow RM: Poikilocytes in otherwise normal blood (elliptical human erythrocytes). *Bull Johns Hopkins Hosp* **34:**390, 1923.
419. Hunter WC, Adams RB: Hematologic study of three generations of a white family showing elliptical erythrocytes. *Ann Intern Med* **2:**1162, 1929.
420. Hunter WC: Further study of a white family showing elliptical erythrocytes. *Ann Intern Med* **6:**775, 1932.
421. Giffin HZ, Watkins CH: Ovalocytosis with features of hemolytic icterus. *Trans Assoc Am Physicians* **54:**355, 1989.
422. Penfold J, Lipscomb JM: Elliptocytosis in man, associated with hereditary haemorrhagic telangiectasis. *Q J Med* **12:**157, 1943.
423. Grzegorzewski H: Über familiäres Vorkommen elliptisher Erythrocyten beim Menschen. *Folia Haematol (Leipz)* **50:**260, 1933.
424. van den Bergh AAH: Elliptische rote Blutköperchen, (Addendum). *Dtsch Med Wochenschr* **54:**1244, 1928.
425. Mason VR: Ovalocytosis (elliptical human erythrocytes), in Downey H (ed): *Handbook of Hematology*. New York, Paul B. Hoeber, 1938, vol 3, p 2351.
426. Lawrence JS: Elliptical and sickle-shaped erythrocytes in the circulating blood of white persons. *J Clin Invest* **5:**31, 1927.
427. Pollock LH, Dameshek W: Elongation of red blood cells in a Jewish family. *Am J Med Sci* **188:**822, 1934.
428. Introzzi P: Anemia ipocromica splenomegalica emolitica con ovalocitosi (ellitticitosi), poichilocitosi ed aumento della resistenza osmotica dei globuli rossi, Splenectomia. *Haematologica* **16:**525, 1935.
429. Wyandt H, Bancroft PM, Winship TO: Elliptic erythrocytes in man. *Arch Intern Med* **68:**1043, 1941.
430. Wolman IJ, Ozge A: Studies on elliptocytosis. I. Hereditary elliptocytosis in the pediatric age period: A review of recent literature. *Am J Med Sci* **234:**702, 1957.
431. Dacie JV: Hereditary elliptocytosis, in *The Hemolytic Anemias, Congenital and Acquired, Part I. The Congenital Anemias,* 2d ed. New York, Grune & Stratton, 1960, p 151.
432. Josephs HW, Avery ME: Hereditary elliptocytosis associated with increased hemolysis. *Pediatrics* **16:**741, 1965.
433. Weiss HJ: Hereditary elliptocytosis with hemolytic anemia. *Am J Med* **35:**455, 1963.
434. Cutting HO, McHugh WJ, Conrad FG, Marlow AA: Autosomal dominant hemolytic anemia characterized by ovalocytosis. A family study of seven involved members. *Am J Med* **39:**21, 1965.
435. McCarty SH: Elliptical red blood cells in man. A report of eleven cases. *J Lab Clin Med* **19:**612, 1934.
436. Goodall HB, Hendry DWW, Lawler SD, Stephen SA: Data on linkage in man: Elliptocytosis and blood groups. II. Family 3. *Ann Eugenet* **17:**272, 1953.

437. Morton NE: The detection and estimation of linkage between the genes for elliptocytosis and the Rh blood type. *Am J Hum Genet* **8**:80, 1956.
438. Bannerman RM, Renwick JH: The hereditary elliptocytoses: Clinical and linkage data. *Ann Hum Genet* **26**:23, 1962.
439. Cook PJL, Noades JE, Newton MS, De Mey R: On the orientation of the Rh El, linkage group. *Ann Hum Genet* **41**:157, 1977.
440. Conboy J, Kan YW, Shohet SB, Mohandas N: Molecular cloning of protein 4.1, a major structural element of the human erythrocyte membrane skeleton. *Proc Natl Acad Sci USA* **83**:9512, 1986.
441. Keats BJB: Another elliptocytosis locus on chromosome 1? *Hum Genet* **50**:227, 1979.
442. Lawler J, Liu SC, Palek J, Prchal J: Molecular defect of spectrin in hereditary pyropoikilocytosis: Alterations in the typsin-resistant domain involved in spectrin self-association. *J Clin Invest* **70**:1019, 1982.
443. Mentzer WC, Turetsky T, Mohandas N, Schrier S, Wu CS: Identification of the hereditary pyropoikilocytosis carrier state. *Blood* **63**:1439, 1984.
444. Lawler J, Liu SC, Palek J, Prchal J: Molecular defect of spectrin in a subgroup of patients with hereditary elliptocytosis: Alteration in the alpha subunit involved in spectrin self association. *J Clin Invest* **73**:1688, 1984.
445. Palek J, Lux SE: Red cell membrane skeletal defects in hereditary and acquired hemolytic anemias. *Semin Hematol* **20**:189, 1983.
446. Florman AL, Wintrobe MM: Human elliptical red corpuscles. *Bull Johns Hopkins Hosp* **63**:209, 1938.
447. Motulsky AG, Singer K, Crosby WH, Smith V: The life span of the elliptocyte. Hereditary elliptocytosis and its relationship to other familial hemolytic diseases. *Blood* **9**:57, 1954.
448. Garrdo-Lacca G, Merino C, Luna G: Hereditary elliptocytosis in a Peruvian family. *N Engl J Med* **256**:311, 1957.
449. Geerdink RA, Helleman PW, Verloop MC: Hereditary elliptocytosis and hyperhaemolysis. A comparative study of 6 families with 145 patients. *Acta Med Scand* **179**:715, 1966.
450. Jensson O, Jonasson TH, Olafsson O: Hereditary elliptocytosis in Iceland. *Br J Haematol* **13**:844, 1967.
451. Trinick RH: Elliptocytosis. *Lancet* **1**:963, 1948.
451a. Coetzer T, Lawler J, Prchal JT, Palek J: Molecular determinants of clinical expression of hereditary elliptocytosis and pyropoikilocytosis. *Blood* **70**:766, 1987.
452. Helz MK, Menten ML: Elliptocytosis, a report of two cases. *J Lab Clin Med* **29**:185, 1944.
453. Gunther H: Die Klinische Bedeutung der Ellipsenformen der Erythrozyten. *Dtsch Arch Klin Med* **162**:215, 1928.
454. Geerdink RA, Nijenhuis LE, Huizinga J: Hereditary elliptocytosis: Linkage data in man. *Ann Hum Genet* **30**:363, 1967.
455. van den Bergh AAH, Rehorst K: A propos des hématies elliptiques (ovalocytose). *Rev Belg Sci Med* **3**:683, 1931.
456. Grech JL, Cachia EA, Calleja F, Pullicino F: Hereditary elliptocytosis in two Maltese families. *J Clin Pathol* **14**:365, 1961.
457. McCurdy PR: Clinical, genetic and physiological studies in hereditary elliptocytosis, in *Proceedings of the IX Congress International Society of Hematology*. Mexico City, Universidad Nacional Autonoma de Mexico, 1964, vol 1, p 155.
458. Ozer L, Mills GC: Elliptocytosis with haemolytic anaemia. *Br J Haematol* **10**:468, 1964.
459. Nkrumah FK: Hereditary elliptocytosis associated with severe haemolytic anaemia and malaria. *Afr J Med Sci* **3**:131, 1972.
460. Kruatrachuo M, Asawapokee N: Hereditary elliptocytosis and Plasmodium falciparum malaria. *Ann Trop Med Parasitol* **66**:161, 1972.
461. Pearson HA: The genetic basis of hereditary elliptocytosis with hemolysis. *Blood* **32**:972, 1968.
462. Blackburn EK, Jordan A, Lytle WJ, Swan HT, Tudhope GR: Hereditary elliptocytic haemolytic anaemia. *J Clin Pathol* **11**:316, 1958.
463. Lane PA, Shew RL, Iarocci TA, Mohandas N, Hays T, Mentzer WC: Unique alpha-spectrin mutant in a kindred with common hereditary elliptocytosis. *J Clin Invest* **79**:989, 1987.
464. Baker SJ, Jacob E, Rajan KT, Gault EW: Hereditary haemolytic anaemia associated with elliptocytosis: A study of three families. *Br J Haematol* **7**:210, 1961.
465. Austin RF, Desforges FJ: Hereditary elliptocytosis: An unusual presentation of hemolysis in the newborn associated with transient morphologic abnormalities. *Pediatrics* **44**:196, 1969.
466. Carpentieri U, Gustavson LP, Haggard ME: Pyknocytosis in a neonate: An unusual presentation of hereditary elliptocytosis. *Clin Pediatr* **16**:76, 1977.
467. Zarkowsky HS: Heat-induced erythrocyte fragmentation in neonatal elliptocytosis. *Br J Haematol* **41**:515, 1979.
468. Lux SE, John KM: Unpublished observations.
469. Torlontano G, Fioritoni G, Salvati AM: Hereditary haemolytic ovalocytosis with defective erythropoiesis. *Br J Haematol* **43**:435, 1979.
470. Lipton EL: Elliptocytosis with hemolytic anemia; the effects of splenectomy. *Pediatrics* **15**:67, 1955.
471. Pryor DS, Pitney WR: Hereditary elliptocytosis: A report of two families from New Guinea. *Br J Haematol* **13**:126, 1967.
472. Nielsen JA, Strunk KW: Homozygous hereditary elliptocytosis as a cause of haemolytic anaemia in infancy. *Scand J Haematol* **5**:486, 1968.
473. Evans JPM, Baines AJ, Hann IM, Al-Hakim I, Knowles SM, Hoffbrand AV: Defective spectrin dimer-dimer association in a family with transfusion dependent homozygous hereditary elliptocytosis. *Br J Haematol* **54**:163, 1983.
474. Garbarz M, LeComte MC, Dhermy D, Féo C, Chaveroche I, Gautero H, Bournier O, Picat C, Goepp A, Boivin P: Double inheritance of an alpha I/65 spectrin variant in a child with homozygous elliptocytosis. *Blood* **67**:1661, 1986.
475. Tchernia G, Mohandas N, Shohet SB: Deficiency of cytoskeletal membrane protein band 4.1 in homozygous hereditary elliptocytosis: Implications for erythrocyte membrane stability. *J Clin Invest* **68**:454, 1981.
476. Zarkowsky HS, Mohandas N, Speaker CB, Shohet SB: A congenital haemolytic anaemia with thermal sensitivity of the erythrocyte membrane. *Br J Haematol* **29**:537, 1975.
477. Wiley JS, Gill FM: Red cell calcium leak in congenital hemolytic anemia with extreme microcytosis. *Blood* **47**:197, 1976.
478. Dacie JV, Mollison PL, Richardson N, Selwyn JG, Shapir I: Atypical congenital haemolytic anaemia. *Q J Med (New Series)* **22**:79, 1953.
479. Coetzer TL, Palek J: Partial spectrin deficiency in hereditary pyropoikilocytosis. *Blood* **67**:919, 1986.
480. Greenberg LH, Tanaka KR: Hereditary elliptocytosis with hemolytic anemia—a family study of five affected members. *Calif Med* **110**:389, 1969.
481. Wilson HE, Long MJ: Hereditary ovalocytosis (elliptocytosis) with hypersplenism. *Arch Intern Med* **95**:438, 1955.
482. Matsumoto N, Ishihara T, Takahashi M, Uchino F, Ono J, Miwa S, Kiyomitsu Y: Fine structure of the spleen in hereditary elliptocytosis. *Acta Pathol Jpn* **26**:533, 1976.
483. Baer A, Lie-Injo LE, Welch QB, Lewis AN: Genetic factors and malaria in the Temuan. *Am J Hum Genet* **28**:179, 1976.
484. Cattani JA: The ovalocytosis polymorphism and malaria resistance in Papua New Guinea: An epidemiological study. PhD dissertation. University of California–Berkeley, 1984, p 1.
485. Fix AG, Baer AS, Lie-Injo LE: The mode of inheritance of ovalocytosis/elliptocytosis in Malaysian Orang Asli families. *Hum Genet* **61**:250, 1982.
486. Castelino D, Saul A, Myler P, Kidson C, Thomas H, Cooke R: Ovalocytosis in Papua New Guinea—dominantly inherited resistance to malaria. *Southeast Asian J Trop Med Public Health* **12**:549, 1981.
487. Liu S-C, Zhai S, Palek J, Golan DE, Amato D, Hassan K, Nurse G, Babona D, Coetzer T, Jarolim P, Zaik M, Borwein S: Molecular defect of the band 3 protein in Southeast Asian ovalocytosis. *N Engl J Med* **323**:1530, 1990.

488. Amato D, Booth PB: Hereditary ovalocytosis in Melanesians. *Papua New Guinea Med J* **20**:26, 1977.
489. Harrison KL, Collins KA, McKenna HW: Hereditary elliptical stomatocytosis; a case report. *Pathology* **8**:307, 1976.
490. Booth PB, Sevjeantson S, Woodfield DG, Amato D: Selective depression of blood group antigens associated with hereditary ovalocytosis among Melanesians. *Vox Sang* **32**:99, 1977.
491. Honig GR, Lacson PS, Maurer HS: A new familial disorder with abnormal erythrocyte morphology and increased permeability of the erythrocytes to sodium and potassium. *Pediatr Res* **5**:159, 1971.
492. Serjeantson S, Bryson K, Amato D, Babona D: Malaria and hereditary ovalocytosis. *Hum Gent* **37**:161, 1977.
493. Kidson C, Lamont G, Saul A, Nurse G: Ovalocytic erythrocytes from Melanesians are resistant to invasion by malaria parasites in culture. *Proc Natl Acad Sci USA* **78**:5829, 1981.
494. Hadley T, Saul A, Lamont G, Hudson DE, Miller LH, Kidson C: Resistance of Melanesian elliptocytes (ovalocytes) to invasion by Plasmodium knowlesi and Plasmodium falciparum malaria parasites in vitro. *J Clin Invest* **71**:780, 1983.
495. Mohandas N, Lie-Injo LE, Friedman M, Mak JW: Rigid membranes of Malayan ovalocytes: A likely genetic barrier against malaria. *Blood* **63**:1385, 1984.
496. Saul A, Lamont G, Sawyer WH, Kidson C: Decreased membrane deformability in Melanesian ovalocytes from Papua New Guinea. *J Cell Biol* **98**:1348, 1984.
497. Miller LH, Mason SJ, Dvorak JA, McGinniss MLT, Rothman IK: Erythrocyte receptors for (Plasmodium knowlesi) malaria: Duffy blood group determinants. *Science* **189**:561, 1975.
498. Perkins M: Inhibitory effects of erythrocyte membrane proteins on the in vitro invasion of the human malarial parasite (Plasmodium falciparum) into its host cell. *J Cell Biol* **90**:563, 1981.
499. Hermentin P, Enders B: Erythrocyte invasion by malaria (Plasmodium falciparum) merozoites: Recent advances in the evaluation of receptor sites. *Behring Inst Mitt* 1984, p 121.
500. Liu SC, Palek J, Prchal J: Defective spectrin dimer-dimer association in hereditary elliptocytosis. *Proc Natl Acad Sci USA* **79**:2072, 1982.
501. Mohandas N, Clark MR, Health BP, Rossi M, Wolfe LC, Lux SE, Shohet SB: A technique to detect reduced mechanical stability of red cell membranes: Relevance to elliptocytic disorders. *Blood* **59**:768, 1982.
502. Chang K, Williamson JR, Zarkowsky HS: Effect of heat on the circular dichroism of spectrin in hereditary pyropoikilocytosis. *J Clin Invest* **64**:326, 1979.
503. Liu SC, Palek J, Prchal J, Castlebury RP: Altered spectrin dimer-dimer association and instability of erythrocyte membrane skeletons in hereditary pyropoikilocytosis. *J Clin Invest* **68**:697, 1981.
504. Knowles WJ, Morrow JS, Speicher DW, Zarkowsky AS, Mohandas N, Mentzer WC, Shohet SB, Marchesi VT: Molecular and functional changes in spectrin from patients with hereditary pyropoikilocytosis. *J Clin Invest* **71**:1867, 1983.
505. Marchesi SL, Knowles WT, Morrow JS, Bologna M, Marchesi VT: Abnormal spectrin in hereditary elliptocytosis. *Blood* **67**:141, 1986.
506. Morlé L, Alloisio N, Ducluzeau MT, Pothier B, Blibech R, Kastally R, Delaunay J: Spectrin Tunis (I/78): A new I variant that causes asymptomatic hereditary elliptocytosis in the heterozygous state. *Blood* **71**:508, 1988.
507. Lawler J, Liu S-C, Palek J, Prchal J: Molecular defect of spectrin in hereditary pyropoikilocytosis: Alterations in the trypsin-resistant domain involved in spectrin self-association. *J Clin Invest* **70**:1019, 1982.
508. Palek J, Liu SC, Liu PY, Prchal J, Castleberry RP: Altered assembly of spectrin in red cell membranes in hereditary pyropoikilocytosis. *Blood* **57**:130, 1981.
509. Lecomte MC, Dhermy D, Garbarz M, Gautero H, Bournier O, Galand C, Boivin P: Hereditary elliptocytosis with spectrin molecular defect in a white patient. *Acta Haematol (Basel)* **71**:235, 1984.
510. Dhermy D, Lecomte MC, Garbarz M, Féo C, Gauter H, Bournier O, Galand C, Herrera A, Gretillat F, Boivin P: Molecular defect of spectrin in the family of a child with congenital hemolytic poikilocytic anemia. *Pediatr Res* **18**:1005, 1984.
511. Dhermy D, Garbarz M, LeComte MC, Féo C, Bournier D, Chareroche I, Gauters H, Galand C, Boivin P: Hereditary elliptocytosis: Clinical, morphogical, and biochemical studies of 38 cases. *Nouv Rev Fr Hematol* **28**:129, 1986.
512. LeComte MC, Dhermy D, Solis C, Ester A, Féo C, Gauters H, Bournier O, Boivin P: A new abnormal variant of spectrin black patients with hereditary elliptocytosis. *Blood* **65**:1208, 1985.
513. Alloisio N, Guetorni D, Morlé L, Pothier B, Duchizeau MT, Soun A, Colonna P, Clerc M, Philippe N, Delaunay J: Sp alpha I/65 hereditary elliptocytosis in North Africa. *Am J Hematol* **23**:113, 1986.
514. Lawler J, Coetzer TL, Mankad VN, Moore RV, Prchal JT, Palek J: Spectrin $\alpha^{I/61}$: A new structural variant of α spectrin in a double heterozygous form of hereditary pyropoikilocytosis. *Blood* **72**:1412, 1988.
515. Lecomte MC, Dhermy D, Garbarz M, Féo C, Gautero H, Bournier O, Picat C, Chareroche I, Ester A, Galard C: Pathologic and non-pathologic variants of the spectrin molecule in two black families with hereditary elliptocytosis. *Hum Genet* **71**:351, 1985.
516. Marchesi SL, Letsinger JT, Speicher DW, Marchesi VT, Agre P, Hyun B, Gulati G: Mutant forms of spectrin alpha-subunits in hereditary elliptocytosis. *J Clin Invest* **80**:191, 1987.
517. Lambert S, Zail S: A new variant of the α subunit of spectrin in hereditary elliptocytosis. *Blood* **69**:473, 1987.
518. Baklouti F, Marechal J, Wilmotte R, Alloisio N, Morlé L, Ducluzeau MT, Denoroy L, Mrad A, Ben Aribia MH, Kastally R, Delaunay J: Elliptocytogenic $\alpha^{I/36}$ spectrin Sfax lacks nine amino acids in helix 3 of repeat 4. Evidence for the activation of a cryptic 5′-splice site in exon 8 of spectrin α-gene. *Blood* **79**:2464, 1992.
519. Morlé L, Morlé F, Roux AF, Godet J, Forget BG, Denoroy L, Garbarz M, Dhermy D, Kastally R, Delaunay J: Spectrin Tunis (Sp $\alpha^{I/78}$), an elliptocytogenic variant, is due to the CGG→TGG codon change (Arg→Trp) at position 35 of the αI domain. *Blood* **74**:828, 1989.
520. Lecomte MC, Garbarz M, Grandchamp B, Féo C, Gautero H, Devaux I, Bournier O, Galand C, d'Auriol L, Galibert F, Sahr KE, Forget BG, Boivin P, Dhermy DL: Sp $\alpha^{I/78}$: A mutation of the αI spectrin domain in a white kindred with HE and HPP phenotypes. *Blood* **74**:1126, 1989.
521. Garbarz M, Lecomte MC, Féo C, Devaux I, Picat C, Lefebvre C, Gailbert F, Gautero H, Bournier O, Galand C, Forget BG, Boivin P, Dhermy D: Hereditary pyropoikilocytosis and elliptocytosis in a white French family with the spectrin $\alpha^{I/74}$ variant related to a CGT to CAT codon change (Arg to His) at position 22 of the spectrin αI domain. *Blood* **75**:1691, 1990.
522. Morle L, Roux AF, Alloisio N, Pothier B, Starck J, Denoroy L, Morle F, Rudigoz RC, Forget BG, Delaunay J, Godet J: Two elliptocytogenic $\alpha^{I/74}$ variants of the spectrin αI domain spectrin Culoz (GGT→GTT; αI 40 Gly→Val) and spectrin Lyon (CTT→TTT; αI 43 Leu→Phe). *J Clin Invest* **86**:548, 1990.
523. Coetzer T, Sahr K, Prchal J, Blacklock H, Peterson L, Koler R, Doyle J, Manaster J, Forget B, Palek J: Four different mutations in codon 28 of α spectrin are associated with structurally and functionally abnormal spectrin $\alpha^{I/74}$ in hereditary elliptocytosis. *J Clin Invest* **88**:743, 1991.
524. Floyd PB, Gallagher PG, Valentino LA, Davis M, Marchesi SL, Forget BG: Heterogeneity of the molecular basis of hereditary pyropoikilocytosis and hereditary elliptocytosis associated with increased levels of the spectrin $\alpha^{I/74}$-kilodalton tryptic peptide. *Blood* **78**:1364, 1991.
525. Lane PA, Shaw RL, Iarocci TA, Mehandas N, Hays T, Mentur WC: Unitque α-spectrin mutant in a kindred with common hereditary elliptocytosis. *J Clin Invest* **79**:989, 1987.
526. Roux AF, Morle F, Guetarni D, Colonna P, Sahr K, Forget BG, Delaunay J, Godet J: Molecular basis of Sp $\alpha^{I/65}$ hereditary elliptocytosis in North Africa: Insertion of a TTG triplet between codons 147 and 149 in the α-spectrin gene from five unrelated families. *Blood* **73**:2196, 1989.

527. Dhermy D, Boulanger L, Silva CJ, et al: Spectrin Ponte de Sor (Gly151→Asp): A mutation of the spectrin α gene associated with Sp $\alpha^{I/65}$ hereditary elliptocytosis. 24th Congress of the International Society of Hematology 143, 1992.
528. Dhermy D, Lecomte MC, Garbarz M, Féo C, Galand C, Bournier O, Gautero H, Boivin P: A new kindred of hereditary elliptocytosis (HE) with a shortened spectrin alpha chain. *Blood (suppl 1)* **70**:52a, 1987.
529. Coetzer T, Palek J, Lawler J, Liu S-C, Jarolim P, Lahav M, Prchal JT, Wang W, Alter BP, Schewitz G, Mankad V, Gallanello R, Cao A: Structural and functional heterogeneity of α spectrin mutations involving the spectrin heterodimer self-association site: Relationships to hematologic expression of homozygous hereditary elliptocytosis and hereditary pyropoikilocytosis. *Blood* **75**:2235, 1990.
530. Hanspal M, Hanspal JS, Sahr KE, Fibach E, Nachman J, Palek J: Molecular basis of spectrin deficiency in hereditary pyropoikilocytosis. *Blood* **82**:1652, 1993.
531. Dhermy D, Lecomte MC, Garbarz M, Bournier O, Galand C, Gauters H, Féo C, Alloisio N, Delaunay J, Boivin P: Spectrin beta-chain variant associated with hereditary elliptocytosis. *J Clin Invest* **70**:707, 1982.
532. Ohanian V, Evans JP, Gratzer WB: A case of elliptocytosis associated with a truncated spectrin chain. *Br J Haematol* **61**:31, 1985.
533. Eber SW, Morris SA, Schröter W, Gratzer WB: Interactions of spectrin in hereditary elliptocytes containing truncated spectrin β-chains. *J Clin Invest* **81**:523, 1988.
534. Garbarz M, Tse WT, Gallagher PG, Picat C, Lecomte MC, Galibert F, Dhermy D, Forget BG: Spectrin Rouen ($\beta^{220/218}$), a novel shortened β-chain variant in a kindred with hereditary elliptocytosis. *J Clin Invest* **88**:76, 1991.
535. Tse WT, Gallagher PG, Pothier B, Costa FF, Scarpa A, Delaunay J, Forget BG: An insertional frameshift mutation of the β-spectrin gene associated with elliptocytosis in spectrin Nice ($\beta^{220/216}$). *Blood* **78**:517, 1991.
536. Garbarz M, Boulanger L, Pedroni S, Lecomte MC, Gautero H, Galand C, Boivin P, Feldman L, Dhermy D: Spectrin β^{TANDIL}, a novel shortened β-chain variant associated with hereditary elliptocytosis is due to a deletional frameshift mutation in the β-spectrin gene. *Blood* **80**:1066, 1992.
537. Kanzaki A, Rabodonirina M, Yawata Y, Wilmotte R, Wada H, Ata K, Yamada O, Akatsuka J, Iyori H, Horiguchi M, Nakamura H, Mishima T, Morle L, Delaunay J: A deletional frameshift mutation of the β-spectrin gene associated with elliptocytosis in spectrin Tokyo ($\beta^{220/216}$). *Blood* **80**:2115, 1992.
538. Gallagher PG, Tse WT, Costa F, Scarpa A, Boivin P, Delaunay J, Forget BG: A splice site mutation of the β-spectrin gene causing exon skipping in hereditary elliptocytosis associated with a truncated β-spectrin chain. *J Biol Chem* **266**:15154, 1991.
539. Yoon SH, Yu H, Eber S, Prchal JT: Molecular defect of truncated β-spectrin associated with hereditary elliptocytosis. β-spectrin Göttingen. *J Biol Chem* **266**:8490, 1991.
540. Takanashi K, Sugawar T, Sakurai K, et al: A trait of hereditary elliptocytosis with truncated β-spectrin (spectrin Yamagata $\beta^{220/210}$). *Jpn J Clin Hematol* **32**:1365a, 1991.
541. Gallagher PG, Tse WT, Mohandas N, Marchesi SL, Forget BG: Spectrin Providence: A defect of erythrocyte beta spectrin ($\beta^{2019\ Ser\text{-}Pro}$) homozygosity for which is associated with fatal hydrops fetalis. *Blood (suppl 1)* **80**:145a, 1992.
542. Sahr KE, Coetzer TL, Moy LS, Derick LH, Chishti AH, Jarolim P, Gallanello R, Cao A, Liu S-C, Palek J: An Ala to Gly substitution in β spectrin associated with spectrin αI/74 in hereditary elliptocytosis (HE) and hereditary pyropoikilocytosis (HPP). *Blood (suppl 1)* **80**:276a, 1992.
543. Leconte C, Fis C, Gantere H, Bournier O, Galand C, Ganbarz M, Boivin P, Dhomy D: Severe recessive poikilocytic anemia with a new spectrin α chain variant. *Br J Haematol* **74**:497, 1990.
544. Gallagher PG, Tse WT, Coetzer T, Lecomte MC, Garbarz M, Zarkowsky HS, Baruchel A, Ballas SK, Dhermy D, Palek J, Forget BG: A common type of the spectrin αI 46-50a-dK peptide abnormality in hereditary elliptocytosis and hereditary pyropoikilocytosis is associated with a mutation distant from the proteolytic cleavage site—evidence for the functional importance of the triple helical model of spectrin. *J Clin Invest* **89**:892, 1992.
545. Sahr K, Tobe T, Scarpa A, Laughinghouse K, Marchesi SL, Agre P, Linnenbach AJ, Marchesi VT, Forget BG: Sequence and exon-intron organization of the DNA encoding the αI domain of human spectrin. Application to the study of mutations causing hereditary elliptocytosis. *J Clin Invest* **84**:1243, 1989.
546. Dalla Venezia N, Alloisio N, Forssier A, Denoroy L, Aymerich M, Vives-Corrons JL, Besalduch J, Besson I, Delaunay J: Elliptopoikilocytosis associated with the α469 His→Pro mutation in spectrin Barcelona ($\alpha^{I/50\text{-}46b}$). *Blood* **82**:1661, 1993.
547. Gallagher PG, Roberts WE, Benoit L, Speicher DW, Marchesi SL, Forget BG: Poikilocytic hereditary elliptocytosis associated with spectrin Alexandria: An $\alpha^{I/50b}$ kd variant that is caused by a single amino acid deletion. *Blood* **82**:2210, 1993.
548. Knowles WJ, Morrow JS, Speicher DW, Zarkowsky AS, Mohandas N, Mentzer WC, Shohet SB, Marchesi VT: Molecular and functional changes in spectrin from patients with hereditary pyropoikilocytosis. *J Clin Invest* **71**:1867, 1983.
549. Alloisio N, Mark L, Dorleai E, Gentilhemme O, Bachier D, Guetarni D, Colenna P, Bost M, Zouaoui Z, Roda L: The heterozygous form of 4.1(-) hereditary elliptocytosis [the 4.1(-) trait]. *Blood* **65**:46, 1985.
550. Alloisio N, Dorléac E, Girot R, Delaunay J: Analysis of the red cell membrane in a family with hereditary elliptocytosis—total or partial absence of protein 4.1. *Hum Genet* **59**:68, 1981.
551. Takakuwa Y, Tchernia G, Rossi M, Benabadji M, Mohandas N: Restoration of normal membrane stability to unstable protein 4.1-deficient erythrocyte membranes by incorporation of purified protein 4.1. *J Clin Invest* **78**:80, 1986.
552. Alloisio N, Morlé L, Bachir D, Guetarni D, Colonna P, Delaunay J: Red cell membrane sialoglycoprotein beta in hemozygous and heterozygous 4.1(-) hereditary elliptocytosis. *Biochim Biophys Acta* **816**:57, 1985.
553. Conboy J, Mohandas N, Tchernia G, Kan YW: Molecular basis of hereditary spherocytosis due to protein 4.1 deficiency. *N Engl J Med* **315**:680, 1986.
554. Féo CJ, Fischer S, Piau JP, Grange MJ, Tchernia G: Première observation de l'absence d'une protéine de la membrane érythrocytaire (band-4_1) dans un cas d'anemie elliptocytaire familiale. *Nouv Rev F Hematol* **22**:315, 1981.
555. Mueller TY, William J, Wang W, Morrison M: Cycloskeletal alterations in hereditary elliptocytocytosis. *Blood* **58**:47a, 1981.
556. Discher DK, Parra M, Conboy JG, Mohandas N: Mechanochemistry of the alternatively spliced spectrin-actin binding domain in membrane skeletal protein 4.1. *J Biol Chem* **268**:7186, 1993.
557. Conboy JG, Chasis JA Winardi R, Tchernia G, Kan YW, Mohandas N: An isoform-specific mutation in the protein 4.1 gene results in hereditary elliptocytosis and complete deficiency of protein 4.1 in erythrocytes but not nonerythroid cells. *J Clin Invest* **91**:77, 1993.
558. Dalla Venezia N, Gilsanz F, Alloisio N, Ducluzeau M-T, Benz EJ Jr, Delaunay J: Homozygous 4.1(-) hereditary elliptocytosis associated with a point mutation in the downstream initiation codon of protein 4.1 gene. *J Clin Invest* **90**:1713, 1992.
559. Reid ME, Takakuwa Y, Conboy J, Tchernia G, Mohandas N: Glycophorin C content of human erythrocyte membranes is regulated by protein 4.1. *Blood* **75**:2229, 1990.
560. Grabarz M, Dhermy D, LeComte MC, Féo C, Chaveroche I, Galand C, Bournier O, Bertrand O, Boivin P: A variant of erythrocyte membrane skeletal protein band 4.1 associated with hereditary elliptocytosis. *Blood* **64**:1006, 1984.
561. Conboy JG, Shitamoto R, Parra M, Winardi R, Kabra A, Smith J, Mohandas N: Hereditary elliptocytosis due to both qualitative and quantitative defects in membrane skeletal protein 4.1. *Blood* **78**:2438, 1991.
562. Marchesi SL, Conboy J, Agre P, Letsinger JT, Marchesi VT, Speicher DW, Mohandas N: Molecular analysis of insertion/deletion mutations in protein 4.1 in elliptocytosis. I.

Biochemical identification of rearrangements in the spectrin/actin binding domain and functional characterization. *J Clin Invest* **86:**516, 1990.

563. Conboy J, Marchesi S, Kim R, Agre P, Kan YW, Mohandas N: Molecular analysis of insertion/deletion mutations in protein 4.1 in elliptocytosis. II. Determination of molecular genetic origins of rearrangements. *J Clin Invest* **86:**524, 1990.
564. Horne WC, Huang S-C, Becker PS, Tang TK, Benz EJ Jr: Tissue-specific alternative splicing of protein 4.1 inserts an exon necessary for formation of the ternary complex with erythrocyte spectrin and actin. *Blood* **82:**2558, 1993.
565. Morlé L, Garbarz M, Alloisio N, et al: The characterization of protein 4.1 Presles, a shortened variant of RBC membrane protein 4.1 *Blood* **65:**1511, 1985.
566. Feddal S, Hayette S, Baklaouti F, Rimokh R, Wilmotte R, Mayaud JP, Maréchal J, Benz EJ Jr, Girot R, Delaunay J, Morlé L: Prevalent skipping of an individual exon accounts for shortened protein 4.1 Presles. *Blood* **80:**2925, 1992.
567. Anstee DJ, Ridgewell K, Tanner MJ, Daniels GL, Parsons SF: Individuals lacking the Gerbich blood-group antigens have alterations in the human erythrocyte membrane sialoglycoproteins beta and gamma. *Biochem J* **221:**97, 1984.
568. Mueller T, Manson M: Glycoconnectin (PAS2) a membrane attachment site for the human erythrocyte cytoskeleton, in Kruckeberg W, Eaton J, Greuner G (eds): *Erythrocyte Membranes 2: Recent Clinical and Experimental Advances*. New York, Alan R. Liss, 1981, p 95.
569. Alloisio N, Wilmotte R, Morlé L, Baklouti F, Maréchal J, Ducluzeau M-T, Denoroy L, Féo C, Forget BG, Kastally R, Delaunay J: Spectrin Jendouba: An $\alpha^{II/31}$ spectrin variant that is associated with elliptocytosis and carries a mutation distant from the dimer self-association site. *Blood* **80:**809, 1992.
570. Alloisio N, Morle L, Pothier B, et al: Spectrin Oran ($\alpha^{II/21}$), a new spectrin variant concerning the αII domain and causing severe elliptocytosis in the homozygous state. *Blood* **71:**1039, 1988.
571. Jarolim P, Rubin HL, Zhai S, Sahr KE, Liu S-C, Mueller TJ, Palek J: Band 3 Memphis: A widespread polymorphism with abnormal electrophoretic mobility of erythrocyte band 3 protein caused by the substitution AAG→GAG (Lys→Flu) in codon 56. *Blood* **80:**1592, 1992.
572. Yannoukakos D, Vasseur C, Driancourt C, et al: Human erythrocyte band 3 polymorphism (band 3 Memphis): Characterization of the structural modification (Lys56→Glu) by protein chemistry methods. *Blood* **78:**1117, 1991.
573. Mueller TJ, Morrison M: Detection of a variant of protein 3, the major transmembrane protein on the human erythrocyte. *J Biol Chem* **252:**6573, 1977.
574. Jarolim P, Palek J, Amato D, Hassan K, Sapak P, Nurse GT, Rubin HL, Zhai S, Sahr KE, Liu S-C: Deletion in erythrocyte band 3 gene in malaria-resistant Southeast Asian ovalocytosis. *Proc Natl Acad Sci USA* **88:**11022, 1991.
575. Mohandas N, Winardi R, Knowles D, Leung A, Parra M, George E, Conboy J, Chasis J: Molecular basis for membrane rigidity of hereditary ovalocytosis—a novel mechanism involving the cytoplasmic domain of band 3. *J Clin Invest* **89:**686, 1992.
576. Liu S-C, Yi SJ, Derick LH, et al: Characterization of the band 3 protein in Southeast Asian ovalocytosis (SAO): Interrelationships among band 3 self-association, ankyrin binding, rotational and lateral mobilities. *Clin Res* **41:**135a, 1993.
577. Moriyama R, Ideguchi H, Lombardo CR, Van Dort HM, Low PS: Structural and functional characterization of band 3 from Southeast Asian ovalocytes. *J Biol Chem* *267:*25792, 1992.
578. Schofield AE, Tanner MJA, Pinder JC, Clough B, Bayley PM, Nash GB, Dluzewski AR, Reardon DM, Cox TM, Wilson RJM, Gratzer WB: Basis of unique red cell membrane properties in hereditary ovalocytosis. *J Mol Biol* **223:**949, 1992.
579. Jones GL, Edmundson HM, Wesche D, Saul A: Human erythrocyte band 3 has an altered N-terminus in malaria-resistant Melanesian ovalocytosis. *Biochim Biophys Acta* **1096:**33, 1991.
580. Kay MMB, Gieljan JC, Bosman GJCG, Lawrence C: Functional topography of band 3: Specific structural alteration linked to functional aberrations in human erythrocytes. *Proc Natl Acad Sci USA* **85:**492, 1988.

580a. Bruce LJ, Kay MM, Lawrence C, Tanner MJ: Band 3 HT, a human red-cell variant associated with acanthocytosis and increased anion transport, carries the mutation Pro868→Leu in the membrane domain of band 3. *Biochem J* **293:**317, 1993.

581. Shneidman D, Kiessling P, Onstad J, Wolf P: Red pulp of the spleen in hereditary elliptocytosis. *Virchows Arch [A]* **372:**337, 1977.
582. Lux SE, Glader BE: Disorders of the red cell membrane, in Nathan DG, Oski FA (eds): *Hematology of Infancy and Childhood*, 2d ed. Philadelphia, Saunders, 1981, p 456.
583. Becker PS, Lux SE: Hereditary spherocytosis and related disorders. *Clin Haematol* **14:**15, 1985.
584. Palek J: Hereditary elliptocytosis and related disorders. *Clin Haematol* **14:**45, 1985.
585. Lecomte MC, Féo C, Gautero H, Bournier O, Galand C, Boivin P, Tchernia G, Dhermy D: Severe hereditary elliptocytosis in two related Caucasian children with a decreased amount of spectrin (Sp) α chain. *J Cell Biochem* **13B:**230, 1989. (abstr)
586. Morlé L, Pothier B, Alloisio N, Ducluzeau M-T, Marques S, Olim G, Martins e Silva T, Féo C, Garbarz M, Chaveroche I, Boivin P, Delaunay J: Red cell membrane alteration involving protein 4.1 and protein 3 in a case of recessively inherited haemolytic anemia. *Eur J Haematol* **38:**447, 1987.
587. Lawler J, Coetzer TL, Palek J, Jacob HS, Luban N: Sp $\alpha^{I/65}$: A new variant of the alpha subunit of spectrin in hereditary elliptocytosis. *Blood* **66:**706, 1985.

Part 16

MEMBRANE TRANSPORT SYSTEMS

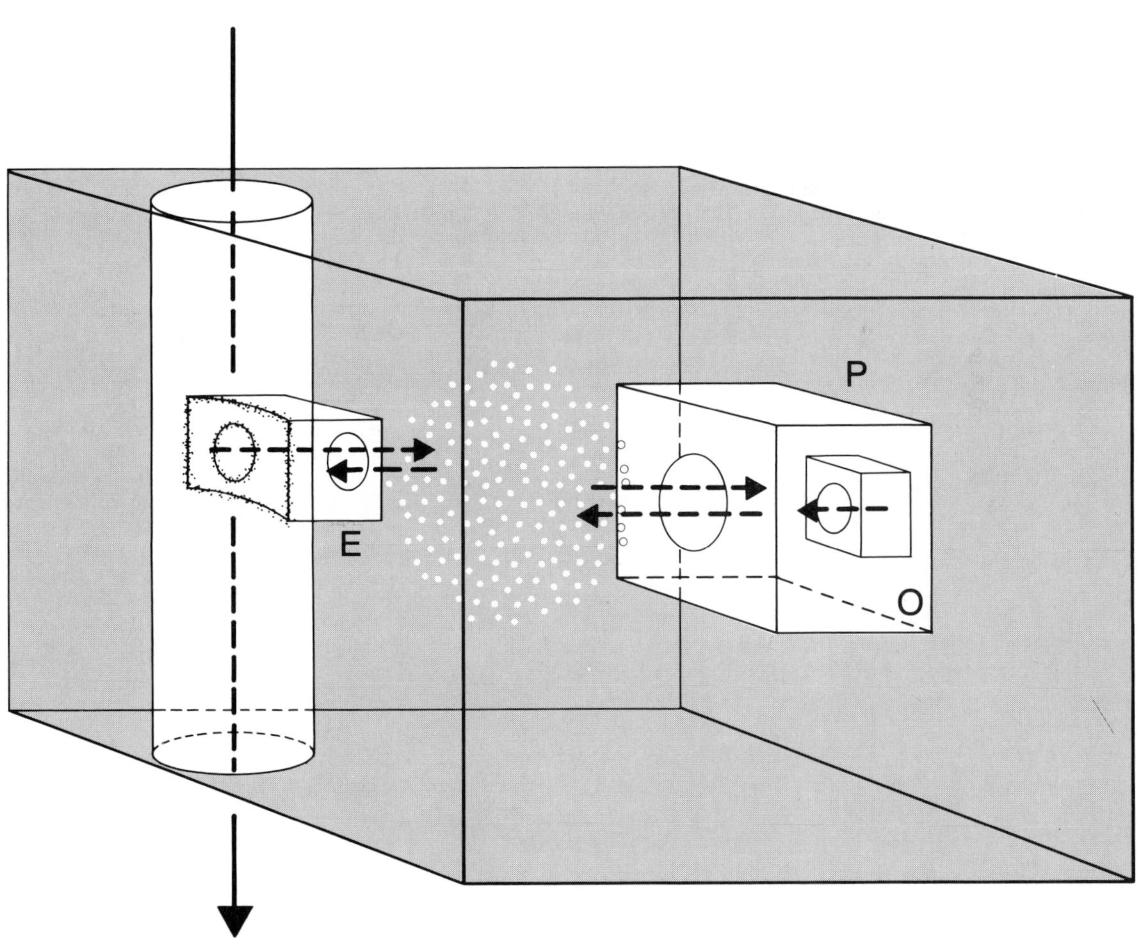

Membrane transport systems affect epithelial cells (E), parenchymal (P) cells, and organelles (O).

CHAPTER 116

Congenital Selective Na^+ D-Glucose Cotransport Defects Leading to Renal Glycosuria and Congenital Selective Intestinal Malabsorption of Glucose and Galactose

Jehan-François Desjeux ▪ Eric Turk ▪ Ernest Wright

1. **Na^+ D-glucose cotransport systems are present in the luminal membrane of epithelial cells in the small intestine and the proximal tubule of the kidney. They are essential for the absorption from lumen to blood of glucose and galactose, but not fructose. Congenital defects of Na^+ D-glucose cotransport systems are expressed in two clinical entities: selective congenital glucose and galactose malabsorption by the small intestine and familial renal glycosuria.**

2. **A minimum of two Na^+ D-glucose cotransporter genes are necessary to explain the clinical findings. Glucose–galactose malabsorption, is characterized by severe impairment of hexose transport in the small intestine with only a small deficit in the proximal tubule. Renal glycosuria, affects reabsorption of glucose by the proximal tubule but does not involve any apparent intestinal defect.**

3. **The intestinal Na^+-D-glucose cotransporter (SGLT1) has been cloned, and the gene was mapped to chromosome 22 (22q13.1). SGLT1 has been expressed in various cell types, and exhibits all the properties of the intestinal brush border Na^+-cotransporter. In two sisters suffering from glucose–galactose malabsorption, the defect has been traced to a single missense mutation (D28N; A → G position 92) in the SGLT1 gene. There is evidence that SGLT1 is expressed in the kidney, but the major cortical low-affinity Na^+-glucose cotransporter has yet to be identified and cloned. The molecular genetics are consistent with the clinical findings regarding the defects in intestinal and renal sugar absorption.**

4. **Glucose–galactose malabsorption is a rare disease characterized by the neonatal onset of severe, watery, acidic diarrhea that quickly leads to severe dehydration. Related gastrointestinal symptoms are uncommon, but intermittent or constant glucosuria is a frequent finding. Intestinal malabsorption of glucose and galactose is easily identified by the hydrogen breath test. Dramatic improvement of the diarrhea with a glucose- and galactose-free diet is typical of the disease. The diagnosis is established by direct determination of selective glucose and galactose intestinal malabsorption. Usually children and adults are able to live once glucose and galactose are removed from the diet.**

5. **Renal glycosuria denotes the renal tubule abnormality displayed by individuals who excrete a variable amount of glucose in their urine with normal levels of blood glucose. Although more frequently encountered than glucose–galactose malabsorption, this condition is not common. It is benign, usually without symptoms or physical consequences.**

6. **The intestinal congenital defect displays only one phenotype, while renal glycosuria is heterogeneous, resulting from several mutations and phenotypes, as indicated by analysis of titration curves for glucose reabsorption. In type A, minimal renal glucose threshold and maximal tubular reabsorption are both reduced; in type B, the threshold is usually reduced, while maximal tubular reabsorption is normal with an increased splay; in type O, tubular reabsorption is virtually absent.**

7. **Comparison of the clinical consequences of defective glucose absorption in the proximal tubule and small intestine may provide insight into the specific roles of the kidney and intestinal tract.**

D-glucose is an important source of energy for most cells of the body, and enters them via the plasma membrane by Na^+-independent transport systems.

In the small intestine and proximal tubule of the kidney, D-glucose is absorbed by epithelial cells that both possess an Na^+–D-glucose cotransport system at luminal membrane level and an Na^+-independent transport system at the baso-

A list of standard abbreviations is located immediately preceding the index in each volume. Additional abbreviations used in this chapter include: F_{minG} = threshold glucose concentration; GGM = glucose–galactose malabsorption; Isc = short circuit current; PD = potential difference; SGLT = sodium-glucose cotransporter; T_{mG} = glucose transport rate.

lateral membrane level. This asymmetric distribution of the D-glucose transport system is essential for the vectorial transport of glucose from lumen to blood via the epithelial cells. The genetic defects of this cotransport system at luminal membrane level are expressed mainly in two clinical entities: selective congenital glucose–galactose malabsorption by the small intestine and familial renal glycosuria. The first is characterized by severe impairment of hexose transport in the small intestine with only a small corrresponding deficit in the proximal tubule; the second is a disorder affecting proximal tubular reabsorption of D-glucose but does not involve any corresponding intestinal transport. At least two mutations at the chromosomal locus, or loci, for Na^+-dependent glucose transport are necessary to explain these clinical findings.

Substantial progress has been made in recent years in the identification of sugar transporters and their genes. There are five major Na^+-independent hexose transporters (GLUT 1 to GLUT 5) and at least two Na^+-dependent sugar transporters (SGLT1 and SGLT2). In the small intestine the major brush border Na^+-glucose cotransporter is SGLT1 and in the kidney, where SGLT1 is of minor importance, another brush border Na^+-glucose cotransporter (SGLT2) is largely responsible for the reabsorption of glucose from the glomerular filtrate. The clinical consequences of mutations in the two Na^+-dependent glucose transporters are very different. A defect in SGLT1 leads to a severe intestinal disease (glucose–galactose malabsorption) and a mild renal glycosuria, while a defect in SGLT2 produces a quantitatively severe but clinically benign renal glycosuria.

GLUCOSE–GALACTOSE MALABSORPTION

Introduction and History

Glucose–galactose malabsorption (GGM) is a rare congenital disease resulting from a selective defect in the intestinal transport of glucose and galactose. It is characterized by the neonatal onset of severe, watery, acidic diarrhea. In the past, it usually resulted in death within the first weeks of life. Now that the disease has been identified, children recover if glucose and galactose are withdrawn from their diet. In 1962, it was simultaneously described in France as an "intolerance to actively transported sugars" by Laplane et al.[1] and in Sweden by Lindquist and Meeuwisse as a "chronic diarrhea caused by monosaccharide malabsorption.[2] Thirty years later, approximately 45 cases have been reported in families of diverse origin, including Europe (from Sweden to the South of France), North America, Morocco, Turkey, Syria, Iraq, Pakistan, Bangladesh, Singapore (Chinese origin) and Japan. Newly diagnosed cases are not often reported now in the medical literature. The number of patients living with the disease at present is probably around 100.[3–29]

In 1987 the rabbit intestinal Na^+-glucose cotransporter (SGLT1) was cloned,[30] expressed, and sequenced, and in 1989 the homologous human intestinal cotransporter was cloned.[31] More recently a missense mutation in SGLT1 was found to cosegregate with the GGM phenotype in one family and to account for the defect in sugar transport.[32,33]

Clinical Description

The clinical history of GGM was almost identical for all patients: watery diarrhea is profuse, acidic, and contains sugar. In affected children given lactose, fecal sugar consists mainly of glucose and galactose, with only a small amount of lactose. For the equivalent amount of sugar given by mouth (2 g per kilogram of body weight), fecal excretion of galactose is much higher than those of glucose.[10] Incidentally, as the low stool pH results from the bacterial metabolism of the sugar in the colon, fecal acidity can be eliminated by antibiotics.[13]

Characteristically, diarrhea develops within 4 days of birth. Occasionally, it may be noticed later, within 2 weeks, or may be diagnosed only in adults.[10,18,26] Diarrhea usually leads to remarkably severe dehydration. Thus, in a series of eight patients, weight losses of 17 to 24 percent were reported.[3] Metabolic acidosis and hyperosmolar dehydration gradually develop with serum protein concentrations of up to 76 g/liter and sodium concentrations of up to 173 meq/liter. Related gastrointestinal signs and symptoms are uncommon. Abdominal distension and vomiting have been noticed. Anorexia is unusual. Apart from signs of severe dehydration, physical examination is normal.

Intermittent or permanent glycosuria after fasting or after a glucose load is a frequent finding. Thus, the combination of reducing sugars in the feces and of slight glycosuria despite a low blood sugar level is highly suggestive of GGM.[10] From the practical point of view, glycosuria may be difficult to detect due to a low quantity of glucose ingested and the small and intermittent appearance of glucose in urine. Thus, absence of glycosuria previously reported in two families[21,29,32] could be interpreted as unnoticed transient glycosuria.

Laboratory tests carried out in order to exclude causes of diarrhea other than GGM are usually consistent with integrity of intestinal mucosa; thus, moderate steatorrhea could be interpreted as a consequence of watery diarrhea. Although normal values for xylose absorption are common in GGM, low or borderline values have sometimes been recorded.[34] The histology of the biopsies taken after diarrhea had stopped was normal under light and electron microscopy. The fact that disaccharidase activities were found within the control range further indicates the integrity of the intestinal mucosa. During an episode of diarrhea, nonspecific alterations in both histologic appearance and disaccharidase activity are sometimes observed.[3,9,10,13]

The abnormality of carbohydrate metabolism is confined to glucose transport in the small intestine and the proximal renal tubule. Glucose entry into the erythrocytes is normal,[35] as is fasting blood glucose. Whereas galactose and glucose disappear from plasma at normal rates after IV infusion,[4,11,14] oral sugar tolerance tests with glucose, galactose, and lactose yield flat blood glucose response curves in most cases. In contrast, blood glucose increases considerably after oral fructose loading. These results are the consequence of selective malabsorption of glucose and galactose. Although these tests are commonly performed, they are not very useful in identifying GGM for three reasons: (1) When glucose or galactose is given at the dose of 2 g per kilogram of body weight, watery diarrhea is usually produced, but this response is not specific to GGM and may aggravate the clinical status. (2) Approximately 25 percent of normal children have a flat blood glucose curve, and what is more, (3) in GGM, not all response curves are flat. The increase in blood glucose within 1 h may reach 1 mmol/liter.[3] From the practical point of view, subjects undergoing oral sugar tests must be closely monitored for dehydration; stools must be collected, weighed, and immediately analyzed for pH, the presence of reducing sugars, and sugar identification.

Malabsorption of glucose and galactose is easily identified by the hydrogen breath test.[36,37] It is safe to perform the first test with a dose of 0.5 g of glucose per kilogram of body weight. Usually, the breath hydrogen concentration exceeds 20 parts per million (ppm) within 3 h of glucose or galactose oral loading (Fig. 116-1)[3,37] However, after several days of glucose feeding, breath hydrogen production may decrease,[36,38] a finding related to adaptive changes in colonic bacterial metabolism induced by prolonged malabsorption of fermentable sugars.

The course of GGM under a glucose- and galactose-free diet is predictable. Very often, the diarrhea stops with IV feeding but resumes with standard oral feeding. An immediate improvement is seen as soon as children are put on a fructose-based milk formula free of glucose and galactose. However, diarrhea may persist on a fructose diet if the amount of fructose exceeds the absorptive capacity of the small intestine (see below). The diagnosis of GGM can be established later by direct determination of selective glucose and galactose intestinal malabsorption.

As affected children grow older and their diet becomes more diversified, the dietary restrictions are increasingly difficult to maintain, and both children and parents learn to "titrate" the symptoms according to carbohydrate tolerance. In older children and adults, tolerance of the offending carbohydrates improves,[3,10,17–19,39] although malabsorption of glucose and galactose in the small intestine remains unchanged. In most cases, growth and mental development have been normal when glucose and galactose were removed from the diet[3]; adults with GGM live relatively normal lives.[10,18,26]

Physiology of Glucose Absorption

Dietary carbohydrates are digested in the gut through the action of pancreatic enzymes and the brush border hydrolases. The final products of digestion are D-glucose and D-galactose in milk-fed infants, and mostly D-glucose, D-galactose and D-fructose in older children and adults. These

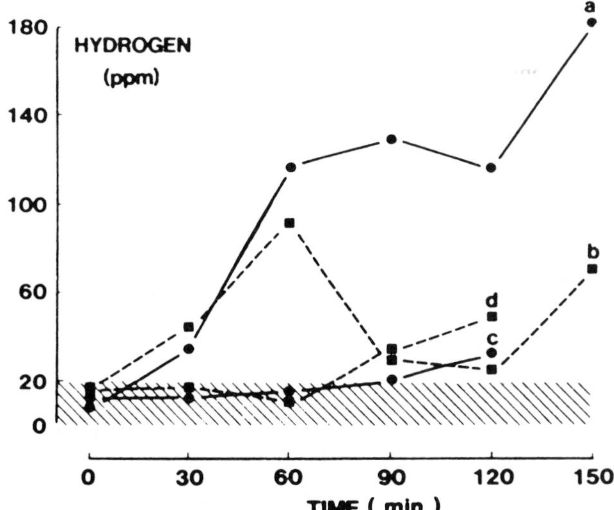

FIG. 116-1 Concentration of hydrogen expired after oral administration of glucose and galactose to two children with GGM. a = O.L., 2 g/kg glucose; b = O.L., 1 g/kg galactose; c = H.F., 0.5 g/kg glucose; d = H.F., 0.5 g/kg galactose. Shaded area shows control range. For greater clarity, the hydrogen expiration recorded after two challenges with 2 g/kg fructose has been omitted, but it never exceeded 20 ppm. *(From Evans et al.[3] Used by permission.)*

monosaccharides are absorbed into the body by the mature enterocytes lining the upper villi of the duodenum and jejunum. Absorption occurs by a two-stage process: cotransport with Na^+ from the gut lumen into the enterocyte across the brush border membrane followed by facilitated transport out of the cell and to blood. D-glucose and D-galactose are accumulated within the cell by the brush border Na^+-glucose cotransporter (SGLT1). The electrochemical potential gradient for Na^+ across the membrane provides the energy for this process (fructose is transported across the brush border by a facilitated transporter).[40] The second stage is the transport of sugar from the enterocyte into the blood across the basolateral membrane. It appears that the facilitated transporter GLUT2 is responsible for the exit of D-glucose, D-galactose and D-fructose from the cell.[40] It follows that a defect in D-glucose and D-galactose absorption, in the presence of normal D-fructose absorption, must be due to a defect in the brush border Na^+-glucose cotransporter.

Over the past 30 years a clear understanding of the mechanism of intestinal sugar absorption has emerged from studies on the intact mucosa, isolated cells, brush border membrane vesicles and basolateral membrane vesicles (see refs. 41 to 44 for reviews of the earlier literature).

One major Na^+-cotransporter exists in the brush border that handles glucose and galactose and all hexoses with an equatorial OH group on carbon 2. At saturating Na^+ concentrations ($\geq$100 m*M*) the K_m for D-glucose is 0.1 to 2 m*M* and the relative affinities for other sugars are D-glucose, D-galactose, and α-methyl-D-glucopyranose > 3-0-methyl-D-glucoside ›› D-allose. Note that α-methyl-D-glucopyranose is not a substrate for facilitated glucose transporters, so this nonmetabolized sugar analogue can be used to dissect out the properties of the cotransporter. Phlorizin is a nontransported competitive inhibitor of Na^+-glucose cotransport with a K_i of 5 to 10 μ*M*. The aglycone, phloretin, is a much more potent inhibitor of the basolateral facilitated sugar transporter than is phlorizin.

The affinity of the cotransporter for sugar is Na^+-dependent. When the Na^+ concentration is reduced below 100 m*M*, the K_m for sugar is increased with little change in V_{max}. In the absence of Na^+ the K_m for glucose is much greater than 10 m*M*. This suggests an ordered binding mechanism in which Na^+ binds first to change the conformation of the transport protein and allow sugar binding. The requirement for Na^+ is quite specific and no other monovalent cation is capable of driving sugar transport.

It is the Na^+ electrochemical potential gradient across the brush border that provides the energy for the accumulation of sugar in the enterocyte: The enterocyte Na^+ activity is less than 20 meq/liter and the membrane potential is about −40 mV. The Na^+ gradient is maintained by the Na^+/K^+ pump located in the basolateral membrane. Consequently, the Na^+ that enters across the brush border through the cotransporter is pumped out of the cell across the basolateral membrane. This accounts for the observation that sugars stimulate salt, and water, absorption across the intestine, and this provides the basis for oral rehydration therapy.[45,46]

The protein responsible for Na^+-glucose cotransport was first identified as a 70 to 75-kDa polypeptide using biochemical techniques.[47] The rabbit transporter (SGLT1) was cloned using a novel expression cloning technique,[30] and a human clone was subsequently isolated by screening a human cDNA library with the rabbit probe.[48] The human protein has 664 amino acid residues, and structural analysis suggests that the hydrophobic protein spans the brush border membrane 12 times. The protein exhibits N-linked glycosylation at Asp

248 and this increases the apparent size by about 15 kDa. The mature protein has an estimated mass of 86 kDa, but it runs on SDS-PAGE with an apparent relative size of ~70 kDa. The rabbit and human proteins are virutally identical (86 percent of the residues are identical and another 10 percent are conservative substitutions). On the basis of western and northern blots,[49] SGLT1 is evidentally conserved in fish, amphibians, birds, and mammals.

The clone coding for SGLT1 has been functionally expressed in Xenopus oocytes, cultured renal, HeLa, and insect ovary cells.[50] The properties of SGLT1 expressed in these cells are virtually identical to those in the native intestinal brush border membranes (kinetics, ion and sugar specificity, and phlorizin sensitivity). A detailed kinetic model of SGLT1 has been presented that quantitatively accounted for the experimental observations.[51] The essential features of this six-state, nonequilibrium model are: (1) the carrier is negatively charged ($Z = -2$); (2) $2Na^+$ ions bind to the carrier at the external face of the membrane; (3) the Na^+-carrier complex has a high affinity for external sugar; (4) the fully loaded sugar-$2Na^+$-carrier complex crosses the membrane to deliver sugar and Na^+ to the cell interior; and (5) the empty carrier reorientates from the internal to external surface of the brush border membrane to complete the reactions cycle. The model predicts that external Na^+ binding to the carrier and the conformation changes of the empty carrier are both voltage-dependent, that is, a normal membrane potential of -40 mV facilitates Na^+ binding at the external surface of the brush border and speeds up the return of the empty carrier from the internal and external surface. Inward sugar transport occurs because the internal Na^+ is low compared with that in the gut lumen, and a steady state is reached only when the sugar concentration gradient (Glc_i/Glc_o) is equal and opposite to the inward Na^+ electrochemical potential gradient (Na_o/Na_i) exp (VF/RT) n, where V is the membrane potential, F, R and T have their usual meaning, and n is the Na^+-sugar coupling ratio. In the absence of sugar exit across the basolateral membrane, and assuming a coupling coefficient of 2, the theoretical sugar concentration gradient is greater than 100.

Additional information is required to understand the symptoms associated with GGM. This information is essentially related to four factors:

(1) D-Glucose and D-galactose produced by lactose hydrolysis are absorbed mainly in the upper part of the small intestine, and the transport capacity for all monosaccharides declines from jejunum to ileum. In healthy breast-fed children, a portion of the carbohydrates they receive are metabolized in the colon, as indicated by increased hydrogen concentration in alveolar breath tests. In preterm and term infants, incomplete lactose absorption appears to be common and presumably is physiological.[52] It constitutes neither a nutritional risk nor a cause of diarrhea, because inadequately absorbed carbohydrates are salvaged by colonic flora.[53-55]

(2) Lactose is not the sole source of carbohydrates in the first months of life. Sucrose, maltose, or maltodextrins may be present in infant formulas. The glucose thus arriving at the brush border membrane is transported by the Na^+-glucose cotransporter. The fructose is transported by another system.[40] Most adult subjects absorb fructose incompletely if the fructose concentration is high.[56] Intestinal perfusion studies in adults whose absorption of disaccharides was compared with that of equivalent amounts of monosaccharide mixtures demonstrated that maltose and sucrose hydrolysis is fast. However, the rate of lactose hydrolysis in vivo is only about half that of sucrose. Hence, contrary to what is observed for sucrose and maltose, hydrolysis of lactose rather than glucose transport is the rate limiting step for glucose assimilation.[57]

(3) There is a close relationship between intestinal absorption of glucose, Na^+, and water.[45] Between meals, water from digestive secretion enters the lumen of the small intestine and is reabsorbed passively following the active absorption of Na^+ by the epithelium covering the villi of the small intestine (Fig. 116-2). Consequently, little water is lost in the stools. After a meal, breast milk or formula, a large amount of water enters the intestinal lumen following the stimulation of digestive secretion. Glucose plays a key role in stimulating the reabsorption of Na^+, and therefore, the reabsorption of water, by the epithelium covering the villi. Fructose, which is not cotransported with Na^+, does not stimulate water reabsorption. The oral rehydration therapy that prevents or cures the dehydration caused by acute diarrhea is based on the relationship between glucose, Na^+, and water.[45,46] The hypernatremia frequently observed in the dehydration phase of GGM might indicate an upper limit for the glucose concentration in the oral rehydration solution used in treating acute diarrhea.[46]

(4) The Na^+-glucose cotransporter has been extensively studied in healthy animals, and it is obviously also present in the jejunum of children. Everted sacs from 10-week-old human fetuses absorb glucose against a concentration gradient. By the age of 16 weeks, this absorption almost triples.[58] Using the transepithelial potential as an index of

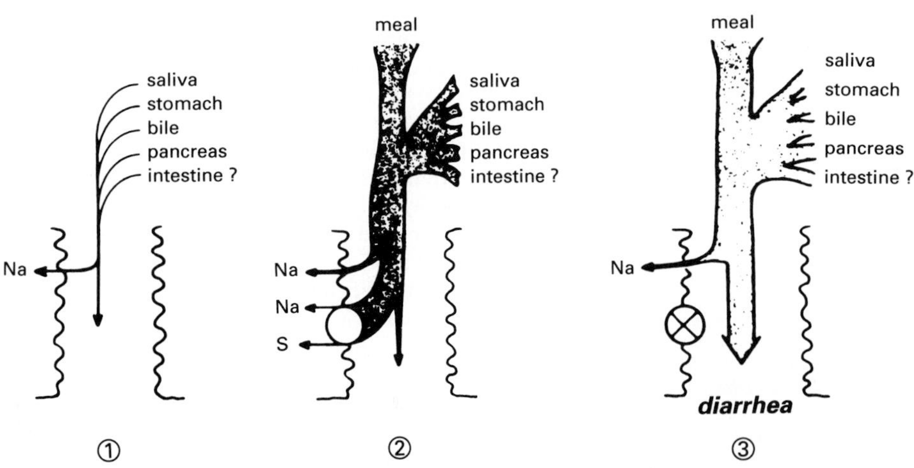

FIG. 116-2 Effect of sodium-solute-coupled transport on sodium and water reabsorption. Between meals (1), digestive secretions are balanced by intestinal sodium absorption. During meals (2), there is a sudden increase in the volume of fluid entering the intestinal lumen. Actively absorbed solutes, sugars, and amino acids present in the meal immediately increase sodium reabsorption by stimulating sodium-solute transport, thereby increasing water reabsorption. In glucose and galactose malabsorption (3), there is no increase in sodium reabsorption during meals. Therefore, water entering the intestine is poorly reabsorbed. *(From Desjeux et al.[45] Used by permission.)*

Na^+ absorption, Levin and Koldovsky demonstrated that glucose stimulates Na^+ absorption in the fetal jejunum as early as the fifteenth week of gestation.[59,60] In addition, the maximal absorption rates for glucose measured in vivo and normalized per centimeter of intestine were four to five times higher in adults than in infants.[61] This increased transport with age is due, at least in part, to the age-related increase in intestinal diameter and hence in surface area.[62]

The Na^+–D-glucose cotransporter can be studied in isolated jejunal epithelium of healthy children.[3,34,63] The use of isotopic D-glucose and Na^+ tracers makes it possible to determine simultaneously the intracellular concentration of D-glucose and Na^+ at the steady state. The method was originally described by Rosenberg et al. for amino acids.[64] Jejunal epithelial cells can accumulate 43 m*M* glucose in the intracellular water when the incubation medium contains 10 m*M* glucose (Table 116-1). With 0.1 m*M* glucose in the medium, the cells can concentrate glucose more than twentyfold. Their ability to concentrate galactose is four times less than their ability to concentrate glucose. In the meantime, the intracellular Na concentration is only one third of the extracellular concentration (Table 116-2). The electrochemical gradient for Na^+ is sufficient to explain the accumulation of glucose or galactose.[63] Ouabain, which inhibits the Na^+/K^+-ATPase, simultaneously reduces the Na^+ and glucose gradients, thus indicating that active glucose transport (against a concentration gradient) is Na^+-dependent (Fig. 116-3).

D-Glucose stimulates Na^+ absorption on the Na^+-glucose cotransporter. This is best studied by measuring the transepithelial potential difference (PD)[60] or the current produced by the active transport of Na^+, called short-circuit current (Isc). The method shows that addition of glucose to the mucosal or luminal side of the tissue is followed by an immediate increase in PD and Isc.[63] Glucose does not stimulate Na^+ absorption by supplying the cell with more energy. Rather, this absorption is stimulated by the structure of D-glucose or its nonmetabolized analogue, 3-O-methylglucose, at the brush border membrane. The importance of the structural role of glucose is further substantiated by the effect of phlorizin, a competitive inhibitor of glucose at the brush border membrane, which reduces glucose and galactose accumulation against a concentration gradient without altering the Na^+ gradient. Phlorizin decreases glucose entry at the luminal membrane, and the Isc stimulated by glucose declines.

The relative permeability to glucose of the brush membrane that contains the Na^+-glucose cotransporter and of the basolateral membrane that contains the facilitated diffusion system can be estimated by measuring the ratio of [^{3}H]glucose entering the brush border membrane from the mucosal solution to the [^{14}C]glucose entering the basolateral mem-

Table 116-1 Intracellular Substrate Concentration at Various Substrate Concentrations in the Medium in Jejunal Biopsies from Children (Expressed as Cellular/Medium Concentration)*

Substrate	Concentration (m*M*)	Controls	GGM (Homozygotes)	GGM (Heterozygotes)	Renal Glycosuria
Glucose	10	4.34±0.61 (42)	0.98±0.11† (9)		
+ Phlorizin	+ 0.5	2.09±1.24 (9)	0.52 (1)		
+ Ouabain	+ 0.1	2.6 ± 1.8 (9)			
Na-free		1.05±0.19 (8)	0.45 (1)		
Glucose	1	12.47±3.15 (5)			
Glucose	0.1	13.69±1.11 (49)	2.31±0.35† (22)	13.2 and 20.4	11.1 (1)
+ Phlorizin	+ 0.5	1.86±1.2 (26)	1.07±0.15 (16)		0.6 (1)
Na-free			1.46±0.43 (7)		
Galactose	10	2.42±0.69 (11)	0.94±0.24† (6)		
Galactose	0.1	5.15±0.73 (15)	2.91±0.38† (5)	1.1 and 1.2	
+ Phlorizin	+ 0.5	0.76±0.17 (6)	0.87±0.11 (5)		
α-Methylglucose	0.1	13.54±5.2 (3)	1.26±0.59† (7)		
+ Phlorizin	+ 0.5	0.79±0.58 (3)			
Alanine	0.8	15.80±3.01 (11)	11.35±1.25 (13)		
Xylose	10	1.1±0.08 (13)	0.92 and 0.93		

*The pieces of jejunum were placed in a beaker containing the oxygenated medium at 37°C for 1 h. The substrate was labeled with ^{14}C and the extracellular marker was ^{3}H polyethylene glycol, 4000 MW. The C:M ratio is the result of steady state uptake from brush border and basolateral membranes. C:M > 1 represents uptake in excess of simple diffusion.

†Significantly different from controls.

Table 116-2 Intracellular Na Concentration (μEq/liter) in Jejunal Biopsies from Children*

Substrate	Controls	GGM (Homozygotes)	GGM (Heterozygotes)
Glucose	45±4 (52)	6±24† (11)	35 and 44
+ Phlorizin	52±8 (11)	29±18†	
+ Ouabain	100±23 (6)		
Galactose	56±10 (19)	23±23† (5)	53
Alanine		38±6 (3)	

*The Na concentration in the incubation medium was 140 mEq/liter. Procedure performed as described in Table 116-1.
†Significantly different from controls.

brane from the blood side.[65] When 10 m*M* glucose is present on both sides of the epithelium, the brush border membrane is twice as permeable as the basolateral membrane (Fig. 116-3) (Table 116-3).

Pathophysiology

In GGM, the diarrhea is a consequence of a selective congenital defect in the absorption of these sugars from lumen to blood in the small intestine. This defect is situated at the brush border membrane, a conclusion essentially reached by means of in vivo intubation studies and investigation of in vitro transport in isolated pieces of jejunum. The

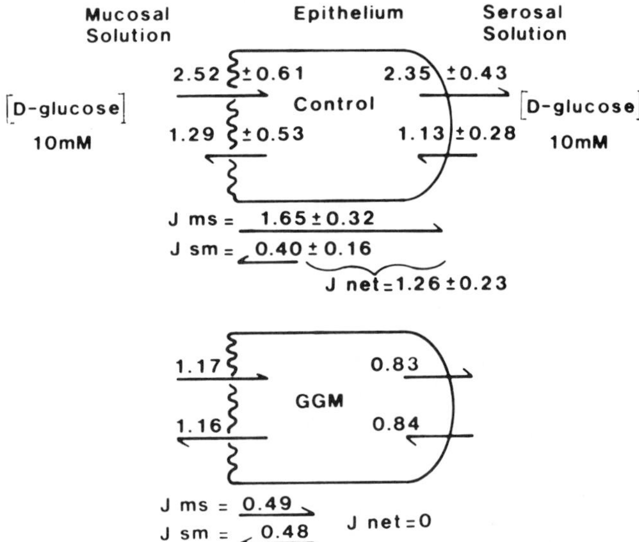

FIG. 116-3 **Schematic representation of steady state unidirectional fluxes of D-glucose, calculated on the same piece of tissue according to Naftalin and Curran,[65] in control epithelium (upper cell) and epithelium from one patient with glucose–galactose malabsorption (GGM, lower cell). In the control epithelium (n = 6) the ratio of influx to efflux values calculated for the luminal membrane provides evidence for an energy-mediated event at the level of this membrane. In GGM (one patient), this ratio did not differ from unity, indicating a loss of the energy-mediated D-glucose transport. Consequently, D-glucose did not accumulate in the cell, and the efflux at basolateral membrane level decreased; the influx did not alter, indicating that the apparent permeability of this membrane remained unchanged.**

intubation studies and investigation of in vitro transport in isolated pieces of jejunum. The main results of these experiments are discussed below.

The intubation studies were performed under various technical conditions. Initially, Meeuwisse and Melin[10] compared the absorption of glucose and fructose after ingestion of a test meal containing the same concentrations of both sugars. Glucose was always absorbed more slowly than fructose. These authors also demonstrated that lactose, sucrose, and maltose were hydrolyzed in the patients tested. In more recent experiments, the jejunum was perfused using either a double-lumen tube[18,22] or a four-lumen tube incorporating an occlusive balloon, in order to isolate effectively a 25-cm segment of bowel distal to the duodenojejunal junction.[26] This study was done in two adults and a 9-month-old child. The results were essentially the same and may be summarized as follows: glucose and galactose were poorly absorbed. At low concentrations of 5.6 m*M* or less, a small amount of glucose was secreted in the lumen (Fig. 116-4). At high concentrations of up to 280 m*M*, glucose absorption was less than 10 percent of the control value. In one patient,[26] the basal potential difference of the jejunal mucosa was normal, but did not respond to the addition of intraluminal glucose, a result that was in agreement with the absence of a functional Na^+–D-glucose cotransporter. The jejunal mucosa secreted electrolytes and fluid, suggesting that under the prevailing experimental conditions, the combined glucose-sodium-water absorption process was defective.[26] Sucrose was hydrolyzed and fructose absorbed, suggesting that malabsorption of glucose and galactose is a selective defect.

The major characteristic of GGM is the lack of intracellular glucose or galactose accumulation against a concentration gradient (see Table 116-1). This has been observed at a low glucose concentration (e.g., 0.1 m*M*) and at a high concentration (e.g., 10 m*M*). In principle, the disappearance of active glucose and galactose transport might be due either to a reduced driving force, that is a less steep Na^+ electrochemical gradient, or to decreased permeability of the brush border membrane to sugar. However, there is no evidence for the first possibility, since when intracellular sodium was measured with isotopic tracers, it was found to be lower, not higher, in patients with GGM than in controls, an observation that may in fact indicate a steeper Na^+ electrochemical gradient (see Table 116-2).

Furthermore, the transport of other solutes such as alanine or leucine via an Na^+-solute cotransporter does not

Table 116-3 Glucose Net Transepithelial Flux and Apparent Permeability across Luminal and Basolateral Membranes of Jejunal Epithelium of Children*

Children	Jnet ($\mu mol \cdot hr^{-1}\ cm^{-2}$)	Pmc/Pcm (Luminal Membrane)	Pcs/Psc (Serosal Membrane)
Control (7)	1.29±0.2	14.3±6.0	0.49±0.04
GGM (1)	−0.06	1.1	0.7

*The pieces of jejunum were placed in an Ussing chamber and the isotopic fluxes of glucose from mucosal (m) to serosal (s) side (Jms) and in the opposite direction (Jsm) were determined. The net flux (Juet) was calculated as the difference Jms − Jsm. In control group, net absorption together with asymmetric permeability across the luminal membrane (entry permeability, Pmc, over exit permeability, Pcm, greater than unity) both are functional expression of Na^+–D-glucose cotransporter. In GGM, the loss of net absorption and asymmetric permeability across the luminal membrane are both an expression of the functional defect of the cotransport.

change.[3,20,66] The autoradiographic studies of Stirling and Kinter et al.[13,67] clearly indicate a defect in glucose uptake at the brush border membrane (Fig. 116-5). The diminished glucose influx across the luminal membrane in intact epithelium (Table 116-4) and isolated brush border membrane vesicles[68] (and Shirazi-Beechey SP, Hirayama B, Walker-Smith J, Wright EM: unpublished observations) and the selective absence of in vivo intestinal potential difference[26] and in vitro short-circuit current stimulation by glucose further substantiate this possibility (Fig. 116-6). Taken together, these experimental findings indicate that the functional activity of the Na^+–D-glucose cotransporter at the brush border membrane is either absent or reduced. However, in three different patients, western blot analysis has shown that the cotransport protein is present in the brush border membrane.[33] In addition, the participation of mutarotase in sugar transport has been suggested, and the absence of this enzyme has been demonstrated in one case of glucose–galactose malabsorption.[69] This later finding is difficult to interpret at present, especially since there is no homology between mutarotase and SGLT1.

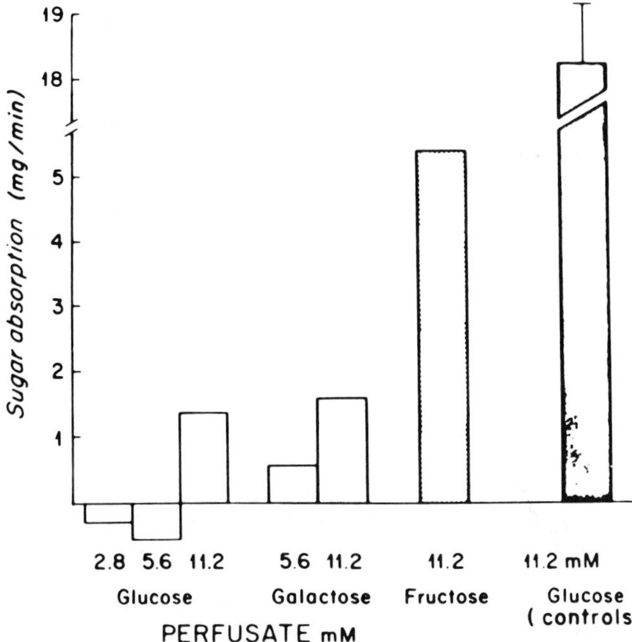

FIG. 116-4 **Absorption of sugars from a 25-cm segment of jejunum in an adult with glucose and galactose malabsorption. Negative values represent secretion of glucose into the jejunum. Mean glucose absorption (±SE) for healthy controls is shown for comparison.** ***(From Phillips and McGill.[26] Used by permission.)***

Genetics

The children affected by GGM are of very diverse origin. Of 39 cases reported, 27 were girls.[3] The high consanguinity rate and the fact that no vertical transmission has been found argue in favor of an autosomal recessive mode of inheritance.[12] Although the proportion of siblings affected (6 of 16) may appear high, the true expression rate is masked by the small sample numbers, and the size of the family concerned cannot be used as an argument against this mode of inheritance. In addition, the high proportion of consanguineous mating implies that the mutant gene is very infrequent.[3]

Attempts to detect heterozygotes with reduced glucose intestinal absorption have been made in three familial studies. Meeuwisse and Dahlqvist[9] found reduced intestinal glucose accumulation in the father of one child, while the results were normal in the mother. Elsas et al.[8] demonstrated, in both parents of an affected child and also in a half-sister, that glucose accumulation dropped to a level intermediate between that of the controls and the proband. However, when we studied the father and mother of three children with GGM (one is reported in ref. 3), they exhibited no

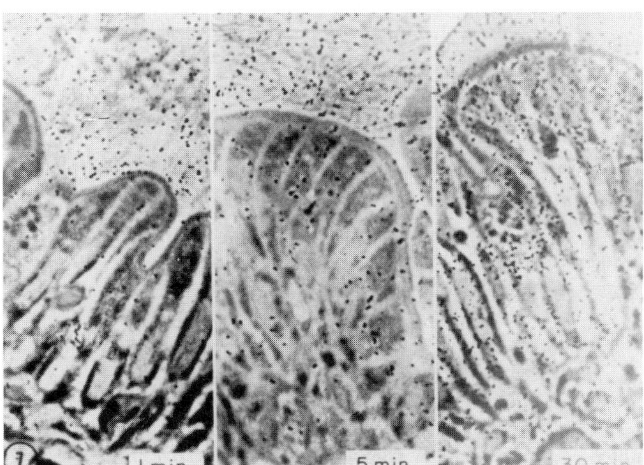

FIG. 116-5 **Galactose-^{3}H radioautographs of columnar epithelium from a patient at 3 years. Small pieces of tissue were incubated for 1, 5, and 30 min in medium containing 1 m*M* labeled galactose. Limited uphill accumulation of galactose inside absorptive cells had occurred by 30 min. ×1300.** ***(From Stirling et al.[67] Used by permission.)***

Table 116-4 Monosaccharide Influx across the Luminal Membrane of Jejunal Biopsies from Children (Jmc in μmol·hr^{-1} cm^{-2})

Substrate	Concentration (m*M*)	Controls	GGM
Glucose	10	3.89±0.98 (14)	0.81±0.26† (4)
+ Phlorizin	+0.5	1.46±0.12 (4)	
Glucose	0.1	0.59±0.17 (8)	0.40 (1)
α-Methylglucose	0.1	0.67±0.26 (8)	0.31±0.07† (3)
+ Phlorizin	+0.5	0.19±0.07 (8)	0.32±0.07 (3)

*Pieces of jejunum were mounted, luminal surface up, on a moistened filter paper placed on a piece of lucite. The block was covered with a thin plate of lucite with an aperture 4 mm in diameter, through which the mucosal surface was directly in contact with the mucosal solution. After a 30-min preincubation into 10 ml Ringer the block was dipped into the incubation solution containing the substrate labeled with ^{14}C and ^{3}H polyethylene glycol 4000 as extracellular marker. After 1 or 2 min the tissue was washed and the radioactivity counted for determination of the flux from mucosal solution to cell (Jmc).

†Significantly different from controls.

clinical symptoms of the disease. Hydrogen breath tests after glucose and galactose were normal. With 50 g of fructose we observed abdominal pain and diarrhea, as well as an increased hydrogen concentration; however, this response was probably physiological.[56] In one family, glucose accumulation in the epithelial jejunal cells was normal (see Table 116-1). These discrepancies may be an expression of the genetic heterogeneity of the disease.

Molecular Genetics

Following the cloning of SGLT1 it was possible to investigate the human genetics of SGLT1 and GGM. The chromosomal location of the SGLT1 gene was first mapped to the distal q arm of chromosome 22 using a human genomic fragment containing an exon from the 5′ end of the coding region of SGLT1 and somatic-cell hybrids.[48] This was confirmed using a fluorescent cosmid probe together with *in situ* hybridization techniques.[70] In addition, the location of the SGLT1 was refined to 22q13.1. Given the size of SGLT1 mRNA (2.3 kb), the gene is large, with 15 exons, and the introns range between 3 and 22 kb (Turk E: unpublished data).

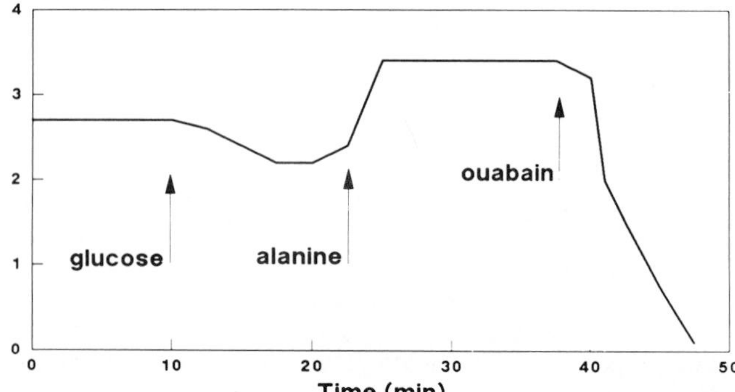

FIG. 116-6 Effects of glucose, alanine, and ouabain on the short-circuit current (Isc), in a tissue sample from a patient with glucose and galactose malabsorption. Isc was recorded after successive addition to the incubation medium, on both sides of the tissue, 33 m*M* glucose, 35 m*M* alanine, and 0.1 m*M* ouabain.

In our family with two daughters diagnosed with GGM, a missense mutation in SGLT1 has been identified as the cause of sugar malabsorption.[71] In both children, oral sugar tolerance tests established malabsorption of glucose and galactose but normal absorption of fructose and xylose. These children are being successfully maintained on a glucose/galactose-free diet.

The approach used to identify the mutation was to isolate RNA from duodenal biopsies, synthesize cRNA by reverse transcriptase, amplify overlapping segments of SGLT1 cDNA using PCR, and then sequence the DNA.[71] A single base change was identified in the entire coding region of one child, and this was confirmed in the other afflicted sister. This was a homozygous guanine-to-adenine base change at position 92. The mutation removed an *Eco*RV restriction site, which permitted an independent confirmation of the mutation in the two probands. *Eco*RV digestion of the parents' genomic DNA showed incomplete cleavage, and sequencing exon 1 revealed both an A and a G at position 92. This established that each parent carried a mutation at position 92 on one chromosome (Fig. 116-7).

The mutation corresponds to the first codon position of amino acid residue 28 in SGLT1, changing an aspartic acid to an asparagine; in the conventional way of naming mutations it is D28N. The position of the residue is at the interface between the cytoplasmic N-terminus and the first hydrophobic membrane spanning segment of the protein. Is this mutation responsible for GGM in these two children? This question was approached by expressing the wild type and mutant proteins in Xenopus oocytes and measuring sugar uptake. The wild type gave normal sugar transport but the mutant protein was unable to function. It was concluded that the D28N mutation caused the defect in intestinal glucose–galactose transport.

To explore the reason for the defect in sugar transport in the D28N mutation, Asp28 was also changed by site-directed mutagenesis to either Glu28 or Ala28.[72] In both cases transport was severely impaired, indicating that Asp28 is required for normal transport activity, possibly by maintaining the tertiary structure of the protein. It is noteworthy that 10 of 15 cloned Na^+-cotransport proteins contain an aspartic acid residue at the cytoplasmic interface between the N-terminus

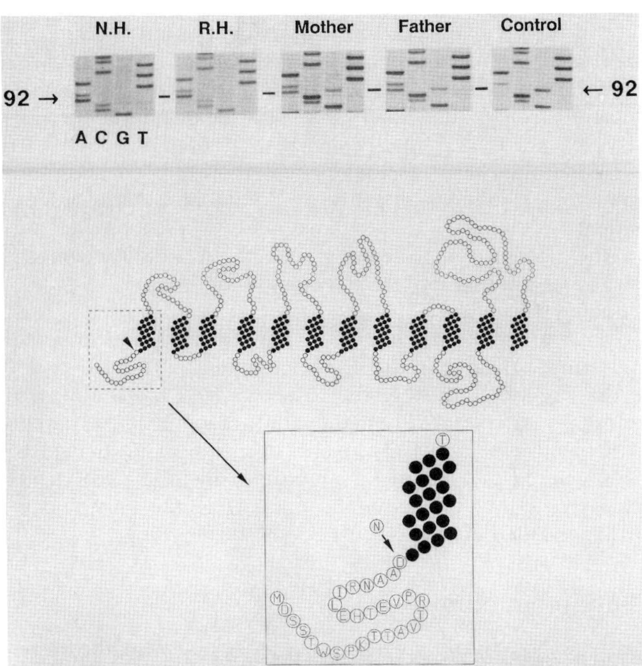

FIG. 116-7 **Identification of a missense mutation in two sisters, N.H., and R.H., afflicted with GGM. *A*. Sequence analysis at base 92 of GGM family members and an unaffected control. *B*. Localization of the $Asp_{28} \rightarrow Asn_{28}$ mutation and a 12-span secondary structure model of the Na^+-glucose cotransporter protein, predicted using the algorithms previously described.[30,31] Transmembrane residues are shown filled in.** ***(From Turk et al.[33] Used by permission.)***

and the first transmembrane spanning domain. This suggests that this residue is important in maintaining functional expression of these transporters.

Molecular genetic studies have been extended to four additional patients with GGM. The experimental approach was to amplify exon 1 of SGLT1 in each patient and test for the D28N mutation. None of the four patients has the mutation, and this suggests that, as expected for an autosomal recessive disease, other mutations account for sugar malabsorption in these four patients. Experiments are in progress to identify these mutations.

Diagnosis

The primary diagnostic criterion is a history of watery diarrhea as soon as milk or sugar water is given. The diarrhea is profuse and acidic and contains reducing substances; it is frequently associated with milk glycosuria; it only improves if glucose and galactose are withdrawn from the diet; and it will reappear within a few hours when ingestion of glucose or galactose (usually in the form of lactose) is resumed.

The diagnosis of GGM is further substantiated by oral sugar loading tests, which we usually start at a dose of 0.5 g of glucose. Loading of glucose or galactose, but not of fructose, is followed by an increase in the output of stools containing the loaded sugar, an enhanced hydrogen concentration in alveolar breath air (more than 20 ppm in 3 h), little or no increase in blood sugar, and mild glycosuria (see Fig. 116-1).

On clinical grounds alone, the following neonatal diseases may be difficult to differentiate from congenital GGM—congenital lactose malabsorption, congenital sucrose–isomaltose malabsorption, familial chloride diarrhea, congenital sodium malabsorption, microvillus atrophy, and infectious diarrheas.[73] Stool analysis for electrolytes and sugars and removal of glucose and galactose from the diet usually supply decisive information strongly suggestive that a child has GGM.

Acquired monosaccharide intolerance may occur after mucosal injury causing villus flattening or damage to the intestinal epithelium.[66,74–76] Disorders that often produce this lesion include infectious enteritis (rotavirus and giardiasis), gluten-sensitive enteropathy, radiation enteritis, drug-induced enteritis, and inflammatory bowel disease. However, this intolerance may also be of unknown origin.[77] Acquired monosaccharide intolerance differs from congenital GGM in that it is not usually present at birth, although its clinical presentation is essentially the same.[78]

Isolated fructose malabsorption has not often been described[79] and does not seem to occur at birth. In fact, isolated fructose malabsorption with diarrhea, abdominal cramps, flatulence, and increased hydrogen production is common after ingestion of 50 g of pure fructose[80] in healthy human subjects. However, fructose malabsorption does not seem to occur at birth probably because children do not receive a high dose of pure fructose. Indeed, the absorption of fructose improves when given with glucose or in the form of sucrose. Similar observations have been made with alcohol-sugars and other related molecules commonly used in soft drinks and candies.[81–83]

The decisive information for the diagnosis of GGM is obtained between the ages of 6 and 12 months, when the child displays no symptoms when on a glucose- and galactose-free diet. The glucose–galactose transport defect is best established in vitro by observing that the piece of jejunal biopsy does not accumulate glucose (and galactose) against a concentration gradient. It is also wise to identify the selectivity of the defect by checking that alanine or leucine is actively transported[3] (see Table 116-1). It should be noted that in acquired monosaccharide malabsorption with flat intestinal mucosa, the concentrative power of the remaining epithelium is still 30 percent that of the control intestine.[66,73] Alternatively, intestinal perfusion *in situ* has been used successfully to assess the diagnosis of GGM by measurement of glucose absorption[18,22,26] or the glucose-dependent potential difference.[26]

Molecular biology is of limited value as a diagnostic tool, since the mutation responsible for GGM has been identified in only one pedigree,[71] and with autosomal recessive diseases many different mutations are to be anticipated (see Fig. 116-7). D28N mutation can be identified by either Southern blots of genomic DNA cleaved with *Eco*RV or by PCR amplification of exon 1,[71] and a positive result would only confirm the diagnosis.

Treatment

Treatment consists of immediate rehydration (oral rehydration solutions that contain glucose must be avoided) and feeding a glucose- and galactose-free diet. In the first 3 months of life, a commercial glucose- and galactose-free formula, such as Galactomine 19 from Nutricia (Zoetermeer, Holland) supplemented with iron and vitamins, may be given. Similarly, the completely carbohydrate-free formula, RCF (Ross Laboratories, Columbus, Ohio) to which 70 g per liter of fructose was added, has proved to be effective in two children with GGM.[84] However, because of the limitation of fructose absorption, even in healthy children, it might be desirable to start with lower quantities of fructose. Alternatively, a special formula may be prepared containing calcium caseinate, 19 to 29 g/liter, fructose, 39 to 59 g/liter, and corn oil, 34 g/liter, to which electrolytes, vitamins, iron and oligoelements should be added.[11] The sugar-free diet formula 3232A (Mead Johnson, Nutritional Division, Evansville, IN) containing 25 g per liter of tapioca starch is not appropriate as an initial diet.[84]

After the age of 3 months, it is probably safe to add other foodstuffs either free of glucose and galactose (e.g., fish, meat, eggs, oil) or containing low quantities of these sugars (e.g., many vegetables and varieties of fruits and cheese). Honey, which children usually like, may also be given. Gradually, the diet can be increasingly varied and can include milk products and potatoes, bread, and other starch products, provided that there are no symptoms such as abdominal cramps or diarrhea not compatible with social life. As stated below, adaptive changes occurring in the colon may explain the improved tolerance to starchy food.

RENAL GLYCOSURIA

Clinical Description

Renal glycosuria denotes the renal tubular abnormality displayed by individuals who excrete a variable amount of glucose in their urine with normal levels of blood glucose.[85] This section deals with the situation in which glucose excretion is the only apparent tubular defect. The following diagnostic criteria, proposed by Marble in 1959, are commonly accepted[86]:

1. Glycosuria is present without hyperglycemia. The amount of glucose excreted may vary from less than 10 g to more than 100 g/24h; it remains essentially stable, except during pregnancy, when it may increase.
2. The degree of glycosuria is largely independent of diet but may fluctuate according to the amount of carbohydrate ingested. In general, all specimens of urine examined, including those collected after an overnight fast, should contain sugar.
3. Levels of blood glucose are only slightly affected by dietary carbohydrates. The oral glucose tolerance curve is normal or slightly flat, and the levels of plasma insulin and free fatty acids are within control limits.[87] The glycosylated hemoglobin fraction is not increased.
4. The sugar excreted is glucose alone, identified by simple specific methods using glucose oxidase. Other sugars are not found (e.g., pentoses, fructose, galactose, lactose, sucrose, maltose, and heptulose).
5. Subjects with renal glycosuria are able to store and utilize carbohydrates normally.

When the above criteria are strictly applied, the condition is not common. For instance, only 94 cases have been observed among the 50,000 cases of melituria seen at the Joslin Clinic.[86] On the other hand, Lawrence proposed that renal glycosuria is proven whenever glycosuria occurs with a normal glucose tolerance test.[88] On the basis of this more liberal definition, he found that 65 percent of 800 selectees with glycosuria fell into this category. According to the same criteria, Lestradet et al.,[87] who reported 103 cases in 24 years, found only 60 with glycosuria after an overnight fast. During that period, the latter authors observed 1700 children with insulin-dependent diabetes.

All the authors agree that renal glycosuria is a benign condition without symptoms or physical consequences, except in type 0 glycosuria, in which dehydration and ketosis may develop during pregnancy or starvation.[85,89] This rare, acute situation may lead to erroneous treatment of diabetic ketacidosis. Although renal glycosuria and insulin-dependent diabetes are two distinct entities, a combination of these two conditions has occasionally been reported.[85] In addition, immunologic abnormalities were found in a series of 11 patients.[90,91]

The age at which renal glycosuria is first recognized varies, depending on the frequency of urinary tests for reducing substances. The number of cases diagnosed seems to reach a peak at the age of military service, and in some countries at the age of the first vaccination; of the 103 cases in the French study referred to above,[87] 25 were detected before 6 years of age. Pregnancy and screening in the family of subjects with renal glycosuria occasioned the diagnosis of seven cases. whereas symptoms, including polyuria, excessive thirst, or abdominal pain, were the only reason for diagnosis in five cases.

Pathophysiology

In renal glycosuria, the presence of glucose in the urine results from a selective congenital defect in proximal tubule glucose reabsorption from the lumen into the blood. This definition is essentially based on four major clinical findings: (1) The metabolism of glucose, including its storage and utilization and insulin secretion, does not change. (2) Glycosuria is present, but not hyperglycemia. (3) The only kidney function that changes is the increase in the urinary excretion of glucose, but there is no increase in the excretion of other solutes. The glomerular filtration, *p*-aminohippuric acid secretion, and phosphate and amino acid reabsorption are normal in patients with glycosuria.[92-94] (4) Renal glycosuria is usually not associated with anatomic abnormality, as assessed by routine histologic exploration, including histochemistry and electron microscopy, thus indicating that the defect involved in renal glycosuria must be examined at the biochemical and biophysical levels. Taken together, these clinical observations strongly suggest that this defect is selectively expressed in the tubular glucose transport system.

At the same time, several observations relative to patients with renal glycosuria and kidney physiology suggest that the pathophysiology of renal glycosuria is more complex than the schematic view just presented. These observations concern three concepts.

The first is that the kidney is the only organ involved. This notion has been questioned, and a possible relationship with diabetes mellitus has been envisaged, because certain patients with an initial diagnosis of renal glycosuria were found to have hyperglycemia when retested after periods of 3 months to 13 years.[95] However, it is now clear that diabetes mellitus and renal glycosuria are two different conditions. Nevertheless, from the clinical point of view, it is important to check for the absence of transient or permanent hyperglycemia before the diagnosis of renal glycosuria is established. In addition to the fasting blood glucose concentration, it might be useful to measure the percentage of glycosylated hemoglobin and the increase in the plasma insulin concentration after glucose loading.

If renal glycosuria is indeed the genetic expression of a defect in the tubular glucose transport system, one would expect to observe symptoms in organs in which the same transport system exists, including, first of all, the small intestine. However, in renal glycosuria, glucose is well absorbed in the small intestine, as assessed in vivo by oral glucose tolerance and in vitro by glucose accumulation against a concentration gradient in the intestinal epithelial cells.[9] This point will be further discussed below.

The second is that structural integrity of the kidney may be in question.[93,96] However, the defects found are too small to explain a significant functional abnormality. Hence, it is probably safe to conclude that defective glucose transport in the proximal tubule is not related to anatomic abnormalities.

The third is that renal glycosuria might be due to an isolated selective defect in tubular glucose reabsorption. However, it is not clear whether this defect constitutes a single entity or is the result of several mutations. Reubi[97] and Bradley et al.[98] orginally proposed that patients with renal glycosuria seemed to fall into two separate groups.

In this connection, data were later obtained by the titration method of Smith,[99] allowing a distinction to be made between the threshold glucose concentration (F_{minG}) and the maximum glucose transport rate (T_{mG}). The threshold concentration was defined as the plasma concentration at which glucose appears in the urine (i.e., for readily detectable concentrations far above normal trace values) and T_{mG}, as the plasma concentration required to saturate the reabsorptive capacity for glucose reabsorption.[100]

Analysis of titration curves for glucose reabsorption suggests that its values are heterogeneous in patients with renal glycosuria (Fig. 116-8). In type A, or classic, renal glycosuria,[97] F_{minG} and T_{mG} are reduced, so that a significant amount of glucose spills over into the urine during fasting. In type B, F_{minG} is usually reduced while T_{mG} is normal but has an increased splay. Type A might well be a mutation reflecting a reduction in the capacity of the transport system. It is best explained by a diffuse defect involving all the nephrons. Type B might constitute a mutation reflected by a decrease in the affinity of the transport system. It may also be a consequence of functional or anatomic nephron heterogeneity.[85,100,101]

Oemar et al.[89] have observed a new type of glycosuria, which they called "type 0," in a 15-year-old boy who had complete absence of tubular glucose reabsorption. Of German origin, the parents, who were distant relatives, had a daily glycosuria of 1.1 g/1.73 m^2 for the father and 2.7 g/1.73 m^2 for the mother. Two of three sibs also had small losses of glucose. The proband's glycosuria was diagnosed when he was 11 years old and complained about persistent enuresis nocturna, polyuria, polydipsia, and episodes of polyphagia. He excreted daily 136 to 160 g/1.73 m^2 of glucose accompanied by normal blood glucose levels between 75 and 105 mg/dl. The endogenous glucose clearance [112 to 160 ml/(min/1.73 m^2)] was nearly identical to inulin clearance [148 to 153 ml/(min/1.73 m^2)]. After IV glucose loading with a blood glucose concentration of 261 to 342 mg/dl, glucose clearance remained in the same range, and tubular glucose reabsorption was virtually absent.

It should be stressed that titration curve analysis is not a simple method allowing constant clear discrimination between type A and type B glycosuria. For example, it is difficult to raise the blood glucose level without producing volume expansion, thus altering tubular sodium reabsorption and hormonal responses.[89] It is also difficult to obtain accurate values for F_{minG} by this method.[102] In conclusion, titration curve analysis underlines the diversity of the phenotypes, thus suggesting that no single defect characterizes all subjects with renal glycosuria.

Physiology of Renal Glucose Transport

Several features should be considered in connection with renal glycosuria:

(1) As glucose is completely filterable at the glomerulus, but it is not normally detectable in voided urine, it must be reabsorbed from lumen to blood in the tubule.[100]

(2) Glucose reabsorption occurs through the epithelial cells of this tubule. Experimentally in the presence of

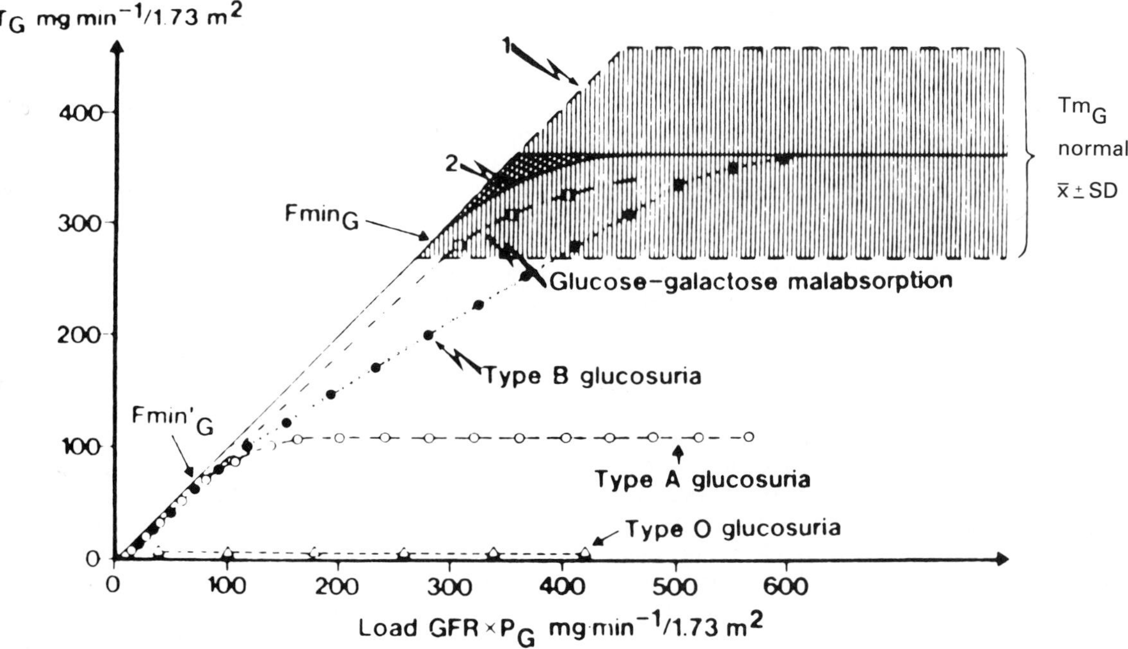

FIG. 116-8 Glucose titration curves showing renal tubular glucose reabsorption (T_G) as a function of filtered load (GFR × P_G). Schematic drawing of normal and pathological states. 1 = theoretical curve; 2 = actual curve found in normal humans; F_{minG} = minimal renal glucose threshold in normal subjects; $F_{\mathrm{min'G}}$ = minimal renal glucose threshold in renal glycosuria. *(From Oemar et al.[89] Used by permission.)*

phlorizin, a specific inhibitor of Na^+-glucose cotransport whose action mimics renal glycosuria, glucose secretion may be demonstrated when the glucose concentration is lower in the tubular fluid than in the plasma.[103]

(3) The proximal tubule is the major site of glucose reabsorption. There is no evidence of glucose reabsorption in the loop of Henle or distal tubule. A small fraction of the filtered glucose may be reabsorbed in the collecting ducts. There are differences in glucose transport by the superficial and deep nephrons.[103,104]

(4) At the cellular level, D-glucose is reabsorbed from the urine in the proximal tubule via a sodium-coupled secondary active transport system located in the brush border membrane. As a result of this process, glucose is concentrated in the proximal tubule cells and subsequently passes down its concentration gradient into the blood via a facilitated transport system (GLUT 2) located in the antiluminal or plasma membrane. The driving force for D-glucose reabsorption is, thus, supplied by the electrochemical gradient for sodium across the brush border membrane. Phlorizin is a potent and highly specific inhibitor of the brush border membrane Na^+–D-glucose transport system. The sodium electrochemical gradient is maintained by the activity of the Na^+/K^+-ATPase in the plasma membrane.

(5) Physiological studies strongly suggest that sodium-dependent D-glucose transport is heterogeneous along the proximal tubule. The transepithelial parameters of glucose transport were studied, using the isolated perfused tubule technique. Barfuss and Schafer[105] examined the properties of glucose transport in tubule segments thought to be representative of the three ultrastructurally defined cell types (S1, S2, and S3) found in the proximal tubule. These cell types predominate in the early proximal convoluted tubule (S1 segment), the early proximal straight tubule of the superficial nephrons (S2 segment), and the late proximal straight tubule (S3 segment). Active reabsorption of glucose was found to occur via a low-affinity, high-capacity system in S1 segments, a higher-affinity, lower-capacity system in S2 segments, and a still higher affinity and lower-capacity system in S3 segments.

The heterogeneity of the sodium-dependent D-glucose system has been further examined by quantitative analysis of glucose transport kinetics in brush border membrane vesicles prepared from the whole cortex of human beings and dogs.[106] The curvilinear Eadie-Hofstee plots in both preparations cannot be accounted for by a single transporter obeying Michaelis-Menten kinetics. Turner and Moran,[107] following the suggestion of Scriver et al.[115a] compared the glucose transport properties of proximal tubule brush border membrane vesicles prepared from two regions of rabbit kidney—the outer cortex, thought to contain S1 and some S2 cell types, and the outer medulla, thought to contain S3 cells types. In the outer cortical preparation, or the pars convoluta of the proximal tubule, the behavior of the sodium-dependent component of the D-glucose flux indicated the presence of a low-affinity transport system with K_m of 6 mM and a V_{max} of 10 mmol/min per milligram of protein, as measured at 17°C under zero-*trans* conditions (i.e., with initial intravesicular concentrations of sodium and glucose of zero). By contrast, in the outer medullary preparation, or pars recta of the proximal tubule, this flux component behaved like a high-affinity system, as its K_m was 0.35 mM and its V_{max} 4 nmol/min per milligram of protein (Table 116-5).

The low-affinity glucose carrier was associated with a high-affinity phlorizin-binding site. The sodium glucose stoichiometry for this system was 1:1. The high-affinity carrier was almost two orders of magnitude less sensitive to inhibition by phlorizin, and its sodium stoichiometry was 2:1.

(6) Similary, the uptake of D-galactose in vesicles from whole cortex seems to be mediated by a low-affinity and a high-affinity transport system.[108] More precisely, the D-galactose uptake from the pars recta was found to be mediated via a high-affinity transport system (K_m = 0.15±0.02 mM) and was strictly Na^+-dependent. In the pars convoluta D-galactose uptake was mediated by a system that had a low affinity (K_m = 15±2 mM) and was Na^+-dependent.

(7) In the inner cortical preparation, the rate of uptake of D-glucose was much higher than that of D-galactose. D-Glucose and D-galactose were transported by a single Na^+-dependent transport by means of a high-affinity system (K_m for galactose and glucose, 0.15±0.02 mM and 0.13±mM, respectively.)

(8) A clone identical to the rabbit intestinal SGLT1 was isolated from rabbit kidney[109] and more recent studies[110,110a] indicate that SGLT1 is the high-affinity, low-capacity transporter found in the inner medulla. A preliminary report on the rat kidney[110] using *in situ* hybridization indicates that SGLT1 is expressed in S3 segments of proximal tubules.

(9) The low-affinity, high-capacity Na^+-glucose cotransporter of the rabbit outer cortex (SGLT2) is predicted to have cDNA and protein sequences different from SGLT1 by more than 20 percent.[110] A candidate SGLT2 clone[111] has been reported to be expressed in rat kidney proximal tubule S1 segments.[112]

Genetics

The preceding section appears to confirm the suggestion that no single defect characterizes all subjects with renal glycosuria. The conflicting data reported in the literature about the pattern of inheritance of renal glycosuria probably result from three factors.

First, in many of the reports describing families, information is incomplete or the techniques for detection are insensitive or inaccurate. Diagnostic criteria include the appearance of glucose in the urine during an otherwise normal glucose tolerance test, in the presence or absence of fasting glycosuria. The use of titration methods does not always allow clear separation of type A and type B glycosuria. Therefore, to define the pattern of inheritance better it seems appropriate to include the search for genetic markers in addition to the renal investigations.[113] Second, the genetic heterogeneity may be related to both the heterozygous and the homozygous state. Third, the genetic defect is not defined at the molecular level and may be heterogeneous, involving, for instance, K_m, V_{max}, different locations on the tubule, and activation of the transporter in the membrane.

In 1937 Hjärne was able to obtain information about 141 of 199 individuals belonging to generations with common ancestors in the eighteenth century.[114] He concluded that the defect was inherited as an autosomal dominant characteristic, in view of the following features: (1) Glycosuria occurred in both male and female members of the family. (2) When neither parent had glycosuria, none of the offspring had it either. (3) When either of the parents had glycosuria, some of the children generally had the defect. Similar conclusions regarding inheritance were reached in subsequent studies.[85]

More recently, De Marchi et al.[113] reported on five unrelated families affected by type A renal glycosuria. After careful examination of 25 patients and 40 healthy relatives

Table 116-5 Characteristics of Na^+–D-Glucose Transport in the Proximal Tubule of Humans and Rabbits

	I Early Proximal (Outer Cortex, Pars Convoluta)	II Late Proximal (Outer Medulla, Pars Recta)
K_m glucose, mM	2.5–5.7	0.13–0.35
J_{max}, nmol/(min·mg)	10	4
Hexose specificity	Glc >> Gala	Glc = Gala
Na^+-glucose	1:1	2:1
Phlorizin inhibition	90%	60%

NOTE: Glc = glucose; Gala = galactose.
SOURCES: Barfuss and Schafer,[105] Turner and Silverman,[106] and Turner and Moran.[107]

(Fig. 116-9) these authors concluded that type A renal glycosuria was transmitted as an autosomal dominant trait because in each family, the gene responsible for the tubular defect was segregated with the HLA complex. Two cases carried intra-HLA recombinant haplotypes, thus providing clues to the location of the abnormal gene on the sixth pair of chromosomes, i.e., closer to the HLA-A locus than to the HLA-B locus. Note that renal glycosuria was not associated with HLA-A, -B, or -C specific antigens.

The autosomal dominant mode of inheritance was queried by Elsas and Rosenberg,[115] who pointed out that the affected members of pedigrees demonstrating a dominant pattern of inheritance might actually be heterozygotes and homozygotes for different mutations in the glucose tranport process. They interpreted their own detailed study of two pedigrees as suggestive of autosomal recessive inheritance of renal glycosuria, with the clinical phenotype resulting from a double dose of the mutant gene. Alternatively, the above results could, in principle, be the consequence of a variety of genetic alterations of a single transporter.

Relationship between Renal Glycosuria and Glucose-Galactose Malabsorption?

On the basis of comparison of renal glycosuria and GGM, Meeuwisse postulated in 1970[11] that two glucose transport systems are present in both the small intestine and proximal renal tubule; the same author also suggested that one of these systems with a similar affinity for galactose and glucose predominates in the intestine (he called it the "intestinal mechanism"), while the other, with little or no affinity for galactose, predominates in the kidney (this he called the "tubular mechanism"). According to Meeuwisse, the genetic defect in the intestine system causes GGM, while the defect in the tubular one causes renal glycosuria.

Accordingly, at high concentrations, glucose is not absorbed in the intestine in GGM, on account of the absence of functional intestinal transport system. However, at low concentrations, glucose should be better absorbed if the tubular transport system is present. This was not found to be the case in perfusion studies.[26] However, the results of in vitro transport studies are consistent with this hypothesis, since when the glucose concentration in the incubation medium was low (0.1 mM) epithelial jejunum from GGM patients accumulated glucose against a concentration gradient (see Table 116-1). Furthermore, addition of phlorizin to the incubation medium containing glucose reduced the intracellular glucose concentration gradient in GGM tissues to a lower level than in phlorizin-free medium. The presence of a minor glucose intestinal transport system was also suggested in a child referred to our department for failure to thrive, although he displayed no gastrointestinal symptoms

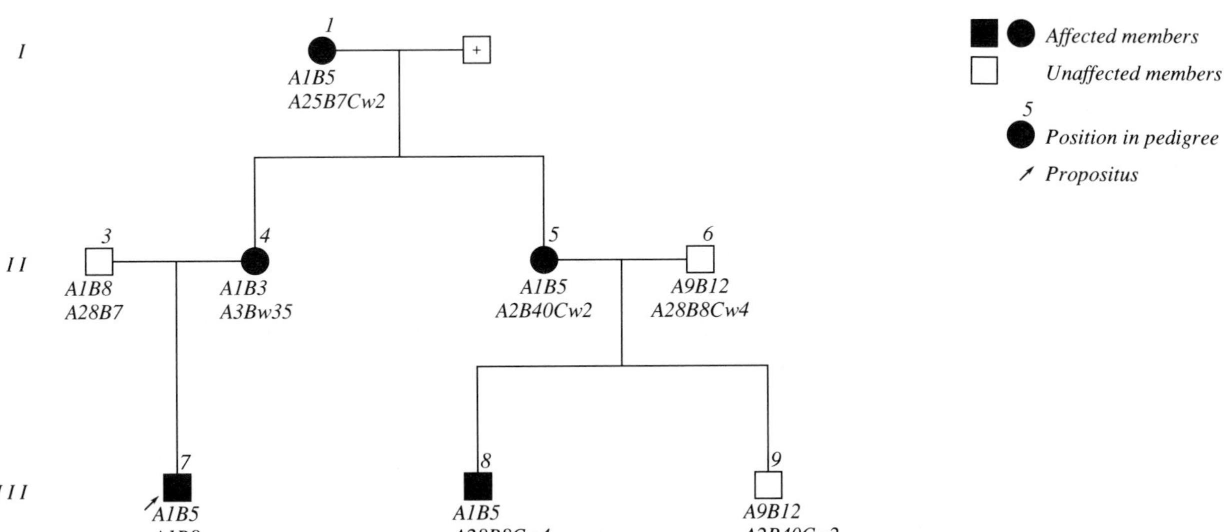

FIG. 116-9 **Pedigree of "Mogl" family with HLA genotypes. All the affected members of the family carry the A1, B5 haplotype.** ***(From De Marchi et al.[90] Used by permission.)***

and normal histology. Study of the child's jejunal mucosa showed a reduced glucose accumulation (C:M = 6.9 at 0.1 m*M* glucose in the medium) but no decrease in galactose accumulation (C:M = 30.4 at 0.1 m*M* galactose in the medium) (unpublished data).

Conversely, a defect in the tubular transport system should be associated with renal glycosuria and the absence of digestive symptoms. This hypothesis is more difficult to test, as defects in a minor glucose transport system in the intestine are difficult to find and have, in fact, have never been detected.[101] The presence in the kidney of a residual glucose transport system (i.e., the intestinal mechanism SGLT1) must be postulated to explain why part of the glucose is reabsorbed in renal glycosuria.[115a]

To sum up, the studies of the two genetic diseases (GGM and renal glycosuria) and of glucose transport in the brush border membrane vesicles of the proximal tubule and small intestine both suggest the presence of at least two Na^+-dependent glucose transport systems (SGLT1 and SGLT2). However, genetic and physiological studies suggest the existence of at least one transport system (SGLT1) common to the intestine and kidney.

Clinical Consequences

Comparison of the clinical consequences of defective glucose absorption in the proximal tubule and small intestine may provide insight into the specific roles of the kidney and intestinal tract. In renal glycosuria, tubular malabsorption of glucose does not cause severe polyuria or dehydration, but both these disorders are constant features in GGM. Moreover, to our knowledge, the consequences of defective tubular transport of glucose have not been specifically studied in renal glycosuria.

Nevertheless, the following sequence of events is conceivable in renal glycosuria: Glucose is filtered together with water and electrolytes through the glomerular membrane. Then, in the proximal tubule, the decreased glucose reabsorption must be associated with diminished sodium and water reabsorption. The failure of this tubule to reabsorb 10 g or 55 mOsm of glucose might result in a 180-ml load in the distal tubule. In principle, water could be selectively reabsorbed in the distal tubule as a consequence of its increased hydraulic conductivity, which is regulated by the antidiuretic hormone vasopressin. However, in the absence of dehydration, there is no reason to suppose that vasopressin secretion is increased. Therefore, 10 g of glucose will be excreted together with an excess volume of urine of about 200 ml.

In the gastrointestinal tract, the situation is more complex, as shown by the following features.[116,117] In GGM, glucose stimulates water and electrolyte loss in the jejunum, as demonstrated by *in situ* perfusion.[22,26] The water loss observed in the absence of perfused sugar was stimulated by the presence of glucose, galactose, maltose, sucrose, and lactose, but not fructose.[26] Sodium, potassium, and chloride were always secreted together with water. However, the mechanism of this loss is not clear, as the osmolarity of the solutions perfused was made isotonic with plasma (300 mOsm/kg). Water loss during perfusion of solutions containing sucrose was also demonstrated by Launiala[118] in a case of sucrase–isomaltase deficiency during perfusion of solutions containing sucrose. It was identical to that observed in normal children during perfusion of mannitol, a poorly absorbed sugar. Thus, water and electrolyte loss is related to the presence of unabsorbed sugar in the intestinal lumen.

Fluid secretion in the lumen of the small intestine is accompanied by a reduction in the transit time of the perfused solution, probably secondary to the increased flow rate in the segment under study.[118] Thus, unusually large amounts of water, electrolytes, and glucose enter the colon.

In contrast to the distal tubule, the colon is known not to reabsorb water under active regulation of hydraulic conductivity.[119] Consequently, the osmolality of fecal water is only slightly greater than than of plasma, and the colon must therefore adjust to acute loads of water and glucose by a mechanism other than hydraulic conductivity.

The role of the colon in handling water was examined in healthy adult volunteers by perfusing the stomach with an isotonic saline solution at an increasing rate.[120] The results indicate that diarrhea appeared when fluid entered the colon at a flow rate of 6.3 ml/min or more (Fig. 116-10). This threshold is about twice the colonic maximal absorption rate of 2.7 ml/min found in the same subjects. Therefore, under these experimental conditions, the colon is able to store about 1 liter of unabsorbed fluid before diarrhea starts.

The consequences of acute loading of glucose and other carbohydrates have been examined experimentally in animals and humans. Stool output was measured in healthy volunteers given an acute load of sugars poorly absorbed by the small intestine.[121] Diarrhea occurred when the load exceeded 120 to 220 mmol of mannitol, 73 to 146 mmol of lactulose, or 80 mmol of raffinose (Fig. 116-11). The significance of a colonic threshold for water and glucose loading is to be found in the three major activities of the colon—motility, absorption, and intraluminal bacterial metabolism. As we know very little about these activities in the human newborn, all we can do is to attempt to draw conclusions from studies performed at different ages. The magnitude and consequences of the osmotic load entering the adult colon

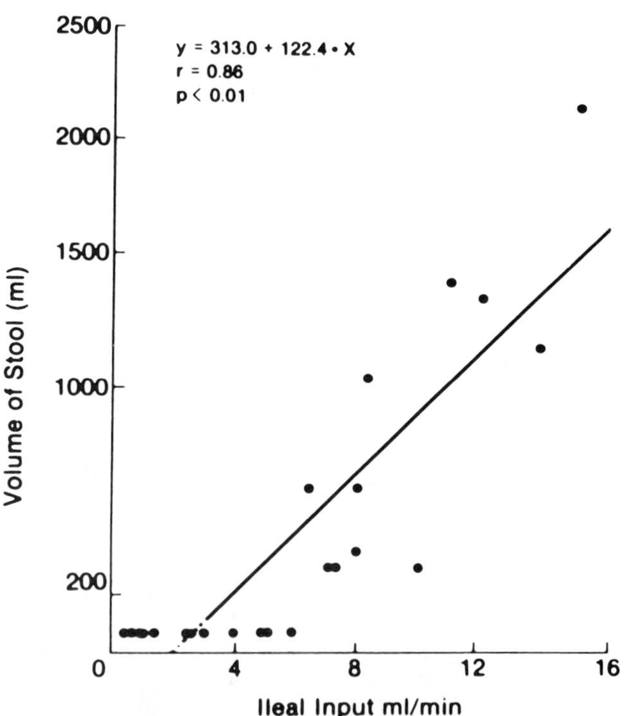

FIG. 116-10 Ileal input into the cecum and volume of stools. A wide range of ileal inputs was observed; diarrhea appeared only when the rate of ileal discharge exceeded the threshold of 6.3 ml/min. ***(From Palma et al.[120] Used by permission.)***

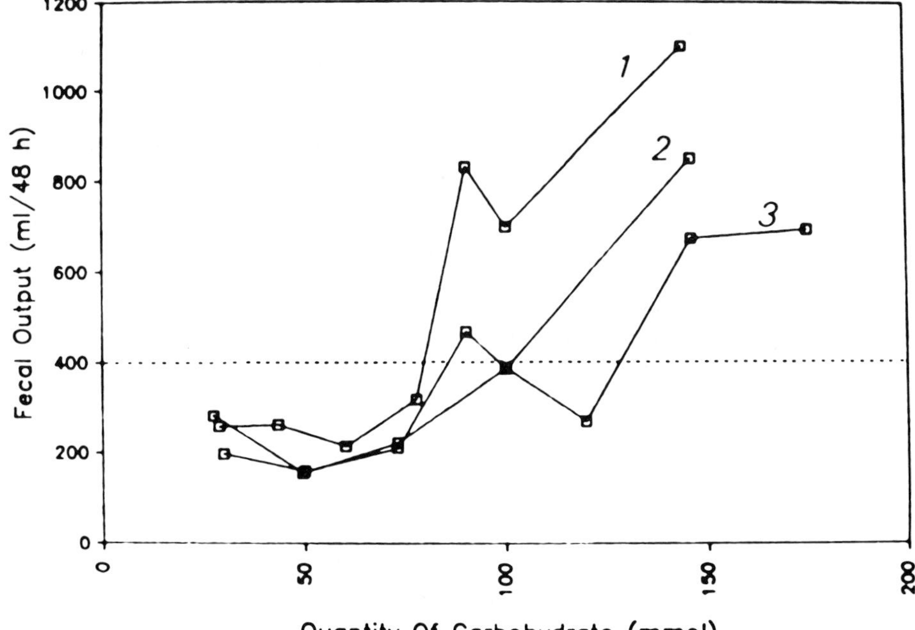

FIG. 116-11 Relationship between stool output and colonic carbohydrate load. 1 = raffinose, 2 = lactulose, 3 = mannitol. Points were obtained experimentally in one adult volunteer who could tolerate 80 to 100 mmol before fecal output of water exceeded 400 ml in 48 h or before test carbohydrate appeared in stools. *(From Saunders and Wiggins.[121] Used by permission.)*

in the form of glucose were examined by Bond and Levitt.[122] Carbohydrates may be broken into short-chain fatty acids by the bacteria that are active under anaerobic conditions of the colon lumen. The short-chain fatty acids not absorbed would then hold in their ionized form an equal number of milliequivalents of cation. Thus, failure to absorb only 10 g or 55 mOsm of glucose in the small bowel could result in a 220-mOsm load in the colon, which is the isotonic equivalent of about 650 ml of fecal water.

In fact, however, the short-chain fatty acids in the colon are absorbed and oxidized by the bacteria, and most of the remaining fecal glucose is converted into a larger molecular form with limited osmotic activity. Thus, the colonic flora benefits the host by reducing the osmotic load of unabsorbed carbohydrate and by salvaging of a large percentage of the calories of carbohydrate not absorbed in the small bowel.[122] When the colonic capacity to remove glucose is exceeded, it is the unfermented carbohydrate as well as the unabsorbed short-chain fatty acids that enhances the output of fecal water.[122–124]

The metabolic adaptation of colonic flora to long-term glucose loading results in an increased capacity to ferment this sugar; it may therefore explain the ability to tolerate larger amounts of dietary glucose as patients with GGM grow older. This mechanism has been examined in transmissible gastroenteritis of 3-day-old and 3-week-old pigs. Infected animals did not absorb fluid and glucose in the small intestine. However, in contrast to the 3-day-old group, the large intestine of the 3-week-old infected pigs increased fluid absorption some six times over the control, and this compensatory response prevented diarrhea in these older animals.[125] This adaptation was further examined in adults given a long-term load of lactulose, a nonabsorbable sugar.[126] After 8 days of a daily load of 20 g, fecal water, and carbohydrate output declined, β-galactosidase activity, short-chain fatty acid, and lactic acid production increased, whereas H_2 excreted in breath decreased. Thus, long-term lactulose loading induced changes in bacterial metabolism and improved the efficiency of the carbohydrate digestion by flora. A similar adaptative mechanism was found in one patient with GGM who was given a moderate amount of glucose.[38]

In conclusion, comparison of the clinical consequences of defective glucose absorption in kidney or intestine stresses the importance of the colon in water economy. The control of the colonic threshold for water and glucose loading is the main compensatory mechanism that prevents diarrhea secondary to glucose malabsorption.

ACKNOWLEDGMENT

Our own work was supported by grants from the National Institutes of Health (Washington, D.C.): Grants DK 19567 and DK 44582.

REFERENCES

1. Laplane R, Polonovski C, Etienne M, Debray P, Lods JC, Pissaro B: L'intolérance aux sucres à transfert intestinal actif. Ses rapports avec l'intolérance au lactose et le syndrome coeliaque. *Arch Fr Pediatr* **19**:895, 1962.
2. Lindquist B, Meeuwisse GW: Chronic diarrhea caused by monosaccharide malabsorption. *Acta Paediatr* **51**:674, 1962.
3. Evans L, Grasset E, Heyman M, Dumontier AM, Beau JP, Desjeux JF: Congenital selective malabsorption of glucose and galactose. *J Pediatr Gastroenterol Nutr* **4**:878, 1985.
4. Abraham JM, Levin B, Oberholzer VG, Russel A: Glucose-galactose malabsorption. *Arch Dis Child* **42**:592, 1967.
5. Jehan P, Jezequel C, Coutel Y: Troubles du transfert actif du glucose. *Quest Med* **31**:479, 1978.
6. Grasset E, Heyman M, Dumontier AM, Lestradet H, Desjeux JF: Possible sodium and D-glucose cotransport in isolated jejunal epithelium of children. *Pediatr Res* **13**:1240, 1979.
7. Gerard-Brochot E, Brochot JL, Bocquet A, Menget A, Schirrer J, Raffi A: Malabsorption congénitale du glucose et du galactose. A propos d'un cas. *Med Hyg* **41**:3897, 1983.
8. Elsas LJ, Hillman RE, Paterson JH, Rosenberg LE: Renal and intestinal hexose transport in familial glucose-galactose malabsorption. *J Clin Invest* **49**:576, 1970.

9. Meeuwisse GW, Dahlqvist A: Glucose-galactose malabsorption. A study with biospy of the small mucosa. *Acta Paediatr Scand* **57**:273, 1968.
10. Meeuwisse GW, Melin K: Glucose-galactose malabsorption. A clinical study of 6 cases. *Acta Paediatr Scand Suppl* **188**:3, 1969.
11. Meeuwisse G: Glucose-galactose malabsorption. An inborn error of carrier-mediated transport. University of Lund, Sweden, 1970, vol. 7.
12. Melin K, Meeuwisse GW: Glucose-galactose malabsorption. A genetic study. *Acta Paediatr Scand Suppl* **188**:19, 1969.
13. Schneider AJ, Kinter WB, Stirling CE: Glucose-galactose malabsorption. Report of a case with autoradiographic studies of a mucosal biopsy. *N Engl J Med* **274**:305, 1966.
14. Pruitt AW, Achord JL, Fales FW, Patterson JH: Glucose-galactose malabsorption complicated by monilial arthritis. *Pediatrics* **43**:106, 1969.
15. Kaijser K, Ockerman PA: Diagnostic problems in glucose-galactose malabsorption. *Acta Paediatr Scand* **59**:214, 1970.
16. Linneweh F, Schaumloffel E, Barthelmai W: Angeborence glucose und galactose-malabsorption. *Klin Wochenschr* **43**:405, 1965.
17. Wimberley PD, Harries JT, Burgess EA: Congenital glucose-galactose malabsorption. *Proc R Soc Med* **67**:755, 1974.
18. Hughes WS, Senior JR: The glucose-galactose malabsorption syndrome in a 23-year-old woman. *Gastroenterology* **68**:142, 1975.
19. Anderson CM, Kerry KR, Townley RRW: An inborn defect of intestinal absorption of certain monosaccharides. *Arch Dis Child* **40**:1, 1965.
20. Eggermont E, Loeb H: Glucose-galactose intolerance. *Lancet* **2**:343, 1966.
21. Dubois R, Loeb H, Eggermont E, Mainguet P: Etude clinique et biochimique d'un cas de malabsorption congénitale du glucose et du galactose. *Helv Paediatr Acta* **6**:577, 1966.
22. Fairclough PD, Clark ML, Dawson AM, Silk DBA, Milla PJ, Harries JT: Absorption of glucose and maltose in congenital glucose-galactose malabsorption. *Pediatr Res* **12**:1112, 1978.
23. Deprettere AJR, Van Acker KJ, Eggermont E, Carchom H, Evens M: Primary glucose-galactose malabsorption. *Acta Paediatr Belg* **33**:121, 1980.
24. Esposito F, Faelli A, Capraro V: Sugar and electrolyte absorption in the rat intestine perfused "in vivo." *Pflugers Arch* **340**:335, 1973.
25. Liu HY, Anderson GJ, Tsao MU, Moore BF, Giday Z: Tm glucose in a case of congenital intestinal and renal malabsorption of monosaccharides. *Pediatr Res* **1**:386, 1967.
26. Phillips SF, McGill DB: Glucose-galactose malabsorption in an adult: Perfusion studies of sugar, electrolyte, and water transport. *Am J Dig Dis* **18**:1017, 1973.
27. Marks JF, Norton JB, Fortran JS: Glucose-galactose malabsorption. *J Pediatr* **69**:225, 1966.
28. Beauvais P, Vaudour G, Desjeux JF, Le Balle JC, Birot JY, Brissaud HE: La malabsorption congénitale du glucose-galactose. Un nouveau cas avec l'étude in vitro de l'absorption intestinale et l'étude du TmG. *Arch Fr Pediatr* **28**:573, 1971.
29. Lebenthal E, Garti R, Mathoth Y, Cohen B, Katzenelson D: Glucose-galactose malabsorption in an Oriental-Iraqi Jewish family. *J Pediatr* **78**:844, 1971.
30. Hediger MA, Coady MJ, Ikeda TS, Wright EM: Expression cloning and cDNA sequencing of the Na^+/glucose cotransporter. *Nature* **330**:379, 1987.
31. Hediger MA, Turk E, Wright EM: Homology of the human intestinal Na^+/glucose and E. coli Na^+/proline cotransporters. *Proc Natl Acad Sci USA* **86**:5748, 1989.
32. Wright E, Turk E, Zabel B, Mundlos S, Dyer J: Molecular genetics of intestinal glucose transport. *J Clin Invest* **88**:1435, 1991.
33. Turk E, Zabel B, Mundlos S, Dyer J, Wright E: Glucose/galactose malabsorption: A defect in the Na^+/glucose cotransporter. *Nature* **350**:354, 1991.
34. Heyman M, Desjeux JF, Grasset E, Dumontier AM, Lestradet H: Relationship between transport of D-xylose and other monosaccharides in jejunal mucosa of children. *Gastroenterology* **80**:758, 1981.
35. Meeuwisse GW: Glucose-galactose malabsorption: A study on the transfer of glucose across the red cell membrane. *Scand J Clin Lab Invest* **25**:145, 1970.
36. Bond JH, Levitt MD: Investigation of small bowel transit time in man utilizing pulmonary hydrogen (H2) measurement. *J Lab Clin Med* **85**:546, 1975.
37. Douwes AC, Van Caillie M, Fernandes J, Bijleveld CMA, Desjeux JF: Interval breath hydrogen test in glucose-galactose malabsorption. *Eur J Pediatr* **137**:273, 1981.
38. Sarles J, Collard Y, Arnaud-Battandier F, Bresson JL, Schmitz J, Ricour C, Rey J: Fermentation acide et production d'hydrogène par la flore colique dans un cas de malabsorption du glucose et du galactose. *Gastroenterol Clin Biol* **10**:848, 1986.
39. Elsas LJ, Lambe DW: Familial glucose-galactose malabsorption: Remission of glucose intolerance. *J Pediatr* **83**:226, 1973.
40. Burant CF, Takeda J, Brot-Laroche E, Bell GI, Davidson NO: Fructose transporter in human spermatozoa and small intestine is GLUT5. *J Biol Chem* **267**:14523, 1992.
41. Schultz SG, Curran PF: Coupled transport of sodium and organic solutes. *Physiol Rev* **50**:637, 1970.
42. Kimmich GA: Intestinal absorption of sugar, in Johnson LR (ed): *Physiology of the Gastrointestinal Tract*. New York, Raven, 1981.
43. Semenza G, Kessler M, Hosang M, Weber J, Schmidt U: Biochemistry of the Na^+ D-glucose cotransporter of the small intestinal brush border membrane. The state of the art in 1984. *Biochim Biophys Acta* **779**:343, 1984.
44. Hopfer U: Membrane transport mechanism for hexoses and amino acids in the small intestine, in Johnson LR (ed): *Physiology of the Gastrointestinal Tract*, 2d ed. New York, Raven, 1987.
45. Desjeux JF, Tannenbaum C, Tai YJ, Curran PF: Effects of sugars and amino acids on sodium movement across small intestine. *Am J Dis Child* **131**:331, 1977.
46. Mahalanabis D, Merson M: Development of an improved formulation of oral rehydration salts (ORS) with antidiarrhoeal and nutritional properties: A "super ORS," in Holmgren J, Lindberg A, Möllby R (eds): *Development of Vaccines and Drugs against Diarrhea, 11th Nobel Conference, Stockholm, 1986* (student literature, Lund, Sweden), p 240.
47. Wright EM: Intestinal sugar transport, in Lebenthal E, Duffey M (eds): *Textbook of Secretory Diarrhea*. New York, Raven, 1989.
48. Hediger MA, Budarf ML, Emanuel BS, Mohandas TK, Wright EM: Assignment of the human intestinal Na^+/glucose cotransporter gene (SGLT1) to the q11.2 → qter region of chromosome 22. *Genomics* **4**:297, 1989.
49. Pajor AM, Hirayama BA, Wright EM: Molecular biology approaches to the comparative study of Na^+/glucose cotransporter. *Am J Physiol* **263**:R489, 1992.
50. Wright EM, Hager KM, Turk E: Sodium cotransport proteins. *Curr Opin Cell Biol* **4**:696, 1992.
51. Parent L, Supplisson S, Loo DF, Wright EM: Electrogenic properties of the cloned Na^+/glucose cotransporter: Part II. A transport model under non rapid equilibrium conditions. *J Membr Biol* **125**:63, 1992.
52. Douwes AC, Oosterkamp RF, Fenandes J, Los T, Jongloed A: Sugar malabsorption in healthy neonates estimated by breath hydrogen. *Arch Dis Child* **55**:512, 1980.
53. Mobassaieh M, Montgomery RK, Biller JA, Grand RJ: Development of carbohydrate absorption in the fetus and neonate. *Pediatrics (suppl)* **75**:160, 1985.
54. Lifschitz CH, O'Brien Smith E, Garza C: Delayed complete functional lactase sufficiency in breast-fed infants. *J Pediatr Gastroenterol Nutr* **2**:478, 1983.
55. Kien CL, Kepner J, Grotjohn K, Ault K, McClead RE: Stable isotope model for estimating colonic acetate production in premature infants. *Gastroenterology* **102**:1458, 1992.
56. Ravich WJ, Bayless TM, Thomas M: Fructose: Incomplete intestinal absorption in humans. *Gastroenterology* **84**:26, 1983.
57. Gray GM, Santiago NA: Disaccharide absorption in normal and diseased human intestine. *Gastroenterology* **51**:489, 1966.
58. Jirosova V, Koldovsky O, Heringova A, Hoskova J, Jirasek J, Uher J: The development of the functions of the small intestine of human fetus. *Biol Neonate* **9**:44, 1966.
59. Levin RJ, Koldovsky O, Hoskova J, Jirsova V, Uher

J: Electrical activity across human foetal small intestine associated with absorption processes. *Gut* **9**:206, 1968.

60. Koldovsky O, Heringova A, Jirsova V, Jirasek JE, Uher J: Transport of glucose against a concentration gradient in everted sacs of jejunum and ileum of human fetuses. *Gastroenterology* **48**:185, 1965.
61. Younoszai MK: Jejunal absorption of hexose in infants and adults. *J Pediatr* **85**:446, 1974.
62. Karasov WH, Diamond JM: Adaptive regulation of sugar and amino acid transport by vertebrate intestine. *Am J Physiol* **245**:G443, 1983.
63. Grasset E, Heyman M, Dumontier AM, Lestradet H, Desjeux JF: Possible sodium and D-glucose cotransport in isolated jejunal epithelium of children. *Pediatr Res* **13**:1240, 1979.
64. Rosenberg LE, Blair A, Segal S: Transport of amino acids by slices of rat-kidney cortex. *Biochim Biophys Acta* **54**:479, 1961.
65. Naftalin R, Curran PF: Galactose transport in rabbit ileum. *J Membr Biol* **16**:257, 1974.
66. Desjeux JF, Sandler L, Sassier P, Lestradet H: Acquired and congenital disorders of intestinal transport of D-glucose in children. *Rev Eur Etud Clin Biol* **16**:364, 1971.
67. Stirling CE, Schneider AJ, Wong MD, Kinter WB: Quantitative radioautography of sugar transport in intestinal biopsies from normal humans and a patient with glucose-galactose malabsorption. *J Clin Invest* **51**:438, 1972.
68. Booth IW, Patel PB, Sule D, Brown GA, Buick R, Beyreiss K: Glucose-galactose malabsorption: Demonstration of specific jejunal brush border membrane defect. *Gut* **29**:1661, 1988.
69. Keston AS, Meeuwisse G, Fredrikson B: Evidence for participation of mutarotase in sugar transport: Absence of the enzyme in a case of glucose-galactose malabsorption. *Biochem Biophys Res Commun* **108**:1574, 1982.
70. Turk E, Klisak I, Bacallao R, Sparkes RS, Wright EM: Assignment of the human Na^+/glucose cotransporter gene SGLT1 to chromosome 22q13.1. *Genomics* **17**:752, 1993.
71. Turk E, Zabel B, Mundlos S, Dyer J, Wright EM: Glucose/galactose malabsorption caused by a defect in the Na^+/glucose cotransporter. *Nature* **350**:354, 1991.
72. Hager KM, Lescale-Matys L, Wright EM: Site directed mutagenesis of the rabbit intestinal Na^+/glucose cotransporter. *FASEB J* **6**:A1769, 1992.
73. Desjeux JF: Congenital transport defects, in Walker WA, Durie PR, Hamilton JR, Walker-Smith JA, Watkins JB (eds): *Pediatric Gastrointestinal Disease*. Philadelphia, B.C. Decker, 1991, pp 668–688.
74. Burke V, Anderson CM: Sugar intolerance as a cause of protracted diarrhea following surgery of the gastrointestinal tract of neonates. *Aust Pediatr* **2**:219, 1966.
75. Lifshitz F, Coello-Ramirez P, Gutierrez-Topete G: Monosaccharide intolerance and hypoglycemia in infants with diarrhea. I. Clinical course of 23 infants. *J Pediatr* **77**:595, 1970.
76. Desjeux JF, Sassier P, Tichet J, Sarrut S, Lestradet H: Sugar absorption by flat jejunal mucosa. *Acta Paediatr Scand* **62**:531, 1973.
77. Lifshitz F, Coello-Ramirez P, Gutierrez-Topete G: Monosaccharide intolerance and hypoglycemia in infants with diarrhea. II. Metabolic studies in 23 infants. *J Pediatr* **77**:604, 1970.
78. Nichols BL: Pathogenesis of glucose malabsorption in acquired monosaccharide intolerance, in Lifshitz F (ed): *Carbohydrate Intolerance in Infancy*. New York, Marcel Dekker, 1982, p 105.
79. Barnes G, McKellar W, Lawrence S: Detection of fructose malabsorption by breath hydrogen test in a child with diarrhea. *J Pediatr* **103**:575, 1983.
80. Truswell AS, Seach JM, Thorburn AW: Incomplete absorption of pure fructose in healthy subjects and the facilitating effect of glucose. *Am J Clin Nutr* **48**:1424, 1988.
81. Beaugerie L, Nath SK, Desjeux JF: Glucose stimulates the absorption of sorbitol through the human jejunal mucosa. *Gastroenterol Clin Biol* **13**:379, 1989.
82. Beaugerie L, Flourié B, Pellier P, Achour L, Franchisseur C, Rambaud JC: Clinical tolerance, intestinal absorption, and energy value of four sugar alcohols taken on an empty stomach. *Gastroenterol Clin Biol* **15**:929, 1991.
83. Beaugerie L, Flourié B, Marteau P, Pellier P, Franchisseur C, Rambaud JC: Digestion and absorption in the human intestine of three sugar alcohols. *Gastroenterology* **99**:717, 1990.
84. Lloyd-Still JD, Listernick R, Buentello G: Complex carbohydrate intolerance: Diagnostic pitfalls and approach to management. *J Pediatr* **112**:709, 1988.
85. Krane SM: Renal glycosuria, in Stanbury JB, Wyngaarden JB, Frederickson DS (eds): *The Metabolic Basis of Inherited Disease*, 4th ed. New York, McGraw-Hill, 1978.
86. Marble A: Non-diabetic melituria, in Joslin EP, Root HF, White P, Marble A (eds): *The Treatment of Diabetes Mellitus*. Philadelphia, Lea & Febiger, 1959.
87. Lestradet H, Labrune B, Duval C, Deschamps I: Le diabète rénal. A propos de 103 observations chez l'enfant. *Arch Fr Pediatr* **36**:760, 1979.
88. Lawrence RD: Symptomless glycosurias: Differentiation by sugar tolerance tests. *Med Clin North Am* **31**:289, 1947.
89. Oemar BS, Byrd DJ, Brodehl J: Complete absence of tubular glucose reabsorption: A new type of renal glucosuria (type O). *Clin Nephrol* **27**:156, 1987.
90. De Marchi S, Cecchin E, Basile A, Proto G, Donadon W, Schinella D, Lengo A, De Paoli P, Jus A, Villalta D, Tesio F, Santini G: Is renal glycosuria a benign condition? *Proc Eur Dial Transplant Assoc* **20**:681, 1983.
91. De Paoli P, Battistin S, Jus A, Reitano M, Villalta D, De Marchi S, Cecchin E, Basile A, Santini G: Immunological characterization of renal glycosuria patients. *Clin Exp Immunol* **56**:289, 1984.
92. Leonardi P, Ruol A, Munari R: Morphologic aspects of renal glycosuria. *Am J Med Sci* **239**:721, 1960.
93. Freeman JA, Roberts KE: A fine structural study of renal glycosuria. *Exp Mol Pathol* **2**:83, 1963.
94. Mudge GH: Clinical patterns of tubular dysfunction. *Am J Med* **24**:785, 1958.
95. Ackerman IP, Fajans SS, Conn JW: The development of diabetes mellitus in patients with nondiabetic glycosuria. *Clin Res Proc* **6**:251, 1958.
96. Monasterio G, Oliver J, Muiesan G, Pardelli G, Marinozzi V, MacDowell M: Renal diabetes as a congenital tubular dysplasia. *Am J Med* **37**:44, 1964.
97. Reubi FC: Glucose titration in renal glycosuria, in Lewis AAG, Wolstenholme GEW (eds): *Ciba Foundation Symposium on the Kidney*. Boston, Little, Brown, 1954.
98. Bradley SE, Bradley GP, Tyson CJ, Curry JJ, Blake WC: Renal function in renal diseases. *Am J Med* **9**:766, 1950.
99. Smith HW: *The Kidney: Structure and Function in Health and Disease*. New York, Oxford University Press, 1958.
100. Mudge GH, Bernt WO, Valtin H: Tubular transport of urea, glucose, phosphate, uric acid, sulfate, and thiosulfate, in Orloff J, Berliner RW (eds): *Renal Physiology, Handbook of Physiology*. Washington, DC, Amrican Physiological Society, 1973.
101. Elsas LJ, Rosenberg LE: Familial renal glycosuria: A genetic reappraisal of hexose transport by kidney and intestine. *J Clin Invest* **48**:1845, 1969.
102. Darmaun D, Robert JJ, Chevrot M, Dieterlen PH, Reach G, Desjeux JF: Filtration glomérulaire et réabsorption tubulaire du glucose dans le diabète insulinodépendant de l'enfant. *Arch Fr Pediatr* **43**:23, 1986.
103. Loeschke K, Bauman K, Renschler H, Ullrich KJ: Differenzierung zwischen aktiver und passiv komponente des D-glucosetransports a proximalen konvolut der ratteuniere. *Arch Ges Physiol* **305**:118, 1969.
104. Hoshi T, Kikuta Y: Effects of organic solute-sodium cotransport on the transmembrane potential resistance parameters of the proximal tubule of Triturus kidney, in Anagnostopoulos T (ed): *Electrophysiology of the Nephron*. Paris, INSERM, 1977, vol 67, p 135.
105. Barfuss DW, Schafer JA: Differences in active and passive glucose transport along the proximal nephron. *Am J Physiol* **240**:F322, 1981.
106. Turner RJ, Silverman M: Sugar uptake into normal human renal brush border vesicles. *Proc Natl Acad Sci USA* **75**:2825, 1977.

107. Turner RJ, Moran A: Heterogeneity of sodium-dependent D-glucose transport sites along the proximal tubule: Evidence from vesicle studies. *Am J Physiol* **242**:F406, 1982.
108. Roigaard-Petersen H, Jacobsen C, Sheikh MI: Characteristics of D-galactose transport systems by luminal membrane vesicles from rabbit kidney. *Biochim Biophys Acta* **856**:578, 1986.
109. Coady MJ, Pajor AM, Wright EM: Sequence homologies among intestinal and renal Na^+/glucose cotransporters. *Am J Physiol* **259**:C605, 1990.
110. Lee WS, Wells RG, Hediger MA: Localization of the rat high affinity Na^+/glucose cotransporter, RNA in the kidney proximal tubule S3 segment. *J Am Soc Nephrol* **3**:830, 1992.
110a. Pajor AM, Hirayama BA, Wright EM: Molecular evidence for two renal Na^+/glucose cotransporters. *Biochim Biophys Acta* **1106**:216, 1992.
111. Wells RG, Kandi Y, Pajor AM, Turk E, Wright EM, Hediger MA: The cloning of a human kidney cDNA with similarity to the sodium/glucose cotransporter. *Am J Physiol* **263**:F459, 1992.
112. Kanai Y, Lee W-S, Hediger MA: Structure and function of the human low affinity Na^+/glucose cotransporter (SGLT2). *J Am Soc Nephrol* **3**:830, 1992.
113. De Marchi S, Cecchin E, Basile A, Proto G, Donadon W, Jengo A, Schinella D, Jus A, Villalta D, De Paoli P, Santini G, Tesio F: Close genetic linkage between HLA and renal glycosuria. *Am J Nephrol* **4**:280, 1984.
114. Hjärne VA: Study of orthoglycaemic glycosuria with particular reference to its hereditability. *Acta Med Scand* **67**:422, 1937.
115. Elsas JJ, Busse D, Rosenberg LE: Autosomal recessive inheritance of renal glycosuria. *Metabolism* **20**:968, 1971.
115a. Scriver CR, Chesney RW, McInnes RR: Genetic aspects of renal tubular transport: Diversity and topology of carriers. *Kidney Int* **9**:149, 1976.
116. Caspary WF: Diarrhoea associated with carbohydrate malabsorption. *Clin Gastroenterol* **15**:631, 1986.
117. Gray GM: Intestinal disaccharidase deficiencies and glucose-galactose malabsorption, in Stanbury JB, Wyngaarden JB, Fredrickson DS (eds): *The Metabolic Basis of Inherited Disease*, 4th ed. New York, McGraw-Hill, 1978.
118. Launiala K: The effect of unabsorbed sucrose and mannitol on the small intestinal flow rate and mean transit time. *Scand J Gastroenterol* **3**:665, 1968.
119. Bridges RJ, Rummel W: Mechanistic basis of alterations in mucosal water and electrolyte transport. *Clin Gastroenterol* **15**:491, 1986.
120. Palma R, Vidon N, Bernier JJ: Maximal capacity for fluid absorption in human bowel. *Dig Dis Sci* **26**:929, 1981.
121. Saunders DR, Wiggins HS: Conservation of mannitol, lactulose and raffinose by the human colon. *Am J Physiol* **241**:G397, 1981.
122. Bond JH, Levitt MD: Fate of soluble carbohydrate in the colon of rats and man. *J Clin Invest* **57**:1158, 1976.
123. Hammer HF, Santa Ana CA, Schiller LR, Fordtran JS: Studies of osmotic diarrhea induced in normal subjects by ingestion of polyethylene glycol and lactulose. *J Clin Invest* **84**:1056, 1989.
124. Hammer HF, Fine KD, Santa Ana CA, Porter JL, Schiller LR, Fordtran JS: Carbohydrate malabsorption. Its measurement and its contribution to diarrhea. *J Clin Invest* **86**:1936, 1990.
125. Argenzio RA, Moon HW, Kemeny LJ, Whipp SC: Colonic compensation in transmissible gastroenteritis of swine. *Gastroenterology* **86**:1501, 1984.
126. Florent C, Flourie B, Leblond A, Rautureau M, Bernier JJ, Rambaud JC: Influence of chronic lactulose ingestion on the colonic metabolism of lactulose in man (an in vivo study). *J Clin Invest* **75**:608, 1985.

CHAPTER 117

Cystinuria

Stanton Segal ▪ Samuel O. Thier

1. **Cystinuria is a disorder of amino acid transport affecting the epithelial cells of the renal tubule and the gastrointestinal tract. The defective transport of cystine, lysine, arginine, and ornithine is transmitted as an autosomal recessive trait. The heterozygous state may reflect true recessive or incompletely recessive inheritance. In the latter state the affected amino acids are excreted in urine in quantities greater than normal but less than in the homozygous state. By use of the intestinal transport system as a sensitive genetic marker, three types of cystinuric homozygotes can be defined, and the evidence is that these types result from allelic mutations.**

2. **The intestinal defect can be demonstrated in vivo by oral loading tests and by intestinal perfusion studies. Complementary data showing the defect have also been obtained by incubations in vitro measuring transport into mucosal biopsies. The dibasic amino acids can be absorbed by cystinuric subjects in a normal fashion as dipeptides.**

3. **The renal lesions for all four amino acids and the mixed disulfide of cysteine–homocysteine can be demonstrated by clearance studies. The clearance of cystine in both humans and dogs with cystinuria frequently exceeds the glomerular filtration rate. This suggests that secretion occurs. Studies in vitro of amino acid transport by renal cortical slices of affected kidneys demonstrate a defect for dibasic amino acids but not for cystine. There exist, in rat renal tubule fragments and isolated brush border membrane vesicles, multiple systems for cystine and lysine transport. Cystine and the dibasic amino acids appear to share the low K_m, high-affinity system that is probably defective in the cystinuric kidney. Microperfusion of rat kidney tubules and studies of rat cortical transport in vivo indicate that there may be an interaction of cystine and dibasic amino acids at the luminal membrane of the renal tubule cells. Cysteine, the intracellular form of cystine, shares a cellular efflux system with dibasic amino acids. This interaction may play an important role in the regulation of cystine transport into renal cortical cells.**

4. **Cystinuria is expressed clinically as urinary tract calculus disease. Radiopaque cystine stones are formed, and hexagonal cystine crystals appear in the urine. Diagnosis may be pursued by testing urine with nitroprusside, high-voltage electrophoresis, or column amino acids analysis. Stones generally form at cystine excretion rates of greater than 300 mg cystine per gram of creatinine in acid urine. Cystinuric patients are susceptible to all complications of stone disease. Treatment is directed at reducing the concentration of cystine in urine by increasing urine volume, increasing cystine solubility by alkalinizing the urine, and reducing cystine excretion by use of D-penicillamine. Although extremely effective, D-penicillamine is not without risk and should be reserved for patients who fail to respond to conservative therapy.**

   Other sulfhydryl-containing compounds, such as mercaptopropionylglycine (MPG) and captopril, have been shown to reduce cystine excretion and stone formation. MPG appears to be quite effective but has a significant frequency of side effects, particularly in patients who have had reactions to D-penicillamine. The place of captopril in the treatment of cystinuria has not been defined.

5. **Models of human cystinuria have been described in animals. Studies of these models may help clarify the cellular defect in cystinuria and may provide a system for testing new drug therapy.**

A list of standard abbreviations is located immediately preceding the index in each volume. An additional abbreviation used in this chapter is: MPG = mercaptopropionylglycine.

Cystinuria is a heritable disorder of amino acid transport affecting the epithelial cells of the renal tubules and gastrointestinal tract. The disease is expressed clinically by the formation of calculi in the urinary tract, with the potential for obstruction, infections, and ultimately renal insufficiency. The disease is characterized primarily by the precipitation of cystine, the least soluble of the naturally occurring amino acids; lysine, arginine, ornithine, and cysteine-homocysteine mixed disulfide are also present in excess in the urine. Since this aminoaciduria occurs with a normal or reduced filtered load of cystine and the dibasic amino acids, it was postulated earlier that cystinuria is a disorder of tubular transport in the kidney. The subsequent demonstration of comparably defective transport in the intestine established the present view of this disorder as an inherited defect in a specific transepithelial transport mechanism, which is expressed in two areas, the kidney and the intestine.

HISTORY

The historical development of a theory of the pathogenesis of cystinuria was anything but orderly. Although the data suggesting renal and intestinal lesions appeared in random order, it is easier to trace the history of the renal lesion before that of the intestinal defect.

In 1810 Wollaston analyzed two stones recovered from urinary bladders and discerned that they differed from all previously described calculi. Because of their bladder origin and supposed chemical nature, they were named cystic oxide stones.[1] In 1824 Stromeyer noted hexagonal platelike crystals in the urine of patients with cystinuria.[2] The finding of cystine crystals served for many years as the chief means of diagnosing the disease and remains helpful even today.

In 1833 Berzelius, recognizing that the compound was not an oxide, renamed the substance "cystine," perpetuating the fallacy that it originated in the bladder.[3] Although improved descriptions of the chemistry of cystine were developed over the next 70 years, it was not until 1902 that Friedman defined the chemical structure of cystine.[4] In his 1908 Croonian lectures, Garrod discussed cystinuria among the inborn errors of metabolism and postulated that a defect in the metabolism of cystine was responsible for the disorder.[5] During the next 40 years, in spite of the reports of increased lysine in the urine of cystinuric subjects, there was little advance in our understanding of the disease. The present concepts of cystinuria emerged after the advent of paper chromatography and development of polarographic and microbiologic assays. With these methods, Yeh et al. demonstrated in 1947 that lysinuria and argininuria also occur in cystinuria,[6] and Stein found that a large quantity of ornithine was also present.[7] Subsequently, Dent et al.[8] and Arrow and Westall[9] noted that plasma levels of cystine and of dibasic amino acids were normal or low. Dent and Rose observed that cystine and the dibasic amino acids had structural similarities, i.e., two amino groups separated by four to six chemical bonds. They postulated that there was a single renal transport mechanism shared by these amino acids and proposed that this mechanism was defective or absent in cystinuria[10] (Fig. 117-1). Although defective uptake of lysine and arginine has been demonstrable in tissue slices from cystinuric subjects, cystine uptake was unimpaired, and cystine did not appear to compete with the dibasic amino acids for transport.[11]

Recent studies with rat renal cortical tubule fragments[12] and isolated brush border membrane vesicles[13] indicate that there are two transport systems for cystine: one with a high affinity that is shared with dibasic amino acids, and another with low affinity that is unshared. It appears that the latter system is the only one observable during in vitro studies with cortical slices, and that the results of cystine uptake experiments with slices do not reveal an important aspect of the transport of this amino acid. The data with isolated brush border membranes[13] support the formulation of Dent and Rose and suggest that cystinuria may result from defective function of a common high-affinity uptake system for cystine and dibasic amino acids. This explanation for the renal defect in cystinuria is complicated, however, by the occurrence of cystine clearances exceeding creatinine clearances in cystinuric patients. This indicates that cystine secretion may contribute to the aminoaciduria.[14–16]

The intestinal defect was not recognized as promptly. Von Udranszky and Baumann in 1889 observed that cadaverine and putrescine, decarboxylation products of lysine and arginine, were present in large amounts in urine of cystinuric subjects.[17] These findings were confirmed by Loewy and Neuberg.[18] Subsequently an increase of urinary cystine excretion was reported in cystinuria in response to protein feeding, but feeding of cystine itself was not observed to increase either serum or urine cystine.[19,20] After half a century these data were finally interpreted by Milne, who had already recognized the intestinal transport defect associated with the renal aminoaciduria in Hartnup disease.[21] Milne performed experiments that demonstrated reduced intestinal absorption of the dibasic amino acids in patients with cystinuria.[22,23] His findings have been confirmed in vitro by studies of transport in jejunal biopsies.[24–26] The question of why malabsorption of an essential amino acid does not result in more serious problems of growth and development has been answered in part by the observation that oligopeptide absorption from the intestine may account for a significant proportion of amino acid absorption.[27,28] Lysine absorption from an oligopeptide may be normal in the same cystinuric subject who has poor absorption of free lysine. On the other hand, a recent biochemical investigation of sulfur amino acid metabolism in cystinuria by Martensson et al.[29] suggests that there may be intracellular cysteine deficiency, as evidenced by decreased leukocyte glutathione and taurine levels, decrease plasma levels of cyst(e)ine and taurine, and lower urinary excretion of mercaptolactate, taurine, thiosulfate, and inorganic sulfate.

CLINICAL ASPECTS

Although cystinuria is thought to be a rare disease because of the estimated prevalence of 1 per 100,000 in Sweden[30] and 1 per 20,000 in England,[31,32] there are populations where homozygous cystinuria is a frequently inherited disorder. The prevalence in Israeli Jews of Libyan origin has been estimated to be 1 in 2500.[33] Screening programs of newborn babies show the prevalence in England to be 1 in 2000[34]; in Australia, 1 in 4000[35]; and in the United States, 1 in 15,000.[36] According to Levy,[37] who summarized the results of newborn screening, the overall prevalence is 1 in 7000, which makes cystinuria one of the most common inherited disorders. The disease occurs equally in both sexes, but males are more severely affected and have a higher mortality rate. The greater severity of the disease in males may be related to urinary tract anatomy, with a greater likelihood of urethral obstruction in males. Although clinical expression of the disease may occur in the first year of life or as late as the ninth decade, the second and third decades appear to be the peak times for expression of cystinuria. Colic, the most common presentation, may be associated with obstruction of the urinary tract, subsequent infection, and eventual loss of function. Infection, hypertension, and renal failure occur occasionally and may cause the patient first to seek medical attention. The belief that cystinuric patients are shorter than the general population[38] has not been substantiated.[39]

Cystine Stones

Both cystine stones and uric acid stones form readily in acid urine, and the two are frequently confused. However, the

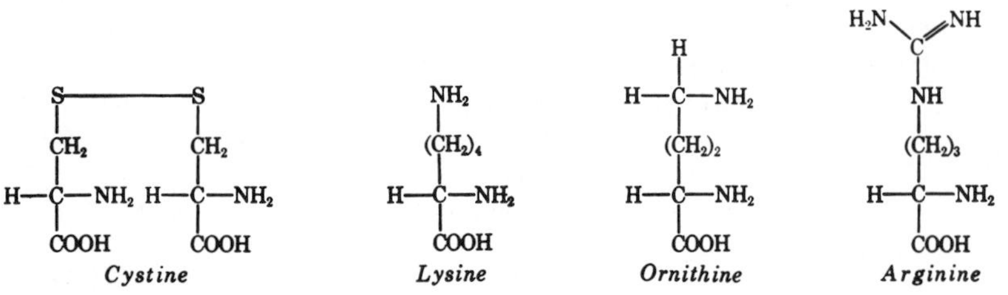

FIG. 117-1 Chemical structures of the amino acids excreted in excessive amounts in the urine in cystinuria.

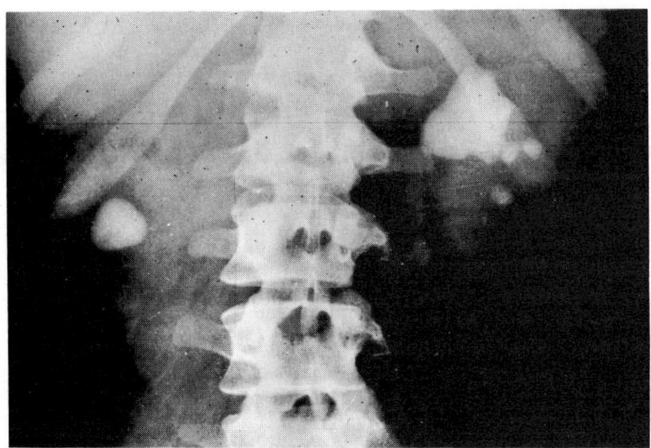

FIG. 117-2 Roentgenogram of the abdomen of a cystinuric patient showing bilateral radiopaque calculi.

cystine stone, with its yellow-brown color and maple sugar crystal surface, is much firmer than uric acid and is radiopaque.[40,41] The radiopacity of cystine is due to the density of the sulfur molecules. On roentgenograms cystine stones appear smooth and are less dense than calcium stones. Cystine calculi tend to occur as staghorn or multiple recurrent stones, frequently necessitating surgery (Fig. 117-2). Calcium and/or magnesium ammonium phosphate (struvite) stones may also be formed as a result of infection secondary to cystine calculi.

DIAGNOSIS

The diagnosis of cystinuria should be entertained in every patient with urinary calculi or with urinary tract symptoms suggestive of calculi. The simplest diagnostic procedure is the microscopic examination of urinary sediment, preferably from the first voiding in the morning or from other concentrated urine, for typical cystine crystals (Fig. 117-3). Acidification of a cooled concentrated urine specimen with acetic acid may precipitate cystine crystals that were not visible in a fresh urine specimen.

The cyanide-nitroprusside test has been widely applied as a chemical screening procedure.[42,43] It is important that the color obtained be compared with that of a specimen of normal urine to which cystine has been added. Since the lower limit of sensitivity of the reaction is about 75 to 125 mg per gram of creatinine, the reaction permits easy detection of homozygous stone formers, who usually excrete more than 250 mg per gram of creatinine.[44,45] Some but not all of the heterozygotes that have increased urinary cystine may also be detected by this procedure. A positive nitroprusside test may be seen in homocystinuria as well as in patients with acetonuria. Patients with crystalluria or a positive cyanide-nitroprusside test should be further studied for identification of urinary amino acids by such methods as thin-layer chromatography[46] or high-voltage electrophoresis.[47] Quantitation of cystine may be made easily following its electrolytic reduction to the thiol, which can be colorimetrically determined.[46] Quantitative ion-exchange chromatography is a commonly used procedure.[48,49] The upper limits of the normal ranges for cystine, lysine, arginine, and ornithine as measured by this method in the adult are 18, 130, 16 and 22 mg per gram of creatinine, respectively.[32] A sophisticated method of liquid chromatography–mass spectrometry for identifying cystine and dibasic amino acids has been described.[50] Urinary cysteine and cystine can be measured quantitatively by high-performance liquid chromatography[51] and by a spectrophotometric method involving oxidation of cysteine by thallium(III) to create fluorescent thallium(I).[52]

Cystinuria has been associated with hyperuricemia,[53] hemophilia,[54] retinitis pigmentosa,[55] muscular dystrophy,[56] muscular hypotonia,[57] mongolism,[58] and hereditary pancreatitis,[59] and it occurs as an isolated aminoaciduria with hypocalcemic tetany.[60] A urinary amino acid excretion pattern consistent with the cystinuric phenotype has been observed in infants with organic acidemias such as propionic,[61] methylmalonic,[62] and isovaleric acidemia.[63] In the latter instance the cystinuric pattern reverted to normal when the acute isovaleric acid toxicity state was successfully treated. Hypercalcuria, hyperuricosuria, and hypocitraturia have been found in a number of cystinuric stone formers. The hypocitraturia was frequently associated with defective urinary acidification.[64]

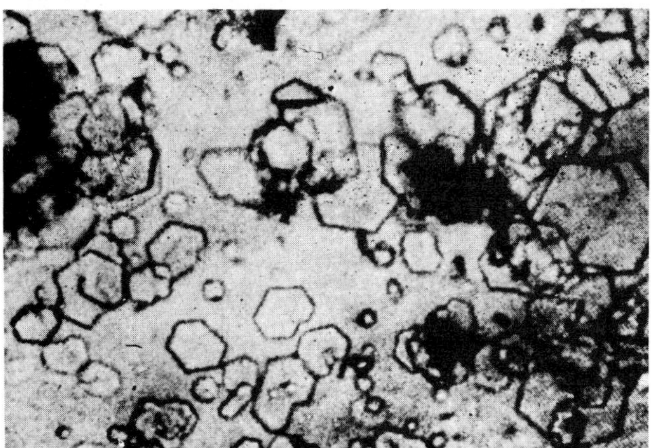

FIG. 117-3 Cystine crystals as they appear in the urinary sediment in cystinuria.

BIOCHEMISTRY OF CYSTINURIA

Consideration of cystinuria as an inborn error of metabolism by Garrod[5] was based on the assumption that an enzyme responsible for cystine catabolism was missing or defective. Although Garrod's concept of a missing enzyme in a metabolic pathway has been substantiated for the other diseases on which his theory was based, this was not the case for cystinuria. Garrod was not truly incorrect about cystinuria, since the modern view that the disease is an inherited disorder of membrane transport supposes the genetic loss of a mechanism located in the membrane and is responsible for movement of extracellular cystine into the confines of the cell. The concept of a membrane transport mechanism involving an amino acid-binding site and genetic control is consistent with the function of a "carrier" protein. What Garrod did not anticipate was the membrane nature of the disorder and the primary involvement of the kidney and intestine.

Garrod's concept stimulated the elucidation of the transsulfuration metabolic pathway. The feeding experiments of Brand and his colleagues demonstrated that methionine[19] and proteins high in methionine[65] resulted in higher cystine excretion, since methionine is converted to cysteine and then to cystine. Feeding of cystine itself did not give rise to

Table 117-1 Intracellular Forms of ^{35}S after Incubation of Rat Kidney Cortex Slices with Labeled L-Cystine and L-Cysteine

			Intracellular Form of ^{35}S as Percent of Intracellular ^{35}S			
Age of Animal	Transported Substrate	Concentration, m*M*	Cystine	Reduced Glutathione	Cysteine	Other
5 days	Cystine	0.07	0	25	62	13
5 days	Cysteine	0.07	6	24	62	8
Adult	Cystine	0.07	0	12	68	20
Adult	Cysteine	0.07	14	20	64	8

SOURCE: From Segal and Smith.[75] Used by permission.

increased amounts of urinary cystine, but giving cysteine did.[20] This can now be interpreted on the basis of an intestinal defect in cystine absorption, which does not involve cysteine (see below). The role of cystathionine as an intermediate was shown in du Vigneaud's laboratory when that compound gave rise to cystine.[66] Most recent observations have been concerned with the enzymes of the pathway in relation to homocystinuria[67] and cystathioninuria.[68] The observation that the body can convert methionine or homocystine to cystine by way of the transsulfuration pathway has relegated cystine to the position of a nonessential amino acid, but the demonstration that cystathionase is not active in fetal tissues implies that cystine may be an essential amino acid in fetal development.[69]

Relatively less seems to be known of the catabolism of cystine or cysteine to sulfate. Oxidation to cysteinesulfonate, taurine, cysteic acid, and sulfite appears to be involved (see Chap. 70).[70,71] Increased urinary sulfate excretion in cystinuric patients fed cystine may involve the oxidation of unabsorbed cystine in the gastrointestinal tract and subsequent absorption of the inorganic ion.[72]

These aspects of cystine catabolism may be more appropriately considered with regard to the human cystine storage disease cystinosis,[73] which should not be confused with cystinuria. Although a generalized aminoaciduria is present with cystinosis, the large amounts of cystine and dibasic amino acids found with cystinuria are absent. Cystine storage disease is associated with deposition of cystine in various tissues; in cystinuria there is no tissue deposition, only urinary loss.

Of importance to a basic understanding of both human diseases involving cystine is the fact that the intracellular form of the amino acid is not the disulfide but the free thiol, cysteine.[74,75] When [^{35}S]cystine is incubated with kidney cortex slices or other tissues, the ^{35}S within the cell is mainly in cysteine or glutathione, little or none being maintained as cystine[75] (Table 117-1). Reduction of cystine to cysteine is believed to take place within the cell by a mechanism mediated by glutathione-cysteine transhydrogenase,[76] since cystine taken up by isolated renal brush border membrane vesicles is not reduced to the free thiol.[13]

RENAL TRANSPORT DEFECTS

Cystinuria is a classic example of a disorder of renal tubular function. In a discussion of aminoaciduria it should be kept clearly in mind that most aminoacidurias are not disorders of tubular function. Normally, amino acids are filtered and are almost entirely reabsorbed in the proximal nephron. The reabsorptive mechanism has a maximal capacity that is exceeded in certain disorders. In most cases of aminoaciduria, an extrarenal metabolic defect leads to the accumulation of an amino acid in the plasma, which is then filtered in amounts exceeding the normal capacity of the nephron for reabsorption. These are not disorders of tubular function. When excessive loss occurs in the face of normal or low plasma levels and diminished filtered loads of the amino acid, then the reabsorptive capacity of the tubule is said to be below normal and tubular dysfunction exists. The latter situation obtains in cystinuria. Excessive urinary losses of cystine and dibasic amino acids occur with normal or less than normal plasma levels of the affected amino acids.[8,9]

Of all amino acids studied, only cystine and the dibasic amino acids are involved in cystinuria. On the basis of this information, Dent and Rose postulated the existence of a single transport mechanism shared by cystine and the dibasic amino acids which is defective in cystinuria.[10] Recent reports of clinical disorders in which cystine and dibasic aminoacidurias occur independently have complicated this interpretation and indicate that there may be separate systems for transport of cystine and lysine by the kidney tubule. Brodehl et al.[60] have found isolated cystinuria without dibasic aminoaciduria, and Stephens and Perrett[77] reported a patient with cystine stones who had minimal dibasic aminoaciduria, a finding in many dogs with cystinuria and urolithiasis.[78] Conversely, dibasic aminoaciduria without cystinuria has been observed.[79,80] Lysinuric protein intolerance is characterized by lysinuria without cystinuria, and defective renal tubular reabsorption of lysine and competition among the dibasic amino acids have been demonstrated (see Chap. 118).[81]

Observations in Vivo

The increase in renal clearance of cystine and the dibasic amino acids reported first by Dent et al.[8] and then by Arrow and Westall[9] has also been found in more recent investigations.[82,83] Although in many patients the cystine clearance is equal to or somewhat less than the glomerular filtration rate, certain patients with cystinuria have a cystine clearance ($C_{cystine}$) greater than glomerular filtration, with a $C_{cystine}/C_{inulin}$ ratio ranging between 1 and 2.[14–16] The clearance of lysine is usually about 50 to 70 percent of the glomerular filtration rate. Arginine and ornithine reabsorption is less defective than lysine resorption.[83]

The hypothesis of Dent and Rose that there is a single shared transport mechanism for cystine and dibasic amino acids leads to the prediction that increasing the filtered load of one amino acid in the group should reduce the reabsorption of the others. Robson and Rose,[84] Lester and Cusworth,[82] and Kato[83] demonstrated that this was indeed true in normal humans. Similar data were derived in studies on normal dogs by Webber et al.[85] While Robson and Rose did not find that infusion of lysine increased cystine excretion by cystinuric subjects, both Lester and Cusworth[82] and Kato[83] observed such an effect on cystine, ornithine, and arginine excretion. Lester and Cusworth showed that lysine infusion caused the clearance of cystine to increase to a value greater than glomerular filtration, with a $C_{cystine}/C_{creatinine}$ ratio of 1.5. Kato[83] infused increasing amounts of arginine into three patients whose tubular reabsorption of cystine ranged from 10 to 50 percent (normal, 99 percent). This reduced the cystine reabsorption to −25 percent.

A careful examination of the data of Webber et al.[85] indicates that lysine infusion in a normal dog caused the cystine clearance to exceed the glomerular filtration rate. Bovee and Segal[86] have reported that infusion of lysine into cystinuric dogs can alter what appears to be a simple reabsorptive defect into cystine clearances greater than the glomerular filtration rate. The data are consistent with secretion of cystine under these conditions and raise the question of bidirectional cystine transport. The dibasic amino acid infusion data imply that these amino acids may not only compete with cystine for reabsorption but that by some enigmatic process they induce cystine secretion. The concept of amino acid secretion has been amply supported by experimental findings employing a variety of techniques.[87–89]

Additional studies in cystinuric patients have revealed a low renal threshold for lysine.[82] When homozygous subjects were infused with increasing amounts of lysine, they were unable to reabsorb the amino acid to any extent above the endogenous capacity until the filtered load was seven- to tenfold higher than the basal state. A further increase in the filtered load was associated with a tubular reabsorption in cystinuric patients that did not differ from the normal rate.[82] These findings are consistent with the functioning of dual systems for lysine transport, a low-capacity system acting at low substrate concentrations, which is defective in cystinurics, and a high-capacity transport system, which dominates at high lysine levels and is unaffected. Such a dual transport system for lysine has been described in human renal cortical slices.[90] The occurrence of multiple systems for cystine and dibasic amino acids is also supported by Brodehl, who found that newborn human infants have diminished reabsorption of cystine and dibasic amino acids and that reabsorption capacity matured at different rates for each of the substrates.[91] Scriver et al.[92] have extended these observations on the urinary amino acid patterns of newborns. Of 340,000 newborns, 730 had increased urinary cystine and dibasic amino acid excretion, which persisted in 191. With further follow-up and matching of infants to their parental phenotypes (see "Genetics" below for explanation of types I, II, and III) it was noted that in heterozygous but not homozygous infants, amino acid excretion fell with age to reach the level of their parental variants. With the exception of type I heterozygotes (who had clearly lower urinary amino acid levels), heterozygotes could not be differentiated from homozygotes during early infancy. These findings have important implications for genetic screening and counseling programs.

Examination of cystine levels in blood flowing through the kidneys of cystinuric patients has revealed minimal arteriovenous differences[93,94] and no alteration from the normal. Assuming that total failure of tubular reabsorption of cystine accounts for cystinuria, a large arteriovenous difference for cystine should be discernible. The inability to demonstrate this has raised the possibility of cystine synthesis de novo or kidney protein catabolism to account for the presence of urinary cystine in the face of normal plasma extraction. Frimpter[95] has attempted to solve this puzzle by comparing the specific activity of plasma and urinary cystine after infusing [^{35}S]cystine. The fact that these activities were the same argues against an endogenous kidney production of cystine, but it is possible that the long infusion period may have labeled the kidney pools of cystine so that the sought-for specific activity differences would not be detected.

The reduced form of cystine, cysteine, may play an important role in the underlying abnormality. Plasma cysteine in cystinuric patients is decreased proportionally more than cystine or the dibasic amino acids, but little cysteine appears in urine, and no increased conversion of cysteine to cystine has yet been demonstrated.[95,96] Frimpter,[93] having found an arteriovenous difference for cysteine but not for cystine across the kidney of a single patient, postulated that urinary cystine may be derived from plasma cysteine. Rosenberg et al.,[94] however, found no increase in cysteine extraction in two patients when compared with controls. An increase in cysteine clearance by the kidney would seem an unlikely source of urinary cystine. The plasma level of cysteine is only about 25 percent that of cystine, too low to explain the large amounts of urinary cystine on the basis of a total loss of filtered cysteine.

Results of microperfusion experiments with rat kidney tubules[97,98] show arginine inhibition of cystine and cysteine removal from the lumen of the tubule. Volkl et al.[99] in later microperfusion studies could not demonstrate saturability of cystine luminal uptake within the range of cystine solubility up to 0.4 m*M*. The fractional reabsorption rate of cystine was inhibited by a number of neutral amino acids, such as alanine, methionine, citrulline, α-aminoisobutyric acid, phenylalanine, and cycloleucine, but only methionine inhibited cysteine uptake.

Although these data suggest an interaction at the luminal membrane and the possibility of a shared transport system, it must be kept in mind that the cystine in the lumen is a resultant of fluxes and that the effect of arginine may not be a simple inhibition of uptake at the luminal membrane. Schafer and Watkins,[100] who examined unidirectional fluxes of [^{35}S]cystine in isolated perfused segments of rabbit proximal straight tubule, found a saturable system of the lumen-to-bath flux with a K_m of 0.2 m*M* but a nonsaturable bath-to-lumen flux. Luminal lysine inhibited the absorptive cystine flux but did not affect bath-to-lumen flux, thus providing evidence for the absence of a shared cystine–lysine transport system in the basolateral membrane.

A series of in vivo studies of lysine and cystine transport in rats attempted to demonstrate bidirectional transport by examining cellular accumulation after ureteral ligation and cessation of glomerular filtration.[101,102] The fact that cellular accumulation was maintained in the presence of ureteral ligation suggested that basolateral uptake had occurred, but this interpretation is open to question, since 1 to 2 h after ureteral obstruction in the rat the single-nephron glomerular filtration rate is only slightly reduced.[103] The interaction of dibasic amino acids and cystine was also examined in the intact rat kidney.[101,102] The injection of a large amount of arginine increased the fractional excretion of lysine, while injection of a lysine load increased the excretion of cystine. An unexplained finding was that during the arginine-induced lysinuria, when less lysine would be thought to be entering the tubule cells from the lumen, the tubule cell content of radioactive lysine was greater than in cells of control rats. A similar type of result occurred during lysine-induced cystinuria, when an increase in tubule cell cysteine, the intracellular form of cystine, was noted. These increases varied with the depth of the cell from the kidney surface and were greatest in cells of the outer medulla. The significance of these observations is not clear, but they suggest a functional heterogeneity of kidney tubule cells with regard to cystine and dibasic amino acids. Schwartzman et al.[104] have reported that lysine inhibits cysteine efflux from renal tubule cells and have postulated an efflux system shared by lysine and cystine. An elevation of intracellular cysteine could result from an inhibition by lysine of the transfer of cysteine into the peritubular capillary at the basolateral aspect of the cell.

Observations in Vitro

Studies in vitro with slices of human renal cortex have demonstrated that the dibasic amino acids lysine, arginine, and ornithine share a common renal transport mechanism.[11] The ability of cortical slices from cystinuric persons to take up lysine and arginine is impaired[11] (Fig. 117-4). The cystinuric tissue has about 50 to 60 percent of the normal capacity to take up lysine. This corresponds to the reabsorptive defect observed during clearance experiments in vivo.[83] Evidence that the shared dibasic amino acid transport system is only partially defective is that the low uptake of lysine can be further suppressed by the addition of arginine. Rosenberg et al.[90] examined the concentration dependence of lysine uptake by normal and cystinuric renal cortex slices. Lineweaver-Burk plots were indicative of the presence of two distinct influx systems, one a high-affinity, low-capacity system and the other a low-affinity, high-capacity system. From the observed K_m and V_{max} parameters it appeared that the V_{max} of the high-affinity, low-K_m system was lower than normal. At a physiologic plasma lysine concentration of 0.1 mM, the major lysine transport ability of normal renal tissue would result in the low-K_m system, and that system appears to have a limited capacity in the cystinuric kidney.

The uptake of neither cystine[11] nor cysteine[105] is impaired in slices of renal cortex from cystinuric patients. Cystine and the dibasic amino acids did not appear to share a common transport system.[11] Although cysteine transport is effected by dual systems in human cortical slices,[105] only one system could be observed for cystine entry into human renal cells.[11] These unexpected findings stimulated an extensive investigation of the characteristics of cystine and dibasic amino acid transport by rat renal cortex slices, isolated tubule fragments, and brush border membrane vesicles.

Numerous experiments have been performed using kidney-slice transport techniques. These clearly demonstrate that the transport systems for lysine and cystine in rat kidney cortex are not the same.[106–110] In addition to the lack of mutual inhibition between these two amino acids and their nonparticipation in heteroexchange diffusion, there are certain biochemical differences in their transport characteristics. Lysine transport is only partially dependent on the presence of sodium ion and aerobic conditions, and over a pH range of 6 to 8.5 there is little change of influx in rats.[108] Cystine transport, on the other hand, is completely dependent on sodium and oxygen and shows marked differences in influx with changes in pH, with an optimum at about pH 7.4.[109] While there is evidence for more than one lysine transport system in rat cortical slices, only one system was evident for cystine, with a K_m of 0.8 mM. Kinetic studies in rat kidney cortex slices have furnished evidence, based on response to alteration of pH, temperature changes, oxygen lack, and sodium deprivation, that the kidney cystine and cysteine transport systems are different.[109] Confirmation of this supposition has come from ontogenetic studies, which show a separate developmental time pattern for cystine and cysteine transport in rat kidney cortex.[75] An examination of the transport interaction of cysteine with dibasic amino acids in vitro showed no mutual inhibition of uptake.[104] Even so, incubation of cysteine with lysine causes an enhanced accumulation of the sulfur amino acid by kidney cortex.[104,107] Schwartzman et al.[104] have explained the lysine-enhanced accumulation of cystine by showing that the dibasic amino acids inhibit the efflux of intracellular cysteine into the incubation fluid. This interaction between the sulfur amino acids and the dibasic amino acids may have physiological importance, since the natural intracellular form is cysteine, even if cystine is the compound being transported.[74,75]

With the recent use of rat tubule fragments[12] and brush border membrane vesicles,[13,111] a more complete picture of cystine and dibasic amino acid transport in the proximal tubule has emerged. Cystine uptake by isolated cortical tubules occurred via two saturable transport systems with K_m values of 0.012 and 0.55 mM. Lysine inhibited cystine uptake via the low-K_m system but appeared not to inhibit

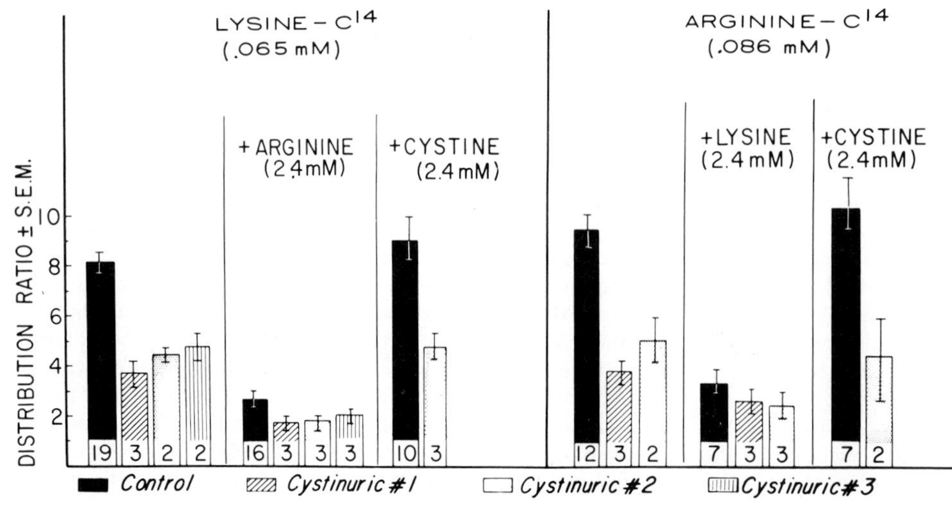

FIG. 117-4 Uptake of lysine and arginine by renal cortex slices from cystinuric and noncystinuric subjects. The distribution ratio is the ratio of radioactivity in counts per minute per milliliter of intracellular fluid to counts per minute per milliliter of incubation media. *(From data in Fox et al.[11])*

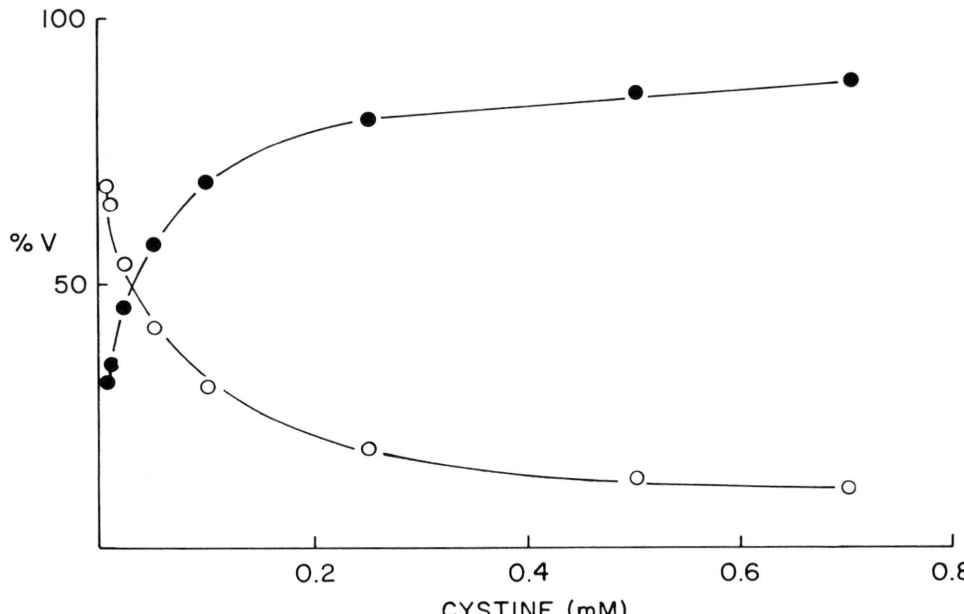

FIG. 117-5 The percentages of total velocity of cystine uptake by rat renal proximal tubules in vitro mediated by the high-K_m (closed circles) and low-K_m (open circles) systems at various cystine concentrations. *(From Foreman et al.*[12] *Used by permission.)*

cystine uptake via the high-K_m mechanism. Cystine inhibited the uptake of lysine by the tubules. Figure 117-5 shows the calculated percentages of cystine uptake mediated by the two systems present in tubule fragments at various cystine concentrations. At a plasma concentration of about 0.05 m*M*, about 50 percent would be handled by each system.[12]

With brush border membrane vesicles, two comparable transport systems for cystine were demonstrated, with dibasic amino acids inhibiting the low-K_m, high-affinity system (Fig. 117-6).[13,111] Heteroexchange diffusion of lysine and cystine was demonstrated by the high-affinity component.[111] In contrast to tubule fragments, where the cystine entering the cell was reduced to cysteine,[12] the intravesicular amino acid was cystine, indicating that the unreduced form was transported across the brush border membrane.[13,111] Also, unlike the findings in tubule cells, where the intracellular cysteine is not bound to proteins, the intravesicular cystine became bound to the membrane. This emphasizes the importance of the intracellular reducing process for maintaining free cysteine within the cell, a process that facilitates unhampered transcellular movement of the amino acid during the reabsorptive process. The renal brush border vesicle system[112,113] has been used to examine the transport of arginine[114–116] and lysine.[112,113] On the basis of inhibition studies, rabbit vesicle lysine uptake appeared to Mircheff et al.[112] to be mediated by two systems, one of which was shared with phenylalanine. On the basis of kinetic data obtained using rat membranes, McNamara et al.[117] concluded that lysine uptake involves only one system, which is not dependent on sodium nor shared with cystine. The same group showed that cystine uptake by rat brush border vesicles was also sodium-independent,[118] and that there was no preferential ionic form of cystine for the carrier-mediated process.[119] In rat and human renal brush border membranes, Furlong and Posen showed the independence of cystine transport from that of cysteine and cysteine-penicillamine mixed disulfide.[120]

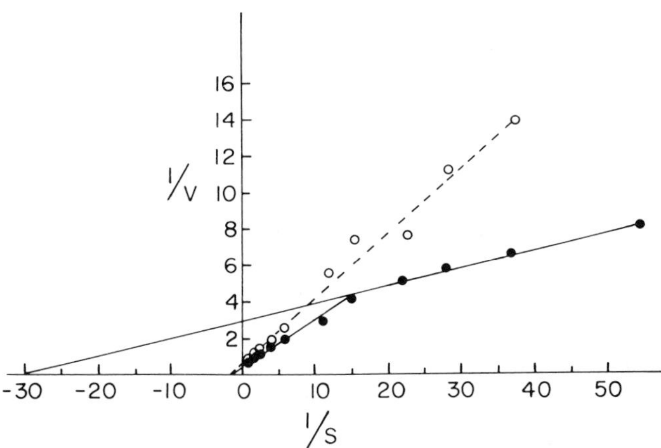

FIG. 117-6 Concentration dependence of cystine on the initial rate of uptake by rat renal brush border membrane vesicles. Closed circles represent uptake of ^{14}C-L-lysine, and open circles show its uptake in the presence of 1 m*M* L-lysine. *(From Segal et al.*[13] *Used by permission.)*

The correlation of the dual cystine transport systems in tubule fragments and in brush border membrane vesicles indicates that transport across the luminal side of the proximal tubule cell can be observed when tubule fragments are studied. With renal cortical slices, only one component of cystine transport is demonstrated, and that corresponds to the high-K_m system observed in both renal cortical tubules and brush border membrane vesicles. Since only the high-K_m system is observed in slice experiments, an interaction between cystine and dibasic amino acids would not be expected; this interaction occurs in the low-K_m shared system. Why the renal slice experiments give a broad picture of dibasic amino acid transport but only a truncated view of cystine transport is at present unclear. Equally enigmatic are the observations that in cultured human renal proximal tubule cells[121] and LLC-PK_1 cells derived from pig renal tubules,[122] the cystine transport system is dissociated from that of the dibasic amino acids and becomes shared with glutamate transport. Such a cystine–glutamate exchange system has been observed in cultured human fibroblasts[123,124] and cultured rat hepatocytes.[125] On the other hand, uptake studies with a continuously growing opossum kidney cell line (OK) indicate the presence of the cystine–dibasic amino acid transport system and absence of the cystine–glutamate system in confluent monolayers.[126] Cystine transport occurs via a high-affinity, sodium-independent process localized to the apical brush border.[126] Primary cultures of dog proximal renal tubular cells maintain the cystine–dibasic amino acid transport process, but, on subsequent passage, the cystine–glutamate system emerges.[127] An excellent review of cystine transport processes has been published by Bannai.[128]

The demonstration of a shared system for cystine and dibasic amino acids in the luminal membrane of the renal tubule cell substantiates the original hypothesis of Dent and Rose[10] that cystinuria results from defective reabsorption by a common transport process. The finding of another unshared system aids in interpreting some of the clinical observations. Figure 117-7 shows a possible model of the carrier systems in the brush border membrane for cystine and dibasic amino acids. A defective low-K_m system would result in excessive amounts of cystine, lysine, arginine, and ornithine in urine, as in classic cystinuria. This is the system whose defective function has been observed in human cystinuric kidney slices when lysine was the transported substrate,[11] and which was inhibited by infusion of large amounts of lysine in humans and dogs.[82–86] Cystinuric patients, who do not have dibasic aminoaciduria, may have a defect in the high-K_m unshared cystine system. Dibasic aminoaciduria without cystinuria[79,80] may be due to a defect in a dibasic transport system unshared with cystine. Remaining to be explained is the apparent secretion of cystine by some cystinuric patients[14–16] and dogs infused with lysine.[86]

Molecular Biology of Cystine Transport

The examination of renal cystine transport using cortical slices, isolated tubule fragments, and membrane vesicles described above has now been augmented by molecular biologic techniques aimed at identifying the cystine transporter. The *Xenopus* oocyte has become the model system for examining the expression of the cystine transporter. Since the first description of this system by McNamara et al.,[129] who injected rat intestinal mRNA and expressed sodium-independent, lysine-inhibited, low-K_m cystine transport, the molecular search for the "cystine carrier" has advanced considerably. Two kidney cortex cDNA clones have been isolated–a rat clone called D2[130] and a rabbit clone called rBAT[131]–whose cRNA, when injected into *Xenopus* oocytes, expresses high-affinity transport of L-dibasic and some neutral amino acids, especially L-leucine, L-methionine and L-phenylalanine, as well as cystine. The expressed cystine uptake is saturable, having a K_m in the micromolar range cDNAs encoding the human ortholog of this protein (designated D2H or human rBAT) also have been isolated[132,133] and the structural gene mapped to 2p.[132] The 2.3 kb mRNA is expressed in kidney cortex and intestinal epithelium and encodes a 663-amino-acid protein with a molecular mass of 78.8 kDa.[132,136] The protein is dissimilar to most transporters in that it is a glycoprotein with only a single putative transmembrane domain. It does resemble the 4F2 cell surface antigen heavy chain protein which induces dibasic amino acid transport without a cystine component.[134,135] The protein encoded by D2H or human rBAT induces cystine uptake that is inhibited by dibasic amino acids.[132] The rBAT protein may activate or regulate the carrier, rather than being the actual cystine–dibasic amino acid transporter itself. The relationship of rBAT and D2H to cystinuria remains to be determined (see Addendum).

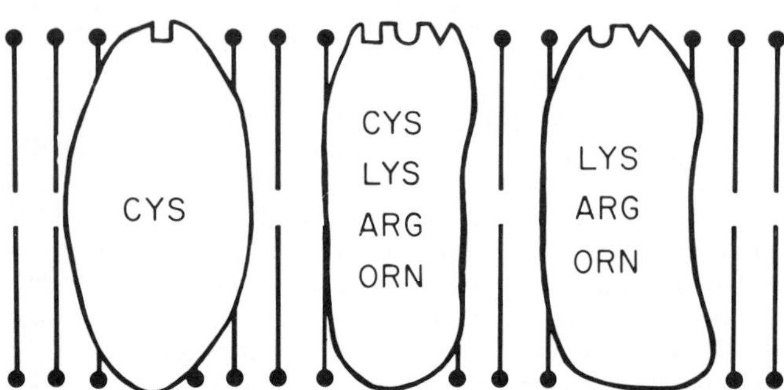

FIG. 117-7 Schematic diagram of a membrane from a renal proximal tubule cell showing the possible diversity of carrier proteins for cystine (CYS), lysine (LYS), arginine (ARG), and ornithine (ORN).

URINARY EXCRETION OF OTHER AMINO ACIDS IN CYSTINURIA

Although hyperexcretion of lysine, arginine, ornithine, and cystine in the urine is the hallmark of cystinuria, other amino acids have been found in higher than normal amounts in the urine of some patients. These include glycine,[14] methionine,[137] cystathionine,[138] and homocysteine-cysteine disulfide[139] (Fig. 117-8). The latter is most consistently present in variable amounts up to 224 mg/24 h,[93] the amount being related directly to the amount of cystine excreted.[140] This mixed disulfide has also been found in the urine of patients with Fanconi syndrome on the basis of Wilson disease, as well as in dogs with cystinuria.[93] Subsequently, the mixed disulfide was demonstrated in normal plasma and in increased amount in the plasma of a patient with homocystinuria.[141] Although it was thought at first to be uniquely associated with cystinuria, homocysteine-cysteine mixed disulfide probably is a normal plasma constituent which is overexcreted because it participates in the renal tubular defect responsible for the loss of cystine.

INTESTINAL TRANSPORT DEFECTS

When an amino acid is eaten, absorption occurs, and the unabsorbed amino acid will be used by the intestinal flora. The less an amino acid is absorbed, the lower the blood levels will be after feeding, and the greater will be the levels of bacterial breakdown products in the stool and perhaps also in plasma and urine. If bacterial flora are suppressed,

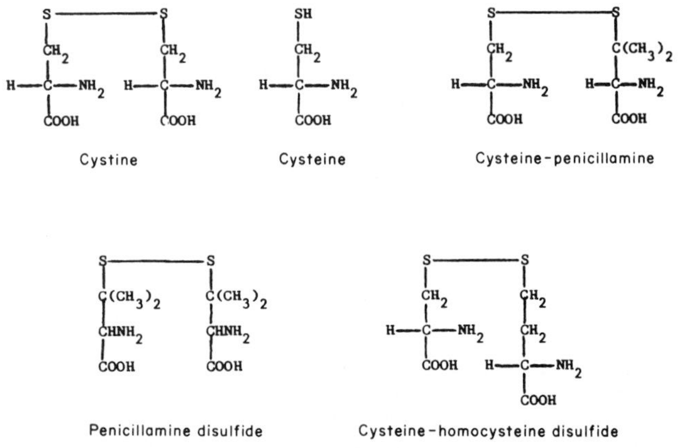

Cystine — Cysteine — Cysteine-penicillamine

Penicillamine disulfide — Cysteine-homocysteine disulfide

FIG. 117-8 The structures of cystine and related compounds.

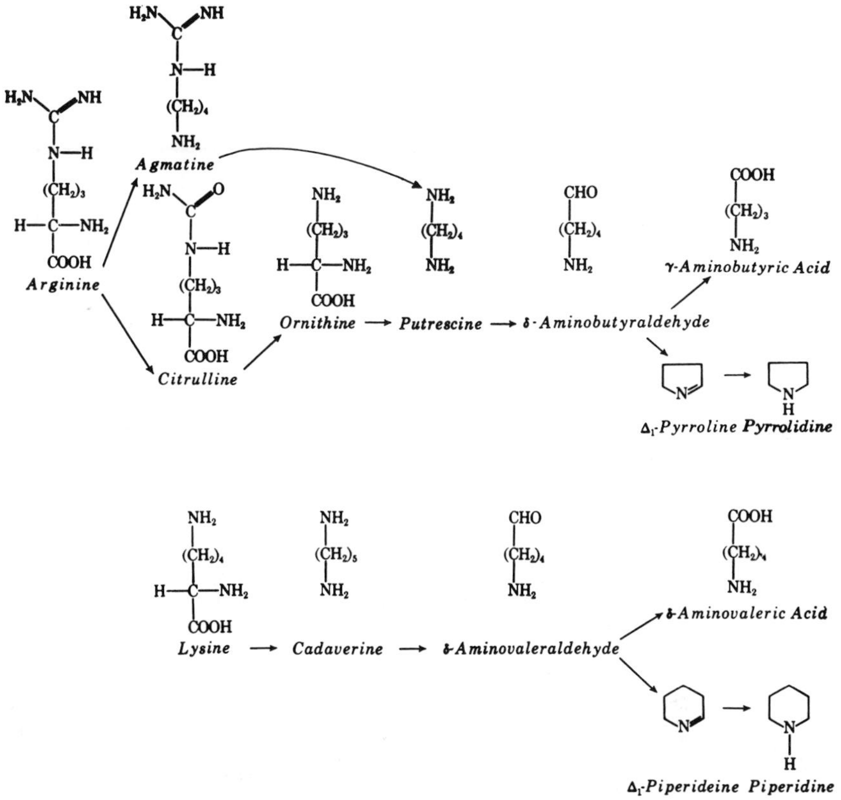

FIG. 117-9 **Formation of putrescine and pyrrolidine from arginine and cadaverine and of piperidine from lysine.** *(After Crawhall and Watts.[31])*

the nonabsorbed amino acid should be demonstrable in the stool. Lysine, arginine, and ornithine are decarboxylated by bacteria in the intestine to the diamines cadaverine, agmatine, and putrescine. Piperidine is formed by lysine breakdown, and pyrrolidine from arginine and ornithine metabolism (Fig. 117-9). These heterocyclic amines are formed from the diamines. As mentioned earlier, the data suggesting an intestinal transport defect in cystinuric patients were available by the late nineteenth century, when diamines were detected in the urine of these patients.[17,18] It was only after Milne and coworkers demonstrated defective tryptophan absorption from the intestine of patients with the neutral aminoaciduria of Hartnup disorder that the data on cystinuria were finally brought into focus.[21] Milne et al. observed increased putrescine and pyrrolidine in the urine after feeding arginine, and increased cadaverine, piperidine, and pyrrolidine after feeding lysine. Since the pyrrolidine could not have been derived from lysine, it was concluded that lysine was competitively inhibiting arginine transport in the intestine. The role of bacterial degradation in this process was proved in patients treated with oral neomycin; pyrrolidine and putrescine decreased in stool and urine, while lysine, arginine, and ornithine increased in the stool of patients so treated.[22,23] Evidence for a failure of cystine absorption was presented by Brand et al.,[19] by Dent et al.,[8] and more recently by London and Foley,[72] Rosenberg et al.,[94] and Silk et al.[142] using ion-exchange chromatography to measure plasma cystine concentration after oral loading. In all these studies, cysteine absorption by cystinuria patients was not impaired.[142,143]

Double-lumen perfusion of the jejunum with low concentrations of lysine demonstrates defective dibasic amino acid transport in vivo, while in the same patient oral administration of a large dose results in a normal increase in the plasma concentration of lysine.[144] The response to a large oral dose of lysine suggests that diffusion or alternate transport routes may protect cystinuric individuals from amino acid malnutrition. Perhaps a better explanation of why there is little evidence of dibasic amino acid malabsorption in cystinuria derives from recent studies indicating that oligopeptide transport is normal in these patients. In fact, in cystinuric individuals, administration of lysylglycine results in a greater increase in plasma lysine than equimolar feeding of free lysine plus glycine. Similarly, casein feeding produces a more rapid increase in plasma arginine and lysine than does feeding a mixture of free amino acids derived from a casein hydrolysate.[145–149]

The concept of impaired intestinal amino acid transport derived from feeding experiments received direct confirmation by the demonstration in vitro of defective amino acid accumulation in specimens of jejunal mucosa obtained by peroral biopsy.[24–26] The results of further studies showed that there were some patients who had total impairment of cystine, lysine, and arginine accumulation, others who had small but detectable cystine transport but no dibasic amino acid transport, and still a third group who had normal or only slightly impaired cystine uptake and demonstrable but diminished lysine and arginine accumulation[150] (Fig. 117-10). Later experiments showed that intestinal mucosa from individuals with the different types of cystinuria had no impairment of cysteine accumulation in vitro.[151] This finding not only established the independence of the cystine and cysteine transport mechanism but when combined with the results of studies of cystine uptake in vitro, explained the many oral feeding experiments previously performed, which showed a rise in plasma and urinary cystine after cysteine feeding but not after cystine feeding.[72,143]

Recent work suggests that mucosal biopsy specimens from cystinuric patients have diminished lysine permeability at the brush border membrane,[152] while biopsied tissues of

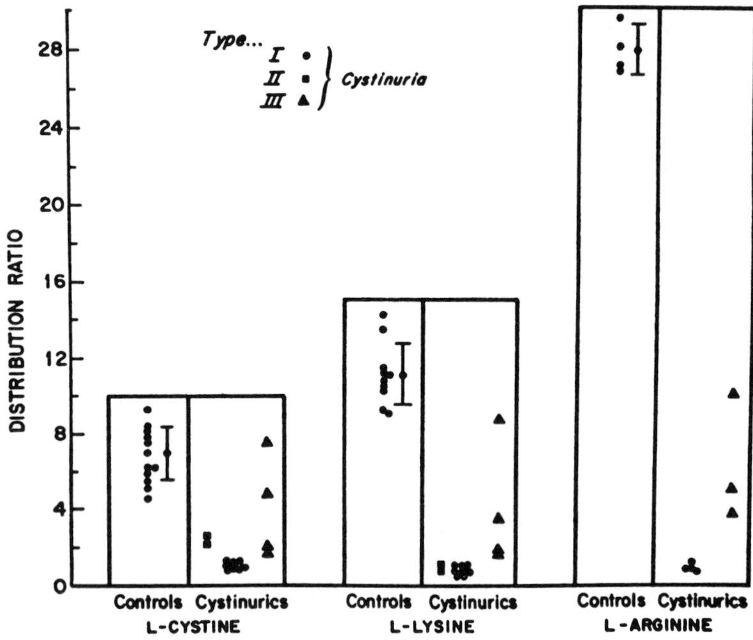

FIG. 117-10 Uptake of cystine, lysine, and arginine by jejunal mucosa from control and cystinuric subjects, expressed as the distribution ratio, i.e., the ratio of radioactive amino acid inside the cell to that in the medium, after a 45-min incubation. *(From Rosenberg et al.[150] Used by permission.)*

patients with lysinuric protein intolerance have an impaired flux of lysine at the basolateral membrane of the epithelial cells.[153] Measurement of cystine fluxes across intestinal biopsy specimens suggests that there is an increased efflux permeability at the luminal membrane, which would explain the defective cystine uptake.[154] Since the intracellular form is cysteine and cysteine transport by biopsied mucosa is unimpaired,[151] the conclusions of Desjeux et al.[153,154] that efflux is increased await further evaluation.

Differences between the characteristics of intestinal and renal transport of lysine in vitro have been clearly demonstrated in the rat. Lysine uptake by intestinal mucosa is sodium- and oxygen-dependent and sensitive to pH changes; that by the kidney is only minimally affected by changes in sodium, oxygen, or pH.[155] Lysine[156] and cystine[157] uptake has been examined in rat intestinal brush border vesicles. A single system for cystine transport is present; it is shared by lysine but inhibited by other amino acids.[157]

Family studies of cystine excretion alone allowed differentiation of phenotypically identical cystinuric subjects into two genetically different groups.[44,158,159] Additional consideration of the intestinal mucosal transport patterns for the dibasic amino acids allows homozygous cystinuric subjects to be differentiated into three groups[150] (Table 117-2). In type I, which includes the majority of patients, there is no accumulation of either cystine or the dibasic amino acids against a gradient, and oral cystine loading fails to raise serum cystine levels (Fig. 117-11). In type II, there is detectable active accumulation of cystine but no accumulation of dibasic amino acids; as in type I, oral loading fails to raise serum cystine levels. In type III, accumulation of cystine and dibasic amino acids does occur, but not to the normal extent; oral cystine loading results in normal elevation of plasma cystine levels.

In an elegant study in which urinary excretion of amino acids, renal clearances, intestinal biopsies, and oral cystine loading were performed, Morin et al.[16] obtained data confirming the existence of type I and II cystinuria. They found no patients, however, with a condition corresponding to type III. Disorders suggestive of type III were found in persons

Table 117-2 Classification of Cases of Cystinuria

Experimental Observations	Type I	Type II	Type III
Intestine:			
In vitro transport	No transport of cystine, lysine, or arginine; normal cysteine transport	No transport of lysine; markedly reduced cystine transport	Transport of cystine reduced but may be normal; lysine variably reduced
Oral cystine administration	No plasma cystine elevation	No plasma cystine elevation	Slow increase in plasma cystine to normal elevation
Kidney:			
In vitro transport, cortical slices	Reduced lysine transport		Reduced lysine transport
Urinary amino acid excretion	Increased cystine, lysine, arginine, ornithine excretion	Increased cystine, lysine, arginine, ornithine excretion	Increased cystine, lysine, arginine, ornithine excretion
Urinary amino acid excretion in heterozygotes	Normal	Cystine and lysine above normal	Cystine and lysine above normal

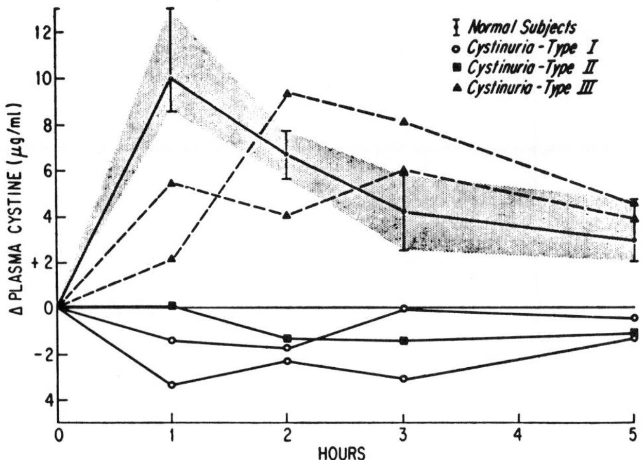

FIG. 117-11 **The change of plasma cystine levels after oral cystine administration of 0.5 μmol/kg.** ***(From Rosenberg et al.[150] Used by permission.)***

produced by the mating of heterozygous carriers of type I and type II. The family studies based on this separation are discussed under "Genetics."

The results of intestinal transport studies in vitro fit the hypothesis of Dent and Rose that cystine and dibasic amino acids share a common transport system. In the intestinal mucosa there is evidence of only a single shared system which in many patients is completely defective in its function.[26,150] That system corresponds to the low-K_m, high-affinity shared component recently demonstrated in renal brush border membranes.[13,111] An important difference is that lysine transport by the cystinuric kidney is only partially impaired.[11] Although this intestinal defect may be of little clinical importance, it has served as an extremely sensitive genetic marker and has paved the way for a new genetic classification of cystinuria. The lack of amino acid transport defects in circulating leukocytes of cystinuric patients has precluded their usefulness for discerning genetic aspects of the disease.[160]

CYSTINURIA AND THE CENTRAL NERVOUS SYSTEM

There have been numerous reports of an association of cystinuria with central nervous system abnormalities. Scriver et al.[161] reported an increase in the prevalence of cystinuria in a group of mentally disturbed patients, and there have been reports of cystinuria patients with spastic paraplegia.[162–164] Mental retardation has been described occasionally in homozygous patients,[165] but testing of a large group of homozygous cystinuric patients for mental deficiency did not reveal an increased prevalence.[166] Smith and Procopis[167] reported a thirteen-fold higher incidence of heterozygous cystinuric subjects than would have been expected in a population of retarded persons in New South Wales, but no instances of homozygous cystinuria were detected. A pertinent question has been whether cystinuric patients are at a greater risk for cerebral dysfunction because there is defective transport into the brain of an essential amino acid such as lysine or, in the neonatal period, cystine,[69] as has been demonstrated in the intestine and kidney of affected subjects.

The relationship of cystine, cysteine, and lysine transport by isolated rat brain synaptosomes has been examined.[168–170] Dual systems for their uptake were described, but there was no inhibition of either mechanism of cystine entry by dibasic amino acids. Cysteine uptake was only slightly inhibited by lysine but was strongly affected by glycine. The low-K_m lysine transport system was shared by other dibasic amino acids but not by cystine, as it is in the kidney and intestines. The uptake of cystine by isolated rat brain capillaries appeared to be independent of dibasic amino acid transport.[171] All the findings in vitro indicate that the systems for entry of these amino acids into brain differ from those of kidney and intestine and make it unlikely that cystinuric subjects are at risk because of transport abnormalities in the central nervous system.

GENETICS

An understanding of the genetics of cystinuria depends on a phenotypic definition of the homozygous state. This state is suggested by (1) the excretion of over 250 mg cystine per gram of creatinine, often with formation of urinary calculi, and (2) the presence of an intestinal absorptive defect for cystine and the dibasic amino acids. In the first large-scale genetic studies, Harris and coworkers divided cystinuric families into two groups, in each of which homozygous subjects were indistinguishable.[159] In one group the disease was transmitted as a true recessive trait; no family members other than the homozygous individual had aminoaciduria. The second group was designated as incompletely recessive; family members frequently excreted excessive amounts of cystine and lysine, although significantly less than homozygotes. The heterozygous incompletely recessive cystinuric subject did not form stones. On the basis of variable patterns of amino acid excretion in homozygous cystinuric patients, Harris and Robson[172] postulated that the condition in this group might be under polygenic influences. The exhaustive analysis by Crawhall et al. of urinary cystine, lysine, and arginine excretion by cystine stone formers, their parents, other relatives, and normal persons seems to support this view.[32] After examining many kindreds, these workers emphasized the wide disparities among the amounts of individual amino acids excreted by different heterozygous and homozygous individuals (Figs. 117-12 and -13). Thus it appears that multiple genetic factors influence the quantities of the various amino acids excreted in the urine and the final phenotypic expression.

The availability of jejunal mucosa led to the recognition that more than one pattern of cystine and dibasic amino acid transport could be recognized in homozygotes, and that these patterns correlated with different modes of inheritance, as suggested by Harris. Homozygotes can now be differentiated without recourse to family studies. The pattern of jejunal mucosal transport discussed above under "Intestinal Transport Defects" is summarized in Table 117-2. Note that three classes of cystinuria may now be developed and that the last two were combined in the incompletely recessive group II of Harris.

With the ability to separate homozygous cystinuric subjects into distinct groups based on intestinal transport, Rosenberg restudied the families of these individuals and found distinctive urinary amino acid patterns.[173] First-degree relatives of type I patients had no abnormal urinary amino acid excretion. Type II and type III heterozygous individuals excreted excessive amounts of cystine and the dibasic amino acids in their urine, and could be distinguished from each other. The quantities excreted were consistently higher in

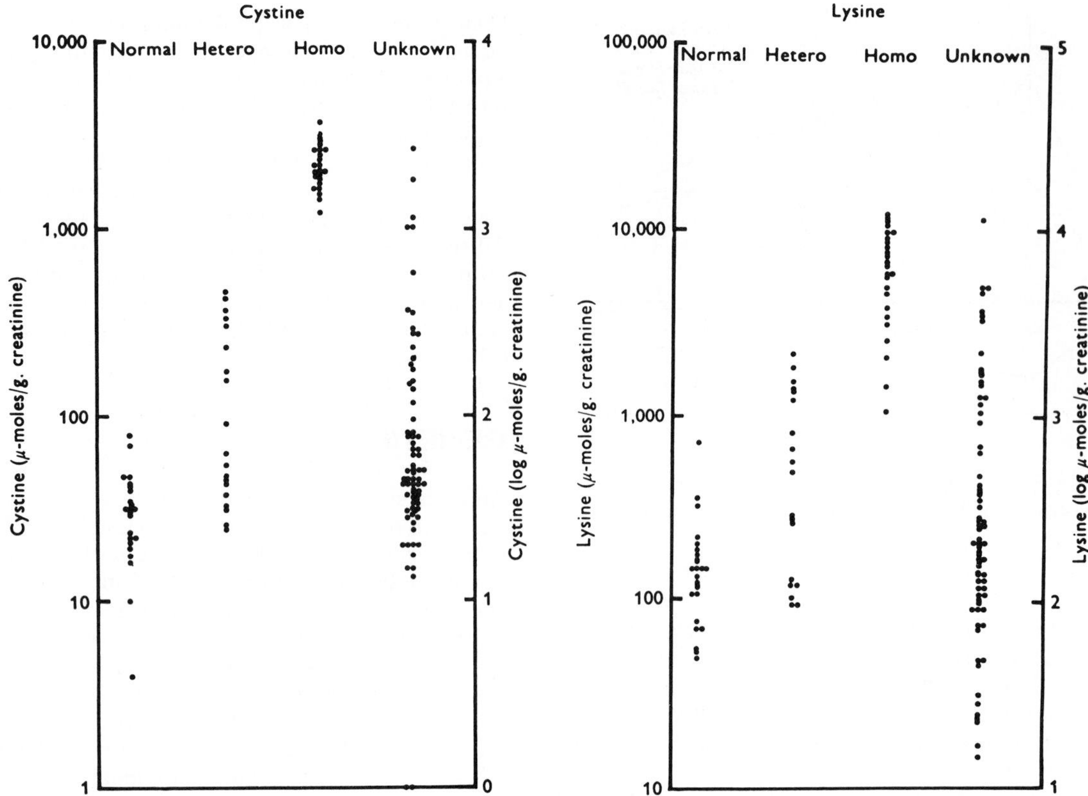

FIG. 117-12 The excretion of cystine and lysine by normal subjects, patients with cystinuria, heterozygotes for cystinuria, and relatives of cystinuric patients. *(From Crawhall et al.[32] Used by permission.)*

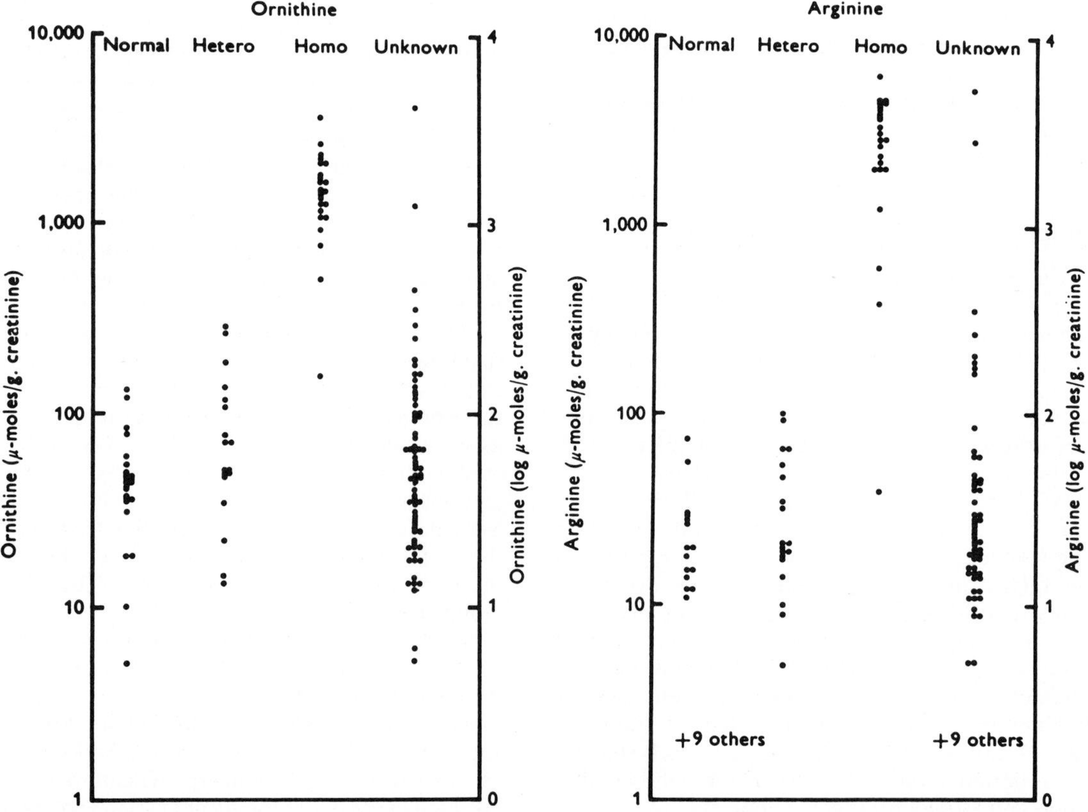

FIG. 117-13 The excretion of arginine and ornithine by normal subjects, cystinuric patients, heterozygotes for cystinuria, and relatives of cystinuric patients. *(From Crawhall et al.[32] Used by permission.)*

type II heterozygotes. Morin et al.,[16] on the other hand, in their study of the urinary amino acid excretion of cystinuric families, did not encounter more than two patterns in heterozygotes. The patterns of excretion that Rosenberg et al.[173] considered to indicate type III heterozygotes correspond to that of type I and type II compound heterozygotes (offspring of the mating of type I and type II carriers) found by Morin et al.[16] By analyzing the type of aminoaciduria in relatives, Byrd et al.[174] were able to classify 25 cystinuric probands as representing of type I, 11 of type II or III, and 3 compound heterozygotes. Goodyer et al.[175] classified parents into three known phenotypes by calculating the sum of urinary cystine, lysine, arginine, and ornithine, and were able to discern that type I//I homozygotes excrete greater amounts of cystine than children who are type I/III genetic compounds.

The presence of at least three distinct genetic types raised the question of whether cystinuria represents a group of diseases with defects in separate steps of amino acid transport or whether it represents different defects in the same genetically controlled step; i.e., are the different types the result of nonallelic or allelic mutations? The results of matings between type I and type II or III heterozygous individuals could provide an answer. If the defects are allelic, a fully expressed homozygous state (a better term is "genetic compound") might appear in the offspring. If the defects are in separate genes, then only the expressed heterozygous state should appear in the offspring. The fact that "homozygous" children are found suggests that the defects are allelic.[176,177] Although studies in vitro of intestinal transport have defined what seem to be three phenotypes,[144] it should be pointed out that within the third type the cystine uptake by mucosal biopsy specimens ranges from normal to an impairment almost as severe as in the first type (Fig. 117-10). The third type may be an expression of an even greater multiplicity of genetic factors involved in the intestinal transport phenotype.

Thus cystinuria is defined as a genetic disorder with a complex recessive mode of inheritance resulting from allelic mutations. At least some of the mutations may be expressed in the heterozygous state, both as an aminoaciduria and in type II and III heterozygotes as an increased risk factor for stone formation.[178] The most sensitive means for differentiating the three types of homozygous cystinuric subjects is the study of the intestinal transport of cystine and the dibasic amino acids in vitro. Similar differentiation can be attempted from studies of urinary amino acid excretion in families of cystinuric subjects. This approach is neither as sensitive nor as direct as the study of transport in vitro.

ANIMAL MODELS OF CYSTINURIA

Several animal models have been suggested for the study of cystinuria. As a result of studies of amino acid excretion patterns of animals in the London Zoo, Harris thought that the blotched genet excreted large amounts of cystine.[179] The genet appeared to be unique in that "cystine" was excreted without the dibasic amino acids, and was excreted in concentrations far greater than would ordinarily remain in solution. Crawhall and Segal subsequently demonstrated that the genet excretes not cystine, but the far more soluble sulfur amino acid S-sulfo-L-cysteine.[180] There is in fact no abnormality of cystine transport in the genet, and this apparent animal model must be discarded.

In 1956 a male mink with large numbers of apparently pure cystine stones was reported. This was a ranch mink on a higher than usual protein intake but otherwise unremarkable.[181] The presence of cystinuria in an animal group already carefully bred and therefore easily studied bears further investigation, but at present little further information is available.

Canine cystinuria represents potentially the most useful model for study. Although cystine stones in dogs were described as early as 1823, it was not until Brand and Cahill bred a group of Irish terriers with cystinuria that any systematic observations were made.[182-186] The expression of cystinuria corresponded to a sex-linked inheritance pattern. As in human beings, their animals responded with rises in cystine excretion after methionine feeding, and had no change after cystine feeding. Most, if not all, canine cystinuria has appeared in males. Though this may be due to the narrow urethra of male dogs, which brings stone production to clinical attention, amino acid chromatography has not revealed the disease in females to date.

The exact amino acid excretion pattern in canine cystinuria is not clear. Isolated cystinuria, cystinuria plus lysinuria, and the full pattern of cystine and all dibasic amino acids appearing in excess in the urine have been reported.[78,187,190] An intestinal defect in amino acid transport has been postulated.[191]

Recent application of transport techniques in vitro to both intestinal and kidney biopsy samples from cystine stone-forming dogs has disclosed a defect neither in cystine nor in lysine accumulation by either tissue.[78] The absence of a demonstrable lysine transport defect in these dog tissues is unlike the findings in human biopsy samples, while the absence of a cystine transport defect is consistent with findings in human beings. It would appear that canine cystinuria is a heterogeneous entity. The presence of large amounts of cystine in the urine of these dogs makes this strain an excellent model for evaluating the nature of hyperexcretion of cystine. Clearance studies have been performed on a group of cystinuric and control dogs.[86,192] What emerges is a striking cystinuria accompanied by variable degrees of dibasic aminoaciduria. The dibasic aminoaciduria does not correlate well with the degree of cystinuria. The extent of the cystinuria is variable and may reach clearances twice creatinine clearance, demonstrating the secretion of cystine. Infusion of lysine into cystinuric dogs may cause secretion of cystine.[86] Plasma concentrations of the cystine precursor methionine were elevated and correlated with plasma cystine levels and with fractional reabsorption of cystine. These observations suggest that canine cystinuria may be a metabolic disorder associated with cystine secretion. The cystinuric dog is also an excellent model for assessment of therapeutic approaches for decreasing the amounts of urinary cystine in human beings. To date, fluid intake, alkalinization, and D-penicillamine have all been observed to alter the clinical course favorably.[193] Mercaptopropionylglycine has also been effective in treatment of cystinuric dogs.[194]

A non-stone-forming cystinuria occurs in the Basenji dog as a component of a Fanconi syndrome. No decrease in uptake of cystine by isolated brush border vesicles was demonstrated in these animals, suggesting that the cystinuria did not have a membrane locus. On the other hand, membrane vesicles from a stone-forming cystinuric dog were shown to have a decrease in cystine uptake, a finding compatible with a membrane transport defect in such animals.[195]

Cystinuria has also been found in the maned wolf of Brazil.[196] Eighty percent of these wolves tested in zoos in the United States and abroad as well as animals whose urine was collected in the Brazilian jungle are affected. Several animals are known to have died in zoos because of cystine stones and urinary tract obstruction. Amino acid clearance studies in five affected wolves revealed variable cystine reabsorptive defects. In one animal there was evidence for secretion not only of cystine but of lysine, arginine, and ornithine as well. Cystinuria has also been observed in a cat.[197]

One human experimental model has been described by Brown.[198] He produced increased urinary excretion of several amino acids (principally cystine, lysine, ornithine, and arginine) in amounts similar to homozygous cystinuria in patients fed the nonmetabolizable amino acid cycloleucine. The rat also shows this response to cycloleucine administration.[199] Holtzapple et al.[200] have shown that cycloleucine is a competitive inhibitor of the transport of both neutral and dibasic amino acids by slices of human kidney cortex. Craan and Bergeron[98] have performed microperfusion experiments with rat renal tubules and have found that cycloleucine inhibits the reabsorption of both cystine and lysine.

Perhaps the most common animal model is the cystinuria that occurs in the neonatal rat[201] and dog[202] as well as in the human.[203] In vitro studies of cystine uptake by isolated dog renal tubules show diminished cellular influx of cystine.[202] The comparable experiments with rat tubules show no impairment of uptake,[201] which may mean that different mechanisms underlie the neonatal cystinuria.

TREATMENT

Were it not for the insolubility of cystine, cystinuria would be a metabolic oddity of no clinical significance except under conditions of critical limitation of protein intake. Therefore treatment is designed to reduce excretion and increase the solubility of cystine. Therapeutic approaches may be divided into three categories: (1) dietary restriction aimed at reducing cystine production and excretion, (2) attempts to increase cystine solubility, and (3) attempts to convert cystine to a more soluble compound. Surgical therapy can be divided into three categories: (1) attempts to dissolve cystine calculi by irrigation, (2) removal of cystine stones by lithotripsy or lithotomy, and (3) renal transplantation to replace kidneys destroyed by cystinuria. Stephens has recently reviewed 25 years of cystinuria treatment at St. Bartholomews Hospital.[204]

Dietary Therapy

Cystine production arises from the essential amino acid methionine. Numerous attempts have been made to design diets low in methionine, yet adequate for nutritional purposes. The results of use of such diets are extremely variable. Disappearance of cystinuria while the patient was on one of these diets has been reported by some investigators, whereas others have been unable to demonstrate any significant reduction in urinary cystine with careful methionine restriction.[205,206] The amount of sulfur amino acids in the diet of rats does not alter the transport of cystine by isolated membrane vesicles.[207] It is probably reasonable to avoid excessive methionine intake, but it is clear that uncomfortable diets are not indicated. High sodium intake will increase urinary amino acid excretion in patients with cystinuria. Low-sodium diets have been shown to decrease cystine excretion in a number of patients and have been recommended as a therapeutic strategy in cystinuric patients.[208–210]

Alteration of Cystine Solubility

At urinary pH values below 7.5, about 300 mg cystine per liter of urine will be in solution. Increasing urine volume provides a progressive reduction in urinary cystine concentration and reduces the likelihood of precipitation. Some reports of stone dissolution on high fluid intake programs have appeared.[211] Many cystinuric subjects excrete in the range of 1 g cystine per day and will require a fluid intake of 4 or more liters per day. Cystine solubility can also be enhanced by providing an alkaline pH, but the solubility does not increase significantly until the pH is above 7.5 (Fig. 117-14). Since the maximum urine pH that can be achieved is about 8, there is little leeway in the alkalinizing program. A regimen of bicarbonate, citrate, and carbonic anhydrase inhibitors has been advocated for improving solubility, but while this approach is theoretically reasonable, it is not clear that it gives practical benefit. Since altering these physical factors—fluid intake and urine pH—is a simple and logical approach to treatment, it should be included in the first therapeutic program in all cystinuric patients. In considering high fluid intake therapy, Dent and Senior[212] pointed out the importance of preventing supersaturation of urine with cystine at night when urine flow is low. The intake of two glasses of water at bedtime repeated at 2 or 3 A.M. is recommended. Dent et al.[211] found hydration therapy to be successful in preventing stone formation in about two-thirds of patients who adhered to it, during a 10-year study. Their therapeutic hydration regimen is well outlined in their paper.

Penicillamine. In spite of the best and most controlled therapeutic efforts, some patients with cystinuria will repeatedly form and pass stones, and a significant number will require surgery for relief of urinary tract obstruction. For those who were apparently not helped by diet, high fluid intake, and urine alkalinization, there was little to be done until Crawhall, Scowen, and Watts introduced the use of D-penicillamine (ββ-dimethylcysteine). Through a disulfide exchange reaction, this drug can produce the mixed disulfide cysteine-penicillamine, which is significantly more soluble than cystine[213,214] (Fig. 117-8). On adequate penicillamine therapy, usually 1 to 2 g/24 h, cystine excretion may be kept below 200 mg/g creatinine, a level at which stone formation

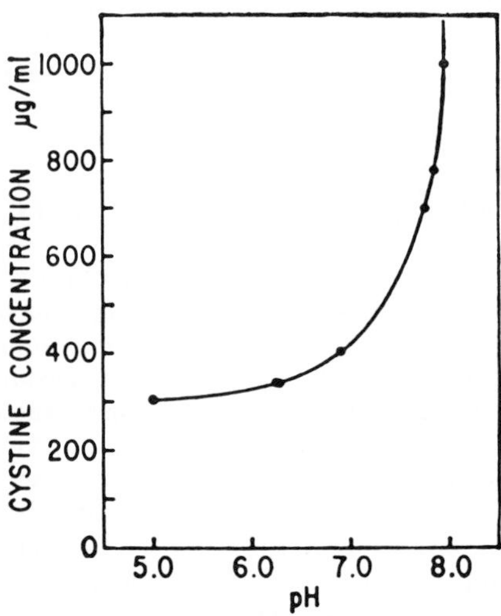

FIG. 117-14 The solubility of cystine in relation to urinary pH. *(From Dent and Senior.[212] Used by permission.)*

is minimal. The reduction of urinary cystine does not appear to be balanced by the amount of cysteine which is combined with penicillamine into the cysteine-penicillamine mixed disulfide. The total molar amount of half-cystine excreted on penicillamine therapy, i.e., the sum of cystine plus the cysteine moiety of the mixed disulfide, is much less than prior to drug treatment. This plus the reduction of plasma cystine levels by the drug suggests another biochemical effect of penicillamine besides disulfide exchange.[215–217] In contrast to the results on cystinuric subjects, the total molar amount of half-cystine in urine of normal individuals given penicillamine is greatly increased.[215] This finding has not been satisfactorily explained.

Although strikingly effective in preventing and dissolving cystine stones,[218,219] penicillamine has certain undesirable side effects. As many as 50 percent of patients receiving the drug will develop allergic reactions, usually fever and rash; rarely arthralgias appear.[215] More severe reactions include development of a nephrotic syndrome[220–222] and of pancytopenia.[223] Proteinuria of more than 500 mg/24 h occurs after several months of therapy in approximately one-third of patients treated with penicillamine. The proteinuria almost invariably clears when the drug is discontinued but usually recurs when the drug is started again.[224] Penicillamine-induced dermatopathy includes epidermolysis,[225–227] pseudoxanthoma elasticum-like skin lesions,[228] hemorrhagic skin lesions with lymphangiectasia,[229] and elastosis performans serpiginosa.[230] Thrombocytosis[231] and loss of taste (hypogeusia) have also been reported.[232] The hypogeusia may be reversed by copper.[233] The chelating property of penicillamine is responsible for increased copper and zinc excretion in the urine. It also has less significant effects on calcium, mercury, and iron excretion.[234–236] Part of the increase in copper excretion is independent of chelation[236] and is as yet unexplained. In addition, a possible problem resulting from inhibition of pyridoxine should be recognized and treated with supplemental pyridoxine phosphate. The possible reaction of penicillamine with pyridoxine to form a thiazolidine led to studies demonstrating a reduced pyridoxal effect in patients on penicillamine therapy (increased kynurenic acid excretion).[237] The hypogeusia may also be reversed by the administration of pyridoxine.[238,239] No interference with growth is seen in children, and pregnancies have been successfully completed in women receiving the drug.[219,240] Most recently the disturbing association of penicillamine therapy with a fatal Goodpasture-like syndrome has been reported.[241]

In view of the drawbacks of D-penicillamine therapy, its use should be restricted to patients in whom more conservative therapy has failed or who have lost one kidney from cystine stone disease. Therapy should be started in the hospital in order to monitor reactions of hypersensitivity. In those patients initially sensitive to the drug, adequate results have been obtained by readministering the medication in gradually increasing doses over a period of 1 to 2 months. A related compound, *N*-acetyl-D-penicillamine, has been developed which is effective in disulfide formation and thus in reducing cystine content; this compound appears to have fewer side effects, perhaps because of the unavailability of an amino group for chemical reaction.[30,242–244] Cross-sensitivity between penicillamine and penicillin has not been a problem.

Mercaptopropionylglycine. Another drug which may be of interest for therapy is mercaptopropionylglycine (MPG), which Timmerman et al.[245] suggested would be useful in dissolving renal calculi by renal pelvic perfusion. King first reported the use of MPG in cystinuria.[246]

Subsequently a number of reports have suggested that oral MPG may substitute for penicillamine in the treatment of cystinuria.[247–253] MPG has a higher oxidation–reduction potential than penicillamine and may be more effective in a disulfide exchange reaction leading to production of a mixed disulfide with cysteine. The pharmacokinetics of MPG have been extensively studied in dogs[254] and in man.[255] In controlled clinical trials, MPG appears to be as effective as D-penicillamine with a similar mechanism of action. Side effects have included skin rash, fever, nausea, and soft feces. Proteinuria and membranous glomerulonephritis can be induced and are not dose-related.[256] The proteinuria may be reversible with cessation of therapy. The nephrotic syndrome[257,258] as well as hyperlipidemia[259] has also been reported in association with MPG therapy. Chronic administration of MPG to cystinuric dogs did not produce the increase in urinary loss of copper, zinc, and iron that is seen in dogs treated with D-penicillamine.[260] Among patients who have a high incidence of untoward reactions to penicillamine, about one-third will have reactions to MPG; the other two-thirds will have tolerable side effects.[261]

Captopril. The sulfhydryl compound captopril is an angiotensin-converting enzyme inhibitor that is effective as an antihypertensive agent. The initial report described its ability to reduce cystine excretion by 70 and 93 percent in two cystinuric patients given 75 and 150 mg/day as treatment for hypertension.[262] Other patients have been successfully managed with the drug.[263–265] However, there have been reported failures of captopril to lower urinary cystine excretion.[266–268] The fall in cystine excretion may take a period of several weeks of therapy. The mechanism of the effect is not understood since the decrease in urinary cystine is greater than can be explained by the conversion of cystine to the more soluble (200-fold) mixed disulfide cysteine—captopril. Why captopril should be unpredictable in its ability to lower urinary cystine, and whether it will prove effective for long periods and will be tolerated by those with allergic reactions to D-penicillamine or MPG, remain unanswered questions.

Pharmacologic Reduction of Cystine Excretion

Glutamine administered orally or intravenously has been reported to reduce cystine excretion in cystinuria. The original report documented the effectiveness of glutamine in a single patient from Japan.[269] Subsequent studies failed to demonstrate reduced cystine excretion in patients receiving glutamine orally[270–271] or intravenously.[272]

Jaeger et al.[208] have clarified some of the confusion about glutamine. In patients in whom cystinuria is enhanced by a high sodium intake, glutamine will lower cystine excretion to the level seen with a low sodium intake. In patients with a low sodium intake, glutamine has no effect on cystine excretion. Thus, glutamine appears to have no therapeutic benefit beyond what can be achieved by avoiding a high sodium intake. The physiological significance of the glutamine–sodium–cystine interaction remains to be elucidated. Diazepoxide has been reported to reduce cystine crystalluria.[273] Whether this drug directly alters cystine solubility is not known, but it bears further investigation.

Surgical Approaches

Catheter Irrigation. Reports of dissolution of cystine stones by irrigation of the urinary tract by ureteral catheters placed by means of a supercutaneous nephrostomy have been encouraging.[274–276] Irrigation with alkaline solution of *N*-acetylpenicillamine, D-penicillamine, or tromethamine has proved successful in dissolving cystine calculi in 1 week to several months. Although infection may be a complication, if this therapeutic approach is successful, surgery should be avoided.

Lithotripsy. The introduction of extracorporeal lithotripsy has not been of great benefit to patients with cystinuria. Cystine stones may be fractured for easier dissolution with alkalinizing solutions, but they are not as readily pulverized as other stones. Percutaneous lithotripsy is more effective, though cystine stones are still among those most resistant to disintegration. A large number of patients have retained stone fragments and require reoperation.[277,278] Lithotripsy has, however, markedly curtailed the need for muscle-splitting lithotomy.

Lithotomy. Surgical removal of obstructing stones or stones causing intractable pain remains a necessary form of treatment for occasional patients with cystinuria. Correct diagnosis, more effective medical treatment, and the judicious use of lithotripsy and/or irrigation should nearly eliminate the need for repeated lithotomies.

Transplantation. Occasionally cystinuria will cause sufficient renal injury to lead to chronic renal failure. In these rare circumstances, renal transplantation may be effective. Since the defect in cystinuria resides in the transport epithelium of the genetically affected person, a kidney from a noncystinuric donor should remain disease-free. Normal amino acid excretion has been documented as long as $3\frac{1}{2}$ years after transplantation for cystinuria.[279]

ADDENDUM

Recent reports confirm a role for the human rBAT (also designated D2H) gene on chromosome 2p in cystinuria.[280–282] Pras and colleagues performed linkage analysis in 17 families of Libyan Jewish, Ashkenazi, Yemenite, Arabic, Persian, and East European origin with multiple affected members with cystinuria.[280] Their results localized the gene responsible for cystinuria in these families to chromosome 2p, the same region as the rBAT gene. Simultaneously, Calonge et al. surveyed the human rBAT gene for mutations in unrelated cystinuric probands.[281] They found 6 missense mutations (R180Q, M467K, M467T, P615T, T652R, L678P) that accounted for about half of the possible mutant alleles. None of these were present on 126 normal chromosomes, and M467T was present in at least 5 additional cystinuric pedigrees mainly of Spanish origin. Expression of the M467T allele in the Xenopus oocyte system showed that the mutant protein had only 20% of normal transport activity. These results confirm a role for the rBAT gene in cystinuria. How the rBAT protein actually functions to achieve cystine transport, what other proteins are involved and how the anticipated molecular data will fit with the wealth of previous transport studies in cystinuria are all exciting questions that remain to be answered.

REFERENCES

1. Wollaston WH: On cystic oxide: A new species of urinary calculus. *Trans R Soc London* **100**:223, 1810.
2. Noehden GH: Scientific notices—chemistry, cystic oxide—communicated in a letter from Dr. Noehden to Mr. Children. *Ann Philos* **7**:146, 1824.
3. Berzelius JJ: Calculus urinaries. *Traite Chem* **7**:424, 1833.
4. Friedman E: Der Kreislauf des Schwefels in der organischen Natur. *Ergebn Physiol* **1**:15, 1902.
5. Garrod AE: Inborn errors of metabolism. *Lancet* 2, 1908. (Lecture I, p 1; Lecture II, p 73; Lecture III, p 142; Lecture IV, p 214.)
6. Yeh HL, Frankl W, Dunn MS, Parker P, Hugher B, Gyorgy P: The urinary excretion of amino acids by a cystinuric subject. *Am J Med Sci* **214**:507, 1947.
7. Stein WH: Excretion of amino acids in cystinuria. *Proc Soc Exp Biol Med* **78**:705, 1951.
8. Dent CE, Senior B, Walshe JM: The pathogenesis of cystinuria. II. Polarographic studies of the metabolism of sulphur-containing amino-acids. *J Clin Invest* **33**:1216, 1954.
9. Arrow VK, Westall RG: Amino acid clearances in cystinuria. *J Physiol* **142**:141, 1958.
10. Dent CE, Rose GA: Amino acid metabolism in cystinuria. *Q J Med* **20**:205, 1951.
11. Fox M, Thier S, Rosenberg LE, Kiser W, Segal S: Evidence against a single renal transport defect in cystinuria. *N Engl J Med* **270**:556, 1964.
12. Foreman JW, Hwang SM, Segal S: Transport interactions of cystine and dibasic amino acids in isolated rat renal tubules. *Metabolism* **29**:53, 1980.
13. Segal S, McNamara PD, Pepe LM: Transport interaction of cystine and dibasic amino acids in renal brush border vesicles. *Science* **197**:169, 1977.
14. Frimpter GW, Horwith M, Furth E, Fellows RE, Thompson DD: Inulin and endogenous amino acid renal clearances in cystinuria: Evidence for tubular secretion. *J Clin Invest* **41**:281, 1962.
15. Crawhall JC, Scowen EF, Thompson CJ, Watts RWE: The renal clearance of amino acids in cystinuria. *J Clin Invest* **46**:1162, 1967.
16. Morin CL, Thompson MW, Jackson SH, Sass-Kortsak A: Biochemical and genetic studies in cystinuria: Observations on double heterozygotes of genotype I/II. *J Clin Invest* **50**:1961, 1971.
17. Von Udranszky L, Baumann E: Ueber das Vorkommen von Diaminen, sogenannten Ptomainen, bei Cystinurie. *Z Physiol Chem* **13**:562, 1889.
18. Loewy A, Neuberg C: Über Cystinurie. *Z Physiol Chem* **43**:338, 1904.
19. Brand E, Cahill GF, Harris MM: Cystinuria. II. The metabolism of cysteine, methionine and glutathione. *J Biol Chem* **109**:69, 1935.
20. Brand E, Cahill GF: Further studies on metabolism on sulfur compounds in cystinuria. *Proc Soc Exp Biol Med* **31**:1247, 1934.
21. Milne MD, Crawford MA, Girao CB, Loughridge LW: The metabolic disorder in Hartnup disease. *Q J Med* **29**:407, 1960.
22. Milne MD, Asatoor AM, Edwards KDG, Loughridge LW: The intestinal absorption defect in cystinuria. *Gut* **2**:323, 1961.
23. Asatoor AM, Lacey BW, London DR, Milne MD: Amino acid metabolism in cystinuria. *Clin Sci* **23**:285, 1962.
24. Thier S, Fox M, Segal S, Rosenberg LE: Cystinuria: In vitro demonstration of an intestinal transport defect. *Science* **143**:482, 1964.
25. McCarthy CF, Borland JL, Lynch HJ, Owen EE, Tyor MPL: Defective uptake of basic amino acids and L-cystine by intestinal mucosa of patients with cystinuria. *J Clin Invest* **43**:1518, 1964.
26. Thier S, Segal S, Fox M, Blair A, Rosenberg LE: Cystinuria: Defective intestinal transport of dibasic amino acids and cystine. *J Clin Invest* **44**:442, 1965.
27. Hellier MD, Perrett D, Holdsworth CD: Dipeptide absorption in cystinuria. *Br Med J* **4**:782, 1970.

28. Silk DBA: Progress report—peptide absorption in man. *Gut* **15**:494, 1974.
29. Martensson J, Denneberg T, Lindell A, Textorius O: Sulfur amino acid metabolism in cystinuria. *Kidney Int* **37**:143, 1990.
30. Bostrom H, Hambraeus L: Cystinuria in Sweden. VII. Clinical histopathological and medico-social aspect of the disease. *Acta Med Scand* suppl **411**:1, 1964.
31. Crawhall JC, Watts RWE: Cystinuria. *Am J Med* **45**:736, 1968.
32. Crawhall JC, Purkiss P, Watts RWE, Young EP: The excretion of amino acids by cystinuric patients and their relatives. *Ann Hum Genet* **33**:149, 1969.
33. Weinberger A, Sperling O, Rabinovitz M, Brosh S, Adam A, De Vries A: High frequency of cystinuria among Jews of Libyan origin. *Hum Hered* **24**:568, 1974.
34. Woolf LI: Large-scale screening for metabolic disease in the newborn in Great Britain, in Anderson JA, Swaiman KF (eds): *Phenylketonuria and Allied Metabolic Disorders*. U.S. Department of Health, Education and Welfare (Children's Bureau), Washington, 1967, pp 50–59.
35. Turner B, Brown DA: Amino acid excretion in infancy and early childhood: A survey of 200,000 infants. *Med J Aust* **1**:62, 1972.
36. Levy HL, Shih VE, Madigan PM: Massachusetts metabolic disorders screening program. I. Technics and results of urine screening. *Pediatrics* **49**:825, 1971.
37. Levy HL: Genetic screening, in Harris H, Hirschhorn K (eds): *Advances in Human Genetics*. New York, Plenum, 1973, vol 4, p 1.
38. Collis JE, Levi AJ, Milne MD: Stature and nutrition in cystinuria and Hartnup disease. *Br Med J* **1**:590, 1963.
39. Smith A, Yu JS, Brown DA: Childhood cystinuria in New South Wales. *Arch Dis Child* **54**:676, 1979.
40. Renander A: The roentgen density of the cystine calculus. *Acta Radiol* suppl 41, 1941.
41. Hambraeus L, Lagergren C: Cystinuria in Sweden. VI, Biophysical and roentgenological studies of urinary calculi from cystinurics. *J Urol* **88**:826, 1962.
42. Brand E, Harris MM, Biloon S: Cystinuria: Excretion of a cystine complex which decomposes in the urine with the liberation of free cystine. *J Biol Chem* **86**:315, 1930.
43. Lewis HB: Cystinuria: A review of some recent investigations. *Yale J Biol Med* **4**:437, 1932.
44. Harris H, Mittwoch U, Robson EB, Warren FL: Pattern of amino acid excretion in cystinuria. *Ann Hum Genet* **19**:196, 1955.
45. Hambraeus L: Comparative studies of the value of two cyanide-nitroprusside methods in the diagnosis of cystinuria. *Scand J Lab Clin Invest* **15**:657, 1963.
46. Crawhall JC, Saunders EP, Thompson CJ: Heterozygotes for cystinuria. *Ann Hum Genet* **29**:257, 1966.
47. Sackett DL: Adaptation of monodirectional high voltage electrophoresis on long papers to the rapid qualitative identification of urinary amino acids. *J Lab Clin Med* **63**:306, 1964.
48. Stein WH: A chromatographic investigation of the amino acid constituents of normal urine. *J Biol Chem* **201**:45, 1953.
49. Soupart P: Free amino acids of blood and urine in the human, in Holden JT (ed): *Amino Acid Pools*. Amsterdam, Elsevier, 1962, p 220.
50. Watanabe H, Sugahara K, Inoue K, Fujita Y, Kodama H: Liquid chromatographic-mass spectrometric analysis for screening of patients with cystinuria, and identification of cystine stone. *J Chromatogr* **568**:445, 1991.
51. Birwe H, Hesse A: High-performance liquid chromatographic determination of urinary cysteine and cystine. *Clin Chim Acta* **199**:33, 1991.
52. Perez-Ruiz T, Martinez-Lozano C, Tomas V, Carpena J: Spectrofluorimetric flow injection method for the individual and successive determination of L-cysteine and L-cystine in pharmaceutical and urine samples. *Analyst* **117**:1025, 1992.
53. Meloni CR, Canary JJ: Cystinuria with hyperuricemia. *JAMA* **200**:169, 1967.
54. Dent CE, Harris H: The genetics of cystinuria. *Ann Hum Genet* **16**:60, 1951.
55. Brooks WDW, Heasman MA, Lovell RRH: Retinitis pigmentosa associated with cystinuria: 2 uncommon inherited conditions occurring in family. *Lancet* **1**:1096, 1949.
56. Hurwitz LJ, Carson NAJ, Allen IV, Fannin TF, Lyttle JA, Neill DW: Clinical, biochemical and histopathological findings in a family with muscular dystrophy. *Brain* **90**:799, 1967.
57. Clara R, Lowenthal A: Familial and congenital lysine-cystinuria with benign myopathy and dwarfism. *J Neurol Sci* **3**:434, 1966.
58. Tanguay RB, Galindo J: Cystinuria associated with mongolism and identification of an abnormal pyrrolidine compound in urine. *Am J Clin Pathol* **46**:442, 1966.
59. Gross JB, Ulrich JA, Jones JD: Urinary excretion of amino acids in a kindred with hereditary pancreatitis and aminoaciduria. *Gastroenterology* **47**:41, 1964.
60. Brodehl J, Gallissen K, Kowalewski S: Isolated cystinuria (without lysine-ornithine-argininuria) in a family with hypocalcemia tetany. *Klin Wochenschr* **45**:38, 1967.
61. Purkiss P, Chalmers RA, Borud O: Combined iminoglycinuria and cystine- and dibasic aminoaciduria in patients with propionic acidaemia and 3-methylcrotonylglycinuria. *J Inherited Metab Dis* **3**:85, 1980.
62. Delvalle JA, Merinero B, Garcia MJ, Ugarte M, Gonzalez M, Gracia R, Peralta A: Biochemical findings in a patient with neonatal methylmalonic acidaemia. *J Inherited Metab Dis* **5**:53, 1982.
63. Segal S: Unpublished data.
64. Sakhaee K, Poindexter JR, Pak CY: The spectrum of metabolic abnormalities in patients with cystine nephrolithiasis. *J Urol* **141**:819, 1989.
65. Brand E, Block RJ, Kassell B, Cahill GF: Cystinuria. V. The metabolism of casein and lactalbumin. *J Biol Chem* **119**:669, 1937.
66. Rachele JR, Reed LJ, Kidwal AR, Ferger MF, Du Vigneaud V: Conversion of cystathionine labeled with S^{35} to cystine *in vivo*. *J Biol Chem* **185**:817, 1950.
67. Schimke RN, McKusick VA, Weilbaecher RG: Homocystinuria, in Nyhan WL (ed): *Amino Acid Metabolism and Genetic Variation*. New York, McGraw-Hill, 1967, pp 297–313.
68. Frimpter GW: Cystathionuria, in Nyhan WL (ed): *Amino Acid Metabolism and Genetic Variation*. New York, McGraw-Hill, 1967, pp 315–523.
69. Sturman JA, Gaull G, Raths NCR: Absence of cystathionase in human fetal liver: Is cystine essential? *Science* **169**:74, 1970.
70. Gaitonde MK, Gaull G: A procedure for the quantitative analysis of the sulphur amino acids of rat tissues. *Biochem J* **102**:959, 1967.
71. Wheldrake JF, Pasternak CA: The oxidation of cystine by mast-cell tumor P815, in culture. *Biochem J* **106**:437, 1968.
72. London DR, Foley TH: Cystine metabolism in cystinuria. *Clin Sci* **29**:133, 1965.
73. Crawhall JC, Lietman PS, Schneider JA, Seegmiller JE: Cystinosis: Plasma cystine and cysteine concentration and effect of D-penicillamine and dietary treatment. *Am J Med* **44**:330, 1968.
74. Crawhall JC, Segal S: The intracellular ratio of cysteine and cystine in various tissues. *Biochem J* **105**:891, 1967.
75. Segal S, Smith I: Delineation of cystine and cysteine transport systems in rat kidney cortex by development patterns. *Proc Natl Acad Sci USA* **63**:926, 1969.
76. States B, Segal S: Distribution of glutathione-cystine transhydrogenase activity in subcellular fractions of rat intestinal mucosa. *Biochem J* **113**:443, 1969.
77. Stephens AD, Perrett D: Cystinuria: A new genetic variant. *Clin Sci Mol Med* **51**:27, 1976.
78. Holtzapple PG, Bovee K, Rea CF, Segal S: Amino acid uptake by kidney and jejunal tissue from dogs with cystine stones. *Science* **166**:1525, 1969.
79. Whelan DT, Scriver CR: Hyperdibasic aminoaciduria: An inherited disorder of amino acid transport. *Pediatr Res* **2**:525, 1968.
80. Oyangi K, Miura R, Yamanoughi T: Congenital lysinuria: A new inherited transport disorder of dibasic amino acids. *J Pediatr* **77**:259, 1970.

81. Simell O, Perheentupa J: Renal handling of diamino acids in lysinuric protein intolerance. *J Clin Invest* **54**:9, 1974.
82. Lester FT, Cusworth DC: Lysine infusion in cystinuria: Theoretical renal thresholds for lysine. *Clin Sci* **44**:99, 1973.
83. Kato T: Renal handling of dibasic amino acids and cystine in cystinuria. *Clin Sci Mol Med* **53**:9, 1977.
84. Robson EB, Rose GA: The effect of intravenous lysine on the renal clearances of cystine, arginine and ornithine in normal subjects, in patients with cystinuria and Fanconi syndrome and their relatives. *Clin Sci* **16**:75, 1957.
85. Webber WA, Brown JL, Pitts RF: Interactions of amino acids in renal tubular transport. *Am J Physiol* **200**:380, 1961.
86. Bovee KC, Segal S: Renal tubular reabsorption of amino acids after lysine loading of cystinuric dogs. *Metabolism* **33**:602, 1984.
87. Bergeron M, Vadeboncoeur M: Antiluminal transport of L-arginine and L-leucine following microinjections in peritubular capillaries of the rat. *Nephron* **8**:355, 1971.
88. Bergeron M, Vadeboncoeur M: Microinjections of L-leucine into tubules and peritubular capillaries of the rat. II. The maleic acid model. *Nephron* **8**:367, 1971.
89. Poulkes BC: Effects of heavy metals on renal appartate transport and the nature of solute movement in kidney cortex slices. *Biochim Biophys Acta* **241**:815, 1971.
90. Rosenberg LE, Albrecht I, Segal S: Lysine transport in human kidney: Evidence for two systems. *Science* **155**:1426, 1967.
91. Brodehl J: Postnatal development of tubular amino acid reabsorption, in Silbernagel S, Lang F, Greger R (eds): *Amino Acid Transport and Uric Acid Transport*. Stuttgart, Georg Thieme, 1975, p 128.
92. Scriver C, Goodyer P, Giguere R: Ontogeny modifies manifestations of cystinuria genes: Implications for counseling. *J Pediatrics* **106**:3, 1985.
93. Frimpter GW: Cystinuria: Metabolism of the disulfide of cysteine and homocysteine. *J Clin Invest* **42**:1956, 1963.
94. Rosenberg LE, Durant JL, Holland IM: Intestinal absorption and renal extraction of cystine and cysteine in cystinuria. *N Engl J Med* **273**:1239, 1965.
95. Frimpter GW: Cystinuria: Intravenous administration of S^{35} cystine and S^{35} cysteine. *Clin Sci* **31**:207, 1966.
96. Stein WH, Moore S: The free amino acids of human blood plasma. *J Biol Chem* **211**:915, 1954.
97. Silbernagl S, Deetjen P: The tubular reabsorption of L-cystine and L-cysteine: A common transport system with L-arginine or not? *Pfluegers Arch* **337**:277, 1972.
98. Craan AG, Bergeron M: Experimental cystinuria: The cycloleucine model. I. Amino acid interactions in renal and intestinal epithelia. *Can J Physiol* **53**:1027, 1975.
99. Volkl H, Silbernagl S, Ascher A: Mutual inhibition of L-cystine/L-cysteine and other neutral amino acids during tubular reabsorption. A microperfusion study in rat kidney. *Pflugers Arch* **395**:190, 1982.
100. Schafer JA, Watkins ML: Transport of L-cystine in isolated perfused proximal straight tubules. *Pflugers Arch* **401**:143, 1984.
101. Ausiello DA, Segal S, Thier SO: Cellular accumulation of L-lysine in rat kidney cortex in vivo. *Am J Physiol* **222**:1473, 1972.
102. Greth WE, Thier SO, Segal S: Cellular accumulation of L-cystine in rat kidney cortex in vivo. *J Clin Invest* **52**:454, 1973.
103. Dal Canton A, Stanziale R, Corradi A, Andreucci VE, Migone L: Effects of acute ureteral obstruction on glomerular hemodynamics in rat kidney. *Kidney Int* **12**:403, 1977.
104. Schwartzman L, Blair A, Segal S: A common renal transport system for lysine, ornithine, arginine and cysteine. *Biochem Biophys Res Commun* **23**:220, 1966.
105. Segal S, Crawhall JC: Transport of cysteine by human kidney cortex. *Biochem Med* **1**:141, 1967.
106. Rosenberg IE, Downing SJ, Segal S: Competitive inhibition of dibasic amino acid transport in rat kidney. *J Biol Chem* **237**:2265, 1962.
107. Schwartzman L, Blair A, Segal S: Exchange diffusion of dibasic amino acids in rat-kidney cortex slices. *Biochim Biophys Acta* **135**:120, 1967.
108. Segal S, Schwartzman L, Blair A, Bertoli D: Dibasic acid transport in rat kidney cortex slices. *Biochim Biophys Acta* **135**:127, 1967.
109. Segal S, Crawhall JC: Characteristics of cystine and cysteine transport in rat kidney cortex slices. *Proc Natl Acad Sci USA* **59**:231, 1968.
110. Segal S, Smith I: Delineation of separate transport systems in rat-kidney cortex for L-lysine and L-cystine by developmental patterns. *Biochem Biophys Res Commun* **35**:771, 1969.
111. McNamara PD, Pepe LM, Segal S: Cystine uptake by renal brush border vesicles. *Biochem J* **194**:443, 1981.
112. Mircheff AK, Kippen I, Hirayama B, Wright EM: Delineation of sodium-stimulated amino acid transport pathways in rabbit kidney brush border vesicles. *Membr Biol* **64**:113, 1982.
113. Stieger B, Stange G, Biber J, Murer H: Transport of L-lysine by rat renal brush border membrane vesicles. *Pflugers Arch* **397**:106, 1983.
114. Hammerman MR: Na^+-independent L-arginine transport in rabbit renal brushborder membrane vesicles. *Biochim Biophys Acta* **685**:17, 1982.
115. Hilden SA, Sacktor B: L-arginine uptake into renal brush border membrane vesicles. *Arch Biochem Biophys* **210**:289, 1981.
116. Jean T, Ripoche P, Poujeol P: A sodium-independent mechanism for L-arginine uptake by rat renal brush border membrane vesicles. *Membr Biochem* **5**:1, 1983.
117. McNamara PD, Rea CT, Segal S: Lysine uptake by rat renal brush-border membrane vesicles. *Am J Physiol* **251**:F734, 1986.
118. McNamara PD, Rea CT, Segal S: Ion dependence of cystine and lysine uptake by rat renal brushborder membrane vesicles. *Biochim Biophys Acta* **1103**:101, 1992.
119. Reynolds RA, Mahoney SG, McNamara PD, Segal S: The influences of pH on cystine and dibasic amino acid transport by rat renal brushborder membrane vesicles. *Biochim Biophys Acta* **1074**:56, 1991.
120. Furlong TJ, Posen S: D-penicillamine and the transport of L-cystine by rat and human renal cortical brushborder membrane vesicles. *Am J Physiol* **258**:F321, 1990.
121. States B, Foreman JW, Lee J, Harris D, Segal S: Cystine and lysine transport in cultured human renal epithelial cells. *Metabolism* **36**:356, 1987.
122. Foreman JW, Lee J, Segal S: Characteristics of cystine uptake by cultured LLC-PK_1 cells. *BBA* **968**:323, 1988.
123. Bannai S, Kitamura E: Transport interaction of L-cystine and L-glutamate in human diploid fibroblasts in culture. *J Biol Chem* **255**:2372, 1980.
124. Bannai S: Exchange of cystine and glutamate across plasma membrane of human fibroblasts. *J Biol Chem* **261**:2256, 1986.
125. Takada A, Bannai S: Transport of cystine in isolated rat hepatocytes in primary culture. *J Biol Chem* **259**:2441, 1984.
126. States B, Segal S: Cystine and dibasic amino acid uptake by opossum kidney cells. *J Cell Physiol* **143**:555, 1990.
127. States B, Reynolds R, Lee J, Segal S: Cystine uptake by cultured cells originating from dog proximal tubule segments. *In Vitro Cell Dev Biol* **26**:105, 1990.
128. Bannai S: Transport of cystine and cysteine in mammalian cells. *Biochim Biophys Acta* **779**:289, 1984.
129. McNamara PD, Rea CT, Segal S: Expression of rat jejunal cystine carrier in *Xenopus* oocytes. *J Biol Chem* **266**:986, 1991.
130. Wells R, Hediger MA: Cloning of a rat kidney cDNA that stimulates dibasic and neutral amino acid transport and has sequence similarity to glucosidases. *Proc Natl Acad Sci USA* **89**:5596, 1992.
131. Bertran J, Werner A, Moore ML, Stange G, Markovich D, Biber J, Testar X, Zorzano A, Palacin M, Murer H: Expression cloning of a cDNA from rabbit kidney cortex that induces a single transport system for cystine and dibasic and neutral amino acids. *Proc Natl Acad Sci USA* **89**:5601, 1992.
132. Lee WS, Wells RG, Sabbah RV, Mohandas TK, Hediger MA: Cloning and chromosomal localization of a human kidney cDNA involved in cystine, dibasic, and neutral amino acid transport. *J Clin Invest* **91**:1959, 1993.
133. Bertran J, Werner A, Chillaron J, Nunes V, Biber J, Testar X, Zorzano A, Estivill X, Murer H, Palacin M: Expression cloning of a human renal cDNA that induces high

affinity transport of L-cystine shared with dibasic amino acids in *Xenopus* oocytes. *Am J Biol Chem* **268**:1482, 1993.
134. Bertran J, Magagnin S, Werner A, Markovich D, Biber J, Testar X, Zorzano A, Kühn LC, Palacin M, Murer H: Stimulation of system y^+-like amino acid transport by the heavy chain of human 4F2 surface antigen in *Xenopus laevis* oocytes. *Proc Natl Acad Sci USA* **89**:5606, 1992.
135. Wells RG, Lee WS, Kanai Y, Leiden JM, Hediger MA: The 4F2 antigen heavy chain induces uptake of neutral and dibasic amino acids in *Xenopus* oocytes. *J Biol Chem* **267**:15285, 1991.
136. Magagnin S, Bertran J, Werner A, Markovich D, Biber J, Palacin M, Murer H: Poly $(A)^+$ RNA from rabbit intestinal mucosa induces $b^{0,+}$ and y^+ amino acid transport activities in *Xenopus laevis* oocytes. *J Biol Chem* **267**:15384, 1992.
137. King JS Jr, Wainer A: Cystinuria with hyperuricemia and methioninuria: Biochemical study of a case. *Am J Med* **43**:125, 1967.
138. Frimpter GW: Cystathioninuria in a patient with cystinuria. *Am J Med* **46**:832, 1969.
139. Frimpter GW: The disulfide of L-cysteine and L-homocysteine in urine of patients with cystinuria. *J Biol Chem* **236**:651, 1961.
140. Hambraeus L: Cystinuria in Sweden: Quantitative studies of urinary amino acid excretion in cystinurics. *Acta Soc Med Ups* **6**:1, 1964.
141. Schneider JA, Bradley KH, Seegmiller JE: Identification and measurement of cysteine-homocysteine mixed disulfide in plasma. *J Lab Clin Med* **71**:122, 1968.
142. Silk DB, Perrett D, Stephens AD, Clark ML, Scowen EF: Intestinal absorption of cystine and cysteine in normal human subjects and patients with cystinuria. *Clin Sci Mol Med* **47**:393, 1974.
143. Foley TH, London DR: Cysteine metabolism in cystinuria. *Clin Sci* **29**:549, 1965.
144. Hellier MD, Holdsworth CD, Perrett D: Dibasic amino acid absorption in man. *Gastroenterology* **65**:613, 1973.
145. Mawer GE, Nixon E: The net absorption of amino acid constituents of a protein meal in normal and cystinuric subjects. *Clin Sci* **36**:463, 1969.
146. Milne MD: Amino acid metabolism in cystinuria. *Proc Biochem Soc* **122**:9P, 1971.
147. Asatoor AM, Crouchman MR, Harrison AR, Light FW, Loughridge LW, Milne MD, Richards AJ: Intestinal absorption of oligopeptides in cystinuria. *Clin Sci* **41**:23, 1971.
148. Hellier MD, Perrett D, Holdsworth CD, Thirumalai C: Absorption of dipeptides in normal and cystinuric subjects. *Gut* **12**:496, 1971.
149. Asatoor AM, Harrison RDW, Milne MD, Prosser DI: Intestinal absorption of an arginine-containing peptide in cystinuria. *Gut* **13**:95, 1972.
150. Rosenberg LE, Downing S, Durant JL, Segal S: Cystinuria: Biochemical evidence of three genetically distinct diseases. *J Clin Invest* **45**:365, 1966.
151. Rosenberg LE, Crawhall JC, Segal S: Intestinal transport of cystine and cysteine in man: Evidence for separate mechanisms. *J Clin Invest* **46**:30, 1967.
152. Coicadan L, Heyman M, Grasset E, Desjeux JF: Cystinuria: Reduced lysine permeability at the brush border of intestinal membrane cells. *Pediatr Res* **14**:109, 1980.
153. Desjeux JF, Simell RJ, Dumontier AM, Perheentupa J: Lysine fluxes across the jejunal epithelium in lysinuric protein intolerance. *J Clin Invest* **65**:1382, 1980.
154. Desjeux JF, Vonlanthen M, Dumontier AM, Simell O, Legrain M: Cystine fluxes across the isolated jejunal epithelium in cystinuria: Increased efflux permeability at the luminal membrane. *Pediatr Res* **21**:477, 1987.
155. Segal S, Lowenstein LM, Wallace A: Comparison of the transport characteristics by rat intestine and kidney cortex. *Gastroenterology* **55**:386, 1968.
156. Cassano G, Leszczynska B, Murer H: Transport of L-lysine by rat intestinal brush border membrane vesicles. *Pflugers Arch* **397**:114, 1983.
157. Ozegovic B, McNamara PD, Segal S: Cystine uptake by rat jejunal brushborder membrane vesicles. *Biosci Rep* **2**:913, 1982.
158. Harris H, Warren FL: Quantitative studies on the urinary cystine in patients with cystine stone formation and their relatives. *Ann Eugen* **18**:125, 1953.
159. Harris H, Mittwoch U, Robson EB, Warren FL: Phenotypes and genotypes in cystinuria. *Ann Hum Genet* **20**:57, 1955.
160. Rosenberg LE, Downing S: Transport of neutral and dibasic amino acids by human leucocytes: Absence of a defect in cystinuria. *J Clin Invest* **44**:1382, 1965.
161. Scriver CR, Whelan DT, Clow CL, Dallaire L: Cystinuria: Increased prevalence in patients with mental disease. *N Engl J Med* **283**:783, 1970.
162. Banerji NK, Millar JHD: Paraplegia associated with cystinuria. *J Neurol Sci* **12**:101, 1971.
163. DeMyer W, Gebhard RL: Subacute combined degeneration of the spinal cord with cystinuria. *Neurology* **25**:994, 1975.
164. Blackburn CR, McLeod JG: CNS lesions in cystinuria. *Arch Neurol* **32**:638, 1977.
165. Berry HK: Cystinuria in mentally retarded siblings with atypical osteogenesis imperfecta. *Am J Dis Child* **97**:196, 1959.
166. Gold RJM, Dobrinski MJ, Gold DP: Cystinuria and mental deficiency. *Clin Genet* **12**:329, 1977.
167. Smith A, Procopis PG: Cystinuria and its relationship to mental retardation. *Med J Aust* **2**:932, 1975.
168. Hwang SM, Segal S: Developmental and other aspects of $[^{35}S]$cysteine transport by rat brain synaptosomes. *J Neurochem* **33**:1303, 1979.
169. Segal S, Hwang SM: L-$[^{35}S]$cystine uptake by rat brain synaptosomes. *J Neurochem* **33**:697, 1979.
170. Hwang SM, Segal S: Developmental and other characteristics of lysine uptake by rat brain synaptosomes. *Biochim Biophys Acta* **557**:436, 1979.
171. Hwang SM, Weiss S, Segal S: Uptake of L-$[^{35}S]$cystine by isolated rat brain capillaries. *J Neurochem* **35**:417, 1980.
172. Harris H, Robson EB: Variation in homozygous cystinuria. *Acta Genet (Basel)* **5**:581, 1955.
173. Rosenberg LE, Durant JL, Albrecht I: Genetic heterogeneity in cystinuria: Evidence for allelism. *Trans Assoc Am Physicians* **79**:284, 1966.
174. Byrd DJ, Lind M, Brodehl J: Diagnostic and genetic studies in 43 patients with classic cystinuria. *Clin Chem* **37**:68, 1991.
175. Goodyer PR, Clow C, Reade T, Girardin C: Prospective analysis and classification of patients with cystinuria identified in a newborn screening program. *J Pediatr* **122**:568, 1993.
176. Rosenberg LE: Genetic heterogeneity in cystinuria, in Nyhan WL (ed): *Amino Acid Metabolism and Genetic Variation.* McGraw-Hill, New York, 1967, p 341.
177. Hershko C, Ben-Ami E, Paciorkovski J, Levin N: Alleomorphism in cystinuria. *Proc Tel-Hashomer Hosp* **4**:21, 1965.
178. Giugliani R, Ferrari I, Greene LJ: Heterozygous cystinuria and urinary lithiasis. *Am J Med Genet* 22, 1986.
179. Datta SP, Harris H: Urinary amino acid patterns of some mammals. *Ann Eugen* **18**:107, 1953.
180. Crawhall JC, Segal S: Sulphocysteine in the urine of the blotched Kenya genet. *Nature* **208**:1320, 1965.
181. Oldfield JE, Allen PH, Adair J: Identification of cystine calculi in mink. *Proc Soc Exp Biol Med* **91**:560, 1956.
182. Lassaigne JL: Observation sur l'existence de l'oxide cystique dans un calcul vésical du chien, et essai analytique sur la composition élémentaire de cette substance particulière. *Ann Chim Phys* 2d ser, **23**:328, 1823.
183. Morris ML, Green DF, Dinkel JH, Brand E: Canine cystinuria. *North Am Vet* **16**:16, 1935.
184. Brand E, Cahill GF: Canine cystinuria. III. *J Biol Chem* **114**:XV, 1936.
185. Brand E, Cahill GF, Kassell B: Canine cystinuria. V. Family history of two cystinuric Irish terriers and cystine determination in dog urine. *J Biol Chem* **133**:431, 1940.
186. Green DG, Morris ML, Cahill GF, Brand E: Canine cystinuria. II. Analysis of cystine calculi and sulfur distribution in the urine. *J Biol Chem* **114**:91, 1936.
187. Crane CW, Turner AW: Amino acid patterns of urine in blood plasma in a cystinuric Labrador dog. *Nature* **177**:237, 1956.
188. Treacher RJ: Amino acid excretion in canine cystine-stone disease. *Vet Rec* **74**:503, 1962.

189. Cornelius CE, Bishop JA, Schaffer MH: A quantitative study of amino aciduria in dachshunds with a history of cystine urolithiasis. *Cornell Vet* 177, April 1967.
190. Goulden BE, Leaver JL: Low voltage paper electrophoresis as a screening test for the diagnosis of canine cystinuria. *Vet Rec* **80**:244, 1967.
191. Treacher RJ: Intestinal absorption of lysine in cystinuric dogs. *J Comp Pathol* **75**:309, 1965.
192. Bovee KC, Thier SO, Rea C, Segal S: Renal clearance of amino acids in canine cystinuria. *Metabolism* **23**:51, 1974.
193. Frimpter GW, Thouin P, Ewalds BH: Penicillamine in canine cystinuria. *J Am Vet Med Assoc* **151**:1084, 1967.
194. Hoppe A, Denneberg T, Kågedal B: Treatment of clinically normal and cystinuric dogs with 2-mercaptopropionylglycine. *Am J Vet Res* **49**:923, 1988.
195. McNamara P, Rea C, Bovee K, Reynolds R, Segal S: Cystinuria in dogs: Comparison of the cystinuric component of the Fanconi syndrome in Basenji dogs to isolated cystinuria. *Metabolism* **38**:8, 1989.
196. Bovee KC, Bush M, Dietz J, Jezyk P, Segal S: Cystinuria in the maned wolf of South America. *Science* **212**:919, 1981.
197. DiBartola SP, Chew DJ, Horton ML: Cystinuria in a cat. *J Am Vet Med Assoc* **198**:102, 1991.
198. Brown RR: Aminoaciduria resulting from cycloleucine administration in man. *Science* **157**:432, 1967.
199. Goyer RA, Reynolds JO Jr, Elston RC: Characteristics of the aminoaciduria resulting from cycloleucine administration in pair fed rats. *Proc Soc Exp Biol Med* **130**:860, 1969.
200. Holtzapple P, Rea C, Genel M, Segal S: Cycloleucine inhibition of amino acid transport in human and rat kidney cortex. *J Lab Clin Med* **75**:818, 1970.
201. Hwang SM, Foreman J, Segal S: Developmental pattern of cystine transport in isolated rat renal tubules. *Biochem Biophys Acta* **690**:145, 1982.
202. Medow MS, Foreman JW, Bovee KC, Segal S: Developmental changes of glycine transport in the dog. *Biochim Biophys Acta* **693**:85, 1982.
203. Brodehl J, Gelissen K: Endogenous renal transport of free amino acids in infancy and childhood. *Pediatrics* **42**:395, 1968.
204. Stephens AD: Cystinuria and its treatment. *J Inherited Metab Dis* **12**:197, 1989.
205. Kolb FO, Earll JM, Harris HA: Disappearance of cystinuria in a patient treated with prolonged low methionine diet. *Metabolism* **16**:378, 1967.
206. Zinneman HH, Jones JE: Dietary methionine and its influence on cystine excretion in cystinuric patients. *Metabolism* **15**:915, 1966.
207. Chesney RW, Gusowski N, Padilla M, Lippincott S: Effect of amino acid intake on brush-border membrane uptake of sulfur amino acids. *Am J Physiol* F125, 1986.
208. Jaeger P, Portmann L, Saunders A, Rosenberg LE, Thier SO: Anticystinuric effects of glutamine and of dietary sodium restriction. *N Engl J Med* **315**:1120, 1986.
209. Norman RW, Manette WA: Dietary restriction of sodium as a means of reducing urinary cystine. *J Urol* **143**:1193, 1990.
210. Peces R, Sanchez L, Gorostidi M, Alvarez J: Effects of variation in sodium intake on cystinuria. *Nephron* **57**:421, 1991.
211. Dent CE, Friedmann M, Green H, Watson LCA: Treatment of cystinuria. *Br Med J* **1**:403, 1965.
212. Dent CE, Senior B: Studies on the treatment of cystinuria. *Br J Urol* **27**:317, 1955.
213. Crawhall JC, Scowen EF, Watts RWE: Effect of penicillamine on cystinuria. *Br Med J* **1**:585, 1963.
214. Crawhall JC, Scowen EF, Watts RWE: Further observations on use of D-penicillamine in cystinuria. *Br Med J* **1**:1411, 1964.
215. Bartter FC, Lotz M, Thier S, Rosenberg LE, Potts JT: Cystinuria: Combined clinical staff conference at the National Institutes of Health. *Ann Intern Med* **62**:796, 1965.
216. Crawhall JC, Thompson CJ: Cystinuria: Effect of D-penicillamine on plasma and urinary cystine concentrations. *Science* **147**:1459, 1965.
217. Lotz M, Potts JT: Quantitation of the effects of penicillamine therapy in cystinuria. *J Clin Invest* **43**:1293, 1964.
218. McDonald JE, Henneman PH: Stone dissolution in vivo and control of cystinuria with D-penicillamine. *N Engl J Med* **273**:578, 1965.
219. Crawhall JC, Scowen EF, Thompson CJ, Watts RWE: Dissolution of cystine stones during D-penicillamine treatment of a pregnant patient with cystinuria. *Br Med J* **1**:216, 1967.
220. Fellers FX, Shahidi NT: The nephrotic syndrome induced by penicillamine therapy. *Am J Dis Child* **98**:669, 1959.
221. Adams DA, Goldman R, Maxwell MH, Latta H: Nephrotic syndrome associated with penicillamine therapy of Wilson's disease. *Am J Med* **36**:330, 1964.
222. Rosenberg LE, Hayslett JP: Nephrotoxic effects of penicillamine in cystinuria. *JAMA* **201**:698, 1967.
223. Corcos JM, Soler-Bechera J, Mayer K, Freyberg RH, Goldstein R, Jaffe I: Neutrophilic agranulocytosis during administration of penicillamine. *JAMA* **189**:265, 1964.
224. Halperin EC, Thier SO, Rosenberg LE: The use of D-penicillamine in cystinuria: Efficacy and untoward reactions. *Yale J Biol Med* **54**:439, 1981.
225. Beer WE, Cooke KB: Epidermolysis bullosa induced by penicillamine. *Br J Dermatol* **79**:123, 1967.
226. Katz R: Penicillamine-induced skin lesions, a possible example of human lathyrism. *Arch Dermatol Syphilol* **95**:196, 1967.
227. Harris ED, Sjoerdsma A: Effect of penicillamine on human collagen and its possible application to treatment of scleroderma. *Lancet* **1**:996, 1966.
228. Bolognia JL, Braverman I: Pseudoxanthoma-elasticum-like skin changes induced by penicillamine. *Dermatology* **184**:12, 1992.
229. Goldstein JB, McNutt NS, Hambrick GW Jr, Hsu A: Penicillamine dermatopathy with lymphangiectases. *Arch Dermatol* **125**:92, 1989.
230. Sahn EE, Maize JC, Garen PD, Mullins SC, Silver RM: D-penicillamine-induced elastosis perforans serpiginosa in a child with juvenile rheumatoid arthritis. *J Am Acad Dermatol* **20**:979, 1989.
231. Fawcett NP, Nyhan WL, Anderson WW: Thrombocytosis during treatment of cystinuria with penicillamine. *J Pediatr* **69**:976, 1966.
232. Keiser HR, Henkin RI, Bartter FC, Sjoerdsma A: Loss of taste during therapy with penicillamine. *JAMA* **203**:381, 1968.
233. Henkin RI, Keiser HR, Jaffe IA, Sternlieb I, Scheinberg IH: Decreased taste sensitivity after D-penicillamine reversed by copper administration. *Lancet* **16**:1268, 1967.
234. Walsh JM, Patston V: Effect of penicillamine on serum iron. *Arch Dis Child* **40**:651, 1965.
235. Bostrom H, Wester PO: Excretion of trace elements in two penicillamine-treated cases of cystinuria. *Acta Med Scand* **181**:475, 1967.
236. McCall JT, Goldstein NP, Randall RV, Gross JB: Comparative metabolism of copper and zinc in patients with Wilson's disease (hepatolenticular degeneration). *Am J Med Sci* **254**:35, 1967.
237. Jaffe IA, Altman K, Merryman P: The antipyridoxine effect of penicillamine in man. *J Clin Invest* **43**:1969, 1964.
238. Gibbs K, Walshe JM: Penicillamine and pyridoxine requirements in man. *Lancet* 175, January 1966.
239. Heddle JG, Mettenry EW, Beaton GH: Penicillamine and vitamin B_6 interrelationships in the rat. *Can J Biochem Physiol* **42**:1215, 1963.
240. Pruzanski W: Cystinuria and cystine urolithiasis in childhood. *Acta Paediatr Scand* **55**:97, 1966.
241. Sternlieb I, Bennett B, Scheinberg IH: D-Penicillamine induced Goodpasture's syndrome in Wilson's disease. *Ann Intern Med* **82**:673, 1975.
242. Stokes GS, Potts JT, Lotz M, Bartter F: A new agent in the treatment of cystinuria: *N*-acetyl-D-penicillamine. *Br Med J* **1**:284, 1968.
243. Stephens AD, Watts RWE: The treatment of cystinuria with *N*-acetyl-D-penicillamine, a comparison with the results of D-penicillamine treatment. *Q J Med* **40**:335, 1971.
244. Mulvaney WP, Quilter T, Mortera A: Experiences with acetylcysteine in cystinuric patients. *J Urol* **114**:107, 1975.
245. Timmerman A, Kallistratos G, Fenner O, Sommer E: A tentative map suggesting the possible role of urinary minerals for the formation of renal stones, in Hodgkinson A, Nordin

BEC (eds): *Renal Stone Research Symposium* (Leeds, 1968). London, J & A Churchill, 1969.
246. King JS: Treatment of cystinuria with α-mercaptopropionylglycine: A preliminary report. *Proc Soc Exp Biol Med* **129**:927, 1968.
247. Kinoshita K, Yachiku S, Kotake T, Takeuchi M, Sonoda T: Treatment of cystinuria with 2-mercaptopropionylglycine (MPG), *Proc 2nd Internat Sympos on Thiola*. Osaka, Santen Pharmaceutical Co, 1972, p 50.
248. Sonoda T, Kinoshita K, Kotake T, Yachiku S, Takeuchi M: Effect of thiola on cystinuria, *Proc Int Symp Thiola*. Osaka, Santern Pharmaceutical Co, 1970, p 231.
249. Nishimura R, Ishido T, Takai S: Studies on cystinuria, *Proc 2nd Internat Sympos on Thiola*. Osaka, Santen Pharmaceutical Co, 1972, p 47.
250. Hautmann R, Terhorst B, Stuhlsatz HW, Lutzeyer W: Mercaptopropionylglycine: A progress in cystine stone therapy. *J Urol* **117**:628, 1977.
251. Kallistratos G, Mita I, Vadaloyka-Kalfakakou V: Management of cystinuric disorders with sulfhydryl drugs, in *The Management of Genetic Disorders*. New York, Alan R. Liss, 1979, pp 255–263.
252. Harbar JA, Cusworth DC, Lawes LC, Wrong OM: Comparison of 2-mercaptoproprionylglycine and D-penicillamine in the treatment of cystinuria. *J Urol* **136**:146, 1986.
253. Hautman RE: Cystine stone-therapy with alpha-mercaptopropionylglycine—ten years experience with forty two patients, in Smith LH, Robertson G, Finlayson B (eds): *Urolithiasis: Clinical and Basic Research*. New York, Plenum, 19XX, p 139.
254. Hoppe A, Denneberg T, Emanuelsson BM, Kagedal B, Lindgren S: Pharmacokinetics and bioavailability of 2-mercaptopropionylglycine administered intravenously and orally in dogs. *J Vet Pharmacol Therap* **14**:374, 1991.
255. Carlsson SM, Denneberg T, Emanuelsson BM, Kågedal B, Lindgren S: Pharmacokinetics of intravenous 2-mercaptopropionylglycine in man. *Eur J Clin Pharmacol* **38**:499, 1990.
256. Lindell A, Denneberg T, Eneström S, Fich C, Skogh T: Membranous glomerulonephritis induced by 2-mercaptopropionylglycine (2-MPG). *Clin Nephrol* **34**:108, 1990.
257. Lupo A, Farraggiana T, Loschiavo C, Parolini C, Maschio G: Nephrotic syndrome during 2-mercaptopropionylglycine (Thiola) therapy. *Nephron* **28**:96, 1981.
258. Rizzoni G, Pavanello L, Dussini N, Chiandetti L, Zacchello G: Nephrotic syndrome during treatment with alpha-mercaptopropionylglycine. *J Urol* **22**:381, 1979.
259. Siskind MS, Popovtzer MM: Hyperlipidemia associated with alpha-mercaptopropionylglycine therapy for cystinuria. *Am J Kidney Dis* **19**:179, 1992.
260. Hoppe A, Denneberg T, Frank A, Kagedals B, Petersson LR: Urinary excretion of metals during treatment with D-penicillamine and 2-mercaptopropionylglycine in normal and cystinuric dogs. *J Vet Pharmacol Therap* **16**:93, 1993.
261. Pak YC, Fuller C, Khashayar S, Zerwekh JE, Adams BV, with investigators from collaborating units: Management of cystine nephrolithiasis with alpha-mercaptopropionylglycine. *J Urol* 136, 1986.
262. Sloand JA, Isso JL, Jr: Captopril reduces urinary cystine excretion in cystinuria. *Arch Intern Med* 147, 1987.
263. Sandroni S, Stevens P, Barraza M, Tolaymat A: Captopril therapy of recurrent nephrolithiasis in a child with cystinuria. *Child Nephrol Urol* **9**:347, 1988.
264. Streem SB, Hall P: Effect of captopril on urinary cystine excretion in homozygous cystinuria. *J Urol* **142**:1522, 1989.
265. Perezella MA, Bullen GK: Successful treatment of cystinuria with captopril. *Am J Kidney Dis* **21**:504, 1993.
266. Dahlberg PJ, Jones JD: Cystinuria: Failure of captopril to reduce cystine excretion. *Arch Intern Med* **149**:713, 1989.
267. Aunsholt NA, Ahlbom G: Lack of effect of captopril in cystinuria. *Clin Nephrol* **34**:92, 1990.
268. Coulthard M, Richardson J, Fleetwood A: Captopril is not clinically useful in reducing the cystine load in cystinuria or cystinosis. *Pediatr Nephrol* **5**:98, 1991.
269. Miyagi K, Nakada S, Ohshiro D: Effect of glutamine on cystine excretion in a patient with cystinuria. *N Engl J Med* **301**:196, 1979.
270. Skovby F, Rosenberg LE, Thier SO: No effect of L-glutamine on cystinuria. Letter to the editor. *N Engl J Med* **302**:236, 1980.
271. Aunsholt NA, Ahlbom G: The effect of L-glutamine and sodium intake in cystinuric patients. *Scand J Urol Nephrol* **24**:281, 1990.
272. Van den Berg CJ, Jones JD, Wilson DM, Smith LH: Glutamine therapy of cystinuria. *Invest Urol* **18**:155, 1980.
273. Fariss BL, Kolb FO: Preliminary communications: Factors involved in crystal formation in cystinuria. *JAMA* **205**:138, 1968.
274. Smith AD, Lange PH, Miller RP, Reinke DB: Dissolution of cystine calculi by irrigation with acetylcysteine through percutaneous nephrostomy. *Urology* **13**:422, 1979.
275. Crissey MM, Gittes RF: Dissolution of cystine ureteral calculus by irrigation with tromethamine. *J Urol* **121**:811, 1979.
276. Stark H, Savir A: Dissolution of cystine calculi by pelviocaliceal irrigation with D-penicillamine. *J Urol* **124**:895, 1980.
277. Knoll LD, Segura JW, Patterson DE, Leroy AJ, Smith LH: Long-term followup in patients with cystine urinary calculi treated by percutaneous ultrasonic lithotripsy. *J Urol* **140**:246, 1988.
278. Hernandez-Graulau JM, Castanda-Zuniga W, Hunter D, Hulbert JC: Management of cystine nephrolithiasis by endourologic methods and shock-wave lithotripsy. *Urology* **34**:139, 1989.
279. Kelly S, Nolan DP: Letter to the editor. *JAMA* **243**:1897, 1980.
280. Pras E, Arber N, Aksentijevich I, Katz G, Schapiro JM, Prosen L, Gruberg L, Harel D, Liberman U, Weissenbach J, Pras M, Kastner DL: Localization of a gene causing cystinuria to chromosome 2p. *Nat Genet* **6**:415, 1994.
281. Calonge MJ, Gasparini P, Chillaron J, Chillon M, Gallucci M, Rousaud F, Zelante L, Testar X, Dallapiccola B, DiSilverio F, Barcelo P, Estivill X, Zorzano A, Nunes V, Palacin M: Cystinuria caused by mutations in *rBAT*, a gene involved in the transport of cystine. *Nat Genet* **6**:420, 1994.
282. Wright EM: Cystinuria defect expresses itself. *Nat Genet* **6**:328, 1994.

CHAPTER 118

Lysinuric Protein Intolerance and Other Cationic Aminoacidurias

Olli Simell

1. **Membrane transport of cationic amino acids lysine, arginine, and ornithine is abnormal in four disease entities: classic cystinuria; lysinuric protein intolerance (hyperdibasic aminoaciduria type 2, or familial protein intolerance); hyperdibasic aminoaciduria type 1; and isolated lysinuria (lysine malabsorption syndrome). Cystinuria, the most common of these, is dealt with in Chapter 117. About 100 patients with lysinuric protein intolerance (LPI) have been reported or are known to me. Almost half of them are from Finland, where the prevalence of this autosomal recessive disease is 1 in 60,000. Autosomal dominant hyperdibasic aminoaciduria type 1 has been described in 13 of 33 members in a French Canadian pedigree, and isolated lysinuria has been described in one Japanese patient.**

   Arginine and ornithine are intermediates in the urea cycle; lysine is an essential amino acid. In lysinuric protein intolerance (LPI), urinary excretion and clearance of all cationic amino acids, especially of lysine, are increased, and these amino acids are poorly absorbed from the intestine. Their plasma concentrations are low, and their body pools become depleted. The patients have periods of hyperammonemia caused by "functional" deficiency of ornithine, which provides the carbon skeleton of the urea cycle. Consequently, nausea and vomiting occur, and aversion to protein-rich food develops. The patients fail to thrive, and symptoms of protein malnutrition are further aggravated by lysine deficiency.

2. **Patients with LPI are usually symptom-free when breast-fed but have vomiting and diarrhea after weaning. The appetite is poor, they fail to thrive, and if force-fed high-protein milk or formulas, they may go into coma. After infancy, they reject high-protein foods, grow poorly, and have enlarged liver and spleen, muscle hypotonia, and sparse hair. Osteoporosis is prominent, and fractures are not uncommon; bone age is delayed. The mental prognosis varies from normal development to moderate retardation; most patients are normal. Four patients have had psychotic periods. The final height in treated patients has been slightly subnormal or low-normal. Pregnancies are risky: Profound anemia develops, platelet count decreases, and severe hemorrhages during labor and a toxemic crisis have occurred, but the offspring are normal if not damaged by delivery-related complications. Acute exacerbations of hyperammonemia have not been a frequent problem in treated patients, but may have been the cause of the sudden death in one adult male after moderate alcohol ingestion. About two thirds of the patients have interstitial changes in chest radiographs. Some patients have developed acute or chronic respiratory insufficiency, which in a few has led to fatal pulmonary alveolar proteinosis and to multiple organ dysfunction syndrome. Patients present with fatigue, cough, dyspnea during exercise, fever, and, rarely, hemoptysis, and may also show signs of nephritis and renal insufficiency. One adult patient with pulmonary symptoms has been treated with high-dose prednisolone and is in remission over 6 years after the occurrence of the symptoms. In another patient, bronchoalveolar lavages have produced immediate relief during several subacute exacerbations.**

3. **In LPI, the concentrations of the cationic amino acids in plasma are subnormal or low-normal, and the amounts of glutamine, alanine, serine, proline, citrulline, and glycine are increased. Lysine is excreted in urine in massive excess, and arginine and ornithine in moderate excess. Daily urine contains a mean amount of 4.13 mmol lysine (range 1.02 to 7.00), 0.36 mmol arginine (0.08 to 0.69) and 0.11 mmol ornithine (0.09-0.13) per 1.73 m^2 body surface area. The mean renal clearances are 25.7, 11.5, and 3.3 ml/min/1.73 m^2, respectively; occasional values suggest net tubular secretion of lysine. Cystine excretion may be slightly increased. Blood ammonia and urinary orotic acid excretion are normal during fasting but are increased after protein meals. The serum urea level is low to normal, and lactate dehydrogenase, ferritin, and thyroid-binding globulin levels are elevated.**

4. **The transport abnormality is expressed in the kidney tubules, intestine, cultured fibroblasts, and probably in the hepatocytes, but not in mature erythrocytes. In vivo and in vitro studies of the handling of cationic amino acids in the intestine and kidney strongly suggest that the transport defect is localized at the basolateral (antiluminal) membrane of the epithelial cells. In vivo, plasma concentrations increase poorly after oral loading with the cationic amino acids, but also if lysine is given as a lysine-containing dipeptide. Dipeptides and other oligopeptides use a different transport mechanism not shared with that of free amino acids. The dipeptide thus crosses the luminal membrane normally, and is hydrolyzed to free amino acids in the**

A list of standard abbreviations is located immediately preceding the index in each volume. Additional abbreviations used in this chapter include: HHH = hyperornithinemia–hyperammonemia–homocitrullinuria; LDH = lactate dehydrogenase; LPI = lysinuric protein intolerance; MCAT-1 and MCAT-2 = mouse cationic amino acid transporter-1 and transporter-2, respectively; TBG = thyroxine-binding globulin.

cytoplasm of the enterocyte. An efflux defect at the basolateral membrane explains why the dipeptide-derived lysine is unable to enter the plasma compartment in LPI. Direct measurements and calculations of unidirectional fluxes of lysine in intestinal biopsy specimens have confirmed that the defect indeed localizes to the basolateral cell surface. Similar cellular localization of the defect in the kidney tubules is suggested by infusions of citrulline, which cause not only citrullinuria but also significant argininuria and ornithinuria. Because citrulline and the cationic amino acids do not share transport mechanisms in the tubules, part of the citrulline is converted to arginine and then to ornithine in the tubule cells during reabsorption. A basolateral transport defect prohibits antiluminal efflux of arginine and ornithine, which accumulate and escape through the luminal membrane into the urine. The genetic mutations in LPI and possibly in all cationic aminoacidurias apparently lead to kinetic abnormalities in the transport protein(s) of the cationic amino acids. This is suggested by the fact that increasing the tubular load of a single cationic amino acid by intravenous infusion increases its tubular reabsorption, but reabsorption remains subnormal even at high loads. The other cationic amino acids are able to compete for the same transport site(s) also in LPI, but an increase in the load of one cationic amino acid frequently leads to net secretion of the others.

The plasma membrane of cultured fibrolasts shows a defect in the trans-stimulated efflux of the cationic amino acids; i.e., their flux out of the cell is not stimulated by cationic amino acids present on the outside of the cell as efficiently as it is in the control fibroblasts. The percent of trans-stimulation of homoarginine efflux in the fibroblasts of the heterozygotes is midway between that of the patients and the control subjects.

5. **The exact cause of hyperammonemia in LPI remains unknown. The enzymes of the urea cycle have normal activities in the liver, and the brisk excretion of orotic acid during hyperammonemia supports the view that *N*-acetylglutamate and carbamyl phosphate are formed in sufficient quantities. Low plasma concentrations of arginine and ornithine suggest that the malfunctioning of the cycle is caused by a deficiency of intramitochondrial ornithine. This hypothesis is supported by experiments in which hyperammonemia after protein or amino nitrogen loading is prevented by intravenous infusion of arginine or ornithine. Citrulline, a third urea cycle intermediate, also abolishes hyperammonemia if given orally, because, as a neutral amino acid, it is well-absorbed from the intestine. Ornithine deficiency in LPI has recently been questioned because cationic amino acids and their nonmetabolized analogues accumulate in higher-than-normal amounts in intestinal biopsy specimens and cultured fibroblasts from LPI patients in vitro and the concentrations of the cationic amino acids in liver biopsy samples are similar or higher in the patients when compared to these concentrations in the control subjects. If hyperammonemia is not due to simple deficiency of ornithine, it could be caused by inhibition of the urea cycle enzymes by the intracellularly accumulated lysine; by a coexisting defect in the mitochondrial ornithine transport necessary for the function of the urea cycle; or by actual deficiency of ornithine in the cytoplasm caused by abnormal pooling of the cationic amino acids into some cell organelle(s), most likely lysosomes. The latter two explanations imply that the transport defect is expressed also in the organelle(s).**

6. **Lysine is present in practically all proteins, including collagen. Lysine deficiency may cause many of the features of the disease that are not corrected by prevention of hyperammonemia, including enlargement of the liver and spleen, poor growth and delayed bone age, and osteoporosis. Oral lysine supplements are poorly tolerated by the patients because of their poor intestinal absorption. ε-*N*-acetyl-L-lysine, but not homocitrulline, efficiently increases plasma concentration of lysine in the patients, but acetyllysine or other neutral lysine analogues have not been used for supplementation.**

7. **Recently, a 622-amino-acid retroviral receptor (murine leukemia viral receptor REC1) with 12 to 14 potential membrane-spanning domains has been cloned. The physiological role of the receptor was soon found to be that of a cationic amino acid transporter at the cell membrane; the protein was hence renamed MCAT-1, mouse cationic amino acid transporter-1. The functional characteristics of the transporter are similar to those of system y^+, a widely expressed Na^+-independent transport system for cationic amino acids. The human counterpart of the mouse REC1 gene, encoding the retroviral receptor–transport protein, has been assigned to chromosome 13q12-q14 and named ATRC1. MCAT-1 (and y^+) activity is not expressed in rodent liver, but two other related cationic amino acid transport proteins, formed presumably as a result of alternative splicing—Tea (T cell early activation; expressed also in activated T and B lymphocytes) and MCAT-2—are probably responsible for the low-affinity transport of cationic amino acids that is characteristic of (mouse) liver. Studies addressing the ATRC1 gene as well as the Tea and MCAT-2 genes as candidate genes for LPI are under way.**

8. **Treatment in lysinuric protein intolerance consists of protein restriction and supplementation with oral citrulline, 3 to 8 g daily during meals. Patients are encouraged to increase their protein intake modestly during citrulline supplementation, but aversion to protein in most patients effectively inhibits them from accepting more than the minimal requirement. The treatment clearly improves the growth and well-being of the patients. Pulmonary complications (interstitial pneumonia, pulmonary alveolar proteinosis, cholesterol granulomas, and respiratory insufficiency) have occasionally responded to early treatment with high-dose prednisolone, or to bronchoalveolar lavages. No therapy is known for the associated renal disease and renal failure.**

9. **The clinical and biochemical findings in other cationic aminoacidurias differ slightly from those in lysinuric protein intolerance. The symptoms of the index case with hyperdibasic aminoaciduria type 1 resemble those of LPI, but the other affected members of the pedigree are clinically healthy. The Japanese patient with isolated lysinuria has severe growth failure, seizures, and mental retardation. Her transport defect is apparently limited to lysine, and hyperammonemia is not a feature of the disease.**

Perheentupa and Visakorpi described the first three patients with "familial protein intolerance with deficient transport of basic amino acids" in 1965.[1] The disease is now called lysinuric protein intolerance (LPI) or "hyperdibasic aminoaciduria type 2."[2-5] Over 100 patients with this autosomal recessive disease have been described or are known to me; 41 of them are Finns or Finnish Lapps.[6-52] The incidence in

Finland is 1 in 60,000 births but varies considerably within the country.[2,53] Patients of black and white American, Japanese, Turkish, Moroccan, Arab, Jewish, Italian, French, Dutch, Irish, Norwegian, Swedish, and Russian origin have also been described. The fascinating combination in the disease of urea cycle failure, expressed as postprandial hyperammonemia, and a defect in the transport of the cationic amino acids lysine, arginine, and ornithine in the intestine and kidney tubules has led to extensive studies of the mechanisms that link these two phenomena. The mechanisms are still partly unresolved, and the sequence of events leading to hyperammonemia is unclear. We can simplify our knowledge by saying that hyperammonemia is caused by "functional deficiency" of the urea cycle intermediates arginine and ornithine in the urea cycle[4,11,14,54] (Fig. 118-1). LPI has also been a productive model for studies of cellular transport: It is the first human disease where the transport defect has been localized to the basolateral (antiluminal) membrane of the epithelial cells.[55-57] Further, in LPI the parenchymal cells show a defect in the trans-stimulated efflux of the cationic amino acids, suggesting that the basolateral membrane of the epithelial cells and the plasma membrane of the parenchymal cells have analogous functions.[58,59]

Recently, the first candidate gene for LPI, ATRC1, encoding a human cationic amino acid transporter, has been mapped to the long arm of chromosome 13 (13q12-q14).[60] Without further proof, it is intriguing to hypothesize how a mutation in this or in a functionally similar gene or in genes encoding regulatory proteins of these transporters might lead to the membrane-selective cationic amino acid transport defect of LPI and to the complicated clinical features of the disease.

Several patients with variant forms of cationic aminoaciduria have been described in which the protein tolerance often is better than in LPI and the selectivity and severity of cationic aminoaciduria differs.[23,25,33,61,62] In the report by Whelan and Scriver[61] only the history of the index case suggested hyperammonemia, but other members of the pedigree have been symptom-free. The inheritance of this hyperdibasic aminoaciduria type 1 is autosomal dominant, implying that the patients are heterozygous for LPI or another type of hyperdibasic aminoaciduria.

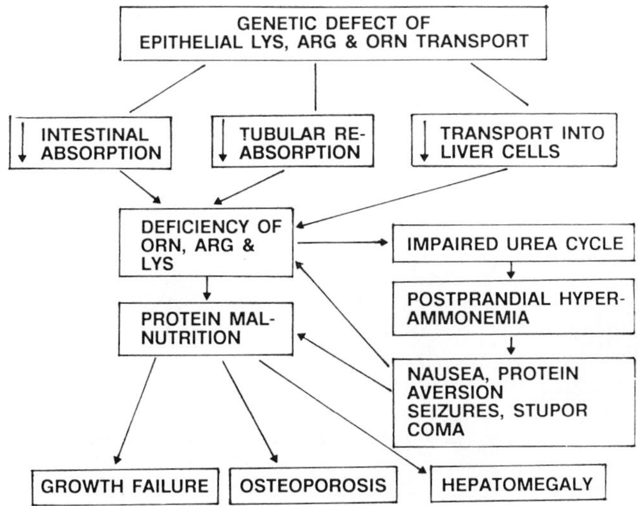

FIG. 118-1. **The suggested pathogenesis of lysine, arginine, and ornithine deficiency, hyperammonemia, and aversion to protein in LPI.**

CLINICAL ASPECTS

Lysinuric Protein Intolerance

Natural Course of the Disease. The gestation and delivery of infants with LPI has been uneventful.[4-6,9-11,35] Breast-fed infants usually thrive because of the low protein concentration in human milk, but symptoms of hyperammonemia may appear during the neonatal period and reflect exceptionally low protein tolerance or a high protein content in the breast milk. Nausea, vomiting, and mild diarrhea appear usually within 1 week of weaning or another increase in the protein content of the meals. Soy-based formulas are perhaps slightly better tolerated than cow's milk. The infants are poor feeders, cease to thrive, and have marked muscular hypotonia. The patient's liver and spleen are enlarged from the neonatal period onward. The association of episodes of vomiting with high protein feeds is not always apparent to the parents and may remain unnoticed even by trained physicians for years. Thus, the diagnosis frequently has been delayed until the school age or even adulthood.[35,47,63]

Around the age of 1 year, most patients begin to reject cow's milk, meat, fish, and eggs. The diet then mainly contains cereals cooked in water, potatoes, rice and vegetables, fruits and juices, bread, butter, and candies. The frequency of vomiting decreases on this diet, but accidental increases in protein intake lead to dizziness, nausea, and vomiting. A few patients have lapsed into coma, to the point where the EEG became isoelectric when the children were tube-fed with high-protein foods.[27,35,40,41,47] Enteral alimentation and total parenteral nutrition may cause symptoms in patients who have remained undiagnosed, because the protein or amino acid loads often exceed patient's tolerance. Prolonged, moderately increased protein intake may lead to dizziness, psychotic periods, chronic abdominal pains, or suspicion of abdominal emergencies.

Bone fractures occur frequently, often after minor trauma.[4,14,30,35,63-66] In a Finnish series, 20 of 29 patients (69 percent) had suffered from fractures of the long bones or of compression fractures of the lumbar spine; ten (34 percent) had had more than two fractures during the 18-year follow-up.[63-65] Most fractures occurred before the age of 5 years. Symptoms of osteoarthrosis often begin at the age of 30 to 40 years. The radiologic signs of osteoporosis are usually severe before puberty but decrease with advancing age. The effect of citrulline therapy on osteoporosis is minimal.

Our accumulating experience with the late complications associated with the disease, together with recent reports of patients from outside Finland, suggest that in a sizeable proportion of the patients the classic symptoms of protein intolerance may remain unnoticed. Instead, the patients may present with interstitial lung disease or respiratory insufficiency, or have renal glomerular or glomerulotubular disease with or without renal insufficiency as the first clinical finding (see "Complications and Autopsy Findings" below).

Physical Findings. Muscular hypotonia and hypotrophy are usually noticeable from early infancy but improve with advancing age.[35] Most patients are unable to perform prolonged physical exercises, but acute performance is relatively good. The body proportions of patients after the first couple of years of life are characteristic: the extremities are thin, but the front view of the body is squarelike with abundant centripetal subcutaneous fat. The hair is thin and sparse, the skin may be slightly hyperelastic, and the nails are normal. The liver is variably enlarged, and the spleen is often palpable and is large by ultrasound.

Patients who have remained undiagnosed until the age of several years have had characteristics typical of protein–calorie malnutrition and frequently resemble patients with advanced celiac disease. The subcutaneous fat may be reduced and the skin "loose" and "too large for the body" (Fig. 118-2).

The ocular fundi have been normal by ophthalmoscopy.[35] Of 20 patients studied, 14 had minute opacities in the anterior fetal Y suture of both lenses. In 10 patients, the opacities were surrounded by minute satellites. The opacities were never large enough to cause visual impairment and have remained stable, in some patients now for over 25 years. The mechanism underlying the lens abnormalities is unknown.[67]

The dentition of the patients has been normal, and the patients do not appear to be especially prone to caries, despite the high carbohydrate content of the diet.

Growth. Birth weights and lengths have been normal for gestational age, and postnatal growth is normal before weaning. The growth curves then begin to deviate progressively from the normal mean, and, at the time of diagnosis, 16 of 20 Finnish patients were more than 2 SD below the mean height, 12 patients were more than 3 SD, 6 patients more than 4 SD, 2 patients more than 5 SD, and 1 patient 6 SD below the mean.[35] Skeletal maturation is considerably delayed.[63,64] The bones usually mature slowly and linearly without a pubertal catch-up spurt, and most patients have not reached skeletal maturity by the age of 20 years. The final height of the patients has almost invariably been closer to the normal than the height measured at the time of diagnosis, because of therapy and the late cessation of growth. The head circumferences have been normal for age.

The body proportions are normal, but with advancing age the moderate centripetal obesity, which is present from early childhood, becomes more obvious.

Skeletal Manifestations and Bone Metabolism. Osteoporosis is often recognizable in skeletal radiogrpahs and has occasionally been the leading sign of LPI.[30,63-65] Two-thirds of the patients have had fractures, half of which have occurred after insignificant trauma. All fractures have healed properly within a normal time. The skull and sella turcica have been normal in roentgenograms.

Over 70 percent of the patients have some skeletal abnormalities, either osteoporosis, deformations, or early osteoarthrosis.[63-65] In radiographs of 29 Finnish patients, osteoporosis was present in 13; the cortices of the long bones were abnormally thin in 5; the vertebrae had endplate impressions in 8; metaphyses were rickets-like in 2; and cartilage showed early destruction in 3. The cortex of the metacarpal bones was characteristically thickened in 7.[64] Morphometric analyses of bone biopsy samples showed moderate to severe osteoporosis in eight of nine patients studied; trabecular bone and osteoid volume were markedly reduced.[65] After double-labeling of bones with tetracycline in vivo, barely identifiable single lines were detected, suggesting poor bone deposition; the findings resembled those in severe malnutrition.[68-74] The number of osteoblasts and osteoclasts was low, and the extent of osteoid along the bone surfaces was low or normal in all specimens studied.

Laboratory tests for evaluation of calcium and phosphate metabolism have given unremarkable results.[35,63-65] Serum calcium and phosphate concentration, urinary excretion of calcium and phosphate, serum magnesium, estradiol, testosterone, thyroid-stimulating hormone, cortisol, vitamin D metabolites [25-$(OH)_2$-D, 1,25-$(OH)_2$-D and 24,25-$(OH)_2$-D], parathyroid hormone, calcitonin, and osteocalcin concentrations have all been within the reference range.

The daily urinary excretion of hydroxyproline is significantly increased during pubertal growth, but half of the adult patients also have supranormal excretion rates (mean of all adults 212 ± 103 $\mu mol/m^2$; adult reference range, 60 to 180 $\mu mol/m^2$).[65] The serum hydroxyproline concentration is in-

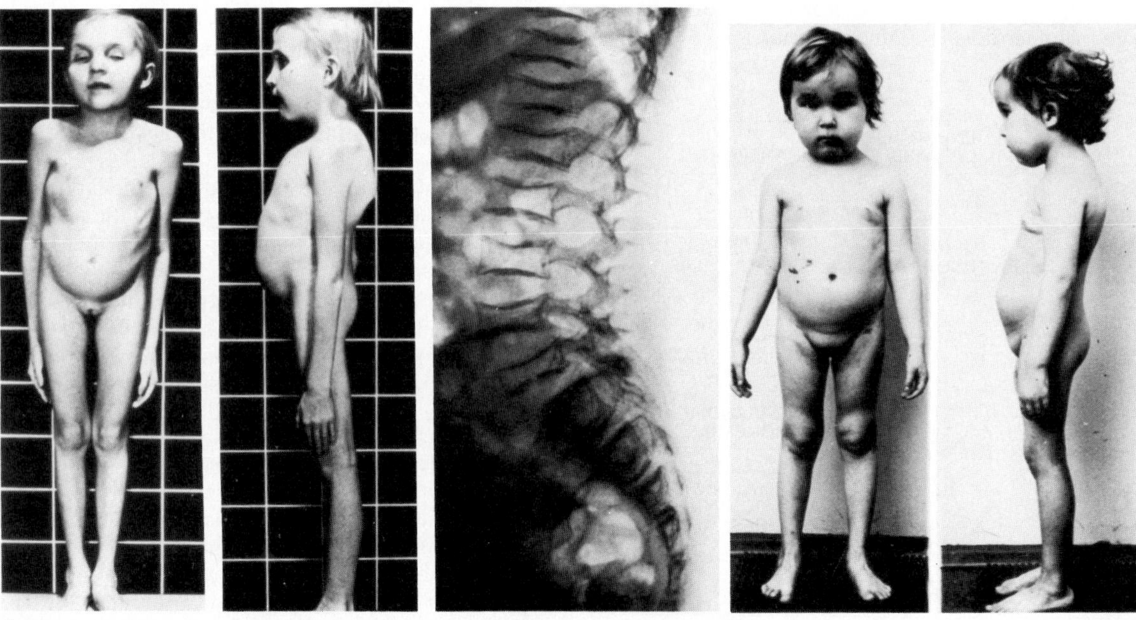

FIG. 118-2. Two children with LPI. The pictures were taken at the time of diagnosis. *A*. Child 12 years old. *B*. Child 6 years old. Note the prominent abdomen, hypotrophic muscles, and "loose" skin. The thorax of the child in *A* is deformed and her trunk shortened because of osteoporosis and pathologic fractures of the vertebrae.

creased in almost all patients irrespective of age. Serum concentrations of the C-terminal propeptide of type I procollagen and of the N-terminal propeptide of type III procollagen have been normal in all pediatric patients, but the concentration of the latter increases during puberty and remains elevated in adult patients.

The incorporation of labeled hydroxyproline into collagen was significantly decreased in cultured LPI fibroblasts as compared with age-matched controls at the ages of 5, 14, and 30 years, but there was no difference at the age of 44 years.[65] Morphometry of the collagen fibrils in electron microscopy showed no differences between patients and controls.

Liver Pathology. In the youngest patients, the histologic findings in liver biopsy specimens have been normal, with only occasional fat droplets in the hepatocytes.[8,35,63,75] In older patients, delimited areas in periportal or central parts of the liver lobules contained hepatocytes with ample pale cytoplasm and small pyknotic nuclei. In these cells the glycogen content is decreased, and glycogen appears in coarse particles. At the borders of the abnormal areas, many nuclei are ghostlike and have central inclusion bodies staining positively with periodic acid-Schiff. Cytoplasmic fat droplets occur especially in the periportal areas. Children who died of alveolar proteinosis with multiple organ dysfunction syndrome have mostly shown extensive fatty degeneration of the liver but minimal or moderate cirrhosis. Inflammatory cells have always been absent in the liver biopsy samples.

Liver changes in LPI may reflect generalized protein malnutrition, because in kwashiorkor liver fat synthesis is increased, apolipoprotein synthesis is decreased, and lipoprotein lipases are inhibited.[76] Similar liver changes have also been induced in rats by lysine and arginine deprivation.[77]

Performance in Adult Life. Mental development is normal in most subjects. Performance is decreased, particularly in patients with known histories of prolonged hyperammonemia. Altogether, about 20 percent of the patients with LPI reported in the literature or otherwise known to me are mentally retarded. Convulsions are uncommon, but periods of stupor have occasionally been misinterpreted as psychomotor seizures.[18] Four patients have had psychotic periods, which have clearly been precipitated by prolonged moderate hyperammonemia.[35]

Neuropsychologic evaluation of the patients suggests that mathematical and other abstract skills are particularly vulnerable to hyperammonemia. Treatment with a low-protein diet and citrulline supplementation[11,14,63] (see "Treatment" below) has significantly improved the life quality of the patients. Episodes of vomiting and other signs of hyperammonemia have become a rare exception. The patients who underwent prolonged periods of hyperammonemia in early infancy and childhood and who appeared severely retarded at the first presentation have considerably and continuously improved their performance during therapy. All Finnish patients are now able to take care of the activities of daily life, and none of them is institutionalized. The most severely retarded patient, who had an IQ of 40 at the age of 12 years, lives now at the age of 40 in the custody of another family and is capable of taking care of her daily activities; she also works in a protected environment outside the home for a few hours a day and helps routinely in the household. She is talkative, happy, and socially active. At the other end of the spectrum, one patient has graduated from a medical school, works successfully as an internist, is married, and is a mother of one. Several other patients have also graduated from high school or other secondary schools and are permanently employed. The physical fitness of the patients is fair, but their capacity for prolonged heavy work and physical endurance is clearly limited. One patient worked as a construction worker in a building company for a few years, but found the job too heavy; another has been an active jogger for years and is capable of running 15 km without problems. The oldest patient in Finland is now 49 years of age and retired 7 years ago because of back problems. He is mentally and physically active and takes care of the household duties of a small farmhouse. A Finnish-born patient in Sweden is now 58 years old.[16,21,29] One male and seven female patients are married.

Pregnancies of the Patients. The seven married women have had fifteen pregnancies. One of the mothers was treated during the pregnancy only with protein restriction; the other received citrulline supplementation (8 to 14 pills containing 0.414 g L-citrulline daily during meals). Anemia (hemoglobin < 8.5 g/dl) occurred in all, and the platelet count decreased to less than $50 \times 10^3/\text{mm}^3$. A severe hemorrhage complicated two deliveries in one patient. Another patient had severe toxemia in her second pregnancy. The blood pressure increased to crisis values and she had prolonged convulsions and unconsciousness, but she recovered totally. In a third patient, an ultrasound-guided amniotic fluid puncture led to a bleed and loss of the fetus at 35 gestational weeks. Despite the mothers' anemia and severely decreased platelet count, other pregnancies and deliveries have been uneventful.

Of the 14 living children born to the patients, 13 are well at the age of 0.5 to 14 years. One child, whose delivery was complicated by a severe maternal hemorrhage, has hemiplegia and slightly delayed mental development, and another one was late in learning to speak but has later developed well.

One male patient has a healthy son.

Complications and Autopsy Findings. Since the first description of LPI in 1965,[1] 4 children and 1 adult of the 39 known Finnish patients have died, and a few pediatric LPI patients have died in other countries. A Moroccan patient died with pulmonary symptoms and autopsy findings similar to those of the four Finnish children (see below),[37] and a Japanese patient has had long-lasting, slowly progressive interstitial changes in the lungs.[36] An American child with LPI presented with interstitial pneumonia at the age of 27 months and later died of pulmonary alveolar proteinosis.[38] More recently, three Italian patients with severe interstitial lung disease have been described.[51] One of them died at the age of 18 months; two others had an accompanying renal glomerular or glomerulotubluar disease. One Arab child had severe respiratory insufficiency as the presenting sign at the age of 11 years, and had had clubbing of the fingers for 5 years.[52] An open lung biopsy showed cholesterol casts surrounded by a granulomatous process and giant cells; there was a small amount of interstitial inflammation and a moderate degree of scarring. Electron microscopy demonstrated cholesterol casts around and within macrophages and within alveolar cells in the alveolar spaces, but no hemorrhage.

Two of the four Finnish children who died had another systemic disease in addition to LPI (SLE; hypothyreosis). In all four, the fatal courses began as acute or subacute respiratory insufficiency, which progressed to multiorgan failure[63,75,78-80]; the symptoms fulfilled the criteria of the multiple organ dysfunction syndrome.[81,82] Progressive fatigue, cough, and mild to high fever were typical, and some children had blood in the sputum.[78-80] Dyspnea with marked air hunger during minimal exercise developed. Hemoglobin and platelet values fell, and the values of serum ferritin and lactate dehydrogenase, which are high in normal circumstances in these patients, increased even further. The sedimentation rate was elevated. Arterial oxygen tension was decreased, and the children had a severe bleeding tendency. The severity of liver, kidney, and pancreas involvement in the multiorgan failure varied. The pulmonary symptoms lasted from 2 weeks to 6 months before death.

The radiologic findings during the acute phase were similar in all patients with a fatal course.[78] Diffuse, reticulonodular densities and, later, signs of rapidly progressing airspace disease appeared in the chest radiographs at the mean age of 5 years (range 1.2 to 10.2 years) (Fig. 118-3). Two children developed acute respiratory insufficiency 2 months after the first radiologic signs of lung involvement, but one patient had densities for over 2 years and another for 12 years before acute exacerbation.

In one patient, a lung biopsy specimen taken at the time of appearance of the reticulonodular densities showed pulmonary alveolar proteinosis (Fig. 118-3C). At autopsy, three of the patients showed pulmonary alveolar proteinosis, and one had pulmonary hemorrhage with cholesterol granulomas. The specimens showed accumulations of myelin-like multilamellar structures, simple vesicles, granules, amorphous material, and crystals in transmission electron microscopy (Fig. 118-4).[79] Samples from the patient with pulmonary cholesterol granulomas contained interstitial and intraalveolar cholesterol crystals and some multilamellar structures. It is interesting that similar pulmonary cholesterol granulomas were described in the lung biopsy sample of the Saudi Arabian child from Israel.[52]

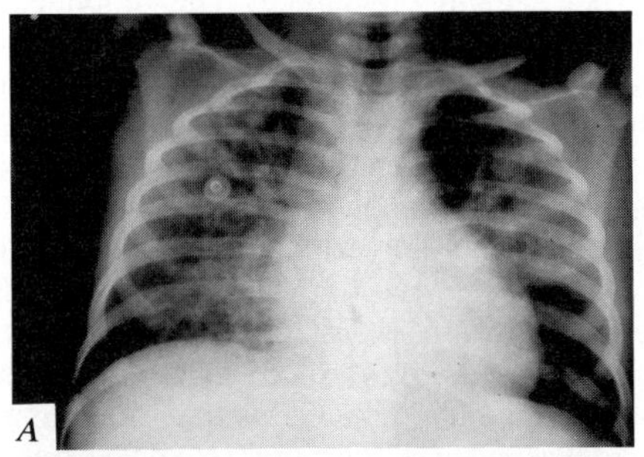

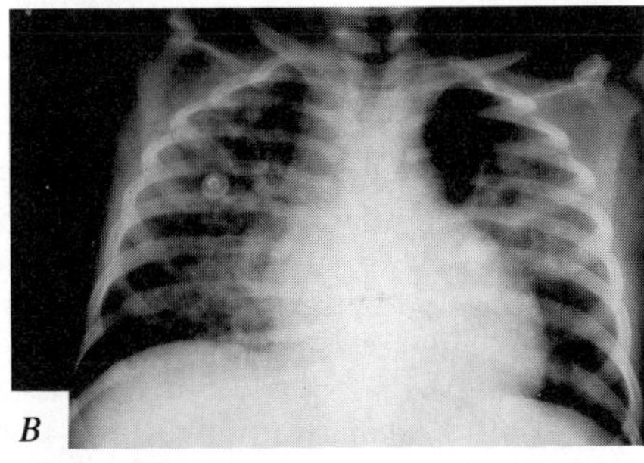

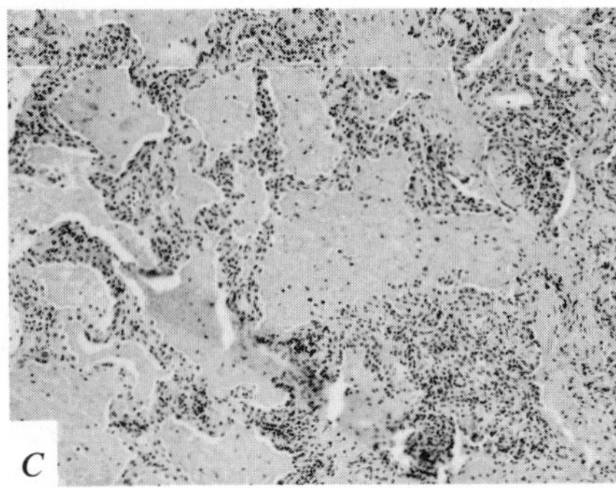

FIG. 118-3. A 13-year-old girl with LPI who developed fatal respiratory insufficiency after a mild respiratory infection. *A*. Chest radiograph at the time of the first respiratory symptoms showed reticulonodular interstitial densities. *B*. Chest radiograph taken two weeks later shows interstitial and alveolar densities. *C*. Pulmonary biopsy specimen shows signs of alveolar proteinosis (hematoxylin-eosin, original magnification ×115). (*From Parto et al.*[78] *Used by permission.*)

One adult patient developed acute respiratory insufficiency with cough, fever, dyspnea, and hemoptysis at the age of 23 years.[78-80] Chest radiographs showed interstitial densities and airspace disease. Pulmonary function tests showed minimal obstruction of the distal airways but normal diffusing capacity. Extensive microbiologic investigations showed no evidence of infection. An open lung biopsy specimen showed bronchiolitis obliterans with signs of interstitial pneumonia. Granulation tissue polyps obstructed bronchiolar lumina, alveolar septa were thickened, and the sample contained a number of infiltrating lymphocytes and macrophages as well as signs of alveolar hemorrhages; no vasculitis nor full-blown alveolar proteinosis were found. The cytocentrifuge preparation made from the lung biopsy specimen showed 57 percent macrophages, 15 percent neutrophils, and 26 percent lymphocytes of the total cell count. The T-helper to T-suppressor cell ratio was 0.81. Symptoms disappeared rapidly and radiologic findings normalized within two months during high-dose prednisolone treatment. Eight months later, the patient relapsed with hemoptysis, but he responded well again to an increased corticosteroid dose. Now, five years later, he is symptom-free; the results of pulmonary function tests, high-resolution computed tomography, and radionuclide imaging are normal, but the proportion of erythrocytes in the bronchoalveolar lavage fluid is increased.

Another patient developed chronic, slowly progressive pulmonary insufficiency with dyspnea, cough, chest pain, and hypoxia at the age of 42 years.[78-80] A bronchoalveolar lavage cured clinical symptoms in hours, and the response has been as good in all of the six relapses that have occurred during the 7 years of follow-up. His chest radiographs show increasing interstitial linear and nodular densities. Six years after the initial symptoms, radionuclide perfusion imaging showed a segmental defect and uneven perfusion, and pulmonary function tests suggested slight restriction but normal diffusing capacity. Bronchoscopy showed signs of chronic bronchitis. The relative proportions of cells in the bronchoalveolar lavage fluid were normal.

It is interesting that one-third of the symptom-free patients studied (8 of 25) had findings in chest radiographs that suggested pulmonary fibrosis, and high-resolution computed tomography suggested pulmonary fibrosis in two-thirds of the patients studied (8 of 14).[78] Most of the symptom-free patients (9 of 12) also showed mild abnormalities in perfusion imaging or in pulmonary function tests (8 of 12).

The total cell count in the bronchoalveolar lavage fluid of three adult LPI patients was normal, but two showed markedly increased lymphocyte and decreased macrophage percentages, suggesting alveolar immunoactivation and subclinical alveolitis, as is common in many systemic diseases (Table 118-1).[83] Similar alterations have also been found in lavage fluid of patients with isolated pulmonary alveolar proteinosis.[84] Furthermore, the LPI lavage fluid also con-

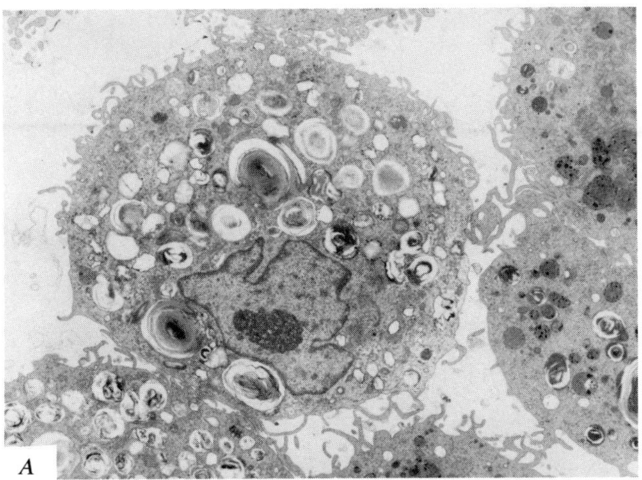

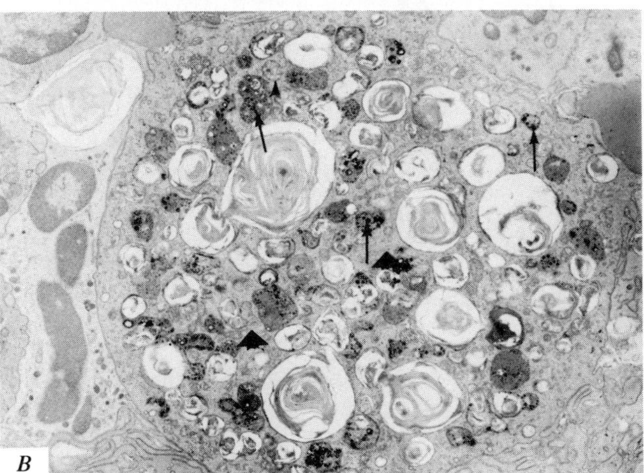

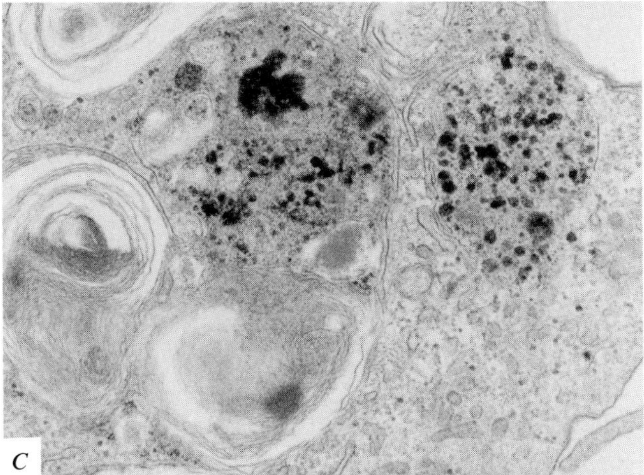

FIG. 118-4. **Pulmonary macrophages of patients with LPI.** ***A*****. An electron micrograph shows macrophage containing multilamellar structures and electron-dense bodies that contain iron (magnification ×3,100).** ***B*****. The same cell at a greater magnification shows characteristic electron-dense areas which, according to the x-ray spectrum, contained mainly iron (×4,600).** ***C*****. Another pulmonary macrophage containing a number of black-staining, iron-containing precipitations (×27,200).** ***(From Parto et al.*[79] *Used by permission.)***

tained multilamellar structures of various sizes and shapes, which were absent in control samples. In one patient, the size of macrophages in the lavage fluid was markedly increased, but the size was normal in the others. Macrophages in all patients were filled with multilamellar structures similar to those in type II pneumocytes (Fig. 118-4). The estimated proportional volume of multilamellar structures in pulmonary macrophages was significantly increased, macrophages contained dense inclusions with iron-like material, and the iron content of the cells was elevated (Table 118-1).[63,79] Whether these changes in alveolar macrophages reflect altered iron or phospholipid metabolism in LPI or are a consequence of repeated subclinical pulmonary hemorrhages is unknown. It is possible that increased concentrations of cationic amino acids in the alveolar lining of LPI patients[85,86] may interfere with phospholipid metabolism, change the composition of the surfactant, and lead to the clinical symptoms. Because of their phagocytic nature, normal pulmonary macrophages contain a multitude of inclusions, including round, dense bodies, lamellae, myelin-like figures, and homogeneous lipid-like bodies.[87,88] Multilamellar structures closely resembling those of alveolar macrophages in LPI have been reported in pulmonary alveolar proteinosis associated with other diseases; in abnormalities of phospholipid metabolism; in a silica-induced animal model of alveolar proteinosis; and after experimental use of amphiphilic cationic drugs.[88-91]

Alveolar proteinosis is less common in children than in adults, but the course is usually more aggressive in childhood. Almost 60 pediatric patients with pulmonary alveolar proteinosis have been described, associated in some with alymphoplasia,[92] decreased IgA levels,[93] or various autoimmune diseases.[94,95] It is interesting that there are 10 pairs of siblings with alveolar proteinosis,[93,96-102] suggesting that genetic factors are important or that some of these patients with pulmonary alveolar proteinosis may also have had LPI.

It is apparent that the cascade leading to pulmonary alveolar proteinosis or cholesterol granulomas is part of the symptomatology of LPI. The pathophysiology remains unknown, but the abnormal content of cationic amino acids in the bronchoalveolar lavage fluid of these patients suggests that the transport of cationic amino acids may be abnormal also in the pulmonary alveolar epithelium (Table 118-1).[63,85,86] The transport defect might influence gas exchange or alter the production, composition, or function of surfactant in the alveoli. High-dose prednisolone treatment and bronchoalveolar lavages may slow down or prevent disease progression if started early. Thus, all patients and their guardians should be warned of the symptoms.

Two of the patients who died had increased serum creatinine or decreased creatinine clearance values during exacerbation of the symptoms. At autopsy, kidney histology and immunohistochemistry unexpectedly showed immune-mediated glomerulonephritis in all four patients.[63,75] The disease was morphologically classified as diffuse, membranous or mesangial proliferative glomerulonephritis. Histologic findings were similar to those commonly seen in systemic lupus erythematosus. It is interesting that two patients also had onion-skin arteries in spleen tissue, another finding often associated with lupus. The glomeruli were hypercellular, the capillaries were narrowed, and the basement membranes were thickened. The tubules contained granular or homogenous periodic acid–Schiff (PAS)-positive material and, occasionally, calcium crystals. Indirect immunofluorescence studies revealed heavy membranous deposits of IgG, IgM, IgA, complement components C3 and C1q, and immunoglobulin κ and λ light chains in the glomeruli, and electron microscopy revealed large subepithelial and mesangial electron-dense deposits, proliferation of Bowman's epithelium, and tubuloreticular structures in the glomerular endothelial cells. The absence of linear deposition

Table 118-1 Cell and Amino Acid Content of Bronchoalveolar Lavage Fluid in Four Adult Patients with Lysinuric Protein Intolerance and in Control Subjects

Case No.	Cell Count × 10^6/liter	Lymphs (%)	Baso (%)	Eos (%)	Polys (%)	Macroph (%)	Eryth (per view)	T_H/T_S	Total Amino Acid Concentration (μM)	Lysine/Total Amino Acids (μmol/μmol)	Arginine/Total Amino Acids (μmol/μmol)	Ornithine/Total Amino Acids (μmol/μmol)	Cross-Sectional Area of Macrophages (mean±SD)	Volume of Multilamellar Structures/Macrophage Volume	Fe/Cl in Intramacrophage Inclusions
Patients with LPI															
1	77	6	0	3	0	89	>20	1.16	950	55.7	31.8	6.0	128.0±39.9	0.27±0.15	1.63±0.95
2	205	46	1	0	1	52	10	0.96	667	11.7	7.8	3.6			
3	96	59	1	1	0	38	5	0.72	1088	60.8	25.7	9.8	215.4±53.1	0.36±0.10	2.88±5.36
4*	237	3	0	0	0	97	0	1.80	1370	28.5	16.7	5.4	162.8±40.1	0.36±0.11	3.86±2.30
4*	113	18	0	0	0	82	0	1.34	1122	67.6	43.9	4.4			
4*	178	22	0	2	5	71	0	0.65	728	7.8	13.9	5.8			
Mean									905	39.7	14.3	5.8	166.0±57.1	0.32±0.18	2.79±3.48
Control Subjects															
1	821	77	0	0	7	16	0		1370	27.0	17.3	11.8	115.2±32.5	0.09±0.07	0.69±0.98
2	70	5	0	3	3	78	0		761	9.1	0	4.6	112.3±24.7	0.06±0.06	0.27±0.31
3	129	1	0	0	5	93	0		1231	15.4	5.9	5.8	160.3±37.8	0.09±0.05	0.19±0.06
4	165	17	0	3	2	78	0		1232	27.7	15.9	7.2	168.1±35.5	0.02±0.03	0.40±0.15
5	NT	16	0	0	3	81	0		867	10.1	7.2	4.0	138.6±41.9	0.05±0.06	0.48±0.42
Mean									1092	17.9	9.3	6.7	141.1±41.7	0.06±0.06	0.41±0.53

*Bronchoalveolar lavage was performed on one patient with LPI on three separate occassions.
NOTE: NT = not tested; T_H = helper T cells; T_S = suppressor T cells.
SOURCE: From Parto[63] and Parto et al.[79] Used by permission.

of IgG in glomerular and pulmonary capillaries in all patients and the lack of anti-glomerular basement membrane (anti-GBM) antibodies in the only patient so studied excluded the anti-GBM disease.[103] Other diseases without anti-GBM antibody in which pulmonary hemorrhage and glomerulonephritis have occurred include SLE, Wegener granulomatosis, systemic necrotizing vasculitis, cryoglobulinemia, immune complex-mediated glomerulonephritis, and idiopathic crescentic glomerulonephritis with negative immunofluorescence.[104-107] The recent report by DiRocco and coworkers[51] confirms that renal glomerular involvement in LPI is not uncommon. In their patients, progression of the renal changes (as well as of the pulmonary changes) occurred despite treatment with high-dose prednisone. At this time, there is no known effective treatment of the renal glomerular disease in LPI.

The pediatric patients who died developed symptoms and signs of hepatic insufficiency in the terminal phase of their disease; the liver showed fatty degeneration and mild to severe cirrhosis at autopsy. Excessive amyloid was found in the lymph nodes and spleen. The pancreas showed acinar atrophy and fibrosis, resembling findings in kwashiorkor, and deficiency of cationic amino acids.[77,108] One patient at autopsy had pancreatic necrotizing inflammation, possibly due to shock, terminal pancreatitis,[109] or plugs in pancreatic ducts. However, the possible association of LPI with familial pancreatitis cases is intriguing, as some patients with familial pancreatitis excrete excessive lysine in the urine.[110] Bone marrow was hypercellular at autopsy, but the amount of megakaryocytes was decreased. None of the Finnish patients showed erythroautophagocytosis or erythroblastophagocytosis in the marrow.[20,32,75] Bone specimens showed osteoporosis.

Five adult Finnish patients (age 27 to 49 years) have developed arterial hypertension, and three have hypercholesterolemia (serum cholesterol > 9.0 mmol/liter), which may represent heterozygous familial cholesterolemia. The one adult Finnish patient who died, died of a cause unrelated to the pulmonary disease.

Other LPI-Associated Features. A few patients with biochemical LPI have had uncommon associated features, which may point to heterogeneity of the syndrome or may be random associations; I have included these patients in the LPI group because of their biochemical identity. A mentally retarded boy with biochemical features typical of LPI showed a peculiar response to phenothiazines, which were prescribed to relieve his hyperactivity.[33] A Japanese 8-year-old girl had a prestage of systemic lupus erythematosus and showed multiple immunologic abnormalities, including impaired function of lymphocyte functioning and the presence of lupus erythematosus cells, anti-nuclear antibodies, and hypergammaglobulinemia.[31] Interestingly, also, one Finnish patient had systemic lupus erythematosus (see "Complications and Autopsy Findings" above), and another patient had anti-nuclear antibody-positive rheumatoid arthritis. Two Italian boys with LPI had striking joint hyperextensibility, and three had prominent autophagy of erythroblasts by granulocytes as well as clusters of degenerated erythroblast nuclei in the bone marrow[20,32,51]; autophagy was found also in a patient of Turkish ancestry.[22] The findings in the bone marrow aspirates are interesting and may be a common phenomenon in the disease, but were not found in several Finnish patients studied so far.[35,63,75] The autophagocytosis might be linked with abnormalities in the peripheral red cells of the patients.[35,111] Two Japanese patients with typical LPI findings also had decreased argininosuccinate synthase activity,[45,50] and one patient had glucose 6-phosphate dehydrogenase deficiency.[49]

Other Cationic Aminoacidurias

The proband described by Whelan and Scriver[61] has many clinical features of LPI, including recurrent vomiting during infancy, poor growth, and delayed bone age. The other affected members of the kindred with the dominantly inherited trait were also below the third percentile in height for normals individuals, but they were otherwise healthy. Whelan and Scriver discuss the possibility that the trait was a heterozygous manifestation of the LPI gene or of some other recessive transport disorder. It is interesting that the obligate heterozygotes in the pedigree of Kihara et al.[33] had urinary excretion values similar to those of the subjects with the dominant trait described by Whelan and Scriver,[61] suggesting that the index case might be homozygous for hyperdibasic aminoaciduria type 1. Further pedigrees with the trait of hyperdibasic-aminoaciduria type 1 are needed before firm conclusions concerning this relationship are possible.

In my opinion, the patients described by Kihara et al.,[33] Oyanagi et al.,[24,25] Brown et al.,[23] and others[13,18,20,22,28] have sufficient clinical and biochemical features to be regarded as patients with LPI. The only significant clinical differences are the less marked protein intolerance,[25,28] less significant growth failure,[18,28] and some peculiar features (see below).[20,31-33] We now know that clinical protein tolerance may vary also in LPI, and that vomiting and aversion to high-protein foods are not always prominent in confirmed patients. This variability may depend on the subject's capacity to handle waste nitrogen via other metabolic routes.[112-120]

Omura and coworkers[62] described a Japanese 21-month-old girl with severe mental retardation, convulsions, marked growth failure, and clear signs of malnutrition. She excreted excessive lysine in the urine, "but arginine excretion was at the upper limit of normal while ornithine excretion was only slightly increased." Her intestinal absorption of lysine was decreased, but arginine, ornithine, and cystine absorption did not differ from that of control subjects. Fasting blood ammonia and values after loading with cow's milk were normal. LPI cannot with certainty be excluded in this patient, but she likely represents another mutation affecting the transport of the cationic amino acids, and the disease should tentatively be regarded as an entity of its own, best called "isolated lysinuria."

BIOCHEMICAL INVESTIGATIONS

Plasma and Urine Amino Acids

Plasma and urinary amino acid concentrations and the renal clearances of plasma amino acids are given in Table 118-2. Plasma concentrations of lysine, arginine, and ornithine are typically one-third to one-half the normal means values, but occasionally may be well within the normal range.[8,14,19,25,33,35,121] The concentrations of serine, glycine, citrulline, proline, and, especially, alanine and glutamine are increased. The accumulation of amino nitrogen in these pools seems to be a regular feature of LPI. The increase in plasma citrulline is noteworthy.

Urinary excretion and renal clearance of lysine is massively increased, and that of arginine and ornithine is moderately increased. Because of the high plasma concentrations

Table 118-2 Plasma Concentration, Urinary Excretion, and Renal Clearance of Free Amino Acids in Patients with Lysinuric Protein Intolerance*

Amino Acid	Plasma Concentration, m*M*			Urinary excretion (mmol/24 h/1.73 m^2)		Renal clearance (ml/min/1.73 m^2)	
	Range in Normal Children†	Patients with LPI					
		Mean	Range	Mean	Range	Mean	Range
Alanine	0.173–0.305	0.772	0.417–1.017	1.068	0.465–1.586	0.953	0.698–1.324
α-amino-adipic acid	0.002	n.m.		0.609	0.405–0.821		
Arginine	0.023–0.086	0.027	0.012–0.058	0.356	0.076–0.687	11.508	3.175–22.300
Aspartic acid	0.004–0.023	n.m.		n.m.		n.m.	
Asparagine and glutamine	0.057–0.467	5.583	3.644–7.161	6.491	4.365–8.542	0.891	0.595–1.628
Citrulline	0.012–0.055‡	0.232	0.141–0.530	0.519	0.155–0.988	1.440	0.762–2.425
Cystine	0.048–0.140‡	0.080	0.057–0.105	0.120	0.059–0.209	0.175	0.050–0.324
Glutamic acid	0.023–0.250	0.049	0.021–0.081	0.047	0.040–0.051	0.853	0.427–0.839
Glycine	0.117–0.223	0.467	0.385–0.530	2.058	1.595–2.808	3.062	2.538–4.067
Histidine	0.024–0.085	0.110	0.084–0.139	0.637	0.155–1.232	4.374	1.184–10.221
Isoleucine	0.028–0.084	0.059	0.029–0.082	0.099	0.071–0.158	1.306	0.598–2.076
Leucine	0.056–0.178	0.090	0.050–0.126	0.101	0.067–0.142	0.830	0.596–1.184
Lysine	0.071–0.151	0.070	0.032–0.179	4.126	1.022–7.000	25.655	11.116–45.877
Methionine	0.011–0.016	0.032	0.021–0.048	0.050	0.038–0.063	1.356	0.976–2.044
Ornithine	0.027–0.086	0.021	0.002–0.083	0.106	0.091–0.134	3.268	2.709–5.357
Phenylalanine	0.026–0.061	0.049	0.033–0.084	0.078	0.056–0.094	1.268	0.574–1.966
Proline	0.068–0.148	0.189	0.158–0.268	n.m.		n.m.	
Serine	0.079–0.112	0.251	0.199–0.246	0.607	0.398–0.878	1.900	1.257–2.628
Threonine	0.042–0.095	0.113	0.030–0.172	0.277	0.111–0.554	1.825	1.235–2.578
Tyrosine	0.031–0.071	0.047	0.030–0.072	0.142	0.125–0.158	2.361	1.202–3.688
Valine	0.128–0.283	0.182	0.132–0.244	0.047	0.035–0.059	0.177	0.167–0.186

*The plasma concentrations were measured after an overnight fast, and the respective 24-h urines were collected when the patients were on a self-chosen hospital diet. The clearance values are calculated from the 24-h urinary excretion and from the fasting plasma concentration. Plasma lysine, arginine, and ornithine concentrations were measured on 33 occasions in 20 patients; the other values are from four patients.

†From Dickenson et al.[278]

‡From Scriver and Davies[279]

NOTE: n.m. = not measurable

SOURCE: From Simell et al.[35] Used by permission.

of serine, glycine, citrulline, proline, alanine, and glutamine, they are also found in excess in the urine, but their renal clearances are within the normal range.

In some patients, lysinuria and arginine-ornithinuria have been missed in the thin-layer or paper chromatograms used for screening of inborn errors of metabolism. The reason for the low excretion in these patients has always been that the plasma concentration of the cationic amino acids has been exceptionally low. In such a situation the molar and relative excretion of the cationic amino acids can be minimal even though the clearances are high. I have seen this phenomenon a few times in older, undiagnosed patients who have spontaneously restricted their protein intake to the extreme, and who also have had clear signs of protein malnutrition. When protein intake has been increased, cationic aminoaciduria has become as prominent as in other patients.

The reabsorption defect in kidney tubules is most marked for lysine; arginine is less affected; and ornithine is absorbed best.[121] The measurements of tubular reabsorption of lysine have in some urine collections suggested net secretion. The reabsorption defect for arginine and ornithine and presumably for lysine remains significant also when plasma concentrations of these amino acids are increased, but at extremely high filtered loads, when plasma concentrations are several millimolar, the tubular reabsorption of arginine and ornithine reabsorption resembles normal. At these very high filtered loads, selective transport probably becomes unimportant and physical diffusion phenomena determine the rate of absorption. A significant increase in plasma concentration and, consequently, in the filtered load of one cationic amino acid leads easily to net tubular secretion of the other two cationic amino acids.

Blood Ammonia, Urinary Orotic Acid Excretion, and Serum Urea

Blood ammonium concentration is normal (<70 μ*M*) during fasting, but is elevated (100 to 560 μ*M*) after regular meals.[8,35] The extent of postprandial hyperammonemia depends on the protein content of the meal. The ammonia values usually return to the normal range 2 to 6 hours later. Frequent ingestion of high-protein foods, extensive fasting, acute infections (especially gastroenteritis), and severe physical or psychological stress increase blood ammonia in the patients and easily cause persisting hyperammonemia, which does not disappear during fasting.

Urinary orotic acid is increased more frequently than blood ammonia, suggesting that orotic acid is a better indicator of urea cycle failure in these patients than hyperammonemia.[13,46,122-125] Urine samples collected during fasting frequently contain normal amounts of orotic acid (<0.03 μmol/kg/h, or <11 μmol/mmol creatinine), but values are increased even during a self-chosen low-protein diet (geometric mean, 0.52; range 0.05 to 3.77 μmol/kg/h in 24-h pooled urine samples) and increase massively if the protein intake is increased.[122] Nitrogen loads given in the form of cow's milk protein (0.5 g/kg), ammonium lactate (2.5 mmol/kg) or intravenous alanine (6.6 mmol/kg during 90 min) can be given without clinical risk to the patients. In healthy subjects, blood ammonia is stable after such loads, but blood ammonia and certainly urinary orotic acid excretion increase in the patients (geometric mean and range in the patients: 4.93; 1.61 to 11.19 μmol/kg/h in 4- to 6-h pooled urine; 0.61; 0.10 to 7.22 in 1.5-h urine; and 3.32, 0.30 to 11.73 in 6-h urine after the three loads, respectively). Another advantage in orotic acid measurement is the stability of the compound: Urine samples can be sent via post at room temperature for orotic acid measurement, but blood ammonia has to be measured immediately.[46,122]

Serum urea concentration has been high-normal or even slightly elevated during the first few months of life, but later it has been consistently below the normal mean and often subnormal, the mean of 126 determinations in the patients being 3.7 μ*M* (range, 1.5 to 8.5 μ*M;* normal, 2 to 7 μ*M*).[35] Serum urea increases slowly after nitrogen loading in the patients.[8,35]

Other Laboratory Tests

Slight normochromic or hypochromic anemia with anisocytosis and poikilocytosis is common.[8,35,63,75,111] Most patients have leukopenia, and the platelet count is decreased, in some young patients not uncommonly to less than $30 \times 10^3/m^3$. Reticulocyte count is often slightly elevated, and the osmotic resistance of the erythrocytes, the red cell indexes, and the serum iron level and iron binding capacity are normal. In some patients, autoerythrophagocytosis or erythroblastophagocytosis has been observed in the bone marrow,[20,22,32,51] and the number of megakaryocytes may be increased; in one patient the marrow was hypoplastic with pathologic megaloblastic erythrocyte precursor forms, and in another the marrow was dyserythropoetic, suggesting ineffective erythropoesis.[75] It is interesting that the changes in the peripheral blood cells decrease in intensity during and after puberty, and values in adults are usually within the range of healthy subjects.

The blood pH and the serum concentrations of sodium, potassium, chloride, calcium, and phosphate are normal. Serum low-density lipoprotein (LDL) and high-density lipoprotein (HDL) cholesterol values are often high in older children and adults, probably because the patients replace a large part of their protein calories by fat in the diet. In animals, high orotic acid concentrations influence lipoprotein metabolism,[126] but the possible link between orotic acidemia and hyperlipidemia in LPI is unclear. The triglycerides are usually slightly elevated in the patients. No constant abnormal peaks have been found in analyses of organic acids in the urine.

Interestingly, several of the patients with different ethnic backgrounds and all the Finnish patients have consistently had significantly increased concentrations of lactate dehydrogenase (LDH) and ferritin in serum.[22,35,127] All LDH isoenzymes, but most significantly the liver isoenzyme, are affected; the values are usually two to five times higher than the upper limit of normal. The LDH and ferritin values increase further during complications of the disease, including pulmonary alveolar proteinosis (see "Complications and Autopsy Findings" above). Thyroxine-binding globulin (TBG) is also elevated in the patients, and, consequently, measurements of total T_4 give high values; free T_4 is normal, and the patients are clinically euthyroid.[34,35,128,129] Whether there is a general increase in hormone carrier proteins or only a specific increase in TBG is not known.

In two Japanese patients, growth hormone responsiveness to glucagon, propranolol, arginine, and insulin was studied as a possible cause for the delayed growth and bone age of the patients.[34] The response to insulin was moderately decreased in the one patient studied before arginine supplementation was started, but all responses were normal when the patients had been on arginine supplementation for 8 months.

Kekomäki and coworkers[130] confirmed that the activities of the urea cycle enzymes in liver biopsy samples of the patients were normal. Glutaminase I activity, once suggested to be the basic defect in patients with LPI,[16,21,29] has since been proven to be normal in both leukocytes and liver.[131] Likewise, the activity of ornithine aminotransferase, the enzyme responsible for the main catabolic pathway of ornithine, has been normal or slightly elevated in the liver and cultured fibroblasts of the patients.[57,132,133] The concentration of *N*-acetylglutamine and the rate of its synthesis have not been measured in the patients, but the efficient production of orotic acid by the patients[13,22,122,134] strongly suggests that this cofactor and regulator of the carbamyl phosphate synthase activity[135] is available in sufficient quantities.

PATHOPHYSIOLOGY

Normal Cellular Transport of Cationic Amino Acids

In normal physiology, cationic and other amino acids reach the body only by passing through the intestinal wall in the process of absorption. They do this mainly as free amino acids but also partly as dipeptides and other small peptides, which then are hydrolyzed to free amino acids at the luminal brush border and, predominantly, in the cytoplasm of the epithelial cells.[136-141] During absorption, the amino acids first cross the luminal membrane of the epithelial cell. A fraction of the amino acids is used in cellular metabolism in the cytoplasm ("metabolic runout"),[142,143] and the remainder must cross the basolateral (antiluminal) membrane of the cell to reach the body. In the cytoplasm, the amino acids may also enter the subcellular organelles (mitochondria, lysosomes, other vesicles, etc.), where some amino acids are metabolized. In adult intestine, only free amino acids, not peptides, are able to cross the whole cell in absorption.

Absorption of the cationic amino acids lysine, arginine, and ornithine has been extensively studied in the kidneys,[136,144-157] intestine,[158-160] and some parenchymal tissues[161-163] of animals and human beings. Most studies have included cyst(e)ine, because in cystinuria the transport of all four amino acids is affected.[148,158,164-179] I·: the kidney, reabsorption occurs along the full length of the nephron. The proximal segment of the tubule receives the highest load of filtered amino acids and, consequently, has to absorb a significant load quickly and efficiently, whereas further down in the tubule a more selective reabsorption system would be more profitable. Such axial heterogeneity[143,180] in absorption has indeed been demonstrated for several amino acids, including the cationic amino acids. The net handling of the cationic amino acids in the kidney and their mutual interactions have been studied by administering amino acid loads and then measuring the urinary excretion and renal clearances of the amino acids.[170,171,174,181-183] Microperfusions of animal nephrons[149,153,177,178] and flux measurements in nephron segments or tubule fragments,[149,150,166,184] in renal cortical slices,[148,151,152,166] in cultured tubule-cells,[185] and in isolated vesicles prepared from the brush border[146,155,172,186,187] or basolateral cell membrane[157] have been performed. The transport of the cationic amino acids across the luminal membrane occurs via a shared, Na^+-dependent system. The system selective for the cationic amino acids in the proximal convoluted tubule has high capacity and low affinity,[150] whereas the system in the proximal straight segment has low capacity and high affinity and is shared with cystine.[149]

At the basolateral membrane in the kidney tubules, the transport of the cationic amino acids is not shared with cystine, and both high- and low-affinity systems are used. The transport from the cell to the pericellular space (efflux) occurs via Na^+-independent exchange diffusion, which may be shared with cystine on the cytoplasmic surface.[143,157,166]

At the brush border of the intestinal epithelium, the cationic amino acids are transported by a single Na^+-dependent system, which has high affinity and is shared by all cationic amino acids and cystine.[188,189]

White and Christensen[162] and others[161,168,185,190] have carefully characterized transport of cationic amino acids in cultured or isolated cells using human fibroblasts,[161,168,191] permanent hepatoma cell lines, rat hepatocytes,[162] and other cells.[185,190] Transport of cationic amino acid into human fibroblasts occurs by a saturable mediation, which they designated "system y^+" (earlier called Ly^+). The system serves the flow of ω-guanidino amino acids and ω, α-diamino acids. The uptake of cationic substrates by system y^+ is Na^+-independent, pH-insensitive, stereoselective, and inhibitable by neutral amino acids in the presence of Na^+ ion. This system is not shared with cystine.[164,168] The uptake and efflux of the substrates are strongly stimulated by cationic amino acids inside and outside the cell, respectively. Arginine and homoarginine accumulate in human fibroblasts and can reach distribution ratios of more than 20 at physiological external amino acid concentrations.[161] The driving force appears to be the transmembrane voltage.

In hepatoma cell lines, the transport of cationic amino acids occurs by the saturable mediation of the system y^+.[162] The influx into hepatoma cells has all the characteristics seen also in the system y^+ of the fibroblasts, including strong stimulation by cationic amino acids inside the cell, i.e., trans-stimulation. In normal hepatocytes, no significant trans-stimulation was observed, suggesting that the y^+ system is absent in these cells. The rate at which arginine is transported at the hepatocyte plasma membrane suggests that transport is the rate-limiting step in hydrolysis of arginine by arginase.

Recently, a more detailed analysis of amino acid transport at diverse cellular membranes has led to the discovery of at least three separate transport systems for the cationic amino acids. Furthermore, direct studies of some cationic amino acid transport proteins has become possible after cloning of the respective genes (see "Genetics" below).

Mutations in the Transport of Cationic Amino Acids

In a long series of studies, Segal and coworkers,[176] States and coworkers,[185] and others[160,164,165,169-175,192] have analyzed the interactions of the cationic amino acids and cystine in transport mutations, especially in the cystinuric kidney (see Chap. 117). Scriver and coworkers have provided a detailed review of current knowledge of the transport mutations in cystinuria and other cationic aminoacidurias.[143]

In classic cystinuria, reabsorption of cystine and the cationic amino acids in the kidney tubules is selectively impaired, occasionally to the extent that measurements show net tubular secretion of cystine or lysine.[154,193] In normal tubules, cystine, lysine, arginine, and ornithine mutually compete for transport. Intravenous loading studies in cystinuria suggest that the residual reclamation of cationic amino acids and cystine follows rules of competition similar to those in the normal tubules.[169,174] An absorption defect has also been found in the intestinal epithelium in vivo[175] and in biopsy samples of the jejunum.[158,160] Measurement of unidirectional and net fluxes of cationic amino acids in intestinal biopsy samples of patients with cystinuria clearly shows that the transport defect is localized at the luminal membrane of the epithelial cells.[188] Most likely, the efflux permeability of the luminal membrane is increased, but the influx is normal.[189]

Is the transport defect in patients with LPI similar to that in cystinuria? In their first report on LPI, Perheentupa and Visakorpi[1] had access only to semiquantitative measurement of plasma and urinary amino acids, and they regarded the urinary amino acid excretion as identical to that in cystinuria. It soon became apparent that cystine was excreted in significantly smaller quantities than in cystinuria, and Kekomäki and coworkers[6,8] suggested that the mechanisms of the transport defects differ in the two diseases. Absorption of the cationic amino acids by the kidneys[10,15,25,121,156] and small intestine[9,23,24,33,55,194-196] in LPI has later been carefully characterized. In both organs, absorption of lysine, arginine, and ornithine is defective. The slight increase in renal cystine losses could be explained by the excessive tubular lysine load and normal competition for absorption in the kidney tubules. Oral loading with the dipeptide lysylglycine increased plasma glycine concentrations properly, but plasma lysine remained almost unchanged in the patients[55] (Fig. 118-5). This was in striking contrast to the control subjects, in whom concentrations of both amino acids of the dipeptide increased in plasma. LPI was thus the first human disease in which a defect in peptide absorption was recognized. Because the transport of oligopeptides is not shared with transport of free amino acids at the luminal membrane of the enterocyte, the lysine-containing dipeptide enters the cell normally in LPI. The absorbed peptides are hydrolyzed to free amino acids mainly in the cytoplasm of the enterocyte,[137,138,197] and they are able to cross the basolateral membrane only as free amino acids. The missing increase in plasma lysine after the lysylglycine load but normal increase in plasma glycine shows that the intracellularly released dipeptide-derived lysine is unable to cross the basolateral (antiluminal) membrane of the enterocyte and strongly suggests that the transport defect in LPI is localized at this membrane in the epithelial cells.

In vitro studies of unidirectional and net transport of cationic amino acids in jejunal biopsy samples of the patients soon proved even more directly that the transport defect is situated at the basolateral (antiluminal) membrane of the epithelial cell.[57] These in vitro results differed clearly from identical experiments in cystinuria,[189] where the abnormality in lysine transport was located at the luminal membrane, and the defect in cystine absorption could perhaps best be explained by increased efflux permeability at the luminal membrane of the epithelium. Interestingly, in an earlier study of cationic amino acid accumulation in jejunal biopsy samples and uptake during intestinal perfusion in LPI, no defects could be found.[194] This failure is understandable now, when the defect in LPI has been localized at the antiluminal membrane, and we know that the epithelial cells in LPI accumulate higher-than-normal concentrations of the cationic amino acids (see below).

Rajantie and coworkers[56] gave patients with LPI prolonged intravenous infusions of citrulline and measured

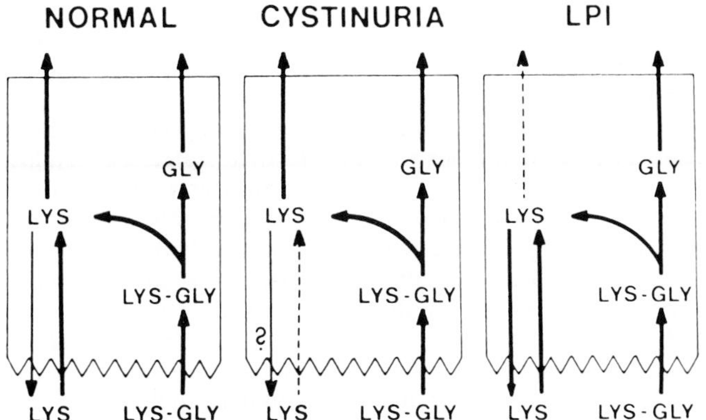

FIG. 118-5. Schematic representation of brush border cells of jejunal mucosa, showing absorption of diamino acids (here lysine, in free and dipeptide form) and suggested sites of defect in cystinuria and LPI. Defective fluxes are indicated by dashed arrows. LYS = lysine. (*From Rajantie et al.*[55] *Used by permission.*)

plasma and urinary amino acids during the loading. Compared with controls, the plasma citrulline concentration of the patients increased normally, but urinary citrulline excretion increased excessively. Rises in plasma arginine and ornithine during the loading were subnormal, but massive argininuria and moderate ornithinuria appeared (Fig. 118-6). The excretion rates of lysine and other amino acids remained practically unaltered, thus excluding mutual competition as the cause for the increases. This finding is compatible with a transport defect at the basolateral membrane of the renal tubule cells and can be explained as follows: Citrulline as a neutral amino acid does not use the cationic amino acid transport system; citrulline is partly converted to arginine and further to ornithine in the tubule cell as an integral part of the reabsorption process; in LPI, formed arginine and ornithine are unable to exit at the antiluminal membrane, their intracellular concentrations increase, and backflux (argininuria and ornithinuria) into the lumen occurs; high intracellular arginine and ornithine concentrations inhibit citrulline metabolism in

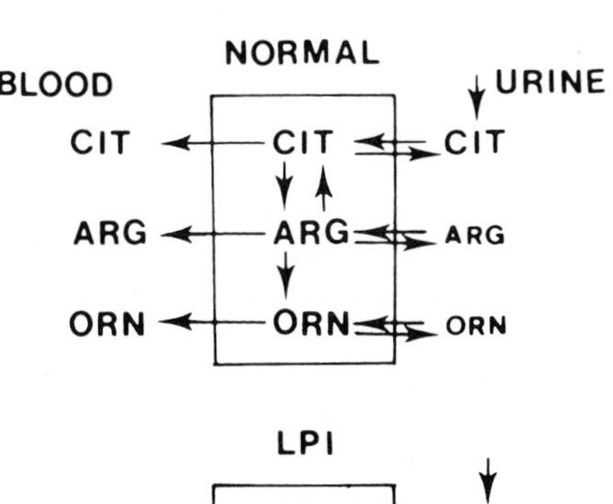

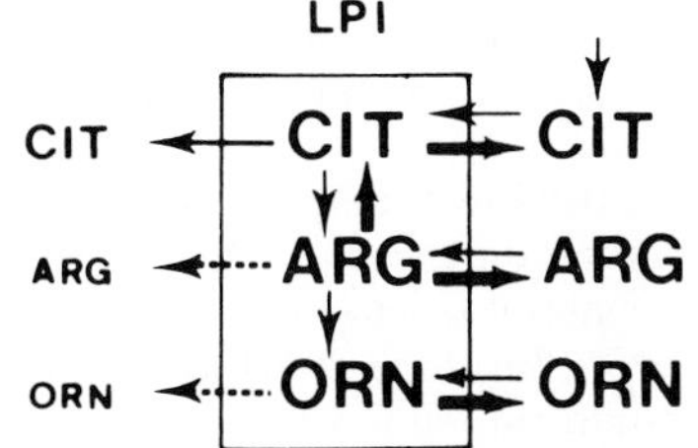

FIG. 118-6. Suggested mechanism of tubular reabsorption of citrulline in human beings and of the pathophysiology of the massive argininuria and moderate citrullinuria and ornithinuria in LPI. Bold type and arrows indicate increased concentrations and fluxes; thin type and dotted arrows indicate decreased concentrations and impaired fluxes. (*From Rajantie et al.*[56] *Used by permission*)

the tubule cell; intracellular citrulline concentration increases, and leads to citrullinuria.

Reabsorption curves for arginine and ornithine have been produced in patients with LPI by increasing the plasma concentration of arginine or ornithine in a stepwise manner and simultaneously measuring tubular filtration rate and plasma concentration and urinary excretion of the two amino acids.[121] The curves were clearly below those of healthy control subjects at all loads except at values close to the tubular reabsorption maxima of the controls, where the patients' curves approached those of the control subjects. It is possible that at such filtered loads (at plasma concentrations of several millimolar), active transport plays a minor part, and physical factors regulate the amount of reabsorption. The extrarenal metabolic clearances of arginine and ornithine by tissues, calculated from the same infusion experiments, were significantly decreased in the patients.[198] This finding suggests that besides the defect in epithelial transport, transport in LPI is abnormal in other tissues as well.[190]

A direct proof of such an extraepithelial transport defect was obtained in studies of Smith and coworkers,[58] who investigated steady-state amino acid concentrations in intact fibroblasts (Table 118-3), and influx (Figs. 118-7 and 118-8), efflux, and trans-stimulation of the transport of lysine and other cationic amino acids and their nonmetabolized analogues[199] in cultured fibroblasts of the patients (Fig. 118-9). In trans-stimulation experiments, the amino acid in question, or another amino acid which uses the same transport system, is present on the other side of the membrane than the labeled amino studied. The influx at the plasma membrane was not different from controls in LPI; trans-stimulated efflux was. A defect in trans-stimulation was found also in fibroblasts of the heterozygotes with values about 50 percent of that in homozygotes suggesting gene-dosage effect (Fig. 118-10). The results also imply that the basolateral membrane of epithelial cells and the plasma membrane of parenchymal cells are functionally analogous at least in transport of cationic amino acids, but it may well be that this analogy is a general physiological principle. Vesicles prepared from LPI fibroblast plasma membranes failed to show a transport defect for cationic amino acids.[200] This finding possibly is explained by the fact that the preparation of the vesicles favored equally formation of inside-out and right-side-out vesicles. If both forms are present in equal quantities, and the defect is only expressed in efflux, the sum effect in the mixture of the vesicles with be the same as in controls.

Table 118-3 Steady-State Amino Acid Concentrations in Intact Cultured Fibroblasts of a Control Subject and a Patient with Lysinuric Protein Intolerance

	Concentration Ratio	
Amino Acid	Control	LPI
Lysine/alanine	0.23±0.007	0.35±0.014
Ornithine/alanine	0.11±0.009	0.19±0.008
Arginine/alanine	0.40±0.024	0.54±0.012
Leucine/alanine	0.30±0.016	0.31±0.015

NOTE: Human skin fibroblasts were maintained in culture medium 24 h prior to harvest with a rubber policeman. Cells were resuspended in 1 ml phosphate-buffered saline, sonicated, and deproteinized. The supernatants were assayed for amino acid content with a Durrum D-500 amino acid analyzer. Values are the mean ± SEM, n = 4. Amino acid values were normalized to fibroblast alanine concentrations, which were 18 ± 1.3 and 17 ± 1.2 pmol/mg protein in control and LPI cells, respectively.

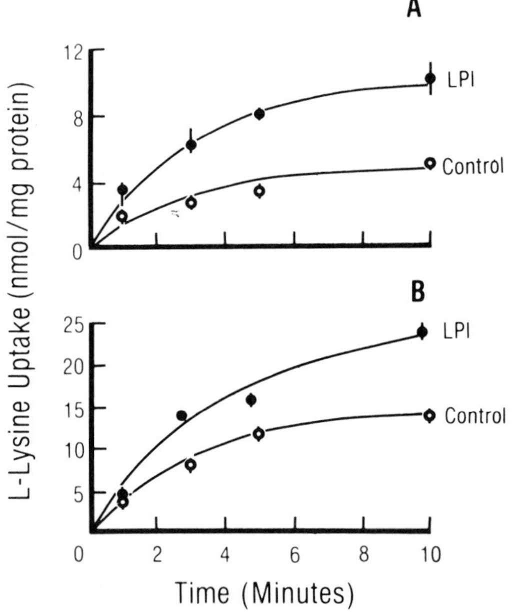

FIG. 118-7. L-lysine uptake by cultured fibroblasts from a control subject (open circles) and a patient with LPI (solid circles). The cells were incubated for 90 min at 37°C in buffer without arginine (*A*) or in buffer containing 1 m*M* arginine (*B*), washed twice with PBS (37°C), and then incubated for 1, 3, 5, or 10 min at 37°C in PBS containing 0.1 m*M* L-[^{3}H]lysine. Data are means and ranges of two or three measurements. (*From Smith et al.*[58] *Used by permission.*)

Smith and others[201] measured transport of the cationic amino acids and their nonmetabolized analogues in isolated erythrocytes of the patients. The mutant erythrocytes had identical transport characteristics with the controls, and the authors concluded that the mutant transporter is not expressed on the surface of mature human erythrocytes.

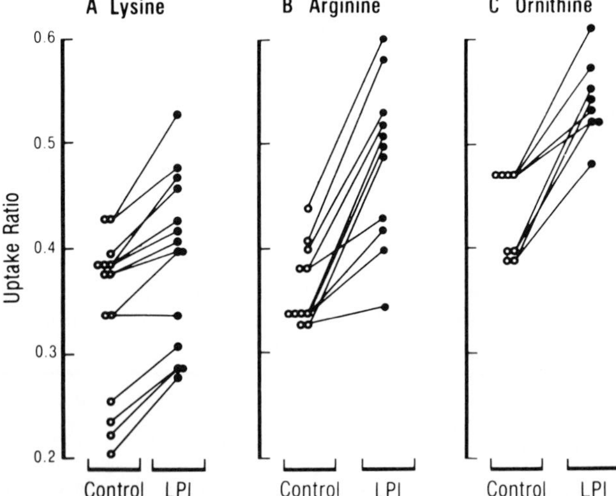

FIG. 118-8. Uptake ratios of the cationic amino acids versus L-leucine at steady state in cultured fibroblasts of control subjects and patients with lysinuric protein intolerance. The cells were incubated for 10 min at 37°C in PBS containing 0.1 m*M* L-[^{3}H]leucine and (*A*) 0.1 m*M* L-[^{14}C]lysine, (*B*) L-[^{14}C]arginine, or (*C*) L-[^{14}C]ornithine. Each point represents a single measurement of the net isotopic molar uptake ratio (cationic amino acid/leucine) in paired control and LPI cell strains. The differences between control and LPI cells for uptake of L-lysine ($n = 13, p < 0.02$), L-arginine ($n = 16, p < 0.01$), and L-ornithine ($n = 8, p < 0.01$) are significant by the Wilcoxon signed rank tests. (*From Smith et al.*[58] *Used by permission.*)

The findings are in agreement with those of Gardner and Levy,[202] who noticed that the transport of dibasic amino acids in human erythrocytes is temperature-dependent, incapable of uphill transport, and not dependent on extracellular sodium or potassium concentrations or on energy derived from cellular metabolism. They further stated that lysine transport in human erythrocytes comprises two saturable, carrier-mediated processes operating in parallel: One is a high-affinity, low-capacity process that predominates at low lysine concentrations; the other is a low-affinity, high-capacity process that predominates at higher lysine concentrations. Further studies on cationic amino acid transport in rabbit reticulocytes[203] and human erythrocytes[204] have clarified details of the transport phenomena in these specialized cells.

Subcellular Transport of Cationic Amino Acids

In the urea cycle, the urea molecule is assembled on an ornithine backbone; cleavage of the urea from arginine regenerates free ornithine. During the cycle, ornithine has to pass from the cytoplasm into the mitochondrial matrix to be carbamylated, and the formed citrulline has to be exported back to the cytoplasm to be further exposed by the enzyme argininosuccinic acid synthase. Whether or not mitochondrial transport processes are involved in the pathophysiology of LPI remains an open question.[205] In rat liver mitochondria and in mitochondria of human cultured fibroblasts, ornithine and citrulline transport has been relatively well characterized. In the classic study of Gamble and Lehninger,[206] the entry of ornithine into the mitochondria of rat liver was mediated by a carrier that was respiratory-dependent and required permeant proton-yielding anions for function.

Ornithine fluxes in mitochondria were earlier measured in the absence of active citrulline synthesis.[207-218] The study of Cohen and coworkers[213] avoided this pitfall: They analyzed the transport phenomena during and without citrulline synthesis in respiring rat liver mitochondria. They were able to characterize both influx of ornithine and efflux of citrulline in the mitochondria. When respiring mitochondria were preloaded with cold ornithine and then incubated in [^{3}H]ornithine, the mitochondria produced citrulline of the same specific activity as that of external ornithine, but ornithine in mitochondrial matrix remained unlabeled. The concentration of ornithine in the matrix was also extremely low when the ornithine concentration in the incubation medium was less than 1 m*M*. Both findings imply that the ornithine molecule is not transported into the matrix randomly, but is channeled to the intramitochondrial enzymes for further processing to citrulline. The importance of ornithine catabolism by the matrix enzyme ornithine aminotransferase for the net movement of ornithine has remained unclear, but the activity in liver mitochondria is such that all ornithine not immediately used in the urea cycle is transaminated (see Chap. 32).

Studies of citrulline transport in rat liver mitochondria have suggested that the transport mechanisms do not depend on respiratory energy or the presence of permeant cations or anions.[206,212,213] Citrulline transport occurs in liver mitochondria but not in mitochondria of the heart.[206] Some studies have also implied that an ornithine–citrulline antiporter exists in the mitochondrial membrane,[210] but this finding may have been an artifact caused by experimental circumstances in which citrulline was not formed.[211,213]

Recently, increasing evidence has accumulated suggesting that mitochondrial ornithine transport is genetically altered

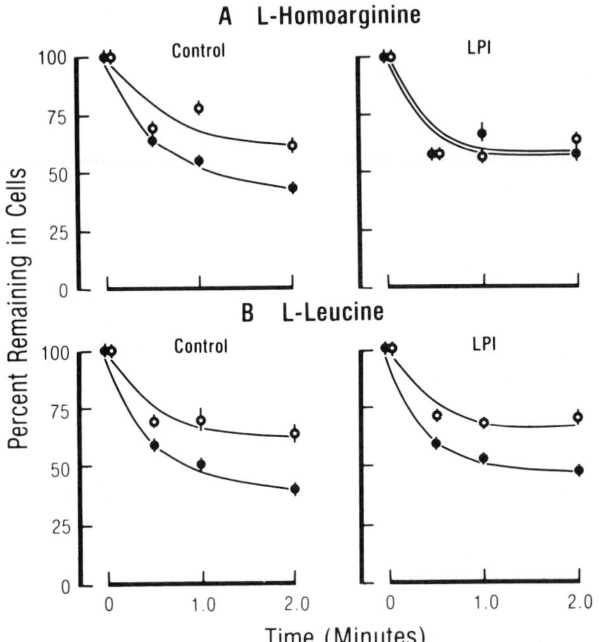

FIG. 118-9. Efflux of L-homoarginine from cultured skin fibroblasts of a control and LPI cell line. The cells were incubated for 40 min at 37°C in buffer containing (*A*) 0.1 m*M* L-[^{3}H]homoarginine and (*B*) 0.1 m*M* L-[^{14}C]leucine. The time course of efflux was measured into unlabeled incubation buffer (trans-zero condition, open circles) or into buffer containing 1 m*M* unlabeled amino acid (trans-stimulated condition, solid circles). Time course for efflux from the cellular pool is shown. Zero-time homoarginine content (100 percent value) was 2.8 ± 0.16 (control) and 2.9 ± 0.29 (LPI) nmol/mg protein; zero-time leucine content was 8.5 ± 0.37 (control) and 9.8 ± 0.59 (LPI) nmol/mg protein. The difference in the zero-time leucine content for LPI and control cells was not significant. Each point represents the mean and SEM of four determinations. (*From Smith et al.*[58] *Used by permission.*)

in another human urea cycle disease, the hyperornithinemia–hyperammonemia–homocitrullinuria (HHH) syndrome[112,215,216,218-226] (see Chap. 31). If the plasma membranes of cultured fibroblasts are made permeable to amino acids by digitonin, accumulation of labeled ornithine can be measured in the particulate fraction of the cells, which mainly contains mitochondria.[223,224] Such studies have suggested that ornithine accumulation in mitochondria is decreased in fibroblasts and liver of patients with the HHH syndrome.[220,221,223,224,227] If cultured HHH fibroblasts are incubated with labeled ornithine, a subnormal fraction of label is found in CO_2, implying that ornithine is unable to enter the mitochondria to be further metabolized.[215,216,218-221,225,227]

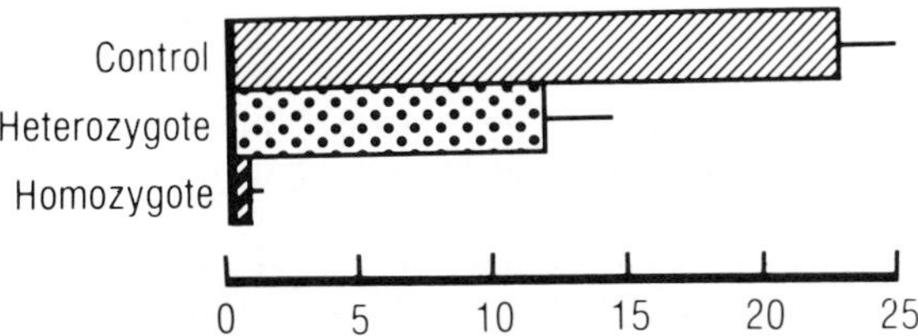

FIG. 118-10. Percent trans-stimulation of homoarginine efflux from cultured skin fibroblasts of control cells and cells from homozygotes and heterozygotes for LPI. The cells were preincubated for 40 min at 37°C in buffer containing 0.1 m*M* L-[^{3}H]homoarginine and 0.1 m*M* L-[^{14}C]leucine. The 1-min efflux of label was measured as described in Figure 118-9. "Trans-stimulation" refers to the difference (increase) between trans-zero and trans-stimulated efflux, normalized to zero-time cellular isotope. Each value represents the mean of three or four determinations on one cell line; error bars indicate the range. (*From Smith et al.*[58] *Used by permission.*)

A mitochondrial transport defect also has been proposed to have a part in the pathophysiology of LPI.[205] This theory has been based on biochemical results that speak against cytoplasmic ornithine deficiency in this disease. First, biopsy samples from the intestinal epithelium accumulate higher-than-normal concentrations of the cationic amino acids in vitro.[57] Second, LPI fibroblasts also accumulate higher-than-normal concentrations of cationic amino acids.[58,59] Third, direct measurements of concentrations of the cationic amino acids in liver biopsy samples of the patients contain normal or elevated concentrations of the cationic amino acids, even though their plasma concentrations are decreased.[24,205] Fourth, there is evidence that citrulline formation is not impaired: Plasma concentration of citrulline is constantly high-normal or elevated in the patients[8,30,31,34,35]; citrulline concentration is high-normal or increased in liver biopsy samples of the patients[24,205]; and the extrarenal metabolic clearance of citrulline and conversion of citrulline to arginine and ornithine are retarded[54,205] (Fig. 118-11).

These conflicting findings have been reconciled in a hypothesis which suggests that in LPI a defect in the efflux of the cationic amino acids exists at the plasma membrane of the liver cells or, if the cells retain polarity, at the basolateral membrane, and that the transport defect is expressed also in the mitochondria.[205] Such a mitochondrial defect would further increase cytoplasmic concentrations

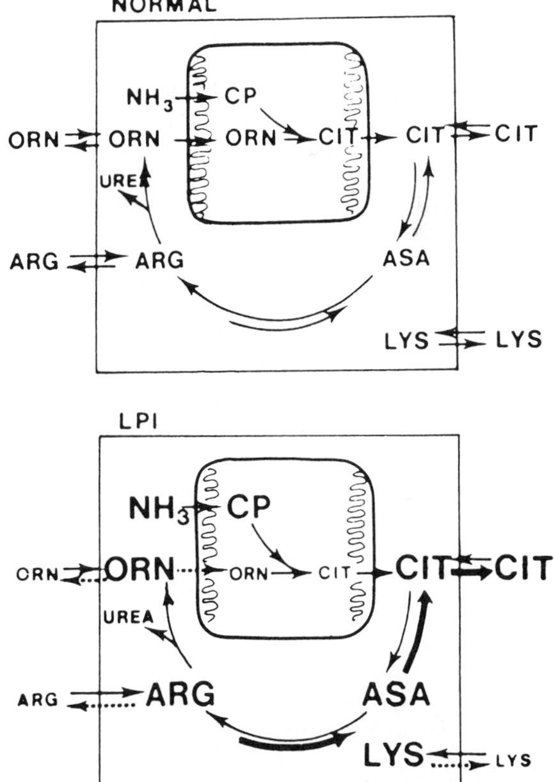

FIG. 118-11. Hypothetical mechanism of the elevated plasma citrulline concentration and the urea cycle failure in LPI. Bold type and arrows indicate supranormal concentrations and fluxes; thin type and dotted arrows, subnormal concentrations and impaired fluxes. For simplicity, only those fluxes are shown that are present at the "basolateral" and mitochondrial membranes of the liver cells. (*From Rajantie et al.*[205] *Used by permission.*)

of arginine and ornithine. Depletion of ornithine in the mitochondria would lead to accumulation of carbamyl phosphate and to hyperammonemia. This theory, though interesting, has recently been questioned because the oxidation of ornithine in cultured LPI fibroblasts proceeds normally.[59]

System y^+ for the cationic amino acids is expressed on the lysosomal membranes and used at least for influx of the cationic amino acids.[228] Normal lysosomes have active and selective efflux mechanisms for cystine, sialic acid, and probably other substances[229-234] (see Chap. 126). Efflux of other amino acids from the lysosomes is strictly limited as is suggested by the disruption of rat liver lysosomes if they are filled by passive diffusion with amino acid methyl esters.[234] These esters are hydrolyzed by lysosomal enzymes, but the liberated amino acids cannot readily escape from the lysosomes, possibly because of their high polarity. They accumulate in the lysosomes and may cause osmotic lysis of the organelles. In LPI, the lysosomes or other vesicular organelles might function as a metabolically excluded pool of lysine and other cationic amino acids, so that the actual cytoplasmic lysine concentration would be relatively normal or even low. No direct proof of such a transport defect has been obtained, but the hypothesis is attractive.

Malfunction of the Urea Cycle

Patients with LPI have decreased nitrogen tolerance and exhibit hyperammonemia after ingestion of even moderate amounts of protein.[8,11,14,35,75,122] The urea cycle failure is clearly less severe than in the "first" enzyme defects of the cycle, i.e., in deficiencies of carbamyl phosphate synthase, ornithine transcarbamylase, and *N*-acetylglutamate synthase, or even in a deficiency of argininosuccinate synthase or lyase (see Chap. 32). The clinical impression is that the tendency to hyperammonemia in LPI closely resembles that seen in patients with the HHH syndrome.[112,219,221-223,226]

Already in the first description of the disease, Perheentupa and Visakorpi[1] noticed that intravenous infusion of ornithine during a loading with protein or intravenous L-alanine prevented the hyperammonemia that otherwise followed the loadings. An identical effect has since been shown with arginine and citrulline when given intravenously.[8,11,14,35,123,195]

Oral supplementation with arginine and ornithine has been only minimally effective in these patients, because both amino acids are poorly absorbed from the intestine and easily produce diarrhea.[10,57,196,235] Obviously the absorption defect is not total because a low-protein diet and arginine or ornithine supplementation have improved growth and decreased hyperammonemia in patients with LPI.[6-8,13,17,28,32,63] A few variant patients tolerate arginine or ornithine supplementation well.[13,17,28,32] Awrich et al.[14] showed that the neutral amino acid citrulline, also an intermediate in the urea cycle, when taken as an oral supplement prevents hyperammonemia. It is well tolerated by LPI patients,[11,30] and its effect of preventing hyperammonemia in LPI has now been well documented.[61,122] As a neutral amino acid, it passes the cell membranes normally in LPI and is rapidly converted in the body to arginine and then to ornithine.

Poor intestinal absorption, excessive loss in the urine, and low plasma concentrations of the cationic amino acids arginine and ornithine strongly suggest that the malfunctioning of the urea cycle is caused by deficiencies of these urea cycle intermediates (Fig. 118-1). The finding that hyperammonemia produced by amino nitrogen or protein loads could effectively be prevented by simultaneous intravenous infusion of arginine or ornithine led to the hypothesis that the malfunctioning of the cycle was caused by a deficiency of ornithine in the liver cell.[1,4,236] Even now, when increasing evidence supports the view that the intracellular concentration of the cationic amino acids is increased in these patients in both epithelial and parenchymal cells,[24,205] the malfunction is best explained as a "functional deficiency" of the intermediates. In reality, it is possible that enzymes of the urea cycle are inhibited by an increased intracellular concentration of lysine (see Chap. 32) or that a transport defect at the inner mitochondrial membrane prevents the entry of ornithine into the mitochondria, just as hypothesized in the HHH syndrome (see Chap. 31). Such a defect would decrease the ornithine concentration in the mitochondrial matrix, decrease transcarbamylation, and slow down urea production. It is also possible that cytoplasmic concentrations of the cationic amino acids actually are diminished because of accumulation of these substances in lysosomes or some other vesicular organelles. In such a case, cytoplasmic ornithine concentration could be temporarily increased by supplementation with arginine or ornithine. Similar genetic defects are known for transporters in lysosomal membranes (see Chap. 126). These defects all cause reduced efflux from the lysosomes; this is the case at least in cystinosis and Salla disease. An efflux defect could theoretically explain pooling and cytoplasmic depletion of the cationic amino acids in LPI, but our knowledge of amino acid movements into and out of the lysosomes is too sparse, and no direct data to confirm the hypothesis of a lysosomal or vesicular efflux defect exist.

Half of the urea nitrogen originates as free ammonium, which enters the urea cycle by way of carbamyl phosphate synthesis, but this nitrogen does not gain access to the liver cell as free ammonium.[237,238] Animal experiments have suggested that the amide nitrogen of glutamine is an important precursor of urea nitrogen; glutamine functions as a transport and storage form of ammonium ion to keep its tissue levels within tolerable ranges via glutamine synthetase.[16] The ammonium for carbamyl phosphate synthesis is released from glutamine by intramitochondrial glutaminase, which was found to be defective in the leukocytes of one patient.[16,21] The suspected defect in glutaminase led to an interesting hypothesis of the mechanism of the transport disorder in LPI,[16] but later studies did not confirm the deficiency of glutaminase in leukocytes or liver biopsy samples of other patients.[131]

It is possible that during large nitrogen inflow—i.e., after protein meals—intrahepatic glutamine synthesis serves to trap free ammonium and amino groups from other amino acids. Plasma glutamine is constantly high in LPI, and its fluctuations seem to be related to the previous nitrogen loading. Exact knowledge of the nitrogen flow in the liver during protein absorption is lacking, and the rate-limiting step in urea formation is not known. It may well be that the rate-limiting step varies and depends on several other factors, including the availability of the substrates.[206,208,213,214,217,239-241]

Patients with LPI efficiently produce orotic acid after nitrogen loading.[22,46,122] This cytoplasmic pathway could theoretically serve as a means to excrete excessive nitrogen from the body via carbamyl phosphate and aspartate, i.e., the same substrates as in the urea cycle.[242,243] The level of renal clearance and urinary excretion of orotic acid is high, but the overall capacity of the pathway is limited, and only relatively small amounts of excess nitrogen can be excreted as orotate even during loading conditions.[134] It is interesting that uracil is also excreted in excess in LPI.[22]

Lysine Deficiency

Despite prevention of hyperammonemia by citrulline supplementation and a low-protein diet, several features of the disease have remained unaltered in treated patients. Growth has not totally normalized, bone age is delayed, liver and spleen are enlarged, and liver pathology is unaltered.[11,35] The hematologic abnormalities have also persisted during therapy, osteoporosis persists, and the patients are prone to develop life-threatening pulmonary alveolar proteinosis or pulmonary cholesterol granulomas. These are possibly signs of a continuing deficiency of lysine, whose bioavailability is significantly reduced by the poor intestinal absorption and heavy renal losses.[4,55,121,196] In addition to the transport defects in the epithelial cells, which lead to poor net reclamation of lysine in the body, the transport defect at the plasma membrane of the parenchymal cells and the proposed transport defects in cell organelles also may contribute to the suspected lysine deficiency.[58,205]

Lysine is an integral part of practically all proteins. Relatively speaking, collagen is especially rich in lysine. The pathophysiological mechanisms of the often prominent osteoporosis in patients with LPI have remained uncertain.[63-65] It may well be that the osteoporosis is caused by lysine deficiency, which delays formation of the bone matrix and is an important factor in poor formation of other essential structural proteins and additional proteins.[244-248] Nothing is known of the acute or long-term effects of intravenous lysine infusions or oral supplementation with absorbable lysine derivatives in osteoporosis in LPI. Rajantie and coworkers found that ε-*N*-acetyllysine but not homocitrulline efficiently increases plasma lysine in patients with LPI.[249] Acetyllysine uses a transport system different from that of the cationic amino acids, making it suitable for oral use. Despite the apparently fast metabolism of acetyllysine to lysine in human beings, its suitability for lysine replacement may be limited. In mice fed synthetic amino acid diets, replacement of L-lysine with ε-*N*-methyl-L-lysine, ε-*N*-dimethyl-L-lysine, or ε-*N*-trimethyl-L-lysine resulted in relative replacement values of about 1/12, 1/20, and 1/25, respectively, of the value obtained with the standard lysine diet.[250] α-*N*-acetyl-L-lysine was not used by mice, and the replacement value of the ε-*N*-acetyllysine was about 3 percent that of lysine. Replacement of the charged ε-amino group in lysine with a sulfur-containing group led to weight reduction. *N*-phosphorylated lysine has not been tested in this system.[251]

Arginine is an essential amino acid in inborn errors of the urea cycle and probably in growing children[114,115] and some animals, at least the cat.[252,253] However, arginine deficiency is unlikely to play a role in the symptoms in LPI because ample amounts of arginine should be available during citrulline supplementation.[11,14,63,195]

Serum Ferritin, LDH, and TBG. Serum concentrations of ferritin, LDH, and TBG have been consistently elevated in these patients.[22,35,75] The cause of the high concentration of ferritin is its decreased catabolism in the liver,[111,127] but the reason for this decrease is not known. High ferritin and LDH values have increased further during acute illnesses (see "Complications and Autopsy Findings" above). The increase in TBG and the associated increase in total T_4 has in some occasions led to suspicion of hyperthyroidism in these patients.

GENETICS

The inheritance of LPI follows a pattern typical for an autosomal recessive disease.[2,53] The incidence of the disease is 1 in 60,000 in Finland, but the birthplaces of the patients' grandparents are unevenly distributed in the country, and at least three large clusters of families can be recognized.[2,4,35,53] Most patients in other countries have been isolated cases[13-15,18,19,22,23,27,28,30,31,33,44-46,48-52] or multiple affected members of one family.[17,20,25,26,32,34,47,51]

Extensive functional studies have suggested that transport of amino acids into mammalian cells is mediated in different cell lines or tissues by a number of carrier proteins with differing characteristics.[161-163,208,254-259] Competition assays have shown that the cationic amino acids lysine, arginine, and ornithine share the same carrier(s), and that the kinetics of cationic amino acid uptake are similar in many tissues.[161-163,258,260] A widely expressed sodium-independent carrier system designated y^+ has been extensively studied[161-163,258,260] Another carrier, system $b^{0,+}$ is also Na^+-independent and accepts both cationic and neutral amino acids.[256,258] Some mammalian cells express a third, Na^+-dependent transport process, designated $B^{0,+}$.[257,258] The degree to which each of these three systems is expressed varies widely among cell types.[258]

Recently, a cDNA encoding a retroviral receptor (murine leukemia viral receptor REC1) was cloned from NIH 3T3 fibroblasts by expression in human bladder carcinoma cells, which are normally resistant to the virus owing to absence of receptor.[261] The cDNA encoded a 622 amino acid protein with 12 to 14 potential membrane-spanning domains. The extent of homology between the retroviral receptor and the arginine-histidine transporters of *Saccharomyces cerevisiae* (permeases CAN-1 and HIP-1)[262-264] raised the possibility that the physiological role of the receptor might be mediating cationic amino acid transport at the cell membrane.[265,266] Indeed, this hypothesis was confirmed by expression in *Xenopus* oocytes,[265,266] where the functional characteristics of the transporter were similar to those of the system y^+. Studies using northern blotting showed expression of mouse transporter RNA in a variety of tissues but not in the liver, again supporting the identity with system y^+.[161,258] This transport protein has now been renamed MCAT-1 (mouse cationic amino acid transporter-1) to better represent its physiological function.[267] Using mouse–human somatic cell hybrids, the human version of the mouse REC-1 gene, ATRC1, was soon assigned to chromosome 13, and in-situ hybridization localized the gene to 13q12-q14.[60] The locus shows restriction fragment length polymorphism with *Taq*I. Pairwise and multilocus linkage analyses have shown that the ATRC1 locus is close to the locus ATP1AL1 (ATPase, Na^+K^+, α-polypeptide-like 1) on one side and to the locus D13S6 on the other side.[60]

MCAT-1 is not expressed in freshly isolated rat hepatocytes or in normal rodent liver.[162,258,259] Furthermore, there are data suggesting that murine hepatocytes are resistant to ecotropic retrovirus infection, further suggesting that system y^+ is not expressed in hepatic tissues.[265,268] However, the liver plays a central role in balancing the peripheral amino acid supply after and between meals, and the flux of amino acids between the liver and other tissues is determined, in part, by the activity of specific transport proteins. Recently, a cDNA was isolated from a murine T cell lymphoma cell line that encoded a protein related to MCAT-1, named Tea

(T cell early activation).[269] Interestingly, the gene encoding Tea was expressed not only in activated T and B lymphocytes but also in liver. Hypothesizing that the Tea-encoded protein might be the hepatic cationic amino acid transporter, Closs and coworkers[267] found another cationic amino acid carrier (MCAT-2), which was closely related to Tea, was expressed in mouse liver, and had the same substrate specificity as the carrier in extrahepatic tissues. Furthermore, the MCAT-2 protein was encoded by the same gene as Tea, but differed in part of its sequence, presumably as a result of alternative splicing. Functional comparisons of the two transporters (the hepatic MCAT-2 and the more widely expressed MCAT-1 or y^+) in *Xenopus* oocytes showed that, unlike in the extrahepatic transporter, arginine uptake mediated by the MCAT-2 transporter is significant only at substrate concentrations that exceed systemic levels in plasma; its function is also less dependent on the intracellular concentration of the cationic amino acids. Thus, the properties of MCAT-2 suggest that it is the low-affinity transporter of cationic amino acids known to be expressed in the rodent (and human)[190] liver. These properties enable hepatocytes expressing this carrier to remove excess cationic amino acids from the blood without interfering with their uptake by extrahepatic tissues.[267]

Cloning by expression in *Xenopus* oocytes has recently resulted in the isolation of kidney and intestine-specific cDNA clones called rat D2,[270] rat NAA-Tr,[271] and rabbit rBAT.[272] These clones have about 80 percent amino acid sequence identity and induce high-affinity uptake into *Xenopus* oocytes of a broad spectrum of amino acids including cystine, and dibasic and neutral amino acids. These transporters are type II membrane glycoproteins and exhibit similarity to α-glucosidases and to 4F2 cell surface antigen heavy chain. The 4F2 protein also induces amino acid uptake into oocytes, but its substrate specificity is different.[270,273-275] It may well be that D2, rBAT, and the 4F2 heavy chain are not transporters as such but belong to a group of regulatory subunits of heterooligomeric transporters or are independent transport regulators.[270,272-274] Isolation of D2H, the human cDNA counterpart of the rat D2, from a human kidney library, and expression of D2H in *Xenopus* oocytes, showed that D2H induces uptake of cystine as well as dibasic and neutral amino acids. Furthermore, northern blot analysis demonstrated strong expression of D2H in human kidney and intestine. Mouse–human somatic cell hybrids showed that the human gene for D2H resides on chromosome 2.[273]

The genes for MCAT-1, MCAT-2 and the transporter regulatory units are strong candidate genes for the LPI mutation(s). Our increasing knowledge of the multiplicity and functional diversity of the cationic amino acid transporter proteins and transport regulatory proteins in mammalian tissues allows me to predict that the LPI phenotype will be split into subgroups based on different mutations in one or several transporters; furthermore, mutations in genes encoding transport regulatory proteins may also be involved in some families.

The hyperdibasic aminoaciduria type 1 described by Whelan and Scriver[61] showed autosomal dominant inheritance. Of the 33 subjects in the kindred, 13 had the trait. The suggestion that the affected members of the kindred are heterozygotes of an autosomal recessive disease seems likely, even though no confirmed homozygotes are known. The possibility exists that the patient of Kihara et al.[33] is a homozygote for the trait, as has been suggested by Bergeron and Scriver,[143] but this remains a hypothesis. The original proposal by the authors that the carriers of the trait could be heterozygous for LPI is at least equally attractive.

The expression of the mutant gene in heterozygotes for LPI has been only partially characterized.[2,53,58] The constant finding of decreased epithelial transport of the cationic amino acids in the homozygotes and, especially, the direct measurement of defective cationic amino acid transport in cultured fibroblasts of homozygotes and heterozygotes for LPI,[58] strongly support the view that the mutation affects the transport protein at the basolateral cell membrane of the epithelial cells and at the plasma membrane of the parenchymal cells. Many LPI heterozygotes excrete slightly increased amounts of the cationic amino acids in the urine, but this has not been a constant finding.[2,53] The fact that the heterozygotes have not shown signs and symptoms of protein intolerance suggests that the urea cycle failure is a secondary consequence of the primary defect.[276]

TREATMENT

Hyperammonemia, which occurs in the patients after high-protein meals, during prolonged fasting, or during severe infections, can now be effectively prevented and treated. A diet in which the protein content has been moderately decreased—in children, to 1.0 to 1.5 g/kg/day and, in adults, to 0.5 to 0.7 g/kg/day—forms the basis of successful treatment.[11,14,35] Acute symptoms disappear when the patients are on this diet, but, in many infants, severe protein aversion leads to minimal energy intake as well, and even though nausea and vomiting can be avoided, pediatric patients usually eat very poorly during the first years of life. Supplementation with arginine or ornithine has been moderately helpful in some patients,[6-8,13,17,28,32] but the decreased intestinal absorption of cationic amino acids limits their usefulness, and supplementation often leads to osmotic diarrhea.[55,195,196] Citrulline is a neutral amino acid and uses another transport mechanism at the cell membrane. It is readily absorbed from the intestine and converted to arginine and then to ornithine in the body, especially in the liver. Citrulline supplementation guarantees an adequate supply of urea cycle intermediates at the site of urea synthesis, and, indeed, oral citrulline supplementation has proved clinically to prevent hyperammonemia as efficiently as intravenous arginine or ornithine.[11,14,122] The dose of citrulline supplementation has been 2.5 to 8.5 g (14 to 48 mmol) daily, divided into three to five doses and taken with meals. The individual doses are first calculated according to the protein content of the meals and then adjusted according to the clinical and biochemical responses of the patients. Most patients quickly learn to know how much citrulline they need for a specific portion of each high-protein food. Citrulline can be given as powder dissolved in juice or as pills (ours have 0.414 g L-citrulline) or capsules.

In acute hyperammonemic crisis in LPI, the best treatment has been total removal of protein and nitrogen from the nutrition. Intravenous glucose should be given to supply as much energy as possible. In hyperammonemia we have also infused ornithine, arginine, or citrulline intravenously, starting with a priming dose of 1 mmol/kg in 5 to 10 min and then infusing at a rate of about 0.5 to 1 mmol/kg/h until the symptoms have subsided. Sodium benzoate and sodium phenylacetate given intravenously or orally[113,116,118,119] appear clinically effective even though they only minimally correct alanine-induced hyperammonemia.[134]

Lysine has been given orally to these patients, but its intestinal absorption is poor and it causes diarrhea and abdominal pains.[11] A few patients have received lysine supplementation for longer periods, but the evidence that lysine can correct signs of protein malnutrition has not been convincing. It is interesting that acute loads of ε-*N*-acetyllysine, a neutral analogue of lysine and a readily absorbed substance, increased plasma lysine concentrations in the patients as well as in the control subjects.[249] Homocitrulline had no effect on plasma lysine. Because of the limited availability and high price of acetyllysine, it has not been used as a long-term supplement in patients.[277] Its usefulness as a replacement for lysine has recently been questioned.[250]

A potentially life-threatening complication of LPI is acute or chronic pulmonary involvement, which may present as interstitial changes on radiographs or as respiratory insufficiency and may progress to pulmonary alveolar proteinosis or cholesterol granulomas[51,52,63,75,78-80] (see "Complications and Autopsy Findings" above). Occasionally, lung involvement may be the presenting sign of the disease.[38,51,52] One adult patient with acute respiratory insufficiency was treated efficiently with high-dose prednisolone immediately after the onset of pulmonary symptoms; the symptoms subsided rapidly after initiation of the therapy. The dose was soon tapered, but a 2.5-mg intermittent-day dose was continued. A relapse 8 months later was again successfully treated by increasing the prednisolone dose. The patient received intermittent-day prednisolone for over 2 years, and has since been symptom-free for over 5 years. However, several pediatric deaths from pulmonary complications suggest either that it is necessary to start the treatment early, or that the response may be variable.[51,52,75,80] Indeed, in two Italian patients aged 5 and 24 years, treatment with prednisolone had no effect on the progression of the pulmonary changes, and the effect was minimal or absent also in an 11-year-old Arab girl.[51,52]

Glomerulonephritis and renal insufficiency, amyloid deposition in the spleen and lymph nodes, and occasionally severe fatty degeneration and cirrhosis of the liver appear to be not uncommon in association with the pulmonary symptoms of LPI; the potentially fatal syndrome fits the criteria of the multiple organ dysfunction syndrome.[81,82] Currently, I have no suggestions for specific treatment of this syndrome in patients with LPI.

ACKNOWLEDGMENTS

This study was supported in part by grants from the Sigrid Juselius Foundation, the Academy of Finland, the Signe and Ane Gyllenberg Foundation, and the University Foundation, Turku, Finland. I am grateful to Dr. Katriina Parto, M.D., Dr. Ilkka Sipilä, M.D., Dr. Jukka Rajantie, M.D., Dr. Martti Kekomäki, M.D., and Prof. Jaakko Perheentupa, M.D., for collaboration, fruitful discussions and help in treating the Finnish patients during a quarter of a century. I want to thank Mrs. Marja Piippo, Mrs. Anneli Enlund, and my wife, Tuula, for help in the processing of the manuscript.

REFERENCES

1. Perheentupa J, Visakorpi JK: Protein intolerance with deficient transport of basic amino acids. *Lancet* **2**:813, 1965.
2. Norio R, Perheentupa J, Kekomäki M, Visakorpi JK: Lysinuric protein intolerance, an autosomal recessive disease. *Clin Genet* **2**:214, 1971.
3. McKusick VA, Francomano CA, Antonarakis SE: *Mendelian Inheritance in Man. Catalogs of Autosomal Dominant, Autosomal Recessive and X-linked Phenotypes*, 10th ed. Baltimore, Johns Hopkins University Press, 1992, p 1336.
4. Simell O, Rajantie J, Perheentupa J: Lysinuric protein intolerance, in Eriksson AW, Forsius H, Nevanlinna HR, Workman PL, Norio RK (eds): *Population Structure and Genetic Disorders*, London, Academic, 1980, p 633.
5. Scriver CR, Simell O: Hyperdibasic-aminoaciduria, in Buyse ML (ed): *Birth Defects Encyclopedia*. Dover, MA, Center for Birth Defects Information Services/Blackwell Scientific, 1990, p 900.
6. Kekomäki M: Familial protein intolerance. Studies on an inborn error of metabolism and related biochemical problems. Thesis, Helsinki, 1969.
7. Kekomäki M, Toivakka E, Häkkinen V, Salaspuro M: Familial protein intolerance with deficient transport of basic amino acids. Report on an adult patient with chronic hyperammonemia. *Acta Med Scand* **183**:357, 1968.
8. Kekomäki M, Visakorpi JK, Perheentupa J, Saxen L: Familial protein intolerance with deficient transport of basic amino acids. An analysis of 10 patients. *Acta Paediatr Scand* **56**:617, 1967.
9. Rajantie J: Lysinuric protein intolerance: Intestinal transport defect and treatment. Thesis, Helsinki, 1980.
10. Simell O: Lysinuric protein intolerance. Thesis. Helsinki, Yliopistokirjapaino, 1975.
11. Rajantie J, Simell O, Rapola J, Perheentupa J: Lysinuric protein intolerance: A two-year trial of dietary supplementation therapy with citrulline and lysine. *J Pediatr* **97**:927, 1980.
12. Perheentupa J, Simell O: Lysinuric protein intolerance. *Birth Defects* **10**(4):201, 1974.
13. Russell A, Slatter M, Ben-Zvi A: Ornithine administration as a therapeutic tool in dibasic aminoaciduric protein intolerance. *Hum Hered* **27**:206, 1977.
14. Awrich AE, Stackhouse J, Cantrell JE, Patterson JH, Rudman D: Hyperdibasicaminoaciduria, hyperammonemia, and growth retardation: Treatment with arginine, lysine, and citrulline. *J Pediatr* **87**:731, 1975.
15. Kato T, Tanaka E, Horisawa S: Hyperdibasicaminoaciduria and hyperammonemia in familial protein intolerance, *Am J Dis Child* **130**:1340, 1976.
16. Malmquist J, Jagenburg R, Lindstedt G: Familial protein intolerance: Possible nature of enzyme defect. *N Engl J Med* **284**:997, 1971.
17. Yoshimura T, Kato M, Goto I, Kuroiwa Y: Lysinuric protein intolerance—two patients in a family with loss of consciousness and growth retardation. *Rinsho Shinkeigaku* **23**:140, 1983.
18. Kitajima I, Goto K, Umehara F, Nagamatsu K, Kanehisa Y: A case of lysinuric protein intolerance with intermittent stupor looking like psychomotor seizure in adulthood. *Rinsho Shinkeigaku* **26**:592, 1986.
19. Carson NAJ, Redmond OAB: Lysinuric protein intolerance. *Ann Clin Biochem* **14**:135, 1977.
20. Andria G, Battaglia A, Sebastio G, Strisciuglio P, Auricchio S: Lysinuric protein intolerance. *Rev Ital Pediatr* **2**:386, 1977.
21. Malmquist J, Hetter B: Leucocyte glutaminase in familial protein intolerance. *Lancet* **2**:129, 1970.
22. Behbehani AW, Gahr M, Schröter W: Lysinuric protein intolerance. *Monatsschr Kinderheilkd* **131**:784, 1983.
23. Brown JH, Fabre LF Jr, Farrell GL, Adams ED: Hyperlysinuria with hyperammonemia. *Am J Dis Child* **124**:127, 1972.
24. Oyanagi K, Sogawa H, Minami R, Nakao T, Chiba T: The mechanism of hyperammonemia in congenital lysinuria. *J Pediatr* **94**:255, 1979.
25. Oyanagi K, Miura R, Yamanouchi T: Congenital lysinuria: A new inherited transport disorder of dibasic amino acids. *J Pediatr* **77**:259, 1970.
26. Kato T, Mizutani N, Ban M: Hyperammonemia in lysinuric protein intolerance. *Pediatrics* **73**:489, 1984.

27. Chan H, Billmeier GJ Jr, Molinary SV, Tucker HN, Shin B-C, Schaffer A, Cavallo K: Prolonged coma and isoelectric electroencephalogram in a child with lysinuric protein intolerance. *J Pediatr* **91**:79, 1977.
28. Endres W, Zoulek G, Schaub J: Hyperdibasicaminoaciduria in a Turkish infant without evident protein intolerance. *Eur J Pediatr* **131**:33, 1979.
29. Jagenburg R, Lindstedt G, Malmquist J: Familjär [?] proteinintolerans med hyperammoniemi. *Läkartidningen* **67**:5255, 1970.
30. Carpenter TO, Levy HL, Holtrop ME, Shih VE, Anast CS: Lysinuric protein intolerance presenting as childhood osteoporosis. Clinical and skeletal response to citrulline therapy. *N Engl J Med* **312**:290, 1985.
31. Nagata M, Suzuki M, Kawamura G, Kono S, Koda N, Yamaguchi S, Aoki K: Immunological abnormalities in a patient with lysinuric protein intolerance. *Eur J Pediatr* **146**:427, 1987.
32. Andria G, Sebastio G, Strisciuglio P, Del Giudice E: Lysinuric protein intolerance: Possible genetic heterogeneity? *J Inherited Metab Dis* **4**:151, 1981.
33. Kihara H, Valente M, Porter MT, Fluharty AL: Hyperdibasicaminoaciduria in a mentally retarded homozygote with a peculiar response to phenothiazines. *Pediatrics* **51**:223, 1973.
34. Goto I, Yoshimura T, Kuroiwa Y: Growth hormone studies in lysinuric protein intolerance. *Eur J Pediatr* **141**:240, 1984.
35. Simell O, Perheentupa J, Rapola J, Visakorpi JK, Eskelin L-E: Lysinuric protein intolerance. *Am J Med* **59**:229, 1975.
36. Yamaguchi S: Personal communication, 1987.
37. Saudubray JM: Personal communication, 1987.
38. Fisher M, Roggli V, Merten D, Mulvihill D, Spock A: Coexisting endogenous lipoid pneumonia, cholesterol granulomas, and pulmonary alveolar proteinosis in a pediatric population: A clinical, radiographic, and pathologic correlation. *Pediat Pathol* **12**:365, 1992.
39. Krasnopolskaia KD, Iakovenko LP, Mazaeva IV, Lebedev BV: Lysinuric protein intolerance, a hereditary defect of amino acid transport. *Pediatriia* **6**:78, 1978.
40. Coude FX, Ogier H, Charpentier C, Cathelineau L, Grimber G, Parvy P, Saudubray JM, Frezal J: Lysinuric protein intolerance: A severe hyperammonemia secondary to L-arginine deficiency. *Arch Fr Pediatr* **38**(suppl. 1):829, 1981.
41. Mori H, Kimura M, Fukuda S: A case of lysinuric protein intolerance with mental-physical retardation, intermittent stupor and hemiparesis. *Rinsho Shinkeigaku* **22**:42, 1982.
42. Mizutani N, Kato T, Maehara M, Watanabe K, Ban M: Oral administration of arginine and citrulline in the treatment of lysinuric protein intolerance. *Tohoku J Exp Med* **142**:15, 1984.
43. Rottem M, Statter M, Amit R, Brand N, Bujanover Y, Yatziv S: Clinical and laboratory study in 22 patients with inherited hyperammonemic syndromes. *Isr J Med Sci* **22**:833, 1986.
44. Takada G, Goto A, Komatsu K, Goto R: Carnitine deficiency in lysinuric protein intolerance: Lysine sparing effect of carnitine. *Tohoku J Exp Med* **153**:331, 1987.
45. Shioya K, Yamamura Y, Kurihara T, Matsukura S: A case of combined lysinuric protein intolerance and hypoactivity of argininosuccinate synthetase (citrullinemia). *Nippon Naika Gakkai Zasshi* **77**:667, 1988.
46. De Parshau L, Vianey-Liaud C, Hermier M, Divry P, Guibaud P: Protein intolerance with lysinuria. Value of orotic aciduria in adjusting treatment with citrulline. *Arch Fr Pediatr* **45**:809, 1988.
47. Shaw PJ, Dale G, Bbates D: Familial lysinuric protein intolerance presenting as coma in two adult sublings. *J Neurol Neurosurg Psychiatry* **52**:648, 1989.
48. Kato T, Sano M, Mizutani N: Homocitrullinuria and homoargininuria in lysinuric protein intolerance. *J Inherited Metab Dis* **12**:157, 1989.
49. Parini R, Vegni M, Pontiggia M, Melotti D, Corbetta C, Rossi A, Piceni-Sereni L: A difficult diagnosis of lysinuric protein intolerance: Association with glucose-6-phosphate dehydrogenase deficiency. *J Inherited Metab Dis* **14**:833, 1991.
50. Ono N, Kishida K, Tokumoto K, Watanabe M, Shimada Y, Yoshinaga J, Fujii M: Lysinuric protein intolerance presenting deficiency of argininosuccinate synthetase. *Intern Med* **31**:55, 1992.
51. DiRocco M, Garibotto G, Rossi GA, Caruso U, Taccone A, Picco P, Borrone C: Role of haematological, pulmonary and renal complications in the long-term prognosis of patients with lysinuric protein intolerance. *Eur J Pediatr* **152**:437, 1993.
52. Kerem E, Elpelg ON, Shalev RS, Rosenman E, Bar Ziv Y, Branski D: Lysinuric protein intolerance with chronic interstitial lung disease and pulmonary cholesterol granulomas at onset. *J Pediatr* **123**:275, 1993.
53. Salonen T: Lysinuric protein intolerance: Finnish pedigrees and the diagnosis of heterozygotes. Master's thesis. Turku, University of Turku, 1991.
54. Sogowa H: Studies on the etiology of hyperammonemia associated with inborn errors of amino acid metabolism, part 2: Etiology of hyperammonemia associated with hyperdibasic aminoaciduria. *Sapporo Med J* **47**:215, 1978.
55. Rajantie J, Simell O, Perheentupa J: Basolateral-membrane transport defect for lysine in lysinuric protein intolerance. *Lancet* **1**:1219, 1980.
56. Rajantie J, Simell O, Perheentupa J: Lysinuric protein intolerance. Basolateral transport defect in renal tubuli. *J Clin Invest* **67**:1078, 1981.
57. Desjeux J-F, Rajantie J, Simell O, Dumontier A-M, Perheentupa J: Lysine fluxes across the jejunal epithelium in lysinuric protein intolerance. *J Clin Invest* **65**:1382, 1980.
58. Smith DW, Scriver CR, Tenenhouse HS, Simell O: Lysinuric protein intolerance mutation is expressed in the plasma membrane of cultured skin fibroblasts. *Proc Natl Acad Sci USA* **84**:7711, 1987.
59. Botschner J, Smith DW, Simell O, Scriver CR: Comparison of ornithine metabolism in hyperornithinemia-hyperammonemia-homocitrullinuria syndrome, lysinuric protein intolerance, and gyrate atrophy fibroblasts. *J Inherited Metab Dis* **12**:33, 1989.
60. Albritton LM, Bowcock AM, Eddy RL, Morton CC, Tseng L, Farrer LA, Cavalli-Sforza LL, Shows TB, Cunninham JM: The human cationic amino acid transporter [ATRC1]: Physical and genetic mapping to 13q12-q14. *Genomics* **12**:430, 1992.
61. Whelan DT, Scriver CR: Hyperdibasicaminoaciduria: An inherited disorder of amino acid transport. *Pediatr Res* **2**:525, 1968.
62. Omura K, Yamanaka N, Higami S, Matsuoka O, Fujimoto A, Issiki G, Tada K: Lysine malabsorption syndrome: A new type of transport defect. *Pediatrics* **57**:102, 1976.
63. Parto K: Skeletal and visceral findings in lysinuric protein intolerance. Thesis. Turku, Grafia, 1993.
64. Svedström E, Parto K, Marttinen M, Virtama P, Simell O: Skeletal manifestations of lysinuric protein intolerance. *Skeletal Radiol* **22**:11, 1993.
65. Parto K, Penttinen R, Paronen I, Pelliniemi L, Simell O: Osteoporosis in lysinuric protein intolerance. *J Inherited Metab Dis* **16**:441, 1993.
66. Lysinuric protein intolerance: A rare cause of childhood osteoporosis. *Nutr Rev* **44**:110, 1986. (no author)
67. Moschos M, Andreanos D: Lysinuria and changes in the crystalline lens. *Bull Mem Soc Fr Ophtalmol* **96**:322, 1985.
68. Neuberger A, Webster TA: The lysine requirements of adult rat. *J Biochem* **39**:200, 1945.
69. Likens R, Bavetta L, Posner A: Calcification in lysine deficiency. *Arch Biochem Biophys* **70**:401, 1957.
70. Jha G, Deo MG, Ramalingaswami V: Bone growth in protein deficiency, a study in rhesus monkeys. *Am J Pathol* **53**:1111, 1968.
71. Garn SM, Guzman MA, Wagner B: Subperiosteal gain and endosteal loss in protein-calorie malnutrition. *Am J Phys Anthropol* **30**:153, 1969.
72. Shieres R, Avioli LV, Bergfeld MA, Fallon MD, Slatopolsky E, Teitelbaum SL: Effects of semistarvation on skeletal homeostasis. *Endocrinology* **107**:1530, 1980.
73. Orwoll E, Ware M, Sstribrska L, Bikle D, Sanchez T, Andon M, Li H: Effects of dietary protein deficiency on mineral metabolism and bone mineral density. *Am J Clin Nutr* **56**:314, 1992.
74. Branca F, Robin SP, Ferro-Luzzi A, Golden MHN:

Bone turnover in malnourished children. *Lancet* **340:**1493, 1992.
75. Parto K, Kallajoki M, Aho H, Simell O: Pulmonary alveolar proteinosis and glomerulonephritis in lysinuric protein intolerance: Case reports and autopsy findings of four pediatric patients. *Hum Pathol* (in press).
76. Dhansay MA, Benade AJ, Donald PR: Plasma lecithin-cholesterol acyltransferase activity and plasma lipoprotein composition and concentrations in kwashiorkor. *Am J Clin Nutr* **53:**512, 1991.
77. Sidransky H, Verney E: Chemical pathology of diamino acid deficiency: Considerations in relation to lysinuric protein intolerance. *J Exp Pathol* **2:**47, 1985.
78. Parto K, Svedström E, Majurin ML, Härkönen R, Simell O: Pulmonary manifestations in lysinuric protein intolerance. *Chest* **104:**1176, 1993.
79. Parto K, Mäki J, Pelliniemi L, Simell O: Abnormal pulmonary macrophages in lysinuric protein intolerance. Ultrastructural, morphometric and x-ray microanalytical study. *Arch Pathol Lab Med* (in press).
80. Simell OG, Sipilä I, Perheentupa J, Rapola J: Lysinuric protein intolerance: Undefined interstitial pneumonia, a lethal or life-threatening complication. Sendai, Japan, The Fourth International Congress of Inborn Errors of Metabolism. 1987, p 38 (abstract).
81. Bone RC, Balk RA, Cerra FB, Dellinger RP, Fein AM, Knaus WA, Schein RMH, Sibbald WJ: Definitions for sepsis and organ failure and guidelines for the use of innovative therapies in sepsis. *Chest* **101:**1644, 1992.
82. Cohen IL: Definitions for sepsis and organ failure—The ACCP/SCCM consensus conference report. *Chest* **103:**656, 1993.
83. Wallaert B: Subclinical alveolitis in immunologic systemic disorders. *Lung* **168**(suppl.):974, 1990.
84. Milleron BJ, Costabel U, Teschler H, Ziesche R, Cadranel JL, Matthys H, Akoun GM: Bronchoalveolar lavage cell data in alveolar proteinosis. *Am Rev Respir Dis* **144:**1330, 1991.
85. Hallman M, Sipilä I: Lysinuric protein intolerance (LPI): A possible defect in diamino acid transport in pulmonary alveolar epithelium. Oslo, Norway, European Society for Pediatric Research, Annual Meeting, 1988 (abstract).
86. Hallman M, Maasilta P, Sipilä I, Tahvanainen J: Composition and function of pulmonary surfactant in adult respiratory distress syndrome. *Eur Respir J* **2**(suppl. 3):104, 1989.
87. Pratt SA, Smith MH, Ladman AJ, Finley TN: The ultrastructure of alveolar macrophages from human cigarette smokers and nonsmokers. *Lab Invest* **24:**331, 1971.
88. Hocking WG, Golde DW: The pulmonary alveolar macrophage. *N Engl J Med* **301:**639, 1979.
89. Heppleston AG: Animal model of human disease. Silica induced pulmonary alveolar lipoproteinosis. *Am J Pathol* **78:**171, 1975.
90. Lullmann H, Lullmann-Rauch R, Wasserman O: Lipidosis induced by amphiphilic cationic drugs. *Biochem Pharmacol* **27:**1103, 1978.
91. Hook GER: Alveolar proteinosis and phospholipidoses of the lung. *Toxicol Pathol* **19:**482, 1991.
92. Colon AR Jr, Lawrence RD, Mills SD, O'Connell EJ: Childhood pulmonary alveolar proteinosis [PAP]. Report of a case and review of the literature. *Am J Dis Child* **121:**481, 1971.
93. Webster JR Jr, Battifora H, Fureay C, Harrison RA, Shapiro B: Pulmonary alveolar proteinosis in two siblings with decreased immunoglobulin A. *Am J Med* **69:**786, 1980.
94. Gray ES: Autoimmunity in childhood pulmonary alveolar proteinosis. *Br Med J* **887:**296, 1973.
95. Samuels MP, Warner JO: Pulmonary alveolar lipoproteinosis complicating juvenile dermatomyositis. *Thorax* **43:**939, 1988.
96. Haworth JC, Hoogstraten J, Taylor H: Thymic alymphoplasia. *Arch Dis Child* **42:**40, 1967.
97. Wilkinson RH, Blanc WA, Hagström JWC: Pulmonary alveolar proteinosis in three infants. *Pediatrics* **41:**510, 1968.
98. Danigelis JA, Markarian B: Pulmonary alveolar proteinosis. Including pulmonary electron microscopy. *Am J Dis Child* **118:**871, 1969.
99. Lippman M, Mok MS, Wasserman K: Anesthetic management for children with alveolar proteinosis using extracorporeal circulation. Report of two cases. *Br J Anesthesiol* **49:**173, 1977.
100. Teja K, Cooper PH, Squires JE, Schnatterly PT: Pulmonary alveolar proteinosis in four siblings. *N Engl J Med* **305:**1390, 1981.
101. Schumacher RE, Marrogi AJ, Heidelberger KP: Pulmonary alveolar proteinosis in a newborn. *Pediatr Pulmology* **7:**178, 1989.
102. Moulton SL, Krous HF, Merritt TA, Odell RM, Gangitano E, Cornish JD: Congenital pulmonary alveolar proteinosis: Failure of treatment with extracorporeal life support. *J Pediatr* **120:**297, 1992.
103. Porter KA: The kidneys, in Symmers WS (ed): *Systemic Pathology*. Edinburgh, Churchill Livingstone, 1992, p 217.
104. Marino CT, Pertschuk LP: Pulmonary hemorrhage in systemic lupus erythematosus. *Arch Intern Med* **141:**201, 1981.
105. Hensley MJ, Feldman NT, Lazarus JM, Galvanek EG: Diffuse pulmonary hemorrhage and rapidly progressive renal failure: An uncommon presentation of Wegener's granulomatosis. *Am J Med* **66:**894, 1979.
106. Thomashow BM, Felton CP, Navarro C: Diffuse intrapulmonary hemorrhage, renal failure, and a systemic vasculitis. *Am J Med* **68:**299, 1980.
107. Loughlin GM, Taussig LM, Murphy SA, Strunk RC, Kohnen PW: Immune complex-mediated glomerulonephritis and pulmonary hemorrhage simulating Goodpasture's syndrome. *J Pediatr* **93:**181, 1978.
108. Davies JNP: The essential pathology of kwashiorkor. *Lancet* **1:**317, 1948.
109. Gmaz-Nikulin E, Nikulin A, Plamenac P, Hegenwald G, Gaon D: Pancreatic lesions in shock and their significance. *J Pathol* **135:**223, 1981.
110. Klujber V, Klujber L: Hereditary pancreatitis. *Orv Hetil* **130:**1777, 1989.
111. Rajantie J, Simell O, Perheentupa J, Siimes M: Changes in peripheral blood cells and serum ferritin in lysinuric protein intolerance. *Acta Paediatr Scand* **69:**741, 1980.
112. Simell O, MacKenzie S, Clow CL, Scriver CR: Ornithine loading did not prevent induced hyperammonemia in a patient with HHH syndrome. *Pediatr Res* **19:**1283, 1985.
113. Coude FX, Coude M, Grimber G, Pelet A, Charpentier C: Potentiation by piridoxilate of the synthesis of hippurate from benzoate in isolated rat hepatocytes. An approach to the determination of new pathways of nitrogen excretion in inborn errors of urea synthesis. *Clin Chim Acta* **136:**211, 1984.
114. Brusilow SW: Arginine, an indispensable amino acid for patients with inborn errors of urea synthesis. *J Clin Invest* **74:**2144, 1984.
115. Visek WJ: Arginine needs, physiological state and usual diets. A reevaluation. *J Nutr* **116:**36, 1986.
116. Brusilow SW, Danney M, Waber LJ, Batshaw M, Burton B, Levitsky L, Roth K, McKeethren C, Ward J: Treatment of episodic hyperammonemia in children with inborn errors of urea synthesis. *N Engl J Med* **310:**1630, 1984.
117. Batshaw ML, Painter MJ, Sproul GT. Schafer IA, Thomas GH, Brusilow S: Therapy of urea cycle enzymopathies: Three case studies. *Johns Hopkins Med* **148:**34, 1981.
118. Brusilow S, Tinker J, Batshaw ML: Amino acid acylation: A mechanism of nitrogen excretion in inborn errors of urea synthesis. *Science* **207:**659, 1980.
119. Smith I: The treatment of inborn errors of the urea cycle. *Nature* **291:**378, 1981.
120. McCormick K, Viscardi RM, Robinson B, Heininger J: Partial pyruvate decarboxylase deficiency with profound lactic acidosis and hyperammonemia: Responses to dichloroacetate and benzoate. *Am J Med Genet* **22:**291, 1985.
121. Simell O, Perheentupa J: Renal handling of diamino acids in lysinuric protein intolerance. *J Clin Invest* **54:**9, 1974.
122. Rajantie J: Orotic aciduria in lysinuric protein intolerance: Dependence on the urea cycle intermediates. *Pediatr Res* **15:**115, 1981.
123. Wendler PA, Blanding JH, Tremblay GC: Interaction between the urea cycle and the orotate pathway: Studies with isolated hepatocytes. *Arch Biochem Biophys* **224:**36, 1983.
124. Milner JA, Prior RL, Visek WJ: Arginine deficiency and

orotic aciduria in mammals. *Proc Soc Exp Biol Med* **150**:282, 1975.

125. Milner JA, Visek WJ: Urinary metabolites characteristic of urea-cycle amino acid deficiency. *Metabolism* **24**:643, 1975.
126. Kelley WN, Greene ML, Fox IH, Rosenbloom FM, Levy RI, Seegmiller JE: Effects of orotic acid on purine and lipoprotein metabolism in man. *Metabolism* **19**:1025, 1970.
127. Rajantie J, Rapola J, Siimes MA: Ferritinemia with subnormal iron stores in lysinuric protein intolerance. *Metabolism* **30**:3, 1981.
128. Lamberg B-A, Simell O, Perheentupa J, Saarinen P: Increase in TBG, T4, FT4 and T3 in the lysinuric protein intolerance. Exerpta Medica Int Congress Series **378**:232, 1975.
129. Lamberg BA, Perheentupa J, Rajantie J, Simell O, Saarinen P, Ebeling P, Welin M-G: Increase in thyroxine-binding globulin [TBG] in lysinuric protein intolerance. *Acta Endocrinol* **97**:67, 1981.
130. Kekomäki M, Räihä NCR, Perheentupa J: Enzymes of urea synthesis in familial protein intolerance with deficient transport of basic amino acids. *Acta Paediatr Scand* **56**:631, 1967.
131. Simell O, Perheentupa J, Visakorpi JF: Leukocyte and liver glutaminase in lysinuric protein intolerance. *Pediatr Res* **6**:797, 1972.
132. Kekomäki MP, Räihä NCR, Bickel H: Ornithine-ketoacid aminotransferase in human liver with reference to patients with hyperornithinaemia and familial protein intolerance. *Clin Chim Acta* **23**:203, 1969.
133. Valle D: Personal communication, 1988.
134. Simell O, Sipilä I, Rajantie J, Valle DL, Brusilow SW: Waste nitrogen excretion via amino acid acylation: Benzoate and phenylacetate in lysinuric protein intolerance. *Pediatr Res* **20**:1117, 1986.
135. Bachmann C, Krahenbuhl S, Colombo JP, Schubiger G, Jaggi KH, Tonz O: *N*-acetylglutamate synthetase deficiency: A disorder of ammonia detoxication. *N Engl J Med* **304**:543, 1981.
136. Hammerman MR: Na^+-independent l-arginine transport in rabbit renal brush border membrane vesicles. *Biochim Biophys Acta* **685**:71, 1982.
137. Adibi SA: Intestinal transport of dipeptides in man: Relative importance of hydrolysis and intact absorption. *J Clin Invest* **50**:2266, 1971.
138. Matthews DM, Adibi SA: Peptide absorption. *Gastroenterology* **71**:151, 1976.
139. Asatoor AM, Groughman MR, Harrison AR, Light FW, Loughridge LW, Milne MD, Richards AJ: Intestinal absorption of oligopeptides in cystinuria. *Clin Sci* **41**:23, 1971.
140. Ganapathy V, Mendicino JF, Leibach FH: Transport of glycyl-l-proline into intestinal and renal brush border vesicles from rabbit. *J Biol Chem* **256**:118, 1981.
141. Ganapathy V, Mendicino J, Pashley DH, Leibach FH: Carrier-mediated transport of glycyl-l-proline in renal brush-border vesicles. *Biochem Biophys Res Commun* **97**:1133, 1980.
142. Scriver CR, McInnes RR, Mohyuddin F: Role of epithelial architecture and intracellular metabolism in proline uptake and transtubular reclamation in PRO/Re mouse kidney. *Proc Natl Acad Sci USA* **72**:1431, 1975.
143. Bergeron M, Scriver CR: Pathophysiology of renal hyperaminoacidurias and glucosuria, in Seldin DW, Giebisch G (eds): *The Kidney. Physiology and Pathophysiology*, 2nd ed. New York, Raven, 1992, p 2947.
144. Wilson OH, Scriver CR: Specificity of transport of neutral and basic amino acids in rat kidney. *Am J Physiol* **213**:185, 1967.
145. Webber WA, Brown JL, Pitts RF: Interactions of amino acids in renal tubular transport. *Am J Physiol* **200**:380, 1961.
146. Steiger B, Stange G, Biber J, Murer H: Transport of l-lysine by rat renal brush border membrane vesicles. *Pflügers Arch* **397**:106, 1983.
147. Scriver CR, Clow CL, Reade TM, Goodyer P, Auray-Blais C, Giguere R, Lemieux B: Ontogeny modifies manifestations of cystinuria genes. Implications for counseling. *J Pediatr* **106**:411, 1985.
148. Schwartzman L, Blair A, Segal S: A common renal transport system for lysine, ornithine, arginine and cysteine. *Biochem Biophys Res Commu* **23**:220, 1966.
149. Schafer JA, Watkins ML: Transport of l-cystine in isolated perfused proximal straight tubules. *Pflügers Arch* **401**:143, 1984.
150. Samarzija I, Fromter E: Electrophysiological analysis of rat renal sugar and amino acid transport. IV. Basic amino acids. *Pflügers Arch* **393**:199, 1982.
151. Rosenberg LE, Downing SJ, Segal S: Competitive inhibition of dibasic amino acid transport in rat kidney. *J Biol Chem* **237**:2265, 1962.
152. Rosenberg LE, Albrecht I, Segal S: Lysine transport in human kidney: Evidence for two systems. *Science* **155**:1426, 1967.
153. Bergeron M, Morel F: Amino acid transport in rat renal tubules. *Am J Physiol* **216**:1139, 1969.
154. Crawhall JC, Scowen EF, Thompson CJ, Watts RWE: The renal clearance of amino acids in cystinuria. *J Clin Invest* **46**:1162, 1967.
155. Hilden SA, Sacktor B: l-Arginine uptake into renal brush brush membrane vesicles. *Arch Biochem Biophys* **210**:289, 1981.
156. Kato T, Mizutani N, Ban M: Renal transport of lysine and arginine in lysinuric protein intolerance. *Eur J Pediatr* **139**:181, 1982.
157. Leopolder A, Burchhardt G, Murer H: Transport of l-ornithine across isolated brush border membrane vesicles from proximal tubule. *Renal Physiol* **2**:157, 1980.
158. McCarthy CF, Borland JL Jr, Lynch HJ Jr, Owen EE, Tyor MP: Defective uptake of basic amino acids and l-cystine by intestinal mucosa of patients with cystinuria. *J Clin Invest* **43**:1518, 1964.
159. Ozegovic B, McNamara D, Segal S: Cystine uptake by rat jejunal brush border membrane vesicles. *Biosci Rep* **2**:913, 1982.
160. Thier SO, Segal S, Fox M, Blair A, Rosenberg LE: Cystinuria: Defective intestinal transport of dibasic amino acids and cystine. *J Clin Invest* **44**:442, 1965.
161. White MF: The transport of cationic amino acids across the plasma membrane of mammalian cells. *Biochim Biophys Acta* **822**:355, 1985.
162. White MF, Christensen HN: Cationic amino acid transport into cultured animal cells. II. Transport system barely perceptible in ordinary hepatocytes, but active in hepatoma cell lines. *J Biol Chem* **257**:4450, 1982.
163. White MF, Gazzola GC, Christensen HN: Cationic amino acid transport into cultured animal cells. I. Influx into cultured human fibroblasts. *J Biol Chem* **257**:4443, 1982.
164. Bannai S: Transport of cystine and cysteine in mammalian cells. *Biochim Biophys Acta* **779**:289, 1984.
165. Dent CE, Rose GA: Aminoacid metabolism in cystinuria. *Q J Med* **79**:205, 1951.
166. Foreman JW, Hwang S-M, Segal S: Transport interactions of cystine and dibasic amino acids in isolated rat renal tubules. *Metabolism* **29**:53, 1980.
167. Foreman JW, Medow MS, Bovee KC, Segal S: Developmental aspects of cystine transport in the dog. *Pediatr Res* **20**:593, 1986.
168. Groth U, Rosenberg LE: Transport of dibasic amino acids, cystine, and tryptophan by cultured human fibroblast: Absence of a defect in cystinuria and Hartnup disease. *J Clin Invest* **51**:2130, 1972.
169. Kato T: Renal handling of dibasic amino acids and cystine in cystinuria. *Clin Sci Molec Med* **53**:9, 1977.
170. Kato T: Renal transport of lysine and arginine in cystinuria. *Tohoku J Exp Med* **139**:9, 1983.
171. Lester FT, Cusworth DC: Lysine infusion in cystinuria: Theoretical renal thresholds for lysine. *Clin Sci* **44**:99, 1973.
172. McNamara D, Pepe M, Segal S: Cystine uptake by rat renal brush border vesicles. *Biochem J* **194**:443, 1981.
173. Morin CL, Thompson MW, Jackson SH, Sass-Kortsak A: Biochemical and genetic studies in cystinuria: Observations on double heterozygotes of genotype I/II. *J Clin Invest* **50**:1961, 1971.
174. Robson EB, Rose GA: The effect of intravenous lysine of the renal clearances of cystine, arginine and ornithine in normal subjects, in patients with cystinuria and Fanconi syndrome and in their relatives. *Clin Sci* **16**:75, 1957.

175. Rosenberg LE: Cystinuria: Genetic heterogeneity and allelism. *Science* **154:**1341, 1966.
176. Segal S, McNamara PD, Pepe CM: Transport interaction of cystine and dibasic amino acids in renal brush border vesicles. *Science* **197:**169, 1977.
177. Volkl H, Silbernagl S: Mutual inhibition of l-cystine/cysteine and other neutral amino acids during tubular reabsorption. A microperfusion study in rat kidney. *Pflügers Arch* **395:**190, 1982.
178. Volkl H, Silbernagl S: Reexamination of the interplay between dibasic amino acids and l-cystine/l-cysteine during tubular reabsorption. *Pflügers Arch* **395:**196, 1982.
179. Thier S, Foc M, Segal S: Cystinuria: In vitro demonstration of an intestinal transport defect. *Science* **143:**482, 1964.
180. Scriver CR, Chesney RW, McInnes RR: Genetic aspects of renal tubular transport. Diversity and topology of carriers. *Kidney Int* **9:**149, 1976.
181. Strauven T, Mardens Y, Clara R, Terheggen H: Intravenous loading with arginine-hydrochloride and ornithine-aspartate in siblings of two families, presenting a familial neurological syndrome associated with cystinuria. *Biomedicine* **24:**191, 1976.
182. Frimpter GW, Horwith M, Furth E, Fellows RE, Thompson DD: Inulin and endogenous amino acid renal clearances in cystinuria: Evidence for tubular secretion. *J Clin Invest* **41:**281, 1962.
183. Bovee KC, Segal S: Renal tubule reabsorption of amino acids after lysine loading of cystinuric dogs. *Metabolism* **33:**602, 1984.
184. Bowring MA, Foreman JW, Lee J, Segal S: Characteristics of lysine transport by isolated rat renal cortical tubule fragments. *Biochim Biophys Acta* **901:**23, 1987.
185. States B, Foreman J, Lee J, Harris D, Segal S: Cystine and lysine transport in cultured human renal epithelial cells. *Metabolism* **36:**356, 1987.
186. Stevens BR, Ross HJ, Wright EM: Multiple transport pathways for neutral amino acids in rabbit jejunal brush border vesicles. *J Membr Biol* **66:**213, 1982.
187. Busse D: Transport of l-arginine in brush border vesicles derived from rabbit kidney cortex. *Arch Biochem Biophys* **191:**551, 1978.
188. Coicadan L, Heyman M, Grasset E, Desjeux J-F: Cystinuria: Reduced lysine permeability at the brush border of intestinal membrane cells. *Pediatr Res* **14:**109, 1980.
189. Desjeux JF, Volanthen M, Dumontier AM, Simell O, Legrain M: Cystine fluxes across the isolated jejunal epithelium in cystinuria: Increased efflux permeability at the luminal membrane. *Pediatr Res* **21:**477, 1987.
190. Simell O: Diamino acid transport into granulocytes and liver slices of patients with lysinuric protein intolerance. *Pediatr Res* **9:**504, 1975.
191. Metoki K, Hommes FA: The uptake of ornithine and lysine by isolated hepatocytes and fibroblasts. *Int J Biochem* **16:**833, 1984.
192. Scriver CR: Cystinuria. *N Engl J Med* **315:**1155, 1986.
193. Frimpter GW: Cystinuria: Metabolism of the disulfide of cysteine and homocysteine. *J Clin Invest* **42:**1956, 1963.
194. Kekomäki M: Intestinal absorption of l-arginine and l-lysine in familial protein intolerance. *Ann Paediatr Fenn* **14:**18, 1968.
195. Rajantie J, Simell O, Perheentupa J: Oral administration of urea cycle intermediates in lysinuric protein intolerance: Effect on plasma and urinary arginine and ornithine. *Metabolism* **32:**49, 1983.
196. Rajantie J, Simell O, Perheentupa J: Intestinal absorption in lysinuric protein intolerance: Impaired for diamino acids, normal for citrulline. *Gut* **21:**519, 1980.
197. Silk DBA: Peptide absorption in man. *Gut* **15:**494, 1974.
198. Simell O, Perheentupa J: Defective metabolic clearance of plasma arginine and ornithine in lysinuric protein intolerance. *Metabolism* **23:**691, 1974.
199. Christensen HN, Cullen AM: Synthesis of metabolism-resistant substrates for the transport system for cationic amino acids; their stimulation of the release of insulin and glucagon, and of the urinary loss of amino acids related to cystinuria. *Biochim Biophys Acta* **298:**932, 1973.
200. Buchanan JA, Rosenblatt DS, Scriver CR: Cultured human fibroblasts and plasma membrane vesicles to investigate transport function and the effects of genetic mutation. *Ann NY Acad Sci* **456:**401, 1985.
201. Smith DW, Scriver CR, Simell O: Lysinuric protein intolerance mutation is not expressed in the plasma membrane of erythrocytes. *Hum Genet* **80:**395, 1988.
202. Gardner JD, Levy AG: Transport of dibasic amino acids by human erythrocytes. *Metabolism* **21:**413, 1972.
203. Christensen HN, Antonioli JA: Cationic amino acid transport in the rabbit reticulocyte. *J Biol Chem* **244:**1497, 1969.
204. Vadgama JV, Christensen HN: Discrimination of Na^+-independent transport systems L, T, and ASC in erythrocytes. Na^+ independence of the latter a consequence of cell maturation? *J Biol Chem* **260:**2912, 1985.
205. Rajantie J, Simell O, Perheentupa J: "Basolateral" and mitochondrial membrane transport defect in the hepatocytes in lysinuric protein intolerance. *Acta Paediatr Scand* **72:**65, 1983.
206. Gamble JG, Lehninger AL: Transport of ornithine and citrulline across the mitochondrial membrane. *J Biol Chem* **248:**610, 1973.
207. Aronson DL, Diwan JJ: Uptake of ornithine by rat liver mitochondria. *Biochemistry* **20:**7064, 1981.
208. Metoki K, Hommes FA: A possible rate limiting factor in urea synthesis by isolated hepatocytes: The transport of ornithine into hepatocytes and mitochondria. *Int J Biochem* **16:**1155, 1984.
209. Hommes FA, Kitchings L, Eller AG: The uptake of ornithine and lysine by rat liver mitochondria. *Biochem Med* **30:**313, 1983.
210. Bradford NM, McGivan JD: Evidence for the existence of an ornithine/citrulline antiporter in rat liver mitochondria. *FEBS Lett* **113:**294, 1980.
211. Raijman L: Citrulline synthesis in rat tissues and liver content of carbamoyl phosphate and ornithine. *Biochem J* **138:**225, 1974.
212. Bryla J, Harris EJ: Accumulation of ornithine and citrulline in rat liver mitochondria in relation to citrulline formation. *FEBS Lett* **72:**331, 1976.
213. Cohen NS, Cheung C-W, Raijman L: Channeling of extramitochondrial ornithine to matrix ornithine transcarbamylase. *J Biol Chem* **262:**203, 1987.
214. Cohen NS, Cheung C-W, Raijman L: The effects of ornithine on mitochondrial carbamyl phosphate synthesis. *J Biol Chem* **255:**10248, 1980.
215. Grays RGF, Hill SE, Pollitt RJ: Studies on the pathway from ornithine to proline in cultured skin fibroblasts with reference to the defect in hyperornithinaemia with hyperammonaemia and homocitrullinuria. *J Inherited Metab Dis* **6:**143, 1983.
216. Grays RGF, Hill SE, Pollitt RJ: Reduced ornithine catabolism in culture fibroblasts and phytohaemagglutinin-stimulated lymphocytes from a patient with hyperornithinaemia, hyperammonaemia and homocitrullinuria. *Clin Chim Acta* **118:**141, 1982.
217. Shih VE: Regulation of ornithine metabolism. *Enzyme* **26:**254, 1981.
218. Shih VE, Mandell R: Defective ornithine metabolism in the syndrome of hyperornithinaemia, hyperammonaemia and homocitrullinuria. J Inherited Metab Dis **4:**95, 1981.
219. Vici CD, Bachmann C, Gambarara M, Colombo JP, Sabetta G: Hyperornithinemia-hyperammonemia-homocitrullinuria syndrome: Low creatine excretion and effect of citrulline, arginine, or ornithine supplement. *Pediatr Res* **22:**364, 1987.
220. Inoue I, Saheki T, Kayanuma K, Uono M, Nakajima M, Takeshita K, Koike R, Yuasa T, Miyatake T, Sakoda K: Biochemical analysis of decreased ornithine transport activity in the liver mitochondria from patients with hyperornithinemia, hyperammonemia and homocitrullinuria. *Biochim Biophys Acta* **964:**90, 1988.
221. Inoue I, Koura M, Saheki T, Kayanuma K, Uono M, Nakajima M, Takeshita K, Koike R, Yuasa T, Miyatake T, Sakoda K: Abnormality of citrulline synthesis in liver mitochondria from patients with hyperornithinaemia, hyperammonaemia and homocitrullinuria. *J Inherited Metab Dis* **10:**277, 1987.
222. Gatfield PD, Taller E, Wolfe DM, Haust DM: Hyperorni-

thinemia, hyperammonemia, and homocitrullinuria associated with decreased carbamyl phosphate synthetase I activity. *Pediatr Res* **9**:488, 1975.

223. Hommes FA, Roesel RA, Metoki K, Hartlage PL, Dyken PR: Studies on a case of HHH-syndrome (hyperammonemia, hyperornithinemia, homocitrullinuria). *Neuropediatrics* **17**:48, 1986.
224. Hommes FA, Ho CK, Roesel RA, Coryell ME: Decreased transport of ornithine across the inner mitochondrial membrane as a cause of hyperornithinaemia. *J Inherited Metab Dis* **5**:41, 1982.
225. Oyanagi K, Tsuchiyama A, Itakura Y, Sogawa H, Wagatsuma K, Nakao T: The mechanism of hyperammonaemia and hyperornithinaemia in the syndrome of hyperornithinaemia, hyperammonaemia with homocitrullinuria. *J Inherited Metab Dis* **6**:133, 1983.
226. Shih VE, Efron ML, Moser HW: Hyperornithinemia, hyperammonemia, and homocitrullinuria. A new disorder of amino acid metabolism associated with myoclonic seizures and mental retardation. *Am J Dis Child* **117**:83, 1969.
227. Koike R, Fujimori K, Yuasa T, Miyatake T, Inoue I, Saheki T: Hyperornithinemia, hyperammonemia, and homocitrullinuria: Case report and biochemical study. *Neurology* **37**:1813, 1987.
228. Pisoni RL, Thoene JG, Christensen HN: Detection and characterization of carrier-mediated cationic amino acid transport in lysosomes of normal and cystinotic human fibroblasts. *J Biol Chem* **260**:4791, 1985.
229. Aula P, Autio S, Raivio KO, Rapola J, Thoden C-J, Koskela S-L, Yamashina I: "Salla Disease". A new lysosomal storage disorder. *Arch Neurol* **36**:88, 1979.
230. Gahl WA, Bashan N, Iteze F, Bernardini I, Schulman JD: Cystine transport is defective in isolated leukocyte lysosomes from patients with cystinosis. *Science* **217**:1263, 1982.
231. Renlund M, Aula P, Raivio KO, Autio S, Sainio K, Rapola J, Koskela S-L: Salla disease: A new lysosomal storage disorder with disturbed sialic acid metabolism. *Neurology* **33**:57, 1983.
232. Renlund M, Kovanen PT, Raivio KO, Aula P, Gahmberg CG, Ehnholm C: Studies on the defect underlying the lysosomal storage of sialic acid in Salla disease. Lysosomal accumulation of sialic acid formed from *N*-acetyl-mannosamine or derived from low density lipoprotein in cultured mutant fibroblasts. *J Clin Invest* **77**:568, 1986.
233. Renlund M, Tietze F, Gahl WA: Defective sialic acid egress from isolated fibroblast lysosomes of patients with Salla disease. *Science* **232**:759, 1986.
234. Reeves JP: Accumulation of amino acids by lysosomes incubated with amino acid methyl esters. *J Biol Chem* **254**:8914, 1979.
235. Desjeux JF, Rajantie J, Simell O, Dumontier AM, Perheentupa J: Flux de lysine a travers l'epithelium du jejunum dans l'intolerance aux proteines avec lysinurie. *Gastroenterol Clin Biol* **4**:31A, 1980.
236. Perheentupa J, Kekomäki M, Visakorpi JK: Studies on amino nitrogen metabolism in familial protein intolerance. *Pediatr Res* **4**:209, 1970.
237. Ratner S: Urea synthesis and metabolism of arginine and citrulline. *Adv Enzymol* **15**:319, 1954.
238. Meister A: Metabolism of glutamine. *Physiol Rev* **36**:103, 1956.
239. Bachmann C, Colombo JP: Computer simulation of the urea cycle: Trials for an appropriate mode. *Enzyme* **26**:259, 1981.
240. Krebs HA, Hems R, Lund P, Halliday D, Read WWC: Sources of ammonia for mammalian urea synthesis. *Biochem J* **176**:733, 1978.
241. Stumph DA, Parks JK: Urea cycle regulation: I. Coupling of ornithine metabolism to mitochondrial oxidative phosphorylation. *Neurology* **30**:178, 1980.
242. Natale PJ, Tremblay GC: On the availability of intramitochondrial carbamylphosphate for the extramitochondrial biosynthesis of pyrimidines. *Biochem Biophys Res Commun* **37**:512, 1969.
243. Pausch J, Rasenack J, Häussinger D, Gerok W: Hepatic carbamoyl phosphate in de novo pyrimidine synthesis. *Eur J Biochem* **150**:189, 1985.
244. Graham GG, MacLean WC Jr, Placko RP: Plasma free amino acids of infants and children consuming wheat-based diets, with and without supplemental casein or lysine. *J Nutr* **111**:1446, 1981.
245. Cree TC, Schalch DS: Protein utilization in growth: Effect of lysine deficiency on serum growth hormone, somatomedins, insulin, total thyroxine [T_4] and triiodothyronine, free T_4 index, and total corticosterone. *Endocrinology* **117**:667, 1985.
246. Borum PR, Broquist HP: Lysine deficiency and carnitine in male and female rats. *J Nutr* **107**:1209, 1977.
247. Jansen GR: Lysine in human nutrition. *J Nutr* **76**:1, 1962.
248. Hwang S-M, Segal S: Developmental and other characteristics of lysine uptake by rat brain synaptosomes. *Biochim Biophys Acta* **557**:436, 1979.
249. Rajantie J, Simell O, Perheentupa J: Oral administration of ε-*N*-acetyllysine and homocitrulline for lysinuric protein intolerance. *J Pediatr* **102**:388, 1983.
250. Friedman M, Gumbmann MR: Bioavailability of some lysine derivatives in mice. *J Nutr* **111**:1362, 1981.
251. Fujitaki JM, Steiner AW, Nichols SE, Helander ER, Lin YC, Smith RA: A simple preparation of *N*-phosphorylated lysine and arginine. *Prep Biochem* **10**(2):205, 1980.
252. Morris JG, Rogers QR: Ammonia intoxication in the near-adult cat as a result of a dietary deficiency of arginine. *Science* **199**:431, 1978.
253. Morris JG, Rogers QR; Arginine: An essential amino acid for the cat. *J Nutr* **108**:1944, 1978.
254. Christensen HN: A transport system serving mono- and diamino acids. *Proc Natl Acad Sci USA* **51**:337, 1964.
255. Christensen HN, Handlogten M, Thomas EL: Na^+ facilitated reactions of neutral amino acids with a cationic amino acid transport system. *Proc Natl Acad Sci USA* **63**:948, 1969.
256. Van Winkle LJ, Christensen HN, Campione AL: Na^+-dependent transport of basic, zwitterionic, and bicyclic amino acids by a broad-scope system in mouse blastocysts. *J Biol Chem* **260**:12118, 1985.
257. Van Winkle LJ, Campione AL, Gorman JM: Na^+-independent transport of basic and zwitterionic amino acids in mouse blastocysts by a shared system and by processes which distinguish between these substrates. *J Biol Chem* **263**:3150, 1988.
258. Kilberg MS, Stevens BR, Novak DA: Recent advances in mammalian amino acid transport. *Ann Rev Nutr* **13**:137, 1993.
259. Metoki K, Hommes FA: The uptake of ornithine and lysine by isolated hepatocytes and fibroblasts. *Int J Biochem* **16**:833, 1984.
260. Christensen HN: Role of amino acid transport and countertransport in nutrition and metabolism. *Physiol Rev* **70**:43, 1990.
261. Albritton LM, Tseng L, Scadden D, Cunningham JM: A putative murine ecotropic retrovirus receptor gene encodes a multiple membrane-spanning protein and confers susceptibility to virus infection. *Cell* **57**:659, 1989.
262. Hoffman W: Molecular characterization of the CAN1 locus in *Saccharomyces cerevisiae*. A transmembrane protein without N-terminal hydrophobic signal sequence. *J Biol Chem* **260**:11831, 1985.
263. Tanaka J, Fink GR: The histidine permease gene (HIP1) of *Saccharomyces cerevisiae*. *Gene* **38**:205, 1985.
264. Weber E, Chevallier M-R, Jund R: Evolutionary relationship and secondary structure predictions in four transport proteins of *Saccharomyces cerevisiae*. *J Mol Evol* **27**:341, 1988.
265. Kim JW, Closs EI, Albritton LM, Cunningham JM: Transport of cationic amino acids by the mouse ecotropic retrovirus receptor. *Nature* **352**:725, 1991.
266. Wang H, Kavanaugh MP, North RA, Kabat D: Cell-surface receptor for ecotropic murine retroviruses is a basic amino-acid transporter. *Nature* **352**:729, 1991.
267. Closs EI, Albritton LM, Kim JW, Cunningham JM: Identification of a low affinity, high capacity transporter of cationic amino acids in mouse liver. *J Biol Chem* **268**:7538, 1993.
268. Jaenisch R, Hoffman E: Transcription of endogenous C-type viruses in resting and proliferating tissues of BALB/Mo mouse. *Virology* **98**:289, 1979.

269. MacLeod CL, Finley K, Kakuda D, Kozak CA, Wilkinson MF: Activated T cells express a novel gene on chromosome 8 that is closely related to the murine ecotropic retroviral receptor. *Mol Cell Biol* **10:**3663, 1990.
270. Wells RG, Hediger MA: Cloning of a rat kidney cDNA that stimulates dibasic and neutral amino acid transport and has sequence similarity to glucosidases. *Proc Natl Acad Sci USA* **89:**5596, 1992.
271. Tate SS, Yan N, Udenfriend S: Expression cloning of a Na^+-independent neutral amino acid transporter from rat kidney. *Proc Natl Acad Sci USA* **89:**1, 1992.
272. Bertran J, Werner A, Moore ML, Stange G, Markovich D, Biber J, Testar X, Zorzano A, Palacin M, Murer H: Expression-cloning of a cDNA from rabbit kidney cortex that induces a single transport system for cysteine, dibasic, and neutral amino acids. *Proc Natl Acad Sci USA* **89:**5601, 1992.
273. Lee W-S, Wells RG, Sabbag RV, Mohandas TK, Hediger MA: Cloning and chromosomal localization of a human kidney cDNA involved in cystine, dibasic, and neutral amino acids transport. *J Clin Invest* **91:**1959, 1993.
274. Bertran J, Magagnin S, Werner A, Markovich D, Biber J, Testar X, Zorzano A, Kuhn LC, Palacin M, Murer H: Stimulation of system y^+-like amino acid transport by the heavy chain of human 4F2 surface antigen in *Xenopus laevis* oocytes. *Proc Natl Acad Sci USA* **89:**5606, 1992.
275. Wells RG, Lee W-S, Kanai Y, Leiden JM, Hediger MA: The 4F2 antigen heavy chain induces uptake of neutral and dibasic amino acids in *Xenopus* oocytes. *J Biol Chem* **267:**15285, 1992.
276. Kacser H, Burns JA: The molecular basis of dominance. *Genetics* **97:**639, 1981.
277. Li-Chan E, Nakai S: Covalent attachment of N^ϵ-acetyl lysine, N^ϵ-benzylidene lysine, and threonine to wheat gluten for nutritional improvement. *J Food Sci* **45**(3):514, 1980.
278. Dickinson JC, Rosenblom H, Hamilton PB: Ion exchange chromatography of the free amino acids in the plasma of the newborn infant. *Pediatrics* **36:**2, 1965.
279. Scriver CR, Davies E: Endogenous renal clearance rates of free amino acids in prepubertal children. *Pediatrics* **36:**592, 1965.

CHAPTER 119

Hartnup Disorder

Harvey L. Levy

1. **Hartnup disorder is an autosomal recessive impairment of neutral amino acid transport limited to the kidneys and small intestine. It is believed to be caused by a genetic defect in a specific system responsible for neutral amino acid transport across the brush-border membrane of renal and intestinal epithelium. Neither the carrier nor the gene responsible for this transport system has been identified, but recent findings with a human cell-surface protein known as 4F2 suggest that it could be involved in such transport. The diagnostic feature is a striking neutral hyperaminoaciduria. Most affected individuals also have increased excretion of indolic compounds, notably indican (indoxyl sulfate). These indoles originate in the gut from bacterial degradation of unabsorbed tryptophan. Reduced intestinal absorption of tryptophan and increased tryptophan loss in the urine lead to reduced availability of tryptophan for the synthesis of niacin.**

2. **Pellagra-like clinical features have been described in patients with Hartnup disorder. These include a photosensitive skin rash, intermittent ataxia, and psychotic behavior. Some affected individuals have also been mentally retarded or mentally subnormal to a mild degree. Treatment with nicotinamide has been associated with clearing of the rash and, on occasion, disappearance of the ataxia. This has led to the theory that the clinical abnormalities are due to niacin deficiency. Most subjects identified by routine newborn screening, however, as well as most affected sibs of probands, have remained clinically normal without treatment. The most plausible explanation for the disparity in clinical expression is that, while the disorder is monogenic, the "disease" is multifactorial and requires the presence of complicating environmental influences, such as poor diet or diarrhea, and perhaps also a polygenic influence, such as a tendency for low plasma amino acid levels.**

3. **The renal and intestinal defects are not always expressed concordantly. Some individuals with the Hartnup hyperaminoaciduria do not have increased urinary excretion of indolic acids, suggesting that they have the renal defect without the intestinal defect. Conversely, one individual with evidence of an intestinal neutral amino acid transport defect but without the Hartnup hyperaminoaciduria has been reported.**

4. **Maternal Hartnup disorder is probably benign to the fetus and to the pregnancy. At least 14 offspring from women with Hartnup disorder are known, and almost all are normal. One man with Hartnup disorder has fathered two normal children.**

Hartnup disorder is a familial disorder of renal and intestinal amino acid transport. Its constant feature is a specific hyperaminoaciduria that is caused by a diminished capacity for renal reabsorption of a group of monoamino-monocarboxylic ("neutral") acids that share a common, and in this case defective, transport system. In most affected individuals there is also reduced intestinal absorption of at least some of the neutral amino acids, notably tryptophan.

This disorder was once considered to be a rare and usually symptomatic "disease."[1] Information derived from newborn urine screening has widened our view. We now know that Hartnup disorder is one of the most frequent of the hyperaminoacidurias, and that most affected individuals remain asymptomatic,[2] but symptoms can occur when certain factors are present.[3,4]

Jepson, the original author of this chapter, accurately described the place that Hartnup disorder occupies in human biology when he stated, "The disorder has a physiologic interest out of all proportion to its rare clinical occurrence. . . . Its study has shed light on general problems of renal absorption, amino acid transport, protein digestion, nicotinamide metabolism, and intestinal bacterial reactions."[1]

An interesting historical note is that the name of the disorder is the surname of the family in which the disorder was first found. In the original report[5] the term "H disease" was used; subsequently, the full surname was applied, apparently with the consent of the family.[1]

THE HARTNUP FAMILY

In 1951, a 12-year-old boy, E. Hartnup, was admitted to the Middlesex Hospital, London, England, with mild cerebellar ataxia and a red, scaly rash on the exposed areas of his body. His mother said he had pellagra, since her eldest daughter (P.H.), with identical symptoms, had been treated for that disease. Although the rash in E.H. was quite consistent with pellagra, other findings were not, and a diagnosis of pellagra as a dietary deficiency was untenable.

Apart from variable cerebellar signs and retarded mental development, the only abnormality detected at that time was in the urinary excretion of free amino acids. Paper chromatography of the urine disclosed an excretion pattern of amino acids quite unlike that seen in any other disease.

At the same time, P.H., then 19 years old, had a recurrence of ataxia (without a rash), similar to the episode she had had in childhood when the pellagra-like rash was most severe. The excretion pattern of amino acids in her urine was identical to that of her brother, E.H.

A list of standard abbreviations is located immediately preceding the index in each volume. Additional abbreviations used in this chapter include: 5-HIAA = 5-hydroxyindoleacetic acid; PET = positron emission tomography.

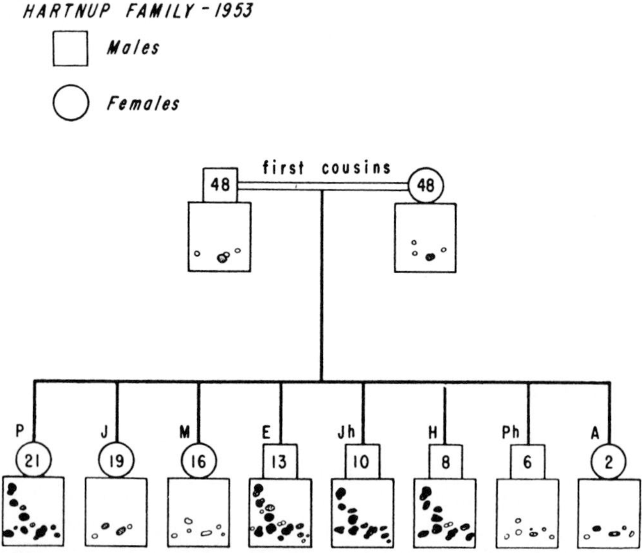

FIG. 119-1 The genealogy of Hartnup disorder as illustrated in the original Hartnup family. The parents were first cousins. The ages of the subjects in 1953 are indicated by the numbers; in the squares are the chromatography patterns of urine samples of two-dimensional chromatograms stained for amino acids.

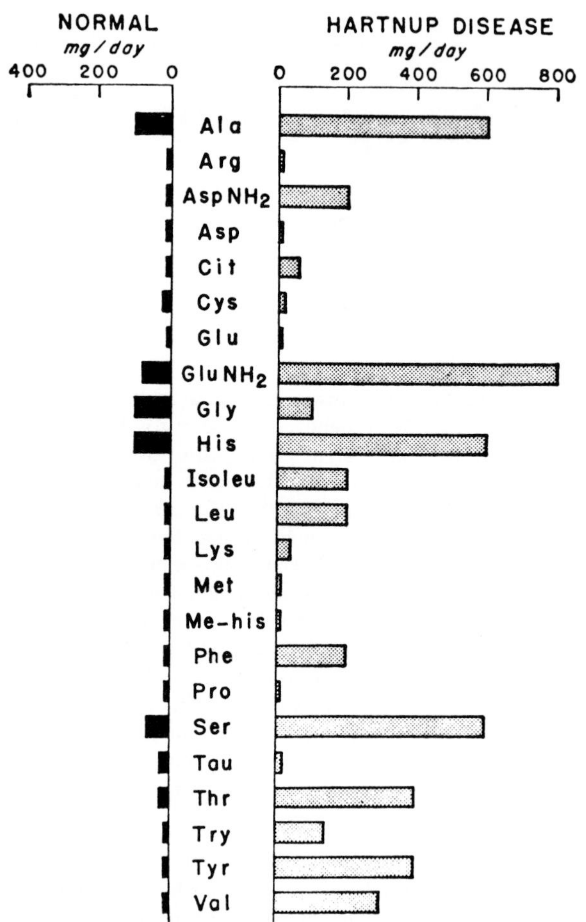

FIG. 119-2 The excretion of free amino acids in the urine of normal subjects and patients with Hartnup disorder.

It was then clear that these two sibs were affected by the same disease. An inherited condition seemed probable when it was learned that the parents were first cousins.

Neither parent and none of their other six children gave a clinical history to suggest that they were similarly affected, although one girl (M.H.) was mentally retarded. Two younger sibs, Jh. H. and H.H., also had gross aminoaciduria with the characteristic chromatographic pattern. No abnormality was detected in the urine of the other four sibs or in either parent. In the affected children, the amino acid excretion persisted unchanged in pattern and amount. The skin and neurologic disturbances gradually lessened in P.H. and E.H. but made a fleeting appearance in the younger boys.

The pedigree of the Hartnup family, with a diagrammatic representation of the amino acid chromatographic findings, is given in Fig. 119-1. No other relatives of the Hartnup parents showed the amino acid abnormality.

The publication that first fully reported this family and the existence of this disorder was entitled "Hereditary pellagra-like skin rash with temporary cerebellar ataxia. Constant renal amino-aciduria. And other bizarre biochemical features."[5] As a description of the fully expressed phenotype of the disorder, this title cannot be bettered.

BIOCHEMICAL PHENOTYPE

The diagnosis of Hartnup disorder is based on biochemical rather than clinical abnormalities. The characteristic pattern of neutral hyperaminoaciduria is the one constant feature and is considered the sine qua non for diagnosis. This pattern is a consequence of the defect in renal amino acid transport. The feces contain increased free amino acids, a consequence of the defect in intestinal amino acid transport. The intestinal defect also accounts for the presence of indoles in the urine. Defective absorption of tryptophan allows bacterial enzymes to degrade tryptophan, releasing indole and related metabolites for absorption and further degradation within the body.

Amino Acids

Renal Defect. The pattern of hyperaminoaciduria in Hartnup disorder is distinctive and quite different from other forms of renal hyperaminoaciduria, such as the generalized hyperaminoaciduria of the Fanconi syndrome, cystinuria, or iminoglycinuria. The neutral hyperaminoaciduria of Hartnup disorder consists of striking increases in the monoamino-monocarboxylic amino acids, including alanine, serine, threonine, valine, leucine, isoleucine, phenylalanine, tyrosine, tryptophan, and histidine, as well as glutamine and asparagine, which are neutral monoaminodicarboxylic amides. These free amino acids are excreted in amounts 5 to 20 times normal (Fig. 119-2). The levels of amino acids in the "acidic" (monoaminodicarboxylic) group, such as glutamic acid and aspartic acid, as well as those in the "basic" (diaminomonocarboxylic) group, such as lysine and ornithine, are usually normal or only slightly increased.[6] Methionine, a sulfur-containing neutral amino acid, is also usually normal, although it may be increased. The β-amino acids, taurine and β-aminoisobutyric acid, are not detected in Hartnup urine. It is worth noting that even the most sensitive methods fail to detect increased amounts of proline, hydroxyproline, or arginine. The absence of proline in particular distinguishes the Hartnup pattern from generalized hyperaminoaciduria.[7] The free amino acids are all of the L configuration.[8]

The hyperaminoaciduria is of renal origin, not an "overflow" phenomenon, since plasma amino acid concentrations are not increased. The renal clearances of the excessively

Table 119-1 Renal Clearance of Amino Acids in Hartnup Disorder

Amino Acid	Excretion in Hartnup Disorder	Clearance (ml/min)*	
		Hartnup	Normal
Total amino acid nitrogen			
Fasting	High	6–22	1.5
Maximum on oral protein load	Very high	25–50	3.0
Threonine	High	70	1.0
Tyrosine	High	66	1.5
Histidine	High	122	6.0
Taurine	Low	1.9	5.0
Proline	Low	0.3	0.1
Cystine	Low	0.4	0.5

*Data from Refs. 10–13.

excreted amino acids are grossly elevated above normal, both in the fasting state[9] and following an oral load of casein,[10] while the clearances of the amino acids that are not excreted in excess are normal or only slightly elevated. Table 119-1 provides data on renal clearances from several studies.[10–13] The clearance of histidine has been reported to be as high as 140 ml/min,[14] approximating the GFR. One patient excreted 17 percent of an intravenous load of L-histidine unchanged within 4 h, while a control excreted only 0.3 percent.[12] For the other amino acids excreted in excess by Hartnup individuals, the tubular reabsorption of the filtered load at physiological concentrations is about 30 to 60 percent, compared to over 95 percent for normal subjects.

These excretion studies indicate a disturbance in the renal tubular transport of a certain group of amino acids, specifically those of the neutral type, which share a common system for renal membrane transport.[15] The quartet of amino acids excreted in cystinuria (cystine, ornithine, lysine, and arginine; see Chap. 117) share another transport system; this system is obviously intact in Hartnup individuals, as is a third distinct transport system, for the glycine-imino acid group, that is defective iminoglycinuria (see Chap. 120). This concept—that Hartnup disorder is one of a trio of genetic disorders each involving only one of the systems for amino acid transport—was first suggested by Milne et al.,[16] who also extended the concept to apply to intestinal transport as well as the renal tubule.

Despite the obvious defect, substantial renal tubular transport of the involved amino acids remains. As noted above, except in rare instances, renal clearances do not approach the GFR. It is possible that the renal tubular defect is far from complete. A more likely explanation is that each amino acid is transported by more than one system.[17] One of these systems transports most of the neutral amino acids. This is most likely a high-capacity system and is defective in Hartnup disorder. Specific low-capacity systems may also exist for each amino acid, as is known to be the case for glycine (see Chap. 120). Thus, in Hartnup disorder, renal tubular reabsorption of neutral amino acids may occur by a combination of specific amino acid transport, passive diffusion, and, perhaps, residual activity of the defective neutral amino acid transport system.

The amino acid excretion pattern is remarkably constant, and is unchanged by nicotinamide or other vitamins, drugs, or antibiotics, despite isolated reports to the contrary.[18,19]

All other tests of renal function have given normal results. One patient was found at autopsy to lack the descending limb of the loop of Henle.[20] This child had unusual features, which included fatty degeneration of the liver with liver failure and terminal myocardial involvement.[21] Microdissection of nephrons was not reported in other patients studied at autopsy.[22,23] The defect is certainly at a subcellular level, but in vitro studies of renal amino acid transport in Hartnup individuals have not yet been performed.

Intestinal Defect. Demonstrating a defect in intestinal absorption of free amino acids analogous to the defect in renal transport has been more difficult than identifying the renal defect, but several studies have shown that (1) feces from Hartnup patients contain increased amounts of the affected amino acids; (2) the rise in plasma concentration of several involved amino acids following an oral load is abnormally low or delayed, although normal concentrations are found after intravenous administration; and (3) bacterial degradation products from unabsorbed amino acids are found in excess in urine. The latter feature has been especially investigated for tryptophan.

The first indication of an intestinal defect in Hartnup disorder was the discovery that intestinal transport of tryptophan is affected.[24] This finding will be discussed below in the section on indole compounds. Following this discovery, Scriver and Shaw[25] and then Scriver[26] described a pattern of increased fecal amino acids that almost mirrored the typical Hartnup urinary pattern. Asatoor and coworkers[27] also found that the feces of patients with Hartnup disorder contained greater quantities of tryptophan, phenylalanine, tyrosine, valine, and leucine/isoleucine than did the feces of normal individuals.

In other studies, however, fecal amino acids were not increased when the patients were on regular diets.[28–30] This seemingly conflicting evidence stimulated investigation of transport with orally administered amino acid loads. These studies demonstrated that intestinal transport of leucine, methionine, phenylalanine, and tyrosine is reduced in the Hartnup disorder,[28–33] whereas proline, glycine, and β-alanine, which have normal renal transport in the Hartnup disorder, also have normal intestinal transport.[29–32] On the other hand, studies of intestinal histidine and lysine transport have not produced consistent results, with evidence for reduced transport in Hartnup disorder in some investigations[28,32] and for normal transport in other studies.[12,28,30,34]

Impaired intestinal transport for several free amino acids has been demonstrated in vitro in Hartnup disorder. Tarlow et al.[33,34] found that jejunal biopsy tissue in one patient showed very little accumulation of histidine when incubated with L-histidine. Shih and coworkers[30] studied the uptake of four amino acids by jejunal mucosa obtained through biopsy from two affected brothers. Tryptophan and methionine uptakes were markedly reduced, while lysine and glycine uptakes were only slightly but significantly diminished. Jejunal mucosa has been histologically normal.[20,22,30,32]

The defective intestinal absorption of certain neutral amino acids seems not to apply to their ketoacid analogues. Scriver[26] found that transport by the gut of indolepyruvic acid, the ketoacid of tryptophan (Fig. 119-3), was normal in Hartnup disorder, in contrast to the defective transport of tryptophan.

The defect also does not involve intestinal absorption of peptides. When histidine was given to a Hartnup subject in the form of oral carnosine (β-alanyl-L-histidine) rather than as free histidine, the plasma histidine response was normal.[31] This subject also absorbed phenylalanine and tryptophan better when they were in the dipeptide form than as the corresponding mixed free amino acids, while the reverse is true in normal individuals.[32] Analogous results were seen in another affected individual after oral administration of glycyl-tyrosine and free tyrosine.[34] When hydrolyzed casein was given to an individual with Hartnup disorder, there was a rise in plasma amino acids, but when an equivalent mixture of amino acids was given, there was no comparable rise.[35] This suggests that amino acid nutrition in Hartnup disorder (and possibly in analogous situations) is maintained more by absorption of small peptides than by essential amino acids in free form.[36]

An intestinal defect in amino acid transport similar to that noted in the classic Hartnup disorder defect can be present without the renal defect. Drummond et al.[37] reported intestinal malabsorption seemingly limited to tryptophan, with normal urine amino acid excretion in one child and, most probably, also in a deceased sib (see below). Hillman and coworkers[38] described an infant with markedly increased neutral amino acids in the stool and normal or near-normal urine amino acids. These cases, in combination with the diversity in intestinal amino acid transport suggested by the studies in patients with the renal defect, indicate a substantial degree of heterogeneity in the linked renal and intestinal transport of neutral amino acids.

Blood Amino Acids. In all cases in which blood amino acids have been analyzed, the levels have been normal or low, the latter as could be anticipated from diminished absorption and increased excretion.[9,39–41] A study of cases identified by routine screening[3] disclosed slightly lower summed plasma values for the "Hartnup" amino acids in 21 Hartnup subjects as compared to 19 age-matched, unaffected sibs (1552 ± 299 μM and 1657 ± 311 μM, respectively; $p = 0.16$ and 0.06 by Student's t-test and ANOVA, respectively). Summed plasma values for the "non-Hartnup" amino acids were also slightly lower in the Hartnup subjects.

Transport in Other Tissues. Sweat and saliva from Hartnup individuals have a normal amino acid composition.[5] Leukocytes[42] and cultured skin fibroblasts[43] from Hartnup patients transport tryptophan normally. These observations emphasize the conclusion that humans have many genetically independent transport mechanisms and that Hartnup disorder affects only one type and only in specific tissues.

Indole Compounds

Tryptophan Metabolism and Nicotinic Acid (Niacin). Among the clinical abnormalities recognized in the first individuals with Hartnup disorder were psychosis, a photosensitive skin rash, and, occasionally, diarrhea.[5,44,45] Since these are features of pellagra, attention was early directed to the

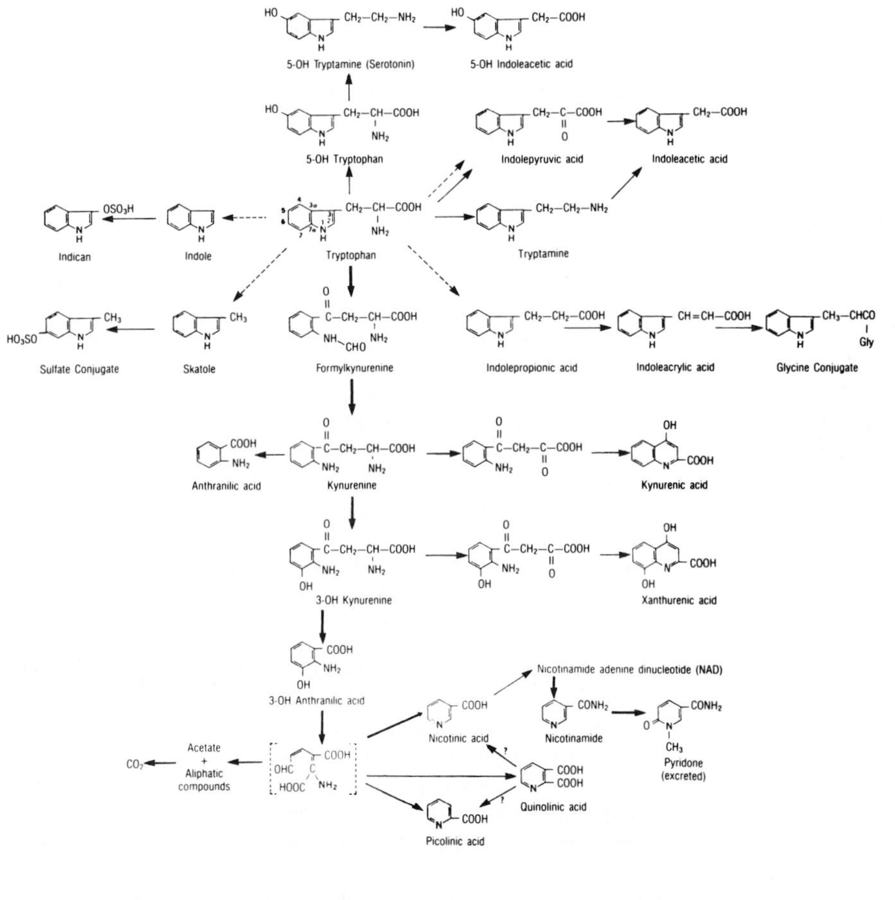

FIG. 119-3 Pathways of tryptophan catabolism. Broken arrows indicate intestinal catabolism by microorganisms.

possible role of niacin deficiency in the disorder. However, these patients did not have a dietary history suggesting pellagra nor a deficiency of nicotinic acid derivatives in the urine. Additional tryptophan did not substantially increase the excretion of nicotinic acid derivatives, as would be expected in pellagra.[5] Furthermore, urine amino acids were normal in a patient with diet-induced pellagra.[5] Nevertheless, frequently there seemed to be a clinical response to nicotinamide treatment.[5,44,45] Thus, a defect in the availability of niacin was suspected.

Nicotinic acid and nicotinamide can be synthesized from tryptophan. Figure 119-3 depicts the pathway for this synthesis, the major tryptophan catabolic pathway, as well as some of the many other pathways along which tryptophan catabolism can proceed. Tryptophan is first converted to formylkynurenine by the liver enzyme tryptophan pyrrolase; activity of this enzyme is stimulated by tryptophan administration or by corticoids.[46,47] Formylkynurenine is hydrolyzed to kynurenine by the liver enzyme kynurenine formylase. Kynurenine is hydroxylated to 3-hydroxykynurenine by the mitochondrial enzyme kynurenine-3-hydroxylase, which can be cleaved by the pyridoxal-requiring enzyme kynureninase to alanine and 3-hydroxyanthranilic acid. The latter product is oxidized to a labile ring-opened aldehyde intermediate. Ring closure and decarboxylation then occur simultaneously, with the formation of either nicotinic acid or picolinic acid, each by its specific enzyme. Nicotinic acid is further metabolized to nicotinamide adenine dinucleotide (NAD) and nicotinamide.

Under normal conditions, very little tryptophan appears to be converted to nicotinic acid. It is estimated that in the human 60 mg tryptophan is required to replace 1 mg dietary nicotinamide in the form of niacin.[48] Nevertheless, tryptophan may be an important source of niacin, particularly in individuals with relatively poor protein diets.[49]

Evidence that tryptophan is an important source of niacin is seen in patients suspected of having a defect in tryptophan degradation. Common clinical features in several of these patients have included characteristics of niacin deficiency such as a photosensitive rash, ataxia, and mental subnormality.[50–53] In addition, they have often had reduced urinary excretion of *N*-methylnicotinamide,[50,52,53] indicating that the block in tryptophan degradation limited nicotinic acid synthesis.

At least 10 such patients have been reported. Snedden and coworkers[54] described two sibs who had markedly increased plasma and urine tryptophan levels and reduced kynurenine. A block in the conversion of tryptophan to kynurenine was postulated, but enzyme studies to confirm the block were not performed. Tada and colleagues[50] and, later, Wong et al.[51] described children with growth and developmental delay, ataxia, and a photosensitive rash who had very mild increases in plasma tryptophan, which were accentuated by tryptophan loading. On the basis of reduced urinary kynurenine after tryptophan loading, they also postulated a block in the conversion of tryptophan to kynurenine, but, again, enzyme studies were not done. Komrower et al.[55] reported a child with borderline intelligence, short stature, and headaches who excreted large amounts of both kynurenine and 3-hydroxykynurenine. They suggested that she had a defect in kynureninase, which catalyzes the conversion of kynurenine to anthranilic acid as well as the degradation of 3-hydroxykynurenine. More recently, Clayton and coworkers[56] described a girl with a photosensitive rash, colitis, intellectual deterioration, and severe emotional symptoms who completely recovered with nicotinamide therapy. The increased excretion of kynurenine and kynurenic acid, which was greatly accentuated by tryptophan loading, and the reduced excretion of 3-hydroxykynurenine led these investigators to propose that the defect was at the level of kynurenine-3-hydroxylase. Other reports include a postulated defect in picolinate carboxylase,[52] a suggested partial defect in kynurenine-3-hydroxylase,[57] the suggestion of an unspecified block proximal to 3-hydroxyanthranilic acid,[53] and an infant with increased tryptophan accompanied by increased blood serotonin who was identified by routine newborn screening.[58]

Other Tryptophan Derivatives. Serotonin (5-hydroxytryptamine), a monoamine neurotransmitter, is an important derivative of tryptophan, although little tryptophan is catabolized in this direction. Serotonin is usually estimated in urine or cerebrospinal fluid as its oxidation product, 5-hydroxyindoleacetic acid (5-HIAA).

Another pathway of tryptophan metabolism is conversion to indolic acids. Normal urine contains a number of indolic acids, the major ones being indoleacetic acid, indolelactic acid, 5-hydroxyindoleacetic acid, and indoleacetylglutamine.[59] The indoleacetic acid is a product of metabolism by intestinal microorganisms and mammalian tissues.[60] This conversion occurs mainly by transamination of tryptophan to indolepyruvic acid, with subsequent decarboxylation to indoleacetic acid. Small amounts of tryptophan are also converted to indoleacetic acid by way of tryptamine. The normal tryptamine excretion by humans is very low, but it can be raised manyfold by the administration of monoamine oxidase inhibitors.[61]

If intestinal absorption of tryptophan is delayed, colonic bacteria can transform tryptophan into indolepropionic acid (Fig. 119-3). This substance is absorbed from the intestine and converted by tissues into indoleacrylic acid, which is excreted as the glycine conjugate.[62,63] Apparently, mammalian tissue cannot produce either indolepropionic acid or indoleacrylic acid directly from tryptophan.

Other important products from the degradation of tryptophan by intestinal microorganisms are indole and skatole (3-methylindole).[64] These microorganisms contain tryptophanase, an enzyme which cleaves tryptophan to indole and pyruvic acid.[65] Indole is absorbed from the intestine, partly oxidized to oxindole and derivatives that are not detectable by standard tests for indoles,[66] and partly hydroxylated in the 3-position to form indoxyl and then its sulfate conjugate (indican). Skatole, the methylated derivative of indole, is converted to 6-hydroxyskatole and likewise conjugated with sulfate for excretion.[67]

Over the years, many correlations have been sought between deranged tryptophan–indole metabolism and mental illness, particularly schizophrenia.[68] Unfortunately, nothing substantial has yet been established.

On the other hand, delayed tryptophan absorption can introduce abnormal urinary excretion of indoles that may mimic metabolic abnormalities.[69] Hartnup disorder is the most extreme of these situations, but many other examples can be found. Africans accustomed to consuming large quantities of matoke (cooked banana) excrete indolylacryloylglycine, presumably because enhanced intestinal motility speeds tryptophan down to colonic bacteria.[70] This effect is also obtained by administering tryptophan orally or per rectum, with a more rapid response by the latter route of administration[71]; sterilization of the gut eliminates this effect.[70,71] Indolylacryloylglycine has also been found in the urine of individuals with unusual intestinal flora.[72,73]

Patients with blind-loop syndrome excrete vast amounts of indican.

A familial and specific intestinal malabsorption of tryptophan known as the "blue diaper syndrome" has been described by Drummond et al.[37] (see above). In this disorder, intestinal bacteria convert much of the unabsorbed tryptophan to indican (the designation "blue diaper" comes from indigotin—or indigo blue—the hydrolytic and oxidation product of indican identified in the urine). Other indolic acids are also excreted in abundance. Unlike Hartnup disorder, the defect affects only tryptophan and is expressed only in the intestine, not in the kidney.

Indoles in Hartnup Disorder

Early in the investigations of the Hartnup family, a high but variable excretion of indoxylsulfate (indican) was apparent among affected members. This led to a survey which disclosed increased urinary excretion of other indole compounds as well.[5] Thus, increased excretion of indolic acids derived from tryptophan was revealed in the Hartnup disorder (Fig. 119-4).

Indican has been the most prominent of these urinary indoles; in some instances, Hartnup probands excreted almost 400 mg/day, compared to approximately 100 mg/day excreted by age-matched normal subjects.[74,75] As with normal individuals, urinary indican disappears when the gut is sterilized with antibiotics.[5,19,76–78] Antibiotics do not alter the urinary amino acid excretion, and the indoluria returns to its high level within a few days after cessation of treatment.

Oral administration of L-tryptophan dramatically raises the indicanuria, even in Hartnup patients showing a reasonably normal indican excretion in the basal state,[24] but intravenous L-tryptophan does not have this effect.[19,79] It was the demonstration of this response to oral tryptophan that led Milne and his group[24] to recognize that the transport defect in Hartnup disorder involves the intestine as well as the kidney. Oral tryptophan in normal subjects produces a slight, variable rise in indican, followed by a fall to normal within 12 h, representing a tryptophan-to-indican conversion of no more than 1.6 percent. By contrast, in Hartnup disorder there is a greatly increased indican excretion, which reaches a maximum after 12 h and persists for more than 24 h, with a conversion of 7 to 13 percent[24,79] (Fig. 119-5). A patient investigated by Srikantia et al.[80] is exceptional in showing a fivefold rise in the urinary indican level within 1 h of an oral tryptophan load; the indican level returned to normal within 3 h but peaked again 3 h later. This patient may have a variant of the intestinal defect in Hartnup disorder. In fact, fecal amino acid values and in vitro studies of intestinal transport indicate considerable heterogeneity in the disorder (see "Intestinal Defect" above).

The urinary indoxyl derivatives are final excretion products, formed in the liver from indole absorbed from the colon. Here they must arise from the action of intestinal microorganisms on tryptophan not absorbed from the jejunum because of the transport defect. Studies of the indole-producing bacteria *(Escherichia coli)* from the feces of Hartnup patients failed to show that chronic exposure to tryptophan alters the colonic flora in type or amount from that normally found.[27] On the other hand, there is little or no excretion of 6-hydroxyskatole sulfate, the final product of intestinal skatole formation that may be seen in malabsorption syndromes.[69]

Other urinary indoles that are increased in Hartnup disorder include indoleacetic acid and its conjugate, indole-

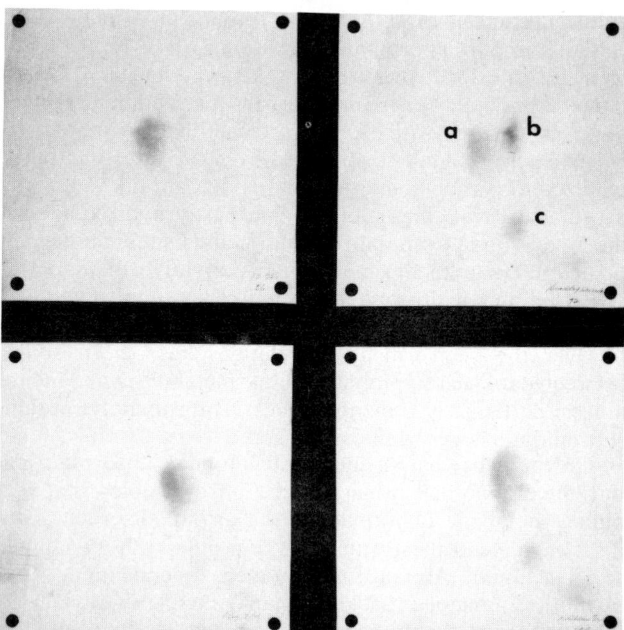

FIG. 119-4 **Urine indole patterns (in standardized aliquots) in a normal control (top left), his Hartnup sib (top right), a Hartnup proband with a variant allele (bottom right), and her control sib (bottom left). The typical pattern shows an excess of indoxyl sulfate and tryptophan. The variant pattern shows an excess of tryptophan only. a = urea; b = indoxyl sulfate; c = tryptophan** ***(Scriver, Clow, and Levy, unpublished data.)***

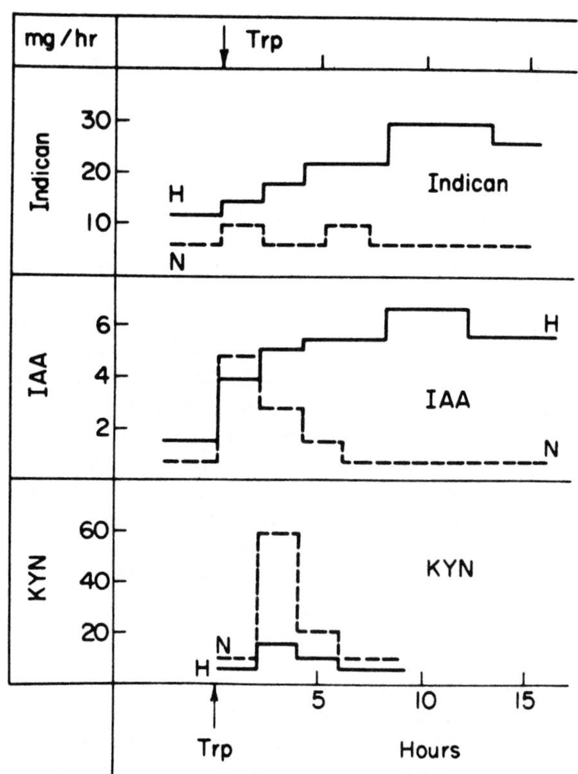

FIG. 119-5 **Urinary excretion (mg/h) of tryptophan derivatives following administration of oral L-tryptophan (about 70 mg per kilogram body weight) administered to normal subjects (N – – –) and to Hartnup patients (H–). These are idealized responses, averaged from the results of several investigators.**

acetylglutamine.[75,81–83] Indolelactic acid and indoleacetylglucuronide, the other possible conjugate of indoleacetic acid, have also been reported, but only in moderate amounts.[83] The excretion of these indolic acids, especially indoleacetic acid, has been particularly prominent during acute bouts of ataxia and rash in some patients.[5,78]

Nevertheless, the urinary indolic acid pattern has been quite variable in Hartnup individuals and has often been normal under usual conditions as well as during acute clinical episodes.[24,31] Under the stimulus of an oral tryptophan load, however, indolic acid production becomes an obvious feature of Hartnup disorder. The oral administration of L-tryptophan to normal subjects in quantities of about 70 mg per kilogram body weight causes a sharp sixfold rise in free and conjugated urine indoleacetic acid.[24] The peak is reached at 2 h, and the excretion returns to its normal low level in 8 h. The total conversion of such a load to urinary indolic acids is about 0.2 percent. In Hartnup patients, the rise is several times larger, does not reach its peak until 8 or 10 h, and persists at a high level for at least 24 h (Fig. 119-5). The total conversion has been calculated at 1.3 to 1.7 percent in these patients.[24]

Hartnup patients on oral tryptophan loading also excrete large quantities of indolylacryloylglycine with the same 8-h lag period that applies to indoleacetic acid production[76,84]; they may even excrete small amounts of indolylacryloylglycine on a normal diet.[78] In contrast, normal individuals never produce indolylacryloylglycine even with a large oral load of tryptophan, provided the usual intestinal transport mechanisms are operative.

As with indoxyl derivatives, other indolic acids are also derived from bacterial catabolism of tryptophan in the gut. This explanation for their origin is supported by two findings. The first of these findings is the effect of intestinal antibiotics in Hartnup patients. Neomycin (with nystatin) not only lowers the excretion of all indolic acids to somewhat less than the usual level but virtually abolishes any rise after oral tryptophan loading.[19,76,78] It is possible that neomycin slightly inhibits tryptophan or indoleacetic acid absorption from the intestine,[85] but this could not account for more than a small part of the dramatic effect. Second, intravenous tryptophan does not increase indolic acid excretion.[79]

Indolepyruvic acid and its decomposition products have not been detected in the urine of Hartnup patients.[86,87] The urinary excretion of tryptamine is within normal limits in these patients.[1] This may only be tryptamine produced in the kidney and might not reflect tryptamine formation in other tissues or in the intestine.[27] Tryptamine is catabolized to indoleacetic acid by way of the corresponding aldehyde. Experiments to see if oxidation could be diverted through a reductive pathway by the administration of ethanol[88] were unsuccessful; no urinary tryptophol or its conjugates were detectable in Hartnup or control subjects, before or after the consumption of large quantities of alcohol.[1]

Indoluria other than increased tryptophan may not be present in infants during the first 6 months of life.[89,90] This may reflect the more rapid transit of food through the gut during these early months, with less time for bacteria to act upon the tryptophan. After age 6 months, children originally identified by newborn urine amino acid screening have almost always had increased excretion of indolic compounds.[3,89]

Indolic Acids in the Blood. Whole-blood indolic acids have been found normal.[75] This finding could be explained by the renal clearance values of indolic acids, which are normally very high.[91] The clearance of indolylacetylglutamine is at least 150 ml/min; the compound may be synthesized, at least in part, from indoleacetic acid in the kidney.[1]

Serotonin Levels. Blood and urine levels for serotonin (5-hydroxytryptamine) have been within normal limits or on the low side of the normal range, in parallel with reduced urinary 5-hydroxyindoleacetic acid excretion.[1,75,77]

Jonas and Butler[41] reported substantially reduced concentrations of 5-hydroxyindoleacetic acid, the oxidation metabolite of serotonin, in the cerebrospinal fluid of a child with Hartnup disorder who had delayed growth and development. Other neurotransmitter metabolite levels were normal. The tryptophan level in cerebrospinal fluid was also reduced, suggesting that this deficiency led to reduced serotonin. Supporting this suggestion was the response to intravenous tryptophan, which increased the level of 5-hydroxyindoleacetic acid in cerebrospinal fluid to a normal value.

Nicotinic Acid Derivatives

The pellagra-like clinical features of some patients with Hartnup disorder led to an early interest in the tryptophan-kynurenine-nicotinic acid pathway.[5] Surprisingly, the urinary excretion of nicotinic acid and derivatives such as nicotinamide and *N*-methylnicotinamide were within normal limits, albeit on the low side. Visakorpi et al.[21] later reported normal niacin concentrations in blood and urine from one patient. Other studies, however, have found that Hartnup subjects may excrete less *N*-methylnicotinamide than normal individuals, both in the basal state[39,42,77,92,93] and after an oral, tryptophan load.[39,42,94]

These data might indicate that the amount of nicotinic acid and its derivatives in Hartnup disorder is not necessarily deficient, perhaps because ingested nicotinic acid is absorbed and metabolized normally,[92] but that less comes from ingested tryptophan than in normal individuals. This is not due to a block in the major pathway of tryptophan catabolism through kynurenine (Fig. 119-3), as was once thought might be the case.[5] Notably, tryptophan administered intravenously to Hartnup subjects produces normally enhanced excretion of kynurenine and *N*-methylnicotinamide.[19,79] Rather, it is due to a lower availability of ingested tryptophan, as evidenced by the formation of much less kynurenine[19,24,31,42,79] and xanthurenic acid[76] than in normal controls. Normal individuals converted 3 to 7 percent of oral L-tryptophan to urinary kynurenine, with a peak excretion rate of about 80 mg/h, while Hartnup patients converted only 0.5 to 1.5 percent to kynurenine, with a maximum excretion rate of 10 mg/h.[24] The reduced availability of ingested tryptophan is presumably a result of the defect in intestinal transport (see "Intestinal Defect" above).

CLINICAL PHENOTYPE

The clinical findings in at least two of the four affected children in the original Hartnup family were so much like those seen in pellagra that the investigators performed amino acid analyses on urine specimens from two other English children who had previously been reported as having pellagra.[44,45] In at least one of these children, the diet was much better than that usually ingested by individuals with pellagra.[44] In both children, the amino acid pattern was like that seen in the affected members of the Hartnup family. Thus, it seemed that Hartnup disorder might be phenotypically similar to pellagra.

Subsequent experience has not confirmed such a close association. In fact, children with Hartnup disorder identified by routine newborn urine screening have almost always remained clinically normal.[3,89] This suggests that Hartnup disorder is usually benign. There is little doubt, however, that some individuals with the Hartnup biochemical phenotype develop clinical abnormalities. The unusual combination of a photosensitive rash and neuropsychiatric manifestations has been more often associated with the Hartnup pattern of neutral hyperaminoaciduria than would be expected from coincidence. The most likely explanation for the wide clinical spectrum, proposed by Scriver et al.[3] and Scriver,[4] is that Hartnup disorder represents a monogenic transport defect with which polygenic and environmental factors interact. When these factors are aberrant, as occasionally they are, disease results. Thus the cause of Hartnup "disease" is multifactorial. Otherwise, the transport disorder is benign.

Skin Lesions

An unusual "pellagra-like" rash has been the most frequent clinical abnormality seen in Hartnup patients. The age of onset has varied from as early as 10 days[95] or three months[5,76,96,97] to as late as 13 years.[39] The photosensitive rash has appeared as "severe sunburn," and the patient becomes known as one who should avoid the sun. After unusual exposure to sunlight, blisters have formed much more readily than in normal individuals. The rash has been exclusively or predominantly on the exposed areas of the body, particularly the face, back of neck, back of hands and wrists, external surfaces of the arms and legs, anterior surfaces of the knees, and dorsal surfaces of the feet. In several individuals the rash has been pruritic[39,78,97] and, on occasion, has had the appearance of eczema.[5,21] In three patients the appearance of umbilicated bullae surrounded by erythematous halos suggested the diagnosis of hydroa vacciniforme.[22,98,99] Following the acute erythematous phase, the skin has frequently desquamated, exposing areas of depigmentation. Subsequently, the skin becomes dry and scaly with peripheral depigmentation. The rash has usually been bilateral. Minor skin manifestations were found at slightly higher frequency in Hartnup persons relative to their control sibs in a prospective study.[3]

Neurologic Manifestations

Ataxia. Intermittent ataxia has been the next most frequent abnormality reported among clinically affected patients and the most frequently noted neurologic abberation. The ataxia has usually appeared as unsteadiness while standing and as an unsteady, wide-based gait. In general, no unilaterality has been noted, although in two patients[5,82] the ataxia was more pronounced on the left side and in another patient[80] there was a tendency to fall to one side. The ataxia has usually begun later than the skin abnormalities, but in one case[14] it was the first clinical abnormality noted and in two other cases[80,82] it appeared at the same time as the rash. It has frequently been accompanied by other abnormalities such as nystagmus, diplopia, and tremors, suggesting a cerebellar origin. The most striking characteristic of the ataxia, however, has been its intermittency. In most instances it was present for only a few days or less at a time and then spontaneously disappeared. Precipitating factors in the ataxic episodes have usually not been identifiable, although *Shigella* dysentery seems to cause an attack in one patient,[5] and exposure to sunlight was implicated in both the rash and ataxia in two other patients.[39]

Mental Development. Although the first two cases identified in the original Hartnup family were mentally retarded, the other two affected members were not retarded.[5] Most of the subsequently reported clinically affected Hartnup patients have not had frank intellectual retardation. School performance has been consistent with intelligence test scores and clinical estimates of intelligence,[5,75,78,87] as have been the types of labor performed.[5,75,82] One of two symptomatic Hartnup patients in a prospective study[3] had delayed cognitive development relative to his non-Hartnup sibs.

Neurologic Signs. Other than the ataxia, there have been few specific neurologic findings. Increased muscle tone and increased deep-tendon reflexes have been reported, usually involving all extremities but, on occasion, only the lower extremities.[39,40,80,93] With the exception of a transient Babinski response in one patient[22] and a persisting response in a child with a progressive encephalopathy,[23] the plantar reflex has been flexor. Pyramidal tract signs have only infrequently been present and when they are present, usually occur during ataxia episodes. One patient had decreased deep tendon reflexes,[42] and another patient had decreased muscle tone.[100]

Electroencephalographic Findings. Electroencephalographic abnormalities have been described in a number of patients, but there has been no consistent pattern of changes. The abnormalities have ranged from nonspecific slowing[87,101] to variable dysrhythmias, and interpretations of the dysrythmias have ranged from "electrical immaturity"[100] to "general cerebral dysrhythmia."[78] Increases in theta,[23,31,75] delta,[94] theta-delta,[39,78] and beta[23,39] activities have been mentioned. The abnormalities have usually been generalized, but localized abnormal activities in the parietotemporal,[78] temporal,[23] posterior temporal,[31] and occipital[94] areas have been recorded.

All patients with abnormal EEGs have had clinical abnormalities referable to the central nervous system. In two patients, these findings have been as nonspecific as increased anxiety and irritability.[75] In another case, ataxia and mental retardation were present,[94] while a recently reported child with encephalographic abnormalities died with a progressive encephalopathy.[23] On the other hand, at least two patients with profound central nervous system disease had normal EEGs,[29,87] as did a child with intermittent dystonia and a declining IQ.[93] Electroencephalographic findings have not been recorded in individuals with Hartnup disorder who have not had neurologic disease.

Other Neurologic Findings. One patient had choreiform movements when ataxia was pronounced.[5] Another patient has had intermittent dystonia.[93] Frequent headaches were noted in two patients.[5,78] A patient who had deaf-mutism and was mentally retarded had a history of generalized seizures during early childhood.[29] One patient was prone to vasovagal attacks.[5]

Neuroimaging and Other Studies. Neuroimaging studies have been performed in a few patients with Hartnup disorder. Cranial CT disclosed a small calcification in a frontal subcortical area in an adult with neuropsychiatric illness[101] and minor brain atrophy in a child with progressive encephalopathy,[23] but has also been normal in a child with neurologic disease.[93] Magnetic resonance imaging (MRI) of the brain has been described as normal in at least two patients,[23,102] but revealed atrophy, delayed myelination, and dysgenesis of the corpus callosum in a child with intermittent ataxia, developmental delay, and growth failure.[103] Positron emission tomography (PET) revealed "possible bifrontal hypoperfusion" in one adult.[101]

Findings in additional neurologic studies in patients with Hartnup disorder have included normal somatosensory evoked potentials and normal nerve conduction velocities in two patients.[93,101] One child with severe neurologic disease had low-normal nerve conduction velocities.[23]

Psychological Changes

Most of the clinically affected Hartnup patients have had no psychiatric disturbances. Abnormalities of a psychiatric nature suggesting psychosis, however, were among the prominent findings in several of the early cases. The boy described by Hersov[44] was "irritable and morose." The first two members of the Hartnup family had marked emotional instability with depression and outbursts of temper accompanying ataxic episodes. Other patients have been "depressed and depersonalized" with suicidal tendencies,[75] severely anxious,[75] nervous and hallucinatory,[39,78] continuously crying,[78,87] severely confused with hypomania, making meaningless utterances and incontinent,[31] having continuous daytime bruxism,[101] and markedly aggressive.[100] These disturbances have always been episodic and frequently were accompanied by ataxia.

General Somatic Abnormalities

Several different somatic abnormalities have been described in patients with Hartnup disorder. It is doubtful that most are related to the basic defect. Visakorpi et al.[21] described edema and hypoproteinemia with fatty degeneration of the liver and death from liver failure in a child whose affected sister had transient hypoproteinemia and urinary calculi but recovered. Edema and hypoproteinemia were also described in another child who was otherwise well.[104] The patient described by Daute et al.[22] had fever, diarrhea, anemia, and leukopenia and eventually died. Wong and Pillai[79] described recurrent vomiting in one patient. Oyanagi et al.[39] recorded fatty liver in one patient.

Two abnormalities may be related to the Hartnup disorder in some patients. The first of these is atrophic glossitis, present in at least six patients.[22,31,44,45,75,76] The second is small stature, noted in many of the reported cases. Although the general experience from prospective studies of cases identified by newborn screening[3,89] does not support the conclusion of Colliss et al.[105] that Hartnup subjects have a significant reduction in height, occasional children identified prospectively have had growth delay.[3] It is possible that either niacin deficiency or a general deficiency of amino acids[3] complicating certain cases of Hartnup disorder could explain the glossitis and growth retardation.

Characteristics of Individuals Identified by Newborn Screening

Wilcken and her coworkers[89] studied 15 children with Hartnup disorder detected through routine newborn urine screening in New South Wales. Most did not receive nicotinamide treatment. Their intelligence and growth were considered normal and comparable to that of their unaffected sibs. None had abnormal neurologic findings, and only one had a photosensitive rash.

Scriver et al.[3] reported the study of 21 affected children who came to attention through routine urine screening in Massachusetts and Quebec, compared to 19 age-matched unaffected sib controls. None had received continual nicotinamide therapy. Two developed major clinical manifestations, considered to be due to factors acting in concert with the Hartnup defect (see "Is Hartnup Disorder a Disease?" below). Among the remaining 19 affected children, five developed skin lesions, which were eczematous in three cases and psoriatic in two but not photosensitive in any; one unaffected sib had eczema ($p = 0.19$). One Hartnup subject had seizures and an abnormal EEG. The mean ± SD full-scale IQ scores for 12 Hartnup subjects and 8 sib controls were 103 ± 10 and 108 ± 12, respectively. The difference was insignificant. School performances were similar for the two groups. Two Hartnup subjects had learning difficulties, and one of them was subsequently found to also have 47,XXX aneuploidy.[106] Somatic growth was normal in the affected children and comparable to that of their sib controls. Thus, it seems that most Hartnup subjects remain clinically normal.

DIAGNOSIS

The only constant feature of Hartnup disorder is the characteristic excretion of free amino acids, and it is on this that the diagnosis must be based.[1,2] The *pattern* of urinary amino acids, rather than the total amino acid excretion, is the determining factor. A simple two-dimensional paper or thin-layer chromatographic system with location reagents for amino acids will reveal this pattern,[107] as will quantitative amino acid analysis by column chromatography. Figure 119-2 indicates the urinary amino acids expected in excess in the Hartnup disorder.

Very little else even remotely resembles the Hartnup pattern. In generalized hyperaminoaciduria, with which the Hartnup pattern is most likely confused, proline is always prominent, and cystine and the dibasic amino acids (lysine and ornithine) are excreted in excess. These compounds, particularly proline, are not increased in Hartnup disorder.[5] Fecal contamination of urine, which has often produced factitious results in newborn screening,[108] causes an amino acid pattern much more like generalized hyperaminoaciduria than one resembling Hartnup disorder.[109]

The indolic excretion is not constant enough to be the basis of a diagnostic test. Even increased excretion of indolic acids after an oral tryptophan load might be misleading, since an intestinal defect similar or identical to that in Hartnup disorder may be present without neutral hyperaminoaciduria.[38] Conversely, Hartnup subjects may have only the renal defect.[3] Thus, Hartnup disorder is not excluded by a normal indole excretion, but all patients with a high indican or other indolic acid excretion should be further examined for Hartnup disorder by urine amino acid analysis.

The only alternative diagnoses for the full clinical expression associated with Hartnup disorder would be pellagra or, possibly, a defect in the major pathway of tryptophan catabolism. In pellagra, amino acid excretion is low or normal.[5] Putative defects in tryptophan catabolism include familial disease with pellagra-like skin rash and ataxia, but renal and intestinal amino acid transport is normal.[50–53,110] Hartnup disorder should be suspected in patients with pellagra-like signs but without gross dietary deficiency; photosensitive rash, especially if accompanied by neurologic changes; intermittent ataxia, especially where sibs are similarly affected; or high excretion of indican or other indolic acids.

TREATMENT

The only rational treatment for this disorder is the administration of nicotinic acid or, better, nicotinamide to patients who have signs suggesting a deficiency of this vitamin. This treatment has been used with dosages from 50 to 300 mg/day administered orally. In many instances the rash has cleared with this therapy.[78,111] Several investigators have also reported cessation of ataxia[39,44,82,94] and amelioration of psychotic-type behavior.[31,39,44,75,78,112] Despite reports to the contrary,[18,19] neither the hyperaminoaciduria nor the intestinal transport defect responds to this treatment.[28,92] In addition to nicotinamide, a high-protein diet or protein supplementation might be beneficial in some instances,[1] particularly for patients with low plasma amino acid values[3] in whom symptomatic Hartnup episodes might be prevented. Intravenous nutrition has been beneficial in correcting an eczematoid rash and hypoproteinemic edema associated with low plasma amino acid levels in one patient.[3]

The efficacy of treatment is difficult to evaluate. Since the clinical abnormalities have generally been intermittent, their disappearance in most cases cannot clearly be designated as a therapeutic result. Furthermore, therapy with nicotinamide has not always achieved the desired result. In one patient the rash disappeared after treatment on one occasion but did not on another occasion.[5] However, it seems that patients with clinical abnormalities associated with Hartnup disorder should be given at least a trial of nicotinamide therapy.

GENETICS

Hartnup disorder has an autosomal recessive inheritance pattern; males and females are about equally represented, sibs are often affected,[1,3,5,89] and parents have normal urine amino acid profiles.[5] Consanguinity between parents, as in the original family,[5] has been reported in a number of families.[1,95,97]

There seems to be widespread distribution of Hartnup disorder with no ethnic predilection. Cases have been found wherever urine amino acid analysis has been conducted, including England, continental Europe, Canada, the United States, Australia, India, Japan, West Africa, and Israel.[113]

Hartnup disorder is not associated with other genetic disorders. Jonxis[14] reported phenylketonuria and Hartnup disorder in one patient. Shih et al.[114] reported the coexistence of Hartnup disorder and methylmalonic aciduria in two families. In one of these families the proband had both Hartnup disorder and methylmalonic aciduria, and a sib had methylmalonic aciduria alone. The methylmalonic aciduria was B_{12}-unresponsive and was considered to be a benign variant of methylmalonyl CoA mutase deficiency.[115] In the second family, an infant died with severe methylmalonic aciduria; his mother was subsequently found to have Hartnup disorder when she was evaluated for recurrent skin rashes. We are aware of 47,XXX aneuploidy in a girl with Hartnup syndrome,[106] and Tarlow et al.[34] described the coexistence of celiac disease and Hartnup disorder in a boy. One girl identified in newborn screening by Wilcken developed juvenile diabetes mellitus.[116] All of these combinations appear to be purely chance occurrences.

Heterozygotes for the Hartnup mutation, including parents and offspring of Hartnup subjects, have shown no evidence of the renal defect.[1,29,117] The mother of the original Hartnup children has a normal amino acid clearance, even in response to a casein load.[10] Tryptophan loading in heterozygotes, however, might elicit evidence of deficient intestinal transport. The parents of two Hartnup patients had a delayed peak for plasma tryptophan following an oral load.[79] Similarly challenged, all the offspring of two Hartnup patients excreted abnormally large amounts of indican, indoleacetic acid, indolylacryloylglycine, indoleacetylglutamine, and indoleacetamide.[29] There may also be a high incidence of photosensitivity among heterozygous individuals.[78,83]

Cellular Phenotype

The specific membrane carrier system responsible for neutral amino acid transport has not been identified. It is apparently located in the brush-border membrane of cells expressing the Hartnup gene[31,32,36]; the gene is not expressed in parenchymal[43] or blood cells.[42] Similarly, the gene that encodes this protein has neither been mapped nor cloned. Hediger and his group, however, have recently found that the heavy chain of a human cell-surface dimeric protein known as 4F2 induces the uptake of dibasic and neutral amino acids in *Xenopus* oocytes.[118,119] Although dibasic amino acid transport does not seem to be involved in Hartnup disorder, it is possible, as they suggest, that this protein is in a family of proteins involved in amino acid transport, functioning as transport activators or regulators or perhaps directly as transporters.

These studies would be greatly facilitated by the availability of an animal model for Hartnup disorder. Unfortunately, no animal model has yet been identified or developed. Schiffer et al.[120] reported a monoaminomonocarboxylic hyperaminoaciduria in males of an inbred mouse strain, but the pattern differed somewhat from the Hartnup hyperaminoaciduria[121] and required testosterone for expression.

SCREENING AND INCIDENCE

Urine amino acid screening of individuals institutionalized for mental retardation has led to the identification of several Hartnup subjects. Among 729 such individuals screened in India, two Hartnup cases were found.[122] Two affected brothers were found among 2,100 mentally defective persons screened in a Massachusetts institution.[30] A single case was discovered among an unspecified number of individuals screened in a New Hampshire institution for the mentally retarded.[29]

The fact that the known cases of Hartnup disorder included only these few plus the relatively small number of others identified as a result of amino acid screening for medical indications led to the belief that Hartnup disorder was very rare and, therefore, that the presence of clinical abnormalities in these individuals was highly significant. Routine newborn urine screening has demonstrated, however, that the Hartnup finding is one of the more frequent amino acid disorders.[107] Newborn screening data include incidences of 1:23,000 among one million screened in Massachusetts,[123] 1:25,000 among one million screened in New South Wales, Australia,[124] 1:32,000 among 193,000 screened in Manitoba,[125] and 1:54,000 among 1.4 million screened in Quebec.[126,127] The combined newborn screening experience is 116 affected infants identified among approximately 3.5 million screened, an incidence of 1:30,000. Additional cases have been identified among sibs of these infants.[3,89] The prevalence of Hartnup disorder seems to be slightly lower than that of cystinuria,[123,127] both of which are about one-half as frequent as phenylketonuria (see Chap. 27).

IS HARTNUP DISORDER A DISEASE?

From prospective and retrospective studies of Hartnup subjects identified by routine newborn screening and followed for many years, most without therapy, it is clear that very few become symptomatic.[3,7,89] On this basis, Hartnup disorder could be considered benign. Furthermore, even the symptomatic few[3] have not had the complete clinical phenotype that was once thought to be characteristic of the Hartnup disorder.[5] These observations and the relatively high frequency of the Hartnup finding in the general population prompt the question of whether the symptoms described in patients with Hartnup disorder might be coincidental and not causally related to the genetic defect.

It is reasonable to propose that this is so. In addition to the preponderance of asymptomatic affected subjects identified by routine screening, the great majority of affected sibs identified by family screening of symptomatic probands have also been clinically normal.[7] Therapeutic correction of niacin deficiency, the factor that is believed to cause clinical abnormalities in the Hartnup disorder, does not always reverse the clinical findings and sometimes produces no benefit whatsoever.[1] Nevertheless, it is difficult to disregard the very striking and unusual pellagra-like phenotype observed in a number of affected individuals.

Attempts to reconcile these quite different observations in Hartnup subjects have produced several hypotheses. The first of these holds that symptomatic cases come from families whose diets are barely adequate for normal individuals or are persons under the stress of temporary malnutrition.[6,128] Thus, a very limited dietary niacin compounds their inherent limited ability to form nicotinamide from its only precursor amino acid, tryptophan.[15] A second hypothesis is that at least the acute attacks of ataxia and, perhaps, psychosis are a result of toxicity to the central nervous system from indolic acids produced in large amounts in some patients by the bacterial degradation of unabsorbed tryptophan in the gut.[24] Supporting this is a report that the ingestion of indoleacetic acid or indolepropionic acid causes irritability and ataxia.[129] In another study, however, indoleacetic acid given in huge quantities did not produce ill effects.[130]

The most recent hypothesis is that of Scriver et al.,[3] which holds that liability to disease in the Hartnup disorder is determined by one or more polygenic factors, notably the associated plasma amino acid value. Accordingly, disease is not likely to occur if the inherent aggregate value for plasma amino acids is normal but will occur, especially in response to environmental stress such as diarrhea, if the aggregate plasma amino acid value is low (Fig. 119-6). In this concept, the cause of disease in the Hartnup disorder is multifactorial.[3] It would seem that this theory is the most reasonable one yet advanced to explain the clinical observations in Hartnup disorder.

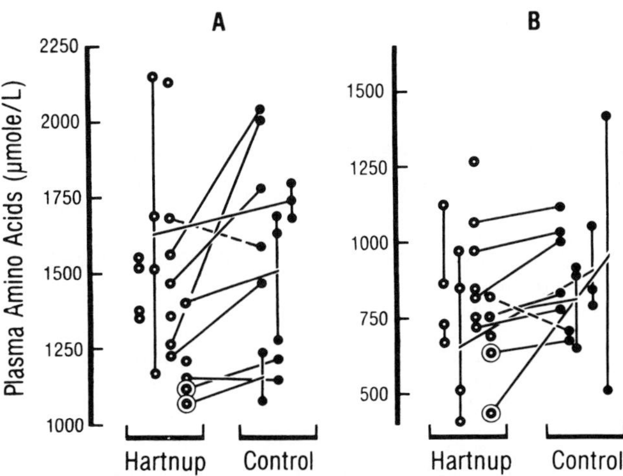

FIG. 119-6 Distributions of plasma amino acid values in Hartnup subjects (circles) and control sibs (black dots). Lines join the corresponding values for sibs (vertical lines, Hartnup vs. Hartnup and control vs. control; solid crossing lines, Hartnup value < control value; interrupted crossing line, Hartnup value > control value). *A.* Aggregate values (μmol/liter) for 10 amino acids (excluding tryptophan) affected by Hartnup mutation. *B.* Aggregate values for the remaining amino acids. Two symptomatic probands are indicated by the bull's-eye symbol. *(From Scriver et al.[3] Used by permission.)*

MATERNAL HARTNUP DISORDER

Eleven offspring have been reported from four women with the Hartnup disorder.[29,114,117] In addition, Seakins[6] mentions two offspring born to affected women who were reported before their pregnancies[31,82] and a woman who had two offspring when reported[117] and has subsequently had a third child. Twelve of these 14 offspring are clinically normal, and none has had the Hartnup disorder. Of the two abnormal offspring, one had a meningomyelocele with hydrocephalus and died at age 3 months.[114] The other had methylmalonic acidemia with severe metabolic acidosis and died during early infancy.[114] Pregnancies have been normal in these women, with the exception of one complicated by placenta previa.[117] It seems likely that Hartnup disorder does not adversely affect pregnancy and is harmless to the fetus. The occurrences of methylmalonic acidemia in one offspring and a neural tube defect in another were almost certainly coincidental.[114,117]

In one pregnancy, the ratios between maternal and umbilical vein amino acids at delivery were normal, suggesting that the neutral amino acid transport defect is not expressed in the placenta when the mother has the Hartnup disorder.[117]

One man with Hartnup disorder has fathered two normal non-Hartnup offspring.[29]

REFERENCES

1. Jepson JB: Hartnup disease, in Stanbury JB, Wyngaarden JB, Fredrickson DS (eds): *The Metabolic Basis of Inherited Disease,* 4th ed. New York, McGraw-Hill, 1978, p 1563.
2. Efron M: Comments in Greer M: Hartnup's syndrome. *Trans Am Neurol Assoc* **90**:53, 1965.
3. Scriver CR, Mahon B, Levy HL, Clow CL, Reade TM, Kronick J, Lemieux B, Laberge C: The Hartnup phenotype: Mendelian transport disorder, multifactorial disease. *Am J Hum Genet* **40**:401, 1987.
4. Scriver CR: Nutrient-gene interactions: The gene is not the disease and vice versa. *Am J Clin Nutr* **48**:1505, 1988.

5. Baron DN, Dent CE, Harris H, Hart EW, Jepson JB: Hereditary pellagra-like skin rash with temporary cerebellar ataxia. Constant renal amino-aciduria. And other bizarre biochemical features. *Lancet* **2**:421, 1956.
6. Seakins JWT: Hartnup disease, in Vinken PJ, Bruyn GW (eds): *Metabolic and Deficiency Diseases of the Nervous System*. Amsterdam, North-Holland, 1977, p 149.
7. Levy HL: Hartnup disease, in Goldensohn ES, Appel SH (eds): *Scientific Approaches to Clinical Neurology*. Philadelphia, Lea & Febiger, 1977, p 75.
8. Bonetti E, Dent CE: The determination of optical configuration of naturally occurring amino acids using specific enzymes and paper chromatography. *Biochem J* **57**:77, 1954.
9. Cusworth DC, Dent CE: Renal clearances of amino acids in normal adults and in patients with aminoaciduria. *Biochem J* 74:550, 1960.
10. Dent CE: The renal aminoacidurias. *Exp Med Surg* **12**:229, 1954.
11. Evered DF: The excretion of amino acids by the human: A quantitative study with ion-exchange chromatography. *Biochem J* **62**:416, 1956.
12. Halvorsen S, Hygstedt O, Jagenburg R, Sjaastad O: Cellular transport of L-histidine in Hartnup disease. *J Clin Invest* **48**:1552, 1969.
13. Tada K, Hirono H, Arakawa T: Endogenous renal clearance rates of free amino acids in prolinuric and Hartnup patients. *Tohoku J Exp Med* **93**:57, 1967.
14. Jonxis JHP: Oligophrenia phenylpyruvica en de hartnupziekte. *Ned Tijdschr Geneeskd* **101**:569, 1957.
15. Scriver CR, Rosenberg LE: *Amino Acid Metabolism and Its Disorders*. Philadelphia, Saunders, 1973.
16. Milne MD, Asatoor A, Loughridge L: Hartnup disease and cystinuria. *Lancet* **1**:51, 1961.
17. Scriver CR, Hechtman P: Human genetics of membrane transport with emphasis on amino acids. *Adv Hum Genet* **1**:211, 1970.
18. Fois A, Lecchini L: Acute cerebellar ataxia associated with some features of the Hartnup syndrome. *Helv Paediatr Acta* **19**:42, 1964.
19. De Laey P, Hooft C, Timmermans J, Snoeck J: Biochemical aspects of Hartnup disease. *Ann Paediatr* **202**:145, 321, 1964.
20. Hjelt L, Paatela M, Visakorpi JK: Autopsy findings in Hartnup disease. *Proc 13th Northern Pediatr Cong*, Copenhagen, 1961.
21. Visakorpi JK, Hjelt L, Lahikainen T, Ohman S: Hartnup disease in two siblings: Clinical observations and biochemical studies. *Ann Paediatr Fenn* **10**:42, 1964.
22. Daute K-H, Dietel K, Ebert W: Das Hartnupsyndrom. Bericht über einen tödlichen Krankheitsverlauf. *Z Kinderheilkd* **95**:103, 1966.
23. Schmidtke K, Endres W, Roscher A, Ibel H, Herschkowitz N, Bachmann C, Plöchl E, Hadorn HB: Hartnup syndrome, progressive encephalopathy and allo-albuminaemia. A clinico-pathological case study. *Eur J Pediatr* **151**:899, 1992.
24. Milne MD, Crawford MA, Girao CB, Loughridge LW: The metabolic disorder in Hartnup disease. *Q J Med* **29**:407, 1960.
25. Scriver CR, Shaw KNF: Hartnup disease: An example of genetically determined defective cellular amino acid transport. *Can Med Assoc J* **86**:232, 1962.
26. Scriver CR: Hartnup disease. A genetic modification of intestinal and renal transport of certain neutral alpha-amino acids. *N Engl J Med* **273**:530, 1965.
27. Asatoor AM, Craske J, London DR, Milne MD: Indole production in Hartnup disease. *Lancet* **1**:126, 1963.
28. Seakins JWT, Ersser RS: Effects of amino acid loads on a healthy infant with the biochemical features of Hartnup disease. *Arch Dis Child* **42**:682, 1967.
29. Pomeroy J, Efron ML, Dayman J, Hoefnagel D: Hartnup disease in a New England family. *N Engl J Med* **278**:1214, 1968.
30. Shih VE, Bixby EM, Alpers DH, Bartsocas CS, Thier SO: Studies of intestinal transport defect in Hartnup disease. *Gastroenterology* **61**:445, 1971.
31. Navab F, Asatoor AM: Studies on intestinal absorption of amino acids and a dipeptide in a case of Hartnup disease. *Gut* **11**:373, 1970.
32. Asatoor AM, Cheng B, Edwards KDG, Lant AF, Matthews DM, Milne MD, Navab F, Richards AJ: Intestinal absorption of two dipeptides in Hartnup disease. *Gut* **11**:380, 1970.
33. Tarlow MJ, Seakins JWT, Lloyd JK, Matthews DM, Cheng B, Thomas AJ: Intestinal absorption and biopsy transport of peptides and amino acids in Hartnup disease. *Clin Sci* **39**:18P, 1970.
34. Tarlow MJ, Seakins JWT, Lloyd JK, Matthews DM, Cheng B, Thomas AJ: Absorption of amino acids and peptides in a child with a variant of Hartnup disease and coexistent coeliac disease. *Arch Dis Child* **47**:798, 1972.
35. Leonard JV, Marrs TC, Addison JM, Burston D, Clegg KM, Lloyd JK, Matthews DM, Seakins JW: Intestinal absorption of amino acids and peptides in Hartnup disorder. *Pediatr Res* **10**:246, 1976.
36. Asatoor AM, Cheng B, Edwards KDG, Lant AF, Matthews DM, Milne MD, Navab F, Richards AJ: Intestinal absorption of dipeptides and corresponding free amino acids in Hartnup disease. *Clin Sci* **39**:1P, 1970.
37. Drummond KN, Michael AF, Ulstrom RA, Good RA: The blue diaper syndrome: Familial hypercalcemia with nephrocalcinosis and indicanuria. *Am J Med* **37**:928, 1964.
38. Hillman RE, Stewart A, Miles JH: Aminoacid transport defect in intestine not affecting kidney. *Pediatr Res* **20**:265A, 1986.
39. Oyanagi K, Takagi M, Kitabatake M, Nakao T: Hartnup disease. *Tohoku J Exp Med* **91**:383, 1967.
40. Nielsen EG, Vedso S, Zimmermann-Nielsen C: Hartnup disease in three siblings. *Dan Med Bull* **13**:155, 1966.
41. Jonas AJ, Butler IJ: Circumvention of defective neutral amino acid transport in Hartnup disease using tryptophan ethyl ester. *J Clin Invest* **84**:200, 1989.
42. Tada K, Morikawa T, Arakawa T: Tryptophan load and uptake of tryptophan by leukocytes in Hartnup disease. *Tohoku J Exp Med* **90**:337, 1966.
43. Groth U, Rosenberg LE: Transport of dibasic amino acids, cystine, and tryptophan by cultured human fibroblasts: Absence of a defect in cystinuria and Hartnup disease. *J Clin Invest* **51**:2130, 1972.
44. Hersov LA: A case of childhood pellagra with psychosis. *J Ment Sci* **101**:878, 1955.
45. Hickish GW: Pellagra in an English child. *Arch Dis Child* **30**:195, 1955.
46. Feigelson P, Feigelson M, Greengard O: Comparison of the mechanisms of hormonal and substrate induction of rat liver tryptophan pyrrolase. *Recent Prog Horm Res* **18**:491, 1962.
47. Schimke RT, Sweeney EW, Berlin CM: The roles of synthesis and degradation in the control of rat liver tryptophan pyrrolase. *J Biol Chem* **240**:322, 1965.
48. Goldsmith GA: Niacin-tryptophan relationships in man and niacin requirements. *Am J Clin Nutr* **6**:479, 1958.
49. Goldsmith GA: The B vitamins: Thiamine, riboflavin, niacin, in Beaton GH, McHenry EW (eds): *Nutrition. A Comprehensive Treatise*. New York, Academic, 1964, vol 2, p 110.
50. Tada K, Ito H, Wada Y, Arakawa T: Congenital tryptophanuria with dwarfism. *Tohoku J Exp Med* **80**:118, 1963.
51. Wong PWK, Forman P, Tabahoff B, Justice P: A defect in tryptophan metabolism. *Pediatr Res* **10**:725, 1976.
52. Salih MAM, Bender DA, McCreanor GM: Lethal familial pellagra-like skin lesion associated with neurologic and developmental impairment and the development of cataracts. *Pediatrics* **76**:787, 1985.
53. Fenton DA, Wilkinson JD, Toseland PA: Family exhibiting cerebellar-like ataxia, photosensitivity, and shortness of stature—A new inborn error of tryptophan metabolism. *J R Soc Med* **76**:736, 1983.
54. Snedden W, Mellor CS, Martin JR: Familial hypertryptophanemia, tryptophanuria and indoleketonuria. *Clin Chim Acta* **131**:247, 1983.
55. Komrower GM, Wilson V, Clamp JR, Westall RG: Hydroxykynureninuria. A case of abnormal tryptophan metabolism probably due to a deficiency of kynureninase. *Arch Dis Child* **39**:250, 1964.

56. Clayton PT, Bridges NA, Atherton DJ, Milla PJ, Malone M, Bender DA: Pellagra with colitis due to a defect in tryptophan metabolism. *Eur J Pediatr* **150**:498, 1991.
57. Price JM, Yess N, Brown RR, Johnson SAM: Tryptophan metabolism. A hitherto unreported abnormality occurring in a family. *Arch Dermatol* **95**:462, 1967.
58. McCoy EE, Ferreira P: Hypertryptophanemia and hyperserotonemia—detection in a newborn screening program for PKU. *Clin Res* **35**:212A, 1987.
59. Armstrong MD, Shaw KNF, Gortatowski MJ, Singer H: The indole acids of human urine. *J Biol Chem* **232**:17, 1958.
60. Weissbach H, King W, Sjoerdsma A, Udenfriend S: Formation of indole-3-acetic acid and tryptamine in animals. *J Biol Chem* **234**:81, 1959.
61. Sjoerdsma A, Oates JA, Zaltzman P, Udenfriend S: Identification and assay of urinary tryptamine. *J Pharmacol Exp Ther* **126**:217, 1959.
62. Smith HG, Smith WRD, Jepson JB: Interconversions of indolic acids by bacteria and rat tissue—possible relevance to Hartnup disorder. *Clin Sci* **34**:333, 1968.
63. Smith HG, Smith WRD, Jepson JB, Sorensen K: The metabolism and excretion of indolylacrylic acid in the rat. *Biochem Pharmacol* **19**:1689, 1970.
64. Fordtran JS, Scroggie WB, Polter DE: Colonic absorption of tryptophan metabolites in man. *J Lab Clin Med* **64**:125, 1964.
65. Happold FC: Trytophanase-tryptophan reaction. *Adv Enzymol* **10**:51, 1950.
66. King LJ, Parke DV, Williams RT: Metabolism of indole-2-^{14}C. *Biochem J* **88**:66P, 1963.
67. Nakao A, Ball M: The appearance of a skatole derivative in the urine of schizophrenics. *J Nerv Ment Dis* **130**:417, 1960.
68. Sprince H: Indole metabolism in mental illness. *Clin Chem* **7**:203, 1961.
69. Scriver CR: Abnormalities of tryptophan metabolism in a patient with malabsorption syndrome. *J Lab Clin Med* **58**:908, 1961.
70. Crawford MA: Degradation of aminoacids in the large gut of East Africans and its possible significance. *East Afr Med J* **41**:228, 1964.
71. Crawford MA: Discussion of indole metabolism in Hartnup disease. *Adv Pharmacol* **6B**:176, 1968.
72. Mellman WU, Barness LA, Tedesco TA, Besselman D: Indolylacryloyl-glycine excretion in a family with mental retardation. *Clin Chim Acta* **8**:843, 1963.
73. Szeinberg A, Bar-Or R, Pollack S, Cohen BE, Jepson JB: Observations on urinary excretion of indolylacryloylglycine. *Clin Chim Acta* **11**:506, 1965.
74. Rodnight R, McIlwain H: Indicanuria and the psychosis of a pellagrin. *J Ment Sci* **101**:884, 1955.
75. Hersov LA, Rodnight R: Hartnup disease in psychiatric practice: Clinical and biochemical features of three cases. *J Neurol Neurosurg Psychiatry* **23**:40, 1960.
76. Shaw KNF, Redlich D, Wright SW, Jepson JB: Dependence of urinary indole excretion in Hartnup disease upon gut flora. *Fed Proc* **19**:194, 1960.
77. Hooft C, De Laey P, Timmermans J, Snoeck J: La maladie de Hartnup. *Acta Paediatr Belg* **16**:281, 1962.
78. Halvorsen K, Halvorsen S: Hartnup disease. *Pediatrics* **31**:29, 1963.
79. Wong PWK, Pillai PM: Clinical and biochemical observations in two cases of Hartnup disease. *Arch Dis Child* **41**:383, 1966.
80. Srikantia SG, Venkatachalam PS, Reddy V: Clinical and biochemical features of a case of Hartnup disease. *Br Med J* **1**:282, 1964.
81. Jepson JB: Indolylacetyl-glutamine and other indole metabolites in Hartnup disease. *Biochem J* **64**:14p, 1956.
82. Henderson W: A case of Hartnup disease. *Arch Dis Child* **33**:114, 1958.
83. Weyers H, Bickel H: Photodermatose mit Aminoacidurie, Indolaceturie und cerebralen Manifestationen (Hartnup-Syndrom). *Klin Wochenschr* **36**:893, 1958.
84. Jepson JB: Indole metabolism in Hartnup disease. *Adv Pharmacol* **6B**:171, 1968.
85. Hvidt S, Kjeldsen K: Malabsorption induced by small doses of neomycin sulfate. *Acta Med Scand* **173**:699, 1963.
86. Jepson JB: Indolylacetamide, a chromatographic artifact from the natural indoles indolylacetylglucosiduronic acid and indolylpyruvic acid. *Biochem J* **69**:22P, 1958.
87. Lopez F, Velez H, Toro G: Hartnup disease in two Colombian siblings. *Neurology* **19**:71, 1969.
88. Davis VE, Brown H, Huff JA, Cashaw JL: Alteration of serotonin metabolism to 5-hydroxytryptophol by ethanol ingestion in man. *J Lab Clin Med* **69**:132, 1967.
89. Wilcken B, Yu JS, Brown DA: Natural history of Hartnup disease. *Arch Dis Child* **52**:38, 1977.
90. Levy HL, Shih VE, MacCready RA: Inborn errors of metabolism and transport. Prenatal and neonatal diagnosis. *Proc 13th Int Cong Pediatrics*. Vienna, 1971, vol 5, p 1.
91. Despopoulos A, Weissbach H: Renal metabolism of 5-hydroxyindoleacetic acid. *Am J Physiol* **189**:548, 1957.
92. Wong PWK, Lambert AM, Pillai PM, Jones PM: Observations on nicotinic acid therapy in Hartnup disease. *Arch Dis Child* **42**:642, 1967.
93. Darras BT, Ampola MG, Dietz WH, Gilmore HE: Intermittent dystonia in Hartnup disease. *Pediatr Neurol* **5**:118, 1989.
94. Albers FH, Wadman SK: Een patiënte met H-ziekte. *Maandschr Kindergeneeskd* **29**:102, 1961.
95. Somasundaram O, Papakumari M: Hartnup disease. A report on two siblings. *Indian Pediatr* **10**:455, 1973.
96. Haim S, Gilhar A, Cohen A: Cutaneous manifestations associated with aminoaciduria. Report of two cases. *Dermatologica* **156**:244, 1978.
97. Strobel M, Fall M, Kuakuvi N, N'Diaye B, Sanokho A, Marchand J-P: Maladie de Hartnup. *Bull Soc Méd Afr Noire Lgue Frse* **23**:118, 1978.
98. Ashurst PJ: Hydroa vacciniforme occurring in association with Hartnup disease. *Br J Dermatol* **81**:486, 1969.
99. Kimmig J: Hartnup-syndrom. *Arch Klin Exp Dermatol* **219**:753, 1964.
100. Guzzetta F, Mazzaglia E: La malattia di Hartnup. *Minerva Pediatr* **22**:480, 1970.
101. Mori E, Yamadori A, Tsutsumi A, Kyotani Y: Adult-onset Hartnup disease presenting with neuropsychiatric symptoms but without skin lesions. *Clin Neurol* **29**:687, 1989.
102. Pomeranz SJ: *Craniospinal Magnetic Resonance Imaging*. Philadelphia, Saunders, 1989, p 479.
103. Erly W, Castillo M, Foosaner D, Bonmati C: Hartnup disease: MR findings. *AJNR* **12**:1026, 1991.
104. Ozalp I, Saatçi U, Hassa R: A case of Hartnup disorder with hypoalbuminemia and edema. *Turk J Pediatr* **19**:73, 1977.
105. Colliss JE, Levi AJ, Milne MD: Stature and nutrition in cystinuria and Hartnup disease. *Br Med J* **1**:590, 1963.
106. Levy HL, Kupke KG: Unpublished data.
107. Levy HL: Genetic screening. *Adv Hum Genet* **4**:1, 1973.
108. Levy HL, Coulombe JT, Shih VE: Newborn urine screening, in Bickel H, Guthrie R, Hammersen G (eds): *Neonatal Screening for Inborn Errors of Metabolism*. Heidelberg, Springer-Verlag, 1980, p 89.
109. Levy HL, Madigan PM, Lum A: Fecal contamination in urine amino acid screening. Artifactual cause of hyperaminoaciduria. *Am J Clin Pathol* **51**:765, 1969.
110. Freundlich E, Statter M, Yatziv S: Familial pellagra-like skin rash with neurologic manifestations. *Arch Dis Child* **56**:146, 1981.
111. Milne MD: Hartnup disease. *Biochem J* **111**:3P, 1969.
112. Bartelheimer HK, Grüttner R, Simon HA: Das Hartnup-Syndrom. I. Diagnose, Therapie und klinischer Verlauf. *Monatsschr Kinderheilkd* **119**:52, 1971.
113. Levy HL: Unpublished data.
114. Shih VE, Coulombe JT, Wadman SK, Duran M, Waelkens JJJ: Occurrences of methylmalonic aciduria and Hartnup disorder in the same family. *Clin Genet* **26**:216, 1984.
115. Ledley FD, Levy HL, Shih VE, Benjamin R, Mahoney MT: Benign methylmalonic aciduria. *N Engl J Med* **311**:1015, 1984.
116. Wilcken B: Personal communication.
117. Mahon BE, Levy HL: Maternal Hartnup disorder. *Am J Med Genet* **24**:513, 1986.
118. Wells RG, Lee W-S, Kanai Y, Leiden JM, Hediger MA: The 4F2 antigen heavy chain induces uptake of neutral and

dibasic amino acids in *Xenopus* oocytes. *J Biol Chem* **267**:15285, 1992.

119. Hediger MA, Kanai Y, Lee W-S, Wells RG: Identification of a new family of proteins involved in amino acid transport, in Reuss L, Russell JM, Jennings ML (eds): *Molecular Biology and Function of Carrier Proteins*. Vol. 48. New York, Rockefeller Univ. Press, 1993, p 301.
120. Schiffer SP, Jezyk PF, Patterson DF, Roderick TH: Characterization of aminoaciduria in P/J mice. *Lab Anim Sci* **36**:586, 1986.
121. Schiffer SP: Personal communication.
122. Rao BS, Narayanan HS, Reddy GN: A clinical and biochemical survey of 729 cases of mental subnormality. *Br J Psychiatry* **118**:505, 1971.
123. Swenson EF, Walraven C, Levy HL: A 25 year experience with newborn urine screening. 9th National Neonatal Screening Symposium. Apr 7-11, Raleigh, NC, 1992, p 69. Abstract.
124. Wilcken B, Smith A, Brown DA: Urine screening for aminoacidopathies: Is it beneficial? *J Pediatr* **97**:492, 1980.
125. Stockl E: Personal communication.
126. Lemieux B, Auray-Blais C, Giguère R, Shapcott D, Scriver CR: Newborn urine screening experience with over one million infants in the Quebec Network of Genetic Medicine. *J Inherited Metab Dis* **11**:45, 1988.
127. Lemieux B: Personal communication.
128. Jepson JB: Hartnup disease, in Benson PF (ed): *Cellular Organelles and Membranes in Mental Retardation*. Edinburgh, Churchill Livingstone, 1971, p 55.
129. Greer M: Hartnup's syndrome. *Trans Am Neurol Assoc* **90**:53, 1965.
130. Mirsky JA: Insulinase, insulinase inhibitors and diabetes mellitus. *Recent Prog Horm Res* **13**:429, 1957.

CHAPTER 120

Iminoglycinuria*

Russell W. Chesney

1. **Familial iminoglycinuria is a benign inborn error of membrane transport. It involves a membrane carrier in the renal tubule with preference for L-proline, hydroxy-L-proline, and glycine resulting in net reabsorption. The iminoglycinuria phenotype is autosomal recessive.**

2. **Homozygotes retain appreciable tubular reabsorption of the imino acids and glycine. The residual transport function is saturated at endogenous concentrations of substrate, and the normal competitive interactions between the imino acids and glycine during tubular reabsorption are absent. These seemingly paradoxical observations can be understood if multiple carriers participate in the reabsorption of imino acids and glycine. Loss of a carrier shared by the imino acids and glycine, and retention of other carriers with preferences for glycine and imino acids individually, could account for the homozygous iminoglycinuric phenotype.**

3. **A variant phenotype in which imino acid reabsorption has a normal T_m value and the defect affects glycine reclamation more than proline probably indicates a K_m variant.**

4. **Impaired intestinal transport of L-proline has been demonstrated in some but not all homozygotes. A transport defect has not been shown in the leukocytes or skin fibroblasts.**

5. **Obligate heterozygotes may be "hyperglycinuric" (incompletely recessive) or "silent" (completely recessive) for expression of the mutant allele. Phenotypic heterogeneity among probands and obligate heterozygotes indicates genetic heterogeneity.**

6. **The different mutations appear to be allelic. Probands inheriting two "silent" mutant alleles, two "hyperglycinuric" alleles, or two different alleles have the same renal phenotype.**

7. **The differential diagnosis of familial iminoglycinuria includes: hyperprolinemia, in which iminoglycinuria occurs by a combined saturation-inhibition mechanism; the Fanconi syndrome, in which iminoglycinuria occurs as part of a generalized disturbance of transport; and the newborn, in whom hyperiminoglycinuria occurs in the first 6 months of life. Neonatal iminoglycinuria involves ontogeny of separate transport systems not controlled by the gene locus involved in hereditary iminoglycinuria.**

8. **Several different forms of renal hyperglycinuria are appreciated which must be distinguished from the hyperglycinuric phenotype of the "incompletely recessive" heterozygote with renal iminoglycinuria.**

A list of standard abbreviations is located immediately preceding the index in each volume.

Familial renal iminoglycinuria is a Mendelian disorder expressed in homozygotes or genetic compounds as a selective hyperaminoaciduria. It is caused by several autosomal alleles, some of which are partially expressed in heterozygotes (incompletely recessive alleles). The disorder is not a disease, although ascertainment of the phenotype in probands with clinical signs suggested to early observers that it might be. Familial iminoglycinuria is significant because it provides evidence for a transport system selective for imino acids† and glycine in the renal tubule and intestine under the control of a single locus. In its medical context, the disorder enters into the differential diagnosis of several hyperaminoacidurias, and because newborn infants have physiological iminoglycinuria, the ontogenetic and Mendelian phenotypes need to be discriminated from each other.

When Dent[4] applied chromatographic methods to the investigation of diseases, he fostered an exponential increase in the discovery of disorders of amino acid metabolism.[5] Renal iminoglycinuria is one of those disorders. Urine was a revealing mirror of metabolic disorders, and chromatography of urine amino acids evinced great interest.[6] It was soon recognized that urine of young infants normally contains a large quantity of the two imino acids proline and hydroxyproline and of the amino acid glycine.[7–10] It then became known that iminoaciduria disappeared as the infant reached about 3 months of age, and therefore the urine normally did not contain detectable amounts of proline or hydroxyproline; the hyperglycinuria had disappeared by about 6 months. Impaired net tubular reabsorption explained neonatal iminoglycinuria (Fig. 120-1).

Persistence of iminoglycinuria beyond 6 months constitutes an abnormality. It occurs under three different clinical situations:

1. As a "combined" aminoaciduria[11] in the presence of hyperprolinemia or hyperhydroxyprolinemia (see Chap. 30).

2. As a component of a generalized disturbance of membrane transport, for example, in the Fanconi syndrome (see Chap. 122).

*Many sections of this chapter remain unaltered. Permission has been obtained from the previous author, Dr. Charles R. Scriver, for publication.

†These compounds are also excreted in bound form as oligopeptides (see Chap. 30). Familial iminoglycinuria is a trait affecting only the free forms of proline, hydroxyproline, and glycine. "Imino acid" is a popular term used to distinguish the configuration of the secondary amino group (RC—NHCH—COOH) of the heterocyclic amino acids from the primary amino group (NH_2—CHR—COOH) of other amino acids. The term *imino acid* is freely used in standard textbooks on the biochemistry and metabolism of amino acids,[1,2] but reservations have been expressed about the accuracy of its use in this way.[3]

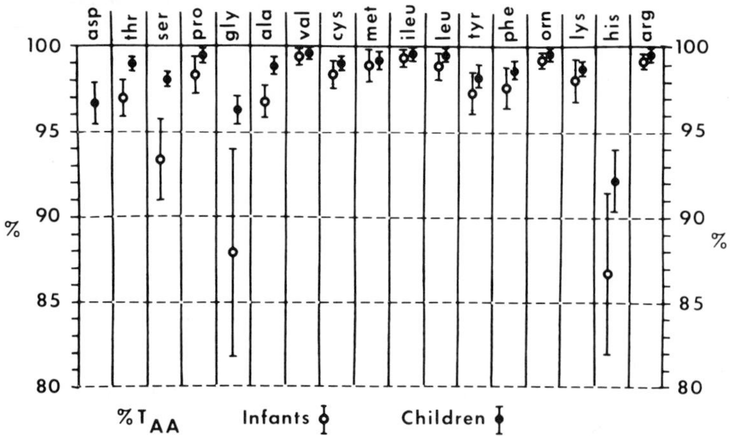

FIG. 120-1 Net tubular reabsorption of amino acids (expressed as percent of filtered load) is less efficient in the newborn human subject than in older subjects. Glycine reabsorption is particularly impaired, and the presence of imino acids in the urine of neonates and young infants is noteworthy. *(Redrawn from Brodehl and Gellissen.[10] Reproduced from* Pediatrics, *with permission.)*

3. As a specific inborn error of membrane transport of amino acids now usually known as familial (renal) iminoglycinuria (the subject of this chapter).

Most of the early reports of pathologic iminoglycinuria[12–34] testify that the condition was discovered during retrospective studies carried out for other purposes. Ascertainment bias is still evident in case reports of iminoglycinuria in which the disorder is found in subjects with retardation, propionic acidemia and 3-methylcrotonylglycinuria.[35,36] The diversity of the clinical abnormalities in probands with familial iminoglycinuria suggests now that there is little or no direct relationship between the inherited disorder of membrane transport and the accompanying illness. It is appropriate to classify familial iminoglycinuria as a benign inborn error of membrane transport,[20–22] a conclusion borne out by the frequent occurrence of healthy iminoglycinuric sibs of probands and by the prospective discovery of probands, through large newborn screening programs,[28,30] in whom follow-up observations have revealed no late-appearing illness.

RENAL TRANSPORT OF IMINO ACIDS AND GLYCINE

Investigation into the cause of iminoglycinuria in another disorder, familial hyperprolinemia[37,38] (see Chap. 30), led to the concept that imino acids and glycine share a specific renal transport system which has preference for these three substrates.[11] Familial renal iminoglycinuria, the phenotype described here, corroborates this hypothesis. Many studies in humans and other mammals indicate that renal transport of amino acids is a complex process apparently involving several carriers, presumably under the control of several genes. Carriers for the imino acids and glycine, of which there are also several, are among them.

Human Studies

There appears to be a maximum rate for net tubular absorption of proline (T_m proline).[38] Hydroxy-L-proline reabsorption also exhibits a T_m value.[39] The capacity of the normal human renal tubule to transport proline and hydroxyproline is shown in Table 120-1. A T_m for glycine has not been demonstrated in human beings, probably because there is extensive paracellular diffusion for glycine in the proximal tubule and because glycine excretion exceeds 2 percent of filtered load (see Fig. 120-1).[40] This relative hyperexcretion of glycine may also be related to the high K_m for the glycine carrier relative to other amino acid transport systems[35] and to the V_{max} for glycine transport.[41] Infusion of one imino acid increases urinary excretion of the other and of glycine in humans[38,39]; this procedure has little or no influence on the excretion of other amino acids.

Patients with familial hyperprolinemia have hyperiminoglycinuria[37,38] directly proportional to the plasma concentration of proline when it exceeds 1 m*M*; this is the level at which proline saturates its own transport system and appears in the urine.[38] The data for imino acid and glycine transport by normal human subjects and by patients with disorders of imino acid catabolism are complementary. They indicate the presence of a renal transport process, selective in its preference for proline, hydroxyproline, and glycine, and finite in its capacity.

Reabsorption of substrate is initiated by events at the brush-border membrane (see "Intracellular Events Influencing Proline Reabsorption" below). Transport of imino acids and glycine has been measured in purified brush-border membrane vesicles prepared from human renal cortex samples obtained at operation.[42] Two saturable uptake systems were identified: one has high affinity and is shared both by imino acids and by glycine; the other has low affinity and is not shared by glycine. The high-affinity system can apparently accommodate most of the imino acid load at physiological concentrations in filtrate, and if it were placed distally in proximal nephron, for instance, in the straight segment, it would explain the absence of iminoaciduria in the mature subject (see "Nonhuman Studies" below).

Nonhuman Studies

Amino acid reabsorption in the mammalian nephron is accomplished by a variety of carriers in the brush-border membrane, with selective preferences for particular amino acids and groups of amino acids.[43,44] There exist an axial heterogeneity of carriers located in the more proximal segments of proximal nephron having higher capacity but broader specificity and lower affinity for substrate and those located more distally having lower capacity but higher affinity and often a narrower specificity.[45] Net reabsorption also uses transport processes that prevent backflux so that the effective concentration of substrate at the luminal pole of the cell is kept lower than the equilibrium concentration; the processes for this situation include intracellular metabolic runout and efflux of substrate at the basolateral pole of the cell by carriers with properties different from those of the

Table 120-1 Renal Clearance, Net Tubular Absorption, and T_m of Amino Acids and Glycine in Familial Iminoglycinuria

	Proline			Hydroxyproline	
Phenotype	Endogenous clearance, ml(min · 1.73 m²)	Reabsorbed, %	T_m µmol(min · 1.73m²)	Endogenous clearance, ml(min · 1.73 m²)	Reabsorbed, %
Normal	0–0.03	>99.8	180–300	0	100
Homozygous mutant* (classic type):					
Mean	6.7			13	
Range	0.5–19.6	77–99.5	10–18	1–33.6	65–99
Heterozygous† ("hyperglycinuric")	0	100	35–117	0	100
Heterozygous‡ ("silent")	0	100	?	0	100
Generic compound (K_m variant)§	~0.3	>99	Normal with "splay"	2–4	<100

*Compiled from Goodman et al.,[18] Scriver,[17] Rosenberg et al.,[21] Hoefnagel and Pomeroy,[19] and Tada et al.[40] Includes genetic compound and homozygous probands.
†Compiled from Goodman et al.,[18] Scriver,[17] Rosenberg et al.,[21] and Hoefnagel and Pomeroy.[19]
‡Compiled from Scriver[17] and Hoefnagel and Pomeroy.[19]
§Compiled from Greene et al.[27]

carriers in the brush-border membrane.[43,45] While the weight of evidence pertaining to reabsorption of imino acids and glycine is concordant with this general scheme, details have yet to be resolved, and it should be kept in mind that findings in the nonhuman nephron may not reflect the human case precisely. In fact, it is not possible from current evidence to develop an accurate taxonomy of the tubular transport systems for imino acids and glycine in human beings.

Selective interactions between imino acids and glycine occur in vivo during renal reabsorption in rats and dogs.[46,47] Microperfusions *in vivo et situ* in the rat confirm this finding.[48–52] The reabsorption process is saturable, stereospecific (for L-proline), and Na^+-dependent. Electrophysiological studies[53] reveal two mechanisms for reabsorption of imino acids and glycine, both located at the renal brush-border membrane of proximal convolutions: one with low affinity, presumably more proximal and apparently a general system shared by many neutral amino acids; the other with high affinity, apparently more specific for the triad of substrates and possibly located more distally in proximal nephron.

In the case of glycine, two Na^+-dependent active transport systems have been demonstrated along the luminal membrane of the isolated perfused proximal tubule: a low-affinity (K_m, 11.8 mM), high-capacity (V_{max}, 28.5 pmol/min/mm tubule length) system in the convoluted segment, and a high-affinity (K_m, 0.7 mM), low-capacity (V_{max}, 2.5 pmol/min/mm) in the straight segment.[54] The latter system, which also operates parallel to a lower apical membrane backflux permeability in the proximal straight tubule,[55] absorbs smaller amounts of glycine against a greater concentration gradient and probably permits the reduction of the luminal glycine concentrations to lower levels than would be achieved in the proximal convoluted tubule.[55] The latter study corroborates earlier findings obtained by the continuous microperfusion technique in rats[50,51] and with the brush-border membrane vesicle preparation from human kidney.[42] The low-capacity, high-affinity system for proline is shared with glycine and hydroxyproline in human kidney.

As noted above, glycine transport has been studied in great detail in the isolated perfused rabbit nephron segment.[56,57] Glycine is transported against the chemical gradient, from lumen to cell, by a saturable Na^+-dependent carrier. Two forms of glycine transport were identified: one in the proximal convoluted segments has high capacity and low affinity; the other in the proximal straight segment has low capacity and high affinity. A paracellular, diffusional bidirectional flux was also found. Glycine uptake from peritubular space to cell across the basolateral membrane is both active and Na^+-dependent. The inward-directed basolateral flux is greater in straight segments relative to convoluted segments. The lumen-to-peritubular transcellular flux exceeds the flux in the reverse direction at physiological concentrations of glycine. No observations were made in this work on interactions of imino acids with glycine during transport.

Studies with purified membrane vesicles segregate membrane events from the intracellular events which influence net reabsorption,[43,45] and they are valuable for this reason, provided one recognizes that vesicle and microperfusion experiments measure different properties.[53] The vesicle studies[58–62] are both informative and confusing. Brush-border and basolateral membranes have Na^+-dependent and Na^+-independent systems respectively for L-proline transport (Fig. 120-2). This indicates that brush-border and basolateral membranes have carriers that are different in their function and therefore, presumably, in the genes that control them. Glycine transport by luminal membrane vesicles is Na^+-dependent[61] (see Fig. 120-2); studies of glycine transport by basolateral membrane vesicles have not yet been reported. Imino acids interact with each other[59] but not with glycine[62] during uptake by rabbit renal brush-border membrane vesicles; on the other hand, imino acids and glycine interact on a shared carrier in rat nephron vesicles.[61] It is unclear whether these functional differences reflect differences in species or in methodology, such as the nephron segment from which vesicles were isolated.

Na^+-proline cotransport by rat renal brush-border membrane vesicles appears to be both chloride-dependent and membrane potential–dependent.[63] Hence, both membrane potential and anion-specific properties govern the uptake of L-proline. The imposition of an extravesicular H^+ gradient stimulates L-proline uptake in rabbit kidney[64] but diminishes uptake by rat kidney.[63] Consistent with these findings, agents

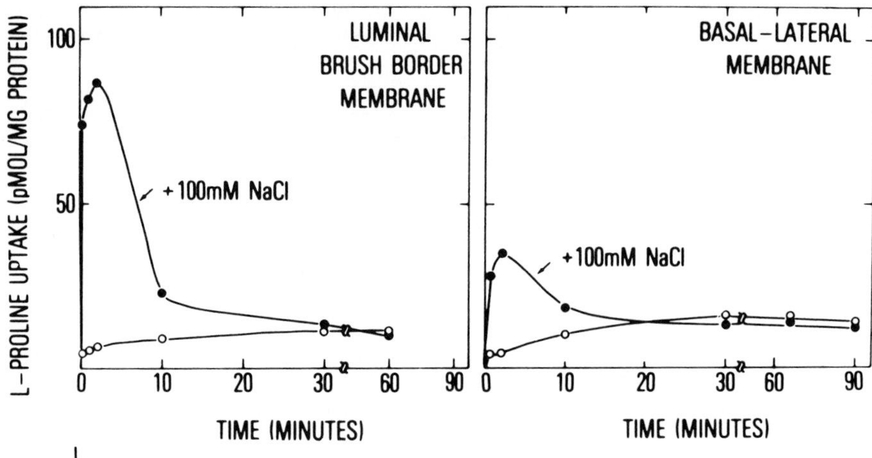

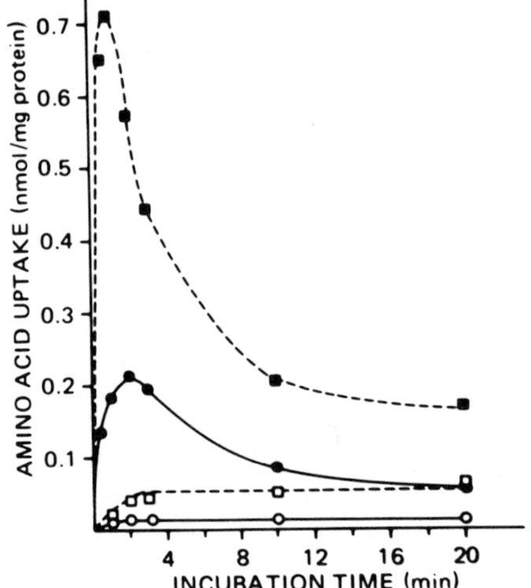

FIG. 120-2 *Upper panels:* Transport of L-proline (25 μM) by rabbit kidney brush-border and basolateral membranes. ● = Na^+ gradient; ○ = Na^+-free medium. *(From Barfuss and Schafer.[56] Used by permission.) Lower panel:* Transport of L-proline and glycine by rat renal brush-border membranes. ■□ = proline; ●○ = glycine, both at 0.06 mM; closed symbols = Na^+ gradient; open symbols = no Na^+ gradient. *(From Slack, Liang, and Sacktor.[58] Used by permission.)* Graphs show sodium-dependent transport for proline and glycine transport at brush-border membrane. Apparent Na^+-dependence for a small component of proline transport in basolateral membranes reflects contamination of membrane fraction by brush borders during preparation.

capable of altering proton accumulation, such as amiloride or carbonyl cyanide p-(trifluoromethoxy)phenyl-hydrazone diminish proline uptake by rabbit kidney but do not influence this process in rat kidney. An inward directed H^+ gradient stimulates glycine transport across rabbit renal brush-border surface, and this H^+-driven glycine uptake is attenuated by carbonyl cyanide m-chlorophenyl-hydrazone.[65] This H^+ glycine in rabbit is both a carrier-mediated electrogenic process whose transport is shared with the imino acids and to a slight degree by β-alanine.

The transport characteristics of D-proline were evaluated in rabbit kidney and were found to depend both on an H^+ flux and to be inhibited by L-proline. Hence D-imino acids and their naturally occurring L-isomers probably share a common transport system along the proximal tubule[66] in rabbits, but not in rats, as noted previously.[63]

Renal transport of imino acids and glycine has been studied in rat cortex slides[67] and in isolated tubule fragments from rabbits.[68,69] The slice preparation preferentially exposes the basolateral membrane,[70,71] while the tubule fragment preparation exposes both luminal and antiluminal membranes. There is heterogeneity of carriers for imino acids and glycine in the basolateral membrane with a high-capacity, low-affinity function shared by the three substrates and separate low-capacity, high-affinity functions for imino acids and glycine, respectively.

These descriptions may represent an oversimplification, particularly when one is trying to understand which carrier in which membrane of which nephron segment is affected by the human iminoglycinuria mutation. The apparent distribution of carriers for imino acids and glycine in proximal nephron is summarized in Table 120-2.

Intracellular Events Influencing Proline Reabsorption

A nonhuman mutation (PRO/Re in mouse) affecting renal proline oxidase activity[72] is informative about the overall mechanism for the reabsorption of L-proline. Mammalian renal cortex has a large capacity for proline oxidation.[67,73,74] This provides metabolic runout of proline[43] which *in vivo et situ* facilitates net reabsorption of the imino acid. Proline oxidation is blocked in the PRO/Re mouse (see Chap. 30), proline content of cortical cells is elevated, and net

Table 120-2 Tentative Classification of Membrane Carriers by Segment, Side of Cell, and Preference for Imino Acids and Glycine in Mammalian Nephron

Segment	Brush-Border Membrane	Basolateral Membrane
PC	P + HP + (G?)	P + HP + G
	G alone?	p + hp + g
PS	p + hp + (g?)*	
	g	g

*System affected in familial renal iminoglycinuria (hypothesis only).
PC = proximal convoluted; PS = proximal straight; upper-case letters = high-capacity, low-affinity; lower-case letters = low-capacity, high-affinity; G and g = glycine; HP and hp = hydroxyproline; P and p = proline.

reabsorption is impaired because backflux from cell to lumen across the brush-border membrane is increased[72] (see Fig. 81-3 in the fifth edition of this book for further details).

cAMP-dependent protein kinase (protein kinase A) also appears to modulate proline transport across the rat brush-border surface.[75] The exogenous addition of a highly purified catalytic subunit of protein kinase A will result in reduced Na^+ and Cl^- linked proline transport across the apical surface. The addition of cAMP reduces proline uptake, which indicates that endogenous protein kinase A activity also influences transport.[76] The activity of both protein kinase C and calmodulin-dependent protein kinase are also found in rat kidney. The activity of both protein kinase C and calmodulin-dependent kinase is reduced in tissue from immature rats;[76] their roles in proline reabsorption is unclear at present.

Ontogeny of Renal Transport of Imino Acids and Glycine

Ontogeny affects renal transport of imino acids and glycine. When ontogeny is combined with Mendelian variation, the findings are informative. Hyperiminoglycinuria in the normal human newborn[6–10] reflects reduced net reabsorption of imino acids and glycine[10,77,78] (see Fig. 120-1). The maturation of tubular transport functions occurs by independent schedules for proline and glycine,[77,78] suggesting that separate carriers are involved. This conclusion is given strong support by findings in probands homozygous for hereditary iminoglycinuria.[78] Such individuals have near-total absence of tubular reabsorption for proline and glycine in the early postnatal period. As tubular function matures, reabsorptive activity for proline appears first, followed by the later appearance of a glycine reabsorptive activity (Fig. 120-3). The profile of maturing proline and glycine transport in the mutant homozygote indicates that there are independent carriers for proline and glycine not controlled by the gene locus affected by the mutation.

Transient postnatal iminoglycinuria is characteristic of mammals in general.[79] Postnatal maturation of membrane transport activities is believed to involve intensification of specific membrane functions,[80] for which an explanation may be improved efficiency in maintaining and coupling the inward-directed Na^+ gradient, which is the driving force for uptake of amino acids at the brush-border membrane.[81]

Although there has been controversy about the process of ontogeny as it involves renal transport of proline and glycine,[82–85] several observations provide an overall insight. First, backflux of amino acids in the immature distal tubule is not a component of postnatal iminoglycinuria.[86] Second, diminished metabolic runout is not a significant cause of diminished net reabsorption.[82–86] Third, postnatal prolinuria in rats is associated with low activity of the high-affinity Na^+-dependent proline transport system in nephron[86,87] in the brush-border membrane.[87] Fourth, cortical tubule fragments[86] and slices[79,82,83] from newborn animals have impaired efflux of proline. Together, these findings suggest that ontogeny is associated with deficient activity of high-affinity systems for imino acids and glycine that do not include the system controlled by the familial iminoglycinuria locus.

An alternate explanation is that Na^+ uptake across the renal brush-border surface is enhanced in younger animals. This rapid entry of Na^+ would tend to reduce the driving force for Na^+-proline or Na^+-glycine uptake and reduce Na^+-dependent organic solute transport in young animals[88,89] (Fig. 120-4).

Renal Reabsorption of Imino Acids and Glycine in Familial Iminoglycinuria

Endogenous renal clearance rates are elevated and net reabsorption is decreased in probands (see Table 120-1). Of note, however, net tubular absorption of imino acids and glycine is not completely eliminated in homozygotes. Also, the abnormal prolinuria may disappear at low plasma proline concentrations in homozygotes (Fig. 120-5). The venous plasma "threshold" for prolinuria is very low in homozygotes (about 0.1 m*M*) as compared with normal subjects (about 0.8 m*M*).

The ability of homozygotes with hereditary iminoglycinuria to retain a considerable fraction of their specific tubular absorptive function is a feature shared by homozygotes with other inborn errors of membrane transport. For example,

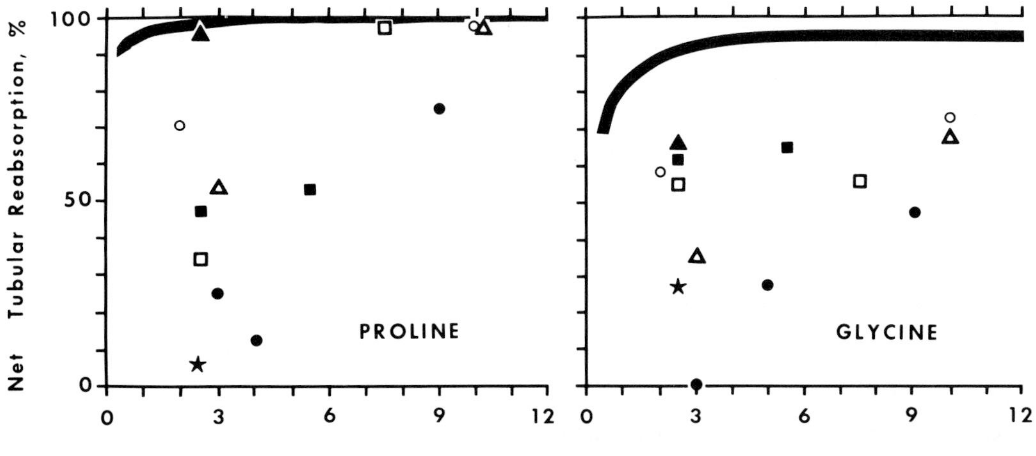

FIG. 120-3 Tubular reabsorption data for proline and glycine in relation to age in seven probands (various symbols, from Lasky and Scriver[78]) with familial renal iminoglycinuria. Shaded region indicates reabsorption values in normal infants. *(From Brodehl.[77] Reproduced from* Pediatric Research, *with permission.)*

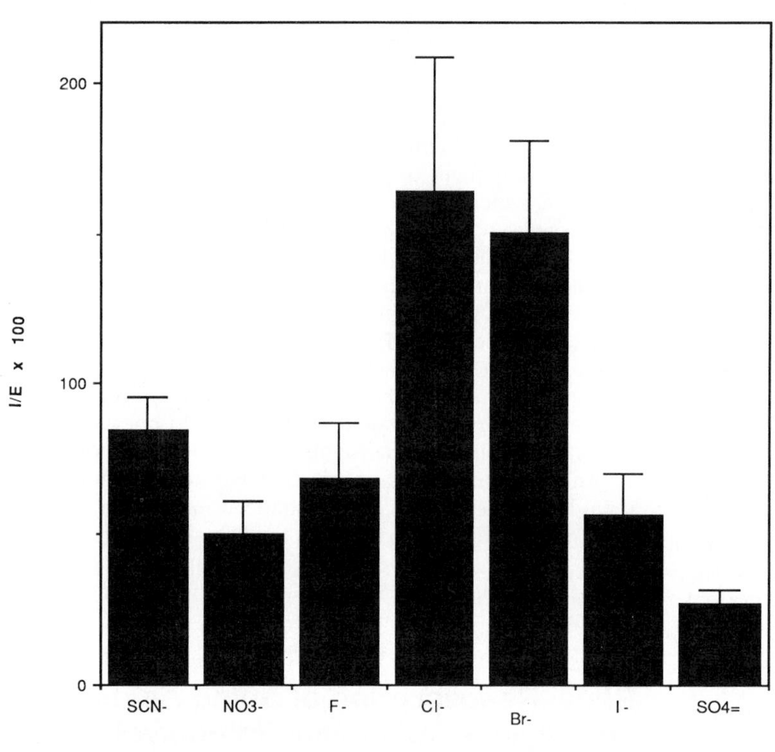

FIG. 120-4 Initial rate/Equilibrium (I/E) values for proline uptake in the presence of external anions with varying membrane permeabilities. Incubation media contained 2 m*M* HEPES/TRIS (pH 7.35), 1 m*M* $MgSO_4$, 50.53 m*M* mannitol, and 100 m*M* NaSCN, $NaNO_3$, NaF, NaCl, NaBr, NaI, or 50 m*M* Na_2SO_4. Data are the mean ±SE of four determinations performed in triplicate. *(From Chesney, Zelikovic, Budreau, and Randle.*[64] *Used by permission of the* Journal of the American Society of Nephrology.*)*

homozygotes with either classic cystinuria, isolated hypercystinuria, or Hartnup disorder usually retain some capacity to transport the relevant amino acids. A similar characteristic is also observed for hexose transport in glucose-galactose malabsorption in regard to renal tubular absorption of glucose.[43] One interpretation of this phenomenon in mutant phenotypes is that more than one type of transport system serves reabsorption of the specific substrate along the nephron, the different systems being controlled by different genes. This theory has not been examined directly.

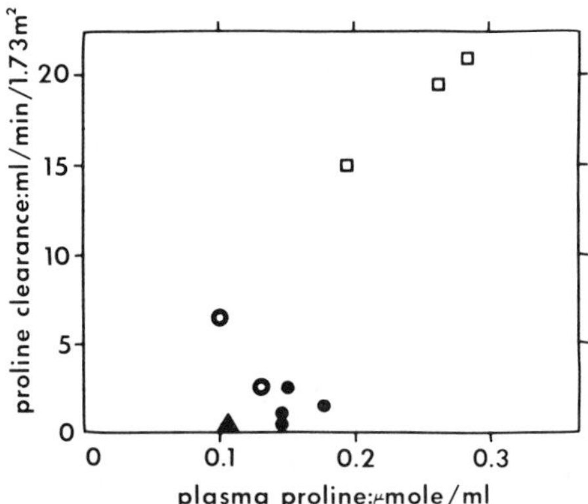

FIG. 120-5 Endogenous renal clearance of L-proline related to its concentration in plasma in homozygotes with familial iminoglycinuria. The "venous plasma threshold concentration" at which prolinuria appears is about 0.1 m*M*; the normal value is about 0.8 m*M*.[38] Abnormal prolinuria disappears in mutant homozygotes at low plasma proline concentration, indicating the existence of a small but efficient tubular capacity to transport proline. *(Redrawn from Scriver,*[17] *with permission of the* Journal of Clinical Investigation, *with data (symbol ○) added from Greene et al.*[27] *and other data (symbol ▲) added from Tada et al.*[40]*)*

Transport at Saturation in the Mutant Iminoglycinuria Phenotype

T_m values have been measured in mutant homozygotes and obligate heterozygotes infused with L-proline and hydroxy-L-proline.[16,17,21] Imino acid transport is present but saturated at normal plasma concentration of proline and hydroxyproline in the mutant homozygotes (Fig. 120-6). The heterozygote has a T_m value intermediate between normal and homozygous mutant values (see Fig. 120-6); imino acid reabsorption is normal at concentrations below the T_m, suggesting that affinity of the available imino acid transport sites is normal in the heterozygote. Taken together, these findings indicate that the mutation causes deletion of a transport system which has a capacity well above the normal concentration of imino acids in filtrate. Another modality of uptake with a small but recognizable capacity and high affinity is retained.

Greene et al.[27] described a proband in whom the mutant allele did not delete the affected transport function but altered its affinity for substrate, so that glycine was very poorly reabsorbed and proline was less avidly transported by the mutant carrier (see Fig. 120-6); a K_m variant was proposed.

Interactions between Imino Acids and Glycine during Tubular Reabsorption in the Mutant Phenotype

Normal adult subjects infused with proline or hydroxyproline show brisk inhibition of glycine reabsorption; mutant homozygotes show no inhibition of the residual activity serving glycine reabsorption[17] (Fig. 120-7). The latter may represent transport of glycine on the high-affinity system in proximal straight tubule or by the diffusional mode in proximal

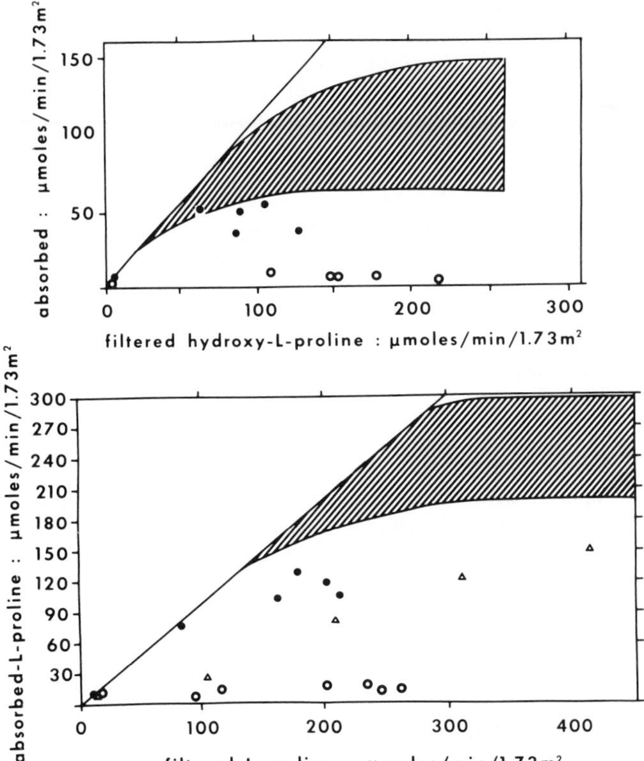

FIG. 120-6 Maximum rates of tubular reabsorption (T_m) of L-proline and hydroxy-L-proline in normal subjects (hatched), heterozygotes (solid circles), and mutant homozygotes (open circles) with classic iminoglycinuria. Data for patient with K_m variant of iminoglycinuria[27] are also shown (△). *(Redrawn from Scriver[17] and Greene et al.[27] Used by permission.)*

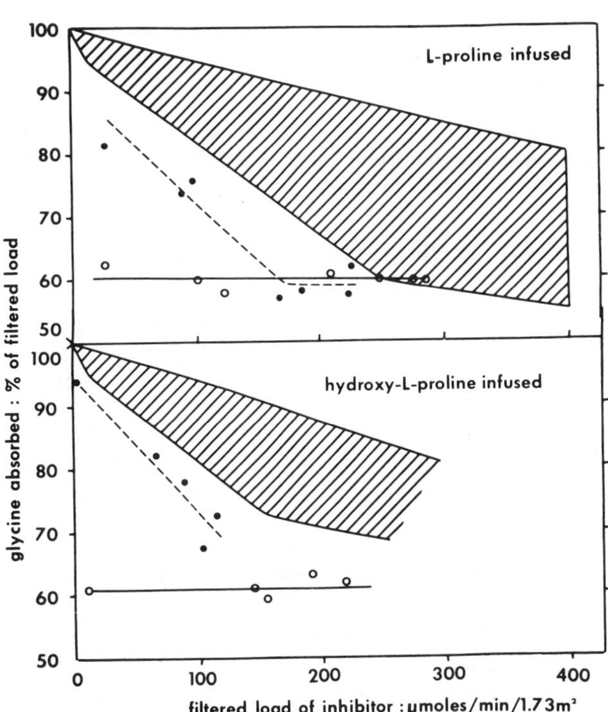

FIG. 120-7 Effect of L-proline and hydroxy-L-proline on net tubular reabsorption of glycine in normal subjects (hatched), heterozygotes (solid circles), and mutant homozygotes with classic iminoglycinuria. *(Redrawn from Scriver[17] and Greene et al.,[27] with permission.)*

nephron.[56] Loss of a portion of the glycine transport activity in the mutant phenotype is somewhat discordant with an opinion[62] that imino acids and glycine do not share a transport system in the brush-border membrane. The latter hypothesis implies that the iminoglycinuria mutation, which is at one locus, affects two transport systems; this could be explained if a polypeptide subunit were common to both carriers.

Infusion of one imino acid also impairs reabsorption of the other in normal subjects and in mutant homozygotes.[17] This finding in the mutant phenotype is compatible with inhibition of residual imino acid transport, on the broad-specificity, high-capacity neutral amino acid system in proximal convolutions.[53]

Imino acids and glycine do share transport on a high-capacity, low-affinity system at the basolateral membrane.[67] However, some heterozygotes have hyperglycinuria at normal plasma glycine concentrations (Figs. 120-6 and 120-7). This finding is compatible with impaired transport activity at the brush-border membrane and less so with impairment at the basolateral membrane (see Scriver and Tenenhouse[90] for explanation). Therefore, although we know that familial iminoglycinuria is a disorder involving a carrier selective for imino acids and glycine, it is still uncertain which transport system or site is affected.

Expression of Phenotype in Nonrenal Tissues

Intestine. Intestinal transport of L-proline has been examined in vivo[14,15,17,18,21] and in intestinal biopsy material.[21] Fecal excretion of amino acids has also been measured.[17,21] Two phenotypes have been identified. Some homozygotes have normal intestinal transport of L-proline and normal fecal excretion,[14,17,21] while others have impaired absorption and increased fecal excretion of proline.[15,18] The association of different intestinal phenotypes with a single renal phenotype suggests that more than one mutant allele is responsible for the iminoglycinuric trait.

The plasma response to glycine loading by mouth is normal in patients with and without demonstrable impairment of proline absorption.[15,18,21] This may indicate that transport by intestine is qualitatively different from that in kidney or that diffusional uptake of glycine, which would be unaffected by mutation, is significant in the intestine.

Leukocytes and Skin Fibroblasts. Net uptake of isotopically labeled proline at low extracellular concentrations (0.05 m*M*) by leukocytes and skin fibroblasts was apparently normal in homozygotes.[91] A negative finding has two interpretations: either the mutant system is not expressed in the plasma membrane of parenchymal cells or the experiment did not test for uptake on the mutant system. The former explanation involves an understanding that plasma membranes of parenchymal cells share homologous transport functions with basolateral membranes of renal and intestinal epithelium but not necessarily with functions in the brush-border membranes,[17,92] and renal iminoglycinuria appears to be a disorder of a brush-border membrane carrier.

DIAGNOSIS

Criteria for Abnormal Iminoglycinuria

Any degree of iminoaciduria after 6 months of age may be considered abnormal. Hyperglycinuria may be recognized on partition chromatograms when the glycine spot is disproportionately intense in comparison with other amino acids. The quantitative criteria for hyperglycinuria are urinary excretion exceeding 150 μmol per gram of total nitrogen,[20] or 150 mg/24 h,[93] or an endogenous clearance rate exceeding 8.6 ml (min · 1.73 m²).[94]

Differential Diagnosis

Hyperprolinemia and Hydroxyprolinemia. Iminoglycinuria occurs by a "combined" mechanism when there is hyperprolinemia in excess of about 0.8 m*M*.[38] Hyperprolinemia, type I or type II (see Chap. 30) is usually accompanied by iminoglycinuria. Patients with hydroxyprolinemia have not exhibited iminoglycinuria because the concentration of hydroxyproline in their plasma has not exceeded 0.4 m*M*; hydroxyproline must be present in plasma at least at this concentration to inhibit tubular absorption of proline and glycine competitively.[39] Hyperprolinemia and hydroxyprolinemia can be ruled out as a cause of iminoglycinuria if the concentration of both imino acids in plasma is normal in subjects with iminoglycinuria.

Fanconi Syndrome. Iminoglycinuria occurs in Fanconi syndrome as part of a generalized hyperaminoaciduria, in contrast to the selective hyperaminoaciduria in familial iminoglycinuria.

Neonatal Iminoglycinuria. The human infant normally has some degree of hyperiminoaciduria until about the third month of postnatal life; the hyperglycinuria subsides by the sixth month.

Renal Glycinuria. There have been numerous reports of hyperglycinuria without iminoaciduria. This phenotype may represent one form of the heterozygote with the iminoglycinuria mutation or the "K_m variant" form of renal iminoglycinuria.[27] Differential diagnosis includes:

1. Dominantly inherited renal hyperglycinuria and nephrolithiasis.[95,96]
2. Autosomal dominant glucoglycinuria.[97] Glucosuria occurs by the type B mechanism of Reubi, that is, the renal threshold for glucosuria is low (79 mg/dl), but the T_{mG} is normal—386 mg (min · 1.73 m²). Of the 44 subjects examined,[97] 13 healthy relatives also had glucoglycinuria; no subjects with glucosuria or glycinuria alone were found.
3. X-linked hypophosphatemia with glucoglycinuria.[98,99] Glucosuria is Reubi type A (low T_m). A glycine carrier, shared with imino acids, is present, but it is operating inefficiently. The glucoglycinuria occurs through a mechanism different from that described in the autosomal dominant condition.[97]

These traits should all be distinguished from the "prerenal" form of hyperglycinuria found in hyperglycinemia.

GENETICS

Familial renal iminoglycinuria is the expressed phenotype of alleles at an autosomal locus which controls a membrane carrier shared by imino acids and glycine. Consanguinity in parents of iminoglycinuria probands has been reported[14,22] (Fig. 120-8).

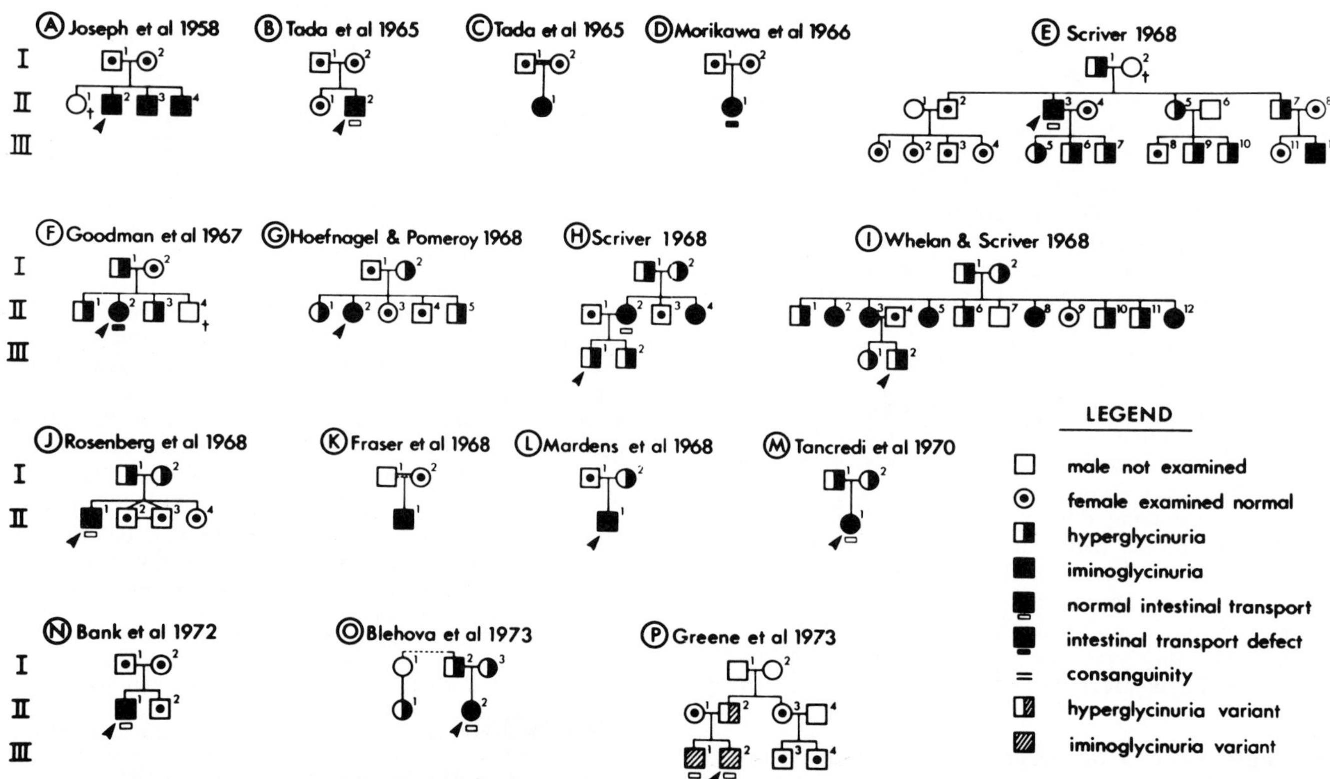

FIG. 120-8 Pedigrees of patients with familial iminoglycinuria. See ref. 12 for pedigree A; ref. 14 for B and C; ref. 15 for D; ref. 17 for E and H; ref. 18 for F; ref. 19 for G; ref. 20 for I; ref. 21 for J; ref. 22 for K; ref. 23 for L; ref. 24 for M; ref. 25 for N; ref. 26 for O; and ref. 27 for P.

Table 120-3 Evidence for Allelic Mutations in Familial Renal Iminoglycinuria. Phenotype Heterogeneity among Homozygotes, "Genetic Compounds," and Obligate Heterozygotes

Presumed Allelic Pair	Renal Phenotype in Homozygote or Compound	Renal Phenotype in Heterozygote	Intestinal Phenotype in Homozygote (or Compound)	Exemplary Pedigrees in Fig. 120-8
I-I	IG	N	Present	D
II-II	IG	N	N	B, N
III-III	IG	G	N	E, H, J, M, O
I-III (or II)	IG	N or G	Present	F
	IG	N or G	Not tested	E, G, L
II-IV	iG(K_m)	N or iG(K_m)	N	P

IG = iminoglycinuria (with loss of "high-K_m" system;) G = glycinuria alone; iG(K_m) = (K_m) variant involving "high-K_m" system affecting glycine more than imino acids; N = normal; "Present" implies defective absorption of proline and/or glycine in test procedure.

In some pedigrees, obligate heterozygotes have hyperglycinuria (see Fig. 120-8). This represents expression of an "incompletely recessive" allele, and the phenotype must be differentiated from other forms of dominantly inherited hyperglycinuria (see "Renal Glycinuria" above). Most heterozygotes for familial iminoglycinuria do not have hyperglycinuria; their mutant allele is "completely recessive." A third allele[27] is apparent in pedigree P (Fig. 120-8), in which a heterozygote and two affected offspring had hyperglycinuria associated with a mutant transport system expressing lowered affinity for glycine.

There are pedigrees (E, F, G, and L in Fig. 120-8) in which one parent is hyperglycinuric and the other is not; their offspring are indistinguishable from homozygotes with two hyperglycinuric parents or with two "silent" parents. When probands with the fully expressed phenotype have parents showing phenotypic heterogeneity (incomplete recessive × silent recessive) the probands are presumed to be genetic compounds for different alleles.

Some mutant homozygotes have impaired intestinal transport of proline (Fig. 120-8), whereas others do not. The intestinal phenotype is not consistently associated with any form of the heterozygous phenotypes. From the various combinations of phenotypes, including the K_m variant,[27] one can postulate four mutant alleles (Table 120-3). There has been no opportunity for analysis by molecular genetic methods to confirm this hypothesis.

Prevalence

Newborn screening data[27-29] indicate that the frequency of the presumed homozygote (or genetic compound) among Caucasians is about 1 in 15,000 livebirths. Of aminoacidurias detected by the screening of 1 million 6-week-old infants, iminoglycinuria was less common than cystinuria, histidinemia, and Hartnup disease.[100] Accordingly, the frequency of heterozygotes in the population is about 2 percent, about half being incompletely recessive (hyperglycinuric phenotype). The corresponding frequencies of specific alleles (silent, incomplete, and K_m variant) are therefore lower than 1 percent. Because these alleles are presumably all neutral in terms of selection, their high frequency may reflect founder effect or high mutation rate at the locus.

TREATMENT

Familial iminoglycinuria is a benign condition involving nonessential amino acids, and no treatment is indicated. The considerable number of healthy subjects in whom iminoglycinuria was discovered quite incidentally (see Fig. 120-8, pedigree E, subjects II.3 and III.12; pedigree H, subjects II.2 and II.4; and all homozygous members of pedigree I) supports this interpretation. The various illnesses that have been associated with the iminoglycinuric trait apparently served only to bring the transport mutation to attention.

REFERENCES

1. Greenstein JP, Winitz M: *Chemistry of the Amino Acid*. New York, John Wiley, 1961.
2. Meister A: *Biochemistry of the Amino Acid*, 2d ed. New York, Academic, 1965.
3. McMillan DE: Letter to the editor. *N Engl J Med* **273**:771, 1965.
4. Dent CE: Detection of amino acids in urine and other fluids. *Lancet* **2**:637, 1946.
5. Scriver CR, Rosenberg LE: *Amino Acid Metabolism and Its Disorders*. Philadelphia, Saunders, 1973.
6. Scriver CR: Hereditary aminoaciduria, in Bearn A, Steinberg AG (eds): *Progress in Medical Genetics*. New York, Grune & Stratton, 1962, vol 2, p 83.
7. Sereni F, McNamara H, Shibuya M, Kretchmer N, Barnett HL: Concentration in plasma and rate of urinary excretion of amino acids in premature infants. *Pediatrics* **15**:575, 1955.
8. Woolf LI, Norman AP: The urinary excretion of amino acids and sugars in early infancy. *J Pediatr* **50**:271, 1957.
9. O'Brien D, Butterfield LJ: Further studies on renal tubular conservation of free amino acids in early infancy. *Arch Dis Child* **38**:437, 1963.
10. Brodehl J, Gellissen K: Endogenous renal transport of free amino acids in infancy and childhood. *Pediatrics* **42**:395, 1968.
11. Scriver CR, Schafer IA, Efron ML: New renal tubular amino acid transport system and a new hereditary disorder of amino acid metabolism. *Nature* **192**:672, 1961.
12. Joseph R, Ribierre M, Job JC, Girault M: Maladie familiale associante des convulsions a debut tres precoce, une hyperalbuminorachie et uen hyperaminoacidurie. *Arch Fr Pediatr* **15**:374, 1958.
13. Mozziconacci P, Boisse J, Lemonnier A, Charpentier C: Les maladies metaboliques des acides amines avec arrieration mentale. Paris, L'Expansion Scientifique Francaise, 1968, p 249.
14. Tada K, Morikawa T, Ando T, Yoshida T, Mirigawa A: Prolinuria: A new renal tubular defect in transport of proline and glycine. *Tohoku J Exp Med* **87**:133, 1965.
15. Morikawa T, Tada K, Ando T, Yoshida T, Yokoyama Y, Arakawa T: Prolinuria: Defect in intestinal absorption of imino acids and glycine. *Tohoku J Exp Med* **90**:105, 1966.

16. Scriver CR, Wilson OH: Amino acid transport in human kidney: Evidence for genetic control of two types. *Science* **155**:1428, 1967.
17. Scriver CR: Renal tubular transport of proline, hydroxyproline and glycine. III. Genetic basis for more than one mode of transport in human kidney. *J Clin Invest* **47**:823, 1968.
18. Goodman SI, McIntyre CA, O'Brien D: Impaired intestinal transport of proline in a patient with familial iminoaciduria. *J Pediatr* **71**:246, 1967.
19. Hoefnagel D, Pomeroy J: Personal communication of unpublished data 1968, 1969.
20. Whelan DT, Scriver CR: Cystathioninuria and renal iminoglycinuria in a pedigree: A perspective on counseling. *N Engl J Med* **278**:924, 1968.
21. Rosenberg IE, Durant JL, Elsas LJ II: Familial iminoglycinuria: An inborn error of renal tubular transport. *N Engl J Med* **278**:1407, 1968.
22. Fraser GR, Friedmann AI, Patton VM, Wade DN, Woolf LL: Iminoglycinuria—a "harmless" inborn error of metabolism? *Humangenetik* **6**:362, 1968.
23. Mardens Y, Andriaenssens K, van Sande M: Glycinurie et iminoacidurie renales associes a une oligophrenie: Etude clinique et biochimique. *J Neurol Sci* **6**:333, 1968.
24. Tancredi F, Guazzi G, Aurichio S: Renal iminoglycinuria without intestinal malabsorption of glycine and imino acids. *J Pediatr* **7**:386, 1970.
25. Bank H, Crispin M, Ehrlich D, Szeinberg A: Iminoglycinuria: A defect of renal tubular transport. *Isr J Med Sci* **8**:606, 1972.
26. Blehová B, Pažoutová N, Hyánek J, Jirásek J: Iminoglycinuria in a child in Czechoslovakia. *Humangenetik* **19**:207, 1973.
27. Greene ML, Lietman PS, Rosenberg LE, Seegmiller JE: Familial hyperglycinuria: New defect in renal tubular transport of glycine and imino acids. *Am J Med* **54**:265, 1973.
28. Levy HL: Genetic screening, in Harris H, Hirschhorn K (eds): *Advances in Human Genetics*. New York, Plenum, 1973, vol 4, p 1.
29. Turner B, Brown DA: Amino acid excretion in infancy and early childhood: A survey of 200,000 infants. *Med J Aust* **1**:62, 1972.
30. Procopis PG, Turner B: Iminoaciduria: A benign renal tubular defect. *J Pediatr* **79**:419, 1971.
31. Paine RS: Evaluation of familial biochemically determined mental retardation in children, with special reference to aminoaciduria. *N Engl J Med* **262**:658, 1966.
32. Jonxis JHP: Personal communication, 1962.
33. Miller M: Familial cirrhosis with hepatoma. *Am J Dig Dis* **12**:633, 1967.
34. Statter M, Ben-Zvi A, Shina A, Schein R, Russell A: Familial iminoglycinuria with normal intestinal absorption of glycine and imino acids in association with profound mental retardation, a possible "cerebral phenotype." *Helv Paediatr Acta* **31**:173, 1976.
35. Purkiss P, Chalmers RA, Borud O: Combined iminoglycinuria and cystine- and dibasic aminoaciduria in patients with propionic acidaemia and 3-methylcrotinylglycinuria. *J Inherited Metab Dis* **3**:85, 1980.
36. Hayasaka S, Mizuno K, Yabata K, Saito T, Tada K: Atypical gyrate atrophy of the choroid and retina associated with iminoglycinuria. *Arch Ophthalmol* **100**:423, 1982.
37. Schafer IA, Scriver CR, Efron ML: Familial hyperprolinemia, cerebral dysfunction and renal anomalies occurring in a family with hereditary nephritis and deafness. *N Engl J Med* **267**:51, 1962.
38. Scriver CR, Efron ML, Schafer IA: Renal tubular transport of proline, hydroxyproline and glycine in health and in familial hyperprolinemia. *J Clin Invest* **43**:374, 1964.
39. Scriver CR, Goldman H: Renal tubular transport of proline, hydroxyproline and glycine. II. Hydroxy-L-proline as substrate and as inhibitor in vivo. *J Clin Invest* **45**:1357, 1966.
40. Tada K, Hirono H, Arakawa T: Endogenous renal clearance rates of free amino acids in prolinuric and Hartnup patients. *Tohoku J Exp Med* **93**:57, 1967.
41. Mitch WE, Chesney RW: Amino acid metabolism by the kidney. *Miner Electrolyte Metab* **9**:190, 1983.
42. Foreman JW, McNamara PD, Pepe LM, Ginkinger K, Segal S: Uptake of proline by brush border vesicles isolated from human kidney cortex. *Biochem Med* **34**:304, 1985.
43. Scriver CR, Chesney RW, McInnes RR: Genetic aspects of renal tubular transport: Diversity and topology of carriers. *Kidney Int* **9**:149, 1976.
44. Schafer JA, Barfuss DW: Membrane mechanisms for transepithelial amino acid absorption and secretion. *Am J Physiol* **238**:F335, 1980.
45. Scriver CR, Tenenhouse HS: Genetics and mammalian transport system. *Ann NY Acad Sci* **456**:384, 1985.
46. Wilson OH, Scriver CR: Specificity of transport of neutral and basic amino acids in rat kidney. *Am J Physiol* **213**:185, 1967.
47. Webber WA: Interactions of neutral and acidic amino acids in renal tubular transport. *Am Physiol* **202**:577, 1962.
48. Bergeron M, Morel F: Amino acid transport in rat renal tubules. *Am J Physiol* **216**:1139, 1969.
49. Dubord L, Bergeron M: Multiplicite des systemes transporteurs a la membrane luminale du nephron chez le rat normal. *Rev Can Biol* **33**:99, 1975.
50. Volkl H, Silbernagl S, Deetjen P: Kinetics of L-proline reabsorption in rat kidney studied by continuous microperfusion. *Pflugers Arch* **382**:115, 1979.
51. Volkl H, Silbernagl S: Molecular specificity of tubular reabsorption of L-proline. A microperfusion study in rat kidney. *Pflugers Arch* **387**:253, 1980.
52. Ulrich KJ, Reimrich G, Kloss S: Sodium dependence of the amino acid transport in the proximal convolution of the rat kidney. *Pflugers Arch* **351**:49, 1974.
53. Somarzija I, Fromter E: Electrophysiological analysis of rat renal sugar and amino acid transport. III. Neutral amino acids. *Pflugers Arch* **393**:199, 1982.
54. Zelikovic I, Chesney RW: Sodium-coupled amino acid transport in renal tubule. *Kidney Int* **36**:351, 1989.
55. Barfuss DW, Schafer JA: Active amino acid absorption by proximal convoluted and proximal straight tubules. *Am J Physiol* **236**:F149, 1979.
56. Barfuss DW, Schafer JS: Active amino acid absorption by proximal convoluted and proximal straight tubules. *Am J Physiol* **236**:F149, 1979.
57. Barfuss DW, Mays JM, Schafer JA: Peritubular uptake and transepithelial transport of glycine in isolated proximal tubules. *Am J Physiol* **238**:F324, 1980.
58. Slack EN, Liang C-CT, Sacktor B: Transport of L-proline and D-glucose in luminal (brush border) and contraluminal (basal-lateral) membrane vesicles from the renal cortex. *Biochem Biophys Res Commun* **77**:891, 1977.
59. Hammerman MR, Scaktor B: Transport of amino acids in renal brush border membrane vesicles. Uptake of L-proline. *J Biol Chem* **252**:591, 1977.
60. McNamara PD, Ozegovic B, Pepe LM, Segal S: Proline and glycine uptake by renal brush border membrane vesicles. *Proc Natl Acad Sci USA* **73**:4521, 1976.
61. McNamara PD, Pepe LM, Segal S: Sodium gradient dependence of proline and glycine uptake in renal brush-border membrane vesicles. *Biochim Biophys Acta* **556**:151, 1979.
62. Hammerman MR, Sacktor B: Na^+-dependent transport of glycine in renal brush border membrane vesicles. *Biochim Biophys Acta* **686**:189, 1982.
63. Schafer JA, Barfuss DW: Membrane mechanisms for transepithelial amino acid absorption and secretion. *Am J Physiol* **238**:F335, 1980.
64. Chesney RW, Zelikovic I, Budreau A, Randle D: Chloride and membrane potential dependence of sodium ion-proline symport. *J Am Soc Nephrol* **2**:885, 1991.
65. Roigaard-Petersen H, Jessen H, Mollerup S, Jorgensen KE, Jacobsen C, Sheikh MI: Proton gradient-dependent renal transport of glycine: Evidence from vesicle studies. *Am J Physiol* **258**:F388, 1990.
66. Radendran VM, Barry JA, Kleinman JG, Ramaswamy K: Proton gradient-dependent transport of glycine in rabbit renal brush-border membrane vesicles. *J Biol Chem* **262**:14974, 1987.
67. Mohyuddin F, Scriver CR: Amino acid transport in mammalian kidney: Identification and analysis of multiple systems for iminoacids and glycine in rat kidney. *Am J Physiol* **219**:1, 1970.
68. Hillman RE, Albrecht I, Rosenberg LE: Identification

and analysis of multiple glycine transport systems in isolated mammalian renal tubules. *J Biol Chem* **243**:5566, 1968.

69. Hillman RE, Rosenberg LE: Amino acid transport by isolated mammalian renal tubules. II. Transport systems for L-proline. *J Biol Chem* **244**:4494, 1969.
70. Wedeen RP, Weiner B: The distribution of p-aminohippuric acid in rat kidney slices. I. Tubular localization. *Kidney Int* **3**:205, 1973.
71. Arthus MF, Bergeron M, Scriver CR: Topology of membrane exposure in the renal cortex slice. Studies of glutathione and maltose cleavage. *Biochim Biophys Acta* **692**:371, 1982.
72. Scriver CR, McInnes RR, Mohyuddin F: Role of epithelial architecture and intracellular metabolism in proline uptake and transtubular reclamation in PRO/Re mouse kidney. *Proc Natl Acad Sci USA* **72**:1431, 1975.
73. Holtzapple P, Genel M, Rea C, Segal S: Metabolism and uptake of L-proline by human kidney cortex. *Pediatr Res* **7**:818, 1973.
74. Greth WE, Thier SO, Segal S: The transport and metabolism of L-proline-^{14}C in the rat and in vivo. *Metabolism* **27**:975, 1978.
75. Roigaard-Petersen H, Jacobsen C, Jessen H, Mollerup S, Sheikh MI: Electrogenic uptake of D-imino acids by luminal membrane vesicles from rabbit kidney proximal tubule. *Biochim Biophys Acta* **984**:231, 1989.
76. Zelikovic I, Przekwas J: cAMP-dependent protein kinase modulates proline transport across the rat renal tubular luminal membrane. *Pediatr Res* **31**:346A, 1992.
77. Brodehl J: Postnatal development of tubular amino acid reabsorption, in Silbernagl S, Lang F, Greger R (eds): *Amino Acid Transport and Uric Acid Transport*. Stuttgart, Thieme, 1976, p 128.
78. Lasley L, Scriver CR: Ontogeny of amino acid reabsorption in human kidney. Evidence from the homozygous infant with familial renal iminoglycinuria for multiple proline and glycine systems. *Pediatr Res* **13**:65, 1979.
79. Baerlocher K, Scriver CR, Mohyuddin F: Ontogeny of iminoglycine transport in mammalian kidney. *Proc Natl Acad Sci USA* **65**:1009, 1970.
80. Christensen HN: On the development of amino acid transport systems. *Fed Proc* **32**:19, 1973.
81. Medow MS, Roth KS, Goldmann DR, Ginkinger K, Hsu BYL, Segal S: Developmental aspects of proline transport in rat renal brush border membranes. *Proc Natl Acad Sci USA* **83**:7561, 1986.
82. Baerlocher KE, Scriver CR, Mohyuddin F: The ontogeny of amino acid transport in rat kidney. II. Kinetics of uptake and effect of anoxia. *Biochim Biophys Acta* **249**:364, 1971.
83. Baerlocher KE, Scriver CR, Mohyuddin F: The ontogeny of amino acid transport in rat kidney. I. Effect on distribution ratios and intracellular metabolism of proline and glycine. *Biochim Biophys Acta* **249**:353, 1971.
84. Roth KS, Hwang S-M, London JW, Segal S: Ontogeny of glycine transport in isolated rat renal tubules. *Am J Physiol* **233**:F241, 1977.
85. Reynolds R, Roth KS, Hwang SM, Segal S: On the development of glycine transport systems by rat renal cortex. *Biochim Biophys Acta* **511**:274, 1979.
86. Scriver CR, Arthus MF, Bergeron M: Neonatal iminoglycinuria: Evidence that the prolinuria originates in selective deficiency of transport activity in proximal nephron. *Pediatr Res* **16**:684, 1982.
87. Goldmann DR, Roth KS, Langfitt TW Jr, Segal S: L-proline transport by newborn rat kidney brush-border membrane vesicles. *Biochem J* **178**:253, 1979.
88. Zelikovic I, Przekwas J: Ca^{++} dependent protein kinases in the rat kidney during development. *Pediatr Res* **31**:346A, 1992.
89. Zelikovic I, Stejskal-Lorenz E, Lohstroh P, Budreau A, Chesney RW: Developmental maturation of Na^+/H^+ exchange in rat renal tubular brush border membrane. *Am J Physiol* **261**:F1017, 1991.
90. Scriver CR, Tenenhouse HS: Mendelian phenotypes as "probes" of renal transport system for amino acids and phosphate, in Windhager EE (ed): *Handbook of Physiology, Section 8: Renal Physiology*. New York, Oxford University Press, 1992, vol II, p 1977.
91. Tada K, Morikawa T, Arakawa T: Prolinuria: Transport of proline by leukocytes. *Tohoku J Exp Med* **90**:189, 1966.
92. Smith DW, Scriver CR, Tenenhouse HS, Simell D: The lysinuric protein intolerance mutation is expressed in plasma membrane of cultured skin fibroblasts. *Proc Natl Acad Sci USA* **84**:7711, 1987.
93. Carver MJ, Paska R: Ion-exchange chromatography of urinary amino acids. I. Normal children. *Clin Chim Acta* **6**:721, 1961.
94. Scriver CR, Davies E: Endogenous renal clearance rates of free amino acids in pre-pubertal children. *Pediatrics* **36**:592, 1965.
95. DeVrics A, Kochwa S, Lazebnik J, Frank M, Djaldetti M: Glycinuria, a hereditary disorder associated with nephrolithiasis. *Am J Med* **23**:408, 1957.
96. Oberiter V, Pureti CZ, Fabe CI, C-Sabadi V: Hyperglycinuria with nephrolithiasis. *Eur J Pediatr* **127**:279, 1978.
97. Kaser H, Cottier P, Antener I: Glucoglycinuria, a new familial syndrome. *J Pediatr* **61**:386, 1962.
98. Scriver CR, Goldbloom RB, Roy CC: Hypophosphatemic rickets with renal hyperglycinuria, renal glucosuria and glycylprolinuria: A syndrome with evidence for renal tubular secretion of phosphorus. *Pediatrics* **34**:357, 1964.
99. Dent CE, Harris H: Hereditary forms of rickets and osteomalacia. *J Bone Joint Surg [Br]* **38**:204, 1956.
100. Wilcken B, Smith A, Brown DA: Urine screening for aminoacidopathies: Is it beneficial? Results of a long-term follow-up of cases detected by screening one million babies. *J Pediatr* **97**:492, 1980.

CHAPTER 121

Renal Tubular Acidosis

Thomas D. DuBose, Jr. ▪ Robert J. Alpern

1. Renal tubular acidosis (RTA) is a clinical syndrome characterized by hyperchloremic metabolic acidosis secondary to an abnormality in renal acidification. The acidification defect may be manifest by an inappropriately high urine pH, bicarbonaturia, and, by definition, reduced net acid excretion. Classical distal renal tubular acidosis and proximal renal tubular acidosis are frequently associated with hypokalemia. Distal renal tubular acidosis can also result from a generalized dysfunction of the distal nephron, in which case it is usually accompanied by hyperkalemia and may be associated with either hypoaldosteronism or aldosterone resistance.

2. Proximal renal tubular acidosis may result from an isolated defect of acidification in the proximal nephron. The isolated defect in acidification could be the result of selective dysfunction of the Na^+/H^+ antiporter, the proximal tubule H^+-ATPase, or the $Na^+/HCO_3^-/CO_3^=$ symporter.

3. More commonly, proximal renal tubular acidosis occurs as one manifestation of a generalized defect in proximal tubule function. Patients with this generalized abnormality—the Fanconi syndrome—usually have glycosuria, aminoaciduria, citraturia, and phosphaturia. The acidification defect associated with this generalized tubular dysfunction may be the result of impairment of cellular ATP generation and/or cellular phosphate depletion.

4. Vitamin D deficiency is associated with the Fanconi lesion. The transport defect may be due to a combination of factors, including reduction in 1,25-dihydroxyvitamin D_3 levels, elevated parathyroid hormone levels, hypocalcemia, and intracellular phosphate depletion.

5. The diagnosis of proximal renal tubular acidosis is based on the demonstration of a chronic hyperchloremic metabolic acidosis frequently associated with an acid urine pH. Correction of the metabolic acidosis with alkali raises the plasma bicarbonate level above the renal threshold and results in prominent bicarbonaturia and an alkaline purine pH. The fractional excretion of bicarbonate may exceed 15 percent of the filtered load in such conditions, and hypokalemia is common. Bone disease, which commonly accompanies this disorder, is expressed as rickets in children and osteopenia in adults.

6. The goal of therapy in proximal renal tubular acidosis is to maintain a near-normal serum bicarbonate concentration while avoiding potassium deficiency. Concomitant administration of thiazide diuretics to reduce intravascular volume and secondarily to reduce the filtered load of bicarbonate is often beneficial.

7. The mechanisms underlying hypokalemic classical distal renal tubular acidosis are not fully understood. The hypokalemia suggests a lesion in the medullary collecting duct or a selective lesion in the cortical collecting tubule. Possible mechanisms include an abnormal leak pathway or "gradient" lesion, or a "rate defect." An example of a leak defect is that induced by amphotericin B in which the urine-blood P_{CO_2} gradient is normal. The observed low urine-blood P_{CO_2} gradient in most patients with distal renal tubular acidosis argues against a gradient lesion and suggests a rate defect (compromise of H^+-ATPase or H^+/K^+-ATPase) as the underlying mechanism for most patients with this disorder.

8. Classical hypokalemic distal renal tubular acidosis (type I RTA) is characterized clinically by an inability to acidify the urine appropriately during metabolic acidosis. Hypokalemia, hypercalciuria, and hypocitraturia frequently accompany this disorder, but proximal tubular reabsorptive function is preserved. Chronic metabolic acidosis results in calcium, magnesium, and phosphate wasting which may be associated with dissolution of bone and nephrocalcinosis.

9. Most patients with classical hypokalemic distal renal tubular acidosis have the condition in association with a systemic illness (acquired). Classical hypokalemic distal renal tubular acidosis also occurs as an isolated defect inherited as an autosomal dominant trait. Hypercalciuria and hypocitraturia may occur, in which case nephrocalcinosis usually develops.

10. Untreated classical distal renal tubular acidosis produces growth retardation which is responsive to alkali therapy. Correction of the acidosis by alkali administration leads to correction of hypokalemia, sodium depletion, and hypercalciuria, and also results in an increase in citrate excretion. Progression of nephrocalcinosis and nephrolithiasis are usually arrested. Restoration of normal growth and prevention of nephrocalcinosis are the major goals of therapy.

11. A generalized dysfunction of the distal nephron produces distal renal tubular acidosis in association with hyperka-

A list of standard abbreviations is located immediately preceding the index in each volume. Additional abbreviations used in this chapter include: CA = carbonic anhydrase; CCT = cortical collecting tubule; FE = fractional excretion; IMCD = inner medullary collecting duct; J-G = juxtaglomerular (apparatus); $JtCO_2$ = bicarbonate transport; OMCT = outer medullary collecting tubule; PD = potential difference; PEPCK = phosphoenolpyruvate carboxykinase; PTH = parathormone; RTA = renal tubular acidosis; TTKG = transtubular potassium gradient; U-B P_{CO_2} = urinary (urine minus blood) P_{CO_2}; UUO = unilateral ureteral obstruction.

lemia. The acidification defect in this disorder may, on occasion, result from a "voltage" defect which limits the rate of proton secretion by the cortical collecting tubule at any given luminal pH. More frequently, this defect involves compromise of the H^+-ATPase and cannot be ascribed merely to inability to generate a negative transepithelial potential difference.

12. **Aldosterone deficiency also results in hyperkalemia and metabolic acidosis by limiting proton secretion by the cortical collecting tubule. The hyperkalemia which invariably accompanies this defect has independent effects on net acid excretion by reducing renal ammoniagenesis and ammonium transport in the thick ascending limb of Henle's loop, thereby impairing ammonium excretion. Mineralocorticoid resistance also causes hyperkalemic-hyperchloremic metabolic acidosis in children and adults.**

13. **Renal insufficiency, especially due to diabetes and tubulointerstitial disease, may be associated with hyperkalemia and evidence of compromise of distal acidification. The hyperkalemia is out of proportion to the reduction in glomerular filtration rate. Underlying this disorder is either mineralocorticoid deficiency or mineralocorticoid resistance. As in primary mineralocorticoid deficiency, metabolic acidosis is secondary, in part, to the hyperkalemia. Simply lowering blood potassium may result in improvement of the acidosis.**

14. **Patients with hyporeninemic hypoaldosteronism and chronic renal insufficiency may require cation exchange resins, alkali therapy, and a loop diuretic to enhance renal potassium and salt excretion. Superphysiological doses of mineralocorticoids may be employed on occasion, but usually must be administered in combination with a loop diuretic in order to avoid volume overexpansion and aggravation of hypertension.**

Renal tubular acidosis (RTA) is a clinical syndrome characterized by a hyperchloremic metabolic acidosis secondary to an abnormality in renal acidification. It can be demonstrated as either an inappropriately high urine pH or bicarbonaturia, but by definition always includes reduced net acid excretion (titratable acid and ammonium excretion). The clinical expression of the defect in acidification depends on the specific nephron segment in which the defect arises. The general types of RTA are summarized in Table 121-1. RTA may occur clinically as a hyperchloremic metabolic acidosis with hypokalemia or hyperkalemia. Classical distal RTA (type I) and proximal RTA (type II) are frequently associated with hypokalemia. In contrast, a generalized dysfunction of the distal nephron, often associated with either hypoaldosteronism or aldosterone resistance, is usually seen in association with hyperkalemia. Lastly, RTA may occur in patients with renal insufficiency associated with a normal serum potassium. Since all varieties of RTA are associated with hyperchloremic metabolic acidosis when they are fully expressed, the differential diagnosis of hyperchloremia with metabolic acidosis and a normal anion gap is discussed first.

Table 121-1 Types of Renal Acidosis

Associated with hypokalemia
Proximal RTA (type II)
Distal RTA (type I)
Associated with hyperkalemia
Aldosterone deficiency or resistance (type IV)
Nonmineralocorticoid voltage defect
Associated with normokalemia
RTA of renal insufficiency

HYPERCHLOREMIC METABOLIC ACIDOSIS

The diverse clinical disorders which may result in a hyperchloremic metabolic acidosis are outlined in Table 121-2. Since a reduced plasma HCO_3^- and elevated Cl^- concentration may also occur in chronic respiratory alkalosis, it is important to confirm an acidemia by measuring arterial pH. In the absence of this information, a slightly elevated anion gap (12 to 15 meq/liter) and/or signs of pulmonary or hepatic disease suggests the presence of respiratory alkalosis. Hyperchloremic metabolic acidosis occurs most often as a result of loss of HCO_3^- from the gastrointestinal tract or as a result of a renal acidification defect. Hypokalemia may accompany both gastrointestinal loss of HCO_3^- and proximal and distal RTA.

Diarrhea results in the loss of large quantities of HCO_3^- and HCO_3^- decomposed by reaction with organic acids.[1] Since diarrheal stools contain a higher concentration of HCO_3^- and decomposed HCO_3^- than plasma, volume depletion and metabolic acidosis will develop. Hypokalemia exists because large quantities of K^+ are lost from stool and because volume depletion causes elaboration of renin and aldosterone, enhancing renal potassium secretion. Instead of an acid urine pH as anticipated with diarrhea, a pH of 6.0 or more may be found.[2] This occurs because metabolic acidosis and hypokalemia increase renal ammonium synthesis and excretion, thus providing more urinary buffer, which causes an increase in urine pH. Metabolic acidosis due to gastrointestinal losses with a high urine pH can be differentiated from RTA, since urinary NH_4^+ excretion is typically low in RTA, while NH_4^+ excretion is high in patients with diarrhea.[3,4] Urinary NH_4^+ levels can be estimated as

Table 121-2 Differential Diagnosis of Hyperchloremic Metabolic Acidosis

Gastrointestinal bicarbonate loss
Diarrhea
External pancreatic or small bowel drainage
Ureterosigmoidostomy, jejunal loop
Drugs
Calcium chloride
Magnesium sulfate
Cholestyramine
Renal acidosis
Proximal RTA (type II)
Distal ("classical") RTA (type I)
Generalized distal nephron dysfunction (type IV)
Mineralocorticoid deficiency
Mineralocorticoid resistance
Nonmineralocorticoid voltage defects
Renal insufficiency
Other
Acid loads (ammonium chloride, arginine chloride, arginine hydrochloride, hyperalimentation, sulfur)
Loss of potential bicarbonate—ketosis with ketone excretion
Dilutional acidosis
Posthypocapnic state

suggested by Halperin and associates[4,5] by calculating the urine net charge (UNC):

$$UNC = [Na^+ + K^+]_u - [Cl]_u$$

Since NH_4^+ can be assumed to be present if the sum of the major cations ($Na^+ + K^+$) is less than the sum of major anions in urine, a negative urine net charge is taken as evidence for ammonium in the urine. This test is only useful in the differential diagnosis of metabolic acidosis. If the patient has ketonuria, or drug excreted as anions in large quantity (penicillins or aspirin), the test will not be reliable. Urine containing little NH_4^+ will have more $Na^+ + K^+$ than Cl^- (urine net charge is positive)[6] and suggests a renal mechanism, such as RTA. Conversely, if the urine Cl^- exceeds the sum of $Na^+ + K^+$ in the urine, an extrarenal cause of the hyperchloremic acidosis should be considered. In addition, the fractional excretion of sodium would be expected to be low (<1 to 2 percent) in patients with HCO_3^- loss from the gastrointestinal tract, but usually exceeds 2 to 3 percent in RTA.[2]

In addition to gastrointestinal tract HCO_3^- loss, external loss of pancreatic and biliary secretions can also cause a hyperchloremic acidosis. Cholestyramine, calcium chloride, and magnesium sulfate ingestion can result in a hyperchloremic metabolic acidosis (see Table 121-2), especially in patients with renal insufficiency, but the plasma potassium is typically normal, not depressed.[2,7]

Severe hyperchloremic metabolic acidosis with hypokalemia may occur on occasion in patients with ureteral diversion procedures. Since the ileum and colon are both endowed with Cl^-/HCO_3^- exchanges, when the Cl^- from the urine enters the gut, the HCO_3^- concentration increases as a result of the exchange process.[8] Moreover, K^+ secretion is stimulated which, together with HCO_3^- loss, can result in a hyperchloremic, hypokalemic metabolic acidosis. This defect is particularly common in patients with ureterosigmoidostomies and is more common with this type of diversion because of the prolonged transit time of urine due to stasis in the colonic segment.[9]

Dilutional acidosis, acidosis due to exogenous acid loads and the posthypocapnic state, can usually be excluded by history. When isotonic saline is infused rapidly, particularly in patients with temporary or permanent renal failure, the plasma bicarbonate will decline reciprocally in relation to chloride.[2] Addition of acid or acid equivalents (arginine HCl, lysine HCl, or NH_4Cl) to blood results in metabolic acidosis.[10] A similar situation may arise from endogenous addition of ketoacids during recovery from ketoacidosis when the sodium salts of ketones may be excreted by the kidneys and lost as potential bicarbonate.

Loss of functioning renal parenchyma by progressive renal disease is known to be associated with metabolic acidosis. Typically, the acidosis is hyperchloremic when the GFR is between 20 and 50 ml/min, but may convert to the typical acidosis of uremia with high anion gap with more advanced renal failure—that is, when the GFR is <15 ml/min.[2,11,12] It is generally assumed that such a progression is observed more commonly in patients with tubulointerstitial forms of renal disease, but hyperchloremic metabolic acidosis can occur with advanced glomerular disease.[13,14] The principal defect in acidification of advanced renal failure is that ammoniagenesis is reduced in proportion to the loss of functional renal mass. In addition, medullary ammonium accumulation and trapping in the outer medullary collecting tubule may be impaired.[4] Because of adaptive increases in potassium secretion by the collecting duct[15] and colon,[16] the acidosis of chronic renal insufficiency is typically normokalemic.[14] Hyperchloremic metabolic acidosis associated with hyperkalemia is almost always associated with a generalized dysfunction of the distal nephron. However, potassium-sparing diuretics, nonsteroidal antiinflammatory drugs, angiotensin-converting enzyme inhibitors, beta blockers, and heparin may mimic or cause this disorder, resulting in hyperkalemia and a hyperchloremic acidosis. Such drugs should be discontinued before the diagnosis of a nonreversible, generalized defect of the distal nephron is considered.

The diverse clinical disorders associated with hyperchloremic metabolic acidosis should be considered and excluded before embarking on an extensive evaluation of renal acidification and the diagnosis of RTA (see Table 121-2).

PROXIMAL RENAL TUBULAR ACIDOSIS

Mechanism and Regulation of Proximal Acidification

The kidney filters approximately 4000 meq of HCO_3^- per day. To maintain acid–base balance and to reabsorb the filtered load of HCO_3^-, the renal tubules must secrete 4000 meq of hydrogen ions. Although the kidney must secrete an additional 50 to 80 meq of hydrogen ions to titrate urinary buffers, the majority of hydrogen ion secretion is involved in the "reclamation" of filtered HCO_3^-. Approximately 80 to 90 percent of filtered HCO_3^- is reabsorbed in the proximal tubule. Thus, while the distal nephron is responsible for the final acidification of the urine and the generation of large pH gradients, the proximal tubule represents a high-capacity system and secretes the majority of hydrogen ions. Defects in proximal tubular reabsorption of HCO_3^- are typically characterized by large amounts of bicarbonaturia.

Mechanism of H^+ Secretion/HCO_3^- Absorption. Reabsorption of HCO_3^- in the proximal tubule depends on active secretion of hydrogen ions across the apical membrane.[17–19] This process is effected mostly by an apical membrane Na^+/H^+ antiporter which results in hydrogen ion secretion into the lumen in exchange for sodium ions entering the cell.[20–26] The driving force for hydrogen ion secretion is provided by the low cell sodium concentration which is generated by the basolateral membrane Na^+/K^+-ATPase. Thus, ATP indirectly drives this active proton secretion.

Sardet et al. have cloned a cDNA for a human Na^+/H^+ antiporter.[27] The Na^+/H^+ antiporter is predicted to be a protein of molecular weight 99,354 with an amino terminal domain containing 10 to 12 transmembrane spanning regions and a carboxyterminal cytoplasmic domain. This clone is believed to correspond to the amiloride-sensitive housekeeping Na^+/H^+ antiporter which is present in nonpolar cells. Based on the sensitivity to amiloride analogues, it is now believed that there are at least two types of Na^+/H^+ antiporters.[28] The housekeeping Na^+/H^+ antiporter, corresponding to the above-described clone and now denoted NHE-1, has been shown to be sensitive to nanomolar concentrations of ethylisopropylamiloride[28] and is located on nonpolar cells and on the basolateral membrane of certain epithelia. The Na^+/H^+ antiporter present on the apical membrane of the proximal tubule is more resistant to amiloride and requires micromolar concentrations of ethylisopropylamiloride. There is now accumulating evidence that this apical membrane Na^+/H^+ antiporter is encoded by a separate isoform of the Na^+/H^+ antiporter gene.[29] Two additional Na^+/H^+

antiporter isoforms have been cloned and are referred to as NHE-2 and NHE-3. These isoforms are partially homologous to NHE-1. It is not clear at present which of these, if either, corresponds to the apical membrane Na^+/H^+ antiporter.

In parallel with the Na^+/H^+ antiporter is an H^+-ATPase which mediates a small fraction of apical membrane H^+ secretion.[26,30,31] This H^+-ATPase is believed to be of the vacuolar type, based on staining of the proximal tubule brush-border membrane with antibodies against subunits of vacuolar H^+-ATPases.[32] The molecular characteristics of H^+ pumps are discussed further under the "H^+ Secretion/ HCO_3 Absorption" heading in the section on Distal Renal Tubule Acidosis below.

The base generated in the cell by these two transporters then exits the cell across the basolateral membrane via an electrogenic $Na^+/HCO_3^-/CO_3^=$ symporter which transports one sodium, one HCO_3^-, and one $CO_3^=$ ion.[33–38] The driving force for this transporter is the negative cell potential.

Carbonic anhydrase is present in the cytoplasm and on both apical and basolateral membranes of the proximal tubule. The cytoplasmic form is very similar to carbonic anhydrase II of red blood cells.[39,40] The membrane-bound form has been named type IV.[39–41] The molecular characteristics of the carbonic anhydrases are described extensively in Chapter 137. Carbonic anhydrase I, the most prevalent red-cell carbonic anhydrase, is not present in the kidney.[42] The major function of carbonic anhydrase (CA) in the proximal tubule (and in the kidney in general) is to accelerate the reaction indicated below:

$$H^+ + HCO_3^- \leftrightarrow H_2CO_3 \overset{CA}{\leftrightarrow} CO_2 + H_2O$$

Since in the lumen of the proximal tubule hydrogen ions are secreted into HCO_3^- containing filtrate, H_2CO_3 is formed. The H_2CO_3 is rapidly dehydrated by luminal carbonic anhydrase (type IV) to form CO_2 and H_2O.[41] The CO_2 is freely diffusible and is reabsorbed. In the cell, carbonic anhydrase (type II) catalyzes the formation of H_2CO_3 from CO_2 and H_2O. H_2CO_3 then dissociates rapidly to H^+ and HCO_3^- which are transported across the apical and basolateral membranes, respectively. Thus, carbonic anhydrase allows transmembrane pH gradients to be minimal and facilitates further proton secretion and HCO_3^- reabsorption.[41]

In parallel with the active H^+ secretory mechanism is a leak through the paracellular pathway. Because luminal HCO_3^- concentration is lower than that of blood, HCO_3^- can back-diffuse into the lumen. While the proximal tubule is a leaky epithelium with relatively high paracellular permeabilities, the HCO_3^- permeability is comparatively small.[43–47] Diffusion of hydrogen ions is even smaller in magnitude.[48] Thus, leak pathways tend to be unimportant under normal conditions.

Other Proximal Tubular Functions. Proximal renal tubular acidosis is usually associated with defects in other proximal tubule function. The proximal tubule is the major site for reabsorption of glucose, amino acids, organic anions, and phosphate. Each of these solutes is reabsorbed across the apical membrane on transporters coupled to sodium transport. The low intracellular sodium concentration and negative cell voltage which are generated by the basolateral membrane Na^+/K^+-ATPase provide the driving force for these transporters to take up these solutes from the lumen actively. Most of these solutes are then either metabolized within the proximal tubular cell or passively exit across the basolateral membrane. These mechanisms lead to low concentrations of these solutes in the lumen, creating a driving force for back-diffusion of these solutes across the paracellular pathway. Once again, under normal conditions, these back-diffusing fluxes are present but small in magnitude.

Of particular relevance to RTA is the proximal tubular transport of citrate. Although citrate is present in plasma in very low concentration, its presence in the urine and tubular fluid is key to the prevention of calcium stones and nephrocalcinosis. Citrate is reabsorbed by the proximal tubule on an Na-coupled transporter which carries numerous dicarboxylic and tricarboxylic acids. After entering the cell, citrate is transported into mitochondria, where it enters the tricarboxylic acid cycle. Because citrate is metabolically equivalent to HCO_3^- (its metabolism leads to the generation of HCO_3^-), citrate excretion in the urine is equivalent to HCO_3^- excretion. Thus, proximal tubular citrate absorption increases in metabolic acidosis, leading to hypocitraturia and a predisposition to kidney stones and nephrocalcinosis. This adaption involves an adaptive increase in apical membrane Na/citrate cotransporter activity.[49]

Proximal absorption of Na^+ and Cl^- is more complex. High rates of HCO_3^- absorption, preferential to Cl^- in the early proximal tubule, lead to an increased concentration of Cl^- in the late proximal tubule. This provides a chemical gradient for Cl^- absorption which drives Cl^- movement and causes a lumen-positive potential difference (PD) that secondarily drives Na^+ absorption. While 50 percent of proximal tubular NaCl absorption occurs by such a passive mechanism, there is an additional active transcellular component of NaCl absorption.[50–53] This, however, also appears to be related to acidification in that the apical membrane mechanism is Na^+/H^+ antiport and Cl^-/base exchange in parallel.[54–57] Figure 121-1 summarizes the transport mechanism present in the proximal tubule. Defects in transporter on the left side of the figure lead to isolated proximal RTA, while defects on the right side of the figure lead to generalized function of the proximal tubule.

Thus, diseases which interfere with HCO_3^- absorption in any manner can interfere secondarily with passive Cl^- absorption by preventing the rise in luminal Cl^- concentrations. In addition, any mechanism which interferes with the Na^+/K^+-ATPase or the Na^+/H^+ antiporter will also interfere with transcellular Cl^- absorption. In theory, if the inhibition of HCO_3^- and Cl^- absorption is in proportion to their plasma concentrations (corrected for differences in volume of distribution), the result will be a decrease in extracellular fluid

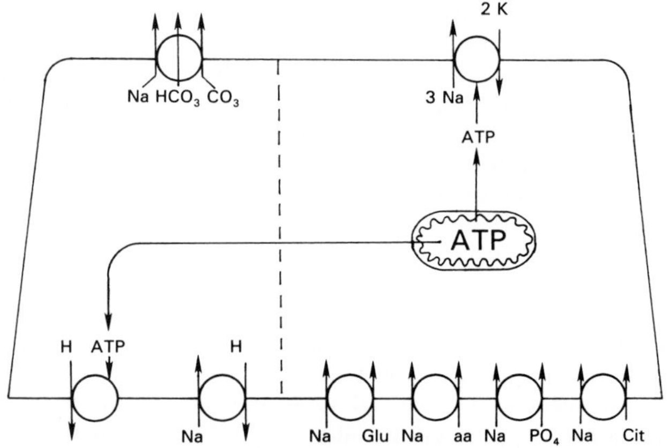

FIG. 121-1 Cell model of proximal tubule. Defects in transporter (left) lead to isolated proximal RTA, while defect on right side of figure leads to generalized dysfunction of the proximal tubule.

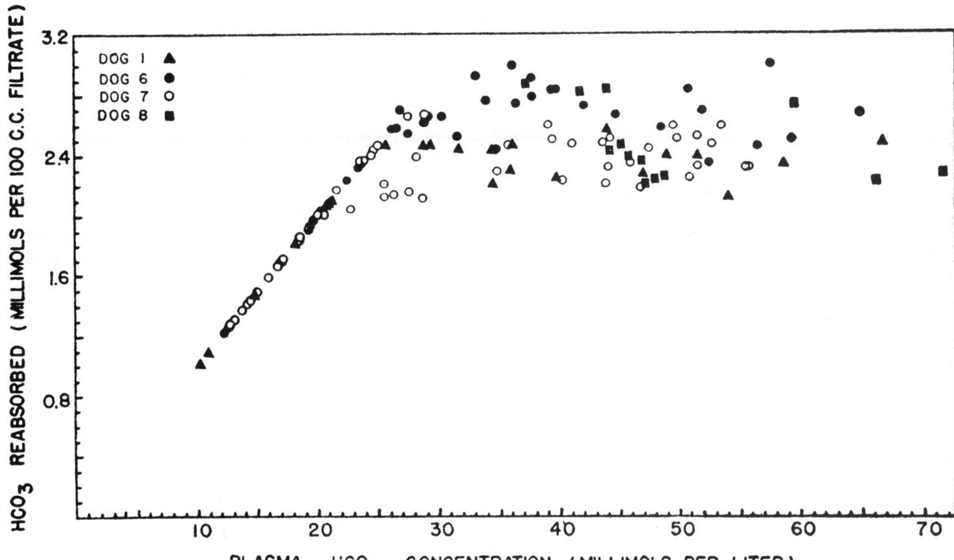

FIG. 121-2 Effect of varying plasma bicarbonate concentration on renal bicarbonate absorption in normal dogs. *(From Pitts and Lotspeich.[58] Used by permission.)*

volume with no change in the concentrations of HCO_3^- or Cl^-. In reality, the inhibition of HCO_3^- absorption in proximal RTA is proportionately greater than that of Cl^- absorption, resulting in a decrease in plasma HCO_3^- concentration and an increase in plasma Cl^- concentration.

Regulation of Proximal Tubular Bicarbonate Absorption. Pitts and Lotspeich[58] examined the effect of an HCO_3^- infusion on renal HCO_3^- absorption and excretion in normal dogs. The results are displayed in Fig. 121-2. As the plasma HCO_3^- concentration rises, renal HCO_3^- absorption also increases. At low plasma bicarbonate concentrations, nearly 100 percent of filtered HCO_3^- is absorbed. However, at higher plasma HCO_3^- concentrations, a threshold is reached at which HCO_3^- first appears in the urine (the threshold for bicarbonaturia). As plasma HCO_3^- concentration increases further, HCO_3^- absorption continues to increase until a maximal level is reached, the so-called T_m for HCO_3^- absorption.

The initial interpretation of these studies was that HCO_3^- absorption was a saturable process such that at low filtered loads of HCO_3^- luminal transporters were able to reabsorb all the HCO_3^-, but as luminal HCO_3^- concentration increased, the transporters became saturated and fractional HCO_3^- absorption decreased. Tubular microperfusion studies have demonstrated that this interpretation is only partly correct.[43,59] While proximal tubular HCO_3^- absorption does saturate as a function of luminal HCO_3^- concentration, a more important regulatory effect is that exerted by the peritubular HCO_3^- concentration. Increases in peritubular HCO_3^- concentration directly inhibit proximal tubular HCO_3^- absorption. Thus, when plasma HCO_3^- is increased, both luminal and peritubular HCO_3^- concentrations are increased. While the increase in luminal HCO_3^- concentration leads toward saturation of the system, the increase in peritubular HCO_3^- concentration markedly inhibits proximal tubular HCO_3^- absorption. The net result produces the curve reported by Pitts and Lotspeich (Fig. 121-2).[58]

The studies of Pitts and Lotspeich form the basis for understanding proximal tubular acidification defects. Patients with proximal RTA have apparently normal rates of renal HCO_3^- absorption at low plasma HCO_3^- concentrations. However, even at these low plasma HCO_3^- concentrations, proximal tubular HCO_3^- absorption is probably still subnormal. However, distal HCO_3^- delivery is low enough that the distal nephron can reabsorb the excess HCO_3^-. Because distal nephron acidification is not impaired, the urine can then be acidified appropriately. As plasma bicarbonate concentration increases, these patients are found to have a low threshold for bicarbonaturia, as shown in Fig. 121-3. At high plasma HCO_3^- concentrations, distal delivery of HCO_3^- exceeds the capacity of the distal nephron for HCO_3^- absorption and there is significant bicarbonaturia. Patients with distal renal tubular acidification defects, on the other hand, may have small degrees of bicarbonaturia but never have large amounts of bicarbonaturia unless the patients are made frankly alkalotic. Figure 121-2 shows a typical HCO_3^- titration curve for a normal patient, a patient with proximal RTA, and a patient with distal RTA.

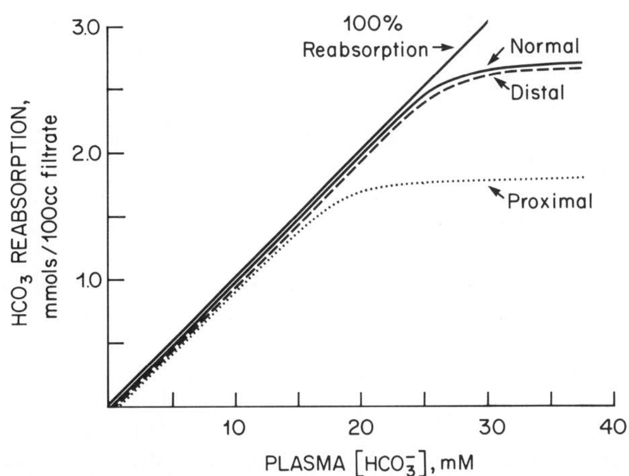

FIG. 121-3 Effect of plasma bicarbonate concentration on renal bicarbonate absorption in normal patients (solid line), patients with hypokalemic distal RTA (broken line), and patients with proximal RTA (dotted line). Bold diagonal line represents 100 percent reabsorption of filtered bicarbonate. Note that in distal RTA, the threshold for bicarbonaturia (i.e., the plasma bicarbonate concentration at which renal bicarbonate absorption is not 100 percent of filtered load) is normal, while in patients with proximal RTA the threshold is decreased.

Pathogenesis of Proximal Renal Tubular Acidosis

Possible Defects. Proximal RTA can be divided into two general categories, one in which acidification is the only defective function and one in which there is a more generalized proximal tubular dysfunction. A generalized proximal tubular defect could occur by one of two mechanisms. First, there could be an increase in the permeability of the paracellular pathway. This would lead to a backleak into the lumen of solutes for which the proximal tubule is the main site of reabsorption and whose concentration is thus low in the lumen. These solutes would include HCO_3^-, phosphate, glucose, amino acids, and organic anions. An alternative mechanism is a generalized disorder of cellular function which would inhibit absorption of all these solutes. For example, any disorder which inhibits ATP production in the proximal tubule would lead to a generalized defect in reabsorption. Similarly, because reabsorption of these solutes as well as acidification are coupled to sodium transport, any disorder in which the Na^+/K^+-ATPase is abnormal would lead to a generalized defect in proximal tubular function.

A proximal tubular defect involving only acidification is rare. Such a disorder would have to involve a selective defect in the Na^+/H^+ antiporter, the H^+-ATPase, or the $Na^+/HCO_3^-/CO_3^=$ symporter. Abnormalities of cell depolarization or abnormalities in carbonic anhydrase could also present in this manner.

Generalized Proximal Tubular Dysfunction. The majority of cases of proximal RTA fit into the category of generalized proximal tubular dysfunction with glycosuria, generalized aminoaciduria, hypercitraturia, and phosphaturia. The generalized failure of proximal tubular function is referred to as the Fanconi syndrome. Because Chap. 122 deals with this syndrome, we will only briefly discuss the Fanconi syndrome as it relates to the mechanism of the acidification defect.

In 1951, Berliner, Kennedy, and Hilton,[60] while examining the capacity of organic acids to serve as effective buffers for acidification, accidentally found that maleic acid infused intravenously into dogs caused a syndrome with proximal RTA and glycosuria. This condition, now referred to as "maleic acid nephropathy," has been subsequently used to study the mechanism of the Fanconi syndrome. Al-Bander et al.,[61] using clearance techniques in dogs undergoing a free-water diuresis, found results suggesting that maleic acid inhibits proximal tubular solute and water absorption. While initial studies raised the possibility of abnormal proximal tubular leaks in the genesis of maleic acid nephropathy,[62] the techniques used were indirect, and the conclusions have not been substantiated by more direct studies performed subsequently. A more recent study which found evidence for renal tubular leakage[63] exposed animals to maleic acid for 20 h prior to studying renal function. In this study, tubules were leaky to lissamine green and inulin, suggesting that nephrotoxicity had approached the level of acute tubular necrosis. Hoppe et al.[64] and Gougoux et al.[65] found that the effect of maleate on bicarbonaturia was additive to that of carbonic anhydrase inhibition, suggesting separate mechanisms. Gmaj et al.[66] found no effect of maleate on renal carbonic anhydrase activity.

In studies in which the lumen of the proximal tubule was microperfused and rates of acidification measured, Bank et al.[67] found that previous maleic acid treatment inhibited the rates of HCO_3^- absorption and of sodium chloride absorption. These investigators found no inulin leak. In addition, in studies in which tubules were perfused in the absence of HCO_3^- and the rate of HCO_3^- entrance was measured (a measure of paracellular HCO_3^- permeability), maleic acid had no effect. Thus, Bank et al. concluded that maleic acid acted by interfering with transcellular active HCO_3^- absorption rather than enhancing HCO_3^- backleak. Similar results were obtained by Reboucas et al.[68] employing split droplet microperfusion. Rates of volume absorption were inhibited. In further studies with a pH electrode in the luminal fluid, these investigators measured the rates of luminal acidification and alkalinization. In tubules perfused with alkaline solutions, the rate of acidification was inhibited, a result consistent with either a transcellular defect or enhanced leak. However, in tubules perfused with very acid solutions, the rate of alkalinization was also inhibited, a result consistent only with an inhibited transcellular flux and not consistent with enhanced leakiness. In addition, in these studies, cell voltage was measured and found to be decreased consistent with inhibition of the Na^+/K^+-ATPase.[68] Günther et al.[69] examined the effect of maleic acid infusion on glycine absorption. Maleic acid infusion inhibited glycine absorption in the microperfused proximal tubule. However, when saturable transcellular glycine absorption was inhibited by excess phenylalanine in the lumen, maleic acid had no effect on glycine absorption.

Salmon and Baum have examined this question utilizing an experimental model of cystinosis.[70] Proximal tubule segments perfused in vitro were incubated with a dimethyl ester of cystine. This compound diffuses into cells, where cytoplasmic esterases cleave the ester groups generating intracellular cystine. Proximal tubules incubated with this compound showed decreased rates of volume absorption, HCO_3^- absorption, and glucose absorption, while tubules incubated with methyl esters of leucine or tryptophan demonstrated no abnormalities. Cystine dimethyl ester had no effect on mannitol or HCO_3^- permeability.

These studies demonstrate that the nephropathies associated with maleic acid and cystine involve disruption of active transcellular absorption of HCO_3^-, amino acids, and other solutes. Such a defect could be due to a generalized disorder of apical membrane transporters, a disorder of the basolateral Na^+/K^+-ATPase, or a metabolic disorder which lowers intracellular ATP concentrations. Addition of maleic acid to isolated brush-border membrane vesicles did not affect Na^+/glucose cotransport.[71] In addition, the Na^+/glucose cotransporter isolated from either control animals or animals treated in vivo with maleic acid were similar in function. Addition of maleic acid to brush-border membranes did not affect transport of α-methylglucoside, alanine, proline, or lysine.[72] Silverman and Huang[73] found that the addition of maleic acid to vesicles did not affect phlorizin binding to the Na^+/glucose cotransporter. Lastly, Le Grimellec et al.[74] found no effect of maleate on the fluidity of the lipids of brush-border membranes. Thus, no abnormality of apical membrane transporters could be demonstrated.

Kramer and Gonick[75] found that maleic acid treatment of rats inhibited Na^+/K^+-ATPase activity in renal cortical homogenates prepared 1.0 h after treatment. There was no effect on Na^+/K^+-ATPase in medullary homogenates. Thus, inhibition of the Na^+/K^+-ATPase provides one mechanism by which all of the transport defects in maleic acid nephropathy and in Fanconi syndrome could be produced.

In addition to the defect in Na^+/K^+-ATPase, Kramer and Gonick found decreased ATP concentrations in renal cortical homogenates. Coor et al. examined the role of ATP depletion and Na^+/K^+-ATPase inhibition in the model of cystinosis discussed above.[76] Proximal tubules incubated with the dimethyl ester of cystine demonstrated a 60 percent decrease in intracellular ATP, with no change in Na^+/K^+-ATPase activity. Incubation of cystine dimethyl ester–treated tubules with exogenous ATP partially ameliorated the transport defect. These authors thus concluded that the major defect was one of ATP depletion rather than an abnormality in the Na^+/K^+-ATPase. One possible explanation for these decreased ATP levels is inhibition of metabolism by maleic acid. Angielski and Rogulski[77] found that maleic acid interferes with the Krebs cycle. While this effect occurs in many tissues, only kidney cells actively accumulated maleate. Another possible cause of decreased ATP levels is sequestration of intracellular phosphate. Al-Bander et al.[78] found that previous phosphate loading in dogs could markedly ameliorate the maleic acid–induced bicarbonaturia, natriuresis, and aminoaciduria. There was no effect of previous phosphate loading on the hypercitraturia. In subsequent studies, Al-Bandar et al.[79] found that prior phosphate loading attenuated the increased renal excretion of low-molecular-weight proteins and lysosomal enzymes seen in maleic acid–treated kidneys.

Production of the Fanconi syndrome by intracellular phosphate depletion has also been proposed in hereditary fructose intolerance where ingestion of fructose leads to accumulation of fructose 1-phosphate in the proximal tubule. Because these patients lack the enzyme fructose 1-phosphate aldolase, the fructose 1-phosphate cannot be further metabolized, and intracellular phosphate is sequestered in this form. The renal lesion is confined to the proximal tubule because this is the only segment in the kidney that possesses the enzyme fructokinase.[80] Administration of large parenteral loads of fructose to rats leads to high intracellular concentrations of fructose 1-phosphate and low concentrations of ATP and GTP, as well as of total adenine nucleotides.[80] Prior phosphate loading prevents the reductions in intracellular ATP, total adenine nucleotides, and phosphate.[81]

A clinical association which has occurred relatively frequently is that of vitamin D deficiency, resistance, or dependence and generalized proximal tubular dysfunction. Numerous investigators have noted an association between vitamin D deficiency and a generalized Fanconi syndrome with proximal RTA, aminoaciduria, and hyperphosphaturia.[82–84] In these studies, correction of the vitamin D deficiency has caused correction of the proximal tubular dysfunction.[82,83] Similar results have been obtained in patients with vitamin D–dependent and vitamin D–resistant rickets treated with dihydrotachysterol.[85,86] While the existence of this association is undisputed, the mechanisms involved in the proximal tubular dysfunction are not yet clear.

Vitamin D deficiency states are associated with low levels of vitamin D, low levels of serum calcium, and high levels of parathormone (PTH). Parathyroid hormone has been demonstrated to be an important inhibitor of proximal tubular bicarbonate absorption.[87–90] This results from inhibition of active transcellular proton secretion, rather than by an increase in bicarbonate backleak.[89,90] Although the mechanism of this inhibition is not yet settled, some studies suggest a direct effect on the Na^+/H^+ antiporter, mediated possibly by the cAMP-dependent protein kinase.[91,92] While such an effect may explain proximal RTA, studies have suggested that chronic PTH administration does not lead to metabolic acidosis but rather to metabolic alkalosis.[93,94] This appears to be due to a stimulation of HCO_3^- absorption in more distal segments, either in the loop of Henle[95] or in the collecting tubule. Some studies have suggested that the increased distal phosphate delivery induced by PTH can stimulate distal nephron acidification.[96] Thus, in spite of the marked inhibitory effect of PTH on proximal tubular absorption of HCO_3^-, the effect on whole kidney HCO_3^- absorption appears to be small and overall there is a small stimulation of acidification.

Extracellular Ca^{2+} concentration is also a regulator of proximal tubular transport, although less potent than PTH. In the in vitro perfused proximal convoluted tubule, increases in extracellular Ca^{2+} concentration stimulate HCO_3^- absorption and decreases in extracellular Ca^{2+} concentration inhibit HCO_3^- absorption.[97] However, in these studies, large changes in Ca^{2+} concentrations produced only small effects on HCO_3^- absorption. Although the effects of vitamin D have not yet been studied in the perfused proximal tubule, clearance studies have found that administration of 25-hydroxyvitamin D stimulates renal absorption of Ca^{2+}, PO_4^{3-}, sodium, and HCO_3^-.[98,99] The exact nephron segment in which this effect occurs has not been established, but is thought to be the proximal tubule.[100]

An additional pathophysiological mechanism for the proximal tubular defect in the Fanconi syndrome could be intracellular phosphate depletion, as discussed above. Intracellular PO_4^{3-} depletion has been proposed as a cause of ATP depletion and the secondary Fanconi syndrome in maleic acid nephropathy and in hereditary fructose intolerance. High levels of PTH will inhibit proximal tubular PO_4^{3-} absorption. In addition, vitamin D may promote proximal tubular phosphate absorption, and its deficiency reduces PO_4^{3-} absorption, secondarily contributing to intracellular phosphate depletion. Gross and Scriver[101] created an experimental model of vitamin D deficiency in the rat and demonstrated hyperphosphaturia and aminoaciduria. These authors noted that aminoaciduria was not prominent until the animals had been on a vitamin D–deficient diet for 6 weeks. In addition, they noted that the aminoaciduria appeared 2 to 4 weeks after hyperphosphaturia, supporting a role for a more complex scheme than mere hormone presence or absence.

Further support for a role of the Ca^{2+}/PO_4^{3-}/PTH/vitamin D system in proximal RTA can be found from the results of Morris et al.,[102] who found that hypoparathyroidism ameliorated the fructose-induced proximal tubular dysfunction in a patient with hereditary fructose intolerance. Administration of PTH to this hypoparathyroid patient enhanced the fructose-induced renal defect. As discussed above, intracellular PO_4^{3-} depletion has been proposed as the cause of Fanconi syndrome in hereditary fructose intolerance. Decreased levels of PTH could protect these patients by enhancing phosphate uptake by the proximal tubule. An alternative explanation is that the inhibiting effect of PTH on acidification is additive to the effect of fructose-induced intracellular phosphate depletion.

The association between Fanconi syndrome and vitamin D disorders may be partially related to decreased 1α-hydroxylase activity in disorders of proximal tubule function. 1α-Hydroxylase, which is present in proximal tubular mitochondria, could be deficient in the Fanconi syndrome. Brewer et al.[103] found that conversion of 25-hydroxyvitamin D_3 to 1,25-hydroxyvitamin D_3 was impaired in maleic acid nephropathy. However, Chesney[104] measured levels of vitamin D metabolites and found them to be normal in three patients with the Fanconi syndrome. In summary, vitamin

D deficiency is clearly associated with the Fanconi syndrome. The defect is related to low levels of 1,25-dihydroxyvitamin D_3, high levels of PTH, and low levels of Ca^{2+}. These findings may be produced in part by intracellular phosphate depletion.

Isolated Proximal Tubular Acidosis. One model for selective inhibition of proximal tubular HCO_3^- absorption is that of lysine infusion. Walker et al.[105] reported that lysine caused marked bicarbonaturia in the dog. Chan and Kurtzman[106] examined the effect of microperfusing rat proximal tubules with lysine. Lysine was found to inhibit HCO_3^- absorption with no effect on volume absorption. This effect was seen only with L-lysine, not with D-lysine, and the dose response for this effect was similar to that of the concentration relationship for lysine absorption from the lumen. Although no specific mechanism for this effect was established, Frömter[107] and Hoshi et al.[108] have found that luminal lysine depolarizes the proximal tubular cell. Such an effect could inhibit HCO_3^- efflux across the basolateral membrane, secondarily alkalinizing the cell and inhibiting apical membrane proton secretion.

Another model for isolated proximal tubular acidosis is inherited carbonic anhydrase deficiency. Sly and associates[109,110] have reported an inherited syndrome with osteopetrosis, cerebral calcification, and RTA due to an inherited deficiency of carbonic anhydrase II. These patients may have a combined proximal and distal RTA, but have no other evidence for proximal tubular dysfunction.[111,112] As discussed above, carbonic anhydrase II is present in the cytoplasm of renal cells; thus, an acidification defect occurring in association with its deficiency is not unexpected. This syndrome is discussed extensively in Chap. 137.

An association between RTA and an aberrant carbonic anhydrase I has also been reported.[113,114] These patients appeared to have a combined proximal and distal RTA. While they had normal amounts of carbonic anhydrase I assayed antigenically, carbonic anhydrase I enzyme activity was decreased. Kondo et al.[113] proposed that this defect may be related to abnormal binding of zinc to carbonic anhydrase I. This association may have been a coincidence and not a causal one, since biochemical studies have failed to demonstrate carbonic anhydrase I in the kidney.[42] In addition, in patients with a syndrome of inherited deficiency of carbonic anhydrase I, there is no disorder of renal function.[115]

Diagnosis of Proximal Renal Tubular Acidosis

The diagnosis of proximal RTA rests initially on the finding of a hyperchloremic metabolic acidosis. These patients will generally present in the steady state with a chronic metabolic acidosis, an acid urine pH, and a small amount of bicarbonate excretion. On HCO_3^- infusion, as the plasma HCO_3^- rises above the threshold in these patients, bicarbonaturia ensues, and the urine becomes alkaline. In its isolated form this metabolic acidosis occurs alone or in association with mild hypokalemia. If bicarbonate intake has been high in an attempt to repair the acidosis, patients will have significant bicarbonaturia on presentation and hypokalemia may be severe.

The diagnosis thus rests on an appropriately acidified urine (pH <5.5) in acidotic patients and a high fractional excretion of HCO_3^- (>10 to 15 percent) in patients with a near-normal serum HCO_3^- concentration. An additional clue to the diagnosis is the difficulty with which the plasma HCO_3^- concentration is corrected. In patients with proximal RTA, large amounts of exogenous HCO_3^- are usually required.

In most patients, this acidification defect is part of a generalized proximal tubular dysfunction called the Fanconi syndrome. These patients have hypophosphatemia, hyperphosphaturia, hypouricemia, hyperuricosuria, glycosuria, aminoaciduria, hypercitraturia, hypercalciuria, and proteinuria. In addition, this syndrome is frequently associated with bone disease which presents as rickets in children or osteopenia in adults.[116] The diagnostic approach to patients with RTA and the use of the fractional excretion of HCO_3^- are discussed later in this chapter in the section on "Distal Renal Tubular Acidosis."

Clinical Spectrum

Table 121-3 lists the causes of proximal RTA. Isolated proximal RTA occurs either as an idiopathic or genetic condition or is related to carbonic anhydrase insufficiency or inhibition. Syndromes of generalized proximal tubular dysfunction will be discussed in depth in a subsequent chapter, but generally fall into the categories of primary defects and those associated with inherited disorders of metabolism, dysproteinemic states, nephrotoxins, interstitial nephritis, or vitamin D–deficiency states.

Associated Findings

Proximal RTA occurs in two forms: (1) as a part of a broader syndrome of proximal tubular dysfunction, namely, the Fanconi syndrome, and (2) as an isolated defect. In the Fanconi syndrome, the pathophysiological consequences are complex because of the multiple tubular defects. In the pure form of proximal RTA, all of the pathophysiological consequences can be explained by inhibition of proximal tubular HCO_3^- absorption.

Rodriquez-Soriano et al.[117] used clearance techniques to examine the distribution of NaCl and volume absorption in patients with proximal RTA. In these studies, the patients were found to have marked inhibition of proximal tubular NaCl and volume absorption with increased distal delivery. Distal NaCl absorption was normal. As discussed above, proximal tubular NaCl absorption is integrally related to proximal tubular acidification mechanisms. First, because proximal tubular bicarbonate absorption establishes the high luminal chloride concentrations which drive passive NaCl absorption, inhibition of acidification will lead to inhibition of passive NaCl absorption. Second, transcellular NaCl absorption is mediated by apical membrane Na^+/H^+ antiport, which may also be defective in proximal RTA.

In patients with proximal RTA who have a significant acidosis but are not excreting HCO_3^-, potassium handling is normal. Indeed, in two clinical studies of isolated proximal RTA, patients were found to have normal serum potassium, presumably because of a lack of significant bicarbonaturia in the steady state.[118,119] Patients with proximal RTA have renal potassium wasting only during bicarbonaturia. In fact, Sebastian et al.[120] found that the magnitude of potassium excretion correlated well with the magnitude of HCO_3^- excretion. The mechanism of the potassium wasting is related to increased distal delivery of sodium with a poorly reabsorbable anion (i.e., bicarbonate). In addition, inhibition of proximal tubular NaCl absorption leads to volume depletion, which leads to increased aldosterone levels and enhanced potassium secretion.

Table 121-3 Disorders Associated with Proximal RTA

Isolated RTA
- Primary (sporadic or familial)
- Carbonic anhydrase
  - Inhibition
    - Acetazolamide
    - Mafenide (Sulfamylon)
  - Deficiency
    - Osteopetrosis with carbonic anhydrase II deficiency
- Pyruvate carboxylase deficiency
- York-Yendt syndrome
- Cyanotic congenital heart disease

Generalized
- Primary (sporadic or familial)
- Genetically transmitted systemic diseases
  - Cystinosis
  - Lowe syndrome
  - Hereditary fructose intolerance (during fructose ingestion)
  - Tyrosinemia
  - Galactosemia
  - Wilson disease
  - Mitochondrial phosphoenolpyruvate carboxykinase deficiency
  - Metachromatic leukodystrophy
  - Glycogen storage disease
  - Cytochrome *c* oxidase deficiency
- Dysproteinemic states
  - Multiple myeloma
  - Light-chain disease
  - Light-chain nephropathy
  - Amyloidosis
- Vitamin D deficiency, dependence, or resistance
- Other renal diseases
  - Sjögren syndrome
  - Medullary cystic disease
  - Renal transplantation rejection (early)
  - Balkan nephropathy
  - Chronic renal vein thrombosis
  - Nephrotic syndrome
  - Paroxysmal nocturnal hemoglobinuria
- Toxins
  - Outdated tetracycline
  - Lead
  - Gentamicin
  - Cadmium
  - Maleic acid
  - Coumarin
  - Streptozocin

There is at present no evidence to suggest that proximal RTA causes hypercalciuria or hyperphosphaturia.[118,119] Phosphate wasting associated with proximal RTA appears to occur only in association with the Fanconi syndrome. The hypercalciuria frequently seen with chronic metabolic acidosis is not observed in this disorder, probably because increased distal HCO_3^- delivery enhances calcium absorption in the distal nephron.[121] In addition, hypercitraturia helps to prevent nephrocalcinosis and nephrolithiasis, which are not seen in proximal RTA. Rickets, which frequently accompanies the Fanconi syndrome, is probably a result of phosphate wasting rather than a result of the proximal RTA per se.

Management and Prognosis

The goal of treatment in proximal RTA is to maintain a normal serum bicarbonate concentration and pH. This can be achieved only by the exogenous administration of large amounts of alkali such as HCO_3^- or an equivalent organic anion such as citrate which consumes H^+ during metabolism in the liver. As described above, such treatment will be associated with massive bicarbonaturia in the form of Na^+-HCO_3^- and K^+-HCO_3^-. Thus, the HCO_3^- or citrate administered should be administered as a mixture of the sodium and potassium salts depending on the moieties excreted (K^+-Shohls) (Table 121-4). One approach to decreasing the magnitude of bicarbonate excretion is to administer thiazide diuretics,[122,123] a maneuver which lowers the filtered load of bicarbonate by decreasing GFR as a result of chronic extracellular fluid volume depletion. Although the prognosis varies according to the specific cause of the proximal tubular dysfunction, proximal RTA per se should not result in major consequences for the patient if the metabolic acidosis is corrected. While growth is stunted in children with isolated proximal RTA, this is corrected by correction of the acidosis and represents one of the major reasons for adequate alkali replacement, especially in children. Some investigators have noted that the tubular defect improves over time in isolated proximal RTA presenting in childhood.

DISTAL RENAL TUBULAR ACIDOSIS

Mechanism and Regulation of Distal Acidification

Most of the filtered HCO_3^- (90 percent) is reabsorbed in the proximal tubule. One of the functions of the distal nephron is to reabsorb the remainder of the filtered HCO_3^- (about 5 to 10 percent). In addition, the distal nephron must secrete a quantity of protons equal to that generated systemically by metabolism in order to maintain acid–base balance. While this quantity of protons, approximately 50 to 80 meq/day, is relatively small, it is necessary to buffer this amount in order to prevent the cumulative development of chronic positive hydrogen ion balance and metabolic acidosis. Proton in the amount of 10 meq/liter would be equivalent to a pH of 2.0 and would expose the urinary tract to extreme acidity if unbuffered. Moreover, to achieve a urine pH of this acidity, proton secretory mechanisms would be required to generate large gradients between blood and tubule fluid. To mitigate the development of limiting pH gradients and increase the rate of acid excretion, protons secreted in the collecting tubule are buffered by ammonia, phosphate, creatinine, and other miscellaneous buffers. Thus, the distal nephron reabsorbs a small fraction of filtered HCO_3^- and secretes 50 to 80 meq of acid per day in the form of NH_4^+ and titratable acid.

Table 121-4 Forms of Alkali Replacement

Shohl's solution	
Na citrate	1 meq/ml
Citric acid	1 meq/ml
$NaHCO_3$	3.9 meq/tablet (325 mg)
Baking soda	60 meq/teaspoon
K-Lyte	25 or 50 meq/tablet
Polycitra (K-Shohl's)	
Na citrate	1 meq/ml
K citrate	1 meq/ml
Citric acid	1 meq/ml

Anatomic and Physiological Components of the Distal Nephron. The mechanisms of acidification have been discussed extensively elsewhere[34] and are reviewed here as pertinent to the distal renal tubular acidoses. For the purpose of this discussion, the distal nephron can be considered to consist of three segments. The first is the cortical collecting tubule (CCT). This segment has three important characteristics. First, it is capable of HCO_3^- absorption and HCO_3^- secretion,[124,125] which are performed by separate cells in this segment.[126] Second, the relative magnitudes of HCO_3^- absorption and secretion can be modulated by the acid–base status of the animal.[126] Third, the CCT actively transports Na^+ and K^+ in addition to H^+-HCO_3^-. The CCT normally has a negative transepithelial voltage due to sodium transport,, which can be modulated by variations in the rate of sodium absorption.

It should be pointed out that considerable research on the mechanism of acidification has been conducted by micropuncture techniques in the superficial distal convoluted tubule of the rat. This segment of the nephron actually includes three distinct morphologic segments: the true distal convoluted tubule, the connecting tubule, and the initial cortical collecting tubule. When studied functionally with respect to acidification, however, this segment appears to have many characteristics which are similar to the cortical collecting tubule. For example, the superficial distal convoluted tubule actively absorbs sodium and secretes potassium and is capable of absorption or secretion of HCO_3^-, depending on the acid–base status of the animal.[127–129] Thus, the superficial distal tubule and the CCT can be viewed as similar segments of the distal nephron.

The second major segment of the distal nephron which is important in acidification is the outer medullary collecting tubule (OMCT). Lombard and colleagues[130] first demonstrated that the OMCT (inner stripe) was capable of high rates of proton secretion. This segment absorbs HCO_3^- at rates exceeding that observed in the CCT. In addition, this segment does not actively transport sodium or potassium[131] and does not secrete HCO_3^-, but only absorbs HCO_3^-.[121] Moreover, the rate of HCO_3^- absorption is unaffected by the chronic acid–base status of the animal.[121] Finally, as a result of these transport characteristics, specifically, active proton secretion, the luminal electrical potential difference is positive in this segment (see below).[130]

The third distal nephron segment involved in acidification is the inner medullary collecting duct (IMCD). Microcatheter and micropuncture studies have demonstrated a declining pH profile along the length of the IMCD in vivo which occurs in parallel with an increase in net acid secretion. Bicarbonate reabsorption by the terminal IMCD has been substantiated both in vivo and in vitro.[132–134] Although it is clear that apical proton secretion mediates bicarbonate absorption, titrates urinary buffers, and "traps" ammonium, the precise cellular mechanisms responsible for luminal acidification in the IMCD have not yet been fully elucidated. Nevertheless, morphological, immunohistochemical, and immunocytochemical studies have helped characterize some features of IMCD cells relevant to acid–base transport, which have been reviewed in detail.[135] At least two subsegments have been identified: the initial IMCD and the terminal IMCD. The initial subsegment is composed of two cell types, the α intercalated cell and a cell unique to this segment, the IMCD cell; but β intercalated cells are not present. In contrast, the predominant cell type in the distal two thirds of the IMCD (terminal subsegment) is the "IMCD-cell."[136]

Thus, acidification in the distal nephron can be viewed as occurring predominantly in three segments. The first segment, represented by the CCT, is a low-capacity segment where acidification can be regulated by sodium transport–dependent changes in potential difference, as well as by long-term systemic acid–base balance. The second segment, represented by the OMCT, has a higher capacity for proton secretion but is unaffected by long-term systemic acid–base changes and, because this segment does not transport sodium actively, should not be affected by sodium delivery. Finally, the IMCD has a low capacity for acidification but is regulated by systemic acid–base status and potassium balance both in terms of net proton secretion and ammonium transport.[135]

H^+ Secretion/HCO_3^- Absorption. The mechanism of HCO_3^- absorption appears to be similar in all the segments of the distal nephron. Studies measuring disequilibrium pH have demonstrated that HCO_3^- absorption in the superficial distal nephron[17,19] and in the medullary collecting duct is mediated by apical membrane secretion of hydrogen ions.[137] Because of the negative cell potential, secretion of hydrogen ions must be an active process which requires energy input. Numerous studies suggest that active proton secretion at the apical membrane is mediated by an ATP-dependent electrogenic proton pump. This conclusion is based on studies which have demonstrated electrogenicity and sodium-independence of HCO_3^- absorption.[138–140] An H^+-ATPase has been demonstrated in vesicles from renal medulla and has been purified.[141–144] This H^+-ATPase is similar to that found in endosomes, clathrin-coated vesicles, Golgi, and endoplasmic reticulum. This type of H^+-ATPase is similar to the F_0-F_1 ATPase of mitochondria in that it is composed of multiple subunits and does not possess a phosphorylated intermediate, but differs in that it is insensitive to oligomycin and is inhibited by *N*-ethylmaleimide.[143] It is referred to as a "vacuolar" pump. The bovine brain clathrin-coated vesicle H^+ pump has been extensively characterized and is a heteroligomer of 500 to 700 kDa composed of nine major polypeptides of 116, 70, 58, 40, 38, 34, 33, 19, and 17 kDa.[145] Similar to the mitochondrial H^+ pump, vacuolar H^+ pumps consist of two components—a transmembranous component and a peripheral component. In the clathrin-coated vesicle H^+ pump, it has been demonstrated that the 70-, 58-, 40-, and 33-kDa polypeptides are required for ATPase activity and most likely contribute to the peripheral component, while the 17-kDa subunit serves as part of a *N*,N′-cyclohexylcarbodiimide (DCCD)-sensitive transmembranous H^+ channel.[145] The kidney H^+ pump lacks the 116-kDa component that is a common feature of other vacuolar H^+ pumps, but it contains the polypeptides of 70, 58, 31, and 17 kDa.[146] Antibodies directed against the purified H^+-ATPases of renal medulla stain the apical membrane of the hydrogen-secreting cells in the CCT and OMCT.[147,148]

Data have suggested the possibility that a second H^+ pump may contribute to apical membrane H^+ secretion in cortical and outer collecting duct cells, an H^+/K^+-ATPase, similar to that present in gastric parietal cells. This pump is of the E_1-E_2 type in that it possesses a phosphoaspartyl intermediate as part of its catalytic cycle and is inhibited by micromolar concentrations of vanadate. Preliminary evidence suggests, however, more similarity between the colonic and kidney H^+/K^+-ATPase than between kidney and gastric cDNAs.[149] The H^+/K^+-ATPase is also inhibited competitively by SCH 28080 and omeprazole. Using measurements of H^+ and K^+ fluxes as well as inhibitor studies, it has been suggested that an H^+/K^+-ATPase in the collecting duct may contribute to H^+ secretion and K^+ absorption.[150]

Moreover, antibodies against the gastric H^+/K^+-ATPase have been demonstrated to stain intercalated cells of the CCT and OMCT of control rat and rabbit kidney slices.[151] The overall contribution of the H^+/K^+-ATPase to proton transport by the collecting duct has not been established. Indeed, a significant contribution of an H^+/K^+-ATPase was discernible only in the isolated perfused rabbit OMCT during diet-induced hypokalemia.[150] Finally, studies suggest that H^+/K^+-ATPase activity, by indirect enzymatic techniques, is decreased during long-term vanadate administration in rats, which was also associated with metabolic acidosis, hypokalemia, and an inappropriately alkaline urine.[152] The pathophysiological role of H^+/K^+-ATPase in other acidification defects has not yet been investigated, however.

Active H^+ secretion by the apical membrane generates base in the cell which must exit the basolateral membrane. The mechanism of base exit appears to be Cl^-–HCO_3^- exchange. This conclusion is based on studies which have demonstrated that chloride is required for HCO_3^- absorption and proton secretion in the turtle urinary bladder and in the OMCT.[153,154] In addition, Cl^-–HCO_3^- exchange has been demonstrated directly on the basolateral membrane of proton secretory cells of the CCT by measuring cell pH.[115] Using antibodies against the red-cell anion exchanger (Cl^-–HCO_3^-), an antigenically similar protein was detected in the basolateral membrane.[155] The cDNA encoding this Cl^-–HCO_3^- exchanger has now been cloned.[156,157] This basolateral membrane Cl^-–HCO_3^- exchanger is encoded by the same gene that encodes the red cell Cl^-–HCO_3^- exchanger. However, the two messenger RNAs differ in that exons 1 to 3 of the red-cell Cl^-–HCO_3^- exchanger are not present in the renal Cl^-–HCO_3^- exchanger—a difference that is due to alternate initiation sites. Chloride, which enters the cell in exchange for bicarbonate, exits the cell through a basolateral membrane chloride conductance.[158] Chloride then diffuses across the tight junction driven by the positive transepithelial voltage. The mechanism of bicarbonate absorption is summarized in Fig. 121-4.

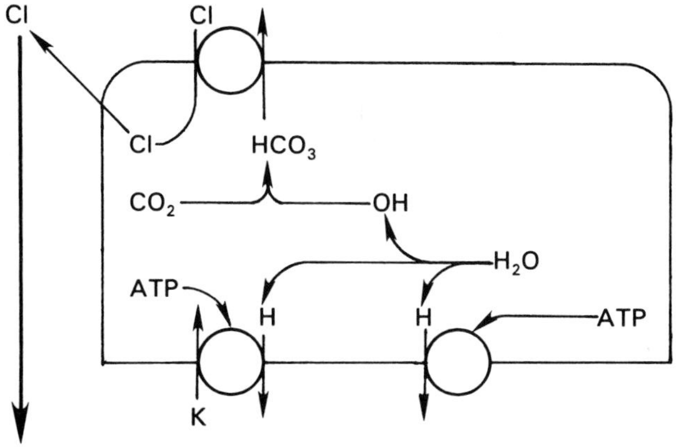

FIG. 121-4 **Cell model for hydrogen ion secretion into the lumen of the collecting tubule (and bicarbonate absorption).**

Bicarbonate Secretion. When animals are pretreated with an alkaline diet, net bicarbonate secretion is observed in the CCT.[159] A similar adaptation occurs in the turtle urinary bladder in which the mechanism of HCO_3^- secretion has been investigated extensively. Subsequent studies in the CCT have suggested that the turtle urinary bladder and the mammalian CCT share similar transport characteristics. As was true for HCO_3^- absorption, HCO_3^- secretion is dependent on the presence of chloride and independent of sodium.[160–162] Under control conditions, HCO_3^- secretion is electroneutral and active.[163] Based on these findings, it appears that HCO_3^- secretion is mediated by a basolateral membrane H^+-ATPase coupled with an apical membrane Cl^-–HCO_3^- exchanger (Fig. 121-5*A* and *B*). It is not clear whether the basolateral membrane H^+-ATPase in bicarbonate-secreting cells is identical to the apical membrane H^+-ATPase in bicarbonate-absorbing cells. However, antibodies raised against purified H^+-ATPase label the basolateral membranes of some CCT cells.[147] While apical membrane Cl^-–HCO_3^- exchange has been demonstrated in HCO_3^- secreting cells by measuring cell pH, antibodies against the red-cell Cl^-–HCO_3^- exchanger do not stain the apical membrane in the CCT. The model which best explains the mechanism of electroneutral HCO_3^- secretion is shown in Fig. 121-5*A*.[22] Here, protons are actively secreted across the basolateral membrane, generating base within the cell. Base then exits across the apical membrane as HCO_3^- in exchange for chloride. The chloride exits across the basolateral membrane chloride conductance. This process is electroneutral, since equal proton and chloride currents flow across the basolateral membrane.

It has been demonstrated clearly in the turtle urinary

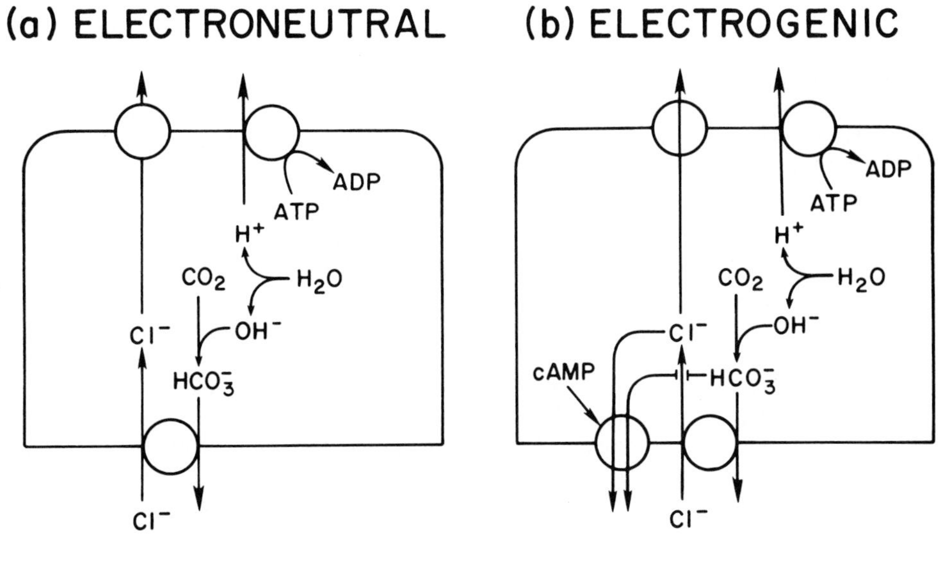

FIG. 121-5 **Cell model for electroneutral *(a)* and electrogenic *(b)* bicarbonate secretion into the lumen of the CCT. Note that the H^+-ATPase is in the basolateral membrane in this model.** ***(Used by permission from R.J. Alpern and F.C. Rector Jr: Renal acidification: Cellular mechanisms of tubular transport and regulation. In:*** **Handbook of Physiology,** ***edited by E.E. Windhager and G. H. Giebisch. Rockville Pike, MD: American Physiological Society, 1992.)***

bladder that increases in intracellular cAMP levels stimulate HCO_3^- secretion and convert it from electroneutral to electrogenic.[164-166] These data are best explained by activation or appearance of an anion channel in the apical membrane which is conductive to chloride or HCO_3^-.[143] This has the effect of accelerating HCO_3^- secretion in several ways. First, an additional mechanism for apical membrane HCO_3^- exit has been added. Second, an additional mechanism for chloride efflux is added which can then allow the Cl^-–HCO_3^- exchanger to proceed at a faster rate. Lastly, addition of a conductance pathway should depolarize the cell, allowing the H^+-ATPase to secrete at a faster rate. The mechanism of electrogenic HCO_3^- secretion is shown in Fig. 121-5*B*. Schuster has demonstrated that cAMP increased HCO_3^- secretion in the CCT perfused in vitro.[159,167] However, electrogenicity was not demonstrated in these studies. It was shown that the receptor responsible for adenylyl cyclase stimulation was β catecholamine.

Buffers. As discussed above, secreted protons must be buffered to prevent extreme luminal acidity. These buffer systems are conveniently divided into two types: closed and open. A closed buffer system is one in which the concentration of total buffer is fixed. Addition of acid to the solution converts the basic form of the buffer to the acidic form. Such buffers are most efficient at the pK level at which 50 percent of the total buffer is in the acid form and 50 percent is in the basic form. Because the total concentration of these buffers is fixed, one can calculate the contribution to renal acid secretion by titrating urine from the urinary pH back to blood pH (to simulate the pH of the fluid entering the renal tubules). This is referred to as titratable acidity and represents the contribution of titrated closed buffers to net acid excretion.

An open buffer system is one in which one of the moieties, the acid or base, can enter or leave the system. The concentration of the other component varies with pH. In biological systems, the component which enters and leaves the system is lipid soluble and capable of rapid transepithelial diffusion. Such systems have greatest buffer capacity when the total buffer concentration is greatest. The contribution of these buffers to acidification is assessed by measuring the concentration in the urine of the impermeable form. One example of such a buffer system is $CO_2/H_2CO_3/HCO_3^-$. The concentration of carbonic acid is essentially fixed in the presence of the enzyme carbonic anhydrase because of rapid dehydration to CO_2 which is highly permeable. Addition of acid merely decreases the concentration of HCO_3^-. However, in the absence of accessibility of tubule fluid at the apical membrane to carbonic anhydrase (type IV carbonic anhydrase), as occurs in the collecting duct, carbonic acid accumulates to concentrations above that predicted if HCO_3^- were in equilibrium with CO_2. Such a condition results in a lower pH *in situ* than at equilibrium (disequilibrium pH).[19]

Ammonium. Another important open buffer system is NH_3/NH_4^+. Since NH_3 permeability is high, proton secretion merely affects the concentration of NH_4^+. This process is referred to as "nonionic diffusion." Addition of acid to the lumen causes NH_3 to be converted to NH_4^+, which lowers the concentration of NH_3 and allows NH_3 to diffuse (by nonionic transport) into the lumen.[168] Moreover, a spontaneous acid disequilibrium pH as prevails in the IMCD favors NH_3 entry from interstitium to tubule lumen.[137] Some studies have demonstrated that the tubular permeability to NH_3 is not as great as was previously thought, so that in some segments, transport of NH_4^+ can lead to gradients of NH_3.[168]

While several nephron segments have been shown to possess ammoniagenic enzymes, the majority of ammonium excreted in the urine is derived from the metabolism of glutamine in proximal tubule cells.[168,169] Ammonium production in the proximal tubule is regulated homeostatically. The rate limiting enzyme steps for ammoniagenesis are glutaminase and phosphoenolpyruvate carboxykinase (PEPCK). In states of chronic acidosis, the activities of both of these enzymes increase, as does the abundance of their respective messenger RNAs.[170,171] The increase in glutaminase messenger RNA is secondary to an increase in the stability of the message, while the increase in PEPCK message is secondary to transcriptional activation.[170,171] The precise promoter elements responsible for transcriptional activation of PEPCK have not been defined.[172] At physiological pH, two ammonium ions and the divalent anion α-ketoglutarate are the major products of glutamine metabolism. α-Ketoglutarate serves as a major substrate for the formation of "new bicarbonate," which is transported across the basolateral membrane to the extracellular fluid. This "new bicarbonate" serves to restore the bicarbonate lost in the extracellular fluid in the buffering of acid products of metabolism. A major portion of the NH_4^+ produced in the proximal tubule will be excreted in the urine. In contrast, any NH_4^+ returned by way of the renal vein to the liver will be consumed to produce urea. Thus, the hydrogen ions produced by ureagenesis in the liver neutralize the bicarbonate produced in the kidney from α-ketoglutarate. Therefore, to be effective in maintaining acid–base balance, the ammonium generated by renal ammoniagenesis must be excreted in the urine to avoid hepatic metabolism.

Ammonium is preferentially secreted into the proximal tubule lumen across the apical membrane.[173-176] Quantitatively, the majority of ammonium secretion is accomplished in the earliest portion of the proximal convoluted tubule. Ammonium may then be absorbed to a small extent in the late proximal tubule. The rate of secretion in both the early and late proximal tubules is a highly regulated process, one that is augmented dramatically by systemic metabolic acidosis. In the S3 segment of the proximal straight tubule, ammonium secretion is enhanced by the presence of an acid disequilibrium pH. The cellular mechanism of ammonium transport involves both NH_3 diffusion and NH_4^+ transport. Direct NH_4^+ secretion may occur via transport of NH_4^+ on the apical membrane Na^+–H^+ exchanger.

As tubule fluid leaves the proximal tubule and enters the loop of Henle, a number of processes lead to ammonium and ammonia efflux and result in high medullary interstitial ammonium concentrations. First, the luminal fluid which issues out of the proximal tubule is alkalinized in the thin descending limb due to water abstraction which concentrates HCO_3^-.[177-179] This alkalinization creates a condition favorable for ammonia efflux by nonionic diffusion. In addition, direct NH_4^+ transport by the thick ascending limb has been demonstrated[180] and is responsive to systemic acid–base, potassium, and sodium homeostasis. Ammonia (NH_3) is capable of reentering the proximal straight tubule from the interstitium,[181] thus leading to countercurrent multiplication, in which the "single effect" involves selective addition of ammonium by the proximal tubule and active ammonium absorption in the ascending limb. The countercurrent system in the loop then multiplies the effect. The net result of this system is a medullary-to-cortical gradient for ammonium with medullary concentrations exceeding cortical concentrations several times.[134,168,184] Ammonium concentrations in the inner medullary interstitium reach greatest amplification over cortical levels during chronic metabolic acidosis.[182] Ammonium is secreted from the medullary interstitium into the medullary collecting ducts by a combination of NH_3 diffusion and active H^+ secretion (H^+-ATPase and the H^+/K^+-ATPase), resulting in high concentrations of ammonium in final urine.[168,182,183] Maintenance of a high excretion rate of ammonium by the kidney minimizes the amount of ammonium which can exit the kidney via the renal veins and be washed into the systemic circulation (where the liver is responsible for conversion of ammonium to glutamine and urea). Such conversion in the liver consumes protons, thus negating the beneficial effects of renal ammoniagenesis, the byproduct of which is bicarbonate from α-ketoglutarate.[168]

Regulation of Distal Acidification. As described above, distal acidification involves both HCO_3^- absorption and HCO_3^- secretion, which may be either electroneutral or electrogenic. These mechanisms are subjected to many forms of regulation which have been reviewed extensively elsewhere.[40] In this section, we will discuss some of the aspects of regulation or bicarbonate absorption which are relevant to distal RTA.

The rate of proton secretion is very sensitive to luminal pH. This has been studied extensively in the turtle urinary bladder, in which the net proton secretory rate has been shown to be related linearly to luminal pH (Fig. 121-6).[184] Because leak pathways are extremely small in the distal nephron, this relationship is due to an effect of luminal pH on active transepithelial proton secretory rate.[184,185]

As discussed above, HCO_3^- absorption or proton secretion is mediated by both an electrogenic mechanism (proton-translocating ATPase) and also by an electroneutral H^+/K^+-ATPase. As such it would be expected that the rate of the former process would be affected by the transepithelial potential difference. This type of dependency has been demonstrated in turtle urinary bladder, where transepithelial voltage and transepithelial pH gradients (see Fig. 121-6)[186] have been found to have similar effects on the rate of proton secretion. In the CCT, changes in transepithelial potential difference which occur secondary to changes in sodium transport affect the rate of proton secretion.[187] This provides a mechanism by which changes in sodium delivery and changes in the sodium avidity of the CCT, possibly related to mineralocorticoid levels, can affect acidification secondarily. Although the OMCT also secretes protons by an electrogenic mechanism, this segment does not actively transport sodium, and, thus, transepithelial voltage would not be expected to be affected by sodium delivery. It is not established at present whether electrogenic HCO_3^- secretion occurs in the CCT. If this were the case, the HCO_3^- secretory rate could also be affected by sodium transport and secondary changes in transepithelial voltage. Lastly, it should be noted that anion gradients may affect the transepithelial potential difference in the CCT or OMCT and thus secondarily affect the rate of proton secretion.

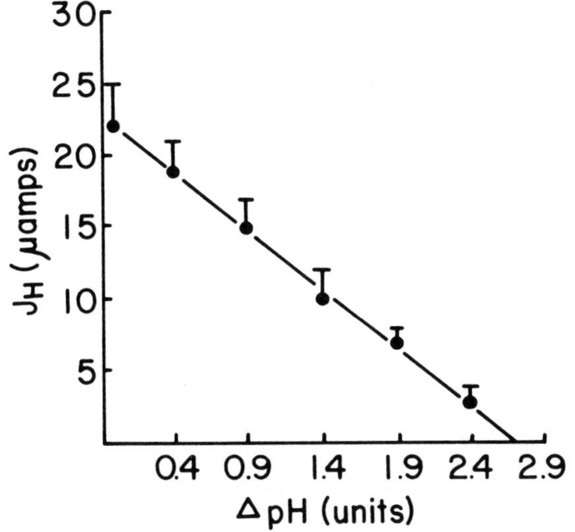

FIG. 121-6 Effect of mucosal pH on rate of hydrogen ion secretion in the turtle urinary bladder. Note that hydrogen secretory rate is linearly related to mucosal pH rather than mucosal hydrogen ion concentration. *(Adapted from Q. Al-Awqati:* **Am J Physiol** *235:F77, 1978. Used by permission.)*

Mineralocorticoid levels have also been demonstrated to be a potent determinant of proton secretory rate. In the CCT, mineralocorticoids stimulate sodium absorption, increasing the lumen negative transepithelial potential and secondarily stimulating electrogenic proton secretion.[188,189] In addition, mineralocorticoids have been demonstrated to stimulate proton secretion directly in the turtle urinary bladder[190,191] and in the cortical, outer, and inner medullary collecting tubules even in the absence of sodium.[138,140,192] Mineralocorticoids do not affect the limiting luminal pH gradient, but rather affect the rate of H^+ secretion at high luminal pH.[190]

Finally, both hypokalemia and hyperkalemia should be regarded as important determinants of the renal response to acid–base balance. While clearance studies have suggested that potassium deficiency stimulates distal proton secretion, more direct studies in perfused segments have been conflicting.[193,194] Potassium status can affect distal nephron acidification by indirect mechanisms. First, the level of potassium is an important determinant of aldosterone elaboration which, as discussed above, is an important determinant of distal acidification. Even more important is the effect of potassium on ammonium synthesis in the proximal tubule[195] and on ammonium excretion.[168] Chronic potassium deficiency stimulates ammonium production, while hyperkalemia suppresses ammoniagenesis.[168,196] These changes in ammonium production may also affect medullary interstitial ammonium concentration and buffer availability.[134] The effects of potassium balance on ammonium transport in proximal tubule and the thick ascending limb of Henle's loop have been elucidated. Hyperkalemia has no effect on ammonium transport in the superficial proximal tubule, but markedly impairs ammonium absorption in the thick ascending limb, reducing inner medullary concentrations of total ammonia and decreasing secretion of NH_3 into the IMCD.[196–198]

Pathogenesis of Distal Renal Tubular Acidosis

Hypokalemia (Classic). The mechanisms involved in the pathogenesis of hypokalemic distal RTA are not yet resolved. There are three important considerations. First, the fact that these patients tend to be hypokalemic (and not hyperkalemic) demonstrates that generalized CCT dysfunction or aldoster-one deficiency are not causative. Other possibilities include some type of lesion in the medullary collecting ducts, or a selective lesion of the CCT.

The second consideration is the inability to acidify the urine maximally (to below pH 5.5), which is often considered a cardinal feature of this entity. This characteristic has resulted in the designation of hypokalemic distal RTA as a "gradient lesion" and suggested to many the possibility of an abnormal leak pathway (see below).[199,200] Some investigators have also employed the response of urine pH to Na_2SO_4 infusion to classify the defect, arguing that an abnormal leak would theoretically respond to Na_2SO_4.[201–203] However, a response to Na_2SO_4 infusion has other interpretations (see below).

The third consideration is the response of the urine P_{CO_2} to $NaHCO_3^-$ infusion in these patients. In patients given large infusions of $NaHCO_3^-$ to produce a high HCO_3^- excretion rate, distal nephron hydrogen ion excretion will lead to the generation of high CO_2 tension in the renal medulla and urine.[204] In fact, the magnitude of the urinary P_{CO_2} (often referred to as the urine-minus-blood P_{CO_2}, or $U-B\ P_{CO_2}$) is quantitatively related to distal nephron hydrogen ion secretion in this setting.[137,205,206] Because of marked bicarbonaturia, the test offers an opportunity to examine distal nephron hydrogen ion secretion in the absence of blood-to-lumen HCO_3^- gradients.

However, it would be incorrect to assume that gradients for H^+ ions, H_2CO_3, and non-HCO_3^- buffers are absent in this setting. Because luminal carbonic anhydrase is not present in the collecting tubule, hydrogen ion secretion increases the concentration of these acid moieties in the lumen. Thus, while the luminal HCO_3^- concentrations may exceed that of the interstitium, gradients may exist for backleak of H^+ ions, H_2CO_3, and acid HCO_3^- buffers out of the lumen. Backleak of any of these moieties or decreased rates of hydrogen ion secretion will lead to a low $U-B\ P_{CO_2}$. While this test has not been routinely performed in all patients with hypokalemic distal RTA, the $U-B\ P_{CO_2}$ is generally subnormal except in amphotericin B–induced distal RTA.[204,205,207]

With this background, we will now explore a number of possible mechanisms for defective distal tubular acidification. We will orient this discussion along the lines of Fig. 121-7. In this figure, the line labeled "normal" represents the usual relationship between proton secretory rate and luminal pH in the collecting tubule, which is presumed to be similar to the relationship in the turtle bladder as displayed in Fig. 121-6. When luminal fluid is alkaline, proton secretion is rapid and leads to luminal acidification. The limiting luminal pH represents the pH at which net proton secretion ceases. In the collecting tubule, leak pathways are normally of only minor significance. Thus, the limiting pH represents the pH at which active transepithelial proton secretion ceases.[186]

In Fig. 121-7 the line labeled "leak" represents an approximation of the expected relationship when an abnormal leak pathway is inserted into the collecting tubule. In the absence of a transepithelial pH gradient, the effect of such a leak would be minimal or absent. However, as luminal pH decreases, the leak would provide a pathway for base addition and acid efflux from the lumen, which would markedly decrease net proton secretion. Thus, a leak would appear as a "gradient" defect, in which abnormal acidification would be most obvious when the filtered load of HCO_3^- is low and the need to excrete a highly acid urine is great.

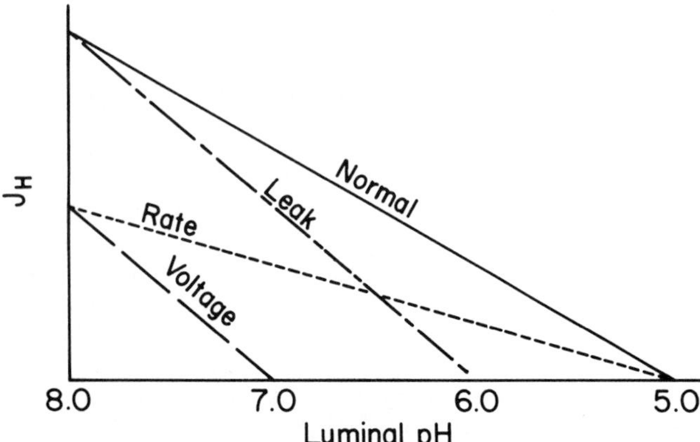

FIG. 121-7 **Theoretical mechanisms for defect in hydrogen ion secretion. Rate of hydrogen ion secretion is expressed as a function of luminal pH. See text for explanation.**

The exact acid–base moiety which would leak is not known but could vary with the type of leak. Possibilities include H^+, OH^- ions, H_2CO_3, HCO_3^-, or nonbicarbonate buffers. Based on Fick's law of diffusion, the rate of diffusion is equal to the permeability times the concentration gradient. The HCO_3^- and non-HCO_3^- buffers, therefore, would be likely moieties to back-diffuse because of the large concentration gradients (millimolar range). Protons, because of high mobility in aqueous solutions, may leak back when the H^+ concentration is sufficiently high (i.e., low luminal pH). Carbonic acid would be unlikely to back-diffuse through an aqueous pore because of the low concentration in lumen and blood (micromolar). However, if the leak pathway were through lipids, possibly due to an alteration in membrane composition, H_2CO_3 diffusion could be important.

Two additional theoretical mechanisms exist by which a gradient distal RTA could occur. First, in the absence of an abnormal leak pathway, an inability to maximally acidify luminal fluid could represent an energetic problem such as an altered ATP or ADP ratio in the cell or an altered stoichiometry of a transporter (i.e., H^+-ATPase or H^+/K^+-ATPase). Such defects would be expected to present as "gradient" lesions and could behave like an abnormal leak (see Fig. 121-7), but have not yet been described. A second possible mechanism of a gradient defect is an enhanced rate of active HCO_3^- secretion. This would lead to an inability to acidify the urine maximally along with lower rates of net hydrogen ion secretion. Such a lesion, however, has not yet been reported. An enhanced rate of HCO_3^- secretion would be associated with a normal $U-B\ P_{CO_2}$, which, when found, has always been associated with insertion of aqueous channels and increased leak pathway (see below). Therefore, we have not considered this possible mechanism in Fig. 121-7.

An alternative to a gradient lesion is denoted in Fig. 121-7 by the line labeled "rate." In the absence of pH gradients, the rate of proton secretion is markedly depressed. However, the epithelium still retains the ability to achieve normal pH gradients and thus achieve maximal acidification. It is important to note that in the presence of a severe rate defect, achievement of maximal pH gradients may require an extremely long contact time, such that maximal acidification is never achieved. Based on the cell model for HCO_3^- absorption, a rate defect could involve an abnormality in the H^+-ATPase, the H^+/K^+-ATPase, the Cl^-–HCO_3^- exchanger, the chloride conductance, or cell metabolism. All of these could be present if there were generalized damage to the H^+-secreting cell.

At present, the best experimental model representative of a "leak" defect is that induced by amphotericin B. Amphotericin B, when inserted into lipid membranes, forms an aqueous channel.[208,209] Animals treated with amphotericin B are unable to acidify their urine maximally under control conditions.[202–205,207–211] However, in response to Na_2SO_4 infusion, urinary pH is maximally acidified.[205,211] During HCO_3^- loading in amphotericin-treated rats, the $U-B\ P_{CO_2}$ is normal.[205,210] In addition, DuBose and Caflisch[205] found a normal ("acid") disequilibrium pH in the papillary collecting duct (also indicating a normal H^+-secretion rate) in association with a papillary P_{CO_2} elevated to levels similar to those achieved in control animals. These studies demonstrated that the hydrogen ion secretory rate is normal in this form of distal RTA and that the characteristically inappropriately alkaline urine pH observed spontaneously, after an NH_4Cl challenge, is the result of back-diffusion of an acid–base moiety. Because amphotericin B is known to form cation selective channels in lipid membranes, the species most likely to backleak is H^+. The occurrence of a normal U − B P_{CO_2} and normal acid disequilibrium pH during $NaHCO_3$ infusion suggests that, in this setting, H^+ gradients are not sufficient to generate significant H^+ backleak. However, when the urine pH is lower, significant backleak occurs. Other toxins such as toluene have been suggested to produce a similar lesion, but this model has not been studied extensively.[212]

Unlike the situation with the amphotericin B defect, the pathophysiology of the acidification defect in classic hypokalemic distal RTA is unresolved. This is partly due to the lack of availability of suitable animal models for this disorder. Under a number of different circumstances, however, including acute acid infusion, patients with classic hypokalemic distal RTA are unable to acidify their urine below pH 5.5.[1,2,14,199,202,207] In most of the reported studies, urine pH remains alkaline after Na_2SO_4 infusion or furosemide administration.[213] In addition, patients with classical hypokalemic distal RTA can enhance net acid excretion in a normal manner in response to buffer infusion. More importantly, patients with classical hypokalemic distal RTA have been reported uniformly to display a low U − B P_{CO_2}.[3,202–204,207,213] This finding is not consistent with an enhanced HCO_3^- leak pathway because such a defect would not affect net proton secretion in the absence of a gradient (high tubular fluid HCO_3^- concentration). Rather, these data are consistent with a rate defect. The inability to acidify the urine below pH 5.5 could be due to the fact that rates of proton secretion are extremely limited in the most distal segments that can normally secrete protons against large gradients and establish a low urine pH. A normal response of net acid secretion to buffer infusion may be due to the fact that the diseased segments contribute little quantitatively to whole-kidney hydrogen ion secretion in the absence of steep gradients.

An alternative, but less likely, explanation for the defect in classical hypokalemic distal RTA is an enhanced leakiness of the epithelium to H^+ ions, H_2CO_3, or HCO_3^- buffer. As discussed above, such a leak would explain the inability of these patients to create maximal pH gradients and acidify their urine below pH 5.5. In addition, this mechanism would explain the normal response in net acid excretion to a buffer infusion.[199] However, as discussed above, such a leak would not explain the low U − B P_{CO_2}. In order for a significant acid backleak to occur in the presence of significant bicarbonaturia, a large acid disequilibrium pH would have to be present, leading to large H^+ gradients. However, the normal U − B P_{CO_2} in the amphotericin model argues against the presence of sufficiently large H^+ gradients in this setting.

Based on evidence supporting the existence of potassium-dependent bicarbonate absorption in the CCT and OMCT[150] which was inhibitable by omeprazole, and of recognition in these same nephron segments by antibodies to the gastric H^+/K^+-ATPase,[151] it is attractive to speculate that a defect in this pump, which would be predicted to result in both hypokalemia and metabolic acidosis, could be an explanation for classical hypokalemic distal RTA. Moreover, some studies have suggested that H^+/K^+-ATPase activity, by indirect enzymatic techniques, is decreased during chronic vanadate administration to rats, which was also associated with metabolic acidosis, hypokalemia, and an inappropriately alkaline urine.[152] An unusually high incidence of hypokalemic distal RTA has been reported in adults and children in northeastern Thailand.[214] This disorder has been assumed to be a result of vanadate contamination of drinking water.[152,215] Vanadate is a well-known inhibitor of a variety of ATPases, including H^+/K^+-ATPase, but not the vacuolar H^+-ATPase. In the studies with chronic vanadate intoxication, CCT H^+/K^+-ATPase enzymatic activity (and H^+/K^+-ATPase) was reduced by 75 percent, while no effect on *N*-ethylmaleimide (NEM)-sensitive (H^+-ATPase) enzymatic activity was observed.[152] This striking effect did not hold for medullary segments, where a significant but only modest reduction was noted. Nevertheless, H^+/K^+-ATPase immunoreactivity has been reported in 32 percent of cells in the rat and rabbit OMCT output, 20 percent in OMCT input, and 20 percent in CCT.[151] However, enzymatic activity and immunoreactivity may not always correlate with transport, and studies are needed to determine the role of H^+/K^+-ATPase in acidification and potassium balance.

Patients with impaired collecting-duct hydrogen-ion secretion and classical distal RTA also exhibit uniformly low excretory rates of ammonium when the degree of systemic acidosis is taken into account.[3–5] Low ammonium excretion equates with inappropriately low renal regeneration of bicarbonate, indicating that the kidney is responsible for causing or perpetuating the chronic metabolic acidosis. Low ammonium excretion in classical hypokalemic distal RTA could result from failure to trap ammonium in the medullary collecting duct, due to higher-than-normal tubular fluid pH in this segment and loss of the disequilibrium pH (pH >6.0).[177] The high urine pH indicates impaired H^+ secretion. However, given the presence of chronic metabolic acidosis and potassium deficiency, it would be expected that rates of ammonium synthesis would be high. In this setting, a urine pH of 5.5 to 6.5 would be sufficient to trap large amounts of ammonium. Since ammonium is normally trapped in the medulla by mechanisms involving the countercurrent system,[168,182] patients with classical distal RTA, who commonly have an associated urinary concentrating defect and/or medullary interstitial disease, could have increased rates of renal ammoniagenesis in the cortex but an inability to trap ammonium in the medullary countercurrent system.[3,216] This defect would reduce the normally favorable ammonia concentration gradient from loop of Henle and medullary interstitium to the OMCT[182] and would be associated with a decrease in NH_4^+ excretion. Whether this type of defect contributes to the reduction in ammonium excretion in classical hypokalemic distal RTA requires further investigation. It seems reasonable, however, that an abnormality in medullary ammonium accumulation could occur in various forms of tubulointerstitial disease involving the medulla.

In summary, hypokalemic distal RTA is characterized by an inability to acidify the urine below pH 5.5. In some patients, this is attributable to an enhanced leak pathway (amphotericin lesion). However, in most patients, the defect cannot be attributed to such a leak. In these patients, a decreased rate of distal proton secretion is the likely mechanism. A defect in a cell secreting H^+ by the H^+/K^+-ATPase might be expected to cause hypokalemia, a reduction in ammonium excretion, and metabolic acidosis.[217] However, if the defect were in a cell secreting H^+ by the H^+-ATPase, hypokalemia could occur secondarily as a result of volume depletion–induced hypereninemic-hyperaldosteronism and acidosis that accompany this disorder. It should be emphasized that only a few reports exist in which patients have been thoroughly evaluated with respect to minimal urine pH, response to Na_2SO_4 (or furosemide), and response of urinary P_{CO_2} to $NaHCO_3$ infusion. Delineation of the pathogenesis of classic hypokalemic distal RTA will require the examination of many more patients, the development of more precise and definitive clinical tests, and, most importantly, clinically relevant animal models.

Hyperkalemia in Association with an Acidification Defect: Generalized Distal Nephron Dysfunction. An additional mechanism by which the proton secretory rate can be affected is an altered transepithelial potential difference in the collecting tubule, which has been referred to as "short circuit" distal RTA or "voltage defect."[218] The expected effect of such a defect on proton secretory rate is denoted by the line in Fig. 121-7 labeled "voltage." As demonstrated in this figure, the effect of transepithelial potential difference and luminal pH are additive. Thus, an altered transepithelial potential will shift the line, thereby affecting both the limiting pH gradient and the rate of proton secretion at any given luminal pH. Any process inhibiting sodium transport in the CCT would be expected to cause such a defect. Moreover, in this setting, K^+ secretion in the CCT should also be decreased.

Three experimental models of "voltage" defects in the collecting tubule have been proposed. The traditional model of such a transport defect is that observed after amiloride administration. This agent inhibits sodium transport in the CCT and in the turtle urinary bladder, decreasing the negative transepithelial voltage in the lumen and secondarily inhibiting proton secretion.[219] The ability to maximally acidify the urine is clearly impaired and does not respond to sodium sulfate.[202,205,220] Micropuncture studies employing microelectrodes to measure disequilibrium pH as an index of proton secretion, as well as P_{CO_2} in the papillary collecting duct in rats with the amiloride defect, have revealed that this lesion is associated with a reduction in proton secretion and, as anticipated, a reduction in P_{CO_2}.[205] Potassium secretion is also decreased secondary to decreased voltage, and may result in hyperkalemia.[205,221] Data from preliminary studies designed to quantitate enzymatic activity in both the cortical and medullary collecting tubules have revealed a decline in H^+-ATPase activity in these segments after amiloride administration.[217] This finding is compatible with the previous results of DuBose[205] which suggested that amiloride inhibits acidification by mechanisms other than by simply impairing sodium-dependent transepithelial voltage. The observation was that amiloride obliterated the acid disequilibrium pH in the IMCD,[205] a segment in which acidification is not dependent on voltage and cannot be dependent, directly or indirectly, on sodium uptake across the apical membrane.[135]

The second defect attributed to a "voltage" lesion is that caused by lithium administration. In contrast to the failure of the amiloride-induced acidification defect to respond to sodium sulfate infusion, the distal RTA produced by lithium administration is characterized by an inappropriately alkaline urine pH which decreases appropriately during sodium sulfate infusion after an acid challenge.[202,205,222] The failure of urinary P_{CO_2} to increase above blood levels during $NaHCO_3$ infusion in animals with lithium-induced distal RTA demonstrates, however, that proton secretion is impaired.[223] However, studies in the turtle urinary bladder under open-circuit conditions revealed that lithium impairs proton secretion by virtue of a detrimental effect on the electrical gradient favoring H^+ secretion.[224] As was noted with the amiloride defect, the disequilibrium pH and papillary P_{CO_2} were also reduced, indicating clearly impaired proton secretion in the lithium defect.[205] In keeping with this observation, studies have demonstrated a decrease in H^+-ATPase activity not only in the cortical but also in the medullary collecting duct after lithium administration.[217,225] This finding is consistent with the observation of obliteration of the disequilibrium pH and reduction in IMCD P_{CO_2} in lithium intoxication in rats,[205] as well as reports that some patients receiving lithium are unable to increase the $U-B$ P_{CO_2} during a bicarbonate infusion.[189] Lithium appears then to impair acidification in both the cortical[217] and medullary[205] collecting tubules by a mechanism other than simply interfering with sodium-dependent voltage generation. Frank metabolic acidosis generally does not develop in patients receiving lithium therapy but who fulfill the criteria for incomplete distal RTA[226] (see below), and hyperkalemia is not observed.

The third experimental model of distal RTA associated with hyperkalemia assumed to be due to a "voltage" defect is that induced by unilateral ureteral obstruction. While findings in the postobstructed kidney are similar in many respects to the amiloride defect,[203,205,213] several lines of evidence indicate clearly that this disorder is the result of a non-voltage-mediated rate defect, not merely a voltage defect. The postobstructed model is associated with an inability to acidify the urine after an acid challenge, a decrease in ammonium excretion, obliteration of the acid disequilibrium pH, and a marked reduction in papillary P_{CO_2}[205]—all compatible with a pump defect. The decrease in ammonium entry into the IMCD appears to be the consequence of the absence of an acid disequilibrium pH. Laski and Kurtzman[187] have reported that the decrease in bicarbonate transport ($JtCO_2$) observed in rabbit collecting ducts perfused in vitro after obstruction appears first in medullary segments. Only after prolonged obstruction was $JtCO_2$ reduced in the CCT. Sabatini and Kurtzman[227] have measured enzymatically the activity of H^+-ATPase in dissected segments of rat collecting ducts 24 h after unilateral ureteral obstruction (UUO). H^+-ATPase activity was reduced to a greater extent in medullary than in cortical segments. With immunocytochemical techniques, Purcell et al.[228] have reported interruption in the cellular distribution of the 31-kDa subunit of H^+-ATPase in rat intercalated cells, suggesting a cytoskeletal defect in UUO and resulting in a failure to insert H^+-ATPase into the apical membrane ("gaps" or "discontinuity"). Moreover, with return of acidification 5 to 10 days after release of UUO, cell convexity and the apical distribution of the proton pump were restored. Sawczuk et al.[229] have observed that UUO is associated with induction of growth-related genes (c-*fos*, c-*myc*, cH-*ras*) in the obstructed kidney. It is conceivable that differences in gene expression between the obstructed and contralateral kidneys may correlate with expression of pump activity. Thus, biochemical in vitro microperfusion and in vivo micropuncture studies support the view that the proton pump is impaired in this defect.

Since the CCT is responsible for sodium reabsorption by an aldosterone-dependent process, which enhances the lumen negative transepithelial potential difference and thereby favors the secretion of potassium and hydrogen, it is not surprising that aldosterone deficiency would cause hyperkalemia[230] and metabolic acidosis.[231] Moreover, aldosterone stimulates potassium secretion in the distal tubule and whole kidney and hydrogen ion secretion in both the turtle urinary bladder[190] and medullary collecting tubule, independent of sodium transport.[140,154] Therefore, a decrease in the relative amount of aldosterone, or alternatively, a decrease in responsiveness of the collecting tubule to aldosterone, could result in a reduction in distal sodium reabsorption which would be expected to impair both potassium and hydrogen ion secretion.

Based on the direct and indirect (sodium transport–dependent voltage changes) effects, two mechanisms exist for defective collecting tubule proton secretion in aldosterone deficiency. When examined along the lines displayed in Fig. 121-7, low aldosterone levels cause a "rate" defect.[228] This type of defect would be associated with the ability to achieve a normal minimal urine pH, but low rates of proton secretion would be observed at higher luminal pH. In contrast, a voltage-dependent lesion would be associated with an inability to achieve a normal minimal urine pH (Fig. 121-7). Whole-kidney studies have revealed that, during conditions associated with low buffer excretion (i.e., decreased ammonium excretion), a normal minimal urine pH can be achieved.[220] Such findings suggest that the "rate" defect is quantitatively more important than the "voltage" defect in hypoaldosteronism and imply that the direct effect of aldosterone on H^+ secretion is quantitatively more important than indirect effects mediated through voltage changes.

Additional evidence in this regard can be deduced from studies which have examined the effect of spironolactone on acidification. In the turtle urinary bladder, spironolactone blocks aldosterone-stimulated sodium absorption, but serves as an agonist for the direct effect of mineralocorticoid on proton secretion.[232] The inability of spironolactone to cause a metabolic acidosis in the intact animal supports the relative unimportance of voltage-mediated changes in mineralocorticoid deficiency–induced distal RTA.[233]

The OMCT also serves as a target organ for aldosterone by increasing net proton secretory capacity independently of sodium transport. Selective aldosterone deficiency in rats has been reported to be associated with impaired H^+ secretion by the IMCD.[192] In this same study, ammonium transfer into the IMCD was markedly impaired so that ammonium excretion was reduced dramatically. Moreover, as a result of impaired ammonium production, ammonium delivery to the loop of Henle was also reduced. Thus, a decrease in inner medullary ammonium accumulation accounted for the reduction in ammonium transfer to the IMCD. Since papillary P_{CO_2} was reduced during bicarbonate loading, the rate of proton secretion was also clearly compromised.

In addition to impaired hydrogen and potassium secretion as a result of decreased activity of aldosterone, the development of hyperkalemia appears to have independent effects on net acid excretion.[234] Hyperkalemia per se inhibits renal ammoniagenesis and is associated with a decrease in excretion of ammonium which contributes to the development of metabolic acidosis.[197,230,235] The importance of hyperkalemia in the development of metabolic acidosis due to mineralocorticoid deficiency has been demonstrated further by correction of hyperkalemia with cation exchange resins. This correction was associated with a significant increase in net acid excretion (ammonium excretion).[234,236] Studies in a rat model of chronic hyperkalemia have affirmed that whole-kidney ammonium excretion is reduced significantly in vivo in chronic hyperkalemia.[196] This decrease in excretion was associated with a marked reduction in whole-kidney ammonium production, which occurred despite coexistent chronic metabolic acidosis. Nevertheless, chronic hyperkalemia had no effect on net secretion of ammonium by the superficial proximal convoluted tubule. Chronic hyperkalemia, at least in part by inhibition of active NH_4^+ absorption by the medullary thick ascending limb,[197] impairs accumulation of ammonium in the inner medulla and significantly compromises the transfer of ammonium into the IMCD.[198]

The importance of mineralocorticoids in the regulation of net acid excretion has also been documented in mineralocorticoid-deficient animals and humans.[237,238] In human subjects who have undergone adrenalectomy, net acid excretion and plasma total CO_2 decreased when mineralocorticoid was selectively discontinued but increased when mineralocorticoid was reinitiated.[238] The change in plasma total CO_2 correlated directly with changes in ammonium excretion, as expected, and inversely with corresponding changes in potassium balance.

Taken together, these findings provide compelling evidence that renal acidification is under the influence of mineralocorticoid and that mineralocorticoid deficiency can cause acidosis and impairment of renal acidification even in the absence of renal disease or glucocorticoid deficiency. The potential for systemic metabolic acidosis in such a setting could be amplified greatly, however, in individuals with renal insufficiency and a decrease in functioning renal mass.

The role of aldosterone deficiency in the pathogenesis of metabolic acidosis in patients with renal insufficiency has been investigated further by the administration of fludrocortisone in the setting of hyperkalemia and hyporeninemic hypoaldosteronism.[236,238] With administration of fludrocortisone in physiological replacement amounts, net acid excretion increased and the hyperkalemia and systemic acidosis improved.[236] Initially, urine pH decreased as a result of mineralocorticoid-mediated enhanced hydrogen ion secretion, but as urinary NH_4^+ excretion increased over several days, urine pH increased as a result of the increase in urinary buffer. Thus, in patients with selective hypoaldosteronism and chronic renal insufficiency, mineralocorticoid administration enhances renal acid excretion directly by increasing renal hydrogen ion secretion and indirectly by correcting hyperkalemia, which allows ammonium production and excretion to increase.[168]

Mineralocorticoid resistance also causes hyperkalemic-hyperchloremic metabolic acidosis in both children and adults. Pseudohypoaldosteronism is more common in children, and two types have been recognized. Classical pseudohypoaldosteronism of infancy (type I pseudohypoaldosteronism) may be familial and is characterized by renal salt wasting and a tendency toward hypotension.[239] Chronic hyperkalemia and metabolic acidosis may occur in the absence of diffuse renal parenchymal disease or a reduction in GFR.[240] Dehydration and hyponatremia due to renal salt wasting and hyperkalemia due to renal potassium retention are typically observed in association with distal RTA.[239,240] Plasma renin activity and plasma aldosterone concentrations are elevated, but deoxycorticosterone and corticosterone concentrations are within the normal range.[240] Supplemental salt administration can reverse the hyponatremia and hyperkalemia and allow improved growth.[240] After infancy the disorder typically abates, permitting reduction or discontinuation of sodium chloride supplements. However, it may recur during periods of salt restriction. This disorder has been attributed to an abnormality in the aldosterone receptor in the CCT.[240] In one patient with type I pseudohypoaldosteronism, binding of aldosterone was normal in mucosal cells obtained from the sigmoid colon.[241] In another patient with pseudohypoaldosteronism, however, mineralocorticoid stimulation of sodium and potassium transport was impaired in multiple target organs, including salivary glands, sweat glands, the colon, and the kidney.[242] Such a defect could be explained by a deficiency of Na^+/K^+-ATPase. Renal Na^+/K^+-ATPase activity was undetectable in either the proximal or distal nephron segments in two studies.[243] This finding does not prove that a deficiency in renal Na^+/K^+-ATPase is the primary defect, since Na^+/K^+-ATPase activity can decrease under circumstances associated with a reduction in net renal sodium reabsorption.[244]

In summary, type I pseudohypoaldosteronism could be the result of a decrease in aldosterone receptor activity or the result of a decrease in Na^+/K^+-ATPase activity. Additional possibilities include a decrease in apical membrane Na^+ transport or a generalized metabolic defect of the CCT. These latter defects would resemble the amiloride lesion.

Type II pseudohypoaldosteronism occurs in older children or adults and is most easily distinguished from type I pseudohypoaldosteronism by the presence of hypertension, volume expansion, and low-to-normal plasma aldosterone levels.[245–249] Three patients in one family have been reported in whom the defect appears to be inherited as an autosomal dominant trait.[250] In contrast to patients with type I pseudohypoaldosteronism, patients with type II pseudohypoaldosteronism respond to diuretics and salt restriction.[246,251] Studies have suggested that the disorder represents a unique abnormality in the distal nephron in which marked avidity for sodium chloride results in volume overexpansion, hypertension, suppressed renin activity, hypoaldosteronism, and reduced potassium secretion.[249] The primary defect appears to be an increase in the reabsorptive avidity for sodium chloride in the connecting tubule,[250] leading to a reduction in sodium delivery to the CCT and impairing potassium and hydrogen ion secretion.[249] The hyperkalemia further impairs urinary acidification by decreasing ammonium production and excretion, resulting in metabolic acidosis.[235] Such patients respond either to salt restriction,[246] which reduces salt delivery to the connecting tubule, or to thiazide diuretics,[253] which reduce electroneutral sodium chloride cotransport in the connecting tubule.[252] Mineralocorticoid replacement is not required.[246,249,251]

Hyporeninemic hypoaldosteronism has been recognized with increasing frequency in adults with chronic renal insufficiency as a cause of hyperkalemic, hyperchloremic metabolic acidosis. Patients with this disorder almost always exhibit mild-to-moderate renal insufficiency and acidosis in association with chronic hyperkalemia in the range of 5.5 to 6.5 meq/liter.[230,254,255] It is important to recognize that both the metabolic acidosis and the hyperkalemia are out of proportion to the level of reduction in GFR. The most frequently associated renal diseases are diabetic nephropathy and tubulointerstitial disease.[255–257] For 80 to 85 percent of such patients, there is a reduction in plasma renin activity that cannot be stimulated by the usual physiological maneuvers.[258] Aldosterone secretion, while low, can be increased by administration of angiotensin II or ACTH.[258] The degree of salt wasting associated with hyporeninemic hypoaldosteronism is generally not severe and is no worse than that seen in patients with chronic renal insufficiency at comparable GFR.[259] Since approximately 30 percent of patients with hyporeninemic hypoaldosteronism are hypertensive,[14] the finding of a low plasma renin in such patients suggests a volume-dependent form of hypertension with physiological suppression of renin elaboration.[260] In general, patients with more advanced renal insufficiency as a result of glomerular disease rather than tubulointerstitial disease (e.g., diabetic nephropathy) more commonly have volume expansion.[14,260] Therefore, because either mild salt wasting or salt retention may occur in this disorder, the precise etiology of the decrease in plasma renin has not been established firmly. Primary destruction of cells in the juxtaglomerular (J-G) apparatus may be observed in diabetic nephropathy.[261,262] Deficient release of renin also occurs in diabetic autonomic insufficiency or in prostaglandin deficiency.[263,264] A defect in conversion of renin precursor to renin was suggested in some patients with diabetes as well.[265]

The pathogenesis of the metabolic acidosis in hyporeninemic hypoaldosteronism is complex. Proximal HCO_3^- reabsorption was shown to be mildly abnormal, and the fractional excretion of HCO_3^- ranges from 3 to 10 percent at a normal plasma HCO_3^- concentration.[230,266] Whether this degree of bicarbonate wasting is a result of a defect in proximal bicarbonate reabsorption is not established. The ability to acidify the urine during metabolic acidosis is intact, but there is typically a reduced rate of net acid excretion and ammonium excretion.[230] As mentioned above and outlined in Table 121-5, impaired ammonium excretion is the combined result of hyperkalemia, impaired ammoniagenesis, a reduction in nephron mass, reduced proton secretion, and impaired transport of ammonium by nephron segments in the inner medulla.[255]

Based on the above discussion, acidification defects in

Table 121-5 Diagnostic Studies in RTA

		Type of RTA	
Finding	Proximal (II)	Classical Distal (I)	Generalized Distal Dysfunction (IV)
Plasma $[K^+]$	Low	Low	High
Urine pH with acidosis	<5.5	>5.5	<5.5 or >5.5
Urine net charge	Positive	Positive	Positive
Fanconi lesion	Present	Absent	Absent
Fractional bicarbonate excretion	>10–15%	<5%	<5–10%
U-B P_{CO_2}	Normal	Low*	Low
Response to therapy	Least readily	Readily	Less readily
Associated features	Fanconi syndrome	Nephrocalcinosis/ hyperglobulinemia	Renal insufficiency

*Except in amphotericin B nephrotoxicity.

the distal nephron can be grouped into three general categories: (1) an abnormal leak pathway resulting in back-diffusion of bicarbonate or hydrogen ions (e.g., amphotericin B defect), (2) a voltage-dependent defect associated with intact proton secretion but suppressed net acidification due to an abnormal transepithelial voltage (e.g., type II pseudohypoaldosteronism), and (3) a rate defect with decreased rates of transepithelial proton secretion (e.g., hypoaldosteronism). Classical hypokalemic distal RTA (excluding the amphotericin-induced gradient defect) appears to be a rate defect in transepithelial proton secretion based on the observed reduction in the U − B P_{CO_2} difference.[24] The inability to acidify the urine maximally is most likely due to a severe rate defect in the terminal portion of the collecting duct, the only segment of the nephron shown to be capable of lowering urine pH below 5.5.

Diagnosis of Type of Defect: Tests of Urinary Acidification

Urinary Net Charge and Ammonium Excretion. All forms of RTA are associated with an inappropriately low excretion of ammonium. Halperin and associates have proposed a means of estimating urinary ammonium excretion by consideration of the urinary net charge.[3–6] This test relies on the assumption that chloride is the most prevalent anion in urine and that urine with a low concentration of NH_4^+ will have more Na^+ + K^+ than Cl^- (net charge will be positive).[5] The urinary ammonium level is estimated by calculating the urine net charge (UNC): [UNC = $(Na_u{}^+ + K_u{}^+ - Cl_u{}^+]$.[5] When the urine chloride concentration is greater than the sum of sodium and potassium, the ammonium level is usually increased appropriately, suggesting an extrarenal cause for the acidosis. After confirming that the ammonium concentration is low, the urine pH should be measured.

Minimal Urine pH and Maximal Acid Excretion. Historically, the measurement of urine pH is the step applied most commonly to assess the ability to acidify the urine in the clinical setting. In the presence of systemic metabolic acidosis, the urine pH should be below 5.5, and is often below 5.0.[3,14,202,213] A urine pH consistently above 5.5 in the presence of systemic metabolic acidosis suggests an acidification defect involving the more distal portions of the nephron. A urine pH below 5.5 is also found in patients with proximal RTA when systemic acidosis is present and the filtered load of bicarbonate is low (i.e., below 15 meq/liter).[267] The explanation for this finding is that when the distal nephron is not impaired, reduced filtered loads of HCO_3^- can be reabsorbed in more distal segments so that HCO_3^- does not appear in the urine.[268] A urine pH below 5.5 is also characteristic of patients with selective aldosterone deficiency.[213] In this disorder, low urinary buffer excretion allows the urine pH to reach a limiting pH gradient more rapidly. These findings emphasize that while urine pH is the most commonly used test of renal acidification, it does not measure total hydrogen ion excretion. Patients with chronic metabolic acidosis and normal renal function (as is seen with chronic diarrhea) may have a higher urine pH as a result of the excretion of large quantities of ammonium.[3] A low urine pH, therefore, does not ensure that the proton secretory mechanism is either intact or appropriate for the level of acidosis, and a high urine pH does not prove an abnormality in acidification. The urine pH should be evaluated in conjunction with an estimate, or precise knowledge, of urine ammonium excretion.[3]

The urine pH should be measured on freshly voided urine collected under mineral oil. In patients with systemic acidosis, there is no need to perform an ammonium chloride loading test. If systemic acidosis is not present at the time of study, ammonium chloride can be given as a single dose orally (0.1 g/kg body weight) along with food, followed by hourly determinations of urine pH for 2 to 8 h.[269,270] The total CO_2 concentration in plasma should decrease by at least 3 to 5 meq/liter, and the urine pH should fall below 5.5.

Fractional Excretion of HCO_3^-. The fractional excretion of HCO_3^- during $NaHCO_3$ loading, or at a time when the plasma HCO_3^- is normal, is a convenient means of distinguishing proximal RTA from other forms. In patients with distal RTA, HCO_3^- reabsorption, while incomplete at low plasma levels of HCO_3^-, increases with increasing plasma HCO_3^- concentrations. The fractional excretion of HCO_3^- ($FE_{HCO_3^-}$ percent), is calculated as the $(U/P_{HCO_3^-} \div U/P_{Cr}) \times 100$. This value is persistently elevated (>10 to 15 percent) in patients with proximal RTA when the plasma HCO_3^- is near the normal range (20 meq/liter).[14,268] Patients with hyperkalemic distal RTA may have an $FE_{HCO_3^-}$ between 5 and 10 percent. By contrast, the $FE_{HCO_3^-}$ is usually less than 5 percent in classical hypokalemic distal RTA patients, except in children, in whom values may exceed 5 to 10 percent.[268,271]

$NaHCO_3$ Administration and U − B P_{CO_2}. The increment in urinary P_{CO_2} during $NaHCO_3$ infusion or oral $NaHCO_3$ administration in amounts which result in excretion of a highly alkaline urine is a reliable and sensitive index of proton secretion by the terminal nephron.[137,204,205,272,274] After sodium bicarbonate loading, the urine P_{CO_2} may reach a value at least 25 mmHg higher than systemic levels. The test is performed by infusing a solution containing 500 meq of sodium bicarbonate at a rate of 3 ml/min into a peripheral vein.[273] Timed urine collections at approximately 15- to 30-min intervals are obtained by having the patient void spontaneously while in the upright position. The test may be terminated after completion of at least three clearance periods when the urine pH is consistently 7.5 or greater. A steady state is usually achieved within 180 to 260 min after initiation of the bicarbonate infusion. Urine should always be collected under mineral oil for measurement of urine pH and P_{CO_2}. Patients with decreased rates of distal hydrogen secretion are expected to display subnormal values during HCO_3^- loading, since the U − B P_{CO_2} gradient will be lower than 10 to 15 mmHg.[204,274] In contrast, patients with a gradient or backleak defect of the type exemplified by the amphotericin B lesion are expected to retain the ability to generate high urinary CO_2 tensions during $NaHCO_3$ loading.[205,210]

Sodium Sulfate Infusion. If normal subjects are reabsorbing sodium avidly, sodium sulfate administration will result in maximal acidification as assessed by a significant decrease in urine pH.[169] This evaluation requires that the patient be placed on a low-salt diet to enhance distal sodium avidity. The delivery of sodium to the distal nephron is then promoted by administration of sodium accompanied by a poorly reabsorbable anion such as sulfate. This may be accomplished by infusion of 500 ml of 4% Na_2SO_4 over 1 h. One milligram of 9α-fludrocortisone administered orally 12 h before Na_2SO_4 infusion is usually required to ensure a sodium-avid state.[213] The typical response to sodium sulfate infusion in control subjects is a decrease in urine pH below 5.5, with or without systemic acidosis.[201,202] Urine collections should be continued for 2 to 3 h after discontinuing the sodium sulfate infusion because of a delayed response in some patients with distal RTA and some with chronic renal insufficiency.[202,213]

Unfortunately, the acidification response to sodium sulfate infusion provides little help in elucidating the mechanisms involved in the acidification defect.[207] A stimulation of proton secretion in response to Na_2SO_4 would be expected in (1) the gradient defect (e.g., amphotericin B lesion), (2) a sodium-responsive voltage lesion (e.g., lithium-induced RTA), or (3) a rate lesion with decreased pump activity in which the remaining activity is voltage sensitive (e.g., hypoaldosteronism). In addition, if the defect does not involve the CCT at all (i.e., confined to deeper medullary structures), the normal transport mechanisms in the CCT could still respond to the associated increase in sodium delivery. The only conditions in which one would not anticipate a response to Na_2SO_4 are those in which either Na_2SO_4 cannot alter voltage (e.g., amiloride defect, medullary collecting duct lesion) or those in which acidification mechanisms in the CCT have been totally eliminated.

Furosemide Administration. Since administration of sodium sulfate is cumbersome in the clinical setting and rarely applied except in clinical research centers, Batlle has suggested that the response of urine pH and potassium excretion to a single oral dose of 80 mg of furosemide can be employed to characterize the defect in collecting tubule acidification in distal RTA.[207] Furosemide is administered orally after completing baseline urine collections. Urine is then collected at hourly intervals (or when convenient for the subject) and pH and potassium concentration are determined. In all instances in which the response to furosemide has been evaluated concomitant with administration of sodium sulfate, the two tests have been shown to give the same result.[207] Batlle has reported that furosemide, when administered to normal subjects, stimulates voltage-dependent hydrogen and potassium secretion in the collecting tubule.[207] Based on such findings, he has suggested that furosemide can be used to disclose the segmental localization of the defect underlying distal RTA. Support for this hypothesis was obtained by observing that the fall in urine pH induced by furosemide was blocked by simultaneous administration of amiloride. In patients with classical hypokalemic distal RTA, furosemide did not produce a decrease in urine pH, but potassium excretion increased normally. In hyperkalemic distal RTA, furosemide failed to lower pH below 5.5 and was associated with a blunted increase in potassium excretion.[207] However, the same reservations about interpreting such data as outlined above for Na_2SO_4 infusion pertain to the furosemide effect on acidification.

Integrated Approach to the Diagnosis of RTA. Whether precise localization of the defect in distal RTA can be discerned by using such provocative tests of urinary acidification in any given patient, especially those with distal RTA, has not yet been tested rigorously. Additional evaluation of these maneuvers in experimental models of distal RTA is necessary before wide application can be extended to the clinical setting. As a result of the inherent limitations of these tests and the difficulties encountered when employing them clinically, some investigators have suggested simplified approaches to the evaluation of patients with a suspected defect in acidification.[2,3,273,275] Such an approach is outlined in Table 121-6. Patients with a hyperchloremic metabolic acidosis which cannot be ascribed to bicarbonate loss from the gastrointestinal tract should be suspected of having a defect in urinary acidification, especially when the urine net charge is positive, suggesting RTA. Patients with either classical distal RTA or proximal RTA usually have hypokalemia, while patients with generalized dysfunction of the distal nephron due to aldosterone deficiency or resistance usually have hyperkalemia. Therefore, the serum potassium may provide a clue to the type of defect. If the urine pH with either spontaneous metabolic acidosis or after an ammonium chloride challenge is less than 5.0, the defect may be in the proximal tubule or may be a result of a generalized defect in distal nephron function with hyperkalemia associated with reduced ammoniagenesis, as occurs in hypoaldosteronism.

A urine pH above 5.5 usually denotes a defect in distal nephron hydrogen ion secretion which can be further exam-

Table 121-6 Disorders Associated with Classical Hypokalemic Distal RTA

Primary
Familial
Sporadic
Acquired (secondary)
Autoimmune disorders
Hyperglobulinemic purpura
Cryoglobulinemia
Sjögren syndrome
Thyroiditis
Fibrosing alveolitis
Chronic active hepatitis
Primary biliary cirrhosis
Polyarthritis nodosa
Hypercalciuria and nephrocalcinosis
Primary hyperparathyroidism
Hyperthyroidism
Medullary sponge kidney
Fabry disease
Vitamin D intoxication
Idiopathic hypercalciuria
Wilson disease
Hereditary fructose intolerance
Drug- and toxin-induced disease
Amphotericin B
Cyclamate
Vanadate
Hepatic cirrhosis
Toluene
Mercury
Lithium
Classical analgesic nephropathy
Tubulointerstitial diseases
Balkan nephropathy
Chronic pyelonephritis
Obstructive uropathy
Renal transplantation
Leprosy
Jejunoileal bypass with hyperoxaluria
Associated with genetically transmitted diseases
Ehlers-Danlos syndrome
Sickle cell anemia
Medullary cystic disease
Hereditary nerve deafness
Hereditary elliptocytosis
Marfan syndrome
Jejunal bypass with hyperoxaluria
Osteopetrosis with carbonic anhydrase II deficiency

ined by evaluating the U − B P_{CO_2} following bicarbonate loading. The U − B P_{CO_2} following bicarbonate loading is typically low in hypokalemic distal RTA of the secretory or rate type, but not of the gradient type. Generalized distal nephron dysfunction is associated with a low U − B P_{CO_2}, while in proximal RTA the U − B P_{CO_2} is normal. Hyperkalemia in association with a low U − B P_{CO_2} suggests simultaneous defects in hydrogen ion secretion and potassium secretion. This combination may be due to a failure to generate a normal transepithelial potential gradient in the collecting tubule due to a voltage defect, a generalized defect in CCT function, a defect in permeability to chloride, or low mineralocorticoid levels.

Observing the difficulty with which systemic metabolic acidosis is corrected may also provide more information about the diagnosis of the type of RTA. Proximal RTA is particularly difficult to correct because bicarbonate administration aggravates bicarbonate wasting and also increases urinary potassium excretion. Classical hypokalemic distal RTA typically responds readily to bicarbonate administration. Selective aldosterone deficiency generally responds more readily than proximal RTA but less readily than classical distal RTA. Finally, the accompanying features of the disorder will often allow the clinician to categorize the general type of lesion. For example, the Fanconi syndrome is seen in association with proximal RTA; nephrocalcinosis and nephrolithiasis with classical hypokalemic distal RTA; and diabetic nephropathy, obstructive uropathy, or tubulointerstitial disease with a generalized dysfunction of the distal nephron associated with hyperkalemia.

Clinical Disorders of Impaired Net Acid Excretion with Hypokalemia: Classical Distal Renal Tubular Acidosis

Historically, the hallmark of classical hypokalemic distal RTA has been an inability to acidify the urine appropriately during spontaneous or chemically induced metabolic acidosis.[276] The defect in acidification by the collecting duct impairs ammonium and titratable acid excretion and results in positive acid balance, hyperchloremic metabolic acidosis, and volume depletion.[269,276] Moreover, medullary interstitial disease, which commonly occurs in conjunction with distal RTA, may impair ammonium excretion by interrupting the medullary countercurrent system for ammonium.[134,168] Hypokalemia and hypercalciuria[277] often accompany this disorder but proximal tubule reabsorptive function is preserved as evidenced by the conspicuous absence of findings compatible with the Fanconi syndrome.[14,278] The dissolution of bone, which may on occasion accompany distal RTA, appears to be the result of chronic positive acid balance, which causes calcium, magnesium, and phosphate wasting.[2,14] Hypercalciuria is, therefore, typical of distal RTA. Since chronic metabolic acidosis also decreases renal production of citrate,[277,279] the resulting hypocitraturia in combination with hypercalciuria creates an environment favorable for urinary stone formation and nephrocalcinosis.[277,280] Nephrocalcinosis appears to be a reliable marker of classical distal RTA since this disorder does not occur in proximal RTA or the generalized dysfunction of the nephron associated with hyperkalemia.[281] Nephrocalcinosis probably aggravates further the reduction in net acid excretion by impairing the transfer of ammonia from the loop of Henle to the collecting duct.[134] Pyelonephritis is one of the most common complications of distal RTA, especially in the presence of nephrocalcinosis, and eradication of the causative organism may be difficult.[268]

The vast majority of patients with distal RTA have it in association with a systemic illness, which is referred to as "secondary" distal RTA. Conversely, distal RTA may occur as a part of an inherited defect in which there is no association with systemic disease. The clinical spectrum of classical distal RTA is outlined in Table 121-6.

Primary Complete or Incomplete Distal RTA: Genetics. Classical distal RTA may occur in the absence of other diseases as an inherited defect (primary distal RTA) which may be intrinsic to the kidney.[282] The majority of cases of isolated distal RTA occur with no prior family history of RTA, but approximately 30 families with classical hypokalemic distal RTA involving over 300 affected individuals have been reported.[268,278,280,283–292] Autosomal dominant and X-linked inheritance are reported, and the mode of inheritance is unclear in some families.[109,278,288,291–294] Among the genetic types of distal RTA, most are associated with hypercalciuria and hypocitraturia, which may give rise to nephrocalcinosis and nephrolithiasis. Other familial forms do not appear to be associated with abnormalities in calcium transport.[277,278,281,291–293] The proposed sequence of events through which genetic defects are expressed is summarized in Fig. 121-8 for four reported kindred studies.[278,283,286,289] The same genetic defect which apparently results in the acidification defect can give rise to nephrocalcinosis.[278,290] Patients with primary distal RTA and nephrocalcinosis most often have hypercalciuria and hypocitraturia.[283–286,290] In seven affected members of kindreds studied in San Francisco (see Fig. 121-8), nephrocalcinosis was present radiographically as early as age 5, even in patients receiving alkali therapy.[283] However, in a later generation of patients in whom high-dose alkali therapy had been initiated prior to 4 years of age, nephrocalcinosis or nephrolithiasis was not detectable for the period of follow-up, which ranged from 10 to 20 years.[290] Moreover, the GFR remained normal during follow-up in these patients.[268] In these children and in other children treated similarly for autosomal dominant classical distal RTA, the hypercalciuria, hypocitraturia, and stunting of growth are invariably corrected by high-dose alkali therapy.[268,290]

Wrong and Davies were the first to observe that patients with acidification defects evidenced by a failure to lower urine pH during an acid challenge did not always display frank metabolic acidosis (incomplete distal RTA). Nephrocalcinosis was already present in some of these patients.[276] Buckalew et al. observed that the genetically transmitted acidification defect of distal RTA can occur without metabolic acidosis in some affected members of certain large kindreds.[280] The studies of Wrong and Buckalew and their colleagues support the view that incomplete distal RTA is a milder form of the disease characterized by preservation of renal function which sustains renal ammonium excretion, thus preventing metabolic acidosis. That few patients with the incomplete form have progressed to the complete form with frank acidosis, supports the proposal of Wrong and Davies. The finding that older family members may exhibit complete distal RTA while younger members exhibit the incomplete form does not document progression unequivocally.[282]

Buckalew and coworkers have reported a 64-member kindred comprising four generations in which hypercalciuria was the primary manifestation of the autosomal dominant defect (Atlanta kindred) in Fig. 121-8.[278] It was proposed by

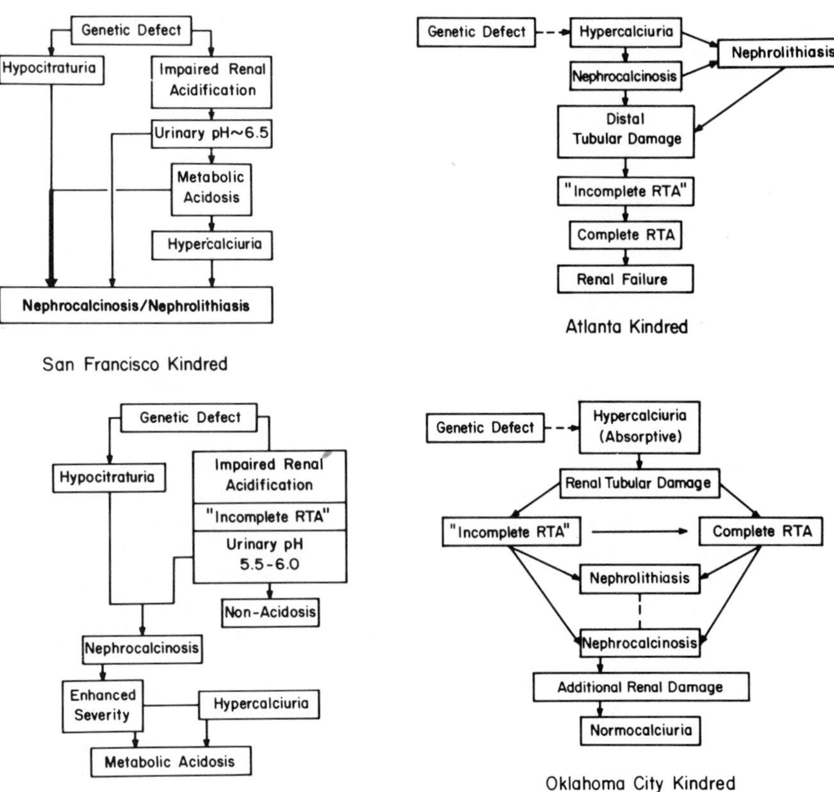

FIG. 121-8 **Pathophysiology of development of distal RTA in four family groups designated by the city in which the investigation was conducted. Pathways depicted by dotted lines are assumed. The major differences in these disorders reflect the relationships between metabolic acidosis and hypercalciuria and the sequence in which full expression of the defect occurs. See text for explanation.** ***(Adapted from Morris and Sebastian.[268] Used by permission.)***

Buckalew that the sequence of hypercalciuria, nephrocalcinosis, and renal damage was necessary for the development of the defect in renal acidification.[278,292] However, the existence of nephrocalcinosis in the complete absence of a demonstrable defect in renal acidification was not documented in other studies of families with an inability to acidify the urine after an acid challenge. In addition, in the patients in whom hypercalciuria was severe, aminoaciduria, lysozymuria, and other features were present, which suggested that the proximal tubule could also be involved. Therefore, the renal defect described in this kindred may be complex.

In a defect described by Norman and colleagues[295] in a kindred from Philadelphia (see Fig. 121-8), incomplete distal RTA was the defect expressed initially which apparently progressed to complete RTA only after the appearance of nephrocalcinosis. As occurs in other patients with hereditary distal RTA, severe hypocitraturia was observed in many affected individuals in the kindred. The extent to which the hypocitraturia was corrected by alkali therapy was variable, despite correction of the acidosis. Although the benefit of correction of hypocitraturia is not established, hypocitraturia in this genotype appears to be critical to the development of nephrocalcinosis.[282]

A similar sequence was reported by Coe and Parks, who found that alkali therapy in amounts adequate to elevate the plasma bicarbonate concentration to normal had little effect on the hypocitraturia, but was associated with correction of hypercalciuria and reduction in the frequency of nephrolithiasis.[277] Thus, the observations of Norman, Coe, and Buckalew and their colleagues suggest that hypocitraturia and hypercalciuria may be primary metabolic manifestations of the disorder, but that hypocitraturia in combination with hypercalciuria may be critical in the pathogenesis of nephrocalcinosis and nephrolithiasis with progression to complete distal RTA.

Finally, Hamed and associates have reported a large kindred from Oklahoma City in which hypercalciuria was the most frequent finding. The disorder was inherited as an autosomal dominant trait through four generations.[291] The hypercalciuria in this kindred was felt to be a result of augmented intestinal absorption, which appeared to precede both RTA and nephrocalcinosis. Thus, it was proposed that sustained hypercalciuria could damage the renal tubule and ultimately impair acidification, setting the stage for further damage and ultimately nephrocalcinosis.

Sly and associates have investigated 18 patients in 11 unrelated families with osteopetrosis, RTA, and cerebral calcification.[109,110] Carbonic anhydrase II has been shown to be virtually absent from red blood cells in all patients studied.[109] Moreover, reduced levels of carbonic anhydrase II were found in heterozygotes. These findings suggested that carbonic anhydrase II deficiency is the enzymatic basis for this autosomal recessive syndrome. The type of RTA present in this disorder has not been clearly delineated. While these patients generally exhibit frank bicarbonate wasting at normal plasma bicarbonate concentrations, suggesting a proximal defect, a number of patients have demonstrated an inability to acidify the urine during sustained systemic acidosis.[296] It is not clear if the bicarbonate wasting seen in such patients is a result of a distal defect alone, as is seen in prepubescent children with typical distal RTA, or if indeed a proximal defect is also present. A more detailed analysis of patients with this interesting syndrome can be found in Chap. 137.

Secondary Distal RTA. The disorders associated with acquired classical distal RTA are outlined in Table 121-6. The frequency with which hypokalemic distal RTA complicates the hyperglobulinemic states is especially striking. Failure to acidify the urine maximally can be demonstrated in up to

50 percent of patients with Sjögren syndrome and hyperglobulinemic purpura.[297–300] Round-cell infiltration of the renal interstitium is frequently found in such disorders and, although it is as yet unproven, the tubular dysfunction may have an immunologic basis (see Addendum). It is not known how dysglobulinemia results in distal RTA, but it is clear that there is no correlation between the class or quantity of the circulating globulin and the renal defect.[297] The autoimmune and hyperglobulinemic states reported to be associated with distal RTA include hyperglobulinemic purpura,[297] cryoglobulinemia,[301] fibrosing alveolitis,[302] Sjögren syndrome,[303–305] thyroiditis and Grave disease,[306] primary biliary cirrhosis,[307] chronic active hepatitis,[308–312] and systemic lupus erythematosus.[313,314]

The distal acidification defect that complicates the major disorders of calcium metabolism is usually, but not always, associated with nephrocalcinosis. Primary hyperparathyroidism, for example, appears to result in distal RTA only after the development of nephrocalcinosis.[315–317] Similarly, in the absence of nephrocalcinosis, distal RTA does not appear to be a characteristic complication of a number of other disorders, such as vitamin D intoxication,[317,318] hyperthyroidism,[319,320] idiopathic hypercalciuria,[321,322] medullary sponge kidney,[323,324] hereditary fructose intolerance,[325] Wilson disease, and Fabry disease.[326] The increased incidence of distal RTA with medullary sponge kidney suggests that cystic dilation of collecting ducts may disrupt acid secretion.[327] Medullary sponge kidney is usually benign, unless complicated by nephrocalcinosis, distal RTA, stones, or infection.[324]

Several drugs and toxins can result in a distal tubular acidification defect, including amphotericin B,[328–330] toluene,[212] lithium carbonate,[226] cyclamate,[331] analgesics,[332,333] and vanadate.[152,215] Amphotericin B, as outlined in the section on "Pathogenesis of Distal Renal Tubular Acidosis," above, alters the permeability of the distal nephron, allowing backleak of hydrogen ions from blood to lumen and a reduction in net hydrogen secretion ("gradient defect").[205] A concentrating defect due to a direct antagonism by lithium of the effect of antidiuretic hormone on the collecting tubule is commonly observed.[213] Lithium also impairs distal acidification in therapeutic doses and may cause structural tubulointerstitial disease with long-term administration.[226] Long-term vanadate administration to rats has been reported to induce a defect compatible with hypokalemic distal RTA.[152] This toxin was associated with a reduction in enzymatic activity of H^+/K^+-ATPase in the cortical and medullary collecting tubules. Interestingly, H^+-ATPase activity was unaffected by vanadate. By analogy with one documented outbreak of hypokalemic distal RTA in Thailand, which was ascribed to vanadate contamination of drinking water,[215] the authors inferred that classical hypokalemic distal RTA in humans might be a result of deranged function of the H^+/K^+-ATPase. Whether this intriguing association can be extended beyond the vanadate model requires additional study. The RTA associated with renal transplantation may be either proximal or distal. The distal variety is more common in association with chronic rejection.[334–336] Other tubulointerstitial diseases associated with distal RTA include leprosy,[337] hyperoxaluria,[338] obstructive uropathy,[339–341] and pyelonephritis secondary to urolithiasis.[342] Finally, distal RTA may occur in association with a variety of genetically transmitted disorders such as Ehlers-Danlos syndrome,[343] hereditary elliptocytosis,[344] hereditary sensorineural deafness,[345] sickle cell disease,[346] medullary cystic disease,[347] and carbonic anhydrase II deficiency.[109]

Bicarbonate Excretion in Adults and Children with Distal RTA. In adults with classical hypokalemic distal RTA, the fractional excretion of bicarbonate is elevated at both normal and reduced plasma bicarbonate concentrations, but is usually less than 5 percent.[268] This contrasts with the typical finding in proximal RTA of frank bicarbonate wasting at a normal plasma bicarbonate concentration (fractional excretion of 10 to 15 percent)[348] (Table 121-6). The finding of a lower fractional excretion in adults with distal RTA implies that reabsorption of bicarbonate in the proximal tubule is normal. Therefore, adult patients with distal RTA characteristically correct the metabolic acidosis if the amount of alkali needed to titrate the acid which enters the extracellular fluid from metabolism is replaced. The average alkali replacement requirement in adults usually amounts to 1 to 1.5 meq/kg.[268] This explains the relative ease with which correction of the acidosis is achieved in distal RTA as compared with proximal RTA (Table 121-6).[2,3,14,268]

In children, however, renal bicarbonate wasting accompanies the otherwise typical features of distal RTA. In infants with distal RTA, frank renal bicarbonate wasting is present initially, but may become apparent only after alkali therapy has been initiated.[283] Endogenous acid production in prepubertal children can be as high as 3 meq/kg/day.[348,349] In older children, renal bicarbonate wasting is often apparent during periods of accelerated growth.[349] McSherry and associates have shown that the fractional excretion of bicarbonate in children with classical distal RTA may range as high as 6 to 14 percent.[283,348] Such findings lead initially to the designation of this defect as type III RTA. It is now clear that children with hereditary distal RTA and bicarbonate wasting have affected parents who do not display renal bicarbonate wasting. Since renal bicarbonate wasting in these children usually subsides after puberty, the designation of type III RTA has been abandoned. Children with distal acidification defect and renal bicarbonate wasting are now felt to have classical distal RTA. The important practical point, however, is that renal bicarbonate wasting should be anticipated in children with distal RTA and that adequate alkali replacement must be provided in order to ensure normal growth and maturation.[283]

Associated Findings in Classical Distal RTA. The pathophysiological basis of the associated clinical features of classical distal RTA are outlined schematically in Fig. 121-9. Abnormal calcium metabolism, as manifested by hypercalciuria, nephrocalcinosis, and nephrolithiasis, is a prominent feature in many patients with classical distal RTA. Low urinary citrate levels are presumed to be the result of chronic metabolic acidosis and to facilitate development of nephrolithiasis and nephrocalcinosis.[350,351] Musculoskeletal complaints are frequent accompanying features of distal RTA, and hypocalcemic tetany may occur during alkali therapy.[352] Salt wasting also occurs in distal RTA and is seen more commonly in association with tubulointerstitial disease or advanced nephrocalcinosis.[353,354] Potassium wasting may be particularly severe during acidosis.[355] On occasion, hypokalemia is severe enough to cause paralysis and respiratory depression, and should always be corrected prior to alkali therapy. Long-term alkali therapy usually corrects the potassium wasting, the hypokalemia, and metabolic acidosis.[356]

Renal ammonium excretion in distal RTA is clearly subnormal for the degree of prevailing systemic acidosis and hypokalemia.[269,270] Aldosterone levels are often elevated because of volume contraction and are especially elevated considering the magnitude of hypokalemia.[268,355] In addition to hypercalciuria, the increased renal clearance of phosphate

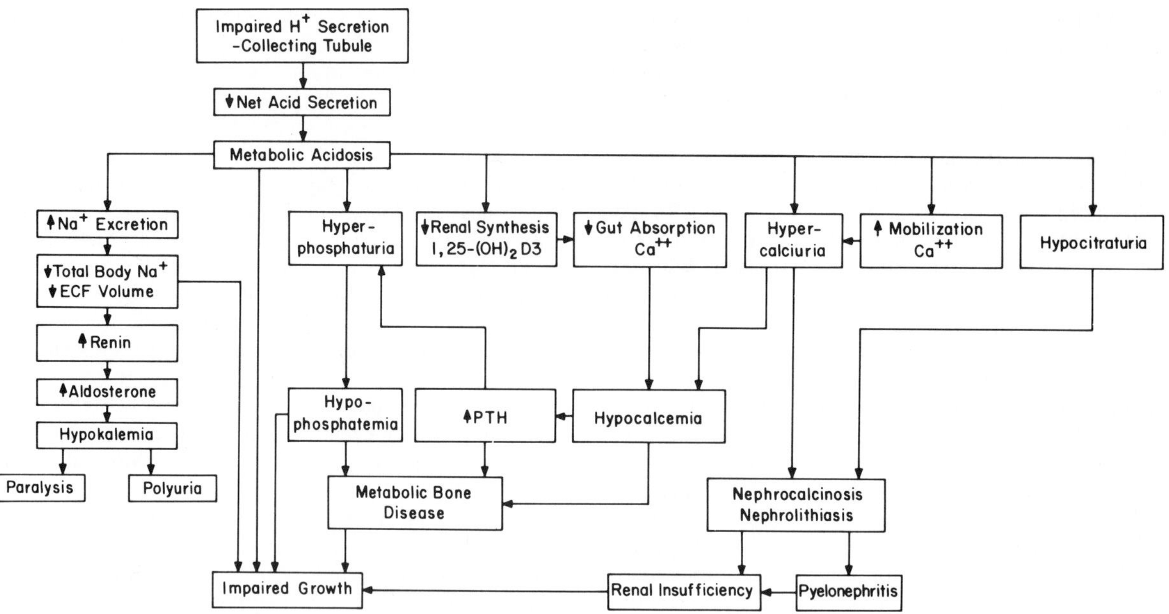

FIG. 121-9 **Pathophysiological basis of the numerous clinical features which may accompany classical hypokalemic distal RTA.** *(Modified and adapted from Morris and Sebastian.[268] Used by permission.)*

occurs predictably during metabolic acidosis.[357] Calcium phosphate might be expected to be the major constituent of urinary stones in patients with classical distal RTA,[277] but calcium oxalate stones were reported with equal frequency in one study.[358] Hypocalcemia and hypophosphatemia, when occurring concomitantly, are usually related to the osteomalacia that may occur with chronic metabolic acidosis.[356,359] Chronic metabolic acidosis results in mobilization of skeletal calcium and inhibition of renal conversion of 25-hydroxyvitamin D_3 to 1,25-dihydroxyvitamin D_3.[360] In one series, radiographic evidence of bone disease was observed in only one of 44 patients with carefully documented classical distal RTA,[281] suggesting that overt bone disease, initially observed commonly in distal RTA, is now less common in this disorder. It has also been emphasized that patients with distal RTA commonly have a urinary concentrating defect, perhaps as a result of tubulointerstitial disease.[361–363] When a significant concentrating defect accompanies classical distal RTA, it appears to result from the underlying defect, such as tubulointerstitial disease or nephrocalcinosis. Thus, both the concentrating defect and impaired ammonium excretion appear to be the result of interruption of the countercurrent system in the inner medulla.

In infants and young children with untreated distal RTA, abnormal growth is often seen.[283] The velocity of growth increases within several weeks after initiating alkali therapy. Within 3 to 6 months normal stature may be attained.[283] Older children may require several years to achieve normal height.[268,290] Renal HCO_3^- wasting tends to occur and increases during periods of increased growth velocity.[283] As a result, in children with hypokalemic distal RTA, alkali therapy should be provided in an amount which allows sustained correction of the underlying metabolic acidosis. When initiated before age 3, it appears that alkali therapy sufficient to sustain correction of acidosis can prevent nephrocalcinosis.[283]

Treatment of Classical Hypokalemic Distal RTA. Correction of chronic metabolic acidosis can usually be achieved in patients with classical distal RTA by administering enough alkali to neutralize the production of metabolic acids derived from the diet. In adult patients with distal RTA, this is usually equal to no more than 1 to 3 meq/kg/day.[14] In growing children, endogenous acid production is often 2 to 3 meq/kg/day. However, in children renal HCO_3^- wasting may even exceed 5 meq/kg/day. Therefore, larger amounts of bicarbonate must be administered to correct the acidosis and maintain normal growth.[283] Most children with distal RTA are able to take $NaHCO_3$ or bicarbonate precursors orally in amounts needed to sustain correction of acidosis.[283,290] The various forms of alkali replacement are outlined in Table 121-4. Most patients, especially children, tolerate Shohl's solution better than $NaHCO_3$ tablets. Compliance in adults is often limited by taste fatigue with Shohl's solution and by gastrointestinal discomfort with $NaHCO_3$ tablets. Alternating therapy among the numerous forms of alkali may be helpful. In patients with distal RTA, correction of acidosis with alkali therapy reduces urinary potassium excretion, and hypokalemia and sodium depletion may resolve with sustained correction of metabolic acidosis.[267,355,362] Therefore, in most patients with distal RTA, potassium supplements are not necessary. Frank wasting of potassium may occur in association with secondary hyperaldosteronism in a minority of patients despite correction of the acidosis by the alkali therapy.[355] In some children, but not most adults, potassium supplementation may be required even after the acidosis is corrected. It may be given as potassium bicarbonate (K-Lyte).

On occasion, strikingly severe hypokalemia, metabolic acidosis, and hypocalcemia may require immediate therapy. This constellation of findings in an emergency setting has occurred often enough to warrant the designation "crisis of distal RTA." Since hypokalemia may be severe enough to result in paralysis and respiratory depression, immediate therapy with potassium replacement is necessary and should always be carried out before administering alkali.

Prognosis. The goal of therapy in distal RTA is to prevent the relentless progression of renal disease. The prognosis of well-treated patients appears to be excellent, but is determined primarily by the severity of the underlying disease.

The GFR should stabilize and remain constant during replacement with alkali therapy, even if it is initially reduced.[364]

Hypercalciuria usually disappears on sustained correction of metabolic acidosis. Citrate excretion may increase, and intestinal reabsorption of calcium increases.[14,351,359,365,366] Moreover, the renal clearance of phosphate decreases and the serum concentration of both phosphate and calcium may reach normal levels.[359] While nephrocalcinosis may persist, nephrolithiasis occurs much less frequently with adequate alkali therapy, which may correlate with correction of the hypocitraturia.[277]

Disorders of Impaired Net Acid Excretion with Hyperkalemia: Generalized Distal Nephron Dysfunction

Generalized distal nephron dysfunction is manifest as a hyperchloremic, hyperkalemic metabolic acidosis in which urinary ammonium excretion is invariably depressed and renal function is often compromised at the time of diagnosis. Although hyperchloremic metabolic acidosis and hyperkalemia occur with regularity in advanced renal insufficiency, patients selected because of severe hyperkalemia (>5.5 meq/liter) with diabetic nephropathy and tubulointerstitial disease have hyperkalemia that is disproportionate to the reduction in GFR. The transtubular potassium gradient (TTKG)[367] is usually low in patients with this disorder, indicating that the collecting tubule is not responding appropriately to the prevailing hyperkalemia. In such patients, a unique dysfunction affecting both potassium and acid secretion by the collecting tubule occurs, which can be attributed in many cases to hypoaldosteronism[254,256] and in others to a decrease in effectiveness of aldosterone.[256] In patients presenting with this constellation of findings, an evaluation of renin-aldosterone elaboration is indicated. A classification of the underlying disorders resulting in a generalized distal tubule dysfunction according to the production of and responsiveness to aldosterone is outlined in Table 121-7. Three general categories of lesions are noted: (1) a primary defect in the adrenal gland as a result of generalized dysfunction of the gland or abnormalities in mineralocorticoid synthesis: (2) defective stimulation of aldosterone elaboration because of suppressed or inadequate renin-angiotensin elaboration; and (3) resistance of the collecting tubule to mineralocorticoid action.

Primary Mineralocorticoid Deficiency. Destruction of the adrenal cortex by hemorrhage, infection, invasion by tumors, or autoimmune processes results in Addison disease. This causes combined glucocorticoid and mineralocorticoid deficiency and is recognized clinically by hypoglycemia, anorexia, weakness, and a failure to respond to stress. These defects can occur in association with renal salt wasting, hyperkalemia, and metabolic acidosis.[234,254–256] The most common congenital adrenal defect in steroid biosynthesis is 21β-hydroxylase deficiency, which is associated with salt wasting, hyperkalemia, and metabolic acidosis in a fraction of the patients.[368] Complete deficiency can be fatal unless diagnosed promptly, while less severe deficiency is compatible with survival without specific therapy. The adrenogenital syndrome occurs as a result of a shift of glucocorticoid precursors to androgen synthesis. 21β-Hydroxylase deficiency accounts for 90 percent of all cases of adrenogenital syndrome. The defect may be isolated to the glucocorticoid pathway, sparing mineralocorticoid synthesis.[368] With the

Table 121-7 Disorders Associated with Aldosterone Deficiency or Resistance

- Primary mineralocorticoid deficiency
  - Combined glucocorticoid and mineralocorticoid deficiency
    - Addison disease
    - Bilateral adrenalectomy
    - Congenital adrenal enzyme defects
      - 21-Hydroxylase deficiency
      - 3-β-Hydroxydehydrogenase deficiency
      - Desmolase deficiency
  - Isolated mineralocorticoid deficiency
    - Familial methyl oxidase deficiency
    - Transient mineralocorticoid deficiency of infancy
    - Chronic idiopathic hypoaldosteronism
    - Chronic heparin administration
- Hyporeninemic hypoaldosteronism
  - Diabetic nephropathy
  - Tubulointerstitial disease
  - Obstructive nephropathy
  - Renal transplantation
  - Systemic lupus nephritis
  - Volume expansion with renal functional impairment
- Angiotensin II—impaired production or reduced sensitivity
  - Converting enzyme inhibitors
  - Impaired angiotensin II production
  - Adrenal insensitivity to angiotensin II (acquired)
  - Impaired production of angiotensinogen
- Aldosterone resistance
  - Type I pseudohypoaldosteronism (infancy)
  - Adult form with renal insufficiency (type II pseudohypoaldosteronism)
  - Salt-wasting nephritis
  - Drugs
    - Spironolactone
    - Amiloride
    - Triamterene
  - 21β-Hydroxylase deficiency secondary to progesterone excess

combined defect, mineralocorticoid deficiency typically results in salt wasting, hyperkalemia, and metabolic acidosis.[369,370]

Hyporeninemic Hypoaldosteronism. In contrast to patients with the primary adrenal disorder, which occurs far less frequently, patients in the hyporeninemic hypoaldosteronism group exhibit low plasma renin activity. Hyperchloremic metabolic acidosis occurs in approximately 50 percent of patients with hyporeninemic hypoaldosteronism. This disorder has been recognized with increasing frequency in adults as a cause of hyperkalemic hyperchloremic metabolic acidosis and is most typically seen in older adults with diabetes mellitus or tubulointerstitial disease and renal insufficiency.[256,266] Patients usually have mild to moderate renal insufficiency and acidosis with a modest elevation in plasma potassium (5.5 to 6.0 meq/liter) and concurrent hypertension and congestive heart failure. Both the metabolic acidosis and the hyperkalemia are out of proportion to the degree of impairment in GFR.[254,256] Drugs may cause a similar syndrome. The nonsteroidal antiinflammatory drugs, in particular, have the ability to produce hyperkalemia with hyperchloremic metabolic acidosis in patients with renal insufficiency.[263,371,372] The principal defect in hyporeninemic hypoaldosteronism is a reduced level of plasma renin activity which appears to be unresponsive to the usual physiological stimuli.[254,258] Aldosterone secretion is low as a result, especially in view of the degree of hyperkalemia.[258] While reduction in plasma potassium by administration of cation exchange resins may reduce aldosterone levels, the beneficial effect of enhanced renal ammoniagenesis improves or corrects the metabolic acidosis and hyperkalemia.[234] The magnitude of salt wasting in hyporeninemic hypoaldosteronism is variable. While the capacity to conserve salt is diminished during salt restriction in patients with hyporeninemic hypoaldosteronism, the degree of salt wasting is no more severe than in patients with chronic renal insufficiency of a comparable magnitude without hyporeninemic hypoaldosteronism.[140,260] Hyponatremia does not usually occur in this setting. Mineralocorticoid replacement with 9α-fludrocortisone improves net acid excretion, but high doses may be required, particularly when some degree of renal tubular unresponsiveness is present, as is often the case.[236]

The means by which renin secretion is reduced has been discussed in the section on "Pathogenesis of Distal Renal Tubular Acidosis" above. The importance of volume expansion in this regard has not yet been established, but hypertensive patients with this disorder are often volume overexpanded, suggesting physiological suppression of renin elaboration.[255] Orthostatic hypotension may accompany autonomic insufficiency in diabetic nephropathy and is not a reliable index of volume contraction. When volume overexpansion is present, diuresis would be expected to reverse the disorder.[260,373] Diuretics alone are frequently not sufficient to correct the abnormalities in acid–base and electrolyte balances.

Resistance to Mineralocorticoid. Mineralocorticoid resistance with hyperkalemia may occur with salt retention or with salt wasting. A number of patients have been reported with hyperkalemia, hyperchloremic metabolic acidosis, hypertension, undetectable plasma renin activity, and low aldosterone levels (type II pseudohypoaldosteronism).[245–249,251,336] These patients generally have not exhibited glomerular or tubulointerstitial disease.[374,375] The acidosis in such patients is mild and can be accounted for by the magnitude of hyperkalemia. Furthermore, renal potassium secretion is resistant to mineralocorticoid administration. Renin and aldosterone levels both increase if volume expansion is corrected by diuretics or salt restriction.[246,249,350] The original patients were described by Paver and Pauline,[375] Arnold and Healy,[245] and Gordon et al.[246] Schambelan et al. have investigated this disorder in detail and have demonstrated that potassium excretion responds to sodium sulfate infusion but not sodium chloride infusion.[249] It has been suggested that a distal tubule "chloride shunt" which was reversed by administration of thiazide diuretics can explain this disorder. Presumably, if chloride shunting is responsible, a distal tubule diuretic such as a thiazide would serve to prevent distal tubule chloride reabsorption. However, based on the response to thiazide diuretics, it is more likely that this disorder is the result of increased activity of the Na^+–Cl^- cotransporter in the connecting tubule which results in an increase in salt absorption and volume expansion. A familial form of this disorder has also been described in children with short stature.[247] Three patients from one family were reported in which type II pseudohypoaldosteronism appeared to be inherited as an autosomal dominant trait.[250]

Mineralocorticoid resistance with salt wasting also results in hyperkalemic-hyperchloremic acidosis because of a decrease in effectiveness of mineralocorticoid at the level of the CCT. Several distinct syndromes have been described and may be due to a primary genetic defect of the aldosterone receptor or a more generalized defect involving CCT function. Idiopathic pseudohypoaldosteronism occurs in young children, usually boys, without accompanying renal pathology.[239–242] While the defect improves as the child matures, high aldosterone levels are required to maintain acid and potassium balance. Patients with type I pseudohypoaldosteronism will require supplemental sodium chloride which can reverse the hyponatremia and hyperkalemia, improve the symptoms, and enhance growth.[255] After infancy, the disorder typically abates enough to permit reduction or discontinuation of sodium chloride supplements, but the findings can recur during periods of dietary salt restriction. Pseudohypoaldosteronism may be acquired in systemic lupus erythematosus,[376] obstructive uropathy,[377] sickle cell disease,[378] drug-induced interstitial nephritis,[379] and in the rejection of a renal transplant.[380]

Finally, Batlle and associates have emphasized that hypoaldosteronism and classical distal RTA may coexist in patients with decreased responsiveness to mineralocorticoid,[202,207] and have designated this disorder "hyperkalemic distal RTA." We prefer to consider the hyperkalemic disorders as a part of a generalized defect in the distal nephron in which the severity of abnormalities in H^+ and K^+ secretion may vary and may progress over time. Therefore, hyperkalemia with an alkaline urine pH may occur as a result of involvement of both the cortical and medullary collecting tubules. Conversely, hyperkalemia, with an appropriately acid urine pH, may be a result of less extensive collecting tubule disease, confined to the cortical and perhaps the outer medullary segments only.

Drugs may also produce mineralocorticoid resistance and result in a clinical constellation which mimics the acidification defect seen in hyperkalemic distal RTA. These drugs and toxins are summarized in Table 121-8. The spironolactones act as competitive inhibitors of aldosterone, and they may cause hyperkalemia and metabolic acidosis when administered to patients with significant renal insufficiency.[233,381] Similarly, amiloride and triamterine may be associated with this disorder.[203,220] Finally, the inhibitors of cyclooxygenase, the pivotal enzyme in the production of prostaglandins from arachidonic acid precursors, can produce hyperkalemia and metabolic acidosis.[371,372] Other drugs, including converting enzyme inhibitors, have been observed by us to be associated with this disorder. Drugs should be ruled out as a cause of hyperkalemia in metabolic acidosis in such patients.

Treatment (Table 121-9). In hyperkalemic-hyperchloremic metabolic acidosis, documentation of the underlying disorder is necessary. Treatment of patients with hyperkalemia and

Table 121-8 Drug-Induced Hyperchloremic Metabolic Acidosis

Hyperkalemia
- Potassium-sparing diuretics (spironolactone, triamterene, amiloride)
- Potassium supplement (KCl, salt substitutes, dietary)
- Nonsteroidal antiinflammatory drugs
- Beta blockers
- Converting enzyme inhibitors
- Heparin in acutely ill patients

Hypokalemia
- Acetazolamide
- Amphotericin B
- Lithium carbonate

Table 121-9 Treatment of Generalized Dysfunction of the Nephron with Hyperkalemia

Alkali therapy
Loop diuretic (furosemide, bumetanide)
Sodium polysterene sulfonate (Kayexalate)
Fludrocortisone (0.1–0.3 mg/day)
Avoid in hypertension, volume expansion, heart failure
Combine with loop diuretic
Avoid drugs associated with hyperkalemia

metabolic acidosis with chronic renal insufficiency is not always necessary, and the decision to treat is often based on the severity of the hyperkalemia. Reduction in serum potassium often improves the metabolic acidosis. Patients with combined glucocorticoid and mineralocorticoid deficiency should receive both adrenal steroids in replacement dosages. Patients with hyporeninemic hypoaldosteronism may respond to a cation exchange resin (sodium polystyrene sulfonate), alkali therapy, or treatment with a loop diuretic to induce renal potassium and salt excretion (Table 121-9). Volume depletion should be avoided unless the patient is volume overexpanded or hypertensive. Supraphysiological doses of mineralocorticoids may be necessary but should be administered cautiously, in combination with a loop diuretic to avoid volume overexpansion and aggravation of hypertension, and to increase potassium excretion.[373] Infants with type I pseudohypoaldosteronism should receive salt supplement in amounts sufficient to correct the syndrome and allow normal growth,[370] while patients with type II pseudohypoaldosteronism should receive thiazide diuretics coupled with dietary salt restriction.[249,250]

ADDENDUM

Recently evidence has shown that in a patient with Sjögren syndrome and distal RTA, the proton secretory defect could be attributed to absence of the H^+-ATPase in intercalated cells. The renal biopsy specimen in this patient was examined by immunocytochemical study with an antibody to the M(r) 31 K subunit of the mammalian kidney vacuolar H^+-ATPase and was compared to normal human kidney. The biopsy sample from the patient was devoid of anti-H^+-ATPase, whereas the control material revealed localization to subvillar invaginations of intercalated cells of the collecting duct.[382]

REFERENCES

1. Teree TM, Mirabal-Font E, Ortiz A, Wallace WM: Stool losses and acidosis in diarrheal disease of infancy. *Pediatrics* **36:**704, 1965.
2. Emmett M, Seldin DW: Clinical syndromes of metabolic acidosis and metabolic alkalosis, in Seldin DW, Giebisch G (eds): *The Kidney: Physiology and Pathophysiology,* 2d ed. New York, Raven, 1992, p 2759.
3. Halperin ML, Goldstein MB, Richardson RMA, Stinebaugh BJ: Distal renal tubular acidosis syndromes: A pathophysiological approach. *Am J Nephrol* **5:**1, 1985.
4. Halperin M, Goldstein MB, Jungas RL, Stinebaugh BJ: Biochemistry and physiology of ammonium excretion, in Seldin DW, Giebisch G (eds): *The Kidney: Physiology and Pathophysiology,* 2d ed. New York, Raven, 1992, p 2645.
5. Goldstein MB, Bear R, Richardson RMA, Marsden PA, Halperin ML: The urine anion gap: A clinically useful index of ammonium excretion. *Am J Med Sci* **292:**198, 1986.
6. Carlisle EJF, Donnelly SM, Halperin ML: Renal tubular acidosis (RTA): *R*ecognize *T*he *A*mmonium defect and pHorget the urine pH. *Pediatr Nephrol* **5:**242, 1991.
7. Kleinman PK: Cholestyramine and metabolic acidosis. *N Engl J Med* **290:**861, 1974.
8. D'Agostino A, Leadbetter WF, Schwartz WB: Alterations in the ionic composition of isotonic saline solution instilled into the colon. *J Clin Invest* **32:**444, 1953.
9. Stamey TA: The pathogenesis and implications of the electrolyte imbalance in ureterosigmoidostomy. *Surg Gynecol Obstet* **103:**736, 1956.
10. Heird WC, Dell RB, Driscoll JM, Grebin B, Winters RW: Metabolic acidosis resulting from intravenous alimentation mixtures containing synthetic amino acids. *N Engl J Med* **287:**943, 1972.
11. DuBose TD Jr: Acid-base balance, in Eknoyan G, Knochel JP (eds): *The Systemic Consequences of Renal Failure.* Orlando, FL, Grune & Stratton, 1984, pp 421–441.
12. Widmer B, Gerhardt RE, Harrington JT, Cohen JJ: The influence of graded degrees of chronic renal failure. *Arch Intern Med* **139:**1099, 1979.
13. Gonick HC, Kleeman CR, Rubini ME, Maxwell MH: Functional impairment in chronic renal failure. *Nephron* **6:**28, 1969.
14. Cogan MG, Rector FC Jr: Acid-base disorders, in Brenner BM, Rector FC Jr (eds): *The Kidney,* 4th ed. Philadelphia, Saunders, 1991, p 737.
15. Fine LG, Yanagaawa N, Schultz RG, Bricker N: Functional profile of the isolated uremic nephron. Potassium adaptation in the rabbit cortical collecting tubule. *J Clin Invest* **64:**1033, 1979.
16. Van Ypersele de Strihou C: Potassium homeostasis in renal failure. *Kidney Int* **11:**491, 1977.
17. Rector FC Jr, Carter NW, Seldin DW: The mechanism of bicarbonate reabsorption in the proximal and distal tubules of the kidney. *J Clin Invest* **44:**278, 1968.
18. Viera FL, Malnic G: Hydrogen ion secretion by rat renal cortical tubules as studied by an antimony microelectrode. *Am J Physiol* **214:**710, 1968.
19. DuBose TD Jr, Pucacco LR, Carter NW: Determination of disequilibrium pH in the rat kidney in vivo: Evidence for hydrogen secretion. *Am J Physiol* **240:**F138, 1981.
20. Alpern RH, Chambers M: Cell pH in the rat proximal convoluted tubule. Regulation by luminal and peritubular pH and sodium concentration. *J Clin Invest* **78:**502, 1986.
21. Murer H, Hopfer U, Kinne R: Sodium/proton antiport in brush-border membrane vesicles isolated from rat small intestine and kidney. *Biochem J* **154:**597, 1976.
22. Warnock DG, Reenstra WW, Yee VJ: Na^+/H^+ antiporter of brush border vesicles: Studies with acridine orange uptake. *Am J Physiol* 238:F733, 1982.
23. Kinsella JL, Aronson PS: Properties of the Na^+-H^+ exchanger in renal microvillus membrane vesicles. *Am J Physiol* **238:**F461, 1980.
24. Schwartz GJ: Na^+-dependent H^+ efflux from proximal tubule: Evidence for reversible Na^+-H^+ exchange. *Am J Physiol* **241:**F380, 1981.
25. Sasaki S, Shiigai T, Takeuchi J: Intracellular pH in the isolated perfused rabbit proximal straight tubule. *Am J Physiol* **249:**F417, 1985.
26. Preisig PA, Ives HE, Cragoe EJ Jr, Alpern RJ, Rector FC Jr: The role of the Na^+/H^+ antiporter in rat proximal tubule bicarbonate absorption. *J Clin Invest* **80:**970, 1987.
27. Sardet C, Franchi A, Poussegur J: Molecular cloning, primary structure, and expression of the human growth factor-activatable Na^+/H^+ antiporter. *Cell* **56:**271, 1989.
28. Haggerty JG, Agarwal N, Reilly RF, Adelberg EA, Slayman CW: Pharmacologically different Na/H antiporters on the apical and basolateral surfaces of cultured porcine kidney cells (LLC-PK_1). *Proc Natl Acad Sci USA* **85:**6797, 1988.
29. Sardet C, Wakayabashi S, Fafournoud P, Counillon L, Pages G, Pouyssegur J: Molecular properties of Na^+/H^+ exchangers, in De Santo NG, Capasso G (eds): *Acid-Base Balance.* Cosenza, Italy, Editoriale Bios, 1991, p 13.
30. Kinne-Saffran E, Beauwens R, Kinne R: An ATP-driven proton pump in brush-border membranes from rat renal cortex. *J Memb Biol* **64:**67, 1982.

31. Chan YL, Giebisch G: Relationship between sodium and bicarbonate transport in the rat proximal convoluted tubule. *Am J Physiol* **240:**F222, 1981.
32. Brown D, Hirsch S, Gluck S: Localization of a proton-pumping ATPase in rat kidney. *J Clin Invest* **82:**2114, 1988.
33. Alpern RJ: Mechanism of basolateral membrane $H^+/OH^-/HCO_3^-$ transport in the rat proximal convoluted tubule. A sodium-coupled electrogenic process. *J Gen Physiol* **86:**613, 1985.
34. Yoshitomi K, Burckhardt B-CH, Frömter E: Rheogenic sodium-bicarbonate cotransport in the peritubular cell membrane of rat renal proximal tubule. *Pflugers Arch* **405:**360, 1985.
35. Boron WF, Boulpaep EL: Intracellular pH regulation in the renal proximal tubule of the salamander: Basolateral HCO_3^- transport. *J Gen Physiol* **81:**53, 1983.
36. Akiba T, Alpern RJ, Eveloff J, Calamina J, Warnock DG: Electrogenic sodium/bicarbonate cotransport in rabbit renal cortical basolateral membrane vesicles. *J Clin Invest* **78:**1472, 1986.
37. Solemani M, Aronson PS: Ionic mechanism of $Na^+/H^+/CO_3^=$ cotransport in rabbit renal basolateral membranes. *J Biol Chem* **264:**18302, 1989.
38. Sasaki S, Shiigai T, Yoshiyama N, Takeuchi J: Mechanism of bicarbonate exit across basolateral membrane of rabbit proximal straight tubule. *Am J Physiol* **21:**F11, 1987.
39. Dobyan DC, Bulger RE: Renal carbonic anhydrase. *Am J Physiol* **243:**F311, 1982.
40. Alpern RJ, Stone DK, Rector FC Jr: Renal acidification mechanisms, in Brenner BM, Rector FC Jr (eds): *The Kidney*, 4th ed. Philadelphia, Saunders, 1991, p 318.
41. Lucci MS, Tinker J, Weiner I, DuBose TD: Function of proximal tubule carbonic anhydrase defined by selective inhibition. *Am J Physiol* **245:**F535, 1983.
42. Wahlstrand T, Wistrand PJ: Carbonic anhydrase C in the human renal medulla. *Ups J Med Sci* **85:**7, 1980.
43. Alpern RJ, Cogan MG, Rector FC Jr: Effect of luminal bicarbonate concentration on proximal acidification in the rat. *Am J Physiol* **243:**F53, 1982.
44. Chan YL, Malnic G, Giebisch G: Passive driving forces of proximal tubular fluid and bicarbonate transport: Gradient-dependence of H^+ section. *Am J Physiol* **245:**F622, 1983.
45. Holmberg C, Kokko JP, Jacobson HR: Determination of chloride and bicarbonate permeabilities in proximal convoluted tubules. *Am J Physiol* **241:**F386, 1981.
46. Sasaki S, Berry CA, Rector FC Jr: Effect of luminal and peritubular HCO_3^- concentrations and PCO_2 on HCO_3^- reabsorption in rabbit proximal convoluted tubules perfused in vitro. *J Clin Invest* **70:**639, 1982.
47. Warnock DG, Yee VJ: Anion permeabilities of the isolated perfused rabbit proximal tubule. *Am J Physiol* **242:**F395, 1982.
48. Hamm LL, Pucacco LR, Kokko JP, Jacobson HR: Hydrogen ion permeability of the rabbit proximal convoluted tubule. *Am J Physiol* **246:**F3, 1984.
49. Jenkins AD, Dousa TP, Smith LH: Transport of citrate across renal brush border membrane: Effects of dietary acid and alkali loading. *Am J Physiol* **249:**F590, 1985.
50. Green R, Bishop JHV, Giebisch G: Ionic requirements of proximal tubular sodium transport. III. Selective luminal anion substitution. *Am J Physiol* **236:**F268, 1979.
51. Jacobson HR: Characteristics of volume reabsorption in rabbit superficial and juxtamedullary proximal convoluted tubules. *J Clin Invest* **63:**410, 1979.
52. Baum M, Berry CA: Evidence for neutral transcellular NaCl transport and neutral basolateral chloride exit in the rabbit proximal convoluted tubule. *J Clin Invest* **74:**205, 1984.
53. Alpern RJ, Howlin KJ, Preisig PA: Active and passive components of chloride transport in the rat proximal convoluted tubule. *J Clin Invest* **76:**1360, 1985.
54. Lucci MS, Warnock DG: Effects of anion-transport inhibitors on NaCl reabsorption in the rat superficial proximal convoluted tubule. *J Clin Invest* **64:**570, 1979.
55. Baum M: Evidence that parallel Na^+-H^+ and Cl^--$HCO_3^-(OH^-)$ antiporters transport NaCl in the proximal tubule. *Am J Physiol* **252:**F338, 1987.
56. Karniski LP, Aronson PS: Chloride/formate exchange with formic acid recycling: A mechanism of active chloride transport across epithelial membranes. *Proc Natl Acad Sci USA* **82:**6362, 1985.
57. Alpern RJ: Apical membrane chloride/base exchange in the rat proximal convoluted tubule. *J Clin Invest* **79:**1026, 1987.
58. Pitts RF, Lotspeich WD: Bicarbonate and the renal regulation of acid-base balance. *Am J Physiol* **147:**138, 1946.
59. Alpern RJ, Cogan MG, Rector FC Jr: Effects of extracellular fluid volume and plasma bicarbonate concentration on proximal acidification in the rat. *J Clin Invest* **71:**736, 1983.
60. Berliner RW, Kennedy TJ, Hilton JG: Effect of maleic acid on renal function. *Proc Soc Exp Biol Med* **75:**791, 1951.
61. Al-Bander HA, Weiss RA, Humphreys MH, Morris RC Jr: Dysfunction of the proximal tubule underlies maleic acid-induced type II renal tubular acidosis. *Am J Physiol* **243:**F604, 1982.
62. Bergeron M, DuBord L, Hausser C: Membrane permeability as a cause of transport defects in experimental Fanconi syndrome. A new hypothesis. *J Clin Invest* **57:**1181, 1976.
63. Maesaka JK, McCaffery M: Evidence for renal tubular leakage in maleic acid-induced Fanconi syndrome. *Am J Physiol* **239:**F507, 1980.
64. Hoppe A, Gmaj P, Metler M, Angielski S: Additive inhibition of renal bicarbonate reabsorption by maleate plus acetazolamide. *Am J Physiol* **231:**1258, 1976.
65. Gougoux A, Lemieux G, Lavoie N: Maleate-induced bicarbonaturia in the dog: A carbonic anhydrase-independent effect. *Am J Physiol* **231:**1010, 1976.
66. Gmaj P, Hoppe A, Angielski S, Rogulski J: Acid-base behavior of the kidney in maleate-treated rats. *Am J Physiol* **222:**1182, 1972.
67. Bank N, Aynedjian HS, Mutz BF: Microperfusion study of proximal tubule bicarbonate transport in maleic acid-induced renal tubular acidosis. *Am J Physiol* **250:**F476, 1986.
68. Reboucas NA, Fernandes DT, Elias MM, De Mello-Aires M, Malnic G: Proximal tubular HCO_3^-, H^+ and fluid transport during maleate-induced acidification defect. *Pflugers Arch* **401:**266, 1984.
69. Günther R, Silbernagl S, Deetjen P: Maleic acid induced aminoaciduria, studied by free flow micropuncture and continuous microperfusion. *Pflugers Arch* **382:**109, 1979.
70. Salmon RF, Baum M: Intracellular cystine loading inhibits transport in the rabbit proximal convoluted tubule. *J Clin Invest* **85:**340, 1990.
71. Silverman M: The mechanism of maleic acid nephropathy: Investigations using brush border membrane vesicles. *Membr Biochem* **4:**63, 1981.
72. Reynolds R, McNamara PD, Segal S: On the maleic acid induced Fanconi syndrome: Effects on transport by isolated rat kidney brush border membrane vesicles. *Life Sci* **22:**39, 1978.
73. Silverman M, Huang L: Mechanism of maleic acid-induced glucosuria in dog kidney. *Am J Physiol* **231:**1024, 1976.
74. Le Grimellec C, Carriere S, Cardinal J, Giocondi MC: Effect of maleate on membrane physical state of brush border and basolateral membranes of the dog kidney. *Life Sci* **30:**1107, 1982.
75. Kramer HJ, Gonick HC: Experimental Fanconi syndrome. I. Effect of maleic acid on renal cortical Na^+-K^+-ATPase activity and ATP levels. *J Lab Clin Med* **76:**799, 1970.
76. Coor C, Salmon RF, Quigley R, Marver D, Baum M: Role of adenosine triphosphate (ATP) and Na^+-K^+ ATPase in inhibition of proximal tubule transport with intracellular cystine loading. *J Clin Invest* **87:**955, 1991.
77. Angielski S, Rogulski J: Effect of maleic acid on the kidney. I. Oxidation of Krebs cycle intermediates by various tissues of maleate intoxicated rats. *Acta Biochim Pol* **9:**357, 1962.
78. Al-Bander H, Etheredge SB, Paukert T, Humphreys MH, Morris RC Jr: Phosphate loading attenuates renal tubular dysfunction induced by maleic acid in the dog. *Am J Physiol* **248:**F513, 1985.
79. Al-Bander HA, Mock DM, Etheredge SB, Paukert TT, Humphreys MH, Morris RC Jr: Coordinately increased lysozymuria and lysosomal enzymuria induced by maleic acid. *Kidney Int* **30:**804, 1987.
80. Burch HB, Choi S, Dence CN, Alvey TR, Cole BR, Lowry OH: Metabolic effects of large fructose loads in different parts of the rat nephron. *J Biol Chem* **255:**8239, 1980.

81. Morris RC Jr, Nigon K, Reed EB: Evidence that the severity of depletion of inorganic phosphate determines the severity of the disturbance of adenine nucleotide metabolism in the liver and renal cortex of the fructose-loaded rat. *J Clin Invest* **61**:209, 1978.
82. Fraser D, Kooh SW, Scriver CR: Hyperparathyroidism as the cause of hyperaminoaciduria and phosphaturia in human vitamin deficiency. *Pediatr Res* **9**:593, 1975.
83. Guignard JP, Torrado A: Proximal renal tubular acidosis in vitamin D deficiency rickets. *Acta Paediatr Scand* **62**:543, 1973.
84. Vainsel M, Manderlier T, Vis HL: Proximal renal tubular acidosis in vitamin D deficiency rickets. *Biomedicine* **22**:35, 1974.
85. Reade TM, Scriver CR, Glorieux FH, Nogrady B, Delvin E, Poirier R, Holick MF, Deluca HF: Response to crystalline 1α-hydroxyvitamin D_3 in vitamin D dependency. *Pediatr Res* **9**:593, 1975.
86. Huguenin M, Schacht R, David R: Infantile rickets with severe proximal renal tubular acidosis, responsive to vitamin D. *Arch Dis Child* **49**:955, 1974.
87. Bank N, Aynedjian HS: A micropuncture study of the effect of parathyroid hormone on renal bicarbonate reabsorption. *J Clin Invest* **58**:336, 1976.
88. Iino Y, Burg MB: Effect of parathyroid hormone on bicarbonate absorption by proximal tubules in vitro. *Am J Physiol* **236**:F387, 1979.
89. McKinney TD, Myers P: PTH inhibition of bicarbonate transport by proximal convoluted tubules. *Am J Physiol* **239**:F127, 1980.
90. McKinney TD, Myers P: Bicarbonate transport by proximal tubules: Effect of parathyroid hormone and dibutyryl cyclic AMP. *Am J Physiol* **238**:F166, 1980.
91. Pollock AS, Warnock DG, Strewler GJ: Parathyroid hormone inhibition of Na^+-H^+ antiporter activity in a cultured renal cell line. *Am J Physiol* **250**:F217, 1986.
92. Weinman EJ, Shenolikar S, Kahn AM: cAMP-associated inhibition of Na^+-H^+ exchanger in rabbit kidney brush-border membranes. *Am J Physiol* **252**:F19, 1987.
93. Hulter HN, Toto RD, Ilnicki LP, Halloran B, Sebastian A: Metabolic alkalosis in models of primary and secondary hyperparathyroid states. *Am J Physiol* **245**:F450, 1983.
94. Mitnick P, Greenberg A, Coffman T, Kelepouris E, Wolf CJ, Goldfarb S: Effects of two models of hypercalcemia on renal acid metabolism. *Kidney Int* **21**:613, 1982.
95. Bichara M, Mercier O, Paillard M, Prigent A: Effects of parathyroid hormone on urinary acidification. *Am J Physiol* **251**:F444, 1986.
96. Mercier O, Bichara M, Paillard M, Prigent A: Effects of parathyroid hormone and urinary phosphate on collecting duct hydrogen section. *Am J Physiol* **251**:F802, 1986.
97. McKinney TD, Myers P: Effect of calcium and phosphate on bicarbonate and fluid transport by proximal tubules in vitro. *Kidney Int* **21**:433, 1982.
98. Peraino RA, Ghafary E, Rouse D, Stinebaugh BJ, Suki WN: Effect of 25-hydroxycholecalciferol on renal handling of sodium, calcium, and phosphate during bicarbonate infusion. *Miner Electrolyte Metab* **1**:321, 1978.
99. Puschett JB, Moranz J, Kurnick WS: Evidence for a direct action of cholecalciferol and 25-hydroxycholecalciferol on the renal transport of phosphate, sodium, and calcium. *J Clin Invest* **51**:373, 1972.
100. Gekle D, Ströder J, Rostock D: The effect of vitamin D on renal inorganic phosphate reabsorption of normal rats, parathyroidectomized rats, and rats with rickets. *Pediatr Res* **5**:40, 1971.
101. Grose JH, Scriver CR: Parathyroid-dependent phosphaturia and aminoaciduria in the vitamin D-deficient rat. *Am J Physiol* **214**:370, 1968.
102. Morris RC Jr, McSherry E, Sebastian A: Modulation of experimental renal dysfunction of hereditary fructose intolerance by circulating parathyroid hormone. *Proc Natl Acad Sci USA* **68**:132, 1971.
103. Brewer ED, Tsai HC, Szeto KS, Morris RC Jr: Maleic acid-induced impaired conversion of $25(OH)D_3$: Implications for Fanconi's syndrome. *Kidney Int* **12**:244, 1977.
104. Chesney RW, Kaplan BS, Phelps M, Deluca HF: Renal tubular acidosis does not alter circulating values of calcitriol. *J Pediatr* **104**:51, 1984.
105. Walker WG, Dickerman H, Jost LJ: Mechanism of lysine-induced kaliuresis. *Am J Physiol* **206**:409, 1964.
106. Chan YL, Kurtzman NA: Effects of lysine on bicarbonate and fluid absorption in the rat proximal tubule. *Am J Physiol* **242**:F604, 1982.
107. Frömter E: Solute transport across epithelia: What can we learn from micropuncture studies on kidney tubules? *J Physiol* **288**:1, 1979.
108. Hoshi T, Sudo K, Suzuki Y: Characteristics of changes in the intracellular potential associated with transport of neutral, dibasic and acidic amino acids in Trituris proximal tubule. *Biochim Biophys Acta* **44**:492, 1976.
109. Sly WS, Whyte MP, Sundaram V, Tashian RE, Hewett-Emmett D, Guibaud P, Vainsel M, Baluarte HJ, Gruskin A, Al-Mosawi M, Sakati N, Ohlsson A: Carbonic anhydrase II deficiency in 12 families with the autosomal recessive syndrome of osteopetrosis with renal tubular acidosis and cerebral calcification. *N Engl J Med* **313**:139, 1985.
110. Sly WS, Hewett-Emmett D, Whyte MP, Yu YSL, Tashian RE: Carbonic anhydrase II deficiency identified as the primary defect in the autosomal recessive syndrome of osteopetrosis with renal tubular acidosis and cerebral calcification. *Proc Natl Acad Sci USA* **80**:2752, 1983.
111. Bregman H, Brown J, Rogers A, Bourke E: Osteopetrosis with combined proximal and distal renal tubular acidosis. *Am J Kidney Dis* **2**:357, 1982.
112. Bourke E, Delaney VB, Mosawi M, Reavey P, Weston M: Renal tubular acidosis and osteropetrosis in siblings. *Nephron* **28**:268, 1981.
113. Kondo T, Taniguchi N, Taniguchi K, Matsuda I, Murao M: Inactive form of erythrocyte carbonic anhydrase B in patients with primary renal tubular acidosis. *J Clin Invest* **62**:610, 1978.
114. Shapira E, Ben-Yoseph Y, Eyal FG, Russell A: Enzymatically inactive red cell carbonic anhydrase B in a family with renal tubular acidosis. *J Clin Invest* **53**:59, 1974.
115. Kendall AG, Tashian RE: Erythrocyte carbonic anhydrase I: Inherited deficiency in humans. *Science* **197**:471, 1977.
116. Brenner RJ, Spring DB, Sebastian A, McSherry EM, Genant HK, Palubinskas AJ, Morris RC Jr: Incidence of radiographically evident bone disease, nephrocalcinosis, and nephrolithiasis in various types of renal tubular acidosis. *N Engl J Med* **307**:217, 1982.
117. Rodriquez-Soriano J, Vallo A, Castillo G, Oliveros R: Renal handling of water and sodium in children with proximal and distal renal tubular acidosis. *Nephron* **25**:193, 1980.
118. Brenes LG, Brenes JN, Hernandez MM: Familial proximal renal tubular acidosis. A distinct clinical entity. *Am J Med* **63**:244, 1977.
119. Nash MA, Torrado AD, Greifer I, Spitzer A, Edelmann CM Jr: Renal tubular acidosis in infants and children. *J Pediatr* **80**:738, 1972.
120. Sebastian A, McSherry E, Morris RC Jr: On the mechanism of renal potassium wasting in renal tubular acidosis associated with the Fanconi syndrome (Type 2 RTA). *J Clin Invest* **50**:231, 1971.
121. Peraino RA, Suki WN: Urine HCO_3^- augments renal Ca^{2+} absorption independent of systemic acid-base changes. *Am J Physiol* **238**:F394, 1980.
122. Callis L, Castello F, Fortuny G, Vallo A, Ballabriga A: Effect of hydrochlorothiazide on rickets and on renal tubular acidosis in two patients with cystinosis. *Helv Paediatr Acta* **6**:602, 1970.
123. Rampini S, Fanconi A, Illig R, Prader A: Effect of hydrochlorothiazide on proximal renal tubular acidosis in a patient with idiopathic "de Toni-Debre-Fanconi syndrome." *Helv Paediatr Acta* **1**:13, 1968.
124. McKinney TD, Burg MG: Bicarbonate transport by rabbit cortical collecting tubules; effect of acid and alkali loads in vivo on transport in vitro. *J Clin Invest* **60**:766, 1977.
125. Atkins JL, Burg MB: Bicarbonate transport by isolated perfused rat collecting ducts. *Am J Physiol* **249**:F485, 1985.
126. Schwartz GJ, Barasch J, Al-Awqati Q: Plasticity of functional epithelial polarity. *Nature* **318**:368, 1985.
127. Lucci MS, Pucacco LR, Carter NW, DuBose TD Jr:

Evaluation of bicarbonate transport in the rat distal tubule: Effects of acid-base status. *Am J Physiol* **243:**F335, 1982.
128. Levine DZ: An in vivo microperfusion study of distal tubule reabsorption in normal and ammonium chloride rats. *J Clin Invest* **75:**588, 1985.
129. Iacovitti M, Nash L, Peterson LN, Rochon J, Levine DZ: Distal tubule bicarbonate accumulation in vivo. Effect of flow and transtubule bicarbonate gradients. *J Clin Invest* **78:**1658, 1986.
130. Lombard WE, Kokko JP, Jacobson HR: Bicarbonate transport in cortical and outer medullary collecting tubules. *Am J Physiol* **244:**F289, 1983.
131. Stokes JB: Na and K transport across the cortical and outer medullary collecting tubule of the rabbit: Evidence for diffusion across the outer medullary portion. *Am J Physiol* **242:**F514, 1982.
132. Ullrich KJ, Papavassiliou F: Bicarbonate reabsorption in the papillary collecting duct of rats. *Pflugers Arch* **289:**271, 1981.
133. Graber ML, Bengele HH, Schwartz JH, Alexander EA: pH and PCO_2 profiles of the rat inner medullary collecting duct. *Am J Physiol* **241:**F659, 1981.
134. DuBose TD Jr, Good DW: Role of the thick ascending limb and inner medullary collecting duct in the regulation of urinary acidification. *Semin Nephrol* **11:**120, 1991.
135. Wall SM, Knepper MA: Acid-base transport in the inner medullary collecting duct. *Semin Nephrol* **10:**148, 1990.
136. Madsen KM, Clapp WL, Verlander JW: Structure and function of the inner medullary collecting duct. *Kidney Int* **34:**441, 1988.
137. DuBose TD Jr: Hydrogen ion secretion by the collecting duct as a determinant of the urine to blood PCO_2 gradient in alkaline urine. *J Clin Invest* **69:**145, 1982.
138. Koeppen BM, Helman SI: Acidification of luminal fluid by the rabbit cortical collecting tubule perfused in vitro. *Am J Physiol* **242:**F521, 1982.
139. McKinney TD, Burg MB: Bicarbonate absorption by rabbit cortical collecting tubules in vitro. *Am J Physiol* **234:**F141, 1978.
140. Stone DS, Seldin DW, Kokko JP, Jacobson HR: Mineralocorticoid modulation of rabbit medullary collecting duct acidification. A sodium-independent acidification. *J Clin Invest* **72:**77, 1983.
141. Gluck S, Al-Awqati Q: An electrogenic proton-translocating adenosine triphosphatase from bovine kidney medulla. *J Clin Invest* **73:**1704, 1984.
142. Stone DK, Xie XS, Racker E: Comparison of the proton ATPase and chloride transporter from bovine clathrin-coated vesicles and renal medullary vesicles. *Kidney Int* **25:**283, 1984. (abstr.)
143. Diaz-Diaz FD, LaBelle EF, Eaton DC, DuBose TD Jr: ATP-dependent proton transport in human renal medulla. *Am J Physiol* **20:**F297, 1986.
144. Kaunitz JD, Gunther RD, Sachs G: Characterization of an electrogenic ATP and chloride-dependent proton translocating pump from rat renal medulla. *J Biol Chem* **260:**11567, 1985.
145. Stone DK, Xie X-S: Proton translocating ATPases: Issues in structure and function. *Kidney Int* **33:**767, 1988.
146. Gluck S, Bastani B: The biochemistry of distal urinary acidification in health and disease, in De Santo NG, Capasso G (eds): *Acid-Base Balance*. Cosenza, Italy, Editoriale Bios, 1991, p 21.
147. Gluck S, Hirsch S, Brown D: Immunocytochemical localization of H^+-ATPase in rat kidney. *Kidney Int* **31:**167, 1987. (abstr.)
148. Silva F, Schulz W, Davis L, Xie X-S, Stone DK: Immunocytochemical localization of the clathrin-coated vesicle proton pump (CCV-PP). *Kidney Int* **31:**416, 1987. (abstr.)
149. Gifford JD, Ware MW, Crowson S, Shull GE: Expression of a putative rat distal colonic H^+-K^+-ATPase mRNA in rat kidney: Effect of respiratory acidosis. *J Am Soc Nephrol* **2:**700, 1991.
150. Wingo CS: Active proton secretion and potassium absorption in the rabbit outer medullary collecting duct. *J Clin Invest* **84:**361, 1989.
151. Wingo CS, Madsen KM, Smolka A, Tisher CC: H-K-ATPase immunoreactivity in cortical and outer medullary collecting duct. *Kidney Int* **38:**985, 1990.
152. Dafnis E, Spohn M, Lonis B, Kurtzman NA, Sabatini S: Vanadate causes hypokalemic distal renal tubular acidosis. *Am J Physiol* **262:**F449, 1992.
153. Fisher JL, Husted RF, Steinmetz PR: Chloride dependence on the HCO_3 exit step in urinary acidification by the turtle bladder. *Am J Physiol* **245:**F564, 1983.
154. Stone DK, Seldin DW, Kokko JP, Jacobson HR: Anion dependence of rabbit medullary collecting duct acidification. *J Clin Invest* **71:**1505, 1983.
155. Schuster VL, Bonsib SM, Jennings ML: Two types of collecting duct mitochondria-rich (intercalated) cells: Lectin and band 3 cytochemistry. *Am J Physiol* **20:**C347, 1986.
156. Kudrycki KE, Shull GE: Primary structure of the rat kidney band 3 anion exchange protein deduced from a cDNA. *J Biol Chem* **264:**8185, 1989.
157. Brosius FC III, Alper SL, Garcia AM, Lodish HF: The major kidney band 3 gene transcript predicts an amino-terminal truncated band 3 polypeptide. *J Biol Chem* **264:**7784, 1989.
158. Koeppen BM: Conductive properties of the rabbit outer medullary collecting duct: Inner stripe. *Am J Physiol* **17:**F500, 1985.
159. Schuster VL: Bicarbonate reabsorption and secretion in the cortical and outer medullary collecting duct. *Semin Nephrol* **10:**139, 1990.
160. Leslie BR, Schwartz JH, Steinmetz PR: Coupling between Cl^- absorption and HCO_3^- secretion in turtle urinary bladder. *Am J Physiol* **225:**610, 1973.
161. Husted RF, Eyman E: Chloride-bicarbonate exchange in the urinary bladder of the turtle: Independence from sodium ion. *Biochim Biophys Acta* **595:**305, 1980.
162. Star RA, Burg MB, Knepper MA: Bicarbonate secretion and chloride absorption by rabbit cortical collecting ducts: Role of chloride/bicarbonate exchange. *J Clin Invest* **76:**1123, 1985.
163. Oliver JA, Himmelstein AS, Steinmetz PR: Energy dependence of urinary bicarbonate secretion in turtle bladder. *J Clin Invest* **55:**1003, 1975.
164. Satake N, Durham JH, Ehrenspeck G, Brodsky WA: Active electrogenic mechanisms for alkali and acid transport in turtle bladders. *Am J Physiol* **13:**C259, 1985.
165. Ehrenspeck G: Effect of 3-isobutyl-1-methylxanthine on HCO_3^- transport in turtle bladder: Evidence of electrogenic HCO_3^- secretion. *Biochim Biophys Acta* **684:**219, 1982.
166. Stetson DL, Beauwens R, Palmisano J, Mitchell PP, Steinmetz PR: A double-membrane model for urinary bicarbonate secretion. *Am J Physiol* **18:**F546, 1985.
167. Schuster VL: Cyclic adenosine monophosphate-stimulate bicarbonate secretion in rabbit cortical collecting tubules. *J Clin Invest* **75:**2056, 1985.
168. DuBose TD Jr, Good DW, Hamm LL, Wall SM: Ammonium transport in the kidney: New physiologic concepts and their clinical implications. *J Am Soc Nephrol* **1:**1193, 1991.
169. Good DW, Burg MB: Ammonia production by individual segments of the rat nephron. *J Clin Invest* **73:**602, 1984.
170. Hwang J-J, Curthoys NP: Effect of acute alterations in acid-base balance on rat renal glutaminase and phosphoenolpyruvate carboxykinase gene expression. *J Biol Chem* **266:**9392, 1991.
171. Kaiser S, Curthoys NP: Effect of pH and bicarbonate on phosphoenolpyruvate carboxykinase and glutaminase in mRNA levels in cultured renal epithelial cells. *J Biol Chem* **266:**9397, 1991.
172. Pollock AS, Long JA: The 5′ region of the rat phosphoenolpyruvate carboxykinase gene confers pH sensitivity to chimeric genes expressed in renal and liver cell lines capable of expressing PEPCK. *Biochem Biophys Res Commun* **164:**81, 1989.
173. Kinsella JL, Aronson PS: Interaction of NH_4^+ and Li^+ with the renal microvillus membrane Na^+-H^+ exchanger. *Am J Physiol* **241:**C220, 1981.
174. Nagami GT, Sonu CM, Kurokawa K: Ammonia production by isolated mouse proximal tubule perfused in vitro. Effect of metabolic acidosis. *J Clin Invest* **78:**124, 1986.
175. Hamm LL, Trigg D, Martin D, Gillespie C, Buerkert J: Transport of ammonia in the rabbit cortical collecting tubule. *J Clin Invest* **75:**478, 1985.

176. Garvin JL, Burg MB, Knepper MA: NH_3 and NH_4^+ transport by rabbit renal proximal straight tubules. *Am J Physiol* **21:**F232, 1987.
177. DuBose TD Jr, Lucci MS, Hogg RJ, Pucacco LR, Kokko JP, Carter NW: Comparison of acidification parameters in superficial and deep nephrons of the rat. *Am J Physiol* **13:**F497, 1983.
178. Buerkert J, Martin D, Trigg D: Segmental analysis of the renal tubule in buffer production and net acid formation. *Am J Physiol* **244:**F442, 1983.
179. Gottschalk CW, Lassiter WE, Mylle M: Localization of urine acidification in the mammalian kidney. *Am J Physiol* **198:**581, 1960.
180. Good DW, Knepper MA, Burge MB: Ammonia and bicarbonate transport by thick ascending limb of rat kidney. *Am J Physiol* **247:**F35, 1984.
181. Kurtz I, Star R, Balaban RS, Garvin JL, Knepper MA: Spontaneous luminal disequilibrium pH in S_3 proximal tubules. Role in ammonia and bicarbonate transport. *J Clin Invest* **78:**989, 1986.
182. Good DW, Caflisch CR, DuBose TD Jr: Transepithelial ammonia concentration gradients in inner medulla of the rat. *Am J Physiol* **252:**F491, 1987.
183. Knepper MA, Good DW, Burg MB: Mechanism of ammonia secretion by cortical collecting ducts of rabbits. *Am J Physiol* **247:**F729, 1984.
184. Steinmetz PR, Lawson LR: Effect of luminal pH on ion permeability and flows of Na^+ and H^+ in turtle bladder. *Am J Physiol* **220:**1573, 1971.
185. Beauwens R, Al-Awqati Q: Active H^+ transport in the turtle urinary bladder: Coupling of transport to glucose oxidation. *J Gen Physiol* **68:**421, 1976.
186. Al-Awqati Q, Muller A, Steinmetz PR: Transport of H^+ against electrochemical gradients in turtle urinary bladder. *Am J Physiol* **233:**F502, 1977.
187. Laski ME, Kurtzman NA: Characterization of acidification in the cortical and medullary collecting tubule of the rabbit. *J Clin Invest* **72:**2050, 1983.
188. O'Neil RG, Helman SI: Transport characteristics of renal collecting tubules: Influences of DOCA and diet. *Am J Physiol* **233:**F544, 1977.
189. Schwartz GJ, Burg MB: Mineralocorticoid effects on cation transport by cortical collecting tubule in vitro. *Am J Physiol* **235:**F576, 1978.
190. Al-Awqati Q, Norby LH, Mueller A, Steinmetz PR: Characteristics of stimulation of H^+ transport by aldosterone in turtle urinary bladder. *J Clin Invest* **58:**351, 1976.
191. Al-Awqati Q: Effect of aldosterone on the coupling between H^+ transport and glucose oxidation. *J Clin Invest* **60:**1240, 1977.
192. DuBose TD Jr, Caflisch CR: Effect of selective aldosterone deficiency on acidification in nephron segments of the rat inner medulla. *J Clin Invest* **82:**1624, 1988.
193. McKinney TD, Davidson KK: Effect of potassium depletion and protein intake in vivo on renal tubular bicarbonate transport in vitro. *Am J Physiol* **21:**F509, 1987.
194. Hays SR, Seldin DW, Kokko JP, Jacobson HR: Effect of K depletion on HCO_3 transport across rabbit collecting duct segments. *Kidney Int* **29:**268A, 1986. (abstr.)
195. Tannen RL, McGill J: Influences of potassium on renal ammonia production. *Am J Physiol* **231:**1178, 1976.
196. DuBose TD Jr, Good DW: Effects of chronic hyperkalemia on renal production and proximal tubule transport of ammonium in the rat. *Am J Physiol* **260:**F680, 1991.
197. Good DW: Active absorption of NH_4^+ by rat medullary thick ascending limb. *Am J Physiol* **255:**F78, 1988.
198. DuBose TD Jr, Good DW: Chronic hyperkalemia impairs ammonium transport and accumulation in the inner medulla of the rat. *J Clin Invest* **90:**1443, 1992.
199. Seldin DW, Wilson JD: Renal tubular acidosis, in Stanbury JB, Wyngaarden JB, Fredrickson DS (eds): *The Metabolic Basis of Inherited Disease,* 3rd ed. New York, McGraw-Hill, 1972, pp 1548–1566.
200. Rector FC Jr: Acidification of the urine, in Orloff J, Berliner RW (eds): *Renal Physiology, Handbook of Physiology.* Baltimore, Williams & Wilkins, 1973, pp 431–454.
201. Schwartz WB, Jenson RL, Relman AS: Acidification of the urine and increased ammonia excretion without change in acid-base equilibrium: Sodium reabsorption as a stimulus to the acidifying process. *J Clin Invest* **34:**673, 1955.
202. Batlle DC, Sehy JT, Roseman MK, Arruda JAL, Kurtzman NA: Clinical and pathophysiologic spectrum of acquired distal renal tubular acidosis. *Kidney Int* **20:**389, 1981.
203. Arruda JAL, Kurtzman NA: Mechanism and classification of deranged distal urinary acidification. *Am J Physiol* **8:**F515, 1980.
204. Halperin ML, Goldstein MB, Haig A, Johnson MD, Steinbaugh BJ: Studies on the pathogenesis of type 1 (distal) renal tubular acidosis as revealed by the urinary PCO_2 tension. *J Clin Invest* **53:**669, 1974.
205. DuBose TD Jr, Caflisch CR: Validation of the difference in urine and blood CO_2 tension during bicarbonate loading as an index of distal nephron acidification in experimental models of distal renal tubular acidosis. *J Clin Invest* **75:**1116, 1985.
206. Berliner RW, DuBose TD Jr: Carbon dioxide tension of alkaline urine, in Seldin DW, Giebisch G (eds): *The Kidney: Physiology and Pathophysiology,* 2d ed. New York, Raven, 1992, p 2681.
207. Batlle DC: Segmental characterization of defects in collecting tubule acidification. *Kidney Int* **30:**546, 1986.
208. Capasso G, Schultz H, Vickermann B, Kinne R: Amphotericin B and amphotericin B methylester: Effect on brush border membrane permeability. *Kidney Int* **30:**311, 1986.
209. Steinmetz PR, Lawson LR: Defect in acidification induced in vitro by amphotericin B. *J Clin Invest* **49:**596, 1970.
210. Garg LC: Lack of effect of amphotericin-B on urine-blood PCO_2 gradient in spite of urinary acidification defect. *Pflugers Arch* **381:**137, 1979.
211. Julka N, Arruda JAL, Kurtzman NA: The mechanism of amphotericin-induced distal acidification defect in rats. *Clin Sci* **56:**555, 1979.
212. Taher SM, Anderson RJ, McCartney R, Popovtzer MM, Schrier RW: Renal tubular acidosis associated with toluene "sniffing." *N Engl J Med* **290:**765, 1974.
213. Kurtzman NA: Acquired distal renal tubular acidosis. *Kidney Int* **24:**807, 1983.
214. Nimmannit S, Malasit P, Chaovakul V, Susaengrat W, Vasuvattakul S, Nilwarangkur S: Pathogenesis of sudden unexplained nocturnal death (lai tai) and endemic distal renal tubular acidosis. *Lancet* **338:**930, 1991.
215. Sitprija V, Tungsanga K, Eiam-Ong S, Leelhaphunt N, Sriboonlue P: Renal tubular acidosis, vanadium, and buffaloes. *Nephron* **54:**97, 1990.
216. DuBose TD Jr: Experimental models of distal renal tubular acidosis. *Semin Nephrol* **10:**174, 1990.
217. Kurtzman NA: Disorders of distal acidification. *Kidney Int* **38:**720, 1990.
218. Kurtzman NA: "Short-circuit" renal tubular acidosis. *J Lab Clin Med* **95:**633, 1980.
219. Husted RF, Steinmetz PR: The effects of amiloride and oubain on urinary acidification by turtle bladder. *J Pharmacol Exp Ther* **210:**264, 1979.
220. Arruda JAL, Subbarayudu K, Dytko G, Mola R, Kurtzman NA: Voltage dependent distal acidification defect induced by amiloride. *J Lab Clin Med* **95:**407, 1980.
221. Hulter HN, Ilnicki LP, Licht JH, Sebastian A: On the mechanism of diminished urinary carbon dioxide tension caused by amiloride. *Kidney Int* **21:**8, 1982.
222. Nascimento L, Rademacker D, Hamburger R, Arruda JAL, Kurtzman NA: On the mechanism of lithium-induced renal tubular acidosis. *J Lab Clin Med* **89:**445, 1977.
223. Roscoe M, Goldstein MB, Halperin MC, Wilson DR, Stinebaugh BJ: Lithium-induced impairment of urine acidification. *Kidney Int* **9:**344, 1976.
224. Arruda JAL, Dytko G, Mola R, Kurtzman NA: On the mechanism of lithium-induced distal renal tubular acidosis: Studies in the turtle bladder. *Kidney Int* **17:**196, 1980.
225. Daphnis E, Kurtzman NA, Sabatini S: On the mechanism of lithium-induced renal tubular acidosis. *Kidney Int* **37:**534A, 1990.
226. Batlle DC, Gaviria M, Grupp M, Arruda JAL, Wynn J,

Kurtzman NA: Distal nephron function in patients receiving chronic lithium therapy. *Kidney Int* **21**:477, 1982.
227. Sabatini S, Kurtzman NA: Enzyme activity in obstructive uropathy: The biochemical basis for salt wastage and the acidification defect. *Kidney Int* **37**:79, 1990.
228. Purcell H, Hastani B, Harris KPG, Hemken P, Klahr S, Gluck S: Cellular distribution of H^+ ATPase following acute unilateral ureteral obstruction in rats. *Am J Physiol* **261**:F365, 1991.
229. Sawczuk I, Hoke G, Olsson C, Connor J, Buttyan R: Gene expression in response to acute unilateral ureteral obstruction. *Kidney Int* **35**:1315, 1989.
230. Schambelan M, Sebastian A, Hulter HN: Mineralocorticoid excess and deficiency syndromes, in Brenner BM, Stein JH (eds): *Contemporary Issues in Nephrology. Acid-Base and Potassium Homeostasis.* New York, Churchill Livingstone, 1978, vol 2, pp 232–268.
231. Hulter HN, Ilnicki LP, Harbottle JA, Sebastian A: Impaired renal H^+ secretion and NH_3 production in mineralocorticoid-deficient glucocorticoid-replete dogs. *Am J Physiol* **326**:F136, 1979.
232. Steinmetz PR: Cellular mechanisms of urinary acidification. *Physiol Rev* **54**:890, 1974.
233. Hulter HN, Bonner EL Jr, Glynn RD, Sebastian A: Renal and systemic acid-base effects of chronic spironolactone administration. *Am J Physiol* **240**:F381, 1981.
234. Szylman P, Better OS, Chaimowitz C, Rosler A: Role of hyperkalemia in the metabolic acidosis of isolated hypoaldosteronism. *N Engl J Med* **294**:361, 1975.
235. Tannen RC: Relationship of renal ammonia production and potassium homeostasis. *Kidney Int* **11**:453, 1977.
236. Sebastian A, Schambelan M, Lindenfeld S, Morris RC Jr: Amelioration of metabolic acidosis with fludrocortisone therapy in hyporeninemic hypoaldosteronism. *N Engl J Med* **297**:576, 1977.
237. Wilcox CS, Cemeriki DA, Giebisch G: Differential effects of acute mineralo- and glucocorticosteroid administration on renal acid elimination. *Kidney Int* **21**:546, 1982.
238. Sebastian A, Sutton JM, Hulter HN, Schambelan M, Poler SM: Effect of mineralocorticoid replacement therapy on renal acid-base homeostasis in adrenalectomized patients. *Kidney Int* **18**:762, 1980.
239. Cheek DB, Perry JW: A salt-wasting syndrome in infancy. *Arch Dis Child* **33**:252, 1948.
240. Donnell GN, Litman N, Roldan M: Pseudohypoadrenalocorticism; renal sodium loss; hyponatremia, and hyperkalemia due to renal tubular insensitivity to mineralocorticoids. *Am J Dis Child* **97**:813, 1959.
241. Postel-Vinay MC, Alberti GM, Ricour C, Limal JM, Rappaport R, Royer P: Pseudohypoaldosteronism: Multiple target organ unresponsiveness to mineralocorticoid hormones. *J Clin Endocrinol Metab* **48**:228, 1979.
242. Oberfield SE, Levine LS, Carey RM, Bejar R, New MI: Pseudohypoaldosteronism: Multiple target organ unresponsiveness to mineralocorticoid hormones. *J Clin Endocrinol Metab* **478**:228, 1979.
243. Bierich JR, Schmidt U: Tubular Na^+ K^+-ATPase deficiency the cause of congenital renal salt-losing syndrome. *Eur J Pediatr* **121**:81, 1976.
244. Westernfelder C, Arevalo GJ, Baranowski RL, Kurtzman NA, Katz AI: Relationship between mineralocorticoids and renal Na^+ K^+-ATPase: Sodium reabsorption. *Am J Physiol* **233**:F593, 1977.
245. Arnold JE, Healy JK: Hyperkalemia, hypertension and systemic acidosis without renal failure associated with a tubular defect in potassium excretion. *Am J Med* **47**:461, 1969.
246. Gordon RD, Geddes RA, Pawsey CGK, O'Halloran MW: Hypertension and severe hyperkalemia associated with suppression of renin and aldosterone and completely reversed by dietary sodium restriction. *Aust Ann Med* **4**:287, 1970.
247. Spitzer A, Edelmann CM Jr, Goldberg LD, Henneman PH: Short stature hyperkalemia and acidosis: A defect in renal transport of potassium. *Kidney Int* **3**:251, 1973.
248. Weinstein SF, Allan DME, Mendoza SA: Hyperkalemia, acidosis, and short stature associated with a defect in renal potassium excretion. *J Pediatr* **85**:255, 1974.
249. Schambelan M, Sebastian A, Rector FC Jr: Mineralocorticoid-resistant renal hyperkalemia without salt wasting (type II pseudohypoaldosteronism): Role of increased renal chloride reabsorption. *Kidney Int* **19**:716, 1981.
250. Take C, Ikeda K, Kurasawa T, Kurokawa K: Increased chloride reabsorption as an inherited renal tubular defect in familial type II pseudohypoaldosteronism. *N Engl J Med* **324**:472, 1991.
251. Lee MR, Ball SG, Thomas TH, Morgan DB: Hypertension and hyperkalemia responding to bendrogluazide. *Q J Med* **48**:245, 1979.
252. Shimizu T, Yoshitomi K, Nakamura M, Imai M: Site and mechanism of action of trichlormethiazide in rabbit distal nephron segments perfused in vitro. *J Clin Invest* **82**:721, 1988.
253. Gordon RD, Hodsman GP: The syndrome of hypertension and hyperkalemia without renal failure: Long term correction by thiazide diuretic. *Scott Med J* **31**:43, 1986.
254. Schambelan M, Sebastian A, Biglieri EG: Prevalence, pathogenesis, and functional significance of aldosterone deficiency in hyperkalemic patients with chronic renal insufficiency. *Kidney Int* **17**:89, 1980.
255. Sebastian A, Schambelan M, Hulter HN, Maher T, Kurtz I, Biglieri EG, Rector FC Jr, Morris RC Jr: Hyperkalemic renal tubular acidosis, in Gonick HC, Buckalew VM Jr (eds): *Renal Tubular Disorders. Pathophysiology, Diagnosis and Management.* New York, Marcel Dekker, 1985, pp 307–356.
256. DeFronzo RA: Hyperkalemia and hyporeninemic hypoaldosteronism. *Kidney Int* **17**:118, 1980.
257. Carrol HJ, Farber SJ: Hyperkalemia and hyperchloremic acidosis in chronic pyelonephritis. *Metabolism* **13**:808, 1964.
258. Schambelan M, Stockigt JR, Biglieri M: Isolated hypoaldosteronism in adults. A renin-deficiency syndrome. *N Engl J Med* **287**:573, 1972.
259. Coleman AJ, Arias M, Carter NW, Rector FC Jr, Seldin DW: The mechanism of salt wastage in chronic renal disease. *J Clin Invest* **45**:1116, 1966.
260. Oh MS, Carrol HJ, Clemmons JE, Vagnucci AH, Levison SP, Whang ESM: A mechanism for hyporeninemic hypoaldosternoism in chronic renal disease. *Metabolism* **23**:1157, 1974.
261. Sparagna M: Hyporeninemic hypoaldosteronism associated with diabetic glomerulosclerosis. *J Steroid Biochem* **5**:369, 1974.
262. Schinder AM, Sommers SC: Diabetic sclerosis of the renal juxtaglomerular apparatus. *Lab Invest* **15**:877, 1966.
263. Tan SY, Shapiro R, Franco R, Stockard H, Mulrow AJ: Indomethacin-induced prostaglandin inhibition with hyperkalemia. A reversible cause of hyperreninemic hypoaldosteronism. *Ann Intern Med* **90**:783, 1979.
264. Norby LH, Ramwell P, Weidig J, Slotkoff L, Flamenbaum W: Possible role for impaired renal prostaglandin production in pathogenesis of hyporeninemic hypoaldosteronism. *Lancet* **2**:1118, 1978.
265. Deleiva A, Christlich AR, Melby JC, Graham CA, Day RP, Luetscher JA, Zager PG: Big renin and biosynthetic defect of aldosterone in diabetes mellitus. *N Engl J Med* **25**:639, 1976.
266. Perez GO, Oster JR, Vaamonde CA: Renal acidosis and renal potassium handling in selective hypoaldosteronism. *Am J Med* **57**:809, 1974.
267. Morris RC Jr: Renal tubular acidosis. Mechanisms, classification and implications. *N Engl J Med* **281**:1405, 1969.
268. Morris RC Jr, Sebastian A: Renal tubular acidosis and Fanconi syndrome, in Stanbury JB, Wyngaarden JB, Fredrickson DS, Goldstein JL, Brown MS (eds): *The Metabolic Basis of Inherited Disease,* 5th ed. New York, McGraw-Hill, 1983, pp 1808–1843.
269. Elkinton JR, Huth EJ, Webster GD Jr, McCance RA: The renal excretion of hydrogen ion in renal tubular acidosis. *Am J Med* **29**:554, 1960.
270. Wrong O: Urinary hydrogen ion excretion. *J Clin Pathol* **18**:520, 1965.
271. Sebastian A, McSherry E, Morris RC Jr: Metabolic acidosis with special reference to renal acidosis, in Brenner BM, Rector FC Jr (eds): *The Kidney,* 2d ed. Philadelphia, Saunders, 1976, pp 615–660.
272. Kurtzman NA, Arruda JAL: Physiologic significance of

urinary carbon dioxide tension. *Miner Electrolyte Metab* **1:**241, 1978.

273. Batlle DC, Kurtzman NA: The defect in distal (type 1) renal tubular acidosis, in Gonick HC, Buckalew VM Jr (eds): *Renal Tubular Disorders. Pathophysiology, Diagnosis and Management.* New York, Marcel Dekker, 1985, pp 281–305.
274. Stinebaugh BJ, Esquenazi R, Schloeder FX, Suki WN, Goldstein MB, Halperin ML: Control of the urine-blood PCO_2 gradient in alkaline urine. *Kidney Int* **17:**31, 1980.
275. Batlle DC, Kurtzman NA: Renal regulation of acid-base homeostasis; Integrated response, in Seldin DW, Giebisch G (eds): *The Kidney: Physiology and Pathophysiology.* New York, Raven, 1985, pp 1539–1565.
276. Wrong O, Davies HE: The excretion of acid in renal disease. *Q J Med* **28:**259, 1959.
277. Coe FL, Parks JH: Stone disease in heredity distal renal tubular acidosis. *Ann Intern Med* **93:**60, 1980.
278. Buckalew VM Jr, Purvis ML, Shulman MG, Herndon CN, Rudman D: Hereditary renal tubular acidosis. Report of a 64 member kindred with variable clinical expression including idiopathic hypercalcemia. *Medicine (Baltimore)* **53:**229, 1974.
279. Simpson DP: Influence of plasma bicarbonate concentration and pH on citrate excretion. *Am J Physiol* **206:**875, 1964.
280. Buckalew VM Jr, McCurdy DK, Ludwig GD, Chaykin LB, Elkinton JR: The syndrome of incomplete renal tubular acidosis. *Am J Med* **45:**32, 1968.
281. Brenner RJ, Spring DB, Sebastian A, McSherry EM, Genant HK, Palubinskas AJ, Morris RC Jr: Incidence of radiographically evident bone disease, nephrocalcinosis, and nephrolithiasis in various types of renal tubular acidosis. *N Engl J Med* **307:**217, 1982.
282. Morris RC Jr, Ives HE: Inherited disorders of the renal tubule, in Brenner BM, Rector FC Jr (eds): *The Kidney,* 4th ed. New York, Saunders, 1991, p 1596.
283. McSherry EM, Morris RC Jr: Attainment and maintenance of normal stature with alkali therapy in infants and children with classic renal tubular acidosis. *J Clin Invest* **61:**509, 1978.
284. Pitts HH, Schulte JW, Smith DR: Nephrocalcinosis in a father and three children. *J Urol* **73:**208, 1955.
285. Randall RE Jr, Targgart WH: Familial renal tubular acidosis. *Ann Intern Med* **54:**1108, 1961.
286. Randall RE Jr: Familial renal tubular acidosis revisited. *Ann Intern Med* **66:**1024, 1967.
287. Seedat YK: Some observations of renal tubular acidosis: A family study. *S Afr Med J* 38:606, 1964.
288. Gyory AZ, Edwards KDG: Renal tubular acidosis: A family with an autosomal dominant genetic defect in renal hydrogen ion transport, with proximal tubular and collecting duct dysfunction and increased metabolism of citrate and ammonia. *Am J Med* **45:**43, 1968.
289. Richards P, Wrong OM: Dominant inheritance in a family with familial renal tubular acidosis. *Lancet* **2:**998, 1978.
290. McSherry EM, Pokroy MV: The absence of nephrocalcinosis in children with type 1 RTA on high dose alkali therapy since infancy. *Clin Res* **26:**470A, 1978.
291. Hamed IA, Czerwinski AW, Coats B, Kaufman C, Altmiller DH: Familial absorptive hypercalciuria and renal tubular acidosis. *Am J Med* **67:**385, 1979.
292. Buckalew VM Jr: Familial renal tubular acidosis. *Ann Intern Med* **69:**1329, 1968.
293. Donckerwolcke RA, Van Stehelenburg GJ, Tiddens HA: A case of bicarbonate-losing renal tubular acidosis with defective carboanhydrase activity. *Arch Dis Child* **45:**769, 1970.
294. Shapira E, Ben-Yoseph Y, Eyal FC, Russel A: Enzymatically inactive red cell carbonic anhydrase B in a family with renal tubular acidosis. *J Clin Invest* **53:**59, 1974.
295. Norman ME, Cohn RM, McCurdy DK: Urinary citrate excretion in the diagnosis of distal renal tubular acidosis. *J Pediatr* **92:**394, 1978.
296. Bourke E, Delaney VB, Mosawi M, Reavy P, Weston M: Renal tubular acidosis and osteopetrosis in siblings. *Nephron* **28:**268, 1981.
297. Morris RC Jr, Fudenberg HH: Impaired renal acidification in patients with hypergammaglobulinemia. *Medicine (Baltimore)* **46:**57, 1967.
298. Cohen A, Way BJ: The association of renal tubular acidosis with hyperglobulinemic purpura. *Australas Ann Med* **11:**189, 1962.
299. Mason AMS, Golding PL: Hyperglobulinaemic renal tubular acidosis: A report of nine cases. *Br Med J* **3:**143, 1970.
300. Marquez-Julio A, Rapoport A, Wilansky DL, Rabinovich S, Chamberlain D: Purpura associated with hypergammaglobulinemia, renal tubular acidosis and osteomalacia. *Can Med Assoc J* **116:**53, 1977.
301. Lospalluto J, Dorward B, Biller W, Ziff M: Cryoglobulinemia based on interaction between a gamma macroglobulin and 7S gamma globulin. *Am J Med* **32:**142, 1962.
302. Mason AMS, McIllmurray MB, Golding PL, Hughes DTD: Fibrosing alveolitis associated with renal tubular acidosis. *Br Med J* **4:**596, 1970.
303. Talal N, Zisman E, Schur PH: Renal tubular acidosis, glomerulonephritis and immunologic factors in Sjögren's syndrome. *Arthritis Rheum* **2:**774, 1968.
304. Talal N: Sjögren's syndrome, lymphoproliferation, and renal tubular acidosis. *Ann Intern Med* **74:**633, 1971.
305. Shioji R, Furuyama T, Onodera S, Saito H, Ito H, Sasaki Y: Sjögren's syndrome and renal tubular acidosis. *Am J Med* **48:**456, 1970.
306. Mason AM, Golding PL: Renal tubular acidosis and autoimmune thyroid disease. *Lancet* **2:**1104, 1970.
307. Golding PL: Renal tubular acidosis in chronic liver disease. *Postgrad Med J* **51:**550, 1975.
308. Bridi GS, Falcon PW, Brackett NC Jr, Still WJS, Sporn IN: Glomerulonephritis and renal tubular acidosis in a case of chronic active hepatitis with hyperimmunoglobulinemia. *Am J Med* **52:**267, 1972.
309. Reade AE, Sherlock S, Harrison CV: Active "juvenile" cirrhosis considered as part of a systemic disease. *Gut* **4:**378, 1963.
310. Seedat YK, Raine ER: Active hepatitis associated with renal tubular acidosis and successful pregnancy. *S Afr Med J* **39:**595, 1965.
311. Golding PL, Smith M, Williams R: Multisystem involvement in chronic liver disease. Studies on the incidence and pathogenesis. *Ann Intern J Med* **55:**772, 1973.
312. Cochrane AM, Tsantoulos DC, Moussouros A, McFarland IG, Eddleston ALWF, Williams R: Lymphocyte cytotoxicity for kidney cells in renal tubular acidosis of autoimmune liver disease. *Br Med J* **2:**276, 1976.
313. Tu WH, Shearn MA: Systemic lupus erythematosis and latent renal tubular dysfunction. *Ann Intern Med* **67:**100, 1967.
314. Jessop S, Rabkin R, Mumford G, Eales L: Renal tubular function in systemic lupus erythematosis. *S Afr Med J* **47:**132, 1973.
315. Reynolds TB, Bethune JE: Renal tubular acidosis secondary to hyperparathyroidism. *Clin Res* **17:**169, 1969.
316. Cohen SI, Fitzgerald MG, Fourman P, Griffiths WJ, Dewardener HE: Polyuria in hyperparathyroidism. *Q J Med* **26:**423, 1957.
317. Ferris T, Kashgarian M, Livitin H, Brandt I, Epstein FH: Renal tubular acidosis and renal potassium wasting acquired as a result of hypercalcemic nephropathy. *N Engl J Med* **265:**924, 1961.
318. Rochman J, Better OS, Winaver J, Chaimovitz C, Carzilai A, Jacobs R: Renal tubular acidosis due to the milk-alkali syndrome. *Isr J Med Sci* **13:**609, 1977.
319. Huth EJ, Mayock RL, Kerr RM: Hyperthyroidism associated with renal tubular acidosis. *Am J Med* **26:**818, 1959.
320. Zisman E, Buccino RA, Gorden P, Bartter FC: Hyperthyroidism and renal tubular acidosis. *Arch Intern Med* **121:**118, 1968.
321. Parfitt AM, Higgins BA, Nassim JR, Collins JA, Hilb A: Metabolic studies in patients with hypercalciuria. *Clin Sci* **27:**463, 1964.
322. Dent CE, Harper CM, Parfit AM: The effect of cellulose phosphate on calcium metabolism in patients with hypercalciuria. *Clin Sci* **27:**417, 1964.
323. Deck MDF: Medullary sponge kidney with renal tubular acidosis: A report of 3 cases. *J Urol* **94:**330, 1965.
324. Morris RC Jr, Yamauchi H, Palubinskas AJ, Howenstine J: Medullary sponge kidney. *Am J Med* **38:**883, 1965.
325. Mass RE, Smith WR, Walsh JR: The association of heredi-

tary fructose intolerance and renal tubular acidosis. *Am J Med Sci* **251**:516, 1966.
326. Yeoh SA: Fabry's disease with renal tubular acidosis. *Singapore Med J* **8**:275, 1967.
327. Higashihara E, Nutahara K, Tago K, Ueno A, Niijima T: Medullary sponge kidney and renal acidification defect. *Kidney Int* **25**:453, 1984.
328. Patterson RM, Ackerman G: Renal tubular acidosis due to amphotericin B nephrotoxicity. *Arch Intern Med* **127**:241, 1971.
329. Douglas JB, Healy JK: Nephrotoxic effects of amphotericin B, including renal tubular acidosis. *Am J Med* **46**:154, 1969.
330. McCurdy DK, Frederic M, Elkinton JR: Renal tubular acidosis due to amphotericin B. *N Engl J Med* **278**:124, 1968.
331. Yong JM, Sanderson KV: Photosensitive dermatitis and renal tubular acidosis after ingestion of calcium cyclamate. *Lancet* **2**:1273, 1969.
332. Steele TW, Gyory AZ, Edwards KDG: Renal function in analgesic nephropathy. *Br Med J* **2**:213, 1969.
333. Steele TW, Edwards KDG: Analgesic nephropathy. *Med J Aust* **1**:181, 1971.
334. Gyory AZ, Stewart JH, George CRP, Tiller DJ, Edwards KDG: Renal tubular acidosis, acidosis due to hyperkalemia, hypercalcaemia, disordered citrate metabolism and other tubular dysfunctions following human renal transplantation. *Q J Med* **38**:231, 1969.
335. Wilson DR, Siddiqui AA: Renal tubular acidosis after kidney transplantation. *Ann Intern Med* **79**:352, 1973.
336. Better OS, Chaimowitz C, Naveh Y, Stein A, Nahir AM, Barzilai A, Erlik D: Syndrome of incomplete renal tubular acidosis after cadaver kidney transplantation. *Ann Intern Med* **71**:39, 1969.
337. Drutz DJ, Gutman RA: Renal tubular acidosis in leprosy. *Ann Intern Med* **75**:475, 1971.
338. Vainder M, Kelly J: Renal tubular dysfunction secondary to jejuno-ileal bypass. *JAMA* **235**:1257, 1976.
339. Better OS, Arieff AI, Massry SG, Kleeman CR, Maxwell MH: Studies on renal function after relief of complete unilateral ureteral obstruction of three months duration in man. *Am J Med* **54**:234, 1973.
340. Earley LE: Extreme polyuria in obstructive uropathy. *N Engl J Med* **255**:600, 1956.
341. Berlyne GM: Distal tubular function in chronic hydronephrosis. *Q J Med* **30**:339, 1961.
342. Cochran M, Peacock M, Smith DA, Nrodin BEC: Renal tubular acidosis of pyelonephritis with renal stone disease. *Br Med J* **2**:721, 1968.
343. Levine AS, Michael AF Jr: Ehler-Danlos syndrome with renal tubular acidosis and medullary sponge kidneys. *J Pediatr* **71**:107, 1967.
344. Bechner RL, Gilchrist GS, Anderson EJ: Hereditary elliptocytosis and primary renal tubular acidosis in a single family. *Am J Dis Child* **115**:414, 1968.
345. Dunger DB, Brenton DP, Cain AR: Renal tubular acidosis and nerve deafness. *Arch Dis Child* **55**:221, 1980.
346. Oster JR, Lespier LE, Lee SM, Pellegrini EL, Vaamonde CA: Renal acidification in sickle-cell disease. *J Lab Clin Med* **88**:389, 1976.
347. Giselson N, Heinegard D, Holmberg CG, Lindberg LG, Lindstedt G, Schersten B: Renal medullary cystic disease or familial juvenile nephronophthisis: A renal tubular disease. Biochemical findings in two siblings. *Am J Med* **48**:174, 1970.
348. McSherry E, Sebastian A, Morris RC Jr: Renal tubular acidosis in infants: The several kinds, including bicarbonate wasting classic renal tubular acidosis. *J Clin Invest* **51**:499, 1972.
349. Rodriquez-Soriano J, Boichis H, Edelman CM Jr: Bicarbonate reabsorption and hydrogen ion excretion in children with renal tubular acidosis. *J Pediatr* **71**:802, 1967.
350. Dedmon RE, Wrong O: The excretion of organic anion in renal tubular acidosis with particular reference to citrate. *Clin Sci* **22**:19, 1962.
351. Morrissey JF, Ochoa M, Lotspeich WD, Waterhouse C: Citrate excretion in renal tubular acidosis. *Ann Intern Med* **58**:159, 1963.
352. Harrington TM, Bunch TW, Van Den Berg C: Renal tubular acidosis. A new look at treatment of musculoskeletal and renal disease. *Mayo Clin Proc* **58**:354, 1983.
353. Sebastian A, McSherry E, Morris RC Jr: Impaired renal conservation of sodium and chloride during sustained correction of systemic acidosis in patients with Type I, classic renal tubular acidosis. *J Clin Invest* **58**:454, 1976.
354. Rodriquez-Soriano J, Vallo A, Castillo G, Oliveros R: Renal handling of water and sodium in children with proximal and distal renal tubular acidosis. *Nephron* **25**:193, 1980.
355. Sebastian A, McSherry E, Morris RC Jr: Renal potassium wasting in renal tubular acidosis (RTA). Its occurrence in type 1 and 2 RTA despite sustained correction of systemic acidosis. *J Clin Invest* **50**:667, 1971.
356. Lightwood R, Payne WW, Black JA: Infantile renal acidosis. *Pediatrics* **12**:628, 1953.
357. Lemann J Jr, Litzow JR, Lemmon EJ: The effects of chronic acid loads in normal man: Further evidence for participation of bone mineral in the defense against chronic metabolic acidosis. *J Clin Invest* **45**:1608, 1975.
358. Backman U, Danielson BG, Johansson G, Ljunghall S, Wikstrom B: Incidence and clinical importance of renal tubular defects in recurrent stone formers. *Nephron* **25**:96, 1980.
359. Albright F, Burnett CH, Parson W, Reifenstein ED Jr, Roos A: Osteomalacia and late rickets: The various etiologies met in the United States with emphasis on that resulting in a specific form of renal acidosis, the therapeutic indications for each etiological sub-group, and the relationship between osteomalacia and Milkman's syndrome. *Medicine (Baltimore)* **25**:399, 1946.
360. Lee SW, Russel JE, Avioli LV: 25-OHD_3 to 1,25-$(OH)_2D_3$ conversion impaired by systemic acidosis. *Science* **195**:944, 1977.
361. Arruda JAL, Nascimento L, Mehta PK, Rademacher DR, Sehy JT, Westenfelder C, Kurtzman NA: The critical importance of urinary concentration ability in the generation of urinary carbon dioxide tension. *J Clin Invest* **60**:922, 1977.
362. Sebastian A, McSherry E, Morris RC Jr: Impaired renal conservation of sodium and chloride during sustained correction of systemic acidosis in patients with type 1, classic renal tubular acidosis. *J Clin Invest* **58**:454, 1976.
363. Rodriquez-Soriano Jr, Vallo A, Castillo G, Oliveras R: Renal handling of water and sodium in children with proximal and distal renal tubular acidosis. *Nephron* **25**:193, 1980.
364. Morris RC Jr, Sebastian A, McSherry E: Therapeutic experience in patients with classic renal tubular acidosis, in *Proceedings of the VII International Congress of Nephrology*. Basel, Karger, 1978, p 345.
365. Harrington TM, Bunch TW, Van Den Berg C: Renal tubular acidosis. A new look at treatment of musculoskeletal and renal disease. *Mayo Clin Proc* **58**:354, 1983.
366. Harrison HE, Chisolm JJ Jr, Harrison HC: Congenital renal tubular acidosis. *Am J Dis Child* **96**:588, 1958.
367. Carlisle EJF, Donnelly SM, Ethier JH, Quagsin SE, Kaiser UB, Vas Uvattakul S, Kamel KS, Halperin MC: Modulation of the secretion of potassium by accompanying anions in humans. *Kidney Int* **39**:1206, 1991.
368. Oetliker OH, Zurbrugg PRP: Renal tubular acidosis in salt-losing syndrome of congenital adrenal hyperplasia (CAH). *J Clin Endocrinol Metab* **31**:447, 1970.
369. Iversen T: Congenital adrenocortical hyperplasia with disturbed electrolyte regulations: "Dysadrenocorticism." *Pediatrics* **16**:875, 1955.
370. New MI, Dupont B, Grumbach K, Levine LS: Congenital adrenal hyperplasia and related conditions, in Stanbury JB, Wyngaarden JB, Fredrickson DS, Goldstein JL, Brown MS (eds): *The Metabolic Basis of Inherited Disease*, 5th ed. New York, McGraw-Hill, 1983, p 973.
371. Henrich WL: Nephrotoxicity of nonsteroidal anti-inflammatory agents. *Am J Kidney Dis* **2**:478, 1983.
372. Dunn MJ: Nonsteroidal antiinflammatory drugs and renal function. *Annu Rev Med* **35**:411, 1984.
373. Sebastian A, Schambelan M, Sutton JM: Amelioration of hyperchloremic acidosis with furosemide therapy in patients with chronic renal insufficiency and type 4 renal tubular acidosis. *Am J Nephrol* **4**:287, 1984.
374. Brautbar N, Levi J, Rosler A, Leitesdorf E, Djaldeti M, Eptstein M, Kleeman CR: Familial hyperkalemia, hy-

pertension and hyporeninemia with normal aldosterone levels. A tubular defect in potassium handling. *Arch Intern Med* **138**:607, 1978.

375. Paver WKA, Pauline GJ: Hypertension and hyperpotassemia without renal disease in a young male. *Med J Aust* **2**:305, 1964.
376. Defronzo RA, Cooke CR, Goldberg M, Cow M, Myers AR, Agus ZS: Impaired renal tubular potassium secretion in systemic lupus erythematosus. *Ann Intern Med* **86**:268, 1977.
377. Batlle DC, Arruda JAL, Kurtzman NA: Hyperkalemic distal renal tubular acidosis associated with obstructive uropathy. *N Engl J Med* **304**:373, 1981.
378. Batlle D, Itsarayoungyven K, Arruda JAL, Kurtzman NA: Hyperkalemic hyperchloremic metabolic acidosis in sickle cell hemoglobinopathies. *Am J Med* **72**:188, 1982.
379. Cogan MG, Arieff AI: Sodium wasting, acidosis and hyperkalemia induced by methicillin interstitial nephritis. Evidence for selective distal tubular dysfunction. *Am J Med* **64**:500, 1978.
380. Defronzo RA, Goldberg M, Cooke CR, Barker C, Grossmann RA, Agus ZS: Investigations into the mechanisms of hyperkalemia following renal transplantation. *Kidney Int* **11**:357, 1977.
381. Gabow PA, Moore S, Schrier RW: Spironalactone-induced hyperchloremic metabolic acidosis in cirrhosis. *Ann Intern Med* **90**:338, 1979.
382. Cohen EP, Bastani B, Cohen MR, Kolner S, Hemkin P, Gluck SL: Absence of H^+-ATPase in cortical collecting tubules of a patient with Sjögen's syndrome and distal renal tubular acidosis. *J Am Soc Neph* **3**:264, 1992.

CHAPTER 122

The Renal Fanconi Syndrome

Michel Bergeron ▪ André Gougoux ▪ Patrick Vinay

1. The renal Fanconi syndrome consists of two components: (1) a generalized dysfunction of the proximal renal tubule leading to impaired proximal reabsorption of amino acids, glucose, phosphate, urate, and bicarbonate, and therefore increased urinary excretion of all these solutes; and (2) a vitamin D–resistant metabolic bone disease—either rickets in growing children or osteomalacia in adults.

2. The renal Fanconi syndrome is either associated with various inborn errors of metabolism or acquired through exposure to various toxic agents. The inherited form may be idiopathic (in the absence of any metabolic disease) or secondary to various primary Mendelian diseases. Cystinosis is the most common cause of a secondary hereditary Fanconi syndrome in children. The degree of cystine accumulation determines three clinical forms of cystinosis: infantile, adolescent, and adult. The Fanconi syndrome disappears in patients with hereditary fructose intolerance, galactosemia, tyrosinemia, and Wilson disease when these disorders are treated by restriction of fructose, galactose, tyrosine, or copper, respectively. Expression of the Fanconi syndrome is linked to the abnormal gene product by way of reversible abnormality of renal metabolism. Other metabolic diseases can also be associated with the Fanconi syndrome: vitamin D dependency, glycogen storage disease, and oculocerebrorenal (Lowe) syndrome.

3. A wide variety of toxic and immunologic tubular injuries may produce the generalized renal dysfunction characteristic of the Fanconi syndrome. Heavy metals (cadmium, uranium, mercury, lead, and platinum), various drugs (especially antibiotics), the urinary excretion of abnormal proteins observed in dysproteinemias, and immunologic disorders are all known to induce a Fanconi syndrome. Maleate and cadmium can be used to produce experimental models in the animal. Finally, the Basenji dog can have a spontaneous Fanconi syndrome.

4. The renal Fanconi syndrome might theoretically result either from multiple transport dysfunctions restricted to the proximal tubule or from concomitant proximal and distal tubular dysfunctions. Some experimental data suggest that, in addition to the proximal disturbance, a distal nephron involvement may play a role in the final production of the aminoaciduria, glycosuria, and phosphaturia observed in the Fanconi syndrome; all these transport defects could result from a decreased entry of molecules into the cell, or an increased efflux at its luminal pole or a combination of both. An impaired mitochondrial production of ATP and a reduced activity of the basolateral membrane Na^+,K^+-ATPase have also been suggested as pathogenetic mechanisms. The presence of physiological intracellular gradients of Na^+, ATP, and ADP may amplify a minor decrease in mitochondrial phosphorylation and translate a modest defect in energy production into a major transport dysfunction. However, further investigation with various experimental models is still needed to clarify: (1) the respective roles of proximal and distal tubule, (2) the contribution of a reduced influx and/or an accelerated efflux of molecules, and (3) the basic cellular defect(s) underlying the disturbed reabsorptive processes.

5. The clinical features of the renal Fanconi syndrome (mostly in affected children) are not specific and result from the renal losses of fluid and electrolytes and the characteristic vitamin D–resistant metabolic bone disease. The most frequent are polyuria, polydipsia, dehydration, hypokalemia, acidosis, impaired growth, and rickets.

In the absence of a specific treatment, the fluids and electrolytes lost have to be replaced, the metabolic bone disease resulting from Fanconi syndrome must be treated, and renal transplantation may be useful when children with nephropathic cystinosis become severely uremic.

A list of standard abbreviations is located immediately preceding the index in each volume.

DEFINITION

The renal Fanconi syndrome (Lignac-de Toni-Debré-Fanconi syndrome) is characterized by two components:

1. A generalized renal tubular dysfunction leading to impaired net proximal reabsorption of amino acids, glucose, phosphate, urate, and bicarbonate and therefore increased urinary excretion of all these solutes.

2. A vitamin D–resistant metabolic bone disease, either rickets in growing children or osteomalacia in adults. Water[1] and solutes, normally reabsorbed by the kidney, could also be lost in the urine: sodium, potassium, calcium, magnesium,[2–5] carnitine,[6] glyceraldehyde,[7] lysozyme,[8,9] and other low-molecular-weight proteins[10] such as peptide hormones, enzymes, and immunoglobulin light chains.

The clinical features are polyuria, dehydration, hypokalemia, acidosis, impaired growth, and rickets.

HISTORICAL SUMMARY

The disease was first recognized in 1903 by Abderhalden,[11] who found cystine crystals in the liver and spleen of a

Table 122-1 Inherited Fanconi Syndrome

IDIOPATHIC (22770, 22780)	
KNOWN PRIMARY MENDELIAN DISEASES IN THE FANCONI SYNDROME:	
Cystinosis (21980, 21990, 22000)	Chap. 126
Hepatorenal tyrosinemia (tyrosinemia type I) (27670)	Chap. 28
Hereditary fructose intolerance (22960)	Chap. 23
Galactosemia (23040)	Chap. 25
Glycogen storage disease type I (23220)	Chap. 24
Wilson disease (27790)	Chap. 68
Vitamin D–dependent rickets (26470)	Chap. 100
Oculocerebrorenal (Lowe) syndrome (30900)	Chap. 123
THE BASENJI DOG	Chap. 122

NOTE: Numbers in parentheses are from the current McKusick catalogues. Inheritance of all disorders is autosomal recessive except Lowe syndrome, which is X-linked recessive. The chapter numbers indicate where these diseases are described in greater detail in this edition.

21-month-old infant and called the disorder a "familial cystine diathesis"—considered an inherited susceptibility conferring chemical individuality. In 1924, Lignac[12] described three similar cases in children with severe rickets, dwarfism, renal disease, and progressive wasting. In 1931, Fanconi described rickets and stunted growth in a child with glucosuria and albuminuria.[13] After de Toni in 1933[14] and Debré et al. in 1934[15] had reported similar cases, Fanconi in 1936 recognized the similarity between these few reported cases and suggested for this syndrome the name of "nephrotic-glycosuric dwarfism with hypophosphatemic rickets."[16] This name, which is sometimes referred to in the literature as the "Lignac-de Toni-Debré-Fanconi syndrome," was reduced to "Fanconi syndrome" by McCune et al.[17] in 1943.

ETIOLOGIC CLASSIFICATION

The Fanconi syndrome can be associated either with various inborn errors of metabolism (Table 122-1) or acquired from a wide variety of experiences (Table 122-2).

Genetic Causes

Idiopathic. This condition occurs in the absence of any recognized inherited metabolic disease, and its diagnosis can be made only when all the possible acquired causes and various inborn errors of metabolism producing Fanconi syndrome can be excluded. Most cases are sporadic in occurrence, but some familial forms have also been described, most often transmitted in an autosomal dominant fashion.[18–22] Various abnormalities of carbohydrate metabolism have been described in some patients with idiopathic Fanconi syndrome.[23,24]

Known Primary Mendelian Diseases in the Fanconi Syndrome. Several inborn errors of metabolism have been reported to induce a Fanconi syndrome, including abnormalities in the metabolism of amino acids (cystinosis, tyrosinemia) and carbohydrates (hereditary fructose intolerance, galactosemia, glycogen storage disease).

Cystinosis. This autosomal recessive disorder associated with the intralysosomal accumulation of cystine in different tissues of the body[25,26] is the inherited metabolic disease most commonly associated with Fanconi syndrome in children.[27] According to the degree of cystine accumulation, three clinical forms of the disease have been recognized:

1. The infantile or nephropathic cystinosis, characterized by onset of signs and symptoms within the first year of life and progressive renal failure leading to terminal uremia toward the end of the first decade.[28,29]
2. The adolescent or intermediate cystinosis appearing during the second decade of life.[30]
3. The adult or benign form of cystinosis without Fanconi syndrome or impaired renal function.[31]

Only the infantile and adolescent forms are accompanied by Fanconi syndrome. Cystinosis is discussed further in Chap. 126.

Table 122-2 Acquired Fanconi Syndrome

Heavy metals
- Cadmium
- Uranium
- Mercury
- Lead
- Platinum

Drugs
- Antibiotics
  - Outdated tetracycline
  - Aminoglycosides: gentamicin and others
- Others
  - Valproate
  - 6-Mercaptopurine
  - Methyl-3-chromone
  - Lysol
  - Paraquat
  - Toluene

Urinary excretion of abnormal proteins
- Multiple myeloma
- Other dysproteinemias

Immunologic disorders
- Nephrotic syndrome
- Interstitial nephritis with antitubular basement membrane antibodies
- Renal transplantation
- Malignancy

Experimental models
- Maleate
- Cadmium
- Cystine dimethylester
- 4-pentenoate
- Fructose (in hereditary fructose intolerance)

Hepatorenal Tyrosinemia (Tyrosinemia Type I). When the ingestion of tyrosine or phenylalanine is not restricted, the Fanconi syndrome is induced in patients with this autosomal recessive disease and will disappear with the dietary restriction of these two amino acids. However, this therapeutic maneuver does not prevent the progressive hepatic failure that is responsible for the death of these children within the first decade of life. In this disease, an increased urinary excretion of succinylacetone is observed, a substance found to decrease the uptake of glucose and amino acids by rat renal brush-border membrane vesicles.[32] The various disorders of tyrosine metabolism are discussed in Chap. 28.

Hereditary Fructose Intolerance. In this autosomal recessive disorder associated with deficient activity of fructose 1-phosphate aldolase, the intravenous infusion of fructose rapidly induces an accumulation of fructose 1-phosphate, an intracellular depletion of inorganic phosphate, and a reversible and complete Fanconi syndrome, with the markedly increased urinary excretion of the characteristic substances.[33,34] The renal toxicity is probably related to the depletion of inorganic phosphate and the reduction of ATP[35] in the renal cortex. Because the infusion of fructose induces within minutes a reversible Fanconi syndrome, this is a very useful experimental model utilized to study the human Fanconi syndrome. Hereditary fructose intolerance is discussed in Chap. 23.

Galactosemia. The autosomal recessively inherited deficiency of galactose 1-phosphate uridyltransferase (catalyzing the transformation of galactose 1-phosphate into glucose 1-phosphate) leads to accumulation of galactose 1-phosphate. It is associated with an incomplete Fanconi syndrome that is reversible with the removal of lactose or galactose from the diet.[36] The toxic product is presumably the accumulated galactose 1-phosphate, which could also deplete the intracellular inorganic phosphate in a fashion similar to that observed in hereditary fructose intolerance. Galactosemia is discussed in Chap. 25.

Glycogen Storage Disease (Type I). The type with autosomal recessive inheritance and galactose intolerance is associated with Fanconi syndrome.[37] Glycogen storage diseases are discussed in Chap. 24.

Wilson Disease. This autosomal recessive disorder of copper metabolism, primarily affecting the liver and the brain (hepatolenticular degeneration), is also accompanied by copper accumulation in the renal cortex and the various tubular defects characteristic of Fanconi syndrome,[38] both of which can be reversed when copper is chelated by penicillamine.[39] The following clinical triad is characteristic of this disease: (1) hepatic cirrhosis; (2) a wide variety of neurologic symptoms; and (3) the Kayser-Fleischer rings in the cornea. Wilson disease is discussed in Chap. 68.

Vitamin D Dependency (Type I). In this autosomal recessive disorder, the 1α hydroxylation of 25-hydroxycholecalciferol in the kidney mitochondria is apparently defective, a phenomenon that induces decreased intestinal absorption of calcium, hypocalcemia, and parathyroid hormone excess. This disease is discussed in Chap. 100.

Oculocerebrorenal (Lowe) Syndrome. Originally described by Lowe and his coworkers in 1952[40] and characterized by a Fanconi syndrome, rickets (or osteomalacia in a few patients), growth retardation, bilateral congenital cataracts, glaucoma, generalized muscular hypotonia, hyporeflexia, and severe mental retardation, this syndrome often becomes apparent during the first year of life (see Chap. 123). In this familial disorder, transmitted as an X-linked recessive trait,[41] the great majority of the cases have been observed in boys, although a few have been reported in girls.[42] Cortical opacities can also be found in the lenses of heterozygotes,[43,44] suggesting the possibility of another mode of inheritance. There are three distinct phases in the natural history of this inborn error of metabolism: (1) during infancy, neurologic and ophthalmologic manifestations predominate, but the various tubular dysfunctions of the Fanconi syndrome may all appear within the first year of life; (2) during childhood, severe rickets, growth failure, and the Fanconi syndrome are obvious; and (3) later, the patient dies from inanition, pneumonia, and chronic renal failure.

Although the specific defect responsible for Lowe syndrome remains unknown, the increased urinary excretion of mucopolysaccharides, chondroitin sulfate, and hydroxyproline[45,46] either suggests an abnormal metabolism in connective tissue or simply reflects the metabolic bone disease. Early in the course of the disease, renal dysfunction is tubular but is followed by a progressive reduction of GFR. The finding that the mitochondrial changes and the functional defects are both proximal suggests a relationship between anatomic and physiological abnormalities.[42] The tubular changes observed with renal biopsy are not specific,[47] whereas variable pathological changes have been described in the central nervous system, the eyes, the skeletal muscles, and other tissues. Since the possible biochemical abnormality underlying this disorder remains unknown, there is no specific diagnostic test and treatment. However, vitamin D therapy is useful to treat the metabolic bone disease, as is the case for the Fanconi syndrome associated with other inborn errors of metabolism.

Spontaneous Animal Model: The Basenji Dog. A spontaneous animal model resembling the human idiopathic Fanconi syndrome has been found in Basenji dogs.[48–51] They show clinical signs analogous to those found in humans: polydipsia, polyuria, dehydration, weight loss, and weakness; renal failure occurs after months or years. Plasma electrolytes in these dogs were normal, with the exception of a moderate metabolic acidosis. Glucosuria, phosphaturia, and a generalized aminoaciduria along with elevated sodium, potassium, and urea excretion were documented in all affected animals. Renal biopsies were normal, but when renal failure was present, various degrees of tubular and glomerular damage were found.

Acquired Causes

Table 122-2 lists a wide variety of toxic and immunologic renal tubular injuries that may produce the generalized impairment of net proximal tubular reabsorption characteristic of the Fanconi syndrome. In contrast to the Fanconi syndrome observed with various inherited metabolic diseases, these acquired Fanconi syndromes are seen primarily in adults, although some can occur at any age.

Heavy Metals. Among the heavy metals that can bind selectively to the proximal tubular cells and induce the reabsorptive dysfunctions characteristic of the Fanconi syndrome, lead was the most frequent cause but now cadmium is the agent most commonly responsible. These induced tubular dysfunctions are reversible when exposure to the toxic environment ceases.

Cadmium. After a prolonged occupational or environmental exposure to cadmium of many years, its excessive accumulation in the kidney is responsible for chronic nephrotoxicity.[52] The increased excretion of the low-molecular-weight β_2 microglobulin, an indicator of renal tubular damage, can allow the early detection of cadmium nephrotoxicity.[53]

Fanconi syndrome appears frequently among workers exposed to cadmium,[54] a finding which has stimulated many investigators to study the experimental cadmium-induced nephropathy in many animal models, including the rabbit[55,56] and the rat.[57–59] Many cases were described after World War II in Japan in middle-aged, postmenopausal, multiparous women; their disease, characterized by severe osteomalacia, is known as the itai-itai, or "ouch-ouch" disease.[60–62] Intoxication came from soil and rice fields contaminated with cadmium in the Jinzu River Basin.

Uranium. Exposure to gaseous uranium compounds has also been associated with Fanconi syndrome. Uranium and cadmium are more toxic than are lead and mercury.[54]

Mercury. The accumulation of mercury in the proximal tubular cells after exposure to inorganic mercury salts or organic mercury compounds (mercurial diuretics) can also produce a reversible Fanconi syndrome.[5]

Lead. In lead poisoning, intranuclear inclusion bodies containing lead bound to a protein appear in proximal tubular cells,[63] and a reversible Fanconi syndrome has been observed, especially in acutely intoxicated children.[64]

Platinum. Cisplatin (*cis*-diaminedichloroplatinum II) is a new and potent chemotherapeutic agent used very effectively in the treatment of many carcinomas, particularly testicular and ovarian. Dose-dependent nephrotoxicity with reduced GFR results from the use of this drug.[65] Among the various tubular dysfunctions observed, the most important clinically is the severe urinary loss of magnesium, inducing severe magnesium depletion and hypomagnesemia.[66]

Drugs. The tubular dysfunctions characteristic of Fanconi syndrome have also been described with the utilization of several drugs and are reversible when the responsible agent is discontinued.

The ingestion of *outdated tetracycline* produces a reversible Fanconi syndrome.[67,68] Among the degradation products of tetracycline, outdated or stored in a moist warm environment, anhydro-4-epi-tetracycline has been shown to be the intoxicating substance responsible for the tubulopathy.[69] In rats this metabolite induces mitochondrial injury in proximal nephron and decreases oxidative enzymatic activity and energy production.[70] Most cases of Fanconi syndrome resulting from *aminoglycoside antibiotics* have been associated with the use of gentamicin. Renal magnesium and potassium wasting with severe hypomagnesemia and hypokalemia have also been observed with aminoglycoside antibiotics,[71,72] substances well known to accumulate selectively in proximal tubular cell.[73] A reversible Fanconi syndrome has been reported with the anticonvulsant *valproate*.[74] Some patients with nephrotic syndrome and receiving *6-mercaptopurine* have also had Fanconi syndrome.[75] It is not easy in these patients to dissociate the respective contribution of the nephrotic syndrome and of the 6-mercaptopurine administration. The accidental ingestion of large amounts of *methyl-3-chromone*, a substance structurally related to tetracycline, has also been reported to induce a reversible Fanconi syndrome.[76] Finally, a Fanconi syndrome has been recognized following an extensive *Lysol* burn,[77] the ingestion of the herbicide *paraquat*,[78] *toluene* inhalation,[79] and ifosfamide chemotherapy.[80]

Urinary Excretion of Abnormal Proteins. *Multiple myeloma* and *other dysproteinemias* are a frequent cause of acquired Fanconi syndrome in adults,[81] which in some patients may even precede by many years the appearance of dysproteinemia.[82] Indeed, this diagnosis of dysproteinemia must be excluded in all adult patients with a Fanconi syndrome of obscure cause. Bence Jones proteinuria is always present[82]; all patients have light chains of the κ variety, except a few with λ light chains.[83] Crystalline inclusion bodies and nonamyloid microfibrils probably representing light-chain accumulation, can be observed in the cytoplasm of proximal tubular cells.[81,82,84] These light chains might therefore be directly toxic to the proximal tubular cells[85] or to a specific enzyme such as Na^+,K^+-ATPase.[86] Renal tubular transport abnormalities can disappear after the successful therapy of multiple myeloma and the disappearance of urinary Bence Jones protein.[87] Amyloidosis,[88,89] light-chain nephropathy, [90–92] and benign monoclonal gammopathy[93] are among the dysproteinemias other than multiple myeloma reported to induce Fanconi syndrome and urinary excretion of monoclonal light chains.

Immunologic Disorders. Fanconi syndrome has been reported in *nephrotic syndrome*,[94] most often with focal and segmental glomerular sclerosis,[95] but the pathogenesis remains uncertain. *Interstitial nephritis with antitubular basement membrane antibodies* (linear deposits along the basement membrane of the proximal tubules) may be accompanied by a Fanconi syndrome. A reversible Fanconi syndrome has also been observed in several patients following *renal transplantation*,[96–98] and the defects of proximal reabsorption, most probably resulting from immunologic tubular injury during acute rejection episodes, seem to disappear during the first year following transplantation. The immunosuppressive drug cyclosporine does not seem to be responsible for the various defects of proximal reabsorption.[99] Some tumors, such as nonossifying fibroma of bone, can also produce Fanconi syndrome, possibly through the release of a humoral factor.[100] Lymphoid *malignancies* with peritubular infiltrates have been associated with a Fanconi syndrome and could result either from immunologic tubular injury or from tubular destruction by tumor infiltration.[101] The simultaneous occurrence of a Fanconi syndrome and other malignancies such as carcinoma of the lung,[102] liver,[103] pancreas,[104] and ovary[105] may be fortuitous.

Experimental Models. *Maleate*, first used by Berliner et al. in the dog,[106] was found by Harrison and Harrison[107] to induce a Fanconi syndrome in rats. Maleate still remains a model widely used to study the mechanisms and pathogenesis of this complex renal tubular dysfunction.[108] *Cadmium* has been utilized extensively[47–50] and *cystine dimethylester* has produced the Fanconi syndrome in rats.[109] *4-Pentenoate* has also been shown to produce an experimental Fanconi syndrome in dogs.[110]

MECHANISMS AND PATHOGENESIS

General Characteristics

The pathogenetic mechanisms underlying the Fanconi syndrome remain to be elucidated as do, more specifically, the respective contributions of the proximal and distal nephron, the organelles involved, the membrane transport defects, or the possibly abnormal enzymatic activities. However, many conclusions can be drawn from study of the hereditary or the acquired diseases as well as of the experimental models.

1. The Fanconi syndrome clearly has *two components*: a multiple renal transport disorder and a metabolic bone disease—rickets in children or osteomalacia in adults. Since the bone disease is not always present, the primary disturbance in this syndrome could be thought to be renal. In fact, some of the etiologic agents might have direct effects on both bone and kidney, whereas others might have an effect only on kidney.

2. Since amino acids, glucose, phosphate, and other molecules are transported into the cells by multiple carriers, it is hard to visualize how point mutations could disturb simultaneously so many of these. It is more likely that the various mutations associated with the Mendelian forms of the Fanconi syndrome affect components of the transport mechanism other than the carrier(s) per se. The modified critical step has to be *global* enough to affect many transport functions. Such a step could be a disruption of the energy source, a generalized nonspecific membrane permeability defect, or a specific organelle pathology.

3. In many cases, the Fanconi syndrome is expressed only when well-defined factors are present, such as the unrestricted intake of tyrosine and phenylalanine in tyrosinemia[111–113] or the ingestion of fructose in hereditary fructose intolerance.[33,34,114] Reciprocally, when galactose is removed in galactosemia,[36,115] fructose in hereditary fructose intolerance,[33,114] or tyrosine and phenylalanine in tyrosinemia,[116–119] the Fanconi syndrome is no longer expressed. These observations demonstrate the *reversibility* of the abnormality leading to the Fanconi syndrome.

4. The *duration of exposure* to the specific agent also appears to be an important element but varies with the disease underlying the Fanconi syndrome. Intravenous injection of small amounts of fructose to patients with hereditary fructose intolerance increases the excretion of amino acids, phosphate, glucose, and other electrolytes in a dose-dependent fashion.[33,34] On the other hand, patients with galactosemia have to ingest galactose for days[36] before the renal dysfunction occurs, whereas, by contrast, hepatic dysfunction can be noted within minutes.[120] Renal tubular dysfunction caused by cadmium occurs after many years of exposure to a polluted environment or to industrial cadmium (pigment, plastic, alloy, accumulator battery, nuclear and electronic industries).[52–55] Lead can induce a Fanconi syndrome in acutely intoxicated children almost exclusively,[64,121] in experimental animals,[122] and, rarely, in chronic states.

5. A *specific biochemical sequence* of events can take place, as illustrated in patients with hereditary fructose intolerance: following a fructose infusion, an accumulation of fructose 1-phosphate in proximal tubular cells is postulated to result from the deficiency of aldolase B activity; a severe depletion of inorganic phosphate, ATP, and total adenine nucleotides ensues and might contribute to the multiple transport disorders of the Fanconi syndrome.[123] Any interruption of this sequence of events could prevent the pathologic manifestations. Since in normal humans, rats, and dogs the administration of large amounts of fructose does not induce a Fanconi syndrome, despite the hepatic and renal cortical accumulation of large amounts of fructose 1-phosphate,[124–126] Morris et al.[123] have suggested that the genetic defect is primary and that abnormalities other than the kinetic deficiency of the enzyme are secondarily involved.

Nephron Segment(s) Involved

In normal mammalian kidneys, the reabsorptive capacity of proximal tubular cells is immense for amino acids since most of the filtered load is reabsorbed within the first few millimeters of the proximal nephron[127]; in fact, less than 2 percent of the filtered load of amino acids will appear in the urine, with the exception of aspartic acid, glycine, and histidine, of which only 94 to 98 percent are reabsorbed.[128] In the Fanconi syndrome, the aminoaciduria is generalized, with the pattern of excretion appearing to be similar to normal.[129] The absence of selective aminoaciduria does not point toward a specific lesion of a carrier or even to a specific segment.

Morphological Changes. A "swan-neck lesion," resulting from cell atrophy in the earliest portion of the proximal tubule, was found at autopsy in a few patients with cystinosis and was thought for many years to be the cause of transport dysfunction.[130] This is not likely, since micropuncture studies have demonstrated that the entire length and not only the early part of the proximal nephron has the capacity to reabsorb amino acids.[127] The popularity of this explanation can be attributed to the beauty of the image given as evidence rather than to a critical assessment of the data: this hypothesis should be forgotten. The cell atrophy observed is most probably secondary, since the emergence of the swan-neck lesion in cystinosis is progressive with age and not related to the transport dysfunction. Nonspecific tubular and glomerular lesions were also documented in renal biopsies of patients with Lowe syndrome.[41,131]

Major morphologic lesions were not found in many reported cases of human Fanconi syndrome such as hereditary tyrosinemia,[113] galactosemia,[36] fructosemia,[123] heavy metal poisoning, and various other forms.[18,132] Renal biopsies from Basenji dogs with the Fanconi syndrome showed normal histology; various degrees of tubular and glomerular damage were found only when renal failure was present.[49,50] It should be pointed out, however, that the absence of morphologic lesions does not mean the absence of functional disturbance; for instance, histologic lesions are seldom observed in most specific transport defects.

In the experimental models of Fanconi syndrome, ultrastructural modifications were always found in the proximal tubule,[9,133–137] but varied from cell to cell: extensive cytoplasmic vacuolization, darkening or swelling of the mitochondrial matrix, enlargement of the lysosomes, disruption of cytoplasmic organization, distension of the granular ER, loss of basolateral membrane infoldings, and even cell necrosis. Maleate and heavy metals are readily filtered, and the early part of the proximal nephron is therefore first exposed to their deleterious effects; for instance, Gonick and Kramer showed that cadmium specifically accumulates in proximal tubular cells of the renal cortex.[59] Toxic compounds containing heavy metals also yielded similar lesions. All these ultrastructural changes are reversible within a few days after cessation of maleate or cadmium administration. Several investigators[133,136,137] have found maleate-induced morphologic injury restricted to proximal tubular cells, with the distal tubule appearing normal. By contrast, the distal nephron was also found to be damaged when larger doses of maleate were given.[134,135]

Functional Changes. Maleate decreases phosphate uptake in rat brush-border membrane vesicles.[138] Evidence of proximal nephron damage is suggested by the significant impairment by maleate of the 1 hydroxylation of 25-hydroxyvitamin D_3 in the mitochondria of proximal cells.[139–141] Maleate also affects the γ-glutamyl transpeptidase, a membrane-bound enzyme of the proximal nephron.[142] However, the Fanconi syndrome might theoretically result either from multiple transport dysfunctions restricted to the proximal tubule or from concomitant proximal and distal tubular dysfunctions.[143] Therefore, based on morphologic alterations and on data obtained with micropuncture studies in rats[143] and dogs,[144] some investigators have suggested that maleate has additional sites of action located more distally than the proximal convoluted tubule, namely the thick ascending limb[145] or other parts of the distal nephron. Similarly, micropuncture and free water clearance studies have shown that maleate,[146,147] like acetazolamide,[148,149] has an effect on the thick ascending limb; while sodium chloride and sodium bicarbonate reabsorption were both inhibited in the proximal nephron, chloride but not bicarbonate was reabsorbed by the thick ascending limb. However, one in vitro study has revealed a marked difference between the metabolic findings in renal cortical tubules and the absence of effect in thick ascending limbs.[150] Bergeron et al.[143,151] have suggested that maleate induces an accelerated cellular efflux of amino acids, glucose, and phosphate into the lumen of both proximal and distal nephron. However, in proximal tubular cells the membrane transport carriers still demonstrate the same structural requirements for their substrates, as observed in experimental animals[143,152,153] as well as in humans in whom a competitive inhibition between glycine and amino acids has been reported.[154] Since they are still functioning, albeit at a reduced rate,[153] both the decreased entry from lumen to cell and the increased efflux from cell to lumen can be partially or totally corrected downstream; such is not the case in the distal nephron, where there is no reabsorption of amino acids[127] and little absorption of phosphate and glucose.[144] Molecules that exit at this distal site are irrevocably lost in the urine. Thus, in addition to the proximal disturbance, a distal nephron involvement may be a major determinant in the final production of the aminoaciduria, glycosuria, and phosphaturia seen in the Fanconi syndrome. This is further suggested by the increased urinary-minus-blood P_{CO_2} gradient[155–158] and the increased kaliuresis in maleate-treated animals,[155] both of which could reflect an accelerated cellular exit of hydrogen and potassium ions into the lumen of the last segments of the nephron.

Membrane Permeability Alteration

Increased urinary excretion of electrolytes and nonelectrolytes does not necessarily mean decreased influx or entry alone. Hyperexcretion could result at the tubular level either from defective entry into the cell or from an increased exit of molecules from the cell at its luminal pole. Both mechanisms appear to act in the maleate model.[143,144,151,153,159,160] The in vitro studies of Rosenberg and Segal,[159] later confirmed by in vivo studies of Bergeron et al.,[143,151] have clearly shown the preponderant role of cellular efflux as opposed to decreased influx in explaining the low intracellular concentration of amino acids and sugars in maleate-treated kidneys.[161,162] These efflux data suggest a maleate-induced impairment of the barrier function of the membrane, as illustrated by the increased cellular exit of amino acids,[143,151,159] sugars,[143,144,160] potassium,[155,163] and bicarbonate[146,155,158,164] (Fig. 122-1).

Maleic anhydride has been shown to react rapidly and specifically with the amino groups associated with the protein fraction of the red-cell membrane: sodium and potassium permeability was increased while that of sulfate and chloride was reduced, suggesting a specific action of maleate on the membrane physicochemical properties.[165] In contrast, in the study of Le Grimellec et al.,[166] maleate did not alter the composition and the physical status of brush-border and basolateral membranes obtained from dog kidney cortex; similarly, vesicles obtained from brush-border membranes of rats[167] and dogs[168] were not influenced by maleate, although this could be explained by the reversibility of the action of maleate.[129] Actually, maleate does not have to modify the physical chemistry of membranes to affect their permeability, since this could also be achieved by its chelating properties.[152,169] The divalent anion maleate could chelate divalent cations (Mg^{2+} and Ca^{2+}) essential to the maintenance of membrane stability. Silverman and Huang[160] have shown that the cytoplasmic face of cell membranes appears to be modified by maleate: by using indicators to localize the interactions of various sugars at either the internal or external side of these membrane surfaces, they concluded that the glycosuria found in maleate-treated dogs could be related to the movement of cytoplasmic glucose back across the brush border into the urine or could be attributed to partial inhibition of glucose movement from the cytoplasm across the antiluminal membrane. In vitro studies of Rosenberg and Segal[159] and in vivo studies of Bergeron et al.,[143] Wen,[144] Maesaka and McCaffery,[170] and Günther et al.[153] are all compatible with such a membrane effect of maleate at the cytoplasmic leaflet. Maleate could thus affect the membrane transfer of amino acids and other molecules at both proximal and distal nephron sites. Studies of the maleate-induced lysozymuria carried out by Christensen and Maunsbach[9] further illustrated the maleate-induced membrane derangement; they demonstrated that, in proximal cells, the transport of lysozyme from endocytic vacuoles to lysosomes was partially inhibited by maleate, leading to an accumulation of these vacuoles in the apical cytoplasm and a disappearance of apical tubules, and suggesting an altered recycling of membranes. The mere volume of these numerous vacuoles observed in all studies certainly contributes to organelle dysfunction; this distension factor has always been underestimated. In fact, Pfaller et al. have shown that these fused apical vesicles reflect an enhanced exocytosis phenomenon of lysosomal, mitochondrial, and cystolic enzymes.[171]

Maleate, cadmium, and tetracyclines all have specific, albeit reversible, effects not only on plasma membranes but also on organelles and their interrelationships.[59,135,136] Mitochondria seem to concentrate cadmium, mercury, and maleate.[57,59] The decreased activity of 25-hydroxyvitamin D_3-1-hydroxylase,[139] an enzyme localized in renal cortical mitochondria,[140] suggests that these chemicals can affect their membranes as well. The ER is also markedly affected

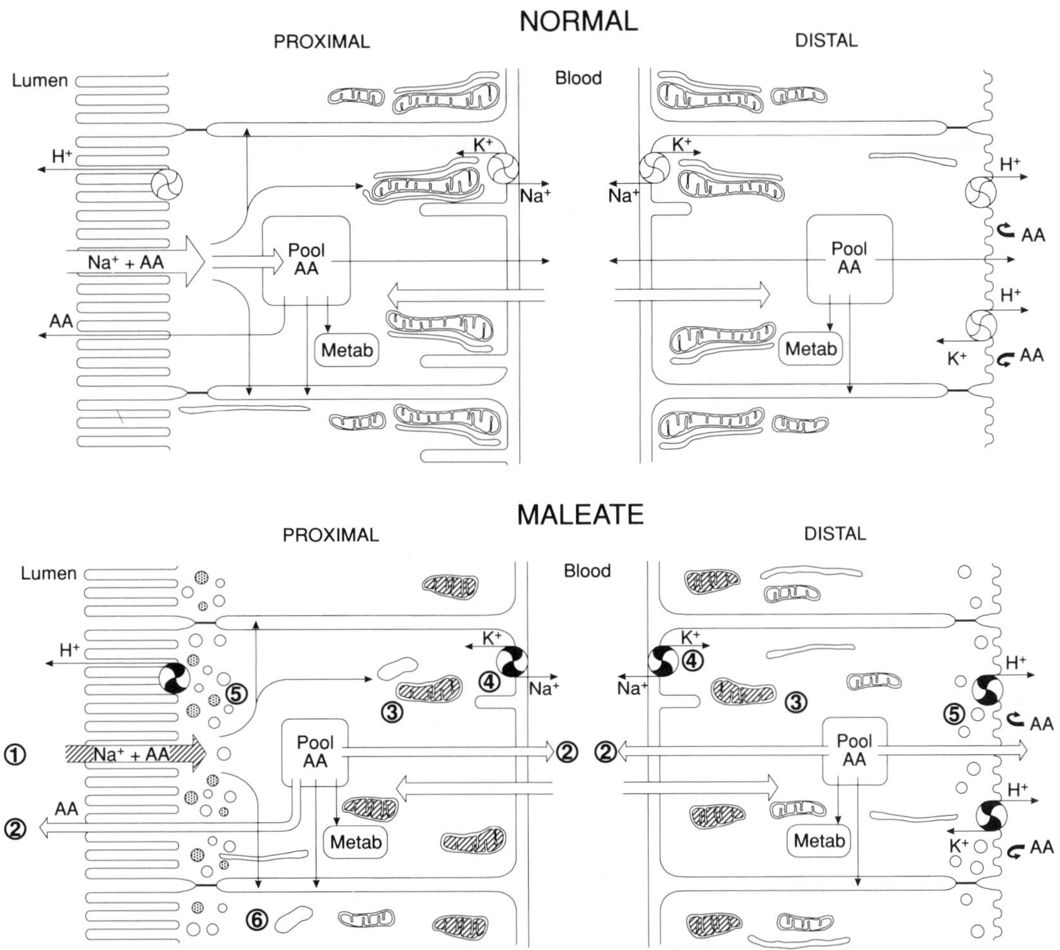

FIG. 122-1 *Upper panel*: Movements of amino acids in the normal nephron. At the level of proximal tubule, amino acids (AA) gain access to the cell through the apical microvilli or through the infoldings of the antiluminal membrane. Intracellular accumulation of amino acids can be against a concentration gradient. At the brush border, uptake is a carrier-mediated process and, when coupled to a sodium gradient (Na^+ output > Na^+ intake), is "secondary active" transport. Efflux can occur at all membranes. Amino acids can also be metabolized (Metab) in the renal tubular cell. In the distal tubule, similar amino acid movements (efflux and influx) occur except that there is no entry from the lumen of amino acids and little, if any, of glucose and phosphate.

In the maleate model (*lower panel*), morphologic changes in renal epithelium are dose-dependent and vary from minor cytoplasmic vacuolization, mitochondrial swelling, and dilatation of ER cisternae, to cell disorganization and even necrosis. Intracellular accumulation of amino acids is decreased, despite reduced but adequate entry at the luminal site. However, efflux of amino acids is markedly increased, offset (partially or totally) in the proximal nephron by the high reabsorption capacity of these cells. Because no absorption takes place at the luminal membrane of the distal nephron, the excessive loss of molecules by efflux is not offset, and they appear in the final urine. This schematic view is based on data of various authors quoted in the text. The renal Fanconi syndrome could be explained by several mechanisms: (1) A defective entry of molecules at the proximal nephron. Most solutes lost in the urine are coupled to luminal reabsorption of sodium. (2) A defective entry in proximal cells coupled with an increased backleak of molecules from both proximal and distal cells. Although backflux can be corrected downstream in the proximal tubule, molecules that exit at the distal nephron sites are irrevocably lost in the urine. This is why a distal nephron involvement, in addition to the defective entry at the proximal apical membrane, may be a major determinant in vivo. (3) An impaired energy production. Maleate, for example, decreases the mitochondrial oxidation of Krebs cycle intermediates (especially the CoA-dependent substrates). (4) A reduced NA^+,K^+-ATPase activity at the basolateral membranes, which could affect the sodium gradient. (5) A derangement at the H^+-ATPase (see Fig. 122-2). (6) Organelle pathology and disorganization (ER, mitochondrion, etc.), a deranged recycling of membrane transport proteins, etc.

by maleate both structurally and chemically. A disturbance of the close association between the ER, the mitochondrion and the basolateral membranes must result in profound effects on cellular metabolism and function. A major modification between mitochondria and the network of perimitochondrial membranes was noted by Bergeron and Laporte[135] in the maleate model and by Gonick and Kramer[59] in the cadmium model.

An experimental model of the Fanconi syndrome has been produced in rats by repeated injections of cadmium chloride and was extensively studied by various investigators.[59,172,173] The signs typical of Fanconi syndrome appeared abruptly after 3 weeks of injection and the total administration of about 2.25 mg of cadmium. Mitochondrial enlargement and loss of basolateral membrane infoldings were the most conspicuous morphologic changes. ATP levels decreased by 38 percent and Na^+,K^+-ATPase activity by 60 percent. Kägi and Vallee[174] described the formation of a low-molecular-weight metalloprotein, metallothionein, which has a high sulfhydryl content (cysteine) and metal content (cadmium and zinc). The cadmium metallothionein is synthesized by the liver, filtered by the glomeruli, and reabsorbed proximally.[175] The proximal tubule appears to be more susceptible to the cadmium–metallothionein[176] or cadmium–

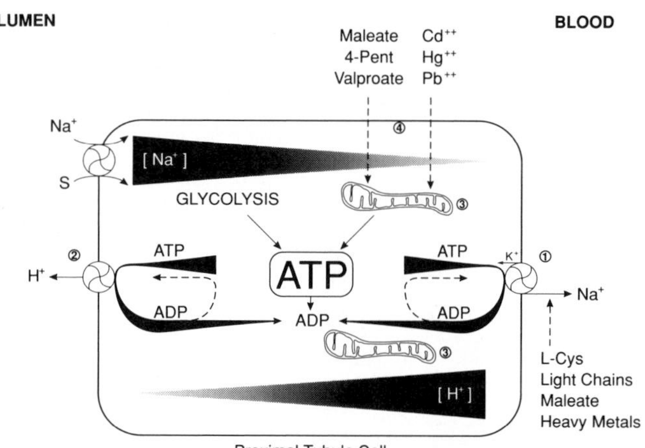

FIG. 122-2 Schematic summary of possible sites of various agents producing the renal Fanconi syndrome. The proximal tubular cell is shown with the intracellular gradients for Na^+ and H^+ (shaded triangles), whose gradients vary in opposite directions and are established by the activity of the basolateral Na^+, K^+-ATPase (1) for the former and by the activity of the apical H^+ ATPase (2) for the latter. Concomitantly ATP and ADP concentration gradients (black arrows) are built up by the compartmentation of membrane ATPases and mitochondrial synthetase (3). The coexistence of Na^+ and ATP gradients may amplify the functional consequences of small changes in ATP:ADP ratio on sodium and proton pumps. Similarly, modest alterations of pump activities induced by various agents which will act at various (4) cell sites (plasma membrane, mitochondria, ER, organelle organization, etc.) may influence markedly the cellular gradients with secondary effects on transepithelial transport.

cysteine[177] complex than to the inorganic cadmium. The protein degradation in the kidney liberates the metal, which is then incorporated into nascent chains of thionein within the kidney. The delayed onset of renal tubular dysfunction seen in cadmium exposure is most likely related to its interaction with the thionein. Raghavan and Gonick[58] offered the hypothesis that the Fanconi syndrome resulted from a saturation of the cadmium-binding capacity of the renal cortical metallothionein; the excess cadmium was then free to "spill" over from the soluble cytoplasmic fraction to other subcellular fractions, in particular the microsomal and mitochondrial fractions containing cadmium-sensitive enzymes. As mentioned above, renal cortical ATP levels and Na^+,K^+-ATPase activities were reduced when the manifestations of the Fanconi syndrome were maximal in these animals (Fig. 122-2).

The Basenji dog model actually suggests a defect only at the substrate entry step. As demonstrated by Bovee et al.,[49] glycine, lysine, and α-methyl-D-glucose uptake were all impaired in slices obtained from renal biopsies of affected dogs. A change in the lipid bilayer of the renal cellular membranes, increasing their fluidity, has been suggested.[178]

Basic Cellular Defect(s)

Maleate could directly inhibit the Na^+,K^+-ATPase activity at the basolateral membrane, a phenomenon which would affect secondarily the electrochemical sodium gradient across the luminal membrane; alternatively, maleate could interfere at some intracellular site (like the mitochondrion) and reduce the production of ATP required for active reabsorption. Either hypothesis could account for all the transport defects observed in the Fanconi syndrome. In this regard, it is of interest that the reabsorption of each solute lost in the urine is coupled to sodium reabsorption across the luminal membrane of proximal cells: Na^+–H^+ exchange (bicarbonate reabsorption), Na^+–glucose cotransport, Na^+–amino acid cotransport, and Na^+–phosphate cotransport.

Reductions in renal cortical ATP concentration[134,163,179] and renal cortical Na^+,K^+-ATPase activity[163] have been reported following maleate administration, but a causal relationship between the decreased ATP level and the inhibited tubular transport of various solutes has not been established unequivocally. Intestinal transport of glucose and amino acids was unaffected by maleate, while sodium absorption and Na^+,K^+-ATPase activity were markedly impaired.[180] Maleate has been shown to decrease markedly the mitochondrial oxidation of Krebs cycle intermediates in the kidney,[181] especially the CoA-dependent substrates such as pyruvate and α-ketoglutarate.[179,182,183] Maleate has also been shown to impair significantly the 1-hydroxylation of 25-hydroxyvitamin D_3 in the mitochondria of proximal tubular cells.[139–141] A decrease in renal cortical ATP concentration has also been observed after the infusion of 4-pentenoate, another metabolic inhibitor inducing an experimental Fanconi syndrome.[110] In the rabbit model of cystinotic Fanconi syndrome, intracellular ATP depletion plays a major role in the inhibition of proximal tubule active transport resulting from intracellular cystine loading.[184,185] Mercury has been shown to be a potent inhibitor of the Na^+,K^+-ATPase,[186] acting primarily on its intracellular side[187] and facilitating release of the α-subunit from the lipid membrane.[188]

The protective effect of acetoacetate on the maleate-induced bicarbonaturia and phosphaturia results from competition between acetoacetate (which is the physiological substrate for succinyl CoA transferase) and maleate for the transfer of CoA.[189] Phosphate loading can also prevent the maleate-induced Fanconi syndrome and decrease the urinary excretion of bicarbonate, amino acids,[190] lysozyme, and lysosomal enzymes.[8] This protective effect of phosphate suggests that a phosphate-dependent metabolic abnormality in proximal tubular cells might play an important role in the pathogenesis of the maleate-induced Fanconi syndrome.

A Physiopathological Hypothesis

The following is our hypothesis to explain the renal Fanconi syndrome: A syndrome in which dysfunction of multiple transport systems is noted may be related to a basic and relatively nonspecific defect. If one considers the special situation of polarized transporting epithelia, such as the proximal tubule, a minor anomaly in the rate of mitochondrial phosphorylation resulting in a minor fall in ATP and a minor rise in ADP may explain the disease. We would like to propose that an amplification of such a defect due to the presence of physiological intracellular gradients of Na^+, ATP, and ADP may translate a modest defect in energy production into a major transport dysfunction (see Fig. 122-2).

Sodium Gradient. Sodium enters proximal cells largely through solute–Na^+cotransport systems located on the luminal membrane. The sodium entry drives the net uptake of cotransported solutes, and this process accumulates sodium inside the luminal membrane. Sodium leaves the cell through expulsion by the basolateral membrane sodium pump. The sodium concentration is therefore higher next to the sodium entry (luminal membrane) and lower close to its exit (basolateral membrane). The sodium ions move across the cell from the point of entry to the point of exit according to a local concentration gradient created in the cytoplasm by the polarization of the cell. This explains why the mean intracellular concentration of sodium in proximal cells is measured at 30 to 50 m*M*,[191-199] that is, well above the saturating sodium concentration for the sodium pump and above the values measured by the direct impalement of the basolateral membrane with specific electrodes.[200,201] Also in accord with this, the sodium pump is able to respond to modest changes in sodium concentration. A small change in the activity of the basolateral sodium pump will increase modestly the resting sodium concentration in the vicinity of the sodium pump, but this may translate into a large increment of sodium concentration close to the luminal membrane with, secondarily, the loss of the driving force energizing all sodium–solute cotransport systems.

ADP/ATP Gradient. ADP is generated in proximal cells largely in the vicinity of the cell membranes where the major ATPases (Na^+,K^+-ATPase for the basolateral and H^+ ATPase for the luminal membrane) consume together over 90 per cent of the ATP synthesized. This ADP is rephosphorylated by the mitochondria, and a low perimitochondrial concentration is thus maintained. A reverse situation applies to ATP synthesized by mitochondria and utilized at the cell membrane. Opposite gradients may thus exist for ATP and ADP in the cells, ensuring the movement of these compounds from the membrane to the mitochondria and back. A small reduction in the mitochondrial capacity to rephosphorylate ADP may thus be translated into a larger accumulation of ADP (and fall in ATP) close to the ion pumps. Since ADP and the ATP:ADP ratio are important regulators of these pumps, a significant inhibition of the basolateral Na^+, K^+ pump[202-204] and of the luminal H^+ pump[205] may be expected.

Thus, by virtue of the amplifying effect of intracellular gradients, a smalll mitochondrial defect may lead to a significant disruption in both sodium-coupled transport systems and ATP-energized systems at the luminal membrane—that is to a large and rather indiscriminate inhibition of transport. It is noteworthy that all models reproducing experimental Fanconi syndrome are capable of producing modest or even large inhibition of mitochondrial ATP synthesis and disrupting the transport even with small changes in tissue ATP.

Because the pathophysiological basis of the Fanconi syndrome remains uncertain, further investigations with various experimental models are needed in order to clarify: (1) the respective roles of the proximal and the distal nephron, (2) the contribution of a reduced influx and/or an accelerated efflux or backleak, and (3) the basic cellular defect(s) underlying the disturbed reabsorptive processes. In this respect the Basenji dog model may shed new light, since the renal tubular defects are a likely consequence of a genetic factor.

CLINICAL SIGNS AND SYMPTOMS

The clinical manifestations of the Fanconi syndrome are not specific and result from the renal losses of fluid and electrolytes and the characteristic vitamin D–resistant metabolic bone disease. The renal loss of other substances such as glucose, amino acids, and uric acid will not induce any clinical signs or symptoms but may contribute in some patients to the diagnosis of Fanconi syndrome.

The age at which a child first becomes symptomatic can provide a clue for the specific inborn error of metabolism. For example, infants with galactosemia or hereditary fructose intolerance can present with acute symptoms within the first few days of life if they ingest galactose or fructose, respectively. Children with nephropathic cystinosis present symptoms only after the age of 6 months. In Wilson disease, symptoms resulting from Fanconi syndrome will not appear before the end of the first decade of life. By contrast, symptoms induced by acquired Fanconi syndrome may appear at any age.

Consequences of Renal Losses of Fluid and Electrolytes

The excessive urinary loss of water resulting from the renal concentration defect will produce polyuria, polydipsia, and, in infants and young children, dehydration, constipation, and unexplained recurrent fever. The chronic hyperchloremic metabolic acidosis resulting from the associated renal proximal tubular acidosis (renal tubular acidosis is discussed extensively in the Chap. 121) can induce anorexia and episodic vomiting. Muscle weakness and even episodic paralysis can result from severe hypokalemia and potassium depletion.

Vitamin D–Resistant Metabolic Bone Disease

Hypophosphatemic rickets (in growing children) or osteomalacia (in adults) is produced at least in part by the exaggerated renal loss of phosphate and may dominate the clinical picture. An impaired renal tubular 1-hydroxylation of 25-hydroxyvitamin D_3 into 1,25-dihydroxyvitamin D_3 may also play a role in the pathogenesis of this metabolic bone disease; indeed this biologically active vitamin D metabolite was not found in the blood of five nonazotemic children with Fanconi syndrome.[139] The child with Fanconi syndrome will fail to grow and may present the characteristic clinical findings of rickets: frontal bossing, rachitic rosary, bowing deformities of the legs, metaphyseal widening at the wrists, knees, or ankles, and waddling gait. By contrast, patients with adult-onset Fanconi syndrome often complain of severe bone pain and spontaneous fractures.

THERAPY

Specific Treatment

Although the clinical management of Fanconi syndrome consists mostly of replacing the renal losses of substances not reabsorbed adequately by the kidney, one must always consider the possibility of a dramatic improvement when the responsible metabolite (in some inborn errors of metabolism) or the toxic agent (in acquired Fanconi syndrome) can be removed.

In the absence of a specific treatment, such as oral dithiothreitol[206] or cysteamine therapy to reduce intracellular cystine levels in nephropathic cystinosis,[207] fluids and electrolytes have to be replaced, the metabolic bone disease resulting from Fanconi syndrome must be treated, and renal transplantation may be useful when children with nephropathic cystinosis are severely uremic. By contrast, no therapy is required for the asymptomatic renal loss of substances such as glucose, amino acids, and uric acid.

Correction of Fluid and Electrolyte Disturbances

First, dehydration resulting from polyuria must be prevented by restoring free water balance. Second, the correction of the hyperchloremic metabolic acidosis usually requires large amounts of alkali (more than 3 and up to 10 to 20 meq/kg/day), a therapeutic maneuver that will aggravate the renal potassium wasting. Extracellular fluid volume contraction may also be induced by the restriction of sodium chloride and water[208] and the long-term administration of hydrochlorothiazide[209] in an attempt to reduce a very large alkali requirement to a level tolerable for the patient. Third, potassium supplements are always necessary in the presence of a severe hypokalemia or during the treatment of metabolic acidosis with alkali therapy. Potassium bicarbonate, citrate, or acetate will simultaneously improve the potassium depletion and the metabolic acidosis.

Treatment of Metabolic Bone Disease

Oral phosphate therapy to replace the renal phosphate loss helps to correct the rickets in children or osteomalacia in adults. Vitamin D therapy, in the form of its more biologically active metabolites, 1,25-dihydroxyvitamin D_3 and 1 α-hydroxyvitamin D_3, is preferred because renal production of hormone could be impaired in patients with Fanconi syndrome.[139]

Renal Transplantation

Long-term dialysis and renal transplantation should be considered when patients with Fanconi syndrome become terminally uremic. Renal transplantation from either a cadaveric or a living related donor has been especially useful to treat young children with nephropathic cystinosis because the transplanted kidney does not have the genetic defect and consequently there is no recurrence of renal cystinosis and Fanconi syndrome.[210,211] However, these transplanted cystinotic patients remain of short stature and often photophobic despite a successful renal transplantation. The severe mental retardation of patients like those with Lowe syndrome may prevent the utilization of long-term dialysis and/or renal transplantation in the treatment of their end-stage renal disease.

ACKNOWLEDGMENTS

This investigation was supported by the Medical Research Council of Canada. We acknowledge the roles our colleagues Alfred Berteloot, Raynald Laprade, Jennifer McLeese, Stanton Segal, and Georges Thiéry have played in the development of the ideas expressed in this chapter; any errors are our sole responsibility, not theirs. The authors acknowledge the skillful assistance of Mrs. G. Grenier and Messrs. D. Cyr and G. Filosi.

REFERENCES

1. Rodriguez-Soriano J, Vallo A, Castillo G, Oliveros R: Renal handling of water and sodium in children with proximal and distal renal tubular acidosis. *Nephron* **25**:193, 1980.
2. Houston IB, Boichis H, Edelmann CM: Fanconi syndrome with renal sodium wasting and metabolic alkalosis. *Am J Med* **44**:638, 1968
3. Sebastian A, McSherry E, Morris RC Jr: On the mechanism of renal potassium wasting in renal tubular acidosis associated with the Fanconi syndrome (type 2 RTA). *J Clin Invest* **50**:231, 1971.
4. Rodriguez Soriano J, Houston IB, Boichis H, Edelmann CM Jr: Calcium and phosphorus metabolism in the Fanconi syndrome. *J Clin Endocrinol Metab* **28**:1555, 1968.
5. Lee DBN, Drinkard JP, Rosen VJ, Gonick HC: The adult Fanconi syndrome: Observations on etiology, morphology, renal function and mineral metabolism in three patients. *Medicine (Baltimore)* **51**:107, 1972.
6. Bernardini I, Rizzo WB, Dalakas M, Bernar J, Gahl WA: Plasma and muscle free carnitine deficiency due to renal Fanconi syndrome. *J Clin Invest* **75**:1124, 1985.
7. Jonas AJ, Lin SN, Conley SB, Schneider JA, Williams JC, Caprioli RC: Urine glyceraldehyde excretion is elevated in the renal Fanconi syndrome. *Kidney Int* **35**:99, 1989.
8. Al-Bander HAJ, Mock MD, Etheredge SB, Paukert TT, Humphreys MH, Morris RC Jr: Coordinately increased lysozymuria and lysosomal enzymuria induced by maleic acid. *Kidney Int* **30**:804, 1986.
9. Christensen EI, Maunsbach AB: Proteinuria induced by sodium maleate in rats: Effects on ultrastructure and protein handling in renal proximal tubule. *Kidney Int* **17**:771, 1980.
10. Dillard MG, Pesce AF, Pollak VE, Boreisha I: Proteinuria and renal protein clearances in patients with renal tubular disorders. *J Lab Clin Med* **78**:203, 1971.
11. Abderhalden F: Familiare Cystindiathese. *Z Physiol Chem* **38**:557, 1903.
12. Lignac GOE: Stooris der Cystine-stofwisseling byj Kinderen. *Ned Tijdschr Geneeskd* **68**:2987, 1924.
13. Fanconi G: Die nicht diabetischen Glykosurien und Hyperglykamien des altern Kindes. *Jahrb Kinderheilk* **133**:257, 1931.
14. De Toni G: Remarks on the relations between renal rickets (renal dwarfism) and renal diabetes. *Acta Paediatr* **16**:479, 1933.
15. Debré R, Marie J, Cleret F, Messimy R: Rachitisme tardif coexistant avec une néphrite chronique et une glycosurie. *Arch Méd Enf* **37**:597, 1934.
16. Fanconi G: Der nephrotisch-glykosurische Zwergwuchs mit Hypophosphatamischer Rachitis. *Dtsch Med Wochenschr* **62**:1169, 1936.
17. McCune DJ, Mason HH, Clarke HT: Intractable hypophosphatemic rickets with renal glycosuria and acidosis (the Fanconi syndrome): Report of a case in which increased urinary organic acids were detected and identified, with a review of the literature. *Am J Dis Child* **65**:81, 1943.
18. Hunt DD, Stearns G, McKinley JB, Froning E, Hicks P, Bonfiglio M: Long-term study of family with Fanconi syndrome without cystinosis (DeToni-Debré-Fanconi syndrome). *Am J Med* **40**:492, 1966.
19. Friedman AL, Trygstad CW, Chesney RW: Autosomal dominant Fanconi syndrome with early renal failure. *Am J Med Genet* **2**:225, 1978.
20. Brenton DP, Isenberg DA, Cusworth DC, Garrod P, Krywawych S, Stamp TCB: The adult presenting idiopathic Fanconi syndrome. *J Inherited Metab Dis* **4**:211, 1981.
21. Tolaymat A, Sakarcan A, Neiberger R: Idiopathic Fanconi syndrome in a family. Part 1. Clinical aspects. *J Am Soc Nephrol* **2**:1310, 1992.
22. Wen SF, Friedman AL, Oberley TD: Two case studies from a family with primary Fanconi syndrome: *Am J Kidney Dis* **13**:240, 1989.
23. Chesney RW, Kaplan BS, Colle E, Scriver CR, McInnes RR, Dupont CH, Drummond KN: Abnormalities of carbohydrate metabolism in idiopathic Fanconi syndrome. *Pediatr Res* **14**:209, 1980.
24. Chesney RW, Kaplan BS, Teitel D, Colle E, McInnes RR, Goldman H, Scriver CR: Metabolic abnormalities in the idiopathic Fanconi syndrome: Studies of carbohydrate metabolism in two patients. *Pediatrics* **67**:113, 1981.
25. Schneider JA, Bradley K, Seegmiller JE: Increased cystine in leukocytes from individuals homozygous and heterozygous for cystinosis. *Science* **157**:1321, 1967.

26. Schneider JA, Rosenbloom FM, Bradley KH, Seegmiller JE: Increased free-cystine content of fibroblasts cultured from patients with cystinosis. *Biochem Biophys Res Commun* **29**:527, 1967.
27. Foreman JW, Roth KS: Human renal Fanconi syndrome—then and now. *Nephron* **51**:301, 1989.
28. Crawhall JC, Lietman PS, Schneider JA, Seegmiller JE: Cystinosis: Plasma cystine and cysteine concentrations and the effect of D-penicillamine and dietary treatment. *Am J Med* **44**:330, 1968.
29. Schneider JA, Wong V, Seegmiller JE: The early diagnosis of cystinosis. *J Pediatr* **74**:114, 1969.
30. Goldman H, Scriver CR, Aaron K, Delvin E, Canlas Z: Adolescent cystinosis: Comparisons with infantile and adult forms. *Pediatrics* **47**:979, 1971.
31. Lietman PS, Frazier PD, Wong VG, Shotton D, Seegmiller JE: Adult cystinosis: A benign disorder. *Am J Med* **40**:511, 1966.
32. Spencer PD, Medow MS, Moses LC, Roth KS: Effects of succinylacetone on the uptake of sugars and amino acids by brush border vesicles. *Kidney Int* **34**:671, 1988.
33. Morris RC Jr: An experimental renal acidification defect in patients with hereditary fructose intolerance. I. Its resemblance to renal tubular acidosis. *J Clin Invest* **47**:1389, 1968.
34. Morris RC Jr: An experimental renal acidification defect in patients with hereditary fructose intolerance. II. Its distinction from classical renal tubular acidosis; its resemblance to the renal acidification defect associated with the Fanconi syndrome of children with cystinosis. *J Clin Invest* **47**:1648, 1968.
35. Morris RC Jr, Nigon K, Reed EB: Evidence that the severity of depletion of inorganic phosphate determines the severity of the disturbance of adenine nucleotide metabolism in the liver and renal cortex of the fructose-loaded rat. *J Clin Invest* **61**:209, 1978.
36. Holzel A, Komrower GM, Schwarz V: Galactosemia. *Am J Med* **22**:703, 1957.
37. Garty R, Cooper M, Tabachnik E: The Fanconi syndrome associated with hepatic glycogenosis and abnormal metabolism of galactose. *J Pediatr* **85**:821, 1974.
38. Morgan HG, Stewart WK, Lowe KG, Stowers JM, Johnstone JH: Wilson's disease and the Fanconi syndrome. *Q J Med* **31**:361, 1962.
39. Elssas LJ, Hayslett JP, Spargo BH Durant JL, Rosenberg LE: Wilson's disease with reversible renal tubular dysfunction: Correlation with proximal tubular ultrastructure. *Ann Intern Med* **75**:427, 1971.
40. Lowe CU, Terrey M, MacLachlan EA: Organic-aciduria, decreased renal ammonia production, hydrophthalmos, and mental retardation: A clinical entity. *Am J Dis Child* **83**:164, 1952.
41. Abbassi V, Lowe CU, Calcagno PL: Oculo-cerebro-renal syndrome: A review. *Am J Dis Child* **115**:145, 1968.
42, Sagel I, Ores RO, Yuceoglu AM: Renal function and morphology in a girl with oculocerebrorenal syndrome. *J Pediatr* **77**:124, 1970.
43. Gardner RJM, Brown N: Lowe's syndrome: Identification of carriers by lens examination. *J Med Genet* **13**:449, 1976.
44. Hittner HM, Carroll AJ, Prchal JT: Linkage studies in carriers of Lowe oculo-cerebro-renal syndrome *Am J Hum Genet* **34**:966, 1982.
45. Akasaki M, Fukui S, Sakano T, Tanaka T, Usui T, Yamashina I: Urinary excretion of a large amount of bound sialic acid and of undersulfated chondroitin sulfate A by patients with the Lowe syndrome. *Clin Chim Acta* **89**:119, 1978.
46. Hayashi S, Nagata T, Kimura A, Tsurumi K: Urinary excretion of acid glycosaminoglycans and hydroxyproline in a patient with oculo-cerebro-renal syndrome. *Tohoku J Exp Med* **126**:215, 1978.
47. Habib R, Bargeton E, Brissaud HE, Raynaud J, Le Ball JC: Constations anatomiques chez un enfant atteint d'un syndrome de Lowe. *Arch Fr Pédiatr* **19**:945, 1962.
48. Easley JR, Breitschwerdt EB: Glycosuria associated with renal tubular dysfunction in three Basenji dogs. *J Am Vet Med Assoc* **168**:938, 1976.
49. Bovee KC, Joyce T, Reynolds R, Segal S: The Fanconi syndrome in Basenji dogs: A new model for renal transport defects. *Science* **201**:1129, 1978.
50. Bovee KC, Joyce T, Reynolds R, Segal S: Spontaneous Fanconi syndrome in the dog. *Metabolism* **27**:45, 1978.
51. McNamara PD, Rea CT, Bovee KC, Reynolds RA, Segal S: Cystinuria in dogs: Comparison of the cystinuric component of the Fanconi syndrome in Basenji dogs to isolated cystinuria. *Metabolism* **38**:8, 1989.
52. Adams RG, Harrison JF, Scott P: The development of cadmium-induced proteinuria, impaired renal function, and osteomalacia in alkaline battery workers. *Q J Med* **38**:425, 1969.
53. Bernard A, Buchet JP, Roels H, Masson P, Lauwerys R: Renal excretion of protein and enzymes in workers exposed to cadmium. *Eur J Clin Invest* **9**:11, 1979.
54. Clarkson TW, Kench JE: Urinary excretion of amino acids by men absorbing heavy metals. *Biochem J* **62**:361, 1956.
55. Axelsson B, Dahlgren SE, Piscator M: Renal lesions in the rabbit after long-term exposure to cadmium. *Arch Environ Health* **17**:24, 1968.
56. Stowe HD, Wilson M, Goyer RA: Clinical and morphologic effects of oral cadmium toxicity in rabbits. *Arch Pathol* **94**:389, 1972.
57. Nishizumi M: Electron microscopic study of cadmium nephrotoxicity in the rat. *Arch Environ Health* **24**:215, 1972.
58. Raghavan SRV, Gonick HC: Experimental Fanconi syndrome. IV. Effect of repetitive injections of cadmium on tissue distribution and protein-binding of cadmium. *Miner Electrolyte Metab* **3**:36, 1980.
59. Gonick HC, Kramer HJ: Pathogenesis of the Fanconi syndrome, in Gonick HC, Buckalew VM Jr (eds): *Renal Tubular Disorders. Pathophysiology, Diagnosis and Management*. New York, Marcel Dekker, 1985, p 545.
60. Nomiyama K, Sugata Y, Murata I, Nakagawa S: Urinary low-molecular-weight proteins in itai-itai disease. *Environ Res* **6**:373, 1973.
61. Saito H, Shioji R, Hurukawa Y, Nagai K, Arikawa T, Saito T, Sasaki Y, Furuyama T, Yoshinaga K: Cadmium-induced proximal tubular dysfunction in a cadmium-polluted area. *Contrib Nephrol* **6**:1, 1977.
62. Brewer ED: The Fanconi syndrome: Clinical disorders, in Gonick HC, Buckalew VM Jr (eds): *Renal Tubular Disorders. Pathophysiology, Diagnosis and Management*. New York, Marcel Dekker, 1985, p 475.
63. Goyer RA, May P, Cates MM, Krigman MR: Lead and protein content of isolated intranuclear inclusion bodies from kidneys of lead-poisoned rats. *Lab Invest* **22**:245, 1970.
64. Chisolm JJ Jr, Harrison HC, Eberlein WR, Harrison HE: Amino-aciduria, hypophosphatemia, and rickets in lead poisoning. *Am J Dis Child* **89**:159, 1955.
65. Blachley JD, Hill JB: Renal and electrolyte disturbances associated with cisplatin. *Ann Intern Med* **95**:628, 1981.
66. Schilsky RL, Anderson T: Hypomagnesemia and renal magnesium wasting in patients receiving cisplatin. *Ann Intern Med* **90**:929, 1979.
67. Frimpter GW, Timpanelli AE, Eisenmenger WJ, Stein HS, Ehrlich LI: Reversible "Fanconi syndrome" caused by degraded tetracycline. *JAMA* **84**:111, 1963.
68. Gross JM: Fanconi syndrome (adult type) developing secondary to the ingestion of outdated tetracycline. *Ann Intern Med* **58**:523, 1963.
69. Benitz KF, Diermeier HF: Renal toxicity of tetracycline degradation products. *Proc Soc Exp Biol Med* **115**:930, 1964.
70. Lindquist RR, Fellers FX: Degraded tetracycline nephropathy: Functional, morphologic, and histochemical observations. *Lab Invest* **15**:864, 1966.
71. Bar RS, Wilson HE, Mazzaferri EL: Hypomagnesemic hypocalcemia secondary to renal magnesium wasting: A possible consequence of high-dose gentamicin therapy. *Ann Intern Med* **82**:646, 1975.
72. Kelnar CJH, Taor WS, Reynolds DJ, Smith DR, Slavin BM, Brook CGD: Hypomagnesaemic hypocalcemia with hypokalaemia caused by treatment with high dose gentamicin. *Arch Dis Child* **53**:817, 1978.
73. Kuhar MJ, Mak LL, Lietman PS: Autoradiographic local-

ization of (^{3}H) gentamicin in the proximal renal tubules of mice. *Antimicrob Agents Chemother* **15**:131, 1979.

74. Lenoir GR, Pérignon JL, Gubler MC, Broyer M: Valproic acid: A possible cause of proximal tubular renal syndrome. *J Pediatr* **98**:503, 1981.
75. Butler HE Jr, Morgan JM, Smythe CM: Mercaptopurine and acquired tubular dysfunction in adult nephrosis. *Arch Intern Med* **116**:853, 1965.
76. Otten J, Vis HL: Acute reversible renal tubular dysfunction following intoxication with methyl-3-chromone. *J Pediatr* **73**:422, 1968.
77. Spencer AG, Franglen GT: Gross amino-aciduria following a Lysol burn. *Lancet* **1**:190, 1952.
78. Vaziri ND, Ness RL, Fairshter RD, Smith WR, Rosen SM: Nephrotoxicity of paraquat in man. *Arch Intern Med* **139**:172, 1979.
79. Moss AH, Gabow PA, Kaehny WD, Goodman SI, Haut LL, Haussler MR: Fanconi's syndrome and distal renal tubular acidosis after glue sniffing. *Ann Intern Med* **92**:69, 1980.
80. Burk CD, Restaino I, Kaplan BS, Meadows AT: Ifosfamide-induced renal tubular dysfunction and rickets in children with Wilms tumor. *J Pediatr* **117**:331, 1990.
81. Costanza DJ, Smoller M: Multiple myeloma with the Fanconi syndrome: Study of a case, with electron microscopy of the kidney. *Am J Med* **34**:125, 1963.
82. Maldondo JE, Velosa JA, Kyle RA, Wagoner RD, Holley KE, Salassa RM: Fanconi syndrome in adults: A manifestation of a latent form of myeloma. *Am J Med* **58**:354, 1975.
83. Walker BR, Alexander F, Tannenbaum PJ: Fanconi syndrome with renal tubular acidosis and light chain proteinuria. *Nephron* **8**:103, 1971.
84. Orfila C, Lepert JC, Modesto A, Bernadet P, Suc JM: Fanconi's syndrome, kappa light-chain myeloma, non-amyloid fibrils and cytoplasmic crystals in renal tubular epithelium. *Am J Nephrol* **11**:345, 1991.
85. Sanders PW, Herrera GA, Galla JH: Human Bence Jones protein toxicity in rat proximal tubule epithelium in vivo. *Kidney Int* **32**:851, 1987.
86. McGeoch J, Smith JF, Ledingham J, Ross B: Inhibition of active transport sodium-potassium-ATPase by myeloma protein. *Lancet* **2**:17, 1978.
87. Uchida S, Matsuda O, Yokota T, Takemura T, Ando R, Kanemitsu H, Hamaguchi H, Miyake S, Marumo F: Adult Fanconi syndrome secondary to κ-light chain myeloma: Improvement of tubular functions after treatment for myeloma. *Nephron* **55**:332, 1990.
88. Finkel PN, Kronenberg K, Pesce AJ, Pollak VE, Pirani CL: Adult Fanconi syndrome, amyloidosis and marked x-light chain proteinuria. *Nephron* **10**:1, 1973.
89. Rochman J, Lichtig C, Osterweill D, Tatarsky I, Eidelman S: Adult Fanconi's syndrome with renal tubular acidosis in association with renal amyloidosis: Occurrence in a patient with chronic lymphocytic leukemia. *Arch Intern Med* **140**:1361, 1980.
90. Harrison JF, Blainey JD: Adult Fanconi syndrome with monoclonal abnormality of immunoglobulin light chain. *J Clin Pathol* **20**:42, 1967.
91. Smithline N, Kassirer JP, Cohen JJ: Light-chain nephropathy. Renal tubular dysfunction associated with light-chain proteinuria. *N Engl J Med* **294**:71, 1976.
92. Rao DS, Parfitt AM, Villanueva AR, Dorman PJ, Kleerekoper M: Hypophosphatemic osteomalacia and adult Fanconi syndrome due to light-chain nephropathy. *Am J Med* **82**:333, 1987.
93. Dahlstrom U, Marftensson J, Lindstrom FD: Occurrence of adult Fanconi syndrome in benign monoclonal gammopathy. *Acta Med Scand* **208**:425, 1980.
94. van Hooft C, Vermassen A: DeToni-Debré-Fanconi syndrome in nephrotic children: A review. *Ann Pediatr (Paris)* **194**:193, 1960.
95. McVicar M, Exeni R, Susin M: Nephrotic syndrome and multiple tubular defects in children: An early sign of focal segmental glomerulosclerosis. *J Pediatr* **97**:918, 1980.
96. Friedman A, Chesney R: Fanconi's syndrome in renal transplantation. *Am J Nephrol* **1**:45, 1981.
97. Vertuno LL, Preuss HG, Argy WP Jr, Schreiner GE: Fanconi syndrome following homotransplantation. *Arch Intern Med* **133**:302, 1974.
98. Vaziri ND, Nellans RE, Brueggemann RM, Barton CH, Martin DC: Renal tubular dysfunction in transplanted kidneys. *South Med J* **72**:530, 1979.
99. Palestine AG, Austin HA, Nussenblatt RB: Renal tubular function in cyclosporine-treated patients. *Am J Med* **81**:419, 1986.
100. Leehey DJ, Ing TS, Daugirdas JT: Fanconi syndrome associated with a non-ossifying fibroma of bone. *Am J Med* **78**:708, 1985.
101. Goldsweig HG, Brisson De Champlain ML, Davidman M: Proximal tubular dysfunction associated with Burkitt's lymphoma. *Cancer* **41**:568, 1978.
102. Weinstein B, Irreverre F, Watkin DM: Lung carcinoma, hypouricemia and aminoaciduria. *Am J Med* **39**:520, 1965.
103. Stowers JM, Dent CE: Studies on the mechanism of the Fanconi syndrome. *Q J Med* **16**:275, 1947.
104. Myerson RM, Pastor BH: The Fanconi syndrome and its clinical variants. *Am J Med Sci* **228**:378, 1954.
105. Clay RD, Darmady EM, Hawkins M: The nature of the renal lesion in the Fanconi syndrome. *J Pathol Bacteriol* **65**:551, 1953.
106. Berliner RW, Kennedy TJ, Hilton JG: Effect of maleic acid on renal function. *Proc Soc Exp Biol Med* **75**:791, 1950.
107. Harrison HE, Harrison HC: Experimental production of renal glycosuria, phosphaturia, and aminoaciduria by injection of maleic acid. *Science* **120**:606, 1954.
108. Shvil Y, Wald H, Popovtzer MM: Effect of bicarbonate and phosphate on renal phosphate leak in experimental Fanconi syndrome. *Am J Physiol* **252**:F310, 1987.
109. Foreman JW, Bowring MA, Lee J, States B, Segal S: Effect of cystine dimethylester on renal solute handling and isolated renal tubule transport in the rat: A new model of the Fanconi syndrome. *Metabolism* **36**:1185, 1987.
110. Gougoux A, Zan N, Dansereau D, Vinay P: Experimental Fanconi's syndrome resulting from 4-pentenoate infusion in the dog. *Am J Physiol* **257**:F959, 1989.
111. Fritzell S, Jagenburg OR, Schnurer LB: Familial cirrhosis of the liver, renal tubular defects with rickets and impaired tyrosine metabolism. *Acta Paediatr* **53**:18, 1964.
112. Halvorsen S, Gjessing LR: Studies on tyrosinosis: 1, Effect of low-tyrosine and low-phenylalanine diet. *Br Med J* **2**:1171, 1964.
113. Harries JT, Seakins JWT, Ersser RS, Lloyd JK: Recovery after dietary treatment of an infant with features of tyrosinosis. *Arch Dis Child* **44**:258, 1969.
114. Levin B, Snodgrass GJAI, Oberholzer VG, Burgess EA, Dobbs RH: Fructosaemia: Observations on seven cases. *Am J Med* **45**:826, 1968.
115. Cusworth DC, Dent CE, Flynn FV: The amino-aciduria in galactosemia. *Arch Dis Child* **30**:150, 1955.
116. Jagenburg R, Lindblad B, De Mare JM, Rodjer S: Hereditary tyrosinemia: Metabolic studies in a patient with partial p-hydroxyphenylpyruvate hydroxylase activity. *J Pediatr* **80**:994, 1972.
117. Aronsson S, Engleson G, Jagenburg R, Palmgren B: Long-term dietary treatment of tyrosinosis. *J Pediatr* **72**:620, 1968.
118. Scriver CR, Silverberg M, Clow CL: Hereditary tyrosinemia and tyrosyluria: Clinical report of four patients. *Can Med Assoc J* **97**:1047, 1967.
119. Kang ES, Gerald PS: Hereditary tyrosinemia and abnormal pyrrole metabolism. *J Pediatr* **77**:397, 1970.
120. Isselbacher KJ: Galactosemia, in Stanbury JB, Wyngaarden JB, Fredrickson DS (eds): *The Metabolic Basis of Inherited Disease*, 2nd ed. New York, McGraw-Hill, 1966, p 178.
121. Chisolm JJ Jr: Aminoaciduria as a manifestation of renal tubular injury in lead intoxication and a comparison with patterns of aminoaciduria seen in other diseases. *J Pediatr* **60**:1, 1962.
122. Goyer RA: The renal tubule in lead poisoning. I. Mitochondrial swelling and aminoaciduria. *Lab Invest* **19**:71, 1968.
123. Morris RC Jr, McInnes RR, Epstein CJ, Sebastian A, Scriver CR: Genetic and metabolic injury of the kidney, in

Brenner BM, Rector FC Jr (eds): *The Kidney*. Philadelphia, Saunders, 1976, p 1193.
124. Burch HB, Lowry OH, Meinhardt L, Max P Jr, Chyu KJ: Effect of fructose, dihydroxyacetone, glycerol, and glucose on metabolites and related compounds in liver and kidney. *J Biol Chem* **245**:2092, 1970.
125. Woods HF, Eggleston LV, Krebs HA: The cause of hepatic accumulation of fructose-1-phosphate on fructose loading. *Biochem J* **119**:501, 1970.
126. Woods HF: Hepatic accumulation of metabolites after fructose loading. *Acta Med Scand Suppl* **542**:87, 1972.
127. Bergeron M, Morel F: Amino acid transport in rat renal tubules. *Am J Physiol* **216**:1139, 1969.
128. Brodehl J, Bickel H: Aminoaciduria and hyperaminoaciduria in childhood. *Clin Nephrol* **1**:149, 1973.
129. Roth KS, Foreman JW, Segal S: The Fanconi syndrome and mechanisms of tubular transport dysfunction. *Kidney Int* **20**:705, 1981.
130. Darmady EM, Stranack F: Microdissection of the nephron in disease. *Br Med Bull* **13**:21, 1957.
131. Witzleben CL, Schoen EJ, Tu WH, McDonald LW: Progressive morphologic renal changes in the oculo-cerebrorenal syndrome of Lowe. *Am J Med* **44**:319, 1968.
132. Schneider JA, Seegmiller JE: Cystinosis and the Fanconi syndrome, in Stanbury JB, Wyngaarden JB, Fredrickson DS (eds): *The Metabolic Basis of Inherited Disease*, 3rd ed. New York, McGraw-Hill, 1972.
133. Worthen HG: Renal toxicity of maleic acid in the rat: Enzymatic and morphologic observations. *Lab Invest* **12**:791, 1963.
134. Scharer K, Yoshida T, Voyer L, Berlow S, Pietra G, Metcoff J: Impaired renal gluconeogenesis and energy metabolism in maleic acid-induced nephropathy in rats. *Res Exp Med (Berlin)* **157**:136, 1972.
135. Bergeron M, Laporte P: Effet membranaire du maléate au niveau du néphron proximal et distal. *Rev Can Biol* **32**:275, 1973.
136. Rosen VJ, Kramer HJ, Gonick HC: Experimental Fanconi syndrome. II. Effect of maleic acid on renal tubular ultrastructure. *Lab Invest* **28**:446, 1973.
137. Verani RR, Brewer ED, Ince A, Gibson J, Bulger RE: Proximal tubular necrosis associated with maleic acid administration to the rat. *Lab Invest* **46**:79, 1982.
138. Guntupalli J, Delaney V, Weinman EJ, Lyle D, Allon M, Bourke E: Effects of maleic acid on renal phosphorus transport: Role of dietary phosphorus. *Am J Physiol* **261**:F227, 1991.
139. Brewer ED, Tsai HC, Szeto KS, Morris RC Jr: Maleic acid-induced impaired conversion of 25 $(OH)D_3$ to $1,25(OH)_2D_3$: Implications for Fanconi's syndrome. *Kidney Int* **12**:244, 1977.
140. Gray RW, Omdahl JL, Ghazarian JG, Deluca HF: 25-hydroxycholecalciferol-1-hydroxylase: Subcellular location and properties. *J Biol Chem* **247**:7528, 1972.
141. Akiba T, Endou H, Koseki C, Sakai F: Localization of 25-hydroxyvitamin D_3-1a-hydroxylase activity in the mammalian kidney. *Biochem Biophys Res Commun* **94**:313, 1980.
142. Tate SS, Meister A: Stimulation of the hydrolytic activity and decrease of the transpeptidase activity of γ-glutamyl transpeptidase by maleate; identity of a rat kidney maleate-stimulated glutaminase and γ-glutamyl transpeptidase. *Proc Natl Acad Sci USA* **71**:3329, 1974.
143. Bergeron M, Dubord L, Hausser C: Membrane permeability as a cause of transport defects in experimental Fanconi syndrome: A new hypothesis. *J Clin Invest* **57**:1181, 1976.
144. Wen SF: Micropuncture studies of glucose transport in the dog: Mechanism of renal glycosuria. *Am J Physiol* **231**:468, 1976.
145. Brewer ED, Senekjian HO, Ince A, Weinman EJ: Maleic acid-induced reabsorptive dysfunction in the proximal and distal nephron. *Am J Physiol* **245**:F339, 1983.
146. Bank N, Aynedjian HS, Mutz BJ: Microperfusion study of proximal tubule bicarbonate transport in maleic acid-induced renal tubular acidosis. *Am J Physiol* **250**:F476, 1986.
147. Al-Bander HA, Weiss RA, Humphreys MH, Morris RC Jr: Dysfunction of the proximal tubule underlies maleic acid-induced type II renal tubular acidosis. *Am J Physiol* **243**:F604, 1982.
148. Rosin JM, Katz MA, Rector FC Jr, Seldin DW: Acetazolamide in studying sodium reabsorption in diluting segment. *Am J Physiol* **219**:1731, 1970.
149. Kunau RT Jr: The influence of the carbonic anhydrase inhibitor, benzolamide (C1-11,366), on the reabsorption of chloride, sodium, and bicarbonate in the proximal tubule of the rat. *J Clin Invest* **51**:294, 1972.
150. Gougoux A, Zan N, Dansereau D, Vinay P: Metabolic effects of 4-pentenoate on isolated dog kidney tubules. *Kidney Int* **42**:586, 1992.
151. Bergeron M, Vadeboncoeur M: Microinjections of L-leucine into tubules and peritubular capillaries of the rat. II. The maleic acid model. *Nephron* **8**:367, 1971.
152. Bergeron M, Dubord L, Laporte P, Hausser C, Alle-Ando L: On the physiopathology of the Fanconi syndrome, in Silbernagl S, Lang F, Greger R (eds): *Amino Acid Transport and Uric Acid Transport*. Stuttgart, Thieme, 1976, p 46.
153. Günther R, Silbernagl S, Deetjen P: Maleic acid induced aminoaciduria, studied by free flow micropuncture and continuous microperfusion. *Pflügers Arch* **382**:109, 1979.
154. Scriver CR, Chesney RW, McInnes RR: Genetic aspects of renal tubular transport: Diversity and topology of carriers. *Kidney Int* **9**:149, 1976.
155. Gougoux A, Lemieux G, Lavoie N: Maleate-induced bicarbonaturia in the dog: A carbonic anhydrase-independent effect. *Am J Physiol* **231**:1010, 1976.
156. Gmaj P, Hoppe A, Angielski S, Rogulski J: Acid-base behavior of the kidney in maleate-treated rats. *Am J Physiol* **222**:1182, 1972.
157. Gmaj P, Hoppe A, Angielski S, Rogulski J: Effects of maleate and arsenite on renal reabsorption of sodium and bicarbonate. *Am J Physiol* **225**:90, 1973.
158. Hoppe A, Gmaj P, Metler M, Angielski S: Additive inhibition of renal bicarbonate reabsorption by maleate plus acetazolamide. *Am J Physiol* **231**:1258, 1976.
159. Rosenberg LE, Segal S: Maleic acid-induced inhibition of amino acid transport in rat kidney. *Biochem J* **92**:345, 1964.
160. Silverman M, Huang L: Mechanism of maleic acid-induced glucosuria in dog kidney. *Am J Physiol* **231**:1024, 1976.
161. Bergeron M: Renal amino acid accumulation in maleate treated rats. *Rev Can Biol* **30**:267, 1971.
162. Ausiello DA, Segal S, Thier SO: Cellular accumulation of L-lysine in rat kidney cortex in vivo. *Am J Physiol* **222**:1473, 1972.
163. Kramer HJ, Gonick HC: Experimental Fanconi syndrome. I. Effect of maleic acid on renal cortical Na-K-ATPase activity and ATP levels. *J Lab Clin Med* **76**:799, 1970.
164. Reboucas NA, Fernandes DT, Elias MM, De Mello-Aires M, Malnic G: Proximal tubular HCO_3^-, H^+ and fluid transport during maleate-induced acidification defect. *Pflügers Arch* **401**:266, 1984.
165. Obaid AL, Rega AF, Garrahan PJ: The effects of maleic anhydride on the ionic permeability of red cells. *J Membr Biol* **9**:385, 1972.
166. Le Grimellec C, Carrière S, Cardinal J, Giocondi MC: Effect of maleate on membrane physical state of brush border and basolateral membranes of the dog kidney. *Life Sci* **30**:1107, 1982.
167. Reynolds R, McNamara PD, Segal S: On the maleic acid induced Fanconi syndrome: Effects on transport by isolated rat kidney brushborder membrane vesicles. *Life Sci* **22**:39, 1978.
168. Silverman M: The mechanism of maleic acid nephropathy: Investigations using brush border membrane vesicles. *Membr Biochem* **4**:63, 1981.
169. Laprade R, Beauchesne G, Bergeron M: Effet membranaire du maléate: Etude à l'aide de membranes artificielles lipidiques, in Proceedings of the VIIth International Congress of Nephrology, 1978, p M-6.
170. Maesaka JK, McCaffery M: Evidence for renal tubular leakage in maleic acid-induced Fanconi syndrome. *Am J Physiol* **239**:F507, 1980.
171. Pfaller W, Joannidis M, Gstraunthaler G, Kotanko P: Quantitative morphological changes of nephron structures and urinary enzyme activity pattern in sodium maleate-induced renal injury. *Renal Physiol Biochem* **12**:56, 1989.
172. Gonick HC, Indraprasit S, Rosen VJ, Neustein H,

Van De Velde R, Raghavan SRV: Experimental Fanconi Syndrome. III. Effect of cadmium on renal tubular function, the ATP-NA$^+$,K$^+$-ATPase transport system and renal tubular ultrastructure. *Miner Electrolyte Metab* **3**:21, 1980.

173. Lee HY, Kim KR, Woo JS, Kim YK, Park YS: Transport of organic compounds in renal plasma membrane vesicles of cadmium intoxicated rats. *Kidney Int* **37**:727, 1990.

174. Kägi JHR, Vallee BL: Metallothionein: A cadmium- and zinc-containing protein from equine renal cortex. *J Biol Chem* **235**:3460, 1960.

175. Foulkes EC: Renal tubular transport of cadmium-metallothionein. *Toxicol Appl Pharmacol* **45**:505, 1978.

176. Nordberg GF, Goyer RA, Nordberg M: Comparative toxicity of cadmium-metallothionein and cadmium chloride on mouse kidney. *Arch Pathol* **99**:192, 1975.

177. Gunn SA, Gould TC, Anderson WAD: Selectivity of organs response to cadmium injury and various protective measures. *J Pathol Bacteriol* **96**:89, 1968.

178. Hsu BYL, McNamara PD, Mahoney SG, Fenstermacher EA, Rea CT, Bovee KC, Segal S: Membrane fluidity and sodium transport by renal membranes from dogs with spontaneous idiopathic Fanconi syndrome. *Metabolism* **41**:253, 1992.

179. Gougoux A. Vinay P, Duplain M: Maleate-induced stimulation of glutamine metabolism in the intact dog kidney. *Am J Physiol* **248**:F585, 1985.

180. Wapnir RA, Exeni RA, McVicar M, De Rosas FJ, Lifshitz F: Inhibition of sodium intestinal transport and mucosal Na$^+$,K$^+$-ATPase in experimental Fanconi syndrome. *Proc Soc Exp Biol Med* **150**:517, 1975.

181. Angielski S, Rogulski J: Effect of maleic acid on the kidney. I. Oxidation of Krebs cycle intermediates by various tissues of maleate intoxicated rats. *Acta Biochim Pol* **9**:357, 1962.

182. Rogulski J, Pacanis A, Adamowicz W, Angielski S: On the mechanism of maleate action on rat kidney mitochondria: Effect on oxidative metabolism. *Acta Biochim Pol* **21**:403, 1974.

183. Gougoux A, Vinay P, Duplain M: Maleate-induced stimulation of glutamine metabolism in dog renal cortical tubules. *Contrib Nephrol* **47**:36, 1985.

184. Salmon RF, Baum M: Intracellular cystine loading inhibits transport in the rabbit proximal convoluted tubule. *J Clin Invest* **85**:340, 1990.

185. Coor C, Salmon RF, Quigley R, Marver D, Baum M: Role of adenosine triphosphate (ATP) and Na$^+$,K$^+$-ATPase in the inhibition of proximal tubule transport with intracellular cystine loading. *J Clin Invest* **87**:955, 1991.

186. Anner BM, Moosmayer M, Imesch E: Mercury blocks Na-K-ATPase by a ligand-dependent and reversible mechanism. *Am J Physiol* **262**:F830, 1992.

187. Anner BM, Moosmayer M: Mercury inhibits Na$^+$,K$^+$-ATPase primarily at the cytoplasmic side. *Am J Physiol* **262**:F843, 1992.

188. Imesch E, Moosmayer M, Anner BM: Mercury weakens membrane anchoring of Na$^+$,K$^+$-ATPase. *Am J Physiol* **262**:F837, 1992.

189. Szczepanska M, Angielski S: Prevention of maleate-induced tubular dysfunction by acetoacetate. *Am J Physiol* **239**:F50, 1980.

190. Al-Bander H, Etheredge SB, Paukert T, Humphreys MH, Morris RC Jr: Phosphate loading attenuates renal tubular dysfunction induced by maleic acid in the dog. *Am J Physiol* **248**:F513, 1985.

191. Beck F, Bauer R, Bauer U, Mason J, Dörge A, Rick R, Thurau K: Electron microprobe analysis of intracellular elements in the rat kidney. *Kidney Int* **17**:756, 1980.

192. Boulanger Y, Vinay P, Boulanger M: NMR monitoring of intracellular sodium in dog and rabbit kidney tubules. *Am J Physiol* **253**:F904, 1987.

193. Field MJ, Bostrom TE, Seow F, Györy AZ, Cockayne DJH: Acute cisplatine nephrotoxicity in the rat. Evidence for impaired entry of sodium into proximal cells. *Pflügers Arch* **414**:647, 1989.

194. Gullans SR, Avison MJ, Ogino T, Giebisch G, Shulman RG: NMR measurements of intracellular sodium in the rabbit proximal tubule. *Am J Physiol* **249**:F160, 1985.

195. Kumar AM, Gupta RK, Spitzer A: Intracellular sodium in proximal tubules of diabetic rats. Role of glucose. *Kidney Int* **33**:792, 1988.

196. Kumar AM, Spitzer A, Gupta RK: ^{23}Na-NMR spectroscopy of proximal tubule suspensions. *Kidney Int* **29**:747, 1986.

197. Pollock CA, Field MJ, Bostrom TE, Györy AZ, Cockayne DJH: Proximal tubular cell sodium concentration in early diabetic nephropathy assessed by microprobe analysis. *Pflügers Arch* **418**:14, 1991.

198. Rick R, Dörge A, Bauer R, Beck F, Mason J, Roloff C, Thurau K: Quantitative determination of electrolyte concentration in epithelial tissues by electron microprobe analysis. *Curr Top Membr Transp* **13**:107, 1980.

199. Thurau K, Dörge A, Mason J, Beck F, Rick R: Intracellular elemental concentrations in renal tubular cells. An electron microprobe analysis. *Klin Wochenschr* **57**:993, 1979.

200. Frömter E: Electrophysiological analysis of the rat renal sugar and amino acid transport. 1. Basic phenomena. *Pflügers Arch* **393**:179, 1982.

201. Yoshimoto K, Frömter E: How big is the electrochemical potential difference of Na$^+$ across rat renal proximal tubular cell membrane *in vivo*? *Pflügers Arch* **405**:S121, 1985.

202. Apell HJ, Nelson MT, Marcus MM, Laüger P: Effects of ATP, ADP and inorganic phosphate on the transport rate of the Na$^+$, K$^+$-pump. *Biochim Biophys Acta* **857**:105, 1986.

203. Garay RP, Garrahan PJ: The interaction of adenosine triphosphate and inorganic phosphate with the sodium pump in red cells. *J Physiol* **249**:51, 1975.

204. Hexum T, Sansom FE, Himes RH: Kinetic studies of membrane (Na$^+$-K$^+$-Mg^{2+})-ATPase. *Biochim Biophys Acta* **212**:322, 1970.

205. Simon BJ, Burckhardt G: Characterization of inside-out oriented H$^+$-ATPase in cholate pretreated renal brush-border membrane vesicles. *J Membr Biol* **117**:141, 1990.

206. Goldman H, Aaron K, Scriver CR, Pinsky L: Use of dithiothreitol to correct cystine storage in cultured cystinotic fibroblasts. *Lancet* **1**:811, 1970.

207. Gahl WA, Reed GF, Thoene JG, Schulman JD, Rizzo WB, Jonas AJ, Denman DW, Schlesselman JJ, Corden BJ, Schneider JA: Cysteamine therapy for children with nephropathic cystinosis. *N Engl J Med* **316**:971, 1987.

208. Arant BS, Greifer I, Edelmann CM, Spitzer A: Effect of chronic salt and water loading on the tubular defects of a child with Fanconi syndrome (cystinosis). *Pediatrics* **58**:370, 1976.

209. Rampini S, Fanconi A, Illig R, Prader A: Effect of hydrochlorothiazide on proximal renal tubular acidosis in a patient with idiopathic "deToni-Debré-Fanconi syndrome." *Helv Paediatr Acta* **23**:13, 1968.

210. Malekzadeh MH, Neustein HB, Schneider JA, Pennisi AJ, Ettenger RB, Uittenbogaart CH, Kogut MD, Fine RN: Cadaver renal transplantation in children with cystinosis. *Am J Med* **63**:525, 1977.

211. West JC, Goodman SI, Schroter GP, Bloustein PA, Hambidge KM, Well R: Pediatric kidney transplantation for cystinosis. *J Pediatr Surg* **12**:651, 1977.

CHAPTER 123

The Oculocerebrorenal Syndrome of Lowe (Lowe Syndrome)

Lawrence R. Charnas ▪ Robert L. Nussbaum

1. **The oculocerebrorenal syndrome of Lowe (OCRL) is a multisystem disorder with major abnormalities in the eyes, the nervous system, and the kidneys. Prenatal development of cataracts is universal, and other ocular abnormalities, including glaucoma, microphthalmos, decreased visual acuity, and corneal keloid formation, are frequent. Neonatal or infantile hypotonia, intellectual impairment, and areflexia are also cardinal features. Mental retardation, although very common, is not universal. Stereotypic behaviors, including tantrums and aggressiveness, are some of the more difficult management problems in the disease. Fanconi syndrome of the renal tubule (bicarbonaturia, renal tubular acidosis, aminoaciduria, phosphaturia, tubular proteinuria, and impaired urine concentrating ability) is also a major feature, but the severity and age of onset of the tubular dysfunction are variable. Slowly progressive renal failure can also occur in the second to fourth decade of life. Musculoskeletal abnormalities such as joint hypermobility, dislocated hips, and fractures may develop as secondary consequences of hypotonia or renal tubular acidosis and hypophosphatemia, but nontender joint swelling and subcutaneous nodules are also frequently seen and may reflect a primary abnormality of excessive connective tissue growth.**

2. **Undersulfation of glycosaminoglycans in the urine and fibroblasts from OCRL patients has been reported and was ascribed to a deficiency of an activated nucleotide which serves as donor of sulfate used in GAG biosynthesis. This finding remains controversial and requires additional confirming data.**

3. **OCRL is an X-linked disorder previously mapped to Xq25-q26. The only significant manifestation in carriers is in the lens. The sensitivity of carrier detection by slit-lamp exam is >90 percent but, as with most X-linked conditions, penetrance is unlikely to ever be 100 percent in female carriers because X-inactivation is random and the proportion of cells in the lens that have an inactivated normal OCRL allele can vary by chance between carriers.**

4. **A gene for OCRL, termed *OCRL-1*, was identified by positional cloning in the Xq25-q26 region of the X chromosome and found to have very strong homology to the gene on chromosome 1p for human inositol polyphosphate-5-phosphatase (INPP5B), an enzyme that removes the 5-phosphate from (1,4,5)-inositol trisphosphate and (1,3,4,5)-inositol tetrakisphosphate, thereby presumably inactivating them as second messengers in the phosphatidylinositol signaling pathway. Although the genetic evidence is conclusive that *OCRL-1* is the gene involved in OCRL, an abnormality in inositol phosphate metabolism is yet to be demonstrated.**

5. **Clinical diagnosis of OCRL depends on the cardinal ophthalmologic, neurologic, and renal abnormalities, while X-linked inheritance is extremely helpful when present. Carrier detection by slit-lamp examination has high but not perfect sensitivity. Molecular diagnosis has been accomplished in a few patients and reveals allelic heterogeneity between families. Prenatal diagnosis and carrier detection can be done by direct detection of mutations when known and by linked markers when the mutation is unknown.**

6. **Treatment includes cataract extraction, refraction for aphakia, control of glaucoma, speech and physical therapy for developmental delay, anticonvulsants if needed, and replacement of urinary bicarbonate, water, and phosphate losses if indicated by the development of acidosis or bone disease.**

The inclusion of the oculocerebrorenal syndrome of Lowe (OCRL) as a separate chapter, rather than as a subheading of a chapter describing renal Fanconi syndrome, reflects the advances in both clinical and molecular medicine that have led to better understanding of this inherited metabolic disease. In this chapter we will review the historical aspects of the disorder, the present state of knowledge about its clinical features, manifestations in carriers, inheritance pattern, and the rapidly evolving understanding of the underlying gene defect and corresponding metabolic disorder.

HISTORICAL FEATURES

OCRL was first described as a discrete entity by Lowe and colleagues in 1952[1] in an infant with organic aciduria, decreased renal ammonia production, hydrophthalmos, and mental retardation. Two elements of the description focused on secondary features of the disorder that are neither uniformly present nor specific for OCRL and which may have allowed inclusion of a heterogenous mix of other

A list of standard abbreviations is located immediately preceding the index in each volume. Additional abbreviations used in this chapter include: GAG = glycosaminoglycans; INPP5B = human platelet inositol polyphosphate-5-phosphatase; NPP = nucleotide pyrophosphatase; OCRL = oculocerebrorenal syndrome of Lowe; *OCRL-1* = candidate gene for OCRL identified by positional cloning; PAPS = adenosine 3′-phosphate 5′-phosphosulfate.

disorders into some reports.[2–4] The renal Fanconi syndrome associated with Lowe syndrome was recognized in 1954,[5] and a number of additional reports confirmed and expanded the clinical phenotype.[6–15]

X-linked recessive inheritance was first suggested in 1957[16] and convincingly demonstrated in 1965.[17] Ocular manifestations that could identify female carriers were identified a decade later.[18–20] The combination of X-linked inheritance and reliable heterozygote detection allowed gene mapping[21,22] and ultimately, gene identification using positional cloning techniques.[23] Current work now focuses on determining the function of the product of the gene for OCRL and the pathogenesis of the phenotype.

CLINICAL FEATURES

The oculocerebrorenal syndrome is named because of the prominent involvement in this disorder of three organ systems: the eye, the central nervous system, and the kidney. However, connective tissue, bone, gonads, muscle, and skin may be involved with what are characteristic and, in some cases, unique clinical features.

Ophthalmologic Abnormalities

The hallmark of this condition is the presence of congenital cataracts, which develop prenatally and are always present prior to birth. Abnormal lens formation in OCRL begins at 7 to 9 weeks' gestation and is due to disordered migration of the embryonic lens epithelium[24] as a primary defect rather than a secondary effect of systemic metabolic imbalance. Pathologic changes in the ocular lens have been described in 20- and 24-week fetuses. In the 20-week fetus, lens size was normal but there was abnormal concavity of the anterior portion of the lens and necrosis of the embryonic lens nucleus with disorganized architecture and swelling of the residual lens cells (M. M. Padilla, personal communication) (Fig. 123-1). In the other fetus studied, a cone-shaped opacity at the posterior pole caused loss of light transmission and additional aberrant developmental changes included disorganized nests of epithelial cells directly beneath the anterior lens capsule and swelling of the anterior lens fibers.[25] Histologically, the posterior lens capsule was incomplete, with protrusion of lens material and a cellular reaction surrounding the protruding material. It is not known if this histologic appearance results from abnormal formation of the lens capsule with secondary protrusion of material or if it is due to primary dysmigration. No glaucomatous changes were found, and the globes and anterior chambers were otherwise unremarkable in both fetuses.

Later in development there is continued protrusion of the posterior polar material through the posterior lens capsule, producing poor demarcation between the lens nucleus and cortex, marked thinning of the lens, and adherence of the vitreous to the posterior pole.[24,26,27] Calcification is frequent, with calcific excrescences of both anterior and posterior capsule, and hyperplasia of capsular epithelium. Changes secondary to lens abnormality include anteriorly displaced ciliary processes[28] and drawn retina, and a narrow anterior chamber angle. Microphthalmia and enophthalmos are also present, and are secondary to the lens abnormality, similar to that seen in transgenic animal models of lens damage.[29]

Glaucoma, either with or without buphthalmos, is quite frequent, occurring in 50 to 60 percent of patients in some series. It is usually bilateral and is a characteristic feature of the disorder rather than a reflection of the surgical technique used for cataract extraction.[1,30,31] Glaucoma is typically detected in the first year of life, but may appear as late as the second or third decade (L. Charnas, unpublished data).

Impaired visual acuity is almost universally present. Corrected visual acuity is rarely better than 20/100 despite optimal management, and the impairment represents both the morphologic changes in the eye caused by congenital cataract and a primary retinal dysfunction caused by the underlying disorder. Nystagmus develops postnatally secondary to the poor visual acuity and is virtually always present in older OCRL patients.

Corneal scarring and keloids are additional features of

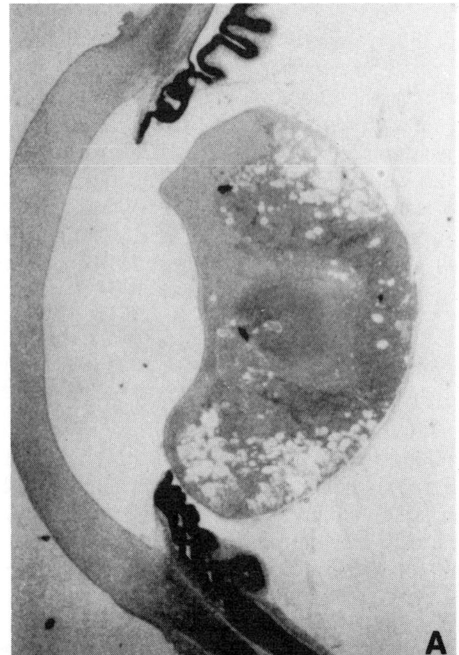

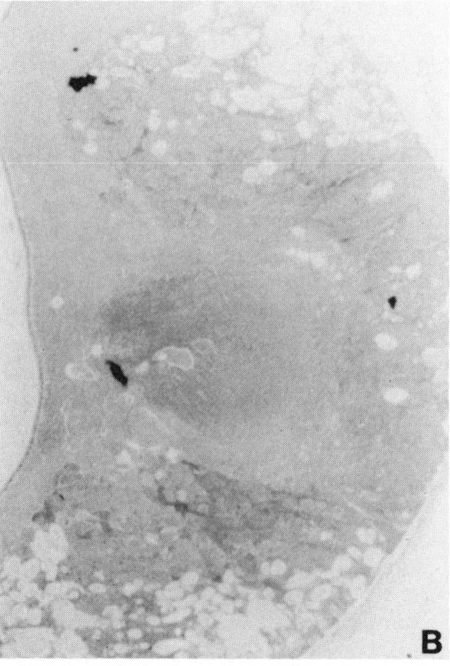

FIG. 123-1 *A*. Coronal section through anterior portion of the eye including cornea, anterior chamber, lens, and ciliary bodies of a 20-week OCRL fetus (mag × 24). *B*. Higher magnification of lens (mag × 40). Note abnormal anterior concave shape with central fluid-filled space and necrotic cells in the fetal lens nucleus location. Remaining lens cells above and below the fetal nucleus are large, frequently swollen, and disorganized, without a regular parallel distribution. *(Courtesy of M.M. Padilla, M.D.)*

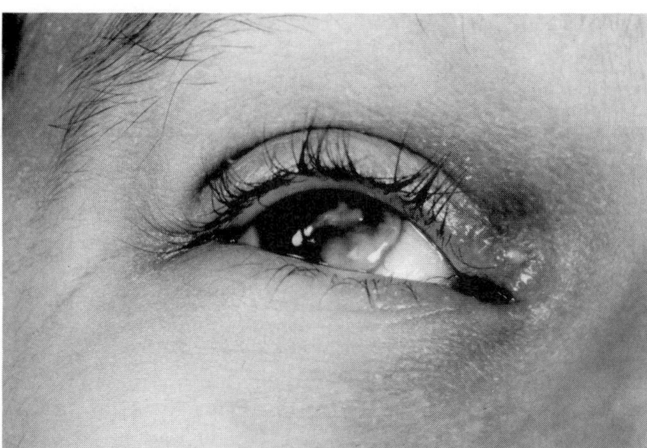

FIG. 123-2 Corneal keloid of the right eye in a 14-year-old boy without known eye-poking behavior or use of contact lenses. The keloid has its densest portion at the limbus and extends centrally to partially obscure central vision in this eye.

OCRL that probably develop spontaneously without trauma[32] (Fig. 123-2). Keloids may develop in up to 25 percent of OCRL patients, usually after age 5, and are bilateral in about half of affected patients.[31] Keloids are often stable and do not interfere with central vision, but they may cause significant visual impairment.

Nervous System Abnormalities

Both the central and the peripheral nervous system are involved in OCRL, and these involvements cause the greatest disease burden of the illness. A prominent feature is cognitive impairment, but neonatal hypotonia with delay in motor milestones is the initial neurologic manifestation and a cardinal feature of the disorder. In addition, areflexia, seizures, neuropathologic and neuroimaging abnormalities, and behavioral disturbances may also be present.

Cognitive Outcome. Mental retardation is common in OCRL patients but is not a cardinal feature because the diagnosis of OCRL is compatible with normal intelligence.[33] A more accurate description of the cognitive outcome is intellectual impairment, i.e., functioning below what would be an individual's predicted intellectual level in the absence of OCRL. This distinction is subtle, but normal intelligence in an otherwise typical OCRL patient has led to the exclusion of the diagnosis of OCRL (L. Charnas, unpublished data). Approximately 10 percent of OCRL patients will have intelligence within the normal range, typically borderline or low normal. The median IQ is in the moderately retarded range, and one third of affected individuals appear to be profoundly retarded. These estimates for intelligence suffer from the use of testing techniques that inappropriately penalize OCRL patients for their visual impairment and for behavioral disturbances that may impair accurate testing.[33] Socioeconomic status, maternal intelligence, MRI findings, and even the specific mutation causing the disorder appear to have little predictive value for intellectual outcome[34] (R. Nussbaum and L. Charnas, unpublished data). Intelligence appears to be stable over the life span of the individual, and deterioration in cognitive performance, occasionally reported in OCRL,[35] most likely represents decline due to progressive renal disease or another intercurrent illness.

Behavioral Abnormalities. Behavioral disturbances may be the most troublesome feature for caregivers. Early reports described a high-pitched scream, head banging, and an unusual mannerism characterized by hand waving between the eyes and a light source (oculodigital phenomenon),[1,17,36] but were dismissed as nonspecific mannerisms in handicapped individuals.[37] Two later studies confirmed a high incidence of stereotypic behavioral disturbances including self-injury, episodic outbursts (Lowe tantrum), aggression, irritability, and repetitive nonpurposeful movements that interfered with function.[31,33] A specific behavioral phenotype for OCRL consisting of stubbornness, temper tantrums, rigidity of thought, and unacceptable stereotypic behavior emerged when age, gender, visual impairment, and cognitive function were controlled for (Kenworthy L, Charnas L, to be published). This behavioral phenotype is reminiscent of the obsessive-compulsive disorder spectrum and warrants further study.

Neuromuscular Abnormalities. Neonatal or infantile hypotonia are cardinal manifestations of OCRL and may persist into childhood. A neuromuscular cause of hypotonia is suggested by the mildly elevated creatine kinase values and areflexia and by isolated reports of nerve and muscle abnormalities,[38–40] but the improvement with age, and the absence of reproducible and significant nerve or muscle pathology in most patients (L. Charnas, unpublished data), is more consistent with a central nervous system origin.

Deep tendon reflexes (areflexia) are uniformly absent after 1 year of age[1,30,37] and may be considered a late cardinal feature. It is unclear if reflexes are present at birth and then lost, or if they are never present. A progressive, axonal neuropathy has been proposed to explain the areflexia, but the small sample size, uncertainty concerning medical treatment, and excessive sampling from a homogeneous genetic population weakens this conclusion.[39,41–43] Another study found no pathologic evidence of an active neuropathy.[40] A much larger, longitudinal study at NIH has found, in general, normal nerve conduction velocities and motor amplitudes, although the "H" reflex, the electrical equivalent of a deep tendon reflex, is uniformly absent when tested (L. Charnas, unpublished data). These data do not support the presence of a progressive peripheral neuropathy in OCRL.

Central Nervous System Abnormalities. Seizures may occur in up to 50 percent of patients with OCRL. There is no characteristic seizure type, and infantile spasms with hypsarrythmia, myoclonic seizures, partial complex seizures, and generalized convulsions have all been reported or observed in the series of OCRL patients studied at the NIH. "Febrile" seizures appear to occur at a higher frequency than in the general population (9 percent versus 1 percent), and approximately one-third of these patients will progress to a true seizure disorder. Most seizures occur before age 6, although some patients have developed seizures as late as age 19. Severe, early-onset seizure disorders carry a poor prognosis for intellectual development and seizure control, as they do in the general population.

Cranial MRI demonstrates mild ventriculomegaly in about a third of patients, as well as areas of increased signal intensity on T_2-weighted scans (which are particularly sensitive for water) in a periventricular and centrum semiovale distribution, without involvement of other myelinated areas (corpus callosum, cortical U-fibers, brainstem, or cerebellum).[37,44] These areas correspond to cysts of variable size and number[45] (Fig. 123-3). The signal is undetectable

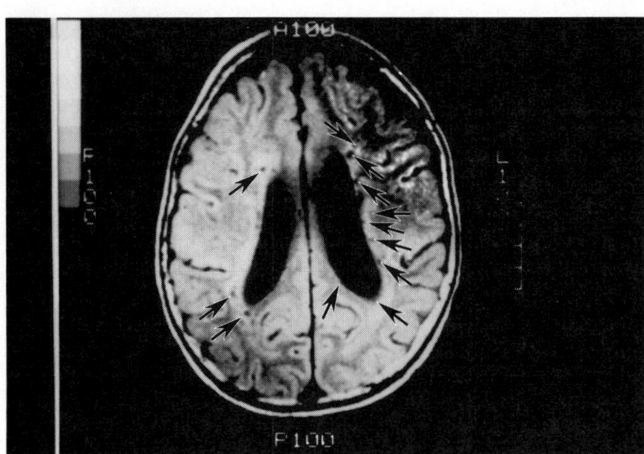

FIG. 123-3 Multiple periventricular cysts and ventriculomegaly in an 18-year-old boy with OCRL, more prominent in left hemisphere in this section.

until cerebral myelination is well advanced, but it is uncertain whether cysts are present at birth and not detectable or whether they develop as myelination proceeds. Cysts appear to be stable in size and location over a several-year observation period, and their size, location, and number have no clinical significance (L. Charnas, unpublished data).

Neuropathologic Features. Results of neuropathologic examination of the brain in OCRL were normal in some reports, while in others a number of different abnormalities were found, such as diffuse or focal myelin pallor without myelin breakdown, ventriculomegaly, mild cerebral abnormalities, isolated cases of subependymal cysts, mesencephalic proencephaly, postencephalitic changes, blunted and foreshortened frontal lobes, acute pontine necrosis, cerebellar hypoplasia, and aberrant neuronal migration.[35,41,42,46–52] Multiple tiny cysts without inflammatory changes were found in the cerebral white matter of one patient with typical evidence of such cysts on MRI (Wendy Shertz, M.D., personal communication).

Renal Manifestations

Tubular Defect. Abnormal kidney function is part of the clinical triad on which the diagnosis of OCRL is based, and its occurrence has been well documented in clinical reports and series.[15,17,30,35,39,41,46,48,53–57] Renal function and histology are apparently normal in utero, although the observation that amniotic fluid and maternal serum alpha-fetoprotein levels are elevated in some affected pregnancies with a male fetus suggests there may be a defect in the fetal kidney with resulting leakage of serum protein.[115] The most striking renal abnormality is found postnatally, with the onset of proximal tubular acidosis, aminoaciduria, phosphaturia, and proteinuria. The renal tubular dysfunction, in contrast to the cataracts, is not always present at birth and may require a few weeks to months to become apparent. Renal tubular dysfunction is quite variable in severity and clinical significance and may not require medical intervention.[57]

Acidosis is clearly of the proximal renal tubular type with bicarbonate wasting,[15,17,53] and leads to the failure to thrive, recurrent infections, and metabolic collapse seen in early case reports when the disease was poorly recognized and untreated. Water resorption is also defective, as reflected in elevated 24-h volumes and low urine osmolality.[57] Clinically significant hypokalemia or hypocalcemia requiring replacement therapy occurs in a minority of patients[57] and may be part of a preterminal exacerbation of tubular dysfunction.[34] The aminoaciduria is generalized, with greater elevations of basic amino acids and cysteine and relative sparing of branched-chain residues, but the profile is variable, with the degree of aminoaciduria (amino acid index) ranging from just above the upper limit of normal to 15 times the upper limit of normal.[15,57] In OCRL, as in other forms of the renal Fanconi syndrome, the pattern of aminoaciduria is not diagnostic of any particular etiology of the renal tubular dysfunction.[58] Proteinuria is very frequently seen, but the amount of urinary protein loss and age of onset are both highly variable. Proteinuria is usually present in infancy but can occur first later in childhood. When present, protein losses can be substantial (1.38 to 10.77 g/m^2/day; normal <0.1 g/m^2/day) and are composed of roughly equal proportions of tubular proteinuria (molecular mass <40 kDa) and albuminuria, with little to no protein of higher molecular weight. Glycosuria is generally not a feature of the renal tubular dysfunction seen in OCRL. Early reports suggested that a transient, severe acidotic phase that could be refractory to therapy[30] was followed by steady improvement of renal tubular dysfunction as renal failure developed. This course has not been observed in later reports,[57] and the renal Fanconi syndrome is usually stable in older patients once established. Occasional patients continue to appear whose acidosis is inexplicably more difficult to control.

Hyperphosphaturia is also frequent but variable, and may lead to osteomalacia, renal rickets, and pathologic fractures if untreated. It probably does not contribute significantly to the short stature seen in the syndrome.[57] In approximately half of patients, fractional excretions of phosphate are elevated despite low-normal serum phosphate levels, and there appears to be a progressive worsening of tubular phosphate wasting with age,[57] which may require nasogastric supplementation if refractory.[59] Severe hypophosphatemia has been detected preterminally in several patients and may have contributed to their demise[34] (L. Charnas, unpublished data). Nephrolithiasis and nephrocalcinosis may occur in OCRL[60] because of hyperphosphaturia and hypercalciuria, but high urinary volume may be partially protective. The frequency with which these complications occur is unknown.

Progressive Renal Failure. In addition to renal tubular dysfunction, gradual loss of creatine clearance reflecting progressive renal failure is a feature seen in OCRL patients in the second and third decades of life. The rate and extent of deterioration of renal function is, however, open to interpretation. In a series of 13 OCRL patients ranging in age from 10 to 31 years of age, a statistically significant straight line can be drawn for reciprocal serum creatinine plotted versus age, a commonly used method of monitoring the rate of loss of renal function in chronic renal failure in children.[61,62] However, the rate of loss of renal function could also be biphasic, with more rapid loss in children under age 15 and relative stability of function after that. Thus, although gradual loss of glomerular filtration has been seen in OCRL, the average age of onset of renal insufficiency and its severity have not been clearly defined in a large enough population of patients.

Renal Pathology. Results of histologic examination by light microscopy are usually normal in very young infants, but dilatation, atrophy, loss of brush border, and accumulation of proteinaceous material in the tubule lumen appear in the first few months of life.[15,17,56,63] These tubular abnormalities have been documented in a number of studies, including some in which serial biopsy specimens from the same patients were examined, and affect predominantly the proximal tubules; some involvement of Henle's loop, the distal tubules, and the conducting system is occasionally reported as well. Glomeruli are frequently normal in young children, even when proximal tubular lesions are present. After the first few years of life, however, glomerular lesions can be seen. These include thickening of basement membranes, focal fibrosis, and sclerosis. By EM, swelling of mitochondria in renal tubules was reported in a 22-month-old who showed no glomerular abnormalities.[15] When the same child was biopsied 7 years later, distinctive glomerular changes, including podocyte fusion and basement membrane thickening, were apparent.[56] Some of the most severe EM abnormalities in glomeruli and proximal tubules were reported in a female patient who did not satisfy current clinical diagnostic criteria for OCRL,[3] raising the question of whether these findings apply to OCRL.

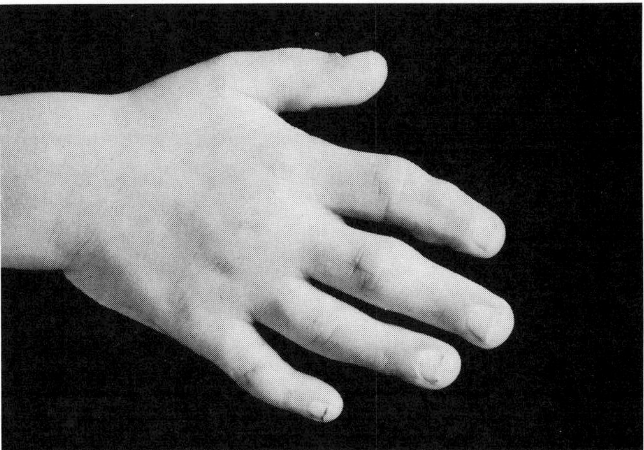

FIG. 123-4 Hand of a 7-year-old boy showing nontender, diffuse swelling of the second and third proximal interphalangeal joints and a subcutaneous nodule on the second digit over the distal interphalangeal joint. There was no history of trauma to this area.

Musculoskeletal Complications

Musculoskeletal complications of OCRL can arise either as complications of cardinal features of the illness—i.e., hypotonia and renal disease—or as specific and possibly unique manifestations of the underlying disorder. Reported complications include joint hypermobility, recurrent fractures, genu valgum, joint contractures, scoliosis, kyphosis, platyspondyly, dislocated and/or subluxated hips, cervical spine anomalies,[64] as well as tenosynovitis and a nonspecific arthropathy.[54,65–67] Hypotonia contributes to joint hypermobility, decreased movement fosters the development of contractures, and inadequately treated rickets can lead to genu valgum deformities. Coxa valga deformity and hip contractures were found in a 16-year-old, profoundly retarded male who lost the ability to walk at age 13 years, but the hips were neither subluxated nor dislocated.[40] Joint laxity leading to varus deformity or hyperextension of the knee has also been seen. Osteopenia can be worsened by untreated renal phosphate wasting, but it is almost always present, with variable severity, despite adequate phosphate replacement, and it appears to be a specific manifestation of OCRL. Some of the patients studied in the NIH series had mildly increased cervical spine mobility without subluxation, and three had asymptomatic bone cysts,[37] but platyspondyly, hip dislocation or subluxation, and cervical spine anomalies are quite uncommon in most series.[37] In contrast, scoliosis is widely reported in OCRL[26,31,40,64] and may be progressive postpubertally, suggesting that it is a specific feature of OCRL.

Tenosynovitis, joint swelling, and arthritis or arthropathy appear to be frequent and striking primary complications of OCRL and probably represent the same underlying disorder of excessive growth of fibroblasts. This manifestation was initially reported as palmar and plantar fibrosis[66] and later as thickened articular joint surfaces with nonspecific tenosynovitis, flexion contractures of the digits, and swelling of the interphalangeal and metacarpophalangeal joints[65]; the first detailed investigation described four additional patients with similar joint manifestations and varying degrees of nontender swelling of multiple joints. In some cases the periarticular areas and joints of the fingers and wrist were involved, with erosion of the carpal bones. Results of laboratory studies were normal. A synovial biopsy found rubbery tissue with loss of the normal glistening surface, sparse synovial lining cells, no inflammatory cell infiltrate, fibrous connective tissue containing mature collagen and thin fibrils, and large amounts of finely fibrillar material and a granular basement membrane-like substance around the small vessels.[54]

Similar diffuse swellings of the fingers, wrists, ankles, and feet without evidence of an inflammatory arthritis and similar joint changes are reported in 50 percent of OCRL patients over 20 years of age.[31] The spectrum of joint involvement is quite broad, presenting as nontender joint swelling involving both small and large joints, focal nodules (Fig. 123-4) on the finger, or bilateral plantar masses (Fig. 123-5). On occasion these masses become painful and require resection.[37] It seems likely that these changes are the manifestation of abnormal, excessive growth of fibroblasts from periarticular tissue or tendons.

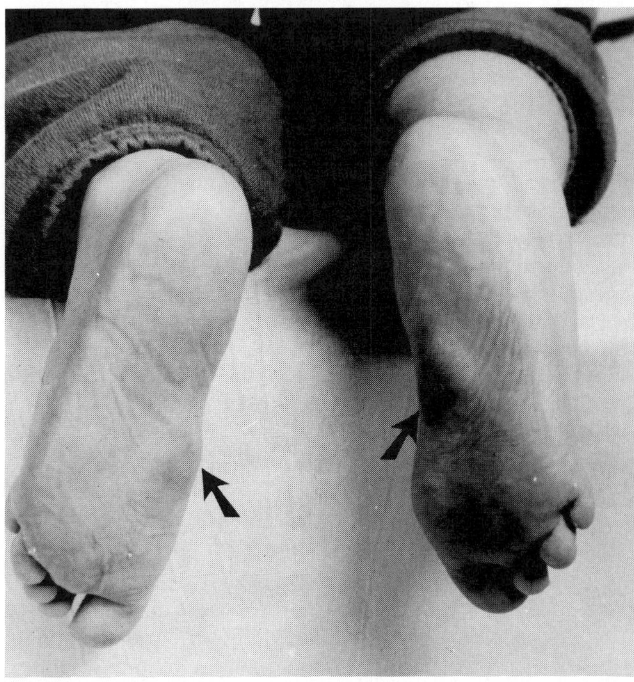

FIG. 123-5 Bilateral plantar masses (arrows) in a 12-year-old boy. The masses are firm and are attached to underlying connective tissue, but they are nontender and do not interfere with ambulation.

Sexual Development

The onset and progression of puberty occurs at a normal age in OCRL patients, producing Tanner V genitalia and axillary and facial hair. Testosterone levels are normal. Sexual interest among older males varies, but there is a notable lack of a strong sexual drive in comparison with other similarly intellectually compromised adults. Fertility may also be reduced owing to the peritubular fibrosis and azoospermia associated with OCRL.[35]

Other Clinical Manifestations

Cryptorchidism is a common occurrence in OCRL, up to 40 percent in one report[30] and 15 percent in a more comprehensive survey.[31] Dental "blue dome" cysts during primary tooth eruption have been reported and, in older individuals, sebaceous cysts on the buttocks and perineum appear to occur frequently (L. Charnas, unpublished data). Constipation of variable severity is frequent in OCRL and usually improves with age,[31] although it may persist and cause a protuberant abdomen or diarrhea with stooling around a fecal impaction (L. Charnas, unpublished data).

Growth

The mean length and weight are within the normal range at birth, typically above the 50th percentile, but fall from the normal curve with age. Mean height falls to the third percentile by three years of age, and continues to show a relative fall throughout adolescence. Mean final height is less than the third percentile, but OCRL patients continue to grow into early adulthood. Bone age lags slightly behind height age, and epiphyses fuse at adult height. Mean weight shows a similar profile, with a late plateau phase into the early twenties and a final weight less than the third percentile. Head circumference of OCRL patients is within the normal range, with a mean adult head circumference at the 50th percentile.[57]

Cause of Death

OCRL patients have been reported to succumb to renal failure or infection in their second or third decade,[30] but infection as a cause of death has become infrequent with more aggressive medical intervention. Other causes of death include status epilepticus, refractory renal tubular wasting of electrolytes, respiratory compromise from scoliosis, and sudden, unexplained death (L. Charnas, unpublished data). The oldest OCRL patient in the United States expired at age 41. The expected lifespan with current medical practice has not been defined.

Laboratory Findings

A few laboratory aberrations are curious concomitants of OCRL.[57] Specifically, serum acid phosphatase, a marker for prostate cancer in adults or lysosomal storage diseases in children, is elevated in most OCRL patients. Serum protein electrophoresis demonstrates a markedly elevated alpha-2 band in two-thirds of patients examined, and total serum protein concentration is frequently elevated in patients over 4 years of age, occasionally to values as high as 9 g/liter, without dehydration. No abnormal proteins or elevations of a particular protein appear to cause the alpha-2 or total protein elevation; these increases appear to be general. Erythrocyte sedimentation rate is increased in over one-third of patients, and is probably a nonspecific effect of renal Fanconi syndrome. Serum T4 may be slightly elevated, in part owing to an elevated thyroid binding globulin level, and thyroid stimulating hormone (TSH) as well as triiodothyronine are in the normal range.

Serum enzyme levels are frequently outside the normal range and serve as a useful confirmation of the clinical diagnosis. Mild elevations of aspartate aminotransferase (AST), lactate dehydrogenase (LDH), and creatine phosphokinase (CPK) activities and minor isoenzyme changes with normal alanine aminotransferase (ALT) are typically found, but the clinical significance of these changes is unknown. In most OCRL patients, serum triglycerides are normal, but total cholesterol is typically elevated, usually owing to increased HDL.[57]

BIOCHEMICAL ABNORMALITIES

A number of biochemical abnormalities have been reported in OCRL patients, including a defect in cellular proline uptake,[68] a deficiency of procollagen synthesis in fibroblasts,[69] disturbances in mitochondrial energy production,[70] and, in some studies, abnormalities in the size distribution and degree of sulfation of glycosaminoglycans (GAG), particularly chondroitin sulfate, in urine[71] and in cultured fibroblasts.[72,73] Undersulfation of GAGs in OCRL fibroblasts was ascribed to a deficiency of a sulfate donor for GAG biosynthesis, adenosine 3′-phosphate 5′-phosphosulfate (PAPS), caused by a three- to eightfold elevation of the levels of nucleotide pyrophosphatase (NPP) (E.C. 3.6.1.9), an enzyme that degrades PAPS,[73–76] although this interpretation has been disputed by other workers.[77] The abnormal sulfation in the urine or cultured fibroblasts of OCRL patients has not been a consistent finding, however, and remains controversial.[9,72,78] The elevation in the activity of NPP[75,76] in many OCRL patients, however, has been confirmed in other laboratories (L. Charnas, unpublished data) but the relationship of the elevated activity of this enzyme to a defect in the gene product of the OCRL candidate gene, *OCRL-1* (see below), is obscure.

GENETICS

From the first, a straightforward analysis of patients with OCRL indicated that the overwhelming majority of patients were male and that the disease was inherited as an X-linked condition, with multiply affected males in pedigrees related to each other through essentially asymptomatic, unaffected female carriers.[17,79–81] A few rare females with features of OCRL have been reported as sporadic occurrences.[4,17,79–83] In some of these patients, portions of the OCRL phenotype were either absent or were included in a wider spectrum of congenital malformations and birth defects that made the diagnosis of OCRL uncertain. In others, the phenotype was consistent with a diagnosis of OCRL, but cytogenetic analysis was not adequate to determine whether there was a chromosomal basis for the disease. Two other interesting groups of female patients, however, have been described. One girl was reported with a progressive multisystem disease reminiscent of OCRL and a deletion of mitochondrial DNA, which raised the possibility that a mitochondrial genocopy for OCRL may exist.[4] In two other females,[83,84] a classic OCRL was seen in association with balanced X;autosome translocations involving, in both cases, the Xq26 region of the X chromosome with two different autosomes. Since the normal X chromosome is generally inactive when there is a balanced X;autosome translocation, females carrying such translocations can develop full expression of an X-linked disorder if the translocation breakpoint disrupts the disease locus. Female patients with translocations proved instrumental in allowing the identification and characterization of the OCRL gene.

The gene for OCRL was isolated by positional cloning[85] in 1992.[23] First, the locus was regionally mapped to the Xq25-q26 region using linkage analysis with RFLP in families with multiply affected individuals.[21,22,86,87] This same region of the X chromosome was implicated in the disease by the findings in two females with classic OCRL and X;autosome translocations, in whom the breakpoint on the X was in the very distal Xq25 or proximal Xq26 region.[82,83] In one of these females, who had an X;3 translocation, yeast artificial chromosomes containing the region of the X chromosome involved in the translocation were isolated and used to identify genes that could be tested as candidates for OCRL.[88–90] A gene termed *OCRL-1* was found that was disrupted by the translocation breakpoints in both females with OCRL and X;autosome translocations.[23] The gene detected a ~5.7-kb transcript in brain and kidney, as well as skeletal muscle, heart, placenta, lung, ovary, testis, and fibroblasts, but showed little or no transcript in peripheral leukocytes, spleen, or thymus. Transcripts for this gene were either absent or aberrant in size in nearly 50 percent of unrelated male patients with the disease.[23] Nonsense mutations in *OCRL-1* in patients with OCRL completed the genetic proof that *OCRL-1* was indeed the disease gene.[34]

The precise function of the gene product of *OCRL-1* is not known. One strong clue, however, is the striking homology to a human enzyme involved in inositol phosphate metabolism, a 75-kDa inositol polyphosphate-5-phosphatase (INPP5B) described in platelets[91,92] and cloned from platelet and placenta cDNA libraries.[93] This enzyme cleaves the 5-phosphate specifically from inositol (1,4,5)-trisphosphate and inositol (1,3,4,5)-tetrakisphosphate and is thought thereby to terminate their activity as second messengers in the phosphatidylinositol signaling pathway.[94] The enzyme appears to act only on soluble inositol phosphates, rather than on phospholipids containing inositol phosphate, since it does not utilize glycerol inositol-5-phosphate as a substrate.[92] The two proteins show 53 percent identity and 71 percent similarity in primary amino acid sequence, but are distinct in their map location, size of transcript, and pattern of expression. INPP5B has a 4.4-kb transcript, much smaller than *OCRL-1*, and, in contrast to *OCRL-1*, is expressed strongly in cells of hematopoietic origin, such as peripheral leukocytes, spleen, and thymus, but not in brain (P. A. Janne and R. L. Nussbuam, unpublished data). INPP5B maps to chromosome 1p,[116] whereas *OCRL-1* is X-linked.[23]

INPP5B is only one of several mammalian inositol (1,4,5)-trisphosphate-5-phosphatases that have been described in different tissues and species, but it is the only one for which the gene has been isolated to date.[51,91,92,95–98] Activity has been found in cell extracts either in the soluble fraction or in the particulate fraction or in both fractions, in a number of different tissues. The various activities differ in estimated molecular mass, ranging from 45 kDa to >160 kDa, and in specificity for substrates such as (1,3,4,5)-inositol tetrakisphosphate, for which the K_m has been measured to be $<1 \mu M$ to $>160 \mu M$. For this reason, it is tempting to hypothesize that *OCRL-1* may encode one of the inositol polyphosphate-5-phosphatases other than INPP5B.[99] That *OCRL-1* encodes another enzymatic activity in inositol metabolism, such as inositol monophosphate phosphatase, is less likely since that enzyme bears no significant amino acid sequence homology with INPP5B or *OCRL-1*.[98,100]

The relationship between the putative involvement of the *OCRL-1* gene in inositol metabolism and the abnormalities in sulfated GAG observed in fibroblasts from OCRL patients is obscure. A tenuous relationship between inositol metabolism and abnormalities in sulfated GAG can be drawn from the facts that reduced sulfated proteoglycan levels have been observed in diabetics[101] and that abnormalities in inositol metabolism have been proposed but not proved to have a role in the pathogenesis of cataracts in galactosemia[102,103] and diabetes mellitus.[104,105] Thus, one could hypothesize that the alteration in GAG seen in OCRL may be secondary to abnormal inositol metabolism. However, a specific defect in inositol polyphosphate-5-phosphatase activity in particular, or in inositol phosphate metabolism more generally, has yet to be demonstrated in an easily accessible tissue from OCRL patients, such as fibroblasts. Whether OCRL is an inborn error of inositol phosphate metabolism awaits direct confirmation or refutation.

DIAGNOSIS AND TREATMENT

Diagnostic Criteria

In the absence of a reproducible biochemical defect or a confirmed family history with an identified molecular defect, diagnosis relies on the cardinal clinical features of OCRL: congenital cataracts, neonatal or infantile hypotonia with later cognitive impairment and areflexia, and, eventually, renal tubular dysfunction. Confirming features include glaucoma (either congenital or developing postoperatively), buphthalmos, megalocornea, cryptorchidism, characteristic appearance, and abnormalities in serum and urine electrolytes and protein (see below). Cataracts are congenital in the strict sense, being present at birth with the characteristic thin lens and complete visual occlusion. Neonatal hypotonia is typically obvious. Demonstration of renal tubular dysfunction may be difficult initially and may require quantitative determination of amino acid or protein excretion as well as of impaired water-concentrating ability.

The differential diagnosis of neonatal hypotonia and dense cataracts is limited to OCRL and congenital rubella. These two disorders may be distinguished by serology, intracranial calcifications, and other clinical features. Congenital myotonic dystrophy presents with severe neonatal hypotonia; lenticular opacities may also be present, but these cataracts are clinically subtle, metachromatic, and easily distinguished from the cataract in OCRL.

Prenatal Diagnosis

Prenatal diagnosis of OCRL can be achieved using linked markers in families or by direct detection of the mutant alleles. Flanking linked markers[22,87] have been used in families known to be at risk for recurrence[106] (R. L. Nussbaum, unpublished data). Because current linked markers have poor polymorphism information content, additional highly polymorphic markers in or around the *OCRL-1* gene itself would be very helpful but have not yet been detected (R. Nussbaum, unpublished data). Direct detection of mutations in *OCRL-1* by PCR analysis of RNA and DNA has just begun and has revealed significant allelic heterogeneity between families[34] (R. Nussbaum, unpublished data), as would be expected when new mutation is the likely explanation for cases of an X-linked lethal equivalent. Molecular diagnosis will require therefore that the mutation be identified in order to provide specific and accurate diagnosis in each family.

In addition to direct molecular diagnosis or diagnosis by linked markers, maternal serum alpha-fetoprotein measurements and fetal ultrasound may be useful adjuncts. In a small series of patients, unexplained elevations of alpha-fetoprotein levels have been reported well above 2 multiples of the median in a minority of pregnancies carrying a fetus affected with OCRL.[115] Ultrasound detection of an abnormal lens in a male fetus at 18 weeks' gestation was reported in a woman who had the typical lens changes of the OCRL carrier state and who had given birth to a previous male child affected with OCRL.[107] Pathologic examination of fetal lens tissue following abortion confirmed the abnormalities seen on ultrasound. However, the sensitivity of ultrasound detection of cataracts in fetuses at risk for OCRL may be low, since directed prenatal ultrasound examination in two similar situations at experienced centers was unsuccessful in identifying the abnormal lens at 18 and 20 weeks, respectively (D. Steele and R. Miller, personal communication).

Carrier Detection

Female carriers of OCRL are usually asymptomatic and have no significant renal or neurologic defects detectable upon clinical or laboratory examination. Ophthalmologic evaluation, however, reveals one of two distinctive lenticular changes in most heterozygotes.[18,20,79,108–110] The most common finding on slit-lamp examination is numerous punctate, white-to-gray opacities, which are present in all layers of the lenticular cortex except the nucleus and are distributed in a radial, spoke-like pattern (Fig. 123-6A). The distribution of opacities just outside the nucleus suggests that the opacities develop very early in life, while the more superficial opacities must arise in adulthood.[110] There are usually more than 15 of these opacities, and there may be hundreds. A few female carriers show a single subcapsular dense cataract in the posterior pole[109] (Fig. 123-6B). This form of cataract may be present congenitally and become clinically more apparent with age eventually requiring surgery.

Controversy exists concerning the specificity of the lens changes in OCRL carrier females compared with the changes that are seen with increasing age in normal individuals.[18,20] Specificity can be markedly improved by taking into account not only the number of such opacities but also their characteristic distribution, particularly if one concentrates on females of child-bearing age, who are likeliest to seek carrier detection for genetic counseling.[108]

The sensitivity (penetrance) of lens opacities for carrier detection has been evaluated in families in whom female carriers were diagnosed using flanking linked markers.[22] In one study, 31 of 33 (94 percent) of carriers could be detected by slit-lamp exam. The presence of cataracts in female carriers suggests that the defect is expressed in a cell-autonomous manner—that is, groups of cells in which the X chromosome carrying the normal OCRL allele is inactivated express the defect and cannot be "cross-corrected" by neighboring cells that have an active normal allele. As with most X-linked conditions, however, expression is likely to be very variable and penetrance unlikely to ever be 100 percent in female carriers because X-inactivation is random

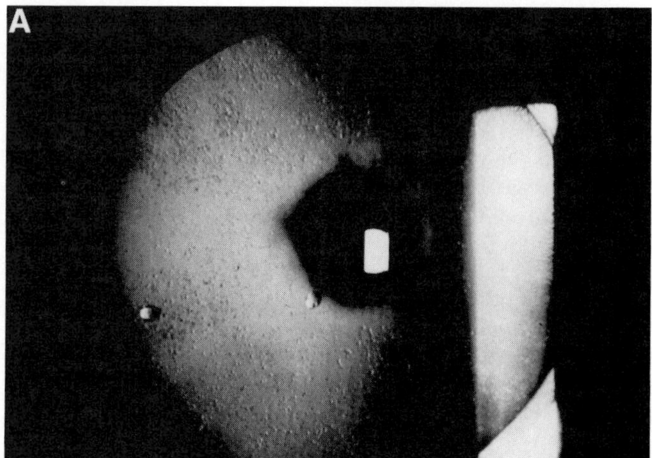

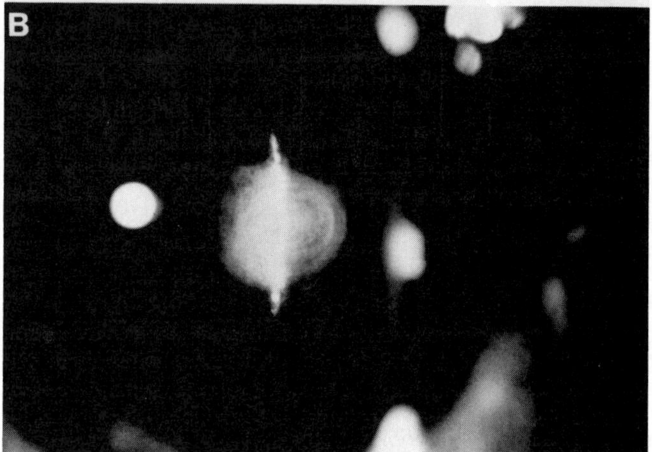

FIG. 123-6 **Slit-lamp examination of female carriers of Lowe's syndrome. *A*. The typical pattern of hundreds of micropunctate, gray opacities in a radial distribution in the lens. *B*. A single dense posterior cataract, as seen in some OCRL heterozygotes. *(Courtesy of R. A. Lewis, M.D.)***

and the proportion of cells in the lens that have inactivated the normal OCRL allele can vary by chance between carriers.

Treatment

Vision. The visual defects in OCRL patients constitute a major obstacle to the ability of these patients to reach their developmental potential. A detailed discussion of ophthalmologic therapy and procedures is beyond the scope of this chapter, and early ophthalmologic consultation and therapy are mandated to aid in diagnosis and institution of therapy.[110] Cataracts should be removed when diagnosed, and the resulting aphakia treated with glasses. Glaucoma, a frequent component of the disease, may be difficult to control medically, and goniotomy or trabeculotomy to control intraocular pressure is often required. Corneal keloid formation is another serious complication that usually develops after age 5. Opinions differ as to whether corneal trauma or the use of contact lenses contributes to keloid development. For this reason, glasses are preferred over contact lenses, especially since younger patients are less likely to lose or damage glasses anyway. The fact that the keloids involve the full thickness of the cornea makes lamellar keratoplasty ineffective. Even with early ophthalmologic intervention, including treatment of cataracts and glaucoma, some degree of impairment of visual acuity is usually present, and nystagmus is a common finding.

Nervous System. The treatment of neurologic manifestations in OCRL is largely symptomatic. Hypotonia and developmental delay are treated with a combination of speech, physical, and occupational therapy beginning at an early age. Such interventions are designed to facilitate the progress of each child according to his ability, and the use of appropriate testing techniques and specialized environments appears to offer a better-than-expected outcome in some cases. Areflexia is a medical curiosity and does not warrant therapy. Seizures are treated according to current standards, depending on the seizure type and precipitating features. Phenobarbital, carbamazepine, phenytoin, and valproic acid, as well as the benzodiazepines, have all been used with success in patients with OCRL.[111]

Stereotypic behaviors that frequently interfere with normal function and the inability to change a pattern without precipitating a temper tantrum (rigidity, stubbornness) are frequently the most difficult treatment issues facing the clinician. Many psychopharmaceuticals (neuroleptics, stimulants, benzodiazepines, antidepressants) have been used without a clear pattern of success. Improvement of stereotypic behavior and stubbornness following treatment with clomipramine, a tricyclic antidepressant that significantly inhibits serotonin reuptake, has been seen (L. Charnas, unpublished data).

Renal Disease. Periodic monitoring for renal complications of OCRL should begin at the first suggestion of the diagnosis and continue every three months in the first 2 years of life in anticipation of development of significant tubular wasting of small molecules. The renal tubular Fanconi syndrome is similar, although less severe, than that seen in cystinosis, and treatment guidelines have been modified from the cystinosis experience (see Chap. 126). All individuals have impaired water-concentrating ability and should have free access to fluids to replace urinary water losses. Alkalinizing therapy to counter renal bicarbonate losses should begin when serum bicarbonate drops below 20 mEq/liter, using either a tricitrate solution (Polycitra, Bicitra) or sodium bicarbonate starting at a dose of 2 to 3 mEq/kg/day given every 6 to 8 h, and adjusted once or twice a week until serum bicarbonate is above 20 mEq/liter. Typically, patients can be corrected to values of 23 to 24 mEq/liter, but more refractory patients may require higher doses and administration every 6 h. Hypokalemia is not usually encountered in OCRL, but administration of Polycitra, with 1 mEq of potassium and 1 mEq of sodium per milliequivalent of citric acid, may avoid this problem. Urinary phosphorus losses are variable and may be elevated without requiring phosphate supplementation.

The easiest and most reliable indicator for phosphorus supplementation is serum alkaline phosphatase, which increases as bone resorption occurs to maintain normal phosphorus levels. Clinical or radiographic evidence of rickets are late findings, and serum phosphate levels are maintained within the normal range until there is severe bone demineralization. Sodium or potassium phosphate administration should be initiated at between 1 to 4 g/day in divided doses, and serum alkaline phosphatase monitored at 2- to 4-month intervals to follow normalization. A vitamin D preparation may be a useful adjunct to increase intestinal phosphate absorption, although it should be used cautiously because of the potential to overstimulate intestinal calcium absorption, leading to increased urinary calcium excretion with the potential for nephrocalcinosis or nephrolithiasis. Calcium replacement is infrequently required in OCRL, and care should be taken to avoid precipitation of calcium phosphate in the renal collecting system.

Limitation of protein intake has been recommended by some nephrologists to decrease the likelihood of renal insufficiency in the long term. Although this approach may be beneficial to adults with chronic renal failure, its efficacy in OCRL has not been demonstrated. Nitrogen losses from proteinuria and aminoaciduria in OCRL are significant, and severe protein restriction without consideration of these losses may lead to a protein intake that is inadequate for growth.

The efficacy of L-carnitine replacement in OCRL has not been systematically studied. Carnitine deficiency defined as plasma values greater than 2 standard deviations below the mean have been documented in OCRL, and a transient clinical benefit from carnitine supplementation has been reported in only one patient.[112] Normalization of plasma carnitine following oral supplementation is easily demonstrated, but there is no objective evidence of benefit. The major complications from L-carnitine supplementation are the expense of the medication, which is frequently available at health food stores, and the social stigma of a fishy odor due to tertiary amine release from carnitine breakdown.

Administration of recombinant human growth hormone (rhGH) to increase linear growth in OCRL should be limited to those individuals who have demonstrable growth hormone deficiency. The use of rhGH in other disorders with renal insufficiency has led to early kidney transplants owing to increased somatic growth without concomitant growth in glomerular filtration,[113] and this is a potential outcome in OCRL.

Acute renal failure, such as acute tubular necrosis from myoglobinuria, has been reported in OCRL and resolves with appropriate medical support.[114] There are no reports of chronic renal dialysis or renal transplantation in OCRL patients.

Musculoskeletal Abnormalities and Other Clinical Findings. The treatment of most of the musculoskeletal problems associated with OCRL is straightforward. Contractures are avoided by maintaining mobility, and osteopenia and fractures can be prevented by astute management of the renal disease. Scoliosis should be anticipated and treated using standard methods, including use of rods. The proper management of joint swelling and fibroid tumors is less clear, but minimizing discomfort, maintaining mobility, and judicious use of surgery for relief of pain are reasonable guidelines. Undescended testes should be managed using standard criteria.

ACKNOWLEDGMENTS

The authors acknowledge the officers and members of the Lowe's Syndrome Association for their support, cooperation, and patience. We also thank W. Shertz, M. Norman, K. Armfield, D. Steele, R. Miller, E. Rawnlsey, M. M. Padilla, and R. A. Lewis for making patient information and photographs available to us. We are very grateful to L. C. Bailey for critical reading of the manuscript and numerous helpful suggestions.

REFERENCES

1. Lowe CU, Terrey M, MacLachan EA: Organic aciduria, decreased renal ammonia production, hydrophthalmos, and mental retardation: A clinical entity. *Am J Dis Child* **83**:164, 1952.
2. McCance RA, Matheson WJ, Gresham GA, Elkington JR: The cerebro-ocular-renal dystrophies: A new variant. *Arch Dis Child* **35**:240, 1960.
3. Sagel I, Ores RO, Yuceoglu AM: Renal function and morphology in a girl with oculocerebrorenal syndrome. *J Pediatr* **77**:124, 1970.
4. Moraes CT, Zeviani M, Schon EA, Hickman RO, Vlcek BW, DiMauro S: Mitochondrial DNA deletion in a girl with manifestations of Kearns-Sayre and Lowe syndromes: An example of phenotypic mimicry? *Am J Med Genet* **41**:301, 1991.
5. Bickel H, Thursby-Pelham DC: Hyper-amino-aciduria in Lignac-Fanconi disease, in galactosaemia and in an obscure syndrome. *Arch Dis Child* **29**:224, 1954.
6. Dent C, Smellie JM: Two children with the oculocerebrorenal syndrome of Lowe, Terrey and Maclachlan. *Proc R Soc Med* **54**:335, 1961.
7. Auricchio AW, Frischkvecht O, Shmerling B: Primare tubulopathien III einfall von oculo-cerebro-renalen syndroms (Lowe syndrome). *Helv Paediatr Acta* **16**:647, 1961.
8. Terslev E: Two cases of amino aciduria, ocular changes and retarded mental and somatic development (Lowe's syndrome). *Acta Paediatr Scand* **49**:635, 1960.
9. Yokoi T, Uozaki T, Kasei M, Sato T, Taniguchi N: Low urinary excretion of heparan sulfate in three patients with Lowe's syndrome. *Clin Chim Acta* **116**:153, 1981.
10. Scholten HG: Een meisje met het syndroom van Lowe. *Maandschr Kindergeneesk* **28**:251, 1960.
11. Donnell GN, Wilson WA, Stowen DS: The oculocerebrorenal syndrome of Lowe. *Am J Dis Child* **100**:707, 1960.
12. Seedorff HH: Ocular changes in certain forms of amino aciduria. *Acta Ophthalmol* **37**:125, 1959.
13. Jagenburg OR: The urinary excretion of free-amino acids and other amino compounds by the human. *Scand J Clin Lab Invest* **11** (Suppl 43):1, 1959.
14. Falls HG: Ocular manifestations of the chronic renal tubular insufficiency syndromes. *Arch Ophthalmol* **62**:188, 1959.
15. Schoen EJ, Young G: "Lowe's syndrome": Abnormalities in renal tubular function in combination with other congenital defects. *Am J Med* **27**:781, 1959.
16. Le Febvre G, Biserte G, Woillez M, Fraismel M, Gosselin J: Etude clinique, genetique et biologique du syndrome de Lowe-Bickel. *Pediatrie* **12**:527, 1957.
17. Richards W, Donnell GN, Wilson WA, Stowens D, Perry T: The oculocerebrorenal syndrome of Lowe. *Am J Dis Child* **109**:185, 1965.
18. Brown N, Gardner RJM: Lowe syndrome: Identification of the carrier state. *Birth Defects* **12**(3):579, 1976.
19. Delleman JW, Bleeker-Wagemakers EM, van Veelen AWC: Opacities of the lens indicating carrier status in the oculo-cerebro-renal (Lowe) syndrome. *J Pediatr Ophthalmol* **14**:205, 1976.
20. Gardner RJM, Brown N: Lowe's syndrome: Identification of carriers by lens examination. *J Med Genet* **13**:449, 1976.
21. Silver DN, Lewis RA, Nussbaum RL: Mapping the Lowe oculocerebrorenal syndrome to Xq24-q26 by use of restriction fragment length polymorphisms. *J Clin Invest* **79**:282, 1987.
22. Reilly DS, Lewis RA, Ledbetter DH, Nussbaum RL: Tightly linked flanking markers for the Lowe oculocerebrorenal syndrome with application to carrier assessment. *Am J Hum Genet* **42**:748, 1988.
23. Attree O, Olivos IM, Okabe I, Bailey LC, Nelson DL, Lewis RA, McInnes RR, Nussbaum RL: The Lowe oculocerebrorenal syndrome gene encodes a novel protein highly homologous to inositol polyphosphate-5-phosphatase. *Nature* **358**:239, 1992.
24. Ginsberg J, Bove KE, Fogelson MH: Pathological features of the eye in the oculocerebrorenal (Lowe) syndrome. *J Pediatr Ophthalmol Strabismus* **18**:16, 1981.
25. Endres W, Schaub J, Stefani FH, Wirtz A, Zahn V: Cataract in a fetus at risk for oculocerebrorenal syndrome. *Klin Wochenschr* **55**:141, 1977.
26. Curtin VT, Joyce EE, Ballin N: Ocular pathology in the oculo-cerebro-renal syndrome of Lowe. *Am J Opthalmol* **64**:533, 1967.
27. Tripathi RC, Cibis GW, Tripathi BJ: Pathogenesis of cataracts in patients with Lowe's syndrome. *Ophthalmology* **93**:1046, 1986.
28. Dufier JL, Dhermay P, Farriaux JP, Amedee-Manesme P, Broyer M, Francois P: Contributeurs au diagnostique antenatal d'un syndrome de Lowe par l'examen histologique des yeux de foetus. *J Fr Ophtalmol* **9**:361, 1986.
29. Klein KL, Klintworth GK, Bernstein A, Breitman ML: Embryology and morphology of microphthalmia in transgenic mice expressing a gamma F-crystallin/diphtheria toxin A hybrid gene. *Lab Invest* **67**:31, 1992.
30. Abbassi V, Lowe CU, Calcagno PL: Oculo-cerebro-renal syndrome. *Am J Dis Child* **115**:145, 1968.
31. McSpadden K: *Report of the Lowe's Syndrome Comprehensive Survey*. Lowe's Syndrome Association, West Lafayette, IN, 1991.
32. Cibis GW, Tripathi RC, Tripathi BJ, Harris DJ: Corneal keloid in Lowe's syndrome. *Arch Ophthalmol* **100**:1795, 1982.
33. Kenworthy L, Park T, Charnas LR: Cognitive and behavioral profile of the oculocerebrorenal syndrome of Lowe. *Am J Med Genet* **46**:297, 1993.
34. Leahey AM, Charnas LR, Nussbaum RL: Nonsense mutations in the OCRL-1 gene in patients with the oculocerebrorenal syndrome of Lowe. *Hum Mol Genet* **4**:461, 1993.
35. Matin MA, Sylvester PE: Clinicopathologic studies of oculocerebrorenal syndrome of Lowe, Terry and MacLachlan. *J Ment Defic Res* **24**:1, 1980.
36. Lamy M, Frezal J, Ray J, Larsen C: Etude metabolique du syndrome de Lowe. *Rev Fr Etud Clin Biol* **7**:271, 1962.
37. Charnas LR, Gahl WA: The oculocerebrorenal syndrome of Lowe. *Adv Pediatr* **31**:75, 1991.
38. Kohyama J, Niimura F, Kawashima K, Iwakawa Y, Nonaka I: Congenital fiber type disproportion myopathy in Lowe syndrome. *Pediatr Neurol* **5**:373, 1989.
39. Kornfeld M, Synder RD, MacGee J, Appenzeller O: The oculo-cerebral-renal syndrome of Lowe: Neuromuscular components. *Arch Neurol* **32**:103, 1975.
40. Charnas L, Bernar J, Pezeshkpour GH, Dalakas M, Harper GS, Gahl WA: MRI findings and peripheral neuropathy in Lowe syndrome. *Neuropediatrics* **19**:7, 1988.
41. Banerjee AK, Allen IV, McKee P: Oculo-cerebro-renal syndrome: Failure to demonstrate specific neuropathological abnormalities in four cases. *Ir J Med Sci* **15**:42, 1982.
42. Hooft C, Valcke R, Herpol J, Van Bogaert L, Guazzi GC: Neurologie et neuropathologie du syndrome de Lowe. *J Neurol Sci* **3**:353, 1966.
43. Chaptal J, Jean R, Grastes de Paulet A, Dossa MD, Ilivier G, Guillaumot J: Etude clinique et biologique d'un enfant atteint d'un syndrome de Lowe. *Arch Franc Pediatr* **16**:849, 1958.
44. Budden S, Meek M, Henighan C: Communication and oral-motor function in Rett syndrome. *Dev Med Child Neurol* **32**:51, 1990.
45. Demmer LA, Wippold FJ II, Dowton SB: Periventricular white matter cystic lesions in Lowe (oculocerebrorenal) syndrome. *Pediatr Radiol* **22**:76, 1992.
46. Chutorian A, Rowland LP: Lowe's syndrome. *Neurology* **16**:115, 1966.
47. Gebert P: Beitrag zum Oculocerebrorenalen Syndrome (Lowe-Syndrome). *Monatsschr Kinderheilkd* **111**:453, 1963.
48. Garzuly F, Jellinger K, Szabo L, Toth K: Morbid changes in oculocerebrorenal syndrome. *Neuropadiatrie* **4**:304, 1973.
49. Martin JJ, Schlote W: Central nervous system lesions in disorders of amino-acid metabolism—A neuropathologic study. *J Neurol Sci* **15**:49, 1972.
50. Habib R, Bargeton E, Brissnad E, Raynaud J, LeBall JC: Constatations anatomiques chez un enfant atteint d'un syndrome de Lowe. *Arch Fr Pediatr* **19**:945, 1962.
51. Downes CP, Mussat MC, Michell RH: The inositol trisphosphate phosphomonoesterase of the human erythrocyte. *Biochem J* **203**:169, 1982.
52. Pueschel SM, Brem AS, Nittoli P: Central nervous system

and renal investigations in patients with Lowe syndrome. *Child Nerv Syst* **8**:45, 1992.

53. Matsuda I, Takeda T, Sugai M, Matsuura N: Oculocerebrorenal syndrome in a child with normal urinary acidification and a defect in bicarbonate reabsorption. *Am J Dis Child* **117**:205, 1969.
54. Athreya B, Schumacher HR, Getz HD, Norman ME, Borden S IV, Witzleben CL: Arthropathy of Lowe's (oculocerebrorenal) syndrome. *Arthritis Rheum* **26**:728, 1983.
55. Gellis SS, Feingold M: Oculocerebrorenal syndrome. *Am J Dis Child* **124**:892, 1972.
56. Witzleben CL, Schoen EJ, Tu WH, McDonald LW: Progressive morphologic renal changes in the oculo-cerebro-renal syndrome of Lowe. *Am J Med* **44**:319, 1968.
57. Charnas L, Bernardini I, Rader D, Hoeg J, Gahl WA: Clinical and laboratory findings in the oculocerebrorenal syndrome of Lowe, with special reference to growth and renal function. *N Engl J Med* **324**:1318, 1991.
58. Manz F, Bremer HJ, Brodehl J: Renal transport of amino acids in children with oculocerebrorenal syndrome. *Helv Paediatr Acta* **33**:37, 1978.
59. Redfield VA, Mimouni F, Strife FC, Tsang RC: Severe rickets in Lowe syndrome: Treatment with continuous nasogastric infusion. *Pediatr Nephrol* **5**:696, 1991.
60. Schaper G, Horstmann W: Lowe syndrom mit hydrocephalus, nephrocalcinose, und nephrolithiasis. *Monatsschr Kinderheilkd* **111**:17, 1963.
61. Arbus GS, Bacheyie GS: Method for predicting when children with progressive renal disease may reach high serum creatinine levels. *Pediatrics* **67**:871, 1981.
62. Reimold EW: Chronic progressive renal failure: Rate of progression monitored by change of serum creatinine concentration. *Am J Dis Child* **135**:1039, 1981.
63. Van Acker KJ, Roels H, Beelaerts W, Pasternack A, Valcke R: The histologic lesions of the kidney in the oculo-cerebro-renal syndrome of Lowe. *Nephron* **4**:193, 1967.
64. Holtgrewe JL, Kalen V: Orthopedic manifestations of the Lowe (oculocerebrorenal) syndrome. *J Pediatr Orthop* **6**:165, 1986.
65. Rosenblatt D, Holmes LB: Development of arthritis in Lowe's syndrome. *J Pediatr* **84**:924, 1974.
66. Phelip X, Bocquet B, Gras JP, Bouvier M, Cabanel G, Lejeune E: Fibrose palmo-plantaire extensive au cours d'un syndrome de Lowe. *Rev Rhum Mal Osteoartic* **40**:597, 1973.
67. Elliman D, Woodley A: Tenosynovitis in Lowe syndrome. *J Pediatr* **103**:1011, 1983.
68. States B, Palmieri MJ, Segal S: Uptake of proline in cultured cells from patients with Lowe's syndrome. *Biochem Biophys Res Commun* **109**:428, 1982.
69. Palmieri MJ, O'Hara J, States B, Segal S: Decreased procollagen production in cultured fibroblasts from patients with Lowe's syndrome. *J Inherit Metab Dis* **8**:187, 1985.
70. Gobernado JM, Lousa M, Gimeno A, Gonsalvez M: Mitochondrial defects in Lowe's oculocerebrorenal syndrome. *Arch Neurol* **41**:208, 1984.
71. Akasaki M, Fukui S, Sakano T, Tanaka T, Usui T, Yamashina I: Urinary excretion of a large amount of bound sialic acid and of undersulfated chondroitin sulfate A by patients with the Lowe syndrome. *Clin Chim Acta* **9**:119, 1978.
72. Wisniewski K, Kieras FJ, French JH, Houck GE, Ramos PL: Ultrastructural, neurological, and glycosaminoglycan abnormalities in Lowe's syndrome. *Ann Neurol* **16**:40, 1984.
73. Fukui S, Yoshida H, Tanaka T, Sakano T, Usui T, Yamashina I: Glycosaminoglycan synthesis by cultured skin fibroblasts from a patient with Lowe's syndrome. *J Biol Chem* **256**:10313, 1981.
74. Fukui S, Yoshida H, Yamashina I: Sulfohydrolytic degradation of 3′-phosphladensoine 5′-phosphosulfate (PAPS) and adenosine 5″-phosphosulfate (APS) by enzymes of a nucleotide pyrophosphatase nature. *J Biochem* **90**:1537, 1981.
75. Yoshida H, Fukui S, Yamashina I, Tanaka T, Sakano T, Usui T, Shimotsuji T, Yabuuchi H, Owada M, Kitagawa T: Elevation of nucleotide pyrophosphatase activity in skin fibroblasts from patients with Lowe's syndrome. *Biochem Biophys Res Commun* **107**:1144, 1982.
76. Horie K, Yano T, Funakoshi I, Yamashina I: Elevated nucleotide pyrophosphatase activity in cultured skin fibroblasts from patients with Lowe's syndrome. *Clin Chim Acta* **177**:41, 1988.
77. Donnelly PV, Reed P, DiFerrante N: Synthesis and sulfation of glycosaminoglycans in fibroblasts from a patient with Lowe's syndrome. *Connect Tissue Res* **13**:89, 1984.
78. Harper GS, Hascall VC, Yanagashita M, Gahl WA: Proteoglycan synthesis in normal and Lowe syndrome fibroblasts. *J Biol Chem* **262**:5637, 1987.
79. Wilson WA, Richards W, Donnell GN: Oculo-cerebro-renal syndrome of Lowe: A review of eight cases noting the genetic inheritance. *Arch Ophthalmol* **70**:5, 1963.
80. Pallisgaard G, Goldschmidt E: The oculocerebrorenal syndrome of Lowe in four generations of one family. *Acta Paediatr Scand* **60**:146, 1971.
81. Holmes GE, Tucker V: Oculo-cerebro-renal syndrome: A four generation family study and case reports of two living children. *Clin Pediatr* **11**:119, 1972.
82. Mueller OT, Hartsfield JK Jr, Gallardo LA, Essig Y-P, Miller KL, Papenhausen PR, Tedesco TA: Lowe oculocerebrorenal syndrome in a female with a balanced X;20 translocation: Mapping of the X chromosome breakpoint. *Am J Hum Genet* **49**:804, 1991.
83. Hodgson SV, Heckmatt JZ, Hughes E, Crolla JA, Dubowitz V, Bobrow M: A balanced de novo X/autosome translocation in a girl with manifestation of Lowe syndrome. *Am J Med Genet* **23**:837, 1986.
84. Inhorn RC, Majerus PW: Properties of inositol polyphosphate 1-phosphatase. *J Biol Chem* **236**:14559, 1988.
85. Collins FS: Positional cloning: Let's not call it reverse anymore. *Nature Genetics* **1**:3, 1992.
86. Wadelius C, Fagerholm P, Pettersson U, Anneren G: Lowe oculocerebrorenal syndrome: DNA-based linkage of the gene to Xq4-626, using tightly linked flanking markers and the correlation to lens examination in carrier diagnosis. *Am J Hum Genet* **44**:241, 1989.
87. Reilly DS, Lewis RA, Nussbaum RL: Genetic and physical mapping of Xq24-q26 markers flanking the Lowe oculocerebrorenal syndrome. *Genomics* **8**:62, 1990.
88. Nelson DL, Ballabio A, Victoria MF, Pieretti M, Bies RD, Gibbs RA, Maley JA, Chinault AC, Webster TD, Caskey CT: *Alu*-primed polymerase chain reaction for regional assignment of 110 yeast artificial chromosome clones from the human X chromosome: Identification of clones associated with a disease locus. *Proc Natl Acad Sci USA* **88**:6157, 1991.
89. Okabe I, Attree O, Bailey LC, Nelson DL, Nussbaum RL: Isolation of cDNA sequences around the chromosomal breakpoint in a female with Lowe syndrome by direct screening of cDNA libraries with yeast artificial chromosomes. *J Inherited Metab Dis* **15**:1992.
90. Attree O, Nelson DL, Caskey CT, Nussbaum RL: Isolation of cross-species conserved DNA sequences in the vicinity of the breakpoint of a Lowe syndrome-associated translocation. *Am J Hum Genet* **47**(suppl.):A 24 (0960), 1990.
91. Connolly TM, Bross TE, Majerus PW: Isolation of a phosphomonoesterase from human platelets that specifically hydrolyzes the 5-phosphate of inositol (1,4,5)-trisphosphate. *J Biol Chem* **260**:7868, 1985.
92. Mitchell CA, Connolly TM, Majerus PW: Identification and isolation of a 75-kDa inositol polyphosphate-5-phosphatase from human platelets. *J Biol Chem* **264**:8873, 1989.
93. Ross TS, Jefferson AB, Mitchell CA, Majerus PW: Cloning and expression of human 75-kDa inositol polyphosphate-5-phosphatase. *J Biol Chem* **266**:20283, 1991.
94. Berridge MJ: Inositol trisphosphate and calcium signalling. *Nature* **361**:315, 1993.
95. Kukita M, Hirata M, Koga T: Requirement of Ca^{2+} for the production and degradation of inositol (1,4,5)-trisphosphate in macrophages. *Biochim Biophys Acta* **885**:121, 1986.
96. Erneux C, Delvaux A, Moreau C, Dumont JE: Characterization of D-myo-inositol (1,4,5)-trisphosphate phosphatase in rat brain. *Biochem Biophys Res Commun* **134**:351, 1986.
97. Hansen CA, Johanson RA, Williamson MT, Williamson JR: Purification and characterization to two types of soluble inositol phosphate 5-phosphomonoesterases from rat brain. *J Biol Chem* **262**:17319, 1987.

98. Storey DJ, Shears SB, Kirk CJ, Michell RH: Stepwise enzymatic dephosphorylation of inositol (1,4,5)-triphosphate to inositol in liver. *Nature* **312**:374, 1984.
99. Irvine R: Seeking the Lowe life. *Nature Genetics* **1**:315, 1992.
100. York JD, Majerus PW: Isolation and heterologous expression of a cDNA encoding bovine inositol polyphosphate 1-phosphatase. *Proc Natl Acad Sci USA* **87**:9548, 1990.
101. Epstein S: Diabetes mellitus and abnormalities of bone and collagen metabolism, in Draznin B, Melmeel S, LeRoith D (eds): *Complications of Diabetes Mellitus*. New York, Alan R. Liss, 1989, p 115.
102. Cammarata PR, Tse D, Yorio T: Sorbinol prevents the hypergalactosemic-induced reduction in [^{3}H]-myo-inositol uptake and decreased [^{3}H]-myo-inositol incorporation into the phosphoinositide cycle in bovine lens epithelial cells in vitro. *Curr Eye Res* **9**:561, 1990.
103. Diehl RE, Whiting P, Potter J, Gee N, Ragan CI, Linemeyer D, Schoepfer R, Bennett C, Dixon RAF: Cloning and expression of bovine brain inositol monophosphatase. *J Biol Chem* **265**:5946, 1990.
104. Greene DA, De Jesus PV Jr, Winegrad AI: Effects of insulin and dietary myoinositol on impaired peripheral motor nerve conduction velocity in acute streptozotocin diabetes. *J Clin Invest* **55**:1326, 1975.
105. Greene DA, Lattimer SA, Sima AAF: Sorbitol, phosphoinositides, and sodium-potassium-ATPase in the pathogenesis of diabetic complications. *N Engl J Med* **316**:599, 1987.
106. Gazit E, Brand N, Harel Y, Lotan D, Barkai G: Prenatal diagnosis of Lowe's syndrome: A case report with evidence of de novo mutation. *Prenat Diagn* **10**:257, 1990.
107. Gaary EA, Rawnsley E, Marin-Padilla JM, Morse CL, Crow HC: In utero detection of fetal cataracts. *J Ultrasound Med* **12**:*234, 1993.*
108. Cibis GW, Waeltermann JM, Whitcraft CT, Tripathi RC, Harris DJ: Lenticular opacities in carriers of Lowe's syndrome. *Ophthalmology* **93**:1041, 1986.
109. Tongue AC: Lowe's syndrome: With particular reference to the carrier state. *Trans Pac Coast Ophthalmol Soc* **53**:219, 1972.
110. Cibis GW, Tripathi RC, Tripathi BJ: Lowe's oculocerebrorenal syndrome, in Gold DH, Weingeist TA (eds): *The Eye in Systemic Disease,* Philadelphia, Lippincott, 1990, p 504.
111. Charnas L: Seizures in the oculocerebrorenal syndrome of Lowe. *Neurology* **39**(Suppl. 1):362, 1989.
112. Bernardini I, Rizzo WB, Dalakas M, Bernar J, Gahl WA: Plasma and muscle free carnitine deficiency due to renal Fancondi syndrome. *J Clin Invest* **75**:1124, 1985.
113. Andersson HC, Markello T, Schneider JA, Gahl WA: Effect of growth hormone treatment on serum creatinine concentration in patients with cystinosis and chronic renal disease. *J Pediatr* **120**:716, 1992.
114. Fivush BA, Racusen LC, Christenson MJ, Olson JL: Acute tubular necrosis associated with Lowe's syndrome: Possible role of rhabdomyolysis. *Am J Kidney Dis* **20**:396, 1992.
115. Miller, RC, Wolf, EJ, Gould, M, Macri C, Charnas LR. Fetal oculocerebrorenal syndrome of Lowe associated with elevated maternal serum and amniotic fluid alpha-tetoprotein. *Obstet Gynecol,* 1994. (In Press)
116. Jänne P, Dutra AS, Dracapoli NC, Charnas L, Puck JM, Nussbaum RL. Localization of a type II inositol polyphosphate-5-phosphatase to human chromosome 1p34. *Cytogenet Cell Genet,* 1994. (In Press)

CHAPTER 124

Mendelian Hypophosphatemias

Howard Rasmussen ■ Harriet S. Tenenhouse

1. Several Mendelian hypophosphatemias have been reported. Each has a decrease in fractional renal tubular phosphate reabsorption as a major underlying abnormality and is associated with rickets and osteomalacia. Some have specific changes in vitamin D metabolism. They differ one from another in clinical and biochemical features and in response to therapy. This chapter describes two of these diseases in detail. A third, autosomal hypophosphatemic bone disease, is mentioned briefly for purposes of differential diagnosis. A discussion of the acquired disorder, oncogenic hypophosphatemic osteomalacia, is included because of the similarity of its manifestations to those of X-linked hypophosphatemia.

2. Hereditary hypophosphatemic rickets with hypercalciuria (HHRH) has a mode of inheritance that is compatible with autosomal recessive inheritance with an incomplete recessive phenotype in the heterozygotes. It is characterized by hypophosphatemia, a reduced tubular maximum for P_i/glomerular filtration rate (TmP/GFR), normocalcemia, hypercalciuria, a high plasma 1,25-dihydroxyvitamin D concentration, a low parathyroid hormone concentration, and elevated plasma alkaline phosphatase activity. These defects are associated with growth retardation, bone pain, muscle weakness, femoral and tibial bowing, and radiologic and histomorphometric evidence of rickets and osteomalacia. A primary defect in renal phosphate transport linked to a secondary stimulation of the renal 25-hydroxyvitamin D_3-1α-hydroxylase appears to account for all the biochemical manifestations of the condition. Treatment with oral phosphate alone (1.0 to 2.5 g/day in divided doses) reduces bone pain, heals rickets, and stimulates skeletal growth. Family members with milder degrees of hypophosphatemia have been found to have hypercalciuria, elevated plasma 1,25-dihydroxyvitamin D and nephrolithiasis without bone disease.

3. The predominant type of familial hypophosphatemic rickets is inherited as an X-linked dominant trait and referred to as X-linked hypophosphatemia (XLH). It has been mapped to Xp22.1-p22.2 and is characterized by hypophosphatemia, normocalcemia, normal to low plasma 1,25-dihydroxyvitamin D concentrations, normal parathyroid function, elevated plasma alkaline phosphatase activity, a reduced TmP/GFR and abnormal regulation of 1,25-dihydroxyvitamin D_3 metabolism. These changes are associated with growth retardation, femoral and tibial bowing, radiologic and histomorphometric evidence of rickets and osteomalacia, but no muscle weakness or tetany. This disease appears to result from a combined defect in renal tubular phosphate transport and abnormal regulation of renal 25-hydroxyvitamin D metabolism, in that plasma 1,25-dihydroxyvitamin D does not increase in response to either increases in parathyroid hormone concentration or to phosphate deprivation. In contrast, there is a normal increase in plasma 1,25-dihydroxyvitamin D in response to the administration of calcitonin. The precise pathogenesis of XLH is not yet clear. It is possible that both renal abnormalities arise as a consequence of an intrinsic defect in the phosphate transport system(s) in renal tubular cells. However, it is more likely that they occur as a consequence of the production of a humoral factor that influences renal cell function. The most effective therapy is a combination of oral phosphate (1.0 to 2.0 g/day in four to five divided doses) and 1,25-dihydroxyvitamin D (1.0 to 3.0 μg/day), but this form of therapy is far from ideal and, if not carefully monitored, can lead to renal failure.

4. Hypophosphatemic rickets in the mouse is caused by mutation at one of two closely linked loci, *Hyp* and *Gy*, on the X chromosome. The more extensively studied *Hyp* phenotype is a murine homologue of XLH and is associated with renal defects in brush-border membrane Na^+-dependent phosphate transport and mitochondrial 25-hydroxyvitamin D metabolism. Furthermore, studies in the *Hyp* mouse provide considerable evidence in support of the view that the defects in renal phosphate transport and vitamin D metabolism result from the production of a humoral factor. Current evidence is compatible with a model in which such a humoral factor acts on receptors on the luminal membrane of proximal tubular cells to alter protein kinase C activity and in this way bring about alterations in both phosphate transport and vitamin D metabolism. The *Gy* phenotype is associated with extreme circling behavior, an inner ear abnormality, and renal defects in brush-border membrane Na^+-dependent phosphate transport and vitamin D metabolism. These mouse mutations have proven useful models to examine the genetic and biochemical mechanisms of XLH and to assess treatment protocols for this condition.

A list of standard abbreviations is located immediately preceding the index in each volume. Additional abbreviations used in this chapter include: calbindin-D_{ak} = intestinal vitamin D–dependent 9-kDa calcium-binding protein; DMD = Duchenne muscular dystrophy; ECF = extracellular fluid; *Gy* = X-linked gyro locus in the mouse; HBD = hypophosphatemic bone disease; HHRH = hereditary hypophosphatemic rickets with hypercalciuria; 1-hydroxylase = 25-hydroxyvitamin D_3-1α-hydroxylase; 24-hydroxylase = 25-hydroxyvitamin D_3-24-hydroxylase; *Hyp* = X-linked hypophosphatemia locus in mice; HYP = X-linked hypophosphatemia locus in humans; IH = idiopathic hypercalciuria; $1,25(OH)_2D$ = 1,25-dihydroxyvitamin D_2 and D_3; $1,25(OH)_2D_3$ = 1,25-dihydroxyvitamin D_3; $24,25(OH)_2D$ = 24,25-dihydroxyvitamin D_2 and D_3; $24,25(OH)_2D_3$ = 24,25-dihydroxyvitamin D_3; 25(OH)D = 25-hydroxyvitamin D_2 and D_3; $25(OH)D_3$ = 25-hydroxyvitamin D_3; OHO = oncogenic hypophosphatemic osteomalacia; PFA = phosphonoformic acid; PTH = parathyroid hormone; TmP/GFR = phosphate transfer maximum per unit volume glomerular filtrate; XLH = X-linked hypophosphatemia.

Inorganic phosphate is an essential nutrient both in terms of cell function and skeletal mineralization. It is essential to the basic processes of glycolysis, gluconeogenesis, and energy metabolism. It serves as the source of phosphate for such organic cell constituents as DNA, RNA, a variety of phosphorylated metabolic intermediates, and the phospholipid constituents of cellular membranes. In addition, phosphorylation of cellular proteins is a major mechanism by which cell function is controlled. The intracellular regulatory functions of the inorganic phosphate anion involve such diverse effects as the control of aerobic metabolism, the control of the O_2 dissociation curve of hemoglobin in the intact red cell, and the regulation of cellular calcium metabolism.

Phosphate is sufficiently abundant in natural foods that dietary phosphate deficiency is unlikely to develop except under conditions of extreme starvation or as a consequence of administration of a class of therapeutic agents, known as phosphate binders, which bind phosphate in the intestinal lumen and prevent its absorption. Furthermore, the major proportion of ingested phosphate (65 to 75 percent), either in the inorganic or organic form, is absorbed in the small intestine, and hormonal regulation of this process plays only a minor role in normal phosphate homeostasis. Absorbed phosphate is either eliminated by the kidney, incorporated into organic forms in proliferating cells, or deposited as a component of bone mineral (hydroxyapatite). Bone deposition accounts for a much larger percentage of retained phosphate during the growth period. However, even in the growing organism only a small percentage of the dietary phosphate is retained. Most of the absorbed phosphate is excreted in the urine. This means that phosphate homeostasis and plasma phosphate concentration depend primarily on the renal mechanisms that regulate tubular phosphate transport. In addition, during times of severe phosphate deprivation, particularly when caloric intake is adequate, the phosphate contained in bone mineral provides the only alternative source of phosphate for the metabolic needs of the organism. Hence, in severe phosphate deficiency, there is a net loss of phosphate from bone due both to an inhibition of the mineralization process and to a stimulation of bone resorption.

In view of the central role of the kidney in phosphate homeostasis, it is not surprising that the tubular mechanisms that determine tubular phosphate reabsorption are complex and are regulated by multiple factors (for reviews, see refs. 1 to 9). Nonetheless, two of these are of overriding importance to this discussion: dietary phosphate intake and circulating parathyroid hormone. Conversely, the renal conversion of 25-hydroxyvitamin D ($25(OH)D_3$) to 1,25-dihydroxyvitamin D ($1,25(OH)_2D$), an active metabolite of vitamin D, is controlled by plasma phosphate concentration or some signal related to plasma phosphate concentration.[10–12] These associations mean that in diseases that involve a renal tubular phosphate leak, a fall in plasma phosphate concentration and associated bone disease will develop and will be accompanied by an alteration in renal vitamin D metabolism. Three well-characterized conditions that exemplify these states will be discussed herein. Two of these conditions—X-linked hypophosphatemia (XLH) and hereditary hypophosphatemic rickets with hypercalciuria (HHRH)—are inherited; the third condition—oncogenic hypophosphatemic osteomalacia (OHO)—is acquired. The latter is included in this discussion because of its possible relevance to our understanding of the pathogenesis of XLH.

In spite of the fact that all three conditions are thought to have a primary renal phosphate leak [i.e., a reduced tubular maximum for P_i/glomerular filtration rate (TmP/GFR) and hypophosphatemia], each leading to rickets and/or osteomalacia, patients with XLH, HHRH, and OHO exhibit different alterations in vitamin D metabolism. They also display different responses to alterations in dietary phosphate intake and parathyroid infusion, and they require different therapeutic measures. In the ensuing discussion, a consideration of phosphate homeostasis and the renal handling of phosphate will be followed by a consideration of the pathogenic mechanisms involved in these three conditions. The clinical features of each syndrome and its treatment will be presented. Emphasis is placed on more recent work that has enhanced both our understanding of phosphate homeostasis and phosphate transport and on the pathogenesis and treatment, particularly of XLH. A major factor that has contributed to this increased understanding is the study of two mouse models of XLH, the *Hyp* mouse and a second related mouse model, the *Gy* mouse. The clinical and physiological manifestations of the altered metabolism of phosphate, vitamin D, and calcium in the *Hyp* mouse and in the human patient are quite similar, so a detailed comparison between the two states forms an important part of the ensuing discussion. For a discussion of earlier work relating to these conditions, the reader is referred to the discussion of XLH and the *Hyp* mouse that appeared in the previous editions of this book.[13,14]

It should be noted that other Mendelian hypophosphatemias have been documented (Table 124-1). However, considerably less information is available about these disorders and, with the exception of hypophosphatemic bone disease (HBD), they will not be discussed here.

PHOSPHATE HOMEOSTASIS

Under most ordinary circumstances, the major determinants of phosphate homeostasis are dietary phosphate intake and the absorption of phosphate from the intestine and its filtration and reabsorption by the renal tubule. The cellular mechanisms underlying transport across the intestinal mucosal cell and the renal tubular cell are quite similar, but their hormonal and dietary controls are quite different.

Normal phosphate intake in the adult human is in the range of 800 to 1600 mg/day. This phosphate is in both the organic and inorganic forms, but the organic forms, except for phytates, are degraded in the intestinal lumen to yield inorganic phosphate, which is the form absorbed. The absorptive rate for phosphate is highest in the jejunum and ileum, with a lower rate in the duodenum. Essentially no absorption occurs in the colon.[15] This pattern contrasts with that of calcium, which is absorbed at the highest rates in duodenum and ileum and at lower rates in both jejunum and colon.

Although intestinal phosphate absorption is regulated by the vitamin D metabolites, 25(OH)D and $1,25(OH)_2D$,[16,17] these hormones play a relatively minor role in normal phosphate homeostasis. Between 65 and 75 percent of ingested phosphate is absorbed regardless of the level of phosphate intake. In vitamin D deficiency, this percentage may fall to 50 to 60 percent due both to a failure to absorb calcium and thereby reduce free phosphate concentration in the lumen and to a direct effect of $1,25(OH)_2D$ on the phosphate transport system in the intestinal mucosal cell.[18]

Over a large range of phosphate intake, plasma phosphate concentration remains normal, while intestinal phosphate absorption increases in proportion to the phosphate content

Table 124-1 Mendelian Hypophosphatemias

		McKusick No.*
Type I	Hereditary hypophosphatemia with hypercalciuria (HHRH)	241530
Type II	Hypophosphatemic bone disease (HBD)	146350
Type III	X-linked hypophosphatemia (XLH)	307800, 307810
Type IV	Autosomal dominant vitamin D resistant rickets (not HBD)	193100
Type V	Autosomal recessive hypophosphatemic rickets	241520

*From McKusick VA.[241]

of the diet.[19-21] This means that the renal excretion of phosphate increases and decreases in direct relation to phosphate intake over a wide range of intake. The mechanism(s) underlying this important renal adaptation to phosphate intake is not completely understood.

Plasma phosphate concentration varies as a function of age in humans: in the range of 3.8 to 5.5 mg/dl (1.23 to 1.77 m*M*) in children and 3.0 to 4.5 mg/dl (0.97 to 1.45 m*M*) in adults. Of interest is the fact that mice and rats have higher normal plasma phosphate values than humans. This difference in plasma phosphate correlates with differences in basal metabolic rate. In both rodent species, the basal metabolic rate is higher than that of humans.[22]

Although long-term changes in plasma phosphate concentration clearly depend on the balance between intestinal absorption and renal excretion, short-term changes in phosphate concentrations can occur as a consequence of the redistribution of phosphate between the extracellular fluid (ECF) and either bone or cell constituents. Since the ECF phosphate represents less than 1 percent of total body phosphate, either the mobilization of phosphate following tissue destruction or the mobilization of phosphate from bone mineral can lead to temporary increases in plasma phosphate concentration.

In measuring plasma phosphate concentration and relating this value to a clinical situation, it is necessary to bear in mind that there is a diurnal variation in plasma phosphate concentration with a nadir at 9:30 to 10:00 AM and a peak at 4 AM.[23] The change in concentration from nadir to peak may be as much as 1 mg/dl, that is, a 25 to 35 percent change in concentration. The factors determining this diurnal variation are not known but probably involve extrarenal mechanisms.

Phosphate Homeostasis in States of Altered Mineral Intake

In considering the mechanisms involved in the pathogenesis of XLH, HHRH, and OHO, it is useful to discuss our current view of how an organism adapts to severe dietary restrictions of either phosphate or calcium.

A discussion of calcium homeostasis within a discussion of disorders of renal phosphate transport is necessary because of: (1) the intimate link between the transport of these ions across the intestine and renal tubule, (2) their coexistence as components of bone mineral, (3) their interrelated effects on the regulation of vitamin D metabolism, and (4) the interrelated changes in their metabolism in response to parathyroid hormone (PTH), calcitonin, and 1,25$(OH)_2$D. The reader is referred to Chap. 100 by Marx in this volume for a more complete discussion of vitamin D metabolism, and to Chap. 99 by Spiegel for a more complete discussion of parathyroid hormone function.

The key tissues involved in calcium and phosphate homeostasis are the gut, kidney, and bone, and the key hormonal regulators are PTH, calcitonin, and 1,25$(OH)_2$D.

Phosphate Deprivation. The changes in phosphate and calcium metabolism that occur as a consequence of severe dietary phosphate restriction are represented schematically in Fig. 124-1.[1-12] A decrease in phosphate intake leads to a prompt fall in renal phosphate excretion due to a renal adaptive response so that within a few days renal phosphate excretion falls nearly to zero. During this transient period, plasma phosphate may fall only minimally, but with continued phosphate restriction, plasma phosphate concentration falls and filtered load decreases. Either a change in the tubular phosphate transport or the change in plasma phosphate concentration leads to an increase in 25(OH)D-1α-hydroxylase (1α-hydroxylase) activity in the proximal renal tubule. As a consequence, the plasma 1,25$(OH)_2$D rises. The fall in plasma phosphate leads to an inhibition of bone mineral deposition, and if bone resorption continues, there is a net shift of phosphate from the skeleton to ECF. The rise in the plasma 1,25$(OH)_2$D concentration provides an additional stimulus to bone resorption.[24] The increase in plasma 1,25$(OH)_2$D also stimulates intestinal phosphate transport by a direct action on the mucosal phosphate transport system, and indirectly by the action of 1,25$(OH)_2$D on intestinal calcium absorption.

As a consequence of the rise in plasma 1,25$(OH)_2$D concentration and the resultant increases in both intestinal calcium absorption and bone resorption, the plasma calcium concentration rises. This change in calcium concentration acts to inhibit PTH secretion. As a consequence, PTH concentration falls and the distal tubular reabsorption of calcium is decreased; the increased influx of calcium into the ECF from bone and gut is thus balanced by an increased renal loss. The decreased effect of PTH on tubular phosphate transport should also contribute to renal phosphate retention, but in fact, the phosphate transport system in the tubules of the phosphate-deprived organism is insensitive to this action of PTH. Hence, even the infusion of PTH will not increase urinary phosphate excretion in the phosphate-deprived organism.

These homeostatic changes lead to a nearly complete renal conservation of phosphate coupled to the mobilization of phosphate from the skeleton to replace extrarenal loss

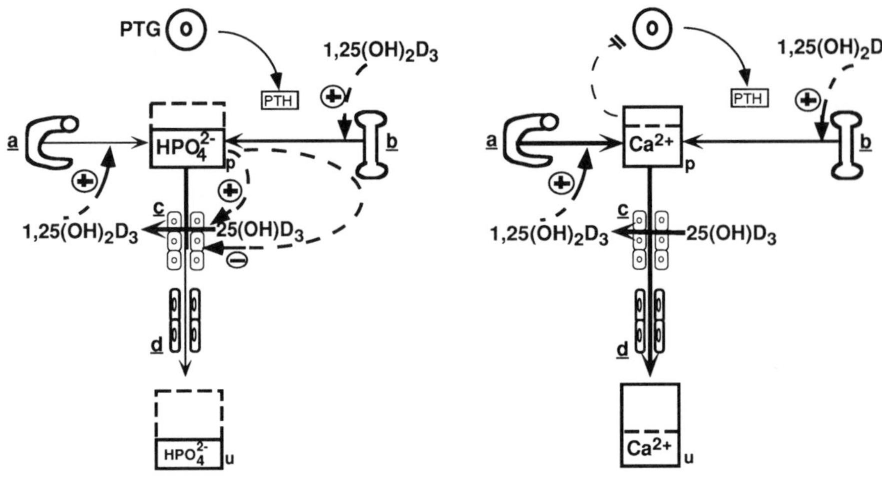

A. PHOSPHATE METABOLISM

B. CALCIUM METABOLISM

FIG. 124-1 **Changes in phosphate and calcium metabolism induced by restriction of dietary phosphate intake.** ***A*****. A decrease in phosphate intake leads to a decrease in intestinal phosphate absorption (a) and eventually to a fall in the plasma phosphate concentration ($\overline{HPO_4}^{2-}$). This fall in plasma phosphate concentration brings about two important changes in proximal renal tubular function (c): an increase in $1,25(OH)_2D_3$ synthesis and a marked increase in the phosphate reabsorption (by a mechanism that is independent of PTH) so that the urinary excretion of phosphate decreases. As a consequence, phosphate virtually disappears from the urine even though the rise in plasma $1,25(OH)_2D_3$ acts to enhance the removal of phosphate from bone (b). The increase in plasma $1,25(OH)_2D_3$ also acts to enhance phosphate absorption from the intestine.** ***B*****. The increase in plasma $1,25(OH)_2D_3$ concentration (caused by the fall in plasma phosphate concentration) enhances the absorption of Ca^{2+} from the intestine (a) and the removal of Ca^{2+} from bone (b). As a consequence, plasma Ca^{2+} concentration $(Ca^{2+})_p$ rises, thereby causing an inhibition of PTH secretion. The resulting fall in plasma PTH concentration leads to a decrease in the distal tubular reabsorption of Ca^{2+} (d) thus minimizing the rise in plasma Ca^{2+} concentration. As a consequence, urinary Ca^{2+} excretion increases even though there is only a small increase in plasma Ca^{2+} concentration.**

(occurring largely via the gastrointestinal tract). These changes in phosphate metabolism are associated with increased intestinal calcium absorption and hypercalciuria.

One would predict that a simple renal phosphate leak should lead to a similar sequence of events and, in particular, to increases in plasma $1,25(OH)_2D$ concentration and intestinal calcium absorption, resulting in hypercalciuria. However, in the case of both XLH and OHO, the renal phosphate leak coexists with a disordered regulation of the renal synthesis of $1,25(OH)_2D$. On the other hand, in HHRH, the phosphate leak is associated with the tetrad of high plasma $1,25(OH)_2D$, low plasma PTH, increased calcium absorption, and hypercalciuria—the same tetrad seen during dietary phosphate restriction in animals or humans.

Calcium Deprivation. The changes in both calcium and phosphate metabolism that occur in response to severe dietary calcium restriction are shown in Fig. 124-2. The decrease in calcium intake leads to a slight fall in plasma calcium concentration, and a stimulation of PTH secretion. The resulting rise in plasma PTH concentration leads to an increase in bone resorption leading to a net loss of calcium from bone, an increase in the distal tubular reabsorption of calcium, and an increase in the rate of $1,25(OH)_2D$ synthesis by the proximal tubule. The resulting rise in plasma $1,25(OH)_2D$ leads to an increased efficiency of intestinal calcium absorption and acts synergistically with PTH to enhance resorption of bone.

As a result of the increases in plasma $1,25(OH)_2D$ concentration, intestinal phosphate absorption and the net removal of phosphate from bone both increase. However, in spite of this increase in the net movement of phosphate into the ECF, the plasma phosphate concentration does not increase, but rather falls slightly due to the inhibitory action of PTH on renal tubular phosphate transport, and thus a decrease in TmP/GFR.

Phosphate Excess. A marked increase in dietary phosphate intake can occur without a marked change in plasma phosphate concentration because of the compensatory increase in renal phosphate clearance. However, with very high phosphate intakes, particularly if associated with a reduced calcium intake, plasma phosphate may rise sufficiently to reduce plasma ionized calcium, leading to an increase in PTH secretion, a rise in plasma PTH, and a further reduction in renal tubular phosphate reabsorption. Under these circumstances, PTH causes less of an increase in $1,25(OH)_2D$ synthesis, but it does stimulate bone turnover. Whether the effect of $1,25(OH)_2D$ leads to a net removal of calcium and phosphate from bone depends on the calcium intake. The key point is that excessive phosphate intake can lead to a state of secondary hyperparathyroidism, an important consideration in the therapeutic use of phosphate in HHRH, XLH, and OHO.

RENAL PHOSPHATE TRANSPORT

The renal excretion of phosphate is determined by the balance between the rates of glomerular filtration and tubular reabsorption.[1-9] There is no convincing evidence for net tubular secretion of phosphate by the mammalian nephron under normal conditions. Not all the phosphate in plasma is ultrafilterable, and the phosphate concentration in the glomerular ultrafiltrate is only approximately 90 percent of that in plasma.[25,26] The percentage of phosphate filtered decreases as the plasma calcium concentration rises above 10.5 mg/dl. At a plasma calcium concentration of 18 mg/dl,

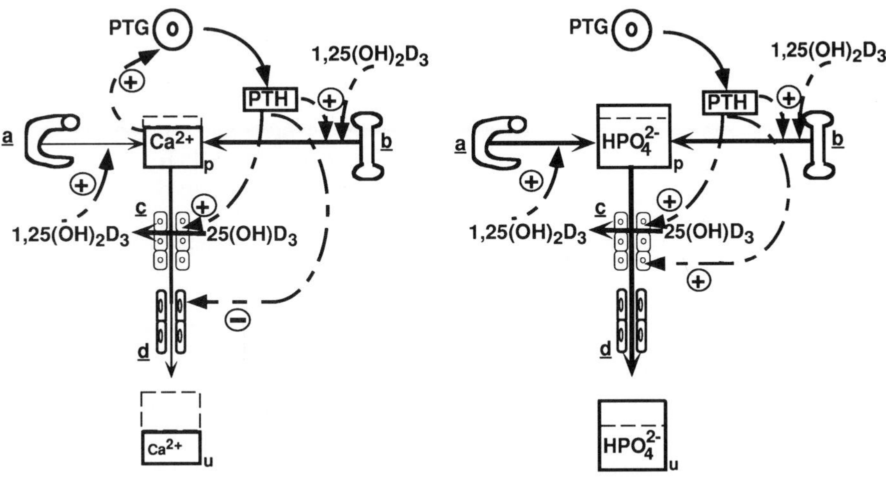

FIG. 124-2 Changes in calcium and phosphate metabolism induced by restriction of dietary calcium intake. *A*. A decrease in the intestinal absorption of Ca^{2+} (a) leads to a slight fall in the plasma Ca^{2+} concentration (Ca^{2+})p. This fall stimulates the secretion of parathyroid hormone (PTH) from the parathyroid glands (PTG). The rise in the plasma PTH concentration acts to increase the net removal of Ca^{2+} from bone (b), enhance the production of $1,25(OH)_2D_3$ from $25(OH)D_3$ in the proximal renal tubule (c), enhance the distal tubular reabsorption of Ca^{2+} (d) leading to a decrease in urinary calcium excretion. As a consequence of the increase in the plasma $1,25(OH)_2D_3$ concentration, intestinal Ca^{2+} absorption is increased. $1,25(OH)_2D_3$ also acts synergistically with PTH to enhance Ca^{2+} removal from bone (b). As a consequence of these changes, the plasma Ca^{2+} concentration is maintained close to its normal value but urinary Ca^{2+} excretion is markedly reduced. *B*. The effect of the same hormonal changes [i.e., an increase in the plasma concentrations of both PTH and $1,25(OH)_2D_3$] on phosphate metabolism are an increase in intestinal phosphate absorption (a) and an increase in the removal of phosphate from bone (b). These changes lead to a net increase in the amount of phosphate entering the plasma and extracellular fluid. However, the plasma phosphate concentration (HPO_4^{2-})p rises only slightly because the increase in PTH concentration acts on the proximal renal tubule (c) to inhibit phosphate reabsorption. As a consequence, the major change in phosphate metabolism is a significant increase in the urinary excretion of phosphate, with only a small rise in plasma phosphate concentration.

only about 75 percent of plasma phosphate appears in the glomerular filtrate.[25]

As in the case of many transport processes, the transcellular transport of phosphate is a carrier-mediated, saturable process. Hence, one might anticipate that a transfer maximum, or T_{max}, for the renal reabsorption of this anion could be determined. However, because of the marked effect of phosphate intake on the renal handling of phosphate, the T_{max} varies considerably as dietary phosphate rises and falls. The best way to estimate the overall capacity of the renal phosphate transport system is to measure the T_{max} for phosphate per unit volume of glomerular filtrate (TmP/GFR) during acute phosphate infusions. In practice, an estimate of TmP/GFR can be made by measuring phosphate and creatinine excretions and plasma phosphate concentrations, and using this information and the nomogram developed by Bijvoet[27,28] (showing the relationship between plasma phosphate concentration and the fractional excretion of phosphate) to derive this value (Fig. 124-3). The use of this nomogram is limited to situations in which there are significant rates of urinary phosphate excretion.

Tubular Sites of Phosphate Reabsorption, Parathyroid Hormone and Calcitonin Action, and 1,25-Dihydroxyvitamin D Synthesis

Considerable information from animal studies has accumulated in the past few years in terms of the tubular sites at which phosphate reabsorption occurs, PTH and calcitonin act, and $1,25(OH)_2D$ synthesis occurs.[29-36] This information is summarized in Table 124-2.

The major site of phosphate reabsorption is in the proximal convoluted tubule. Reabsorption at this site normally accounts for approximately 60 percent of the filtered load. A second site, accounting for another 15 to 20 percent, is the proximal straight tubule. The importance of phosphate reabsorption in the distal tubule is difficult to define because of considerable heterogeneity between the ability of deep and superficial nephrons to conserve phosphate.

When the tubular locations of PTH-sensitive adenylate cyclase are mapped, this enzyme is found at all three sites of phosphate transport—proximal convoluted tubule, proximal straight tubule, and distal tubule.[34,35] There is also clear evidence that PTH (or cAMP) will decrease phosphate reabsorption in both proximal convoluted tubule and proximal straight tubule. From these observations, it has been concluded that PTH inhibits phosphate transport in each of these tubular segments via a cAMP-dependent process. Further, PTH stimulates 1α-hydroxylase by a cAMP-dependent mechanism in the proximal convoluted tubule[36] and inhibits Na^+/H^+ exchange in this nephron segment.[37,38] Finally, PTH stimulates distal tubular calcium reabsorption by a mechanism that may not involve cAMP.[39,40]

In contrast to PTH, calcitonin-sensitive adenylate cyclase is localized in the medullary and cortical thick ascending limbs and in the distal tubule,[41] but the calcitonin-sensitive 1α-hydroxylase is localized in the proximal straight tubule.[36] Calcitonin acts in the proximal convoluted tubule, and possibly in proximal straight tubule, to inhibit phosphate reabsorption. From the facts that calcitonin acts on both phosphate reabsorption and 1α-hydroxylase activity in nephron segments that do not possess calcitonin-sensitive adenylate cyclase,[41] it has been concluded that calcitonin regulates

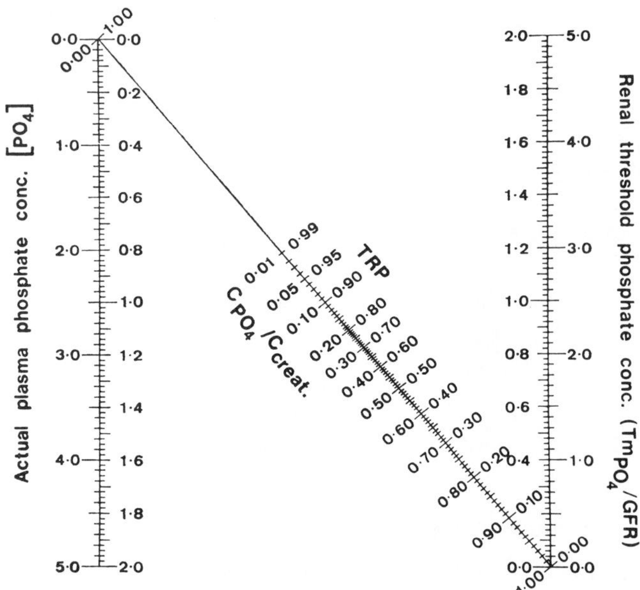

FIG. 124-3 Nomogram for derivation of renal threshold phosphate concentration (Tm_{PO_4}/GFR. A straight line through the appropriate plasma phosphate and TRP (fractional reabsorption of filtered phosphate load, i.e., phosphate/creatinine clearance) values passes through the corresponding values of Tm_{PO_4}/GFR. The scales and units of the figures are arbitrary, provided consistent dimensions are used. *(From Walton and Bijvoet.[28] Used by permission.)*

these processes by a cAMP-independent mechanism. The nature of this mechanism remains to be defined. Calcitonin also acts on the medullary thick ascending limb to increase calcium reabsorption presumably by a cAMP-dependent mechanism. The action of calcitonin on the distal tubule remains undefined, even though this is the segment that expresses the most abundant calcitonin-sensitive cyclase.

During dietary phosphate deprivation there is an increase in phosphate transport in all nephron segments and probably an increase in 1α-hydroxylase in the proximal convoluted tubule but not in the proximal straight tubule.

Cellular Mechanism of Phosphate Transport

The most detailed studies of the cellular mechanism for phosphate transport have been done in proximal tubules and cultured cells derived from them.[1–9] In these cells and tissues, the process is essentially a unidirectional transport from luminal- to basal-cell surface. Based on current information, a model of phosphate transport can be constructed (Fig. 124-4) in which HPO_4^{2-} entry into the cell from the tubular fluid across the brush-border membrane involves the secondary active transport of phosphate driven by the Na^+ gradient. The transport occurs via a Na^+/HPO_4^{2-} cotransport system in which $2Na^+$ ions enter with each phosphate. This means that when HPO_4^{2-} is the predominant species, the process is electroneutral, but when the species is $H_2PO_4^{1-}$, transport is electrogenic. The rate of phosphate transport is dependent on the magnitude of the Na^+ gradient maintained across the luminal membrane, which, in turn, depends on the activity of the $Na^+/14^+$-ATPase or sodium pump on the basolateral membrane. Inhibition of this pump leads to an inhibition of phosphate transport. Further, the rate limiting step in transcellular transport is probably the Na^+-dependent entry of phosphate across the luminal membrane. This process has a low K_m for luminal phosphate (0.1 m*M* or less), so it is possible for phosphate transport to be highly efficient.

An additional order of complexity has been introduced by the findings of multiple Na^+-dependent phosphate transport processes in the brush-border membranes of proximal tubular cells from pigs[42] and mice.[43] In the early proximal convoluted tubule, there appears to be two such systems—one of low affinity and high capacity, which appears to be responsible for the reabsorption of the bulk of the filtered load, and a high-affinity, low-capacity system, which is responsible for the remainder. In the proximal straight tubule, a single high-affinity system is found. Studies with isolated proximal tubular segments derived from rabbit kidney also revealed two phosphate transport systems—a PTH-insensitive high-capacity system in the proximal convoluted tubule and a PTH-sensitive low-capacity system in the proximal straight tubule.[44]

The phosphate that enters the cell is in rapid exchange with intracellular phosphate. There does not appear to be a separate transport pool. The efflux of phosphate out of the cell across the basolateral membrane appears to be a passive process driven by the electrical gradient existing across this membrane and occurring via an anion-exchange mechanism. In addition, there appears to be a small component of Na^+-linked secondary active influx of phosphate across the basolateral membrane that has a V_{max} only 10 percent of the luminal process.[45] This process can be distinguished from that in the brush-border membrane because it has a lower K_M for phosphate (0.014 m*M*), is insensitive to pH, and is more electrogenic. However, this Na^+-dependent entry of phosphate across the basolateral membrane appears to be insufficient to maintain normal intracellular phosphate concentrations in the absence of luminal phosphate entry (see "Regulation by Dietary Phosphate" below).

Table 124-2 Renal Tubular Site of Phosphate Transport, 1α-Hydroxylase, and Hormone-Sensitive Adenylate Cyclase

	Phosphate Transport	PTH-Sensitive Adenylate Cyclase	PTH-Sensitive 1α-hydroxylase	CT-Sensitive Adenylate Cyclase	CT-Sensitive 1α-hydroxylase
PCT	+ + +	+ +	+ + + +	−	−
PST	+ +	+	−	−	+ + +
MTAL	−	−	−	+	−
CTAL	−	+ + + +	−	+ + +	−
DT	+	+ + +	−	+ + + +	−
CT	−	−	−	+ +	−

PCT = proximal convoluted tubule; PST = proximal straight tubule; MTAL = medullary thick ascending limb; CTAL = cortical thick ascending limb; DT = distal tubule; CT = collecting tubule.

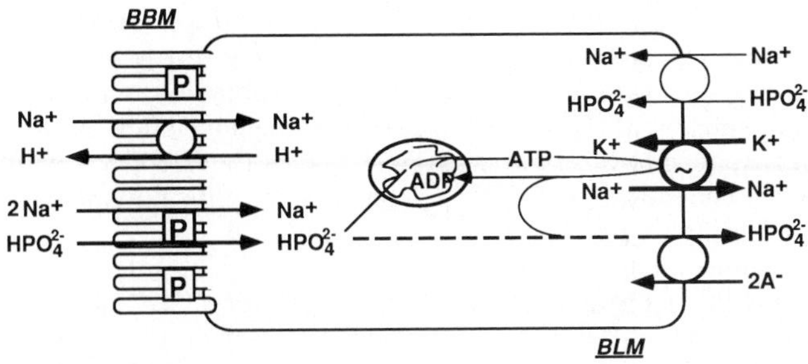

FIG. 124-4 Model of the process of transcellular transport of inorganic phosphate (HPO_4^{2-}) in the cell of the proximal convoluted tubule of the mammalian kidney. The luminal or brush-border membrane (BBM) is depicted on the left and the basolateral membrane (BLM) on the top, bottom, and right, and the only intracellular organelle depicted is the mitochondrion. Both a Na^+/H^+ exchanger and a $2Na^+/HPO_4^{2-}$ cotransporter operate in the luminal membrane. The HPO_4^{2-}, which enters the cell across the luminal surface mixes with the metabolic pool of phosphate in the cell and is eventually transported out of the cell across the basolateral membrane via an anion (A −) exchange mechanism. There is also a Na^+/HPO_4^{2-} cotransporter on the basolateral membrane, and a Na^+/K^+-ATPase on this membrane. The ATPase transports the Na^+ (which enters the cell on its luminal side) out of the cell, thereby maintaining the Na^+ gradient driving force for luminal phosphate entry.

The difficulties in defining the transcellular transport process are an inability to measure the intracellular inorganic phosphate concentration accurately and the inability to use tracer methods effectively to study the transcellular transport process because of the rapid mixing of the tracer with the metabolically active organic phosphate pools within the cell. Estimates of intracellular inorganic phosphate concentration range from 0.7 to 2.0 m*M*, with the former value obtained by MRI spectroscopy.[46] A value between 0.6 and 1.0 m*M* is likely to be close to the true value.

Because intracellular phosphate is of key importance to cellular energy metabolism (and its concentration is one factor determining the phosphate potential of the cell [ATP]/[ADP][P_i]), one might anticipate that some type of functional coupling exists between the transport processes across the two cell surfaces so that large changes in free phosphate concentration do not occur as a result of large changes in phosphate load.[5] However, the existence of such a homeostatic mechanism has not been clearly demonstrated. Under extreme nonphysiological circumstances, removal of phosphate from tubular lumen in a perfused kidney leads to a fall in total cellular inorganic phosphate but to a sustained near-normal transcellular transport of Na^+ and an intracellular free phosphate concentration measured by ^{31}P-MRI spectroscopy of 0.7 m*M*[46]. In isolated perfused proximal tubules, removal of phosphate from the luminal but not the peritubular fluid leads to an inhibition of net fluid absorption, that is, a decrease in transcellular Na^+-transport that can be reversed by removal of glucose from the medium (the phosphorylation of intracellular glucose and the resulting increase in the content of phosphorylated glycolytic intermediates). Together with a reduced luminal entry of phosphate this process can lead to a fall in intracellular phosphate concentration sufficient to cause a decrease in the rate of oxidative ATP synthesis.[5]

Hormonal Regulation

Phosphate reabsorption by the kidney can be modulated by a variety of peptide and steroid hormones.[3–9] Growth hormone, insulin-like growth factor I, insulin, epidermal growth factor, thyroid hormone and 1,25(OH)$_2$D all stimulate renal phosphate reabsorption, while PTH, PTH-related peptide, calcitonin, atrial natriuretic factor, transforming growth factor-α and glucocorticoids inhibit renal phosphate reclamation. From in vitro studies using cultured renal epithelial cells, there is evidence of a direct action of these hormones on the kidney (Table 124-3). The exception is growth hormone, which appears to increase phosphate transport by virtue of its ability to stimulate production of insulin-like growth factor I. Although the mechanisms for hormonal regulation of renal phosphate transport are not entirely clear, the target for regulation appears to be the high-affinity Na^+-phosphate cotransport system on the apical surface of renal proximal tubular cells. Because of the physiological importance of PTH in the regulation of renal phosphate reabsorption, and the vast literature devoted to this subject, the following discussion will focus on the cellular mechanisms whereby PTH inhibits phosphate uptake in renal epithelial cells.

The original model of PTH action on proximal tubular phosphate transport was one in which the interaction of

Table 124-3 Hormonal Regulation of Phosphate Transport: Evidence from Studies in Cultured Renal Epithelial Cells

Hormone	Target Cells	Direction of Change	Reference
PTH	OK cells	↓	59
	Mouse primary cultures	↓	265
Glucocorticoids	Chick primary cultures	↓	266
PTHrP	OK cells	↓	267
ANF	OK cells	↓	268
TGFα	OK cells	↓	269
1,25(OH)$_2$D$_3$	Chick primary cultures	↑	270
T_3	Chick primary cultures	↑	271
EGF	LLC-PK$_1$ cells	↑	272
IGF-I	OK cells	↑	273
Insulin	OK cells	↑	274

PTHrP = parathyroid hormone related peptide; ANF = atrial natriuretic factor; TGFα = transforming growth factor-α; EGF = epidermal growth factor; IGF-I = insulin-like growth factor I; LLC-PK$_1$ = porcine kidney epithelial cell line; OK = opossum kidney epithelial cell line.

PTH with its receptor on the basolateral membrane leads to the activation of adenylate cyclase. This results in an increase in intracellular cAMP, which diffuses across the cell and inhibits Na^+-phosphate cotransport by catalyzing protein kinase A–dependent phosphorylation of one or more proteins in the brush-border membrane. More recently, however, this mechanism has been questioned by Cole et al.,[47] who demonstrated a discrepancy between dose–response curves for PTH-dependent inhibition of Na^+-phosphate cotransport and PTH-dependent activation of cAMP production in opossum kidney (OK) cells, a cell line that expresses several differentiated functions of the proximal tubule.[47] They showed that whereas half-maximal inhibition of phosphate transport is observed at 5×10^{-11} M PTH, a concentration of 10^{-8} M PTH is required to achieve half-maximal stimulation of cAMP production. These findings raise the possibility that at low PTH concentrations, another regulatory cascade is involved in triggering the PTH-dependent reduction in phosphate transport. Indeed, dose–response curves performed in OK cells provide firm evidence for a phospholipase C–dependent pathway in PTH action that occurs at much lower concentrations of PTH than those required for activation of adenylate cyclase[48,49]; PTH concentrations less than 10^{-10} M were sufficient to elicit a concomitant increase in inositol triphosphate, diacylglycerol, and cytosolic calcium.

Further support for the involvement of the phospholipase C–protein kinase C signal transduction pathway in PTH regulation of phosphate transport is provided by the following observations. (1) PTH is unable to inhibit phosphate transport in protein kinase C–down-regulated cells.[50] (2) PTH is unable to inhibit phosphate transport in an OK cell line apparently lacking PTH-dependent phospholipase C–dependent activation.[51] (3) Activation of protein kinase C with phorbol myristic acid (PMA) elicits an inhibition of phosphate transport in OK cells[47] and in freshly isolated renal tubules.[52]

The involvement of the phospholipase C signaling pathway in the action of PTH on phosphate transport does not preclude the participation of the adenylate cyclase signaling pathway. Indeed, an intact cAMP–protein kinase A pathway appears to be required for PTH inhibition of phosphate transport in OK cells.[53] Moreover, dose–response curves show that PTH activation of protein kinase A is more closely correlated to phosphate transport inhibition than to cAMP production in OK cells.[54] The findings to date, therefore, suggest that both signal transduction pathways are involved in PTH regulation of renal phosphate transport, with the phosphoinositide pathway operating at low PTH concentrations (10^{-8} to $10^{-10}M$). Consistent with this hypothesis is the demonstration that the pattern of apical membrane protein phosphorylation in response to PMA, an activator of protein kinase C, resembles that obtained with low concentrations of PTH, whereas the phosphorylation pattern in response to 8-bromo-cAMP resembles that obtained with high concentrations of PTH.[55] The identity of the phosphorylated proteins remains to be determined.

Some studies have provided some insight into events following PTH activation of the regulatory cascades discussed above. It was demonstrated that interference with the endocytotic pathway, either by the microtubule-disrupting agent colchicine or high-medium osmolarity, is associated with reduced PTH inhibition of phosphate transport in OK cells.[56,57] Moreover, a concomitant change in PTH stimulation of cAMP production was not apparent under these conditions.[56,57] These results suggest that endocytosis of cell-surface transporters may be involved in PTH inhibition of phosphate uptake. Because recovery of Na^+-phosphate cotransport activity following PTH inhibition requires protein synthesis,[58] it has been suggested that phosphate transporters are degraded following PTH-induced endocytosis.

It has generally been accepted that PTH action on renal phosphate transport is initiated by PTH binding to its receptor on the basolateral membrane. Yet, in confluent renal epithelial cell cultures grown in plastic dishes, apically administered PTH, that is, PTH added to the culture medium, is able to elicit a rapid inhibition of phosphate transport.[59] These results are consistent with the presence of PTH receptors on the apical surface. To establish whether apical localization of PTH receptors is or is not an artifact of incomplete differentiation and functional polarization associated with cell growth on a solid impermeable surface,[60] studies were performed in OK cells grown to confluence on permeable, collagen-coated filters under conditions permitting cell polarization.[61] Results from these studies demonstrate that PTH inhibition of phosphate transport is approximately 100 times more sensitive to apical PTH application ($K_d \approx 5 \times 10^{-12}$ M) than to basolateral PTH application ($K_d \approx 5 \times 10^{-10}$ M) (Fig. 124-5).[61] Because this difference in PTH sensitivity could not be attributed to either a diffusional leak of PTH to the opposing surface or to differential degradation of PTH, the authors concluded that receptors for PTH are present on both apical and basolateral surfaces of OK cell monolayers grown on permeant supports.[61] In the same study, it was demonstrated that the inhibitory effect of PTH is restricted to the high-affinity Na^+-dependent phosphate transport system on the apical surface of OK cells.[61] The low-affinity, Na^+-dependent and Na^+-independent phosphate

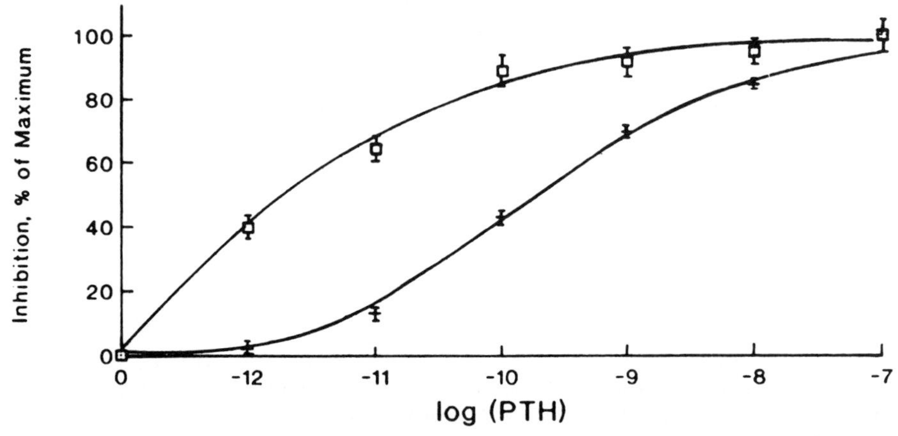

FIG. 124-5 Polarity of PTH effect on phosphate transport in opossum kidney cells. The effect of increasing concentrations of either apical (square) or basolateral (cross) application of PTH on initial rate of apical Na^+-phosphate cotransport was measured. The percent of maximum PTH inhibition is shown. (*From Reshkin et al.*[61] *Used by permission.*)

transport systems, which are only expressed on the basolateral surface of OK cells, are not sensitive to PTH inhibition.[61]

Notwithstanding the use of conditions to promote cellular differentiation and polarization, the findings in OK cells do not exactly reflect results of Na^+-phosphate cotransport in renal brush-border membrane vesicles derived from control and PTH-treated rats.[62,63] First, apical membrane vesicles prepared from intact kidney express both high-affinity and low-affinity Na^+-dependent phosphate transport systems,[42,43] while the apical surface of OK cells expresses only a high-affinity system.[64] Second, both phosphate transport systems are significantly inhibited in brush-border membrane vesicles after the in vivo administration of PTH,[62,63] while only the apical high-affinity system is inhibited in PTH-treated OK cells.[61]

Clearly, further work is required to resolve these discrepancies and to obtain direct evidence for PTH receptor localization in renal brush-border membranes isolated from intact kidney. In this regard, it is noteworthy that both phospholipase C[65] and protein kinase C[66,67] activities have been identified in purified preparations of renal brush-border membranes, thereby demonstrating the presence of signaling pathway machinery on the apical surface. Moreover, receptors for angiotensin II, a peptide hormone that regulates fluid reabsorption, have been found to be distributed on both brush-border and basolateral surfaces.[68] It is also of interest that evidence for PTH binding to the luminal surface of proximal tubular cells was obtained from studies in intact rats receiving intravenously administered, radiolabeled PTH.[69] PTH binding was highest in segment I of the proximal tubule, where labeling at the luminal surface (high-capacity binding) far exceeded that at the basolateral surface (low-capacity binding).[69] However, because luminal binding of filtered hormone appeared to be associated with the apical vacuolar system, the authors suggested that high-capacity luminal binding of PTH is related to hormone degradation, while low-capacity basolateral binding of hormone delivered from the peritubular capillary plexus was likely associated with PTH action.[69]

Regulation by Dietary Phosphate

Dietary phosphate intake is an important determinant of renal phosphate reabsorption. The adaptive response in the proximal tubule is associated with an alteration in Na^+-phosphate cotransport across the brush-border membrane. The increase in phosphate transport following phosphate restriction involves an increase in apparent V_{max} of both the high-capacity, low-affinity and the low-capacity, high-affinity Na^+-phosphate cotransport systems; the apparent affinity of the cotransporters is not affected by phosphate deprivation.[43] Although protein synthesis is required for the adaptive response,[70] it is not clear whether the increase in phosphate transport involves *de novo* synthesis of additional transport units, recruitment of preformed transport units to the brush-border surface, or activation of transport units already associated with the brush-border membrane. Contrary to earlier speculation, it is now evident that the alteration in phosphate transport is not secondary to changes in brush-border membrane fluidity or lipid composition, which are apparent following phosphate depletion.[71]

Although the signal for the adaptive increase in phosphate transport in response to a low-phosphate diet is not yet known, studies using MRI spectroscopy demonstrated a reciprocal relationship between intracellular phosphate concentration and brush-border membrane phosphate transport and suggested that low cytosolic phosphate may serve as an important cellular signal in mediating the transport response.[72] Studies in OK-cell monolayers grown on permeant supports demonstrated that the adaptive increase in Na^+-phosphate cotransport was apparent when cells were exposed to the low-phosphate medium on apical surface but not when the monolayers were incubated with the low-phosphate medium on the basolateral surface.[73] These findings suggest that apical Na^+-dependent phosphate influx is also important in signaling the adaptive response to low extracellular phosphate[73] (see "Cellular Mechanism of Phosphate Transport" above).

Structural Identification of a Renal Brush-Border Membrane Na^+-Phosphate Cotransport System

Until recently, there was very little information about the molecular structure of the phosphate transporter, since traditional approaches for its solubilization, purification, and reconstitution met with limited success because of enormous technical difficulties.[8] Strategies to identify the transporter using inhibitors of transport function such as phosphonoformic acid[74] and *N*-ethylmaleimide[75] or amino acid–specific reagents such as *N*-acetylimidazole[76] and phenylglyoxal,[77] in the presence and absence of excess Na^+ and phosphate, have also been used with limited success. A Na^+-phosphate cotransport system from rabbit kidney cortex has been cloned[78] using a novel approach that does not require protein purification. The method involves expression cloning in *Xenopus laevis* oocytes and was successfully used to clone the intestinal Na^+-glucose cotransporter.[79] Werner et al. demonstrated that size-fractionated mRNA prepared from rabbit kidney was able to stimulate Na^+-dependent phosphate transport in injected oocytes.[80] Moreover, the kinetic properties of the expressed transporter in mRNA-injected oocytes were indistinguishable from the renal brush-border membrane Na^+-phosphate cotransporter and distinct from the endogenous oocyte phosphate transporter.[80] Using this approach, a size-fractionated cDNA library from rabbit kidney cortex was screened, and a single clone with a 1.9-kb insert was identified. The clone stimulated expression of Na^+-dependent phosphate transport approximately 700 times as compared with total rabbit kidney mRNA.[78] The cDNA encodes a 465 amino acid protein with a molecular weight of approximately 52 kDa. The cloned renal Na^+-phosphate cotransporter does not share sequence homology with other cloned phosphate transport systems, from mitochondria or *Escherichia coli*, or with other proteins in the current protein data banks. The transporter does, however, contain a consensus motif shared by other Na^+-dependent transport systems.[78] Hydropathy analysis of the deduced amino acid sequence suggests that the cloned cDNA codes for a membrane protein with at least six, and perhaps eight, transmembrane segments, with N- and C-termini located at the cytoplasmic surface of the membrane.[78]

CLINICAL DISORDERS OF PHOSPHATE TRANSPORT

The three clinical states to be discussed are HHRH, XLH and OHO (Table 124-4). Even though the latter is an acquired disease, its discussion is warranted because of the similarity of its manifestations to those of XLH.

Table 124-4 **Comparison of the Inherited Hypophosphatemic Rickets with Oncogenic Hypophosphatemic Osteomalacia**

	XLH	HHRH	OHO
Inheritance	X-linked	AR	–
Age of onset	Early childhood	Early childhood	Any age
Clinical features			
Short stature	+ +	+ +	+ +
Bone pain	+ +	+ + +	+ + +
Femoral bowing	+ +	+ +	+ +
Muscle weakness	–	+ +	+ +
Radiologic signs			
Rickets	+ +	+ +	+ +
Pseudofracture	+	+ +	+ +
Coarse trabeculi	+ +	+ +	+ +
Dental abnormalities	+ +	?	–
Calcium metabolism			
Serum Ca^{2+}	N-LN	N-HN	N-LN
iPTH	N-HN	LN	N-HN
Ca_u	L	H	L
Ca absorption	L	H	L
Phosphate metabolism			
Serum phosphate	L	L	L
TmP/GFR	L	L	L
Alkaline phosphatase	H	H	H
Vitamin D metabolism			
Serum 25(OH)D	N	N	N
Serum $1,25(OH)_2D$	N-LN	H	LN-L
25(OH)D 1α-hydroxylase			
Response to phosphate	Abnormal	Normal	Abnormal

AR = autosomal recessive; N-LN = normal to low normal; iPTH = immunoreactive parathyroid hormone; N-HN = normal to high normal; LN = low normal; L = low; H = high; LN-L = low normal to low.

HEREDITARY HYPOPHOSPHATEMIC RICKETS WITH HYPERCALCIURIA

HHRH was first reported in closely related members of a single Bedouin tribe in which intermarriage has been widely practiced for many generations.[81,82]

Clinical Features

Presumed Homozygotes. The major clinical features of the condition are bone pain, skeletal deformities, short stature, and muscle weakness with x-ray signs of rickets and osteomalacia occurring during infancy and childhood. The biochemical findings include a reduced serum phosphate concentration, a reduced TmP/GFR, a normal serum calcium concentration, low or low normal serum PTH and urinary cAMP concentrations, an elevated serum alkaline phosphatase, normal serum 25-hydroxyvitamin D [25(OH)D] and 24,25-dihydroxyvitamin D [$24,25(OH)_2D$] concentrations, but an elevated serum $1,25(OH)_2D$ concentration associated with a marked increase in urinary calcium excretion.

The patient's response to either an oral calcium-loading or a phosphate-loading test shows that there is hyperabsorption of both calcium and phosphate from the intestine. These changes are indicative of the fact that the intestinal mucosa in these patients is normally responsive to $1,25(OH)_2D$. The IV injection of parathyroid extract is found to reduce TmP/GFR even further and to increase urinary cAMP excretion.

Presumed Heterozygotes. In an extensive study of 59 closely related members of this Bedouin tribe, nine individuals were identified with the characteristics just described. However, an additional 21 members were found to be clinically healthy but to display idiopathic hypercalciuria (IH) with slightly reduced plasma phosphate concentrations, elevated plasma $1,25(OH)_2D$ concentrations, and elevated urinary calcium excretion. The values seen in the patients with IH are intermediate between normal members of the same tribe and members with HHRH: urinary calcium concentration 0.43 ± 0.14 mg/mg of creatinine for HHRH, 0.34 ± 0.07 for IH, and 0.14 ± 0.5 for normal individuals; plasma $1,25(OH)_2D$, 303 pg/ml for HHRH, 145 pg/ml for IH, and 95 pg/ml for normal individuals; TmP/GFR was 3.05 SD units below the mean in HHRH and 1.15 below the mean in IH. Thus, the IH patients appear to have a milder metabolic defect characterized by elevated plasma $1,25(OH)_2D$ concentrations and hypercalciuria without evidence of bone disease or growth retardation. They often present with nephrolithiasis.

Bone Morphology

An examination of transilial biopsies from children with HHRH provides unequivocal evidence for osteomalacia in this disorder.[83] All patients display irregular mineralization fronts, markedly elevated osteoid surface and seam width, increased number of osteoid lamellae and prolonged mineralization lag time. A significant inverse relationship is evident between plasma phosphate concentration and osteoid parameters, suggesting that hypophosphatemia is a significant cause for osteomalacia in HHRH.[83] Osteoid parameters of hypercalciuric but otherwise asymptomatic, age-matched family members are within the normal range.[83]

Pathogenesis

From the point of view of pathophysiology, these patients appear to have the biochemical and physiological responses appropriate to chronic phosphate deprivation, but have high rates of urinary phosphate excretion and a low TmP/GFF. These latter two changes are not compatible with phosphate deprivation, but indicate instead that the primary defect is the renal handling of phosphate leading to an appropriate increase in $1,25(OH)_2D$ synthesis, the hyperabsorption of both calcium and phosphate from the gastrointestinal tract, and a suppression of PTH secretion. As a consequence, persistent hypophosphatemia develops of a sufficient degree to lead to a reduction in the rate of bone mineralization and bone growth. The fact that these patients respond to oral phosphate therapy with an increase in plasma PTH, a fall in plasma $1,25(OH)_2D$ concentration, a fall in bone turnover, bone growth, and a healing of the rickets fits with this pathogenic mechanism. Unresolved is the location of the tubular segment that expresses the disorder in phosphate reabsorption. It is presumed to be the proximal tubule.

Genetics

The genetic relationship in a single Bedouin tribe in which 9 individuals have HHRH and 21 have IH without clinical evidence of bone disease is shown in Fig. 124-6. The interrelationships emphasize the considerable intermarriage seen within the extended kindred. On the basis of this family tree, it is logical to assume that patients with HHRH and IH share a common inherited defect that leads to a milder degree of phosphate leak and the attendant changes in vitamin D and calcium metabolism in patients with IH than in those with HHRH. The data are compatible with autosomal recessive inheritance of a single mutant allele with an incomplete recessive phenotype in the heterozygotes (as in cystinuria [Chap. 117] and familial iminoglycinuria [Chap. 120]).

It is not clear whether patients with IH and nephrolithiasis with a so-called phosphate leak who have been reported in this country and Europe[84–86] have the same disease as the subjects with IH seen in the HHRH kindred. There is a report of a single case of hypophosphatemic rickets with hypercalciuria from Japan.[87] This case did not respond to therapy with 1α-hydroxyvitamin D_3 but did respond to phosphate treatment. It seems quite likely that this patient has HHRH.

Treatment

Administration of 1 to 2.5 g of neutral phosphate daily, given in five divided doses, leads to an increase in growth rate, disappearance of bone pain and muscle weakness. and disappearance of the radiologic signs of rickets. The plasma phosphate concentration rises; the plasma $1,25(OH)_2D$ concentration falls, as do the plasma calcium and alkaline phosphatase concentrations. Likewise, urinary calcium excretion falls, the urinary cAMP rises, but TmP/GFR does not change. Bone biopsy of a treated subject reveals healing of osteomalacia.

X-LINKED HYPOPHOSPHATEMIA

XLH is the most common inherited abnormality of renal tubular phosphate transport (see Table 124-4). It is inherited as an X-linked dominant trait. It is also known as vitamin D resistant rickets, familial hypophosphatemic rickets, or hypophosphatemic vitamin D resistant rickets.

Clinical Features in Children

The most common features of XLH are short stature and femoral and/or tibial bowing presenting early in life (1 to 2 years) without muscle weakness, tetany, or convulsions.[13,14,88–93] The degree of growth retardation and of skeletal

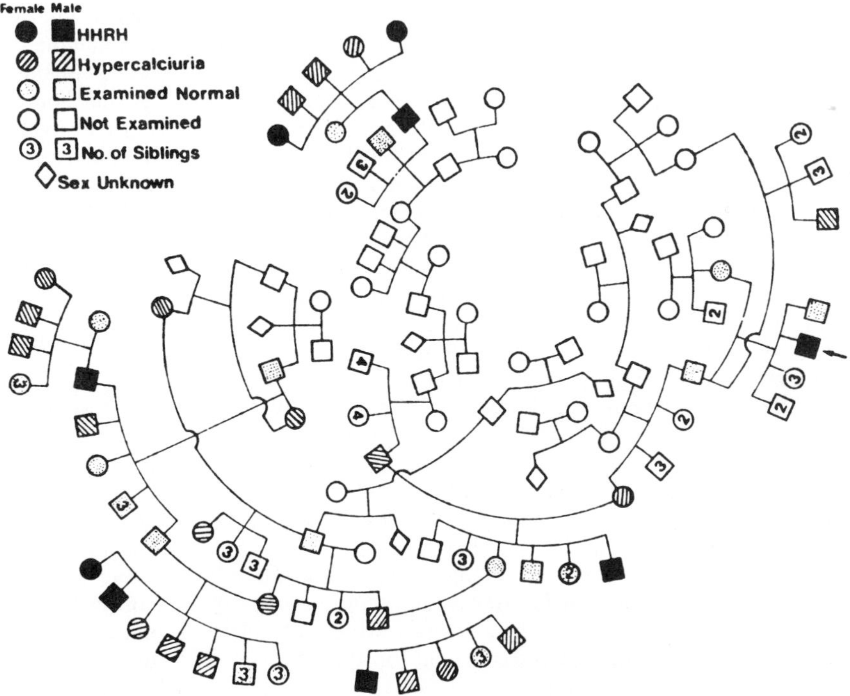

FIG. 124-6 Genetic relationship of 9 patients with hereditary hypophosphatemic rickets and hypercalciuria and 21 subjects with 'idiopathic' hypercalciuria alone. Arrow indicates index case. (*From Tieder et al.*[82] *Used by permission.*)

abnormalities is quite variable within a given kindred. Females often have less severe bone disease than do males. This difference has been ascribed to sex hormone-dependent modulation of mutant gene expression and/or to the presence of lyonization in the heterozygous female. However, even in affected males, there is a considerable variability in the severity of the bone disease and of the growth retardation. Of particular importance, there is no correlation between the severity of bone disease and the serum phosphate concentration.

The diagnosis of XLH in suspected patients during early infancy is difficult even in known kindreds. The plasma phosphate concentration may be normal at birth and is likely to remain so for 6 to 9 months. The most reliable early sign of the disease is an elevation of plasma alkaline phosphatase activity, which may occur as early as 4 to 6 months of age and is usually associated with early but definite radiologic signs of rickets. By 1 year of age, some retardation of growth usually occurs with established hypophosphatemia, elevated plasma alkaline phosphatase, and definite radiologic signs of rickets. Coarse trabeculation of bone consistent with osteomalacia is also seen. There may also be some retardation of bone age.

Other early manifestations of the disease are late dentition and recurrent dental abscesses. These may be associated with cranial synostosis. Fractures or pseudofractures in the growing child practically never occur even in untreated patients, but in such cases, there is progressive femoral and/or tibial bowing, usually resulting in genu valgum; genu varum is also seen in some cases. Growth retardation and the radiologic signs are more apparent in the lower than upper extremity. These findings have led to the suggestion that growth failure is limited to the lower extremities. However, when upper segment height is measured, it too has shown growth retardation.[94]

Clinical Features in Adults

An earlier view of the natural history of this condition was that once the patient had gone through puberty and further skeletal growth had stopped, the disease did not progress.[14,95,96] However, this view is clearly incorrect. A more systematic study of adults of various ages has shown persistent and often progressive evidence of disease, as well as mechanical complications arising from the skeletal deformities acquired during childhood and adolescence.[96]

The persistence of disease is evident by the facts that: (1) many but not all adults have some elevation in plasma alkaline phosphatase; (2) every adult in whom transiliac crest biopsy has been appraised by histomorphometric analysis has unequivocal osteomalacia[97]; (3) nearly all the patients have radiologic evidence of pseudofractures[98]; and (4) a third of patients have bone pain, and a majority have radiologic signs of bone and/or joint abnormalities. It is clear that osteomalacia of some degree persists throughout life, as does the defect in phosphate transport.[96] Paradoxically, total bone mass is often increased,[97] as is the rate of bone turnover, assessed by measurements of hydroxyproline excretion and serum osteocalcin.[96] Serum osteocalcin levels are also increased in the *Hyp* mouse homologue of the human disorder[99] (see below).

It is of interest that even though plasma $1,25(OH)_2D$ concentrations are normal in these adults, both severity of bone pain and severity of osteomalacia were negatively correlated with plasma $1,25(OH)_2D$ concentration.[96]

Two other common manifestations of XLH in adults are repeated dental abscesses[100–103] and radiologic evidence of enthesopathy (ossification of tendon, ligaments, and joint capsules).[97,98,104,105] In addition, a large and increasing number of patients complain of joint pain (as distinct from bone pain) and have clinical and radiologic evidence of osteoarthritis, particularly of the joints in the lower extremities. In general, the more evident the bowing of the lower limbs, the greater the degree of osteoarthritis and the greater the joint pain.

Laboratory Findings

The two most reliable markers for XLH are a reduced plasma phosphate concentration and a reduced TmP/GFR with otherwise normal renal tubular function. These findings are associated with normal to slightly low plasma calcium concentration, normal to slightly high PTH, elevated plasma alkaline phosphatase, low or low normal plasma $1,25(OH)_2D$ and normal 25(OH)D concentration, and reduced urinary calcium excretion (see Table 124-4). On administration of an oral calcium load, there is a very small increase in either plasma calcium concentration or urinary calcium excretion, implying a secondary defect in the absorption of calcium from the gastrointestinal tract. The serum $24,25(OH)_2D$ levels are reported to be low in untreated children[12] and normal after treatment with ergocalciferol.[12,106]

Dental Findings

Spontaneous dental abscesses are common both in early and late childhood.[101–103,107] Hypomineralization of the enamel associated with a defect in dentin maturation with enlarged pulp chambers is commonly seen in XLH.[108,109] Under normal circumstances, the dentin matrix calcifies by the formation of calcospheres containing calcium phosphate crystals. These coalesce to form a uniformly calcified dentin. In patients with XLH, the calcospheres fail to coalesce normally so that a distinct pattern of interglobular dentin forms and persists throughout life.

In a study of teeth forming secondary dentin, it was reported that dental pulp space is highest in treated XLH males, intermediate in treated XLH females, and lowest in age-matched controls, despite near-normal serum phosphate levels in both groups of treated XLH patients.[110] On the assumption that extracellular phosphate was maintained at normal levels during the long period of tooth development in the treated XLH patients, the demonstration of a gene dose effect in teeth implies that the mutant gene is expressed in tooth-forming cells. The gene product and the developmental process are unknown (see "Bone Phenotype" under "The *Hyp* Mouse" below).

Radiologic Findings

Early in life, the predominant changes are the characteristic signs of rickets with fraying, widening, and cupping of the metaphyseal ends of the proximal and distal tibia, the distal femur, and the ulna and radius. As the child grows older the changes at the wrist become minimal. Those at the knee become more pronounced and become associated with a widening of the metaphysis. During late childhood and adolescence the shafts of the long bones display thickened cortices and coarse, unusually dense trabecular bone. Bone mineral analysis usually reveals a normal value, which means that total bone (mineralized and unmineralized) is greater than normal, but there is a marked increase in incompletely mineralized bone. Parenthetically, successful treatment often leads to a remodeling of the skeleton, and a decrease in cortical thickness and trabecular bone volume.

Bone Morphology

Transileal biopsies have been performed in a number of patients,[111-113] showing evidence of osteomalacia in both the cortical and trabecular bone with an increase in osteoid volume, osteoid surface, and mean osteoid seam width. Using the technique of double tetracycline labeling, it has been possible to demonstrate a decrease in calcification rate and a prolongation of mineralization lag time (the time between bone matrix deposition and its eventual calcification). In association with these changes, there are areas of hypomineralization around osteocytes in the lamellar cortical bone, which are characteristic of this type of osteomalacia.[114]

Given the finding of a nearly normal amount of mineralized bone as determined both by bone mineral analysis in vivo and in bone biopsy material in vitro, the question arises as to why bowing of the longbones, particularly the tibias and femora, occurs. The answer appears to lie in the fact that areas of osteomalacia are not confined simply to bone surfaces, but are distributed throughout the cortical bone so that the structural properties of the whole organ are adversely affected. The increase in total bone volume can be viewed as an effort to compensate for this lack of structural integrity at the organ level.

Genetics

A more complete discussion of the genetics of XLH is given in the previous editions of this work.[13,14] XLH is inherited as an X-linked dominant trait.[115] One feature that is not simply accounted for in XLH is the apparent lower incidence of bone disease in females as compared with males, despite the fact that both sexes exhibit a similar degree of hypophosphatemia. Two possible explanations have been offered to account for the relative immunity of the female from severe bone disease: (1) There is an intrinsic bone defect that is independent of serum phosphate and both normal and mutant alleles are expressed in females as a consequence of X-chromosome inactivation. (2) There is a sex-linked factor independent of gene dose that confers a relative immunity to the effects of the abnormal gene. This latter possibility is supported by the observation that ovariectomy causes the appearance of more severe bone changes in female *Hyp* mice[116] (see "General Phenotype" under "The *Hyp* Mouse," below).

Neither the human (symbol HYP, formerly HPDR) nor the mouse (*Hyp*) loci have been cloned, nor have their products been identified. However, some progress has been made in determining the locus of the human and mouse genes. The hypophosphatemia region is in one of five conserved segments that have taken up different orientations and physical order during the evolution of human and mouse X chromosomes[117,118] (Fig. 124-7). The human gene has been mapped to the short arm of the X chromosome (Xp22.1-p.22.2) in the region extending from Duchenne muscular dystrophy (DMD) to steroid sulfatase (see Fig. 124-7). The locus lies somewhere between markers DXS43 and DXS41 which are, respectively, telomeric and centromeric to HYP,[119-122] and is linked to the glycine receptor.[123] The polymorphic markers DXS207 and DXS197 are telomeric to

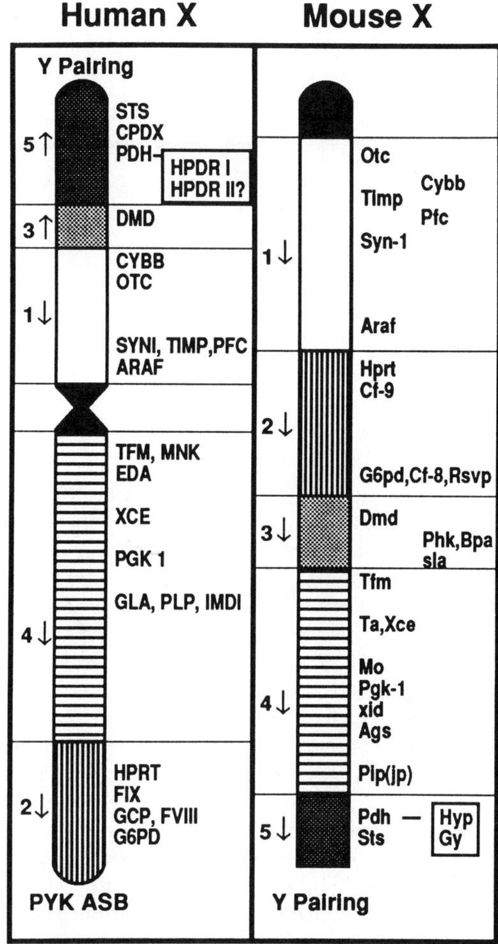

FIG. 124-7 **Homologous linkage groups and rearrangements on human and mouse X chromosomes. HPDR-1 and HPDR-II, now known as HYPI and HYPII,[241] are putative human homologues of *Hyp* and *Gy*, respectively. Conserved segments and their orientation are depicted.** ***(Adapted from Searle et al.***[118] ***and reproduced from Scriver and Tenenhouse***[227] ***by permission.)***

HYP and may be useful alternative markers.[124] Some studies localized the HYP gene between tightly linked flanking markers DXS257 (telomeric) and DXS274 (centromeric), which are approximately 3.5 cM apart[125,126] (Fig. 124-8). These findings will facilitate attempts to localize further and eventually clone the HYP gene.[127]

A molecular genetic approach to map the mouse gene has also been reported.[128] To facilitate the detection of restriction fragment length polymorphisms (RFLP), an interspecific backcross between two evolutionary divergent species, *Mus spretus* and *Mus musculus domesticus* (carrying the *Hyp* mutation), was established by in vitro fertilization.[128] Using a variety of X-linked mouse probes, the most likely gene order in the distal portion of the mouse X chromosome is Pgk-1-DXSmh43-*Hyp*-Cbx-rs1-Amg, from proximal to distal. The distance between DXSmh43 and *Hyp* is approximately 2.5 cM and that between *Hyp* and Cbx-rs1 1.98 cM.[128]

Pathogenesis

A discussion of the pathogenesis of the human disease will be considered below in the context of a discussion of the *Hyp* and *Gy* mouse models.

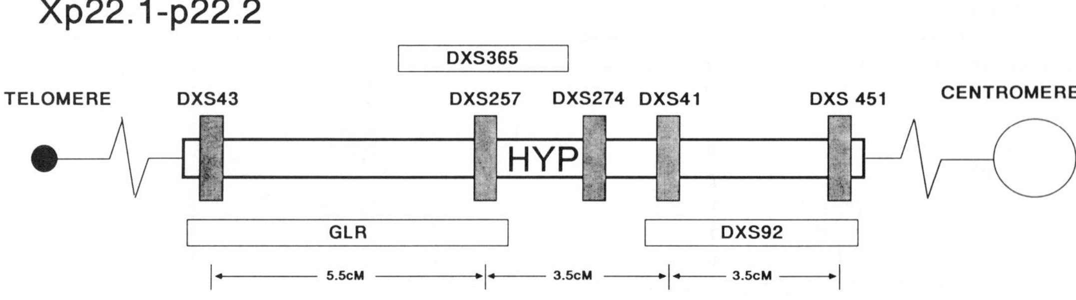

FIG. 124-8 **Map position of HYP relative to human X-chromosome polymorphic probes.** (*The figure was provided by M.J. Econs and is based on data in refs.*125 and 126.)

The *Hyp* Mouse

A major advance in the study of the pathophysiology of XLH was the discovery of a mutation in the laboratory mouse that exhibits many of the phenotypic features of XLH.[129] The *Hyp* mouse is characterized by hypophosphatemia, decreased growth rate, rickets and osteomalacia, and reduced net tubular reabsorption of phosphate without hypocalcemia and secondary hyperparathyroidism. Moreover, the trait in the *Hyp* mouse is inherited as an X-linked dominant and has been mapped to the distal part of the X chromosome (see "Genetics," above). Because the *Hyp* locus on the mouse X chromosome is part of a syntenic group that is conserved,[117] and because phenotypic expression of *Hyp* is similar to that of XLH, it is likely that the X-linked mutations causing hypophosphatemia in mice and humans involve homologous genes. Accordingly, the *Hyp* mouse appears to be an appropriate model for the human disease, XLH. The ensuing discussion of pathophysiology considers data derived both from human and mouse studies. Before undertaking this discussion, a brief description of the mouse phenotype is given.

General Phenotype. Heterozygous *Hyp* females (*Hyp*/+) and hemizygous *Hyp* males (*Hyp*/Y) can be distinguished from their normal littermates (+/+ and +/y) by their shortened hind limbs and tail and reduced body weight. These features persist throughout life and become more obvious with age. Kyphosis of the thoracic vertebrae, rachitic rosary, and prominent bowing of the femur develop with age in mutant mice, and bone ash is significantly reduced.[129,130] The skeletal abnormalities are more uniformly severe in the hemizygous males as compared with the heterozygous females,[129,130] as in the case of the human disease, XLH.

Although the basis for the sex difference in bone disease was thought to be the result of random X-chromosome inactivation in females, some studies have suggested that gonadal hormones contribute to the sexual dimorphism.[116] Gonadectomy of hemizygous mutant males and heterozygous mutant females abolished the sex difference in bone mineral content.[116] Moreover, in spite of two mutant alleles, bone parameters in homozygous mutant females (*Hyp*/*Hyp*) are more similar to heterozygous mutant females than to hemizygous mutant males.[131,132]

The plasma concentration of inorganic phosphate is significantly reduced in both *Hyp* males and *Hyp* females as compared with that of normal littermates.[129] These differences are apparent by 20 to 49 days of age and persist up to and beyond 400 days of age. Plasma calcium concentration is slightly but significantly reduced in *Hyp* males and *Hyp* females. Urinary phosphate excretion, in relation to plasma phosphate, is significantly elevated in *Hyp* mice. Mutant mice appear to live a normal life span. *Hyp*/+ females are fertile and raise their young but not all *Hyp*/Y males can sire offspring.

Renal Phenotype. ***Phosphate Transport.*** The defect in phosphate reabsorption in *Hyp* mice has been localized to the proximal tubule by micropuncture studies.[133,134] The defect persists after parathyroidectomy of *Hyp* mice[134,135] and is expressed in the luminal membrane.[136,137] The specificity of the brush-border membrane phosphate transport defect in *Hyp* mice was established by the demonstration of normal Na^+-dependent glucose,[136,137] alanine,[138] proline,[139] and sulfate[140] uptake in luminal vesicle preparations derived from mutant mouse kidney. Moreover, the phosphate transport defect in *Hyp* mice cannot be attributed to alterations in renal Na^+-transport,[141] brush-border membrane fluidity,[142] or lipid composition.[142]

Kinetic studies in isolated brush-border membrane vesicles demonstrate that while both low-affinity, high-capacity and high-affinity, low-capacity Na^+-phosphate cotransport systems are expressed in *Hyp* mice, only the high-affinity system is impaired by the mutation, with a 50 percent decrease in apparent V_{max} and no change in apparent K_m for phosphate.[43] These findings underscore the relative importance of the high-affinity phosphate transport system in the overall maintenance of phosphate homeostasis and suggest that a perturbation of this transport system is sufficient cause for the significant hypophosphatemia that characterizes the *Hyp* mutation.

The mechanism for reduced phosphate transport on the high-affinity system in *Hyp* mice is not understood. Half-normal V_{max} values are compatible with either fewer phosphate transport units or with malfunction of a normal number of carriers. The first possibility was tested by measuring the effect of the *Hyp* mutation on binding of phosphonoformic acid (PFA)—a putative probe for the Na^+-phosphate cotransporter[74]—to luminal membrane vesicles. The mutation altered neither Na^+-dependent PFA binding nor its phosphate-displaceable component, suggesting that the number of Na^+-phosphate cotransporters is not decreased in renal brush-border membranes of *Hyp* mice.[143] However, because PFA does not interact exclusively with the Na^+-phosphate cotransporter,[144] PFA binding to sites other than the Na^+-phosphate cotransporter may have masked a difference in cotransporter number in *Hyp* mice.

The second possibility was tested by comparing the effects of Na^+, membrane potential, and pH on Na^+-phosphate cotransport in renal brush-border membrane vesicles of normal and mutant mice. Affinity for Na^+, number of Na^+ ions interacting with the high-affinity phosphate transport system, and response of the cotransporter to membrane potential and pH were not different from normal in *Hyp* mice, thereby ruling out these mechanisms for decreased intrinsic activity of the Na^+-phosphate cotransporter in the mutant strain.[145]

Radiation inactivation analysis demonstrated that the molecular size of protein(s) mediating Na^+-dependent phosphate transport is similar in brush-border membranes isolated from normal mice (242±16 kDa) and *Hyp* littermates (227±39 kDa).[143] Because Na^+-solute cotransporters function as multimeric protein complexes, these results indicate that aggregation of monomeric subunits that form the phosphate carrier is normal in the mutant *Hyp* strain.

Dietary phosphate deprivation elicits a striking suppression in renal fractional excretion of phosphate and a significant rise in Na^+-dependent phosphate transport in renal brush-border membrane vesicles in male[146] and female[147] mice bearing the X-linked *Hyp* mutation. The adaptive increase in transport is associated with an increase in V_{max} of the high-affinity Na^+-phosphate cotransport process in renal brush-border membranes of normal and *Hyp* mice[43] (Fig. 124-9). The genotypic difference in phosphate transport between normal and *Hyp* mice is still maintained under these conditions[43,146,147] (see Fig. 124-9). In vivo assessment of tubular adaptation to phosphate deprivation, by estimation of maximal net phosphate reabsorption per unit volume of glomerular filtrate, indicates that *Hyp* mice exhibit a blunted adaptive response as compared to normal littermates.[148] These findings suggest that targets other than the high-affinity Na^+-phosphate cotransport system in the brush-border membrane may contribute to the adaptive response in *Hyp* mice.[148a]

Expression studies in microinjected *Xenopus laevis* oocytes demonstrate that poly(A)$^+$RNA from kidneys of normal mice, but not *Hyp* mice, elicit a significant increase in oocyte Na^+-phosphate cotransport.[149] However, it is difficult to explain why *Hyp* kidney, which retains a significant fraction of Na^+-phosphate cotransport function, should be devoid of mRNA capable of mediating phosphate transport in injected oocytes.[149] The cloning of a renal epithelial Na^+-phosphate cotransporter cDNA by Werner et al.[78] will permit expression studies to determine the abundance of Na^+-phosphate cotransporter mRNA in *Hyp* mouse kidney. In addition, chromosomal mapping studies will establish whether the cotransporter cDNA maps to the X chromosome and is thus a candidate gene for the transport system affected by the *Hyp* mutation (see "Addendum").

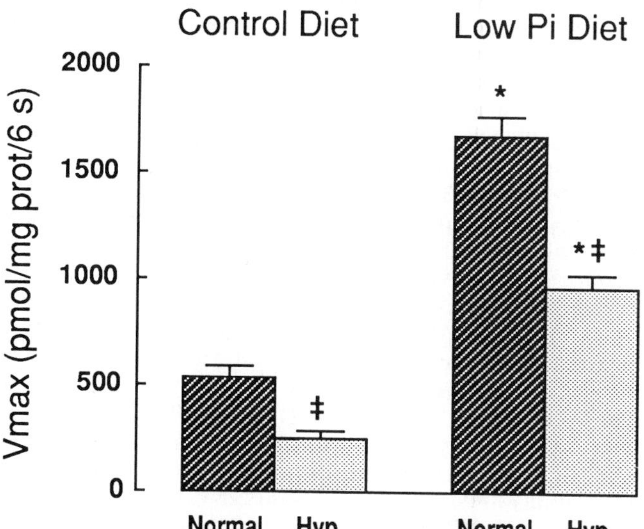

FIG. 124-9 **Effect of phosphate deprivation on apparent V_{max} of the high-affinity Na^+-phosphate cotransport system in renal brush-border membrane vesicles prepared from normal and *Hyp* mice. V_{max} values were estimated from Eadie-Hofstee plots of initial-rate phosphate uptake measured over a phosphate concentration range of 10 to 500 μM.[43] Under these conditions, transport is almost exclusively mediated by the high-affinity, low-capacity Na^+-phosphate cotransport process. The data show that while both normal and *Hyp* mice exhibit an increase in phosphate transport V_{max}, phosphate transport is significantly reduced in brush-border membranes from *Hyp* mice under both dietary conditions. (*Data redrawn from Boneh and Tenenhouse,[228] with permission.*)**

Vitamin D Metabolism. The regulation of renal $25(OH)D_3$ metabolism is impaired in the X-linked *Hyp* mouse, as it is in the XLH human. The plasma concentration of $1,25(OH)_2D$ and the renal production of $1,25(OH)_2D$ in *Hyp* mice, although similar to that observed in normal littermates, are inappropriate for the degree of hypophosphatemia.[150,151] Moreover, the renal 1α-hydroxylase response to a variety of regulatory factors is abnormal in the mutant strain. Phosphate restriction which stimulates $1,25(OH)_2D$ production in normal mice[150-152] decreases hormone synthesis in mutant mice.[150,152] On the other hand, phosphate supplementation which inhibits $1,25(OH)_2D$ production in normal mice[152,153] dramatically stimulates hormone synthesis in *Hyp* mice.[152,153] *Hyp* mice exhibit a significantly blunted renal 1α-hydroxylase response to vitamin D deficiency[154,155] and calcium restriction.[156] Reduced synthesis of $1,25(OH)_2D$ in vitamin D deficient *Hyp* mice is independent of genotype differences in serum calcium[154] and parathyroid hormone levels[155] and is associated with a decrease in the apparent V_{max} for 1α-hydroxylase, with no change in apparent K_m.[155,157] *Hyp* mice also exhibit a significantly reduced renal 1α-hydroxylase response to infusion of PTH,[158] cAMP,[159] and PTH-related peptide.[160] Patients with XLH also show similar blunted 1α-hydroxylase responses to both lowered plasma phosphate concentration[161] and elevated PTH concentration.[162]

It is of interest that renal 1α-hydroxylase is appropriately stimulated by calcitonin infusion in *Hyp* mice.[163] Moreover, calcitonin elicited a comparable increase in the serum concentration of $1,25(OH)_2D$ in XLH patients and in controls.[164] The differences between the effects of PTH[158,162] and calcitonin[163,164] on 1α-hydroxylase activity in *Hyp* mice and XLH patients provides genetic confirmation of the previously reported existence of two anatomically distinct, independently regulated renal 1α-hydroxylase systems in mammalian kidney (see Table 124-2)—a PTH-regulated system in the proximal convoluted tubule and a calcitonin-stimulated system in the proximal straight tubule.[165,166]

The *Hyp* mutation is also characterized by increased catabolism of $1,25-(OH)_2D$. In addition to in vivo clearance studies,[167] degradation of the hormone in *Hyp* mice was assessed by measurement of renal mitochondrial 24-hydroxylase, an enzyme that catalyzes the first of a series of reactions, known collectively as the C-24 oxidation or side-chain cleavage pathway, that converts $1,25(OH)_2D_3$ to its final inactivation product, calcitroic acid.[168-171] The 24-hydroxylation of $1,25(OH)_2D_3$ and its $25(OH)D_3$ precursor are significantly elevated in *Hyp* mice.[172] Moreover, using ^3H-labeled $24,25(OH)_2D_3$ as substrate, it was demonstrated that the second reaction in the catabolic sequence (24-oxidation) is also elevated in renal mitochondria of *Hyp* mice.[173] These results may explain why the plasma concentration of $24,25-(OH)_2D$ is not elevated in the mutant strain.[174]

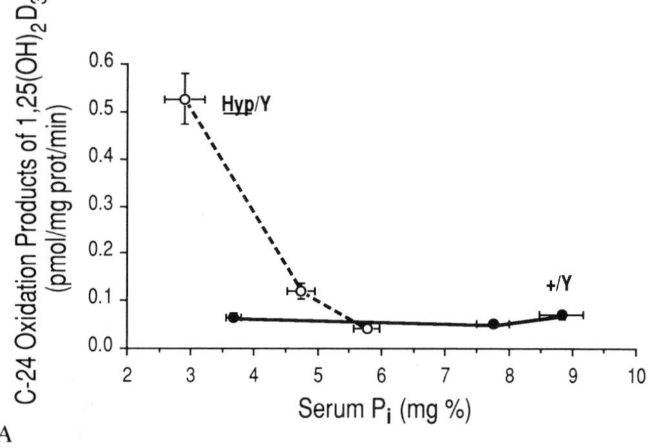

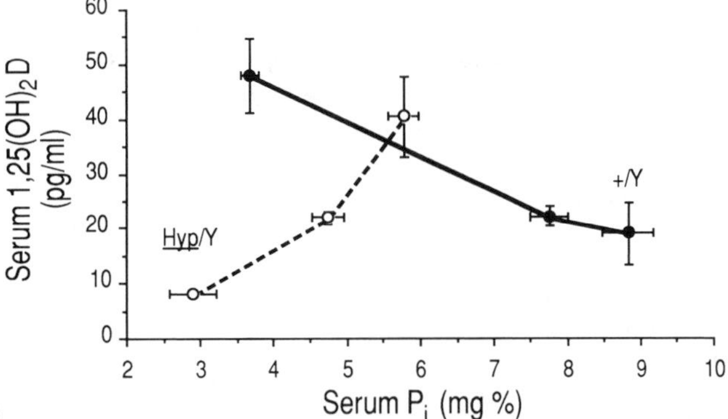

FIG. 124-10 **Relationship between serum phosphate concentration and (A) the rate of formation of C-24 oxidation products from $1,25(OH)_2D_3$ by isolated renal mitochondria and (B) the steady state serum concentration of $1,25(OH)_2D$ in normal and *Hyp* mice. ● = +/Y mice; o = *Hyp*/Y mice. (*From Tenenhouse and Jones.*[175] *Used by permission.*)**

Comparable data on catabolism of $1,25(OH)_2D$ in patients with XLH are not yet available.

Regulation of the catabolic pathway by dietary phosphate is also abnormal in *Hyp* mice.[175] In contrast to normal mice in which phosphate intake does not appear to influence renal 24-hydroxylase activity, *Hyp* mice respond to phosphate deprivation with increased $1,25(OH)_2D$ catabolism and to phosphate supplementation with decreased hormone catabolism[175] (see Fig. 124-10A). The increase in $1,25(OH)_2D$ catabolism in phosphate-deprived *Hyp* mice is associated with an increase in the abundance of renal 24-hydroxylase mRNA which is evident as early as 1 day after the administration of the low-phosphate diet.[176] In addition, the plasma concentration of $1,25(OH)_2D$ is inversely correlated with renal 24-hydroxylase activity in *Hyp* mice[175] (Fig. 124-10B). These findings suggest that (1) the renal catabolic pathway is a more important determinant of plasma $1,25(OH)_2D$ levels in *Hyp* mice than in normal littermates, (2) the reported deficit in net renal $1,25(OH)_2D$ synthesis in *Hyp* mice can be attributed both to increased hormone catabolism and reduced hormone synthesis, and (3) the disorder in renal vitamin D metabolism in the mutant strain is secondary to the perturbation in phosphate homeostasis, since correction of the defect can be achieved by phosphate supplementation of *Hyp* mice.[152,153,175] There is no evidence to show that a similar increase in $1,25(OH)_2D$ synthesis occurs in response to phosphate supplementation in XLH patients.

Tissue Phosphate. The precise relationship between the defect in brush-border membrane phosphate transport and mitochondrial 25(OH)D metabolism in *Hyp* mice is poorly understood. One possibility is that the abnormalities in $1,25(OH)_2D$ synthesis and catabolism are due to altered renal cell phosphate concentration. Although reduced renal cortical ribonucleoside triphosphate pools in *Hyp* mice have been reported,[177] both chemical and ^{31}PMRI methods have failed to demonstrate genotype differences in the intracellular concentration of inorganic phosphate and phosphorylated compounds.[129,146,178] Moreover, the demonstration of normal phosphate uptake in isolated renal mitochondria derived from *Hyp* mice, under conditions in which renal 25(OH)D metabolism is disturbed, suggests that mitochondrial phosphate transport does not contribute to the problems in the regulation of $1,25(OH)_2D$ synthesis and catabolism.[157]

PTH Status and Response to PTH. The persistence of the renal phosphate transport leak after parathyroidectomy of X-linked *Hyp* mice firmly establishes that the brush-border membrane phosphate transport defect is not secondary to hyperparathyroidism.[134,135] The PTH status of *Hyp* mice is, nevertheless, a controversial issue, and both normal[129,155] and elevated levels of PTH[179,180] have been reported. It is noteworthy that humans with XLH have either normal or elevated plasma PTH concentrations (see above).

Although the relative contribution of hyperparathyroidism to the mutant renal phenotype is difficult to ascertain, genotype differences in brush-border membrane phosphate transport persist after comparable diet-induced hyperparathyroidism in normal and mutant subjects.[181]

The effect of the *Hyp* mutation on the renal response to PTH has also been investigated. No evidence for hypersensitivity to PTH was documented, thereby ruling out one of the postulated mechanisms for this disorder.[181,182] Moreover, renal cAMP-dependent protein kinases[183] and the pattern of cAMP-dependent brush-border membrane protein phosphorylation and dephosphorylation[184] are similar in normal and *Hyp* mice.

Intestinal Phenotype. Whereas there is unequivocal evidence for normal intestinal phosphate absorption in adult *Hyp* mice,[185,186] juvenile *Hyp* mice exhibit a significant impairment in jejunal phosphate absorption.[186] *Hyp* mice who are 3 to 6 weeks old also exhibit intestinal calcium malabsorption[187,188] accompanied by decreased levels of intestinal vitamin D–dependent 9-kDa calcium-binding protein (calbindin-D_{9k}).[189] Based on the findings that juvenile *Hyp* mice have significantly lower plasma levels of $1,25(OH)_2D$ relative to normal mice[190] and that the abnormal intestinal phenotype can be corrected by $1,25(OH)_2D$ infusion of juvenile *Hyp* mice,[191] it is likely that intestinal abnormalities in juvenile *Hyp* mice are secondary to abnormal renal metabolism of $1,25(OH)_2D$.[150,151,156,172,175] The reduced calcium absorption seen in young XLH patients may have a similar basis.

Studies of intestinal phosphate uptake by jejunal biopsies derived from patients with XLH have demonstrated both deficient[192] and normal uptake.[193] Genetic heterogeneity between cases and ages of patients studied are possible explanations for the disparate findings.

The effect of the *Hyp* mutation on intestinal $1,25(OH)_2D$ receptor function has also been investigated. While genotype differences in receptor number and receptor affinity for $1,25(OH)_2D$ are not apparent in juvenile[188] and adult[194] *Hyp* mice, decreased nuclear uptake of $1,25(OH)_2D_3$ by duodenal mucosal cells was reported in adult *Hyp* mice.[195] The demonstration that phosphate supplementation of *Hyp* mice corrects the defect in nuclear $1,25(OH)_2D_3$ binding[196] suggests that hypophosphatemia may play a role in vitamin D resistance in *Hyp* mice and may account for low levels of intestinal calbindin-D_{28k} in adult mutant mice.[197]

Bone Phenotype. In addition to the skeletal features described above (see "General Phenotype"), *Hyp* mice exhibit craniosynostosis due to premature fusion of the coronal suture[198] and abnormal skull morphology arising mainly from deficient linear growth of the nasal bone.[199] Analytical and histomorphometric methods reveal a shorter than normal vertebral length associated with a wider epiphyseal growth plate in *Hyp* mice.[200] Moreover, impaired endosteal bone mineralization is present in the mutants as demonstrated by excessive osteoid surface and thickness, and decreased extent of the mineralization front.[200]

Some studies have suggested that abnormal bone formation in *Hyp* mice is determined not only by the hypophosphatemic environment arising from the renal phosphate leak[201,202] but also by an intrinsic osteoblast defect in the mutant strain.[202–204] In these studies, osteoid seam thickness and osteoid volume were used as indices of bone formation 2 weeks after transplantation of bone cells derived from either normal mice or *Hyp* mice into the gluteal muscle of either normal or *Hyp* mouse recipients. Bone cells isolated from normal and *Hyp* mice produce abnormal bone when transplanted intramuscularly into mutant mice[202] or into phosphate-deprived normal mice,[204] suggesting that the low-phosphate environment significantly contributes to abnormal bone formation. When bone cells from *Hyp* mice are transplanted into normal mice[202] or into phosphate-supplemented *Hyp* mice,[204] parameters of bone formation are significantly improved, but not normalized. In contrast, normal bone formation is apparent when bone cells from normal mice, with comparable diet-induced hypophosphatemia, are transplanted into normal mice.[203] These findings support the hypothesis that bone cells from *Hyp* mice may express an intrinsic mineralization defect and that osteoblast dysfunction cannot be corrected by a normal phosphate environment (see "Dental Findings" under "X-Linked Hypophosphatemia" above).

The precise mechanism for abnormal osteoblast function, whether secondary to hypophosphatemia alone or determined also by an intrinsic bone defect in *Hyp* mice, is not known. Both Na^+-phosphate cotransport[205,206] and $1,25(OH)_2D$ receptor number and affinity[207] are normal in cultured osteoblasts derived from *Hyp* mice. However, the alkaline phosphatase and proliferative responses to $1,25(OH)_2D$ are inappropriately regulated by phosphate in osteoblasts derived from the mutant strain.[208] Moreover, the content of complexed acidic phospholipids is significantly reduced in bones of *Hyp* mice.[209]

Hyp mice exhibit dental abnormalities similar to those reported in patients with XLH.[210–213] The molars of *Hyp*/Y mice tend to have rather large pulp chambers and a wider predentin band than +/Y controls, with mutant dentin showing prominent interglobular areas of deficient mineralization. Normalization of serum phosphate in *Hyp* mice by feeding a high-calcium, high-phosphate diet for 30 days did not affect the appearance of interglobular dentin in the mutant strain.[214] In addition to these dental abnormalities, exposure of the dental pulp occurs frequently in *Hyp* mice as a result of developmental deficiency of the dentin.

Other Phenotypic Characteristics. Although the phosphate concentration of breast milk was reported to be low in two mothers with XLH,[215,216] the phosphate content of milk from lactating normal and *Hyp*/+ females is not significantly different.[217] The data in mice suggest that mutant females can accumulate a normal amount of phosphate in milk despite significant hypophosphatemia and provide evidence for the absence of a phosphate transport defect in mammary glands.[217] Although the phosphate concentration is lower than normal in saliva from *Hyp* mice, salivary phosphate levels in *Hyp* mice are similar to that of normal mice with a comparable degree of diet-induced hypophosphatemia, suggesting that the phosphate transport defect, which is expressed in the renal brush-border membrane, is not expressed in the salivary gland.[218] In addition, Na^+-phosphate cotransport is not depressed in cultured skin fibroblasts derived from patients with XLH as compared with age-matched controls.[219]

Food consumption and metabolic rate are elevated in *Hyp* mice.[220] However, T_4 levels are normal,[139] and increased oxygen consumption in *Hyp* mice is not affected by serum phosphate.[220] It is not yet known whether metabolic rate is elevated in patients in XLH.

Hyp mice do not exhibit the normal rise in serum phosphate following fasting.[221] This failure has been attributed to their apparent failure to adapt to phosphate deprivation.[148] It has been proposed that the hyperphosphatemic response to fasting is related to the adaptive renal response, which prevents phosphate, mobilized from body stores during fasting, from being excreted in the urine. However, the demonstration of adaptation to phosphate deprivation at the renal brush-border membrane of *Hyp* mice[43,146,147] casts doubt on the validity of this hypothesis.

Origin of the Mutant Renal Phenotype—Evidence for a Humoral Basis

The assumption has been made that the genetic defect in XLH leads to either an altered phosphate transport protein in the renal proximal tubule, and possibly in bone, or to a decrease in the amount of a normal phosphate transport protein. However, evidence has indicated that this assumption may not be correct. This conclusion is based on four types of evidence: studies in parabiotic mice, studies of renal transplantion in mice, the absence of gene dose effect in *Hyp* and XLH, and the similarity in the metabolic changes seen in patients with OHO and those with XLH.

Parabiosis

When normal mice are surgically joined to *Hyp* mice, significant hypophosphatemia and decreased renal phosphate reabsorption develop in the normal animals. Furthermore, when brush-border membranes are prepared from the kidneys of these "normal" animals who have undergone parabiosis, a defect in Na^+-dependent phosphate transport, but not in Na^+-dependent glucose transport, is seen in these vesicles.[222] No such changes in renal phosphate handling are seen in normal-normal animals who have undergone parabiosis.[222]

The changes in renal phosphate handling in normal mice after parabiosis to *Hyp* mice are not dependent on PTH because similar results were obtained in parathyroidectomized normal-*Hyp* pairs.[222] Also, the changes in tubular phosphate handling are reversed on the reestablishment of separate circulations in normal mice of normal-*Hyp* pairs.[223] The response to hypophosphatemia also differs in normal mice of normal-normal pairs and normal-*Hyp* pairs. Phosphate restriction leads to enhanced Na^+-phosphate cotransport in renal brush-border membrane vesicles of the normal-normal mouse pairs.[224] In contrast, no increase in Na^+-phosphate cotransport is evident in vesicles obtained from normal mice rendered hypophosphatemic by parabiosis to *Hyp* mice.[222]

The simplest interpretation of these results is that a transacting humoral factor derived from the *Hyp* mouse is perfusing the kidney of the normal animal in the normal-*Hyp* pairs. This factor induces changes in renal phosphate handling both in vivo and in brush-border vesicle studies in vitro. These changes are the same as those seen in *Hyp* mice.

Renal Transplantation

Strong supporting evidence for a transacting humoral factor has come from the studies of Nesbitt and colleagues.[225] They have carried out cross-transplantation experiments between normal and *Hyp* mice. When a kidney from a *Hyp* mouse donor is transplanted into a normal mouse recipient, this kidney functions normally in terms of phosphate handling, and hypophosphatemia does not develop in the recipient mouse.[225] In contrast, when a normal mouse is the donor animal, and the *Hyp* mouse the recipient, the previously normal kidney does not transport phosphate normally, and the animal displays persistent hypophosphatemia.[225]

The data obtained from these renal transplant studies in mice are of particular interest in view of the report that transplantation of a kidney from a normal donor (an unaffected sister) into a 47-year-old man with XLH did not correct the abnormalities in phosphate homeostasis.[226] Hypophosphatemia and disordered renal phosphate handling persisted in the normal kidney after transplantation in the XLH recipient.

Absence of Gene Dose Effect

A humoral basis for X-linked hypophosphatemia is also compatible with the failure to demonstrate expected gene dose effects in *Hyp* mice and in patients with XLH. Serum phosphate values and renal brush-border membrane Na^+-dependent phosphate transport are similar and half of normal in heterozygous (*Hyp*/+) and homozygous (*Hyp*/*Hyp*) mutant female mice.[227,227a] Moreover, serum phosphate values and brush-border membrane phosphate transport are similar in mutant hemizygous males and mutant heterozygous females.[227,227a] Male and female patients with XLH also have similar age-specific serum phosphate values.[115] If the gene dose effect were conventional, heterozygotes should have values intermediate to age-specific values for affected males and unaffected individuals.

X-Linked Hypophosphatemia and Oncogenic Hypophosphatemic Osteomalacia

As discussed below, there is an acquired condition (OHO) in which a humoral factor (derived from a variety of tumors) can induce in previously normal patients (in terms of phosphate metabolism and bone morphology) persistent hypophosphatemia, a decrease in TmP, and osteomalacia without secondary hyperparathyroidism. Furthermore, all these changes are reversible on removal of the tumor. Hence, in most respects the characteristics of the acquired disease (OHO) are the same as those of the inherited one (XLH). Furthermore, if overproduction of a humoral factor does account for the disease in both cases, other manifestations of the disease (e.g. in bones and teeth) may result not only from the persistent hypophosphatemia but also from the action of this humoral factor on cells in other tissues.

Consideration of Pathogenesis in Light of Current Data

The combined data from human and mouse renal transplantation studies, the similarities between OHO and XLH, and the lack of a gene dose effect in mice and humans, provide strong evidence for the hypothesis that XLH and *Hyp* may arise from either the overproduction of a normal phosphaturic hormone or the production of an abnormal phosphaturic hormone. Such a hypothesis raises the interesting possibility that there is a phosphaturic hormone, other than PTH, that plays a role in normal phosphate homeostasis. The hypothesis also predicts that the gene locus on the X chromosome that is associated with XLH and *Hyp* will not be the gene encoding the renal brush-border membrane Na^+-phosphate cotransporter (see Addendum).

A variety of data clearly show that this postulated humoral factor is not PTH. In particular, hypophosphatemia and decreased renal brush-border membrane phosphate transport persist in normal mice who have undergone parabiosis to *Hyp* mice following parathyroidectomy.[222] Moreover, in spite of a marked reduction in renal phosphate reabsorption in XLH, there is no increase in nephrogenous cAMP—a hallmark of increased PTH activity. Furthermore, the reduction in phosphate transport is not associated with an increase in plasma $1,25(OH)_2D$—another hallmark of PTH action.

Of particular interest are the differences seen in patients with HHRH and those with XLH. Patients with HHRH have increased plasma $1,25(OH)_2D$ concentrations, hyperabsorption of calcium, and hypercalciuria. All these changes are what one would predict from a persistent fall in plasma phosphate concentration. Hence, the simplest model to account for the findings in HHRH is either an abnormality in the renal Na^+-dependent phosphate transporter or a decrease in the amount of this transporter. On the other hand, the pathogenesis of XLH must result from a different mechanism, because, in addition to a phosphate transport defect, there is a disorder of $1,25(OH)_2D$ metabolism in the proximal tubule.

Since, in XLH there is both an alteration in renal phosphate transport and in $1,25(OH)_2D$ metabolism, it has been difficult to relate two defects in any simple way to a single genetic defect, particularly as it was thought to be at the level of phosphate transport. But this may not be the case when one considers the evidence suggesting that the alterations in tubular function arise from the action of a humoral agent. Furthermore, two features of tubular phosphate transport and PTH action provide new insights of particular value in considering XLH.

The first feature is the evidence suggesting that PTH inhibition of phosphate transport occurs by endocytosis, that is, that phosphate transporters originally in the brush-border membrane are translocated to a vesicular compartment in the cytosol.[56,57] On removal of PTH, transporter-containing vesicles would become reincorporated in the brush-border membrane. It has been suggested, however, that the vesicular transporters undergo degradation, since restoration of brush-border membrane phosphate transport following PTH inhibition requires protein synthesis—that is, the synthesis of new transporters.[58]

The second feature is that there are specific receptors for PTH on both the basolateral and brush-border membranes of OK cells and that activation of the brush-border receptors by low doses of PTH inhibits phosphate entry across this membrane and thereby inhibits transcellular phosphate transport.[61] There is no evidence to suggest that PTH binding to the brush-border membrane receptor stimulates adenylate cyclase. Rather, it would appear that PTH acts to enhance either calcium entry and/or protein kinase C activation. It is noteworthy that a considerable percentage of renal protein kinase C is constitutively associated with the brush-border membrane,[66,67] that renal protein kinase C activity is increased in the *Hyp* mouse,[183,228] and that treatment of normal mouse proximal tubules with phorbol ester activators of protein kinase C causes an inhibition of both renal Na^+-phosphate cotransport[52] and $1,25(OH)_2D$ synthesis[229] as well as a stimulation of renal 24-hydroxylase activity.[229,230] Given these facts, the action of a humoral factor on a brush-border membrane receptor in the renal tubule that is linked in some way to the activation of protein kinase C in the same membrane could induce the changes in phosphate transport and vitamin D metabolism characteristic of the *Hyp* mouse and XLH human (Fig. 124-11).

An observation not fully accounted for by this hypothesis is that renal epithelial cells from *Hyp* mice continue to display abnormal phosphate transport and vitamin D metabolism after several days in culture in a hormonally defined medium,[231] whereas when a normal circulation is restored

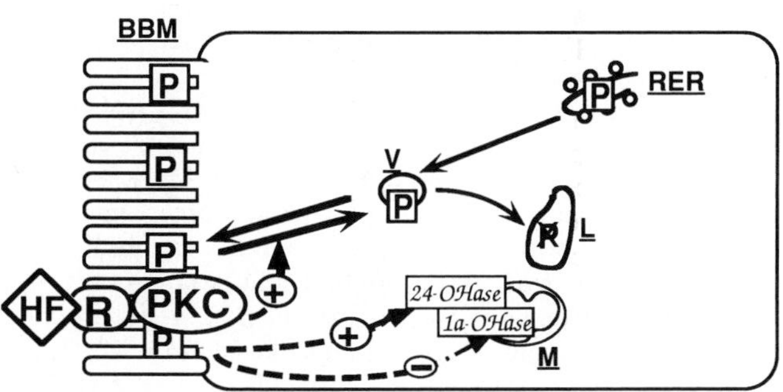

FIG. 124-11 Pathogenesis of the alterations in proximal renal tubular function in XLH and *Hyp*. A proximal tubular cell is represented schematically with the brush-border membrane (BBM) on the apical surface on the left and the Na^+-phosphate cotransporters (P) in either the brush-border membrane or an intracellular vesicular (V) compartment. The phosphate transporters can shuttle between the brush-border membrane and the vesicular compartment, and, at a slower rate, can be incorporated into the lysosomal (L) compartment, where they undergo degradation. The synthesis of new phosphate transporters takes place in the RER, from which they enter the vesicular pool. In addition, the mitochondrion (M) is represented as the site of 1α-hydroxylase (1-OHase) and 24-hydroxylase (24-OHase) activities. It is postulated that a humoral factor (HF) acting on an apical receptor (R) causes the phosphate transporters to translocate from the brush-border membrane to the vesicular compartment, and that when its action is prolonged, lysosomal degradation of phosphate transporters occurs. As a consequence, the content of phosphate transporters in both compartments decreases. The postulate is that activation of the receptor leads, by an undefined mechanism, to the activation of protein kinase C (PKC). Activation of this kinase is linked both to the redistribution of the phosphate transporters, and to the inhibition of 1α-hydroxylase and stimulation of 24-hydroxylase in the mitochondria.

to a normal mouse, after separation from a *Hyp* mouse, the renal phosphate transport defect disappears.[223] However, given the evidence that protein synthesis (i.e., synthesis of new phosphate transporters) is required to reestablish normal phosphate transport in OK cells previously treated with PTH,[58] it is quite possible that under the particular culture conditions, the renal cells from the *Hyp* mouse do not synthesize phosphate transporters normally, and hence the defect persists even though the humoral factor is no longer present.

A second set of observations not easily explained by the model in Fig. 124-11 relate to the effects of phosphate supplementation on vitamin D metabolism in *Hyp* mice. It has been shown that phosphate supplementation increases renal 1α-hydroxylase[152,153] and decreases renal 24-hydroxylase activities[175]—that is, corrects the defects in $1,25(OH)_2D$ metabolism in *Hyp* mice. These data could be accounted for if one assumed that the primary defect in *Hyp* and XLH is a protein kinase C–mediated inhibition of luminal phosphate entry and that the defects in mitochondrial $1,25(OH)_2D$ synthesis and catabolism are the consequence of altered phosphate entry rather than activation of protein kinase C, as depicted in Fig. 124-11.

Treatment

Dietary phosphate supplementation of *Hyp* mice from weaning prevents the appearance of severe skeletal abnormalities.[129] Histomorphometric analysis of bone demonstrates that phosphate normalizes endochondral calcification but does not correct endosteal bone mineralization, as evidenced by a decreased mineralization front and increased mean osteoid seam thickness in treated *Hyp* males as compared with controls.[200] Secondary hyperparathyroidism arising from phosphate therapy appears to stimulate osteoblastic and osteoclastic recruitment and activity and thereby increase endosteal bone turnover.[200] A similar development of secondary hyperparathyroidism occurs in children treated with phosphate alone. However, in contrast to the *Hyp* mouse, phosphate treatment of children with XLH improves endochondral mineralization but does not lead to its normalization.[232] Whether the differences between mice and humans are due to a more uniform and sustained increase in plasma phosphate concentration in mice remains to be determined.[200]

Because phosphate supplementation raises plasma $1,25(OH)_2D$ levels in *Hyp* mice by stimulating renal hormone synthesis[152,153] and inhibiting renal hormone catabolism,[175] it may be that the effects of phosphate supplementation on endochondral calcification are attributable in part to the phosphate-induced rise in the plasma $1,25(OH)_2D$ concentration. However, both in the *Hyp* mouse and the XLH patient, correction of the mineralization defect in endosteal bone requires the administration of $1,25(OH)_2D$ along with phosphate. Using this regimen, secondary hyperparathyroidism does not develop and, as a consequence, bone turnover rate does not increase as it does in animals or humans treated with phosphate alone. Neither 25(OH)D nor $24,25(OH)_2D$ can substitute for $1,25(OH)_2D$ in normalizing endosteal bone mineralization in the *Hyp* mouse.[233]

Improvement in phosphate homeostasis can be achieved by the continuous subcutaneous administration of $1,25(OH)_2D$ to *Hyp* mice. This improvement can be attributed to increased intestinal absorption of phosphate.[234] Everted gut sacs prepared from all segments of the small intestine of $1,25(OH)_2D$-treated *Hyp* mice exhibited significantly higher phosphate transport activity than sacs from untreated mutants. In contrast, 1,25$(OH)_2$D treatment had no effect on the renal brush-border membrane phosphate transport defect.[234] However, there are data from studies in XLH patients suggesting that 1,25$(OH)_2$D may increase renal phosphate retention.[235,236] Thus, it is possible that there is not always a one-to-one correspondence between phosphate handling by the intact kidney and phosphate uptake in isolated renal brush-border membrane vesicles. Furthermore, there is an important difference between phosphate homeostasis in mouse and humans: The plasma phosphate concentration is normally maintained at a higher value in mice than in humans. The basis for this difference is not known. Nor is it clear how this difference might affect the expression of a similar genetic defect in the two species.

Hyp mice exhibit a slight elevation in serum magnesium and a lower than normal bone magnesium content.[130] The effect of magnesium supplementation was therefore assessed to establish whether reduced skeletal magnesium is involved in the pathogenesis of the bone disease in the mutant mice. Magnesium therapy restores osteoclastic bone resorption and improves bone mineralization in *Hyp* mice.[237] In the same study, lactose supplementation was found to induce a partial inhibition of bone resorption and to improve renal phosphate conservation, probably through a calcium-induced suppression of PTH secretion. These studies suggest that secondary hyperparathyroidism contributes to the renal phosphate leak in *Hyp* mice.

Treatment of *Hyp* mice with thyroid hormone (T_3 or T_4) leads to a rise in serum phosphate, a decrease in urinary phosphate excretion and a stimulation of renal brush-border membrane Na^+-dependent phosphate transport.[139] The effect of thyroid hormone appears to be specific, since the transport of proline in the same brush-border membrane preparation remains unchanged. Although the cellular mechanism for the effect of thyroid hormone on renal phosphate transport is not understood, the response appears to be independent of PTH and calcitonin. Because there is no evidence to suggest that *Hyp* mice are hypothyroid,[139,220] this treatment should be recognized as a pharmacologic maneuver that is not feasible in patients with the homologous disorder.

The *Gy* Mouse

Another X-linked mutation (gene symbol, *Gy*) in the mouse also perturbs phosphate homeostasis.[138] The *Gy* gene maps to an independent locus close to *Hyp* (see Fig. 124-7) and confers a phenotype (designated *Gyro*) characterized by hypophosphatemia, dwarfism, rickets, extreme circling behavior, hyperactivity, abnormalities of the inner ear, and deafness. *Gy* females have craniofacial abnormalities that are similar to those of *Hyp* females.[132]

Gy males exhibit a specific impairment in renal brush-border membrane Na^+-dependent phosphate transport and, like *Hyp* males, have 50 percent of the activity of normal littermates.[138] Kinetic studies in *Gy* females demonstrated that the apparent V_{max} of the high-affinity Na^+-phosphate cotransport system is significantly decreased in *Gy* mice, whereas the affinity of the cotransporter for phosphate is unchanged in the mutant strain.[238] *Gy* mice adapt to phosphate deprivation with a threefold increase in renal brush-border membrane Na^+-dependent phosphate transport.[238] Neither dietary phosphate nor the *Gy* mutation alter Na^+-dependent glucose transport in renal brush-border membranes.[238]

Studies of vitamin D metabolism in *Gy* mice have led to conficting data. Davidai et al.[239] demonstrated that serum levels of 1,25$(OH)_2$D and renal production of 1,25$(OH)_2D_3$ are significantly elevated in *Gy* mice as compared with normal littermates, suggesting that *Gy* mice respond appropriately to endogenous hypophosphatemia. Moreover, both *Gy* and normal mice exhibited a comparable increase in renal 1,25$(OH)_2D_3$ synthesis in response to either PTH or calcitonin infusion, again suggesting that regulation of renal 1,25$(OH)_2$D synthesis is intact in the mutant strain.[239] The same group demonstrated that although down-regulation of renal 1α-hydroxylase activity by a high-calcium diet, 1,25$(OH)_2D_3$ infusion, or a high-phosphate diet appears to be incomplete in *Gy* mice relative to normal littermates, renal 1,25$(OH)_2$D synthesis under these conditions is appropriately correlated to serum phosphate concentration in the mutant strain.[153]

However, a more recent study demonstrates that the plasma concentration of 1,25$(OH)_2$D is not elevated in *Gy* mice relative to normal littermates, despite significant hypophosphatemia, and that the circulating level of 1,25$(OH)_2$D in *Gy* mice is significantly lower than that of normal mice with comparable hypophosphatemia.[238] Moreover, *Gy* mice do not exhibit an adaptive increase in plasma 1,25$(OH)_2$D in response to phosphate deprivation.[238] Rather, the plasma concentration of 1,25$(OH)_2$D falls to undetectable levels when *Gy* mice are fed low-phosphate diets—a response similar to that previously reported in X-linked *Hyp* mice.[150,175] The demonstration that the renal 1,25$(OH)_2$D degradative pathway is elevated in *Gy* mice and further increased on phosphate deprivation[238] suggests that depressed plasma 1,25$(OH)_2$D levels in the mutant strain can be attributed to increased hormone catabolism.[238] These results are consistent with the original findings of Lyon et al.,[138] who demonstrated that urine calcium-to-creatinine ratios are not elevated in *Gy* mice, suggesting that the vitamin D endocrine system in the mutant strain is not responding appropriately to hypophosphatemia. The basis for the difference between these findings[138,238] and those described above[153,239] is not clear.

The *Gy* mutation reveals that there are two closely linked loci on the X chromosome (*Gy* and *Hyp*) that play a role in the maintenance of phosphate homeostasis. Moreover, it is of interest that perturbation of phosphate homeostasis itself is not the cause of the inner-ear lesion in the *Gy* mouse. The nature of the *Gy* translation product that is common to the inner ear and the kidney is unknown. The gene products encoded by these gene loci remain to be identified.

A gyro counterpart in patients with XLH has been reported.[240] This entity, distinguished by audiometric findings, is designated HYPII (formerly HPDRII, McKusick No. 307810)[241] (see Fig. 124-7).

Treatment of XLH

Children. At present there is no completely satisfactory treatment for XLH.[242–247] Improvement in growth rate and the associated skeletal abnormalities can be achieved with combination therapy with 1,25$(OH)_2$D or 1α(OH)D (0.5 to 2.0 μg/day) and inorganic phosphate (1–2 g/day in four to five divided doses). However, long-term compliance with this regimen is difficult. Even with good compliance and conscientious parents, it is rare that complete healing of the rickets occurs. Two persistent radiologic signs are commonly observed: a widening or flaring of the distal end of the femora and of the proximal end of the tibia and a weblike abnormality of the medial segments of the growth plate, particularly of the distal femoral epiphyses. Both are indicators of a lack of complete normalization of the events at the growth plate.

One study evaluated the factors associated with a favorable growth response during 3 years of therapy with $1,25(OH)_2D$ and phosphate in 20 prepubertal and nonsurgically treated children with XLH.[248] The patients fell into two groups with respect to their linear growth response to therapy. Both groups were similar in mean age, dietary calcium, dose of $1,25(OH)_2D$ and phosphate, and compliance with therapy. However, the group that grew well had a high serum phosphate and a higher TmP/GFR before the initiation of treatment and contained a disproportionate number of girls (10 of 12) as compared with the group that grew poorly (3 of 8). The finding that heterozygous females appear to respond better than hemizygous males to $1,25(OH)_2D$ and phosphate therapy is consistent with a gene dose effect in the expression of this X-linked dominant disorder.

In employing combined therapy, careful follow-up is required because the two agents balance each other's effects. Administration of phosphate alone leads invariably to secondary hyperparathyroidism, and administration of $1,25(OH)_2D$ alone commonly leads to hypercalciuria and hypercalcemia. Hence, a patient on combined therapy can contract hypercalciuria either as a consequence of too much $1,25(OH)_2D$ or too little phosphate. Because of this balance, anytime it becomes necessary to interrupt phosphate administration, it is necessary to discontinue $1,25(OH)_2D$ therapy as well. The objectives of therapy are to enhance growth rate, correct bone pathology, suppress parathyroid function, and avoid hypercalciuria and hypercalcemia. These are difficult objectives to achieve because the needs for both $1,25(OH)_2D$ and phosphate are high in infancy (or in older children when therapy is first started), are less during the childhood years, and increase again during the adolescent growth spurt.

Of equal concern is the fact that there can be several serious complications of therapy. The most common is the development of nephrocalcinosis.[96,242,245–247,249] Its occurrence appears to be related to phosphate dosage. With the widespread use of renal ultrasonography, this abnormality has been noted with increasing frequency—it is seen in over 60 percent of patients. In most cases, the nephrocalcinosis is observed without evident changes in GFR. In a few patients, progressive nephrocalcinosis with renal failure has been reported. Kidney biopsy specimens from three treated patients with nephrocalcinosis showed that renal calcifications are located mainly intratubularly and are composed exclusively of calcium phosphate.[250] What has yet to be determined are the long-term consequences of this nephrocalcinosis, because combined therapy with $1,25(OH)_2D$ and phosphate has been employed for only the past 15 years or so.

A second, much rarer complication is the development of tertiary hyperparathyroidism.[13,14,251] In patients with this state, a progressive decrease in GFR is seen, and combined therapy must be discontinued, leading to the redevelopment or worsening of the bone disease. A small number of such patients have undergone total parathyroidectomy with autotransplantation to the forearm. In a number of these cases, the transplanted tissue has shown a propensity to proliferate and lead to the redevelopment of tertiary hyperparathyroidism. Removal of this hyperplastic tissue from the forearm site leads to a reduction in PTH levels. A therapeutic option that may be a better alternative is total parathyroidectomy followed by treatment with $1,25(OH)_2D$ and phosphate and, if necessary, very small doses of human PTH. At present, however, there is insufficient experience with this approach to recommend its use.

Because of the failure to obtain complete healing of rickets, the difficulty with combined therapy, and the complications attributable, in part at least, to therapy, additional therapeutic options are being explored. These include the use of human growth hormone[252] and thiazide diuretic therapy.[95] Neither is an alternative to combined therapy, but each has been employed as adjuvant therapy.

The rationale for using growth hormone is based on the well-known ability of this agent to increase renal phosphate retention. In nine children given biosynthetic human growth hormone for 6 months (0.05 mg/kd/day), there was an increase in serum insulin-like growth factor I, phosphate, osteocalcin, and alkaline phosphatase, and these changes were associated with an increase in growth velocity.[252] Few side effects were noted, and no assessment of radiologic changes was reported. Nonetheless, a longer-term assessment of this therapy appears to be warranted.

The rationale for the use of thiazide diuretics and amiloride as adjuvant therapy is that by reducing extracellular fluid volume, tubular reabsorption of phosphate is increased, and that by giving the thiazide one enhances tubular calcium reabsorption.[95] Again, preliminary data indicate that growth rate increases and the radiologic appearance of the epiphyses improves. However, long-term consequences of this very complicated therapeutic program are not yet known.

Adults. There is less experience with long-term therapy in adults with XLH. However, it is now clear that nearly all untreated adults have osteomalacia on bone biopsy, even though in many such patients, the plasma alkaline phosphatase activity is normal. Also, many patients have bone pain. The results of treatment of 16 adults with XLH has been reported.[253] Administration of $1,25(OH)_2D$ and phosphate led to a reduction in bone pain and a healing of osteomalacia, as evidenced by a reduction in both osteoid volume and osteoid thickness on histomorphometric examination of iliac bone biopsies.[253] However, even with a mean duration of therapy of 4.2 years, these values did not return completely to normal. Of particular note, this therapy was effective without significant complications. There was no evidence of renal impairment, and tertiary hyperparathyroidism developed in only one case. Based on this experience, treatment of adults with XLH using combined therapy seems warranted.[253]

A continued search for better therapeutic agents is needed because it is increasingly clear that the present-day combined therapy is not curative and is accompanied by a high complication rate, a rate such that some experts argue that until a better treatment is established, it may be better not to treat these patients.[247] Based on a variety of data,[106,111,112,232,236,254] this view is not shared by us because if therapy with combined phosphate and $1,25(OH)_2D$ is carefully monitored, growth rates increase, rickets is corrected, and bowing of the low extremities is significantly reduced.

ONCOGENIC HYPOPHOSPHATEMIC OSTEOMALACIA

OHO is a rare, acquired form of hypophosphatemia that is of importance both because it may be confused with XLH and because the changes in proximal tubular function seen in XLH and OHO are so similar.[14,255–260]

Clinical Features

The disease is characterized by an insidious onset of fatigability, bone pain, and skeletal deformities, and in children, growth retardation. Proximal muscle weakness causing a waddling gait is also a prominent feature in contrast to the lack of this sign in XLH. Age of onset is usually in adult life but has been reported in patients ranging in age from 5 to 70 years.

The patients have the same key triad of abnormal laboratory findings as seen in XLH: a reduced TmP/GFR, hypophosphatemia, and a low plasma $1,25(OH)_2D$. The reduction in serum phosphate and $1,25(OH)_2D$ concentrations are usually more severe than those seen in the typical XLH patient. The presence of muscle weakness in OHO has been ascribed to the more profound hypophosphatemia. The serum calcium and 25(OH)D concentrations are normal or low normal with a mildly elevated PTH, but high PTH with aminoaciduria and glycosuria have been reported. On bone biopsy, osteomalacia is present. Radiologic examination reveals decreased mineral density, occasional rib fractures or pseudofractures at other sites, and, in children, rickets.

The differentiation between XLH and OHO is relatively easy since, in most cases, OHO first appears later in life and leads to progressive disease. Usually, the opposite is the case in XLH. It is rare for a patient with XLH who has minimal disease during childhood and adolescence to then display signs of severe disease in adult life. Even when OHO appears in children, its differentiation from sporadic XLH is usually possible based on the facts that XLH is considerably more likely than OHO, the signs of XLH appear usually within the first 2 to 3 years of life, and the plasma $1,25(OH)_2D$ is higher in XLH than in OHO.

Pathogenesis

The most intriguing feature of OHO is its association with small mesenchymal tumors. These have been described as hemangiopericytoma, odontogenic tumor of the maxilla, fibroma, angiosarcoma, oat-cell carcinoma, myoma, angiofibroma, sclerosing hemangioma, ossifying mesenchymal tumor, or osteoblastoma. In spite of this variety of designations, the majority have been reported to have prominent vascularity and often osteoclastlike multinucleated giant cells. Additionally, patients with the linear sebaceous nevus syndrome have been found to have as a component of their disease a variant of this syndrome. The tumors have been found in the skin, subcutaneous tissue, the nasopharynx, the bone, the paranasal sinuses, the palm of the hand, and the sole of the foot.

The tumor is usually small and may be extremely difficult to locate. Nevertheless, if found and successfully removed, the manifestations of the disease disappear completely. There is a restoration of normal renal function, the TmP/GFR becomes normal, plasma $1,25(OH)_2D$ rises to supranormal values within a few days of the surgical removal of the tumor and then falls slowly to normal values, and with time the osteomalacia heals completely. The working hypothesis is that the tumor produces a humoral factor(s) that acts specifically on the proximal renal tubule to bring about the same, or nearly the same, abnormalities in tubular phosphate transport and $1,25(OH)_2D$ synthesis as seen in XLH. The hypothesis is supported by the observation that transplantation of such a human tumor into a nude mouse leads to the development of hypophosphatemia in the mouse.[261] The humoral factor may also act directly on bone.

Treatment

The obvious therapy for patients with OHO is the surgical removal of the tumor that is the source of the presumed humoral factor. The difficulty is often that of finding the tumor. If no tumor can be found, then the alternative is treatment with combined phosphate and $1,25(OH)_2D$. These agents may ameliorate some of the signs and symptoms of the disease and may cause a partial healing of the osteomalacia, but they do not normally lead to a complete cure, and often are quite ineffective.

HYPOPHOSPHATEMIC BONE DISEASE

Hypophosphatemic bone disease (HBD) is another hypophosphatemic phenotype with modest shortening of stature, bowing of lower limbs, and osteomalacic bone disease.[262] Several features distinguish this disorder from XLH: rickets is rarely present in patients with HBD; fractional tubular reabsorption of phosphate is normal at endogenous levels of filtered phosphate (a decrease in TmP/GFR is apparent only after infusion of phosphate); the phosphaturic response to PTH is not blunted; the mode of inheritance does not appear to be X-linked; and patients with HBD respond to therapy with $1,25(OH)_2D$ alone.[263] The demonstration of normal plasma levels of $1,25(OH)_2D$[264] and normal urinary calcium excretion (Scriver CR: personal communication) in patients with HBD suggests that this hypophosphatemic phenotype may also be distinct from HHRH.[81,82] However, the precise relationship between the mutant genes associated with HBD and HHRH will require further study.

ADDENDUM

Homologous cDNAs encoding high affinity, renal-specific Na^+-phosphate cotransporters have recently been cloned from rat (NaPi-2) and human (NaPi-3) kidney cortex by expression cloning in *Xenopus laevis* ooctyes.[275] Using immunohistochemical techniques and the reverse transcriptase/polymerase chain reaction, it was established that NaPi-2 is expressed exclusively in the brush-border membrane of the proximal tubule of rat kidney.[276]

The NaPi-2 cDNA probe and an antibody raised against a C-terminal NaPi-2 peptide were used to examine the mechanism for the reduction in V_{max} of the high affinity Na^+-phosphate cotransport system in the renal brush-border membrane of X-linked *Hyp* mice.[277] The abundance of both Na^+-phosphate cotransporter mRNA and protein was significantly reduced in kidneys of *Hyp* mice when compared to that of normal littermates.[277] Moreover, Na^+-phosphate cotransport, but not Na^+-sulphate cotransport, was significantly decreased in Xenopus oocytes injected with renal mRNA isolated from *Hyp* mice when compared to an equivalent amount of renal mRNA from normal mice.[277] Hybrid depletion experiments documented that renal mRNA-dependent expression of Na^+-dependent phosphate transport in Xenopus oocytes was indeed related to NaPi-2.[277] These findings demonstrate that the number of high-affinity Na^+-phosphate cotransport sites is significantly reduced in the renal brush-border membrane of *Hyp* mice by a mechanism that may involve either decreased Na^+-phosphate cotransporter gene transcription or increased mRNA turnover.

To understand the relationship between the decrease in renal Na^+-phosphate cotransporter gene expression and the

X-linked mutation in mice (*Hyp*) and humans (HYP), recent studies were undertaken to determine the chromosomal localization of the renal-specific Na^+-phosphate cotransporter gene.[278] Using high resolution fluorescence *in situ* hybridization of a biotinylated, full length NaPi-3 cDNA probe to metaphase and prometaphase chromosomes derived from peripheral blood lymphocytes, the Na^+-phosphate cotransporter gene was mapped to human chromosome 5q35.[278] This map assignment excludes the renal-specific Na^+-phosphate cotransporter gene as a candidate gene for X-linked hypophosphatemia and suggests that the gene at the HYP (*Hyp*) locus may be involved in the regulation of renal Na^+-phosphate cotransporter gene expression. These genetic findings lend further support to the hypothesis that the renal phenotype in both mouse and man is due to the generation of a humoral factor that alters renal phosphate transport and vitamin D metabolism. These findings also suggest that mutations in the renal-specific Na^+-phosphate cotransporter gene may be responsible for Mendelian hypophosphatemias that are autosomally inherited (Table 124-1).

REFERENCES

1. Dennis VW, Brazy PC: Divalent anion transport in isolated renal tubules. *Kidney Int* **22**:498, 1982.
2. Murer H, Burckhardt G: Membrane transport of anions across epithelia of mammalian small intestine and kidney proximal tubule. *Rev Physiol Biochem Pharmacol* **96**:1, 1983.
3. Bonjour J-P, Caverzasio J: Phosphate transport in the kidney. *Rev Physiol Biochem Pharmacol* **100**:161, 1984.
4. Mizgala CL, Quamme GA: Renal handling of phosphate. *Physiol Rev* **65**:431, 1985.
5. Gmaj P, Murer H: Cellular mechanisms of inorganic phosphate transport in kidney. *Physiol Rev* **66**:36, 1986.
6. Hammerman MR: Phosphate transport across renal proximal tubular cell membranes. *Am J Physiol* **251**:F385, 1986.
7. Biber J: Cellular aspects of proximal tubular phosphate reabsorption. *Kidney Int* **36**:360, 1989.
8. Murer H, Werner A, Reshkin S, Wuarin F, Biber J: Cellular mechanisms in proximal tubular reabsorption of inorganic phosphate. *Am J Physiol* **260**:C885, 1991.
9. Berndt TJ, Knox FG: Renal regulation of phosphate excretion, in Seldin DW, Giebisch G (eds): *The Kidney, Physiology and Pathophysiology*. New York, Raven, 1992, p 2511.
10. Haussler M, Hughes M, Baylink D, Littlekide ET, Cork D, Pitt M: Influence of phosphate depletion on the biosynthesis and circulating level of 1-α-25-dihydroxyvitamin D. *Adv Exp Med Biol* **31**:233, 1977.
11. Tanaka Y, Deluca HF: The control of 25-hydroxyvitamin D metabolism by inorganic phosphorus. *Arch Biochem Biophys* **154**:566, 1973.
12. Mason RS, Rohl PG, Lissner D, Posen S: Vitamin D metabolism in hypophosphatemic rickets. *Am J Dis Child* **136**:909, 1982.
13. Rasmussen H, Anast C: Familial hypophosphatemic rickets and vitamin D-dependent rickets, in Stanbury JB, Wyngaarden JB, Fredrickson DS, Goldstein JL, Brown MS (eds): *The Metabolic Basis of Inherited Disease*, 5th ed. New York, McGraw-Hill, 1983, p 1743.
14. Rasmussen H, Tenenhouse HS: Hypophosphatemias, in Scriver CR, Beaudet AL, Sly WS, Valle D (eds): *The Metabolic Basis of Inherited Disease*, 6th ed. New York, McGraw-Hill, 1989, vol 2, p 2581.
15. Walling MW: Intestinal Ca and phosphate transport: Differential responses to vitamin D_3 metabolites. *Am J Physiol* **233**:E488, 1977.
16. Lee DBN, Walling MW, Brautbar N: Intestinal phosphate absorption: Influence of vitamin D and non-vitamin D factors. *Am J Physiol* **250**:G369, 1986.
17. Rizzoli R, Fleisch H, Bonjour J-P: Role of 1,25-dihydroxyvitamin D_3 on intestinal phosphate absorption in rats with a normal vitamin D supply. *J Clin Invest* **60**:639, 1977.
18. Matsumoto T, Fontaine O. Rasmussen H: Effects of 1,25-dihydroxyvitamin D_3 on phosphate uptake into chick intestinal brush border membrane vesicles. *J Biol Chem* **256**:3354, 1981.
19. Brazy P, McKeown JW, Harris RH, Dennis VW: Comparative effects of dietary phosphate, unilateral nephrectomy, and parathyroid hormone on phosphate transport by the rabbit proximal tubule. *Kidney Int* **17**:788, 1980.
20. Frick A: Reabsorption of inorganic phosphate in the rat kidney. I. Saturation of transport mechanism. II. Suppression of fractional phosphate reabsorption due to expansion of extracellular fluid volume. *Pflugers Arch* **304**:351, 1968.
21. Steele TH, Deluca HF: Influence of dietary phosphorus on renal phosphate reabsorption in the parathyroidectomized rat. *J Clin Invest* **57**:867, 1976.
22. Sestoft L: Is the relationship between the plasma concentration of inorganic phosphate and the rate of oxygen consumption of significance in regulating energy metabolism in mammals? *Scand J Clin Invest* **39**:191, 1979.
23. Markowitz M, Rotkin L, Rosen JF: Circadian rhythms of blood minerals in humans. *Science* **213**:672, 1981.
24. Baylink D, Wergedal J, Staeffer M: Formation, mineralization and resorption of bone in hypophosphatemic rats. *J Clin Invest* **50**:2519, 1971.
25. Harris CA, Sutton RA, Dirks JH: Effects of hypercalcemia and tubular calcium and phosphate ultrafilterability on tubular reabsorption in the rat. *Am J Physiol* **233**:F201, 1977.
26. Legrimellec C: Micropuncture study along the proximal convoluted tubule. Electrolyte reabsorption in the first convolutions. *Pflugers Arch* **354**:133, 1975.
27. Bijvoet O: The importance of the kidney in phosphate homeostasis, in Avioli L, Bordier P, Fleisch H, Massry S, Slatopolsky E (eds): *Phosphate Metabolism, Kidney and Bone*. Paris, Armour-Montagu, 1976, p 421.
28. Walton RJ, Bijvoet OLM: Nomogram for the derivation of renal threshold phosphate concentration. *Lancet* **2**:309, 1975.
29. Strickler JC, Thompson DD, Klose RM, Giebisch G: Micropuncture study of inorganic phosphate excretion in the rat. *J Clin Invest* **43**:1596, 1964.
30. Kuntziger H, Amiel C, Gaudebout C: Phosphate handling by the rat nephron during saline diuresis. *Kidney Int* **2**:318, 1972.
31. Legrimellec C, Roinel N, Morel F: Simultaneous Mg, Ca, P, K, Na and Cl analysis in the rat tubular fluid. I. During perfusion of either inulin or ferrocyanide. *Pflugers Arch* **304**:181, 1973.
32. Wen S-F: Micropuncture studies of phosphate transport in the proximal tubule of the dog. The relationship to sodium reabsorption. *J Clin Invest* **53**:143, 1974.
33. Greger RF, Lang FC, Marchand G, Knox FG: Site of renal phosphate reabsorption: Micropuncture and microinfusion study. *Pflugers Arch* **369**:111, 1977.
34. Morel F: Sites of hormone action in the mammalian nephron. *Am J Physiol* **240**:F159, 1981.
35. Knox FG, Haramati A: Renal regulation of phosphate excretion, in Seldin DW, Giebisch G (eds): *The Kidney: Physiology and Pathophysiology*. New York, Raven, 1985, p 1381.
36. Kawashima H, Kurokawa K: Metabolism and sites of action of vitamin D in the kidney. *Kidney Int* **29**:98, 1986.
37. McKinney TD, Myers P: Bicarbonate transport by proximal tubules; effect of parathyroid hormone and dibutyryl cyclic AMP. *Am J Physiol* **238**:F166, 1980.
38. Hammerman MR, Klarh S, Cohn DE: Renal failure, metabolic acidosis, and parathyroidectomy in the dog increase Na^+H^+ exchange in isolated renal brush border membrane vesicles, in Forte J, Rector F (eds): *Hydrogen Ion Transport in Epithelia*. New York, John Wiley, 1983, p 139.
39. Suki WN: Calcium transport in the nephron. *Am J Physiol* **237**:F1, 1979.
40. Imai M: Effect of parathyroid hormone and N^6, O^2-dibutyryl cyclic AMP on Ca transport across the rabbit distal nephron segments perfused *in vitro*. *Pflugers Arch* **390**:145, 1981.
41. Berndt TJ, Knox FG: Proximal tubule site of inhibition of phosphate reabsorption by calcitonin. *Am J Physiol* **246**:F927, 1984.
42. Walker JJ, Yan TS, Quamme GA: Presence of multiple sodium-dependent phosphate transport processes in proximal brush-border membranes. *Am J Physiol* **252**:F226, 1987.

43. Tenenhouse HS, Klugerman AH, Neal JL: Effect of phosphonoformic acid, dietary phosphate and the *Hyp* mutation on kinetically distinct phosphate transport processes in mouse kidney. *Biochim Biophys Acta* **984:**207, 1989.
44. Dennis VW, Bello-Reuss E, Robinson RR: Response of phosphate transport to parathyroid hormone in segments of rabbit nephron. *Am J Physiol* **233:**F29, 1977.
45. Schwab SJ, Klahr S, Hammerman MR: Na^+ gradient-dependent Pi uptake in basolateral membrane vesicles from dog kidney. *Am J Physiol* **246:**F633, 1984.
46. Freeman D, Bartlett S, Radda G, Ross B: Energetics of sodium transport in the kidney. Saturation transfer ^{31}P-NMR. *Biochim Biophys Acta* **762:**325, 1983.
47. Cole JA, Eber AL, Poelling RE, Thorne PK, Forte LR: A dual mechanism for regulation of kidney phosphate transport by parathyroid hormone. *Am J Physiol* **253:**E221, 1987.
48. Quamme G, Pfeilschifter J, Murer H: Parathyroid hormone inhibition of Na^+-phosphate cotransport in OK cells: Generation of second messengers in the regulatory cascade. *Biochem Biophys Res Commun* **158:**951, 1989.
49. Dunlay R, Hruska K: PTH receptor coupling to phospholipase C is an alternate pathway of signal transduction in bone and kidney. *Am J Physiol* **258:**F223, 1990.
50. Quamme G, Pfeilschifter J, Murer H: Parathyroid hormone inhibition of Na^+/phosphate cotransport in OK cells: Requirement of protein kinase C-dependent pathway. *Biochim Biophys Acta* **1013:**159, 1989.
51. Miyauchi A, Dobre V, Rickmeyer J, Cole J, Forte LR, Hruska KA: Stimulation of transient elevations of Ca^{2+} is related to inhibition of Pi transport in OK-cells. *Am J Physiol* **259:**F485, 1990.
52. Boneh A, Mandla S, Tenenhouse HS: Phorbol myristate acetate activates protein kinase C, stimulates the phosphorylation of endogenous proteins and inhibits phosphate transport in mouse renal tubules. *Biochim Biophys Acta* **1012:**308, 1989.
53. Segal JH, Pollack AS: Transfection-mediated expression of a dominant cAMP-resistant phenotype in the opossum (OK) cell line prevents parathyroid hormone-induced inhibition of Na-phosphate cotransport. *J Clin Invest* **86:**1442, 1990.
54. Martin KJ, McConkey CL, Garcia JC, Montani D, Betts CR: Protein kinase A and the effects of parathyroid hormone on phosphate uptake in opossum kidney cells. *Endocrinology* **125:**295, 1989.
55. Reshkin SJ, Murer H: Parathyroid hormone regulation in opossum kidney cells: In situ protein phosphorylation reactions involving protein kinase A, protein kinase C and GTP-binding proteins. *Cell Physiol Biochem* **1:**143, 1991.
56. Kempson SA, Ying AL, McAteer JA, Murer H: Endocytosis and Na^+/solute cotransport in renal epithelial cells. *J Biol Chem* **264:**18451, 1989.
57. Kempson SA, Helmle C, Abraham MI, Murer H: Parathyroid hormone action on phosphate transport is inhibited by high osmolality. *Am J Physiol* **258:**F1336, 1990.
58. Malstrom K, Murer H: Parathyroid hormone regulates phosphate transport in OK cells via an irreversible inactivation of a membrane protein. *FEBS Lett* **216:**257, 1987.
59. Caverzasio J, Rizzoli R, Bonjour J-P: Sodium-dependent phosphate transport inhibited by parathyroid hormone and cyclic AMP stimulation in an Opossum kidney cell line. *J Biol Chem* **261:**3233, 1986.
60. Handler JS, Preston AS, Steel RE: Factors affecting the differentiation of epithelial transport and responsiveness to hormones. *Fed Proc* **43:**2221, 1984.
61. Reshkin SJ, Forgo J, Murer H: Functional asymmetry in phosphate transport and its regulation in opossum kidney cells: Parathyroid hormone inhibition. *Pflugers Arch* **416:**624, 1990.
62. Sartori L, Insogna KL, Barrett PQ: Renal phosphate transport in humoral hypercalcemia of malignancy. *Am J Physiol* **255:**F1078, 1988.
63. Quamme GA: Effect of parathyroid hormone and dietary phosphate on phosphate transport in renal outer cortical and outer medullary brush-border membrane vesicles. *Biochim Biophys Acta* **1024:**122, 1990.
64. Reshkin SJ, Forgo J, Murer H: Functional asymmetry of phosphate transport and its regulation in opossum kidney cells: Phosphate transport. *Pflugers Arch* **416:**554, 1990.
65. Schwertz DW, Kreisberg JI, Venkatachalam MA: Characterization of rat kidney proximal tubule brush border membrane-associated phosphorylinositol phosphodiesterase. *Arch Biochem Biophys* **224:**555, 1983.
66. Barrett PQ, Zawalich K, Rasmussen H: Protein kinase C activity in renal microvillus membranes. *Biochem Biophys Res Comm* **128:**494, 1985.
67. Boneh A, Tenenhouse HS: Protein kinase C in mouse kidney: Subcellular distribution and endogenous substrates. *Biochem Cell Biol* **66:**262, 1988.
68. Douglas JG: Angiotensin receptor subtypes of the kidney cortex. *Am J Physiol* **253:**F1, 1987.
69. Rouleau MF, Warshawsky H, Goltzman D: Parathyroid hormone binding *in vivo* to renal, hepatic, and skeletal tissues of the rat using a radioautographic approach. *Endocrinology* **118:**919, 1986.
70. Shah SV, Kempson SA, Northrup TE, Dousa TP: Renal adaptation to a low phosphate diet in rats. Blockade by actinomycin D. *J Clin Invest* **64:**955, 1979.
71. Levine BS, Knibloe KA, Golchini K, Hashimoto S, Kurtz I: Renal adaptation to dietary phosphate deprivation: Role of proximal tubule brush-border membrane fluidity. *Am J Physiol* **260:**F613, 1991.
72. Barac-Nieto M, Dowd TL, Gupta RK, Spitzer A: Changes in NMR-visible kidney cell phosphate with age and diet: Relationship to phosphate transport. *Am J Physiol* **261:**F153, 1991.
73. Reshkin SJ, Forgo J, Biber J, Murer H: Functional asymmetry of phosphate transport and its regulation in opossum kidney cells: Phosphate "adaptation." *Pflugers Arch* **419:**256, 1991.
74. Szczepanska-Konkel M, Yusufi ANK, Dousa TP: Interactions of [^{14}C]Phosphonoformic acid with renal cortical brush-border membranes. Relationship to the Na^+-phosphate cotransporter. *J Biol Chem* **262:**8000, 1987.
75. Vizel EJ, Tenenhouse HS, Scriver CR: Effect of the X-linked *Hyp* mutation on N-ethylmaleimide labelling of proteins in renal brush border membrane. *J Inherited Metab Dis* **10:**243, 1987.
76. Wuarin F, Wu K, Murer H, Biber J: The Na/Pi cotransporter of OK cells: Reaction and tentative identification with N-acetylimidazole. *Biochim Biophys Acta* **981:**185, 1989.
77. Peerce BE: Identification of the intestinal Na-phosphate cotransporter. *Am J Physiol* **256:**G645, 1989.
78. Werner A, Moore ML, Mantei N, Biber J, Semenza G, Murer H: Cloning and expression of cDNA for a Na/Pi cotransport system of kidney cortex. *Proc Natl Acad Sci USA* **88:**9608, 1991.
79. Hediger MA, Coady MJ, Ikeda TS, Wright EM: Expression cloning and cDNA sequencing of the Na^+/glucose cotransporter. *Nature* **330:**379, 1987.
80. Werner A, Biber J, Forgo J, Palacin M, Murer H: Expression of renal transport systems for inorganic phosphate and sulfate in *Xenopus laevis* oocytes. *J Biol Chem* **265:**12331, 1990.
81. Tieder M, Modai D, Samuel R, Arie R, Halabe A, Bab I, Gabizon D, Lieberman UA: Hereditary hypophosphatemic rickets with hypercalciuria. *N Engl J Med* **312:**611, 1985.
82. Tieder M, Modai D, Shaked U, Samuel R, Arie R, Halabe A, Maor J, Weissgarten J, Averbukh Z, Cohen N, Edelstein S, Lieberman UA: "Idiopathic" hypercalciuria and hereditary hypophosphatemic rickets. *N Engl J Med* **316:**125, 1987.
83. Gazit D, Tieder M, Liberman UA, Passi-Even L, Bab IA: Osteomalacia in hereditary hypophosphatemic rickets with hypercalciuria: A correlative clinical-histomorphometric study. *J Clin Endocrinol Metab* **72:**229, 1991.
84. Broadus AE, Insogna KL, Lang R, Ellison AF, Dreyer BE: Evidence for disordered control of 1,25-dihydroxyvitamin D production in absorptive hypercalciuria. *N Engl J Med* **311:**73, 1984.
85. Tieder M, Stark H, Shainkin-Kastenbaum R: Pathophysiologic studies in idiopathic hypercalciuria presenting in childhood. *Int J Pediatr Nephrol* **4:**197, 1983.
86. Broadus AE, Insogna KL, Lang R, Mallette LE, Oren OA, Gertner JM, Kliger AS, Ellison AF: A consideration

of the hormonal basis and phosphate leak hypothesis of absorptive hypercalciuria. *J Clin Endocrinol Metab* **58**:161, 1984.
87. Nishiyama S, Inoue F, Makuda I: A single case of hypophosphatemic rickets with hypercalciuria. *J Pediatr Gastroenterol Nutr* **5**:826, 1986.
88. Lapatsanes PD, Sbyrakis S, Megreli CHR, Edelstein S: The management of siblings with familial hypophosphatemic rickets. *Helv Paediatr Acta* **38**:373, 1983.
89. Chan JC, Alon U, Hirschman GM: Renal hypophosphatemic rickets. *J Pediatr* **106**:533, 1985.
90. Schimert G, Fanconi A: Early history of familial hypophosphatemic vitamin D-resistant rickets. *Helv Paediat Acta* **38**:383, 1983.
91. Herweijer TJ, Steendijk R: The relation between attained adult height and the metaphyseal lesions in hypophosphatemic vitamin D-resistant rickets. *Acta Paediatr Scand* **74**:196, 1985.
92. Harrison HE: Primary hypophosphatemic rickets and growth retardation. *Growth Genet Horm* **2**:1, 1986.
93. Scriver CR, Tenenhouse HS, Glorieux FH: Commentary. X-linked hypophosphatemia: An appreciation of a classic paper and a survey of progress since 1958. *Medicine (Baltimore)* **70**:218, 1991.
94. Steendijk R, Herweijer TJ: Height, sitting height and leg length in patients with hypophosphatemic rickets. *Acta Paediatr Scand* **73**:181, 1984.
95. Hanna JD, Niimi K, Chan JCM: X-linked hypophosphatemia. Genetic and clinical correlates. *Am J Dis Child* **145**:865, 1991.
96. Reid IR, Hardy DC, Murphy WA, Teitelbaum SL, Bergfeld MA, Whyte MP: X-linked hypophosphatemia: A clinical, biochemical, and histopathologic assessment of morbidity in adults. *Medicine (Baltimore)* **68**:336, 1989.
97. Reid IR, Murphy WA, Hardy DC, Teitelbaum SL, Bergfeld MA, Whyte MP: X-linked hypophosphatemia: Skeletal mass in adults assessed by histomorphometry, computed tomography, and absorptiometry. *Am J Med* **90**:63, 1991.
98. Hardy DC, Murphy WA, Seigel BA, Reid IR, Whyte MP: X-linked hypophosphatemia in adults: Prevalence of skeletal radiographic and scintigraphic features. *Radiology* **171**:403, 1989.
99. Gundberg CM, Clough ME, Carpenter TO: Development and validation of a radioimmunoassay for mouse osteocalcin: Paradoxical response in the *Hyp* mouse. *Endocrinology* **130**:1909, 1992.
100. Larmas M, Hietala EL, Similia S, Pajari U: Oral manifestations of familial hypophosphatemic rickets after phosphate therapy: A review of the literature and report of a case. *J Dent Child* **58**:328, 1991.
101. Abe K, Ooshima T, Tong SML, Yasufuku Y, Sobue S: Structural deformities of deciduous teeth in patients with hypophosphatemic vitamin D-resistant rickets. *Oral Surg* **65**:191, 1988.
102. McWhorter AG, Seale NS: Prevalence of dental abcess in a population of children with vitamin D-resistant rickets. *Pediatr Dent* **13:91, 1991.**
103. Seow WK: The effect of medical therapy on dentin formation in vitamin D resistant rickets. *Pediatr Dent* **13**:97, 1991.
104. Greene WB, Kahler SG: Surgical aspects of limb deformity in hypophosphatemic rickets. *South Med J* **78**:1185, 1985.
105. Rubinovitch M, Said SE, Glorieux FH, Cruess RL, Royala E: Principles and results of connective lower limb osteotomies for patients with vitamin D-resistant hypophosphatemic rickets. *Clin Orthop* **237**:264, 1988.
106. Chesney RW, Mazess RB, Rose P, Hamstra AJ, Deluca HF Breed AL: Long-term influence of calcitriol (1,25-dihydroxyvitamin D) and supplemental phosphate in X-linked hypophosphatemic rickets. *Pediatrics* **71**:559, 1983.
107. Tulloch EN, Andrews FFH: The association of dental abscesses with vitamin D-resistant rickets. *Br Dent J* **154**:136, 1983.
108. Rakocz M, Keating J III, Johnson R: Management of the primary dentition in vitamin D-resistant rickets. *Oral Surg* **54**:166, 1982.
109. Herbert FL: Hereditary hypophosphatemic rickets: An important awareness for dentists. *J Dent Child* **53**:223, 1986.
110. Shields ED, Scriver CR, Reade T, Fujiwara TM, Morgan K, Chiampi A, Schwartz S: X-linked hypophosphatemia: The mutant gene is expressed in teeth as well as in kidney, *Am J Hum Genet* **46**:434, 1990.
111. Drezner MK, Lyles KW, Haussler MR, Harrelson JM: Evaluation of a role for 1,25-dihydroxyvitamin D_3 in the pathogenesis and treatment of X-linked hypophosphatemic rickets and osteomalacia. *J Clin Invest* **66**:1020, 1980.
112. Rasmussen H, Pechet M, Anast C, Mazur H, Gertner J, Broadus AE: Long-term treatment of familial hypophosphatemic rickets with oral phosphate and 1 α-hydroxyvitamin D_3. *J Pediatr* **99**:16, 1981.
113. Marie PJ, Glorieux FH: Histomorphometric study of bone remodelling in hypophosphatemic vitamin D-resistant rickets. *Metab Bone Dis Rel Res* **3**:31, 1981.
114. Choufoer JH, Stindjik R: Distribution of the perilacuna Hypomineralized areas in cortical bone of patients with familial hypophosphatemic (vitamin D-resistant) rickets. *Calcif Tissue Int* **27**:101, 1979.
115. Winters RW, Graham JB, Williams TF, McFalls VW, Burnett CH: A genetic study of familial hypophosphatemia and vitamin D-resistant rickets with a review of the literature. *Medicine (Baltimore)* **37**:97, 1958.
116. Soener RA, Meyer MH, Meyer RA Jr: Ovariectomy abolishes the normalization of femoral mineral content in 40-week-old female X-linked hypophosphatemic mice. *Miner Electrolyte Metab* **14**:321, 1988.
117. Lyon MF: X-chromosome inactivation and the location and expression of X-linked genes. *Am J Hum Genet* **42**:8, 1988.
118. Searle AG, Peters J, Lyon MF, Hall, JG, Evans EP, Edwards JH, Buckle VJ: Chromosome maps of man and mouse. IV. *Ann Hum Genet* **53**:89, 1989.
119. Read AP, Thakker RV, Davies KE, Mountford RC, Brenton DP, Davies M, Glorieux F, Harris R, Hendy GN, King A, McGlade S, Peacock CJ, Smith R, O'Riordan JLH: Mapping of human X-linked hypophosphatemic rickets by multilocus linkage analysis. *Hum Genet* **73**:267, 1986.
120. Mächler M, Frey D, Gal A, Orth U, Wienker TF, Fanconi A, Schmid W: X-linked dominant hypophosphatemia is closely linked to DNA markers DXS41 and DXS43 at Xp22. *Hum Genet* **73**:271, 1986.
121. Thakker RV, Read AP, Davies KE, Whyte MP, Weksberg R, Glorieux F, Davies M, Mountford RC, Harris R, King A, Kim GS, Fraser D, Kooh SW, O'Riordan JLH: Bridging markers defining the map position of X linked hypophosphatemic rickets. *J Med Genet* **24**:756, 1987.
122. Rowe PS, Read AP, Mountford R, Benham F, Kruse TA, Camerino G, Davies KE, O'Riordan JL: Three DNA markers for hypophosphatemic rickets. *Hum Genet* **89**:539, 1992.
123. Econs MJ, Pericak-Vance MA, Betz H, Bartlett RJ, Speer MC, Drezner MK: The human glycine receptor: A new probe that is linked to the X-linked hypophosphatemic rickets gene. *Genomics* **7**:439, 1990.
124. Thakker RV, Davies KE, Read AP, Tippett P, Wooding C, Flint T, Wood S, Kruse TA, Whyte MP, O'Riordan JLH: Linkage analysis of two cloned DNA sequences, DXS197 and DXS207, in hypophosphatemic rickets families. *Genomics* **8**:189, 1990.
125. Econs MJ, Barker DF, Speer MC, Pericak-Vance MA, Fain PR, Drezner MK: Multilocus mapping of the X-linked hypophosphatemic rickets gene. *J Clin Endocrinol Metab* **75**:201, 1992.
126. Econs MJ, Fain PR, Norman M, Speer MC, Pericak-Vance MA, Becker PA, Barker DF, Taylor A, Drezner MK: Flanking markers define the X-linked hypophosphatemic rickets locus. *J Bone Miner Res* **8**:1149, 1993.
127. Collins FS: Positional cloning: Let's not call it reverse anymore. *Nature Genet* **1**:3, 1992.
128. Kay G, Thakker RV, Rastan S: Determination of a molecular map position for *Hyp* using a new interspecific backcross produced by *in vitro* fertilization. *Genomics* **11**:651, 1991.
129. Eicher EM, Southard JL, Scriver CR, Glorieux FH: Hypophosphatemia: Mouse model for human familial hypophosphatemic (vitamin D-resistant) rickets. *Proc Natl Acad Sci USA* **73**:4667, 1976.

130. Meyer RA Jr, Jowsey J, Meyer MH: Osteomalacia and altered magnesium metabolism in the X-linked hypophosphatemic mouse. *Calcif Tissue Int* **27:**19, 1979.
131. Brault BA, Meyer MH, Meyer RA Jr, Iorio RJ: Mineral uptake by the femora of older female *Hyp* mice but not older male *Hyp* mice. *Clin Orthop Rel Res* **222:**289, 1987.
132. Shetty NS, Meyer RA Jr: Craniofacial abnormalities in mice with X-linked hypophosphatemic genes (*Hyp* or *Gy*). *Teratology* **44:**463, 1991.
133. Giasson SD, Brunette MG, Danan G, Vigneault N, Carriere S: Micropuncture study of renal phosphorus transport in hypophosphatemic vitamin D resistant rickets mice. *Pflugers Arch* **371:**33, 1977.
134. Cowgill LD, Goldfarb S, Lau K, Slatopolsky E, Agus ZS: Evidence for an intrinsic renal tubular defect in mice with genetic hypophosphatemic rickets. *J Clin Invest* **63:**1203, 1979.
135. Kiebzak GM, Meyer RA, Mish PM: X-linked hypophosphatemic mice respond to thyroparathyroidectomy. *Miner Electrolyte Metab* **6:**153, 1981.
136. Tenenhouse HS, Scriver CR, McInnes RR, Glorieux FH: Renal handling of phosphate in vivo and in vitro by the X-linked hypophosphatemic male mouse: Evidence for a defect in the brush border membrane. *Kidney Int* **14:**236, 1978.
137. Tenenhouse HS, Scriver CR: The defect in transcellular transport of phosphate in the nephron is located in brush-border membranes in X-linked hypophosphatemia (Hyp mouse model). *Can J Biochem* **56:**640, 1978.
138. Lyon MF, Scriver CR, Baker LRI, Tenenhouse HS, Kronick J, Mandla S: The *Gy* mutation: Another cause of X-linked hypophosphatemia in mouse. *Proc Natl Acad Sci USA* **83:**4899, 1986.
139. Kiebzak GM, Dousa TP: Thyroid hormones increase renal brush border membrane transport of phosphate in X-linked hypophosphatemic (*Hyp*) mice. *Endocrinology* **117:**613, 1985.
140. Tenenhouse HS, Lee J, Harvey N: Renal brush-border membrane Na^+-sulfate cotransport: Stimulation by thyroid hormone. *Am J Physiol* **261:**F420, 1991.
141. Brunette MG, Mernissi GE, Doucet A: Renal sodium transport in vitamin D resistant hypophosphatemic rickets. *Can J Physiol Pharmacol* **63:**1339, 1985.
142. Ford DM, Molitoris BA: Abnormal proximal tubule apical membrane protein composition in X-linked hypophosphatemic mice. *Am J Physiol* **260:**F317, 1991.
143. Tenenhouse HS, Lee J, Harvey N, Potier M, Jette M, Beliveau R: Normal molecular size of the Na^+-phosphate cotransporter and normal Na^+-dependent binding of phosphonoformic acid in renal brush border membranes of X-linked *Hyp* Mice. *Biochem Biophys Res Commun* **170:**1288, 1990.
144. Tenenhouse HS, Lee J: Sulfate inhibits 14C-phosphonoformic acid binding to renal brush-border membranes. *Am J Physiol* **259:**F286, 1990.
145. Harvey N, Tenenhouse HS: Renal Na^+-phosphate cotransport in X-linked *Hyp* mice responds appropriately to Na^+-gradient, membrane potential and pH. *J Bone Miner Res* **7:**563, 1992.
146. Tenenhouse HS, Scriver CR: Renal brush border membrane adaptation to phosphorus deprivation in the *Hyp*/Y mouse. *Nature* **281:**225, 1979.
147. Tenenhouse HS, Scriver CR: Renal adaptation to phosphate deprivation in the Hyp mouse with X-linked hypophosphatemia. *Can J Biochem* **57:**938, 1979.
148. Muhlbauer RC, Bonjour J-P, Fleisch H: Abnormal tubular adaptation to dietary Pi restriction in X-linked hypophosphatemic mice. *Am J Physiol* **242:**F353, 1982.
148a. Tenenhouse HS, Martel J: Renal adaptation to phosphate deprivation: Lessons from the X-linked *Hyp* mouse. *Ped Nephrol* **7:**312, 1993.
149. Nakagawa N, Arab N, Ghishan FK: Characterization of the defect in the Na^+-phosphate transporter in vitamin D-resistant hypophosphatemic mice. *J Biol Chem* **266:**13616, 1991.
150. Meyer RA Jr, Gray RW, Meyer MH: Abnormal vitamin D metabolism in the X-linked hypophosphatemic mouse. *Endocrinology* **107:**1577, 1980.
151. Lobaugh B, Drezner MK: Abnormal regulation of renal 25-hydroxyvitamin D-1α-hydroxylase activity in the X-linked hypophosphatemic mouse. *J Clin Invest* **71:**400, 1983.
152. Yamaoka K, Seino Y, Satomura K, Tanaka Y, Yabuuchi H, Haussler MR: Abnormal relationship between serum phosphate concentration and renal 25-hydroxycholecalciferol-1-alpha-hydroxylase activity in X-linked hypophosphatemic mice. *Miner Electrolyte Metab* **12:**194, 1986.
153. Davidai GA, Nesbitt T, Drezner MK: Variable phosphate-mediated regulation of vitamin D metabolism in the murine hypophosphatemic rachitic/osteomalacic disorders. *Endocrinology* **128:**1270, 1991.
154. Tenenhouse HS: Abnormal renal mitochondrial 25-hydroxyvitamin D3-1-hydroxylase activity in the vitamin D and calcium deficient X-linked *Hyp* mouse. *Endocrinology* **113:**816, 1983.
155. Tenenhouse HS: Investigation of the mechanism for abnormal renal 25-hydroxyvitamin D_3-1-hydroxylase activity in the X-linked *Hyp* mouse. *Endocrinology* **115:**634, 1984.
156. Tenenhouse HS: Metabolism of 25-hydroxyvitamin D_3 in renal slices from the X-linked hypophosphatemic (*Hyp*) mouse: Abnormal response to fall in serum calcium. *Cell Calcium* **5:**634, 1984.
157. Carpenter TO, Shiratori T: Renal 25-hydroxyvitamin D-1 alpha-hydroxylase activity and mitochondrial phosphate transport in *Hyp* mice. *Am J Physiol* **259:**E814, 1990.
158. Nesbitt T, Drezner MK, Lobaugh B: Abnormal parathyroid hormone stimulation of 25-hydroxy vitamin D-1α-hydroxylase activity in the hypophosphatemic mouse: Evidence for a generalized defect of vitamin D metabolism. *J Clin Invest* **77:**181, 1986.
159. Nesbitt T, Davidai GA, Drezner MK: Abnormal adenosine 3′,5′-monophosphate stimulation of renal 1,25-dihydroxyvitamin D production in *Hyp* mice: Evidence that 25-hydroxyvitamin D-1 α-hydroxylase dysfunction results from aberrant intracellular function. *Endocrinology* **124:**1184, 1989.
160. Nesbitt T, Drezner MK: Abnormal parathyroid hormone-related peptide stimulation of renal 25-hydroxyvitamin D-1-hydroxylase in *Hyp* mice: Evidence for a generalized defect of enzyme activity in the proximal convoluted tubule. *Endocrinology* **127:**843, 1990.
161. Insogna KL, Broadus AL, Gertner JM: Impaired phosphorus conservation and 1,25-dihydroxyvitamin D generation during phosphorus deprivation in familial hypophosphatemic rickets. *J Clin Invest* **71:**1562, 1983.
162. Lyles KW, Drezner MK: Parathyroid hormone effects on serum 1,25-dihydroxyvitamin D levels in patients with X-linked hypophosphatemic rickets: Evidence for abnormal 25-hydroxyvitamin D-1-hydroxylase activity. *J Clin Endocrinol Metab* **54:**638, 1982.
163. Nesbitt T, Lobaugh B, Drezner MK: Calcitonin stimulation of renal 25-hydroxyvitamin D-1α-hydroxylase activity in hypophosphatemic mice. Evidence that the regulation of calcitriol production is not universally abnormal in X-linked hypophosphatemia. *J Clin Invest* **79:**15, 1987.
164. Econs MJ, Lobaugh B, Drezner MK: Normal calcitonin stimulation of serum calcitriol in patients with X-linked hypophosphatemic rickets. *J Clin Endocrinol Metab* **75:**408, 1992.
165. Kawashima H, Torikai S, Kurokawa K: Calcitonin selectively stimulates 25-hydroxyvitamin D_3-1α-hydroxylase in proximal straight tubule of rat kidney. *Nature* **291:**327, 1981.
166. Kawashima H, Torikai S, Kurokawa K: Localization of 25-hydroxyvitamin D_3 1α-hydroxylase and 24-hydroxylase along the rat nephron. *Proc Natl Acad Sci USA* **78:**1199, 1981.
167. Seino Y, Yamaoka K, Ishida M, Tanaka Y, Kurose H, Yabuuchi H, Tohira Y, Fukushima M, Nishii Y: Plasma clearance for high doses of exogenous 1,25-dihydroxy [23,24(n)-^{3}H] cholecalciferol in X-linked hypophosphatemic mice. *Biomed Res* **3:**683, 1982.
168. Kumar R: Metabolism of 1,25-dihydroxyvitamin D_3. *Physiol Rev* **64:**478, 1984.
169. Jones G, Vriezen D, Lohnes D, Palda V, Edwards NS: Side chain hydroxylation of vitamin D_3 and its physiological implications. *Steroids* **49:**29, 1987.
170. Makin G, Lohnes D, Byford V, Ray R, Jones G: Target cell metabolism of 1,25-dihydroxyvitamin D_3 to calcitroic acid. Evidence for a pathway in kidney and bone involving 24-oxidation. *Biochem J* **262:**173, 1989.
171. Reddy SG, Tserng K: Calcitroic acid, end product of

renal metabolism of 1,25-dihydroxyvitamin D_3 through C-24 oxidation pathway. *Biochemistry* **28**:1763, 1989.

172. Tenenhouse HS, Yip A, Jones G: Increased renal catabolism of 1,25-dihydroxyvitamin D_3 in murine X-linked hypophosphatemic rickets. *J Clin Invest* **81**:461, 1988.
173. Jones G, Yip A, Tenenhouse HS: Side-chain oxidation of vitamin D_3 in mouse kidney mitochondria: Effect of the *Hyp* mutation and 1,25-dihydroxyvitamin D_3 treatment. *Biochem Cell Biol* **65**:853, 1987.
174. Cunningham J, Coldwell RD, Jones G, Tenenhouse HS, Trafford DJ, Makin HL: Plasma 24,25-dihydroxyvitamin D_3 concentrations in X-linked hypophosphatemic mice: Studies using mass fragmentographic and radioreceptor assays. *J Bone Miner Res* **5**:173, 1990.
175. Tenenhouse HS, Jones G: Abnormal regulation of renal vitamin D catabolism by dietary phosphate in murine X-linked hypophosphatemic rickets. *J Clin Invest* **85**:1450, 1990.
176. Roy S, Martel J, Ma S, Tenenhouse HS: Inherited renal 25-hydroxyvitamin D_3-24-hydroxylase mRNA and immunoreactive protein in phosphate-deprived *Hyp* mice: A mechanism for accelerated 1,25-dihydroxyvitamin D_3 catabolism in X-linked hypophosphatemic rickets. *Endocrinology* **134**:1994. (In press.)
177. Sabina RL, Drezner MK, Holmes EW: Reduced renal cortical ribonucleoside triphosphate pools in three different hypophosphatemic animal models. *Biochem Biophys Res Commun* **109**:649, 1982.
178. Brown CE, Wilkie CA, Meyer MH, Meyer RA Jr: Response of tissue phosphate content to acute dietary phosphate deprivation in the X-linked hypophosphatemic mouse. *Calcif Tissue Int* **37**:423, 1985.
179. Kiebzak GM, Roos BA, Meyer RA Jr: Secondary hyperparathyroidism in X-linked hypophosphatemic mice. *Endocrinology* **111**:650, 1982.
180. Posillico JT, Lobaugh B, Muhlbaier LH, Drezner MK: Abnormal parathyroid function in the X-linked hypophosphatemic mouse. *Calcif Tissue Int* **37**:418, 1985.
181. Tenenhouse HS, Veksler A: Effect of the *Hyp* mutation and diet-induced hyperparathyroidism on renal parathyroid hormone- and forskolin-stimulated adenosine 3′5′-monophosphate production and brush border membrane phosphate transport. *Endocrinology* **118**:1047, 1986.
182. Kiebzak GM, Meyer RA Jr: X-linked hypophosphatemic mice are not hypersensitive to parathyroid hormone. *Endocrinology* **110**:1030, 1982.
183. Tenenhouse HS, Henry HL: Protein kinase activity and protein kinase inhibitor in mouse kidney: Effect of the X-linked *Hyp* mutation and vitamin D status. *Endocrinology* **117**:1719, 1985.
184. Hammerman MR, Chase LR: Pi transport, phosphorylation, and dephosphorylation in renal membranes from *Hyp*/Y mice. *Am J Physiol* **245**:F701, 1983.
185. Tenenhouse HS, Fast DK, Scriver CR, Koltay M: Intestinal transport of phosphate anion is not impaired in the *Hyp* (hypophosphatemic) mouse. *Biochem Biophys Res Commun* **100**:537, 1981.
186. Brault BA, Meyer MH, Meyer RA Jr: Malabsorption of phosphate by the intestines of young X-linked hypophosphatemic mice. *Calcif Tissue Int* **43**:289, 1988.
187. Meyer MH, Meyer RA Jr, Iorio RJ: A role for the intestine in the bone disease of juvenile X-linked hypophosphatemic mice: Malabsorption of calcium and reduced skeletal mineralization. *Endocrinology* **115**:1464, 1984.
188. Meyer RA Jr, Meyer MH, Erickson PR, Korkor AB: Reduced absorption of ^{45}Calcium from isolated duodenal segments "in vivo" in juvenile but not adult X-linked hypophosphatemic mice. *Calcif Tissue Int* **38**:95, 1986.
189. Bruns ME, Meyer RA Jr, Meyer MH: Low levels of intestinal vitamin D-dependent calcium binding protein in juvenile X-linked hypophosphatemic mice. *Endocrinology* **115**:1459, 1984.
190. Meyer RA Jr, Meyer MH, Gray RW, Bruns ME: Evidence that low plasma 1,25-dihydroxyvitamin D causes intestinal malabsorption of calcium and phosphate in juvenile X-linked hypophosphatemic mice. *J Bone Miner Res* **2**:67, 1987.
191. Bruns ME, Christakos S, Huang YC, Meyer MH, Meyer RA Jr: Vitamin D-dependent calcium binding proteins in the kidney and intestine of the X-linked hypophosphatemic mouse: Changes with age and responses to 1,25-dihydroxycholecalciferol. *Endocrinology* **121**:1, 1987.
192. Short EM, Binder HJ, Rosenberg LE: Familial hypophosphatemic rickets: Defective transport of inorganic phosphate by intestinal mucosa. *Science* **179**:700, 1973.
193. Glorieux FH, Morin CL, Travers R, Delvin EE, Poirier R: Intestinal phosphate transport in familial hypophosphatemic rickets. *Pediatr Res* **10**:691, 1976.
194. Seino Y, Sierra RI, Ichikawa M, Avioli LV: 1,25-Dihydroxyvitamin D_3 receptor in the X-linked hypophosphatemic mouse. *Endocrinology* **111**:329, 1982.
195. Yamamoto T, Seino Y, Yamaoka K, Yabuuchi H: Decreased nuclear uptake of 1,25-dihydroxyvitamin D_3 by duodenal mucosal cells in the X-linked hypophosphatemic mouse. *Endocrinology* **117**:2252, 1985.
196. Yamamoto T, Seino Y, Tanaka H, Yamaoka K, Kurose H, Ishida M, Yabuuchi H: Effects of the administration of phosphate on nuclear 1,25-dihydroxyvitamin D_3 uptake by duodenal mucosal cells of *Hyp* mice. *Endocrinology* **122**:576, 1988.
197. Tohmon M, Fukase M, Fujita T: Low levels of intestinal calbindin-D28K in X-linked hypophosphatemic mice. *Bone Miner* **6**:15, 1989.
198. Roy WA, Iorio RJ, Meyer RA Jr: Craniosynostosis in vitamin D-resistant rickets. A mouse model. *J Neurosurg* **55**:265, 1981.
199. Mostafa YA, El-Mangoury NH, Meyer RA Jr, Iorio RJ: Deficient nasal bone growth in the X-linked hypophosphatemic (*Hyp*) mouse and its implication in craniofacial growth. *Arch Oral Biol* **27**:311, 1982.
200. Marie PJ, Travers R, Glorieux FH: Healing of rickets with phosphate supplementation in the hypophosphatemic male mouse. *J Clin Invest* **67**:911, 1981.
201. Yoshikawa H, Masuhara K, Takaoka K, Ono K, Tanaka H, Seino Y: Abnormal bone formation induced by implantation of osteosarcoma-derived bone-inducing substance in the X-linked hypophosphatemic mouse. *Bone* **6**:235, 1985.
202. Ecarot-Charrier B, Glorieux FH, Travers R, Desbarats M, Bouchard F, Hinek A: Defective bone formation by transplanted *Hyp* mouse bone cells into normal mice. *Endocrinology* **123**:768, 1988.
203. Ecarot B, Glorieux FH, Desbarats M, Travers R, Labelle L: Defective bone formation by *Hyp* mouse bone cells transplanted into normal mice: Evidence in favor of an intrinsic osteoblast defect. *J Bone Miner Res* **7**:215, 1991.
204. Ecarot B, Glorieux FH, Desbarats M, Travers R, Labelle L: Effect of dietary phosphate deprivation and supplementation of recipient mice on bone formation by transplanted cells from normal and X-linked hypophosphatemic mice. *J Bone Miner Res* **7**:523, 1992.
205. Ecarot B, Caverzasio J, Desbarats M, Bonjour JP, Glorieux FH: Phosphate transport in osteoblasts isolated from normal and *Hyp* mice. *J Bone Miner Res* **6**:839, 1991.
206. Rifas L, Halstead LL, Cheng S-L, Scott MJ, Fausto A, Roberts M, Avioli LV: Na^+-dependent phosphate transport in normophosphatemic and hypophosphatemic osteoblasts in an X-linked hypophosphatemic mouse model. *J Bone Miner Res* **6**:437, 1991.
207. Delvin EE, Richard P, Desbarats M, Ecarot-Charrier B, Glorieux FH: Cultured osteoblasts from normal and hypophosphatemic mice: Calcitriol receptors and biological response to the hormone. *Bone* **11**:87, 1990.
208. Yamamoto T, Ecarot B, Glorieux FH: Abnormal response of osteoblasts from *Hyp* mice to 1,25-dihydroxyvitamin D_3. *Bone* **13**:209, 1992.
209. Boskey AL, Gilder H, Neufeld E, Ecarot B, Glorieux FH: Phospholipid changes in the bones of the hypophosphatemic mouse. *Bone* **12**:345, 1991.
210. Iorio RJ, Bell WA, Meyer MH, Meyer RA Jr: Radiographic evidence of craniofacial and dental abnormalities in the X-linked hypophosphatemic mouse. *Ann Dent* **38**:31, 1979.
211. Iorio RJ, Bell WA, Meyer MH, Meyer RA Jr: Histologic evidence of calcification in teeth and alveolae bone of mice with X-linked dominant hypophosphatemia (VDRR). *Ann Dent* **38**:38, 1979.
212. Sofaer JA, Southam JC: Naturally-occurring exposure of

the dental-pulp in mice with inherited hypophosphatemia. *Arch Oral Biol* **27:**701, 1982.

213. Abe K, Ooshima T, Masatomi Y, Sobue S, Moriwaki Y: Microscopic and crystallographic examinations of the teeth of the X-linked hypophosphatemic mouse. *J Dent Res* **68:**1519, 1989.
214. Abe K, Masatomi Y, Nakajima Y, Shintani S, Moriwaki Y, Sobue S, Ooshima T: The occurrence of interglobular dentin in incisors of hypophosphatemic mice fed a high-calcium and high-phosphate diet. *J Dent Res* **71:**478, 1992.
215. Reade TM, Scriver CR: Hypophosphatemic rickets and breast milk. *N Engl J Med* **300:**1397, 1979.
216. Jonas AJ, Dominguez B: Low breast milk phosphorus concentration in familial hypophosphatemia. *J Pediatr Gastroenterol Nutr* **8:**541, 1989.
217. Delzer PR, Meyer RA Jr: Normal milk composition in lactating X-linked hypophosphatemic mice despite continued hypophosphatemia. *Calcif Tissue Int* **35:**750, 1983.
218. Delzer PR, Meyer RA Jr: Normal handling of phosphate in the salivary glands of X-linked hypophosphatemic mice. *Arch Oral Biol* **29:**1009, 1984.
219. Escoubet B, Silve C, Balsan S, Amiel C: Phosphate transport by fibroblasts from patients with hypophosphatemic vitamin D-resistant rickets. *J Endocrinol* **133:**301, 1992.
220. Vaughn LK, Meyer RA Jr, Meyer MH: Increased metabolic rate in X-linked hypophosphatemic mice. *Endocrinology* **118:**441, 1986.
221. Muhlbauer RC, Bonjour J-P, Fleisch H: Abnormal hyperphosphatemic response to fasting in X-linked hypophosphatemic mice. *Miner Electrolyte Metab* **10:**362, 1984.
222. Meyer RA Jr, Tenenhouse HS, Meyer MH, Klugerman AH: The renal phosphate transport defect in normal mice parabiosed to X-linked hypophosphatemic mice persists after parathyroidectomy. *J Bone Miner Res* **4:**523, 1989.
223. Meyer RA Jr, Meyer MH, Gray RW: Parabiosis suggests a humoral factor is involved in X-linked hypophosphatemia in mice. *J Bone Miner Res* **4:**493, 1989.
224. Meyer RA Jr, Tenenhouse HS, Gray RW, Meyer MH: Normal mice joined by parabiosis adapt to phosphate restriction. *J Bone Miner Res* **5:**528, 1990.
225. Nesbitt T, Coffman TM, Griffiths R, Drezner MK: Cross-transplantation of kidneys in normal and *Hyp* mice: Evidence that the *Hyp* phenotype is unrelated to an intrinsic renal defect. *J Clin Invest* **89:**1453, 1992.
226. Morgan JM, Hawley WL, Chenoweth AI, Retan WJ, Diethelm AG: Renal transplantation in hypophosphatemia with vitamin D-resistant rickets. *Arch Intern Med* **134:**549, 1974.
227. Scriver CR, Tenenhouse HS: Conserved loci on the X chromosome confer phosphate homeostasis in mice and humans. *Genet Res Camb* **56:**141, 1990.
227a. Qui ZQ, Tenenhouse HS, Scriver CR: Parental origin of mutant allele does not explain absence of gene dose effect in X-linked *Hyp* mice. *Genet Res Camb* **63:**39, 1993.
228. Boneh A, Tenenhouse HS: Protein kinase C in mouse kidney: Effect of the *Hyp* mutation and phosphate deprivation. *Kidney Int* **37:**682, 1990.
229. Henry HL: Influence of a tumor promoting phorbol ester on the metabolism of 25-hydroxyvitamin D_3. *Biochem Biophys Res Commun* **139:**495, 1986.
230. Mandla S, Boneh A, Tenenhouse HS: Evidence for protein kinase C involvement in the regulation of renal 25-hydroxyvitamin D_3-24-hydroxylase. *Endocrinology* **127:**2639, 1990.
231. Bell CL, Tenenhouse HS, Scriver CR: Primary cultures of renal epithelial cells from X-linked hypophosphatemic (*Hyp*) mice express defects in phosphate transport and vitamin D metabolism. *Am J Hum Genet* **43:**293, 1988.
232. Glorieux FH, Marie PJ, Pettifor JM, Delvin EE: Bone response to phosphate salts, ergocalciferol, and calcitriol in hypophosphatemic vitamin D-resistant rickets. *N Engl J Med* **303:**1023, 1980.
233. Marie PJ, Travers R, Glorieux FH: Bone response to phosphate and vitamin D metabolites in the hypophosphatemic male mouse. *Calcif Tissue Int* **34:**158, 1982.
234. Tenenhouse HS, Scriver CR: Effect of 1,25-dihydroxyvitamin D_3 on phosphate homeostasis in the X-linked hypophosphatemic (*Hyp*) mouse. *Endocrinology* **109:**658, 1981.
235. Alon U, Chan JCM: Effects of PTH and $1,25(OH)_2D_3$ on tubular handling of phosphate in hypophosphatemic rickets. *J Clin Endocrinol Metab* **58:**671, 1984.
236. Harrell RM, Lyles KW, Harrelson JM, Friedman NE, Drezner MK: Healing of bone disease in X-linked hypophosphatemic rickets/osteomalacia. *J Clin Invest* **75:**1858, 1985.
237. Marie PJ, Travers R: Effects of magnesium and lactose supplementation on bone metabolism in the X-linked hypophosphatemic mouse. *Metabolism* **32:**165, 1983.
238. Tenenhouse HS, Meyer RA Jr, Mandla S, Meyer MH, Gray RW: Renal phosphate transport and vitamin D metabolism in X-linked hypophosphatemic *Gy* mice: Responses to phosphate deprivation. *Endocrinology* **131:**51, 1992.
239. Davidai GA, Nesbitt T, Drezner MK: Normal regulation of calcitriol metabolism in Gy mice. Evidence for biochemical heterogeneity in the X-linked hypophosphatemic diseases. *J Clin Invest* **85:**334, 1990.
240. Boneh A, Reade TM, Scriver CR, Rishikof E: Audiometric evidence for two forms of X-linked hypophosphatemia in humans, apparent counterparts of *Hyp* and *Gy* mutations in mouse. *Am J Med Genet* **27:**997, 1987.
241. McKusick VA: *Mendelian Inheritance in Man*, 10th ed. Baltimore, Johns Hopkins University Press, 1992.
242. Verge CF, Lam A, Simpson JM, Cowell CT, Howard NJ, Silink M: Effects of therapy in X-linked hypophosphatemic rickets. *N Engl J Med* **325:**1843, 1991.
243. Glorieux FH: Rickets, the continuing challenge. *N Engl J Med* **325:**1875, 1991.
244. Tsuru N, Chan JCM, Chinchilli VM: Renal hypophosphatemic rickets. *Am J Dis Child* **141:**108, 1987.
245. Balsan S, Tieder M: Linear growth in patients with hypophosphatemic rickets: Influence of treatment regimen and parental height. *J Pediatr* **116:**365, 1990.
246. Bettinelli A, Bianchi ML, Mazzucchi E, Gandolini G, Appiani AC: Acute effects of calcitriol and phosphate salts on mineral metabolism in children with hypophospatemic rickets. *J Pediatr* **118:**372, 1991.
247. Stickler GB, Morgenstern BZ: Hypophosphataemic rickets: Final height and clinical symptoms in adults. *Lancet* **2:**902, 1989.
248. Petersen DJ, Boniface AM, Schranck FW, Rupich RC, Whyte MP: X-linked hypophosphatemic rickets: A study (with literature review) of linear growth response to calcitriol and phosphate therapy. *J Bone Miner Res* **7:**583, 1992.
249. Goodyer PR, Kronick JB, Jequier S, Reade TM, Scriver CR: Nephrocalcinosis and its relationship to treatment of hereditary rickets. *J Pediatr* **111:**700, 1987.
250. Alon U, Donaldson DL, Hellerstein S, Warady BA, Harris DJ: Metabolic and histologic investigation of the nature of nephrocalcinosis in children with hypophosphatemic rickets and in the *Hyp* mouse. *J Pediatr* **120:**899, 1992.
251. Futh RG, Giant CS, Riggs BL: Development of hypercalcemic hyperparathyroidism after long-term phosphate supplementation in hypophosphtemic osteomalacia. *Am J Med* **78:**669, 1985.
252. Wilson DM, Lee PD, Morris AH, Reiter EO, Gertner JM, Marcus R, Quarmby VE, Rosenfeld RG: Growth hormone therapy in hypophosphatemic rickets. *Am J Dis Child* **145:**1165, 1991.
253. Sullivan W, Carpenter T, Glorieux F, Travers R, Insogna K: A prospective trial of phosphate and 1,25-dihydroxyvitamin D_3 therapy in symptomatic adults with X-linked hypophosphatemic rickets. *J Clin Endocrinol Metab* **75:**879, 1992.
254. Costa T, Marie PJ, Scriver CR, Cole DEC, Reade TM, Nogrady B, Glorieux FH, Delvin EE: X-linked hypophosphatemia: Effect of calcitriol on renal handling of phosphate, serum phosphate, and bone mineralization. *J Clin Endocrinol Metab* **52:**463, 1981.
255. Weidner N: Review and update: Oncogenic osteomalacia-rickets. *Ultrastruct Pathol* **15:**317, 1991.
255a. Drezner MK: Tumor-associated rickets and osteomalacia, in Favus MJ (ed): *Primer on the Metabolic Bone Diseases and Disorders of Mineral Metabolism,* 2d ed. New York, Raven, 1993, p 282.
256. Uchida H, Yokoyama S, Kashima K, Nakayama I, Shimizu K, Masumi S: Oncogenic vitamin D resistant

hypophosphatemic osteomalacia (benign ossifying mesenchymal tumor of bone): Case report. *Jpn J Clin Oncol* **21**:218, 1991.

257. McGuire MH, Merenda JT, Etzkorn JR, Sundaram M: Oncogenic osteomalacia. A case report. *Clin Orthop* **244**:305, 1989.
258. Schultze G, Delling G, Faensen M, Haubold R, Loy V, Molzahn M, Pommer W, Semler J, Trempenau B: Oncogenic hypophosphatemic osteomalacia. *Dtsch Med Wochenschr* **114**:1073, 1989.
259. Nuovo MA, Dorfman HD, Sun CC, Chalew SA: Tumor-induced osteomalacia and rickets. *Am J Surg Pathol* **13**:588, 1989.
260. Leicht E, Biro G, Langer HJ: Tumor-induced osteomalacia: Pre-and postoperative biochemical findings. *Horm Metab Res* **22**:640, 1990.
261. Miyauchi A, Fukase M, Tsutsumi M, Fujita T: Hemangiopericytoma-induced osteomalacia. Tumor transplantation in nude mice causes hypophosphatemia and tumor extracts inhibit renal 25-hydroxyvitamin D 1-hydroxylase activity. *J Clin Endocrinol Metab* **67**:46, 1988.
262. Scriver CR, MacDonald W, Reade T, Glorieux FH, Nogrady B: Hypophosphatemic non-rachitic bone disease: An entity distinct from X-linked hypophosphatemia in the renal defect, bone involvement and inheritance. *Am J Med Genet* **1**:101, 1977.
263. Scriver CR, Reade T, Halal F, Costa T, Cole DEC: Autosomal hypophosphatemic bone disease responds to 1,25-$(OH)_2D_3$. *Arch Dis Child* **56**:203, 1981.
264. Scriver CR, Reade TM, Deluca HF, Hamstra AJ: Serum 1,25-dihydroxyvitamin D levels in normal subjects and in patients with hereditary rickets or bone disease. *N Engl J Med* **299**:976, 1978.
265. Kinoshita Y, Fukase M, Miyauchi A, Takenaka M, Nakada M, Fujita T: Establishment of a parathyroid hormone-responsive phosphate transport system *in vitro* using cultured renal cells. *Endocrinology* **119**:1954, 1986.
266. Noronha-Blob L, Sacktor B: Inhibition by glucocorticoids of phosphate transport in primary cultured renal cells. *J Biol Chem* **261**:2164, 1986.
267. Pizurki L, Rizzoli R, Moseley J, Martin TJ, Caverzasio J, Bonjour J-P: Effect of synthetic tumoral PTH-related peptide on cAMP production and Na-dependent Pi transport. *Am J Physiol* **255**:F957, 1988.
268. Nakai M, Fukase M, Kinoshita Y, Fujita T: Atrial natriuretic factor inhibits phosphate uptake in opossum kidney cells: As a model of renal proximal tubules. *Biochem Biophys Res Commun* **152**:1416, 1988.
269. Pizurki L, Rizzoli R, Caverzasio J, Bonjour J-P: Effect of transforming growth factor-α and parathyroid hormone-related protein on phosphate transport in renal cells. *Am J Physiol* **259**:F929, 1990.
270. Liang CT, Barnes J, Balakir R, Cheng L, Sacktor B: *In vitro* stimulation of phosphate uptake in isolated chick renal cells by 1,25-dihydroxycholecalciferol. *Proc Natl Acad Sci USA* **79**:3532, 1982.
271. Noronha-Blob L, Lowe V, Sacktor B: Stimulation by thyroid hormone of phosphate transport in primary cultured renal cells. *J Cell Physiol* **137**:95, 1988.
272. Goodyer PR, Kachra Z, Bell C, Rozen R: Renal tubular cells are potential targets for epidermal growth factor. *Am J Physiol* **255**:F1191, 1988.
273. Caverzasio J, Bonjour J-P: Insulin-like growth factor I stimulates Na-dependent P_i transport in cultured kidney cells. *Am J Physiol* **257**:F712, 1989.
274. Abraham MI, McAteer JA, Kempson SA: Insulin stimulates phosphate transport in opossum kidney epithelial cells. *Am J Physiol* **258**:F1592, 1990.
275. Magagnin S, Werner A, Markovich D, Sorribas V, Stange G, Biber J, Murer H: Expression cloning of human and rat renal cortex Na/Pi cotransport. *Proc Natl Acad Sci USA* **90**:5979, 1993.
276. Biber J, Custer M, Kaissling B, Lotscher M, Murer H: Molecular localization of Na/Pi-cotransport (NaPi-2) in the nephron of rat kidney. *J Am Soc Nephrol* **4**:703, 1993. (abstr)
277. Tenenhouse HS, Werner A, Biber J, Ma S, Martel J, Roy S, Murer H: Renal Na^+-phosphate cotransport in murine X-linked hypophosphatemic rickets: Molecular characterization. *J Clin Invest* **94**:671, 1994.
278. Kos CH, Tihy F, Econs MJ, Murer H, Lemieux N, Tenenhouse HS: Localization of a renal sodium phosphate cotransporter gene to human chromosome 5q35. *Genomics* **19**:176, 1994.

CHAPTER 125

Hereditary Renal Hypouricemia

Oded Sperling

1. **Hereditary renal hypouricemia is an inborn error of membrane transport, presumably in urate reabsorption in the proximal tubule. It is inherited in an autosomal recessive mode. In homozygotes, it is manifest as hypouricemia and increased renal urate clearance. Heterozygosity may be detected by moderately decreased serum urate levels and moderately but significantly increased renal urate clearance.**
2. **The homozygosity is associated with moderate or excessive uricosuria, reflecting the diversion of intestinal urate elimination to urinary urate excretion consequent to the hypouricemia. There is no evidence for purine overproduction. Hypercalciuria, probably of the hyperabsorptive type, is associated with renal hypouricemia in about 21 percent of the propositi. The mechanism for this abnormality is not yet clarified. The hyperuricosuria and/or hypercalciuria are etiologic factors in uric acid or calcium oxalate urolithiasis, occurring in about 25 percent of the propositi.**
3. **Transport of urate through the intestinal wall and through the erythrocyte membrane appears to be normal.**
4. **The differential diagnosis of hereditary renal hypouricemia includes familial conditions, in which the defective renal urate transport is one component in a generalized transport abnormality, such as in Hartnup syndrome or in the group of diseases with the Fanconi renal tubulopathy (Wilson disease, cystinosis, galactosemia, and hereditary fructose intolerance).**
5. **The model of the renal handling of urate in humans includes four components: free glomerular filtration, net early proximal tubular reabsorption (segment S_1), net tubular secretion (segment S_2), and net postsecretory tubular reabsorption (segment S_3). It is assumed that reabsorption and secretion of urate in the proximal tubule occur simultaneously and that the manifestation of net reabsorption or secretion at the various segments reflects different intensities of the two processes. The residual urinary urate in the S_1 region derives originally from filtration, whereas that in the S_3 segment arises from secretion in the S_2 segment.**
6. **Several types of renal hypouricemia may be distinguished according to the nature and site of the transport defect, as reflected in the fractional clearance of urate and the effects on this parameter of pyrazinamide (inhibiting urate secretion) and probenecid (inhibiting urate reabsorption). In hereditary renal hypouricemia, the most common type appears to be that of a presecretory reabsorption defect. Some of the cases may have a total transport defect (no reabsorption, no secretion) or total reabsorption defect. A postsecretory reabsorption defect has not been documented in hereditary renal hypouricemia, but was found to characterize acquired renal hypouricemia and familial conditions in which renal hypouricemia is a part of a generalized tubular reabsorption defect (Fanconi syndrome). A hypersecretion defect was suggested in one family with hereditary renal hypouricemia and in three cases of isolated renal hypouricemia without evidence for familiality.**

INTRODUCTION

It is common knowledge that a certain proportion of the inborn errors of metabolism in humans represent extremely rare and benign diseases. Yet, the discovery and study of such defects are very often of utmost importance in that the work contributes to the understanding of the metabolic pathways or processes occurring in the normal human cell or organ. In humans, the renal handling of urate, the final waste product of purine metabolism, is complex; its exact nature has not been conclusively clarified. Hereditary renal hypouricemia is a rare, almost harmless (except for urolithiasis in some of the patients), inborn error in membrane urate transport in the kidney. It represents "experiments of nature" in the renal handling of urate in humans, furnishing valuable information on urate handling in the normal kidney. Indeed, the first case reported in 1950 to be affected with this syndrome, although lacking conclusive evidence for familiality,[1] furnished the first indication of renal tubular secretion of urate in humans. The study of the 28 cases with true hereditary renal hypouricemia, first documented in 1972, provided data supporting the four-component model of the renal handling of urate in humans that is accepted at present. Furthermore, the results of these studies suggested that the two reabsorption components in the model—namely, the presecretory and the postsecretory—are controlled by different genes.

DEFINITION AND DIFFERENTIAL DIAGNOSIS

Hereditary renal hypouricemia refers to the hereditary condition of increased renal urate clearance (see Table 125-2 for normal values), caused by a specific (isolated) inborn error of membrane transport for urate in the renal proximal tubule. This condition is manifested by hypouricemia as defined by

A list of standard abbreviations is located immediately preceding the index in each volume. Additional abbreviations used in this chapter are: FC_{ur} = fractional urate clearance; PAH = para-aminohippuric acid; SITS = 4-acetamido-4′-isothiocyanostilbene-2,2′-disulfonic acid; T_m = maximal rate for net tubular absorption.

a serum urate less than 149 μ*M* (2.5 mg/dl) for adult males and less than 125 μ*M* (2.1 mg/dl) for adult women using a colorimetric determination.[2-5] Hereditary renal hypouricemia should be differentiated from other hereditary conditions of renal hypouricemia, in which the urate transport defect is only one component in a generalized disturbance of membrane transport, e.g., Fanconi (see Chap. 122)[6-8] and Hartnup (see Chap. 119)[9] syndromes. It should also be distinguished from genetically determined metabolic hypouricemia, such as in xanthinuria (see Chap. 54)[10,11] and in purine nucleoside phosphorylase deficiency (see Chap. 52).[12] In the latter conditions, decreased production of uric acid due to specific enzyme abnormalities is manifested by very low uric acid levels in both serum and urine.

According to the above definition, subjects with persistent hypouricemia with normal or somewhat excessive (see below) urinary excretion of uric acid, that is, increased renal urate clearance, should be investigated for hereditary renal hypouricemia. Hypouricemia is a relatively rare condition; study of hospital populations ranging from 2990 to 27,987 patients revealed a rate of from 0.57 to 1 percent.[13-18] In an apparently normal Japanese population (11,499 subjects) only 0.18 percent could be classified as hypouricemic.[19] The frequency of idiopathic renal hypouricemia is even lower—0.12 percent of 3258 Japanese outpatients.[20] In all reported cases of hereditary renal hypouricemia, the classification of hereditary isolated renal hypouricemia was established by demonstration of familiality and by refuting the presence of other renal tubular reabsorption defects. In order to establish the familiality of the defect, sibs and other family members should be screened for hypouricemia (see "Genetics" below). Finding of an additional affected hypouricemic (homozygous) sib is proof of familiality. Finding of parents or offspring with intermediate blood levels of uric acid (148 to 208 μ*M*) associated with significantly increased renal urate clearance may be taken to indicate heterozygosity. When familial renal hypouricemia is established, the isolated type can be verified by ruling out the presence of other tubular abnormalities. The presence of the following hereditary diseases should be excluded: Wilson disease,[21-24] cystinosis,[25] galactosemia,[26] and hereditary fructose intolerance[27] (see Chaps. 68, 126, 25 and 23, respectively). All these diseases are associated with the Fanconi syndrome, in which uric acid reabsorption in the proximal tubule is decreased along with other crystalloid solutes. Renal hypouricemia is also part of the Hartnup syndrome, which should also be excluded (see Chap. 119).[9]

Subjects with persistent renal hypouricemia, who have no sibs or other relatives, may be classified as having suspected hereditary renal hypouricemia if they are proved to have the isolated defect in uric acid transport and when the presence of acquired renal hypouricemia is excluded beyond doubt. Acquired renal hypouricemia may accompany conditions of extracellular fluid volume expansion, such as in inappropriate antidiuretic hormone secretion,[28-30] and in various malignancies, such as multiple myeloma,[31] lymphomas,[32,33] and pulmonary neoplasms.[34-37] In some of the neoplasms, the renal hypouricemia is part of a broader, Fanconi-like tubulopathy, whereas in others, like Hodgkin disease, it appears as an isolated defect. In the latter disease, the degree of renal urate clearance was found to correlate with the activity of the neoplastic process.[32,33] Renal hypouricemia may also occur in heavy metal intoxication[38,39] and following use of outdated tetracyclines.[40] In both conditions, the renal hypouricemia is part of a general tubulopathy of the type of the Fanconi syndrome. It can also occur in liver disease, such as jaundice,[41] in which the degree of renal urate clearance was shown to improve (decrease) with recovery, and cirrhosis,[42] in which an inverse correlation was found between serum bilirubin and urate.

Further support (but by no means proof) for the presence of hereditary renal hypouricemia in subjects with persistent renal hypouricemia, who have no evidence for acquired conditions, but who lack conclusive evidence for familiality, may be obtained by demonstration of the presecretory reabsorption type of defect in renal urate handling. This is because of the apparently characteristic presence of this type of defect in subjects with hereditary renal hypouricemia (see below).

HISTORY

True hereditary renal hypouricemia, due to an isolated tubular defect for urate transport, was first described in humans by Greene et al. in 1972.[43] This condition was described by Praetorius and Kirk[1] in 1950, but in their patient there was no evidence of genetic transmission. The second true case of hereditary renal hypouricemia was documented in 1973 by Khachadurian and Arslanian.[44] In 1974, Sperling et al. reported a new hereditary syndrome which included hypouricemia, hypercalciuria, and decreased bone density.[45] Since then, another 25 families have been documented[46-64] with true hereditary renal hypouricemia. Many more cases which could fit with this category were reported,[1,47,65-72] but the genetic transmission was not established.

RENAL HANDLING OF URATE IN NORMAL HUMANS

Since hereditary renal hypouricemia is believed to be caused by a primary defect in the renal handling of urate, the present knowledge of the normal handling of urate in the human kidney is reviewed first. The exact nature of the renal handling of urate in humans has not been clarified conclusively. This is due in part to the lack of an animal model in which the renal handling of urate is identical to that in humans. Experiments in humans were limited to the study of the effects of urate loading[73,74] and of various drugs[74-77] on uric acid excretion. In addition, important information was furnished by the "experiments of nature"—that is, the inborn defects in renal urate reabsorption, the subject of this chapter. In constructing a plausible model for the renal handling of urate in humans, the animal information was selected according to its compatibility with the information obtained for humans. Data were obtained from a wide range of laboratory animals, such as reptiles, rats, dogs, Cebus monkeys, and chimpanzees. In these animals, stop-flow, micropuncture and microperfusion experiments in vivo, as well as vesicle studies in vitro, furnished the basic information on the renal handling of urate and the mechanism of renal urate transport.[78] The species which were found to resemble humans most closely were the chimpanzee and the Cebus monkey.[79] The first study on urate transport in the proximal tubule of human kidney was published in 1991[80] (and see below).

Components of Renal Handling of Urate

Glomerular Filtration of Uric Acid. Urate is probably bound to plasma proteins, the amount of binding being approximately 5 to 10 percent.[81,82] However, the data regarding binding are conflicting. Practically, urate is freely filtered at the glomerulus, since the binding of urate to plasma proteins is offset by the plasma negative Gibbs-Donnan potential generated across the glomerular membrane.[83] Indeed, determinations of the concentration of urate in glomerular ultrafiltrate and plasma water indicate that they are almost equal.[84-86]

Reabsorption of Uric Acid. In a number of species, the fraction of filtered urate excreted in the urine is less than 100 percent, indicating net reabsorption. This is true for cats, some monkeys, rats, mongrel dogs, the Cebus monkey, chimpanzees, and humans.[79] In humans, the fractional clearance of urate, in relation to that of inulin or creatinine, is about 7 to 10 percent, indicating very efficient reabsorption. In all animals in which urate reabsorption has been localized, including the Cebus monkey,[87] it was found to occur largely in the proximal tubules, although it is possible that some degree of urate reabsorption may occur in some animals in more distal segments. Urate reabsorption may proceed by two mechanisms, a saturable mediated pathway through the cell and a nonsaturable-noninhibitible pathway across the tight junction.[88] That urate reabsorption is an active transport process is evident from several findings. In free-flow, micropuncture studies, the ratio between urate concentration in the proximal tubule fluid to that in plasma was shown to be less than 1.[89] Similar results were obtained also in microperfusion studies.[90] In addition, in nonhuman primates and in humans, diuresis and inhibition of urate secretion by pyrazinoate caused the concentration of urate in urine to approach 10 percent of the plasma concentration.[91] In chimpanzees and monkeys, urate concentration in the tubular fluid was found to be from 20 to 60 percent of plasma urate concentration.[92] The relationship between the active absorption of urate and the intraluminal concentration of urate was found to follow first-order kinetics.[88] The urate reabsorption process was found to be affected by alterations in the reabsorption of sodium,[93] but could be dissociated from that of the sodium by pharmacologic agents[94,95] and by expansion of the extracellular fluid volume.[96] That urate and sodium reabsorption are not linked intimately was also confirmed in vesicle studies.[97,98] Studies in rats in vivo and in vesicles in vitro demonstrated that urate reabsorption is inhibited by a number of substances, such as probenecid, furosemide, para-aminohippuric acid (PAH) and the anion exchange inhibitors 4-acetamido-4′-isothiocyanostilbene-2,2′-disulfonic acid (SITS), and 4,4′-diisothiocyanostilbene-2,2′-disulfonic acid, and thus that urate reabsorption is mediated by an anion-exchange mechanism.

Secretion of Uric Acid. The first evidence for tubular urate secretion in humans was found in 1950,[1] in the first subject with renal hypouricemia, in whom the fractional urate clearance (FC_{ur}; urate:inulin clearance ratio) was 1.46. This early evidence for the bidirectional tubular transport of urate was subsequently augmented by studies in humans, in which the FC_{ur} was increased artificially to as high as 1.23 by use of urate loading, mannitol diuresis, and probenecid.[74] In humans, the exact localization of urate secretion has not been conclusively established. In one study,[99] the proximal nephron was found to transport urate to the tubular fluid, whereas the distal nephron was unable to do so. Net secretion of urate occurs in many species, such as birds, reptiles, guinea pigs, Dalmatian coach hounds, some individual rabbits, and certain species of monkeys. In virtually all these animals, there is evidence for bidirectional urate transport. In rats, urate secretion occurs by both saturable transcellular and nonsaturable paracellular pathways.[100] The relationship between the mediated secretory flux of urate and the urate concentration in the peritubular capillaries demonstrates first-order kinetics.[100] In vivo microperfusion and microinjection studies indicated that, similar to the reabsorption of urate, the secretory process is a result of an anion-exchange mechanism. The secretory flux of urate was inhibited by probenecid, *p*-chloromercuribenzoate, SITS, PAH, and pyrazinoate.[100-102] Accordingly, it was concluded that the secretory urate exchanger has affinity for PAH and pyrazinoate. Several experiments indicated the presence of an uphill transport step for urate in the rat proximal tubule, probably at the basolateral membrane. When rat kidney slices were incubated in a medium containing urate, the slice-to-medium urate ratio was 0.71.[103] Intravenous loading of rats with urate accompanied by administration of the uricase inhibitor oxonate resulted in a mean fractional delivery of urate to the early proximal tubule of 130 percent.[89] Also in the rabbit, an uphill transport site for urate secretion was firmly implicated in the proximal tubule[104,105] at the basolateral membrane.[103,106] An interesting finding in rabbits is that urate secretion is modulated by a serum protein which affects the basolateral transporter by allosteric modification.[105] This finding may be taken to suggest that abnormalities in renal urate handling may also reflect primary defects in such modulators of secretion or reabsorption (see below). In rabbits, urate secretion was demonstrated to increase markedly with plasma urate concentration.[107,108]

Urate Transport in the Proximal Tubule of Human Kidney. Studies have demonstrated in human brush-border vesicles that urate is exchanged for Cl^-. This exchange was shown to be saturable and to be *cis*-inhibited by pyrazinoic acid, probenecid, and L-lactate. This transport mechanism differs from that found in rats and dogs, mainly in having a very low affinity for PAH.[80]

A Model for Urate Transport. The studies with renal brush-border and basolateral membrane vesicles from rats and brush-border vesicles from dogs[108-115] led Kahn and Weinman[83] to construct a model for the bidirectional transport of urate in the proximal tubules of rats. According to this model (Fig. 125-1), urate reabsorption from the lumen to the cell is mediated by the brush-border anion exchanger, exchanging urate for intracellular anions. Anions such as hydroxyl or bicarbonate are above electrochemical equilibrium within the cell; thus, their exchange with urate allows uphill reabsorption of urate. Other anions—such as lactate, pyruvate, and succinate—may also exchange with urate. These anions may either be produced in the cell or transported from the lumen via a sodium cotransport system. The transport of urate from the cell into the interstitium could occur by simple diffusion or through an anion-exchange mechanism (e.g., for chloride). According to this model of urate reabsorption, compounds such as probenecid, PAH, or furosemide inhibit urate reabsorption from the lumen to the proximal tubule cell by blocking the brush-border anion exchanger. In the secretion process, urate transport from plasma to cell through the basolateral membrane is mediated via anion exchange with cellular chloride or other anions not yet identified. These cellular anions should be above electrochemical equilibrium with respect to the interstitium, to allow uphill urate secretion. Another transport mechanism that could mediate uphill urate transport from interstitium to the cell is a sodium-urate transport system. However,

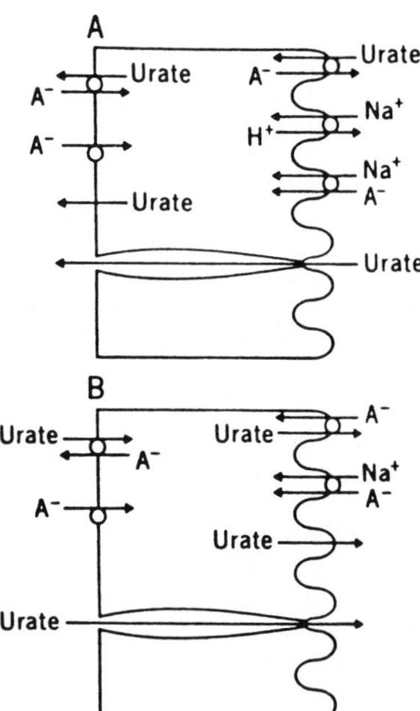

FIG. 125-1 Proposed scheme for urate reabsorption (*A*) and secretion (*B*) in the proximal tubules of rats. The luminal surface is to the right. (*From Kahn and Weinman.*[83] *Used by permission.*)

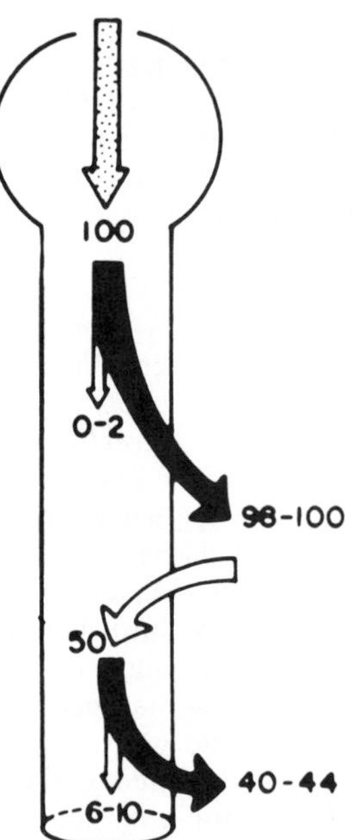

FIG. 125-2 Model for the renal handling of urate in humans. The size and direction of arrows indicate intensity and direction of urate transport. The stippled arrow represents filtered urate; the solid arrow, urate reabsorption; and the open arrow, urate secretion or urate remaining in tubular fluid after reabsorption. Numerical values indicate hypothetical orders of magnitude of the transport processes (*From Rieselbach and Steele.*[121] *Used by permission.*)

this system has not as yet been demonstrated. The flux of urate from the tubule cell to the lumen could occur by simple diffusion or could be mediated by an anion exchanger, most likely with chloride.

Models for Urate Handling in Humans

Studies on renal handling of urate in humans generated models of a two-, a three-, and finally a four-component system. The first model, suggested in 1950 by Berliner et al.,[73] included glomerular filtration followed by extensive, though incomplete, tubular reabsorption. Eleven years later, following the demonstration of uric acid secretion in humans, this third component was added by Gutman and Yu.[116] More recently, a fourth component, that of postsecretory reabsorption, was added in order to explain the effects of pyrazinamide in some patients or conditions which otherwise, according to the three-component model, could only be interpreted as enhanced tubular secretion of urate. These effects of pyrazinamide included the suppression of the increased uric acid clearance in patients with Wilson disease[24] and Hodgkin disease[32,33] and the suppression in normal subjects, by pretreatment with pyrazinamide, of the probenecid-induced uricosuria, of the uricosuric response to intravenous chlorothiazide,[116] and of the increased urate clearance in volume expansion associated with hypertonic sodium chloride administration.[117] The four-component model (Fig. 125-2) was suggested in 1973 by Steele and Boner,[118] Steele,[119] and Diamond and Paolino,[120] and in 1974 by Rieselbach and Steele.[121] It includes glomerular filtration, early proximal reabsorption, later proximal secretion, and extensive postsecretory reabsorption, which could occur at the same location as the secretion, separate and distal to it, or both. Evidence for the existence of the postsecretory reabsorption site with a different mechanism than that of the presecretory reabsorption site was obtained in several patients with renal hypouricemia (see below), in whom the increased urate clearance was attributed to a defect in postsecretory reabsorption.[8,24,32,122,123]

Another model has been proposed (Fig. 125-3).[124] It is similar to the former model, including the same four components, but according to which, reabsorption and secretion of urate occur simultaneously along all the proximal tubule, each at different intensities at the different segments of the tubule. The model suggests a higher density of reabsorption transporters at the S_1 segment, as compared with S_2 and S_3, and a higher intensity of secretion at the S_2 region of the tubule. These differences in the intensities of reabsorption and secretion along the tubule result in initial net reabsorption of urate in the S_1 segment, followed by net secretion in the S_2 segment and by net reabsorption in the S_3 segment. According to both models the residual urinary urate in the S_1 region is derived originally from filtration, whereas that in the S_3 segment arises from secretion in the S_2 segment.

Factors That Affect Renal Handling of Urate in Humans

Age and Sex. Urate excretion becomes less efficient with age.[125-127] Accordingly, plasma urate levels increase with age. This change with maturation was attributed to increased urate reabsorption, rather than a decrease in urate secretion.[127] The mean clearance of urate is 1.2 to 2.3 ml/min higher in females than in males.[128,129] Exogenous estrogen was found to produce a significant increase in urate clearance in transsexual males.[130]

Extracellular Fluid Volume and Urine Flow Rate. The extracellular fluid volume or, more precisely, the volume of the effective arterial circulation is one of the most dominant

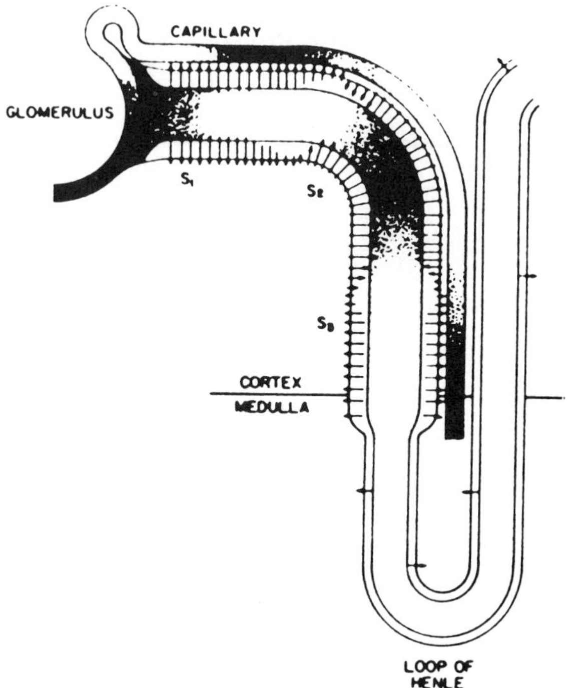

FIG. 125-3 Mode of renal handling of urate in humans. The size and direction of arrows indicate intensity and direction of urate transport. The density of shading in the tubule and the capillary indicates the relative amounts of urate (not concentration) in the lumina; see text for details. (*From Grantham and Chonko.*[124] *Used by permission.*)

factors in renal urate handling.[93,131-137] Volume expansion (like that associated with administration of isotonic or hypertonic saline) increases urate clearance, whereas volume contraction (like that associated with restricted sodium chloride intake) decreases urate clearance. Presumably, these effects of changes in extracellular volume are mediated through alterations in urate reabsorption in the proximal tubule.[93,134,135] The rate of urinary flow affects urinary urate concentration and therefore may affect the back-diffusion of urate in the relatively impermeable terminal renal tubules.[136,137] Nevertheless, these effects are probably minor in relation to those of the extracellular fluid volume, as can be judged from the values of renal urate clearance in patients with inappropriate secretion of antidiuretic hormone and in patients with nephrogenic diabetes insipidus. In the former patients with expanded extracellular fluid volume, renal urate clearance is high despite slow urinary flow rate.[28,29,138] In the latter patients with contracted extracellular fluid volume, urinary urate clearance is decreased despite rapid urinary flow rate.[139]

Drugs. Many drugs affect renal urate excretion.[124,140] A biphasic effect (different effect at low and high concentration of the drug) was documented for some of the drugs and suggested for all others.[140] Pyrazinamide, probenecid, phenylbutazone, and salicylate inhibit urate secretion at low doses, but inhibit urate reabsorption at high doses.[85,116,141,142] Diuretic drugs are initially uricosuric by direct inhibition of urate reabsorption, but their long-term administration is associated with contraction of the extracellular fluid volume, resulting in antiuricosuria.[116,143-147] An additional property of some of the diuretic drugs is their tendency to compete with tubular urate secretion, decreasing further urate excretion.[145]

RENAL HANDLING OF URATE IN HEREDITARY RENAL HYPOURICEMIA

Renal Clearance of Urate

The data on the renal handling of urate in the propositi of the 28 families documented to be affected with the true hereditary renal hypouricemia are summarized in Table 125-1. As can be seen from the table, all the propositi have significantly decreased plasma urate levels, ranging from 12 to 119 μM. Indeed, these markedly low serum urate values were unexpected in almost all cases, being found during investigation for unrelated medical problems (to exclude urolithiasis, see below). Urinary urate excretion in the propositi is normal or excessive, renal urate clearance is markedly elevated (ranging from 39.5 to 173 ml/min), and the fractional clearance of urate (FC_{ur}) ranges from 36 to 169 percent. However, the FC_{ur} was found to exceed 100 percent in only 4 of the 28 propositi. Twenty of the propositi were male and eight were female; their ages at diagnosis ranged from 3 to 74 years.

The group of subjects with renal hypouricemia in whom no conclusive evidence for familiality could be obtained[1,47,65-72] had similar levels of uric acid in serum and urine as in the propositi with the familial disorder.

Two normouricemic subjects were reported[67,77] to have a renal defect for uric acid handling, which was manifested as increased renal urate clearance only under conditions of purine load. The familiality of this type of defect in the renal handling of urate is not clarified.

Nature of the Renal Transport Defect

Increased renal urate clearance could be caused by defective reabsorption or by increased secretion. Based on the models of urate transport in the proximal tubule (see Fig. 125-1) and of renal handling of urate in humans (see Figs. 125-2 and 125-3), as presented above, five main possibilities of specific abnormalities in the active urate transport processes should be considered as causing renal hypouricemia (Fig. 125-4):

A. Total transport defect (no reabsorption and no secretion)

B. Total reabsorption defect

C. Presecretory reabsorption defect

D. Postsecretory reabsorption defect

E. Increased secretion

Being an inborn error, this classification depends of course on the genetic control of each of the active transport processes. Accordingly, possibility A is based on the assumption of a common genetic control for all transport processes (i.e., reabsorption and secretion of urate in the renal proximal tubules reflect only inverse positioning of the same mechanism), possibility B on the assumption of a common genetic control for all reabsorption processes, and possibilities C and D on the assumption of separate genetic control for the two reabsorption processes.

Effect of Pyrazinamide and of Probenecid on FC_{ur}. According to the simple model of the renal handling of urate in humans, as depicted in Fig. 125-2, one may distinguish between the above types of transport defects by use of drugs inhibiting urate reabsorption or secretion. In the localization of the tubular defect in renal hypouricemia, two drugs, probenecid

Table 125-1 Data on Renal Handling of Urate in Hereditary Renal Hypouricemia

First author	Year	Propositus: Age at Diagnosis	Propositus: Sex	Plasma Urate, μM	Urinary Urate, mmol/24 h	C_{ur} ml/min	FC_{ur} (C_{ur}/GFR), %
1. Greene[43]	1972	23	M	53	3.80	46	38
2. Khachadurian[44]	1973	57	M	12	4.74	173	148
3. Sperling[45]	1974	53	M	35	4.11	55	70.6
4. Akaoka[46]	1975	28	M	24	4.11	88.5	107.3
5. Akaoka[47]	1977	40	M	32	3.55	99	75
6. Akaoka[47]	1977	41	M	28	3.73	114	95
7. Benjamin[48]	1977	37	F	65	3.94	39.5	37.6
8. Benjamin[49]	1978	48	M	71	4.46	553	38.5
9. Frank[50]	1979	39	M	59	5.95	80	47.9
10. Frank[50]	1979	37	M	59	5.95	60	45
11. Weitz[51]	1980	8	M	41	2.11	35.2	43.7
12. Hedley[52]	1980	63	M	77	6.20	—	169
13. Fujiwara[53]	1980	24	M	53	5.72	74.1	56.8
14. Delevelle[54]	1980	74	M	25	3.13	85	80
15. Garty[55]	1981	10	M	89	1.70	45.8	36
16. Matsuda[56]	1982	43	F	29	3.97	83	91.7
17. Tachibana[57]	1982	35	M	24	—	—	—
18. Vinay[58]	1983	43	F	18	6.19	144	77
19. Takeda[59]	1985	3	F	47	3.94	75	90
20. Takeda[59]	1985	10	M	59	7.79	117	88
21. Takeda[59]	1985	12	F	41	9.10	93	102
22. Takeda[59]	1985	4	M	47	6.79	102	146
23. Nakajima[60]	1987	36	M	119	—	31.2	31.9
24. Shichiri[61]	1987	25	F	12	—	54.9	45.2
25. Shichiri[61]	1987	40	F	55	—	74.6	60.6
26. Hisatome[62]	1988	22	M	65	3.55	31.9	46
27. Gafter[63]	1989	60	F	59	4.79	60.5	65.5
28. Tofuku[64]	1990	16	M	41	4.58	76.4	—

NOTE: Values given for serum urate are the lowest or average values reported for each subject. Values given for urinary urate excretion, for urate clearance (C_{ur}) and for FC_{ur} are the highest or average values reported for each subject.

and pyrazinamide, are employed. Probenecid is the generic name for 4-[(dipropylamino)sulfonyl] benzoic acid and has a dual action on urinary urate excretion. When administered by the oral or intravenous route, at the usual "high" doses, it increases renal urate clearance markedly[43,123,148] (Table 125-2). On the other hand, at low doses, the drug causes a so-called paradoxical urate retention.[148] While the increase of renal urate clearance at a high dose of probenecid appears to be due solely to inhibition of tubular reabsorption, the paradoxical urate retention at low doses has been explained by inhibition of tubular secretion. In any event, the net effect of a high probenecid dose (2 to 3 g orally) is a substantial rise in urate excretion. There are several reasons for the assumption that probenecid inhibits tubular urate reabsorption chiefly at the postsecretory site. First, in the plasma, probenecid is largely bound to albumin[149]; thus the amount filtered is relatively small. Second, probenecid appears in the urine chiefly by tubular secretion, possibly by the same mechanism as uric acid.[150] The tubular secretion of probenecid would explain both its paradoxical urate-retaining action (at low doses) by competition with urate at the secretory site, and its reabsorption inhibitory action (at high dose) at a postsecretory tubular site.

Whether and to what extent probenecid also inhibits presecretory tubular reabsorption is still an open question. Evidently, the manyfold increase of urate clearance in response to probenecid in normal subjects is compatible with the dominance of postsecretory absorption in the normal regulation of renal urate excretion. On the other hand, in subjects with renal hypouricemia, the probenecid response should be attenuated, its magnitude depending on the tubular site of the defect, whether postsecretory or presecretory or both. In the case in which the defect is exclusively postsecretory and complete (type D), probenecid will have no effect on urinary urate excretion. However, in cases in which the defect is presecretory (type C), the probenecid response will be maintained but may be of lesser magnitude than normal. When the defect in tubular urate reabsorption is combined presecretory and postsecretory (type B), the probenecid response will be nil.

The separation between the reabsorption sites, as well as the very existence of the postsecretory site, were postulated according to data obtained by the use of pyrazinamide, although the exact effect of this drug on renal urate handling is still under dispute. Following administration of pyrazinamide, urinary uric acid is transiently reduced to very low levels, without change of GFR (Table 125-2).[151,152] This effect may be attributed to inhibition of urate secretion, a property demonstrated for this drug in dogs[153] and rats.[154] Indeed, this property has been extensively used as a pharmacologic aid in quantitating urate reabsorption and secretion. The pyrazinamide suppression test in humans[119] is based on the assumption that pyrazinamide blocks completely and specifically only urate secretion. It is performed by determining uric acid excretion before and immediately after administration of pyrazinamide, in a dose sufficient to give maximal suppression of uric acid excretion (usually 3 g, administered orally). The difference between the amount of

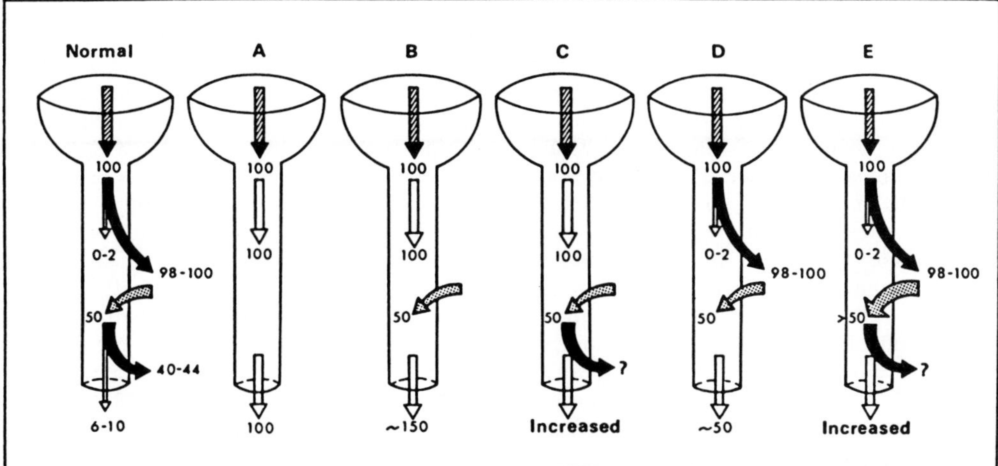

FIG. 125-4 Model for the renal handling of urate in normal humans and the five possible defects (*A* to *E*) that may cause renal hypouricemia. See text for detailed explanation. The size and direction of arrows indicate intensity and direction of urate transport. The hatched arrows represent filtered urate; the solid arrows, urate reabsorption; the dotted arrows, urate secretion; and the open arrows, urate remaining in the tubular fluid after reabsorption. Numerical values indicate hypothetical order of magnitude of the transport process. The normal model is based on the model suggested by Rieselbach and Steele.[121] (*From Sperling, Contributions to Nephrology, 100:1, 1992. Used by permission.*)

urate filtered and that excreted under maximal effect of the drug is taken to represent urate reabsorption, which was found to be 98 to 99 percent complete in normal humans. On the other hand, the decrement in uric acid excretion, observed under maximal effect of pyrazinamide, is taken to represent tubular urate secretion. The latter was found to account for 80 to 85 percent of excreted urate in normal subjects.[151,155] Data obtained in vivo and in vitro indicate, however, that attribution of the suppression of uric acid excretion by pyrazinamide to a specific effect of blocking tubular urate secretion is an oversimplification. Evidence was first obtained that the effect of pyrazinamide depends

Table 125-2 **Effect of Pyrazinamide and Probenecid on FC_{ur} in Control Subjects and Differentiation by These Effects between the Various Types of Renal Hypouricemia***

No. of Control Subjects	FC_{ur} %	Effect on FC_{ur}, %: Pyrazinamide	Probenecid
10[a]	9.8±3.4	Decrease to 2.15±1.7	
14[b]	10.3±4	Decrease to 1.2±1.1	
10[c]	8.2±0.6	Decrease to 1.8	Increase to 40.4±8
10[d]	9.3±2.6	Decrease to 1.13±0.35	
5[e]	8.4±2.7		Increase to 46.7±8.3
Type of renal hypouricemia			
A. Total transport defect (reabsorption and secretion)	100	No effect	No effect
B. Total reabsorption defect	>100	Attenuated effect Decreasing FC_{ur} to 100%	No effect
C. Presecretory reabsorption defect	?	Attenuated effect	Attenuated effect
D. Postsecretory reabsorption defect	<100	Normal effect	No effect
E. Increased secretion	<100	Normal effect	Normal effect

*Values represent means ±SD.

SOURCES OF DATA: a = Steele and Rieselbach[151]; b = Tofuku et al.[68]; c = Meisel and Diamond[8] (values represent C_{ur} in ml/min instead of FC_{ur} with 1 g probenecid administered intravenously); d = Akaoka et al.,[47] Kawabe et al.,[66] Fujiwara et al.,[53] and Shichiri et al.[69]; e = Fujiwara et al.[53] and Shichiri et al.[69]

on its concentration and that at high concentrations it also inhibits urate reabsorption, increasing urate excretion.[156] Support for the dual effect of the drug was indicated by the findings that pyrazinamide inhibited the precession of [^{14}C]urate relative to [^{3}H]inulin into the urine when both compounds were simultaneously injected into a peritubular capillary,[101] and that pyrazinoate inhibited the reabsorption of [^{14}C]urate injected into the rat proximal tubule.[157] In addition to its inhibitory effect on urate reabsorption and secretion, pyrazinamide was also found to enhance urate reabsorption.[158] Thus, the suppression effect of pyrazinamide on urate excretion may reflect both inhibition of urate secretion and enhancement of urate reabsorption. Studies in isolated membranes have indicated that pyrazinoate has affinity for the urate anion exchanger in the brush-border membrane.[98,113,159] Accordingly, when in the lumen this drug will inhibit urate reabsorption, but when in the cell it will enhance urate reabsorption. These effects have been demonstrated in studies with dog brush-border vesicles.[83]

Although, in view of the foregoing data, the interpretation of the pyrazinamide effect in normal subjects, as well as subjects with increased renal urate clearance, should be done with reservation and regarded as tentative, the pyrazinamide response may be still interpreted as mainly reflecting the inhibitory effect of the drug on tubular urate secretion, even though the magnitude of the response need not be an exact measure of it. In normal subjects in whom tubular secretion is the main source of urinary urate, pyrazinamide response is expected to be of great magnitude (see Table 125-2). On the other hand, in subjects with increased urate clearance due to a defect in tubular urate reabsorption, the pyrazinamide response could vary according to the site of the defect, whether presecretory or postsecretory. In case of a postsecretory defect in urate reabsorption (type D), pyrazinamide will markedly reduce urinary urate excretion, bringing it to a level similar to that reached in pyrazinamide-treated normal subjects. In the case of a presecretory defect (type C), however, the pyrazinamide response will be attenuated. In the case of combined presecretory and postsecretory defective tubular urate reabsorption (type B), in which the clearance of urate exceeds the GFR, pyrazinamide will reduce the elevated urate clearance to a value close or equal to GFR. In patients with a total transport defect (type A), pyrazinamide will have no effect, but in case of increased secretion (type E), the effect of the drug will be normal.

According to the above considerations on the renal urate handling and the action of pyrazinamide and probenecid, the five types of renal hypouricemia would be expected to conform to the following responses (see Table 125-2): In a total transport defect (type A), FC_{ur} should be about 100 percent, and this value should not be altered by administration of pyrazinamide or probenecid. In a total reabsorption defect (type B)—that is, absence of reabsorption at both the presecretory and postsecretory sites, but presence of normal secretion—FC_{ur} should be greater than 100 percent. In such a defect, blocking secretion by pyrazinamide will result in an attenuated decrease in FC_{ur}, which should approach 100 percent. Administration of probenecid will not alter FC_{ur}. In a presecretory reabsorption defect (type C), FC_{ur} cannot be estimated, since the maximal rate for net tubular absorption (T_m) for urate at the postsecretory site is unknown. If indeed the excreted urate represents the amount of secreted urate escaping reabsorption at the postsecretory reabsorption site, one can expect a substantial proportion, probably the majority of the filtered load (not reabsorbed at the presecretory site) to escape the postsecretory reabsorption too. If this is the case, then FC_{ur} in a presecretory reabsorption defect will be greater than 100 percent. In a presecretory reabsorption defect, administration of pyrazinamide will decrease FC_{ur} and administration of probenecid will increase this parameter, but both effects will be attenuated. In defective reabsorption at the postsecretory site (type D), FC_{ur} will be less than 100 percent, if the amount secreted is less than that filtered. In the presence of such a defect, administration of pyrazinamide will decrease FC_{ur} to normal levels, but administration of probenecid will have no effect. In the case of a defect manifested in increased secretion (type E), FC_{ur} will probably be less than 100 percent (unless the secretion is increased to such a level that its fraction escaping reabsorption will exceed the amounts of filtered urate). In such a defect, the administration of pyrazinamide and of probenecid will result in a normal response.

Type of Defect in Hereditary Renal Hypouricemia

The greatest proportion of the propositi—15 subjects—had FC_{ur} values between 36 and 85 percent and exhibited an attenuated response to the administration of pyrazinamide and probenecid. These propositi[43,45,47-51,53,54,56,62,63,64] may be classified as type C—affected with presecretory reabsorption defect. In some of these subjects,[50-52] the effect of pyrazinamide was somewhat greater than in the others, but the lowest FC_{ur} values, obtained under the maximal effect of the drug, did not reach the normal level.

Two patients studied by Akaoka et al.,[47] one studied by Matsuda et al.,[56] and three studied by Takeda et al.,[59] had FC_{ur} values close to 100 percent, which were not affected significantly by administration of pyrazinamide and probenecid. These six cases may fit with either type C or A. In only three of the propositi, FC_{ur} values were clearly greater than 100 percent. In two of them, the pyrazinamide and probenecid tests were not done. In the third patient, a 4-year-old Japanese boy,[59] the tests were done, but under different conditions than those adopted by all other investigators. In this boy, pyrazinamide had almost no effect, whereas benzbromarone (employed instead of probenecid) had an inverse effect, decreasing FC_{ur}. This case could fit with total reabsorption defect (type B). Two brothers reported by Nakajima et al.[60] exhibited normal response to pyrazinamide and probenecid and, therefore, were classified with type E (increased secretion). Two cases reported by Shichiri et al.[61] exhibited resistance to both pyrazinamide and probenecid administration and, therefore, were suggested to represent a subtotal defect in urate transport (subtotal type A). None of the propositi could be conclusively classified with type D. Thus, of the 22 propositi studied for the effects of the drugs, 14 could definitely be classified with type C (presecretory reabsorption defect), 6 with type C or A (total transport defect), 1 with type B (total reabsorption defect), 1 with type A, and 1 with type E. None of the propositi could be classified with type D (postsecretory reabsorption defect).

Nature of the Defect in Other Conditions of Renal Hypouricemia

The pyrazinamide and probenecid tests were done in patients with the Fanconi syndrome,[8] Wilson disease,[24] Hodgkin disease,[32,33] and hyperparathyroidism.[123] In some of these patients, the renal hypouricemia was part of a generalized tubular reabsorption defect, such as in the Fanconi syndrome, whereas in the others it represented an isolated defect. Interestingly, most if not all of these subjects could be classified as type D (postsecretory reabsorption defect), which was not found in the subjects with hereditary isolated renal hypouricemia. One subject with Hodgkin disease was classified as type D,[33] but two other subjects with Hodgkin disease exhibited a normal response to pyrazinamide and were classified as having increased secretion.[32] Nevertheless, the probenecid effect was not studied in these patients; therefore, the normal pyrazinamide effect could also be interpreted to reflect a postsecretory reabsorption defect. The subjects reported with isolated renal hypouricemia but without proof for familiality represent a heterogeneous group. One of these subjects,[68] could be classified as type D. Three subjects[69,70] could be classified as type E. They had moderately increased FC_{ur} values, which were normally affected by both pyrazinamide and probenecid or sulfinpyrazone.[70] Three such patients, studied by Gaspar et al.,[72] exhibited a normal response to pyrazinamide and were classified as affected with impaired postsecretory reabsorption. An additional subject in this group, who demonstrated a normal response to pyrazinamide but also the usual response to probenecid, was classified as affected with enhanced tubular secretion. In two other subjects, studied by Shichiri et al.,[160] administration of probenecid and of pyrazinamide did not affect FC_{ur}. These subjects were classified, therefore, as type A—that is, with total transport defect, including both reabsorption and secretion. Only three of the subjects[68,71] could be classified as type C, the most common type in the group with hereditary renal hypouricemia. In the rest of the subjects of this group, the results of the pyrazinamide and probenecid tests did not allow classification.

In the two normouricemic subjects, in whom increased FC_{ur} was found only following purine load,[67,77] the effect of pyrazinamide was normal. In one of these subjects,[67] the defect was suggested to be at the postsecretory reabsorption site, in view of an attenuated response of FC_{ur} to administration of benzbromarone (given instead of probenecid). In the other subject,[77] a high rate of secretion was demonstrated following RNA administration, but the probenecid test was not performed.

The above data may be taken to suggest that type C, the presecretory reabsorption defect, is the most common (if not the only type) among the subjects with hereditary (isolated) renal hypouricemia, whereas type D (postsecretory reabsorption defect) is the most common in patients with acquired renal hypouricemia and in patients with hereditary renal hypouricemia associated with a generalized renal tubular reabsorption defect. According to the foregoing discussion, in subjects who from all possible aspects appear to be affected with the true hereditary renal hypouricemia, but who lack familiality, demonstration of a presecretory reabsorption defect may be taken to support this classification, whereas demonstration of the postsecretory reabsorption defect may be taken to refute it.

Urate Transport in Nonrenal Tissues

Assuming that deletion of a specific carrier is the primary abnormality leading to the defective reabsorption of urate in the renal tubule of the subjects with hereditary renal hypouricemia, the tissue specificity of this defect was investigated.[58,161]

Erythrocytes. Uric acid transport into normal human erythrocytes has been shown to be partially inhibited by hypoxanthine,[162] and this is presumed to represent active uric acid transport mediated by an enzymatic system. This active system was suggested to be lacking in the Dalmatian coach hound,[163] but found later to be normal in these dogs.[58] Uric acid transport into erythrocytes was studied in five hypouricemic subjects.[58,161] In all these subjects, urate uptake by the erythrocytes—total uptake as well as that inhibited by hypoxanthine—was normal (Figs. 125-5 and 125-6). The lack of expression of the transport defect in the erythrocytes is expected, since to our knowledge the respective transport defect cannot be demonstrated in erythrocytes in any of the known renal tubular transport disorders.

Intestine. Active urate transport through the normal intestinal wall has not been demonstrated.[164,165] Nevertheless, the intestinal uptake of urate was studied in one hypouricemic subject,[161] since genetically determined renal transport defects are often expressed also in the intestinal mucosa, as in cystinuria,[166] iminoglycinuria,[167] and the Hartnup syndrome.[168] The intestinal absorption of uric acid was gauged by the 7 days' cumulative urinary excretion of [^{14}C], following oral administration of [^{14}C]urate (in the presence of bacteriostasis). The value in the hypouicemic subject was similar to that obtained in two control subjects (Fig. 125-7). The apparently accelerated urinary excretion of labeled uric acid

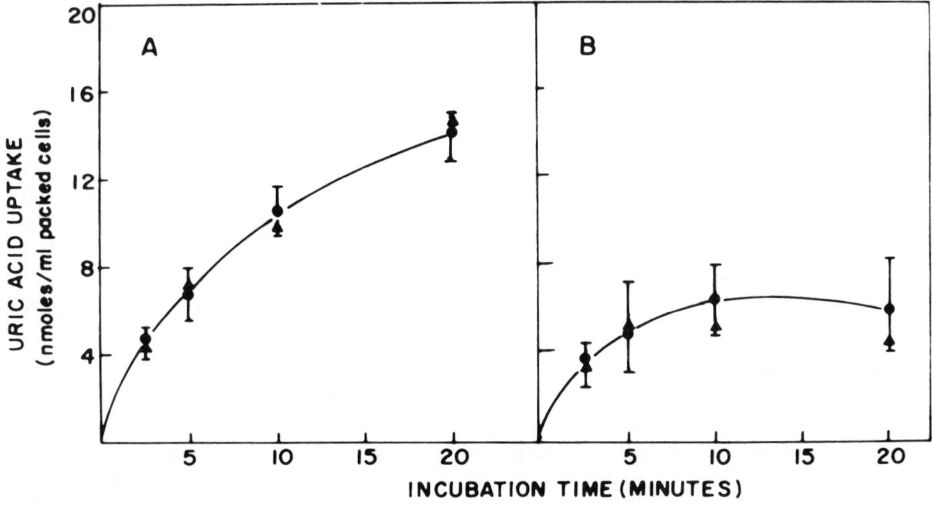

FIG. 125-5 Uptake of uric acid by erythrocytes. The range and mean for five normal subjects (●) and the mean of two experiments for a patient with renal hypouricemia (▲) are presented. *A*, total uptake; *B*, hypoxanthine-inhibited uptake. (*From Sperling et al.*[161] *Used by permission.*)

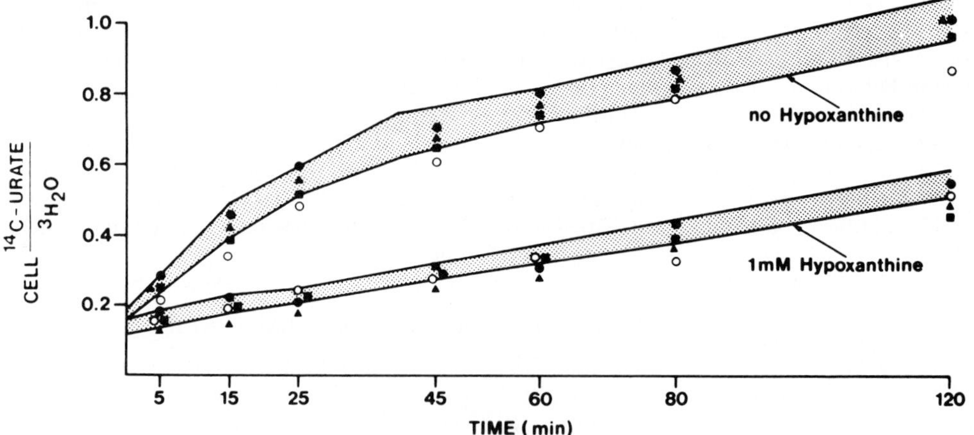

FIG. 125-6 Transport of urate into erythrocytes. The transport is the ratio of [^{14}C]labeled urate space to tritiated water space, with and without hypoxanthine in the buffer. Hatched areas represent ranges for normal controls; symbols represent values for four hypouricemic patients. (*From Vinay et al.*[58] *Used by permission.*)

in the patient may be taken to reflect his increased uric acid clearance.

Presence of an Endogenous Uricosuric Agent

In all the above considerations, the existence of an inborn primary renal tubular urate transport defect was presumed. However, in making this assumption and the above interpretations as to the location of the tubular defect, caution should be exercised in view of the possibility that the renal tubular abnormalities may be secondary to an abnormal metabolite produced elsewhere in the body or to qualitative or quantitative alterations in modulators affecting urate transport processes. The presence of a humoral uricosuric factor may be possible in some conditions with acquired renal hypouricemia, in which the transitory nature of the defect was demonstrated. In Hodgkin disease, serum uric acid and renal uric acid clearance became normal following chemotherapy, but the hypouricemia and increased renal clearance of urate reappeared with recrudescence of disease.[24,33] Similarly, in severe burns, the increased renal urate clearance was found to decrease to normal with recovery.[169] Nevertheless, there is no experimental evidence to date for the presence of a uricosuric agent in the plasma of patients with acquired or hereditary renal hypouricemia. Infusing the plasma of a hypouricemic patient with Hodgkin disease into a *Cebus albifrons* monkey did not affect urate clearance.[170] Furthermore, unpublished studies in our laboratory in rabbit kidney slices failed to detect any abnormal uricosuric agent in the plasma of several subjects with renal hypouricemia.

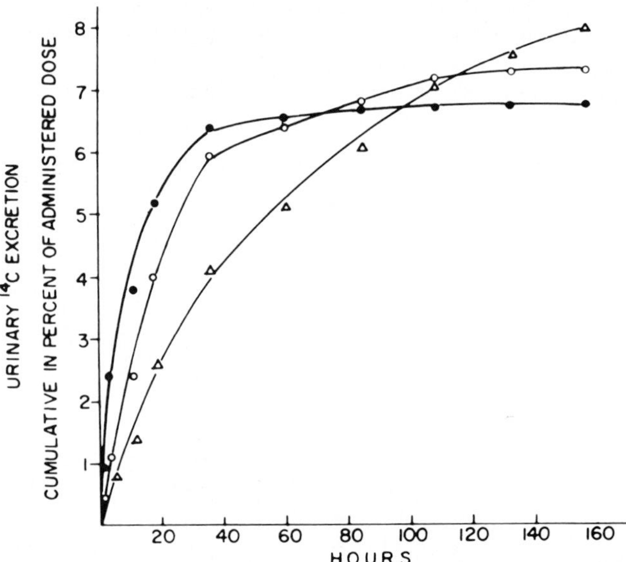

FIG. 125-7 Urine excretion of orally administered [^{14}C]labeled uric acid. Symbols are (●) for a patient with hereditary renal hypouricemia and (○) and (Δ) for normal subjects. (*From Sperling et al.*[161] *Used by permission.*)

The Dalmatian Coach Hound. This breed of dogs differs from others in that they are relatively hyperuricemic and hyperuricosuric and exhibit increased renal urate clearance.[171-178] The relative hyperuricemia–hyperuricosuria in this breed of dogs was demonstrated to reflect a defective uric acid transport into hepatocytes, the uricase-containing tissue.[179] On the other hand, the reason for the increased renal urate clearance has not yet been clarified. It could reflect a urate transport defect in the kidney or in all tissues.[171,180] Moreover, data are available suggesting that the increased renal urate clearance in this breed of dog reflects the presence of a uricosuric substance produced in the Dalmatian liver. The results of the liver transplantation experiments performed by Kuster et al.[180,181] support this hypothesis. These investigators found that when non-Dalmatian dogs received Dalmatian livers, the renal clearance and excretion of uric acid increased to values typical of Dalmatians and that when Dalmatians received non-Dalmatian livers, the above parameters diminished to those typical for non-Dalmatians. These results were taken to indicate that the Dalmatian liver is responsible for both the increased amount of excreted urate, as well as the increased renal urate clearance. According to the results of this study, the increased renal urate clearance in the Dalmatian is caused by an abnormal metabolite produced in the liver.

An additional support for the possibility that a humoral substance may affect renal urate transport and therefore that abnormality in such a substance may be the primary defect in hereditary renal hypouricemia may be drawn from the finding that in the rabbit, a serum protein was found to modulate, by allosteric modification, the basolateral transporter associated with urate secretion (see above).[105]

CLINICAL SIGNIFICANCE

The hypouricemia in the syndrome is generally discovered during screening procedures, mainly for investigation of various diseases such as osteoporosis, familial hypercholesterolemia, urolithiasis, polyarthralgia, stomatitis, neurologic disorders, glomerulonephritis, idiopathic edema, noncongenital colloid goiter, etc. All these diseases, except for urolithiasis, are unrelated to the renal hypouricemia.

Hypouricemia. The hypouricemia as such has, as far as is known, no clinical significance. Indeed, speculatively, the hypouricemia might be advantageous in avoiding the risks associated with hyperuricemia, mainly the various clinical manifestations of urate crystal deposition disease.

Hyperuricosuria. In three patients with hereditary renal hypouricemia, the hypouricemia was associated with a marked hyperuricosuria, the urinary uric acid excretion exceeding 5.95 mmol/day. Furthermore, hyperuricosuria, although moderate, was present in many of the other hypouricemic propositi. Thus, hyperuricosuria appears to be a constant feature of isolated renal hypouricemia. Principally, the hyperuricosuria might reflect purine overproduction or diversion of intestinal urate elimination to urinary urate excretion consequent to the hypouricemia. There is no evidence in the hypouricemic hyperuricosuric subjects for purine overproduction. Incorporation of [^{14}N]glycine into urinary uric acid was measured in one such patient and was found to be moderately excessive,[47] probably reflecting the decreased intestinal urate disposal. Normal [^{15}N]glycine incorporation was found in another hypouricemic uric acid stone–forming patient as well as in two hypouricemic patients in whom familiality was not proven.[66]

Hypercalciuria. Hypercalciuria was associated with the renal hypouricemia in six of the propositi.[43,45,50,51] In all these subjects, in whom there was no detectable etiology for the hypercalciuria, it may be classified as "idiopathic hypercalciuria." In three of these,[43,50] the hypercalciuria was proven to be of the hyperabsorptive type—that is, secondary to increased intestinal calcium absorption. Thus far, evidence has not been obtained for a primary abnormality in renal calcium handling in any of these hypouricemic-idiopathic hypercalciuric patients. Thus, at this stage of knowledge, the renal tubular defect leading to hypouricemia may be considered as an isolated tubular abnormality in these subjects until proven otherwise. The apparently frequent association between the renal defect for urate handling and the intestinal calcium hyperabsorption is as yet unexplained.

Urolithiasis. Seven of the 28 propositi with inborn isolated renal hypouricemia[43,48,50,52,57] had urinary calculi. Three had uric acid stones, three had calcium oxalate stones, and one had a stone of unidentified composition. In four other propositi,[59] urolithiasis was present in other family members. The high prevalence of urolithiasis among the subjects with hereditary renal hypouricemia may be explained by the occurrence of hyperuricosuria and of hypercalciuria among these subjects. Indeed, the patients who had uric acid stones had the most significant hyperuricosuria (more than 5.95 mmol/day). It is not surprising that only some of the hypouricemic patients had evidence of urolithiasis, since hyperuricosuria or hypercalciuria are important but are not the only determinants in the causation of stone formation.

Of interest is the series of four subjects with idiopathic renal hypouricemia (no evidence for familiality or associating abnormalities) reported by Gaspar et al.[72] In this group, four had hyperuricosuria, three had hypercalciuria, and three had calcium oxalate nephrolithiasis.

Uric Acid Nephropathy. Acute uric acid nephropathy may occur in the presence of massive uricosuria, such as in the tumor lysis syndrome. More rarely it may occur also in some gouty subjects with excessive purine overproduction, especially in association with inborn errors of metabolism, such as the Lesch-Nyhan syndrome (see Chap. 50) and phosphoribosylpyrophosphate synthetase superactivity (see Chap. 49).

In view of the prevalence of hyperuricosuria in renal hypouricemia, the possibility of acute uric acid nephropathy in this syndrome should be taken into consideration, especially under conditions of temporary increased urate excretion (increased purine intake, increased ATP breakdown, etc). Such cases were first reported in nonhereditary renal hypouricemia. One patient[182] required hemodialysis due to oliguric renal failure. Renal biopsy showed amorphous uric acid crystals in some of the tubular lumina and mild-to-moderate interstitial inflammation. In this case the hyperuricosuria was attributed to the increased tubular uric acid secretion. Mild acute renal failure induced by exercise in three subjects with renal hypouricemia, one of whom had familial renal hypouricemia, was reported from Japan.[183] The clinical manifestations in these patients resembled very much the acute renal failure syndrome described by this group in 1982.[184] This syndrome, characterized by patchy renal vasoconstriction, is usually mild and nonoliguric, appears in young healthy subjects, and has a good prognosis. There is only mild to moderate rise in CK, suggesting that massive rhabdomyolysis does not occur. It has been suggested[183,184] that in the three reported subjects, the renal failure is caused by the precipitation of uric acid. Nevertheless, this could not be demonstrated in the affected patients. An additional case of familial renal hypouricemia associated with acute renal failure has been reported by Tofuku et al.[64] The authors speculated that the urinary urate excretion could have been accelerated in the patient due to the increased production of uric acid during physical exercise.

Decreased Bone Density. Decreased bone density was found to be associated with the hypercalciuria in two renal hypouricemic sibs[45] and osteoporosis was found in a 4-year-old boy with hereditary renal hypouricemia.[59] Similar abnormalities have not been observed in the other reported hypouricemic families. The association between renal hypouricemia and decreased bone density remains unexplained.

Genetics

Hereditary renal hypouricemia occurs when two mutant autosomal alleles occur at the locus which controls the urate transport site. Known consanguinity in parents of hypouricemic children in 5 of the 28 families[44-47,51] demonstrates the recessive mode of inheritance of the trait (Fig. 125-8). A dominant mode was suggested in one family,[52] in view of the finding that the propositus had three hypouricemic daughters, without consanguinity, and in another family,[60] due to the finding of borderline hypouricemia and increased urate clearance in the mother of two hypouricemic sons. Nevertheless, in the first family[52] serum uric acid levels reported for these daughters (119, 130, and 142 μM), could very well represent heterozygosity rather than homozygosity. The same is true for the mother of the second family.[60] There is no evidence for X-linkage in the reported pedigrees. In one family,[63] a pseudodominant transmission of a recessive disease was postulated. In at least six of the pedigrees,[44-46,49,50,62] both sexes were affected.

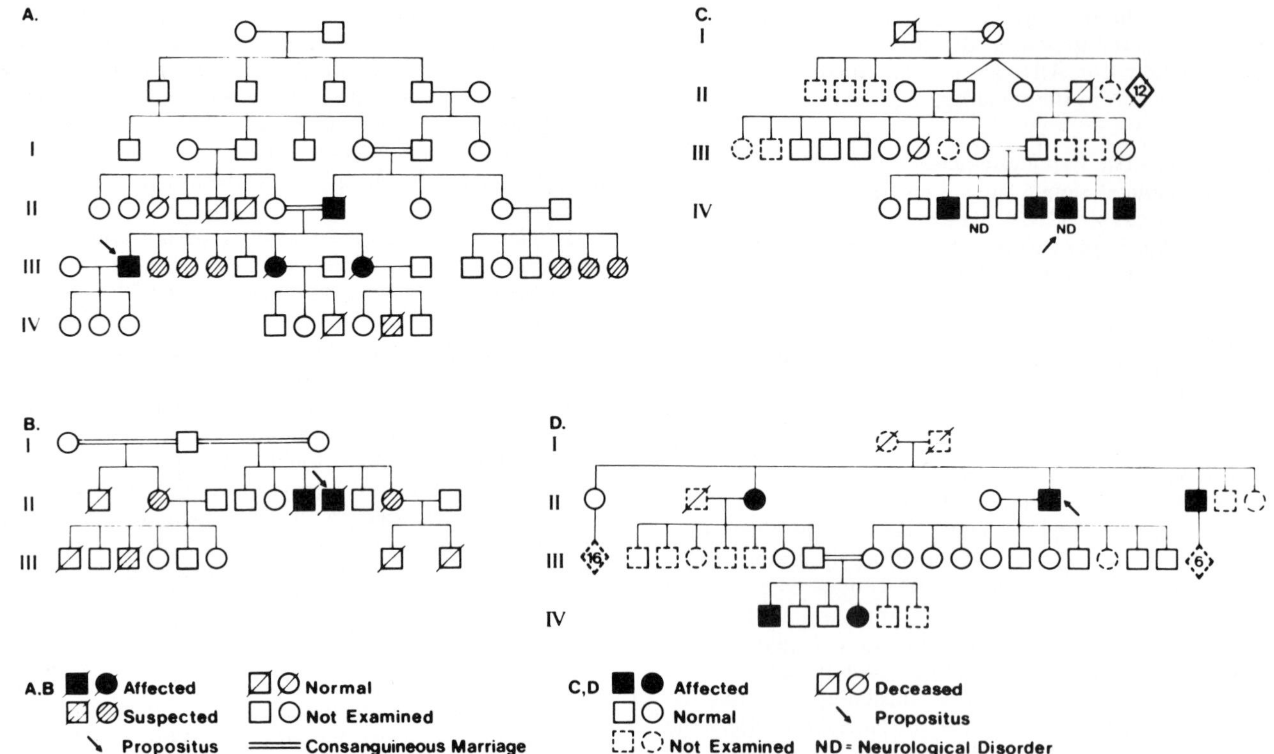

FIG. 125-8 Pedigrees of consanguineous families with hereditary renal hypouricemia. (A *from Akaoka et al.*[46]; B *from Akaoka et al.*[47]; C *from Weitz and Sperling;*[51] D *from Sperling et al.*[45] *All used by permission.*)

It is of interest that, in addition to exhibiting the same mode of inheritance, the vast majority of patients with hereditary renal hypouricemia were classified as being affected with the same type of reabsorption defect—at the presecretory site. Moreover, in none of the families with hereditary renal hypouricemia could an isolated defect for the postsecretory reabsorption site be demonstrated, although such a defect was suggested in other conditions of renal hypouricemia (see above). These findings may be taken to suggest that the presecretory and postsecretory reabsorption sites for urate in the proximal tubule are controlled by different genes.

Another point of interest is that all cases of hereditary renal hypouricemia reported from Israel[45,48-51,55,63] were Jews of non-Ashkenazic (i.e., Sephardic) origin: six were Iraqi, one was Libyan, and one was Turkish. It appears likely, therefore, that hereditary renal hypouricemia is relatively common among non-Ashkenazic Jews.

Treatment

As indicated above, urolithiasis is the only clinical manifestation which may be associated with hereditary renal hypouricemia. The urolithiasis is probably the result of the hyperuricosuria and the hypercalciuria found to be common in these patients. Thus, it is advisable to study the affected subjects carefully for these parameters and to treat them accordingly. High fluid intake and control of urinary pH may suffice to prevent uric acid stones.[185] In some cases, in which uric acid excretion is markedly excessive, allopurinol may be needed to reduce uric acid excretion. For prevention of calcium stones, patients exhibiting marked hypercalciuria should be treated by conventional means.

REFERENCES

1. Praetorius E, Kirk JE: Hypouricemia with evidence for tubular elimination of uric acid. *J Lab Clin Med* **35**:856, 1950.
2. Mikkelsen WM, Dodge HJ, Valkenburg H: The distribution of serum uric acid values in a population unselected as to gout or hypouricemia. *Am J Med* **39**:242, 1965.
3. Ramsdell CM, Kelley WN: The clinical significance of hypouricemia. *Ann Intern Med* **73**:239, 1973.
4. Dwosh IL, Roncari DAK, Marliss E, Fox IH: Hypouricemia in disease: A study of different mechanisms. *J Lab Clin Med* **90**:153, 1977.
5. Wyngaarden JB, Kelley WN: Miscellaneous forms of hypouricemia, in *Wyngaarden JB, Kelley WN (eds): Gout and Hyperuricemia*. New York, Grune & Stratton, 1976, p 411.
6. Wallis IA, Eagle RI: The adult Fanconi syndrome. II. Review of eighteen cases. *Am J Med* **22**:13, 1957.
7. Lee DBN, Drinkard JP, Rosen VJ, Gnick HC: The adult Fanconi syndrome: Observation on etiology, morphology, renal functions and mineral metabolism in three patients. *Medicine (Baltimore)* **51**:107, 1972.
8. Meisel AD, Diamond HS: Hyperuricosuria in the Fanconi syndrome. *Am J Med Sci* **274**:109, 1977.
9. Baron DN, Dent CE, Harris H, Hard EW, Jebson JB: Hereditary Pellagra-like skin rash with temporary cerebellar ataxia, constant renal aminoaciduria and other bizarre biochemical features. *Lancet* **2**:421, 1956.
10. Dent CE, Philpot GR: Xanthinuria, an inborn error (or deviation) of metabolism. *Lancet* **1**:182, 1954.
11. Holmes EW, Wyngaarden JB: Hereditary xanthinuria, in Stanbury JB, Wyngaarden JB, Fredrickson DS, Goldstein JL, Brown MS (eds): *The Metabolic Basis of Inherited Diseases*, 5th ed. New York, McGraw-Hill, 1983, p 1192.
12. Giblett ER, Amman AJ, Sandman R, Wara DW, Diamond LK: Nucleoside phosphorylase deficiency in a child with severely defective T-cell immunity and normal B-cell immunity. *Lancet* **1**:1010, 1975.

13. Cass E, Serrano C, Daimiel E, Michan A, Mateos F, Garcia Puig J: Prevalence, physiopathology and conditions associated with hypouricemia in a hospital population; analysis of 27,987 analytical determinations. *Rev Clin Esp* **186**:211, 1990.
14. Diaz Curiel M, Zea Mendoza A, Rapado A, Gonzalez Villasante J: Significacion clinica de la hipouicemia en 14,865 determinaciones del autoanalizador. *Rev Clin Esp* **139**:365, 1975.
15. Mikkelsen WM, Dodge HJ, Valkenburg H: The distribution of serum uric acid values in a population unselected as to gout or hyperuricemia. Tecumseh, Michigan 1959-1960. *Am J Med* **39**:242, 1965.
16. Ramsdell CM, Kelley WN: The clinical significance of hypouricemia. *Ann Intern Med* **24**:239, 1975.
17. Sperling O, Weinberger A, Pinkhas J, de Vries A: Frequency and causes of hypouricemia in hospital patients. *Isr J Med Sci* **13**:529, 1977.
18. van Pennen HJ: Causes of hypouricemia. *Ann Intern Med* **78**:977, 1973.
19. Yanasze M, Nakahama H, Mikami H, Fukuhara Y, Orita Y, Yoshikawa H: Prevalence of hypouricemia in apparently normal population. *Nephron* **48**:80, 1988.
20. Hisatome I, Ogino K, Kotake H, Ishiko R, Saito M, Hasegawa J, Mashiba H, Nakamoto S: Cause of persistent hypouricemia in outpatients. *Nephron* **51**:13, 1989.
21. Morgan HG, Steewart WK, Lowe KG, Stowers JM, Johnstone JH: Wilson's disease and the Fanconi syndrome. *Q J Med* **31**:361, 1962.
22. Leu ML, Strickland GT, Gutman RA: Renal function in Wilson's disease: Response to penicillamine therapy. *Am J Med Sci* **250**:381, 1970.
23. Elsas LJ, Hayslett JP, Spargo BH, Durant JL, Rosenberg LE: Wilson's disease with reversible renal tubular dysfunction. *Ann Intern Med* **75**:127, 1971.
24. Wilson DB, Goldstein NP: Renal urate excretion in patients with Wilson's disease. *Kidney Int* **4**:331, 1973.
25. Schneider JA, Schulman JD, Seegmiller JE: Cystinosis and the Fanconi syndrome, in Stanbury JB, Wyngaarden JB, Fredrickson DS (eds): *The Metabolic Basis of Inherited Disease,* 4th ed. New York, McGraw-Hill, 1978, p 1660.
26. Cusworth DC, Dent CE, Flynn FV: The amino-aciduria in galactosaemia. *Arch Dis Child* **30**:150, 1955.
27. Lamiere N, Mussche M, Bacle G, Kint J, Ringoir S: Hereditary fructose intolerance: A difficult diagnosis in the adult. *Am J Med* **65**:416, 1978.
28. Beck IH: Hypouricemia in the syndrome of inappropriate secretion of antidiuretic hormone. *N Engl J Med* **301**:528, 1979.
29. Osterlind K, Hansen M, Dombernowsky P: Hypouricemia and inappropriate secretion of antidiuretic hormone in small cell bronchogenic carcinoma. *Acta Med Scand* **209**:289, 1981.
30. Weinberger A, Santo M, Solomon F, Shalit M, Pinkhas J, Sperling O: Abnormality in renal urate handling in the syndrome of inappropriate secretion of antidiuretic hormone. *Isr J Med Sci* **18**:711, 1982.
31. Smithline N, Kassirer JP, Cohen JJ: Light-chain nephropathy. *N Engl J Med* **294**:71, 1976.
32. Bennett JS, Bond J, Singer I, Gottlieb AJ: Hypouricemia in Hodgkin's disease. *Ann Intern Med* **76**:751, 1972.
33. Tykarski A: Mechanism of hypouricemia in Hodgkin's disease. Isolated defect in postsecretory reabsorption of uric acid. *Nephron* **50**:217, 1988.
34. Weinstein B, Irreverre F, Watkin DM: Lung carcinoma, hypouricemia and aminoaciduria. *Am J Med* **39**:520, 1965.
35. Cooper DS: Oat-cell carcinoma and severe hypouricemia. *N Engl J Med* **288**:321, 1973.
36. Gorshein D, Asbell S: Ectopic production of hormones in tumors. *JAMA* **235**:2716, 1976.
37. Weinberger A, Pinkhas J, Sperling O, de Vries A: Frequency and causes of hypouricemia in hospital patients. *Isr J Med Sci* **13**:529, 1977.
38. Chisholm JJ Jr, Harrison HC, Everlein WR, Harrison HE: Amino-aciduria, hypophosphatemia and rickets in lead poisoning. *Am J Dis Child* **89**:159, 1955.
39. Clarkson TW, Kench JE: Urinary excretion of amino acids by men absorbing heavy metals. *Biochem J* **62**:361, 1965.
40. Gross JM: Fanconi syndrome (adult type) developing secondary to the ingestion of outdated tetracycline. *Ann Intern Med* **48**:523, 1963.
41. Schlosstein L, Kippen I, Bluestone R, Whitehouse MW, Klinenberg JR: Association between hypouricemia and jaundice. *Ann Rheum Dis* **33**:308, 1974.
42. Michelis MF, Warms PC, Fusco RD, Davis BB: Hypouricemia and hyperuricosuria in Laennec cirrhosis. *Arch Intern Med* **134**:681, 1974.
43. Greene ML, Marcus R, Aurbach GD, Kazam ES, Seegmiller JH: Hypouricemia due to isolated renal tubular defect. *Am J Med* **53**:361, 1972.
44. Khachadurian AK, Arslanian MJ: Hypouricemia due to renal uricosuria. *Ann Intern Med* **78**:547, 1973.
45. Sperling O, Weinberger A, Oliver I, Liberman UA, de Vries A: Hypouricemia, hypercalciuria and decreased bone density: A hereditary syndrome. *Ann Intern Med* **80**:482, 1974.
46. Akaoka I, Nishizawa T, Yano E, Takeuchi A, Nishida Y, Yoshimura T, Horiuchi Y: Familial hypouricemia due to renal tubular defect of urate transport. *Ann Clin Res* **7**:318, 1975.
47. Akaoka I, Nishizawa T, Yano E, Kamatani N, Nishida T, Sasaki S: Renal urate excretion in five cases of hypouricemia with an isolated renal defect of urate transport. *J Rheumtol* **4**:86, 1977.
48. Benjamin D, Sperling O, Weinberger A, Pinkhas J, de Vries A: Familial hypouricemia due to isolated renal tubular defect. *Nephron* **18**:220, 1977.
49. Benjamin D, Sperling O, Weinberger A, Pinkhas J: Familial hypouricemia due to isolated renal tubular defect. *Biomedicine* **29**:54, 1978.
50. Frank M, Many M, Sperling O: Familial renal hypouricemia: Two additional cases with uric acid lithiasis. *Br J Urol* **51**:88, 1979.
51. Weitz R, Sperling O: Hereditary renal hypouricemia: Isolated tubular defect of urate reabsorption. *J Pediatr* **96**:850, 1980.
52. Hedley JM, Phillips PJ: Familial hypouricemia and uric acid calculi: Case report. *J Clin Pathol* **33**:971, 1980.
53. Fujiwara J, Takamitsue J, Ueda N, Orita Y, Abe H: Hypouricemia due to an isolated defect in renal tubular urate reabsorption. *Clin Nephrol* **13**:44, 1980.
54. Delevelle F, Trombert JC, Bouvier MF, Canarelli G: Hypouricemie renale idiopathique: 1 observation. *Nouv Presse Med* **35**:2578, 1980.
55. Garty BZ, Nitzan M, Sperling O: Inborn hypouricemia due to isolated defect in renal tubular uric acid transport. *Isr J Med Sci* **17**:295, 1981.
56. Matsuda O, Shiigai T, Ito Y, Aonuma K, Takenchi J: A case of familial renal hypouricemia associated with increased secretion of PAH and idiopathic edema. *Nephron* **30**:178, 1982.
57. Tachibana S, Wakatsuki A, Kamei O, Ochi K, Takeuchi M: A case of idiopathic hypouricemia with recurrent renal stones. *Nish J Urol* **44**:795, 1982.
58. Vinay P, Gatterean A, Moulin B, Gougoux A, Lemieux G: Normal urate transport into erythrocytes in familial renal hypouricemia and in Dalmatian dog. *Can Med Assoc J* **128**:545, 1983.
59. Takeda E, Kuroda T, Ito M, Toshima K, Watanabe T, Ito M, Naiko E, Yokota I, Huwang TJ, Miyao M: Hereditary renal hypouricemia in children. *J Pediatr* **107**:71, 1985.
60. Nakajima H, Gomi M, Iida S, Kono N, Moriwaki K, Tarui S: Familial renal hypouricemia with intact reabsorption of uric acid. *Nephron* **45**:40, 1987.
61. Shichiri M, Iwamoto H, Maeda M, Kanayama M, Shiigai J: Hypouricemia due to subtotal defect in the urate transport. *Clin Nephrol* **28**:300, 1987.
62. Hisatome I, Ogino K, Saito M, Miyamoto J, Hasegawa J, Kotake H, Mashiba H, Nakamoto S: Renal hypouricemia due to an isolated renal defect of urate transport. *Nephron* **49**:81, 1988.
63. Gafter U, Zuta A, Frydman M, Lewinski UH, Levi J: Hypouricemia due to familial isolated renal tubular uricosuria—

evaluation with the combined pyrazinamide-probenecid test. *Minerva Electrol Metab* **15:**309, 1989.
64. Tofuku Y, Ito M, Takasaki H, Koni I, Takeda R: A case of familial renal hypouricemia associated with acute renal failure. *Pur Pyrimid Metabol (Jpn)* **14:**8, 1990.
65. Simkin PA, Skeith DA, Healy LA: Suppression of uric acid secretion in a patient with renal hypouricemia. *Adv Exp Med Biol* **41B:**723, 1974.
66. Kawabe K, Murayama T, Akaoka I: A case of uric acid renal stone with hypouricemia caused by tubular reabsorption defect of uric acid. *J Urol* **116:**690, 1976.
67. Soerensen LB, Levinson DJ: Isolated defect in postsecretory reabsorption of uric acid. *Ann Rheum Dis* **39:**180, 1980.
68. Tofuku Y, Kuroda M, Tekada R: Hypouricemia due to renal urate wasting. *Nephron* **30:**39, 1982.
69. Shichiri M, Matsuda O, Shugai T, Takeuchi J, Kanayama M: Hypouricemia due to an increment in renal tubular urate secretion. *Arch Intern Med* **142:**1855, 1982.
70. Dumont I, Decaux G: Hypouricemia related to a hypersecretional tubulopathy. *Nephron* **34:**256, 1983.
71. Smetana SS, Bar-Khayim J: Hypouricemia due to renal tubular defect: A study with the probenecid-pyrazinamide test. *Arch Intern Med* **145:**1200, 1985.
72. Gaspar GA, Puig TG, Mateos FA, Oria CR, Gomez MEM, Gil AA: Hypouricemia due to renal urate wasting: Different types of tubular transport defects. *Adv Exp Med Biol* **195A:**357, 1986.
73. Berliner RW, Hilton JG, Yu TF, Kennedy TJ Jr: The renal mechanism for urate excretion in man. *J Clin Invest* **29:**396, 1950.
74. Gutman AB, Yu TF, Berger L: Tubular secretion of urate in man. *J Clin Invest* **38:**1778, 1959.
75. Yu TF, Berger L, Stone DJ, Wolf J, Gutman AB: Effect of pyrazinamide and pyrazinoic acid on urate clearance and other discrete renal functions. *Proc Soc Exp Biol Med* **96:**264, 1957.
76. Yu TF, Berger L, Gutman AB: Suppression of tubular secretion of urate by pyrazinamide in the dog. *Proc Soc Exp Biol Med* **107:**905, 1961.
77. Steele TH, Rieselbach RE: The renal mechanism for urate homeostasis in normal man. *Am J Med* **43:**868, 1967.
78. Roch-Ramel F, Werner D: Urate transport in mammalian nephron, in Hatano M (ed): *Nephrology, Proceedings of the 11th International Congress of Nephrology.* Berlin, Springer-Verlag, 1991, p 1399.
79. Weiner IM: Urate transport in the nephron. *Am J Physiol* **237:**F85, 1979.
80. Werner D, Guisan B, Roch-Ramel F: Urate transport in the proximal tubule of human kidney. *Adv Exp Med Biol* **309A:**177, 1991.
81. Abramson RG, Levitt MF: Micropuncture study of uric acid in rat kidney. *Am J Physiol* **228:**1597, 1975.
82. Wyngaarden JB, Kelley WN: Gout, in Stanbury JB, Wyngaarden JB, Fredrickson DS, Goldstein JL, Brown MS (eds): *The Metabolic Basis of Inherited Disease,* 5th ed. New York, McGraw-Hill, 1983, p 1043.
83. Kahn AM, Weinman EJ: Urate transport in the proximal tubule: *in-vivo* and vesicle studies. *Am J Physiol* **249:**F789, 1985.
84. Roch-Ramel F, Chomety-Diez F, De Rougemont D, Tellier M, Widmer J, Peters G: Renal excretion of uric acid in the rat: A micropuncture and microperfusion study. *Am J Physiol* **230:**768, 1976.
85. Roch-Ramel F, Diez-Chomety F, Roth L, Weiner IM: A micropuncture study of urate excretion by Cebus monkeys employing high performance liquid chromatography with amperometric detection of urate. *Pflugers Arch* **383:**203, 1980.
86. Weinman EJ, Steplock D, Sansom SC, Knight TF, Senekjian HO: Use of high-performance liquid chromatography for determination of urate concentrations in nanoliter quantities of fluid. *Kidney Int* **19:**83, 1981.
87. Roch-Ramel F, Weiner IM: Excretion of urate by the kidney of Cebus monkeys: A micropuncture study. *Am J Physiol* **224:**1369, 1973.
88. Sansom SC, Senekjian HO, Knight TF, Babino H, Steplock D, Weinman EJ: Determination of the apparent transport constants for urate absorption in the rat proximal tubule. *Am J Physiol* **240:**F406, 1981.
89. de Rougement D, Henchoz M, Roch-Ramel F: Renal urate excretion at various plasma concentrations in the rat: A free-flow micropuncture study. *Am J Physiol* **231:**387, 1976.
90. Weinman EJ, Senekjian HO, Sansom SC, Steplock D, Sheth A, Knight TF: Evidence for active and passive urate transport in the rat proximal tubule. *Am J Physiol* **240:**F90, 1981.
91. Fanelli GM Jr, Weiner IM: Pyrazinoate excretion in the chimpanzee: Relation to urate disposition and the actions of uricosuric drugs. *J Clin Invest* **52:**1946, 1973.
92. Weiner IM, Fanelli GM Jr: Renal urate excretion in animal models. *Nephron* **14:**33, 1975.
93. Weinman EJ, Eknoyan G, Suki WN: The influence of the extracellular fluid volume on the tubular reabsorption of uric acid. *J Clin Invest* **55:**283, 1975.
94. Weinman EJ, Knight TF, McKenzie R, Eknoyan G: Dissociation of urate from sodium transport in the rat proximal tubule. *Kidney Int* **10:**295, 1976.
95. Weinman EJ, Steplock D, Suki WN, Eknoyan G: Urate reabsorption in proximal convoluted tubule of the rat kidney. *Am J Physiol* **231:**509, 1976.
96. Senekjian HO, Knight TF, Sansom SC, Weinman EJ: Effect of flow rate and the extracellular fluid volume on proximal urate and water absorption. *Kidney Int* **17:**155, 1980.
97. Kahn AM, Aronson PS: Urate transport via anion exchange in dog renal microvillus membrane vesicles. *Am J Physiol* **244:**F56, 1983.
98. Kahn AM, Branham S, Weinman EJ: Mechanism of urate and p-aminohippurate transport in rat renal microvillus membrane vesicles. *Am J Physiol* **245:**F151, 1983.
99. Podevin R, Ardaillou R, Paillard F, Fontannele J, Richet G: Etude chez l'homme de la cinetique d'apparition dans purine de l'acide urique 2 ^{14}C. *Nephron* **5:**134, 1968.
100. Weinman EJ, Sansom SC, Steplock DA, Sheth AU, Knight TF, Senekjian HO: Secretion of urate in the proximal convoluted tubule of the rat. *Am J Physiol* **239:**F383, 1980.
101. Kramp RA, Lenoir RH: Characteristics of urate influx in the rat nephron. *Am J Physiol* **229:**1654, 1975.
102. Weinman EJ, Sansom SC, Bennett S, Kahn AM: Effect of anion exchange inhibitors and para-aminohippurate on the transport of urate in the rat proximal tubule. *Kidney Int* **23:**832, 1983.
103. Platts MM, Mudge GH: Accumulation of uric acid by slices of kidney cortex. *Am J Physiol* **200:**387, 1961.
104. Senekjian HO, Knight TF, Weinman EJ: Urate transport by the isolated perfused S_2 segment of the rabbit. *Am J Physiol* **240:**F530, 1981.
105. Shimomura A, Chonko A, Tanner RM, Edwards R, Grantham JJ: Nature of urate transport in isolated rabbit proximal tubules. *Am J Physiol* **241:**F565, 1981.
106. Tanner EJ, Chonko AM, Edwards RM, Grantham JJ: Evidence for an inhibitor of renal urate and PAH secretion in rabbit blood. *Am J Physiol* **244:**F590, 1983.
107. Moller JV: The relation between secretion of urate and p-aminohippurate in the rabbit kidney. *J Physiol (Lond)* **192:**505, 1967.
108. Poulsen H, Praetorius E: Tubular excretion of uric acid in rabbits. *Acta Pharm Toxicol* **10:**371, 1954.
109. Abramson RG, King VF, Reif MC, Leal-Pinto E, Baruch SB: Urate uptake in membrane vesicles of rat renal cortex: Effect of copper. *Am J Physiol* **242:**F158, 1982.
110. Abramson RG, Lipkowitz MS: Carrier-mediated concentrative urate transport in rat renal membrane vesicles. *Am J Physiol* **248:**F574, 1985.
111. Blomstedt JW, Aronson PS: pH Gradient-stimulated transport of urate and p-aminohippurate in dog renal microvillus membrane vesicles. *J Clin Invest* **65:**931, 1980.
112. Boumendil-Podevin EF, Podevin RA, Priol C: Uric acid transport in brush border membrane vesicles isolated from rabbit kidney. *Am J Physiol* **236:**F519, 1979.
113. Guggino SE, Aronson PS: Paradoxical effects of pyrazinoate (PZA) on urate transport in dog renal brush border membrane vesicles (BBMV). *Kidney Int* **23:**256, 1983.
114. Kippen I, Hirayama B, Klinenberg JR, Wright EM:

Transport of p-aminohippuric acid and glucose in highly purified rabbit renal brush border membranes. *Biochim Biophys Acta* **556:**161, 1979.
115. Nord E, Wright SH, Kippen IM, Wright EM: Pathways for carboxylic acid transport by rabbit renal brush border membrane vesicles. *Am J Physiol* **243:**F456, 1982.
116. Gutman AB, Yu TF: A three-component system for regulation of renal excretion of uric acid in man. *Trans Assoc Am Physicians* **74:**353, 1961.
117. Manuel MA, Steele TH: Pyrazinamide suppression of the uricosuric response to sodium chloride infusion. *J Lab Clin Med* **83:**417, 1974.
118. Steele TH, Boner G: Origins of the uricosuric response. *J Clin Invest* **52:**1368, 1973.
119. Steele TH: Urate secretion in man: The pyrazinamide suppression test. *Ann Intern Med* **79:**734, 1973.
120. Diamond HS, Paolino JS: Evidence for a post-secretory reabsorptive site for uric acid in man. *J Clin Invest* **52:**1491, 1973.
121. Rieselbach RE, Steele TH: Influence of the kidney upon urate homeostasis in health and disease. *Am J Med* **56:**665, 1974.
122. Sorensen LB, Levinson DJ: Isolated defect in post-secretory reabsorption of uric acid. *Ann Rheum Dis* **39:**180, 1980.
123. Gibson T, Sims HP, Jimenez SA: Hypouricemia and increased renal urate clearance associated with hyperparathyroidism. *Ann Rheum Dis* **35:**372, 1976.
124. Grantham JJ, Chonko AM: Renal handling of organic anions and cations; metabolism and excretion of uric acid, in Brenner BM (ed): *The Kidney,* 3d ed. Philadelphia, Saunders, 1986, p 663.
125. Harknes RA, Nicol AD: Plasma uric acid levels in children. *Arch Dis Child* **44:**773, 1969.
126. Stapelton FB, Linshawm MA, Hassancin K, Gruskin AB: Uric acid excretion in normal children. *J Pediatr* **92:**911, 1978.
127. Stapelton FB: Renal uric acid clearance in human neonates. *J Pediatr* **103:**290, 1983.
128. Wolfson WO, Hunt HJ, Levine E, Gutterman HS, Cohn C, Rosenberg EF, Huddlestun B, Kadota IC: The transport and excretion of uric acid in man V. A sex differential in urate metabolism; with a note on clinical and laboratory findings in gouty women. *J Clin Exp* **9:**749, 1949.
129. Scott JT, Pollard AC: Uric acid excretion in relatives of patients with gout. *Ann Rheum Dis* **29:**397, 1970.
130. Nicholls S, Snaith MZ, Scott JT: Effect of estrogen therapy on plasma and urinary levels of uric acid. *Br Med J* **1:**449, 1973.
131. Steele TH: Evidence for altered renal urate reabsorption during changes in volume of the extracellular fluid. *J Lab Clin Med* **74:**288, 1969.
132. Cannon PJ, Svahn DS, Demartini FF: The influence of hypertonic saline infusions upon the fractional reabsorption of urate and other ions in normal and hypertensive man. *Circulation* **41:**97, 1970.
133. Diamond H, Meisel A: Influence of volume expansion, serum sodium and fractional excretion of sodium on urate excretion. *Pflugers Arch* **356:**47, 1975.
134. Steele TH, Oppenheimer S: Factors affecting urate excretion following diuretic administration in man. *Am J Med* **47:**564, 1969.
135. Steele TH, Manuel MA, Boner G: Diuretics, urate excretion and sodium reabsorption: A test of acetazolamide and urinary alkalinization. *Nephron* **11:**48, 1975.
136. Engle JE, Steele TH: Variation of urate excretion with urine flow in normal man. *Nephron* **16:**50, 1976.
137. Meisel A, Diamond H: Effect of vasopressin on uric acid excretion: Evidence for distal nephron reabsorption of urate in man. *Clin Sci Mol Med* **51:**33, 1976.
138. Mees EJD, van Assendelft PB, Nieuvenhuis MG: Elevation of uric acid clearance caused by inappropriate antidiuretic hormone secretion. *Acta Med Scand* **189:**69, 1971.
139. Gordon P, Robertson GL, Seegmiller JE: Hyperuricemia, a concomitant congenital vasopressin-resistant diabetes insipidus in the adult. *N Engl J Med* **284:**1057, 1971.
140. Emmerson BT: Abnormal urate excretion associated with renal and systemic disorders, drugs and toxins, in Kelley WN, Weiner IM (eds): *Handbook of Experimental Pharmacology, Uric Acid.* Berlin, Springer-Verlag, 1978, vol 51, p 287.
141. Yu TF, Gutman AB: Paradoxical retention of uric acid by uricosuric drugs in low dosage. *Proc Soc Exp Biol Med* **90:**542, 1955.
142. Yu TF, Gutman AB: Study of the paradoxical effects of salicylate in low, intermediate and high dosage on the renal mechanisms for excretion of urate in man. *J Clin Invest* **38:**1298, 1959.
143. Manuel MA, Steele TH: Changes in renal urate handling after prolonged thiazide treatment. *Am J Med* **57:**741, 1974.
144. Demartini FE: Hypouricemia induced by drugs. *Arthritis Rheum* **8:**823, 1965.
145. Stewart RJ, Chonko AM: Pharmacologic inhibition of urate transport across perfused and non-perfused rabbit proximal straight tubules. *Kidney Int* **19:**258, 1981.
146. Reese OG Jr, Steele TH: Renal transport of urate during diuretic-induced hypouricemia. *Am J Med* **60:**973, 1978.
147. Nemati M, Kyle MC, Freis ED: Clinical study of ticrynafen. *JAMA* **237:**652, 1977.
148. Grobner TO, Zollner N: Uricosuria, in Zollner N, Grobner W (eds): *Gicht, Handbuch der Inn Med,* 5th ed. Berlin, Springer, 1976, vol 7 (Stoff wechsel krankheiten), part 3, p 491.
149. Dayton PG, Yu TF, Chen W, Berger L, Westm LA, Gutman AB: The physiological disposition of probenecid, including renal clearance in man, studied by an improved method for its estimation in biological material. *J Pharmacol Exp Ther* **140:**278, 1963.
150. de Vries A, Sperling O: Implications of disorders of purine metabolism for the kidney and the urinary tract, in *Purine and Pyrimidine Metabolism.* Ciba Foundation Symposium. Amsterdam, Elsevier, 1977, vol 48 (new series), p 179.
151. Steele TH, Rieselbach RE: The renal mechanism for urate homeostasis in normal man. *Am J Med* **43:**868, 1967.
152. Yu TF, Berger L, Stone DJ, Wolf J, Gutman AB: Effects of pyrazinamide and pyrazinoic acid on urate clearance and other discrete renal functions. *Proc Soc Exp Biol Med* **96:**264, 1957.
153. Yu TF, Berger L, Gutman AB: Suppression of the tubular secretion of urate by pyrazinamide in the dog. *Proc Soc Exp Biol Med* **107:**905, 1961.
154. Davis BB, Field JB, Rodnan GP, Kedes LH: Localization and pyrazinamide inhibition of distal transtubular movement of uric acid-2-^{14}C with a modified stop-flow technique. *J Clin Invest* **44:**716, 1965.
155. Gutman A, Yu TF, Berger L: Renal function in gout III. Estimation of tubular secretion and reabsorption of uric acid by use of pyrazinamide (pyrazinoic acid). *Am J Med* **47:**575, 1969.
156. Weiner IM, Tinker JP: Pharmacology of pyrazinamide: Metabolic and renal function studies related to the mechanism of drug-induced urate retention. *J Pharmacol Exp Ther* **180:**411, 1972.
157. Kramp RA, Lassiter WE, Gottschalk CW: Urate-2-^{14}C transport in the rat nephron. *J Clin Invest* **50:**35, 1971.
158. Frankfurt SJ, Weinman EJ: Pyrazinoic acid and urate transport in the rat. *Proc Soc Exp Biol Med* **159:**16, 1978.
159. Guggino SE, Aronson PS: Paradoxical effects of pyrazinoate and nicotinate on urate transport in dog renal microvillus membranes. *J Clin Invest* **76:**543, 1985.
160. Shichiri M, Itoh H, Iwamoto H, Hirata Y, Marumo F: Renal tubular hypouricemia: Evidence for defect of both secretion and reabsorption. *Nephron* **56:**421, 1990.
161. Sperling O, Boer P, Weinberger A, de Vries A: Transport into erythrocytes and intestinal absorption of uric acid in hereditary renal hypouricemia. *Biomedicine* **23:**157, 1975.
162. Hansen KO, Lassen UV: Active transport of uric acid through the human erythrocyte membrane. *Nature* **4685:**553, 1959.
163. Harvey AM, Christensen HN: Uric acid transport system. Apparent absence in erythrocytes of Dalmatian coach hounds. *Science* **145:**826, 1964.
164. Oh JH, Dossetor JB, Beck IT: Kinetics of uric acid

transport and its production in rat small intestine. *Can J Physiol Pharmacol* **45:**121, 1967.
165. Wilson DW, Wilson HC: Studies "in vitro" of the digestion and absorption of purine ribonucleotides by the intestine. *J Biol Chem* **237:**1643, 1962.
166. Thier SO, Segal S: Cystinuria, in Stanbury JB, Wyngaarden, JB, Fredrickson DS (eds): *The Metabolic Basis of Inherited Disease,* 3d ed. New York, McGraw-Hill, 1972, p 1504.
167. Scriver CR: Familial iminoglycinuria, in Stanbury JB, Wyngaarden JB, Fredrickson DS (eds): *The Metabolic Basis of Inherited Disease,* 3d ed. New York, McGraw-Hill, 1972, p 1520.
168. Jepson JB: Hartnup disease, in Stanbury JB, Wyngaarden JB, Fredrickson DS (eds): *The Metabolic Basis of Inherited Disease,* 3d ed. New York, McGraw-Hill, 1972, p 1486.
169. Weinberger A, Weinberger A, Sperling O, Ben-Bassat M, Kaplan I, Pinkhas J: Increased uric acid clearance in patients with burns. *Biomedicine* **27:**277, 1977.
170. Kay NE, Gotlieb AJ: Hypouricemia in Hodgkin's disease: Report of an additional case. *Cancer* **32:**1508, 1973.
171. Briggs OM, Sperling O: Uric acid metabolism in the Dalmatian coach hound. *J S Afr Vet Assoc* **53:**201, 1982.
172. Friedman M, Byers SD: Observations concerning the causes of the excess excretion of uric acid in the Dalmatian dog. *J Biol Chem* **175:**727, 1948.
173. Kessler RH, Hierholzer K, Gurd RS: Localization of urate transport in the nephron of mongrel and Dalmatian dog kidney. *Am J Physiol Ther* **197:**601, 1959.
174. Mudge GH, Gucchi J, Platts M, O'Connell JMB, Berndt WO: Renal excretion of uric acid in the dog. *Am J Physiol* **215:**404, 1968.
175. Mudge GH, Berndt WO, Valtin H: Tubular transport of urea, glucose, phosphate, uric acid, sulphate and thiosulphate, in Orloff J, Berliner BW (eds): *Handbook of Physiology: Section 8 Renal Physiology*. Washington, DC, American Physiological Society, 1973, chap. 19, p 587.
176. Myers VC, Hanzal RF: The metabolism of methylanthine and their related methyluric acids. *J Biol Chem* **162:**309, 1946.
177. Young EG, Conway CF, Crandall WA: On the purine metabolism of the Dalmatian coach hound. *Biochem J* **32:**1138, 1938.
178. Zins GR, Weiner IM: Bidirectional urate transport limited to the proximal tubule in dogs. *Am J Physiol* **215:**411, 1968.
179. Klemperer FW, Trimble HC, Hastings AB: The uricase of dogs, including the Dalmatian. *J Biol Chem* **125:**445, 1938.
180. Kuster G, Shorter RG, Dawson B, Hallenbeck GA: Uric acid metabolism in Dalmatian and other dogs. *Arch Intern Med* **129:**492, 1972.
181. Kuster G, Shorter RG, Dawson B, Hallenbeck GA: Effect of allogenic hepatic transplantation between Dalmatian and mongrel dogs on urinary excretion of uric acid. *Surg Forum* **18:**360, 1967.
182. Erley CMM, Hirschberg RR, Hoefer W, Schaefer K: Acute renal failure due to uric acid nephropathy in a patient with renal hypouricemia. *Klin Wochenschr* **67:**308, 1989.
183. Ishikawa I, Sakurai Y, Masuzaki S, Sugishita N, Shinoda A, Shikura N: Exercise-induced acute renal failure in 3 patients with renal hypouricemia. *Jpn J Nephrol* **32:**923, 1990.
184. Ishikawa I, Onoudi Z, Yuri T, Saito Y, Shinoda A, Yamamoto I: Acute renal failure with severe loin pain and patchy renal vasoconstrictions, in Eliahou HE (ed): *Acute Renal Failure*. London, Libbey, 1982, p 224.
185. Sperling O: Uric acid nephrolithiasis, in Wickham JEA, Buck AC (eds): *Renal Tract Stone, Metabolic Basis and Clinical Practice*. London, Churchill Livingstone, 1990, p 349.

CHAPTER 126

Lysosomal Transport Disorders: Cystinosis and Sialic Acid Storage Disorders

William A. Gahl ▪ Jerry A. Schneider ▪ Pertti P. Aula

1. **Cystinosis and the sialic acid storage diseases are rare lysosomal disorders resulting from defective carrier-mediated transport of the amino acid cystine and the charged monosaccharide sialic acid, respectively, across the lysosomal membrane. The major clinical manifestation of cystinosis is renal failure at approximately 9 to 10 years of age. Sialic acid storage diseases are characterized by various degrees of psychomotor retardation. Both are autosomal recessively inherited disorders whose genes have not been isolated.**
2. **In cystinosis, free, nonprotein cystine accumulates to 10 to 1000 times normal levels and forms crystals within the lysosomes of most tissues, which are damaged at different rates. The diagnosis is made by demonstrating an elevated cystine content in polymorphonuclear leukocytes or cultured fibroblasts or by slit-lamp examination showing corneal crystals which are generally present in patients over 1 year of age. Cystinosis can be diagnosed in utero by cystine measurements in amniocytes or chorionic villi or at birth by cystine measurements of the placenta.**
3. **Children with cystinosis are normal at birth but signs of the renal tubular Fanconi syndrome develop, usually between 6 and 12 months of age. These include dehydration, acidosis, vomiting, electrolyte imbalances, hypophosphatemic rickets, and failure to grow. Weight is proportional to height. Head circumference and intelligence are spared. Other manifestations of cystinosis include photophobia, hypothyroidism, and decreased ability to sweat. Renal glomerular damage progresses inexorably, requiring dialysis or transplantation at 6 to 12 years of age.**
4. **Cystine storage does not occur in the donor kidney, but continued accumulation in the host tissue can result in retinal blindness, corneal erosions, diabetes mellitus, a distal myopathy, swallowing difficulties, pancreatic insufficiency, and primary hypogonadism in patients 13 to 35 years old. Neurologic deterioration has been seen in a significant number of postrenal transplant patients.**
5. **Therapy for cystinosis includes replacement of renal losses due to the Fanconi syndrome, provision of thyroxine, insulin, pancreatic enzymes, and testosterone for deficient patients, and symptomatic care of ophthalmic complaints. Long-term cystine-depleting therapy with the aminothiol cysteamine significantly lowers leukocyte and parenchymal cystine levels and improves growth. Oral cysteamine therapy preserves renal function and, if initiated in the first 2 years of life, can allow for a net increase in the GFR. Side effects include nausea and vomiting. Cysteamine eyedrops can dissolve corneal crystals in young children and remove the haziness from the corneas of older patients.**
6. **The clinical course and severity of cystine accumulation in cystinosis varies in different kindreds, from benign cystinosis in adults with corneal crystals but no renal disease, to intermediate cystinosis in adolescents with late-onset renal deterioration, and finally to classic nephropathic cystinosis in infants. Heterozygotes for all types of cystinosis are clinically normal.**
7. **The free sialic acid storage disorders include Salla disease and the more severe infantile free sialic acid storage disease (ISSD). Patients with Salla disease, a disorder largely of the Finnish population, are normal at birth, but psychomotor delay and ataxia develop in infancy. Intelligence is moderately to severely impaired, and life span is slightly reduced. In contrast, patients with ISSD can present at birth and often die in the first year of life. They have failure to thrive, hepatosplenomegaly, and severe mental and motor retardation and often have coarse facial features and dysostosis multiplex. Intermediate phenotypes have been reported. There are approximately 100 Salla disease patients known and 15 ISSD cases reported.**
8. **Patients with Salla disease and ISSD store approximately tenfold and one hundredfold normal amounts of free (unbound) *N*-acetylneuraminic acid in their tissues, respectively, and excrete 10 and 100 times normal amounts in the urine. Glucuronic acid also accumulates in Salla disease and ISSD fibroblasts, since the lysosomal acid monosaccharide carrier defective in these disorders recognizes both sialic acid and glucuronic acid.**

*A list of standard abbreviations is located immediately preceding the index in each volume. Additional abbreviations used in this chapter include: CCCP = carbonyl cyanide *m*-chlorophenylhydrazone; DIDS = 4,4′-diisothiocyanatostilbene-2,2–disulfonate; FRTL-5 = functional rat thyroid cells; GluAc = glucuronic acid; ISSD = infantile free sialic acid storage disease; ManNAc = *N*-acetylmannosamine; NeuAc = *N*-acetylneuraminic acid, or sialic acid; NICHD = National Institute of Child Health and Human Development; PRC_{10} = predicted reciprocal serum creatinine at age 10 years; rhGH = recombinant human growth hormone; TSH = thyrotropin.

9. Sialic acid storage disorders can be diagnosed based on increased urinary free sialic acid and histologic evidence of lysosomal storage. Prenatal diagnosis is available. Only symptomatic therapy can be offered for patients with these diseases.

Cystinosis and sialic acid storage diseases are lysosomal storage disorders resulting from defective transport of cystine and sialic acid (Fig. 126-1), respectively, across the lysosomal membrane. The term *cystinosis* can refer to one of several variants of the disease but, unless specified, here denotes nephropathic cystinosis, which results in renal failure at approximately 9 to 10 years of age. Salla disease, a disorder most prevalent in Finland, represents the most common inborn error associated with lysosomal storage of free sialic acid; patients with more extensive clinical and biochemical involvement are considered to have infantile free sialic acid storage disease (ISSD). All patients with lysosomal sialic acid storage disorders suffer some degree of psychomotor retardation. Cystine and sialic acid serve as prototypes for amino acids and monosaccharides, having carriers within the lysosomal membrane, and cystinosis and free sialic acid storage diseases represent examples of metabolic disorders due to defective integral lysosomal membrane transport proteins.

CYSTINOSIS

Historical Aspects

The current understanding of cystinosis as an inherited, multisystemic disease resulting from failure of lysosomal cystine transport follows from more than eight decades of both clinical and laboratory research. Over this time, a number of basic issues were addressed: (1) What is the clinical phenotype of the disease? (2) Is cystinosis different from renal Fanconi syndrome and cystinuria? (3) Where in the cell is the cystine stored? (4) Do the crystals form *in situ* or are they phagocytosed from preformed crystals in the extracellular fluid? (5) What is the source of the stored cystine? (6) Why does the cystine accumulate? (7) What causes the renal failure in cystinosis? (8) How can the disease be treated? The answers to these questions are now known, but with various degrees of certitude.

The first known description of cystinosis appeared in 1903 in an article in the *Zeitschrift fur Physiologie Chemie* by Emil Abderhalden; a family from Basel was described.[1] The propositus was a 21½-month-old boy who died of inanition and whose organs had a grossly white appearance with punctate lesions throughout. Classic chemical analysis demonstrated an identity between the stored material and the amino acid cystine. Two sibs had died of inanition similar to the index case. Two other children and a grandfather were reported to excrete excessive amounts of cystine in the urine. If correct, this might be explained by the possibility that the genes for both cystinosis and cystinuria were present in this family.

Lignac's report in 1924 of cystine deposits in each of three infants with rickets, dwarfism, renal disease, and wasting provided some delineation of the clinical expression of cystinosis.[2] Additional aspects emerged from the association of rickets and stunted growth in a child with glycosuria and albuminuria described by Fanconi in 1931.[3] Vitamin D–resistant rickets with spontaneous fractures was described in 1933 by deToni in a dwarfed child who also had hypophosphatemia, acidosis, albuminuria, and glycosuria.[4] A report of a similar child by Debré et al. in 1934[5] led Fanconi in 1936 to propose a syndrome of "nephrotic-glycosuric dwarfism with hypophosphatemic rickets."[6] At that time this condition was termed the *deToni-Debré-Fanconi syndrome*.

The hypothesis that this syndrome and cystinosis were but two aspects of the same entity was proposed by Beumer and Wepler in 1937, when they found cystine crystals in the glomeruli of a patient with this condition.[7] This possibility was supported by the demonstration of cystine crystals in the tissues at autopsy of one of Fanconi's original patients.[8] A detailed study of a larger series of patients by Bickel and colleagues[9] in 1952 provided further evidence of the association of cystinosis with the Fanconi syndrome and progressive glomerular damage.

The aminoaciduria in this condition was extensively studied by Dent who, in 1947, also quantified the extent of polyuria, glucosuria, phosphaturia, and proteinuria.[10] Dent also noted that the generalized aminoaciduria in cystinosis was not due to "overflow" of plasma amino acids and that no obvious error of sulfur amino acid metabolism was present in these patients. The clear distinction between cystinosis and cystinuria was first provided in 1949,[11] when the familial nature of both diseases was recognized and the rarity of cystine stones in patients with cystinosis was appreciated. Further details on the early investigations of this disorder are available elsewhere.[12–14]

The precise location of the cystine crystals was difficult to ascertain, but Baar[15] and Bickel concluded correctly that they were primarily intracellular and within reticuloendothelial cells. Clay and colleagues demonstrated in histological studies of cystinotic kidney that many nephrons were hypotrophic, particularly in the proximal convoluted tubules, with narrowing in the first part of the tubule forming a "swan-neck" lesion.[16] Darmady and others showed that these lesions are not specific for cystinosis, but are seen in other renal conditions as well.[9,17] In 1962, electron microscopy of

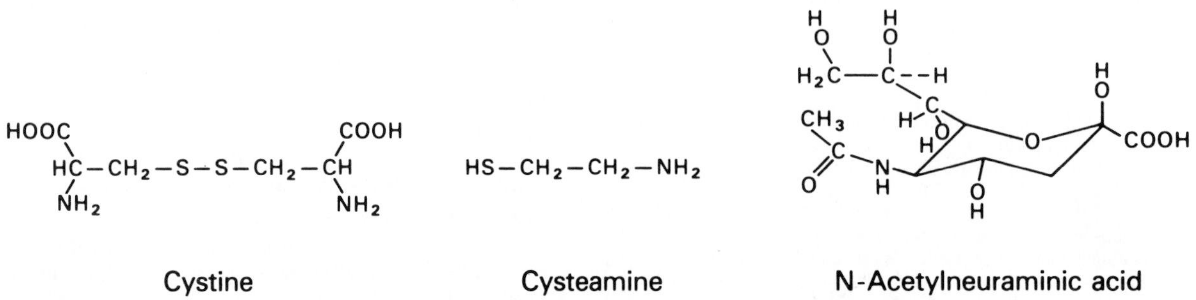

Cystine   Cysteamine   N-Acetylneuraminic acid

FIG. 126-1 Structures of the disulfide amino acid cystine, which is stored in cystinosis; the aminothiol cysteamine, which depletes cells of cystine; and the charged sugar *N*-acetylneuraminic acid, which is stored in free sialic acid storage disorders.

renal biopsy specimens demonstrated hexagonal crystals between tubules in the kidney, and the pathognomonic "swan neck" deformity of the proximal tubule was confirmed on light microscopy.[18] Vacuolation and swelling of the ER were noted, and cytoplasmic bodies were found in the apical and central portions of the cell, frequently with coarse granules in the proximal convoluted tubule. It was concluded that crystallization of cystine between cells, secondary to some unknown primary metabolic or enzymatic defect, led to the renal pathology.

The modern era of clinical investigation into cystinosis began in 1967 when the intracellular location of the stored cystine was identified as the lysosome. This was demonstrated by differential centrifugation of leukocyte[19] and fibroblast[20] subcellular fractions, by electron microscopy in lymph node cells,[21] histiocytes,[22] and rectal mucosal cells,[23] by ferritin labeling,[24] by sucrose density gradients,[25] and by exposure of cystinotic fibroblasts to L-cysteine-D-penicillamine disulfide to selectively induce vacuolation.[26] Next, the metabolism and plasma membrane transport of cysteine and cystine were investigated in cystinotic fibroblasts and leukocytes, with no consistent demonstration of a defect as compared with normal.[27] In particular, enzymes involved in cyst(e)ine and glutathione redox reactions were not impaired in cystinotic tissues and cells.[27,28]

These findings, detailed previously,[27] set the stage for pursuit of the hypothesis that transport of small molecules across the lysosomal membrane was carrier-mediated.[29] To investigate this possibility for cystine directly, normal polymorphonuclear leukocytes were loaded to very high cystine concentrations by exposure to cystine dimethylester, which like other amino acid methylesters[30,31] was specifically hydrolyzed within lysosomes to methanol and free cystine. This ingenious technique, suggested by Dr. Frank Tietze and exploited in Dr. Joseph Schulman's laboratory in the early 1980s, allowed normal and cystinotic leukocytes to be equivalently loaded with cystine. Subsequent whole-cell egress studies, using either [^{35}S]cystine or nonradioactive cystine, revealed rapid losses of cystine from normal cells ($t_{1/2}$ approximately 45 min) and slow losses from cystinotic cells ($t_{1/2}$ approaching infinity).[32] At the same time, investigators in Dr. Jerry Schneider's laboratory were loading cultured fibroblasts with cystine by exposing them to 30 m*M* cysteine-glutathione mixed disulfide for 24 h. With low but roughly equal initial loadings, the normal cells lost half their cystine in 20 min, while the cystinotic cells lost none in 90 min.[33]

Experiments using isolated leukocyte lysosomes verified the whole-cell results, with 13 normal granular fractions having a mean $t_{1/2}$ for [^{35}S]cystine of 26.1±1.4 SEM min and 12 cystinotic granular fractions having a mean $t_{1/2}$ of 80.8±0.7 min.[34] Nonradioactive experiments gave similar results, regardless of the initial level of cystine loading.[34] Epstein-Barr-virus–transformed lymphoblasts, loaded using cystine dimethylester, showed a rate of cystine efflux which was two to three times greater in normal as compared with cystinotic granular fractions.[35] Comparable experiments in fibroblasts using either [^{35}S]cystine[36,37] or nonradioactive cystine[37] also revealed short half-times for cystine egress from normal lysosomes and very long half-times using cystinotic lysosomes.

A major advance was the expression of egress rates as initial velocities,[38] which increased linearly with loading of normal lysosomes and then leveled off (Fig. 126-2), indicating saturation kinetics, a hallmark of carrier-mediated transport. Cystinotic granular fractions displayed negligible velocities of cystine egress, regardless of the level of cystine loading.

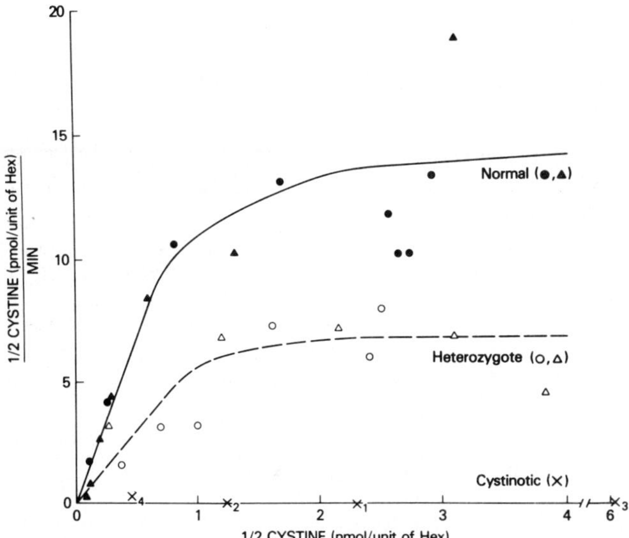

FIG. 126-2 Initial velocity of cystine transport as a function of lysosomal cystine loading using human leukocytes. Normal egress velocity increased with loading and then plateaued, indicating saturation kinetics. Heterozygotes for cystinosis followed a similar pattern but reached only half the normal maximal velocity. Cystinosis patients displayed negligible egress velocity regardless of the level of loading. Values were normalized to the activity of hexosaminidase, a lysosomal enzyme. *(From Gahl et al.: "Cystine Transport is Defective in Isolated Leukocyte Lysosomes from Patients with Cystinosis,"* **Science,** *Sept. 24, 1982, vol. 217, pp. 1263–1265. Copyright 1982 by the American Association for the Advancement of Science.)*

Heterozygotes for cystinosis exhibited a V_{max} half that of normal individuals.[38]

Finally, the carrier-mediated nature of lysosomal cystine transport was proven definitively by the demonstration of cystine countertransport, or transstimulation. In countertransport, tracer amounts of a radiolabeled substance will cross a membrane at an increased rate if there is a substantial concentration of the nonradioactive substance on the opposite side of the membrane.[39] Thus, normal leukocyte lysosomes loaded with nonradioactive cystine took up [^{3}H]cystine (present in tracer concentrations) more rapidly than lysosomes not loaded with cystine,[40] proving that a carrier for cystine was present in the lysosomal membrane. Cystinotic granular fractions took up virtually no [^{3}H]cystine, regardless of the level of loading.[40] Obligate heterozygotes for cystinosis exhibited half the normal [^{3}H]cystine countertransport.[41]

As described in some detail previously,[27,42] impaired transport of cystine across the lysosomal membrane gradually became accepted as the cause of cystinosis, largely because experiments were performed using several different cell types (polymorphonuclear leukocytes, Epstein-Barr-virus–transformed lymphoblasts, and cultured fibroblasts) in several different laboratories. These studies created a new class of inborn errors of metabolism and provided the basis for a rational approach to treating a lysosomal storage disease by depletion of the stored product. In this respect, cystinosis still serves as a model for the interaction of basic and clinical research, each advancing the other in discrete steps.

Cystine

Chemical Properties. Cystine, the disulfide of the amino acid cysteine, has a molecular weight of 240.3. Cystine and cysteine participate in a reversible oxidation-reduction reaction whose redox potential is −0.22 eV[43] or even more negative.[44] In the presence of oxygen, cysteine is rapidly oxidized to cystine. Cystine's two carboxyl groups and two amine residues have pKa's of <1, 1.7, 7.48, and 9.02, respectively[45]; its net charge at physiological pH is zero, and its pI is 4.60.[45] The disulfide's solubility in water at 25°C approximates 0.5 m*M* at pH 7.0,[46] but heating or the use of small volumes of dilute (0.01 *N*) acid or alkali facilitates crystal dissolution. The poor solubility of cystine in aqueous solution explains the formation of urinary crystals and renal calculi in cystinuria, a defect of tubular reabsorption of cystine and dibasic amino acids (see Chap. 117). Human plasma at 37°C and pH 7.3 can dissolve approximately 1.67 m*M* cystine.[12] Cystine's insolubility in alcohol provides the basis for the preservation of cystine crystals in cystinotic tissue by alcohol fixation; the use of aqueous solutions can dissolve the intracellular crystals.

Metabolism. Cystine forms largely by the direct oxidation of two cysteine molecules. Cysteine is both a precursor in protein synthesis and a product of protein hydrolysis. It is also synthesized *de novo*, deriving its sulfur atom from the essential amino acid methionine. The transsulfuration of methionine yields homocysteine, which combines with serine to form cystathionine, the proximate precursor of cysteine through the enzymatic activity of cystathionase (see Chap. 35). In conditions in which cystathionine β-synthase or cystathionase is deficient[47] (e.g., in homocystinuria or cystathioninuria, or in normal human fetuses and neonates[48]), cysteine becomes an essential amino acid. Cysteine (or cystine) is also required for the growth of normal human fibroblasts[49] but not normal human lymphoid cells[50] in culture. In vivo, cysteine is oxidized to inorganic sulfate by one of several pathways[14] for excretion in the urine. It can also be incorporated into free thiols such as glutathione (GSH, γ-glutamylcysteinylglycine), through the γ-glutamyl cycle (see Chap. 43).

Because of the many cystine-reducing systems present in the cytosol, most cellular cyst(e)ine exists in the free thiol form. It is maintained as cysteine by GSH-disulfide transhydrogenases[51] acting in concert with high cellular concentrations of reduced glutathione (up to 10 m*M*[52]). Cystine and GSH participate in a disulfide interchange reaction[53] to form cysteine and cysteine–GSH mixed disulfide; a second reaction between reduced GSH and the mixed disulfide produces cysteine and oxidized glutathione. The same type of disulfide interchange reaction provides the basis for the reduction of cystine by cysteamine (see "Mechanism of Cystine Depletion by Cysteamine" below). These disulfide interchange reactions and their products occur within the cytosol, and isolated reports of lysosomal cystine-reducing systems[54] have not been supported in subsequent investigations.[28]

Methods of Assay. Cystine can be reduced to cysteine and measured qualitatively by the cyanide–nitroprusside reaction.[55] Semiquantitative assays employ paper[56] or thin-layer[57] chromatography. The routine quantitation of cystine in plasma or urine involves separation from other amino acids by ion-exchange chromatography and identification by ninhydrin staining.[58] The procedure measures total cystine plus cysteine; it cannot differentiate the two. This explains the conventional use of "half-cystine" to express amounts of the disulfide. Most current research employs the *Escherichia coli* cystine-binding protein assay[59] to measure specifically picomole quantities of cystine in protein-free extracts. This assay, which utilizes *N*-ethylmaleimide to form a cysteine adduct and prevent spontaneous oxidation of cysteine to cystine, also allows physicians to diagnose cystinosis and follow cystine depletion by cysteamine. The assay involves competition by unknown quantities of nonradioactive cystine for [^{14}C]cystine bound to the protein, with trapping of protein-bound radioactivity on nitrocellulose filters. The less radioactivity trapped, the greater the competing nonradioactive cystine.

Cystine Storage in Cystinosis. Plasma cystine concentrations are normal in cystinosis.[12] Intestinal absorption of cystine is normal, and urinary cystine levels are no more elevated than those of other amino acids, differentiating cystinosis from cystinuria (see Chap. 117). Rather, cystine storage in cystinosis is intracellular (Fig. 126-3), with crystal formation in the kidney,[60] liver,[61] lung, pancreas,[62] intestine,[63,64] appendix,[65] spleen,[66] conjunctiva and cornea,[67] retina,[68] lymph node,[21] polymorphonuclear leukocyte and monocyte,[69] bone marrow,[70] thyroid,[71] thymus,[72] muscle,[73] placenta,[74] choroid plexus,[75,76] and meninges.[73] Pure cystine crystals can be rectangular (in which case they are birefringent[12]) or hexagonal. Cystine hydrochloride crystallizes as prismatic needles[77]; this describes the corneal crystals in cystinosis. Various peripheral leukocyte populations[78] and all cells in culture remain devoid of crystals but accumulate 5 to 500 times normal amounts of cystine (Table 126-1). Cystine accumulation and crystal formation occur according to a tissue-specific chronology, with considerable variation among individual patients. Corneal crystals may not be present until 1 year of age, yet crystals have been identified in the Kupffer cells of a 22-week fetus.[79] The brain white and gray matter may be entirely spared of cystine accumulation in a young cystinosis patient,[80] yet show cystine levels increased several times in a 25-year-old woman with cystinosis.[81] Both muscle and liver cystine levels increase with age in cystinosis patients who have not received cystine-depleting therapy.[82,83] The reasons for variable rates of cystine accumulation among different tissues are unknown, but may be related to different rates of protein degradation and cell turnover.

Circulating leukocytes from cystinosis patients exhibit normal morphology and normal cysteine concentrations.[19] Cystinotic polymorphonuclear leukocytes, as well as cultured fibroblasts, myoblasts, corneal cells, and renal epithelial and tubular cells, contain fiftyfold to one hundredfold normal amounts of cystine (see Table 126-1). Leukocyte cystine values are generally greater in older than in younger patients. Thirteen children under 3 years of age averaged 6.5±3.5 nmol of half-cystine per milligram of protein as compared with a mean value of 9.9±4.1 nmol of half-cystine per milligram of protein for 18 patients 15 to 28 years old.[84]

Lysosomal Cystine Transport. Early studies using polymorphonuclear leukocytes delineated several characteristics of lysosomal cystine transport. For example, since *N*-ethylmaleimide did not affect the egress of cystine from normal lysosomes,[38] it was clear that cystine was not being reduced to cysteine and reoxidized to cystine during the transport process; cystine itself was the transported ligand. Moreover, the fact that cystinotic granular fractions cleared tryptophan and methionine in a normal fashion[34] meant that the lysosomal cystine carrier exhibited some specificity.

That specificity was investigated using the powerful technique of countertransport. In particular, normal, cystine-loaded granular fractions did not countertransport other

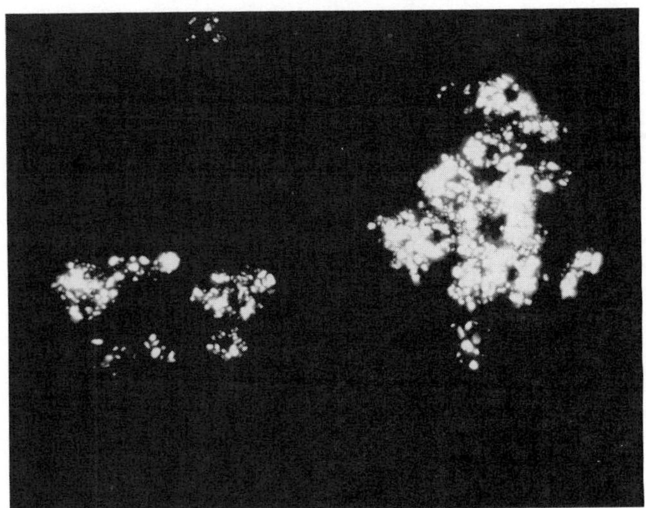

A

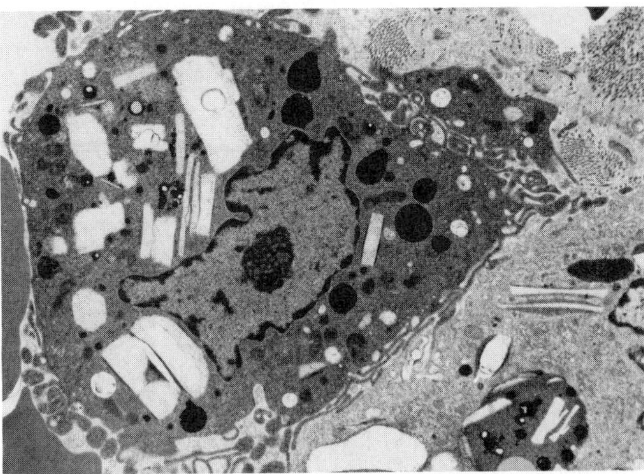

B

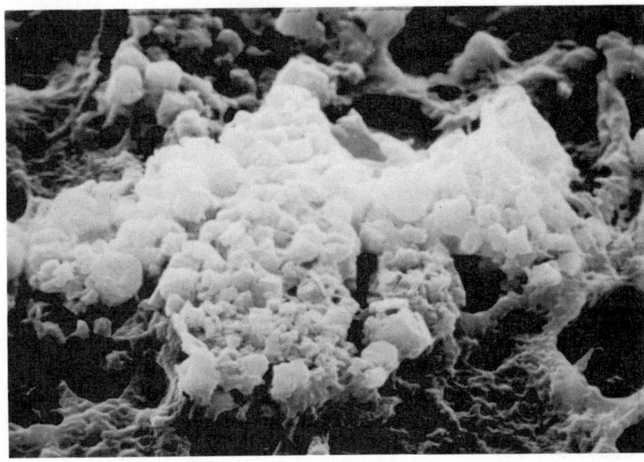

C

FIG. 126-3 Cystine crystals in the liver of a cystinosis patient. *A*. Light microscopy showing crystals under cross-polarizing light; ×530. *B*. Electron micrograph of hexagonal cystine crystals within lysosomes of a Kupffer cell, ×14,500. *C*. Scanning electron micrograph showing crystals protruding from the surface of a Kupffer cell; ×2500. ***(Courtesy of K.G. Ishak, M.D., Ph.D., Armed Forces Institute of Pathology, Washington, D.C.)***

amino acids such as [^{35}S]homocystine except, to a certain extent, [^{35}S]cystathionine.[40] Extralysosomal nonradioactive L-cystine, but not D-cystine, competed with [^{3}H]cystine for uptake into cystine-loaded normal granular fractions,[40] establishing the stereospecificity of the carrier for the L isomer. Certain sulfur compounds resembling cystine, such as cystathionine and cystamine, were presumably also recognized by the carrier since they competed with cystine for countertransport.[40] Since the dibasic amino acid arginine did not compete with cystine, the carrier was presumed to be different from the plasma membrane carrier for dibasic amino acids in renal tubular and intestinal epithelial cells (see Chap. 117). The lysosomal cystine carrier did not recognize glutamate,[40] indicating that it was genetically distinct from the plasma membrane cystine carrier of fibroblasts, which transports both cystine and glutamate.[85] Several other amino acids—methionine, alanine, tryptophan, tyrosine, and homocystine—as well as β-carboxyethyl-L-thiocysteine and other cystine analogues, also did not compete with cystine for transport.[40] The cystine carrier appeared specific for compounds of chain length 6 (not 8) sulfur or methylene units having an amine (but not necessarily a carboxyl) group at each end. Similar ligand preferences have been demonstrated for lysosome cystine transport in mouse L-929 cells, in which it was also shown that selenium could substitute for sulfur, and the carrier's recognition site for cystine was dominated by hydrophobic interactions.[86] There were no net charge requirements for ligand binding, but the binding site had both polar and apolar domains. The apolar domain could accommodate branching on the carbon-3 of cystine.

The kinetic properties of lysosomal cystine transport have been loosely defined in at least two different systems. In leukocyte lysosomes, the K_m approximated 0.5 mM with respect to L-cystine,[40] and the V_{max} for egress was approximately 23 pmol of half-cystine per unit of hexosaminidase per minute.[38] (Hexosaminidase is a lysosomal enzyme whose activity provides a denominator for expressing transport rates per lysosome.) The Q_{10} approximated 2.0 with an energy of activation of 11.4 kcal/mol.[40] In mouse L-929 cells, the K_m was 0.27 mM, and there appeared to be a component of cystine uptake that could not be saturated.[86]

Normal cystine countertransport, studied in leukocyte lysosomes, was relatively independent of the extralysosomal sodium or potassium ion concentration.[40] However, cystine efflux was greatly enhanced when lysosomal membranes were made permeable to potassium ions either by an ionophore such as valinomycin or by the presence of a permeant anion.[87] The potassium–valinomycin effects were present in cystinotic lysosomes as well, suggesting that they were not mediated through the carrier system deficient in cystinosis. Moreover, the valinomycin effect was not observed in fibroblast lysosomes,[88] and valinomycin–potassium pretreatment did not enhance cystine egress from rat liver lysosomes.[89] Magnesium chloride did stimulate leukocyte lysosomal cystine transport in a concentration-dependent fashion up to 5 mM at pH 5.5.[90]

Table 126-1 Cystine Content of Cystinotic Tissue and Cells

	Cystinotic			Normal			
	N	x̄ ± SD	Range	N	x̄ ± SD	Range	Reference
Tissues		*nmol half-cystine/mg wet weight*			*nmol half-cystine/mg wet weight*		
Kidney	1	25.6					84
	4	94.8±79.7	24.6–29.5	1	0.25	—	80
	5	51.4±32.6	16.7–101.7	?	—	<0.29	239
	3	64.7±22.2	39.2–80.0	—			366
	1	—	19.8, 21.0	—			246
Conjunctiva	7	117.9±115.3	5.2–314.0	13	—	<0.38	183, 367
Muscle	10	0.77±0.53	0.05–1.94	10	0.023±0.003	—	82
	3	0.31±0.23	0.06–0.95	1	0.003	—	191
	12	2.27±3.35	0.23–12.30	1	0.004	—	73, 83
Brain	2	—	0.02–0.08	1	0.17	—	80
	1	—	0.05–0.20	—			246
	1	—	0.80–4.0	—			73
Lung	1	44.5		—			84
Pancreas	1	35.8		—			84
	1	40.2		—			73
Liver	3	73.0±35.0	45.8–112.5	2	—	0.58, 0.92	366
	1	69.1		—			84
	1	—	34.5, 42.4	—			246
	4	—	2.0–360.0	4	0.04±0.04	0.02–0.10	83
Spleen	1	132.7		—			73
	1	119.0		—			83
Cells		*nmol half-cystine/mg protein*			*nmol half-cystine/mg protein*		
Polymorphonuclear leukocytes	9	6.4±2.8	4.0–13.2	9	0.08±0.06	<0.2	19, 20, 213
	3	—	6.9–10.0	2	—	<0.1	214
	29	8.9±4.7	2.6–23.1	29	0.14±0.06	0.04–0.28	41, 84
Cultured fibroblasts	6	8.4±1.3	6.6–10.6	9	0.07±0.05	<0.2	20, 213
	6	—	6.7–14.3	3	—	<0.1	214
Cultured leukocytes	3	—	0.31–3.10	3	—	<0.03	368
Epstein-Barr-virus–transformed lymphoblasts	3	0.46±0.10	—	3	0.10±0.02	—	35
Cultured myoblasts/ myotubes	1*	29.8±10.8	16.7–41.2	1	0.31	—	191
Cultured cornea	1	23.2±14.1	11.0–38.7	1	0.27†	—	268
Cultured renal cells	1	8.0±0.6	—	1‡	0.06±0.02	—	369
Cultured renal tubular cells	1	3.5	—	1	0.06	—	301

*When a single individual's cells were studied, the mean ±SD for at least three separate cultures is given.
†Another reported normal value is ≤0.40.[370]
‡Madin-Darby canine kidney epithelial cells; human renal cells in culture were not available.

The interpretation of ATP effects on lysosomal cystine transport has been complicated by the fact that ATP not only provides energy but also effects lysosomal acidification through a divalent cation–dependent proton pump.[91] ATP did stimulate normal lysosomal cystine transport twofold in polymorphonuclear leukocytes,[38] but the effect required the presence of both 90 m*M* potassium chloride and 2 m*M* magnesium chloride.[90] The possibility that ATP's stimulation of cystine egress was due to lysosomal acidification was examined by measuring cystine transport in the presence of the protonophore, CCCP (carbonyl cyanide *m*-chlorophenylhydrazone), the alkalinizing agents ammonium chloride and methylamine, the anion transport inhibitor DIDS (4,4′-diisothiocyanatostilbene-2,2′-disulfonate), and an inhibitor of ATP-dependent acidification NN′-dicyclohexylcarbodiimide, all of which diminish the proton gradient across the lysosomal membrane.[92–94] None of these reagents decreased cystine transport either in the absence or in the presence of Mg-ATP.[90]

In Epstein-Barr-virus–transformed human lymphoblasts, 2 m*M* Mg-ATP stimulated the loss of cystine from normal granular fractions, but the stimulation was inhibited by CCCP[35,95] and the nonhydrolyzable ATP analogue 5-adenylylimidophosphate.[35] This study showed that nucleotides such as ITP, GTP, and UTP, which acidified lysosomes by at least 0.2 pH units, stimulated cystine efflux to exactly the same extent as ATP; ADP and AMP, which did not acidify lysosomes, did not stimulate cystine egress.[95] Inhibition of acidification by reagents such as *N*-ethylmaleimide also correlated with inhibition of cystine efflux. At the same time, ATP-dependent acidification and ATPase activity of lymphoblast lysosomes[95] and the intralysosomal pH of fibroblast lysosomes[96] were demonstrated to be normal in cystinotic cells.

In rat liver lysosomes purified eighty-nine-fold, Mg-ATP stimulated lysosomal acidification and, in separate preparations, stimulated the efflux of cystine, but not leucine, methionine, or tyrosine.[89] Divalent cations also stimulated cystine efflux, and the calcium ionophore A23187, which altered the lysosomal membrane potential, inhibited the cation-stimulated cystine efflux. Ionophores such as CCCP and alkalinizing agents such as chloroquine and ammonium chloride, which reduced the proton gradient across the lysosomal membrane, also decreased cystine efflux rates. These results, as well as normal fibroblast lysosome studies showing decreased cystine egress in the presence of CCCP or *N*-ethylmaleimide, have led to the conclusion that both decreased membrane potentials and increased pH gradients stimulate lysosomal cystine transport.[88] Cystine loading itself may affect the membrane potential, and it would be informative to measure the extent to which the membrane potential is altered by ionophores using cystine-loaded lysosomes.

The differences between the findings in human leukocytes and lymphoblasts may be related to technical aspects of the studies or to properties intrinsic to the two cell types.[97,98] ATP may stimulate cystine exodus from leukocyte granular fractions only at low levels of cystine loading and in the absence of *N*-ethylmaleimide. Standard leukocyte experiments were performed at high levels of cystine loading in the presence of *N*-ethylmaleimide but not magnesium chloride, and the appearance of cystine outside highly loaded lysosomes was measured. Lymphoblast experiments were done at low levels of cystine loading in the absence of *N*-ethylmaleimide but with magnesium chloride present, and the disappearance of cystine from lysosomes was measured. The leukocyte and lymphoblast may also differ in lysosomal pH or level of endogenous ATP retained after preparation of the granular fraction. The issue of whether cystine transport requires lysosomal acidification may only be resolved when the cystine carrier is isolated, incorporated into liposomes, and studied under defined conditions. At present, there is no evidence for a direct energy requirement for lysosomal cystine transport, and all systems tested exhibit some lysosomal cystine transport in the absence of *added* Mg-ATP. Since any cystine that leaves the lysosome is rapidly reduced to cysteine in the cytoplasm, cystine would be expected always to move down its concentration gradient, and energy might not be required for this process.

I-cell fibroblasts, which lack the Golgi enzyme necessary for placement of the mannose 6-phosphate recognition marker on lysosomal enzymes (see Chap. 79), store cystine in their lysosomes.[99,100] I-cell granular fractions have prolonged half-times for cystine clearance,[37] perhaps because optimal cystine carrier function requires lysosomal processing by enzymes deficient in I-cell disease.

Several miscellaneous properties of lysosomal cystine transport have been reported. Polyamines have been shown to stimulate cystine egress from rat liver lysosomes.[101] Stearylamine enhances cystine efflux from cystinotic lysosomes, probably through its detergent properties.[102] Cystinotic fibroblasts lose cystine at above-normal temperatures,[103,104] perhaps because of increased membrane fluidity or because another carrier recognizes cystine at elevated temperatures. Lysosomal cystine transport does not appear to be mediated by γ-glutamyltranspeptidase, since a patient deficient in this enzyme had normal lysosomal cystine transport.[105]

Finally, lysosomal cystine transport has been described in functional rat thyroid (FRTL-5) cells in culture[106] and in *Saccharomyces cerevisiae* yeast acidic vacuoles.[107]

Mechanism of Cystine Depletion by Cysteamine. Cysteamine, or β-mercaptoethylamine, is an aminothiol that was demonstrated in 1976 to lower the cystine content of cystinotic fibroblasts rapidly and extensively.[108] It was suggested that cysteamine reacted with cystine to form cysteine and cysteine–cysteamine mixed disulfide (Fig. 126-4). The cysteine would leave cystinotic lysosomes freely,[34] perhaps via a specific lysosomal membrane carrier.[109] The mixed disulfide would also exit the lysosome because its molecular mass was less than 220 daltons, the accepted upper limit for free movement of amino acids and dipeptides and tripeptides across the lysosomal membrane.[110] Subsequent work demonstrated that because cysteine–cysteamine mixed disulfide resembles lysine structurally and because cystinotic fibroblasts have an intact lysosomal transport system for lysine, the mixed disulfide was transported across cystinotic lysosomal membranes in a carrier-mediated fashion, by the intact lysine porter.[36] In fact, experiments in leukocytes demonstrated that cysteine–cysteamine mixed disulfide was cleared at a significant rate from cystinotic granular fractions, in contrast to cystine, which remained trapped inside the lysosomes.[111] These two studies essentially verified the hypothesis put forth several years earlier concerning the mechanism of cystine depletion by cysteamine.[108]

Several other reagents have also been investigated for their cystine-depleting ability, including many which were enclosed in liposomes for presentation to cells.[112] Dithiothreitol lowered the cystine content of intact cystinotic fibroblasts[113] and of leukocyte granular fractions,[111] presumably by penetrating the lysosome and reducing cystine to cysteine. Ascorbic acid caused a 50 percent decrease in the cystine content of cultured fibroblasts, perhaps by its effects on properties of the lysosomal membrane.[114] Several other compounds apparently act by producing cysteamine itself. Pantethine, which depletes intact cystinotic fibroblasts[115] but not leukocyte granular fractions of cystine,[111] is degraded to cysteamine by pantetheinase,[116] an enzyme present in human fibroblasts.[117] The aminothiol WR 1065, or *N*-(2′-mercaptoethyl)-1,3-propanediamine, and WR 638, or phosphocysteamine, were also proposed to produce cysteamine as the active cystine-depleting agent.[118,119] Mercaptoethylgluconamide has been shown to lower the cystine content of cystinotic cells,[120] again by its breakdown to the active compound cysteamine.

Source of Lysosomal Cystine in Cystinosis. The intralysosomal cystine crystals in cystinotic cells are thought to form because of saturating concentrations of cystine within lysosomes[24] rather than the phagocytosis of preformed crystals.[15] In cultured cells, the source of intralysosomal cystine appears to be cystine itself in the presence of exogenous cystine and to be protein catabolism in the absence of exogenous cystine.[121–123] When exogenous cystine serves as the source of lysosomal cystine in cystinotic fibroblasts,[122,124] it may enter via two routes.[125] One is rapid, low-capacity, chloroquine inhibitable, and involves movement through the plasma membrane, cytosol, and lysosomal membrane. The

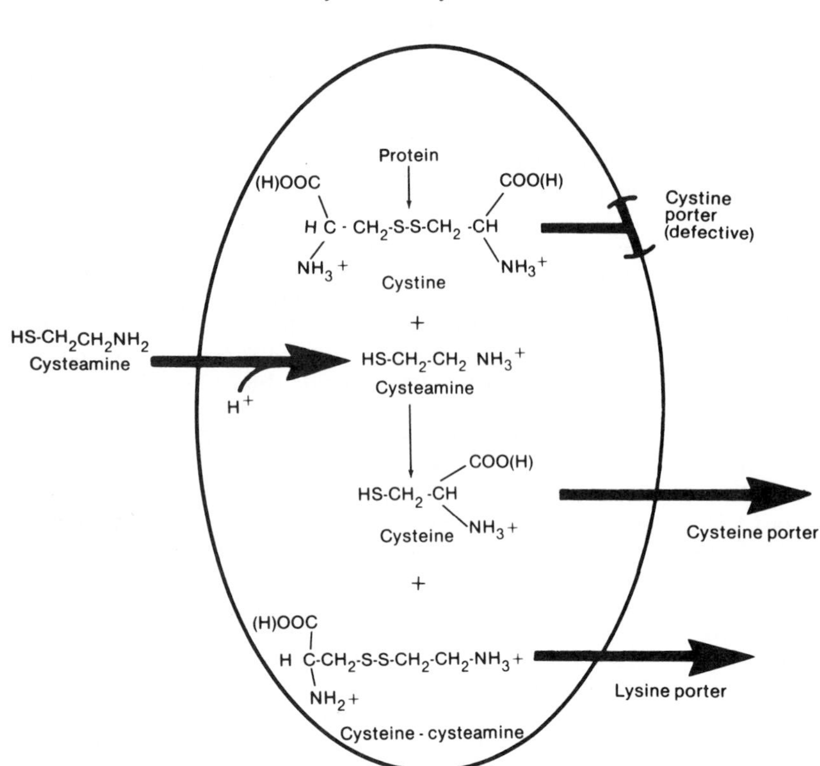

FIG. 126-4 **Mechanism of cystine depletion by cysteamine. Cystine is stored inside the cystinotic lysosome because the cystine carrier in the lysosomal membrane is defective. Cysteamine traverses the lysosomal membrane by virtue of its neutral amine group, which acquires a positive charge within the acidic lysosome. Cysteamine then reacts with cystine, producing cysteine and the mixed disulfide cysteine–cysteamine, by disulfide interchange. Cysteine leaves the cystinotic lysosome, perhaps via a cysteine carrier system. The mixed disulfide cysteine–cysteamine is structurally analogous to lysine, and exits the cystinotic lysosome via a lysosomal lysine carrier, which remains functional in cystinosis cells.**

other is slow, high-capacity, stimulated by chloroquine and low medium pH, and might involve pinocytosis, with fusion of pinosomes and lysosomes. There is also evidence that cystine entering fibroblasts is reduced in the cytoplasm to cysteine,[126] which could enter the lysosome by a known cysteine carrier in the lysosomal membrane.[109] Protein catabolism also gives rise to lysosomal cystine; the lysosomal cystine content has been shown to vary directly with the concentration in the medium of the cystine-rich protein, bovine serum albumin.[127] The process consists of pinocytosis of proteins followed by proteolysis, the rate of which is normal in cystinotic fibroblasts.[127,128] Glutathione may[129] or may not[123] be a source of lysosomal cystine in cystinosis. However, *de novo* cysteine synthesis through the cystathionine β-synthase pathway has been shown not to be the source of stored cystine in cystinosis.[123,130]

We currently do not know why cystine is lost from cystinotic fibroblasts when they are placed at acid pH,[131] in chloroquine-containing medium,[132] at an elevated temperature,[103] or when they are labeled with [^{35}S]cystine and placed in cystine-free medium. This latter occurrence may be due to exocytosis, since the kinetics of [^{35}S]cystine egress resemble those of tritiated sucrose and tritiated mannitol, fluid-phase markers of endocytosis and exocytosis.[27]

Genetics

All forms of cystinosis display autosomal recessive patterns of inheritance. Genetic heterogeneity of this disease is suggested by the variations in severity among different families and by the similar clinical expression of the disease within a given family. Several variants of cystinosis are recognized (see "Cystinosis Variants" below.) One study in which somatic cell hybrids were prepared between cells from patients with different types of cystinosis suggests that the various forms of cystinosis are allelic.[133]

There are no published reports of any heterozygote for cystinosis having cystine crystals in any tissue or cell or exhibiting any clinical manifestations of the renal Fanconi syndrome. Nevertheless, their polymorphonuclear leukocytes contain an increased amount of nonprotein cystine,[134] and peripheral leukocytes of obligate heterozygotes exhibit approximately half-normal rates of lysosomal cystine egress[38] and countertransport.[41] Surprisingly, the free-cystine content of cultured skin fibroblasts from obligate heterozygotes is not significantly different from that found in normal control fibroblasts.[133]

Patients with the late-onset variant of cystinosis represent part of the spectrum of different types of cystinosis. These individuals may be compound heterozygotes who have inherited a gene for the infantile nephropathic variant from one parent, and a second gene for the benign variant from the other parent. Patients with various degrees of severity of classic cystinosis may also be compound heterozygotes, but for two more debilitating allelic mutations.

In North America, the incidence of infantile nephropathic cystinosis is approximately 1 per 100,000 to 1 per 200,000 live births, with a carrier frequency of roughly 1 in 200 in the general population. An estimated 300 to 400 children in the United States have the disease, but ascertainment is suspected to be grossly incomplete, with many undiagnosed infants dying of dehydration. The incidence is higher in certain subpopulations. The French province of Brittany, for example, has an estimated incidence of 1 in 26,000, while in the rest of France the incidence is 1 per 326,440.[135] The incidence of infantile and adolescent cystinosis in the Federal Republic of Germany is approximately 1 per 179,000 live births; of 101 registered patients, 95 had infantile type cystinosis, 5 had the adolescent type, and 1 had the adult type.[136] In the past there appeared to be a slight preponderance of males, but as more patients have been identified, the sex ratio has approached unity.

Cystinosis is often considered a disease of fair-skinned individuals of European descent, but it is known to occur in blacks, Hispanics, and people of Middle Eastern descent, and has also been described in at least one Chinese and several Japanese patients. It is likely that most cases of nonnephropathic (i.e., benign) cystinosis are never diagnosed; thus, one can only speculate on the incidence of this type of cystinosis.

No linkage between cystinosis and HLA loci has been found,[137] and the chromosomal location of the cystinosis gene has not been determined. Cystinosis and Fabry disease have been reported in the same family.[138] Cystinosis and cystic fibrosis have been diagnosed in the same patient, who died at 6 years of age.[139] Studies indicated that this child inherited a mutant allele for both diseases independently from each parent.

Clinical Features and Pathology

Presentation and General Course (Fig. 126-5). A composite history for a typical child with cystinosis has been published previously.[140] As for most lysosomal storage disorders, patients with nephropathic cystinosis are entirely normal at birth, except perhaps for lighter skin and hair pigmentation than their sibs. Development proceeds normally until the second half of the first year of life, when an affected infant generally fails to grow and gain weight, eats poorly, appears fussy, urinates and drinks excessively, and suffers isolated or recurrent episodes of acidosis and dehydration. These findings all result from renal tubular Fanconi syndrome; glucosuria may also eventually lead to a diagnosis of cystinosis. For 55 patients seen at the National Institutes of Health between 1960 and 1980, the median age at diagnosis was 20 months; for 44 patients seen between 1980 and 1992, the median age at diagnosis was 14 months.[141] The age at diagnosis is constantly decreasing because of increased physician awareness, but some children probably still escape diagnosis when they succumb to severe dehydration during an acute diarrheal illness.

The natural history of cystinosis after infancy dictates that an affected child will manifest normal intelligence but continue to grow poorly. Photophobia will develop, and gradually renal glomerular function is lost, requiring renal transplantation at approximately 9 to 10 years of age. The child will not have a predisposition to infections, although certain abnormalities in phagocytic cells have been reported in children with cystinosis.[142] After kidney transplantation, renal function is normalized, but the inexorable accumulation of cystine in other organs creates newly recognized threats to their proper functioning.[140]

Renal Tubular Involvement. The kidney appears particularly susceptible to the adverse effects of cystine accumulation in cystinosis. Initially, the renal abnormality consists of the Fanconi syndrome, or failure of the tubules to properly reabsorb small molecules. The pathological correlate of the Fanconi syndrome appears to be the "swan-neck" deformity of the proximal convoluted tubule[16] and the disorganized and poorly developed tubules, seen in a cystinosis patient's kidney even prior to the onset of frank Fanconi syndrome.[143] Cystinosis represents the most common identifiable cause of renal tubular Fanconi syndrome in children, although tyrosinemia, Wilson disease, Lowe syndrome, galactosemia, and glycogen storage disease are part of the differential diagnosis.

The Fanconi syndrome results in excessive urinary losses of glucose, amino acids, phosphate, calcium, magnesium, sodium, potassium, bicarbonate, carnitine, water, and, undoubtedly, other small molecules yet to be identified. Children with cystinosis may initially receive a diagnosis of Bartter syndrome, nephrogenic diabetes insipidus, or pseudohypoaldosteronism.[144–146] A "tubular" proteinuria, in which

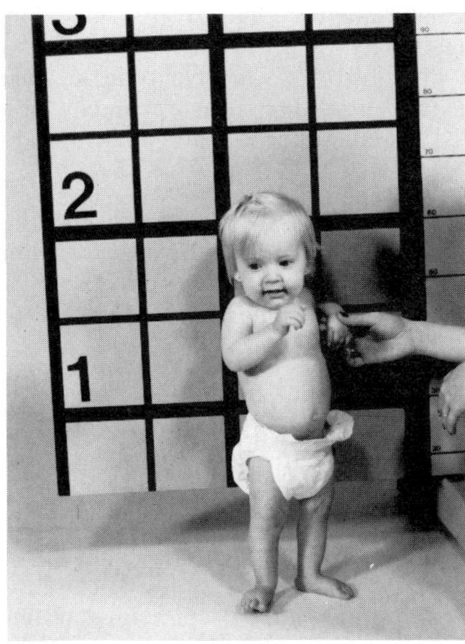

A

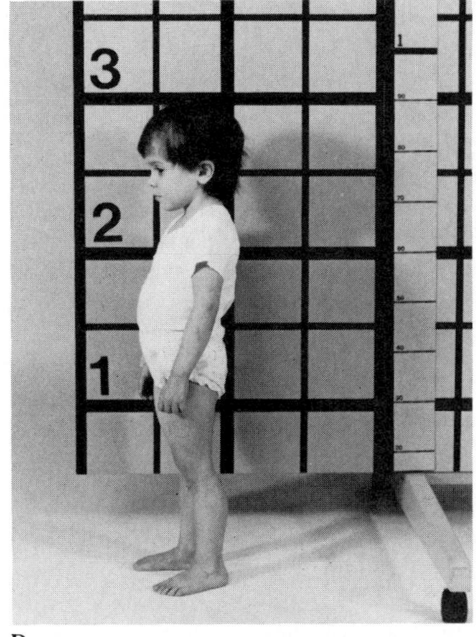

B

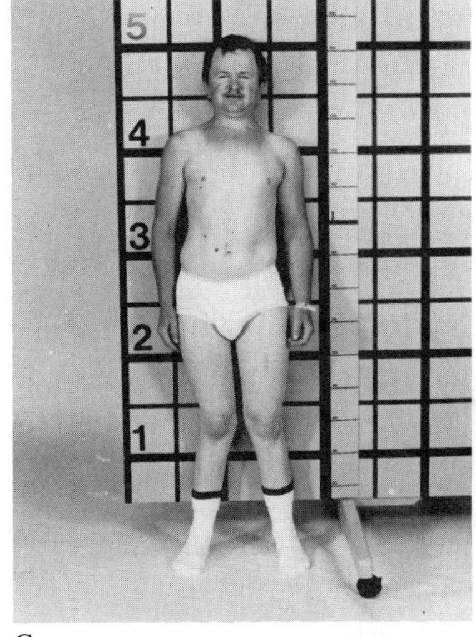

C

FIG. 126-5 **Patients with nephropathic cystinosis. *A.* A 12-month-old girl with typical blonde hair and blue eyes. *B.* A 3⁸⁄₁₂-year-old girl with well-pigmented hair but severe short stature. *C.* A 25-year old patient posttransplantation with evidence of photophobia and renal osteodystrophy (genu valgum). *(Courtesy of National Institutes of Health Clinical Center.)***

proteins of molecular weight 10 to 50,000 are excreted in fiftyfold normal amounts, can also develop.[147] Total protein excretion can be up to 2 g/day.[84] Microscopic hematuria is occasionally present. Renal calculi of urate and calcium oxalate have been reported in cystinosis.[148] Although blood glucose levels are normal, glucosuria and polyuria can lead to the mistaken diagnosis of juvenile onset diabetes mellitus. The polyuria consists of daily excretion of 2 to 6 liters of dilute urine (less than 300 mOsm/liter), and may contribute to persistent enuresis or be life-threatening in an infant suffering acute gastroenteritis. Dehydration in such a patient is rapid and can be associated with a mild chronic fever. Acidosis can be profound due to renal losses of bicarbonate. Hyponatremia and hypokalemia, with its risk of arrhythmias, also occur. Hypocalcemia, and occasionally hypomagnesemia, can result in tetany, especially when acidosis is acutely reversed by alkali therapy or when phosphate supplements bind ionized calcium. Phosphaturia leads to hypophosphatemic rickets with typical metaphyseal widening, rachitic rosary, frontal bossing, genu valgum, and failure to walk. Elevated heat-labile serum alkaline phosphatase levels reflect active rickets. Vitamin D metabolites are normal in cystinosis.[149] A generalized aminoaciduria results in excretion of, on average, over 1 mmol/kg/day of 21 measurable amino acids; this is over tenfold the normal amino acid excretion.[150] The mean fractional excretions of individual amino acids vary widely,[151] ranging from 0.10 for arginine to 0.71 for histidine[152]; normally, 94 to 99 percent of each amino acid is reabsorbed. Carnitine, a small molecule required for transport of free fatty acids into mitochondria for subsequent energy production, is normally 97 percent reabsorbed. However, because of their Fanconi syndrome, cystinosis patients reabsorb only 70 percent of their carnitine, resulting in plasma and muscle carnitine deficiency.[150] Consequently, lipid droplets accumulate in the muscle, which may appear weak and poorly developed. The full ramifications of the Fanconi syndrome in cystinosis have not yet been determined, but they include the failure to thrive characteristic of this disorder.

Glomerular Damage. The glomerular deterioration that provides the clinical hallmark of cystinosis proceeds inexorably in untreated patients. Pathologically, the cystinotic kidney manifests different stages of destruction,[153] with giant-cell transformation of the glomerular epithelium,[154] hyperplasia and hypertrophy of the juxtaglomerular apparatus,[14,82] and occasional "dark" cells and cytoplasmic inclusions.[60] The ultimate result remains a classic end-stage kidney with scarring and fibrosis, chronic interstitial nephritis, and tubular degeneration.[75,155] Crystals, identified as L-cystine,[18] are abundant, but renal stones do not form, as in cystinuria. Clinically, most patients have proteinuria and many have granular casts and microscopic hematuria. Measured creatinine clearances fall monotonically from infancy in untreated patients,[156] although in individual patients renal reserve may prevent the serum creatinine from rising above 1.0 mg/dl before approximately 5 years of age. As for other renal disease,[157] the reciprocal of serum creatinine decreases linearly with age, predicting renal failure in cystinosis at 9.1[156] or 10.7[158] years of age. For 205 European patients, the mean age of renal death was 9.2 years.[159] Many patients approaching renal failure continue to waste large volumes of fluids and electrolytes despite low filtration rates. In others, the Fanconi syndrome appears to improve with the reduced filtration. Some patients have unexplained plateaus in their renal function lasting months to years; others suffer a rapid deterioration of renal function with the onset of an acute infection, acute poststreptococcal glomerulonephritis, or in infants, hypoperfusion secondary to dehydration. Cystinosis patients with uremia can die in congestive heart failure.

Growth. Growth retardation represents a significant part of the clinical picture of nephropathic cystinosis, yet it does not commence in utero. Length and weight are normal at birth. During the first year of life, linear growth begins to decrease. Height falls to the third percentile by 1 year of age. In patients who do not receive cystine depletion, growth proceeds at only 50 to 75 percent of the normal rate, so that an 8-year-old patient has the height of a normal 4-year-old.[160] Bone age follows height age, which soon lags years behind chronological age.[140,161,162] Since height and weight are equally delayed, the children appear proportional except for a relative macrocephaly caused by sparing of head circumference.

Growth and final height of cystinosis patients after renal transplantation are extremely variable.[82] Mean heights for posttransplant patients age 10 to 18 are 20 to 30 cm below the 50th percentile for age.[163] Of 25 patients aged 18 to 33 seen at the National Institute of Child Health and Human Development (NICHD), the tallest male was 177 cm and the shortest was 129 cm (mean ±SD, 146±12 cm); the mean was more than 30 cm below the average normal adult height. Among females, the range was 126 to 149 cm, with a mean ±SD of 137±8cm, or 26 cm below the mean adult height. While children who undergo transplantation before adolescence have some chance of realizing a growth spurt and achieving near-normal height, this prospect appears remote for patients who undergo grafting after 16 years of age, despite a bone age several years delayed.[162] Daily steroids and other immunosuppressive agents may impair growth in these patients.

The pathogenesis of the growth retardation in cystinosis remains unresolved. Children with renal failure due to other causes generally do not show the profound impairment of growth exhibited by patients with cystinosis. Renal failure, chronic acidosis, and renal rickets result in growth delays, but even cystinosis patients without these complications grow poorly. Cystine storage in other organs, including growth plates of long bones and developing myofibrils, may inhibit growth, which improves with chronic cystine depletion.[160] Single growth hormone measurements[164] and somatomedin C levels[161] are normal in patients with cystinosis.

Ocular Damage. Cystinosis eventually affects most of the structures[165] and many of the functions of the eye, but with variable rates of progression. Several reviews have detailed the early[166,167] and late[68,82,162] ocular findings in cystinosis.

Retina. A characteristic peripheral retinopathy, consisting of a patchy depigmentation of the retina with pigment clumps of various sizes, typifies nephropathic cystinosis.[168] This finding is not present at birth, although vacuolization of retinal pigment epithelial cells has been reported in a 21-week cystinotic fetus.[169] A pigment retinopathy has been reported in a 5-week-old girl subsequently diagnosed as having cystinosis.[70] Despite the "blond fundus" resulting from degeneration of the retinal pigment epithelium, visual acuity, visuals fields, night vision, and electroretinography have been normal in young children with cystinosis.[167] But posttransplant patients, whose retinas have accumulated cystine for one to three decades, exhibit a disconcerting frequency of visual impairment. Although visual acuity was subjectively normal in a series of 10 patients aged 11 to 19, electroretinography was abnormal in one individual.[170] Of 16 patients in a French study, 3 exhibited marked visual impairment and 8 had abnormal electroretinography.[82] In a survey of 80 patients over the age of 10 in North America, one-third had decreased visual acuity.[171] It is clear that the frequency and severity of visual impairment increase with age. Of six patients over age 30 examined at the National Eye Institute, five had visual acuities of 20/200 or worse, with color vision and dark adaptation deficits as well.[162] Electroretinography confirmed the clinical findings in affected patients,[68,162] and retinal crystals were documented by photography in one individual.[68] Color vision deficits appear to precede problems with acuity.

Cornea. Corneal crystals, first described in cystinosis in 1941,[172] are pathognomonic of the disorder when seen on slit-lamp examination by a trained ophthalmologist. Descriptions of the pathology of the corneal tissue in cystinosis are numerous.[166,167,173–175] Fusiform crystals involve the anterior portion of the central cornea but occupy the full thickness of the peripheral cornea.[67,167] They are absent at birth and at 3 months of age[67] but are generally present by 1 year of age.[167] A patchy pattern is occasionally observed between 1 and 2 years of age, and the presence of crystals not apparent on slit-lamp examination in a moving infant can sometimes be documented by photography. By 3 or 4 years, cystinotic corneas are packed with crystals, and by 10 to 20 years of age, corneas often develop a characteristic haziness.[68] At this time, exquisitely painful corneal erosions, documented by fluorescein testing (Fig. 126-6*A*), can recur several times a month and seriously interfere with normal activities.[68,162,176] Decreased tearing, documented by Schirmer testing,[177] can exacerbate this condition. In one patient whose cornea was examined immunohistologically, an inflammatory component appeared to be involved.[178] Of 50 patients over 16 years of age examined at the National Eye Institute, 8 had some degree of band keratopathy. One 15-year-od girl exhibited such plaque formation that she was blind to all light perception.[177] Corneal thickness has been reported to be increased in cystinosis.[179] A keratopathy has been described in rabbits fed L-cystine.[180]

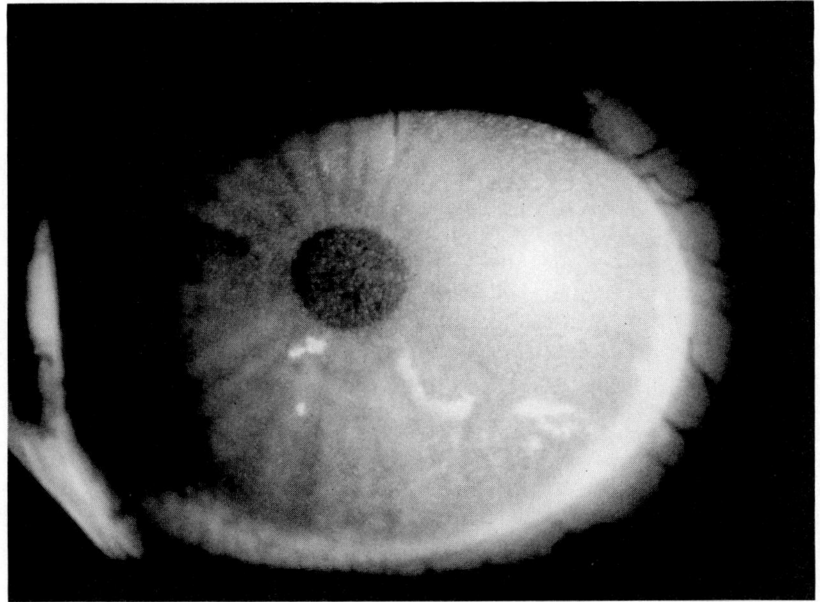

A

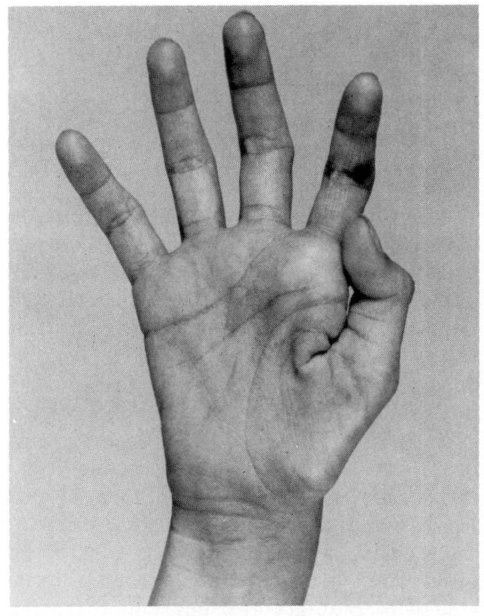

B

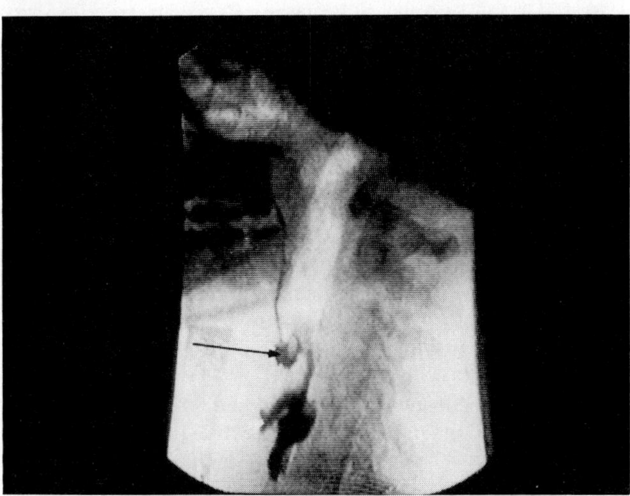

C

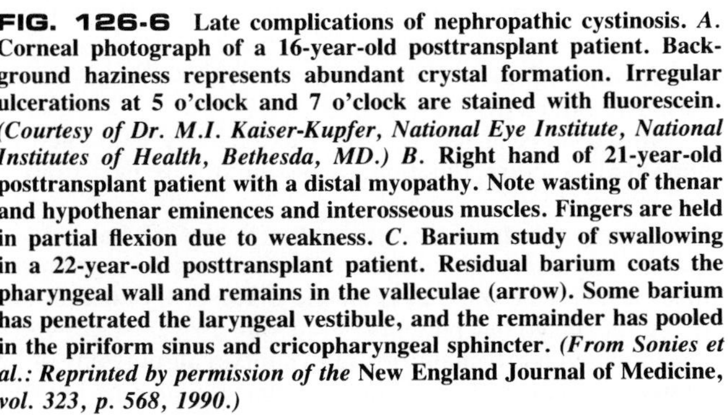

FIG. 126-6 **Late complications of nephropathic cystinosis. *A*. Corneal photograph of a 16-year-old posttransplant patient. Background haziness represents abundant crystal formation. Irregular ulcerations at 5 o'clock and 7 o'clock are stained with fluorescein. *(Courtesy of Dr. M.I. Kaiser-Kupfer, National Eye Institute, National Institutes of Health, Bethesda, MD.) B*. Right hand of 21-year-old posttransplant patient with a distal myopathy. Note wasting of thenar and hypothenar eminences and interosseous muscles. Fingers are held in partial flexion due to weakness. *C*. Barium study of swallowing in a 22-year-old posttransplant patient. Residual barium coats the pharyngeal wall and remains in the valleculae (arrow). Some barium has penetrated the laryngeal vestibule, and the remainder has pooled in the piriform sinus and cricopharyngeal sphincter. *(From Sonies et al.: Reprinted by permission of the* New England Journal of Medicine, *vol. 323, p. 568, 1990.)***

Photophobia of variable onset produces various degrees of discomfort in children with cystinosis,[68,181] who often avoid sunlight. The photophobia probably results from reflections of light off corneal and conjunctival crystals, since it decreases with cysteamine eyedrop therapy[177] and progresses in severity if left untreated.[68]

Conjunctiva. The conjunctiva and uvea contain birefringent hexagonal and rectangular crystals[67] shown by x-ray diffraction studies to be made of L-cystine.[175] These can produce a ground-glass appearance on slit-lamp examination, but do not cause inflammation.[167] Electron microscopy of conjunctival tissue has been used to demonstrate the lysosomal location of the crystals.[182] Cystine measurements in conjunctival biopsies have been suggested for the early diagnosis of cystinosis,[183] but leukocyte assays are less invasive.

Other Ocular Tissues. Cystine crystals are present in the uvea and sclera of cystinosis patients.[167] The irides also contain crystals, especially in older individuals,[68] and crystals have been documented overlying the lenses of posttransplant patients.[68,176] The presence of crystals in these locations may give rise to tissue reactions which result in posterior synechiae, observed in nine National Eye Institute patients 16 to 34 years old.[68,162,177] This complication may in turn lead to glaucoma, which has been observed in two patients 19 and 27 years old.[68,162,182] Refractory blepharospasm, apparently a result of constant guarding against painful photophobia, has been found in a few older individuals.[68,162]

Endocrine Involvement. Primary hypothyroidism, with atrophy and crystal formation in follicular cells, frequently develops in children with cystinosis.[71] This apparently reduces the thyroid's functional reserve and causes compensated hypothyroidism—i.e., an increase in thyrotropin (TSH) prior to the onset of frank hypothyroidism.[164,184] In particular, the α subunit of TSH is often elevated.[185] Hypothyroidism clearly represents an age-related phenomenon. In one study, 3 of 15 patients examined before age 13 years were clinically hypothyroid.[71] Fifteen of 27 cystinotic French children of all ages were hypothyroid.[82] More than 70 percent of 80 North American patients over 10 years of age required thyroid replacement, with an average age of 10 years at the initiation of therapy.[171] Hypothyroidism in cystinosis may be associated with pituitary resistance to thyroid hormone,[186] and histologic studies of cystinotic pituitary glands have revealed occasional hyperplasia of thyrotrophs and refractile crystals.[71] However, growth hormone,[164] somatomedin C,[161] and cortisol response to ACTH[164] appear normal in children with cystinosis.

The pancreas may also be affected by longstanding cystine accumulation. Although nonsuppressible insulinlike activity is normal in young children with cystinosis,[164] insulin-dependent diabetes mellitus has developed in several patients after the age of 10.[62,82,187] Poor glucose tolerance results from impaired insulin production,[62] and is exacerbated by antirejection steroid therapy. Diabetes mellitus has been reported in a 13-month-old infant with cystinosis,[188] and β-cell hyperplasia has been found in cystinotic pancreases examined post mortem.[189]

Female patients with cystinosis undergo pubertal events in a normal sequence,[162] but at ages which range from normal to late—16 to 17 years of age. To date, most affected girls have undergone renal transplantation prior to puberty, meaning that either uremia or immunosuppressive therapy or both have interfered with normal development. Nevertheless, virtually all eventually progress,[163] and one 20-year-old woman with cystinosis and a renal transplant gave birth to a normal boy in late 1986.[74]

Male patients with cystinosis have delayed puberty (with a normal sequence of progression), again with some influence exerted by renal failure and transplantation.[190] None of 10 male patients aged 15 to 28 years studied at the NICHD reached Tanner stage 5 of pubertal development. Three had decreased testosterone and seven had elevated follicle-stimulating and luteinizing hormone levels.[190] These findings suggest primary hypogonadism, and the occurrence of crystals and fibrosis in the testes of a 22-year-old patient is consistent with this diagnosis. Older male patients can experience erections, but three patients who produced a semen sample all proved to be azoospermic.[84,190] To our knowledge, no cystinosis patient has fathered a child.

Myopathy. Although muscle was long considered to be spared in cystinosis, it has become apparent that the continued accumulation of cystine in this tissue leads to structural changes and functional impairment. Not only do cystinotic myotubes in culture store cystine,[191] but the cystine content of biopsied muscle increases with age to values 1000 times normal.[73,82,83] The clinical characteristics of the muscle involvement in cystinosis were first recognized in a 22-year-old man with generalized muscle wasting.[73] Hypophonia and dysphagia developed in this posttransplant patient at age 20, weakness and wasting progressed, and the patient died of aspiration 2 years later. He had normal nerve conduction studies, but electromyography showed low-amplitude, brief-duration, polyphasic motor unit potentials consistent with a myopathy. Muscle biopsy sealed the diagnosis with the appearance of type I fiber atrophy, variation in fiber size, and numerous ring fibers. Cystine crystals were apparent in fibroblastoid cells in the perimysial and endomysial spaces adjacent to muscle fibers.[73] To date at least five other patients seen at the National Institutes of Health (NIH) have had clinically documented myopathies, supported by electrophysiological evidence.[192] One 21-year-old woman with severe wasting of her hand muscles (Fig. 126-6*B*) underwent a biopsy of one of her abductor digiti minimi muscles, which showed striking vacuolization and a cystine concentration elevated over one hundredfold.[192] A case of myopathy and corneal crystals reported in the ophthalmic literature appears to represent cystinosis with muscle involvement.[193]

The severe swallowing difficulties observed in older cystinosis patients probably result from impaired muscle function.[194] Affected individuals have decreased tongue and lip strength, hypophonic speech, and abnormal oral structure and anatomy. Swallowing studies (Fig. 126-6*C*) show pooling of barium in the valleculae and piriform sinuses, and some penetration of the laryngeal vestibule, with a significantly increased duration of swallowing. The severity of oral motor dysfunction increased with age. One patient died of his swallowing difficulty,[73] and at least two others have been seriously affected.

Cardiac muscle has not been extensively examined for abnormal structure, function, or cystine storage in cystinosis.

Nervous System Involvement. Although the central nervous system has also been considered to be spared in cystinosis, this may be true only early in the disease. Cystine storage is limited in young patients,[80] but one 25-year-old woman accumulated large quantities of cystine in all portions of her central nervous system,[81] and a 28-year-old man had cystine crystals within white matter parenchymal cells.[195] The clinical correlates of central nervous system storage include cerebral atrophy on CT scan, seen in 3 cystinosis patients in chronic renal failure,[196] in 7 of 9[197] and 11 of 17 posttransplant patients,[163] in a group of 10 cystinosis patients with neurologic symptoms such as seizures, tremor, mental retardation, or pyramidal syndrome,[198] in 13 of 14 unselected cystinosis patients aged 13 to 25,[199] and in 10 of 11 cystinosis children and adolescents.[200] Cerebral cortical atrophy can be observed in pediatric patients with end-stage renal disease,[201] but the frequency in cystinosis seems excessive, and one study controlled for this.[198] Other cerebral involvement in cystinosis includes nonabsorptive hydrocephalus,[202] demyelination of the internal capsule and brachium pontis,[76] and cystic necrosis with calcification, spongy change, and vacuolization.[195] The patient with the latter problem, a man in his midtwenties with a renal transplant for 14 years, had difficulty swallowing, slow speech, loss of recent memory, extremity weakness, and a gait disturbance confining him to a wheelchair.[195,199] Deficits of short-term visual memory, not based on ophthalmologic abnormalities, have also been reported in cystinosis.[203] Despite the cerebral atrophy seen on CT scan, most cystinosis patients have normal neurologic examinations.[199] Neurophysiological testing of the peripheral nervous system has been normal in cystinosis.[204]

Hepatic and Gastrointestinal Complications. Hepatomegaly has been reported in 7 of 16 dialysis and transplant patients with cystinosis[82] and in 42 percent of 80 cystinosis patients over the age of 10.[171] Many children under age 5 also have hepatomegaly, the etiology of which is unknown. In general, it is not associated with elevated serum liver enzymes or clinical abnormalities. Esophageal varices in two patients[82] and bleeding gastric varices in another[205] did result from portal hypertension. Hypersplenism syndrome has occasionally been seen,[82,162] and the incidence of splenomegaly among patients over age 10 is 27 percent.[171]

Liver pathology has demonstrated crystals[61] and hepatic venoocclusive disease[205] but not cirrhosis.[82] The liver has a normal acinar architecture with hypertrophy of Kupffer cells and, to a lesser extent, portal macrophages as a result of cystine crystal formation[206] (see Fig. 126-3*A*). The affected Kupffer cells are haphazardly distributed, but may be clustered around terminal hepatic venules in zone 3. There is usually no inflammatory response and little or no fibrosis. Hepatocytes, perisinusoidal lipocytes (Ito cells), bile ducts, and blood vessels usually show no pathological changes.[206]

Cystine crystals also occur in the appendix,[65] rectal mucosa,[63] and intestinal mucosa.[64] Their presence may contribute to the morning nausea and vomiting observed among some children with cystinosis, many of whom are also poor eaters with penchants for hot, spicy foods.[140] One 7-year-old boy with severe cystinosis has been diagnosed with ulcerative colitis,[207] and a 17-year-old woman[208] as well as a 21-year-old man[84] had objective evidence of pancreatic exocrine insufficiency.

Other Clinical and Laboratory Abnormalities. Caucasian (not Hispanic or black) patients with cystinosis have skin and hair pigmentation noticeably lighter than their unaffected sibs. We speculate that pigment formation may be impaired in the melanosomes, which are the melanocyte counterparts of lysosomes. Young patients with cystinosis have average intelligence and school performance.[209] Psychosocial problems occur because of their chronic illness, and adjusting to a life of short stature often proves difficult.[140] Some children avoid school and others fail to extricate themselves from dependence on their parents.

Most children with nephropathic cystinosis display an inability to produce a normal volume of sweat, although sweat electrolyte concentrations are normal.[210] This deficiency results in heat intolerance and avoidance, flushing, hyperthermia, and vomiting in small children. The cause is unknown. Stimulated salivary flow rates were also decreased below the normal range in 10 of 18 cystinosis patients tested.[211]

Polyneuropathy and pulmonary fibrosis have been reported in individual posttransplant patients.[212]

For reasons that remain mysterious, several laboratory values are often chronically elevated in cystinosis, including the sedimentation rate, total serum cholesterol (including VLDL and HDL subfractions), and platelet count.[140,162] The platelet count normalizes after renal transplantation.[162] A mild anemia becomes severe with the onset of uremia, with a hematocrit of 15 to 20 percent accompanying a serum creatinine of 3 to 8 mg/dl. The anemia, not due to iron deficiency, may result from decreased erythropoietin production by a damaged kidney and, later, from uremia. Posttransplant patients have normal hematocrits.[162]

Cystinosis as an Adult Disease. Renal allograft procedures have changed the face of cystinosis from a fatal childhood disease followed by pediatric nephrologists to an adult disorder challenging internists and other specialists. The imprint of cystinosis appears immediately on the prematurely aged, jowled faces of young adults, who often have slow, raspy speech,[84] and who almost always have short stature.[162] The associated problem of poor self-image is exacerbated in males by the prospect of infertility. Medical catastrophes are also threatening. Of 27 patients over age 20 seen at the NIH, 13 have either a severe myopathy, blindness, central nervous system involvement, or pancreatic insufficiency. None received prior cysteamine therapy (see "Oral Cysteamine Therapy" below). One of the enigmas of cystinosis is why certain patients suffer severe involvement of a single organ, with sparing of other systems, and other patients suffer complications of a different organ system.

Diagnosis

Postnatal. The first individual diagnosed as having nephropathic cystinosis in a family generally is diagnosed because of suspicion aroused by the presenting renal abnormalities. In patients over 3 months old with failure to thrive, a random urine creatinine test may point the way to the diagnosis. All cystinosis patients seen at the NIH had a urine creatinine below 25 mg/dl, and 90 percent had a value below 15 mg/dl. The diagnosis is confirmed by measuring the white-cell cystine content. Leukocytes are prepared from as little as 3 ml of heparinized blood by acid citrate–dextran sedimentation, followed by hypotonic lysis of erythrocytes. Cystine is then measured either with an automated amino acid analyzer using column chromatography or by utilizing a specific cystine-binding protein in an isotope dilution assay.[59] In normal control individuals the cystine content of mixed leukocyte preparations is less than 0.2 nmol of half-cystine per milligram of protein. In infantile nephropathic cystinosis the value averages approximately 8 nmol of one half-cystine per milligram of protein[19,20,41,213,214] (see Table 126-1). In other forms of cystinosis the value may be lower, but is generally greater than 2 nmol of one half-cystine per milligram of protein.

Cultured skin fibroblasts also store cystine to levels between 6 and 14 nmol of half-cystine per milligram of protein[20,213,214] (see Table 126-1). The fibroblast cystine content of cystinosis patients varies somewhat with cell preparation and storage,[215] cell passage number and confluency,[130] and the cystine and protein content of the culture medium.[122,127]

Cystinosis can also be diagnosed immediately by ophthalmologic examination, revealing the typical crystalline keratopathy in children over 1 year of age[216] and/or the salt-and-pepper retinopathy in infants even younger.[70] Abnormal eye findings were also reported in an aborted fetus affected with cystinosis.[169] Detection of the typical retinopathy requires use of an indirect ophthalmoscope and generally is successfully accomplished in the newborn only by an ophthalmologist using anesthesia. Since diagnosis can now be directly accomplished by measuring the leukocyte cystine content, use of anesthesia for this purpose is only of historical interest. Other methods used in the past included study of conjunctival biopsy,[67] rectal mucosal biopsy,[63] or most often bone marrow aspirate, in which the hexagonal and monoclinic cystine crystals are obvious under crossed polarizing prisms.[70]

The first case of benign cystinosis in a family is always detected by an ophthalmologist who is doing a slit-lamp examination for some other reason. Once again, the diagnosis can be verified by white-cell cystine assay. Because late-onset cystinosis has been diagnosed in two sisters with glomerular disease at age 25 years, it would seem appropriate to rule out cystinosis in young adults who present with glomerular failure for which other causes cannot be demonstrated.

There is no newborn screening program for cystinosis because of the labor-intensive nature of current diagnostic tests.

Prenatal. Prenatal diagnosis can be performed on either cultured amniocytes following amniocentesis at 14 to 18 weeks of gestation[169] or on chorionic villus samples obtained at 6 to 8 weeks of gestation.[217,218] For chorionic villus samples affected with cystinosis, direct measurement of the cystine contents gave values of 34.7, 3.3, and 17.98 nmol of half-cystine per milligram of protein.[217,219] Normal cystine levels, using chorionic villi of at least 5 mg wet weight, are 0.102 ± 0.011 (SEM)[220] or 0.12 ± 0.02 (SD)[219] nmol of half-cystine per milligram of protein. Cells cultured from three affected chorionic villus samples contained 9.7, 3.1, and 7.3 nmol of half-cystine per milligram of protein (normal, 0.14 ± 0.04).[219] Both amniocytes and chorionic villus cells can also be grown in [^{35}S]cystine and the intracellular fate of this isotope studied.[56,221] With improved techniques for growing these cells it is now usually possible to grow enough cells for direct measurement of intracellular free cystine. The amniotic fluid cystine concentration was normal in an affected pregnancy.[169]

Because of the success with cysteamine therapy (see "Oral Cysteamine Therapy" below), many families now refuse prenatal diagnosis but ask that the diagnosis be made immediately at birth so that treatment with cysteamine or phosphocysteamine can be started as soon as possible. This can be done by measuring the cystine content of cord blood leukocytes or of the placenta.[222] The placental cystine concentrations of five affected pregnancies were 2.3, 2.9, 4.2, 4.8, and 70.0 nmol of half-cystine per milligram of protein, as compared with a mean $\pm$SD of 0.18 ± 0.12 nmol of half-cystine per milligram of protein for 14 normal controls.

Heterozygotes. Leukocytes from obligate heterozygotes for cystinosis contain, on average, four to five times more free cystine per milligram of protein than normal control individuals.[19] However, approximately 10 percent of heterozygotes have values that fall into the normal range when mixed populations of leukocytes are measured.[134] This occurs because most of the cystine is found in the polymorphonuclear cells and monocytes, and very little in the lymphocytes.[78] When polymorphonuclear cells were prepared by centrifugation through a discontinuous Ficoll-Hypaque gradient, 29 obligate heterozygotes were all clearly distinguished from 18 control subjects on the basis of the cystine content of these cells.[134] This very tedious procedure is not suitable for general screening, although it can be performed for members of families at risk.

Therapy

Symptomatic. In infants with cystinosis, the renal Fanconi syndrome causes severe electrolyte imbalances which can result in fatal dehydration, particularly during summer months and during episodes of gastroenteritis. These acute, life-threatening imbalances must be promptly treated with enormous IV replacement of fluids and electrolytes. Daily losses during periods of health are managed by oral replacement therapy. Patients vary widely in their needs; estimates of appropriate amounts of intravenous and oral supplements are discussed elsewhere.[140] Electrolyte supplementation is usually accomplished by some combination of sodium and potassium bicarbonate. Polycitra provides 1 meq of sodium and 1 meq of potassium, along with 2 meq of bicarbonate anion (as citrate) in each milliliter.[223] In patients with normal potassium, sodium citrate alone (Bicitra) may be substituted. Citrate compounds have been the usual form of alkali replacement in cystinosis patients, but physicians should keep in mind that gastrointestinal aluminum absorption is enhanced in patients receiving citrate. Although this is primarily a problem for uremic patients receiving aluminum hydroxide to control phosphorus levels, some physicians may prefer to use the bicarbonate anion for long-term correction of acidosis.[224] Patients whose bicarbonate wastage is less severe than other electrolyte losses may require only sodium or potassium chloride. Children with cystinosis may have extreme polyuria secondary to their renal tubular damage, so that free access to large amounts of water is essential during both day and night. Salt craving is also commonly observed in cystinosis patients, who regulate themselves well if given access to salty food or, in many cases, plain table salt.

Progressive urinary losses of phosphate lead to rickets and can be replaced using sodium phosphate (Nutraphos), which contains 765 mg of phosphate in 2.5 oz. If gastrointestinal disturbances do not interfere with the administration of the phosphate preparation, any existing rickets can be corrected. In practice, however, most patients require supplementation with vitamin D. This is usually done with dihydrotachysterol or 1,25-dihydroxycholecalciferol. A typical dose of the latter might be 0.25 μg every other day, but the dose must be individualized for each patient. Although children with cystinosis have generalized and profound aminoaciduria, nitrogen wastage has not been documented.[225]

Poor appetite and eating disorders are common in cystinosis, but placement of nasogastric or gastrostomy tubes should be approached with caution. We know of three children in whom long-term tube placement has extinguished the swallowing reflex, and these children must now relearn how to eat.

Many European medical centers find indomethacin extremely helpful in treating children with cystinosis.[226–229] Properly used, it markedly reduces the abnormal urinary losses.[230] The decreased need for water ingestion may lead to an increased appetite and improved growth.[231] The dose of indomethacin (2 to 3 mg/kg/day) is individualized for each patient so as not to decrease the GFR. Any decrease in GFR appears to be reversible when the drug dose is lowered.[232] The mechanism of indomethacin's action appears to be related to an inhibition of prostaglandin synthesis.[229,230]

Carnitine deficiency due to Fanconi syndrome can be treated with oral L-carnitine replacement.[150] Plasma carnitine levels return promptly to normal, but because of enormous ongoing urinary losses, the muscle compartment may take years to replete—at least at 100 mg/kg/day of L-carnitine given in divided doses every 6 h.[233] Several cystinosis patients, treated from infancy with oral L-carnitine, have had normal muscle carnitine levels when biopsied at 5 to 6 years of age.[234]

As renal failure supervenes, the basic aspects of medical care are similar to those for any uremic patient. Care must be taken to manage serum concentrations of calcium, phosphate, and potassium properly. However, cystinosis patients have some unique problems. Hypothyroidism often develops by the end of the first decade of life,[164,171] but responds well to standard doses of L-thyroxine.[235] Similarly, insulin-deficient patients are benefited by insulin therapy.[62] Rarely, incapacitating corneal erosions require a penetrating keratoplasty. The cornea has been reported to be clear of crystals following this procedure in one patient[176] and to have reaccumulated cystine crystals (presumably by migration of host cells) in another patient.[236]

Renal Allografts. The natural history of infantile nephropathic cystinosis treated symptomatically is one of unremitting progression of glomerular damage, eventually leading to death in uremia before puberty. In a large European study the mean age of "renal death" was approximately 9 years.[159] Once uremia ensues in cystinosis, dialysis or renal transplantation becomes essential. Hemodialysis of a boy with cystinosis was first reported in 1966[237] and rapidly became part of the standard of care for uremic patients. It has since been supplanted in some areas by peritoneal dialysis, which can be continuous or intermittent, inpatient or ambulatory. Dialysis represents a temporizing measure for patients awaiting renal transplantation.

Since the primary abnormality leading to renal failure in cystinosis is a genetically determined defect of the intracellular environment, cells without this genetic defect transplanted into a cystinosis patient do not accumulate intralysosomal cystine. This knowledge and the success of the procedure has led to the widespread use of transplantation in cystinosis patients.[82,159,162,163,235,238] Indeed, renal transplantation in cystinosis patients has been just as successful as,[163] or more successful than,[82,163] renal transplantation in children with other chronic renal diseases. Transplanted kidneys do not develop the series of functional changes typical of cystinosis,[238,239] but they may reaccumulate some cystine, which electron microscopic studies suggest is largely and perhaps entirely confined to interstitial and mesangial cells, presumably of host origin.[240] This phenomenon occurs in both heterozygous and cadaver donor kidneys. In spite of theoretical concerns that heterozygote donor kidneys might be more prone than cadaver kidneys to cystine reaccumulation,[241] there is no evidence for this, and heterozygotes are widely accepted as kidney donors. The best immunologic match should always be sought. In one sampling of 14 posttransplant patients with cystinosis, kidneys from living related donors performed better and longer than cadaveric kidneys.[162]

Specific Treatment to Reduce Cystine Storage. Dietary restriction of methionine and cystine to reduce cystine storage has proven of no benefit in cystinosis.[12,225,242] In retrospect, this seems logical, since intracellular protein serves as an abundant source of cystine in cystinotic fibroblasts.[123]

Specific drug therapy has been directed toward the reduction of cystine to cysteine. In 1961, penicillamine was proposed to serve this function,[243] but subsequent clinical trials demonstrated a conclusive lack of efficacy.[242,244] It was later apparent that penicillamine did not efficiently deplete either cystinotic fibroblasts[108] or leukocyte granular fractions[111] of cystine, probably because its size or configuration prevents entry into lysosomes.

Dithiothreitol was the first thiol-reducing agent shown to be an effective cystine-depleting agent in cultured fibroblasts.[113] The cystine could be mobilized by either dithiothreitol disulfide or free thiol.[245] Although oral dithiothreitol therapy produced moderate reductions in leukocyte cystine content in two children treated for 8 months,[246] longer-term stabilization of renal function has not been demonstrated, and dithiothreitol has not been widely used during the past 20 years.

Ascorbic acid reduced the cystine content of cultured cystinotic fibroblasts by 50 percent,[114] but did not benefit renal function in 32 cystinosis patients treated for 28 months in a placebo-controlled clinical trial.[247]

Oral Cysteamine Therapy. The largest and best experience with cystine-depleting drugs in cystinosis involves cysteamine* (β-mercaptoethylamine), whose mechanism of action has already been described (see "Mechanism of Cystine Depletion" above). In 1976, in vitro experiments demonstrating cystine-depleting efficacy in cystinotic fibroblasts provided the basis for in vivo administration of the drug.[108] A cystinosis patient with end-stage renal disease tolerated up to 90 mg/kg/day of cysteamine hydrochloride with marked cystine depletion in circulating leukocytes, but suffered a seizure, presumably due to her advanced renal failure.[108] That trial was discontinued, but other workers treating a small number of cystinosis patients with advanced renal failure for a relatively short time noted no significant improvement.[248] Other anecdotal reports of short-term cysteamine use are referred to in a previous edition of this chapter.[14]

In 1978, a multicentered collaborative trial was begun at the University of California, San Diego, the University of Michigan, and the NICHD. In this study, 93 children with infantile nephropathic cystinosis were treated with oral cysteamine (mean dose, 51.3 mg free-base per kilogram of body weight per day) for up to 73 months.[160] The drug was given every 6 h because of its short duration of cystine-depleting action.[108] The mean depletion of cystine from leukocytes was 82 percent. When the patients were studied at age 6, 17 of 27 children treated with cysteamine for at least a year had a serum creatinine of less than 88 μmol/liter (1.0 mg/dl), as compared with only 2 of 17 in a historical

*This drug had not been approved by the Food and Drug Administration at the time of writing.

control group not treated with cysteamine ($p = 0.002$). When the study was terminated, the mean creatinine clearance was 0.64±0.04 ml/s (38.5±2.5 ml/min) per 1.73 m^2 for cysteamine-treated patients and 0.50±0.03 ml/liter (29.7±2.0 ml/min) per 1.73 m^2 for patients not receiving cysteamine ($p = 0.015$). In addition, significant improvement of growth was noted during the first year on cysteamine and every year thereafter. Between 2 and 3 years of age, patients treated with cysteamine had 93.1 percent of the normal growth velocity, whereas in untreated children growth was only 53.5 percent of normal. There was no improvement seen in the symptoms of the Fanconi syndrome which all patients had before they entered the study.[160]

The data of the above study were analyzed using the predicted reciprocal serum creatinine at age 10 years (PRC_{10}), a parameter based on the linear relationship between reciprocal serum creatinine and age. The higher the PRC_{10}, the better the expected renal function. The PRC_{10} increased with duration of cysteamine therapy and with the degree of leukocyte cystine depletion achieved,[158] confirming the value of early therapy and good compliance. Conversely, the PRC_{10} decreased as the initial serum creatinine rose, suggesting that renal damage already present was irreversible.

In a second national collaborative study,[249] cystinosis patients received either a "standard dose" of cysteamine or phosphocysteamine (1.3 g/m^2/day of the free-base), given every 6 h, or a dose 50 percent higher (1.95 g/m^2/day). The dose of 1.3 g/m^2 is equivalent to 60 mg/kg in the typical cystinosis child at age 4 years. The dosage was changed to be based on surface area because some patients were growing so large that a dosage based on weight was not tolerated. Data analysis after 24 months showed no statistical differences in the calculated creatinine clearances or the height standard scores between the two drugs or the two dose levels. The mean creatinine clearance was 1.06±0.040 ml/s (63.3±2.3 ml/min) per 1.73 m^2 at admission and 1.13±0.095 ml/s (67.7±2.8 ml/min) per 1.73 m^2 after 24 months in these 95 patients. These creatinine clearances are much better than in the previous study,[160] in which the mean creatinine clearance for 93 patients was 0.64±0.03 ml/liter (38.4±2.0 ml/min) per 1.73 m^2 at admission and 0.64±0.04 ml/s (38.5±2.5 ml/min) per 1.73 m^2 after 34 months. The differences may be because patients in the second study began cystine depleting therapy at 28.1±2.1 months of age as compared with 46.7±3.0 months in the previous study. Also, the patients in the more recent study were more compliant, with average leukocyte cystine values 21 percent lower than in the previous study. On admission, the 95 patients in the more recent study had height standard scores of −2.87±0.13 from the mean. At 24 months the height standard score was −2.90±0.14. This indicates a normal growth rate, but lack of catch-up growth. Patients not receiving cystine-depleting drugs fall further from the normal growth curve with time. This study also found that cysteamine and phosphocysteamine have a wide therapeutic dose range.[249]

Thirty years of experience involving 76 cystinosis patients at the NIH have been reviewed.[156] Over 2000 24-h urine collections were performed, and creatinine clearances were measured. Patients who never received cysteamine lost renal function monotonically, reaching renal failure at 9 to 10 years of age. Seventeen patients were considered well-treated with oral cysteamine, since they began treatment prior to age 2 years and achieved good leukocyte cystine depletion. These children, selected without knowledge of their ultimate renal function results, exhibited the same slow decline in reciprocal serum creatinine (Fig. 126-7) that normal

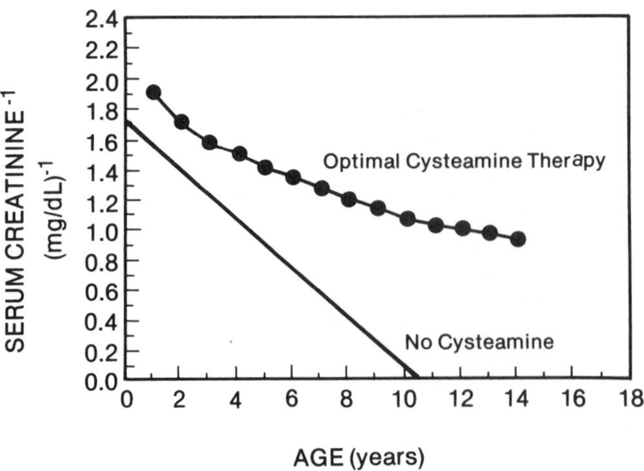

FIG. 126-7 Relationship between reciprocal serum creatinine and age in nephropathic cystinosis. The straight line represents the natural history of renal deterioration in cystinosis, with end-stage renal disease predicted at 10.1 years of age.[158] Each point of the curved line represents the reciprocal of the mean serum creatinine value for 17 cystinosis patients optimally treated with cysteamine and followed at the National Institute of Child Health and Human Development over the past 14 years. Renal function is well maintained by early, diligent cysteamine therapy.

individuals display. The well-treated patients were predicted to maintain adequate renal function past 25 years of age. Moreover, they exhibited an *increase* in creatinine clearance in the first 3 years of life, consistent with the natural growth of renal function during this period. This increase in GFR translated into vastly prolonged maintenance of renal function later in life, emphasizing the value of early therapy and bolstering hope that some patients may never require a renal allograft procedure. Patients treated less well or later with cysteamine therapy displayed renal function results which were intermediate between those of well-treated patients and those of patients not treated with cysteamine. Well-treated patients grew at approximately a normal rate, approaching the fifth percentile for normal children and growing parallel to it (Fig. 126-8).

Life-table analysis has been performed on cysteamine-treated cystinosis patients for comparison with 205 European patients who never received cysteamine. The untreated group had a median age at renal death of approximately 9 years[159] as compared with over 15 years for 142 American patients treated with cysteamine.[219]

Other promising results have come from measurements of parenchymal cell cystine concentrations in patients treated for several years with oral cysteamine.[83] In particular, the mean muscle cystine content for 15 patients treated for 4 to 11 years with cysteamine therapy was one-eighth the mean value for 11 patients the same age but not treated with cysteamine. Moreover, a single 9-year-old boy treated from age 1 with oral cysteamine had cystine values in his kidney, liver, lung, and pancreas which were fiftyfold to one hundredfold less than those of an age-matched cystinosis patient who never received cysteamine. The treated patient also had no crystals in his liver. The combined findings of parenchymal organ cystine depletion and functional improvement in growth and GFR provide powerful evidence for the efficacy of systemic cysteamine therapy as the treatment of choice for nephropathic cystinosis. The value of early diagnosis cannot be overemphasized, since intervention with

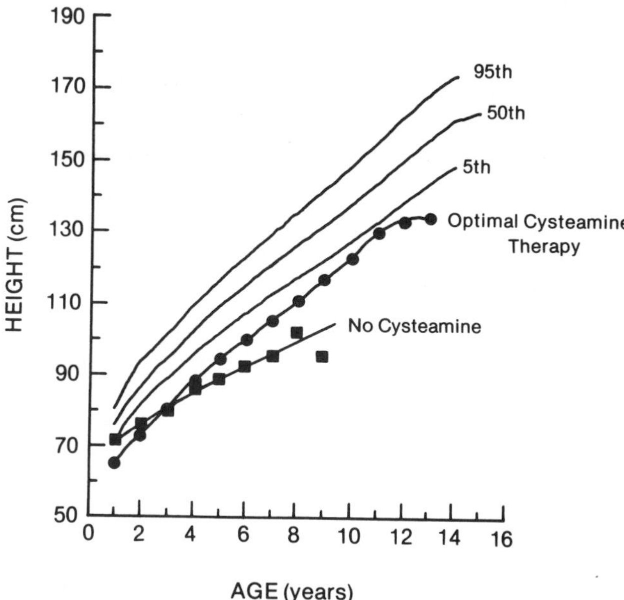

FIG. 126-8 **Growth in nephropathic cystinosis with and without cysteamine therapy. Solid squares give the natural history of growth in cystinosis without cysteamine therapy. The 5th, 50th, and 95th percentiles for the heights of normal children are given for comparison. Children with cystinosis grow at 50 to 60 percent of the normal rate.[160] The circles represent mean heights of 17 cystinosis children well treated with cysteamine at the National Institute of Child Health and Human Development.**

cysteamine in the first 2 years of life can allow for critical growth in absolute renal function.

A British study found that cysteamine could be given rectally.[250] A mean peak plasma cysteamine concentration of 17.2 μM was attained following a rectal dose of 0.13 mmol cysteamine per kilogram of body weight, and the plasma concentration was 36.4 μM following an equimolar oral dose of phosphocysteamine. The half-life of plasma cysteamine was 0.78±0.46 h (mean±SD) following rectal administration and 1.59±1.48 h following oral administration. The mean leukocyte cystine content was 8.09 nmol of half-cystine/milligram of protein at time zero, 3.26 at 3 h, and 4.93 at 12 h. Since the leukocyte cystine values at 12 h were significantly lower than at time zero, this group of investigators recommend that phosphocysteamine can be given every 12 h.[250] We disagree, and think this altered dosage schedule requires much more study before it can be adopted. The 13 years of clinical experience which has shown cysteamine–phosphocysteamine to be highly effective was based on patients receiving medication every 6 h. Before changing to an every-12-h schedule, there should be convincing evidence that this regimen results in leukocyte cystine depletion to levels below 1.0 nmol of half-cystine/milligram of protein at the 12-h time point.

Cysteamine has served as a duodenal ulcerogen in rats,[251] and it depletes somatostatin[252,253] and pituitary prolactin[254] in rats given doses much larger than those used in humans. (Blood levels of cysteamine in treated cystinosis children reach only 30 to 80 μM 1 h after a dose.[255,256]) Long-term cysteamine administered intraperitoneally to mice has not altered hepatic microsomal aryl hydrocarbon hydroxylase activity as compared with controls.[257] Standard treatment of patients with cysteamine has revealed inhibition of glycine turnover,[258] blunting of a prolactin response in thyrotropin-releasing hormone,[259] and conversion of apolipoprotein E_3 to an apolipoprotein E_4 phenotype on isoelectric focusing,[260] but no clinical ramifications have accompanied these laboratory findings. Three patients whose cysteamine dose was abruptly started at up to 70 mg/kg/day experienced a Stevens-Johnson–like rash, central nervous system disorientation and lethargy, or neutropenia; all these resolved on discontinuing the drug.[261] With the gradual incremental dosing over 6 to 8 weeks used in the long-term studies, the only significant side effects were nausea and vomiting observed in approximately 14 percent of patients.[160] Cysteamine, a free thiol, has the odor and taste of rotten eggs. The hepatic venoocclusive disease reportedly due to cysteamine therapy[205] appears more likely to be a complication of cystinosis itself.[262] Hepatomegaly is no more frequent among patients treated with cysteamine than among those who never received cysteamine.[171]

One issue is whether cystinosis patients treated from early childhood with oral cysteamine will experience normal puberty. We are now following a 14-year-old male, treated from age 4, who is Tanner stage III, and a 14-year-old girl, treated for 12 years, who has undergone thelarche and menarche. More time and patients are required to determine if puberty can always progress normally after long-term oral cysteamine therapy.

Most cystinosis patients are diagnosed after the Fanconi syndrome develops. However, a 4-week-old asymptomatic infant was diagnosed with cystinosis because his sib had the disease.[263] Cysteamine treatment was begun at 5 weeks of age; at 10 years of age the patient had normal growth and normal renal tubular and glomerular function.[264] The patient had corneal cystine crystals, and an elevated cystine content in his cultured skin fibroblasts confirmed a typical level for cystinosis. Since the three major types of cystinosis appear allelic, this child is presumed to have the same type of cystinosis as his brother, who had typical infantile cystinosis. We have now started three cystinosis patients on phosphocysteamine shortly after birth.[265] Although the Fanconi syndrome has developed in all three, their clinical courses have been milder than their affected sibs. The fact that our three patients have not had as successful a response to early cysteamine therapy as the earlier case is probably because of genetic heterogeneity in cystinosis.

In utero therapy with cysteamine might seem reasonable because cystine accumulation begins early in fetal life,[169] but the risks of teratogenic effects of the free thiol appear prohibitive at this time. Animal studies may alter this conclusion.

The use of cysteamine is now being considered to prevent the late nonrenal complications of cystinosis. Perhaps the best gauge of the efficacy of cysteamine in this population will be provided by a comparison of the frequency of nonrenal involvement among current patients aged 10 to 30 and future patients the same age who will have been treated for 10 to 15 years with cysteamine.

Because of cysteamine hydrochloride's foul taste and odor, other means of delivering the free thiol have been pursued. Cysteamine in gelatin capsules using 0.2 percent silicic acid as a desiccant has been recommended.[266] Pantetheine, when degraded by pantetheinase,[117] produces cysteamine, but pantetheine's cystine-depleting efficacy appears inferior to that of cysteamine.[267] Phosphocysteamine, the phosphate ester (phosphorothioester) of cysteamine, has cystine-depleting effects similar to cysteamine, but does not have cysteamine's repulsive taste and smell.[119] Phosphocysteamine is rapidly hydrolyzed to cysteamine in the gut and leads to blood levels of cysteamine identical to those achieved with equimolar amounts of cysteamine.[256]

Cysteamine Eyedrops. Despite years of oral cysteamine therapy, children with cystinosis continued to accumulate corneal crystals, causing painful erosions and ulcerations in older patients. One 12-year-old boy had such debilitating corneal pain that he underwent a penetrating keratoplasty,[176] with marked improvement in his quality of life. The epithelial cells of his cornea were cultured; they exhibited both cystine storage and susceptibility to depletion by cysteamine.[268] This meant that cystinotic corneal cells were intrinsically capable of responding to cysteamine therapy, and that low cysteamine concentrations in the avascular cornea were most likely responsible for the failure of oral cysteamine to lower the corneal crystal content. Delivery might be readily achieved using topically administered cysteamine.

After demonstrating the safety of cysteamine eyedrops in rabbit eyes,[268,269] two cystinosis patients under age 2 years were enrolled in a randomized, double-blind clinical trial involving a placebo (normal saline) for one eye and 10 m*M* (0.1 percent) cysteamine plus normal saline for the other eye.[268] Eyedrops were administered every hour while awake, with a marked diminution in corneal crystals in the treated eyes after 4 to 5 months of therapy. By 1990, 29 patients up to 31 years of age had entered the double-masked, randomized, placebo-controlled protocol, which then employed 50 m*M* (0.5 percent) cysteamine in normal saline. Eight of 18 patients under 42 months of age, and 2 of 11 patients 4 to 31 years of age showed marked clearing in one eye, which was subsequently shown to be the cysteamine-treated eye.[270] After breaking the randomization code, both eyes were treated with cysteamine eyedrops. Currently, over 100 patients are on this protocol, and there have been no side effects attributable to this therapy. The formulation now contains preservative, and modifications are being considered in order to bring the preparation to the New Drug Approval stage.

Some generalizations can be drawn concerning the use of cysteamine eyedrops. First, compliance determines the outcome. When drops are given 10 to 14 times per day, a marked decrease in crystal density is apparent within 4 to 8 months. If given three to four times per day, no benefit is evident.[271] Second, young patients with fewer crystals (Fig. 126-9*A*, *B*) respond better and faster than older ones with packed corneas. Several children are now approximately 6 years old with no crystals visible in their corneas. Older patients can lose the haziness to their corneas (Fig. 126-9*C*, *D*) and can experience improved visual acuity. Third, crystal formation appears to be a reversible process. Crystals can be removed at any age, and stopping therapy or reducing the frequency of administration (e.g., to every 4 h) results in recurrence of corneal crystals. Fourth, since the concentration of cysteamine has not been pushed to toxicity, the optimal concentration has not yet been determined. Finally, virtually all compliant patients experience relief of their photophobia.

Use of Growth Hormone. The use of cysteamine–phosphocysteamine has markedly improved the growth of cystinosis patients.[160] After starting therapy, patients tend to have a normal growth rate, but do not exhibit "catch-up" growth. Thus, most patients remain below the third percentile for height. There is some evidence that indomethacin also has a positive influence on growth.[231] The short-term efficacy of recombinant human growth hormone (rhGH) for short stature in patients with chronic renal disease has been established,[272–275] although its effect on final adult height has not yet been demonstrated. Several patients with cystinosis have received rhGH because of its salutary effect on short stature, even in the absence of growth hormone deficiency.[273,275,276] In one of these studies the growth rate of one patient went from 4.8 to 10.0 cm/year, while another improved from 3.5 to 6.4 cm/year with rhGH therapy.[276] In a study from England, six prepubertal children with chronic renal failure, six prepubertal children with renal transplants (including two cystinosis patients), and six pubertal children with renal transplants were all treated with rhGH.[274] Mean growth velocity increased in all three groups. However, there was no improvement in height SD score for bone age in any group. In another study, three patients who had been treated for many years with cysteamine or phosphocysteamine had a twofold to fourfold increase in growth velocity when treated with rhGH.[277] Unfortunately, this was accompanied by an accelerated rate of rise of their serum creatinine concentrations, hastening renal transplantation in one patient and the anticipated need for transplantation in another.

In patients with chronic renal disease who have good growth responses to rhGH, the potential deleterious renal effect may vary according to the etiology of the renal disease. The majority of patients with chronic renal disease who have received growth hormone treatment have had congenital anatomic lesions, whereas patients with cystinosis have a metabolic disease in all cells of their kidneys with progressive cystine accumulation and, perhaps, some degree of ongoing damage.[277] Cystinosis patients with significant chronic renal disease who undergo rhGH treatment, and their families, should consider that by increasing body mass and accelerating the production of creatinine and other waste products, they may hasten their need for renal transplantation and thus trade pretransplant time for increased height.

Family Support Group. The Cystinosis Foundation[278] has been active since 1983 in supporting families, physicians, and investigators involved in cystinosis.

Cystinosis Variants

There are two basic cystinosis phenotypes—nephropathic and nonnephropathic. The nephropathic form can be further subdivided, based on age of presentation, as shown in Table 126-2. Each type appears to represent a different, but allelic, mutation, and there likely exists a continuum of disease severity.

The infantile nephropathic form, described above, is the most common and devastating variant of cystinosis, with presentation in the first year or two of life. In the late-onset forms of nephropathic cystinosis, the age of presentation ranges from 2 to 26 years.[214,279–285] Age of onset and symptoms are usually similar in affected sibs or in members of a family. The most common age of presentation has been 12 to 15

Table 126-2 Different Forms of Cystinosis

Nephropathic	Nonnephropathic
Infantile (6–18 months)	Benign (formerly, adult)
Late-onset	
Child (4–5 years)	
Adolescent (12–15 years)	
Adult-onset (26 years)	

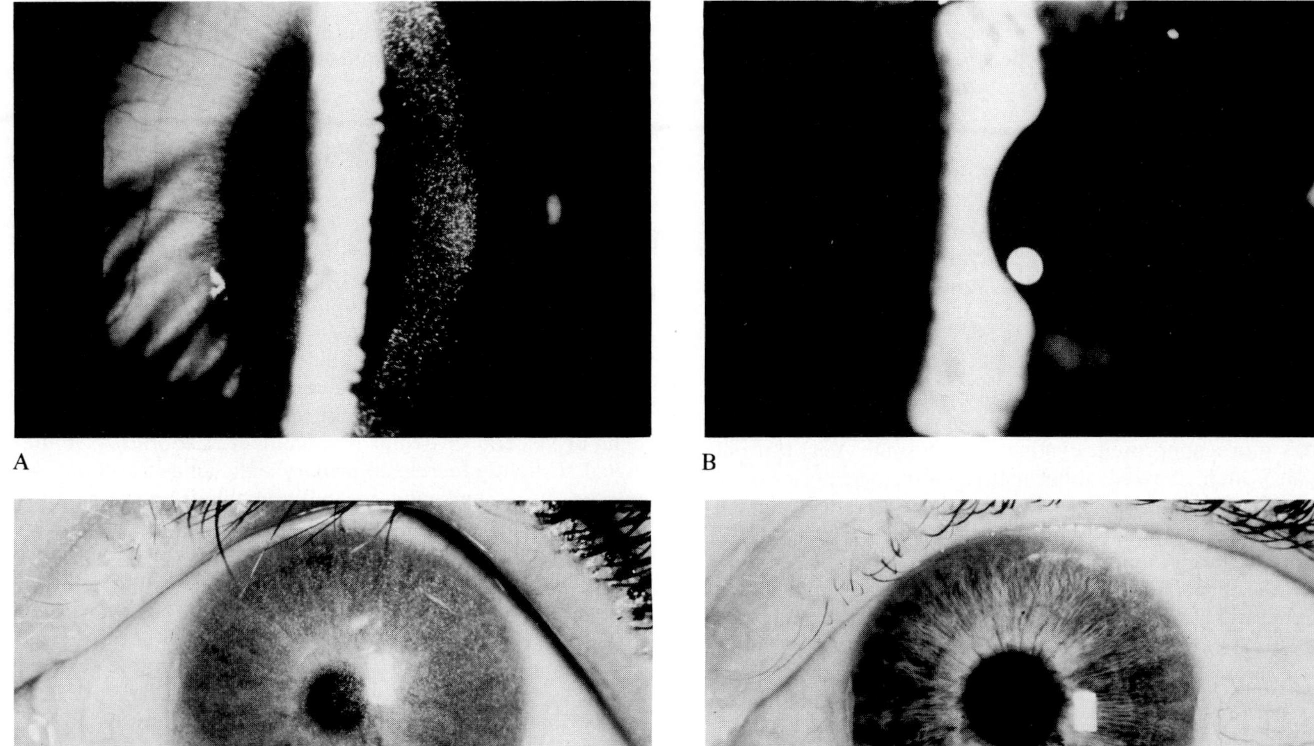

FIG. 126-9 Slit-lamp photographs of corneal cystine crystals before and after cysteamine eyedrop therapy in cystinosis patients. *A*. Right eye of a 2 4/12-year-old boy before topical cysteamine therapy, showing abundant crystals. *B*. Same eye after 7 months of 0.5% cysteamine eyedrops administered 8 to 12 times per day, with clearing of corneal crystals. *C*. Left eye of 21-year-old woman prior to cysteamine eyedrop therapy. Uniform haziness typifies appearance of cornea at this age. *D*. Left eye after several months of diligent therapy with 0.5% cysteamine eyedrops. Cornea is clear to inspection, although crystals remain visible on slit-lamp examination. *(Courtesy of Dr. M.I. Kaiser-Kupfer, National Eye Institute, National Institutes of Health, Bethesda, MD.)*

years.[285] These patients have crystalline deposits in the cornea and conjunctiva, and have cystine crystals within bone marrow aspirates. The complete Fanconi syndrome often does not develop in patients with late-onset cystinosis, but their renal disease may progress to end-stage renal failure within a few years of diagnosis. In one family, two sisters were found to have proteinuria during a routine medical examination at age 25.[286] The older sister had rapid deterioration of glomerular function and required a renal transplant at age 30. No specific diagnosis was made at that time. The younger sister had a similar course, also requiring a transplant at 30 years of age. However, the younger sister had a renal biopsy at age 26 which demonstrated cystine crystals. Both patients were found to have late-onset cystinosis.

Other patients have a benign or nonnephropathic form of cystinosis that is usually discovered by serendipity when an ophthalmologic examination reveals crystalline opacities within the cornea and conjunctiva. This was first reported in 1957,[287] and since then many more cases have been reported.[213,288-293] These patients may suffer from photophobia similar to that of patients with the nephropathic forms of cystinosis, but their photophobia may not begin until middle age and is usually not debilitating. Since the only patients found to have this condition are those who have had a slit-lamp examination, it is possible that many individuals with this form of cystinosis have no eye symptoms and are never diagnosed. Patients with benign cystinosis have crystalline deposits in their bone marrow and leukocytes, but never have renal disease. They appear to have a normal life expectancy, but since some patients with late-onset cystinosis do not have renal dysfunction until their midtwenties, patients with presumably benign cystinosis must be followed diligently.

Patients with benign cystinosis do not appear to accumulate cystine crystals in their kidneys,[289,292] which may explain their lack of kidney pathology. Also, retinopathy does not develop. Patients with benign cystinosis tend to have lower levels of leukocyte cystine than do patients with late-onset cystinosis, who in turn have lower levels than patients with infantile nephropathic cystinosis.[213,214] However, there is much overlap among these values, and the measurements were performed using mixed leukocyte preparations, without regard for the fact that the cystine is stored primarily in polymorphonuclear leukocytes.[78]

Lysosomes from a patient with late-onset cystinosis have deficient cystine-transporting ability. One patient with benign cystinosis had 9 percent and 29 percent residual lysosomal cystine-transporting capacity in two different experiments.[293] These experiments were repeated with lysosomes from different patients with late-onset and benign cystinosis in a different laboratory with the same results.[294] Thus, it appears that the transport defect is most severe in infantile nephropathic cystinosis and least severe in benign cystinosis.

Future Research

The major research goals in cystinosis are understanding the pathophysiology of cystine damage, improving current therapy, and cloning the cystinosis gene.

We do not yet understand why different organs are affected by cystine storage at different times. When a 20-week-old fetus was studied, all organs contained 50 to 100 times more nonprotein cystine than normal. Yet, the only organ which showed abnormalities histologically was the retina.[169] In infants at risk for infantile nephropathic cystinosis, the first renal tubular abnormalities have been observed at 4 to 6 months of age.[70,295] Yet two sibs, aged 5 and 7, with corneal cystine crystals and completely normal tubular and glomerular function had severe glomerular damage 8 years later.[285] Their diagnoses changed from benign to late-onset cystinosis. We do not even know if cystine crystals or only elevated cystine levels per se are responsible for the damage in cystinosis.

Advances in understanding the tubular damage caused by cystine have been made using both in vivo and in vitro models. Investigators have created the Fanconi syndrome in rats by parenteral administration of cystine dimethylester,[296] which loads lysosomes with cystine. Cystine dimethylester loading has also been used to study the effects of cystine loading on plasma membrane transport processes in cultured renal epithelial cells.[297] In other studies, cystine dimethylester loading impaired the transport of small molecules in both rat cortical tubule fragments[296,298] and rabbit proximal convoluted tubules.[299] The latter effect appears to be due to ATP depletion.[300] Other investigators have cultured renal tubular cells from the urine of cystinosis patients[301] for future studies of plasma membrane transport function. These models provide the opportunity for more in-depth studies of the exact causes of cystine toxicity in individual cells.

Cystinosis therapy might be advanced by determining if indomethacin in infants or growth hormone in young children assists growth and well-being without injuring glomerular function. We also need to know if cysteamine depletes the central nervous system of cystine, and we need to develop a better delivery system for both oral and topical cysteamine. Cystinosis should be diagnosed earlier, perhaps by obtaining urine creatinine determinations on all patients with failure to thrive, so that therapy can be initiated early. Long-term cysteamine therapy should be assessed for its ability to preserve nonrenal organ functions.

At the bench, cloning the cystinosis gene will enable investigators to classify the cystinosis variants in a meaningful way (see "Genetics" above). This may be especially helpful in evaluating therapy, since patients with different mutant alleles may have different prognoses and may respond differently to various drugs. The availability of the cystinosis gene should allow the synthesis of the lysosomal cystine transporter, which could then be studied in model membrane systems. It should also permit the determination of how an integral membrane protein (i.e., the cystine carrier) is processed, targeted, and incorporated into the lysosomal membrane. At present the cystinosis gene has not even been mapped to its chromosome. The report of a system which selectively kills cystinotic but not normal control fibroblasts may be an important stimulus to the search for this gene.[302]

SIALIC ACID STORAGE DISORDERS

Historical Aspects

Sialic acid storage disorders have a relatively short history. In 1979 three mentally retarded brothers and their female cousin from northeastern Finland were found to suffer from a hitherto unknown lysosomal storage disorder which was named "Salla disease" after the birthplace of the patients.[303] The clinical presentation included early onset of developmental delay, ataxia, and minor dysmorphic features without signs of visceral or ocular involvement. Laboratory studies revealed slightly increased urinary sialic acid excretion, and enlarged lysosomal vacuoles in lymphocytes and skin biopsy fibroblasts, but normal activities of several lysosomal enzymes. Subsequent studies on the urine of the original four patients and nine other patients with similar clinical presentations revealed a tenfold to fifteenfold increase in free sialic acid but no other abnormal oligosaccharides.[304] Studies on cultured fibroblasts indicated that the material stored in the lysosomes was also free sialic acid. A large number of patients, mainly from northeastern Finland, were subsequently detected. Detailed clinical studies enabled the course of the disease to be delineated, from the hypotonia of a newborn baby to the severely disabled adult with a nearly normal life span.

In 1982, another phenotype was described in severely ill infants with similar, although more pronounced, abnormalities in sialic acid metabolism.[305,306] These infants were characterized by failure to thrive, visceral enlargement, edema, and early death. The disease, called "infantile free sialic acid storage disease," or ISSD, is less frequent than Salla disease and has no ethnic predilection. Only 15 patients with ISSD have been reported in the literature,[307,308] in contrast to 87 Salla disease patients from Finland and a few cases from elsewhere. A series of studies since 1986 has led to the conclusion that both diseases are caused by a genetic defect of lysosomal membrane transport of free sialic acid.

The Basic Defect

Sialic Acid Metabolism. The sialic acids are a family of over 30 compounds derived from neuraminic acid, with many biologic roles.[309,310] In humans, the predominant sialic acid is *N*-acetylneuraminic acid (see Fig. 126-1), a negatively charged compound of molecular weight 309 and pK 2.6, which we refer to as sialic acid. While a small portion of total sialic acid is free in tissues and body fluids, most is bound by an α-glycosidic linkage to glycoconjugates. Sialic acid provides these macromolecules with a negatively charged terminal sugar that serves many functions,[311] but no direct biologic role has been attributed to unbound sialic acid. Human plasma has a low concentration of free sialic acid—0.80 nmol/ml (±0.28) according to one study.[312] The same study also demonstrated that free sialic acid is filtered by renal glomeruli, but not reabsorbed or secreted by tubules. Free sialic acid clearance parallelled creatinine clearance in individuals with normal as well as impaired renal function.

The synthesis of sialic acid begins with glucose, which undergoes several modifications to become activated UDP-*N*-acetyl-D-glucosamine (Fig. 126-10). This central metabo-

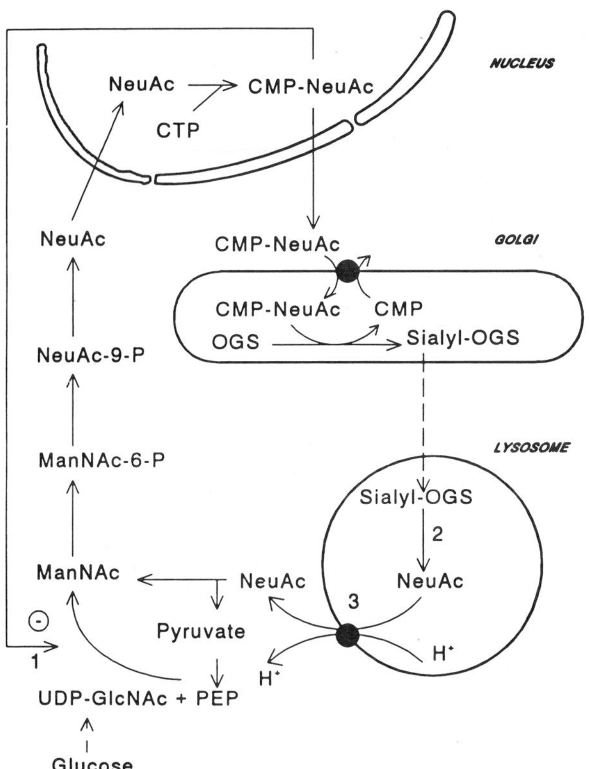

FIG. 126-10 Metabolism of sialic acid. UDP-GLcNAc = Uridine-diphosphate-*N*-acetylglucosamine; ManNAc = *N*-acetylmannosamine; PEP = phosphoenolpyruvate; OGS = oligosaccharide. 1, 2, and 3 point to sites of genetic errors of sialic acid metabolism: 1. UDP-GlcNAc-2-epimerase; 2. lysosomal sialidase; 3. lysosomal sialic acid carrier. *(From Mancini GMS.[307] Used by permission of Erasmus University, Rotterdam, The Netherlands.)*

lite is converted to *N*-acetylmannosamine (ManNac) in a reaction that is subject to feedback inhibition by CMP sialic acid.[313,314] ManNac is modified in stepwise fashion to produce *N*-acetylmannosamine-6-phosphate, *N*-acetylneuraminic acid-9-phosphate, and *N*-acetylneuraminic acid (sialic acid) in reactions apparently not subject to feedback inhibition.[313,315] Sialic acid is then incorporated into glycoconjugates by a trans-Golgi process utilizing CMP as a carrier.

The degradation of sialoglycoconjugates occurs within lysosomes by sequential hydrolysis of terminal glycosidic linkages, usually initiated by the removal of one or more sialic acid residues by an acid sialidase. A genetic deficiency of this enzyme leads to accumulation of undegraded sialoglycoconjugates and to an increase of bound sialic acid in sialidosis and galactosialidosis (see Chap. 81). The free sialic acid produced by the action of sialidase can be reutilized or degraded by *N*-acetylneuraminate lyase,[316] a cytoplasmic enzyme apparently not present within lysosomes.[317,318] This suggests that sialic acid must be removed from the lysosomes for further metabolism. Prior to the discovery of free sialic acid storage disorders the requirement for such a transport process was unrecognized.

Sialic Acid Metabolism in Salla Disease and ISSD. Recognition of free sialic acid as the storage compound prompted metabolic studies of the turnover of this molecule. Using cultured fibroblasts and liver from normal and affected individuals, it was shown that the major enzymes involved in the metabolism of sialic acid were normal. These studies included assays of *N*-acetylneuraminate lyase, sialidase, CMP-*N*-acylneuraminate phosphodiesterase, and acylneuraminate cytidylyltransferase.[317,319] In fibroblasts, the activity of sialidase was reported to be normal by most investigators, although two authors reported threefold to fivefold increases.[320,321] Sialidase was also reportedly increased in the lymphocytes of one patient with Salla disease.[322] All other lysosomal enzymes studied have been normal in ISSD and Salla disease.

Sialic Acid Transport. Several studies in which cultured fibroblasts were loaded with sialic acid demonstrated retention of sialic acid in mutant cells, providing indirect evidence that a defective function of the transport system is the primary cause of sialic acid storage disorders. In these experiments, sialic acid precursors,[319] LDL,[323] the methylester of sialic acid,[324] fetuin,[325] or *N*-acetylneuraminic acid itself[326,327] were used to load the lysosomes with sialic acid. In each case, retention of free sialic acid in the lysosomal fraction could be shown in the cell strains from sialic acid storage disease patients, suggesting a block in the efflux of free sialic acid through the lysosomal membrane. The rate of egress of free sialic acid from the lysosomes was characterized in more detailed studies with isolated lysosomal fractions from fibroblasts preloaded with ManNac to yield equal sialic acid concentrations in the lysosomes of normal and mutant cell strains.[328,329] The initial velocity of egress from normal lysosomes increased linearly with loading; the Q_{10} for sialic acid transport was 2.4, suggesting a carrier-mediated mode of transport. Patient cell strains displayed a negligible egress velocity regardless of the initial sialic acid loading. These findings, obtained both with Salla disease[328] and ISSD cell strains,[329] reflect a defective lysosomal membrane transport function in the mutant cells.

More direct evidence for a specific carrier to facilitate the efflux of free sialic acid from the lysosomes has been presented in experiments using radiolabeled sialic acid uptake studies in resealed lysosomal membrane vesicles.[330] These studies have unequivocally proven that a genetic defect of the sialic acid transport system, presumably a protein, is the primary cause of the sialic acid storage disorders. Resealed vesicles from purified rat liver lysosomes and impermeable buffers were employed to produce a pH difference across the lysosomal membrane, thereby mimicking in vivo lysosomal conditions. Cotransport of sialic acid with protons produced by an ATP-dependent proton pump provided the physiological mechanism for sialic acid transport. The K_m for sialic acid transport under the experimental conditions was about 0.2 m*M*. The sialic acid transport system exhibited the properties of both *trans*-stimulation and *cis*-inhibition, demonstrating that it was carrier-mediated. Interestingly, it was found that glucuronic acid (GluAc) and some other acidic monosaccharides act under similar experimental conditions as competitive substrates for the carrier (Table 126-3).

An identical carrier for acidic monosaccharides was subsequently demonstrated in resealed lysosomal vesicles from cultured human fibroblasts and lymphoblasts.[331] The transport could be inhibited to the same extent by the addition of either unlabeled GluAc or *N*-acetylneuraminic (sialic) acid (NeuAc). Lysosomal vesicle preparations from cell strains of patients with sialic acid storage disorders were almost completely devoid of the transport activity both with sialic acid and glucuronic acid (Table 126-4). No differences were observed between the transport activities of Salla disease and ISSD cell strains. Further evidence that deficient carrier-mediated transport of sialic acid is the primary genetic

Table 126-3 Substrate Specificity of the Sialic Acid Carrier*

	% of Uninhibited Rate
Sialic acid analogues	
No addition	100
Sialic acid	10
Glycolylneuraminic acid	12
N-acetylneuraminic acid methylester	49
4-Methylumbelliferyl-α-D-acetylneuraminic acid	58
2-Deoxy-2,3-dehydro-*N*-acetylneuraminic acid	50
Other monosaccharides, acidic amino acids	
Glucuronate	10
Gluconate	14
Galacturonate	34
Galactonate	36
Pyruvate	50
Glucose	80
N-Acetylglucosamine	100
N-Acetylmannosamine	100
Gulonolactone	88
Mannuronolactone	86
Aspartate	89
Glutamate	86

**Cis*-inhibition of NeuAc uptake into lyosomal membrane vesicles by sialic acid analogues, other monosaccharides, and acidic amino acids. Uptake of 0.15 m*M* [^{14}C]NeuAc into lysosome membrane vesicles was studied in the presence of the inhibitors (7 m*M*) under conditions given in Mancini et al.[330] Uptake in the presence of inhibitor is expressed as a percentage of the uninhibited rate for duplicate determinations.

SOURCE: From Mancini et al.[330] Used by permission of the American Society for Biochemistry and Molecular Biology.

defect in these diseases came from studies of obligate heterozygotes. Transport activity in lysosomal preparations from lymphoblast cell strains of Salla disease parents demonstrated intermediate transport rates for glucuronic acid (Fig. 126-11).

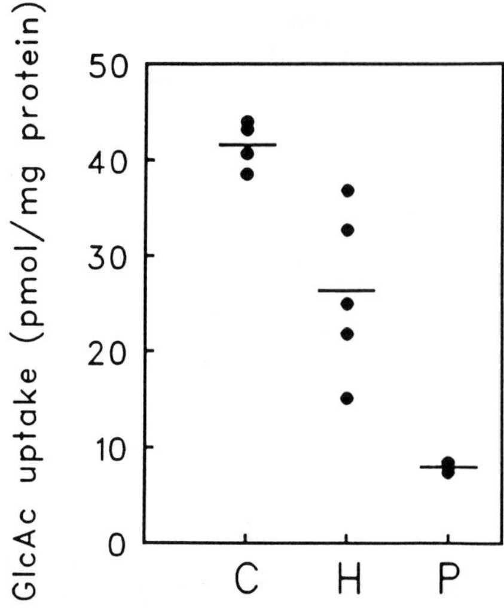

FIG. 126-11 Intermediate glucuronic acid transport of obligate carriers of Salla disease. Lysosomal membrane vesicles from controls (C), from patients with Salla disease (P), and from unrelated parents of Salla disease patients (H) were assayed for transport capacity of 0.055 m*M* [^{3}H]GluAc (3 μCi) under conditions given in Mancini et al.[331] *(From the* Journal of Clinical Investigation, *1991, vol. 87, pp. 1329–35 by copyright permission of the American Society for Clinical Investigation.)*

The significance of defective lysosomal transport of glucuronic acid to the pathogenesis of sialic acid storage diseases remains unknown. Lysosomal accumulation of GluAc as well as reduced egress from isolated lysosomal fractions in cell strains from both Salla disease and ISSD patients has been reported.[332] The amount of glucuronic acid accumulated in the mutant cells averaged only 5 percent of the corresponding amount of free sialic acid. Whether glucuronic acid also accumulates in tissues of patients and is excreted in excess in urine has not yet been investigated.

Development of the experimental assay system for sialic acid transport has created possibilities to isolate the carrier protein. To this end, transport activity has been successfully reconstituted in proteoliposomes using phospholipids and

Table 126-4 Defective Sialic Acid and Glucuronic Acid Transport in Different Clinical Types of Sialic Acid Storage Disease*

	Uptake rate pmol/30 s/mg protein	
Cell line	**[^{3}H]NeuAc**	**[^{3}H]GluAc**
Control 698	20.9	24.6
Control 540	12.6	17.4
Control 53	23.6	35.0
Infantile sialic acid storage disease		
Patient A.Z.	1.1	0
Patient D.R.	0.4	0
Salla disease		
Patient S.P.	0	0
Patient 9015	0	0
Intermediate non-Finnish phenotype		
Patient E.P.	0.5	1.4
Patient E.B.	0.7	0

*Proton-driven transport of NeuAc and GluAc in fibroblast membrane vesicles, expressed as an uptake rate.[331]

SOURCE: From the *Journal of Clinical Investigation,* 1991, vol. 87, pp. 1329-35, by copyright permission of the American Society for Clinical Investigation.

Table 126-5 Urinary Free Sialic Acid in Salla Disease, ISSD and Sialuria Patients

Disease	n	Free Sialic Acid (nmol/mg creatinine)	Reference
Salla	22	700–2100	363
ISSD	10	1071–14,230	306, 321, 326, 345, 348
		6002 (mean)	364
Sialuria	2	123–894	351
		75–221	348
Controls			
Adults	24	7–28	304
Children	74	100–650	342

detergents.[333] Transport properties in proteoliposomes were essentially identical to those of resealed lysosomal membrane vesicles, offering a promising starting point for further purification and molecular characterization of the carrier protein. Purification of the protein and determination of its amino acid sequence should eventually lead to cDNA cloning and identification of the gene defect(s) causing the sialic acid storage disorders.

Storage of Sialic Acid in Salla Disease and ISSD. A constant finding in both types of sialic acid storage diseases is the urinary excretion (Table 126-5) and increased cellular concentration of free sialic acid (Table 126-6). Exhaustive characterization of both the urinary excretion product and the storage material in cells has almost exclusively identified NeuAc.[304,305,317,319,320,334] Studies in liver, brain, kidney, placenta, and leukocytes, as well as cultured fibroblasts and amniotic fluid cells, have all given identical results.

In Salla disease, the urinary excretion of free sialic acid is fivefold to twentyfold normal and the cellular concentration tenfold to thirtyfold compared with age-matched controls, while in ISSD there is a twentyfold to two hundredfold increase both in urine and tissues (see Tables 126-5 and 126-6). In contrast, bound sialic acid levels in the urine and cells of patients have been in the range of controls or only marginally elevated.

Lysosomal accumulation of free sialic acid has been documented both morphologically and biochemically. Intralysosomal localization of sialic acid was first indicated by immunohistochemical methods using the sialic acid–specific lectin *Limulus polyphemus* agglutinin in cultured fibroblasts from Salla disease patients.[335] Several studies employing cell

Table 126-6 Free Sialic Acid in Cultured Cells and Tissues of Patients with Salla Disease, ISSD, and Sialuria

		Free Sialic Acid (nmol/mg prot)			
Sample Disease	n	Mean	SD	Range	Reference
Fibroblasts					
Salla disease	11			6–33	27, 363
ISSD	12	75		10–269	27, 321, 345, 348, 364, 365
Sialuria	3	143		75–273	354
Control	10	1.1	1.0		329
Liver					
Salla	2			0.9–1.1	27
ISSD	1	18			
Control	3			0.03–0.09	
Chorionic villus sampling (direct)					
ISSD	1	30.6			339
Control	12	11.2		1.4–19.1	
Chorionic villus sampling (culture)					
ISSD	1			22.8, 64.6	348
Control	12	2.2		0–4.5	
Amniocyte culture					
Salla	1	2.6			349
ISSD	1	111.0			348
ISSD	1	25.0			338
Control	19			0.4–0.5	363

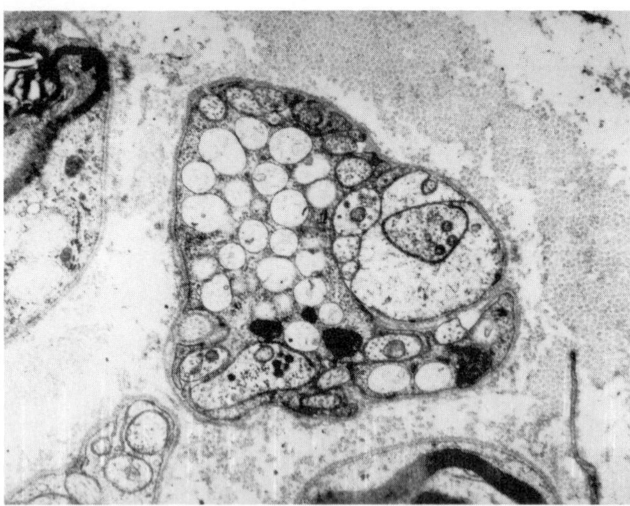

FIG. 126-12 **Electron photomicrograph of unmyelinated dermal nerve Schwann cell from a skin biopsy of a patient with Salla disease. Enlarged single membrane-bound vesicles are filled with amorphous fibrillogranular material, × 11,220.** *(From* Archives of Neurology, *1979, vol. 36, pp. 88–94, copyright 1979, American Medical Association.)*

fractionation of fibroblasts from Salla disease and ISSD patients have demonstrated that the free sialic acid accumulated in the cells cosediments with the lysosome-enriched fraction.[27]

In EM studies, typical single membrane-bound vacuoles containing amorphous fibrillogranular material have been detected in several organs and in various cells types,[303,306,321,322,336,337] including fibrocytes, histiocytes, perithelial cells of capillaries, exocrine and myoepithelial cells of sweat glands, and Schwann cells of peripheral nerves (Fig. 126-12). Lymphocytes and bone marrow cells as well as hepatocytes and Kupffer cells in hepatic biopsies have displayed similar storage lysosomes. In two cases of fetuses affected by ISSD, EM studies of chorionic villus biopsies have shown enlarged lysosomal vacuoles, supporting the biochemical diagnosis.[338,339] Enlarged lysosomes were not present in an 11-week chorionic villus sample obtained for prenatal diagnosis in a family with Salla disease.[339]

Although intralysosomal accumulation of free sialic acid in several organs of patients has been clearly documented, its role in the pathogenesis of the diseases is still largely unknown. Future studies must explain the connection between the severe dysfunction of the brain and free sialic acid storage in the lysosomes.

Genetics and Epidemiology

The mode of inheritance in Salla disease and ISSD is autosomal recessive. This is supported by genealogical studies of Salla disease in Finnish families,[340] by the high rate of consanguineous families with ISSD, and by the demonstration of half-normal sialic acid transport activity in the lysosome membrane preparations of obligate heterozygotes for Salla disease.[331]

The gene coding for the transport protein has not yet been cloned. A genetic linkage study in Finnish families, including 35 patients with Salla disease and 98 healthy family members, has excluded more than 50 percent of the genome, but the disease locus is still to be defined.[341]

Salla disease displays a strong clustering in the Finnish population, whereas no ethnic predilection exists in the more rare phenotype of ISSD. At present, 87 Salla disease patients from 58 Finnish families are known. Most of the families originate from a northeastern area, but occasionally families come from other areas of the country. An analysis of the birthplace of the grandparents in 45 families with one or more Salla disease patients revealed that 78 of 172 grandparents (45 percent) originated from a region approximately 100 km in diameter with a present population of approximately 37,000. Several of these families can be traced back to common ancestors.

A total of 11 isolated cases (eight families) with the Salla disease phenotype have been described from other countries with a variety of ethnic backgrounds.[307] Some of these patients had intermediate types of sialic acid storage disorder, with clinical findings typical of both the Salla disease and ISSD phenotype. Since the first description of ISSD in 1982, 15 patients from 10 families have been reported in the literature.[307] Most patients come from Caucasian families with a wide geographic distribution.

Clinical Findings

Salla Disease. Detailed clinical observations of Salla disease patients have been described from 34 adult[340] and 6 pediatric cases.[342] Additional data, less systematically collected, are available from the rest of the 87 Finnish Salla disease patients. These observations have allowed a delineation of the clinical course of the disease (Table 126-7) from the normal-appearing newborn to a severely mentally and physically disabled adult.

The pregnancy and newborn period are uneventful for Salla disease patients. The first clinical signs of the disease

Table 126-7 **Clinical Findings and Course of Disease in Patients with Salla Disease**

Neonatal period	
Normal	6/6
Infancy	
Hypotonia	5/6
Ocular nystagmus	4/6
Ataxia	6/6
Sitting at 8 months	1/6
Walking at 2 years	1/6
Words at 15 months	2/6
Childhood	
Developmental delay	34/34
Impaired speech	34/34
Unable to walk	8/34
Growth retardation (<−2 SD)	18/34
Adult	
Severe mental ratardation	
IQ 20–40	7/34
IQ <20	27/34
Ataxia	34/34
Athetosis	22/34
Abnormal tendon reflexes	29/34
Exotropia	17/34
Convulsions	9/34
Age at death (12 patients)	36 years (range, 4–70 years)

SOURCE: Adapted from Renlund et al.[340] and Renlund.[342]

are muscular hypotonia and ataxia, which usually appear at 6 to 9 months of age. Ocular horizontal nystagmus has frequently been seen even earlier, only to be replaced later by a divergent squint in about half the cases. One patient exhibited horizontal nystagmus as early as 3 weeks of age.[340] The ataxia can be truncal as well as in the extremities. The general health of the infants with Salla disease has been unremarkable, with no increased susceptibility to infections or gastrointestinal disturbances. After the age of 1 year several patients have brisk tendon reflexes and spasticity in the lower limbs. Motor development is always clearly delayed, and approximately one-third of the patients never learn to walk. Ataxia is commonly accompanied by athetosis. Speech development is regularly delayed and impaired. The majority of patients have learned single words or even short sentences during the first years of life, but approximately a third lose speech later. In addition, the speech of all patients is characterized by dysarthria and dyspraxia; the ability to produce words is affected more than comprehension.

The development of Salla disease patients is severely delayed initially, so that by adulthood patients are mentally retarded, with IQs in the range of 20 to 40. The inexorable progression of symptoms which characterizes many lysosomal diseases is not a prominent finding in Salla disease, except in the late stages of the disease.

Somatic growth is often retarded. Eighteen of 34 patients had a height more than 2 SD below the expected height calculated on the basis of parental height and population averages.[340] Two sibs 21 and 17 years of age exhibited extreme growth retardation, with heights 8.4 and 5.2 SD below expected. These patients also showed virtually undeveloped secondary sexual features, although most patients have normal pubertal development.

Somatic findings in addition to growth retardation and neurologic abnormalities are limited. Facial features (Fig. 126-13) may be coarse at later stages of the disease but to a much lesser extent than in aspartylglucosaminuria and other lysosomal storage disorders. Skeletal dysplasias and other radiologic abnormalities have not been encountered, with the exception of a thickened calvarium present in many patients. Liver and spleen enlargement do not occur, despite an abundance of storage lysosomes and excess amounts of free sialic acid in these organs.

Corneal clouding and fundal changes, frequent manifestations of lysosomal storage disorders, are absent in Salla disease. A constant finding in Salla disease patients over 10 years of age has been a low-voltage-type electroencephalographic recording. The severity of the symptoms and the age of the patients was correlated with the decrease in amplitude. Spike waves were recorded in Salla disease patients who had convulsions. Generalized convulsions are not common in Salla disease but absence type episodes of short duration (formerly called petit mal seizures) have occasionally been seen. Electroretinograms, visual evoked potentials, and nerve conduction velocities have been normal in all cases studied. Cranial CT has revealed cortical and basal atrophy, more pronounced in older than in younger patients.

The life span of patients with Salla disease is relatively long. The oldest patient known to us was 72 at the time of his death. The mean age at death for 12 patients has been 34.6 years, but in several cases the cause of death (e.g., accidents or infections) has been only indirectly related to the disease.

The neuropathology of two patients who died of pneumonia at age 41 has been reported.[343] The cerebral white matter was severely reduced in both cases, with marked loss of axons and myelin sheaths. Abnormally large amounts of a lipofuscin-like material were seen in the perikaryons of the neurons, particularly in the deep cortical layers. The cerebellum also showed degenerative features and loss of Purkinje cells.

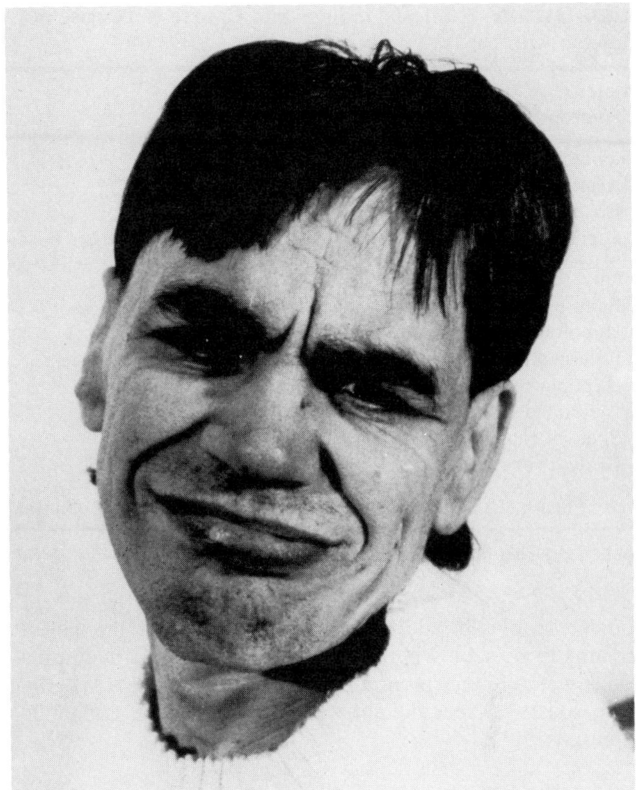

FIG. 126-13 **Salla disease patient, 40 years of age and severely retarded.**

ISSD. The clinical presentation of ISSD is more fulminant than that of Salla disease and leads to death during the first years of life. The main features and the course of the disease are outlined in Table 126-8 as compiled from the data of the 15 cases of ISSD so far reported.[307,308] Four patients manifested the clinical disease at birth, presenting with ascites, hepatosplenomegaly, and coarse facial features. By the age of 3 months, ISSD patients showed failure to thrive, generalized hypotonia, enlarged liver and spleen, mild bone dysplasias, and coarse facial features with hypopigmented skin and fair hair. Psychomotor development of the patients was markedly delayed. The age at death in 10 cases reported in the literature has ranged from 1 month to 5 years (mean, 18.1 months). Autopsy reports in two cases have described severe involvement of the central nervous system.[308,344] Widespread neuronal storage was detected with myelin loss, axonal spheroids, and gliosis. Staining with the sialic acid–specific lectin, wheat germ agglutinin, gave direct evidence for sialic acid accumulation in neuronal cells.[308] Cardiac muscle cells, renal tubular cells, fat cells, and macrophages from several organs also contained clear vacuoles with electron-lucent material. A unique presentation of ISSD was seen in two Austrian sibs, whose sialic acid storage disease was associated with a steroid-resistant congenital nephrosis.[345] On EM of a kidney biopsy, the podocytes, mesangial cells, and endothelial cells displayed numerous membrane-

Table 126-8 Clinical Findings and Course of Disease of Patients with ISSD

In utero	
Hydrops fetalis	2/15
Neonatal period	
Ascites and edema	4/15
Enlarged liver	8/15
Facial dysmorphism	8/15
Infancy	
Failure to thrive	15/15
Hypotonia	8/15
Enlarged liver/spleen	15/15
Hypopigmentation of skin/hair	10/15
Skeletal changes	4/15
Growth retardation	9/9
Age at death (10 patients)	10 months (range, 1–42 months)

SOURCE: Adapted from Mancini[307] and Pueschel et al.[308]

bound vacuoles in addition to typical nephrotic changes. It remains to be seen whether lysosomal sialic acid accumulation can lead to basement membrane dysfunction or whether there exists a specific subtype of ISSD with congenital nephrosis.

Intermediate Phenotypes. A few cases of sialic acid storage disease have been reported with a phenotype intermediate between classic Salla disease and ISSD.[322,334,346] Considerable variation in the severity of the clinical manifestations has also been observed among the Finnish Salla disease patients. The most severely affected patients are characterized by early-onset muscular hypotonia, leading to spasticity in the lower extremities in more advanced stages, severe growth retardation, absent pubertal development, and profound mental retardation. Only biochemical and molecular studies on the transport protein or the corresponding gene will reveal whether such cases represent specific entities (e.g., allelic mutations) or simply reflect variable clinical manifestations of the same basic defect.

Diagnosis

The precise diagnosis of both Salla disease and ISSD is based on (1) clinical findings, (2) increased urinary excretion of free sialic acid, and (3) the presence of storage lysosomes in various types of cells and tissues. The distinct and early clinical findings and rapid progression in ISSD easily focus the diagnostic studies toward lysosomal diseases. In Salla disease, however, the paucity of clinical findings and the very slow or even absent rate of progression of the disease often hamper the specific diagnosis. Several patients, particularly those with no affected sibs, have come to adult age before diagnostic studies have been undertaken. The association of mental retardation, spasticity, and ataxia has often been attributed to brain damage caused by an episode of perinatal asphyxia.

Urinary free sialic acid is most commonly demonstrated with thin-layer chromatography.[347] Patients constantly excrete excess free sialic acid, which has been found in the urine of one patient with Salla disease as early as 3 days of age. The enhanced free sialic acid spot of the patient's sample is usually distinctive enough for diagnosis. Normal newborn infants may also show a pronounced sialic acid spot warranting further studies. More-sophisticated techniques need to be applied for quantitative assays of urinary free sialic acid, but for diagnostic purposes such methods are only rarely needed.

ISSD patients excrete approximately 10 times the free sialic acid that Salla disease patients excrete, and the intermediate types fall between the two. There appears to be a correlation between the severity of the clinical manifestations and the level of sialic acid excretion. A similar correlation has been seen between the severity of clinical disease and the amount of sialic acid stored in tissues.

Lysosomal accumulation of free sialic acid can be demonstrated by finding vacuolated lymphocytes or enlarged lysosomes on EM of a skin or conjunctival biopsy. Vacuolated lymphocytes may not always be present in Salla disease; younger patients, in particular, may not have them.[342] In ISSD, vacuolated lymphocytes are almost always present.

A skin or conjunctival biopsy serves diagnostic purposes very well because of the variety of cell types present in the specimen. Electron-lucent single membrane-bound lysosomes containing fibrillogranular material with some membrane fragments and occasional dark globules have been seen in fibrocytes, Schwann cells, sweat gland cells, myoepithelial cells, and capillary epithelial cells. The morphology of the enlarged lysosomes in sialic acid storage disorders is similar to that in other glycoproteinoses such as mannosidosis and aspartylglucosaminuria and in various types of mucopolysaccharidoses.

Prenatal. Elevation of intracellular free sialic acid concentrations allows prenatal detection of both Salla disease and ISSD. In addition, the presence of vacuoles on EM study of a first-trimester chorionic villus specimen can support the biochemical diagnosis of ISSD but not of Salla disease.

The first prenatal diagnosis of sialic acid storage diseases was reported in 1986 in a family with two previous children affected by ISSD.[338] Free sialic acid in cultured amniotic fluid cells was increased approximately seventyfold (25.0 nmol/mg protein) that in control cultures. The cell-free amniotic fluid had a sixfold increase of free sialic acid. The pregnancy was terminated, and the diagnosis was confirmed by a ninefold to two hundredfold elevation of free sialic acid in cultured fibroblasts, liver, brain, and kidney of the aborted fetus. Several tissues, including placental trophoblasts, had typical storage lysosomes on EM. At least two other prenatal diagnoses of ISSD have been reported,[339,348] and in one of them the increase of free sialic acid was also shown in an uncultured first-trimester chorionic villus sample.[339]

Chorionic villus cells had numerous vacuoles on EM. Salla disease is also amenable to intrauterine diagnosis by free sialic acid assay of cultured amniotic fluid cells or of a chorionic villus sample, but the moderate elevation of intracellular free sialic acid renders the diagnosis more difficult. A fivefold increase of free sialic acid was seen in cultured amniotic fluid cells in a pregnancy which led to delivery of a child in whom the first signs of Salla disease developed shortly after birth.[349] The amniotic fluid supernatant had sialic acid in the range of controls. In one case, a twentyfold increase of free sialic acid was seen in a chorionic villus sample of a pregnancy in which the fetus had both biochemical and EM evidence for Salla disease after termination.[350]

Heterozygotes. Heterozygotes for Salla disease and ISSD have no clinical manifestations, and their urinary excretion of free sialic acid is within normal limits. The assay of transport activity with resealed lysosomal vesicles from cultured cells can differentiate between the carriers and normals, but the method is not feasible for clinical purposes.[331] The observation of an intermediate free sialic acid level in the granulocyte subpopulation of peripheral blood leukocytes in obligate heterozygotes of Salla disease and ISSD[346] requires confirmation in a larger series of individuals.

Differential. Four clinical entities present with intracellular accumulation and urinary excretion of sialic acid: (1) ISSD and Salla disease are probably allelic mutations of a gene coding for a lysosome membrane transport protein. (2) Sialuria is a genetic error of impaired feedback inhibition in the synthesis of sialic acid. (3) Sialidosis is due to deficiency of lysosomal neuraminidase leading to storage of undegraded sialyloligosaccharides, or bound sialic acid. (4) Galactosialidosis is due to deficiency of a 32-kDa protective protein, and affected patients also excrete sialyloligosaccharides in urine (see Chap. 91).

Distinction between ISSD and Salla disease is straightforward in typical cases. The severity of the clinical course of the disease and the difference in the amount of sialic acid excreted in the urine and stored in the tissues usually identify the type of the disease. Atypical patients, however, may pose diagnostic difficulties. Visceromegaly, dysmorphic features, and hypopigmentation of the skin point to ISSD because these findings have not been described in Salla disease patients.

Sialuria, originally described in 1968 in a mentally retarded French boy, is another inborn error of sialic acid metabolism.[351] Three other patients with the same biochemical and clinical presentation have subsequently been identified.[352–355] The clinical presentation is characterized by varying degrees of developmental delay, hepatosplenomegaly, and coarse facial features. Patients excrete massive amounts of free sialic acid in their urine, ranging up to several grams a day. The cellular concentration of free sialic acid is also increased, but the accumulation is in the cytosol and not in the lysosomal fraction as in Salla disease and ISSD. Studies have revealed that sialic acid overproduction and excretion in these patients is caused by defective feedback inhibition of the rate limiting step in the synthesis of sialic acid.[354,356] UDP-GlcNAc-2-epimerase, which converts UDP-*N*-acetylglucosamine to *N*-acetylmannosamine, is normally feedback-inhibited by CMP-NeuAc, but this feedback is strongly impaired in sialuria patients. Still another case of sialuria has been reported with cytosolic accumulation and urinary excretion of free sialic acid but without biochemical characterization of the metabolic defect.[357]

The other group of inborn errors of sialic acid metabolism causing sialic acid excretion in urine is the genetic deficiency of neuraminidase, the lysosomal enzyme cleaving sialic acid from the sialyloligosaccharides.[358] Sialidosis patients show evidence of lysosomal accumulation, but the storage material as well as the urinary excretion is bound, not free sialic acid. Definitive diagnosis of sialidosis can be made by assay of neuraminidase activity in leukocytes or cultured fibroblasts (see Chap. 81).

The clinical presentations of infantile sialidosis (type II), galactosialidosis, and ISSD may be very similar during the neonatal period, with hepatosplenomegaly, ascites, edema, and dysmorphic features. Cherry-red spots, which are typical ocular findings in sialidosis and galactosialidosis, are not yet detectable at this early age. Assay of urinary oligosaccharides and enzyme activities in leukocytes or cultured cells usually leads to the correct diagnosis.

Therapy

At present, no specific treatment is available for patients with Salla disease or ISSD. No therapeutic trials with bone marrow transplantation are known. Detailed molecular characterization of the transport mechanism at the lysosomal membrane may pave the way to specific therapeutic modalities.

OTHER DISORDERS OF LYSOSOMAL MEMBRANE TRANSPORT

A disorder of lysosomal storage of vitamin B_{12} has been described as resulting from impaired transport of cobalamin across the lysosomal membrane.[359] Two affected patients had methylmalonic acidemia, one with developmental delay and the other with homocystinuria.[359,360] Fibroblast studies indicate that free cobalamin accumulates in lysosomes after dissociation from a transcobalamin II–vitamin B_{12} complex.[359,361] The defect has been termed the *cobalamin F mutation* (see Chap. 102).

Many other small molecules, produced by the intralysosomal degradation of macromolecules, can be salvaged by transport across the lysosome and into the cytoplasm; deficiency of this mechanism could result in lysosomal storage. Candidate small molecules include calcium, phosphate, sulfate, nucleosides, carbohydrates, various amino acids, and vitamins, especially since lysosomal membrane carrier systems have been described for many of these compounds.[42,362] Patients with signs of lysosomal storage, in whom all known defects have been ruled out, might appropriately be investigated for defects of lysosomal membrane transport. Still other patients may present with product deficiency, if salvage of the stored compound is essential.

ADDENDUM

Cystinosis

In the past 10 years, 36 adult patients with nephropathic cystinosis were evaluated at the National Institutes of Health.[371] The 1-year and 5-year graft survival rates for 30 cadaveric allografts were 90 percent and 75 percent, respectively. Seven patients are deceased, five are legall blind, and three others have severely impaired vision in one eye. Twelve patients have a distal myopathy, and eight have cerebral calcifications on CT scan. None of the severely affected individuals has received significant cystine-depleting therapy.

In September 1993, an application for New Drug Approval was submitted to the FDA for a capsule preparation of cysteamine. At the time of this writing (February 1994) a decision on its disposition remains pending.

A controlled clinical trial of indomethacin is being initiated to determine whether the decreased urinary output effected by this drug will increase caloric intake and growth without decreasing renal function.

A consortium of cystinosis investigators is currently engaged in linkage analysis to determine the chromosomal location of the cystinosis gene.

Free Sialic Acid Storage Diseases

MRI of the central nervous system was recently performed on six Salla disease patients aged 2 to 39 years with varying degrees of clinical involvement.[372] Mature myelination was present only in the brainstem, cerebellar peduncles, cerebral hemispheres, and the thalamus. In all cases, the subcortical white matter of the cerebrum had failed to myelinate. Hypoplasia of the corpus callosum, cerebellar atrophy, and cortical and central cerebral atrophy were present in older patients. The pattern of myelination in Salla disease resembled that seen during the normal newborn period.

The locus for Salla disease has recently been assigned to the long arm of chromosome 6 using linkage analysis of 35 Finnish patients with Salla disease and 98 healthy family members. The highest lod score (8.95) was obtained with a microsatellite marker of locus D6S286 at zero recombination fraction.[373] Allelic association between the disease locus and specific alleles of the linked markers was observed, suggesting that one major mutation is responsible for enrichment of the disease in the Finnish population. The assignment of the gene locus for Salla disease now offers the possibility of prenatal diagnosis using analysis of linked markers at 6q. Carrier detection in families with previously affected individuals is also feasible with the aid of linked markers.

REFERENCES

1. Abderhalden E: Familiäre cystindiathese. *Z Physiol Chem* **38**:557, 1903.
2. Lignac GOE: Über storung des cystinstoffwechsels bei kindern. *Deutsch Arch Klin Med* **145**:139, 1924.
3. Fanconi G: Die nicht diabetischen glykosurien und hyperglykämien des ältern kindes. *Jahrb Kinderheilkd* **133**:257, 1931.
4. deToni G: Remarks on the relations between renal rickets (renal dwarfism) and renal diabetes. *Acta Paediatr* **16**:479, 1933.
5. Debré R, Marie J, Clétet F, Messimy R: Rachitisme tardif coexistent avec une néphrite chronique et une glycosurie. *Arch Med Enf* **37**:597, 1934.
6. Fanconi G: Der nephrotisch-glykosurische zwergwuchs mit hypophosphatämischer rachitis. *Dtsch Med Wochenschr* **62**:1169, 1936.
7. Beumer H, Wepler W: Über die cystinkrankheit der ersten lebenzeit. *Klin Wochenschr* **16**:8, 1937.
8. Fanconi G, Bickel H: Die chronische aminoacidurie (aminosäurediabetes oder nephrotisch-glukosurischer zwergwuchs) bei der glykogenose und der cystinkrankheit. *Helv Paediatr Acta* **4**:359, 1949.
9. Bickel H, Baar HS, Astley R, Douglas AA, Finch E, Harris H, Harvey CC, Hickmans EM, Philpott MG, Smallwood WC, Smellie JM, Teall CG: Cystine storage disease with aminoaciduria and dwarfism (Lignac-Fanconi Disease). *Acta Paediatr Upps Suppl* **90**:1, 1952.
10. Dent CE: The amino-aciduria in Fanconi syndrome. A study making extensive use of techniques based on paper partition chromatography. *Biochem J* **41**:240, 1947.
11. Freudenberg E: Cystinosis: Cystine disease (Lignac's disease) in children. *Adv Pediatr* **4**:265, 1949.
12. Seegmiller JE, Friedmann T, Harrison HE, Wong V, Schneider JA: Cystinosis. Combined clinical staff conference at the National Institutes of Health. *Ann Intern Med* **68**:883, 1968.
13. Schulman JD: Historical perspective, in Schulman JD (ed): *Cystinosis*. Washington, DC, Government Printing Office, 1973, DHEW publication no (NIH) 72-249, pp 1–9.
14. Schneider JA, Schulman JD: Cystinosis, in Stanbury JB, Wyngaarden JB, Fredrickson DS, Goldstein JL, Brown MS (eds): *The Metabolic Basis of Inherited Disease*, 5th ed. New York, McGraw-Hill, 1983, pp 1844–1867.
15. Baar HS: Pathologie des aminosären-diabetes. *Monatsschr Kinderheilk* **99**:35, 1951.
16. Clay RD, Darmady EM, Hawkins M: The nature of the renal lesion in the Fanconi syndrome. *J Pathol Bacteriol* **65**:551, 1953.
17. Darmady EM: The renal changes in some metabolic diseases, in Mostofi FK, Smith DE (eds): *The Kidney*. Baltimore, Williams & Wilkins, 1966, p. 253.
18. Jackson JD, Smith FG, Litman NN, Yuile CL, Latta H: The Fanconi syndrome with cystinosis. Electron microscopy of renal biopsy specimens from five patients. *Am J Med* **33**:653, 1962.
19. Schneider JA, Bradley K, Seegmiller JE: Increased cystine in leukocytes from individuals homozygous and heterozygous for cystinosis. *Science* **157**:1321, 1967.
20. Schneider JA, Rosenbloom FM, Bradley K, Seegmiller JE: Increased free-cystine content of fibroblasts cultured from patients with cystinosis. *Biochem Biophys Res Commun* **29**:527, 1967.
21. Patrick AD, Lake BD: Cystinosis: Electron microscopic evidence of lysosomal storage of cystine in lymph node. *J Clin Pathol* **21**:571, 1968.
22. Wong VG, Kuwabara T, Brubaker R, Olson W, Schulman J, Seegmiller JE: Intralysosomal cystine crystals in cystinosis. *Invest Ophthalmol* **9**:83, 1970.
23. Hummeler K, Zajac BA, Genel M, Holtzapple PG, Segal S: Human cystinosis: Intracellular deposition of cystine. *Science* **168**:859, 1970.
24. Schulman JD, Wong V, Olson WH, Seegmiller JE: Lysosomal site of crystalline deposits in cystinosis as shown by ferritin uptake. *Arch Pathol* **90**:259, 1970.
25. Schulman JD, Bradley KH, Seegmiller JE: Cystine: Compartmentalization within lysosomes in cystinotic leukocytes. *Science* **166**:1152, 1969.
26. Schulman JD, Bradley KH: Cystinosis: Selective induction of vacuolation in fibroblasts by L-cysteine-D-penicillamine disulfide. *Science* **169**:595, 1970.
27. Gahl WA, Renlund M, Thoene JG: Lysosomal transport disorders: Cystinosis and sialic acid storage disorders, in Scriver CR, Beaudet AL, Sly WS, Valle D (eds): *The Metabolic Basis of Inherited Disease*, 6th ed. New York, McGraw-Hill, 1989, vol 2, p 2619.
28. Tietze F, Bradley KH, Schulman JD: Enzymic reduction of cystine by subcellular fractions of cultured and peripheral leukocytes from normal and cystinotic individuals. *Pediatr Res* **6**:649, 1972.
29. Lucy JA: Lysosomal membranes, in Dingle JT, Fell HB (eds): *Lysosomes in Biology and Pathology*. New York, Elsevier, 1969, vol 2, p 313.
30. Goldman R, Kaplan A: Rupture of rat liver lysosomes mediated by L-amino acid esters. *Biochim Biophys Acta* **318**:205, 1973.
31. Reeves JP: Accumulation of amino acids by lysosomes incubated with amino acid esters. *J Biol Chem* **254**:8914, 1979.
32. Steinherz R, Tietze F, Gahl WA, Triche TJ, Chiang H, Modesti A, Schulman JD: Cystine accumulation and clearance by normal and cystinotic leukocytes exposed to cystine dimethyl ester. *Proc Natl Acad Sci USA* **79**:4446, 1982.
33. Jonas AJ, Greene AA, Smith ML, Schneider JA: Cystine accumulation and loss in normal, heterozygous, and cystinotic fibroblasts. *Proc Natl Acad Sci USA* **79**:4442, 1982.
34. Gahl WA, Tietze F, Bashan N, Steinherz R, Schulman JD: Defective cystine exodus from isolated lysosome-rich fractions of cystinotic leucocytes. *J Biol Chem* **257**:9570, 1982.
35. Jonas AJ, Smith ML, Schneider JA: ATP-dependent lysosomal cystine efflux is defective in cystinosis. *J Biol Chem* **257**:13185, 1982.
36. Pisoni RL, Thoene JG, Christensen HN: Detection and characterization of carrier-mediated cationic amino acid transport in lysosomes of normal and cystinotic human fibroblasts. *J Biol Chem* **260**:4791, 1985.
37. Tietze F, Rome LH, Butler JD, Harper GS, Gahl WA: Impaired clearance of free cystine from lysosome-enriched granular fractions of I-cell-disease fibroblasts. *Biochem J* **237**:9, 1986.
38. Gahl WA, Bashan N, Tietze F, Bernardini I, Schulman JD: Cystine transport is defective in isolated leukocyte lysosomes from patients with cystinosis. *Science* **217**:1263, 1982.
39. Christensen HN: *Biological Transport*, 2nd ed. Reading, MA; Benjamin, 1975.
40. Gahl WA, Tietze F, Bashan N, Bernardini I, Raiford D, Schulman JD: Characteristics of cystine counter-transport

in normal and cystinotic lysosome-rich leucocyte granular fractions. *Biochem J* **216**:393, 1983.
41. Gahl WA, Bashan N, Tietze F, Schulman JD: Lysosomal cystine counter-transport in heterozygotes for cystinosis. *Am J Hum Genet* **36**:277, 1984.
42. Gahl WA: Lysosomal cystine transport, in Thoene JG (ed): *Pathophysiology of Lysosomal Transport*. Boca Raton, FL, CRC, 1992 pp 45–71.
43. Jocelyn PC: The standard redox potential of cysteine-cystine from the thiol-disulphide exchange reaction with glutathione and lipoic acid. *Eur J Biochem* **2**:327, 1967.
44. Gorin G, Doughty G: Equilibrium constants for the reaction of glutathione with cystine and their relative oxidation-reduction potentials. *Arch Biochem Biophys* **126**:547, 1968.
45. Meister A: *Biochemistry of the Amino Acids*. New York, Academic, 1965.
46. Lewis H: The metabolism of sulfur IX. The effect of repeated administration of small amounts of cystine. *J Biol Chem* **65**:187, 1925.
47. Brenton DP, Cusworth DC, Dent DE, Jones EE: Homocystinuria: Clinical and dietary studies. *Q J Med* **35**:325, 1966.
48. Sturman JA, Gaull G, Raiha NCR: Absence of cystathionase in human fetal liver: Is cystine essential? *Science* **169**:74, 1970.
49. Eagle H, Piez KA, Oyama VI: The biosynthesis of cystine in human cell cultures. *J Biol Chem* **236**:1425, 1961.
50. Iglehart JD, York RM, Modest AP, Lazarus H, Livingston DM: Cystine requirement of continuous human lymphoid cell lines of normal and leukemic origin. *J Biol Chem* **252**:32767, 1977.
51. Tietze F: Enzymic reduction of cystine and other disulfides, in Schulman JD (ed): *Cystinosis*. Washington, DC, Government Printing Office, 1973, DHEW publication no (NIH) 72-249, p 147.
52. Jocelyn PC: Glutathione metabolism in animals, in Crook EM (ed): *Glutathione*. Cambridge, England, Cambridge University Press, 1959, p. 43.
53. Eldjarn L, Phil A: Equilibrium constants and oxidation-reduction potentials of some thiol-disulfide systems. *J Biol Chem* **79**:4589, 1957.
54. States B, Segal S: Distribution of glutathione-cystine transhydrogenase activity in subcellular fractions of rat intestinal mucosa. *Biochem J* **113**:443, 1969.
55. Brand E, Harris MM, Biloon S: Cystinuria. The excretion of a cystine complex which decomposes in the urine with the liberation of free cystine. *J Biol Chem* **86**:315, 1930.
56. Schneider JA, Bradley KH, Seegmiller JE: Transport and intracellular fate of cysteine-35S in leukocytes from normal subjects and patients with cystinosis. *Pediatr Res* **2**:441, 1968.
57. States B, Segal S: Thin-layer chromatographic separation of cystine and the N-ethylmaleimide adducts of cysteine and glutathione. *Anal Biochem* **27**:323, 1969.
58. Lee PLY: Single-column systems for accelerated amino acid analysis of physiological fluids using five lithium buffers. *Biochem Med* **10**:107, 1974.
59. Oshima RG, Willis RC, Furlong CE, Schneider JA: Binding assays for amino acids. The utilization of a cystine binding protein from Escherichia coli for the determination of acid-soluble cystine in small physiological samples. *J Biol Chem* **249**:6033, 1974.
60. Spears GS, Slusser RJ, Tousimis AJ, Taylor CG, Schulman JD: Cystinosis: An ultrastructural and electron-probe study of the kidney with unusual findings. *Arch Pathol* **9**:206, 1971.
61. Scotto JM, Stralin HG: Ultrastructure of the liver in a case of childhood cystinosis. *Virchows Arch [A]* **377**:43, 1977.
62. Fivush B, Green OC, Porter CC, Balfe JW, O'Regan S, Gahl WA: Pancreatic endocrine insufficiency in posttransplant cystinosis. *Am J Dis Child* **141**:1087, 1987.
63. Holtzapple PG, Genel M, Yakovac WC, Hummeler K, Segal S: Diagnosis of cystinosis by rectal biopsy. *N Engl J Med* **281**:143, 1969.
64. Morecki R, Paunier L, Hamilton JR: Intestinal mucosa in cystinosis. A fine structure study. *Arch Pathol* **86**:297, 1968.
65. Schneider JA, Nolan SP, Seegmiller JE: Appendicitis in a child with cystinosis. *Arch Surg* **97**:565, 1968.
66. Gross U, Masshoff W, Korz R: Die milz in allgemein pathologischer sicht. *Internist (Berl)* **9**:1, 1968.
67. Cogan DG, Kuwabara T: Ocular pathology of cystinosis, with particular reference to the elusiveness of the corneal crystals. *Arch Ophthalmol* **63**:51, 1960.
68. Kaiser-Kupfer MI, Caruso RC, Minkler DS, Gahl WA: Long-term ocular manifestations in nephropathic cystinosis. *Arch Ophthalmol* **104**:706, 1986.
69. Korn D: Demonstration of cystine crystals in peripheral white blood cells in a patient with cystinosis. *N Engl J Med* **262**:545, 1960.
70. Schneider JA, Wong V, Seegmiller JE: The early diagnosis of cystinosis. *J Pediatr* **74**:114, 1969.
71. Chan AM, Lynch MJ, Bailey JD, Ezrin C, Fraser D: Hypothyroidism in cystinosis. A clinical, endocrinologic and histologic study involving sixteen patients with cystinosis. *Am J Med* **48**:678, 1970.
72. Casey TP: Cystine storage disease. A case report with a note on the extraction of cystine from formalin-fixed tissues. *Aust Ann Med* **15**:61, 1966.
73. Gahl WA, Dalakas MC, Charnas L, Chen KT, Pezeshkpour GH, Kuwabara T, Davis SL, Chesney RW, Fink J, Hutchison HT: Myopathy and cystine storage in muscles in a patient with nephropathic cystinosis. *N Engl J Med* **319**:1461, 1988.
74. Reiss RE, Kuwabara T, Smith ML, Gahl WA: Successful pregnancy despite placental cystine crystals in a woman with nephropathic cystinosis. *N Engl J Med* **319**:223, 1988.
75. Baar HS, Bickel H: Morbid anatomy, histology,and pathogenesis of Lignac-Franconi disease. *Acta Paediatr Upps Suppl* **90**:171, 1952.
76. Levine S, Paparo G: Brain lesions in a case of cystinosis. *Acta Neuropathol (Berl)* **57**:217, 1982.
77. *Merck Index*, 10th ed. Rahway, NJ, Merck, 1983.
78. Schulman JD, Wong VG, Kuwabara T, Bradley KH, Seegmiller JE: Intracellular cystine content of leukocyte populations in cystinosis. *Arch Intern Med* **125**:660, 1970.
79. Harnes MD, Carter RF, Pollard AC, Carey WF: Light and electron microscopy of infantile and fetal tissues in cystinosis. *Micron* **11**:443, 1980.
80. Schulman JD: Cystine storage disease: Investigations at the cellular and subcellular levels, in Carson NAJ, Raine DN (eds): *Inherited Disorders of Sulphur Metabolism*. Edinburgh, Churchill Livingstone, 1971, pp 123–140.
81. Jonas AJ, Conley SB, Marshall R, Johnson RA, Marks M, Rosenberg H: Nephropathic cystinosis with central nervous system involvement. *Am J Med* **83**:966, 1987.
82. Broyer M, Guillot M, Gubler MC, Habib R: Infantile cystinosis: A reappraisal of early and late symptoms. *Adv Nephrol* **10**:137, 1981.
83. Gahl WA, Charnas LR, Markello TC, Bernardini IM, Ishak KG, Dalakas MC: Parenchymal organ cystine depletion with long term cysteamine therapy. *Biochem Med Metab Biol* **48**:275, 1992.
84. Gahl WA: Unpublished data.
85. Bannai S, Kitamura E: Transport interaction of L-cystine and L-glutamine in human diploid fibroblasts in culture. *J Biol Chem* **255**:2372, 1980.
86. Greene AA, Marcusson EG, Pintos Morell G, Schneider JA: Characterization of the lysosomal cystine transport system in mouse L-929 fibroblasts. *J Biol Chem* **265**:9888, 1990.
87. Bashan N, Gahl WA, Tietze F, Bernardini I, Schulman JD: The effect of ions and ionophores on cystine egress from human leucocyte lysosome-rich granular fraction. *Biochim Biophys Acta* **777**:267, 1984.
88. Smith ML, Greene AA, Potashnik R, Mendoza SA, Schneider JA: Lysosomal cystine transport. Effect of intralysosomal pH and membrane potential. *J Biol Chem* **262**:1244, 1987.
89. Jonas AJ: Cystine transport in purified rat liver lysosomes. *Biochem J* **236**:671, 1986.
90. Gahl WA, Tietze F: pH effects on cystine transport in lysosome-rich leucocyte granular fractions. *Biochem J* **228**:263, 1985.
91. Okhuma S, Moriyama Y, Takano T: Identification and characterization of a proton pump on lysosomes by fluorescein isothiocyanate-dextran fluorescence. *Proc Natl Acad Sci USA* **79**:2758, 1982.

92. Schneider DL: ATP-dependent acidification of intact and disrupted lysosomes. Evidence for an ATP-driven proton pump. *J Biol Chem* **256**:3858, 1981.
93. Stone DK, Xie X, Racker E: An ATP-driven proton pump in clathrin coated vesicles. *J Biol Chem* **258**:4059, 1983.
94. Xie X, Stone DK, Racker E: Determinants of clathrin coated vesicle acidification. *J Biol Chem* **258**:14834, 1983.
95. Jonas AJ, Smith ML, Allison WS, Laikind PK, Greene AA, Schneider JA: Proton-translocation ATPase and lysosomal cystine transport. *J Biol Chem* **258**:1727, 1983.
96. Oude-Elferink RP, Harms E, Strijland A, Tager JM: The intralysosomal pH in cultured human skin fibroblasts in relation to cystine accumulation in patients with cystinosis. *Biochem Biophys Res Commun* **116**:154, 1983.
97. Smith ML, Greene AA, Schneider JA, Pisoni RL, Christensen HN: Cystine exodus from lysosomes: Cystinosis. *Methods Enzymol* **174**:154, 1989.
98. Greene AA, Clark KF, Smith ML, Schneider JA: Cystine exodus from normal leukocytes is stimulated by MgATP. *Biochem J* **246**:547, 1987.
99. Tietze F, Butler JD: Elevated cystine levels in cultured skin fibroblasts from patients with I-cell disease. *Pediatr Res* **13**:1350, 1979.
100. Greene AA, Jonas AJ, Harms E, Smith ML, Pellett OL, Bump EA, Miller AL, Schneider JA: Lysosomal cystine storage in cystinosis and mucolipidosis type II. *Pediatr Res* **19**:1170, 1985.
101. Jonas AJ, Symons LJ, Speller RJ: Polyamines stimulate lysosomal cystine transport. *J Biol Chem* **262**:16391, 1987.
102. Jonas AJ, Speller RJ: Stearylamine permeabilizes the lysosomal membrane to cystine and sialic acid. *Biochim Biophys Acta* **984**:257, 1989.
103. Lemons RM, Pisoni RL, Christensen HN, Thoene JG: Elevated temperature produces cystine depletion in cystinotic fibroblasts. *Biochim Biophys Acta* **884**:429, 1986.
104. Forster S, Scarlett L, Lloyd JB: The effects of decreased growth temperature on the cystine content of cystinotic fibroblasts. *Biochim Biophys Acta* **1013**:7, 1989.
105. Schulman JD, Patrick AD, Goodman SI, Tietze F, Butler J: Gamma-glutamyl transpeptidase (GGTPase): Investigations in normals and patients with inborn errors of sulfur metabolism. *Pediatr Res* **9**:355, 1975.
106. Harper GS, Kohn LD, Bernardini I, Bernar J, Tietze F, Andersson HC, Gahl WA: Thyrotropin stimulation of lysosomal tyrosine transport in rat FRTL-5 thyroid cells. *J Biol Chem* **263**:9320, 1988.
107. Idriss JM, Jonas AJ: Cystine transport by yeast acidic vacuoles. *Am J Hum Genet* **47**:A159/0621, 1990.
108. Thoene JG, Oshima RG, Crawhall JC, Olson DL, Schneider JA: Cystinosis. Intracellular cystine depletion by aminothiols in vitro and in vivo. *J Clin Invest* **58**:180, 1976.
109. Pisoni RL, Acker TL, Lisowski KM, Lemons RM, Thoene JG: A cysteine-specific lysosomal transport system provides a major route for the delivery of thiol to human fibroblast lysosomes: Possible role in supporting lysosomal proteolysis. *J Cell Biol* **110**:327, 1990.
110. Ehrenreich BA, Cohn ZA: The fate of peptides pinocytosed by macrophages *in vitro*. *J Exp Med* **129**:227, 1969.
111. Gahl WA, Tietze F, Butler JD, Schulman JD: Cysteamine depletes cystinotic leucocyte granular fractions of cystine by the mechanism of disulphide interchange. *Biochem J* **228**:545, 1985.
112. Butler JD: Depletion of cystine in cystinotic fibroblasts by homocysteine. Synergism of cysteamine with various reducing agents in depletion of cystine from cystinotic fibroblasts. *Biochem Pharmacol* **40**:879, 1990.
113. Goldman H, Scriver CR, Aaron K, Pinsky L: Use of dithiothreitol to correct cystine storage in cultured cystinotic fibroblasts. *Lancet* **1**:811, 1970.
114. Kroll WA, Schneider JA: Decrease in free cystine content of cultured cystinotic fibroblasts by ascorbic acid. *Science* **186**:1040, 1974.
115. Butler JD, Zatz M: Pantethine depletes cystinotic fibroblasts of cystine. *J Pediatr* **102**:796, 1983.
116. Butler JD, Zatz M: Pantethine and cystamine deplete cystine from cystinotic fibroblasts via efflux of cysteamine-cysteine mixed disulfide. *J Clin Invest* **74**:411, 1984.
117. Orloff S, Butler JD, Towne D, Mukherjee AB, Schulman JD: Pantetheinase activity and cysteamine content in cystinotic and normal fibroblasts and leukocytes. *Pediatr Res* **15**:1063, 1981.
118. Butler JD, Gahl WA, Tietze F: Cystine depletion by WR-1065 in cystinotic cells. Mechanism of action. *Biochem Pharmacol* **34**:2179, 1985.
119. Thoene JG, Lemons R: Cystine depletion of cystinotic tissues by phosphocysteamine (WR638). *J Pediatr* **96**:1043, 1980.
120. Pisoni RL, Lisowski KM, Lemons RM, Thoene JG: Utilization of mercaptoethylgluconamide for depleting human cystinotic fibroblasts of their accumulated lysosomal cystine. *Pediatr Res* **26**:73, 1989.
121. Danpure CJ: The effect of chloroquine on the metabolism of [^{35}S]cystine in normal and cystinotic human skin fibroblasts. *Biochem J* **200**:555, 1981.
122. Thoene JG, Lemons RM: Cystine accumulation in cystinotic fibroblasts from free and protein-linked cystine but not cysteine. *Biochem J* **208**:823, 1982.
123. Thoene JG, Oshima RG, Ritchie DG, Schneider JA: Cystinotic fibroblasts accumulate cystine from intracellular protein degradation. *Proc Natl Acad Sci USA* **74**:4505, 1977.
124. Schulman JD, Bradley KH: Cystinosis: Therapeutic implications of in vitro studies of cultured fibroblasts. *J Pediatr* **78**:833, 1971.
125. Danpure CJ, Jennings PR, Fyfe DA: Further studies on the effect of chloroquine on the uptake, metabolism and intracellular translocation of [^{35}S]cystine in cystinotic fibroblasts. *Biochim Biophys Acta* **885**:256, 1986.
126. Forster S, Scarlett L, Lloyd JB: Mechanism of cystine reaccumulation by cystinotic fibroblasts in vitro. *Biosci Rep* **10**:225, 1990.
127. Thoene JG, Lemons R: Modulation of the intracellular cystine content of cystinotic fibroblasts by extracellular albumin. *Pediatr Res* **14**:785, 1980.
128. Kooistra T, Lloyd JB: Pinocytosis and degradation of exogenous proteins by cystinotic fibroblasts. *Biochim Biophys Acta* **887**:182, 1986.
129. Butler JD, Spielberg SP: Accumulation of cystine from glutathione-cysteine mixed disulfide in cystinotic fibroblasts; blockade by an inhibitor of gamma-glutamyl transpeptidase. *Life Sci* **31**:2563, 1982.
130. Crawhall JC, Oshima RG, Schneider JA: Factors controlling the nonprotein cystine content of cystinotic fibroblasts. *Pediatr Res* **11**:41, 1977.
131. Ritchie DG, Jonas AJ, Oshima RG, Neal P, Schneider JA: Cystinotic fibroblasts are depleted of free-cystine by acid pH medium. *Pediatr Res* **15**:1492, 1981.
132. States B, Lee J, Segal S: Effect of chloroquine on handling of cystine by cystinotic fibroblasts. *Metabolism* **32**:272, 1983.
133. Pellett OL, Smith ML, Greene AA, Schneider JA: Lack of complementation in somatic cell hybrids between fibroblasts from patients with different forms of cystinosis. *Proc Natl Acad Sci USA* **85**:3531, 1988.
134. Smolin LA, Clark KF, Schneider JA: An improved method for heterozygote detection of cystinosis using polymorphonuclear leukocytes. *Am J Hum Genet* **41**:266, 1987.
135. Bois E, Feingold J, Frenay P, Briard ML: Infantile cystinosis in France: Genetics, incidence, geographic distribution. *J Med Genet* **13**:434, 1976.
136. Manz F, Gretz N: Cystinosis in the Federal Republic of Germany. Coordination and analysis of the data. *J Inherited Metab Dis* **8**:2, 1985.
137. Steinherz R, Raiford D, Mittal KK, Schulman JD: Association of certain human leukocyte antigens with nephropathic cystinosis in the absence of linkage between these loci. *Am J Hum Genet* **33**:227, 1981.
138. Gahl WA, Adamson M, Kaiser-Kupfer I, Ludwig IH, O'Connell HJ, Cohen W, Barranger J: Biochemical phenotyping of a single sibship with both cystinosis and Fabry disease. *J Inherited Metab Dis* **8**:127, 1985.
139. Smith ML, Pellett OL, Cahill TC, David DN, Kaskel FJ, Smolin LA, Greene AA, Weissbecker K, Dean M, Schneider JA: Biochemical and genetic analysis of a child with cystic fibrosis and cystinosis. *Am J Med Genet* **39**:84, 1991.

140. Gahl WA: Cystinosis coming of age. *Adv Pediatr* **33**:95, 1986.
141. Markello TC: Unpublished data.
142. Morell GP, Niaudet P, Jean G, Descamps-Latscha B: Altered oxidative metabolism, motility, and adherence in phagocytic cells from cystinotic children. *Pediatr Res* **19**:1318,1985.
143. Teree TM, Friedman AB, Kest LM, Fetterman GH: Cystinosis and proximal tubular nephropathy in siblings. Progressive development of the physiological and anatomical lesion. *Am J Dis Child* **119**:481, 1970.
144. Lemire J, Kaplan BS, Scriver CR: Presentation of cystinosis as Bartter's syndrome and conversion to Fanconi syndrome on indomethacin treatment. *Pediatr Res* **12**:544, 1978.
145. O'Regan S, Mongeau JG, Robitaille P: A patient with cystinosis presenting with the features of Bartter syndrome. *Acta Paediatr Belg* **33**:51, 1980.
146. Lemire J, Kaplan BS: The various renal manifestations of the nephropathic form of cystinosis. *Am J Nephrol* **4**:81, 1984.
147. Bûrki VE: Ueber die cystinkrankheit im klienkindesalter under besonderes berûcksichtigung des augenbefundes. *Ophthalmologica* **101**:257, 1941.
148. Black J, Stapleton FB, Roy S 3d, Ward J, Noe HN: Varied types of urinary calculi in a patient with cystinosis without renal tubular acidosis. *Pediatrics* **78**:295, 1986.
149. Steinherz R, Chesney RW, Schulman JD, DeLuca HF, Phelps M: Circulating vitamin D metabolites in nephropathic cystinosis. *J Pediatr* **102**:592, 1983.
150. Bernardini I, Rizzo WB, Dalakas M, Bernar J, Gahl WA: Plasma and muscle free carnitine deficiency due to renal Fanconi syndrome. *J Clin Invest* **75**:1124, 1985.
151. Brodehl J, Bickel H: Aminoaciduria and hyperaminoaciduria in childhood. *Clin Nephrol* **1**:149, 1973.
152. Charnas LR, Bernardini I, Rader D, Hoeg JM, Gahl WA: Clinical and laboratory findings in the oculocerebrorenal syndrome of Lowe, with special reference to growth and renal function. *N Engl J Med* **324**:1318, 1991.
153. Spear GS: The pathology of the kidney, in Schulman JD (ed): *Cystinosis*. Washington, DC, Government Printing Office, 1973, DHEW publication no (NIH) 72-249, p 37.
154. Spear GS, Slusser RJ, Schulman JD, Alexander F: Polykaryocytosis in the visceral glomerular epithelium in cystinosis with description of an unusual clinical variant. *Johns Hopkins Med J* **129**:83, 1971.
155. Spear GS: Pathology of the kidney in cystinosis. *Pathol Annu* **9**:81,1974.
156. Markello TC, Bernardini IM, Gahl WA: Improved renal function in children with cystinosis treated with cysteamine. *N Engl J Med* **328**:1157, 1993
157. Leumann EP: Progression of renal insufficiency in pediatric patients: Estimation from serum creatinine. *Helv Paediatr Acta* **33**:25, 1978.
158. Gahl WA, Schneider JA, Schulman JD, Thoene JG, Reed GF: Predicted reciprocal serum creatinine at age 10 years as a measure of renal function in children with nephropathic cystinosis treated with oral cysteamine. *Pediatr Nephrol* **4**:129, 1990.
159. Gretz N, Manz F, Augustin R, Barrat TM, Bender-Götze C, Brandis M, Bremer HJ, Brodehl J, Broyer M, Bulla M, Callis L, Chantler C, Diekmann L, Dillon MJ, Egli F, Ehrich JH, Endres W, Fanconi A, Feldhoff C, Geisert J, Gekle D, Geschöll-Bauer B, Grote K, Grüttner R, Hagge W, Haycock CB, Hennemann H, Klare B, Leupold D, Löhr H, Michalk D, Oliveira A, Ott F, Pistor K, Rau J, Schärer K, Schindera F, Schmidt H, Schulte-Wissermann H, Verrier-Jones K, Weber HP, Willenbockel U, Wolf H: Survival time in cystinosis. A collaborative study. *Proc Eur Dial Transplant Assoc* **19**:582, 1983.
160. Gahl WA, Reed, GF, Thoene JG, Schulman JD, Rizzo WB, Jonas AJ, Denman DW, Schlesselman JJ, Corden BJ, Schneider JA: Cysteamine therapy for children with nephropathic cystinosis. *N Engl J Med* **316**:971, 1987.
161. Bercu BB, Rizzo WB, Corden BJ, Reed GF, Schulman JD: Circulating somatomedin-C levels in nephropathic cystinosis. *Isr J Med Sci* **20**:236, 1984.
162. Gahl WA, Kaiser-Kupfer MI: Complications of nephropathic cystinosis after renal failure. *Pediatr Nephrol* **1**:260, 1987.
163. Ehrich JHH, Brodehl J, Byrd DI, Hossfeld S, Hoyer PF, Leipert K-P, Offner G, Wolff G: Renal transplantation in 22 children with nephropathic cystinosis. *Pediatr Nephrol* **5**:707, 1991.
164. Lucky AW, Howley PM, Megyesi K, Spielberg SP, Schulman JD: Endocrine studies in cystinosis: Compensated primary hypothyroidism. *J Pediatr* **91**:204, 1977.
165. Sanderson PO, Kuwabara T, Stark WJ, Wong VG, Collins EMK: Cystinosis: A clinical, histopathologic, and ultrastructural study. *Arch Ophthalmol* **91**:270, 1974.
166. Francois J, Hanssens M, Coppleters R, Evens L: Cystinosis. A clinical and histopathologic study. *Am J Ophthalmol* **73**:643, 1972.
167. Wong VG: The eye and cystinosis, in Schulman JD (ed): *Cystinosis*. Washington, DC, Government Printing Office, 1973, DHEW publication no (NIH) 72-249, p 23.
168. Wong VG, Lietman PS, Seegmiller JE: Alterations of pigment epithelium in cystinosis. *Arch Ophthalmol* **77**:361, 1967.
169. Schneider JA, Verroust FM, Kroll WA, Garvin AJ, Horger EO 3rd, Wong VG, Spear GS, Jacobson C, Pellett OL, Becker FL: Prenatal diagnosis of cystinosis. *N Engl J Med* **290**:878, 1974.
170. Yamamoto GK, Schulman JD, Schneider JA, Wong VG: Long-term ocular changes in cystinosis: Observations in renal transplant recipients. *J Pediatr Ophthalmol Strabismus* **16**:21, 1979.
171. Gahl WA, Schneider JA, Thoene JG, Chesney R: Course of nephropathic cystinosis after age 10 years. *J Pediatr* **109**:605, 1986.
172. Bürki VE: Ueber die cystinkrankheit im klienkindesalter unter besonderer Berücksichtigung des Augenbefundes. *Ophthalmologica* **101**:257, 1941.
173. Cogan DG, Kuwabara T, Kinoshita J, Sudarsky D, Ring H: Ocular manifestations of systemic cystinosis. *Arch Ophthalmol* **55**:36, 1956.
174. Kenyon ER, Sensenbrenner JA: Electron microscopy of cornea and conjunctiva in childhood cystinosis. *Am J Ophthalmol* **78**:68, 1974.
175. Frazier PD, Wong VG: Cystinosis. Histologic and crystallographic examination of crystals in eye tissue. *Arch Ophthalmol* **80**:87, 1968.
176. Kaiser-Kupfer MI, Datiles MB, Gahl WA: Corneal transplant in a twelve-year-old boy with nephropathic cystinosis. *Lancet* **1**:331, 1987.
177. Kaiser-Kupfer MI, Gahl WA: Unpublished data.
178. Kaiser-Kupfer MI, Chan CC, Rodrigues M, Datiles MB, Gahl WA: Nephropathic cystinosis: Immunohistochemical and histopathologic studies of cornea, conjunctiva and iris. *Curr Eye Res* **6**:617, 1987.
179. Katz B, Melles RB, Schneider JA, Rao NA: Corneal thickness in nephropathic cystinosis. *Br J Ophthalmol* **73**:665, 1989.
180. Weber U, Sons HU, Bernsmeier H, Lenz W: Experimentally induced cystine keratopathy in rabbits. *Graefes Arch Clin Exp Ophthalmol* **224**:443, 1986.
181. Richler M, Milot J, Quigley M, O'Regan S: Ocular manifestations of nephropathic cystinosis. The French-Canadian experience in a genetically homogeneous population. *Arch Ophthalmol* **109**:359, 1991.
182. Wan WL, Minckler DS, Rao NA: Pupillary-block glaucoma associated with childhood cystinosis. *Am J Ophthalmol* **101**:700, 1986.
183. Schulman JD, Wong VG, Bradley KH, Seegmiller JE: A simple technique for the biochemical diagnosis of cystinosis. *J Pediatr* **76**:289, 1970.
184. Burke JR, El-Bishti MM, Maisey MN, Chantler C: Hypothyroidism in children with cystinosis. *Arch Dis Child* **53**:947, 1978.
185. Bercu BB, Schulman JD: Pituitary secretion of alpha and beta subunits of thyroid: stimulating hormone (TSH) in nephropathic cystinosis. *Isr J Med Sci* **20**:179, 1984.
186. Bercu BB, Orloff S, Schulman JD: Pituitary resistance to thyroid hormone in cystinosis. *J Clin Endocrinol Metab* **51**:262, 1980.

187. Chantler C, Carter JE, Bewick M, Counahan R, Cameron JS, Ogg CS, Williams DG, Winder E: 10 years' experience with regular haemodialysis and renal transplantation. *Arch Dis Child* **55**:435, 1980.
188. Ammenti A, Grossi A, Bernasconi S: Infantile cystinosis and insulin-dependent diabetes mellitus. *Eur J Pediatr* **145**:548, 1986.
189. Milner RD, Wirdnam PK: The pancreatic beta cell fraction in children with errors of amino acid metabolism. *Pediatr Res* **16**:213, 1982.
190. Chik CL, Friedman A, Merriam GR, Gahl WA: Pituitary-testicular function in nephropathic cystinosis. *Ann Intern Med* **119**:568, 1993.
191. Harper GS, Bernardini I, Hurko O, Zuurveld J, Gahl WA: Cystine storage in cultured myotubes from patients with nephropathic cystinosis. *Biochem J* **243**:841, 1987.
192. Charnas LR, Luciano CA, Dalakas M, Gilliatt RW, Bernardini I, Ishak K, Cwik VA, Fraker D, Brushart TA, Gahl WA: Distal vacuolar myopathy in nephropathic cystinosis. *Ann Neurol* **35**:181, 1994.
193. Arnold RW, Stickler GB, Bourne WM, Mellinger JF: Corneal crystals, myopathy, and nephropathy: A new syndrome: *J Pediatr Ophthalmol Strabismus* **24**:151, 1987.
194. Sonies BC, Ekman EF, Andersson HC, Adamson MD, Kaler SG, Markello TC, Gahl WA: Swallowing dysfunction in nephropathic cystinosis. *N Engl J Med* **323**:565, 1990.
195. Vogel DG, Malekzadeh MH, Cornford ME, Schneider JA, Shields WD, Vinters HV: Central nervous system involvement in nephropathic cystinosis. *J Neuropathol Exp Neurol* **49**:591, 1990.
196. Ehrich JHH, Stoeppler L, Offner G, Brodehl J: Evidence for cerebral involvement in nephropathic cystinosis. *Neuropaediatrie* **10**:128, 1979.
197. Brodehl J, Ehrich JHH, Krohn JP, Offner G, Byrd D: Kidney transplantation in nephropathic cystinosis, in Brodehl J, Ehrich JHH (eds): *Pediatric Nephrology*. Berlin, Springer-Verlag, 1984, p 172.
198. Cochat P, Drachman R, Gagnadoux MF, Pariente D, Broyer M: Cerebral atrophy and nephropathic cystinosis. *Arch Dis Child* **61**:401, 1986.
199. Fink JK, Brouwers P, Barton N, Malekzadeh MH, Sato S, Hill S, Cohen WE, Fivush B, Gahl WA: Neurologic complications in long-standing nephropathic cystinosis. *Arch Neurol* **46**:543, 1989.
200. Nichols SL, Press GA, Schneider JA, Trauner DA: Cortical atrophy and cognitive performance in infantile nephropathic cystinosis. *Pediatr Neurol* **6**:379, 1990.
201. Schnaper HW, Cole BR, Hodges FJ, Robson AM: Cerebral cortical atrophy in pediatric patients with end-stage renal disease. *Am J Kidney Dis* **2**:645, 1983.
202. Ross DL, Strife CF, Towbin R, Bove KE: Nonabsorptive hydrocephalus associated with nephropathic cystinosis. *Neurology* **32**:1330, 1982.
203. Trauner DA, Chase CH, Scheller JM, Fontanesi J, Katz B, Schneider JA: Neurologic and cognitive deficits in cystinosis. *Pediatr Res* **21**:498A, 1987.
204. Swenson MR, Rimmer S, Schneider JA, Melles RB, Trauner DA, Katz B: Neurophysiologic studies of the peripheral nervous system in nephropathic cystinosis. *Arch Neurol* **48**:528, 1991.
205. Avner ED, Ellis D, Jaffe R: Veno-occlusive disease of the liver associated with cysteamine treatment of nephropathic cystinosis. *J Pediatr* **102**:793, 1983.
206. Ishak K: Personal communication, March 9, 1992.
207. Treem WR, Rusnack EJ, Ragsdale BD, Seikaly MG, DiPalma JS: Inflammatory bowel disease in a patient with nephropathic cystinosis. *Pediatrics* **81**:584, 1988.
208. Fivush B, Flick JA, Gahl WA: Pancreatic exocrine insufficiency in a patient with nephropathic cystinosis. *J Pediatr* **112**:49, 1988.
209. Wolff G, Ehrich JHH, Offner G, Brodehl J: Psychosocial and intellectual development in 12 patients with infantile nephropathic cystinosis. *Acta Paediatr Scand* **71**:1007, 1982.
210. Gahl WA, Hubbard VS, Orloff S: Decreased sweat production in cystinosis. *J Pediatr* **104**:904, 1984.
211. Fox PC, Baum BJ, Gahl WA: Unpublished data.
212. Almond PS, Morel P, Troppmann C, Matas A, Najarian JS, Chavers B: Progression of infantile cystinosis after renal transplantation. *Transplant Proc* **23**:1386, 1991.
213. Schneider JA, Wong V, Bradley K, Seegmiller JE: Biochemical comparisons of the adult and childhood forms of cystinosis. *N Engl J Med* **279**:1253, 1968.
214. Goldman H, Scriver CR, Aaron K, Delvin E, Canlas Z: Adolescent cystinosis: Comparisons with infantile and adult forms. *Pediatrics* **47**:979, 1971.
215. Kroll WA, Becker FL, Schneider JA: Measurement of intracellular amino acids in cultured skin fibroblasts. The effect of storage on cystine recovery and evaluation of three methods of cell preparation. *Biochem Med* **10**:368, 1974.
216. Wong VG: Ocular manifestations in cystinosis. *Birth Defects* **12**:181, 1976.
217. Smith ML, Pellett OL, Cass MMJ, Kennaway NG, Buist NRM, Buckmaster J, Golbus M, Spear GS, Schneider JA: Prenatal diagnosis of cystinosis utilizing chorionic villus sampling. *Prenat Diagn* **6**:195, 1986.
218. Patrick AD, Young EP, Mossman J, Warren R, Kearney L, Rodeck CH: First trimester diagnosis of cystinosis using intact chorionic villi. *Prenat Diagn* **7**:71, 1987.
219. Schneider A: Unpublished data.
220. Gahl WA, Dorfmann A, Evans MI, Karson EM, Landsberger FJ, Fabro SE, Schulman JD: Chorionic biopsy in the prenatal diagnosis of nephropathic cystinosis, in Fraccaro M, Simmoni G, Brambti B (eds): *First Trimester Fetal Diagnosis*. Springer-Verlag, 1985, p. 260.
221. Schulman JD, Fujimoto WY, Bradley KH, Seegmiller JE: Identification of heterozygous genotype for cystinosis in utero by a new pulse-labeling technique: Preliminary report. *J Pediatr* **77**:468, 1970.
222. Smith ML, Clark KF, Davis SE, Greene AA, Marcusson EG, Chen Y-J, Schneider JA: Diagnosis of cystinosis with use of placenta. *N Engl J Med* **321**:397, 1989.
223. Schneider JA: Clinical aspects of cystinosis, in Schulman JD (ed): *Cystinosis*. Washington, DC, Government Printing Office, 1973, DHEW publication no (NIH) 72-249, pp 11–22.
224. Molitoris BA, Froment DH, Mackenzie TA, Huffer WH, Alfrey AC: Citrate: A major factor in the toxicity of orally administered aluminum compounds. *Kidney Int* **36**:949, 1989.
225. Bickel H, Lutz P, Schmidt H: The treatment of cystinosis with diet or drugs, in Schulman JD (ed): *Cystinosis*. Washington, DC, Government Printing Office, 1973, DHEW publication no (NIH) 72-249, pp 199–224.
226. Bëtend B, David L, Vincent M, Hermier M, François R: Successful indomethacin treatment of two paediatric patients with severe tubulopathies. A boy with an unusual hypercalciuria and a girl with cystinosis. *Helv Paediatr Acta* **34**:339, 1979.
227. Haycock GB, Al-Dahhan J, Mak RH, Chantler C: Effect of indomethacin on clinical progress and renal function in cystinosis. *Arch Dis Child* **57**:934, 1982.
228. Betend B, Pugeaut R, David L, Hermier M, François R: Pediatric cystinosis: An experience with indomethacin therapy for nearly 4 years. *Pediatrie* **37**:31, 1982.
229. Parchoux B, Guibaud P, Louis JJ, Benzoni D, Larbre F: Urinary prostaglandins and effect of indomethacin therapy in cystinosis. *Pediatrie* **37**:19, 1982.
230. Usberti M, Pecoraro C, Federico S, Cianciaruso B, Guida B, Romano A, Grumetto L, Carbonaro L: Mechanism of action of indomethacin in tubular defects. *Pediatrics* **75**:501, 1985.
231. Broyer M, Tete MJ: Treatment of cystinosis using cysteamine. *Ann Pediatr (Paris)* **37**:91, 1990.
232. Lemire J, Kaplan BS: Prolonged use of indomethacin in cystinosis. *Pediatr Res* **15**:696, 1981. (abstr.)
233. Gahl WA, Bernardini I, Dalakas M, Rizzo WB, Harper GS, Hoeg JM, Hurko O, Bernar J: Oral carnitine therapy in children with cystinosis and renal Fanconi syndrome. *J Clin Invest* **81**:549, 1988.
234. Gahl WA, Bernardini IM, Dalakas MC, Markello TC, Krasnewich DM, Charnas LR: Muscle carnitine repletion by long-term carnitine supplementation in nephropathic cystinosis. *Pediatr Res* **34**:115, 1993.
235. Malekzadeh MH, Neustein HB, Schneider JA, Pennisi AJ, Ettenger RB, Uittenbogaart CH, Kogut MD, Fine

RN: Cadaver renal transplantation in children with cystinosis. *Am J Med* **63**:525, 1977.
236. Katz B, Melles RB, Schneider JA: Recurrent crystal deposition after keratoplasty in nephropathic cystinosis. *Am J Ophthalmol* **104**:190, 1987.
237. Mahoney CP, Manning GB, Hickman RO: Hemodialysis in a patient with cystinosis. Effects on amino acid and bone metabolism. *Am J Dis Child* **112**:65, 1966.
238. Mahoney CP, Striker GE, Hickman RO, Manning GB, Marchioro TL: Renal transplantation for childhood cystinosis. *N Engl J Med* **283**:397, 1970.
239. Goodman SI, Hambidge KM, Mahoney CP, Striker GE: Renal homotransplantation in the treatment of cystinosis, in Schulman JD (ed): *Cystinosis*. Washington, DC, Government Printing Office, DHEW publication no (NIH) 72-249, 1973, pp 225–232.
240. Spear GS, Gubler MC, Habib R, Broyer M: Renal allografts in cystinosis and mesangial demography. *Clin Nephrol* **32**:256, 1989.
241. West JC, Goodman SI, Schřoter GP, Bloustein PA, Hambidge KM, Weil R 3d: Pediatric kidney transplantation for cystinosis. *J Pediatr Surg* **12**:651, 1977.
242. Crawhall JC, Lietman PS, Schneider JA, Seegmiller JE: Cystinosis. Plasma cystine and cysteine concentrations and the effect of D-penicillamine and dietary treatment. *Am J Med* **44**:330, 1968.
243. Clayton BE, Patrick AD: Use of dimercaprol or penicillamine in the treatment of cystinosis. *Lancet* **2**:909, 1961.
244. Hambraeus L, Broberger O: Penicillamine treatment of cystinosis. *Acta Paediatr Scand* **56**:243, 1967.
245. Lancaster GA, Scriver CR: Cystinotic and normal fibroblasts: Differential protection in cystine-free medium by dithiothreitol. *Pediatr Res* **16**:86, 1982.
246. Depape-Brigger D, Goldman H, Scriver CR, Delvin E, Mamer O: The in vivo use of dithiothreitol in cystinosis. *Pediatr Res* **11**:124, 1977.
247. Schneider JA, Schlesselman JJ, Mendoza SA, Orloff S, Thoene JG, Kroll WA, Godfrey AD, Schulman JD: Ineffectiveness of ascorbic acid therapy in nephropathic cystinosis. *N Engl J Med* **300**:756, 1979.
248. Yudkoff M, Foreman JW, Segal S: Effects of cysteamine therapy in nephropathic cystinosis. *N Engl J Med* **304**:141, 1981.
249. Clark KF, Franklin PS, Reisch JS, Hoffman HJ, Gahl WA, Thoene JG, Schneider JA: Effect of cysteamine-HCl and phosphocysteamine dosage on renal function and growth in children with nephropathic cystinosis. *Clin Res* **40**:113A, 1992.
250. van't Hoff WG, Baker T, Dalton RN, Duke LC, Smith SP, Chantler C, Haycock GB: The effects of oral phosphocysteamine and rectal cysteamine in cystinosis. *Arch Dis Child* **66**:1434, 1991.
251. Selye H, Szabo S: Experimental model for production of perforating duodenal ulcers by cysteamine in the rat. *Nature* **244**:458, 1973.
252. Szabo S, Reichlin S: Somatostatin in rat tissues is depleted by cysteamine administration. *Endocrinology* **109**:2255, 1981.
253. Szabo S, Reichlin S: Somatostatin depletion by cysteamine: Mechanism and implication for duodenal ulceration. *Fed Proc* **44**:2540, 1985.
254. Scammell JG, Dannies PS: Depletion of pituitary prolactin by cysteamine is due to loss of immunological activity. *Endocrinology* **114**:712, 1984.
255. Jonas AJ, Schneider JA: Plasma cysteamine concentrations in children treated for cystinosis. *J Pediatr* **100**:321, 1982.
256. Smolin LA, Clark KF, Thoene JG, Gahl WA, Schneider JA: A comparison of the effectiveness of cysteamine and phosphocysteamine in elevating plasma cysteamine concentration and decreasing leukocyte free cystine in nephropathic cystinosis. *Pediatr Res* **23**:616, 1988.
257. Peterson TC: Effect of chronic cysteamine treatment on mouse liver aryl hydrocarbon hydroxylase activity. *Can J Physiol Pharmacol* **66**:1433, 1988.
258. Yudkoff M, Nissim I, Schneider A, Segal S: Cysteamine inhibition of [^{15}N]-glycine turnover in cystinosis and of glycine cleavage system in vitro. *Metabolism* **30**:1096, 1981.
259. Gahl WA, Bercu BB: Blunted prolactin response to thyrotropin-releasing hormone stimulation in cystinotic children receiving cysteamine. *J Clin Endocrinol Metab* **60**:793, 1985.
260. Gahl WA, Gregg RE, Hoeg JM, Fisher E: In vivo alteration of a mutant human protein using the free thiol cysteamine. *Am J Med Genet* **20**:409, 1985.
261. Corden BJ, Schulman JD, Schneider JA, Thoene JG: Adverse reactions to oral cysteamine use in nephropathic cystinosis. *Dev Pharmacol Ther* **3**:25, 1981.
262. Gahl WA, Schulman JD, Thoene JG, Schneider J: Hepatotoxicity of cysteamine? (letter). *J Pediatr* **103**:1008, 1983.
263. da Silva VA, Zurbrugg RP, Lavanchy P, Blumberg A, Suter H, Wyss SR, Luthy CM, Oetliker OH: Long-term treatment of infantile nephropathic cystinosis with cysteamine. *N Engl J Med* **313**:1460, 1985.
264. Oetliker O: Personal communication, February 24, 1992.
265. Reznik VM, Adamson M, Adelman RD, Murphy JL, Gahl WA, Clark KF, Schneider JA: Treatment of cystinosis with cysteamine from early infancy. *J Pediatr* **119**:491, 1991.
266. Bergonzi E, Herren A, Lavanchy P, Bühlmann C, Wyss SR, Lüthy C, Oetliker O: Treatment of cystinosis with cysteamine. A pilot study determining dose and form of application. *Helv Paediatr Acta* **36**:437, 1981.
267. Wittwer CT, Gahl WA, Butler JD, Zatz M, Thoene JG: Metabolism of pantethine in cystinosis. *J Clin Invest* **76**:1665, 1985.
268. Kaiser-Kupfer MI, Fujikawa L, Kuwabara T, Jain S, Gahl WA: Removal of corneal crystals by topical cysteamine in nephropathic cystinosis. *N Engl J Med* **316**:775, 1987.
269. Jain S, Kuwabara T, Gahl WA: Range of toxicity of topical cysteamine in rabbit eyes. *J Ocul Pharmacol* **4**:127, 1988.
270. Kaiser-Kupfer MI, Gazzo MA, Datiles MB, Caruso RC, Kuehl EM, Gahl WA: A randomized placebo-controlled trial of cysteamine eye drops in nephropathic cystinosis. *Arch Ophthalmol* **108**:689, 1990.
271. MacDonald IM, Noel LP, Mintsioulis G, Clarke WN: The effect of topical cysteamine drops on reducing crystal formation within the cornea of patients affected by nephropathic cystinosis. *J Pediatr Ophthalmol Strabismus* **27**:272, 1990.
272. Koch VH, Lippe BM, Nelson PA, Boechat MI, Sherman BM, Fine RN: Accelerated growth after recombinant human growth hormone treatment of children with chronic renal failure. *J Pediatr* **115**:365, 1989.
273. Tönshoff B, Mehis O, Heinrich U, Blum WF, Ranke MB, Schauer A: Growth-stimulating effects of recombinant human growth hormone in children with end-stage renal disease. *J Pediatr* **116**:561, 1990.
274. Rees L, Rigden SP, Ward G, Preece MA: Treatment of short stature in renal disease with recombinant human growth hormone. *Arch Dis Child* **65**:856, 1990.
275. Johansson G, Sietnieks A, Janssens F, Proesmans W, Vanderschueren-Lodeweyckx M, Holmberg C, Sipilä I, Broyer M, Rappaport R, Albertsson-Wikland K, Berg U, Jodal U, Rees L, Rigden SPA, Preece MA: Recombinant human growth hormone treatment in short children with chronic renal disease, before transplantation or with functioning renal transplants: An interim report on five European studies. *Acta Paediatr Scand Suppl* **370**:36, 1990.
276. Wilson DP, Jelly D, Stratton R, Coldwell JG: Nephropathic cystinosis: Improved linear growth after treatment with recombinant human growth hormone. *J Pediatr* **115**:758, 1989.
277. Andersson HC, Markello T, Schneider JA, Gahl WA: Effect of growth hormone treatment on serum creatinine concentration in patients with cystinosis and chronic renal disease. *J Pediatr* **120**:716, 1992.
278. 1212 Broadway, Suite 830, Oakland, CA 94612.
279. Aaron K, Goldman H, Scriver CR: Cystinosis; new observations: 1. Adolescent (type III) form. 2. Correction of phenotypes in vitro with dithiothreitol, in Carson NAJ, Raine DN (eds): *Inherited Disorders of Sulphur Metabolism*. Edinburgh, Churchill Livingstone, 1971, pp 150–161.
280. Hooft C, Carton D, DeSchrijver F, Delbeke MJ, Samijn W, Kint J: Juvenile cystinosis in two siblings, in Carson NAJ, Raine DN (eds): *Inherited Disorders of Sulphur Metabolism*. Edinburgh, Churchill Livingstone, 1971, pp 141–149.
281. Hauglustaine D, Corbeel L, van Damme B, Serrus M, Michielsen P: Glomerulonephritis in late-onset cystinosis.

Report of two cases and review of the literature. *Clin Nephrol* **6**:529, 1976.
282. Pabico RC, Panner BJ, McKenna BA, Bryson MF: Glomerular lesions in patients with late-onset cystinosis with massive proteinuria. *Renal Physiol* **3**:347, 1980.
283. Dale RT, Rao GN, Aquavella JV, Metz HS: Adolescent cystinosis: A clinical and specular microscopic study of an unusual sibship. *Br J Ophthalmol* **65**:828, 1981.
284. Manz F, Harms E, Lutz P, Waldherr R, Scharer K: Adolescent cystinosis: Renal function and morphology. *Eur J Pediatr* **138**:354, 1982.
285. Langman CB, Moore ES, Thoene JG, Schneider JA: Renal failure in a sibship with late-onset cystinosis. *J Pediatr* **107**:755, 1985.
286. Schneider JA, Katz B, Melles RB: Cystinosis. *AKF Nephrol Lett* **7**:22, 1990.
287. Cogan DG, Kuwabara T, Kinoshita J, Sheehan L, Merola L: Cystinosis in an adult. *JAMA* **164**:394, 1957.
288. Cogan DG, Kuwabara T, Hurlbut CS Jr, McMurray V: Further observations on cystinosis in the adult. *JAMA* **166**:1725, 1958.
289. Lietman PS, Frazier PD, Wong VG, Shotton D, Seegmiller JE: Adult cystinosis—a benign disorder. *Am J Med* **40**:511, 1966.
290. Brubaker RF, Wong VG, Schulman JD, Seegmiller JE, Kuwabara T: Benign cystinosis. The clinical, biochemical and morphologic findings in a family with two affected siblings. *Am J Med* **49**:546, 1970.
291. Kraus E, Lutz P: Ocular cystine deposits in an adult. *Arch Ophthalmol* **85**:690, 1971.
292. Dodd MJ, Pusin SM, Green WR: Adult cystinosis. A case report. *Arch Ophthalmol* **96**:1054, 1978.
293. Gahl WA, Tietze F: Lysosomal cystine transport in cystinosis variants and their parents. *Pediatr Res* **21**:193, 1987.
294. Greene AA, Schneider JA: Unpublished data.
295. Bickel H: Die entwicklung der biochemischen läsion bei der Lignac-Fanconischen krankheit. *Helv Paediatr Acta* **10**:259, 1955.
296. Foreman JW, Bowring MA, Lee J, States B, Segal S: Effect of cystine dimethylester on renal solute handling and isolated renal tubule transport in the rat: A new model of the Fanconi syndrome. *Metabolism* **36**:1185, 1987.
297. Moran A, Ben-Nun A, Potashnik R, Bashan N: Renal cells in culture as a model for cystinosis. *J Basic Clin Physiol Pharmacol* **1**:357, 1990.
298. Foreman JW, Benson LL: Effect of cystine loading on substrate oxidation by rat renal tubules. *Pediatr Nephrol* **4**:236, 1990.
299. Salmon RF, Baum M: Intracellular cystine loading inhibits transport in the rabbit proximal convoluted tubule. *J Clin Invest* **85**:340, 1990.
300. Coor C, Salmon RF, Quigley R, Marver D, Baum M: Role of adenosine triphosphate (ATP) and NaK ATPase in the inhibition of proximal tubule transport with intracellular cystine loading. *J Clin Invest* **87**:955, 1991.
301. Racusen LC, Fivush BA, Andersson H, Gahl WA: Culture of renal tubular cells from the urine of patients with nephropathic cystinosis.*J Am Soc Nephrol* **1**:1028, 1991.
302. Pisoni RL, Lemons RM, Thoene JG: Description of a selection method highly cytotoxic for cystinotic human fibroblasts but not normal human fibroblasts. *Clin Res* **37**:542A, 1989.
303. Aula P, Autio S, Raivio KO, Rapola J, Thoden CJ, Koskela SL, Yamashina I: "Salla disease": A new lysosomal storage disorder. *Arch Neurol* **36**:88, 1979.
304. Renlund M, Chester AM, Lundblad A, Aula P, Raivio KO, Autio S, Koskela SL: Increased urinary excretion of free N-acetylneuraminic acid in thirteen patients with Salla disease. *Eur J Biochem* **101**:245, 1979.
305. Hancock LW, Thaler MM, Horwitz AL, Dawson G: Generalized N-acetylneuraminic acid storage disease: Quantitation and identification of the monosaccharide accumulating in brain and other tissues. *J Neurochem* **38**:803, 1982.
306. Tondeur M, Libert J, Vamos E, Van Hoff F, Thomas GH, Strecker G: Infantile form of sialic acid storage disorder: Clinical, ultrastructural and biochemical studies in two siblings. *Eur J Pediatr* **139**:142, 1982.
307. Mancini GM: Lysosomal membrane transport. Physiological and pathological events. Thesis. Rotterdam, the Netherlands, Erasmus Universiteit, 1991. (abstr.)
308. Pueschel SM, O'Shea PA, Alroy J, Ambler MW, Dangond F, Daniel PF, Kolodny EH: Infantile sialic acid storage disease associated with renal disease. *Pediatr Neurol* **4**:207, 1988.
309. Schauer R: *Sialic Acids: Chemistry, Metabolism and Function*. New York, Springer-Verlag, 1982.
310. Schauer R: Sialic acids: Chemistry, metabolism and functions of sialic acids. *Adv Carbohydr Chem Biochem* **40**:131, 1982.
311. Schauer R: Sialic acids and their role as biological masks. *Trends Biochem Sci* **10**:357, 1985.
312. Seppala R, Renlund M, Bernardini I, Tietze F, Gahl WA: Renal handling of free sialic acid in normal humans and patients with Salla disease or renal disease. *Lab Invest* **63**:197, 1990.
313. Kornfeld S, Kornfeld R, Neufeld EF, O'Brien PJ: The feedback control of sugar nucleotide biosynthesis in liver. *Proc Natl Acad Sci USA* **52**:371, 1964.
314. Sommar KM, Ellis DB: Uridine diphosphate N-acetyl-D-glucosamine 2-epimerase from rat liver. Catalytic and regulatory properties. *Biochim Biophys Acta* **268**:581, 1972.
315. Thomas GH, Scocca J, Miller CS, Reynolds LW: Accumulation of N-acetylneuraminic acid (sialic acid) in human fibroblasts cultured in the presence of N-acetylmannosamine. *Biochim Biophys Acta* **846**:37, 1985.
316. Kolisis FN, Hervagault JF: Theoretical and experimental studies on the competition of NAN-aldolase and cytidine-5'-monophosphate synthetase for their common substrate N-acetylneuraminic acid. *Biochem Int* **13**:493, 1986.
317. Renlund M, Chester AM, Lundblad A, Parkkinen J, Krusius T: Free N-acetylneuraminic acid in tissues in Salla disease and the enzymes involved in its metabolism. *Eur J Biochem* **130**:39, 1983.
318. Brunetti P, Jourdian GW, Roseman S: The sialic acids. III. Distribution and properties of animal N-acetylneuraminic acid aldolase. *J Biol Chem* **237**:2447, 1962.
319. Hancock LW, Horwitz AL, Dawson G: N-acetylneuraminic acid sialoglycoconjugate metabolism in fibroblasts from a patient with generalized N-acetylneuraminic acid storage disease. *Biochim Biophys Acta* **760**:42, 1983.
320. Thomas GH, Scocca J, Libert J, Vamos E, Miller CS, Reynolds LW: Alterations in cultured fibroblasts of sibs with an infantile form of a free (unbound) sialic acid storage disease. *Pediatr Res* **17**:307, 1983.
321. Stevensson RE, Lubinsky M, Taylor HA, Wenger DA, Schroer RJ, Olmstead PM: Sialic acid storage disease with sialuria: Clinical and biochemical features in the severe infantile type. *Pediatrics* **72**:441, 1983.
322. Ylitalo V, Hagberg B, Rapola J, Mansson JE, Svennerholm L, Sanner G, Tonnby B: Salla disease variants. Sialoylaciduric encephalopathy with increased sialidase activity in two non-Finnish children. *Neuropediatrics* **17**:44, 1986.
323. Renlund M, Kovanen PT, Raivio KO, Aula P, Gahmberg CG, Ehnholm C: Studies on the defect underlying the lysosomal storage of sialic acid in Salla disease. *J Clin Invest* **77**:568, 1988.
324. Mancini GMS, Verheijen FW, Galjaard H: Free N-acetylneuraminic acid (NANA) storage disorders: Evidence for defective NANA transport across the lysosomal membrane. *Hum Genet* **73**:214, 1986.
325. Mendla K, Baumkotter J, Rosenau C, Ulrich-Bott B, Cantz M: Defective lysosomal release of glycoprotein-derived sialic acid in fibroblasts from patients with sialic acid storage disease. *Biochem J* **250**:261, 1988.
326. Paschke E, Hofler G, Roscher A: Infantile sialic acid storage disease: The fate of biosynthetically labeled N-acetyl(^{3}H) neuraminic acid in cultured human fibroblasts. *Pediatr Res* **20**:773, 1986.
327. Jonas AJ: Studies of lysosomal sialic acid metabolism: Retention of sialic acid by Salla disease lysosomes. *Biochem Biophys Res Commun* **137**:175, 1986.
328. Renlund M, Tietze F, Gahl WA: Defective sialic acid egress from isolated fibroblast lysosomes of patients with Salla disease. *Science* **232**:759, 1986.

329. Tietze F, Seppala R, Renlund M, Hopwood JJ, Harper GS, Thomas GH, Gahl WA: Defective lysosomal egress of free sialic acid (N-acetylneuraminic acid) in fibroblasts of patients with infantile free sialic acid storage disease. *J Biol Chem* **264**:15316, 1989.
330. Mancini GMS, De Jong HR, Galjaard H, Verheijen FW: Characterization of a proton-driven carrier for sialic acid in the lysosomal membrane. Evidence for a group-specific transport system for acidic monosaccharides. *J Biol Chem* **264**:15247, 1989.
331. Mancini GMS, Beerens CEMT, Aula PP, Verheijen FW: Sialic acid storage diseases. A multiple lysosomal transport defect for acidic monosaccharides. *J Clin Invest* **87**:1329, 1991.
332. Blom HJ, Andersson HC, Seppala R, Tietze F, Gahl WA: Defective glucuronic acid transport from lysosomes of infantile free sialic acid storage disease fibroblasts. *Biochem J* **268**:621, 1990.
333. Mancini GMC, Beerens CEMT, Galjaard H, Verheijen FW: Functional reconstitution of the lysosomal sialic acid carrier into proteoliposomes. *Proc Natl Acad Sci USA* **89**:6609, 1992.
334. Baumkötter J, Cantz M, Mendla K, Baumann W, Frieboli H, Gehler J, Spranger J: N-acetylneuraminic acid storage disease. *Hum Genet* **71**:155, 1985.
335. Virtanen I, Ekblom P, Laurila P, Nordling S, Raivio KO, Aula P: Characterization of storage material in cultured fibroblasts by specific lectin binding in lysosomal storage disease. *Pediatr Res* **14**:1199, 1980.
336. Echenne B, Vidal M, Maire I, Michalski JC, Baldet P, Astruc J: Salla disease in one non-Finnish patient. *Eur J Pediatr* **124**:320, 1986.
337. Wolburg-Bucholz K, Scholte W, Baumkötter J, Cantz M, Holder H, Harzer K: Familial lysosomal storage disease with generalized vacuolization and sialic aciduria. Spodaric Salla disease. *Neuropediatrics* **16**:67, 1985.
338. Vamos E, Libert J, Elkhazen N, Jauniaux E, Hustin J, Wilkin P: Prenatal diagnosis and confirmation of infantile sialic acid storage disease. *Prenat Diagn* **6**:437, 1986.
339. Lake BD, Young EP, Nicolaides K: Prenatal diagnosis of infantile sialic acid storage disease in a twin pregnancy. *J Inherited Metab Dis* **12**:152, 1989.
340. Renlund M, Aula PP, Raivio KD, Autio S, Sainio K, Rapola J, Koskela SL: Salla disease: A new lysosomal storage disorder with disturbed sialic acid metabolism. *Neurology* **33**:57, 1983.
341. Haataja L, Schleutker J, Renlund M, Palotie A, Peltonen L, Aula P: Exclusion map of Salla disease: Attempts to localize the disease gene using a computer program. *Hum Genet* **88**:298, 1992.
342. Renlund M: Clinical and laboratory diagnosis of Salla disease in infancy and childhood. *J Pediatr* **104**:232, 1984.
343. Autio-Harmainen H, Oldfors A, Sourander P, Renlund M, Dammert K, Similä S: Neuropathology of Salla disease. *Acta Neuropathol (Berl)* **75**:481, 1988.
344. Stevenson RE, Lubinsky M, Taylor HA, Wenger DA, Schroer RJ, Olmstead PM: Sialic acid storage disease with sialuria: Clinical and biochemical features in the severe infantile type. *Pediatrics* **72**:441, 1983.
345. Sperl W, Gruber W, Quatacker J, Monnens L, Thoenes W, Fink FM, Paschke E: Nephrosis in two siblings with infantile sialic acid storage disease. *Eur J Pediatr* **149**:477, 1990.
346. Mancini GMS, Hu P, Verheijen FW, Van Diggelen OP, Janse HC, Kleijer WJ, Beemer FA, Jennekens FGI: Salla disease variant in a Dutch patient. Potential value of polymorphonuclear leukocytes for heterozygote detection. *Eur J Pediatr* **151**:590, 1992.
347. Humbel R, Collart M: Oligosaccharides in the urine of patients with glycoprotein storage diseases. Rapid detection by thin-layer chromatography. *Clin Chim Acta* **60**:143, 1975.
348. Clements PR, Taylor JA, Hopwood JJ: Biochemical characterization of patients and prenatal diagnosis of sialic acid storage disease for three families. *J Inherited Metab Dis* **11**:30, 1988.
349. Renlund M, Aula P: Prenatal detection of Salla disease based upon increased free sialic acid in amniocytes. *Am J Med Genet* **28**:377, 1987.
350. Renlund M: Unpublished data.
351. Fontaine G, Biserte G, Montreuil J, Dupont A, Ferriaux JP, Strecker G, Spik G, Puvion E, Puvion-Dutilleul F, Sezille G, Piquie MT: La sialurie: Un trouble metabolique original. *Helv Paediatr Acta (suppl 17)* **23**:3, 1968.
352. Wilcken B, Don N, Greenaway R, Hammond J, Sosula L: Sialuria: A second case. *J Inherited Metab Dis* **10**:97, 1987.
353. Don NA, Wilcken B: Sialuria: A follow-up report. *J Inherited Metab Dis* **14**:942, 1991.
354. Seppala R, Tietze F, Krasnewich D, Weiss P, Ashwell G, Barsh G, Thomas GH, Packman S, Gahl WA: Sialic acid metabolism in sialuria fibroblasts. *J Biol Chem* **266**:7456, 1991.
355. Krasnewich DM, Tietze F, Krause W, Pretzlaff R, Wenger DA, Diwadkar V, Gahl WA: Clinical and biochemical studies in an American child with sialuria. *Biochem Med Metab Biol* **49**:90, 1993
356. Weiss P, Tietze F, Gahl WA, Seppala R, Ashwell G: Identification of the metabolic defect in sialuria. *J Biol Chem* **264**:17635, 1989.
357. Palo J, Rauvala H, Finne J, Haltia M, Palmgren K: Hyperexcretion of free N-acetylneuraminic acid. A novel type of sialuria.*Clin Chim Acta* **145**:237, 1985.
358. Beaudet AL, Thomas GH: Disorders of glycoprotein degradation: Mannosidosis, fucosidosis, sialidosis, and aspartylglycosaminuria, in Scriver CR, Beaudet AL, Sly WS, Valle D (eds): *The Metabolic Basis of Inherited Disease*, 6th ed. New York, McGraw Hill, 1989, p 1603.
359. Rosenblatt DS, Hosack A, Matiaszuk NV, Cooper BA, Laframboise R: Defect in vitamin B12 release from lysosomes: Newly described inborn error of vitamin B12 metabolism. *Science* **228**:1319, 1985.
360. Rosenblatt DS, Laframboise R, Pichette J, Langevin P, Cooper BA, Costa T: New disorder of vitamin B12 metabolism (cobalamin F) presenting as methylmalonic aciduria. *Pediatrics* **78**:51, 1986.
361. Vassiliadis A, Rosenblatt DS, Cooper BA, Bergeron JJM: EM autoradiography of cbl F fibroblasts: Demonstration of vitamin B12 in lysosomes. *Am J Hum Genet* **43**:A17, 1988.
362. Gahl WA: Lysosomal membrane transport in cellular nutrition. *Annu Rev Nutr* **9**:39, 1989.
363. Tietze F: Lysosomal transport of sugars: Normal and pathological, in Thoene JG (ed): *Pathophysiology of Lysosomal Transport*. Boca Raton, FL: CRC, 1992.
364. Cameron PD, Dobowitz V, Besley GTM, Fensoma H: Sialic acid storage disease. *Arch Dis Child* **65**:314, 1990.
365. Cooper A, Sardharwalla IB, Thornley M, Ward KP: Infantile sialic acid storage disease in two siblings. *J Inherited Metab Dis* **2**:259, 1988.
366. Patrick AD: Deficiencies of -SH-dependent enzymes in cystinosis. *Clin Sci* **28**:427, 1965.
367. Wong VG, Schulman JD, Seegmiller JE: Conjunctival biopsy for the biochemical diagnosis of cystinosis. *Am J Ophthalmol* **70**:278, 1970.
368. Schulman JD, Bradley KH, Berezesky IK, Grimley PM, Dodson WE, Al-Aish MS: Biochemical, morphologic, and cytogenetic studies of leukocytes growing in continuous culture from normal individuals and from patients with cystinosis. *Pediatr Res* **5**:501, 1971.
369. Pellet OL, Smith ML, Thoene JG, Schneider JA, Jonas AJ: Renal cell culture using autopsy material from children with cystinosis. *In Vitro* **20**:53, 1984.
370. Harms E, Krauss-Mackiw E, Lutz P: Cystine concentration of cultivated cells from skin and cornea. *Metab Pediatr Ophthalmol* **3**:157, 1979.
371. Theodoropoulos DS, Krasnewich D, Kaiser-Kupfer MI, Gahl WA: Classical nephropathic cystinosis as an adult disease. *JAMA* **270**:2200, 1993.
372. Haataja L, Sonninen PH, Parkkola RK, Aarimaa T, Aula P: Unpublished data.
373. Haataja L, Schleutker J, Laine A-P, Renlund M, Savontaus M-L, Dib C, Weissenbach J, Peltonen L, Aula P: The genetic locus for free sialic acid storage disease maps to the long arm of chromosome 6. *Am J Hum Genet* **54**:1042, 1994.

CHAPTER 127

Cystic Fibrosis

Michael J. Welsh ▪ Lap-Chee Tsui
Thomas F. Boat ▪ Arthur L. Beaudet

1. **Cystic fibrosis (CF) is the most common fatal autosomal recessive disease affecting Caucasian populations, with an incidence of 1 in 2000 to 3000 births in various groups.**

2. **The most life-threatening clinical features of CF are pulmonary obstruction and infection. Thick mucous secretions are associated initially with chronic obstructive lung disease, predominantly involving the small airways. Recurrent and persistent infections, especially with *Pseudomonas* and *Staphylococcus,* lead to bronchiectasis and respiratory failure, often accompanied by cor pulmonale and death. In the majority of cases, exocrine pancreatic dysfunction begins in utero and causes postnatal steatorrhea and failure to thrive. Neonatal meconium ileus occurs in 10–20 percent of newborns and is highly suggestive of CF. Other manifestations include cirrhosis of the liver; diabetes mellitus; infertility, especially in males; and abnormally high levels of sodium and chloride in sweat.**

3. **The diagnosis is suggested by the clinical features of chronic obstructive lung disease, persistent pulmonary infection (particularly with mucoid strains of *Pseudomonas*), meconium ileus, pancreatic insufficiency with failure to thrive, or a positive family history. In the presence of such features, the diagnosis is confirmed by a sweat chloride concentration greater than 60 meq/liter or by the presence of pathologic CF mutations on both chromosomes. Newborn screening is possible using dried blood specimens for quantitation of immunoreactive trypsin in combination with mutation analysis, but screening has not become universal because of lack of definitive evidence that early diagnosis improves long-term outcome.**

4. **Treatment involves a comprehensive approach to provide postural drainage with chest percussion, inpatient and outpatient antibiotics, pancreatic enzyme replacement, proper nutrition, and psychosocial support. Aerosolized recombinant DNase is a new treatment aimed at improved airway clearance. Somatic gene therapy for CF is the focus of research efforts. The prognosis has improved greatly, with a median survival of 28.2 years for females and 30.6 for males.**

5. **The CF gene was mapped to chromosome 7q31.2 and was cloned in 1989 using a positional cloning strategy. The gene contains 27 coding exons spread over 230 kb and produces as mRNA of 6.5 kb. The protein encoded by the CF gene is designated cystic fibrosis transmembrane conductance regulator (CFTR) and contains 1480 amino acids with a molecular mass of about 170,000. CFTR is a member of the ATP-binding cassette family of transporter proteins and contains five domains: two membrane-spanning domains (MSD), each composed of six transmembrane segments; an R domain, which contains several consensus phosphorylation sequences; and two nucleotide-binding domains (NBD), which interact with ATP.**

6. **The major mutation causing CF is a 3-basepair deletion causing loss of phenylalanine 508 (ΔF508). This mutation had a unique origin and is found on about 70 percent of CF chromosomes worldwide, the percentage being higher in northern Europe and lower in southern and eastern Europe. At least 350 other pathologic CF mutations and numerous benign variations are known; only 7 or 8 of the other pathologic mutations represent more than one half percent of CF chromosomes worldwide, although they may occur at higher frequencies in selected populations as exemplified by the W1282X mutation on 60 percent of Ashkenazic CF chromosomes.**

7. **CF epithelia are characterized by defective electrolyte transport, and defective Cl^- transport has been demonstrated in the apical membrane of epithelial cells from sweat gland, airway, pancreas, and intestine. CFTR functions as a cAMP-regulated Cl^- channel, and expression studies indicate that the membrane-spanning domains contribute to the channel pore and that the phosphorylation of specific residues in the R domain opens the channel.**

8. **Mutations causing CF have been classified as follows: class I mutations have defective protein production (includes many severe, null alleles); class II mutations have defective protein processing (includes ΔF508); class III mutations show defective regulation of the channel; and class IV mutations show defective conduction through the channel (includes numerous milder alleles).**

A list of standard abbreviations is located immediately preceding the index in each volume. Additional abbreviations used in this chapter include: ABC = ATP-binding cassette; AMP-PNP = 5-adenylylimidodiphosphate; ATPγS = adenosine 5′−3-*O*-(thio)triphosphate; CBAVD = congenital bilateral absence of the vas deferens; CF = cystic fibrosis; CFTR = cystic fibrosis transmembrane conductance regulator; cGK = cyclic GMP-dependent protein kinase; DIDS = 4,4′ -diisothio-cyanato-stilbene-2,2′ -disulphonic acid; EC_{50} = effective concentration, 50%; FEV_1 = forced expiratory volume in one second; FVC = forced vital capacity; I-V = current-voltage; MDR = multiple drug resistance protein; *met* or *MET* = *met* oncogene or gene symbol for same; MSD = membrane spanning domain; mV = millivolt; 8-N_3ATP = β-azidoadenosine 5′ -triphosphate; NBD = nucleotide binding domain; NPPB = 5-nitro-2-(3-phenylpropylamino) benzoic acid; Pa_{CO_2} = partial pressure (arterial) CO_2; Pa_{O_2} = partial pressure (arterial) O_2; PI = pancreatic insufficient; PKA = cAMP-dependent protein kinase; PKC = protein kinase C; P_o = open state probability; pS = picosiemens; PS = pancreatic sufficient; Sa_{O_2} = saturation (arterial) O_2; STE6 = sterile 6 protein/gene of yeast; Ω = olm electrical resistance. Missense and nonsense mutations are designated in single letter code; e.g., glycine to aspartic acid at codon 551 = G551D and glycine to stop at codon 542 = G542X. See Beaudet and Tsui for additional details on mutation nomenclature.[502]

9. **The correlation of genotype with phenotype is substantial for pancreatic function with 85 percent of patients being pancreatic insufficient and having two severe mutations while pancreatic sufficient patients have one or two mild mutations. Genotype does not correlate well or allow prediction of phenotype for pulmonary involvement or survival for most patients with a classic phenotype. A few mutations may be associated with milder pulmonary disease, and some particularly mild mutations are found in males with congenital bilateral absence of the vas deferens without classic CF.**

10. **Molecular diagnosis for CF now relies primarily on mutation analysis and is highly reliable for prenatal diagnosis and carrier detection within families. Although interpretation is complex, DNA analysis is also useful for evaluating fetal echogenic bowel and in diagnosing atypical CF phenotypes. Pilot programs evaluating population-based carrier screening are in progress, but it is not clear how widespread such programs may become and what the effect might be on the prevalence of CF.**

INTRODUCTION AND HISTORICAL PERSPECTIVES

Cystic fibrosis (CF) is a single-gene disorder with a complex phenotype. It affects children, many of whom now live into adulthood, and is characterized chiefly by chronic obstruction and infection of the respiratory tract, exocrine pancreatic insufficiency and its nutritional consequences, and elevated levels of sweat electrolytes. This condition represents the most common life-threatening recessive genetic trait in the Caucasian population. Dysfunction of exocrine glands appears to be the predominant pathogenetic mechanism and is responsible for a broad and variable array of presenting manifestations and subsequent complications.

CF is an important medical problem. It is the most prevalent cause of severe, progressive lung disease in children and has become an important cause of lung-related morbidity and mortality in young adults. CF is responsible for most of the exocrine pancreatic insufficiency of childhood and early adulthood and for much of the nasal polyposis, pansinusitis, rectal prolapse, nonketotic insulin-dependent hyperglycemia, and biliary cirrhosis seen at these ages. Therefore, CF enters into the differential diagnosis of many pediatric and young adult patients. Finally, researchers recently have identified and cloned the CF gene, described many of the structural and functional properties of its product (cystic fibrosis transmembrane conductance regulator, or CFTR), detected a large number of mutations in this gene, and made striking progress toward understanding the related epithelial cell pathophysiology. These advances have fostered the proposal and testing of an array of new therapeutic strategies. Thus, CF provides a model for achieving rapid advances in understanding genetic disease pathogenesis and translating this understanding into potentially important clinical interventions.

CF was first described as a distinct clinical entity in the late 1930s. However, numerous references to infants and children with meconium ileus and typical pancreatic and lung disease are sprinkled through the literature from as early as 1650. Of interest are references in European folklore to the association of salty skin and early demise.[1] In 1936, Fanconi reported a child with the clinical features of CF but failed to recognize the scope or importance of this syndrome.[2] Anderson is usually credited with the first comprehensive description of CF, published in 1938.[3] She coined the term "cystic fibrosis of the pancreas." In 1945, Farber suggested that CF is a disease of exocrine glands, characterized largely by failure to clear their mucous secretory product.[4] He introduced the term *mucoviscidosis*, which was popular in the medical literature for a number of years. Chronic infection of the lungs was recognized early as a major contributing factor, and antibiotics were first used for the treatment of CF in the 1940s. At that time, an autosomal recessive inheritance pattern for CF was suggested by Anderson and Hodges.[5] In 1953, di Sant' Agnese and colleagues investigated salt depletion in children with CF during a summertime heat wave and concluded that excessive loss of salt occurred via the sweat.[6] They subsequently documented that sodium and chloride levels in sweat are elevated in virtually all individuals with CF. This observation led to a description by Gibson and Cooke of the pilocarpine iontophoresis method for sweat testing,[7] a method that remains the diagnostic standard to this day. By the late 1950s, CF was reported occasionally in older children and young adults. Soon thereafter, comprehensive and aggressive approaches to the care of patients were instituted in many treatment centers, and these measures are credited with a steadily increasing survival to adulthood of CF patients. In the past 35 years, a progressively more refined description of the CF syndrome and its complications has emerged.

Two sets of observations in the early 1980s set the stage for rapid progress toward understanding the molecular defect. Knowles and coworkers described altered electrical properties of CF respiratory epithelium, associated with abnormalities of both sodium and chloride transport.[8] Soon thereafter, Quinton and colleagues demonstrated chloride impermeability in CF sweat gland ducts.[9] These observations focused attention on a pathogenetic role for electrolyte and water movement across CF epithelia and for the first time offered a plausible explanation both for the previously noted water deficits in mucous secretions[10,11] and for dysfunction of multiple organs. Subsequent work with epithelial cells and their membranes identified dysfunction of a cAMP-dependent activation of chloride channels as the primary pathophysiologic lesion. Following the identification and cloning of the CF gene,[12–14] it soon became apparent that its product, CFTR, was in fact a chloride channel that is dysfunctional in CF epithelia.[15,651,674] Ongoing investigations target structure–function relationships of the normal and altered gene product, the contribution of different mutations to the heterogeneity of the CF phenotype, and strategies for circumventing the molecular abnormality in CF epithelia. These investigations are now aided by the creation of transgenic animal models of CF.[16]

PATHOLOGIC AND CLINICAL FEATURES OF CLASSIC CF

Classic CF presents in many different ways and mimics a number of other clinical entities; see "Atypical CF Phenotypes" below for other presentations. Usual presentations include persistent cough and recurrent or refractory lung infiltrates and also reflect gastrointestinal disturbance, including meconium ileus in approximately 10 percent of patients as well as failure to thrive with steatorrhea. A number of individuals escape detection in the first decade or two of life, often because symptoms are unusual, subtle, or even absent. It is now widely accepted that some of the disease variation has a genetic basis, although nongenetic

Table 127-1 Unusual Presentations of Cystic Fibrosis

Respiratory
- Bronchiolitis/asthma
- *Pseudomonas aeruginosa* colonization of the respiratory tract
- Staphylococcal pneumonia
- Nasal polyposis
- Sinusitis

Gastrointestinal
- Meconium plug syndrome
- Rectal prolapse
- Recurrent abdominal pain and/or right lower quadrant mass
- Hypoproteinemic edema
- Prolonged neonatal jaundice
- Biliary cirrhosis with portal hypertension
- Pseudotumor cerebri
- Vitamin deficiency states (A, D, E, K)
- Acrodermatitis enteropathica-like eruption with fatty acid and zinc deficiency
- Recurrent pancreatitis
- Volvulus in fetal life

Genitourinary
- Discovery of absent vas deferens early in life
- Male infertility
- Female infertility

Other
- Hypochloremic, hyponatremic alkalosis
- Mother of a child with cystic fibrosis

factors are also important. A list of unusual presentations is compiled in Table 127-1. Recognition of the protean manifestations of CF and a high index of suspicion are required to detect all cases, particularly at early stages, before extensive lung injury.

Respiratory Tract

Pathology. Mucous obstruction and infection, the major pathologic events in the lung, are confined, at least initially, to the conducting airways. In fact, the earliest consistent pathologic lesion is said to be mucous obstruction of bronchioles with accompanying bronchiolar wall inflammation.[17] It is clear that conducting airways disease is acquired postnatally. The airways of children with CF who have died within the first days of life display no obvious abnormalities.[18] For example, the numbers and distribution of mucus-producing goblet cells and the numbers and sizes of submucosal glands appear to be within the normal range at birth. A careful morphometric analysis of CF airways early in life has demonstrated dilated acinar and duct lumens in submucosal glands before reaction to chronic infection would be expected.[19] This finding suggests either hypersecretion or accumulation of secretions with abnormal properties at an early age and provides strong evidence that the primary pathogenetic event is accumulation of secretions rather than infection.

With progression of lung disease, evidence for bronchiolitis and bronchitis becomes more prominent, the submucosal glands hypertrophy, and goblet cells not only increase in number but extend distally into the bronchioles. Focal areas of squamous metaplasia develop and may impair clearance of mucus. Some small airways are obstructed completely by secretions (Fig. 127-1). Bronchiolectasis and then bronchiectasis result from repetitive cycles of obstruction and infection. Extensive bronchiectasis is a usual finding by the second decade of life but is often noted much earlier. Pneumonia, when present, generally is distributed in a peribronchial pattern.[20]

Detailed pathologic descriptions of lung disease are based on examination of lungs at autopsy and reflect advanced lung disease. Bronchiectatic cysts, initially most prominent in the upper lobes, occupy as much as 50 percent of the cross-sectional area of the lung.[21] In addition to dilation, bronchioles undergo stenosis or even obliteration.[22] At autopsy, the lungs also show extensive overinflation of air spaces. Scattered areas of destructive emphysema (Fig. 127-1) are seen in patients who have lived for two or three decades.[23] Absence of more extensive alveolar wall destruction can be explained by effective confinement of chronic infection to conducting airways. Several patterns of interstitial pneumonia also have been described.[24] Peribronchiolar and peribronchial fibrosis accelerates with time and contributes to the restrictive lung function pattern that is superimposed on obstruction in advanced lung disease.

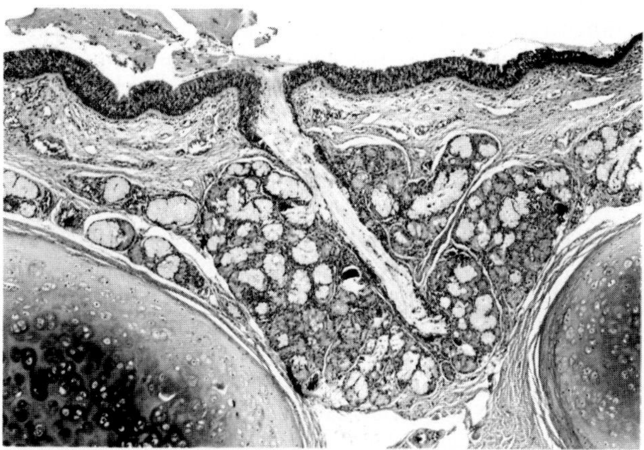

A.

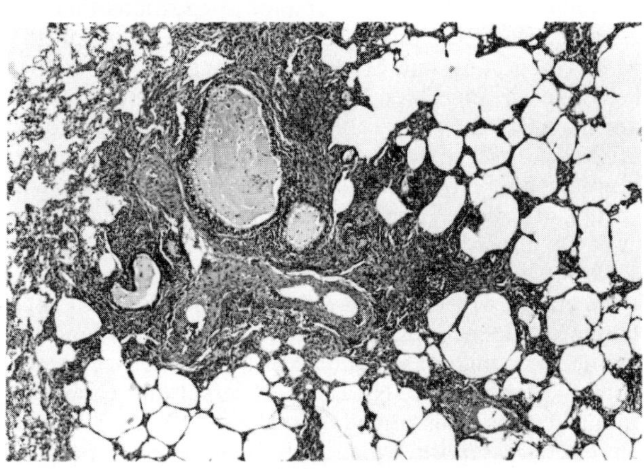

B.

FIG. 127-1 Tracheobronchial pathology in CF. *A*. Hypertrophied submucosal gland in the trachea of an 18-year-old woman with CF. Mucus-containing acini are distended. The duct lumen is distended with secretions, which contain inflammatory and/or epithelial cells. H & E, ×42 (original magnification). *B*. Large and small bronchioles in the lungs of a 21-year-old man with CF. These airways are completely obstructed with secretions and display chronic inflammation of the walls and surrounding tissues. Peribronchiolar fibrosis also can be demonstrated with appropriate stains. Air space enlargement is prominent *(right)*, but more normal-appearing peripheral lung is present *(left)*. H & E, ×42.

Subpleural cysts eventually occur on the mediastinal surfaces of the upper lobes and seem to be related to the occurrence of pneumothorax in patients with advanced lung disease.[25] Bronchial arteries become large and tortuous,[26] contributing to a propensity for hemoptysis in ectatic airways. Pulmonary arteries display varying degrees of change, reflecting secondary pulmonary hypertension.[27]

Hypertrophy and hyperplasia of secretory elements, mucus accumulation, and chronic inflammatory changes also are characteristic of paranasal sinuses and the nasal passages. A common feature of nasal pathology is inflammatory edema of the mucosa with subsequent pedunculation and formation of polyps.[28]

Pathogenesis of Lung Infection. While mucous obstruction is likely to be the primary pathophysiological event, chronic infection in the respiratory tract appears to be the more destructive process. The chronic airways infection of CF may be unique, particularly with respect to its confinement to the endobronchial space and the organisms involved, primarily *Staphylococcus aureus* and *Pseudomonas aeruginosa*. Once established, infection of the lungs is nearly impossible to eradicate. Bacterial infection extending beyond the lungs is distinctly uncommon. Therefore, local rather than general host defense mechanisms must be compromised.

A possible reason for failure of lung defense and bacterial colonization of airways is defective mucociliary clearance. However, mucus transport velocity in the central airways is not consistently or profoundly diminished.[29] Clearance from the more peripheral airways, where mucus first accumulates, has not been assessed directly. Studies to date suggest that the morphology and frequency of beating of cilia are normal.[30,31] Therefore, most investigators assume that abnormal physical properties or overabundance of secretions are responsible for retention of mucus. No matter what the basis, failure to clear secretions is likely to provide an environment that is conducive to the establishment of chronic endobronchial infection.

The role played by *P. aeruginosa* and *S. aureus* in endobronchial infection has prompted suggestions that surface properties of CF airways are altered in a fashion that promotes their adhesion. Studies of *S. aureus* have failed to find unique or increased numbers of receptors for this organism on CF respiratory epithelial cell surfaces. However, *S. aureus* recovered from CF airways are more adherent than organisms recovered from airways of individuals with other lung disorders.[32] It has been proposed that the environment of CF airways induces bacterial adhesins. In contrast, *P. aeruginosa* binds more avidly to CF buccal cells[33] and primary cultures of CF airway cells[34] than to control cells. Preliminary evidence suggests that a ΔF508/ΔF508 genotype is particularly linked to increased binding properties of respiratory epithelial cells. These observations cannot be reproduced using transformed CF and control cells.[34] Mucoid strains of *P. aeruginosa*, which are frequently recovered from CF lungs, appear to have enhanced adherence properties.[35]

Pulmonary immunology has also been investigated extensively in an effort to identify host defense abnormalities. There is little reason to believe that a primary deficiency state exists. Although CF subjects tend to have low levels of serum IgG in the first decade of life, these levels increase dramatically as chronic infection is established.[36] Secretory antibody levels appear to be normal or enhanced.[37] IgG harvested from the serum of patients with CF lacks a full complement of sugars on the termini of oligosaccharide chains. However, this alteration may reflect enhanced deglycosylation rather than a biosynthetic abnormality.[38] Antibody responses specific for infecting organisms in the respiratory tract are brisk.[39] Numbers of B lymphocytes and B cells that differentiate into immunoglobulin-secreting cells are not depressed.[40] T-lymphocyte numbers are adequate, and these lymphocytes proliferate in response to nonspecific mitogens.[41] With advancing severity of pulmonary disease, lymphocytes of CF patients proliferate less briskly when challenged with *P. aeruginosa* and other gram-negative organisms.[42] Blood lymphocytes of CF patients who are experiencing exacerbation of lung infection also display depressed production of interleukin-2.[43] These acquired dysfunctions can be reversed in some patients by intensive antibiotic treatment for *P. aeruginosa* but may contribute to antimicrobial therapy failures associated with end-stage lung disease.

Neutrophils and alveolar macrophages are plentiful in CF airways. Interleukin-8 (IL-8) is generated in large amounts by infection and acts as a potent chemoattractant for neutrophils.[44] IL-8[44] and bacterial endotoxins or immune complexes[45] in CF sputum appear to prime neutrophils for enhanced oxidative function. However, investigators have examined the possibility that phagocytic cells are not fully functional in CF lungs. This idea gained credence from observations that CF serum inhibits the phagocytosis of *P. aeruginosa* organisms (but not of several other bacteria) by rabbit and human alveolar macrophages when removed from their usual environment.[46,47] The putative phagocytic defect in cystic fibrosis appears to be related to deficient opsonic activity, is seen only in patients who have established *P. aeruginosa* infection, and may be caused by proteolytic fragmentation of IgG.[48] In addition, recent work suggests that the major subclass of IgG in serum and lungs and attached to lung organisms of CF subjects is IgG_2. Because alveolar macrophages have receptors largely for other subclasses of IgG, a preponderance of IgG_2 would be expected to interfere with opsonin-mediated phagocytic clearance.[49] In all phagocytic studies, abnormalities appear to be secondary to chronic lung infection rather than a primary contributor.

Whole complement activity is normal in CF. Decreased activity of the alternative complement pathway has been documented, and circulating immune complexes are present, mainly in patients with severe lung disease.[50] The roles of complement abnormalities and immune complexes in the pathogenesis of lung disease are uncertain. Neither is likely to be primary. A number of investigators have attempted to relate *S. aureus* infection of CF lungs to a deficiency of fatty acids, particularly linoleic acid.[51] Fatty acid deficiency is most likely secondary to the fat maldigestion resulting from exocrine pancreatic insufficiency. Although CF patients who maintain exocrine pancreatic function experience less rapid progression of lung disease,[52] there is no evidence that this subpopulation avoids *S. aureus* colonization and infection of the airways.

The mechanisms by which chronic infection produces airways obstruction and destruction of airways walls have received attention. Increasingly, the role of proteinases has been considered. Both leukocyte and bacterial elastases are known to generate C5a nonimmunologically in CF secretions.[53] High levels of this chemotactic factor may contribute to the brisk polymorphonuclear leukocyte response characteristic of infected CF airways. Elastases and other proteases are potent stimulators of secretion by goblet cells[54] and mucus gland cells.[55] Furthermore, proteolytic enzymes introduced into the airways of animals produce marked hyperplasia of mucus-secreting cells in the surface epithelium.[56] Airways secretions of CF patients with chronic lung disease contain large amounts of uninhibited proteolytic enzyme activity.[57] Therefore, it is likely that these enzymes play a role in the development and perpetuation of the striking hypersecretion of mucus in CF. Proteinases also are capable of interfering with ciliary function[58] and enhance bacterial adherence to epithelial cells.[59] Furthermore, proteolytic injury to airway walls may be a factor contributing to structural damage and the development of widespread bronchiolectasis and bronchiectasis. The fact that destructive emphysema is not a prominent feature of cystic fibrosis lungs, especially early in the course of lung disease, may be attributed to confinement of infection to endobronchial spaces in mild to moderate lung disease. Detrimental chronic inflammatory reactions in conducting airways may be fueled by immunologic responses to microbial residents.[60] Conducting airways tissue may also be injured by oxidative products of inflammatory cells.[61]

Clinical Manifestations. The earliest manifestation of CF lung disease is generally cough. At first it is intermittent, coinciding with episodes of acute respiratory tract infection but persisting longer than expected. With time, the cough becomes a daily event. It is often worse at night and on arising in the morning. With progression of lung disease, the cough becomes productive and then paroxysmal. Sputum is usually tenacious, purulent, and often green, the latter reflecting *P. aeruginosa* infection. Hyperinflation of the lungs is noted early in the progression of lung disease. Wheezing may occur, especially during the first 2 years of life, owing to inflammation and edema in small airways. Wheezing also may be associated with evidence for atopy, which, according to some observers, is more frequent in CF.[62] Lung sounds are often unremarkable for long periods, sometimes years. Not infrequently, a diminution in the intensity of breath sounds may be the only abnormality noted, usually correlating with the extent of hyperinflation. Coarse crackles frequently are heard first over the right upper lobe but eventually achieve general distribution.

CF patients may have only bronchitic symptoms for long periods, in some cases for a decade or two, but eventually periods of relative stability are punctuated with exacerbations of symptoms, including increased intensity of cough, tachypnea, shortness of breath, decreased activity and appetite, and weight loss. These exacerbations may be triggered by acute respiratory infections, perhaps of viral or mycoplasmal origin, although studies differ concerning evidence for these infections during early stages of increasing lung symptoms.[63,64] Intensive antibiotic therapy and assistance with clearance of mucus are usually required to control exacerbations of lung symptoms and to improve lung function. Exacerbations characteristically occur with increasing frequency. However, frank limitation of activity is associated only with end-stage lung disease and heralds a sequence of terminal events including substantial hypoxemia, pulmonary hypertension, cor pulmonale, and death. Rate of progression of lung disease is not a direct function of genotype; acquired factors seem to play a prominent role.

Most patients with cystic fibrosis have chronic rhinitis with increased volumes of upper airways secretions and moderate airflow obstruction. Nasal polyps occur in 15 to 20 percent of patients and are most common toward the end of the first decade and during the second decade of life.[65] Manifestations include severe or complete obstruction of airflow, profuse rhinorrhea, and, occasionally, widening of the bridge of the nose. Even though all sinuses usually display roentgenographic opacification, symptoms of acute or chronic sinusitis are infrequent. Nevertheless, sinus disease has occasionally been the presenting manifestation of CF.[66] Cultures of the maxillary antra in 20 patients were remarkable for the presence of *P. aeruginosa* in 13 and the lack of recovery of *S. aureus*.[67] Mucocele of the paranasal sinuses is an infrequent finding and can be complicated by infection[68] with erosion of bone.[68a] A preliminary report suggests that drainage procedures for symptomatic sinusitis can reduce subsequent hospitalizations.[68b] Middle ear disease is surprisingly uncommon.[69]

Microbiology. The airways of individuals with CF are colonized early with bacteria, and, once established, infection is rarely if ever eradicated. *S. aureus* and *Haemophilus influenzae* are often the first organisms detected.[70] *P. aeruginosa* characteristically is cultured from respiratory secretions months to years later, although this organism is present at diagnosis with increasing frequency. With progression of lung disease, *P. aeruginosa* is often the only organism recovered from sputum, and it may be present in several colonial forms, all with different antibiotic sensitivity patterns. Typically, one of these types is mucoid, due to elaboration of large amounts of alginate, a polyuronic acid. Mucoid properties were first thought to be associated with more rapid progression of lung disease. However, they seem to have little effect on antibiotic susceptibility[71] or clearance from guinea pig lungs.[72] Alginate may provide a physical barrier to antibiotics and phagocytic cells. The recovery of *P. aeruginosa*, particularly the mucoid form, from the lower respiratory tract of a child or young adult with chronic lung symptoms is virtually diagnostic of CF. Recently, other species of *Pseudomonas* have been recovered from CF lungs with increasing frequency, particularly *P. cepacia* and *Xanthamonas maltophilia*. The former is now recovered from a substantial number of patients, and is particularly difficult to control because of its resistance to most antimicrobial agents.[73,74] Occasionally other gram-negative rods are present in sputum, including a mucoid *Escherichia coli*, *Klebsiella*, and *Proteus*. Anaerobes or microaerophilic organisms have been recovered from CF lung tissue and may be undetected pathogens; on rare occasions they are found in large abscess cavities.[75] Sputum bacteriology correlates reasonably well with specimens obtained directly from the lower respiratory tract. Quantitative bacteriology may be particularly useful for determining the relative contributions of the multiple organisms isolated.[76] A large number of sputum specimens contain yeast and *Aspergillus fumigatus*. Neither organism is often a serious pathogen, although the latter occasionally causes the symptoms of allergic bronchopulmonary aspergillosis. Infection of lungs with *Mycobacterium tuberculosis*[77] is unusual. However, rapidly growing mycobacteria are recovered in the sputum of up to 20 percent of older patients, and occasionally this organism is considered a pathogenic factor.[78,79]

The frequency of respiratory tract infections with viruses, mycoplasma, and chlamydia does not appear to be increased.[63,80] However, the severity and duration of accompanying symptoms may be greater. One hypothesis states that CF airways function relatively well until an initial insult, such as the first respiratory syncytial virus infection, is encountered.

Radiology. The earliest radiographic change is usually hyperinflation of the lungs.[70] As bronchitis progresses, peribron-

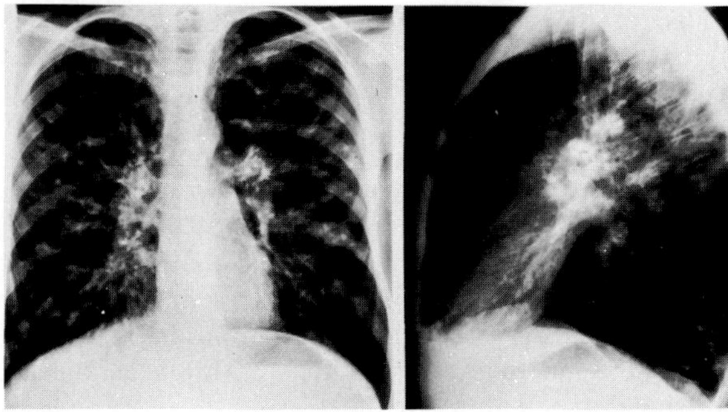

FIG. 127-2 **Advanced changes of CF seen on this chest radiograph include: hyperinflation, bronchial wall thickening due to bronchiectasis, mucus plugs, and enlarged hila probably due to large pulmonary arteries.**

chial cuffing becomes increasingly prominent, creating linear densities in the lung fields (Fig. 127-2). Impaction of mucus in airways may be seen as branching, finger-like shadows. Evidence for bronchiectasis such as enlarged ring shadows and cysts is common by 5 to 10 years of age. Frequently, peripheral rounded densities appear during acute exacerbations and may clear with treatment, leaving residual cysts. For reasons that remain unexplained, the right upper lobe usually displays the earliest and most severe changes. With advancing disease, the pulmonary artery segments are increasingly prominent. A relatively small and vertical cardiac shadow enlarges appreciably with evidence for right heart failure. Hilar adenopathy is rarely prominent radiographically. Lobar or segmental atelectasis is uncommon.

Roentgenographic improvement with intensive treatment is not readily appreciated because of the fixed nature of changes in the airways. The most striking evidence for improvement often is diminished inflation of the lungs, which tends to make the fixed markings more prominent. Chest roentgenogram scoring may be useful for clinical studies and to chart the course of lung injury.[81] A recent scoring system was designed to be more sensitive to early changes.[81a]

Bronchograms are no longer useful, even when lobectomy is considered. Computed tomography (CT) of the chest is preferable for documenting localization of bronchiectasis. Some centers have begun to use periodic chest CT evaluation to follow the course of lung changes. The cost is high, as is the radiation exposure, and the resolution of lung structures in young patients who cannot hold their breath has been poor. With the advent of rapid scanning (0.1 s) and the use of a limited number of thin slices, these obstacles can be surmounted wherever equipment with this capacity is available. Bronchial wall thickening, mild bronchiectasis, and mucoid impaction can be observed at all ages.[82] CT scanning detects these lesions even when radiographs are nearly normal. The severity of bronchiectasis has been graded for older patients.[83]

Magnetic resonance imaging (MRI) can also identify peribronchial thickening, mucoid impaction, and bronchiectasis but has no well-documented advantage over CT scans.[84] MRI may be superior for distinguishing hilar adenopathy and prominent pulmonary vessels, the latter showing as tubular structures.[85]

Lung Function. Newborns are thought to have normal lung function. However, within weeks to months, many infants with CF show evidence for increased airways resistance, gas trapping, and diminished flow rates.[70] When children become old enough to cooperate, more complete testing first demonstrates obstruction of small airways, as evidenced by reduced maximum midexpiratory flow rates, reduced flows at low lung volumes, and elevation of the ratio of residual volume to total lung capacity (RV/TLC).[86] Another sensitive indicator of lung pathology is an increased alveolar–arterial oxygen gradient, reflecting ventilation–perfusion inequalities.[70] The tests used most often to follow the course of pulmonary function include spirometry, lung volume measurements, and measures of oxygenation. In general, patients progress from initial reductions in maximum midexpiratory flow rates to reductions in FEV_1/FVC and then to diminished vital capacity and total lung volumes. This progression from peripheral airways obstruction to more generalized obstruction to acquisition of a restrictive component is illustrated in Table 127-2.

By the time a diagnosis is made, many children with CF display mild decrements of Pa_{O_2}. Oxygenation declines slowly throughout life. As a rule, patients who maintain satisfactory oxygenation continue to do well clinically, independent of the extent of the obstructive lesion. When Pa_{O_2} values dip below 55 mmHg on a sustained basis, symptomatic pulmonary hypertension should be expected.[87] Nocturnal and postural desaturation experienced by CF individuals may be a contributing factor.[88,89] Hypoxemia generally is not accompanied by polycythemia, at least in part owing to an expanded plasma volume and, in some individuals, also to suppressed erythropoiesis secondary to chronic infection.[90] Tissue oxygenation appears to be further compromised by failure of CF erythrocytes to adequately increase their 2,3-diphosphoglycerate levels as pulmonary involvement progresses.[91] Elevation of Pa_{CO_2} generally occurs with FEV_1 values less than 30 percent predicted and is an end-stage event for most patients; thereafter, survival averages 2 years.[92]

Airway reactivity is a common feature of CF lung disease. Up to 68 percent of the CF population demonstrates decreased flows after histamine administration, and flows improve in as many as 40 percent of patients with aerosolized bronchodilators.[93,94] In contrast to cross-sectional studies,

Table 127-2 **Representative Pulmonary Function Test Results from Three Young Adult Men with Mild (A), Moderate (B) and Severe (C) Lung Disease**

	Patients		
	A	B	C
FVC	98	72	48
FEV_1	92	46	34
FEV_1/FVC	(.81)	(.70)	(.64)
MMEF	83	15	6
V_{max}, 50%	91	19	11
V_{max}, 25%	52	10	5
FRC	162	112	75
RV	189	200	120
TLC	131	105	62
RV/TLC	(.29)	(.45)	(.50)
Pa_{O_2} (room air)	[87]	[74]	[48]

NOTE: Values are the percent of the predicted value, except those in parentheses, which are simple ratios, and those in brackets, which are torr. Patient A coughs several times a day, occasionally produces sputum, and shows no restriction of activity. Patient B coughs frequently, expectorates moderately large amounts of mucus, but is able to jog 3 miles daily and is a full-time student in a professional school. Patient C has chronic right heart failure but is able to work daily as a hair stylist.

tests every 1 to 3 months for a year have demonstrated bronchodilator responsiveness at least once in 95 percent of subjects.[95] Responsiveness seems to be more prevalent during winter months and diminishes with exacerbations of lung disease. The pathogenesis of bronchial reactivity in CF is unclear.

Exercise tolerance is related to the severity of airway obstruction.[96] Oxygen desaturation with exercise is generally not a problem but was noted in 12 of 29 patients with an FEV_1 below 50 percent of FVC.[97] Ventilatory muscle endurance is higher than expected but does not augment exercise performance.[98] Exercise does improve cardiorespiratory fitness but does not improve results of pulmonary function testing.[99] Maximum oxygen consumption during exercise appears to be a better predictor of survival than routine pulmonary function testing.[100]

Resting energy expenditure is elevated in CF. Onset and magnitude are variable. Some have claimed that certain CFTR mutations are associated with genetically determined increases in energy expenditure, for example, owing to increased ATP hydrolysis.[101] It is more likely that increased work of breathing is responsible.[102]

Complications of Respiratory Tract Disease. Lobar or segmental *atelectasis* occurs in approximately 5 percent of patients.[103] This complication is most common in the first 5 years of life. Many episodes occur in conjunction with an exacerbation of clinical symptoms, but silent atelectasis has been noted. Occasionally, volume loss is associated with allergic aspergillosis and endobronchial mucus plugging from other causes. However, in most instances, a discrete mucus plug is not evident on bronchoscopy.

Pneumothorax is a more frequent complication and, in contrast to atelectasis, has an increasing incidence with age.[25] In the 1960s, pneumothorax occurred in approximately 5 percent of all patients. There are now strong indications that this problem occurs more frequently, probably related to the prolonged course of chronic lung disease. Pneumothorax occurs equally often in both sexes and is more frequent in the right chest. Not uncommonly, a small asymptomatic pneumothorax may be discovered at the time of routine chest roentgenographic examination. More commonly, patients present with acute onset of shortness of breath, chest pain, and hemoptysis. The incidence of tension is probably higher in CF than in patients with less severe or no lung disease, and, under these circumstances, the accumulation of pleural air may become a life-threatening event. Simultaneous bilateral pneumothoraces have been described and constitute a crisis. Once an initial pneumothorax has been recognized, the rate of recurrence is high.[104]

Hemoptysis is a common event in older CF patients and correlates with clinical and radiologic evidence for bronchiectasis. In most cases, hemoptysis is not associated with vigorous activity, trauma to the chest, or other suspected contributory factors. Most frequently, only blood streaking of the mucus occurs. A few patients will occasionally cough up a mouthful of blood. Massive hemoptysis occurs in approximately 5 percent of individuals.[105] There is a strong correlation between the occurrence of both small- and large-volume hemoptysis and exacerbation of lung infection. Patients with relatively large-volume hemoptysis may be able to localize the site of bleeding by describing a bubbling or gurgling sensation in one area of the chest. However, localization usually is difficult. Bronchoscopy seldom identifies the source of blood loss. Patients who experience massive hemoptysis originally were considered to have a poor prognosis.[106] The immediate mortality may be as high as 10 percent, but a more recent analysis suggests that massive hemoptysis usually is not a harbinger of terminal events.[105]

In one study, more than 50 percent of patients with CF had precipitating antibodies to *A. fumigatus* in their serum, and this organism can be recovered from the sputum with a similar frequency.[107] A small number of patients develop the syndrome of allergic bronchopulmonary aspergillosis, including new lung infiltrates, increased cough, respiratory distress, and often wheezing. The expectoration of rusty brown plugs of sputum suggests this diagnosis. Occasionally, plugging of bronchi with hyphae-laden mucus causes lobar or segmental atelectasis.

Digital *clubbing* occurs in virtually all patients with cystic fibrosis and is usually present early in the course of symptomatic lung disease. The etiology is unknown, but the extent of clubbing seems to correlate with the severity of lung disease.[108] *Hypertrophic pulmonary osteoarthropathy* occurs in as many as 15 percent of older adolescents and adults.[109] If roentgenographic evidence for periostitis is used as the definition, the incidence is 8 percent. The most common sites are the distal aspects of the tibia, fibula, radius, and ulna. Signs and symptoms include pain, bone tenderness, swelling, and warmth over the involved areas. Effusions in nearby joints may occur. Often there is discomfort with ambulation. Symptoms of hypertrophic pulmonary osteoarthropathy frequently intensify with pulmonary exacerbations and tend to subside when control of pulmonary disease is achieved.

Pleural disease is uncommon in cystic fibrosis. Occasionally, pleuritic symptoms and signs may accompany exacerbations of lung infection. Sympathetic effusions are distinctly uncommon, even during episodes of frank pneumonia. Staphylococcal empyema has been described in a rare patient,[110] but, by and large, respiratory tract infections spare the pleural space.

Respiratory failure and *cor pulmonale* are late events. While progressive hypoxemia is characteristic of this disease, hypercapnea usually occurs only weeks to months before death. Similarly, liver congestion and peripheral edema associated with pulmonary hypertension appear on average 8 months before death,[111] although occasionally patients may live with systemic venous congestion for 5 or more years. Unless associated with a reversible event such as a severe virus infection, hypercapnea and cor pulmonale generally persist once they have been detected.

Gastrointestinal Tract

Symptoms related to the gastrointestinal tract may predominate, although they are rarely life-threatening if properly treated.

Pathology. Changes in the intestinal tract itself are not prominent.[112] Brunner's glands of the duodenum are hypertrophied, with dilated ducts and acinar lumens filled with mucus. There is little if any primary change of the small intestinal tract mucosa. The appendix frequently displays goblet-cell hyperplasia of the epithelium and accumulation of secretions within crypts and in the lumen, changes which may be diagnostic of CF. In the past, a number of investigators have claimed to be able to diagnose CF by rectal biopsy on the basis of goblet-cell hyperplasia and accumulation of mucus in the crypts. However, subsequent studies have demonstrated that these findings are not consistent in CF rectal mucosa.[113]

Clinical Manifestations. Meconium ileus occurs in 10–20 percent of newborns with CF and is virtually diagnostic.[112] Its pathogenesis has been ascribed to failure of pancreatic enzyme secretion and, thus, of digestion of intralumenal contents in utero. However, dehydration of intestinal contents[114] due to epithelial transport dysfunction in utero is more likely to be causal. These infants fail to pass meconium in the first day or two of life, develop abdominal distention, and proceed to bilious emesis. Occasionally, perforation occurs, and peritonitis accompanied by shock intervenes. Flat and upright abdominal films reveal multiple dilated loops of intestine with fluid levels (Fig. 127-3). The lower abdomen often takes on a granular appearance, representing accumulated meconium containing small air bubbles. Barium enema demonstrates a small, unexpanded colon, and, if contrast material can be refluxed into the ileum, the point of ileal obstruction is identified. Occasionally, in-utero perforation results in peritoneal and scrotal calcifications. For other newborns, obstruction may occur in the large intestine and only delay passage of meconium. This condition is termed the "meconium plug syndrome" and is less specific for CF.[115]

Beyond the newborn period, small bowel obstruction may occur for a variety of reasons. Perhaps the most common (occurring in 20 percent of patients) has been called "meconium ileus equivalent" or the "distal intestinal obstruction syndrome."[112,116] As with meconium ileus of the newborn, obstruction occurs in the terminal ileum and is usually associated with voluminous, sticky, incompletely digested intestinal contents. Complete obstruction is associated with failure to pass stools, abdominal distention, and vomiting. In some instances, a partial obstruction occurs, accompanied only by intermittent abdominal pain. A mobile right lower quadrant mass may be palpable. These episodes of obstruction often follow ingestion of large, fatty meals or else result from noncompliance with pancreatic enzyme replacement therapy. Other causes of abdominal pain associated with obstruction include intussusception and intestinal adhesions from previous abdominal surgery, the latter being a particular problem for individuals with CF. Lower abdominal pain also may attend low-grade appendicitis (partially suppressed by antibiotic therapy) and periappendiceal abscess.[117] Nonfilling of the appendix on contrast enema is frequent in CF, even in the absence of appendicitis[118] and is due to accumulation of secretions.[119] Diverticulosis of the appendix has been reported in 14 percent of autopsy and surgical cases, a much greater incidence than is found in control populations.[120] Duodenal irritation, caused by failure to buffer gastric acid, may be responsible for recurrent epigastric pain and radiographic changes such as thickened, redundant mucosal folds in this area.[121]

Rectal prolapse occurs in nearly 20 percent of children, but it is an infrequent event for adults with cystic fibrosis.[122] In fact, CF is one of the most common causes of rectal prolapse in the United States. Factors contributing to rectal prolapse include the presence of bulky, sticky stools, which adhere to the rectal mucosa, loss of perirectal fat, which normally supports the rectum, and an increased frequency of high intraabdominal pressure due to paroxysmal coughing. Pneumatosis coli has been reported in association with rectal prolapse in an 18-year-old with CF.[123]

Pancreatic Disease

Exocrine pancreatic insufficiency is present from birth in the great majority of patients with CF.[124] Loss of pancreatic function occasionally occurs in childhood, attended by symptoms of pancreatitis.[125] It occurs almost uniformly in patients homozygous for the ΔF508 mutation, and much less commonly in the absence of this or similarly severe mutations (see "Genotype/Phenotype Correlations" below).

Pathology. The pancreas is abnormal in almost all cases and is virtually destroyed in most cases at autopsy (Fig. 127-4).[124] Obstruction of ducts by inspissated secretions is an early feature, followed by dilation of secretory ducts and acini and flattening of the epithelium. Loss of acinar cells is widespread, and areas of destruction are replaced by fibrous tissue and fat. Intralumenal calcifications may occur and be noted roentgenographically. Small cysts are common and generally represent dilated ducts. Inflammatory changes are not prominent. The islets of Langerhans are relatively spared, at least for extended periods. Late changes of the islets include distortion by fibrous tissue which may disrupt blood flow or provide a barrier between hormone-secreting cells and the vascular spaces.[126] Changes in the distribution of

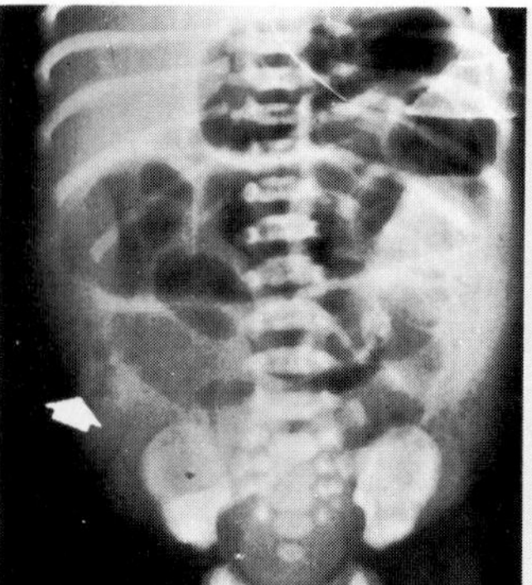
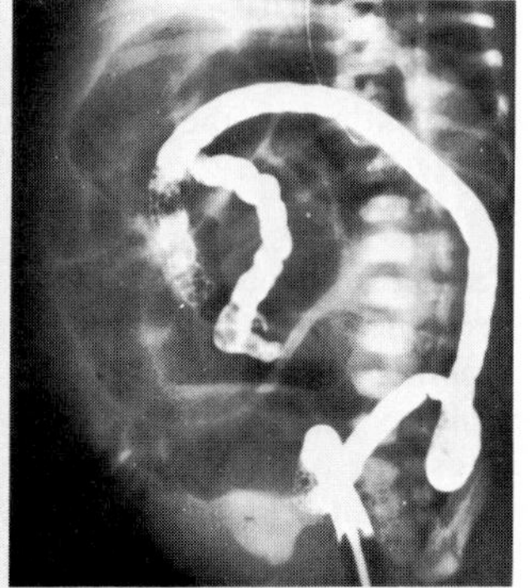

FIG. 127-3 Newborn with intestinal obstruction. Abdomen film *(left)* shows distended bowel loops with "bubbly" pattern of inspissated meconium in terminal ileum *(arrow)*. Barium enema *(right)* shows a microcolon from disuse secondary to intrauterine obstruction.

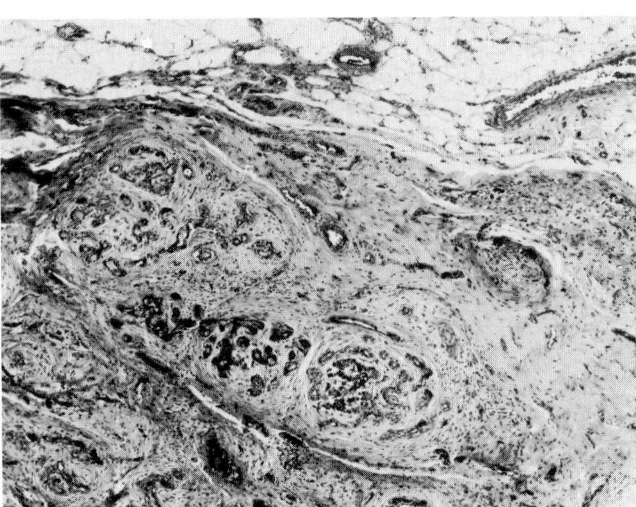

FIG. 127-4 Histologic section of pancreas from a 12-year-old girl, showing changes typical of CF, including extensive fibrosis of acini, dilation of ductules, plugs within acini, and focal acinar calcifications. H & E, × 310.

islet cell types also have been noted.[127] Pathologic changes in the pancreas are used occasionally to make a postmortem diagnosis in atypical or missed cases of CF.

Clinical Manifestations. Pancreatic enzyme deficiency causes fat and protein maldigestion, producing a distended abdomen and frequent, bulky, greasy, foul-smelling stools. Uncorrected maldigestion results in failure to gain weight and, ultimately, in a failure of linear growth. However, poor growth also may be associated with increased expenditure of energy to accomplish the work of breathing, a point that is often overlooked in the assessment of patients who are short or excessively thin. Fat loss in stools may be low, or as high as 50 to 70 percent of total intake. Residual lipolytic activity has been ascribed to lingual lipase.[128] This lipase has a low pH optimum (5.4) for activity and can act in the stomach as well as the duodenum. In fact, its activity in the CF duodenum may be enhanced because of diminished bicarbonate secretion from the pancreas. Nitrogen malabsorption is roughly comparable or perhaps somewhat less severe. In general, carbohydrate digestion is not severely impaired in CF.[129] Deficient absorption of fat-soluble vitamins occasionally produces symptoms. Vitamin A deficiency, which once was a prominent part of the CF syndrome, is now rare, occurring only in patients who do not take supplementary vitamins or pancreatic enzymes. Increased intracranial pressure, xerophthalmia, and night blindness may result. Vitamin D-deficiency rickets is rarely seen, but serum levels of 25-hydroxyvitamin D may be reduced. Bone demineralization is present in up to 40 percent of all patients and is most prevalent in older females.[130] Diminished bone density seems to occur largely after the first decade of life. Calcitriol levels in serum of older CF patients vary seasonally and appear to correlate with extent of sun exposure.[131] Osteomalacia has been reported in an adult with CF and biliary cirrhosis.[132] Vitamin E deficiency is common in unsupplemented patients, but only rarely causes detectable abnormalities such as neuroaxonal dystrophy[133] or decreased red blood cell survival due to low-grade hemolysis.[134] Additional evidence for vitamin E deficiency seen at autopsy includes focal necrosis of striated muscle and ceroid pigment deposition in intestinal smooth muscle.[135] Vitamin K-dependent coagulation factors may also be deficient, occasionally resulting in a severe hemorrhagic diathesis.[136] More commonly, vitamin K deficiency results in depression of factor II (prothrombin) coagulant activity without changes of antigen level or of the prothrombin time.[137] In addition to fat malabsorption, frequent use of antimicrobials and hepatic dysfunction may be contributing factors. While severe hemorrhagic problems have occurred in young children, bleeding problems associated with vitamin K deficiency, such as hemoptysis, are occasionally seen in older patients. Vitamin B_{12} deficiency occurs infrequently and can be corrected by administration of pancreatic enzymes.[138] More often, serum vitamin B_{12} levels are high, probably owing to hepatic dysfunction.[139] Pyridoxal 5′-phosphate levels also may be low in the plasma of CF patients, correlating inversely with liver function test values,[140] but there are no currently recognized adverse consequences. An acrodermatitis-type rash has been reported in an infant with Zn^{2+} deficiency. Both the deficiency state and the skin problem cleared when pancreatic enzyme therapy was started.[141]

Increased fecal losses of bile acids also appear to contribute to fat maldigestion. CF patients with steatorrhea have substantial decreases in bile acid absorption in the ileum. Interruption of the enterohepatic circulation can be explained largely by binding of bile acids to undigested intestinal contents, including proteins as well as lipids.[142] Kinetic studies show that bile acid synthesis is accelerated and the bile acid pool contracted in CF, and that the bile acid pool increases with pancreatic enzyme therapy.[143] However, pancreatic enzymes do not normalize bile acid excretion,[143] an expected finding because exogenous enzyme therapy rarely eliminates steatorrhea. Ileal reabsorption and hepatic secretion of conjugated bile acids in response to cholecystokinin and secretin seem to be intact.[144] The functional consequence is that intralumenal solubilization of lipid may be deficient and may contribute to the fat malabsorption characteristic of CF. For reasons that are not clear, fecal loss of bile acids diminishes with age.[145]

Severe maldigestion and malnutrition during the first 6 months of life may induce hypoproteinemia and anasarca.[146] This syndrome, accompanied in some cases by hemolytic anemia and hepatic steatosis,[147] may be the presenting manifestation in up to 8 percent of patients with CF. In many instances, the introduction of a soy-protein-based formula has preceded development of profound hypoproteinemia,[147] suggesting that these formulas are a suboptimal source of protein for CF infants. Hypoalbuminemia at diagnosis may[146] or may not[149] serve as a marker for a subsequent severe respiratory course.

It is now recognized that symptoms of pancreatitis are encountered in a small percentage of adolescent or adult CF patients, especially those who have retained some exocrine pancreatic function.[150] The genesis of this problem is probably ongoing ductal obstruction and extravasation of secreted enzymes, causing pancreatic cell damage and secondary inflammation. Pancreatic calcifications are occasionally seen roentgenographically but do not seem to correlate with symptomatic pancreatitis.

Diabetes. Endocrine pancreatic dysfunction has a predilection for older CF patients, although it has presented in the first year of life. This complication was noted in the first comprehensive description of CF in 1938.[3] A study of patients 12 years old and older demonstrated a 57 percent incidence of abnormal glucose tolerance.[151] Other studies using different populations and criteria for impaired tolerance have identified this abnormality in 27 and 42 percent of study patients.[126] Surveys of two populations including 536 patients older than 11 years have found an 8 percent incidence of fasting hyperglycemia, glycosuria, and a requirement for insulin therapy.[116,151]

Insulin responses to an oral glucose load are delayed in nearly all subjects with CF. Individuals with glucose intolerance have a response that is even more delayed and is variably subnormal.[126] Responses to tolbutamide, glucagon, and intravenous arginine are more prompt but clearly meager.[126,152] Responses of glucagon to arginine may be variable[153] but frequently are diminished.[152] Glucose administration does not suppress plasma glucagon levels. Insulin and glucagon responses of CF subjects with fasting hyperglycemia differ from those of patients with typical insulin-dependent diabetes mellitus, who demonstrate more profound insulinopenia and an increased response of glucagon to arginine stimulation.[151]

Functional assessments of pancreatic islets in CF correlate well with morphometric analyses of cell types in islets of CF patients at autopsy.[127] β cells occupy 28 percent of the islet surface area, compared with less than 10 percent in insulin-dependent diabetes mellitus and more than 50 percent in control subjects. The surface area occupied by glucagon-producing cells is normal, not increased as in people with type I diabetes. Somatostatin-producing cells are increased in all CF subjects, with and without hyperglycemia. These figures must be interpreted in the light of other observations that the number of islets is diminished in most CF pancreases, so that the total number of β cells, for example, may be profoundly diminished. Islet cell antibodies or anti-insulin antibodies, frequently observed in type I diabetes mellitus, are not characteristic of CF endocrine pancreatic dysfunction.[154]

Insulin receptors on circulating monocytes are increased in number but have impaired insulin affinity.[155] This does not seem to be true for CF red cells.[151] One study suggests that peripheral tissue in CF subjects without diabetes has an increased sensitivity to insulin that may compensate for impaired insulin secretion.[156] However, another study has demonstrated decreased peripheral response to insulin by CF subjects with fasting hyperglycemia.[151]

The presentation of symptomatic hyperglycemia is the same for subjects with CF and type I diabetes mellitus, namely, abrupt onset of thirst, polyuria, and weight loss. The hyperglycemia of CF does induce microvascular changes in the retina and the kidney if the course of the metabolic disorder is sufficiently long.[157,158] A striking feature of CF-associated endocrine pancreatic insufficiency is the virtual absence of ketoacidosis.[151] The reason for this difference from type I diabetes mellitus is unknown, but may be related to the relatively better preservation of insulin secretion as well as a less brisk glucagon response. Even though glucagon responses are diminished, patients recover normally from hypoglycemia.[159]

Considerable discussion has surrounded the question of the effects of fasting hyperglycemia and glycosuria on progression of CF-related organ dysfunction. While the appearance of a diabetes-like state complicates therapy and may be psychologically devastating, reports differ concerning the effect of insulin-dependent hyperglycemia on the rate of deterioration of pulmonary function[160,161] and therefore, presumably, longevity. However, diabetes may have a more profound influence on the well-being of individuals with CF if survival is extended substantially.

Hepatobiliary Disease

Liver changes are variable. In 25 percent or more of all autopsies, islands of relatively normal parenchyma are surrounded by fibrotic bands, creating a distinctive multilobular appearance.[162] Microscopically (Fig 127-5), this focal biliary cirrhosis is characterized by inspissation of secretions within the bile ductules, biliary duct proliferation, periportal inflammatory reaction and fibrosis, and little evidence for bile stasis.[163] In living patients, focal biliary cirrhosis may be identifiable only by an elevated level of hepatic alkaline phosphatase in serum.[164,165] Occasionally, prolonged neonatal jaundice with cirrhosis is encountered.[166] Thereafter, symptomatic biliary cirrhosis occurs in 2 to 5 percent of patients and presents with hyperbilirubinemia, ascites and peripheral edema, or massive hematemesis due to esophageal varices.[167] Evidence for hypersplenism is frequent in these cases. The presence of hepatosplenomegaly is virtually diagnostic for cirrhosis with portal hypertension. Bleeding from esophageal varices is the most feared complication of CF-related hepatobiliary disease and may even be the presenting manifestation of CF.[168] At times, the lobulation of the liver that is characteristic of the multilobular biliary cirrhosis can be appreciated by palpation. The frequency of liver disease does not appear to segregate according to genotype.[169] Especially early in life, a large liver may be due to massive fatty infiltration.[170] Infiltration by fat often is a response to inadequate nutrition and can be detected as increased radiolucency of the liver.[171] Unlike focal biliary cirrhosis, this condition responds favorably to dietary treatment.

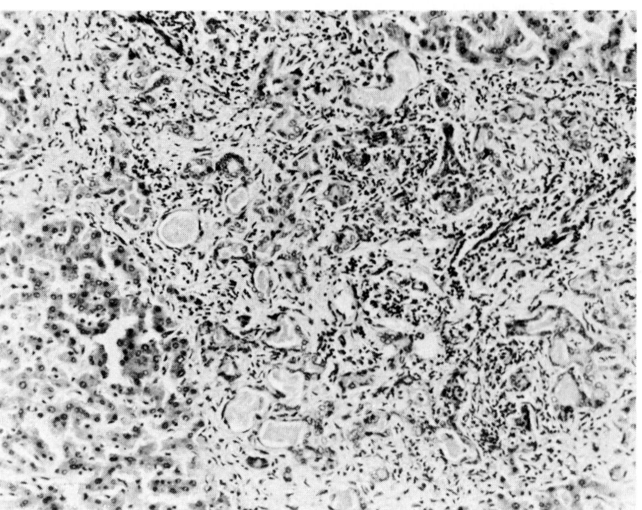

FIG. 127-5 Histologic section of liver from a 12-year-old girl with CF, showing focal biliary cirrhosis. The periportal area shows fibrosis, chronic inflammation, and bile duct proliferation with intracanalicular bile plugs. H & E, × 620.

Cholelithiasis, sometimes with biliary colic, is diagnosed before death in up to 12 percent of older patients[172] and has been detected as early as at 3 years of age.[173] Radiolucent stones are found in both extrahepatic and intrahepatic sites.[174] At autopsy, the gallbladder is abnormal in many more cases.[175] Alterations include hypoplasia (microgallbladder), calculi, and a content of thick, colorless mucus (white bile). In one study, calculi, nonvisualization, or structural abnormalities were noted in 45 percent of cholecystograms.[176] Bile in patients with CF who are not receiving pancreatic enzyme supplements has been considered lithogenic because of a high content of cholesterol,[177] but recent spectroscopic analyses suggest the presence of calcium bilirubinate and proteins rather than cholesterol in CF stones.[178] Gallbladder emptying and plasma cholecystokinin responses to meals are well preserved in CF adults.[179]

Genitourinary Tract

More than 95 percent of male patients with cystic fibrosis have altered Wolffian duct structures.[180–183] The vas deferens, tail and body of the epididymis, and seminal vesicles are atrophic, fibrotic, or completely absent. The pathogenesis of these structural changes probably relates to early, often intrauterine, obstruction of the genital tract with inspissated secretions.[181] Developmental failure cannot be excluded at this time. A relatively high incidence of inguinal hernia, hydrocele, and undescended testis has also been noted.[184] Failure of reproductive function does not become an issue until well into the second decade of life. Because 2 to 3 percent of males with cystic fibrosis are fertile, a semen analysis should be performed on all males at an appropriate time after puberty. The volume of ejaculate is usually one-third to one-half of normal. There is complete absence of spermatozoa, and a number of chemical abnormalities of semen have been demonstrated, including increased acidity, decreased fructose concentration, and increased levels of citric acid and acid phosphatase. These chemical changes reflect the absence of secretions from the seminal vesicles.[182] A testicular biopsy will demonstrate spermatogenesis,[185] indicating that the functional CF genitourinary abnormality should be termed "azoospermia." However, it is not necessary to perform a biopsy unless a diagnosis of cystic fibrosis is still in question after the usual diagnostic criteria are examined.[186] Sexual function is usually normal and is only limited by physical stamina and psychological factors.[187] Male infertility can be the major or only presenting feature in mild or atypical forms of CF, as discussed under "Atypical CF Phenotypes" below.

Fertility in women with CF is most likely greater than 10 percent,[188] but reliable figures are not available. Menstrual irregularity and oligomenorrhea are common.[189] Many women with CF are anovulatory because of poor nutrition and chronic lung infection. Another major obstacle to conception may be the presence of a plug of thick, tenacious mucus in the cervical os, which is very difficult to dislodge. The cervical mucus in CF patients is dehydrated and has abnormal electrolyte concentrations, preventing the usual ferning at midcycle and perhaps impeding normal sperm migration.[190] Endocervicitis and polyp formation are also commonly noted.

The U.S. Cystic Fibrosis Registry recorded pregnancies in 275 women between 1986 and 1990.[190a] A survey of cystic fibrosis centers in 1980 documented 129 pregnancies in 100 patients.[191] Of these pregnancies, 75 percent were completed, and 89 percent of the completed pregnancies produced a viable infant. Five percent of pregnancies resulted in spontaneous abortion, and one maternal death occurred during pregnancy. Therapeutic abortion was carried out in approximately 20 percent. A subsequent report of 38 pregnancies noted only 2 therapeutic abortions and 34 completed pregnancies.[192] The incidence of prematurity was low, and mothers tolerated the pregnancies well. Women with CF can breast-feed successfully. Analysis of CF breast milk has demonstrated essentially normal protein and electrolyte composition,[193] and minor variations in phospholipid composition, similar to the differences found in blood.[194]

Delayed onset of puberty is common in both males and females with CF. Reproductive endocrine function is intact, and delays in age-related increments of follicle-stimulating hormone (FSH) and luteinizing hormone (LH) secretion are thought to be consequences of chronic lung disease and inadequate nutrition. Most patients with cystic fibrosis do complete sexual maturation, sometimes at an appropriate age but frequently with a 2- to 4-year delay.[189,195] Height is in the normal range for more than 90 percent of adults, although mean height is somewhat below that of the normal population.[116]

Sweat Glands

The most consistent functional alteration in CF has been elevated concentrations of chloride, sodium, and potassium in eccrine sweat. The number of sweat glands is normal.[196] Sweat rates are stimulated as in normal subjects by cholinomimetic drugs, but the usual response to β-adrenergic agonists is missing.[197] However, the pathophysiology of the sweat electrolyte disturbance relates primarily to a failure to reabsorb chloride along the sweat gland duct (see "Sweat Gland Duct" under "Epithelial Transport Abnormalities" below). There is no structural abnormality of eccrine sweat glands.[198] In contrast, apocrine sweat glands of children with CF are more dilated and filled with retained secretions than glands of control subjects.[199]

Children with CF may "taste salty" or have salt crystals on their skin following profuse sweating. Excessive loss of salt in the sweat provokes both the release of aldosterone and attempts at salt retention by the kidneys.[200] The CF sweat gland is relatively refractory to mineralocorticoids.[201] Young children are predisposed to salt depletion episodes, especially at times when there is extra salt loss due to vomiting or diarrhea. These children develop profound hypochloremia, less impressive hyponatremia, and alkalosis.[202] They present with lethargy, anorexia, and hypochloremic alkalosis, an occurrence that is more common in warm, arid zones.[203] Hypochloremic alkalosis is rarely seen in older children and adults. Hypokalemia is not commonly recognized even though increased amounts of potassium are also present in sweat. Young adults with CF have on average lower systolic and diastolic blood pressures than age- and sex-matched controls, perhaps owing to chronic, low-grade salt depletion.[204]

Other Manifestations

A number of other minor or infrequent pathologic and clinical manifestations of CF include enlarged submandibular, sublingual, and submucosal salivary glands with scattered histologic evidence for diluted ducts, inspissated secretions, and eventual atrophy of acini.[173] The parotid glands, which are not mucus-secreting, show no morphologic change. Other reported findings include seronegative, nondisabling arthritis,[205] painful subcutaneous nodules,[206] palpable purpura,[207] brain abscess,[208] and inappropriate antidiuretic hormone (ADH) secretion.[209] Several neoplasms have been reported.[210,211] Although carcinoma of the pancreas and ileum are infrequent, there may be an increased incidence.[211a] Amyloidosis, a recognized complication of chronic infection, has now been reported in a number of older individuals with CF.[212]

DIAGNOSIS AND COURSE OF DISEASE

A diagnosis of classic CF is based on carefully defined clinical criteria and analysis of sweat chloride levels. Accepted diagnostic criteria are listed in Table 127-3. Any one of the major clinical features of CF, if accompanied by a sweat chloride level >60 meq/liter or by pathologic mutations on both chromosomes (see "Molecular Diagnosis" below) is sufficient to make the diagnosis. Nonclassic phenotypes are discussed under "Atypical CF Phenotypes" below. A number of individuals with sweat chloride values persistently in the diagnostic range but without clinical features of CF or a family history have been identified. As long as they remain symptom-free, a diagnosis of CF cannot be made. Other clinical entities may be accompanied by elevated sweat chloride concentrations. These are listed in Table 127-4.

Table 127-3 Criteria for Diagnosis of Cystic Fibrosis

1. Typical pulmonary manifestations, and/or
2. Typical gastrointestinal manifestations, and/or
3. A history of cystic fibrosis in the immediate family, plus
4. Sweat chloride concentration >60 meq/liter or pathologic CFTR mutations on both chromosomes

Table 127-4 Conditions Other than Cystic Fibrosis Associated with Elevated Sweat Chloride Levels

Adrenal insufficiency	Mucopolysaccharidoses
Pseudohypoaldosteronism	Fucosidosis
Hypothyroidism	Malnutrition
Hypoparathyroidism	Mauriac syndrome
Nephrogenic diabetes insipidus	Familial cholestasis syndrome
Ectodermal dysplasia	Pancreatitis
Glycogen storage disease (type I)	Prostaglandin E_1 administration
	Hypogammaglobulinemia

None of these disorders is easily confused with CF. It is now recognized that a very small percentage of individuals with CF have sweat chloride values in a range that is intermediate (40 to 60 meq/liter) or even frankly normal.[213]

For the 1 to 2 percent of patients with compatible clinical features but normal sweat chloride levels, several approaches to the diagnosis have been proposed. Demonstration of azoospermia in sexually mature males may be of considerable value.[186] Demonstration of pancreatic insufficiency by collecting duodenal fluid following stimulation with secretin and pancreozymin is also informative but has fallen into disfavor because of the extraordinary time and technical expertise required and the discomfort to the individual being tested. Alternatively, exocrine pancreatic function can be assessed by calculating the percentage of ingested fat in a 72-hour stool collection. Other tests of pancreatic function are more easily performed but less direct and specific. For example, serum trypsinogen levels may be abnormal in 80 to 85 percent of individuals with CF, but these values only correlate with pancreatic function after 7 years of age.[214] The discovery that bioelectrical potential differences across respiratory epithelia are more negative in individuals with CF at all ages[215] offers an additional diagnostic test that may be useful in evaluating atypical patients.[216] DNA analysis may be particularly useful in these situations. For one splicing mutation (3849 + 10kbC→T), 50 percent or more of patients with the mutation have normal sweat chloride values.[217]

The authors' experience at North American CF Centers indicates that DNA analysis for 20 to 30 of the most prevalent CF mutations will identify the defect on about 90 percent of chromosomes associated with classic CF. That implies that both mutations can be detected in about 81 percent of patients, one mutation in about 18 percent of patients, and neither mutation in about 1 percent of patients. These figures would differ for populations where mutation detection is more or less effective. Until better alternatives are available, the sweat test remains the diagnostic standard. A single methodology is recognized as adequate for the definitive diagnosis of CF. This test involves collection of sweat by pilocarpine iontophoresis coupled with chemical determination of the chloride concentration.[218] Simultaneous analysis of sodium levels does not provide further information. The procedure must be carried out meticulously to avoid errors, which frequently contribute to misleading values. As many as 40 percent of patients referred to CF centers are inaccurately diagnosed because of false positive or false negative sweat test results.[219] In addition to frequent laboratory errors, faulty values can be obtained if the sweat rate is not sufficiently high. At least 50 mg of sweat must be collected in a 45-min period. Potential pitfalls in interpretation include the presence of hypoproteinemic edema, failure to consider age-related effects, and concurrent administration of corticosteroids. Though a value above 60 meq/liter of chloride in sweat appears to discriminate nearly all adults with cystic fibrosis from those with other lung conditions,[220] normal values of sweat chloride do increase with age, and some workers insist on using sweat chloride levels in excess of 80 meq/liter as the criterion for diagnosing CF in adults.

Sweat electrolyte levels are elevated even in the first days of life. However, collecting sufficient amounts of sweat in newborns is frequently a problem. In addition, sweat electrolyte levels may be elevated for normal infants on the first day or two of life.[221] Therefore, testing is usually delayed for several weeks, unless diagnostic information is urgently needed.

Newborn screening for CF can be carried out using dried blood specimens for analysis of immunoreactive trypsin,[222] as discussed further under "Newborn Screening" below. Although this test identifies most newborns with CF,[223] routine screening has not been recommended up to the present.[224] However, if new therapies are introduced that can unequivocally delay the early progression of lung disease, routine newborn screening would be justified (see "Newborn Screening" below).

CF runs a highly variable course, ranging from death in the first days of life caused by complications of meconium ileus or death in the first few months from severe respiratory tract problems to essentially asymptomatic existence for 10 to 20 years[168] and protracted survival. Individuals with CF do live into the sixth and seventh decades of life.[225] More than 6000 (33 percent) of the individuals in the 1992 United States CF patient registry were 18 years of age or older.

At most care centers, patients with CF are monitored by general clinical assessment, which often involves the use of a scoring system,[80,226,227] periodic monitoring of respiratory tract pathogens, periodic chest roentgenograms, serial pulmonary function testing, and ongoing nutritional assessment. Initial intensive treatment is often followed by improvement of chest roentgenograms and pulmonary function as well as substantial improvement of weight-to-height ratios and accelerated linear growth. Following initial improvement and/or stabilization, there is often an extended period of stable lung function which may last 5, 10, or 15 years. However, longitudinal patterns of pulmonary function in older individuals with CF, while highly variable,[228,229] usually show slow deterioration.

Statistics from the U.S. Cystic Fibrosis Foundation indicate that 50 percent of patients can be expected to survive to 29 years of age. These data were generated on all patients under care in cystic fibrosis-sponsored centers in 1991 (Fig. 127-6). Analyses of survival curves over the years have suggested that survival has increased steadily to the present time. Some of the improvement in survival may have resulted from the diagnosis of milder forms of the disease. However, improved symptomatic therapy undoubtedly also has contributed to better survival.

Multiple factors determine the prognosis for individuals with CF.[230] Data from all U.S. cystic fibrosis centers suggest that survival is better for patients living in northern climates as compared with those in the South. On average, males live 2–3 years longer than females. Blacks who survive the first several years of life may have a better prognosis than whites. Age at diagnosis has not emerged as a clear determinant of survival. However, a study of sibling pairs suggests that a younger sibling who is diagnosed before 1 year of age, prior to the onset of symptoms, usually has better pulmonary function at 7 years of age than the older sibling diagnosed because of symptoms.[231] Outcome analyses

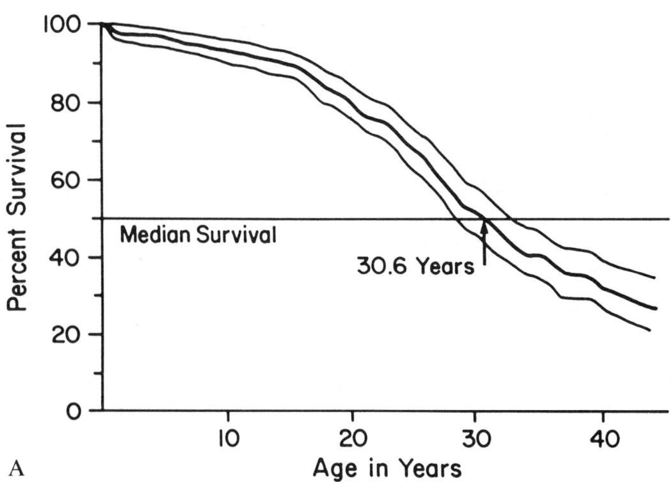

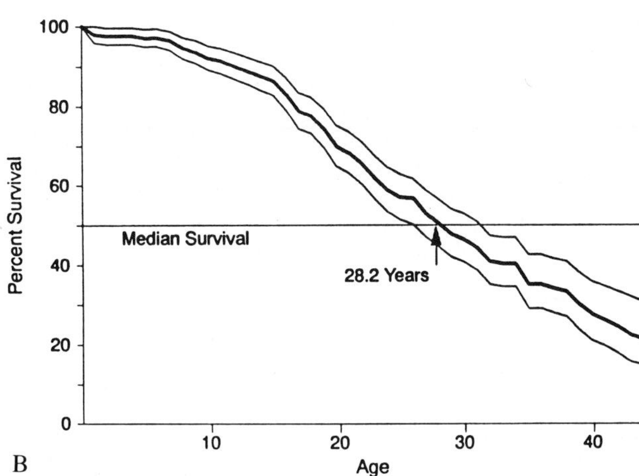

FIG. 127-6 **Survival curves for male *(A)* and female *(B)* CF patients followed in all U.S. Centers, 1991 data. These curves demonstrate that the age to which 50 percent of the population may be expected to survive exceeds 30 years for males and 28 years for females. Aggregate median survival is 29.4 years.** ***(Data from the Patient Registry, Cystic Fibrosis Foundation, Bethesda, Maryland. Courtesy of S. Fitzsimmons.)***

of patients who were identified at birth by screening procedures and those who were diagnosed after onset of symptoms should provide more definitive evidence for the efficacy of early diagnosis and treatment. Several studies suggest that clinical features at presentation do make a difference. Patients who present only with steatorrhea and failure to thrive generally improve remarkably upon treatment and do well for extended periods. On the other hand, patients who present with respiratory tract symptoms, particularly wheezing early in life, usually continue to have respiratory tract manifestations, more abnormal pulmonary function, and a less favorable prognosis.[232,233] When the entire CF population is considered, those patients who retain pancreatic function display a slower progression of pulmonary disease.[52] Meconium ileus does not influence longevity if the patient survives the first months of life.[52] Claims that CF patients with allergic manifestations have improved survival cannot be substantiated.[234] There are numerous indicators of poor prognosis once lung disease has been established, including colonization of the respiratory tract with *P. aeruginosa*[234] or *P. cepacia*[235] and the occurrence of pulmonary complications such as hemoptysis.[236] Because lung disease progression is not closely related to genotype, longevity is also not directly linked to genotype. On the other hand, several reported genotypes[237,238] appear to be associated with mild disease, and these individuals appear to live well into adulthood (see "Genotype/Phenotype Correlations" below).

Little is known about the influence of medical care on longevity. Individuals followed at established care centers appear to have a greater median survival than those who receive care in nonspecialized settings.[239] In addition, recent evidence suggests that center-to-center variation in survival of patients is directly related to frequency of monitoring, use of antibiotics, and hospitalization for treatment of pulmonary exacerbations.[240]

Finally, psychosocial factors undoubtedly play a prominent role in outcome, although this is difficult to document. The role of a supportive family is crucial. Suicide is uncommon. However, it is widely recognized that a substantial number of adolescent and adult patients do not comply fully with therapy regimens because of denial, unresolved dependence–independence issues, and depression. Clearly, attitude and the ability to cope with a fatal illness during maturation and early adulthood do influence quality of life and survival.[241]

Even though faced with a life-threatening illness and burdened with staggering demands on time, energy, and financial resources to comply with therapy, many adolescents and young adults are coping admirably and are able to achieve a satisfactory quality of life. Meaningful relationships, an advanced education, and full occupation are frequently achieved, indicating that independent lifestyles and substantial participation in life events are attainable goals for many.[242]

TREATMENT

The primary objectives of CF treatment are to control infection, promote mucus clearance, and improve nutrition. In addition, experience has repeatedly demonstrated that attention to preventive aspects of lung care and psychosocial factors is important. The efficacy of new therapeutic approaches has become the focus of several collaborative studies.

Ambulatory Care

At diagnosis, most patients are introduced to a care program including postural drainage with chest percussion, administration of antimicrobials as indicated, and a nutritional regimen including pancreatic enzymes and fat-soluble vitamins. Other types of treatment are prescribed on an individualized basis.

Postural Drainage with Chest Percussion. This approach to clearance of mucus is based on the idea that coughing clears mucus from large airways but vibrations are necessary to remove secretions from the small airways, where expiratory flow rates are low. Pulmonary function evaluations before and after this procedure sometimes have and sometimes have not shown improvements in airflow.[243,244] Postural drainage alone may be helpful.[245] The most compelling argument for the use of this therapeutic modality comes from a study of older children with mild to moderate airflow limitation.[246] When these patients were receiving chest physical therapy on a regular basis, little effect could be demonstrated from a single therapy session. However, after 3 weeks without chest physical therapy, when both forced vital capacity and flow rates were significantly reduced, lung function could be improved by reinstituting therapy. Most care centers prescribe this treatment one to four times a day, depending on the severity of illness. A question has been raised about the advisability of chest physical therapy for patients who have minimal cough and no apparent sputum production. Experimental results are not available to answer this question. Several studies in the literature suggest that voluntary coughing,[247] positive expiratory pressure,[248] special breathing maneuvers (autogenic drainage), or repeated forced expiratory maneuvers, and vigorous exercise[249] may substitute for chest physical therapy. In the absence of definitive supporting data, others have suggested that these should be considered adjunct therapies.

Antimicrobials. Lung infection is the major source of morbidity and mortality in CF. Therefore, antibiotic therapy is the mainstay of treatment designed to control progression of disease. In general, antibiotic therapy should be based on the presence of symptoms and guided by the identification of organisms from the lower respiratory tract. There is evidence that early and vigorous use of antibiotics produces better results than administration of antibiotics after symptoms are well-developed or advanced.[250] Some have advocated the early use of continuous antibiotic therapy.[251] Data justifying this approach are lacking. Another principle of antimicrobial therapy in cystic fibrosis is that dosages need to be higher than for non-CF-related chest infections. Both total-body clearance and volume of distribution are considerably greater for CF than for other patients.[252] In addition, large doses are needed to achieve therapeutic levels in infected and mucus- or pus-filled endobronchial spaces. Sputum levels achieved are highly variable, ranging from less than 10 percent to nearly 50 percent of levels measured in serum.[253] Experience has also led many caretakers of CF patients to use longer-than-usual courses of antibiotics, e.g., courses of at least 2 to 4 weeks. Continuous coverage is dictated by repeated, prompt increase in lung symptoms after antibiotic therapy is discontinued.

The choice of antibiotics optimally should be based on the results of sputum culture and appropriate sensitivity testing. If *S. aureus* is present or expected, the choice may include a semisynthetic penicillin, a combination of ampicillin and clavulanic acid, a cephalosporin, clindamycin, or chloramphenicol. Drugs and dosages are listed in Table 127-5. *Haemophilus* infections are best treated with ampicillin, trimethoprim-sulfamethoxazole, or chloramphenicol. In most cases, these antibiotics will temporarily eradicate *S. aureus* and *H. influenzae* from the airways. In older children and adults, tetracyclines may provide useful empirical therapy. Ciprofloxacin appears to control symptoms in patients harboring *P. aeruginosa* and reduces numbers of these organisms in CF airways. Its usefulness is limited by rapid emergence of resistant organisms.[254]

Because the treatment of *Pseudomonas* with oral antibiotics is frequently ineffective, intravenous preparations of aminoglycosides or other antibiotics have been delivered to the lower respiratory tract by aerosol. Several studies now suggest that symptoms can be controlled better and numbers of hospitalizations can be reduced with this approach.[255–257] Surprisingly, emergence of resistant organisms has not been a great problem with aerosolized antibiotic therapy.

Aerosol Therapy. Other solutions given by aerosol have the objective of providing water to hydrate inspissated mucus secretions. One frequently used solution contains 0.45 percent saline. The efficacy of this approach has not been substantiated. In the past, patients were encouraged to sleep in mist tents. This treatment has been largely abandoned because evidence that it is beneficial is lacking and it is aggravating for patients and their families. New approaches to the hydration of airway secretions, e.g., regulation of salt and water movement across the respiratory epithelium, are currently experimental (see "Other Respiratory Therapies").

There have been several trials of treatment with human recombinant DNase in patients with moderate suppurative lung disease.[258,259] The rationale for this treatment—that lysis of polymorphonuclear cells contributes viscous DNA to CF airway secretions, further impairing their clearance properties—appears to be supported by rapid improvement of FVC and FEV_1 following once or twice daily aerosolization. In short-term studies comparing various doses to placebo, recombinant DNase improved lung function and was well tolerated.[260,261] The recommended dose is 2.5 mg by aerosol once daily. The cost of therapy is high, and the potential for long-term benefit requires further evaluation.

Bronchodilators. As detailed above in "Clinical Manifestations" under "Respiratory Tract," many patients demonstrate bronchial lability, prompting frequent use of bronchodilators, particularly β-adrenergic agonists.[95] While the immediate effectiveness of this treatment can be demonstrated in the pulmonary function laboratory, overall improvement or long-term benefit has not been established. Indications for the use of bronchodilators include troublesome wheezing or a demonstrated improvement in pulmonary function, e.g., at least a 15 percent improvement of FEV_1. β-adrenergic agonists can be nebulized, administered from meter-dosed inhalers, or given orally. The aerosol route is clearly superior. Caution should be exercised concerning long-term therapy with these agents, because animal studies show that administration of large amounts of β-adrenergic agonists causes submucosal gland hypertrophy and, presumably, a hypersecretory state.[262] Theophylline preparations also may be effective in some cases. However, CF patients seem to be less tolerant of theophylline than normal because of frequent gastrointestinal irritation.[263] Inhaled atropine improves airflow in CF patients,[94] but systemic side effects prohibit its clinical use. Newer, poorly absorbed, inhaled anticholinergics, such as ipratropium bromide, may provide similar benefit without adverse consequences. Cromolyn sodium has also been used, but claims of efficacy are only anecdotal. This preparation has the advantage of avoiding the adverse effects of other bronchodilators.

Corticosteroids. A small, double-blind controlled study of alternate-day corticosteroid administration demonstrated better maintenance of pulmonary function and fewer exacerbations of lung disease requiring hospitalization over a 4-year period in the treatment group.[264] A large multicenter study of corticosteroid treatment has not supported this conclusion.[265] Alternate-day prednisone (2 mg/kg) was attended by adverse effects (growth failure, hyperglycemia, cataracts), requiring that this arm of the study be discontinued. At 1 mg/kg on alternate days, prednisone provided little if any benefit and still produced unacceptable side effects. Long-term use of corticosteroids cannot be advocated at this time. Time-limited courses for allergic broncho-

Table 127-5 Antimicrobial Agents Used to Treat CF Lung Infection

Organism	Agent	Dose: Pediatric, mg/(kg·day)	Dose: Adult, g/day	Doses/day
Oral Route				
S. aureus	Cloxacillin	50–100	2–4	3–4
	Cefaclor	40–60	3–4	3
	Clindamycin	20	0.6–1.2	3–4
	Erythromycin	50–100	2	3–4
	Amoxicillin/clavulanate	40	2	3
H. influenzae	Amoxicillin	50–100	2	3
	Trimethoprim–sulfamethoxazole (trimethoprim)	20	0.32–0.64	2–4
	Chloramphenicol	50–100	2	3–4
P. aeruginosa	Ciprofloxacin	—	1.5–2.25	3
Empirical	Tetracycline	50–100	2	3–4
Intravenous Route				
S. aureus	Oxacillin	150–200	*	4
P. aeruginosa	Gentamicin or tobramycin	8–20	*	3
	Amikacin	15–30	*	2–3
	Netilmicin	6–12	*	2–3
	Carbenicillin or ticarcillin	250–500	*	4–6
	Piperacillin, mezlocillin, or azlocillin	250–450	*	4–6
	Ticarcillin/clavulanate	250–450	*	4–6
	Imipenim/cilastatin	45–90	4	3–4
P. aeruginosa and *P. cepacia*	Ceftazidime	150	4–6	3
Aerosol Route		**mg/dose**	**mg/dose**	
P. aeruginosa	Gentamicin	40–80	80–160	2–4
	Tobramycin	40–80	80–160	2–4
	Carbenicillin	—	2000–4000	2–4

*Usually dosed by mg/(kg·day), as with children.

pulmonary aspergillosis and other forms of reversible airway obstruction may be helpful.

Other Respiratory Therapies. Mucolytics, expectorants, and cough suppressants have been used for relief of chest symptoms. In general, coughing is an important mechanism for clearance of mucus in patients with CF and should not be suppressed. Currently formulated expectorants, which, by definition, should increase the amount of water in secretions, probably do not achieve that objective. Rather than being helpful, long-term administration of iodides to patients with CF has been associated with a high incidence of goiter and hypothyroidism.[266] Mucolytics such as *N*-acetylcysteine are injurious to respiratory epithelium and, when used regularly, promote bronchitis. Therefore, aerosols of this substance should be used selectively and only for short periods.

Exercise is generally considered to be beneficial for patients with CF and should be encouraged for all but those with the most severe lung disease. In one study, 12 of 29 patients with an FEV_1 <50 percent of FVC experienced a reduction of Sa_{O_2} below 90 percent with peak exercise, compared with no reduction in patients with less obstruction.[97] A 12-week exercise program consisting of three 1-h sessions a week during which jogging produced a heart rate averaging 70 to 85 percent of peak heart rate has been shown to increase exercise tolerance and cardiorespiratory fitness, probably by increasing respiratory muscle endurance.[99] However, this program did not improve pulmonary function. Weight training appears to be safe and may promote weight gain as well as strength.[267] Most caretakers of patients with CF feel that regular, vigorous exercise promotes a positive self-image and increases the perception of wellness. Although CF patients have normal thermoregulatory responses to exercise, they do lose more salt through the skin, and with exercise plus heat stress their serum sodium and chloride concentrations drop.[268] Furthermore, failure to achieve hyperosmolarity under these conditions may preclude the usual thirst stimulus and place CF subjects at greater risk for dehydration.[269] Therefore, exercise programs should include attention to salt and water replacement.

Experimental therapies include the use of aerosolized antiproteinases to counteract the presence of free elastase and other proteinase activities in CF airways,[270] aerosolized amiloride[271] to block excessive sodium reabsorption, and aerosolized UTP[272] to augment chloride secretion by CF respiratory epithelial cells. The latter two agents may be particularly effective in combination to increase salt and water within the airway lumen.

Somatic gene therapy has emerged as a serious possibility for treatment of CF,[273] as discussed in the last section of this chapter.

Nutrition. Approximately 90 percent of patients with cystic fibrosis require pancreatic enzyme supplementation. This is accomplished by mealtime administration of an enzyme extract, usually in the form of encapsulated microspheres coated with acid-resistant material to promote delivery to the small intestine. Enzyme replacement diminishes but does not normalize the amount of fat and nitrogen excreted in stools.[274] One to four capsules per meal or snack generally is adequate. The number of capsules taken should be adjusted on the basis of weight gain or loss, the presence or absence of abdominal cramping, and the character of stools. Because postprandial pH is low in the CF duodenum, the encapsulated spheres may not dissolve optimally in the proximal small intestine.[275] Complications of pancreatic enzyme replacement therapy include oral and perianal ulcerations, hyperuricosuria,[276] and proximal colonic stricture[276a] when large amounts of pancreatic extract are given. Vitamins A and D are generally supplied by a daily multiple-vitamin preparation. Vitamin E, 100 to 200 units daily, also is recommended, because serum levels are generally low in unsupplemented patients. Vitamin K usually is given sporadically to treat bleeding complications or to correct prolonged prothrombin times. Some caregivers prescribe 5 mg of water-miscible vitamin K twice weekly. Other vitamins and trace minerals may be deficient and require supplementation on a selective basis. Adequate administration of carotenoids and vitamin E are suggested to combat oxidative stresses imposed by chronic lung infection.[61,277]

Many individuals with CF have a higher than normal caloric need because of the increased work of breathing. In general, patients should be encouraged to eat a balanced diet including at least a moderate amount of fat. When the anorexia of chronic infection supervenes, failure to gain weight or weight loss occurs. Further encouragement to eat high-calorie foods may be helpful. Supplementation with elemental dietary preparations by mouth is unlikely to be sustained over an extended period. Some CF care centers have begun to administer supplementary elemental feedings nocturnally by nasogastric tube or by percutaneous gastrostomy or duodenostomy.[278] While short-term benefits such as increased weight gain can be achieved, long-term benefits, including effects on pulmonary function and psychological status, have not been established. A preliminary study of slow-growing older children without glycosuria and mild to moderate lung disease demonstrated much-improved growth with the administration of tolbutamide, 750 mg per day.[279]

Patients with CF who retain exocrine pancreatic function and maintain good nutrition experience a slower decline of pulmonary function than those with no demonstrable pancreatic function.[52] This observation has been used as a reason for emphasizing nutritional interventions. However, it may be more efficacious to maintain good nutrition by preventing progression of lung disease than to maintain good lung function by emphasizing nutritional therapy. A combination of these approaches is probably best. The better pulmonary function in patients who retain pancreatic function probably reflects the presence of a set of mutations including R117H that determine an overall milder phenotype.

Salt and Water. During the hot-weather season, children require extra salt. In general, this can be achieved by salting their food liberally and providing access to salt. In fact, infant formulas now contain enough salt to avoid the depletion seen in the past. Specific attention to salt intake may be warranted by strenuous activity in warm environments. Recent work suggests that CF children who are active during hot weather should also have enforced rather than voluntary fluid intake, because they are unable to generate a hyperosmolar body fluid stimulus for thirst.[269]

Psychosocial Factors. As with any chronic disease, compliance with therapy and ability to function fully depend highly on patient attitude. Therefore, approaches that promote a positive self-concept, foster the ability of individuals to take control of their medical management, and allow them to participate fully in life events are likely to promote well-being and perhaps longevity. However, caretakers of patients with CF must recognize that these individuals may participate in harmful behaviors, such as substance abuse,[280] just like their healthy peers. Medical care that provides continuity and fosters trust may pay large dividends. Personnel who specifically provide psychosocial support are important contributors to CF care teams.

Prevention of Lung Disease. Rubeola, pertussis, and influenza infections are particularly injurious to CF lungs and may trigger a downward spiral of lung function. Adequate immunization early in life for pertussis and measles is mandatory. In addition, patients of all ages should be adequately immunized for influenza virus infection on a yearly basis. The early use of amantidine for acute respiratory illnesses during epidemics of influenza A infections may further prevent adverse consequences of this infection. There is no evidence that administration of the pneumococcal vaccine is useful. Cigarette smoke[281] and other air pollutants are likely to have adverse effects, but their specific role in the decline of lung function is undetermined. Evidence is accumulating that *P. cepacia* and perhaps *P. aeruginosa* are acquired by patient-to-patient transmission.[282,283] Avoidance of close contact between colonized and noncolonized patients, such as at camps or on hospital inpatient units, has been recommended.

Hospital Therapy

Indications for hospitalization and intensive pulmonary therapy include increased cough or wheezing, respiratory distress with decreased activity tolerance, weight loss, sustained downward trend in pulmonary function, increasing hypoxemia, or one of the pulmonary complications of CF. Although all the modalities of therapy can be intensified in the hospital, the major advantage of hospitalization has been the ability to administer intravenous antimicrobial agents that control *Pseudomonas* infection.

Antibiotics for intravenous administration should be selected on the basis of respiratory tract cultures and susceptibility studies. Two-drug treatment of *Pseudomonas* infection is the rule. A third antibiotic may be added as necessary for control of *S. aureus* or other organisms. Drugs and dosages currently used for intravenous therapy are listed in Table 127-5. A response often is not seen for 4 to 7 days after initiation of therapy. In general, a 2-week course provides good improvement in pulmonary function[284] and more sustained benefit. With refractory infection, treatment for 3 or more weeks is not unusual. Some advocate intensive therapy until pulmonary function has returned to previous baseline or until improvement has reached a plateau. Prolonged courses of antibiotic therapy should include weekly monitoring of respiratory tract organisms and their sensitivities, as shifts in either are not uncommon. In general, determination of minimum inhibitory concentrations provides more useful informaton about susceptibility of *Pseudomonas* organisms than do disk methods of sensitivity testing.

Aminoglycosides have been the mainstay of anti-*Pseudomonas* therapy for more than 20 years. A major advantage of these drugs is the ability to monitor and adjust their blood levels. For gentamicin or tobramycin, thrice-daily administration to achieve peak blood levels in the range of 10 μg/ml seems to be optimal. The same daily dose of aminoglycosides can be given once or twice daily, and the high peak levels achieved under these conditions are well tolerated.[285] Patients should be monitored during aminoglycoside therapy for nephrotoxicity and ototoxicity. An aminoglycoside is usually paired with one of the penicillin derivatives or with ceftazidime.

Individuals with cystic fibrosis, particularly those who are in school or holding full-time jobs, may opt to administer intravenous antibiotics at home for all or part of the treatment course. Properly administered intravenous therapy at home appears to be nearly as effective as in-hospital treatment.[286] For patients requiring long-term home antibiotic therapy, central intravenous catheters have been surgically placed.

Interest in bronchial lavage as a therapeutic modality has been tempered by the realization that it is unlikely to give long-term benefits and that acute deterioration of lung function is a possible outcome.[287] In fact, there is no evidence that bronchoscopy and lavage, whether whole-lung, lobar, or segmental, is superior to intensive antibiotic therapy and chest percussion.

Treatment of Complications

Respiratory. The most feared complications of CF lung disease are pulmonary hypertension with right heart failure and respiratory failure. Low-flow oxygen is effective in alleviating nocturnal hypoxemia and does not cause clinically important hypercapnea.[288] However, there is no evidence that this approach is effective in preventing pulmonary hypertension or postponing the onset of symptomatic right heart failure, as may be the case with older patients who have chronic bronchitis. If systemic venous congestion is present, furosemide, 1 mg/kg, administered intravenously usually results in brisk diuresis and reduced fluid retention.[289] If needed, long-term diuretic therapy with spironolactone prevents potassium depletion and seems to be helpful. Digitalis is not effective in the face of pure right-sided heart failure, but it may be useful when there is associated left-sided dysfunction.[290] Acute pharmacologic relief of high pulmonary artery pressures has been achieved with tolazoline[291] but not with other pulmonary vasodilators.[292] Evidence for sustained improvement with drug therapy has not been forthcoming. The most effective approach to relieving right heart failure is improving oxygenation through intensive pulmonary therapy. A moderate limitation of salt intake, i.e., 2 g sodium per day, may be helpful. Carbenicillin and related drugs may promote fluid retention because of their relatively high sodium content.

Respiratory failure is best managed with vigorous medical therapy of lung disease. All evidence to date suggests that respiratory insufficiency in a patient who has experienced slow deterioration in lung function over months to years will not be reversed by assisted ventilation. In fact, the usual outcome of intubation and ventilatory assistance is prolonged ventilator dependence.[293] For this reason, assisted ventilation has been recommended only for patients who have had at least moderately good lung function and who have experienced rapid deterioration because of a reversible insult to the lungs, such as influenza virus infection. More recently, assisted ventilation has also been used in anticipation of a lung transplant.

Atelectasis is best treated with vigorous antibiotic therapy and frequent chest percussion and drainage. Corticosteroids may be helpful in the face of severe reactive airways disease or evidence for allergic aspergillosis. There is no evidence that bronchoscopy and lavage hasten the expansion of collapsed segments or lobes.[103] However, fiber-optic bronchoscopy and the sampling of secretions from an atelectatic area of the lung for cytologic and microbiologic assessment may be helpful.

Pneumothorax can be handled by observation if it is small (<10 percent of the hemithorax cross-sectional area) and asymptomatic. Because of a tendency toward persistent air leakage and a high recurrence rate, many advocate instilling a sclerosing agent such as Atabrine or performing a limited thoracotomy with both oversewing of obvious areas of leakage and pleural abrasion or stripping.[104] In general, these interventions are well tolerated by patients and shorten rather than lengthen hospitalization for pneumothorax.

Small-volume hemoptysis requires no specific therapy other than aggressive treatment of lung infection and vitamin K supplements if indicated. Large-volume hemoptysis usually subsides spontaneously[105] but, if persistent, has been treated successfully by bronchial artery embolization.[294] Allergic aspergillosis usually responds to systemic corticosteroid therapy and is self-limiting.[295] For refractory cases, itraconazole or aerosolized amphotericin B may be helpful. There is no specific therapy for hypertrophic osteoarthropathy. Symptoms usually wane as lung infection comes under control. Gastroesophageal reflux has been documented in about 20 percent of infants and children with cystic fibrosis[296,297] and is probably caused by increased intraabdominal pressure owing to obstructive lung disease and frequent coughing. It may contribute to airways obstruction and lung infiltrates by reflex mechanisms or aspiration. Medical therapy for reflux reduces symptoms in most of these patients, but several have required fundoplication.[296] Use of bethanechol to treat reflux has resulted in marked deterioration of lung function,[298] presumably owing to enhanced bronchospasm and secretion of mucus.

Gastrointestinal Complications. Meconium ileus can often be relieved with enemas using Gastrografin or other contrast materials, which are refluxed into the terminal ileum under fluoroscopy.[299] If this fails, or if there is evidence of perforation, surgical intervention is required. Distal intestinal obstruction syndrome also can be relieved with contrast enemas that reach the terminal ileum.[299] Some success is also claimed for oral administration of *N*-acetylcysteine[300] and perioral lavage with large volumes of physiological fluids containing polyethylene glycol.[301] Occasionally, surgical intervention is necessary. Older patients usually can reduce rectal prolapse voluntarily by using their abdominal, perianal, and gluteal muscles, but in small children the prolapse must be reduced manually by continuous gentle pressure with the patient in the knee-chest position.[122] Sedation may be helpful. Adequate pancreatic enzyme therapy, decreased fat in the diet, and control of pulmonary infection usually eliminate recurrences. A few patients require surgical stabilization of the rectum. Cirrhosis is generally focal and usually does not require specific therapy. Bleeding varices usually can be managed with sclerotherapy. In the past, significant bleeding has been treated successfully with portal–systemic shunting.[168] Splenorenal anastomoses have been most effective, and hepatic encephalopathy has not been a problem. Occasionally, pronounced hypersplenism may require splenectomy. Liver failure and ascites are treated as in other patients. Liver transplantation is now an option, and lung function remains surprisingly stable after transplant.[302] Similarly, pancreatitis, when it occurs in adolescents or young adults with CF, is treated with standard regimens.

Hyperglycemia attending cystic fibrosis can occur at any age but is generally a problem of the second and third decades of life. Ketoacidosis is rare. When blood glucose levels are only intermittently elevated and glycosuria does not intervene, no treatment is necessary. With the advent of sustained glycosuria, insulin treatment should be instituted. Oral hypoglycemic agents may or not be effective. Vascular disease affecting the retina and the kidneys has been documented in CF patients with prolonged hyperglycemia. Therefore, consistent control of blood sugar levels is desirable, although caution must be exercised with insulin therapy, in that CF subjects frequently become hypoglycemic.[151]

Many of the complications of CF are iatrogenic. A number of therapy-related medical problems are listed in Table 127-6.

Surgical Therapy. The most common reason for surgery in cystic fibrosis is nasal polypectomy. Surgery may be required when the nasal passages are completely obstructed, when rhinorrhea is particularly bothersome, or if the polyps cause internal pressure and widen the bridge of the nose. Elective operations should be avoided during exacerbations of lung disease. Intensive pulmonary therapy for several days before surgery may be useful, and careful monitoring postoperatively is essential for preventing postanesthetic problems.[28] Polyps do tend to recur after surgical removal, but the incidence of polyposis wanes after the second decade of life. Removal of lung segments or lobes because of chronic atelectasis or severe focal lung disease is attempted infrequently. In carefully selected patients, this approach may provide additional years with fewer symptoms. However, lobectomy should be undertaken with the knowledge that postoperative complications are not uncommon and that removal of any functioning lung tissue may be detrimental, given that the patients have a progressive, generalized pulmonary disease. Furthermore, intrathoracic procedures may be an obstacle to later options for lung transplantation.

Table 127-6 Complications of Therapy for CF

Complication	Agent
Renal dysfunction	
Tubular	Aminoglycosides
Interstitial nephritis	Semisynthetic penicillins
Hearing loss	Aminoglycosides
Peripheral neuropathy and/or optic atrophy	Chloramphenicol (prolonged course)
Hypomagnesemia	Aminoglycosides
Hyperuricemia, colonic stricture	Pancreatic extracts (very large doses)
Goiter	Iodine-containing expectorants
Gynecomastia	Spironolactone
Enamel hypoplasia/staining	Tetracyclines (used in first 8 years of life)

NOTE: Common hypersensitivity reactions to drugs are not included.

Abdominal surgery for intestinal obstruction, appendicitis, or cholelithiasis is occasionally indicated and usually is well tolerated if attention is paid to care of the lungs.

Heart–lung and double-lung transplants have been attempted in many care centers. Initial results have been encouraging, with more than half of recipients surviving for one or more years.[303,304] The epithelium of transplanted lungs retains the electrochemical properties of normal tissue,[305] and the infections typical of CF reportedly are not a problem in transplanted lungs. The lung function of survivors has approached normal. However, bronchiolitis obliterans and other complications of lung rejection are frequently encountered. An FEV_1 <30 percent of predicted qualifies CF patients for transplant consideration.[306]

BIOCHEMICAL ABNORMALITIES OF MACROMOLECULAR SECRETION

Following Farber's report of mucus obstruction in many exocrine glands, a search was initiated for abnormal macromolecules that might change the physical properties of CF exocrine secretions. This line of investigation has produced no candidate for a general pathogenetic mechanism. Once the CFTR gene product was identified and its contribution to the CF chloride transport abnormality defined, attention shifted to the role played by salt and water in the generation of secretions with altered clearance properties. However, several issues relating to the solids of CF mucus deserve attention.

Hypersecretion of glycoproteins and perhaps other glycoconjugates contributes extensively to the obstructive events in CF lungs and perhaps other organs. A primary abnormality in the control of mucus secretion has not been identified, and the rate of secretion of glycoproteins by CF airway explants and cultured cells is not increased.[307–309] The apparent increase in glycoproteins may be a response to airway inflammation. Compositional or structural abnormalities of glycoconjugates secreted by CF cells are difficult to confirm or exclude because of the extensive heterogeneity of these substances. Initial claims of increased fucosylation and decreased sialylation have not been consistently confirmed,[310] but they deserve continuing attention in light of recent claims that defective conductance of Cl^- into intracellular organelles diminishes acidification and consequently sialylation of glycoconjugates.[311] Yet another proposed abnormality of glycoconjugate biosynthesis—increased sulfation—might relate to anion conductance abnormalities.[309] CF respiratory tract mucins purified from sputum and intestinal mucins are oversulfated.[312,313] Both glycoproteins and proteoglycans secreted by CF respiratory epithelial cells in primary culture also are excessively sulfated.[309] Furthermore, the cell-surface glycoconjugates of these cells are strikingly oversulfated.[309] The reason for enhanced sulfation is unclear. CF cell lines and primary cells from respiratory epithelium have normal sulfate influx and efflux as well as normal intracellular concentrations of inorganic sulfate.[314] Sulfate activation or sulfation of glycoconjugates in the Golgi must be enhanced. The notion that these changes could be related to the adherence of *P. aeruginosa* to CF respiratory epithelial cells[34] or to the rheologic properties of secretions deserves consideration.

Several investigators have claimed that an elevated calcium content of CF exocrine secretions plays a pathogenetic role. The calcium content of CF epithelial and other cells is elevated.[315,316] Although calcium transport via ATPase-dependent mechanisms is probably intact[317] and calmodulin levels are normal,[318] excess amounts of calcium are secreted into several body fluids, including submandibular saliva and nasal secretions.[310,319] Conflicting data have been reported concerning calcium concentrations in tracheobronchial secretions.[310] Interactions between calcium and a small phosphoprotein result in precipitation of this protein and turbidity of CF submandibular saliva. This interaction can be explained entirely by the high calcium levels in CF saliva and the fact that the solubility product for calcium and the phosphoprotein is exceeded.[320] Turbidity of CF submandibular saliva appears to have no adverse consequences. Thus, there is no evidence that calcium plays a primary role in obstructive events within other organs.

A full understanding of the pathogenesis of mucus clearance deficits in CF awaits systematic studies of the water content, glycoconjugate content and composition, and rheologic properties of these secretions.

CF GENE AND MUTATIONS

Gene Mapping

Mapping of a disease gene without knowledge of the biochemical defect, now known as positional cloning, became an attractive approach when the concept of polymorphic DNA markers was introduced in the early 1980s. A major challenge in mapping and cloning the CF locus was the lack of any known chromosomal deletions or translocations associated with the disease. Thus, the approach required the exclusive use of linkage analysis. The abundance of families suitable for linkage analysis compensated for the small size of individual families, the latter being related to the recessive nature and severity of CF. The first genetic marker that was found linked to *CF* was paraoxonase (*PON*), estimated to be 10 cM from *CF*.[321,322] The linkage information was not immediately useful for CF gene cloning work because the chromosomal location of paraoxonase had yet to be determined, and it could not be mapped as readily as for DNA markers.

The demonstration of linkage between *CF* and the DNA marker *D7S15* (formerly D0CRI-917) was an important milestone in the mapping of the CF gene.[323] *D7S15* was found to be about 15 cM from *CF*, and the localization of this marker on chromosome 7[324,325] provided the information needed to search for additional, closer markers. Further information on the localization of *CF* was derived from the almost simultaneous discovery of close linkage between *CF* and two other markers, the *met* oncogene (*MET*)[326] and *D7S8*.[327] Both of these markers were estimated to be about 1 cM from *CF*, and subsequently they were found to flank the locus.[328–330] In addition to their utility in serving as two closely linked reference points for isolation of the CF gene, *MET* and *D7S8* proved remarkably useful as markers for genetic diagnosis.

The linkage data using very close markers also strongly suggested that there was a single locus for the CF gene,[328] and there has not been any evidence to date in support of a second locus causing CF.[325,331] A number of other genetic markers known to be on chromosome 7 were also examined for possible linkage to *CF*, but most of them were found to be more distant from *CF* than *MET* or *D7S8*.[330,332,333] Attempts were also made to screen for deletions located in the CF region with the use of pulsed-field gel electrophoresis, but none were found.[334]

Gene Cloning

Many different molecular cloning techniques and strategies were employed in attempts to isolate the gene for CF. The general principle was to narrow the region of interest using additional DNA markers; clone the DNA segments from the region; identify candidate genes; and analyze these genes for possible disease-causing mutations. The strategies included isolation of DNA segments from flow-sorted libraries,[335–339] from cell lines generated by chromosome-mediated gene transfer,[340–343] from pulsed-field gel electrophoresis,[344,345] from chromosome jumping libraries,[346,347] from microdissected chromosome fragments,[348,349] and from chromosome walking.[12,345,350–352] These efforts resulted in the isolation of several DNA fragments that were crucial for the eventual cloning of the CF gene. The XV-2c and KM.19 probes of the *D7S23* locus[340,341] were isolated through chromosome-mediated gene transfer and enrichment for CpG islands; *D7S340* and *D7S122*[336] were selected from a flow-sorted chromosome 7-specific library.

The positioning of the CF gene was guided by long-range restriction maps of the region,[12,353–355] by study of recombination events near the CF locus,[14,328,329,356–360] and by analysis of linkage disequilibrium.[328,356,361–363] Striking linkage disequilibrium was detected for two RFLP markers at the *D7S23* locus, XV-2c and KM.19. For example, 88 percent (157/178) of CF chromosomes were found to carry the common CF haplotype, which was present on only 29 percent (50/175) of the normal chromosomes in one study.[364] Further, it was shown that the common haplotype ("B") for these two markers accounted for 85 percent of CF chromosomes but only 16 percent of normal chromosomes. Similar observations were made for these and other DNA markers by many other investigators.[352,365–371] The strong linkage disequilibrium suggested that these markers were probably quite close to the CF gene.[12,341,372]

In 1989, the gene responsible for CF was identified through a series of molecular cloning experiments.[12–14] A 280-kb DNA region was isolated through "chromosome walking" and "jumping" from the DNA markers *D7S122* and *D7S340*.[336] Small DNA segments from this region were purified and tested for the presence of genes by their ability to detect evolutionarily conserved sequences, transcripts on northern blots, or cDNA clones. Several candidate genes, including one reported earlier,[341] were identified, and one of these was proven, largely on the basis of the discovery of a common mutation, to be the CF gene.[12]

CFTR Gene Structure

The CF gene spans approximately 230 kb of DNA and contains at least 27 exons.[12,373] The encoded mRNA is about 6.5-kb long and can be detected by northern blotting in a variety of affected tissues including lung, pancreas, sweat glands, liver, nasal polyps, salivary gland, and colon.[13] The deduced polypeptide was termed cystic fibrosis transmembrane conductance regulator (CFTR), and it contains 1,480 amino acid residues with a calculated molecular mass of about 170,000. The sequence data may be obtained from GenBank with accession numbers M55106-M55131. The entire CF gene locus has also been isolated subsequently in yeast artificial chromosomes.[374,375]

The primary sequence shows that CFTR contains two similar halves, each of which consists of a domain capable of spanning the membrane six times and another containing the consensus sequence for nucleotide(ATP)-binding domains (NBD). The predicted protein also has a high proportion of charged amino acid residues in an unusual region, called the R-domain, linking the two halves of the protein (Fig. 127-7). The R domain is thought to have a regulatory function.[13] In overall structure, this protein resembles many other prokaryotic and eukaryotic transport proteins, most notably the mammalian P-glycoprotein. Further discussion of the function of CFTR is presented under "Function of CFTR" below.

Multiple transcription initiation sites have been described for the CFTR gene. While the first study suggested that transcription is probably initiated from locations close to the reported +1 position of the cDNA sequence,[13] subsequent analyses show that there are additional transcription initiation sites at the +60, +70, and +100 regions[376,377] (J. Rommens et al., personal communication). DNA transfection studies demonstrated that the basal promoter of the CFTR gene lies between nucleotide positions −228 and +48, although there are probably multiple positive and negative elements involved in regulating the transcription of this gene.[378] Other groups have not detected the negative regulatory-element.[376,377]

The use of multiple initiation sites probably reflects the lack of a TATA sequence in the promoter region. Furthermore, different initiation sites are found for RNA prepared from different sources; however, the major product appears to be initiated from the +60 region in both the colonic carcinoma cell line T84 and the pancreas.[377,379] In the T84 cell line, a second class of transcripts, accounting for about 3 to 4 percent of the total population, is found to initiate from an upstream region; these transcripts contain at least two upstream exons, designated exons 1a and 1b, in place of the originally designated exon 1.[377,379] The biological relevance of these putative transcripts is unknown, particularly since they do not contain any open reading frame contiguous with the remaining exons; the next available methionine codon in CFTR after the one located in exon 1 is in exon 4.

Alternative Splicing. Absence of exons in transcripts of the CFTR gene has been found particularly with the use of the sensitive reverse transcriptase-polymerase chain reaction (RT-PCR) method.[380–383] Sequences corresponding to exons 4, 9, 12, or a portion of 13 are apparently absent in a fraction of the RNA isolated from some tissues and cell lines. A wide variation in the relative amount of transcripts lacking exon 9 has been detected among normal (non-CF) control subjects[381]; the proportion of this shorter mRNA in bronchial or nasal epithelial samples varies from 0 to 92 percent.[384,385] The difference is apparently due to the length of the polythymidine tract at the exon 9 splice branch/acceptor site.[384] There is less variation among CF chromosomes. It has been suggested, however, that alternative splicing is one possible mechanism to bypass nonsense and frameshift mutations in certain coding regions of CFTR,[386] although clear evidence supporting this hypothesis has not been available to date. There is evidence that the efficiency of the exon 9 splicing in *cis* with the R117H mutation can influence disease severity[387] (see "Genotype/Phenotype Correlations" below). *Trans*-splicing of CFTR transcripts has also been noted; PCR data showed that exon 10 and 11 sequences were spliced in front of exon 2.[379] The significance of the latter finding is unclear.

Exon 9 minus transcripts and transcripts representing the

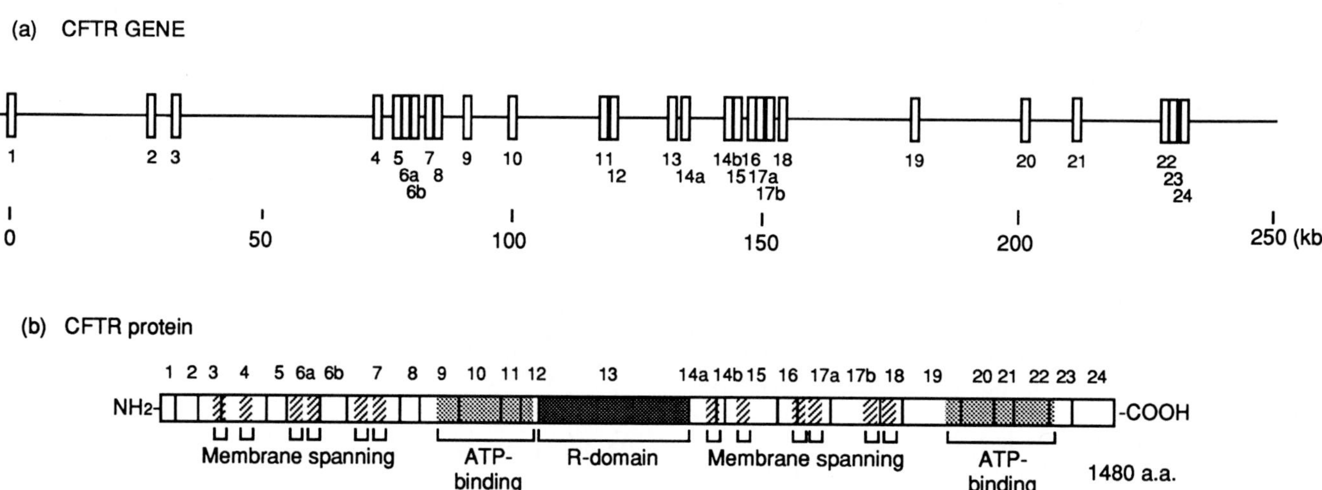

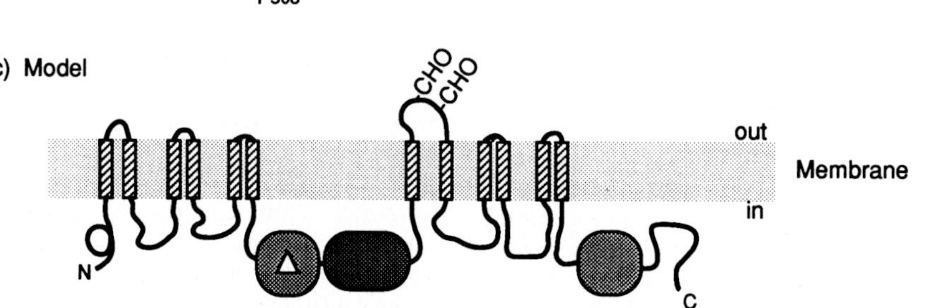

FIG. 127-7 The CFTR gene and its encoded polypeptide. *(From Tsui and Buchwald.[379] Used by permission of* Advances in Human Genetics.)

complete deletion of exons 4 and 12 have also been detected by RT-PCR in human intestine, kidney, lung, liver, placenta, and a small number of cell lines.[382,383] Evaluation of the relative amounts of the transcript variants indicated that the exon 4 minus transcripts constituted <2 percent of the total, and exon 12 minus constituted 5 to 30 percent. The finding that mice have a different pattern of alternative splicing (deletion of exon 5, exon 4/5, and exon 11) indicates that splicing is not conserved across species, and this argues against a physiological role for the alternative splicing.[388]

The Major CF Mutation—ΔF508

The major CF mutation, named ΔF508, is a 3-bp deletion that removes the phenylalanine residue at amino acid position 508 of CFTR[14]; this mutation accounts for about 70 percent of mutant chromosomes worldwide. There are remarkable differences in the proportion of CF chromosomes with the ΔF508 among different populations,[389] as described in 39 articles in a special journal issue.[390] A generally higher frequency is observed for northern Europeans in comparison to southern European populations,[391–393] ranging from 30 to 35 percent in the Ashkenazic Jewish population[394,395] to 87 percent in Denmark.[396]

Haplotype analysis of DNA markers closely linked to the CF gene has shown that there is a strict association of one haplotype group ("Ia" using markers very close to the gene) with the ΔF508-bearing chromosomes, suggesting that all the ΔF508 alleles originated from a single mutational event.[14] Similar analyses have also been performed for additional ΔF508-bearing chromosomes with DNA markers more distantly linked to the mutation.[393] The results of these studies show that, while there is a strong association between ΔF508 and a particular extended haplotype ("B"), the mutation is also found on chromosomes with other haplotypes. The latter observation likely reflects recombination events between the mutation and these more distant DNA markers (KM.19 and XV-2c).[397]

The observed southeast-to-northwest gradient of the relative frequency of ΔF508 has allowed the European Working Group[393] to hypothesize that there was a diffusion of this mutation during the Neolithic Age, at a time when immigration of early farmers started from the Middle East and slowly progressed toward the northwest of Europe.[398] A selective advantage of this mutation or an allele at a tightly linked locus may have contributed to the spread of this mutation. The biochemical and functional aspects of the ΔF508 protein are discussed below under "Class II Mutations: Defective Protein Processing."

Other CF Mutations

More than 400 sequence variations have been detected in the CFTR gene in the 4 years since its isolation. Of these alterations, about 350 are presumed to be pathologic mutations (Table 127-7 and Fig. 127-8), while others are likely benign sequence variations (Table 127-8 and Fig. 127-8). The rapid accumulation of mutation data partly represents the collaborative effort of the CF Genetic Analysis Consortium. Many more mutations are likely to be found in the coming years, as 10 to 20 percent of the mutant alleles have yet to be defined in several different populations. The large number of mutations has thus provided a rich source of information about the structure and function of CFTR. Unfortunately, however, many of the reported mutations have only been described at the DNA sequence level and have not been studied at the biochemical and functional level. The functional consequence of many of the presumed pathologic mutations is therefore unclear.

Different types of mutations have been identified in the CFTR gene (Fig. 127-8). About half of the reported CFTR mutations are amino acid substitutions (missense mutations). Other types of mutations—nonsense, frameshift, and mRNA splicing mutations—constitute the remainder. There are a few single-amino-acid deletions, one large in-frame deletion, and a single case of a large, complex deletion in which exons 4 through 7 and 11 through 18 are deleted but exons 8 through 10 apparently are intact.[490] No promoter mutations have been described. As expected, most of the mutations are found among patients of Caucasian ancestry, but some are apparently unique to populations of non-Caucasian origin (see "Ethnic/Geographic Distribution" below for further discussion).

To date, more than 35,000 mutant chromosomes have been examined worldwide, and 68 percent of them were found to carry the ΔF508 mutation (data of the CF Genetic Analysis Consortium). The relative frequencies of the other mutations vary among different populations, and most of the mutations are rare; only eight other mutant alleles are represented by more than 100 chromosomes found worldwide, and about 25 additional ones by more than 10 chromosomes; many mutations have only been reported once. Some of the mutations, such as A455E,[441] G542X,[441] G551D,[454] R553X,[454] W1282X,[466] N1303K,[487] and 621 + 1G→T[237] may individually account for as high as 10 percent of CF chromosomes in certain populations. The system used for mutation nomenclature is described in detail elsewhere.[502]

The distribution of mutations in different regions of the gene appears to be nonrandom (Fig. 127-8). There are clearly mutation "hotspots," and different substitutions for a single base pair can be found in many places in the gene. One region of exon 11, which corresponds to NBD1 of the protein, seems to have the highest density of mutations, with at least 11 different sequence alterations clustered within five codons. These include four different sequence alterations for the AGT codon for serine at position 549 in exon 11.[441,453,454] The equivalent position in NBD2 does not seem to have a high density of mutations. In addition, the frequencies for several mutations in exon 11 also appear to be relatively high in most populations.[503]

As has been demonstrated for ΔF508, the more frequent CF mutations have been found to have a unique DNA marker haplotype for each, suggesting that they too are derived from single origins.[441,454,504] Nevertheless, at least two different DNA marker haplotypes have been described for R553X[505] and R117H,[387] indicating possible recurrent events at the same nucleotide position for each of these mutations. There has been only one example of a de novo mutation, R851X.[467]

Examples have been found indicating that two independent mutations can coexist on the same chromosome. An additional mutation, R553Q, found together on the same chromosome with ΔF508, was thought to have an attenuating effect on the disease.[457] It is of interest to note that this intragenic complementation phenomenon was independently observed in a chimeric protein assay system involving CFTR and the yeast mating factor transporting protein sterile 6 (STE6).[506] In another example, the S1251N mutation was always found together with F508C,[483] although the latter could exist by itself as a benign sequence variation.[491]

Table 127-7 Cystic Fibrosis Disease Mutations*

Name	Location (Exon)	Nucleotide Change	CFTR Domain†	Consequence (e.g., Amino Acid Change)	Reference
M1V	1	A$\rightarrow$G at 133		No initiation codon	399
M1K	1	T$\rightarrow$A at 134		No initiation codon	400
Q2X (linked to R3W?)	1	C$\rightarrow$T at 136		Gln$\rightarrow$Stop at codon 2	401
R3W (linked to Q2X?)	1	A$\rightarrow$T at 139		Arg$\rightarrow$Trp at codon 3	401
S4X	1	C$\rightarrow$A at 143		Ser$\rightarrow$Stop at 4	402
182delT	1	Deletion of T at 182		Frameshift	403
185+4A$\rightarrow$T	Intron 1	A$\rightarrow$T at 185+4		mRNA splicing mutation?	404
G27X	2	G$\rightarrow$T at 211		Gly$\rightarrow$Stop at 27	405
G27E	2	G$\rightarrow$A at 212		Gly$\rightarrow$Glu at 27	406
Q30X	2	C$\rightarrow$T at 220		Gln$\rightarrow$Stop at 30	407
R31L	2	G$\rightarrow$T at 224		Arg$\rightarrow$Leu at 31	408
241delAT	2	Deletion of AT from 241		Frameshift	409
Q39X	2	C$\rightarrow$T at 247		Gln$\rightarrow$Stop at 39	410
D44G	2	A$\rightarrow$G at 263		Asp$\rightarrow$Gly at 44	409
296+12T$\rightarrow$C	Intron 2	T$\rightarrow$C at 296+12		mRNA splicing mutation?	H. Cuppens et al., personal communication
W57X	3	G$\rightarrow$A at 302		Trp$\rightarrow$Stop at 57	411
E60X	3	G$\rightarrow$T at 310		Glu$\rightarrow$Stop at 60	G. Malone et al., personal communication
R74W	3	C$\rightarrow$T at 352		Arg$\rightarrow$Trp at 74	400
G85E	3	G$\rightarrow$A at 386	TM1	Gly$\rightarrow$Glu at 85	237
394delTT	3	Deletion of TT from 394	TM1	Frameshift	400
L88X(T$\rightarrow$A)	3	T$\rightarrow$A at 395	TM1	Leu$\rightarrow$Stop at 88	401
L88X(T$\rightarrow$G)	3	T$\rightarrow$G at 395	TM1	Leu$\rightarrow$Stop at 88	412
G91R	3	G$\rightarrow$A at 403	TM1	Gly$\rightarrow$Arg at 91	413
405+1G$\rightarrow$A	Intron 3	G$\rightarrow$A at 405+1	TM1	mRNA splicing mutation	414
406−6T$\rightarrow$C	Intron 3	T$\rightarrow$C at 406−6	TM1	mRNA splicing mutation (?)	400
E92K	4	G$\rightarrow$A at 406	TM1	Glu$\rightarrow$Lys at 92	415
435insA	4	Insertion of A after 435		Frameshift	416
441delA	4	Deletion of A at 441 and T$\rightarrow$A at 486		Frameshift	408
457TAT$\rightarrow$G	4	TAT$\rightarrow$G at 457		Frameshift	417; C. Férec et al., personal communication
444delA	4	Deletion of A at 444		Frameshift	418
D110H	4	G$\rightarrow$C at 460		Asp$\rightarrow$His at 110	238
R117H	4	G$\rightarrow$A at 482	TM2	Arg$\rightarrow$His at 117	238
A120T	4	G$\rightarrow$A at 490	TM2	Ala$\rightarrow$Thr at 120	407
Y122X	4	T$\rightarrow$A at 498	TM2	Tyr$\rightarrow$Stop at 122	419
541delC	4	Deletion of C at 541		Frameshift	420
556delA	4	Deletion of A at 556		Frameshift	237
557delT	4	Deletion of T at 557		Frameshift	421
574delA	4	Deletion of A at 574		Frameshift	409
I148T	4	T$\rightarrow$C at 575		Ile$\rightarrow$Thr at 148	422
Q151X	4	C$\rightarrow$T at 583		Gln$\rightarrow$Stop at 151	423
621+1G$\rightarrow$T	Intron 4	G$\rightarrow$T at 621+1		mRNA splicing mutation	237
621+2T$\rightarrow$G	Intron 4	T$\rightarrow$G at 621+2		mRNA splicing mutation	400
622−2A$\rightarrow$C	Intron 4	A$\rightarrow$C at 622−2		mRNA splicing mutation	424
G178R	5	G$\rightarrow$A at 664		Gly$\rightarrow$Arg at 178	237
681delC	5	Deletion of C at 681		Frameshift	408

Table 127-7 Cystic Fibrosis Disease Mutations* *(Continued)*

Name	Location (Exon)	Nucleotide Change	CFTR Domain†	Consequence (e.g., Amino Acid Change)	Reference
711+1G→T	Intron 5	G→T at 711+1		mRNA splicing mutation	237
H199Q	6a	T→G at 729	TM3	His→Gln at 199	M. Dean et al., personal communication
P205S	6a	C→T at 745	TM3	Pro→Ser at 205	425
L206W	6a	T→G at 749	TM3	Leu→Trp at 206	400
Q207X	6a	C→T at 751		Gln→Stop at 207	J. Zielenski et al., personal communication
Q220X	6a	C→T at 790		Gln→Stop at 220	403; M. Schwartz & L. Holmberg, personal communication
C225R	6a	T→C at 805	TM4	Cys→Arg at 225	409
G239R	6a	G→A at 847		Gly→Arg at 239	J. Zielenski et al., personal communication
852del22	6a	Deletion of 22 bp from 852		Frameshift	426
875+1G→C	Intron 6a	G→C at 875+1		mRNA splicing mutation	J. Zielenski et al., personal communication
876−14del12	Intron 6a	Deletion of 12 bp from 876−14		mRNA splicing mutation?	411
977insA	6b	Insertion of A after 977		Frameshift	427
R297Q	7	G→A at 1022		Arg→Gln at 297	428
ΔF311	7	Deletion of 3 bp between 1059 and 1069	TM5	Deletion of Phe310, 311 or 312	429
F311L	7	C→G at 1065	TM5	Phe→Leu at 311	430
G314E	7	G→A at 1073	TM5	Gly→Glu at 314	431
1078delT	7	Deletion of T at 1078	TM5	Frameshift	432
R334W	7	C→T at 1132	TM6	Arg→Trp at 334	433
I336K	7	T→A at 1139	TM6	Ile→Lys at 336	424
T338I	7	C→T at 1145	TM6	Thr→Ile at 338	434
1154insTC	7	Insertion of TC after 1154	TM6	Frameshift	435
1161delC	7	Deletion of C at 1161	TM6	Frameshift	M. Schwarz et al., personal communication
L346P	7	T→C at 1169	TM6	Leu→Pro at 346	436
R347H	7	G→A at 1172	TM6	Arg→His at 347	420
R347L	7	G→T at 1172	TM6	Arg→Leu at 347	411
R347P	7	G→C at 1172	TM6	Arg→Pro at 347	238
M348K	7	T→A at 1175	TM6	Met→Lys at 348	437
A349V	7	C→T at 1178	TM6	Ala→Val at 349	411
R352Q	7	G→A at 1187		Arg→Gln at 352	420
Q359K/T360K	7	C→A at 1207 and C→A at 1211		Glu→Lys at 359 and Thr→Lys at 360	438
1213delT	7	Deletion of T at 1213		Frameshift	435
1221delCT	7	Deletion of CT from 1221		Frameshift	430
W401X	8	G→A at 1335		Trp→Stop at 401	424
1342−2A→C	Intron 8	A→C at 1342−2		mRNA splicing mutation	439
1342−1G→C	Intron 8	G→C at 1342−1		mRNA splicing mutation	410
Q414X	9	C→T at 1372		Gln→Stop at 414	440
1461ins4	9	Insertion of AGAT after 1461		Frameshift	408
A455E	9	C→A at 1496	NBD1	Ala→Glu at 455	441
V456F	9	G→T at 1498	NBD1	Val→Phe at 456	440

(Continues)

Table 127-7 Cystic Fibrosis Disease Mutations* (*Continued*)

Name	Location (Exon)	Nucleotide Change	CFTR Domain†	Consequence (e.g., Amino Acid Change)	Reference
G458V	9	G→T at 1505	NBD1	Gly→Val at 458	442
1525 − 1G→A	Intron 9	G→A at 1525 − 1	NBD1	mRNA splicing mutation	443
S466X	10	C→G at 1529	NBD1	Ser→Stop at 466	444
G480C	10	G→T at 1570	NBD1	Gly→Cys at 480	445
S492F	10	C→T at 1607	NBD1	Ser→Phe at 492	430
Q493X	10	C→T at 1609	NBD1	Gln→Stop at 493	441
1609delCA	10	Deletion of CA from 1609	NBD1	Frameshift	446; 447
Q493R	10	A→G at 1610	NBD1	Gln→Arg at 493	401
E504Q	10	G→C at 1642	NBD1	Glu→Gln at 504	V. Baranov, personal communication
I506S	10	T→G at 1649	NBD1	Ile→Ser at 506	444
ΔI507	10	Deletion of 3 bp between 1648 and 1653	NBD1	Deletion of Ile506 or Ile507	441; 448
ΔF508	10	Deletion of 3 bp between 1652 and 1655	NBD1	Deletion of Phe508	14
1677delTA	10	Deletion of TA from 1677	NBD1	Frameshift	449
V520F	10	G→T at 1690	NBD1	Val→Phe at 520	450
C524X	10	C→A at 1704	NBD1	Cys→Stop at 524	450
Q525X	10	C→T at 1705	NBD1	Gln→Stop at 525	403
1706del17	10	Deletion of 17 bp from 1706	NBD1	Deletion of splice site	451
1717 − 8G→A	Intron 10	G→A at 1717 − 8	NBD1	mRNA splicing mutation?	401
1717 − 1G→A	Intron 10	G→A at 1717 − 1	NBD1	mRNA splicing mutation	441; 452
A534E	11	C→A at 1733	NBD1	Ala→Glu at 534	411
G542X	11	G→T at 1756	NBD1	Gly→Stop at 542	441
S549R(A→C)	11	A→C at 1777	NBD1	Ser→Arg at 549	453
S549N	11	G→A at 1778	NBD1	Ser→Asn at 549	454
S549I	11	G→T at 1778	NBD1	Ser→Ile at 549	441
S549R(T→G)	11	T→G at 1779	NBD1	Ser→Arg at 549	441
G551S	11	G→A at 1783	NBD1	Gly→Ser at 551	455
G551D	11	G→A at 1784	NBD1	Gly→Asp at 551	454
1784delG	11	Deletion of G at 1784	NBD1	Frameshift	456
Q552X	11	C→T at 1786	NBD1	Gln→Stop at 552	456
R553X	11	C→T at 1789	NBD1	Arg→Stop at 553	454
R553Q	11	G→A at 1790	NBD1	Arg→Gln at 553 (associated with ΔF508; "mild")	457
L558S	11	T→C at 1805	NBD1	Leu→Ser at 558	M. Goossens et al., personal communication
A559T	11	G→A at 1807	NBD1	Ala→Thr at 559	454
R560K	11	G→A at 1811	NBD1	Arg→Lys at 560	430
R560T	11	G→C at 1811	NBD1	Arg→Thr at 560; mRNA splicing mutation	441
1811 + 1.2kbA→G	Intron 11	A→G at 1811 + 1.2 kb	NBD1	Creation of splice donor site	X. Estivill & M. Chillón et al., personal communication
1812 − 1G→A	Intron 11	G→A at 1812 − 1	NBD1	mRNA splicing mutation	407
Y563N	12	T→A at 1819	NBD1	Tyr→Asn at 563	441
P574H	12	C→A at 1853	NBD1	Pro→His at 574	441

Table 127-7 Cystic Fibrosis Disease Mutations* (*Continued*)

Name	Location (Exon)	Nucleotide Change	CFTR Domain†	Consequence (e.g., Amino Acid Change)	Reference
E585X	12	G→T at 1885	NBD1	Glu→Stop at 585	420
1898+1G→A	Intron 12	G→A at 1898+1		mRNA splicing mutation	458
1898+1G→C	Intron 12	G→C at 1898+1		mRNA splicing mutation	424
1898+5G→T	Intron 12	G→T at 1898+5		mRNA splicing mutation	J. Zielenski et al., personal communication
1898+73T→G	Intron 12	T→G at 1898+73		mRNA splicing mutation?	L. Smit et al., personal communication
1918delGC	13	Deletion of GC from 1918	R	Frameshift	459
1949del84	13	Deletion of 84 bp from 1949	R	Deletion of 28aa (Met607 to Gln634)	460
D614G	13	A→G at 1973	R	Asp→Gly at 614	437
G628R(G→A)	13	G→A at 2014	R	Gly→Arg at 628	409
G628R(G→C)	13	G→C at 2014	R	Gly→Arg at 628	424
2043delG	13	Deletion of G at 2043	R	Frameshift	409
2118del4	13	Deletion of AACT from 2118	R	Frameshift	459
2143delT	13	Deletion of T at 2143	R	Frameshift	461
2183AA→G	13	A→G at 2183 and deletion of A at 2184	R	Frameshift	422
2184delA	13	Deletion of A at 2184	R	Frameshift	F. Chevalier & D. Bozon, T. Dörk et al., personal communication
2184insA	13	Insertion of A after 2184	R	Frameshift	A Kälin et al., personal communication
F693L	13	T→C at 2209	R	Phe→Leu at 693	437
K710X	13	A→T at 2260	R	Lys→Stop at 710	409
K716X	13	AA→GT at 2277 and 2278	R	Lys→Stop at 716	411
2307insA	13	Insertion of A after 2307	R	Frameshift	462
E730X	13	G→T at 2320	R	Glu→Stop at 730	424
2372del8	13	Deletion of 8 bp from 2372	R	Frameshift	459
R792X	13	C→T at 2506	R	Arg→Stop at 792	400
2522insC	13	Insertion of C after 2522	R	Frameshift	418
2556insAT	13	Insertion of AT after 2556	R	Frameshift	463
E822K	13	G→A at 2596	R	Glu→Lys at 822	464
E827X	13	G→T at 2611	R	Glu→Stop at 827	430
K830X	13	A→T at 2620	R	Lys→Stop at 830	464
2622+1G→A	Intron 13	G→A at 2622+1		mRNA splicing mutation	411
W846X1	14a	G→A at 2669		Trp→Stop at 846	465
W846X	14a	G→A at 2670		Trp→Stop at 846	466
R851X	14a	C→T at 2683		Arg→Stop at 851	467
2721del11	14a	Deletion of 11 bp from 2721		Frameshift	424
C866Y	14a	G→A at 2729	TM7	Cys→Tyr at 866	C. Feréc et al., personal communication
2789+5G→A	Intron 14b	G→A at 2789		mRNA splicing mutation	217
Q890X	15	C→T at 2800		Gln→Stop at 890	468
S912X	15	C→A at 2867	TM8	Ser→Stop at 912	434
2869insG	15	Insertion of G after 2869	TM8	Frameshift	469; 470
Y913C	15	A→G at 2870	TM8	Tyr→Cys at 913	466

(*Continues*)

Table 127-7 **Cystic Fibrosis Disease Mutations*** *(Continued)*

Name	Location (Exon)	Nucleotide Change	CFTR Domain†	Consequence (e.g., Amino Acid Change)	Reference
Y919C	15	A→G at 2888	TM8	Tyr→Cys at 919	401
2907delTT	15	Deletion of TT from 2907		Frameshift	417
2909delT	15	Deletion of T at 2909		Frameshift	456
S945L	15	C→T at 2966		Ser→Leu at 945	400
G970R	15	G→C at 3040		Gly→Arg at 970	424
3041delG	16	Deletion of G at 3041		Frameshift	403
3120G→A	16	G→A at 3120	TM9	mRNA splicing mutation	J. Zielenski et al., personal communication
3120+1G→A	Intron 16	G→A at 3120+1	TM9	mRNA splicing mutation	M. Macek et al., personal communication
3195del6	17a	Deletion of AGTGAT from 3195 to 3200	TM10	Deletion of Val1022 and Ile1023	471
3272−26A→G	Intron 17a	A→G at 3272−26		mRNA splicing mutation?	409
3272−1G→A	Intron 17a	G→A at 3272−1		mRNA splicing mutation	472
F1052V	17b	T→G at 3286		Phe→Val at 1052	472
H1054D	17b	C→G at 3292		His→Asp at 1054	473
G1061R	17b	G→C at 3313		Gly→Arg at 1061	472
3320ins5	17b	Insertion of CTATG after 3320		Frameshift	430
W1063X	17b	G→A at 3321		Trp→Stop at 1063	409
L1065P	17b	T→C at 3326		Leu→Pro at 1065	M. Goossens et al., personal communication
R1066C	17b	C→T at 3328		Arg→Cys at 1066	409
R1066H	17b	G→A at 3329		Arg→His at 1066	430
R1066L	17b	G→T at 3329		Arg→Leu at 1066	472
A1067T	17b	G→A at 3331		Ala→Thr at 1067	430
G1069R	17b	G→A at 3337		Gly→Arg at 1069	401
R1070Q	17b	G→A at 3341		Arg→Gln at 1070	472
3359delCT	17b	Deletion of CT from 3359		Frameshift	472
L1077P	17b	T→C at 3362		Leu→Pro at 1077	422
H1085R	17b	A→G at 3386		His→Arg at 1085	472
W1089X	17b	G→A at 3398		Trp→Stop at 1089	T. Shoshani et al., personal communication
Y1092X	17b	C→A at 3408		Tyr→Stop at 1092	422
W1098R	17b	T→C at 3424		Trp→Arg at 1098	408
M1101K	17b	T→A at 3434		Met→Lys at 1101	474
M1101R	17b	T→G at 3434		Met→Arg at 1101	472
E1104X	17b	G→T at 3442	TM11	Glu→Stop at 1104	408
3601−17T→C	Intron 18	T→C at 3601−17		mRNA splicing mutation?	411
3601−2A→G	Intron 18	A→G at 3601−2		mRNA splicing mutation	443
R1158X	19	C→T at 3604		Arg→Stop at 1158	475
R1162X	19	C→T at 3616		Arg→Stop at 1162	433
3659delC	19	Deletion of C at 3659		Frameshift	441
3662delA	19	Deletion of A at 3662		Frameshift	410
3667del4	19	Deletion of 4 bp from 3667		Frameshift	407
3667ins4	19	Insertion of TCAA after 3667		Frameshift	476
S1196X	19	C→G at 3719		Ser→Stop at 1196	477
3724delG	19	Deletion of G at 3724		Frameshift	478

Table 127-7 Cystic Fibrosis Disease Mutations* (*Continued*)

Name	Location (Exon)	Nucleotide Change	CFTR Domain†	Consequence (e.g., Amino Acid Change)	Reference
3732delA	19	Deletion of A at 3732 and A→G at 3730		Frameshift and Lys→Glu at 1200	409
3737delA	19	Deletion of A at 3737		Frameshift	479
W1204X	19	G→A at 3743		Trp→Stop at 1204	400
3750delAG	19	Deletion of AG from 3750		Frameshift	464
3821delT	19	Deletion of T at 3821		Frameshift	418
I1234V	19	A→G at 3832	NBD2	Ile→Val at 1234	479
S1235R	19	T→G at 3837	NBD2	Ser→Arg at 1235	424
Q1238X	19	C→T at 3844	NBD2	Gln→Stop at 1238	411
3849G→A	19	G→A at 3849	NBD2	mRNA splicing mutation?	410
3849 + 1G→A	Intron 19	G→A at 3849 + 1	NBD2	mRNA splicing mutation	480
3849 + 10kbC→T	Intron 19	C→T in a 6.2 kb *Eco*RI fragment 10 kb from 19	NBD2	Creation of splice acceptor site	217
3849 + 4A→G	Intron 19	A→G at 3849 + 4	NBD2	mRNA splicing mutation?	475
3850 − 1G→A	Intron 19	G→A at 3850 − 1	NBD2	mRNA splicing mutation	411
3850 − 3T→G	Intron 19	T→G at 3850 − 3	NBD2	mRNA splicing mutation	443
3860ins31	20	Insertion of 31 bp after 3860	NBD2	Frameshift	481
G1244E	20	G→A at 3863	NBD2	Gly→Glu at 1244	456
G1244V	20	G→T at 3863	NBD2	Gly→Val at 1244	482
S1251N	20	G→A at 3884	NBD2	Ser→Asn at 1251	483; 464
S1255P	20	T→C at 3895	NBD2	Ser→Pro at 1255	484
S1255X	20	C→A at 3896 and A→G at 3739 in exon 19	NBD2	Ser→Stop at 1255 and Ile→Val at 1203	386
3898incC	20	Insertion of C after 3898	NBD2	Frameshift	411
3905insT	20	Insertion of T after 3905	NBD2	Frameshift	N. Malik et al., personal communication
D1270N	20	G→A at 3940	NBD2	Asp→Asn at 1270	485
W1282R	20	T→C at 3976	NBD2	Trp→Arg at 1282	477
W1282X	20	G→A at 3978	NBD2	Trp→Stop at 1282	466
R1283M	20	G→T at 3980	NBD2	Arg→Met at 1283	486
F1286S	20	T→C at 3989	NBD2	Phe→Ser at 1286	I. Dorvel et al., personal communication
Q1291H	20	G→C at 4005	NBD2	Gln→His at 1291; mRNA splicing mutation (?)	450
4005 + 1G→A	Intron 20	G→A at 4005 + 1	NBD2	mRNA splicing mutation	430
4006 − 19del3	Intron 20	Deletion of 3 bp from 4006 − 19	NBD2	mRNA splicing mutation?	N. Malik et al., personal communication
4010del4	21	Deletion of 4 bp from 4010	NBD2	Frameshift	T. Shoshani et al., personal communication
4016insT	21	Insertion of T at 4016	NBD2	Frameshift	427
N1303H	21	A→C at 4039	NBD2	Asn→His at 1303	479
N1303K	21	C→G at 4041	NBD2	Asn→Lys at 1303	487
W1310X	21	G→A at 4061	NBD2	Trp→Stop at 1310	424
Q1313X	21	C→T at 4069	NBD2	Gln→Stop at 1313	411
W1316X	21	G→A at 4079	NBD2	Trp→Stop at 1316	386

(*Continues*)

Table 127-7 Cystic Fibrosis Disease Mutations* (*Continued*)

Name	Location (Exon)	Nucleotide Change	CFTR Domain†	Consequence (e.g., Amino Acid Change)	Reference
4114ATA→TT	22	ATA→TT from 4114	NBD2	Ile→Leu at 1328 and frameshift	488
G1349D	22	G→A at 4178	NBD2	Gly→Asp at 1349	489
4218insT	22	Insertion of T after 4218	NBD2	Frameshift	424
E1371X	22	G→T at 4243	NBD2	Glu→Stop at 1371	410
4271delC	23	Deletion of C at 4271	NBD2	Frameshift	403
4374+1G→A	Intron 23	G→A at 4374+1		mRNA splicing mutation	409
4374+1G→T	Intron 23	G→T at 4374+1		mRNA splicing mutation	443
4382delA	24	Deletion of A at 4382		Frameshift	400
CF50kbdel#1	4–7, 11–18	Complex deletion involving exons 4–7 and 11–18		Complex deletion	490

*This table lists mutations published or communicated to the CF Genetic Analysis Consortium through April 6, 1994; a complete list may be obtained from the Consortium through L.-C. Tsui. The nucleotide and amino acid numbering systems follow Riordan et al.[13] and the nomenclature is explained in Beaudet and Tsui.[502]

†Domains are NBD for nucleotide binding domains 1 and 2 and TM for transmembrane segments 1 to 12.

Benign Sequence Variations

Many nonpathologic nucleotide substitutions have been detected in various parts of the CFTR gene (Table 127-8). Approximately half of these result in amino acid substitutions as well, but they are regarded as non-disease-causing because they have been found in healthy compound heterozygotes with another known CF mutation. These benign sequence variations may help in elucidating the structure and function of CFTR.

The distinction between a disease-causing mutation and a normal sequence variant is uncertain in some cases. For example, one of these variations occurs at amino acid residue 508, where the phenylalanine codon has been changed to a cysteine codon (F508C). This change is found on both presumed normal[491] and CF[373] alleles, although the evidence

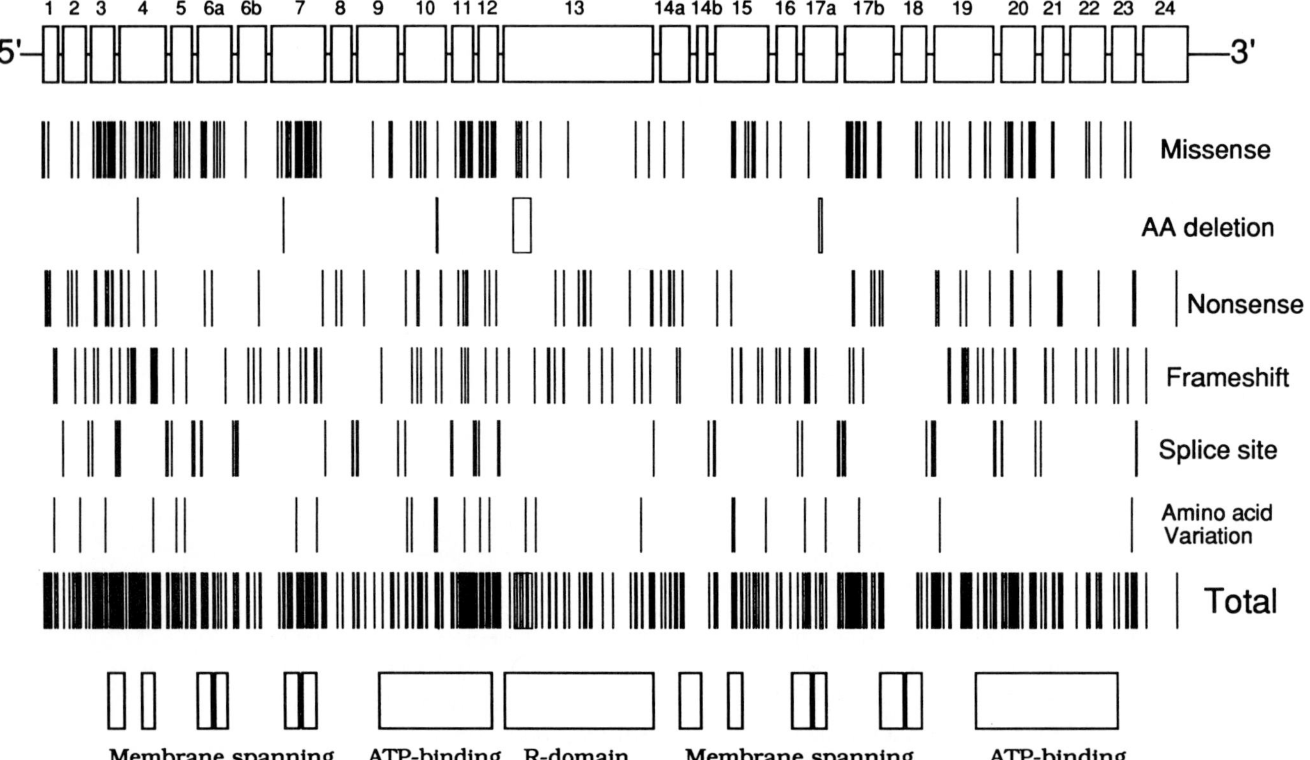

FIG. 127-8 Distribution of cystic fibrosis mutations and amino acid polymorphisms. The schematic diagram contains unpublished data from the CF Genetic Analysis Consortium through April 6, 1994. "Amino acid variation" refers to presumed benign polymorphisms; the other mutations are thought to be pathologic. See Tables 127-7 and 127-8 for more detail.

Table 127-8 Examples of DNA Sequence Polymorphisms and Variations in the CF Gene*

I. Nucleotide Substitutions within the Coding Regions

Name of Nucleotide Substitution	Exon	Amino Acid Change	Reference
263A/T	2	Asp or Val at 44	409
356G/A	3	Arg or Gln at 75	373
873C/T	6a	No change (Tyr at 247)	433
1184C/G	7	Thr or Ser at 351	464
1531C/T	10	Leu or Phe at 467	N. Ghanem et al., personal communication
1540A/G	10	Met or Val at 470	441
1648A/G	10	Ile or Val at 506	491; M. Vidaud et al., personal communication
1651A/G	10	Ile or Val at 507	492
1655T/G	10	Phe or Cys at 508	491
1713A/G	10	No change (Glu at 527)	410
1716G/A	10	No change (Glu at 528)	441
1773A/T	11	No change (Thr at 547)	433
1816G/A	12	Val or Ile at 562	409
1859G/C	12	Gly or Ala at 576	409
2134C/T	13	Arg or Cys at 668	409
2694T/G	14a	No change (Thr at 854)	373
2736G/A	14a	No change (Val at 868)	409; C. Verlingue et al., personal communication
2867C/T	15	Ser or Leu at 912	N. Ghanem et al., personal communication
3030G/A	15	No change (Thr at 966)	493
3032T/C	15	Leu or Ser at 967	400
3123G/C and 3212T/C	17a	Leu or Phe at 997 and Ile or Thr at 1027	409
3332C/T	17b	Ala or Val at 1067	468
3617G/T	19	Arg or Leu at 1162	409
3726G/T	19	No change (Val at 1198)	400
3867A/G	20	No change (Arg at 1245)	P.F. Pignatti, personal communication
4002A/G	20	No change (Pro at 1290)	477; C. Férec et al., personal communication
4029A/G	21	No change (Thr at 1299)	409
4404C/T	24	No change (Tyr at 1424)	T. Shoshani et al., personal communication
4521G/A	24	No change (Gln at 1463)	433

II. DNA Sequence Polymorphisms in the Noncoding Regions

Name of Nucleotide Substitution	Location	Reference
125G/C	G or C at position 125, 5′UT region	410
129G/C	G or C at position 129, 5′UT region (C in strong association with R117H)	237; D. Markiewicz et al., personal communication

(*Continues*)

Table 127-8 Examples of DNA Sequence Polymorphisms and Variations in the CF Gene* (*Continued*)

II. DNA Sequence Polymorphisms in the Noncoding Regions

Name of Nucleotide Substitution	Location	Reference
405 + 46G/T	G or T at position +46 of intron 3	400
875 + 40A/G	A or G at position +40 of intron 6a	409
IVS6 TTGA repeat	Variable number of copies (5–7) in the 5′ flanking region of exon 6b	494; 495; T. Horn et al., personal communication
1001 + 11C/T	C or T at position +11 of intron 6b	424; 409
1001 + 12C/T	C or T at position +12 of intron 6b	V. Nunes & X. Estivill, personal communication
1248 + 17C/T	C or T at position +17 of intron 7	A. Harris, personal communication
IVS8 GT repeat	Variable number of copies of GT repeats (~17) in intron 8 (at around 1342 − 265 to −310)	496
IVS8 GT/T repeat	Variable number of copies of GT repeats (8–10) and T tract (5–9) in intron 8 (at around 1342 − 12 to −35)	381; Chu et al. 1991
1525 − 61A/G	A or G at position −61 of intron 9	T. Ivaschenko et al., personal communication
1525 − 60G/A	G or A at position −60 of intron 9	M. Chillón et al., personal communication
1716 + 12T/C	T or C at position +12 of intron 10	477
dup1716 + 51→61	Duplication of 11 bp in intron 10	446
1898 + 152T/A	T or A at position +152 of intron 12	497
3041 − 71G/C	G or C at position −71 of intron 15	C. Férec et al., personal communication
3121 − 92A12/13	12A or 13A at position −82 of intron 16	417
3271 + 42A/T	A or T at position +42 of intron 17a	424
3272 − 93T/C	T or C at position −93 of intron 17a	417
3499 + 45T/C	T or C at position +45 of intron 17b	J. Zielenski et al., personal communication
IVS17b CA and TA repeats	TA repeats (>25 alleles) and CA repeats (>7 alleles) in intron 17b	498; 499
3500 − 140A/C	A or C at position −140 of intron 17b	R. Parad & C. Gerard, personal communication
3600 − 65C/A	C or A at position −65 of intron 18	500
4005 + 117T/G	T or G at position +117 of intron 20	424; I. Greil et al., personal communication
4006 − 199G/A	G or A at position −199 of intron 20	501

*See footnote to Table 127-7.

favors the interpretation that it is a benign variation that is sometimes present coincidentally on CF chromosomes carrying a pathologic mutation.[507,507a] Another example is R75Q sequence variation[373] that has also been found on a CF chromosome (C. Férec, personal communication). Given the large number of pathologic and benign mutations, it is to be expected that a CF chromosome might easily carry one of each on a coincidental basis.

A sequence variation near the splice donor site in intron 8 is thought to play a role in moderating the splicing efficiency of exon 9.[381] This variation affects the phenotypic severity of the R117H mutation, as described under "Genotype/Phenotype Correlations" below.

EPITHELIAL TRANSPORT ABNORMALITIES

Defective electrolyte transport, particularly defective Cl^- transport, is the hallmark abnormality in CF epithelia. The work that led to this realization was promoted by two clinical aspects of the disease. First, the organs classically involved by CF—sweat glands, airways, pancreas, salivary glands, epididymis, and intestine—are all composed of epithelia. Second, the secretions from several organs appear to be abnormally thick and dehydrated, in consequence of which they obstruct gland ducts. These observations led to basic studies of electrolyte transport by CF epithelia. The resultant findings of abnormal electrolyte transport provided a unifying hypothesis about the biologic defect in numerous organs involved by CF, related the tissue and cellular abnormalities to the genetic defect, and began to provide some insight into the pathophysiology. The following discussion considers abnormalities of electrolyte transport in each organ system.

Sweat Gland Duct

The sweat gland is composed of two different regions, the secretory coil and the reabsorptive duct; Fig. 127-9 shows a schematic representation. The secretory coil produces nearly isotonic fluid. Then, as the sweat passes up through the water-impermeable duct, NaCl is absorbed, and a hypotonic fluid emerges at the surface of the skin. In the secretory coil, active Cl^- transport drives fluid and electrolyte secretion; in the duct, active Na^+ transport drives fluid and electrolyte absorption. In each case, the counterion appears to follow passively.

The clinical observation that Cl^- and Na^+ concentrations are increased in CF sweat led Quinton and colleagues to examine the ion transport properties of the sweat duct.[9,508–511] They found that CF ducts, both in vivo and in vitro, had a higher transepithelial voltage than normal ducts. Normal isolated, perfused ducts generated a voltage of about −7 mV, whereas CF ducts had a voltage of −76 mV (lumen voltage with respect to bath). When luminal Cl^- (or NaCl) concentration was reduced in normal ducts, luminal voltage became more negative; this finding indicates that Cl^- transport is electrically conductive. In contrast, when luminal Cl^- was decreased in CF ducts, transepithelial voltage became more positive. These results indicate that the CF sweat duct is impermeable to Cl^- and suggest that the increased transepithelial voltage results from normal mechanisms for absorption of Na^+ in the presence of impermeability to Cl^-.

Studies of transepithelial electrical conductance support and extend the conclusion that the sweat duct is impermeable to Cl^-.[512] Normal sweat ducts have a transepithelial conductance of approximately 100 to 125 mS/cm^2, 90 percent of which results from a Cl^- conductance. Studies with intracellular microelectrodes indicate that conductive Cl^- flow is predominantly through the cells (transcellular) rather than between the cells through the tight junctions (paracellular). In contrast to normal ducts, CF ducts have a conductance of 10 to 20 mS/cm^2 because Cl^- conductance is low or absent.

Electrophysiological studies of isolated, perfused sweat gland ducts provided insight into the site of the Cl^- permeability defect.[509,513] The results suggested that the Cl^-

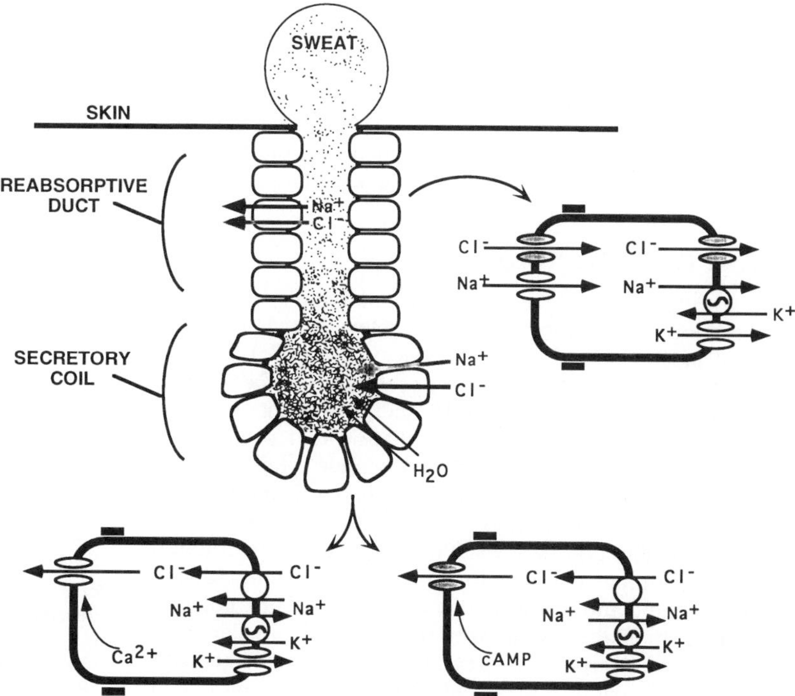

FIG. 127-9 Schematic representation of sweat production and electrolyte transport by the sweat gland. Reabsorptive duct and secretory coil are indicated. Insets show cellular mechanisms of electrolyte transport by duct and coil epithelial cells. Note that cAMP-dependent and Ca^{2+}-dependent Cl^- secretion appear to occur in two different types of cells in the secretory coil. The CFTR Cl^- channel that is defective in CF is indicated by shading; all other channels, transporters, and pumps are indicated by open symbols.

permeability of the apical cell membrane was greatly reduced, as occurs in CF secretory epithelia (see "Defective Transport by CF Airway" below). But, in addition, the basolateral membrane had a significant Cl^- permeability that was reduced in CF. Thus, in the sweat gland duct, Cl^- is transported down its electrochemical gradient across both the apical and basolateral membranes, and Cl^- conductance is reduced at both membranes in CF (Fig. 127-9).[509,511,514–516] The immunocytochemical localization of CFTR to both cell membranes[517,518] supports this interpretation of the electrophysiological abnormalities.

Na^+ absorption in the sweat duct occurs by Na^+ entry into the cell across the apical membrane, driven by a favorable electrochemical gradient (Fig. 127-9). Na^+ then exits across the basolateral membrane in exchange for K^+ via the Na^+, K^+-adenosine triphosphatase (ATPase). K^+ that enters the cell is predominantly recycled via basolateral membrane K^+ channels. These processes establish the ion concentration and voltage gradients that drive Cl^- absorption. Cl^- absorption occurs through channels that are more permeable to Cl^- than to I^-.[519]

Under basal conditions, Cl^- channels at both cell membranes appear to be constitutively open. However, studies with intracellular microelectrodes[516] and halide-specific fluorescent dyes,[520] as well as studies of ducts in which the basolateral membrane had been permeabilized with *Staphylococcus aureus* α-toxin,[521] indicate that the Cl^- conductance is stimulated by agents that increase cellular levels of cAMP. The fact that Cl^- conductance is high in sweat duct epithelia even under basal conditions has suggested either that basal levels of cAMP are relatively high, thereby stimulating kinase activity and phosphorylation of Cl^- channels, or that there is little specific phosphatase activity, so that the Cl^- channels remain in a phosphorylated and activated state.[516]

In addition to regulation by intracellular levels of cAMP, intracellular ATP is required for the Cl^- conductance.[521] Activation of the Cl^- conductance (CFTR Cl^- channels) required millimolar concentrations of ATP. ATP appeared to be required by a process different from phosphorylation, which requires only low levels of ATP. It was speculated that the coupling of Cl^- conductance and thus transepithelial ion transport to cellular ATP levels might provide an adaptive mechanism to protect the epithelium from damage resulting from excessive energy depletion.[521]

In the sweat gland duct, the decreased Cl^- conductance explains the pathophysiology; Cl^- cannot follow Na^+ absorption; hence, NaCl absorption is prevented, and the Na^+ and Cl^- concentrations in the sweat are increased.

Sweat Gland Secretory Coil

The secretory coil of the CF sweat gland can secrete fluid in response to secretagogues that elevate two different second messengers.[522–524] Cholinergic (muscarinic) agonists increase the intracellular Ca^{2+} concentration, $[Ca^{2+}]_c$, and stimulate sweat production. β-Adrenergic agonists increase cellular levels of cAMP and stimulate sweat production, although the rate is less than with cholinergic agonists. Ca^{2+}-dependent secretion is normal in CF, whereas isoproterenol, a β-adrenergic agonist, fails to stimulate secretion in CF. The abnormality does not result from a defective interaction between hormone and receptor, since isoproterenol-induced cAMP accumulation is normal in CF glands.[525] In studies of β-agonist-stimulated sweat secretion in vivo, the glands of normal subjects produced sweat, the glands of subjects with CF failed to sweat, and the glands of heterozygotes produced approximately half as much sweat as those of normal subjects.[526,527]

The secretory coil of the sweat gland contains at least two cell types that are involved in the production of sweat: morphologically, there are clear cells and dark cells, and functionally there are cells that respond to cAMP and β-adrenergic agonists and cells that respond to muscarinic cholinergic agonists (Fig. 127-9, bottom).[528–530] Although the relationship between morphologic appearance and function is not yet certain, it is clear that only cAMP-stimulated secretion is abnormal in CF. The cellular mechanisms of cAMP-stimulated secretion are not as well understood as those of electrolyte absorption in the duct, but they appear to conform to a model for other secretory epithelia[531] (Fig. 127-10).

Airway Epithelium

Cystic fibrosis involves the epithelia lining the airways of the lung. The proximal airway epithelium is a pseudostratified columnar epithelium composed of ciliated cells, goblet cells, and basal cells.[532] The distal airway epithelia is predominantly composed of ciliated and nonciliated bronchiolar (Clara) cells.[533] In addition, the proximal epithelium contains submucosal glands that are composed of both serous and mucous cells and have a duct that is composed of cuboidal ciliated and nonciliated cells.[534,535]

An important function of the airway epithelium is mucociliary clearance, the removal of inhaled particulate material and toxins from the lung (Fig. 127-10). At least three components are required to effect mucociliary clearance. (1) The cilia provide the mechanical force to propel mucus up the airways and out of the lung. (2) The submucosal glands and, to a lesser extent, goblet cells, produce the mucus, which has the viscoelastic properties required to trap inhaled particulate material. (3) The epithelium performs transepithelial electrolyte transport, which controls the quantity and composition of the respiratory tract fluid and may contribute to hydration of the mucus. In CF airways, the primary abnormality in electrolyte transport is thought to alter the quantity of the respiratory tract fluid and possibly the properties of the mucus, so that the mucociliary defense system is impaired.

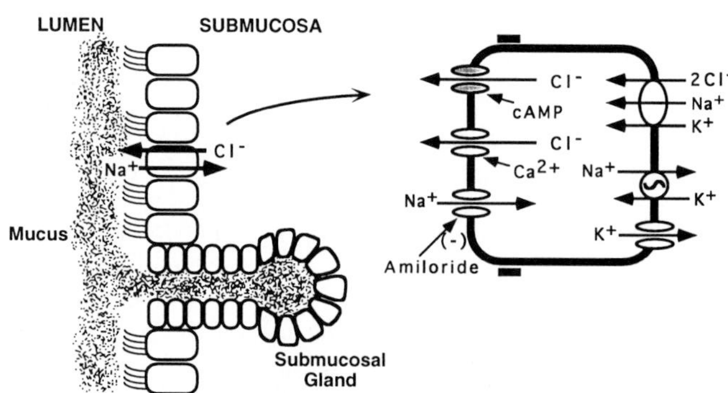

FIG. 127-10 **Schematic representation of mucociliary clearance and electrolyte transport by airway epithelia. Inset shows cellular mechanisms of electrolyte transport by surface epithelial cells; similar mechanisms are used by submucosal gland cells. Serous and mucous cells of the submucosal glands are not shown. Note that cAMP-dependent and Ca^{2+}-dependent Cl^- secretion and amiloride-sensitive Na^+ absorption appear to occur in the same cell type. The CFTR Cl^- channel that is defective in CF is indicated by shading; all other channels, transporters, and pumps are indicated by open symbols.**

Figure 127-10 schematically represents the airway epithelium and the mechanisms of electrolyte transport.[536–539] Human airway epithelium studied in vitro generates a transepithelial electrical potential difference of approximately -10 to -30 mV, with the lumen electrically negative relative to the submucosal surface.[540–542] This value is in good agreement with values measured in vivo.[543–545] The transepithelial electrical resistance ranges from approximately 150 to 1000 $\Omega \cdot cm^2$. When the epithelium is studied in vitro in Ussing chambers and transepithelial voltage is clamped to 0 mV, the resulting current (the short-circuit current) is accounted for by the absorption of Na^+ from the mucosal to the submucosal surface and by secretion of Cl^- from the submucosal to the mucosal surface. Under short-circuit conditions, with no agents added to the bathing solutions, the relative magnitude of net Na^+ and Cl^- transport varies substantially from one species to another and within a species from one airway region to another.[537] However, in humans, electrogenic absorption of Na^+ makes a much greater contribution to the short-circuit current than does secretion of Cl^-. In fact, definite identification of Cl^- secretion in human airway epithelia requires inhibition of Na^+ absorption and stimulation of Cl^- secretion.

In airway epithelia it appears that the ciliated surface cells most likely have the capacity for both Na^+ absorption and Cl^- secretion (Fig. 127-10). The most direct evidence to support this contention comes from intracellular microelectrode studies. During impalement of a single cell, investigators have observed the characteristic electrophysiological responses to agents that alter either the rate of Na^+ transport or the rate of Cl^- secretion.[546] Alternatively, it is possible that a specific cell type absorbs Na^+ and a different cell type secretes Cl^-, but that the cells are electrically coupled. Thus, the electrophysiologic characteristics of both transport processes would be observed during a recording from a single cell. At least in cultured epithelia, there is evidence for functional cell–cell coupling,[547] and gap junctions have been observed microscopically in cultured and native airway epithelia.[548–552]

Regulation of Electrolyte Transport. A variety of neurohumoral and pharmacologic agents regulate the rate of transepithelial electrolyte transport by the airway epithelia.[536] Extracellular signals regulate two main second messengers: cAMP and $[Ca^{2+}]_c$. An increase in the cAMP level activates cAMP-dependent protein kinase, which phosphorylates and thereby regulates specific membrane transport processes. An increase in $[Ca^{2+}]_c$ may have direct effects on transport proteins, as well as activating $[Ca^{2+}]_c$- and calmodulin-dependent kinases. An increase in $[Ca^{2+}]_c$ and diacylglycerol may also activate protein kinase C (PKC), which can modulate transepithelial electrolyte transport.

Most agents that increase intracellular levels of cAMP increase the apical membrane Cl^- permeability and, in many cases, stimulate transepithelial Cl^- secretion.[536] β-Adrenergic agonists were the first agents found to induce secretion and have been some of the most extensively studied.[553–558] When β-adrenergic agonists bind to their receptors, they activate G proteins, which then stimulate adenylate cyclase and increase intracellular levels of cAMP. Cellular levels of cAMP are also increased by a number of other agents, including vasoactive intestinal peptide[559] and adenosine.[560] Prostaglandins appear to be particularly important regulators of transepithelial transport. The airway epithelium produces prostaglandins, which in turn interact with receptors on the epithelium to regulate cellular levels of cAMP.[556,561–563] Moreover, prostaglandin production is regulated by a number of neurotransmitters and inflammatory mediators.

Other agonists stimulate secretion by increasing $[Ca^{2+}]_c$; bradykinin is an example.[564–568] When bradykinin binds to its receptor, it stimulates the hydrolysis of phosphatidylinositol 4,5-bisphosphate, which generates inositol 1,4,5-trisphosphate (IP_3),[566,568] which in turn increases $[Ca^{2+}]_c$. A number of other extracellular agents are also known to increase $[Ca^{2+}]_c$, including substance P,[569] leukotrienes,[570] and nucleotides including ATP.[272,571,572] Extracellular nucleotides are of particular interest, because they interact with receptors on the apical surface of the epithelium and, by activating Ca^{2+}-activated Cl^- channels (see "Ca^{2+}-Activated Cl^- Channels" below), they stimulate transepithelial Cl^- secretion even in CF airway epithelia (Fig. 127-10).

Much less is known about how Na^+ transport is regulated. Under some conditions, cAMP may stimulate Na^+ absorption,[537,573–577] and an increase in $[Ca^{2+}]_c$ may inhibit transport. As in a variety of other Na^+-absorbing epithelia, aldosterone may also regulate Na^+ absorption, although the effects appear to be variable. More work is required to understand the control of Na^+ transport in airway epithelia.

Fluid Transport by Airway Epithelia. Although many studies have examined transepithelial electrolyte transport by airway epithelia, current knowledge of the composition of the respiratory tract fluid and how electrolyte transport generates and regulates fluid transport is inadequate. This is a particular problem because such knowledge might influence approaches to therapy of CF. The paucity of knowledge results, in large part, from the inaccessibility of the respiratory tract fluid. Sputum has been collected and analyzed,[578,579] but sputum also contains mucus and may be modified by cellular debris, bacteria, and saliva, especially in subjects with increased respiratory secretions.[10,580] Collection of sheep and human airway surface fluid in vivo has allowed an analysis of electrolyte concentrations.[581,582] The rate of fluid transport has also been studied in cultured human airway epithelial cells.[583] As predicted from the electrolyte transport data described above, active Na^+ absorption appears to be responsible for fluid absorption under baseline conditions. When the epithelium is treated with amiloride and agonists that increase cellular levels of cAMP, fluid secretion ensues.

The rate of fluid transport that has been measured in a number of studies suggests that fluid transport could easily modify the respiratory tract fluid.[583,584] If it is estimated that the aqueous layer of surface fluid in vivo is approximately 5 μm in depth, one would predict a volume of 500 nl of fluid over each square centimeter of epithelium. Measurements of the rate of fluid transport under basal conditions correspond to the absorption of several times this volume over a 24-h period. In contrast, when epithelia are stimulated to secrete, the rate of fluid secretion would yield at least 10 times this volume in a 24-h period. These results suggest that electrolyte transport can easily modify the surface fluid and that the inability of CF epithelia to modify the rate of ion transport may significantly alter the quantity and composition of the respiratory tract fluid.

Cellular Mechanisms of Electrolyte Transport. Figure 127-10 shows a model that describes our current understanding of how airway epithelial cells secrete Cl^- and absorb Na^+; more extensive discussions are available.[536–539,585] The main features of the model are as follows. (1) Cl^- enters the cell across the basolateral membrane via an electrically neutral cotransport process, coupled to Na^+ and K^+. The entry of Na^+ provides the driving force for accumulation of Cl^- against its electrochemical gradient. (2) Cl^+ exits passively through an apical membrane Cl^- channel, moving down a favorable electrochemical gradient. The regulation of the apical membrane Cl^- permeability controls, in part, the rate of transepithelial secretion. As discussed below, there are at least two types of apical Cl^- channels: those activated by an increase in $[Ca^{2+}]_c$ and those activated when intracellular levels of cAMP increase. The latter are CFTR Cl^- channels. (3) Na^+, which enters the cell at the basolateral membrane coupled to Cl^-, exits across the basolateral membrane via the Na^+,K^+-ATPase. This enzyme provides the energy for transepithelial Cl^- secretion by maintaining a low intracellular Na^+ concentration. The Na^+,K^+-ATPase also accumulates K^+ inside the cell. (4) K^+ exits passively through a basolateral membrane K^+ channel. The basolateral K^+ conductance and the K^+ gradient hyperpolarize the cell, providing the electrical driving force for Cl^- exit and part of the driving force for Na^+ entry at the apical membrane. (5) Na^+ enters the cell passively through an apical membrane Na^+ channel, moving down a favorable electrochemical gradient.

Defective Transport by CF Airway. The clinical observation that CF airway secretions appear thick and dehydrated led Knowles and colleagues to study electrolyte transport by CF respiratory epithelia.[8] They and then others[215,543,586,587] found that, in vivo, the voltage across upper and lower airway epithelia was higher in CF patients (−50 mV, lumen with respect to submucosa) than in normal subjects or diseased control subjects (−20 to −25 mV). This observation suggested a defect in electrolyte transport. The results of subsequent in vivo Cl^- substitution studies and the observation that transepithelial Cl^- fluxes are decreased in excised airway epithelia as well as in CF airway epithelia cultured on permeable supports indicated that CF airway epithelium is relatively impermeable to Cl^-.[541,542,574,586,588–591] Intracellular microelectrode measurements, combined with ion substitution studies, then localized the CF Cl^- impermeability to the cellular pathway and, specifically, to the apical membrane. Thus, in CF epithelia there is a failure of cAMP agonists to activate Cl^- channels in the apical membrane. As a result, cAMP-stimulated Cl^- secretion is abolished.

In contrast, Ca^{2+}-activated Cl^- secretion (Fig. 127-10) remains intact in CF airway epithelia[571,588,590–593] because a different apical membrane Cl^- channel is involved in the response to Ca^{2+} (see "Ca^{2+}-Activated Cl^- Channels" below).

CF airway epithelia also manifest abnormal Na^+ absorption. In excised nasal epithelia and airway epithelial cells grown on permeable supports, the rate of transepithelial Na^+ absorption was two- to threefold greater than in non-CF epithelia.[573–576,589] In addition, cAMP agonists stimulated Na^+ absorption in CF epithelia.[573] The opposite was found in normal epithelia: cAMP either did not change or decreased the rate of Na^+ absorption. The abnormally increased Na^+ transport in CF airway epithelia is due to an increased apical membrane Na^+ permeability. The Na^+ permeability can be inhibited by the addition of amiloride to the apical surface; this observation has formed the basis of studies directed at using inhaled amiloride as therapeutic intervention in patients with CF.[271]

It is thought that the increased rate of Na^+ transport and the decreased Cl^- permeability combine to produce an abnormal, dehydrated respiratory tract fluid. Of note, studies of ion transport by cells cultured from human submucosal glands show defects in Cl^- transport similar to those observed in the surface epithelium.[594,595] At present the relative contribution of abnormal ion transport by the surface epithelium and by the gland epithelium to the pathogenesis and pathology of the disease is uncertain.

Pancreas

The pancreatic secretory system appears to be composed of at least two functionally distinct systems: the acinar system and the pancreatic ducts. The acinar system secretes a relatively low volume of enzyme in response to stimulation by cholecystokinin and acetylcholine. The small pancreatic ducts are thought to secrete fluid to increase both the volume and the HCO_3^- content of the luminal fluid. Kopelman and colleagues[11] studied pancreatic secretions from CF subjects before total organ failure developed and from control subjects with similar levels of pancreatic acinar function. In CF secretions, they found higher concentrations of protein than in controls, primarily because the CF pancreas secreted less fluid at all levels of pancreatic function. This work suggested that the site of the CF defect in the pancreas was in the ducts. Of note, immunocytochemical studies have supported this conclusion by localizing CFTR to the small pancreatic ducts.[596]

In the apical membrance of the ducts, Cl^- channels are thought to work in parallel with Cl^-, HCO_3^- exchangers to secrete a HCO_3^--rich fluid. Cl^- is thought to enter the lumen through Cl^- channels. It is then recycled back across the apical membrane into the cell in exchange for intracellular HCO_3^-. The Cl^- channel responsible for apical Cl^- transport has been identified by patch-clamp analysis.[597–600] An increase in cellular levels of cAMP opens apical Cl^- channels that have a low conductance (~5 pS), have a linear current–voltage (I-V) relationship, are not blocked by 4,4′-diisothiocyanato-stilbene-2,2′-disulphonic acid (DIDS), are blocked by 5-nitro-2-(3-phenylpropylamino)benzoic acid (NPPB), and are more permeable to Cl^- than to I^-. These properties are similar to those observed for Cl^- channels in airway epithelia and in cells expressing recombinant CFTR (see "Evidence that CFTR is a Cl^- Channel" below).

The loss of cAMP-stimulated fluid secretion in CF pancreatic ducts is thought to produce fluid that is abnormally dehydrated. As a result, the ducts become plugged by thick secretions, and obstruction may lead to destruction of the organ.

Intestine

The intestine exhibits a large diversity of absorptive and secretory processes both along its length and in specific regions. The most consistent abnormality observed in CF has been the loss of cAMP-stimulated Cl^- secretion.[601–606] The cellular mechanism of intestinal Cl^- secretion appears to be similar to that of airway epithelium (Fig. 127-10), with Cl^- entry at the basolateral membrane via a $Na^+,K^+,2Cl^-$ cotransport process and Cl^- exit across the apical membrane via Cl^- channels. The ion channels that are activated when cellular levels of cAMP increase have been most extensively studied in Cl^--secreting cell lines derived from intestinal tumors. In T84 cells, HT29 cells, and Caco-2 cells, the Cl^- channels that mediate cAMP-dependent secretion[592,607–612] have properties similar to those generated by expression of CFTR (see "Function of CFTR" below): they are activated by an increase in cellular levels of cAMP or by cAMP-dependent protein kinase (PKA) in excised patches of membrane; they have a small single-channel conductance (4 to 10 pS); the I-V relationship is linear; they are more permeable to Cl^- than to I^-; they show little in the way of time-dependent voltage effects; they are variably blocked by NPPB; and they are not blocked by DIDS. In T84 cells, it has been shown that they are also dependent on cytosolic ATP.[613]

In contrast to the airway, where Ca^{2+}-dependent Cl^- secretion is similar in normal and CF epithelia, Ca^{2+}-stimulated Cl^- secretion is defective in intestinal epithelium. Although this observation initially suggested that there might be tissue-specific regulation of apical Cl^- channels in CF, it now appears that the observation is explained by the lack of apical membrane Ca^{2+}-activated Cl^- channels in at least some intestinal epithelia (see "Ca^{2+}-Activated Cl^- Channels" below).

Because the amiloride-sensitive Na^+ current is increased in airway epithelia, absorptive processes have been studied in the intestine. Glucose-coupled Na^+ transport is normal in CF.[601–603] The amiloride-inhibitable component of electrogenic Na^+ transport also appears to be normal in CF.[603,614]

The abnormal electrolyte transport by CF intestinal epithelia may lead to an alteration of the composition of the lumenal contents. The lack of Cl^- secretion to counterbalance intestinal absorptive processes could reduce the fluid content in the intestinal lumen, causing dehydration and hence impaction.[602] Thus, it may cause the meconium ileus and distal intestinal obstruction found in patients with CF.

Male Genital Tract

The observation that most males with CF are sterile and observations of histologic changes in the epididymis and vas deferens have suggested that ion transport abnormalities in these ducts may occur in CF. Studies of the epididymis from rats have shown that the epithelium secretes Cl^- and HCO_3^-.[615,616] The mechanism of secretion is most likely similar to that observed in airway epithelia and in pancreatic ducts, with anion accumulation processes at the basolateral membrane and anion channels at the apical membrane.

Studies of epididymal cells using the patch-clamp technique have demonstrated the presence of a low-conductance Cl^- channel (3 to 5 pS) that was activated by addition of cAMP agonists to the cells.[617] The channel showed only slight time-dependent voltage effects and was more permeable to Cl^- than to HCO_3^-. This channel most likely represents the CFTR Cl^- channel. It has been suggested that dysfunction of this channel in CF may result in thickened secretions that plug the small ducts of the male genital tract, thereby producing the pathology and sterility in males with CF.

THE CFTR PROTEIN

Predicted Structure of CFTR and Relationship to Other Proteins

Identification of the primary sequence of CFTR[13] allowed the prediction of a potential structure. In large part, predictions were based on a comparison of CFTR with a family of proteins named the traffic ATPases[618] or ABC (ATP-binding cassette) transporters.[619] As shown in Fig. 127-11, CFTR was predicted to contain five domains: two membrane-spanning domains (MSD), each composed of six transmembrane segments; an R domain, which contains several consen-

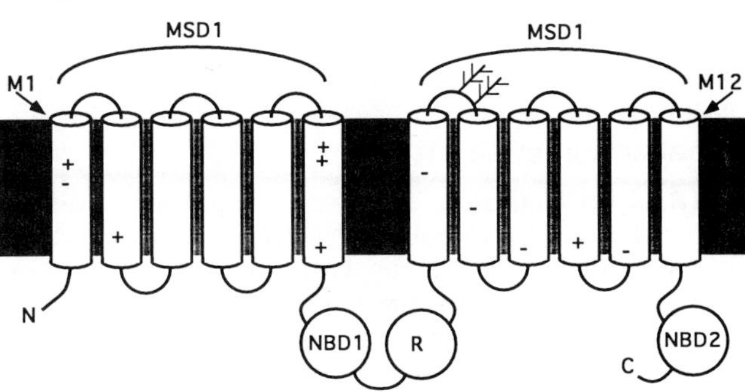

FIG. 127-11 Model showing the proposed domain structure of CFTR. MSD refers to the membrane-spanning domains and NBD refers to the nucleotide-binding domains. The membrane is represented by the shaded area. Sites of charged residues in the MSD are indicated by + and −. Glycosylation sites between M7 and M8 are indicated as branched structures.

sus phosphorylation sequences; and two nucleotide-binding domains (NBD), which were predicted to interact with ATP. Sequence similarity in the two NBDs, the prediction of two membrane-spanning domains, and the overall topology were features that placed CFTR in the traffic ATPase/ABC transporter family. That family includes periplasmic permeases in prokaryotes, such as the histidine and maltose transport systems; STE6, involved in the secretion of A mating factor in yeast; and P-glycoprotein, responsible for multidrug resistance. The R domain, with its many potential phosphorylation sites and multiple charged amino acids, is a unique feature of CFTR, not shared by other members of the family. The primary sequence of CFTR did not resemble that of any known ion channels.

Topology of CFTR

The identification of stretches of hydrophobic residues within its sequence suggested that CFTR was a membrane protein. The development of antibodies that recognize CFTR and the expression of recombinant CFTR in vitro and in vivo showed that this prediction was correct: CFTR is a membrane-associated glycoprotein.[620]

Although present knowledge is incomplete, several findings have provided preliminary information about the topology of CFTR (Fig. 127-11). Studies with antibodies in permeabilized and nonpermeabilized cells have placed the loop between M1 and M2 on the extracellular surface, and the R domain and C-terminus on the intracellular surface.[621] As will be described below, functional studies also place the R domain and the two NBDs on the cytosolic side of the membrane. Because there is no signal sequence, the N-terminus is probably intracellular.[13] Thus, it is likely that M1 spans the bilayer. Asparagines 894 and 900 between M7 and M8 are glycosylated[622,623]; thus, they presumably lie on the extracellular surface. These results also suggest that M7 spans the bilayer, because it lies between the intracellular R domain and the extracellular glycosylation sites.

Thus, present data about the topology of CFTR agree with predictions made from the primary sequence. The actual topology may not, however, be exactly as predicted. For example, in contrast to the original predictions that they would have 12 membrane-spanning sequences, two other members of the traffic ATPase/ABC transporter family—the P-glycoprotein[624,625] and the histidine transport system[626]—probably contain only 10 membrane-spanning sequences. In addition to knowledge of its topology, it will be important to learn if CFTR functions as a monomer or as a multimer; at present there are no data that directly address this issue.

Localization of CFTR

CFTR is predominately expressed in epithelia. Northern blot analysis of CFTR mRNA suggested it was expressed in the epithelia affected by CF.[13] Studies using in-situ hybridization confirmed and extended the assignment of CFTR to epithelial tissues,[627–630] including the pancreatic ductal cells, salivary glands, intestine (where the crypts express more than the villus), lung (where submucosal glands express more than the airway surface epithelium), testis, and endometrium. In the human fetus, CFTR has been detected in the airway epithelium of the lung.[631] RT-PCR, which provides a very sensitive assay, has also allowed detection of CFTR transcripts in lymphocytes, monocytes, neutrophils, and fibroblasts,[632,633] although the biologic and clinical significance of expression in these cells is uncertain. CFTR has also been detected by PCR and functional analysis in the heart.[634,635]

A number of antibodies have been used in immunocytochemical studies to localize CFTR to the apical region of polarized epithelia cells, including small pancreatic ducts, intestinal crypts, sweat gland ducts, airway epithelia (where submucosal glands contained more than the surface epithelia), Cl^--secreting epithelial cell lines, and kidney tubules.[517,518,596,621,636–643] Figure 127-12 shows an example of the localization of CFTR to the apical region of the T84 intestinal cell line.

Evidence that CFTR is located *within* the apical membrane has come from two kinds of studies. In one study, an antibody directed against an extracellular epitope labeled the apical membrane of unpermeabilized intestinal epithelial cell lines and primary cultures of airway epithelia.[621,637] In contrast, antibodies directed against intracellular epitopes of CFTR could only label the protein after the cells had been permeabilized. In other studies, CFTR was biochemically labeled from the extracellular surface using a hydrazide reagent to biotinylate the protein.[644] Although most studies show CFTR localized at the apical membrane, functional[509,513] and immunohistochemical[517,518] studies suggest that in the sweat gland duct epithelium, CFTR may be localized at the basolateral membrane as well as the apical membrane. This result suggests the presence of cell-specific factors that can direct the targeting of CFTR.

CFTR is also located within intracellular vesicles beneath the apical membrane. Labeling of cell-surface CFTR suggested that only half the protein was available for labeling and that the other half was intracellular.[644] Light-level immunocytochemical studies have also suggested the presence of subapical CFTR but have been unable to convincingly characterize it.[517,621,636–639] Immunoelectron photomicrographs have shown CFTR on intracellular vesicles,[639] but the identity of the vesicles and the quantitative distribution of the protein are not yet certain. Preliminary studies suggest that much of the intracellular CFTR may be located on clathrin-coated vesicles.[645] Studies of cells expressing recombinant CFTR suggest that CFTR on endosomes is functionally active.[646]

Localization of CFTR to the apical membrane places it in a position where it can directly mediate Cl^- transport. In the apical membrane, it serves as a pathway by which Cl^- moves from the cell into the lumen, and, in so doing, it regulates the rate of transepithelial Cl^- movement. The function of CFTR on intracellular membranes is less certain; it may function in parallel with H^+ pumps to acidify intracellular vesicles.[311] By changing the degree of vesicle acidification, the presence or absence of CFTR Cl^- channels might alter pH-sensitive enzymatic processes. It is also possible that CFTR, located either in the apical membrane or on intracellular vesicles, may regulate vesicle endocytosis or exocytosis.[647] Additional work is required to provide further insight into the function of CFTR on intracellular vesicles.

It is interesting to note that the epithelia lining the pulmonary airways express little CFTR,[627,630,637,648] yet the Cl^- channel function (and its absence in CF) is easily measured, and the airway epithelia are a site of disease. The Cl^- channel function of CFTR is readily measured because ion chennels are very efficient, with an ability to transport 10^6 to 10^7 ions/s. Thus, a relatively small number of CFTR molecules are sufficient to support transepithelial Cl^- transport.

FUNCTION OF CFTR

Evidence that CFTR Is a Cl^- Channel

In the first functional studies, CFTR cDNA was expressed in CF airway and pancreatic epithelial cells.[620,649,650] Expression of wild-type CFTR corrected the defect in cAMP-regulated Cl^- premeability. This observation demonstrated a causal relationship between mutations in the CFTR gene and the CF phenotype. But those results did not identify the function of CFTR. Data obtained since then provide compelling evidence that CFTR is a Cl^- channel.

Expression of CFTR Generates Cl^- Channels. The first evidence that CFTR was a Cl^- channel came from studies in which CFTR was expressed in cells that do not normally contain cAMP-regulated Cl^- channels and express little or no endogenous CFTR. CFTR has been expressed in a number of mammalian and nonmammalian cells, including NIH 3T3 fibroblasts, Chinese hamster ovary cells, HeLa cells, mouse L cells, Vero cells, CF-PAC cells, IEC-6 intestinal cells, Sf9 insect cells, and *Xenopus* oocytes.[15,651–662] In each case, expression of CFTR generated a unique Cl^- current that was activated by cAMP agonists.

CFTR Is in the Apical Membrane. As indicated above, both CFTR and the cAMP-regulated Cl^- channels that are defective in CF are located in the apical membrane. Colocalization is necessary but not in itself sufficient to support the hypothesis that CFTR is a Cl^- channel.

Cl^- Channels from Recombinant CFTR and from Endogenous CFTR in Epithelia Have Identical Properties. The regulatory and biophysical properties of Cl^- currents are the same in cells expressing recombinant CFTR, in epithelial cells expressing endogenous CFTR,[591,607,608,663,664] and in the apical membrane of Cl^- secretory epithelia.[591] One defining property is channel regulation. Under baseline conditions, there is little, if any, Cl^- current. But following addition of cAMP agonists, there is a dramatic increase in Cl^- current measured with either the whole-cell or the single-channel patch-clamp technique. An increase in intracellular Ca^{2+} does not activate CFTR Cl^- channels.

Figure 127-13*A* shows an example of single-channel traces from a CFTR Cl^- channel; Fig. 127-13*B* shows the corres-

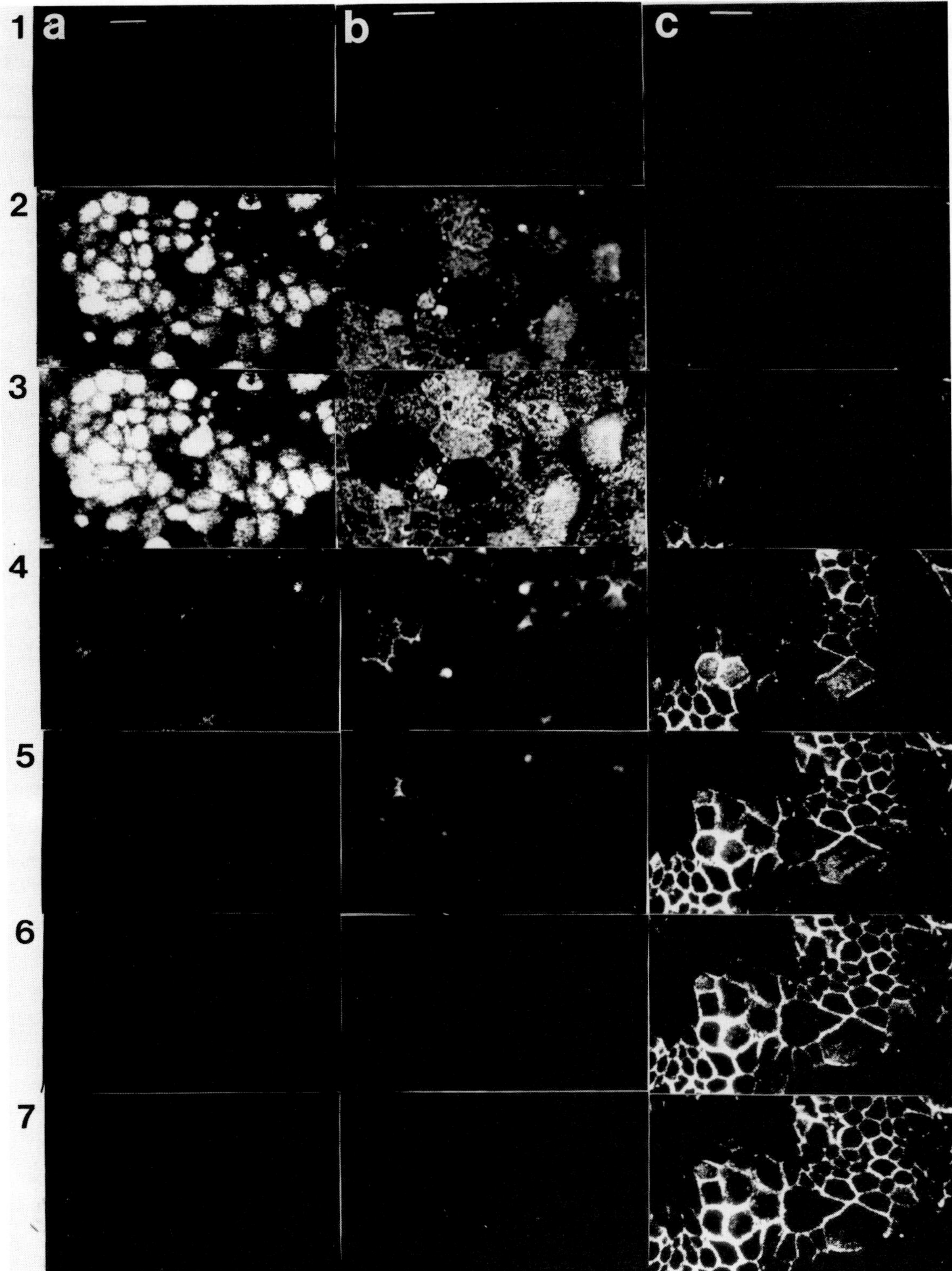

FIG. 127-12 **Comparison of the immunofluorescence staining pattern of CFTR with the patterns for apical and basolateral membrane proteins in polarized monolayers of T84 cells. A series of confocal images were collected, starting above the cell monolayer and moving toward the filter support in 2 μm increments. Cells were stained with an antibody against the C-terminus of CFTR (*a* 1–7), or with FITC-conjugated streptavidin after membrane-specific biotinylation of the apical (*b* 1–7) or basolateral (*c* 1–7) surface of the cells. Bars, 10 μm. (*From Denning et al.*[621] *Used by permission of the* Journal of Clinical Investigation.)**

ponding current–voltage (I-V) relationship. The channel has a small conductance (6 to 10 pS) and a linear I-V relationship, and is selective for anions over cations. In studies of the apical membrane, as well as in whole-cell and single-channel studies, time-dependent voltage effects are slight or absent. The anion permeability sequence is $Br^- > Cl^- > I^-$. This sequence is a distinguishing feature of CFTR Cl^- currents, because it differs from the reported anion selectivity sequences of many although not all other epithelial and nonepithelial Cl^- channels.[609,612,665]

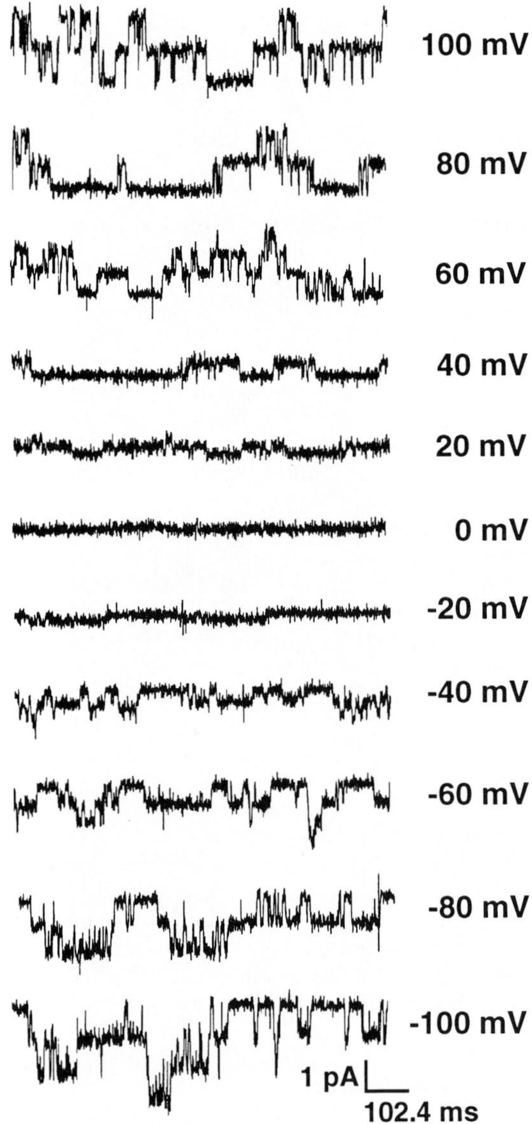

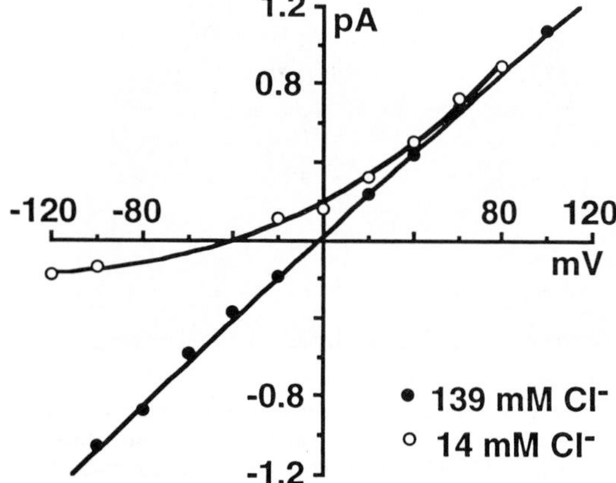

FIG. 127-13 Single-channel current traces from an excised, inside-out patch of membrane. *A*. Patch contains at least three active channels. Patch was obtained from a 3T3 fibroblast expressing CFTR, and the cytosolic surface of the membrane was exposed to PKA and 1 m*M* ATP. Voltages are indicated. I-V relationship is shown in *B*. Pipette contained 140 m*M* Cl^-; bath Cl^- concentration was 139 m*M* in *A* and as indicated in *B*. *(From Berger et al.*[653] *Used by permission of the* Journal of Clinical Investigation.)

Alteration of Specific Residues in CFTR Alters the Properties of Cl^- Channels. CFTR contains six positively charged amino acids in the putative membrane-spanning sequences (Fig. 127-11). These residues are conserved across species, suggesting conservation of function. Four of the basic residues were individually converted to acidic residues[651]; it was reasoned that, if CFTR is itself a Cl^- channel, then altering the charge on residues that might contribute to the ion conduction pathway could alter the channel's properties. Similar strategies have identified amino acid sequences that contribute to the pore of voltage-dependent K^+ channels,[666,667] the nicotinic acetylcholine receptor,[668] and the mitochondrial voltage-dependent anion-selective channel.[669]

Many properties of CFTR were unchanged by the mutations. In each mutant, cAMP-dependent channel regulation was intact, and selectivity for Cl^- over Na^+ was unaltered. Thus, the mutations did not cause a general disruption of channel structure. Yet two mutations, K95D and K335E, each altered anion selectivity. With both mutations, the permeability sequence was converted from $Br^- > Cl^- > I^-$ to $I^- > Br^- > Cl^-$. The two mutations were not, however, equivalent: unlike the changes in permeability, only K335E changed the conductivity sequence from $Br^- \geq Cl^- > I^-$ to $Br^- > I^- > Cl^-$. Mutation of two other basic residues, R347E and R1030E, did not change the selectivity sequence. It is interesting that in the topological model of CFTR (Fig. 127-11), both K95 and K335 are predicted to lie toward the outer half of the channel, whereas R347 and R1030 lie toward the inner half of the channel.

CFTR variants containing three different missense mutations that are associated with CF[238,670–672]—R117H, R334W, and R347P—also produced regulated Cl^- channels that had altered conduction properties.[673] Patch-clamp analysis revealed that all three mutants had reduced single-channel conductances. In addition, R117H exhibited altered sensitivity to external pH and had altered single-channel kinetics. The ability of mutations in residues R117, R334, and R347 to alter the properties of the Cl^- channel supports the conclusion that CFTR is a Cl^- channel.

Incorporation of Purified CFTR into Planar Lipid Bilayers Produces Cl^- Channels. CFTR was purified from Sf9 cells, reconstituted into proteoliposomes, and fused with bilayers.[674] Addition of PKA and ATP to the bathing solution activated low-conductance, Cl^--selective channels that had a linear I-V relationship and showed no appreciable time-dependent voltage effects. These properties were the same as those observed in the native cell membrane. These data indicate that CFTR is a Cl^- channel and argue that the channel does not require loosely associated factors for regulation or function. Similar results have been obtained when membrane vesicles from cells expressing high levels of CFTR have been fused with bilayers.[674,675]

The Membrane-Spanning Domains May Contribute to the Channel Pore. In CFTR, M1 through M12 are predicted to form membrane-spanning alpha helices. Because mutation of residues R334, K335, and R347 altered specific properties of the pore and because all these residues are located in the putative M6, M6 may contribute to the pore of the CFTR Cl^- channel. The finding that mutations in M1 (K95) and at the external surface of M2 (R117) also alter specific pore properties suggests that the permeation pathway may also involve these regions of CFTR. However, current data are insufficient to provide much insight into which sequences actually line the pore and which are involved in interactions with regions that line the pore.

In voltage-gated K^+ channels, a hydrophobic sequence between S5 and S6 appears to contribute to the pore, perhaps as a β sheet as reviewed elsewhere.[676] Could an unsuspected part of the CFTR sequence contribute to the pore? Perhaps—but, in contrast to the *Shaker* K^+ channel, where hydrophobic residues led to the prediction that the sequence between S5 and S6 contributes to the pore, no similar sequence has been identified in CFTR. Work with the histidine transport system, another member of the traffic ATPase/ABC transporter family, yields a particularly intriguing suggestion.[677] In that system, *HisP*—the protein analogous to the NBD of CFTR—may interact with the membrane via interactions with *HisQ* and *HisM*, the proteins analogous to the MSD of CFTR. Could either or both of the NBDs of CFTR interact with the MSDs, thereby contributing to the formation of a pore[678]? Such an interaction could potentially provide a mechanism for coupling the activity of the NBDs (see "Regulation by Intracellular Nucleotides" below) with ion flow through the pore.

Other Functions of CFTR

The conclusion that CFTR is a Cl^- channel does not exclude the possibility that it has additional functions. Two lines of reasoning argue that CFTR must have additional functions other than those of a Cl^- channel. First, most members of the traffic ATPase/ABC transporter family appear to actively transport substrate across membranes. Thus, it is possible that CFTR might, under some circumstances, actively transport as yet unidentified substances. This possibility is given credence by the observation that expression of the P-glycoprotein or multiple drug resistance (MDR) protein is associated with volume-regulated Cl^- channels, as well as with transport of hydrophobic drugs out of cells.[679,680] (Note, however, that at present there is no definite evidence that MDR is itself a Cl^- channel.) Second, numerous phenotypic abnormalities have been observed in CF epithelia, including increased electrogenic Na^+ absorption, increased sulfation of glycoconjugates, and abnormal regulation of outwardly-rectifying Cl^- channels. It is not currently understood how these multiple phenotypic abnormalities could be produced solely by a defect in a Cl^- channel, and, thus, additional functions for CFTR have been proposed.

The rejoinder to these contentions is the following. First, the observation that some members of the traffic ATPase/ABC transporter family actively transport substrate does not necessarily mean that CFTR also performs active transport, just as the observation that CFTR is an ion channel does not mean that other proteins in this family are also ion channels. Second, unexplained phenotypic abnormalities in CF might be secondary to loss of Cl^- channel function, although the mechanisms involved are at present obscure. By analogy, CF is not the only human disease in which mutation of a single gene encoding a Cl^- channel can produce multiple phenotypic abnormalities in affected cells: mutations of the ClC-1 skeletal-muscle Cl^- channel cause autosomal recessive generalized myotonia (Becker disease), yet alterations in both Cl^- and Na^+ currents have been reported in muscle cells.[681] Thus, it is possible that a single-gene defect may produce a number of secondary manifestations. Clearly, additional research is required to explore these issues and to understand how the loss of CFTR function· produces multiple phenotypic abnormalities.

Several studies have suggested that CFTR may affect the endocytosis and exocytosis of membrane vesicles. In the T84 colonic epithelial cell line which expresses CFTR, intracellular cAMP-regulated membrane recycling occurs.[682,683] In CF pancreatic epithelial cells, expression of recombinant CFTR conferred cAMP-dependent plasma membrane recycling. In CF cells expressing wild-type CFTR, but not in the uncorrected cells, cAMP agonists inhibited endocytosis and stimulated exocytosis.[647] At present, it is not clear how CFTR controls membrane recycling. However, it is possible that Cl^- channel function either in the plasma membrane or in the membrane of endosomes could influence the insertion and retrieval of membrane. The identity of the intracellular vesicles that contain CFTR has not yet been extensively investigated, but they likely include clathrin-coated vesicles.[645]

Although CFTR may regulate endocytosis and exocytosis, the fusion of vesicles with the plasma membrane is not required for the activation of an apical membrane Cl^- conductance and for stimulation of Cl^- secretion. CFTR is present in the apical membrane of T84 intestinal epithelia[621,644] and primary cultures of airway epithelia[637] even in the absence of cAMP-dependent stimulation. Moreover, insertion of channels by fusion of vesicles with the apical membrane was not required for a cAMP-mediated increase in apical membrane Cl^- conductance,[621] nor did cAMP agonists appear to increase the amount of CFTR in the plasma membrane.[644]

One hypothesis about how Cl^- channel dysfunction could cause multiple phenotypic abnormalities in CF involves the suggestion that CFTR Cl^- channels located on endosomal vesicles of epithelia are involved in acidification of the vesicle interior. Some intracellular vesicles are acidified by a proton pump and a Cl^- channel, located in parallel on the vesicular membrane. The proton pump provides the driving force for acidification, and the Cl^- channel provides both a pathway for anion movement (to maintain electroneutrality) and a means to regulate acidification. In some cases, the proton pump is constitutively active and the opening and closing of Cl^- channels regulates acidification. It has been proposed[311] that CFTR Cl^- channels are located on such vesicles and that the loss of CFTR Cl^- channel function in endosomes leads to defective acidification of intracellular compartments. Defective acidification of the trans-Golgi complex, endosomes, and prelysosomes in CF airway epithelia might alter the activity of pH-sensitive trans-Golgi enzymes, such as sialyltransferases. As a result, sialylation of glycoproteins and glycolipids and protein sulfation might be altered in CF.[313,684–686] Altered processing of surface proteins might in turn contribute to the colonization and adherence of microorganisms on the airway epithelium. This intriguing hypothesis has not yet been proven, although studies have shown that CFTR can function as a regulated Cl^- channel on intracellular vesicles.[646]

Relationship of CFTR to Other Cl^- Channels

Outwardly-Rectifying Cl^- Channels. Early patch-clamp studies of epithelial cells identified a Cl^- channel with a characteristic outwardly-rectifying I-V relationship in excised membrane patches bathed by symmetrical Cl^- solutions. The slope conductance measured at 0 mV was in the range 25 to 50 pS. This channel has been identified in many epithelia and, interestingly, has also been found in nonepithelial tissues, including fibroblasts and lymphocytes.[687,688] Its biophysical properties have been characterized in detail, as reviewed elsewhere.[609,689] The channel is more permeable to I^- than to Cl^-, and it is inhibited by DIDS, diphenylamine 2-carboxylic acid (DPC), and a large number of newly developed blockers.[690–692] The channel is also inhibited by

HEPES and related biological buffers[693]; such inhibition may contribute, in part, to the outward rectification of the I-V relationship. Variable effects of membrane potential on channel open-state probability (P_o) have been reported.[694–698]

A curious and distinguishing feature of the outwardly-rectifying channel was that in excised membrane patches it could often be activated by sustained strong membrane depolarization.[699–702] However, membrane depolarization only activated the channel in excised, cell-free patches of membrane; in cell-attached membrane patches, depolarization failed to activate the outward rectifier.[694,702] The channel could also be activated by a number of other interventions, including increasing temperature (37°C vs. 20 to 23°C[702,703]), application of trypsin to the internal membrane surface,[702] bathing the internal surface with solutions containing high salt concentrations, increasing pH,[701] and altering the electrolyte composition of the solution.[701] Many of these maneuvers may somehow alter the stability of the channel protein.

Several studies of the outwardly-rectifying Cl^- channel indicated that it can be activated by adding the catalytic subunit of PKA or PKC in excised, inside-out patches of membrane from airway or intestinal epithelia.[605,694,695,697,699,700,703–709] Moreover, such regulation was reported to be defective in CF cells. Regulation of this channel by PKA has not, however, been consistent or always reproducible[696,701,710] and, at least in the cell-attached mode, appeared to occur in only a small percentage of patches.[706,710]

Because its regulation was found to be defective in CF, a great deal of attention was focused on the outwardly-rectifying Cl^- channel. It was an attractive hypothesis that this channel might be the product of the CFTR gene. However, it is now clear that the CFTR Cl^- channel and the outwardly-rectifying Cl^- channel are two different proteins. Specifically, (1) they manifest very different biophysical properties, including anion selectivity, single-channel conductance, rectification, and sensitivity to blockers[612]; (2) they have very different regulatory properties[612]; (3) there is no correlation between the presence of CFTR transcripts and the presence of outwardly-rectifying Cl^- channels[711]; and (4) outwardly-rectifying Cl^- channels are observed in epithelia from mice in which the gene for CFTR has been disrupted.[712] Nevertheless, the studies in CF epithelia that were described above suggest that expression of CFTR in some way influences the regulation of outwardly-rectifying Cl^- channels. That suggestion was supported by two additional studies. First, when wild-type CFTR was expressed in CF airway epithelial cells, outwardly-rectifying Cl^- channels were activated by PKA.[713] Second, in airway epithelial cells from mice in which the CFTR gene was disrupted, outwardly-rectifying Cl^- channels were not activated by PKA, whereas they were opened by PKA in normal mice.[712]

What then is the physiological function of the outwardly-rectifying Cl^- channel? There are several points to consider. First, because its properties are different from those of the cAMP- and Ca^{2+}-activated apical membrane Cl^- currents, it is not directly involved in the transepithelial Cl^- secretion stimulated by these second messengers. Second, because it shares many properties with volume-activated Cl^- channels, the two may be one and the same.[714] Third, the location of the channel in polarized epithelia is not known; such knowledge is essential for any attempt to decipher its physiological function in epithelia. Fourth, the channel may not have a function unique to epithelia; this speculation might explain the fact that the channel is observed in a wide variety of nonepithelial cells.

Ca^{2+}-Activated Cl^- Channels. Ca^{2+}-activated Cl^- channels are also different from CFTR Cl^- channels; for a review, see Anderson et al.[612] In contrast to cAMP-stimulated Cl^- secretion, Ca^{2+}-stimulated Cl^- secretion is preserved in CF airway epithelia and, thus, has the potential to bypass the CF Cl^- secretory defect. One potential therapeutic strategy for bypassing the CF Cl^- secretory defect is to activate endogenous apical membrane Ca^{2+}-regulated Cl^- channels. That has been the goal of studies directed at the use of extracellular ATP to stimulate Cl^- secretion in CF airway epithelia.[272,571,572] Ca^{2+}-activated Cl^- channels are present in the apical membrane of airway but not intestinal epithelia.[591] This observation explains the initially puzzling observation that Ca^{2+}-stimulated Cl^- secretion is intact in CF airway epithelium[588,593] but defective in CF intestine,[602,606,716] because the Ca^{2+}-activated Cl^- channels that could circumvent the Cl^- secretory defect in the CF airway are missing from the apical membrane of intestinal epithelia. In normal intestine, an increase in $[Ca^{2+}]_i$ activates basolateral membrane K^+ channels.[717] The resulting hyperpolarization increases the driving force for Cl^- exit across the apical membrane, apparently through CFTR Cl^- channels. Because some apical Cl^- channels are open under basal conditions in the intestine, Cl^- secretion results.

In a number of reports, cells grown on impermeable supports (where cell polarity is undefined) have been studied with the patch-clamp technique in an attempt to identify Ca^{2+}-activated Cl^- channels. In whole-cell and single-channel patch-clamp studies of airway or intestinal cells,[591,663,718–721] Ca^{2+}-activated Cl^- currents have a linear I-V relationship, are more permeable to I^- than to Cl^-, and are inhibited by DIDS. These properties are the same as those of Ca^{2+}-activated Cl^- currents located in the apical membrane of airway epithelia.[591] However, two observations hint that Ca^{2+}-activated Cl^- channels in the apical membrane may be different from those in cells grown on impermeable supports. First, a striking property of Ca^{2+}-activated Cl^- channels in cells grown on impermeable supports is the time-dependent increase in current seen at depolarizing voltages.[591,663,718,719] In contrast, Ca^{2+}-activated Cl^- currents located in the apical membrane did not display any time-dependent voltage effects.[591] Second, although a number of researchers have reported Ca^{2+}-activated Cl^- channels in intestinal cells grown on impermeable supports (where the Ca^{2+}-activated currents had properties similar to those found in airway epithelia), these currents are not present in the apical membrane of polarized intestinal epithelia.[591] It has been speculated that this particular Ca^{2+}-activated Cl^- channel may not be expressed in the apical or basolateral membrane of polarized intestinal or airway epithelial cells. Such a conclusion would be consistent with the observation that the expression of many epithelial proteins depends on the growth substrate. These observations raise an important question: Are the Ca^{2+}-activated Cl^- channels studied in the plasma membrane of airway epithelial cells grown on impermeable supports, the same as those in the apical membrane of airway epithelia grown on permeable filters? At present, the data are insufficient to answer the question.

Volume-Regulated Cl^- Channels. Whole-cell patch-clamp studies of single airway and intestinal epithelial cells grown on impermeable supports identified a large Cl^- current that exhibited voltage-dependent inactivation at depolarizing voltages.[698,714,722,723] These currents were augmented by hypo-osmotic solutions and inhibited by hyperosmotic extracellular solutions. Although the corresponding changes in cell volume have not been measured, these effects presumably result from cell swelling and shrinkage, respectively. A number of properties distinguish the volume-regulated Cl^- channels from CFTR Cl^- channels. The volume-regulated Cl^- channels display a permeability sequence of $I^- > Cl^-$, an outwardly-rectifying I-V relationship, block by DIDS, and time-dependent current inactivation at depolarizing voltages. Single-channel studies of volume-regulated Cl^- channels showed an outwardly-rectifying I-V relationship and inactivation by depolarizing voltages. The single-channel conductance was approximately 50 pS at 0 mV.[698,714] This volume-regulated Cl^- channel may exist in the apical membrane, although other interpretations are possible.[698,724] Recent work raises the possibility that volume-regulated Cl^- channels may result from expression of the P-glycoprotein MDR.[679,680]

REGULATION OF CFTR Cl^- CHANNELS

Regulation by Phosphorylation

The suggestion that CFTR might be regulated by phosphorylation was made at the time the primary sequence was discovered. The suggestion was based on the observation that the R domain contains multiple consensus sequences for phosphorylation by PKA and PKC[13] and on the finding that cAMP-stimulated Cl^- secretion is defective in CF airway epithelia. That knowledge, plus the ability of intracellular cAMP to stimulate Cl^- secretion and activate CFTR Cl^- channels, suggested that phosphorylation of the R domain might open the CFTR Cl^- channel.

Subsequent studies of CFTR showed that addition of cAMP agonists in vivo, or of PKA and ATP in vitro, phosphorylated CFTR.[620,725] Then investigators found that in excised, cell-free patches of membrane, addition of the catalytic subunit of PKA and ATP to the cytosolic solution activated the channel.[653,658] Similar results were obtained with CFTR in planar lipid bilayers.[674,675]

CFTR is Regulated by Kinases and Phosphatases. Control of CFTR Cl^- channel activity depends on the balance of kinase and phosphatase activity in the cell. Although PKA appears to be the primary kinase responsible for regulation, other kinases can also phosphorylate and open the channel. Both Ca^{2+}-independent and Ca^{2+}-dependent isoforms of PKC phosphorylate and activate CFTR Cl^- channels, although only to 15 percent of the level observed with PKA.[726] However, pretreatment with PKC increased the speed and extent of channel activation when PKA was subsequently applied.[658] It has been speculated that cyclic-GMP-dependent protein kinase (cGK) might be involved in stimulating Cl^- secretion in the intestine, thereby producing watery diarrhea. But, although cGK can phosphorylate CFTR, it may not activate the channel; some studies suggest that cGK does not open CFTR,[726,727] but other work suggests that it may have some role.[728] Thus, if cGK phosphorylates CFTR in vivo, it may do so at sites not involved in PKA-dependent channel activation. Alternatively, if cGMP regulates endogenous CFTR in intestinal epithelia, it may do so through a different isoform of cGK.[729] In contrast, the multifunctional Ca^{2+}/calmodulin-dependent protein kinase failed either to activate or to phosphorylate CFTR Cl^- channels, suggesting that it has no direct effect on CFTR.[726] This result is consistent with evidence suggesting that an increase in cell Ca^{2+} concentration does not regulate CFTR.

Protein phosphatases dephosphorylate CFTR and close the channel. Protein phosphatase 2A (PP2A) dephosphorylated PKA-phosphorylated CFTR and inactivated the channel in excised patches of membrane.[726] In contrast, neither protein phosphatases 1 nor 2B dephosphorylated or inactivated PKA-phosphorylated channels. Some but not all preparations of alkaline phosphatase may regulate the channel.[658,726] Thus, specific protein phosphatases reverse the effect of kinases and terminate channel activity.

The balance between kinase and phosphatase activity will determine channel activity and, thus, the rate of transepithelial ion transport. The differences in second messenger levels and in the amount and localization of kinases and phosphatases in different cells may account for the different basal and stimulated levels of channel activity. For example, it has been speculated that low levels of a specific phosphatase in the sweat gland duct may account for the fact that these epithelial cells have a high Cl^- conductance, even under basal conditions.

Phosphorylation of Specific Residues in the R Domain Opens the Channel. The R domain contains a number of potential phosphorylation sites for PKA.[13] PKA favors the consensus phosphorylation sequence R-R/K-X-S*/T*, where X is any amino acid, and the phosphoacceptor is indicated by an asterisk (for a review see Kennelly and Krebs[730]). There are 10 such sequences within CFTR: eight serines plus one threonine in the R domain and one serine positioned just prior to the first nucleotide binding domain. However, PKA does not phosphorylate all 10 consensus phosphorylation sites[725,731]: Neither the threonine located in the R domain (T788) nor the one consensus serine located outside the R domain (S422) were phosphorylated in vitro by PKA or in vivo following addition of cAMP agonists. Moreover, in contrast to most of the consensus serines in the R domain, neither T788 nor S422 are well conserved in CFTR from different species. Site-directed mutagenesis and tryptic phosphopeptide maps were used to show that PKA phosphorylates four or five serines in the R domain in vivo[725,731,732]; those serines are S660, S700, S737, S795, and S813.

Regulation of CFTR by phosphorylation of the R domain is complex and not yet completely understood. Studies of CFTR variants that contain site-directed mutations in which the phosphorylated serines are mutated to alanine indicate that PKA-dependent phosphorylation of multiple different serines in the R domain can open the channel.[715,725,731,732] Moreover, as the total number of phosphoserines was decreased by mutation, the open state probability (P_o) of the channels decreased, indicating a reduction in channel activity. A surprising observation was that PKA still opened the channel when all of the serines that are phosphorylated in vivo or all of the potential phosphoserines and phosphothreonines were mutated to alanine.[715,725,732] This result suggests that there may be additional cryptic phosphorylation sites in the R domain that are substrates for PKA. Which phosphorylation sites are the most important for regulation of channel activity? For two reasons, it has been proposed that S660, S737, S795, S813, and perhaps S700 are the major regulatory sites for cAMP-dependent phosphorylation in vivo. First, those sites were phosphorylated in vivo following stimulation by cAMP agonists.[725,731,732] Even when phosphorylation of those serines was prevented by mutation to alanine, no additional phosphorylation sites were detected by tryptic phosphopeptide mapping. Second, most of the decrease in P_o occurred with simultaneous mutation of S660, S737, S795, and S813. Mutation of additional serines produced only a small additional decrement in P_o.[715,732]

Additional evidence that the R domain serves to regulate

the channel comes from studies in which the R domain was partially deleted. Deletion of part of the R domain (residues 708 through 835, CFTRΔR) produced Cl^- channels that were constitutively open.[733] More extensive deletions in the R domain failed to generate functional CFTR Cl^- channels.[734] The R domain of CFTR was originally defined as the 241 amino acids (residues 590 through 830) encoded by exon 13.[13] While such exon/intron boundaries provide a convenient way to define the R domain, they do not necessarily reflect the boundaries of the corresponding functional domain in CFTR. An alignment of CFTR with sequences from the human P-glycoprotein MDR and the yeast STE6 A-mating pheromone transporter shows that amino acid sequence similarity extends beyond the exon 13 exon/intron boundary.[734] The portion of protein that could be deleted without destroying function corresponds to sequences that are not conserved in related proteins.

Although CFTRΔR formed a channel that was active even without phosphorylation, PKA-dependent phosphorylation produced a further increase in P_o.[732] This effect was ascribed to S660, which remains in the sequence of CFTRΔR and is a substrate for PKA-dependent phosphorylation. When S660 in CFTRΔR was mutated to alanine, the effect of PKA was abolished.

How does phosphorylation of the R domain regulate the CFTR Cl^- channel? Current data suggest that the R domain regulates CFTR by keeping the channel closed (Fig. 127-14). Phosphorylation or deletion of part of the R domain may relieve the inhibitory effect. The effect of phosphorylation can be mimicked by substituting six or more negatively charged aspartates for serines in the R domain; such substitutions generated Cl^- channels that were open without phosphorylation by PKA. This result suggests that electrostatic interactions within the protein may be important for channel activation. Perhaps negative charge generates charge–charge interactions between the R domain and another part of the protein to either push or pull the R domain away from the pore and open the channel. Alternatively, charge-induced conformational changes in the R domain may open the channel. In either case, it is unclear which is more important—the number of charges introduced by aspartate addition or PKA phosphorylation or the charge density in the R domain. Additional questions remain about the sequence in which the various sites are phosphorylated, about the effect of phosphorylation of individual sites on P_o, and about interactions between phosphorylation by PKA and other kinases.

Why is regulation of CFTR by the R domain so complex? It has been speculated that graded phosphorylation of CFTR may be a way to provide graded CFTR Cl^- channel activity and hence graded Cl^- secretion. Multiple phosphorylation sites may also provide the means for slightly different regulation in specific tissues. Finally, it is also possible that the abundance of sites may allow for interactions between a number of different regulatory kinases and phosphatases so as to provide both precise quantitative and precise temporal control of the channel.

Regulation by Intracellular Nucleotides

In the traffic ATPase/ABC transporter family, the NBDs appear to be the site of ATP hydrolysis. In some members of the family, the energy released during ATP hydrolysis is used to actively transport substrate across the cell membrane. In CFTR, the function of the NBDs was an enigma. On the one hand, the NBDs provided the conserved feature that brought CFTR into the family. On the other hand, why should an ion channel contain a domain that might hydrolyze

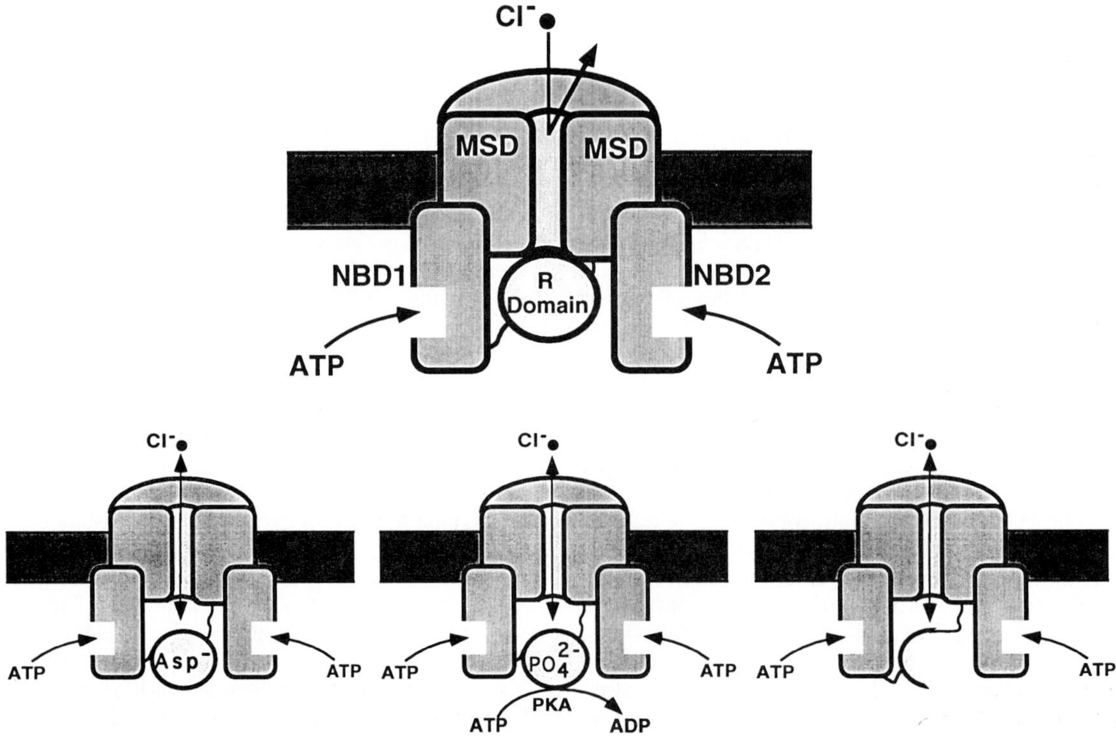

FIG. 127-14 **Model of regulation of CFTR Cl^- channels by the R domain. The channel is shown as opening when the R domain moves, but it is not known whether that is actually the case. The channel can be opened by phosphorylation of the R domain, by substitution of phosphoserines by aspartates, or by deletion of part of the R domain. In all three cases, ATP is required for channel activity.**

ATP? Adding to the mystery, the NBDs are the site of many CF-associated mutations.

Intracellular ATP Regulates the Channel. Because the NBDs were predicted to interact with ATP and because CFTR formed a regulated Cl^- channel, Anderson et al. tested the hypothesis that ATP would regulate channel activity.[652] Figure 127-15 shows an experiment in which Cl^- channel currents were measured in an excised, inside-out patch of membrane. Addition of ATP alone to the cytosolic surface had no effect, but the combination of ATP plus PKA activated Cl^- channels. When PKA and ATP were removed, the channels closed. Then, readdition of ATP reactivated the channel. These results indicate that ATP regulates the channel, but only when the channel has first been phosphorylated by PKA. Several additional studies have indicated that ATP had a direct effect, not due to reversible phosphorylation. (1) Once the channel was phosphorylated by PKA, reversible regulation by ATP was not affected by a number of kinase and phosphatase inhibitors. (2) CFTR Cl^- channels in which the R domain had been deleted still required ATP for activity. (3) ATPγS is an ATP analog that can serve as a substrate for protein kinases, but because it is slowly hydrolyzed, it does not substitute for ATP in many proteins where the rate of ATP hydrolysis is directly coupled to the protein's function. Addition of ATPγS plus PKA to the cytosolic surface of excised membrane patches produced little channel activity. However, after PKA and ATPγS were removed, addition of ATP increased the current.

Evidence that ATP interacts with both the NBDs of CFTR came from studies of CFTR variants containing site-directed mutations in each NBD: mutations at critical residues altered the relation between ATP concentration and channel activity.[735] However, the specific effect of ATP interaction with each of the two NBDs is still unknown.

ATP Hydrolysis May Be Required to Open the Channel. ATP hydrolysis is required for the function of some members of the traffic ATPase/ABC transporter family. Although it has not been directly tested in CFTR, hydrolysis may be required for channel activation, because nonhydrolyzable nucleotides and Mg^{2+}-free ATP were unable to substitute for ATP in activating the channel.[652] The nucleoside triphosphate potency was rather broad (at 1 m*M* relative to ATP): ATP (1.00) > GTP (0.65) > ITP (0.49) ≈ UTP (0.42) > CTP (0.25). This broad specificity contrasts with the high specificity for ATP observed for a number of kinases and the Na^+,K^+-ATPase. ATP increased Cl^- channel activity in a dose-dependent manner with an EC_{50} of 250 to 300 μ*M*. Again, this value is much higher than that for kinases or G proteins. The broad nucleoside triphosphate specificity and high EC_{50} are reminiscent of results of studies on other members of the traffic ATPase/ABC transporter family.

ADP, the product of ATP hydrolysis, did not stimulate channel activity.[735] However, in the presence of ATP, increasing concentrations of ADP progressively inhibited the channel.[735] The data suggested that ADP was a competitive antagonist. In contrast to the effect of ATP, nonhydrolyzable analogs, including 5-adenylylimidodiphosphate (AMP-PNP) were either unable to support channel activity or were much less efficient.[634,652,736] However, there are suggestions that AMP-PNP might interact with CFTR in a nonhydrolytic manner and allosterically control the channel. In sweat gland duct epithelia in which the basolateral membrane had been permeabilized by *Staphylococcus aureus* α-toxin, AMP-PNP could stimulate apical membrane Cl^- channels (i.e., CFTR).[521] However, stimulation only occurred in the presence of ATP. These data suggested that nonhydrolyzable analogs might interact with and activate CFTR Cl^- channels by a nonhydrolytic mechanism in the presence of ATP. That suggestion was supported indirectly by observations on the P-glycoprotein MDR-1, which is associated with a volume-regulated Cl^- channel[679] and also with drug transport.[737] Although drug transport requires ATP hydrolysis, the channel function associated with MDR-1 appears to be supported by nonhydrolyzable analogs of ATP, including AMP-PNP.[680]

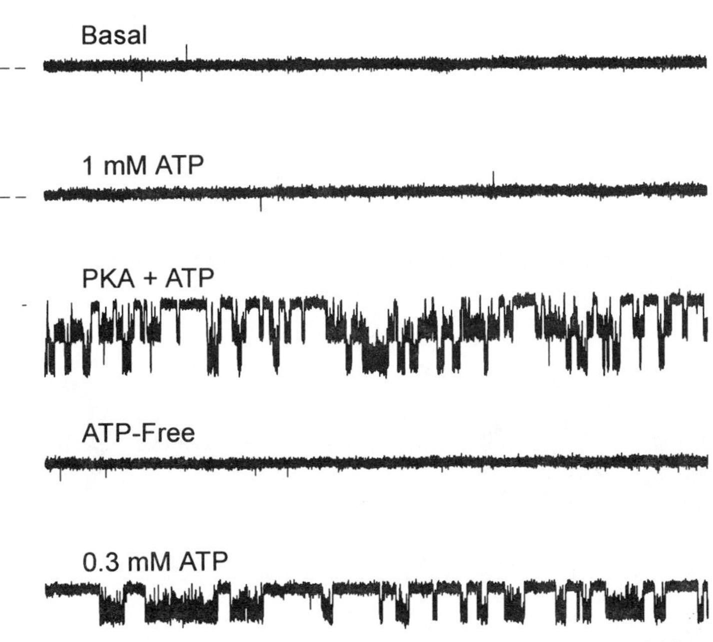

FIG. 127-15 Effect of ATP on CFTR Cl^- channel activity. Data points are current at −90 mV from an excised, inside-out patch containing two channels. ATP (1 m*M*) and PKA (75 n*M*) were present during the times indicated. Then both were removed, and 0.3 m*M* ATP was present during the time of the fifth trace. *(Courtesy of Dr. David N. Sheppard and Michael J. Welsh.)*

ATP Binds to CFTR NBD. A synthetic peptide containing 67 amino acids from NBD1[738,739] and a larger peptide containing a substantial amount of NBD1 sequence[740] were shown to bind nucleotide analogs. Intact CFTR studied in membranes of Sf9 insect cells[741] was also specifically photolabeled by [γ-^{32}P]β-azidoadenosine 5′-triphosphate (8-N_3ATP), a photo-activatable ATP analog. 8-N_3ATP also substituted for ATP in activating CFTR Cl^- channels, indicating that it interacts with the active site(s) in CFTR. Both ATP and GTP prevented photolabeling with half-maximal inhibition at approximately 1 m*M*. ADP and AMP-PNP prevented photolabeling, but at much higher concentrations, whereas AMP did not inhibit photolabeling at concentrations of up to 100 m*M*. These results support the conclusion that the NBDs of CFTR interact directly with nucleotides at concentrations similar to those that regulate CFTR Cl^- channel activity.

Phosphorylation of CFTR by PKA had little effect on 8-N_3ATP photolabeling, suggesting that phosphorylation of the R domain may not be required for nucleotide binding. Although cytosolic Mg^{2+} was required for ATP to open CFTR Cl^- channels,[652] Mg^{2+} was not required for ATP binding to either intact CFTR or to peptides corresponding to NBD1.[738,740,741] Similarly, *HisP* (a bacterial histidine transporter related to CFTR) can bind 8-N_3ATP in the absence of Mg^{2+}[742] but requires Mg^{2+} for ATP-dependent transport. Additional studies are required to determine whether or not ATP hydrolysis is required for the opening of CFTR Cl^- channels.

How does ATP regulate the channel? Present knowledge is insufficient to answer this question. If it should be shown that CFTR hydrolyzes ATP, then it is possible that the energetically favorable conformation of the channel is the inactivated (or closed) state, and that energy input (from ATP hydrolysis) is required for the transition to and/or maintenance of the activated (or open) state. In either case, the observation that CFTR forms a Cl^- channel that passively transports Cl^- down its electrochemical gradient indicates that the energy of ATP hydrolysis or binding is not used to generate a Cl^- concentration gradient and that there is not a stoichiometric relationship between the interaction of the channel with ATP and the number of transported ions.

MOLECULAR MECHANISMS OF CFTR Cl^- CHANNEL DYSFUNCTION

Mutations in the gene encoding CFTR can disrupt CFTR function in a number of different ways. Although insights into the mechanism of dysfunction have been obtained for only a few of the many CF-associated mutations shown in Table 127-7, four general mechanisms have been described.[743] Figure 127-16 shows a schematic diagram of the mechanisms, and Table 127-9 gives a few examples.

Class I Mutations: Defective Protein Production

Table 127-7 shows that there are many reports of mutations that produce premature termination signals owing to splice-site abnormalities, frameshifts caused by insertions or deletions, or nonsense mutations. CFTR genes bearing these mutations are all predicted to fail to synthesize full-length protein. In some cases (such as R553X), the mutation generates an unstable mRNA and no detectable protein.[744] In other cases, a truncated protein or an aberrant protein missing part of the normal sequence or containing novel amino acid sequences may be produced. However, such proteins are often unstable and would usually either be degraded relatively rapidly or have little or no function. To date, naturally occurring truncated or aberrant versions of protein have not been detected in CF cells. It is possible that mutations in the gene promoter could also be responsible for the loss of protein.

Table 127-9 groups together in class I all mechanisms of mutation that would lead to defective protein production. However, future studies may yield data that will allow subclassification of mutations in this class. Since all mutants in class I are expected to produce little or no full-length protein, it follows that they would cause a loss of CFTR Cl^- channel function in affected epithelia.

Another form of CFTR variant, alternatively spliced transcripts, has been reported in vivo in normal individuals, as discussed under "Alternative Splicing" above. Skipping

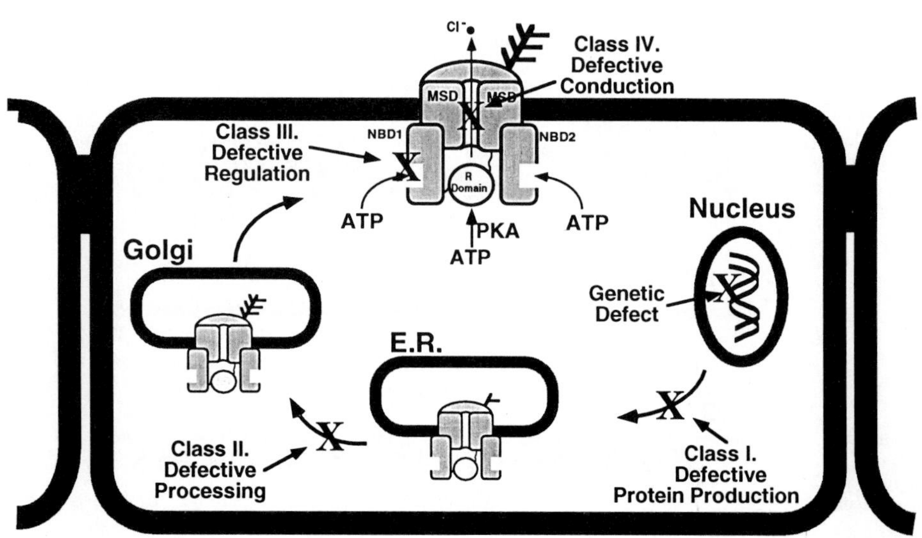

FIG. 127-16 Diagram of the biosynthesis and function of CFTR in an epithelial cell and of mechanisms of dysfunction associated with CF mutations. *(From Welsh and Smith.[743] Used by permission of* Cell.)

Table 127-9 Classes of Mutations That Cause CF

Class	Defect	Examples	Domain	Frequency	Clinical
I	Defective protein production				
	Nonsense	G542X	NBD1	3.4	PI
	Frameshift	3905insT	NBD2	2.1	PI
	Splice	621+1G→T	MSD1	1.3	PI
II	Defective processing				
		ΔI507	NBD1	0.5	PI
		ΔF508	NBD1	67.2	PI
		S549R	NBD1	0.3	
		A559T	NBD1	—	PI
		N1303K	NBD2	1.8	
					PI
III	Defective regulation				
		G551D	NBD1	2.4	PI
		G551S	NBD1	—	PS
		G1244E	NBD2	—	PI
		S1255P	NBD2	—	PI
		G1349D	NBD2	—	PI
IV	Defective conduction				
		R117H	MSD1	0.8	PS
		R334W	MSD1	0.4	PS
		R347P	MSD1	0.5	PS

NOTE: PI and PS refer to pancreatic insufficiency and pancreatic sufficiency, respectively. The approximate frequencies of mutations as a percent of CF chromosomes are taken from Tsui.[503] Dashes indicate a rare mutation. Examples shown account for about 81 percent of CF chromosomes.
SOURCE: *From Welsh and Smith.*[743] *Used by permission of* Cell.

of exon 9 is particularly common, with low levels of exon 9 minus mRNA in most individuals, but four normal individuals were found to have 73 to 92 percent of transcripts with absence of exon 9.[381,384,385] Expression of CFTR lacking exon 9 failed to generate functional Cl^- channels because the protein was defectively processed.[388,388a] The observation that some apparently normal individuals have only a small percentage of normal transcripts and that most of their transcripts do not produce functional protein suggests that only a small amount of functional CFTR is sufficient for normal epithelial function.

Class II Mutations: Defective Protein Processing

Several CF-associated mutations, including the most common, ΔF508, fail to traffic to the correct cellular location. The failure of CFTR mutants to progress through the biosynthetic pathway can be followed by assessing their state of glycosylation. In cells producing recombinant protein, CFTR containing the ΔF508 mutation fails to mature to the fully glycosylated form (Fig. 127-17).[622,623] Instead, following its production, the partially glycosylated mutant protein is degraded. As a result, the ΔF508 protein cannot be detected at the cell surface. The initial studies showing mislocalization of CFTRΔF508 were performed on heterologous cells expressing recombinant protein.[622,623] Studies on CF epithelia expressing endogenous CFTR have shown that CFTRΔF508 is similarly mislocalized in CF airway epithelial cells,[637] in sweat gland duct cells,[517] and in airway submucosal gland cells.[630] Table 127-9 lists examples of some other CF-associated mutants that also appear to be mislocalized. Mutations in this class affect most CF chromosomes because the ΔF508 mutation is so common.

The reason that these mutant forms of CFTR fail to traffic correctly has not been established. However, experience with other proteins suggests that the mutation prevents CFTR from adopting its correct conformation: that is, the nascent protein folds incorrectly and is recognized as abnormal by cellular "quality control" mechanisms that mark the protein for degradation rather than movement to the plasma membrane.[622,739] An alternative is that CFTR mutants such as ΔF508 are recognized as different only by cellular proteases.

Although CFTRΔF508 is mislocalized in cells grown at 37° C, when the incubation temperature is reduced to 23°C to 30°C, the mutant protein escapes from the endoplasmic reticulum, is fully glycosylated in the Golgi complex, and is delivered to the cell membrane.[745] Presumably, the folding process is able to occur, at least partially, at the reduced temperature. Once delivered to the cell membrane, CFTRΔF508 retains some function: the Cl^- conductive properties and regulation by phosphorylation appeared to be intact. However, some[654,655,745] but not all[746] reports suggest that the activity of CFTR Cl^- channels is reduced to approximately one-third that of wild type CFTR.

It is possible that additional class II mutations may be identified for which the protein is processed through the Golgi complex yet fails to traffic to the apical membrane, perhaps instead residing on some intracellular membrane or in the basolateral membrane.

Class III Mutations: Defective Regulation

Analysis of the mutant proteins that do reach the plasma membrane indicates that several have mutations in the

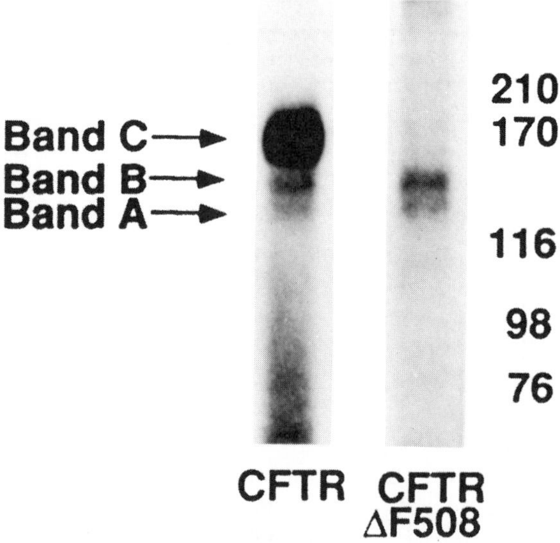

FIG. 127-17 Immunoprecipitation of CFTR and CFTRΔF508. Immunoprecipitates were phosphorylated with PKA and [^{32}P]ATP and separated by gel electrophoresis. The unglycosylated protein is labeled *band A*, the core glycosylated form is *band B*, and the fully glycosylated form is *band C*. Recombinant CFTR or CFTRΔF508 was expressed in 3T3 fibroblasts. *(Courtesy of Dr. Lynda S. Ostegaard and Michael J. Welsh.)*

NBDs. Because intracellular ATP regulates the opening of CFTR Cl^- channels, it is perhaps not surprising that mutations in these domains could alter channel function. Several abnormalities have been observed: in some NBD mutants (such as G551D) there is very little function, in some (such as S1255P), ATP is less potent at stimulating activity, and in others (such as G551S, G1244E, and G1349D), the absolute activity is reduced.[654,735] The defective regulation of such mutants and the resulting decrease in net Cl^- channel activity is likely to be responsible for the defective epithelial Cl^- permeability in patients bearing these mutations.

CFTR is also regulated by phosphorylation of the R domain. Although a few missense mutations have been reported to occur in exon 13, in what was originally defined as the R domain, it is not yet known how they cause CFTR Cl^- channel dysfunction. It is possible that some might cause defective regulation.

Class IV Mutations: Defective Conduction

The membrane-spanning domains (MSD) are thought to contribute to the channel pore, and a number of CF-associated missense mutations have been identified there. Three mutations in MSD1 (R117H, R334W, and R347P) affect arginine residues located in putative membrane-spanning sequences. When these mutant CFTRs were expressed in heterologous epithelial cells, all three were correctly processed, were present in the apical membrane, and generated cAMP-regulated apical membrane Cl^- currents.[673] Moreover, regulation by PKA-dependent phosphorylation and intracellular ATP appeared similar to that of wild-type CFTR. Nevertheless, the amount of current was reduced, with wild-type CFTR > R347P > R117H > R334W. An analysis of single channels in excised, inside-out membrane patches indicated that these proteins generate less Cl^- current because the rate of ion flow through a single open channel is reduced. In addition, the amount of time that the channel was open was reduced to one-third that of wild type CFTR, at least for R117H.

Although the grouping of mutations into different classes is useful for understanding the mechanism of dysfunction, it is probably inappropriate to apply it rigidly. For example, a single mutation could cause more than one type of abnormality, and hence fall into multiple classes. As mentioned above for ΔF508, although mislocalization is the major abnormality, defective regulation of function has also been demonstrated. Likewise, R117H has a reduced single channel conductance but also shows a reduced open state probability P_o.

GENOTYPE–PHENOTYPE CORRELATIONS

Classic Cystic Fibrosis Phenotype

As described in previous sections, the presentation of CF is complex; the disease affects multiple organs; and the symptoms vary among different patients. Genotype–phenotype correlations are of value to provide both better understanding of the function of CFTR and improved diagnosis, prognosis, and management for patients. Although the role of CFTR in the function of various epithelia may be elucidated through analysis of patients' genotypes and their corresponding phenotypes, it is necessary to examine the affected organs separately before any correlation emerges.[503] In general, the phenotypic features of CF may be divided into three categories.

The first category includes the symptoms that are common to most, if not all, CF patients, regardless of the types of mutations. For example, abnormal electrolyte composition of sweat is common to virtually all patients with classic CF. Although some genotype groups may show values different from those of typical CF patients, these values are usually significantly different from those of normal control subjects.[671,747] This fact suggests that CFTR plays a major role in chloride transport by the sweat gland ducts and that the requirement for the function or regulation of CFTR is more stringent in this tissue than in others. Sweat chloride levels are often abnormal even with atypical phenotypes.

The second category of phenotypic features in CF includes symptoms that show a good correlation with genotype. This category is best represented by the pancreatic function of patients. Two groups of patients can be clearly identified,[748] and there is a remarkable concordance of the levels of exocrine pancreatic function among affected members of the same sibship.[749] The latter finding provides a strong indication that the pancreatic phenotype—pancreatic insufficiency (PI) versus pancreatic sufficiency (PS)—is determined primarily by the genotype at the CFTR locus. Specific mutations have also been found to correlate with congenital bilateral absence of the vas deferens (CBAVD) as the only major finding (see "Atypical Cystic Fibrosis Phenotypes" below) and with atypical chloride levels in sweat in patients with CF.

The third category of phenotypic features includes the symptoms that do not show significant correlation with genotype or good concordance within a sibship. The pulmonary status of CF patients is a good example of this category, in which the severity of disease is affected by other genetic and nongenetic factors. Other symptoms, such as meconium ileus, pancreatitis, and liver disease, may also belong in this category.

Chloride Levels in Sweat. Three specific mutations (G551S),[455] 2789+5G→A (personal communication, W.E. Highsmith et al.), 3849+10kbC→T[217,750] were found in association with normal or closer-to-normal sodium and chloride concentration in the sweat in patients diagnosed with CF. A difference in the mean chloride concentration in the sweat is also generally observed between PS and PI patients; the former group has levels significantly lower than those of the latter, although there is an overlap of values.[671,747]

Pancreatic Enzyme Secretion. Besides the remarkable familial concordance for the status of pancreatic function among the affected members of the same family,[749,751] DNA marker haplotype analysis also predicted that the mutations leading to PI were different from those conferring PS.[14,752–755] With the identification of the major ΔF508 mutation, the hypothesis of "severe" and "mild" mutations was introduced; patients in whom both CF chromosomes carry a "severe" mutation are expected to have the PI phenotype and those with one or two "mild" mutations would be PS.[14,441] A remarkable correlation between genotype and phenotype has been observed.[14,441,672,754,756,757] As 85 percent of CF patients are PI and 15 percent are PS, it can be calculated that over 90 percent of the CF chromosomes carry mutations belonging to the "severe" group (including ΔF508), and less than 10 percent have mutations belonging to the "mild" group. Patients with PI are diagnosed at an earlier age, have poorer lung function, and have higher sweat chloride concentrations than PS patients.[671,747,758]

As a general rule, all mutations classified as nonsense, frameshift, splice-site affecting the consensus AG/GT sequences, or amino acid deletions, and most missense mutations, are "severe" and confer the PI phenotype.[672] Only a small fraction of missense mutations and splicing defects (usually outside the AG/GT consensus) can be correlated with PS; examples of the "mild" alleles are G91R,[413] E92K,[415] R117H,[441,672] P205S,[425] R334W,[441,672] R347H,[411] R347P,[441,672] A455E,[441,672] G551S,[455] Y563N,[441,672] P574H,[441,672] and 3849+10kbC→T.[217,750] Many of these mutations affect amino acid residues in or near the predicted transmembrane domain of CFTR[503] and appear to result in normal regulation of the chloride channel but altered ion permeability.[673] Additional description of this subject is provided above (see "Class IV Mutations: Defective Conduction"). The splicing mutations that confer PS presumably allow a low percentage of normal splicing of transcripts from the mutant allele.[217] These observations suggest that a low level of CFTR function is sufficient to allow proper pancreatic function. The PI and PS phenotypes thus may directly reflect the function of mutant CFTR protein.

There are a few exceptions reported in the literature with regard to the genotype–phenotype correlation in exocrine pancreatic function. Five out of 300 homozygous ΔF508 patients were reported to be PS in one study,[756] but pancreatic function was only determined by clinical course and history. Another study cited two homozygous ΔF508 patients with borderline pancreatic function.[759] Two of the 150 homozygous ΔF508 patients who were found to be PS in an initial study[671] were found to have only borderline pancreatic enzyme levels (personal communication, P. Kristidis et al.). It is well documented that 10 to 20 percent of patients initially diagnosed as PS may show deterioration of pancreatic function at an older age.[760]

Meconium Ileus. An allelic association was detected for meconium ileus with the DNA marker D7S8 but not with more closely linked markers XV-2c and KM.19.[761,762] It was suggested that some CF mutation was responsible for this phenotype, but the recurrence risk of meconium ileus for sibs was only 30 to 40 percent. Several other groups were unable to confirm this association.[763–765] Since patients with PI appeared to be more likely to develop meconium ileus, it was proposed that meconium ileus might be a severe variant of PI.[14] An increased risk for meconium ileus was detected with the G542X mutation,[672] but this observation was not statistically significant in a larger study,[747] where 57 of 394 (14.5 percent) ΔF508 homozygotes and 35 of 147 (23.8 percent) ΔF508/G542X compound heterozygotes had meconium ileus. In contrast, G551D was found to have a negative correlation with meconium ileus, and patients with G551D also develop PI at a later-than-average age.[766]

Lung Disease. Attempts to correlate genotype and phenotype with respect to the severity of pulmonary disease have been hampered by the lack of a simple measure of lung function and by the influence of other genetic and environmental factors. Measurements such as chest radiograph scores, FVC, FEV_1, and age of *Pseudomonas* colonization have been used. Absence of genotype–phenotype correlation is generally reported when ΔF508/ΔF508, ΔF508/non-ΔF508, and non-ΔF508/non-ΔF508 patients are compared.[671,756,767–769] All patient groups showed an inverse relationship between lung function and age. When patients are separated according to the pancreatic status, however, the PS patients as a group generally show much better lung function than the PI group.[671,756] The R117H mutation is in the "mild" group associated with PS and has been associated with mild lung disease.[747,768] It is unclear if the better lung function detected in the PS group is a consequence of a better nutritional status. The different approach of looking at older adult patients with classic CF has led to reports of a possible elevated frequency of certain mutations, such as A455E,[770] and a low frequency of homozygosity for ΔF508, with the presence of other possibly milder mutations.[771] In the case of the 3849+10kbC→T mutation, no decreased severity of pulmonary function could be detected despite evidence that this was a milder mutation on the basis of later age at diagnosis, more normal sweat chloride values, and often a PS phenotype.[217,750]

Several patients with nonsense mutations on both CF chromosomes (e.g., homozygous G542X) were reported to have relatively mild lung disease.[386,772,773] It was argued that truncation or total absence of CFTR might be associated with near-normal lung function. As additional data became available, a wider spectrum of lung disease was found, and no difference was noted between patients with two nonsense mutations and those homozygous for ΔF508.[747,774–776] Moreover, the difference in pulmonary function may be correlated with the age at which medical intervention for the disease takes place.[231] It is also of interest that three patients homozygous for R553X presented with a two-stage course of lung disease—mild progression before *P. aeruginosa* infection and a severe course after infection.[777]

One study suggested that a specific DNA haplotype (that found with ΔF508) is associated with severe pulmonary involvement.[778] Since PI patients as a group have more severe pulmonary problems, the latter observation may simply reflect the association of the specific haplotype group with "severe" mutations. It has been shown that the age-specific rates of colonization with *P. aeruginosa* were significantly lower in patients with PS ("mild" missense and splice-site mutations) than in those with PI.[779] Another study based on infants identified through neonatal screening showed that infants who were asymptomatic and homozygous for ΔF508 have early evidence of airway obstruction not detected in other genotype groups.[780]

Other Manifestations. An increased incidence of diabetes mellitus has been detected in patients homozygous for ΔF508, but there is no absolute correlation between the two, and the effect is thought to be secondary to the increased pancreatic degeneration in these patients.[781] There is a significant incidence of liver disease in CF patients,[782] and one study found an increased frequency of homozygosity for ΔF508 among 20 adult patients with liver involvement.[783] Other studies have found no significant correlation between genotype and liver disease.[169]

Total body water in CF patients was measured, but no correlation could be detected for ΔF508.[784] One report described a significant difference between the energy expenditure of patients homozygous for ΔF508 and those who did not carry this mutation.[101] No difference was observed in another study in which only patients with relatively good lung function (FEV_1>75 percent) were included.[785] The latter investigators suggested that the difference observed in the early study was probably due to differences in lung function among the patient groups in the study.

Atypical Cystic Fibrosis Phenotypes

Congenital Bilateral Absence of the Vas Deferens (CBAVD). CBAVD is virtually uniformly present in males with a diagnosis of classic CF. It is now well established that healthy males with CBAVD have a high frequency of CF mutations and a high incidence of the R117H defect.[485,786–790] When CBAVD males are tested for known CF mutations, 60 to 65 percent are positive, about 10 percent being compound heterozygotes and the remainder being heterozygotes. It is generally assumed that most of the CBAVD males who are heterozygous for a known mutation have a second mutation on the other chromosome, but it has been difficult to identify these mutations in the coding region, leading to the suggestion that promoter or other regulatory mutations might be involved.[791] Although subclinical lung disease has been reported in some cases,[787] most studies report complete absence of pulmonary disease or other major symptoms of classic CF in these males. Males with CBAVD may have normal or abnormal sweat chloride values, and chronic sinusitis is frequently reported. Nasal epithelial ion transport studies in CBAVD males suggest that ion transport is abnormal but that the findings are distinct from those in classic CF patients.[791] CBAVD is sometimes seen in association with unilateral renal agenesis (not a feature of CF), and unilateral absence of the vas deferens occurs with and without unilateral renal agenesis. CF mutations have also been reported in patients with unilateral absence of the vas deferens.[792] It seems likely that more than half of patients with CBAVD have a phenotype caused by mutations in CFTR, while another group have other etiologies, perhaps particularly the patients with associated renal agenesis.

It is possible to treat the infertility in men with CBAVD by using microsurgical epididymal sperm aspiration (MESA) and in vitro fertilization.[793] One study found substantially lower fertilization rates for CBAVD men with CF mutations than for those without CF mutations; pregnancy rates were 23 percent and 48 percent, respectively, for the two groups.[794] In advising men with CBAVD, it is appropriate to offer mutation analysis to their partners, and the option of prenatal or preimplantation diagnosis may arise if the partner is a carrier. Depending on the mutations present, it may or may not be possible to predict a phenotype of classic CF or CBAVD in the fetus. Females with a genotype that might be associated with CBAVD in males presumably are phenotypically normal except for the possibility of chronic sinusitis[387] (see "The R117H Mutation" below).

Young syndrome is characterized by chronic sinopulmonary infections and obstructive azoospermia.[795] It is possible that there is an increased frequency of CF mutations in patients with Young syndrome,[796] but it is unlikely that most of these patients have CF mutations.[797]

The R117H Mutation. The R117H mutation is frequently seen in combination with a severe mutation such as ΔF508 in patients with classic CF and in CBAVD, although the classic CF patients often have a milder phenotype. There is now a satisfying explanation for the phenotypic difference.[387] The R117H mutation may have occurred twice; it is found with two slightly different chromosomal haplotypes, in one case with a more efficient splice-site variation preceding exon 9 and in the other with a less efficient splice-site sequence. R117H is a class IV mutant with normal channel regulation but altered conduction properties. Although further studies are needed, it appears that patients with R117H on a chromosome with an inefficient splice site and a severe mutation on the other chromosome develop classic (although possibly milder) CF whether male or female. In the case of individuals who have the R117H mutation on a chromosome with the efficient splice site and a severe mutation on the other chromosome, the phenotype is most often CBAVD in males and normal or chronic sinusitis in females. This means that the phenotypic implications of the R117H mutation, particularly when found during carrier testing, must be interpreted with caution, and only after correlating the data with clinical and family information and determining whether the mutation occurs on a chromosome with the efficient or inefficient splice site.

Pulmonary and Other Phenotypes. It was once speculated that some adult phenotypes such as chronic obstructive pulmonary disease might represent mild forms of CF. CFTR mutations have been found in patients with bronchiectasis,[798] but some of these patients may meet the criteria for a diagnosis of classic CF. Direct DNA sequencing analysis of patients with bronchiectasis in Japan revealed two novel mutations in the CFTR gene.[799] One study found CF mutations in 7 of 28 unrelated patients (a ninefold increase) with chronic obstructive pulmonary disease, but six of the seven patients with mutations had bronchiectasis.[800] It appears likely that most patients with chronic obstructive pulmonary disease do not have a CF-related etiology, but that CF mutations are more likely to be found in patients with bronchiectasis or with *Pseudomonas* colonization.

Other possible phenotypic associations, including allergic bronchopulmonary aspergillosis, chronic *Pseudomonas* bronchitis, neonatal transient hypertrypsinemia, and nasal polyposis, are discussed elsewhere.[801]

Genotype–Phenotype Correlation and Mechanism of Dysfunction

The clearest correlation of genotype and phenotype with mechanism of dysfunction involves pancreatic function.

Patients with PI have two severe mutations. Since class I and II mutations result in the absence of protein from the correct cellular location, they would be expected to have a severe effect on function. Indeed, to date all class I and II mutations have been associated with the severe PI phenotype. In contrast, all class III and IV mutants result in proteins that are correctly localized, and some of these proteins retain significant residual function, although others have little measurable activity. In the case of those class IV mutants where channel regulation appears intact but ion flow through an open Cl^- channel is reduced, the residual activity may be sufficient to confer a PS phenotype. In fact, some individuals with these mutations (e.g., R117H) do not exhibit classic CF symptoms as discussed above. Some individuals with class III mutants (e.g., G551S) are also PS,[455] whereas most others (e.g., those with G551D) are PI.[454] Presumably, this difference must relate to the degree of abnormal regulation, but, at present, its molecular basis is not understood.

Assessing Prognosis from Genotype

It would probably be inappropriate to try to base a prognosis on genotype at this time in most cases. Obviously, parents of infants diagnosed with classic CF will have the greatest interest in the prognosis for pulmonary disease and for survival. As discussed above, the correlation of pulmonary disease with genotype is very poor, and predictions of this type are generally inappropriate. Indeed, since there is evidence based on lack of concordance in sibs that other genetic and nongenetic factors are of major importance, it is likely that it will remain impossible to predict the severity of pulmonary involvement on the basis of CF genotype alone.

There are some instances where genotype–phenotype information can be of significant prognostic value. Patients with two severe mutations should be followed carefully for pancreatic insufficiency if they are free of such findings initially, whereas patients with at least one mild mutation can be expected to be more likely to maintain pancreatic sufficiency. A few mutations may be associated with an overall milder course, and some mutations may more likely be associated with CBAVD in males or a more normal phenotype in females, as discussed above. Prognostications in patients with the R117H mutation must take into account whether the mutation is on a chromosome with the efficient or inefficient splice-site variation.

GENETICS

Although alternative hypotheses were put forward over the years, cystic fibrosis became well accepted as an autosomal recessive disorder with an unusually high incidence. With the cloning of the CF gene and the characterization of hundreds of mutations, the genetic basis of the disorder is now clear, and the possibility of a second locus is eliminated. One genetic curiosity is the occurrence of CF and short stature in two patients with maternal uniparental disomy for chromosome 7[802,803] (see Chap. 7). Detailed discussions of the genetics of CF prior to the identification of the gene are available elsewhere.[804–806]

Classic Genetics

Although older questions such as the possibility of multiple loci and the number of CF alleles are now resolved, the question remains as to whether some form of selective advantage accounts for the high incidence of CF in Caucasian populations. The debate is long-standing as to whether a genetic advantage is associated with CF or whether the high frequency can be explained by chance factors such as genetic drift and founder effects. Increased fertility or higher reproductive capacity for heterozygotes has been suggested as a possible mechanism for increased frequency.[807–809] Although increased resistance to tuberculosis in CF heterozygotes has been suggested as a possible mechanism,[810,811] no data support this hypothesis. It was first proposed by P. Quinton and colleagues that CF heterozygotes might be protected against the life-threatening diarrhea of cholera, and this attractive but unproven hypothesis has been reviewed in detail.[811a] Any hypothesis to explain the high incidence of CF must take into account the dramatic differences in ethnic/geographic distribution. In addition, any hypothesis must carefully consider the available mutation and haplotype data. The frequency of the ΔF508 mutation alone is sufficient to account for the unusual incidence of CF, as the incidence in European populations would be quite unremarkable (about 1 in 30,000) without the contribution of the ΔF508 mutation. In general, populations with the highest proportion of the ΔF508 mutation also have the highest incidence, and vice versa.

The hypothesis of some form of selective advantage is favored by the finding of the same extended haplotype on chromosomes carrying the more common CF mutations.[812–814] The finding of the same extended haplotype (including markers flanking the CFTR gene) with different CF mutations suggests that it might be not the mutation itself that is associated with selective advantage but, rather, some other allelic difference within the gene or at an adjacent locus. The possibility of a hitchhiking effect, which was discussed many years ago,[815] is compatible with the data showing that the same extended haplotype is present with numerous common mutations.

A selective advantage for CF might involve differential fitness of heterozygotes, segregation distortion (meiotic drive), or some other mechanism. The magnitude of any advantage need only be very small, and might not be detectable given the samples available. It has been estimated that a sample of approximately 26,000 offspring of carriers would be required to detect at the 5 percent level a differential fitness or segregation distortion accounting for an equilibrium frequency of 1 in 40 for the CF gene.[816] There is an unusual and unexplained observation involving distortion of segregation of CF alleles to unaffected children born to CF carrier couples.[817,818] There is a statistically significant excess of homozygous normal girls and a reciprocal excess of heterozygous boys. Analysis of individual sperm from a male heterozygous for the ΔF508 mutation did not demonstrate a preferential association of either CF allele with the presence of an X or Y chromosome.[819] It is still possible that sperm carrying a mutant allele and a Y chromosome, and those carrying a normal allele and an X chromosome, could fertilize eggs preferentially over the other genotype associations. Alternatively, there could be selective survival of certain genotypes after fertilization. The relationship of these observations to any possible selective advantage associated with CF is not clear.

A selective advantage for the CF gene in Caucasian populations is not proven. Rao and Morton[820] pointed out that large deviations in the incidence of genetic diseases are not improbable and could be caused by chance alone. Presumably, a founder effect and inbreeding can account for the very high incidence in some populations, as in Brittany,[821] Southwest Africa,[822] and American Amish populations.[823] More recent mutation data confirm the role of founder effects in these populations.

Incidence

CF is the most common autosomal recessive fatal disorder in Caucasians, with an incidence of 1 in 1700 to 1 in 6500 reported in various larger populations (Table 127-10). Most older studies represent epidemiologic surveys; data based on newborn screening has been available only within the last 15 years. Estimates based on molecular screening for heterozygotes are feasible now.[850,851] Epidemiologic data and newborn screening data from Australia have yielded similar incidences (approximately 1 in 2500).[807,824,844] A moderately wide range of incidence has been reported in the United States, and newborn screening data indicate a slightly lower incidence than epidemiologic studies (Table 127-10). The incidence in North American Hispanic and black populations reflects European/Native American and European/African admixture, respectively, as indicated by mutation data. Only rough estimates of incidence are available for Mexico, for other North American Hispanics, and for American blacks, and incidence may vary within the groups. Examples of higher incidence presumably due to random genetic drift and founder effects have been reported from smaller populations with incidences of 1 in 377 in parts of Brittany,[821] 1 in 640 to 1 in 1200 in an American Amish population,[823] 1 in 891 in one portion of the French-Canadian population,[852] and 1 in 1192 in Southwest Africa.[822] The disease is rare in Finland.[853] The disease has been reported but is definitely much less frequent in American Indians,

Table 127-10 The Incidence of Cystric Fibrosis in Various Populations

Country	Incidence	References
Epidemologic Studies		
Australia	1 in 2450; 1 in 2550	807, 824
Czechoslovakia	1 in 2600; 1 in 3300	825, 826
Brittany, France	1 in 1800	821
Germany	1 in 3300	827
Israel	1 in 5000	828
Italy	1 in 2000	829
South Africa	1 in 6500	822
Sweden	1 in 7700	830
England: Caucasian	1 in 2400 to 1 in 3000	831–833
England: Asian	1 in 10,000	834
Northern Ireland	1 in 1700; 1 in 1900	835, 836
United States: Caucasian	1 in 1900 to 1 in 3700	837–840
United States: blacks	1 in 17,000	841
Mexico	1 in 8000 to 1 in 9000	See in 842
Hawaii: Caucasian	1 in 3800	843
Hawaii: Original	1 in 90,000	843
Newborn Screening		
Australia: New South Wales	1 in 2564	844
New Zealand	1 in 4140	845
United States: Colorado	1 in 3827	846
United States: Wisconsin	1 in 3431	847
Italy: Veneto	1 in 3944	223, 848
England: Peterboro	1 in 3190	223
England: East Anglia	1 in 2234	849
Average newborn screening	1 in 3190	223

Africans, and Asians (see refs. 805 and 806 for further bibliographies). Reliable incidence figures are not available for most non-Caucasian groups, with the exception of Hawaiian Orientals in whom Wright and Morton[843] estimated a frequency of 1 in 90,000.

Ethnic/Geographic Distribution

As is obvious from the preceding section, the incidence of CF varies markedly among different populations. As mentioned above, the frequency would be no different from that of an ordinary autosomal recessive disease were it not for the ΔF508 mutation.[379] Across Europe, there is a clear gradient in the relative frequency of ΔF508, from peak values in the Northwest (e.g., 88 percent in Denmark and part of England) to low values in the Southeast (30 percent in Turkey as well as Israel).[393,854] It is suggested that the spread of ΔF508 might have accompanied the migration of early farmers from the Middle East progressing toward the northwest of Europe.[397] One analysis of haplotype data was interpreted to indicate that the ΔF508 mutation arose more than 52,000 years ago and spread throughout Europe in distinct expansions.[854a]

Variation is also observed for the relative frequencies of some of the more common CF mutations other than ΔF508 (Fig. 127-18). A founder effect is apparent for several of the mutant alleles. While 88 percent of the CF mutations detected in the Danish population are ΔF508,[396,855] this mutation accounts for only about 30 percent of the CF chromosomes in the Ashkenazic Jewish population, in which the W1282X mutation is much more frequent, at 60 percent.[774,850] The G542X mutation is more common in Spain[504] and in Ashkenazic Jews[856] than in other populations. R1162X is frequent in a northern part of Italy.[433,857] Y122X is unique as well as frequent in the French population of Reunion Island (A. Kitzis and J. C. Chomel, personal communication). M1101K and ΔF508 are the only two mutations among one group of Hutterites.[474] A report of the distribution of mutations is available from the CF Genetic Analysis Consortium.[857a]

Newborn Screening

Early attempts at newborn screening for CF involved assessment of the albumin content of meconium. In 1979 it was found that newborns with CF had elevated immunoreactive trypsin in the blood and that dried blood samples already being collected for newborn screening could be tested using a radioimmunoassay to quantitate trypsin.[222,858] Subsequently, enzyme-linked immunoassays using monoclonal antibodies have been developed and adapted for high-volume screening.[859,860] Excellent reviews of newborn screening are available,[223,861,862] and there is evidence that at least 95 percent of CF patients can be detected by this strategy, although false negative results do occur.[863] Approximately 1 in 200 screening subjects require repeat sampling using immunoreactive trypsin determinations alone, but mutation analysis can be applied to initial positive samples to increase the specificity without significant increase in cost.[861,862,864]

The potential benefits and risks of newborn screening for CF have been reviewed[223,224,861,862,865,866] (see particularly ref. 862 and the editorial and concluding remarks in ref. 861). Although newborn screening for CF meets most of the criteria for such programs, it is not yet clear that screening significantly improves long-term prognosis. A position paper from an ad hoc force of the United States Cystic Fibrosis Foundation,[224] subsequently endorsed by the American

	Total CF chromosomes screened	G853	R117H	621+1G→T	711+1G→T	1078delT	R334W	R347P	A455E	Δ1507	ΔF508	1717-1G→T	G542X	S549N	G551D	R553X	R560T	1898+1G→A	2184delA	2789+5G→A	R1162X	3659delC	3849+10kbC→	W1282X	N1303K	Fraction of mutations detected
Europe, North	21,154	30	62	97	15	53	18	55	35	57	14,866	160	439	18	356	165	40	41	14	27	36	39	23	120	209	80.2 (%)
Europe, South	7,281	14	3	37	13	2	21	24	0	5	4,007	65	259	2	37	44	0	10	7	10	68	1	8	43	179	66.7
America, North	10,438	16	61	154	21	1	12	26	27	20	6,900	44	234	5	206	96	24	2	8	17	19	14	57	245	130	79.9
America, South Central	758									2	342		38	1	1	5									11	52.8
Australasia	3,095		7	27		1	2	1		9	2,309	12	56	3	117	11	3				2			6	23	83.7
Asia, mainly Middle East	608	7	0							0	173	3	27	0	0	0	0						16	120	29	61.7
Africa	515										351		9	1		1								2	8	72.2
Totals	43,849	67	133	315	49	57	53	106	62	93	28,948	284	1,062	30	717	322	67	53	29	54	125	54	104	536	589	77.3
Relative frequency	%	0.2	0.3	0.7	0.1	0.1	0.1	0.2	0.1	0.2	66.0	0.6	2.4	0.1	1.6	0.7	0.1	0.1	0.1	0.1	0.3	0.1	0.2	1.2	1.3	

FIG. 127-18 **Common cystic fibrosis mutations. The frequency distribution is shown by continent.** *(From a report of the CF Genetic Analysis Consortium.*[857a]*)*

Academy of Pediatrics,[865] said in 1983 that "until sufficient information related to these and other issues can be obtained, the task force strongly recommends that no mass population screening for cystic fibrosis be implemented, even if a valid and reliable test is available." A statement in 1986 by some directors of major screening programs[223] concluded as follows: "All in all we feel that the case for screening is now strong." This conclusion was based in part on evidence of short-term benefits such as reduced hospitalization costs in the first year of life and on the presumption that early diagnosis will lead to improved reproductive counseling, particularly since reliable prenatal diagnosis had become available. However, after 5 years of randomized screening in Wisconsin, it still has not been possible to document any pulmonary benefits of screening,[862] and the case for newborn screening remains in doubt. Current programs are continuing, but newborn screening is performed in a minority of states and countries.

Molecular Diagnosis

General Issues. Diagnosis of classic CF continues to rely primarily on clinical findings and the sweat test. The preferred method for molecular diagnosis is mutation analysis, although linkage analysis may still be needed in a small percentage of cases for prenatal diagnosis or carrier detection within CF families, if mutations cannot be identified. Numerous methods are available for analyzing the more common mutations including forward or reverse hybridization with allele-specific oligonucleotides (ASO), allele-specific amplification, ligase amplification or analysis, primer extension sequencing, and restriction enzyme analysis (including artificial introduction of restriction enzyme sites)[867] (see examples in Chap. 1). For identification of rare unknown mutations, available methods include ribonuclease cleavage, denaturing gradient-gel electrophoresis (DGGE), carbodiimide modification, chemical cleavage of mismatches, single-strand conformation polymorphism (SSCP) analysis, heteroduplex analysis, and sequencing of DNA.[867,868] The ΔF508 mutation can be detected by simple gel electrophoresis to separate the wild-type and mutant PCR products.[869] Almost all the routine diagnostic procedures begin with amplification of genomic DNA from blood samples, dried blood spots,[870] oral samples, or fetal cells. Although blood samples are most widely used, reliable procedures for collecting oral samples include buccal scraping with brushes or swabs and mouthwash collection.[871,872] Amplification can also be performed from paraffin blocks, although this is less important with mutation analysis where family members can be tested directly than was the case earlier with linkage analysis.

Most laboratories now test routinely for from 10 to over 30 of the more common CF mutations using forward or reverse ASO methods[872–876] or variations of allele-specific amplification.[877–879] These procedures generally involve multiplex steps for amplification and/or mutation analysis using partial automation in some cases. The reverse ASO method[876] and one version of allele-specific amplification designated the "amplification refractory mutation system" (ARMS)[877] have been developed as laboratory kits. Solid-phase methods based on ligation detection, single-base sequencing, and other strategies offer great promise for the development of highly automated procedures for the economical analysis of dozens of mutations simultaneously.[880] Use of DNA fixed on biological chips may provide a competitive technology.[881,882]

The number of mutations that should be tested for routine diagnostic purposes is a point of considerable interest. The sensitivity for detection of CF chromosomes shows diminishing improvement as mutations are added after the 10 to 15 mutations most common in any given population (Fig. 127-19), but some laboratories routinely offer analysis of 20 to over 30 mutations, which is attractive if the additional information can be available at trivial increased cost through

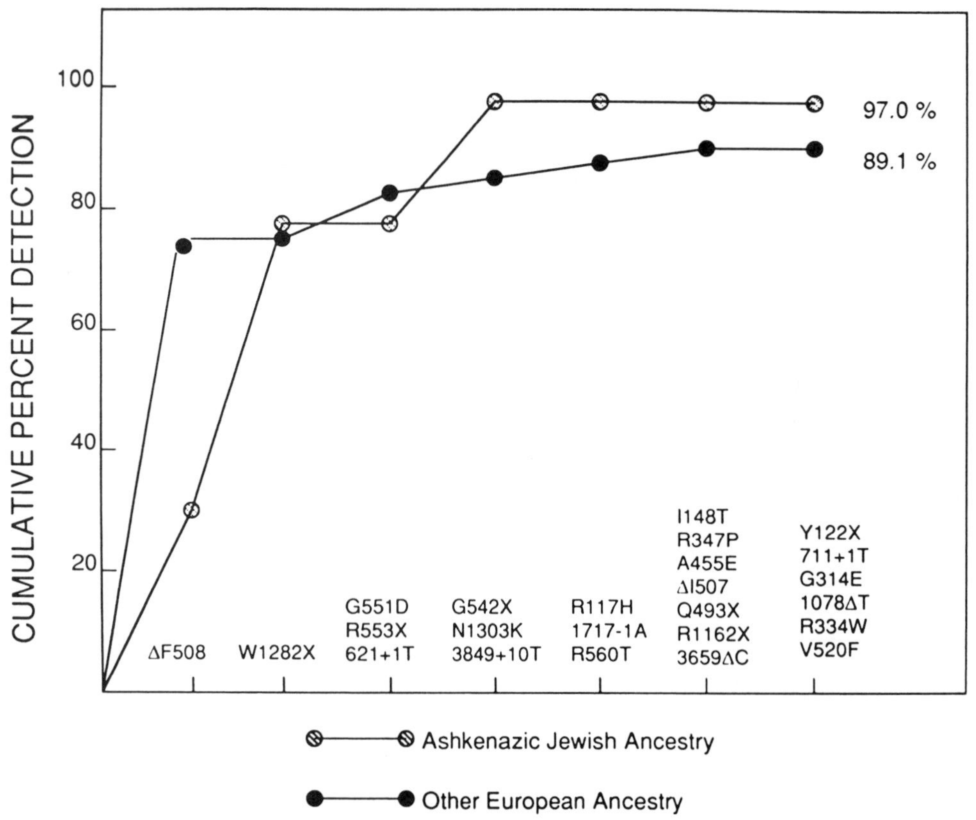

FIG. 127-19 Cumulative percent detection of CF chromosomes using analysis of 24 mutations in North Americans of Ashkenazic or other European ancestry. The mutation groups are added to the cumulative total progressing from left to right. *(From DeMarchi et al.[874] Used by permission.)*

the use of multiplexing and automation. Since mutation analysis is ordinarily based on the most common mutations causing classic CF in populations of European descent, the percentage detection of mutant chromosomes is substantially lower in other populations, such as Asians, Africans, American blacks, Hispanics, and native Americans.[857a] Detection is also lower for atypical phenotypes, as discussed above for CBAVD. In general it is desirable to analyze for the maximum number of mutations available without excessive expense. Any mutational analysis can be tailored to fit the mutational profile of different ethnic populations (Fig. 127-18), but a single panel for analysis is adequate in the vast majority of circumstances if 20 to 30 mutations are analyzed. Analysis of 20 to 30 mutations detects the defect on about 89 percent of North American CF chromosomes associated with a classic phenotype[874]; this proportion varies considerably, with higher percentages in Northern Europe and lower percentages in Southern Europe. Calculations of sensitivity for carrier detection should be based on unbiased populations of CF patients, and pooled data from many laboratories must be interpreted with caution, since biases of ascertainment and tabulation may occur; compare numbers elsewhere from the CF Genetic Analysis Consortium[503,857a] to the totals in Fig. 127-18. These numbers cannot be used to calculate *precisely* the sensitivity for carrier detection in any given population. For risk calculations, the percentage detection in a given family must take into account the ethnic background; some North American individuals know their European ancestry (e.g., Italian or Irish), whereas others are of mixed or unknown European ancestry.

Numerous laboratories have used procedures such as SSCP, DGGE, and direct sequencing to identify the rarer mutations in CF patients,[468,883] and the great majority of mutations have been detected in various populations, including 94 and 98 percent in Belgium,[424,464] 98 percent in a Celtic population,[430] and 99 percent in Wales.[399] It may be desirable to have a two-tiered strategy for mutation detection,[884] with a more economical first step and a more elaborate method for detecting all mutations in CF patients and for use in carrier screening of partners of known carriers. While methods for identifying rare mutations are available, they are generally restricted to research laboratories and are not available on a routine diagnostic basis. Mutations occurring outside the coding exons and their boundaries are more difficult to identify and interpret.

Although mutation analysis is adequate for almost all molecular diagnosis for CF, it is occasionally necessary to resort to linkage analysis for prenatal diagnosis or carrier detection in families where the CF mutation cannot be identified. It is now possible to use polymorphic dinucleotide and tetranucleotide repeats in the CF gene,[494,496,498] so there is a negligible risk of diagnostic errors due to recombination. Older flanking markers can be used if necessary, and essentially all families can be made informative by these methods. Linkage analysis is not relevant to carrier screening in the general population, to assessment of pregnancies with abnormal ultrasound results, or to the resolution of diagnostic problems regarding CF.

Diagnostic Pitfalls. All the routine hazards of molecular diagnosis apply in the case of CF, including the risk of sample mix-ups, contamination of PCR reactions, and clerical and other human errors. In any PCR reaction, there is the possibility of failing to obtain a PCR product owing to polymorphisms at primer sites.[885] There is also the possibility of failing to obtain a PCR product owing to deletions; at least one large deletion is known in the CF gene,[490] and others are unreported. There is also the general problem of polymorphisms at the site of ASO hybridization causing misleading results. This is a substantial concern in the case of the common ΔF508 mutation, since polymorphisms are known that can lead to apparent homozygosity for ΔF508 when the individual has a genotype such as ΔF508/F508C.[491] Such individuals are revealed as heterozygous for the ΔF508 mutation when the size of the PCR product is assessed by gel electrophoresis,[869] but they erroneously appear homozygous by ASO analysis. The occurrence of CF deletions and polymorphisms such as F508C emphasize the need to interpret any homozygous mutation result with caution, particularly homozygosity for ΔF508, whether in a CF patient or in a normal individual. Although the vast majority of CF patients who appear to have a homozygous ΔF508 genotype by ASO analysis do have this genotype, it is important to detect the occasional exception in order to avoid diagnostic errors in prenatal diagnosis and carrier detection. Although analysis of putative ΔF508 homozygotes by gel electrophoresis identifies ΔF508/F508C heterozygotes, it would not distinguish uniparental disomy or ΔF508/deletion compound heterozygotes, and analysis of parents is the most definitive approach. Compound heterozygous genotypes are more straightforward to interpret, if both mutations are identified and known to be pathologic.

Analysis by loss of a restriction enzyme site is not specific for a particular mutation, and at least one prenatal diagnostic error was uncovered on this basis (S. Richards and A.L. Beaudet, unpublished). Prenatal diagnostic errors can occur particularly through overgrowth of maternal cells with cultured chorionic villus sampling (CVS). For this reason, it is recommended that maternal cell contamination be assessed routinely by DNA polymorphisms at least for cultured CVS samples. Identity correlation of fetal and maternal samples can also be used to monitor for sample mix-ups.

Index Cases with a Classic Phenotype. In most cases, a diagnosis of CF will be established by conventional clinical criteria and the sweat test. The question arises as to whether all newly diagnosed CF patients should be genotyped, and it seems likely that this will become routine for a variety of reasons. First, the genotype permits some additional delineation of the diagnosis and may have some prognostic relevance, although prognoses on this basis must be made with great care, as discussed above under "Assessing Prognosis from Genotype." Second, and perhaps most compelling, is the fact that the genotypic information will be important for carrier detection among relatives. Carrier testing for relatives should be performed by mutation analysis if the mutation is known on the relevant side of the family, but must be performed by linkage analysis if the mutation cannot be identified. Third, if the family should desire prenatal diagnosis for a future pregnancy, it is important to know in advance whether mutation analysis will provide a complete diagnosis. Fourth, a large fraction of CF patients participate in clinical research trials, and interpretation of all information regarding CF patients is best subdivided by genotype. The cost of mutation analysis is small relative to the total cost of caring for a CF patient.

Occasionally, DNA analysis will be used to establish a diagnosis of CF in the absence of a sweat test, most frequently in the case of newborns with meconium ileus, who are too young for a reliable sweat test. DNA analysis has significant but limited value in the case of patients who are suspected of having a CF-related disorder but do not meet the conventional diagnostic criteria. This frequently involves patients with some combination of chronic bronchitis, *Pseudomonas* colonization, borderline sweat test results, pancreatic insufficiency, or other features. The identification of pathologic mutations on both chromosomes establishes a diagnosis of a CF-related disorder in these cases. The identification of one pathologic mutation makes a CF-related phenotype more likely but does not establish a diagnosis, because such individuals might be coincidental carriers for CF and have an unrelated phenotype. Finally, the failure to identify any pathologic mutation in individuals with possible CF makes a CF-related phenotype much less likely but does not eliminate the possibility. Individuals with atypical phenotypes or with non-European ethnicity are more likely to carry less common mutations that will not be included in the routine analyses, and this must be taken into account when interpreting mutation data.

Atypical Phenotypes/CBAVD. The interpretation of mutational data for individuals with atypical phenotypes is similar to that discussed immediately above for patients with possible diagnoses of CF. In the case of CBAVD, it is presumed that a substantial fraction of the CF chromosomes carry unidentified mutations, because of the high incidence of heterozygotes for known mutations, and it is likely that additional mutations will be identified in this group. Males with CBAVD and one CF mutation are generally presumed to have a CF-related phenotype, while those in whom no mutation is identified are less likely to have a CF-related phenotype, perhaps particularly if additional malformations such as renal agenesis are present.

Fetal Echogenic Bowel. There is a significant incidence of increased echogenicity of the bowel in fetuses affected with CF, but the great majority of fetuses found to have echogenic bowel on a coincidental basis with a negative family history do not have CF. There is considerable uncertainty regarding the exact probability that a fetus coincidentally found to have echogenic bowel will be affected with CF. First it is important to define the precise circumstances and findings. The probability of serious pathology is different if echogenic abnormalities are discovered during the second trimester than during the third trimester. Additional diagnostic procedures such as DNA analysis for CF and cytogenetic analysis are relevant in either case, although the focus may be on the option of pregnancy termination during the second trimester and on obstetrical and postnatal management during the third trimester. Findings of echogenic bowel should not be grouped with circumstances of intraabdominal or intrahepatic calcification. There are reports that 4 of 30 fetuses[886] and 2 of 4 fetuses[887] with echogenic bowel discovered during the second trimester proved to have CF, but this almost certainly represents a substantial bias of reporting. The experience of laboratories performing analysis for CF on fetuses or parents where the fetus is coincidentally found to have echogenic abnormalities during the second trimester indicates that the vast majority of these fetuses are not affected with CF, and most are born healthy.[874,886] Most laboratories find that certainly below 15 percent and possibly below 5 percent of fetuses with echogenic bowel discovered coincidentally during the second trimester prove to be affected with CF[874] (personal observation, A.L. Beaudet). Despite this relatively low risk, it is appropriate to perform mutational studies in such circumstances, starting with the fetus if samples are already incidentally available or with the parents if they are not. Obviously the finding of two pathologic mutations in the fetus is diagnostic of CF. The finding of one pathologic mutation in the fetus creates a very difficult counseling situation. A Bayesian calculation can be performed regarding the possibility that the fetus is affected with CF.

If one assumes (1) a 5 to 15 percent prior probability that a fetus with echogenic bowel discovered incidentally during the second trimester will have CF, (2) an incidence of 1 in 2500 for CF, and (3) a sensitivity of 89 percent for detection of CF chromosomes by mutation analysis, then a fetus with one known CF mutation and an echogenic bowel during the second trimester has a probability of 21 to 47 percent of being affected with CF. Using similar assumptions, the probability that a fetus with a second-trimester echogenic bowel but no identifiable mutation is affected is between 1 in 453 and 1 in 1516.

The circumstances are different during the third trimester, with one report that 5 of 15 fetuses found to have an echogenic bowel at 30 weeks gestation or later were affected with CF and an additional 7 of these fetuses had bowel obstruction due to other causes. Fetuses with echogenic abnormalities late in pregnancy appear much more likely to have significant pathology. Many fetuses with echogenic findings have chromosomal abnormalities such as trisomy 21 or trisomy 18.[888] Findings are more typical for duodenal atresia and/or Down syndrome if a double-bubble appearance is present. Other findings such as imperforate anus, increased risk of perinatal death, and fetal growth retardation may be associated with echogenic abnormalities of the fetal abdomen.[886,889]

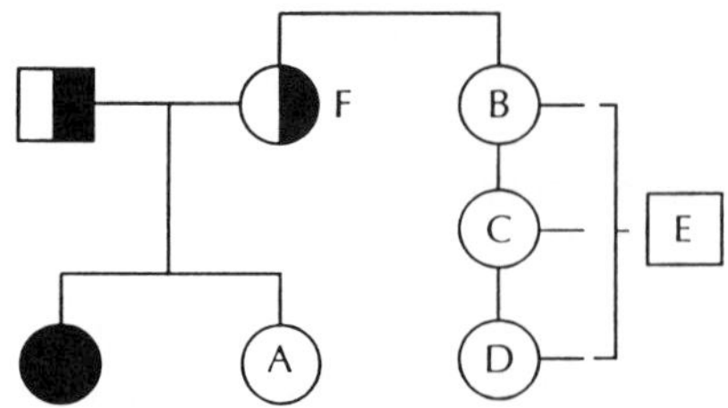

Individual CF Carrier Risk

Individual	Prior to Testing	With Negative Mutation Result When: F Not Tested	F Tested; Mutation Identified	F Tested; Mutation Not Identified
A	2/3	1/5.5	...	...
B	1/2	1/10	1/917	1/2.0
C	1/3.8	1/27	1/394	1/4.0
D	1/6.8	1/54	1/305	1/7.9
E	1/25.5	1/224	...	...

FIG. 127-20 Risk analysis for relatives of CF patients. Analysis assumes a sensitivity of 89 percent for carrier detection by mutation analysis and an incidence of 1 in 2500; a gene frequency (*q*) of 1 in 50 yields a carrier frequency (2 *pq*) of 1 in 25.5. Values were derived using the risk analysis program MLINK. *(From DeMarchi et al.[874] Used by permission.)*

Carrier Detection in CF Families. Carrier detection should be offered to relatives of CF patients who are considering reproduction. Similarly, a history regarding the occurrence of CF or carrier status should be obtained as part of routine primary or obstetrical care, and testing should be offered to those with a positive family history. Increasingly, individuals may have a history that a relative was identified as a carrier through population screening. Carrier testing should be performed by mutation analysis and, if that is not informative, by linkage analysis. In practice, couples where one partner is a definite carrier and the other partner has a negative mutation analysis will remain at a slightly increased risk relative to the general population.[394] Such couples generally proceed with reproduction without undue anxiety, and prenatal diagnosis is not useful in such circumstances. Numerous couples with a 1 in 4 risk of producing a CF child have been identified by offering testing in this setting to relatives of CF patients.[874] In attempts to economize, couples may choose to test only the partner with a negative family history or only the partner with a positive family history initially, but it is generally better to test both partners if one has a family history of CF. Individuals with a positive family history of CF and a negative mutation analysis can have a carrier risk calculated using Bayesian methods taking into account available information regarding the mutation on that side of the family, the exact relationship to the propositus, and the ethnic background[874] (Fig. 127-20). If linkage analysis is required because of the presence of an undetectable mutation, or if samples are not readily available for mutation analysis from the index family members, a couple may be satisfied to know that no mutation is found for the partner with the negative family history.

Prenatal Diagnosis. Prenatal diagnosis for pregnancies at a 1 in 4 risk is now performed routinely using primarily mutation analysis with linkage analysis added as needed. Earlier methods based on measurement of microvillar intestinal enzymes in amniotic fluid are rarely if ever used. Prenatal diagnosis is usually of little relevance except in the case of pregnancies known to be at a 1 in 4 risk. To maximize diagnostic accuracy, it is recommended that mutation analysis be performed on the propositus and parents. Analysis of parents generally will uncover unusual circumstances such as uniparental disomy in the propositus or the kinds of errors described under "Diagnostic Pitfalls" above. Parental analysis does raise the risk of uncovering nonpaternity. In addition to conventional prenatal diagnosis using cultured amniotic fluid cells or chorionic villus sampling, preimplantation diagnosis is possible.[890–893]

Quantitative data are not available for different populations regarding what proportion of CF families choose to avoid recurrence through the use of prenatal diagnosis and selective termination of pregnancy. A significant fraction of families decline prenatal diagnosis, and, of those who use the procedure, some choose to terminate affected pregnancies and others do not. There has been concern regarding pregnancy termination related to population-based screening, particularly in cases where a fetus has inherited one CF mutation. There is substantial experience with such fetuses among relatives of CF patients. Although there are reports of pregnancy termination if a fetus inherits one CF mutation,[894] this is exceedingly rare in the experience of most laboratories.[874,895]

Population-Based Carrier Screening. Immediately upon the cloning of the CF gene, intensive discussions began regarding the appropriateness of offering carrier testing on a population basis to individuals of high-risk ethnic background. There were some recommendations that carrier testing be relatively widely and immediately available[896–898]; others emphasized concerns and hazards[899,900]; and American professional genetic groups recommended that screening be postponed.[901–903] There is a general consensus that carrier testing should be offered to anyone with a positive family history, and it seems prudent to require that sperm or egg donors be tested. Numerous studies have been completed that assess attitudes and knowledge in the community.[904–910] Many groups have developed educational materials and leaflets.[911–913] Many recent commentaries, discussions, and reviews of the complex issues are available, some advocating screening and some expressing concerns.[914-921] The importance of cascade testing (preferentially offering carrier testing to relatives of known carriers) has been emphasized.[919,922] Numerous pilot studies have been performed, and reports are beginning to appear.[913,919,923-928] Groups such as the World Health Organization[929] and the United States Office of Technology Assessment[930,931] have published statements.

There was an initial focus on the question of what sensitivity might be achieved using mutation analysis for carrier detection.[902] Present data suggest that the sensitivity can be well above 90 percent in some Northern European populations and in Ashkenazic Jews, is about 89 percent for North American populations of heterogeneous European descent, and is well below 90 percent for Southern European populations (see "General Issues" under "Molecular Diagnosis" above). The risks for couples and individuals being tested are calculated readily.[394]

Numerous other issues which have been discussed include the educational level and readiness of the population for screening, the knowledge of health professionals, the availability of counseling services, the possibilities of psychological harm, the risk of discrimination regarding insurance or employment, the obligation to inform the public of the availability of carrier testing, the potential for major therapeutic breakthroughs for CF, justification of the cost of carrier screening within a health care system, the need to explain the burden of CF to screening subjects before and/or after testing, and other topics. Readers are referred to the bibliography in this section for more detailed discussions. Pilot screening programs are expanding in many European countries and to a lesser extent in North America, and it appears likely that population-based carrier screening will increase at some unpredictable rate. Some groups have offered couples routine fetal testing for CF when prenatal diagnosis is being performed for an incidental reason such as advanced maternal age,[894,932] but this practice is not widespread. Once individuals are identified as carriers, whether by the occurrence of the disease in their family or by population screening, this information will be passed on to their offspring, such that most carriers in future generations may be aware of their risks because of the known carrier status of a parent. It is difficult to predict the relative roles for prevention versus definitive treatment for future generations.

MOUSE MODELS

The long-awaited animal model for CF arrived in 1992 through the use of gene targeting in mice. Numerous mutant mice have been produced using this strategy.[16,933-937] All these mice appear to have null mutations except one,[934] which has a milder phenotype and presumably produces small amounts of normal CFTR related to skipping of the mutated exon in a gene duplication. The mice with null mutations have severe intestinal involvement, which is very similar to meconium ileus and results in death due to intestinal obstruction in a high proportion of CF mice. Disappointingly, the initial reports found very subtle if any pulmonary disease in mice, but there is hope that crossing the mutation on to other genetic backgrounds, exposing the mice to CF pathogens, introducing additional mutations, protecting against early death through transgenic expression of CFTR in the intestine, and other strategies will make the mice more useful for assessing treatments of pulmonary disease. The mice also have very limited if any pancreatic involvement, in sharp contrast to the human phenotype. Electrophysiological abnormalities very similar to those seen in human CF are readily demonstrated in the intestine and some other epithelia. Some of the differences between the human and mouse phenotypes may be related to tissue-specific patterns of expression of CFTR. In addition, the differences in disease severity may relate to the expression of an alternative plasma membrane Cl^- conductance.[938]

SOMATIC GENE THERAPY

There is considerable hope that the use of somatic gene therapy will provide a definitive treatment for the pulmonary disease and perhaps other abnormalities in CF. After the cloning of the gene, expression of CFTR in cultured cells was shown to correct the electrophysiological defect.[649,650] Attention has focused on the use of adenoviral vectors and DNA–liposome complexes for gene delivery, but other approaches, such as adeno-associated viral vectors and DNA–ligand complexes, are also being evaluated. Numerous phase I clinical trials are being initiated in the United States and Europe using adenoviral vectors or DNA–liposome delivery. Numerous reviews of gene therapy for CF are available,[273,939-943] including a detailed bibliography as of early 1994 and a tabulation of most clinical trials.[273]

It has been shown that administration of adenoviral vectors to the human nasal epithelium will correct the electrophysiological defect.[944] There is substantial evidence that adenoviral vectors can cause inflammatory responses in animal models[945,946] and humans,[273] although there are some reports of minimal inflammation and ability to readminister vectors to animals.[947] The first generation of adenoviral vectors are typically deleted for the E1 gene of the virus and often deleted for the E3 region. These vectors express low levels of viral proteins, and either introduction of mutations in the E2 region to further cripple viral protein expression or immunosuppression of the host may minimize the host response and prolong the duration of expression.[948,949] There is less in vivo data in animals for the use of DNA–liposome delivery,[950-952] and even less information regarding the in vivo use of adeno-associated viral vectors[953] or DNA–ligand complexes. Airway instillation of an adenoviral vector and aerosol delivery of DNA–liposome complexes have been reported to correct the electrophysiological defect in CF mice.[954,955]

The advantages and disadvantages of various delivery systems as well as many other aspects of gene therapy for CF are discussed in the available reviews.[273,939-943,956] It is obvious that information on gene therapy will evolve extremely rapidly, and the most recent reviews as well as the primary literature will need to be consulted for up-to-date information. CF patients and their families are intensely interested in this approach and expect clinicians to provide them with up-to-date information.

Remarkable resources are being marshalled to develop a definitive treatment for CF, and great benefits are likely to ensue. It should be kept in mind that patients with advanced lung disease may not benefit from gene therapy and that CF patients protected from pulmonary disease will remain susceptible to other complications such as diabetes mellitus. Until the complete success is achieved, a combination of intense commitment, cautious optimism, and avoidance of false guarantees will be needed.

REFERENCES

1. Taussig LM: Cystic fibrosis: An overview, in Taussig LM (ed): *Cystic Fibrosis*. New York, Thieme-Stratton, 1984, p 1.
2. Fanconi G, Uehlinger E, Knauer C: Das coeliakiesyndrom be: Angeborener zysticher pancreas fibromatose und bronkiektasien. *Wien Med Wochenschr* **86**:753, 1936.
3. Anderson DH: Cystic fibrosis of the pancreas and its relation to celiac disease: A clinical and pathological study. *Am J Dis Child* **56**:344, 1938.
4. Farber S: Some organic digestive disturbances in early life. *J Mich Med Soc* **44**:587, 1945.
5. Anderson DH, Hodges RG: Celiac syndrome. V. Genetics of cystic fibrosis of the pancreas with a consideration of etiology. *Am J Dis Child* **72**:62, 1946.
6. di Sant'Agnese PA, Darling RC, Perrera GA, Shea E: Abnormal electrolytic composition of sweat in cystic fibrosis of the pancreas. Clinical significance and relationship of the disease. *Pediatrics* **12**:549, 1953.
7. Gibson LE, Cooke RE: A test for concentration of electrolytes in sweat in cystic fibrosis of the pancreas utilizing pilocarpine by iontophoresis. *Pediatrics* **23**:545, 1959.
8. Knowles M, Gatzy J, Boucher R: Increased bioelectric potential difference across respiratory epithelia in cystic fibrosis. *N Engl J Med* **305**:1489, 1981.
9. Quinton PM, Bijman J: Higher bioelectric potentials due to decreased chloride absorption in the sweat glands of patients with cystic fibrosis. *N Engl J Med* **308**:1185, 1983.
10. Matthews LW, Spector S, Lemm J, Potter UL: Studies on pulmonary secretions. The overall chemical composition of pulmonary secretions from patients with cystic fibrosis, bronchiectasis, and laryngectomy. *Am Rev Respir Dis* **88**:199, 1963.
11. Kopelman H, Durie P, Gaskin K, Weizman Z, Forstner G: Pancreatic fluid secretion and protein hyperconcentration in cystic fibrosis. *N Engl J Med* **312**:329, 1985.
12. Rommens JM, Iannuzzi MC, Kerem B, Drumm ML, Melmer G, Dean M, Rozmahel R, Cole JL, Kennedy D, Hidaka N, Zsiga M, Buchwald M, Riordan JR, Tsui L-C, Collins FS: Identification of the cystic fibrosis gene: Chromosome walking and jumping. *Science* **245**:1059, 1989.
13. Riordan JR, Rommens JM, Kerem B, Alon N, Rozmahel R, Grzelczak Z, Zielenski J, Lok S, Plavsic N, Chou J-L, Drumm ML, Iannuzzi MC, Collins FS, Tsui L-C: Identification of the cystic fibrosis gene: Cloning and characterization of complementary DNA. *Science* **245**:1066, 1989.
14. Kerem B, Rommens JM, Buchanan JA, Markiewicz D, Cox TK, Chakravarti A, Buchwald M, Tsui L-C: Identification of the cystic fibrosis gene: Genetic analysis. *Science* **245**:1073, 1989.
15. Anderson MP, Rich DP, Gregory RJ, Smith AE, Walsh MN: Generation of cAMP-activated chloride currents by expression of CFTR. *Science* **251**:679, 1991.
16. Snouwaert JN, Brigman KK, Latour AM, Malouf NN, Boucher RC, Smithies O, Koller BH: An animal model for cystic fibrosis made by gene targeting. *Science* **257**:1083, 1992.
17. Zuelzer WW, Newton WA Jr: The pathogenesis of fibrocystic disease of the pancreas. A study of 36 cases with special reference to the pulmonary lesions. *Pediatrics* **4**:53, 1949.
18. Sturgess J, Imprie J: Quantitative evaluations of the development of tracheal submucosal glands in infants with cystic fibrosis and control infants. *Am J Pathol* **106**:303, 1982.
19. Sturgess J: Morphologic characteristics of the bronchial mucosa in cystic fibrosis, in Quinton P, Martinez R, Hopfer U (eds): *Fluid and Electrolyte Abnormalities in Exocrine Glands in Cystic Fibrosis*. San Francisco, San Francisco Press, 1982, p 254.
20. Bedrossian CWM, Greenberg SD, Singer DB, Hansen JJ, Rosenberg HS: The lung in cystic fibrosis. *Hum Pathol* **7**:195, 1976.
21. Tomashefski JF Jr, Bruce M, Goldberg HI, Dearborn DG: Regional distribution of macroscopic lung disease in cystic fibrosis. *Am Rev Respir Dis* **133**:535, 1986.
22. Sobonya RE, Taussig LM: Quantitative aspects of lung pathology in cystic fibrosis. *Am Rev Respir Dis* **134**:290, 1986.
23. Tomashefski JF Jr, Bruce M, Stern RC, Dearborn DG, Dahms B: The pathology of pulmonary air cysts in cystic fibrosis. Relation to radiologic findings and history of pneumothorax. *Hum Pathol* **16**:253, 1985.
24. Tomashefski JF Jr, Konstan MW, Bruce M: The pathology of interstitial pneumonia in cystic fibrosis. *Am Rev Respir Dis* **133**:A365, 1986.
25. Boat TF, di Sant'Agnese PA, Warwick W, Handwerger S: Pneumothorax in cystic fibrosis. *JAMA* **209**:1498, 1969.
26. Mack JF, Moss AF, Harper WW, O'Loughlin BJ: The bronchial arteries in cystic fibrosis. *Br J Radiol* **38**:422, 1965.
27. Ryland D, Reid L: The pulmonary circulation in cystic fibrosis. *Thorax* **30**:285, 1975.
28. Stern RC, Boat TF, Wood RE, Matthews LW, Doershuk CF: Treatment and prognosis of nasal polyps in cystic fibrosis. *Am J Dis Child* **126**:1067, 1982.
29. Wood RE, Wanner A, Hirsch J, Farrell PM: Tracheal mucociliary transport in patients with cystic fibrosis and its stimulation by terbutaline. *Am Rev Respir Dis* **111**:733, 1975.
30. Katz SM, Holsclaw DS: Ultrastructural features of respiratory cilia in cystic fibrosis. *Am J Clin Pathol* **73**:682, 1980.
31. Rutland J, Cole PJ: Nasal mucociliary clearance and ciliary beat frequency in cystic fibrosis compared with sinusitis and bronchiectasis. *Thorax* **36**:654, 1981.
32. Schwab UE, Wold AE, Carson JL, Leigh MW, Cheng PW, Gilligan PH, Boat TF: Increased adherence of *Staphlococcus aureus* from cystic fibrosis lungs to airway epithelial cells. *Am Rev Respir Dis* **148**:365, 1993.
33. Woods DE, Bass JA, Johanson WG, Straus DC: Role of adherence in the pathogenesis of *Pseudomonas aeruginosa* lung infection in cystic fibrosis patients. *Infect Immun* **30**:694, 1980.
34. Saiman L, Cacalano G, Gruenert D, Prince A: Comparison of adherence of *Pseudomonas aeruginosa* to respiratory epithelial cells from cystic fibrosis patients and healthy subjects. *Infect Immun* **60**:2808, 1992.
35. Ramphal R, Pier GB: Role of *Pseudomonas aeruginosa* mucoid exopolysaccharide in adherence to tracheal cells. *Infect Immun* **47**:1, 1985.
36. Matthews WJ, Williams M, Oliphant B, Geha R, Colten RH: Hypogammaglobulinemia in patients with cystic fibrosis. *N Engl J Med* **302**:245, 1980.
37. Gugler E, Pallavicini JD, Swerdlow TL: Immunological studies of submaxillary saliva from patients with cystic fibrosis. *J Pediatr* **73**:548, 1982.
38. Margolies R, Gray B, Boat TF: Identification of a major heparin-precipitable protein in human serum and its relationship to cystic fibrosis. *Pediatr Res* **16**:181, 1982.
39. Baltimore RS, Fick RB, Fino L: Antibody to multiple mucoid strains of *Pseudomonas aeruginosa* in patients with cystic fibrosis, measured by an enzyme-linked immunosorbent assay. *Pediatr Res* **16**:181, 1986.
40. Sorensen R, Ruuskanen O, Miller K, Stern RC: B-lymphocyte function in cystic fibrosis. *Eur J Respir Dis* **64**:524, 1983.
41. Sorensen RU, Stern RC, Polmar SH: Cellular immunity to bacteria: Impairment of in vitro lymphocyte response to *Pseudomonas aeruginosa* in cystic fibrosis patients. *Infect Immun* **18**:735, 1977.
42. Sorensen RU, Stern RC, Chase P, Polmar SH: Defective cellular immunity to gram-negative bacteria in cystic fibrosis patients. *Infect Immun* **23**:398, 1979.
43. Miller TJ, Olds LC: Interleukin-2 production by lymphocytes from blood of children with arthritis is less suppressed than in systemic lupus or cystic fibrosis. *J Rheumatol* **14**:736, 1987.
44. Richman-Eisenstat J, Jorens PG, Ueki I, Nadel JA: Interleukin-8 accounts for the majority of the neutrophil chemotactic activity in sputum of patients with chronic inflammatory airways disease. *Am Rev Respir Dis* **147**:A29, 1993.
45. Kharazmi A, Rechnitzer C, Schietz PO, Jensen R, Baek L, Hoiby N: Priming of neutrophils for enhanced oxidative burst by sputum from cystic fibrosis patients with *Pseudomonas aeruginosa* infection. *Eur J Clin Invest* **17**:256, 1987.
46. Thomassen MJ, Demko CA, Wood RE, Kuchenbrod PJ, Dearborn DG, Wood RE: Inhibitory effect of cystic fibrosis serum on *Pseudomonas* phagocytosis by rabbit and human alveolar macrophages. *Pediatr Res* **13**:3085, 1979.
47. Thomassen MJ, Demko CA, Wood RE, Tandler B,

Dearborn DG, Boxerbaum B, Kuchenbrod PJ: Ultrastructure and function of alveolar macrophages from cystic fibrosis patients. *Pediatr Res* **14**:715, 1980.

48. Fick RB, Naegel GP, Squier SU, Wood RE, Gee BL, Reynolds HY: Proteins of the cystic fibrosis respiratory tract: Fragmented immunoglobulin G opsonic antibody causing defective opsonophagocytosis. *J Clin Invest* **74**:236, 1984.
49. Fick RB, Olcholski J, Squier SU, Merrill WW, Reynolds HY: Immunoglobulin-G subclasses in cystic fibrosis: IgG2 response to *Pseudomonas aeruginosa* lipopolysaccharide. *Am Rev Respir Dis* **133**:418, 1986.
50. Wisnieski JJ, Todd EW, Fuller RK, Jones PK, Dearborn DG, Boat TF, Naff GB: Immune complexes and complement abnormalities in patients with cystic fibrosis. *Am Rev Respir Dis* **132**:770, 1986.
51. Campbell IM, Crozier DN, Silver J, Buivids IA: The effect of fatty acids on *Staphylococcus aureus* in vitro, in Sturgess JM (ed): *Perspectives in Cystic Fibrosis*. Mississauga, Ontario, Canada, Imperial Press, 1980, p 359.
52. Gaskin K, Gurwitz D, Durie P, Corey M, Levison H, Forstner G: Improved respiratory prognosis in patients with cystic fibrosis with normal fat absorption *J Pediatr* **100**:857, 1982.
53. Fick RB Jr, Robbins RV, Squier SU, Robbins PA, Schoderbek WE, Russ WO: Complement activation in cystic fibrosis respiratory fluids: In vivo and in vitro generation of C5a and chemotactic activity. *Pediatr Res* **20**:1258, 1986.
54. Klinger JD, Tandler B, Liedtke CM, Boat TF: Proteinases of *Pseudomonas aeruginosa* evoke mucin release by tracheal epithelium. *J Clin Invest* **74**:1669, 1984.
55. Nadel J: Role of mast cell and neutrophil proteases in airway secretion. *Am Rev Respir Dis* **144**:548, 1991.
56. Christensen TG, Korthy AL, Snider GL, Hayes JA: Irreversible bronchial goblet cell metaplasia in hamsters with elastase induced panacinar emphysema. *J Clin Invest* **59**:1669, 1977.
57. Goldstein W, Doring G: Lysosomal enzymes with polymorphonuclear leukocytes and proteinase inhibitors in patients with cystic fibrosis. *Am Rev Respir Dis* **134**:49, 1986.
58. Hingley ST, Hastie AT, Kueppers F, Higgins ML: Disruption of respiratory cilia by proteases including those of *Pseudomonas aeruginosa*. *Infect Immun* **54**:379, 1986.
59. Niederman MS, Merrill WW, Polomski LM, Reynolds HY, Gee BL: Influence of sputum IgA and elastase on tracheal cell bacterial adherence. *Am Rev Respir Dis* **133**:255, 1986.
60. Schoitz PO, Nielsen H, Hoiby N, Glikmann G, Svehag SE: Immune complexes in the sputum of patients with cystic fibrosis suffering from chronic *Pseudomonas aeruginosa* lung infection. *Acta Pathol Microbiol Scand* **86**:37, 1978.
61. Langley SC, Brown RR, Kelly FJ: Reduced free-radical trapping capacity and altered plasma antioxidant status in cystic fibrosis. *Pediatr Res* **33**:247, 1993.
62. Talamo RC, Schwartz RH: Immunologic and allergic manifestations, in Taussig LM (ed): *Cystic Fibrosis*. New York, Thieme-Stratton, 1984, p 175.
63. Wang EEL, Prober CG, Manson B, Corey M, Levison H: Association of respiratory viral infections with pulmonary deterioration of patients with cystic fibrosis. *N Engl J Med* **311**:1653, 1984.
64. Peterson NT, Hoiby N, Mordhorst CH, Lind K, Flensboro EW, Brunn B: Respiratory infections in cystic fibrosis patients caused by virus, chlamydia, and mycoplasma: Possible synergism with *Pseudomonas aeruginosa*. *Acta Paediatr Scand* **70**:623, 1981.
65. Stern RC, Boat TF, Wood RE, Matthews LW, Doershuk CF: Treatment and prognosis of nasal polyps in cystic fibrosis. *Am J Dis Child* **136**:1067, 1982.
66. Wiatrik BJ, Myer CM, Cotton RT: Cystic fibrosis presenting with sinus disease in children. *Am J Dis Child* **147**:258, 1993.
67. Shapiro ED, Milmoe GJ, Wald ER, Rodman JB, Bowen A: Bacteriology of the maxillary sinuses in patients with cystic fibrosis. *J Infect Dis* **146**:589, 1982.
68. Strauss RG, West PJ, Silverman FN: Unilateral proptosis in cystic fibrosis and hearing loss. *Arch Otolaryngol* **105**:338, 1979.

68a. Sharma GD, Doershuk CF, Stern RC: Erosion of the wall of the frontal sinus caused by mucopyocele in cystic fibrosis. *J Pediatr* **124**:745, 1994.

68b. Umetsu DT, Moss RB, King VV, Lewiston NJ: Sinus disease in patients with severe cystic fibrosis: Relation to pulmonary exacerbation. *Lancet* **335**:1077, 1990.

69. Forman-Franco B, Abramson AL, Gorvoy JD, Stein T: Cystic fibrosis and hearing loss. *Arch Otolaryngol* **105**:338, 1979.
70. Taussig LM, Landau LI, Marks MI: Respiratory system, in Taussig LM (ed): *Cystic Fibrosis*. New York, Thieme-Stratton, 1984, p 115.
71. Demko CA, Thomasen MJ: Effect of mucoid property on antibiotic susceptibility of *Pseudomonas aeruginosa*. *Curr Microbiol* **4**:69, 1980.
72. Blackwood L, Pennington JE: Influence of mucoid coating on clearance of *Pseudomonas aeruginosa* from lungs. *Infect Immun* **32**:443, 1981.
73. Isles A, Maclusky I, Corey M, Gold R, Prober C, Fleming P, Levison H: *Pseudomonas cepacia* infection in cystic fibrosis: An emerging problem. *J Pediatr* **104**:206, 1984.
74. Thomassen MJ, Demko AC, Klinger JD, Stern RC: *Pseudomonas cepacia* colonization among patients with cystic fibrosis. *Am Rev Respir Dis* **131**:791, 1985.
75. Lester LA, Egge A, Hubbard VS, di Sant'Agnese PA: Aspiration and lung abscess in cystic fibrosis. *Am Rev Respir Dis* **127**:786, 1983.
76. Kilbourn JP, Campbell RA, Grach JL: Quantitative bacteriology of sputum. *Am Rev Respir Dis* **98**:810, 1968.
77. Wood RE, Boat TF, Doershuk CF: State of the art: Cystic fibrosis. *Am Rev Respir Dis* **113**:833, 1976.
78. Boxerbaum B: Isolation of rapidly growing mycobacteria in patients with cystic fibrosis. *J Pediatr* **96**:689, 1980.
79. Kilby JM, Gilligan PH, Yankaskas JR, Highsmith WE, Edwards LJ, Knowles MR: Nontuberculous mycobacteria in adult patients with cystic fibrosis. *Chest* **102**:70, 1992.
80. Ramsey BW, Gore EJ, Smith AL, Cooney MK, Redding G, Foy H: The effect of respiratory viral infections on patients with cystic fibrosis. *Am J Dis Child* **143**:662, 1989.
81. Brasfield D, Hicks G, Soong S, Peters J, Tiller R: Evaluation of a scoring system of chest radiographs in cystic fibrosis: A collaborative study. *Pediatrics* **63**:24, 1979.

81a. Weatherly MR, Palmer CGS, Peters ME, Green CG, Fryback D, Langhough R, Farell PM: Wisconsin cystic fibrosis chest radiograph scoring system. *Pediatrics* **91**:488, 1993.

82. Nathanson I, Conboy K, Murphy S, Afshani E, Kuhn JP: Ultrafast computerized tomography of the chest in cystic fibrosis: A new scoring system. *Pediatr Pulmonol* **11**:81, 1991.
83. Bhalla M, Turcois N, Aponte V, Jenkins M, Leitman BS, McCauley DI, Naidich DP: Cystic fibrosis: Scoring system with the thin section CT. *Radiology* **179**:783, 1991.
84. Gooding CA, Lallemand DP, Brasch RC, Wesley GE, Davis B: Magnetic resonance imaging in cystic fibrosis. *J Pediatr* **105**:384, 1984.
85. Kinsella D, Hamilton A, Goddard P, Duncan A, Carswell F: The role of magnetic resonance imaging in cystic fibrosis. *Clin Radiol* **44**:23, 1991.
86. Levison H, Godfrey S: Pulmonary aspects of cystic fibrosis, in Mangos JA, Talamo RE (eds): *Cystic Fibrosis: Projections into the Future*. New York, Stratten Intercontinental Medical Books, 1976, p 3.
87. Siassi B, Moss AJ, Dooley RR: Clinical recognition of cor pulmonale in cystic fibrosis. *J Pediatr* **78**:794, 1971.
88. Francis PWJ, Muller NL, Gurwitz D, Milligan DWA, Levison H, Bryan AC: Hemoglobin desaturation. Its occurrence during sleep in patients with cystic fibrosis. *Am J Dis Child* **134**:734, 1980.
89. Stokes DC, Wohl ME, Khaw KT, Strieder DJ: Postural hypoxemia in cystic fibrosis. *Chest* **87**:785, 1985.
90. Wagener JS, McNeil GC, Taussig LM, Corrigan JJ, Lemen R: Ferrokinetic and hematologic studies in cystic fibrosis patients. *Am J Pediatr Hematol Oncol* **5**:153, 1983.
91. Rosenthal A, Khaw KT, Shwachman H: Hemoglobin-oxygen equilibrium in cystic fibrosis. *Pediatrics* **59**:919, 1977.
92. Wagener JS, Taussig LM, Burrows B, Hernreid L, Boat T: Comparison of lung infection and survival patterns between

cystic fibrosis and emphysema or chronic bronchitis patients, in Sturgess JM (ed): *Perspectives in Cystic Fibrosis*. Mississauga, Ontario, Canada, Imperial Press, 1980, p 236.

93. Haluszka J, Scislicki A: Bronchial lability in children suffering from some diseases of the bronchi. *Respiration* **32**:217, 1975.
94. Larsen GL, Barron RJ, Cotten EK, Brooks JG: A comparative study of inhaled atropine sulfate and isoproterenol hydrochloride in cystic fibrosis. *Am Rev Respir Dis* **119**:399, 1979.
95. Hordvik NL, Konig P, Morris D, Kreutz C, Barbero GF: A longitudinal study of bronchodilator responsiveness in cystic fibrosis. *Am Rev Respir Dis* **131**:889, 1985.
96. Godfrey S, Mearns M: Pulmonary function and response to exercise in cystic fibrosis. *Arch Dis Child* **46**:144, 1971.
97. Henke KG, Orenstein DM: Oxygen saturation during exercise in cystic fibrosis. *Am Rev Respir Dis* **129**:708, 1984.
98. Asher MI, Pardy RL, Coates AL, Thomas E, Macklem PT: The effects of inspiratory muscle training in patients with cystic fibrosis. *Am Rev Respir Dis* **126**:855, 1982.
99. Orenstein DM, Franklin BA, Doreshuk CF, Hellerstein HK, German KF, Horowitz FG, Stern RC: Exercise conditioning and cardiopulmonary fitness in cystic fibrosis. *Chest* **80**:392, 1981.
100. Nixon PA, Orenstein D: Prognostic value of exercise testing in patients with cystic fibrosis. *N Engl J Med* **327**:1785, 1992.
101. O'Rawe A, McIntosh I, Dodge JA, Brock DJH, Redmond AOB, Ward R, MacPherson AJS: Increased energy expenditure in cystic fibrosis is associated with specific mutations. *Clin Sci* **82**:71, 1992.
102. Davies PSW, Bronstein MN: Energy expenditure of infants with cystic fibrosis. *Pediatr Pulmonol* **58**:175, 1992.
103. Stern RC, Boat TF, Orenstein DM, Wood RE, Matthews LW, Doershuk CF: Treatment and prognosis of lobar and segmental atelectasis in cystic fibrosis. *Am Rev Respir Dis* **118**:821, 1978.
104. Stowe SM, Boat TF, Mendelson H, Stern RC, Tucker AS, Doershuk CF, Matthews LW: Open thoracotomy for pneumothorax in cystic fibrosis. *Am Rev Respir Dis* **111**:611, 1975.
105. Stern RC, Wood RE, Boat TF, Matthews LW, Tucker AS, Doershuk CF: Treatment and prognosis of massive hemoptysis in cystic fibrosis. *Am Rev Respir Dis* **117**:825, 1978.
106. Holsclaw DS, Grand RJ, Shwachman H: Massive hemoptysis in cystic fibrosis. *J Pediatr* **76**:829, 1970.
107. Schonheyder H, Jensen T, Hoiby N, Andersen P, Koch C: Frequency of *Aspergillus fumigatus* isolates and antibodies to aspergillus antigens in cystic fibrosis. *Acta Pathol Microbiol Immunol Scand* **93**:105, 1985.
108. Lemen RJ, Gates AJ, Mathe AA, Waring WW, Hyman AL, Kadowitz PD: Relationships among digital clubbing, disease severity, and serum prostaglandins $F_{2\alpha}$ and E concentrations in cystic fibrosis patients. *Am Rev Respir Dis* **117**:639, 1978.
109. Cohen AM, Yulish BS, Wasser KB, Vignos PJ, Jones PK, Sorin SB: Evaluation of pulmonary hypertrophic osteoarthropathy in cystic fibrosis. *Am J Dis Child* **140**:74, 1986.
110. Taussig LM, Belmonte M, Beaudry PH: *Staphylococcus aureus* empyema in cystic fibrosis. *J Pediatr* **84**:724, 1974.
111. Stern RC, Borkat G, Hirschfield SS, Boat TF, Matthews LW, Liebman G, Doershuk CF: Heart failure in cystic fibrosis. *Am J Dis Child* **134**:267, 1980.
112. di Sant'Agnese PA, Hubbard VS: The gastrointestinal tract, in Taussig LM (ed): *Cystic Fibrosis*. New York, Thieme-Stratton, 1984, p 212.
113. Neutra MR, Trier JS: The rectal mucosa in cystic fibrosis: Morphologic features before and after short term organ culture. *Gastroenterology* **75**:701, 1978.
114. Kopito L, Shwachman H: Mineral composition of meconium. *J Pediatr* **68**:313, 1966.
115. Rosenstein BJ, Langbaum TS: Incidence of meconium abnormalities in newborn infants with cystic fibrosis. *Am J Dis Child* **134**:72, 1980.
116. di Sant'Agnese PA, Davis PB: Cystic fibrosis in adults: 75 cases and a review of 232 cases in the literature. *Am J Med* **66**:121, 1979.
117. McCarthy VP, Mischler EJ, Hubbard VS, Chernick MS, di Sant'Agnese PA: Appendiceal abscess in cystic fibrosis: A diagnostic challenge. *Gastroenterology* **86**:564, 1984.
118. Fletcher BD, Abramowsky CR: Contrast enemas in cystic fibrosis: Implications of appendiceal nonfilling. *AJR* **137**:323, 1981.
119. Dolan TF, Meyers A: Mild cystic fibrosis presenting as an asymptomatic distended appendiceal mass: A case report. *Clin Pediatr* **14**:862, 1975.
120. George DH: Diverticulosis of the vermiform appendix in patients with cystic fibrosis. *Hum Pathol* **18**:75, 1987.
121. Taussig LM, Saldine RM, di Sant'Agnese PA: Radiographic abnormalities of the duodenum and small bowel in cystic fibrosis of the pancreas. *Radiology* **106**:369, 1973.
122. Stern RC, Izant RJ, Boat TF, Wood RE, Matthews LW, Doershuk CF: Treatment and prognosis of rectal prolapse in cystic fibrosis. *Gastroenterology* **82**:707, 1982.
123. Wood RE, Herman CJ, Johnson KW, di Sant'Agnese PA: Pneumatosis coli in cystic fibrosis. Clinical, radiologic and pathologic features. *Am J Dis Child* **129**:246, 1975.
124. di Sant'Agnese PA, Hubbard VS: The pancreas, in Taussig LM (ed): *Cystic Fibrosis*. New York, Thieme-Stratton, 1984, p 230.
125. Atlas AB, Orenstein SR, Orenstein DM: Pancreatitis in young children with cystic fibrosis. *J Pediatr* **120**:756, 1992.
126. Handwerger S, Roth J, Gorden P, di Sant'Agnese PA, Carpenter DF, Peter G: Glucose intolerance in cystic fibrosis. *N Engl J Med* **281**:451, 1969.
127. Abdul-Karim FW, Dahms BB, Velasco ME, Rodman HM: Islets of Langerhans in adolescents and adults with cystic fibrosis. *Arch Pathol Lab Med* **110**:602, 1986.
128. Abrams CK, Hamosh M, Hubbard VS, Datta SK, Hamosh P: Lingual lipase in cystic fibrosis. *J Clin Invest* **73**:374, 1984.
129. Hoffman RD, Isenberg JN, Powell GK: Carbohydrate malabsorption is minimal in school-age cystic fibrosis children. *Dig Dis Sci* **32**:1071, 1987.
130. Mischler EH, Chesney PJ, Chesney RW, Mazess RB: Demineralization in cystic fibrosis. *Am J Dis Child* **133**:632, 1979.
131. Reiter EO, Brugman SM, Pike JW, Pitt M, Dokoh S, Haussler MR, Gerstle RS, Taussig LM: Vitamin D metabolites in adolescents and young adults with cystic fibrosis. *J Pediatr* **106**:21, 1985.
132. Friedman HZ, Langman CB, Favus MJ: Vitamin D metabolism and osteomalacia in cystic fibrosis. *Gastroenterology* **38**:803, 1985.
133. Elias E, Muller DPR, Scott J: Association of spinocerebellar disorders with cystic fibrosis or chronic childhood cholestasis and very low serum vitamin E. *Lancet* **2**:1319, 1981.
134. Farrell PM, Bieri JG, Fratantoni JF, Wood RE, di Sant'Agnese PA: The occurrence and effects of human vitamin E deficiency: A study in patients with cystic fibrosis. *J Clin Invest* **60**:233, 1977.
135. Blanc WA, Reid JD, Anderson DH: Avitaminosis E in cystic fibrosis of the pancreas. *Pediatrics* **22**:494, 1958.
136. Torstenson OL, Humphrey GB, Edson JR: Cystic fibrosis presenting with severe hemorrhage due to vitamin K malabsorption: A report of three cases. *Pediatrics* **45**:857, 1970.
137. Corrigan JJ, Taussig LM, Beckerman R, Wagener JS: Factor III (prothrombin) coagulant activity and immunoreactive protein: Detection of vitamin K deficiency and liver disease in patients with cystic fibrosis. *J Pediatr* **99**:254, 1981.
138. Deren JJ, Arora B, Toskes PP, Hansell J, Sibinga MD: Malabsorption of crystalline vitamin B_{12} in cystic fibrosis. *N Engl J Med* **288**:949, 1973.
139. Lindemans J, Abels J, Neijens HJ, Kerrebijn KF: Elevated serum vitamin B_{12} in cystic fibrosis. *Acta Paediatr Scand* **73**:768, 1984.
140. Faraj BA, Caplan DB, Camp VM, Pilzer E, Kutner W: Low levels of pyridoxal 5′-phosphate in patients with cystic fibrosis. *Pediatrics* **78**:278, 1986.
141. Hansen RC, Lemen R, Revsin B: Cystic fibrosis manifesting with acrodermatitis enteropathica-like eruption. *Arch Dermatol* **129**:51, 1983.
142. Weber A, Roy CC, Morin CL, Lasalle R: Malabsorption

of bile acids in children with cystic fibrosis. *N Engl J Med* **289**:1001, 1973.

143. Watkins JB, Tercyak AM, Szczepanik P, Klein PD: Bile salt kinetics in cystic fibrosis: Influence of pancreatic enzyme replacement. *Gastroenterology* **73**:1023, 1977.
144. Robb TA, Davidson GP, Kirubakaron C: Conjugated bile acids in serum and secretions in response to cholecystokinin-secretin stimulation in children with cystic fibrosis. *Gut* **26**:1246, 1985.
145. di Sant'Agnese PA, Hubbard VS: The hepatobiliary system, in Taussig LM (ed): *Cystic Fibrosis*. New York, Thieme-Stratton, 1984, p 296.
146. Fleischer DA, DiGeorge AM, Barnes LA, Cornfield D: Hypoproteinemia and edema in infants with cystic fibrosis of the pancreas. *J Pediatr* **64**:341, 1964.
147. Lee PA, Roloff DW, Howatt WF: Hypoproteinemia and anemia in infants with cystic fibrosis. *JAMA* **228**:585, 1974.
148. Abman SH, Reardon MC, Accurso FJ: Hypoalbuminemia at diagnosis as a marker for severe respiratory course in infants with cystic fibrosis identified by newborn screening. *J Pediatr* **107**:933, 1985.
149. Reisman J, Petrou C, Corey M, Stringer D, Durie P, Levison H: Hypoalbuminemia at initial examination in patients with cystic fibrosis. *J Pediatr* **115**:755, 1989.
150. Shwachman H, Lebenthal E, Khaw KT: Recurrent acute pancreatitis in patients with cystic fibrosis with normal pancreatic enzymes. *Pediatrics* **55**:86, 1975.
151. Rodman HM, Matthews LW: Hyperglycemia in cystic fibrosis: A review of the literature and our own patient experience, in Warwick WJ (ed): *1000 Years of Cystic Fibrosis*, Minneapolis, MN, University of Minnesota Press, 1981, p 67.
152. Lippe B, Sperling MA, Dooley RR: Pancreatic alpha and beta cell functions in cystic fibrosis. *J Pediatr* **90**:751, 1977.
153. Redmond AO, Buchman KD, Trimble ER: Insulin and glucagon response to arginine infusion in cystic fibrosis. *Acta Paediatr Scand* **66**:199, 1977.
154. Geffner ME, Lippe BM, Maclaren NK, Riley WJ: Role of autoimmunity in insulinopenia and carbohydrate derangements associated with cystic fibrosis. *J Pediatr* **112**:419, 1988.
155. Lippe BM, Kaplan SA, Neufeld ND, Smith A, Scott W: Insulin receptors in cystic fibrosis: Increased receptor number and altered affinity. *Pediatrics* **65**:1018, 1980.
156. Wilmshurst EG, Soeldner JS, Holsclaw DS, Kaufman RL, Shwachman H, Aski TT, Gleason RE: Endogenous and exogenous insulin responses in patients with cystic fibrosis. *Pediatrics* **55**:75, 1975.
157. Rodman HM, Waltman SR, Krupin T, Lee AT, Frank KE, Matthews LW: Quantitative vitreous fluorophotometry in insulin-treated cystic fibrosis patients. *Diabetes* **32**:505, 1983.
158. Allen JL: Progressive nephropathy in a patient with cystic fibrosis and diabetes. *N Engl J Med* **315**:764, 1986.
159. Moran A, Diem P, Klein DJ, Levitt MD, Robertson RP: Pancreatic endocrine function in cystic fibrosis. *J Pediatr* **118**:715, 1991.
160. Rodman HM, Doershuk CF, Roland JM: The interaction of two diseases: Diabetes mellitus and cystic fibrosis. *Medicine* **65**:389, 1986.
161. Finkelstein SM, Wielinski CL, Elliott GR, Warwick WJ, Barbosa J, Wu SC, Klein DJ: Diabetes mellitus associated with cystic fibrosis. *J Pediatr* **112**:373, 1988.
162. di Sant'Agnese PA, Blanc WA: A distinctive type of biliary cirrhosis of the liver associated with cystic fibrosis of the pancreas. *Pediatrics* **188**:387, 1956.
163. Craig JM, Haddad H, Shwachman H: The pathologic changes in the liver in cystic fibrosis of the pancreas. *Am J Dis Child* **93**:357, 1957.
164. Kattwinkel J, Taussig LM, Statland BE, Verter JI: The effects of age on alkaline phosphatase and other serologic liver function tests in normal subjects and patients with cystic fibrosis. *J Pediatr* **82**:234, 1973.
165. Boat TF, Doershuk CF, Stern RC, Matthews LW: Serum alkaline phosphatase in cystic fibrosis. *Clin Pediatr* **13**:505, 1974.
166. Valman HV, France NE, Wallis PG: Prolonged neonatal jaundice in cystic fibrosis. *Arch Dis Child* **46**:805, 1971.
167. Stern RC, Stevens DP, Boat TF, Doershuk CF, Izant RF, Matthews LW: Symptomatic hepatic disease in cystic fibrosis: Incidence, course, and outcome of portal systemic shunting. *Gastroenterology* **70**:645, 1976.
168. Stern RC, Boat TF, Doershuk CF, Tucker AS, Miller RB, Matthews LW: Cystic fibrosis diagnosed after age 13. *Ann Intern Med* **87**:188, 1977.
169. Duthie A, Doherty DG, Williams C, Scott-Jupp R, Warner JO, Tanner MS, Williamson R, Mowat AP: Genotype analysis for ΔF508, G551D and R553X mutations in children and young adults with cystic fibrosis with and without chronic liver disease. *Hepatology* **15**:660, 1992.
170. Schwartz HP, Kraemer R, Thurnheer U, Rossi E: Liver involvement in cystic fibrosis: A report of 9 cases. *Helv Paediatr Acta* **33**:351, 1978.
171. Griscom NT, Capitanio MA, Wagoner ML, Culham G, Morris L: The visibly fatty liver. *Radiology* **117**:385, 1975.
172. L'Heureux PR, Isenberg JN, Sharp HL, Warwick WJ: Gallbladder disease in cystic fibrosis. *Am J Roentgenol* **128**:953, 1977.
173. Oppenheimer EH, Esterly JR: Pathology of cystic fibrosis: Review of the literature and comparison with 146 autopsied cases. *Perspect Pediatr Pathol* **2**:241, 1975.
174. Esterly JR, Oppenheimer EH: Observation in cystic fibrosis. 1. The gall bladder. *Bull Johns Hopkins Hosp* **110**:247, 1962.
175. Bass S, Connon JJ, Ho CS: Biliary tree in cystic fibrosis. *Gastroenterology* **84**:1592, 1985.
176. Isenberg JN, L'Hereux PR, Warwick WJ, Sharp HL: Clinical observations on the biliary system in cystic fibrosis. *Am J Gastroenterol* **65**:134, 1976.
177. Roy CC, Weber AM, Morin CL, Combes JJC, Nussle D, Megevand A, LaSalle R: Abnormal biliary lipid composition in cystic fibrosis: Effect of pancreatic enzymes. *N Engl J Med* **297**:1301, 1977.
178. Angelico M, Gandin C, Canuzzi P, Bertasi S, Cantafora A, DeSantis A, Quattrucci S, Antonelli M: Gallstones in cystic fibrosis: A critical appraisal. *Hepatology* **14**:769, 1991.
179. Van Haren EJH, Hopman WPM, Hansen JBMJ, Rosenbusch G, Lamers CBHW, Van Herwaarden CLA: Increased plasma cholecystokinin levels and small gallbladders in adult patients with cystic fibrosis. *Clin Sci* **81**:85, 1991.
180. Landing BH, Wells TR, Wang CI: Abnormality of the epididymis and vas deferens in cystic fibrosis. *Arch Pathol* **88**:570, 1969.
181. Taussig LM, Lobeck CC, di Sant'Agnese PA, Ackerman DR, Kattwinkel J: Fertility in males with cystic fibrosis. *N Engl J Med* **287**:586, 1972.
182. Kaplan E, Shwachman H, Perlmutter AD, Rule A, Khaw KT, Holsclaw DS: Reproductive failure in males with cystic fibrosis. *N Engl J Med* **279**:65, 1968.
183. Valman HB, France NE: The vas deferens in cystic fibrosis. *Lancet* **2**:566, 1969.
184. Holsclaw DS, Shwachman H: Increased incidence of inguinal hernia, hydrocele, and undescended testicle in males with cystic fibrosis. *Pediatrics* **48**:442, 1971.
185. Denning CR, Sommers SC, Quigley HJ Jr: Infertility in male patients with cystic fibrosis. *Pediatrics* **41**:7, 1968.
186. Stern RC, Boat TF, Doershuk CF: Obstructive azoospermia as a diagnostic criterion for the cystic fibrosis syndrome. *Lancet* **1**:1401, 1982.
187. Levine SB, Stern RC: Sexual function in cystic fibrosis. *Chest* **81**:422, 1982.
188. Shwachman H, Kowalski M, Khaw KT: Cystic fibrosis: A new outlook. *Medicine* (Baltimore) **56**:129, 1977.
189. Neinstein LS, Stewart D, Wang CI, Johnson I: Menstrual dysfunction in cystic fibrosis. *J Adolesc Health Care* **4**:153, 1983.
190. Kapito LE, Losasky HJ, Shwachman H: Water and electrolytes in cervical mucus from patients with CF. *Fertil Steril* **24**:512, 1973.

190a. FitzSimmons SC: The changing epidemiology of cystic fibrosis. *J Pediatr* **122**:1, 1993.

191. Cohen LF, di Sant'Agnese PA, Friedlander J: Cystic fibrosis and pregnancy: A national survey. *Lancet* **2**:842, 1980.
192. Canny GJ, Corry M, Livingstone RA, Carpenter S, Green L, Levison H: Pregnancy and cystic fibrosis. *Obstet Gynecol* **37**:850, 1991.

193. Alpert SE, Cormier AD: Normal electrolyte and protein content in milk from mothers with cystic fibrosis. *J Pediatr* **102**:77, 1983.
194. Bitman J, Hamosh M, Wood DL, Freed LM, Hamosh P: Lipid composition of milk from mothers with cystic fibrosis. *Pediatrics* **80**:927, 1987.
195. Mitchell-Heggs P, Mearns M, Batten JC: Cystic fibrosis in adolescents and adults. *Q J Med* **179**:479, 1976.
196. Gibson LE, di Sant'Agnese PA: Studies of salt excretion in sweat. *J Pediatr* **62**:855, 1963.
197. Sato K, Sato F: Defective beta-adrenergic response of cystic fibrosis sweat glands in vivo and in vitro. *J Clin Invest* **73**:1763, 1984.
198. Munger B, Brusilow S, Cooke R: An electron microscopic study of eccrine sweat glands in patients with cystic fibrosis of the pancreas. *J Pediatr* **59**:497, 1961.
199. Esterly NB, Oppenheimer EH, Esterly JR: Observations on cystic fibrosis of the pancreas: The apocrine sweat gland. *Am J Dis Child* **123**:200, 1972.
200. Simopoulous AP, Lapey A, Boat TF, di Sant'Agnese PA, Bartter FC: The renin-angiotensin-aldosterone system in patients with cystic fibrosis of the pancreas. *Pediatr Res* **5**:626, 1971.
201. Grand RJ, di Sant'Agnese PA, Talamo RC, Pallavicinni JC: The effects of exogenous aldosterone on sweat electrolytes. II. Patients with cystic fibrosis of the pancreas. *J Pediatr* **70**:357, 1967.
202. Nussbaum E, Boat TF, Wood RE, Doershuk CF: Cystic fibrosis with acute hypoelectrolytemia and metabolic acidosis in infancy. *Am J Dis Child* **133**:965, 1979.
203. Beckerman RC, Taussig LM: Hyperelectrolytemia and metabolic alkalosis in infants with cystic fibrosis. *Pediatrics* **63**:580, 1979.
204. Lieberman J, Rodbard S: Low blood pressure in young adults with cystic fibrosis. *Ann Intern Med* **82**:806, 1975.
205. Newman AJ, Ansell BM: Episodic arthritis in children with cystic fibrosis. *J Pediatr* **94**:594, 1979.
206. Schidlow DV, Goldsmith DP, Palmer J, Huang NN: Arthritis in cystic fibrosis. *Arch Dis Child* **59**:377, 1984.
207. Soter NA, Mihm MC, Colten HR: Cutaneous necrotizing venulitis in patients with cystic fibrosis. *J Pediatr* **95**:197, 1979.
208. Fischer EG, Shwachman H, Wepsie JG: Brain abscess and cystic fibrosis. *J Pediatr* **95**:385, 1979.
209. Cohen LF, di Sant'Agnese PA, Taylor A, Gill JR: The syndrome of inappropriate antidiuretic hormone secretion as a cause of hyponatremia in cystic fibrosis. *J Pediatr* **90**:574, 1977.
210. Miller RW: Childhood cancer and congenital defects: A study of U.S. death certificates during the period 1960–1966. *Pediatr Res* **3**:389, 1969.
211. Abdul-Karim FW, King TA, Dahms BB, Gauderer MW, Boat TF: Carcinoma of extrahepatic biliary system in an adult with cystic fibrosis. *Gastroenterology* **82**:758, 1982.
211a. Neglia JP, Wielinski CL, Warwick WJ: Cancer risk among patients with cystic fibrosis. *J Pediatr* **119**:764, 1991.
212. Castile R, Shwachman H, Travis W, Hadley CA, Warwick W, Missmahl HP: Amyloidosis as a complication of cystic fibrosis. *Am J Dis Child* **139**:728, 1985.
213. Stern RC, Boat TF, Abramowsky CR, Matthews LW, Wood RE, Doershuk CR: Intermediate-range sweat chloride concentration and *Pseudomonas* bronchitis. A cystic fibrosis variant with preservation of exocrine pancreatic function. *JAMA* **239**:2676, 1978.
214. Durie PR, Forstner GG, Gaskin KJ, Moore DJ, Cleghorn GD, Wong SS, Corey ML: Age-related alterations of immunoreactive pancreatic cationic trypsinogen in sera from cystic fibrosis patients with and without pancreatic insufficiency. *Pediatr Res* **20**:209, 1986.
215. Gowen CW, Lawson EE, Gingras-Leatherman J, Gatzy JT, Boucher RC, Knowles MR: Increased nasal potential difference and amiloride sensitivity in neonates with cystic fibrosis. *J Pediatr* **108**:517, 1986.
216. Sauder RA, Chesrown SE, Loughlin GM: Clinical application of transepithelial potential difference measurements in cystic fibrosis. *J Pediatr* **111**:353, 1987.
217. Highsmith WE, Burch LH, Zhou Z, Olsen JC, Boat TE, Spock A, Gorvoy JD, Quittell L, Friedman KJ, Silverman LM, Boucher RC, Knowles MR: Cystic fibrosis gene mutation in patients with normal sweat chloride concentrations. *N Engl J Med* 1994 (in press).
218. Denning CR, Huang NN, Cusay LR, Shwachman H, Tocci P, Warwick WJ, Gibson LE: Cooperative study comparing three methods of performing sweat tests to diagnose cystic fibrosis. *Pediatrics* **66**:752, 1980.
219. Rosenstein BJ, Langbaum TS: Diagnosis, in Taussig LM (ed): *Cystic Fibrosis*. New York, Thieme-Stratton, 1984, p 85.
220. Davis PB, Del Rio S, Munts JA, Diekman L: Sweat chloride concentration in adults with pulmonary disease. *Am Rev Respir Dis* **138**:34, 1983.
221. Hardy JD, Davison SHH, Higgins MU, Polycarpou PN: Sweat tests in the newborn period. *Arch Dis Child* **48**:316, 1973.
222. Crossley JR, Elliott RB, Smith PA: Dried-blood spot screening for cystic fibrosis in the newborn. *Lancet* **1**:472, 1979.
223. Hammond K, Naylor E, Wilcken B: Screening for cystic fibrosis, in Therrell BL (ed): *Advances in Neonatal Screening*. New York, Excerpta Medica, 1987, p 377.
224. Ad Hoc Task Force on Neonatal Screening, Cystic Fibrosis Foundation: Neonatal screening for cystic fibrosis: Position paper. *Pediatrics* **72**:741, 1983.
225. Sanders JS, Proyer TD, Wedel MK: Prolonged survival in an adult with cystic fibrosis. *Chest* **77**:226, 1980.
226. Shwachman H, Kulczycki LL: Long-term study of 105 patients with cystic fibrosis. Studies made over a 5 to 14 year period. *Am J Dis Child* **96**:6, 1958.
227. Taussig LM, Kattwinkel J, Friederwald WT, di Sant'Agnese PA: A new prognostic score and clinical evaluation system for cystic fibrosis. *J Pediatr* **82**:380, 1973.
228. Fink RJ, Doershuk CF, Tucker AS, Stern RC, Boat TF, Matthews LW: Pulmonary function and morbidity in 40 adult patients with cystic fibrosis. *Chest* **74**:643, 1978.
229. Corley M, Levison H, Crozier D: Five-to-seven year course of pulmonary function in cystic fibrosis. *Am Rev Respir Dis* **114**:1085, 1976.
230. Wood RE: Prognosis, in Taussig LM (ed): *Cystic Fibrosis*. New York, Thieme-Stratton, 1984, p 434.
231. Orenstein DM, Boat TF, Stern RC, Tucker AS, Charnock EL, Matthews LW, Doershuk CF: The effect of early diagnosis and treatment on the progression of the pulmonary disease in cystic fibrosis. *Am J Dis Child* **131**:973, 1977.
232. Katz JN, Horowitz RI, Dolan TF, Shapiro ED: Clinical features as predictors of functional status in children with cystic fibrosis. *J Pediatr* **108**:352, 1986.
233. Kerem E, Reisman J, Corey M, Bentur L, Canny G, Levison H: Wheezing in infants with cystic fibrosis: Clinical course, pulmonary function and survival analysis. *Pediatrics* **90**:703, 1992.
234. Wilmott WR, Tyson SL, Matthew DJ: Cystic fibrosis survival rates: The influences of allergy and *Pseudomonas aeruginosa*. *Am J Dis Child* **139**:669, 1985.
235. Toblan OC, Martore WJ, Doershuk CF, Stern RC, Thomasen MJ, Klinger JD, White JW, Carson LA, Jarvis WR: Colonization of the respiratory tract with *Pseudomonas cepacia* in cystic fibrosis. *Chest* **91**:527, 1987.
236. Knoke JD, Stern RC, Doershuk CF, Boat TF, Matthews LW: Cystic fibrosis: The prognosis for five-year survival. *Pediatr Res* **12**:676, 1978.
237. Zielenski J, Bozon D, Kerem B, Markiewicz D, Durie P, Rommens JM, Tsui L-C: Identification of mutations in exons 1 through 8 of the cystic fibrosis transmembrane conductance regulator (CFTR) gene. *Genomics* **10**:229, 1991.
238. Dean M, White MB, Amos J, Gerrard B, Stewart C, Khaw KT, Leppert M: Multiple mutations in highly conserved residues are found in mildly affected cystic fibrosis patients. *Cell* **61**:863, 1990.
239. Hill DJS, Martin AJ, Davidson GP, Smith GS: Survival of cystic fibrosis patients in South Australia. *Med J Aust* **143**:230, 1985.
240. Wood RE: Determinants of survival in cystic fibrosis. *CF Club Abstracts* **26**:69, 1985.
241. Denning CR, Gluckson MM: Psychosocial aspects of cystic fibrosis, in Taussig LM (ed): *Cystic Fibrosis*. New York, Thieme-Stratton, 1984, p 461.

242. Lewiston NJ: Psychosocial impact of cystic fibrosis. *Semin Respir Med* **6**:321, 1985.
243. Zinman R: Cough versus chest physiotherapy: A comparison of the acute effects on pulmonary function in patients with cystic fibrosis. *Am Rev Respir Dis* **129**:182, 1984.
244. Zapletal A, Stefanova J, Horak J, Vavrova V, Samanek M: Chest physiotherapy and airway obstruction in patients with cystic fibrosis—A negative report. *Eur J Respir Dis* **64**:426, 1983.
245. Wong JW, Keens TG, Wannamaker EM, Crozier DN, Levison H, Aspin J: Effects of gravity on tracheal mucus transport rates in normal subjects and in patients with cystic fibrosis. *Pediatrics* **60**:146, 1977.
246. Desmond KJ, Schwenk F, Thomas E, Beaudry PH, Coates AL: Immediate and long-term effects of chest physiotherapy in patients with cystic fibrosis. *J Pediatr* **103**:538, 1983.
247. De Boeck C, Zinman R: Cough versus chest physiotherapy: A comparison of the acute effects on pulmonary function in patients with cystic fibrosis. *Am Rev Respir Dis* **129**:182, 1984.
248. Falk M, Kelstrup M, Anderson JB, Kinoshita T, Falk P, Stovring S, Gothgen I: Improving the ketchup bottle method with positive expiratory pressure, PEP, in cystic fibrosis. *Eur J Respir Dis* **65**:423, 1984.
249. Blemquist M, Freyschuss U, Wiman L-G, Strandvik B: Physical activity and self-treatment in cystic fibrosis. *Arch Dis Child* **61**:362, 1986.
250. Szaff M, Hoiby N, Flensberg EW: Frequent antibiotic therapy improves survival of cystic fibrosis patients with chronic *Pseudomonas aeruginosa* therapy. *Acta Paediatr Scand* **72**:651, 1983.
251. Lawson D, Potter J: Serum precipitins against respiratory tract pathogens in 522 "normal" children and 48 cases of cystic fibrosis treated with cloxacillin. *Arch Dis Child* **51**:890, 1976.
252. Bosso JA, Townsend PL, Herbst JJ, Matsen JM: Pharmacokinetics and dosage requirements of netilmicin in cystic fibrosis. *Antimicrob Agents Chemother* **28**:829, 1985.
253. Mendelman PM, Smith AL, Levy J, Weber A, Ramsey B, Davis R: Aminoglycoside penetration, inactivation, and efficacy in cystic fibrosis sputum. *Am Rev Respir Dis* **132**:761, 1985.
254. LeBel M, Bergeron MG, Vallee F, Fiset C, Chasse G, Bigonesse P, Rivard G: Pharmacokinetics and pharmacodynamics of ciprofloxacin in cystic fibrosis patients. *Antimicrob Agents Chemother* **30**:260, 1986.
255. Hodson ME, Penketh ARL, Batten JC: Aerosol carbenicillin and gentamicin treatment of *Pseudomonas aeruginosa* infection in patients with cystic fibrosis. *Lancet* **2**:1137, 1981.
256. Wall MA, Terry AB, Eisenberg J, McNamara M: Inhaled antibiotics in cystic fibrosis. *Lancet* **1**:1325, 1983.
257. Ramsey BW, Dorkin HL, Eisenberg JD, Gibson RL, Harwood IR, Kravitz RM, Schidlow DV, Wilmott RW, Astley SJ, McBurnie MA, Wentz K, Smith AL: Efficacy of aerosolized tobramycin in patients with cystic fibrosis. *N Engl J Med* **328**:1740, 1993.
258. Hubbard RC, McElvaney NG, Birrer P, Shak S, Robinson WW, Wu CJM, Chernick MS, Crystal RG: A preliminary study of aerosolized recombinant human deoxyribonuclease I in the treatment of cystic fibrosis. *N Engl J Med* **326**:812, 1992.
259. Aitken ML, Burke W, McDonald G, Shak S, Montgomery AB, Smith A: Recombinant human DNase inhalation in normal subjects and patients with cystic fibrosis. *JAMA* **267**:1947, 1992.
260. Ranasinha C, Assoufi B, Shak S, Christiansen D, Fuchs H, Empey D, Geddes D, Hodson M: Efficacy and safety of short-term administration of aerosolised recombinant human DNase I in adults with stable stage cystic fibrosis. *Lancet* **342**:199, 1993.
261. Ramsey BW, Astley SJ, Aitken ML, Burke W, Colin AA, Dorkin HL, Eisenberg JD, Gibson RL, Harwood IR, Schidlow DV, Wilmott RW, Wohl ME, Meyerson LJ, Shak S, Fuchs H, Smith AL: Efficacy and safety of short-term administration of aerosolized recombinant human deoxyribonuclease in patients with cystic fibrosis. *Am Rev Respir Dis* **148**:145, 1993.
262. Sturgess J, Reid L: The effect of isoprenaline and pilocarpine on a) bronchial mucus-secreting tissue and b) pancreas, salivary glands, heart, thyroid, liver, and spleen. *Br J Exp Pathol* **54**:388, 1973.
263. Shapiro GG, Bamman J, Kanarek P, Bierman CW: The paradoxical effect of adrenergic and methylxanthine drugs in cystic fibrosis. *Pediatrics* **58**:740, 1976.
264. Auerbach HS, Williams M, Kirkpatrick JA, Colten HR: Alternate-day prednisone reduces morbidity and improves pulmonary function in cystic fibrosis. *Lancet* **2**:686, 1985.
265. Rosenstein BJ, Eigen H, Schidlow DV: Alternate day prednisone in patients with cystic fibrosis. *Pediatr Res* **31**:A2289, 1993.
266. Donlan TF, Gibson LE: Complications of iodide therapy in patients with cystic fibrosis. *J Pediatr* **79**:684, 1971.
267. Strauss GD, Osher A, Wang C-I, Goodrich E, Gold F, Colman W, Stabile M, Dobrenchuk A, Keens TG: Variable weight training in cystic fibrosis. *Chest* **92**:273, 1987.
268. Orenstein DM, Henke KG, Costill DL, Doershuk CF, Lemon PT, Stern RD: Exercise and heat stress in cystic fibrosis patients. *Pediatr Res* **17**:267, 1983.
269. Bar-Or D, Blimkie CJR, Hay JA, MacDougall JD, Ward DS, Wilson WM: Voluntary dehydration and heat intolerance in cystic fibrosis. *Lancet* **339**:696, 1992.
270. Meyer KC, Lewandeski JR, Zimmerman JJ, Nunley D, Calhoun WJ, Dopico GA: Human neutrophil elastase and elastase/alpha$_1$-antiprotease complex in cystic fibrosis. *Am Rev Respir Dis* **144**:580, 1991.
271. Knowles MR, Church NL, Waltner WE, Yankaskas JR, Gilligan P, King M, Edwards LJ, Helms R, Boucher RC: A pilot study of aerosolized amiloride for the treatment of lung disease in cystic fibrosis. *N Engl J Med* **322**:1189, 1990.
272. Knowles MR, Clarke LL, Boucher RC: Activation by extracellular nucleotides of chloride secretion in the airway epithelia of patients with cystic fibrosis. *N Engl J Med* **325**:533, 1991.
273. O'Neal WK, Beaudet AL: Somatic gene therapy for cystic fibrosis. *Hum Mol Genet* 1994. (In Press)
274. Lapey A, Kattwinkel J, di Sant'Agnese PA, Lester L: Steatorrhea and azotorrhea and their relation to growth and nutrition in adolescents and young adults with cystic fibrosis. *J Pediatr* **84**:328, 1974.
275. Youngberg CA, Bernardi RR, Howatt WF, Hyneck ML, Avidon GL, Meyer JH, Dressman JB: The comparison of gastrointestinal pH in cystic fibrosis and healthy subjects. *Dig Dis Sci* **32**:472, 1987.
276. Stapleton FB, Kennedy J, Nousia-Arvanitakis S, Lindshaw MA: Hyperuricosuria due to high-dose pancreatic extract therapy in cystic fibrosis. *N Engl J Med* **295**:246, 1976.
276a. Smyth RL, van Velzen D, Smyth AR, Lloyd DA, Heaf DP: Strictures of ascending colon in cystic fibrosis and high-strength pancreatic enzymes. *Lancet* **343**:85, 1994.
277. Homnick DN, Cox JH, DeLoof MJ, Ringer TV: Carotenoid levels in normal children and in children with cystic fibrosis. *J Pediatr* **122**:703, 1993.
278. Bertrand JM, Morin CL, Lasalle R, Patrick R, Coates AL: Short-term clinical, nutritional, and functional effects of continuous elemental enteral alimentation in children with cystic fibrosis. *J Pediatr* **104**:41, 1984.
279. Zipf WB, Kien CL, Horswill KS, McCoy KS, O'Dorisio T, Pinyerd BL: Effects of tolbutamide on growth and body composition of nondiabetic children with cystic fibrosis. *Pediatr Res* **30**:309, 1991.
280. Stern RC, Byard PJ, Tomashefski JF, Doershuk CF: Recreational use of psychoactive drugs by patients with cystic fibrosis. *J Pediatr* **111**:293, 1987.
281. Campbell PW, Parker RA, Roberts BT, Krishnamani MRS, Philips JA: Association of poor clinical status and heavy exposure to tobacco smoke in patients with cystic fibrosis who are homozygous for the F508 deletion. *J Pediatr* **120**:261, 1992.
282. LiPuma JJ, Dasen SE, Nielson DW, Stern RC, Stull TL: Person-to-person transmission of *Pseudomonas cepacia* between patients with cystic fibrosis. *Lancet* **226**:1094, 1990.
283. Tummler B, Koopman U, Grothues D, Weillbrodt H, Steinkamp G, van der Hardt H: Nosocomial acquisition of *Pseudomonas aeruginosa* by cystic fibrosis patients. *J Clin Microbiol* **29**:1265, 1991.
284. Redding GJ, Restuccia R, Cotton EK, Brooks JG: Serial

changes in pulmonary functions in children hospitalized with cystic fibrosis. *Am Rev Respir Dis* **126**:31, 1982.

285. Powell SH, Thompson WL, Luthe MA, Stern RC, Grossniklaus DA, Bloxham DD, Groden DL, Gacolos MR, Discenna AO, Cash HA, Klinger JD: One daily vs. continuous aminoglycoside dosing: Efficacy and toxicity in animal and clinical studies of gentamicin, netilmicin, and tobramycin. *J Infect Dis* **147**:918, 1983.
286. Donati MA, Guenette G, Auerbach H: Prospective controlled study of home and hospital therapy of cystic fibrosis pulmonary disease. *J Pediatr* **111**:28, 1987.
287. Braunstein MS, Fleegler B: Failure of bronchopulmonary lavage in cystic fibrosis. *Chest* **66**:96, 1974.
288. Spier S, Rivlin J, Hughes D, Levison H: The effect of oxygen on sleep, blood gases and ventilation in cystic fibrosis. *Am Rev Respir Dis* **129**:712, 1984.
289. Whitman V, Stern RC, Bellet P, Doershuk CF, Liebman Z, Boat TF, Borkat G, Matthews LW: Studies on cor pulmonale in cystic fibrosis: 1. Effects of diuresis. *Pediatrics* **55**:83, 1975.
290. Benson LN, Newth CJL, Olley PM: Radionuclide assessment of right and left ventricular function during bicycle exercise in young patients with cystic fibrosis. *Am Rev Respir Dis* **130**:987, 1984.
291. Liebman J, Lucas RV, Moss A, Rosenthal A: Cor pulmonale and related cardiovascular effects of cystic fibrosis, in Mangos JA, Talamo RC (eds): *Cystic Fibrosis: Projections into the Future*. New York, Stratton Intercontinental Medical Books, 1976, p 41.
292. Geggel RL, Dozor AJ, Fyler DC, Reid LM: Effect of vasodilators at rest and during exercise in young adults with cystic fibrosis and chronic cor pulmonale. *Am Rev Respir Dis* **131**:531, 1985.
293. Davis PB, di Sant'Agnese PA: Assisted ventilation for patients with cystic fibrosis. *JAMA* **239**:1851, 1978.
294. Fellows KE, Khaw K-T, Schuster S, Shwachman H: Bronchial artery embolization in cystic fibrosis. Technique and long-term results. *J Pediatr* **95**:959, 1979.
295. Voss MJ, Bush RK, Mischler EH, Peters ME: Association of allergic bronchopulmonary aspergillosis and cystic fibrosis. *J Allergy Clin Immunol* **69**:539, 1982.
296. Vincour CD, Marmon L, Shidlow DV, Weintraub WH: Gastroesophageal reflux in the infant with cystic fibrosis. *Am J Surg* **149**:182, 1985.
297. Scott RB, O'Loughlin EV, Gall DG: Gastroesophageal reflux in patients with cystic fibrosis. *J Pediatr* **106**:223, 1985.
298. Dolly T, Rothberg RM, Lester LA: Cystic fibrosis and gastroesophageal reflux in infancy. *Am J Dis Child* **139**:66, 1985.
299. O'Halloran SM, Gilbert J, McKendrick OM, Carty HML, Heaf DP: Gastrografin in acute meconium ileus equivalent. *Arch Dis Child* **61**:1128, 1986.
300. Lillibridge CB, Docter JM, Eidelman S: Oral admission of N-acetylcysteine in the prophylaxis of meconium ileus equivalent. *J Pediatr* **71**:887, 1967.
301. Cleghorn GJ, Forstner GG, Stringer DA, Durie PR: Treatment of distal intestinal obstruction syndrome in cystic fibrosis with a balanced intestinal lavage solution. *Lancet* **1**:8, 1986.
302. Mieles LA, Orenstein D, Teperman L, Podesta L, Koneru B, Starzl TE: Liver transplantation in cystic fibrosis. *Lancet* **1**:1073, 1989.
303. Madden BP, Hodson ME, Tsang V, Radley-Smith R, Khaghani A, Yacoub MY: Intermediate-term results of heart-lung transplantation for cystic fibrosis. *Lancet* **339**:1583, 1992.
304. Shernib H, Noirclerc M, Ernst P, Metras D, Mulder DS, Guidicelli R, Lebel F, Duman J-F: Double-lung transplantation for cystic fibrosis. *Ann Thorac Surg* **54**:27, 1992.
305. Alton EWFW, Batten J, Hodson M, Wallwork J, Higgenbottom T, Geddes DW: Measurement of lower airways' potential difference in CF following heart-lung transplantation. *Pediatr Pulmonol* **S1**:111, 1987.
306. Kerem E, Reisman J, Corey M, Canny GJ, Levison H: Prediction of mortality in patients with cystic fibrosis. *N Engl J Med* **326**:1187, 1992.
307. Neutra MR, Grand RJ, Trier JS: Glycoprotein synthesis, transport, and secretion by epithelial cells of human rectal mucosa: Normal and cystic fibrosis. *Lab Invest* **36**:535, 1977.
308. Boat TF, Cheng PW: Mucus glycoproteins, in Mangos JA, Talamo RC (eds): *Cystic Fibrosis: Projection into the Future*. Miami, Symposia Specialists, 1976, p 165.
309. Cheng P-W, Boat TF, Cranfill K, Yankaskas JR, Boucher RC: Increased sulfation of glycoconjugates by cultured nasal epithelial cells from patients with cystic fibrosis. *J Clin Invest* **84**:68, 1989.
310. Boat TF, Dearborn DG: Etiology and pathogenesis, in Taussig LM (ed): *Cystic Fibrosis*. New York, Thieme-Stratton, 1984, p 25.
311. Barasch J, Kiss B, Prince A, Saiman L, Gruenert D, Al-Awqati Q: Defective acidification of intracellular organelles in cystic fibrosis. *Nature* **352**:70, 1991.
312. Boat TF, Cheng PW, Iyer R, Carlson DM, Polony I: Human respiratory tract secretions: Mucous glycoproteins of nonpurulent tracheobronchial secretions and sputum of patients with bronchitis and cystic fibrosis. *Arch Biochem Biophys* **177**:95, 1976.
313. Wesley A, Forstner J, Qureshi R, Mantle M, Forstner G: Human intestinal mucin in cystic fibrosis. *Pediatr Res* **17**:65, 1983.
314. Mohapatra NK, Cheng P-W, Parker JJC, Paradiso AM, Yankaskas JR, Boucher RC, Boat TF: Sulfate transport and concentrations are not altered in CF airway epithelial cells. *Pediatr Pulmonol* (Suppl) **8**:283, 1992.
315. Roomans GM: Calcium and cystic fibrosis. *Scanning Electron Microsc* **1**:165, 1986.
316. Schoni MH, Schoni-Affolter F, Jeffery D, Katz S: Intracellular free calcium levels in mononuclear cells of patients with cystic fibrosis and normal controls. *Cell Calcium* **8**:53, 1987.
317. Dearborn DG, Wityk RJ, Johnson LR, Poncz L, Stern RC: Calcium-ATPase activity in cystic fibrosis erythrocyte membranes: Decreased activity in patients with pancreatic insufficiency. *Pediatr Res* **18**:890, 1984.
318. Tallant EA, Wallace RW: Altered binding of ^{125}I-labeled calmodulin to a 46-kilodalton protein in skin fibroblasts cultured from patients with cystic fibrosis. *J Clin Invest* **79**:643, 1987.
319. Gugler E, Pallavicini JC, Swerdlow H, di Sant'Agnese PA: The role of calcium in submaxillary saliva of patients with cystic fibrosis. *J Pediatr* **71**:585, 1967.
320. Boat TF, Weisman UN, Pallavicini JC: Purification and properties of the calcium precipitable protein in submaxillary saliva of normal and cystic fibrosis subjects. *Pediatr Res* **8**:531, 1974.
321. Eiberg H, Mohr J, Schmiegelow K, Nielsen LS, Williamson R: Linkage relationships of paraoxonase *(PON)* with other markers: Indication of *PON*-cystic fibrosis synteny. *Clin Genet* **28**:265, 1985.
322. Schmiegelow K, Eiberg H, Tsui L-C, Buchwald M, Phelan PD, Williamson R, Warwick W, Niebuhr E, Mohr J, Schwartz M, Koch C: Linkage between the loci for cystic fibrosis and paraoxonase. *Clin Genet* **29**:374, 1986.
323. Tsui L-C, Buchwald M, Barker D, Braman JC, Knowlton R, Schrumm JW, Eiberg H, Mohr J, Kennedy D, Plavic N: Cystic fibrosis locus defined by a genetically linked polymorphic DNA marker. *Science* **230**:1054, 1985.
324. Knowlton RG, Cohen-Haguenauer O, Cong NV, Frézal J, Brown VA, Barker D, Braman JC, Schumm JW, Tsui L-C, Buchwald M, Donis-Keller H: A polymorphic DNA marker linked to cystic fibrosis is located on chromosome 7. *Nature* **318**:380, 1985.
325. Tsui L-C, Zengerling S, Willard HF, Buchwald M: Mapping of the cystic fibrosis locus on chromosome 7. *Cold Spring Harbor Symp Quant Biol* **51**:325, 1986.
326. White W, Woodward W, Leppert M, O'Connell PO, Hoff M, Herbst F, Lalouel FM, Dean M, Vande Woude G: A closely linked genetic marker for cystic fibrosis. *Nature* **318**:382, 1985.
327. Wainwright BJ, Scambler PJ, Schmidtke J, Watson EA, Law H-Y, Farrell M, Cooke HJ, Eiberg H, Williamson R: Localization of cystic fibrosis locus to human chromosome 7 cen-q22. *Nature* **318**:384, 1985.
328. Beaudet A, Bowcock A, Buchwald M, Cavalli-Sforza

L, Farrall M, King M-C, Klinger K, Lalouel J-M, Lathrop G, Naylor S, Ott J, Tsui L-C, Wainwright B, Watkins P, White R, Williamson R: Linkage of cystic fibrosis to two tightly linked DNA markers: Joint report from a collaborative study. *Am J Hum Genet* **39**:681, 1986.

329. White R, Leppert M, O'Connell P, Nakamura Y, Woodward S, Hoff M, Herbst J, Dean M, Vande Woude G, Lathrop GM, Lalouel J-M: Further linkage data on cystic fibrosis: The Utah study. *Am J Hum Genet* **39**:694, 1986.
330. Lathrop GM, Farrall M, O'Connell P, Wainwright B, Leppert M, Nakamura Y, Lench N, Kruyer H, Dean M, Park M, Vande Woude G, Lalouel J-M, Williamson R, White R: Refined linkage map of chromosome 7 in the region of the cystic fibrosis gene. *Am J Hum Genet* **42**:38, 1988.
331. Tsui L-C, Buchwald M: No evidence for genetic heterogeneity in cystic fibrosis. *Am J Hum Genet* **42**:184, 1988.
332. Barker D, Green P, Knowlton R, Schumm J, Lander E, Oliphant A, Willard H, Akots G, Brown V, Gravius T, Helms C, Nelson C, Parker C, Rediker K, Rising M, Watt D, Weiffenbach B, Donis-Keller H: Genetic linkage map of human chromosome 7 with 63 DNA markers. *Proc Natl Acad Sci USA* **84**:8006, 1987.
333. Lathrop GM, O'Connell P, Leppert M, Nakamura Y, Farrall M, Tsui L-C, Lalouel J, White R: Twenty-five loci form a continuous linkage map of markers for human chromosome 7. *Genomics* **5**:866, 1989.
334. Morreau J, Sinaasappel M, Oostra BA, Halley DJJ: Cystic fibrosis: Screening for a DNA deletion by field inversion gel electrophoresis. *Hum Genet* **79**:64, 1988.
335. Scambler PJ, Wainwright BJ, Watson E, Bates G, Bell G, Williamson R, Farrall M: Isolation of a further anonymous informative DNA sequence from chromosome seven closely linked to cystic fibrosis. *Nucleic Acids Res* **14**:1951, 1986.
336. Rommens JM, Zengerling S, Burns J, Melmer G, Kerem B, Plavsic N, Zsiga M, Kennedy D, Markiewicz D, Rozmahel R, Riordan JR, Buchwald M, Tsui L-C: Identification and regional localization of DNA markers on chromosome 7 for the cloning of the cystic fibrosis gene. *Am J Hum Genet* **43**:645, 1988.
337. Melmer G, Sood R, Rommens J, Rego D, Tsui L-C, Buchwald M: Isolation of clones on chromosome 7 that contain recognition sites for rare-cutting enzymes by oligonucleotide hybridization. *Genomics* **7**:173, 1990.
338. Burns J, Melmer G, Rommens JM, Riordan JR, Buchwald M: Identification of sequences of chromosome 7 that are expressed in sweat gland epithelial cells. *Hum Genet* **85**:151, 1990.
339. Jobs A, Klein-Bolting D, Jandel AS, Driesel A, Olek K, Grzeschik K-H: Regional assignment of 41 human DNA fragments on chromosome 7 by means of a somatic cell hybrid panel. *Hum Genet* **84**:147, 1990.
340. Scambler PJ, Law H-Y, Williamson R, Cooper CS: Chromosome mediated gene transfer of six DNA markers linked to the cystic fibrosis locus on human chromosome seven. *Nucleic Acids Res* **14**:7159, 1986.
341. Estivill X, Farrall M, Scambler PJ, Bell GM, Hawley KMF, Lench NJ, Bates GP, Kruyer HC, Frederick PA, Stanier P, Watson EK, Williamson R, Wainwright J: A candidate for the cystic fibrosis locus isolated by selection for methylation-free islands. *Nature* **326**:840, 1987.
342. Dorin JR, Inglis JD, Porteous DJ: Selection of precise chromosomal targeting of a dominant marker by homologous recombination. *Science* **243**:1357, 1989.
343. Porteous DJ, Dorin JR, Wilkinson MM, Fletcher JM, Emslie E, van Heyningen V: SV40-mediated tumor selection and chromosome transfer to enrich for cystic fibrosis region. *Somat Cell Mol Genet* **16**:29, 1990.
344. Michiels F, Burmeister M, Lehrach H: Derivation of clones close to *met* by preparative field inversion gel electrophoresis. *Science* **236**:1305, 1987.
345. Ramsey M, Wainwright BJ, Farrall M, Estivill X, Sutherland H, Ho M-F, Davies R, Halford S, Tata F, Wicking C, Lench N, Bauer I, Ferec C, Farndon P, Kruyer H, Stanier P, Williamson R, Scambler PJ: A new polymorphic locus, D7S411, isolated by cloning from preparative pulsed-field gels is close to the mutation causing cystic fibrosis. *Genomics* **6**:39, 1990.
346. Collins FS, Drumm ML, Cole JL, Lockwood WK, Vande Woude GF, Iannuzzi MC: Construction of a general human chromosome jumping library, with application to cystic fibrosis. *Science* **235**:1046, 1987.
347. Iannuzzi MC, Dean M, Drumm ML, Hidaka N, Cole JL, Perry A, Stewart C, Gerrard B, Collins FS: Isolation of additional polymorphic clones from the cystic fibrosis region using chromosome jumping from D7S8. *Am J Hum Genet* **44**:695, 1989.
348. Kaiser R, Weber J, Grzeschik K-H, Edström JE, Driesel A, Zengerling S, Buchwald M, Tsui L-C, Olek K: Microdissection and microcloning of the long arm of human chromosome 7. *Mol Biol Rep* **12**:3, 1987.
349. Weber J, Weith A, Kaiser R, Grzeschik K-H, Olek K: Microdissection and microcloning of human chromosome 7q22-32 region. *Somat Cell Mol Genet* **16**:123, 1990.
350. Dean M, O'Connell P, Leppert M, Park M, Amos JA, Phillips DG, White R, Vande Woude GF: Three additional DNA polymorphisms in the *met* gene and D7S8 locus: Use in prenatal diagnosis of cystic fibrosis. *J Pediatr* **111**:490, 1987.
351. Scambler PJ, Estivill X, Bell G, Farrall M, McLean C, Newman R, Little PFR, Frederick P, Hawley K, Wainwright BJ, Williamson R, Lench NJ: Physical and genetic analysis of cosmids from the vicinity of the cystic fibrosis locus. *Nucleic Acids Res* **15**:3639, 1987.
352. Estivill X, McLean C, Nunes V, Casals T, Gallano P, Scambler P, Williamson R: Isolation of a new DNA marker in linkage disequilibrium with cystic fibrosis, situated between J3.11 (D7S8) and IRP. *Am J Hum Genet* **44**:704, 1989.
353. Poustka A, Lehrach H, Williamson R, Bates G: A long-range restriction map encompassing the cystic fibrosis locus and its closely linked genetic markers. *Genomics* **2**:337, 1988.
354. Drumm ML, Smith CL, Dean M, Cole JL, Iannuzzi MC, Collins FS: Physical mapping of the cystic fibrosis region by pulsed-field gel electrophoresis. *Genomics* **2**:346, 1988.
355. Fulton TR, Bowcock AM, Smith DR, Daneshvar L, Green P, Cavalli-Sforza LL, Donis-Keller H: A 12 megabase restriction map at the cystic fibrosis locus. *Nucleic Acids Res* **17**:271, 1989.
356. Tsui L-C, Buetow K, Buchwald M: Genetic analysis of cystic fibrosis using linked DNA markers. *Am J Hum Genet* **39**:720, 1986.
357. Farrall M, Watson E, Bates G, Bell G, Bell J, Davies KE, Estivill X, Kruyer H, Law H-Y, Lench N, Lissens W, Simon P, Scambler P, Stanier P, Vassart G, Worrall C, Williamson R, Wainwright BJ: Further data supporting linkage between cystic fibrosis and the *met* oncogene and haplotype analysis with *met* and pJ3.11. *Am J Hum Genet* **39**:713, 1986.
358. Berger W, Hein J, Gedschold J, Bauer I, Speer A, Farrall M, Williamson R, Coutelle C: Crossovers in two German cystic fibrosis families determine probe order for MET, 7C22 and XV-2c/CS.7. *Hum Genet* **77**:197, 1987.
359. Farrall M, Wainwright BJ, Feldman GL, Beaudet A, Sretenovic Z, Halley D, Simon M, Dickerman L, Devoto M, Romeo G, Kaplan J-C, Kitzis A, Williamson R: Recombinations between IRP and cystic fibrosis. *Am J Hum Genet* **43**:471, 1988.
360. Devoto M, Ronchetto P, Romano L, Romeo G: Analysis of delta F508 does not confirm a previously reported recombination in a cystic fibrosis family. *Am J Hum Genet* **46**:1004, 1990.
361. Mathy L, Kampmann W, Higuchi M, Schwartenbeck G, Bartholomé K, Driesel AJ, Grzeschik K-H, Olek K: Cystic fibrosis: Typing 48 German families with linked DNA probes. *Hum Genet* **75**:359, 1987.
362. Schmidtke J, Krawczak M, Schwartz M, Alkan M, Bonduelle M, Büchler E, Chemke M, Darnedde T, Domagk J, Engel W, Frey D, Fryburg K, Halley D, Hundrieser J, Ladanyi L, Libaers I, Lissens W, Mächler M, Malik NJ, Morreau J, Neubauer V, Oostra B, Pape B, Pincin JE, Schinzel A, Simon P, Trefz FK, Tümmler B, Vassart G, Ross R: Linkage relationships and allelic associations of the cystic fibrosis locus and four marker loci. *Hum Genet* **76**:337, 1987.

363. McMillan SA, Hills AJ, Graham CA, Nevin NC, Fay AC: T cell receptor beta chain polymorphisms are associated with cystic fibrosis. *J Med Genet* **26**:431, 1989.
364. Estivill X, Scambler PJ, Wainwright BJ, Hawley K, Frederick P, Schwartz M, Baiget M, Kere J, Williamson R, Farrall M: Patterns of polymorphism and linkage disequilibrium for cystic fibrosis. *Genomics* **1**:257, 1987.
365. Beaudet AL, Spence JE, Montes M, O'Brien WE, Estivill X, Farrall M, Williamson R: Experience with new DNA markers for the diagnosis of cystic fibrosis. *N Engl J Med* **318**:50, 1988.
366. Weber J, Aulehla-Scholz C, Kaiser R, Eigel A, Neugebauer M, Horst J, Olek K: Cystic fibrosis: Typing 89 families with linked DNA probes. *Hum Genet* **81**:54, 1988.
367. Maciejko D, Bal J, Mazurczak T, te Meerman G, Buys C, Oostra B, Halley D: Different haplotypes for cystic fibrosis-linked DNA polymorphisms in Polish and Dutch populations. *Hum Genet* **83**:220, 1989.
368. Hill AJM, Graham CA, Kelly ED, Morrison PJ, Nevin NC: Linkage disequilibrium and CF allele segregation analysis in cystic fibrosis families in Northern Ireland. *Hum Genet* **83**:391, 1989.
369. Lucotte G, Barrè E, David F: Linkage disequilibrium between cystic fibrosis and linked DNA polymorphisms at two DNA markers, XV-2c and KM.19, in North African families. *Am J Hum Genet* **45**:635, 1989.
370. Vidaud M, Kitzis A, Ferec C, Bozon D, Dumur V, Giraud G, David F, Pascal O, Auvinet M, Morel Y, Andre J, Chomel JC, Salem JP, Farriaux JP, Roussel P, Labbé A, Dastugue B, Lucotte G, Munnier N, Foucaud P, Goossens M, Feingold J, Kaplan JC: Confirmation of linkage disequilibrium between haplotype B (XV-2c, allele 1; KM-19, allele 2) and cystic fibrosis allele in the French population. *Hum Genet* **81**:183, 1989.
371. Fernandez E, Benitez J, Villamar M, Ramos C: Linkage disequilibrium between cystic fibrosis locus and three DNA markers, KV-2c, KM19 and MP6d-9, in 43 Spanish families. *Hum Genet* **84**:379, 1990.
372. Weir BS: Locating the cystic fibrosis gene on the basis of linkage disequilibrium with markers? *Prog Clin Biol Res* **329**:81, 1989.
373. Zielenski J, Rozmahel R, Bozon D, Kerem B, Grzelczak Z, Riordan JR, Rommens J, Tsui L-C: Genomic DNA sequence of the cystic fibrosis transmembrane conductance regulator (CFTR) gene. *Genomics* **10**:214, 1991.
374. Green ED, Olson MV: Chromosome region of the cystic fibrosis gene in yeast artificial chromosomes: A model for human genome mapping. *Science* **250**:94, 1990.
375. Anand R, Ogilvie DJ, Butler R, Riley JH, Finniear RS, Powell SJ, Smith JC, Markham AF: A yeast artificial chromosome contig encompassing the cystic fibrosis locus. *Genomics* **9**:124, 1991.
376. Trapnell BC, Zeitlin PL, Chu C-S, Yoshimura K, Nakamura H, Guggino WB, Bargon J, Banks TC, Dalemans W, Pavirani A, Lecocq J-P, Crystal RG: Down-regulation of cystic fibrosis gene mRNA transcript levels and induction of the cystic fibrosis chloride secretory phenotype in epithelial cells by phorbol ester. *J Biol Chem* **266**:10319, 1991.
377. Koh J, Sferra TJ, Collins FS: Characterization of the cystic fibrosis transmembrane conductance regulator promoter region: Chromatin context and tissue-specificity. *J Biol Chem* **268**:15912, 1993.
378. Chou J-L, Rozmahel R, Tsui L-C: Characterization of the promoter region of the cystic fibrosis transmembrane conductance regulator gene. *J Biol Chem* **266**:24471, 1991.
379. Tsui L-C, Buchwald M: Biochemical and molecular genetics of cystic fibrosis. *Adv Hum Genet* **20**:153, 1991.
380. Strong TV, Koh J, Tsui L-C, Collins FS: Analysis of CFTR transcription. *Pediatr Pulmonol* (Suppl) **5**:195, 1990.
381. Chu C-S, Trapnell BC, Murtagh JJ Jr, Moss J, Dalemans W, Jallat S, Mercenier A, Pavirani A, Lecocq J-P, Cutting GR, Guggino WB, Crystal RG: Variable deletion of exon 9 coding sequences in cystic fibrosis transmembrane conductance regulator gene mRNA transcripts in normal bronchial epithelium. *EMBO J* **10**:1355, 1991.
382. Chu C-S, Trapnell BC, Murtagh JJ Jr, Moss J, Dalemans W, Jallat S, Mercenier A, Pavirani A, Lecocq J-P, Cutting GR, Guggino WB, Crystal RG: Cystic fibrosis transmembrane conductance regulator (CFTR) gene transcripts. *EMBO J* **11**:379, 1992.
383. Bremer S: Quantitative expression patterns of multidrug-resistance P-glycoprotein (MDR1) and differentially spliced cystic fibrosis transmembrane-conductance regulator mRNA transcripts in human epithelia. *Eur J Biochem* **206**:137, 1992.
384. Chu CS, Trapnell BC, Curristin S, Cutting GR, Crystal RG: Genetic basis of variable exon 9 skipping in cystic fibrosis transmembrane conductance regulator mRNA. *Nat Genet* **3**:151, 1993.
385. Chu CS, Trapnell BC, Curristin SM, Cutting GR, Crystal RG: Extensive posttranscriptional deletion of the coding sequences for part of nucleotide-binding fold 1 in respiratory epithelial mRNA transcripts of the cystic fibrosis transmembrane conductance regulator gene is not associated with the clinical manifestations of cystic fibrosis. *J Clin Invest* **90**:785, 1992.
386. Cutting GR, Kasch LM, Rosenstein BJ, Tsui L-C, Kazazian HH Jr, Antonarakis SE: Two patients with cystic fibrosis, nonsense mutations in each cystic fibrosis gene, and mild pulmonary disease. *N Engl J Med* **323**:1685, 1990.
387. Kiesewetter S, Macek M Jr, Davis C, Curristin SM, Chu C-S, Graham C, Shrimpton AE, Cashman SM, Tsui L-C, Mickle J, Amos J, Highsmith WE, Shuber A, Witt DR, Crystal RG, Cutting GR: A mutation in CFTR produces different phenotypes depending on chromosomal background. *Nat Genet* **5**:274, 1993.
388. Delaney SJ, Rich DP, Thomason SA, Hargrave MR, Welsh MJ, Wainwright BJ: CFTR splice variants are not conserved and fail to produce Cl^- channels. *Nat Genet* **4**:426, 1993.
388a. Strong TV, Wilkinson DJ, Mansoura MK, Devor DC, Henze K, Yang Y, Wilson JM, Cohn JA, Dawson DC, Frizzell RA, Collins FS: Expression of an abundant alternatively spliced form of the cystic fibrosis transmembrane conductance regulator (CFTR) gene is not associated with a cAMP-activated chloride conductance. *Hum Mol Genet* **2**:335, 1993.
389. The Cystic Fibrosis Genetic Analysis Consortium: Worldwide survey of the delta F508 mutation—Report from the Cystic Fibrosis Genetic Analysis Consortium. *Am J Hum Genet* **47**:354, 1990.
390. Romeo G, Devoto M: Population analysis of the major mutation in cystic fibrosis. *Hum Genet* **85**:391, 1990.
391. Estivill X, Chilton M, Casals T, Bosch A, Morral N, Nunes V, Gasparini P, Seia A, Pignatti PF, Novelli G, Dallapicolla B, Fernandez E, Benitez J, Williamson R: Delta F508 gene deletion in cystic fibrosis in southern Europe. *Lancet* **2**:1404, 1989.
392. McIntosh I, Lorenzo ML, Brock DJH: Frequency of the delta F508 mutation on CF chromosomes in UK. *Lancet* **2**:1404, 1989.
393. European Working Group on CF Genetics: Gradient of distribution in Europe of the major CF mutation and of its associated haplotype. *Hum Genet* **85**:436, 1990.
394. Lemna WK, Feldman GL, Kerem B, Fernbach SD, Zevkovich EP, O'Brien WE, Riordan JR, Collins FS, Tsui L-C, Beaudet AL: Mutation analysis for heterozygote detection and the prenatal diagnosis of cystic fibrosis. *N Engl J Med* **322**:291, 1990.
395. Lerer I, Cohen S, Chemke M, Sanilevich A, Rivlin J, Golan A, Yahav J, Friedman A, Abeleiovich D: The frequency of the delta F508 mutation on cystic fibrosis chromosomes in Israeli families: Correlation to CF haplotypes in Jewish communities and Arabs. *Hum Genet* **85**:416, 1990.
396. Schwartz M, Johansen HK, Kock C, Brandt NJ: Frequency of the delta F508 mutation on cystic fibrosis chromosomes in Denmark. *Hum Genet* **85**:427, 1990.
397. Serre JL, Simon-Buoy B, Mornet E, Jaume-Roig B, Balassopoulou A, Schwartz M, Taillandier A, Boué J, Boué A: Studies of RFLP closely linked to the cystic fibrosis locus throughout Europe lead to new considerations in population genetics. *Hum Genet* **84**:449, 1990.
398. Ammerman AJ, Cavalli-Sforza LL: *The Neolithic Transition and the Genetics of Populations in Europe,* Princeton, Princeton University Press, 1984.

399. Cheadle JP, Goodchild MC, Meredith AL: Direct sequencing of the complete CFTR gene: The molecular characterization of 99.5% of CF chromosomes in Wales. *Hum Mol Genet* **2**:1551, 1993.
400. Claustres M, Maguelone L, Desgeorges M, Giansily M, Culard JF, Rapakatsara G, Gerrard B, Demaille J: Analysis of the 27 exons and flanking regions of the cystic fibrosis gene: 40 different mutations account for 91.2% of the mutant alleles in southern France. *Hum Mol Genet* **2**:1209, 1993.
401. Savov A, Mercier B, Kalaydjieva L, Férec C: Identification of six novel mutations in the CFTR gene of patients from Bulgaria by screening the twenty-seven exons and exon/intron boundaries using DGGE and direct DNA sequencing. *Hum Mol Genet* **3**:57, 1994.
402. Glavac D, Ravnik-Glavac M, Dean M: Identification of a rare cystic fibrosis mutation (S4X) in a Slovenian population. *Hum Mol Genet* **2**:315, 1993.
403. Shackleton S, Hull J, Dear S, Seller A, Thomson A, Harris A: Identification of rare and novel mutations in the CFTR genes of CF patients in southern England. *Hum Mutat* **3**:141, 1994.
404. Culard JF, Desgeorges M, Romey MC, Malzac P, Demaille J, Claustres M: A novel splice site mutation in the first exon of the cystic fibrosis transmembrane conductance regulator (CFTR) gene identified in a CBAVD patient. *Hum Mol Genet* **3**:369, 1994.
405. Shackleton S, Harris A: G27X: A novel mutation in exon 2 of the CFTR gene. *Hum Mol Genet* **1**:445, 1992.
406. Bienvenu T, Cazaneuve C, Beldjord C, Dusser D, Kaplan JC, Hubert D: A new missense mutation (G27E) in exon 2 of the CFTR gene in a mildly affected cystic fibrosis patient. *Hum Mol Genet* **3**:365, 1994.
407. Chillón M, Casals T, Giménez J, Nunes V, Estivill X: Analysis of the CFTR gene in the Spanish population: SSCP-screening for 60 known mutations and identification of four new mutations (Q30X, A120T, 1812-1G→A, and 3667del4). *Hum Mutat* **3**:223, 1994.
408. Zielenski J, Markiewicz D, Chen HS, Schappert K, Seller A, Durie P, Corey M, Tsui L-C: Identification of six mutations (R31L, 441delA, 681delC, 1461ins4, W1098R, E1104X) in the cystic fibrosis transmembrane conductance regulator (CFTR) gene. *Hum Mutat* 1994. (In press)
409. Fanen P, Ghanem N, Vidaud M, Besmond C, Martin J, Costes B, Plassa F, Goossens M: Molecular characterization of cystic fibrosis: 16 novel mutations identified by analysis of the whole cystic fibrosis transmembrane conductance regulator (CFTR) coding regions and splice site junctions. *Genomics* **13**:770, 1992.
410. Cutting GR, Curristan SM, Nash E, Rosenstein BJ, Lerer I, Abeliovich D, Hill A, Graham C: Analysis of four diverse population groups indicates that a subset of cystic fibrosis mutations occurs in common among Caucasians. *Am J Hum Genet* **50**:1185, 1992.
411. Audrézet MP, Mercier B, Guillermit H, Quéré I, Verlingue C, Rault G, Férec C: Identification of 12 novel mutations in the CFTR gene. *Hum Mol Genet* **2**:51, 1993.
412. Macek M, Hamosh A, Kiesewetter S, McIntosh I, Rosenstein BJ, Cutting GR: Identification of a novel nonsense mutation (L88X) in exon 3 of the cystic fibrosis transmembrane conductance regulator gene in a native Korean cystic fibrosis chromosome. *Hum Mutat* **1**:501, 1992.
413. Guillermit H, Fanem P, Férec C: A novel mutation in exon 3 of the CFTR gene. *Hum Genet* **92**:233, 1993.
414. Dörk T, Will K, Demmer A, Tümmler B: A donor splice mutation (405 + 1G→A) in cystic fibrosis associated with exon skipping in epithelial CFTR mRNA. *Hum Mol Genet* **3**:1965, 1993.
415. Nunes V, Chillón M, Dörk T, Tümmler B, Casals T, Estivill X: A new missense mutation (E92K) in the first transmembrane domain of the CFTR gene causes a benign cystic fibrosis phenotype. *Hum Mol Genet* **2**:79, 1993.
416. Kälin N, Dörk T, Bozon D, Tümmler B: A novel frameshift mutation in exon 4 of the cystic fibrosis gene (435insA) demonstrates the ambiguity of restriction analysis for mutation screening. *Hum Mol Genet* **1**:545, 1992.
417. Ravnik-Glavac M, Galvac D, Komel R, Dean M: Single-strand conformation polymorphism analysis of the CFTR gene in Slovenian cystic fibrosis patients: Detection of mutations and sequence variations. *Hum Mutat* **2**:286, 1993.
418. White MB, Krueger LJ, Holsclaw DS, Gerrard B, Stewart C, Quittell L, Dolganov G, Baranov V, Ivaschenko T, Kapronov NI, Sebastio G, Castiglione O, Dean M: Detection of three rare frameshift mutations in the cystic fibrosis gene in an African-American (CF444delA), Italian (CF2522insC), and a Soviet (CF3821delT). *Genomics* **10**:266, 1991.
419. Chevalier-Porst F, Chomel JC, Hillaire D, Kitzis A, Kaplan JC, Goutaland R, Mathieu M, Bozon D: A nonsense mutation in exon 4 over the cystic fibrosis gene frequent among the population of the Reunion Island. *Hum Mol Genet* **1**:647, 1992.
420. Cremonesi L, Ferrari M, Belloni E, Magnani C, Seia M, Ronchetto P, Raddy M, Russo MP, Romeo G, Devoto M: Four new mutations of the CFTR gene (541delC, R347H, R352Q, E585X) detected by DGGE analysis in Italian CF patients, associated with different clinical phenotypes. *Hum Mutat* **1**:314, 1992.
421. Graham CA, Goon PKC, Hill AJM, Nevin NC: Identification of a frameshift mutation (557delT) in exon 4 of the CFTR gene. *Genomics* **12**:854, 1992.
422. Bozon D, Zielenski J, Rininsland F, Tsui L-C: Identification of four new mutations in the cystic fibrosis transmembrane conductance regulator gene: I148T, L1077P, Y1092X, 2183AA→G. *Hum Mutat* **3**:330, 1994.
423. Shackleton S, Beards F, Harris A: Detection of a novel and rare mutation in exon 4 of the cystic fibrosis gene by SSCP. *Hum Mol Genet* **1**:439, 1992.
424. Cuppens H, Marymen P, DeBoeck C, Cassiman JJ: Detection of 98.5% of the mutations in 200 Belgian cystic fibrosis alleles by reverse dot-blot and sequencing on the complete coding region and exon/intron junctions of the CFTR gene. *Genomics* **18**:693, 1993.
425. Chillón M, Casals T, Nunes V, Giménez J, Ruiz EP, Estivill X: Identification of a new missense mutation (P205S) in the first transmembrane domain of the CFTR gene associated with a mild cystic fibrosis phenotype. *Hum Mol Genet* **2**:1741, 1993.
426. Dean M, White MB, Gerrard B, Amos J, Milunsky A: A 22 basepair deletion in the coding region of cystic fibrosis gene. *Genomics* **13**:235, 1992.
427. Cheadle JP, Al-Jader LN, Meredith AL: Two novel frame-shift mutations: 977insA in exon 6B, and 4016insT in exon 21, of the cystic fibrosis transmembrane conductance regulator (CFTR) gene. *Hum Mol Genet* **2**:317, 1994.
428. Graham CA, Goon PKC, Hill AJM, Cutting GR, Curristan S, Nevin NC: Identification of a new mutation (R297Q) in exon 7 of the CFTR gene in a Northern Ireland family. *J Med Genet* **28**:571, 1991.
429. Meitinger T, Golla A, Döner C, Deufel A, Aulehla-Scholz C, Bölm I, Reinhardt D, Deufel T: In frame deletion (delta F311) within a short trinucleotide repeat of the first transmembrane region of the cystic fibrosis gene. *Hum Mol Genet* **2**:2173, 1993.
430. Férec C, Audrézet MP, Mercier B, Guillermit H, Moullier P, Quéré I, Verlingue C: Systematic screening for mutations in the cystic fibrosis gene: New implications for carrier detection. *Nat Genet* **1**:188, 1992.
431. Golla A, Deufel A, Aulehla-Scholz C, Böhm I, Hilz B, Meitinger T, Deufel T: Identification of a novel missense mutation (G314E) in exon 7 of the cystic fibrosis transmembrane conductance regulator gene identified in a CF patient with pancreatic sufficiency. *Hum Mutat* **3**:67, 1994.
432. Claustres M, Gerrard B, White MB, Desgeorges M, Kjellberg P, Rollin B, Dean M: A rare mutation (1078delT) in exon 7 of the CFTR gene in a southern French adult with cystic fibrosis. *Genomics* **13**:907, 1992.
433. Gasparini P, Nunes V, Savoia A, Dognini M, Morral N, Gaona A, Bonizzato A, Chillon M, Sangiuolo F, Novelli G, Dallapiccola B, Pignatti PF, Estivill X: The search for south European cystic fibrosis mutations: Identification of two new mutations, four variants, and intronic sequences. *Genomics* **10**:193, 1991.
434. Saba L, Leoni GB, Meloni A, Faa V, Cao A, Rosatelli

MC: Two novel mutations in the transmembrane domain of the CFTR gene in subjects of Sardinian descent. *Hum Mol Genet* **2**:1739, 1993.
435. Iannuzzi MC, Stern RC, Collins FS, Tom Hon C, Hidaka N, Strong T, Becker L, Drumm M, White MB, Gerrard B, Dean M: Two frameshift mutations in the cystic fibrosis gene. *Am J Hum Genet* **48**:227, 1991.
436. Boteva K, Papageorgiou E, Georgiou C, Angastiniotis M, Middleton L, Constantinou-Deltas CD: Novel cystic fibrosis mutation associated with mild disease in Cypriot patients. *Hum Genet* **93**:529, 1994.
437. Audrézet MP, Novelli G, Mercier B, Sangiuolo F, Maceratesi P, Férec C, Dallapiccola B: Identification of three novel cystic fibrosis mutations in a sample of Italian cystic fibrosis patients. *Hum Hered* **43**:295, 1993.
438. Shoshani T, Berkun Y, Yahav Y, Augarten A, Bashan N, Rivlin Y, Gazit E, Seret H, Kerem E, Kerem B: A new mutation in the cystic fibrosis gene, comprised of two adjacent DNA alterations, is common among Georgian Jews. *Genomics* **15**:236, 1992.
439. Dörk T, Fislage R, Rappen U, Tümmler B: Severe splice site mutation preceding exon 9 of the CFTR gene. *Hum Mol Genet* **2**:1313, 1993.
440. Dörk T, Fislage R, Neumman T, Wulf B, Tümmler B: Exon 9 of the CFTR gene: splice site haplotypes and cystic fibrosis mutations. *Hum Genet* **93**:67, 1994.
441. Kerem B, Zielenski J, Markiewicz D, Bozon D, Gazit E, Yahaf J, Kennedy D, Riordan JR, Collins FS, Rommens J, Tsui L-C: Identification of mutations in regions corresponding to the 2 putative nucleotide (ATP)-binding folds of the cystic fibrosis gene. *Proc Natl Acad Sci USA* **87**:8447, 1990.
442. Cuppens H, Marynen P, DeBoeck C, DeBaets F, Eggermont E, Van den Berghe H, Cassiman JJ: A child, homozygous for a stop codon in exon 11, shows milder cystic fibrosis symptoms than her heterozygous nephew. *J Med Genet* **27**:717, 1990.
443. Dörk T, Wulbrand U, Tümmler B: Four novel cystic fibrosis mutations in splice junction sequences affecting the CFTR nucleotide binding folds. *Genomics* **15**:688, 1993.
444. Deufel A, Deufel T, Golla A, Achatz H, Bertele-Harms R, Roscher AA, Meitinger T: Three novel mutations (I506S, S466X, 1651A→T) in exon 10 of the cystic fibrosis transmembrane conductance regulator (CFTR) detected in patients of southern German descent. *Hum Mutat* **3**:64, 1994.
445. Smit L, Strong T, Cole J, Knowles M, Turpin S, Iannuzzi M, Petty T, Tsui L-C, Collins FS: Identification of 5 new CF mutations by chemical mismatch cleavage, including a missense mutation in two mildly affected sisters with normal sweat electrolyte levels. *Pediatr Pulmonol* (Suppl) **6**:244, 1991.
446. Cuppens H, Loumi O, Marynen P, Cassiman JJ: Identification of a new frameshift mutation and a duplication polymorphism in the CFTR gene in the Algerian population. *Hum Mol Genet* **1**:283, 1992.
447. Chillón M, Palacio A, Nunes V, Casals T, Giménez J, Estivill X: Identification of a frameshift mutation (1609delCA) in exon 10 of the CFTR gene in seven Spanish cystic fibrosis patients. *Hum Mutat* **1**:75, 1992.
448. Schwarz M, Summers C, Heptinstall L, Newton C, Markham A, Cain R, Super M: A deletion mutation of the cystic fibrosis transmembrane conductance regulator (CFTR) locus: Delta I507. *Adv Exp Med Biol* **290**:393, 1991.
449. Ivaschenko E, White MB, Dean M, Baranov VS: A deletion of two nucleotides in exon 10 of the CFTR gene in a Soviet family with cystic fibrosis causing early infant death. *Genomics* **10**:298, 1991.
450. Jones CT, McIntosh I, Keston M, Ferguson A, Brock DJH: Three novel mutations in the cystic fibrosis gene detected by chemical cleavage: Analysis of variant splicing and a nonsense mutation. *Hum Mol Genet* **1**:11, 1992.
451. Leoni GB, Rosatelli MC, Cossu G, Pischedda MC, DeVirgilis S, Cao A: A novel cystic fibrosis mutation: Deletion of seventeen nucleotides at the exon 10–intron 10 boundary of the CFTR gene, in a Sardinian patient. *Hum Mol Genet* **2**:83, 1993.
452. Guillermit H, Fanem P, Férec C: A 3′ splice site consensus sequence mutation in the cystic fibrosis gene. *Hum Genet* **85**:450, 1990.
453. Sangiuolo F, Novelli G, Murru S, Dallapiccola B: A serine to arginine (AGT to CTG) mutation in codon 549 of the CFTR gene in an Italian patient with severe cystic fibrosis. *Genomics* **9**:788, 1991.
454. Cutting GR, Kasch LM, Rosenstein BJ, Zielenski J, Tsui L-C, Antonarakis SE, Kazazian HH Jr: A cluster of cystic fibrosis mutations in the first nucleotide binding fold of the cystic fibrosis conductance regulator protein. *Nature* **346**:366, 1990.
455. Strong TV, Smit LS, Turpin SV, Cole JL, Hon CT, Markiewicz D, Petty TL, Craig MW, Rosenow EC, Tsui L-C, Iannuzzi MC, Knowles MR, Collins FS: Cystic fibrosis gene mutation in two sisters with mild disease and normal sweat electrolyte levels. *N Engl J Med* **325**:1630, 1991.
456. Devoto M, Ronchetto P, Fanen P, Telleria Orriols JJ, Romeo G, Goossens M, Ferrari M, Magnani C, Seia M, Cremonesi L: Screening for non delta F508 mutations in 5 exons of the CFTR gene in Italy. *Am J Hum Genet* **48**:1127, 1991.
457. Dörk T, Wulbrand U, Richter T, Neumman T, Wolfes H, Wulf B, Maab G, Tümmler B: Cystic fibrosis with three mutations in the cystic fibrosis transmembrane conductance regulator gene. *Hum Genet* **87**:441, 1991.
458. Strong TV, Smit LS, Nasr S, Wood DL, Cole JL, Iannuzzi MC, Stern RC, Collins FS: Characterization of an intron 12 splice donor mutation in the cystic fibrosis transmembrane conductance regulator (CFTR) gene. *Hum Mutat* **1**:380, 1992.
459. Chevalier-Porst F, Mathieu M, Bozon D: Identification of three rare frameshift mutations in exon 13 of the cystic fibrosis gene: 1918delGC, 2118del14 and 2372del8. *Hum Mol Genet* **2**:1071, 1993.
460. Granell J, Solera J, Carrasco S, Molano J: Identification of a nonframeshift 84-bp deletion in exon 13 of the cystic fibrosis gene. *Am J Hum Genet* **50**:1022, 1992.
461. Dörk T, Kälin N, Stuhrmann M, Schmidtke J, Tümmler B: A termination mutation (2143delT) in the CFTR gene of German cystic fibrosis patients. *Hum Genet* **90**:279, 1992.
462. Smit LS, Nasr SZ, Iannuzzi MC, Collins FS: An African-American cystic fibrosis patient homozygous for a novel frameshift mutation associated with reduced CFTR mRNA levels. *Hum Mutat* **2**:148, 1993.
463. White MB, Amos J, Hsu JMC, Gerrard B, Finn P, Dean M: A frameshift mutation in the cystic fibrosis gene. *Nature* **344**:665, 1990.
464. Mercier B, Lissens W, Audrezet MP, Bonduelle M, Liebaers I, Férec C: Detection of more than 94% cystic fibrosis mutations in a sample of Belgian population and identification of four novel mutations. *Hum Mutat* **2**:16, 1993.
465. Cheadle JP, Al-Jader LN, Meredith AL: A novel nonsense mutation, W8846X1 (amber termination), in exon 14a of the cystic fibrosis transmembrane conductance regulator (CFTR) gene. *Hum Mol Genet* **2**:1067, 1993.
466. Vidaud M, Fanen P, Martin J, Ghanem N, Nocolas S, Goossens M: Three mutations in the CFTR gene in French cystic fibrosis patients: Identification by denaturing gradient gel electrophoresis. *Hum Genet* **85**:446, 1990.
467. White MB, Leppert M, Nielsen D, Zielenski J, Gerrard B, Stewart C, Dean M: A de novo cystic fibrosis mutation: CGA (Arg) to TGA (stop) at codon 851 of the CFTR gene. *Genomics* **11**:778, 1991.
468. Costes B, Fanen P, Goossens M, Ghanem N: A rapid and sensitive assay for simultaneous detection of multiple cystic fibrosis mutations. *Hum Mutat* **2**:185, 1993.
469. Gasparini P, Bonizzato A, Dognini M, Pignatti PF: Restriction site generating polymerase chain reaction (PR-PCR) for the probeless detection of hidden genetic variation: Application to the study of some common cystic fibrosis mutations. *Mol Cell Probes* **6**:1, 1992.
470. Nunes V, Bonizzato A, Gaona A, Dognini M, Chillón M, Casals T, Pignatti PF, Novelli G, Estivill X: A frameshift mutation (2869insG) in the second transmembrane domain of the CFTR gene. Identification, regional distribution, and clinical presentation. *Am J Hum Genet* **50**:1140, 1992.

471. Claustres M, Laussel M, Desgeorges M, Demaille J: Identification of a 6 bp deletion (3195del6) in exon 17a of the cystic fibrosis (CFTR) gene. *Hum Mol Genet* **3**:371, 1994.
472. Mercier B, Lissens W, Novelli G, Kalaydjieva L, De Arce M, Kapranov N, Klain NC, Lenoir G, Chauveau P, Lenaerts C, Rault G, Cashman S, Sangiuolo F, Audrézet MP, Dallapiccola B, Guillermit H, Bonduelle M, Liebaers I, Quéré I, Verlingue C, Férec C: Identification of eight novel mutations in a collaborative analysis of a part of the second transmembrane domain of the CFTR gene. *Genomics* **16**:296, 1993.
473. Férec C, Verlingue C, Guillermit H, Quéré I, Raguénès O, Feigelson J, Audrézet MP, Mercier B: Genotype analysis of adult cystic fibrosis patients. *Hum Mol Genet* **2**:1557, 1993.
474. Zielenski J, Fujiwara TM, Markiewicz D, Paradis AJ, Anacleto AI, Richards B, Schwartz RH, Klinger KW, Tsui L-C, Morgan K: Identification of the M1101K mutation in the cystic fibrosis transmembrane conductance regulator (CFTR) gene and complete detection of cystic fibrosis mutations in the Hutterite population. *Am J Hum Genet* **52**:609, 1993.
475. Ronchetto P, Telleria Orriols JJ, Fanen P, Cremonesi L, Ferrari M, Magnani C, Seia M, Goossens M, Romeo G, Devoto M: A nonsense mutation (R1158X) and a splicing mutation (3849+4A→G) in exon 19 of the cystic fibrosis transmembrane conductance regulator gene. *Genomics* **12**:417, 1992.
476. Sangiuolo F, Lo Cicero S, Maceratesi P, Quattrucci S, Novelli G, Dallapiccola B: Molecular characterization of a frameshift mutation in exon 19 of the CFTR gene. *Hum Mutat* **2**:422, 1993.
477. Ivaschenko TI, Baranov VS, Dean M: Two new mutations detected by single-strand conformation analysis in cystic fibrosis from Russia. *Hum Genet* **91**:63, 1993.
478. Bienvenu T, Lenoir G, Fonknechten N, Descalux-Arramond F, Kaplan JC, Beldjord C: Identification of a new frameshift mutation (3724delG) in exon 19 of the CFTR gene. *Hum Mutat* **3**:69, 1994.
479. Claustres M, Gerrard B, Kjellberg P, Desgeorges M, Demaille J, Dean M: Screening for mutations in southern France: Identification of a frameshift mutation and two missense variations. *Hum Mutat* **1**:310, 1992.
480. Greil I, Wagner K, Rosenkranz W: Identification of a new splice site mutation (3849+1G→A) in the intron 19 of the CFTR gene. *Hum Mol Genet* **2**:2171, 1993.
481. Chillón M, Casals T, Nunes V, Giménez J, Estivill X: Identification of a 31-bp insertion (3860ins31) in exon 20 of the cystic fibrosis (CFTR) gene. *Hum Mol Genet* **2**:1317, 1993.
482. Savov A, Jordanova A, Gavrilov D, Angelicheva D, Kalaydjieva L: G1244V: A novel missense mutation in exon 20 of the CFTR gene in a Bulgarian cystic fibrosis patient. *Hum Mol Genet* **3**:513, 1994.
483. Kälin N, Dörk T, Tümmler B: A cystic fibrosis allele encoding missense mutations in both nucleotide binding folds of the cystic fibrosis transmembrane conductance regulator. *Hum Mutat* **1**:204, 1992.
484. Lissens W, Bonduelle M, Malfroot A, Dab I, Liebaers I: A serine to proline substitution (S1255P) in the second nucleotide binding fold of the cystic fibrosis gene. *Hum Mol Genet* **1**:441, 1992.
485. Anguiano A, Oates RD, Amos JA, Dean M, Gerrard B, Stewart C, Maher TA, White MB, Milunsky A: Congenital bilateral absence of the vas deferens: A primary genital form of cystic fibrosis. *JAMA* **267**:1794, 1992.
486. Cheadle JP, Meredith AL, Al-Jader LN: A new missense mutation (R1283M) in exon 20 of the cystic fibrosis transmembrane conductance regulator gene. *Hum Mol Genet* **1**:123, 1992.
487. Osborne L, Knight RA, Santis G, Hodson M: A mutation in the second nucleotide binding fold of the cystic fibrosis gene. *Am J Hum Genet* **48**:608, 1991.
488. Dörk T, Fislage R, Tümmler B: A complex mutation (4114ATA→TT) in exon 22 of the CFTR gene. *Hum Mutat* **2**:489, 1993.
489. Beaudet AL, Feldman GL, Kobayashi K, Lemna WK, Fernbach SD, Knowles MR, Boucher RC, O'Brien WE: Mutation analysis for cystic fibrosis in a North American population, in Tsui L-C, Romeo G, Greger R, Gorini S (eds): *The Identification of the CF (Cystic Fibrosis) Gene—Recent Progress and New Research Strategies*. New York, Plenum, 1991, p 53.
490. Morral N, Nunes V, Casals T, Cobos N, Asensio O, Dapena J, Estivill X: Uniparental inheritance of microsatellite alleles of the cystic fibrosis gene (CFTR): Identification of a 50 kilobase deletion. *Hum Mol Genet* **2**:677, 1993.
491. Kobayashi K, Knowles MR, Boucher RC, O'Brien WE, Beaudet AL: Benign missense variations in the cystic fibrosis gene. *Am J Hum Genet* **47**:611, 1990.
492. Will K, Stuhrmann M, Ellemunter H, Hoffknecht N, Schmidtke J: Missense variation of the CFTR gene codon 507. *Hum Mutat* **1**:165, 1992.
493. Chillón M, Palacio A, Nunes V, Estivill X: A rare DNA variant in exon 15 of the cystic fibrosis transmembrane conductance regulator (CFTR) gene. *Hum Genet* **90**:474, 1992.
494. Gasparini P, Dognini M, Bonizzato A, Pignatti PF, Morral N, Estivill X: A tetranucleotide repeat polymorphism in cystic fibrosis gene. *Hum Genet* **86**:625, 1991.
495. Chehab EF, Johnson J, Louie E, Goossens M, Kawasaki E, Erlich H: A dimorphic 4-bp repeat in the cystic fibrosis gene is in absolute linkage disequilibrium with the delta F508 mutation: Implications for prenatal diagnosis and mutation origin. *Am J Hum Genet* **48**:223, 1991.
496. Morral N, Nunes V, Casals T, Estivill X: CA/GT microsatellite alleles within the cystic fibrosis transmembrane conductance regulator (CFTR) gene are not generated by unequal crossing over. *Genomics* **10**:692, 1991.
497. Chillón M, Nunes V, Estivill X: SSCP-polymorphism in intron 12 of the CFTR gene recognized by *Bcl*I. *Nucleic Acids Res* **19**:6343, 1991.
498. Zielenski J, Markiewicz D, Rininsland F, Rommens JR, Tsui L-C: A cluster of highly polymorphic dinucleotide repeats in intron 17b of the CFTR gene. *Am J Hum Genet* **49**:1256, 1991.
499. Morral N, Girbau E, Zielenski J, Nunes V, Casals T, Tsui L-C, Estivill X: Dinucleotide (CA/GT) repeat polymorphism in intron 17b of the cystic fibrosis transmembrane conductance regulator gene. *Hum Genet* **88**:356, 1992.
500. Dörk T, Wulbrand U, Tümmler B: A *Hinf*I polymorphism in the cystic fibrosis gene CFTR. *Nucleic Acids Res* **19**:2517, 1991.
501. Quere I, Guillermit H, Mercier B, Audrezet MP, Ferec C: A polymorphism in intron 20 of the CFTR gene. *Nucleic Acids Res* **19**:5453, 1991.
502. Beaudet AL, Tsui L-C: A suggested nomenclature for designating mutations. *Hum Mutat* **2**:245, 1993.
503. Tsui L-C: The spectrum of cystic fibrosis mutations. *Trends Genet* **8**:392, 1992.
504. Casals T, Nunes V, Palacio A, Gimenez J, Gaona A, Ibanez N, Morral N, Estivill X: Cystic fibrosis in Spain: High frequency of mutation G542X in the Mediterranean coastal area. *Hum Genet* **91**:66, 1993.
505. Reiss J, Cooper DN, Bal J, Slomski R, Cutting GR, Krawczak M: Discrimination between recurrent mutation and identity by descent: Application to point mutations in exon 11 of the cystic fibrosis (CFTR) gene. *Hum Genet* **87**:457, 1991.
506. Teem JL, Berger HA, Ostedgaard LS, Rich DP, Tsui L-C, Welsh MJ: Identification of revertants for the cystic fibrosis delta F508 mutation using STE6-CFTR chimeras in yeast. *Cell* **73**:335, 1993.
507. Meschede D, Eigel A, Horst J, Nieschlag E: Compound heterozygosity for the delta F508 and F508C cystic fibrosis transmembrane conductance regulator (CFTR) mutations in a patient with congenital bilateral aplasia of the vas deferens. *Am J Hum Genet* **53**:292, 1993.
507a. Desgeorges M, Kjellberg P, Demaille J, Claustres M: A healthy male with compound and double heterozygosities for ΔF508, F508C, and M470V in exon 10 of the cystic fibrosis gene. *Am J Hum Genet* **54**:384, 1994.
508. Quinton PM: Chloride impermeability in cystic fibrosis. *Nature* **301**:421, 1983.
509. Quinton PM: Cystic fibrosis: A disease in electrolyte transport. *FASEB J* **4**:2709, 1990.

510. Bijman J, Quinton P: Permeability properties of cell membranes and tight junctions of normal and cystic fibrosis sweat ducts. *Pflügers Arch* **408**:505, 1987.
511. Reddy MM, Quinton PM: Localization of Cl^- conductance in normal and Cl^- impermeability in cystic fibrosis sweat duct epithelium. *Am J Physiol* **257**:C727, 1989.
512. Quinton PM: Missing Cl conductance in cystic fibrosis. *Am J Physiol* **251**:C649, 1986.
513. Quinton PM: Abnormalities in electrolyte secretion, in Quinton PM, Martinez JR, Hopfer U (eds): *Cystic Fibrosis Sweat Glands Due to Decreased Anion Permeability*. San Francisco, San Francisco Press, 1982, p 53.
514. Reddy MM, Quinton PM: Intracellular potentials of microperfused human sweat duct cells. *Pflügers Arch* **410**:471, 1987.
515. Reddy MM, Quinton PM: Altered electrical potential profile of human reabsorptive sweat duct cells in cystic fibrosis. *Am J Physiol* **257**:C722, 1989.
516. Reddy MM, Quinton PM: cAMP activation of CF-affected Cl^- conductance in both cell membranes of an absorptive epithelium. *J Membr Biol* **130**:49, 1992.
517. Kartner N, Augustinas O, Jensen TJ, Naismith AL, Riordan JR: Mislocalization of delta F508 CFTR in cystic fibrosis sweat gland. *Nat Genet* **1**:321, 1992.
518. Cohn JA, Melhus O, Page LJ, Dittrich KL, Vigna SR: CFTR: Development of high affinity antibodies and localization in sweat gland. *Biochem Biophys Res Commun* **181**:36, 1991.
519. Bell CL, Reddy MM, Quinton PM: Reversed anion selectivity in cultured cystic fibrosis sweat duct cells. *Am J Physiol* **262**:C32, 1992.
520. Ram SJ, Weaver ML, Kirk KL: Regulation of Cl^- permeability in normal and cystic fibrosis sweat duct cells. *Am J Physiol* **259**:C842, 1990.
521. Quinton PM, Reddy MM: Control of CFTR chloride conductance by ATP levels through non-hydrolytic binding. *Nature* **360**:79, 1992.
522. Sato K, Sato F: Relationship between quin2-determined cytosolic $[Ca^{2+}]$ and sweat secretion. *Am J Physiol* **254**:C310, 1988.
523. Sato K: *Fluid and Electrolyte Abnormalities in Exocrine Glands in Cystic Fibrosis*. San Francisco, San Francisco Press, 1982, p 35.
524. Sato K, Saga K, Sato F: Membrane transport and intracellular events in control and cystic fibrosis eccrine sweat glands, in Mastella G, Quinton PM (eds): *Cellular and Molecular Basis of Cystic Fibrosis*. San Francisco, San Francisco Press, 1988, p 171.
525. Alder J, Lu B, Valtorta F, Greengard P, Poo MM: Calcium-dependent transmitter secretion reconstituted in *Xenopus* oocytes: requirement for synaptophysin. *Science* **257**:657, 1992.
526. Behm JK, Hagiwara G, Lewiston NJ, Quinton PM, Wine JJ: Hyposecretion of β-adrenergically induced sweating in cystic fibrosis heterozygotes. *Pediatr Res* **22**:271, 1987.
527. Sato K, Sato F: Variable reduction in β-adrenergic sweat secretion in cystic fibrosis heterozygotes. *J Lab Clin Med* **111**:511, 1988.
528. Takemura T, Sato F, Saga K, Suzuki Y, Sato K: Intracellular ion concentrations and cell volume during cholinergic stimulation of eccrine secretory coil cells. *J Membr Biol* **119**:211, 1991.
529. Reddy MM, Bell CL, Quinton PM: Evidence of two distinct epithelial cell types in primary cultures from human sweat gland secretory coil. *Am J Physiol* **262**:C891, 1992.
530. Reddy MM, Quinton PM: Electrophysiologically distinct cell types in human sweat gland secretory coil. *Am J Physiol* **262**:C287, 1992.
531. Frizzell RA, Field M, Schultz SG: Sodium-coupled chloride transport by epithelial tissues. *Am J Physiol* **236**:F1, 1979.
532. Breeze RG, Wheeldon RB: The cells of the pulmonary airways. *Am Rev Respir Dis* **116**:705, 1977.
533. Plopper CG, Hill LL, Mariassy AT: Ultrastructure of the nonciliated bronchiolar epithelial (Clara) cell of mammalian lung. III. A study of man with comparison of 15 mammalian species. *Exp Lung Res* **1**:171, 1980.
534. Reid L, deHaller R: The bronchial mucous glands—their hypertrophy and change in intracellular mucus. *Mod Prob Pediatr* **10**:195, 1966.
535. Basbaum CB, Jany B, Finkbeiner WE: The serous cell. *Annu Rev Physiol* **52**:97, 1990.
536. Welsh MJ, Basbaum C: Mucus secretion and ion transport in airways, in Nadel J (ed): *Textbook of Respiratory Medicine*. Philadelphia, Saunders, 1993.
537. Welsh MJ: Electrolyte transport by airway epithelia. *Physiol Rev* **67**:1143, 1987.
538. Boucher RC, Knowles MR, Stutts MJ, Gatzy JT: Epithelial dysfunction in cystic fibrosis lung disease. *Lung* **161**:1, 1983.
539. Frizzell RA, Halm DR, Rechkemmer G, Shoemaker RL: Chloride channel regulation in secretory epithelia. *Fed Proc* **45**:2727, 1986.
540. Knowles M, Murray G, Shallai J, Askin F, Ranga V, Gatzy J: Bioelectric properties and ion flow across excised human bronchi. *J Appl Physiol* **56**:868, 1984.
541. Knowles MR, Stutts MJ, Spock A, Fischer N, Gatzy JT, Boucher RC: Abnormal ion permeation through cystic fibrosis respiratory epithelium. *Science* **221**:1067, 1983.
542. Widdicombe JH, Welsh MJ, Finkbeiner WE: Cystic fibrosis decreases the apical membrane chloride permeability of monolayers cultured from cells of tracheal epithelium. *Proc Natl Acad Sci USA* **82**:6167, 1985.
543. Knowles MR, Buntin WH, Bromberg PA, Gatzy JT, Boucher RC: Measurements of transepithelial electric potential differences in the trachea and bronchi of human subjects in vivo. *Am Rev Respir Dis* **126**:108, 1982.
544. Knowles MR, Carson JL, Collier AM, Gatzy JT, Boucher RC: Measurements of nasal transepithelial electric potential differences in normal human subjects in vivo. *Am Rev Respir Dis* **124**:484, 1981.
545. Widdicombe JH, Coleman DL, Finkbeiner WE, Tuet IK: Electrical properties of monolayers cultured from cells of human tracheal mucosa. *J Appl Physiol* **58**:1729, 1985.
546. Welsh MJ, Smith PL, Frizzell RA: Chloride secretion by canine tracheal epithelium. III. Membrane resistances and electromotive forces. *J Membr Biol* **71**:209, 1983.
547. Johnson LG, Olsen JC, Sarkadi B, Moore KL, Swanstrom R, Boucher RC: Efficiency of gene transfer for restoration of normal airway epithelial function in cystic fibrosis. *Nat Genet* **2**:21, 1992.
548. Gordon RE, Lane BP, Marin M: Regeneration of rat tracheal epithelium: Changes in gap junction during specific phases of the cell cycle. *Exp Lung Res* **3**:47, 1982.
549. Inoue A, Hogg JC: Freeze-etch study of the tracheal epithelium of normal guinea pigs with particular reference to intercellular junction. *J Ultrastruct Res* **61**:89, 1977.
550. Marin ML, Lane BP, Gordon RE, Drummond E: Ultrastructure of rat tracheal epithelium. *Lung* **156**:223, 1979.
551. Schneeberger EE: Heterogeneity of tight junction morphology in extrapulmonary and intrapulmonary airways of the rat. *Anat Rec* **198**:193, 1980.
552. Welsh MJ: Ion transport by primary cultures of canine tracheal epithelium: Methodology, morphology, and electrophysiology. *J Membr Biol* **88**:149, 1985.
553. Davis B, Marin MG, Yee JW, Nadel JA: Effect of terbutaline on movement of Cl^- and Na^+ across the trachea of the dog in vitro. *Am Rev Respir Dis* **120**:547, 1979.
554. Al-Bazzaz FJ, Cheng E: Effect of catecholamines on ion transport in dog tracheal epithelium. *J Appl Physiol* **47**:397, 1979.
555. Liedtke CM, Tandler B: Physiological responsiveness of isolated rabbit tracheal epithelial cells. *Am J Physiol* **247**:C441, 1984.
556. Smith PL, Welsh MJ, Stoff JW, Frizzell RA: Chloride secretion by canine tracheal epithelium. I. Role of intracellular cAMP levels. *J Membr Biol* **70**:217, 1982.
557. Welsh MJ: Adrenergic regulation of ion transport by primary cultures of canine tracheal epithelium: Cellular electrophysiology. *J Membr Biol* **91**:121, 1986.
558. Boucher RC, Gatzy JT: Regional effects of autonomic agents on ion transport across excised canine airways. *J Appl Physiol* **52**:893, 1982.
559. Nathanson I, Widdicombe JH, Barnes PJ: Effect of vasoactive intestinal peptide on ion transport across dog tracheal epithelium. *J Appl Physiol* **55**:1844, 1983.
560. Pratt AD, Clancy G, Welsh MJ: Mucosal adenosine stimu-

lates chloride secretion in canine tracheal epithelium. *Am J Physiol* **251**:C167, 1986.

561. Widdicombe JH, Ueki IF, Emery D, Margolskee D, Yergey J, Nadel JA: Release of cyclooxygenase products from primary cultures of tracheal epithelia of dog and human. *Am J Physiol* **257**:L361, 1989.
562. Liedtke CM: Interaction of epinephrine with isolated rabbit tracheal epithelial cells. *Am J Physiol* **251**:C209, 1986.
563. Lazarus SC, Basbaum CB, Gold WM: Prostaglandins and intracellular cyclic AMP in respiratory secretory cells. *Am Rev Respir Dis* **130**:262, 1984.
564. Leikauf GD, Ueki IF, Nadel JA, Widdicombe JH: Bradykinin stimulates Cl secretion and prostaglandin E2 release by canine tracheal epithelium. *Am J Physiol* **248**:F48, 1985.
565. Clarke LL, Paradiso AM, Mason SJ, Boucher RC: Effects of bradykinin on Na^+ and Cl^- transport in human nasal epithelium. *Am J Physiol* **262**:C644, 1992.
566. McCann JD, Bhalla RC, Welsh MJ: Release of intracellular calcium by two different second messengers in airway epithelium. *Am J Physiol* **257**:L116, 1989.
567. Smith JJ, McCann JD, Welsh MJ: Bradykinin stimulates airway epithelial Cl^- secretion via two second messenger pathways. *Am J Physiol* **258**:L369, 1990.
568. Denning GM, Welsh MJ: Polarized distribution of bradykinin receptors on airway epithelial cells and independent coupling to second messenger pathways. *J Biol Chem* **266**:12932, 1991.
569. Al-Bazzaz FJ, Kelsey JG, Kaage WD: Substance P stimulation of chloride secretion by canine tracheal mucosa. *Am Rev Respir Dis* **131**:86, 1985.
570. Leikauf GD, Ueki IF, Widdicombe JH, Nadel JA: Alteration of chloride secretion across canine tracheal epithelium by lipoxygenase products of arachidonic acid. *Am J Physiol* **250**:F47, 1986.
571. Mason SJ, Paradiso AM, Boucher RC: Regulation of transepithelial ion transport and intracellular calcium by extracellular ATP in human normal and cystic fibrosis airway epithelium. *Br J Pharmacol* **103**:1649, 1991.
572. Clarke LL, Boucher RC: Chloride secretory response to extracellular ATP in human normal and cystic fibrosis nasal epithelia. *Am J Physiol* **263**:C348, 1992.
573. Boucher RC, Stutts MJ, Knowles MR, Cantley L, Gatzy JT: Na^+ transport in cystic fibrosis respiratory epithelia. Abnormal basal rate and response to adenylate cyclase activation. *J Clin Invest* **78**:1245, 1986.
574. Boucher RC, Cotton CU, Gatzy JT, Knowles MR, Yankaskas JR: Evidence for reduced Cl^- and increased Na^+ permeability in cystic fibrosis human primary cell cultures. *J Physiol (Lond)* **405**:77, 1988.
575. Willumsen NJ, Boucher RC: Sodium transport and intracellular sodium activity in cultured human nasal epithelium. *Am J Physiol* **261**:C319, 1991.
576. Willumsen NJ, Boucher RC: Transcellular sodium transport in cultured cystic fibrosis human nasal epithelium. *Am J Physiol* **261**:C332, 1991.
577. Cullen JJ, Welsh MJ: Regulation of sodium absorption by canine tracheal epithelium. *J Clin Invest* **79**:73, 1987.
578. Adams GK, Aharanson EF, Reasor MJ, Proctor DF: Collection of normal canine tracheobronchial secretions. *J Appl Physiol* **40**:247, 1979.
579. Boat TF, Cheng PW: Biochemistry of airway mucus secretions. *Fed Proc* **39**:3067, 1980.
580. Cherniak WS, Barbero GJ: Composition of tracheobronchial secretions in cystic fibrosis of the pancreas and bronchiectasis. *Pediatrics* **24**:739, 1959.
581. Mentz WM, Brown JB, Friedman M, Stutts MJ, Gatzy JT, Boucher RC: Deposition, clearance, and effects of aerosolized amiloride in sheep airways. *Am Rev Respir Dis* **134**:938, 1986.
582. Joris L, Quinton PM: Concentration of elements in airway surface fluid. *Med Sci Res* **15**:855, 1987.
583. Smith JJ, Welsh MJ: Fluid and electrolyte transport by cultured human airway epithelia. *J Clin Invest* **91**:1590, 1993.
584. Welsh MJ, Widdicombe JH, Nadel JA: Fluid transport across canine tracheal epithelium. *J Appl Physiol* **49**:905, 1980.
585. Liedtke CM: Electrolyte transport in the epithelium of pulmonary segments of normal and cystic fibrosis lung. *FASEB J* **6**:3076, 1992.
586. Knowles M, Gatzy J, Boucher R: Relative ion permeability of normal and cystic fibrosis nasal epithelium. *J Clin Invest* **71**:1410, 1983.
587. Alton EW, Currie D, Logan-Sinclair R, Warner JO, Hodson ME, Geddes DM: Nasal potential difference: A clinical diagnostic test for cystic fibrosis. *Eur Respir J* **3**:922, 1990.
588. Widdicombe JH: Cystic fibrosis and β-adrenergic response of airway epithelial cell cultures. *Am J Physiol* **251**:R818, 1986.
589. Cotton CU, Stutts MJ, Knowles MR, Gatzy JT, Boucher RC: Abnormal apical cell membrane in cystic fibrosis respiratory epithelium. An in vitro electrophysiologic analysis. *J Clin Invest* **79**:80, 1987.
590. Boucher RC, Cheng EH, Paradiso AM, Stutts MJ, Knowles MR, Earp HS: Chloride secretory response of cystic fibrosis human airway epithelia. Preservation of calcium but not protein kinase C- and A-dependent mechanisms. *J Clin Invest* **84**:1424, 1989.
591. Anderson MP, Welsh MJ: Calcium and cAMP activate different chloride channels in the apical membrane of normal and cystic fibrosis epithelia. *Proc Natl Acad Sci USA* **88**:6003, 1991.
592. Hartmann T, Kondo M, Mochizuki H, Verkman AS, Widdicombe JH: Calcium-dependent regulation of Cl secretion in tracheal epithelium. *Am J Physiol* **262**:L163, 1992.
593. Willumsen NJ, Boucher RC: Activation of an apical Cl^- conductance by Ca^{2+} ionophores in cystic fibrosis airway epithelia. *Am J Physiol* **256**:C226, 1989.
594. Yamaya M, Finkbeiner WE, Widdicombe JH: Altered ion transport by tracheal glands in cystic fibrosis. *Am J Physiol* **261**:L491, 1991.
595. Yamaya M, Finkbeiner WE, Widdicombe JH: Ion transport by cultures of human tracheobronchial submucosal glands. *Am J Physiol* **261**:L485, 1991.
596. Marino CR, Matovcik LM, Gorelick FS, Cohn JA: Localization of the cystic fibrosis transmembrane conductance regulator in pancreas. *J Clin Invest* **88**:712, 1991.
597. Gray MA, Harris A, Coleman L, Greenwell JR, Argent BE: Two types of chloride channel on duct cells cultured from human fetal pancreas. *Am J Physiol* **257**:C240, 1989.
598. Gray MA, Greenwell JR, Argent BE: Secretin-regulated chloride channel on the apical plasma membrane of pancreatic duct cells. *J Membr Biol* **105**:131, 1988.
599. Gray MA, Pollard CE, Harris A, Coleman L, Greenwell JR, Argent BE: Anion selectivity and block of the small-conductance chloride channel on pancreatic duct cells. *Am J Physiol* **259**:C752, 1990.
600. Gray MA, Plant S, Argent BE: cAMP-regulated whole cell chloride currents in pancreatic duct cells. *Am J Physiol* **264**:C591, 1993.
601. Taylor CJ, Baxter PS, Hardcastle J, Hardcastle PT: Failure to induce secretion in jejunal biopsies from children with cystic fibrosis. *Gut* **29**:957, 1988.
602. Berschneider HM, Knowles MR, Azizkhan RG, Boucher RC, Tobey NA, Orlando RC, Powell DW: Altered intestinal chloride transport in cystic fibrosis. *FASEB J* **2**:2625, 1988.
603. Veeze HJ, Sinaasappel M, Bijman J, Bouquet J, De-Jong HR: Ion transport abnormalities in rectal suction biopsies from children with cystic fibrosis. *Gastroenterology* **101**:398, 1991.
604. Goldstein JL, Shapiro AB, Rao MC, Layden TJ: In vivo evidence of altered chloride but not potassium secretion in cystic fibrosis rectal mucosa. *Gastroenterology* **101**:1012, 1991.
605. De-Jong HR, Van Den Berghe N, Tilly BC, Kansen M, Bijman J: (Dys)regulation of epithelial chloride channels. *Biochem Soc Trans 17*:816, 1989.
606. De-Jong HR, Bijman J, Sinaasappel M: Relation of regulatory enzyme levels to chloride transport in intestinal epithelial cells. *Pediatr Pulmonol* (Suppl) **1**:54, 1987.
607. Tabcharani JA, Low W, Elie D, Hanrahan JW: Low-conductance chloride channel activated by cAMP in the epithelial cell line T84. *FEBS Lett* **270**:157, 1990.
608. Bear CE, Reyes EF: cAMP-activated chloride conductance in the colonic cell line, Caco-2. *Am J Physiol* **262**:C251, 1992.

609. Frizzell RA, Halm DR: Chloride channels in epithelial cells. *Curr Top Membr Transp* **37**:247, 1990.
610. Kubitz R, Warth R, Allert N, Kunzelmann K, Greger R: Small-conductance chloride channels induced by cAMP, Ca^{2+}, and hypotonicity in HT29 cells: Ion selectivity, additivity and stilbene sensitivity. *Pflügers Arch* **421**:447, 1992.
611. Kunzelmann K, Grolik M, Kubitz R, Greger R: cAMP-dependent activation of small conductance Cl^- channels in HT29 colon carcinoma cells. *Pflügers Arch* **421**:230, 1992.
612. Anderson MP, Sheppard DN, Berger HA, Welsh MJ: Chloride channels in the apical membrane of normal and cystic fibrosis airway and intestinal epithelia. *Am J Physiol* **263**:L1, 1992.
613. Bell CL, Quinton PM: Regulation of CFTR Cl^- conductance in secretion by cellular energy levels. *Am J Physiol* **264**:C925, 1993.
614. Goldstein JL, Nash NT, Al-Bazzaz F, Layden TJ, Rao MC: Rectum has abnormal ion transport but normal cAMP-binding proteins in cystic fibrosis. *Am J Physiol* **254**:C719, 1988.
615. Wong PYD: Mechanism of adrenergic stimulation of anion secretion in cultured rat epididymal epithelium. *Am J Physiol* **254**:F121, 1988.
616. Cuthbert AW, Wong PYD: Anion secretion in cultured rat epididymal epithelium. *J Physiol* **378**:335, 1986.
617. Pollard CE, Harris A, Coleman L, Argent BE: Chloride channels on epithelial cells cultured from human fetal epididymis. *J Membr Biol* **124**:275, 1991.
618. Ames GF-L, Minura CS, Shyamala V: Bacterial periplasmic permeases belong to a family of transport proteins operating from *Escherichia coli* to human: Traffic ATPases. *FEMS Microbiol Rev* **75**:429, 1990.
619. Hyde SC, Emsley P, Hartshorn MJ, Mimmack MM, Gileadi U, Pearce SR, Gallagher MP, Gill DR, Hubbard RE, Higgins CF: Structural model of ATP-binding proteins associated with cystic fibrosis, multidrug resistance and bacterial transport. *Nature* **346**:362, 1990.
620. Gregory RJ, Cheng SH, Rich DP, Marshall J, Paul S, Hehir K, Ostedgaard L, Klinger KW, Welsh MJ, Smith AE: Expression and characterization of the cystic fibrosis transmembrane conductance regulator. *Nature* **347**:382, 1990.
621. Denning GM, Ostedgaard LS, Cheng SH, Smith AE, Welsh MJ: Localization of cystic fibrosis transmembrane conductance regulator. *J Clin Invest* **89**:339, 1992.
622. Cheng SH, Gregory RJ, Marshall J, Paul S, Souza DW, White GA, O'Riordan CR, Smith AE: Defective intracellular transport and processing of CFTR is the molecular basis of most cystic fibrosis. *Cell* **63**:827, 1990.
623. Gregory RJ, Rich DP, Cheng SH, Souza DW, Paul S, Manavalan P, Anderson MP, Welsh MJ, Smith AE: Maturation and function of cystic fibrosis transmembrane conductance regulator variants bearing mutations in putative nucleotide-binding domains 1 and 2. *Mol Cell Biol* **11**:3886, 1991.
624. Zhang JT, Ling V: Study of membrane orientation and glycosylated extracellular loops of mouse P-glycoprotein by *in vitro* translation. *J Biol Chem* **266**:18224, 1991.
625. Skach WR, Calayag MC, Lingappa VR: Evidence for an alternate model of human P-glycoprotein structure and biogenesis. *J Biol Chem* **268**:6903, 1993.
626. Kerppola RE, Ames GF: Topology of the hydrophobic membrane-bound components of the histidine periplasmic permease. Comparison with other members of the family. *J Biol Chem* **267**:2329, 1992.
627. Trezise AE, Buchwald M: In vivo cell-specific expression of the cystic fibrosis transmembrane conductance regulator. *Nature* **353**:434, 1991.
628. Trezise AE, Romano PR, Gill DR, Hyde SC, Sepulveda FV, Buchwald M, Higgins CF: The multidrug resistance and cystic fibrosis genes have complementary patterns of epithelial expression. *EMBO J* **11**:4291, 1992.
629. Trezise AEO, Linder CC, Grieger D, Thompson EW, Meunier H, Griswold MD, Buchwald M: CFTR expression is regulated during both the cycle of the seminiferous epithelium and the oestrous cycle of rodents. *Nat Genet* **3**:157, 1993.
630. Engelhardt JF, Yankaskas JR, Ernst SA, Yang Y, Marion CR, Boucher RC, Cohn JA, Wilson JM: Submucosal glands are the predominant site of CFTR expression in the human bronchus. *Nat Genet* **2**:240, 1992.
631. McCray PBJ, Wohlford-Lenane CL, Snyder JM: Localization of cystic fibrosis transmembrane conductance regulator mRNA in human fetal lung tissue by in situ hybridization. *J Clin Invest* **90**:619, 1992.
632. Yoshimura K, Nakamura H, Trapnell BC, Chu CS, Dalemans W, Pavirani A, Lecocq JP, Crystal RG: Expression of the cystic fibrosis transmembrane conductance regulator gene in cells of non-epithelial origin. *Nucleic Acids Res* **19**:5417, 1991.
633. McDonald TV, Nghiem PT, Gardner P, Martens CL: Human lymphocytes transcribe the cystic fibrosis transmembrane conductance regulator gene and exhibit CF-defective cAMP-regulated chloride current. *J Biol Chem* **267**:3242, 1992.
634. Nagel G, Hwang T-C, Nastiuk KL, Nairn C, Gadsby DC: The protein kinase A-regulated cardiac Cl^- channel resembles the cystic fibrosis transmembrane conductance regulator. *Nature* **360**:81, 1992.
635. Levesque PC, Hart PJ, Hume JR, Kenyon JL, Horowitz B: Expression of cystic fibrosis transmembrane regulator Cl^- channels in heart. *Circ Res* **71**:1002, 1992.
636. Crawford I, Maloney PC, Zeitlin PL, Guggino WB, Hyde SC, Turley H, Gatter KC, Harris A, Higgins CF: Immunocytochemical localization of the cystic fibrosis gene product CFTR. *Proc Natl Acad Sci USA* **88**:9262, 1991.
637. Denning GM, Ostedgaard LS, Welsh MJ: Abnormal localization of cystic fibrosis transmembrane conductance regulator in primary cultures of cystic fibrosis airway epithelia. *J Cell Biol* **118**:551, 1992.
638. Dalemans W, Hinnrasky J, Slos P, Dreyer D, Fuchey C, Pavirani A, Puchelle E: Immunocytochemical analysis reveals differences between the subcellular localization of normal and delta Phe508 recombinant cystic fibrosis transmembrane conductance regulator. *Exp Cell Res* **201**:235, 1992.
639. Puchelle E, Gaillard D, Ploton D, Hinnrasky J, Fuchey C, Boutterin MC, Jacquot J, Dreyer D, Pavirani A, Dalemans W: Differential localization of the cystic fibrosis transmembrane conductance regulator in normal and cystic fibrosis airway epithelium. *Am J Respir Cell Mol Biol* **7**:485, 1992.
640. Morris AP, Cunningham SA, Frizzell RA: CFTR targeting in epithelial cells. *J Bioenerg Biomembr* **25**:21, 1993.
641. Cohn JA, Nairn AC, Marino CR, Melhus O, Kole J: Characterization of the cystic fibrosis transmembrane conductance regulator in a colonocyte cell line. *Proc Natl Acad Sci USA* **89**:2340, 1992.
642. Hoogeveen AT, Keulemans J, Willemsen R, Scholte BJ, Bijman J, Edixhoven MJ, DeJong HR, Galjaard H: Immunological localization of cystic fibrosis candidate gene products. *Exp Cell Res* **193**:435, 1991.
643. McCray PBJ, Bettencourt JD, Bastacky J, Denning GD, Welsh MJ: Expression of CFTR and a cAMP-stimulated chloride secretory current in cultured human fetal alveolar epithelial cells. *Am J Respir Cell Mol Biol* **9**:578, 1993.
644. Prince LS, Tousson A, Marchase RB: Cell surface labeling of CFTR in T84 cells. *Am J Physiol* **264**:C491, 1993.
645. Bradbury NA, Cohn JA, Venglarik CJ, Bridges RJ: The cystic fibrosis gene product (CFTR) is in endocytic clathrin coated vesicles. *Proc Int Union Physiol Sci* **32**:30, 1993.
646. Lukacs GL, Chang XB, Kartner N, Rotstein OD, Riordan JR, Grinstein S: The cystic fibrosis transmembrane regulator is present and functional in endosomes. Role as a determinant of endosomal pH. *J Biol Chem* **267**:14568, 1992.
647. Bradbury NA, Jilling T, Berta G, Sorscher EJ, Bridges RJ, Kirk KL: Regulation of plasma membrane recycling by CFTR. *Science* **256**:530, 1992.
648. Trapnell BC, Chu CS, Paakko PK, Banks TC, Yoshimura K, Ferrans VJ, Chernick MS, Crystal RG: Expression of the cystic fibrosis transmembrane conductance regulator gene in the respiratory tract of normal individuals and individuals with cystic fibrosis. *Proc Natl Acad Sci USA* **88**:6565, 1991.
649. Rich DP, Anderson MP, Gregory RJ, Cheng SH, Paul S, Jefferson DM, McCann JD, Klinger KW, Smith AE, Welsh MJ: Expression of cystic fibrosis transmembrane

conductance regulator corrects defective chloride channel regulation in cystic fibrosis airway epithelial cells. *Nature* **347**:358, 1990.

650. Drumm ML, Pope HA, Cliff WH, Rommens JM, Marvin SA, Tsui L-C, Collins FS, Frizzell RA, Wilson JM: Correction of the cystic fibrosis defect in vitro by retrovirus-mediated gene transfer. *Cell* **62**:1227, 1990.
651. Anderson MP, Gregory RJ, Thompson S, Souza DW, Paul S, Mulligan RC, Smith AE, Welsh MJ: Demonstration that CFTR is a chloride channel by alteration of its anion selectivity. *Science* **253**:202, 1991.
652. Anderson MP, Berger HA, Rich DP, Gregory RJ, Smith AE: Nucleoside triphosphates are required to open the CFTR chloride. *Cell* **67**:775, 1991.
653. Berger HA, Anderson MP, Gregory RJ, Thompson S, Howard PW: Identification and regulation of the cystic fibrosis transmembrane conductance regulator. *J Clin Invest* **88**:1422, 1991.
654. Drumm ML, Wilkinson DJ, Smit LS, Worrell RT, Strong TV, Frizzell RA, Dawson DC, Collins FS: Chloride conductance expressed by delta F508 and other mutant CFTRs in *Xenopus* oocytes. *Science* **254**:1797, 1991.
655. Dalemans W, Barbry P, Champigny G, Jallat S, Dott K, Dreyer D, Crystal RG, Pavirani A, Lecocq JP, Lazdunski M: Altered chloride ion channel kinetics associated with the delta F508 cystic fibrosis mutation. *Nature* **354**:526, 1991.
656. Bijman J, Dalemans W, Kansen M, Keulemans J, Verbeek E, Hoogeveen A, De-Jong H, Wilke M, Dreyer D, Lecocq JP: Low-conductance chloride channels in IEC-6 and CF nasal cells expressing CFTR. *Am J Physiol* **264**:L229, 1993.
657. Bear CE, Duguay F, Naismith AL, Kartner N, Hanrahan JW, Riordan JR: Cl^- channel activity in *Xenopus* oocytes expressing the cystic fibrosis gene. *J Biol Chem* **266**:19142, 1991.
658. Tabcharani JA, Chang X-B, Riordan JR, Hanrahan JW: Phosphorylation-regulated Cl^- channel in CHO cells stably expressing the cystic fibrosis gene. *Nature* **352**:628, 1991.
659. Kartner N, Hanrahan JW, Jensen TJ, Naismith AL, Sun S, Ackerley CA, Reyes EF, Tsui L-C, Rommens JM, Bear CE, Riordan JR: Expression of the cystic fibrosis gene in non-epithelial invertebrate cells produces a regulated anion conductance. *Cell* **64**:681, 1991.
660. Rommens JM, Dho S, Bear CE, Kartner N, Kennedy D, Riordan JR, Tsui L-C, Foskett JK: cAMP-inducible chloride conductance in mouse fibroblast lines stably expressing the human cystic fibrosis transmembrane conductance regulator. *Proc Natl Acad Sci USA* **88**:7500, 1991.
661. Cliff WH, Schoumacher RA, Frizzell RA: cAMP-activated Cl channels in CFTR-transfected cystic fibrosis pancreatic epithelial cells. *Am J Physiol* **262**:C1154, 1992.
662. Cunningham SA, Worrell RT, Benos DJ, Frizzell RA: cAMP-stimulated ion currents in *Xenopus* oocytes expressing CFTR cRNA. *Am J Physiol* **262**:C783, 1992.
663. Cliff WH, Frizzell RA: Separate Cl^- conductances activated by cAMP and Ca^{2+} in Cl^--secreting epithelial cells. *Proc Natl Acad Sci USA* **87**:4956, 1990.
664. Haws C, Krouse ME, Xia Y, Gruenert DC, Wine JJ: CFTR channels in immortalized human airway cells. *Am J Physiol* **263**:L692, 1992.
665. Gogelein H: Chloride channels in epithelia. *Biochim Biophys Acta* **947**:521, 1988.
666. Yool AJ, Schwarz TL: Alteration of ionic selectivity of a K^+ channel by mutation of the H5 region. *Nature* **349**:700, 1991.
667. Stevens CF: Making a submicroscopic hole in one. *Nature* **349**:657, 1991.
668. Leonard RJ, Labarca CG, Charnet P, Davidson N, Lester HA: Evidence that the M2 membrane-spanning region lines the ion channel pore of the nicotinic receptor. *Science* **242**:1578, 1988.
669. Blachly-Dyson E, Peng S, Colombini M, Forte M: Selectivity changes in site-directed mutants of the VDAC ion channel: Structural implications. *Science* **247**:1233, 1990.
670. Tsui L-C: Mutations and sequence variations detected in the cystic fibrosis transmembrane conductance regulator (CFTR) gene: A report from the Cystic Fibrosis Genetic Analysis Consortium. *Hum Mutat* **1**:197, 1992.
671. Kerem E, Corey M, Kerem B-S, Rommens J, Markiewicz D, Levison H, Tsui L-C, Durie P: The relation between genotype and phenotype in cystic fibrosis—analysis of the most common mutation (delta F508). *N Engl J Med* **323**:1517, 1990.
672. Kristidis P, Bozon D, Corey M, Markiewicz D, Rommens J, Tsui L-C, Durie P: Genetic determination of exocrine pancreatic function in cystic fibrosis. *Am J Hum Genet* **50**:1178, 1992.
673. Sheppard DN, Rich DP, Ostedgaard LO, Gregory RJ, Smith AE, Welsh MJ: Mutations in CFTR associated with mild-disease-form Cl^- channels with altered pore properties. *Nature* **362**:160, 1993.
674. Bear CE, Li C, Kartner N, Bridges RJ, Jensen TJ, Ramjeesingh M, Riordan JR: Purification and functional reconstitution of the cystic fibrosis transmembrane conductance regulator (CFTR). *Cell* **68**:809, 1992.
675. Tilly BC, Winter MC, Ostedgaard LS, O'Riordan C, Smith AE: cAMP-dependent protein kinase activation of CFTR chloride channels in planar lipid bilayers. *J Biol Chem* **267**:9470, 1992.
676. Miller C: 1990: *Annus mirabilis* of potassium channels. *Science* **252**:1092, 1991.
677. Mimura CS, Holbrook SR, Ames GF: Structural model of the nucleotide-binding conserved component of periplasmic permeases. *Proc Natl Acad Sci USA* **88**:84, 1991.
678. Arispe N, Rojas E, Hartman J, Sorscher EJ, Pollard HB: Intrinsic anion channel activity of the recombinant first nucleotide binding fold domain of the cystic fibrosis transmembrane regulator protein. *Proc Natl Acad Sci USA* **89**:1539, 1992.
679. Valverde MA, Diaz M, Sepulveda FV, Gill DR, Hyde SC, Higgins CF: Volume-regulated chloride channels associated with the human multidrug-resistance P-glycoprotein. *Nature* **355**:830, 1992.
680. Gill DR, Hyde SC, Higgins CF, Valverde MA, Mintenig GM, Sepulveda FV: Separation of drug transport and chloride channel functions of the human multidrug resistance P-glycoprotein. *Cell* **71**:23, 1992.
681. Koch MC, Steinmeyer K, Lorenz C, Ricker K, Wolf F, Otto M, Zoll B, Lehmann-Horn F, Grzeschik KH, Jentsch TJ: The skeletal muscle chloride channel in dominant and recessive human myotonia. *Science* **257**:797, 1992.
682. Sorscher EJ, Fuller CM, Bridges RJ, Tousson A, Marchase RB, Brinkley BR, Frizzell RA, Benos DJ: Identification of a membrane protein from T84 cells using antibodies made against a DIDS-binding protein. *Am J Physiol* **262**:C136, 1992.
683. Bradbury NA, Jilling T, Kirk KL, Bridges RJ: Regulated endocytosis in a chloride secretory epithelial cell line. *Am J Physiol* **262**:C752, 1992.
684. Boat TF, Kleinerman JI, Carlson DM, Maloney WH, Matthew LW: Human respiratory tract secretions. *Am Rev Respir Dis* **110**:428, 1974.
685. Frates RCJ, Kaizu TT, Last JA: Mucus glycoproteins secreted by respiratory epithelial tissue from cystic fibrosis patients. *Pediatr Res* **17**:30, 1983.
686. Scanlin TF, Wang YM, Glick MC: Altered fucosylation of membrane glycoproteins from cystic fibrosis fibroblasts. *Pediatr Res* **19**:368, 1985.
687. Bear CE: Phosphorylation-activated chloride channels in human skin fibroblasts. *FEBS Lett* **237**:145, 1988.
688. Chen JH, Schulman H, Gardner P: A cAMP-regulated chloride channel in lymphocytes that is affected in cystic fibrosis. *Science* **243**:657, 1989.
689. Welsh MJ: Abnormal regulation of ion channels in cystic fibrosis epithelia. *FASEB J* **4**:2718, 1990.
690. Singh AK, Afink GB, Venglarik CJ, Wang RP, Bridges RJ: Colonic Cl channel blockade by three classes of compounds. *Am J Physiol* **261**:C51, 1991.
691. Tilmann M, Kunzelmann K, Frobe U, Cabantchik I, Lang HJ, Englert HC, Greger R: Different types of blockers of the intermediate-conductance outwardly rectifying chloride channel in epithelia. *Pflügers Arch* **418**:556, 1991.
692. Wangemann P, Wittner M, Di-Stefano A, Englert HC,

Lang HJ, Schlatter E, Greger R: Cl^- channel blockers in the thick ascending limb of the loop of Henle. Structure–activity relationship. *Pflügers Arch* **407(Suppl)2**:S128, 1986.

693. Hanrahan JW, Tabcharani JA: Inhibition of an outwardly rectifying anion channel by HEPES and related buffers. *J Membr Biol* **116**:65, 1990.
694. Halm DR, Rechkemmer GR, Schoumacher RA, Frizzell RA: Apical membrane chloride channels in a colonic cell line activated by secretory agonists. *Am J Physiol* **254**:C505, 1988.
695. Hayslett JP, Gogelein H, Kunzelmann K, Greger R: Characteristics of apical chloride channels in human colon cells (HT29). *Pflügers Arch* **410**:487, 1987.
696. Giraldez F, Murray KJ, Sepulveda FV, Sheppard DN: Characterization of a phosphorylation-activated Cl^- selective channel in isolated *Necturus* enterocytes. *J Physiol (Lond)* **416**:517, 1989.
697. Hanrahan JW, Tabcharani JA: Possible role of outwardly rectifying anion channels in epithelial transport. *Ann NY Acad Sci* **574**:30, 1989.
698. McCann JD, Li M, Welsh MJ: Identification and regulation of whole-cell chloride currents in airway epithelium. *J Gen Physiol* **94**:1015, 1989.
699. Li M, McCann JD, Liedtke CM, Nairn AC, Greengard P, Welsh MJ: Cyclic AMP-dependent protein kinase opens chloride channels in normal but not cystic fibrosis airway epithelium. *Nature* **331**:358, 1988.
700. Schoumacher RA, Shoemaker RL, Halm DR, Tallant EA, Wallace RW, Frizzell RA: Phosphorylation fails to activate chloride channels from cystic fibrosis airway cells. *Nature* **330**:752, 1987.
701. Tabcharani JA, Hanrahan JW: On the activation of outwardly rectifying anion channels in excised patches. *Am J Physiol* **261**:G992, 1991.
702. Welsh MJ, Li M, McCann JD: Activation of normal and cystic fibrosis Cl^- channels by voltage, temperature, and trypsin. *J Clin Invest* **84**:2002, 1989.
703. Kunzelmann K, Pavenstadt H, Greger R: Properties and regulation of chloride channels in cystic fibrosis and normal airway cells. *Pflügers Arch* **415**:172, 1989.
704. Frizzell RA, Rechkemmer G, Shoemaker RL: Altered regulation of airway epithelial cell chloride channels in cystic fibrosis. *Science* **233**:558, 1986.
705. Welsh MJ: An apical membrane chloride channel in human tracheal epithelium. *Science* **232**:1648, 1986.
706. Welsh MJ: Single apical membrane anion channels in primary cultures of canine tracheal epithelium. *Pflügers Arch* **407**:S116, 1986.
707. Hwang TC, Lu L, Zeitlin PL, Gruenert C, Huganir R, Guggino WB: Cl^- channels in CF: Lack of activation by protein kinase C and cAMP-dependent protein kinase. *Science* **244**:1351, 1989.
708. Jetten AM, Yankaskas JR, Stutts MJ, Willumsen NJ, Boucher RC: Persistence of abnormal chloride conductance regulation in transformed cystic fibrosis epithelia. *Science* **244**:1472, 1989.
709. Greger R: Epithelial chloride channels, in Wong PYD, Young JA (eds): *Exocrine Secretion*. Hong Kong, Hong Kong University Press, 1988, p 81.
710. Wine JJ, Brayden DJ, Hagiwara G, Krouse ME, Law TC, Muller UJ, Solc CK, Ward CL, Widdicombe JH, Xia Y: Cystic fibrosis, the CFTR, and rectifying Cl^- channels, in Tsui L-C (ed): *Identification of the CF Gene*. New York, Plenum, 1991, p 253.
711. Ward CL, Krouse ME, Gruenert DC, Kopito RR, Wine JJ: Cystic fibrosis gene expression is not correlated with rectifying Cl^- channels. *Proc Natl Acad Sci USA* **88**:5277, 1991.
712. Gabriel SE, Clarke LL, Boucher RC, Stutts MJ: CFTR and outward rectifying chloride channels are distinct proteins with a regulatory relationship. *Nature* **363**:263, 1993.
713. Egan M, Flotte T, Afione S, Solow R, Zeitlin PL, Carter BJ, Guggino WB: Defective regulation of outwardly rectifying Cl^- channels by protein kinase A corrected by insertion of CFTR. *Nature* **358**:581, 1992.
714. Solc CK, Wine JJ: Swelling-induced and depolarization-induced Cl^- channels in normal and cystic fibrosis epithelial cells. *Am J Physiol* **261**:C658, 1991.
715. Chang XB, Tabcharani JA, Hou YX, Jensen TJ, Kartner N, Alon N, Hanrahan JW, Riordan JR: Protein kinase A (PKA) still activates CFTR chloride channel after mutagenesis of all 10 PKA consensus phosphorylation sites. *J Biol Chem* **268**:11304, 1993.
716. Campbell IM, Crozier DN, Trim A, Sigrist J: Cystic fibrosis and bacterial conversion of oleic acid to a cathartic, 10-hydroxystearic acid. *Lancet* **2**:107, 1987.
717. Devor DC, Simasko SM, Duffey ME: Carbachol induces oscillations of membrane potassium conductance in a colonic cell line, T84. *Am J Physiol* **258**:C318, 1990.
718. Wagner JA, Cozens AL, Schulman H, Gruenert DC, Stryer L, Gardner P: Activation of chloride channels in normal and cystic fibrosis airway epithelial cells by multifunctional calcium/calmodulin-dependent protein kinase. *Nature* **349**:793, 1991.
719. Worrell RT, Frizzell RA: CaMKII mediates stimulation of chloride conductance by calcium in T84 cells. *Am J Physiol* **260**:C877, 1991.
720. Morris AP, Frizzell RA: Ca^{2+}-dependent Cl^- channels in undifferentiated human colonic cells (HT-29). I. Single-channel properties. *Am J Physiol* **264**:C968, 1993.
721. Morris AP, Frizzell RA: Ca^{2+}-dependent Cl^- channels in undifferentiated human colonic cells (HT-29). II. Regulation and rundown. *Am J Physiol* **264**:C977, 1993.
722. Schoppa N, Shorofsky SR, Jow F, Nelson DJ: Voltage-gated chloride currents in cultured canine tracheal epithelial cells. *J Membr Biol* **108**:73, 1989.
723. Worrell RT, Butt AG, Cliff WH, Frizzell RA: A volume-sensitive chloride conductance in human colonic cell line T84. *Am J Physiol* **256**:C1111, 1989.
724. Butt AG, Clapp WL, Frizzell RA: Potassium conductances in tracheal epithelium activated by secretion and cell swelling. *Am J Physiol* **258**:C630, 1990.
725. Cheng SH, Rich DP, Marshall J, Gregory RJ, Welsh MJ: Phosphorylation of the R domain by cAMP-dependent protein kinase. *Cell* **66**:1027, 1991.
726. Berger HA, Travis SM, Welsh MJ: Regulation of the cystic fibrosis transmembrane conductance regulator Cl^- channel by specific protein kinases and protein phosphatases. *J Biol Chem* **268**:2037, 1993.
727. Forte LR, Thorne PK, Eber SL, Krause WJ, Freeman RH, Francis SH, Corbin JD: Stimulation of intestinal Cl^- transport by heat-stable enterotoxin: activation of cAMP-dependent protein kinase by cGMP. *Am J Physiol* **263**:C607, 1992.
728. Lin M, Nairn AC, Guggino SE: cAMP-dependent protein kinase regulation of a chloride channel in T84 cells. *Am J Physiol* **262**:C1304, 1992.
729. van-Dommelen FS, De-Jonge HR: Cyclic-GMP and cyclic AMP induced intestinal ion secretion: Analysis at the level of brush border membrane vesicles. *Adv Cycl Nucl Prot Phosphor Res* **17**:303, 1984.
730. Kennelly PJ, Krebs EG: Consensus sequences as substrate specificity determinants for protein kinases and protein phosphatases. *J Biol Chem* **266**:15555, 1991.
731. Picciotto MR, Cohn JA, Bertuzzi G, Greengard P, Nairn AC: Phosphorylation of the cystic fibrosis transmembrane conductance regulator. *J Biol Chem* **267**:12742, 1992.
732. Rich DP, Berger HA, Cheng SH, Travis SM, Saxena M, Smith AE, Welsh MJ: Regulation of the cystic fibrosis transmembrane conductance regulator Cl^- channel by negative charge in the R domain. *J Biol Chem* **268**:20259, 1993.
733. Rich DP, Gregory RJ, Anderson MP, Manavalan P, Smith AE: Effect of deleting the R domain on CFTR-generated chloride channels. *Science* **253**:205, 1991.
734. Rich DP, Gregory RJ, Cheng SH, Smith AE, Welsh MJ: Effect of deletion mutations on the function of CFTR chloride channels. *Recept Chan* **1**:221, 1993.
735. Anderson MP, Welsh MJ: Regulation by ATP and ADP of CFTR chloride channels that contain mutant nucleotide-binding domains. *Science* **257**:1701, 1992.
736. Carson MR, Welsh MJ: 5′ adenylylimidodphosphate (AMP-PNP) does not activate CFTR chloride channels in free patches of membrane. *Am J Physiol* **265**:L27, 1993.
737. Gottesman MM, Pastan I: The multidrug transporter, a double-edged sword. *J Biol Chem* **263**:12163, 1988.

738. Thomas PJ, Shenbagamurthi P, Ysern X, Pedersen PL: Cystic fibrosis transmembrane conductance regulator: Nucleotide binding to a synthetic peptide. *Science* **251**:555, 1991.
739. Thomas PJ, Shenbagamurthi P, Sondek J, Hullihen JM, Pedersen PL: The cystic fibrosis transmembrane conductance regulator. Effects of the most common cystic fibrosis causing mutation on the secondary structure and stability of a synthetic peptide. *J Biol Chem* **267**:5727, 1992.
740. Hartman J, Huang Z, Rado RA, Peng S, Jilling T, Muccio DD, Sorscher EJ: Recombinant synthesis, purification, and nucleotide binding characteristics of the first nucleotide binding domain of the cystic fibrosis gene product. *J Biol Chem* **267**:6455, 1992.
741. Travis SM, Carson MR, Ries DR, Welsh MJ: Interaction of nucleotides with membrane associated cystic fibrosis transmembrane conductance regulator. *J Biol Chem* **268**:15336, 1993.
742. Hobson AC, Weatherwax R, Ames GF-L: ATP-binding sites in the membrane components of histidine permease, a periplasmic transport system. *Proc Natl Acad Sci USA* **81**:7333, 1984.
743. Welsh MJ, Smith AE: Molecular mechanisms of CFTR chloride channel dysfunction in cystic fibrosis. *Cell* **73**:1251, 1993.
744. Hamosh A, Trapnell BC, Zeitlin PL, Montrose-Rafizadeh C, Rosenstein BJ, Crystal RG, Cutting GR: Severe deficiency of cystic fibrosis transmembrane conductance regulator messenger RNA carrying nonsense mutations R553X and W1316X in respiratory epithelial cells of patients with cystic fibrosis. *J Clin Invest* **88**:1880, 1991.
745. Denning GM, Anderson MP, Amara J, Marshall J, Smith AE, Welsh MJ: Processing of mutant cystic fibrosis transmembrane conductance regulator is temperature-sensitive. *Nature* **358**:761, 1992.
746. Li C, Ramjeesingh M, Reyes E, Jensen T, Chang X, Rommens JM, Bear CE: The cystic fibrosis mutation (delta F508) does not influence the chloride channel activity of CFTR. *Nat Genet* **3**:311, 1993.
747. The Cystic Fibrosis Genotype-Phenotype Consortium: Correlation between genotype and phenotype in patients with cystic fibrosis. *N Engl J Med* **329**:1308, 1993.
748. Gaskin KJ, Durie PR, Lee L, Hill R, Forstner GG: Colipase and lipase secretion in childhood-onset pancreatic insufficiency: Delineation of patients with steatorrhea secondary to relative colipase deficiency. *Gastroenterology* **86**:1, 1984.
749. Corey M, Durie P, Moore D, Forstner G, Levison H: Familial concordance of pancreatic function in cystic fibrosis. *J Pediatr* **115**:274, 1989.
750. Augarten A, Kerem B-S, Yahav Y, Noiman S, Rivlin Y, Tal A, Blau H, Ben-Tur L, Szeinberg A, Kerem E, Gazit E: Mild cystic fibrosis and normal or borderline sweat test in patients with the 3849 + 10 kb C→T mutation. *Lancet* **342**:25, 1993.
751. Corey M, McLaughlin FJ, Williams M, Levison H: A comparison of survival, growth, and pulmonary function in patients with cystic fibrosis in Boston and Toronto. *J Clin Epidemiol* **41**:583, 1988.
752. Devoto M, DeBenedetti L, Seia M, Piceni-Sereni L, Ferrari M, Bonduelle ML, Malfroot A, Lissens W, Balassopoulou A, Adam G, Loukopoulos D, Cochaux P, Vassart G, Szibor R, Hein J, Grade K, Berger W, Wainwright B, Romeo G: Haplotypes in cystic fibrosis patients with or without pancreatic insufficiency from four European populations. *Genomics* **5**:894, 1989.
753. McConkie-Rosell A, Chen YT, Harris D, Speer MC, Perciak-Vance MA, Ding JH, Highsmith WE Jr, Knowles M, Kahler SG: Mild cystic fibrosis linked to chromosome 7q22 markers with an uncommon haplotype. *Ann Intern Med* **111**:797, 1989.
754. Borgo G, Mastella G, Gasparini P, Zorzanello A, Doro R, Pignatti PF: Pancreatic function and gene deletion F508 in cystic fibrosis. *J Med Genet* **27**:665, 1990.
755. Ferrari M, Antonelli M, Bellini F, Borgo G, Castiglione O, Curcio L, Dallapiccola B, Devoto M, Estivill X, Gasparini P, Giunta A, Marianelli L, Mastella G, Novelli G, Pignatti P, Romano L, Romeo G, Seia M, Williamson R: Genetic differences in cystic fibrosis patients with and without pancreatic insufficiency. An Italian collaborative study. *Hum Genet* **84**:435, 1990.
756. Stuhrmann M, Macek M Jr, Reis A, Schmidtke J, Tümmler B, Dörk T, Vavrova V, Macek M, Krawczak M: Genotype analysis of cystic fibrosis patients in relation to pancreatic sufficiency. *Lancet* **335**:638, 1990.
757. Lanng S, Schwartz M, Thorsteinsson B, Koch C: Endocrine and exocrine pancreatic function and the delta F508 mutation in cystic fibrosis. *Clin Genet* **40**:345, 1991.
758. Johansen HK, Nir M, Hoiby N, Koch C, Schwartz M: Severity of cystic fibrosis in patients homozygous and heterozygous for delta F508 mutation. *Lancet* **337**:631, 1991.
759. Kopelman H, Rozen R: Genetic analysis and pancreatic function in cystic fibrosis. *Lancet* **335**:1601, 1990.
760. Waters DL, Dorney SFA, Gaskin KJ, Gruca MA, O'Halloran M, Wilcken B: Pancreatic function in infants identified as having cystic fibrosis in a neonatal screening program. *N Engl J Med* **322**:303, 1990.
761. Mornet E, Simon-Buoy B, Serre JC, Estivill X, Farrall M, Williamson R, Bove J, Bove A: Genetic difference between cystic fibrosis with and without meconium ileus. *Lancet* **1**:376, 1988.
762. Simon-Bouy B, Serre JL, Mornet E, Tallandier A, Bove J, Bove A: Genetic heterogeneity between 2 clinical forms of cystic fibrosis evidenced by familial analysis and linked DNA probes. *Clin Genet* **35**:81, 1989.
763. Auvinet M, Morel Y, Chambon V, Andre J, Vidaud M, Goossens M, Bellon G, Gily R: Cystic fibrosis with and without meconium ileus. *Lancet* **1**:161, 1989.
764. Curtis A, Jackson J, Keston M, Brock DJ: Genetic differences between cystic fibrosis with and without meconium ileus. *Lancet* **1**:1078, 1989.
765. Kerem E, Corey M, Kerem B, Durie P, Tsiu L-C, Levison H: Are there clinical and genetical differences between cystic fibrosis with and without meconium ileus? *J Pediatr* **114**:767, 1989.
766. Hamosh A, King TM, Rosenstein BJ, Corey M, Levison H, Durie P, Tsiu L-C, McIntosh L, Keston M, Brock DJH, Macek M Jr, Zemková D, Krásnicanová H, Vávrová V, Macek M Sr, Golder N, Schwarz MJ, Super M, Watson EK, Williams C, Bush A, O'Mahoney SM, Humphries P, DeArce MA, Reis A, Bürger J, Stuhrmann M, Schmidtke J, Wulbrand U, Dörk T, Tümmler B, Cutting GR: Cystic fibrosis patients bearing both the common missense mutation Gly→Asp at codon 551 and the delta F508 mutation are clinically indistinguishable from delta F508 homozygotes, except for decreased risk of meconium ileus. *Am J Hum Genet* **51**:245, 1992.
767. Burke W, Aitken ML, Chen S-H, Scott CR: Variable severity of pulmonary disease in adults with identical cystic fibrosis mutations. *Chest* **102**:506, 1992.
768. Al-Jader LN, Meredith AL, Ryley HC, Cheadle JP, Maguire S, Owen G, Goodchild MC, Harper PS: Severity of chest disease in cystic fibrosis patients in relation to their genotypes. *J Med Genet* **29**:883, 1992.
769. Lester LA, Kraut J, Lloyd-Still J, Karrison T, Mott C, Billstrand C, Lemke A, Ober C: Delta F508 genotype does not predict disease severity in an ethnically diverse cystic fibrosis population. *Pediatrics* **93**:114, 1994.
770. Gan KH, Heijerman HGM, Bakker W: Correlation between genotype and phenotype in patients with cystic fibrosis. *N Engl J Med* **333**:365, 1994.
771. Férec C, Verlingue C, Guillermit H, Quéré I, Raguénès O, Feigelson J, Audrézet M-P, Moullier P, Mercier B: Genotype analysis of adult cystic fibrosis patients. *Hum Mol Genet* **2**:1557, 1993.
772. Cuppens H, Marynen P, DeBoeck C, Cassiman JJ: Study of the G542X and G458V mutations in a sample of Belgian patients. *Pediatr Pulmonol Suppl* **5**:203, 1990.
773. Bal J, Stuhrmann M, Schloesser M, Schmidtke J, Reiss J: A cystic fibrosis patient homozygous for the nonsense mutation R553X. *J Med Genet* **28**:715, 1991.
774. Shoshani T, Augarten A, Gazit E, Bashan N, Yahav Y, Rivlin Y, Tal A, Seret H, Yaar L, Kerem E, Kerem B-S: Association of a nonsense mutation (W1282X), the most

common mutation in the Ashkenazi Jewish cystic fibrosis patients in Israel, with presentation of severe disease. *Am J Hum Genet* **50**:222, 1992.

775. Beaudet AL, Perciaccante RG, Cutting GR: Homozygous nonsense mutation causing cystic fibrosis with uniparental disomy. *Am J Hum Genet* **48**:1213, 1991.
776. Wine JJ: No CFTR: are CF symptoms milder? *Nat Genet* **1**:10, 1992.
777. Liechti-Gallati S, Bonsall I, Malik N, Schneider V, Kraemer LG, Ruedeberg A, Moser H, Kraemer R: Genotype/phenotype association in cystic fibrosis: Analyses of the delta F508, F553X, and 3905insT mutations. *Pediatr Res* **32**:175, 1992.
778. Santamaria F, Salvatore D, Castiglione O, Raia V, deTitis G, Sebastio G: Lung involvement, the delta F508 mutation and DNA haplotype analysis in cystic fibrosis. *Hum Genet* **88**:639, 1992.
779. Kubesch P, Dörk T, Wulbrand U, Kälin N, Neumman T, Wulf B, Geerlings H, Weibbrodt H, von Der Hardt H, Tümmler B: Genetic determinants of airways' colonisation with *Pseudomonas aeruginosa* in cystic fibrosis. *Lancet* **341**:189, 1993.
780. Mahon RT, Wagener JS, Abman SH, Seltzer WK, Accurso FJ: Relationship of genotype to early pulmonary function in infants with cystic fibrosis identified through neonatal screening. *J Pediatr* **122**:550, 1993.
781. Hamdi I, Payne SJ, Barton DE, McMahon R, Green M, Shneerson JM, Hales CN: Genotype analysis in cystic fibrosis in relation to the occurrence of diabetes mellitus. *Clin Genet* **43**:186, 1993.
782. Nagel RA, Westaby D, Javaid A, Kavani J, Meire HB, Lombard MG, Wise A, Williams R, Hodson ME: Liver disease and bile duct abnormalities in adults with cystic fibrosis. *Lancet* **2**:1422, 1989.
783. De Arce M, O'Brien S, Hegarty J, O'Mahoney SM, Cashman SM, Martinez A, Delgado M, Fitzgerald MX: Deletion of delta F508 and clinical expression of cystic fibrosis-related liver disease. *Clin Genet* **42**:271, 1992.
784. Azcue M, Fried M, Pencharz PB: Use of bioelectrical impedance analysis to measure total body water in patients with cystic fibrosis. *J Pediatr Gastroenterol Nutr* **16**:440, 1993.
785. Fried MD, Durie PR, Tsui L-C, Corey M, Levison H, Pencharz PB: The cystic fibrosis gene and resting energy expenditure. *J Pediatr* **119**:913, 1991.
786. Dumur V, Gervais R, Rigot J-M, Lafitte J-J, Manouvrier S, Biserte J, Mazeman E, Roussel P: Abnormal distribution of CF delta F_{508} allele in azoospermic men with congenital aplasia of epididymis and vas deferens. *Lancet* **336**:512, 1990.
787. Bienvenu T, Beldjord C, Adjiman M, Kaplan JC: Male infertility as the only presenting sign of cystic fibrosis when homozygous for the mild mutation R117H. *J Med Genet* **30**:797, 1993.
788. Patrizio P, Asch RH, Handelin B, Silber SJ: Aetiology of congenital absence of vas deferens: Genetic study of three generations. *Hum Reprod* **8**:215, 1993.
789. Gervais R, Dumur V, Rigot J-M, Lafitte J-J, Roussel P, Clausteres M, Demaille J: High frequency of the R117H cystic fibrosis mutation in patients with congenital absence of the vas deferens. *N Engl J Med* **328**:446, 1993.
790. Williams C, Mayall ES, Williamson R, Hirsh A, Cookson H: A report on CF carrier frequency among men with infertility owing to congenital absence of the vas deferens. *J Med Genet* **30**:973, 1993.
791. Osborne LR, Lynch M, Middleton PG, Alton EWFW, Geddes DM, Pryor JP, Hodson ME, Santis GK: Nasal epithelial ion transport and genetic analysis of infertile men with congenital bilateral absence of the vas deferens. *Hum Mol Genet* **2**:1605, 1993.
792. Mickle JE, Oster RD, Colin A, Maher TA, Milunsky A, Amos JA: Increased frequency of cystic fibrosis (CF) mutation in males with unilateral absence of the vas deferens (UAVD). *Am J Hum Genet Suppl* **53**:1204, 1993.
793. Silber SJ, Ord T, Balmaceda J, Patrizio P, Asch RH: Congenital absence of the vas deferens. The fertilizing capacity of human epididymal sperm. *N Engl J Med* **323**:1788, 1990.
794. Patrizio P, Ord T, Silber SJ, Asch RH: Cystic fibrosis mutations impair the fertilization rate of epididymal sperm from men with congenital absence of the vas deferens. *Hum Reprod* **8**:1259, 1993.
795. Handelsman DJ, Conway AJ, Boylan LM, Turtle JR: Young's syndrome: Obstructive azoospermia and chronic sinopulmonary infections. *N Engl J Med* **310**:3, 1984.
796. Hirsh A, Williams C, Williamson C: Young's syndrome and cystic fibrosis mutation delta F508. *Lancet* **342**:118, 1993.
797. Friedman KJ, Teichtahl H, Robinson JM, Silverman LM, Highsmith WE Jr, Boucher RC, Knowles MR: Screening Young's syndrome patients for CFTR mutations. *Pediatr Pulmonol Suppl* **9**:236, 1993.
798. Poller W, Faber J-P, Scholz S, Olek K, Müller K-M: Sequence analysis of the cystic fibrosis gene in patients with disseminated bronchiectatic lung disease. *Klin Wochenschr* **69**:657, 1991.
799. Nukiwa T, Seyama K: Personal communication.
800. Pignatti PF, Bombieri C, Marigo C, Luisetti M: Cystic fibrosis gene mutations in adults with chronic obstructive pulmonary disease. *Hum Mol Genet* (in press, 1994.)
801. Pignatti PF: Cystic fibrosis, in Humphries S, Malcom S (eds): *From Genotype to Phenotype*. Oxford, Bios Scientific Publishers, 1994.
802. Spence JE, Perciaccante RG, Greig GM, Willard HF, Ledbetter DH, Hejtmancik JF, Pollack MS, O'Brien WE, Beaudet AL: Uniparental disomy as a mechanism for human genetic disease. *Am J Hum Genet* **42**:217, 1988.
803. Voss R, Ben-Simon E, Avital A, Zlotogora Y, Dagan J, Godrey S, Tikochinski Y, Hillil J: Isodisomy of chromosome 7 in a patient with CF: Could uniparental disomy be common in humans? *Am J Hum Genet* **45**:373, 1989.
804. Nadler HL, Girimaji JS, Rao JS, Taussig LM: Cystic fibrosis, in Stanbury JB, Wyngaarden JB, Fredrickson DS (eds): *The Metabolic Basis of Inherited Disease,* 4th ed. New York, McGraw-Hill, 1978, p 1683.
805. Nadler HL, Ben-Yoseph Y: Genetics, in Taussig LM (ed): *Cystic Fibrosis. New York, Thieme-Stratton, 1984, p 10.*
806. Thompson MW: Genetics of cystic fibrosis, in Sturgess JM (ed): *Perspectives in Cystic Fibrosis*. Mississauga, Ontario, Canada, Imperial Press, 1980, p 281.
807. Danks DM, Allan J, Anderson CM: A genetic study of fibrocystic disease of the pancreas. *Ann Hum Genet* **28**:323, 1965.
808. Conneally PM, Merritt AD, Yu P: Cystic fibrosis: Population genetics. *Tex Rep Biol Med* **31**:639, 1973.
809. Knudsen AG Jr, Wayne L, Hallett WY: On selective advantage of cystic fibrosis heterozygotes. *Am J Hum Genet* **19**:388, 1967.
810. Crawford MD: A genetic study including evidence for heterosis in cystic fibrosis of the pancreas. *Heredity* **29**:126, 1972.
811. Meindl RS: Hypothesis: A selective advantage for cystic fibrosis heterozygotes. *Am J Phys Anthropol* **74**:39, 1987.
811a. Morral N, Bertranpetit J, Estivil X, Nunes V, Časals T, Giménez, Reis A, Varon-Mateeva R, Macek M Jr, Kalaydjieva L, Angelicheva D, Dancheva R, Romeo G, Russo MP, Garnerone S, Restagno G, Ferrari M, Magnani C, Claustres M, Desgeorges M, Schwartz M, Schwarz M, Dallapiccola B, Novelli G, Ferec C, de Arce M, Nemeti M, Kere J, Anvret M, Dahl N, Kadasi L: The origin of the major cystic fibrosis mutation (ΔF508) in European populations. *Nat Genet* **7**:169, 1994.
812. Sereth H, Shoshani T, Bashan N, Kerem B: Extended haplotype analysis of cystic fibrosis mutations and its implications for the selective advantage hypothesis. *Hum Genet* **92**:289, 1993.
813. Morral N, Nunes V, Casala T, Chillón M, Giménez J, Bertranpetit J, Estivill X: Microsatellite haplotypes for cystic fibrosis: Mutation frameworks and evolutionary tracers. *Hum Mol Genet* **2**:1015, 1993.
814. Cuppens H, Teng H, Raeymaekers P, De Boeck C, Cassiman J-J: CFTR haplotype backgrounds on normal and mutant CFTR genes. *Hum Mol Genet* **3**:607, 1994.
815. Wagener DK, Cavalli-Sforza LL: Ethnic variation in genetic disease: Possible roles of hitchhiking and epistasis. *Am J Hum Genet* **27**:348, 1975.
816. Bowcock AM, Crandall J, Daneshvar L, Lee GM, Young B, Zunzunegui V, Craik C, Cavalli-Sforza LL,

King M-C: Genetic analysis of cystic fibrosis: Linkage of DNA and classical markers in multiplex families. *Am J Hum Genet* **39**:699, 1986.

817. Kitzis A, Chomel JC, Kaplan JC, Giraud G, Labbe A, Dastugue B, Dumur V, Farriaux JP, Roussel P, Williamson R, Feingold J: Unusual segregation of cystic fibrosis allele to males. *Nature* **333**:215, 1988.
818. Kitzis A, Chomel JC, Haliassos A, Tesson L, Kaplan JC, Feingold J, Giraud G, Labbe A, Dastugue B, Dumur V, Farriaux JP, Roussel P, Ferec C, Vidaud M, Goossens M, Bozon D, Auvinet M, Chambon V, Andre J, Lissens W, Bonduelle M, Liebaers I, Cochaux P, Vassart G, Willems P, Duckworth-Raysiecki G, Kerem B, Tsui L-C, Ray PN, Krawczak M, Schmidtke J, Novelli G, Dallapiccola B, Gasparni G, Pignatti PF, Seia M, Ferrari M, Devoto M, Romeo G, Schwarz M, Super M, Ivinson A, Read AP, Meredith L, Curtis A, Williamson R, Beaudet AL, Feldman GL, O'Brien WE, Bowcock AM, Cavilli-Sforza LL, Gilbert F, Braman J, King MC: Unusual segregation of cystic fibrosis alleles. *Nature* **336**:316, 1992.
819. Williams C, Davies D, Williamson R: Segregation of delta F508 and normal CFTR alleles in human sperm. *Hum Mol Genet* **2**:445, 1993.
820. Rao DC, Morton NE: Large deviations in the distribution of rare genes. *Am J Hum Genet* **25**:594, 1973.
821. Bois E, Feingold J, Demenais F, Runavot Y, Jehanne M, Toudic L: Cluster of cystic fibrosis cases in a limited area of Brittany (France). *Clin Genet* **14**:73, 1978.
822. Super M: Factors influencing the frequency of cystic fibrosis in southwest Africa. *Monogr Paediatr* **10**:106, 1979.
823. Klinger KW: Cystic fibrosis in the Ohio Amish: Gene frequency and founder effect. *Hum Genet* **65**:94, 1983.
824. Danks DM, Allan J, Phelan PD, Chapman C: Mutations at more than one locus may be involved in cystic fibrosis—Evidence based on first-cousin data and direct counting of cases. *Am J Hum Genet* **35**:838, 1983.
825. Houstek J, Vávrová V: Notre expérience à propos de la mucoviscidose. *Rev Med Liegè* 22:421, 1967.
826. Brunecky Z: The incidence and genetics of cystic fibrosis. *J Med Genet* **9**:33, 1972.
827. Vivell VO, Jacobi H, Münchbach K: Zur mucoviscidosis im kindesalter. *Monatsschr Kinderheilkd* **111**:62, 1963.
828. Levin S: Fibrocystic disease of the pancreas, in Goldschmidt E (ed): *Genetic of Migrant and Isolate Populations*. Baltimore, Williams & Wilkins, 1963, p 294.
829. Romeo G, Bianco M, Devoto M, Menozzi P, Mastella G, Giunta AM, Micalizzi C, Antonelli M, Battistini A, Santamaria F, Castello D, Marianelli A, Marchi AG, Manca A, Miano A: Incidence in Italy, genetic heterogeneity, and segregation analysis of cystic fibrosis. *Am J Hum Genet* **37**:338, 1985.
830. Selander P: The frequency of cystic fibrosis of the pancreas in Sweden. *Acta Paediatr* **51**:65, 1962.
831. Carter CO: Genetic aspects of cystic fibrosis of the pancreas. *Mod Probl Pediatr* **10**:372, 1967.
832. Pugh RJ, Pickup JD: Cystic fibrosis in Leeds region: Incidence and life expectancy. *Arch Dis Child* **42**:544, 1967.
833. Hall BD, Simpkiss MJ: Inheritance of fibrocystic disease in Wessex. *J Med Genet* **5**:262, 1968.
834. Goodchild MC, Insley J, Rushton DI, Gaze H: Cystic fibrosis in 3 Pakistani children. *Arch Dis Child* **49**:739, 1974.
835. Stevenson AC: The load of hereditary defect in human populations. *Radiat Res Suppl* **1**:306, 1959.
836. Nevin GB, Nevin NC, Redmond AD: Cystic fibrosis in Northern Ireland. *J Med Genet* **16**:122, 1979.
837. Steinberg AG, Brown DC: On the incidence of cystic fibrosis of the pancreas. *Am J Hum Genet* **12**:416, 1960.
838. Kramm ER, Crane MM, Sirkin MG, Brown ML: A cystic fibrosis pilot survey in three New England states. *Am J Public Health* **52**:2041, 1962.
839. Merritt AD, Hanna BL, Todd CW, Myers TL: Incidence and mode of inheritance of cystic fibrosis. *J Lab Clin Med* **52**:2041, 1962.
840. Sultz HA, Schlesinger ER, Moshe WE: The Erie County survey of long term childhood illness. *Am J Public Health* **56**:1461, 1966.
841. Kulczycki IL, Schauf V: Cystic fibrosis in blacks in Washington, D.C. *Am J Dis Child* **127**:64, 1974.
842. Grebe TA, Seltzer WK, DeMarchi J, Silva DK, Doane WW, Gozal D, Richter SF, Bowman CM, Norman RA, Rhodes SN, Hernried LS, Murphy S, Harwood IR, Accurso FJ, Jain KD: Genetic analysis of Hispanic individuals with cystic fibrosis. *Am J Hum Genet* **54**:443, 1994.
843. Wright SE, Morton NE: Genetic studies on cystic fibrosis in Hawaii. *Am J Hum Genet* **20**:157, 1968.
844. Wilcken B, Brown ARD: Screening for cystic fibrosis in New South Wales, Australia: Evaluation of the results of screening 400,000 babies, in Therrell BL (ed): *Advances in Neonatal Screening*. New York, Excerpta Medica, 1987, p 385.
845. Lyon ICT, Webster DR: Newborn screening for cystic fibrosis. *Pediatrics* **87**:954, 1991.
846. Hammond KB, Abman SH, Sokol RJ, Accurso FJ: Efficacy of statewide neonatal screening for cystic fibrosis by assay of trypsinogen concentrations. *N Engl J Med* **325**:769, 1991.
847. Gregg RG, Wilfond BS, Farrell PM, Laxova A, Hassemer D, Mischler EH: Application of DNA analysis in a population-screening program for neonatal diagnosis of cystic fibrosis (CF): Comparison of screening protocols. *Am J Hum Genet* **52**:616, 1993.
848. Pederzini F, Armani P, Barbato A, Borgo G: Newborn screening for cystic fibrosis. Two methods compared on 229,626 newborns tested in 8 years in the Veneto region. *Ital J Pediatr* **9**:445, 1983.
849. Green MR, Weaver LT, Heeley AF, Nicholson K, Kuzemko JA, Barton DE, McMahon R, Payne SJ, Austin S, Yates JRW, Davis JA: Cystic fibrosis identified by neonatal screening: Incidence, genotype, and early natural history. *Arch Dis Child* **68**:464, 1993.
850. Abeliovich D, Lavon IP, Lerer I, Cohen T, Springer C, Avital A, Cutting GR: Screening for five mutations detects 97% of cystic fibrosis (CF) chromosomes and predicts a carrier frequency of 1:29 in the Jewish Ashkinazi population. *Am J Hum Genet* **51**:951, 1992.
851. Zamostiano R, Nolman S, Yahav J, Schonberg A, Kerem B, Gazit E: Screening for carriers of cystic fibrosis mutations in Ashkenazi volunteers. *Harefuah* **124**:202, 1993.
852. Rozen R, De Braekeleer M, Daigneault J, Ferreira-Rajabi L, Gerdes M, Lamoureux L, Aubin G, Simard F, Fujiwara TM, Morgan K: Cystic fibrosis mutations in French Canadians: Three CFTR mutations are relatively frequent in a Quebec population with an elevated incidence of cystic fibrosis. *Am J Med Genet* **42**:360, 1992.
853. Norio R, Nevalinna HR, Perheentupa J: Hereditary diseases in Finland: Rare flora in rare soil. *Ann Clin Res* **5**:109, 1973.
854. Lucotte G, Loirat F: A more detailed map of the cystic fibrosis mutation delta F508 frequencies in Europe. *Hum Biol* **65**:503, 1993.
854a. Rodman DM, Zamudio S: The cystic fibrosis hererozygote—advantage in surviving cholera? *Med Hypotheses* **36**:253, 1991.
855. Schwartz M, Brandt NJ, Koch C, Lanng S, Schiotz PO: Genetic analysis of cystic fibrosis in Denmark. Implications for genetic counseling, carrier diagnosis and prenatal diagnosis. *Acta Paediatr* **81**:522, 1992.
856. Lerer I, Sagi M, Cutting GR, Abeliovich D: Cystic fibrosis mutations delta F508 and G542X in Jewish patients. *J Med Genet* **29**:131, 1992.
857. Gasparini P, Borgo G, Mastella G, Bonizzato A, Dognini M, Pignatti PF: Nine cystic fibrosis patients homozygous for the CFTR nonsense mutation R1162X have mild or moderate lung disease. *J Med Genet* **29**:558, 1992.
857a. The Cystic Fibrosis Genetic Analysis Consortium: Population variation of common cystic fibrosis mutations. *Hum Mutat* **4**:167, 1994.
858. King DN, Heeley AF, Walsh M, Kuzemko JA: Sensitive trypsin assay for dried blood specimens as a screening procedure for early detection of cystic fibrosis. *Lancet* **2**:1217, 1979.
859. Bowling FG, Brown ARD: Newborn screening for cystic fibrosis using an enzyme linked immunoabsorbent assay (ELISA) technique. *Clin Chim Acta* **171**:257, 1988.
860. Ryall RG, Gjerde EM, Gerace RL, Ranieri E: Modifying

an enzyme immunoassay of immunoreactive tripsinogen to use time-resolved fluorescence. *Clin Chem* **39**:224, 1993.
861. Dodge JA: IVth International Conference on Newborn Screening for Cystic Fibrosis. *Pediatr Pulmonol Suppl* **7**:1, 1991.
862. Farrell PM, Mischler EH: Newborn screening for cystic fibrosis. *Adv Pediatr* **39**:35, 1992.
863. Henry RL, Boulton TJC, Roddick LG: False negative results on newborn screening for cystic fibrosis. *J Paediatr Child Health* **26**:150, 1990.
864. Spence WC, Paulus-Thomas J, Orenstein DM, Naylor EW: Neonatal screening for cystic fibrosis: Addition of molecular diagnostics to increase specificity. *Biochem Med Metab Biol* **49**:200, 1993.
865. Holtzman NA: Routine screening of newborns for cystic fibrosis: Not yet. *Pediatrics* **73**:98, 1984.
866. Farrell PM: Early diagnosis of cystic fibrosis: To screen or not to screen—An important question. *Pediatrics* **73**:115, 1984.
867. Cotton RGH: Current methods of mutation detection. *Mutat Res* **285**:125, 1993.
868. Grompe M: The rapid detection of unknown mutations in nucleic acids. *Nat Genet* **5**:111, 1993.
869. Rommens J, Kerem B, Greer W, Chang P, Tsui L-C, Ray P: Rapid nonradioactive detection of the major cystic fibrosis mutation. *Am J Hum Genet* **46**:395, 1990.
870. McCabe ERB, Huang S, Seltzer WK, Law ML: DNA microextraction from dried blood spots on filter paper blotters: Potential applications to newborn screening. *Hum Genet* **75**:213, 1987.
871. Lench N, Stanier P, Williamson R: Simple non-invasive method to obtain DNA for gene analysis. *Lancet* **1**:1356, 1988.
872. Richards B, Skoletsky J, Shuber AP, Balfour R, Stern RC, Dorkin HL, Parad RB, Witt D, Klinger KW: Multiplex PCR amplification from the CFTR gene using DNA prepared from buccal brushes/swabs. *Hum Mol Genet* **2**:159, 1993.
873. Shuber AP, Skoletsky J, Stern R, Handelin BL: Efficient 12-mutation testing in the CFTR gene: A general model for complex mutation analysis. *Hum Mol Genet* **2**:153, 1993.
874. DeMarchi JM, Beaudet AL, Caskey CT, Richards CS: Experience of an academic reference laboratory using automation for analysis of cystic fibrosis mutations. *Arch Pathol Lab Med* 118:26, 1994.
875. DeMarchi JM, Richards CS, Fenwick RG, Pace R, Beaudet AL: A robotics-assisted procedure for large scale cystic fibrosis mutation analysis. *Hum Mutat* (in press, 1994.)
876. Kawasaki E, Saiki R, Erlich H: Genetic analysis using polymerase chain reaction amplified DNA and immobilized oligonucleotide probes: Reverse dot-blot typing. *Methods Enzymol* **218**:369, 1993.
877. Ferrie RM, Schwarz MJ, Robertson NH, Vaudin S, Super M, Malone G, Little S: Development, multiplexing, and application of ARMS test for common mutations in the CFTR gene. *Am J Hum Genet* **51**:251, 1992.
878. Gilfillan A, Axton R, Brock DJH: Mass screening for cystic fibrosis heterozygotes: Two assay systems compared. *Clin Chem* **40**:197, 1994.
879. Fortina P, Conant R, Monokian G, Dotti G, Parrella T, Hitchcock W, Kant J, Scanlin T, Rappaport E, Schwartz E, Surrey S: Non-radioactive detection of the most common mutations in the cystic fibrosis transmembrane conductance regulator gene by multiplex allele-specific polymerase chain reaction. *Hum Genet* **90**:375, 1992.
880. Syvänen A-C, Landegren U: Detection of point mutations by solid-phase methods. *Hum Mutat* **3**:172, 1994.
881. Barinaga M: Will "DNA chip" speed genomic initiative? *Science* **253**:1489, 1991.
882. Fodor SPA, Rava RP, Huang XC, Pease AC, Holmes CP, Adams CL: Multiplexed biochemical assays with biological chips. *Nature* **364**:555, 1993.
883. Ravnik-Glavac M, Glavac D, Chernick M, di Sant'Agnese P, Dean M: Screening for CF mutations in adult cystic fibrosis patients with a directed and optimized SSCP strategy. *Hum Mutat* **3**:231, 1994.
884. Beaudet AL, O'Brien WE: Advantages of a two step laboratory approach for cystic fibrosis carrier screening. *Am J Hum Genet* **50**:439, 1992.
885. Fujimura F, Northrup H, Beaudet AL, O'Brien WE: Genotyping errors with the polymerase chain reaction. *N Engl J Med* **322**:61, 1990.
886. Dicke JM, Crane JP: Sonographically detected hyperechoic fetal bowel: Significance and implications for pregnancy management. *Obstet Gynecol* **80**:778, 1992.
887. Hogge WA, Hogge JS, Boehm CD, Sanders RC: Increased echogenicity in the fetal abdomen: Use of DNA analysis to establish a diagnosis of cystic fibrosis. *J Ultrasound Med* **12**:451, 1993.
888. Scioscia AL, Pretorius DH, Budorick NE, Cahill TC, Axelrod FT, Leopold GR: Second-trimester echogenic bowel and chromosomal abnormalities. *Am J Obstet Gynecol* **167**:889, 1992.
889. Estroff JA, Parad RB, Benacerraf BR: Prevalence of cystic fibrosis in fetuses with dilated bowel. *Radiology* **183**:677, 1992.
890. Verlinksy Y, Rechitsky S, Evsikov S, White M, Cieslak J, Lifchez A, Valle J, Moise J, Strom CM: Preconception and preimplantation diagnosis for cystic fibrosis. *Prenat Diagn* **12**:103, 1992.
891. Handyside AH, Lesko JG, Tarín JJ, Winston RML, Hughes MR: Birth of a normal girl after in vitro fertilization and preimplantation diagnostic testing for cystic fibrosis. *N Engl J Med* **327**:905, 1992.
892. Simpson JL, Carson SA: Preimplantation genetic diagnosis. *N Engl J Med* **327**:951, 1992.
893. Liu J, Lissens W, Devroey P, Van Steirteghem A, Liebaers I: Polymerase chain reaction analysis of the cystic fibrosis delta F508 mutation in human blastomeres following oocyte injection of a single sperm from a carrier. *Prenat Diagn* **13**:873, 1993.
894. Brambati B, Tului L, Fattore S: First-trimester fetal screening of cystic fibrosis in low-risk population. *Lancet* **342**:624, 1993.
895. Black SH, Bick DP, Maddalena A, Schulman JD, Jones SL, Fallon L, Cummings E, Menapace-Drew G: Pregnancy screening for cystic fibrosis. *Lancet* **342**:1112, 1993.
896. Goodfellow PN: Steady steps lead to the gene. *Nature* **341**:102, 1989.
897. Brock D: Population screening for cystic fibrosis. *Am J Hum Genet* **47**:164, 1990.
898. Schulman JD, Maddalena A, Black SH, Bick DP: Screening for cystic fibrosis carriers. *Am J Hum Genet* **47**:740, 1990.
899. Billings PR: Mutation analysis in cystic fibrosis. *N Engl J Med* **323**:62, 1990.
900. Wilfond BS, Fost N: The cystic fibrosis gene: Medical and social implications for heterozygote detection. *JAMA* **2777**:2783, 1990.
901. Caskey CT, Kaback MM, Beaudet AL: The American Society of Human Genetics statement on cystic fibrosis screening. *Am J Hum Genet* **46**:393, 1990.
902. Workshop on Population Screening for the Cystic Fibrosis Gene: Statement from the National Institutes of Health Workshop on population screening for the cystic fibrosis gene. *N Engl J Med* **323**:70, 1990.
903. American Society of Human Genetics: Statement of The American Society of Human Genetics on Cystic Fibrosis Carrier Screening. *Am J Hum Genet* **51**:1443, 1992.
904. Wertz DC, Janes SR, Rosenfield JM, Erbe RW: Attitudes toward the prenatal diagnosis of cystic fibrosis: Factors in decision making among affected families. *Am J Hum Genet* **50**:1077, 1992.
905. Watson EK, Marchant J, Bush A, Williamson B: Attitudes towards prenatal diagnosis and carrier screening for cystic fibrosis among the parents of patients in a paediatric cystic fibrosis clinic. *J Med Genet* **29**:490, 1992.
906. Botkin JR, Alemagno S: Carrier screening for cystic fibrosis: A pilot study of the attitudes of pregnant women. *Am J Public Health* **82**:723, 1992.
907. Decruyenaere M, Evers-Kiebooms G, Denayer L, Van den Berghe H: Cystic fibrosis: Community knowledge and attitudes towards carrier screening and prenatal diagnosis. *Clin Genet* **41**:189, 1992.
908. Mennie ME, Gilfillan A, Compton ME, Liston WA, Brock DJH: Prenatal cystic fibrosis carrier screening: Factors

in a woman's decision to decline testing. *Prenat Diagn* **13**:807, 1993.

909. Mennie M, Compton M, Gilfillan A, Axton RA, Liston WA, Pullen I, Whyte D, Brock DJH: Prenatal screening for cystic fibrosis: Attitudes and responses of participants. *Clin Genet* **44**:102, 1993.
910. Rowley PT, Loader S, Levenkron JC, Phelps CE: Cystic fibrosis carrier screening: Knowledge and attitudes of prenatal care providers. *Am J Prev Med* **9**:261, 1993.
911. Mennie ME, Liston WA, Brock DJH: Prenatal cystic fibrosis carrier testing: Designing an information leaflet to meet the specific needs of the target population. *J Med Genet* **29**:308, 1992.
912. Myers MF, Bernhardt BA, Tambor ES, Holtzman NA: Involving consumers in the development of an educational program for cystic fibrosis carrier screening. *Am J Hum Genet* **54**:719, 1994.
913. Livingstone J, Axton RA, Mennie M, Gilfillan A, Brock DJH: A preliminary trial of couple screening for cystic fibrosis: Designing an appropriate information leaflet. *Clin Genet* **43**:57, 1993.
914. Danks DM: Carrier testing for cystic fibrosis. *Med J Aust* **159**:148, 1993.
915. Wilfond BS, Nolan K: National policy development for the clinical application of genetic diagnostic technologies: Lessons from cystic fibrosis. *JAMA* **270**:2948, 1993.
916. Burns J: Screening for cystic fibrosis in primary care: Family practice at last? *Br Med J* **306**:1558, 1993.
917. Bekker H, Modell M, Denniss G, Silver A, Mathew C, Bobrow M, Marteau T: Uptake of cystic fibrosis testing in primary care: Supply push or demand pull? *Br Med J* **306**:1585, 1993.
918. Stevenson J: Screening for cystic fibrosis: Patients don't want it. *Br Med J* **307**:262, 1993.
919. Williamson R: Universal community carrier screening for cystic fibrosis? *Nat Genet* **3**:195, 1993.
920. Haan EA: Screening for carriers of genetic disease: Points to consider. *Med J Aust* **158**:419, 1993.
921. Scriver CR, Fujiwara TM: Cystic fibrosis genotypes and views on screening are both heterogeneous and population related. *Am J Hum Genet* **51**:943, 1992.
922. Turner G, Meagher W, Willis C, Colley P: Cascade testing for carrier status in cystic fibrosis in a large family. *Med J Aust* **159**:163, 1993.
923. Kaplan F, Clow C, Scriver CR: Cystic fibrosis carrier screening by DNA analysis: A pilot study of attitudes among participants. *Am J Hum Genet* **49**:240, 1991.
924. Mitchell J, Scriver CR, Clow CL, Kaplan F: What young people think and do when the option for cystic fibrosis carrier testing is available. *J Med Genet* **30**:538, 1993.
925. Mennie ME, Gilfillan A, Compton M, Curtis L, Liston WA, Pullen I, Whyte DA, Brock DJH: Prenatal screening for cystic fibrosis. *Lancet* **340**:214, 1992.
926. Harris H, Scotcher D, Hartley N, Wallace A, Craufurd D, Harris R: Cystic fibrosis carrier testing in early pregnancy by general practitioners. *Br Med J* **306**:1580, 1993.
927. Mennie ME, Compton ME, Gilfillan A, Liston WA, Pullen I, Whyte DA, Brock DJH: Prenatal screening for cystic fibrosis: Psychological effects on carriers and their partners. *J Med Genet* **30**:543, 1993.
928. Grody WW, Kronquist KE, Lee EU, Edmond J, Rome LH: PCR-based cystic fibrosis (CF) carrier screening in a first-year medical student biochemistry laboratory. *Am J Hum Genet* **53**:1352, 1993.
929. Dodge JA, Boulyjenkov V: New possibilities for population control of cystic fibrosis. *Bull WHO* **70**:561, 1992.
930. Nishimi RY: Cystic fibrosis and DNA tests—The implications of carrier screening. *JAMA* **269**:1921, 1993.
931. U.S. Congress Office of Technology Assessment: *Cystic Fibrosis and DNA Tests: Implications of Carrier Screening*. Publication OTA-BA-532, Washington, DC, U.S. Government Printing Office, 1992.
932. Bick DP, Maddalena A, Black SH, Headrick EG, Cummings E, Jones SL, Costakos D, Becker R, Schulman JD: Prenatal screening for delta F508 mutation in population not selected for cystic fibrosis. *Lancet* **336**:1324, 1990.
933. Clarke LL, Grubb BR, Gabriel SE, Smithies O, Koller BH, Boucher RC: Defective epithelial chloride transport in a gene-targeted mouse model of cystic fibrosis. *Science* **257**:1125, 1992.
934. Dorin JR, Dickinson P, Alton EWFW, Smith SN, Geddes DM, Stevenson BJ, Kimber WL, Fleming S, Clarke AR, Hooper ML, Anderson L, Beddington RSP, Porteous DJ: Cystic fibrosis in the mouse by targeted insertional mutagenesis. *Nature* **359**:211, 1992.
935. Colledge WH, Ratclif R, Foster D, Williamson R, Evans MJ: Cystic fibrosis mouse with intestinal obstruction. *Lancet* **340**:680, 1992.
936. Ratcliff R, Evans MJ, Cuthbert AW, MacVinish LJ, Foster D, Anderson JR, Colledge WH: Production of a severe cystic fibrosis mutation in mice by gene targeting. *Nat Genet* **4**:35, 1993.
937. O'Neal WK, Hasty P, McCray PB Jr, Casey B, Rivera-Pérez J, Welsh MJ, Beaudet AL, Bradley A: A severe phenotype in mice with a duplication of exon 3 in the cystic fibrosis locus. *Hum Mol Genet* **2**:1561, 1993.
938. Clarke LL, Grubb BR, Yankaskas JR, Cotton CU, McKenzie A, Boucher RC: Relationship of a non-cystic fibrosis transmembrane conductance regulator-mediated chloride conductance to organ-level disease in CFTR (−/−) mice. *Proc Natl Acad Sci USA* **91**:479, 1994.
939. Coutelle C, Caplan N, Hart S, Huxley C, Williamson R: Gene therapy for cystic fibrosis. *Arch Dis Child* **68**:437, 1993.
940. Flotte TR: Prospects for virus-based gene therapy for cystic fibrosis. *J Bioenerg Biomembr* **25**:37, 1993.
941. Porteous DJ, Dorin JR: Gene therapy for cystic fibrosis—Where and when? *Hum Mol Genet* **2**:211, 1993.
942. Porteous DJ, Alton EW: Cystic fibrosis: Prospects for therapy. *BioEssays* **15**:485, 1993.
943. Wilson JM: Vehicles for gene therapy. *Nature* **365**:691, 1993.
944. Zabner J, Couture LA, Gregory RJ, Graham SM, Smith AE, Welsh MJ: Adenovirus-mediated gene transfer transiently corrects the chloride transport defect in nasal epithelia of patients with cystic fibrosis. *Cell* **75**:207, 1993.
945. Simon RH, Engelhardt JF, Yang Y, Zepeda M, Weber-Pendleton S, Grossman M, Wilson JM: Adenovirus-mediated transfer of the CFTR gene to lung of nonhuman primates: Toxicity study. *Hum Gene Ther* **4**:771, 1993.
946. Yei S, Mittereder N, Wert S, Whitsett JA, Wilmott RW, Trapnell B: In vivo evaluation of the safety of adenovirus-mediated transfer of the human cystic fibrosis transmembrane conductance regulator cDNA to the lung. *Hum Gene Ther* **5**:731, 1994.
947. Zabner J, Petersen DM, Puga AP, Graham SM, Couture LA, Keyes LD, Lukason MJ, St. George JA, Gregory RJ, Smith AE, Welsh MJ: Safety and efficacy of repetitive adenovirus-mediated transfer of CFTR cDNA to airway epithelia of primates and cotton rats. *Nat Genet* **6**:75, 1994.
948. Yang Y, Nunes FA, Berencsi K, Furth EE, Gönczöl E, Wilson JM: Cellular immunity to viral antigens limits E1-deleted adenoviruses for gene therapy. *Proc Natl Acad Sci USA* **91**:4407, 1994.
949. Engelhardt JF, Ye X, Doranz B, Wilson JM: Ablation of E2a recombinant adenoviruses improves transgene persistence and decreases inflammatory response in mouse liver. *Proc Natl Acad Sci USA* **91**:6196, 1994.
950. Stribling R, Brunette E, Liggitt D, Gaensler K, Debs R: Aerosol gene delivery in vivo. *Proc Natl Acad Sci USA* **89**:11277, 1992.
951. Yoshimura K, Rosenfeld MA, Nakamura H, Scherer EM, Pavirani A, Lecocq J-P, Crystal RG: Expression of the human cystic fibrosis transmembrane conductance regulator gene in the mouse lung after in vivo intratracheal plasmid-mediated gene transfer. *Nucleic Acids Res* **20**:3233, 1992.
952. Logan JJ, Bebok Z, Walker LC, Peng S, Felgner PL, Siegal GP, Frizzell RA, Dong J, Howard M, Matalon S, Duvall M, Sorscher EJ: Catonic lipids for CFTR gene transfer. *Gene Ther* (in press, 1994.)
953. Flotte TR, Afione SA, Conrad C, McGrath SA, Solow R, Oka H, Zeitlin PL, Guggino WB, Carter BJ: Stable in vivo expression of the cystic fibrosis transmembrane conductance regulator with an adeno-associated virus vector. *Proc Natl Acad Sci USA* **90**:10613, 1993.

954. Hyde SC, Gill DR, Higgins CF, Trezise AEO, MacVinish LJ, Cuthbert AW, Ratcliff R, Evans MJ, Colledge WH: Correction of the ion transport defect in cystic fibrosis transgenic mice by gene therapy. *Nature* **362**:250, 1993.

955. Alton EWFW, Middleton PG, Caplen NJ, Smith SN, Steel DM, Munkonge FM, Jeffery PK, Geddes DM, Hart SL, Williamson R, Fasold KI, Miller AD, Dickinson P, Stevenson BJ, McLachlan G, Dorin JR, Porteous DJ: Non-invasive liposome-mediated gene delivery can correct the ion transport defect in cystic fibrosis mutant mice. *Nat Genet* **5**:135, 1993.

956. Mulligan RC: The basic science of gene therapy. *Science* **260**:926, 1993.

Part 17

DEFENSE AND IMMUNE MECHANISMS

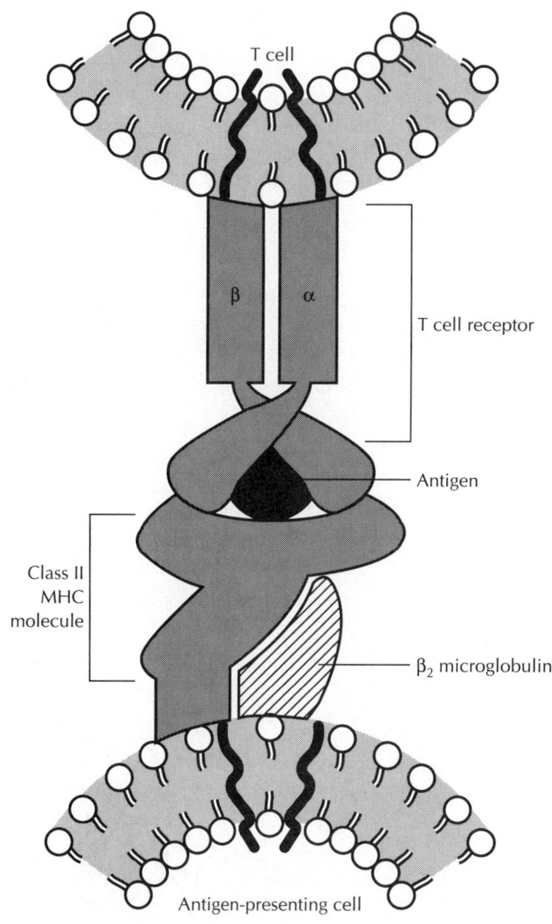

CHAPTER 128

Antibody Deficiency Diseases

Douglas J. Barrett ▪ Joseph L. Butler ▪ Max D. Cooper

1. Antibodies are protein molecules that specifically recognize and bind to antigens to protect the host from microbial infection. They can be divided into five immunoglobulin classes based on their physicochemical or serologic properties: IgG, IgM, IgA, IgD, and IgE. There are four subclasses of IgG that are numbered according to their relative abundance in the circulation: IgG1>IgG2>IgG3>IgG4. There are two subclasses of IgA—IgA1 and IgA2. Thus, there are nine different isotypes of antibodies, each of which has special biologic advantages.

2. B cells are produced in the bone marrow where stem-cell progeny may undergo an orderly developmental sequence to become recognizable precursors of B cells (pre–B cells), and then mature B cells. Newly formed B cells are seeded to the spleen and other peripheral lymphoid tissues, where they may respond to antigen stimulation and T-cell help to become antibody-secreting plasma cells. Aberrations in normal B-cell development and differentiation lead to diseases characterized by antibody deficiency. The level of the B-cell differentiation arrest influences the clinical and laboratory characteristics of the immunodeficiency disease.

3. Primary antibody deficiency diseases may be inherited in X-linked recessive or autosomal recessive transmission patterns. In some cases, a mode of inheritance is not apparent. The hallmark of these diseases is recurrent infections, primarily of bacterial etiology. Treatment by antibody replacement reduces the number and severity of infections in many of these immunodeficient patients. When abnormal T-cell function accompanies the B-cell deficiency, bone marrow transplantation may result in normal immunologic function.

The immune system consists of four major components that productively interact to protect the individual against microbes and other agents capable of producing disease. These components consist of the antibody (or humoral) immune system, the cellular immune system, the complement system, and the phagocytic system. Abnormalities in the development of function of any one of these components may lead to altered immune responsiveness manifested by immunodeficiency or autoimmunity.

In this chapter, we discuss deficiencies of antibody-mediated immunity. First, the structure and function of the immunoglobulin classes are considered. Next, we review the generation of B cells from stem-cell precursors and the steps involved in their terminal differentiation into antibody-secreting plasma cells. Particular attention is given to immunoglobulin gene rearrangement and isotype switching and to the events involved in B-cell activation. This information is incorporated into a model of normal B-cell development and differentiation.

Using this developmental model, we review the antibody deficiency diseases. The inherited and acquired defects in B-cell development that produce these diseases are discussed. The clinical and laboratory features of each disease are considered, and useful diagnostic tests are outlined. Finally, we provide an overview of treatment options, with emphasis on antibody replacement.

IMMUNOGLOBULIN STRUCTURE AND FUNCTION

Immunoglobulin molecules are multichain glycoproteins composed of 80 to 95 percent polypeptide and 5 to 18 percent carbohydrate. The biologic properties of the molecules are determined primarily by their polypeptide moieties, but the function of the carbohydrate components is poorly understood. In their monomeric form, immunoglobulin molecules are composed of two identical heavy chains and two identical light chains, as shown in Fig. 128-1.[1] Antigen differences reflecting the primary structural characteristics of the heavy chains can be used to separate immunoglobulins into the five major isotypes: G, M, A, D, and E. Similarly, light chains can be divided into κ and λ types. An individual antibody molecule has either κ or λ chains, but not both, and the usual κ:λ ratio of Ig molecules is 65:35 in human beings. This ratio may vary for antibodies with different antigen-binding specificities, suggesting that changes in the κ and λ constituents may be important in recognition of certain antigens. Both types of light chains consist of a single 23-kDa polypeptide structure. Interchain disulfide bonds formed between cysteine residues are essential to the development of a stable three-dimensional structure. Intrachain bonds separate the chains into domains of relatively constant size, each containing approximately 100 amino acid residues. Greater variability in the amino acid sequence occurs in the N-terminal portion of each chain. These domains, termed the "variable regions" of heavy and light chains, contribute to the antigenic specificity of the immunoglobulin molecule.[2] The C-terminal domains are designated as constant regions and are responsible for secondary biologic properties such as transmembrane transport, histamine release from mast cells, and complement fixation.

A list of standard abbreviations is located immediately preceding the index in each volume. Additional abbreviations used in this chapter include: C1 = first component of complement; CVID = common variable immunodeficiency; PNP = purine nucleoside phosphorylase; SCID = severe combined immunodeficiency; XLA = X-linked agammaglobulinemia.

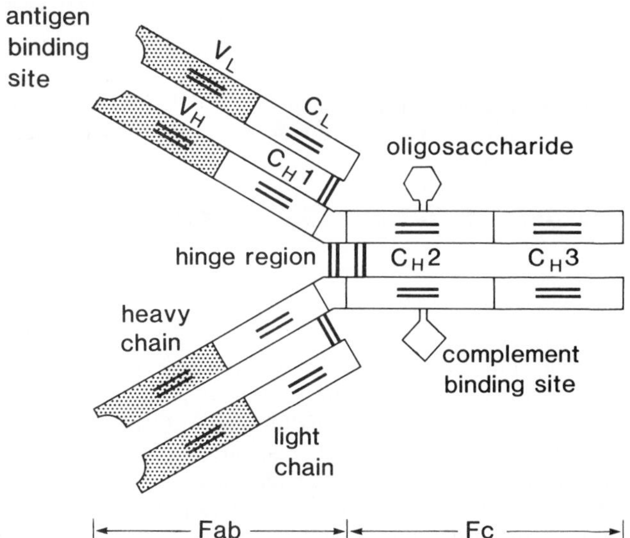

FIG. 128-1 A simplified schematic model for an IgG human antibody molecule. Heavy double lines symbolize inter- and intrachain disulfide bonds; V_L and V_H indicate the variable region of light and heavy chains, respectively. C denotes the constant region. Only one of the two antigen-binding sites is indicated.

Studies elucidating immunoglobulin structure were facilitated by the discovery that enzymes could be used to cleave the molecule at specific sites. Treatment with papain cleaves the molecules on the N-terminal side of the disulfide bonds connecting the heavy chains.[3] Three fragments of similar size are produced: one crystallizable fragment (Fc) consisting of the C-terminal ends of the heavy chains and two antibody-binding fragments (Fab) made up of the N-terminal portions of the heavy and light chains. The two Fab fragments from an antibody molecule are identical, and their variable regions make them uniquely suited to recognize and bind the antigenic determinant. The Fc fragment contains binding sites for components of the classic complement system and for surface receptors (Fc receptor) on neutrophils, macrophages, and monocytes. If IgG is digested with pepsin, the molecule is cleaved on the C-terminal side of the interchain disulfide bonds, producing a large $F(ab)'_2$ fragment,[2] while the Fc fragment is extensively digested.

The immunoglobulins represent a wide variety of proteins that share structural similarities, but exhibit diverse antigenic specificity and biologic functions. Differences in the sequence of amino acids produce structural changes in the molecule which, in turn, dictate the biologic properties. The characteristic properties of each immunoglobulin isotype are summarized in Table 128-1.

Immunoglobulin G

IgG is the most plentiful and widely distributed immunoglobulin, accounting for 70 to 80 percent of the total serum immunoglobulins. The four IgG subclasses are designated IgG1 to IgG4 on the basis of their relative concentrations in the serum: IgG1, 60 to 70 percent; IgG2, 15 to 20 percent; IgG3, 5 to 8 percent; and IgG4, 1 to 5 percent of the total IgG (Table 128-2).[2] The constant region of each IgG subclass is encoded by a separate gene, yet they share greater than 95 percent homology in amino acid sequence.[4] Sequence differences are found primarily in the hinge region of the molecule. The hinge of IgG3 is expanded to more than 100 amino acid residues, accounting for the higher molecular weight of IgG3 as compared with other subclasses.[5] Unlike other isotypes, all the IgG subclasses are passively transferred across the placenta. The half-life of IgG is inversely related to the pool size, but normally is about 4 weeks. Maternally derived IgG thus constitutes the majority of the newborn's serum immunoglobulins until endogenous IgG production becomes prevalent at 4 to 6 months of age. Physiological hypogammaglobulinemia occurs during this transitional period, but is rarely of clinical significance.

On initial antigen exposure, production of IgM antibodies precedes IgG antibody production. Subsequent exposure to antigen induces a rapid and prolonged IgG response, with most of the antibodies produced in the secondary response being IgG. This anamnestic response and the long half-life of IgG make it well suited for prolonged immunity. All four subclasses participate in this antibody response, but with some selectivity. The IgG1 and IgG3 subclasses contain most of the antibodies to protein antigens. If the antigen is a carbohydrate, IgG2 is the predominant antibody produced.[6,7] IgG1, IgG2, and IgG3 can bind the classic complement components via their interaction with a specific complement-binding region located in CH2 domain. IgG4 lacks this ability but may be able to activate the alternate complement pathway. In addition to complement-mediated killing, IgG

Table 128-1 Properties of the Human Immunoglobulin Classes

Property	IgG	IgM	IgA	IgD	IgE
Chains:					
Heavy	γ	μ	α	δ	ε
Light	κ,λ	κ,λ	κ,λ	κ,λ	κ,λ
Number of subclasses	4	2	2	0	0
Molecular weight	150,000	900,000	160–500,000	180,000	200,000
Sedimentation coefficient (S)	6–7	19	7	7–8	8
Percent carbohydrate	4	15	10	18	18
Serum concentration, approximate, in mg/dl	658–1522	54–238	52–364	1–3	0.01–0.05
Serum half-life, days	23	5	6	2–8	1–5
Placental transfer	+	0	0	0	0
Complement fixation (classic pathway)	+	+ + + +	0	0	0
Opsonization	+	+ +	0	0	0
Agglutination	+	+ +	0	0	0
Reaginic activity	0	0	0	0	+ + + +

Table 128-2 Properties of the Human IgG Subclasses

Property	IgG1	IgG2	IgG3	IgG4
Molecular weight	146,000	146,000	165,000	146,000
Percent of total IgG	60–70	15–20	5–8	1–5
Serum half-life, days	23–25	23	9–11	21–25
Placental transfer	+	+	+	+
Complement fixation (classic pathway)	+ + + +	+ +	+ + + +	0
Reactivity with staphylococcal protein A	+	+	0	+
Lymphocyte receptors	+	+	+	+
Monocyte receptors	+	0	+	0
Neutrophil receptors	+	+	+	+

antibodies promote microbial opsonization, as macrophages and neutrophils bear receptors for the Fc portion of the IgG complexes. The IgG1 and IgG3 antibody–antigen complexes bind to these cells with greater affinity than do IgG2 and IgG4 complexes. The binding site on the IgG molecule resides in the CH3 domain, and its interaction with the target cell may result in up-regulation of chemotaxis, phagocytosis, mediator release, and cytotoxicity. All IgG1, IgG2, and IgG4 antibodies (but not IgG3) bind to protein A, present in the cell walls of staphylococci, but the biologic significance of this phenomenon is unknown.

Immunoglobulin M

IgM is the largest of the polymeric immunoglobulins. It normally exists in a 900-kDa pentameric form in the serum, but is expressed as a monomer on the surface of most B cells and in the serum in various hypergammaglobulinemic conditions. The five structural monomers that compose pentameric IgM antibodies are arranged in a radial distribution, connected by interchain disulfide bonds and a joining (J) chain. The J chain is a 15-kDa polypeptide associated with all polymeric immunoglobulin molecules.[2]

IgM constitutes approximately 10 percent of the total immunoglobulin in serum and is the first antibody produced during fetal life. As the first antibody to be produced after antigen exposure, IgM provides the initial line of humoral defense against infections. Passive transfer of IgM to the fetus does not occur, and consequently, elevated levels of IgM in newborns have been used as an indicator of congenital infection.[8] Its short half-life precludes its ability to provide sustained immunity in the absence of long-term antigen exposure. Stimulation with polysaccharide antigens induces high levels of serum IgM, as exemplified by the antibody response to erythrocyte ABO antigens and endotoxins of gram-negative bacteria.

Each pentameric IgM molecule has 10 antigen-combining sites, making it very effective in the opsonization and agglutination of bacteria. These properties lead to increased clearance of antigens by the reticuloendothelial system. IgM is also the most efficient complement-fixing antibody. Through its interaction with the first component of complement (C1), one molecule of IgM can activate the classic complement pathway. This property provides an important biologic advantage in the eradication of bacterial infection, but it may also be detrimental, as in the case of complement-mediated autoimmune hemolytic anemias. Pentameric IgM is more efficient than the monomeric form in antigen agglutination and complement fixation. Approximately 80 percent of the total IgM is localized to the intravascular space, but exocrine secretions also contain IgM. Secretory levels are particularly high in selective IgA-deficient individuals, which may help to explain why some individuals with total absence of secretory IgA are asymptomatic.

Immunoglobulin A

IgA antibodies are an important component of the mucosal immune system, being the major immunoglobulin isotype in body secretions.[2] IgA1 exists as a monomer of 160 kDa and predominates in the circulation, while polymeric IgA2 may be more prevalent in secretions. Dimeric IgA is by far the most common polymer in exocrine secretions. Secretory IgA is composed of two IgA immunoglobulin molecules connected by a J chain and a secretory component. The secretory component or polymeric Ig receptor, which is produced by the epithelial cells of mucosal surfaces, binds specifically to dimeric IgA1 and IgA2 molecules. This 60-kDa polypeptide recognizes IgA dimers and transports them through epithelial cells to the mucous membrane surface. IgA-producing plasma cells are abundant in the laminae propriae of the intestinal and respiratory tracts, and most of the IgA found in secretions is synthesized locally by these cells.

IgA is rarely produced in the fetus in the absence of a congenital infection, and it is the last immunoglobulin to reach adult levels (by the age of 12 to 14 years). IgA antibodies do not activate complement through the classic pathway but may have antibacterial activity in body secretions through blocking their interaction with epithelial receptors and thus preventing entry into the body. Other bacterial or viral inhibition activities of secretory IgA may also be important. IgA is important in the immune response to orally or nasally administered vaccines such as polio and may be similarly crucial to naturally encountered infectious agents. The primary functions of IgA antibodies may be to prevent the entry of antigen via the mucosal surfaces and to remove antigens from the circulation. The latter function is achieved via the interaction of IgA-antigen complexes with Fc-α receptors on neutrophils and monocytes. Its inability to initiate inflammation by complement activation also makes IgA ideal for removing antigens that have leaked into the circulation from the gut or respiratory tract. Otherwise, a different class of antibody could bind to the antigen and induce a harmful inflammatory reaction through the formation of immune complexes and the activation of complement. The high incidence of autoantibody production and autoimmune diseases in IgA-deficient individuals supports this view.

Immunoglobulin D

IgD is coexpressed with IgM on the surface of most B cells but is present in very low concentrations in human serum. The mature B cell represents the first stage of differentiation at which IgD expression occurs.[9] Expression of IgD ceases following B-cell activation and progression toward terminal plasma-cell differentiation. The specific function of IgD is unknown. Cell-surface IgD can serve as a functional antigen receptor through its ability to bind antigen.[10,11] Stimulation of B cells with anti-IgD antibodies produces increased intracellular concentrations of free calcium and inositol phospholipids, both of which are indicative of early cell activation.[12,13] Thus, IgD may function on the B-cell surface as an important component of the clonal activation mechanism. The small amount of IgD present in the serum makes the investigation of its role as a circulatory antibody difficult, but it could serve an immunoregulatory role.

Immunoglobulin E

IgE constitutes only a small fraction of the total serum immunoglobulins (0.05 mg/ml); the majority is bound to basophils and mast cells and exists as a 190-kDa monomer. The fetus does not receive maternal IgE but is capable of limited endogenous synthesis. The low levels of IgE in the newborn gradually increase to adult values before 10 years of age. IgE has the shortest serum half-life of any immunoglobulin class (approximately 2.5 days) and the lowest rate of synthesis (4 to 5 μg per kilogram of body weight per day). The wide distribution of IgE-producing plasma cells in the lymphoid tissue of the gut and respiratory tract suggests that IgE may function in local mucosal immunity. Unlike other species, IgE responses in human beings are long-lived.

IgE antibodies are increased in individuals with allergic diseases and play an important role in hypersensitivity through their characteristic property of binding to the high-affinity Fc receptors on basophils and mast cells.[14] Cross-linkage of this cell-surface–bound IgE by antigens such as ragweed or insect venom induces the release of pharmacologic mediators capable of producing wheal-and-flare skin reactions, bronchospasm, and even fatal anaphylaxis.[15] In addition to its activity in immediate hypersensitivity diseases, IgE is produced in response to parasitic diseases, particularly helminthic infestations. The role that it plays in the immune response to parasites is unclear, but its serum concentration is significantly increased in areas of the world where parasitic diseases are endemic and varies proportionally to the level of parasitic infestation. IgE is similarly increased in selective IgA deficiency and in immunodeficiency diseases characterized by defective T-cell function (DiGeorge, Wiskott-Aldrich, hyper-IgE, and acquired immunodeficiency syndromes).[16,17]

GENERATION OF B CELLS

The development of B-lineage cells involves a progressive series of differentiative steps that can be divided conveniently into two distinct phases: an antigen-independent pre–B-cell phase and an antigen-dependent B-cell phase (Fig. 128-2). Abortive B-cell development may result from inherited or acquired defects at specific points along this differentiation

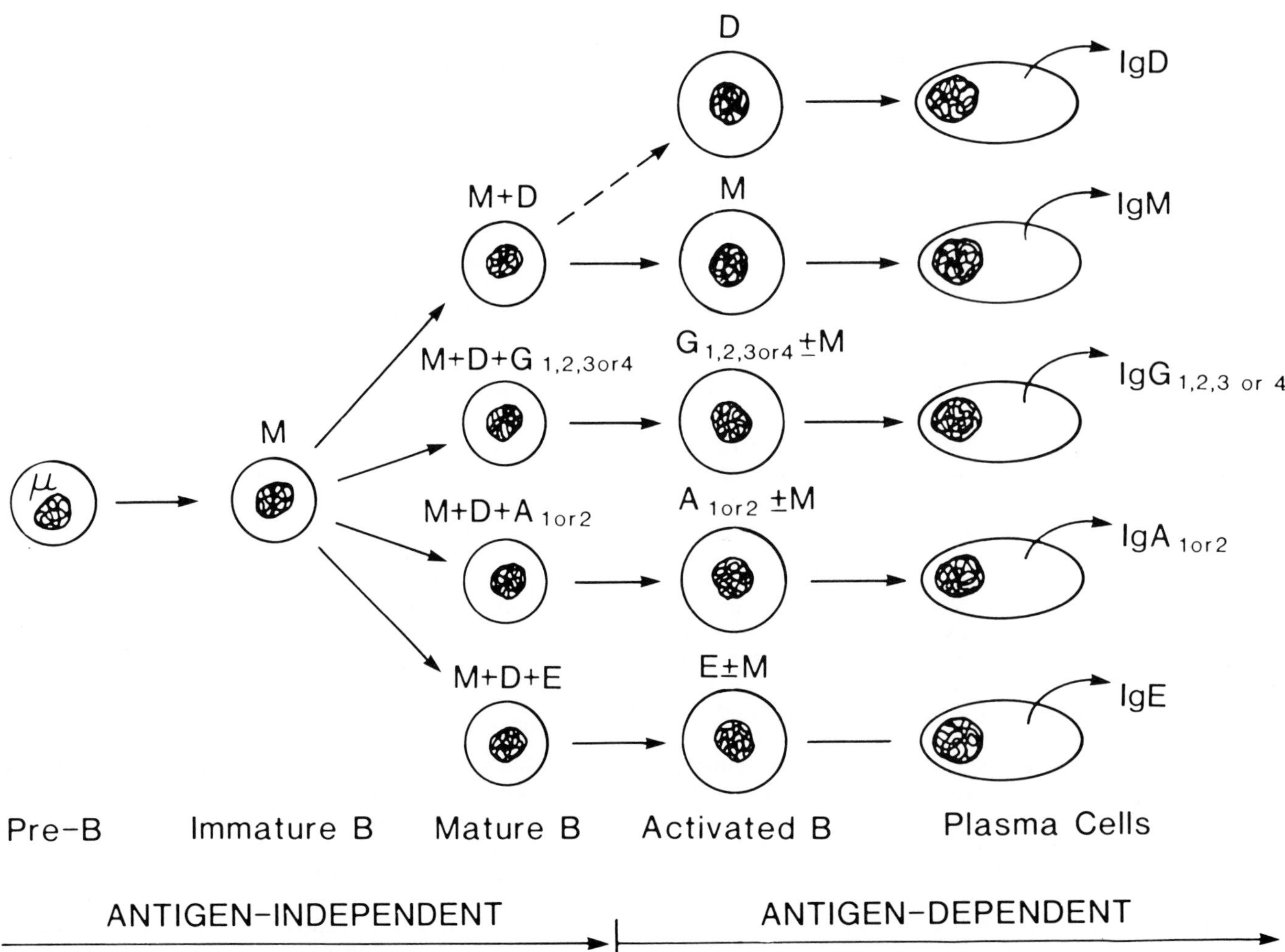

FIG. 128-2 **The development of B-lineage cells showing the early antigen-independent and the later antigen-dependent phases. μ indicates μ heavy chain in the cytoplasm of a pre-B cell. Uppercase letters denote immunoglobulin isotypes, and subclasses are indicated by numbers. Secreted immunoglobulin is symbolized by curved arrows.** *(Adapted by permission of M.D. Cooper, New England Journal of Medicine, in press.*

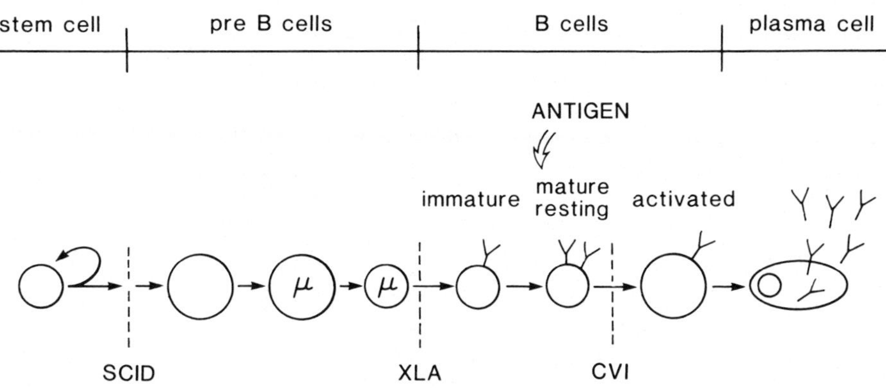

FIG. 128-3 A model of B-cell differentiation. μ indicates cytoplasmic μ heavy chain in pre-B cells; Y denotes immunoglobulin molecules. Dashed lines symbolize points along the differentiation pathway where defects may occur in severe combined immunodeficiency (SCID), X-linked agammaglobulinemia (XLA), and common variable immunodeficiency (CVI). (*Adapted by permission of M.D. Cooper, New England Journal of Medicine, in press*).

continuum, as shown in Fig. 128-3. Therefore, the analysis of antibody deficiency diseases depends on an understanding of the normal development and differentiation of B-lineage cells.

Pluripotential stem cells of mesenchymal origin initially give rise to erythroid and myeloid cells in blood islands of the yolk sac. At approximately 8 weeks of gestation, these cells migrate to the fetal liver, where differentiation along the B lineage begins.[18,19] The bone marrow is then populated by stem cells and soon becomes the primary site of B-cell hemopoiesis for the remainder of life. Development of B cells begins when stem cells give rise to large lymphoid cells that do not express immunoglobulin heavy or light chains, but express other B-lineage markers in the form of cell-surface glycoproteins.[20] The subsequent development of clonally diverse B cells in large numbers is dependent on two processes that take place during the antigen-independent phase. The first is an organized sequence of immunoglobulin variable region gene rearrangements and expression. The second is polyclonal cell proliferation.

IMMUNOGLOBULIN GENE REARRANGEMENTS

Individuals can produce millions of antibodies, each with different antigenic specificity. If every antibody molecule were encoded by a separate gene, much of the entire human genome would have to be committed to antibody production. This apparent paradox is explained through an understanding of the pattern of arrangement of genetic information for antibodies in vertebrates. The nucleic acid message for antibody structure is arranged into patches of DNA coding sequences separated by intervening noncoding segments. These split genes, encompassing both DNA coding and intervening sequences, are first transcribed into RNA. The intervening segments are removed by splicing, and the pertinent coding sequences are joined to form messenger RNA from which the antibody molecule is synthesized. The variable recombination of the gene pieces allows remarkable diversity in the antibody repertoire within the constraints of the genetic information available.

Immunoglobulin heavy and light chains are encoded by genes located on different chromosomes. The heavy-chain genes are present on chromosome 14, κ light-chain genes are on chromosome 2, and λ light-chain genes are on chromosome 22. As shown in Fig. 128-4, heavy-chain variable region genes on chromosome 14 are selected for the first DNA rearrangements by translocation of one of the 20 or more diversity (D) genes to juxtaposition with one of six joining (J_H) genes and deletion of the interposed DNA.[21] Next, the complete variable region of the heavy chains is encoded by translocating one of the 100 to 200 variable region (V_H) genes on one chromosome to the downstream DJ_H segment to form a VDJ complex. Such an arrangement allows transcriptional enhancer sequences located within the intervening sequence between the J_H and Vμ genes to influence the promoter DNA sequence located 5′ to the transposed V_H leader sequence.[22,23] The constant region (Cμ) gene complex is then transcribed and the transcript processed into μ-chain mRNA. A "nonproductive" VDJ_H rearrangement occurs when a defective V_H gene is transposed or the V-DJ splicing is defective. To prevent an individual B cell from making two heavy chains with different antibody specificities, the V_H rearrangement process stops when a productive VDJ_H rearrangement occurs on one chromosome. The successful completion of heavy-chain gene rearrangement is reflected by the expression of μ heavy chains in the cytoplasm of large pre–B cells.[24–26]

The rearrangement of light-chain variable region genes usually begins in the κ gene loci on chromosome 2 after productive VDJ_H rearrangement occurs in the postmitotic pre–B cells.[27] The pattern of VJ_L rearrangement and expression is comparable to that described for the VDJ_H gene complex. Transcription begins when a productive VJ_L rearrangement occurs in one light-chain gene locus. When light-chain mRNA is formed from the transcript, further VJ_L rearrangements on other chromosomes stop. If a productive VJ_K rearrangement fails on both chromosomes, the rearrangement mechanism proceeds to the λ locus on chromosome 22.

When the V_L genes are transposed, transcriptional enhancers located between the J_L and C_L genes influence the V_L promoter sequence to make it receptive to binding by regulatory nuclear proteins to initiate transcription of the light-chain gene. When this process is successful, light chains are assembled, and the pre–B cell is converted to an immature B cell expressing IgM molecules on its surface. The expression of surface immunoglobulin molecules is necessary for B-cell activation and clonal selection by antigen. Thus, light-chain synthesis heralds the antigen-dependent B-cell phase.

A late pre–B-cell phase has been recognized during which the pre–B cell expresses low levels of a novel cell-surface receptor composed of μ chains together with a surrogate light-chain complex. The surrogate light chains are encoded by the V pre–B and 14.1/λ5 genes that are expressed without rearrangement in pre–B cells.[28] The precise function of the μ/surrogate light-chain receptor is unknown, but its expression is essential for efficient progression to the B-cell stage.

Normal individuals generate approximately 10^9 B cells in

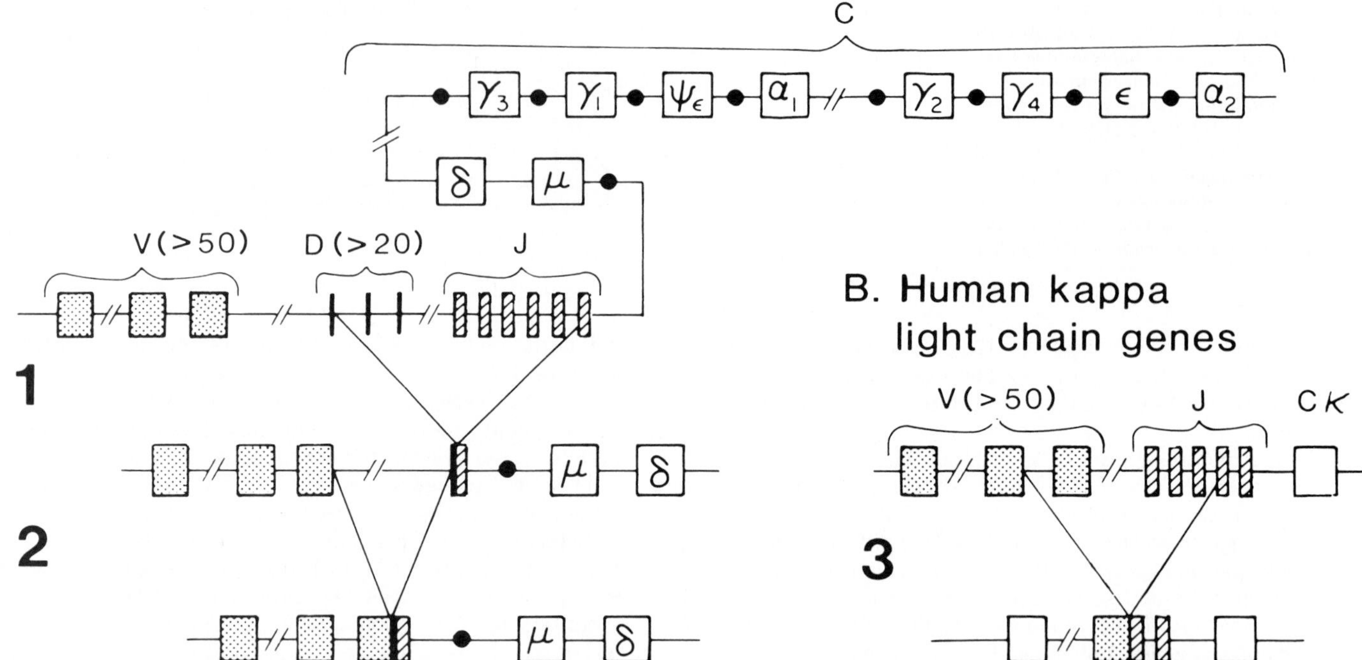

FIG. 128-4 Schematic representation of rearrangement of the human (A) heavy- and (B) light (κ)-chain genes. Open squares indicate the constant (C) region exons; stippled squares symbolize the variable (V) regions; hatched squares and heavy lines denote the joining (J) and diversity (D) segments, respectively. Heavy-chain isotype switch sequences are indicated by solid circles. In Step 1, one of the D genes is translocated in proximity to a J gene with deletion of the intervening DNA. Step 2 is completed when a V-region gene combines with the DJH segment to form a VDJ_H complex. Step 3 shows a productive VJ_L rearrangement in one κ light-chain locus. (*Adapted by permission of M.D. Cooper, New England Journal of Medicine, in press.*)

the bone marrow each day. Each clone differs in its utilization of immunoglobulin heavy- and light-chain genes and in the antigenic specificity of the antibody molecule that these genes determine. Newly formed B cells leave the bone marrow microenvironment and migrate to the spleen, lymph nodes, and other lymphoid tissues.

ISOTYPE SWITCHING

Isotype switching is the phenomenon by which members of each B-cell clone undergo a change in the heavy-chain class of their antibodies from IgM to the production of a different isotype (see Fig. 128-2). Switching, which does not result in a loss or change in antigenic specificity, involves two major molecular pathways. The first is used by all mature B cells to express IgD on their surface and requires the production of a long VDJ-Cμ-Cδ transcript.[29,30] The transcript is differentially spliced into VDJ-Cμ and VDJ-Cδ messenger RNAs that are used to produce intact μ and δ heavy chains. Mature B cells use this mechanism to express surface IgM and IgD molecules with identical antigenic specificity. The second isotype switch mechanism can be used by members of each B-cell clone in the last step in the sequence of immunoglobulin gene rearrangements. Repetitive DNA sequences in a switch (S) region 5′ of the Cμ gene are recombined with an S region 5′ of the downstream C_H gene to be expressed next [31,32] This recombination event results in the transient coexpression of surface IgM and non-IgM isotypes in B cells undergoing an isotype switch. Relatively few B cells successfully complete the switch from IgM to IgD by deletion of the Cμ gene because there is now well-formed switch sequence 5′ to the Cδ genes. T cells are essential for efficient isotype switching and differentiation of non-IgM-producing plasma cells. T-cell control of the switch process is mediated by the secretion of cytokines which may influence the isotype.

B-CELL ACTIVATION AND DIFFERENTIATION

The end product of the humoral immune response is the generation of specific antibody molecules by antigen-stimulated B cells. However, only a small number of the approximately 10^9 B cells produced daily participate in this response. B-cell clones that encounter antigens are selected for survival and clonal expansion on the basis of their antibody specificity. During this clonal expansion in germinal centers of peripheral lymphoid tissues, in addition to isotype switching, somatic mutations occur in the VDJ_H and VJ_L genes. In this way, the B-cell progeny expressing antibodies with higher affinity for the antigen are selected. Memory B cells thus generated are available for the production of antibodies of relatively high affinity in secondary responses.

Surface immunoglobulin molecules also provide the recognition link between the B cell, its specific antigen, and the helper T cell.[33] Antigen bound to surface antibody molecules is internalized, partially degraded, and reexpressed on the cell surface in association with class II molecules of the MHC. Helper T cells recognize the antigenic peptide–MHC class II aggregate with their antigen receptor and thus are stimulated to produce B-cell growth and differentiation factors.[34,35] A second activation signal for the T cell is received via the interaction of its CD28 and CTL4 receptors with the B7/BB1 molecule on activated B cells. In turn, the B cell receives an activation signal via its CD40 receptor when it binds its ligand on T cells (CD40L).

Cell-surface immunoglobulins have short intracytoplasmic tails and thus require associated transmembrane proteins for efficient signal transduction. The associated proteins, called α and β chains, are encoded by the mb-1 and B29 genes, respectively. These are present as covalently linked heterodimers that are noncovalently associated with surface Ig to form a signal-transducing antigen receptor complex on B cells that is comparable with the TCR/CD3 receptor complex on T cells.[36,37] Antigen binding results in cross-linkage of the B-cell receptor units and acts as a stimulus to drive the small, resting B cell into the cell cycle. One of the first steps in the cell-activation process is the activation of a series of protein tyrosine kinases, such as $p56^{blk}$, $p59^{fyn}$, $p72^{syk}$, $p56^{lck}$, and $p53/56^{lyn}$.[38–40] One of the important substrates is phospholipase C.[41,42] This enzyme catalyzes the metabolism of membrane inositol phospholipids to inositol triphosphate and diacylglycerol. These metabolites trigger the mobilization of calcium from intracellular stores, leading to a rapid increase in intracellular free calcium.[42] This may amplify the activity of protein kinase C or modulate the hydrolysis of phosphatidylinositol to induce increased production of diacylglycerol and secondary activation of protein kinase C. B-cell mitogens such as lipopolysaccharide and phorbol esters may bypass the activation pathway used by ligands that crosslink surface immunoglobulin.[43,44] They interact with the B cell to activate protein kinase C without affecting phospholipid metabolism and intracellular calcium concentrations. The resultant phosphorylation of intracellular proteins leads to the transmission of external signals to the nuclear genome.

A variety of other cell-surface receptors are expressed during B-cell activation and differentiation. These integral membrane molecules serve as communication links between the B cell, antigen–antibody complexes, and other immunocompetent cells to facilitate antibody production. B cells express receptors for soluble factors produced by activated T helper cells such as interleukins 2, 4, and 6 and transforming growth factor beta.[36,45,46] These lymphokines may induce isotype switching, enhance B-cell proliferation, and induce the expression of receptors for additional growth and differentiation factors such as transferrin and interferon γ. Complement receptors CR1 and CR2 serve to trap antigen–antibody complexes associated with the C3b and C3d fragments of the third complement component (C3) (see Chap. 30). CR2 receptors loaded with an antigen–antibody C3d complex interact with the CD19 transmembrane protein and other cell-surface molecules to facilitate B-cell triggering via the Ig receptor units. These B-cell receptors may have binding sites for multiple ligands. As an example, the C3d receptor also binds the Epstein-Barr virus.[47]

As differentiation proceeds toward the mature plasma-cell stage, the expression of cell-surface immunoglobulin, HLA-DR, and complement receptors decline with the onset of high-rate synthesis and secretion of immunoglobulin molecules (10^3/s). Plasma cells rarely divide and usually survive for only a few days, so their B-cell precursors must be continuously replaced by lymphopoiesis in the bone marrow and replication in peripheral lymphoid tissues.

Some members of the activated B-cell clones do not immediately undergo terminal plasma-cell differentiation. These cells, termed *memory B cells*, are characterized by their relatively long life span and heightened antibody responses on secondary exposure to antigen.[48,49]

Maturational changes in the overall B-cell population reflect the age of the individual and the pattern of exposure to environmental antigens. This complex pattern of increasing maturation of an individual's B-cell population is best illustrated by age-related changes in the ability to generate antibodies to polysaccharide antigens. The capacity to synthesize IgG2, the predominant antibody to these antigens produced, is acquired relatively late in infancy.[6,50,51] Immunization with carbohydrate antigens before the age of 2 years produces an IgM antibody response that does not result in durable immunity. Immune responses requiring IgA antibodies are the last to mature. This developmental pattern is reflected in the sequential attainment of adult levels of serum immunoglobulins: IgM at 1 year, IgG at 5 to 6 years, and IgA at 10 to 14 years. While the immunoglobulin levels then remain high throughout life, a gradual decline may occur in the antibody responsiveness of elderly individuals, who often exhibit the same nonresponsiveness to polysaccharide antigens as do infants.

IMMUNOGLOBULIN DEFICIENCY SYNDROMES

Antibody deficiency diseases range from asymptomatic selective deficiency of a single immunoglobulin class to panhypogammaglobulinemia associated with severe, recurrent infections (Table 128-3). This broad spectrum of clinical expression results from variability in the nature and extent of the defect in B-cell development and function. In general, individuals with lower levels of serum immunoglobulins have an increased risk of recurrent infections with bacterial, viral, and protozoan pathogens. Fungal infections are uncommon unless a defect in T-cell function accompanies the hypogammaglobulinemia. The diagnosis of antibody deficiency disease requires measurement of serum immunoglobulins and antibody responses to antigenic challenge. When these tests are coupled with evaluation of B and T cells in the peripheral blood and bone marrow, the stage of the B-cell developmental defect can be determined. Effective antibody replacement therapy for many of these diseases is available in the form of intravenous immunoglobulin infusion.

Congenital X-Linked Agammaglobulinemia

Bruton's report in 1952 of a young boy with profound hypogammaglobulinemia and recurrent bacterial infections provided the first clinical description of an immunodeficiency disease.[52] Males with X-linked agammaglobulinemia (XLA) generally have very low levels of serum immunoglobulins. They have bone marrow pre–B cells in reasonable numbers, but a paucity of B cells in the circulation and peripheral lymphoid tissues. Analysis of the B-lineage cells in the bone marrow indicates a bottleneck in the pre-B to B-cell stages in differentiation.[53–56] Epstein-Barr virus infection of bone marrow cells from affected individuals generates cell lines resembling each stage of B-cell development, with the greatest frequency represented by pre–B cells.[57,58] While abnormal Ig gene rearrangements with truncated Cμ and incomplete V-D-J_H rearrangement, or failure of light-chain gene rearrangements have been reported, other studies indicate that the program of immunoglobulin gene re-

Table 128-3 Antibody Deficiency Diseases

Nomenclature	Presumed pathogenic defect	Serum immunoglobulin levels	B-cell number	Inheritance*
X-linked agammaglobulinemia	Block in differentiation from pre-B to B cell	Decrease in all isotypes	Reduced to absent	XL
X-linked agammaglobulinemia with growth hormone deficiency	Unknown	Decrease in all isotypes	Reduced to absent	XL
Common variable immunodeficiency	Low B-cell numbers; B-cell maturation arrest; defective T-cell help; autoantibodies to B and T cells	Decrease in multiple isotypes	Normal, increased, or decreased	AR, autosomal dominant, or unknown
Selective IgA deficiency	Failure of IgA-B cells to undergo terminal differentiation	Decrease in IgA1 and/or IgA2 +/− IgG subclass deficiency	Normal but with immature phenotype	Unknown
IgG subclass deficiency	Defect in Ig heavy-chain genes or in isotype switching	Variable decreases in IgG1, IgG2, IgG3, and IgG4	Normal	Unknown
Immunodeficiency with elevated IgM	Defective isotype switching	Elevated IgM and IgD; low IgG and IgA	Reduced IgG- and IgA-bearing cells	XL,AR
Severe combined immunodeficiency†	Defective stem-cell differentiation	Decrease in all isotypes	Decreased	XL,AR
Light-chain deficiencies	Intrinsic B-cell defect	Decreased Ig (κ or λ); IgA deficiency in some cases	Normal or decreased	Unknown
Immunodeficiency with thymoma	Intrinsic B-cell defect in some; lack of T-cell help in others	Decrease in all isotypes	Decreased	Unknown

*XL = X-linked; AR = autosomal recessive.
† Severe combined immunodeficiency is classified as a combined immunodeficiency but is included as an important cause of panhypogammaglobulinemia. Transient hypogammaglobulinemia of infancy has been excluded from this list.

arrangement and expression is intact.[58–62] Linkage analyses have localized the XLA locus to the long arm of the X chromosome in the region of Xq21.3-Xq22.[63–65] The responsible gene was predicted to encode a product important for precursor B-cell growth and differentiation. A novel gene encoding a protein tyrosine kinase called *atk* has been identified as the XLA gene; *atk* is a member of the *src* family of protooncogenes. The *atk* gene maps to Xq21.3-Xq22, is expressed in B-cell, but not T-cell, lineages, and is structurally abnormal in XLA families.[66]

Mothers of patients with XLA, who are obligate heterozygotes for the defective gene on the X chromosome, have normal numbers of B cells and normal antibody levels. However, all of their B cells utilize the X chromosome bearing the normal XLA gene as the active X chromosome.[67,68] Thus, expression of a mutant XLA gene in a pre–B cell intrinsically limits its maturation into a B cell[54,60,69] (see Fig. 128-3).

Patients with XLA are usually asymptomatic during the first 6 months of life. A pattern of recurrent infections then ensues when the infant's passively transferred maternal IgG reaches its nadir. Over 90 percent of XLA patients have infections of the respiratory tract and the gastrointestinal tract, often in combination.[70] The majority of these infections are accounted for by otitis media, sinusitis, pneumonia, and gastroenteritis. *Streptococcus pneumoniae* and *Haemophilus influenzae* are the most common bacterial isolates. A few patients have central nervous system infections at the time of diagnosis. Young infants may present with sepsis due to Pseudomonas. In unusual cases, pneumonia is caused by *Pneumocystis carinii*.[71] The repeated respiratory infections result in chronic pulmonary disease and bronchiectasis, unless these patients are adequately treated with immunoglobulin replacement.[70]

Individuals with XLA usually have intact cellular immunity and can recover normally from infections with viruses such as varicella and rubeola. Certain viruses, however, pose particular hazards to the patient with XLA. Severe and chronic enteroviral infection manifests as gastroenteritis with malabsorption, oligoarthritis, meningoencephalitis, hepatitis, or a dermatomyositis-like syndrome.[70] Poliomyelitis has occurred following live-virus vaccination in some patients[72]; consequently, only killed vaccines should be used. Hepatitis B virus infection may be either self-limited or progressive and fatal. Other causes of chronic diarrhea and malabsorption in patients with XLA include *Giardia lamblia* infestation[73] and rotavirus infection.[74] Arthritis develops in 20 percent of children with agammaglobulinemia, clinically resembling juvenile chronic arthritis.[75,76] In the majority of these patients no organism is identified, but in some patients enteroviruses, *Ureaplasma urealyticum*, and pyogenic bacteria can be isolated from the joint fluid.[70,77]

Physical findings in patients with XLA include poor growth, evidence of chronic dermatitis due to pyogenic infection of the skin, small tonsils, and small lymph nodes.

The characteristic laboratory abnormalities in XLA include extremely low levels of serum immunoglobulins. IgG is usually less than 200 mg/dl, and IgM, IgA, IgD, and IgE are low to undetectable. Since the presence of maternal IgG may obscure the diagnosis of agammaglobulinemia in infants less than 6 months of age, the measurement of IgM and IgA is especially useful. Demonstrating a failure to produce specific antibody following antigenic challenge helps to confirm the diagnosis. Pre–B cells are present in the bone marrow of affected individuals, but circulating B cells are rare. T cells are present in normal numbers, and their subset distribution is usually normal. Intact cellular immunity is evidenced by positive delayed hypersensitivity skin tests and normal lymphocyte proliferative responses to T-cell mitogens and recall antigens. Lymph node biopsies, though unnecessary for diagnostic purposes, demonstrate a lack of primary and secondary follicles.

The treatment of choice to prevent recurrent bacterial infections is antibody replacement by intravenous infusion of γ-globulin in doses of 400 mg/kg given every 3 to 4 weeks. Trough levels of serum IgG should be maintained around 500 to 600 mg/dl to prevent chronic sinopulmonary complications.[78,79] Adverse reactions to γ-globulin administration include a symptom complex of diaphoresis, musculoskeletal pain, tachycardia, and hypotension.[80,81] These immediate reactions, which are thought to be mediated by aggregates of IgG or biologically active cytokines in the γ-globulin preparations, can often be avoided by slowing the infusion rate or changing to another commercial source. It should be emphasized that commercial γ-globulin does not contain infectious viruses, in particular the human immunodeficiency virus. Infusion of fresh plasma was used in the past in some patients who failed to respond to maximum doses of intramuscular γ-globulin. This therapy has the advantage of replacing IgM and IgA, but has the major disadvantage of potentially transmitting viruses that can produce devastating infections.

Prophylactic antibiotics are necessary in some patients, particularly those with chronic sinopulmonary disease and bronchiectasis. Provision of good pulmonary toilet by vigorous and regular chest percussion and postural drainage is an important part of the treatment of these individuals.

X-Linked Hypogammaglobulinemia with Growth Hormone Deficiency

The syndrome of isolated growth hormone deficiency and X-linked hypogammaglobulinemia with antibody deficiency has been described in patients with recurrent sinopulmonary infections, short stature, delayed puberty, and retarded bone age.[82,83] Marked reduction of all immunoglobulin isotypes is usually present, but normal serum levels of IgM and IgA have been seen in these and other patients with XLA. Circulating B cells are rare, and immunization fails to induce an antibody response. Cellular immunity is normal, suggesting an isolated B-cell defect. Growth hormone levels are reduced in response to insulin–arginine or insulin–levodopa stimulation. A common developmental or biochemical defect explaining the coexistence of antibody deficiency and growth hormone deficiency has not been elucidated, since the genes encoding growth hormone and its receptor do not map to the X chromosome, but this defect apparently maps to the same region of the X chromosome as XLA.[84]

Common Variable Immunodeficiency

Common variable immunodeficiency (CVID) includes a heterogeneous group of disorders in antibody synthesis that may affect both males and females of all ages. Antibody deficiency usually extends to all immunoglobulin isotypes, but can be limited to IgG and IgA deficiency. Often there is no obvious pattern of genetic transmission, but a recessive mode of inheritance is evident in certain families.[85–87] CVID and IgA deficiency (see below) frequently occur in members of the same family and are associated with certain extended MHC haplotypes, suggesting that these are related disorders.[88]

CVID is associated with an arrest of B-cell maturation into plasma cells[89–91] (Fig. 128-3). Immunoglobulin levels in the serum are low, but variable. IgM levels are usually less than 10 to 20 mg/dl, but can be normal. IgG values are usually less than 250 mg/dl; IgA is usually very low; and specific antibody responses are greatly reduced. Most patients have normal numbers of clonally diverse B cells that are phenotypically immature,[90] although occasionally patients with CVID have reduced numbers of circulating B cells.[87] CVID B cells activated by pokeweed mitogen, Epstein-Barr virus, or anti-IgM plus interleukin-2 may be induced to become IgM-secreting cells, but rarely IgG- and IgA-producing cells.[91,92] The B cells in some patients fail to proliferate normally when cell-surface immunoglobulins are crosslinked by anti-IgM antibodies, but they may be activated normally by phorbol esters and calcium ionophores.[93,94] This suggests that an intrinsic abnormality in B-cell activation via surface immunoglobulin may sometimes account for the defective plasma-cell differentiation. The Ig heavy-chain gene locus appears to be normal in CVID patients,[95,96] but abnormalities in the genes encoding *trans*-acting factors involved with the Ig enhancer, switch factors, or other factors involved in the induction of B-cell maturation remain candidates.[96,97] Abnormalities of cellular immunity, manifested by absent delayed hypersensitivity skin test responses, alterations in the distribution of T-cell subpopulations, reduced T-cell proliferation to mitogens, and excessive T-cell suppression have each been demonstrated in individuals with CVID.[87,98] Rarely, patients with CVID may have an absence of CD4+ helper T cells which leads to failure of B-cell differentiation.[99] Autoantibodies to B or T cells is another rare association. Deficient production of, or responsiveness to, B-cell active lymphokines such as interleukin-2, interleukin-4, interleukin-5, and interferon gamma[97,100–103] have also been reported, raising the question of cytokine replacement therapy.[101,104,105]

CVID becomes clinically evident usually during the second to the fourth decades of life, although the disorder has been described in early childhood.[87] The pattern of recurrent infections that ensues is similar to that seen in XLA. Respiratory infections predominate and often lead to bronchiectasis if inadequately treated. Recurrent or chronic infection with *G. lamblia* produces chronic diarrhea, malabsorption, and malnutrition in some patients. The block in B-cell differentiation may result in the accumulation of large numbers of activated B cells in antigen-stimulated lymphoid tissues, and this is manifested by marked lymphadenopathy, splenomegaly, and nodular lymphoid hyperplasia of the gastrointestinal tract. Autoimmune diseases such as pernicious anemia, autoimmune hemolytic anemia, idiopathic thrombocytopenic purpura, autoimmune hepatitis, endocrinopathies, rheumatoid arthritis, systemic lupus erythematosus, or dermatomyositis develop in one-fourth of CVID patients.[87,106] Similar autoimmune disorders occur with high frequency in first-degree relatives. Cancers such as lymphoma and adenocarcinoma may develop in as many as 15 percent of patients with CVID.[87,107]

The same treatment principles outlined for XLA apply to this antibody deficiency disease. Most patients respond well to adequate intravenous immunoglobulin therapy, but individualized management with constant vigilance is required for optimal care.

Selective IgA Deficiency

IgA deficiency is defined usually by a serum IgA concentration of less than 5 mg/dl with normal or increased IgG and IgM levels. This is the most common primary immunodeficiency, but the frequency varies among different populations. IgA deficiency occurs in approximately 1 in 700 Caucasians of European ancestory, but it is much less common in African Americans and Asians. The incidence is 1 in 18,500 in Japanese.[108,109] Many instances of familial IgA deficiency have been reported, and IgA deficiency is often seen in immediate relatives of individuals with CVID.

The underlying pathogenesis of IgA deficiency is still unclear, but affected individuals have IgA-bearing B cells, demonstrating the presence and expression of both the $C\alpha_1$ and $C\alpha_2$ genes. The IgA B cells often coexpress IgM, an immature phenotype that is seen in normal neonates.[110] Thus, as in CVID, the cellular defect involves a failure of immature IgA B cells to undergo terminal differentiation. IgA deficiency and CVID may represent different manifestations of the same basic defect. In support of this hypothesis, both IgA deficiency and CVID are often associated with inheritance of the same small number of extended MHC haplotypes.[88] These two patterns of arrested B-cell maturation may reflect a common susceptibility gene(s) located within the MHC class region. Two groups of investigators have provided evidence that the defect may be in the class III region of the MHC, perhaps involving the C4A gene, while other investigators point to the class II MHC region, and the DQ β-chain gene in particular.[88,111] However, family studies indicate that the MHC susceptibility genes alone are not sufficient for manifestation of IgA deficiency or CVID. Environmental factors that may serve as cofactors for IgA deficiency include drugs, such as phenytoin,[112,113] and congenital intrauterine infection with rubella, toxoplasmosis, or cytomegalovirus.[114]

The clinical manifestations of IgA deficiency are highly varied.[115] Many affected individuals are asymptomatic in spite of their inability to make either IgA1 or IgA2 antibodies. In contrast, others have sinopulmonary and gastrointestinal infections as would be anticipated from the role of IgA in mucosal immunity. Respiratory tract infections include otitis media, sinusitis, bronchitis, and pneumonia. Systemic infections may also occur in IgA deficiency, but in general, infections are less severe than in patients with XLA or CVID, and chronic pulmonary disease with bronchiectasis is less common. Inflammatory gastrointestinal diseases range from occasional diarrhea to a syndrome of malabsorption and weight loss resulting from gluten-sensitive enteropathy.[116] Infections are more frequent in IgA-deficient patients who also have IgG2 and IgG4 subclass deficiency and reduced antibody response to polysaccharide antigens.[117–119] IgA-deficient patients have a high incidence of IgE-mediated asthma and other allergic diseases.[120,121] Autoimmune diseases such as systemic lupus erythematosus, rheumatoid arthritis, type I diabetes, thyroiditis, dermatomyositis, Sjögren syndrome, Addison disease, primary biliary cirrhosis, chronic active hepatitis, idiopathic thrombocytopenic purpura, and hemolytic anemia all occur with increased frequency in IgA-deficient individuals.[108,114,115,117]

Laboratory evaluation indicates that serum and secretory forms of IgA are very low or absent, while the levels of IgM and IgG are usually normal. Circulating B cells are normal in number, but the IgA-bearing cells appear immature in that they coexpress IgM.[110] In some individuals with IgA deficiency, the IgG2 and IgG4 subclasses are also diminished. These patients are more likely to have diminished responses to polysaccharide antigens.[118,119] IgE levels are usually normal, but these vary from increased levels in patients with atopy to reduced levels in nonatopic patients.[122]

There is no definitive treatment for IgA deficiency. Treatment of the associated disorders and especially the early use of antibiotics for suspected bacterial infection remain the mainstay of therapy. Intravenous immunoglobulin may be useful in patients with combined IgA-IgG2/4 deficiency and serious infections who fail to respond to appropriate antibiotic therapy.[117–119] However, extreme care must be taken in administering immunoglobulin (or any IgA-containing blood products) to IgA-deficient patients since they have an increased risk of anaphylaxis mediated by anti-IgA antibodies.[121,123]

IgG Subclass Deficiency

Antibody deficiency resulting from isolated deficiencies in one or more IgG subclasses may be associated with recurrent infections.[86,114] Serum IgG subclass abnormalities may occur in monoclonal gammopathies[124] and in other primary immunodeficiency diseases, notably IgA deficiency, CVID, Wiskott-Aldrich syndrome, and ataxia-telangiectasia.[118,125–128]

Recurrent sinopulmonary infections with the encapsulated bacteria *S. pneumoniae* and *H. influenzae* are common in individuals with IgG2 deficiency. IgG antibodies to the protein antigens are primarily IgG1 and IgG3, while antibodies to the carbohydrate antigens are found predominantly in the IgG2 subclass.[2,129,130] Therefore, IgG2 subclass deficiency may be associated with an impaired antibody response to immunization with the purified capsular polysaccharide of these organisms.[128,131] Chronic lung disease and progressive impairment in pulmonary function tests have been documented in patients with IgA and IgG2 and/or IgG3 subclass deficiencies.[115] Nonatopic children with chronic lower respiratory symptoms may have reduced levels of IgG1, IgG2, and IgG4.[132]

The pathogenesis of IgG subclass deficiency is usually unclear, but a regulatory defect may underlie the aberrant differentiation of IgG-producing cells.[128] Since immunoglobulin isotype distribution is influenced by T cells and their lymphokine products, such as interleukin-4, interleukin-5, and interleukin-6, a specific deficiency in interleukin secretion or interleukin receptor expression could be responsible in some cases. The only precisely defined basis for IgG subclass deficiency, with or without IgA1 deficiency, is the homozygous deletion of immunoglobulin heavy-chain C_H genes on chromosome 14[95,133] (Fig. 128-5). However, most individuals with multigene deletion haplotypes reported to date have been healthy.[134] Thus, this form of gene deletion does not appear to be a common basis for IgG subclass deficiency.

Quantitation of the IgG subclasses should be performed in individuals with recurrent pyogenic infections and low IgG and/or IgA levels. Treatment of the symptomatic individual requires appropriate antibiotics and, in many cases, intravenous immunoglobulin replacement.

Transient Hypogammaglobulinemia of Infancy

Maternal IgG antibodies are selectively transported across the placental barrier into the fetus during the latter months of gestation. Consequently, full-term newborns have adult levels of serum IgG. The serum IgG levels fall to 300 mg/dl

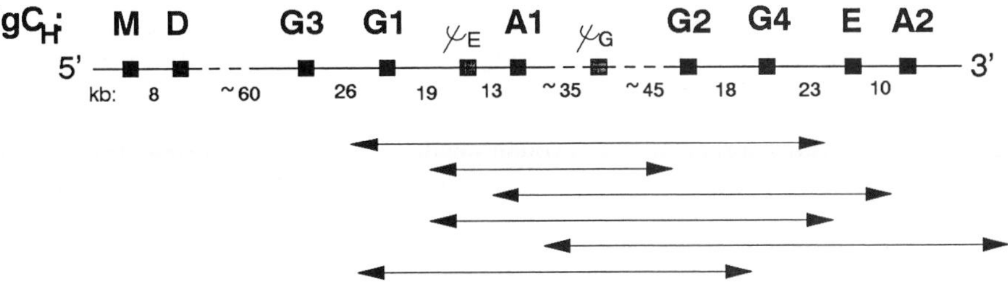

FIG. 128-5 Deletions in the human immunoglobulin heavy chain constant region gene locus. Six patterns of multigene deletions (↔) in the IgC_H region have been described.[6,134] Most of these deletions were detected in healthy individuals who lacked several immunoglobulin subclasses and who were found to be homozygous for one type of deletion or heterozygous for two overlapping deletions.

between 3 and 6 months of postnatal life as passively transferred maternal IgG is actively catabolized (IgG half-life is approximately 3 to 4 weeks) and before endogenous IgG levels accrue. Transient hypogammaglobulinemia of infancy is an exaggerated form of this normal physiological hypogammaglobulinemia. Because of the difficulty in discerning a true delay in immune system development, the actual number of well-documented cases is small, although the reported incidence is highly variable.[135,136] Some of the affected infants have had immediate relatives with other types of immunodeficiency.[137,138]

IgG levels in infants with transient hypogammaglobulinemia may remain low for a variable period of time, but typically recover during the first 2 years of life. Despite the transiently low levels of IgG, a characteristic feature is that immunization induces normal serum antibody responses in these infants. There is often no deficiency of IgM and IgA, and the number of circulating B cells is normal. Numerical and functional abnormalities in CD4+ helper T cells have been reported, but not confirmed.[139] Careful immunologic assessment and periodic reevaluation are essential to differentiate this form of antibody deficiency. A few individuals with this diagnosis may acquire IgA deficiency, but most recover spontaneously.[140]

Treatment includes appropriate antibiotics for infections. Immunoglobulin replacement is unnecessary, except in rare cases with unusually severe and recurrent infections.

Immunoglobulin Deficiency with Increased IgM (Hyper-IgM Syndrome)

This immunodeficiency syndrome is characterized by increased serum IgM levels and the absence of serum IgG, IgA, and IgE. It can be inherited in X-linked, autosomal dominant, or autosomal recessive patterns.[128,141] This immunodeficiency pattern may also follow congenital rubella infections or may be acquired later in life.[142] B cells are essentially normal in number except for an absence of IgG- and IgA-bearing B-cell subpopulations. Evidence for a defect in T cells responsible for Ig-class switching ("switch T cells") has been presented, but normal T-cell function is found in most patients with this syndrome.[143,144] Defective regulatory mechanisms for the isotype switch are presumed to be responsible since the heavy-chain genes and their switch regions appear normal.[144,145] The gene encoding the CD40 ligand (gp 39) on T cells has been mapped to the X chromosome and has been found to be defective in males with this syndrome.

The pattern of recurrent pyogenic infections in this isotype switch disorder is similar to that seen in other antibody deficiency diseases. Specific IgM antibodies are produced following immunization, and IgM antibodies to naturally occurring carbohydrate blood group antigens may be elevated, but antibodies of other isotypes are not made. Neutropenia may complicate the antibody deficiency, and this may lead to increased severity of infections. Hemolytic anemia, aplastic anemia, and lymphoid malignancy have been associated with this immunodeficiency. Treatment principles for the recurrent infections are similar to those discussed for XLA. Intravenous immunoglobulin replacement and appropriate antibiotic therapy may reverse the neutropenic state, suggesting that the neutrophil maturational arrest is secondary.

Severe Combined Immunodeficiency

Severe combined immunodeficiency disease (SCID) is the result of profound functional impairment in both humoral and cell-mediated immunity.[128,141,146] Affected individuals begin to have severe life-threatening infections with a wide variety of bacteria, viruses, fungi, and protozoans very early in infancy. Several forms of SCID can be distinguished by mode of inheritance, identification of enzyme deficiency, or level of faulty cellular differentiation. SCID may occur sporadically or can be inherited in either X-linked or autosomal recessive fashion.[141,146] Because of the severity of the immune deficit, survival beyond 1 year of age is unusual without treatment.

The "Swiss type" of SCID (classical SCID) is inherited as an autosomal recessive disease characterized by severe reduction in the numbers of B and T cells. The defect results from faulty differentiation of lymphoid stem-cell precursors (see Fig. 128-3). Transplantation of normal bone marrow can permanently correct the T- and B-cell defects in this disease.

Deficiency of either ADA[147] or purine nucleoside phosphorylase (PNP)[148] due to deletions or point mutations in the ADA[149] or PNP genes results in SCID forms that are transmitted in an autosomal recessive fashion. The ADA gene is located on the long arm of chromosome 20 and the PNP gene on the long arm of chromosome 14. The purine salvage pathway enzymes encoded by these genes are necessary for the normal catabolism of purines. Individuals deficient in these enzymes accumulate metabolic products that are toxic for lymphoid cells (see Chap. 52 for a detailed description of these enzyme deficiencies). As a consequence, DNA synthesis is impaired, and variable degrees of cellular and humoral immunodeficiency are the result. ADA deficiency leads to impaired development of both T and B cells, while PNP deficiency typically affects T-cell development more than B-cell development. Hence, the clinical manifestations of the latter are usually much less severe. Natural killer cell activity appears normal in these patients.

Another autosomal recessive form of SCID results from an inability to express MHC class II molecules on B lymphocytes and other types of cells that normally present antigens to T cells. This condition, also known as the "bare lymphocyte syndrome," is clinically and immunologically heterogeneous.[150] T cells are usually reduced in number because of a selective deficit in CD4+ helper T cells, whereas B cells are normally present but functionally immature.[151] The primary defect may affect the synthesis of a DNA-binding protein, RF-X, or another nuclear protein needed for RF-X to bind to the MHC class II promoter region in order to activate gene transcription.[146]

Reticular dysgenesis is a rare autosomal recessive form of SCID that is manifested as an early maturational defect of T cells, B cells, and cells of myeloid lineage. Without phagocytic cells or specific immune responsiveness, the affected newborns rapidly succumb to overwhelming infection unless the defect is repaired immediately by bone marrow transplantation.

An X-linked form of SCID is associated with a marked reduction in circulating T cells in the presence of normal or near-normal B-cell numbers. The primary cellular defect appears to be in the bone marrow–derived precursors of T cells, since the defect can be corrected by bone marrow transplantation.

There are a variety of other SCID forms, some of which are associated with the expression of phenotypically immature or otherwise abnormal T cells. These include patients with CD4+ T-cell deficiency,[146,152] circulating lymphocytes that resemble immature thymocytes (CD2+,CD3−, CD4−,CD8−), circulating lymphocytes that resemble common thymocytes (CD2+,CD3+,CD4+,CD8+), impaired cell-surface expression of the T-cell receptor–CD3 complex due to low CD3-ζ-chain or CD3-δ-chain expression, and defective lymphocyte activation due to an abnormality in T-cell receptor signal transduction.[146,153–156]

Patients with SCID usually die in infancy from overwhelming infections with "low-grade" pathogens such as *Pneumocystis carinii* or *Candida albicans*. Bacterial infections are less common during the first few months of life because of the protective effect of maternal IgG antibodies. Subsequently, when profound panhypogammaglobulinemia develops, bacterial infections become a major problem.

SCID can be treated successfully by transplantation of histocompatible bone marrow, usually obtained from a sib.[157] Graft-versus-host disease may develop following bone marrow transplantation or after blood transfusion in untreated patients. However, HLA-nonidentical transplants of bone marrow depleted of T cells may offer an alternative for immunologic reconstitution in patients who lack a matched sib.[157] Reconstitution of cellular immunity occurs within weeks after transplantation, while normal antibody production may be delayed for 1 to 3 years. Intravenous immunoglobulin replacement may provide protection from recurrent pyogenic infections until normal humoral immunity is established. Due to the wide variety of infections in these infants, aggressive diagnostic measures should be used to establish a specific pathogen to ensure that appropriate treatment is given. SCID patients should also receive antibiotic prophylaxis for Pneumocystis until cellular immunity is reconstituted. Patients with ADA deficiency may respond to polyethylene glycol–stabilized ADA enzyme replacement. Gene replacement therapy by insertion of human recombinant ADA into cultured autologous lymphocytes promises to be the best therapeutic approach for patients with ADA deficiency (see Chap. 52).

Light-Chain Deficiencies

Rare instances of inherited abnormalities of light-chain synthesis have been reported. Both κ-chain and λ-chain deficiencies have been described.[128,158] Point mutations in the κ-chain gene locus at chromosome 2p11 can produce this deficiency, but a regulatory defect in B-lineage cells may also account for the disease. The numbers of antibody-producing cells in bone marrow and gastrointestinal tract are decreased, and there are diminished serum antibody responses. Affected individuals may experience recurrent respiratory infections, diarrhea, achlorhydria, and megaloblastic anemia. One patient with κ-chain deficiency and selective IgA deficiency also had cystic fibrosis and malabsorption.

Immunodeficiency with Thymoma

The association of hypogammaglobulinemia with thymoma has long been recognized,[142] but the pathogenic link between the two is still unknown. In contrast to most patients with CVID, patients with thymoma and immunodeficiency have reduced numbers of circulating B cells. They also have a significant deficit of pre–B cells in their bone marrow.[142,159] Differentiation defects in erythroid and myeloid cell lineages (especially eosinophils) are frequent. These features suggest that the immunodeficiency may result from defective stem-cell differentiation. Most of the affected individuals have reduced levels of all classes of immunoglobulins, and they respond poorly to antigenic stimulation. The number of circulating T cells is usually normal, but functional tests of cell-mediated immunity, such as skin graft rejection and positive delayed hypersensitivity skin tests, are often abnormal, suggesting a compromise in the functional pool of T cells. The importance of B cells in antigen presentation to T cells could be a factor in the T-cell dysfunction.

Recurrent sinopulmonary infections are the most common consequence of hypogammaglobulinemia. Chronic diarrhea, urinary tract infection, dermatitis, stomatitis, and arthritis may also occur. Hematologic abnormalities include thrombocytopenia, anemia, leukopenia, and the characteristic feature of profound eosinopenia. Myasthenia gravis is sometimes associated with the thymoma.

Treatment with intravenous immunoglobulin replacement may prevent recurrent pyogenic infections. Removal of the thymoma or steroid treatment may result in improvement of the associated red-cell aplasia or myasthenia gravis, but does not affect the immunodeficiency. However, regeneration of B-lineage cells occurred in one such individual several years after thymectomy. Hemopoietic growth factor deficiencies could play a role in the pathogenesis of this syndrome.

REFERENCES

1. Wasserman RL, Capra JD: Immunoglobulins, in Pigman W, Horowitz MI (eds): *The Glycoproteins*. New York, Academic, 1977, p 323.
2. Paul WE: *Fundamental Immunology*, 2d ed. New York, Raven, 1989.
3. Porter RR: The hydrolysis of rabbit γ-globulin and antibodies with crystalline papain. *Biochem J* **73**:119, 1959.
4. Ellison J, Hood L: Linkage and sequence homology of two human immunoglobulin gamma heavy chain constant region genes. *Proc Natl Acad Sci USA* **79**:1984, 1982.
5. Michaelsen TE, Frangione B, Franklin EC: Primary structure of the "hinge" region of human IgG3. *J Biol Chem* **252**:883, 1977.
6. Barrett DJ, Ayoub EM: IgG2 subclass restriction of antibody to pneumococcal polysaccharides. *Clin Exp Immunol* **63**:127, 1986.

7. Siber GR, Schur PH, Aisenberg AC, Weitzman SA, Schiffman G: Correlation between serum IgG2 concentrations and the antibody response to bacterial polysaccharide antigens. *N Engl J Med* **303**:178, 1980.
8. Alford CA Jr, Wu LYF, Blanco A, Lawton, AR: Developmental humoral immunity and congenital infections in man, in Neter E, Milgrom F (eds): *The Immune System and Infectious Diseases*. Basel, Karger, New York, 1974, p 42.
9. Vitetta ES, Uhr JW: Cell surface immunoglobulin. XV. The presence of IgM and IgD-like molecule on the same cell in murine lymphoid tissue. *Eur J Immunol* **6**:140, 1976.
10. Sieckmann DG, Scher I, Asofsky R, Mosier DE, Paul WE: Activation of mouse lymphocytes by anti-immunoglobulin. II. A thymus-independent response by a mature subset of B lymphocytes. *J Exp Med* **148**:1628, 1978.
11. Scott DW, Layton JE, Nossal GJ: Role of IgD in the immune response and tolerance. I. Anti-delta pretreatment facilitates tolerance induction in adult B cells in vitro. *J Exp Med* **146**:1473, 1977.
12. Pozzan T, Arslan P, Tsien RY, Rink TJ: Anti-immunoglobulin, cytoplasmic free calcium, and capping in B lymphocytes. *J Cell Biol* **94**:335, 1982.
13. Coggeshall KM, Cambier JC: B cell activation. VIII. Membrane immunoglobulins transduce signals via activation of phosphatidylinositol hydrolysis. *J Immunol* **133**:3382, 1984.
14. Ishizaka K, Ishizaka T, Lee EH: Biologic function of the Fc fragments of E myeloma protein. *Immun Chem* **7**:687, 1970.
15. Ishizaka K, Ishizaka T: Immune mechanisms of reversed type reaginic hypersensitivity. *J Immunol* **103**:588, 1969.
16. Polmar SH, Waldmann TA, Balestra ST, Jost MC, Terry WD: Immunoglobulin E in immunologic deficiency diseases. *J Clin Invest* **51**:326, 1972.
17. Buckley RH, Fiscus SA: Serum IgD and IgE concentrations in immunodeficiency diseases. *J Clin Invest* **55**:157, 1975.
18. Gathings WE, Lawton AR, Cooper MD: Immunofluorescent studies of the development of pre-B cells, B lymphocytes and immunoglobulin isotype diversity in humans. *Eur J Immunol* **7**:804, 1977.
19. Kamps WA, Cooper MD: Microenvironmental studies of pre-B and B cell development in human and mouse fetuses. *J Immunol* **129**:526, 1982.
20. Landreth KS, Rosse C, Clagett J: Myelogenous production and maturation of B lymphocytes in the mouse. *J Immunol* **127**:2027, 1981.
21. Tonegawa S: Somatic generation of antibody diversity. *Nature* **302**:575, 1983.
22. Perry RP, Kelley DE, Coleclough C, Kearney JF: Organization and expression of immunoglobulin genes in fetal liver hybridomas. *Proc Natl Acad Sci USA* **78**:247, 1981.
23. Staudt LM, Lenardo MJ: Immunoglobulin gene transcription. *Immunol Rev* **9**:373, 1991.
24. Wabl MR, Burrows PD: Expression of immunoglobulin heavy chain at a high level in the absence of a proposed immunoglobulin enhancer element in cis. *Proc Natl Acad Sci USA* **81**:2452, 1984.
25. Raff MC, Megson M, Owen JJ, Cooper MD: Early production of intracellular IgM by B-lymphocyte precursors in mouse. *Nature* **259**:224, 1976.
26. Levitt D, Cooper MD: Mouse pre-B cells synthesize and secrete μ heavy chains but not light chains. *Cell* **19**:617, 1980.
27. Hieter PA, Korsmeyer SJ, Waldmann TA, Leder P: Human immunoglobulin Kappa light-chain genes are deleted or rearranged in lambda-producing B cells. *Nature* **290**:368, 1981.
28. Burrows PD, Cooper MD: B-cell development in man. *Curr Opin Immunol* **5**:201, 1993.
29. Blattner FR, Tucker PW: The molecular biology of immunoglobulin D. *Nature* **307**:417, 1984.
30. Maki R, Roeder W, Traunecker A, Sidman C, Wabl M, Raschke W, Tonegawa S: The role of DNA rearrangement and alternative RNA processing in the expression of immunoglobulin delta genes. *Cell* **24**:353, 1981.
31. Davis MM, Kim SK, Hood LE: DNA sequences mediating class switching in alpha-immunoglobulins. *Science* **209**:1360, 1980.
32. Honjo T: Immunoglobulin genes. *Annu Rev Immunol* **1**:499, 1983.
33. Raff MC, Owen JJ, Cooper MD, Lawton AR III, Megson M, Gathings WE: Differences in susceptibility of mature and immature mouse B lymphocytes to anti-immunoglobulin-induced immunoglobulin suppression *in vitro*: Possible implications for B-cell tolerance to self. *J Exp Med* **142**:1052, 1975.
34. Reinherz EL, Schlossman SF: The differentiation and function of human T lymphocytes. *Cell* **19**:821, 1980.
35. Acuto O, Fabbi M, Bensussan A, Milanese C, Campen TJ, Royer HD, Reinherz EL: The human T-cell receptor. *J Clin Immunol* **5**:141, 1985.
36. Reth M: Antigen receptors on B lymphocytes. *Annu Rev Immunol* **10**:97, 1992.
37. Van Noesel CJ, Brouns GS, van Schijndel GM, Bende RJ, Mason DY, Borst J, van Lier RA: Comparison of human B-cell antigen receptor complexes: Membrane-expressed forms of immunoglobulin (Ig) M, IgD, and IgG are associated with structurally related heterodimers. *J Exp Med* **175**:1511, 1992.
38. Yamanashi Y, Fukui Y, Wongsasant B, Kinoshita Y, Ichimori Y, Toyoshima K, Yamamoto T: Activation of Src-like protein-tyrosine kinase *Lyn* and its association with phosphatidylinositol 3-kinase upon B-cell antigen receptor-mediated signaling. *Proc Natl Acad Sci USA* **89**:1118, 1992.
39. Lin J, Justement LB: The MB-1/B29 heterodimer couples the B-cell antigen receptor to multiple src family protein tyrosine kinases. *J Immunol* **149**:1548, 1992.
40. Campbell MA, Sefton BM: Association between B lymphocyte membrane immunoglobulin and multiple members of the src family of protein tyrosine kinases. F. *Mol Cell Biol* **12**:2315, 1992.
41. Michell RH: Inositol phospholipids and cell surface receptor function. *Biochim Biophys Acta* **415**:81, 1975.
42. Hirata F, Toyoshima S, Axelrod J, Waxdal MJ: Phospholipid methylation: A biochemical signal modulating lymphocyte mitogenesis. *Proc Natl Acad Sci USA* **77**:862, 1980.
43. Freedman MH: Early biochemical events in lymphocyte activation. I. Investigations on the nature and significance of early calcium fluxes observed in mitogen-induced T and B lymphocytes. *Cell Immunol* **44**:290, 1979.
44. Suzuki T, Butler JL, Cooper MD: Human B cell responsiveness to B cell growth factor after activation by phorbol ester and monoclonal anti-μ antibody. *J Immunol* **134**:2470, 1985.
45. Rabin EM, Ohara J, Paul WE: B cell stimulatory factor 1 activates resting B cells. *Proc Natl Acad Sci USA* **82**:2935, 1985.
46. Miyawaki T, Suzuki T, Butler JL, Cooper MD: Interleukin-2 effects on human B cells activated in vivo. *J Clin Immunol* **7**:277, 1987.
47. Fingeroth JD, Weis JJ, Tedder TF, Strominger JL, Biro PA, Fearon DT: Epstein-Barr virus receptor of human B lymphocytes is the C3d receptor CR2. *Proc Natl Acad Sci USA* **81**:4510, 1984.
48. Askonas BA, Williamson AR: Factors affecting the propagation of a B cell clone forming antibody to the 2,4-dinitrophenyl group. *Eur J Immunol* **2**:487, 1972.
49. Black SJ, Tokushia T, Herzenberg LA, Herzenberg LA: Memory B cells at successive stages of differentiation: Expression of surface IgD and capacity for self renewal. *Eur J Immunol* **10**:846, 1980.
50. Adderson EE, Johnston JM, Shackelford PG, Carroll WL: Development of the human antibody repertoire. *Pediatr Res* **32**:257, 1992.
51. Barrett DJ, Lee CG, Ammann AJ, Ayoub EM: IgG and IgM pneumococcal polysaccharide antibody responses in infants. *Pediatr Res* **18**:1067, 1984.
52. Bruton OC: Agammaglobulinemia. *Pediatrics* **9**:722, 1952.
53. Cooper MD, Lawton AR: Circulating B-cells in patients with immunodeficiency. *Am J Pathol* **69**:513, 1972.
54. Conley ME: B cells in patients with X-linked agammaglobulinemia. *J Immunol* **134**:3070, 1985.
55. Pearl ER, Vogler LB, Okos AJ, Crist WM, Lawton AR, Cooper MD: B lymphocyte precursors in human bone marrow: An analysis of normal individuals and patients with antibody-deficiency states. *J Immunol* **120**:1169, 1978.
56. Tedder TF, Crain MJ, Kubagawa H, Clement LT, Cooper MD: Evaluation of lymphocyte differentiation in

primary and secondary immunodeficiency diseases. *J Immunol* **135**:1786, 1985.

57. Schwaber J, Lazarus H, Rosen FS: Bone marrow-derived lymphoid cell lines from patients with agammaglobulinemia. *J Clin Invest* **62**:302, 1978.
58. Levitt D, Ochs H, Wedgwood RJ: Epstein-Barr virus-induced lymphoblastoid cell lines derived from the peripheral blood of patients with X-linked agammaglobulinemia can secrete IgM. *J Clin Immunol* **4**:143, 1984.
59. Ichihara Y, Matsuoka H, Tsuge I, Okada J, Torii S, Yasui H, Kurosawa Y: Abnormalities in DNA rearrangements of immunoglobulin gene loci in precursor B cells derived from X-linked agammaglobulinemia patient and a severe combined immunodeficiency patient. *Immunogenetics* **27**:330, 1988.
60. Leickley FE, Buckley R: Variability in B cell maturation and differentiation in X-linked agammaglobulinemia. *Clin Exp Immunol* **65**:90, 1986.
61. Mensink E, Schuurman R, Schot J, Thompson A, Alt F: Immunoglobulin heavy chain gene rearrangements in X-linked agammaglobulinemia. *Eur J Immunol* **16**:963, 1986.
62. Schwaber J, Molgaard H, Orkin SH, Gould HJ, Rosen FS: Early pre-B cells from normal and X-linked agammaglobulinemia produce Cμ without an attached V_h region. *Nature* **304**:355, 1983.
63. Mensink EJ, Thompson A, Schot JD, van de Greef WM, Sandkuyl LA, Schuurman RK: Mapping of a gene for X-linked agammaglobulinemia and evidence for genetic heterogeneity. *Hum Genet* **73**:327, 1986.
64. Kwan SP, Kunkel L, Bruns G, Wedgwood RJ, Latt S, Rosen FS: Mapping of the X-linked agammaglobulinemia locus by the use of restriction fragment-length polymorphismnos. *J Clin Invest* **77**:649, 1986.
65. Malcolm S, de Saint Basile G, Arveiler B, Lan YL, Szabo P, Fischer A, Griscelli C, Debre M, Mandel JL, Callord RE: Close linkage of random DNA fragments from Xq 21.3-22 to X-linked agammaglobulinemia (XLA). *Hum Genet* **77**:172, 1987.
66. Vetrie D, Vorechovsky I, Sideras P, Holland J, Davies A, Flinter F, Hammarstrom L, Kinnon C, Levinsky R, Bobrow M, Edvard Smith CI, Bentley DR: The gene involved in X-linked agammaglobulinemia is a member of the src family of protein-tyrosine kinases. *Nature* **361**:226, 1993.
67. Conley ME, Brown P, Pickard A, Buckley R, Miller DS, Raskind WH, Singer JW, Fialkow PJ: Expression of the gene defect in X-linked agammaglobulinemia. *N Engl J Med* **315**:564, 1986.
68. Fearon ER, Winkelstein JA, Civin CI, Pardoll DM, Vogelstein B: Carrier detection in X-linked agammaglobulinemia agammaglobulinemia by analysis of X-chromosome inactivation. *N Engl J Med* **316**:427, 1987.
69. Schwaber J, Koenig N, Girard J: Correction of the molecular defect in B lymphocytes from X-linked agammaglobulinemia by cell fusion. *J Clin Invest* **82**:1471, 1988.
70. Lederman HM, Winkelstein JA: X-linked agammaglobulinemia: An analysis of 96 patients. *Medicine-Baltimore* **64**:145, 1985.
71. Saulsbury FT, Bernstein MT, Winkelstein JA: *Pneumocystis carinii* pneumonia as the presenting infection in congenital hypogammaglobulinemia. *J Pediatr* **95**:559, 1979.
72. Wright PF, Hatch MH, Kasselberg AG, Lowry SP, Wadlington WB, Karzon DT: Vaccine-associated poliomyelitis in a child with sex-linked agammaglobulinemia. *J Pediatr* **91**:408, 1977.
73. Ochs HD, Ament ME, Davis SD: Giardiasis with malabsorption in X-linked agammaglobulinemia. *N Engl J Med* **287**:341, 1972.
74. Saulsbury FT, Winkelstein JA, Yolken RH: Chronic rotavirus infection in immunodeficiency. *J Pediatr* **97**:61, 1980.
75. Janeway CA, Gitlin D, Craig JM, Grice DS: Collagen disease in patients with congenital agammaglobulinemia. *Trans Assoc Am Physicians* **69**:93, 1956.
76. Good RA, Rotstein J: Rheumatoid arthritis and agammaglobulinemia. *Bull Rheum Dis* **10**:203, 1960.
77. Stuckey M, Quinn PA, Gelfand EW: Identification of *Ureaplasma urealyticum* (T-strain mycoplasma) in patient with polyarthritis. *Lancet* **2**:917, 1978.
78. Ochs HD, Fisher SH, Wedgwood RJ, Wara DW, Cowan MJ, Ammann AJ, Saxon A, Budinger MD, Allred RU, Rousell RH: Comparison of high-dose and low-dose intravenous immunoglobulin therapy in patients with primary immunodeficiency diseases. *Am J Med* **76(3A)**:78, 1984.
79. Roifman CM, Levison H, Gelfand EW: High-dose versus low-dose intravenous immunoglobulin in hypogammaglobulinemia and chronic lung disease. *Lancet* **1**:1075, 1987.
80. Barandun S, Kistler P, Jeunet F, Isliker H: Intravenous administration of human gamma globulin. *Vox Sang* **7**:157, 1962.
81. Alving BM, Tankersley DL, Mason BL, Rossi F, Aronson DL, Finlayson JS: Contact activated factors: Contaminants of immunoglobulin preparations with coagulant and vasoactive properties. *J Lab Clin Med* **96**:334, 1980.
82. Fleisher TA, White RM, Broder S, Nissley SP, Blaese RM, Mulvihill JJ, Olive G, Waldmann TA: X-linked hypogammaglobulinemia and isolated growth hormone deficiency. *N Engl J Med* **302**:1429, 1980.
83. Sitz KV, Burks AW, Williams LW, Kemp SF, Steele RW: Confirmation of X-linked hypogammaglobulinemia with isolated growth hormone deficiency as a disease entity. *J Pediatr* **116**:292, 1990.
84. Conley ME, Burks AW, Herrod HG, Puck JM: Molecular analysis of X-linked agammaglobulinemia with growth hormone deficiency. *J Pediatr* **119**:392, 1991.
85. Wollheim FA, Belfrage S, Coster C, Lindholm H: Primary "acquired" hypogammaglobulinemia, clinical and genetic aspects of nine cases. *Acta Med Scand* **176**:1, 1964.
86. Rosen FS, Wedgwood RJ, Eibl M, Aiuti F, Cooper MD, Good RA, Criscelli C, Hanson LA, Hitzig WH, Matsumoto S, Seligmann M, Soothill JF, Waldmann TA: Primary immunodeficiency diseases. *Clin Immunol Immunopathol* **40**:166, 1986.
87. Cunningham-Rundles C: Clinical and immunologic analyses of 103 patients with common variable immunodeficiency. *J Clin Immunol* **9**:22, 1989.
88. Volanakis JE, Zhu ZB, Schaffer FM, Macon KJ, Palermos J, Barger BO, Go R, Campbell RD, Schroeder HW, Cooper MD: Major histocompatibility complex class III genes and susceptibility to immunoglobulin A deficiency and common variable immunodeficiency. *J Clin Invest* **89**:1914, 1992.
89. Cooper MD, Lawton AR, Bockman DE: Agammaglobulinemia with B lymphocytes: Specific defect of plasma-cell differentiation. *Lancet* **2**:791, 1971.
90. Preud'Homme JL, Griscelli C, Seligmann M: Immunoglobulins on the surface of lymphocytes in fifty patients with primary immunodeficiency diseases. *Clin Immunol Immunopathol* **1**:241, 1973.
91. Bryant A, Calver NC, Toubi E, Webster ADB, Farrant J: Classification of patients with common variable immunodeficiency by B cell secretion of IgM and IgG in response to anti-IgM and interleukin-2. *Clin Immunol Immunopathol* **56**:239, 1990.
92. Mayer L, Fu SM, Cunningham-Rundles C, Kunkel HG: Polyclonal immunoglobulin secretion in patients with common variable immunodeficiency using monoclonal B cell differentiation factors. *J Clin Invest* **74**:2115, 1984.
93. Chien M, Yokoyama W, Ashman R: Abnormal membrane depolarization response to anti-μ plus B cell growth factor (BCGF) in B cells from patients with common variable hypogammaglobulinemia. *Fed Proc* **45**:982, 1986.
94. Saxon A, Giorgi JV, Sherr EH, Kagan JM: Failure of B cells in common variable immunodeficiency to transit from proliferation to differentiation is associated with altered B cell surface-molecule display. *J Allergy Clin Immunol* **84**:44, 1989.
95. Olsson G, Hofker MH, Walter MA, Smith S, Hammarstrom L, Edvard-Smith CI, Cox DW: Ig H chain variable and C region genes in common variable immunodeficiency: Characterization of two new deletion haplotypes. *J Immunol* **147**:2540, 1991.
96. Kaneko H, Kondo N, Motoyoshi F, Mori S, Kobayashi Y, Inoue Y, Orii T: Expression of immunoglobulin genes in common variable immunodeficiency. *J Clin Immunol* **11**:262, 1991.
97. Matheson DS, Weisdorf DJ: Impaired responsiveness to

B cell growth factor in a patient with common variable hypogammaglobulinemia. *J Immunol* **138**:2469, 1987.

98. Waldmann TA, Durm M, Broder S, Blackman M, Blaese RM, Strober W: Role of suppressor cells in the pathogenesis of common variable hypogammaglobulinemia. *Lancet* **2**:609, 1974.
99. Reinherz EL, Cooper MD, Schlossman SF, Rosen FS: Abnormalities of T cell maturation and regulation in human beings with immunodeficiency disorders. *J Clin Invest* **68**:699, 1981.
100. Saeki O, Shimizu M, Saeki Y, Kishimoto S, Kishimoto T: Dissociation in the production of B cell stimulating factors (BCGF and BCDF) and interleukin 2 by T cells from a common variable immunodeficient patient. *J Immunol* **133**:1920, 1984.
101. Spickett GP, Farrant J: The role of lymphokines in common variable hypogammaglobulinemia. *Immunol Today* **10**:192, 1989.
102. Rump JA, Schlesier M, Brugger W, Drager R, Melchers I, Andreesen R, Peter HH: Possible role of IL-2 deficiency for hypogammaglobulinemia in common variable immunodeficiency (CVI) patients, in Chapel HM, Levinsky RJ, Webster ADB (eds): *Progress in Immune Deficiency*, 3rd ed. Royal Society of Medicine Services, London; New York, 1991, p 77.
103. Sneller MC, Strober W: Abnormalities of lymphokine gene expression in patients with common variable immunodeficiency. *J Immunol* **144**:3762, 1990.
104. Stohl W, Cunningham-Rundles C, Mayer L: *In vitro* induction of T cell-dependent B cell differentiation in patients with common varied immunodeficiency. *Clin Immunol Immunopathol* **49**:273, 1988.
105. Cunningham-Rundles C, Mayer L, Sapira E, Mendelsohn L: Restoration of immunoglobulin secretion *in vitro* in common variable immunodeficiency by *in vivo* treatment with polyethylene glycol conjugated human recombinant interleukin-2. Clin Immunol Immunopathol **64**:46, 1992.
106. Conley ME, Park CL, Douglas SD: Childhood common variable immunodeficiency with autoimmune disease. *J Pediatr* **108**:915, 1986.
107. Cunningham-Rundles C, Siegal FP, Cunningham-Rundles S, Lieberman P: Incidence of cancer in 98 patients with common varied immunodeficiency. *J Clin Immunol* **7**:294, 1987.
108. Ammann AJ, Hong R: Selective IgA deficiency: Presentation of 30 cases and a review of the literature. *Medicine* (Baltimore) **50**:223, 1971.
109. Ropars C, Muller A, Paint N, Beige D, Avenard G: Large scale detection of IgA deficient blood donors. *J Immunol Methods* **54**:183, 1982.
110. Conley ME, Cooper MD: Immature IgA B cells in IgA-deficient patients. *N Engl J Med* **305**:495, 1981.
111. Olsson PG, Hammarstrom L, Cox DW, Smith CI: Involvement of both HLA and Ig heavy chain haplotypes in human IgA deficiency. *Immunogenetics* **36**:389, 1992.
112. Seager J, Jamison DL, Wilson J, Hayward AR, Soothill JF: IgA deficiency, epilepsy, and phenytoin treatment. *Lancet* **2**:632, 1975.
113. Dosch H-M, Jason J, Gelfand EW: Transient antibody deficiency and abnormal T suppressor cells induced by phenytoin. *N Engl J Med* **306**:406, 1982.
114. Rosen FS: Immune deficiencies: An overview, in Gelfand EW, Dosch H-M (eds): *Biological Basis of Immunodeficiency*. New York, Raven, 1980, p 1.
115. Plebani A, Ugazio AG, Monafo V, Burgio GR: Clinical heterogeneity and reversibility of selective immunoglobulin A deficiency in 80 children. *Lancet* **1**:829, 1986.
116. Mann JG, Brown WR, Kern F: The subtle and variable clinical expressions of gluten-induced enteropathy (adult celiac disease, non-tropical sprue): An analysis of twenty-one consecutive cases. *Am J Med* **48**:357, 1970.
117. Hanson LA, Bjorkander J, Carlsson B, Roberton D, Soderstrom T: The heterogeneity of IgA deficiency. *J Clin Immunol* **8**:159, 1988.
118. Oxelius V-A, Laurell A-B, Lindquist B, Golebiowska H, Axelsson U, Bjorkander J, Hanson LA: IgG subclasses in selective IgA deficiency: Importance of IgG2-IgA deficiency. *N Engl J Med* **304**:1476, 1981.
119. Ugazio AG, Out TA, Plebani A, Duse M, Monafo V, Nespoli L, Burgio GR: Recurrent infections in children with "selective" IgA deficiency: Association with IgG2 and IgG4 deficiency. *Birth Defects* **19**:169, 1983.
120. Bjorkander J, Bake B, Oxelius V-A, Hanson LA: Impaired lung function in patients with IgA deficiency and low levels of IgG2 or IgG3. *N Engl J Med* **313**:720, 1985.
121. Vyas GN, Perkins HA, Fudenberg HH: Anaphylactoid transfusion reactions associated with anti-IgA. *Lancet* **2**:312, 1968.
122. Zeiss CR: Immunologic aspects of immediate hypersensitivity, in Patterson R (ed): *Allergic Diseases*. Philadelphia, Lippincott, 1985, p 52.
123. Burks AW, Sampson HA, Buckley RH: Anaphylactic reactions after gamma globulin administration in patients with hypogammaglobulinemia. *N Engl J Med* **314**:560, 1986.
124. Schur PH, Kyle RA, Bloch KJ, Hammack WS, Rivers SL, Sargent A, Ritchie RF, McIntyre OR, Moloney WC, Wolfson L: IgG subclasses: Relationship to clinical aspects of multiple myeloma and frequency distribution among M-components. *Scand J Haematol* **12**:60, 1974.
125. Yount WJ, Hong R, Seligmann M, Good R, Kunkel HG: Imbalances of gamma globulin subgroups and gene defects in patients with primary hypogammaglobulinemia. *J Clin Invest* **49**:1957, 1970.
126. Oxelius V-A: Quantitative and qualitative investigations of serum IgG subclasses in immunodeficiency diseases. *Clin Exp Immunol* **36**:112, 1979.
127. Oxelius V-A, Berkel AI, Hanson LA: IgG2 deficiency in ataxia-telangiectasia. *N Engl J Med* **306**:515, 1982.
128. Cooper MD, Butler JL: Primary immunodeficiency diseases, in Paul WE (ed): *Fundamental Immunology*, 2d ed. New York, Raven, 1989, p 1033.
129. Hammarstrom L, Granstrom M, Oxelius V, Persson MAA, Smith CIE: IgG subclass distribution of antibodies against *S. aureus* teichoic acid and alpha-toxin in normal and immunodeficient donors. *Clin Exp Immunol* **55**:593, 1984.
130. Stevens R, Dichek D, Keld B, Heiner D: IgG1 is the predominant subclass of in vivo- and in vitro-produced anti-tetanus toxoid antibodies and also serves as the membrane IgG molecule for delivering inhibitory signals to anti-tetanus toxoid antibody-producing B cells. *J Clin Immunol* **3**:65, 1983.
131. Umetsu DT, Ambrosino DM, Quinti I, Siber GR, Geha RS: Recurrent sinopulmonary infection and impaired antibody response to bacterial capsular polysaccharide antigen in children with selective IgG subclass deficiency. *N Engl J Med* **313**:1247, 1985.
132. Smith TF, Morris EC, Bain RP: IgG subclasses in nonallergic children with chronic chest symptoms. *J Pediatrics* **105**:896, 1984.
133. Lefranc MP, Hammarstrom L, Smith CI, Lefranc G: Gene deletions in the human immunoglobulin heavy chain constant region locus: Molecular and immunological analysis. *Immunodefic Rev* **2**:265, 1991.
134. Smith CI, Hammarstrom L, Henter JI, de-Lange GG: Molecular and serologic analysis of IgG1 deficiency caused by new forms of the constant region of the Ig H chain gene deletions. *J Immunol* **142**:4514, 1989.
135. Hayakawa H, Iwata T, Yata J, Kobayashi N: Primary immunodeficiency syndrome in Japan. I. Overview of a nationwide survey on primary immunodeficiency syndromes. *J Clin Immunol* **1**:31, 1981.
136. Tiller TL Jr, Buckley RH: Transient hypogammaglobulinemia of infancy: Review of the literature, clinical and immunologic features of 11 new cases, and long-term follow-up. *J Pediatr* **92**:347, 1978.
137. Soothill JF: Immunoglobulins in first-degree relatives of patients with hypogammaglobulinemia: Transient hypogammaglobulinemia: A possible manifestation of heterozygocity. *Lancet* **1**:1001, 1968.
138. Rieger CHI, Nelson LA, Peri BA, Lustig JV, Newcomb RW: Transient hypogammaglobulinemia of infancy. *J Pediatr* **91**:601, 1977.
139. Siegel RL, Issekutz T, Schwaber J, Rosen FS, Geha RS: Deficiency of T helper cells in transient hypogammaglobulinemia of infancy. *N Engl J Med* **305**:1307, 1981.
140. McGeady SJ: Transient hypogammaglobulinemia of infancy:

Need to reconsider name and definition. *J Pediatr* **110**:47, 1987.

141. Rosen FS, Cooper MD, Wedgwood RJP: The primary immunodeficiencies. *N Engl J Med* **311**:235, 1984.
142. Jeunet FS, Good RA: Thymoma, immunologic deficiencies and hematological abnormalities, in Bergsma D, Good RA (eds): *Immunologic Deficiency Diseases in Man*, published: New York, National Foundation-March of Dimes, 1968, p 192.
143. Mayer L, Kwan SP, Thompson C, Ko HS, Chiorazzi N, Waldmann T, Rosen F: Evidence for a defect in "Switch" T cells in patients with immunodeficiency and hyperimmunoglobulinemia M. *N Engl J Med* **314**:409, 1986.
144. Levitt D, Haber P, Rich K, Cooper MD: Hyper IgM immunodeficiency: A primary dysfunction of B lymphocyte isotype switching. *J Clin Invest* **72**:1650, 1983.
145. Burrows PD, Kubagawa H, Borzillo GV, Cooper MD: Immunoglobulin isotype switching in humans, in Singhal SK, Delovitch TL (eds): *Mediators of Immune Regulation and Immunotherapy*. New York, Elsevier, 1986, p 158.
146. Fischer A: Severe combined immunodeficiencies. *Immundefic Rev* **3**:83, 1992.
147. Hirschhorn R: Adenosine deaminase deficiency. *Immundefic Rev* **2**:175, 1990.
148. Markert ML: Purine nucleoside phosphorylase deficiency. *Immundefic Rev* **3**:45, 1991.
149. Kashii S, Ito K, Monden S, Sasai Y, Tsuchida K, Fujita M, Kawamoto H, Norioka M, Okuma M: Adenosine deaminase deficiency due to heterozygous abnormality consisting of a deletion of exon 7 and the absence of enzyme mRNA. *J Cell Biochem* **47**:49, 1991.
150. Clement LT, Plaeger-Marshall S, Haas A, Saxon A, Martin AM: Bare lymphocyte syndrome: Consequences of absent class II major histocompatibility antigen expression for B lymphocyte differentiation and function. *J Clin Invest* **81**:669, 1988.
151. Clement LT, Giorgi JV, Plaeger-Marshall S, Haas A, Stiehm ER, Martin AM: Abnormal differentiation of immunoregulatory T-lymphocyte subpopulations in the major histocompatibility complex (MHC) class II antigen deficiency syndrome. *J Clin Immunol* **8**:503, 1988.
152. Sleasman JW, Tedder TF, Barrett DJ: Combined immunodeficiency due to the selective absence of CD4 inducer T lymphocytes. *Clin Immunol Immunopathol* **55**:401, 1990.
153. Chatila T, Wong R, Young M, Miller R, Terhorst C, Geha RS: An immunodeficiency characterized by defective signal transduction in T lymphocytes. *N Engl J Med* **320**:696, 1989.
154. Arnaiz-Villena A, Timon M, Corell A, Perez-Aciego P, Martin-Villa JM, Regueiro JR: Brief report: Primary immunodeficiency caused by mutations in the gene encoding the CD3-y subunit of the T-lymphocyte receptor. *N Engl J Med* **327**:529 1992.
155. Alarcon B, Terhorst C, Arnaiz-Villena A, Perez-Aciego P, Ramon-Regueiro J: Congenital T-cell receptor immunodeficiencies in man. *Immundefic Rev* **2**:1, 1990.
156. Perez-Aciego P, Alarcon B, Arnaiz-Villena A, Terhorst C, Timon M, Segurado OG, Regueiro JR: Expression and function of a variant T-cell receptor complex lacking CD3-gamma. *J Exp Med* **174**:319, 1991.
157. Fischer A, Landais P, Friedrich W, Morgan G, Gerritsen B, Fasth A, Porta F, Griscelli C, Goldman SF, Levinsky R, Vossen J: European experience of bone-marrow transplantation for severe combined immunodeficiency. *Lancet* **336**:850, 1990.
158. Zegers BJM, Maertzdorf WJ, Van Loghem E, Mul NAJ, Stoop JW, Van Der Laag J, Vossen JJ, Ballieux RE: Kappa-chain deficiency. An immunoglobulin disorder. *N Engl J Med* **294**:1026, 1976.
159. Litwin SD: Immunodeficiency with thymoma: Failure to induce Ig production in immunodeficiency lymphocytes cocultured with normal T cells. *J Immunol* **122**:728, 1979.

CHAPTER 129

Genetic Immunodeficiency Syndromes with Defects in Both T- and B-Lymphocyte Function

R. Michael Blaese

1. **During the development of mature T- and B-lymphocyte populations, similar molecular mechanisms are involved in the assembly of receptors from discontinuous genetic elements coding for variable and constant regions of these receptor molecules. In addition to expression of these unique receptors for antigen, an appropriate specific immune response depends on a complex network of cellular interactions and communication involving multichain cell surface receptors and secreted biologically active regulatory molecules (cytokines), multichain recognition and antigen presentation molecules of the major histocompatibility complex (MHC), and adhesion molecules and integrins involved in cell migration, interaction and communication. When T cells or B cells fail to function appropriately, distinct clinical disorders occur which are characterized by increased infections with different classes of microorganisms.**

2. **Severe combined immunodeficiency (SCID) is a heterogenous group of disorders characterized by profound functional deficiency in both cellular (T-cell) and humoral (B-cell) immunity. SCID may be inherited as an autosomal recessive or X-linked trait. The X-linked form, which accounts for 40 to 60 percent of cases of SCID, is caused by a defect in the γ chain of the cellular receptor for the cytokine interleukin-2. About 30 percent of SCID is associated with deficiency of the purine catabolic enzyme adenosine deaminase (ADA). Other cases of SCID are associated with defective expression of class II MHC molecules on the surface membranes of lymphocytes as well as epithelial and endothelial cells. These cells from these patients lack a nuclear transcription factor, RF-X, which binds to the class II promoter region and is essential for expression of the protein. Combined immunodeficiency may also occur in association with defects in IL-2 production and defects in the multichain T-cell receptor (TCR). Carrier heterozygotes with ADA deficiency can be identified because they express only half-normal ADA levels. Carriers of X-linked SCID can also be detected by analysis of the γ chain IL2 receptor gene and because these females demonstrate unbalanced X chromosome inactivation in their peripheral T cells.**

3. **Ataxia telangiectasia (AT) is an autosomal recessive multisystem disorder consisting of profound neurologic disability, oculocutaneous telangiectasia, and variable immunologic deficiency. The patients develop disabling cerebellar ataxia and chorioathetosis early in life, with recurrent infections appearing somewhat later and correlating with the degree of immunodeficiency. Both humoral and cellular immune responses may be defective, and the patients have a high incidence of neoplasia. The thymus is embryonic in appearance, and patients have persistent production of α-fetoprotein. Fibroblasts from AT patients have a markedly reduced colony-forming ability in vitro following x-irradiation and are presumed to have a defect in DNA repair. There is a very high incidence of chromosomal translocations and breaks in T-cell leukemias and lymphoblastoid cell lines from AT patients, centered in areas of the T-cell receptor genes and the immunoglobulin genes, genetic segments known to undergo breaks, rearrangements, deletions, and repair of DNA. The AT gene has been mapped to chromosome 11q22-23.**

4. **The Wiskott-Aldrich syndrome is an X-linked disease defined by the triad of recurrent infections with all classes of microorganisms, hemorrhage secondary to dual-system immunodeficiency with selective defects in both the T- and B-cell systems as well as selective functional defects in monocytes, granulocytes, and platelets. Their selective inability to produce antibodies to polysaccharide antigens is an immunologic defect unique to this disease. Autoimmune disease is a major complicating factor, and malignancy also occurs in high frequency. Splenectomy corrects the thrombocytopenia and results in conversion of the platelets from small to normal size, indicating that this part of the "classic" triad is a secondary phenomenon. The primary defect is unknown. Defects in expression of the cell membrane glycoprotein sialophorin (CD43) have been demonstrated in some situations, but this protein does not map to the X chromosome, and the possibility that these defects are also secondary phenomena have not been excluded. Carriers can be detected because they demonstrate a nonrandom pattern of X-chromosome inactivation in their T cells, B cells, and granulocytes.**

A list of standard abbreviations is located immediately preceding the index in each volume. Additional abbreviations used in this chapter include: AT = ataxia telangiectasia; GVHD = graft-versus-host disease; SCID = severe combined immunodeficiency; TCR = T cell receptor; WAS = Wiskott-Aldrich syndrome.

The genetic immunodeficiency diseases were unrecognized until the seminal report by Bruton in 1952[1] of the presence of agammaglobulinemia in a boy with recurrent infections. For the next decade, immunodeficiency remained an ill-defined explanation for patients who were experiencing an increased susceptibility to infections. Confusion existed because agammaglobulinemia was found only in some of these patients and because classes of infectious agents that seemed to dominate the clinical picture in one patient appeared to cause no difficulty at all for another patient. Understanding of the immunodeficiency diseases was greatly enhanced when the two-component makeup of the immune system was delineated in the 1960s. Studies in mice and chickens established the presence of two distinct and complementary systems, the T-cell, or cellular, immune system, and the B-cell, or humoral, immune system.[2]

The T-cell population consists of lymphocytes that arise from precursor cells migrating to the thymus, an epithelial structure embryonically derived from the third and fourth pharyngeal pounches. T cells mature into subsets that perform an array of different functions, ranging from the killing by cytotoxic cells of virus-infected host tissues or foreign tissue grafts to the synthesis and secretion of biologically active mediator molecules (the cytokines) to important immunoregulatory functions such as helper and suppressor activities.

B cells arise in the bursa of Fabricius in birds and in the fetal liver and bone marrow in mammals and mature into cells specialized for antibody secretion. The T-cell system and the B-cell system interact in an exquisitely complex dance involving positive and negative regulatory effects and resulting in the final expression of immunity. Because of the complexity of the interactions involved, there are many sites where defects that lead to altered immune function can occur.

Study of patients with severe T-cell defects revealed an increased incidence of serious infections with agents such as *Monilla, Pneumocystis carinii*, herpes zoster, cytomegalovirus, and other "opportunistic organisms." These patients experience chronic thrush, interstitial pneumonitis, and intractable diarrhea. They frequently develop generalized vaccinia following smallpox vaccination and generalized BCGosis if immunized with viable bacille Calmette-Guérin. By contrast, patients with defective antibody production experience recurrent infections with high-grade encapsulated organisms such as pneumococci and *Hemophilus influenzae*. These patients present with recurrent otitis media, sinusitis, bronchitis, and pneumonia. Fulminant bacterial sepsis and meningitis are commonly seen, whereas significant infection with herpesviruses such as varicella-zoster virus or cytomegalovirus are not.

CELLULAR AND MOLECULAR COMPONENTS

The normal, functioning immune system involves an extremely complex orchestra of cells, signal and recognition molecules, and receptors. During the 1960s and 1970s, great advances in understanding the cellular components of the system were made. In the 1980s and 1990s, an explosion of information concerning the details of many of the molecular mechanisms involved in the functioning of the immune system has become available. With this burgeoning understanding, the defects responsible for many of the primary immunodeficiency diseases are just beginning to be identified.

A comprehensive survey of the basic molecular mechanisms of the immune system are beyond the scope of this chapter. Antibody-producing cells develop through a series of differentiation stages that mirror the molecular events leading to the expression of immunoglobulin molecules.[3] Hematopoietic precursors differentiate to become cells containing μ immunoglobulin heavy-chain molecules in their cytoplasm.[4] These pre-B cells lack surface-expressed immunoglobulin molecules and, therefore, are not directly stimulated by antigens in their environment. Next, the cells express genes encoded as part of the immunoglobulin light-chain locus, and these combine with the μ heavy chains to form complete multichain molecules. With further differentiation of the B cell, including mechanisms involving alternative splicing of the IgM mRNA transcript, some immunoglobulin molecules are expressed as a part of the cell membranes of the developing B cells. This allows these cells to interact with antigenic determinants that have selective binding affinity for this particular rearranged immunoglobulin, which further stimulates these cells to divide and differentiate. Additional molecular mechanisms, some involving the direct membrane interaction or secretion of cytokine molecules by other lymphoid cells in the immediate environment of the responding B cell, induce switching of the class of immunoglobulin being expressed and secreted by the B cell.

The genes that specify the structure of each antibody (or T-cell receptor, TCR) are not present as such in the germ line. They are found as discontinuous DNA segments in the nonlymphoid cells of the body.[5-9] During the differentiation of precursor stem cells into antibody-producing cells, a series of rearrangements of the immunoglobulin genes occurs that both activates these genes and serves to amplify the diversity of the resulting gene products. Individual mutations also increase the diversity of B-cell products, such that millions of different distinct immunoglobulin molecules can be generated by the B-cell system. In T cells, genes encoding the antigen receptor are also shuffled as precursor cells develop into mature T lymphocytes, resulting in diversity of these immune receptors in a similar fashion.

The detailed account of immunoglobulin gene rearrangement and activation has been presented in Chap. 128. The immunoglobulin chain genes are located at band q32 of chromosome 14, the κ light-chain genes at band p11 of chromosome 2, and the λ light-chain genes at band q11 on chromosome 22.[10-13] As the precursor stem cells differentiate to pre-B cells, DNA rearrangement occurs, bringing the separate gene segments found in the germ line into continuity. The heavy chain gene family contains several hundred variable region (V_H) genes, which encode the first 95 amino acids of the variable portion of the heavy chain, more than 20 diversity region (D) genes, which encode the next few amino acids, six joining region (J_H) genes, which encode the final 13 amino acids of the variable region, and then a series of nine functional constant region (C_H genes).[14] As the initial event, a single D_H segment is combined with a single J_H segment through a process of DNA rearrangement. Following DJ_H joining, a single V_H element is combined with this DJ segment. As a consequence of this VDJ_H joining, a promoter sequence present 5′ to the V_H segment is brought close to a tissue-specific enhancer sequence located 3′ to the J region, between the J and C genes.[15,16] This ten activates the gene complex, increasing transcription of mRNA for the heavy-chain gene utilizing the first of the C_H gene segments, the one for μ. This results in production of cytoplasmic μ chain and thus the appearance of the pre-B cell.

Following an effective heavy-chain gene rearrangement,

the light-chain genes rearrange, and this event is followed by the eventual assembly of complete IgM molecules and their expression on the cell surface. B cells and their progeny produce only one of the two possible light-chain types. However, B cells can produce both IgM and IgD simultaneously and are capable of switching subsequently to produce other immunoglobulin isotypes. The simultaneous production of IgM and IgD as well as the transition from membrane-bound Ig to the production of the secreted form involves alternative mRNA splicing.[17,18] The conversion of a B cell expressing IgM and IgD to a B cell expressing another isotype involves a process known as heavy-chain class switching.

In class switching, an area known as the switch region located 5′ to each C_H gene is spliced to the switch region of the downstream heavy-chain C region to be expressed.[19,20] During this recombination, deletion of the DNA between the two switch regions occurs, allowing a new constant region to be transcribed with the preexisting VDJ_H recombined variable region gene. Failure of class switching occurs in the primary immunodeficiency known as immunodeficiency with hyper-IgM, recently shown to be associated with a defect in the expression of CD40 ligand on the helper T cell.[21,22]

T cells are also derived from pluripotent stem cells, which mature and differentiate under the influence of the microenvironment of the thymus. During maturation, T cells express a variety of cell membrane glycoproteins, which correlate with the functional properties of the differentiated cells.[23,24] The most primitive cells in the thymus express CD7. Subsequently, thymocytes coexpress CD4 and CD8 and, finally, they express CD3 as well as the TCR for antigen. Mature T cells leaving the thymus express CD4 or CD8, but usually not both, and these cell populations represent distinct functional classes of cells. While the immunoglobulin receptors on B cells can recognize free antigen, T lymphocytes recognize only antigens that have been "processed" or degraded and that are presented on the surface of macrophages and other "antigen-presenting cells" in conjunction with membrane molecules of the major histocompatibility locus (MHC). Helper T cells co-recognize antigen in association with MHC class II (HLA-DR, -DS, -DQ) molecules, with the T-cell CD4 molecules involved in this class-II-restricted recognition process. Thus, most helper T cells are included in the CD4 T-cell subpopulation.[25,26] Cytotoxic T cells also recognize foreign antigens associated with MHC. In those cases in which the cytotoxic T cell responds to antigens in association with class I MHC molecules (HLA-A, -B, -C), the CD8 T-cell subpopulation is involved.[26] When the cytotoxic T cell recognizes antigens in association with class II MHC molecules, the T cells are in the CD4 subset.

The TCR for antigen is a disulfide-linked heterodimer consisting of a 45- to 50-kDa α subunit and a 40-to 45-kDa β subunit.[27–29] Both α and β chains consist of constant and variable domains, and these two chains are part of a macromolecular complex that includes the five nonpolymorphic polypeptides making up the CD3 complex. The α and β chains recognize antigen, while the CD3 complex transduces the signal to nucleus, initiating cellular activation. An alternative TCR employing γ and δ instead of α and β chains is used on a significantly smaller subpopulation of T cells with a more restricted variable-chain repetoire.[30–32]

The recombinatorial processes for the generation of the T-cell antigen receptor are similar (Fig. 129-1) to those used by the B-cell immunoglobulin genes, and a common recombinase performs all of the variable-region gene-assembly events of both B and T cells.[33]

SEVERE COMBINED IMMUNODEFICIENCY

Severe combined immunodeficiency (SCID) is the most extreme form of the inherited primary immunodeficiency diseases. It is characterized by profound defects in both the humoral and cell-mediated immune systems. A positive family history is obtained in about 50 percent of cases with SCID. Within this disease classification are several distinct disorders that have different modes of inheritance and different patterns of cellular deficiency. Both autosomal

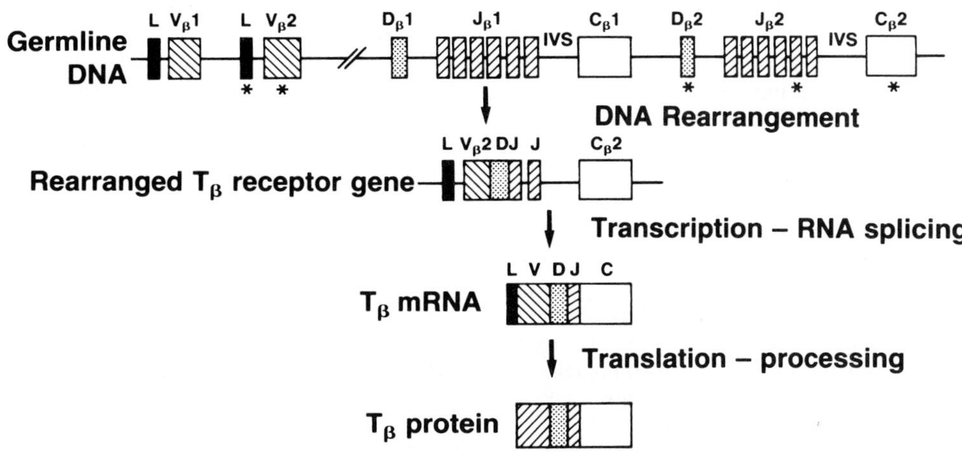

FIG. 129-1 The arrangement of the human T-cell receptor β-chain gene locus. Multiple variable (V_{β}) regions exist, each with one associated leader (L) sequence. There are two alternative diversity (D_{β}) segments and two sets of six alternative joining (J_{β}) segments encoding the remainder of the variable region. There are also two alternative constant (C_{β}) region elements per allele. DNA rearrangements lead to the joining of a single V with a single D and a single J element. When the gene is activated, RNA is transcribed, and the intervening sequences (IVS) are removed by RNA splicing. The leader sequence is removed after translation and the processed protein is inserted into the T-cell surface membrane in association with the T-cell receptor α-chain protein and the molecules of the T3 complex. In this example, the germ line elements marked (*) have rearranged to form the active gene.

recessive and X-linked modes of inheritance have been demonstrated in SCID.[34,35] By definition, SCID is a disorder of infancy, since the immune deficit is so profound that children usually die of infection in the first weeks or months of life.

Clinical Features

Infants with SCID present with infections within the first weeks of life. Recurrent pneumonia, failure to thrive, chronic diarrhea, and persistent *Candida* infection of the mouth, esophagus, and skin of the face and diaper area are common. These children are susceptible to infections with all types of microorganisms, but infections with opportunistic pathogens tend to dominate the clinical picture. Death has resulted from generalized chickenpox, measles with Hecht pneumonia, and cytomegalovirus and adenovirus infection. In addition to infections, many children with SCID have developed graft-versus-host disease (GVHD) following transfusions of whole blood containing immunocompetent T lymphocytes from adult donors. Maternal lymphocytes entering the fetal circulation during labor and delivery or during gestation have also caused GVHD in infants with SCID.[36] When smallpox vaccination was routinely employed, inoculated SCID infants regularly developed generalized vaccinia. Paralytic poliomyelitis also has occurred following administration of live attenuated polio vaccine to infants with SCID.

The physical examination of infants with SCID shows evidence of acute and chronic infection and failure to thrive. Lymph nodes are not palpable, and the tonsils and adenoids are absent. Chest radiographs may show evidence of infection but will also reveal the absence of a thymic shadow.

Immunologic Defects

SCID is a dual-system immune deficiency disease with severe functional defects in both the T- and B-cell immune systems. Careful laboratory evaluation may disclose considerable heterogeneity, with certain portions of the immune system preserved essentially intact in some patients. The levels of serum IgM, IgA, and IgG are usually extremely low, but a few patients have been found with normal amounts of one or more of the immunoglobulin isotypes.[37] Antibody responses, however, have been almost universally absent. B lymphocytes may be absent in some SCID patients, while others may have almost normal numbers of B cells. In these patients, B cells may account for all the circulating lymphocytes, since T-cell deficiency is the norm for this disease.

All tests of cell-mediated immunity give abnormal results in SCID. Numbers of peripheral blood T cells are depressed to less than 10 percent of normal in 90 percent of SCID patients.[38] All patients are anergic to recall skin test antigens and cannot be sensitized to new antigens. They are even unresponsive to intradermal administration of phytohemagglutinin and have a profound defect in skin allograft rejection.[38] In vitro T-cell function tests show marked impairment, with defective proliferative responses to mitogens, lack of cytotoxic T-cell activity, and absent T-cell immunoregulatory activity.

Genetics and Pathogenesis

SCID is a diagnostic category containing a heterogeneous group of disorders that have dual-system immunodeficiency as the common feature; therefore, no single pathogenic mechanism is operative in all cases. There are autosomal recessive as well as X-linked forms of SCID. As more and more data on the molecular mechanisms of these disorders have appeared, it has become apparent that they include a much broader spectrum of clinical presentations than previously recognized. Classic SCID is now seen as representing the extreme end of the spectrum of clinical presentations of several of these dual-system or combined immunodeficiency syndromes.

X-Linked SCID, XSCID. Forty to sixty percent of SCID occurs in male infants with an X-linked pattern of inheritance. XSCID patients are deficient in both T cells and B cells, but female carriers of this mutant gene, it is interesting to note, are immunologically normal. Studies of the pattern of X chromosome inactivation in the peripheral T cells from obligate carriers of XSCID have shown an unbalanced pattern of X-chromosome inactivation, indicating that the XSCID gene defect results in failure of normal T-cell development in the cells that use this gene.[40] Mature B cells from these obligate carriers also demonstrate a skewed pattern of X inactivation, with the normal X as the active X, while immature B cells and monocytes show a balanced X chromosome use.[41,42] These observations suggest that the gene defect in XSCID does not affect the primitive lymphohematopoietic stem cell but, rather, involves a later stage of lymphoid development so that there is selection against cells whose active X bears the mutant gene.

Recently, studies of three unrelated patients with XSCID have found a defect in the gene for the γ chain of the interleukin-2 (IL-2) receptor.[43] IL-2 and IL-2 receptors are critical in the regulation of the duration and magnitude of the antigen-induced T-cell immune response.[44] The receptor for IL-2 is expressed to different degrees on T cells, B cells, NK cells, and monocytes. It is a multichain receptor, and different combinations of the IL-2 receptor′, β, and γ chains result in the formation of different IL-2 receptors with different cellular distributions and IL-2 binding affinities. Low-affinity IL-2 receptors contain IL-2R′ alone, while intermediate-affinity receptors contain IL-r β and γ but not IL-2R. High-affinity receptors contain all three chains. Intermediate- and high-affinity receptors are important for IL-2 signaling. The IL-2R γ chain gene spans 4.2 kb at Xq13 and is organized in 10 exons and 9 introns. Direct sequencing of the gene in these three patients showed that each contained a different point mutation resulting in a different premature stop codon and predicted C-terminal truncation of the protein.[43]

The development of SCID in patients with defects in the IL-2R γ gene suggests that IL-2R γ is critical for thymic maturation of lymphoid stem cells. Cases of combined immunodeficiency have been previously observed in patients with defective IL-2 production or signal transduction,[45–48] suggesting that mutations in components of the IL-2/IL-2R system should be carefully explored as the cause of other cases of combined or cellular immunodeficiency. The identification of this gene defect as a cause of XSCID should permit development of more accurate tests for carrier detection as well as prenatal diagnosis. The potential for gene therapy for this disease is now also being actively studied.

SCID with Adenosine Deaminase Deficiency, ADA(−)SCID. ADA(−)SCID was the first of the primary immunodeficiency diseases in which the specific enzyme defect was identified.[49] The disorder (discussed in detail in Chap. 52) is inherited as an autosomal recessive trait and is indistinguishable clinically from cases of SCID with normal ADA.[50,51] The diagnosis is usually made by measuring the ADA concentration in red blood cells. ADA activity is present in fetal cells, so prenatal diagnosis of ADA deficiency is possible.[52–54]

ADA is a 38-kDa enzyme coded for by a gene on chromosome 20. The enzyme catalyzes the conversion of adenosine and deoxyadenosine to inosine and deoxyinosine, respectively. The mechanism by which ADA deficiency results in immune deficiency is not completely understood, but it is probably related to the accumulation of ADA substrates rather than to a deficiency of a product of ADA enzyme action (Fig. 129-2). The ADA substrates, adenosine and 2′-deoxyadenosine, accumulate in high concentrations, and both compounds are toxic to lymphocytes, particularly T cells.[55–68] Many mechanisms have been proposed, but none alone adequately explains all the findings in this disorder. ADA deficiency can result in elevated levels of cyclic AMP, pyrimidine starvation, diminished cellular phosphoribosyl pyrophosphate, inhibition of ribonucleotide reductase and S-adenosylhomocystine hydrolase, and accelerated poly (ADP)ribose synthesis with NAD and ATP depletion. Other effects are also likely, and probably several mechanisms cooperate in the pathophysiology of this disease.

ADA deficiency has a unique combination of features that led to its selection as an early candidate for gene therapy. The gene was cloned in 1983,[69–71] and its function has been extensively characterized. Although ADA is expressed to different degrees in various cells and organs, the gene's expression is not under tight regulation (for example, it does not depend on the phase of the cell cycle or other critical variables). Individuals with ADA levels ranging from less than one-tenth of the normal mean to over 50 times normal have normal immune function,[72,73] further indicating that precise control of the inserted gene's expression should not be necessary and suggesting that unwanted side effects would be an unlikely consequences of moderate over- or under-expression of the replaced gene. The disease is curable by transplantation with lymphoid cells from normal donors, suggesting that ex-vivo genetic correction of the patient's own lymphoid cells could similarly be effective treatment. This is in contrast to another disorder of purine metabolism, the Lesch-Nyhan syndrome (see Chap. 50), in which bone marrow transplantation does not cure the neurologic defects, and, therefore, ex vivo gene therapy of the bone marrow would also not be expected to be successful therapy. Since the lymphoid system is very dependent on cellular proliferation for appropriate functioning, a gene-transfer technique achieving stable integration of the inserted gene is necessary for long-term genetic correction. In addition, since bone marrow transplantation can result in immunoreconstitution in this disease without using preparative cytoreductive conditioning, it is expected that the autologous gene-corrected cells will also have a significant survival advantage, permitting the use of gene transfer techniques that are less than completely efficient in correcting every lymphoid cell.

Combined Immunodeficiency with Defective Expression of MHC Class II Genes. A unique form of combined immunodeficiency is associated with the lack of expression of cell membrane MHC class II[74–78] cell-surface antigens. Since T cells "see" antigen after it is processed and then presented in association with MHC antigens, the lack of MHC expression cripples the T-cell recognition process. Quite unlike the other disorders having profound functional defects in responses to foreign antigens, this disorder is characterized by the continued presence of normal numbers of both T cells and B cells. Almost all of the bone marrow-derived cells, including lymphocytes and monocytes as well as epithelial and endothelial cells, lack expression of all HLA class II (DR, DQ, DS) molecules. This disorder is transmitted as an autosomal recessive trait, but inheritance is not linked to genes on chromosome 6, the chromosomal location of the MHC genes. HLA Class II´ and β chains are not synthesized, leading to the idea that this disease results from a general MHC class II regulatory defect. The binding of nuclear proteins to the promoter region of the HLA class II genes was evaluated. Individual proteins known to bind to either the Y-box, the TRE/CRE element, or the X-box were studied in detail in these patients' cells.[78] These studies clearly demonstrated that RF-X, a factor that binds to the X-box motif common to all HLA class II promoters, is abnormal in this disorder. There is a family of RF-X factors. Two of the cloned RF-X genes have been mapped to the short arm of chromosome 19,[79] but the particular X-box binding protein

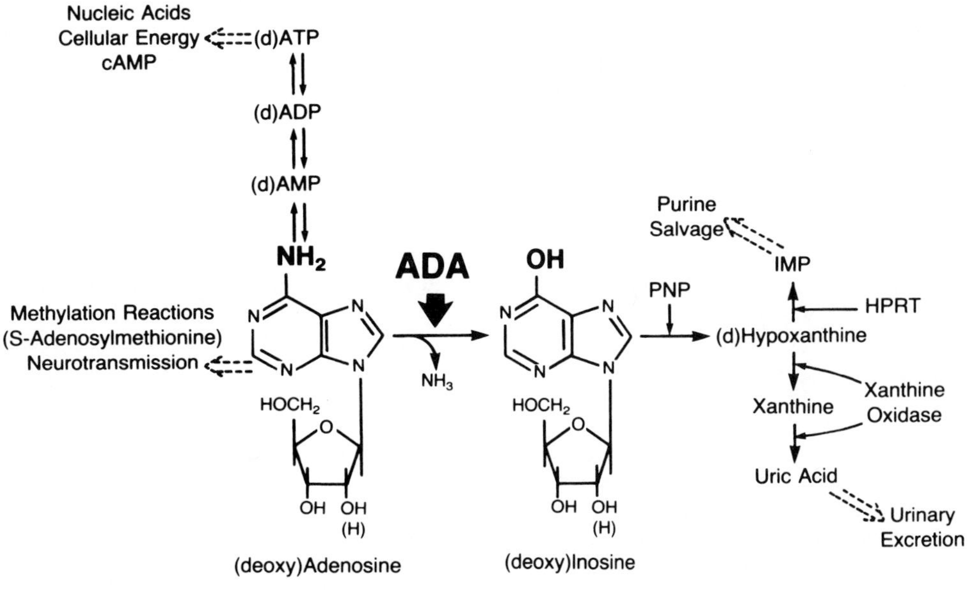

FIG. 129-2 **The pathway of purine metabolism, illustrating the site of action of adenosine deaminase (ADA). The accumulation of deoxyadenosine and dATP as a consequence of the ADA deficiency leads to lymphocytotoxicity and subsequent combined T-cell and B-cell immunodeficiency.**

responsible for the defective regulation in MHC class II deficiency has not yet been identified. This disease represents one of the first examples of a genetic defect involving a DNA-binding regulatory protein.

Congenital T-Cell Receptor Immunodeficiency. TCR is a transmembrane complex of at least seven polypeptide chains. Two chains form a heterodimer that determines antigen specificity (/β, γ/δ). The CD3 monomorphic components are involved in signal transduction (γ, δ, ε η, ζ). Defects in both portions of the TCR complex have been described and can result in impaired T-cell activation.[80–84] These are mild and severe phenotypes of immunodeficiency, which appear to correlate roughly with differences in the levels of TCR surface expression and T-cell function in vivo. Not enough is yet known about the fundamental genetic defect in most instances to define a specific disorder. The biochemical basis of one of the cases is a selective inherited deficiency of the CD3 γ component, which is suggested to cause impaired association of the CD3 ζ chain with the other chains of the CD3–TCR complex.[84] The fact that both normal children and children with SCID in the same family can manifest the defective cell membrane phenotype suggests that the deficiency is more complicated than merely the malfunctioning of a gene encoding one of the polypeptide chains of the receptor complex.

Other Types of SCID. SCID has been described in several other contexts, but clear metabolic or genetic data concerning these disorders has not yet been developed. *SCID with generalized hematopoietic hypoplasia (reticular dysgenesis)* is the most severe form of SCID, since it is characterized by agranulocytosis as well as profound dual-system immunodeficiency. These patients die of overwhelming infection within hours or days of birth because they lack both specific immunity and a critical nonspecific defense agent, the polymorphonuclear leukocyte.[85–88] *SCID with failure of lymphoid stem cell development (Swiss type)* is a name used for a rare autosomal recessive disorder in which infants lack both T and B lymphocytes.[89] It is unclear whether this disease classification actually represents a distinct entity or a combination of several even rarer defects. Similarly, *SCID with normal B cells* is a general diagnostic grouping that probably will disappear as specific molecular defects responsible for disease are described for subgroups of patients in this category. In many of these cases, the primary defect is probably a failure of T-cell development, with the lack of B-lymphocyte maturation occurring as a secondary event. Defects at the level of the prethymic T-lymphocyte precursor, the intrathymic T lymphocyte, and the postthymic T-cell precursor have all been demonstrated.[90,91] B cells from some of these patients have been shown to produce IgG and IgA as well as IgM in response to stimulation with pokeweed mitogen in vitro when cocultured with T cells from a normal individual. In this case, the normal T cells provided appropriate helper T-cell activity, which permitted the patient's B cells to function normally.

Treatment of SCID

The need to develop effective treatment for these desperately ill children has been one of the greatest challenges for clinical immunology. In 1968, bone marrow transplantation was introduced to clinical medicine when an infant with SCID was given bone marrow from a histocompatible sibling.[92] The transplanted marrow effected total immunologic reconstitution in this infant and opened a new era in therapy for this and many other immunologic and hematologic disorders. In the two decades since its introduction, bone marrow transplantation has been performed in several hundred infants with SCID. When the donor was a genotypically identical HLA-matched sibling and the transplant was performed when the infant was free of serious infection, over 80 percent of SCID recipients have had long-lasting immunologic reconstitution.

Since only a minority of patients have an HLA-matched sibling donor, many alternative transplantation strategies have been tried. Transplantation with whole bone marrow from HLA-incompatible donors has been almost universally unsuccessful because of the development of fatal GVHD. To avoid this, transplants with embryonic lymphoid tissues such as fetal thymus and fetal liver have been attempted. Initially the rate of immunologic reconstitution in SCID recipients of fetal tissue was less than 20 percent and was frequently limited to partial T-cell recovery without any B-cell reconstitution. Recently it has been found that children maintained in a germ-free environment for several months after fetal liver transplantation have a better rate of immune reconstitution, perhaps because of the slow pace of repopulation of the lymphoid population when fetal grafts are used.

More recently, reconstitution using HLA-nonidentical bone marrow treated to remove mature T lymphocytes has shown very promising results.[93] In this approach, parents are used as marrow donors, so that at least 50 percent identity is maintained between the donor and recipient to enhance MHC-dependent interactions between the donor immune cells and the host tissues. T cells in the donor marrow are eliminated by treatment either with lectins, monoclonal antibodies, and complement or with immunotoxins to remove the cells capable of causing GVHD.[94,95] The success rate with this technique in infants with SCID is now approaching that of transplants using HLA-identical siblings as the marrow donors, offering potential cure to almost every infant with this disease. With the establishment of large international databases of individuals who have been HLA typed, the possibility of finding an HLA-matched unrelated donor have increased dramatically over the past decade. Matched-unrelated bone marrow transplantation has now been used successfully in several forms of SCID and will be increasingly used as the number of potential donors in the various databases increases.

Bone marrow transplantation has been successful in the treatment of both ADA(+) and ADA(−) SCID.[96] Enzyme replacement has also been attempted in the treatment of ADA(−)SCID. Initially, exchange tranfusions with irradiated whole blood were used, since erythrocytes are a rich source of ADA.[97] In practice, erythrocyte transfusions have not been very effective in correcting the immunodeficiency in ADA(−)SCID patients. They have, however, resulted in transient improvement in lymphocyte functioning in vitro and correction of the levels of deoxyadenosine in the blood and deoxy-ATP in the lymphoid cells of these patients. In 1985, Herschfield and colleagues administered large amounts of bovine ADA conjugated to polyethylene glycol (PEG-ADA) to ADA(−)SCID patients.[98] The PEG conjugation renders the bovine enzyme nonimmunogenic and increases its half-life in blood from just minutes to several hours. Weekly or twice-weekly intramuscular injections of PEG-ADA have resulted in a modest to striking improvement in the biochemical and immunologic defects seen in many ADA(−) patients. It is unclear why the degree of immune reconstitution achieved by enzyme replacement in different patients has been so varied, but clearly many patients have been helped significantly by this treatment.

The primary immunodeficiency diseases as a group are among the best initial candidates for gene therapy because many of these disorders are cured by allogeneic bone marrow transplantation. If one can cure the disease by providing normal bone marrow stem cells, there is reason to hope that genetic correction of the patients' own stem cells would also be effective treatment.[90–101] In this regard, gene therapy has been successfully used to treat several patients with ADA deficiency. In the initial trial begun in 1990,[102] two children achieving less than complete immune reconstitution with PEG-ADA treatment were treated with repeated infusions of autologous, cultured, expanded ADA gene-corrected T cells. These children showed significant objective improvements in lymphocyte counts, cellular and humoral immune responses, and general well-being.[103] Second-generation gene therapy trials for ADA deficiency employing various strategies for lymphohematopoietic stem cell gene correction are currently under way, including treatment of autologous CD34 selected cord blood stem cells of affected newborns identified by prenatal testing.

ATAXIA TELANGIECTASIA

Ataxia telangiectasia (AT) is an autosomal recessive disorder characterized by variable immunodeficiency, oculocutaneous telangiectasia, and cerebellar ataxia. Onset of the neurologic deficit typically occurs in early childhood and dominates the clinical picture throughout.[104,105]

Clinical Features

Neurologic symptoms are the usual presenting problem in these patients, with difficulty in learning to walk commonplace. The early manifestation of cerebellar dysfunction as ataxia is followed somewhat later by chorioathetosis, myoclonic jerking, and oculomotor abnormalities. The telangiectases characteristic of this disease usually appear by to 7 years of age. They initially appear on the bulbar conjunctiva (Fig. 129-3) and develop later on the skin in exposed areas and areas of trauma such as the nasal bridge, the ears, and the flexor folds on the neck and extremities. Other cutaneous manifestations include vitiligo, café au lait spots, an early loss of subcutaneous fat, and premature graying of the hair. Endocrine abnormalities are also very common and may

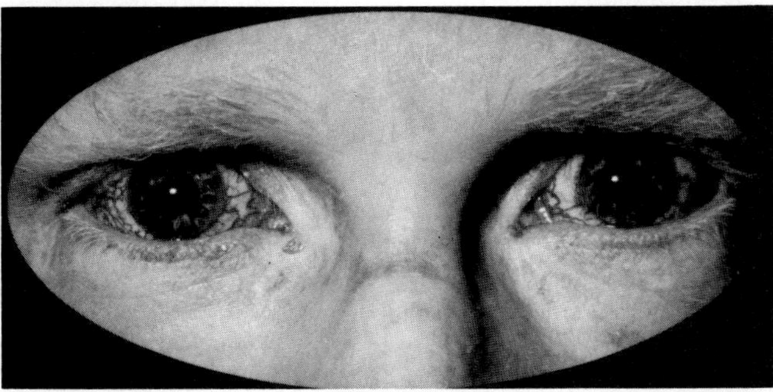

FIG. 129-3 Telangiectatic blood vessels on the bulbar conjunctiva and nasal bridge of a 22-year-old patient with ataxia telangiectasia. The recognition of these vascular abnormalities is frequently the initial clue leading to the correct diagnosis in a child being evaluated for cerebellar ataxia.

involve multiple organs. More than 50 percent of patients display glucose intolerance.[106] Delayed or absent development of secondary sexual characteristics in females is associated with absent or hypoplastic ovaries. Hypogonadism is a less consistent finding in males. Half the patients have mild elevations in liver enzymes, which is usually associated with fatty infiltration and round-cell accumulation in the portal areas.

An increased incidence of cancer is a feature of several of the primary immunodeficiency diseases and is prominent in AT, with up to 15 percent of the patients ultimately dying of malignancy.[107,108] Non-Hodgkins lymphomas predominate in childhood AT patients, as they do in other primary immunodeficiency diseases. Adult male patients have an estimated seventy fold higher incidence of carcinoma of the stomach than the general population. It is interesting that these cases of carcinoma all have occurred in AT patients who lack serum IgA, although IgA deficiency is seen in only 70 percent of ataxia telangiectasia patients overall.[109] Rare forms of lymphoid leukemia have been observed, including subacute T-cell lymphocytic leukemia and T-cell chronic lymphocytic leukemia. In these T-cell malignancies, chromosomal translocations have been defined for several patients with a high incidence of breakpoints clustered on chromosomes 14a11, 7p13-15, and 7q32-35.[110–113] These are the chromosomal regions that undergo rearrangement to generate active TCR genes. In addition, breaks and translocations involving chromosome 14q32, the site of the immunoglobulin heavy-chain genes, are frequent in AT.

Recurrent infections are a major feature in some patients, while other patients seem to have little problem with infection. In general there is a good correlation between the severity of infectious illnesses and the immunologic status of the patient.[104] Sinopulmonary infections are the most common problem. Chronic pulmonary disease, which is contributed to by both the immune deficiency and recurrent aspiration of oral secretions secondary to the neurologic deficit, results in pulmonary failure as a common terminal event.

Immunologic Defects

AT has a variable pattern of immunodeficiency, with considerable differences from patient to patient even within the same family. Defects in both humoral and cellular immunity have been described, but few of the abnormalities occur in all or even most patients.[104,114] The most consistent B-lymphocyte defects are an absence of serum IgA in about 75 percent and of serum IgE in about 85 percent of patients. The IgA and IgE deficiencies may occur independently of one another, and siblings within a family may have different patterns of immunoglobulin deficiency. IgG2 and IgG4 may also be deficient in this disorder.[115] In addition, 80 percent of patients have serum IgM in a monomeric 7S form rather than as the pentameric 19S molecule usually found in serum. Total B lymphocyte numbers are normal, as are numbers of IgA-bearing B cells. Antibody responses to a variety of specific antigens have been variable, with no consistent pattern of deficiency present. Autoantibodies to self-antigens are common in AT. Included are antibodies to mitochondria, basement membranes, muscle, thyroid, and even immunoglobulins.[116]

The cellular immune system also shows variable degrees of impairment. Many patients are anergic to delayed hypersensitivity skin testing, and a few have had delayed skin allograft rejection. Half of the patients have depressed lymphocyte proliferative responses to mitogens, and even more have defective proliferative and cytotoxic T-cell responses to viral pathogens.[117] Immunoregulatory T-cell function has also been variable, with defects in helper T-cell function and in vitro immunoglobulin production observed in more than half the patients studied.[118]

Pathogenesis

The fundamental biochemical defect underlying AT is unknown. However, the constellation of findings in the patients has led to two major hypotheses. One of the most striking and consistent pathologic features of this disease is that the thymus is small or absent, lacks Hassall corpuscles, and is embryonic in appearance.[119] This observation led to the proposal that the disorder is a consequence of a defect in tissue differentiation.[120] Auerbach[121] first showed that thymic development depends on the interaction of ectodermal and mesodermal elements. The proposed defect in AT involved a failure in the development and maturation of tissues that require an essential interaction between primitive mesoderm and ectoderm. Supporting this hypothesis was the observation that AT patients have high circulating concentrations of oncofetal antigens, which are ordinarily found only with immaturity. α-Fetoprotein, a protein produced normally by the fetal liver, was shown to be elevated in 59 of 60 AT patients but not in their parents or in patients with other immunodeficiency diseases (Fig. 129-4).[122] AT patients have been reported also to have elevated levels of carcinoembryonic antigen.[123] As an additional correlative observation, ovarian agenesis is frequently seen in these patients.

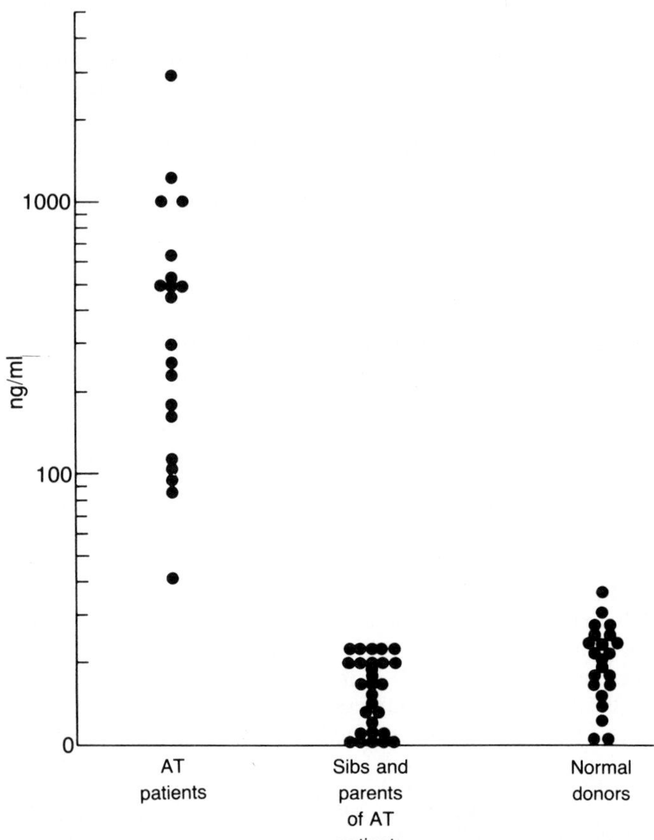

FIG. 129-4 The levels of α-fetoprotein in the serum of patients with ataxia telangiectasia (AT), their normal sibs and parents, and a group of normal donors. Elevated α-fetoprotein is one of the most consistent findings in this disorder and may be useful in early diagnosis of affected patients. (*Courtesy of Dr. Thomas A. Waldmann.*)

Another hypothesis advanced to explain some of the manifestations of this disease was developed after it was observed that patients with AT have an increased sensitivity to ionizing radiation and radiomimetic drugs.[124,125] Furthermore, cultured fibroblasts from AT patients have a markedly reduced colony-forming ability after x-irradiation but are not unusually sensitive to ultraviolet irradiation, in contrast to cells from patients with xeroderma pigmentosum. There is presumably a defect in DNA repair after x-irradiation in these cells, but convincing evidence for a specific biochemical defect has not been presented.[126–128] Fibroblasts from different patients have been fused and found to cross-correct the defect in x-ray sensitivity. At least five complementation groups have been defined by this technique.[129,130] The AT cells examined failed to pause sufficiently after x-ray for DNA repair to be completed. Rather, they launch directly into DNA replication. As mentioned, there is a high incidence of chromosomal translocations in the leukemia cells of these patients as well as in cultured lymphocyte lines established from AT patients. These translocations usually involve chromosomes 7 and 14, the sites of the T-cell receptor genes and the immunoglobulin heavy-chain genes. These are chromosomal regions that undergo DNA rearrangements, deletions, and repair to generate active receptor genes. Further, site-specific DNA breaks and subsequent repair are involved in immunoglobulin heavy chain class switching. If such breaks are not normally repaired in AT patients, they could contibute to both the immune deficiency and the neoplasia observed. For example, AT patients frequently have reduced or absent IgA, IgG2, IgG4, and IgE, the immunoglobulins encoded by the genes at the 3′ end of the heavy-chain gene cluster.[115,131] These Ig classes are dependent on additional steps of site-specific DNA breaking and rejoining to generate an active gene and could be expected to be more severely affected by an abnormality in this cellular mechanism.

The seemingly unrelated multisystem biological defects that are characteristic of AT—including thymic dystrophy, chromosomal instability radiosensitivity, Purkinje cell degeneration, and telangiectasia—are difficult to reconcile with any particular hypothesis, and true understanding will most likely await the cloning and characterization of the gene involved. Linkage studies[132] have clearly localized the AT gene to a 3-cM region of chromosome 11q22-23. Although the presence of several complementation groups suggests that more than one AD gene may exist, convincing evidence for another locus has not been found by linkage studies of more than 150 AT families.[132]

Treatment

No form of therapy has proved to be effective either in preventing progression of the neurologic disability or in reconstituting the immune system defects in this disease. Immunoglobulin replacement therapy and blood transfusions have been associated with severe and even fatal episodes of anaphylaxis in IgA-deficient AT patients. The mechanism of this anaphylaxis is the spontaneous production of anti-IgA antibodies in these patients, which then react with IgA in the infused blood products, resulting in the systemic allergic response.

WISKOTT-ALDRICH SYNDROME

Wiskott-Aldrich syndrome (WAS) is an X-linked condition characterized by the clinical triad of recurrent infections with all types of microorganisms, hemorrhages secondary to thrombocytopenia, and eczema of the skin.[133,134] Symptoms typically commence during the first 6 months of life with the appearance of petechiae and the development of infections such as otitis media.[135]

Clinical Features

Boys affected with WAS have a great variety of clinical problems. The severity of their immune deficiency is second only to that in SCID, leading to infections with high-grade encapsulated organisms such as *Hemophilus influenzae* and pneumococci as well as with opportunistic pathogens such as *Pneumocystis carinii*, cytomegalovirus, and *Candida albicans*. WAS patients have died with disseminated herpes simplex infections, and varicella has also been fatal, particularly in patients treated with corticosteroids.

The thrombocytopenia is often profound, with platelet counts averaging in the 15,000 to 30,000 cells per microliter range. Bleeding accounts for about 30 percent of the mortality in this disease, with intracranial hemorrhage the greatest threat. The thrombocytopenia is unique because WAS is the only disease regularly associated with small-sized platelets.[136] The mean platelet volume in idiopathic thrombocytopenic purpura, by contrast, is increased.

In addition to eczema, the third component of the classic clinical triad, these patients have a high incidence of severe autoimmune disease. This autoimmunity may take the form of Coombs'-positive hemolytic anemia, a juvenile rheumatoid arthritis-like syndrome with hectic fever and joint involvement, a leukocytoclastic vasculitis primarily involving the legs, and large-vessel vasculitis affecting the coronary or cerebral arteries. An autoimmune thrombocytopenia with high levels of platelet-associated IgG may be superimposed on the preexisting low platelet count or may be the cause of the reappearance of thrombocytopenia following splenectomy. High levels of circulating immune complexes may be found intermittently. The development of this aggressive autoimmune disorder may be an ominous sign of clinical deterioration.

Another striking feature of this disease is a high incidence of malignancy.[137,138] In some series over 20 percent of the patients develop cancer, usually a form of nonHodgkin lymphoma. Almost 50 per cent of these patients have lymphoma involving the brain, sometimes as the primary site. It appears that the incidence of lymphoma has lessened since the introduction of splenectomy and routine antibiotic prophylaxis. A confusing clinical issue is the frequent development of marked peripheral lymphadenopathy in these boys. These isolated nodes almost never contain lymphoma unless widely disseminated cancer is present.

Immunologic Defects

WAS has selective defects involving parts of each of the major host defense systems, in contrast to SCID, where more global defects are found.[139,140] The patients may have normal immunoglobulin levels, but the most common pattern is normal IgG, high levels of IgA and IgE, and IgM levels about half normal. Antibody responses to many antigens are normal, while responses to others are completely absent. WAS is the only described disorder in which patients fail to produce antibodies to an entire class of antigens, the polysaccharides. Therefore, these patients have low or absent isohemagglutinins. They produce antibodies to tetanus toxoid, a protein antigen, but not to the capsular polysaccharides of *H. influenzae* or pneumococcus.[141] This unique defect explains their susceptibility to infection with these encapsulated organisms despite normal or elevated total immunoglobulin levels in the serum.

Another unique abnormality in WAS is the observation that these patients hypercatabolize their serum immunoglobulins and albumin. The serum half-life of IgG, IgM, IgA, and albumin is shortened to one-third to one-half of normal. Therefore, to maintain normal serum levels, WAS patients actually synthesize immunoglobulin and albumin at far greater than normal rates.[142]

The cellular immune system also shows selective defects. The boys are generally anergic when tested for cutaneous delayed hypersensitivity, and even have prolonged survival of skin allografts.[141] However, they have nearly normal absolute T-lymphocyte numbers and a normal ratio of CD4 to CD8 cells. In vitro, their lymphocytes can proliferate well when stimulated with mitogens such as phytohemagglutinin[143] and produce substantial amounts of the lymphokines IL-I and IL-2. Nevertheless, their T cells proliferate very poorly in response to antigens or allogeneic cells, and these patients do not develop self-restricted virus-specific cytotoxic T cells even though they may produce antibody to the same virus.

The lymphocytes from WAS patients have been reported to have a characteristic appearance by scanning electron microscopy, which may be useful as a diagnostic test for this disease.[144] Carefully performed size analysis of platelets found a mean platelet volume more than 3 SD below the mean normal volume in 17 of 18 of our patients. This is probably the most reliable single test to confirm the diagnosis of WAS.[136]

The polymorphonuclear leukocytes from WAS patients have been reported to have a defect in chemotactic responsiveness, as do the monocytes from these patients[145,146] Their monocytes also have a defect in killer activity in antibody-dependent cellular cytotoxicity (ADCC) and in cytotoxicity mediated via the mannosylfucosyl membrane receptor.[147,148]

Pathogenesis and Genetics

The fundamental defect responsible for the diverse manifestations of WAS is unknown. At least seven distinct immunodeficiency diseases are inherited as X-linked traits, and each of the ones studied by linkage analysis has mapped to a different region of the X chromosome. WAS is most tightly linked to markers that map near the centromere on the short arm of X at Xp11.2-Xp11.3.[149]

The selective defects in cellular function involving T cells, B cells, granulocytes, platelets, and the mononuclear phagocytes demonstrate that this disorder is not the result of a defect in differentiation of just a single immune cellular element. Parkman and colleagues have described a defect in a cell membrane glycoprotein, GP115, on lymphocytes from some WAS patients as well as from another immunodeficient subject.[150-154] This molecule, sialophorin or CD43, is encoded by an intronless gene on chromosome 16 as a 400-amino-acid transmembrane protein with 90 *O*-linked and one *N*-linked oligosaccharide side chains. The mature protein contains 50 per cent carbohydrate by weight and appears in two predominant isoforms, a 115-kDa molecule found on T cells, thymocytes, and monocytes, and a 135-kDa molecule found on polymorphonuclear neutrophils, platelets, and B cells.[155] The intracytoplasmic portion has 123 amino acids, with a number of potential phosphorylation sites that might mediate signal transduction. CD43 has been proposed to play a role as a costimulatory molecule in T-cell activation as well as a potential participant in cell adhesion. Unfortunately, the nature of the CD43 defect in WAS has not been elucidated. It has been suggested that CD43 in WAS patients may be abnormal in that some sialic acid residues are more labile than normal and are thus lost from the surface of WAS cells more rapidly than from normal cells.[156] Given that the sialophorin gene does not map to the X chromosome but rather to chromosome 16,[157] this molecule can be involved centrally in the defect of WAS only if the involvement is indirect, occurring perhaps through a defect in a gene that regulates *O*-linked glycosylation or a similar trans-acting process. It has also been suggested that perhaps the WAS defect involves a defective glycosyltransferase that is involved in posttranslational modification of the CD34 molecule's carbohydrate side chains. Two groups have reported studies of this question with totally conflicting conclusions.[158,159] Our laboratory has used two different monoclonal anti-CD43 antibodies to study CD43 expression by FACS analysis of peripheral cells from 12 splenectomized WAS patients, and the results of this analysis were indistinguishable from the profiles found on the cells of normal control subjects. The possibility that the apparent defect in CD43 is a secondary event similar to the thrombocytopenia in WAS needs to be ruled out.

As with most X-linked immunodeficiency diseases, the carriers of WAS are immunologically and hematologically normal, demonstrating none of the defects found in the affected males. Carrier identification therefore has not been possible except for a few situations in large families where linkage analysis using RFLP markers has been successful.[149] Since females are mosaics for genes encoded on the X chromosome, some defect in immune or platelet function might be detectable in the blood of WAS heterozygotes. This should be possible unless there is selection against cells whose active X bears the mutant WAS gene so that all surviving peripheral cells use the X bearing the normal WAS gene as their active X chromosome; or, if both types of cells are present but the cells expressing the normal gene are somehow able to correct the defect in cells expressing the mutant gene. Because X inactivation is random and occurs in the very early embryo, essentially all cell lineages in the female body have the same ratio of cells in which each of the parental X chromosomes is active. Under average conditions, approximately 50 percent of a female's cells use the maternally derived X chromosome and the remaining half use the paternally derived X. Using RFLPs for the genes phosphoglycerol kinase and hypoxanthine-phosphoribosyl transferase to distinguish the maternally and paternally derived X chromosomes and methylation-sensitive restriction endonucleases to distinguish the active from inactive chromosomes, it has been possible to evaluate the pattern of X inactivation in the peripheral blood cells of WAS carriers. Skin biopsies from the carriers showed a normal random pattern of X inactivation. However, all T cells, B cells, and granulocytes in each of the carriers had a nonrandom pattern of X inactivation such that one homologue was used preferentially as the active X[160,161] (Fig. 129-5). This strikingly unbalanced pattern was seen in each of the 14 informative carriers studied and was not observed in any of over 80 normal female controls subjects. In the one family studied where linkage phase could be determined, the X bearing the normal allele at the WAS locus was used as the active X. Gealy and colleagues[162] have shown that a similar unbalanced X-chromosome utilization occurs in carrier platelets by evaluating isozymes of glucose 6-phosphate dehydrogenase in rare double heterozygotes for both glucose 6-phosphate dehydrogenase deficiency and WAS. These results provide the basis for carrier identification and also give unique insights into the extent of the cell lineages affected by the WAS genetic defect.

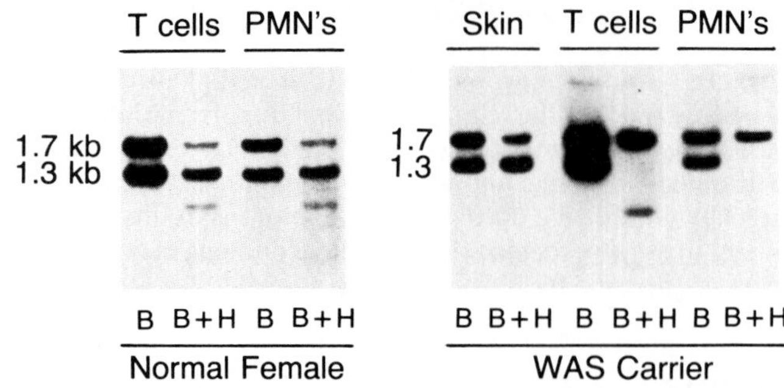

FIG. 129-5 **Unbalanced X-chromosome inactivation in a carrier of the Wiskott-Aldrich syndrome (WAS). A probe for the X-linked gene phosphoglycerate kinase (PKG) was hybridized to DNA extracted from various cell populations from normal females and carriers of the disease. B indicates DNA samples digested with the restriction endonuclease *BglI*, which is used to identify females who are heterozygous for a RFLP at this locus (1.7-kb and 1.3-kb alleles). In heterozygous females, another aliquot of DNA was further digested with *HpaII* (B + H). Methylated PGK gene segments are resistant to digestion by *HpaII*, and, therefore, the extent of digestion of the two alleles by *HpaII* indicates the relative proportion of methylated (i.e., inactive) to unmethylated (i.e., active) DNA. In the T cells and granulocytes (PMNs) of normal females, HpaII digestion, as expected, affects both alleles with a reduction in the intensity of both the 1.7- and the 1.3-kb bands and generation of fragments of smaller size. Similarly, the skin sample from the WAS carrier also shows a balanced pattern of X inactivation. By contrast, the DNA from the T cells and PMNs from the WAS carrier show a striking unbalanced pattern of X inactivation, with the 1.3-kb allele totally digested (i.e., active) and the 1.7-kb allele unchanged (i.e., inactive). This pattern indicates that all of the peripheral blood T cells and granulocytes from this carrier have the same X chromosome active, in contrast to the mixed usage seen with her skin cells or in the T cells and granulocytes of the normal female.**

Treatment

There are several potential forms of therapy for the WAS. HLA-matched bone marrow transplantation has a higher rate of success in this disease than in any other condition.[163,164] In over 30 patients treated, the level of cure exceeds 90 percent. Interestingly, after successful transplantation, all of the immune and hematologic abnormalities are corrected, as is the eczema.

The choice of treatment for patients lacking an HLA-matched sibling donor is more complex. T cell-depleted haploidentical bone marrow transplantation has been successful in less than 40 percent of cases, with failure of engraftment or B-cell lymphoma a fatal complication in several. Splenectomy cures the thrombocytopenia in over 90 percent of cases and has had a major impact on the patient's quality of life and on the medical management of this disease.[165] It is interesting, that the platelet size also normalizes after splenectomy.[136] Early experience with splenectomy was very poor, because many of the patients experienced overwhelming infections.[166] The use of routine prophylactic antibiotics and/or intravenous γ-globulin to prevent infections with high-grade pathogens has been essential to the successful use of splenectomy and seems to result in an overall lessened problem with infection as well. A recent review of our experience with 62 WAS patients showed an expected survival for nontransplanted, splenectomized patients of 25 years, while nonsplenectomized WAS patients had a mean survival of less than 5 years.[167]

The autoaggressive syndrome[168] that frequently complicates WAS may be very difficult to treat. Bone marrow transplantation has been used in this setting and has been successful. The thrombocytopenia that occasionally appears after splenectomy most commonly resolves without specific treatment. Corticosteroids, high-dose intravenous γ-globulin, and vinblastine have all been used with success in treating more prolonged episodes of this thrombocytopenia. The juvenile rheumatoid arthritis-like syndrome frequently responds to nonsteroidal anti-inflammatory treatment, but occasionally high-dose steroid therapy may be needed to control severe vasculitis. As with all cases of severe T-cell deficiency, all blood and platelets for transfusion should be irradiated to prevent GVHD.

ADDENDUM

Two very recent reports describe the basic defect in an autosomal recessive form of SCID.[169,170] The SCID phenotype was associated with an unusual T-cell subset distribution in blood; all patients in two unrelated families had virtually absent $CD8^+$ cells with normal to elevated numbers of $CD4^+$ cells. Although present, the $CD4^+$ cells did not respond normally to mitogenic stimuli such as phytohemagglutinin and concanavalin A. Functional studies suggested a defect in the coupling of activated TCR to cytoplasmic protein tyrosine kinases, an obligatory step in T-cell activation. Immunoblot analysis of multiple protein tyrosine kinases in leukocyte extracts showed a selective deficiency of ZAP-70. Molecular analysis in the two families led to the discovery of three ZAP-70 mutant alleles: a missense mutation involving a highly conserved serine, S518R; an intronic nucleotide substitution that alters splice site selection and causes insertion of three residues (-LEQ-) in the catalytic domain of the enzyme; and a 13-bp deletion that frameshifts translation after codon 503 in the kinase domain. Expression studies showed that all three mutations inactivate catalytic function.

REFERENCES

1. Bruton OC: Agammaglobulinemia. *Pediatrics* **9**:722, 1952.
2. Cooper MD, Peterson RDA, South MA, Good RA: The functions of the thymus system and the bursa system in chickens. *J Exp Med* **123**:75, 1966.
3. Cooper MD: Pre B cells: Normal and abnormal development. *J Clin Immunol* **1**:81, 1981.
4. Cooper MD, Kearney I, Scher I: B lymphocytes, in Paul WE (ed): *Fundamental Immunology*. New York, Raven, 1984, p 43.
5. Leder P: The genetics of antibody diversity. *Sci Am* **246**:102, 1982.
6. Honjo T: Immunoglobulin genes. *Annu Rev Immunol* **1**:499, 1983.
7. Tonegawa S: Somatic generation of antibody diversity. *Nature* **302**:575, 1983.
8. Hood LE, Weissman IL, Wood WB, Wilson JH: *Immunology*, 2d ed. Menlo Park, CA, Benjamin/Cummings, 1984, p 81.
9. Waldmann TA: The arrangement of immunoglobulin and T cell receptor genes in human lymphoproliferative disorders. *Adv Immuno* **40**:247, 1987.
10. Croce CM, Shander M, Martins J, Cicurel L, D'Ancona GG, Dolby TW, Koprowski H: Chromosomal locations of the human genes for immunoglobulin heavy chains. *Proc Natl Acad Sci USA* **76**:3416, 1979.
11. Erikson J, Martinis J, Croce CM: Assignment of the genes for human γ immunoglobulin chains to chromosome 22. *Nature* **295**:173, 1981.
12. Malcolm S, Barton P, Murphy C, Ferguson-Smith MA, Bentley DL, Rabbits TH: Localization of human immunoglobulin κ light chain variable region genes to the short arm of chromosome 2 by in situ hybridzation. *Proc Natl Acad Sci USA* **79**:4957, 1982.
13. McBride OW, Hieter PA, Hollis GF, Swan D, Otey MC, Leder P: Chromosomal location of human kappa and lambda immunoglobulin light chain constant region genes. *J Exp Med* **155**:1480, 1982.
14. Early P, Huang H, Davis M, Calame K, Hood L: An immunoglobulin heavy chain variable region gene is generated from three segments of DNA: V_H, D and J_H. *Cell* **19**:981, 1980.
15. Gillis SD, Morrison SL, OI VT, Tonegawa A: A tissue-specific transcription enhancer element is located in the major intron of a rearranged immunoglobulin heavy chain gene. *Cell* **33**:717, 1983.
16. Queen C, Baltimore D: Immunoglobulin gene transcription is activated by downstream sequence elements. *Cell* **33**:741, 1983.
17. Early P, Rogers J, Davis M, Calame K, Bond M, Wall R, Hood L: Two mRNAs can be produced from a single immunoglobulin μ gene by alternative RNA processing pathways. *Cell* **20**:313, 1980.
18. Moore KW, Rogers J, Hunkapiller T, Early P, Nottenburg C, Weiss Man J, Bazin H, Wall R, Hood LE: Expression of IgD may use both DNA rearrangement and RNA splicing mechanisms. *Proc Natl Acad Sci* USA **78**:1800, 1981.
19. Davis MM, Kim SK, Hood LE: DNA sequences mediating class switching in α-immunoglobulins. *Science* **209**:1360, 1980.
20. Marcu KB, Cooper MD: New views of the immunoglobulin heavy-chain switch. *Nature* **298**:327, 1982.
21. Korthauer U, Graf D, Mages HW, Briere F, Padayachee M, Malcolm S, Ugazio AG, Notarangelo LD, Levinsky RJ, Kroczek RA: Defective expression of T-cell CD40 ligand causes X-linked immunodeficiency with hyper-IgM. *Nature* **361**:539, 1993.
22. DiSanto JP, Bonnefoy JY, Gauchat JF, Fischer A, de Saint Basile G: CD40 ligand mutations in X-linked immunodeficiency with hyper-IgM. *Nature* **361**:541, 1993.
23. Reinherz EL, Schlossman SF: The differentiation and function of human T lymphocytes. *Cell* **19**:821, 1980.
24. Reinherz EL, Schlossman SF: The characterization and function of human immunoregulatory T lymphocyte subsets. *Immunol Today* **2**:69, 1981.
25. Moretta L, Mingari MC, Sekaly PR, Moretta A, Chapuis B, Cerottini C: Surface markers of cloned human T cells with various cytolytic activities. *J Exp Med* **154**:569, 1981.
26. Engleman EG, Benike CJ, Grumet FC, Evans RL: Activation of human T-lymphocyte subsets: Helper and suppressor/cytotoxic T cells recognize and respond to distinct histocompatibility antigens. *J Immunol* **127**:2124, 1981.
27. Allison JP, McIntyre RW, Bloch D: Tumor-specific antigen of murine T lymphoma defined with monoclonal antibody. *J Immunol* **129**:2293, 1982.
28. Meuer SC, Fitzgerald KA, Hussey RE, Hodgdon JC Schlossman SF, Reinherz EL: Clonotypic structures involved in antigen-specific human T-cell function. *J Exp Med* **157**:705, 1983.
29. Haskins K, Kubo R, White J, Pigeon M, Kappler J, Marrack P: The major histocompatibility complex-restricted antigen receptor on T cells. Isolations with a monoclonal antibody. *J Exp Med* **157**:1149, 1983.

30. Chien YH, Becker DM, Lindsten T, Okamuras M, Cohen DI, Davis MM: A third type of murine T-cell receptor gene. *Nature* **312**:31, 1984.
31. Hedrick SM, Nielsen EA, Kavaler J, Cohen DI, Davis MM: Sequence relationships between putative T-cell receptor polypeptides and immunoglobulins. *Nature* **308**:153, 1984.
32. Saito H, Kranz DM, Takagaki Y, Hayday AC, Eisen HN, Tonegawa S: A third rearranged and expressed gene in a clone of cytotoxic T lymphocytes. *Nature* **312**:36, 1984.
33. Yancopoulos GD, Blackwell TK, Suh H, Hood L, Alt FW: Introduced T cell receptor variable region gene segments recombine in pre-B cells; evidence that B and T cells use a common recombinase. *Cell* **44**:251, 1986.
34. Hitzig WH: Congenital thymic and lymphocytic deficiency disorders, in Stiehm ER, Fulginiti V (eds): *Immunologic Disorders in Infants and Children*. Philadelphia, WB Saunders, 1973.
35. Hoyer JR, Cooper MD, Gabrielson AE, Good RA: Lymphopenic forms of congenital immunologic deficiency diseases. *Medicine* **47**:201, 1968.
36. Pollack MS, Kirkpatrick D, Kapoor N, Dupont B, O'Reilly R: Identification by HLA typing of intrauterine derived maternal T cells in four patients with severe combined immunodeficiency. *N Engl J Med* **307**:662, 1982.
37. Pahwa SG, Pahwa RN, Good RA: Heterogeneity of B lymphocyte differentiation in severe combined immunodeficiency disease. *J Clin Invest* **66**:543, 1980.
38. Hitzig WH: Portean appearances of immunodeficiencies: Syndromes and inborn errors involving other systems which express associated primary immunodeficiency, in Wedgwood R, Rosen FS, Paul NW (eds): *Primary Immunodeficiency Diseases*. New York, Alan R Liss, 1983, p 307.
39. Blaese RM, Weiden PL, Oppenheim JJ, Waldmann TA: Phytohemagglutinin as a skin test for the evaluation of cellular immune competence in man. *J Lab Clin Med* **81**:538, 1973.
40. Puck JM, Nussbaum RL, Conley ME: Carrier detection in X-linked severe combined immunodeficiency based on patterns of X chromosome inactivation. *J Clin Invest* **79**:1395, 1987.
41. Conley MA, Lavoie A, Briggs C, Brown P, Guerra C, Puck JM: Nonrandon X inactivation in B cells from carriers of X chromosome-linked severe combined immunodeficiency *Proc Natl Acad Sci USA* **85**:3090, 1988.
42. Conley MA: X-linked severe combined immunodeficiency, in Gupta S, Griscelli C (eds): *New Concepts in Immunodeficiency Diseases*. Chichester, John Wiley, 1993, p. 159.
43. Noguchi M, Huafang Y, Rosenblatt HM, Filipovich AH, Adelstein S, Modi WS, McBride OW, Leonard WJ: Interleukin-2 receptor γ chain mutation results in X-linked severe combined immunodeficiency in humans. *Cell* **73**:147, 1993.
44. Leonard WJ: The interleukin-2 receptor: structure, function, intracellular messengers and molecular regulation, in Waxman J, Balkwill (eds): *Interleukin-2*. Oxford, Blackwell Scientific, 1992, p 29.
45. Weinberg K, Parkman R: Severe combined immunodeficiency due to a specific defect in the production of interleukin-2. *N Engl J Med* **322**:1718, 1990.
46. Castigli E, Geha RS, Chatila T: Severe combined immunodeficiency with selective T-cell cytokine genes. *Pediatr Res* **33**:S20, 1993.
47. Chatila T, Castigili E, Pahwa R, Pahwa S, Chirmule N, Oyaizu N, Good RA, Geha RS: Primary combined immunodeficiency resulting from defective transcription of multiple T-cell lymphokine genes. *Proc Natl Acad Sci USA* **87**:10033, 1990.
48. Chatila T, Wong R, Young M, Miller R, Terhorst C, Geha R: An immunodeficiency characterized by defective signal transduction in T lymphocytes. *N Engl J Med* **320**:696, 1989.
49. Giblett ER, Anderson JE, Cohen F, Pollara B, Meuwissen HJ: Adenosine deaminase deficiency in two patients with severely impaired cellular immunity. *Lancet* **2**:1067, 1972.
50. Meuwissen HJ, Pollara B, Pickering RJ: Combined immunodeficiency disease associated with adenosine deficiency. *J Pediatr* **86**:169, 1975.
51. Wara DW, Ammann AJ: Laboratory data, in Meuwissen HJ, Pickering RJ, Pollara B, Porter IH (eds): *Combined Immunodeficiency Disease and Adenosine Deaminase Deficiency, a Molecular Defect*. New York, Academic, 1975.
52. Chen S-H, Scott CR, Swedberg KR: Heterogeneity for adenosine deaminase deficiency: Expression of the enzyme in cultured skin fibroblasts and amniotic fluid cells. *Am J Hum Genet* **27**:46, 1975.
53. Hirschhorn R, Beratis N, Rosen FS: Characterization of residual enzyme activity in fibroblasts from patients with adenosine deaminase deficiency and combined immunodeficiency: Evidence for a mutant enzyme. *Proc Natl Acad Sci USA* **73**:213, 1976.
54. Carson DA, Goldblum R, Seegmiller JE: Quantitative immunoassay for adenosine deaminase in combined immunodeficiency disease. *J Immunol* **118**:270, 1977.
55. Cohen A, Hirschhorn R, Horowitz SD, Rubenstein A, Polmar SH, Hong R, Martin DW: Deoxyadenosine triphosphate as a potentially toxic metabolite in adenosine deaminase deficiency. *Proc Natl Acad Sci USA* **75**:472, 1978.
56. Gelfand EW, Cohen A: Disorders of purine metabolism and immunodeficiency, in Gallin JI, Fauci AS (eds): *Advances in Host Defense Mechanisms*. New York, Raven, 1983, vol 2.
57. Kredick NM: The methylation hypothesis of adenosine toxicity. *Ciba Found Symp* **68**:153, 1979.
58. Carson DA, Kaye J, Seegmiller JE: Lymphospecific toxicity in adenosine deaminase deficiency and purine nucleoside phosphorylase deficiency: Possible role of nucleoside kinase(s). *Proc Natl Acad Sci USA* **24**:5677, 1977.
59. Carson DA, Kaye J, Seegmiller JE: Differential sensitivity of human leukemia T cell lines and B cell lines to growth inhibition by deoxyadenosine. *J Immunol* **121**:1726, 1978.
60. Mitchell BS, Mejias E, Daddona PE, Kelley WN: Purinogenic immunodeficiency diseases: Selective toxicity of deoxyribonucleosides for T cells. *Proc Natl Acad Sci USA* **75**:5011, 1978.
61. Wilson JM, Mitchell BS, Daddona PE, Kelley WN: Purinogenic immunodeficiency diseases: Differential effects of deoxyadenosine and deoxyguanosine on DNA synthesis in human T-lymphoblasts. *J Clin Invest* **64**:1475, 1979.
62. Mejias E, Mitchell B, Cassidy J, Kelley WN: Deoxyribonucleotide pools in immunodeficiency states. III. International Symposium on Purine Metabolism in Man. *Clin Res* **27**:331A, 1979.
63. Hershfield MS, Kredich NM, Ownby DR, Ownby H, Buckley R: In vivo inactivation of erythrocyte S-adenosylhomocysteine hydrolase by 2′deoxyadenosine in adenosine deaminase-deficient patients. *J Clin Invest* **63**:807, 1979.
64. Carson DA, Seto S, Wasson DB: Lymphocyte dysfunction after DNA damage by toxic oxygen species: A model of immunodeficiency. *J Exp Med* **163**:746, 1986.
65. Markert ML, Hershfield MS, Wiginton DA, States JC, Ward FE, Bigner SH, Buckely RH, Kaufman RE, Hutton JJ: Identification of a deletion in the adenosine deaminase gene in a child with severe combined immunodeficiency. *J Immunol* **138**:3203, 1987.
66. Hirschhorn R, Ellenbogen A: Genetic heterogeneity in adenosine deaminase (ADA) deficiency: Five different mutations in five new patients with partial ADA deficiency. *Am J Hum Genet* **38**:13, 1986.
67. Akeson AL, Wiginton DA, States JC, Perme CM, Dusing CM, Hutton JJ: Mutations in the human adenosine deaminase gene that affect protein structure and RNA splicing. *Proc Natl Acad Sci USA* **84**:5947, 1987.
68. Carson DA, Wasson DB, Lakow E, Kamatani N: Possible metabolic basis for the different immunodeficient states associated with genetic deficiencies of adenosine deaminase and purine nucleoside phosphorylase. *Proc Natl Acad Sci USA* **79**:3848, 1982.
69. Orkin SH, Dadonna PE, Shewach DS, Markham AF, Bruns GA, Goff SC, Kelley W: Molecular cloning of human adenosine deaminase gene sequences. *J Biol Chem* **258**:12753, 1983.
70. Valerio D, Duyvesteyn MGC, Merra Khan P, Geurts Van Kessel A, deWaard A, van der Eb AJ: Isolation of cDNA clones for human adenosine deaminase. *Gene* **25**:231, 1983.
71. Wiginton DA, Adrian GS, Friedman RL, Suttle DP,

Hutton JJ: Cloning of cDNA sequences of human adenosine deaminase. *Proc Natl Acad Sci USA* **80**:7481, 1983.

72. Daddonna PE, Mitchell BS, Meuwissen HG, Davidson BL, Wilson JM, Koller CA: Adenosine deaminase deficiency with normal immune function. *J Clin Invest* **72**:483, 1993.
73. Valentine WN, Paglia DE, Tartaglia AP, Gilsanz F: Hereditary hemolytic anemia with increased adenosine deaminase (45-70 fold) and decreased adenosine triphosphates. *Science* **195**,783, 1977.
74. Touraine J-L, Betuel H, Souilet G, Jeune M: Combined immunodeficiency disease associated with absence of cell-surface HLA-A and -B antigens. *J Pediatr* **93**:47, 1978.
75. Schuurman PKB, van Rood JJ, Vossen JM, Schellekens PTA, Feltkamp-Vroom TM, Doyer E, Gmelig-Meyling F, Visser HKA: Failure of lymphocyte-membrane HLA A and B expression in two siblings with combined immunodeficiency. *Clin Immunol Immunopathol* **14**:418, 1979.
76. DePreval C, Lisowska-Grospierre B, Loche M, Griscelli C, Mach B: A transacting class II regulatory gene unlinked to the MHC control expression of HLA class II genes. *Nature* **318**:291, 1985.
77. Griscelli C, Fischer A, Durandy A, Lisowska-Grospierre B, Bremard C, Cerf-Bensussan N, Le Deist F, Marcadet A, De Preval C: Defective synthesis of HLA class I and II molecules associated with combined immunodeficiency, in Eibl MM, Rosen ES (eds): *Primary Immunodeficiency Diseases* Amsterdam, Elsevier, 1986.
78. Griscelli C, Lisokska-Grospierre, Mach B: Combined immunodeficiency with defective expression of MHC class II genes, in Gupta S, Griscelli C (eds): *New Concepts in Immunodeficiency Diseases*. Chichester, John Wiley, 1993, p 177.
79. Pugliattil, Derre J, Berger R, Ucla C, Reigh WQ, Mach B: The genes for MHC class II regulatory factors RFX1 and RFX2 are located on the short arm of chromosome 19. *Genomics* **13**:1307, 1992.
80. Arnaiz-Villena A, Timon M, Corell A, Periez-Aciego P, Martin-Villa JM, Rogueiro JR: Primary immunodeficiency caused by mutations in the gene encoding the CD3-gamma subunit of the T-lymphocyte receptor. *N Engl J Med* **327**:529, 1992. Brief report.
81. Alarcon B, Regueiro JR, Arnaiz-Villena A, Terhorst C: Familial defect in the surface expression of the T-cell receptor-CD3 complex. *N Engl J Med* **319**:1203, 1988.
82. LeDeist F, de Saint Basile G, Mazerolles F, *et al.*: Primary membrane T cell immunodeficiencies. *Clin Immunol Immunopathol* **61**:S56, 1991.
83. Alarcon B, Terhorst C: Congenital T-cell receptor immunodeficiencies in man. *Immunodefic Rev* **2**:1, 1990.
84. Alarcon B, Terhorst C, Arnaiz-Villena A, Perez-Aciego P, Regueiro JR: Congenital T-cell receptor immunodeficiencies in man. In Rosen FS and Seligmann M (eds): *Immunodeficiencies*. Chur, Switzerland, Harwood, 1993, p 155.
85. Devaal OM, Skynhaeve V: Reticular dysgenesia. *Lancet* **2**:1123, 1959.
86. Haas RJ, Niethammer D, Goldman SF, Heit W, Bienzle U, Kleihauer E: Congenital immunodeficiency and agammaglobulinemia (reticular dysgenesis). *Acta Paediatr Scand* **66**:279, 1977.
87. Levinsky RJ, Tiedeman K: Successful bone-marrow transplantation for reticular dysgenesis. *Lancet* **1**:671, 1983.
88. Ownby DR, Pizzo S, Blackmon L, Gall SA, Buckley RH: Severe combined immunodeficiency with leukopenia (reticular dysgenesis) in siblings: Immunologic and histopathologic findings. *J Pediatr* **89**:382, 1876.
89. Hitzig WH, Landolt R, Miller G, Bodmer P: Heterogeneity of phenotypic expression in a family with Swiss-type agammaglobulinemia: Observations on the acquisition of agammaglobulinemia. *J Pediatr* **78**:986, 1971.
90. Pyke KW, Dosch HM, Ipp MM, Gelfand EW: Demonstration of an intrathymic defect in a case of severe combined immunodeficiency disease. *N Engl J Med* **193**:424, 1975.
91. Incefy GS, O'Reilly RI, Kapoor N, Iwata T, Good RA: In vitro differentiation of human marrow T cell precursors by thymic factors in severe combined immunodeficiency. *Transplantation* **32**:299, 1981.
92. Gatti RA, Allen HD, Meuwissen HJ, Hong R, Good RA: Immunological reconstitution of sex-linked lymphopenic immunological deficiency. *Lancet* **2**:1366, 1968.
93. Reisner Y, Kapoor N, Kirkpatrick D, Pollack MS, Dupont B, Good RA, O'Reilly RJ: Transplantation of acute leukemia with HLA-A and B identical parental marrow cells fractionated with soybean and sheep red blood cells. *Lancet* **2**:327, 1981.
94. O'Reilly RJ, Kapoor N, Kirkpatrick D, Flomenberg N, Pollack MS, Dupont B, Good RA, Reisner Y: Transplantation of hematopoietic cells for lethal congenital immunodeficiencies, in Wedgwood R, Rosen FS, Paul NW (eds): *Primary Immunodeficiency Diseases*. New York, Alan R Liss, 1983, p 307.
95. Fischer A, Griscelli C, Blanche S, LeDeist F, Veber F, Lopez M, Delaage M, Olive D, Mawas C, Janossy G: Prevention of graft failure by an anti-HLFA-I monoclonal antibody in HLA-mismatched bone marrow transplantation. *Lancet* **2**:1058, 1986.
96. Markert ML, Hershfield MS, Schiff RI, Buckley RH: Adenosine deaminase and purine nucleoside phosphorylase deficiencies: Evaluation of therapeutic interventions in eight patients. *J Clin Immunol* **7**:389, 1987.
97. Polmar SH, Stern RC, Schwartz AL, Wetzler EM, Chase PA, Hirsch Horn R: Enzyme replacement therapy for adenosine deaminase deficiency and severe combined immunodeficiency. *N Engl J Med* **295**:1337, 1976.
98. Hershfield MS, Buckley RH, Greenberg ML, Melton AL, Schiff R, Hatem C, Kurtzberg J, Markert ML, Kobayashi RH, Kobayashi AL, et al: Treatment of adenosine deaminase deficiency with polethylene glycol-modified adenosine deaminase. *N Engl J Med* **136**:589, 1987.
99. Anderson WF: Prospects for human gene therapy. *Science* **226**:401, 1984.
100. Kantoff PW, Kohn DB, Mitsuya H, Armentano D, Sieberg M, Zwiebel JA, Eglitis MA, McLachlin JR, Wiginton DA, Hutton JJ, Horowitz SD, Gilboa E, Blaese RM, Anderson WF: Correction of adenosine deaminase deficiency in cultured human T and B cells by retrovirus-mediated gene transfer. *Proc Natl Acad Sci USA* **83**:6563, 1986.
101. Blaese RM, Culver KW: Gene therapy for primary immunodeficiency. *Immunodeficiency Rev* **3**:329, 1992.
102. Blaese RM, Anderson WF, Culver KW: The ADA human gene therapy clinical protocol. *Hum Gene Therap* **1**:327, 1990.
103. Blaese RM: Development of gene therapy for immunodeficiency: Adenosine deaminase deficiency. *Pediatr Res* 33(Suppl.):S49, 1993.
104. McFarlin DE, Strober W, Waldmann TA: Ataxia-telangiectasia. *Medicine* **51**:281, 1972.
105. Boder E: Ataxia-telangiectasia: Some historic, clinical and pathologic observations, in Bergsma D, Good RA, Finstad J, Paul NW (eds): *Immunodeficiency in Man and Animals*. Sunderland, MA, Sinauer, 1975, p 255.
106. Bar RS, Levis WR, Rechler MM, Harrison LC, Siebert C, Podskalny J, Roth J, Muggeo M: Extreme insulin resistance in ataxia telangiectasia: Defect in affinity of insulin receptors. *N Engl M Med* **298**:164, 1978.
107. Waldmann TA, Strober W, Blaese RM: Immunodeficiency disease and malignancy. *Ann Intern Med* **77**:605, 1972.
108. Spector BD, Perry GS, Kersey JH: Genetically determined immunodeficiency disease and malignancy: Report from the immunodeficiency-Cancer Registry. *Clin Immunol Immunopathol* **11**:12, 1978.
109. Filipovich AH, Zerbe D, Spector B, Kersey J: Lymphomas in persons with naturally occurring immune deficiency disorders, in MaGrath IT, O'Connor GT, Ramot B (eds): *Pathogenesis of Leukemias and Lymphomas: Environmental Influences*. New York, Raven, 1984, p 225.
110. Cohen MM, Shaham M, Dagan J, Shmueli E, Kohn G: Cytogenetic investigations in families with ataxia-telangiectasia. *Cytogenet Cell Genet* **15**:338, 1975.
111. McCaw BK, Hecht F, Harnden DG, Teplitz KL: Somatic rearrangement of chromosome 14 in human lymphocytes. *Proc Natl Acad Aci USA* **72**:2071, 1975.
112. Oxford JM, Harnden DG, Parrington JM, Delhanty JDA: Specific chromosome aberrations in ataxia-telangiectasia. *J Med Genet* **12**:251, 1975.

113. Hecht F, Hecht BK: Chromosome changes connect immunodeficiency and cancer in ataxia-telangiectasia. *Am J Pediatr Hematol Oncol* **9**:185, 1987.
114. McFarlin DE, Oppenheim JJ: Impaired lymphocyte transformation in ataxia-telangiectasia in part due to a plasma inhibitory factor. *J Immunol* **103**:1212, 1969.
115. Oxelius VA, Berkel AI, Hansen LA: IgG2 deficiency in ataxia-telangieclasia. *N Engl J Med* **306**:515, 1982.
116. Ammann AJ, Hong R: Autoimmune phenomena in ataxia telangiectasia. *Pediatr* **78**:821, 1971.
117. Waldmann TA, Misiti J, Nelson D, Kraemer KH: Ataxia telangiectasia: A multi-system hereditary disease with immunodeficiency, impaired organ maturation, x-ray hypersensitivity, and a high incidence of neoplasia. A combined staff conference of the NIH. *Ann Intern Med* **99**:367, 1983.
118. Waldmann TA, Broder S, Goldman CK, Frost K, Korsmeyer SJ, Uedici MA: Disorders of B cells and helper T cells in the pathogenesis of the immunoglobulin deficiency of patients with ataxia-telangiectasia. *J Clin Invest* **71**:282, 1983.
119. Peterson RDA, Kelly WD, Good RA: Ataxia-telangiectasia: Its association with a defective thymus, immunological-deficiency disease and malignancy. *Lancet* **1**:1189, 1964.
120. Peterson RDA, Cooper MD, Good RA: Lymphoid tissue abnormalities associated with ataxia-telangiectasia. *Am J Med* **41**:342, 1966.
121. Auerbach R: Morphogenetic interactions in the development of the mouse thymus gland. *Dev Biol* **2**:271, 1960.
122. Waldmann TA, McIntire KR: Serum alpha-fetoprotein levels in patients with ataxia-telangiectasia. *Lancet* **2**:1112, 1972.
123. Sugimoto T, Sawada T, Tozawa M, Kidowaki T, Kusunoki T, Yamaguchi N: Plasma levels of carcinoembryonic antigen in patients with ataxia-telangiectasia. *J Pediatr* **92**:436, 1978.
124. Gotoff SP, Amirmokri E, Liebner EJ: Ataxia telangiectasia: Neoplasia, untoward response to x-irradiation and tuberous sclerosis. *Am J Dis Child* **114**:617, 1967.
125. Cunliffe PN, Mann JR, Cameron AH, Roberts KD, Ward HWC: Radiosensitivity in ataxia telangiectasia. *Br J Radiol* **48**:374, 1975.
126. Taylor AMR, Harnden DG, Arlett CF, Harcourt SA, Lehmann AR, Stevens S, Bridges BA: Ataxia telangiectasia: A human mutation with abnormal radiation sensitivity. *Nature* **258**:427, 1975.
127. Bridges BA: Some DNA repair-deficient human syndromes and their implications for human health. *Proc R Soc Lond [Biol]* **212**:263, 1981.
128. Taylor AMR, Metcalfe JA, Oxford JM, Harnden DG: Is chromatid-type damage in ataxia telangiectasia after irradiation at G_0 a consequence of defective repair? *Nature* **260**:441, 1976.
129. Jaspers NGJ, Bootsma D: Genetic heterogeneity in ataxia-telangiectasia studied by cell fusion. *Proc Natl Acad Sci USA* **79**:2641, 1982.
130. Murnane JP, Painter RB: Complementation of the defects in DNA synthesis in irradiated and unirradiated ataxis-telangiectasia cells. *Proc Natl Acad Sci USA* **79**:1960, 1982.
131. Pyun KH, Ochs HD, Xang X, Wedgwood RJ: Antibody deficiency in ataxia-telangiectasia, a defect in heavy chain constant gene rearrangement. *Clin Res* **35**:218A, 1987.
132. Gatti R: Ataxia-telangiectasia: genetic studies, in Gupta S, Griscelli C (eds): *New Concept in Immunodeficiency Diseases*. Chichester, John Wiley, 1993, p 203.
133. Aldrich RA, Steinberg AG, Campbell DC: Pedigree demonstrating a sex-linked recessive condition characterized by draining ears, eczematoid dermatitis and bloody diarrhea. *Pediatrics* **13**:133, 1954.
134. Krivit W, Good RA: Aldrich's syndrome (thrombocytopenia, eczema and infection) in infants. *Am J Dis Child* **97**:137, 1959.
135. Perry GS III, Spector BD, Schuman LM, Mandel JS, Anderson E, McHugh RB, Hanson MR, Fahlstorm SM, Krivit W, Kersey JH: The Wiskott-Aldrich syndrome in the United States and Canada (1982-1979). *J Pediatr* **97**:72, 1980.
136. Corash L, Shafer B, Blaese RM: Platelet-associated immunoglobulin, platelet size, and the effect of splenectomy in the Wiskott-Aldrich syndrome. *Blood* **65**:1439, 1985.
137. Blaese RM: Defects in the afferent limb of the immune system, in Waldmann TA (moderator): Immunodeficiency disease and malignancy. *Ann Intern Med* **77**:605, 1972.
138. Cotelingham D, Witebsky FG, Hsu SM, Blaese RM, Gaffe ES: Malignant lymphoma in patients with the Wiskott-Aldrich syndrome. *Cancer Invest* **3**:515, 1985.
139. Blaese RM, Strober W, Waldmann TA: Immunodeficiency in the Wiskott-Aldrich syndrome, in Bergsma D (ed): *Immunodeficiency in Man and Animals. Birth Defects*. Sunderland, MA, Sinauer, 1975, p 250.
140. Cooper MD, Chase HP, Lowman JT, Krivit W, Good RA: Wiskott-Aldrich syndrome: An immunologic deficiency disease involving the afferent limb of immunity. *Am J Med* **44**:499, 1968.
141. Blaese RM, Strober W, Brown RS, Waldmann TA: The Wiskott-Aldrich syndrome. A disorder with a possible defect in antigen processing or recognition. *Lancet* **1**:1056, 1968.
142. Blaese RM, Strober W, Levy AL, Waldmann TA: Hypercatabolism of IgG, IgA, IgM and albumin in the Wiskott-Aldrich syndrome. *J Clin Invest* **50**:2331, 1971.
143. Oppenheim JJ, Blaese RM, Waldmann TA: Defective lymphocyte transformation and delayed hypersensitivity in Wiskott-Aldrich syndrome. *J Immunol* **104**:835, 1970.
144. Kenney D, Cairns L, Remold-O'Donnell E, Peterson J, Rosen FS Parkman R: Morphological abnormalities in the lymphocytes of patients with the Wiskott-Aldrich syndrome. *Blood* **68**:1329, 1986.
145. Ochs HD, Slichter SJ, Harker LA, Von Behrens WE, Clark RA, Wedgwood RJ: The Wiskott-Aldrich syndrome: Studies of lymphocytes, granulocytes, and platelets. *Blood* **55**:243, 1980.
146. Altman LC, Synderman R, Blaese RM: Abnormalities of chemotactic lymphokine synthesis and mononuclear leukocyte chemotaxis in Wiskott-Aldrich syndrome. *J Clin Invest* **54**:486, 1974.
147. Poplack DG, Bonnard GD, Holiman BI, Blaese RM: Monocyte-mediated antibody-dependent cellular cytotoxicity: A clinical test of monocyte function. *Blood* **48**:809, 1976.
148. Blaese RM, Muchmore AV, Lawrence EC, Poplack DG: The cytolytic effector function of monocytes in immunodeficiency disease, in Seligmann M, Hitzig W (eds): *Primary Immunodeficiencies*. Amsterdam, Elsevier/North Holland, 1980, p 391.
149. Kwan SP, Lehner Y, Lu B, Raghu G, Blaese M, Sandkuyl L, Ott J, Fraser N, Boyd Y, Craig I, Fischer S, Rosen FS: Localization of the gene for Wiskott-Aldrich syndrome between two flanking markers TIMP and DXS255 on Xp11.2-11.3. Human Gene Mapping 10. *Cytogenet Cell Genet* **51**:1027, 1989.
150. Parkman R, Kenney DM, Remold-O'Donnell PS, Rosen FS: Surface protein abnormalities in lymphocytes and platelets from patients with Wiskott-Aldrich syndrome. *Lancet* **2**:1387, 1982.
151. Reisinger D, Parkman R: Molecular heterogeneity of a lymphocyte glycoprotein in immunodeficient patients. *J Clin Invest* **79**:595, 1987.
152. Remold-O'Donnell E, Kenney DM, Parkman R, Cairns L, Savage B, Rosen FS: Characterization of a human lymphocyte surface sialoglycoprotein that is defective in Wiskott-Aldrich syndrome. *J Exp Med* **159**:1705, 1984.
153. Remold-O'Donnell E, Zimmerman C, Kenney D, Rosen FS: Expression on blood cells of sialophorin, the surface glycoprotein that is defective in Wiskott-Aldrich syndrome. *Blood* **70**:104, 1987.
154. Rosenstein Y, Park JK, Bierer BA, Burakoff SJ: The Wiskott-Aldrich syndrome: An immunodeficiency associated with defects of the CD43 molecule, in Gupta S, Griscelli C (eds): *New Concepts in Immunodeficiency Diseases*. Chichester, John Wiley, 1993, p 258.
155. Remold-O'Donnell E, Zimmerman C, Kenney D, Rosen FS: Expression on blood cells of sialophorin, the surface glycoprotein that is defective in Wiskott-Aldrich syndrome. *Blood* **70**:104, 1987.
156. Remold-O'Donnell E, Rosen FS: Proteolytic fragmentation of sialophorin (CD43):Localization of the activation-inducing site and examination of the role of sialic acid. *J Immunol* **145**:3372, 1990.

157. Pallant A, Eskenazi A, Mattei MG, Fournier RE, Carlsson SR, Fukuda M, Frelinger JG: Characterization of cDNAs encoding human leukosialin and localization of the leukosialin gene to chromosome 16. *Proc Natl Acad Sci USA* **86**:1328, 1989.
158. Pillar F, Pillar V, Fox RI, Fukuda. Human T-lymphocyte activation is associated with changes in *O*-glycan biosynthesis. *J Biol Chem* **263**:15146, 1988.
159. Higgins EA, Siminovitch KA, Zhuang D, Brockhausen I, Dennis JW: Abberant *O*-linked oligosaccharide biosynthesis in lymphocytes and platelets from patients with the Wiskott-Aldrich syndrome. *J Biol Chem* **266**:6280, 1991.
160. Kohn DB, Fearon ER, Winkelstein JA, Vogelstein B, Blaese RM: Wiskott-Aldrich carrier detection by X-chromosome inactivation analysis. *Pediatr Res* **21**:838, 1987.
161. Fearon ER, Kohn DA, Winkelstein JA, Vogelstein B, Blaese RM: Carrier detection and cell population analysis in the Wiskott-Aldrich syndrome by studies of maternal X-chromosome inactivation. *Blood* **72**:1735, 1988.
162. Gealy WI, Dwyer JM, Harley J: Allelic exclusion of glucose-6-phosphate dehydrogenase in platelets and T lymphocytes from a Wiskott-Aldrich syndrome carrier. *Lancet* **1**:63, 1980.
163. Parkman R, Rappeport J, Geha R, Belli J, Cassidy R, Levey R, Nathan DG, Rosen FS: Complete correction of the Wiskott-Aldrich syndrome by allogeneic bone marrow transplantation. *N Engl J Med* **298**:921, 1978.
164. Kapoor N, Kirkpatrick D, Blaese RM, Oleske J, Hilgartner MH, Chaganti RSK, Good RA, O'Reilly RI: Reconstitution of normal megakaryocytopoiesis and immunologic functions in Wiskott-Aldrich syndrome by marrow transplantation following myeloablation and immunosuppression with busulfan and cyclophosphamide. *Blood* **57**:692, 1981.
165. Lum LG, Tubergen DG, Corash L, Blaese RM: Splenectomy in the management of the thrombocytopenia of the Wiskott-Aldrich syndrome. *N Engl J Med* **302**:892, 1980.
166. Weiden PL, Blaese RM: Hereditary thrombocytopenia: Relation to the Wiskott-Aldrich syndrome with special reference to splenectomy. *J Pediatr* **80**:226, 1972.
167. Mullen CA, Anderson KD, and Blaese RM: Splenectomy and/or bone marrow transplantation in the management of the Wiskott-Aldrich Syndrome: long-term follow-up of 62 cases. *Blood* **82**:2961, 1993.
168. Filipovich AH, Krivit W, Kersey IH, Burke BA: Fatal arteritis as a complication of Wiskott-Aldrich syndrome. *J Pediatr* **95**:742, 197.
169. Elder ME, Lin D, Clever J, Chan AC, Hope TJ, Weiss A, Parslow TG: Human severe combined immunodeficiency due to a defect in ZAP-70, a T cell tyrosine kinase. *Science* **264**:1596, 1994.
170. Chan AC, Kadlecek TA, Elder ME, Filipovich AH, Kuo W-L, Iwashima M, Parslow TG, Weiss A: ZAP-70 deficiency in an autosomal recessive form of severe combined immunodeficiency. *Science* **264**:1599, 1994.

CHAPTER 130

Genetically Determined Disorders of the Complement System

Jerry A. Winkelstein ▪ Kathleen E. Sullivan
Harvey R. Colten

1. **The complement system is composed of a series of plasma proteins and membrane receptors, which, when functioning in an ordered and integrated fashion, serve as important mediators of host defense and inflammation. In order for the individual components of complement to subserve their biologic functions, however, they must first be activated. Activation of the complement system can occur via either the classical activating pathway or the alternative activating pathway. Once activated, individual components act as opsonins, possess chemotactic activity, are potent anaphylatoxins, and can assemble into the membrane attack complex and generate cytolytic activity. In addition, the complement system is important in the processing of immune complexes and the generation of a normal antibody response.**

2. **Some of the complement genes have been grouped into supergene families based on similarities in their structure, function, and chromosomal location. For example, the genes encoding C2, factor B, and C4 constitute the class III genes of the MHC on chromosome 6; the products of these genes are constituents of the enzymes that activate C3 and C5. The genes for C4-binding protein, factor H, decay-accelerating factor, membrane cofactor protein, and two of the receptors for C3 cleavage products make up another family of complement genes located on the long arm of chromosome 1; the products of these genes share their ability to interact with the activation products of C4 and C3. The synthesis of a number of components of complement is regulated by cytokines such as interleukins 1 and 6, tumor necrosis factor and γ-interferon, and by endotoxic lipopolysaccharide.**

3. **Genetically determined deficiencies have been described for most of the individual components of complement. The usual mode of inheritance is as an autosomal recessive disorder with only two exceptions; C1-inhibitor deficiency is inherited as an autosomal dominant disorder, and properdin deficiency is inherited as an X-linked recessive disorder. The clinical manifestations of individuals with complement deficiencies has varied. Most individuals have had either an increased susceptibility to infection, rheumatic disorders, or angioedema. Patients with a deficiency of C3, or with a deficiency of a component in either of the two pathways necessary for the activation of C3, have an increased susceptibility to infection with encapsulated bacteria for which C3b-dependent opsonization is an important host defense. Patients with deficiencies of terminal components C5 through C9 are markedly susceptible to systemic neisserial infections, since serum bactericidal activity is an important host defense against these organisms. The prevalence of rheumatic disorders is highest in patients who are deficient in components of the classical activating pathway (C1, C4, and C2) and C3. They include systemic lupus erythematosus, vasculitis, membranoproliferative glomerulonephritis, and dermatomyositis. The pathophysiological basis for the occurrence of these disorders in complement-deficient patients is unclear. Finally, patients with C1-inhibitor deficiency present with angioedema.**

The complement system was first described around the turn of the century as a cytolytic mechanism responsible for lysing bacteria or erythrocytes sensitized with antibody.[1] The term "complement" was used since the cytolytic principle "complemented" the action of antibody. Nearly 100 years later, it is now appreciated that the complement system is composed of a series of proteins that, when functioning in an ordered and integrated fashion, serve as important mediators of host defense and inflammation.[2] In addition to its cytolytic function, the complement system subserves a variety of other biologically significant functions. Individual components of the complement system act as opsonins, possess chemotactic activity, or are potent anaphylatoxins.

A list of standard abbreviations is located immediately preceding the index in each volume. Additional abbreviations used in this chapter include: AP_{50} = alternative pathway 50; Ba = the smaller cleavage product of factor B; Bb = the larger cleavage product of factor B; CH_{50} = total serum hemolytic complement; C1-INH = C1 esterase inhibitor; C1q, C1r, C1s = the subcomponents of C1; $C1\bar{r}$ = activated C1r; $C1\bar{s}$ = activated C1s; C1 to C9 = the first through ninth components of complement; C2a = the larger cleavage product of C2; C2b = the smaller cleavage product of C2; C3a = the smaller cleavage fragment of C3; C3b = the larger cleavage fragment of C3; C3, Bb = the priming C3 convertase; C3b,Bb = the amplification C3 convertase = the C3a-desArg = the molecule produced by removal of the C-terminal Arg from C3a; $\overline{(C3b)_2,Bb}$ = the alternative pathway C5 convertase; C4a = the smaller cleavage product of C4; C4b = the larger cleavage product of C4; C4b,2a = the C3 convertase produced by the classical pathway; $\overline{C4b,2a,3b}$ = the C5 convertase produced by the classical pathway; C4-bp = C4-binding protein; C4c = the large cleavage product of C4b; C4d = the small cleavage product of C4b which remains bound to the cell surface; C5a = the smaller cleavage fragment of C5; C5a-desArg = the molecule produced by removal of the C-terminal Arg from C5a; CRI-4 = receptors for C3b and its cleavage products; DAF = decay-accelerating factor; GPI = glycosyl-phosphaidylinositol anchor; HAE = hereditary angioedema; C3b = inactive C3b; IFN-γ = γ-interferon; LFA-1 = lymphocyte function–associated antigens; MCP = membrane cofactor protein; 21-OH = steroid 21-hydroxylase; *QO = a null allele at a complement component locus; SERPIN = serine protease inhibitor; SLE = systemic lupus erythematosus; TNF = tumor necrosis factor/cachectin.

In addition, the complement system plays an important role in the processing of immune complexes and the generation of a normal antibody response. When its activation is controlled, and directed against invading microorganisms, the complement system is an important mechanism of defense and is beneficial to the host. However, when its activation proceeds in an uncontrolled manner, or is directed against the host, the complement system is an important mediator of immunopathological damage and is detrimental to the host.

The first description of an individual with a genetically determined deficiency of one of the components of complement appeared in 1960.[3] Since then, genetically determined deficiencies of nearly all of the components of the complement system have been described in humans.[4,5] The discovery of individuals with genetically determined abnormalities of the complement system has not only identified a new group of patients with inborn errors of metabolism, but the elucidation of pathophysiology in these patients has led to a better understanding of the physiological role of complement in normal individuals.

This chapter will review the biochemistry, biology, and molecular genetics of the normal complement system and relate these to the genetically determined disorders of the complement system in humans.

BIOCHEMISTRY OF THE COMPLEMENT SYSTEM

The complement system is composed of a series of individual proteins (Table 130-1). The majority of the biologically significant effects of the complement system are mediated by C3 and the terminal components, C5, C6, C7, C8, and C9. In order to subserve their biologic functions, however, C3 and C5 to C9 must first be activated. Activation of C3 and C5 to C9 may occur through at least two mechanisms, the classical pathway and the alternative pathway (Fig. 130-1).

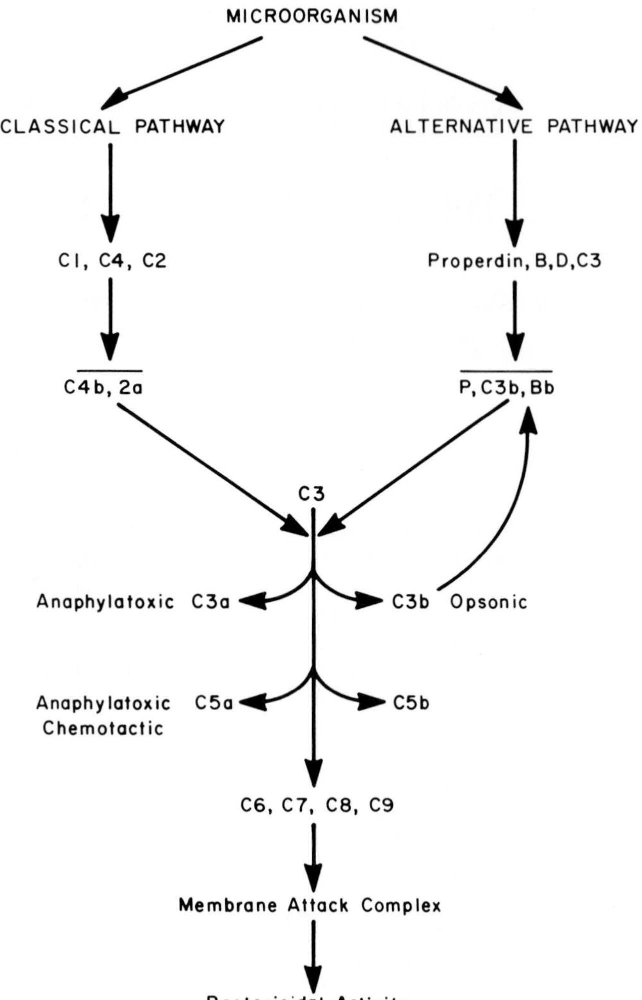

FIG. 130-1 Activation of C3 and the terminal components (C5 to C9) of complement by the classical and alternative pathways.

The Classical Pathway

Activation of the classical pathway is usually initiated by antigen–antibody complexes (Fig. 130-2). Antibodies of the appropriate class (IgG and IgM) or subclass (IgG1, IgG2, IgG3) combine with an antigen to form an immune complex, which is then capable of binding and activating the first component of complement (C1) (reviewed in Porter and Reid[6]). Only one molecule of pentameric IgM is needed for activation of C1, but the IgM molecule must combine with the antigen through more than one of its Fab arms. In contrast, two IgG molecules must be in close proximity in order for C1 to bind and activation to occur. The requirements for an IgG doublet greatly reduces the efficiency of immune complexes composed of IgG, as compared with IgM, to activate C1 and the classical pathway.

In its native state, a single molecule of C1 is a macromolecular Ca^{2+}-dependent complex composed of three distinct subcomponents, designated C1q, C1r, and C1s,[7] which are present in a molar ratio of 1:2:2, respectively.[8] It is the C1q that binds to the immunoglobulin molecules in the immune complex.[9] Binding of C1q to the immune complex results in the activation of C1r. Presumably, a conformational change in C1r exposes a proteolytic site that initiates the autocatalytic cleavage of C1r and thereby converts the single chain zymogen to the disulfide-linked heterodimer that is the active enzyme ($\overline{\text{C1r}}$).[10,11] A serine esterase, $\overline{\text{C1r}}$ then converts C1s to its active form, $\overline{\text{C1s}}$. Native C1s is present in serum as a single polypeptide chain and is similar in molecular mass and amino acid sequence to C1r. On activation by $\overline{\text{C1r}}$, C1s is cleaved into two disulfide-linked chains and its serine esterase activity is expressed.[12,13]

Activated $\overline{\text{C1s}}$ then activates its natural substrate, the fourth component of complement (C4) by cleavage. Native C4 is composed of three disulfide-linked chains (α, β, and γ).[14] Activation of C4 is accomplished by cleaving a peptide (C4a) of 6 kDa from the N-terminal portion of the α chain, the largest of the three chains.[14] This exposes an intrachain reactive thiolester bond in the remaining portion of the α chain of the larger cleavage product (C4b). The nascent C4b is then able to bind covalently to cell surfaces or to immunoglobulins through either esterification of hydroxyl groups on polysaccharides or amidation of amino groups on proteins by the acyl group of the reactive thiolester.[15,16] The internal thiolester bond of the C4b is highly labile, however, and if transesterification or amidation does not occur quickly, the C4b is inactivated by hydrolysis in the fluid phase and unable to bind to the cell surface or immunoglobulin. It is the lability of the reactive thiolester that confines the binding of the nascent C4b to the immediate vicinity of the immune complex and thereby helps to restrict the activation of the

Table 130-1 Components of Human Complement

Component	Chromosomal Location	Approximate Molecular Weight (kDa)	Chains
Classical pathway			
Clq	1p34.1-36.3	460	6A, 6B, 6C
Clr	12p13	83	Single
Cls	12p13	83	Single
C4	6p	200	1 alpha, 1 beta, 1 gamma
C2	6p	102	Single
Alternative pathway			
Factor D	?	25	Single
Factor B	6p	93	Single
C3 and terminal components			
C3	19p	185	1 alpha, 1 beta
C5	9q32-34	190	1 alpha, 1 beta
C6	5q13	128	Single
C7	5q13	120	Single
C8	1p3.2	163	1 alpha, 1 beta
	9q		1 gamma
C9	5p13	79	Single
Control proteins			
Cl inhibitor	11q	105	Single
C4-binding protein	1q4	550	7 to 8 identical
Factor H	1q	150	Single
Factor I	4q2	100	1 alpha, 1 beta
Properdin	Xp11.23-21	223	4 identical
Membrane cofactor protein (CD46)	1q	58	Single
Membrane inhibitor of reactive lysis (CD59)(HRF20)	11p13-14	20	Single
Membrane/receptor proteins			
Decay accelerating factor (CD55)	1q	70	Single
CR1 (CD35)	1q	250	Single
CR2 (CD21)	1q	145	Single
CR3 (CD11b/18)	16p	250	1 alpha
	21q		1 beta
CR4 (CD11c/18)		150	1 alpha, 1 beta

complete cascade to the area in which it was initiated. The reaction continues with the cleavage of the second component (C2) by the $C\overline{1s}$.[17] In order for the most efficient activation of native C2 to occur, however, the C2 must first form a complex, through Mg^{2+}-dependent binding, with C4b molecules that are in close proximity to $C\overline{1s}$. Cleavage of C2 results in the liberation of a small peptide (C2b). The larger fragment, C2a, remains in a complex with the C4b to form a bimolecular enzyme, $C\overline{4b,2a}$, which is responsible for activating C3[18] and initiating the assembly of the terminal components (C5 through C9) into the membrane attack complex.

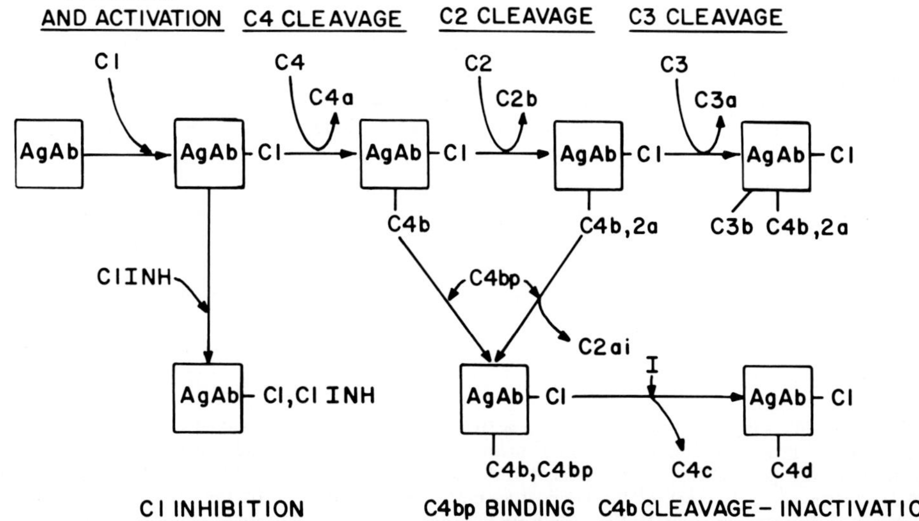

FIG. 130-2 Classical pathway of C3 activation. Activation of the pathway is initiated by immune complexes (AgAb), which activate C1. Activated C1 then cleaves C4 and C2, generating cleavage products that form a bimolecular complex, C4b,2a, which is the classical pathway C3 convertase. The generation and expression of the C3 convertase is regulated by the control proteins, C1 inhibitor (C1-INH), C4-binding protein (C4-bp), and factor I (I). *(Modified from* The Metabolic Basis of Inherited Disease, *5th ed.)*

If the activation of the classical pathway were to proceed in an uncontrolled fashion, then the generation of the $\overline{C4b,2a}$ enzyme would lead to the continuous activation of C3, C5, and the other terminal components. This, in turn, could result in the generation of excessive amounts of the phlogistic fragments of complement, which could cause widespread immunopathological damage to the host. Fortunately, a number of mechanisms act to control the assembly and expression of the classical pathway C3 convertase, $\overline{C4b,2a}$. First, the $\overline{C4b,2a}$ enzyme is very labile at physiological temperatures and undergoes spontaneous decay with release of C2a and loss of enzymatic activity. Second, the enzymatic actions of $C\overline{1r}$ and $C\overline{1s}$ can be inhibited by a control protein, C1 inhibitor (C1-INH).[19] The C1-INH is a naturally occurring glycoprotein, which binds covalently to $C\overline{1r}$ and $C\overline{1s}$, leading to dissociation of the C1 macromolecular complex.[20] Third, another regulatory protein, C4-binding protein (C4-bp), inhibits the $\overline{C4b,2a}$ enzyme by limiting the uptake of C2 by the C4b, by accelerating the decay/dissociation of the C2a once it has formed a complex with the C4b, and by enhancing the ability of yet another inhibitor, factor I (C3b/C4b inactivator), to cleave and inactivate C4b.[21,22] Factor I is a serine protease that inhibits the activity of the C4b of the classical pathway C3-cleaving enzyme but also inhibits the C3b of the alternative pathway C3-cleaving enzyme (see below). In the case of C4b, factor I cleaves the α chain so as to release a large cleavage product (C4c) of the C4b into the fluid phase, leaving a smaller fragment of the α chain (C4d) still covalently attached to the cell surface but no longer able to bind native C2.[22] Finally, a fourth inhibitor, decay accelerating factor (DAF), a membrane protein found in erythrocytes and a variety of other cells, also accelerates the release of C2a from the $\overline{C4b,2a}$ enzyme.[23] Thus, in the usual situation, the assembly and expression of the $\overline{C4b,C2a}$ enzyme, and the activation of C3, proceeds in a controlled fashion and is limited to the immediate vicinity of the initiating substance (e.g., a microbial surface or an immune complex).

Activation of the classical pathway is usually initiated by antigen–antibody complexes and, therefore, is considered to be especially important in acquired immunity. However, some enveloped RNA viruses,[24] some mycoplasma species,[25] and certain strains and species of both gram-negative[26] and gram-positive bacteria[27] can bind C1q directly and activate the classical pathway. Thus, under some circumstances, the classical pathway may be activated in an antibody-independent fashion and function in "natural" immunity (reviewed in Winkelstein[28]).

The Alternative Pathway

Activation of the alternative pathway begins with the C3 molecule (reviewed in Fearon[29]) (Fig. 130-3). Like C4 (see above), native C3 contains an internal thiolester in its α chain.[30] Under normal physiological conditions, this internal thiolester undergoes continuous low-grade hydrolysis to create a C3b-like molecule.[31] The "C3b-like" C3 then can bind native factor B and allow its cleavage by a serine protease, factor D.[32] Two cleavage products of factor B are generated, a larger C-terminal product, Bb, and a smaller, N-terminal product, Ba. The association of the hydrolyzed C3 with Bb then creates a C3-cleaving enzyme, $\overline{C3,Bb}$, (termed the "priming" C3-convertase),[29] which is responsible for a continuous, low-grade cleavage of C3 and, hence, the generation of nascent C3b. As with the activation of C4, the cleavage of native C3 exposes the reactive thiolester, allowing transesterification with, or amidation of, suitable acceptor sites on the cell surface. Should a suitable surface not be available, then hydrolysis of the thiolester results in an inactive C3b molecule. On the other hand, if the nascent C3b binds covalently to a suitable surface, it forms an Mg^{2+}-dependent, reversible complex with native factor B, which is then cleaved by factor D to create a highly efficient C3-cleaving enzyme, $\overline{C3b,Bb}$, termed the "amplification" C3-convertase.[29]

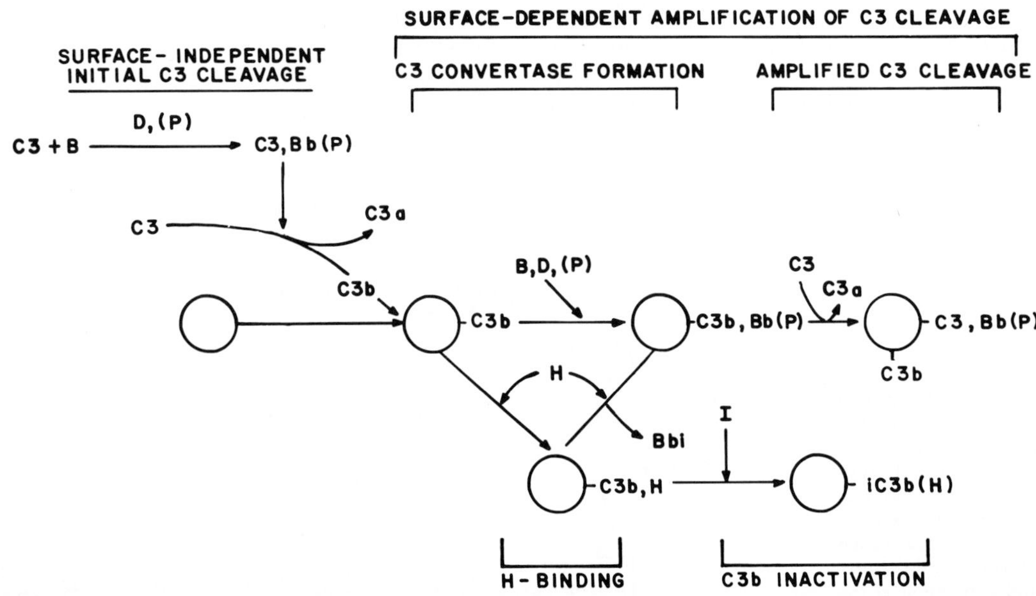

FIG. 130-3 Alternative pathway of C3 activation. There is a continuous, low-grade generation of C3b by a "priming" C3 convertase (C3,Bb,P) in the fluid phase. If the nascent C3b attaches to a cell surface that is an "activator" of the alternative pathway, then the amplification C3 convertase (C3b,Bb,P) is formed, additional C3 is cleaved and more C3b is deposited on the surface. However, if the nascent C3b attaches to a "nonactivating" surface, then the control proteins, factors H and I, act to prevent the generation and expression of the amplification C3 convertase. *(Modified from* The Metabolic Basis of Inherited Disease, *5th ed.)*

Two points regarding the relationship of the classical and alternative pathways to the activation of C3 and C5 through C9 deserve emphasis. First, since C3b is both the product of the alternative pathway C3-convertase and also forms part of the alternative pathway C3-convertase, the activation of C3 via the alternative pathway creates a positive-feedback amplification loop (see Fig. 130-1). Second, activation of the classical pathway, by creating nascent C3b, can lead to activation of the alternative pathway. Thus, the alternative pathway can act to amplify the action of the classical pathway.

As with the classical pathway, a number of opposing factors influence the activity of the alternative pathway C3 convertase.[29] The $\overline{C3b,Bb}$ enzyme is relatively labile, and under physiological conditions rapidly undergoes intrinsic decay through dissociation of the Bb. One of the proteins of the alternative pathway, properdin (P), stabilizes the binding of Bb to C3b, and thereby retards its intrinsic decay.[33] Two other control proteins—factor H and factor I—act to inhibit the generation and/or expression of the $\overline{C3b,Bb}$ enzyme. Factor H not only competes with B for binding to C3b in the assembly of the alternative pathway C3 convertase,[34] but it also can displace Bb from the $\overline{C3b,Bb}$ complex once the C3 convertase has formed.[35] Factor I inhibits the alternative pathway C3 convertase by inactivating cell-bound C3b through proteolytic cleavage, creating iC3b (Fig. 130-4). The rate of inactivation of C3b by factor I is markedly accelerated by factor H[36] and by an integral membrane protein termed "membrane cofactor protein" (MCP).[37]

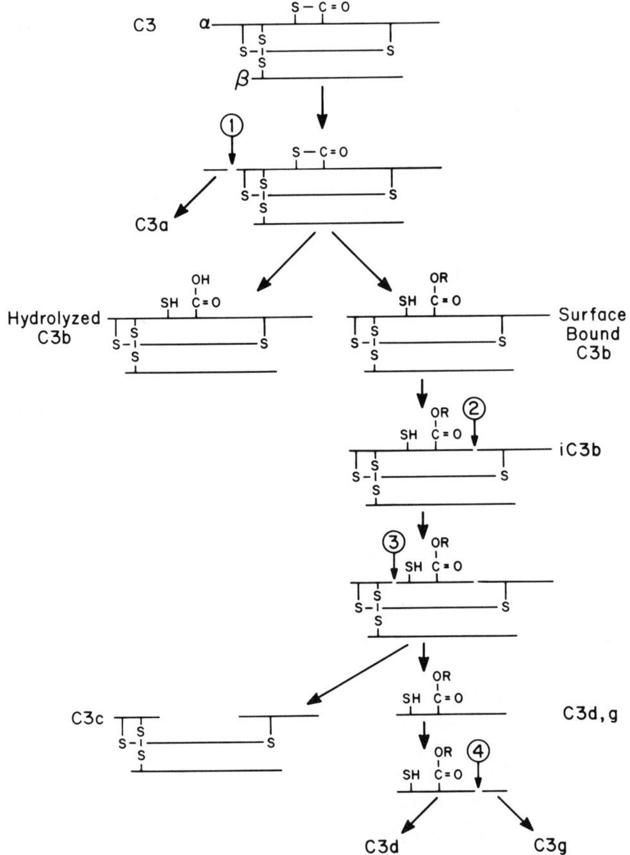

FIG. 130-4 **Proteolytic cleavage of C3. Step 1 involves the cleavage of the α chain by either the alternative pathway or classical pathway C3 convertases. Step 2 results from the action of factor I with factor H or the CR1 (C3b) receptor serving as cofactors. Step 3 is also mediated by factor I and CR1. Step 4 involves cleavage by plasmin, trypsin, leukocyte elastase and cathepsin G.** ***(From* The Metabolic Basis of Inherited Disease, *6th ed.)***

Certain particles, such as yeast cells,[38] rabbit erythrocytes,[39] and some bacteria,[28,40] are potent activators of the alternative pathway. They do so, in part, by virtue of their ability to bind nascent C3b and to protect the $\overline{C3b,Bb}$ enzyme from the inhibitory actions of factors H and I.[41] At least one molecular mechanism by which a particle protects the alternative pathway C3 convertase from these control proteins has been elucidated. The binding of factor H to a particle, and thus its inhibitory effects on the alternative pathway C3-cleaving enzyme, is favored by the presence of sialic acid residues on the particle.[34,42]

Antibody is not required for the activation of the alternative pathway, and thus, the alternative pathway is generally viewed as an important mechanism of natural immunity (reviewed in Winkelstein[28]). However, antibody can enhance the activation of the alternative pathway by a variety of particles, including bacteria-[40,43,44] and virus-infected cells,[45] although the mechanism differs depending on the nature of the initiating particle and class of antibody involved.[44,46,47] Thus, the alternative pathway can also participate in "acquired" immunity.

Activation of C3

Whether C3 is activated via the classical or alternative pathway, the α chain of the C3 is cleaved, generating two fragments of unequal size, C3a and C3b (see Fig. 130-4). In the classical pathway C3 convertase ($\overline{C4b,2a}$), the C2a contains the active site,[18] while in the alternative pathway C3 convertase ($\overline{C3b,Bb}$), the Bb contains the active site.[48] The activation of C3 by either of the two C3-convertases represents an amplification step, since many hundreds of C3 molecules can be cleaved by one C3 convertase. Cleavage of native C3 by either convertase releases a small peptide (C3a) from the α chain into the fluid phase, where it acts as an anaphylatoxin (see below). Most of the nascent C3b is also released into the fluid phase, where it rapidly is inactivated through hydrolysis. Other molecules of C3b, however, bind covalently to the cell surface or immunoglobulins through transesterification with hydroxyl groups of polysaccharides or amidation of amino groups of proteins (reviewed in Hostetter and Gordon[49]). The cell-bound C3b may then be degraded by factor I and other proteases, yielding a variety of cleavage products (see Fig. 130-4). If the cell-bound C3b is not degraded, it is then able to combine with either of the C3 convertases to create two new enzymes—the alternative pathway and classical pathway C5 convertases.

Activation of the Terminal Components (C5 through C9)

The classical pathway C5 cleaving enzyme is composed of $\overline{C4b,2a,3b}$.[50] In this complex, the C3b acts to bind native C5, while the C2a carries the active enzymatic site. In the alternative pathway, the C5 cleaving enzyme is composed of $\overline{(C3b)_2,Bb}$.[51] The two C3b molecules in the $\overline{(C3b)_2Bb}$ enzyme serve different functions in the trimolecular complex. One C3b molecule binds Bb in the proper configuration for expression of its enzymatic activity, while the other C3b serves to bind native C5 in the proper location for cleavage by Bb.

Activation of C5 by either the alternative or classical pathway C5 convertases results in cleavage of the α chain of the native molecule to create a low-molecular-weight product, C5a, and a high-molecular-weight product, C5b. The smaller cleavage product, C5a, is released into the fluid phase, where it, like C3a, can act as an anaphylatoxin (see below). In addition, C5a possesses potent chemotactic activity (see below). If the C5b combines with native C6 while it is still attached to the C5 convertase, it is stabilized and can initiate formation of the membrane attack complex, a multimolecular assembly of C5b, C6, C7, C8, and C9 that is capable of cytolytic activity.[1,52] The initial event is stabilization of the nascent C5b by C6.[53] Addition of C7 to form the C5b,6,7 complex leads to insertion of hydrophobic domains of this trimolecular complex into the cell membrane and results in stable binding to the cell membrane.[54–56] The addition of C8 leads to further insertion of the complex and the generation of small and unstable pores in the membrane through which small molecules can pass.[52,57] On reaction of C5b-8 with C9, and polymerization of C9, a large and stable transmembrane channel is formed, leading to accelerated lysis of the target cell.[58]

Just as there are regulatory proteins affecting the classical and alternative pathways, there are proteins that regulate the assembly of the membrane attack complex. For example, a protein, termed HRF20 or CD59, inhibits, in a species-specific fashion, cell lysis mediated by C8 and C9.[59]

Complement Receptors

Receptors for many of the cleavage products of individual components of complement exist on a variety of cells (reviewed in Fearon and Wong[60]). In general, two types of receptors exist: receptors that bind low-molecular-weight, diffusible fragments, such as C3a, C4a, and C5a, and receptors that bind high-molecular-weight fragments, primarily C3b and its degradation products, which have become fixed to the activating material.

Receptors for C3a, C4a, and C5a are present on mast cells, and receptors for C5a are also found on neutrophils, monocytes, and macrophages.[61] The interactions of C3a, C4a, and C5a with these receptors are capable of initiating the anaphylatoxic and chemotactic responses of these cells.

There are four distinct receptors for C3b and its cleavage products. The CR1 receptor (C3b/C4b receptor) (CD35) is found on polymorphonuclear leukocytes, eosinophils, monocytes, macrophages, mast cells, glomerular podocytes, B lymphocytes, and some T lymphocytes (reviewed in Fearon and Wong[60]). In addition, it is found on the erythrocytes of primates, including humans.[62] Although C3b is the primary ligand for the CR1 receptor, it is also capable of binding C4b. One of the more important functions of the CR1 receptor is to enhance the phagocytosis of particles opsonized with C3b.[63] In addition, its presence on erythrocytes allows them to bind circulating immune complexes bearing C3b and transport the immune complexes to cells of the reticuloendothelial system.[64] Finally, CR1 can act to dissociate Bb from the $\overline{\mathrm{C3b,Bb}}$ enzyme and act as a cofactor in the factor I–mediated cleavage of C3b to iC3b,[65] functions it holds in common with factor H. In an analogous fashion, it can facilitate dissociation of C2a from the $\overline{\mathrm{C4b,2a}}$ enzyme and act as cofactor in the cleavage of C4b to iC4b by factor I.[66]

The CR2 receptor (CD21) is found on B lymphocytes and follicular dendritic cells. It binds C3d,g and C3d (see Fig. 130-4) and the Epstein-Barr virus. The CR2 receptor on B cells appears to be important in mediating the role of C3 in enhancing B-cell responses to antigens.[67] The CR3 receptor (CD11b/18) is a member of the integrin family. It is found on the same cells as the CR1 receptor, and its primary ligand appears to be iC3b. Since iC3b is one of the C3-degradation products formed in the presence of serum, the CR3 receptor also plays an important role in ingestion of opsonized particles. The CR4 receptor (CD11c/18) is also a member of the integrin family. It is found on monocytes, polymorphonuclear leukocytes, and macrophages and its primary ligand also appears to be iC3b. Its function has not been clearly delineated.

BIOLOGIC CONSEQUENCES OF COMPLEMENT ACTIVATION

Anaphylatoxic Activity

The smaller cleavage products of both C3 and C5 (C3a and C5a), possess anaphylatoxic activity.[68] Each of these small polypeptides (9 and 11 kDa, respectively) is cleaved from the NH_2-terminal portion of the α-chain of their respective parent molecules. When compared on a molar basis, C5a is a more potent anaphylatoxin than C3a.[69] Both of these anaphylatoxins are subject to attack by a serum carboxypeptidase. This enzyme rapidly cleaves the C-terminal arginine that is common to both, creating a new molecule (C3a-desArg and C5a-desArg, respectively) that is significantly less potent as an anaphylatoxin than the parent molecule. It should also be noted that C4a also possesses some anaphylatoxic activity but with a specific activity much less than either C3a or C5a[70]; the biologic significance of C4a as an anaphylatoxin is unclear.

Complement-derived anaphylatoxins possess a variety of activities of biologic importance. They were originally identified through their ability to cause histamine release from basophils and certain tissue mast cells, to promote smooth muscle contraction, and to increase vascular permeability (reviewed in Hugli[61]). More recently, these peptides have been shown to promote the aggregation of platelets and the subsequent release of arachidonic acid metabolites.[69] In addition, they can cause neutrophils to aggregate and degranulate, generate arachidonic acid metabolites, produce toxic oxygen radicals, and discharge their granular enzymes.

Chemotactic Activity

The smaller cleavage product of C5, C5a, is also a potent chemotactic factor, which causes the directed movement of polymorphonuclear leukocytes and monocytes as well as eosinophils and basophils (reviewed in Snyderman and Goetzl[71]). When the terminal arginine is removed by the action of carboxypeptidase-B, producing C5a-desArg, the molecule loses approximately 90 percent of its biologic activity because of its decreased affinity for the C5a receptor.[72] In addition to its role in attracting mobile phagocytic cells to foci of complement activation, C5a also promotes adherence of phagocytic cells to vascular endothelium via its capacity to alter surface expression of adhesion molecules,[73] a necessary prerequisite to their exit from the intravascular compartment. A variety of in vivo studies have demonstrated that C5a plays an important role in attracting phagocytic cells to local sites of microbial invasion or immune complex deposition.[74,75]

Opsonic Activity

The larger cleavage products of C3—C3b and iC3b—act as potent opsonins when fixed to the surface of a microorganism.[76] It appears that they subserve different opsonic functions depending on the nature of the phagocytic cell and its state of activation. In the case of neutrophils and nonactivated macrophages, C3b promotes attachment of the particle, whereas immunoglobulin G acts to promote ingestion.[77] In the case of activated macrophages, C3b serves to aid in both attachment and ingestion.[78]

There is a great deal of data to suggest that C3-dependent opsonic activity is one of the more important activities of the complement system. Studies in experimental animals have shown that C3 is an important opsonin in the nonimmune host,[79] as well as in hosts who have high levels of antibody.[80]

Bactericidal Activity

The generation of complement-mediated serum bactericidal activity requires the participation of the entire terminal complement sequence (reviewed in Muschel and Fong[81]). Although bactericidal activity can occur in the absence of C9, killing proceeds at a very much slower rate.[82] Only gram-negative bacteria can be killed by complement. Although protoplasts of gram-positive organisms are susceptible to lysis by complement,[83] intact gram-positive organisms are not, suggesting that their thick cell wall somehow interferes with the bactericidal action of C5 through C9. The site of action of C5 through C9 appears to be the outer lipid membrane of gram-negative organisms.[84]

Processing of Immune Complexes

The complement system also appears to play an important role in the processing of immune complexes (reviewed in Schifferli et al.[85]). There are a number of mechanisms by which the complement system could modify the structure and/or influence the biologic activities of immune complexes. First, opsonically active C3b or iC3b can enhance the uptake of immune complexes by phagocytic cells.[86] Second, the activation of C3 via the classical pathway can retard the formation of large complexes and prevent, to some degree, their precipitation from serum.[87] Third, once complexes are formed, they can be solubilized by the complement system.[88] Apparently, it is much easier to prevent immune precipitation than it is to solubilize the complexes once they have formed. The mechanisms by which complement modifies the structure of immune complexes are incompletely understood. Clearly, the covalent binding of C3b to the immune complex is important in both the prevention of precipitation and the solubilization of preformed complexes. The biologic significance of the role of C3 in the inhibition and/or solubilization of immune complexes in vivo is not fully understood. However, in an experimental model of serum sickness, C3 has been shown to be necessary for the efficient removal of immune complexes in the kidney, suggesting that C3 may play an important role of solubilization of immune complexes in vivo.[89]

Primates have an additional complement-mediated mechanism available for handling immune complexes. They possess the CR1 receptor for C3b on their erythrocytes,[60,62] and circulating immune complexes bearing C3b will fix to erythrocytes through these receptors.[64] The erythrocyte-bound complexes are then transported to the liver, where they are transferred to Kupffer cells and the erythrocytes are returned to the circulation.[64] In this manner, erythrocytes serve to capture immune complexes, prevent their deposition in organs such as the kidney, and enhance their clearance by organs of the reticuloendothelial system.

Role of Complement in Antibody Formation

Interest in the role of complement in antibody formation has been stimulated by a number of independent but related observations. Monocytes/macrophages, B lymphocytes, and a subset of T lymphocytes all have receptors for C3 and/or C5 cleavage products[60]; it is therefore possible that their participation in the generation of a normal antibody response could be influenced by the complement system. In fact, a variety of in vitro studies have shown that cleavage products of both C3 and C5 can either enhance or inhibit a number of cellular functions important in the generation of a normal antibody response (reviewed in Weiler et al.[90]). The in vivo significance of these in vitro studies has been difficult to predict since the inhibitory/enhancing effects of these different C3 and C5 cleavage products operate at different steps in a complex series of cell-to-cell interactions.

In vivo studies, however, using experimental animals pharmacologically depleted of C3,[91] or using animals with genetically determined deficiencies of C4,[92] C2,[93] or C3,[94] have clearly shown the complement system to be important in the generation of a normal antibody response. The antibody response to T-dependent antigens is relatively more dependent on an intact complement system than is the response to T-independent antigens. In addition, an intact complement system facilitates the isotype switch from IgM to IgG in the normal immune response.

MOLECULAR GENETICS OF COMPLEMENT

Gene Families

The complement genes have been grouped into supergene families on the basis of similarities in structure, function, and chromosomal localization.[95] For instance, the genes encoding C2, factor B, and C4 constitute the class III genes of the MHC on human chromosome 6 (Fig. 130-5).[96] The 3′ terminus of the C2 gene is just 421 bp upstream of the factor B gene.[97] Factor B and C2 are similar in structural and functional features, suggesting that the genes were derived from a common ancestral gene.[98] The two C4 genes (C4A and C4B) lie approximately 30 kb centromeric from the C2 and factor B genes. The C4 loci are separated by 10 kb, and each has a cytochrome P_{450} steroid 21-hydroxylase (21-OH) gene within 1.5 kb of the 3′ terminus.[100–102] The order of the genes in the direction of transcription is C2-BF-C4A-210HA-C4B-210HB, and they have been mapped within a 0.7-cM region between HLA-B and HLA-DR.[99–101] The topology of these MHC class III genes is highly conserved in evolution as shown in several studies of the syntenic region in mice.[98,103] Other genes in this region include the newly described RING 4, 10, 11, and 12 genes, which are involved in antigen processing, tumor necrosis factor genes A and B, and the heat shock protein 70 gene. This region apparently contains an unusually high density of transcribed genes and there are many other genes in this region for which a function has yet to be determined (reviewed in Trowsdale et al.[104]).

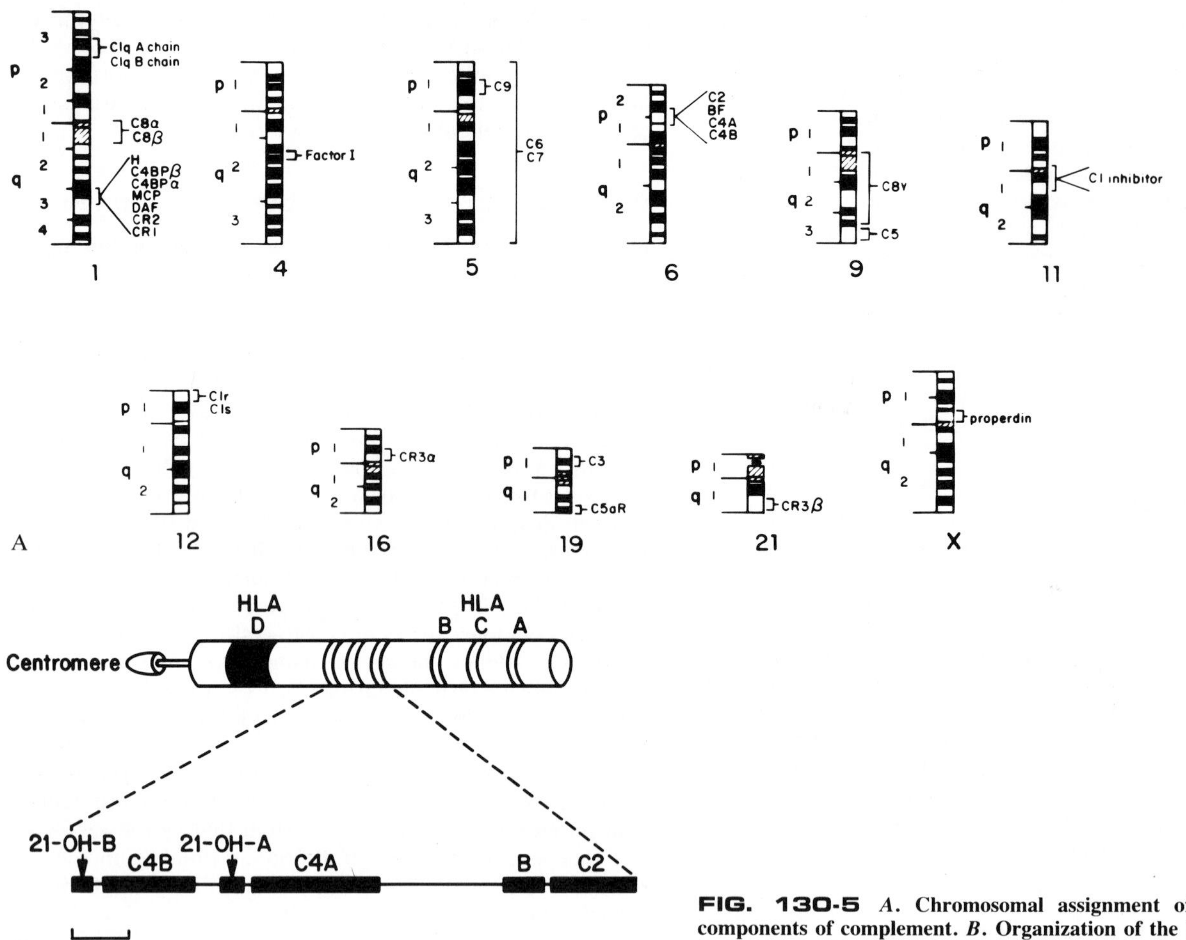

FIG. 130-5 *A*. **Chromosomal assignment of the individual components of complement.** *B*. **Organization of the human MHC on chromosome 6p. Classes I, II, and III genes are shown.**

The genes encoding complement receptors CR1 and CR2, C4-bp, factor H, MCP, and DAF are members of another supergene family, the RCA family (regulators of complement activation).[95] They are closely clustered on the long arm of chromosome 1,[105–110] and their products share several structural and functional characteristics. These six genes share the capacity to act as cofactors for factor I, bind C3b, and modulate C3 convertase activity. Direct sequence analyses of genes within this family have demonstrated repeating homology units of approximately 60 amino acids.[105] These repeating units, termed "short consensus repeats" (SCR), are also seen in the sequence of C2,[111] factor B,[104,112] and C1r/s.[113] One property common to all the complement proteins that have these highly conserved repeating homology units is their capacity to bind fragments of C3 and C4. Therefore, the complement regulatory genes on chromosome 1 and the genes encoded in the class III region of the MHC on chromosome 6 may be considered parts of a larger supergene family related because of their capacity to interact with the activation fragments of C3 and C4 (reviewed in refs. 95 and 113). These repeating homology units are also found in noncomplement proteins such as the interleukin-2 (IL-2) receptor, β_2-glycoprotein 1, the haptoglobin α chain, and the herpes simplex virus glycoprotein C—all proteins that do not interact with C3 or C4.

The genes for complement proteins C3, C4, and C5 have been described as a family that share structural and functional properties at the protein level with α_2-macroglobulin, α_1-inhibitor 3, and the pregnancy zone protein.[95,114] These genes all encode multichain disulfide-linked molecules. Except for C5, a thiolester reactive site is a distinct characteristic of this family. These genes do not appear to be clustered in a specific chromosomal region, however.

Based on primary sequence homologies, several of the proteins of the membrane attack complex also appear to be members of a large gene family[95,115–117] that also includes other proteins with pore-forming functions. That is, C6, C7, C8 α chain, C8 β chain, C9, perforin, mellitin, and the pore-forming protein of *Trypanosoma cruzi* all share sequence and domain homologies.

C1 inhibitor shares structural and functional characteristics with several other serine proteinase inhibitors so that it is often included in the SERPIN (serine proteinase inhibitor) supergene family. The chromosomal localization of several SERPIN genes has been determined, and they are dispersed throughout the genome. For example, C1 inhibitor maps to human chromosome 11,[118] whereas another member of this family, α_1-proteinase inhibitor, is localized on chromosome 14.

Protein Polymorphisms

Many of the individual components of complement demonstrate protein polymorphisms (reviewed in refs. 119 and 120). Polymorphic variants of C3 were the first to be identified because the relatively high concentration of C3 in serum permitted direct visualization of C3 variants in prolonged agarose-gel electrophoresis. The common C3 variants (C3 fast and C3 slow) are found in all major racial groups. In addition, about 20 rare C3 variants have been detected in one or several populations. Polymorphic variants of other complement proteins, such as factor B, C2, C4, C6, C7, C8, and factor D[120] have also been detected. In some instances the structural basis for this genetic variation has been determined by sequence analysis of cDNA clones[121,122] or genomic DNA.[122]

Considerable attention has been given to an analysis of the complement proteins encoded by genes within the MHC. Studies of protein polymorphisms of the C2, factor B, C4A, and C4B loci, together with typing of the MHC class I and class II genes, have generated the concept of "extended" haplotypes.[123,124] This concept derives from data in haplotypes showing a decreased frequency of recombinant events extending over a 7×10^6- to 14×10^6-bp region of chromosome 6. Taken together, the extended haplotypes account for nearly 30 percent of haplotypes in normal Caucasian populations studied this far.

Regulation of Complement Gene Expression

The delicate balance between the activation of the complement system and inhibition of activation is controlled to a certain extent by the production and local concentrations of the individual components and regulatory proteins. Particularly for the components present in the serum in small amounts, the capacity to synthesize those components at local sites may be critical for host defense and inflammation. Transcription, splicing, translation, and posttranslational modification may all play a role in controlling the local production of complement components. In general, quantitative control of production occurs at the level of transcription, which in turn is regulated by the tissue specificity, developmental pattern, and cytokine responsiveness of the individual genes.

The majority of the complement components found in serum are derived predominantly from liver synthesis. For example, the majority of serum factor B, C4, and C3 have been shown to be produced by the liver.[125–127] Monocytes, macrophages, fibroblasts, and certain endothelial cells also make small amounts of certain soluble complement components (reviewed in Colten[128]). Additionally, C3 has been detected in epithelial cells of uterus, kidney, small intestine, lung, and vascular endothelium and neutrophils.[129,130] However, the functional importance of extrahepatic sources of complement has not been established.

Production of many of the complement components is influenced by various endogenous mediators such as cytokines and hormones and exogenous agents such as endotoxin (reviewed in Colten[128]). In general, control of complement gene expression is unique for each, even among those that encode subunits of single multisubunit complement proteins (e.g., C1 and C8). Nevertheless, common *cis* regulatory motifs and similar or identical *trans*-acting nuclear transcription factors impact on the expression of several. For instance, the regulated expression of C3 and factor B by the cytokines IL-1 and IL-6 depend on members of the C/EBP and NFkB transcriptional regulatory protein families interacting with *cis*-acting sequences 5′ to the corresponding genes.[131,132] Moreover, cellular specificity of complement gene regulation is a consequence of a number of variables, including cell-surface signaling events (e.g., estrogen/progesterone regulation of C3 in uterine epithelium but not liver)[133] and *cis* and *trans* elements as in the genetic and tissue-specific expression of factor B.[134]

COMPLEMENT DEFICIENCIES: GENERAL CONSIDERATIONS

Genetically determined deficiencies have been described for nearly all of the individual components of the complement system[4,5] (Table 130-2). The usual mode of inheritance is as an autosomal recessive trait with only two known exceptions. Deficiency of C1 inhibitor has an autosomal dominant mode of inheritance, while properdin deficiency is inherited as an X-linked recessive disorder.

Diagnosis

Most of the genetically determined deficiencies of the classical activating pathway (C1, C4, and C2), of C3, and of the terminal components (C5, C6, C7, C8, and C9) can be detected using antibody-sensitized sheep erythrocytes in a total serum hemolytic complement (CH_{50}) assay. Since this assay depends on the functional integrity of C1 through C9, severe deficiencies of any of these components lead to a marked reduction or absence of total hemolytic complement activity. There is one exception; the lysis of sensitized erythrocytes can occur in the absence of C9,[57] although at a much slower rate and to a lesser extent than in the presence of C9. Therefore, patients with C9 deficiency do have some serum hemolytic complement activity, but it is reduced to between one third and one-half of the lower limit of normal.[135]

Deficiencies of factor H, factor I, and properdin of the alternative activating pathway can be detected by a hemolytic assay that assesses lysis of rabbit erythrocytes mediated by the alternative pathway.[136] Rabbit erythrocytes are potent activators of the alternative pathway,[39] due in part to the fact that they have very low levels of surface sialic acid.[29] Obviously, the serum of patients with deficiencies of C3 or C5 through C9 will also be abnormal when tested in the rabbit erythrocyte assay (as well as in the CH_{50} assay), since the lysis of rabbit erythrocytes depends on these components as well as on components of the alternative activating pathway.

The identification of the specific component that is deficient usually rests on both functional and immunochemical tests. Highly specific functional assays have been developed for each of the individual components.[137] They usually depend on reagents that lack the specific component in question, but possess the other components of the hemolytic pathway in excess. Monospecific antibodies are also available for each of the individual components, allowing for their detection by immunochemical techniques. In most cases, either functional or immunochemical assessment of the specific component will identify the deficiency. There are some exceptions, however. For example, one form of C1 inhibitor deficiency[138] and one form of C1q deficiency[139] are characterized by dysfunctional proteins that can be detected by using immunochemical assays but are markedly reduced in functional activity. In addition, patients with C8 deficiency lack either one (C8β) or two (C8α and C8γ) chains of the complete three-chain molecule.[140] This too may lead to the detection of C8 antigen in the serum of such patients while their C8 function is markedly reduced.

Individuals who are heterozygous for a deficiency of a single component usually have normal CH_{50} levels since this assay is not sensitive enough to detect reliably mild to moderate reductions in a single component. As a group, individuals who are heterozygous-deficient usually have levels of the specific component that are approximately one

Table 130-2 Genetically Determined Deficiencies of Complement in Humans

Deficiency	Inheritance	Approximate Number Patients/Kindreds	Major Clinical Manifestations
Clq	Autosomal recessive	24/14	Rheumatic disorders and pyogenic infections
Clr/s	Autosomal recessive	11/7	Rheumatic disorders
C4	Autosomal recessive	21/17	Rheumatic disorders and pyogenic infections
C2	Autosomal recessive	109/79	Rheumatic disorders and pyogenic infections
C3	Autosomal recessive	19/14	Pyogenic infections and rheumatic disorders
C5	Autosomal recessive	27/17	Meningococcal sepsis and meningitis
C6	Autosomal recessive	77/49	Meningococcal sepsis and meningitis
C7	Autosomal recessive	73/50	Meningococcal sepsis and meningitis
C8	Autosomal recessive	73/52	Meningococcal sepsis and meningitis
C9	Autosomal recessive	18/15	Asymptomatic
Factor H	Autosomal recessive	13/8	Hemolytic uremic syndrome
Factor I	Autosomal recessive	14/12	Pyogenic infections
Properdin	X-linked recessive	70/23	Meningococcal sepsis and meningitis
Factor D	Unknown	3/2	Meningococcal sepsis and meningitis/ sinopulmonary infections
C4-bp	Unknown	1/1	Behçet's disease and angioedema
DAF	Unknown	2/2	Inab phenotype
CD59	Unknown	1/1	Paroxysmal nocturnal hemoglobinuria
C1 inhibitor	Autosomal dominant	100s/100s	Angioedema

Some data from Ross and Densen[4] and Figueroa and Densen.[5]

third to one-half the average level of normals. Assignment of a given individual as a heterozygote may be difficult, since the range of values for normals may be quite wide and the levels in some heterozygotes may overlap the lower limit of normal. In some instances, such as in C2 deficiency[141] and C4 deficiency,[142] the gene for the deficiency is closely linked to the MHC and often is associated with a specific extended haplotype, thus allowing family members of deficient individuals to be assigned provisionally as heterozygotes based on HLA typing.[143,144] Studies that have identified the molecular genetic basis for some of the complement deficiencies (e.g., C2 and C4 deficiency) will allow for more precise detection of heterozygous deficient individuals.[145]

Clinical Presentation

The clinical presentation of individuals with genetically determined deficiencies of complement components is variable. Some individuals are asymptomatic, but most present with either increased susceptibility to infection, a variety of rheumatic diseases, or angioedema.[4,5]

Among those with an increased susceptibility to infection, the kinds of infections reflect the biologic functions of the missing component.[4,5] C3 is an important opsonic ligand in both the nonimmune and the immune host. Therefore, patients with a deficiency of C3, or with a deficiency of a component in either of the two pathways necessary for the activation of C3, have an increased susceptibility to encapsulated bacteria for which opsonization is the primary host defense, (e.g. the pneumococcus and *Haemophilus influenzae*). Similarly, C5 through C9 form the membrane attack complex and are therefore responsible for the bactericidal/bacteriolytic functions of complement. Thus, patients with deficiencies of C5 to C9 can opsonize bacteria normally and are not unduly susceptible to infection by bacteria for which opsonization is the primary host defense. These patients are, however, markedly susceptible to Neisseria species, since serum bactericidal activity is an important host defense against these organisms.

Patients with complement deficiencies not only have an increased frequency of infections, but the infections may also have features that differ from those in the normal population. For example, sepsis and meningitis caused by unencapsulated "avirulent" meningococci rarely occurs in normal hosts[146] but is well described in complement-deficient individuals.[147,148] Patients with deficiencies of terminal components have a higher risk for recurrence of systemic meningococcal infections, but with a lower mortality rate.[4,5]

Patients with complement deficiencies also have a variety of clinical phenotypes that can best be characterized as rheumatic disorders.[4,5] These include systemic lupus erythematosus (SLE), discoid lupus, glomerulonephritis, dermatomyositis, anaphylactoid purpura, and vasculitis. The prevalence of these inflammatory disorders is highest in patients with deficiencies of the classical activating pathway (C1, C4, and C2) and of C3. For example, approximately 80 percent of patients with C1 deficiency and 50 percent of patients with C2 deficiency have presented with a rheumatic disorder.[4,5] In contrast, patients with deficiencies of terminal complement components infrequently have rheumatic disorders.[4,5]

There are some interesting and important differences between the rheumatic diseases seen in complement-deficient patients and their counterparts in "normal" non-complement-deficient individuals. For example, the SLE seen in complement-deficient individuals is usually characterized by an early onset (often in childhood), prominent annular photosensitive skin lesions resembling discoid lupus (Fig. 130-6), relatively limited renal and pleuropericardial involvement, and a relatively infrequent occurrence of immunoglobulin and C3 in the skin.[4,5] In addition, complement-deficient individuals with SLE usually have absent or relatively low titers of both antinuclear antibodies and antinative DNA antibodies, and their lupus preparations are often negative.[143,149,150] In contrast, the incidence of anti-Ro(SSA) antibodies is significantly higher in complement-deficient patients with lupus than it is in non-complement-deficient patients with lupus.[149,150] Thus, both with respect to some of their clinical manifestations and with respect to their serologic findings, complement-deficient patients with lupus bear a striking resemblance to a subgroup of lupus patients who are "ANA-negative."[151,152]

The pathophysiological basis for the association between rheumatic disorders and complement deficiencies is unclear, but a number of possibilities exist. First, several studies have shown that components of the complement system can neutralize and/or lyse certain viruses in vitro (reviewed in Hirsch[153]), while other studies in experimental animals have shown that C3 and C5 are important mechanisms of antiviral host defense in vivo.[154,155] Thus, in some instances, the rheumatic disorders seen in complement-deficient patients might be the consequence of an altered host response to recurrent or chronic viral infections, although this has never been documented. Second, the genes for three of the individual components of complement (C4, C2, and factor B) are located within the MHC and are in linkage disequilibrium with specific HLA haplotyes (reviewed in refs. 120, 156, and 157). It is possible, therefore, that in some instances,

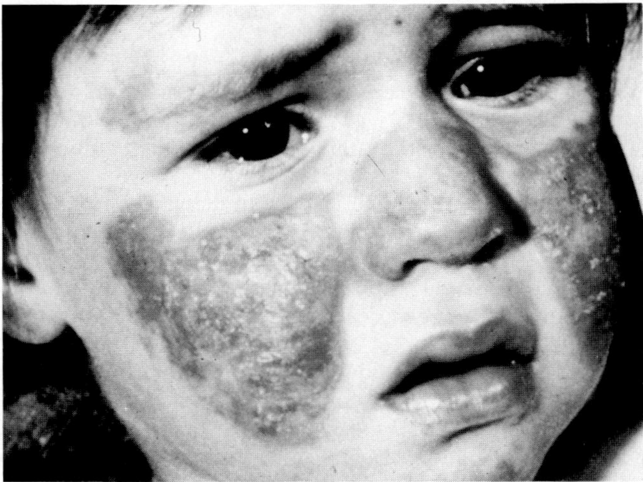

FIG. 130-6 Photosensitive skin lesions on the face of a child with C4 deficiency. ***(Courtesy of Dr. Georges Hauptmann.)***

the rheumatic disorders seen in complement-deficient patients are due in part to other genes within the MHC, which in some manner influence immune function, rather than the mutant complement alleles, per se. Third, since the complement system appears to play some role in the generation of a normal antibody response,[90–94] the rheumatic diseases seen in complement-deficient patients could result from disordered humoral immunity.

Perhaps, the most attractive hypothesis linking rheumatic diseases and complement deficiency diseases has to do with the role of the complement system in the clearance and processing of immune complexes (see above). A number of studies have shown that patients with complement deficiencies have altered and/or reduced abilities to process immune complexes. For example, serum from patients with genetically determined deficiencies of C1q, C4, C2, and C3 fails to prevent the precipitation of immune complexes as they are forming,[87,158] has a reduced ability to resolubilize complexes once they have formed,[158–160] and does not support the binding of preformed immune complexes to CR1 receptors on human erythrocytes.[161] In addition, a single in vivo study showed that a C2-deficient individual was unable to clear radiolabeled immune complexes normally from the circulation.[162] In contrast, in instances in which they have been tested, the serums of patients with deficiencies of terminal components (C5 through C9) are normal with respect to these activities. Thus, for a given complement deficiency disease, there appears to be an excellent correlation between the inability of the patient to process immune complexes normally and their susceptibility to rheumatic diseases.

Epidemiology

Given the limited manifestations of complement deficiencies, a number of studies have examined series of patients with specific clinical disorders in order to determine the frequency of genetically determined complement deficiencies in these clinical settings and to evaluate the utility of screening for complement deficiencies.

A number of studies have shown that the prevalence of genetically determined complement deficiencies is significantly higher in children or adults with systemic meningococcal infections than in the general population. Prospective studies have estimated the frequency of complement deficiencies in unselected cases of meningococcal sepsis and/or meningitis to be between 0 and 15 percent,[163–167] the range probably reflects the different populations that have been studied. In general, the prevalence is higher among sporadic cases than it is in epidemic cases.[4,5] The prevalence is also higher in patients who present with unusual serotypes. For example, two different studies have shown that between 20 and 50 percent of patients with uncommon meningococcal serotypes—such as serotypes X, Y, Z, W135, or 29E—have an inherited deficiency of a component of complement system.[168,169] Similarly, the prevalence is also higher among patients with recurrent meningococcal disease, or a positive family history of meningococcal disease.[168] For example, as many as 40 percent of patients with recurrent meningococcal disease, and as many as 10 percent of patients with a positive family history of meningitis, have genetically determined complement deficiencies.[168]

Although, a relatively large number of complement-deficient patients have presented with bacteremia and/or meningitis due to pneumococcus, streptococcus, and *H. influenzae*,[4,5] the prevalence of inherited disorders of the complement system does not appear to be markedly elevated in these infections.[166,167,170] To date, only one study has identified complement-deficient patients in such a series of patients; in that series of 389 patients only one was found to have a complement deficiency.[167]

A number of studies have examined the frequency of complement deficiencies in a variety of rheumatic diseases. However, only a few studies have examined a large enough series of patients with a single rheumatic disorder in order to yield meaningful information.[143,171,172] The prevalence of homozygous C2 deficiency in the general population has been estimated at 1 in 10,000 (0.01 percent).[143,173] In contrast, the prevalence of homozygous C2 deficiency in large series of patients with SLE has varied between 0.4 and 2.0 percent.[143,171,172] Attempts have also been made to determine whether there is an increased frequency of heterozygotes for C2 deficiency in SLE. In one study, the prevalence of heterozygotes for C2 deficiency was estimated (based on C2 levels and HLA typing) to be 5 percent,[143] a figure approximately five times the estimate in the general population. A 28-bp deletion in the C2 gene has been found to account for over 90 percent of C2 null alleles.[145,174] This mutation has allowed the precise identification of C2 null alleles in a large cohort of lupus patients and controls.[174] Among white SLE patients, although the frequency of homozygous C2-deficiency was increased, the frequency of heterozygotes was not.[174]

The most common complement deficiency found in lupus patients is a deficiency of one of the isotypes of C4. The fourth component of complement is encoded by two closely linked genes that give rise to two proteins or isotypes—C4A and C4B—[175,176] which differ by only 12 of their 1706 residues. Although complete C4 deficiency is uncommon, deficiencies of one or the other isotype are not unusual; approximately 1 percent of normal individuals are homozygous C4A-deficient and 3 percent of normal individuals are homozygous C4B-deficient.[176,177] A number of studies have demonstrated that both homozygous and heterozygous C4A deficiency are associated with SLE.[178–180] In one of these studies, the association of C4A deficiency with SLE was found to be independent of other MHC associations and represented a distinct risk factor.[180] Additionally, the association of C4A null alleles with SLE is seen in many ethnic groups, although the mutations are distinct in the different ethnic groups. Having a C4A null allele also appears to predispose individuals to the development of hydralazine-induced lupus.[181]

COMPLEMENT DEFICIENCIES: SPECIFIC DISORDERS

Clq Deficiency

Molecular Biology. As noted earlier, C1 is a macromolecule consisting of three noncovalently bound subcomponents (C1q, C1r, and C1s), which are the products of five genes—three for C1q (A, B, and C chains) and one each for C1r and C1s. The three different polypeptides that constitute the C1q molecule are encoded by three highly homologous, tightly linked genes on the long arm of chromosome 1 (1p34.1-36.3) in the order A-C-B (5′ → 3′).[182] Each 2.6-kb gene is comprised of two exons. The region coding for a collagenlike domain interrupts the sequence exactly at the site at which the triple helix of C1q bends when viewed in the electron microscope.

Pathophysiology and Clinical Expression. Only a limited number of individuals with C1q deficiency have been described.[4,5,183] In instances in which a genetic basis has been determined, the deficiency appears to be inherited as an autosomal recessive trait. Individuals with C1q deficiency have markedly reduced levels of both CH_{50} and C1 functional activity in their serum. Serum levels of the other components of complement, including C1r and C1s, are generally normal. There appear to be at least two distinct forms of C1q deficiency.[183] In one form, no C1q can be detected by either functional or immunochemical analysis.[184–186] In the other form, immunochemical C1q is present, but it lacks functional activity (i.e. dysfunctional C1q).[139,187–189] Studies of the dysfunctional C1q in two different families have shown that it is antigenically deficient as compared with normal C1q.[139,187] The dysfunctional C1q does not bind to immunoglobulin,[187,188] nor does it interact with C1r and C1s.[188] The dysfunctional C1q found in one family is distinct from that in the other since the abnormal molecules differ in molecular mass from each other as well as from normal C1q[187,188]; that is, the deficiency is genetically heterogeneous.

The predominant clinical presentation associated with either form of C1q deficiency has been lupus.[4,5,183] Although the disease has varied from patient to patient (both between and within families), skin lesions, fevers, arthralgias, and nephritis have been relatively common. As with other genetically determined complement deficiencies in which lupus develops, antinuclear antigen (ANA) and anti-DNA antibodies are absent, or present in low titers, and lupus preparations may be negative. Some patients with C1q deficiency also have an increased susceptibility to infection. In fact, four C1q-deficient patients have had sepsis and/or meningitis.

Molecular Genetic Defects. Among the several kindreds with little or no C1q protein thus far reported, the molecular defect has been defined in only two.[190,191] In one family, a stop codon interrupts B-chain translation.[190] The mutation also alters a restriction site (loss of a TAQ1 site) allowing for carrier detection. In a second family, the mutation generates a stop signal in the A chain of C1q and also yields a *Pvu*II RFLP.[191] The precise molecular defect(s) accounting for the dysfunctional form of C1q deficiency are unknown, but defects in the C chain and B chain are found in different kindreds with this variant of C1q deficiency.[187–189] Interestingly, in one kindred with dysfunctional C1q, fibroblasts from affected individuals produced normal functional C1q in vitro.[192]

Clr/Cls Deficiency

Molecular Biology. The genes encoding C1r and C1s map to 12p13.[193,194] They are separated by 9.5 kb and oriented tail to tail. The C1r and C1s genes are highly homologous, and although they share the same pattern of tissue expression, each is separately regulated.[195] C1r and C1s are expressed predominantly in the liver, but extrahepatic tissues also produce low levels of both C1r and C1s.[194,195]

Pathophysiology and Clinical Expression. An inherited deficiency of C1r has been described in which C1r is markedly reduced (<1 percent of normal) and C1s is moderately reduced (between 20 and 50 percent of normal).[4,5,183] The disorder is inherited in an autosomal recessive fashion. Patients with C1r/C1s deficiency have markedly reduced CH_{50} and C1 functional activity in their serum. Their C1q levels are normal. The basis for the association of the moderately reduced levels of C1s with the absence of C1r in these patients is unknown, but may be related to the close proximity of the two genes or to an effect of C1r metabolism on C1s expression. Interestingly, a single case of C1s deficiency has been described in which C1s was undetectable while C1r was present at approximately 50 percent of normal levels.[196]

The clinical features of C1r/C1s deficiency are similar to those found in the other deficiencies of the classical activating pathway. Rheumatic disorders resembling lupus and glomerulonephritis have each been seen. In addition, some patients ascertained as part of family studies have been clinically well.

Molecular Genetic Defects. Thus far, the molecular basis for C1r/C1s deficiency has not been determined.

C4 Deficiency

Molecular Biology. C4 is synthesized as a single polypeptide of 1706 amino acids, which is proteolytically processed into a three-subunit (α, 95 kDa; β, 75 kDa; γ, 30 kDa) disulfide-linked glycoprotein. There are two C4 genes (C4A and C4B), both located in the MHC on chromosome 6p. Although the protein products (isotypes) of the two genes differ by only 12 of their 1706 residues and share functional, structural, and antigenic characteristics that identify them as C4, they vary in electrophoretic mobility,[176] molecular weight of the α chain,[197] specific epitopes,[198] and functional hemolytic activity.[197,199] The differences between the two C4 proteins with respect to functional activity relates to their different abilities to transacylate with either hydroxyl or amino groups after activation. Nascent C4A is much more efficient transacylating with amino groups of proteins, while nascent C4B is more efficient transacylating with hydroxyl groups of carbohydrates.[197,199] Four of the 12 amino acid variations between C4A and C4B account for the difference in hemolytic activity of the two proteins.[121] These occur near the active site, the thiolester region of the C4 α chain; substitution of Asp_{1106} (C4A) to His (C4B) by site-directed mutagenesis has established that this residue is particularly critical for the functional differences between the C4A and C4B.[200]

The complete nucleotide sequences of the two human C4 genes—C4A and C4B—have been determined.[201,202] The C4A gene is 22 kb in size. A variation in size of the C4B gene (16 kb in some individuals and 22 kb in others) is a result of the presence or absence of a 6.8-kb intron toward the 5′ terminus of the C4B gene.[203,204] The variation in sequence between C4A and C4B does not explain the apparent 2-kDa difference in α-chain size between the two isotypes.[205] A relatively high frequency of duplications, deletions, and rearrangements leads to polymorphic variation in the human C4 genes.[177] Thus far, some 35 allotypic variants of C4 have been described. Many of the variants and null alleles ascribed to these genes are based on electrophoretic mobility of the C4 protein. By direct analysis of gene structure, several additional polymorphic variations have been defined and estimates of the frequency of homoduplications and deletions have been revised.[121,206,207]

Hepatic synthesis of the 185-kDa single-chain precursor of C4 pre-pro-C4[208,209] is directed by a polyadenylated mRNA of approximately 5 kb.[207,210] A C4 message has also been detected in mononuclear phagocytes, as well as in thyroid folliculare epithelial cells, salivary gland ductal epithelial cells, renal tubular epithelial cells, brain, and small intestine.[211] There has been speculation that C4 has a physiological role in epithelial cell function. Posttranslational modification involves proteolytic excision of two inter-subunit-linking peptides[212,213] sulfation,[214] modification of residues generating the thiolester reactive site,[215] and glycosylation of the α and β subunits.[216,217] There is also a specific proteolytic cleavage of a C-terminal fragment of the C4 α chain that is mediated by a metalloenzyme.[218,219]

Pathophysiology and Clinical Expression. Since there are two loci controlling the synthesis of C4, patients with total C4 deficiency are homozygous for a double null C4 haplotype, C4A*QO, C4B*QO.[177] As expected, the deficiency is closely linked to other genes of the MHC.[142]

Patients with C4 deficiency usually have severely depressed serum levels of both antigenic and functional C4 (<1 percent). Individuals who are heterozygous for C4 deficiency, at either or both of the C4 loci, as a group will have serum C4 levels that generally reflect the number of active genes.[220,221] However, assignment of a given individual as a heterozygote for the deficiency is complicated by the fact that the range of C4 levels in normal individuals is quite wide and a deficiency of C4 at one or the other locus is relatively common in normal persons.[176,177] Accordingly, assignment of an individual as heterozygous for the deficiency is usually based on kindred analysis using HLA linkage,[142] DNA Southern blot analysis,[206] or electrophoretic analysis of C4 allotypes in serum.[176]

Patients with complete C4 deficiency have a markedly decreased ability to activate C3 via the classical pathway; thus, their CH_{50} activity is virtually absent. In contrast, serum activities that can be mediated via the alternative pathway, such as opsonic, chemotactic, and bactericidal activities, are present, although usually reduced because of a lack of an intact classical pathway.[222,223]

The predominant clinical manifestation of complete C4 deficiency has been SLE.[4,5,177] Although most of the patients have had many of the clinical features of SLE, such as photosensitive skin rashes, renal disease, and occasionally arthritis, they have rarely had ANA antibodies in their serum, and if present they have been of relatively low titer. Biopsies of the affected skin have shown histologic features characteristic of lupus.[224] Although some of the patients have demonstrated an increased susceptibility to infection, these have been patients in whom SLE was also present.[4,5] As with many of the other complement deficiency diseases, there have been a few asymptomatic C4-deficient patients ascertained as the result of family studies.

Although complete C4 deficiency is extremely rare, individuals who are homozygous-deficient for either C4A or C4B are quite common.[176,177] There is a relatively high frequency of null alleles at either the C4A or C4B locus among both African Americans[225] and Caucasians.[176] For example, the frequency of C4A*QO among Caucasians has been estimated as between 13 and 14 percent and that of C4B*QO as between 15 and 16 percent. The corresponding frequencies of homozygous-null individuals at each locus would be just over 1 percent for C4A and just under 3 percent for C4B. These are clearly minimal estimates as revealed by direct studies of the C4A and C4B genes by Southern blotting.[206]

Because of the differences in functional activity between C4A and C4B, it has been suggested that individuals who are homozygous-deficient in one isotype or the other might be predisposed to certain illnesses. For example, individuals with homozygous C4A deficiency lack the isotype that interacts most efficiently with proteins. They, therefore, might not be able to process protein-containing immune complexes as well as individuals who possess this isotype, and as a consequence they might be at an increased risk for immune complex diseases such as SLE. In fact, a number of studies have shown that the prevalence of homozygous C4A deficiency in SLE varies between 10 and 15 percent, a figure 10 to 15 times higher than the prevalence in the general population.[178–180] Individuals with homozygous C4B deficiency lack the isotype that is most efficient in interacting with polysaccharides. They, therefore, might not be able to assemble the classical pathway C3-cleaving enzyme ($\overline{C4b,2a}$), and deposit opsonically active C3b, on the polysaccharide capsules of pathogenic bacteria, which in turn might predispose them to bloodborne bacterial infections. In fact, there is an increased prevalence of homozygous C4B deficiency in children with bacteremia and meningitis.[170,226]

Molecular Genetic Defects. Most of the C4A null genes are the results of deletions or mutations interrupting transcription or translation.[177,227] In contrast, most of the C4B null genes examined so far appear to be due to a gene conversion—that is, mutations that produce a C4A-like product at the C4B locus.[177,227] Complete C4 deficiency, in the cases that have been evaluated, is genetically heterogeneous. Various combinations of deletions and pseudogenes have been identified.[228,229] In no case to date has a large deletion involving both loci been identified.

C2 Deficiency

Molecular Biology. The C2 gene, consisting of 18 exons within a 14-kb span, is quite similar in overall structure to the closely linked factor B gene, and their products display 35 percent homology in the derived amino acid sequences.[96,98,111] The 3′ terminus of the C2 gene is approximately 500 bp upstream of the factor B gene. As a result, critical transcriptional control elements included in the regulation of factor B expression are embedded within the region encoding the 3′ untranslated region of the C2 mRNA.

C2 mRNA programs the translation of three distinct polypeptides.[230] The three forms of C2 are probably derived from differential transcription or posttranscriptional processing. Translation of the most abundant C2 mRNA (2.8 kb) generates an 84-kDa product that is further modified and secreted within 30 to 60 min. Two forms of C2 of lower molecular mass remain cell-associated. These multiple forms of C2 have also been detected in murine L cells transfected with a genomic fragment bearing the human C2 and factor B genes,[231] but their significance is not yet appreciated. Preliminary data suggest that at least one of these cell-associated C2 forms is generated by an alternative splicing mechanism.[232]

Polymorphic variation in C2 and factor B is much less frequent than in C4 or the class I and class II MHC gene products. Nevertheless, several allelic forms of these two proteins have been defined by electrophoretic techniques[120,156] and by restriction endonuclease digestion.[233–235]

Pathophysiology and Clinical Expression. Genetically determined C2 deficiency is the most common of the inherited complement deficiencies.[4,5,236] The frequency of the gene for C2 deficiency has been estimated at between 1 and 1.5 percent in the normal population,[143,174,237] with homozygous deficiency occurring as frequently as 1 in 10,000.[236] Individuals homozygous for C2 deficiency generally have less than 1 percent of the normal amount of C2 functional activity and undetectable C2 by immunochemical analysis.[238] Heterozygotes for C2 deficiency generally have C2 levels between 30 and 70 percent of the average values for normal individuals.[238] The wide range of C2 levels in both normal individuals and individuals who are heterozygous for C2 deficiency makes assignment of heterozygous status based on C2 levels alone difficult.

Complement-mediated serum activities, such as opsonization and chemotaxis, are present in patients with C2 deficiency, presumably because their alternative pathway is intact.[239–241] However, when assessed carefully and compared to normals these activities are not generated as quickly or to the same degree as in individuals with an intact classical pathway.[76,241–243]

The clinical manifestations of C2 deficiency have varied from individuals who are asymptomatic to individuals who are clinically affected with either an increased susceptibility to infection and/or rheumatic diseases.[4,5,236] There appears to be no correlation between the C2-deficient genotype and phenotype,[145,174] but additional studies will be required to establish this conclusion definitively. A number of C2-deficient patients have had an increased susceptibility to bacterial infections. For the most part, the infections have been bloodborne and systemic (e.g., sepsis, meningitis, arthritis, and osteomyelitis) and caused by encapsulated organisms (e.g., pneumococcus, *H. influenzae*, and meningococcus).[4,5,236,240,244–246]

A variety of rheumatic diseases have also been seen in association with C2 deficiency.[4,5,236] The most common of these are SLE and discoid lupus. Although these patients possess many of the characteristic clinical features of SLE, there are some distinctions. In general, although fulminant glomerulonephritis can occur,[247] progressive nephritis and renal failure are uncommon.[236] Similarly, although there are reports of central nervous system involvement, it is relatively uncommon. Arthralgias may be present, but frank arthritis is rare. Cutaneous lesions are seen relatively often among C2-deficient patients with lupus, and many patients have characteristic annular photosensitive lesions.[248] In addition, unlike the situation in typical SLE, biopsies of uninvolved skin do not show deposits of C3 or immunoglobulin at the dermal–epidermal junction.[236,248] The incidence of anti-DNA and ANA antibodies is relatively low in C2-deficient patients with lupus.[143,149] However, they do have a high incidence of anti-Ro(SSA) antibody (75 percent).[149,150] Thus, based on both clinical and serologic criteria, C2-deficient patients with lupus resemble non-complement-deficient patients with "ANA-negative" SLE[151] and/or subacute cutaneous lupus erythematosus.[152] A number of other rheumatic diseases have been described in patients with C2 deficiency.[4,5,236] Chief among these have been glomerulonephritis,[249] dermatomyositis,[250] anaphylactoid purpura,[251] and vasculitis.[241]

Molecular Genetic Defects. A number of studies have shown that null alleles for C2 deficiency (C2*QO) are in linkage disequilibrium with a number of the products of the MHC.[141,144,237,253–256] Thus, the C2*QO allele is often part of an extended haplotype consisting of HLA-A25, B18, C2QO, BfS, C4A4, C4B2, and DR2.[236,256,257] This haplotype is typically associated with one (type I) of two recognized molecular defects that produce C2 deficiency. In the type I defect, a 28-bp deletion from the 3′ end of exon 6 leads to loss of a donor splice site, a loss of exon 6 (134 bp) in the C2 mRNA, and a frameshift stop codon.[145] Hence, although C2 mRNA is generated, no stable C2 protein is translated.[145,258] Type I deficiency accounts for more than 90 percent of C2-deficient patients.[145,174] Type II deficiency is characterized by a block in C2 secretion with accumulation of intracellular C2 with an aberrant molecular weight.[258] The molecular details of the type II deficiency are not known. Individuals homozygous for type I C2 deficiency generally have no detectable serum C2 protein, and serum from type II–deficient individuals contains less than 1 percent of the normal amount of C2 functional activity and protein.[258]

C3 Deficiency

Molecular Biology. The human C3 gene consists of 41 exons spanning 42 kb[259] on chromosome 19.[260] The 5.2-kb mature mRNA[261] encodes the pre-pro-C3 primary translation product.[262] C3 is synthesized primarily in hepatocytes,[262–264] with lesser amounts produced by monocytes, fibroblasts, endothelium, and epithelial cells of several organs.[128–130] Cotranslational and posttranslational processing includes cleavage of the signal peptide and the interchain linking peptide and glycosylation to generate the heterodimeric disulfide-linked C3 protein. The thiolester bridge is generated by isomerization of a lactam to yield a thiolactone perhaps facilitated by a specific enzyme.[265]

Pathophysiology and Clinical Expression. Genetically determined C3 deficiency is inherited as an autosomal recessive trait.[4,5] Although rare, it has been observed in many different ethnic groups throughout the world. Genetic studies using allotypic analysis have shown that mutations in the structural gene for C3 are responsible for C3 deficiency.[266–268] These patients have severely depressed levels of serum C3 (<1 percent of normal)[269]; in some, low levels of C3 antigen and function can be detected using highly sensitive techniques,[269] whereas in others, no C3 protein is detected even when using extremely sensitive assay systems.[270]

Serum functions directly or indirectly dependent on C3 because of its role in the activation of C5 through C9, are also markedly reduced. That is, serum opsonic, chemotactic, and bactericidal activities are either absent or markedly diminished in patients with C3 deficiency.[269–275]

The clinical manifestations of C3 deficiency in humans have included both an increased susceptibility to infection and rheumatic disorders. Patients with C3 deficiency have had a variety of infections, including pneumonia, bacteremia, meningitis and osteomyelitis, caused by encapsulated pyogenic bacteria, such as the pneumococcus, meningococcus, *Klebsiella pneumoniae* and *Escherichia coli*.[4,5,269,270,273–277] To date, no patient with C3 deficiency has been reported to have an unusually severe or recurrent viral or fungal infection.

A variety of rheumatic diseases have also been seen in C3-deficient patients. A number of patients have presented with arthralgias and vasculitic skin rashes.[272,273] Two sisters had a clinical picture of SLE with arthritis, alopecia, malar rash, and photosensitivity.[273] Although certain clinical features of lupus are present in some patients with C3 deficiency, as with other complement-deficient patients, they may not have serologic evidence of lupus. Renal disease has also been seen in C3-deficient patients.[268,278,279] Histologically, the lesions most closely resemble membranoproliferative glomerulonephritis and are often characterized by mesangial-cell proliferation, an increased mesangial matrix, and electron-dense deposits in both the mesangium and the subendothelium of capillary loops.[278,279] Immunofluorescence studies have revealed all major immunoglobulin classes to be present in the deposits but not C3. In one of the cases of renal disease, as well as in some of the cases of vasculitis or lupus in which there was no apparent renal disease, circulating immune complexes have been found in the serum.[273,275,278] Finally, Sweet's syndrome (febrile neutrophilic dermatitis) has also been described in association with C3 deficiency.[280]

C3 is highly polymorphic, with at least 20 allelic variants having been identified[119,120] by electrophoretic techniques. The two most common alleles, C3 Fast (C3*F) and C3 Slow (C3*S), are found in over 98 percent of the population. Two rare variants have been described that are indistinguishable from C3*S and C3*F by electrophoretic mobility, respectively, but with reduced amounts in serum. Termed hypomorphic C3 slow (C3*s) and hypomorphic C3 fast (C3*f), these variants have been identified in patients with a variety of rheumatic disorders. Hypomorphic C3*f has been described in patients with glomerulonephritis and arthritis,[281] cutaneous vasculitis,[282] and recurrent hemolytic-uremic syndrome,[283] as well in normal individuals.[284] Hypomorphic C3*s has been described in a patient with nephritis as well as in his asymptomatic family members.[285]

Molecular Genetic Defects. The molecular basis for C3 deficiency is heterogeneous.[270,286,287] In some families, mutant alleles with frame shifting deletions have been described.[270,286] In other kindreds, there is expression of reduced amounts of normal-sized C3 mRNA, with production of decreased amounts of apparently normal C3 protein.[287,288]

C5 Deficiency

Molecular Biology. C5 is encoded by a 79-kb gene with 41 exons on chromosome 9q.[289,290] The 6.0-kb mature C5 mRNA programs synthesis of pre-pro-C5.[291–293] C5 mRNA undergoes alternative splicing, but the consequences of this at the level of protein function is unknown.[289] Pre-pro-C5 undergoes cotranslational and posttranslational processing to generate the two-chain disulfide-linked mature protein (190 kDa). C5 is synthesized in liver hepatocytes, as well as in alveolar epithelium and mononuclear phagocytes.

Pathophysiology and Clinical Expression. Genetically determined C5 deficiency has been identified in several families.[4,5,294] The deficiency is inherited as an autosomal recessive trait. Homozygous-deficient individuals usually have markedly reduced levels of C5 activity (<1 percent) and antigen. One patient had 1 to 2 percent of normal C5 activity, although her affected sister had less than 0.1 percent.[295] Heterozygotes usually have one-third to one-half normal serum levels. The serums of patients with C5 deficiency are unable to generate normal chemotactic or bactericidal activity,[296,297] but serum opsonic activity is intact, because activation of C3 can proceed without the participation of C5.[296,298]

Although the first patient with C5 deficiency had SLE and membranoproliferative glomerulonephritis,[295] subsequent patients have had either meningococcal meningitis or disseminated gonococcal infections.[296–299] A few asymptomatic C5-deficient patients have been ascertained as part of family studies.

Molecular Genetic Defects. The molecular genetic defects causing C5 deficiency are not known.

C6 Deficiency

Molecular Biology. C6 is a single-chain glycoprotein encoded by a gene on chromosome 5q13.[300] The C6 mRNA is approximately 6.6 kb and is produced primarily in the liver.[301] Cotranslational and posttranslational processing produces a protein of 128 kDa. Circular dichroism spectroscopy and transmission electron microscopy show that the C6 protein has a sickle shape with a small "hook" on one end.[302] The structure also contains several thrombospondin repeat motifs that are believed to function in protein–protein and protein–phospholipid interactions during assembly of the membrane attack complex.

Pathophysiology and Clinical Expression. Deficiency of C6 is inherited as an autosomal recessive trait.[4,5,303] Studies on several probands have shown that the mutations causing C6 deficiency are "null" alleles of the C6 structural gene.[304] Individuals who are homozygous-deficient generally have less than 1 percent of the normal amount of C6 antigen and activity.[304] The only functional abnormality relating to their serum complement system is a marked deficiency of serum bactericidal activity.[305–308] The remainder of their complement-mediated serum activities depend only on the activation of C3 and C5 (e.g., opsonic activity and chemotactic activity) and are normal.[305–308]

The major clinical manifestation of C6 deficiency is susceptibility to disseminated neisserial infections.[4,5] While most patients have had meningococcal sepsis and meningitis, others have had disseminated gonococcal infections. One patient with C6 deficiency has presented with a lupuslike syndrome.[309]

Two unrelated patients with a genetically determined deficiency of both C6 and C7 have been described.[310,311] Both had low levels of both C6 (1 to 5 percent of normal) and C7 (3 to 9 percent of normal). In one, serum C6 was smaller (110 kDa) than normal (140 kDa) and antigenically deficient, while C7 appeared normal.[310] The second patient had no detectable C6, even in a concentrated serum sample, although small amounts of normal C7 were present.[311]

Molecular Genetic Defects. The molecular basis of C6 deficiency is not known.

C7 Deficiency

Molecular Biology. The gene for C7 is closely linked to the gene for C6 on chromosome 5q13.[300]

Pathophysiology and Clinical Expression. Only a few patients with C7 deficiency have been identified.[4,5,312] The defect appears to be inherited as an autosomal recessive trait. For the most part, homozygous-deficient individuals have severely reduced (<1 percent) levels of C7 antigen and activity in serum. In one case, however, the patient's serum level of functionally active C7 varied over time, reaching levels as high as 3.5 percent of normal.[313] At the apex of C7 functional levels, C7 antigen also was detected. C7-deficient patients have little if any CH_{50} activity in their serum. Similarly, serum bactericidal activity is markedly reduced.[314–316]

A number of clinical phenotypes have been associated with C7 deficiency.[4,5,312] As with deficiencies of other terminal components, systemic meningococcal infections and/or disseminated gonococcal infections have predominated. C7-deficient patients also have presented with lupus,[317] rheumatoid arthritis,[318] scleroderma,[313] and pyoderma gangrenosum.[319] Some C7-deficient individuals have been asymptomatic.

Molecular Genetic Defects. Genetic defects causing C7 deficiency have not been elucidated.

C8 Deficiency

Molecular Biology. C8 is composed of three polypeptide chains (α, β, and γ),[320] each encoded by separate genes (C8A, C8B, and C8G).[115,116,322] The α and γ chains are covalently joined to form one subunit (C8, α, γ), which is joined to the β chain (C8 β) noncovalently.[321] C8A and C8B map to 1p3.2 and C8G maps to 9q.[323] The C8A and C8B genes each encode 2.4-kb mRNAs. Although closely linked, they are independently regulated. C8A and C8B contain several thrombospondin repeat motifs that are common to many of the terminal complement components. The precursors of the three C8 polypeptides are translated in liver, cotranslationally and posttranslationally processed, assembled, and secreted.[324] The rates of α- and γ-chain synthesis are equal, but exceed that for β-chain synthesis so that some free α-γ is found in plasma.[325]

Pathophysiology and Clinical Expression. Several variants of C8 deficiency have been recognized. In one form of C8 deficiency, patients lack the C8 α-γ subunit, while in the other form, the C8 β subunit is deficient.[326,327]

Two types of C8 β subunit deficiency have been identified. In one, the β chain is apparently dysfunctional[326,328]; in the other, C8 β-chain expression is markedly decreased,[329] presumably by a pretranslational mechanism (i.e., either decreased transcription or increased catabolism of C8 β mRNA). In all variants, C8 functional activity is markedly reduced (<1 percent of normal). In the case of C8 β subunit deficiency, C8 antigen can be detected in the serum of affected individuals using standard immunodiffusion techniques, but it lacks antigenic determinants present in the intact C8 molecule.[330] Isolation of the C8 antigen from the serum of patients with C8 β subunit deficiency has shown it to be identical to the normal C8 α-γ subunit.[331,332] Addition of C8 β subunit, purified from normal C8, restores C8 functional activity, offering additional evidence that the C8 α-γ subunit in these patients' serums is normal.[331,332]

In the case of C8 α-γ deficiency, initial analyses of serum from these patients using standard immunodiffusion techniques failed to detect any C8 antigen.[333,334] However, when serum from these patients is immunoprecipitated with antiserum to C8 and the precipitates examined using SDS-PAGE analysis, the C8 β subunit can be detected.[327] Addition of purified C8 α-γ from normal serum restores C8 functional hemolytic activity.[327] As expected, when C8 α-γ subunit–deficient serum is mixed with C8 β–deficient serum, hemolytic activity is also restored.[327]

The only functional defect in C8-deficient serum is a marked reduction in bacteriolytic activity.[333,335] Other complement-mediated serum activities, such as opsonization, are intact.

The clinical presentation of C8 deficiency is similar to the other deficiencies in terminal complement components.[4,5,326] Meningococcemia, meningococcal meningitis, and disseminated gonococcal infections predominate. SLE has also been seen.

Molecular Genetic Defects. The molecular genetic basis for C8 deficiency is not known.

C9 Deficiency

Molecular Biology. C9 is a 70-kDa glycoprotein with sequence homology to C8 α and β, perforin (a product of cytotoxic lymphocytes), and the LDL receptor.[336–338] The C9 structural gene is comprised of 11 exons spanning 80 kb[339] on chromosome 5p13.[340] C9 is produced primarily by the liver.

Pathophysiology and Clinical Expression. Only a few patients with C9 deficiency have been identified in Occidentals,[4,5,341] but it appears to be the most common complement deficiency in Japan.[342] In patients in which family members have been available for testing, the disease appears to be inherited as an autosomal recessive trait.

Most affected individuals have markedly reduced levels of C9, whether tested immunochemically or by functional analysis. In one case, however, the patient had trace amounts of C9 antigen detectable in her serum, and between 10 and 15 percent of the normal amount of C9 functional hemolytic activity.[343] The hemolysis of sensitized erythrocytes can be mediated by a membrane attack complex composed of C5b-8 and is not, therefore, strictly dependent on C9.[57] As a result, patients with C9 deficiency have some total hemolytic complement activity although it is usually no more than one third and one half of the lower limit of normal.[344,345] Similarly, their serums have some bactericidal activity, although the rate of killing is significantly reduced.[343]

Like patients with deficiencies of other terminal components, patients with C9 deficiency have an increased susceptibility to systemic meningococcal infections.[4,5,341] Although the first few individuals with C9 deficiency were asymptomatic, subsequent patients with C9 deficiency have presented with systemic meningococcal infections.[4,5,346] In addition, an epidemiologic study of C9 deficiency in Japan has firmly established a relationship between C9 deficiency and meningococcal sepsis and meningitis.[347]

Molecular Genetic Defects. The molecular genetic basis for C9 deficiency is not known.

Factor I Deficiency

Molecular Biology. Factor I is a heterodimer composed of disulfide-linked 50- and 38-kDa subunits; 11 to 20 percent of its mass is contributed by asparagine-linked carbohydrate. The light chain has homology with the classic serine proteases, especially the plasminogen activators. In human hepatoma cells factor I is synthesized as a single precursor polypeptide (pro-I) and undergoes posttranslational proteolysis to generate the mature protein.[348] It is also synthesized in human mononuclear phagocytes and endothelial cells.[349] cDNA clones for factor I have been isolated and the gene localized to chromosome 4.[350]

Pathophysiology and Clinical Expression. Genetically determined factor I deficiency has been described in only a few families.[4,5] It is inherited as an autosomal recessive trait, with about half-normal levels of factor I in heterozygotes.

Patients with factor I deficiency have an uncontrolled activation of C3 via the alternative pathway.[351–354] There is continuous low-grade generation of an alternative pathway C3-cleaving enzyme, $\overline{C3b,Bb}$, which is inhibited by factors H and I. In the absence of factor I there is no control imposed on the formation and expression of the alternative pathway C3 convertase; as a result there is continued activation and cleavage of C3.[355] Patients with factor I deficiency, therefore, have a secondary consumption of native C3 with markedly reduced levels of antigenic C3 in their serum, most of which is not in the form of native C3 but rather in the form of the cleavage product C3b.[351] Serum levels of other components of the alternative pathway—factors B, factor H, and properdin—are also reduced, reflecting continuing activation of the alternative pathway.[354] As expected, serum activities that depend on C3, either directly or indirectly, such as bactericidal activity, opsonic activity, and chemotactic activity, are reduced in patients with factor I deficiency.[351]

In at least one instance, purified factor I has been infused into a patient with factor I deficiency.[354] Levels of factor B and properdin rose within 24 h of the infusion. The level of the C3 cleavage product C3b fell and was followed by a rise in the level of native C3. Apparently, the replacement of factor I corrected the metabolic defect by reestablishing control of the alternative pathway and stopping the activation and consumption of native C3. As a result, the patient's serum hemolytic and opsonic activities also became normal.

The most common clinical expression of factor I deficiency is an increased susceptibility to infection.[351,356–359] As with primary C3 deficiency, infections have included both localized infections on mucosal surfaces and systemic infections. The organisms most commonly responsible for these infections have been encapsulated pyogenic bacteria, such as streptococcus, pneumococcus, meningococcus, and *H. influenzae*—organisms for which C3 is an important opsonic ligand. In addition to problems with infection, some patients have had elevated levels of circulating immune complexes.[357,358] There have been no reports of chronic renal disease developing in patients with factor I deficiency as has been seen in C3 deficiency. However, one patient had a transient illness resembling serum sickness characterized by fever, rash, arthralgia, hematuria, and proteinuria.[357]

Molecular Genetic Defects. Little is known about the molecular defect in factor I deficiency but sequence polymorphisms linked to the factor I gene have been identified in several families that permit carrier detection.[360]

Factor H Deficiency

Molecular Biology. Factor H is a 150-kDa monomeric glycoprotein that regulates the activity of the C3b, Bb enzyme. The protein is composed of 20 homologous repeating units (SCR), which are also found in C4-bp, DAF, MCP, CR1, and CR2.[107] Additional factor H–related cDNAs and proteins have been characterized. Four factor H–related mRNAs are produced in human liver. The 4.4-kb message encodes the 150-kDa factor H protein. A 1.8-kb factor H mRNA is a splice variant that encodes a protein with factor H activity.[361] Two other genes encode factor H–related proteins that do not exhibit cofactor activity and consist of five SCR units, three of which are highly homologous to those found in factor H. All four mRNAs are constitutively expressed in liver. The two mRNAs derived from the factor H gene are also found in fibroblasts, endothelial cells, and monocytes. The short factor H–related mRNAs are found only in liver.[362] The factor H structural gene maps to the RCA region of chromosome 1.

Pathophysiology and Clinical Expression. Genetically determined factor H deficiency has been described in only a few families.[363–365] The deficiency appears to be inherited as an autosomal recessive trait. In two families, the parents were first cousins and had approximately half the normal level of factor H, as did some of the other family members.[364,365] In probands from two families, factor H was undetectable,[363,366] while in probands from two other families factor H was detectable but reduced to less than 10 percent of normal.[363,364] The levels of the alternative pathway components factor B and properdin are also reduced, but not to the same degree as factor H. Similarly, the serum levels of C3 are reduced, and the majority of the C3 present is in the form of an activation/cleavage product. Presumably, the markedly reduced level of factor H leads to continuous activation of the alternative pathway, with resultant depletion of C3 and other proteins of the alternative pathway.

The clinical manifestations of factor H deficiency have included glomerulonephritis, hemolytic uremic syndrome, SLE, and systemic meningococcal infections.[363–366] In addition, some asymptomatic individuals with factor H deficiency have been ascertained in family studies.[365]

Molecular Genetic Defects. The molecular basis of factor H deficiency is not known.

Factor D Deficiency

Molecular Biology. Factor D is a 24-kDa serine protease. A factor D cDNA has been cloned and sequenced and found to be identical to adipsin.[367] Unlike other complement components, factor D is not synthesized in hepatocytes, but in adipocytes, muscle cells, lung, and macrophages/monocytes.[367]

Pathophysiology and Clinical Expression. Two kindreds with factor D deficiency have been described. In one, twins presented with recurrent sinopulmonary infections and were found to have 8 percent of the normal levels of factor D.[368] In the second kindred, factor D was undetectable in the male proband and present in approximately half-normal levels in the mother and sister. As expected, the CH_{50} in the patients was mildly depressed, while the AP_{50} was 0 to 5 percent of normal. Antigenic factor D was not detected in the serum of the second patient.[369]

The clinical manifestations of factor D deficiency have been recurrent neisserial infections and recurrent sinopulmonary infections.[368,369]

Molecular Genetic Defects. The molecular basis for factor D deficiency is unknown.

Properdin Deficiency

Molecular Biology. The gene for properdin maps to Xp11.23-21.1 and produces a 1.5-kb mRNA.[370] The complete primary structure of properdin has been elucidated.[371] The protein appears as a bent rod on electron microscopy and is comprised of six thrombospondin repeat motifs, which are common to many of the terminal complement components. Properdin is produced by activated macrophages.[372] Some studies indicate that liver and lung may also synthesize properdin. Properdin circulates as polydispersed aggregates of 56-kDa polypeptide subunits.

Pathophysiology and Clinical Expression. Properdin deficiency is inherited as an X-linked recessive trait.[4,5] In some families, affected males have markedly reduced levels of properdin (<1 percent of normal),[373,374] while in others the properdin level is as high as 10 percent of normal.[375,376] A third form of properdin deficiency has been described, in which properdin is present in normal concentrations but is dysfunctional.[377] To date, there is no evidence that the dysfunctional properdin differs from normal properdin with respect to subunit size or polymerization.[377] In all cases in which it has been tested, the ability to activate C3 via the alternative pathway has been markedly reduced.[373–379]

The most common clinical manifestation of properdin deficiency has been fulminant meningococcemia and meningococcal meningitis.[4,5] SLE and discoid lupus have also been seen.[4,5,378]

Molecular Genetic Defects. The molecular defects responsible for properdin deficiency are not known.

C4b Binding Protein Deficiency

Molecular Biology. C4b binding protein is composed of seven elongated α chains extending from a central β chain. The α chain is translated from a 2.5-kb mRNA and the β chain from a 1.0-kb mRNA. The α chains each contain eight SCR units, while the β chain contains three SCR as well as a region homologous to the α chain. The β chain is believed to contain the binding site for the vitamin K–dependent protein S.[380] C4b binding protein is expressed primarily in liver and monocytes.[381]

Pathophysiology and Clinical Expression. C4b binding protein controls classical pathway C3 convertase activity by serving as a cofactor for factor I. A single kindred with a deficiency of C4b binding protein has been identified.[382] The proband presented with Behçet's disease and angioedema. C4b binding protein was present at 15 percent of normal levels. Her father and sister had approximately 25 percent of normal levels and were clinically healthy. Another sister had normal C4b binding protein levels.

Molecular Genetic Defects. The molecular basis of C4b binding protein deficiency is not known.

Decay Accelerating Factor

Molecular Biology. DAF is composed of four SCR units and a tail 70 amino acids long. It is encoded by a 35-kb gene that maps to the RCA region on chromosome 1.[106] Expression of DAF is limited to blood components and vascular endothelial cells.[383] There is also high-level expression on the cornea. DAF is attached to the cell membrane by a glycosylphosphatidylinositol (GPI) anchor. The GPI anchor is a posttranslational modification. The GPI anchor associates with SRC family protein tyrosine kinases and may transduce membrane signals.[384]

Pathophysiology and Clinical Expression. Genetically determined deficiency of DAF has been associated with the Inab phenotype.[385,386] Individuals who possess the Inab phenotype lack all blood group antigens of the Cromer complex, antigens that reside in DAF. Acquired DAF deficiency is a manifestation of paroxysmal nocturnal hemoglobinuria in which a series of GPI-anchored proteins are lost from the cell surface, leaving cells abnormally sensitive to lysis by complement. In contrast, the Inab phenotype is not associated with hemolysis. DAF is completely lacking in Inab patients, and in spite of increased deposition of C3, hemolysis is not observed.[385] Two patients with the Inab phenotype have had severe protein-losing enteropathies.[386]

Molecular Genetic Defects. The molecular cause of DAF deficiency is not known.

CD59 Deficiency

Molecular Biology. CD59 (HRF 20, membrane inhibitor of reactive lysis [MIRL]) is a 20-kDa glycoprotein whose structural gene maps to chromosome 11p13-14. CD59 is widely expressed on erythrocytes, leukocytes, and other cells. Like DAF, it is anchored to the cell membrane by a GPI moiety. Also in common with DAF, it appears to subserve a T-cell activation function.[387]

Pathophysiology and Clinical Expression. A single patient with CD59 deficiency, the product of a consanguineous marriage, has been described.[388] He presented with hemolytic anemia as a child and had positive Ham and sucrose tests for paroxysmal nocturnal hemoglobinuria. He also suffered recurrent cerebral infarctions. Studies of four GPI-anchored proteins typically lost in paroxysmal nocturnal hemoglobinuria revealed normal levels of all except for CD59. CD59 was consistently undetectable on the surface of his erythrocytes and fibroblasts. His mother and father had half-normal levels of expression, suggesting autosomal recessive inheritance.[388]

Molecular Genetic Defects. The molecular cause of CD59 deficiency is not known.

C1 Inhibitor Deficiency

Molecular Biology. Genetically determined deficiency of C1-INH is responsible for the clinical disorder termed hereditary angioedema (HAE).[389] C1-INH is a 105-kDa glycoprotein with a total carbohydrate content of 33 percent.[390] The C1-INH gene spans 17 kb on chromosome 11q.[118,391,392] The liver is the major source of plasma C1-INH,[393–396] but mononuclear phagocytes and fibroblasts also synthesize and secrete it.[397–399]

The primary sequence of C1-INH is known.[391,392] It has 20 percent homology with serine protease inhibitors α_1-proteinase inhibitor, α_1-antichymotrypsin, antithrombin III, and angiotensinogen.

Pathophysiology and Clinical Expression. Hereditary angioedema is an autosomal dominant trait. There are at least two forms of C1-INH deficiency.[138,400] The most common (type I), accounts for approximately 85 percent of patients; the serum of affected individuals is deficient in both C1-INH protein (5 to 30 percent of normal) and activity.[389,400–402] In the other, less common, form (type II), a dysfunctional protein is present in normal or elevated concentrations, but the functional activity of C1-INH is markedly reduced.[138,400–402] In patients with type I HAE the diagnosis can be established easily by demonstrating a decrease in serum C1-INH protein when assessed by immunochemical techniques. However, in patients with type II HAE, the diagnosis must rest on demonstrating a decrease in C1-INH functional activity. In either case, C4 levels and C2 levels are usually reduced well below the lower limit of normal during attacks,[401,403,404] due to their uncontrolled cleavage by C1s. The level of C4 in serum is also reduced between attacks, making its measurement useful as a diagnostic clue.[401,404]

A number of studies have examined the dysfunctional C1-INH molecules from different families and found that they differ from normal C1-INH and from each other. Although they appear to be immunochemically identical to normal C1-INH,[138,400,405,406] some, but not all, have a different electrophoretic mobility than normal.[400] In addition, they differ from normal C1-INH, and from each other, with respect to their ability to bind to C1s and their ability to inhibit the cleavage of a synthetic substrate, *N*-acetyl-tyrosine-ethyl-ester by C1s.[400,407] Normal C1-INH also inhibits plasma kallikrein, activated Hageman factor, and plasmin. In one study comparing the dysfunctional C1-INH molecules from eight different kindreds, each dysfunctional C1-INH was unique with respect to its spectrum of inhibitory activities against these enzymes,[407] although none of the dysfunctional proteins inhibited plasmin.

The levels of normal C1-INH function in patients with either type of HAE are lower than one might expect in a hemizygote—5 to 30 percent of normal in type I C1-INH deficiency and little to none in type II C1-INH deficiency. In addition, the levels of the dysfunctional protein in the type II disorder are usually equivalent to or higher than normal, rather than the expected 50 percent of normal. In an attempt to explain this apparent discrepancy, metabolic studies using both normal and dysfunctional proteins have been performed in both normal and deficient subjects.[408] As expected, the synthesis of the normal C1-INH in the type I disorder was reduced, findings consistent with earlier studies showing reduced content of the normal protein in the livers of patients with C1-INH deficiency.[396] The fractional catabolic rate of normal C1-INH in both types of patients with HAE was significantly elevated. Finally, the fractional catabolic rates of two different dysfunctional C1-INH proteins were different from each other and from normal; in one, the fractional catabolic rate was near normal and in the other it was strikingly reduced. These studies have been used to create a model to explain the low levels of C1-INH found in the type I disorder and the elevated levels of dysfunctional protein found in the type II disorder.[409] The model proposes that there are two catabolic routes for normal C1-INH, one in which the inhibitor forms a complex with the enzymes with which it reacts in vivo, and another independent of inhibitor–enzyme complexes and representing the normal catabolism of any serum protein. Thus, it has been suggested that in the type I disorder the markedly lowered levels of C1-INH are the result of both decreased synthesis and increased catabolism consequent to the complexing of the normal C1-INH with the activated enzymes that it normally inhibits. Similarly, it has been suggested that the low levels of normal C1-INH and elevated levels of dysfunctional C1-INH in the type II disorder are the result of decreased synthesis and increased catabolism of the normal C1-INH and, at least in some cases, decreased catabolism of the dysfunctional C1-INH consequent to its inability to complex with C1 and other enzymes.

The pathophysiological mechanism(s) by which the absence of C1-INH activity leads to the angioedema characteristic of the disorder are still incompletely understood. Neither the mediators responsible for producing the edema nor the mechanisms initiating their production have been clearly identified. There is a great deal of evidence implicating complement in the pathogenesis of the edema. Clearly, C$\overline{1s}$ activity is present in the serum of patients during an attack.[410] Furthermore, when purified C$\overline{1s}$ is injected into either normal or HAE patients' skin, angioedema is produced.[411] The intradermal response to C$\overline{1s}$ in C2-deficient individuals is markedly diminished, while it is preserved in C3-deficient individuals, suggesting the direct involvement of C2 in the production of the angioedema.[411] Other evidence suggests that the plasma kallikrein system may also be involved in the generation of the edema. However, there has been no evidence to support a role for bradykinin. C1-INH is capable of inhibiting the ability of activated Hageman factor to initiate kinin generation, fibrinolysis, and coagulation.[412] It also inhibits kallikrein of the kinin system, plasma thromboplastin antecedent (factor XIa) of the clotting system, and plasmin of the fibrinolytic system (reviewed in Frank et al.[401]). It is possible, therefore, that products of the kinin system could be involved in the edema formation. In fact, blister fluids from HAE patients contain active plasma kallikrein,[413] and their serum has decreased amounts of prekallikrein and kininogen,[414] suggesting activation of the kinin system during attacks of edema.

Clinical Expression. Although isolated cases of angioedema were described as early as the midnineteenth century, the first complete clinical description and the familial nature of the disorder were published in 1888 by Sir William Osler.[415] Since that time a number of reports have summarized the clinical manifestations as well as confirmed the hereditary nature of the disorder.[401,402,416,417]

The clinical symptoms of HAE are the result of submucosal or subcutaneous edema. The lesions are characterized by noninflammatory edema associated with capillary and venule dilation.[418] The postcapillary venule also demonstrates gaps between the endothelial cells.[418] The three most prominent areas of involvement are the skin, respiratory tract, and gastrointestinal tract.[401,402,416,417] Although symptoms during attacks may relate to only one of these areas they are not mutually exclusive and may be seen in combination.

Attacks involving the skin may involve an extremity, the face, or genitalia (Fig. 130-7). In some instances, there may be changes immediately preceding the edema, such as mottling, a transient serpinginous erythema, or frank erythema marginatum. The edema usually expands centripetally from a single site and may vary in size from a few centimeters to involvement of a whole extremity. The lesions are pale rather than red, are usually not warm, and are characteristically nonpruritic. There may be, however, a feeling of tightness in the skin due to the accumulation of subcutaneous fluid. Attacks usually progress for 1 to 2 days and resolve over an additional 2 to 3 days.

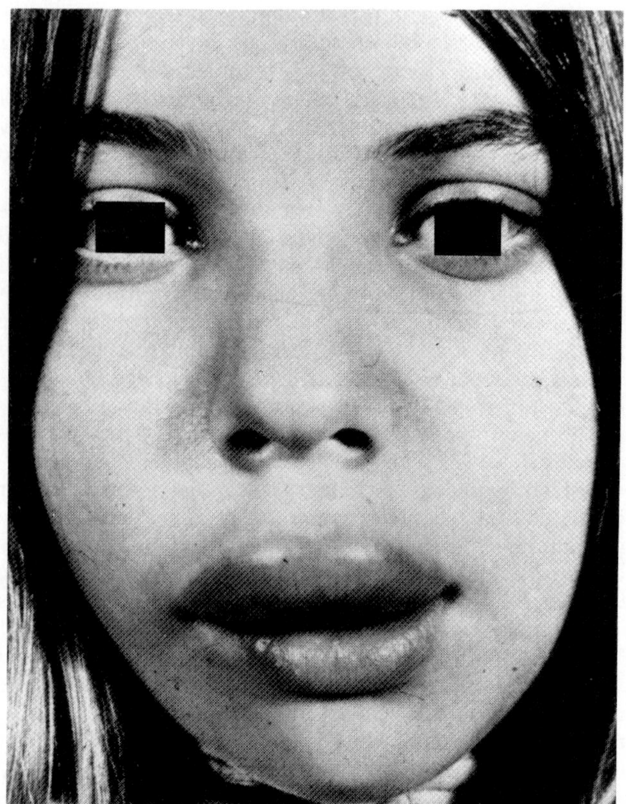

FIG. 130-7 Patient with C1 inhibitor deficiency during an attack of angioedema. *(Courtesy of Dr. Fred S. Rosen.)*

Attacks involving the upper respiratory tract represent a serious threat to the patient with HAE. In one series, pharyngeal edema had occurred at least once in nearly two thirds of the patients.[401] The patient may initially experience a "tightness" in the throat, and swelling of the tongue, buccal mucosa, and oropharynx follows. In some instances laryngeal edema, accompanied by hoarseness and stridor occurs, progresses to respiratory obstruction, and represents a life-threatening emergency. In fact, in one series, tracheostomies had been performed in one of every six patients with HAE.[401]

The gastrointestinal tract can also be affected by HAE. Symptoms are probably related to edema of the bowel wall and may include anorexia, dull aching of the abdomen, vomiting, and in some cases crampy abdominal pain. Abdominal symptoms can occur in the absence of concurrent cutaneous or pharyngeal involvement. In some instances, abdominal symptoms may be the only symptoms the patient has ever had, leading to difficulty in diagnosis.

The onset of symptoms referable to HAE occurs in over half the patients before adolescence,[401,402] but in some patients, their first symptoms do not occur until they are well into adult life. Although in just over half the patients no specific events can be clearly identified as initiating attacks, trauma and anxiety and/or stress are frequently cited.[401,402,417] Dental extractions and tonsillectomy can initiate edema of the upper airway, and cutaneous edema may follow trauma to an extremity. Some patients report attacks following the use of tight-fitting clothing or shoes, while others have related cold exposure to the onset of symptoms.

The therapy of HAE can be conveniently considered to fall into three categories: (1) the long-term prophylaxis of attacks, (2) the short-term prophylaxis of attacks, (3) and the treatment of acute attacks. In patients who have had laryngeal obstruction or have suffered frequent and debilitating attacks that have interfered with work or other responsibilities, the long-term prevention of attacks may be indicated. Antifibrinolytic agents, such as epsilon aminocaproic acid (EACA) or its cyclic analogue, tranexamic acid, have been used with some success in the long-term prevention of attacks.[419,420] Improvement consisted of a decreased frequency of attacks in most patients and a decrease in severity in the others. The mechanisms by which they exert their protective effect is unclear.

More recently, "impeded" androgens, such as danazol and stanozolol, which have attenuated androgenic potential, have been found to be useful in the long-term prophylaxis of HAE.[421] The basis for their use lies in an earlier observation that methyltestosterone therapy was effective in HAE.[422] During a double-blind controlled study of danazol, only 1 of 46 courses of danazol therapy were accompanied by attacks of angioedema, while 44 of 47 courses of placebo therapy were interrupted by an attack.[421] Danazol therapy appears to be effective for extended periods, but because of dose-related adverse reactions (e.g., weight gain, abnormal liver function tests, microscopic hematuria, and altered libido), therapy needs to be closely monitored.[423] Danazol increases serum concentrations of the normal C1-INH in these patients, whether they have the form of the disease characterized by low levels of C1-INH (type I) or the form characterized by a dysfunctional protein (type II).[421,424]

In some instances, patients may need short-term prophylactic therapy, such as before oral surgery. In these circumstances danazol therapy may be initiated 1 week before surgery or EACA the day before surgery. There is some controversy concerning the use of fresh frozen plasma during an acute attack, since the plasma not only supplies the missing C1-INH but also C1 enzyme and substrates such as C4 and C2. Nevertheless, the use of plasma transfusions 12 h before elective surgery may prevent morbidity from the procedure.[425] Preparations of purified C1 inhibitor are now available for use in experimental protocols.

A number of drugs have been used in an attempt to interrupt an attack of HAE once it has begun. Epinephrine, antihistamines and corticosteroids are of no proven benefit. Trials with partially purified C1-INH have been encouraging. Infusion of C1-INH has been accompanied by resolution of edema and symptoms within a few hours.[426]

Molecular Genetic Defects. Among patients with type II HAE missense mutations for residues at or near the active site are most common. Substitutions of His[427] and Cys[428] for Arg_{444} have been identified. The latter variant leads to a disulfide bridge between C1 inhibitor and albumin accounting for the electrophoretic differences in the mutant protein. Several mutations just N-terminal to the active site apparently generate changes in the stressed loop confirmation of the C1-INH SERPIN,[429–431] and one located more distantly leads to an abnormal glycosylation signal.[432]

Multiple molecular mechanisms have also been revealed in type I HAE. For example, the presence of several Alu sequences toward the 5′ end of the C1 inhibitor gene generate many different recombinants in this region.[433–435] Informative RFLP[436,437] detect interruptions in the coding sequences. In addition, point mutations generating a premature stop codon, thereby interrupting translation of C1 inhibitor, have also been observed in type I patients.[438]

Studies of a kindred with HAE type I due to an exon VII deletion has provided direct evidence for a novel molecular mechanism accounting for the lower levels of normal (wild-type) C1 inhibitor. The presence of the mutant gene product (mRNA, protein or both) apparently exerts a *trans*-inhibitory effect on the translation of normal C1 inhibitor in cells from the affected individual.[439]

REFERENCES

1. Mayer MM: Complement: Historical perspectives and current issues. *Complement* **1**:2, 1984.
2. Frank MM: The complement system in host defense and inflammation. *Rev Infect Dis* **1**:483, 1979.
3. Silverstein AM: Essential hypocomplementemia: Report of a case. *Blood* **16**:1338, 1960.
4. Ross SC, Densen P: Complement deficiency states and infection: Epidemiology, pathogenesis and consequences of Neisserial and other infections in an immune deficiency. *Medicine (Baltimore)* **63**:243, 1984.
5. Figueroa JE, Densen P: Infectious diseases associated with complement deficiencies. *Clin Microbiol Rev* **4**:359, 1991.
6. Porter RR, Reid KBM: The biochemistry of complement. *Nature* **275**:699, 1978.
7. Lepow IH, Naff GB, Todd EW, Pensky J, Hinz CF: Chromatographic resolution of the first component of complement into three activities. *J Exp Med* **117**:983, 1963.
8. Gigli I, Porter RR, Sim RB: The unactivated form of the first component of human complement, C1. *Biochem J* **157**:541, 1976.
9. Muller-Eberhard HJ, Kunkel H: Isolation of a thermolabile serum protein which precipitates gammaglobulin aggregates and participates in immune hemolysis. *Proc Soc Exp Biol Med* **106**:291, 1961.
10. Lin TY, Fletcher DS: Activation of human complement C1 by the third subcomponent C1q. *J Biol Chem* **255**:7756, 1980.
11. Ziccardi RJ, Cooper NR: Activation of C1r by proteolytic cleavage. *J Immunol* **116**:504, 1976.
12. Valet G, Cooper NR: Isolation of the proenzyme forms of C1r and C1s from human serum. *J Immunol* **111**:292, 1973.
13. Sakai K, Stroud RM: Purification, molecular properties and activation of C1 proesterase, C1. *J Immunol* **110**:1010, 1973.
14. Schreiber RD, Muller-Eberhard HJ: Fourth component of human complement: Description of a three polypeptide chain structure. *J Exp Med* **140**:1324, 1974.
15. Law SK, Lichtenberg NA, Holcombe FH, Levine RP: Interaction between the labile binding sites of the fourth and fifth components of complement and erythrocyte cell membranes. *J Immunol* **125**:634, 1980.
16. Tack BF: The beta-cys-gamma-glu thiolester bond in C4, C3, and $alpha_2$-macroglobulin. *Springer Semin Immunopathol* **6**:259, 1983.
17. Nagasawa S, Stroud RM: Cleavage of C2 by C1s into antigenically distinct fragments, C2a and C2b: Demonstration of binding of C2a to C4b. *Proc Natl Acad Sci USA* **74**:2998, 1977.
18. Shin HS, Mayer MM: The third component of the guinea pig complement system. II. Kinetic study of the reaction of EAC 4,2a with guinea pig C3. *Biochemistry* **7**:2997, 1968.
19. Pensky J, Levy LR, Lepow IH: Partial purification of a serum inhibitor of C′1-esterase. *J Biol Chem* **236**:1674, 1961.
20. Harpel PC, Cooper NR: Studies on human plasma C1 inactivator-enzyme interactions. I. Mechanisms of interactions with C1s, plasmin, and trypsin. *J Clin Invest* **55**:593, 1975.
21. Gigli I, Fujita T, Nussenzweig V: Modulation of the classical pathway C3 convertase by the plasma proteins, C4-binding protein and C3b inactivator. *Proc Natl Acad Sci USA* **76**:6596, 1979.
22. Nagasawa S, Ichibara C, Stroud RM: Cleavage of C4b by C3b inactivator: Production of a nicked form of C4b, C4b′, as an intermediate cleavage product of C4b by C3b inactivator. *J Immunol* **125**:578, 1980.
23. Nicholson-Weller A, Burge J, Fearon DT, Weller PF, Austen KF: Isolation of a human erythrocytes membrane glycoprotein with decay-accelerating activity for C3 convertases of the complement system. *J Immunol* **129**:184, 1982.
24. Hirsch RL, Winkelstein JA, Griffin DE: The role of complement in viral infections. III. Activation of the classical and alternative pathways by Sindbis virus. *J Immunol* **124**:2507, 1980.
25. Bredt W, Wellek B, Brunner H, Loos M: Interactions between *Mycoplasma pneumoniae* and the first component of complement. *Infect Immun* **15**:7, 1977.
26. Loos M, Wellek B, Thesen R, Opferkuch W: Antibody-independent interaction of the first component of complement with gram-negative bacteria. *Infect Immunol* **22**:5, 1978.
27. Eads ME, Levy NJ, Kasper DL, Baker CJ, Nicholson-Weller A: Antibody-independent activation of C1 by type 1a group B streptococci. *J Infect Dis* **146**:665, 1982.
28. Winkelstein JA: Complement and natural immunity. *Clin Immunol Allergy* **3**:421, 1983.
29. Fearon DT: Activation of the alternative complement pathway. *Crit Rev Immunol* **1**:1, 1979.
30. Tack BF, Harrison RA, Janotova J, Thomas ML, Prahl JW: Evidence for presence of an internal thiolester bond in third component of human complement. *Proc Natl Acad Sci USA* **77**:5764, 1980.
31. Pangburn MK, Muller-Eberhard HJ: Relation of a putative thioester bond in C3 to activation of the alternative pathway and the binding of C3b to biological targets of complement. *J Exp Med* **152**:1102, 1980.
32. Fearon DT, Austen KF: Initiation of C3 cleavage in the alternative complement pathway. *J Immunol* **115**:1357, 1975.
33. Fearon DT, Austen KF: Properdin: Binding to C3b and stabilization of the C3b-dependent C3 convertase. *J Exp Med* **142**:856, 1975.

34. Kazatchkine MD, Fearon DT, Austen KF: Human alternative complement pathway: Membrane-associated sialic acid regulates the competition between B and B1H for cell-bound C3b. *J Immunol* **122**:75, 1979.
35. Weiler JM, Daha MR, Austen KF, Fearon DT: Control of the amplification convertase of complement by the plasma protein, B1H. *Proc Natl Acad Sci USA* **73**:3268, 1976.
36. Whaley K, Ruddy S: Modulation of the alternative complement pathway by B1H globulin. *J Exp Med* **144**:1147, 1976.
37. Lublin DN, Atkinson JP: Decay-accelerating factor and membrane cofactor protein. *Curr Top Microbiol Immunol* **153**:124, 1989.
38. Pillemer L, Blum L, Lepow IH, Ross OA, Todd EW, Wardlaw AC: The properdin system and immunity. I. Demonstration and isolation of a new serum protein, properdin, and its role in immune phenomena. *Science* **120**:279, 1954.
39. Platts-Mills TAE, Ishizakah K: Activation of the alternate pathway of human complement by rabbit cells. *J Immunol* **113**:348, 1974.
40. Winkelstein JA, Shin HS, Wood WB Jr: Heat labile opsonins to pneumococcus. III. Participation of immunoglobulin and of the alternative pathway of C3 activation. *J Immunol* **108**:1681, 1972.
41. Fearon DT, Austen KF: Activation of the alternative complement pathway due to resistance of zymosan-bound amplification convertase to endogenous regulatory mechanisms. *Proc Natl Acad Sci USA* **74**:1683, 1977.
42. Fearon DT: Regulation by membrane sialic acid of B1H-dependent decay. Dissociation of amplification C3 convertase of the alternative pathway. *Proc Natl Acad Sci USA* **75**:1971, 1978.
43. Winkelstein JA, Shin HS: The role of immunoglobulin in the interaction of pneumococci and the properdin pathway: Evidence for its specificity and lack of requirement for the Fc portion of the molecule. *J Immunol* **112**:1635, 1974.
44. Edwards MS, Nicholson-Weller A, Baker CJ, Kasper DL: The role of specific antibody in alternative complement pathway mediated opsonophagocytosis of type III, group B streptococcus. *J Exp Med* **151**:1275, 1980.
45. Perrin LH, Joseph BS, Cooper NR, Oldstone MBA: Mechanism of injury of virus-infected cells by antiviral antibody and complement: Participation of IgG, $F(ab')_2$ and the alternative pathway. *J Exp Med* **143**:1027, 1976.
46. Moore FD Jr, Fearon DT, Austen KF: IgG on mouse erythrocytes augments activation of the human alternative complement pathway by enhancing deposition of C3b. *J Immunol* **126**:1805, 1981.
47. Nicholson-Weller A, Daha MR, Austen KF: Different functions for specific guinea pig IgG1 and IgG2 in the lysis of sheep erythrocytes by C4-deficient guinea pig serum. *J Immunol* **126**:1800, 1981.
48. Fearon DT, Austen KF, Ruddy S: Formation of a hemolytically active cellular intermediate by the interaction between properdin factors B and D and the activated third component of complement. *J Exp Med* **138**:1305, 1973.
49. Hostetter MK, Gordon DL: Biochemistry of C3 and related thiolester proteins in infection and inflammation. *Rev Infect Dis* **9**:97, 1987.
50. Shin HS, Pickering RJ, Mayer MM: The fifth component of the guinea pig complement system. II. Mechanisms of SAC1,4,2,3,5b formation and C5 consumption by EAC1,4,2,3. *J Immunol* **106**:473, 1971.
51. Daha MR, Fearon DT, Austen KF: C3 requirements for formation of alternative pathway C3 convertase. *J Immunol* **117**:630, 1976.
52. Mayer MM, Michaels DW, Ramm LE, Shin ML, Whitlow MB, Willoughby JB: Membrane damage by complement. *Crit Rev Immunol* **2**:133, 1981.
53. Thompson RA, Lachman PJ: Reactive lysis: The complement mediated lysis of unsensitized cells. II. The characterization of activated reactor as C5b and the participation of C8 and C9. *J Exp Med* **131**:643, 1970.
54. Shin ML, Paznekas WA, Abromovitz AS, Mayer MM: On the mechanism of membrane damage by complement: Exposure of hydrophobic sites on activated complement proteins. *J Immunol* **119**:1358, 1977.
55. Hammer CH, Nicholson A, Mayer MM: On the mechanism of cytotysis by complement: Evidence on insertion of C5b and C7 subunits of the C5b,6,7 complex into phospholipid bilayers of erythrocyte membranes. *Proc Natl Acad Sci USA* **72**:5076, 1975.
56. Hu VW, Esser SF, Podack ER, Wisnieshis BJ: The membrane attack mechanism of complement: Photolabelling reveals insertion of terminal proteins into target membranes. *J Immunol* **27**:380, 1981.
57. Stolfi RL: Immune lytic transformation. A state of irreversible damage generated as a result of the reaction of the eighth component in the guinea pig complement system. *J Immunol* **100**:46, 1968.
58. Tschopp J, Podack ER, Muller-Eberhard HJ: The membrane attack complex of complement: C5b-8 complex as accelerator of C9 polymerization. *J Immunol* **134**:495, 1985.
59. Lachman PJ: The control of homologous lysis. *Immunol Today* **12**:312, 1991.
60. Fearon DT, Wong WW: Complement ligand-receptor interactions that mediate biological responses. *Annu Rev Immunol* **1**:243, 1983.
61. Hugli TE: The structural basis for anaphylatoxin and chemotactic functions of C3a, C4a and C5a. *Crit Rev Immunol* **2**:321, 1981.
62. Fearon DT: Identification of the membrane glycoprotein that is the C3b receptor of the human erythrocyte, polymorphonuclear leukocyte, B lymphocyte and monocyte. *J Exp Med* **152**:20, 1980.
63. Ehlenberger AG, Nussenzweig V: The role of membrane receptors for C3b and C3d in phagocytosis. *J Exp Med* **145**:357, 1977.
64. Cornacoff JB, Hebert LA, Smead WL, Van Aman ME, Birmingham DJ, Waxman FJ: Primate erythrocyte-immune complex-clearing mechanism. *J Clin Invest* **71**:236, 1983.
65. Fearon DT: Regulation of the amplification C3 convertase of human complement by an inhibitory protein isolated from human erythrocyte membranes. *Proc Natl Acad Sci USA* **76**:5867, 1979.
66. Iida K, Nussenzweig V: Complement receptor is an inhibitor of the complement cascade. *J Exp Med* **153**:1138, 1981.
67. Hebell T, Ahearn JM, Fearon DT: Suppression of the immune response by a soluble complement receptor of B lymphocytes. *Science* **254**:102, 1991.
68. Cochrane CG, Muller-Eberhard HJ: The derivation of two distinct anaphylatoxins from the third and fifth components of human complement. *J Exp Med* **127**:371, 1968.
69. Vogt W: Anaphylatoxins: Possible roles in diseases. *Complement* **3**:177, 1986.
70. Gorski J, Hugli TE, Muller-Eberhard HJ: C4a: The third anaphylatoxin of the human complement system. *Proc Natl Acad Sci USA* **76**:5299, 1979.
71. Snyderman R, Goetzl EJ: Molecular and cellular mechanisms of leukocyte chemotaxins. *Science* **213**:830, 1981.
72. Perez HD, Goldstein IM, Chernoff D, Webster RO, Henson PM: Chemotactic activity of C5a des arg: Evidence of a requirement for an anionic peptide "helper factor" and inhibition by a cationic protein in serum from patients with systemic lupus erythematosis. *Mol Immunol* **17**:163, 1980.
73. Hoover RL, Briggs RT, Karnovsky MJ: The adhesive interaction between polymorphonuclear leukocytes and endothelial cells in vitro. *Cell* **14**:423, 1978.
74. Snyderman R, Phillips JK, Mergenhagen SE: Biological activity of complement *in vivo*: Role of C5 in the accumulation of polymorphonuclear leukocytes in inflammatory exudates. *J Exp Med* **134**:1131, 1971.
75. Larsen GL, Mitchell BC, Henson PM: The pulmonary response of C5 sufficient and deficient mice to immune complexes. *Am Rev Respir Dis* **123**:434, 1981.
76. Johnston RB Jr, Klemperer MR, Alper CA, Rosen FS: The enhancement of bacterial phagocytosis by serum. The role of complement components and two co-factors. *J Exp Med* **129**:1275, 1969.
77. Mantovani B, Rabinovitch M, Nussenzweig V: Phagocytosis of immune complexes by macrophages. Different roles of the macrophage receptor sites for complement (C3) and for immunoglobulin (IgG). *J Exp Med* **135**:780, 1972.
78. Bianco C, Griffin FM Jr, Silverstein SC: Studies on the macrophage complement receptor: Alteration of receptor

function upon macrophage activation. *J Exp Med* **141**:1278, 1975.
79. Winkelstein JA, Smith MR, Shin HS: The role of C3 as an opsonin in the early stages of infection. *Proc Soc Exp Biol Med* **149**:397, 1975.
80. Hosea SW, Brown EJ, Frank MM: The critical role of complement in experimental pneumococcal sepsis. *J Infect Dis* **142**:903, 1980.
81. Muschel LH, Fong JSC: Serum bactericidal activity and complement, in Day NK, Good RA (eds): *Comprehensive Immunology*. Plenum, New York, 1977, p 137.
82. Haniman GR, Esser AF, Podack ER, Wunderlich AC, Braude AI, Lint TF, Curd JG: The role of C9 in complement-mediated killing of Neisseria. *J Immunol* **127**:2386, 1981.
83. Saulsbury FT, Winkelstein JA: Activation of the alternative complement pathway by L-phase variants of gram-positive bacteria. *Infect Immun* **23**:711, 1979.
84. Wright SD, Levine RP: How complement kills E. coli. I. Location of the lethal lesion. *J Immunol* **127**:1146, 1981.
85. Schifferli JA, Ng YC, Peters DK: The role of complement and its receptor in the elimination of immune complexes. *N Engl J Med* **315**:488, 1986.
86. Van Snick JL, Masson PL: The effect of complement on the ingestion of soluble antigen-antibody complexes and IgM aggregates by mouse peritoneal macrophages. *J Exp Med* **148**:903, 1978.
87. Schifferli JA, Bartolotti SR, Peters DK: Inhibition of immune precipitation by complement. *Clin Exp Immunol* **42**:387, 1980.
88. Miller GW, Nussenzweig V: A new complement function: Solubilization of antigen-antibody aggregates. *Proc Natl Acad Sci USA* **72**:418, 1975.
89. Bartolotti SR, Peters DK: Delayed removal of renal-bound antigen in decomplemented rabbits with acute serum sickness. *Clin Exp Immunol* **32**:199, 1978.
90. Weiler JB, Ballas ZK, Needleman BW, Hobbs MV, Feldbush TL: Complement fragments suppress lymphocyte immune responses. *Immunol Today* **3**:238, 1982.
91. Pepys MB: The role of complement in induction of antibody production in vivo. *J Exp Med* **140**:126, 1974.
92. Ochs HD, Wedgewood RJ, Frank MM, Heller SR, Hosea, SW: The role of complement in the induction of antibody responses. *Clin Exp Immunol* **53**:208, 1983.
93. Bottger EC, Hoffmann T, Hadding V, Bitter-Suermann D: Influence of genetically inherited complement deficiencies on humoral immune response in guinea pigs. *J Immunol* **135**:4100, 1985.
94. O'Neil KM, Ochs HD, Heller SR, Cork LC, Winkelstein JA: Deficient humoral immunity in C3-deficient dogs. *J Immunol* **140**:1939, 1988.
95. Farries TC, Atkinson JP: Evolution of the complement system. *Immunol Today* **12**:295, 1991.
96. Carroll MC, Campbell RD, Bentley DR, Porter RR: A molecular map of the human major histocompatibility complex class III region linking complement genes C4, C2 and factor B. *Nature* **307**:237, 1984.
97. Wu L-C, Morley BJ, Campbell RD: Cell specific expression of the human complement protein factor B gene: Evidence for the role of two distinct 5′ flanking elements. *Cell* **48**:331, 1987.
98. Ishikawa N, Nonaka M, Wetsel RA, Colten HR: Murine complement C2 and factor B genomic and cDNA cloning reveals different mechanisms for multiple transcripts of C2 and B. *J Biol Chem* **265**:19040, 1990.
99. Carroll MC, Campbell RD, Porter RR: Mapping of steroid 21-hydroxylase genes adjacent to complement component C4 genes in HLA, the major histocompatibility complex in man. *Proc Natl Acad Sci USA* **82**:521, 1985.
100. White PC, Grossberger D, Onufer BJ, Chaplin DD, New MI, Dupont B, Strominger JL: Two genes encoding 21-hydroxylase are located near the genes encoding the fourth component of complement in man. *Proc Natl Acad Sci USA* **82**:5111, 1985.
101. Olaisen B, Teisberg R, Jonassen R, Thorsby E, Gedde-Dahl T: Gene order and gene distance in the HLA regions studied by the haplotype method. *Am J Hum Genet* **47**:285, 1983.
102. Whitehead AS, Colten HR, Chang CC, Demars R: Localization of MHC-linked complement genes between HLA-B and HLA-DR by using HLA mutant cell lines. *J Immunol* **134**:641, 1985.
103. Chaplin DD, Woods DE, Whitehead AS, Goldberger G, Colten HR, Seidman JG: Molecular map of the murine S region. *Proc Natl Acad Sci USA* **80**:6947, 1985.
104. Trowsdale J, Ragoussis J, Campbell RD: Map of the human MHC. *Immunol Today* **12**:443, 1991.
105. Klickstein LB, Wong WW, Smith JA, Morton C, Fearon DT, Weis JH: Identification of long homologous repeats in human CR1. *Complement* **2**:44, 1985.
106. Lublin DM, Lemons RS, Lebeau MM, Holers VM, Tykocinski ML, Medof ME, Atkinson JP: The gene encoding decay-accelerating factor is located in the complement regulator locus on the long arm of chromosome 1. *J Exp Med* **165**:1731, 1987.
107. Rodriquez De Cordoba S, Lublin DM, Rubinstein P, Atkinson JP: Human genes for 3 complement components that regulate the activation of C3 are tightly linked. *J Exp Med* **161**:1189, 1985.
108. Kristensen T, Wetsel RA, Tack BF: Structural analysis of human complement protein H: Homology with C4b binding protein, beta-2-glycoprotein 1 and Ba fragment of B. *J Immunol* **136**:3407, 1986.
109. Weis JH, Morton CC, Bruns GAP, Weis JJ, Klickstein LB, Wong WW, Fearon DT: A complement receptor locus: Genes encoding C3b/C4b receptor and C3d/Epstein-Barr virus receptor map to 1q32. *J Immunol* **138**:312, 1987.
110. Campbell RD, Dunham I, Sargent CA: Molecular mapping of the HLA-linked complement genes and the RCA linkage group. *Exp Clin Immunogenet* **5**:81, 1988.
111. Bentley DR: Primary structure of human complement component C2. Homology to two unrelated protein families. *Biochem J* **239**:339, 1986.
112. Morley BJ, Campbell RD: Internal homologies of the Ba fragment from human complement component factor B, a class III MHC antigen. *EMBO J* **3**:153, 1984.
113. Reid KBM, Bentley DR, Campbell RD, Chung LP, Sim RB, Kristensen T, Tack BF: Complement system proteins which interact with C3b or C4b. A super family of structurally related proteins. *Immunol Today* **7**:230, 1986.
114. Suttrup-Jenson L, Stepanik TM, Kristensen T, Conblad PB, Jones CM, Wierzbicki DM, Magnusson S, Domdey H, Wetsel R, Lundwall A, Tack BF, Fey GH: Common evolutionary origin of α_2 macroglobulin and complement components C3 and C4. *Proc Natl Acad Sci USA* **82**:9, 1985.
115. Rao AG, Howard OMZ, Ng S, Whitehead AS, Colten HR, Sodetz JM: cDNA and derived amino acid sequence of the alpha subunit of human complement protein C8: Evidence for the existence of separate alpha subunit mRNA. *Biochemistry* **26**:3556, 1987.
116. Howard OMZ, Rao AG, Sodetz JM: cDNA and derived amino acid sequence of the beta subunit of human complement protein C8: Identification of a close structural and ancestral relationship to the alpha subunit and C9. *Biochemistry* **26**:3565, 1987.
117. Stanley KK, Kocher HP, Luzio JP, Jackson P, Tschopp J: The sequence and topology of human complement component C9. *EMBO J* **4**:375, 1985.
118. Davis AE, Whitehead AS, Harrison RA, Dauphinais A, Bruns GAP, Cicardi M, Rosen FS: Human inhibitor of the first component of complement, C1: Characterization of cDNA clones and localization of the gene to chromosome 11. *Proc Natl Acad Sci USA* **83**:3161, 1986.
119. Morgan BP: *Complement: Clinical Aspects and Relevance to Disease*. San Diego, CA, Academic Press, 1990.
120. Raum D, Donaldson VH, Rosen FS, Alper CA: Genetics of complement. *Curr Top Hematol* **3**:111, 1980.
121. Yu CY, Belt KT, Giles CM, Campbell RD, Porter RR: Structural basis of the polymorphism of human complement components C4A and C4B: Gene size, reactivity and antigenicity. *EMBO J* **5**:2873, 1986.
122. Daurinche C, Abbal M, Clerc A: Molecular characterization of human complement factor B subtypes. *Immunogenetics* **32**:309, 1990.
123. Awdeh ZL, Raum D, Yunis EJ, Alper CA: Extended HLA/complement allele haplotypes: Evidence for T/t-like complex in man. *Proc Natl Acad Sci USA* **80**:259, 1983.

124. Awdeh ZL, Alper CA, Eynon E, Alosco SM, Stein R, Yunis EJ: Unrelated individuals matched for MHC extended haplotypes and HLA-identical siblings show comparable responses in mixed lymphocyte culture. *Lancet* **2**:853, 1985.
125. Alper CA, Raum D, Awdeh ZL, Peterson BH, Taylor PD, Starzl TE: Studies of hepatic synthesis in vivo of plasma proteins, including orosomucoid, transferrin, α-antitrypsin, C8 and factor B. *Clin Immunol Immunopathol* **16**:84, 1980.
126. Wolpl A, Robin-Winn M, Picklmayr R, Goldmann SF: Fourth component of complement (C4) polymorphism in human orthoptic liver transplantation. *Transplantation* **40**:154, 1985.
127. Alper CA, Johnson AM, Birtch AG, Moore FD: Human C3: Evidence for the liver as the primary site of synthesis. *Science* **163**:286, 1969.
128. Colten HR: Tissue specific regulation of inflammation. *J Appl Physiol* **72**:1, 1992.
129. Sundstrom SA, Komm BS, Xu Q, Boundy V, Lyttle CR: The stimulation of uterine complement component C3 gene expression by antiestrogens. *Endocrinology* **126**:1449, 1990.
130. Botto M, Lissandrini D, Sorio C, Walport MD: Biosynthesis and secretion of complement component C3 by activated human polymorphonuclear leukocytes. *J Immunol* **149**:1348, 1992.
131. Wilson DR, Juan TSC, Wilde MD, Fey GH, Darlington GJ: A 58-base pair region of the human C3 gene confers synergistic inducibility by interleukin-1 and interleukin-6. *Mol Cell Biol* **10**:6181, 1990.
132. Kawamura N, Singer L, Wetsel RA, Colten HR: Cis- and transacting elements required for constitutive and cytokine regulated expression of the mouse complement C3 gene. *Biochem J* **283**:705, 1992.
133. Sundstrom SA, Komm BS, Ponce-De-Leon H, Yi Z, Teuscher C, Lyttle CR: Estrogen regulation of tissue-specific expression of complement C3. *J Biol Chem* **264**:16941, 1989.
134. Garnier G, Ault B, Kramer M, Colten HR: Cis and trans elements differ among mouse strains with high and low extrahepatic complement factor B gene expression. *J Exp Med* **175**:471, 1992.
135. Lint TF, Zeitz HJ, Gewurz H: Inherited deficiency of the ninth component of complement in man. *J Immunol* **125**:2252, 1980.
136. Polhill RB Jr, Pruitt KM, Johnston RB Jr: Kinetic assessment of alternative pathway activity in a hemolytic system. I. Experimental and kinetic analysis. *J Immunol* **121**:363, 1978.
137. Nelson RA Jr, Jensen J, Gigli I, Tamura N: Methods for the separation, purification and measurement of the nine components of the hemolytic complement in guinea pig serum. *Immunochemistry* **3**:111, 1966.
138. Rosen FS, Charache P, Pensky J, Donaldson V: Hereditary angioneurotic edema: Two genetic variants. *Science* **148**:957, 1965.
139. Thompson RA, Haeney R, Reid KBM, Davies JG, White RHR, Cameron AH: A genetic defect of the C1q subcomponent of complement associated with childhood (immune complex) nephritis. *N Engl J Med* **303**:22, 1980.
140. Tedesco F, Densen P, Villa MA, Petersen BH, Sirchia G: Two types of dysfunctional eighth component of complement (C8) molecules in C8 deficiency in man: Reconstitution of normal C8 from the mixture of two abnormal C8 molecules. *J Clin Invest* **71**:183, 1983.
141. Fu SM, Kunkel HG, Brusman HP, Allen FH Jr, Fotino M: Evidence for linkage between HL-A histocompatibility genes and those involved in the synthesis of the second component of complement. *J Exp Med* **140**:1108, 1975.
142. Ochs HD, Rosenfeld SI, Thomas ED, Giblett ER, Alper CA, Dupont B, Schaller JG, Gilliland BC, Hansen JA, Wedgewood RJ: Linkage between the gene (or genes) controlling synthesis of the fourth component of complement and the major histocompatibility complex. *N Engl J Med* **296**:470, 1977.
143. Glass D, Raum D, Gibson D, Stillman JS, Schur P: Inherited deficiency of the second component of complement: Rheumatic disease associations. *J Clin Invest* **58**:853, 1976.
144. Gibson DJ, Glass D, Carpenter CB, Schur PH: Hereditary C2 deficiency: Diagnosis and HLA gene complex associations. *J Immunol* **116**:1065, 1976.
145. Johnson CA, Densen P, Hurford R, Colten HR, Wetsel RA: Type I human complement C2 deficiency: A 28 basepair gene deletion causes skipping of exon 6 during RNA splicing. *J Biol Chem* **267**:9347, 1992.
146. Devoe IW: The meningococcus and mechanisms of pathogenicity. *Microbiol Rev* **162**:46, 1982.
147. Hummel DS, Mocca LF, Frasch CE, Winkelstein JA, Jean-Baptiste HJJ, Canas JA, Leggiardro RJ: Meningitis caused by a nonencapsulated strain of Neisseria meningitidis in twin infants with a C6 deficiency. *J Infect Dis* **155**:815, 1987.
148. Kemp AS, Vernon J, Muller-Eberhard HJ, Bau DCK: Complement C8 deficiency with recurrent meningococcemia. *Aust Pediatr J* **21**:169, 1985.
149. Provost TT, Arnett FC, Reichlin M: Homozygous C2 deficiency, lupus erythematosis, and anti-Ro (SSA) antibodies. *Arthritis Rheum* **26**:1279, 1983.
150. Meyer O, Hauptmann G, Tappeiner G, Ochs HD, Mascart-Lemone F: Genetic deficiency of C4, C2 or C1q and lupus syndromes. Association with anti-Ro (SS-A) antibodies. *Clin Exp Immunol* **62**:678, 1985.
151. Maddison PJ, Provost TT, Reichlin M: Serologic findings in patients with "ANA-negative" SLE. *Medicine (Baltimore)* **60**:87, 1981.
152. Sontheimer RD, Stastny P, Maddison P, Reichlin M, Gilliam JN: Serologic and HLA associations in subacute cutaneous lupus erythematosis (SCLE): A clinical subset of lupus erythematosis. *Ann Intern Med* **97**:664, 1982.
153. Hirsch RL: The complement system: Its importance in the host response to viral infection. *Microbiol Rev* **46**:71, 1982.
154. Hirsch RL, Griffin DE, Winkelstein JA: The effect of complement depletion on the course of sindbis virus infection in mice. *J Immunol* **121**:1276, 1978.
155. Hicks JT, Ennis FA, Kim E, Verbonitz M: The importance of an intact complement pathway in recovery from a primary viral infection. Influenza in decomplemented and in C5-deficient mice. *J Immunol* **121**:1437, 1978.
156. Alper CA: Complement and the MHC, in Dorf ME (ed): *The Role of the Major Histocompatibility Complex in Immunology*. New York, Garland, 1981, p 173.
157. Colten HR: Genetics and synthesis of components of the complement system, in Ross GD (ed): *Immunobiology of the Complement System*. New York, Academic, 1986, p 163.
158. Schifferli JA, Steiger G, Hauptmann G, Spaeth PJ, Sjoholm AG: Formation of soluble immune complexes by complement in sera of patients with various hypocomplementemic states. *J Clin Invest* **76**:2127, 1985.
159. Czop J, Nussenzweig V: Studies on the mechanisms of solubilization of immune precipitates by serum. *J Exp Med* **143**:615, 1976.
160. Takahaski M, Takahaski M, Brade V, Nussenzweig V: Requirements for solubilization of immune aggregates by complement. *J Clin Invest* **62**:349, 1978.
161. Paccaud JP, Steiger G, Sjoholm AG, Spaeth PJ, Schifferli JA: Tetanus toxoid-anti-tetanus toxoid complexes: A potential model to study the complement transport system for immune complex in humans. *Clin Exp Immunol* **69**:468, 1987.
162. Davies KA, Erlandsson K, Benyon HLC, Peters AM, Steinsson K, Valdimarsson H, Walport MJ: Splenic uptake of immune complexes in man is complement-dependent, *J Immunol* **151**:3866, 1993.
163. Ellison RT, Kohler PH, Curd JG, Judson FN, Reller LB: Prevalence of congenital and acquired complement deficiency in patients with sporadic meningococcal disease. *N Engl J Med* **308**:913, 1983.
164. Merino J, Rodriquez-Valverde V, Lamelas JA: Prevalence of deficits of complement components in patients with recurrent meningococcal infections. *J Infect Dis* **148**:331, 1983.
165. Leggiadro RJ, Winkelstein JA: Prevalence of complement deficiencies in children with systemic meningococcal infections. *Pediatr Infect Dis* **6**:75, 1987.
166. Rasmussen JM, Brandslund I, Teisner B, Isager H, Suehag S-E, Maarup L, Willumsen L, Ronne-Rasmussen JO, Permin H, Andersen PL, Skovmann O, Sorensen H: Screening for complement deficiencies in unselected patients with meningitis. *Clin Exp Immunol* **68**:437, 1987.

167. Densen P, Sanford M, Burke T, Densen E, Wintermeyer L: Prospective study of the prevalence of complement deficiency in meningitis. 30th Interscience Conference on Antimicrobial Agents and Chemotherapy, 1990. (abstr. 320)
168. Nielsen HE, Koch C, Magnussen P, Lind I: Complement deficiencies in selected groups of patients with meningococcal disease. *Scand J Infect Dis* **21**:389, 1989.
169. Fijen CA, Juijper EJ, Hannema AJ, Sjoholm AG, Van Putten JPM: Complement deficiencies in patients over ten years old with meningococcal disease due to uncommon serogroups. *Lancet* **2**:585, 1989.
170. Rowe PC, McLean RH, Wood RA, Leggiardro RJ, Winkelstein JA: Association of homozygous C4B deficiency with bacterial meningitis. *J Infect Dis* **160**:448, 1989.
171. Hartung K, Fontana A, Klar M, Krippner H, Jorgens K, Lang B, Peter HH, Pichler WJ, Schendel D, Robin-Winn M: Association of class I, II, and III MHC gene products with systemic lupus erythematosis. *Rheumatol Int* **9**:13, 1989.
172. Petri M, Watson R, Winkelstein JA, McLean RH: Clinical expression of systemic lupus in patients with C4A deficiency. *Medicine (Baltimore)* **72**:236, 1993.
173. Ruddy S: Component deficiencies: The second component. *Prog Allergy* **39**:250, 1986.
174. Sullivan KE, Petri M, Bias WB, McLean R, Schmeckpepper B, Winkelstein JA: Prevalence of a mutation which causes C2 deficiency in a population of patients with SLE. *J Rheumat* (in press)
175. O'Neill GJ, Yang SY, Dupont B: Two HLA-linked loci controlling the fourth component of human complement. *Proc Natl Acad Sci USA* **75**:5165, 1978.
176. Awdeh ZL, Alper CA: Inherited structural polymorphism of the fourth component of human complement. *Proc Natl Acad Sci USA* **77**:3576, 1978.
177. Hauptmann G, Tappeiner G, Schifferli JA: Inherited deficiency of the fourth complement. *Immunodefic Rev* **1**:3, 1988.
178. Christiansen FT, Dawkins RL, Uko G, McClusky J, Kay PH, Zilko PJ: Complement allotyping in SLE: Association with C4A null. *Aust N Z J Med* **13**:483, 1983.
179. Fiedler AHL, Walport MJ, Batchelor JR, Rynes RI, Black CM, Dodi IA, Hughes GRV: Family study of the major histocompatibility complex in patients with systemic lupus erythematosis: Importance of null alleles of C4A and C4B in determining disease susceptibility. *Br Med J* **286**:425, 1983.
180. Howard PF, Hochberg MC, Bias B, Arnett FC, McLean RH: Relationship between C4 null genes, HLA-D region antigens, and genetic susceptibility to systemic lupus erythematosis in caucasian and black Americans. *Am J Med* **81**:187, 1986.
181. Speirs C, Fielder AHL, Chapel H, Davey NJ, Batchelor JR: Complement system protein C4 and susceptibility to hydralazine-induced systemic lupus erythematosis. *Lancet* **1**:922, 1989.
182. Sellar GC, Blake DJ, Reid KBM: Characterization and organization of the genes encoding the A-, B- and C-chains of human complement subcomponent C1q. *Biochem J* **272**:481, 1991.
183. Loos M, Heinz HP: Component deficiencies: The first component: C1q, C1r, C1s. *Prog Allergy* **39**:212, 1986.
184. Berkel AI, Loos M, Sanal O, Ersoy F, Yegin O: Selective complete C1q deficiency: Report of two cases. *Immunol Lett* **2**:263, 1981.
185. Leyva-Cobian F, Moneo I, Mampaso R, Sanchez-Boyle M, Ecija JL: Familial C1q deficiency associated with renal and cutaneous disease. *Clin Exp Immunol* **44**:173, 1981.
186. Starsia Z, Buc M, Dluholucky S, Tomicova E, Zitnan D, Niks M, Toth J, Stefanovic J: Inherited deficiency of C1 component of complement in members of gypsy families associated with SLE-like symptoms. *Complement* **3**:28, 1986.
187. Chapuis RM, Hauptmann G, Grosshans E, Isliker H: Structural and functional studies in C1q deficiency. *J Immunol* **129**:1509, 1982.
188. Reid KBM, Thompson RA: Characterization of a non functional form of C1q found in patients with a genetically linked deficiency of C1q activity. *Mol Immunol* **20**:117, 1983.
189. Hannema AJ, Kluin-Nelemans JC, Hack CE, Erenberg-Belmer AJM, Mallee C, Van Helden HPT: SLE-like syndromes and functional deficiency of C1q in members of a large family. *Clin Exp Immunol* **55**:106, 1984.
190. McAdam RA, Goundis D, Reid KBM: A homozygous point mutation results in a stop codon in the C1q B chain of a C1q deficient patient. *Immunogenetics* **27**:259, 1988.
191. Petry F, Le DT, Kirschfink M, Starsia Z, Loos M: Molecular characterization of the C1q genes of patients with various types of C1q deficiency. III International Workshop on C1, Mainz, Germany, November 6–9, 1992. (abstr.)
192. Skok J, Solomon E, Reid KBM, Thompson RA: Distinct genes for fibroblast and serum C1q. *Nature* **292**:549, 1981.
193. Tosi M, Duponchel C, Meo T, Julier C: Complement C1s sequence and linkage to C1r. *Biochemistry* **26**:8516, 1987.
194. Kusumoto H, Hirosawa S, Salier JP, Hagen FS, Kurachi K: Human genes for complement components C1r and C1s in a close tail-to-tail arrangement. *Proc Natl Acad Sci USA* **85**:7307, 1988.
195. Bensa JC, Reboul A, Colomb MG: Biosynthesis in vitro of complement subcomponents C1q, C1s and C1 inhibitor by resting and stimulated human monocytes. *Biochem J* **216**:385, 1983.
196. Suzuki Y, Ogura Y, Otsubo O, Akagi K, Fujita T: Selective deficiency of C1s associated with a systemic lupus-like syndrome. *Arthritis Rheum* **35**:576, 1992.
197. Isenman DE, Young JR: The molecular basis for the difference in immune hemolysis activity of the Chido and Rogers isotypes of human complement components C4. *J Immunol* **132**:3019, 1984.
198. O'Neill GJ, Yang SY, Tegoli J, Berger R, Dupont B: Chido and Rogers blood groups are distinct antigenic components of human complement C4. *Nature* **273**:668, 1978.
199. Law SKA, Dodds AW, Porter RR: A comparison of the properties of two classes, C4A and C4B of the human complement components C4. *EMBO J* **3**:1819, 1984.
200. Carroll MC, Fathallah DM, Bergamaschini L, Alicot EM, Isenman DE: Substitution of a single amino acid (aspartic acid for histidine) converts the functional activity of C4B to C4A. *Proc Natl Acad Sci USA* **87**:6868, 1990.
201. Belt KT, Carroll MC, Porter RR: The structural basis of the multiple forms of human complement component C4. *Cell* **36**:907, 1984.
202. Belt KT, Yu CY, Carroll MC, Porter RR: Polymorphism of the human complement component C4. *Immunogenetics* **21**:173, 1985.
203. Carroll MC, Palsdottir A, Belt KT, Porter RR: Deletion of complement C4 and steroid 21-hydroxylase genes in the HLA class III region. *EMBO J* **4**:2547, 1985.
204. Prentice HL, Schneider PM, Strominger JL: C4B gene polymorphism detected in human cosmid clone. *Immunogenetics* **23**:274, 1986.
205. Roos MH, Mollenhauer E, Demant P, Rittner CH: A molecular basis for the two locus model of human complement component C4. *Nature* **298**:854, 1982.
206. Schneider PM, Carroll MC, Alper CA, Rittner C, Whitehead AS, Yunis EJ, Colten HR: Polymorphism of the human complement C4 and steroid 21-hydroxylase gene. Restriction fragment length polymorphisms revealing structural deletions, homoduplications and size variants. *J Clin Invest* **78**:650, 1986.
207. Whitehead AS, Woods DE, Fleishnick E, Chin JE, Katz AJ, Gerald PS, Alper CA, Colten HR: DNA polymorphism of the C4 gene: A new marker for analysis of the major histocompatibility complex. *N Engl J Med* **310**:88, 1984.
208. Hall RE, Colten HR: Cell-free synthesis of the fourth component of guinea pig complement (C4): Identification of a precursor of serum C4 (pro-C4). *Proc Natl Acad Sci USA* **74**:1707, 1977.
209. Roos MH, Atkinson JP, Shreffler DC: Molecular characterization of SS and Slp (C4) proteins of the mouse H-2 complex subunit composition, chain size, polymorphism and an intracellular (pro-Ss) precursor. *J Immunol* **121**:1106, 1978.
210. Ogata R, Shreffler D, Sepich D, Lilly S: cDNA clone spanning the alpha-gamma subunit junction in the precursor of the murine fourth complement component. *Proc Natl Acad Sci USA* **80**:5061, 1983.
211. Witte DP, Welch TR, Beischel LS: Detection and cellular localization of human C4 gene expression in the renal tubular

epithelial cells and other extrahepatic epithelial sources. *Am J Pathol* **139**:717, 1991.

212. Goldberger G, Colten HR: Precursor complement protein (pro-C4) is converted in vitro by plasmin. *Nature* **286**:514, 1980.
213. Goldberger G, Abraham GN, Williams J, Colten HR: Amino terminal sequence analysis of pro-C4, the precursor of the fourth component of guinea pig complement. *J Biol Chem* **250**:7071, 1980.
214. Karp DR: Post-translational modification of the fourth component of complement. Sulfation of the alpha chain. *Biol Chem* **258**:12745, 1983.
215. Karp DR: Post-translational modification of the fourth component of complement. Effect of tunicamycin and amino acid analogs on the formation of the internal thiolester and disulfide bonds. *J Biol Chem* **258**:14490, 1983.
216. Matthews WJ, Goldberger G, Marino JT, Einstein LP, Gash DJ, Colten HR: Complement proteins C2, C4 and factor B: Effect of glycosylation on their secretion and catabolism. *Biochem J* **204**:839, 1982.
217. Roos MH, Kornfeld S, Shreffler DC: Characterization of the oligosaccharide units of the fourth component of complement (Ss protein) synthesized by murine hepatocytes. *J Immunol* **124**:2860, 1980.
218. Chan AC, Mitchell KR, Munns TW, Karp DR, Atkinson JP: Identification and partial characterization of the secreted form of the fourth component of human complement: Evidence that it is different from the major plasma form. *Proc Natl Acad Sci USA* **80**:268, 1983.
219. Hortin G, Change AS, Fok KF, Strauss AW, Atkinson JP: Sequence analysis of the COOH terminus of the alpha chain of the fourth component of human complement: Identification of the site of its extracellular cleavage. *J Biol Chem* **261**:9065, 1986.
220. Awdeh ZL, Ochs HD, Alper CA: Genetic analysis of C4 deficiency. *J Clin Invest* **67**:260, 1981.
221. Welch TR, Beischel L, Berry A, Forristal J, West CD: The effect of null C4 alleles on complement function. *Clin Immunol Immunopathol* **34**:316, 1985.
222. Clark RA, Klebanoff SJ: Role of the classical and alternative complement pathways in chemotaxis and opsonization: Studies of human serum deficient in C4. *J Immunol* **120**:1102, 1978.
223. Mascart-Lemone F, Hauptmann G, Goetz J, Duchateau J, Delespesse G, Vray B, Dab I: Genetic deficiency of C4 presenting with recurrent infections and a SLE-like disease. *Am J Med* **75**:295, 1983.
224. Tappeiner G, Hintner H, Scholz S, Albert E, Linert J, Wolff K: Systemic lupus erythematosis in hereditary deficiency of the fourth component of complement. *J Am Acad Dermatol* **7**:66, 1982.
225. Budowle B, Roseman JM, Go RCP, Louv W, Barger BO, Acton RT: Phenotypes of the fourth component (C4) in black Americans from the southeastern United States. *J Immunogenet* **10**:199, 1983.
226. Biskof NA, Welch TR, Beischel LS: C4B deficiency: A risk factor for bacteremia with encapsulated organisms. *J Infect Dis* **162**:248, 1990.
227. Braun L, Schneider PM, Giles CM, Bertrams J, Rittner C: Null alleles of human complement C4. Evidence for pseudogenes at the C4A locus and gene conversion at the C4B locus. *J Exp Med* **171**:129, 1990.
228. Fredrikson GN, Truedsson L, Sjoholm AG, Kjellman M: DNA analysis in a MHC heterozygous patient with complete C4 deficiency—homozygosity for C4 gene deletion and C4 pseudogenes. *Exp Clin Immunogenet* **8**:29, 1991.
229. Uring-Lambert B, Mascart-Lemone F, Tongio M-M: Molecular basis of complement C4 deficiency. A study of three patients. *Hum Immunol* **24**:125, 1989.
230. Perlmutter DH, Cole FS, Goldberger G, Colten HR: Distinct primary translation products from human liver mRNA give rise to secreted and cell-associated forms of complement C2. *J Biol Chem* **259**:10380, 1984.
231. Perlmutter DH, Colten HR, Grossberger D, Strominger J, Seidman JD, Chaplin DD: Expression of complement proteins C2 and factor B in transfected L cells. *J Clin Invest* **76**:1449, 1985.
232. Johnson CA, Wetsel RA, Colten HR: Unpublished data.
233. Cross SJ, Edwards JM, Bentley DR, Campbell RD: DNA polymorphism of the C2 and factor B genes. Detection of a restriction fragment length polymorphism which subdivides haplotypes carrying the C2C and factor B F alleles. *Immunogenetics* **21**:39, 1985.
234. Falus A, Wakeland EK, McConnell TJ, Gitlin J, Whitehead AS, Colten HR: DNA polymorphism of MHC class III genes in inbred and wild mouse strains. *Immunogenetics* (in press)
235. Woods DE, Edge MD, Colten HR: Isolation of a cDNA clone for the human complement protein C2 and its use in identification of a restriction fragment length polymorphism. *J Clin Invest* **74**:634, 1984.
236. Ruddy S: Component deficiencies: The second component. *Prog Allergy* **39**:250, 1986.
237. Rhynes RI, Britten AF, Pickering RJ: Deficiency of the second component of complement association with the HLA haplotype A10, B18 in a normal population. *Ann Rheum Dis* **41**:93, 1982.
238. Ruddy S, Klemperer MR, Rosen FS, Austen KF, Kumate J: Hereditary deficiency of the second component of complement in man: Correlation of C2 hemolytic activity with immunochemical measurements of C2 protein. *Immunology* **18**:943, 1970.
239. Johnson FR, Agnello V, Williams RC Jr: Opsonic activity in human serum deficient in C2. *J Immunol* **109**:141, 1971.
240. Sampson HA, Walchner AM, Baker PJ: Recurrent pyogenic infections in individuals with absence of the second component of complement. *J Clin Immunol* **2**:39, 1982.
241. Friend P, Rapine J, Kim Y, Clawson CC, Michael AF: Deficiency of the second component of complement (C2) with chronic vasculitis. *Ann Intern Med* **83**:813, 1975.
242. Repine JE, Clawson CC, Friend PS: Influence of a deficiency of the second component of complement on the bactericidal activity of neutrophils in vitro. *J Clin Invest* **59**:802, 1977.
243. Geibink GS, Verhoeff J, Peterson PK, Quie PG: Opsonic requirements for phagocytosis of streptococcus pneumoniae types VI, XVIII, XXIII and XXV. *Infect Immun* **18**:291, 1977.
244. Newman SL, Vogler LB, Feigen RD, Johnston RB Jr: Recurrent septicemia associated with congenital deficiency of C2 and partial deficiency of factor B of the alternative pathway. *N Engl J Med* **299**:290, 1978.
245. Hyatt AC, Altenburger KM, Johnston RB Jr, Winkelstein JA: Increased susceptibility to severe pyogenic infections in patients with an inherited deficiency of the second component of complement. *J Pediatr* **98**:417, 1981.
246. Fasano MB, Hamosh A, Winkelstein JA: Recurrent systemic bacterial infections in homozygous C2 deficiency. *Pediatr Allergy Immunol* **1**:46, 1990.
247. Gewurz A, Lint TF, Roberts JL, Zeitz H, Gewurz H: Homozygous C2 deficiency with fulminant lupus erythematosus. Severe nephritis via the alternative complement pathway. *Arthritis Rheum* **21**:28, 1978.
248. Levy SB, Pinnell SR, Meadows L, Snyderman R, Ward FE: Hereditary C2 deficiency associated with cutaneous lupus erythematosus. *Arch Dermatol* **115**:57, 1979.
249. Kim Y, Friend PS, Dresner IG, Yunis EJ, Michael AF: Inherited deficiency of the second component of complement (C2) with membranoproliferative glomerulonephritis. *Am J Med* **62**:765, 1977.
250. Leddy JP, Griggs RC, Klemperer MR, Frank MM: Hereditary complement (C2) deficiency with dermatomyositis. *Am J Med* **58**:83, 1975.
251. Gelfand EW, Clarkson JO, Minta JO: Selective deficiency of the second component of complement in a patient with anaphylactoid purpura. *Clin Immunol Immunopathol* **4**:269, 1975.
252. Revielle JD, Bias WB, Winkelstein JA, Provost TT, Dorsch CA, Arnett FC: Familial systemic lupus erythematosis: Immunogenetic studies in eight families. *Medicine (Baltimore)* **62**:21, 1983.
253. Fu SM, Stern R, Kunkel HG, Dupont B, Hansen JA, Day NK, Good RA, Jersild C, Fotino M: Mixed lymphocyte culture determinants and C2 deficiency. LD-7a associated with C2 deficiency in four families. *J Exp Med* **142**:495, 1975.
254. Day NK, L'Esperance P, Good RA, Michael AF, Hansen JA, Dupont B, Jersild C: Hereditary C2 deficiency.

Genetic studies and association with the HL-A system. *J Exp Med* **141**:1464, 1975.

255. Wolski KP, Schmid FR, Mittal K: Genetic linkage between the HL-A system and a deficiency of the second component (C2) of complement. *Science* **188**:1020, 1975.
256. Awdeh ZL, Raum DD, Glass D, Agnello V, Schur PH, Johnston RB Jr, Gelfand EW, Ballow M, Yunis E, Alper CA: Complement-human histocompatibility antigen haplotypes in C2 deficiency. *J Clin Invest* **67**:581, 1981.
257. Hauptmann G, Tongio MM, Goetz J, Mayer S, Fauchet R, Sobel A, Griscel C, Berthoux F, Rivat C, Rother U: Association of the C2-deficiency gene (C2*Q0) with the C4A*4, C4B*2 genes. *J Immunogenet* **9**:127, 1982.
258. Johnson CA, Densen P, Wetsel RA, Cole FS, Goeken NE, Colten HR: Molecular heterogeneity of C2 deficiency. *N Engl J Med* **326**:871, 1992.
259. Vik DP, Amiguet P, Moffat GJ, Fey M, Amiguet-Barras F, Wetsel R, Tack BF: Structural features of the human C3 gene: Intron/Exon organization, transcriptional start site, and promoter region sequence. *Biochemistry* **30**:1080, 1991.
260. Whitehead AS, Solomon E, Chambers S, Bodmer WF, Povey S, Fey G: Assignment of the structural gene for the third component of human complement to chromosome 19. *Proc Natl Acad Sci USA* **79**:5021, 1982.
261. De Bruijn MHL, Fey G: Human complement component C3: cDNA coding sequence and derived primary structure. *Proc Natl Acad Sci USA* **82**:708, 1985.
262. Morris KM, Goldberger G, Colten HR, Aden DP, Knowles BB: Biosynthesis and processing of a human precursor complement protein, pro-C3, in a hepatoma-derived cell line. *Science* **215**:399, 1982.
263. Alper CA, Johnson AM, Birtch AG, Moore RD: Human C3: Evidence for the liver as the primary site of synthesis. *Science* **163**:286, 1969.
264. Ramadori G, Tedesco F, Bitter-Buermann D, Meyer ZUM, Buschenfelde KH: Biosynthesis of the third (C3), eighth (C8), and ninth (C9) complement components by guinea pig hepatocyte primary cultures. *Immunobiology* **170**:203, 1985.
265. Iijima M, Tobe T, Sakamoto T, Tomita M: Biosynthesis of the internal thioester bond of the third component of complement. *J Biochem* **96**:1539, 1984.
266. Alper CA, Propp RP, Klemperer MR, Rosen FS: Inherited deficiency of the third component of complement (C3). *J Clin Invest* **48**:553, 1969.
267. Alper CA, Colten HR, Gear JSS, Robson AR, Rosen FS: Homozygous human C3 deficiency: The role of C3 in antibody production, C1s-induced vasopermeability, and cobra venom-induced passive hemolysis. *J Clin Invest* **57**:222, 1976.
268. Pussell BA, Bourke E, Nayef M, Morris S, Peters DK: Complement deficiency and nephritis: A report of a family. *Lancet* **1**:675, 1980.
269. Davis AE III, Davis JS IV, Robson AR, Osofsky SG, Colten HR, Rosen FS, Alper CA: Homozygous C3 deficiency: Detection of C3 by radioimmunoassay. *Clin Immunol Immunopathol* **8**:543, 1977.
270. Botto M, Fong KY, So AK, Rudge A, Walport MJ: Molecular basis of hereditary C3 deficiency. *J Clin Invest* **86**:11581, 1990.
271. Ballow M, Shira JE, Harden L, Yang SY, Day NK: Complete absence of the third component of complement in man. *J Clin Invest* **56**:703, 1975.
272. Osofsky SG, Thompson BH, Lint TF, Gewurz H: Hereditary deficiency of the third component of complement in a child with fever, skin rash, and arthralgias: Response to transfusion of whole blood. *J Pediatr* **90**:180, 1977.
273. Roord JJ, Daha M, Kuis W, Verbrugh HA, Verhoef J, Zegers BJM, Stoop JW: Inherited deficiency of the third component of complement associated with recurrent pyogenic infections, circulating immune complexes, and vasculitis in a dutch family. *Pediatrics* **71**:81, 1983.
274. Hsieh K-H, Lin C-Y, Lee T-C: Complete absence of the third component of complement in a patient with repeated infections. *Clin Immunol Immunopathol* **20**:305, 1981.
275. Sano Y, Nishinukai H, Kitamura H, Nagaki K, Inai S, Hamasaki Y, Maruyama I, Igata A: Hereditary deficiency of the third component of complement in two sisters with systemic lupus erythematosis-like symptoms. *Arthritis Rheum* **24**:1255, 1981.
276. Alper CA, Colten HR, Rosen FS, Robson AR, MacNab GM, Gear JSS: Homozygous deficiency of C3 in a patient with repeated infections. *Lancet* **2**:1179, 1972.
277. Grace HJ, Brereton-Stiles GG, Vos GH, Schonland M: A family with partial and total deficiency of complement C3. *S Afr Med J* **50**:139, 1976.
278. Berger M, Balow JE, Wilson CB, Frank MM: Circulating immune complexes and glomerulonephritis in a patient with congenital absence of the third component of complement. *N Engl J Med* **308**:1009, 1983.
279. Borzy MS, Houghton D: Mixed-pattern immune deposit glomerulonephritis in a child with inherited deficiency of the third component of complement. *Am J Kidney Dis* **5**:54, 1985.
280. Weiss RM, Schuz ES: Complement deficiency in Sweet's Syndrome. *Br J Dermatol* **121**:413, 1989.
281. McLean RH, Weinstein A, Damjanov I, Rothfield N: Hypomorphic variant of C3, arthritis, and chronic glomerulonephritis. *J Pediatr* **93**:937, 1978.
282. McLean RH, Weinstein A, Chapitis J, Lowenstein M, Rothfield N: Familial partial deficiency of the third component of complement (C3) and the hypocomplementemic cutaneous vasculitis syndrome. *Am J Med* **68**:549, 1980.
283. Wyatt RJ, Jones D, Stapleton FB, Roy S, Odom TW, McLean RH: Recurrent hemolytic-uremic syndrome with the hypomorphic fast allele of the third component of complement. *J. Pediatr* **107**:564, 1985.
284. Alper CA, Rosen FS: Studies of a hypomorphic variant of human C3. *J Clin Invest* **50**:324, 1971.
285. McLean RH, Bryan RK, Winkelstein JA: Hypomorphic variant of the slow allele of C3 associated with hypocomplementemia and hematuria. *Am J Med* **78**:865, 1985.
286. Botto M, So AK, Fong KY, Barlow R, Routier R, Morley BJ: Homozygous hereditary C3 deficiency due to a partial gene deletion. *Complement Inflamm* **8**:130A, 1991.
287. Singer L, Kramer J, Borzy MS, Wetsel RA: Evidence of molecular heterogeneity causing inherited human C3 deficiency. XIV Int Complement Workshop. *Complement Inflamm* **8**:224A, 1991.
288. Einstein LP, Hansen PJ, Ballow M, Davis AE III, Davis JS, Alper CA, Rosen FS, Colten HR: Biosynthesis of the third component of complement (C3) in vitro by monocytes from both normal and homozygous C3 deficient humans. *J Clin Invest* **60**:963, 1977.
289. Carney DF, Haviland DL, Noack D, Wetsel RA, Vik DP, Tack BF: Structural aspects of the human C5 gene: Intron/exon organization, 5′ flanking features, and characterization of two truncated cDNA clones. *J Biol Chem* **266**:18786, 1991.
290. Wetsel RA, Barnum SR: Molecular biology and biochemistry of the third (C3) and fifth (C5) complement components, in Sim RB (ed): *Biochemistry and Molecular Biology of Complement*. Lancaster, England, MTP (in press)
291. Ooi YM, Colten HR: Biosynthesis and post-synthetic modification of a precursor (Pro-C5) of the fifth component of mouse complement (C5). *J Immunol* **123**:2494, 1979.
292. Patel F, Minta JO: Biosynthesis of a single chain pro-C5 by normal mouse liver mRNA: Analysis of the molecular basis of C5 deficiency in AKR/J mice. *J Immunol* **123**:2408, 1979.
293. Lundwall AB, Wetsel RA, Kristensen T, Whitehead AS, Woods DE, Ogden RL, Colten HR, Tack BF: Isolation of a cDNA clone encoding the fifth component of human complement. *J Biol Chem* **260**:2108, 1985.
294. McCarty GA, Snyderman R: Component deficiencies. The fifth component. *Prog Allergy* **39**:271, 1986.
295. Rosenfeld SI, Kelly ME, Leddy JP: Hereditary deficiency of the fifth component of complement in man. I. Clinical, immunochemical, and family studies. *J Clin Invest* **57**:1626, 1976.
296. Rosenfeld SI, Baum J, Steigbigel RT, Leddy JP: Hereditary deficiency of the fifth component of complement in man. II. Biological properties of C5-deficient human serum. *J Clin Invest* **57**:1635, 1976.
297. Snyderman R, Durack DT, McCarty GA, Ward FE, Meadows L: Deficiency of the fifth component of complement in human subjects. Clinical genetic and immunologic studies in a large kindred. *Am J Med* **67**:638, 1979.

298. McLean R, Peter G, Gold R, Guerra L, Yunis EJ, Kruetzer DL: Familial deficiency of C5 in humans: Intact but deficient alternative complement pathway activity. *Clin Immunol Immunopathol* **21**:62, 1981.
299. Peter G, Weigert MB, Bissel AR, Gold R, Kreutzer D, McLean RH: Meningococcal meningitis in familial deficiency of the fifth component of complement. *Pediatrics* **67**:882, 1981.
300. Jeremiah SJ, West LF, Abbott CM, Murad Z, Povey S, Thomas HJ, Solomon E, Discipio R, Fey GH: Three genes coding for late acting components of complement assigned to chromosome 5. *Cytogenet Cell Genet* **51**:1019A, 1989.
301. Haefliger JA, Tschopp J, Vial N, Jenne DE: Complete primary structure and functional characterization of the sixth component of the human complement system. *J Biol Chem* **264**:18041, 1989.
302. Di Scipio RG, Hugli TE: The molecular architecture of human complement component C6. *J Biol Chem* **264**:16197, 1989.
303. Rother U: Component deficiencies. The sixth component. *Prog Allergy* **39**:283, 1986.
304. Glass D, Raum D, Balavitch D, Kagan E, Robson A, Schur PH, Alper CA: Inherited deficiency of the sixth component of complement: A silent or null gene. *J Immunol* **120**:538, 1978.
305. Leddy JP, Frank MM, Gaither T, Baum J, Klemperer MR: Hereditary deficiency of the sixth component of complement in man. I. Immunochemical, biologic, and family studies. *J Clin Invest* **53**:544, 1974.
306. Lim D, Gewurz Z, Lint TF, Ghaze M, Sephari B, Gewurz H: Absence of the sixth component of complement in a patient with repeated episodes of meningococcal meningitis. *J Pediatr* **89**:42, 1976.
307. Vogler LB, Newman SL, Stroud RM, Johnston RB Jr: Recurrent meningococcal meningitis with absence of the sixth component of complement: An evaluation of underlying immunologic mechanisms. *Pediatrics* **64**:465, 1979.
308. Lee TJ, Snyderman R, Patterson J, Rauchbach AS, Folds JD, Yount WJ: Neisseria meningitidis bacteremia in association with deficiency of the sixth component of complement. *Infect Immun* **24**:656, 1979.
309. Tedesco F, Silvani CM, Agelli M, Giovanetti AM, Bombardieri S: A lupus-like syndrome in a patient with deficiency of the sixth component of complement. *Arthritis Rheum* **24**:1438, 1981.
310. Lachman PJ, Hobart MJ, Woo P: Combined genetic deficiency of C6 and C7 in man. *Clin Exp Immunol* **33**:193, 1978.
311. Morgan BP, Vara SP, Bennett AJ, Thomas SP, Mathews N: A case of hereditary combined deficiency of complement components C6 and C7 in man. *Clin Exp Immunol* **75**:396, 1989.
312. Zeitz HJ, Lint TF, Gewurz A, Gewurz H: Component deficiencies. 7. The seventh component. *Prog Allergy* **39**:289, 1986.
313. Boyer JT, Gall EP, Norman ME, Nilsson UR, Zimmerman TS: Hereditary deficiency of the seventh component of complement. *J Clin Invest* **56**:905, 1975.
314. Wellek B, Opferkuch W: A case of deficiency of the seventh component of complement in man: Biological properties of a C7-deficient serum and description of a C7-inactivating principle. *Clin Exp Immunol* **19**:223, 1975.
315. Lee TJ, Utsinger PD, Snyderman R, Yount WJ, Sparling PF: Familial deficiency of the seventh component of complement associated with recurrent bacteremic infections due to Neisseria. *J Infect Dis* **138**:359, 1978.
316. Loirat C, Buriot D, Peltier AP, Berche P, Aujard Y, Griscelli C, Mathieu H: Fulminant meningococcemia in a child with hereditary deficiency of the seventh component of complement and proteinuria. *Acta Paediatr Scand* **69**:553, 1980.
317. Zeitz HJ, Miller GW, Lint TF, Ali MA, Gewurz H: Deficiency of C7 with systemic lupus erythematosis. Solubilization of immune complexes in complement-deficient sera. *Arthritis Rheum* **24**:87, 1981.
318. Alcalay M, Bontoux D, Peltier A: C7 deficiency, abnormal platelet aggregation and rheumatoid arthritis. *Arthritis Rheum* **24**:102, 1981.
319. Friduss SR, Sadoff WI, Hern AE, Fivenson DP: Fatal pyoderma gangrenosum in association with C7 deficiency. *J Am Acad Dermatol* **27**:356, 1992.
320. Kolb WP, Muller-Eberhard HJ: The membrane attack mechanism of complement. The three polypeptide chain structure of the eighth component (C8). *J Exp Med* **143**:1131, 1976.
321. Steckel EW, York RG, Monahan JB, Sodety JM: The eighth component of human complement. Purification and physicochemical characterization of its unusual subunit structure. *J Biol Chem* **255**:11997, 1980.
322. Rittner C, Schneider PM: Genetics and polymorphism of the complement components, in Rother K, Till GO (ed): *The Complement System*. Heidelberg, Springer-Verlag 1993.
323. Kaufman KM, Snider JV, Spurr NK, Schwartz CE, Sodety JM: Chromosomal assignments of genes encoding the α, β, γ subunits of human complement protein C8: Identification of a close physical linkage between the α and β loci. *Genomics* **5**:475, 1989.
324. Ng SC, Sodetz JM: Biosynthesis of C8 by hepatocytes: Differential expression and intracellular association of the α-γ and β subunits. *J Immunol* **139**:3021, 1987.
325. Densen P, McRill CM: Differential expression of C8 subunits: Primary role of C8 beta. *Clin Res* **35**:613A, 1987.
326. Tedesco F: Component deficiencies. 8. The eighth component. *Prog Allergy* **39**:295, 1986.
327. Tedesco F, Densen P, Villa MA, Petersen BH, Sirchia G: Two types of dysfunctional eighth component of complement (C8) molecules in C8 deficiency in man: Reconstitution of normal C8 from the mixture of the two abnormal C8 molecules. *J Clin Invest* **71**:183, 1983.
328. Tschopp J, Penea F, Schifferli J, Spath P: Dysfunctional C8 beta chain in patients with C8 deficiency. *Scand J Immunol* **24**:715, 1986.
329. Warnick PR, Densen P: Reduced C8β messenger RNA expression in families with hereditary C8β deficiency. *J Immunol* **146**:1052, 1991.
330. Tedesco F, Bardare M, Giovanetti AM, Sirchia G: A familial dysfunction of the eighth component of complement (C8). *Clin Immunol Immunopathol* **16**:180, 1980.
331. Tschopp J, Esser AF, Spira TJ, Muller-Eberhard HJ: Occurrence of an incomplete molecule in homozygous C8 deficiency in man. *J Exp Med* **154**:1599, 1981.
332. Tedesco F, Villa MA, Densen P, Sirchia G: Beta chain deficiency in three patients with dysfunctional C8 molecules. *Mol Immunol* **20**:47, 1983.
333. Petersen BH, Graham JA, Brooks GF: Human deficiency of the eighth component of complement. The requirement of C8 for serum Neisseria gonorrhoeae bactericidal activity. *J Clin Invest* **57**:283, 1976.
334. Jasin HE: Absence of the eighth component of complement in association with system lupus erythematosis-like disease. *J Clin Invest* **60**:709, 1977.
335. Nicholson A, Lepow I: Host defense against Neisseria meningitidis requires a complement-dependent bactericidal activity. *Science* **205**:298, 1979.
336. Discipio RG, Gehring MR, Podack ER, Kan CC, Hugli TE, Fey GH: Nucleotide sequence of human complement component C9. *Proc Natl Acad Sci USA* **81**:7298, 1984.
337. Stanley KK, Luzio JP: Construction of a new family of high efficiency bacterial expression vectors: Identification of cDNA clones for human liver proteins. *EMBO J* **3**:11429, 1984.
338. Stanley KK, Kocher HP, Luzio JP, Jackson P, Tschopp J: The sequence and topology of human complement component C9. *EMBO J* **4**:375, 1985.
339. Marazziti D, Eggersten G, Stanley KK, Fey G: Evolution of the cysteine-rich domains of C9. *Complement* **4**:189, 1987.
340. Abbott C, West L, Povey S, Jeremiah S, Murad Z, Discipio R, Fey G: The gene for human complement component C9 mapped to chromosome 5 by polymerase chain reaction. *Genomics* **4**:606, 1989.
341. Lint TF, Gewurz H: Component deficiencies. The ninth component. *Prog Allergy* **39**:307, 1986.
342. Yoshimura K, Fukumori Y, Ohnoki S, O Kubo Y, Yamaguchi H, Tanaka M, Akagaki Y, Inai S: Studies on complement deficiencies in blood donors in Osaka area of Japan. *Jpn J Hum Genet* **28**:120, 1983.

343. Harriman GR, Esser AF, Podack ER, Wunderlich AC, Braude AI, Lint TF, Curd JG: The role of C9 in complement-mediated killing of Neisseria. *J Immunol* **127**:2386, 1981.
344. Inai S, Kitamura H, Hiramatsu S, Nagaki K: Deficiency of the ninth component of complement in man. *J Clin Lab Immunol* **2**:85, 1979.
345. Lint TF, Zeitz HJ, Gewurz H: Inherited deficiency of the ninth component of complement in man. *J Immunol* **125**:2252, 1980.
346. Fine DP, Gewurz H, Griffis M, Lint TF: Meningococcal meningitis in a woman with inherited deficiency of the ninth component of complement. *Clin Immunol Immunopathol* **28**:413, 1983.
347. Nagata M, Hara T, Aoki T, Mizuno Y, Akeda H, Inaba S, Tsumoto K, Veda K: Inherited deficiency of the ninth component of complement: An increased risk of meningococal meningitis. *J Pediatr* **114**:260, 1989.
348. Goldberger G, Arnaout MA, Aden D, Kay R, Rits M, Colten HR: Biosynthesis and postsynthetic processing of human C3b/C4b inactivator (factor I) in three hepatoma cell lines. *J Biol Chem* **259**:6492, 1984.
349. Whaley K: Biosynthesis of complement components and the regulatory proteins of the alternative complement pathway by human peripheral blood monocytes. *J Exp Med* **151**:501, 1980.
350. Goldberger G, Bruns GA, Rits M, Edge MD, Kwiatkowski DJ: Human complement factor I: Analysis of cDNA-derived primary structure and assignment of its gene to chromosome 4. *J Biol Chem* **262**:10065, 1987.
351. Alper CA, Abramson N, Johnston RB Jr, Jandl JH, Rosen FS: Increased susceptibility to infection associated with abnormalities of complement-mediated functions and of the third component of complement (C3). *N Engl J Med* **282**:349, 1970.
352. Alper CA, Abramson N, Johnston RB, Jandl JH, Rosen FS: Studies in vivo and in vitro on an abnormality in the metabolism of C3 in a patient with increased susceptibility to infection. *J Clin Invest* **49**:1975, 1970.
353. Abramson N, Alper CA, Lachmann PJ, Rosen FS, Jandl JH: Deficiency of C3 inactivator in man. *J Immunol* **107**:19, 1971.
354. Zeigler JB, Alper CA, Rosen FS, Lachmann PJ, Sherington L: Restoration by purified C3b inactivator of complement-mediated function in vivo in a patient with C3b inactivator deficiency. *J Clin Invest* **55**:668, 1975.
355. Nicol PAE, Lachmann PJ: The alternative pathway of complement activation. The role of C3 and its inactivator (KAF). *Immunology* **24**:259, 1973.
356. Wahn V, Rother V, Rauterberg EW, Day NK, Laurell AB: C3b inactivator deficiency: Association with an alpha-migrating factor H. *J Clin Immunol* **1**:228, 1981.
357. Solal-Celigny P, Laviolette M, Hebert J, Atkins PC, Sirois M, Brun G, Lehner-Netsch G, Delage JM: C3b inactivator deficiency with immune complex manifestations. *Clin Exp Immunol* **47**:197, 1982.
358. Teisner B, Brandslund I, Folkerson J, Rasmussen JM, Paulsen LO, Svehog SE: Factor I deficiency and C3 nephritic factor: Immunochemical findings and association with Neisseria meningitidis infection in two patients. *Scand J Immunol* **20**:291, 1984.
359. Thompson RA, Lachmann PJ: A second case of human C3b inhibitor (KAF) deficiency. *Clin Exp Immunol* **27**:23, 1977.
360. Kolble K, Buckle V, Lefranc G, Halbawachs-Mecarelli L, Moller-Rasmussen J, Sim RB, Spath P, Svehag SE, Teisner B, Wahn V: Physical mapping of complement factor I gene in normal and deficient genomes. *Complement Inflamm* **6**:355, 1989.
361. Skerka C, Timmann C, Horstmann RD, Zipfel PE: Two additional human serum proteins structurally related to complement factor H. *J Immunol* **148**:3313, 1992.
362. Feifel E, Prodinger WM, Molgg M, Schwaeble W, Schonitzer D, Koistinen V, Misasi R, Dierich MP: Polymorphism and deficiency of human factor H-related proteins p39 and p37. *Immunogenetics* **36**:104, 1992.
363. Nielsen HE, Christensen KC, Koch C, Thomsen BS, Heegaard NHH, Tranum-Jensen J: Hereditary, complete deficiency of complement factor H associated with recurrent meningococcal disease. *Scand J Immunol* **30**:711, 1989.
364. Levy M, Halbwachs-Mecarelli L, Gubler MC, Kohout G, Bensenouci A, Niaudet P, Hauptmann G, Lesavre P: H deficiency in two brothers with atypical dense intramembranous deposit disease. *Kidney Int* **30**:949, 1986.
365. Thompson RA, Winterborn MH: Hypocomplementaemia due to a genetic deficiency of Beta-1H globulin. *Clin Exp Immunol* **46**:110, 1981.
366. Brai M, Misiano G, Maringhini S, Cutaja I, Hauptmann G: Combined homozygous factor H and heterozygous C2 deficiency in an Italian family. *J Clin Immunol* **8**:50, 1988.
367. White RT, Damm D, Hancock N, Rosen BS, Lowell BB, Usher P, Flier JS, Spiegelman BM: Human adipsin is identical to complement Factor D and is expressed at high levels in adipose tissue. *J Biol Chem* **267**:9210, 1992.
368. Kluin-Nelemans HC, Van Velzen-Blad H, Van Helden HPT, Daha MR: Functional deficiency of complement factor D in a monozygous twin. *Clin Exp Immunol* **58**:724, 1984.
369. Hiemstra PS, Langeler E, Compier B, Keepers T, Leijh PCS, Van Den Barselaar MT, Overbosch D, Daha MR: Complete and partial deficiencies of complement factor D in a Dutch family. *J Clin Invest* **84**:1957, 1989.
370. Goundis D, Holt SM, Boyd Y, Reid KBM: Localization of the properdin structural locus to Xp11.23-Xp21.1. *Genomics* **5**:56, 1989.
371. Robson KJH, Halt JRS, Jennings MW, Harris TJR, Marsh K, Newbold CI, Tate VE, Weatherall DJ: A highly conserved amino-acid sequence in thrombospondin, properdin and in proteins from sporozoites and blood stages of a human malarial parasite. *Nature* **335**:79, 1988.
372. Nolan KF, Schwaeble W, Kaluz S, Dierich MP, Reid KBM: Molecular cloning of the cDNA coding for properdin, a positive regulator of the alternative pathway of human complement. *Eur J Immunol* **21**:771, 1991.
373. Sjoholm AG, Braconier JH, Soderstrom C: Properdin deficiency in a family with fulminant meningococcal infections. *Clin Exp Immunol* **50**:291, 1982.
374. Densen P, Weiler JM, Griffiss JM, Hoffmann LG: Familial properdin deficiency and fatal meningococcemia: Correction of the bactericidal defect by vaccination. *N Engl J Med* **316**:922, 1987.
375. Nielson HE, Kock C: Congenital properdin deficiency and meningococcal infection. *Clin Immunol Immunopathol* **44**:134, 1987.
376. Sjoholm AG, Soderstrom C, Nilsson LA: A second variant of properdin deficiency: The detection of properdin at low concentrations in affected males. *Complement Inflamm* **5**:130, 1988.
377. Sjoholm AG, Kuijper EJ, Tijssen CC, Jansz A, Bol P, Spanjaard L, Zanen HC: Dysfunctional properdin in a Dutch family with meningococcal disease. *N Engl J Med* **319**:33, 1988.
378. Holme ER, Veitch J, Johnston A, Hauptmann G, Uring-Lambert B, Seywright M, Docherty V, Morley WN, Whaley K: Familial properdin deficiency associated with chronic discoid lupus erythematosus. *Clin Exp Immunol* **76**:76, 1989.
379. Gelfand DW, Rao CP, Minta JO, Ham T: Inherited deficiency of properdin and C2 in a patient with recurrent bacteremia. *Am J Med* **82**:671, 1987.
380. Hillarp A, Dahlback B: Cloning of cDNA coding for the β chain of human complement component C4b-binding protein: Sequence homolog with the α chain. *Proc Natl Acad Sci USA* **87**:1183, 1990.
381. Lappin DF, Guc D, Hill A, McShane T, Whaley K: Effect of interferon-γ on complement gene expression in different cell types. *Biochem J* **281**:437, 1992.
382. Trapp RG, Fletcher M, Forristal J, West CD: C4 binding protein deficiency in a patient with atypical Bechet's disease. *J Rheumatol* **14**:135, 1987.
383. Ewulonu UK, Ravi L, Medof ME: Characterization of the Decay-Accelerating Factor gene promoter region. *Proc Natl Acad Sci USA* **88**:4675, 1991.
384. Shenoy-Scaria AM, Kwong J, Fujita T, Olszowy MW, Shaw AS, Lublin DM: Signal transduction through Decay-Accelerating Factor. *J Immunol* **149**:3535, 1992.
385. Holguin MH, Martin CB, Bernshaw NJ, Parker CJ: Analysis of the effects of activation of the alternative pathway

of complement on erythrocytes with an isolated deficiency of Decay Accelerating Factor. *J Immunol* **148**:498, 1992.

386. Telen MJ, Green AM: The Inab phenotype: Characterization of the membrane protein and complement regulatory defect. *Blood* **74**:437, 1989.
387. Okada H, Nagami Y, Takahash IK, Okada N, Hideshima T, Takizawa H, Kondo J: 20 kDa homologous restriction factor of complement resembles T cell activating protein. *Biochem Biophys Res Commun* **162**:1553, 1989.
388. Yamashina M, Ueda E, Kinoshita T, Takami T, Ojima A, Ono H, Tanaka H, Kondo N, Orii T, Okada N, Okada H, Inoue K, Kitani T: Inherited complete deficiency of 20 kilodalton homologous restriction factor (CD59) as a cause of paroxysmal nocturnal hemoglobinuria. *N Engl J Med* **323**:1184, 1990.
389. Donaldson VH, Evans RR: A biochemical abnormality in hereditary angioneurotic edema. Absence of serum inhibitor of C1-esterase. *Am J Med* **35**:37, 1963.
390. Harrison RA: Human C1 inhibitor: Improved isolation and preliminary structural characterization. *Biochemistry* **22**:5001, 1983.
391. Carter PE, Duponchel C, Tosi M, Fothergill JE: Complete nucleotide sequence of the gene for human C1 inhibitor with an unusually high density of Alu elements. *Eur J Biochem* **197**:301, 1991.
392. Bock SC, Skriver K, Neilson E, Thogersen HC, Wiman B, Donaldson VH, Eddy RL, Muarinan J, Rodziejewska E, Huber R, Shows TB, Magnusson S: Human C1 inhibitor: Primary structure, cDNA cloning and chromosomal localization. *Biochemistry* **25**:4294, 1986.
393. Morris KM, Aden DP, Knowles BB, Colten HR: Complement biosynthesis by the human hepatoma-derived cell line, HepG2. *J Clin Invest* **70**:906, 1982.
394. Colten HR: Ontogeny of the human complement system: in vitro biosynthesis of individual complement components by fetal tissues. *J Clin Invest* **51**:725, 1972.
395. Gitlin D, Biasucci A: Development of gamma G, gamma A, gamma M, beta-1-C/beta-1-A, C1 esterase inhibitor, ceruloplasmin, transferrin, hemopexin, haptoglobin, fibrinogen, plasminogen, $alpha_1$ antitrypsin, orosomucoid, beta-lipoprotein, $alpha_2$ macroglobulin and prealbumin in the human conceptis. *J Clin Invest* **48**:1433, 1969.
396. Johnson AM, Alper CA, Rosen FS, Craig JM: Immunofluorescent hepatic localization of complement proteins: Evidence for a biosynthetic defect in hereditary angioneurotic edema (HANE). *J Clin Invest* **50**:50a, 1971.
397. Bensa JC, Reboul A, Colomb MG: Biosynthesis in vitro of complement subcomponents C1q, C1s, and C1 inhibitor by resting and stimulated human monocytes. *Biochem J* **216**:385, 1983.
398. Yeung-Laiwah AC, Jones L, Hamilton AD, Whaley K: Complement subcomponent-C1 inhibitor synthesis by human monocytes. *Biochem J* **226**:199, 1985.
399. Kramer J, Katz Y, Rosen FS, Davis AW, Strunk RC: Synthesis of C1 inhibitor in fibroblasts from patients with type I and type II hereditary angioneurotic edema. *J Clin Invest* **87**:1614, 1991.
400. Rosen FS, Alper CA, Pensky J, Klemperer MR, Donaldson VH: Genetically determined heterogeneity of the C1 esterase inhibitor in patients with hereditary angioneurotic edema. *J Clin Invest* **50**:2143, 1971.
401. Frank MM, Gelfand JA, Atkinson JP: Hereditary angioedema: The clinical syndrome and its management. *Ann Intern Med* **84**:580, 1976.
402. Cicardi M, Bergamaschini L, Marasini B, Boccassini G, Tucci A, Agostini A: Hereditary angioedema: An appraisal of 104 cases. *Am J Med Sci* **284**:2, 1982.
403. Austen KF, Sheffer AL: Detection of hereditary angioneurotic edema by demonstration of a reduction in the second component of human complement. *N Engl J Med* **272**:649, 1965.
404. Pickering RJ, Gewurz H, Kelly JR, Good RA: The complement system in hereditary angioneurotic oedema—A new perspective. *Clin Exp Immunol* **3**:423, 1968.
405. Rosen FS, Alper CA, Pensky J, Klemperer MR, Donaldson VH: Genetically determined heterogeneity of C1 esterase inhibitor in patients with hereditary angioneurotic edema. *J Clin Invest* **50**:2143, 1971.
406. Harpel PC, Hugli TE, Cooper NR: Studies on human plasma C1 inactivator-enzyme interactions: II Structural features of an abnormal C1 inactivator from a kindred with hereditary angioneurotic edema. *J Clin Invest* **55**:605, 1975.
407. Donaldson VH, Harrison RA, Rosen FS, Being DH, Kindness G, Canar J, Wagner CJ, Awad S: Variability in purified dysfunctional C1-inhibitor proteins from patients with hereditary angioneurotic edema. Functional and analytical gel studies. *J Clin Invest* **75**:124, 1985.
408. Quastel M, Harrison R, Cicardi M, Alper CA, Rosen FS: Behavior in vivo of normal and dysfunctional C1 inhibitor in normal subjects and patients with hereditary angioneurotic edema. *J Clin Invest* **83**:1041, 1983.
409. Lachman PJ, Rosen FS: The catabolism of C1-Inhibitor and the pathogenesis of hereditary angio-edema. *Acta Pathol Microbiol Immunol Scand* **92**:35, 1984.
410. Donaldson VH, Rosen FS: Action of complement in hereditary angioneurotic edema: Role of C1-esterase. *J Clin Invest* **43**:2204, 1964.
411. Klemperer MR, Donaldson VH, Rosen FS: Effect of C1 esterase on vascular permeability in man: Studies in normal and complement-deficient individuals and in patients with hereditary angioneurotic edema. *J Clin Invest* **47**:604, 1968.
412. Schreiber AP, Kaplan AP, Austen KF: Inhibition by C1INH of Hageman factor fragment activation of coagulation, fibrinolysis, and kinin generation. *J Clin Invest* **52**:1402, 1973.
413. Curd JG, Progais LJ Jr, Cochrane CG: Detection of active kallikrein in induced blister fluids of hereditary angioedema patients. *J Exp Med* **152**:742, 1980.
414. Schapira M, Silver LD, Scott CF, Schmaier AH, Prograis LJ, Curd JG, Colman RW: Prekallikrein activation and high-molecular-weight kininogen consumption in hereditary angioedema. *N Engl J Med* **308**:1050, 1983.
415. Osler W: Hereditary angioneurotic aedema. *Am J Med Sci* **95**:362, 1888.
416. Landerman NS: Hereditary angioneurotic edema. I. Case reports and review of the literature. *J Allergy* **33**:316, 1962.
417. Donaldson VH, Rosen FS: Hereditary angioneurotic edema: A clinical survey. *Pediatrics* **37**:1017, 1966.
418. Sheffer AL, Craig JM, Willms-Kretschmer K, Austen KF, Rosen FS: Histopathological and ultrastructural observations on tissues from patients with hereditary angioneurotic edema. *J Allergy* **47**:292, 1971.
419. Sheffer AL, Austen KF, Rosen FS: Tranexamic acid therapy in hereditary angioneurotic edema. *N Engl J Med* **287**:452, 1972.
420. Frank MM, Sergent JS, Kane MA, Alling DW: Epsilon aminocaproic acid therapy of hereditary angioneurotic edema: A double blind study. *N Engl J Med* **286**:808, 1972.
421. Gelfand JA, Sherins RJ, Alling DW, Frank MM: Treatment of hereditary angioedema with danazol: Reversal of clinical and biochemical abnormalities. *N Engl J Med* **295**:1444, 1976.
422. Spaulding WB: Methyltestosterone therapy for hereditary episodic edema (hereditary angioneurotic edema). *Ann Intern Med* **53**:739, 1960.
423. Hosea SW, Santaella ML, Brown EJ, Berger M, Katusha K, Frank MM: Long-term therapy of hereditary angioedema with danazol. *Ann Intern Med* **93**:809, 1980.
424. Gadek JE, Hosea SW, Gelfand JA, Frank MM: Response of variant hereditary angioedema phenotypes to danazol therapy. *J Clin Invest* **64**:280, 1979.
425. Jaffe CJ, Atkinson JP, Gelfand JA, Frank MM: Hereditary angioedema: The use of fresh frozen plasma for prophylaxis in patients undergoing oral surgery. *J Allergy Clin Immunol* **55**:386, 1975.
426. Gadek JE, Hosea SW, Gelfand JA, Santaella M, Wickerhauser M, Triantaphyllopoulos DC, Frank MM: Replacement therapy in hereditary angioedema: Successful treatment of acute episodes of angioedema with partly purified C1 inhibitor. *N Engl J Med* **304**:542, 1980.
427. Aulak KS, Pemberton PA, Rosen FS, Carrell RW, Lachmann PJ, Harrison RA: Dysfunctional C1 inhibitor (At), isolated from type II hereditary angioedema plasma,

contains a P1 "reactive centre" (Arg 444-His) mutation. *Biochem J* **253**:615, 1988.

428. Skriver K, Radziejewska E, Silbermann JA, Donaldson VH, Bock SC: Mutations in CpG dinucleotide change reactive site arginine 444 to cysteine in dysfunctional C1 inhibitor Da and histidine in dysfunctional C1 inhibitor Ri. *J Biol Chem* **264**:3066, 1989.
429. Levy NJ, Ramesh N, Cicardi M, Harrison RA, David AE: Type II hereditary angioneurotic edema that may result from a single nucleotide change in the codon for alanine-436 in the C1 inhibitor gene. *Proc Natl Acad Sci USA* **87**:265, 1990.
430. Skriver K, Wikoff WR, Patston PA, Tausk F, Schapira M, Kaplan AP, Bock SC: Substrate properties of C1 inhibitor Ma (alanine 434-glutamic acid). General and structural evidence suggesting that the P12-region contains critical determinants of serine protease inhibitor/substrate status. *J Biol Chem* **266**:9216, 1991.
431. Davis AE, Aulak KS, Parad RB, Stecklein HP, Eldering E, Hack CG, Kramer J, Strunk RC, Rosen FS: Characterization and expression of C1 inhibitor non-reactive center mutations. *Complement Inflamm* **8**:138A, 1991.
432. Parad RB, Kramer J, Strunk RC, Rosen FS, Davis AE: Dysfunctional C1 inhibitor Ta: Deletion of Lys-251 results in acquisition of an N-glycosylation site. *Proc Natl Acad Sci USA* **87**:6786, 1990.
433. Stoppa-Lyonnet D, Carter PE, Meo T, Tosi M: Clusters of intragenic Alu repeats predispose the human C1 inhibitor locus to deleterious rearrangements. *Proc Natl Acad Sci USA* **87**:1551, 1990.
434. Ariga T, Carter PE, Davis AE: Recombination between Alu repeat sequences that result in partial deletions with the C1 inhibitor gene. *Genomics* **8**:607, 1990.
435. Stoppa-Lyonnet D, Duponchel C, Meo T, Laurent J, Carter PE, Arala-Chaves M, Cohen JH, Dewald G, Goetz J, Hauptmann G, et al: Recombinational biases in the rearranged C1-inhibitor genes of hereditary angioedema patients. *Am J Hum Genet* **49**:1055, 1991.
436. Stoppa-Lyonnet D, Tosi M, Laurent J, Sobel A, Lagrue G: Altered C1 inhibitor genes in type I hereditary angioedema. *N Engl J Med* **317**:1, 1987.
437. Cicardi M, Igarashi T, Kim MS, Frangi D, Agostoni A, Davis AE: Restriction fragment length polymorphism of the C1 inhibitor gene in hereditary angioneurotic edema. *J Clin Invest* **80**:1640, 1987.
438. Frangi D, Cicardi M, Sica A, Colotta F, Agostini A, Davis AE: Nonsense mutations affect C1 inhibitor mRNA levels in patients with type I hereditary angioneurotic edema. *J Clin Invest* **88**:755, 1991.
439. Kramer J, Rosen FS, Strunk RC: Trans inhibition of normal C1 inhibitor net synthesis in exon VII deleted type I C1 inhibitor deficiency. *Complement Inflamm* **8**:177, 1991.

CHAPTER **131**

Immotile-Cilia Syndrome (Primary Ciliary Dyskinesia), Including Kartagener Syndrome

Björn A. Afzelius ▪ Björn Mossberg

1. **The immotile-cilia syndrome is a genetically determined disorder characterized by dysmotility or even complete immotility of the cilia in the airways and elsewhere. Usually spermatozoa are also either immotile or poorly motile.**

2. **Kartagener syndrome is a subgroup of the immotile-cilia syndrome and is further characterized by situs inversus viscerum. Situs inversus, bronchiectasis, and chronic sinusitis form the classic Kartagener triad.**

3. **The reason for the ciliary immotility or dysmotility can usually be seen with an electron-microscopic investigation of a ciliated mucosal biopsy or of the spermatozoa of an ejaculate. Certain specific defects in the ciliary axoneme are regarded to be pathognomonic of the syndrome, principally a lack of dynein arms. Cilia and sperm tails normally exhibit the same defects in the same patient. Motility can be evaluated by light-microscopic examination of living cilia or spermatozoa, and the functional capacity of cilia by measurement of mucociliary transport.**

4. **The clinical consequences of the immotile-cilia syndrome include chronic cough and expectoration, bronchiectasis, chronic rhinitis and nasal polyposis, chronic or recurrent sinusitis, and often an agenesis of the frontal sinuses. Otosalpingitis and otitis are common. Obstructive lung disease may develop and is expressed as chronic airflow limitation. Most clinical manifestations date from early childhood. Neonatal asphyxia often occurs.**

5. **Males are usually sterile. Females may be fertile or infertile.**

6. **Treatment is symptomatic and directed against complications in the upper and lower respiratory tract. Physiotherapy with postural drainage should probably be started early in life. With modern care and abstinence from smoking the prognosis in the immotile-cilia syndrome is good.**

7. **The immotile-cilia syndrome clearly is a genetically heterogeneous disease, although its clinical profile is fairly uniform. Many genes participate in the construction of a cilium, and an error in any one of them will prevent the cilia from working properly. The inheritance in most cases is autosomal recessive. In families in which the immotile-cilia syndrome occurs, on average half the affected sibs have situs inversus. Presumably, chance alone decides between situs inversus and situs solitus in homozygotes of the syndrome.**

In a paper in 1933 Manes Kartagener published the case histories of four persons who all had situs inversus totalis, bronchiectasis, and chronic sinusitis.[1] Siewert had previously described one such case.[2] This combination of symptoms later came to be known as *Kartagener syndrome* or *Kartagener triad.* It is caused by a structural and generalized abnormality of cilia, making the cilia immotile, feebly motile, or dysmotile[3,4] and, hence, nonfunctional. Ciliary dysmotility is associated with situs inversus in only about half the cases. Because situs inversus per se usually has no serious implications, this chapter will treat the immotile-cilia syndrome in its entirety and will include Kartagener syndrome as a subgroup of the immotile-cilia syndrome.

PREVALENCE

Most authors estimate the prevalence of Kartagener syndrome at 1 in 30,000 to 1 in 60,000.[5,6] Different frequencies will be found depending on how strictly the investigator adheres to the original definition. The prevalence of the immotile-cilia syndrome can be estimated from the following data. Situs inversus has been estimated to have a prevalence in Europe and the United States of 1 in 8000 to 1 in 25,000.[5,7,8] Roughly one fourth to one fifth of all persons with situs inversus also have bronchiectasis and chronic sinusitus.[7] A somewhat higher fraction has generalized bronchitis but not (yet) bronchiectasis. This gives a figure of the prevalence of Kartagener syndrome on the order of 1 in 40,000 to 1 in 120,000. If it is true, as assumed,[3] that half the patients with the immotile-cilia syndrome have situs inversus, then the prevalence of this syndrome will be twice that of Kartagener syndrome, or about 1 in 20,000 to 1 in 60,000.

Geographic and Racial Distribution

Kartagener syndrome has been described in all major races and from most countries with medical journals. Detailed pedigrees have been published from Austria,[9] Canada,[10] France,[11] Germany,[12,13] Great Britain,[14] Israel,[15] Japan,[16]

A list of standard abbreviations is located immediately preceding the index in each volume.

Sweden,[17] Switzerland,[18] the United States,[19-21] and other countries. In all these publications it was remarked that one or several sibs of the propositus had the same bronchial and sinusoidal symptoms as the propositus but had no situs inversus. Sometimes these sibs have been claimed to have an ''incomplete Kartagener syndrome.'' The seemingly equal number of affected sibs with and without situs inversus supports the idea that the immotile-cilia syndrome is inherited as a recessive disorder and that chance alone determines whether the viscera take up the normal or the reversed position during embryogenesis.[3]

The Polynesian population of New Zealand may be a special case: Bronchiectasis is relatively common, and ciliary ultrastructure in the affected persons has been shown to range from normal to abnormal with a deficiency in dynein arms.[22,23] There seems to be no connection to situs inversus. The Polynesian bronchiectasis may either be an acquired defect or a genetic defect that becomes manifest late in development.

Reports from Nonhuman Species

Several canine cases of Kartagener syndrome or of the immotile-cilia syndrome in the dog have been reported.[24-28] The symptoms are the same as in humans: cilia are defective and as a result, chronic rhinitis and bronchopneumonia develop. About half the cases have situs inversus. The nasal turbinals are poorly developed. In some cases the brain ventricles have been shown to be considerably enlarged,[25] and in others hydrocephalus is fully developed.[25-27] Six sibs of pigs with immotile-cilia syndrome have also been reported[29] with defective cilia and two with situs inversus.

Some strains of laboratory animals have been described as suitable ''animal models'' of this disease: Male WIC-Hyd rats have cilia devoid of dynein arms, have situs inversus in half the cases, and will have hydrocephalus; they do not suffer from bronchiectasis.[30] Similarly, mice of the Hpy/Hpy mutant are deficient in dynein arms and are prone to hydrocephalus (and polydactyly),[31] whereas those of the iv/iv mutant,[32] although they have healthy cilia and respiratory tracts, have situs inversus in 50 percent of the cases.

The model organism for ciliary (or flagellar) mutants otherwise is the unicellular alga Chlamydomonas, in which a great variety of mutants have been isolated.[33-37] Biochemical and genetic studies of this organism have shown that ciliary (or, more properly, flagellar) immotility is a heterogeneous condition involving one of several different genes.[36] Ciliary mutants have also been described from other organisms, as reviewed by Afzelius.[38]

CILIA IN THE HUMAN BODY

The symptoms of the immotile-cilia syndrome and of its subgroup, Kartagener syndrome, cannot be understood without a knowledge of the distribution in the body of cilia and of the normal ciliary anatomy. Cilia and sperm tails are outgrowths from centrioles (basal bodies) with an architecture as shown in Figs. 131-1 to 131-3. The central axis is called the axoneme and consists of nine microtubular doublets in a ring around two single microtubules. These 11 units are joined by three types of bonds:

1. Two rows of dynein arms along each doublet, which are instrumental in microtubular sliding and ciliary undulation. Cilia or spermatozoa with no outer dynein arms are capable of slow beatings, whereas the inner arms seem to be indispensable for ciliary movements.[35,39]
2. Nexin links, which are responsible for the maintenance of axoneme structure during sliding. They seem to limit the sliding by being stretchable only to a certain degree.
3. Spokes, which extend from the outer doublets to a central sheath around the two central microtubules and that participate in the mechanism for converting sliding into bending.

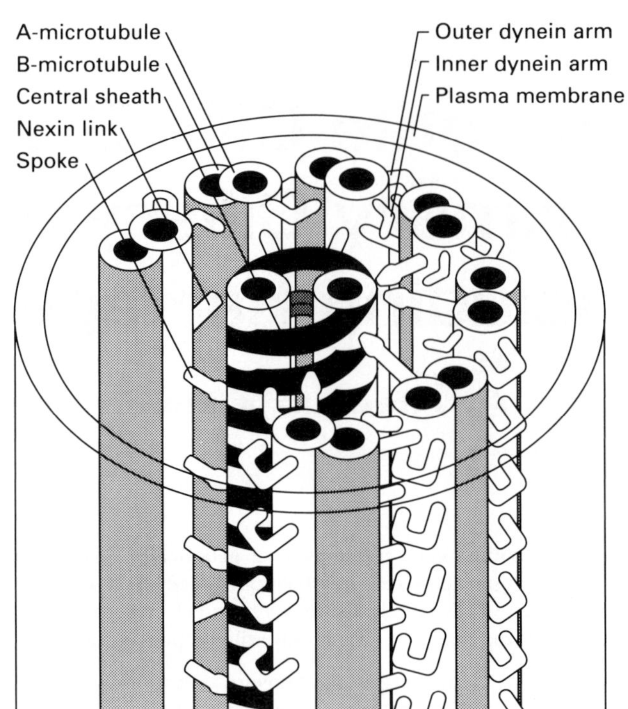

FIG. 131-1 **Three-dimensional reconstruction of the cilium.** *(From Klaus Hausmann. Reproduced by permission of* **Biologie in unserer Zeit.***)*

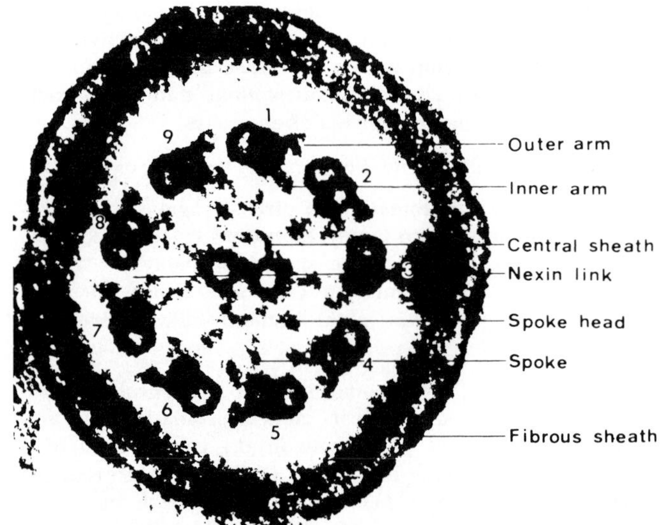

FIG. 131-2 **Electron micrograph of a transversely sectioned human sperm tail from a healthy man. The central part of the sperm tail has the same structure as that of a cilium. There are nine outer microtubular doublets in a ring around two central microtubules. The terms used for some of the components are given.** ***(From Afzelius and Eliasson.[45] Used with permission.)***

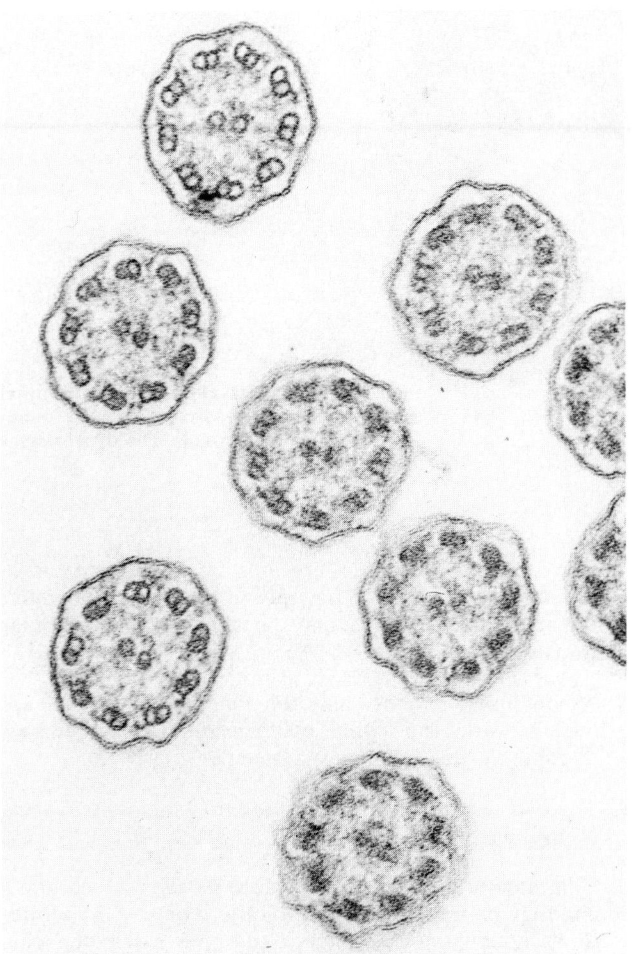

FIG. 131-3 **Cilia from the bronchial mucosa of a person who has normal cilia. Note that the cilia have a fairly ordered orientation best seen in the two central microtubules.**

Further details of the ciliary machinery and its mode of action can be found in refs. 5 and 39 to 44.

Ciliated epithelia are found in the following places in the human body: the upper airways (i.e., nasal passages, paranasal sinuses, eustachian tubes, middle ear mucosa, and nasopharynx); the trachea and bronchi down to respiratory bronchioles; the lacrimal sac; the ependymal lining of the brain and central canal of the spinal cord; the endometrial lining of the deeper parts of the cervix; the fallopian tubes; and the ductuli efferentes on the border between testis and epididymis.

Some epithelia have a single cilium per cell (a primary cilium), for instance, the thyroid gland,[45] the inner corneal endothelium, the trabecular meshwork, and the choroid of the eye,[46] as do several of the embryonic epithelia.[5] Such primary cilia have been found to beat, but whether their beatings can perform work is unknown.[47] Certain sensory cells carry a sensory hair that is a modified cilium. The tail of the human spermatozoon has an axoneme, with the typical structure of a cilium, although it is much longer and has a flagellar beat. Cilia are about 6 μm long, sperm tails about 40 μm.

The cilia of the airway epithelia beat in a layer of serous fluid which is about 5 μm thick (the sol layer). Overlying this layer and at the level of the ciliary tips is a mucous or gel layer that may be either patchy or continuous.[40] Most cilia are oriented in the same general direction, which determines the direction of their effective strokes. The cilia are mechanically coordinated into short metachronal waves and transport the mucous layer with its entrapped inhaled particles and endogenous debris toward the pharynx with a speed of about 2 mm/min in the central bronchi and trachea. The role of cilia in the fallopian tubes, the ductuli efferentes, and the ependyma of the central nervous system is largely speculative.

Ultrastructure of Cilia and Sperm Tails in the Immotile-Cilia Syndrome

The essential feature of the immotile-cilia syndrome, including Kartagener syndrome, is the abnormal structure and function of cilia. Usually an immotility or a dysmotility can be detected by light microscopic videorecording, and an abnormal ciliary ultrastructure can be seen by electron microscopy. Most—possibly all—clinical data of this syndrome can be explained by defective ciliary work. Cilia and sperm tails from hundreds of persons have been examined as to their motility or immotility and ultrastructure and the data from different laboratories are in essential agreement. It is evident that the immotile-cilia syndrome is a heterogeneous disease and that several subgroups can be found:

1. Dynein arms are practically absent in both rows[3,5,48–60] (Figs. 131-4 and 131-5).
2. Both outer and inner dynein arms are reduced in number, often to about half normal.[17,57–61]
3. The outer dynein arms are short, and the inner dynein arms may be missing.[49,53,62–64]
4. Only outer dynein arms are missing[49,50,56–58,60,65] (Fig. 131-6).
5. Only inner dynein arms are missing.[57,60,62,63,67]
6. The entire spokes or the spoke heads as well as the central sheath are missing; the two inner microtubules often are off-center ("the spoke defect"[5,50,51,55,60,68]) (Fig. 131-7).

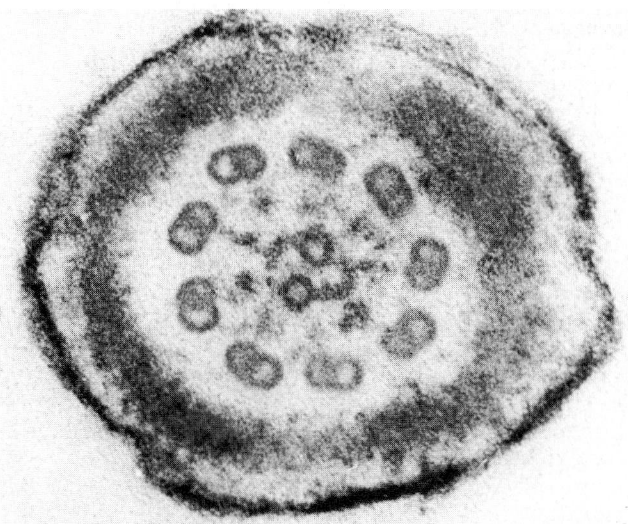

FIG. 131-4 **Sperm tail of a man with the immotile-cilia syndrome. In this man the sperm tails and the cilia are characterized by a total or nearly total lack of both the outer and inner dynein arms.**

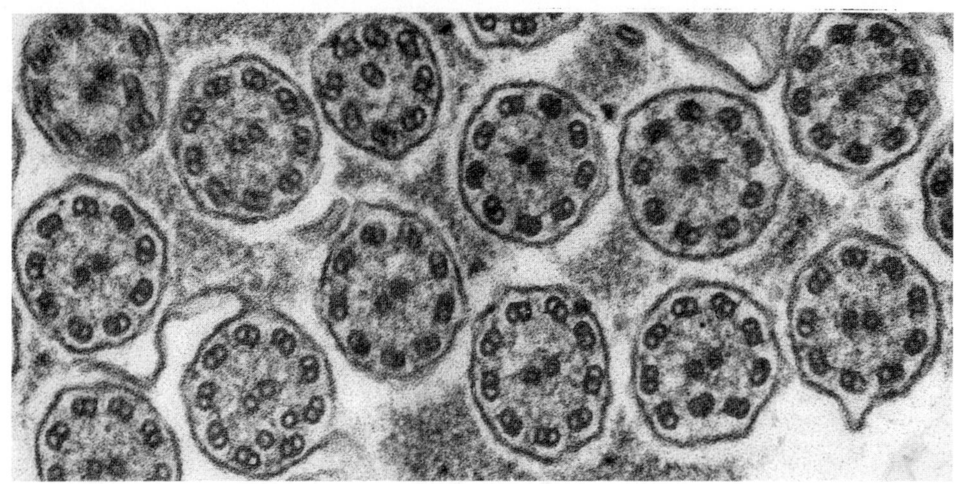

FIG. 131-5 Cilia from the nasal epithelium of a woman with the immotile-cilia syndrome. The dynein arms are missing.

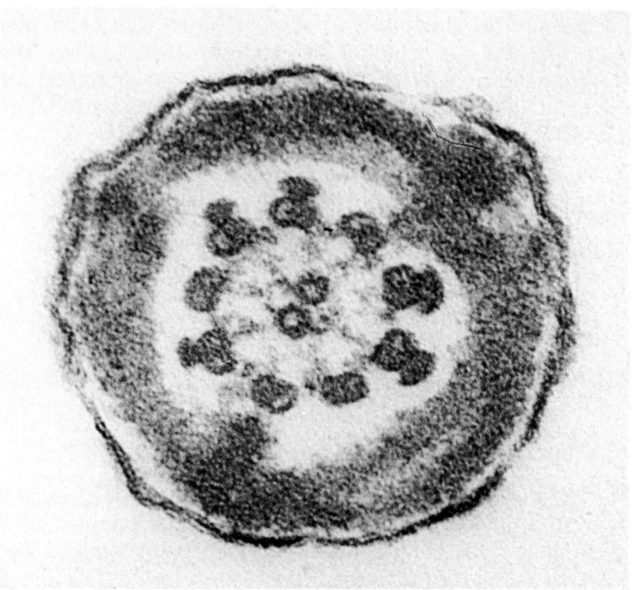

FIG. 131-6 Sperm tail of a man with the immotile-cilia syndrome and characterized by the presence of inner dynein arms but no, or very few, outer dynein arms. The spermatozoa had some degree of motility.

7. The central microtubules are short or absent, and microtubular doublet no. 1 is transposed to a central position; the inner dynein arms may be absent (''microtubular transposition defect''[52,55,60,69]).

8. Nexin links, spokes, and the inner dynein arms are missing, and the circle of microtubular doublets is disrupted (''disorganized'' axoneme[50,53,66]).

9. The two central microtubules and the inner dynein arms are missing.[70]

10. Cilia have a normal ultrastructure as seen in sections[60] and may be immotile,[71,72] dysmotile,[59] or are ''hypermotile'' though nonfunctional.[73] In some cases, the cilia have approximately twice the normal length.[74]

11. Cilia and basal bodies may be completely lacking. Ciliated cells in the nasal epithelium only or in the nasal epithelium and tracheobronchial tree may be replaced by cells that have long microvilli[60,75,77]; these cells may be undifferentiated mucous cells or brush cells.[49,78–81] It should be noted here that viral or bacterial infections tend to reduce the number of ciliated cells, and that it thus may be difficult to distinguish between inherited and acquired diseases.[82]

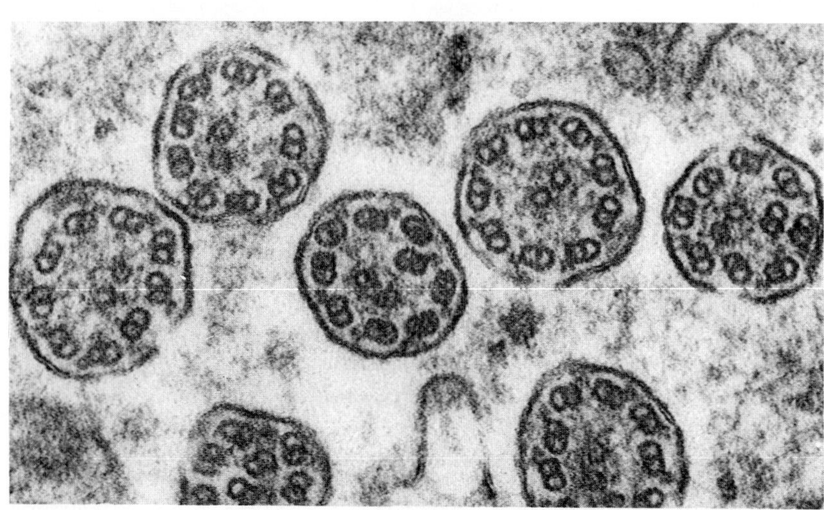

FIG. 131-7 Cilia from the nasal epithelium of a woman with the immotile-cilia syndrome. The inner microtubules are off-center presumably because of defective spokes.

Other subgroups may well exist. In many of the patients in subgroups 1 to 7 the cilia are further characterized by the presence of supernumerary or missing microtubules in the axoneme. Cilia also tend to be rather poorly aligned[83-86]; the range of orientation of the basal feet[83] or of the two central microtubules[84-86] thus is wider than in controls. Although it seems that a very accurate alignment of mucus-propelling cilia may be unnecessary, a random orientation of cilia would exclude coordinated activity. About half the cases in most of these subgroups have situs inversus. Cilia from different types of epithelia of the same patient usually have the same ultrastructure, indicating that the defect is a generalized one.[49,51,87,88] It is possible, however, that focal abnormalities may make the diagnosis uncertain; it is hence recommended that cilia from two or more sites are evaluated. One case has been reported in which cilia at one site of the bronchi had microtubular transposition to a high percentage and at other sites were close to normal.[89] Chronic nasal obstruction may reduce the number of ciliated cells,[90] as may viral airway infections.[91,92] In studies in which repeated biopsies were taken from the same patient, the cilia usually were found to have the same ultrastructure,[93] but in three cases an anomaly (short dynein arms) was found in a first but not a second biopsy.[60,62]

Cilia and sperm tails tend to display the same type of defect in the same patient, although the spermatozoa may be completely devoid of dynein arms in men who have cilia with a few dynein arms.[3,87,94,95] There are also a few published cases with only the spermatozoa immotile and lacking dynein arms[61,96] or in which only the cilia display these features.[97] The difference in axonemal ultrastructure between cilia and spermatozoa from the same patient could be due either to a mosaicism, to a separate genetic control of their structural component, or to a variable penetrance.

Some of the ciliary abnormalities listed above, and in particular defects other than the listed ones, have been described in patients with infections, allergies, or chemical treatment.[62,98,99] These include the clumping of several axonemes within a common limiting membrane (into "compound cilia") or the presence of supernumerary microtubular doublets or singlets or a deficiency in their number.[98-101] These types of ciliary defects hence are not diagnostic of the immotile-cilia syndrome.

Motility of Cilia and Sperm Tails

The immotile-cilia syndrome is due to a lack of cilia[76] or to the cilia being completely immotile,[48,49,102] being feebly motile,[61] or displaying erratic movements.[103-105] Because a good correlation usually exists between ciliary motility and spermatozoal motility, an examination of the spermatozoa can be made for diagnostic purposes.[87] Sperm immotility may be due also to other factors: exposure of the ejaculate to cold, immobilization by antibodies, necrospermia (i.e., dead spermatozoa), and certain disorders in which the spermatozoa are grossly abnormal.[87] In order to observe the motility or immotility of cilia, ciliated cells have to be removed and observed in vitro. Cilia from persons with the immotile-cilia syndrome may be immotile or may have an abnormal and inefficient motility. Several variants of abnormal motility have been described: reduced beat frequency, hyperfrequent low-amplitude vibrations, "windshield wiper-movement," multiplanar "egg-beater–like rotations," "corkscrewlike rotation," slow-grabbing movements of the distal portion, and flagella-like undulation.[103-107] Certain dysmotilities can be correlated to specific ultrastructural defects.[108] However, the functional capacity of the cilia measured by mucociliary clearance is absent; this is a hallmark of the syndrome.[57,92,109-112]

Biopsies or brushings from a ciliated epithelium can be examined with phase contrast or interference contrast microscopy.[102,103,106,113] It is difficult, however, to distinguish between normal and erratic types of ciliary beatings with an unaided eye, and analysis has to be performed either with an oscillographic technique[104,105,114] or by making videorecordings which can be studied in slow motion.[115]

A complete motility study should include three parameters: ciliary beat frequency, ciliary beat coordination, and ciliary beat amplitude.[115] Sometimes, even such a complete study will not be enough. In one patient with immotile spermatozoa and with a reduced number of dynein arms in his cilia, ciliary motility in vitro was not affected, although mucociliary clearance in vivo was, possibly because of the increased load of mucus in vivo.[61] It was noticed that cilia started beating properly in vitro only after the mucus had been washed away.

Some investigators have objected to the term *immotile-cilia syndrome* for patients who have some degree of ciliary motility[103-105] or who evidently lack cilia and have suggested terms such as *primary ciliary dyskinesia,* the *dyskinetic cilia syndrome,* or the *acilia syndrome.* A clinical investigation will not distinguish between immotile and dysmotile cilia or a lack of cilia, however, and hence it is impractical to have different names for different subgroups. Ciliary motility, when present, is ineffective and represents a functionally immotile state; therefore the term *immotile-cilia syndrome* seems appropriate. In a clinical context the disease is an entity.

Situs Inversus and Embryonic Cilia

The following explanation has been suggested for the association between ciliary immotility and situs inversus.[3] Embryonic epithelia often carry a single cilium per cell. In the normal course of events these cilia are assumed to beat and, by their beatings, cause the heart to be moved to the left side, whereupon the liver goes to the right side of the body. With no ciliary work, chance alone will decide whether the visceral asymmetry will be normal or reversed. The validity of this hypothesis can be tested only when suitable animal models are examined, such as the rat strain WIC-Hyd[30] or the mouse strain iv/iv.[32] Layton and colleagues assume that the action of the mutated gene for the animal model or for the immotile-cilia syndrome is due to a loss of the developmental control of the entire cytoskeleton[116,117]; other hypotheses have been proposed as well.[118] Attempts have been made to isolate a polypeptide that has been suggested to be a candidate for determination of laterality.[119]

GENETIC CONSIDERATIONS

An examination of published pedigrees[9-21] indicates that the immotile-cilia syndrome is inherited as an autosomal recessive trait. Heterozygotes have a normal ciliary ultrastructure, as was shown by an examination of parents of the affected children.[120,121] On average, half the affected persons have situs inversus. As a consequence, the offspring of a mating between two heterozygotes each has a one-eighth chance of having situs inversus. Careful segregation analyses of proband sibships in cases of situs inversus[122] or of the immotile-cilia syndrome[68] have been consistent with this mode of inheritance. Approximately 1 in 60 among the population would be a heterozygous carrier if the syndrome were genetically homogeneous.[68] The risk of having a child with the immotile-cilia syndrome is apparently not increased with higher age of the mother.[68] One of the pedigrees published by Katsuhara et al. is more consistent with a dominant mode of inheritance than with the recessive one.[16] A dominant mode of inheritance can be expected when a structural protein is involved but there is no evidence of an autosomal dominant mode of inheritance in this disease,[68] in spite of the fact that the cilium contains many structural proteins.

The primary gene products may be the proteins that are seen to be missing in the cilia: dyneins, nexins, spoke proteins, etc.[33] or proteins that are responsible for the binding of them to the microtubules. Nearly 200 different polypeptides have been identified within the ciliary axoneme of lower organisms,[33] and 85 ciliary loci have been identified by over 270 independent mutations.[37] It is likely that various genes responsible for different subgroups of the immotile-cilia syndrome are located on most chromosomes in humans. Previous attempts to localize the (assumed single) gene for Kartagener syndrome have been unsuccessful. Conclusive results will probably be obtained only when studies are restricted to one family, and these results will not necessarily be valid in other families.

Males and females are equally affected. Most males with the syndrome have immotile spermatozoa and are sterile. Male sterility can also be observed in most, but not all[21,123] published pedigrees. In rare cases, a Kartagener patient may have normally motile spermatozoa and be capable of fathering a healthy child.[97]

In a Norwegian population 5 percent of all children with Kartagener syndrome had first-cousin parents, and 16 percent had second-cousin parents.[124] Among the control population, 0.5 percent of parents are first cousins.

CLINICAL FEATURES

Diagnosis

Diagnosis of the immotile-cilia syndrome can be performed by electron microscopy, if specific ultrastructural defects of cilia or sperm tails are found in persons with a clinical picture compatible with the syndrome. Alternatively, diagnosis requires the demonstration of immotility or severe dysmotility of cilia or spermatozoa. Possibly with the exception of sperm motility investigations, such tests are too complicated to be suited as a first-line screening. Measurements of airway mucociliary clearance may be valuable in excluding the diagnosis, since an absence of mucociliary clearance is a hallmark of the syndrome.[109,125] The measurement of the tracheobronchial clearance of inhaled, radioactively tagged test particles is also a complicated and expensive method, which moreover has to be interpreted with caution since coughing will often obscure the impaired mucociliary clearance in these patients.[112,125] As a first screening method the saccharin test of nasal mucociliary clearance is much more applicable.[126–128] Saccharin particles are placed on the inferior nasal turbinate about 10 mm from its anterior end and the time measured for the sweet taste to appear. A greatly prolonged time—usually to more than 60 min—is found in patients with nonfunctioning cilia. A reduced mucociliary clearance is, however, found also in some other diseases and may be an acquired condition.

Samples of ciliated cells are easily obtained from the inferior nasal turbinate by gentle scraping with a curette or better still with a cytology brush, a procedure that does not require anesthesia.[103,106,113] Alternatively, mucosal biopsies may be obtained by bronchoscopy. Ciliary motility may then be analyzed in vitro, by light microscopy and oscillometry or videoscreen recording, by which methods the characteristic immotility or dysmotility may be accurately assessed.[73,104,129] The ciliary material may also be prepared for electron microscopy, which is diagnostic in typical cases, such as those with a severe deficiency of dynein arms.[5] In cases with more discrete types of defects, the EM evaluation is more problematic and may require quantitative analysis.[130]

A demonstration of specific defects of ciliary ultrastructure and/or motility is unnecessary for purely clinical purposes. The diagnosis may be regarded as established with a sufficient degree of reliability in the following situations: (1) patients with complete Kartagener syndrome, (2) men with the typical clinical signs (chronic bronchitis and rhinitis since early childhood) who have immotile or poorly motile but otherwise normal spermatozoa, and (3) patients with the same clinical signs concerning airway disease and who have a sib who fulfills the criteria of (1) or (2). It should be kept in mind that most persons with situs inversus do not have chronic respiratory tract disease and thus do not have the immotile-cilia syndrome, and cases with situs inversus accompanied by other types of respiratory tract disease, such as asthma and atopic rhinitis, should not be confused with the immotile-cilia syndrome. Cases fulfilling the criteria of Kartagener syndrome but without any ciliary defects whatsoever have been described,[131] which is expected, since causes of chronic respiratory disease other than ciliary defects must occasionally occur in persons with situs inversus. However, such cases probably are rare.

The immotile-cilia syndrome has many features in common with cystic fibrosis, for instance, male infertility. Mucociliary clearance may be retarded in cystic fibrosis but often is present in spite of the airway disease; this disease, nevertheless, has a more serious prognosis than in the immotile-cilia syndrome, and the cilia have a normal ultrastructure.[132] Patients with immunoglobulin deficiency may also have a rather similar clinical profile, with mucociliary clearance retarded secondary to the chronic infections; again ciliary ultrastructure has been found normal.[133] Another differential diagnosis is Young syndrome, defined as obstructive azoospermia and chronic sinopulmonary infections[134,135]; this condition is the most common cause of the combination of male infertility and chronic airway infections. The respiratory tract disease seems to be generally less severe here than in the immotile-cilia syndrome.[135]

Respiratory Tract

Although the immotile-cilia syndrome is a heterogeneous condition with regard to ultrastructure, and hence genetics, the clinical profile seems to be fairly or even remarkably uniform—perhaps not surprising when one considers the absence of mucociliary clearance as a common denominator. Characteristically, the respiratory tract disease can be traced back to early childhood or even infancy—often to the very day of birth.[55,57,73,112,136] Neonatal respiratory distress is not uncommon.[136,137] Chronic cough and expectoration of mucoid, mucopurulent, or at times purulent sputum is generally present and often tends to increase during the day rather than being most prominent in the morning as in smoker's chronic bronchitis. Atelectasis and pneumonia are fairly common.

Rhinitis with discharge of a mostly rather thin secretion is also almost universally present, and it is not infrequently complicated by nasal polyposis.[64,82,136] Chronic or recurrent sinusitis is present, affecting both maxillary and ethmoidal sinuses; the frontal sinuses often fail to develop. The mastoid cells are poorly aerated. Chronic secretory otitis media is constantly present in childhood, with bouts of more acute otitis superimposed.[17,57,82,88,138–140] In most patients there is a conductive hearing loss of moderate degree—10 to 40 dB.[17,82,138] The ear and nose symptoms usually peak in childhood and adolescence, often with numerous surgical interventions, with a considerable improvement by adult age.[17]

Common colds do not seem to have a much more severe course in the immotile-cilia syndrome than in normal subjects. When there is no apparent acute infection, sedimentation rate and serum immunoglobulins are usually normal.[112] Sputum cultures may fail to reveal specific pathogens; when such are found, *Haemophilus influenzae* is a common finding.[60,73,88]

Bronchiectasis is probably never present at birth but often develops during childhood and adolescence (Figs. 131-8 and 131-9). It occurs in dependent parts of the lungs, may be cylindrical or saccular, and on histologic examination shows nonspecific inflammation. The changes are identical to bronchiectasis from other causes.[141,142] When bronchiectasis develops, there may be a marked worsening of the previously often rather discrete endobronchial symptoms, with increased expectoration, infectious episodes with fever, hemoptysis, and development of finger clubbing. The respiratory tract disease of Kartagener syndrome has traditionally been described in terms of bronchiectasis and sinusitis, but now it appears clear that a generalized bronchitis and rhinitis are the more primary features.

Lung function evaluated by spirometry may be normal or show an obstructive impairment of ventilation; in a few cases there may be a restrictive impairment as well,

FIG. 131-8 Chest radiograph of a 32-year-old woman with Kartagener syndrome. Changes suggesting bronchiectasis are seen behind the heart. Note the transposition of the heart and also of the abdominal viscera with part of the colon to the right and the liver to the left.

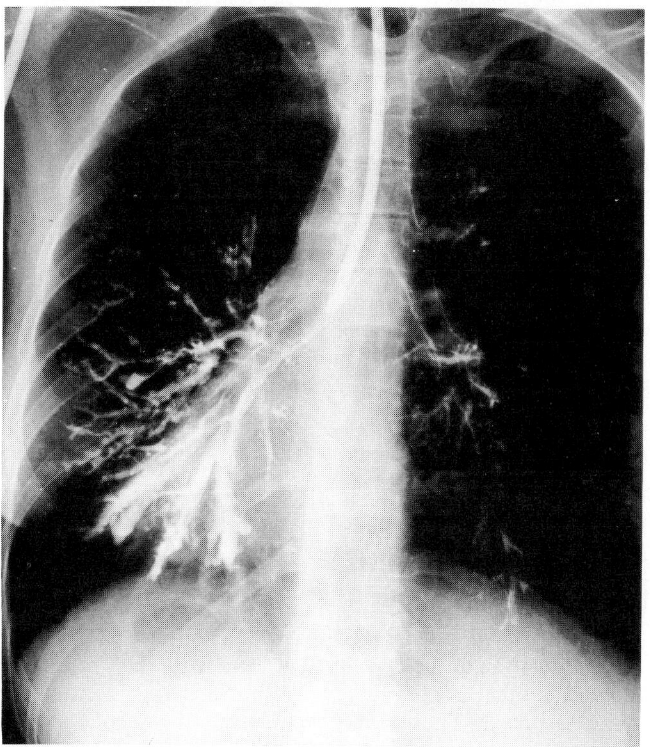

A.

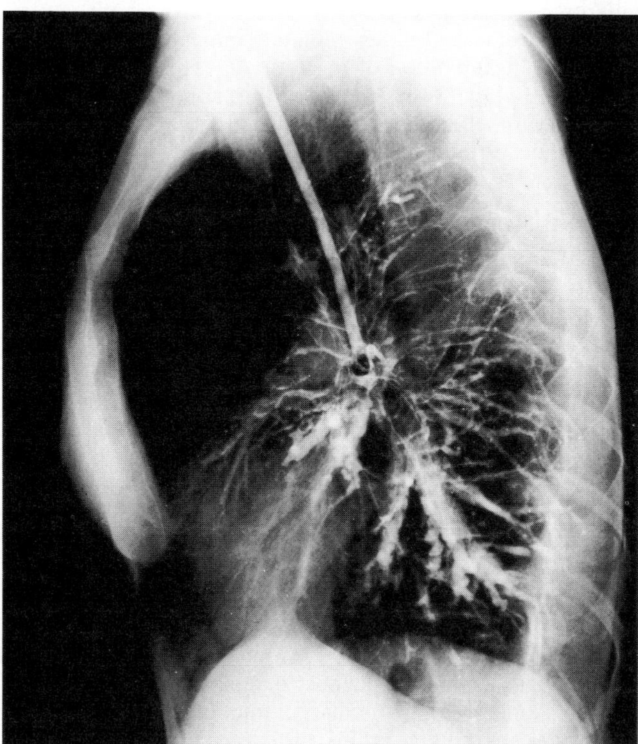

B.

FIG. 131-9 *A* and *B*. Bronchography of the right lung from the same patient as in Fig. 131-7. Large bronchiectasis is seen in the lower lobe and in the right-sided lingula segment of the upper lobe.

attributable to resectional surgery for bronchiectasis or to generally stiff lungs.[112,143] When obstruction occurs, it is usually of moderate degree and does not seem to progress much over the years.[55,57,112,136,144] In spite of this, there may be a tendency to slight arterial desaturation.[55] At times, there may be severe airflow obstruction with effort dyspnea by the third decade, and it seems that smokers are at a particular risk.[136] Usually there is little reversibility of airflow obstruction, although significant bronchospasm is occasionally present.[88,112,136,143] In a series of 35 adult persons with the syndrome (age range, 19 to 65 years), forced expiratory volume in 1 s (FEV_1) averaged 67±21 percent (mean ±SD) of predicted normal value (range, 24 to 112 percent), with no correlation to age. Corresponding values for vital capacity were 79±14 percent (range, 47 to 116 percent).[144]

When significant airways obstruction is present, it is usually expressed as effort dyspnea; asthmatic attacks are not a prominent feature.[136,144] On lung auscultation crackles are usually heard, wheezing to a lesser extent. On chest radiography a moderate degree of hyperinflation is often observable, in children as well as in adults.[57,145]

Sensory Organs

For otologic aspects of the immotile-cilia syndrome, see the discussion above. The sense of balance seems not to be affected in the majority of cases,[4] although about 10 percent of patients claim that they have a less than a good sense of balance. Most subjects with inborn ciliary immotility are anosmic or have a decreased sense of smell.[5,138]

Examination of the eyes of 10 patients with the syndrome showed corneal abnormalities in 9 but no other consistent abnormalities.[146] These abnormalities may be secondary to a developmental disturbance. It may be remembered that the corneal endothelium is a monociliated epithelium. Some patients have been described who suffer from both Kartagener syndrome and either retinitis pigmentosa[60,147–151] or a pigmented degeneration of the retina.[148] This is interesting because Fox et al.[152] have claimed that abnormalities in the ultrastructure of human nasal cilia are found in persons suffering from retinitis pigmentosa.

Central Nervous System

Some patients suffer from dull headaches, endogeneous depression,[5] or schizophrenia.[153] In the Swedish case reports two thirds of the patients complained of chronic headaches, and many had sought medical advice for this complaint. The headaches persisted even during periods free of sinusitis or other infections. Schizophrenia was not seen to be more common than in the general population.

It is likely that patients with the immotile-cilia syndrome run a higher-than-normal risk of neonatal hydrocephalus. Occasionally, patients with the immotile-cilia syndrome have had hydrocephalus.[60,77,147,154] Hydrocephalus developed in one baby at the age of 2 weeks due to exit foramina obstruction, but was treated by a ventricular atrial shunt followed by a ventricular peritoneal shunt; the child grew up with normal intelligence.[155] It may be that ependymal cilia normally keep the aqueduct patent and that the risk of stenosis is increased with ciliary immotility.

In one study, the brains of seven persons with the immotile-cilia syndrome have been examined by means of CT, and a slight enlargement of the ventricular system and the sulci was found in two cases.[5] In another seven persons, no changes were noted.[156] The brain does not seem to be mirrored in persons with Kartagener syndrome; only 3 of 36 patients (8 percent) were left-handed.[5]

Reproductive Organs

It has already been remarked that nearly all men with the immotile-cilia syndrome are sterile because of immotility or poor motility of their spermatozoa, but that some men have motile spermatozoa and are fertile. In typical cases, the volume of the ejaculate and the values for sperm number are within the normal range. Similarly, sperm morphology evaluated by light microscopy is normal. The question arises: Will the spermatozoa be capable of fertilization in an in vitro fertilization test? The answer seems to be negative, although immotile human spermatozoa are capable of entering zonaless hamster eggs.[157] The zona pellucida of a human egg seems, however, to form a barrier to the immotile spermatozoa.[158] An immotile spermatozoon can be injected into the egg. Some patients have hydrocele,[159] oligospermia,[66,104] or azoospermia.[160,161] In one patient, the amount of carboxylmethylase has been measured in spermatozoa and found to be decreased.[162] This enzyme plays a role in chemotactic responses in bacteria and may also be involved in animal-cell motility.

Women with the immotile-cilia syndrome may or may not be fertile.[144,163–165] In a Swedish series, 9 of 19 women had been unsuccessful in their attempts to become pregnant, 5 had conceived, and 4 had not attempted to become pregnant.[144] In a British study, four of seven women were infertile.[58] The fertility of a woman with immotile cilia in the oviduct has been demonstrated by Bleau et al.,[164] whereas in another case, a woman who had never conceived had oviductal cilia that were completely immotile.[166] It has been suggested that femal fertility varies in the different subgroups of the immotile-cilia syndrome,[166] but evidence for this hypothesis has not yet been provided. A priori it would seem likely that women with the immotile-cilia syndrome experience a greater than normal risk of ectopic pregnancies, but no evidence of this has been found.[5,6,164,167] No increased risk of salpingitis been found so far.

Cardiovascular System

As mentioned above, half the persons with the immotile-cilia syndrome have situs inversus and may be classified as having Kartagener syndrome. Most of these patients have a complete transposition of the thoracic and abdominal viscera that form a mirror image of the normal condition. Usually no other congenital malformations of the heart or other organs are apparent in Kartagener syndrome, as is common in cases of isolated dextrocardia.[168,169] Occasional malformations of the heart have been recorded in Kartagener syndrome, as well as cases of incomplete situs inversus.[6,73]

Leukocytes

The capacity of the leukocytes to orient and to migrate in a chemotactic gradient has been examined in an attempt to find out whether defects in cell motility are restricted to spermatozoa and ciliated cells or have a more general occurrence. It has then been reported that the chemotactic migration indeed is significantly reduced in some, but not all, persons investigated, and also, that the capacity to orient is hampered.[170–173] Whether the decreased chemotactic migration is a primary phenomenon or a consequence of the chronic infections is at present unknown. Most persons with the immotile-cilia syndrome do not appear to have an increased incidence of infections at sites outside the airways, although one such case has been reported.[174]

Developmental Anomalies

An extensive list of malformations and diseases that have been observed in patients suffering from Kartagener syndrome is found in Rott.[6] It is likely that the simultaneous occurrence of a certain disease and the syndrome in most cases is purely coincidental. In some instances a disease or an anomaly may be a direct or indirect consequence of the ciliary malfunction. If so, one might expect to find the anomaly in several patients and a similar defect in the animal models. Some of the congenital cardiac malformations may belong to this category. So may polydactyly, which has been noted in some patients[175,176] and which also is characteristic of hpy/hpy mice, a strain in which cilia are abnormal.[31]

TREATMENT AND PROGNOSIS

Treatment is symptomatic and directed against complications in the upper and lower respiratory tract. There is no method available to restore ciliary and spermatozoal motility *in situ*. Antibiotics or chemotherapeutic agents may be given when there are signs of bacterial infections such as increased purulence of sputum or bouts of sinusitis or otitis. The value of mucolytics is uncertain, but they may be tried in selected cases with tenacious secretions. Bronchodilators (β-adrenergics, methylxanthines, or anticholinergics) may be valuable in cases in which there is airway obstruction with a bronchospastic component.

Physiotherapy with postural drainage is often important and, if started early in life, might possibly prevent or delay the evolution of bronchiectasis and atelectasis. Abandonment of smoking is a most important preventive measure, since smoking probably accelerates deterioration of lung function.

Surgical interventions against maxillary sinusitis, nasal polyposis, and middle ear disease are often repeatedly performed in these patients (e.g., endonasal trepanation, Caldwell-Luc operation, polypectomy, tympanostomy). Such operations may doubtless be necessary in certain cases, but a certain amount of conservatism has been advocated in this context, as there often is a spontaneous remission in adulthood.[17,138]

Thoracic surgical intervention against bronchiectasis is sometimes indicated, although the choice may be difficult in individual cases. In a series of 35 adult patients, bronchiectasis had been demonstrated by bronchography in 22 cases, of whom 16 had undergone operation; half of these improved with surgery.[144] The symptoms of chronic bronchitis are not to be expected to be cured by resectional surgery. A heart–lung transplantation has been performed in one patient suffering from the complete Kartagener syndrome.[177]

Without access to antibiotics the average life span may be somewhat reduced owing to severe respiratory tract infections particularly in childhood and adolescence. The rather frequent occurrence of chronic obstructive pulmonary disease with the risk of development of respiratory insufficiency probably also tends to reduce life span somewhat, although airways obstruction might not be very progressive in most cases. Whether there is an increased risk of lung cancer in the syndrome is not known.

Most persons with the syndrome seem to live an active life.[136] General physical and mental development is usually not retarded by the chronic disease. Situs inversus is usually not combined with congenital malformations. Kartagener syndrome has been described in old age.[178] With modern medical care and abstinence from smoking the prognosis may therefore be encouraging or even excellent.

REFERENCES

1. Kartagener M: Zur Pathogenese der Bronchiektasien: Bronchiektasien bei Situs viscerum inversus. *Beitr Klin Tuberk* **83**:489, 1933.
2. Siewert AK: Ueber einen Fall von Bronchiektasie bei einem Patienten mit Situs inversus viscerum. *Berl Klin Wochenschr* **41**:139, 1904.
3. Afzelius BA: A human syndrome caused by immotile cilia. *Science* **193**:317, 1976.
4. Eliasson R, Mossberg B, Camner P, Afzelius BA: The immotile-cilia syndrome. A congenital ciliary abnormality as an etiologic factor in chronic airway infections and male sterility. *N Engl J Med* **297**:1, 1977.
5. Afzelius BA: The immotile-cilia syndrome and other ciliary diseases. *Int Rev Exp Pathol* **19**:1, 1979.
6. Rott H-D: Kartagener's syndrome and the syndrome of immotile cilia. *Hum Genet* **46**:249, 1979.
7. Adams R, Churchill ED: Situs inversus, sinusitis and bronchiectasis. *J Thorac Surg* **7**:206, 1937.
8. Svartengren M, Floderus-Myrhed B, Mossberg B, Camner P: Defekta försvarsmekanismer i lungorna. *Hjarta Karl Lungor (Stockh)* **3**:81, 1983.
9. Falser N: Anomalies of kinocilia in Kartagener's syndrome. *Laryngol Rhinol Otol* **62**:128, 1983.
10. Gibney RTN, Herbert FA: Kartagener's syndrome. *Ir Med J* **73**:87, 1980.
11. Monnet P: Situs inversus and bronchopulmonary disease in the neonatal period. *Arch Fr Pediatr* **35**:607, 1978.
12. Weinaug P: Ein Fall von Kartagener-Syndrom bei Geschwistern. *Z Erkr Atmungsorgane* **134**:454, 1971.
13. Rott H-D, Warnatz H, Pasch-Hilgers R, Weikl A: Kartagener's syndrome in sibs. Clinical and immunological investigations. *Hum Genet* **43**:1, 1978.
14. Knox G, Murray S, Strang L: A family with Kartagener's syndrome: Linkage data. *Ann Hum Genet* **24**:137, 1960.
15. Guggenheim F: Kartagener's syndrome in an Arab family. *Isr J Med Sci* **7**:1079, 1971.
16. Katsuhara K, Kawamoto S, Wakabayashi T, Belsky JL: Situs inversus totalis and Kartagener's syndrome in a Japanese population. *Chest* **61**:56, 1972.
17. Ernstson S, Afzelius BA, Mossberg B: Otological manifestations of the immotile-cilia syndrome. *Acta Otolaryngol (Stockh)* **97**:83, 1984.
18. Kartagener M, Horlacher A: Zur Pathogenese der Bronchiektasien, Situs viscerum inversus and Polyposis nasi in einem Falle familiarer Bronchiektisien. *Beitr Klin Tuberk* **87**:331, 1935.
19. Perone PM: Situs viscerum inversus, bronchiettasie e sinusiti: Tre casi di sindrome di Kartagener. *Arch Ital Otolaryngol* **67**:653, 1956.
20. Overholt EL, Banman DF: Variants of Kartagener's syndrome in the same family. *Ann Intern Med* **48**:547, 1958.
21. Logan WD, Abbott OA, Hatcher CR: Kartagener's triad. *Dis Chest* **48**:613, 1965.
22. Wakefield SJ, Waite D: Abnormal cilia in Polynesians with bronchectasis. *Am Rev Respir Dis* **121**:1003, 1980.
23. Waite DA, Wakefield SJ, Moriarty KM, Lewis ME, Cuttance PC, Scott AG: Polynesian bronchectasis. *Eur J Respir Dis (Suppl 127)* **64**:31, 1983.
24. Afzelius BA, Carlsten J, Karlsson S: Clinical, pathologic, and ultrastructural features of situs inversus and immotile-cilia syndrome in a dog. *J Am Vet Med Assoc* **184**:560, 1984.
25. Randolph JF, Castleman WL: Immotile cilia syndrome in 2 old-English sheepdog littermates. *J Small Anim Pract* **25**:679, 1984.

26. Dhein CR, Prieur DJ, Riggs MW, Potter KA, Widders PR: Suspected ciliary dysfunction in Chinese shar pei pups with pneumonia. *Am J Vet Res* **50**:439, 1990.
27. Edwards DF, Kennedy JR, Patton CS, Toal RL, Daniel GB, Lothrop CD: Familial immotile-cilia syndrome in English springer spaniel dogs. *Am J Med Genet* **33**:290, 1989.
28. Wilsman NJ, Morrison WB, Farnum CE, Fox LE: Microtubular protofilaments and subunits of the outer dynein arm in cilia from dogs with primary ciliary dyskinesia. *Am Rev Respir Dis* **135**:137, 1987.
29. Roperto F, Galati P, Troncone A, Rossacco P, Campofreda M: Primary ciliary dyskinesia in pigs. *J Submicrosc Cytol* **23**:233, 1991.
30. Torikata C, Kijimoto C, Koto M: Ultrastructure of respiratory cilia of WIC-Hyd male rats. An animal model for human immotile cilia syndrome. *Am J Pathol* **138**:341, 1991.
31. Bryan JHD: Abnormal cilia in male-sterile mutant mice. *Virchows Arch [A]* **400**:77, 1983.
32. Layton WM: Random determination of a developmental process. *J Hered* **67**:336, 1976.
33. Luck DJL, Huang B, Piperno G: Genetic and biochemical analysis of the eukaryotic flagellum. *Soc Exp Biol Symp* **35**:399, 1982.
34. Jarvik JW, Chojnacki B: Flagellar morphology in stumpy-flagella mutants of Chlamydomonas reinhardtii. *J Protozool* **32**:649, 1985.
35. Kamiya R, Okamoto M: A mutant of Chlamydomonas reinhardtii that lack the flagellar outer dynein arm but can swim. *J Cell Sci* **74**:181, 1985.
36. Barsel S-E, Wexler DE, Lefebre PA: Genetic analysis of long-flagella mutants of Chlamydomonas rheinhardtii. *Genetics* **118**:637, 1988.
37. Dutcher SK, Lux FG: Genetic interactions of mutations affecting flagella and basal bodies in Chlamydomonas. *Cell Motil Cytoskeleton* **14**:104, 1989.
38. Afzelius BA: Genetic disorders of cilia, in Schweiger HC (ed): *International Cell Biology 1980–1981*. Berlin, Springer-Verlag, 1981, p 440.
39. Weaver A, Hard R: Isolation of newt lung ciliated cell models. *Cell Motil* **5**:355, 1985.
40. Sleigh M, Blake JR, Liron N: The propulsion of mucus by cilia. *Am Rev Respir Dis* **137**:726, 1988.
41. Satir P: Dynein as a microtubule translocator in ciliary motility. *Cell Motil Cytoskeleton* **10**:263, 1988.
42. Sturgess J: Mucous secretion in the respiratory tract. *Pediatr Clin North Am* **26**:481, 1979.
43. Warner FD, Satir P, Gibbons IR (eds): *Cell Movement, The Dynein ATPases*. New York, Alan R. Liss, 1989, vol 1.
44. Goodenough UW, Heuser JE: Outer and inner dynein arms of cilia and flagella. *Cell* **41**:341, 1985.
45. Fujita H: Fine structure of the thyroid gland. *Int Rev Cytol* **40**:197, 1975.
46. Svedbergh B, Bill A: Scanning electron microscopic studies of the corneal epithelium in man and monkeys. *Acta Ophthalmol (Copenh)* **50**:321, 1972.
47. Odor DL, Blandau RJ: Observations on the solitary cilium of rabbit oviductal epithelium. Its motility and ultrastructure. *Am J Anat* **174**:437, 1985.
48. Grimfeld JA, Tournier G, Jouannet P, Bisson JP, Salomon JL, Baculard A, Gerbeaux J: Immotile cilia syndrome in infants and children. *Thorax* **34**:709, 1979.
49. Jahrsdoerfer R, Feldman PS, Rubel EW, Guerrant JL, Eggleston PA, Selden RF: Otitis media and the immotile cilia syndrome. *Laryngoscope* **89**:769, 1979.
50. Afzelius BA, Eliasson R: Flagellar mutants in man: On the heterogeneity of the immotile-cilia syndrome. *J Ultrastruct Res* **69**:43, 1979.
51. Sturgess JM, Chao J, Turner JAP: Cilia with defective radial spokes. A cause of human respiratory disease. *N Engl J Med* **300**:53, 1979.
52. Sturgess JM, Chao J, Turner JAP: Transposition of ciliary microtubules. Another cause of impaired ciliary motility. *N Engl J Med* **303**:318, 1980.
53. Schneeberger EE, McCormack J, Issenberg H, Schuster SR, Gerald PS: Heterogeneity of ciliary morphology in the immotile-cilia syndrome in man. *J Ultrastruct Res* **73**:34, 1980.
54. Pedersen H, Rebbe H: Absence of arms in the axoneme of immobile human spermatozoa. *Biol Reprod* **12**:541, 1975.
55. Corkey CWB, Levison H, Turner JAP: The immotile cilia syndrome—A longitudinal survey. *Am Rev Respir Dis* **124**:544, 1981.
56. Escalier D, Jouannet P, David G: Abnormalities of the ciliary axonemal complex in children. *Biol Cell* **44**:271, 1982.
57. Levison H, Mindorff CM, Chiao J, Turner JAP, Sturgess JM, Stringer DA: Pathophysiology of the ciliary motility syndromes. *Eur J Respir Dis (suppl 127)* **64**:102, 1983.
58. Greenstone M, Dewar A, Mackay I, Cole PJ: Primary ciliary dyskinesia—cytological and clinical features. *Q J Med* **67**:40, 1988.
59. Van Der Baan S, Veerman AJP, Bezemer PD, Feenstra L: Primary ciliary dyskinesia. *Ann Otol Rhinol Laryngol* **96**:264, 1987.
60. Barlocco EG, Valletta EA, Canciano M, Lungarella G, Gardi C, de Santi MM, Mastella G: Ultrastructural ciliary defects in children with recurrent infections of the lower respiratory tract. *Pediatr Pulmonol* **10**:17, 1991.
61. Wilton LJ, Teichtahl H, Temple-Smith PD, De Kretser DM: Kartagener's syndrome with motile cilia and immotile spermatozoa. *Am Rev Respir Dis* **134**:1233, 1986.
62. Corbeel L, Cornille F, Lauweryns J, Boel M, Van Den Berghe G: Ultrastructural abnormalities of bronchial cilia in children with recurrent airway infections and bronchiectasis. *Arch Dis Child* **56**:929, 1981.
63. David G, Serres C, Escalier D: Cinématique du spermatozoide humain. *Ann Endocrinol (Paris)* **42**:391, 1982.
64. Woodring JH, Royer JM, McDonagh D: Kartagener's syndrome. *JAMA* **247**:2814, 1982.
65. Nielsen MH, Pedersen M, Christensen B, Mygind N: Blind quantitative electron microscopy of cilia from patients with primary ciliary dyskinesia and from normal subjects. *Eur J Respir Dis (suppl 127)* **64**:19, 1983.
66. Escalier D, David G: Pathology of the cytoskeleton of the human sperm flagellum. *Biol Cell* **50**:37, 1984.
67. Chabrolle JP, Euziere P, Bigel P, Blondet P: Syndrome d'immotilité ciliaire chez un enfant de 10 ans. *Arch Fr Pediatr* **39**:235, 1982.
68. Sturgess JM, Thompson MW, Czegledy-Nagy E, Turner JAP: Genetic aspects of immotile cilia syndrome. *Am J Med Genet* **25**:149, 1986.
69. Neustein HB, Nickerson B, O'Neil M: Kartagener's syndrome with absence of inner dynein arms of respiratory cilia. *Am Rev Respir Dis* **122**:979, 1980.
70. Salomon JL, Grimfeld A, Tournier G, Baculard A, Escalier D, Jouannet P, David G: Ciliary disorders of the bronchi in children. *Rev Fr Malad Respir* **11**:645, 1983.
71. Herzon FS, Murphy S: Normal ciliary ultrastructure in children with Kartagener's syndrome. *Ann Otol Rhinol Laryngol* **89**:81, 1980.
72. Greenstone MA, Dewar A, Cole PJ: Ciliary dyskinesia with normal ultrastructure. *Thorax* **38**:875, 1983.
73. Pedersen M, Stafanger G: Bronchopulmonary symptoms in primary ciliary dyskinesia. *Eur J Respir Dis (suppl 127)* **64**:118, 1983.
74. Afzelius BA, Gargani G, Romano C: Abnormal length of cilia as a cause of defective mucociliary clearance. *Eur J Respir Dis* **66**:173, 1985.
75. Dudley JP, Waelch MJ, Carney JM, Stiehm ER, Soderber M: Scanning and transmission electron microscopic aspects of the nasal acilia syndrome. *Laryngoscope* **92**:297, 1982.
76. de Santi MM, Gardi C, Barlocco G, Canciani M, Mastella G, Lungarella G: Cilia-lacking respiratory cells in ciliary aplasia *Biol Cell* **64**:67, 1988.
77. de Santi MM, Magni A, Valletta EA, Gardi C, Lungarella G: Hydrocephalus, bronchiectasis, and ciliary aplasia. *Arch Dis Child* **65**:543, 1990.
78. Fonzi L, Lungarella G, Palatresi R: Lack of kinocilia in the nasal mucosa. *Eur J Respir Dis* **63**:558, 1982.
79. Götz M, Stockinger L: Aplasia of respiratory tract cilia. *Lancet* **1**:1283, 1983.
80. Gordon RE, Kattan M: Absence of cilia and basal bodies with predominance of brush cells in the respiratory mucosa from a patient with immotile cilia syndrome. *Ultrastruct Pathol* **6**:45, 1984.

81. Cereso L, Price G: Absence of cilia and basal bodies with predominance of brush cells in the respiratory mucosa from a patient with immotile cilia syndrome. *Ultrastruct Pathol* **8**:381, 1985.
82. Mygind NG, Pedersen M, Toremalm NG: Lazy cilia make the otologist busy. *Clin Otolaryngol* **8**:148, 1983.
83. Holley MC, Afzelius BA: Alignment of cilia in immotile-cilia syndrome. *Tissue Cell* **18**:521, 1986.
84. de Iongh R, Rutland J: Orientation of respiratory tract cilia in patients with primary ciliary dyskinesia, bronchiectasis, and in normal subjects. *J Clin Pathol* **42**:613, 1989.
85. Rautiainen M, Collan Y, Nuutinen J, Afzelius BA: Ciliary orientation in the immotile cilia syndrome. *Eur Arch Otorhinolaryngol* **247**:100, 1990.
86. Rutland J, de Iongh RU: Random ciliary orientation. *N Engl J Med* **323**:1681, 1990.
87. Camner P, Afzelius BA, Eliasson R, Mossberg B: Relation between abnormalities of human sperm flagella and respiratory tract disease. *Int J Androl* **2**:211, 1979.
88. Turner JAP, Corkey CWB, Lee JYC, Levison H, Sturgess JM: Clinical expression of immotile cilia syndrome. *Pediatrics* **67**:805, 1981.
89. Fox B, Bull TB, Makey AR, Rawbone R: The significance of ultrastructural abnormalities of human cilia. *Chest (suppl)* **80**:796, 1981.
90. Hilding AC: The relation of ciliary insufficiency to death from asthma and other respiratory diseases. *Ann Otol Rhinol Laryngol* **52**:5, 1943.
91. Camner P, Jarstrand C, Philipson K: Tracheobronchial clearance in patients with influenza. *Am Rev Respir Dis* **108**:131, 1973.
92. Pedersen M, Sakakura Y, Winther B, Brofeldt S, Mygind N: Nasal mucociliary transport, number of ciliated cells, and beating pattern in naturally acquired colds. *Eur J Respir Dis (suppl 128)* **64**:355, 1983.
93. Pedersen M: Specific types of abnormal ciliary motility in Kartagener's syndrome and analogous respiratory disorders. *Eur J Respir Dis (suppl 127)* **64**:78, 1983.
94. Lungarella G, Fonzi L, Burrini AG: Ultrastructural abnormalities in respiratory cilia and sperm tails in a patient with Kartagener's syndrome. *Ultrastruct Pathol* **3**:319, 1982.
95. Escudier E, Escalier D, Pinchon MC, Boucherat M, Bernaudin JF, Fleuryfeith J: Dissimilar expression of axonemal anomalies in respiratory cilia and sperm flagella in infertile men. *Am Rev Respir Dis* **142**:674, 1990.
96. Walt H, Campana A, Balerna M, Domenighetti G, Hedinger C, Jakob M, Pescia G, Sulmoni A: Mosaicism of dynein in spermatozoa and cilia and fibrous sheath aberrations in an infertile man. *Andrologia* **15**:295, 1983.
97. Jonsson MS, McCormick JR, Gillies CG, Gondos B: Kartagener's syndrome with motile spermatozoa. *N Engl J Med* **307**:1131, 1982.
98. Afzelius BA: Immotile-cilia syndrome and ciliary abnormalities induced by infection and injury. *Am Rev Respir Dis* **124**:107, 1981.
99. Cornille FJ, Lauweryns JM, Corbeel L: Atypical bronchial cilia in children with recurrent respiratory tract infections. *Pathol Res Pract* **178**:595, 1984.
100. Konradova V, Hlouskova Z, Tomanek A: Atypical kinocilia in human epithelium from large bronchus. *Folia Morphol (Praha)* **23**:293, 1975.
101. Takasaka T, Sato M, Onodera A: Atypical cilia in the human mucosa. *Ann Otol Rhinol Laryngol* **89**:37, 1980.
102. Veerman AJP, van Delden L, Feenstra L, Leene W: The immotile cilia syndrome—Phase contrast light microscopy, scanning and transmission electron microscopy. *Pediatrics* **65**:698, 1980.
103. Rutland J, Cole PJ: Non-invasive sampling of nasal cilia for measurement of beat frequency and study of ultrastructure. *Lancet* **2**:564, 1980.
104. Rossman CM, Forrest JB, Lee RMKW, Newhouse MT: The dyskinetic cilia syndrome—Ciliary motility in immotile cilia syndrome. *Chest* **78**:580, 1980.
105. Pedersen M, Mygind N: Ciliary motility in the immotile cilia syndrome. *Br J Dis Chest* **74**:239, 1980.
106. Sturgess JM, Turner JAP: Ultrastructural pathology of cilia in the immotile cilia syndrome. *Perspect Pediatr Pathol* **8**:133, 1984.
107. Rossman CM, Forrest JB, Lee RMKW, Newhouse AF, Newhouse MT: The dyskinetic cilia syndrome. *Chest* **80**:860, 1981.
108. Rossman CM, Lee RMKW, Forrest JB, Newhouse MT: Nasal ciliary ultrastructure and function in patients with primary ciliary dyskinesia compared with that in normal subjects and in subjects with various respiratory diseases. *Am Rev Respir Dis* **129**:161, 1984.
109. Camner P, Mossberg B, Afzelius BA: Evidence for congenitally non-functioning cilia in the tracheobronchial tract in two subjects. *Am Rev Respir Dis* **112**:807, 1975.
110. Palmblad J, Mossberg B, Afzelius BA: Ultrastructural, cellular, and clinical features of the immotile-cilia syndrome. *Annu Rev Med* **35**:481, 1984.
111. Nuutinen J, Kärjä J, Karjalainen P: Measurements of impaired mucociliary activity in children. *Eur J Respir Dis* **64**:454, 1983.
112. Mossberg B, Afzelius BA, Eliasson R, Camner P: On the pathogenesis of obstructive lung disease: A study in the immotile-cilia syndrome. *Scand J Respir Dis* **59**:55, 1978.
113. Boat TF, Wood RE, Tandler B, Stern RC, Orenstein DM, Doershuk CF: A screening test for the immotile cilia syndrome. *Pediatr Res* **13**:531, 1979.
114. Pedersen M, Nielsen MH, Mygind N: Primary ciliary dyskinesia. *Mod Probl Paediatr* **21**:68, 1982.
115. Van Der Baan S, Veerman AJP, Wulffraat N, Bezemer PD, Feenstra L: Primary ciliary dyskinesia. *Acta Otolaryngol (Stockh)* **102**:274, 1986.
116. Layton WM: Heart malformation in mice homozygous for a gene causing situs inversus, in *Normal Morphogenesis of the Heart. Birth Defects* Orig Art Series. Washington, DC, National Foundation, 1978, vol 14, p 277.
117. Hanzlik AJ, Binder M, Layton WM, Rowe L, Layton M, Taylor BA, Osemlak MM, Richards JE, Kurnit DM, Stewart GD: The murine situs inversus viscerum (iv) gene responsible for visceral asymmetry is linked tightly to the Igh-C cluster on chromosome 12. *Genomics* **7**:389, 1990.
118. Brown NA, McCarthy A, Wolpert L: Development of handed body asymmetry in mammals. *Ciba Found Symp* **162**:182, 1991.
119. Van Keuren ML, Layton WM, Iacob RA, Kurnit DM: Situs inversus in the developing mouse. *Mol Reprod Dev* **29**:136, 1991.
120. Eavey RD, Nadol JB, Holmes LB, Laird NM, Lapey A, Joseph MP, Strome M: Kartagener's syndrome. A blinded, controlled study of cilia ultrastructure. *Arch Otolaryngol Head Neck Surg* **112**:646, 1986.
121. Antonelli M, Modesti A, Quattrini A, De Angelis M: Supernumerary microtubules in the respiratory cilia of two sibs. *Eur J Respir Dis* **64**:607, 1983.
122. Moreno A, Murphy EA: Inheritance of Kartagener syndrome. *Am J Med Genet* **8**:305, 1981.
123. Heuckenkamp PU, Marshall M, Meier J, Parrisius G, Zollner N: Das Kartagener-syndrom. *Dtsch Med Wochenschr* **97**:1458, 1972.
124. Torgersen J: Genic factors in visceral asymmetry and in the development and pathologic changes of lungs, heart and abdominal organs. *Arch Pathol* **47**:566, 1949.
125. Camner P, Mossberg B, Afzelius BA: Measurements of tracheobronchial clearance in patients with immotile-cilia syndrome and its value in differential diagnosis. *Eur J Respir Dis (suppl 127)* **64**:57, 1983.
126. Andersen I, Proctor DF: Measurement of nasal mucociliary clearance. *Eur J Respir Dis (suppl 127)* **64**:37, 1983.
127. Stanley P, McWilliam L, Greenstone M, Mackay I, Cole PJ: Efficacy of a saccharin test for screening to detect abnormal mucociliary clearance. *Br J Dis Chest* **78**:62, 1984.
128. Canciani M, Barlocco EG, Mastella G, de Santi MM, Gardi C, Lungarella G: The saccharin method for testing mucociliary function in patients suspected of having primary ciliary dyskinesia. *Pediatr Pulmonol* **5**:210, 1988.
129. Burgersdijk FJA, De Groot JCMJ, Graamans K, Rademakers LHPM: Testing ciliary activity in patients with chronic and recurrent infections of the upper airways. *Laryngoscope* **96**:1029, 1986.
130. Nielsen MH, Pedersen M, Christensen B, Mygind N: Blind quantitative electron microscopy of cilia from patients

with primary ciliary dyskinesia and from normal subjects. *Eur J Respir Dis (suppl 127)* **64:**19, 1983.
131. Greenstone M, Rutman A, Pavia D, Lawrence D, Cole PJ: Normal axonemal ultrastructure and function in Kartagener's syndrome: An explicable paradox. *Thorax* **40:**956, 1985.
132. Kollberg H, Mossberg B, Afzelius BA, Philipson K, Camner P: Cystic fibrosis compared with the immotile cilia syndrome. A study of mucociliary clearance, ciliary ultrastructure, clinical picture and ventilatory function. *Scand J Respir Dis* **59:**297, 1978.
133. Mossberg B, Björkander J, Afzelius BA, Camner P: Mucociliary clearance in patients with immunoglobulin deficiency. *Eur J Respir Dis* **63:**570, 1982.
134. Neville E, Brewis R, Yeates WK, Burridge A: Respiratory tract disease and obstructive azoospermia. *Thorax* **38:**929, 1983.
135. Handelsman DJ, Conway AJ, Boylan LM, Turtle JR: Young's syndrome. Obstructive azoospermia and chronic sinopulmonary infections. *N Engl J Med* **310:**3, 1984.
136. Mossberg B, Camner P, Afzelius BA: The immotile-cilia syndrome compared to other obstructive lung diseases: A clue to their pathogenesis. *Eur J Respir Dis (suppl 127)* **64:**129, 1983.
137. Whitelaw A, Evans A, Corrin B: Immotile cilia syndrome: A new cause of neonatal respiratory distress. *Arch Dis Child* **56:**432, 1981.
138. Mygind N, Pedersen M: Nose-, sinus-, and ear-symptoms in 27 patients with primary ciliary dyskinesia. *Eur J Respir Dis (suppl 127)* **64:**96, 1983.
139. Van Der Baan S: Primary ciliary dyskinesia and the middle ear. Laryngoscope **101:**751, 1991.
140. Pedersen M, Mygind N: Rhinitis, sinusitis and otitis media in Kartagener's syndrome. *Clin Otolaryngol* **7:**373, 1983.
141. Kartagener M, Stucki P: Bronchiectasis with situs inversus. *Arch Pediatr* **79:**193, 1962.
142. Mossberg B, Hanngren Å: Kartagener's syndrome—A ciliary immotility syndrome. *Mt Sinai J Med* **44:**837, 1977.
143. Evander E, Arborelius M, Jonson B, Simonsson BG, Svensson G: Lung function and bronchial reactivity in six patients with immotile cilia syndrome. *Eur J Respir Dis (suppl 127)* **64:**137, 1983.
144. Mossberg B, Afzelius BA, Camner P: Mucociliary clearance in obstructive lung diseases. Correlations to the immotile-cilia syndrome. *Eur J Respir Dis (suppl 146)* **69:**295, 1986.
145. Nadel HR, Stringer DA, Levison H, Turner JAP, Sturgess J: The immotile cilia syndrome: Radiological manifestations. *Radiology* **154:**651, 1985.
146. Svedbergh B, Johnsson V, Afzelius BA: Immotile-cilia syndrome and the cilia of the eye. *Graefes Arch Klin Exp Ophthalmol* **215:**265, 1981.
147. Bonneau D, Raymond F, Kremer C, Klossek JM, Kaplan J, Patte F: Usher syndrome type-1 associated with bronchiectasis and immotile nasal cilia in two brothers. *J Med Genet* **30:**253, 1993.
148. Segal P, Kikiela M, Mrzyglod B, Zeromska-Zbierska I: Kartagener's syndrome with familial eye changes. *Am J Ophthalmol* **55:**1043, 1963.
149. Hunter DG, Fishman GA, Kretzer FL: Abnormal axonemes in X-linked retinitis pigmentosa. *Arch Ophthalmol* **106:**362, 1988.
150. Ohga H, Suzuki T, Fujiwara H, Furutani A, Koga H: A case of immotile cilia syndrome accompanied by retinitis pigmentosa. *Acta Soc Ophthalmol Jpn* **89:**795, 1991.
151. Van Dorp DB, Wright AF, Carothers AD, Bleeker-Wagemakers EM: A family with RP3 type of X-linked retinitis pigmentosa. An association with ciliary abnormalities. *Hum Genet* **88:**331, 1992.
152. Fox B, Bull TB, Arden GB: Variations in the ultrastructure of human nasal cilia including abnormalities found in retinitis pigmentosa. *J Clin Pathol* **33:**327, 1980.
153. Glick ID, Graubert DN: Kartagener's syndrome and schizophrenia: A report of a case with chromosomal studies. *Am J Psychol* **121:**603, 1964.
154. Bergstrom WH, Cook CD, Scannell JG, Berenberg W: Situs inversus, bronchiectasis and sinusitis. *Pediatrics* **6:**573, 1950.
155. Greenstone MA, Jones RWA, Dewar A, Neville BGR: Hydrocephalus and primary ciliary dyskinesia. *Arch Dis Child* **59:**481, 1984.
156. Roth Y, Baum GL, Tadmor R: Brain dysfunction in primary ciliary dyskinesia? *Acta Neurol Scand* **78:**353, 1988.
157. Williamson RA, Koehler JK, Smith WD, Karp LE: Entry of immotile spermatozoa into zona-free hamster ova. *Gamete Res* **10:**319, 1984.
158. Aitken RJ, Ross A, Lees MM: Analysis of sperm function in Kartagener's syndrome. *Fertil Steril* **40:**696, 1983.
159. Pellnitz D, Heyland S: Beitrag zur Kartagenerschen Trias (Situs inversus, Bronchiektasis und Nasenpolypen). *HNO* **3:**41, 1952.
160. Bashi S, Khan MA, Guirjis A, Joharjy IA, Abid MA: Immotile-cilia syndrome with azoospermia—A case report and review of the literature. *Br J Dis Chest* **82:**194, 1988.
161. Matwijiw I, Thliveris JA, Faiman C: Aplasia of nasal cilia with situs inversus, azoospermia and normal sperm flagella: A unique variant of the immotile cilia syndrome. *J Urol* **137:**522, 1987.
162. Gagnon C, Sherins RJ, Mann T, Bardin W, Amelar RD, Dubin L: Deficiency of protein carboxyl-methylase in spermatozoa of necrospermia patients, in Steinberger A, Steinberger E (eds): *Testicular Development, Structure, and Functions*. New York, Raven, 1980, p 491.
163. Afzelius BA, Camner P, Mossberg B: On the function of cilia in the female reproductive tract. *Fertil Steril* **29:**72, 1978.
164. Bleau G, Richer C-L, Bousquet D: Absence of dynein arms in cilia of endocervical cells in a fertile woman. *Fertil Steril* **30:**362, 1978.
165. Lurie M, Tur-Kaspa I, Weill S, Katz I, Rabinovici J, Goldenberg S: Ciliary ultrastructure of respiratory and fallopian tube epithelium in a sterile woman with Kartagener's syndrome. *Chest* **95:**578, 1989.
166. McComb P, Langley L, Villalon M, Verdugo P: The oviductal cilia and Kartagener's syndrome. *Fertil Steril* **46:**412, 1986.
167. Mouriquand P: Dyskinésie ciliaire primitive. Une revue générale. Consequences sur la fertilité. Thesis. University of Lyon, 1985.
168. Cockayne EA: The genetics of transposition of the viscera. *Q J Med* **7:**479, 1938.
169. Miller RD, Divertie MB: Kartagener's syndrome. *Chest* **62:**130, 1972.
170. Afzelius BA, Ewetz L, Palmblad J, Uden A-M, Venizelos N: Structure and function of neutrophil leukocytes from patients with the immotile-cilia syndrome. *Acta Med Scand* **208:**145, 1980.
171. Walter RJ, Malech HL, Oliver JM: Cell motility and microtubules in cultured fibroblasts from patients with Kartagener's syndrome. *Cell Motil* **3:**185, 1983.
172. Valerius NH, Knudsen BB, Pedersen M: Defective neutrophil motility in patients with primary ciliary dyskinesia. *Eur J Clin Invest* **13:**489, 1983.
173. Wolburg H, Dopfer R, Schieferstein G, Thiel E: Immotile cilia syndrome: Reduced chemotaxis and reduced number of intramembranous particles in granulocytes. *Klin Wochenschr* **62:**1044, 1984.
174. Brenner S, Tur E, Fishel B, Alkan M, Topilsky M: Cutaneous manifestations and impaired chemotaxis of polymorphonuclear leukocytes associated with Kartagener's syndrome. *Dermatologica* **183:**251, 1991.
175. Conway DJ: A congenital factor in bronchiectasis. *Arch Dis Child* **26:**253, 1951.
176. Sielicka-Zuber L, Ficer J: Zespół Kartagener. *Przegl Dermatol* **61:**171, 1974.
177. Miralles A, Muneretto C, Gandjbakhch I, Lecompte Y, Pavie A, Rabago G, Bracomonte L, Desruennes M, Cabrol A, Cabrol C: Heart-lung transplantation in situs inversus—A case report in a patient with Kartagener's syndrome. *J Thorac Cardiovasc Surg* **103:**307, 1992.
178. Amjad H, Richburg FD, Adler E: Kartagener's syndrome. Case report in an elderly man. *JAMA* **227:**1420, 1974.

CHAPTER 132

Leukocyte Adhesion Deficiency and Other Disorders of Leukocyte Adherence and Motility

Donald C. Anderson ■ Takashi Kei Kishimoto
C. Wayne Smith

1. **Mobility is essential to the function of neutrophils in host defense against bacterial infection, and the fact that neutrophils accumulate at sites of inflammation has been known for over 100 years. Two major determinants account for the ability of neutrophils to localize at sites of injury or infection. Each is necessary, and neither is sufficient. The first is the ability to adhere to endothelial cells with sufficient strength to resist the drag forces of flowing blood, and the second is the ameboid locomotion that allows adherent cells to migrate through the endothelium and perivascular tissues. Both adhesion and locomotion can be evaluated in vitro using a variety of well-characterized assays. Cell locomotion is most clearly seen in response to chemotactic stimulation.**

2. **The adhesive mechanisms that account for leukocyte emigration involve at least three families of glycoproteins—the β_2 (CD18) integrins, CD11a/CD18 (LFA-1) and CD11b/CD18 (Mac-1); one member of the Ig superfamily, intercellular adhesion molecule-1 (ICAM-1); and the selectins (L-selectin, P-selectin and E-selectin), a family of lectins that recognize carbohydrate structures related to sialyl Lewis X. Current evidence indicates that there are at least four distinct adhesive steps in the process by which neutrophils localize at an inflammatory site. (1) The initial margination where neutrophils first roll along the luminal surface of venular endothelium is supported by each member of the selectin family. When endothelial cells are activated by interleukin-1 (IL-1), tumor necrosis factor (TNF), or endotoxin, they acquire the ability to catch previously unstimulated neutrophils flowing by the endothelium at shear rates found in venules. This rolling adhesion depends on L-selectin on the neutrophil and on newly expressed E-selectin on the endothelial cells. When endothelial cells are stimulated with histamine or thrombin, they rapidly mobilize P-selectin to the luminal surface from Weibel-Palade bodies, and thereby acquire the ability to catch flowing neutrophils. (2) Rolling neutrophils often stop on the luminal surface of the endothelium. This stationary adhesion appears to depend on CD18 integrins and ICAM-1 and is potentiated by stimulation of the neutrophil with chemotactic factors. (3) Homotypic aggregation of neutrophils often occurs at the luminal surface of the endothelium. Aggregation requires stimulation of the neutrophil with chemotactic factors and depends on CD11b/CD18 (Mac-1). (4) Transendothelial migration is largely dependent on CD18 integrins, and both CD11a/CD18 (LFA-1) and CD11b/CD18 (Mac-1) are involved. ICAM-1 serves as a ligand for both LFA-1 and Mac-1. The source of chemotactic factors needed to activate the adhesive functions of CD18 integrins and the ameboid locomotion involved in transendothelial migration is currently poorly defined, but recent evidence indicates that endothelial-derived interleukin-8 (IL-8) and platelet activating factor (PAF) are involved.**

3. **Aberrations in adhesive mechanisms or neutrophil motility account for several clinical syndromes that involve a markedly increased susceptibility to bacterial infection. The most thoroughly characterized of these syndromes is leukocyte adhesion deficiency (LAD), an autosomal recessive trait in humans, dogs, and Holstein cattle resulting from heterogeneous mutations in the gene for CD18 (the β subunit of the β_2 integrins). Affected individuals exhibit profound reductions of all three members of the CD18 integrins on the surface of leukocytes and, consequently, profound deficits in the cellular functions requiring CD18 integrins, the most striking being deficient extravasation of neutrophils at sites of infection. The severity of clinical infectious complications among humans with LAD appears to be directly related to the degree of glycoprotein deficiency. Two phenotypes, designated "severe" and "moderate" deficiency, have been defined. Patients with the severe phenotype have no detectable CD18 on their leukocytes**

A list of standard abbreviations is located immediately preceding the index in each volume. Additional abbreviations used in this chapter include: C = complement (e.g., C5a); CD = T cell differentiation antigens (e.g., CD11, CD18, etc.); CHS = Chediak-Higashi syndrome; CR = complement receptor (e.g., CR1, CR3, etc.); Fc = constant immunoglobulin fragment; GM-CSF granulocyte/monocyte-colony stimulating factor; HEV = high-endothelial venule; HUVEC = human umbilical-vein endothelial cell; ICAM = intercellular adhesion molecule, also ICAM-1, ICAM-2, etc.; IFN = interferon, also IFN-γ; LAD = leukocyte adhesion deficiency; LFA-1 = lymphocyte function-associated antigen-1; Mac-1 = macrophage-1; MoMuLV = Moloney murine leukemia virus; NCAM = neural cell adhesion molecule; NK cell = natural killer cell; PAF = platelet activating factor; PMA = phorbol myristate acetate; sLe^x = sialyl Lewis X; TNF = tumor necrosis factor; VCAM = vascular cell adhesion molecule; VLA = very late activation antigen, also VLA-4, etc.

and often succumb to infections before age 2 years. Patients with the moderate phenotype have up to 10 percent of normal levels of CD18 expression and often survive into the second or third decades of life. An array of CD18 mutations has been defined, and patients are often compound heterozygotes, deriving different mutations from the maternal and paternal alleles. The relative success of allogeneic bone marrow transplantation in treating patients with LAD indicates that the hematopoietic stem cell would be an appropriate target for CD18 gene transfer. Preliminary efforts toward somatic cell gene therapy of human LAD have been reported recently.

4. **Reduced adhesion is apparently linked to reduced resistance to bacterial infections in three clinical syndromes in addition to LAD. Development-related inflammatory deficits observed in human and animal neonates appear to involve defects of neutrophil localization or emigration at sites of inflammation. The quantitative and qualitative changes in CD11b/CD18 (Mac-1) necessary for adherence-dependent cell motility are significantly reduced in neonatal neutrophils, and the surface levels of L-selectin on circulating neutrophils are significantly reduced. Consequently, neonatal neutrophils are markedly deficient in the ability to adhere to endothelial cells under conditions of flow and to emigrate through endothelial monolayers. Necessary quantitative changes in Mac-1 are also abnormal in specific granule deficiency. Indirect evidence implicates abnormalities of the regulation of gene expression during granulopoiesis, resulting in a failure to activate a cassette of genes normally expressed at the myelocyte–metamyelocyte stage of maturation. Leukocytes from these patients are deficient in specific granules and in many of the proteins that are packaged in both these and azurophilic granules. Since specific granules represent an intracellular pool from which Mac-1 can be mobilized to the plasma membrane during chemotaxis, neutrophils in patients with this syndrome are deficient in this regard. The Rambon-Hasharon syndrome represents a third condition in which increased bacterial infections are associated with reduced adhesive functions in neutrophils. These patients fail to incorporate fucose into cell-surface carbohydrates and thus lack the carbohydrate ligands for the selectin family of adhesion molecules. Consequently, their neutrophils are markedly deficient in the ability to adhere to endothelial cells under conditions of flow.**

5. **Inappropriate or excessive acute inflammation results in tissue damage. Intercellular adhesion is involved in these injurious events, not only because the localization and infiltration of leukocytes in inflamed tissues is determined by specific adhesion molecules but also because the adhesion of leukocytes to biologic substrates (i.e., other cells or matrix proteins) primes or amplifies their cytotoxic functions (e.g., oxidative or secretory processes). Neutrophil- or monocyte-mediated vascular and tissue injury has been implicated in a number of clinical entities in which the induction of leukocyte or endothelial adhesion mechanisms have been demonstrated or inferred. These include ischemia–reperfusion states (including hypovolemic shock with multiple organ injury), allograft rejection, and various acute and chronic inflammatory conditions. Numerous studies in animal models demonstrate a beneficial effect of systemic administration of monoclonal antibodies that block the functions of each of the specific adhesion molecules that play a role in leukocyte extravasation. The most profound antiinflammatory effect is produced by anti-CD18 monoclonal antibodies, but tissue- and stimulus-specific factors apparently influence the relative contributions of different adhesion pathways.**

6. **A number of clinical syndromes have associated reductions in the motility of neutrophils as measured in chemotaxis assays in vitro. These changes are usually transient, and little evidence suggests that they are of pathogenic significance. However, in several syndromes the evidence more clearly supports the conclusion that the defect in neutrophil motility is a major contributing factor to increased infectious susceptibility. Chediak-Higashi syndrome, type 1b glycogen storage disease, mannosidosis, periodontitis syndrome, Schwachman-Diamond syndrome, and hyperimmunoglobulin E syndrome all have associated defects in the chemotactic or chemokinetic motility of neutrophils, though in no case has a molecular mechanism accounting for the defect been defined.**

HISTORICAL ACCOUNT

The important role of phagocytic cells in host defense was recognized a century ago by Elie Metchnikoff. Historic findings by this jobless Russian zoologist in 1882 were among the first scientific evidence of phagocyte–host defense interactions. Several years later Metchnikoff described this conceptual breakthrough as follows[1]:

> **One day when the family had gone to a circus to see some extraordinary performing apes, I remained alone at my microscope, observing the life in the mobile cells of a transparent starfish larva, when a new thought suddenly flashed across my brain. It struck me that similar cells might serve in the defense of the organism against intruders. Feeling that there was in this something of surpassing interest, I felt so excited that I began striding up and down the room and even went to the seashore in order to collect my thoughts.**
>
> **I said to myself that, if my supposition was true, a splinter introduced into the body of a starfish larva, devoid of blood vessels or of a nervous system, should soon be surrounded by mobile cells as is to be observed in a man who runs a splinter into his finger. This was no sooner said than done.**
>
> **I was too excited to sleep that night in the expectation of the result of my experiment, and very early the next morning I ascertained that it had fully succeeded.**
>
> **That experiment formed the basis of the phagocyte theory, to the development of which I devoted the next twenty-five years of my life.**

What Metchnikoff had described in the starfish experiment was not phagocytosis itself but rather a more complex process involving the localized accumulation of cells at a point of injury. Further evidence that phagocytes undergo a tropic migration was provided in 1888 by Theodore Leber, a German ophthalmologist.[2] He demonstrated for the first time migration of leukocytes toward chemical stimuli, a response later termed "chemotaxis" when observed in vitro. He wrote at that time[2]:

> **The property of the leukocyte to tropic migration by substances foreign to the organism is of the greatest importance in making possible an extensive counteraction of the organism against external factors, since only in this way is the accumulation of a large number of leukocytes at the site of noxa assured.**

Since the time of these early landmark observations, the critical and multifaceted functions of phagocytes in inflammation have been described in a voluminous scientific literature. However, an understanding of the clinical relevance of these many observations largely awaited the recognition of pathologic disorders in the functions of human phagocytes. In 1954, Janeway and associates[3] described a group of patients with severe recurrent soft tissue infections. Approximately a decade later, Quie and coworkers[4] demonstrated a profound defect of intracellular microbicidal activity of phagocytic cells from these patients, and Holmes and coworkers[5] subsequently demonstrated a defect of oxidative metabolism in this disorder, now termed chronic granulomatous disease of childhood (see Chap. 133). Subsequent to the recognition of this syndrome, a rapid succession of reports[6–11] described a heterogeneous group of patients with severe, recurrent sinopulmonary infections and/or staphylococcal soft tissue abscesses. Abnormal or diminished motility of neutrophils and/or monocytes was suggested as a major pathogenic mechanism accounting for these infectious complications.

Early Studies of Leukocyte Motility

The locomotion of leukocytes is regulated by a complex cellular apparatus responsive to many environmental stimuli.[12–15] Leukocytes demonstrate essentially no movement in vitro in the absence of specific stimuli, but a diverse array of chemotactic factors may modify substantially the speed and direction of locomotion. Stimulated migration with no directional component is termed "chemokinesis" or "random locomotion."[13] When under the influence of concentration gradients of chemotactic factors, however, cells migrate toward the stimulating agent, and individual leukocytes demonstrate a rather uniform orientation toward the origin of the chemotactic gradient.[16,17]

A variety of techniques have been used to evaluate the migratory properties of myeloid or lymphoid cells. Evaluations of the kinetics and extent of the mobilization of leukocytes in various tissues of human subjects are limited to histopathologic assessments and applications of "skin-window" techniques initially described by Rebuck and Crowley.[17a] The skin-window technique and several more quantitative modifications[18] have proved of limited value for several reasons. Difficulties encountered in creating uniform skin lesions, in addition to the pain and possible infectious complications associated with the use of abrasive techniques, limit their overall suitability for clinical application. Findings of large numbers of one or more types of leukocytes in tissue exudates does not exclude the possibility of defective mobility since these cells may have infiltrated too late to prevent the establishment of infections.[19] As a result of these concerns, evaluations of the migratory functions of leukocytes in clinical samples are most commonly performed in vitro.

Assays of chemotaxis include those evaluating the effect of chemoattractants on a population of cells. Each of these assays, in principle, represents a modification of the micropore filter method[20] originally described by Boyden,[21] in which a test cell population migrates into or through a micropore filter toward a test reagent placed in an adjacent stimulant compartment. A modification of the micropore filter method[17] distinguishes chemotaxis from chemokinesis. This is accomplished by using protocols in which a range of concentrations of a stimulant reagent are added independently to the cell and stimulant compartments of a culture chamber.[22]

Direct observations have revealed that leukocytes, particularly neutrophils, are relatively fast-moving cells compared, for instance, to fibroblasts.[16,23,24] Most descriptions of the morphology of leukocytes during locomotion in vitro indicate that they assume a characteristic bipolar shape[16] (Fig. 132-1). This involves the appearance of veil-like, flattened membranes or lamellipodia at the anterior end of the cell. Migrating cells also generally demonstrate a uropod or tail-like structure with retraction fibers developing as a cell migrates. To study the effects of chemotactic factors on these events, it is necessary to establish experimental conditions that allow cells to be exposed to stable and continuous chemical gradients. Under such conditions, effects on both the rate and direction of cell orientation or movement can be observed. Most investigators have used microbial point sources, such as bacterial clumps or yeast spores, or specially designed orientation chambers for applications in visual assays.[15,16,23,24] A conceptually similar technique in which leukocytes migrate toward a chemoattractant source on plastic or glass under agarose[25] has also proved useful.

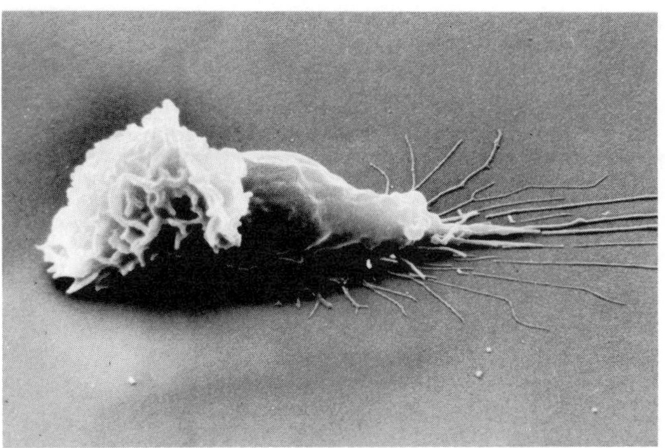

FIG. 132-1 **Scanning electron micrograph of a human neutrophil following activation by a chemotactic factor. The polarized morphology is characteristic of migrating neutrophils. The leading edge of the cell has numerous ruffles and the trailing uropod has numerous retraction fibers resulting from previous attachment sites on the protein-coated glass surface on which this cell was crawling. The rate of migration averages 10 to 15 μm/sec when cells are incubated with chemotactic factors at 37°C.** ***(From Hughes et al.[449] Used by permission.)***

The bipolar shape seen in migrating cells also occurs if neutrophils[20] and monocytes[26] are exposed to chemotactic stimuli in suspension. Thus, the cells need not be attached to a surface in order to assume a bipolar shape. Using this morphologic change as a sensitive indicator of chemotactic stimulation, abnormal cellular responses have been identified in clinical conditions characterized by increased infections, and the inhibitory action of selected pharmacologic agents has been assessed.[27–29]

MOLECULAR MECHANISMS REGULATING ADHESIVENESS OF LEUKOCYTES

The mobility of neutrophils clearly depends on two major factors in addition to the intrinsic ameboid locomotion that is visible after chemotactic stimulation. The first is the flow of blood transporting unstimulated neutrophils throughout the vascular system. The second is the adhesion of neutrophils to endothelial cells at sites of leukocyte emigration. This adhesion must be sufficiently strong first to withstand the shear forces of flowing blood and then to control the movement of neutrophils through the blood vessel wall. Recent advances in understanding these adhesive mechanisms reveal a cascade of events in which different classes of adhesion molecules play distinct and critical roles that ultimately lead to the emigration of neutrophils at sites of inflammation. The discussion that follows will present some details regarding the molecules involved and their respective roles.

The CD18 Integrins

LFA-1, Mac-1 and p150,95 are structurally related αβ heterodimers that share a common β subunit[30] (Table 132-1). The CD18 integrins are in turn related to a larger family of integrin adhesion molecules, which includes primarily extracellular matrix receptors, such as the fibronectin receptor, vitronectin receptor, and platelet glycoprotein IIb/IIIa. The α subunits of the CD18 integrins, like other integrins, contain multiple divalent cation-binding domains, which are similar to the Ca^{2+}-binding domains of calmodulin and troponin C.[31-34] Not surprisingly, CD18 adhesion functions are Mg^{2+}- and Ca^{2+}-dependent. In contrast to members of other integrin families, except for VLA-2, the leukocyte integrin α subunits contain a unique domain, designated the "I" or "inserted" domain, which is homologous to similar domains found in von Willebrand factor, complement proteins C2 and B, and cartilage matrix protein. The leukocyte integrin β subunit, like other integrin β subunits, is a cysteine-rich transmembrane protein with a fourfold repeat of an unusual cysteine motif.[35,36]

CD18 integrin expression is restricted to white blood cells. LFA-1 is expressed by lymphocytes, monocytes, and granulocytes, while Mac-1 and p150,95 are primarily

Table 132-1 Cellular Distribution and Functional Activities of β_2 Integrin Heterodimers

	LFA-1 (CD11a/CD)	Mac-1 (CD11b/CD18)	p150,95 (CD11c/CD18)
Leukocyte distribution	T and B lymphocytes, large granular lymphocytes, monocytes, and granulocytes	Granulocytes, monocytes, macrophages, large granular lymphocytes	Macrophages, monocytes, granulocytes
Myeloid cells functions*	Natural killing Antibody-dependent cellular cytotoxicity Adhesion to endothelium or other mesenchymal or epithelial cells expressing ICAM-1, ICAM-2, and ICAM-3	Complement receptor type 3 functions: iC3b binding Phagocytosis and intracellular killing or cytolysis of complement-opsinized microorganisms or sheep red blood cells Binding of microbial determinants (*Leishmania* gp63, *Bordetella* filamentous hemagglutin) promoting phagocytosis Homotypic aggregation Adhesion to endothelium or protein substrates (fibronectin, fibrinogen, ICAM-1, keyhole limpet hemocyanin) Adhesion-dependent potentiation of oxidative burst and degranulation Chemotaxis, random migration Antibody-dependent cellular cytotoxicity	iC3b binding (complement receptor type 4 activity?) Adhesion to endothelium or protein substrates Chemotaxis, phagocytosis, and aggregation (?)
Lymphoid cells functions*	Cytolytic T lymphocyte mediated killing Natural killing Antigen, mitogen, or alloantigen induced proliferation Phorbal ester elicited T & B lymphocyte aggregation T helper cell responses (i.e., for immunoglobulin or γ-interferon production)	Cytotoxicity by large granular lymphocytes	Cytolytic T cell-target cell conjugation?

*Determined by subunit-specific monoclonal antibody inhibition studies and/or observations of LAD leukocyte functions in vitro.

restricted to myeloid cells, although they are also expressed by some lymphocytes and natural killer (NK) cells. The CD18 integrins have a broad role in many leukocyte adhesion-related functions. LFA-1 has been implicated in cell-mediated cytolysis, antigen presentation, lymphocyte homotypic aggregation, and leukocyte adhesion to a variety of cytokine-activated cells, including endothelial cells (reviewed in Kishimoto et al.[30]). Mac-1 has been implicated in neutrophil homotypic aggregation, adhesion to substrates, binding and phagocytosis of iC3b-coated particles, the adhesion-dependent respiratory burst, neutrophil locomotion, and leukocyte adhesion to cytokine-activated cells.

Both LFA-1 and Mac-1 mediate adhesion through multiple ligands. LFA-1 binds to the intercellular adhesion molecules—ICAM-1,[37] ICAM-2,[38] and ICAM-3.[39] Mac-1 also binds to ICAM-1,[40] although at a site distinct from that of LFA-1.[41] In addition, Mac-1 recognizes a wide spectrum of unrelated molecules, including the iC3b fragment of complement, fibrinogen, factor X, and several microbial antigens. The molecular basis for the promiscuous nature of ligand recognition is not well defined.[30]

CD18 Regulation. The broad range of functions that the CD18 integrins mediate requires that the functional activity of these receptors be closely regulated to prevent inappropriate adhesion. Mac-1 (CD11b/CD18) can be regulated both quantitatively and qualitatively. It is stored in intracellular granules of neutrophils and monocytes,[42] and stimulation with low levels of chemotactic agents cause it to be rapidly recruited to the cell surface, resulting in a 3- to 10-fold increase in the quantity of Mac-1 on the cell surface. In addition, the functional activity of Mac-1 is qualitatively regulated by chemoattractant-induced activation of neutrophils.[43,44] On resting neutrophils, Mac-1, LFA-1 (CD11a/CD18), and possibly p150,95 (CD11c/CD18) are in an inactive state, but after stimulation with chemotactic factors the CD18 integrins undergo a conformational change. This conformational change is transient, allowing adherent leukocytes to detach,[45–47] an event that appears to be necessary for optimal cellular locomotion or repeated target binding in cell-mediated cytolysis. This active state can be recognized and possibly induced by some monoclonal antibodies, which bind to either the α or β subunit and can hold the CD18 integrins in an active conformation in the absence of cellular activation.[48] In addition, the β_2 integrins have been implicated in signaling directly or co-signaling through other receptors. For example, signaling through the T cell receptor is markedly enhanced by co-ligation of LFA-1,[49,50] and Mac-1 (CD11b/CD18) signals the neutrophil for markedly enhanced hydrogen peroxide production.[51]

Intercellular Adhesion Molecules (ICAM). All three members of the ICAM family were originally functionally defined as ligands for LFA-1. ICAM-1, ICAM-2, and ICAM-3 are known to be structurally related members of the immunoglobulin supergene family. They are most closely related to other Ig-like adhesion molecules such as VCAM-1 and NCAM. ICAM-1 has five Ig-like domains, with a short hinge region separating the third and fourth Ig-like domains.[52,53] ICAM-1 is a ligand for Mac-1 as well as LFA-1. It is interesting that the binding sites for LFA-1 and Mac-1 are distinct. LFA-1 binds to domains 1 and 2,[54] while Mac-1 binds to domain 3.[41] ICAM-1 also serves as receptor for rhinovirus[55] and malaria-infected red blood cells. ICAM-2, in contrast, has only two Ig-like domains, which are most closely related to domains 1 and 2 of ICAM-1.[38] ICAM-3 is defined by monoclonal antibodies[39] and is a member of the Ig superfamily, with a five-domain structure similar to that of ICAM-1.

The distribution and regulation of the ICAM molecules are quite distinct. ICAM-1 is expressed basally only at low levels on some vascular endothelial cells and on lymphocytes.[37,56] However, ICAM-1 expression can be induced to high levels on a variety of cells by stimulation with inflammatory cytokines, such as interleukin-1 (IL-1), tumor necrosis factor (TNF), and γ-interferon (IFN-γ).[56] Induced or greatly increased expression of ICAM-1 has been reported on vascular endothelial cells, keratinocytes, epithelial cells, hepatocytes, and myocytes. In addition, ICAM-1 expression is increased on activated lymphocytes. Induction of ICAM-1 requires de novo synthesis. As a counter-receptor for LFA-1, ICAM-1 has been implicated in guiding leukocyte migration, in cell-mediated cytolysis, in antigen presentation, and in lymphocyte homotypic aggregation. In addition, ICAM-1 as a receptor for Mac-1 is involved in neutrophil–endothelial cell interactions, transendothelial migration, and the adhesion-dependent respiratory burst.

ICAM-2 expression, in contrast to that of ICAM-1, is constitutive and is restricted to endothelial cells and mononuclear leukocytes.[39,57] Functionally it is not clear what role ICAM-2 plays in the inflammatory response. ICAM-3 is even more restricted in expression. It is expressed only on monocytes, lymphocytes, and granulocytes.[58] It is interesting that ICAM-3 is the only ICAM molecule expressed by neutrophils.

The Selectins

All three members of the selectin family (Table 132-2) share common structural features[59–65]—most prominently an N-terminal C-type lectin domain. As discussed below, the lectin domain is central to the carbohydrate-binding properties of all three selectins. The lectin-domain motif belongs to the C-type lectin family described by Drickamer.[66] This Ca^{2+}-dependent lectin domain accounts at least in part for the requirement of Ca^{2+} in adhesion mediated by all three selectins. The lectin domain is followed by a domain homologous to epidermal growth factor (EGF); by a variable number of complement regulatory repeat sequences, which constitute a motif found in many complement regulatory proteins; by a conventional transmembrane domain; and by a C-terminal cytoplasmic domain. Much of the size difference between the selectins is accounted for by the number of complement regulatory repeats: L-selectin, the smallest member, has two copies, E-selectin has six, and P-selectin has alternatively spliced forms with eight and nine. This is a highly conserved gene family, with over 60 percent amino acid identity in lectin and EGF domains.

L-selectin was first described as a lymphocyte homing molecule involved in tissue-specific migration to peripheral lymph nodes (reviewed in Yednock and Rosen[67]). More recently, L-selectin has been demonstrated on myeloid cells and is involved in neutrophil–endothelial cell and monocyte–endothelial cell interactions at sites of inflammation. Monoclonal antibodies against L-selectin reduce neutrophil adhesion to cytokine-stimulated endothelial cell cultures. It is interesting that L-selectin-mediated adhesion appears to be most readily measured when neutrophils are subjected to shear stress[68–70] (see below). A role for carbohydrate binding by L-selectin was demonstrated by Rosen and colleagues[67] many years before the lectin domain structure was elucidated by gene cloning.

E-selectin was first defined as a cytokine-inducible adhe-

Table 132-2 Molecular Ligand Receptor Pairs Involved in Leukocyte Adhesion to Vascular Endothelium

Leukocyte Determinants			Endothelial Ligands or Counterreceptors			
Molecule	Structure	Cell Distribution	Molecule	Structure	Cell Distribution	Regulatory Factors
Mac-1 (CD11b/CD18)	β_2 Integrin	Neutrophils, eosinophils, and monocytes	ICAM-1	Ig	Unstimulated and activated endothelial cells, other cell types	LPS,* interferon-γ, IL-1, and TNFα
LFA-1 (CD11a/CD11b)	β_2 Integrin	Neutrophils, monocytes, and lymphocytes	ICAM-1	Ig	Activated endothelial cells, other cell types	LPS, interferon-γ, IL-1, and TNFα
			ICAM-2	Ig	Unstimulated endothelial cells	—
p150,95 (CD11c/CD11d)	β_2 Integrin	Neutrophils, monocytes	Unknown		—	—
VLA-4 ($\alpha_4\beta_1$)	β_1 Integrin	Lymphocytes, monocytes, and eosinophils	VCAM-1	Ig	Activated endothelial cells	LPS, IL-1, and TNFα
L-selectin (CD62L)	Selectin	Neutrophils, eosinophils, monocytes, and lymphocytes	GLYCAM-1, CD34	Mucin-type glycoprotein	High-endothelial venules of peripheral lymph nodes (mouse)	
Sialyl Lewis X bearing glycoprotein(s)	Sialydated and fucosylated lactosaminoglycan	Neutrophils, monocytes, and lymphocyte subsets	E-selectin (CD62E)	Selectin	Activated endothelial cells	LPS, IL-1, and TNFα
Sialyl Lewis X bearing glycoprotein(s)	Sialydated and fucosylated lactosaminoglycan	Neutrophils, monocytes, eosinophils, and lymphocyte subsets	P-selectin (CD62P)	Selectin	Activated endothelial cells and platelets	Histamine, thrombin, H_2O_2, IL-1, and LPS

*LPS = lipopolysaccharide.

sion molecule on endothelial cells.[71] Monoclonal antibodies against E-selectin specifically block adhesion of neutrophil and myeloid cell lines (HL-60) to endothelial cells stimulated with IL-1 and TNF.[71,72] Expression of E-selectin is prominent in acute inflammatory lesions in vivo and correlates with the large influx of neutrophils.[73–77] Although E-selectin appears to be primarily associated with acute inflammatory lesions and in this context can be induced almost anywhere, recent studies have shown E-selectin expression in some chronic inflammatory lesions, notably inflamed skin[76,78] and the synovium from patients with arthritis.[79] Furthermore, a small subset of memory T lymphocytes, defined by HECA-452 (a monoclonal antibody that recognizes a ligand for E-selectin), bind specifically to E-selectin.[78] These studies indicate that, in some circumstances, E-selectin can mediate lymphocyte traffic to chronic inflammatory sites.

P-selectin was first defined as a marker for activated platelets.[80,81] P-selectin was localized to the α-granules of platelets[82,83] and later to the Weibel-Palade bodies of endothelial cells.[84–86] In both cell types, cell activation results in a rapid recruitment of these granules to the cell surface.[82,83,86] P-selectin is involved in mediating neutrophil–platelet interactions[87–89] and in neutrophil–endothelial cell interactions in vitro.[90–92] These results indicate that P-selectin may play a central role in bridging hemostasis and acute inflammation very early in the response to vascular injury or insult.

Selectin Ligands. Since L-selectin was first described as a lymphocyte homing receptor, the most intense search for an L-selectin ligand has been on high-endothelial venules (HEV) of lymph nodes. In a series of elegant studies, Rosen and colleagues demonstrated a clear role for carbohydrates in L-selectin-mediated adhesion.[67] Lymphocyte adhesion to HEV of peripheral lymph nodes is sensitive to neuraminidase treatment of the HEV.[93,94] Charged sugars, such as mannose 6-phosphate, and polymers of charged sugars such as PPME (phosphomannosyl-rich core polysaccharide from yeast) and fucoidin (fucose-sulfate-rich) bind specifically to L-selectin and block lymphocyte adhesion to HEV.[95,96] Rosen, Lasky, and colleagues have recently used soluble L-selectin, in the form of a bivalent L-selectin–IgG chimeric molecule, to immunopurify a 50-kDa protein from lymph node tissue. This protein is heavily glycosylated and contains sulfated sugars.[97] In a parallel line of research, Butcher and colleagues have developed a monoclonal antibody, MECA-79, that specifically stains peripheral lymph node HEV but not mucosal HEV and that blocks lymphocyte adhesion to peripheral-node HEV.[98] The MECA-79 is an IgM and appears to recognize a carbohydrate determinant. Western blot analysis and immunoaffinity purification of reactive antigen shows several distinct bands—a major band of 105 kDa and minor bands of 65, 90, 150, and 200 kDa. The purified MECA-79 antigen supports tissue-specific lymphocyte binding, which is blocked by both MECA-79 and by anti-L-selectin monoclonal antibodies. The major 50-kDa product isolated with the L-selectin–IgG chimeric molecule by Rosen et al. also immunoreacts with the MECA-79. Current evidence indicates that the 50-kDa ligand in mice is a mucin-like molecule now called GlyCAM-1 (glycosylation-dependent cell adhesion molecule) that is rich in *O*-linked, highly sulfated carbohydrates.[99] In addition, a 90-kDa ligand for L-selectin on lymph-node HEV in mice is CD34, another mucin-like molecule rich in *O*-linked, sulfated carbohydrates (L. A. Laskey and S. Rosen, personal communication).

A ligand for L-selectin on stimulated human umbilical-vein endothelial cells (HUVEC) has not been defined. The MECA-79 monoclonal antibody, which cross-reacts with human lymph-node HEV, does not appear to stain stimulated HUVEC. Yet L-selectin-dependent adhesion of neutrophils to stimulated HUVEC has been demonstrated by several independent groups. There is a consensus that L-selectin-dependent neutrophil adhesion to HUVEC occurs only with cytokine stimulation of the endothelium.[68–70] The adhesion occurs readily at low temperature and appears to withstand the shear forces found in small venules.[68–70]

The identification of a lectin domain in the E-selectin structure led to an intense, focused search for a carbohydrate ligand expressed by myeloid cells. Numerous independent groups reported that sialyl Lewis X (sLe^x) or related sialylated, fucosylated sugars serve as specific ligands for E-selectin. sLe^x is appropriately expressed by neutrophils and monocytes. Several complementary lines of evidence support these claims. Phillips et al. demonstrated that liposomes composed of glycolipids containing the sLe^x structure are capable of inhibiting E-selectin-mediated adhesion.[100] Furthermore, the LEC11 cell line, a variant CHO cell, expresses sLe^x and binds to HUVEC in an E-selectin-dependent manner. Monoclonal antibodies against the sLe^x determinant inhibit E-selectin-mediated adhesion.[100,101] Transfection of a 1,3-fucosyltransferase into COS or CHO cells confers on these cells the ability to synthesize sLe^x and to bind E-selectin.[102,103] Brandley and colleagues purified glycolipids from myeloid cells and identified fractions that support E-selectin adhesion.[104] More recently, sialyl Lewis A, an sLe^x-related carbohydrate, has been implicated as a ligand for E-selectin.[105,106] Computer modeling suggests that the sialic acid and fucose residues are oriented in the same manner in sLe^x and sialyl Lewis A. Both sLe^x and sialyl Lewis A are recognized by HECA-452, the monoclonal antibody that defines a subpopulation of lymphocytes capable of binding to E-selectin.[105]

A similar search for carbohydrate ligands of P-selectin followed the recognition that P-selectin possessed an N-terminal lectin domain. Initially it was reported that Lewis X antigen (CD15) was a major ligand for P-selectin.[89] However, several groups have shown that P-selectin-dependent adhesion is sensitive to neuraminidase treatment of the target cell, suggesting a requirement for sialic acid.[107–109] Indeed, P-selectin shows significantly higher affinity for sialyl Lewis X than for Lewis X.[106] Although both E-selectin and P-selectin bind to sLe^x, the binding characteristics are distinct.[106] Thus E-selectin and P-selectin are not identical in ligand specificity. More recently, Aruffo et al.[110] reported that soluble P-selectin–IgG chimeric molecules bind specifically to sulfatides (3-sulfated galactosylceramides) derived from myeloid cells and some tumor cell lines. Treatment of HL-60 cells with selenate, an inhibitor of sulfation, reduces binding to P-selectin but not to E-selectin. These studies suggest that sulfatides may be a biologically significant ligand for P-selectin.

While it is clear that sLe^x on either proteins or lipids can support E-selectin-mediated adhesion in vitro, it appears that not all the sLe^x on the neutrophil cell surface binds with equal efficiency and affinity to E-selectin. One possibility is that sLe^x may be added to a variety of proteins and lipids, but only a subset is presented in a favorable conformation, thus creating a hierarchy where E-selectin preferentially binds to a subset of the total available sLe^x. This hierarchy might reflect the accessibility of the sLe^x or of the protein sequences adjacent to the sLe^x. Alternatively, some proteins may be presented on microvilli and pseudopods, which are more likely to mediate cell–cell contact.[111] Picker et al.[112] have shown that L-selectin is concentrated on the tips of microvillus-like projections from the surface of unstimulated neutrophils. In addition, they found that L-selectin isolated from neutrophils but not from lymphocytes bears the sLe^x carbohydrate and can support E-selectin-dependent adhesion. L-selectin on neutrophils may have a dual role, presenting the sLe^x ligand for E-selectin-dependent adhesion and using its lectin domain for binding to some as yet unidentified ligand on activated endothelial cells. A third binding mechanism was suggested by Siegelman et al.[113] They hypothesized that while the lectin domain of the selectins provides the carbohydrate specificity, the EGF domain may bind to protein determinants.

Selectin Regulation. L-selectin is constitutively expressed on resting neutrophils in a seemingly functional form. However, within minutes of exposure of neutrophils to low levels of chemotactic factors, L-selectin is rapidly down-regulated from the cell surface.[114] Near-complete down-regulation of L-selectin can be detected within minutes in vitro. A large fragment of L-selectin can be recovered from the supernatant of activated cells, suggesting that L-selectin is proteolytically clipped close to the transmembrane domain.[114] A broad range of activating agents, including complement component 5a (C5a), f-Met-Leu-Phe, TNF, granulocyte/monocyte-colony stimulating factor (GM-CSF), and interleukin-8 (IL-8) are effective at inducing this response,[68,114–116] and the rapid shedding of L-selectin follows the kinetics of Mac-1 up-regulation from intracellular stores. Analysis of neutrophils recovered from inflamed peritoneum in vivo[115] and immunohistologic analysis of neutrophils in inflamed skin sites[114] reveal that this inverse regulation of adhesion molecules occurs in vivo as well. These observations led to the proposal of a two-step adhesion model (see below).

E-selectin is normally absent from endothelial cells. However, on stimulation with inflammatory cytokines, endothelial cells express E-selectin within several hours. E-selectin is synthesized de novo, and its expression is blocked by protein synthesis inhibitors.[71] This up-regulation of E-selectin is similar to that seen with other endothelial adhesion molecules, such as ICAM-1 and VCAM-1. However, in contrast to these other adhesion molecules, which remain highly expressed for over 24 hours, E-selectin expression peaks at 3 to 4 h and then is down-modulated over a period of 8 to 24 h in vitro.[71,117] The mechanism of E-selectin down-modulation is not well characterized. The time course of E-selectin expression is similar to the time course of neutrophil infiltration into acute inflammatory sites in vivo. These results suggest that E-selectin is involved primarily in the acute inflammatory response. E-selectin expression in vivo is also rapidly inducible and coincides with the influx of neutrophils.[73–77,118] However, in some chronic inflammatory lesions, notably some inflamed skin and synovial sites, E-selectin expression is quite prominent.[73,78,79,118]

P-selectin, like E-selectin, is expressed by activated endothelium. However, the activation signals and the kinetics of expression are completely different for these two events. P-selectin is stored in intracellular Weibel-Palade bodies.[84–86] Stimulation of endothelial cells with histamine or thrombin induces a rapid recruitment of Weibel-Palade bodies to the cell surface, resulting in surface expression of P-selectin within minutes after stimulation. Similarly, P-selectin is also stored in the α granules of platelets, which are recruited to the cell surface within seconds of platelet activation.[82,83] This near-instantaneous up-regulation of P-selectin suggests it plays a critical role in the earliest events of inflammation and hemostasis. Surface expression of P-selectin on endothelium is also extremely transient. Within 30 min, P-selectin is down-modulated, apparently by receptor endocytosis rather than surface proteolysis.

A Model for Neutrophil–Endothelial Cell Interactions

In 1989, a two-step adhesion model for neutrophil interaction with endothelium was proposed, based primarily on the observation that Mac-1 and L-selectin are inversely regulated by exposure to chemotactic factors.[114,115,119] The rapid down-regulation of L-selectin with a concomitant up-regulation of Mac-1 suggested that these adhesion molecules mediate distinct but complementary adhesion events. In this model (Fig. 132-2), L-selectin mediates the initial interaction of the resting, circulating neutrophil with the activated endothelium, thus guiding the unstimulated neutrophil to the appropriate site of inflammation. This initial binding or rolling event would slow the neutrophil and expose it to the low levels of chemotactic factors released at the site of inflammation. The chemoattractants would provide the signal for the neutrophil to enter the inflamed tissue and would trigger the transition from L-selectin-mediated adhesion to CD18-mediated adhesion. The CD18 integrins, LFA-1 and Mac-1, are largely responsible for subsequent adhesion strengthening, neutrophil aggregation, and transendothelial migration. Data from a number of independent investigators support and extend this model, and the currently recognized adhesion-deficiency syndromes in humans are also consistent with this model (see below).

As presented in Table 132-3, at least four distinct adhesive steps are involved in the emigration of neutrophils to sites of inflammation. Neutrophils in circulation must resist the fluid drag forces of flowing blood in order to stop along the vascular endothelium. The phenomenon of neutrophil rolling (the initial margination step) was observed over a century ago in classic intravital microscopy studies.[120] Neutrophils

Table 132-3 Proposed Steps in Neutrophil Emigration at Sites of Inflammation

Step	Adhesion Molecules Involved	Regulatory Factors
Rolling, initial margination	L-selectin, sLe^x-like saccharides	Active on unstimulated neutrophils
	P-selectin	Histamine, bradykinin, thrombin
	E-selectin	IL-1, TNF, LPS*
Stopping on endothelium	CD18 integrins	Chemotactic factors such as IL-8 or PAF
	ICAM-1	IL-1, TNF, LPS
Neutrophil–neutrophil adhesion on the endothelium	CD11b/CD18	Chemotactic factors such as IL-8 or PAF
Transendothelial migration	CD11b/CD18, CD11a/CD18	Chemotactic factors such as IL-8 or PAF
	ICAM-1	IL-1, TNF, LPS

*LPS = lipopolysaccharide

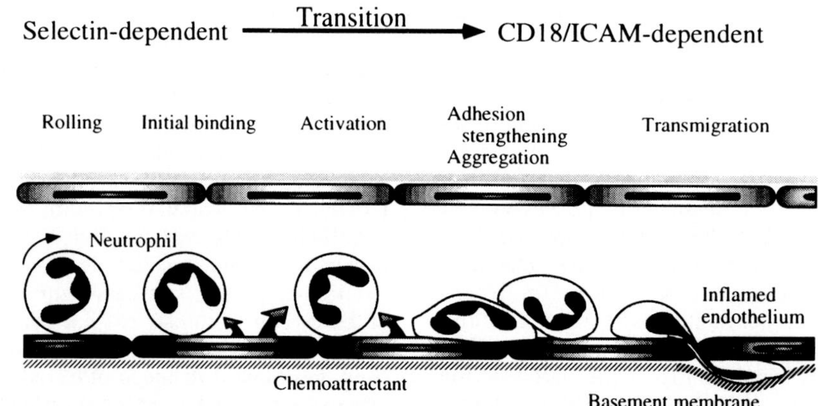

FIG. 132-2 A dynamic model for neutrophil interaction with inflamed endothelium. Neutrophil localization and activation is a multistep process.[40,72,115] Endothelial cells adjacent to a site of inflammation are stimulated by cytokines (such as TNF and IL-1) to synthesize E-selectin and ICAM-1. These inducible adhesion molecules provide position-specific information for leukocytes. L-selectin on the neutrophil[450] and E-selectin on the endothelium[123] mediate the initial interaction between the unactivated neutrophil and the stimulated endothelium. This interaction guides the neutrophil to the appropriate site. The transiently bound neutrophil is exposed to low concentrations of chemoattractants. Free-flowing neutrophils are not activated. This activation event induces a rapid transition in neutrophil morphology and adhesiveness. There is a transient increase in L-selectin-mediated adhesion[451] followed by a rapid shedding of the cell-surface L-selectin.[72,450] Simultaneously, there is activation of Mac-1 adhesiveness[43,44] accompanied by a rapid increase in cell-surface Mac-1 expression from intracellular stores.[42,182] Thus, activation rapidly shuts down one adhesion pathway (L-selectin) and turns on another adhesion pathway (Mac-1).[72] Engagement of Mac-1 results in adhesion strengthening, neutrophil aggregation, and transendothelial migration.

can be seen to roll and stop along venules but not in small arteries or arterioles. In vitro, neutrophils exhibit rolling and sticking behavior under conditions of flow, but only on cytokine-stimulated endothelium, not on unstimulated endothelium.[121] Studies using specific monoclonal antibodies in vitro reveal that L-selectin accounts for 60 to 70 percent of the rolling adhesion under flow,[68,122] and that E-selectin accounts for up to 40 percent of this adhesion.[123] P-selectin also supports rolling adhesion of neutrophils when isolated and inserted in a planar membrane,[124] and the rolling adhesion that occurs when endothelial monolayers are stimulated with histamine to mobilize P-selectin from the Weibel-Palade bodies can be completely blocked by anti-P-selectin monoclonal antibodies.[125] Intravital microscopy studies have confirmed the role of L-selectin and P-selectin in vivo in rolling adhesion of neutrophils in small venules.[126–128]

The transition from selectin-mediated adhesion to CD18-mediated adhesion occurs rapidly in vitro. A variety of chemotactic factors can cause quantitative down-regulation of L-selectin at the same time that Mac-1 is up-regulated. This transition is reflected in neutrophil adhesion to endothelial cells in vitro. Under static conditions, where no shear stress is applied, resting neutrophil adhesion is partially selectin-dependent and partially CD18/ICAM-1-dependent.[68,70,72,111] Upon activation of the neutrophil, the adhesion becomes almost entirely CD18/ICAM-1-dependent.[129,130] Under conditions of flow in vitro the velocity of rolling on cytokine-activated endothelial cell monolayers is greatly increased by anti-CD18 monoclonal antibody,[123] and the ability of neutrophils to stop at wall shear stresses in the venular range is markedly inhibited by anti-CD18 monoclonal antibodies.[125] Similarly, activated neutrophils bind poorly under conditions of flow.[130] The physiologically relevant trigger of this transition in vivo is unknown. It is likely that there are multiple mediators, perhaps used in different types of inflammatory events. It would be most efficient if the stimulated endothelial cells, themselves, could produce the appropriate chemoattractant. This would ensure appropriate localization of the neutrophil to the inflammatory site. Endothelial cells are capable of producing several neutrophil chemoattractants, including IL-8, GM-CSF, and platelet activating factor (PAF). Huber et al.[131] and Kuijpers et al.[132] reported that anti-IL-8 antibodies significantly blocked neutrophil transmigration across stimulated endothelial cells. Immunolocalization of IL-8 demonstrates association with both the endothelial cells and the underlying collagen gel matrix. These results suggest that in endothelial cultures stimulated for 3 to 4 h, IL-8 is the major chemotactic factor involved. Zimmerman, McIntyre, and colleagues have studied the role of PAF in neutrophil adhesion and activation.[133,134] Both PAF and P-selectin are induced within minutes on thrombin- or histamine-activated endothelium, correlating with increased neutrophil adhesiveness.[135,136] These results suggest that in the earliest events in vascular insult, PAF and P-selectin may function cooperatively to mediate neutrophil localization. These investigators propose that P-selectin acts as a tether to stop the circulating neutrophil, allowing PAF to induce the transition to CD18-dependent transmigration.[92]

Following chemotactic stimulation of the neutrophil, CD18 integrins apparently undergo a conformational change resulting in a transient increase in affinity for ligand.[47,137] This increased adhesiveness strengthens the interaction of neutrophils with the endothelium. At the same time, these activated neutrophils show increased adhesiveness for each other, resulting in neutrophil aggregation. Some vessels at sites of inflammation are so filled with neutrophils that they are occluded. This neutrophil aggregation presumably helps to slow blood flow and permit further neutrophil accumulation. Neutrophil aggregation is a Mac-1-dependent event.[138]

Neutrophils enter the inflamed tissue by migrating first between endothelial junctions and then through the basement membrane. Both neutrophil aggregation and transendothelial migration[40,72,139] (reviewed in Smith[140]) are CD18 integrin-dependent events. Neutrophils treated with anti-CD18 monoclonal antibodies and neutrophils isolated from CD18-deficient patients (see below) fail to aggregate or transmigrate in vitro. Thus, these later stages of neutrophil localization to inflammatory sites require CD18 function. These events require distinct CD18 ligands, since monoclonal antibodies against ICAM-1 block neutrophil transendothelial migration but do not affect neutrophil aggregation, and, in contrast to homotypic aggregation, transendothelial migration is inhibited to a significant degree by monoclonal antibodies against CD11a (i.e., LFA-1).[40,140,141]

CLINICAL DISORDERS OF LEUKOCYTE MOBILITY

General Considerations

The rapid localization of phagocytes to sites of microbial invasion or trauma represents a first-line defense mechanism of particular importance in nonimmune hosts. Quantitative or qualitative aberrations of either the cellular or the humoral contributions to these adaptive responses may impair inflammatory defenses, and, thus, increase infectious susceptibility. Early studies[19] demonstrated a critical 2 to 4 h period after cutaneous invasion by bacterial pathogens during which phagocytic cells must arrive at a site of invasion in order to prevent establishment of an infection. Recurrent bacterial or fungal infections of the skin or mucous membranes are prominent in patients with quantitative deficiencies of peripheral blood leukocytes.[142] Such infections are also evident in patients with qualitative disorders resulting in insufficient accumulation of phagocytes at inflammatory sites, despite normal numbers of leukocytes in the peripheral blood.[143,144] Among both patient groups, common pathogens such as *Staphylococcus aureus, Pseudomonas,* other gram-negative enteric species, and *Candida albicans* account for most infectious complications. Infected tissues in these patients are characteristically gangrenous or necrotic, are devoid of pus, and contain few granulocytes when examined microscopically. Local inflammatory signs or symptoms in such patients may be minimal although the infection may lead to the destruction of cutaneous, subcutaneous, periodontal, or other submucosal tissues.

Among early reports of clinical disorders typified by susceptibility to recurrent soft tissue infections were reports of patients with abnormalities of leukocyte migration in vitro and/or of tissue mobilization of leukocytes in vivo.[8,9,145–147] In contrast to observations in patients with chronic granulomatous disease (described in Chap. 133), studies of granulocytes or monocytes in these patients demonstrated neither abnormalities of microbicidal functions nor granulomatous inflammation in infected tissues. Initially, at least for purposes of comparison of individual patients, a distinct subclassification of disorders of leukocyte motility or chemotaxis seemed justified. However, an explosion of literature followed in which defects of chemotaxis in vitro were associated with a wide array of clinical disorders or conditions. Such reports clearly implied but rarely documented that diminished chemotaxis in vitro was associated with diminished availability or delayed infiltration of phagocytes into inflamed tissues. Correlations between abnormalities of cellular motility in vitro and altered exudation in tissues of human subjects have been infrequent because of the imprecisions in the techniques used to evaluate cellular infiltration in vivo in humans (e.g., skin-window techniques).

A reliable interpretation of leukocyte functions in vitro must take into consideration the clinical status of the individual patient, since it is important to determine whether abnormal functions result in increased susceptibility to infection or simply reflect other factors surrounding the patient's condition. Certain pharmacologic agents, as well as the nutritional status of the patient, may transiently influence selected functions tested in vitro.[28,148] Blood samples obtained for study during the course of infections may contain an increased percentage of immature myeloid cells, which function suboptimally.[149] Also, many investigators have reported enhanced, diminished, or otherwise abnormal motility, phagocytosis, oxidative metabolism, and/or other functions of leukocytes in patients with clinical bacterial infections.[150–153] In most cases these abnormalities are found to be transient and probably reflect cellular influences of inflammatory mediators[148,154–156] or products of the infecting organisms. Certain bacterial toxins exert significant inhibitory effects on cellular locomotion as well as other functions in vitro.[148] Some, such as cholera toxin and certain enterotoxins of *E. coli,* exert primarily intracellular effects (for example, activating adenyl cyclase and elevating intracellular cyclic AMP levels).[157,158] Others preferentially perturb cell-membrane properties; these toxins include streptolysin O, the clostridial toxins perfringolysin and phospholipase C, a diverse group of staphylococcal toxins (sphingomyelinase C and leukocidin), and proteases (alkaline protease, elastase) elaborated by pathogenic strains of *Pseudomonas aeruginosa.*[159,160] Suggested pathogenic mechanisms related to microbial toxin exposure include the disruption of receptors for chemotactic factors, complement fragments, or the Fc portion of IgG; alteration of membrane fluidity; and inhibition of cytoskeletal protein assembly. Finally, certain microbial proteases or other products act directly on humoral mediators of cellular locomotion. For example, elastases elaborated by *Pseudomonas aeruginosa* cleave C5 (as well as other serum complement proteins), thereby generating complement-derived chemotactic moieties in vitro or in vivo.[159]

The molecular pathogenesis has been defined for a limited number of genetic or secondary disorders characterized by defective migration of leukocytes. The heritable deficiency of the β_2 integrin subfamily (described below) is an example in which the molecular pathogenesis is clearly defined. In most other primary or acquired disorders of leukocyte motility, molecular pathogenesis has not been clearly defined. Investigation of these clinical syndromes has provided important insights concerning the physiological and pathologic significance of leukocyte trafficking in vivo as well as the molecular determinants of these events.

Leukocyte Adhesion Deficiency

Identification of CD18 Deficiency in Human, Dog, and Cow—Early Reports. An autosomal recessive trait characterized by recurrent bacterial infections, impairment of pus formation and wound healing, and a broad spectrum of functional abnormalities of myeloid and lymphoid cells results from heterogenous mutations of the β subunit of CD18 (β_2) integrins. These mutations result in defective biosynthesis of each of three heterodimeric glycoproteins of the β_2 subfamily: LFA-1 (CD11a/CD18), Mac-1 (CD11b/CD18), and p150,95 (CD11c/CD18).

Before 1980, several reports documented a group of human patients with recurrent bacterial and fungal infections, defective leukocyte motility and phagocytosis, impaired wound healing, and/or delayed umbilical cord severance.[161–169] Crowley et al.[170] first proposed that defects of neutrophil chemotaxis and associated infectious susceptibility were caused by underlying defects of cell adhesion. Moreover, lysates of blood neutrophils in their patient lacked a high-molecular-weight cell-surface glycoprotein termed gp110. Later reports described similar patients lacking leukocyte surface glycoproteins ranging from 130 to 180 kDa.[171,172] This M_r range for deficient glycoproteins was consistent with that of Mac-1, which had been described by that time in mouse and human as an αβ complex with subunits of M_r 165,000 (α) and 95,000 (β) that is present on macrophages, monocytes, neutrophils, and large granular lymphocytes.[173,174] Studies in 1984 by Dana et al.,[175] Anderson et al.,[176] Beatty et al.,[177] and Springer et al.[178] revealed that the α and β subunits of Mac-1 (also designated Mo-1 or CR3) were both deficient on patient leukocytes. Anderson et al.,[176] Springer et al.,[178] and Arnaout et al.[179] also showed that the LFA-1 αβ complex, which had a β subunit identical to that of Mac-1,[173] was deficient on patient neutrophils and lymphocytes. A third type of αβ complex, designated p150,95, was also deficient on patient cells.[180] These findings led to the proposal that the primary defect in this disorder was related to the β subunit, and that biosynthesis of the β subunit was necessary for surface expression of each of the α subunits.[178]

After these early reports appeared, numerous patients with similar clinical features were shown to lack the Mac-1, LFA-1, and p150,95 glycoproteins on neutrophils, monocytes, lymphocytes, and/or transformed B lymphoblasts or T cell lines[42,168,170–172,175,178–202] (reviewed in Anderson et al.[167]). This group of patients who shared similar clinical features and had the same molecular defect clearly defined a distinct pathologic disorder. Because it was identified in several independent laboratories, it was variably referred to as "Mac-1, LFA-1 deficiency disease," "Mo-1 deficiency," "Leu-cam deficiency," or "CR3 deficiency." In the interests of brevity and comprehensiveness, the term "leukocyte adhesion deficiency" (LAD) was proposed in 1987.[167] Very similar clinical disorders recognized in Irish Setter dogs[203,204] and Holstein cattle[205–208] were subsequently described and shown to be due to defects of the β_2 integrin subunit. Thus, the terms "canine LAD" and "bovine LAD" have been adopted.

Bovine LAD was discovered during efforts by the United States Department of Agriculture to develop new methods to prevent mastitis in periparturient dairy cows.[209] As part of these studies, Kehrli et al.[205] identified a Holstein heifer calf who exhibited marked and progressive blood leukocytosis. Analysis of this animal revealed chronic neutrophilia (exceeding 100,000/mm^3) associated with the development of fever and chronic diarrhea leading to death at 48 days of age. Prior to death, in vitro studies of blood neutrophils of the calf revealed several functional abnormalities. As the clinical features of this calf were similar to those of human patients with LAD, further postmortem assessments were performed, including immunoblot analyses of neutrophil lysates, which revealed a total deficiency of Mac-1. Further immunofluorescent analyses indicated diminished amounts of CD18 on blood neutrophils of the calf's dam and sire and diminished amounts of CD18 on neutrophils of 8 of 15 paternal half-siblings, findings consistent with an autosomal recessive disorder.[205] Genealogic studies revealed that the affected proband calf was related to previously reported Holsteins with bovine granulocytopathy syndrome (reviewed in Kehrli et al.[205]), and all of which shared a common ancestor. With the aid of cDNA probes for bovine CD18,[210] it was later shown that a single mutant CD18 allele was prevalent among Holstein cattle worldwide (see below). Bovine LAD represents one of several genetic disorders identified in dairy cattle as a result of highly regulated breeding practices (reviewed in Shuster et al.[210]).

Clinical and Histopathologic Features of Leukocyte Adhesion Deficiency. Clinical and histopathologic features of LAD are remarkably similar among affected human, canine, and bovine subjects.[167,182,203,206] Recurrent necrotic and indolent infections of soft tissues, primarily involving the skin, mucous membranes, and intestinal tract, are the clinical hallmarks of this disease (Fig. 132-3). Superficial infections on body surfaces may invade locally or systemically. Typical small, erythematous, nonpustular skin lesions often progress to large, well-demarcated, ulcerative craters, or "pyoderma gangrenosa" lesions, which heal slowly or with dysplastic eschars.[167,182] Staphylococci or gram-negative enteric bacteria may be cultured from such lesions for up to several weeks despite antimicrobial therapy.

Fulminant progression of soft-tissue of gas gangrene in a distal extremity in one patient prompted surgical amputation as a life-saving measure.[172] Septicemia progressing from omphalitis associated with delayed umbilical cord severance has been observed in several families.[162,163,167,182] Perirectal abscess or cellulitis leading to peritonitis and/or septicemia has been reported in many patients, and facial or deep neck cellulitis has been observed to develop from ulcerative mucous membrane lesions of the oral cavity.[171,172,182] Recurrent invasive candidal esophagitis, erosive gastritis, acute appendicitis, and necrotizing enterocolitis have been reported in many human patients.[167] Recurrent or chronic diarrhea is a common and often lethal complication in affected Holstein cattle.[209] Recurrent otitis media is common, and progression to mastoiditis and facial nerve paralysis has been reported. Other common respiratory infections include severe bacterial (pseudomonal) laryngotracheitis, recurrent pneumonitis, and sinusitis.[167] Severe gingivitis and/or periodontitis is a major feature among all patients who survive infancy. Acute gingivitis always appears during the eruption of the primary dentition. Subsequently, all human and bovine subjects develop characteristic features of a severe, progressive, generalized periodontitis, including gingival proliferation, defective recession, mobility, pathologic migration, and advanced alveolar bone loss associated with periodontal pocket formation and partial or total loss of both the deciduous and permanent dentitions.[182,202,208]

The recurrent infections observed in affected patients appear to reflect a profound impairment of leukocyte mobilization into extravascular inflammatory sites. Skin windows as well as biopsy samples of infected tissues demonstrate inflammatory infiltrates totally devoid of neutrophils.[172,182,196,207] This histopathologic feature is particularly striking considering that marked peripheral blood leukocytosis (5 to 20 times normal values) is a constant feature of this disorder.[182,203,209] Transfusions of leukocytes result in the appearance of donor neutrophils and monocytes in skin windows and in skin chambers.[172] The impaired healing of traumatic or surgical wounds

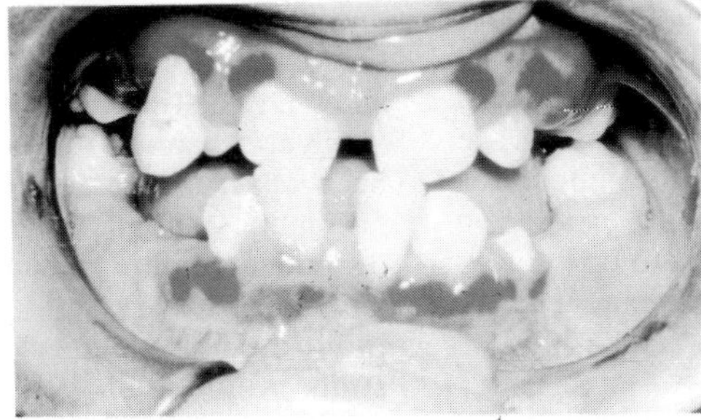
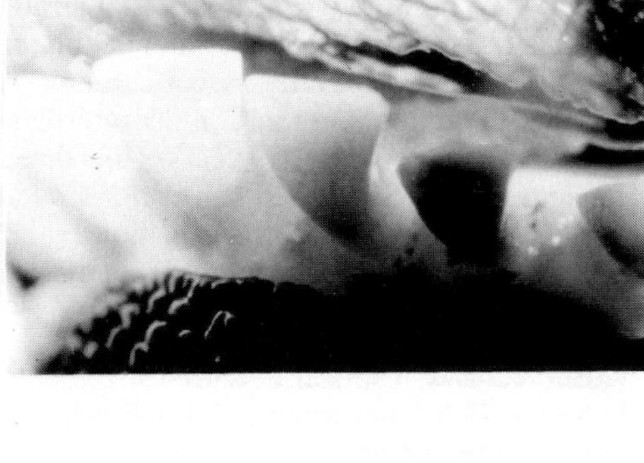
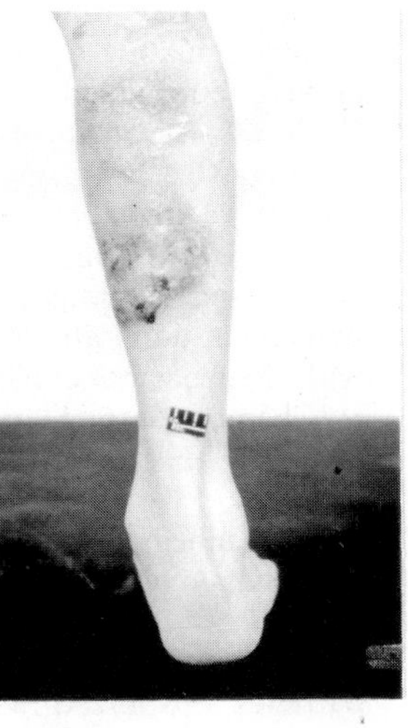
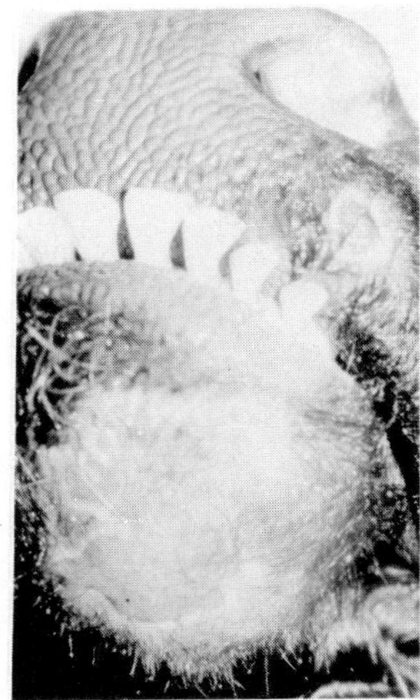
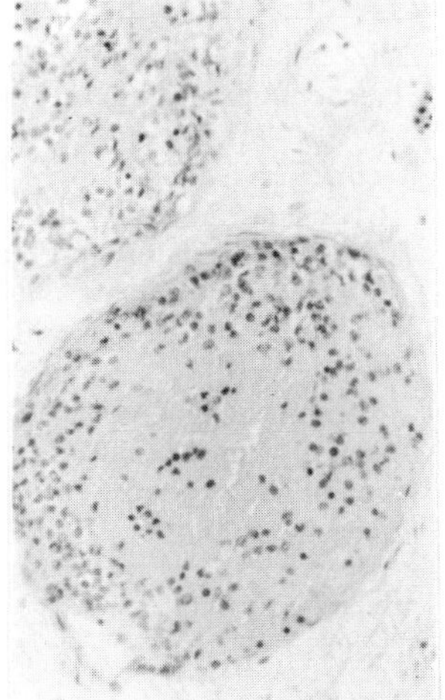

FIG. 132-3 Clinical-pathological characteristics of human or bovine leukocyte adhesion deficiency. Severe gingivitis and periodontal disease involving the permanent dentition of a 9-year-old child (top left) or 9-month-old Holstein heifer (top right) are illustrated. Gingivae exhibit acute inflammation, proliferation, recession, and periodontal pocket formation. Of remaining teeth not prematurely lost or extracted, all exhibit severe mobility. Typical necrotic cutaneous lower extremity ulcers (lower left panel), and ulcers of the cutaneous–mucous membrane junction (lower middle, bovine) are illustrated. *Pseudomonas maltophilia* was culturally isolated from the lower extremity lesions, which failed to heal despite administration of intravenous antibiotics for several weeks. A dysplastic eschar resulted from the chronic superficial infection. Submucosal vessels in an ulcerated and infected region of human ileum that was surgically resected at 18 months of age are shown in the lower right panel. Numerous neutrophils are present in dilated veins, but only a minimal infiltrate of neutrophils is evident in the extravascular connective tissues (H&E; original magnification × 300).

observed in several patients represents a clinical feature not generally observed in patients with neutropenia or dysfunctional neutrophils. Unusual paper-thin or dysplastic cutaneous scars have been found in some patients.[182,211] These may reflect the lack of sufficient monocyte infiltration and the lack of inflammatory contributions to healing, such as the elaboration of angiogenesis factors.[182] A wide spectrum of gram-positive and gram-negative bacterial and fungal infectious microorganisms[167,212] is also characteristic of patients with primary neutropenia syndromes. These patients also demonstrate insufficient tissue leukocyte infiltration. However, the deep-seated granulomatous infections typical of chronic granulomatous disease and other examples of oxidative or nonoxidative intracellular killing deficits have not been observed in LAD.

Some evidence suggests that human patients with LAD have an increased susceptibility to viral infection. Most patients have demonstrated normal, self-limiting courses of varicella or other viral respiratory infections, and five of ten patients in one report[182] showed no untoward reactions to live viral vaccine administration. However, one patient died of an overwhelming infection with picornavirus involving the oropharynx, glottis, trachea, and lungs, and three patients of the same series had one or more episodes of aseptic (presumably viral) meningitis.[182]

The severity of clinical infectious complications among humans with LAD appears to be directly related to the degree of glycoprotein deficiency. Two phenotypes, designated "severe deficiency" and "moderate deficiency," have been defined (Table 132-4 and Fig. 132-4).[167,182,200] As measured by immunofluorescence flow cytometry and verified by radioimmunoassay and immunoprecipitation techniques, four severely deficient patients had essentially undetectable expression of all three complexes[182] on their neutrophils. Six moderately deficient patients expressed 2.5 to 6 percent of all three αβ complexes. Patients with severe deficiency have either died in infancy or have demonstrated a susceptibility to severe, life-threatening systemic infections (peritonitis, septicemia, pneumonitis, aseptic meningitis). In contrast, among the six patients with moderate deficiency (mean age 25 years, range 12 to 43 years), life-threatening infections have been infrequent[182] (Table 132-4). Patients in a given kindred have a similar life span. For example, in one study, three related patients with moderate disease died at ages 22, 19, and 32 years.[213] In other studies of patients with severe disease, five died in their first year and one died at 3 years of age.[163,214,215] In some moderately affected patients, skin lesions may disappear after the first few years of life, recurring only with occasional infections. Severe gingivitis is always observed in these patients and may be the presenting symptom.[202] Delayed umbilical cord separation is more common in patients with the severe phenotype but is not found universally. Heterozygous carriers of alleles with CD18 mutations in human kindreds or Holstein cattle do not show any distinctive clinical features.

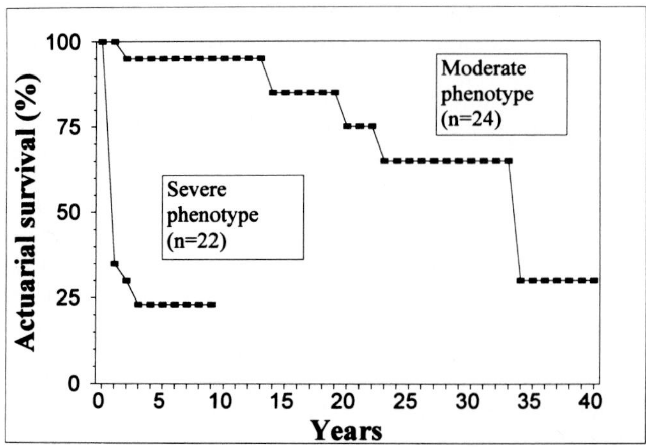

FIG. 132-4 Actuarial survival of patients with LAD. Patients who have undergone bone marrow transplantation are not included. Patients with the severe phenotype were described by Kishimoto et al.[452] (five patients), Brandley et al.[453] (four patients), Ruoslahti and Pierschbacher[454] (one patient), Sheppard et al.[455] (four patients), Phillips et al.[456] (two patients), Erle et al.[457] (one patient), Vogel et al.[458] (two patients), Ginsburg et al.[459] (one patient), and Kunicki et al.[460] (seven patients), and one case from Paris is unpublished. *(From Fisher et al.[200])*

Table 132-4 Clinical Features of Patients with Leukocyte Adhesion Deficiency among Texas Kindreds

Clinical Features	Severe*	Moderate†
Delayed umbilical cord severance	3/4	0/6
Persistent granulocytosis (15,000–161,000/mm³)	4/4	6/6
Recurrent infections:		
Cutaneous abscess or cellulitis	4/4	6/6
Perirectal cellulitis with sepsis	4/4	0/6
Stomatitis and facial cellulitis	4/4	3/6
Gingivitis and periodontitis	4/4	6/6
Pneumonitis	4/4	2/6
Necrotizing enterocolitis, peritonitis	2/4	0/6
Impaired wound healing	3/4	2/6
Parental consanguinity	2/4	3/6
Age range (years)	1 to 14	11 to 44

*Leukocytes from these four patients had less than 0.3 percent normal amounts of Mac-1 on their surfaces.

†Leukocytes from these six patients had 2.5 to 6 percent normal amounts of Mac-1 on their surfaces.

Overall, more profound functional abnormalities have been observed among severely deficient patients.[167,182] Abnormalities of adherence to substrates and of adhesion-dependent functions including chemotaxis and/or aggregation have been observed in almost all patients studied.[143,167,170,182] In vitro, CD18-deficient neutrophils and monocytes demonstrate profound abnormalities of adhesion to and migration through endothelial cell monolayers.[40,130,139,216,217] These abnormalities reflect deficits of the adhesive interactions of Mac-1 and LFA-1 with ICAM-1 and other ligands expressed on vascular endothelial cells[40,139] (see "Molecular Mechanisms Regulating Adhesiveness of Leukocytes" above). The in vivo consequences of these deficits are illustrated in Table 132-4. Deficits of neutrophil transendothelial migration as well as of egress into experimental inflammatory sites are directly related to the degree of CD18 deficiency observed among severe, moderate, and heterozygote patient groups. The finding that heterozygotes have relatively normal neutrophil emigration into experimental skin windows is consistent with their normal clinical status.[167,182,202]

Chemotaxis appears to be affected because it requires adhesion,[182,218] and abnormalities of chemotaxis by CD18-deficient cells are most evident when assay systems that require adhesion for directed migration are used.[218] Binding and phagocytosis of iC3b-opsonized particles is also deficient, in agreement with the identity of the complement receptor type-3 (CR3) with Mac-1.[219] In addition, since particles opsonized with iC3b are phagocytosed poorly, they fail to trigger the respiratory burst or degranulation normally.[162,165,171,176,182,213,220] Abnormalities of neutrophil or monocyte antibody-dependent cellular cytotoxicity have also been observed in several human patients and cattle.[143,182,184,208] In contrast, the adherence-independent cellular functions of CD18-deficient cells elicited by chemotactic factors or phorbol esters are generally normal. These include cell bipolarization,[176] complement receptor type-1 (CR1) up-regulation,[176] L-selectin down-regulation,[68] specific granule release,[176,182] superoxide production induced by phorbol esters,[182] and actin polymerization.[168] Intracellular microbicidal activity (e.g., the ability to kill *Staphylococcus aureus*) is relatively normal in most reported human patients,[172,176,182,213] although diminished killing of this test organism was reported in studies of one cow with bovine LAD.[205] This may reflect the fact that receptors other than CR3 (e.g., FcγR or CR1) are sufficient to promote a normal level of phagocytosis and intracellular killing in these in vitro assays.[176,178,182,221]

In vitro assessments of bovine CD18-deficient neutrophils have shown diminished phagocytosis-associated oxidative and secretory functions during ingestion of iC3b opsonized zymosan, findings similar to those with CD18-deficient human neutrophils. Endocytosis of IgG-opsonized *Staphylococcus aureus* by bovine CD18-deficient neutrophils is significantly reduced, a phenomenon similar to the reported deficiency of IgG-Fc receptor-mediated endocytosis by human CD18-deficient neutrophils. It has been hypothesized that FcγR and Mac-1 interact cooperatively.[185,222] The predominance of recurrent bacterial (as opposed to viral or fungal) infections in patients with LAD implies that the functions of neutrophils or monocytes are more profoundly affected than those of lymphocytes. However, T lymphocyte-mediated killing, proliferative responses, natural killing, and antibody-dependent killing by patients' lymphocytes are deficient compared to those of adult controls.[143,162,184,187,190,197,223,224] In primary mixed lymphocyte cultures, lymphocytes in several studies have demonstrated profoundly diminished cytotoxic and proliferative responses and diminished interferon production.[164,177,187,190] After further stimulation, though, these responses increase to nearly normal levels.[187] This may be due to compensatory mechanisms, perhaps alternative accessory adhesion molecules, and may account for the relatively normal functioning of B and T lymphocytes observed in most patients. Delayed cutaneous hypersensitivity reactions are normal in most patients tested, and most individuals demonstrate normal specific antibody synthesis.[176,193] However, T lymphocyte-dependent antibody responses in vivo (for example, responses to repeated vaccination with tetanus, diphtheria toxoids, and poliovirus) were impaired in some cases, and antibody production in vivo or in vitro in response to influenza virus was found to be abnormal in one patient.[189] Thus, responses of lymphocytes in vivo may be deficient only in patients whose β subunit mutation is particularly deleterious to the expression of LFA-1.

Collectively, these findings imply that in vivo functions of granulocytes and monocytes, including hyperadherence, aggregation, and adhesion-primed cytotoxic functions, are facilitated by an increase in surface expression or functional activation and/or by alterations of the receptor-density distribution for Mac-1 (and presumably for LFA-1 and p150,95) in response to inflammatory mediators. The profound inability of CD18-deficient cells to localize and function normally in inflamed tissues would appear to reflect their inability to up-regulate and/or activate the β_2 heterodimers normally required for avid binding with ICAM-1 and other endothelial ligands or substrates (see "Molecular Mechanisms Regulating Adhesiveness of Leukocytes" above). However, CD18-deficient cells appear capable of normal vascular margination–demargination in vivo,[188] findings indicating that CD18-independent adherence determinants interact with vascular endothelium to mediate this physiological process.

Definition of the Molecular Basis of LAD. Before recombinant DNA reagents for genotypic assessment of LAD patients and their kindreds became available, several lines of evidence supported an autosomal recessive pattern of inheritance for this disorder. Both male and female patients were described in initial reports, and applications of monoclonal antibodies to CD18 subunits in family studies showed heterozygous male and female carriers who expressed $\approx$50 percent of the normal amount of these proteins on their neutrophils and lymphoid cells.[176,182] In three reported families, all the clinically unaffected mothers and fathers and some of the siblings were shown to express intermediate levels of CD18 on their leukocytes.[182] In one family spanning three generations, an affected son was born to heterozygous parents. The affected son married a heterozygote, and the couple bore an affected son and daughter and two heterozygous daughters. These findings, together with the overall equal numbers of male and female patients recognized worldwide[164,182,194,213,214,220] and a frequent history of consanguineous marriages[162,165,182,190,193,215] strongly suggested that LAD is inherited as an autosomal trait. In one kindred,[171,179] X-linked inheritance was suggested, but no definitive evidence for an X-linked form of LAD now exists.

Clinical studies showed that patients with LAD were uniformly deficient in the expression of all three leukocyte integrins,[167] suggesting that a primary defect in the common β subunit of Mac-1, LFA-1, and p150,95 accounted for this disease. To date, none of the reported individuals (human, canine, or bovine) with LAD has demonstrated a selective deficiency of a single β_2 integrin heterodimer. The existence of a defect of the β_2 (CD18) subunit was also suggested by initial biosynthesis studies that used available monoclonal antibodies directed at both subunits of LFA-1. As shown in studies using B lymphocytes transformed with Epstein-Barr virus (EBV) or mitogen-stimulated T-lymphocyte cell lines, normal individuals synthesize LFA-1α (CD11a) and β (CD18) precursors, which associate prior to further carbohydrate processing and transport of $\alpha\beta$ complexes to the cell surface. In contrast, lymphoblasts of patients with LAD synthesize an apparently normal LFA-1α subunit precursor, but this precursor does not undergo normal carbohydrate processing, does not associate with a β precursor, and is never expressed on the cell surface. Such findings indicated that the α subunit of LFA-1 is apparently degraded in the absence of a normal β subunit.[178]

Somatic cell complementation studies further indicated a pathologic role of the β subunit in LAD.[183] In hybrids of human and mouse lymphocytes, human LFA-1α and β subunits from healthy individuals associated with mouse LFA-1$\alpha\beta$ subunits to form interspecies hybrid $\alpha\beta$ complexes. In hybrids of patient and mouse lymphocytes, however, the human α subunit (CD11a) but not β subunit (CD18) was rescued by the formation of interspecies complexes that were expressed on the surface of hybrid cells. Thus, the α subunit of LFA-1 in CD18-deficient cells is competent for biosynthesis and surface expression in the presence of the mouse β_2 (CD18) subunit. These same complementation protocols facilitated mapping of the β_2 subunit to chromosome 21.

Heterogeneity among patients with LAD was first described with respect to the extent of β_2 integrin deficiency on leukocyte surfaces, as shown by flow cytometric or radiolabeled antibody binding assays.[182] As previously discussed, the severity of the clinical features and the magnitude of the functional deficits observed in individual patients is directly related to the degree of protein deficiency[182] (Table 132-4), but the underlying molecular basis for this heterogeneity remained largely undefined. The availability of the CD18 subunit cDNA[35,36] and a rabbit antiserum reactive with the CD18 precursor[225] made possible more precise evaluations of the CD18 subunit of patients. These revealed several distinct phenotypes of CD18 expression and structure among patients previously designated as having the severe or moderate phenotype on the basis of protein expression and clinical features.[182] In one study of six unrelated patients and four related patients plus members of their kindred, the following five distinct variations in CD18 were identified[225]: (1) The CD18 subunit mRNA and protein precursor were undetectable; (2) the quantities of CD18 mRNA and protein precursor were diminished; (3) there was an aberrantly large CD18 subunit precursor, possibly as a result of an extra glycosylation site; (4) there was an aberrantly small CD18 subunit owing to a polypeptide chain defect; and (5) no gross abnormality in the CD18 subunit mRNA or protein precursor was detectable. Findings similar to the latter phenotype were evident in studies of four other patients reported by Dana et al.[226] and one patient described by Dimanche-Boitrel.[227] Despite the presence of apparently normal CD11a and CD18 precursors in this group of patients, neither subunit is processed normally or transported to the cell surface. It is unclear why some of these patients have the moderate and some the severe phenotype.[225–229]

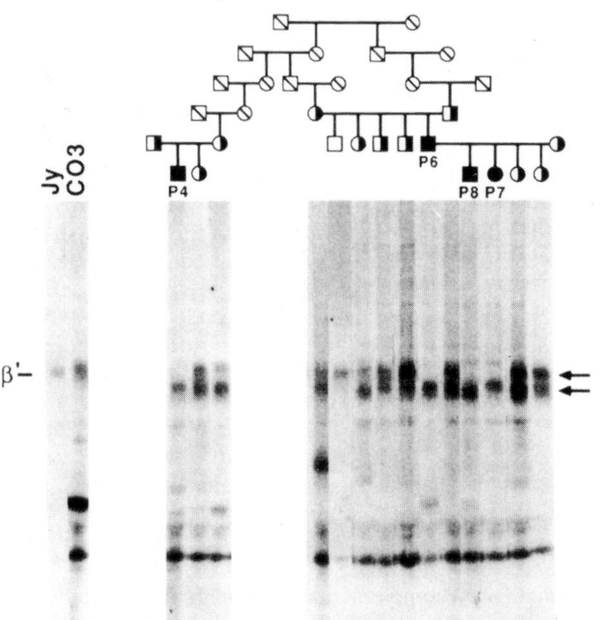

FIG. 132-5 Inheritance of an aberrantly small β (CD18) precursor within a kindred with moderate leukocyte adhesion deficiency. Homozygous deficient patients (P4, 6, 7, and 8, closed symbols), heterozygotes (half-filled symbols), or homozygous noncarriers (open symbols) demonstrate only abnormal β precursor, abnormal and normal β precursor, or only normal precursor, respectively. EBV-transformed cells from a control cell line and from patients with LAD and their kin were pulse-labeled with ^{35}S-methionine. The β subunit precursors were immunoprecipitated with rabbit anti-CD18 serum and protein A-Sepharose. Samples were subjected to SDS-PAGE and autoradiography with fluorography. The normal CD18 precursor and the aberrantly small precursor are indicated by arrows *(From Kishimoto et al.[225] Used by permission.)*

Detailed studies of an extended West Texas kindred including four "unrelated" patients with the moderate phenotype revealed an aberrantly small CD18 precursor of identical size in all of them[230] (Fig. 132-5). Of 10 relatives of this kindred, nine were typed as heterozygous on the basis of protein expression.[182] Each of these showed both the normal and the abnormally small type of CD18 precursor. One noncarrier relative with normal neutrophil surface protein values showed only the normal CD18 precursor. Endoglycosidase H digestion of the *N*-linked carbohydrate from the small CD18 precursor showed that the deficit was in the protein backbone rather than in glycosylation.

Detailed assessments of this kindred by Kishimoto[230] confirmed that an aberrantly small CD18 precursor is synthesized and degraded in patient cells prior to transport to and processing in the Golgi apparatus. However, studies employing large numbers of ^{125}I-labeled patient lymphoblasts revealed that small amounts of normal-sized LFA-1αβ complexes were synthesized and transported to the cell surface, consistent with a moderate phenotype.[182] S1 nuclease protection studies revealed a 90-nucleotide deletion in the CD18 subunit mRNA. Sequence analysis of PCR-amplified cDNA indicated a 90-bp deletion resulting in an in-frame deletion of 30 amino acids in the extracellular domain (Fig. 132-6). Analysis of genomic DNA showed that this 90-bp region is encoded by a single exon (exon 9) in both patients and normal subjects. Sequence analysis of patient genomic DNA revealed a single G-to-C substitution in the third base of the intron following exon 9, suggesting aberrant RNA splicing. A small amount of apparently normally spliced message was detected (by PCR amplification) in patient cells and appears to encode a normal CD18 subunit. This accounts for the low but detectable levels (≈3 to 6 percent of normal) of CD11/CD18 expression in affected patients.

It is significant that the 30-amino-acid deletion recognized in this kindred is located in a 241-amino-acid region of the extracellular domain of CD18 that is highly conserved in evolution. For example, the β subunit of a *Drosophila* integrin shares 35 percent amino acid identity over the whole CD18 subunit but shows 50 percent identity in this sequence,[231] and this sequence, in turn, shares 63 percent amino acid identity with the corresponding region of the fibronectin receptor.[230] It is worth noting that a high percentage of CD18 mutations identified among currently reported kindreds with LAD are contained in this highly conserved segment (Fig. 132-6). Domains within this segment (such as the deleted 30-amino-acid domain described above) are presumably required for αβ precursor association and biosynthesis and may represent critical contact sites between the α and β chain precursors. It is notable that the corresponding region of the β_3 integrin has been directly implicated in binding to peptides containing Arg-Gly-Asp (RGD) sequences. Moreover, a mutation in this region of the β_3 integrin causes Glanzmann thrombasthenia. Patients with this mutation have normal expression of IIb/IIIa on platelets but have defective ligand binding. Thus, this region of the integrin β subunit appears to be critical for both αβ association and ligand binding.

Studies in another patient with a moderate phenotype (patient 10 in Anderson et al.[182])[232] defined distinct mutant alleles of paternal and maternal origin (Fig. 132-6). The paternal allele involves an ATG-to-AAG substitution in the

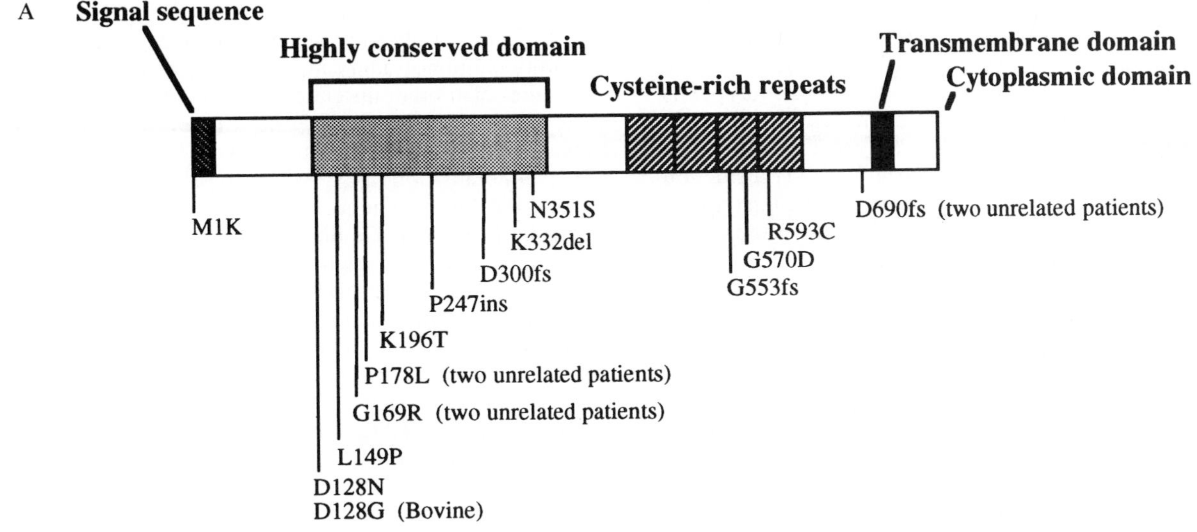

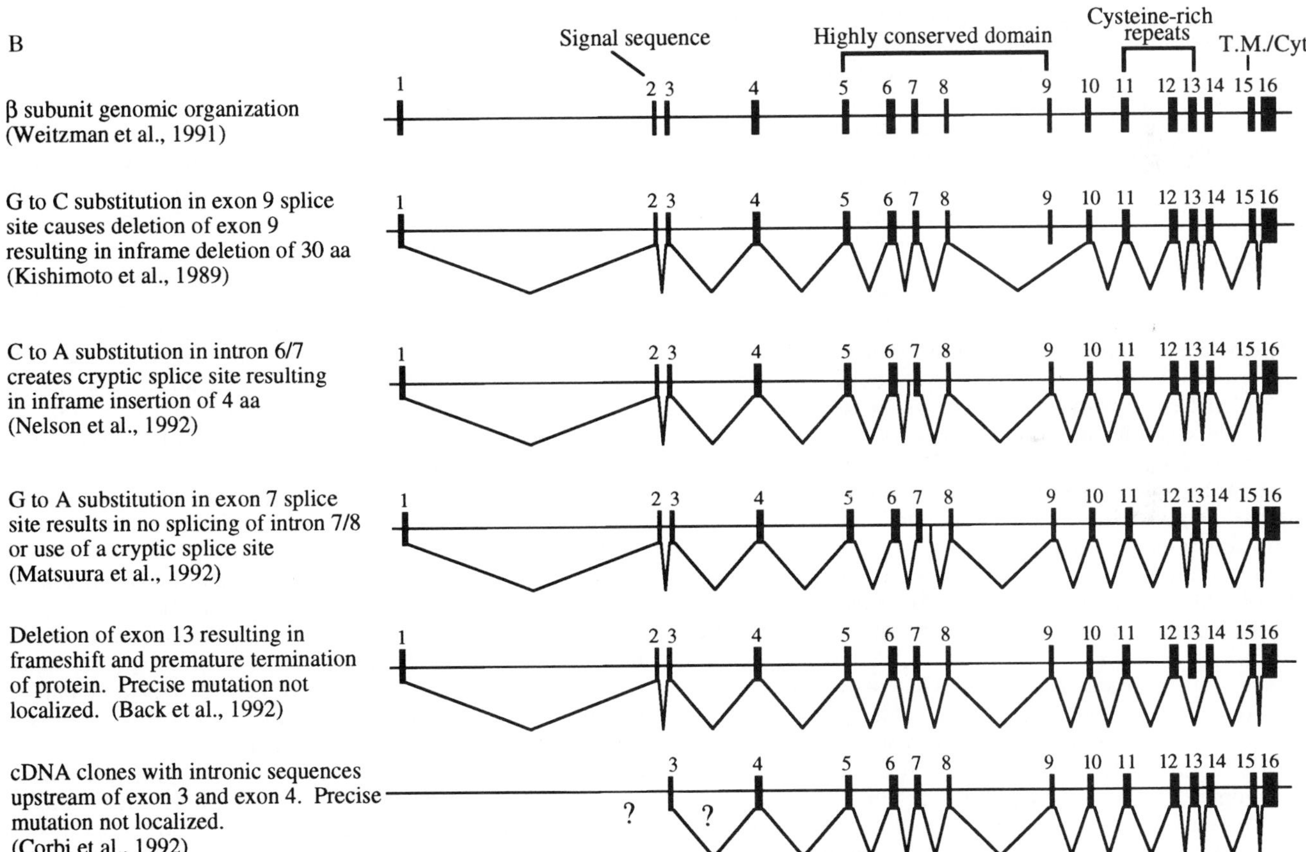

FIG. 132-6 **Mutations in the CD18 gene associated with either severe or moderate phenotypes of leukocyte adhesion deficiency.**

initiation codon of the CD18 mRNA (M1K), and the maternal allele (D690fs, where fs means "frameshift") results from a single T deletion in codon 690 (GAT → GA), 31 nucleotides 5′ to the beginning of the transmembrane domain. (Nucleotide and amino acid numbering for the human is according to Kishimoto et al.[35] although some authors have numbered nucleotides beginning at the start codon.) Studies in expression systems have not yet defined which mutant allele accounts for low levels of apparently normal CD18 protein expression. However, the paternal allele (M1K) most probably allows for low levels of mRNA translation and low-level protein expression. This possibility is suggested by the fact that an alternative translation initiation codon consistent with criteria of Kozak[233] is created by the paternal allelic substitution. Translation via this codon could result in low amounts of an essentially normal-sized message and CD18 protein subunit, as shown in studies of this case by Kishimoto.[225] The predicted result of the maternal mutation is a frameshift in the CD18 subunit mRNA resulting in a premature termination codon and biosynthesis of an aberrantly small CD18 subunit lacking a transmembrane domain and a cytoplasmic tail. Such an "anchorless" subunit might be secreted from the cell, but this possibility has not been confirmed. That the D690fs mutation (maternal allele) does not allow for any biosynthesis of LFA-1 (and therefore cannot account for the patient's moderate phenotype) is strongly supported by the recognition of an identical mutation in another (unrelated) compound heterozygote with a severe phenotype (patient 2 in Anderson et al.[182]).[232] Transfection studies employing each mutant cDNA in mammalian expression systems should permit formal confirmation of the extent to which one or both are capable of promoting CD18 biosynthesis.

Studies in other severe- or moderate-phenotype patients have defined point mutations in the coding region of the CD18 subunit mRNA[228,229,234–236] (Fig. 132-6). Two point mutations were described by Arnaout,[229] one lying in the fourth cysteine-rich repeat [substitution of Cys for Arg at position 593 (R593C)] and the other lying in the 247-amino-acid highly conserved region [substitution of Thr for Lys at position 196 (K196T)]. Each mutant cDNA inhibits expression of LFA-1αβ complexes in COS cells, either completely or partially. Studies of two patients by Wardlaw et al.,[228] one with a moderate phenotype (patient 14 in Anderson et al.[182]) and one with a severe phenotype (patient 2 in Anderson et al.[182]), both of whom had previously been shown to have a normal-sized CD18 subunit precursor, have identified two additional point mutations in an adjacent region of the CD18 subunit cDNA. RNAse mapping and sequence analyses revealed a T-to-C difference (CTA → CCA) resulting in a substitution of Pro for Leu at position 149 (L149P) in one case (patient 14) and a G-to-A transition (GGG → AGG) at amino acid position 169 in another patient (patient 2) substituting an Arg for a Gly (G169R). These mutations are contained in a region of the CD18 subunit cDNA that is highly conserved among the β subunits of the integrin family, as described above. Cotransfection of the CD18 subunit cDNA of patient 2 with wild-type LFA-1α (CD11a) cDNA in COS cells results in no expression of mature protein, whereas similar studies with the CD18 subunit cDNA of patient 14 show detectable but markedly diminished expression of a defective LFA-1 protein (i.e., moderate phenotype). Loss of functional activity as a result of both of these CD18 subunit mutations, as shown with site-directed mutagenesis protocols, suggests that they lie in a site critical for association with α subunit precursors and subsequent biosynthetic events.

Corbi et al.[235] have also identified a Gly-to-Arg substitution at position 169 (G169R) in another patient with severe phenotype. Although detailed phenotypic studies of the patient's family members are not yet available, the known consanguinity in this case and the detection of identical mutations on all analyzed cDNA clones and RT-PCR (reverse-transcriptase polymerase chain reaction) products among this kindred strongly suggest homozygosity of the patient for this CD18 allele. Based on their findings, these investigators emphasized that the highly conserved CD18 domain in which this mutation and several others exist may be critical to CD18 functions, including α chain association and possibly ligand binding. The precise relationship between the kindred identified by Corbi et al. and the one reported by Wardlaw et al.[228] remains uncertain. The former is a Spanish kindred and the latter a Texas kindred of Hispanic origin. Initial genealogic investigations have not found a common inheritance. Studies by Corbi et al.[235] have identified additional abnormalities in some cDNA clones of their patient, including an abnormal sequence immediately 5′ to nucleotide 131, which does not correspond to the 3′ sequence of the intron between exons 2 and 3 of CD18. This suggests the possibility of aberrant splicing in the 5′ region of CD18, an additional abnormality not reported by Wardlaw et al.[228]

Studies of another unrelated compound heterozygote with severe phenotype by Back et al.[234] (previously reported by Bowen[172] and Beatty[177]) identified two CD18 alleles including a 605C→T transition (CCG→CTG) resulting in a substitution of Leu for Pro at amino acid position 178 (P178L). This mutation also lies in the highly conserved region of integrin β subunits. The other mutant allele involves the deletion of 220 base pairs in the cDNA coding for a portion of the extracellular domain and results in a frameshift leading to a premature stop codon. The deleted region (base pairs 1730 through 1950) corresponds to exon 13 of the CD18 gene (Fig. 132-6). It is of considerable interest that the former mutant allele (P178L) has also been identified in an unrelated patient in Japan with a severe phenotype.[236,237] The CD18 mRNA in that patient's B cells was of normal size but was diminished in quantity, to about half normal levels. Sequencing of CD18 cDNA revealed the 605C→T transition and the P178L substitution; this allele was heterozygous in patient genomic DNA and was shown to be of maternal origin. Only limited numbers of transcripts of another allele (lacking the P178L substitution) were detectable. Northern blot analyses revealed reduced CD18 mRNA levels in the patient's father and brother, suggesting that the paternal allele in this compound heterozygote patient causes defective expression of mRNA. Considered together, studies in this patient and that of Back[234] indicate that the P178L allele does not allow for any CD18 biosynthesis.

Still another report by Nelson et al.[238] emphasizes the critical nature of the highly conserved domain in CD18. These investigators identified two distinct mutant maternal alleles in a patient with moderate phenotype. These were (1) a 12-bp insertion in the cDNA that added four amino acids (Pro-Ser-Ser-Gln between Pro 247 and Glu 248) and arose from a single C-to-A transversion in the 3′ terminus of an intron, which generated an aberrant splice receptor site, and (2) an 1828C→T nucleotide transition (CGG→TGG) resulting in an Arg-to-Trp substitution at position 586 (R586W) (Fig. 132-6). A third mutation, an 1124A→G1124 nucleotide transition (AAT→AGT) resulting in an N351S amino acid substitution, was a de novo mutation not found in either parent. To determine the molecular basis of the moderate-deficiency phenotype, these investigators transfected COS cells with normal CD11b cDNA and mutant CD18 cDNAs. The maternal double mutant allele allowed for virtually no surface expression of CD11b/CD18 complex on COS cells. Further analysis showed that this phenotype is due to the four-amino-acid insertion: the R586W mutation alone allowed near-normal expression of CD11b/CD18, suggesting that this may be benign polymorphism. The third mutation, N351S, allowed 22 percent of normal CD11b/CD18 expression as measured by one anti-CD18 monoclonal antibody (60.3), although a second monoclonal antibody (TS1/18) showed no detectable expression. Taken together, these results suggest that the N351S mutation may account for the moderate-deficiency phenotype. It is interesting that the critical insertion mutation and the N351S mutations are in the highly conserved region of the β subunit.

Matsuura et al.[239] described distinct mutant CD18 alleles in two additional patients with the severe phenotype of LAD. In one patient the mutant gene expressed an aberrant mRNA, 1.2 kb longer than usual, resulting from a G-to-A substitution at the splice donor site of a 1.2-kb intron (between exons 7 and 8). Several aberrantly spliced messages arising from cryptic donor sites were also noted. These mutations apparently result in premature termination of translation and abolish CD18 biosynthesis. In a second patient,[240] they identified a G-to-A transition at nucleotide 454 resulting in a substitution of Asn for Asp at position 128 (D128N) and a complete disruption of CD18 biosynthesis. The Asp128 residue is the site of another point mutation resulting in bovine LAD (described below) and is also located in the conserved domain of β integrins.

Investigations prompted by the recognition of bovine LAD[205] led to the identification of a single mutant allele prevalent among Holstein cattle.[208–210] Two point mutations were identified by Shuster et al.[210] in the gene encoding CD18 in a Holstein calf afflicted with this disorder. One mutation causes an Asp-to-Gly substitution at amino acid position 128 (D128G) in the highly conserved region of the extracellular domain of CD18, in which several human mutations have also been identified (Fig. 132-6). A second mutation is silent. Twenty calves with clinical symptoms of LAD were subsequently shown to be homozygous for the D128G allele, and two calves who were shown to be homozygous for this allele by random DNA testing were subsequently shown to exhibit the clinical syndrome. Widespread DNA testing has revealed that the carrier frequency for the D128G allele is approximately 15 percent among Holstein bulls and 6 percent among Holstein cows in the United States. This high carrier rate predicts an incidence of 0.2 percent among Holstein calves in this country. Moreover, many calves with this phenotype have been identified in Europe and Japan.[205] All cattle shown to carry the D128G allele are related to one bull who, through the use of artificial insemination, sired many thousands of calves in the 1950s and 1960s. As predicted based on available breeding records, the D128G mutation is prevalent among Holstein cattle worldwide. However, the organization of the dairy industry and the availability of a rapid DNA diagnostic tool should permit rapid eradication of LAD from Holstein populations.

The currently recognized human mutant CD18 alleles as well as the bovine LAD point mutation are summarized in Fig. 132-6 and Table 132-5. Identified alleles span most of

Table 132-5 Mutations in CD18 Identified in LAD Kindreds*

Nucleotide	Protein	Phenotype	Reference
1155+3G→C Homozygous	Skip exon 9	Moderate Four in kindred	230
518T→C (CTA→CCA) Not determined	L149P ?	Moderate	228
577G→A (GGG→AGG) Homozygous or other allele not expressed	G169R ?	Severe	228
1849C→T (CGT→TGT) 659A→C (AAA→ACA)	R593C K196T	Moderate	229
74T→A (ATG→AAG) 2142delT (GAT→GA)	M1K D690 frameshift	Moderate	232
2142delT (GAT→GA) Not determined	D690 frameshift ?	Severe	232
605C→T (CCG→CTG) Genomic not determined	P178L Skip exon 13	Severe	234
1124A→G (AAT→AGT) de novo 1828C→T (CGG→TGG) and 814-14C→A	N351S R586W (?benign) and splice insertion of four amino acids	Moderate	238
605C→T (CCG→CTG) Transcriptional defect	P178L Absent mRNA	Severe	236, 237
577G→A (GGG→AGG) Probably homozygous, possible splicing	G169R	Severe	235
969+1G→A Homozygous	Splicing truncation	Severe	239
454G→A (GAC→AAC) Homozygous	D128N ?	Severe	239
1781G→A (GGC→GAC) Not determined	G570D ?	Severe	245a
383G→A (GAC→GGC) Homozygous	D128G	Cattle; severe	210

*Each entry represents a patient or kindred, with both alleles indicated separately where known. Nucleotide and amino acid numbering for human is according to Kishimoto et al.,[35] although some authors have numbered nucleotides beginning at the start codon. Style for mutation nomenclature is according to Beaudet and Tsui.[471]

the coding region of the extracellular domain of CD18 and include mutations of exonic as well as intronic sequences. At least four examples of identical mutant alleles have been recognized among apparently unrelated kindreds. It is significant that a disproportionate number of mutant alleles are found in the 241-amino-acid domain that is highly conserved among β integrin subunits (exons 5 through 9) or in a segment encoded by exon 13. The cluster of mutations occurring in the former (conserved) domain includes six distinct single-amino-acid substitutions, which are variably deleterious to CD18 expression. It is of interest that mutations in this domain associated with severe (complete) deficiency involve amino acid residues conserved in all other integrin β subunits,[210,228,234,238] while some alleles associated with a moderate phenotype involve nonconserved amino acids (e.g., L149P and K196T).[228,229]

In addition to these alleles, three splicing mutations have been defined in the conserved domain of CD18. They include an in-frame addition of four amino acids,[238] an in-frame deletion of 30 amino acids (exon 9),[230] and a G-to-A substitution in the exon 7 splice site resulting in aberrant splicing and premature chain termination.[239] These findings provide indirect evidence that this region may be critical to common structural and functional characteristics of β integrin subunits, including the associations of α and β precursors. Electron microscopic studies of $\alpha_5\beta_1$ and other integrins indicate that such subunit associations involve N-terminal domains.[241,242] Moreover, this domain in the β_3 integrin (gpIIb) contains an RGD binding site,[243] a fibrinogen binding site,[244] and a putative divalent cation binding site,[245] each of which is implicated in gpIIb/IIIa ligand binding. A point mutation resulting in an Asp-to-Tyr substitution in β_3 has been shown to underlie deficient RGD binding by gpIIb/IIIa in a patient with Glanzmann thrombasthenia.[245]

A cluster of mutations is evident in the CD18 segment encoded by exon 13, including three different single-amino-acid substitutions and a skipping of exon 13 that results in a loss of reading frame.[229,234,238,245a] Of the three point mutations, two involve amino acids conserved in all β integrins (R593C and G570D), and the third (R586W), which may not be deleterious, involves an amino acid that is not conserved among β integrins. Transfection studies indicate that the R586W mutation allows near-normal expression of CD18[238] but that the R593C mutation abolishes receptor expression.[229] The mechanisms by which exon 13 mutations impair CD11/CD18 expression are uncertain, but this region is a component of the cysteine-rich repeats proposed to impart structural rigidity to β integrin subunits. Mutations involving this region may impede heterodimer formation by introducing conformational changes that preclude stable association of these and other CD18 domains with those of CD11 subunits.

This spectrum of CD18 mutations provides an incomplete explanation for the considerable heterogeneity recognized among patients with LAD. In addition to quantitative abnormalities of expression, relative functional defects of CD18-deficient cells are probably also caused by structural alterations of expressed proteins in certain cases. Studies reported by Wardlaw et al.[228] and Nelson et al.[238] suggest the presence of such structural modifications in certain epitopes, as shown by the finding that selected anti-CD18 monoclonal antibodies fail to bind to expressed mutant protein. Similar studies may prove useful in further defining structural relationships of CD18.

Prospects for Somatic Cell Gene Replacement Therapy for LAD. The introduction of a normal CD18 subunit gene into hematopoietic cells should cure LAD. The relative success of allogenic bone marrow transplantation in treating patients with LAD indicates that the hematopoietic stem cell would be an appropriate target for CD18 gene transfer.[200,247] Studies by Marlin[183] showed that the mouse β (CD18) subunit can complex with and rescue surface expression of human LFA-1α subunits in patient/mouse lymphocyte hybrids. More recent studies by Hibbs et al.[248] demonstrated normal expression of CD11a/CD18 (LFA-1) on EBV-transformed lymphoblasts from CD18-deficient patients following transfection with a normal CD18 subunit cDNA contained in an EBV-based vector. Transfections resulted in stable expression of near-normal levels of functional LFA-1 in cells of four patients with distinct phenotypes. These studies unequivocally confirmed that the primary defect in LAD is in the β_2 subunit.

Wilson et al.[249] described the use of recombinant retroviruses to correct the genetic and functional defects in lymphocytes from a patient with CD18-deficiency. EBV-transformed, CD18-deficient lymphocytes were infected with CD18-expressing retroviruses and enriched for cells that expressed LFA-1 on the cell surface using monoclonal antibodies and fluorescence-activated cell sorting. Enrichment of LFA-1-bearing cells was associated with a coordinate enrichment in the frequency of proviral sequences and the amount of viral-directed CD18 RNA, findings indicating that the selected phenotype resulted from the expression of the retroviral-induced CD18 gene. Moreover, the proportion of cells expressing LFA-1 accurately predicted the frequency of retroviral infection, as shown by Southern blot analysis. Expression on the surface of infected cells of functional LFA-1 was shown by the fact that phorbol myristate acetate (PMA) elicited LFA-1-dependent homotypic aggregation.[37]

Similar studies have been reported by Back et al.[234,250] Those investigators used an alternative amphotropic retroviral vector to transfect the CD18 cDNA in K562 human myeloid leukemia cells and into EBV-transformed B lymphoblasts from a child with LAD. Transfer of the LCD18SN retroviral construct, which expresses the CD18 cDNA from the Moloney murine leukemia virus long terminal repeat (MoMuLV LTR), into K562 cells resulted in relatively high levels of CD18 mRNA and intracellular protein. Retroviral-mediated transfer of CD18 into lymphoblasts from a patient with LAD resulted in low levels of surface expression (5 percent of normal) of CD11a/CD18. Wilson et al.[251] also constructed a retroviral vector expressing CD18 with the MoMuLV LTR as the promoter, and both high-titer ecotropic and amphotropic producer cell lines were isolated. Infection of CD18-deficient lymphoblasts resulted in expression of immunodetectable CD18 at 35 to 40 percent of normal levels in 55 to 60 percent of cells and the restoration of CD 18-dependent aggregation (Fig. 132-7). This relatively high level of expression, as compared to that reported by Wilson[249] and Back et al.[250] is probably due to a high viral titer, which was determined based on expression of the CD18 antigen in 3T3/CD11a cells.

The successful transfer of CD18 into CD18-deficient lymphoblasts prompted further studies in murine models to evaluate the potential for somatic cell gene therapy of LAD.[251,253] Retroviral infection of murine bone marrow cells was first reported by Krauss et al.[253] They employed two retroviral vectors (one with a chicken β-actin promoter and one with the same promoter plus a CMV enhancer) to infect mouse bone marrow cells. Wilson et al. used the ecotropic virus eco-hCD18 for the same purpose.[251] Krauss et al. achieved expression in a variable percentage of granulocytes

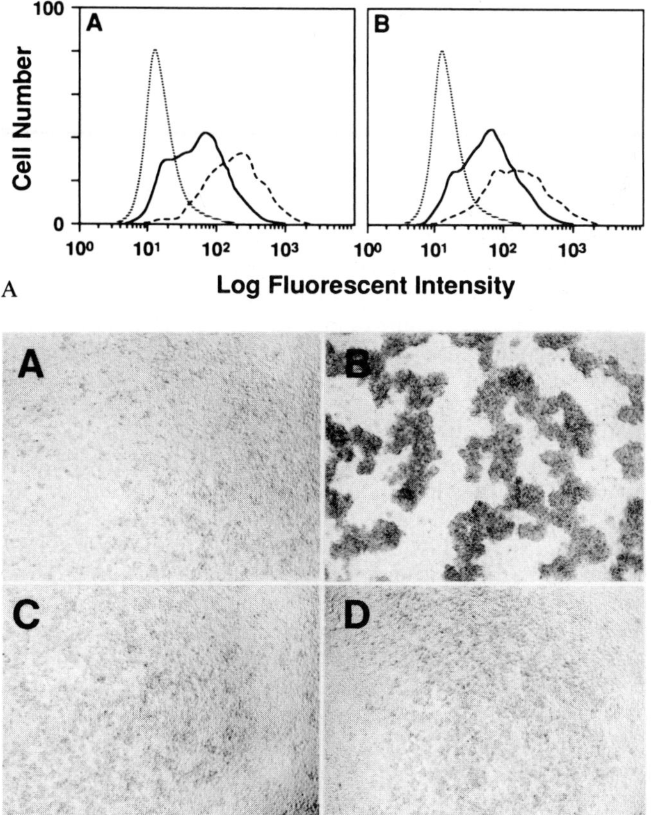

FIG. 132-7 **Studies of somatic cell gene therapy of human LAD in vitro.** ***(A)*** **Immunofluorescent flow cytometry of EBV lymphoblasts from an LAD patient after infection with pΔNN2-hCD18. EBV lymphoblasts from a severely deficient LAD patient expressing no detectable cell surface CD18 were infected by co-cultivation with am-hCD18 and then stained with monoclonal antibody to human CD11a (*panel A*), or CD18 (*panel B*). Dashed line is normal human control EBV-lymphoblasts, solid line is LAD EBV-lymphoblasts infected with pΔNN2-hCD18, and dotted line is LAD EBV-lymphoblasts treated by mock infection.** ***(B)*** **PMA-induced aggregation of LAD EBV lymphoblasts. LAD EBV lymphoblasts were infected with pΔNN2-hCD18 by co-cultivation with am-hCD18, then treated with PMA to induce self-aggregation. Mock-infected cells (*panel A*) failed to aggregate, while pΔNN2-hCD18-infected cells aggregated in large clumps (*panel B*). The PMA-induced aggregation was blocked by incubation of infected cells with monoclonal antibodies to CD11a (TS1/22) (*panel C*) or to CD18 (R15.7) (*panel D*), demonstrating that the aggregation was CD18-dependent.**

at 6 weeks after transplantation with no detectable expression in 60 percent of the animals and only two of 60 animals expressing in >25 percent of cells. The latter investigators observed expression in 17 to 36 percent of granulocytes in all of 16 animals at two weeks after transplantation, with a significant decrease to 7 to 18 percent of cells 4 weeks after transplantation. The exact level of expression of human CD18 in mouse cells is of limited significance since the human β_2 subunit must compete with the mouse β_2 subunit to combine with various α subunits. The failure to elicit expression in mouse lymphocytes in both studies may reflect (1) low expression of the mouse CD11a subunit, (2) poor ability of the human β_2 subunit to compete with the mouse subunit, (3) technical difficulties in detecting low-level CD18 expression in lymphocytes versus granulocytes, or (4) decreased expression from the viral LTR in lymphocytes. Nonetheless, the observations of both groups indicate the feasibility of retroviral expression of CD18 in mouse bone marrow cells, but high efficiency for transfection of stem cells and for long-term expression have not yet been achieved. As one approach, Wilson et al.[254] have used homologous recombination to obtain mice deficient in CD18 for applications as a model for gene therapy.

Preliminary efforts toward somatic cell gene therapy of human LAD have been recently reported by Yorifuji et al.[255] Retroviral producer clones were obtained using the GP + envAm12 amphotropic cell lines. Amphotropic virus was used to infect bone marrow cells from normal volunteers and from patients with LAD. Ficoll–Hypaque-separated bone marrow cells were infected with virus and plated in long-term culture using bone marrow stromal cell feeder layers. PCR analysis of CFU-C colonies initiated after 5 weeks in culture indicated that 30 to 70 percent of the granulocyte/monocyte (GM) colonies contained the provirus. Similar results were observed when infection was performed by cocultivation for 72 h or by addition of viral supernatant. When bone marrow cells of a patient with a severe phenotype were infected, CD18 was expressed on the surface of ≈20 percent of "floating" cells after 10 days in culture, indicating that the virus produced CD18 heterodimers not detectable on bone marrow cells of this patient prior to infection.

Other Disorders Characterized by Diminished Adhesion

Abnormalities of Mac-1 (CD11b/CD18) and L-Selectin in Neonates. Inflammatory deficits related to development that have been observed in human and animal neonates appear to involve defects of neutrophil localization or emigration at sites of inflammation.[256–259] These functional aberrations have important implications with respect to host defenses or inflammatory injury in neonates. Since specific immunity is limited in the immediate postpartum period, the inflammatory functions of phagocytic cells are especially important for host defense against microbial invasion.[256] Several lines of investigation suggest that both quantitative and functional deficits of neutrophils/monocytes contribute to susceptibility to infection.[217,260–262] As these functional deficits are observed commonly among healthy neonates, such abnormalities may play a physiological role in limiting inflammatory responses that might be deleterious in immature hosts.[262]

The most consistently observed functional abnormalities of neonatal neutrophils are those involving chemotactic responses in vitro. Neonatal neutrophils exhibit impaired responses to numerous chemotactic factors, including those released by growing *Staphylococcus aureus* and *E. coli* (e.g., f-Met-peptides), and those generated in plasma by antigen–antibody complexes (e.g., the C5a component of complement).[27,263] Visual assays demonstrate that neonatal cells are significantly impaired not only in their migration but in their ability to orient toward a gradient of chemotactic factors.[27,264] Depressed chemotaxis has been found in healthy neonates 1 to 5 days old,[265,266] although more striking abnormalities have been reported in premature infants. In addition, there is diminished generation of chemotactic activity (chemotaxigenesis) by virulent type III group B streptococci in neonatal sera; the defect is directly related to diminished levels of both type-specific anticapsular antibody and serum complement activity.[267]

Evidence exists that impaired chemotactic functions of neonatal neutrophils are functionally linked to abnormalities in cell adherence.[27,217,259,261,262,264,268–271] At least two distinct abnormalities of neutrophil adhesion to endothelial cells or protein substrates in vitro have been recognized. Chemotactic factors fail to stimulate adhesion of neonatal neutrophils to artificial or endothelial substrates,[27,217,270,272] apparently as a result of a reduction of the up-regulation and/or functional activation of the Mac-1 heterodimer normally elicited by chemotactic factors or phorbol esters.[270-275] Transendothelial migration by neonatal neutrophils in vitro is diminished but not absent as observed with CD18-deficient neutrophils, apparently because expression of LFA-1 on neonatal cells is normal and contributes to both adhesion and migration.[40,217]

Neonatal neutrophils also exhibit diminished adhesion to IL-1-stimulated endothelial cells when studied under conditions of flow (wall shear stress ≈ 2 dynes/cm^2) that select for CD18-independent adhesion mechanisms.[262,276] This abnormality apparently results from markedly diminished surface levels of L-selectin on circulating blood neutrophils or eosinophils of healthy, term human neonates.[262,276] A similar deficiency has been found on blood neutrophils of neonatal rabbits.[277] Monoclonal antibodies recognizing L-selectin fail to significantly inhibit adhesion of neonatal neutrophil suspensions under these experimental conditions, in contrast to their potent inhibitory effects when incubated with normal neutrophils. The basis for these findings is not yet defined but may relate to high levels of GM-CSF (and/or other plasma factors), as demonstrated in umbilical cord blood and placental tissues in some studies.[278] GM-CSF, like chemotactic factors, stimulates the shedding of L-selectin from blood neutrophils in vitro and significantly diminishes neutrophil emigration into experimental skin windows of adult volunteers.[279] In studies of cord blood or neonatal neutrophils, Koenig et al.[280] have shown that diminished levels of neutrophil L-selectin are inversely related to total blood neutrophil count, and similar relationships have been reported in neonatal rabbits.[277]

Deficits of Mac-1 as well as L-selectin may contribute to diminished leukocyte sequestration in neonates, but direct evidence for this is currently lacking. Inflammatory responses in human newborns have been quantitated via Rebuck skin window studies.[281,282] Such assessments have failed to demonstrate strikingly diminished neutrophil mobilization but did show two other abnormalities—(1) a slower and less pronounced shift from the early granulocyte to later mononuclear cell predominance and (2) a marked eosinophilia in some infants 2 to 21 days old. Strikingly diminished leukocyte mobilization in neonatal rats inoculated intraperitoneally with bacteria or chemotactic agents has been reported.[257] Recent studies in neonatal rabbits also indicate a reduction in both CD18-dependent and L-selectin-dependent neutrophil accumulation in inflamed peritoneum, as indirectly shown using monoclonal antibodies administered intravenously before thioglycolate instillation.[283]

Specific Granule Deficiency. Neutrophils contain subpopulations of granules.[284] Azurophil or primary granules appear early in neutrophil development and contain lysosomal enzymes, including lysozyme and myeloperoxidase. Specific or secondary granules develop later and contain a different set of constituents (e.g., chemotactic receptors, lactoferrin, CD11b/CD18).[285,286] The first example of a deficiency of specific granules was recognized in 1972,[287] and other cases have been subsequently reported by several laboratories.[221,285,288-294] One patient[287] appeared to have an acquired deficiency (associated with a myeloproliferative syndrome), while all others appeared to have genetically determined disease. Each has demonstrated susceptibility to recurrent and severe infections of the skin, mucous membranes, and lung, most commonly due to *Staphylococcus aureus, Pseudomonas aeruginosa,* other enteric pathogens, and *Candida albicans*. Detailed descriptions of the histopathology of infected tissues have not been reported in all patients, but skin window studies demonstrated diminished leukocyte sequestration in tissues of some individuals who were not neutropenic.[285,288] The prognosis for patients with this disorder is not well defined, but most individuals have survived childhood with supportive and antimicrobial therapy.

Neutrophils from each patient studied have shown distinct morphologic abnormalities, including a severe or total deficiency of specific granules and a variety of nuclear abnormalities, including bilobed or multilobed nuclei and nuclear blebs, clefts, or pockets. The membrane marker alkaline phosphatase has been shown to be diminished or absent in neutrophils of all but one reported patient, and the total cellular content and/or release of the secondary granule markers (lactoferrin, B_{12} transport protein, cytochrome b, and lysozyme) has been shown to be diminished in most patients. Neutrophils of these patients also lack defensins, localized to the azurophil granules.[295] Azurophil granules of patient cells show a lower density on sucrose gradients than azurophil granules of normal neutrophils.[285] In addition, patients with this disorder have abnormal platelet α granules and lack eosinophil-specific granules (J.I. Gallin, unpublished observations). Thus, functional abnormalities in this disorder are not limited to neutrophils, and the secretory proteins absent from patient neutrophils are not limited to specific granules.

Somewhat heterogenous abnormalities of in vitro neutrophil functions have been observed. Defects of chemotaxis and intracellular microbicidal activity are most consistently reported. The basis of impaired neutrophil locomotion in vitro or diminished accumulation in skin windows in vivo is uncertain. However, in studies of two patients,[221,285,288] defective neutrophil chemotaxis appeared to be functionally related to abnormalities of adherence. One patient's neutrophils showed diminished adherence to nylon fibers and endothelial cells as well as impaired homotypic aggregation in response to f-Met-Leu-Phe.[288] Neutrophils of another patient failed to enhance CR3 (Mac-1) expression in response to f-Met-Leu-Phe, although up-regulation of the CR1 was normal.[221] Immunoprecipitation studies employing monoclonal antibodies against CD11b and CR1 showed that Mac-1 (but not CR1) cosediments with specific granule fractions of normal neutrophils. CR1 is apparently associated with unique microvesicular bodies in neutrophils, which are not associated with specific granules.

The molecular basis for the complex cellular abnormalities of these patients is undefined. Indirect evidence implicates abnormalities of the regulation of gene expression during granulopoiesis resulting in a failure to activate a cassette of genes normally expressed at the myelocyte–metamyelocyte stage of maturation.[295,296] For example, studies of two patients showed no detectable lactoferrin biosynthesis in neutrophils and only trace amounts of lactoferrin transcripts in bone marrow cells.[297] However, lactoferrin biosynthesis in nasal secretory glands and other nonmyeloid tissues was normal in these patients, indicating that the abnormality of lactoferrin gene expression is tissue-specific and limited to cells of myeloid lineage.

Rambon-Hasharon Syndrome. Frydman et al.[298] recently described two male Arab patients (ages 5 and 3) who were both born of unrelated consanguineous matings. Distinctive clinical features of these patients included craniofacial dysmorphism, neurologic deficits (microcephaly, cortical atrophy, central hypotonia, seizures, and developmental delay), recurrent respiratory infections, and striking peripheral blood neutrophilia. That these patients represent examples of a new, presumably autosomal recessive, syndrome was suggested by the finding that both patients lack the red-blood-cell H antigen and manifest the Bombay (hh) phenotype. This phenotype is due to a homozygosity for a rare recessive (h) allele. Individuals with this phenotype generally lack the H antigen, an intermediate in the production of A and B antigens of red blood cells. The H gene product is an α2 fucosyltransferase which catalyzes the addition of a GDP fucose to *N*-acetylgalactosamine to produce the H antigen.[299,300] The Hh system is genetically heterogeneous, and both complete (Bombay) and incomplete (para-Bombay) deficiencies are recognized. In contrast to the patients described here, individuals with these phenotypes do not have any distinctive clinical features.

The findings of markedly elevated blood neutrophil counts (60 to 150 $\times$ $10^3/mm^3$) in the patients reported by Frydman prompted studies of leukocyte functions in vitro. These revealed significant defects of random and directed neutrophil migration and diminished homotypic aggregation of neutrophils. In contrast, opsonophagocytic and bactericidal activities of patient neutrophils were normal, as were lymphocyte proliferation and natural killer cell activities. Unlike the leukocytes of patients with LAD, the leukocytes of these patients showed normal levels of surface CD18.

Several features of this syndrome suggest the possibility of a glycosylation defect that might influence the expression of sialyl-Lewis X (sLe^X) [NeuAcα2,3Galβ1,4(Fucα1,3)GlcNac], a carbohydrate ligand of the endothelial adhesion molecules E-selectin and P-selectin. In addition to this rare Bombay phenotype, both patients were nonsecretors and Lewis negative, blood groups associated with Fucα2,Gal and Fucα1,3/4GlcNac linkages, respectively.[102,301] Since each of these carbohydrate structures contain fucose, Etzioni et al.[302] tested the possibility that patient leukocytes were deficient in sLe^X, which also contains fucose. Flow-cytometric studies using an anti-sLe^X monoclonal antibody confirmed a complete absence of this determinant on neutrophils of both patients. Additional studies demonstrated profoundly diminished adherence of patient neutrophils to IL-1-stimulated endothelial monolayers bearing high levels of E-selectin. These findings suggest that the clinical features of neutrophilia and recurrent pulmonary infections in this syndrome reflect leukocyte adherence defects caused by a lack of the sLe^X-bearing ligands required for selectin-mediated adhesion to endothelial cells. This concept is supported by intravital microscopic studies of patient neutrophils in rabbit mesenteric venules primed for 4 h with IL-1, a situation in which human neutrophils normally demonstrate rolling margination in vivo.[303] Isolated patient neutrophils exhibit markedly reduced rolling adhesion in this model, a finding consistent with the concept that lectin–carbohydrate interactions are necessary for this phase of localization (Fig. 132-2 and Table 132-3; see "Molecular Mechanisms Regulating Adhesiveness of Leukocytes" above).

Studies of this novel syndrome provide strong evidence for important adhesive interactions of sLe^X-bearing ligands and E-selectin in neutrophil migration and recruitment at sites of inflammation in vivo. This possibility is also supported by in vitro investigations and in vivo animal model studies demonstrating that selectins mediate adhesion of neutrophils (and presumably other leukocyte cell types) to vascular endothelium under flow conditions in postcapillary venules.[100,107,123,124,127,304,305] Since P-selectin has also been shown to recognize sLe^X-containing ligands,[107] it is possible that neutrophils of these patients will be defective in P-selectin-mediated adherence functions. It is uncertain whether sLe^X deficiency underlies other neutrophil defects, but the observed defects of homotypic aggregation may reflect the requirement for L-selectin (which is decorated with this carbohydrate ligand) in this process, as recently proposed by Simon.[306] Future studies to elucidate the specific biochemical defects and resulting functional and pathologic consequences in this syndrome should lead to additional insights concerning the physiological roles of selectin-dependent adhesion reactions.

Inflammatory Disorders Characterized by Enhanced Adhesion

As is well illustrated by the patients with CD18 deficiency, the localization and functional activities of blood neutrophils and mononuclear leukocytes normally provide for immunologic host defense and repair of tissues. However, these cells can mediate tissue injury.[307–309] Intercellular adhesion is also involved in these proinflammatory injurious events, not only because the localization and infiltration of leukocytes in inflamed tissues is determined by specific interactions of adhesion molecules, but, in addition, because adhesion to biologic substrates (i.e., other cells or matrix proteins) appears to prime or amplify the cytotoxic functions of leukocytes (e.g., oxidative or secretory processes).[51,310–312] Neutrophil- or monocyte-mediated vascular and tissue injury has been implicated in a number of clinical entities in which the induction of leukocyte or endothelial adhesion mechanisms have been demonstrated or inferred.[307,313] Among these are ischemia–reperfusion states (including hypovolemic shock with multiple organ injury), allograft rejection, and various acute and chronic inflammatory conditions.

Two lines of evidence in vivo are consistent with the concept that β_2 integrins participate in inflammatory tissue injury. These are (1) observations of elevated levels of Mac-1 on circulating and tissue leukocytes and of elevated levels of ICAM-1 in tissues in inflammatory models or clinical disorders and (2) observations of potent antiinflammatory effects of monoclonal antibodies directed at CD11/CD18 subunits or their ligands in animal models of inflammation (see below and Table 132-6). The participation of CD18 adhesion molecules in these pathologic conditions is not unexpected, considering that diverse inflammatory mediators are capable of regulating the expression and functions of these proteins and, thus, promoting elevated leukocyte adherence to endothelial cells and other cell types in vitro.[314]

Early work using experimental animals showed that elevated serum or tissue levels of biologically active complement fragments may stimulate the adherence of circulating neutrophils and, as a consequence, promote their sequestration in tissues.[315–318] This sequence of events was proposed to contribute to the acute respiratory symptoms, multiple organ injury, and relative leukopenia associated with gram-negative septicemia and other complement activation states of human patients.[315–317,319–321] Current data support the likely participation of β_2 integrins in these pathologic entities. Increased expression of Mac-1 on circulating leukocytes has been demonstrated in human patients undergoing hemodialysis[322] or after thermal injury.[323] Quantitative up-regulation of Mac-1 appears to represent a marker of disease activity in

Table 132-6 Investigations of Anti-Adherence Protein Monoclonal Antibodies in Animal Models of Vascular and Tissue Injury*

Animal Model	Experimental Observations/Effects of MAb Administration	Antigens (MAb)	Investigator (reference)
A. Skin Inflammation			
Intradermal administration of chemotactic factors in rabbits	Diminished PMN emigration and vascular permeability	CD18 (60.3)	Arfors (326)
Intradermal implantation of endotoxin-laden sponges in rabbits	Prevented PMN accumulation in sponge	CD18 (60.3)	Price (328)
Intradermal injection of Zymosan-saturated serum	Diminished PMN accumulation, vascular permeability	CD18 (60.3, 7E4)	Lindbom (327)
Intradermal injection of heat-killed *Mycobacterium tuberculosis* in rabbits	Diminished tissue edema associated with DTH reaction	CD18 (60.3, IB4)	Lindbom (461)
Rabbit model of thermal injury	Prevented progression of second-degree to third-degree burns	CD18	Bucky (329)
B. Lung Inflammation			
Rabbit model of lung injury induced by PMA	Diminished accumulation of PMN in pulmonary lavage fluids	CD11a (R3.1), CD18 (R3.3), CD54 (R6.5)	Barton (334)
Rabbit model of lung injury (intrabronchial instillation of PMA/LPS)	Diminished PMN emigration into pulmonary tissue	CD18 (60.3)	Doerschuk (352)
Rabbit model of lung injury (intrabronchial instillation of *S. pneumoniae, E. coli,* endotoxin, HCl, and PMA)	Markedly inhibited neutrophil emigration into pulmonary airspaces elicited by *E. coli,* LPS or PMA (but not *S. pneumoniae*/HCl)	CD18 (60.3)	Doerschuk (358)
Rat model of isolated–perfused lung injury by activated human neutrophils	Diminished lung injury and leukocyte sequestration	CD11b (Mo-1)	Ismail (353)
Primate model of *Ascaris*-induced asthma	Diminished eosinophil emigration, tissue necrosis, and sensitivity to allergen	CD54 (R6.5D6)	Wegner (354)
Mouse model of oxygen-induced lung injury	Attenuated lung injury (edema), dysfunction (carbon monoxide diffusion), and PMN sequestration	CD54 (UN/1.7)	Wegner (355)
Rabbit model of lung injury induced by hindlimb ischemia	Diminished lung permeability, edema, and PMN sequestration following ischemia/reperfusion	CD18 (R15.7)	Welbourn (356)
Primate model of antigen-induced asthma	Diminished acute neutrophil influx and late-phase airway bronchoconstriction	E-selectin (CL-2)	Gundel (360)
Rat model of IgG immune-complex-induced lung (skin) injury	Markedly reduced vascular injury and neutrophil recruitment	E-selectin (CL-3)	Mulligan (359)
Rat model of CVF-induced lung (skin) injury	Markedly reduced vascular injury and neutrophil recruitment	CD11b (Mab 17), CD18 (CL26)	Mulligan (357)
Rat model of IgA immune-complex-mediated lung injury	Reduced vascular injury and neutrophil recruitment	CD11a (WT-1), CD11b (1B6), VLA-4 (TA-2), CD54 (1A29)	Mulligan (314)
Rat model of CVF-induced lung injury	Diminished neutrophil emigration and associated pulmonary vascular injury	CD62 (PB1.3)	Mulligan (361)
C. Ischemia and Reperfusion (I/R) Models			
Cat model of intestinal I/R	Diminished leukocyte sequestration and vascular permeability	CD18 (60.3)	Hernandez (337)
Canine model of myocardial I/R	Diminished myocardial infarct size and leukocyte sequestration	CD11b (904)	Simpson and Todd (339)

Table 132-6 **Investigations of Anti-Adherence Protein Monoclonal Antibodies in Animal Models of Vascular and Tissue Injury* (Continued)**

Animal Model	Experimental Observations/Effects of MAb Administration	Antigens (MAb)	Investigator (reference)
C. Ischemia and Reperfusion (I/R) Models—Continued			
Canine model of myocardial I/R	Diminished sequestration of radiolabeled neutrophils into ischemic tissue segments	CD18 (R15.7)	Dreyer (341)
Rabbit model of I/R transected ear	Diminished tissue injury	CD18 (60.3)	Vedder (346)
Rabbit model of hemorrhagic shock and resuscitation	Diminished vascular and tissue injury	CD18 (60.3)	Vedder (347)
Primate model of hemorrhagic shock	Diminished tissue injury and mortality	CD18 (60.3)	Mileski (348)
Dog model of skeletal muscle I/R injury	Attenuated microvascular dysfunction (increased permeability and resistance) following I/R	CD18 (IB_4)	Carden (349)
Rabbit model of spinal cord injury associated with reversible aortic occlusion	Significantly reduced neurologic defects	CD18 (R3.3)	Clark (350)
Rat model of mesenteric I/R injury	Diminished leukocyte adhesion and emigration in mesenteric venules associated with I/R	CD18 (IB_4), CD11b (LM2), CD11a (R7.1), CD54 (RR1/1)	Granger (338)
Rabbit model of pulmonary artery occlusion and reperfusion	Diminished pulmonary vascular permeability, edema, and neutrophil sequestration	CD18 (IB_4)	Horgan (463)
Rabbit model of tissue hypothermia and rewarming (frostbite)	Diminished tissue edema and injury	CD18 (60.3)	Mileski (351)
Primate model of myocardial I/R injury	Diminished myocardial necrosis and dysfunction	CD18 (R15.7)	Winquist (343)
Primate model of myocardial I/R injury	Diminished myocardial necrosis and dysfunction	CD54 (R6.5D6)	Winquist (343)
Cat model of myocardial I/R injury	Diminished myocardial necrosis and neutrophil sequestration and preserved response of LAD coronary rings to acetylcholine and A23187	CD18 (R15.7)	Ma (342)
D. Graft Rejection and Other Immunologic Models			
Primate model of renal allograft rejection	Prevented or reversed graft rejection and renal dysfunction	CD54 (R6.5D6)	Cosimi (464)
Primate model of cardiac allograft rejection	Prolonged allograft survival	CD54 (R6.5D6)	Flavin (465)
Mouse model of DTH	Diminished PMN and monocyte emigration and edema at cutaneous sites of antigen administration	CD11b (5C6)	Rosen (331)
Rabbit model of chronic antigen-induced arthritis	Diminished synovial fluid leukocyte sequestration 2 and 4 weeks after antigen administration	CD18 (R157)	Jasin (466)
Mouse model of autoimmune insulin-dependent diabetes mellitus	Prevented intra-islet infiltration by macrophages and T cells and the development of insulin-dependent diabetes mellitus	CD11b (5C6)	Hutchings (467)
Mouse ectopic myocardial transplant	Markedly prolonged graft survival	CD11a (KBA), CD54 (YN1/1.7)	Isobe (468)

(*Continues*)

Table 132-6 Investigations of Anti-Adherence Protein Monoclonal Antibodies in Animal Models of Vascular and Tissue Injury* (Continued)

Animal Model	Experimental Observations/Effects of MAb Administration	Antigens (MAb)	Investigator (reference)
E. Miscellaneous Models of Acute Inflammation			
Mouse model of peritonitis	Diminished inflammatory ascites in an additive manner	L-selectin (Mel 14), CD11b (M1/70)	Jutila (115)
Rabbit model of indomethacin-induced gastritis	Prevented hemorrhagic vascular injury and leukocyte margination in gastric mucosa	CD18 (IB_4)	Wallace (333)
Mouse model of listeriosis	Exacerbated clinical course and dissemination of listeriosis	CD11b (5C6)	Rosen (469)
Rabbit model of bacterial meningitis	Reduced PMN/monocyte spinal fluid emigration, central nervous system damage, and mortality	CD18 (IB_4)	Tuomanen (332)
Mouse model of sciatic nerve regeneration	Prevented Wallerian degeneration following sectioning of sciatic nerve	CD11b (5C6)	Lunn (470)
Mouse models of lymphocyte homing and inflammatory ascites	Diminished (1) lymphocyte localization in peripheral and mesenteric lymph nodes and (2) neutrophil peritoneal exudation	L-selectin (Mel-14) or soluble L-selectin–IgG chimaera	Watson (368)
Dog model, evaluation of "spontaneous" rolling of neutrophils in mesenteric venules	Diminished number of rolling leukocytes	P-selectin (MD6)	Doré (128)
Rat model of leukocyte rolling in mesenteric venules	Diminished number of rolling leukocytes	L-selectin (polyclonal antibody) or soluble receptor	Ley (305)
Rabbit model of leukocyte rolling or mesenteric venules	Diminished rolling	L-selectin (DREG 200)	von Andrian (127)

*Abbreviations: CVF = cobra venom factor; DTH = delayed-type hypersensitivity; I/R = ischemia/reperfusion; LPS = lipopolysaccharide; MAb = monoclonal antibody; and PMN = polymorphonuclear leukocyte.

patients with systemic lupus erythematosus,[324] and abnormalities of Mac-1 expression are generally reversible in patients with thermal injuries or lupus during clinical resolution.

The role of β_2 integrins in neutrophil/monocyte localization or tissue injury has been extensively evaluated in animal models of inflammation relevant to human disease (Table 132-6). The use of monoclonal antibodies recognizing one or more β_2 integrin subunits or their ligands in these models has resulted in considerable insight concerning the roles of these molecules and their mechanisms of action in vivo. While these studies convincingly support the concept that neutrophil localization and emigration is β_2 integrin-dependent in many tissues or models, they also suggest that these glycoproteins cooperate with other leukocyte adhesion molecules (e.g., L-selectin) in this process. Moreover, several recent studies indicate that adherence-independent mechanisms play an important role in inflammatory cell sequestration in selected tissues and/or in response to certain inflammatory mediators. These experimental studies support the possibility that blocking cellular adhesion will reduce inflammatory injury in a number of human disorders. Currently, the use of murine or humanized monoclonal antibodies represents a plausible therapeutic approach to acute disorders such as myocardial infarction, hypovolemic shock, traumatic or thermal injury, and acute allograft rejection. Therapy for chronic inflammatory disorders will most likely require the development of antiadhesive drugs other than antibodies, since long-term administration of antibodies, especially of murine origin, will cause problems. Studies to define the safety of such regimens and their potential deleterious effects on host defenses will also be required. Experience to date with anti-CD18 monoclonal antibodies in an animal model reveals some increased susceptibility to bacterial infection, a finding consistent with the clinical course of patients with LAD. The potential adverse effects of profound, long-term inhibition of each of the adhesion molecules will require careful evaluation.

Several monoclonal antibodies capable of binding to functional epitopes of β_2 integrin subunits have been shown to be potential inhibitors of neutrophil or monocyte localization or emigration in response to experimental inflammatory stimuli (Table 132-6) (see reviews 313 and 325). Systemically administered anti-CD18 monoclonal antibodies profoundly inhibit (by >90 percent) neutrophil emigration elicited by chemotactic factors,[326,327] endotoxin,[328] or thermal injury[329] in rabbit skin. In a similar fashion, the intravenous administration of anti-CD11b monoclonal antibodies in mice profoundly inhibits the recruitment of neutrophils and monocytes in thioglycolate-elicited peritoneal exudate[330] as well as the T-lymphocyte-dependent recruitment of myelomonocytic cells to cutaneous sites of antigen challenge in sensitized animals.[331] Anti-CD18 monoclonal antibodies have been reported to reduce neutrophil and monocyte emigration and inflammatory injury associated with experimental bacterial meningitis.[332] Indomethacin-induced gastritis[333] in rabbits is also significantly reduced by anti-CD18 monoclonal antibodies. In one additional study, monoclonal antibodies directed at CD18 as well as at CD11a and ICAM-1 significantly reduced the accumulation of neutrophils in a rabbit model of acute lung injury.[334] These findings are consistent with histopathologic observations in LAD,[182,335] and they emphasize the general importance of CD11/CD18 and ICAM-1 in the process of neutrophil emigration at sites of acute inflammation in vivo.

Monoclonal antibodies directed at β_2 integrin subunits in animal models of ischemia–reperfusion injury substantially reduce neutrophil localization, microvascular permeability, and tissue injury (Table 132-6). These protective effects are not surprising, since inflammatory mediators capable of up-regulating Mac-1 on neutrophils and monocytes as well as ICAM-1 and other adherence determinants on vascular endothelial cells are elaborated in ischemic tissues.[336] As shown in several independent studies, anti-CD11/CD18 monoclonal antibodies (1) diminish leukocyte sequestration and vascular permeability in models of intestinal ischemia in cats[337,338]; (2) reduce leukocyte sequestration and/or infarct size and myocardial dysfunction in dog,[339–341] cat,[341,342] nonhuman primate,[343] or rabbit models[344,345]; (3) prevent or limit tissue injury and edema in transected rabbit ears[346]; (4) diminish hepatic and other organ injury and mortality in rabbit and primate models of hemorrhagic shock and resuscitation[347,348]; (5) reduce microvascular dysfunction associated with skeletal muscle ischemia in dogs[349]; (6) reduce spinal cord injury associated with aortic artery occlusion in rabbits[350]; and (7) diminish tissue edema and injury associated with hypothermia and rewarming in rabbits.[351]

Diverse animal models have been used to document the importance of CD11/CD18-adherence proteins in acute lung inflammation.[334,352–357] (Table 132-6). However, several recent studies emphasize an important role for CD18-independent mechanisms of neutrophil emigration into pulmonary airspaces and associated tissue injury. In rabbit models, Doerschuk[352,358] initially showed that pulmonary recruitment by *Streptococcus pneumonia* organisms (in contrast to endotoxin, *E. coli* organisms, PMA) is only minimally influenced by the anti-CD18 monoclonal antibody 60.3, even though recruitment into inflamed peritoneum is almost totally abolished by this monoclonal antibody in the same experimental animals. Consistent with these findings, autopsy studies in a patient with LAD who died with gram-negative bacterial pneumonia demonstrated vigorous neutrophil recruitment into pulmonary airspaces, as opposed to diminished recruitment in several other inflamed tissues.[335] As shown in other experimental models, selected immunologic stimuli elicit CD18-independent ligands in inflamed pulmonary tissues. For example, IgG immune complexes elicit E-selectin in rat lung, and the anti-E-selectin monoclonal antibody CL3 reduces neutrophil accumulation and lung injury in this experimental model.[359] The monoclonal antibody CL2 (anti-E-selectin) attenuates *Ascaris*-antigen-induced neutrophil influx and late-phase airway bronchoconstriction in primates.[360] Cobra venom factor-induced lung injury in rats involves the participation of P-selectin as well as CD-18-dependent ligands.[361] These observations indicate (1) that neutrophil emigration into inflamed lung (and possibly other tissues) may be stimulus-specific, (2) that the mechanisms of inflammatory emigration may be tissue-specific, and (3) that the relative participation of selected adhesion receptor–ligand pairs in various tissues as well as influences of locally elaborated cytokines may determine these specificities.

Results of still other studies employing monoclonal antibodies suggest that adhesion-independent mechanisms account for pulmonary localization of neutrophils.[362] For example, systemic administration of chemotactic factors in rabbits promotes a rapid (<30 min) sequestration of neutrophils in the pulmonary vasculature and, as a consequence, neutropenia. This localization is not influenced by pretreatment of experimental animals with the anti-CD11b monoclonal antibody 60.3, a reagent previously shown to totally inhibit neutrophil emigration elicited by intradermal administration of chemotactic factors.[326] This appears to be true even though Mac-1 on circulating blood neutrophils is significantly up-regulated in this experimental setting.[362] There is evidence that this CD18-independent phenomenon is related to mechanical trapping. Because of their relatively great diameter (~7.5 μm), neutrophils must deform in order to pass through capillary circuits (~5.5 μm average diameter) such as in lung.[363,364] This process is influenced by rheologic factors as well as by intrinsic properties of neutrophils.[365,366] Worthen et al.[364] have shown that passage of neutrophils through 5-μm-diameter micropore filters is markedly reduced by chemotactic factors, a process independent of cell adhesiveness but directly related to the stiffness of the cells (i.e., a lack of deformability). Thus the rapid pulmonary sequestration of neutrophils in response to intravenously administered chemotactic factors (or endotoxin) may result in part from physical trapping of neutrophils.

A role for L-selectin in conjunction with β_2 integrins in neutrophil emigration has been supported by studies in mice using the MEL-14 monoclonal antibody directed at murine L-selectin.[115,367] Systemic administration of this monoclonal antibody prevents neutrophil emigration in skin after implantation of endotoxin-laden sponges,[367] or into inflammatory ascites elicited by thioglycolate.[115] In the latter studies, anti-LFA-1, anti-Mac-1, and the Mel-14 monoclonal antibody (anti-L-selectin) suppressed neutrophil accumulation in inflamed peritoneum (to 38 percent, 30 percent, 31 percent of control levels, respectively) without influencing levels of circulating neutrophils. Peritoneal exudate neutrophils of control animals exhibited high levels of surface Mac-1 and very low levels of surface binding sites for Mel-14, in contrast to low Mac-1-high L-selectin patterns of circulating cells.[115] These findings indicate that, during the process of extravasation, inflammatory stimuli induce shedding of neutrophil L-selectin and up-regulation of Mac-1, findings similar to those elicited by chemotactic factors in vitro.[114] More recent studies by Watson et al.[368] also showed that both MEL-14 and a soluble L-selectin–IgG chimera significantly diminish neutrophil accumulation in inflammatory ascites when systemically administered in mice.

Clinical Disorders Associated with Incompletely Defined Defects of Leukocyte Mobility

Chediak-Higashi Syndrome. Chediak-Higashi syndrome (CHS) is an autosomal recessive disorder of mink, cattle, beige mice, and humans characterized clinically by partial oculocutaneous albinism, the presence of giant lysosomal granules in all granular cell types, susceptibility to bacterial infection, and an accelerated lymphoma-like proliferative phase generally occurring in the first decade of life.[369–371] Infectious complications are attributable both to neutropenia and to functional deficits of neutrophils, monocytes, and/or natural killer (NK) cells. Among 56 affected individuals reviewed by Blume and Wolff[369] in 1972, 33 died before reaching age 10. Among 27 patients for which a cause of death could be determined, infections represented the sole cause in 17 and were a contributing factor in another nine. Pulmonary, cutaneous, subcutaneous, and upper respiratory infections (due to *Staphylococcus aureus*, group A *Streptococcus*, gram-negative enteric organisms, *Aspergillus*, and *Candida* species) were the most common.

Neutrophils, monocytes, and lymphocytes from CHS patients show the large intracellular inclusions or granules that are the pathologic hallmark of the disease. These are most easily demonstrated in leukocytes but are also present in renal tubular epithelium, gastric mucosa, pancreas, thyroid, neural tissue, and melanocytes.[369] In neutrophils, they contain both azurophilic and specific granule markers.[372] Analysis of bone marrow samples from CHS patients suggests that abnormal granules are formed during granulocyte maturation by the progressive aggregation and fusion of azurophilic and specific granules. Such findings are consistent with a proposed membrane abnormality.[372,373]

Several functional abnormalities of neutrophils, monocytes, and NK cells of these patients have been identified in vitro. Neutrophils demonstrate delayed and diminished intracellular killing of both gram-positive and gram-negative bacteria and a normal or elevated oxidative burst.[369,374] Microbicidal abnormalities are attributed to impaired postphagocytic phagolysosomal fusion.[374] A rather selective impairment of the functions of NK cells (as opposed to other leukocytes) has been reported[375–378] and may account for the ultimate development of an aggressive lymphoproliferative syndrome in most patients. Successful bone marrow transplantation with reversal of the defect in NK activity has been reported in one case.[379]

Chemotaxis in vitro and leukocyte mobilization in vivo, as assessed by the "skin window" technique, are also abnormal.[370] In Boyden chamber assays, the large granular structures of CHS neutrophils may mechanically impede their migration through micropore filters. However, diminished directed migration of CHS neutrophils under agarose[25] and diminished stimulated adhesion to protein substrates have also been found (D.C. Anderson, unpublished observations). It has been proposed that the diminished motility and other functional abnormalities of CHS leukocytes are a result of defective microtubule function and/or cyclic nucleotide metabolism, but no direct evidence supports this possibility.[380–386]

Definitive preventative or therapeutic strategies for CHS will require an understanding of its molecular pathogenesis. It has been proposed that the beige (*bg*) mutation in the mouse represents the homologue of human CHS.[387] Support for this hypothesis stems from recent studies of a structural protein of basement membrane termed "nidogen/entactin," which may be relevant to the pathogenesis of CHS. Nidogen exists in an equimolar complex with laminin and binds type IV collagen and cells. There is evidence that it may play a role in various cellular functions, including adhesion, migration, and differentiation.[388] The cDNAs for both human and mouse nidogen have been cloned, and the human nidogen locus has been assigned to chromosome 1q43. Because of the possible homology of human chromosome 1q with mouse chromosome 13 and the possibility that the *bg* defect in mouse is homologous with CHS, Jenkins et al.[388] predict that the CHS gene is located in the telometric region of human chromosome 1q. It will now be possible to perform linkage studies among CHS families using human chromosome 1q probes to test this hypothesis.

Type 1b Glycogen Storage Disease. The association of neutropenia, impaired neutrophil migration, and recurrent infection in type 1b glycogen storage disease was first reported in 1980.[389] Most clinical features of type 1b glycogen storage disease are similar to those of type 1a glycogen storage disease, including hepatomegaly, fasting hypoglycemia, lactic acidosis, short stature, hyperlipidemia, and the occurrence of hepatomas with potential for malignant degeneration (see Chap. 24). Patients with type 1a glycogen storage disease demonstrate a deficiency of glucose 6-phosphatase activity in liver, kidney, and intestine. In contrast, type 1b glycogen storage disease patients demonstrate normal glucose 6-phosphatase activity.

A review of the clinical and laboratory features of 21 patients with type 1b glycogen storage disease[390] indicated that most suffered from a variety of moderate to severe bacterial infections, including pneumonitis, recurrent otitis media, subcutaneous abscesses, generalized pyoderma, cellulitis, wound infections, and osteomyelitis, usually caused by *Staphylococcus aureus*. Most patients exhibited chronic neutropenia, which, in some patients, was associated with demonstrable serum inhibitors of myeloid stem cell proliferation, abnormalities of myeloid maturation, and/or decreased peripheral marginating pools. Functional abnormalities, including diminished random or directed migration of neutrophils in vitro, were found in 8 of 11 patients tested, and deficient chemotactic modulation of adherence was observed in two patients.[29,390] In contrast, microbicidal activity of neutrophils and phagocytosis-associated oxidative metabolic activity have been shown to be normal in most patients with type 1b glycogen storage disease.[390]

The biochemical basis for the quantitative and qualitative abnormalities of neutrophils and mononuclear leukocytes is uncertain. However, glucose 6-phosphatase activity in liver homogenates from patients with type 1b glycogen storage disease was normal only when assayed in the presence of detergents (e.g., Triton X-100).[389,391] The high latency (90 percent) indicates that detection of this activity depends on the disruption of microsomes by detergent. Further studies in one patient[392] identified a defect of glucose 6-phosphatase translocase, one of three integral membrane components of the hepatic microsomal glucose 6-phosphatase system. A physiological role of glucose 6-phosphate transport in neutrophils has not been defined, and, thus, a causal relationship between aberrant glucose 6-phosphate transport and impaired neutrophil migration cannot yet be established.

Mannosidosis. Mannosidosis is a lysosomal storage disease characterized by psychomotor retardation, facial dysmorphology similar to that of Hurler syndrome, dysostosis multiplex, hepatosplenomegaly, hearing loss, and recurrent soft tissue infections (see Chap. 81). This autosomal recessive disease is due to a deficiency of acidic α-mannosidase A and B activity resulting in an accumulation of mannose-rich oligosaccharide in lysosomes of circulating leukocytes and in neural and visceral tissues. A defect of chemotaxis and phagocytosis in neutrophils and diminished lymphocyte transformation were described in one child with systemic mannosidosis.[393] The adherence properties of neutrophils in patients with this disorder have not been reported. It has been suggested that functional defects result from abnormal mannose catabolism, and that partially degraded oligosaccharides, glycopeptides, glycoproteins, and terminal α-D-mannose residues may bind to leukocyte plasma membranes as well as accumulating in lysosomal granules.

A review of 17 cases of mannosidosis reported that 13 patients experienced significant or recurrent infections, including chronic otitis media, upper respiratory infections, severe or progressive pneumonia, and cutaneous inflammatory lesions. While most of the reported infections were bacterial, these individuals were also susceptible to viral infections, reflecting, in part, impairment of cell-mediated immunity in this disease. One patient died of overwhelming adenoviral pneumonia.[393] A diagnosis of mannosidosis as suggested by typical clinical features can be confirmed by demonstrating deficient acidic α-mannosidase activity in plasma, peripheral blood leukocytes, or cultured skin fibroblasts.

Periodontitis Syndrome. Experimental and clinical evidence has demonstrated the important protective role of phagocytic cells, particularly neutrophils, in tissues of the oral cavity.[394] The infiltration of neutrophils into gingival tissues early in the development of gingivitis is thought to provide a first-line defense against invasion by pathogenic oral microflora.[395] Individuals with developmental, genetic, or acquired disorders involving either quantitative deficiencies of peripheral blood phagocytes or functional abnormalities of neutrophils commonly present with oral complications.[29,172,182,221,373,394–402] Primary or secondary agranulocytosis and cyclic neutropenia syndromes are typified by severe ulceration, necrosis, and chronic inflammation of gingival or periodontal tissues.[397] Patients with severe disorders, such as chronic granulomatous disease,[401] Chediak-Higashi syndrome,[399] or LAD[182] present with systemic as well as oral infections. Individuals with milder leukocyte functional deficits, as observed in localized juvenile periodontitis, postlocalized juvenile periodontitis, or generalized juvenile periodontitis syndromes, generally have no systemic complications.

Defective neutrophil chemotaxis is thought to represent a major pathogenic mechanism in individuals with periodontitis syndromes.[202,394,400,403–408] Of 183 patients with localized juvenile periodontitis studied by multiple investigators,[389,394,398,405,407,409,410] 132 (71 percent) have been reported to exhibit defective chemotaxis. Most patients exhibit intrinsic cellular defects, but cell-directed serum inhibitors, chemotactic factor inactivators, or abnormalities of chemotaxigenesis have been reported in a small proportion of patients tested. The pathogenic mechanisms accounting for impaired chemotaxis have not been defined. De Nardin et al.[411] demonstrated differences in binding of specific monoclonal antibodies to f-Met-Leu-Phe receptors of neutrophils of juvenile periodontitis patients, findings that suggest defects of chemotactic factor receptors underlying diminished cell migration. Perez et al. further showed that f-Met-Leu-Phe receptors of some of these patients are of normal molecular weight but are more resistant to papain cleavage.[412] Two-dimensional electrophoresis of neutrophil extracts showed decreased amounts of f-Met-Leu-Phe receptor isoforms in patient cells, findings not yet corroborated in other patient populations with periodontitis syndromes.

Epidemiologic or clinical associations of certain periodontopathic bacterial organisms with some periodontitis syndromes suggest that cellular constituents or extracellular factors elaborated by these microorganisms may secondarily alter leukocyte functions.[396,413–416] The pathogenic roles of gram-negative oral bacteria, including *Actinobacillus actinomycetemcomitans,* species of *Bacteroides,* and species of *Capnocytophaga,* have been increasingly appreciated.[413,416] A leukocytotoxin elaborated by *Actinobacillus actinomycetemcomitans* that has been identified in vitro may contribute to diminished chemotactic functioning.[417–420]

Despite intensive study, the molecular pathogenesis of juvenile periodontitis syndromes remains undefined. The fact that familial aggregation is often observed in juvenile periodontitis suggests that the disease may have a genetic basis.[402,421] Defects of chemotaxis associated with juvenile periodontitis appear to have a familial distribution, and, in some cases, both functional defects of leukocytes and clinical features of periodontitis are identified in multiple family members.[402] It has not been determined whether the familial occurrence of juvenile periodontitis results from Mendelian inheritance, from multifactorial inheritance, and/or from environmental factors.[421–423] Determination of the mode of genetic transmission of specific periodontitis syndromes awaits the identification of molecular markers of disease.

Schwachman-Diamond Syndrome. Clinical features of a syndrome first described by Schwachman and Diamond include exocrine pancreatic insufficiency, bone marrow hypoplasia with associated neutropenia, metaphyseal chondrodysplasia, growth retardation, and recurrent soft tissue infections.[424–427] Otitis media, bronchial pneumonia, osteomyelitis, dermatitis, and septicemia occurred in 17 (85 percent) of a group of 21 patients,[427] and 3 of these patients (15 percent) died of these causes. Neutropenia was intermittent in most patients in this and other series.[428] Bone marrow aspiration has demonstrated absent myeloid precursors or maturation arrest with variable degrees of hypoplasia.[426–428] Normal bone marrow aspirates in neutropenic patients have also been described, suggesting that marrow hypoplasia is patchy in distribution.[425] Diminished neutrophil chemotaxis without other functional abnormalities was found in 12 of 14 patients with this syndrome.[424] Nine of these patients were neutropenic, and four demonstrated low levels of serum IgA or IgM without other immunologic abnormalities. Parents of some of these individuals showed intermediate abnormalities of neutrophil chemotaxis, suggesting that they were heterozygotes and that this abnormality is inherited as an autosomal recessive trait. The pathogenic basis for the hematologic and other features of this multisystem disease has not been determined, and the relative contributions of impaired cellular motility (as opposed to neutropenia) to infectious susceptibility in affected patients is uncertain.

Hyperimmunoglobulin E and Other Immunologic Disorders Characterized by Defective Leukocyte Motility. Primary immunodeficiency syndromes are described in Chaps. 128 and 129. In some of these disorders, abnormalities of cellular motility have been described. The contributions of these abnormalities to infectious susceptibility in each disorder is uncertain. Possibly the first report of a clinical defect of chemotaxis[145] was a description of two female patients with fair skin, reddish hair, severe eczema, dystrophic fingernails, sinopulmonary infections, and recurrent staphylococcal abscesses (termed Job syndrome). Although the soft-tissue inflammatory lesions in these patients were large, they demonstrated minimal erythema or tenderness. In 1972, two male patients with essentially the same syndrome were described.[9] The patients exhibited a peculiar coarse facies, eczematoid rashes, cold abscesses, and recurrent sinopulmonary infections due to *Staphylococcus aureus* or *Haemophilus influenzae.* Both demonstrated hyperimmunoglobulin E and a variety of additional subtle immunologic abnormalities.

A group of 20 patients with hyperimmunoglobulin E included 13 males and 8 blacks, thus eliminating the concept that Job syndrome affects only red-haired females.[429] All had eczematoid dermatitis, and in seven instances a familial occurrence was noted. Serum IgE levels in unaffected relatives were normal. These patients consistently demonstrated poor delayed hypersensitivity responses as well as poor anamnestic responses to tetanus and diphtheria antigens. Almost all demonstrated diminished lymphocyte proliferation in vitro to specific antigens such as *Candida albicans* or tetanus toxoid, but proliferative responses to lectins were generally normal. Other reports documented deficient suppressor T lymphocytes and increased IgE synthesis in culture.[430,431] Collectively, these reports suggest that a defect of immune regulation is the primary pathogenic basis of this syndrome.[432] The heterogeneity in the chemotactic functions of neutrophils and monocytes observed in patients with Job syndrome suggests that these abnormalities do not reflect a primary cellular dysfunction and that they may be related to high tissue levels of histamine or other inflammatory mediators.[11,433] Histamine significantly inhibits the chemotactic response of normal neutrophils in vitro. Cytophilic IgE directed against invading bacteria could mediate a local release of histamine, thereby diminishing the chemotaxis of circulating neutrophils. Patients with Job syndrome have been found to have high levels of serum IgE directed against antigens of *Staphylococcus aureus* and *Candida albicans*.[434,435]

It has been suggested that patients with hyperimmunoglobulin E have a relative deficiency of IFN-γ production.[329,436] Current evidence indicates that the magnitude of the IgE response to a given stimulus is regulated, in part, by opposing influences of IL-4 and IFN-γ. When T lymphocytes of hyperimmunoglobulin E patients are exposed to mitogenic stimuli in vitro, they produce normal amounts of IL-4, but exhibit deficient IFN-γ production.[436,437] Moreover, IFN-γ production in skin blisters of these patients is also deficient (J. Gallin, unpublished observations). B lymphocytes from some hyperimmunoglobulin E patients show elevated spontaneous IgE production, which can be suppressed by addition of exogenous IFN-γ.[438] Moreover, in short-term trials of IFN-γ administration in hyperimmunoglobulin E patients, a significant decrease in in vitro spontaneous IgE production was seen in each of five patients, and, in two of these, a fall in serum IgE was also observed.[438] Deficient local production of IFN-γ may also account for abnormal neutrophil chemotaxis. In one study, in vitro exposure of patient neutrophils to IFN-γ resulted in a significant increase in chemotactic function.[439] These findings support the idea that exogenous IFN-γ should be evaluated for the clinical management of hyperimmunoglobulin E patients.

One large patient group that must be carefully differentiated from individuals with Job syndrome includes those individuals with atopic eczema who are frequently colonized by *Staphylococcus aureus* and later acquire secondary staphylococcal infections. These patients may demonstrate chemotactic defects,[440] but generally they do not have recurrent sinopulmonary infections or characteristic "cold" abscesses. Still other patients with a prominent allergic history develop recurrent infections that coincide with exacerbations of atopic symptoms.[441]

Defects in chemotaxis have also been described in selected patients with chronic mucocutaneous candidiasis, and these may or may not be accompanied by lymphocyte dysfunction.[10,146,442,443] Diminished chemotaxis of neutrophils associated with marked elevation of IgE was reported in one mother–daughter pair,[444] and abnormal mononuclear leukocyte chemotaxis associated with abnormal production of lymphocyte-derived chemotactic factor was reported in another patient.[146] A plasma inhibitor of neutrophil motility was detected in one patient with chronic mucocutaneous candidiasis. Partial characterization of this inhibitor revealed that it had several properties in common with IgG.[443]

A cellular defect of chemotaxis, phagocytosis, and intracellular bactericidal activity was reported in a 3-year-old boy with agammaglobulinemia, recurrent cutaneous abscesses, and episodes of pneumonia. Similar defects were found in an adult with hypogammaglobulinemia and in another child with gammaglobulin deficiency associated with recurrent sinopulmonary infections.[144] Diminished chemotaxis occurred in 9 of 10 patients with serum IgA deficiency and in 6 of 10 patients with hypogammaglobulinemia.[445,446] Diminished chemotaxis has also been observed in selected patients with severe combined immune deficiency disease.[447] The pathogenic basis and consequences of the abnormal cellular motility described in these reports are uncertain.

In addition to complex immunologic abnormalities, patients with Wiskott-Aldrich syndrome have been reported to show diminished chemotaxis of monocytes in association with abnormal production of a lymphocyte-derived chemotactic factor.[448] These findings suggest that lymphocytes in Wiskott-Aldrich syndrome may release soluble factors that diminish the responsiveness of monocytes to chemotactic stimuli. The pathogenic significance of these limited findings is uncertain.

REFERENCES

1. Metchnikoff E: Immunity in Infectious Diseases (F.G. Binnie), in. London, Cambridge University Press, 1905.
2. Leber T: Ueber die Entstehung der Entzundung die Wirkung der entzundungse-regendon Schadlichkeiten. *Fortsch Med* **6**:460, 1888.
3. Janeway CA, Craig J, Davidson M, Downey W, Gitlin D, Sullivan JC: Hypergammaglobulinemia associated with severe recurrent and chronic nonspecific infection. *Am J Dis Child* **88**:388, 1954.
4. Quie PG, White JG, Holmes B, Good RA: In vitro bactericidal capacity of human polymorphonuclear leukocytes: Diminished activity in chronic granulomatous disease of childhood. *J Clin Invest* **46**:668, 1967.
5. Holmes B, Page AR, Good RA: Studies of the metabolic activity of leukocytes from patients with a genetic abnormality of phagocytic function. *J Clin Invest* **46**:1422, 1967.
6. Alexander JW, Ogle CK, Stinnet JD, MacMillan BG: A sequential, prospective analysis of immunologic abnormalities and infection following severe thermal injury. *Ann Surg* **188**:809, 1978.
7. Ward PA, Johnson KJ, Kreutzer DL: Regulatory dysfunction leukotaxis. *Am J Pathol* **88**:701, 1977.
8. Miller ME, Oski FA, Harris MB: Lazy-leukocyte syndrome: A new disorder of neutrophil function. *Lancet* **1**:665, 1971.
9. Buckley RH, Wray BB, Belmaker EZ: Extreme hyperimmunoglobulinemia E and undue susceptibility to infection. *Pediatrics* **49**:59, 1972.
10. Clark RA, Root RK, Kimball HR, Kirkpatrick CH: Defective neutrophil chemotaxis and cellular immunity in a child with recurrent infections. *Ann Intern Med* **78**:515, 1973.
11. Hill HR, Quie PG: Raised serum IgE levels and defective neutrophil chemotaxis in three children with eczema and recurrent bacterial infections. *Lancet* **1**:183, 1974.
12. Wilkinson PC: The locomotion of leukocytes: Definitions and descriptions, in Wilkinson PC (ed): *Chemotaxis and Inflammation.* New York, Churchill Livingstone, 1982, p 1.

13. Keller HU, Wilkinson PC, Abercrombie M, Becker EL, Hirsch JG, Miller ME, Ramsey WS, Zigmond SH: A proposal for the definition of terms related to locomotion of leukocytes and other cells. *Clin Exp Immunol* **27**:377, 1977.
14. Keller HU, Wilkinson PC, Abercrombie M, Becker EL, Hirsch JG, Miller ME, Ramsey WS, Zigmond SH, Austen KF, Baum J, Borel JF, Curtis ASG, Dunn GA, Gallin JI, Goetzl EJ, Harris AK, Humbert JR, Sorkin E, Trinkaus JP, Vasiliey JM, Weiss L, Wissler JH: A proposal for the definition of terms related to locomotion of leukocytes and other cells. *Bull WHO* **58**:505, 1980.
15. Ramsey WS: Analysis of individual leukocyte behavior during chemotaxis. *Exp Cell Res* **70**:129, 1972.
16. Zigmond SH, Hirsch JG: Leukocyte locomotion and chemotaxis. New methods for evaluation and demonstration of a cell-derived chemotactic factor. *J Exp Med* **137**:387, 1973.
17. Zigmond SH, Levitsky HI, Kreel BJ: Cell polarity: An examination of its behavioral expression and its consequences for polymorphonuclear leukocyte chemotaxis. *J Cell Biol* **89**:585, 1981.
17a. Rebuck JW, Crowley JH: A method of studying leukocyte function in vivo. *Ann NY Acad Sci* **59**:757, 1955.
18. Solberg CO, Halstensen A, Digranes A, Hellum KB: Penetration of antibiotics into human leukocytes and dermal suction blisters. *Rev Infect Dis* **5**:S468, 1983.
19. Miles AA, Miles EM, Burke J: The value and duration of defense reactions of the skin to the primary lodgement of bacteria. *Br J Exp Pathol* **38**:79, 1957.
20. Smith CW, Hollers JC, Patrick RA, Hassett C: Motility and adhesiveness in human neutrophils: Effects of chemotactic factors. *J Clin Invest* **63**:221, 1979.
21. Boyden S: The chemotactic effect of mixtures of antibody and antigen on polymorphonuclear leukocytes. *J Exp Med* **115**:453, 1962.
22. Wilkinson PC, Allan RB: Assay systems for measuring leukocyte locomotion: An overview, in Gallin JI, Quie PG (eds): *Leukocyte Chemotaxis*. New York, Raven Press, 1978, p 1.
23. McCutcheon M: Chemotaxis in leukocytes. *Physiol Rev* **26**:319, 1946.
24. Allan RB, Wilkinson PC: A visual analysis of chemotactic and chemokinetic locomotion of human neutrophil leukocytes. *Exp Cell Res* **111**:191, 1978.
25. Nelson RD, Quie PG, Simmons RL: Chemotaxis under agarose: A new and simple method for measuring chemotaxis and spontaneous migration of human polymorphonuclear leukocytes and monocytes. *J Immunol* **115**:1650, 1975.
26. Verghese MW, Smith CD, Charles LA, Jakoi L, Snyderman RA: A guanine nucleotide regulatory protein controls polyphosphoinositide metabolism, Ca^{2+} mobilization and cellular responses to chemoattractants in human monocytes. *J Immunol* **137**:271, 1986.
27. Anderson DC, Hughes BJ, Smith CW: Abnormal mobility of neonatal polymorphonuclear leukocytes. Relationship to impaired redistribution of surface adhesion sites by chemotactic factor or colchicine. *J Clin Invest* **68**:863, 1981.
28. Anderson DC, Krishna GS, Hughes BJ, Mace ML, Smith CW, Nichols BL: Impaired polymorphonuclear leukocyte motility in malnourished infants: Relationship to functional abnormalities of cell adherence. *J Lab Clin Med* **101**:881, 1983.
29. Anderson DC, Mace ML, Brinkley BR, Martin RR, Smith CW: Recurrent infection in glycogenosis type 1b: Abnormal neutrophil motility related to impaired redistribution of adhesion sites. *J Infect Dis* **143**:447, 1981.
30. Kishimoto TK, Anderson DC: The role of integrins in inflammation, in Gallin JI, Goldstein IM, Snyderman R (eds): *Inflammation. Basic Principles and Clinical Correlates*. New York, Raven, 1992, p 353.
31. Corbi AL, Miller LJ, O'Connor K, Larson RS, Springer TA: cDNA cloning and complete primary structure of the alpha subunit of a leukocyte adhesion glycoprotein, p150,95. *EMBO J* **6**:4023, 1987.
32. Corbi AL, Kishimoto TK, Miller LJ, Springer TA: The human leukocyte adhesion glycoprotein Mac-1 (complement receptor type 3, CD11b) alpha subunit: Cloning, primary structure, and relation to the integrins, von Willebrand factor and factor B. *J Biol Chem* **263**:12403, 1988.
33. Arnaout MA, Gupta SK, Pierce MW, Tenen DG: Amino acid sequence of the alpha subunit of human leukocyte adhesion receptor Mo1 (complement receptor type 3). *J Cell Biol* **106**:2153, 1988.
34. Larson RS, Corbi AL, Berman L, Springer TA: Primary structure of the LFA-1 alpha subunit: An integrin with an embedded domain defining a protein superfamily. *J Cell Biol* **108**:703, 1989.
35. Kishimoto TK, O'Connor K, Lee A, Roberts TM, Springer TA: Cloning of the beta subunit of the leukocyte adhesion proteins: Homology to an extracellular matrix receptor defines a novel supergene family. *Cell* **48**:681, 1987.
36. Law SKA, Gagnon J, Hildreth JEK, Wells CE, Willis AC, Wong AJ: The primary structure of the beta-subunit of the cell surface adhesion glycoproteins LFA-1, CR-3 and p150,95 and its relationship to the fibronectin receptor. *EMBO J* **6**:915, 1987.
37. Rothlein R, Dustin ML, Marlin SD, Springer TA: A human intercellular adhesion molecule (ICAM-1) distinct from LFA-1. *J Immunol* **137**:1270, 1986.
38. Staunton DE, Dustin ML, Springer TA: Functional cloning of ICAM-2, a cell adhesion ligand for LFA-1 homologous to ICAM-1. *Nature* **339**:61, 1989.
39. de Fougerolles AR, Stacker SA, Schwarting R, Springer TA: Characterization of ICAM-2 and evidence for a third counter-receptor for LFA-1. *J Exp Med* **174**:253, 1991.
40. Smith CW, Marlin SD, Rothlein R, Toman C, Anderson CD: Cooperative interactions of LFA-1 and Mac-1 with intercellular adhesion molecule-1 in facilitating adherence and transendothelial migration of human neutrophils in vitro. *J Clin Invest* **83**:2008, 1989.
41. Diamond MS, Staunton DE, Marlin SD, Springer TA: Binding of the integrin Mac-1 (CD11b/CD18) to the third immunoglobulin-like domain of ICAM-1 (CD54) and its regulation by glycosylation. *Cell* **65**:961, 1991.
42. Todd RF III, Arnaout MA, Rosin RE, Crowley CA, Peters WA, Babior BM: Subcellular localization of the large subunit of Mo1 ($Mo1_1$; formerly gp110), a surface glycoprotein associated with neutrophil adhesion. *J Clin Invest* **74**:1280, 1984.
43. Buyon JP, Abramson SB, Philips MR, Slade SG, Ross GD, Weissmann G, Winchester RJ: Dissociation between increased surface expression of Gp165/95 and homotypic neutrophil aggregation. *J Immunol* **140**:3156, 1988.
44. Vedder NB, Harlan JM: Increased surface expression of CD11b/CD18 (Mac-1) is not required for stimulated neutrophil adherence to cultured endothelium. *J Clin Invest* **81**:676, 1988.
45. Hughes BJ, Hollers JC, Crockett-Torabi E, Smith CW: Recruitment of CD11b/CD18 to the neutrophil surface and adherence-dependent cell locomotion. *J Clin Invest* **90**:1687, 1992.
46. Dustin ML, Springer TA: T-Cell receptor cross-linking transiently stimulates adhesiveness through LFA-1. *Nature* **341**:619, 1989.
47. Robinson MK, Andrew D, Rosen H, Brown D, Ortlepp S, Stephens P, Butcher EC: An antibody against the Leu-CAM beta chain (CD18) promotes both LFA-1 and CR3 dependent adhesion events. *J Immunol* **148**:1080, 1992.
48. Keizer GD, Visser W, Vliem M, Figdor CG: A monoclonal antibody (NKL-L16) directed against a unique epitope on the alpha-chain of human leukocyte function-associated antigen 1 induces homotypic cell-cell interactions. *J Immunol* **140**:1393, 1988.
49. Wacholtz MC, Patel SS, Lipsky PE: Leukocyte function-associated antigen 1 is an activation molecule for human T cells. *J Exp Med* **170**:431, 1989.
50. Van Seventer GA, Shimizu Y, Horgan KJ, Shaw S: The LFA-1 ligand ICAM-1 provides an important costimulatory signal for T cell receptor-mediated activation of resting T cells. *J Immunol* **144**:4579, 1990.
51. Shappell SB, Toman C, Anderson DC, Taylor AA, Entman ML, Smith CW: Mac-1 (CD11b/CD18) mediates adherence-dependent hydrogen peroxide production by human and canine neutrophils. *J Immunol* **144**:2702, 1990.
52. Staunton DE, Marlin DC, Stratowa C, Dustin ML, Springer TA: Primary structure of intercellular adhesion molecule 1 (ICAM-1) demonstrates interaction between mem-

bers of the immunoglobulin and integrin supergene families. *Cell* **52:**925, 1988.
53. Simmons D, Makgoba MW, Seed B: ICAM, an adhesion ligand of LFA-1, is homologous to the neural cell adhesion molecule NCAM. *Nature* **331:**624, 1988.
54. Staunton DE, Dustin ML, Erickson HP, Springer TA: The arrangement of the immunoglobulin-like domains of ICAM-1 and the binding sites for LFA-1 and rhinovirus. *Cell* **61:**243, 1990.
55. Staunton DE, Merluzzi VJ, Rothlein R, Barton R, Marlin SD, Springer TA: A cell adhesion molecule, ICAM-1, is the major surface receptor for rhinoviruses. *Cell* **56:**849, 1989.
56. Dustin ML, Rothlein R, Bhan AK, Dinarello CA, Springer TA: Induction by IL-1 and interferon-gamma: Tissue distribution, biochemistry, and function of a natural adherence molecule (ICAM-1). *J Immunol* **137:**245, 1986.
57. Nortamo P, Salcedo R, Timonen T, Patarroyo M, Gahmberg CG: A monoclonal antibody to the human leukocyte adhesion molecule intercellular adhesion molecule-2. Cellular distribution and molecular characterization of the antigen. *J Immunol* **146:**2530, 1991.
58. deFougerolles AR, Springer TA: Intercellular adhesion molecule 3, a third adhesion counter-receptor for lymphocyte function-associated molecule 1 on resting lymphocytes. *J Exp Med* **175:**185, 1992.
59. Johnston GI, Cook RG, McEver RP: Cloning of GMP-140, a granule membrane protein of platelets and endothelium: Sequence similarity to proteins involved in cell adhesion and inflammation. *Cell* **56:**1033, 1989.
60. Lasky LA, Singer MS, Yednock TA, Dowbenko D, Fennie C, Rodriguez H, Nguyen T, Stachel S, Rosen SD: Cloning of a lymphocyte homing receptor reveals a lectin domain. *Cell* **56:**1045, 1989.
61. Siegelman MH, Van de Rijn M, Weissman IL: Mouse lymph node homing receptor cDNA clone encodes a glycoprotein revealing tandem interaction domains. *Science* **243:**1165, 1989.
62. Bevilacqua MP, Stengelin S, Gimbrone MA Jr, Seed B: Endothelial leukocyte adhesion molecule 1: An inducible receptor for neutrophils related to complement regulatory proteins and lectins. *Science* **243:**1160, 1989.
63. Siegelman MH, Weissman IL: Human homologue of mouse lymph node homing receptor: Evolutionary conservation at tandem cell interaction domains. *Proc Natl Acad Sci USA* **86:**5562, 1989.
64. Tedder TF, Isaacs CM, Ernst TJ, Demetri GD, Adler DA, Disteche CM: Isolation and chromosomal localization of cDNAs encoding a novel human lymphocyte cell surface molecule, LAM-1. Homology with the mouse lymphocyte homing receptor and other human adhesion proteins. *J Exp Med* **170:**123, 1989.
65. Bowen BR, Nguyen T, Lasky LA: Characterization of a human homologue of the murine peripheral lymph node homing receptor. *J Cell Biol* **109:**421, 1989.
66. Drickamer K: Two distinct classes of carbohydrate-recognition domains in animal lectins. *J Biol Chem* **263:**9557, 1988.
67. Yednock TA, Rosen SD: Lymphocyte homing. *Adv Immunol* **44:**313, 1989.
68. Smith CW, Kishimoto TK, Abbassi O, Hughes BJ, Rothlein R, McIntire LV, Butcher E, Anderson DC: Chemotactic factors regulate lectin adhesion molecule 1 (LECAM-1)-dependent neutrophil adhesion to cytokine-stimulated endothelial cells in vitro. *J Clin Invest* **87:**609, 1991.
69. Hallmann R, Jutila MA, Smith CW, Anderson DC, Kishimoto TK, Butcher EC: The peripheral lymph node homing receptor, LECAM-1, is involved in CD-18-independent adhesion of human neutrophils to endothelium. *Biochem Biophys Res Commun* **174:**236, 1991.
70. Spertini O, Luscinskas FW, Kansas GS, Munro JM, Griffin JD, Gimbrone MA, Tedder TF: Leukocyte adhesion molecule-1 (LAM-1, L-selectin) interacts with an inducible endothelial cell ligand to support leukocyte adhesion. *J Immunol* **147:**2565, 1991.
71. Bevilacqua MP, Pober JS, Mendrick DL, Cotran RS, Gimbrone MA Jr: Identification of an inducible endothelial-leukocyte adhesion molecule. *Proc Natl Acad Sci USA* **84:**9238, 1987.
72. Luscinskas FW, Brock AF, Arnaout MA, Gimbrone MA Jr: Endothelial-leukocyte adhesion molecule-1-dependent and leukocyte (CD11/CD18)-dependent mechanisms contribute to polymorphonuclear leukocyte adhesion to cytokine-activated human vascular endothelium. *J Immunol* **142:**2257, 1989.
73. Cotran RS, Gimbrone MA Jr, Bevilacqua MP, Mendrick DL, Pober JS: Induction and detection of a human endothelial activation antigen in vivo. *J Exp Med* **164:**661, 1986.
74. Munro JM, Pober JS, Cotran RS: Recruitment of neutrophils in the local endotoxin response: Association with *de novo* endothelial expression of endothelial leukocyte adhesion molecule-1. *Lab Invest* **64:**295, 1991.
75. Redl H, Dinges HP, Buurman WA, van der Linden CJ, Pober JS, Cotran RS, Schlag G: Expression of endothelial leukocyte adhesion molecule-1 in septic but not traumatic/hypovolemic shock in the baboon. *Am J Pathol* **139:**461, 1991.
76. Munro JM, Pober JS, Cotran RS: Tumor necrosis factor and interferon-gamma induce distinct patterns of endothelial activation and associated leukocyte accumulation in skin of *Papio anubis*. *Am J Pathol* **135:**121, 1989.
77. Leung DYM, Pober JS, Cotran RS: Expression of endothelial-leukocyte adhesion molecule-1 in elicited late phase allergic reactions. *J Clin Invest* **87:**1805, 1991.
78. Picker LJ, Kishimoto TK, Smith CW, Warnock RA, Butcher EC: ELAM-1 is an adhesion molecule for skin-homing T-cells. *Nature* **349:**796, 1991.
79. Koch AE, Burrows JC, Haines GK, Carlos TM, Harlan JM, Leibovich SJ: Immunolocalization of endothelial and leukocyte adhesion molecules in human rheumatoid and osteoarthritic synovial tissues. *Lab Invest* **64:**313, 1991.
80. McEver RP, Martin MN: A monoclonal antibody to a membrane glycoprotein binds only to activated platelets. *J Biol Chem* **259:**9799, 1984.
81. Hsu-Lin S-C, Berman CL, Furie BC, August D, Furie B: A platelet membrane protein expressed during platelet activation and secretion. Studies using a monoclonal antibody specific for thrombin-activated platelets. *J Biol Chem* **259:**9121, 1984.
82. Stenberg PE, McEver RP, Shuman MA, Jacques YV, Bainton DF: A platelet alpha granule membrane protein (GMP-140) is expressed on the plasma membrane after activation. *J Cell Biol* **101:**880, 1985.
83. Berman CL, Yeo EL, Wencel-Drake JD, Furie BC, Ginsberg MH, Furie B: A platelet alpha granule membrane protein that is associated with the plasma membrane after activation. *J Clin Invest* **78:**130, 1986.
84. McEver RP, Beckstead JH, Moore KL, Marshall-Carlson L, Bainton DF: GMP-140, a platelet alpha-granule membrane protein, is also synthesized by vascular endothelial cells and is localized in Weibel-Palade bodies. *J Clin Invest* **84:**92, 1989.
85. Bonfanti R, Furie BC, Furie B, Wagner DD: PADGEM (GMP140) is a component of Weibel-Palade bodies of human endothelial cells. *Blood* **73:**1109, 1989.
86. Hattori R, Hamilton KK, Fugates RD, McEver RP, Sims PJ: Stimulated secretion of endothelial von Willebrand factor is accompanied by rapid redistribution to the cell surface of the intracellular granule membrane protein GMP-140. *J Biol Chem* **264:**7768, 1989.
87. Hamburger SA, McEver RP: GMP-140 mediates adhesion of stimulated platelets to neutrophils. *Blood* **75:**550, 1990.
88. Larsen E, Celi A, Gilbert GE, Furie BC, Erban JK, Bonfanti R, Wagner DD, Furie B: PADGEM protein: A receptor that mediates the interaction of activated platelets with neutrophils and monocytes. *Cell* **59:**305, 1989.
89. Larsen E, Palabrica T, Sajer S, Gilbert GE, Wagner DD, Furie BC, Furie B: PADGEM-dependent adhesion of platelets to monocytes and neutrophils is mediated by a lineage-specific carbohydrate, LNF III (CD15). *Cell* **63:**467, 1990.
90. Geng JG, Bevilacqua MP, Moore KL, McIntyre TM, Prescott SM, Kim JM, Bliss GA, Zimmerman GA, McEver RP: Rapid neutrophil adhesion to activated endothelium mediated by GMP-140. *Nature* **343:**757, 1990.
91. Patel KD, Zimmerman GA, Prescott SM, McEver RP, McIntyre TM: Oxygen radicals induce human endothelial cells to express GMP-140 and bind neutrophils. *J Cell Biol* **112:**749, 1991.
92. Lorant DE, Patel KD, McIntyre TM, McEver RP,

Prescott SM, Zimmerman GA: Coexpression of GMP-140 and PAF by endothelium stimulated by histamine or thrombin: A juxtacrine system for adhesion and activation of neutrophils. *J Cell Biol* **115**:223, 1991.

93. Rosen SD, Singer M, Yednock TA, Stoolman LM: Involvement of sialic acid on endothelial cells in organ-specific lymphocyte recirculation. *Science* **228**:1005, 1985.

94. True DD, Singer MS, Lasky LA, Rosen SD: Requirement for sialic acid on the endothelial ligand of a lymphocyte homing receptor. *J Cell Biol* **111**:2757, 1990.

95. Yednock TA, Butcher EC, Stoolman LM, Rosen SD: Receptors involved in lymphocyte homing: Relationship between a carbohydrate-binding receptor and the Mel-14 antigen. *J Cell Biol* **104**:725, 1987.

96. Stoolman LM, Tenforde TS, Rosen SD: Phosphomannosyl receptors may participate in the adhesive interaction between lymphocytes and high endothelial venules. *J Cell Biol* **99**:1535, 1984.

97. Imai Y, Singer MS, Fennie C, Lasky LA, Rosen SD: Identification of a carbohydrate-based endothelial ligand for a lymphocyte homing receptor. *J Cell Biol* **113**:1213, 1991.

98. Streeter PR, Rouse BT, Butcher EC: Immunohistologic and functional characterization of a vascular addressin involved in lymphocyte homing into peripheral lymph nodes. *J Cell Biol* **107**:1853, 1988.

99. Lasky LA, Singer MS, Dowbenko D, Imai Y, Henzel WJ, Grimley C, Fennie C, Gillett N, Watson SR, Rosen SD: An endothelial ligand for L-selectin is a novel mucin-like molecule. *Cell* **69**:927, 1993.

100. Phillips ML, Nudelman E, Gaeta FCA, Perez M, Singhal AK, Hakomori S, Paulson JC: ELAM-1 mediates cell adhesion by recognition of a carbohydrate ligand, sialyl-Le^{X}. *Science* **250**:1130, 1990.

101. Walz G, Aruffo A, Kolanus W, Bevilacqua MP, Seed B: Recognition by ELAM-1 of the sialyl-Le^{X} determinant on myeloid and tumor cells. *Science* **250**:1132, 1990.

102. Lowe JB, Stoolman LM, Nair RP, Larsen RD, Berhend TL, Marks RM: ELAM-1-dependent cell adhesion to vascular endothelium determined by a transfected human fucosyltransferase cDNA. *Cell* **63**:475, 1990.

103. Goelz SE, Hession C, Goff D, Griffiths B, Tizard R, Newman B, Chi-Rosso G, Lobb R: ELFT: A gene that directs the expression of an ELAM-1 ligand. *Cell* **63**:1349, 1990.

104. Tiemeyer M, Swiedler SJ, Ishihara M, Moreland M, Schweingruber H, Hirtzer P, Brandley BK: Carbohydrate ligands for endothelial-leukocyte adhesion molecule-1. *Proc Natl Acad Sci USA* **88**:1138, 1991.

105. Berg EL, Robinson MK, Mansson O, Butcher EC, Magnani JL: A carbohydrate domain common to both sialyl Lea and sialyl LeX is recognized by the endothelial cell leukocyte adhesion molecule ELAM-1. *J Biol Chem* **266**:14869, 1991.

106. Tyrrell D, James P, Rao N, Foxall C, Abbas S, Dasgupta F, Nashed M, Hasegawa A, Kiso M, Asa D, Kidd J, Brandley BK: Structural requirements for the carbohydrate ligand of E-selectin. *Proc Natl Acad Sci USA* **88**:10372, 1991.

107. Polley MJ, Phillips ML, Wayner E, Nudelman E, Singhal AK, Hakomori SI, Paulson JC: CD62 and endothelial cell-leukocyte adhesion molecule 1 (ELAM-1) recognize the same carbohydrate ligand, sialyl-Lewis x. *Proc Natl Acad Sci USA* **88**:6224, 1991.

108. Moore KL, Varki A, McEver RP: GMP-140 binds to a glycoprotein receptor on human neutrophils: Evidence for a lectin-like interaction. *J Cell Biol* **112**:491, 1991.

109. Corral L, Singer MS, Macher BA, Rosen SD: Requirement for sialic acid on neutrophils in a GMP-140 (PADGEM) mediated adhesive interaction with activated platelets. *Biochem Biophys Res Commun* **172**:1349, 1990.

110. Aruffo A, Kolanus W, Walz G, Fredman P, Seed B: CD62/P-selectin recognition of myeloid and tumor cell sulfatides. *Cell* **67**:35, 1991.

111. Kishimoto TK, Warnock RA, Jutila MA, Butcher EC, Lane CL, Anderson DC, Smith CW: Antibodies against human neutrophil LECAM-1 (LAM-1/Leu-8/DREG-56 antigen) and endothelial cell ELAM-1 inhibit a common CD18-independent adhesion pathway in vitro. *Blood* **78**:805, 1991.

112. Picker LJ, Warnock RA, Burns AR, Doerschuk CM, Berg EL, Butcher EC: The neutrophil selectin LECAM-1 presents carbohydrate ligands to the vascular selectins ELAM-1 and GMP-140. *Cell* **66**:921, 1991.

113. Siegelman MH, Cheng IC, Weissman IL, Wakeland EK: The mouse lymph node homing receptor is identical with the lymphocyte cell surface marker Ly-22: Role of the EGF domain in endothelial binding. *Cell* **61**:611, 1990.

114. Kishimoto TK, Jutila MA, Berg EL, Butcher EC: Neutrophil Mac-1 and MEL-14 adhesion proteins inversely regulated by chemotactic factors. *Science* **245**:1238, 1989.

115. Jutila MA, Rott L, Berg EL, Butcher EC: Function and regulation of the neutrophil MEL-14 antigen in vivo: Comparison with LFA-1 and MAC-1. *J Immunol* **143**:3318, 1989.

116. Griffin JD, Spertini O, Ernst TJ, Belvin MP, Levine HB, Kanakura Y, Tedder TF: Granulocyte-macrophage colony-stimulating factor and other cytokines regulate surface expression of the leukocyte adhesion molecule-1 on human neutrophils, monocytes, and their precursors. *J Immunol* **145**:576, 1990.

117. Pober JS, Gimbrone MA Jr, Lapierre LA, Mendrick DL, Fiers W, Rothlein R, Springer TA: Overlapping patterns of antigenic modulation by interleukin 1, tumor necrosis factor and immune interferon. *J Immunol* **137**:1893, 1986.

118. Norris P, Poston RN, Thomas DS, Thornhill M, Hawk J, Haskard DO: The expression of endothelial leukocyte adhesion molecule-1 (ELAM-1), intercellular adhesion molecule-1 (ICAM-1), and vascular cell adhesion molecule-1 (VCAM-1) in experimental cutaneous inflammation: A comparison of ultraviolet B erythema and delayed hypersensitivity. *J Invest Dermatol* **96**:763, 1991.

119. Kishimoto TK: A dynamic model for neutrophil localization to inflammatory sites. *J NIH Res* **3**:75, 1991.

120. Cohnheim J: *Lectures on General Pathology: A Handbook for Practitioners and Students*. London: The New Sydenham Society, 1989.

121. Lawrence MB, Smith CW, Eskin SG, McIntire LV: Effect of venous shear stress on CD18-mediated neutrophil adhesion to cultured endothelium. *Blood* **75**:227, 1990.

122. Abbassi O, Lane CL, Krater SS, Kishimoto TK, Anderson DC, McIntire LV, Smith CW: Canine neutrophil margination mediated by lectin adhesion molecule-1 (LECAM-1) in vitro. *J Immunol* **147**:2107, 1991.

123. Abbassi O, Kishimoto TK, McIntire LV, Smith CW: Neutrophil adhesion to endothelial cells. *Blood Cells* **19**:245, 1993.

124. Lawrence MB, Springer TA: Leukocytes roll on a selectin at physiologic flow rates: Distinction from and prerequisite for adhesion through integrins. *Cell* **65**:859, 1991.

125. Jones DA, Abbassi O, McIntire LV, McEver RP, Smith CW: Neutrophil-endothelial adherence under conditions of flow: P-selectin supports leukocyte rolling. *Circulation* **86**:I-161, 1992.

126. Ley K, Gaehtgens P, Fennie C, Singer MS, Lasky LA, Rosen SD: Lectin-like cell adhesion molecule 1 mediates leukocyte rolling in mesenteric venules in vivo. *Blood* **77**:2553, 1991.

127. von Andrian UH, Chambers JD, McEvoy LM, Bargatze RF, Arfors K-E, Butcher EC: Two step model of leukocyte-endothelial cell interaction in inflammation: Distinct roles for LECAM-1 and the leukocyte beta-2 integrins in vivo. *Proc Natl Acad Sci USA* **88**:7538, 1991.

128. Doré M, Korthuis RJ, Granger DN, Entman ML, Smith CW: P-selectin mediates spontaneous leukocyte rolling in vivo. *Blood* **82**:1308, 1993.

129. Dobrina A, Carlos TM, Schwartz BR, Beatty PG, Ochs HD, Harlan JM: Phorbol ester causes downregulation of a CD11/CD18-independent mechanism of neutrophil adherence to endothelium. *Immunology* **69**:429, 1990.

130. Smith CW, Marlin SD, Rothlein R, Lawrence MB, McIntire LV, Anderson DC: Role of ICAM-1 in the adherence of human neutrophils to human endothelial cells in vitro, in Springer TA, Anderson DC, Rosenthal AS, Rothlein R (eds): *Leukocyte Adhesion Molecules: Structure, Function, and Regulation*. New York, Springer-Verlag, 1989, p 170.

131. Huber AR, Kunkel SL, Todd RF III, Weiss SJ: Regula-

tion of transendothelial neutrophil migration by endogenous interleukin-8. *Science* **254**:99, 1991.

132. Kuijpers TW, Hakkert BC, Hart MHL, Roos D: Neutrophil migration across monolayers of cytokine-prestimulated endothelial cells: A role for platelet-activating factor and IL-8. *J Cell Biol* **117**:565, 1992.
133. Prescott SM, Zimmerman GA, McIntyre TM: Human endothelial cells in culture produce platelet-activating factor (1-alkyl-2-acetyl-sn-glycero-3-phosphocholine) when stimulated with thrombin. *Proc Natl Acad Sci USA* **81**:3534, 1984.
134. Zimmerman GA, McIntyre TM, Mehra M, Prescott SM: Endothelial cell-associated platelet-activating factor: A novel mechanism for signaling intercellular adhesion. *J Cell Biol* **110**:529, 1990.
135. Zimmerman GA, McIntyre TM: Neutrophil adherence to human endothelium in vitro occurs by CDw18 (Mo1, MAC-1/LFA-1/GP150,95) glycoprotein-dependent and independent mechanisms. *J Clin Invest* **81**:531, 1988.
136. Zimmerman GA, McIntyre TM, Prescott SM: Thrombin stimulates the adherence of neutrophils to human endothelial cells in vitro. *J Clin Invest* **76**:2235, 1985.
137. Dransfield I, Cabanas C, Craig A, Hogg N: Divalent cation regulation of the function of the leukocyte integrin LFA-1. *J Cell Biol* **116**:219, 1992.
138. Anderson DC, Miller LJ, Schmalstieg FC, Rothlein R, Springer TA: Contributions of the Mac-1 glycoprotein family to adherence-dependent granulocyte functions: Structure-function assessments employing subunit-specific monoclonal antibodies. *J Immunol* **137**:15, 1986.
139. Smith CW, Rothlein R, Hughes BJ, Mariscalco MM, Schmalstieg FC, Anderson DC: Recognition of an endothelial determinant for CD18-dependent human neutrophil adherence and transendothelial migration. *J Clin Invest* **82**:1746, 1988.
140. Smith CW: Transendothelial migration, in Harlan JM, Liu DY (eds): *Adhesion. Its Role in Inflammatory Disease*. New York, Freeman, 1992, p 85.
141. Furie MB, Tancinco MCA, Smith CW: Monoclonal antibodies to leukocyte integrins CD11a/CD18 and CD11b/CD18 or intercellular adhesion molecule-1 (ICAM-1) inhibit chemoattractant-stimulated neutrophil transendothelial migration in vitro. *Blood* **78**:2089, 1991.
142. Howard MW, Strauss RG, Johnston RB Jr: Infections in patients with neutropenia. *Am J Dis Child* **131**:788, 1977.
143. Kohl S, Loo LS, Schmalstieg FC, Anderson DC: The genetic deficiency of leukocyte surface glycoprotein Mac-1, LFA-1, p150,95 in humans is associated with defective antibody-dependent cellular cytotoxicity in vitro and defective protection against herpes simplex virus in vivo. *J Immunol* **137**:1688, 1986.
144. Gallin JI: Abnormal phagocyte chemotaxis: Pathophysiology, clinical manifestations, and management of patients. *Rev Infect Dis* **3**:1196, 1981.
145. Davis SD, Schaller J, Wedgwood RJ: Job's syndrome: Recurrent "cold" staphylococcal abscesses. *Lancet* **1**:1013, 1966.
146. Snyderman R, Altman LC, Frankel A, Blaese RM: Defective mononuclear leukocyte chemotaxis: A previously unrecognized immune dysfunction. *Ann Intern Med* **78**:509, 1973.
147. Ward PA, Schlegel RJ: Impaired leucotactic responsiveness in a child with recurrent infections. *Lancet* **2**:344, 1969.
148. Wilkinson PC: Leukocyte locomotion and chemotaxis: Effects of bacteria and viruses. *Rev Infect Dis* **2**:293, 1980.
149. Boner A, Zeligs BJ, Bellanti JA: Chemotactic responses of various differentiational stages of neutrophils from human cord and adult blood. *Infect Immun* **35**:921, 1982.
150. Hill HR, Gerrard JM, Hogan NA: Hyperactivity of neutrophil leukotactic responses during active bacterial infections. *J Clin Invest* **53**:996, 1974.
151. Hill HR, Warwick WJ, Dettloff J, Quie PG: Neutrophil granulocyte function in patients with pulmonary infection. *J Pediatr* **84**:55, 1974.
152. McCall CE, Caves J, Cooper R, DeChatelet LR: Functional characteristics of human toxic neutrophils. *J Infect Dis* **124**:68, 1971.
153. Movat AG, Baum J: Polymorphonuclear leukocyte chemotaxis in patients with bacterial infections. *Br Med J* **3**:617, 1971.
154. Gallin JI, Buescher ES: Abnormal regulation of inflammatory skin responses in male patients with chronic granulomatous disease. *Inflammation* **7**:227, 1983.
155. Grinsburg I, Quie PG: Modulation of human polymorphonuclear leukocyte chemotaxis by leukocyte extracts, bacterial products, inflammatory exudates, and polyelectrolytes. *Inflammation* **4**:301, 1980.
156. Hill HR: Clinical disorders of leukocyte functions. *Curr Top Immunol* **12**:345, 1984.
157. Bergman M, Guerrant F, Murad R, Richardson SH, Weaver D, Mandell GL: Interaction of polymorphonuclear neutrophils with *E. coli:* Effects of enterotoxin on phagocytosis, killing, chemotaxis and cyclic AMP. *J Clin Invest* **61**:227, 1978.
158. Bourne HR, Lehrer RI, Lichtenstein LM, Weissmann G, Zurier R: Effects of cholera enterotoxin on adenosine 3′,5′-monophosphate and neutrophil function: Comparison with other compounds which stimulate leukocyte adenyl cyclase. *J Clin Invest* **52**:698, 1973.
159. Fick RB, Robbins RA, Squier SU, Schoderbek WE, Russ WD: Complement activation in cystic fibrosis respiratory fluids: In vivo and in vitro generation of C5a and chemotactic activity. *Pediatr Res* **20**:1258, 1986.
160. Berger M, Dearborn D, Legris G, Doring G, Sorensen R: Complement receptor expression on neutrophils (PMN) in the lung in cystic fibrosis (CF). *Pediatr Res* **20**:305a, 1986.
161. Boxer LA, Hedley-Whyte T, Stossel TP: Neutrophil actin dysfunction and abnormal neutrophil behavior. *N Engl J Med* **291**:1093, 1974.
162. Fischer A, Descamps-Latscha B, Gerota I, Scheinmetzler C, Virelizier JL: Bone marrow transplantation for inborn error of phagocytic cells associated with defective adherence, chemotaxis, and oxidative response during opsonized particle phagocytosis. *Lancet* **2**:473, 1983.
163. Hayward AR, Leonard J, Wood CBS, Harvey BAM, Greenwood MC, Soothill JF: Delayed separation of the umbilical cord, widespread infections, and defective neutrophil mobility. *Lancet* **1**:1099, 1979.
164. Davies EG, Isaacs D, Levinsky RJ: Defective immune interferon production and natural killer activity associated with poor neutrophil mobility and delayed umbilical cord separation. *Clin Exp Immunol* **50**:454, 1982.
165. Harvath L, Andersen BR: Defective initiation of oxidative metabolism in polymorphonuclear leukocytes. *N Engl J Med* **300**:1130, 1979.
166. Dedhar S, Ruoslahti E, Pierschbacher MD: A cell surface receptor complex for collagen type I recognizes the Arg-Gly-Asp sequence. *J Cell Biol* **104**:585, 1987.
167. Anderson DC, Springer TA: Leukocyte adhesion deficiency: An inherited defect in the Mac-1, LFA-1 and p150,95 glycoproteins. *Annu Rev Med* **38**:175, 1987.
168. Southwick FS, Howard TH, Holbrook T, Anderson DC, Stossel TP, Arnaout MA: The relationship between CR3 deficiency and neutrophil actin assembly. *Blood* **73**:1973, 1989.
169. Abramson JS, Mills EL, Sawyer MK, Regelmann WR, Nelson JD, Quie PG: Recurrent infections and delayed separation of the umbilical cord in an infant with abnormal phagocytic cell locomotion and oxidative response during particle phagocytosis. *J Pediatr* **99**:887, 1981.
170. Crowley CA, Curnutte JT, Rosin RE, Andre-Schwartz J, Gallin JI, Klempner M, Snyderman R, Southwick FS, Stossel TP, Babior BM: An inherited abnormality of neutrophil adhesions: Its genetic transmission and its association with a missing protein. *N Engl J Med* **302**:1163, 1980.
171. Arnaout MA, Pitt J, Cohen HJ, Melamed J, Rosen FS, Colten HR: Deficiency of a granulocyte-membrane glycoprotein (gp150) in a boy with recurrent bacterial infections. *N Engl J Med* **306**:693, 1982.
172. Bowen TJ, Ochs HD, Altman LC, Price TH, Van Epps DE, Brautigan DL, Rosin RE, Perkins WD, Babior BM, Klebanoff SJ, Wedgwood RJ: Severe recurrent bacterial infections associated with defective adherence and chemotaxis in two patients with neutrophils deficient in a cell-associated glycoprotein. *J Pediatr* **101**:932, 1982.

173. Springer TA: The LFA-1, Mac-1 glycoprotein family and its deficiency in an inherited disease. *Fed Proc* **44:**2660, 1985.
174. Springer TA, Galfre G, Secher DS, Milstein C: Mac-1: A macrophage differentiation antigen identified by a monoclonal antibody. *Eur J Immunol* **9:**301, 1979.
175. Dana N, Todd RF III, Pitt J, Springer TA, Arnaout MA: Deficiency of a surface membrane glycoprotein (Mo1) in man. *J Clin Invest* **73:**153, 1983.
176. Anderson DC, Schmalstieg FC, Kohl S, Arnaout MA, Hughes BJ, Tosi MF, Buffone GJ, Brinkley BR, Dickey WD, Abramson JS, Springer TA, Boxer LA, Hollers JM, Smith CW: Abnormalities of polymorphonuclear leukocyte function associated with a heritable deficiency of high molecular weight surface glycoproteins (GP138): Common relationship to diminished cell adherence. *J Clin Invest* **74:**536, 1984.
177. Beatty PG, Ochs HD, Harlan JM: Absence of a monoclonal antibody-defined protein complex in a boy with abnormal leukocyte function. *Lancet* **1:**535, 1984.
178. Springer TA, Thompson WS, Miller LJ, Schmalstieg FC, Anderson DC: Inherited deficiency of the Mac-1, LFA-1, p150,95 glycoprotein family and its molecular basis. *J Exp Med* **160:**1901, 1984.
179. Arnaout MA, Spits H, Terhorst C, Pitt J, Todd RF III: Deficiency of a leukocyte surface glycoprotein (LFA-1) in two patients with Mo1 deficiency. *J Clin Invest* **74:**1291, 1984.
180. Springer TA, Miller LJ, Anderson DC: p150,95, the third member of the Mac-1, LFA-1 human leukocyte adhesion glycoprotein family. *J Immunol* **136:**240, 1986.
181. Miller LJ, Bainton DF, Borregaard N, Springer TA: Stimulated mobilization of monocyte Mac-1 and p150,95 adhesion proteins from an intracellular vesicular compartment to the cell surface. *J Clin Invest* **80:**535, 1987.
182. Anderson DC, Schmalstieg FC, Finegold MJ, Hughes BJ, Rothlein R, Miller LJ, Kohl S, Tosi MF, Jacobs RL, Waldrop TC, Goldman AS, Shearer WT, Springer TA: The severe and moderate phenotypes of heritable Mac-1, LFA-1, p150,95 deficiency: Their quantitative definition and relation to leukocyte dysfunction and clinical features. *J Infect Dis* **152:**668, 1985.
183. Marlin SD, Morton CC, Anderson DC, Springer TA: LFA-1 immunodeficiency disease: Definition of the genetic defect and chromosomal mapping of alpha and beta subunits by complementation in hybrid cells. *J Exp Med* **164:**855, 1986.
184. Kohl S, Springer TA, Schmalstieg FC: Defective natural killer cytotoxicity and polymorphonuclear leukocyte antibody dependent cellular cytotoxicity in patients with LFA-1/OKM-1 deficiency. *J Immunol* **133:**2972, 1984.
185. Arnaout MA, Todd RF III, Dana N, Melamed J, Schlossman SF, Colten HR: Inhibition of phagocytosis of complement C3—or immunoglobulin G—coated particles and of C3bi binding by monoclonal antibodies to a monocyte-granulocyte membrane glycoprotein (Mo1). *J Clin Invest* **72:**171, 1983.
186. Issekutz AC, Lee KY, Bigger WD: Combined abnormality of neutrophil chemotaxis and bactericidal activity in a child with chronic skin infections. *Clin Immunol Immunopathol* **14:**1, 1979.
187. Krensky AM, Mentzer SJ, Clayberger C, Anderson DC, Schmalstieg FC, Burakoff SJ, Springer TA: Heritable lymphocyte function-associated antigen-1 deficiency: Abnormalities of cytotoxicity and proliferation associated with abnormal expression of LFA-1. *J Immunol* **135:**3102, 1985.
188. Buchanan MR, Crowley CA, Rosin RE, Gimbrone MA Jr, Babior BM: Studies on the interaction between GP-180 deficient neutrophils and vascular endothelium. *Blood* **60:**160, 1982.
189. Fischer A, Durandy A, Sterkers G, Griscelli C: Role of the LFA-1 molecule in cellular interactions required for antibody production in humans. *J Immunol* **136:**3198, 1986.
190. Fischer A, Seger R, Durandy A, Grospierre B, Virelizier JL, LeDeist F, Griscelli C, Fischer E, Kazatchkine MD, Bohler MC, Descamps-Latscha B, Trung PH, Springer TA, Oliver D, Mavas C: Deficiency of the adhesive protein complex lymphocyte function antigen 1, complement receptor type 3, glycoprotein p150,95 in a girl with recurrent bacterial infections. *J Clin Invest* **76:**2385, 1985.
191. Lisowska-Grospierre B, Bohler MCh, Fischer A, Mawas C, Springer TA, Griscelli C: Defective membrane expression of the LFA-1 complex may be secondary to the absence of the beta chain in a child with recurrent bacterial infections. *Eur J Immunol* **16:**205, 1986.
192. Ross GD: Characterization of phagocytic and cytotoxic abnormalities in patients who have an inherited deficiency of neutrophil complement receptor type three (CR3) and the related membrane antigens LFA-1 and p150,95, in Aiuti F, Rosen F, Cooper MD (eds): *Recent Advances in Primary and Acquired Immunodeficiencies*. New York, Raven Press, 1986, p 119.
193. Buescher ES, Gaither T, Nath J, Gallin JI: Abnormal adherence-related functions of neutrophils, monocytes, and EB virus-transformed B cells in a patient with C3bi receptor deficiency. *Blood* **65:**1382, 1985.
194. Fujita K, Kobayashi K, Uchida M, Kajii T: Neutrophil adhesion abnormality with deficient surface membrane proteins (gp110 and p98): The effect of their antibodies on the function of normal neutrophils. *Pediatr Res* **20:**361, 1986.
195. Reinherz EL: Human myeloid and hematopoietic cells, in Reinherz EL, Haynes BF, Nadler LM, Bernstein ID (eds): *Leukocyte Typing II*. New York, Springer-Verlag, 1986.
196. Weisman SJ, Berkow RL, Plautz G, Torres M, McGuire WA, Coates TD, Haak RA, Floyd A, Jersild R, Baehner RL: Glycoprotein-180 deficiency: Genetics and abnormal neutrophil activation. *Blood* **65:**696, 1985.
197. Weisman SJ, Berkow RL, Plautz G, Torres M, McGuire WA, Coates TD, Haak RA, Floyd A, Jersild R, Baehner RL: Glycoprotein-180 deficiency: Genetics and abnormal neutrophil activation. *Blood* **65:**696, 1985.
198. Fischer A, Blanche S, Veber F, LeDeist F, Gerota I, Lopez M, Durandy A, Griscelli C: Correction of immune disorders by HLA matched and mismatched bone marrow transplantation, in Gale RP (ed): *Recent Advances in Bone Marrow Transplantation*. New York, Alan R. Liss, 1986,
199. Todd RF III, Freyer DR: The CD11/CD18 leukocyte glycoprotein deficiency. *Hematol Oncol Clin North Am* **2:**13, 1988.
200. Fischer A, Lisowska-Grospierre B, Anderson DC, Springer TA: The leukocyte adhesion deficiency: Molecular basis and functional consequences. *Immunodefic Rev* **1:**39, 1988.
201. Arnaout MA: Leukocyte adhesion molecule deficiency: Its structural basis, pathophysiology and implications for modulating the inflammatory response. *Immunol Rev* **114:**145, 1990.
202. Waldrop TC, Anderson DC, Hallmon WW, Schmalstieg FC, Jacobs RL: Periodontal manifestations of the heritable Mac-1, LFA-1 deficiency syndrome—clinical, histopathologic and molecular characteristics. *J Periodont* **58:**400, 1987.
203. Giger U, Boxer LA, Simpson PJ, Lucchesi BR, Todd RF III: Deficiency of leukocyte surface glycoproteins Mo1, LFA-1, and Leu M5 in a dog with recurrent bacterial infections: An animal model. *Blood* **69:**1622, 1987.
204. Trowald-Wigh G, Hakansson L, Johannisson A, Norrgren L, af Segerstad CH: Leucocyte adhesion protein deficiency in Irish Setter dogs. *Vet Immunol Immunopathol* **32:**261, 1992.
205. Kehrli ME, Jr, Schmalstieg FC, Anderson DC, Van Der Maaten MJ, Hughes BJ, Ackermann MR, Wilhelmsen CL, Brown GB, Stevens MG, Whetstone CA: Molecular definition of the bovine granulocytopathy syndrome: Identification of a deficiency of the Mac-1 (CD11b/CD18) glycoprotein. *J Am Vet Med Assoc* **51:**1826, 1990.
206. Gilbert RO, Rebhun WC, Kim CA, Kehrli ME Jr, Shuster DE, Ackermann MR: Clinical manifestations of leukocyte adhesion deficiency in cattle: 14 cases (1987–1991). *J Am Vet Med Assoc* **202:**445, 1993.
207. Kehrli ME Jr, Ackermann MR, Shuster DE, Van Der Maaten MJ, Schmalstieg FC, Anderson DC, Hughes BJ: Animal model of human disease. Bovine leukocyte adhesion deficiency. Beta$_2$ integrin deficiency in young Holstein cattle. *Am J Pathol* **140:**1489, 1992.
208. Kehrli ME Jr, Shuster DE, Ackermann M, Smith CW, Anderson DC, Dore M, Hughes BJ: Clinical and immunological abnormalities associated with bovine leukocyte adhesion deficiency, in Lipsky PE, Rothlein R, Kishimoto TK, Faanes RB, Smith CW (eds): *Structure and Function of Molecules Involved in Leukocyte Adhesion II*. New York, Springer-Verlag, 1993, p 314.

209. Kehrli ME Jr, Shuster DE, Ackermann MR: Genetic abnormalities in leukocyte adhesion deficiency among Holstein cattle. *Cornell Vet* **82**:103, 1992.
210. Shuster DE, Kehrli ME Jr, Ackermann MR, Gilbert RO: Identification and prevalence of a genetic defect that causes leukocyte adhesion deficiency in Holstein cattle. *Proc Natl Acad Sci USA* **89**:9225, 1992.
211. Ross GD, Thompson RA, Walport MJ, Springer TA, Watson JV, Ward RHR, Lida J, Newman SL, Harrison RA, Lachmann PJ: Characterization of patients with an increased susceptibility to bacterial infections and a genetic deficiency of leukocyte membrane complement receptor type 3 and the related membrane antigen LFA-1. *Blood* **66**:882, 1985.
212. Root RK, Metcalf J, Oshino N, Chance B: H_2O_2 release from human granulocytes during phagocytosis. I. Documentation, quantitation, and some regulating factors. *J Clin Invest* **55**:945, 1975.
213. Weening RS, Roos D, Weemaes CMR, Homan-Muller JWT, vanSchaik MLJ: Defective initiation of the metabolic stimulation of phagocytizing granulocytes: A new congenital defect. *J Lab Clin Med* **88**:757, 1976.
214. Bissenden JG, Haeney MR, Tarlow MJ, Thompson RA: Delayed separation of the umbilical cord, severe widespread infections and immunodeficiency. *Arch Dis Child* **57**:397, 1981.
215. Niethammer D, Dieterle U, Kleihauer E, Wildfeuer A, Haferkamp O, Hitzig WH: An inherited defect in granulocyte function: Impaired chemotaxis, phagocytosis and intracellular killing of microorganisms. *Helv Paediatr Acta* **30**:537, 1975.
216. Tonnesen MG, Smedly LA, Henson PM: Neutrophil-endothelial cell interactions: Modulation of neutrophil adhesiveness induced by complement fragments C5a and $C5a_{desArg}$ and formyl-methionyl-leucyl-phenylalanine in vitro. *J Clin Invest* **74**:1581, 1984.
217. Anderson DC, Rothlein R, Marlin SD, Krater SS, Smith CW: Impaired transendothelial migration by neonatal neutrophils: Abnormalities of Mac-1 (CD11b/CD18)-dependent adherence reactions. *Blood* **78**:2613, 1990.
218. Schmalstieg FC, Rudloff HE, Hillman GR, Anderson DC: Two dimensional and three dimensional movement of human polymorphonuclear leukocytes: Two fundamenally different mechanisms of location. *J Leuk Biol* **40**:677, 1986.
219. Beller DI, Springer TA, Schreiber RD: Anti-Mac-1 selectively inhibits the mouse and human type three complement receptor. *J Exp Med* **156**:1000, 1982.
220. Thompson RA, Candy DCA, McNeish AS: Familial defect of polymorph neutrophil phagocytosis associated with absence of a surface glycoprotein antigen (OKM1). *Clin Exp Immunol* **58**:229, 1984.
221. O'Shea JJ, Brown EJ, Seligmann BE, Metcalf JA, Frank MM, Gallin JI: Evidence for distinct intracellular pools of receptors for C3b and C3bi in human neutrophils. *J Immunol* **134**:2580, 1985.
222. Gresham HD, Graham IL, Anderson DC, Brown EJ: Leukocyte adhesion deficient (LAD) neutrophils fail to amplify phagocytic function in response to stimulation: Evidence for CD11b/CD18-dependent and -independent mechanisms of phagocytosis. *J Clin Invest* **88**:588, 1991.
223. Rich KC, Neumann CG, Stiehm ER: Neutrophil chemotaxis in malnourished Ghanaian children, in Suskind RM (ed): *Malnutrition and Immune Response*. New York, Raven Press, 1977, p 271.
224. Mentzer SJ, Bierer BE, Anderson DC, Springer TA, Burakoff SJ: Abnormal cytolytic activity of lymphocyte function-associated antigen-1-deficient human cytolytic T lymphocyte clones. *J Clin Invest* **78**:1387, 1986.
225. Kishimoto TK, Hollander N, Roberts TM, Anderson DC, Springer TA: Heterogenous mutations of the beta subunit common to the LFA-1, Mac-1, and p150,95 glycoproteins cause leukocyte adhesion deficiency. *Cell* **50**:193, 1987.
226. Dana N, Clayton LK, Tennen DG, Pierce MW, Lachmann PJ, Law SA, Arnaout MA: Leukocytes from four patients with complete or partial Leu-CAM deficiency contain the common beta-subunit precursor and beta-subunit messenger RNA. *J Clin Invest* **79**:1010, 1987.
227. Dimanche-Boitrel MT, LeDeist F, Fischer A, Arnaout MA, Giscelli C, Lisowska-Grospierre B: LFA-1 beta-chain synthesis and degradation in patients with leukocyte adhesive protein deficiency. *Eur J Immunol* **17**:417, 1987.
228. Wardlaw AJ, Hibbs ML, Stacker SA, Springer TA: Distinct mutations in two patients with leukocyte adhesion deficiency and their functional correlates. *J Exp Med* **172**:335, 1990.
229. Arnaout MA, Dana N, Gupta SK, Tenen DG, Fathallah DM: Point mutations impairing cell surface expression of the common beta subunit (CD18) in a patient with leukocyte adhesion molecule (Leu-CAM) deficiency. *J Clin Invest* **85**:977, 1990.
230. Kishimoto TK, O'Connor K, Springer TA: Leukocyte adhesion deficiency: Aberrant splicing of a conserved integrin sequence causes a moderate deficiency phenotype. *J Biol Chem* **264**:3588, 1989.
231. MacKrell AJ, Blumberg B, Haynes S, Fessler J: The lethal myospheroid gene of *Drosophila* encodes a membrane protein homologous to vertebrate integrin beta subunits. *Proc Natl Acad Sci USA* **85**:2633, 1988.
232. Sligh JE Jr, Hurwitz MY, Zhu C, Anderson DC, Beaudet AL: An initiation codon mutation in CD18 in association with the moderate phenotype of leukocyte adhesion deficiency. *J Biol Chem* **267**:714, 1992.
233. Kozak M: Context effects and inefficient initiation at non-AUG codons in eucaryotic cell-free translation systems. *Mol Cell Biol* **9**:5073, 1989.
234. Back AL, Kwok WW, Hickstein DD: Identification of two molecular defects in a child with leukocyte adherence deficiency. *J Biol Chem* **267**:5482, 1992.
235. Corbi AL, Vara A, Ursa A, Garcia-Rodriguez MC, Fontan G, Sanchez-Madrid F: Molecular basis for a severe case of leukocyte adhesion deficiency. Simultaneous occurrence of a point mutation and aberrant splicing. *Eur J Immunol* **22**:1877, 1992.
236. Ohashi Y, Yambe T, Tsuchiya S, Kikuchi H, Konno T: Familial genetic defect in a case of leukocyte adhesion deficiency. *Hum Mutat* **2**:458, 1993.
237. Konno T, Tsukamoto J, Terasawa M, Tsuchiya S, Tachibana T: OKM-1(Mol)/LFA-1 deficiency in a Japanese infant with recurrent infection, in Eible MM, Rosen FS (eds): *Primary Immunodeficiency Disease*. Amsterdam, Excerpta Medica, 1986, p 315.
238. Nelson C, Rabb H, Arnaout MA: Genetic cause of leukocyte adhesion molecule deficiency: Abnormal splicing and a missense mutation in a conserved region of CD18 impair cell surface expression of beta-2 integrins. *J Biol Chem* **267**:3351, 1992.
239. Matsuura S, Kishi F, Tsukahara M, Nunoi H, Matsuda I, Kobayashi K, Kajii T: Leukocyte adhesion deficiency: Identification of novel mutation in two Japanese patients with a severe form. *Biochem Biophys Res Commun* **184**:1460, 1992.
240. Nunoi H, Yanabe Y, Higuchi S, Tsuchiya H, Yamamoto J, Matsuda I, Naito M, Takahashi K, Fujita K, Uchida M, Kobayashi K, Jono M, Malech H: Severe hypoplasia of lymphoid tissues in Mo1 deficiency. *Hum Pathol* **19**:753, 1988.
241. Kelly T, Molony L, Burridge K: Purification of two smooth muscle glycoproteins related to integrin. *J Biol Chem* **262**:17189, 1987.
242. Nermut MV, Green NM, Eason P, Yamada SS, Yamada KM: Electron microscopy and structural model of human fibronectin receptor. *EMBO J* **7**:4093, 1988.
243. D'Souza SE, Ginsberg MH, Burke TA, Lam SC-T, Plow EF: Localization of an Arg-Gly-Asp recognition site within an integrin adhesion receptor. *Science* **242**:91, 1988.
244. Kieffer N, Phillips DR: Platelet membrane glycoproteins: Functions in cellular interactions. *Annu Rev Cell Biol* **6**:329, 1990.
245. Loftus JC, O'Toole TE, Plow EF, Glass A, Frelinger AL III, Ginsberg MH: A beta3 integrin mutation abolishes ligand binding and alters divalent cation-dependent conformation. *Science* **249**:915, 1990.
247. LeDeist F, Blanche S, Keable H, Descamps-Latscha B, Pham HT, Wahn V, Griscelli C, Fischer A: Successful

HLA nonidentical bone marrow transplantation in three patients with the leukocyte adhesion deficiency. *Blood* **74**:512, 1989.

248. Hibbs ML, Wardlaw AJ, Stacker SA, Anderson DC, Lee A, Roberts TM, Springer TA: Transfection of cells from patients with leukocyte adhesion deficiency with an integrin β subunit (CD18) restores lymphocyte function-associated antigen-1 expression and function. *J Clin Invest* **85**:674, 1990.
249. Wilson JM, Ping AJ, Krauss JC, Mayo-Bond L, Rogers CE, Anderson DC, Todd RF III: Correction of CD18-deficient lymphocytes by retrovirus-mediated gene transfer. *Science* **248**:1413, 1990.
250. Back AL, Kwok WW, Adam M, Collins SJ, Hickstein DD: Retroviral-mediated gene transfer of the leukocyte integrin CD18 subunit. *Biochem Biophys Res Commun* **171**:787, 1990.
251. Wilson RW, Yorifuji T, Lorenzo I, Smith CW, Anderson DC, Belmont JW, Beaudet AL: Expression of human CD18 in murine granulocytes and improved efficiency for infection of deficient human lymphoblasts. *Hum Gene Ther* **4**:25, 1993.
253. Krauss JC, Bond LM, Todd RF III, Wilson JM: Expression of retroviral transduced human CD18 in murine cells: An in vitro model of gene therapy for leukocyte adhesion deficiency. *Hum Gene Ther* **2**:221, 1991.
254. Wilson RW, Ballantyne CM, Smith CW, Montgomery C, Bradley A, O'Brien WE, Beaudet AL: Gene targeting yields a partially CD18-deficient mouse for study of inflammation. *J Immunol* **151**:1571, 1993.
255. Yorifuji T, Wilson RW, Lorenzo I, Hughes BJ, Smith CW, Anderson DC, Beaudet AL: Towards gene therapy of leukocyte adhesion deficiency. *Pediatr Res* **3**:137A, 1992.
256. Wilson CB: Immunologic basis for enhanced susceptibility of the neonate to infection. *J Pediatr* **108**:1, 1986.
257. Schuit KE, Homisch L: Inefficient in vivo neutrophil migration in neonatal rats. *J Leuk Biol* **35**:583, 1984.
258. Martin TR, Rubens CE, Wilson CB: Lung antibacterial defense mechanisms in infant and adult rats: Implications for the pathogenesis of group B streptococcal infections in the neonatal lung. *J Infect Dis* **157**:91, 1988.
259. Lodge-Patch L: The ageing of cardiac infarcts, and its influence on cardiac rupture. *Br Heart J* **13**:37, 1951.
260. Christensen RD, Rothstein G: Exhaustion of mature marrow neutrophils in neonates with sepsis. *J Pediatr* **97**:316, 1980.
261. Anderson DC: Neonatal neutrophil dysfunction. *Am J Pediatr Hematol Oncol* **11**:224, 1989.
262. Anderson DC, Abbassi O, Kishimoto TK, Koenig JM, McIntire LV, Smith CW: Diminished lectin-, epidermal growth factor-, complement binding domain-cell adhesion molecule-1 on neonatal neutrophils underlies their impaired CD18-independent adhesion to endothelial cells in vitro. *J Immunol* **146**:3372, 1991.
263. Miller ME: Chemotactic function in the human neonate: Humoral and cellular aspects. *Pediatr Res* **5**:487, 1971.
264. Anderson DC, Hughes BJ, Wible LJ, Perry GJ, Smith CW, Brinkley BR: Impaired motility of neonatal PMN leukocytes: Relationship to abnormalities of cell orientation and assembly of microtubules in chemotactic gradients. *J Leuk Biol* **36**:1, 1984.
265. Pahwa SG, Pahwa R, Grimes E, Smithwick E: Cellular and humoral components of monocyte and neutrophil chemotaxis in cord blood. *Pediatr Res* **11**:677, 1977.
266. Klein RB, Fischer TJ, Gard SE, Biberstein M, Rich KC, Stiehm ER: Decreased mononuclear and polymorphonuclear chemotaxis in human newborns, infants, and young children. *Pediatrics* **60**:467, 1977.
267. Anderson DC, Hughes BJ, Edwards MS, Buffone GJ, Baker CJ: Impaired chemotaxigenesis by type III group B streptococci in neonatal sera: Relationship to diminished concentrations of specific anticapsular antibody and abnormalities of serum complement. *Pediatr Res* **17**:496, 1983.
268. Krause PJ, Maderazo EG, Scroggs M: Abnormalities of neutrophil adherence in newborns. *Pediatrics* **69**:184, 1982.
269. Krause PJ, Herson VC, Boutin-Lebowitz J, Eisenfeld L: Polymorphonuclear leukocyte adherence and chemotaxis in stressed and healthy neonates. *Pediatr Res* **20**:296, 1986.
270. Anderson DC, Freeman KLB, Heerdt B, Hughes BJ, Jack RM, Smith CW: Abnormal stimulated adherence of neonatal granulocytes: Impaired induction of surface Mac-1 by chemotactic factors or secretagogues. *Blood* **70**:740, 1987.
271. Anderson DC: Neonatal neutrophils. *J Lab Clin Med* **120**:816, 1992.
272. Jones DH, Schmalstieg FC, Dempsey K, Krater SS, Nannen DD, Smith CW, Anderson DC: Subcellular distribution and mobilization of Mac-1 (CD11b/CD18) in neonatal neutrophils. *Blood* **75**:488, 1990.
273. Bruce MC, Bailey JE, Medvik K, Berger M: Impaired surface membrane expression of C3bi, but not C3b receptors in neonatal neutrophils. *Pediatr Res* **21**:306, 1987.
274. Ambruso DR, Bentwood B, Henson PM, Johnston RB Jr.: Oxidative metabolism of cord blood neutrophils: Relationship to content and degranulation of cytoplasmic granules. *Pediatr Res* **18**:1148, 1984.
275. Jones DH, Schmalstieg FC, Hawkins HK, Burr BL, Rudloff HE, Krater SS, Smith CW, Anderson DC: Characterization of a new mobilizable Mac-1 (CD11b/CD18) pool that co-localizes with gelatinase in human neutrophils, in Springer TA, Anderson DC, Rosenthal AS, Rothlein R (eds): *Leukocyte Adhesion Molecules: Structure, Function, and Regulation.* New York, Springer-Verlag, 1989, p 106.
276. Smith JB, Kunjummen RD, Kishimoto TK, Anderson DC: Neonatal eosinophils and neutrophils have similar abnormalities of expression of leukocyte-endothelial cell adhesion molecule-1 (LECAM-1). *Pediatr Res* **29**:278, 1991.
277. Fortenberry JD, Mariscalco MM, Marolda JR, Smith CW, Anderson DC: Diminished surface levels of LECAM-1 on neonatal lapine neutrophils. *Pediatr Res* **29**:274A, 1991.
278. Laver J, Duncan E, Abboud M, Gasparetto C, Sahdev I, Warren D, Bussel J, Auld P, O'Reilly RJ, Moore MAS: High levels of granulocyte and granulocyte-macrophage colony-stimulating factors in cord blood of normal full-term neonates. *J Pediatr* **116**:627, 1990.
279. Peters WP, Stuart A, Affronti ML, Kim CS, Coleman RE: Neutrophil migration is defective during recombinant human granulocyte-macrophage colony-stimulating factor infusion after autologous bone marrow transplantation in humans. *Blood* **72**:1310, 1988.
280. Koenig JM, Anderson DC, Smith CW: Surface levels of LECAM-1 on neonatal neutrophils are further diminished at 24 hours of life. *Pediatr Res* **29**:276A, 1991.
281. Bullock JD, Robertson AF, Bodenbender JG, Kontras SB, Miller CE: Inflammatory response in the neonate reexamined. *Pediatrics* **44**:58, 1969.
282. Eitzman DV, Smith RT: The nonspecific inflammatory cycle in neonatal infants. *Am J Dis Child* **97**:326, 1974.
283. Fortenberry JD, Mariscalco MM, Marolda JR, Smith CW, Anderson DC: Diminished CD18-dependent neutrophil emigration in neonatal lapine peritonitis. *Pediatr Res* **29**:275A, 1991.
284. Baehner RL, Nathan DG: Quantitative nitroblue tetrazolium test in chronic granulomatous disease. *N Engl J Med* **278**:971, 1968.
285. Gallin JI, Fletcher MP, Seligmann BE, Hoffstein S, Cehr K, Mounessa N: Human neutrophil-specific granules deficiency: A method to access the role of neutrophil-specific granules in the evolution of the inflammatory response. *Blood* **59**:1317, 1982.
286. Gallin JI, Wright DG, Schiffmann E: Role of secretory events in modulating human neutrophil chemotaxis. *J Clin Invest* **62**:1364, 1978.
287. Spitznagel JK, Cooper MR, McCall AE, DeChatelet LR, Welsh IRH: Selective deficiency of granules associated with lysozyme and lactoferrin in human polymorphs (PMN). *J Clin Invest* **51**:93A, 1972.
288. Boxer LA, Coates TD, Haak RA, Wolach JB, Hoffstein S, Baehner RL: Lactoferrin deficiency associated with granulocyte function. *N Engl J Med* **307**:404, 1982.
289. Gallin JI: Neutrophil specific granule deficiency. *Annu Rev Med* **36**:263, 1985.
290. Parmley RT, Ogawa M, Darby CP Jr, Spicer SS: Congenital neutropenia: Neutrophil proliferation with abnormal maturation. *Blood* **46**:723, 1975.
291. Komiyama A, Morosawa H, Nakahata T, Miyagawa Y,

Akabane T: Abnormal neutrophil maturation in a neutrophil defect with morphologic abnormality and impaired function. *J Pediatr* **94:**19, 1979.

292. Breton-Gorius J, Mason DY, Buriot D, Vilde JL, Griscelli C: Lactoferrin deficiency as a consequence of a lack of specific granules in neutrophils from a patient with recurrent infections. *Am J Pathol* **99:**413, 1980.
293. Strauss RG, Bove KE, Jones JF, Mauer AM, Fulginiti VA: An anomaly of neutrophil morphology with impaired function. *N Engl J Med* **290:**478, 1974.
294. Borregaard N, Boxer LA, Smolen JE, Tauber AI: Anomalous neutrophil granule distribution in a patient with lactoferrin deficiency: Pertinence to the respiratory burst. *Am J Hematol* **18:**255, 1985.
295. Gant T, Metcalf JA, Gallin JI, Boxer LA, Lehrer RI: Microbial/cytotoxic proteins of neutrophils are deficient in two disorders: Chediak-Higashi syndrome and "specific" granule deficiency. *J Clin Invest* **82:**552, 1988.
296. Lomax KJ, Malech HL, Gallin JI: The molecular biology of selected phagocyte defects. *Blood Rev* **3:**94, 1989.
297. Lomax KJ, Gallin JI, Rotrosen D, Raphael GD, Kalinir MA, Benz EJ, Boxer LA, Malech HL: Selective defect in myeloid cell lactoferrin gene expression in neutrophil specific granule deficiency. *J Clin Invest* **83:**514, 1989.
298. Frydman M, Etzioni A, Eidlitz-Markus T, Avidov I, Varsano I, Shecter Y, Orlin JB, Gershoni-Baruch R: Rambam-Hasharon syndrome of psychomotor retardation, short stature, defective neutrophil motility, and Bombay phenotype. *Am J Med Genet* **44:**297, 1992.
299. Yunis EJ, Svardal JMK, Bridges RA: Genetics of the Bombay phenotype. *Blood* **33:**124, 1969.
300. Watkins WH: Biochemistry and genetics of the ABO, Lewis, and P blood group systems. *Adv Hum Genet* **10:**1, 1980.
301. Le Pendu J, Cartron JP, Lemieux RU, Oriol R: The presence of at least two different H-blood-group-related beta-D-Gal-alpha-2-L-fucosyltransferases in human serum and the genetics of blood group H substances. *Am J Hum Genet* **37:**749, 1985.
302. Etzioni A, Frydman M, Pollack S, Avidor I, Phillips ML, Paulson JC, Gershoni-Barugh R: Brief report: Recurrent severe infections caused by a novel leukocyte adhesion deficiency. *N Engl J Med* **327:**1789, 1992.
303. von Andrian UH, Berger EM, Chambers JD, Ramezani L, Ochs H, Harlan JM, Paulson JC, Etzioni A, Arfors K-E: In vivo behavior of neutrophils from two patients with distinct inherited leukocyte adhesion deficiency syndromes. *J Clin Invest* **91:**2893, 1993.
304. Butcher EC: Leukocyte-endothelial cell recognition: Three (or more) steps to specificity and diversity. *Cell* **67:**1033, 1991.
305. Ley K, Gaehtgens P, Fennie C, Singer MS, Lasky LA, Rosen SD: LEC-CAM 1 mediates leukocyte rolling in mesenteric venules in vivo. *Blood* **77:**2553, 1991.
306. Simon SI, Rochon YP, Lynam EB, Smith CW, Anderson DC, Sklar LA: Beta$_2$-integrin and L-selectin are obligatory receptors in neutrophil aggregation. *Blood* **82:**1097, 1993.
307. Carlos TM, Harlan JM: Membrane proteins involved in phagocyte adherence to endothelium. *Immunol Rev* **114:**5, 1990.
308. Smith CW, Anderson DC, Taylor AA, Rossen RD, Entman ML: Leukocyte adhesion molecules and myocardial ischemia. *Trends Cardiovasc Med* **1:**167, 1991.
309. Weiss SJ: Tissue destruction by neutrophils. *N Engl J Med* **320:**365, 1989.
310. Nathan CF: Respiratory burst in adherent human neutrophils: Triggering by colony-stimulating factors CSF-GM and CSF-G. *Blood* **73:**301, 1989.
311. Simchowitz L, Fishbein LC, Spilberg I, Atkinson JP: Induction of a transient elevation in intracellular levels of adenosine 3′,5′-cyclic monophosphate by chemotactic factors: An early event in human neutrophil activation. *J Immunol* **124:**1482, 1980.
312. Nathan CF, Srimal S, Farber C, Sanchez E, Kabbash L, Asch A, Gailit J, Wright SD: Cytokine-induced respiratory burst of human neutrophils: Dependence on extracellular matrix proteins and CD11/CD18 integrins. *J Cell Biol* **109:**1341, 1989.
313. Harlan JM, Winn RK, Vedder NB, Doerschuk CM, Rice CL: In vivo models of leukocyte adherence to endothelium, in Harlan JM, Liu DY (eds): *Adhesion. Its Role in Inflammatory Disease*. New York, W. J. Freeman, 1992, p 117.
314. Mulligan MS, Warren JS, Smith CW, Anderson DC, Ward PA: Lung injury following deposition of IgA immune complexes: Requirements for CD11b, CD18 and L-arginine. *J Immunol* **148:**3086, 1992.
315. Craddock PR, Hammerschmidt DE, White JG, Dalmasso AP, Jacob HS: Complement (C5a)-induced granulocyte aggregation in vitro: A possible mechanism of complement-mediated leukostasis and leukopenia. *J Clin Invest* **60:**260, 1977.
316. Hammerschmidt DE, Harris P, Wayland JH, Jacob HS: Intravascular granulocyte (PMN) aggregation in live animals: A complement (C) mediated mechanism of ischemia. *Blood* **52**(Suppl):125, 1978.
317. Hammerschmidt DE, Craddock PR, McCullough J, Kronenberg RS, Dalmasso AP, Jacob HS: Complement activation and pulmonary leukostasis during nylon fiber filtration leukapheresis. *Blood* **51:**721, 1978.
318. Sacks T, Moldow CF, Craddock PR: Oxygen radicals mediate endothelial cell damage by complement-stimulated granulocytes: An in vitro model of immune vascular damage. *J Clin Invest* **61:**1161, 1978.
319. Hammerschmidt PE, White JG, Craddock PR, Jacob HS: Corticosteroids inhibit complement-induced granulocyte aggregation: A possible mechanism for their efficacy in shock states. *J Clin Invest* **63:**798, 1979.
320. Hammerschmidt PE, Bowers TK, Kammi-Kepfe CJ, Jacob HS, Craddock PR: Granulocyte aggregometry: A sensitive technique for the detection of C5a and complement activation. *Blood* **55:**898, 1980.
321. O'Kell RT, Axon LL: Leukocyte alkaline phosphatase in the newborn infant. *Am J Obstet Gynecol* **93:**1181, 1965.
322. Arnaout MA, Hakim RM, Todd RF III, Dana N, Colten HR: Increased expression of an adhesion-promoting surface glycoprotein in the granulocytopenia of hemodialysis. *N Engl J Med* **312:**457, 1985.
323. Nelson RD, Hasslen SR, Ahrenholz DH, Haus E, Solem LD: Influence of minor thermal injury on expression of complement receptor CR3 on human neutrophils. *Am J Pathol* **125:**563, 1986.
324. Buyon JP, Shadick N, Berkman R, Hopkins P, Dalton J, Weissmann G, Winchester R, Abramson SB: Surface expression of Gp165/95, the complement receptor type 3, CR3, as a marker of disease activity in systemic lupus erythematosis. *Clin Immunol Immunopathol* **46:**141, 1988.
325. Van Epps DE, Williams RC: Serum inhibitors of leukocyte chemotaxis and their relationship to skin test anergy, in Gallin JI, Quie PG (eds): *Leukocyte Chemotaxis*. New York, Raven Press, 1978, p 237.
326. Arfors KE, Lundberg C, Lindbom L, Lundberg K, Beatty PG, Harlan JM: A monoclonal antibody to the membrane glycoprotein complex CD18 inhibits polymorphonuclear leukocyte accumulation and plasma leakage in vivo. *Blood* **69:**338, 1987.
327. Lindbom L, Lundberg C, Prieto J, Raud J, Nortamo P, Gahmberg CG, Patarroyo M: Rabbit leukocyte adhesion molecules CD11/CD18 and their participation in acute and delayed inflammatory responses and leukocyte distribution in vivo. *Clin Immunol Immunopathol* **57:**105, 1990.
328. Price TH, Beatty PG, Corpuz SR: In vivo inhibition of neutrophil function in the rabbit using monoclonal antibody to CD18. *J Immunol* **139:**4174, 1987.
329. Bucky LP, Vedder NB, Hong CHZ, May JW Jr, Ehrlich HP: A monoclonal antibody which blocks neutrophil adhesion prevents second degree burns. *Proc Am Burn Assoc* **23:**133, 1991.
330. Rosen H, Gordon S: Monoclonal antibody to the murine type 3 complement receptor inhibits adhesion of myelomonocytic cells in vitro and inflammatory cell recruitment in vivo. *J Exp Med* **166:**1685, 1987.
331. Rosen H, Milon G, Gordon S: Antibody to the murine type 3 complement receptor inhibits T lymphocyte-dependent recruitment of myelomonocytic cells in vivo. *J Exp Med* **169:**535, 1989.

332. Tuomanen EI, Saukkonen K, Sande S, Cioffe C, Wright SD: Reduction of inflammation, tissue damage, and mortality in bacterial meningitis in rabbits treated with monoclonal antibodies against adhesion-promoting receptors of leukocytes. *J Exp Med* **170:**959, 1989.
333. Wallace JL, Arfors KE, McNight GW: A monoclonal antibody against the CD18 leukocyte adhesion molecule prevents indomethacin-induced gastric damage in the rabbit. *Gastroenterology* **100:**878, 1991.
334. Barton RW, Rothlein R, Ksiazek J, Kennedy C: The effect of anti-intercellular adhesion molecule-1 on phorbol-ester-induced rabbit lung inflammation. *J Immunol* **143:**1278, 1989.
335. Hawkins HK, Heffelfinger S, Anderson DC: Leukocyte adhesion deficiency: Clinical and postmortem observations. *Pediatr Pathol* **12:**119, 1991.
336. Dreyer WJ, Smith CW, Michael LH, Rossen RD, Hughes BJ, Entman ML, Anderson DC: Canine neutrophil activation by cardiac lymph obtained during reperfusion of ischemic myocardium. *Circ Res* **65:**1751, 1989.
337. Hernandez LA, Grisham MB, Twohig B, Arfors KE, Harlan JM, Granger DN: Role of neutrophils in ischemia-reperfusion-induced microvascular injury. *Am J Physiol* **238:**H699, 1987.
338. Granger DN, Russell J, Arfors KE, Rothlein R, Anderson DC: Role of CD11/CD18 and ICAM-1 in ischemia-reperfusion induced leukocyte adherence and emigration in mesenteric venules. *FASEB J* **5:**A1753, 1991.
339. Simpson PJ, Todd RF III, Fantone JC, Mickelson JK, Griffin JD, Lucchesi BR: Reduction of experimental canine myocardial reperfusion injury by a monoclonal antibody (anti-Mo1, anti-CD11b) that inhibits leukocyte adhesion. *J Clin Invest* **81:**624, 1988.
340. Todd RF III, Simpson PJ, Lucchesi BR: Anti-inflammatory properties of monoclonal anti-Mo1 (CD11b/CD18) antibodies in vitro and in vivo, in Springer TA, Anderson DC, Rosenthal AS, Rothlein R (eds): *Leukocyte Adhesion Molecules: Structure, Function, and Regulation.* New York, Springer-Verlag, 1989, p 125.
341. Dreyer WJ, Michael LH, West MS, Smith CW, Rothlein R, Rossen RD, Anderson DC, Entman ML: Neutrophil accumulation in ischemic canine myocardium: Insights into the time course, distribution, and mechanism of localization during early reperfusion. *Circulation* **84:**400, 1991.
342. Ma XL, Johnson G III, Tsao PS, Lefer AM: Antibody to CD-18 beta-chain preserves endothelium and myocardium in myocardial ischemia and reperfusion. *Circulation* (Suppl) **82:**III-701, 1992.
343. Winquist R, Frei P, Harrison P, McFarland M, Letts LG, Van G, Andrews L, Rothlein R, Hintze T: An anti-CD18 MAb limits infarct size in primates following myocardial ischemia and reperfusion. *Circulation* (Suppl) **82:**III-701, 1992.
344. Seewaldt-Becker E, Rothlein R, Dammgen JW: CDw18 dependent adhesion of leukocytes to endothelium and its relevance for cardiac reperfusion, in Springer TA, Anderson DC, Rosenthal AS, Rothlein R (eds): *Leukocyte Adhesion Molecules: Structure, Function, and Regulation.* New York, Springer-Verlag, 1989, p 138.
345. Williams FM, Collins PD, Nourshargh S, Williams TJ: Suppression of 111In-neutrophil accumulation in rabbit myocardium by MoA ischemic injury. *J Mol Cell Cardiol* **20:**S33, 1988.
346. Vedder NB, Winn RK, Rice CL, Chi EY, Arfors KE, Harlan JM: Inhibition of leukocyte adherence by anti-CD18 monoclonal antibody attenuates reperfusion injury in the rabbit ear. *Proc Natl Acad Sci USA* **87:**2643, 1990.
347. Vedder NB, Winn RK, Rice CL, Chi EY, Arfors KE, Harlan JM: A monoclonal antibody to adherence-promoting leukocyte glycoprotein, CD18, reduces organ injury and improves survival from hemorrhagic shock and resuscitation in rabbits. *J Clin Invest* **81:**939, 1988.
348. Mileski WJ, Winn RK, Vedder NB, Pohlman TK, Harlan JM, Rice CL: Inhibition of CDW18-dependent neutrophil (PMN) adherence reduced organ injury following hemorrhagic shock in primates. *Surgery* **108:**206, 1990.
349. Carden DL, Smith JK, Korthuis RJ: Neutrophil-mediated microvascular dysfunction in postischemic canine skeletal muscle. Role of granulocyte adherence. *Circ Res* **66:**1436, 1990.
350. Clark WM, Madden KP, Rothlein R, Zivin JA: Reduction of central nervous system ischemic injury in rabbits using leukocyte adhesion antibody treatment. *Stroke* **22:**877, 1991.
351. Mileski WJ, Harlan JM, Heimbach D, Rice CL: Inhibition of neutrophil (PMN) adherence with monoclonal antibody 60.3 reduced tissue loss following frostbite. *Proc Am Burn Assoc* **22:**164, 1990.
352. Doerschuk CM, Winn RK, Harlan JM: Mechanisms of neutrophil emigration, in Springer TA, Anderson DC, Rosenthal AS, Rothlein R (eds): *Leukocyte Adhesion Molecules: Structure, Function, and Regulation.* New York, Springer-Verlag, 1989, p 87.
353. Ismail G, Morganroth ML, Todd RF III, Boxer LA: Prevention of pulmonary injury in isolated perfused rat lungs by activated human neutrophils preincubated with anti-Mo1 monoclonal antibody. *Blood* **69:**1167, 1987.
354. Wegner CD, Gundel RH, Reilly P, Haynes N, Letts LG, Rothlein R: Intercellular adhesion molecule-1 (ICAM-1) in the pathogenesis of asthma. *Science* **247:**456, 1990.
355. Wegner CD, Wolyniec WW, LaPlante AM, Marschman K, Lubbe K, Haynes N, Rothlein R, Letts LG: Intercellular adhesion molecule-1 contributes to pulmonary oxygen toxicity in mice: Role of leukocytes revised. *Lung* **170:**267, 1992.
356. Welbourn R, Goldman G, Hill J, Lindsay T, Shepro D, Hechtman HB: Lung injury following hindlimb ischemia is mediated by neutrophil CD18 adherence receptors. *FASEB J* **5:**A1492, 1991.
357. Mulligan MS, Varani J, Warren JS, Till GO, Smith CW, Anderson DC, Todd RF III, Ward PA: Roles of beta-2 integrins of rat neutrophils in complement- and oxygen radical-mediated acute inflammatory injury. *J Immunol* **148:**1847, 1992.
358. Doerschuk CM, Winn RK, Coxson HO, Harlan JM: CD18-dependent and independent mechanisms of neutrophil emigration in the pulmonary and systemic microcirculation of rabbits. *J Immunol* **144:**2327, 1990.
359. Mulligan MS, Varani J, Dame MK, Lane CL, Smith CW, Anderson DC, Ward PA: Role of endothelial-leukocyte adhesion molecule 1 (ELAM-1) in neutrophil-mediated lung injury in rats. *J Clin Invest* **88:**1396, 1991.
360. Gundel RH, Wegner CD, Torcellini CA, Clarke CC, Haynes N, Rothlein R, Smith CW, Letts LG: Endothelial-leukocyte adhesion molecule-1 mediates antigen-induced acute airway inflammation and late-phase airway obstruction in monkeys. *J Clin Invest* **88:**1407, 1991.
361. Mulligan MS, Polley MJ, Bayer RJ, Nunn MF, Paulson JC, Ward PA: Neutrophil-dependent acute lung injury: Requirement for P-selectin (GMP-140). *J Clin Invest* **90:**1600, 1992.
362. Lundberg C, Wright SD: Relation of the CD11/CD18 family of leukocyte antigens to the transient neutropenia caused by chemoattractants. *Blood* **76:**1240, 1990.
363. Schmid-Schonbein GW: Capillary plugging by granulocytes and the no-reflow phenomenon in the microcirculation. *Fed Proc* **46:**2397, 1987.
364. Worthen GS, Schwab B III, Elson EL, Downey GP: Mechanics of stimulated neutrophils: Cell stiffening induces retention in capillaries. *Science* **245:**183, 1989.
365. Bagge U, Amundson B, Lauritzen C: White blood cell deformability and plugging of skeletal muscle capillaries in hemorrhagic shock. *Acta Physiol Scand* **108:**159, 1980.
366. Bagge U, Johansson B, Olofsson J: Deformation of white blood cells in capillaries. *Adv Microcirc* **7:**29, 1977.
367. Lewinsohn DM, Bargatze RF, Butcher EC: Leukocyte-endothelial cell recognition: Evidence of common molecular mechanism shared by neutrophils, lymphocytes, and other leukocytes. *J Immunol* **138:**4313, 1987.
368. Watson SR, Imai Y, Fennie C, Geoffroy JS, Rosen SD, Lasky LA: A homing receptor-IgG chimera as a probe for adhesive ligands of lymph node high endothelial venules. *J Cell Biol* **110:**2221, 1990.
369. Blume RS, Wolff SM: The Chediak-Higashi syndrome. Studies in four patients and a review of the literature. *Medicine* **51:**247, 1972.
370. Clark RA, Kimball HR: Defective granulocyte chemotaxis in the Chediak-Higashi syndrome. *J Clin Invest* **50:**2645, 1971.

371. Wolff SM, Dale DC, Clark RA, Root RK, Kimball HR: The Chediak-Higashi syndrome: Studies of host defenses. *Ann Intern Med* **76:**293, 1972.
372. Rausch PG, Pryzwansky KB, Spitznagel JK: Immunocytochemical identification of azurophilic and specific granule markers in the giant granules of Chediak-Higashi neutrophils. *N Engl J Med* **298:**693, 1978.
373. Haak RA, Ingraham LM, Baehner RL, Boxer LA: Membrane fluidity in human and mouse Chediak-Higashi leukocytes. *J Clin Invest* **64:**138, 1979.
374. Root RK, Rosenthal AS, Balestra DJ: Abnormal bactericidal, metabolic, and lysosomal functions of Chediak-Higashi syndrome leukocytes. *J Clin Invest* **51:**649, 1972.
375. Klein M, Roder J, Haliotis T, Koter J, Jett RB, Herberman B, Katz P, Fauci AS: Chediak-Higashi gene in humans. II. The selectivity of the defect in natural-killer and antibody-dependent cell-mediator cytotoxicity function. *J Exp Med* **151:**1049, 1980.
376. Abo T, Roder JC, Abo W, Cooper MD, Balch CM: Natural killer (HNK-1$^+$) cells in Chediak-Higashi patients are present in normal numbers but are abnormal in function and morphology. *J Clin Invest* **70:**193, 1982.
377. Katz P, Zaytoun AM, Fauci AS: Deficiency of active natural killer cells in the Chediak-Higashi syndrome. *J Clin Invest* **69:**1231, 1982.
378. Argyle JC, Kjeldsberg CR, Marty J, Shigeoka AO, Hill HR: T-cell lymphoma and the Chediak-Higashi syndrome. *Blood* **60:**672, 1982.
379. Virelizier JL, Lagrue A, Durandy A, Arenzana F, Oury C, Griscelli C: Reversal of natural killer defect in a patient with Chediak-Higashi syndrome after bone marrow transplatation. *N Engl J Med* **306:**1055, 1982.
380. Boxer LA, Rister M, Allen JM, Baehner RL: Improvement of Chediak-Higashi leukocyte function by cyclic guanosine monophosphate. *Blood* **49:**9, 1977.
381. Boxer LA, Watanabe AM, Rister M, Besch HR, Allen J, Baehner RL: Correction of leukocyte function in Chediak-Higashi syndrome by ascorbate. *N Engl J Med* **295:**1041, 1976.
382. Oliver JM, Zurier RB: Correction of characteristic abnormalities of microtubule function and granule morphology in Chediak-Higashi syndrome with cholinergic agonists. *J Clin Invest* **57:**1239, 1976.
383. Oliver JM, Zurier RB, Berlin RD: Concanavalin A cap formation on polymorphonuclear leukocytes of normal and beige (Chediak-Higashi) mice. *Nature* **253:**471, 1975.
384. Malech HL, Root RK, Gallin JI: Structural analysis of human neutrophil migration: Centriole, microtubule, and microfilament orientation and function during chemotaxis. *J Cell Biol* **75:**666, 1977.
385. Anderson DC, Hughes BJ, Wible LJ, Brinkley BR: Normal microtubule assembly of Chediak-Higashi PMNs. *Pediatr Res* **936:**252a, 1984.
386. Nath J, Flavin M, Gallin JI: Tubulin tyrosinolation in human polymorphonuclear leukocytes: Studies in normal subjects and in patients with the Chediak-Higashi syndrome. *J Cell Biol* **95:**519, 1980.
387. Brandt EJ, Elliott RW, Swank RT: Defective lysosomal enzyme secretion in kidneys of Chediak-Higashi (beige) mice. *J Cell Biol* **67:**774, 1975.
388. Jenkins NA, Justice MJ, Gilbert DJ, Chu M-L, Copeland NG: Nidogen/entactin (Nid) maps to the proximal end of mouse chromosome 13 linked to beige (bg) and identifies a new region of homology between mouse and human chromosomes. *Genomics* **9:**401, 1991.
389. Beaudet AL, Anderson DC, Michels VV, Arion WJ, Lange AJ: Neutropenia and impaired neutrophil migration in type 1B glycogen storage disease. *J Pediatr* **97:**906, 1980.
390. Ambruso DR, McCabe ERB, Anderson DC, Beaudet A, Brandt IK, Brown B, Coleman R, Friedman HS, Haymond MW, Keating JP, Kinney TR, Leonard JV, Mahoney DH Jr, Matalon R, Roe TF, Simmond P, Slomin A: Infectious and bleeding complications in patients with glycogenosis 1b: Relationship to neutrophil and platelet function. *Am J Dis Child* **139:**691, 1985.
391. Narisowa K, Igarashi Y, Otomo H, Tada K: A new variant of glycogen storage disease type I probably due to a defect in the glucose-6-phosphate transport system. *Biochim Biophys Res Commun* **83:**1360, 1978.
392. Lange AJ, Arion WJ, Beaudet AL: Type 1b glycogen storage disease is caused by a defect in the glucose-6-phosphate translocase of the microsomal glucose-6-phosphatase system. *J Biol Chem* **255:**8381, 1980.
393. Desnick RJ, Sharp HL, Grabowski GA, Brunning RD, Quie PG, Sung JH, Gorlin RJ, Ikonne JU: Mannosidosis: Clinical, morphologic, immunologic, and biochemical studies. *Pediatr Res* **10:**985, 1976.
394. VanDyke TE, Horoszewicz HU, Cianciola LJ: Neutrophil chemotaxis dysfunction in human periodontitis. *Infect Immun* **27:**124, 1980.
395. Page RC, Schroeder HE: "Pathogenesis of Localized Juvenile Periodontitis," *Periodontitis In Man and Other Animals*. Karger, Basel, 1982, p 1.
396. Shurin SB, Socransky SS, Sweeney E, Stossel TP: A neutrophil disorder induced by *Capnocytophaga,* a dental microorganism. *N Engl J Med* **301:**849, 1979.
397. Cohen DW, Morris AL: Periodontal manifestations of cyclic neutropenia. *J Periodontol* **32:**159, 1961.
398. VanDyke TE, Horoszewicz HU, Genco RJ: The polymorphonuclear leukocyte (PMNL) locomotor defect in juvenile periodontitis: Study of random migration, chemokinesis and chemotaxis. *J Periodontol* **53:**682, 1982.
399. Tempel TR, Kimball HR, Kakenashi S, Amen CR: Host factors in periodontal disease: Periodontal manifestations of Chediak-Higashi syndrome. *J Periodont Res* 7(Suppl 10):26, 1972.
400. Page RC, Bowen T, Altman LC, Vandesteen E, Ochs H, MacKenzie P, Osterberg S, Engle LD, Williams BL: Prepubertal periodontitis. 1. Definition of a clinical disease entity. *J Periodontol* **54:**257, 1983.
401. Quie PG: Chronic granulomatous disease of childhood. *Adv Pediatr* **16:**287, 1969.
402. VanDyke TE, Schweinebraten I, Cianciola LJ, Offenbacher S, Genco RJ: Neutrophil chemotaxis in families with localized juvenile periodontitis. *J Periodont Res* **20:**503, 1985.
403. Page RC, Schroeder HE: Pathogenesis of inflammatory periodontal disease. *J Lab Invest* **33:**234, 1976.
404. VanDyke TE: Role of the neutrophil in oral disease. Receptor deficiency in leukocytes from patients with juvenile periodontitis. *Rev Infect Dis* **7:**419, 1985.
405. Clark RA, Page RC, Wilde G: Defective neutrophil chemotaxis in juvenile periodontitis. *Infect Immun* **18:**694, 1977.
406. Chusid MJ, Bujak JS, Dale DC: Defective polymorphonuclear leukocyte metabolism and function in canine cyclic neutropenia. *Blood* **46:**921a, 1975.
407. Lavine WS, Maderazo EG, Stolman J, Ward A, Cogen RB, Greenblatt I, Robertson PB: Impaired neutrophil chemotaxis in patients with juvenile and rapidly progressing periodontitis. *J Periodont Res* **14:**10, 1979.
408. Genco PS, VanDyke TE, Park B: Neutrophil chemotaxis impairment in juvenile periodontitis for evaluation of specificity, adherence, deformability and serum factors. *J Reticul Soc* **28:**815, 1980.
409. Ranney RR, Debski BF, Tew JG: Pathogenesis of gingivitis and periodontal disease in children and young adults. *Pediatr Dent* **3:**89, 1981.
410. Suzuki JB, Colison C, Falker WF, Newman RK: Immunologic profile of juvenile periodontitis. II. Neutrophil chemotaxis, phagocytosis and spore germination. *J Periodontol* **55:**461, 1984.
411. De Nardin E, De Luca C, Lefine MJ, Genco RJ: Antibodies directed to the chemotactic factor receptor detect differences between chemotactically normal and defective neutrophils from LJP patients. *J Periodontol* **61:**609, 1990.
412. Perez HD, Kelly E, Elman F, Armitage G, Winkler J: Defective polymorphonuclear leukocyte formyl peptide receptors in juvenile periodontitis. *J Clin Invest* **87:**971, 1991.
413. Zambon JJ: *Actinobacillus actinomycetemcomitans* in human periodontal disease. *J Clin Periodontol* **12:**1, 1985.
414. Slots J, Genco RJ: Black-pigmented *Bacteroides sp., Capnocytophage sp., Actinobacillus actinomycetemcomitans* in human periodontol disease. Virulence factors in colonization, survival and tissue destruction. *J Dent Res* **63(3):**412, 1984.

415. Zambon JJ, Christersson LA, Slots J: *Actinobacillus actinomycetemcomitans* in human periodontal disease: Prevalence in patient groups and distribution of biotypes and serotypes within families. *J Periodontol* **54**:707, 1983.
416. Genco RJ, Slots J, Mauton J, Marran P: Systemic immune responses to oral anaerobic organisms, in Lambe DW, Genco RJ, Mayberry-Carson KJ (eds): *Anaerobic Bacteria: Selected Topics*. New York, Plenum 1980, p. 242.
417. Wood DD, Ihrie EJ, Dinarello CA, Cohen PL: Isolation of an interleukin-1-like factor from human joint effusions. *Arthritis Rheum* **26**:975, 1983.
418. Tsai C-C, McArthur WP, Baehni PC, Hammond BF, Taichman NS: Extraction and partial characterization of a leukotoxin from a plaque-derived gram-negative microorganism. *Infect Immun* **25**:427, 1979.
419. Tsai C-C, Taichman NS: Dynamics of infection by leukotoxic strains of *Actinobacillus actinomycetemcomitans* in juvenile periodontitis. *J Clin Periodontol* **13**:303, 1986.
420. Tsai C-C, McArthur WP, Baehni PC, Evian C, Genco RJ, Taichman NS: Serum neutralizing activity against *Actinobacillus actinomycetemcomitans* leukotoxin in juvenile periodontitis. *J Clin Periodontol* **8**:338, 1981.
421. Beaty TH, Boughman JA, Yang P, Astemborski JA, Suzuki JB: Genetic analysis of juvenile periodontitis in families ascertained through an affected proband. *Am J Hum Genet* **40**:443, 1987.
422. Saxen L, Nevenalinna HR: Autosomal recessive inheritance of juvenile periodontitis: Test of a hypothesis. *Clin Genet* **25**:332, 1984.
423. Melnick M, Shilds ED, Bixler D: Periodontitis: A phenotypic and genetic analysis. *Oral Surg Oral Med Oral Pathol* **42**:32, 1976.
424. Agget PJ, Harries JT, Harvey BAM: An inherited defect of neutrophil mobility in Schwachman syndrome. *J Pediatr* **94**:391, 1979.
425. Brueton MJ, Mavromichalis J, Goodchild MC: Hepatic dysfunction in association with pancreatic insufficiency and cyclical neutropenia. *Arch Dis Child* **52**:76, 1977.
426. Schwachman H, Diamond LK, Oski FA, Khaw K-T: The syndrome of pancreatic insufficiency and bone marrow dysfunction. *J Pediatr* **65**:645, 1964.
427. Aggett PJ, Cavanagh NPC, Matthew DJ, Pincott JR, Sutcliffe J, Harries JT: Schwachman's syndrome: A review of 21 cases. *Arch Dis Child* **55**:331, 1980.
428. Burke V, Colebatch JH, Anderson CM, Simons MJ: Association of pancreatic insufficiency and chronic neutropenia in childhood. *Arch Dis Child* **42**:147, 1967.
429. Buckley RH, Becker WG: Abnormalities in the regulation of human IgE synthesis. *Immunol Rev* **41**:288, 1978.
430. Church JA, Frenkel LD, Wright DG, Bellanti JA: T lymphocyte dysfunction, hyperimmunoglobulinemia E, recurrent bacterial infections, and defective neutrophil chemotaxis in a Negro child. *J Pediatr* **88**:982, 1976.
431. Geha RS, Reinherz E, Leung D, McKee KT Jr, Schlossman S, Rosen FS: Deficiency of suppressor T cells in the hyperimmunoglobulin E syndrome. *J Clin Invest* **68**:783, 1981.
432. Donabedian H, Gallin JI: The hyperimmunoglobulin E recurrent infection (Job's) syndrome: A review of the NIH experience and the literature. *Medicine* **62**:195, 1983.
433. Hill HR, Quie PG, Pabst HF, Ochs HD, Clark RA, Klebanoff SJ, Wedgwood RJ: Defect in neutrophil granulocyte chemotaxis in Job's syndrome of recurrent "cold" staphylococcal abscesses. *Lancet* **2**:617, 1974.
434. Schopfer K, Douglas SD, Wilkinson BJ: Immunoglobulin E antibodies against *Staphylococcus aureus* cell walls in the sera of patients with hyperimmunoglobulinemia E and recurrent staphylococcal infection. *Infect Immun* **27**:563, 1980.
435. Berger M, Kirkpatrick CH, Goldsmith PK, Gallin JI: IgE antibodies to *Staphylococcus aureus* and *Candida albicans* in patients with the syndrome of hyperimmunoglobulin E and recurrent infections. *J Immunol* **125**:2437, 1980.
436. Del Prete G, Tiri A, Maggi E: Defective in vitro production of gamma-interferon and tumor necrosis factor by circulating T cells from patients with hyperimmunoglobulin E syndrome. *J Clin Invest* **84**:1830, 1989.
437. Paganelli R, Scala E, Capobianchi MR: Selective deficiency of interferon-gamma production in the hyper-IgE syndrome. *Clin Exp Immunol* **84**:28, 1991.
438. King CL, Gallin JI, Malech HL, Abramson SL, Nutman TB: Regulation of immunoglobulin production in hyperimmunoglobulin E recurrent-infection syndrome by interferon gamma. *Proc Natl Acad Sci USA* **86**:10085, 1989.
439. Jeppson JD, Jaffe HS, Hill HR: Use of recombinant human interferon gamma to enhance neutrophil chemotactic responses in Job syndrome of hyperimmunoglobulin E and recurrent infections. *J Pediatr* **118**:383, 1991.
440. Radermecker M, Maldague MP: Depression of neutrophil chemotaxis in atopic individuals: An H_2 histamine receptor response. *Int Arch Allergy Appl Immunol* **65**:144, 1981.
441. Hill HR, Estensen RD, Hogan NA, Quie PG: Severe staphylococcal disease associated with allergic manifestations, hyperimmunoglobulinemia E, and defective neutrophil chemotaxis. *J Lab Clin Med* **88**:796, 1976.
442. Fischer TJ, Gard SE, Rachelefsky GS, Klein RB, Borut TC, Stiehm ER: Monocyte chemotaxis under agarose: Defects in atopic disease, aspirin therapy, and mucocutaneous candidiasis. *Pediatr Res* **14**:242, 1980.
443. Twomey JJ, Waddell CC, Krantz S, O'Reilly R, L'Esperance P, Good RA: Chronic mucocutaneous candidiasis with macrophage dysfunction, a plasma inhibitor, and coexistent aplastic anemia. *J Lab Clin Med* **85**:968, 1975.
444. VanScoy RE, Hill HR, Ritts RE, Quie PG: Familial neutrophil chemotaxis defect, recurrent bacterial infections, mucocutaneous candidiasis, and hyperimmunoglobulinemia E. *Ann Intern Med* **82**:766, 1975.
445. D'Amelio R, LeMoli S, Rossi P, Aiuti F: Neutrophil chemotaxis defect in IgA deficiency evaluated by migration agarose method. *Scand J Immunol* **11**:471, 1980.
446. D'Amelio R, Rossi P, LeMoli S, Aiuti F: Defective neutrophil chemotaxis in hypogammaglobulinemia and selective IgA deficiency. *Clin Immunol Immunopathol* **16**:287, 1980.
447. Aiuti F, Businco M, Fiorilli M: Fetal liver transplantation in two infants with severe combined immunodeficiency. *Transplant Proc* **11**:230, 1979.
448. Altman LC, Snyderman R, Blaese RM: Abnormalities of chemotactic lymphokine synthesis and mononuclear leukocyte chemotaxis in Wiskott-Aldrich syndrome. *J Clin Invest* **54**:486, 1974.
449. Hughes BJ, Hollers JC, Smith CW: Mac-1 (CD11b/CD18) and adherence-dependent neutrophil locomotion, in Lipsky PE, Rothlein R, Kishimoto TK, Faanes RB, Smith CW (eds): *Structure and Function of Molecules Involved in Leukocyte Adhesion* II. New York, Springer-Verlag, 1993, p 45.
450. Colditz IG, Kerlin RL, Watson DL: Migration of neutrophils and their role in elaboration of host defense. *Crit Rev Physiol* **7**:62, 1987.
451. Arnaout MA, Remold-O'Donnell E, Pierce MW, Harris P, Tenen DG: Molecular cloning of the alpha subunit of human and guinea pig leukocyte adhesion glycoproteins Mo1: Chromosomal localization and homology to the alpha subunits of integrins. *Proc Natl Acad Sci USA* **85**:2776, 1988.
452. Kishimoto TK, Larson RS, Corbi AL, Dustin ML, Staunton DE, Springer TA: Leukocyte integrins, in Springer TA, Anderson DC, Rosenthal AS, Rothlein R (eds): *Leukocyte Adhesion Molecules. Structure, Function, and Regulation*. New York, Springer-Verlag, 1989, p 7.
453. Brandley BK, Swiedler SJ, Robbins PW: Carbohydrate ligands of the LEC cell adhesion molecules. *Cell* **63**:861, 1990.
454. Ruoslahti E, Pierschbacher MD: New perspectives in cell adhesion: RGD and integrins. *Science* **238**:491, 1987.
455. Sheppard D, Rozzo C, Starr L, Quaranta V, Erie DJ, Pytela RP: Complete amnio acid sequence of a novel integrin beta subunit (B6) identified in epithelial cells using the polymerase chain reaction. *J Biol Chem* **265**:11502, 1990.
456. Phillips DR, Charo IF, Parise L, Fitzgerald LA: The platelet membrane glycoprotein IIb-IIIa complex. *Blood* **71**:831, 1988.
457. Erle DJ, Ruegg C, Sheppard D, Pytela R: Complete amino acid sequence of an integrin beta subunit (beta7) identified in leukocytes. *J Biol Chem* **266**:11009, 1991.

458. Vogel BE, Tarone G, Giancotti FG, Gailit J, Ruoslahti E: A novel fibronectin receptor with an unexpected subunit composition ($\alpha_v\beta_1$). *J Biol Chem* **265:**5934, 1990.
459. Ginsberg MH, Loftus JC, Plow EF: Cytoadhesins, integrins, and platelets. *Thromb Haemost* **59:**1, 1988.
460. Kunicki TJ, Pidard D, Rosa JP, Nurden AT: The formation of calcium-dependent complexes of platelet membrane glycoproteins IIb and IIIa in solution as determined by crossed immunoelectrophoresis. *Blood* **58:**268, 1981.
461. Weller A, Isenmänn S, Vestweber D: Cloning of mouse endothelial selectins. Expression of both E- and P-selectin is inducible by tumor necrosis factor-alpha. *J Biol Chem* **267:**15176, 1992.
462. Lipsky PE, Jasin HE, Lightfoot E, Mileski WJ: The role of CD11a/CD18-CD54 interactions in the evolution of animal models of tissue injury, in Lipsky PE, Rothlein R, Kishimoto TK, Faanes RB, Smith CW (eds): *Structure, Function and Regulation of Molecules Involved in Leukocyte Adhesion* II. New York, Springer-Verlag, 1993, p 273.
463. Horgan MJ, Wright SD, Malik AB: Antibody against leukocyte integrin (CD18) prevents reperfusion-induced lung vascular injury. *J Immunol* **143:**1278, 1989.
464. Cosimi AB, Geoffrian C, Anderson T, Conti D, Rothlein R, Colvin RB: Immunosuppression of cynomolgus recipients of renal allografts by R6.5, a monoclonal antibody to ICAM-1, in Springer TA, Anderson DC, Rosenthal AS, Rothlein R (eds): *Leukocyte Adhesion Molecules: Sructure, Function, and Regulation.* New York, Springer-Verlag, 1989, p 274.
465. Flavin T, Ivens K, Rothlein R, Faanes R, Clayberger C, Billingham M, Starnes VA: Monoclonal antibodies against intercellular adhesion molecule 1 prolong cardiac allograft survival in cynomolgus monkeys. *Transplant Proc* **23:**533, 1991.
466. Jasin HE, Lightfoot E, Kavanaugh A, Rothlein R, Faanes RB, Lipsky PE: Successful treatment of chronic antigen-induced arthritis in rabbits with monoclonal antibodies to leukocyte adhesion molecules. *Arthritis Rheum* **33:**S34, 1990.
467. Hutchings P, Rosen H, O'Reilly L, Simpson E, Gordon S, Cook A: Transfer of diabetes in mice prevented by blockade of adhesion-promoting receptor on macrophages. *Nature* **346:**639, 1990.
468. Isobe M, Yagita H, Okumura K, Ihara A: Specific acceptance of cardiac allograft after treatment with antibodies to ICAM-1 and LFA-1. *Science* **255:**1125, 1992.
469. Rosen H, Gordon S, North RJ: Exacerbation of murine listeriosis by a monoclonal antibody specific for the type 3 complement receptor of myelomonocytic cells. *J Exp Med* **170:**27, 1989.
470. Lunn ER, Perry VH, Brown MC, Rosen H, Gordon S: Absence of Wallerian degeneration does not hinder regeneration in peripheral nerve. *Eur J Neurosci* **1:**27, 1989.
471. Beaudet AL, Tsui L-C: A suggested nomenclature for designating mutations. *Hum Mutat* **2:**245, 1993.

CHAPTER 133

Inherited Disorders of Phagocyte Killing

John R. Forehand ▪ William M. Nauseef
John T. Curnutte ▪ Richard B. Johnston, Jr.

1. Phagocytic cells provide the body with a first line of defense against microbial infection. This protective capacity depends on both oxygen-dependent and oxygen-independent killing mechanisms. The latter group includes the release of an array of proteins from cytoplasmic granules into the phagolysosome. Oxygen-dependent microbial killing by phagocytes relies on the phagocytosis-initiated generation of toxic oxygen products from molecular oxygen through a series of single electron transfers. This process is mediated by a multicomponent NADPH oxidase that assembles in the plasma membrane during ingestion of microorganisms. Granules also release myeloperoxidase into the phagolysosome, and the enzyme catalyzes production of the microbicidal agent, hypochlorous acid. These oxygen-dependent events do not occur normally in phagocytes from patients with chronic granulomatous disease, myeloperoxidase deficiency, or deficiency of the enzymes glucose 6-phosphate dehydrogenase (G-6-PD), glutathione synthetase, or glutathione reductase.

2. Congenital absence or structural mutation of one of the four major components of the NADPH oxidase complex in phagocytes results in the clinical syndrome of chronic granulomatous disease, associated with recurrent pyogenic infections of the skin, soft tissues, liver, spleen, lymph nodes, and respiratory tract. Catalase-positive bacteria and fungi are the common pathogens. Phagocytes from these patients ingest organisms normally but display impaired microbial killing, which is the basis of the clinical syndrome. Chronic granulomatous disease is a heterogeneous disorder with regard to mode of inheritance, since the four major oxidase components are encoded at different chromosomal locations (1q25, 7q11.23, 16p23, and Xp21.1). The disease is also heterogeneous with regard to severity of clinical presentation since the mutations in the gene encoding the most commonly affected component (the major subunit of cytochrome b, encoded on the X chromosome) can lead to varying degrees of residual function and, consequently, variability in the capacity to kill ingested microorganisms.

3. Severe G-6-PD deficiency in neutrophils, which leads to impaired hexose monophosphate shunt activity, can mimic chronic granulomatous disease. Affected neutrophils are unable to generate the NADPH required to sustain activity of the respiratory burst oxidase and as a result display a defect in intracellular killing.

4. Myeloperoxidase, present in the azurophilic granules of mature neutrophils, catalyzes the formation of hypochlorous acid from chloride ion and H_2O_2 generated by the respiratory burst. The partial or complete absence of myeloperoxidase affects about 1 in 2000 apparently healthy individuals. Myeloperoxidase deficiency is usually not associated with clinically significant infections, with the exception of invasive fungal disease in individuals with concomitant diabetes mellitus.

5. Glutathione synthetase and glutathione reductase activities are required to maintain adequate intracellular levels of reduced glutathione. This sulfhydryl-containing tripeptide protects the cell from oxidative injury. Deficiency of either of these enzymes permits autooxidative damage, which is associated with abnormal microbicidal activity.

NORMAL MICROBICIDAL MECHANISMS OF PHAGOCYTIC CELLS

The role of phagocytes in host defense against invading microbes has been recognized since Metchnikoff reported his observations in 1883.[1–3] His pioneering studies were made with wandering mesothelial cells from starfish. In the human, phagocytosis is performed efficiently and rapidly by circulating polymorphonuclear neutrophils, eosinophils, and monocytes, and by fixed tissue macrophages, which are the progeny of monocytes.[4] These professional phagocytes provide the body with a first line of defense against infection. When phagocytes, in response to chemotactic stimuli, migrate to sites of infection and contact invading microorganisms, ingestion ensues.

Once microorganisms are ingested, they are retained in intracellular vacuoles (phagosomes), where they are exposed to cell-generated antimicrobial factors and killed. Neutrophils use several methods to destroy invading microbes; these methods can be broadly classified as independent of or dependent on molecular oxygen.

A list of standard abbreviations is located immediately preceding the index in each volume. Additional abbreviations used in this chapter include: CAP = cationic antimicrobial protein, also CAP37 and CAP57; CGD = chronic granulomatous disease; EPO = eosinophil peroxidase; GDI = GDP dissociation inhibitor; IP_3 = inositol 1,4,5-trisphosphate; LPO = lactoperoxidase; NBT = nitroblue tetrazolium; *phox* = phagocyte oxidase; PIP_2 = phosphatidylinositol 4,5-bisphosphate; PKC = protein kinase C; PMA = phorbol myristate acetate; TMP-SMX = trimethoprim/sulfamethoxazole; TPO = thyroid peroxidase.

Table 133-1 Bactericidal Proteins of Human Neutrophils

Bactericidal Protein	Molecular Weight	Chromosomal Location	Granule Location	Susceptible Species
Cationic antimicrobial protein, 37 kDa (CAP37, azurocidin)	~37,000	19pter[9]	Azurophil	Gram-negative bacteria
Bactericidal/ permeability-increasing protein (BPI, CAP57*)	~55,000	20q11-q12[9a]	Azurophil	Gram-negative bacteria
Defensins	~3,000-4,000	8p23[10]	Azurophil	Gram-positive and gram-negative bacteria, many fungi, certain viruses
Cathepsin G	~25,000	14q11.2[11]	Azurophil	Gram-positive and gram-negative bacteria, certain fungi
Lysozyme	~14,500	12[12]	Azurophil and specific	Certain gram-positive bacteria, *Candida albicans*

*Cationic antimicrobial protein, 57 kDA

Oxygen-Independent Mechanisms

It is difficult to determine the effectiveness of nonoxidative killing by neutrophils. However, several lines of evidence support a role for microbicidal activity that occurs in the absence of oxygen. First, the efficacy of oxygen-independent mechanisms can be demonstrated by the bactericidal activity of neutrophils in oxygen-depleted systems.[5–7] The inability to achieve complete anoxia in these systems precludes proof for nonoxidative killing. Secondly, neutrophils from patients with chronic granulomatous disease, which are unable to generate microbicidal oxygen metabolites, can kill at least some of an inoculum of most bacteria.[8] Thirdly, constituents of both major neutrophil granules, the primary (azurophilic) and secondary (specific) granules, have bactericidal capacity (Table 133-1).

Included in the family of neutrophil azurophilic granule-associated serine proteases (possessing chymotryptic activity) are 27-kDa cathepsin G,[13] a 37-kDa cationic antimicrobial protein termed "CAP37,"[14] and azurocidin (AZU).[15] CAP37 and azurocidin appear to be the same protein.[16] Microbial killing by these agents proceeds in vitro in the presence of proteolytic inhibitors suggesting a nonenzymatic mechanism of action. Experiments with purified CAP37 and azurocidin show antimicrobial activity against a variety of gram-negative bacterial as well as *Streptococcus faecalis* and *Candida albicans*.[13]

Cathepsin G, one of the first neutrophil-derived proteolytic enzymes noted to exhibit antibacterial properties, is active against fungi and gram-negative and gram-positive bacteria.[17] Digests of cathepsin G retain antimicrobial activity. Synthetic peptides, copied from two cathepsin G–digest sequences IIGGR and HPQYNQR, show a pattern of killing similar to that of the intact cathepsin G molecule.[18]

Also extracted from the azurophilic granule and possessing antimicrobial activity are bactericidal/permeability factor and the family of defensins. Bactericidal/permeability factor is specific for gram-negative bacteria and its functional domain is contained in a 25-kDa fragment of the N-terminus.[19] Its specificity for gram-negative organisms may lie in its affinity for the lipopolysaccharide outer coating of the bacterial cell wall.[19a] Based on sequence analysis, bactericidal/permeability factor and a cationic antimicrobial protein of 57 kDa (CAP57) are likely identical.[20,21]

The most abundant antimicrobial proteins are four low-molecular-weight peptides (<4000 molecular weight), the defensins.[13] Killing studies indicate a broad spectrum of activity against multiple species of gram-positive and gram-negative bacteria, fungi, and enveloped viruses.[13]

Studied in greater detail is the 14.5-kDa cationic protein lysozyme. This bacteriolytic agent is found in both the azurophilic and specific granules of neutrophils and is secreted constitutively by monocytes and macrophages.[22] The bacteriolytic activity of lysozyme may be enhanced in the presence of complement.[23] It acts by cleaving the $\beta1 \rightarrow 4$ linkage between *N*-acetylmuramic acid and *N*-acetylglucosamine in the glycan backbone of the bacterial cell-wall peptidoglycan.[24] The contribution of lysozyme to the microbicidal activity of the neutrophil is not clear. However, the digestion of bacteria within phagolysosomes correlates with their susceptibility to in vitro lysozyme activity.[24]

Optimal neutrophil antimicrobial activity is also likely to depend on the intraphagolysosomal pH. Microorganisms often do not survive in a low pH environment,[25] and granule-associated antibacterial products that are released into the phagolysosome function within an acid pH range.[24]

Oxygen-Dependent Mechanisms

Respiratory Burst. During phagocytosis, neutrophils undergo a burst of oxidative metabolism[26–31] that is summarized in Table 133-2. This impressive event begins with a marked increase in oxygen uptake and includes increased utilization of glucose via the hexose monophosphate shunt and release

Table 133-2 Components of the Respiratory Burst

1. Increased oxygen consumption
2. Enhanced glucose utilization through the hexose monophosphate shunt
3. Generation of O_2^-, H_2O_2, and ·OH
4. Chemiluminescence
5. Turnover of NADPH and reduced gluthathione

of the bactericidal oxygen metabolites superoxide anion (O_2^-),[32,33] hydrogen peroxide (H_2O_2),[34] hydroxyl radical (·OH),[33–37] and, perhaps, singlet oxygen.[38,39] This cyanide-insensitive[40] increase in oxidative metabolic activity is commonly termed the "respiratory burst." Associated with this burst in oxidative metabolism is the phagocyte's ability to emit low levels of light (chemiluminescence).[38]

The enhanced oxygen consumption in response to phagocytosis was first described over 50 years ago but was thought to be associated with mitochondrial respiration normally required for energy-dependent cellular activity.[26] The observation that the phagocytosis-associated increase in oxygen consumption occurred in the presence of the inhibitor cyanide (CN^-) led to the conclusion in 1959 that mitochondrial energy metabolism was unnecessary for phagocytosis.[40] The significance of the enhanced oxygen uptake was unclear. Two years later it was observed that phagocytosing neutrophils produce H_2O_2, previously recognized for its toxicity to *Escherichia coli*.[41] This finding provided a plausible basis for the microbicidal nature of phagocytosis. H_2O_2 was shown to interact with halide ions in the presence of the granule protein myeloperoxidase to generate microbicidal hypohalites, especially hypochlorite anion (OCl^-).[42] In 1973, phagocytosing neutrophils were reported to release O_2^-,[32] and data were later presented to suggest intraphagosomal generation of hydroxyl radical (·OH).[33]

O_2^-, now recognized to be the initial conversion product of the consumed oxygen, is generated through activity of a plasma membrane-associated enzyme complex termed "NADPH oxidase." This complex reduces oxygen univalently using NADPH as electron donor:[30]

$$2O_2 + NADPH \xrightarrow{\text{NADPH oxidase}} 2O_2^- + NADP^+ + H^+$$

Most of this O_2^- is thought to react with itself in a dismutation reaction (either spontaneously or more rapidly in the presence of superoxide dismutase) to form the second product of the respiratory burst, H_2O_2:

$$2O_2^- + 2H^+ \xrightarrow{\text{superoxide dismutase}} H_2O_2 + O_2$$

The list of oxygen metabolites generated in the phagocytosis-dependent respiratory burst now includes OCl^-[43] and hydroxyl radical (·OH).[33,35–37] ·OH is a highly potent oxidant formed by the interaction between O_2^- and H_2O_2 in the presence of iron or other heavy metal (Haber-Weiss reactions), summarized as follows:

$$O_2^- + Fe^{3+} \rightarrow Fe^{2+} + O_2$$
$$Fe^{2+} + H_2O_2 \rightarrow Fe^{3+} + HO^- + \cdot OH$$

or by the interaction between H_2O_2 and Fe^{2+} (Fenton reaction above).[37] This latter reaction is accelerated by the presence of O_2^-.[44] The physiological role of hydroxyl radical and control of its production are still being elucidated.[45,46] It is generally recognized that what is symbolized to exist as ·OH may, in fact, exist at least partially as one or another potent oxidative radical (i.e., ·OR) formed in the above reactions.

More recently identified as indirect products of the respiratory burst are chloramines, formed by the reaction of hypochlorite with ammonia or amines.[47,48] Other microbicidal products of the reduction of oxygen may be formed by phagocytes, but their roles have not yet been substantiated.

That the respiratory burst is critical for killing of microorganisms by phagocytes was demonstrated convincingly by the occurrence of the inherited disorder chronic granulomatous disease (CGD). Neutrophils from patients with CGD lack a respiratory burst and exhibit markedly deficient killing of most bacteria,[49,50] which is manifested clinically as frequent and life-threatening infections with those bacteria.[51]

Activation. The onset of the respiratory burst requires that an appropriate signal be generated to activate the normally dormant NADPH oxidase into an active state capable of catalyzing the conversion of oxygen to O_2^-.

Specific in vitro stimuli of the respiratory burst include microorganisms opsonized with IgG antibody, complement component 3, or both[33]; phorbol esters, especially phorbol myristate acetate (PMA)[52]; synthetic, bacteria-derived, and complement-derived chemotactic peptides[53–57]; calcium ionophores[58,59]; plant lectins[60]; certain inert particles[33]; fluoride ion[61,62]; immune complexes[63]; products of arachidonic acid metabolism[64–66]; structural analogues of inositol[67,68] and diacylglycerol, especially 1-oleoyl-2-acetyl-glycerol[69]; detergents[70,71]; antineutrophil antibodies[72,73]; the fungal alkaloid cytochalasin E[74]; phospholipase C[75,76]; platelet-activating factor[77]; and platelet-derived growth factor.[78] A typical time course of the release of O_2^- from neutrophils and monocytes exposed to PMA or opsonized yeast particles (zymosan) is shown in Fig. 133-1.

The respiratory burst associated with phagocytosis in normal neutrophils begins 30 to 60 s after initial contact is made between the opsonized microorganism and the phagocytic cell membrane.[79] This delay, or "lag time" (see Fig. 133-1), is presumably the result of the biochemical steps (signal transduction, stimulus-response coupling) required to link ligand-receptor interaction (stimulation) with modification of the NADPH oxidase to an active state (activation).

When specific cell-surface receptors are occupied by ligands such as the chemotactic peptide *N*-formylmethionyl-leucylphenylalanine (f-Met-Leu-Phe), a rapid hydrolysis of plasma membrane phosphatidylinositol 4,5-bisphosphate (PIP_2) is induced via the activation of the phosphodiesterase phospholipase C through an interaction with certain pertussis toxin-sensitive 40-kDa guanine nucleotide regulatory proteins (G proteins).[80] The hydrolytic breakdown of membrane PIP_2 generates inositol 1,4,5-trisphosphate (IP_3) and 1,2-diacylglycerol, molecules that probably serve as dual second messengers.[81,82] IP_3 triggers the release of nonmitochondrial stores of Ca^{2+},[83] which, in turn, may activate calmodulin and thereby stimulate calmodulin-dependent kinases.[84] An increase in intracellular free Ca^{2+} has been linked to the control of a variety of metabolic and cellular activities: enhancement of phospholipase D activity with the release of phosphatidic acid from membrane phospholipid,[85,86] the opening of Ca^{2+}-dependent K^+ channels in the plasma membrane with a resulting change in the membrane potential,[87,88] the facilitation of secretory granule fusion with the phagolysosomal membrane,[89] and shape change secondary to actin rearrangement. Diacylglycerol and Ca^{2+} activate the Ca^{2+} and phospholipid-dependent protein kinase C (PKC)[90] or related enzymes,[91] and Ca^{2+} promotes adherence of

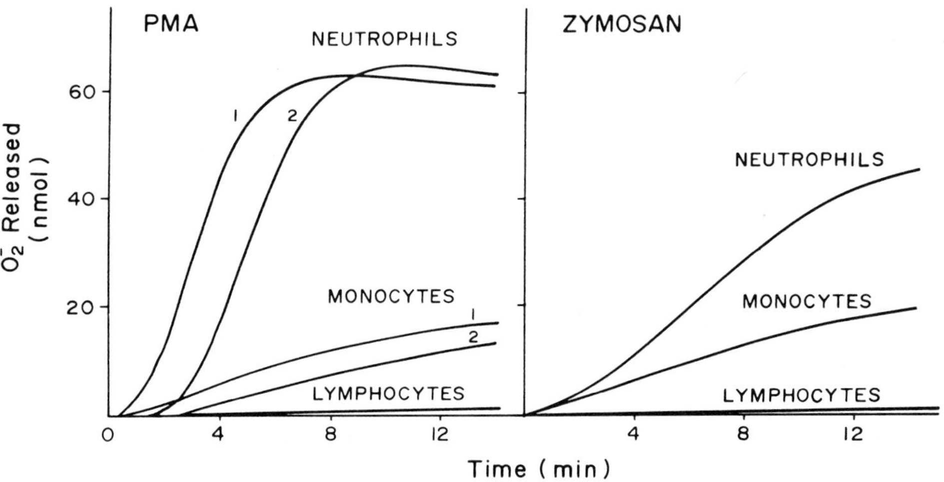

FIG. 133-1 Stimulation of the respiratory burst. Time course of O_2^- generation by 2.5 × 10^6 neutrophils, monocytes, or lymphocytes on contact at 0 min with phorbol myristate acetate (PMA) at concentrations of 67 (*1*) or 33 (*2*) ng/ml (*left*) or with opsonized zymogen (*right*). Actual tracings of the recordings spectrophotometer are represented. Note the typical, more vigorous respiratory burst in neutrophils as compared with monocytes. *(Adapted from data of Johnston and Lehmeyer.[78a] Used by permission.)*

PKC to the plasma membrane.[92] Other signal transduction pathways to stimulate the respiratory burst have been proposed.[93–96]

NADPH Oxidase. The agonist-dependent burst in oxidative activity is catalyzed by an NADPH-dependent oxidase, first described over 30 years ago.[97,98] This multicomponent enzyme is unassembled and inactive in the resting neutrophil and becomes assembled and active when neutrophils are stimulated with an appropriate agonist.[99–102] Knowledge of the number and identity of the components in this oxidase has been greatly extended by the development of a cell-fraction system in which the activation of the oxidase can be studied under defined conditions.[71,103–105] In this system, homogenates of resting neutrophils are first separated into cytosol and plasma membrane fractions.[106] The cytosol is then combined with the plasma membrane fraction in the presence of magnesium, GTP, and NADPH, after which superoxide production is initiated by the addition of a detergent (e.g., sodium dodecyl sulfate or arachidonic acid). Under these conditions, the oxidase possesses biochemical properties similar to those seen for the NADPH-dependent oxidase of intact neutrophils. The observation using this system that superoxide generation requires both membrane and cytosol fractions provided the first firm evidence that not all the oxidase components reside in the membrane fraction of resting neutrophils. Studies using this system have identified the factors necessary for optimal activity of the respiratory burst NADPH oxidase, although the precise functions of some of the components have not been defined.

Components of the NADPH Oxidase. In disrupted resting neutrophils, components of the oxidase are recovered from both the plasma membrane and cytosol fractions. There appears to be a single membrane-associated component, a transmembrane protein known as cytochrome b_{558} or cytochrome b_{-245}, and at least three cytosolic components.

Membrane Component. Cytochrome *b* is a heme-containing glycoprotein with a very low midpoint potential of −245 mV (hence, cytochrome b_{-245}) and a characteristic absorption band at 558 nm when examined spectrophotometrically in its reduced state (hence, cytochrome b_{558}). It is an integral membrane protein of 100 to 135 kDa,[107] which exists as a heterodimer composed of chains of 22kDa (α subunit) and 91 kDa (β subunit).[107,108] Relatively high amounts of cytochrome b_{558} are present in neutrophils, monocytes, eosinophils, and macrophages,[109,110] and low levels are detectable in human glomerular mesangial cells[111] and EBV-transformed B lymphocytes.[112] Complementary DNA (cDNA) for both of the subunits have been cloned and sequenced.[109,110,113,114] The cDNA for the β subunit encodes a 570 amino acid peptide with a number of suitable sites for *N*-linked glycosylation. Direct studies using glycosylation inhibitors and endoglycosidases confirmed the presence of extensive glycosylation on the β subunit, the extent of which varies among phagocytic cells. In contrast, the 195-amino-acid α subunit is not glycosylated. It appears that one heme group binds to each of the two subunits of cytochrome *b*.[115] Although the expression of mRNA for the β subunit is largely restricted to phagocytic cells, the mRNA for the α subunit is constitutively expressed in a variety of cell types, suggesting that β-chain synthesis regulates assembly of the heterodimer.[110]

The unique redox properties of cytochrome *b* make it an excellent candidate for an electron carrier.[116,117] To participate in the conversion of molecular oxygen to superoxide anion, cytochrome b_{558} must undergo sequential reduction and oxidation (i.e., transfer of electrons) during stimulation of intact neutrophils. Phorbol ester stimulation of neutrophils in the absence of oxygen results in the reduction of cytochrome *b*.[118] In like fashion, isolated neutrophil plasma membrane exposed to NADPH—the physiological intracellular substrate for the respiratory burst oxidase—reduces cytochrome *b*.[119] Taken together, these results suggest that cytochrome b_{558} participates in the enzymatic reduction of oxygen to superoxide anion. However, reduced cytochrome *b* is unable to accept directly the two electrons derived per molecule of NADPH, indicating that cytochrome *b* is not the proximal component of the respiratory burst oxidase. In contrast, reduced cytochrome *b* binds reversibly with carbon monoxide and is quickly reoxidized in the presence of oxygen.[116,120] These findings indicate that the cytochrome *b* catalyzes the reduction of molecular oxygen to superoxide anion and that the heme component of the cytochrome is the terminal component of the electron transport chain and interacts directly with oxygen.

As stated earlier, the respiratory burst oxidase of neutrophils is NADPH-dependent. There are extensive experimental data indicating that the nucleotide-binding protein in the oxidase is an FAD containing flavoprotein.[121–126] A major focus of research related to the NADPH oxidase of neutrophils has been the identity and subcellular location of the associated flavoprotein. FAD can accept reducing equivalents directly from NADPH, thereby making it a suitable candidate for the proximal electron carrier in the oxidase. Addition of FAD to membrane preparations of activated oxidase enhances the superoxide-generating activity of the system,[121] whereas inactive FAD analogues and inhibitors decrease activity.[127–129] The level of FAD is diminished by half or more in membranes from neutrophils of some patients with X-linked CGD,[123–126,130] supporting the physiological importance of FAD in this oxidase.

Considerable controversy has existed as to the identity of the flavoprotein and its subcellular location within the resting neutrophil. Two independent studies provide evidence that the FAD redox center of the NADPH-dependent oxidase is contained within the gp91-*phox* subunit of cytochrome b_{558}.[130,131] The experimental data indicate that cytochrome *b* binds both heme and FAD in a molar ratio of 2:1 and that only fully flavinated cytochrome *b* is active in the broken cell superoxide-generating system. In addition, analysis of the amino acid sequence of the β subunit of cytochrome *b* reveals areas of homology with members of the ferredoxin-NADP$^+$ reductase family of reductases. Of note, the observed homology is in the putative NADPH and FAD-binding sites, suggesting that cytochrome *b* is a flavocytochrome. Thus, current evidence suggests that cytochrome *b* is the only membrane-bound enzymatic component of the NADPH-dependent respiratory burst oxidase of neutrophils. By the model, distinct domains within this single protein provide both the heme component and the FAD binding site, which together encompass the membrane component of the enzymatically active NADPH-dependent oxidase.

Cytosolic Components. Cytosolic components are also necessary for optimal oxidase activity. Full oxidase activity can be reconstituted in vitro by combining purified cytochrome b_{558} with only three cytosolic factors, p47-*phox*, p67-*phox*, and a low-molecular-weight G protein (Rac1 or Rac2).[130–133]

p47-*phox* and p67-*phox* [protein 47 kDa (or 67 kDa) *ph*agocyte *ox*idase] were isolated from the cytosol of resting neutrophils by their affinity for GTP-agarose.[134] Both proteins are required for optimal oxidase activity, and the absence of either results in CGD (see below). Despite the absolute requirement of these two proteins for a functioning oxidase, the specific role of each of these proteins is unknown. When neutrophils are stimulated, both p47-*phox* and p67-*phox* translocate from cytosol to the plasma membrane in a fashion that is directly dependent on the concentration of agonist and on the extent of stimulation.[135,136] These proteins apparently dock at the plasma membrane of stimulated cells via an interaction with the cytoplasmic domain of the β subunit of cytochrome *b*, since translocation does not occur when the plasma membrane is deficient in cytochrome b_{558},[137,138] and activation is inhibited by introduction into neutrophils prior to stimulation of a synthetic peptide mimicking a region of the cytoplasmic domain of cytochrome b_{558} (21).[139]

The factors important in regulation of translocation and subsequent assembly of the oxidase are not known. Pretreatment of neutrophils with staurosporine, which inhibits PKC, prior to stimulation with phorbol ester blocks phosphorylation of p47-*phox*, translocation of p47-*phox* to the plasma membrane, and generation of superoxide anion.[136] Translocation of p47-*phox* is a prerequisite for the translocation of p67-*phox*, since p67-*phox* does not translocate in neutrophils of p47-*phox*-deficient patients, whereas p47-*phox* translocates in neutrophils of p67-*phox*-deficient patients.[137] It is not known if p47-*phox* and p67-*phox* are associated as a complex in the cytosol and together become membrane-associated or if they translocate sequentially to the plasma membrane, p47-*phox* being the first to dock at the cytoplasmic domain of the β subunit of cytochrome *b*.

Neither p47-*phox* nor p67-*phox* appears to function enzymatically in the respiratory burst oxidase and more likely serve a regulatory role, perhaps directing or modulating some aspect of assembly of the functioning oxidase at the plasma membrane. The cDNA for each protein has been cloned and sequenced[140–143]: neither sequence provided strong evidence for enzymatically important domains (e.g., NADPH or GTP binding). Nonetheless, the predicted amino acid sequences of both p47-*phox* and p67-*phox* contain two regions of homology with the SH3 domain of the *src* family of proteins. This segment of homology is shared with regions in fodrin and myosin I, two proteins associated with a membrane cytoskeleton.[144] Plasma membrane vesicles from neutrophils contain fodrin,[145] and both p47-*phox* and p67-*phox* are associated with the cytoskeleton of stimulated neutrophils.[136,146] Thus, the SH3 domains may mediate functionally important interactions between these cytosolic NADPH oxidase components and the submembranous cytoskeleton of neutrophils, thereby directing the assembly of the active oxidase at the appropriate site in the plasma membrane.

Recombinant p47-*phox* and p67-*phox* expressed in baculovirus fail to generate superoxide in the presence of membrane,[147] suggesting the existence of at least one more cytosolic factor. A variety of studies demonstrating augmentation of the superoxide-generation system by guanine nucleotides and fluoride[135,148,149] implicated a role for G proteins in the oxidase. In fact, GTP has now been shown to be required for oxidase activity in the cell-fraction system.[150,151] Investigators at three laboratories have demonstrated that a *ras*-related low-molecular-weight G protein is a third cytosolic factor in the oxidase.[132,152,153] Disagreement exists as to whether Rac1 or Rac2, which are 92 percent homologous, is the specific G protein involved in vivo, with sound experimental evidence to support a role for each.[132,152,153] To be active the G protein must be in the GTP-bound form,[153] and posttranslational isoprenoid modification is required for full activity.[154–156] Experimental evidence suggests that in resting neutrophils, isoprenylated Rac2 is complexed with a GDP dissociation inhibitor (GDI), a novel regulatory protein that interacts with GDP-bound forms of *rho* proteins,[157] and thereby the Rac2 remains cytosolic. With activation, the GTP-bound form of Rac2 releases GDI and interacts with the other oxidase components at the plasma membrane. Full oxidase activity can be reconstituted with recombinant p47-*phox*, recombinant p67-*phox*, GTP-bound recombinant Rac1 or Rac2, a detergent and a source of cytochrome b_{558}.[132,158] It thus appears that either Rac1 or Rac2 can support oxidase activity and that processing is important for GDP/GTP nucleotide exchange. Further evidence for the key role of these G proteins in NADPH oxidase function is the finding that the superoxide-generating activity of stimulated EBV-transformed B lymphocytes is inhibited by introduction of antisense oligonucleotides encoding regions shared by Rac1 and Rac2.[159]

Other Putative Factors. Although full oxidase activity can be reconstituted by combining recombinant forms of the three cytosolic proteins described above with plasma membranes or lipidated cytochrome b_{558}, other proteins, both cytosolic and membrane-associated, may participate in regulating the oxidase. The low-molecular-weight G protein Rap1A is associated with cytochrome b_{558}[160] and shares the same

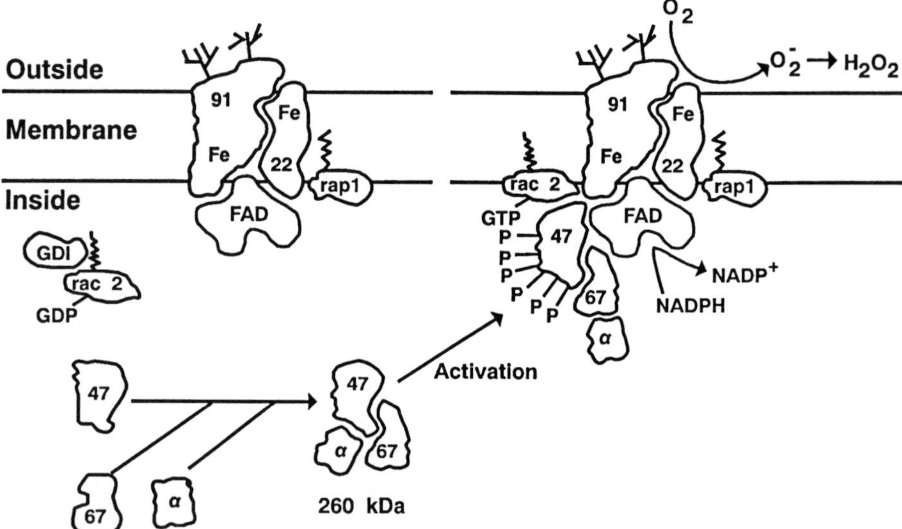

FIG. 133-2 Model of NADPH oxidase activation. In unstimulated neutrophils, NADPH oxidase is in a dormant state and its components are recovered from both the plasma membrane and cytosolic fractions of disrupted cells. As shown on the left side of the figure, the plasma membrane contains the low-potential cytochrome *b* with its p22-*phox* and glycosylated gp91-*phox* subunits, the Rap1a low-molecular-weight GTP-binding protein, and an FAD redox center. The redox center is shown here as a separate subunit, but there is some evidence to suggest that the FAD is part of the gp91-*phox* subunit.[130,131] The cytosolic components include p47-*phox* and p67-*phox*, which appear to exist in a preformed complex of 260 kDa. It is likely that this complex contains at least one other component (as yet undetermined), labeled in this model as "α." The low-molecular-weight GTP-binding protein, Rac2, is also present in the cytosol and is complexed with a GDP dissociation inhibitor (GDI). The p47-/p67-*phox* complex translocates to the membrane. This process may be under the control of the GTP-bound form of Rac2 and further regulated by the phosphorylation of the p47-*phox*. In its active state (right side of figure), the oxidase catalyzes the transfer of electrons from NADPH to molecular oxygen through its FAD and heme redox centers. These electron transfer steps appear to be controlled by p67-*phox* and p47-*phox*.

subcellular distribution as the cytochrome.[161,162] Similarly, isolation of Rac2 from neutrophil cytosol resulted in copurification of two members of the S-100 family of proteins, MRP-8 and MRP-14.[163]

Location and Regulation of the NADPH Oxidase. Resting neutrophils do not consume oxygen; the NADPH-dependent oxidase is unassembled and inactive. On neutrophil activation, the cytosolic factors translocate to the plasma membrane and there assemble into an active oxidase with the NADPH-binding site oriented toward the cytosol and the oxygen-binding and O_2^- releasing component directed extracellularly (and, therefore, into a phagocytic vacuole) (Fig. 133-2).[164,165] Concomitant with activation, neutrophils degranulate, thereby releasing the granule contents extracellularly and fusing granule membranes with the plasma membrane. The membranes of specific granules contain a variety of surface receptors as well as cytochrome b_{558}.[99,166] Thus, degranulation serves to recruit into the plasma membrane a variety of functionally important molecules, including additional cytochrome b_{558}, presumably to participate in the continued assembly and activation of the oxidase.

The genes encoding the individual components of the oxidase are separately regulated. In cultured human cell lines derived from patients with myeloid leukemia, both p47-*phox* and p67-*phox* protein are low constitutively but inducible with dimethyl sulfoxide, retinoic acid, tumor necrosis factor, and interferon-γ.[140–143,167] Constitutive levels of mRNA for the known oxidase components are low but increase when neutrophils are cultured in vitro.[168,169] In contrast, mRNA encoding for gp91-*phox* decreases when monocytes become monocyte-derived macrophages in culture.[170] Lipopolysaccharide, an agent known to prime neutrophils for activation,[171,172] up-regulates mRNA for gp91-*phox* but down-modulates that for p47-*phox*.[170] Neutrophils cultured in the presence of interferon-γ demonstrate enhanced oxidase activity[173] and concomitantly have up-regulation of mRNA for both gp91-*phox* and p47-*phox*.[170] The protein kinase inhibitor staurosporine depresses constitutive and interferon-stimulated levels of mRNA for p47-*phox* and gp91-*phox*, whereas dexamethasone inhibits only mRNA encoding gp91-*phox*,[168] suggesting that the pathways for transcriptional regulation of the various oxidase components are independent. The issue of cytokine-mediated modulation of gene expression of these factors has special clinical implications since recombinant interferon-γ therapy has been used very effectively for prophylaxis against infection in patients with chronic granulomatous disease.[174] Nevertheless, interferon-γ therapy prophylaxis has had no demonstrable effect on the oxidase activity of neutrophils from treated CGD patients.[175]

Antixoidant Mechanisms. Products of the respiratory burst are released into the phagolysosome, where they participate in the destruction of the ingested particle. Figure 133-3 illustrates the biochemical events associated with the respiratory burst and the enzymes required to catalyze the reactions. As toxic oxygen metabolites can harm other circulating cells and adjacent tissues as well as the stimulated phagocyte, it is important that the site of action be concentrated in the phagolysosome. Neutrophils possess protective mechanisms to neutralize and rid the cell of oxygen metabolites not consumed in the microbicidal process.

Superoxide dismutase, which is found in the cytoplasm as a copper–zinc-containing enzyme and in the mitochondria as a manganoprotein, is the principal scavenger of O_2^-.[176–178] This enzyme catalyzes the conversion (dismutation) of two O_2^- molecules to H_2O_2 and oxygen. The copper-containing plasma protein ceruloplasmin may also aid in the removal of O_2^- at sites of inflammation.[179]

Several cytoplasmic systems exist to protect phagocytes

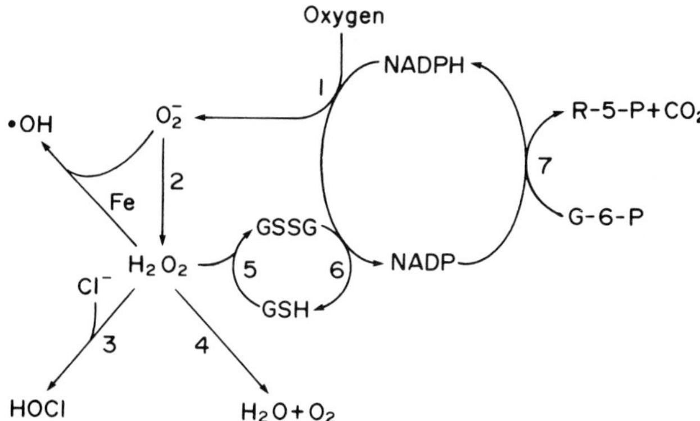

FIG. 133-3 The respiratory burst and associated reactions. Enzymes active in the burst or in protection against its toxic products are indicated by numerals, as follows: 1 = NADPH oxidase; 2 = superoxide dismutase; 3 = myeloperoxidase; 4 = catalase; 5 = glutathione peroxidase; 6 = glutathione reductase; 7 = G-6-PD and 6-phosphogluconate dehydrogenase.

against the potential oxidative injury of H_2O_2. Glutathione, a tripeptide found in all tissues, serves to scavenge H_2O_2 in a reaction catalyzed by glutathione peroxidase.[189] Intracellular glutathione also serves as a source of low-molecular-weight thiols, which interact with protein sulfhydryl groups in the presence of H_2O_2 to form mixed disulfides.[180a] This reversible process, termed "*S*-thiolation," may prevent protein denaturation. Catalase enzymatically converts H_2O_2 to H_2O and oxygen.[181,182] Pyruvate, a product of aerobic glycolysis, can increase the survival of cells in tissue culture and has been proposed as an H_2O_2 scavenger.[183]

Other low-molecular-weight compounds found in cells or plasma can serve as detoxifying agents of harmful oxidants produced by the respiratory burst. Vitamin E (α-tocopherol) reacts with toxic oxygen radicals and preserves cell membranes from oxidative damage.[184] Vitamin C (ascorbic acid) combines with oxygen free radicals to form harmless byproducts[185] and can react with vitamin E radicals to regenerate vitamin E.[186] The nonessential amino acid taurine is a scavenger of hypochlorous acid (HOCl), with the formation of innocuous monochloramine taurine.[187–189]

Myeloperoxidase-Catalyzed System. Since Agner first described myeloperoxidase (MPO) in 1941,[190] numerous investigators have characterized the function and structure of this enzyme.[191–193] MPO is located in the azurophilic granules of neutrophils and in the primary lysosomes of monocytes and is biochemically and immunologically distinct from eosinophil peroxidase.[194]

Oxygen-dependent killing of microorganisms[41,195–197] and tumor cells[198,199] can be mediated by the MPO-dependent system. Stimulated neutrophils release the products of the respiratory burst and the contents of the granules, including MPO, into the phagolysosome or the extracellular space. The combination of MPO, H_2O_2, and halide ions (the MPO-H_2O_2-halide system) results in the production of hypohalous acid and other intermediates that produce cytotoxicity. Hypochlorous acid and the monochloramines, the long-lived oxidants derived from HOCl, have been best studied in this regard.[46,200–210] The actual mechanisms for the cytocidal activity have not been established, but likely possibilities include destruction of bacterial electron transport,[211] ablation of the bacterial adenine nucleotide pool,[211] or oxidation of iron and sulfur centers critical for bacterial viability.[212,213]

MPO could modify the neutrophil-mediated inflammatory response in other ways. MPO-deficient neutrophils or monocytes produce larger amounts of oxygen-derived reactive species than do phagocytes with normal amounts of MPO,[214–222] which supports a role for MPO in terminating the burst as described above.

MPO also influences several features of the inflammatory response not directly related to the respiratory burst. For example, the MPO-dependent system inactivates a number of biologically important proteins,[223] including secreted granule products form neutrophils,[224–226] chemotaxins,[227–231] and α_1-antitrypsin.[232–234] In addition, the MPO-H_2O_2-halide system decreases the binding of chemotactic peptides to chemotactic factor receptors[235] and down-regulates natural killer cell activity.[236] Each of these activities could modulate the intensity or duration of the inflammatory response.

Each molecule of MPO (140 kDa) is composed of two large α subunits (59 kDa) and two smaller β subunits (13 kDa).[237–242] Native MPO can be cleaved by reductive alkylation into a 78-kDa product with one α and one β subunit. This cleavage product, hemi-MPO, retains the same specific activity as native MPO.[243] Analytic ultracentrifugation of native and hemi-MPO indicate that the α and β subunits are linked along their long axes, most likely by a disulfide bond between the two α chains[238] or two β chains.[239] The x-ray crystal structure of canine MPO has been determined[244] and confirms the symmetric organization of native MPO, with the identical halves of the molecule joined by a disulfide bond. In addition to the interchain disulfide bonds, there are six intrachain disulfide bonds, five in the heavy subunit and one in the light subunit. The preliminary crystallographic structure of human MPO has also been described.[245]

MPO binds calcium ions with high affinity and in an equimolar ratio to iron.[246] Although the functional significance of this property is not understood, it is noteworthy that the calcium-binding loop, a structural feature shared by four mammalian peroxidases [MPO, eosinophil peroxidase (EPO), thyroid peroxidase (TPO), and lactoperoxidase (LPO)] influences the protein conformation near the heme binding site in MPO.[244] When calcium is chelated from purified MPO, MPO precipitates from solution.[246]

The presence and significance of various forms of MPO is an unsettled issue. Early studies suggested there were as many as 10 isozymes,[247–250] but more recent studies have failed to reach a consensus on the presence of isozymic variation.[237,251,252] Using cation-exchange chromatography during purification, a number of investigators have identified multiple forms of mature MPO that differ in the size of the α chain[242,253–256] or in the susceptibility to inhibition with 3-aminotriazole,[255] or in both. Three forms of MPO have been recovered from crystalline MPO[254] and may represent biosynthetic intermediates distributed in different subcellular organelles or artifacts produced during purification.[237,257]

There are two iron molecules in each molecule of MPO, each iron bound to the α subunit. Electron spin resonance studies suggest that iron exists linked to a chlorin group and that the chlorin groups are identical.[258–260] However a number of studies have suggested that the prosthetic group is a formyl-substituted porphyrin, akin to that in LPO, rather than a chlorin.[261–263] The region of heme binding has been difficult to characterize clearly[264] using the techniques of physical chemistry but appears to contain five α helixes and a paucity of β sheets.[244]

Expression of cDNA for MPO in baby hamster kidney cells[265] and in S59 insect cells[266] results in synthesis of immunochemically reactive MPO without enzymatic activity. In contrast, expression of MPO cDNA in CHO cells produces MPO precursor with spectral and enzymatic properties similar to those of mature, fully processed native MPO.[267,268] A site-directed mutant with His 502 mutated to Ala (H502A) loses all enzymatic activity, whereas a cDNA with His 416 mutated to Ala (H416A) is fully active in this system.[269] Crystallographic analysis of mutants derived in this fashion should provide important insights into the structure–function domains in MPO, which in turn may be especially relevant to the biochemical basis for hereditary MPO deficiency (see below).

INHERITED DISORDERS OF PHAGOCYTIC KILLING

Chronic Granulomatous Disease

Definition and History. CGD is a heterogeneous group of genetic disorders characterized by recurrent, severe bacterial and fungal infections usually involving the skin, soft tissues, respiratory tract, lymph nodes, liver, and spleen.[270–276] CGD can be inherited in either an X-linked or an autosomal recessive fashion. Infectious episodes can be fatal, and therapy may require weeks to months of parenteral antibiotics in order to clear a deep-seated infection. Phagocytes from individuals with CGD can ingest normally, but they do not undergo a phagocytosis-associated respiratory burst, which is the basis for the defect in bactericidal activity. This defect has been demonstrated in neutrophils,[277] monocytes,[278,279] and eosinophils.[280]

CGD was first reported independently by Good and colleagues[281] and by Landing and Shirkey in 1957.[282] The former report described four boys with suppurative granulomas in biopsy and autopsy specimens. In the latter paper, recurrent suppurative infections in two boys were associated with infiltration of viscera by pigmented lipid-laden histiocytes. The pathogenesis remained in question until the abnormal phagocytosis-associated metabolic and bactericidal defects of patients' neutrophils were described a decade later.[41,42,277] The metabolic defects were found to be accompanied by a failure of neutrophils to reduce the redox dye nitroblue tetrazolium (NBT), which led to the widespread use of phagocytic NBT dye reduction as an aid in diagnosing CGD.[49]

All the initially reported cases were male, suggesting an X-linked pattern of inheritance. However, in 1968, two papers appeared describing CGD in females.[283,284] One report noted the lack of abnormalities in parents, and an autosomal recessive mode of inheritance was proposed.[283] Defective O_2^- generation by CGD phagocytes was reported in 1974,[285] followed by evidence that the basic abnormality was a defect in NADPH-dependent O_2^- generation.[286–288] Cytochrome *b* activity in neutrophils and its absence in CGD were described in 1978,[289] and the link between the lack of detectable cytochrome *b* and X-linked CGD was reported in 1983.[290] The gene that is abnormal in X-linked CGD was cloned in 1986[291] and was subsequently determined to code for the β subunit of cytochrome *b*.[113,114]

Within 2 years the molecular identity of the various autosomally inherited forms of CGD was known. Neutrophils from patients inheriting CGD in an autosomal pattern, which have normal amounts of cytochrome *b*,[290] were found to lack either of the cytosolic components, p47-*phox* or p67-*phox*.[134,292] Mutations in the gene for the 22-kDa α (light) chain of cytochrome *b* (p22-*phox*) were described in three unrelated patients (two female and one male) who apparently had autosomal recessive CGD but whose neutrophils lacked cytochrome *b*.[293]

Table 133-3 Clinical Findings in 168 Patients with Chronic Granulomatous Disease

Finding	Number of Patients Involved
Marked lymphadenopathy	137
Pneumonitis	134
Dermatitis	120
Hepatomegaly	114
Onset by age 1 year	109
Suppuration of nodes	104
Splenomegaly	95
Hepatic-periphepatic abscess	69
Osteomyelitis	54
Onset with dermatitis	42
Onset with lymphadenitis	38
Facial periorificial dermatitis	35
Persistent diarrhea	34
Septicemia or meningitis	29
Perianal abscess	28
Conjunctivitis	27
Death from pneumonitis	26
Persistent rhinitis	26
Ulcerative stomatitis	26

SOURCE: Johnston and Newman.[294] Used by permission.

Clinical Presentation. CGD should be considered in any individual with recurrent purulent infections caused by fungi or catalase-positive bacteria. A typical presentation would be a male infant with a history of fever, infected dermatitis, pneumonia, lymphadenitis, and hepatosplenomegaly (Table 133-3). Since the condition is congenital, CGD is usually recognized in the affected individual before the first birthday, and the disease has been known to manifest itself as early as the first week of life. Suspected cases, in families with a history of CGD, have been diagnosed in utero with fetal blood,[295–297] amniocytes,[298] or chorionic villus samples obtained by transcervical biopsy (see below).[299,300] In patients with X-linked CGD whose diagnosis is made after age 1 year, a typical history of early onset of recurrent infections can usually be obtained. Patients with certain variant forms of CGD,[270] and perhaps those with the autosomally inherited form,[301] may have less severe symptoms and may be recognized later in life.[302,303]

Any organ system can be affected. Nonetheless, cutaneous and mucous membrane surfaces are sites that are normally colonized with bacteria and fungi, making these structures and their underlying tissues a common target of microbial invasions. Therefore, skin and soft tissues and the respiratory and gastrointestinal tracts are frequently involved. Patients occasionally have recurrent infections at the same anatomic sites.[304] Acute invasion and direct extension into adjacent tissues or hematogenous dissemination lead to suppurative complications and abscess formation, and chronic infections result in the development of characteristic noncaseating granulomas.

The most frequent sites of serious infection are in the mononuclear phagocyte system (spleen, liver, lymph nodes, lung).[294,305] This reflects the accumulation of infecting microorganisms by phagocytic cells that cannot kill them.[294] Cervical and other lymph node groups can become enlarged early in the course of the disease; spontaneous rupture and drainage can follow. *Staphylococcus aureus* and enteric bacteria are the organisms most often cultured from material

Table 133-4 Infecting Organisms in 168 Patients with Chronic Granulomatous Disease*

Organism	Number of Patients Involved*
Staphylococcus aureus	87
Klebsiella-Aerobacter organisms	29
Escherichia coli	26
Serratia marcescens	16
Pseudomonas organisms	15
Staphylococcus albus	13
Aspergillus organisms	13
Candida albicans	12
Salmonella organisms	10
Proteus organisms	9
Streptococci	9
Nocardia organisms	4
Mycobacteria	4
Paracolobactrum organisms	4
Actinomyces organisms	2
Other enteric organisms	9

*The number of patients from whom each organism was cultured from blood, cerebrospinal fluid, or purulent focus is shown.
SOURCE: Johnston and Newman.[294] Used by permission.

taken from these sites (Table 133-4).[275,294,305] Chronically inflamed lymph nodes become infiltrated with lipid-laden pigmented macrophages and granulomas.[306]

Hepatomegaly and splenomegaly are prominent, and liver involvement may progress to abscess formation (most commonly with *S. aureus*) requiring surgical intervention.[294] The occurrence of such abscesses, rare in children, should suggest CGD.[307]

Recurrent skin and soft-tissue infections often occur and include pyogenic dermatitis, furunculosis, and subcutaneous abscesses.[294,305,308] An eczematoid dermatitis involving the eyelids and the area around the nares and mouth may be seen early in the course of the illness.[294] Dermatologic findings can be prominent in adults with otherwise mild disease.[309] The cutaneous involvement may provide the first clue of an underlying immunodeficiency in a patient with CGD. Discoid lupus has been recognized in patients with autosomal recessive CGD[310–312] and in carriers of X-linked CGD.[313–315]

Infections of the lower respiratory tract with *S. aureus*, enteric bacteria, and Aspergillus species are common. Pulmonary infections with aspergillus may invade adjacent bone or soft tissues of the chest wall.[307,316–318] The pattern of pneumonia may be lobar, bronchial, or diffuse and generalized (Fig. 133-4) and may be accompanied by consolidation and hilar lymphadenopathy.[307,319,320] Chronic lung disease with granulomatous infiltration of the lung and pulmonary fibrosis has been noted both in adult and pediatric patients.[302,307] In the upper airway, persistent rhinitis and otitis media are common.

The oropharynx and gastrointestinal tract[321] are frequent sites of infectious complications. Ulcerative stomatitis and gingivitis can be recurrent, and esophagitis may result in strictures and regurgitation.[294,322–325] Involvement of the lower gastrointestinal tract also may mimic pyloric stenosis,[326] eosinophilic gastroenteritis,[321] gastrointestinal dysmotility,[327] inflammatory bowel disease,[328] or peritonitis.[329] Granulomatous inflammation of the stomach can lead to a characteristic luminal narrowing of the gastric antrum, as shown in Fig. 133-5, with persistent vomiting.[270,326,330,331] Similar lesions in the small or large bowel may result in diarrhea, malabsorption, or frank obstruction, and may require surgical intervention.[321,332,333] Rectal abscesses, perianal abscesses, and fistulas are not uncommon.[321]

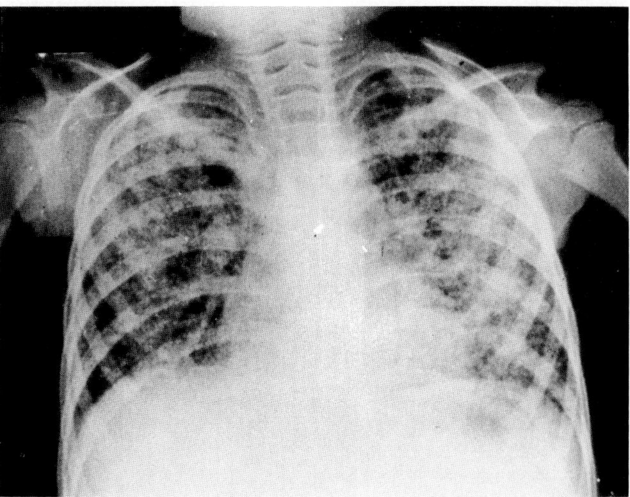

FIG. 133-4 Lower respiratory tract involvement in a boy with CGD. The chest x-ray film shows a diffuse reticulonodular interstitial pattern with superimposed alveolar densities in the left midlung field.

Osteomyelitis has been described in about one-third of patients.[294,305,318,334,335] There is a peculiar predilection for the metacarpals, metatarsals, spine, and ribs. *Serratia marcescens*, *S. aureus*, and Aspergillus species are the most commonly isolated organisms. Body involvement often follows a primary infection in lymph nodes, lung, or the gastrointestinal tract.[318]

Urinary tract involvement ranged from 7 to 48 percent of patients in three published series.[294,336,337] Cystitis or obstructive uropathy may result from granulomatous involvement of the bladder wall (Fig. 133-6).[270,305,338–340] Urinary tract infections and glomerulonephritis,[337,341,342] renal abscesses,[343] and granulomatous inflammation of the kidney parenchyma have also been reported.[344] Gonadal involvement has been noted with tuboovarian abscesses in girls and testicular granulomas reported in a boy.[307]

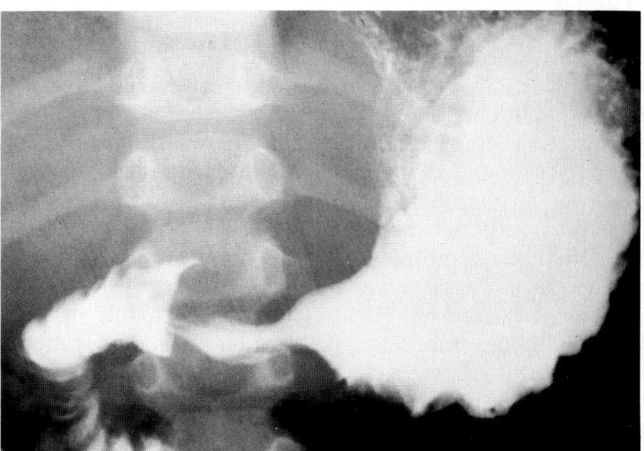

FIG. 133-5 Gastrointestinal involvement in CGD. A 5-year-old boy with X-linked CGD experienced the gradual onset of recurrent vomiting and weight loss. An upper gastrointertinal series showed annular narrowing of the antral lumen, nodular irregularities of the distal greater curvature of the stomach, and delayed gastric emptying.

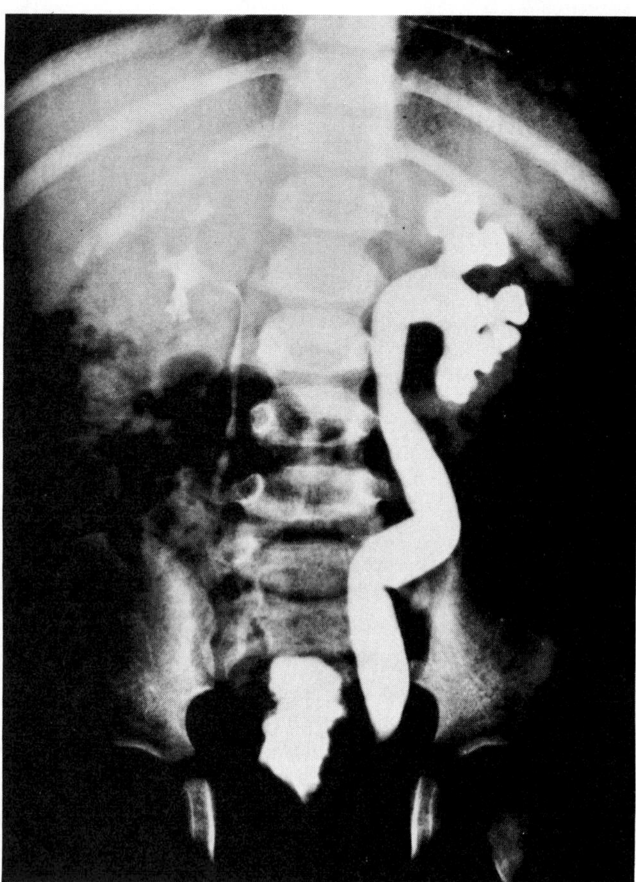

FIG. 133-6 Obstructive uropathy in a patient with CGD. IV pyelogram of a boy with X-linked CGD demonstrating hydronephrosis and hydroureter on the left side. The obstruction was due to compression by a large inflammatory mass in the pelvis between the rectum and the bladder.

Disseminated infection, with bacteremia or meningitis (or both), was reported in 29 (17 percent) of 168 early cases described in detail.[294,345] Salmonella was the most commonly isolated organism from the blood and from fatal infectious episodes.[346] Other complications include destructive chorioretinitis,[347] conjunctivitis,[294] thyroiditis,[348] pericarditis,[294] brain abscess,[294] and granulomatous involvement of the brain or spinal cord.[307,349]

In early surveys of children with CGD (1971 and 1977), one-half to three-fourths of patients had died before the age of 7.[50,294] Although there is still no specific cure for CGD, prophylactic antibiotics and the aggressive management of suppurative complications have greatly reduced deaths from infectious complications. A more recent review of 19 patients disclosed an overall mortality of 5 percent.[270] Although these 19 patients experienced no serious staphylococcal infections once they began antibiotic prophylaxis, the number of gram-negative isolates did not change while on antibiotic therapy.

Typical carriers of X-linked CGD are not unduly susceptible to infection, since about half of their phagocytes function normally; but there is an association with discoid lupus erythematosus and aphthous stomatitis.[310–315] Infiltrative and plaquelike lesions involving the face and distal extremities occur in these individuals. Of 14 carriers of X-linked CGD with discoid lupus erythematosus, none had serologic or clinical evidence of systemic lupus erythematosus.[310–315] One carrier mother was chronically infected with salmonella.[350]

Pathological Findings. The infectious complications of CGD result in characteristic tissue abnormalities. Specimens from acutely infected sites show a necrotic inflammatory process associated with suppuration. If the infection has been prolonged, granulomas are present, with multinucleated giant cells, macrophages, lymphocytes, and plasma cells.[319] The formation of these granulomas appears to be secondary to the prolonged intracellular residence of microorganisms.[351]

The abundance of mononuclear phagocytes in the liver, spleen, lungs, and lymph nodes makes these organs particularly susceptible to the formation of granulomatous lesions. When multiplying organisms are released from one phagocyte, they are ingested by another. This process recruits additional phagocytes with the eventual formation of granulomatous masses. Pigmented lipid-laden macrophages are also commonly seen. The lipid material is yellow or tan in color (hematoxylin and eosin stain) and may result from incomplete degradation of ingested material.[305,306]

Laboratory Findings. Except for studies of phagocyte function, laboratory findings reflect the presence of a chronic inflammatory disorder. During infections, a neutrophilic leukocytosis is frequent and may be associated with an elevated erythrocyte sedimentation rate. Anemia appears to be secondary to chronic infections; resolution usually occurs during disease-free intervals, and patients may benefit from iron therapy.[270,294] A polyclonal hypergammaglobulinemia is present, with elevated serum concentrations of IgG, IgM, and IgA.[51] Other tests of immune function are normal, with the rare exception of abnormal lymphocyte transformation or chemotaxis.[352,353] If the phagocytic load is large, ingestion may be even greater in CGD than normal neutrophils that undergo autooxidation and subsequent decline in function.[354]

Infecting Organisms. Individuals with CGD are susceptible to infections with catalase-producing organisms,[355] including bacteria, Candida, Aspergillus,[356] Nocardia,[357–359] and mycobacteria species.[360,361] The relative frequency of the various species isolated is shown in Table 133-4. The most frequent species associated with infection at almost any site are *S. aureus*, enteric bacteria, and aspergillus, although patients maintained on antimicrobial prophylaxis with trimethoprim/sulfamethoxazole (TMP-SMX) (see below) are infected much less often with *S. aureus*.[270] Unusual organisms, not customarily associated with human disease also have been isolated from sites of infection. Particularly striking is the emergence of *Pseudomonas cepacia* as a cause of lung infection.[362] Other bacterial species include *Legionella gormanii,*[363] *Corynebacterium aquaticum,*[364] *Exophiala dermatitidis,*[365] *Pseudallescheria boydii,*[366] *Paecilomyces lilacinus,*[367] *Chromobacterium violaceum,*[368] Pseudomonas species,[369] *Francisella philomiragia,*[370] *Aspergillus nidulans* var. *echinulatus,*[317] and *Paecilomyces varioti.*[371] Conspicuously absent are the encapsulated streptococcal and Haemophilus species, common pathogens in pediatric pyogenic infections. These latter species do not produce catalase, which degrades H_2O_2, and they fall victim to their own H_2O_2, which can be released into the phagocytic vacuole and converted to HOCl or ·OH.

Diagnosis. CGD should be suspected on examining an individual with recurrent bacterial abscess formation, especially involving the skin and subcutaneous tissues, lymph nodes, and the respiratory tract. In vitro tests of neutrophil bactericidal and respiratory burst activity should follow. The histochemical NBT test remains a reliable screening test for

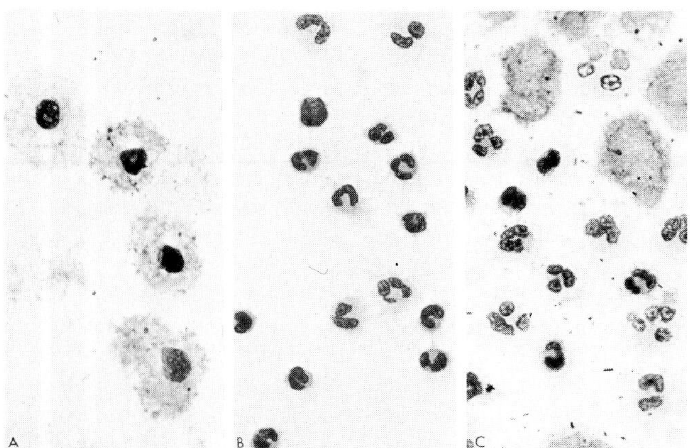

FIG. 133-7 NBT slide test for the diagnosis of CGD. A drop of blood is placed on an endotoxin-coated coverslip and incubated to allow the granulocytes and monocytes to adhere to the glass surface. The coverslip is then incubated with a solution of serum, PMA, and NBT dye and then washed, fixed, counterstained, and mounted. *A*. Normal control; all the granulocytes are NBT-positive and appear as large, degenerated cells with pale-blue cytoplasm. *B*. CGD patient; none of the granulocytes are NBT-positive. The neutrophils retain their typical morphologic appearance and contain no blue (reduced) dye. *C*. Carrier of CGD. Two populations of cells coexist. Some granulocytes are NBT-positive and others are NBT-negative.

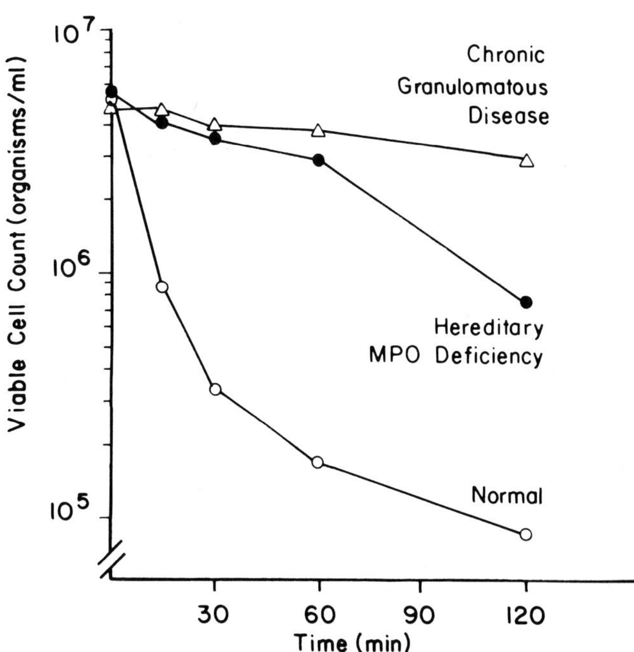

FIG. 133-8 Bactericidal activity against *S. aureus* in neutrophils from a normal individual, a patient with myeloperoxidase deficiency, and a patient with chronic granulomatous disease.

CGD (Fig. 133-7).[51,372] A positive NBT test occurs when yellow, soluble NBT is reduced by O_2^- to blue, insoluble formazan. The assay should be performed so that 100 percent of a normal control's cells on the coverslip reduce the NBT.[373] This method will better ensure that "variants" with minimal respiratory burst activity and carriers of X-linked CGD can be identified.[373,374] A false reading of normality can be avoided by realizing that rare variants of CGD may retain some activity of the respiratory burst, expressed as homogeneous faint blue staining.

An abnormal result in the NBT test should be substantiated by measurement of phagocytic bactericidal activity (Fig. 133-8)[50] and quantitative assay of the respiratory burst, for example, by measurement of O_2^-,[375,376] chemiluminescence,[33] oxygen consumption,[377] or hydrogen peroxide production.[378]

Prenatal diagnosis can be achieved with the NBT test using fetal blood obtained by percutaneous umbilical or placental vessel puncture.[295–297,379] This procedure is deemed relatively safe if performed after 17 weeks of gestation.[380,381] The prenatal diagnosis of X-linked CGD (based on cytochrome *b* abnormality) also has been made by DNA analysis of samples from chorionic villus or amniocytes using RFLP and gene analysis.[298,300,382] These tests offer the advantage of an earlier diagnosis (tenth week of gestation)[383] and no requirement for fetal blood sampling. At present, for this approach to be most informative the suspected genetic defect (e.g., that of an older sib or relative) and the mother's carrier status need to be known.

Treatment. In the infection-free patient, treatment is aimed at preventing the onset of an infectious process. Successful prophylaxis with TMP-SMX has been reported in several series.[270,384,385] In a retrospective study of 18 patients, treatment with TMP-SMX, 5 mg/kg/day led to increased infection-free periods (3.7 months before therapy, 10.7 months during therapy), primarily by eliminating *S. aureus* infections.[270] The improvement of patients on TMP-SMX may be the result of the cell's ability to concentrate the agents in the phagocytic vacuole.[386–388] Twenty patients with autosomal CGD and 16 with X-linked disease followed at the National Institutes of Health since the 1970s experienced a 2.9-fold ($p < 0.01$) and 2.3-fold ($p = 0.06$) decrease respectively in nonfungal infections while being treated with TMP-SMX.[384] There were also less frequent infections with fungal organisms. A retrospective multicenter experience with 34 CGD patients showed similar results, with the average annual incidence of infection per patient improving from 2.06 to 0.43.[385] Patients hypersensitive to TMP-SMX can be treated alternatively with a systemic penicillinase-resistant penicillin.[389]

Interferon-γ is a known immunomodulator of respiratory burst activity in normal phagocytic cells.[390,391] In early studies, phagocytes from seven patients with different genetic forms of CGD who had been given interferon-γ by injection exhibited an enhanced respiratory burst and improved in killing of *S. aureus*.[392–394] Some patients' phagocytes also had a detectable up-regulation of mRNA for the heavy chain (β subunit) of cytochrome *b*.[393,394] B .sed on these observations, a larger multicenter randomized double-blind placebo-controlled study of 128 patients was undertaken to test the effectiveness of subcutaneous administration of interferon-γ to control infectious complications common to CGD.[174] Seventy-seven percent of patients receiving interferon-γ, 1.5 μg/kg (body surface area <0.5 m^2) or 50 μg/m^2 (body-surface area ≥ 0.5 m^2) by subcutaneous injection three times weekly remained free of serious infection after 12 months of therapy as compared with only 30 percent of those receiving placebo. Toxicity was limited to headache, fever and chills, and redness at the injection site. Unlike the preliminary investigations, the reported clinical benefit from interferon-γ was not accompanied by a measurable improvement in phagocytic respiratory burst activity in a majority of patients.[174,175,395] The improvement in the killing of *S. aureus* and *Aspergillus fumigatus* in vitro[396,397] may reflect an alteration in myeloperoxidase-dependent antimicrobial activity. Although the precise mechanism of action of interferon-γ remains unknown, NBT-positive monocytes (but not neutrophils) were described in six of eight patients treated with interferon-γ from the multicenter study, raising the possibility that interferon-γ may act in part by enhancing the respiratory burst activity of a subset of monocytes.[175]

Granulocyte transfusions have been administered to patients with serious systemic infections, including pneumonia, liver abscesses, and an intramural ileal abscess, all apparently refractory to prolonged administration of parenteral antibiotics.[398–404] Transfusions usually were given as daily infusions of approximately 10^{10} to 10^{11} granulocytes, and recipients tolerated up to 8 weeks of granulocyte therapy without untoward reactions. Careful separation of contaminating red blood cells from donor granulocytes can increase the likelihood of a successful transfusion when compatible blood is not available.[405] The efficacy of granulocyte transfusions is still in question, as the majority of patients were also receiving parenteral antibiotics or were recovering from surgical intervention, and the studies were not controlled.

Patients with CGD and the K_0 or McLeod phenotypes are susceptible to sensitization by Kell antigens when given blood. One patient with the McLeod phenotype experienced a hemolytic reaction after the sixth leukocyte transfusion.[406]

In most cases, prolonged antibiotic therapy clears the obstruction created by inflammatory granulomatous lesions of the gastrointestinal or genitourinary tract. In patients with protracted severe narrowing of the gastric antrum, esophagus, and urinary tract, corticosteroids in conjunction with antibiotics and nasogastric or IV nutritional supplementation can reverse the obstruction.[407–409] The response to corticosteroids can be prompt, but relapse is not uncommon. Two patients with progressive respiratory insufficiency responded favorably to corticosteroid therapy.[410]

Marrow transplantation has been attempted in patients with CGD with mixed results.[411–419] There are four known cases of successful sustained engraftment (Di Bartolomeo P: personal communication).[417–419] Three of the four boys were transplanted after experiencing recurrent severe infections. A boy who underwent transplantation at 5 months of age has continued to show chimerism (presence of NBT-positive neutrophils) and has remained asymptomatic for over 5 years.[419] Two boys are doing well 2 years[418] and 6 years[417] after transplantation. A boy who experienced repeated soft-tissue infections and aspergillus pneumonia with chest-wall involvement was transplanted with marrow from his HLA-identical sister. He remains fully engrafted and free of infection 41 months later (Di Bartolomeo P: personal communication). However, failure to engraft is common. Several recipients experienced transplant rejection after initial engraftment.[412,418] One 15-year-old boy succumbed to graft-versus-host disease and sepsis 3 months after transplantation.[414]

Research on more effective therapeutic approaches continues. Antistaphylococcal antibiotics incorporated into liposomes were taken up and delivered to the phagocytic vacuole of CGD neutrophils, with resultant improvement in killing of ingested staphylococci.[420] It has been proposed that liposomes might be employed in gene therapy to replace missing genes in bone marrow–derived stem cells of patients with CGD or to substitute a recombinant cytosolic NADPH oxidase constituent in place of a defective one.[391]

The successful in vitro replacement of a missing cytosolic protein in p47-*phox*-deficient CGD has been reported.[421,422] In these experiments B lymphocytes from patients with this deficiency were transformed by EBV and then infected with a retrovirus containing the p47-*phox* DNA. After a 3- to 6-week incubation recombinant p47-*phox* protein was detectable in retrovirally infected but not uninfected cells.[421,422] One of these studies demonstrated the release of superoxide anion in response to PMA from the patient's EBV-transformed p47-*phox*-positive B lymphocytes. (Normal B-lymphocyte cell lines can release small amounts of O_2^- on exposure to PMA.)[422]

Molecular Basis of CGD. As discussed above, the finding that NADPH oxidase is composed of multiple subunits each encoded by a distinct gene locus provides the molecular explanation for the previously confusing genetic heterogeneity of CGD. To date, defects in four of the oxidase components (gp91-*phox*, p22-*phox*, p47-*phox*, and p67-*phox*) have been identified in patients analyzed at the biochemical or molecular genetic level. Defects in Rap1A, Rac1, Rac2, GDI, or a distinct FAD-containing subunit have not been reported. Based on these considerations, a modern consensus classification scheme for CGD has been formulated that subdivides the disease according to the specific gene defect (Table 133-5). Nomenclature has also been adopted for an abbreviated designation within each major group that includes the mode of inheritance, oxidase component by molecular weight, and level of *phox* protein expression.

In two large series of CGD patients comprised of a total of 121 kindreds, defects in the X-linked gene for the gp91-*phox* subunit of cytochrome *b* account for approximately 65 percent of the cases[423] (Scripps Clinic, 65 kindreds with 71 total patients) (see Table 133-5). Of these, the majority are characterized by undetectable levels of O_2^- production, cytochrome *b*, and NBT reduction (termed "X91^0 CGD"). The X91$^-$ subtype is a variant form of CGD usually characterized by a uniform population of neutrophils that exhibit a low level of oxidase activity roughly proportional to the level of cytochrome *b* expressed.[424] In the NBT test, 80 to 100 percent of the neutrophils stain weakly. An unusual variant form of X-linked CGD has also been described in which 5 to 10 percent of the neutrophils are strongly positive on the NBT test while the remaining cells are devoid of activity.[425,426] In X91$^+$ CGD, cytochrome *b* is present at normal levels but has either a greatly diminished or absent activity. The molecular genetic basis for these "classic" and "variant" forms of CGD is discussed below. Autosomal recessive inheritance is observed in 35 percent of CGD families and is most commonly caused by mutations in the gene encoding p47-*phox*, located on chromosome 7q11.23 (see Table 133-5). Mutations in the gene for the p22-*phox* (chromosome 16p24) and p67-*phox* (chromosome 1q25)[427] each account for 6 percent of the total number of CGD cases.

The gp91-*phox* gene (termed "CYBB") that encodes the large glycosylated subunit of cytochrome *b* contains 13 exons and spans approximately 30 kb in the Xp21.1 region of the X chromosome.[291,428–430] Over 50 distinct mutations in this gene have been identified in X-linked CGD patients (Table 133-6).[291,303,382,426,429–436] There are roughly equal numbers of deletions, frameshifts, splice site, nonsense, and missense mutations that are more or less randomly distributed throughout the gene. To date, only two putative regulatory mutations have been reported. In most cases, the mutations are family-specific. In several cases, however, two or more unrelated kindreds have been found with the same mutation (e.g., cases 14, 26, 27, 29, and 39 in Table 133-6).

Relatively large deletions in Xp21.1 involving the gp91-

Table 133-5 Classification of Chronic Granulomatous Disease

Component Affected	Chro-mosome	Inher-itance	Subtype Designa-tion*	NBT Score (% Positive)	O_2^- Pro-duction (% Normal)	Cytochrome *b* Spectrum (% Normal)	Defect in Cell-free System	Families Evaluated		Frequency§ (% of Cases)
								Scripps†	Europe‡	
gp91-*phox*	Xp21.1	XL	X91⁰	0	0	0	Membrane	33	35	56
			X91⁻	80–100 (weak)	3–30	3–30	Membrane	4	2	5
			X91⁻	5–10	5–10	5–10	Membrane	2	0	2
			X91⁺	0	0	100	Membrane	2	0	2
p22-*phox*	16p24	AR	A22⁰	0	0	0	Membrane	4	3	6
			A22⁺	0	0	100	Membrane	1	0	1
p47-*phox*	7q11.23	AR	A47⁰	0	0–1	100	Cytosol	15	13	23
p67-*phox*	1q25	AR	A67⁰	0	0–1	100	Cytosol	4	3	6

XL = X-linked inheritance; AR = autosomal recessive inheritance.
*In this nomenclature, the first letter represents the mode of inheritance [X-linked (X) or autosomal recessive (A)] while the number indicates the *phox* component that is genetically affected. The superscript symbols indicate whether the level of protein of the affected component is undetectable (⁰), diminished (⁻), or normal (⁺) as measured by immunoblot analysis.
†This group represents 65 kindreds with 71 total patients.
‡Cooperative study reported in 1992[423] represents 56 kindreds and 61 patients.
§Frequency within the combined 121 families.

phox gene and other adjacent loci have been described (cases 1 to 4 in Table 133-6). In each of these types of deletions, the patients have both CGD and the McLeod phenotype (a mild hemolytic anemia associated with depressed levels of Kell antigens due to defects in the red-cell antigen K_x). In a minority of these cases, the patient may also be afflicted with Duchenne muscular dystrophy and X-linked retinitis pigmentosa.[291,429,432,439] The apparent order of these genes (from centromere to telomere) is retinitis pigmentosa, CGD, McLeod, and Duchenne muscular dystrophy with the McLeod and CGD loci located most closely to each other.[382,431,440] Small deletions involving all (case 5) or part (cases 6 to 8) of the gp91-*phox* gene have also been identified. The mutation in patient 8 in Table 133-6 is of interest since it is associated with partial retention of cytochrome *b* and respiratory burst activity (25 percent of normal). There is a deletion of three nucleotides in exon 9 that results in an in-frame loss of Lys315. This patient has an extremely mild clinical phenotype.

Frameshift mutations caused by the insertion or deletion of 1 to 5 nucleotides have been described in a number of patients (cases 9 to 16 in Table 133-6). These frameshifts predict premature stop codons downstream with the production of a truncated gp91-*phox* protein. In the cases in which it has been examined, however, no protein has been detected, due either to the instability of the mRNA or the abnormal polypeptide.

Mutations involving both the 5′ and 3′ splice sites of several of the introns in the gp91-*phox* gene have been identified in some X-linked CGD patients. Generally, these mutations result in the loss of one or more exons and a severe clinical phenotype. In one patient, however, a splice mutation at the 3′ end of intron XI was associated with mild disease. In fact, the patient was not diagnosed until the age of 69 when he presented with *Pseudomonas cepacia* sepsis after having been in excellent health his entire life.[303] Neutrophils from the patient contained normal levels of cytochrome *b* (with normal spectral characteristics) and were able to generate small amounts of superoxide (6 percent of normal). Analysis of the gp91-*phox* cDNA from the patient revealed that only the first 30 nucleotides in exon 12 were deleted due to a cryptic acceptor site in the exon. This splicing defect predicts the deletion of 10 amino acids in the middle of the large intracytoplasmic C-terminal domain of gp91-*phox* (Fig. 133-9). The loss of this segment of the polypeptide apparently does not influence the stability or spectral characteristics of the cytochrome, but does markedly impair its function.

Nonsense mutations in which amino acid codons are changed to stop codons are relatively common in X-linked CGD (cases 26 to 35 in Table 133-6). A frequent mutation is C → T in which a CGA codon (encoding an arginine) is changed to TGA (encoding a stop). As with the frameshift mutations discussed above, these nonsense mutations predict the synthesis of truncated forms of gp91-*phox*, but protein is not detected presumably because of either unstable mRNA or protein. Thus, this group of patients tends to have more clinically severe CGD since their neutrophils fail to express cytochrome *b* and to undergo a respiratory burst.

Mutations resulting in substitution of one amino acid for another (missense mutations) have been identified relatively commonly in X-linked patients and account for some of the variant forms of the disease. In most cases, the predicted amino acid substitutions apparently result in markedly unstable proteins and undetectable levels of cytochrome *b* (e.g., case 36 in Table 133-6). In cases 38, 41, and 42, mutations involving histidine residues that may serve as axial ligands for the heme groups in cytochrome *b*[441] also adversely affect protein stability and result in undetectable levels of cytochrome *b*. In contrast, other missense mutations result in the expression of low levels of cytochrome *b* and superoxide production (e.g., cases 40 and 45 in Table 133-6). Apparently, these amino acid substitutions (which are not necessarily conservative, as in case 45) are at least minimally tolerated and permit some degree of gp91-*phox* expression (see Fig. 133-9). Finally, missense mutations affecting Pro 415 (case 49)[436] and Arg 54 (case 37) result in the normal expression of nonfunctional forms of cytochrome *b*. In both cases, translocation of p47-*phox* and p67-*phox* to the membrane remains intact.[137] These mutations appear to disrupt the flow of electrons between NADPH and molecular oxygen.

Mutations in the regulatory regions of the gp91-*phox* gene are apparently unusual and have been described in just two kindreds.[426] The mutations were only two nucleotides apart and each was associated with a highly unusual biochemical

Table 133-6 Summary of gp91*phox* Mutations in CGD

Type of Mutation	Exon(s) Affected	Nucleotide Change*	Predicted Amino Acid Change	CGD Type	Comments	References†
Deletion						
1	1–13+	~5000 kb deletion	No gp91-*phox*	$X91^0$	Severe with DMD, RP, McLeod	429
2	1–13+	~4000 kb deletion	No gp91-*phox*	$X91^0$	Severe with DMD and McLeod	291, 428, 439
3	1–13+	~1000 kb deletion	No gp91-*phox*	$X91^0$	Severe with McLeod Seen in 5 kindreds	431, 438
4	1–13+	Not known	No gp91-*phox*	$X91^0$	Severe with McLeod and RP	432
5	1–13+	≥ 30 kb deletion	No gp91-*phox*	$X91^0$	No McLeod	382
6	11–13	>4 kb deletion	Deletion of I439-F570	$X91^0$	—	438
7	13	~1 kb deletion	Deletion of ~T530-F570	$X91^0$	Severe CGD	291
8	9	Deletion of G954, A955, A956	Deletion of K315	$X91^-$	In-frame deletion; clinically mild	438
Frameshift						
9	3	Insert G207	Stop in exon 4	$X91^0$	Severe	438
10	3	Delete 263	Stop in exon 4	$X91^0$	Multiple abnormally spliced mRNA	438
11	5	Insert A455	Stop in exon 5	$X91^0$	—	438
12	7	Delete A713 and G714	Stop in exon 7	($X91^0$)	—	438
13	7	Delete A728-T732	Stop in exon 7	$X91^0$	Severe CGD	438
14	7	Insert A754	Stop in exon 8	$X91^0$	Seen in 3 unrelated kindreds; severe CGD	438
15	7	Insert A772	Stop in exon 8	$X91^0$	Severe CGD	438
16	9	Delete G975	Stop in exon 9	$X91^0$	—	438
Splice						
17	Intron XI (3′)	AG→GG	Delete A488-E497	$X91^+$	Cryptic splice site with In-frame deletion; mild CGD	303
18	Intron VII (5′)	GT→GA	Delete exon 7 then frameshift	$X91^0$	—	433
19	Intron V (5′)	GTA→GTT	Delete exon 5 then stop	$X91^0$	—	433
20	Intron III (5′)	GTAAG→GTAAA	Delete exon 3	$X91^0$	In-frame deletion	433
21	Intron I (3′)	AG→AA	Delete exon 2	$X91^0$	In-frame deletion	433
22	Intron II (5′)	GT→TT	Delete exon 2	$X91^0$	Severe CGD	438
23	Intron II (3′)	AG→GG	Delete exon 3	$X91^0$	Severe CGD	438

phenotype in which 5 to 10 percent of the neutrophils were strongly positive by NBT testing. Levels of cytochrome *b* expression and superoxide production were also 5 to 10 percent of normal. It has been hypothesized that these putative regulatory mutations adversely affect cytochrome *b* expression in the majority, but not all, of the circulating neutrophils.[426]

Mutations in the gene for the p22-*phox* subunit of cytochrome *b* cause approximately 6 percent of the cases of CGD (see Table 133-5). The p22-*phox* gene (termed "CYBA") resides at 16q24 and contains six exons that span 8.5 kb.[293] The genetic defects that have been identified are heterogenous (Table 133-7) just as in the case of defects of the gp91-*phox* subunit. The mutations range from large interstitial gene deletions (case 1) to point mutations associated with missense, frameshift, or RNA splicing defects (cases 2 to 7 in Table 133-7). In all but one case, the patients are homozygous for the mutant allele due to consanguinity in the parents.[293,442] Analogous to the cases of $X91^+$ described above, a point mutation in the p22-*phox* gene associated with normal levels of cytochrome *b* and a dysfunctional oxidase has been reported ($A22^+$ CGD, case 6 in Table 133-7).[443] The mutation predicts the substitution of Gln for Pro 156 (P156Q) in the intracytoplasmic C-terminus of p22-*phox*. The patient's neutrophils have undetectable levels of O_2^- production despite the presence of a spectrally normal cytochrome *b*. The underlying mechanism for this profound respiratory burst defect remains unknown.

The map location and gene organization for the cytosolic components are now known. The p47-*phox* gene (NCF1) is mapped to chromosome 7q11.23 and consists of 9 exons spanning 18 kb.[444] The 40 kb p67-*phox* gene (NCF2) contains

Table 133-6 Summary of gp91*phox* Mutations in CGD (Continued)

Type of Mutation	Exon(s) Affected	Nucleotide Change*	Predicted Amino Acid Change	CGD Type	Comments	References†
24	Intron V (5′)	GT→GC	Not determined	($X91^0$)	—	438
25	Intron IX (5′)	GTGC deleted	Not determined	$X91^0$	Severe CGD	438
Nonsense						
26	3	C229→T	stop→R73X	$X91^0$	2 kindreds	434, 438
27	4	C283→T	stop→R91X	$X91^0$	2 kindreds	438
28	5	C454→T	stop→R148X	($X91^0$)	—	438
29	5	C481→T	stop→R157X	$X91^0$	2 kindreds	438
30	7	C688→T	stop→R226X	$X91^0$	Heterozygous female with severe CGD	435
31	8	C880→T	stop→R290X	$X91^0$	Severe CGD	438
32	9	G1018→T	stop→E336X	$X91^0$	Severe CGD	438
33	11	C1332→A	stop→Y440X	($X91^0$)	—	438
34	11	G1341→A	stop→W443X	$X91^0$	—	438
35	12	C1531→T	stop→Q507X	$X91^0$	Severe CGD	438
Missense						
36	2	G70→C	G20R	$X91^0$	Severe CGD	438
37	3	G173→C	R54S	$X91^+$	Nonfunctional cytochrome	438
38	4	A314→G	H101R	$X91^0$	—	434
39	5	G478→A	A156T	$X91^0$	2 kindreds	434, 438
40	5	A494→G	K161R	$X91^-$	Low levels O_2^-; mild CGD	438
41	6	C637→T	H209Y	$X91^0$	Same residue as case 42	434
42	6	T639→A	H209Q	$X91^0$	See case 41	438
43	7	T742→C	C244R	($X91^0$)	Same residue as case 44	438
44	7	G743→C	C244S	$X91^-$	See case 43	434
45	9	C937→A	E309K	$X91^-$	Low levels O_2^-; mild CGD	438
46	9	T1009→C	S333P	($X91^0$)	—	438
47	9	G1151→A	W380R	$X91^0$	Mild CGD	438
48	10	G1178→C	G389A	$X91^-$	—	434
49	10	C1256→A	P415H	$X91^+$	Nonfunctional cytochrome	436
Regulatory						
50	5′ Regulatory	−57A→C	Not applicable	$X91^-$	5–10% of cells NBT-positive	426
51	5′ Regulatory	−55T→C	Not applicable	$X91^-$	Similar to case 50	426

DMD = Duchenne muscular dystrophy; RP = X-linked retinitis pigmentosa; McLeod = McLeod erythrocyte phenotype.
*Nucleotide residues are numbered according to the cDNA sequence described by Orkin.[437]
†Boldface type indicates cases analyzed at The Scripps Research Institute and reported in abstract form.[438]

16 exons at its chromosomal location on 1q25.[444a] In contrast to the diversity of mutations seen in patients with cytochrome *b* deficiency are the relatively limited number identified so far in CGD patients with p47-*phox*[444,445] or p67-*phox*[445a] deficiency. Six of the nine patients lacking p47-*phox* reported to date have been homozygous for a mutant allele with a GT deletion at the beginning of exon 2 that predicts a premature stop codon following amino acid residue 50. The other three patients were compound heterozygotes each having one allele with the GT deletion. In one of these three individuals, the other allele had an A → G substitution at nucleotide 179 that predicts the incorporation of an alanine instead of a threonine at residue 53 (T53A). In the other two patients, an A → G mutation at nucleotide 425 was identified that predicts a Lys 135 to Glu (K135E) substitution. Mutations involving p67-*phox* have not been extensively characterized. One patient has been found to be homozygous for a G → A substitution at nucleotide 233 that predicts a nonconservative Gly 78 to Glu (G78E) replacement in exon 3.[445a]

Glucose-6-Phosphate Dehydrogenase Deficiency

Leukocyte G-6-PD deficiency can be associated with a phagocytic bactericidal defect as the result of a subnormal respiratory burst, and the clinical presentation can mimic CGD.[446–449] Patients with erythrocyte G-6-PD deficiency suffer bouts of hemolytic anemia as a result of exposure to certain drugs and foods (see Chap. 111). G-6-PD catalyzes the first step in the hexose monophosphate shunt, which is necessary to maintain normal amounts of cellular NADPH.

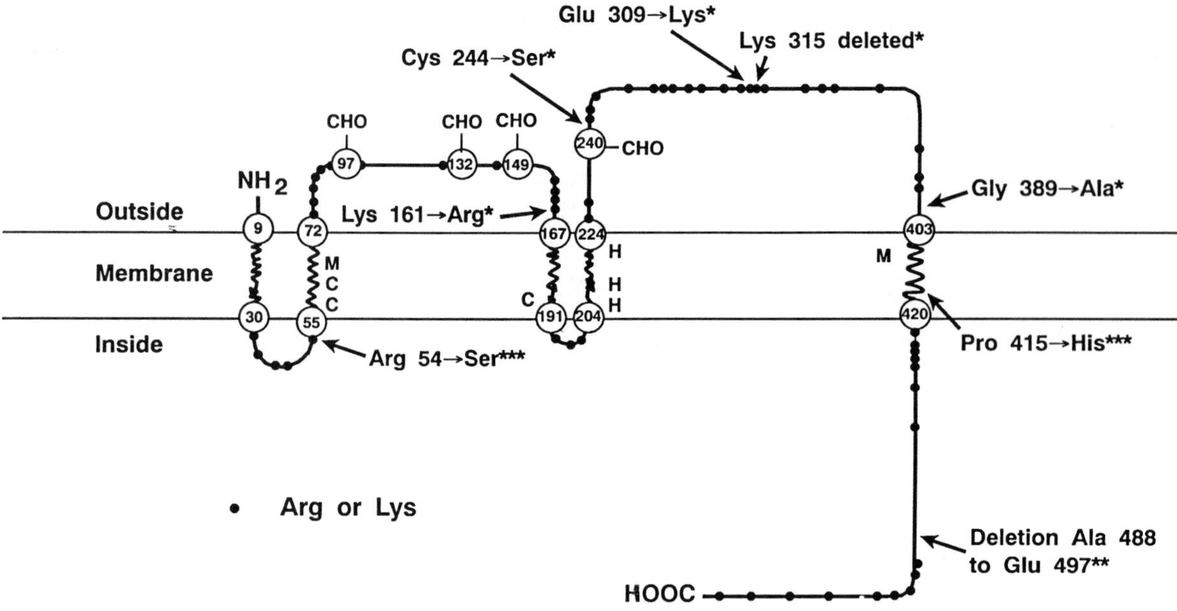

FIG. 133-9 Proposed protein conformation of gp91-*phox*. The locations of predicted amino acid changes in patients with variant forms of X-linked CGD are shown. As indicated by the footnotes, the mutations result in either normal or diminished levels of cytochrome *b*, which may, in turn, be associated with either undetectable or diminished levels of NADPH oxidase activity. Numbers in circles indicate amino acid residue numbers. In the transmembrane domains, M = methionine, C = cysteine, and H = histidine.

Cells, particularly erythrocytes, that lack adequate levels of NADPH are unable to maintain glutathione in a reduced state (GSH) and, thus are susceptible to oxidative damage on exposure to oxidants in drugs or foods. The disorder is inherited in an X-linked fashion, and affected individuals are usually male, although homozygous affected females are not rare in certain populations and heterozygous females can express the disorder (see Chap. 111).

G-6-PD activity is present in normal neutrophils and appears to be required to generate the NADPH used as a

Table 133-7 Summary of p22-*phox* Mutations in CGD

Type of Mutation	Exon(s) Affected	Nucleotide Change[1]	Predicted Amino Acid Change	CGD Type	Comments	References
Deletion						
1	1–6+	>10 kb deletion	No p22-*phox*	A22⁰	Homozygous†; severe CGD	283, 293
Frameshift						
2	4	Delete C272	Stop in exon 6	A22⁰	See case 3 for mutation in other allele	284, 293
Missense						
3	4	G297→A	R90Q	A22⁰	Homozygous in one kindred†; heterozygous in a second kindred (see case 2)	284, 293, 442
4	4	A309→G	H94R	A22⁰	Homozygous†	442
5	5	C382→A	S118R	A22⁰	Homozygous†	293
6	6	C495→A	P156Q	A22⁺	Homozygous†; nonfunctional cytochrome	443
Splice						
7	Intron IV	GT→AT	Delete exon 4	A22⁰	Homozygous†	442

*Nucleotide residues are numbered according to the cDNA sequence described by Orkin.[437]
†In these cases, homozygosity of the mutant allele was due to consanguinity in the parents.

substrate for the respiratory burst oxidase.[446] Patients whose neutrophils are severely deficient in G-6-PD (with less than 5 percent of normal activity) do not undergo a respiratory burst and suffer recurrent and sometimes fatal bacterial infections.[446–449] On the other hand, individuals with as little as 25 percent of normal G-6-PD activity have not shown an unusual susceptibility to infection.[446] Like neutrophils from individuals with CGD, G-6-PD-deficient neutrophils are unable to reduce NBT and demonstrate an in vitro killing defect against catalase-producing microorganisms. CGD and G-6-PD deficiency can be distinguished by exposing neutrophils to methylene blue, an oxidizing agent that converts NADPH to NADP, thereby activating the hexose monophosphate shunt in CGD but not in G-6-PD deficiency.

Myeloperoxidase Deficiency

Description. Until the late 1970s hereditary deficiency of MPO had been infrequently reported; there were descriptions in the literature of only 15 patients from 12 families.[450–457] However, the diagnosis became common with the widespread application in clinical hematology laboratories of automated flow cytochemistry to quantitate peroxidase activity as a means to enumerate neutrophils in peripheral blood. Application of this technique revealed the true prevalence of MPO deficiency to be approximately 1 in 2000 apparently healthy individuals.[218,458] Histochemical studies of peripheral blood from such individuals revealed an absence of peroxidase staining in neutrophils and monocytes, whereas there was normal staining of the peroxidase in eosinophils, consistent with previous understanding that eosinophil peroxidase is a different protein. Other prominent neutrophil granule proteins, including β-glucuronidase, elastase, vitamin B_{12}-binding protein, and lysozyme, are present in normal amounts in MPO-deficient cells.

Clinical Course. Most individuals with MPO deficiency are healthy. In accord with the inability of MPO-deficient neutrophils to kill species of Candida, however, four of the six reported patients with MPO deficiency who have had significant infection had disseminated or visceral candidiasis.[451,455,456,458] Of these four patients, three[451,455,458] had concomitant diabetes mellitus. In some cases, MPO deficiency has been part of more complex clinical pictures; some of these have included associated defects in chemotaxis,[459] normal chemotaxis but recurrent and severe skin infection,[460] acne vulgaris,[221] and pustular psoriasis.[461] The contribution of the deficiency of MPO to the clinical syndrome is not clear in these cases. MPO-dependent oxidants appear to be particularly important for the killing of Candida species,[47] but there are additional antimicrobial systems that adequately protect the host in most situations. In the absence of MPO, more subtle defects in host defense, such as those present in the antifungal defenses of some diabetics, become clinically significant.

In addition to the inherited form of MPO deficiency, there are numerous causes of acquired MPO deficiency. These include pregnancy,[462] lead poisoning,[463] Hodgkin's disease,[464] sepsis,[465] megaloblastic anemia,[466–468] ceroid lipofuscinosis,[469,470] and acute nonlymphocytic leukemias, particularly of the M2 to M4 types.[471–477] The last cause of MPO deficiency is especially noteworthy in that some patients have acquired MPO deficiency in the preleukemic phase of the disease.[478,479]

Laboratory Diagnosis. Neutrophils and monocytes from individuals with MPO deficiency appear completely normal under the microscope. Thus, the clinician must consider the possibility of MPO deficiency in order to alert the hematology laboratory to do the appropriate studies. Recurrent, invasive, or disseminated fungal disease in the absence of clearly identifiable risk factors should suggest the possibility of MPO deficiency.

The diagnosis can be easily made by quantitation of the peroxidase activity of isolated cells or by histochemical analysis of peroxidase activity of neutrophils or monocytes in peripheral blood smears. Peroxidase activity can be quantitated using a variety of different substrates,[480–482] but none differentiate eosinophil from neutrophil monocyte peroxidase. If MPO is quantitated in a population of leukocytes, the presence of a disproportionate number of eosinophils could obscure the diagnosis of MPO deficiency,[483] since eosinophils contain fourfold more peroxidase than do neutrophils,[484] and eosinophil peroxidase is more active than MPO.[485] The diagnosis can be established simply and directly by examining peripheral blood smears stained for peroxidase activity. Currently, substrates such as 3-amino-9-carbazole[486] and 4-chloro-1-naphthol[487] are recommended over the previous standard benzidine dihydrochloride, which is carcinogenic.[488]

Numerous investigators have characterized the in vitro behavior of MPO-deficient neutrophils and monocytes. These cells have an exuberant respiratory burst, manifested by greater than normal oxygen consumption, O_2^- and H_2O_2 release (Fig. 133-10), and hexose monophosphate shunt activity.[43,215,216,429] MPO-deficient neutrophils have normal amounts of catalase and glutathione peroxidase,[214] indicating that the detection of supernormal amounts of oxygen products is due to increased production and not decreased catabolism. In addition, the increase in production is due to a failure in termination of the oxygen burst (see above and Fig. 133-10).

Phagocytosis by MPO-deficient neutrophils of a variety of particles has been normal.[216,455,458,489] Release of granule products to a variety of stimuli has been reported to be normal or increased.[490] There is increased recovery of granule products from MPO-deficient neutrophils,[224–226] since the proteins are not oxidized and inactivated by the MPO-H_2O_2-halide system.

The microbicidal activity of MPO-deficient cells is defective (see Fig. 133-8). MPO-deficient cells kill *S. aureus*,[216,218,455,458,489,491,492] Serratia,[455] and *Escherichia coli*[217,493] significantly more slowly than do normal cells. However, after 1 h of incubation, MPO-deficient cells have killed the same number of organisms as have normal cells. This may reflect the sustained respiratory burst present in MPO-deficient cells and the amplified systems that compensate for the MPO deficiency.[491]

Most striking in vitro is the inability of MPO-deficient cells to kill a variety of species of fungi, including the clinically significant *Candida albicans* and *C. tropicalis*[216,455,456,458,489,494] and hyphal forms of *Aspergillus fumigatus*.[495,496] In contrast *T. glabrata*,[459] *C. parapsilosis*,[497] *C. pseudotropicalis*,[498] and the spores of *A. fumigatus* and of *Rhizopus oryzae*[499] are killed normally by MPO-deficient cells.

Biochemical Defect. The biochemical defect in MPO deficiency is the lack of peroxidase activity in the azurophilic granules of neutrophils and in the primary lysosomes of monocytes. Immunochemical analysis of neutrophils from

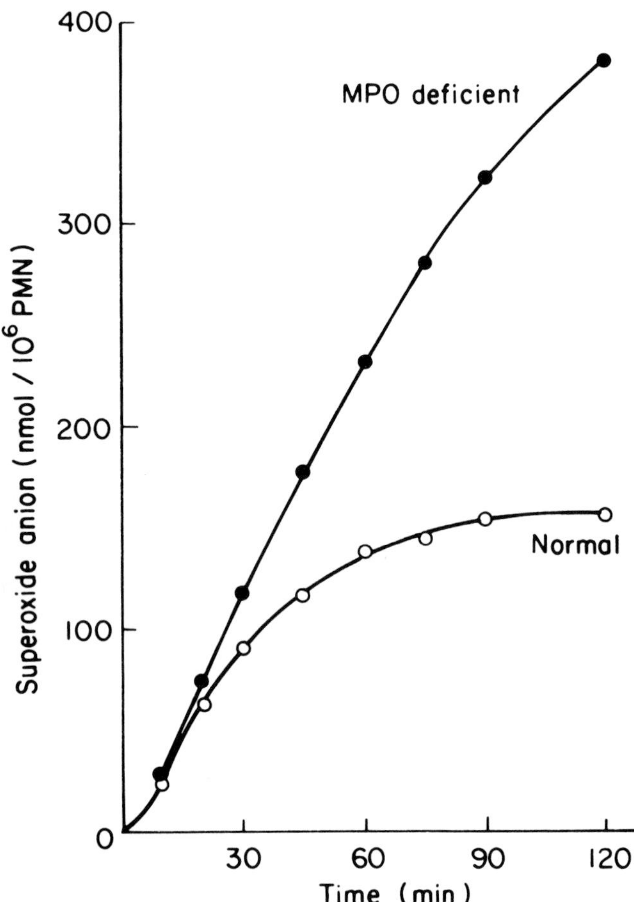

FIG. 133-10 The time course of O_2^- production by neutrophils from a patient with myeloperoxidase deficiency.

affected individuals reveals that the cells lack the subunits of MPO.[240] However, both normal and MPO-deficient neutrophils contain an immunochemically related protein of a higher molecular weight that has characteristics consistent with its being proMPO.

MPO synthesis is under the control of a single gene, although there is evidence of multiple mRNA species in cultured myeloid cells such as the HL-60 cell line,[500] presumably the result of alternative splicing.[501] Expression of mRNA encoding for MPO is restricted to myeloid cells, with other cultured hematopoietic precursors expressing essentially no MPO.[502] Chemical induction of HL-60 cells results in rapid cessation of MPO expression coincident with differentiation into more mature myeloid cells,[503] indicating that transcription of the MPO gene is tightly regulated and temporally linked to myeloid differentiation.[500,503-505] Both demethylation and DNase I hypersensitivity of the MPO gene are associated with MPO gene expression during myeloid differentiation.[506] There are regions 5′ to the transcription initiation site in the MPO gene that share sequence homology with 5′ promoter region of the c-*myc* protooncogene[507] and with 5′ flanking regions of the murine lactoferrin gene,[508] although the specific MPO promoter has not been defined and the significance of these homologies has not been established.

Studies using cultured myeloid cell lines have provided a great deal of information regarding the biosynthesis, processing, and intracellular transport of MPO.[509-516] There is a single primary translation product of approximately 80 kDa, which undergoes cotranslational glycosylation to generate apoproMPO, the enzymatically inactive, heme-free precursor of MPO. Early in biosynthesis, apoproMPO is converted to proMPO,[517] presumably within the ER.[516,518] Subsequently, proMPO undergoes proteolytic processing into the mature heterodimer, assembly into dimeric MPO, and subcellular transport to the azurophilic granules. It is clear that inhibition of heme synthesis by addition of succinyl acetone to the culture medium blocks proteolytic maturation into mature MPO,[516,518] suggesting that insertion of the iron-containing prosthetic group and generation of proMPO is necessary for subsequent processing into MPO. Little is known about the factors that mediate this proteolytic processing or the subcellular compartment in which it takes place. Likewise, the mechanism by which MPO is directed to the azurophilic granule is not defined. ProMPO does not bind to a mannose 6-phosphate receptor affinity column,[516] confirming considerable indirect evidence that MPO lysosomal targeting is independent of the mannose 6-phosphate receptor system.

MPO shares sequence homology with a variety of other peroxidases, including EPO, TPO, and LPO. The sequence homology among these proteins is most striking in the immediate region around the heme.[244,519,520] Thus, these proteins may be evolutionarily related members of a peroxidase superfamily, each with distinctly different physiological functions as determined by the particular cell type expressing the peroxidase.

Although the genetic basis for MPO deficiency has not been defined,[521] it has been proposed that the underlying abnormality in MPO deficiency is in the posttranslational processing of proMPO.[522] This could result from a mutation in the prosequences of the MPO gene, a change akin to that seen in the Z variant of α_1-antitrypsin deficiency.[523] In that disorder, single base changes result in proproteins that are not processed normally into mature proteins. Bone marrow from an MPO-deficient subject contains the same amount and size of MPO mRNA as does control bone marrow.[522] In addition, restriction endonuclease digests of genomic DNA from numerous individuals with MPO deficiency demonstrate a *Bgl*II site not present in genomic DNA from individuals with normal amounts of MPO, although the significance of this additional restriction site has not been defined. In addition to the evidence favoring a posttranslational defect underlying MPO deficiency, one individual has been described with MPO deficiency whose defect is likely pretranslational.[524]

Gene Defect. The gene for MPO is located on chromosome 17 at q22-23,[525,526] near the breakpoint for the 15;17 translocation of promyelocytic leukemia.[527,528] Partial sequence of the MPO gene reveals 12 exons and 11 introns with consensus sequences present for both splice donor and acceptor sites.[507] The genomic sequence spans 14 kb and the full-length cDNA is approximately 3.3 kb, with an open reading frame of 2.2 kb (encoding 745 amino acids). Northern blots of RNA from HL-60 cells or bone marrow cells from humans or mice demonstrate mRNA for MPO at 3.0 to 3.3 kb and 3.5 to 4.0 kb. The significance of the multiple species likely reflects alternative splice sites.

The molecular basis of the clinical disorder is not established for most cases at this time. However, some forms are due to a missense mutation at nucleotide 8089, which results in a substitution of tryptophan for arginine at codon 569 (R569W).[528a] Although a number of studies have suggested an autosomal recessive mode of inheritance,[194,216,217,455,483,489] other studies have suggested variable expression of the gene[218] or defects in structural as well as regulatory genes.[458]

Treatment. There is no specific therapy for MPO deficiency. Given the predilection of diabetics with MPO deficiency for severe fungal infections, it would be prudent to avoid factors that predispose to fungal superinfection (e.g., prolonged use of broad-spectrum antibiotics) and to treat presumed fungal infections earlier in such patients.

Glutathione Synthetase Deficiency

Glutathione (*N*-[*N*-L-γ-glutamyl-L-cysteinyl]glycine) can be found in high concentrations in most cell types. The ratio of GSH (reduced glutathione) to GSSG (oxidized glutathione) in normal cells is approximately 500:1.[529,530] Its biosynthesis from γ-glutamylcysteine and glycine is catalyzed by the enzyme glutathione synthetase. In the neutrophil, glutathione protects cellular structures from the harmful effects of H_2O_2 and, perhaps, other oxidizing radicals generated during the phagocytosis-associated respiratory burst. A reduction in the synthesis or regeneration of glutathione in the phagocyte leads to increased oxidative stress and loss of function.[180,531]

Glutathione synthetase deficiency with 5-oxoprolinuria has been described in a 2-year-old boy with two episodes of neutropenia associated with otitis media (see Chap. 43).[531] Hemolytic anemia had been noted at birth. Erythrocytes, leukocytes, and cultured skin fibroblasts had diminished glutathione synthetase activity (5 to 10 percent of normal) and intracellular glutathione content (10 to 20 percent of normal). There was no history of unusual infections. Neutrophil chemotaxis, phagocytosis, and NBT reduction all occurred normally. However, neutrophil bactericidal capacity and iodination were impaired. These defects were thought to be due to deficiency of glutathione, which would be expected to permit accumulation of H_2O_2 intracellularly after stimulation. The resultant increase in oxidative stress was shown to damage the patient's neutrophil membranes and microtubules and to impair phagolysosomal formation.[531]

The oxidant scavenger vitamin E (α-tocopherol), 400 IU/day, increased red-cell survival, corrected both the bactericidal and iodination defects, and eliminated the neutropenia that had accompanied certain intercurrent illnesses.[532]

Congenital glutathione synthetase deficiency appears to be inherited in an autosomal recessive fashion.

Glutathione Reductase Deficiency

A 22-year-old female of parents who were first cousins suffered bouts of hemolysis in association with eating fava beans (see also Chap. 43). Diminished glutathione reductase activity was noted in her erythrocytes and granulocytes. Two sibs with an identical defect of glutathione metabolism were also identified.

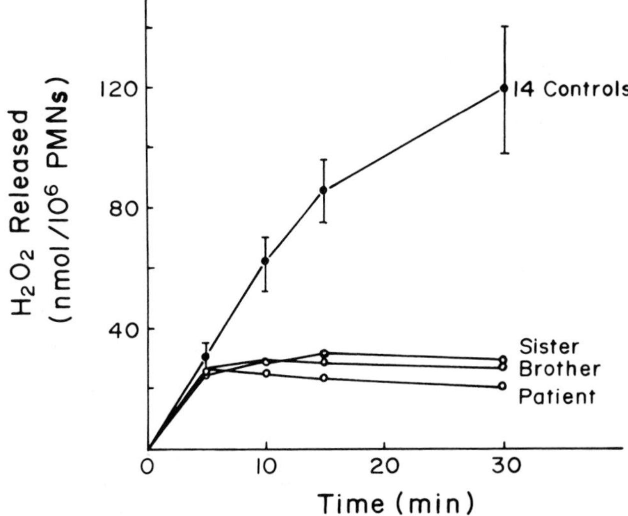

FIG. 133-11 The time course of zymosan-triggered H_2O_2 release by neutrophils from 14 controls and 3 individuals with glutathione reductase deficiency. *(From Roos et al.[180] Used by permission.)*

There was no history of repeated infections in any of the three.[533] Chemotaxis, phagocytosis of opsonized *S. aureus*, and degranulation proceeded normally.[180] Intracellular killing appeared normal at low bacteria:phagocyte ratios, but higher ratios gave defective bacterial killing. The patient's neutrophils phagocytosed opsonized zymosan normally, and oxygen consumption and H_2O_2 production occurred at a normal rate for 5 to 10 min. However, this was followed by complete cessation of respiratory burst activity (Fig. 133-11). Hexose monophosphate shunt activity stopped after 10 min of phagocytosis with a subnormal initial rate.

Glutathione reductase catalyzes the reduction of glutathione disulfide to reduced glutathione, using electrons from NADPH (Fig. 133-12). Absence of glutathione reductase leads to defective generation of reduced glutathione, which permits oxidative damage to the stimulated neutrophil as described above in "Antioxidant Mechanisms." In contrast to other aspects of the respiratory burst, the release of O_2^-, measured as the reduction of cytochrome *c*, proceeded normally. Cytochrome *c* added in vitro scavenges the electrons from O_2^-, which prevents H_2O_2 formation from the dismutation reaction, protecting the cell from oxidative damage.

There is no specific therapy for glutathione reductase deficiency, but avoiding foods and drugs containing potent oxidants will lessen the chance of depleting cellular levels of glutathione. The pattern of inheritance is unknown.

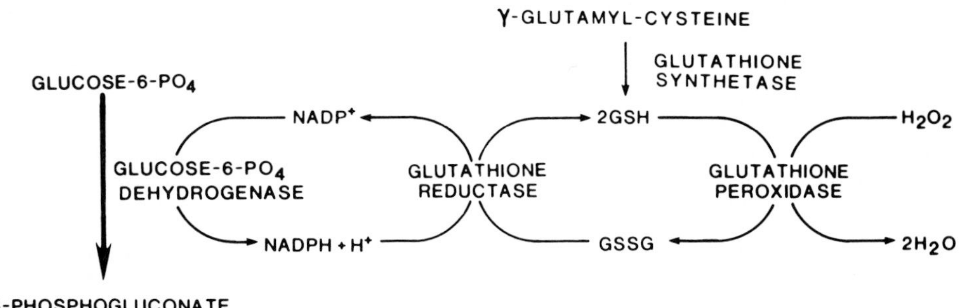

FIG. 133-12 Schematic representation of the glutathione oxidation-reduction cycle. GSH = reduced glutathione; GSSG = oxidized glutathione. *(From Johnston.[534] Used by permission.)*

ACKNOWLEDGMENTS

Supported in part by USPHS grants AI 24748, AI 24838, AI 20866 and HL 34327. Dr. Nauseef is a Clinical Investigator in the Department of Veterans Affairs.

REFERENCES

1. Metchnikoff E: Untersuchungen über die intracelluläre Verdauung bei wirbellosen Thieren. *Arb Zool Inst Univ Wien* **5**:141, 1883.
2. Metchnikoff E: Ueber die Beziehung der Phagocyten zu Milzbrandbacillen. *Virchows Arch [A]* **97**:502, 1884.
3. Metchnikoff E: *Immunity in Infective Diseases*. New York, Cambridge University Press, 1905.
4. Johnston RB Jr: Current concepts: Immunology—Monocytes and macrophages. *N Engl J Med* **318**:747, 1988.
5. Mandell GL: Bactericidal activity of aerobic and anaerobic polymorphonuclear neutrophils. *Infect Immun* **9**:337, 1974.
6. Okamura N, Spitznagel JK: Outer membrane mutants of *Salmonella typhimurium* LT2 lipopolysaccharide have resistance to the bactericidal activity of anaerobic human neutrophils. *Infect Immun* **36**:1086, 1982.
7. Vel WA, Namavar F, Verweij AM, Pubben AN, Maclaren DM: Killing capacity of human polymorphonuclear leukocytes in aerobic and anaerobic conditions. *J Med Microbiol* **62**:65, 1984.
8. Weiss J, Victor M, Stendahl O, Elsbach P: Killing of gram-negative bacteria by polymorphonuclear leukocytes. *J Clin Invest* **69**:959, 1982.
9. Zimmer M, Medcalf RL, Fink TM, Mattmann C, Lichter P, Jenne DE: Three human elastase-like genes coordinately expressed in the myelomonocyte lineage are organized as a single genetic locus on 19pter. *Proc Natl Acad Sci USA* **89**:8215, 1992.

9a. Gray PW, Corcorran AE, Eddy RL Jr, Byers MG, Shows TB: The genes for the lipopolysaccharide binding protein (LBP) and the bactericidal permeability increasing protein (BPI) are encoded in the same region of human chromosome 20. *Genomics* **15**:188, 1993.

10. Sparks RS, Kronenberg M, Heinzmann C, Daher KA, Klisak I, Ganz T, Mohandas T: Assignment of defensin gene(s) to human chromosome 8p23. *Genomics* **5**:240, 1989.
11. Hohn PA, Popescu NC, Hanson RD, Salvesen G, Ley TJ: Genomic organization and chromosomal localization of the human cathepsin G gene. *J Biol Chem* **264**:13412, 1989.
12. Peters CW, Kruse U, Pollwein R, Grzeschik KH, Sippel AE: The human lysozyme gene. Sequence organization and chromosomal localization. *Eur J Biochem* **182**:507, 1989.
13. Lehrer RI, Ganz T: Antimicrobial polypeptides of human neutrophils. *Blood* **76**:2169, 1990.
14. Morgan JG, Sukiennicki T, Pereira HA, Spitznagel JK, Guerra ME, Larrick JW: Cloning of the cDNA for the serine protease homolog CAP37/azurocidin, a microbicidal and chemotactic protein from human granulocytes. *J Immunol* **147**:3210, 1991.
15. Almeida RP, Melchior M, Campanelli D, Nathan C, Gabay JE: Complementary DAN sequence of human neutrophil azurocidin, an antibiotic with extensive homology to serine proteases. *Biochem Biophys Res Commun* **177**:688, 1991.
16. Spitznagel JK: Antibiotic proteins of human neutrophils. *J Clin Invest* **86**:1381, 1990.
17. Gabay JE, Scott RW, Campanelli D, Griffith J, Wilde C, Marra MN, Seeger M, Nathan CF: Antibiotic proteins of human polymorphonuclear leukocytes. *Proc Natl Acad Sci USA* **86**:5610, 1989.
18. Bangalore N, Travis J, Onunka VC, Pohl J, Shafer WM: Identification of the primary antimicrobial domains in human neutrophil cathepsin G. *J Biol Chem* **265**:13584, 1990.
19. Ooi CE, Weiss J, Elsbach P, Frangione B, Mannion B: A 25-kDa NH_2-terminal fragment carries all the antibacterial activities of the human neutrophil 60-kDa bactericidal/permeability-increasing protein. *J Biol Chem* **262**:14891, 1987.

19a. Marra MN, Wilde CG, Collins MS, Snable JL, Thornton MB, Scott RW: The role of bactericidal/permeability-increasing protein as a natural inhibitor of bacterial endotoxin. *J Immunol* **148**:532, 1992.

20. Gray PW, Flaggs G, Leong SR, Gumina RJ, Weiss J, Ooi CE, Elsbach P: Cloning of the cDNA of a human neutrophil bactericidal protein. Structural and functional correlations. *J Biol Chem* **264**:9505, 1989.
21. Pereira HA, Spitznagel JK, Winton EF, Shafer WM, Martin LE, Guzman GS, Pohl J, Scott RW, Marra MN, Kinkade JM Jr: The ontogeny of a 57-kd cationic antimicrobial protein of human polymorphonuclear leukocytes: Localization to a novel granule population. *Blood* **76**:825, 1990.
22. Strominger JL, Ghuysen JM: Mechanisms of enzymatic bacteriolysis. *Science* **156**:213, 1967.
23. Wilson LA, Spitznagel JK: Molecular and structural damage of *Escherichia coli* produced by antibody, complement and lysozyme systems. *J Bacteriol* **96**:1339, 1968.
24. Spitznagel JK: Nonoxidative antimicrobial reactions of leukocytes, *Contemp Top Immunobiol* **14**:283, 1984.
25. Avery OT, Cullen GE: Hydrogen ion concentration of cultures of pneumococci of the different types of carbohydrate media. *J Exp Med* **30**:359, 1919.
26. Baldridge CW, Gerald RW: The extra respiration of phagocytosis. *Am J Physiol* **103**:235, 1933.
27. Karnovsky ML: Metabolic basis of phagocytic activity. *Physiol Rev* **42**:143, 1962.
28. Badwey JA, Karnovsky ML: Active oxygen species and the functions of phagocytic leukocytes. *Annu Rev Biochem* **49**:695, 1980.
29. Klebanoff SJ: Oxygen metabolism and the toxic properties of phagocytes. *Ann Intern Med* **93**:480, 1980.
30. Babior BM: The respiratory burst of phagocytes. *J Clin Invest* **73**:599, 1984.
31. Karnovsky ML, Badwey JA: Respiratory burst during phagocytosis: An overview. *Methods Enzymol* **132**:353, 1986.
32. Babior BM, Kipnes RS, Curnutte JT: Biological defense mechanisms: The production by leukocytes of superoxide, a potential bactericidal agent. *J Clin Invest* **52**:741, 1973.
33. Johnston RB Jr, Keele BB, Misra HP, Lehmeyer JE, Webb LS, Baehner RL, Rajagopalan KV: The role of superoxide anion generation in phagocytic bactericidal activity: Studies with normal and chronic granulomatous disease leukocytes. *J Clin Invest* **55**:1357, 1975.
34. Klebanoff SJ: Antimicrobial mechanisms in neutrophilic polymorphonuclear leukocytes. *Semin Hematol* **12**:117, 1975.
35. Tauber AL, Babior BM: Evidence for hydroxyl radical production by human neutrophils. *J Clin Invest* **60**:374, 1977.
36. Weiss SJ, King GW, Lobuglio AF: Evidence for hydroxyl radical generation by human monocytes. *J Clin Invest* **60**:370, 1977.
37. Weiss SJ, Rustagi PK, Lobuglio AF: Human granulocyte generation of hydroxyl radical. *J Exp Med* **147**:316, 1978.
38. Allen RC, Stjernholm RL, Steele RH: Evidence for the generation of an electronic excitation state(s) in human polymorphonuclear leukocytes and its participation in bactericidal activity. *Biochem Biophys Res Commun* **47**:679, 1972.
39. Krinsky NI: Singlet excited oxygen as a mediator of the antibacterial action of leukocytes. *Science* **186**:363, 1974.
40. Sbarra AJ, Karnovsky ML: The biochemical basis of phagocytosis. 1. Metabolic changes during the ingestion of particles by polymorphonuclear leukocytes. *J Biol Chem* **234**:1355, 1959.
41. Iyer GYN, Islam MF, Quastfl JH: Biochemical aspects of phagocytosis. *Nature* **192**:535, 1961.
42. Klebanoff SJ: A peroxidase-mediated antimicrobial system in leukocytes. *J Clin Invest* **46**:1078, 1967.
43. Klebanoff SJ, Hamon CB: Role of myeloperoxidase-mediated antimicrobial systems in intact leukocytes. *J Reticuloendothel Soc* **12**:170, 1972.
44. Halliwell B: Oxidants and human disease: Some new concepts. *FASEB J* **1**:358, 1987.
45. Cohen MS, Britigan BE, Hassett DJ, Rosen GM: Do human neutrophils form hydroxyl radicals? Evaluation of an unresolved controversy. *J Free Radical Biol Med* **5**:81, 1988.
46. Ramos CL, Pou S, Britigan BE, Cohen MS, Rosen GM: Spin trapping evidence for myeloperoxidase-dependent

hydroxyl radical formation by human neutrophils and monocytes. *J Biol Chem* **267**:8307, 1992.

47. Thomas EL: Myeloperoxidase-hydrogen peroxide-chloride antimicrobial system: Effect of exogenous amines on antibacterial action against *Escherichia coli*. *Infect Immun* **25**:110, 1979.
48. Maródi L, Forehand JR, Johnston RB Jr: Mechanisms of host defense against *Candida* species. II. Biochemical basis for the killing of *Candida* by mononuclear phagocytes. *J Immunol* **146**:2790, 1991.
49. Baehner RL, Nathan DG: Leukocyte oxidase: Defective activity in chronic granulomatous disease. *Science* **155**:835, 1967.
50. Quie PC, White JC, Holmes D, Good RA: In vitro bactericidal capacity of human polymorphonuclear leukocytes: Diminished activity in chronic granulomatous disease of childhood. *J Clin Invest* **46**:668, 1967.
51. Johnston PB Jr, Baehner RL: Chronic granulomatous disease: Correlation between pathogenesis and clinical findings. *Pediatrics* **48**:730, 1971.
52. Dechatelet LR, Shirley PS, Johnston RB Jr: Effect of phorbol myristate acetate on the oxidative metabolism of human polymorphonuclear leukocytes. *Blood* **47**:545, 1976.
53. Goldstein IM, Roos D, Kaplan HB, Weissann G: Complement and immunoglobulins stimulate superoxide production by human leukocytes independently of phagocytosis. *J Clin Invest* **56**:1155, 1975.
54. Boxer LA, Yoder M, Bonsib S, Schmidt M, Ho P, Jersild R, Baehner R: Effects of a chemotactic factor, N-formylmethionyl peptide, on adherence, superoxide anion generation, phagocytosis, and microtubule assembly of human polymorphonuclear leukocytes. *J Lab Clin Med* **93**:506, 1979.
55. Lehmeyer JE, Snyderman R, Johnston RB Jr: Stimulation of neutrophil oxidative metabolism by chemotactic peptides: Influence of calcium ion concentration and cytochalasin B and comparison with stimulation by phorbol myristate acetate. *Blood* **54**:35, 1979.
56. Simchowitz L, Atkinson JP, Spilberg I: Stimulus-specific deactivation of chemotactic factor-induced cyclic AMP response and superoxide generation by human neutrophils. *J Clin Invest* **66**:736, 1980.
57. Webster RO, Hong SR, Johnston RB, Henson PM: Biological effects of the human complement fragments C5a and $C5a_{des\ Arg}$ on neutrophil function. *Immunopharmacology* **2**:201, 1980.
58. Pozzan T, Lew DP, Wollheim CB, Tsien RY: Is cytosolic ionized calcium regulation neutrophil activation? *Science* **221**:1413, 1983.
59. Kitagawa S, Ohta M, Nojiri H, Kakinuma K, Saito M, Takaku F, Miura Y: Functional maturation of membrane potential changes and superoxide-producing capacity during differentiation of human granulocytes. *J Clin Invest* **73**:1062, 1984.
60. Cohen HJ, Whitin JC, Chovaniec ME, Tape E, Simons E: Is activation of the granulocyte by concanavalin A a reversible process? *Blood* **63**:114, 1984.
61. Curnutte JT, Babior BM, Karnovsky ML: Fluoride-mediated activation of the respiratory burst in human neutrophils. *J Clin Invest* **63**:637, 1979.
62. Gabler WL, Creamer HR, Bullock WW: Modulation of the kinetics of induced neutrophil superoxide generation by fluoride. *J Dent Res* **65**:1159, 1986.
63. Johnston RB Jr, Lehmeyer JE: Elaboration of toxic oxygen by-products by neutrophils in a model of immune complex disease. *J Clin Invest* **57**:836, 1976.
64. Serhan CN, Radin A, Smolen JE, Korchak H, Samuelsson B, Weissmann G: Leukotriene B_4 is a complete secretagogue in human neutrophils: A kinetic analysis. *Biochem Biophys Res Commun* **107**:1006, 1982.
65. Samuelsson B: Leukotrienes: Mediators of immediate hypersensitivity reactions and inflammation. *Science* **20**:568, 1983.
66. Curnutte JT, Badwey JA, Robinson JM, Karnovsky MJ, Karnovsky ML: Studies on the mechanism of superoxide release from human neutrophils stimulated with arachidonate. *J Biol Chem* **259**:11851, 1984.
67. English D, Schell M, Siakotos A, Gabig TG: Reversible activation of the neutrophil superoxide generation system by hexachlorocyclohexane: Correlation with effects on a subcellular superoxide-generation fraction. *J Immunol* **137**:283, 1986.
68. Kuhns DB, Kaplan SS, Basford RE: Hexachlorocyclohexanes, potent stimuli of O_2^- production and calcium release in human polymorphonuclear leukocytes. *Blood* **168**:535, 1986.
69. Penfield A, Dale MM: Synergism between A23187 and 1-oleoyl-2-acetyl-glycerol in superoxide production by human neutrophils. *Biochem Biophys Res Commun* **125**:332, 1984.
70. Graham RC, Karnovsky MJ, Shafer AW, Glass EA, Karnovsky ML: Metabolic and morphological observations on the effect of surface-active agents on leukocytes. *J Cell Biol* **32**:629, 1967.
71. Bromberg Y, Pick E: Activation of NADPH-dependent superoxide production in a cell-free system by sodium dodecyl sulfate. *J Biol Chem* **260**:13539, 1985.
72. Rossi F, Zatti M, Partiarca P, Cramer R: Stimulation of the respiration of polymorphonuclear leucocytes by antileucocyte antibodies. *Experientia* **26**:491, 1970.
73. Boxer LA, Stossel TP: Effects of anti-human neutrophil antibodies in quantitative studies. *J Clin Invest* **53**:1534, 1974.
74. Nakagawara A, Minakami S: Generation of superoxide anions by leukocytes treated with cytochalasin E. *Biochem Biophys Res Commun* **64**:760, 1975.
75. Patriarca P, Zatti M, Cramer R, Rossi F: Stimulation of the respiration of polymorphonuclear leucocytes by phospholipase C. *Life Sci* **9**:841, 1970.
76. Patriarca P, Cramer R, Marussi M, Moncalvo S, Rossi F: Phospholipid splitting and metabolic stimulation in polymorphonuclear leukocytes. *J Reticuloendothel Soc* **10**:251, 1971.
77. Ingraham LM, Coates TD, Allen JM, Higgins CP, Baehner RL, Boxer LA: Metabolic, membrane and functional responses of human polymorphonuclear leukocytes to platelet-activation factor. *Blood* **59**:1259, 1982.
78. Tzeng DY, Deuel TF, Huang IS, Senior RM, Boxer LA, Baehner RL: Platelet-derived growth factor promotes polymorphonuclear leukocyte activation. *Blood* **64**:1123, 1984.

78a. Johnston RB Jr, Lehmeyer JE: The involvement of oxygen metabolites from phagocytic cells in bactericidal activity and inflammation, in Michelson AM, McCord JM, Fridovich I (eds): *Superoxide and Superoxide Dismutases*. New York, Academic, 1977, p 291.

79. Newman SL, Johnston RB Jr: Role of binding through C3b and IgG in polymorphonuclear neutrophil function: Studies with trypsin-generated C3b. *J Immunol* **123**:1839, 1979.
80. Cockcroft S: G-protein regulated phospholipases C, D, and A_2-mediated signalling in neutrophils. *Biochim Biophys Acta* **1113**:135, 1992.
81. Berridge MJ: Inositol trisphosphate and diacylglycerol as second messengers. *Biochem J* **220**:345, 1984.
82. Berridge MJ, Irvine RF: Inositol trisphosphate, a novel second messenger in cellular signal transduction. *Nature* **312**:315, 1984.
83. Krause K-H, Lew PD: Subcellular distribution of Ca^{2+} pumping sites in human neutrophils. *J Clin Invest* **80**:107, 1987.
84. Rasmussen H: The calcium messenger system. *N Engl J Med* **314**:1094, 1986.
85. English D: Involvement of phosphatidic acid, phosphatidate phosphohydrolase, and inositide-specific phospholipase D in neutrophil stimulus-response pathways. *J Lab Clin Med* **120**:520, 1992.
86. Agwu De, McPhail LC, Sozzani S, Bass DA, McCall CE: Phosphatidic acid as a second messenger in human polymorphonuclear leukocytes. Effects on activation of NADPH oxidase. *J Immunol* **88**:531, 1991.
87. Gallin EK: Calcium- and voltage-activated potassium channels in human macrophages. *Biophys J* **46**:821, 1984.
88. Peterson OH, Maruyama Y: Calcium-activated potassium channels and their role in secretion. *Nature* **307**:693, 1984.
89. Smolen JE: Neutrophil signal transduction: Calcium, kinases and fusion. *J Lab Clin Med* **120**:527, 1992.
90. Tauber AI: Protein kinase C and the activation of the human neutrophil NADPH oxidase. *Blood* **69**:711, 1987.
91. Majumdar S, Rossi MW, Fujiki T, Phillips WA, Disa S, Queen CF, Johnston RB Jr, Rosen OM, Corkey BE, Korchak HM: Protein kinase C isotypes and signaling in neutrophils. Differential substrate specificities of a translocatable calcium- and phospholipid-dependent beta-protein kinase

C and a phospholipid-dependent protein kinase which is inhibited by long chain fatty acyl coenzyme A. *J Biol Chem* **266**:9285, 1991.

92. Phillips WA, Fujiki T, Rossi MW, Korchak HM, Johnston RB Jr: Influence of calcium on the subcellular distribution of protein kinase C in human neutrophils. Extraction conditions determine partitioning of histone-phosphorylating activity and immunoreactivity between cytosol and particulate fractions. *J Biol Chem* **264**:8361, 1989.
93. Maridonnear-Parini I, Tringale SM, Tauber AI: Identification of distinct activation pathways of the human neutrophil NADPH-oxidase. *J Immunol* **137**:2925, 1986.
94. Agwu De, McPhail LC, Daniel LW, McCall CE: A novel FMLP-activated phospholipase C hydrolyzed 1-0-alkyl-2-acyl-GPC in human neutrophils. *Fed Proc* **46**:605, 1987.
95. Channon JY, Leslie CC, Johnston RB Jr: Zymosan-stimulated production of phosphatidic acid by macrophages: Relationship to release of superoxide anion and inhibition by agents that increase intracellular cyclic AMP. *J Leukoc Biol* **41**:450, 1987.
96. Korchak HM, Vosshall LB, Haines KA, Wilkenfeld C, Lundquist KF, Weissmann G: Activation of the human neutrophil by calcium-mobilizing ligands. II. Correlation of calcium, diacylglycerol, and phosphatidic acid generation with superoxide anion generation. *J Biol Chem* **263**:11098, 1988.
97. Iyer GYN, Quastrel JH: NADPH and NADH oxidation by guinea pig polymorphonuclear leucocytes. *Can J Biochem Physiol* **41**:427, 1963.
98. Rossi R, Zatti M: Biochemical aspects of phagocytosis in polymorphonuclear leucocytes. NADPH oxidation by the granules of resting and phagocytosing cells. *Experientia* **20**:21, 1964.
99. Borregaard N: The respiratory burst of phagocytosis: Biochemistry and subcellular localization. *Immunol Lett* **11**:165, 1985.
100. Babior BM: The nature of the NADPH oxidase, in Gallin JI, Fauci AS (eds): *Advances in Host Defense Mechanisms*. New York, Raven, 1983, p 91.
101. Gabig TG, Lefker BA: Activation of the human neutrophil NADPH oxidase results in coupling of electron carrier function between ubiquinone-10 and cytochrome b_{559}. *J Biol Chem* **260**:3991, 1985.
102. Gabig TG, Lefker BA: NADPH oxidase from polymorphonuclear cells. *Methods Enzymol* **132**:355, 1986.
103. Heyneman, RA Vercauteren RE: Activation of a NADPH-dependent oxidase from horse polymorphonuclear leukocytes in a cell-free system. *J Leukoc Biol* **36**:751, 1984.
104. Curnutte JT: Activation of human neutrophil nicotinamide adenine dinucleotide phosphate, reduced (triphosphopyridine nucleotide, reduced) oxidase by arachidonic acid in a cell-free system. *J Clin Invest* **75**:1740, 1985.
105. McPhail LC, Shirley PS, Clayton CC, Snyderman R: Activation of the respiratory burst enzyme from human neutrophils in a cell-free system: Evidence for a soluble cofactor. *J Clin Invest* **75**:1735, 1985.
106. Borregaard N, Heiple JM, Simons ER, Clark RA: Subcellular localization of the b-cytochrome component of the human neutrophil microbicidal oxidase: Translocation during activation. *J Cell Biol* **97**:52 1983.
107. Parkos CA, Allen RA, Cochrane CG, Jesaitis AJ: Purified cytochrome b from human granulocyte plasma membrane is comprised of two polypeptides with relative molecular weights of 91,000 and 22,000. *J Clin Invest* **80**:732, 1987.
108. Segal AW: Absence of both cytochrome b_{-245} subunits from neutrophils in X-linked chronic granulomatous disease. *Nature* **326**:88, 1987.
109. Segal AW, Garcia R, Goldstone AG, Cross AR, Jones OTG: Cytochrome b_{-245} of neutrophils is also present in human monocytes, macrophages eosinophils. *Biochem J* **194**:599, 1981.
110. Parkos CA, Dinauer MC, Walker LE, Allen RA, Jesaitis AJ, Orkin SH: The primary structure and unique expression of the 22-kDa light chain of human neutrophil cytochrome b. *Proc Natl Acad Sci USA* **85**:3319, 1988.
111. Radeke HH, Cross AR, Hancock JT, Jones OTG, Nakamura M, Kaever V, Resch K: Functional expression of NADPH oxidase components (α- and β-subunits of cytochrome b_{558} and 45-kDa flavoprotein) by intrinsic human glomerular mesangial cells. *J Biol Chem* **266**:21025, 1991.
112. Volkman DJ, Buescher ES, Gallin JI, Fauci AS: B cell lines as models for inherited phagocytic diseases: Abnormal superoxide generation in chronic granulomatous disease and giant granules in Chediak-Higashi syndrome. *J Immunol* **133**:3006, 1984.
113. Dinauer MC, Orkin SH, Brown R, Jesaitis AJ, Parkos CA: The glycoprotein encoded by the X-linked chronic granulomatous disease locus is a component of the neutrophil cytochrome b complex. *Nature* **327**:717, 1987.
114. Teahan C, Rowe P, Parker P, Totty N, Segal AW: The X-linked chronic granulomatous disease gene codes for the β-chain of cytochrome b_{-245}. *Nature* **327**:720, 1987.
115. Quinn MT, Mullen ML, Jesaitis AJ: Human neutrophil cytochrome *b* contains multiple hemes. Evidence for heme associated with both subunits. *J Biol Chem* **267**:7303, 1992.
116. Segal AW: Superoxide generation, cytochrome b_{-245} and chronic granulomatous disease. *Adv Inflam Res* **8**:55, 1983.
117. Gabig TG, Schervish EW, Santiaga JT: Functional relationship of the cytochrome b to the superoxide-generating oxidase of human neutrophils. *J Biol Chem* **257**:4114, 1982.
118. Segal AW, Jones OTG: Reduction and subsequent oxidation of cytochrome b of human neutrophils after stimulation with phorbol myristate acetate. *Biochem Biophys Res Commun* **88**:130, 1979.
119. Cross AR, Higson FK, Jones OTG, Harper AM, Segal AW: The enzymic reduction and kinetics of oxidation of cytochrome b_{-245} of neutrophils. *Biochem J* **204**:479, 1982.
120. Cross AR, Jones OTG, Harper AM, Segal AW: Oxidation reduction properties of the cytochrome b found in the plasma-membrane fraction of human neutrophils. *Biochem J* **194**:599, 1981.
121. Babior BM, Kipnes RS: Superoxide-forming enzyme from human neutrophils: Evidence for a flavin requirement. *Blood* **50**:517, 1977.
122. Babior BM, Peters WA: The O_2^--producing enzyme of human neutrophils: Further properties. *J Biol Chem* **256**:2321, 1981.
123. Cross AR, Jones OTG, Garcia R, Segal AW: The association of FAD with the cytochrome b_{-245} of human neutrophils. *Biochem J* **208**:759, 1982.
124. Gabig TG: The NADPH-dependent O_2^--generating oxidase from human neutrophils: Identification of a flavoprotein component that is deficient in a patient with chronic granulomatous disease. *J Biol Chem* **258**:6352, 1983.
125. Gabig TG, Lefker BA: Deficient flavoprotein component of the NADPH-dependent O_2^--generating oxidase in the neutrophils from three patients with chronic granulomatous disease. *J Clin Invest* **73**:701, 1984.
126. Bohler M-C, Seger RA, Mouy R, Vilmer E, Fischer A, Griscelli C: A study of 25 patients with chronic granulomatous disease: A new classification by correlating respiratory burst, cytochrome b, and flavoprotein. *J Clin Immunol* **6**:136, 1986.
127. Light DR, Walsh C, O'Callaghan AM, Goetzl EJ, Tauber AI: Characteristics of the cofactor requirements for the superoxide-generating NADPH oxidase of human polymorphonuclear leukocytes. *Biochemistry* **20**:1468, 1981.
128. Cross AR: The inhibitory effects of some iodonium compounds on the superoxide generating system of neutrophils and their failure to inhibit diaphorase activity. *Biochem Pharmacol* **36**:489, 1987.
129. Cross AR: Inhibitors of the leukocyte superoxide generating oxidase. *Free Radic Biol Med* **8**:71, 1990.
130. Segal AW, West I, Wientjes F, Nugent JHA, Chavan AJ, Haley B, Garcia RC, Rosen H, Scrace G: Cytochrome b_{-245} is a flavocytochrome containing FAD and the NADPH-binding site of the microbicidal oxidase of phagocytes. *Biochem J* **284**:781, 1993.
131. Rotrosen D, Yeung CL, Leto TL, Malech HL, Kwong CH: Cytochrome b_{558}: The flavin-binding component of the phagocyte NADPH oxidase. *Science* **256**:1459, 1992.
132. Abo A, Boyhan A, West I, Thrasher AJ, Segal AW: Reconstitution of neutrophil NADPH oxidase activity in the cell-free system by four components: p67-*phox*, p47-*phox*, p21*rac*1, and cytochrome b_{245}. *J Biol Chem* **267**:16767, 1992.

133. Uhlinger DJ, Inge KL, Kreck ML, Tyagi SR, Neckelmann N, Lambeth JD: Reconstitution and characterization of the human neutrophil respiratory burst oxidase using recombinant p47-*phox*, p67-*phox* and plasma membrane. *Biochem Biophys Res Commun* **186**:509, 1992.
134. Volpp BD, Nauseef WM, Clark RA: Two cytosolic neutrophil NADPH oxidase components absent in autosomal chronic granulomatous disease. *Science* **242**:1295, 1988.
135. Clark RA, Volpp BD, Leidal KG, Nauseef WM: Two cytosolic components of the human neutrophil respiratory burst oxidase translocate to the plasma membrane during cell activation. *J Clin Invest* **85**:714, 1990.
136. Nauseef WM, Volpp BD, McCormick S, Leidal KG, Clark RA: Assembly of the neutrophil respiratory burst oxidase. Protein kinase C promotes cytoskeletal and membrane association of cytosolic oxidase components. *J Biol Chem* **266**:5911, 1991.
137. Heyworth PG, Curnutte JT, Nauseef WM, Volpp BD, Pearson DW, Rosen H, Clark RA: Neutrophil nicotinamide adenine dinucleotide phosphate oxidase assembly. Translocation of p47-*phox* and p67-*phox* requires interaction between p47-*phox* and cytochrome b_{558}. *J Clin Invest* **87**:352, 1991.
138. Kleinberg ME, Malech HL, Rotrosen D: The phagocyte 47-kilodalton cytosolic oxidase protein is an early reactant in activation of the respiratory burst. *J Biol Chem* **265**:15577, 1990.
139. Rotrosen D, Kleinberg ME, Nunoi H, Leto T, Gallin JI, Malech HL: Evidence for a functional cytoplasmic domain of phagocyte oxidase cytochrome b558. *J Biol Chem* **265**:8745, 1990.
140. Volpp BD, Nauseef WM, Donelson JE, Moser DR, Clark RA: Cloning of the cDNA and functional expression of the 47-kilodalton cytosolic component of human neutrophil respiratory burst oxidase. *Proc Natl Acad Sci USA* **86**:7195, 1989.
141. Leto TL, Lomax KJ, Volpp BD, Nunoi H, Sechler JMG, Nauseef WM, Clark RA, Gallin JI, Malech HL: Cloning of a 67-kD neutrophil oxidase factor with similarity to a noncatalytic region of $p60^{c\text{-}src}$. *Science* **248**:727, 1990.
142. Rodaway ARF, Teahan CG, Casimir CM, Segal AW, Bentley DL: Characterization of the 47-kilodalton autosomal chronic granulomatous disease protein: Tissue-specific expression and transcriptional control by retinoic acid. *Mol Cell Biol* **10**:5388, 1990.
143. Lomax KJ, Leto TL, Nunoi H, Gallin JI, Malech HL: Recombinant 47-kilodalton cytosol factor restores NADPH oxidase in chronic granulomatous disease. *Science* **245**:409, 1989.
144. Mayer BJ, Baltimore D: Signalling through SH2 and SH3 domains. *Trends Cell Biol* **3**:8, 1993.
145. Stevenson KB, Clark RA, Nauseef WM: Fodrin and band 4.1 in a plasma membrane-associated fraction of human neutrophils. *Blood* **74**:2136, 1989.
146. Woodman RC, Ruedi JM, Jesaitis AJ, Okamura N, Quinn MT, Smith RM, Curnutte JT, Babior BM: Respiratory burst oxidase and three of four oxidase-related polypeptides are associated with the cytoskeleton of human neutrophils. *J Clin Invest* **87**:1345, 1991.
147. Leto TL, Garrett MC, Fujii H, Nunoi H: Characterization of neutrophil NADPH oxidase factors p47-*phox* and p67-*phox* from recombinant baculoviruses. *J Biol Chem* **266**:19812, 1991.
148. Gabig TG, English D, Akard LP, Schell MJ: Regulation of neutrophil NADPH oxidase activation in a cell-free system by guanine nucleotides and fluoride. *J Biol Chem* **262**:1685, 1987.
149. Doussiere J, Pilloud MC, Vignais PV: Activation of bovine neutrophil oxidase in a cell free system. GTP-dependent formation of a complex between a cytosolic factor and a membrane protein. *Biochem Biophys Res Commun* **152**:993, 1988.
150. Peveri P, Heyworth PG, Curnutte JT: Absolute requirement for GTP in the activation of the human neutrophil NADPH oxidase in a cell-free system: Role of ATP in regenerating GTP. *Proc Natl Acad Sci USA* **89**:2494, 1992.
151. Uhlinger DJ, Burnham DN, Lambeth JD: Nucleoside triphosphate requirements for superoxide generation and phosphorylation in a cell-free system from human neutrophils: Sodium dodecyl sulfate and diacylglycerol activate independently of protein kinase C. *J Biol Chem* **266**:20990, 1991.
152. Knaus UG, Heyworth PG, Evans T, Curnutte JT, Bokoch GM: Regulation of phagocyte oxygen radical production by the GTP-binding protein Rac 2. *Science* **254**:1512, 1991.
153. Mizuno T, Kaibuchi K, Ando S, Musha T, Hiraoka K, Takaishi K, Asada M, Nunoi H, Matsuda I, Takai Y: Regulation of the superoxide-generating NADPH oxidase by a small GTP-binding protein and its stimulatory and inhibitory GDP/GTP exchange proteins. *J Biol Chem* **267**:10215, 1992.
154. Bokoch GM, Prossnitz V: Isoprenoid metabolism is required for stimulation of the respiratory burst oxidase of HL-60 cells. *J Clin Invest* **89**:402, 1992.
155. Didsbury JR, Iyer S, Menard L, Casey P, Tomhave E, Snyderman R, Clark RA, Nauseef WM: Activation of the NADPH oxidase system in human neutrophils by the ras-related GTP-binding protein RAC1. *Clin Res* **40**:192A, 1992.
156. Ando S, Kaibuchi K, Sasaki T, Hiraoka K, Nishiyama T, Mizuno T, Asada M, Nunoi H, Matsuda I, Matsuura Y, Polakis P, McCormick F, Takai Y: Post-translational processing of rac p21s is important both for their interaction with the GDP/GTP exchange proteins and for their activation of NADPH oxidase. *J Biol Chem* **267**:25709, 1992.
157. Ueda T, Kikuchi A, Ohga N, Yamamoto J, Takai Y: Purification and characterization from bovine brain cytosol of a novel regulatory protein inhibiting the dissociation of GDP from and the subsequent binding of GTP to rhoB p20, a ras p21-like GTP binding protein. *J Biol Chem* **265**:9373, 1990.
158. Heyworth PG, Knaus UG, Xu XM, Uhlinger DJ, Conroy L, Bokoch GM, Curnutte JT: Requirement for posttranslational processing of Rac GTP-binding proteins for activation of human neutrophil NADPH oxidase. *Mol Biol Cell* **4**:261, 1993.
159. Dorseuil O, Vazquez A, Lang P, Bertoglio J, Gacon G, Leca G: Inhibition of superoxide production in B lymphocytes by Rac antisense oligonucleotides. *J Biol Chem* **267**:20540, 1992.
160. Quinn MT, Parkos CA, Walker L, Orkin SH, Dinauer MC, Jesaitis AJ: Association of a ras-related protein with cytochrome b of human neutrophils. *Nature* **342**:198, 1989.
161. Quinn MT, Mullen ML, Jesaitis AJ, Linner JG: Subcellular distribution of the Rap1A protein in human neutrophils: Colocalization and cotranslocation with cytochrome b_{559}. *Blood* **79**:1563, 1992.
162. Bokoch GM, Quilliam LA, Bohl BP, Jesaitis AJ, Quinn MT: Inhibition of Rap1A binding to cytochrome b_{558} of NADPH oxidase by phosphorylation of Rap1a. *Science* **254**:1794, 1991.
163. Knaus UG, Heyworth PG, Kinsella BT, Curnutte JT, Bokoch GM: Purification and characterization of Rac 2. *J Biol Chem* **267**:23575, 1992.
164. Dewald B, Baggiolini M, Curnutte JT, Babior BM: Subcellular localization of the superoxide-forming enzyme in human neutrophils. *J Clin Invest* **63**:21, 1979.
165. Babior GL, Rosin RE, McMurrich BJ, Peters WA, Babior BM: Arrangement of the respiratory burst oxidase in the plasma membrane of the neutrophil. *J Clin Invest* **67**:1724, 1981.
166. Segal AW, Jones OTG: The subcellular distribution and some properties of the cytochrome b component of the microbicidal oxidase system in human neutrophils. *Biochem J* **182**:181, 1979.
167. Gupta JW, Kubin M, Hartman L, Cassatella MA, Trinchieri G: Induction of expression of genes encoding components of the respiratory burst oxidase during differentiation of human myeloid cell lines induced by tumor necrosis factor and γ-interferon. *Cancer Res* **52**:2530, 1992.
168. Amezaga MA, Bazzoni F, Sorio C, Rossi F, Cassatella MA: Evidence for the involvement of distinct signal transduction pathways in the regulation of constitutive and interferon gamma-dependent gene expression of NADPH oxidase components (gp91-phox, p47-phox, and p22-phox) and high-affinity receptor for IgG (FcgammaR-I) in human polymorphonuclear leukocytes. *Blood* **79**:735, 1992.
169. Baneyx F, Gatenby AA: A mutation in GroEL interferes with protein folding by reducing the rate of discharge of sequestered polypeptides. *J Biol Chem* **267**:11637, 1992.
170. Cassatella MA, Bazzoni F, Flynn RM, Dusi S, Trinchieri G, Rossi F: Molecular basis of interferon-γ and

lipopolysaccharide enhancement of phagocyte respiratory burst capability: Studies on the gene expression of several NADPH oxidase components. *J Biol Chem* **265**:20241, 1990.

171. Guthrie LA, McPhail LC, Henson PM, Johnston RB Jr: Priming of neutrophils for enhanced release of oxygen metabolites by bacterial lipopolysaccharide: Evidence for increased activity of the superoxide-producing enzyme. *J Exp Med* **160**:1656, 1984.
172. Forehand JR, Pabst MJ, Phillips WA, Johnston RB Jr: Lipopolysaccharide priming of human neutrophils for an enhanced respiratory burst: Role of intracellular free calcium. *J Clin Invest* **83**:74, 1989.
173. Cassatella MA, Della Bianca V, Berton G, Rossi F: Activation by gamma interferon of human macrophage capability to produce toxic oxygen molecules is accompanied by decreased Km of the superoxide-generating NADPH oxidase. *Biochem Biophys Res Commun* **132**:908, 1985.
174. International Chronic Granulomatous Disease Study Group: A controlled trial of interferon gamma to prevent infection in chronic granulomatous disease. *N Engl J Med* **324**:509, 1991.
175. Woodman RC, Erickson RW, Rae J, Jaffe HS, Curnutte JT: Prolonged recombinant interferon-gamma therapy in chronic granulomatous disease: Evidence against enhanced neutrophil oxidase activity. *Blood* **79**:1558, 1992.
176. McCord JM, Fridovich I: Superoxide dismutase: An enzymic function for erythrocuprein (hemocuprein). *J Biol Chem* **244**:6049, 1969.
177. Dechatelet LR, McCall CE, McPhail LC, Johnston RB Jr: Superoxide dismutase activity in leukocytes. *J Clin Invest* **53**:1197, 1974.
178. Michelson AM, McCord JM, Fridovich I: *Superoxide and Superoxide Dismutases*. New York, Academic, 1977.
179. Goldstein IM, Kaplan HB, Edelson HS, Weissmann G: Ceruloplasmin: A scavenger of superoxide anion radicals. *J Biol Chem* **254**:4040, 1979.
180. Roos D, Weening RS, Voetman AA, van Schaik MLJ, Bot AAM, Meerhof LJ, Loos JA: Protection of phagocytic leukocytes by endogenous glutathione: Studies in a family with glutathione reductase deficiency. *Blood* **53**:851, 1979.
180a. Rokutan K, Thomas JA, Johnston RB Jr: Phagocytosis and stimulation of the respiratory burst by phorbol diester initiate S-thiolation of specific proteins in macrophages. *J Immunol* **147**:260, 1991.
181. Chance B, Sies H, Boveris A: Hydroperoxide metabolism in mammalian organs. *Physiol Rev* **59**:527, 1979.
182. Roos D, Weening RS, Wyss SR, Aebi HE: Protection of human neutrophils by endogenous catalase: Studies with cells from catalase-deficient individuals. *J Clin Invest* **65**:1515, 1980.
183. O'Donnell-Tormey J, Nathan CF, Lanks K, De Boer CJ, de la Harpe J: Secretion of pyruvate: An antioxidant defense of mammalian cells. *J Exp Med* **165**:500, 1987.
184. Lucy J: Functional and structural aspects of biological membranes: A suggested structural role of vitamin E in the control for membrane permeability and stability. *Ann NY Acad Sci* **203**:4, 1972.
185. Bigley RH, Stankova L: Uptake and reduction of oxidized and reduced ascorbate by human leukocytes. *J Exp Med* **139**:1084, 1974.
186. Packer JE, Slater TJ, Willson RL: Direct observation of a free radical interaction between vitamin E and vitamin C. *Nature* **278**:737, 1979.
187. Naskalski JW: Myeloperoxidase inactivation in the course of catalysis of chlorination of taurine. *Biochim Biophys Acta* **485**:291, 1977.
188. Grisham MB, Jefferson MM, Melton DF, Thomas EL: Chlorination of endogenous amines by isolated neutrophils: Ammonia-dependent bactericidal, cytotoxic, and cytolytic activities of the chloramines. *J Biol Chem* **259**:10404, 1984.
189. Green TR, Fellman JH, Eicher AL, Pratt KL: Antioxidant role and subcellular location of hypotaurine and taurine in human neutrophils. *Biochim Biophys Acta* **1073**:91, 1991.
190. Agner K: Verdoperoxidase: A ferment isolated from leukocytes. *Acta Physiol Scand* Suppl **2**:1, 1941.
191. Schultz J: Myeloperoxidase, in Sbarra AJ, Strauss RR (eds): *The Reticuloendothelial System, Biochemistry and Metabolism*. New York, Plenum, 1980, vol 2, p 231.
192. Nauseef WM, Olsson I, Stromberg-Arnljots K: Biosynthesis and processing of myeloperoxidase: A marker for myeloid cell differentiation. *Eur J Haematol* **40**:97, 1988.
193. Zgliczynski JM: Characteristics of MPO from neutrophils and other peroxidases from different cells, in Sbarra AJ, Strauss RR (eds): *The Reticuloendothelial System, Biochemistry and Metabolism*. New York, Plenum, 1980, vol 2, p 255.
194. Salmon SE, Cline MI, Schultz J, Lehrer RI: Myeloperoxidase deficiency: Immunologic study of a genetic leukocyte defect. *N Engl J Med* **282**:250, 1970.
195. Klebanoff SJ: Myeloperoxidase-halide-hydrogen peroxide antibacterial system. *J Clin Invest* **50**:2226, 1971.
196. Lehrer RI: Antifungal effects of peroxidase systems. *J Bacteriol* **95**:2131, 1968.
197. Belding ME, Klebanoff SJ, Ray CG: Peroxidase-mediated viricidal systems. *Science* **167**:195, 1970.
198. Clark RA, Klebanoff SJ: Neutrophil-mediated tumor cell cytotoxicity: Role of the preoxidase system. *J Exp Med* **141**:1442, 1975.
199. Clark RA, Klebanoff SJ, Einstein AB: Peroxidase-H_2O_2-halide system: Cytotoxic effect on mammalian tumor cells. *Blood* **45**:161, 1975.
200. Grisham MB, Jefferson MM, Thomas EL: Role of monochloramines in the oxidation of erythrocyte hemoglobin by stimulated neutrophils. *J Biol Chem* **259**:6757, 1984.
201. Thomas EL, Fishman M: Oxidation of chloride and thiocyanate by isolated leukocytes. *J Biol Chem* **261**:9694, 1986.
202. Thomas EL, Jefferson MM, Grisham M: Myeloperoxidase-catalyzed incorporation of amino acids into proteins: Role of hypochlorous acid and chloramines. *Biochemistry* **21**:6299, 1982.
203. Test ST, Lampert MB, Ossanna PJ, Thoene JG, Weiss SJ: Generation of nitrogen-chlorine oxidants by human phagocytes. *J Clin Invest* **74**:1341, 1984.
204. Weiss SJ, Peppin G, Ortiz X, Ragsdale C, Test ST: Oxidative autoactivation of latent collagenase by human neutrophils. *Science* **227**:747, 1985.
205. Weiss SJ, Regiani S: Neutrophils degrade subendothelial matrices in the presence of alpha-1-protease inhibitor. *J Clin Invest* **73**:1297, 1984.
206. Weiss SJ, Klein R, Slivka A, Wei M: Chlorination of taurine by human neutrophils. *J Clin Invest* **70**:598, 1982.
207. Weiss SJ, Slivka A: Monocyte and granulocyte-mediated tumor cell destruction. *J Clin Invest* **69**:225, 1982.
208. Zgliczynski JM, Stelmaszynska T: Chlorinating ability of human phagcytosing leucocytes. *Eur J Biochem* **56**:157, 1975.
209. Zgliczynski JM, Stelmaszynska T, Domanski J, Ostrowski W: Chloramines as intermediates of oxidation reaction of amino acids by myeloperoxidase. *Biochim Biophys Acta* **235**:419, 1974.
210. Harrison JE, Schultz J: Studies on the chlorinating activity of myeloperoxidase. *J Biol Chem* **251**:1371, 1976.
211. Albrich IM, McCarthy CA, Hurst JK: Biological reactivity of hypochlorous acid and implications for microbicidal mechanism of leukocyte myeloperoxidase. *Proc Natl Acad Sci USA* **78**:210, 1981.
212. Rosen H, Klebanorf SJ: Oxidation of microbial iron-sulfur centers by the MPO-H_2O_2-halide antimicrobial system. *Infect Immun* **47**:613, 1985.
213. Rosen H, Klebanoff SJ: Oxidation of *Escherichia coli* iron centers by the myeloperoxidase-mediated microbicidal system. *J Biol Chem* **257**:13731, 1982.
214. Nauseef WM, Metcalf JA, Root RK: Role of myeloperoxidase in the respiratory burst of human neutrophils. *Blood* **61**:483, 1983.
215. Stendahl O, Coble DI, Dahlgren C, Hed J, Molin L: Myeloperoxidase modulates the phagocytic activity of polymorphonuclear neutrophil leukocytes: Studies with cells from a myeloperoxidase-deficient patient. *J Clin Invest* **73**:366, 1984.
216. Cech P, Papathanassiou A, Boreaux G, Roth P, Miescher PA: Hereditary myeloperoxidase deficiency. *Blood* **53**:403, 1979.
217. Craner R, Soranzo MR, Dri P, Rottini GD, Bramezza M, Cirielli S: Incidence of myeloperoxidase deficiency in an area of northern Italy: Histochemical, biochemical, and functional studies. *Br J Haematol* **51**:81, 1982.
218. Kitahara M, Eyre HJ, Simonian Y, Atkin CL, Hasstedt

SJ: Hereditary myeloperoxidase deficiency. *Blood* **57**:888, 1981.

219. Klebanoff SJ, Pincus SH: Hydrogen peroxide utilization in myeloperoxidase-deficient leukocytes: A possible microbicidal control mechanism. *J Clin Invest* **50**:2226, 1971.
220. Patriarca P, Cramer R, Tedesco F, Kukinuma K: Studies on the mechanism of metabolic stimulation in polymorphonuclear leukocytes during phagocytosis. *Biochim Biophys Acta* **385**:387, 1975.
221. Rosen H, Klebanoff SJ: Chemiluminescence and superoxide production by myeloperoxidase-deficient leukocytes. *J Clin Invest* **58**:50, 1976.
222. Locksley RM, Wilson CR, Klebanoff SJ: Increased respiratory burst in myeloperoxidase-deficient monocytes. *Blood* **62**:902, 1983.
223. Clark RA: Extracellular effect of the myeloperoxidase-hydrogen peroxide-halide system, *Adv Infect Res* **5**:107, A83.
224. Clark RA, Borregaard N: Neutrophils autoinactivate secretory products by myeloperoxidase-catalyzed oxidation. *Blood* **65**:375, 1985.
225. Kobayashi M, Tanaka T, Usui T: Inactivation of lysosomal enzymes by the respiratory burst of polymorphonuclear leukocytes: Possible involvement of myeloperoxidase-H_2O_2-halide system. *J Lab Clin Med* **100**:896, 1982.
226. Voetman AA, Weening RS, Hamers MN, Meerhof LJ, Bot AAAM, Roos D: Phagocytosing human neutrophils inactivate their own granular enzymes. *J Clin Invest* **67**:1541, 1981.
227. Clark RA, Szot S: Chemotactic factor inactivation by stimulated human neutrophils mediated by myeloperoxidase-catalyzed methionine oxidation. *J Immunol* **128**:1507, 1982.
228. Clark RA: Chemotactic factors trigger their own oxidative inactivation by human neutrophils. *J Immunol* **129**:2725, 1982.
229. Clark RA, Szot S, Venkatasubramanian K, Schiffmann R: Chemotactic factor inactivation by myeloperoxidase-mediated oxidation of methionine. *J Immunol* **124**:2020, 1980.
230. Clark RA, Klebanoff SJ: Chemotactic factor inactivation by the myeloperoxidase-hydrogen peroxide-halide system. *J Clin Invest* **64**:913, 1979.
231. Tsan M-F, Denison RC: Oxidation of n-forinyl methionyl chemotactic peptide by human neutrophils. *J Immunol* **126**:1387, 1981.
232. Clark RA, Stone P, El-Hag A, Calore JD, Franzblau C: Myeloperoxidase-catalyzed inactivation of α_1-protease inhibitor by human neutrophils. *J Biol Chem* **256**:3348, 1981.
233. Matheson NR, Wong PS, Schuyler M, Travis J: Interaction of human alpha-1-proteinase inhibitor with neutrophil myeloperoxidase. *Biochemistry* **20**:331, 1981.
234. Matheson NR, Wong PS, Travis J: Enzymatic inactivation of human alpha-1-proteinase inhibitor by neutrophil myeloperoxidase. *Biochem Biophys Res Commun* **88**:402, 1979.
235. Lane TA, Lamkin GE: Myeloperoxidase-mediated modulation of chemotactic peptide binding to human neutrophils. *Blood* **61**:1203, 1983.
236. El-Hag A, Clark RA: Down-regulation of human natural killer activity against tumors by the neutrophil myeloperoxidase system and hydrogen peroxide. *J Immunol* **133**:3291, 1984.
237. Andersen M, Atkin CL, Eyre HJ: Intact form of myeloperoxidase from normal human neutrophils. *Arch Biochem Biophys* **214**:273, 1982.
238. Andrews PC, Krinsky NI: The reductive cleavage of myeloperoxidase in half, producing enzymatically active hemi-myeloperoxidase. *J Biol Chem* **256**:4211, 1981.
239. Harrison JE, Pabalan S, Schultz J: The subunit structure of crystalline canine myeloperoxidase. *Biochim Biophys Acta* **493**:247, 1977.
240. Nauseef WM, Root RK, Malech HL: Biochemical and immunologic analysis of hereditary myeloperoxidase deficiency. *J Clin Invest* **71**:1297, 1983.
241. Olsson I, Olofsson T, Odeber H: Myeloperoxidase-mediated iodination in granulocytes. *Scand J Haematol* **9**:483, 1972.
242. Yamada M, Mori M, Sugimura T: Purification and characterization of small molecular weight myeloperoxidase forms from human promyelocytic leukemia HL-60 cells. *Biochemistry* **20**:766, 1981.
243. Andrews PC, Parnes C, Krinsky NI: Comparison of myeloperoxidase and hemi-myeloperoxidase with regard to catalysis, regulation, and bactericidal activity. *Arch Biochem Biophys* **228**:439, 1984.
244. Zeng J, Fenna RE: X-ray crystal structure of canine myeloperoxidase at 3 Å resolution. *J Mol Biol* **226**:185, 1992.
245. Sutton BJ, Little C, Olsen RL, Willassen NP: Preliminary crystallographic analysis of human myeloperoxidase. *J Mol Biol* **199**:395, 1988.
246. Booth KS, Kimura S, Lee HC, Ikeda-Saito M, Caughey WS: Bovine myeloperoxidase and lactoperoxidase each contain a high affinity binding site for calcium. *Biochem Biophys Res Commun* **160**:897, 1989.
247. Feldberg NT, Schultz J: Evidence that myeloperoxidase is composed of isoenzymes. *Arch Biochem Biophys* **148**:407, 1972.
248. Himmelhock SR, Evans WH, Mage MG, Peterson EA: Purification of myeloperoxidases from the bone marrow of the guinea pig. *Biochemistry* **8**:914, 1969.
249. Schultz J, Feldberg J, John S: Myeloperoxidase. VIII. Separation into ten components by free-flow electrophoresis. *Biochem Biophys Res Commun* **28**:543, 1967.
250. Strauven TA, Armstrong D, James GT, Austin JH: Separation of leukocyte peroxidase isoenzymes by agarose-acrylamide disc electrophoresis. *Age* **1**:111, 1978.
251. Nauseef WM, Malech HL: Immunochemical analysis of myeloperoxidase in normal and MPO-deficient neutrophils and a human promyelocytic cell line. *Clin Res* **30**:560A, 1982.
252. Taylor KL, Guzman GS, Pohl J, Kinkade JM Jr: Distinct chromatographic forms of human hemi-myeloperoxidase obtained by reductive cleavage of the dimeric enzyme. Evidence for subunit heterogeneity. *J Biol Chem* **265**:15938, 1990.
253. Miyasaki KT, Wilson ME, Cohen E, Jones PC, Genco RJ: Evidence for and partial characterization of three major and three minor chromatographic forms of human neutrophil myeloperoxidase. *Arch Biochem Biophys* **246**:751, 1986.
254. Morita Y, Iwamoto H, Aibara S, Kobayashi T, Hasegawa E: Crystallization and properties of myeloperoxidase from normal human leukocytes. *J Biochem* **99**:761, 1986.
255. Pember SO, Fuhrer-Krsi SM, Barnes KC, Kinkade JM: Isolation of three native forms of myeloperoxidase from human polymorphonuclear leukocytes. *FEBS Lett* **140**:103, 1982.
256. Suzuki K, Ota H, Sasagawa S, Sakatani T, Fujikura T: Assay method for myeloperoxidase in human polymorphonuclear leukocytes. *Anal Biochem* **132**:345, 1983.
257. Atkin CL, Andersen MR, Eyre HJ: Abnormal neutrophil myeloperoxidase from a patient with chronic myelogenous leukemia. *Arch Biochem Biophys* **214**:284, 1982.
258. Babcock GT, Ingle RT, Oertling WA, Davis JC, Averill BA, Hulse CL, Stufkens DJ, Bolscher BGJM, Wever R: Raman characterization of human leukocyte myeloperoxidase and bovine spleen haemoprotein: Insight into chromophore structure and evidence that the chromophores of myeloperoxidase are equivalent. *Biochim Biophys Acta* **828**:58, 1985.
259. Ikeda-Saito M, Argade PV, Rousseau DL: Resonance evidence of chloride binding to the heme iron in myeloperoxidase. *FEBS Lett* **184**:52, 1985.
260. Sibbetts S, Hurst JK: Structural analysis of myeloperoxidase by resonance Raman spectroscopy. *Biochemistry* **23**:3007, 1984.
261. Dugad LB, La Mar GN, Lee HC, Ikeda-Saito M, Booth KS, Caughey WS: A nuclear Overhauser effect study of the active site of myeloperoxidase. Structural similarity of the prosthetic group to that on lactoperoxidase. *J Biol Chem* **265**:7173, 1990.
262. Wever R, Oertling WA, Hoogland H, Bolscher BGJM, Kim Y, Babcock GT: Denaturation and renaturation of myeloperoxidase. Consequences for the nature of the prosthetic group. *J Biol Chem* **266**:24308, 1991.
263. Sono M, Bracete AM, Huff AM, Ikeda-Saito M, Dawson JH: Evidence that a formyl-substituted iron porphyrin is the prosthetic group of myeloperoxidase: Magnetic circular dichroism similarity of the peroxidase to *Spirographis* heme-reconstituted myoglobin. *Proc Natl Acad Sci USA* **88**:11148, 1991.
264. López-Garriga JJ, Oertling WA, Kean RT, Hoogland H, Wever R, Babcock GT: Metal-ligand vibrations of cyanoferric myeloperoxidase and cyanoferric horseradish per-

oxidase: Evidence for a constrained heme pocket in myeloperoxidase. *Biochemistry* **29**:9387, 1990.

265. Cully J, Harrach B, Hauser H, Harth N, Robenek H, Nagata S, Hasilik A: Synthesis and localization of myeloperoxidase protein in transfected BHK Cells. *Exp Cell Res* **180**:440, 1989.
266. Taylor KL, Uhlinger DJ, Kinkade JM Jr: Expression of recombinant myeloperoxidase using a baculovirus expression system. *Biochem Biophys Res Commun* **187**:1572, 1992.
267. Moguilevsky N, Garcia-Quintana L, Jacquet A, Tournay C, Fabry L, Piérard L, Bollen A: Structural and biological properties of human recombinant myeloperoxidase produced by Chinese hamster ovary cell lines. *Eur J Biochem* **197**:605, 1991.
268. Jacquet A, Deby C, Mathy M, Moguilevsky N, Deby-Dupont G, Thirion A, Goormaghtigh E, Garcia-Quintana L, Bollen A, Pincemail J: Spectral and enzymatic properties of human recombinant myeloperoxidase: Comparison with the mature enzyme. *Arch Biochem Biophys* **291**:132, 1991.
269. Jacquet A, Deleersnyder V, Garcia-Quintana L, Bollen A, Moguilevsky N: Site-directed mutants of human myeloperoxidase: A topological approach to the heme-binding site. *FEBS Lett* **302**:189, 1992.
270. Forrest CB, Forehand JR, Axtell RA, Roberts RL, Johnston RB Jr: Clinical features and current management of chronic granulomatous disease. *Hematol Oncol Clin North Am* **2**:253, 1988.
271. Babior BM, Woodman RC: Chronic granulomatous disease. *Semin Hematol* **27**:247, 1990.
272. Baehner RL: Chronic granulomatous disease of childhood: Clinical, pathological, biochemical, molecular, and genetic aspects of the disease. *Pediatr Pathol* **10**:143, 1990.
273. Dinauer MC, Orkin SH: Chronic granulomatous disease. *Annu Rev Med* **43**:117, 1992.
274. Segal AW: Chronic granulomatous disease. *Clin Exp Allergy* **21**:195, 1991.
275. Curnutte JT: Disorders of granulocyte function and granulopoiesis, in Nathan DG, Oski FA (eds): *Hematology of Infancy and Childhood*, 4th ed. Philadelphia, Saunders, 1992.
276. Hopkins PJ, Bemiller LS, Curnutte JT: Chronic granulomatous disease: Diagnosis and classification at the molecular level. *Clin Lab Med* **12**:277, 1992.
277. Holmes B, Page AR, Good RA: Studies of the metabolic activity of leukocytes from patients with a genetic abnormality of phagocytic function. *J Clin Invest* **46**:1422, 1967.
278. Davis WC, Huber H, Douglas SD, Fudenberg HH: A defect in circulating mononuclear phagocytes in chronic granulomatous disease of childhood. *J Immunol* **101**:1093, 1968.
279. Rodey GE, Park BH, Windhorst DB, Good RA: Defective bactericidal activity of monocytes in fatal granulomatous disease. *Blood* **33**:813, 1969.
280. Lehrer RI: Measurement of candidacidal activity of specific leukocyte types in mixed cell populations. II Normal and chronic granulomatous disease eosinophils. *Infect Immun* **3**:800, 1971.
281. Berendes H, Bridges RA, Good RA: Fatal granulomatosis of childhood: Clinical study of new syndrome. *Minn Med* **40**:309, 1957.
282. Landing BH, Shirkey HS: Syndrome of recurrent infection and infiltration of viscera by pigmented lipid histiocytes. *Pediatrics* **20**:431, 1957.
283. Beahner RL, Nathan DG: Quantitative nitroblue tetrazolium test in chronic granulomatous disease. *N Engl J Med* **278**:971, 1968.
284. Quie PG, Kaplan EL, Page AR, Gruskay FL, Malawista SE: Defective polymorphonuclear-leukocyte function and chronic granulomatous disease in two female children. *N Engl J Med* **278**:976, 1968.
285. Curnutte JT, Whitten DM, Babior BM: Defective superoxide production by granulocytes from patients with chronic granulomatous disease. *N Engl J Med* **290**:593, 1974.
286. Curnutte IT, Kipnes RS, Barior BM: Defect in pyridine nucleotide-dependent superoxide production by a particulate fraction from the granulocytes of patients with chronic granulomatous disease. *N Engl J Med* **293**:628, 1975.
287. Hohn DC, Lehrer RI: NADPH oxidase deficiency in X-linked chronic granulomatous disease. *J Clin Invest* **55**:707, 1975.
288. McPhail LC, Dechatelet LR, Shirley PS, Wilfert C, Johnston RB Jr, McCall CE: Deficiency of NADPH oxidase activity in chronic granulomatous disease. *J Pediatr* **90**:213, 1977.
289. Segal AW, Jones OTG: Novel cytochrome b system in phagocytic vacuoles of human granulocytes. *Nature* **276**:515, 1978.
290. Segal AW, Cross AR, Garcia RC, Borregaard N, Valerius NH, Soothill JF, Jones OTG: Absence of cytochrome b_{-245} in chronic granulomatous disease: A multicenter European evaluation of its incidence and relevance. *N Engl J Med* **308**:245, 1983.
291. Royer-Pokora B, Kunkel LM, Monaco AP, Goff SC, Newburger PE, Baehner RL, Cole FS, Curnutte JT, Orkin SH: Cloning the gene for an inherited human disorder—chronic granulomatous disease—on the basis of its chromosomal location. *Nature* **322**:32, 19986.
292. Nunoi H, Rotrosen D, Gallin JI, Malech HL: Two forms of autosomal chronic granulomatous disease lack distinct neutrophil cytosol factors. *Science* **242**:1298, 1988.
293. Dinauer MC, Pierce EA, Bruns GAP, Curnutte JT, Orkin SH: Human neutrophil cytochrome *b* light chain (p22-*phox*): Gene structure, chromosomal location, and mutations in cytochrome-negative autosomal recessive chronic granulomatous disease. *J Clin Invest* **86**:1729, 1990.
294. Johnston RB Jr, Newman SL: Chronic granulomatous disease. *Pediatr Clin North Am* **24**:365, 1977.
295. Newburger PE, Cohen HJ, Rothchild SB, Hibbins JC, Malawista SE, Mahoney MJ: Prenatal diagnosis of chronic granulomatous disease. *N Engl J Med* **300**:178, 1979.
296. Matthay KY, Golbus MS, Wara DW, Mentzer WC: Prenatal diagnosis of chronic granulomatous disease. *Am J Med Genet* **17**:731, 1984.
297. Levinsky R, Harvey B, Nicolaides K, Rodeck C: Antenatal diagnosis of chronic granulomatous disease. *Lancet* **1**:504, 1986.
298. Lindlof M, Kere J, Ristola M, Repo H, Leirisalo-Repo M, Von Koskull H, Ammala P, de la Chapelle A: Prenatal diagnosis of X-linked chronic granulomatous disease using restriction fragment length polymorphism analysis. *Genomics* **1**:87, 1987.
299. Nakamura M, Imajoh-Ohmi S, Kanegasaki S, Kurozumi H, Sato K, Kato S, Miyazaki Y: Prenatal diagnosis of cytochrome-deficient chronic granulomatous disease (letter). *Lancet* **336**:118, 1990.
300. De Boer M, Bolscher BGJM, Sijmons RH, Scheffer H, Weening RS, Roos D: Prenatal diagnosis in a family with X-linked chronic granulomatous disease with the use of the polymerase chain reaction. *Prenat Diagn* **12**:773, 1992.
301. Weening RS, Adriaansz LH, Weemaes CMR, Lutter R, Roos D: Clinical differences in chronic granulomatous disease in patients with cytochrome b-negative or cytochrome b-positive neutrophils. *J Pediatr* **107**:102, 1985.
302. Dilworth JA, Mandell GL: Adults with chronic granulomatous disease of "childhood." *Am J Med* **63**:233, 1977.
303. Schapiro BL, Newburger PE, Klempner MS, Dinauer MC: Chronic granulomatous disease presenting in a 69-year-old man. *N Engl J Med* **325**:1786, 1991.
304. Gallin JI, Buescher ES, Seligmann BE, Nath J, Gaither T, Katz P: Recent advances in chronic granulomatous disease. *Ann Intern Med* **99**:67, 1983.
305. Tauber AL, Borregaard N, Simons E, Wright J: Chronic granulomatous disease: A syndrome of phagocyte oxidase deficiencies. *Medicine (Baltimore)* **62**:286, 1983.
306. Hadfield MG, Ghatak NR, Laine FJ, Myer EC, Massie FS, Kramer WM: Brain lesions in chronic granulomatous disease. *Acta Neuropathol (Berl)* **81**:467, 1991.
307. Donowitz GR, Mandell GL: Clinical presentation and unusual infections in chronic granulomatous disease. *Adv Host Defen Mech* **3**:55, 1983.
308. Windhorst DG, Good RA: Dermatologic manifestations of fatal granulomatous disease of childhood. *Arch Dermatol* **103**:351, 1971.
309. Barriere H, Litoux P, Stadler JF, Buriot C, Hakim J:

Chronic granulomatous disease: Late onset of skin lesions only, in two siblings. *Arch Dermatol* **17**:683, 1981.

310. Stalder JF, Dreno B, Bureau B, Hadim J: Discoid lupus erythematosus-like lesions in an autosomal form of chronic granulomatous disease. *Br J Dermatol* **114**:251, 1986.
311. Strate M, Brandrup R, Wand R: Discoid lupus erythematosus-like skin lesions in a patient with autosomal recessive chronic granulomatous disease. *Clin Genet* **30**:184, 1986.
312. Sillevis-Smitt JH, Bos JD, Weening RS, Krieg SR: Discoid lupus erythematosus-like skin changes in patients with autosomal recessive chronic granulomatous disease (letter). *Arch Dermatol* **126**:1656, 1990.
313. Barton LI, Johnson CR: Discoid lupus erythematosus and X-linked chronic granulomatous disease. *Pediatr Dermatol* **3**:376, 1986.
314. Garioch JJ, Sampson JR, Seywright M, Thomson J: Dermatoses in five related female carriers of X-linked chronic granulomatous disease. *Br J Dermatol* **121**:391, 1989.
315. Yeaman GR, Froebel K, Galea G, Ormerod A, Urbaniak SJ: Discoid lupus erythematosus in an X-linked cytochrome-positive carrier of chronic granulomatous disease. *Br J Dermatol* **126**:60, 1992.
316. Kawashima A, Kuhlman JE, Fishman EK, Tempany CM, Magid D, Lederman HM, Winkelstein JA, Zerhouni EA: Pulmonary *Aspergillus* chest wall involvement in chronic granulomatous disease: CT and MRI findings. *Skeletal Radiol* **20**:487, 1991.
317. White CJ, Kwon-Chung KJ, Gallin JI: Chronic granulomatous disease of childhood. An unusual case of infection with *Aspergillus nidulans* var. echinulatus. *Am J Clin Pathol* **90**:312, 1988.
318. Sponseller PD, Malech HL, McCarthy EF Jr, Horowitz SF, Jaffe G, Gallin JI: Skeletal involvement in children who have chronic granulomatous disease. *J Bone Joint Surg [Am]* **73**:37, 1991.
319. Wolfson JJ, Quie PG, Laxdal SD, Good RA: Roentgenologic manifestations in children with a genetic defect of polymorphonuclear leukocyte function. *Radiology* **91**:37, 1968.
320. Gold RH, Douglas SD, Preger L, Steinbach HI, Fudenberg HH: Roentgenographic features of the neutrophil dysfunction syndrome. *Radiology* **92**:1045, 1969.
321. Ament ME, Ochs HD: Gastrointestinal manifestations of chronic granulomatous disease. *N Engl J Med* **288**:382, 1974.
322. Kelleher D, Bloomfield FJ, Lenehan T, Griffin M, Geighery C, McCann SR: Chronic granulomatous disease presenting as an oculomucocutaneous syndrome mimicking Behcet's syndrome. *Postgrad Med J* **62**:489, 1986.
323. Cohen MS, Leong PA, Simpson DM: Phagocytic cells in periodontal defense. Periodontal status of patients with chronic granulomatous disease of childhood. *J Periodontol* **56**:611, 1985.
324. Dusi S, Poli G, Berton G, Catalano P, Fornasa CV, Peserico A: Chronic granulomatous disease in an adult female with granulomatous cheilitis. Evidence for an X-linked pattern of inheritance with extreme lyonization. *Acta Haematol (Basel)* **84**:49, 1990.
325. Renner WR, Johnson JF, Lichtenstein JE, Kirks DR: Esophageal inflammation and stricture: Complication of chronic granulomatous disease of childhood. *Radiology* **178**:189, 1991.
326. Dickerman JD, Colletti RB, Tampas JP: Gastric outlet obstruction in chronic granulomatous disease of childhood. *Am J Dis Child* **140**:567, 1986.
327. Granot E, Matoth I, Korman SH, Ludomirsky A, Lax-E: Functional gastrointestinal obstruction in a child with chronic granulomatous disease. *J Pediatr Gastroenterol Nutr* **5**:321, 1986.
328. Fisher JE, Khan AR, Heitlinger L, Allen JE, Afshani E: Chronic granulomatous disease of childhood with acute ulcerative colitis: A unique association. *Pediatr Pathol* **7**:91, 1987.
329. Rossi TM, Cumella J, Baswell D, Park B: Ascites as a presenting sign of peritonitis in chronic granulomatous disease of childhood. *Clin Pediatr (Phila)* **26**:544, 1987.
330. Griscom NT, Kirkpatrick JA, Girdany BR, Berson WE, Grand RJ, Mackie GG: Gastric antral narrowing in chronic granulomatous disease of childhood. *Pediatrics* **54**:456, 1974.
331. Bowen A III, Gibson MD: Chronic granulomatous disease with gastric antral narrowing. *Pediatr Radiol* **10**:119, 1980.
332. Sty JR, Chusid MJ, Babbitt DP, Werlin SL: Involvement of the colon in chronic granulomatous disease of childhood. *Radiology* **132**:618, 1979.
333. Mulholland MW, Delaney JP, Simmons RL: Gastrointestinal complications of chronic granulomatous disease: Surgical implications. *Surgery* **94**:569, 1983.
334. Wolfson JJ, Kane WJ, Laxdal SD, Good RA, Quie PG: Bone findings in chronic granulomatous disease of childhood. *J Bone Joint Surg [Am]* **51**:1573, 1969.
335. Heinrich SD, Finney T, Craver R, Yin L, Zembo MM: Aspergillus osteomyelitis in patients who have chronic granulomatous disease. Case report. *J Bone Joint Surg [Am]* **73**:456, 1991.
336. Aliabadi H, Gonzalez R, Quie PG: Urinary tract disorders in patients with chronic granulomatous disease. *N Engl J Med* **321**:706, 1989.
337. Walther MM, Malech H, Berman A, Choyke P, Venzon DJ, Linehan WM, Gallin JI: The urological manifestations of chronic granulomatous disease. *J Urol* **147**:1314, 1991.
338. Cyr WL, Johnson H, Balfour J: Granulomatous cystitis as a manifestation of chronic granulomatous disease of childhood. *J Urol* **110**:3537, 1973.
339. Young AK, Middleton RG: Urologic manifestations of chronic granulomatous disease of infancy. *J Urol* **123**:119, 1980.
340. Kontras SB, Bodenbender JG, McClave CR, Smith JP: Interstitial cystitis as a manifestation of chronic granulomatous disease. *Clin Exp Immunol* **43**:390, 1981.
341. van Rhenen DJ, Koolen MI, Feltkamp-Vroom TM, Weening RS: Immune complex glomerulonephritis in chronic granulomatous disease. *Acta Med Complex* **206**:233, 1979.
342. Frifelt JJ, Schonheyder H, Valerius NH, Strate M, Starklint H: Chronic granulomatous disease associated with chronic glomerulonephritis. *Acta Paediatr Scand* **74**:152, 1985.
343. Forbes GS, Hartman GW, Burke EC, Segura JW: Genitourinary involvement in chronic granulomatous disease of childhood. *Am J Roentgenol* **127**:683, 1976.
344. Bloomberg SD, Neu HC, Ehrlich RM, Blanc WA: Chronic granulomatous disease of childhood with renal involvement. *Urology* **4**:193, 1974.
345. Fleischmann J, Church JA, Lehrer RI: Case report: Primary *Candida* meningitis and chronic granulomatous disease. *Am J Med Sci* **291**:334, 1986.
346. Lazarus GM, Heu HC: Agents responsible for infection in chronic granulomatous disease of childhood. *J Pediatr* **86**:415, 1975.
347. Martyn LJ, Lischner HW, Pilaggi AJ, Harley RD: Chorioretinal lesions in familial chronic granulomatous disease of childhood. *Am J Ophthalmol* **73**:403, 1972.
348. Halazun JF, Lukens JN: Thyrotoxicosis associated with aspergillus thyroiditis in chronic granulomatous disease. *J Pediatr* **80**:106, 1972.
349. Walker DH, Okiye G: Chronic granulomatous disease involving the central nervous system. *Pediatr Pathol* **1**:159, 1983.
350. Moellering RC, Weinberg AN: Persistent .almonella infection in a female carrier for chronic granulomatous disease. *Ann Intern Med* **73**:595, 1970.
351. Johnston RB Jr: Unusual forms of an uncommon disease (chronic granulomatous disease). *J Pediatr* **88**:172, 1976.
352. Ward PA, Schlegel RJ: Impaired leucotactic responsiveness in a child with recurrent infections. *Lancet* **2**:344, 1969.
353. Clark RA, Klebanoff SJ: Chronic granulomatous disease: Studies of a family with impaired neutrophil chemotactic, metabolic and bactericidal function *Am J Med* **65**:941, 1978.
354. Baehner RL, Boxer LA, Davis J: The biochemical basis of nitroblue tetrazolium reduction in normal human and chronic granulomatous disease polymorphonuclear leukocytes. *Blood* **48**:309, 1976.
355. Mandell GL, Hook EW: Leukocyte bactericidal activity in chronic granulomatous disease: Correlation of bacterial hydrogen peroxide production and susceptibility to intracellular killing. *J Bacteriol* **100**:531, 1969.
356. Kelly JK, Pinto AR, Whitelaw WA, Rorstad OF, Bowen TJ, Matheson DS: Fatal aspergillus pneumonia in chronic granulomatous disease. *Am J Clin Pathol* **86**:668, 1986.

357. Bujak JS, Ottesen EA, Dinarello CA, Brenner VJ: Nocardiosis in a child with chronic granulomatous disease. *J Pediatr* **83**:98, 1973.
358. Curry WA: Human nocardiosis: A clinical review with selected case reports. *Arch Intern Med* **140**:818, 1980.
359. Casale TB, Macher AM, Fauci AS: Concomitant pulmonary aspergillosis and nocardiosis in a patient with a chronic granulomatous disease of childhood. *South Med J* **77**:274, 1984.
360. Chusid MJ, Parrillo JE, Fauci AS: Chronic granulomatous disease: Diagnosis in a 27-year old man with *Mycobacterium fortuitum*. *JAMA* **233**:1295, 1975.
361. Kobayashi Y, Komazawa Y, Kobayashi M, Matsumoto T, Sakura N, Ishikawa K, Usui T: Presumed BCG infection in a boy with chronic granulomatous disease. A report of a case and a review of the literature. *Clin Pediatr* **23**:586, 1984.
362. O'Neil KM, Herman JH, Modlin JF, Moxon ER, Winklestein JA: *Pseudomonas cepacia:* An emerging pathogen in chronic granulomatous disease. *J Pediatr* **108**:940, 1986.
363. Ephros M, Engelhard D, Maayan S, Bercovier H, Avital A, Yatsiv I: *Legionella gormanii* pneumonia in a child with chronic granulomatous disease. *Pediatr Infect Dis J* **8**:726, 1989.
364. Kaplan A, Israel F: *Corynebacterium aquaticum* infection in a patient with chronic granulomatous disease. *Am J Med Sci* **296**:57, 1988.
365. Kenney RT, Kwon-Chung KJ, Waytes AT, Melnick DA, Pass HI, Merino MJ, Gallin JI: Successful treatment of systemic *Exophiala dermatitidis* infection in a patient with chronic granulomatous disease. *Clin Infect Dis* **14**:235, 1992.
366. Phillips P, Forbes JC, Speert DP: Disseminated infection with *Pseudallescheria boydii* in a patient with chronic granulomatous disease: Response to gamma-interferon plus antifungal chemotherapy. *Pediatr Infect Dis J* **10**:536, 1991.
367. Silliman CC, Lawellin DW, Lohr JA, Rodgers BM, Donowitz LG: *Paecilomyces lilacinus* infection in a child with chronic granulomatous disease. *J Infect* **24**:191, 1992.
368. Sorensen RU, Jacobs MR, Shurin SB: *Chromobacterium violaceum* adenitis acquired in the northern United States as a complication of chronic granulomatous disease. *Pediatr Infect Dis J* **4**:701, 1985.
369. Trotter JA, Kuhls TL, Pickett DA, Reyes De La Rocha S, Welch DF: Pneumonia caused by a newly recognized pseudomonad in a child with chronic granulomatous disease. *J Clin Microbiol* **28**:1120, 1990.
370. Wenger JD, Hollis DG, Weaver RE, Baker CN, Brown GR, Brenner DJ, Broome CV: Infection caused by *Francisella philomiragia* (formerly *Yersinia philomiragia*). A newly recognized human pathogen. *Ann Intern Med* **110**:888, 1989.
371. Williamson PR, Kwon Chung KJ, Gallin JI: Successful treatment of *Paecilomyces varioti* infection in a patient with chronic granulomatous disease and a review of *Paecilomyces* species infections. *Clin Infect Dis* **14**:1023, 1992.
372. Ochs HD, Igo RP: The NBT slide test: A simple screening method for detecting chronic granulomatous disease and female carriers. *J Pediatr* **83**:77, 1973.
373. Johnston RB III, Hardeck RJ, Johnston RB Jr: Recurrent severe infections in a girl with apparently variable expression of mosaicism for chronic granulomatous disease. *J Pediatr* **106**:50, 1985.
374. Meerhof J, Roos D: Heterogeneity in chronic granulomatous disease detected with an improved nitroblue tetrazolium slide test. *J Leukoc Biol* **39**:699, 1986.
375. Johnston RB Jr: Measurement of O_2^- secreted by monocytes and macrophages. *Methods Enzymol* **105**:365, 1984.
376. Markert M, Andrews PC, Babior BM: Measurement of O_2^- production by human neutrophils. The preparation and assay of NADPH oxidase-containing particles from human neutrophils. *Methods Enzymol* **105**:358, 1984.
377. Absolom DR: Basic methods for the study of phagocytosis. *Methods Enzymol* **132**:147, 1987.
378. Baggiolini M, Ruch W, Cooper PH: Measurement of hydrogen peroxide production by phagocytes using homovanillic acid and horseradish peroxidase. *Methods Enzymol* **132**:395, 1987.
379. Huu TP, Dumez Y, Marquetty C, Durandy A, Boue J, Hakim J: Prenatal diagnosis of chronic granulomatous disease (CGD) in four high risk male fetuses. *Prenat Diagn* **7**:253, 1987.
380. Daffos F, Capella-Pavlovsky M, Forestier F: Fetal blood sampling during pregnancy with use of a needle guided by ultrasound: A study of 606 consecutive cases. *Am J Obstet Gynecol* **153**:655, 1985.
381. Golbus MS, McGonigle KF, Goldberg JD, Filly RA, Callen PW, Anderson RL: Fetal tissue sampling. The San Francisco experience with 190 pregnancies. *West J Med* **150**:423, 1989.
382. Pelham A, O'Reilly M-AJ, Malcolm S, Levinsky RJ, Kinnon C: RFLP and deletion analysis for X-linked chronic granulomatous disease using the cDNA probe: Potential for improved prenatal diagnosis and carrier determination. *Blood* **76**:820, 1990.
383. D'Alton ME, Decharney AH: Prenatal diagnosis. *N Engl J Med* **328**:114, 1993.
384. Margolis DM, Melnick DA, Alling DW, Gallin JI: Trimethoprim-sulfamethoxazole prophylaxis in the management of chronic granulomatous disease. *J Infect Dis* **162**:723, 1990.
385. Mouy R, Fischer A, Vilmer E, Seger R, Griscelli C: Incidence, severity, and prevention of infections in chronic granulomatous disease. *J Pediatr* **114**:555, 1989.
386. Johnston RB Jr, Wilfert CM, Buckley RH, Webb LS, Dechatelet LR, McCall CE: Enhanced bactericidal activity of phagocytes from patients with chronic granulomatous disease in the presence of sulfisoxazole. *Lancet* **1**:824, 1975.
387. Gmünder FJ, Segar RA: Chronic granulomatous disease: Mode of action of sulfamethoxazole/trimethoprim. *Pediatr Res* **15**:1533, 1981.
388. Ezer G, Soothill JF: Intracellular bactericidal effects of refampicin in both normal and chronic granulomatous disease polymorphs. *Arch Dis Child* **49**:463, 1974.
389. Philippart AI, Colodny AH, Baehner RL: Continuous antibiotic therapy in chronic granulomatous disease: Preliminary communication. *Pediatrics* **50**:923, 1972.
390. Steinbeck MJ, Roth JA: Neutrophil activation by recombinant cytokines. *Rev Infect Dis* **11**:549, 1989.
391. Gallin JI, Malech HL: Update on chronic granulomatous diseases of childhood: Immunotherapy and potential for gene therapy. *JAMA* **263**:1533, 1990.
392. Ezekowitz AF, Orkin SH, Newburger PE: Recombinant interferon gamma augments phagocyte superoxide production and X-linked chronic granulomatous disease gene expression in X-linked variant chronic granulomatous disease. *J Clin Invest* **80**:1009, 1987.
393. Ezekowitz RA, Dinauer MC, Jaffe HS, Orkin SH, Newberger PG: Partial correction of the phagocyte defect in patients with X-linked chronic granulomatous disease by subcutaneous interferon gamma. *N Engl J Med* **319**:146, 1988.
394. Sechler JMG, Malech HL, White CJ, Gallin JI: Recombinant human interferon-γ reconstitutes defective phagocyte function in patients with chronic granulomatous disease of childhood. *Proc Natl Acad Sci USA* **85**:4874, 1988.
395. Mühlebach TJ, Gabay J, Nathan CF, Erny C, Dopfer G, Schroten H, Wahn V, Seger RA: Treatment of patients with chronic granulomatous disease with recombinant human interferon-gamma does not improve neutrophil oxidative metabolism, cytochrome b_{558} content or levels of four antimicrobial proteins. *Clin Exp Immunol* **88**:203, 1992.
396. Rex JH, Bennett JE, Gallin JI, Malech HL, Melnick DA: Normal and deficient neutrophils can cooperate to damage *Aspergillus fumigatus* hyphae. *J Infect Dis* **162**:523, 1990.
397. Bernhisel-Broadbent J, Camargo EE, Jaffe HS, Lederman HM: Recombinant human interferon-gamma as adjunct therapy for Aspergillus infection in a patient with chronic granulomatous disease. *J Infect Dis* **163**:908, 1991.
398. Chusid MJ, Tomasulo PA: Survival of transfused normal granulocytes in a patient with chronic granulomatous disease. *Pediatrics* **61**:556, 1978.
399. Pedersen FK, Johansen KS, Rosenkvist J, Tygstrup I, Valerius NH: Refractory *Pneumocystis carinii* infection in chronic granulomatous disease: successful treatment with granulocytes. *Pediatrics* **64**:935, 1979.
400. Chusid MJ, Shea ML, Sarff LD: Determination of post-transfusion granulocyte kinetics by chemiluminescence in chronic granulomatous disease. *J Lab Clin Med* **95**:168, 1980.

401. Tomtovian R, Abramson J, Quie P, McCullough J: Granulocyte transfusion therapy in chronic granulomatous disease: Report of 2 patients and review of the literature. *Transfusion* **21**:739, 1981.
402. Buescher ES, Gallin JI: Leukocyte transfusions in chronic granulomatous disease. Persistence of transfused leukocytes in sputum. *N Engl J Med* **307**:800, 1982.
403. Elliot GR, Clay ME, Mills EL, Abramson JS, McCullough J, Quie PG: Granulocyte transfusion kinetics measured by chemiluminescence, nitroblue tetrazolium reduction, and recovery of Indium-111-labeled granulocytes. *Transfusion* **27**:23, 1987.
404. Quie PG: The white cells: Use of granulocyte transfusions. *Rev Infect Dis* **9**:189, 1987.
405. Depalma L, Leitman SF, Carter CS, Gallin JI: Granulocyte transfusion therapy in a child with chronic granulomatous disease and multiple red cell alloantibodies. *Transfusion* **29**:421, 1989.
406. Brzica SM, Rhodes KH, Pineda AA, Taswell HF: Chronic granulomatous disease and the McLeod phenotype: Successful treatment of infection with granulocyte transfusions resulting in subsequent hemolytic transfusion reaction. *Mayo Clin Proc* **52**:153, 1977.
407. Chin TW, Steim ER, Falloon J, Gallin JI: Corticosteroid in treatment of obstructive lesions of chronic granulomatous disease. *J Pediatr* **111**:349, 1987.
408. Collman RJ, Dickerman JD: Corticosteroids in the management of cystitis secondary to chronic granulomatous disease. *Pediatrics* **85**:219, 1990.
409. Danziger RN, Goren AT, Becker J, Greene JM, Douglas SD: Outpatient management with oral corticosteroid therapy for obstructive conditions in chronic granulomatous disease. *J Pediatr* **122**:303, 1993.
410. Quie PG, Belani KK: Corticosteroids for chronic granulomatous disease. *J Pediatr* **111**:393, 1987.
411. Goudemand J, Aussens R, Delams-Marsalet Y, Farriaux JP, Fontaine D: Attempt to treat a case of chronic familial granulomatous disease by allogeneic bone marrow transplantation. *Arch Fr Pediatr* **33**:121, 1976.
412. Westminster Hospital Bone-Marrow Transplant Team: Bone-marrow transplant from an unrelated donor for chronic granulomatous disease. *Lancet* **1**:210, 1977.
413. Anderson JM, Barrett AJ, Byrom N, Foroozanfar N, Gabriel C, Henry K, Hobbs JR, High-Jones K, Humble JG, James DCO, Mawle A, Selwyn S, Watson G, Yamamura M: Clinical results of bone marrow transplantation in SCID and other immunodeficiency states. *Pathol Biol (Paris)* **26**:23, 1978.
414. Rappeport JM, Newburger PE, Goldblum PM, Goldman AS, Nathan DG, Parkman R: Allogeneic bone marrow transplantation for chronic granulomatous disease. *J Pediatr* **101**:952, 1982.
415. Kamani N, August CS, Douglas SD, Burkry E, Etzioni A, Lischner HW: Bone marrow transplantation in chronic granulomatous disease. *J Pediatr* **105**:42, 1984.
416. Kamani N, August CS, Rausen AR, D'Angio G, Douglas SD: Marrow transplantation (BMT) form a heterozygous carrier donor in chronic granulomatous disease (CGD). *Pediatr Res* **19**:276A, 1985.
417. Di Bartolomeo P, Di Girolamo G, Angrilli F, Schettini F, De Mattia D, Manzionna MM, Dragani A, Iacone A, Torlontano G: Reconstitution of normal neutrophil function in chronic granulomatous disease by bone marrow transplantation. *Bone Marrow Transplant* **4**:695, 1989.
418. Hobbs JR, Monteil M, McCluskey DR, Jurges E, El Tumi M: Chronic granulomatous disease: 100% corrected by displacement bone marrow transplantation from a volunteer unrelated donor. *Eur J Pediatr* **151**:806, 1992.
419. Kamani N, August CS, Campbell DE, Hassan NF, Douglas SD: Marrow transplantation in chronic granulomatous disease: An update, with 6-year follow-up. *J Pediatr* **113**:697, 1988.
420. Roesler J, Hockertz S, Vogt B, Lohmann-Matthes ML: Staphylococci surviving intracellularly in phagocytes from patients suffering from chronic granulomatous disease are killed in vitro by antibiotics encapsulated in liposomes. *J Clin Invest* **88**:1224, 1991.
421. Cobbs CS, Malech HL, Leto TL, Freeman SM, Blaese RM, Gallin JI, Lomax KJ: Retroviral expression of recombinant p47-phox protein by Epstein-Barr virus-transformed B lymphocytes from a patient with autosomal chronic granulomatous disease. *Blood* **79**:1829, 1992.
422. Thrasher A, Chetty M, Casimir C, Segal AW: Restoration of superoxide generation to a chronic granulomatous disease-derived B-cell line by retrovirus mediated gene transfer. *Blood* **80**:1125, 1992.
423. Casimir C, Chetty M, Bohler M-C, Garcia R, Fischer A, Griscelli C, Johnson B, Segal AW: Identification of the defective NADPH-oxidase component in chronic granulomatous disease: A study of 57 European families. *Eur J Clin Invest* **22**:403, 1992.
424. Roos D, De Boer M, Borregaard N, Bjerrum OW, Valerius NH, Seger RA, Muhlebach T, Belohradsky BH, Weening RS: Chronic granulomatous disease with partial deficiency of cytochrome b_{558} and incomplete respiratory burst: Variants of the X-linked, cytochrome b_{558}-negative form of the disease. *J Leukoc Biol* **51**:164, 1992.
425. Woodman R, Newburger P, Mayo L, Erickson R, Curnutte J: A new X-linked variant of chronic granulomatous disease (CGD) characterized by a normal clone of phagocytic cells and an associated cytosol factor (CF) deficiency. *Blood* **74**:108a, 1989.
426. Hopkins PJ, Skalnik DG, Eklund EA, Newburger PE, Curnutte JT: Mutations in the gp91-*phox* gene promoter region result in clonal expression of cytochrome b_{558} and symptomatic chronic granulomatous disease. *Blood* **80**:251a, 1992.
427. Francke U, Hsieh C-L, Foellmer BE, Lomax KJ, Malech HL, Leto TL: Genes for two autosomal recessive forms of chronic granulomatous disease assigned to 1q25 (NCF2) and 7q11.23 (NCF1). *Am J Hum Genet* **47**:483, 1990.
428. Baehner RL, Kunkel LM, Monaco AP, Haines JL, Conneally PM, Palmer C, Heerema N, Orkin SH: DNA linkage analysis of X chromosome-linked chronic granulomatous disease. *Proc Natl Acad Sci USA* **83**:3398, 1986.
429. Francke U, Ochs HD, De Martinville B, Giacalone J, Lindgren V, Distèche C, Pagon RA, Hofker MH, Van Ommen G-JB, Pearson PL, Wedgweood RJ: Minor Xp21 chromosome deletion in a male associated with expression of Duchenne muscular dystrophy, chronic granulomatous disease, retinitis pigmentosa, and McLeod syndrome. *Am J Hum Genet* **37**:250, 1985.
430. Skalnik DG, Strauss EC, Orkin SH: CCAAT displacement protein as a repressor of the myelomonocytic-specific gp91-*phox* promoter. *J Biol Chem* **266**:16736, 1991.
431. Frey D, Machler M, Seger R, Schmid W, Orkin SH: Gene deletion in a patient with chronic granulomatous disease and McLeod Syndrome: Fine mapping of the Xk gene locus. *Blood* **71**:252, 1988.
432. De Saint-Basile G, Bohler MC, Fischer A, Cartron J, Dufier JL, Griscelli C, Orkin SH: Xp21 DNA microdeletion in a patient with chronic granulomatous disease, retinitis pigmentosa, and McLeod phenotype. *Hum Genet* **80**:85, 1988.
433. De Boer M, Bolscher BGJM, Dinauer MC, Orkin SH, Smith CIE, Ahlin A, Weening RS, Roos D: Splice site mutations are a common cause of X-linked chronic granulomatous disease. *Blood* **80**:1553, 1992.
434. Bolscher BGJM, De Boer M, De Klein A, Weening RS, Roos D: Point mutations in the β-subunit of cytochrome b_{558} leading to X-linked chronic granulomatous disease. *Blood* **77**:2482, 1991.
435. Curnutte JT, Hopkins PJ, Kuhl W, Beutler E: Studying X inactivation. *Lancet* **339**:749, 1992.
436. Dinauer MC, Curnutte JT, Rosen H, Orkin SH: A missense mutation in the neutrophil cytochrome *b* heavy chain in cytochrome-positive X-linked chronic granulomatous disease. *J Clin Invest* **84**:2012, 1989.
437. Orkin SH: Molecular genetics of chronic granulomatous disease. *Annu Rev Immunol* **7**:277, 1989.
438. Hopkins PJ, Kuruto R, Curnutte JT: Molecular genetic analysis of X-linked chronic granulomatous disease. *Am J Hum Genet* **51(4)**:A37, 1992.
439. Kousseff B: Linkage between chronic granulomatous disease

and Duchenne's muscular dystrophy? *Am J Dis Child* **135**:1149, 1981.

440. Bertelson CJ, Pogo AO, Chaudhuri A, Marsh WL, Redman CM, Banerjee D, Symmans WA, Simon T, Frey D, Kunkel LM: Localization of the McLeod Locus (XK) within Xp21 by deletion analysis. *Am J Hum Genet* **42**:703, 1988.
441. Hurst JK, Loehr TM, Curnutte JT, Rosen H: Resonance Raman and electron paramagnetic resonance structural investigations of neutrophil cytochrome b_{558}. *J Biol Chem* **266**:1627, 1991.
442. De Boer M, De Klein A, Hossle J-P, Seger R, Corbeel L, Weening RS, Roos D: Cytochrome b_{558}-negative, autosomal recessive chronic granulomatous disease: Two new mutations in the cytochrome b_{558} light chain of the NADPH oxidase (p22-*phox*). *Am J Hum Genet* **51**:1127, 1992.
443. Dinauer MC, Pierce EA, Erickson RW, Muhlebach TJ, Messner H, Orkin SH, Seger RA, Curnutte JT: Point mutation in the cytoplasmic domain of the neutrophil p22-*phox* cytochrome *b* subunit is associated with a nonfunctional NADPH oxidase and chronic granulomatous disease. *Proc Natl Acad Sci USA* **88**:11231, 1991.
444. Chanock SJ, Barrett DM, Curnutte JT, Orkin SH: Gene structure of the cytosolic component, *phox*-47 and mutations in autosomal recessive chronic granulomatous disease. *Blood* **78**:165a, 1991.
444a. Kenney RT, Malech HL, Epstein ND, Roberts RL, Leto TL: Characterization of the p67-*phox* gene: Genomic organization and restriction fragment length polymorphism analysis for prenatal diagnosis in chronic granulomatous disease. *Blood* **82**:3739, 1993.
445. Casimir CM, Bu-Ghanim HN, Rodaway ARF, Bentley DL, Rowe P, Segal AW: Autosomal recessive chronic granulomatous disease caused by deletion at a dinucleotide repeat. *Proc Natl Acad Sci USA* **88**:2753, 1991.
445a. de Boer M, Hilarius-Stokman P, Hossle J-P, Verhoeven AJ, Graf N, Kenney RT, Seger R, Roos D: Autosomal recessive chronic granulomatous disease with absence of the 67-kD cytosolic NADPH oxidase component: Identification of mutation and detection of carriers. *Blood* **83**:531, 1994.
446. Baehner RL, Johnston RB Jr, Nathan DG: Comparative study of the metabolic and bactericidal characteristics of severely glucose-6-phosphate dehydrogenase deficient polymorphonuclear leukocytes from children with chronic granulomatous disease. *J Reticuloendothel Soc* **12**:150, 1972.
447. Cooper MR, Dechatelet LR, McCall CE, Lavia MF, Spurr CL, Baehner RL: Complete deficiency of leukocyte glucose-6-phosphate dehydrogenase with defective bactericidal activity. *J Clin Invest* **51**:769, 1972.
448. Gray GR, Klebanoff SJ, Stamatayannopoulos G, Austin T, Naiman SC, Yoshida A, Kliman MR, Robinson GC: Neutrophil dysfunction, chronic granulomatous disease and non-spherocytic haemolytic anaemia caused by complete deficiency of glucose-6-phosphate dehydrogenase. *Lancet* **2**:530, 1973.
449. Mamlok RJ, Mamlok V, Mills GC, Daeschner CW, Schmalstieg FC, Anderson DC: Glucose-6-phosphate dehydrogenase deficiency, neutrophil dysfunction and *Chromobacterium violaceum* sepsis. *J Pediatr* **111**:852, 1987.
450. Jandl RC, Andre-Schwartz J, Borges-DuBois L, Kipnes RS, McMurrich BJ, Babior BM: Termination of the respiratory burst in human neutrophils. *J Clin Invest* **61**:1176, 1978.
451. Cech P, Stalder IT, Widmann, Rohner A, Meischer PA: Leukocyte myeloperoxidase deficiency and diabetes mellitus associated with *Candida albicans* liver abscess. *Am J Med* **66**:149, 1979.
452. Grignaschi VJ, Sperperato AM, Etcheverry MI, Macario AJ: An nuevo cuadio cito guimico: Negativad espontanea de las reacciones de peroxidas, oxidas y lipido en la progenia neutrophilia y en los monocitos de dos hermanos. *Rev Assoc Med Argent* **77**:218, 1963.
453. Huhn D, Belohradsky BH, Haas R: Familiärer myeloperoxidascdefekt und akute myeloische leukämie. *Acta Haematol (Basel)* **59**:129, 1978.
454. Kitahara M, Stimonian Y, Eyre HJ: Neutrophil myeloperoxidase: A simple reproducible technique to determine activity. *J Lab Clin Med* **93**:232, 1979.
455. Lehrer RI, Cline MJ: Leukocyte myeloperoxidase deficiency and disseminated candidiasis: The role of myeloperoxidase in resistance to Candida infection. *J Clin Invest* **48**:14788, 1969.
456. Moosmann K, Bojanowsky A: Rezidivierende Candidiosis bei myeloperoxidase-mangel. *Monatsschr Kinderheilkd* **123**:408, 1975.
457. Undritz E: Die Alius-Grignaschi-anomalie: der erblich konstitutionelle peroxydasedefekt der neutrophilen und monocyten. *Blut* **14**:129, 1966.
458. Parry MF, Root RK, Metcalf JA, Delaney KK, Kaplow LS, Richar WJ: Myeloperoxidase deficiency: Prevalence and clinical significance. *Ann Intern Med* **95**:293, 1981.
459. Robertson CF, Thong YH, Hodge GL, Cheney K: Primary myeloperoxidase deficiency associated with impaired neutrophil margination and chemotaxis. *Acta Paediatr Scand* **68**:915, 1979.
460. Kussenbach G, Rister M: Der Myeloperoxidase-Mangel als Ursache rezidivierende Infektionen. *Klin Padiatr* **197**:443, 1985.
461. Stendahl O, Lindgren S: Function of granulocytes with deficiency of myeloperoxidase-mediated iodination in a patient with generalized pustular psoriasis. *Scand J Haematol* **16**:144, 1976.
462. El-Maallem H, Fletcher J: Impaired neutrophil function and myeloperoxidase deficiency in pregnancy. *Br J Haematol* **44**:375, 1980.
463. Caldwell KC, Taddeini L, Woodburn RL, Anderson GL, Lobell M: Induction of myeloperoxidase deficiency in granulocytes in lead-intoxicated dogs. *Blood* **53**:588, 1979.
464. Lehrer RI, Cline MJ: Leukocyte candidacidal activity and resistance to system candidiasis in patients with cancer. *Cancer* **27**:1211, 1971.
465. Graham GS: The neutrophilic granules of the circulating blood in health and in disease: A preliminary report. *NY State J Med* **20**:46, 1920.
466. Arakawa T, Wada Y, Hayashi T, Kakizaki R, Chiba N, Chida R, Konno T: Uracil-uric refractory anemia with peroxidase negative neutrophils. *Tohoku J Exp Med* **87**:52, 1965.
467. Higashi O, Katsuyama N, Satodate R: A case with hematological abnormalities characterized by the absence of peroxidase activity in blood polymorphonuclear leukocytes. *Tohoku S Exp Med* **87**:77, 1965.
468. Lehrer RI, Goldberg LS, Apple MA, Rosenthal NP: Refractory megaloblastic anemia with myeloperoxidase-deficient neutrophils. *Ann Intern Med* **76**:447, 1972.
469. Armstrong D, Dimmit S, van Wormer DE: Studies in Batten disease I: Peroxidase deficiency in granulocytes. *Arch Neurol* **30**:144, 1974.
470. Bozdech MJ, Bainton DF, Mustacchi P: Partial peroxidase deficiency in neutrophils and eosinophils associated with neurological disease. *Am J Clin Pathol* **73**:409, 1980.
471. Bendix-Hansen K: Myeloperoxidase-deficient polymorphonuclear leukocytes (VII): Incidence in untreated myeloproliferative disorders. *Scand J Haematol* **36**:8, 1986.
472. Bendix-Hansen K: Myeloperoxidase-deficient polymorphonuclear leukocytes. Longitudinal study during preremission–and the remission phase in acute myeloid leukemia. *Blut* **52**:237, 1986.
473. Bendix-Hansen K, Kerndrup G, Pedersen B: Myeloperoxidase-deficient polymorphonuclear leukocytes (VI): Relation to cytogenetic abnormalities in primary myelodysplastic syndromes. *Scand J Haematol* **36**:3, 1986.
474. Bendix-Hansen K, Kerndrup G: Myeloperoxidase-deficient polymorphonuclear leukocytes (V): Relation to FAB classification and neutrophil alkaline phosphatase activity in primary myelodysplastic syndromes. *Scand J Haematol* **35**:197, 1985.
475. Bendix-Hansen K, Nielsen HK: Myeloperoxidase-deficient polymorphonuclear leukocytes I: Incidence in untreated myeloid leukemia, lymphoid leukemia, and normal humans. *Scand J Haematol* **30**:415, 1983.
476. Bendix-Hansen K, Nielsen HK: Myeloperoxidase-deficient polymorphonuclear leukocytes II: Longitudinal study in acute myeloid leukemia, untreated, in remission, and in relapse. *Scand J Haematol* **31**:5, 1983.
477. Bendix-Hansen K, Nielsen HK: Myeloperoxidase-defi-

cient polymorphonuclear leukocytes IV: Relation to FAB classification in acute myeloid leukemia. *Scand J Haematol* **35**:174, 1985.

478. Cech P, Schneider P, Bachmann F: Partial myeloperoxidase deficiency. *Acta Haematol (Basel)* **67**:180, 1982.
479. Cech P, Markert M, Perrin LH: Partial myeloperoxidase deficiency in preleukemia. *Blut* **47**:21, 1983.
480. Baggiolini M, Hirsch JG, Deduve C: Resolution of granules from rabbit heterophil leukocytes into distinct populations by zonal sedimentation. *J Cell Biol* **40**:529, 1969.
481. Chance B, Mahely AC: Assay of catalases and peroxidases, **2**:764, 1955.
482. *Worthington Enzyme Manual*. Freehold, NJ, Worthington Biochemical Corporation, 1972, p 43.
483. Dri P, Cramer R, Soranzo MR, Comin A, Miotti V, Patriarca P: New approaches to the detection of myeloperoxidase deficiency. *Blood* **60**:323, 1982.
484. Wever R, Hamers MN, Weening RS, Roos D: Characterization of the peroxidase in human eosinophils. *Eur J Biochem* **108**:491, 1980.
485. Bos AJ, Wever R, Hamers MN, Roos D: Some enzymatic characteristics of eosinophil peroxidase from patients with eosinophilia and from healthy donors. *Infect Immun* **32**:427, 1981.
486. Kaplow LS: Substitute for benzidine in myeloperoxidase staining. *Am J Clin Pathol* **63**:451, 1975.
487. Elias JM: A rapid, sensitive myeloperoxidase stain using 4-chloro-1-naphthol. *Am J Clin Pathol* **73**:797, 1980.
488. Kaplow LS: Simplified myeloperoxidase stain using benzidine dihydrochloride. *Blood* **26**:215, 1965.
489. Larrocha C, Fernandez de Castro M, Fontan G, Viloria A, Fernandez-Chacon JL, Jimenez C: Hereditary myeloperoxidase deficiency: Study of 12 cases. *Scand J Haematol* **29**:389, 1982.
490. Dri P, Cramer R, Menagazzi R, Patriarca P: Increased degranulation of human myeloperoxidase-deficient polymorphonuclear leukocytes. *Br J Haematol* **59**:115, 1985.
491. Klebanoff SJ: Myeloperoxidase: Contribution to the microbicidal activity of intact leukocytes. *Science* **169**:1095, 1970.
492. Lehrer RI, Hanifin J, Cline MJ: Defective bactericidal activity in myeloperoxidase-deficient human neutrophils. *Nature* **223**:78, 1969.
493. Bos AJ, Weening, Hamers MN, Wever R, Behrendt H, Roos D: Characterization of hereditary partial myeloperoxidase deficiency. *J Lab Clin Med* **99**:589, 198.
494. Root RK, Metcalf JA: The role of iodide versus chloride-dependent reactions in myeloperoxidase-mediated microbicidal activity of human neutrophils. *Clin Res* **29**:534A, 1981.
495. Diamond RD, Krzesicki R: Mechanisms of attachment of neutrophils to *Candida albicans* pseudohyphae in the absence of serum, and of subsequent damage to pseudohyphae by microbicidal processes in neutrophils in vitro. *J Clin Invest* **61**:360, 1978.
496. Diamond RD, Clark PA, Haudenschild CC: Damage to albicans hyphae and pseudohyphae by the myeloperoxidase system and oxidative products of neutrophil metabolism in vitro. *J Clin Invest* **66**:908, 1980.
497. Lehrer RI, Ladra KM, Hake RB: Nonoxidative fungicidal mechanisms of mammalian granulocytes: Demonstration of components with candidacidal activity in human, rabbit, and guinea pig leukocytes. *Infect Immun* **11**:1226, 1975.
498. Lehrer RI: Functional aspects of a second mechanism of candidacidal activity by human neutrophils. *J Clin Invest* **51**:2566, 1972.
499. Levitz SM, Diamond RD: Killing of *Aspergillus fumigatus* spores and *Candida albicans* yeast phase by the iron-H_2O_2-I_2 cytotoxic system: Comparison with MPO-H_2O_2-halide system. *Infect Immun* **43**:1100, 1984.
500. Johnson KR, Nauseef WM: Molecular biology of myeloperoxidase, in Everse J, Everse K, Grisham M (eds): *Peroxidases in Chemistry and Biology*. Boca Raton, FL, CRC, 1991, pp 63–82.
501. Hashinaka K, Nishio C, Hur SJ, Sakiyama F, Tsunasawa S, Yamada M: Multiple species of myeloperoxidase messenger RNAs produced by alternative splicing and differential polyadenylation. *Biochemistry* **27**:5906, 1988.
502. Meier RW, Chen T, Friis RR, Tobler A: Myeloperoxidase is a primary response gene in HL60 cells, directly regulated during hematopoietic differentiation. *Biochem Biophys Res Commun* **176**:1345, 1991.
503. Tobler A, Miller CW, Johnson KR, Selsted M, Rovera G, Koeffler HP: Regulation of gene expression of myeloperoxidase during myeloid differentiation. *J Cell Physiol* **136**:215, 1988.
504. Sagoh T, Yamada M: Transcriptional regulation of myeloperoxidase gene expression in myeloid leukemia HL-60 cells during differentiation into granulocytes and macrophages. *Arch Biochem Biophys* **262**:599, 1988.
505. Rosmarin AG, Weil SC, Rosner GI, Griffin JD, Arnaout MA, Tenen DG: Differential expression of CD11b/CD18(Mo1) and myeloperoxidase genes during myeloid differentiation. *Blood* **73**:131, 1989.
506. Lübbert M, Miller CW, Koeffler HP: Changes of DNA methylation and chromatin structure in the human myeloperoxidase gene during myeloid differentiation. *Blood* **78**:345, 1991.
507. Morishita K, Tsuchiya M, Asano S, Kaziro Y, Nagata S: Chromosomal gene structure of human myeloperoxidase and regulation of its expression by granulocyte colony-stimulating factor. *J Biol Chem* **262**:15208, 1987.
508. Shirsat NV, Bittenbender S, Kreider BL, Rovera G: Structure of the murine lactotransferrin gene is similar to the structure of other transferrin-encoding genes and shares a putative regulatory region with the murine myeloperoxidase gene. *Gene* **110**:229, 1992.
509. Hasilik A, Pohlmann R, Olsen RL, Von Figura K: Myeloperoxidase is synthesized as a larger phosphorylated precursor. *EMBO J* **3**:2671, 1984.
510. Koeffler HP, Ranyard J, Pertcheck M: Myeloperoxidase: Its structure and control of its gene expression during myeloid differentiation. *Blood* **65**:484, 1984.
511. Nauserf WM: Myeloperoxidase biosynthesis by a human promyelocytic leukemia cell line: Insight into myeloperoxidase deficiency. *Blood* **67**:865, 1986.
512. Strömberg K, Persson AM, Olsson I: The processing and intracellular transport of myeloperoxidase. *Eur J Cell Biol* **39**:424, 1986.
513. Yamada M: Myeloperoxidase precursors in human myeloid leukemia HL-60 cells. *J Biol Chem* **257**:5980, 1982.
514. Hur SJ, Toda H, Yamada M: Isolation and characterization of an unprocessed extracellular myeloperoxidase in HL-60 cell cultures. *J Biol Chem* **264**:8542, 1989.
515. Taylor KL, Guzman GS, Burgess CA, Kinkade JM Jr: Assembly of dimeric myeloperoxidase during posttranslational maturation in human leukemic HL-60 cells. *Biochemistry* **29**:1533, 1990.
516. Nauseef WM, McCormick S, Yi H: Roles of heme insertion and the mannose-6-phosphate receptor in processing of the human myeloid lysosomal enzyme, myeloperoxidase. *Blood* **80**:2622, 1992.
517. Strömberg K, Olsson I: Myeloperoxidase precursors incorporate heme. *J Biol Chem* **262**:10430, 1987.
518. Castañeda VL, Parmley RT, Pinnix IB, Raju SG, Guzman GS, Kinkade JM Jr: Ultrastructural, immunochemical, and cytochemical study of myeloperoxidase i . myeloid leukemia HL-60 cells following treatment with succinylacetone, an inhibitor of heme biosynthesis. *Exp Hematol* **20**:916, 1992.
519. Kimura S, Ikeda-Saito M: Human myeloperoxidase and thyroid peroxidase, two enzymes with separate and distinct physiological functions, are evolutionarily related members of the same gene family. *Proteins* **3**:113, 1988.
520. Kimura S, Kotani T, McBride OW, Umeki K, Hirai K, Nakayama T, Ohtaki S: Human thyroid peroxidase: Complete cDNA and protein sequence, chromosome mapping, and identification of two alternatively spliced mRNAs. *Proc Natl Acad Sci USA* **84**:5555, 1987.
521. Nauseef WM: Myeloperoxidase deficiency. *Hematol Pathol* **4**:165, 1990.
522. Nauseef WM: Aberrant restriction endonuclease digests of DNA from subjects with hereditary myeloperoxidase deficiency. *Blood* **73**:290, 1989.
523. Verbanec KM, Health EC: Biosynthesis, processing, and secretion of M and Z variant human α-1-antitrypsin. *J Biol Chem* **261**:9979, 1986.
524. Tobler A, Selsted ME, Miller CW, Johnson KR, No-

votny MJ, Rovera G, Koeffler HP: Evidence for a pretranslational defect in hereditary and acquired myeloperoxidase deficiency. *Blood* **73**:1980, 1989.

525. van Tuinen P, Johnson KR, Ledbetter SA, Nussbaum RL, Merry DE, Rovera G, Ledbetter DH: Localization of myeloperoxidase to the long arm of human chromosome 17: Relationship to the 15, 17 translocation of acute promyelocytic leukemia. *Oncogene* **1**:319, 1987.
526. Inazawa J, Inoue K, Nishigaki H, Tsuda S, Taniwaki M, Misawa S, Abe T: Assignment of the human myeloperoxidase gene (MPO) to bands q21.3→q23 of chromosome 17. *Cytogenet Cell Genet* **50**:135, 1989.
527. Chang KS, Schroeder W, Siciliano MJ, Thompson LH, McCredie K, Beran M, Freireich EJ, Liang JC, Trujillo JM, Stass SA: The localization of the human myeloperoxidase gene is in close proximity to the translocation breakpoint in acute promyelocytic leukemia. *Leukemia* **1**:458, 1987.
528. Liang JC, Chang KS, Schroeder WT, Freireich EJ, Stass SA, Trujillo JM: The myeloperoxidase gene is translocated from chromosome 17 to 15 in a patient with acute promyelocytic leukemia. *Cancer Genet Cytogenet* **30**:103, 1988.

528a. Nauseef WM, Brigham S, Cogley M: Hereditary myeloperoxidase deficiency due to a missense mutation of arginine 569 to tryptophan. *J Biol Chem* **269**:1212, 1994.

529. Meister A: Biochemistry of glutathione, in Greenberg DM (ed): *Metabolism of Sulfur Compounds*. New York, Academic, 1975, pp 101–288.
530. Meister A, Tate SS: Glutathione and related gamma-glutamyl compounds: Biosynthesis and utilization. *Annu Rev Biochem* **45**:559, 1976.
531. Spielberg SP, Boxer LA, Oliver JM, Allen JM, Schulman JD: Oxidative damage to neutrophils in glutathione synthetase deficiency. *Br J Haematol* **42**:215, 1979.
532. Boxer LA, Oliver JM, Spielberg SP, Allen JM, Schulman JD: Protection of granulocytes by vitamin E in glutathione synthetase deficiency. *N Engl J Med* **301**:901, 1979.
533. Loos JA, Roos D, Weening RS, Houwerzijl J: Familial deficiency of glutathione reductase in human blood cells. *Blood* **48**:53, 1976.
534. Johnston RB Jr: Biochemical defects of polymorphonuclear and mononuclear phagocytes associated with disease, in Sbarra AJ, Strauss R (eds): *The Reticuloendothelial System*. New York, Plenum, 1980, vol 2, p 397.

Part 18

CONNECTIVE TISSUES

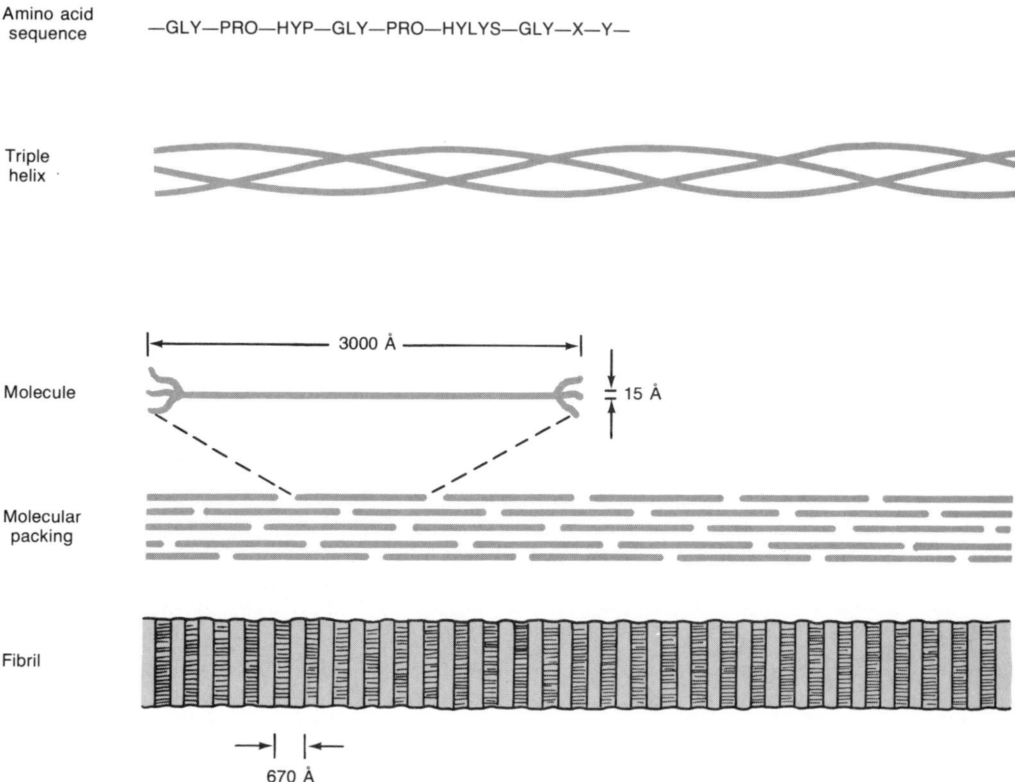

Fibrillar collagen

CHAPTER 134

Disorders of Collagen Biosynthesis and Structure

Peter H. Byers

1. **Collagen is the most abundant protein family in the mammalian body. More than 28 dispersed genes encode the protein products that form more than 16 different types of collagens, which are distributed in a characteristic fashion among tissues.**
2. **Collagens are proteins that contain three chains wound in a triple helix. The biosynthesis is complex. Individual precursor chains are synthesized on membrane-bound polyribosomes. During transfer of the growing chain into the lumen of the rough endoplasmic reticulum (RER), certain prolyl and lysyl residues in the triple-helical domain are hydroxylated and some hydroxylysyl residues are glycosylated. Assembly of the three chains in the RER is mediated by structures in the C-terminal propeptide domains of each chain, and folding of the triple-helix occurs from the C-terminal end of the molecule. Transport through the Golgi apparatus is accompanied by modification of oligosaccharide groups. After secretion, limited proteolysis leads to removal of the N- and C-terminal propeptide extensions. Collagen molecules are stabilized in fibrillar structures or other meshworks through lysine-derived covalent intermolecular crosslinks.**
3. **Disorders currently known to result from alterations in the structure and function of collagens affect the genes of collagens type I, II, III, IV, and VII, and the enzymes lysyl hydroxylase and type I procollagen *N*-proteinase involved in the posttranslational modification of collagens.**
4. **The clinical heterogeneity apparent in the osteogenesis imperfecta (OI) phenotypes is a reflection of the underlying molecular heterogeneity. Mutations that affect the synthesis of the proα1(I) chains of type I collagen generally result in the relatively mild OI type I phenotype. Multiple-exon deletions or insertions in the COL1A1 and COL1A2 genes that encode the chains of type I collagen generally result in the lethal OI type II phenotype. The phenotypic effects of point mutations that result in substitutions for glycine residues in the triple-helical domains of proα1(I) of proα2(I) chains depend on the chain in which the mutation occurs, the location of the substitution within the chain, and the nature of the substituting amino acid.**
5. **The molecular basis of the Ehlers-Danlos syndrome (EDS) is heterogeneous. EDS type IV results from mutations that affect the synthesis, structure, or secretion of type III collagen. EDS type VI is a recessively inherited disorder that results from lack of lysyl hydroxylation. EDS type VII usually results from loss of the substrate sequence for the N-terminal procollagen protease in one of the chains of type I procollagen. Although ultrastructural studies suggest that many of the other forms of EDS result from mutations that affect collagen aggregation in tissue, the molecular basis of most forms is not known.**
6. **Mutations that affect type II collagens give rise to chondrodysplasia, including spondyloepiphyseal dysplasia, achondrogenesis, and Stickler syndrome. The nature of the phenotypic effect of these mutations depends on the character and location of the mutation, in a manner similar to that seen in OI, but the array of mutations available for analysis is smaller.**
7. **Alport syndrome arises from mutations in the COL4A5 gene.**
8. **Mutations in type VII collagen result in the dystrophic forms of epidermolysis bullosa.**
9. **The clinical consequences of mutations in collagen genes reflect the effects of the mutations on biosynthesis, assembly, posttranslational modification, secretion, fibrillogenesis, and interaction with other components of a complex extracellular matrix in which there is considerable molecular interaction.**

The collagens form a multigene family with more than 28 members, the genes for which are known to be dispersed to at least 12 chromosomes (Table 134-1). The products of these genes share important structural properties: they all form molecules that contain three chains (either heterotrimers or homotrimers, depending on collagen type) that have a triple-helical domain characterized by the repeating amino acid sequence (Gly-X-Y)$_n$; they have an abundance of the special amino acids hydroxyproline and hydroxylysine, and they play a structural role in tissues.[1–4] Some other proteins—including acetylcholinesterase,[5] the C1q component of the complement cascade,[6] a pulmonary surfactant protein,[7] bullous pemphigoid antigen-2,[8] and a mannose-binding protein in serum[9,10]—have appropriated stretches of the triple-helical

A list of standard abbreviations is located immediately preceding the index in each volume. Additional abbreviations used in this chapter include: DI = dentinogenesis imperfecta; EB = epidermolysis bullosa; EDS = Ehlers-Danlos syndrome; OI = osteogenesis imperfecta; SED = spondyloepiphyseal dysplasia. See legend to Table 134-1 for collagen nomenclature. Missense mutations are designated by the single letter codes (e.g., glycine to cysteine at codon 244 is indicated as G244C).

By convention, missense mutations within the triple-helical domain of collagen chains are referred to with the reference point being the first glycine of the triple helix. Thus, in the above example, G244C refers to the glycine at position 244 of the triple helix.

Table 134-1 Collagen Types, Tissue Distribution, Molecular Structure, and Gene Location*

Collagen Type	Chain	Gene	Chromosomal Location	Molecules	Tissue Distribution
Fibrillar collagens					
I	α1(I)	COL1A1	17q21–q22	$[\alpha 1(I)]_2\alpha 2(I)$	Skin, bone, tendon, arteries
	α2(I)	COL1A2	7q21–q22	$[\alpha 1(I)]_3$	Skin, bone, tendon, arteries, tumors, amniotic fluid cells
II	α1(II)	COL2A1	12q13–q14	$[\alpha 1(II)]_3$	Cartilage, vitreous humor
III	α1(III)	COL3A1	2q31–q32	$[\alpha 1(III)]_3$	Skin, vessels, uterus
V	α1(V)	COL5A1	9p	$[\alpha 1(V)]_3$	Skin, placenta, vessels chorion, uterus
	α2(V)	COL5A2	2q31–q32	$[\alpha 1(V)]_2\alpha 2(V)$	
	α3(V)	COL5A3		α1(V)α2(V)α3(V)	
XI	α1(XI)	COL11A1	1p21	α1(XI)α2(XI)α1(II)	Cartilage
	α2(XI)	COL11A2			
Basement-membrane collagens					
IV	α1(VI)	COL4A1	13q33–q34	$[\alpha 1(VI)]_2\alpha 2(IV)$	Basement membranes
	α2(VI)	COL4A2	13q33–q34		
	α3(VI)	COL4A3	2	Others uncertain	
	α4(VI)	COL4A4	2		
	α5(VI)	COL4A5	X		
Fibril-associated collagens with interrupted triple helixes [FACIT]					
IX	α1(IX)	COL9A1	6q12–q14	α1(IX)α2(IX)α3(IX)	Cartilage
	α2(IX)	COL9A2			
	α3(IX)	COL9A3			
XII	α1(XII)	COL12A1	6q12–q14	$[\alpha 1(XII)]_3$	Soft tissues
XIV	α1(XIV)	COL14A1			Ubiquitous
Network-forming collagens					
VIII	α1(VIII)	COL8A1	3		Cornea, vessels
	α2(VIII)	COL8A2	1		
X	α1(X)	COL10A1	6q21–q22	$[\alpha 1(X)]_3$	Cartilage
Long-chain, anchoring-fibril collagen with interrupted triple helix					
VII	α(VII)	COL7A1	3q	$[\alpha(VIII)]_3$	Anchoring fibrils

*The nomenclature for collagens is as follows. The individual chain of each molecule is referred to as an α chain. The type of collagen is designated by a Roman numeral in parentheses—for example, (I)—and the chains of a collagen type are numbered in Arabic numerals from 1 upward. The chains of type I collagen were originally numbered by their chromatographic elution during Cm-cellulose column chromatography, α1(I) and α2(I), respectively. This convention no longer applies, and the numbering depends on priority of identification. The precursor chains are designated as preproα chains (with the signal sequence intact) and proα chains once the signal sequence has been removed. Proα chains from which the C-terminal, non-triple-helical precursor-specific domain has been removed are called pNα chains and those from which the N-terminal precursor-specific extension has been removed are called pCα chains. β-Components (sometimes referred to as chains in the older literature) contain two α chains, generally crosslinked by lysine-derived covalent crosslinks; τ-components are three α chains similarly linked. These terms do not refer to individual, genetically distinct chains, as they often do in other protein families. The genes encoding collagen chains are referred to in the following manner: COL1A2 indicates the gene that encodes the α2 (A2) chain of type I collagen (COL1).

structure, perhaps as a structural domain. Since the last edition of this chapter was written, the genes that encode most of the human collagens that had been identified at the protein level have been isolated and partially characterized; a number of collagen genes have been identified by screening of cDNA libraries, necessitating a search for function and distribution of the encoded protein; there has been increasing emphasis on understanding how mutations generate phenotype; and transgenic animals containing altered collagen genes have been used to define the role of those collagens and to identify candidate disorders for those genes. The emphasis on characterization of mutations in the genes that encode the collagen proteins has continued.[11-15] Although mutations in several genes have been identified and shown to result in human genetic disease (osteogenesis imperfecta, forms of Ehlers-Danlos syndrome, several chondrodysplasias, Alport syndrome, and dystrophic forms of epidermolysis bullosa), virtually all our understanding of the effects of these mutations on protein behavior concerns those that affect the genes that encode the proteins of type I collagen. While these studies serve as models for mutations in fibrillar collagen genes,[16,17] they probably fall short in helping to understand how mutations in some of the more complex collagen genes alter molecular behavior and produce disease phenotypes.

As a family of proteins, the collagens are the most abundant in the body. The vast majority of collagen in the body is type I collagen (Fig. 134-1), which is ubiquitously distributed and is the major protein in bone, skin, tendon, ligament, sclera, cornea, blood vessels, and hollow organs. Mutations that affect the structure or processing of the chains of type I collagen are often expressed as generalized connective-tissue disorders, although the specific tissue in which the major effect is seen may vary and determines the clinical phenotype (e.g., osteogenesis imperfecta and forms of the Ehlers-Danlos syndrome all result from mutations in type I collagen genes). With the exception of types III, V, and VI collagen, which are also distributed in virtually all tissues (little type III collagen is found in bone and cartilage), most other collagens have a tissue-specific or structure-

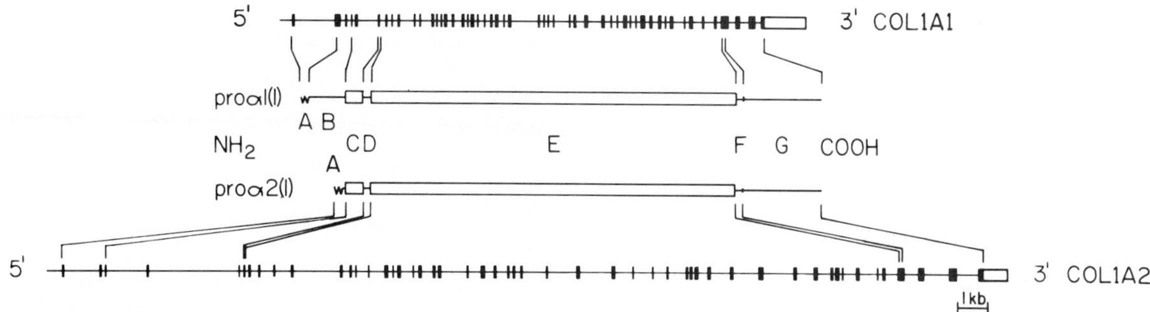

FIG. 134-1 **Fibrillar collagen gene structure. The intron–exon structure of the prototype fibrillar collagen genes [COL1A1 and COL1A2, which encode the proα1(I) and proα2(I) chains of type I procollagen, respectively] are represented. The exons are designated by the solid boxes or vertical lines. All the exons that encode sequences in triple-helical domain (exons 7 to 48) contain 45, 54, 99, 108, or 162 nucleotides; start with a glycine codon; and end with the codon for the Y-position amino acid. The organization of the other fibrillar collagen genes is similar and intron–exon boundaries and exon sizes are maintained throughout. The structure of the genes that encode the nonfibrillar collagens differs considerably. The domains in the polypeptide chains (see also, Fig. 134-2) are: A = signal sequence; B = N-terminal propeptide globular domain; C = N-terminal propeptide triple-helical domain; D = N-terminal telopeptide; E = triple helix; F = C-terminal telopeptide; and G = C-terminal propeptide.** *(Adapted and redrawn from Ramirez et al.,* Ann NY Acad Sci *460:117, 1985. Used by permission.)*

specific distribution. Types II, IX, X, and XI collagens are found in hyaline cartilage and the vitreous of the eye,[18–22] type IV collagens are found in basement membranes,[23,24] and type VII collagen is found at some epithelial–mesenchymal junctions in anchoring fibril structures.[25] With the exception of collagen types I, III, V, and VI, most collagens are expressed by a limited array of fully differentiated cell types, but it is not unusual for one cell to synthesize a group of collagen types. For example, chondrocytes may express types II, IX, X, and XI but not types I and III to any appreciable extent. While the mechanisms of such control are of great interest, there is little understanding of how cell- and tissue-specific control of expression of collagens is achieved.

As a consequence of differences in structure, expression, and tissue distribution, the collagens perform different functions; in different tissues the same collagen may perform different functions. For example, type I collagen provides tensile strength in bone, skin, and tendon but is mineralized only in bone under normal circumstances; it provides or facilitates transparency of the cornea (in part as a consequence of its fibril structure), while the sclera is opaque; and it forms hollow tubes as part of blood vessels but solid structures as part of tendons. Type IV collagen provides the major structural protein of basement membrane, does not form fibril structures, and acts as a filtration barrier in the kidney and at the dermal–epidermal junction. The functions of types II, IX, X, and XI collagens in cartilage are less clear, although in the absence of type II collagen bone does not grow normally. Similarly, the functions of the fibrillar collagens (types III and V) are not clear, although analysis of the phenotypic effects of mutations in type III collagens indicates its essential nature in the formation of intact tissues. Thus, collagens function in a number of ways, to provide tensile strength, to facilitate transparency, to provide form during embryonic and fetal development, to interact with other proteins to build tissues and organs, to separate cell layers during and after development, and to provide filtration barriers between spaces. It is likely that some of the functions are achieved as a direct result of collagen structure, while others depend on interactions with additional matrix macromolecules.

This chapter details the molecular basis of varieties of osteogenesis imperfecta (type I collagen genes); the Ehlers-Danlos syndrome (types I and III collagen genes and post-translational enzymes); several chondrodysplasias including achondrogenesis, hypochondrogenesis, spondyloepiphyseal dysplasia, and Stickler syndrome (type II collagen genes); Alport syndrome (type IV collagen genes); and dystrophic forms of epidermolysis bullosa (type VII collagen genes) (Table 134-2). To put these in perspective, the chapter begins with a review of the nature of the collagen gene family and of the biosynthesis of collagens, using type I collagen as the example. Following that, there is detailed information about each disorder, including clinical presentation, genetics and natural history, and the molecular basis of the clinical phenotype.

Table 134-2 **Collagen Genes and Their Disorders**

Gene	Disorder
COL1A1	Osteogenesis imperfecta
	Type I
	Type II
	Type III
	Type IV
	Ehlers-Danlos syndrome type VIIA
COL1A2	Osteogenesis imperfecta
	Type I
	Type II
	Type III
	Type IV
	Ehlers-Danlos syndrome type II
	Ehlers-Danlos syndrome type VIIB
COL2A1	Stickler syndrome
	Spondyloepiphyseal dysplasia
	Hypochrondrogenesis
	Achondrogenesis
COL3A1	Ehlers-Danlos syndrome type IV
COL4A5	Alport syndrome
COL7A1	Epidermolysis bullosa
	Recessive dystrophic
	Dominant dystrophic

COLLAGEN GENES

Collagen Gene and Protein Structure

On the basis of structure there appear to be several classes of collagen genes[26]:

1. The fibrillar collagens [COL1A1, COL1A2, COL2A1, COL3A1, COL5A1, COL5A2, COL5A3, COL11A1, and COL11A2];
2. The basement-membrane collagens [COL4A1, COL4A2, COL4A3, COL4A4, and COL4A5];
3. The fibril-associated collagens with interrupted triple helixes (FACIT) collagens, [COL9A1, COL9A2, COL9A3, and COL12A1];
4. Network collagens [COL8A1, COL8A2, and COL10A1];
5. Collagens of microfibrils [COL6A1, COL6A2, and COL6A3];
6. The long-chain collagen of anchoring fibrils with an interrupted triple helix [COL7A1].

Genes That Encode the Fibrillar Collagens

The genes that encode the chains of collagen types I, II, III, V, and XI (a total of 10 distinct genes) constitute the family of fibrillar collagen genes[27–33] (see Table 134-1). Each protein is characterized by an unbroken triple-helical domain (Gly-X-Y) containing approximately 1000 amino acids, and the genes encode this structure with a set of 42 exons that contain 45, 54, 99, 108, or 162 base pairs (Fig. 134-2). There are transition exons at both ends of the triple-helical domains that encode the regions that contain the sites of proteolytic cleavage at the N-terminal and C-terminal ends of the triple helix. The triple-helical domain of the N-terminal propeptide extension is contained in a single exon. All the exons in the triple-helical domain begin with a glycine codon and thus end with the codon for the Y-position amino acid; exons in non-triple-helical domains may contain interrupted codons.

The organization of the genes for each of the fibrillar collagens is similar. The intron–exon structure is maintained, and the differences in the sizes of the genes are accounted for by variation in intron size. The gene encoding the proα1(I) chain (COL1A1) is about 18 kb in length, while those encoding the proα2(I) chain (COL1A2), the proα1(II) chains (COL2A1), the proα1(III) chain (COL3A1), and the proα1(V) chain (COL5A1) are each about 40 kb in size. The similar gene structure and homologies in amino acid sequence (see Table 134-1 for a compilation of collagen types, their constituent chains, collagen gene size, and their chromosomal locations) provide strong evidence for the divergence of collagen types following the evolutionary setting of gene structure. The fibrillar collagen gene structure is present in birds and mammals, dating the emergence of the structure of the fibrillar collagen genes prior to the radiation of those two groups, more than 50 million years ago. This concept is supported by analysis of deletion and insertion mutations that affect the genes of type I collagen and demonstrate their lethal nature when only a single allele is involved (see "Osteogenesis Imperfecta" below).

The genes that encode the chains of the fibrillar collagens are widely dispersed among the chromosomes: COL1A1 is on chromosome 17[34,35]; COL1A2 on 7[32,36]; COL2A1 on chromosome 12[37]; COL3A1 on chromosome 2[38,39]; and COL5A2 on chromosome 2 (in the same region as COL3A1).[35,36]

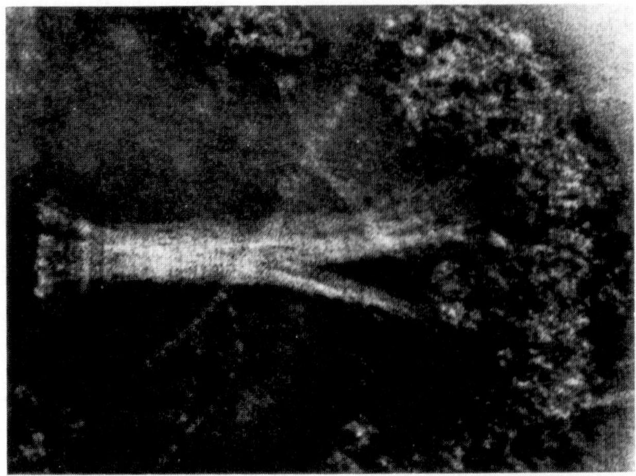

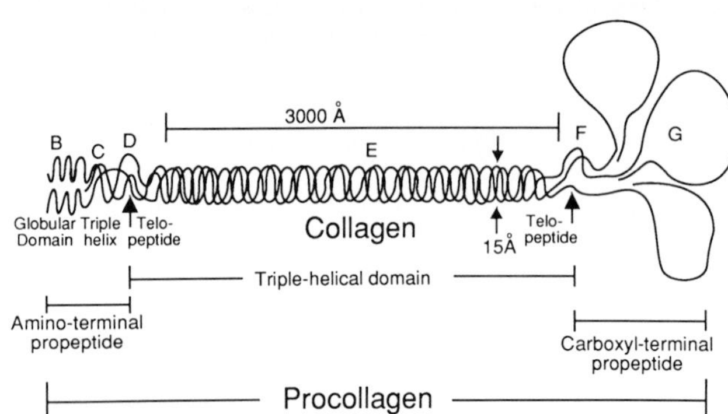

FIG. 134-2 EM of segment-long-spacing (SLS) aggregates of type I procollagen (*top*) and a model of a type I procollagen molecule (*bottom*). SLS aggregates were made by lateral aggregation of procollagen molecules that had been synthesized and secreted into culture medium by normal fibroblasts. Arrayed in a side-to-side orientation, the molecules are precipitated, stained, and then examined in the EM. The model of type I procollagen represents the major domains of the molecule. Designations for domains B through G are as for Fig. 134-1. The signal sequence is not shown for either chain. *(Micrograph courtesy of Dr. Lynne T. Smith, University of Washington.)*

Basement Membrane Collagen Genes—Type IV

The genes that encode the basement membrane nonfibrillar collagens are similar in size to those that encode fibrillar collagens but differ somewhat in organization.[40,41] The exons that encode the largely triple-helical domains vary more widely in size, do not always begin with a glycine codon or end with a codon for a Y-position amino acid, frequently split codons, and encode interruptions of the triple-helix. The interruptions of triple-helical sequence when compared to the fibrillar collagen genes could be explained by small deletions, single nucleotide substitutions, and mutations at former splice junctions. Five genes that encode basement membrane collagens have been isolated and appear to encode similar mRNA, to have similar gene structures, and to have a remarkable organization. Two genes, COL4A1 and COL4A2, are located in a head-to-head array on the distal long arm of chromosome 13[42–48] and share promoter sequences while being transcribed from opposite DNA strands. Two other genes, COL4A3 and COL4A4, are closely linked on chromosome 2,[49,50] while the fifth member of the group is located on the X chromosome.[51,52] Given the current structural relationship among basement-membrane collagen genes and the fibrillar collagen genes, it seems likely that there was a single ancestral gene that duplicated and then each of those genes diverged independently to produce the two arms.

Fibril-Associated Collagens with Interrupted Triple Helixes [FACIT]—Types IX, XII, and XIV

Distinct from both the fibrillar and basement membrane genes are those that encode collagenous proteins that appear to become associated with fibrillar collagens. The first of these recognized was type IX collagen, now known to comprise three genes, each of which encodes chains that contain three triple-helical domains with interruptions. The COL9A1 gene is located on chromosome 6,[53] but the COL9A2 and COL9A3 genes have not yet been mapped. Based on models developed in other species, each chain consists of about 900 amino acids divided into seven distinct domains: three domains that contain triple-helical Gly-X-Y repeat motifs (COL1, COL2, and COL3 domains that contain 134, 339, and 137 amino acids, respectively) and four noncollagenous domains (NC1, NC2, NC3, and NC4 that contain about 20, 30, 12, and 243 amino acids, respectively). The NC1 domain is the most C-terminal region of each chain, the NC2 domain separates COL1 and COL2, and the NC3 domain separates COL2 and COL3. The COL3 domain contains one imperfection and the COL1 domain contains two. Type IX collagen genes are expressed in concert with those of type II collagen and the proteins are found together in cartilage and the vitreous humor of the eye. The α2(IX) chain contains an attachment site for a glycosaminoglycan side chain that may facilitate interactions between collagens and proteoglycans in cartilage matrix.[54]

There are at present two additional members of the FACIT gene family, COL12A1 and COL14A1. The gene that encodes the chains of type XII collagen is located on chromosome 6 in the same region as the COL9A1 gene[55,56]; the COL14A1 gene has not been mapped. The type XII collagen gene draws attention to the complexity of some of the collagen-related genes in that the collagenous domains are quite small in relation to the content of other domains shared by matrix proteins; this gene also introduces the complexity of relationships that exist between collagens and other matrix proteins.[57–59] Type XII collagen is a homotrimer of α1(XII) chains and is ubiquitously distributed, paralleling the distribution of the fibrillar collagens, which has suggested that it may act in a manner similar to that of type IX collagens in interacting with type II collagen in cartilage in which covalent crosslinks that contain sequences from both types of collagen confirm their proximity. The difference in the mass of the N-terminal end of type XII collagen compared to type IX must raise some question about the precise correspondence of the two classes of molecules.

Filament-Producing Collagen—Type VI

The genes for human collagens type VI[60] have been isolated and their chromosomal locations determined.[61,62] The COL6A1 and COL6A2 genes reside on the long arm of chromosome 21, while the COL6A3 gene is located on chromosome 6. These genes encode three chains that have a 335 or 336 amino acid triple helix, with two imperfections embedded within noncollagenous sequences. The COL6A1 and COL6A2 proteins encode an NC2 (N-terminal) peptide of about 235 residues and an NC1 (C-terminal) peptide of about 430 residues. The COL3A1 gene encodes a protein with a homologous collagenous domain but a large (1800 amino acids) NC2 (N-terminal) domain and a NC1 domain that is twice the size of the peptides in the other two type VI collagens. The NC1 domain of the α3(VI) chain contains more than six repeats of a von Willebrand factor domain while the C-terminal noncollagenous domain contains repeats of other types. Type VI collagen is assembled as a trimer of all three chains, although there are some suggestions that other forms may exist. The monomers form partially overlapping head-to-tail structures that interact with other similar structures to produce tetramers, the base unit for forming beaded microfilaments in the matrix. These, in turn, form microfibrillar arrays in extracellular matrix of virtually all tissues and in cultured cells in vitro. The microfibrillar network formed by type VI collagen is probably distinct from that which contains fibrillin (see Chap. 135). The function of these microfibrillar structures is unknown.

Network-Forming Collagens—Types VIII and X

Types VIII and X collagens have very similar gene structures and appear to encode proteins that form meshworks, similar, perhaps to the meshwork produced by type IV collagens in basement membranes. The structure of these genes is, however, markedly at variance with those of the type IV collagen family. Type VIII collagen was originally isolated from endothelial cells but has more recently been recognized to be an abundant component of Descemet's membrane, which separates corneal epithelium and corneal stroma. Two genes of type VIII collagen have been partially characterized and localized to chromosome 3 for COL8A1[63] and to chromosome 1 for COL8A2.[64]

Type X collagen is a component of hypertrophic cartilage, and although a role for endochondral bone formation has been postulated, its function remains uncertain.[65] Only a single gene has yet been isolated that encodes type X collagen chains.[66]

These three genes have a remarkably compact structure and encode chains that are very similar. The two COL8 genes encode chains that have a core triple-helical domain of 454 (COL8A1) and 457 residues (COL8A2) bounded by an NC1 domain (C-terminal) of 173 and 167 residues, respectively, and a slightly smaller NC2 domain (N-terminal). The genes contain three exons with the triple helix and NC1 domains encoded by a single exon, and the NC2 domain is divided between the remaining two exons. The structure of the COL10A1 gene is similar, differing only in the size of the respective domains. The type X collagen protein appears to exist as a homotrimer, and it is likely that the type VIII protein is a heterotrimer of the two gene products, with the precise proportions uncertain.

Anchoring-Fibril Collagen—Type VII

Type VII collagen is confined to anchoring fibrils at the dermal–epidermal junction and at some other basement membranes that separate epithelial and mesenchymal structures. The protein has been partially characterized and shown to be large with a single-chain precursor-size collagen-like domain of approximately 170 kDa. Partial gene sequence now indicates that this is a composite protein with both triple-helix and multiple domains similar to those of other matrix proteins. The gene is located on the long arm of chromosome 3.[67]

COLLAGEN PROTEIN STRUCTURE

Domain Structure of Type I Procollagen

Type I procollagen, a heterotrimer that contains two proα1(I) chains encoded by COL1A1 and one proα2(I) chain (encoded by COL1A2), contains seven distinct domains, each of which has one or more functions (Fig. 134-3). Each preproα chain is synthesized with a signal sequence of approximately 20 residues that facilitates passage across the RER membrane and is cleaved during transit.[68] The proα1(I) chain contains a cysteine-rich globular extension of 86 residues, the function of which is not known; a similar sequence is missing from the proα2(I) chain. Both chains contain a 36-residue domain (of repeating Gly-X-Y triplets) that forms a triple helix in the intact procollagen molecule. This short triple helix has a relatively high denaturation temperature and may stabilize the N-terminal end of the molecule. There is a short, non-triple-helical domain that contains the site of proteolytic cleavage of the N-terminal propeptide extension and lysyl residues, which become involved in intermolecular crosslink formation. The major triple-helical domain of both chains is 1014 residues in length and is characterized by glycine in every third position $(Gly\text{-}X\text{-}Y)_{338}$; hydroxyproline occupies the Y position in about a third of the triplets and is often preceded by proline. Some lysyl residues in the Y-position are also hydroxylated but the extent of this modification is highly dependent on the collagen type. Hydroxyproline and hydroxylysine are found only in the Y-position of the triple helix, while all phenylalanine residues and virtually all leucine residues (with one exception) are found in the X position, apparently because of severe steric hindrance to the formation of the triple helix when these residues occur in the Y position.[69] The basic residue, arginine, occurs preferentially in the Y-position, while the acidic residue (glutamic acid) is found usually in the X position, a distribution that may facilitate charge–charge interactions and increase triple-helix thermal stability. A 28-residue telopeptide at the C-terminal end of the triple helix contains a lysyl residue in proα1(I) that is absent from proα2(I) which is involved in interchain crosslink formation; the telopeptide also contains the site at which the C-terminal procollagen peptidase cleaves. The final 220 residues of the proα chains form globular structures that contain intrachain and interchain disulfide bonds. This domain facilitates chain assembly, determines the chain specificity for assembly of the type I procollagen molecule, and provides intracellular solubility.

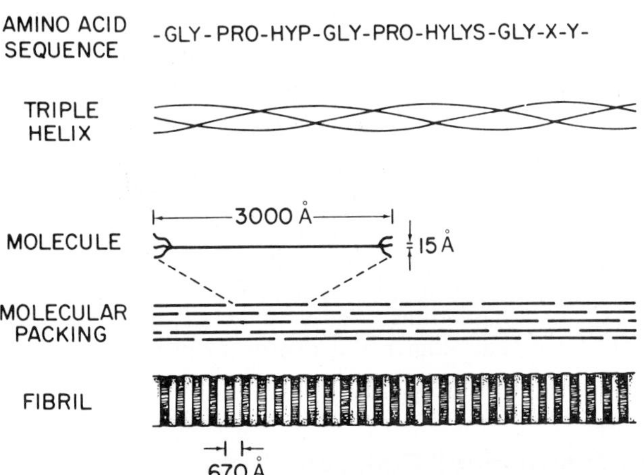

FIG. 134-3 **Hierarchical structure and organization of fibrillar collagens. The α chains of fibrillar collagens contain a core triple-helical domain of slightly more than 1000 residues that is characterized by the repeating triplet, Gly-X-Y (*top*) and in which each chain forms a left-handed helix with a pitch of 3.6 nm. Three chains form a triple-helical molecule in which they are wound in a right-handed spiral. Molecules in the matrix aggregate in an ordered fashion staggered by about a quarter of the length of the triple-helical domain. The staggered order contributes an ordered pattern of electron-dense and electron-lucent regions in fibrils as seen in the EM and reflected in the 670 Å repeating band pattern (*bottom*).**

STRUCTURE OF THE COLLAGEN TRIPLE HELIX

By virtue of the triple-helical structure, collagen has a number of unique features. The primary sequence of the α chains can be written $(Gly\text{-}X\text{-}Y)_{338}$, where X and Y can be most amino acids except for tryptophan and cysteine, which are excluded from the triple helix in both chains of type I collagen; tyrosine is excluded from the triple helix of α1(I) but there is one residue in α2(I). Hydroxyproline and hydroxylysine are found only in the Y-position as a consequence of enzymatic posttranslational modification (see below). The individual α chains assume a left-handed extended polyproline-like helical structure (minor helix) that has a distance of approximately 9.5 Å between residues in equivalent position (pitch). Three chains associate in parallel to form a right-handed triple-helical structure (major helix) that has a pitch of approximately 100 Å (Fig. 134-4). Glycine as the smallest amino acid with no side chains is required in every third position of each chain because space does not exist in the structure for side chains. The side chains on any substituting residue would point toward the center of the helix and disrupt the triple helix (see below in discussion of osteogenesis imperfecta). The side chains of residues in the X and Y positions are arrayed toward the external surface of the molecule. The chains are associated in such a way that the glycine residues are staggered one residue with respect to the next chain. The stability of the triple helix is provided by interchain hydrogen bonds between the amide group of glycine and the oxygen of the carbonyl group of an X-position residue on an adjacent chain.[70] Additional hydrogen bonds that involve the hydroxyl group of hydroxyproline and the carbonyl backbone of the chain further stabilizes the molecule. In the absence of hydroxylation, the triple helix of type I collagen denatures at about 27°C[71,72]; with complete hydroxylation the denaturation temperature is about 42°C (the precise denaturation temperature depends on the manner in which it is measured). Triple-helical structure is one of the requirements for transport of type I collagen beyond the RER[73,74]; thus, in its absence little or no normal collagen is secreted at normal body temperatures. It is likely that other factors, especially charge–charge interactions, contribute to the stability of the triple helix and, although recognized for some time, their importance is often overlooked.

The triple-helical structure of collagen provides resistance to degradation by most proteases, the exceptions being the specific collagenases synthesized by mesenchymal (and some epithelial) cells, and collagenases synthesized by a number of microorganisms.[75,76] The resistance of the triple-helix to proteases allows collagens to provide an extremely stable structure in the extracellular environment. Once denatured, the chains are exquisitely sensitive to most proteases, which ensures normal turnover.

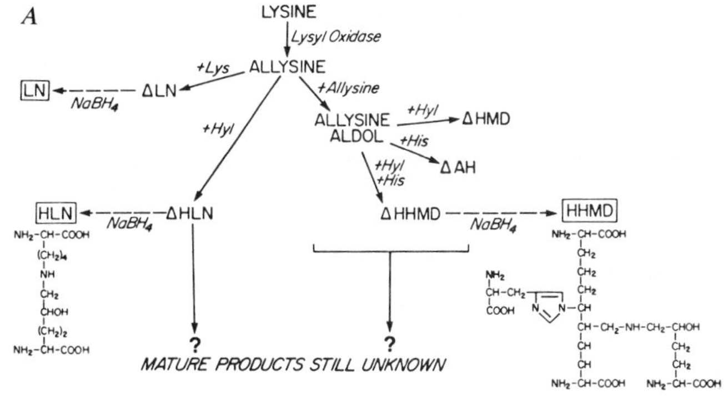

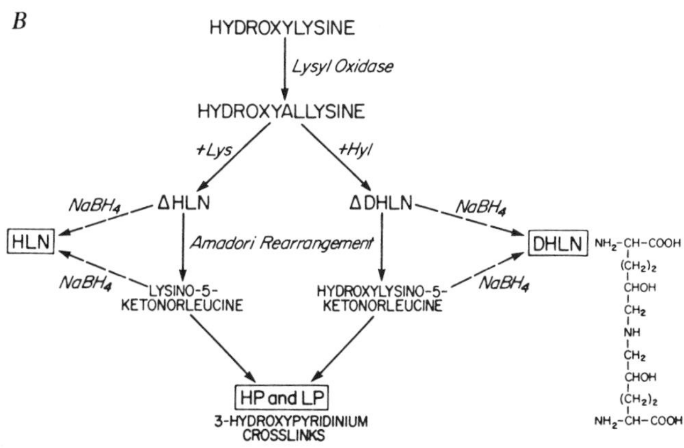

C

HP LP

FIG. 134-4 **Collagen crosslinks. *A*. Crosslinks derived from oxidation of lysyl residues by lysyl oxidase. The oxidation of lysyl residues in collagen peptide linkage begins the minor crosslink pathway. The first product is allysine, which may condense with a lysyl group, an additional allysine, or hydroxylysyl to form bivalent compounds that go on to form other more complex products by the addition of histidine or other residues. The structures of some compounds are known; others have not yet been identified. The intermediates can be trapped by reduction with borohydride to produce the stable products indicated. *B*. The major pathway of crosslink formation begins with the oxidation of hydroxylysyl residues in peptide linkage by lysyl oxidase to form hydroxyallysine, which may condense with lysyl or hydroxylysyl residues on other chains, rearrange, and then as shown in *C*, add a third group to form the fluorescent 3-hydroxypyridinium (HP) and lysyl pyridinium (LP) crosslinks. LN = lysinonorleucine; HLN = hyroxylysinonorleucine; HMD = hydroxymerodesmosine; HHMD = histidinylhydroxymerodesmosine; DHLN = dehydrolysinonorleucine. *(Courtesy of Dr. David Eyre, University of Washington.)***

BIOSYNTHESIS OF COLLAGEN

The biosynthesis, processing, and secretion of collagens is remarkably complex, beginning with coordinated transcription of genes for multiple chains, through posttranslational modifications, to secretion and degradation[77] (Table 134-3).

Control of Collagen Biosynthesis

Collagen biosynthesis is controlled at many levels and the mechanisms by which control is exerted are not completely understood. The genes of type I collagen (COL1A1 and COL1A2) are located on different chromosomes, and their physical relationship during the cell cycle is not known. They are present in equal numbers (one copy per haploid genome) but are transcribed with different efficiencies; COL1A1 produces twice the steady state mRNA levels as COL1A2.[78] The difference results from transcriptional efficiency, not mRNA stability, and is probably not accounted for by the size of the genes. The expression of the genes is almost always coordinated and ultimately results in the synthesis of two proα1(I) chains for each proα2(I) chain. Nucleotide sequences in the first intron of the COL1A1 and COL1A2 genes of type I collagen provide enhancers and direct tissue-specific expression of the genes.[79–82] Upstream regions also provide positive control regions, and there is emerging evidence that those regions, and regions in the first intron, may provide negative control.[83,84] The expression of collagen genes can be altered by a variety of growth factors[85,86] and by the presence or absence of ascorbic acid.[87] Sequences between the transcription start sites and the first translated domain of the mRNA can form stem–loop structures, which appear to influence the efficiency of translation.[88,89] Under some circumstances, for example, in chondrocytes placed in culture, the mRNA for proα2(I) chains is transcribed but inefficiently translated, apparently as a result of translational arrest.[90] There is evidence that control of translation of some collagen mRNA can be influenced by peptides derived from the N-terminal extension of type I procollagen chains[91,92] and by sequences derived from the C-terminal propeptide extension.[93] An additional level of control is provided once the proα chains are synthesized. For heterotrimeric molecules, like type I procollagen, the relative ratios of the two chains determines the amount of the correct molecule available and because molecular stability is determined, at least in part, by prolyl hydroxylation, the activity of the enzyme can be linked to the rate of synthesis of collagen. Finally, there is a constant level of intracellular degradation of collagenous proteins that appears to function to edit out abnormal molecules.[94,95] Thus, the control of collagen production occurs at many levels, some of which function in an "on–off" fashion while others provide a more delicate level of variation.

Nuclear Events

Like virtually all eukaryotic mRNA that encode secreted proteins, those encoding collagen chains are synthesized as precursors that are then spliced to remove intervening sequences,[96] capped, polyadenylated, and transported to the cytoplasm.

Translation

Little is known about the control of translation of collagen mRNA species. As indicated above, the formation of stem–

Table 134-3 Nature and Location of Events During Collagen Biosynthesis

Event	Enzyme	Location
Transcription	Many	Nucleus
Splicing	"Splicesome-complex"	Nucleus
Transport	Unknown	Nucleus-cytoplasm
Translation	Many	Cytoplasm/RER
Signal cleavage	Signal peptidase	RER membrane
Prolyl hydroxylation	Proline 4-hydroxylase	RER lumen
	Proline 3-hydroxylase	RER lumen
Lysyl hydroxylation	Lysyl hydroxylase	RER lumen
Hydroxylysyl glycosylation	Collagen glycosyltransferase	RER lumen
Heterosaccharide addition and modification	Collagen galactosyltransferase	RER lumen
Intrachain disulfide bond formation	Disulfide isomerase	RER lumen
Chain assembly	Not known	RER lumen
Interchain disulfide bond formation	Disulfide isomerase	RER lumen
Triple-helix propagation	Prolyl *cis-trans* isomerase	RER lumen
Transport to Golgi	Many (unknown)	RER/Golgi
Modification of heterosaccharide	Many	Golgi
Sulfation	Sulfotransferase	Golgi
Exocytosis	Many	Cell surface
N-terminal processing	Procollagen aminoprotease	ECM
C-terminal processing	Lysyl oxidase	ECM

*ECM = extracellular matrix.

loop structures in mRNA for some collagens appears to influence the efficiency of translation. The observations that cells from patients and animals with defects in cleavage of the N-terminal propeptide of type I procollagen[97] synthesized less type I procollagen than control cells led to attempts to determine if the decrease in synthesis resulted from feedback regulation. Isolated N-terminal propeptide extension from proα1(I) decreased the translational efficiency of proα1(I), and proα2(I) and proα1(II) nRNA in vitro.[91] A short peptide from the pN domain of proα1(I) can virtually abolish translation at relatively high concentrations but blocks translation of all messages.[91] Evidence has also been presented that suggests that peptides derived from the C-terminal propeptide may also affect the efficiency of translation.[93]

Posttranslational Modification and Events in the Rough Endoplasmic Reticulum

Signal Sequence. The mRNA is translated on ribosomes that become membrane-bound. The signal sequences of preproα1(I) and preproα2(I) are cleaved during elongation of the chains as they are transported through the membrane into the lumen of the RER.

Hydroxylation of Prolyl and Lysyl Residues. During translation, lagging about 300 residues behind assembly, prolyl and lysyl residues N-terminal to glycyl residues in the major and minor triple-helical sequences are hydroxylated by the enzymes prolyl 4-hydroxylase and lysyl hydroxylase, respectively.[98,99] In addition, some prolyl residues in the sequence -Gly-Pro-4Hypro-Gly- are hydroxylated in the 3-position by the enzyme prolyl 3-hydroxylase, a distinct protein.[100] The usual substrates for these reactions are the nascent chain and the free proα chains; for prolyl 4-hydroxylase, the minimum sequence requirement is an -X-Pro-Gly- triplet. The extent of hydroxylation is regulated, in part, by substrate availability because the fully hydroxylated triple helix has a melting temperature of 42°C and chains in triple-helical conformation are not substrates for the hydroxylases.[101] Prolyl 4-hydroxylase, located either in the lumen of the RER or in the inner membrane,[102] is a tetramer that contains two α subunits and two β subunits.[103] The subunits have molecular weight of 64,000 (α) and 60,000 (β) and are the products of different genes. A cDNA for the β-subunit has been isolated and sequenced demonstrating the identity of the protein with protein disulfide isomerase,[104] an enzyme that facilitates disulfide exchange in folding proteins.[105] Like some other molecules that reside in the lumen of the RER, the β-subunit has the C-terminal amino acid sequence Lys-Asp-Glu-Leu (KDEL, using the single letter amino acid code). In some proteins, this sequence appears to confer the ability to reside permanently in the RER.[106]

Lysyl hydroxylase is a homodimer, the monomer of which has a molecular weight of 85 kDa.[107] The gene encoding this enzyme has been isolated and localized to human chromosome 1p36.3-p36.2, the cDNA has been sequenced.[108,109] Despite very similar enzymatic mechanisms, there appears to be relatively little sequence similarity between prolyl 4-hydroxylase and lysyl hydroxylase.[110]

Prolyl 3-hydroxylase has a molecular weight of about 160 kDa, but the subunit composition has not been determined.[111] It is likely that there are not collagen type-specific modifying enzymes, although the extent of posttranslational modification of prolyl and lysyl residues in different collagen types does differ substantially. For example, the relative degree of lysyl hydroxylation in type IV collagen is very high (more than 90 percent of the residues in the Y position are hydroxylated), while in types I and III about 15 percent of such lysyl residues are hydroxylated. The amount of 3-

hydroxyproline differs markedly among collagen types, and the mechanisms that control the extent of modification have not been determined.

The three collagen hydroxylases require Fe^{2+}, 2-oxoglutarate, molecular oxygen (O_2), and ascorbate. The 2-oxoglutarate is decarboxylated and oxidized to succinate[112]; the other member of the oxygen molecule is incorporated into the prolyl residue at the 3- or 4-position or into the lysyl residue at the 5-position. The function of the ascorbate is not clear[113]; it can be replaced by some other reducing agents,[114] and it is thought that ascorbate may keep the Fe^{2+} atom reduced. Ascorbate is not used stoichiometrically during reactions, and there is evidence that it is important during noncoupled oxidation of 2-oxoglutarate. The role of ascorbate in providing a reducing agent for the disulfide exchange portion of prolyl 4-hydroxylase is not known.

The hydroxylation of proline in the 4-position is essential to provide thermal stability to the triple helix. The modification of the chains occurs during elongation and terminates with the formation of a stable triple helix. Hydroxylation of lysyl residues provides substrates for glycosylation and, in addition, the hydroxylysyl residues form more stable covalent crosslinks than lysyl residues and are important determinants of tissue tensile strength.[115] The function of 3-hydroxyproline is unknown.

Assembly of the Molecule. The hydroxylation reactions begin while the chains are being synthesized and are completed when the molecule is assembled and the triple helix is stable. Following completion of synthesis, the globular domains of the proα chains fold and are stabilized by intrachain disulfide bonds.[116] This process is facilitated by a disulfide exchange enzyme, probably the β subunit of prolyl 4-hydroxylase. Once intrachain disulfide bonding is completed, the two proα1(I) chains and single proα2(I) chain associated through domains created by the correct folding of the C-terminal propeptide sequences,[117] and this interaction is stabilized by the formation of interchain disulfide bonds. Triple-helix formation begins at the C-terminal end of the molecule and is propagated toward the N-terminal end.[118] There is a random distribution of *cis*-and *trans*-peptide bonds involving the prolyl residues along the chains in random coil configuration. The propagation of the triple-helical structure requires isomerization to the *trans* form, and it is likely that this is accomplished, in part, by the enzyme peptidyl prolyl *cis–trans* isomerase.[119]

Hydroxylysyl Glycosylation. The glycosylation of hydroxylysyl residues in collagen requires two enzymes—hydroxylysyl galactosyltransferase and galactosylhydroxylysyl glucosyltransferase.[120] The former transfers UDP-galactose to the oxygen on the 5-carbon of hydroxylysine in peptide linkage; Mn^{2+} is probably a cofactor for the enzyme. The latter transfers UDP-glucose, also in the presence of the metal cofactor. The distribution of monosaccharide and disaccharide is influenced by collagen type, probably by the amino acid sequence in the region of the hydroxylysyl residue. The reaction is carried out only on a non-triple-helical substrate. The functions of the carbohydrate on collagens are unknown. Carbohydrate modification may influence fibril formation, may affect collagen–cell interaction and collagen interactions with other macromolecules, and may protect modified hydroxylysyl residues from oxidation to crosslink precursors.

Glycosylation of Asparagine Residues in the Propeptide Extensions. Type I procollagen contains a single asparagine-linked carbohydrate group on the C-terminal propeptide of each chain.[121,122] Other procollagens may contain more units and they may be located in both non-triple-helical extension regions.[123] The carbohydrate units are synthesized on a dolichol lipid intermediate in the membrane of the RER and transferred intact to the proα chains.[124–126] There is initial cleavage of the terminal units while the chains are in the RER and additional trimming and resynthesis of the structure in the Golgi apparatus, which results in a high-mannose unit.[127]

Modifications Beyond the Rough Endoplasmic Reticulum and Secretion

Procollagen molecules are translocated to the Golgi and then packaged in secretory vesicles that fuse with the cell membrane and release their contents into the extracellular environment. The manner in which the molecule is transported from the RER to the Golgi and the structural determinants of that movement are unclear. The importance of triple-helical conformation has been known for many years, but the mechanism by which a cell senses this structure and the nature of the structure that is recognized is not known. Agents that disrupt microtubule function interfere with secretion of procollagen, but this may result from general disruption of cell structure rather than collagen-specific mechanisms.[128–130]

In the Golgi, heterosaccharide is trimmed, and synthesis of a high-mannose structure occurs on each chain of type I procollagen. In addition, some collagens, notably type V, probably type III, and possibly type I, undergo sulfation of some tyrosine residues in the N-terminal propeptide extension[131,132]; phosphorylation of certain serine residues of the extension of proα1(I) occurs in bone.[133] The function of the glycosylation, sulfation, and phosphorylation is not known. Inhibition of glycosylation with tunicamycin does not appear to alter the efficiency of secretion of type I procollagen, as it does with some other matrix macromolecules, notably fibronectin.

Extracellular Events

Once outside the cell, procollagens undergo proteolytic conversion to collagen, form fibrils, interact with noncollagen and collagenous proteins, are stabilized by intermolecular crosslinks, and are degraded.

Cleavage of the N-Terminal and C-Terminal Propeptides. The conversion of procollagen to collagen occurs in the extracellular space. The peptides are removed by two enzymes, procollagen N-proteinase and procollagen C-proteinase.[134–136] The N-proteinases are probably collagen type specific, and there is evidence that those that cleave type I and type III procollagen are distinct enzymes. In type I collagen the enzyme cleaves a Pro-Gln bond in the proα1(I) chains and an Ala-Gln bond in the proα2(I) chain; in both cases cyclization of the glutamine forms the N-terminal residue, pyroglutamic acid. The enzyme is an endopeptidase that requires all three chains of type I procollagen to be in register to form the substrate.[137] The propeptide is removed en bloc without further degradation. Some is detectable in plasma, but the site of further degradation and the half-life of the molecule in plasma are not known. In the procollagen molecule the propeptide probably acts to prevent or delay fibril formation, and the minor triple helix may stabilize the N-terminal end of the major triple helix. The enzyme functions in the extracellular environment, probably close to the cell surface. The activity is maximal at neutral pH, and the enzyme requires a divalent cation for function. Cleavage is sequential in chains without apparent specificity as to the first reaction.

Cleavage at the C-terminal site occurs at an Ala-Asp bond in both proα1(I) and proα2(I). In contrast to cleavage at the N-terminal site, this reaction does not require an intact trimer. The enzyme requires a divalent cation, such as Ca^{2+}. There does not appear to be a preferred order for cleavage of the termini, and intermediates that contain either end intact can be found in tissues and in cultured cells. Some collagens are probably not processed in tissues and some may be cleaved only at one end.

Fibril Formation. Once cleaved, collagen molecules rapidly aggregate into ordered structures. Aggregation occurs in concert with proteolytic processing of the propeptide extensions very close to the cell membrane in invaginations of the cell surface.[138] Under these conditions, the high concentration of collagen molecules would drive the formation of fibrils. It has been proposed, on the basis of EM of cultured cells and of cells in tissues, that procollagen molecules aggregate in an ordered fashion in secretory vesicles and are then reordered following secretion and cleavage of the propeptides.[139] However, this concept is not widely accepted. Fibril formation results from aggregation of molecules. The interaction of molecules is determined largely by the distribution of charged and hydrophobic groups at the surface.[140] Collagen molecules aggregate in an ordered parallel overlapping lateral array such that adjacent molecules are staggered by slightly less than a quarter of a molecule in length (see Fig. 134-3). Fibril formation is a nonenzymatic process, and the nature of the interactions that govern fibril diameter is not completely understood. Interactions with collagens other than type I (e.g., types III and V) or with proteoglycans or other glycoproteins are thought to control the rate of fibrillogenesis and ultimate fibril diameter.[141] That is certainly true of collagens in cartilage[142]; the absence of fibrils in basement membrane is accounted for in part by the absence of conversion of procollagen to collagen, by the interactions of type IV collagen with other components of the basement membrane, and by the interrupted nature of the triple helix.

Formation, Structure, and Function of Crosslinks. Collagen molecules in fibrillar array become substrates for the enzyme lysyl oxidase that oxidatively deaminates certain lysyl and hydroxylysyl residues in collagen and elastin[143,144] (see Fig. 134-4). There are four principal crosslinking loci in molecules of type I, II, and III collagens—a lysyl residue located nine residues from the N-terminal end of the triple helix of the chain in the telopeptide, an hydroxylysyl residue (usually glycosylated at triple-helical residue 87), a glycosylated hydroxylysyl residue at triple-helical position 930, and hydroxylysyl residue 16 amino acids from the C-terminal end of the triple helix in C-terminal telopeptide.[115] The two non-triple-helical sites are the substrate positions of the enzymes. Because the sequences around the triple-helical residues are highly conserved among species and are virtually identical at the two sites, it is thought that this region represents the attachment site for the enzyme and thus explains the need for the fibrillar substrate. The relative positioning of the triple-helical residues and those in the telopeptide extensions in the collagen fibril place the relevant lysyl or hydroxylysyl residues in appropriate proximity. Lysyl oxidase activity results in formation of a reactive aldehyde (allysine or hydroxyallysine if the substrate residues are lysine or hydroxylysine, respectively) that condenses with lysyl or hydroxylysyl residues in adjacent molecules to form divalent crosslinks. The enzyme does not recognize the glycosylated hydroxylysyl residues as substrate, explaining one possible function of that modification. Although divalent crosslinks are first formed, there is rapid formation of more complex crosslinks that stabilize collagen structures in tissues. The complex products may involve histidine or additional lysyl and hydroxylysyl residues to form three-membered crosslinks among amino acids that stabilize interactions among three chains.

Lysyl oxidase functions as a monomeric enzyme, which is a glycoprotein with a molecular weight of approximately 32kDa.[145,146] It requires pyridoxyl and copper as cofactors, the latter probably for stability.[147,148] The human gene encoding lysyl oxidase has been isolated and assigned to chromosome 5q23.3-q31.2.[149] Multiple transcripts are generated from the same gene and, surprisingly, there is extensive homology of the human lysyl oxidase sequence with that of the murine *ras* recision gene, a gene that can reverse the *ras* phenotype in mouse NIH 3T3-transformed cells.[150,151] The consequences of these homologies are unclear at present.

Crosslinking is vitally important to provide tensile strength to tissues. Several defects that affect crosslink formation demonstrate the importance of this aspect of collagen metabolism. Indeed, virtually any mutation that alters the ability of collagens to form fibrils probably affects stabilization of collagens and thus interferes with normal tissue function.

INHERITED DISORDERS OF COLLAGEN BIOSYNTHESIS AND STRUCTURE

Inheritance

Because of the complexity of collagen processing and the stringent requirements for maintenance of many structural motifs in collagen molecules, a variety of mutations that affect collagen structure or modifications are likely to result in recognizable phenotypic alterations.[152] Most mutations in the processing enzymes would be expected to result in clinically apparent phenotypes only when the defect is present in the homozygous state, as is true of most other enzymatic disorders. In contrast, most mutations that affect the structural collagen genes would be expected to be phenotypically apparent in the heterozygous state. Because collagens are polymeric proteins, the effect of mutations in one allele may be amplified beyond the initial expectations. For example, a mutation in a single α2(I) allele would be represented in 50 percent of all type I collagen molecules synthesized (assuming that the defective chains are incorporated into molecules with normal efficiency); a mutation in a single α1(I) allele would be represented in 75 percent of all type I collagen molecules synthesized; but a mutation in a α1(II) or α1(III) allele would be represented in 87.5 percent of all molecules produced (because they are homotrimeric molecules). Fibrillar collagens are the building blocks of extensive fibrils that depend on the uniformity of the components for their integrity. Thus, if even some of the abnormal molecules are incorporated into fibrils, the effects on structure can be dismayingly dramatic, further emphasizing the "dominant negative" mode of action of these mutations. In contrast, the effect of having a nonfunctional (or nonexpressed) allele is far less deleterious and would be expected to have fewer clinical consequences (see "Osteogenesis Imperfecta Type I" below, for example).

Screening and Methods of Analysis

The first disorders of collagen processing were identified almost 20 years ago and were recognized because of the differences in the size of collagen chains in skin in the case of dermatosparaxis in cattle[153] or because of altered posttranslational modification of collagen in skin in the case of Ehlers-Danlos syndrome type VI.[154] Measurements of the relative amounts of collagens in skin were instrumental in suggesting that decreased production of type I collagen could result in the phenotypes of osteogenesis imperfecta (OI).[155] Ultrastructural examination of tissues from individuals with EDS type IV suggested that structural mutations that affect secretion of collagens could produce disease following observation of markedly dilated RER in dermal fibroblasts.[156]

Because of the need to isolate and characterize abnormal collagen molecules, characterization of macromolecules synthesized by cultured dermal fibroblastic cells rapidly became the method of choice to identify mutations that affected collagen molecules synthesized by those cells. This has demonstrated utility in some of the Ehlers-Danlos syndrome (EDS) phenotypes and in many of the OI phenotypes, because skin fibroblasts synthesize types I and III collagens in abundance. The ease with which mutations can be identified depends on the effect they have on molecular structure and processing. For example, large rearrangements in the genes that result in longer than normal or shorter than normal chains are readily apparent when radiolabeled proteins are examined (see below). Certain single amino acid substitutions can also be identified in this manner, either by specific labeling (e.g., with cysteine to identify substitutions within the triple-helical domain of type I collagen) or by their effect on posttranslational modification. Cultured dermal fibroblasts are less valuable in screening for some processing mutations (e.g., mutations that affect extracellular processing—cleavage of the N- and C-terminal propeptides and crosslinking—and some varieties of intracellular modification), unless specific tests for those defects are used. Dermal fibroblasts cannot be used to identify mutations in genes that are not expressed by those cells.

For disorders that affect genes not expressed by fibroblast cells and to determine which type I collagen gene carries a mutation in dominantly inherited disorders, genetic linkage studies have been extremely valuable. Linkage studies with polymorphic markers in the genes for type I collagen have confirmed that mutations in both genes of type I collagen—COL1A1 and COL1A2—can account for dominantly inherited forms of OI. Linkage studies have excluded candidate genes in certain disorders. For example, studies of inheritance of polymorphic markers in the COL2A1 gene have excluded mutations in type II collagen in families with dominantly inherited achondroplasia.[157] Chromosomal localization of collagen genes has, in some cases, excluded genes as candidates in disorders for which they might reasonably be considered—for example, type IV collagen in Alport syndrome, a disorder affecting the basement membranes of the ear and the kidney. Localization of the genes for type IV collagen on chromosome 13 has excluded them as candidates in the X-linked form of the disorder.

Linkage studies in dominantly inherited disorders of type I and type III collagen genes (in OI types I and IV and in EDS type IV) have identified the genes affected and have facilitated prenatal diagnosis and gene isolation. Linkage studies have also excluded mutations in both type I collagen genes in some of the rare families with autosomal recessive forms of severe OI.[158,159]

OSTEOGENESIS IMPERFECTA

OI is a heterogeneous group of inherited disorders characterized by bone fragility that is accompanied by other evidence of connective-tissue malfunction, including abnormalities in teeth (dentinogenesis imperfecta), hearing loss, alterations in scleral hue, and evidence of soft-tissue dysplasia[160] (Table 134-4). The vast majority of individuals with OI have mutations that affect the structure of genes encoding the chains of type I collagen.[161-164] The clinical heterogeneity is extensive, ranging from death in the perinatal period through marked short stature and severe bone deformity, to normal life span with only mild decrease in bone mass.[165] This heterogeneity led to many efforts to devise a classification of OI that would predict natural history (with the attendant needs for medical intervention), determine the mode of genetic transmission, and facilitate a biochemical approach to this group of disorders. An initial attempt to classify OI divided affected individuals into those with fractures and/or deformity at birth (OI congenita) and those in whom fractures or deformity did not develop until later (OI tarda).[166] This scheme was later amended to add a second tarda group to distinguish between the severe and often lethal group and those that survived.[167] Although often helpful in predicting long-term morbidity, this division frequently provided a false sense of security because it could be difficult, several years later, to distinguish some individuals initially classified in the tarda group from those in the congenita group. Nonetheless, this classification became the standard nomenclature for most physicians. Efforts by Ibsen[168] in Denmark expanded the classification based on the additional criterion of the mode of inheritance of the condition. Beginning in the late 1970s Sillence and his colleagues, using radiographic, genetic, and clinical criteria, developed the classification currently in use.[169] Although this classification of OI into four major types (I to IV) was rapidly adopted by the geneticists, it has not achieved similar popularity with orthopedic surgeons because of the difficulty in classifying many patients and the sense that natural history was not a major determinant in developing the classification. The Sillence modification of the Ibsen classification has been used to categorize most of the patients who have been investigated at the biochemical and genetic levels. The biochemical studies themselves and the recent linkage studies generally support the validity of the classification but emphasize that it is, in some respects, incomplete. Ultimately the biochemical and genetic studies will provide the basis of the most rational classification. It is likely, however, that even the biochemical classification will never be entirely adequate for prediction of natural history because of the confounding effects of other matrix components in regulating the phenotypic expression of the primary mutation.

Osteogenesis Imperfecta Type I (Dominant Inheritance with Blue Sclerae)

Genetics and Natural History. OI type I is inherited in an autosomal dominant fashion, and affected individuals typically have blue sclerae, normal teeth, and normal or near-normal stature; they may experience a few or more than 50 fractures (usually of long bones) prior to puberty.[170]

Table 134-4 Clinical Heterogeneity and Biochemical Defects in Osteogenesis Imperfecta

OI Type	Clinical Features	Inheritance*	Biochemical Defects
I	Normal stature, little or no deformity; blue scleras, hearing loss in about 50 percent of individuals; dentinogenesis imperfecta rare and may distinguish a subset	AD	Decreased production of type I procollagen; substitution for residue other than glycine in triple helix of α1(I)
II	Lethal in the perinatal period, minimal calvarial mineralization, beaded ribs, compressed femurs, marked long bone deformity, platyspondyly	AD (new mutation) AR (rare)	Rearrangements in the COL1A1 and COL1A2 genes; substitutions for glycyl residues in the triple-helical domain of the α1(I) or α2(I) chain; small deletion in α2(I) on the background of a null allele
III	Progressively deforming bones, usually with moderate deformity at birth; scleras variable in hue, often lighten with age; dentinogenesis common, hearing loss common; stature very short	AD AR	Point mutation in the α1(I) or α2(I) chain Frameshift mutation that prevents incorporation of proα2(I) into molecules (noncollagenous defects)
IV	Normal scleras, mild to moderate bone deformity; variable short stature; dentinogenesis common; hearing loss occurs in some	AD	Point mutations in the α2(I) chain; rarely, point mutations in the α1(I) chain; small deletions in the α2(I) chain.

*AD = autosomal dominant; AR = autosomal recessive.

It has been suggested that this group of patients could be subdivided on the basis of the absence (type IA) or presence (type IB) of dentinogenesis imperfecta (DI).[171] Because the presence of DI usually indicates the synthesis of abnormal collagen molecules, the OI type IB group would better fit in the OI type IV group if distinction between groups is made on biochemical findings (see below).

Individuals with this type of OI rarely have fractures in the perinatal period, although intrauterine femoral bowing and fractures at birth can be the initial presentation. Fractures may occur first within the weeks following birth associated with diaper changing but more commonly occur as children begin to walk. The most frequent bones broken are the long bones of the arms and legs, the ribs, and the small bones of the hands and feet. The fracture frequency remains steady through childhood and then decreases following the onset of puberty, suggesting the hormonal and other factors alter bone strength. Fractures heal rapidly with evidence of good callus formation, and without deformity.

The frequency of this form of OI has been estimated at between 1 in 15,000 and 1 in 20,000 but because of the relatively mild presentation, it may be more frequent. There appears to be no decrease in fertility or longevity in affected individuals. At birth, blue sclerae are readily apparent and may be darkly colored, lightening gradually to the blue-gray present in affected adults. Radiographic bone morphology is generally normal, although mild osteopenia may be present on radiographs and can be documented by densitometry. Height of affected individuals is usually within the normal range, although affected individuals may be shorter than their unaffected family members. Vertebral body morphology in the adult is normal initially but often develops the classic "codfish" appearance that is accompanied by loss of height in the later decades. Fracture frequency often increases following the menopause in women and in the sixth to eighth decades for men. In about half the families with OI type I, affected individuals have early-onset hearing loss, beginning in the late teens, and leading gradually to profound loss by the end of the fourth to fifth decades.[172–174] Although the hearing loss is mixed in type, advances in design and replacement of the fractured and fused bones of the middle ear have provided significant restoration of hearing for many affected individuals.[175] Early hearing loss is typically high-frequency in type, and tympanometry results in a characteristic bifid compliance curve. Additional clinical findings often include mild joint hypermobility and increased bruising. A variety of nonskeletal problems have been identified in individuals with OI type I, including mitral-valve and aortic valvular problems but it is likely that these are not significantly more frequent than in the general population; however, a small group of patients have been identified with slightly larger than normal aortic root diameters, without the risk of dissection.[176]

Biochemical Basis of OI Type I

Null Alleles (Silent Alleles or Mutations That Lead to Excluded Proteins) Are Most Common. Several forms of OI were among the earliest of the inherited disorders of collagen biosynthesis and structure to be studied using cultured dermal fibroblasts from affected individuals.[177,178] Cells cultured from patients who, in retrospect, would be considered to have OI type I, synthesized less type I procollagen than did controls, but the mechanism by which production was decreased was not determined. These studies were extended from culture to tissue when it was found that skin from most individuals with OI, including those with mild, dominantly inherited OI and blue sclerae, had a low ratio of type I to type III collagen.[179] These results could be explained by decreased synthesis of type I procollagen or by an increase in the synthesis of type III collagen. Shortly thereafter it became clear that the synthesis of type I procollagen by cells cultured from individuals with OI type I was about half the normal level, while that of type III procollagen was normal[180] (Fig. 134-5). The structure of the secreted type I procollagen was normal, and the decrease in type I procollagen production resulted from synthesis of only half the usual amount of the proα1(I) chains of type I procollagen.

The mechanism by which the synthesis of proα1(I) chains is decreased has come under increasing scrutiny but has, nonetheless, proved to be a difficult problem. A variety of

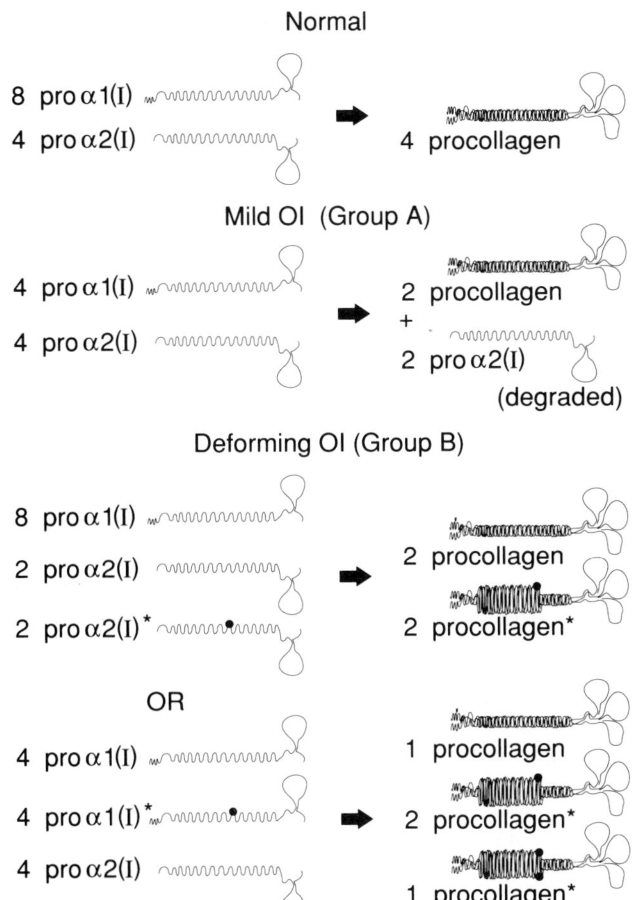

FIG. 134-5 Molecular basis of OI. In the mild dominantly inherited form of OI, OI type I, several defects in the structure of the COL1A1 gene can lead to a decrease in the synthesis of proα1(I) chains and thus to production of less than normal amounts of type I procollagen (*top*). In contrast, in the other forms of OI in which bone deformity and short stature are common features, mutations within the COL1A1 or COL1A2 lead to the synthesis of abnormal molecules that may be poorly secreted but often interfere with the formation of a normal fibrillar structure.

mutations that result in decreased synthesis of proα1(I) chains, such as deletion of an allele, promoter and enhancer mutations, splicing mutations, premature termination, as well as other mutations that result in the inability of proα1(I) chains to assemble into molecules, would presumably result in the same biochemical picture and the same clinical phenotype. In some individuals, the decreased production of proα1(I) by fibroblasts results from about half-normal steady state levels of the mRNA.[181] Genovese and Rowe[182] have suggested that in at least one family there is a defect in splicing of the pre-mRNA of COL1A1 that prohibits transport of the product of the mutant allele to the cytoplasm, but the precise molecular defect has not yet been characterized.[183] Examination of genomic DNA from 15 individuals with OI type I demonstrated no evidence of change in copy number of the COL1A1 gene in individuals[184] but demonstrated that the products of one COL1A1 allele were virtually absent from the cytoplasm of cultured fibroblasts. Further, linkage studies in 38 additional families has demonstrated no evidence of deletion of those regions of the COL1A1 gene used for linkage analysis[185,186] and confirmed that most individuals with the OI type I phenotype have mutations linked to the COL1A1 gene. In some families a similar phenotype is thought to result from mutations in the COL1A2 gene, but the clinical criteria by which the diagnosis of OI type I was made are not always clear.[185–187]

The most completely characterized mutation in the COL1A1 gene that results in defective production of type I procollagen is a 5-bp deletion near the 3′ end of one COL1A1 allele.[188] The mutation results in a reading frameshift 12 amino acid residues from the normal terminus of the chain, and predicts an extension of 84 amino acids beyond the normal termination site. Although the abnormal mRNA can be translated in vitro, it has proved extremely difficult to identify the abnormal chains in cells; it appears that although the mRNA is present in near-normal quantities, the protein product is unstable. In other individuals with OI type I, a variety of mutations result in the *de novo* appearance of a premature stop codon that may be detected by a nuclear scanning mechanism and prohibit exit of the abnormal mRNA.

These mutations provide models of how many different mutations in the COL1A1 gene could produce the OI type I phenotype by resulting in the synthesis of half the normal amount of a functional proα1(I) chain. In each instance, the synthesis of proα2(I) chains would be expected to be normal, but about half of them could not be incorporated into intact molecules, because the excess proα2(I) chains cannot associate into trimeric molecules and thus would be degraded.

Decreased production of proα1(I) is not the only way to decrease the secretion of type I procollagen without secreting abnormal molecules, however. For example, the synthesis of a proα2(I) chain that could be incorporated into molecules normally, but then resulted in rapid and complete intracellular degradation of all such molecules, could have a similar effect; no such mutations have yet been identified.

Structural Mutations in COL1A1 and COL1A2 Can Also Produce OI Type I. Although less common than "null" allele mutations, there are several examples in which synthesis of abnormal type I procollagen molecules can produce the OI type I phenotype (Fig. 134-6). In one family,[189] cells cultured from the affected mother and son, but not the normal daughter, synthesized α1(I) chains bearing a cysteine residue within the protease-resistant domain of the collagen molecule, a region from which that residue is normally absent. Although it was initially thought that the substitution could be for a nonglycine residue in the triple helix,[190] peptide sequence analysis and sequence of the cDNA demonstrated that the mutation resulted in the substitution of a glycine by cysteine three amino acid residues C-terminal to the end of the triple helix.[191] Other substitutions of cysteine for glycine within the triple helix of the α1(I) chain, including G19C,[192] G43C,[193] G46C (unpublished observations), and G94C,[194] also produce very mild forms of OI, compatible with OI type I.

One patient, with blue sclerae, a height of 4 ft. 10 in., deformity as a result of a poor orthopedic result, and hearing loss was the only affected member of her family. Her cultured dermal fibroblasts synthesized a proα2(I) chain in which approximately 30 amino acid residues were deleted from the triple-helical domain.[195] Subsequent studies indicated that a point mutation resulted in the skipping of exon 12 (amino acids 91 to 108) from about half the COL1A2 transcripts, as a result of a point mutation at the consensus splice donor site.[183]

These last findings suggest that other point mutations in the COL1A1 gene, and perhaps in the COL1A2 gene (as

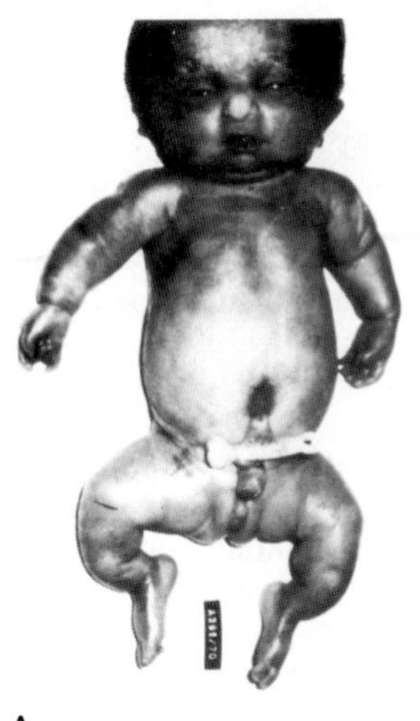

A.

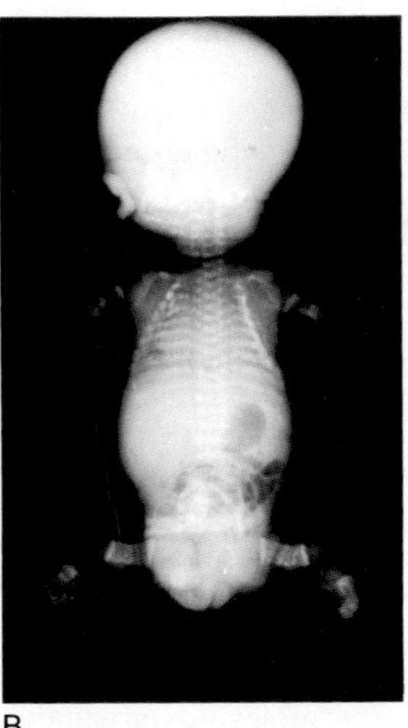

B.

FIG. 134-7 Clinical (*A*) and radiographic (*B*) appearance of an infant with the perinatal lethal form of osteogenesis imperfecta (OI type II). Infants with OI type II have large soft calvaria, a small thoracic cavity, short extremities with marked angulation of the lower legs, and generally have their legs in a flexed and abducted position. X-ray films demonstrate virtual absence of calvarial mineralization, shortened and markedly undermineralized bones, block-shaped femurs, bowed tibias, and markedly flattened vertebral bodies.

There has been some uncertainty about the mode of inheritance of OI type II. Seedorf[166] identified some instances of sib recurrence of OI type II in which parents were not related. Sillence et al.[165,203] identified one family with multiple affected children born to normal but consanguineous parents. Using the formula of multiple, independent ascertainment, they calculated a segregation ratio of close to 0.25, consistent with autosomal recessive inheritance. They were, in addition, able to cite a number of other instances of sib recurrences, with consanguineous matings in some, to support the hypothesis of autosomal recessive inheritance of OI type II.

It now appears that the initial assessment of the mode of inheritance of OI type II was either incorrect or incomplete. Analysis of more than 100 families into which a proband with OI type II was born[199,204,205] indicated that new dominant mutation was the explanation for the phenotype in almost all instances. Although there were no instances of recurrence of OI type II in two studies, there were five in the third. While autosomal recessive inheritance could not be excluded as an explanation for recurrence in one family, biochemical analysis and the structure of one of the other four families, suggested that parental germ-line mosaicism for a mutation in one type I collagen allele was the best explanation for recurrence of OI type II in most families (see below).

The largest study of OI type II found a recurrence risk of 6 to 7 percent among sibs.[199] The recurrence results from parental mosaicism for the mutation that is lethal in the infant who is heterozygous for the same mutation.[206] More than 14 families have been identified in which recurrence of OI type II is explained by parental mosaicism.[207] In the seven families in which the mutation was identified, one parent was mosaic in both germ-line and somatic cells, indicating that the mutation had occurred early in embryogenesis, prior to the allocation of cells to different lineages. On the basis of results to date, it appears that the mutation occurs equally in male and female embryos. In some instances, the extent of mosaicism is sufficient to result in mild features of OI (often compatible with OI type IV, see below) in the mosaic parent.[208–211]

The hypothesis that OI type II was inherited in an autosomal recessive fashion reflected the attempt to explain recurrence of severe OI phenotypes among sibs and the presence of consanguinity in some of the families. In retrospect, the radiologic phenotype of some infants in recurrent families is reminiscent of OI type III,[212,213] in which recessive inheritance can be documented, but in which some instances of recurrence can be attributed to parental mosaicism.

It is worth noting that the subdivision of OI type II into groups A, B, and C[203] and the identification of four groups with OI type II[199] each demand too much of the supporting data. In short, virtually all instances of OI type II represent the results of dominant mutations in the genes of type I collagen, and recurrence of the phenotype among sibs is accounted for by parental mosaicism for the mutation. Several options for prenatal diagnosis in subsequent pregnancies can now be offered to all families who have had a child with OI type II (see below).

OI type II needs to be differentiated from other lethal skeletal dysplasias (especially thanatophoric dysplasia [McKusick no. (MIM) 187600] and achondrogenesis (MIM 200600)[214,215] and the autosomal recessive form of hypophosphatasia (see Chap. 136). While the radiographic picture of OI type II is characteristic, the ultrasound features early in pregnancy may be difficult to distinguish from other lethal forms of skeletal dysplasia. The characteristic rib abnormalities and markedly decreased calvarial mineralization are the most helpful features. Experienced pediatric radiologists generally have little trouble with the diagnosis in newborns although evaluation of x-ray films of early fetuses may present problems. Nonetheless, many referral centers can provide diagnostic assistance. If there is any doubt, the diagnosis of OI type II can be confirmed by examination of the collagens synthesized by cultured fibroblast cells from any of several tissues. Alternatively, if no fibroblasts are available to study, pathological examination with the finding of undermineralized bone, osteoblastic cells with dilated RER, and increased osteoid can help to confirm the diagnosis.[216]

Treatment and Prenatal Diagnosis. OI type II is a lethal condition with a life expectancy ranging from minutes to months. Death may result from pulmonary insufficiency, congestive heart failure, or infection. The most difficult treatment decisions occur at the birth of an affected infant, when the diagnosis may not be clear and the infant has marked pulmonary insufficiency. Ordinarily, when the diagnosis is known, infants are offered supportive care and parental bonding is encouraged. Many affected infants can leave the hospital, and supportive care in the home is essential. Bedding that contains soft foam can decrease fracture frequency. Because of respiratory insufficiency, many of these infants have feeding problems, and it is often difficult to maintain adequate caloric intake.

Prenatal diagnosis of OI type II has been accomplished by ultrasound screening of pregnancies between 14 and 18 weeks of gestation (see above). By that age femurs are short, the thoracic cage is small, and calvarial mineralization is minimal. Analysis of chorionic villi for the presence of abnormal collagens and of collagens synthesized by cells grown from chorionic villi can be used to exclude the diagnosis and to identify an affected fetus. We have studied more than 30 pregnancies at risk for recurrence of the OI type II phenotype and have correctly predicted the outcome in all (unpublished data). It should be noted, however, that with advances in ultrasound scanning, particularly the use of vaginal probes, the gestational age at which an abnormal fetus can be identified is getting earlier. For example, in one recent pregnancy in which a gene-based diagnosis of OI type II was made, ultrasound studies at 12 to 13 weeks of gestation revealed abnormal limb length and morphology.[217] If the mutation in the family is not known, then the time from CVS biopsy to diagnosis is about 3 to 4 weeks (time to culture the cells and time to examine the proteins synthesized by those cells). Thus, with new sonographic techniques, the need for CVS may be reduced.

Biochemical Basis of OI Type II. OI type II is the most extensively studied variety of OI and the best characterized at both the biochemical and molecular genetic levels. Cells from more than 200 affected infants have been studied in culture,[199,218–220] and the molecular basis of OI type II has been established in more than three dozen infants.[161,162,221] A surprisingly wide array of mutations produces the OI type II phenotype—point mutations in the triple-helical domain that result in substitutions for glycine (probably largely in the COL1A1 gene), multiple-exon rearrangements, small deletions (usually the result of splicing defects) in the triple-helical domain of either chain, and mutations in the C-terminal propeptide that interfere with molecular assembly (see Table 134-2 and Fig. 134-6). In almost all instances, the affected individual is heterozygous for the lethal mutations.

Rearrangements. All multiple-exon rearrangements within the COL1A1 or the COL1A2 genes have proved to be lethal. Among the cells initially studied by Pentinnen and his colleagues[178] was one from an infant identified to have the lethal form of OI.[222] Although it was recognized that the cells did not produce type I procollagen efficiently, the nature of the defect was unclear. Studies, by others, of the same cell strain led to the recognition that decreased production was a consequence of inefficient secretion of molecules that contained one or more proα1(I) chains from which the 84 amino acids from 327 to 411 of the triple-helical domain (encoded by exons 23 to 25) had been deleted.[223–225] The shortened chain resulted from an intron-to-intron deletion of approximately 650 bp in one COL1A1 allele that removed three exons.[226,227] The deletion may have been mediated through a short inverted repeat at the ends of the deleted fragment.[226] Because the deletion end points were within introns, the resulting proα1(I) chain was predicted to have an intact Gly-X-Y triplet structure, 84 residues shorter than the product of the normal allele. Cells from this infant synthesized three populations of type I procollagen molecules—normal molecules and those that contained either one or two of the short chains. Molecules that contained the shortened chain had a decreased thermal stability (about 32°C compared to the normal of 42°C)[224] and virtually none of these molecules was secreted.[224] The deletion from the COL1A1 allele probably is sufficient to produce the lethal phenotype, but this cell strain does secrete type III procollagen, the chains of which have been excessively modified following translation (perhaps reflecting the secretion block resulting from accumulation of the abnormal type I procollagen).

Although the identification of a multiple-exon deletion among the first few cell strains from infants with OI type II to be studied created the expectation that such mutations would be encountered frequently, study of more than 200 cell strains in several laboratories has produced only two additional published examples of multiple-exon rearrangements within the type I collagen genes. In the first, a 600-bp insertion within one COL1A1 allele[228] that resulted from a recombinational event involving exons 17 and 14 produces a COL1A1 allele that encoded a proα1(I) chain in which 60 amino acids were duplicated.[229] The abnormal molecules synthesized by these cells were secreted only slightly less efficiently than the normal molecules so that the lethal effect was probably the consequence of the presence of molecules in the matrix that could not copolymerize with the normal molecules to form fibrils.

The other rearrangement identified was a 4.5-kb, seven-exon deletion from one COL1A2 allele. About half the proα2(I) chains synthesized lacked 180 amino acids of the triple helix, residues 586 to 765.[230,231] Molecules that contained the shortened chain were not secreted, but remained in the lumen of the RER for several hours, during which time the molecules gradually acquired a protease-resistant configuration and became overmodified N-terminal to the domain of the mutation.[231] Thus, although the deletion resulted in maintenance of the triplet motif of the triple helix (Gly-X-Y), the molecules that contained the abnormal chain underwent a marked increase in posttranslational modification, but only N-terminal to the deletion junction. This suggested that the triple helix N-terminal to the junction was compromised, presumably because interactions other than those involving hydroxyproline residues normally contributed to helix stability. It was further surprising that the secretion of, at best, very small amounts of the abnormal molecule was sufficient to result in the OI type II phenotype. If the block to secretion were complete, the phenotype would be expected to be OI type I (see above), suggesting that other factors may play a role in the generation of phenotype.

Point Mutations. It soon became clear that multiple-exon rearrangements in the genes encoding the chains of type I collagen were rare and that other mutations were commonly the molecular basis of the OI type II phenotype. The majority of cells from infants with OI type II are heterozygous for point mutations that result in the substitution for single glycine residues within the triple helix of either the proα1(I) or proα2(I) chains. These mutations decrease triple-helix stability, interfere with secretion, and affect the formation of fibrils in the extracellular matrix (Figs. 134-6 and 134-8).

The first demonstration that point mutations in the triple helix of the proα1(I) chain might be significant came with the recognition that cells from an infant with OI type II contained a cysteine residue within the triple-helical domain of the α1(I) chain.[232] Because cysteine is excluded from the triple-helical domain of normal α1(I), the presence of cysteine within the triple helix could be recognized by the formation of an α1(I) chain dimer that resulted from interchain–intramolecular disulfide bonds. The cysteine residue was located within the C-terminal 200 amino acids, and when that domain of both COL1A1 alleles was isolated and sequenced, one was found to contain a single nucleotide substitution that changed the glycine codon at position 988 in the triple helix to that for a cysteine.[233] All molecules that contained either one or two copies of the chain were less efficiently secreted than the normal molecules, had undergone increased posttranslational modification (lysyl hydroxylation and hydroxylysyl glycosylation) along the entire length of the molecule, and were less stable to thermal denaturation; they melted at 38°C instead of the normal 42°C. A similar pattern of behavior of abnormal molecules

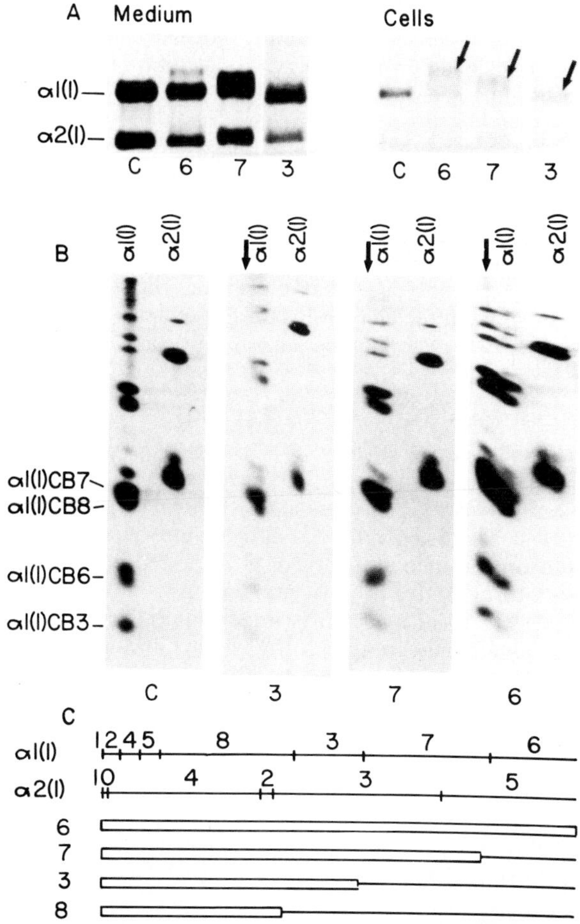

FIG. 134-8 Altered electrophoretic mobility of the chains of type I collagen synthesized by cells for infants with OI type II. *A*. Chains of type I collagen secreted into the medium or retained with the cells were separated by SDS-PAGE under nonreducing conditions following treatment with pepsin to remove the non-triple-helical domains of procollagen. The arrows in the cell portion of the figure indicate the abnormal, slowly migrating α1(I) chains. Lane marker C designates control; 6, 7, and 3 indicate cell strains in which overmodification begins in α1(I)CB6, α1(I)CB7, and α1(I)CB3, respectively. *B*. Cyanogen bromide peptide maps of normal and abnormal type I collagen chains. The section of the gel represented in part *A* was resected; the chains in the gel were treated with cyanogen bromide, which cleaves proteins at methionyl residues; and the resultant peptides were then separated in a second-dimension gel on top of which the gel fragment had been placed. The arrows at the top of each panel indicate the positions of the abnormal, slowly migrating α1(I) chain indicated in part *A*. In panel 3 the mobilities of α1(I)CB8 and α1(I)CB3 from the abnormal chain are slow; in panel 7 the mobilities of α1(I)CB8, α1(I)CB3, and α1(I)CB7 are slow; and in panel 6 the mobility of each of the cyanogen bromide peptides is slow. The delay in electrophoretic mobility results from increased posttranslational modification along all (panel 6) or part (panels 3 and 7) of the chain. *C*. Diagrammatic representation of the extent of increased posttranslational modification along the type I collagen molecule with the triple-helical domain of each α chain. Vertical lines = positions of methyionyl residues; numbers = cyanogen bromide peptides; open bars indicate the extent of increased posttranslational modification along the molecule. *(From Byers et al.* Am J Hum Genet *42:237, 1988. Used by permission of the* American Journal of Human Genetics.*)*

was noted in other cell strains from infants with OI type II in which the mutation had not been characterized.[218–220]

Because of the importance of glycine in every third position for the propagation and stability of the triple helix, it was postulated (as a result of these studies) that substitutions of most glycyl residues in the triple-helical domain of the α1(I) chain would most likely result in the same phenotype, provided they interfered sufficiently with stability. It is now clear that although most substitutions for glycine within the triple-helical domain of either proα1(I) or proα2(I) chains do result in the clinical picture of OI, the severity of the phenotype is a reflection of the chain in which the mutation appears, the location of the mutation in that chain, and the nature of the substituting residue (see Fig. 134-6).

More than 20 point mutations have now been characterized from infants with the lethal OI phenotype. Single nucleotide substitutions in each of the four glycine codons (GGN) give rise to codons for serine, arginine, cysteine, tryptophan, and a stop codon (first position), or aspartic acid, glutamic acid, valine, and alanine (second position), in proportion to the codon usage for glycine. Of these substitutions, tryptophan and glutamic acid would be expected infrequently, and a stop codon would be expected to produce a "null" allele effect and thus an OI type I phenotype. To date, substitutions of glycine by tryptophan or glutamic acid have not been observed in OI type II. The lethal phenotype has resulted from substitutions in the α1(I) chain of glycine by alanine,[234,235] serine,[236–239] cysteine,[194,210,232,233,240–242] arginine,[208,235,243–246] aspartic acid,[161,206,247] and valine.[235,248,249] Fewer lethal mutations have been identified in the COL1A2 gene that result in substitutions for glycine in the triple-helical domain. These include substitutions of glycine by serine,[235] cysteine,[211,240] arginine,[250,251] and aspartic acid.[252–255]

Exon-Skipping Mutations and Small Deletions. Heterozygosity for exon-skipping defects currently comprises the second largest group of mutations that produce the OI type II phenotype (see Fig. 134-6). In general, they occur as a result of point mutations in the splice-donor or splice-acceptor sequences. Skipping of the sequences in the proα1(I) chain encoded by exons 14,[256] 27, 44, and 47[161] in the COL1A1 gene and of the sequences in the proα2(I) chain encoded by exons 28[257–259] or 33[260] of the COL1A2 gene have each resulted in the OI type II phenotype. The infant with the mutation that interferes with splicing of exon 14 in the COL1A1 gene is homozygous for the mutant allele probably as a result of paternal uniparental disomy for all or a portion of chromosome 17 (see below). Furthermore, the infant with the exon 28 skipping mutation in COL1A2 may have a null allele in addition (see below).

Deletions of a single Gly-X-Y triplet in the proα1(I) chain, for example, residues 732 to 734 (Willing MC, Atkinson M, and Byers PH: unpublished data), residues 868 to 870,[261] or residues 874 to 876[262] have also been identified in infants with the perinatal lethal form of OI. Like the other mutations, they alter the extent of posttranslation modification of the triple helix N-terminal to the site of the mutation, alter its thermal stability, and interfere with secretion. The clinical phenotype produced by exon-skipping mutations or small genomic deletions is indistinguishable from those that result from multiple-exon deletions or substitutions for single glycine residues in the triple-helical domain of either chain.

Mutations Outside the Triple-Helical Domain. Although far less common than any of the other mutations, alterations in the sequence of the C-terminal propeptide of the proα1(I) chain are now being recognized as causes of the OI type II phenotype. In one instance, the insertion of a single nucleotide results in a shift in reading frame and premature termination, alters the ability of the molecules to be secreted, and, in effect, acts as a sink for normal chains.[263] Thus, the secretion of normal type I procollagen is reduced to about 25 percent of the normal amount, apparently insufficient to sustain normal bone formation. In other infants, a point mutation results in substitution of a charged amino acid (arginine) for a hydrophobic residue (leucine) in a conserved region of the C-terminal propeptide,[264] substitution of aspartic acid for histidine in a second conserved domain, or a 6-bp and 2 amino acid in-frame deletion.[265] These mutations all appear to alter the ability of the abnormal chains to form stable trimers; the molecules that do result are poorly secreted.

Homozygosity or Compound Heterozygosity in the OI Type II Phenotype Is Rare. Although the vast majority of infants with OI type II appear to be heterozygous for mutations in one of the genes that encode the chains of type I procollagen, there is emerging biochemical and molecular genetic information that suggests that, in some situations, two mutant alleles may be necessary to produce the phenotype. In one instance, biochemical data suggested that the OI type II phenotype resulted from compound heterozygosity for different mutations in the two COL1A2 alleles.[257] The first mutation, new in the family, resulted in deletion of the amino acids encoded by exon 28 as the result of a splice-junction mutation.[259] In addition, the infant apparently received a "null" COL1A2 allele from one parent, although a transcript was synthesized from that copy.[259] As a result, all the proα2(I) chains synthesized (half the normal amount) were abnormal and the cells secreted a trimer of proα1(I) chains.[257]

A more recent example of homozygosity for a mutation provides additional insight into the mechanisms by which OI type II may be produced.[256] The affected infant had two copies of an allele in which there was a point mutation at position +6 in intron 14, just beyond the requisite GT dinucleotide that identifies the beginning of the intron. In cells, there was alternative splicing in both alleles so that the normal and the abnormally spliced mRNA appeared in equal proportion. Thus, although the cells were homozygous for a point mutation that resulted in abnormal splicing of the allele, the result of the mutation was that about half the mRNA derived from each allele had the normal structure while the remainder lacked the sequence of exon 14. In this instance, the asymptomatic father was mosaic for the mutation and the mother lacked it altogether. Further studies indicated that the infant represented an instance of uniparental disomy for all or a portion of chromosome 17 (Bonadio J: personal communication). In this instance, the recurrence risk for OI type II should be negligible, but there would still be concern about the effect of heterozygosity for the mutant allele (see "Osteogenesis Imperfecta Type I" above) in an offspring.

Biochemical-Pathological Correlation. Not yet clear is how such mutations result in lethal disease and why such diverse mutations result in a similar phenotype. From a pathological perspective, bone is markedly undermineralized.[266] Osteoblastic cells with dilated RER are common, and increased osteoid is observed.

The known lethal point mutations in COL1A1 are all between residues 97 and 1014 of the triple helix (see Fig. 134-6). In each case, assembly of the triple helix appears to be normal to the point of the mutation, but the stability of the molecule between the mutation and the N-terminal end of the triple helix is decreased. Further, this portion of the molecule is subjected to increased posttranslational modification. In all known point mutations and in the rearrangements, overmodification occurs N-terminal to the defect, yet modification is generally normal C-terminal to the site. It has been proposed that propagation of the triple-helical structure is very slow through the domain carrying the mutation and that, as a result, the chains remain accessible for further modification. Alternatively, the structure of the triple helix formed may not be as stable as the normal structure, a concept supported by the findings in collagens synthesized with the large deletion from proα2(I) described above. The amount of the abnormal molecule needed in the matrix to produce the phenotype is not clear but, on the basis of studies of some of the cell strains described here and animal models (see below), it may be surprisingly small.

Osteogenesis Imperfecta Type III

Genetics and Natural History. OI type III, the progressive deforming variety, is usually recognized at birth because of short stature and deformities resulting from in utero fractures (Fig. 134-9). There are well-documented autosomal recessive and autosomal dominant forms of OI type III, although the recessive form is rare in most populations.[267–269] Radiologically, at birth the calvarium is undermineralized, the ribs are thin, long bones are thin with evidence of fracture, and the skeleton is osteopenic. If no fractures are present at birth, they usually occur during the first year of life, and deformity becomes apparent during that period. Beginning

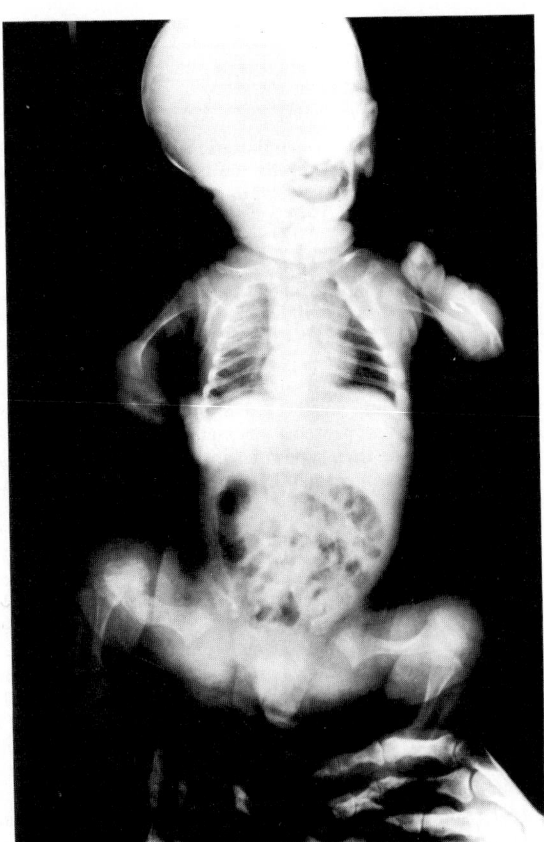

FIG. 134-9 Radiographic features of the progressive deforming OI type III phenotype in the newborn period. Calvarial mineralization is adequate; there is deformity of the long bones and rare fractures of the thin ribs. The infant pictured in this radiograph was heterozygous for mutation that resulted in substitution of cysteine for glycine at position 526 in the COL1A1 gene. *(X-ray film courtesy of Dr. Lester Weiss, Henry Ford Hospital, Detroit, MI.)*

between 2 and 5 years of age, unusual "cystic" structures form in the epiphyseal region of some of the long bones, especially of the femurs.[270] These are areas in which the growth plate is markedly disrupted, probably by recurrent microfractures. As a result, bone growth is poor and marked shortening of stature results. Because of markedly thin cortex, fracture of long bones is frequent. Angulation deformities of the tibias and the femurs reduce the efficiency of weight bearing and increase the likelihood of fracture. Treatment is directed toward providing a more functional anatomy, and it is this group of children in which placement of intramedullary rods in long bones improves prognosis and may facilitate walking in some.[271,272] For some children, bone fragility makes independent ambulation difficult in all but the most restricted circumstances, and motorized wheelchairs provide the most mobility. Growth in these children is limited, and adult height between 3 ft and 4 ft 6 in. is common. Because of the bone fragility and deformity, many of these children develop significant kyphoscoliosis and may progress to pulmonary insufficiency. Sclerae are often pale blue at birth and become nearly normal by puberty. DI is common; the frequency of hearing loss is not known. No medical therapy reliably decreases fracture frequency or increases growth and bone density.[273]

Initially described as an autosomal recessive condition, the OI type III phenotype is genetically heterogeneous. The autosomal recessive phenotype is the unusual form in most populations but among South African blacks, it may be the most common form of OI. In families of most children with the severe deforming varieties of OI, recurrence is rare, which suggests that while there may be some recessive families, in others the condition probably results from new dominant mutations. This has been confirmed in some families by birth of affected children to affected individuals and by biochemical studies (see below).

Treatment and Prenatal Diagnosis. The clinical treatment of children and adults with OI type III represents the most difficult challenge to physicians and others caring for individuals with OI. The primary objectives of therapy should always be to provide an affected individual with the maximum likelihood of enjoying a satisfying and productive life. The major complications are markedly short stature, severe bone fragility and deformity, and severe progressive scoliosis, which may result in life-threatening cardiopulmonary decompensation. The bone fractures and deformity can be managed by a combination of splinting, usual orthopedic treatment of fractures, and intramedullary rodding to provide anatomic positioning of extremities. Because of fragility, independent ambulation may be beyond the capabilities of some affected individuals. If that is the case, then efforts to provide mobility within the home and independence outside the home should be the thrust of therapy. Scoliosis may be difficult to treat because of the compliant nature of bones of the ribs and their deformation with external bracing. In some instances surgical intervention can ameliorate scoliosis, while in others it is of little long-term benefit.

Prenatal diagnosis of OI type III by ultrasound examination of fetuses during the second trimester has been documented.[274,275] If the specific biochemical defect is known in an individual hoping to have children (in the case of the dominantly inherited forms) or in a child in a family seeking to have additional children (with recessively inherited forms or with dominantly inherited forms), the mutations can be detected in collagens synthesized by chorionic villus cells or in the DNA isolated from the tissue directly. If families so choose, prenatal diagnosis by direct analysis of gene structure or by analysis of collagen synthesized by cultured cells can be achieved within 2 to 3 weeks of CVS. Because ultrasound diagnosis may not be feasible until considerably later (20 to 22 weeks), direct diagnosis is probably preferable when it is known that the mutation or the effects of the mutation can be detected.

Biochemical and Molecular Genetic Studies. OI type III has been a particularly difficult disorder to characterize biochemically because in many instances cultured cells appear to synthesize only normal type I procollagen molecules. There are several plausible explanations for these findings. First, the primary mutations may occur in noncollagen proteins; second, the mutations in type I collagen genes may be difficult to detect by the screening studies normally used; and third, mutations may occur in collagen genes other than those that encode the chains of type I collagen. It is likely that all these explanations are correct.

Autosomal Recessive OI Type III. The molecular basis of recessively inherited OI type III has been determined in only one family. The proband was born to phenotypically normal first-cousin parents and recognized to have OI at birth. He had marked bone fragility, short stature, decreased calvarial mineralization, and moderate bone deformity that increased as he grew older.[276,277] Type I collagen isolated from the skin of the proband was comprised solely of α1(I) chains. Cells cultured from the child secreted type I procollagen molecules that contained only proα1(I) chains; the cells synthesized proα2(I) chains that were not incorporated into procollagen molecules.[278,279] Both COL1A2 alleles contained the same 4-bp deletion near the end of the exon that encodes the C-terminal end of the proα2(I) chain.[280,281] The frameshift changed the sequence of the final 33 residues of the chain. In addition to changing the composition, this mutation resulted in the loss of a cysteine in C-terminal propeptide position 245 that normally bonds with a cysteine at position 80 to stabilize the structure of the peptide. The change in sequence and the presumed change in tertiary structure of the C-terminal propeptide extension of the proα2(I) chain alters the ability of the chain to be recognized and incorporated in a type I procollagen mollecule. Although formation of proα1(I) homotrimers is less favored than that of heterotrimers that contain proα1(I) and proα2(I) chains, in the absence of the normal proα2(I) chains, the homotrimers form. The chains in these molecules are overmodified along their entire length, although their thermal stability is normal, and they are secreted more slowly than the normal type I procollagen. About two-thirds the normal amount of type I procollagen would be synthesized and secreted, if the stability of the molecules is normal. It is not clear if the relatively severe phenotype results from the presence in the matrix of molecules that are overmodified, the absence of the α2(I) chain, or the presence of only abnormal molecules. This mutation was surprising in demonstrating that the absence of α2(I) chains in type I collagen can be tolerated.

Autosomal Dominant OI Type III. The OI type III phenotype can result from mutations in both COL1A1 and COL1A2 genes. The first evidence of alterations in type I collagen leading to the phenotype came from studies of skin and bone collagen from an infant who died within 2 months of birth and had a radiologic phenotype compatible with OI type III.[282] Protease digestion of collagen isolated from skin and bone cleaved about 120 residues from the N-terminal end of the triple helix of some of the α1(I) chains. Such instability probably resulted from a mutation that destabilized the triple-helical domain of the type I collagen in that region.

Like most infants with OI type II, individuals with OI type III have mutations that result in the substitution of individual glycine residues within the triple-helical domain of either the proα1(I) or proα2(I) chains of type I procollagen. Only a relatively small number of mutations that produce OI type III have been characterized (see Fig. 134-6). In the COL1A1 gene, these mutations include G844S,[283] G526C,[194] and two examples of G154R.[239] In the COL1A2 gene, the G259C mutation[284,285] produces the OI type III phenotype. In all these instances, molecules that contained one or two abnormal proα chains were assembled and secreted (albeit less efficiently than normal molecules) but were less stable than the normal molecules synthesized and were overmodified N-terminal to the site of the mutation.

Osteogenesis Imperfecta Type IV

Genetics and Natural History. OI type IV is a dominantly inherited disorder characterized by normal or grayish sclerae, mild to moderate deformity, and variable stature, which may be short[286] (Fig. 134-10). DI is common, but hearing loss may affect fewer than half of the affected individuals; when present, both features are familial, like the stature of affected individuals, although they may vary considerably in expression. Some infants with OI type IV have fractures and deformity at birth while others have only mild to moderate femoral bowing. Birth length is usually normal, but by the age of 2 years height may be at or below the 25th percentile (frequently below the 10th percentile), and growth is generally along the lower percentile tracks thereafter. As in the other forms of OI, fracture frequency decreases at the time of puberty only to increase in the older age group, especially postmenopausal women. Progressive scoliosis is seen in about a third of individuals with OI type IV and may compromise pulmonary function if severe.

Although thought to be rare initially,[165] OI type IV may be one of the more common varieties of OI.[287] Both sporadically affected individuals and large families are seen, and there is significant intrafamilial and interfamilial variation. The intrafamilial variation probably results from variation in the genetic background on which the primary mutation is expressed, although none of the other genes that account for the variability have yet been identified, and the interfamilial variation represents molecular heterogeneity within the phenotype. The intrafamilial variability can be striking (such that it may be difficult to decide whether the family is most appropriately classified on clinical grounds as OI type III, OI type IV, or OI type I). My colleagues and I and others have identified three families in which affected parents with OI type IV have had children with a lethal OI phenotype as a consequence of parental mosaicism for the lethal mutation. Such extreme variability is rare but must be considered in counseling.

Treatment and Prenatal Diagnosis. The objectives of treatment of the complications of OI type IV are to provide maximum independence and mobility. The major complications of DI (fracture and excessive wear of very fragile teeth) can be treated by capping teeth with more solid materials. Advances in the use of hard polymers to coat and shape teeth suggest that treatment of DI may be facilitated by such agents. Hearing loss can be managed initially by

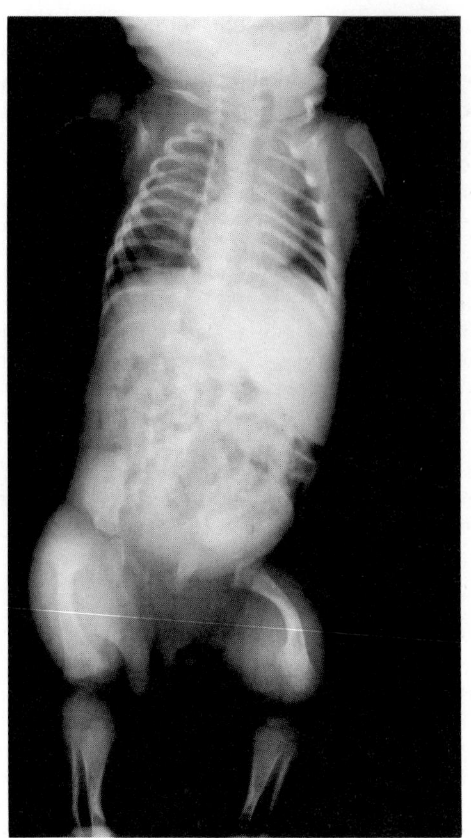

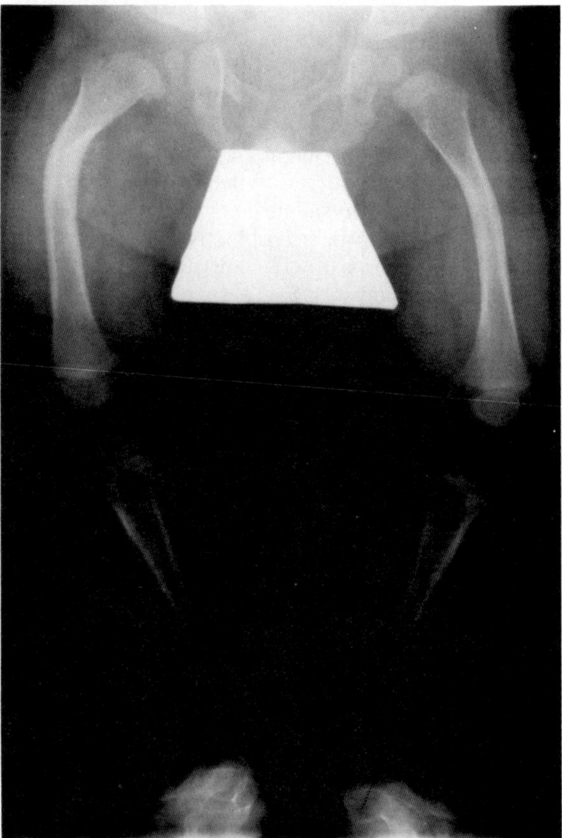

FIG. Fig. 134-10 **Radiographic features of OI type IV in the newborn period (*A*) and at 8 months (*B*). The most notable feature is the bowing of femurs, which gradually lessens during the first year.** ***(This patient is described in detail by Wenstrup et al.,*** **Hum Genet** ***74:47, 1986. X-ray films courtesy of Dr. Alasdair Hunter, Ottawa.)***

aids, but frequently requires surgery to replace the ossicular structures.

Prenatal diagnosis by linkage in the dominant families has been reported using DNA obtained by CVS biopsy to exclude the presence of the mutant allele.[288] Analysis of the collagens synthesized by the mesenchymal cells grown from the biopsy can provide similarly useful information and would be useful in small families in which the linkage phase cannot be determined and for sporadic individuals who wish to have unaffected children.

Biochemical and Molecular Genetic Studies. OI type IV was the first of the OI phenotypes to be studied by linkage analysis, and the initial studies demonstrated that the phenotype usually resulted from mutations in or near the COL1A2 gene.[289] Subsequently linkage heterogeneity was recognized within the dominant OI phenotypes.[290] Although OI type IV was usually linked to COL1A2 polymorphic markers and OI type I to COL1A1, there are some OI type IV families in which linkage to COL1A1 is found and, conversely, some OI type I families in which linkage to COL1A2 is seen. Unfortunately, the clinical phenotypes of these families are not clearly presented in some studies, and the differentiation of the two phenotypes may rest solely on the presence of minor features (subtlety of scleral hue) rather than major features of bone deformity and stature.

Linkage studies have been used to guide biochemical and molecular genetic studies in some families with OI type IV. In the first family in which linkage to COL1A2 could be demonstrated, cells from affected individuals synthesized and secreted normal type I procollagen and synthesized a population of molecules that was retained within cells.[291] These molecules became overmodified asymmetrically within the triple-helical domain and were then degraded. The retained molecules contained a proα2(I) chain that carried a small deletion (10 to 20 amino acids) from the triple-helical domain. Molecules that contained the abnormal chain had a markedly lowered thermal stability. The precise nature of the deletion has not been determined. Although difficult to detect, it seems likely either that the cells secrete some of the abnormal molecules or that the intracellular accumulation affects the manner in which the cell facilitates fibril formation.

In an additional family with OI type IV, cells from the affected members synthesized and secreted normal type I procollagen molecules and molecules that were overmodified along the entire length of the triple helix. The abnormal molecules incorporated a proα2(I) chain that, as the result of a single nucleotide change, substituted glycine 1012 (the last of the triple-helical glycine residues) by arginine.[292] Subsequently, three families have been identified in which the appearance of cysteine within the triple-helical domain of the α2(I) chain (from which it is normally excluded) results in the OI type IV phenotype.[285] Because the molecules that contain the abnormal α2(I) chains are overmodified along a portion of their length, it is likely that the residue substitutes for a glycine. There is marked clinical variation within these families, in one of which an affected male fathered two children with a lethal phenotype.[211]

The linkage heterogeneity identified in OI type IV is reflected in the biochemical studies. For example, at least three families have been identified in which the appearance of cysteine in the triple-helical domain of α1(I), between residues 123 and 400 of the triple helix, leads to a phenotype compatible with OI type IV[293] (and Byers PH: unpublished data).

Other Forms of Osteogenesis Imperfecta

The Sillence classification does not adequately describe all individuals with OI, a point that has become increasingly clear with the sophisticated biochemical and molecular genetic studies done to identify the molecular basis for brittle bone diseases. For example, in one family, affected individuals presented with clinical findings that represent a combination of features of OI and EDS.[294] The absence of amino acid residues encoded by exon 11 from about half the proα2(I) chains synthesized, as a result of a 19-bp deletion that removes a splice junction, appears to account for some of the phenotypic findings.[295] The mutation removes one of the lysyl residues involved in intermolecular crosslink formation: affects the structure of the N-terminal end of the triple helix, where interaction with matrix mineralizing elements may occur; and changes the organization of the N-terminal propeptidase cleavage site.[296] Thus, a small deletion of protein sequence affects multiple functions of the molecule, and the clinical phenotype that results reflects, to some extent, the disruption of several functional domains of the type I procollagen molecule.

Other clinical phenotypes that share similarities to OI include the osteoporosis-glioma syndrome[297-299] (which has been described as a variant of OI), juvenile osteoporosis,[300] and maturity-onset osteoporosis. In each instance, these disorders are characterized by marked osteopenia of unknown cause. There are no biochemical studies that provide clues about the nature of the mutations that result in these conditions.

Isolated DI is genetically distinct from the DI that accompanies some forms of OI.[301] Linkage studies have confirmed that the mutant gene is in close proximity to the Gc locus on chromosome 4,[302] a region devoid of known fibrillar collagen genes. Teeth from individuals with isolated DI have been shown to lack a glycoprotein in dentin.[303] Although the molecular mechanism by which DI is produced is not known, identification of a candidate protein distinct from a collagen suggests that mutations that affect the interaction of the two proteins could result in the phenotype. Thus, mutations that alter collagen structure may produce OI and DI, while mutations that affect the glycoprotein could produce DI but not interfere with other functions of the collagen molecule.

Animal Models. Three naturally occurring animals models of OI are known and, in addition, experiments in transgenic mice and in mice homozygous for retroviral inserts in genomic DNA have demonstrated two further mechanisms for the production of OI in animals.

Two herds of cattle, one first isolated in Australia[304] and a second identified in New Zealand (Thompson K: personal communication), produced calves with a severe form of OI that was lethal in the first few weeks of life. In each herd it was clear that the affected animals were sired by a single bull (i.e., one bull in each herd). In the Australian herd about 45 percent of calves born as a result of insemination of cows with sperm from the progenitor bull had OI, although the bull was phenotypically normal. Outbreeding to different herds confirmed that there was not a high-frequency recessive allele that gave rise to the phenotype and indicated clearly that the bull was mosaic in the germ line for the mutation. Analysis of bone collagen from one of the calves[305] was compatible with the mutation being in a collagen gene because of the presence of normal collagen molecules and collagen molecules that were overmodified; the presence of the two populations of molecules was also consistent with heterozygosity for a mutation in a collagen gene. No molecular genetic studies have been published. In the second herd there were also multiple recurrences of the moderately severe phenotype among calves sired by a single phenotypically normal bull. No biochemical studies have yet been completed.

A recessively inherited form of OI in mice has been known for some time, and the underlying mutation has been characterized.[306] In those animals the insertion of a single T near the end of the coding region of the COL1A2 gene results in a frameshift, and alteration of the sequence of the chain nears the C-terminal end. Although synthesized, the abnormal chain cannot be incorporated into molecules resulting in secretion of molecules that contain only proα1(I) chains. This mouse does provide a model for the very similar human variant of OI and provides animals in which to test a variety of therapies.

A strain of mice has been created in which a retrovirus fortuitously inserted itself into the first intron of one COL1A1 allele.[307,308] Mice heterozygous for the insertion, known as the Mov13 mutation, are apparently asymptomatic, although tissues contain about half the normal amount of COL1A1 mRNA. Embryos homozygous for the insertion die at about 12 days' gestation from rupture of the heart and arterial vessels.[309] Tissues contain no demonstrable type I collagen, and it has been surmised that death results from mechanical failure of the organs. Attempts to rescue the homozygous embryos by insertion of the normal COL1A1 mouse gene into fertilized eggs has not yet proved successful. Transfection of the normal COL1A1 gene into cells grown from the embryos homozygous for the Mov13 mutation rescues proα2(I) chains, which are otherwise rapidly degraded following synthesis.[310] Transfection of Mov13 cells with a gene that contained a point mutation that resulted in substitution for a single glycine resulted in rescue of proα2(I) chains but overmodification of all the molecules synthesized.[311]

An additional transgenic mouse model of OI has been created by insertion of a COL1A1 "minigene" in which a substantial portion of the triple-helical domain was excised.[312] Because some molecules are synthesized that contain the abnormal chain, this mouse may serve to test reagents that alter the production of the abnormal chain or modify the effect of incorporation of the abnormal molecules into fibrils.

Translation of Mutation to Phenotype. The phenotypic consequences of mutations in type I collagen genes reflect the gene in which the mutation occurred, the nature and location of the mutation, and its effect on the behavior of the abnormal chain and molecules that contain it. Sykes[313] proposed that mutations could be considered in two major categories, those that resulted in exclusion of the product of the mutant allele from the mature molecule (i.e., "excluded mutations") and those that permitted the incorporation of a structurally abnormal chain ("included mutations"). Heterozygosity for such mutations would be expected to have different consequences than homozygosity.

Excluded mutations can be thought of in two ways: as failure to synthesize the product of an allele and as failure of the synthesized chain to be incorporated into the protein. Both appear to result in mild phenotypes in the heterozygote and are generally found in individuals with the OI type I phenotype[313] (see Fig. 134-5). In the homozygote, such mutations appear to be lethal in the case of COL1A1[314] but only moderately severe in the case of COL1A2.[277] Very few of the "excluded" mutations identified have yet been characterized at the molecular level. Because the expression of the abnormal (or null) allele may be low, the mutations must be identified at the genomic DNA level, a still difficult task with genes that encompass 18 kb and 38 kb, and have more than 50 exons apiece. Nonetheless, the phenotypic effects of having too little collagen in bone are apparently far milder than those resulting from the presence of molecules that contain abnormal chains.

The effects on tissue strength of decreased production of type I procollagen are not well understood. In the mouse there is a marked decrease in bone strength, compatible with a tissue that has decreased amounts of type I collagen.[315] It is not clear, however, that a decreased mass of collagen is the only effect. The striking morphology of collagen fibrils in skin of individuals with OI type I, similar to those seen in skin from people with EDS type I,[316] suggests that altered ratios of the major components of the matrix may contribute to abnormal tensile strength. Thus, even the simplest of mutations is likely to have complex effects on extracellular matrix, forcing us to recognize the interrelationships of the numerous macromolecules in the tissue.

On the whole, the phenotypic effects of mutations that result in the generation of abnormal type I procollagen molecules are more deleterious than those of "null" mutations. There is, however, an enormous range in the clinical presentation of these mutations, which appears to reflect the gene (chain) in which the mutation occurs, the nature of the mutation, the location of the abnormal sequence in the protein, and the effects of the mutation on the behavior of the chain and of the mature molecule into which it is incorporated.

If an abnormal chain leads to very rapid intracellular degradation of molecules that incorporate the chain, the clinical consequences should differ depending on the gene in which the mutation occurs. Mutations in the COL1A1 gene may be highly deleterious, and even lethal, because the abnormal chain will be found in three-fourths of all the type I procollagen molecules synthesized; half of all molecules will contain one abnormal proα1(I) chain and one-fourth will contain two abnormal proα1(I) chains (see Fig. 134-5). In contrast, a similar mutation in the COL1A2 gene would result in the loss of only half the molecules made and so might be similar in effect to a null COL1A1 allele; that is, only half the normal amount of type I procollagen molecules would be completed in each case. If none of the abnormal protein is secreted but is not rapidly degraded, the effects of intracellular accumulation of these proteins cannot be overlooked; the effects on hepatic function of stored abnormal α_1AT presents just such an example (see Chap. 138).

The effects of mutations reflect the domain of the procollagen molecule in which they occur and, within that domain, the way in which the specific mutation alters function. For point mutations in the COL1A1 gene that result in the substitution of glycine residues within the triple-helical domain of the chain, there is a broad "phenotypic gradient" such that defects near the C-terminal end are generally more severe than those near the N-terminal end of the chain (see Fig. 134-6). This gradient is modified by the nature of the substituting amino acid, so that some may be lethal along the entire domain (e.g., aspartic acid) while others may have a lethal to nonlethal transition in the C-terminal half of the chain (e.g., cysteine).

Point mutations that substitute for glycine residues have several effects on the protein. First, almost all molecules that contain chains with mutations in the triple-helical domains are less stable than their normal counterparts (i.e., they display a reduced thermal stability). Second, the molecules that result are asymmetric in that they fold normally to the site of the mutant sequence and then appear either to fold slowly or to form a subtly different triple-helical structure N-terminal to it. Third, as a result of the change in structure or in the rate of propagation of the triple helix, the chains in the molecules remain accessible to the posttranslationally modifying enzymes and undergo additional hydroxylation of lysyl residues in the triple helix and additional hydroxylysyl glycosylation, further accentuating the asymmetric character of the molecules. Fourth, these molecules often have a long residence time in the RER, where increased posttranslational modification occurs. The dilation of the RER, which in some instances may be striking, could alter the architecture of the cell to distort other functions of the cell, including (but not limited to) secretion of other proteins and activation of the intracellular response to stress. Fifth, the N-terminal propeptide of the abnormal molecules that are secreted may not be cleaved as efficiently as those from the normal molecules[317,318] with the result that partially processed molecules can interfere with the normal fibril nucleation and growth. Sixth, abnormal fibrils are probably poor substrates for mineralization. Finally, the relative tissue specificity of the effects of these mutations in type I collagen genes may reflect more stringent requirements of bone than skin and other soft tissues for aspects of molecular structure that can be altered by helix-altering mutations.

Point mutations and deletions (large or small) affect the processing of molecules in much the same way. N-terminal to the mutant sequence, all the chains of molecules that contain a shortened abnormal chain are overmodified. This finding provided some of the most convincing evidence that the triple helix must be stabilized by forces beyond those conventionally considered to be important and that charge interactions, and possibly hydrophobic interactions, might be significant. Also, such findings suggested that a registration shift in the triple-helical domain of molecules with, for example, chains that have substitutions of single glycine residues could explain the apparently slower propagation of the abnormal structure along the full length of the triple helix. Other models, which propose a more local disturbance in structure[319] would be more compatible with a model in which the mutation produces a delay in folding the triple helix to account for prolonged accessibility of modifying enzymes. It is likely that different mutations have different effects on molecular assembly that can be identified only by more detailed experimental study.

EHLERS-DANLOS SYNDROME

The Ehlers-Danlos syndrome (EDS) is a heterogeneous group of generalized connective-tissue disorders, the major manifestations of which are skin fragility, skin hyperextensibility, and joint hypermobility[320,321] (Table 134-5). During the past several years genetic and biochemical studies have defined more than 10 types of EDS, and the molecular bases of several of them have been identified. It is important to identify correctly the type of EDS with which a patient is affected, because the natural history and mode of inheritance differ among the types. For example, EDS type IV is often complicated by bowel and arterial rupture leading to a shortened life expectancy, while most other types are generally more benign. Unfortunately, much of the older literature does not differentiate among the types clearly, and the complications of EDS type IV often are cited as characteristic of the syndrome as a whole.

This group of disorders has been recognized for many years, but the first formal medical descriptions appeared near the turn of the century.[322-324] The early reports concentrated on the unusual features of the skin and on ocular abnormalities. The heterogeneity began to be appreciated about 30 years ago, and the modern classification was developed by Barabas,[325] extended by Beighton[326] in the late 1960s on the basis of analysis of patients with these phenotypes and then later amplified wiith the insights provided by biochemical and molecular genetic studies. On clinical and genetic grounds, Beighton identified five separate types of EDS. Subsequent biochemical studies identified a sixth[154] and seventh type,[97] and further clinical and biochemical studies identified additional families with diverse findings prompting the expansion of the syndrome.

EDS type VI was the first of the human disorders for which the abnormalities of collagen molecules were identified[154] and is one of the few known in which the defect is in the posttranslational modification of the collagen molecules.

Ehlers-Danlos Syndrome Type I (Gravis Variety), Ehlers-Danlos Syndrome Type II (Mitis Variety), and Ehlers-Danlos Syndrome Type III (Familial Hypermobility)

Clinical Presentations, Genetics, and Natural History. EDS type I is inherited in an autosomal dominant fashion, and affected individuals have markedly soft, velvety hyperextensible skin; impressive joint hypermobility; easy bruising; and formation of thin, atrophic, "cigarette-paper" scars following trauma (Fig. 134-11). Trauma often results in gaping wounds that bleed less than expected. Areas of repeated trauma (elbows, knees, and shins) generally have pigment deposition in addition to scarring. Molluscoid pseudotumors, small accumulations of connective tissue, form in the skin, and some individuals have palpable subcutaneous calcified nodules. Varicose veins are common. As many as half the infants with EDS type I are born 4 to 8 weeks prematurely,[327] usually because of premature rupture of the membranes. The diagnosis of EDS type I can be made in newborns but more often is not considered until children begin to crawl and stand. At that time joint hypermobility may become apparent and lead to concern about delay in motor development in some children because of a delay in walking. Early trauma from falling characteristically leads to scars on the forehead, shins, knees, elbows, and the undersurface of the chin. Because of repeated trauma, easy bruising, and skin fragility, the families of children with EDS type I (and several other forms of EDS and OI) may be evaluated by social service agencies for evidence of child abuse. Many individuals with EDS type I have evidence of mitral prolapse and a few may be symptomatic.[328] Structural cardiac defects are probably not more common than in the general population. Scoliosis is uncommon and usually limited to the lumbar spine. The increased joint mobility is often associated with early degenerative joint disease, apparently because of the alteration in the joint mechanics, the most effective therapy for which is non-weight-bearing exercises and mild antiinflammatory agents.

Surgery in individuals with EDS type I may be complicated by increases in tissue friability and bleeding. Sutures should be left in about twice as long as usual to facilitate

Table 134-5 Ehlers-Danlos Syndrome

Type	Clinical Features	Inheritance	Biochemical Defect
I: Gravis	Soft, velvety, hyperextensible skin; easy bruising; "cigarette paper" scars; hypermobile joints; varicose veins; prematurity	AD	Not known
II A: Mitis	Similar to EDS type I but less severe	AD	Not known
B: Recessive	Similar phenotype; aortic dilatation	(AR, rare)	COL1A2 "null" alleles
III: Familial hypermobility	Soft skin, no scarring, marked large and small joint hypermobility	AD	Not known
IV: Arterial	Thin, translucent skin with visible veins; marked bruising; skin and joints have normal extensibility; arterial, bowel, and uterine rupture	AD	Mutations in the COL3A1 gene that affect type III procollagen synthesis, secretion, or structure
V: X-linked	Similar to EDS type II	XLR	Not known
VI: Ocular	Soft, velvety, hyperextensible skin; hypermobile joints, scoliosis; ocular fragility and keratoconus	AR	Lysyl hydroxylase deficiency due to mutation in the LOH gene
VII: A and B Arthrochalasis multiplex congenita	Congenital hip dislocation, joint hypermobility; soft skin with normal scarring	AD	A: COL1A1 exon 6 skipping mutation that deletes N-proteinase cleavage site B: COL1A2 exon 6 skipping mutation that deletes N-proteinase cleavage site
C: Dermatosparaxis	Very soft, fragile skin; excessive bruising; umbilical hernia; marked joint laxity	AR	C: N-proteinase deficiency
VIII: Periodontal	Generalized periodontitis; skin similar to EDS type II	AD	Not known
IX: X-linked cutis laxa, occipital horn syndrome	Soft, extensible, lax skin; bladder diverticulae and rupture; short arms, limited pronation and supination, broad clavicles, occipital horns	XLR	Copper utilization defect with abnormal copper enzymes, particularly lysyl oxidase; allelic to Menkes syndrome
X: Fibronectin defect	Similar to EDS type II	AR	Defects in fibronectin

AD = autosomal dominant; AR = autosomal recessive; XLR = X-linked recessive.

healing and decrease the likelihood of abnormal scar formation. The precise incidence of EDS type I is not known; estimates are on the order of 1 per 20,000. The life expectancy for individuals with EDS type I is normal.

EDS type II, also a dominantly inherited disorder, is characterized by joint laxity and by soft, hyperextensible, fragile skin. The phenotypic presentation is generally less severe than in EDS type I; prematurity is rare, varicose veins are less frequent, and the skin fragility is less. Mitral-valve prolapse is common, and premature degenerative arthritis develops in some individuals with EDS type II. The biochemical basis of this disorder is not understood, but the morphologic alterations in dermal collagen fibers and fibrils are similar to those seen in EDS type I. It is not clear whether EDS types I and II are allelic mutations or mutations in different genes (for example, mutations in COL1A1 and COL1A2 that interfere with C-terminal propeptide cleavage). Linkage studies and additional biochemical investigations will be necessary before the molecular basis of these disorders can be elucidated.

EDS type III is a dominantly inherited disorder characterized by marked joint hypermobility, recurrent joint dislocation, and soft but not hyperextensible or fragile skin. Affected infants may be slow to walk because of joint laxity. The major complications of EDS type III are recurrent joint dislocation, which may require surgery for stabilization, and early-onset degenerative joint disease. Mitral-valve prolapse is frequently seen. EDS type III is probably the most common type of EDS but precise figures are lacking and discrimination from variants of normal is often difficult.

Treatment. There is no specific therapy for these three types of EDS. Dietary supplementation with ascorbic acid has been recommended with anecdotal reports of decreased bruising and a trend toward normalization of joint hypermobility. However, because joint mobility usually decreases with age, these reports are difficult to evaluate.

The major differential diagnosis for EDS types I and II includes EDS types V, VI, VIII, and X (see below). EDS type III is most commonly confused with a variant of normal.

Biochemical, Genetic, and Structural Studies. The biochemical basis of EDS types I, II, and III are not known. Genetic linkage studies using polymorphic endonuclease restriction sites in COL1A1, COL1A2, and COL2A1 have excluded those genes as sites of mutations in some families.[329] Nonetheless, biomechanical studies of skin fragments are suggestive of abnormal collagen in dermis.[330] EM studies of dermis have demonstrated larger than normal collagen fibrils, frequent composite fibrils, and smaller than normal bundles[331,332] (Fig. 134-12). While these studies indicate an abnormality in the formation of the usual dermal collagen structures they do not identify the specific biochemical abnormality.

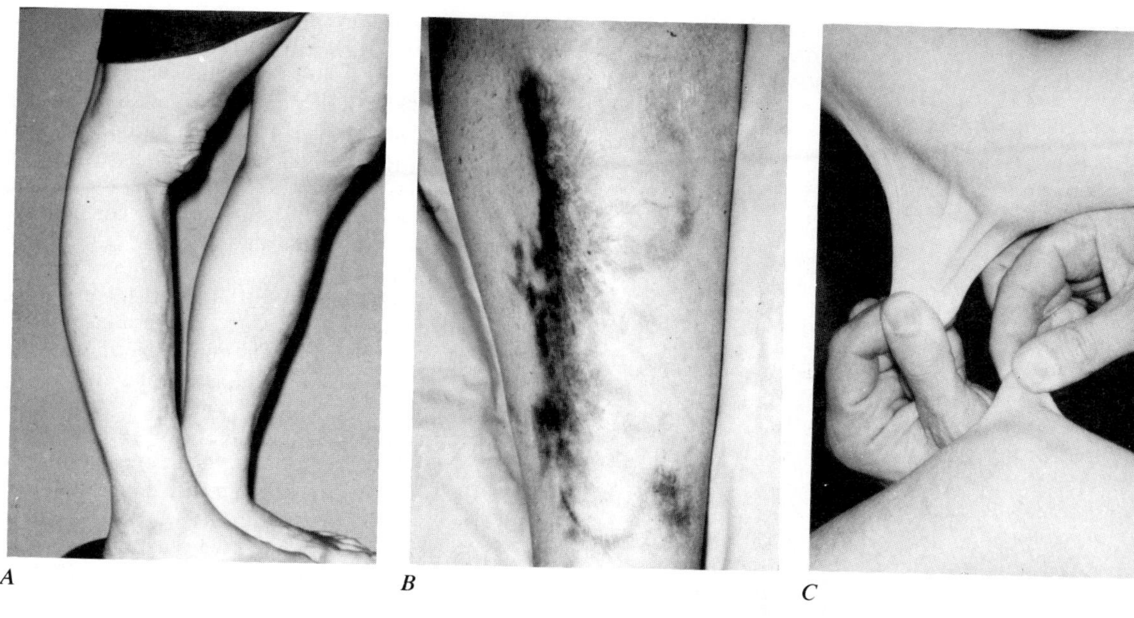

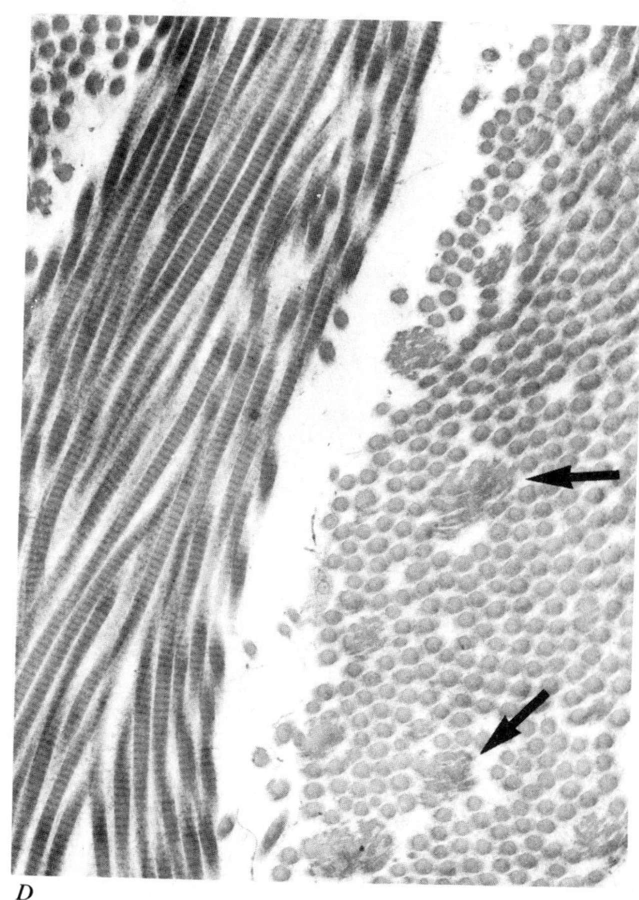

FIG. 134-11 Clinical and EM characteristics of EDS type I. *A.* Large joint hypermobility. *B.* Cigarette paper scars and pigment accumulation in areas of repeated trauma; *C.* Skin hyperextensibility (*top*) with control (*bottom*). (*From P. Bornstein and P. H. Byers, Collagen Metabolism, Kalamazoo, MI: Upjohn, 1980.*) *D.* Morphological appearance of collagen fibrils in skin of an individual with EDS type I. Fibrils are larger than control, and there are frequent "composite" structures (*arrows*). The morphologic appearance of collagen in skin from individuals with EDS types II, III, VI, and X is similar to that shown here. The abnormal fibrils may be seen in other conditions. (*Courtesy of Dr. Karen A. Holbrook, University of Washington.*)

Cells from one patient with EDS type I were found to have abnormalities in the biosynthesis of proteoglycans and in the conversion of type I procollagen to collagen.[333] However, it is not clear whether failure of cleavage is the result of an abnormal enzyme, a defective substrate, or biologic variation. Two patients have been described who have joint hypermobility, hyperextensible skin, and mild aortic root dilatation whose cultured dermal fibroblasts failed to synthesize proα2(I) chains, and as a result, the cells secreted proα1(I) trimers.[334] These are particularly intriguing patients because of the previous description of a child with OI type III and a similar molecular phenotype. The cells from the individuals with EDS did not synthesize any proα2(I) chains, whereas those from the boy with OI type III synthesized chains that were not incorporated into molecules. Failure to synthesize proα2(I) chains appears to be rare among individuals with EDS types I and II; the presence of aortic dilatation suggests that this clinical entity may have

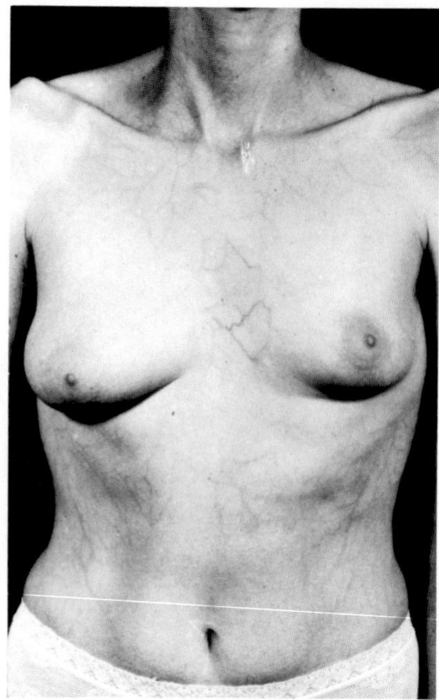

A.

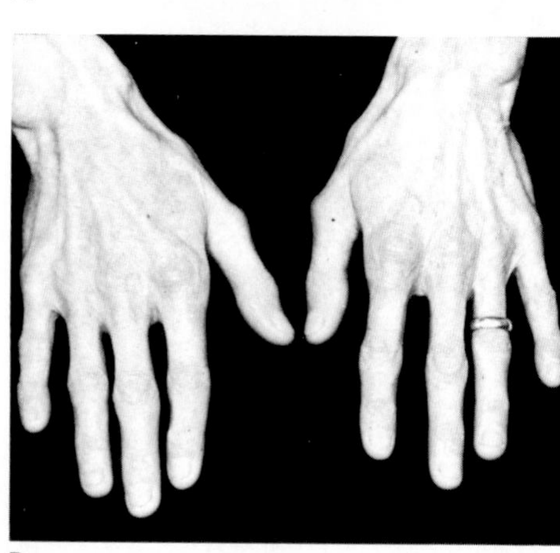

B.

FIG. 134-12 Clinical features of EDS type IV. *A.* Venous vasculature of the chest and abdomen is remarkably apparent in this 26-year-old woman with EDS type IV. *B.* Her hands have the aged appearance of acrogeria. *(From Byers et al.* Hum Genet *47:141, 1979. Used by permission of* Human Genetics.)

a different prognosis. Further, it is likely due to compound heterozygosity for mutations in the COL1A2 gene or homozygosity for mutations that lead to a null allele.

The ultrastructural appearance of dermal collagen from individuals with EDS types II and III is similar to that from patients with EDS type I. There are no biochemical or linkage studies that provide further clues to the nature of the biochemical defects in these disorders. Candidate genes might include COL12A1 because of its role in interacting with type I collagen in fibril formation.

Ehlers-Danlos Syndrome Type IV, Vascular or Ecchymotic Type

Clinical Presentation, Genetics, and Natural History. EDS type IV was recognized as a distinct entity by Barabas in 1966[327] although Sack[335] and Gottron[336] probably described the same entity a quarter of a century earlier. The biochemical basis of the disorder was first recognized in 1975.[337] This is a rare form of EDS, and estimates of its prevalence range from 1 in 100,000 to less than one in 1 million.[338] The disorder is the result of heterozygosity for mutations in the COL3A1 gene, and while generally inherited in an autosomal dominant fashion,[339] it is common to encounter the first affected individuals in a family. While it has been proposed that autosomal recessive forms also exist,[340,341] these are rare, if they exist at all.

Affected individuals have thin, translucent skin through which the venous pattern over the trunk, abdomen, and extremities is visible; minimal joint hypermobility that may be limited to the small joints of the hands and feet; and marked bruising (Fig. 134-13). The skin over the face often has a parchmentlike appearance, and in some individuals there is an aged or "acrogeric" character to the hands and feet; in the older European literature some individuals with "acrogeria" probably have EDS type IV. There is an "EDS type IV facies" that is characterized by a "stare," a very thin nose, and the tight-skinned appearance.[338] Venous varicosities are frequent, may be severe, and appear at a young age. Even in families in which children are known to be at 50 percent risk, it is often difficult to make the diagnosis on clinical grounds in childhood unless bruising is severe or the venous pattern is particularly noticeable. Many individuals with EDS type IV are first thought to have disorders of coagulation because of the marked bruising.

The major clinical complications of EDS type IV are arterial rupture, spontaneous rupture of the colon, and

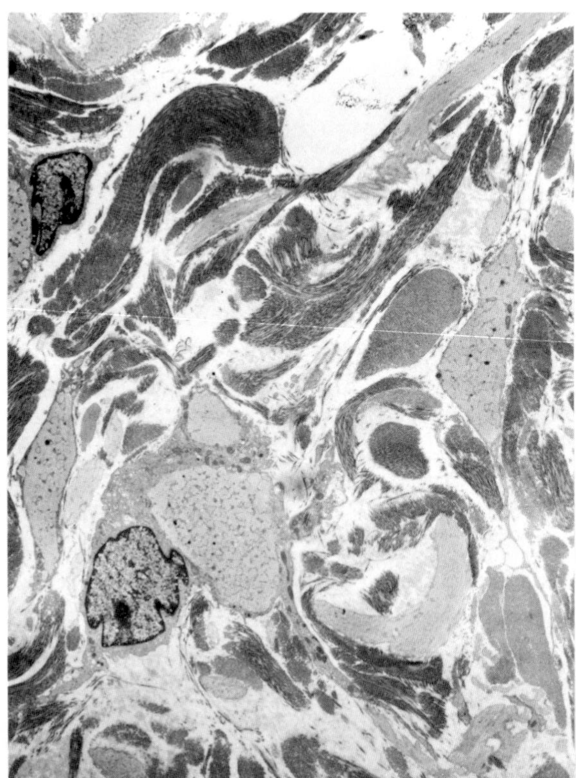

FIG. 134-13 Morphologic appearance of fibroblasts in skin of the woman with EDS type IV shown in Fig. 134-12. There is marked dilatation of the RER with a form of type III procollagen that cannot be secreted. *(Courtesy of Dr. Karen A. Holbrook, University of Washington.)*

rupture of the gravid uterus,[342,343] and some individuals may experience all three. There does not appear to be a familial predilection for gastrointestinal complications, arterial rupture, or uterine tears, and the age of first involvement may vary from late childhood to the seventh decade, although deaths from complications in the third and fourth decade are most common.

The location of arterial hemorrhage determines the presenting symptoms: stroke, intraabdominal or intrathoracic bleeding, or limb compartmental syndrome. The most common locations of arterial bleeding are in the abdominal cavity and involve the smaller arteries rather than the aorta itself. In some individuals there is evidence of aneurysm formation, while in others the vessels appear normal by angiography. Arterial rupture accounts for most deaths in EDS type IV because of its frequency, the involvement of vessels from which hemorrhage is rapid, and because of the difficulty in repairing the markedly friable tissues. Surgical repair is possible but depends on early recognition of the cause of hypotension, the ability to distinguish arterial bleeding from gastrointestinal tract rupture, and rapid and appropriate intervention.

Several individuals with EDS type IV have been described with carotid-cavernous sinus fistula formation and resultant unilateral exophthalmos.[343–348] Surgical repair or embolization has been attempted with success in some.

Rupture of the distal colon, usually in the sigmoid, is the most common of the bowel problems.[343] In some individuals it has been possible to identify diverticulae on the antimesenteric border, but in most the bowel surface appears normal. The clinical presentation of bowel rupture is similar to that in individuals without EDS type IV, and the surgical approach should be the same. Tissue friability and soiling of the peritoneal space are the major impediments to repair and rapid recovery. The degree of tissue friability differs among individuals and even in the same individual with aging. Descriptions of tissues with the physical characteristics of wet blotting paper are common surgical reports. Assiduous attention to surgical technique and lavage of the peritoneal cavity with instillation of antibiotics and parenteral antibiotic therapy frequently permit rapid recovery. Following repair, recurrence of bowel rupture has been seen in some individuals, and the likelihood of repeated episodes can be minimized by removal of the distal two-thirds of the colon.

Rupture of the small bowel is very rare but recurrent abdominal pain during childhood, adolescence, and adult life may result from mural hemorrhage. Bowel function is generally not compromised by these episodes, although occasionally regions of mural fibrosis are observed at surgery or at autopsy in individuals with EDS type IV.

Uterine rupture is a relatively rare complication of EDS type IV and generally occurs in the last 2 months of pregnancy or during labor.[342] Uterine rupture in labor is accompanied by a marked increase in abdominal pain, rapid loss of vascular volume, virtual cessation of labor, and loss of fetal heart tones. Prompt surgical intervention is the only lifesaving technique, and rapid recognition of the condition is necessary. More commonly, uterine rupture is not recognized and leads to maternal and infant death. Although infrequent, the possibility of this occurrence warrants close following of all pregnancies in women with EDS type IV and delivery in tertiary care medical centers with careful monitoring during labor. The complications of pregnancy, in addition to vascular rupture and uterine rupture, include tearing of vaginal tissues during delivery. In one series,[342] almost 20 percent of the women with EDS type IV who became pregnant died as a result of pregnancy complications. In an extension of that series, in which 137 individuals with EDS type IV were identified, 4 of the 16 deaths among women were the result of uterine rupture.[343] The absence of such complications in another series suggested that pregnancy complications may vary in frequency in different populations[349] and makes it difficult to estimate the overall frequency of pregnancy-related deaths.

Other complications of EDS type IV include keratoconus,[343,350] and periodontal disease.

The life span of individuals with EDS type IV is generally shorter than that of their unaffected sibs, with the mean age of death being in the early 30s for women and slightly older for men.[343] Deaths in the third through the fifth decades are the rule, with survival beyond 50 years of age being rare. My colleagues and I have documented the condition in a man who died at 60 during attempted coronary artery bypass surgery.

Although initially proposed to be an autosomal recessive disorder,[340] EDS type IV is inherited in an autosomal dominant fashion or appears as a *de novo* mutation in the proband. Asymptomatic parental mosaicism for the mutation has now been documented in three families, so the frequency of mosaicism is probably similar to that seen in forms of OI (see above), even though there have been no sibships with recurrence of the disorder among children born to unaffected parents.[351–353] Of the more than 80 individuals we have identified through biochemical testing, about half have had family histories compatible with EDS type IV, and the remainder are the first affected individuals in their families.[343] The range of biochemical abnormalities in the two groups is similar. Because of the autosomal dominant mode of transmission, segregation studies using polymorphic restriction sites in the COL3A1 gene, can be used to identify individuals with the affected allele and has the potential for use in prenatal diagnosis.[339] Analysis of the type III collagen synthesized and secreted by cells from chorionic villus biopsies may facilitate prenatal diagnosis in pregnancies in which linkage studies are not informative.

Treatment. When suspected, the diagnosis of EDS type IV can be confirmed by measuring the amount of type III collagen in skin or by examining the biosynthesis of type III procollagen by cultured dermal fibroblasts. The differentiation of this type of EDS from others is important because of the nature of the complications and the importance of prompt surgical intervention. It is unfortunate that the complications that characterize EDS type IV are sometimes cited in textbooks as characteristic of other types of EDS. No medical treatment is currently available to increase the production of normal type III collagen. The important elements of clinical treatment are prompt recognition of the major complications of the disorder, patient education, and clear communication between the patient and physician. We often provide patients with a letter that summarizes the important complications and urge that they carry the letter on extended travel out of their local area.

Biochemical and Ultrastructural Findings. EDS type IV results from abnormalities in the structure, synthesis, or secretion of type III procollagen. At the ultrastructural level, tissues (especially dermis and vessels) from most individuals with EDS type IV have abnormal collagen fibrils and fiber bundles.[354] The dermis is often thin, collagen fiber bundles are small, and fibril diameters are either uniformly small or characterized by marked variation.[335] Elastic fibers are abundant because of the decreased amount of collagen in the dermis. In many patients, dermal fibroblasts have dilated RER that contains the abnormal, poorly secreted type III procollagen species[355,356] (Fig. 134-14). The biochemical abnormalities are heterogeneous. Cells from some individuals in some families synthesize an apparently normal amount of type III procollagen but secrete about 10 to 15 percent of the normal amount.[357,358] The nonsecreted type III procollagen is sequestered within the RER, where it is overmodified (in a manner similar to the handling of abnormal type I procollagen molecules synthesized by cells from infants with OI type II) and very slowly degraded. There is virtual exclusion of the abnormal molecules from the extracellular space, and the abnormal molecules have a decreased thermal stability. Studies of cell strains from other individuals[359] demonstrate a marked reduction in the extracellular accumulation of type III collagen and procollagen but little accumulation of abnormal procollagen within the cells. A plausible explanation for such findings is the instability of the molecules that contain one or more mutant chains and their rapid intracellular degradation. Because type III procollagen is a homotrimer, such a mechanism would result in loss of 85 percent of the newly synthesized protein if all molecules that contained at least one mutant chain were degraded.

Molecular Genetics. EDS type IV results from point mutations that produce substitution of glycine residues within the triple-helical domain, from exon-skipping mutations within the triple-helical domain, and from mutliple-exon deletions, all within the COL3A1 gene. Substitutions for glycine at triple-helix positions 619 by arginine[360]; at 790 by serine[361-363]; at 847 or 1006 by glutamic acid[364-366]; at 833, 1003, or 1018 by aspartic acid[351,352,365,367]; and at 910 or 1000 by valine[365,368] have been reported. An additional point mutation that results in the substitution of glycine at position 136 by arginine[369] has been identified in an individual with arterial aneurysms, but additional clinical details are not available. Among mutations identified in the COL3A1 gene to date, exon-skipping events are almost as common as point mutations, in contrast to the relative infrequency of such mutations in the type I collagen genes. The reported mutations affect the efficiency of incorporation of exons 16,[370] 20,[370-372] 25,[373] 27,[374] 37,[375] 41,[376,377] and 42.[370] Small genomic deletions entirely within an exon,[378,379] and multiple-exon deletions[353,380,381] have been identified.

In contrast to multiple-exon deletions in the COL1A1 and COL1A2 genes, the phenotypic consequences of those in the COL3A1 gene are not demonstrably more severe than other types of mutations in the gene. Perhaps this lack of a more severe effect reflects the homotrimeric nature of the protein, allowing formation of "minimolecules," which, although deleterious in their presence, may be less so than molecules that are substantially overmodified. Multiple-exon deletions result in inefficient secretion of the molecules that contain both the normal and the shortened chain, and there is a decrease in thermal stability of those molecules.[382] Incubation of the cells at 30°C can increase the secretion of molecules that contain the abnormal chain for some but not all mutations.[382]

The molecular findings in EDS type IV parallel those in the several forms of OI. Because of difficulty in quantitating the synthesis and secretion of type III procollagen, it is not clear that the EDS type IV phenotype can result from mutations that result in "functional deletion" of one COL3A1 allele. In other respects, however, it is remarkable that many different types of mutations in the COL3A1 gene result in a single phenotype that exhibits little clinical variability. This contrasts with the wide range of variability seen in OI with different mutations in the COL1A1 and COl1A2 genes. It is possible that certain mutations in the COL3A1 genes are not clinically apparent early in life and lead to mild phenotypes that are difficult to ascertain or, alternatively, appear as arterial aneurysms in later life.[383]

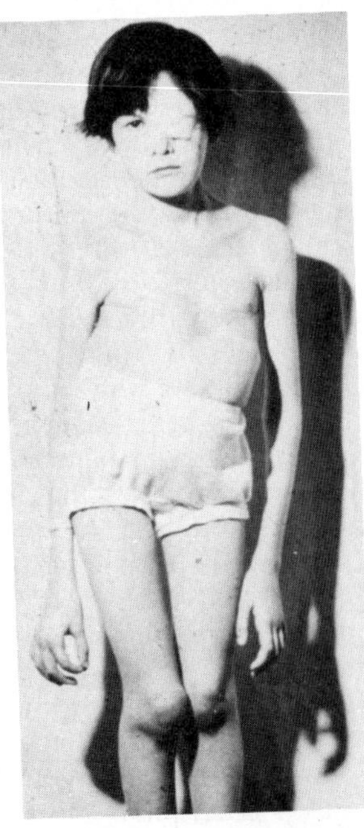

FIG. 134-14 Clinical appearance of the index patient with EDS type VI. *(Courtesy of Dr. Sheldon Pinnell, Duke University.)*

Ehlers-Danlos Syndrome Type V

Clinical Features, Genetics, and Natural History. EDS type V has been used to describe two families in which the inheritance of a phenotype clinically similar to EDS type II except that intramuscular hemorrhage is a common finding[384,385] could be explained by X-linked recessive inheritance rather than variable expression of an autosomal dominant phenotype. The original authors suggested that the disorder is rare; Steinmann et al.[386] have suggested that this entity does not currently warrant a distinct designation.

Biochemical Studies. There has been considerable confusion concerning the molecular basis of this disorder. In one family thought to have a variant of EDS type V, lysyl oxidase activity in the medium of cultured dermal fibroblasts from two of the patients was found to be decreased[387]; however, the methods used to measure the enzyme were probably not reliable. In studies of cells from members of the two original families with EDS type V, the activity of lysyl oxidase in the medium was normal.[388] Close linkage to the Xg blood group (short arm of the X chromosome) and to the loci for color blindness (long arm of the X chromosome) have both been excluded.[384]

Ehlers-Danlos Syndrome Type VI

Clinical Features, Genetics, and Natural History. Individuals with EDS type VI, an autosomal recessive condition,[154,389] often have soft, hyperextensible skin, joint hypermobility, scoliosis, ocular fragility, and a marfanoid habitus (Fig. 134-15). Microcornea and recurrent intraocular bleeding, with resultant blindness, are major features in some patients. Some children have been identified because of delay in reaching major motor milestones—the result of marked joint laxity.[390] Others have been identified by screening sporadically affected individuals with EDS for decreased amounts of hydroxylysine in skin. The disorder is uncommon, and about two dozen individuals have been identified, including some sib pairs.[154,389–397]

Because of the relatively small number of affected individuals identified so far, the natural history of the disorder is not well understood. Three major complications have been identified: severe kyphoscoliosis, which may be resistant to external bracing or surgical intervention; blindness from globe rupture or repeated retinal hemorrhage; and morbidity or death from vascular rupture.[390] Kyphoscoliosis is common among children diagnosed because of a delay in motor development, but it does not represent a universal accompaniment of the biochemical disorder. When severe, the kyphoscoliosis can lead to cardiopulmonary failure, and death has been reported in the third decade.[395] One of the index patients with EDS type VI suffered ocular globe rupture from minimal trauma[154] and retinal hemorrage and gastrointestinal hemorrhage have been known to affect others with EDS type VI. The proband in the second family identified with EDS type VI died in her sixth decade, probably as a result of intraabdominal arterial rupture.[398]

The phenotype may be genetically heterogeneous because at least one family has been identified in which two affected male sibs, with normal parents, have skin and joint manifestation of EDS and are blind from retinal hemorrhage yet both have normal levels of lysyl hydroxylation in skin collagen and have normal levels of lysyl hydroxylase enzyme in cultured cells.[399]

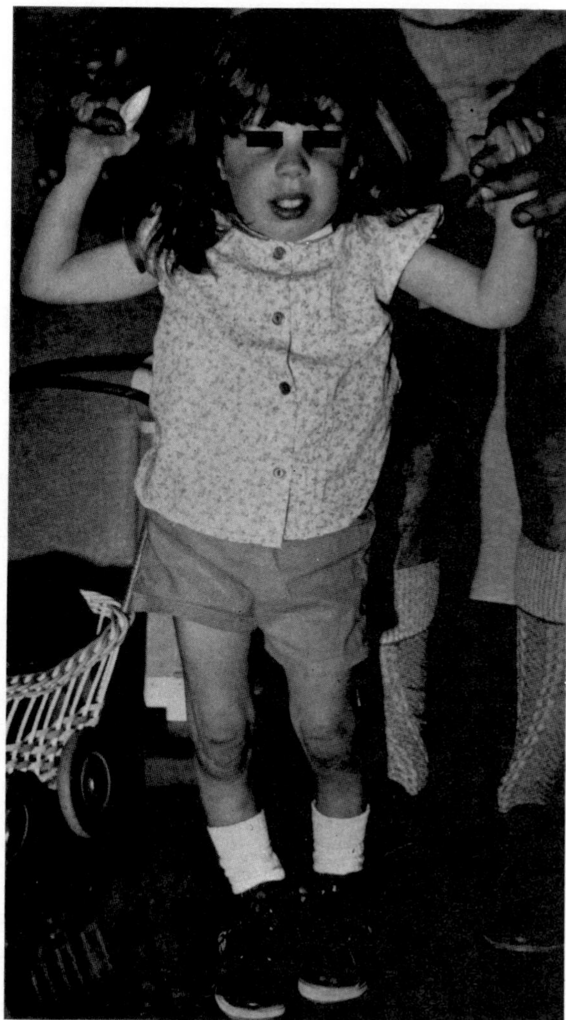

A.

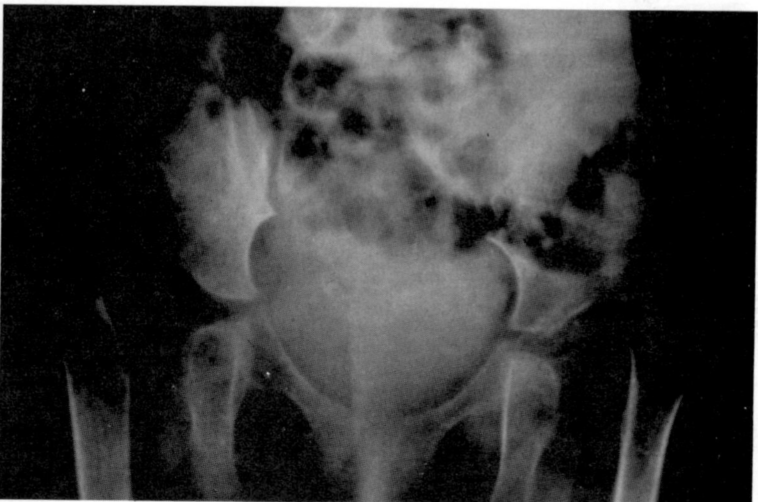

B.

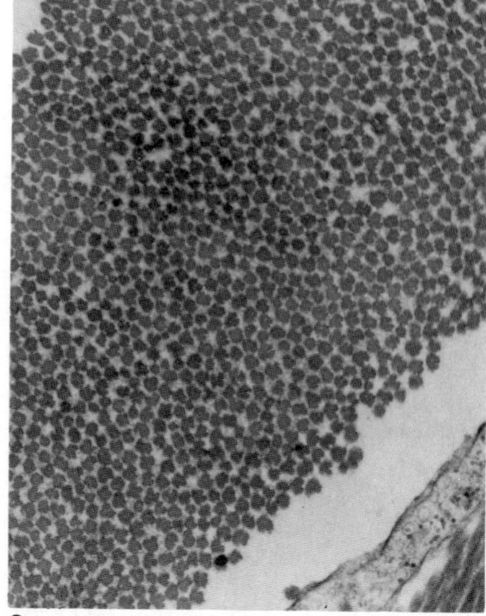

C.

FIG. 134-15 Ehlers-Danlos syndrome type VII. *A*. Clinical features of young girl with EDS type VIIA that results from heterozygous deletion of the amino acid sequences encoded by exon 6 of the COL1A1 gene; the deletion removes the N-terminal procollagen protease cleavage site. She has mild midface hypoplasia and markedly lax ligaments. *B*. Radiograph of bilateral hip dislocation. *C*. Morphologic appearance of collagen fibrils in the child's skin in which the fibrils have an irregular shape. *(Courtesy of Dr. William Cole, Royal Children's Hospital, Melbourne.)*

Clinical Treatment and Prenatal Diagnosis. Because of the apparent frequency of severe kyphoscoliosis and accompanying cardiorespiratory complications, the complications of ocular globe fragility and retinal hemorrhage, and the autosomal recessive mode of inheritance of EDS type VI, it is important that this diagnosis be considered in all sporadic individuals with a compatible phenotype (e.g., EDS type II, V, X) and that appropriate testing be undertaken. The orthopedic management of scoliosis should follow accepted orthopedic practice. The efficacy of bracing and of surgical intervention is not yet established. Routine eye examinations should be recommended because of the relatively high incidence of intraocular bleeding, globe fragility, and keratoconus. While no specific therapy has been demonstrated to be effective, the use of pharmacologic doses of ascorbic acid, a cofactor for lysyl hydroxylase, has been advocated, and an increase in urinary excretion of hydroxylysine has been found following long-term treatment with the vitamin.[392]

Prenatal diagnosis by measurement of lysyl hydroxylase enzyme activity in amniotic fluid cells has been attempted in one family at risk, and the birth of an unaffected but heterozygous infant was corrently predicted.[393] Amniotic fluid cells synthesize amounts of lysyl hydroxylase that are roughly equivalent to those synthesized by dermal fibroblasts.[393]

Biochemical Studies. The EDS type VI phenotype results from markedly decreased activity of the enzyme lysyl hydroxylase.[154] The posttranslational hydroxylation of lysyl residues in types I and III collagens in skin is markedly reduced, but that of type II collagen in cartilage is normal or near normal in tissues from affected individuals in whom it has been measured.[154,394] The residual enzyme appears to be almost normally efficient in the hydroxylation of lysyl residues in type IV collagen.[400] Alternatively, differential lysyl hydroxylation of collagen types in individuals with EDS type VI could be explained by different affinities of a single enzyme for the specific collagens or by the presence of collagen type-specific lysyl hydroxylases.

Residual enzyme activity in the cells of affected individuals ranges from virtually unmeasurable to 10 to 15 percent of normal.[401] Enzyme levels in cells from obligate heterozygotes range from about 40 to 70 percent of control levels. Levels of lysyl hydroxylation of skin collagen also vary, although in most individuals fewer than 5 percent of available hydroxylatable lysyl residues are modified.

Molecular Genetics. The range of enzyme activities in the cells from affected individuals and the range of substrate modifications in skin suggests that the disorder is heterogeneous in the nature of mutations in the enzyme. Furthermore, because consanguinity is not a common feature of families with EDS type VI, it is likely that most affected individuals are compound heterozygotes for mutations in the gene that encodes lysyl hydroxylase. In two families, apparent homozygosity for mutations is probably consistent with parental consanguinity. In one[402] there was homozygosity for a stop codon at residue 319 (R319X), and in the other[403] there was an internal duplication of 180 bp within the coding sequence of the cDNA that apparently led to a marked decrease in enzyme function.

Decreased hydroxylation of lysyl residues in type I collagen interferes with the formation of normal crosslinks among collagen molecules.[404] Although crosslinks form in the absence of lysyl hydroxylation, the lysine-derived crosslinks are not as stable as those derived from hydroxylysine and do not mature as readily to the multiple-component intermolecular links that stabilize molecular interactions at a larger scale. Presumably, the clinical phenotype results from the absence of the more complex crosslinks.

The diagnosis of EDS type VI is established by demonstration of a decreased content of hydroxylysine in dermal collagen and is confirmed by assay of lysyl hydroxylase in cultured dermal fibroblasts. It is very difficult to demonstrate a decrease in hydroxylation of lysyl residues by cultured fibroblasts, because the level of collagen hydroxylation in cultured cells is higher than that in vivo. The lack of collagen hydroxylation does not appear to affect the stability of the transport of procollagen through the cell machinery or into the extracellular space, and although the enzymes have similar substrate requirements, there is no effect on prolyl hydroxylation. The defective hydroxylation does appear to affect the normal incorporation of type I collagen into fibrils that, in skin, have the bizarre branching organization, similar to that seen in EDS type I.

Ehlers-Danlos Syndrome Type VII

Genetics and Natural History. EDS type VII is used to designate disorders in which there are defects in the conversion of type I procollagen to collagen, either because of defects in the substrate (EDS types VIIA and VIIB), or because of defects in the converting enzyme, procollagen N-protease (EDS type VIIC or dermatosparaxis).

EDS types VIIA and VIIB, also known as arthrochalasis multiplex congenita, are characterized by marked joint hypermobility, multiple joint dislocations, and congenital hip dislocation that is usually bilateral (Fig. 134-16). The hip dislocation is often difficult to reduce, even with surgery. Mild to moderate short stature is seen in some individuals in whom mild midface hypoplasia is present. The precise prevalence of the condition is not known but it is probably uncommon. Congenital hip dislocation is one of the more frequent birth defects in the general population (with an incidence of approximately 1 in 500 live births), but only a small proportion of those infants have EDS type VII. All but one of the described individuals are sporadic in the family; there are two examples of autosomal dominant inheritance,[405,406] but all the biochemical studies are entirely compatible with the disorder being the result of dominant mutations (see below).

The major complications of EDS type VIIA and VIIB are those that result from long-term instability of joints and failure to make a normal hip joint. There is insufficient follow-up of the children known to be affected to determine if the degenerative joint disease is sufficient to warrant early hip replacement. Bone fracture may be increased in some families with EDS type VIIA or VIIB.

Biochemical and Molecular Genetic Studies. Initially, EDS type VII was thought to result from abnormalities in the enzyme that cleaves the N-terminal propeptide extension from type I procollagen,[97] analogous to a recessively inherited disorder in cattle, sheep, and cats.[153,407–409] Restudy of some of the original patients and detailed study of collagens synthesized by cells from several new patients has demonstrated that, instead, the mutations involve the cleavage sites of the substrate proα1(I) and proα2(I) chains.[410–413] In all nine patients with EDS type VIIA or VIIB in which the mutation has been characterized, the mRNA from the mutant allele lacks all or most of the sequence of exon 6, the domain that encodes the cleavage site for the N-proteinase. At the

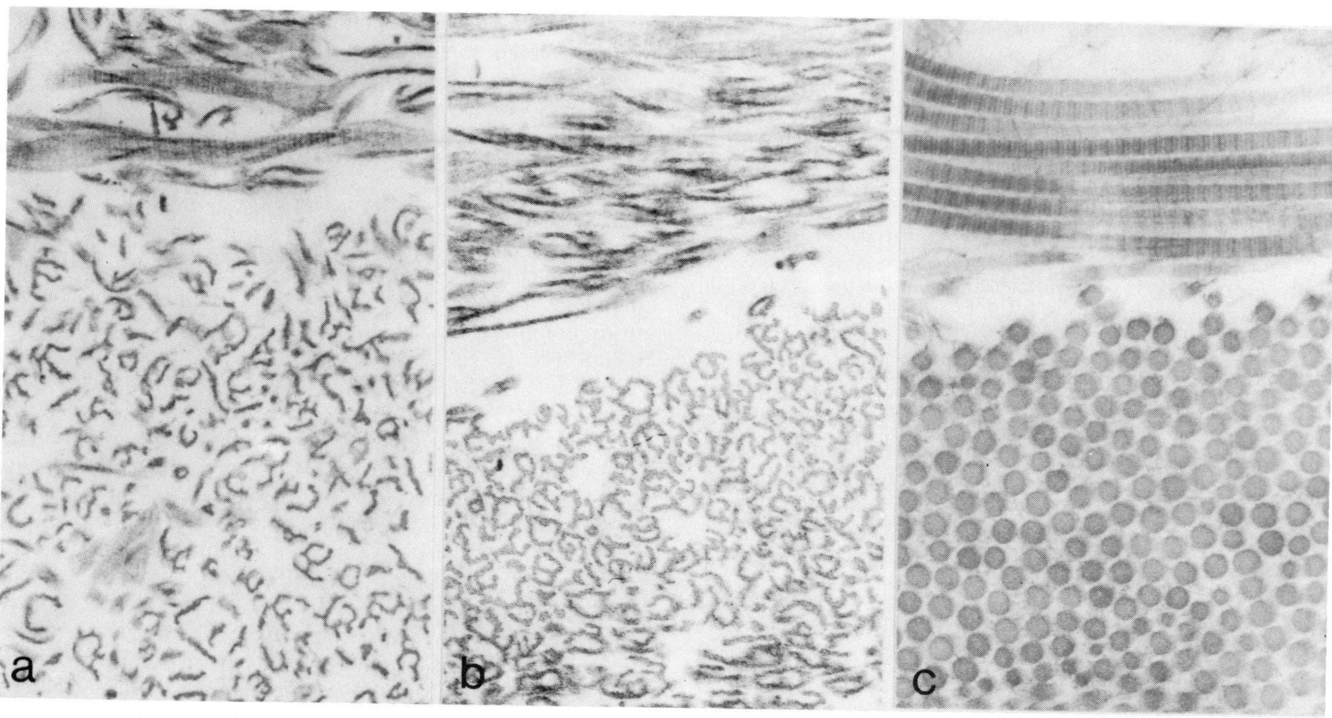

FIG. 134-16 EM of skin from two children (*a* and *b*) with EDS type VIIC. The collagen fibrils form ribbonlike structures that have a hieroglyphic character when seen in cross section, in contrast to those from the normal child (*c*). (*Reprinted from Smith et al.,* Am J Hum Genet *51:235, 1992. Used by permission.*)

genomic level, the mutations are heterogeneous, but all interfere with the normal splicing of exon 6. In six, substitutions in the consensus GT-dinucleotide of the splice-donor domain of intron 6 of the COL1A2 gene[414–418] are the cause, while in two others the mutation is in the COL1A1 gene.[419] In cultured cells it is possible to recognize a defect in the rate of conversion of procollagen to collagen and retention of molecules that contain N-terminal propeptide extensions. In general, in order to identify such an abnormality it is necessary to add agents such as polyethylene glycol or dextran sulfate to the culture medium to concentrate the procollagen and increase the normal rate of conversion.[420] The mutations that delete the exon that contains the substrate site have an anomalous effect on the protein when treated with pepsin because the deletion fuses the minor and major triple helixes and removes the pepsin-sensitive site, causing failure to cleave the chain. Deletion of the exon that encodes the N-terminal procollagen peptidase cleavage site has several effects on the molecule: it deletes the site of cleavage in one chain, it throws into disarray the N-terminal cleavage site in molecules that incorporate the abnormal chain, and it removes a lysyl residue in the telopeptide extension that is frequently hydroxylated and involved in intermolecular crosslinks. When the mutation occurs in the COL1A2 gene, there appears to be relatively little effect on fibril formation in the dermis. In contrast, a mutation in the COL1A1 gene results in formation of more irregular fibrils[421] (see Fig. 134-16). It is likely that the phenotypic effect of the mutations derives from alterations in crosslink formation and fibrillogenesis that result in decreased tensile strength of most tissues made up principally of type I collagen.

EDS Type VIIC, Dermatosparaxis. Search for the recessively inherited EDS type VIIC in humans came to fruition more than 20 years after the disorder was first identified in animals.[422–424] In the space of 2 years, three affected children have been identified. All three have a very similar clinical picture—skin fragility with easy bruising, extremely soft, doughy skin, marked joint laxity with delayed motor milestones, blue sclerae, micrognathia, large umbilical hernia, and mild hirsutism. Intellectual development is normal. One child has had a central nervous system hemorrhage. None is yet older than 3 years so the long-term prognosis is uncertain. The picture in the affected animals is one of marked skin friability, infection, and early death from sepsis, in some settings.

In skin from the affected children, there is accumulation of the precursors to type I procollagen that contain the N-terminal propeptides. Although some apparently "normal" chains are present, it is not known if the site of cleavage is correct or if alternate cleavage has occurred with another matrix protease. Cultured cells from the children fail to remove the N-terminal propeptides from either the proα1(I) or proα2(I) chains of type I procollagen, but the abnormal molecules are processed normally by normal cells.[422] Thus, although it has been suggested that the condition in cattle, dermatosparaxis, may result from a more generalized defect in processing of proteins destined for extracellular transport,[425] the N-terminal propeptidase among them, it appears that the defect in humans is the consequence of an abnormal N-proteinase alone.

Prenatal Diagnosis. Prenatal diagnosis for any form of EDS type VII has not been reported. If the mutation is known, DNA-based diagnosis is straightforward. If there is a defect that results in deletion of the sequences encoded by exon 6 of either type I collagen gene, the defect should be readily identified at the protein level in cultured chorionic villus cells, but not in amniocytes. Alternatively, in families in which the condition is inherited in an autosomal dominant fashion, segregation studies with the appropriate gene markers could be of diagnostic value. Because chorionic villus cells convert type I procollagen relatively inefficiently and may fail to cleave the majority of N-terminal propeptides, even in the presence of dextran sulfate, prenatal diagnosis of EDS type VIIC may be difficult.

Ehlers-Danlos Syndrome Type VIII

EDS type VIII is characterized by bruising, soft, and hyperextensible skin, hypermobile joints, and periodontal disease.[426,427] The disorder is inherited in an autosomal dominant fashion, and loss of teeth, as a result of marked periodontal involvement, is common by the third decade. EDS type VIII is probably uncommon; no prevalence figures are available, and only a few families have been described. No biochemical defects have been identified. Because gingival disease may occur in EDS type IV, it is important to exclude that diagnosis. Biochemical and genetic studies have suggested that EDS type VIII does not result from mutations in COL3A1.[428,429]

Ehlers-Danlos Syndrome Type IX (Occipital Horn Syndrome)

Genetics and Natural History. EDS type IX is a rare X-linked recessive disorder characterized by lax and soft skin at birth, development of bladder diverticulae during childhood that may be complicated by hydronephrosis and hydroureter (Fig. 134-17), and appearance of bony occipital horns develop during adolescence.[430–432] The bladder diverticulae may rupture, and some patients have required low-pressure drainage to maintain bladder integrity. Although the males with this disorder are of normal height, skeletal deformities, including short humeri, partial radioulnar synostosis that limits pronation and supination, and short broad clavicles are apparent on clinical and radiologic examination. Most affected males have a mild chronic diarrhea that appears to result from a defect in bowel motility, and some have orthostatic hypotension that may be symptomatic. Intellect is generally measured as normal (when reported), but some of the affected males have required educational assistance, and in at least one male moderate mental retardation was apparent.[433] Carrier females have, so far, been unaffected by any of the phenotypic manifestations of the condition. Life span is probably normal, although one of the members of the first family described died in his early 50s from complications of transitional-cell carcinoma of the bladder.[434]

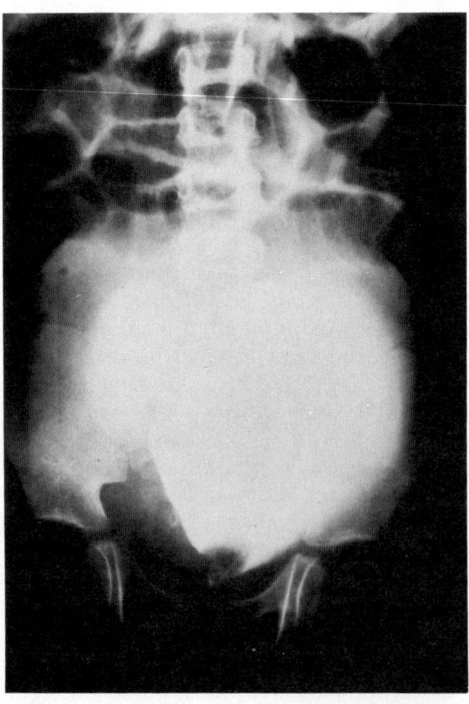

FIG. 134-17 Bladder diverticula in a 6-year-old boy with EDS type IX.

Biochemical Findings. Precise mutations in EDS type IX have not been determined, but like infants with the Menkes kinky hair syndrome, affected males have a defect in distribution of intracellular copper to the apoenzymes into which it is integrated.[435–437] Low levels of mRNA for the Menkes gene product have been found, indicating definitively that the disorders are allelic.[441] In EDS type IX, the major effect of this defect is a decrease in the activity of the copper-dependent enzyme lysyl oxidase, which catalyzes the oxidation of lysyl residues in collagen and elastin to form crosslink precursors. Cells from these patients have a normal rate of copper uptake, but have very high intracellular levels and do not permit the normal efflux of copper bound to copper enzymes. Lysyl oxidase levels and activity in extracellular fluid are extremely low, and the formation of crosslinks in collagen and elastin is correspondingly decreased. The virtually unmeasurable lysyl oxidase in tissue from some patients may reflect the marked instability of the apoenzyme in the absence of copper. No other enzymes have been measured in cells or tissues of affected individuals, but it is likely that defects in other copper-dependent enzymes will be found to account for the altered bowel motility and the orthostatic hypotension.

The diagnosis of EDS type IX is generally suspected on clinical grounds and confirmed when serum copper and ceruloplasmin levels are found to be well below the normal range.

There have been no studies on therapeutic intervention but all such studies in the Menkes syndrome, with which EDS type IX may be allelic, have been of marginal success (see Chap. 68). Prenatal diagnosis in candidate families can probably be achieved by measurement of copper uptake and release by amniotic fluid cells, and the potential exists for linkage analysis in some families. The isolation and characterization of the Menkes syndrome gene as a copper-transporting ATPase,[438–440] permitted testing in some of the families with X-linked cutis laxa. On the basis of those studies it appears that the disorders do result from mutations in the same gene.[441]

Ehlers-Danlos Syndrome Type X

EDS type X is inherited in an autosomal recessive fashion and characterized by mild joint hypermobility and easy bruising. The disorder appears to result from an alteration in fibronectin that interferes with normal platelet aggregation.[442] Only one family has been identified to date.

Approach to Patients with EDS

Many patients with EDS-like clinical findings do not fit the general classification scheme and, as more biochemical studies are completed, it is likely that the classification will expand. From the clinical point of view, the important considerations are whether the patient has a condition inherited in an autosomal dominant, autosomal recessive, or X-linked fashion, and whether the natural history can be predicted from family studies or biochemical studies. It is vital to distinguish the known, well-characterized recessively inherited disorder EDS type VI, because prenatal diagnosis is available and because orthopedic and ophthalmologic management differ from those in other varieties. It is important to identify patients with EDS type IV so that clear discussion of pregnancy risks and of problems in surgery can proceed outside the setting of emergency care. Biochemical studies of collagens synthesized by fibroblastic cells cultured from dermal punch biopsies can identify patients with EDS type IV, EDS type VI, and some patients with EDS type VII. Low serum copper and ceruloplasmin levels identify patients with EDS type IX. It is likely that in the near future, defects in collagen processing, or of the structure or synthesis of other matrix macromolecules, will be identified in patients with EDS types I and II, and research in these areas is under way.

Animal Models of EDS

Mink, cats, and dogs with clinical features of the EDS type I phenotype have been identified and studied in several laboratories.[433–445] These animals have lax joints and hyperextensible skin. Fibril structure in dermal collagen is similar to that in people with EDS type I in that mean fibril diameter is large, most fibrils are irregular, and there is an abundance of composite fibrils. The disorder is inherited in an autosomal dominant fashion in all species; the molecular basis of the disorder is not known.

Dermatosparaxis, an autosomal recessive disorder of the conversion of type I procollagen to collagen, has been identified in cattle, sheep, and cats (see above, EDS type VII). Dermatosparaxis in cattle was the first disorder of collagen processing that was identified and led, first, to the recognition that collagens were initially synthesized as precursors; second, to the isolation, characterization, and sequence determination of the N-terminal propeptide extensions of the proα1(I) and proα2(I) chains; and third, to the suggestion that the propeptides may be involved in feedback regulation of collagen synthesis.[97]

Mice with several alleles at the X-chromosomal *mottled* locus have defects in copper metabolism and connective-tissue abnormalities[446,447] (see also, Chap. 68). One group dies within a few days of birth as a result of severe central nervous system abnormalities and appears to be similar to infants with the Menkes syndrome.[448] In others, there is a gradient of connective-tissue abnormalities that is similar to those identified in individuals with EDS type IX.[449,450] Lysyl oxidase deficiency and alteration in collagen crosslink formation have been demonstrated in mice with the *viable brindle* and *tortoise* alleles.[447] In all mice there are defects in the redistribution of copper from cells, and the different phenotypes probably reflect the efficiency with which copper is provided to the various apoenzymes.[451] The phenotypic diversity probably reflects the clinical spectrum seen in EDS type IX and Menkes syndrome.

Integrating Mechanisms

The clinical heterogeneity within EDS is explained, in part, by the nature of the mutation and the molecules in which mutations occur. EDS type IV is readily distinguished from all the other varieties by the clinical presentation and natural history, and it is the only type that results from mutations in the genes that encode the chains of type III collagen. In contrast to the different forms of OI, the nature and location of the mutations in the COL3A1 gene are not reflected as clearly in clinical heterogeneity.

The clinical phenotypes of EDS types VI, VII, and IX reflect the disruption in formation of fibrils and of intermolecular crosslinks. In EDS type VI the phenotype reflects the differential stability of crosslinks that contain hydroxylysine instead of lysine in addition to a collagen-specific effect of the deficiency of lysyl hydroxylase enzyme activity. In EDS type VII deletion of a lysyl residue involved in crosslink formation is additive with deletion of the propeptide cleavage sequence, and both contribute to a phenotype. Finally, in EDS type IX, defective crosslink formation because of aberrant enzyme activity (which results from lack of available copper) occurs on the background of other enzymatic deficiencies involving copper-dependent enzymes.

In all other forms of EDS the underlying abnormalities are unknown, but the physical properties of tissues suggest that there are alterations in the effective formation of normal crosslinks. It is likely that mutations in genes that encode the chains of type I collagen and in those that encode proteins that interact with collagens in tissues will both result in similar phenotypes.

Because of the heterogeneity of the molecular species that are important to normal fibril formation and to the production of normal tissue tensile strength, it is not possible to derive "molecular rules" in the same way that can be done for OI.

CHONDRODYSPLASIAS: CANDIDATE DISORDERS OF TYPE II COLLAGEN GENES

Chondrodysplasias

More than 150 varieties of chondrodysplasia, disorders of bone growth and structure, have been identified using radiologic, clinical, genetic, and pathological features.[452–456] It is clear that this is a highly heterogeneous group of disorders in which genes encoding any of the many structural proteins of cartilage, the enzymes involved in posttranslational modification, or proteins involved in growth regulation (among others) could harbor mutations leading to these phenotypes. Within this relatively large array of candidate genes and candidate disorders only a few (some forms of achondrogenesis, of spondyloepiphyseal dysplasia, of the Stickler syndrome, and of the Kniest syndrome) appear to result from mutations in the COL2A1 gene that encodes the chains of type II collagen. As Spranger has pointed out,[455] these disorders appear to form one continuous clinical spectrum from a radiologic and clinical perspective. They share abnormalities of the articular cartilage and of the vitreous humor of the eye, both tissues rich in type II collagen.

Stickler Syndrome

Stickler syndrome, hereditary arthroophthalmodystrophy, is an autosomal dominant disorder characterized by early degenerative joint disease in the presence of a mild skeletal epiphyseal dysplasia, and vitreal degeneration, including moderate to severe myopia with retinal detachment in some individuals.[457] In some individuals cleft palate and/or Pierre-Robin anomaly make diagnosis in the newborn period more apparent, but often, in the absence of family history, the diagnosis is delayed. There has been an ongoing concern about the relationship between the Stickler syndrome, the Wagner syndrome, the Marshall syndrome, and other disorders in which both ocular and joint manifestations are present (see discussions elsewhere).[458–461] Linkage studies in families with the Stickler syndrome indicate genetic heterogeneity, with linkage apparent to the COL2A1 locus in some[462–465] and not in others.[463,466] Mutations in the COL2A1 gene have now been identified in four families with the Stickler syndrome, three of which result in stop codons[467–469] and the fourth substitutes aspartic acid for the glycine residue at position 67 of the triple helix.[470]

These findings suggest that a diminished amount of type II collagen in cartilage may be sufficient to produce the Stickler syndrome, that in some instances the presence of mutations near the N-terminal end of the α1(II) chain can result in the phenotype, but that mutations in other genes may also produce the syndrome. Other candidate genes must include those that encode the large cartilage proteoglycan and the chains of type IX collagen, a protein that interacts directly with type II collagen fibrils in tissue.

Spondyloepiphyseal Dysplasia (SED)

SED is a group of chondrodysplasias in which the radiologic features include abnormal epiphyses, flattened vertebral bodies, and frequently, ocular involvement that ranges from myopia to vitreoretinal degeneration. There is a very marked range of clinical expression from mild short stature to very severe short stature, pulmonary compromise, and death in infancy. Analysis of type II collagen in articular cartilage from individuals with different forms of SED has demonstrated alterations in the amount and electrophoretic mobilities of the α1(II) chains in those tissues, compatible with mutations in the COL2A1 gene.[471] Linkage studies are compatible with heterogeneity in the gene in which mutations occur with both presence[472] and absence[473] of cosegregation between polymorphic markers in the COL2A1 gene having been demonstrated. Analysis of the COL2A1 gene from several individuals with different forms of SED has identified mutations that include partial duplication of exon 48 with the resultant addition of 15 amino acids (duplication of residues 970 to 948 of the triple helix),[474] deletion of exon 48 from one allele,[475] substitution of the glycine at position 997 in the triple helix by serine,[476] a splice-junction mutation that results in skipping the sequences of exon 20,[477] and surprisingly, a substitution of cysteine for arginine at position 75 in the triple-helical domain.[478] Because the electrophoretic mobility of the α1(II) chains from tissue is slower than normal, and because the extent of lysyl hydroxylation within the triple-helical domain is increased, it is likely that the mutations that alter the triplet (Gly-X-Y) motif interfere with formation of a stable triple helix.[471] The introduction of free sulfhydryl groups within cartilage by the mutation that substitutes cysteine for arginine no doubt also alters intermolecular interactions.

Achondrogenesis/Hypochondrogenesis

The most severe end of the spectrum of chondrodysplasias in which there is evidence of involvement of the COL2A1 gene is the achondrogenesis/hypochondrogenesis group. Infants with achondrogenesis have severe short-limbed dwarfism and die in the immediate perinatal period or in utero. There has been considerable effort to define subsets within this group[455,479–483] on the basis of the radiologic picture, histopathology, and clinical genetics. The genetics of this group of disorders has been uncertain, with both autosomal recessive inheritance and new dominant mutations proposed. The former was proposed because of recurrences noted within families, but it now seems likely that in at least some of these families parental mosaicism for a dominant mutation accounted for recurrence. EM studies of cartilage from infants or fetuses with achondrogenesis/hypochondrogenesis have demonstrated marked dilation of the RER with electron-dense material and a paucity of fibrils in the extracellular matrix.[484,485] Analysis of the collagen in cartilage from infants with achondrogenesis/hypochondrogenesis demonstrated a paucity of type II collagen in some instances[484,486] or the presence of abnormal molecules in tissues.[487] Several point mutations in the COL2A1 gene have now been identified in this disorder that result in substitution for glycine residues at 574 or 943 by serine,[488,489] or at 853 by glutamic acid.[490] Comparison of these mutations with those that produce the milder SED phenotypes makes it clear that too few mutations in the COL2A1 gene have been identified to permit systematic genotype/phenotype analysis.

ALPORT SYNDROME

Alport syndrome is characterized by progressive hereditary nephritis and sensorineural deafness, which in some families is associated with ocular abnormalities, particularly lenticonus and macular changes.[491,492] The condition is inherited in an X-linked fashion, with both hearing loss and renal dysfunction likely to develop earlier in males than in females in the same family. Indeed, women in some instances do not progress to renal failure but may have mild hematuria for most of their lives. The renal basement membrane shows a characteristic array of findings that include splitting and thinning of the glomerular basement membrane. These findings prompted the suggestion that Alport syndrome reflected abnormalities in type IV collagen,[493] but subsequent data indicating that the known type IV collagen genes were at autosomal loci (see above) excluded the COL4A1 and COL4A2 genes as candidates for mutations that result in the X-linked condition. Linkage studies demonstrated and then confirmed the location of the Alport gene[494–496] at Xq13, and shortly thereafter a type IV collagen gene (COL4A5) was identified and mapped to the same location.[497–500] To date, in all families with X-linked nephritis, with or without significant deafness, the condition has been linked to the COL4A5 gene locus.

The mutational spectrum in the COL4A5 gene is similar to that seen in other collagen genes and, to date, has included multiple-exon deletions,[501,502] point mutations within the triple-helical domain that substitute for glycine residues,[503,504] and mutations within the noncollagenous carboxyl-propeptide domain.[505] Because of the role of the C-terminal propeptide in directing chain aggregation during the early stages of type IV procollagen assembly, the presence of deletions within the portion of the gene encoding that domain appear to be particularly deleterious in that in addition to producing the Alport syndrome, they apparently expose affected individuals to the risk of antibodies developing against the COL4A5 propeptide following renal transplantation.

Extensive deletions involving the 5′ end of the COL4A5 gene and a variable but yet undefined extent of upstream sequence can result in a characteristic form of Alport syndrome in which the renal disease is accompanied by diffuse esophageal leiomyomatosis.[506] Esophageal leiomyomatosis may appear as an isolated disorder, generally inherited in an autosomal dominant manner, or in a variety of syndromic settings; only in the Alport syndrome is the molecular defect identified, although the responsible gene is not yet defined.

DYSTROPHIC FORMS OF EPIDERMOLYSIS BULLOSA, DEFECTS IN TYPE VII COLLAGEN

Epidermolysis bullosa (EB) is a highly heterogeneous group of disorders in which blistering of the skin is the common unifying theme. Blistering occurs within the epidermis (simplex forms of EB), at the dermal–epidermal junction (junctional forms of EB), or within the dermis below the basement membrane (dystrophic forms of EB).[507] Within the past 3 years, several forms of simplex EB have been shown to result from mutations in keratin genes expressed at different levels of the epidermis, apparently accounting for the alterations in cell structure, clumping of keratin filaments at different levels in the epidermis, and the fragility of cells at those levels[508–512] (see Chap. 149). It should be noted that one form of simplex EB initially proposed to result from deficiency of galactosylhydroxylysyl glucosyltransferase,[513] then thought to have a mutation on chromosome 1,[514] has been shown to have the disorder linked to the keratin gene cluster on chromosome 12.[510] Several candidate genes for the junctional varieties of EB have been identified, including epiligrin[515] or kalinin,[516] and the bullous pemphigoid antigens BPAG1 (a 230-kDa noncollagenous protein located in the hemidesmosome[517]) and BPAG2 (a 180-kDa protein with an extensive collagen domain[518–521]).

Dystrophic Forms of Epidermolysis Bullosa

Dominantly inherited forms of dystrophic EB may be generalized in their distribution (blistering occurs early and is generalized with a later involvement of the limbs and scars forming with healing) or more localized over the extremities with a preference for sites of trauma and generally most severe during the first 5 years of life.[507,522] Morphologic studies of skin indicated that individuals with dominant dystrophic forms of EB have abnormalities in the structure and/or amount of anchoring fibrils—structures that course from the basement membrane zone into the upper portion of the papillary dermis and appear to be involved in maintaining dermal–epidermal integrity.[523] Anchoring fibrils consist largely, if not exclusively, of type VII collagen.[524–526] With the identification of polymorphic sites within the COL7A1 gene, it has been shown that in some families with abnormal anchoring fibrils, the disorder is linked to the COL7A1 gene.[527] Thus, the most likely reservoir of mutations leading to the dominant dystrophic forms of EB is the COL7A1 gene, but direct demonstration of mutations and determination of the relation of the limited and generalized form of the disorder are awaited.

Recessive Dystrophic Forms of Epidermolysis Bullosa

The severe recessive dystrophic forms of EB are characterized by generalized blistering in the newborn period; this is often present at birth. Dermal scarring, progressive syndactyly from scarring of the skin of the fingers, and mucosal involvement that leads to esophageal strictures and dysphagia lead to profound disability. Protein and fluid loss through areas of chronic erosion of the skin and mucosal surfaces may lead to infection and malnutrition. Survival is limited both by infection and the consequences of involvement of the gastrointestinal tract. Early ultrastructural studies demonstrated abnormalities at the dermal–epidermal junction,[528] which subsequent analysis showed to reflect absence or markedly diminished number of anchoring fibrils[529–531] (Fig. 134-18). Subsequent studies with antibodies later shown to react with type VII collagen showed that staining at the dermal–epidermal junction was markedly diminished.[532,533] In some individuals, accumulation of type VII collagen within the basal epidermal cells serves to reinforce the idea that type VII collagen is the primary gene in which mutations produce the severe recessive dystrophic phenotype.[534] Studies in 25 families with more than one child with recessive dystrophic EB have failed to demonstrate a single instance in which the sibs do not share the same COL7A1 genotype, compatible with recessive inheritance of mutations in the COL7A1 gene producing the phenotype.[535] No mutations have yet been identified, and it is not known whether mutations in the collagenous or noncollagenous sequences will be more likely to result in this phenotype. It had been suspected on the basis of analysis of collagenase activity in skin from affected individuals that defects in the synthesis or specific activity of this enzyme might result in the recessive dystrophic EB phenotype.[536,537] Genetic linkage studies, using polymorphic markers in the collagenase gene in families with multiple sibs with recessive dystrophic EB, excluded this gene as the one in which mutations result in the phenotype.[538]

SUMMARY

Like many other fields, the investigation of the genetic disorders of collagen metabolism was revolutionized by the introduction of molecular genetic techniques. These techniques have facilitated the analysis of mutations in collagen genes and in the genes that encode processing enzymes, and permitted the creation of mice bearing mutations in some collagen genes (particularly COL1A1, COL2A1, COL3A1, COL9A1, and COL10A1) in attempts to identify candidate phenotypes for mutations in those genes. These approaches have facilitated prenatal diagnosis of a variety of disorders and enabled investigators to explore further the effects of these mutations on the abnormal proteins, both within and outside the cell. Thus, the molecular pathogenesis of some collagen gene disorders, particularly some forms of OI and EDS type IV, is becoming increasingly well understood. Furthermore, the molecular studies have shown that the enormous range in severity of identifiable disorders such as OI, EDS type IV, and some chondrodysplasias, suggest that some forms of far more common disorders such as osteoporosis, arterial aneurysms, and degenerative arthropathies could be due to mutations in the same genes. Hailed as a road to therapy for some of the severe collagen gene disorders, the molecular understanding

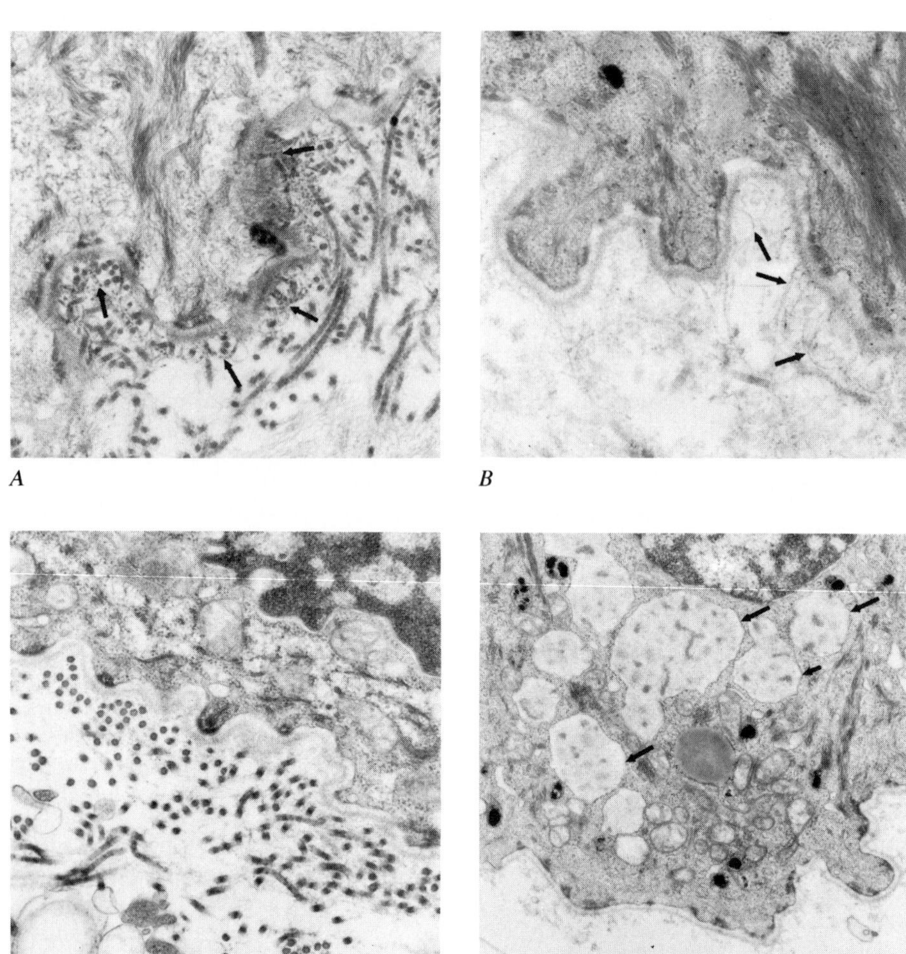

FIG. 134-18 EM of the dermal–epidermal junction in normal skin (*A*), skin from an adult with dominant dystrophic EB (*B*), skin from an infant with recessive dystrophic EB (*C*), and skin from an infant with recessive dystrophic EB whose epidermal cells store type VII collagen (*arrow* in *D*). Anchoring fibrils have an abnormal structure in dominant dystrophic EB and are virtually absent in recessive dystrophic EB. *(Micrographs courtesy of Dr. Lynne Smith, University of Washington.)*

of these disorders has, to date, provided few, if any, insights into productive therapies. The prospect of specific gene-based therapy, either by targeted replacement or inhibition of expression of mutant alleles, seems remote and limited by the often generalized nature of the disorders and the necessity to affect only the mutant allele. With much of the work accomplished to identify mutations in many collagen gene disorders and the recognition of the nature of these disorders, it seems likely that attention could be profitably shifted to an analysis of productive therapies that can use the information currently being generated about the mechanisms of disease.

ACKNOWLEDGEMENTS

Original investigations were supported in part by grants from the National Institutes of Health (AR 21557 and AR 41223) and funds from the Osteogenesis Imperfecta Foundation.

REFERENCES

1. Bornstein P, Traub W: Collagen, in Neurath HG, Hill RL (eds): *The Proteins*, 3rd ed. New York, Academic, 1979, p 411.
2. Mayne R, Burgeson RE (eds): *Structure and Function of Collagen Types*. Orlando, FL, Academic, 1987.
3. Bornstein P, Sage H: Structurally distinct collagen types. *Annu Rev Biochem* **49**:957, 1980.
4. Fleischmajer R, Olsen BR, Kuhn K (eds): Biology, chemistry and pathology of collagen. *Ann NY Acad Sci* **460**:1, 1985.
5. Mays C, Rosenberry TL: Characterization of pepsin-resistant collagen-like tail subunit fragments of 18S and 14S acetylcholinesterase from *electrophorus electricus*. *Biochemistry* **20**:2810, 1981.
6. Reid KBM: Complete amino acid sequences of the three collagen-like regions present in subcomponent C1q of the first component of human complement. *Biochem J* **179**:367, 1979.
7. Bhattacharyya SN, Passero MA, Diaugustine RP, Lynn WS: Isolation and characterization of two hydroxyproline-containing glycoproteins from normal animal lung lavage and lamellar bodies. *J Clin Invest* **55**:914, 1975.
8. Li KH, Sawamura D, Giudice GJ, Diaz LA, Mattei MG, Chu M-L, Uitto J: Genomic organization of collagen domains and chromosomal assignment of human 190-kDa bullous pemphigold antigen-2, a novel collagen of stratified squamous epithelium. *J Biol Chem* **266**:24064, 1991.
9. Taylor ME, Brickell PM, Craig RK, Summerfield JA: Structure and evolutionary origin of the gene encoding a human serum mannose-binding protein. *Biochem J* **262**:763, 1989.
10. Sastry K, Herman GA, Day L, Deignan E, Bruns G, Morton CC, Ezekowitz RA: The human mannose-binding protein gene. Exon structure reveals its evolutionary relationship to a human pulmonary surfactant gene and localization to chromosome 10. *J Exp Med* **170**:1175, 1989.
11. Prockop DJ, Kivirikko KI: Heritable diseases of collagen. *N Engl J Med* **311**:376, 1984.
12. Byers PH, Bonadio JF: The molecular basis of clinical heterogeneity in osteogenesis imperfecta: Mutation in type I collagen genes have different effects on collagen processing, in Lloyd J, Scriver CR (eds): *Metabolic and Genetic Disease in Pediatrics*. London Butterworths, 1985.
13. Cheah KSW: Collagen genes and inherited connective tissue disease. *Biochem J* **229**:287, 1985.

14. Tsipouras P, Ramirez F: Genetic disorders of collagen. *J Med Genet* **24**:2, 1987.
15. Sykes B: Genetics cracks bone disease. *Nature* **330**:607, 1987.
16. Byers PH, Bonadio JF: The nature, characterization and phenotypic effects of mutations that affect collagen structure and processing, in Olsen BR, Nimni M (eds): *Collagen: Biochemistry, Biotechnology, and Molecular Biology*. Boca Raton, FL, CRC, 1989, vol 4.
17. Byers PH, Holbrook KA: Molecular basis of clinical heterogeneity in the Ehlers-Danlos syndrome. *Ann NY Acad Sci* **460**:298, 1985.
18. Miller EJ, Matukas VJ: Chick cartilage collagen: A new type of α1 chain not present in bone or skin of the species. *Proc Natl Acad Sci USA* **64**:1264, 1969.
19. Kuhn K: The classical collagens, in Mayne R, Burgeson RE (eds): *Structure and Function of Collagen Types*. Orlando, FL, Academic, 1987, p 1.
20. van der Rest M, Mayne R: Type IX collagen, in Mayne R, Burgeson RE (eds): *Structure and Function of Collagen Types*. Orlando, FL, Academic, 1987, p 195.
21. Schmid TM, Linsenmayer TF: Type X collagen, in Mayne R, Burgeson RE (eds). *Structure and Function of Collagen Types*. Orlando, FL, Academic, 1987, p 223.
22. Eyre D, Wu J-J: Type XI or 1α2α3α collagen, in Mayne R, Burgeson RE (eds): *Structure and Function of Collagen Types*. Orlando, FL, Academic, 1987, p 261.
23. Kefalides NA, Alper R, Clark CC: Biochemistry and metabolism of basement membranes. *Int Rev Cytol* **61**:167, 1979.
24. Glanville R: Type IV collagen, in Mayne R, Burgeson RE (eds): *Structure and Function of Collagen Types*. Orlando, FL, Academic, 1987, p 43.
25. Burgeson RE: Type VII collagen, in Mayne R, Burgeson RE (eds): *Structure and Function of Collagen Types*. Orlando, FL, Academic, 1987, p 145.
26. van der Rest M, Garrone R: Collagen family of proteins. *FASEB J* **5**:2814, 1991.
27. De Wet W, Bernard M, Benson-Chanda V, Chu M-L, Dickson L, Weil D, Ramirez F: Organization of the human pro-α2(I) collagen gene. *J Biol Chem* **262**:16032, 1987.
28. Barsh GS, Roush CL, Gelinas RE: DNA and chromatin structure of the human α1(I) collagen gene. *J Biol Chem* **259**:14906, 1984.
29. Chu M-L, De Wet W, Bernard M, Ding J-F, Morabito M, Myers J, Williams C, Ramirez F: Human proα1(I) collagen gene structure reveals evolutionary conservation of a pattern of introns and exons. *Nature* **310**:337, 1984.
30. Sangiorgi FO, Benson-Chanda V, De Wet WJ, Sobel ME, Tsipouras P, Ramirez F: Isolation and partial characterization of the entire human proα1(I) collagen gene. *Nucleic Acids Res* **13**:2207, 1985.
31. Cheah KSE, Stoker NG, Griffin JR, Grosveld FG, Solomon E: Identification and characterization of the human type II collagen gene (COL2A1). *Proc Natl Acad Sci USA* **82**:2555, 1985.
32. Chu M-L, Weil D, De Wet W, Bernard M, Sippola M, Ramirez F: Isolation of cDNA and genomic clones encoding human proα1(III) collagen. *J Biol Chem* **260**:4357, 1985.
33. Myers JC, Loidl HR, Stolle CA, Seyer JM: Partial covalent structure of the human α2 type V collagen chain. *J Biol Chem* **260**:5533, 1985.
34. Sunderraj CV, Church RL, Klobucher LA, Ruddle FH: Assignment of the gene for human type I procollagen to chromosome 17 by analysis of cell hybrids and microcell hybrids. *Proc Natl Acad Sci USA* **74**:4444, 1977.
35. Huerre C, Junien C, Weil D, Chu M-L, Morabito M, Van Cong M, Myers JC, Foubert C, Gross M-S, Prockop DJ, Vove A, Kaplan J-C, De La Chapelle A, Ramirez F: Human type I procollagen genes are located on different chromosomes. *Proc Natl Acad Sci USA* **79**:6627, 1982.
36. Solomon E, Hiorne L, Dalgleish R, Tolstoshev P, Crystal R, Sykes B: Regional localization of the human α2(I) collagen gene on chromosome 7 by molecular hybridization. *Cytogenet Cell Genet* **35**:64, 1983.
37. Strom CM, Eddy RL, Shows TB: Localization of human type II procollagen gene (COL2A1) to chromosome 12. *Somat Cell Mol Genet* **10**:651, 1984.
38. Emanuel BS, Cannizzaro LA, Seyer JM, Myers JC: Human α1(III) and α2(V) procollagen genes are located on the long arm of chromosome 2. *Proc Natl Acad Sci USA* **82**:3385, 1985.
39. Huerre-Jeanpiere C, Henry I, Bernard M, Gallano P, Weil D, Grzeschik K-H, Ramirez F, Junien C: The pro α2(V) collagen (COL5A2) maps to 2q14→2q32, syntenic to the pro α1(III) collagen locus (COL3A1). *Hum Genet* **73**:64, 1986.
40. Kurkinen M, Bernard MP, Barlow DP, Chow LT: Characterization of 64-, 123- and 182-base-pair exons in the mouse α2(IV) collagen gene. *Nature* **317**:177, 1985.
41. Sakurai Y, Sullivan M, Yamada Y: α1 type IV collagen gene evolved differently from fibrillar collagen genes. *J Biol Chem* **261**:6654, 1986.
42. Solomon E, Hiorns LR, Spurr N, Kurkinen M, Barlow D, Hogan BLM, Dalgleish R: Chromosomal assignments of the genes coding for human type II, III, and IV collagen: A dispersed gene family. *Proc Natl Acad Sci USA* **82**:3330, 1985.
43. Emanuel BS, Sellinger BT, Gudas LJ, Myers JC: Localization of the human procollagen α1(IV) gene to chromosome 13q34 by in situ hybridization. *Am J Hum Genet* **38**:38, 1986.
44. Griffen CA, Emanuel BS, Hansen JR, Cavenee WK, Myers JC: Human collagen genes encoding basement membrane α1(IV) and α2(IV) chains map to the distal long arm of chromosome 13. *Proc Natl Acad Sci USA* **84**:512, 1987.
45. Bowcock AM, Hebert JM, Christiano AM, Wijsman E, Cavalli-Sforza LL, Boyd CD: The proα1(IV) collagen gene is linked to the D13S3 locus at the distal end of human chromosome 13q. *Cytogenet Cell Genet* **45**:234, 1987.
46. Solomon E, Hall V, Kurkinen M: The human α2(IV) collagen gene, COL4A2, is syntenic with the α1(IV) gene, COL4A1, on chromosome 13. *Ann Hum Genet* **51**:125, 1987.
47. Boyd CD, Toth-Fejel S, Gadi IK, Litt M, Condon MR, Kolbe M, Hagen IK, Kurkinen M, Mackenzie JW, Magenis E: The genes coding for human pro α1(IV) collagen and pro α2(IV) collagen are both located at the end of the long arm of chromosome 13. *Am J Hum Genet* **42**:309, 1988.
48. Cutting GR, Kazazian HH Jr, Antonarakis SE, Killen PD, Yamada Y, Francomano CA: Macrorestriction mapping of COL4A1 and COL4A2 collagen genes on human chromosome 13q34. *Genomics* **3**:256, 1988.
49. Morrison KE, Mariyama M, Yang-Feng TL, Reeders ST: Sequence and localization of a partial cDNA encoding the human alpha 3 chain of type IV collagen. *Am J Hum Genet* **49**:545, 1991.
50. Mariyama M, Zheng K, Yang-Feng TL, Reeders ST: Colocalization of the genes for the α3(IV) and α4(IV) chains of type IV collagen to chromosome 2 band q35-q37. *Genomics* **13**:809, 1992.
51. Hostikka SL, Eddy RL, Byers MG, Hoeyhtyae M, Shows TB, Tryggvason K: Identification of a distinct type IV collagen α chain with restricted kidney distribution and assignment of its gene to the locus of X chromosome-linked Alport syndrome. *Proc Natl Acad Sci USA* **87**:1606, 1990.
52. Myers JC, Jone TA, Pohjolainen ER, Kadri AS, Goddard AD, Sheer D, Solomon E, Pihlajaniemi T: Molecular cloning of α5(IV) collagen and assignment of the gene to the region of the X chromosome containing the Alport syndrome locus. *Am J Hum Genet* **46**:1024, 1990.
53. Kimura T, Mattei MG, Stevens JW, Goldring MB, Ninomiya Y, Olsen BR: Molecular cloning of rat and human type IX collagen cDNA and localization of the α1(IX) gene on the human chromosome 6. *Eur J Biochem* **179**:71, 1989.
54. van der Rest M, Mayne R: Type IX collagen proteoglycan from cartilage is covalently cross-linked to type II collagen. *J Biol Chem* **263**:1615, 1988.
55. OH SP, Taylor RW, Gerecke DR, Rochelle JM, Seldin MF, Olsen BR: The mouse α1(XII) and human α1(XII)-like collagen genes are localized on mouse chromosome 9 and human chromosome 6. *Genomics* **14**:225, 1992.
56. Yoshioka H, Zhang H, Ramirez F, Mattei M-G, Moradi-Ameli M, van der Rest M, Gordon MK: Synteny between the loci for a novel FACIT-like collagen locus (D6S228E) and α1(IX) collagen (COL9A1) on 6q12-q14 in humans. *Genomics* **13**:884, 1992.

57. Dublet B, Oh S, Sugrue SP, Gordon MK, Gerecke DR, Olsen BR, van der Rest M: The structure of avian type XII collagen. Alpha 1(XII) chains contain 190-kDa non-triple-helical amino-terminal domains and form homotrimeric molecules. *J Biol Chem* **264**:13150, 1989.
58. Gordon MK, Gerecke DR, Dublet B, van der Rest M, Olsen BR: Type XII collagen. A large multidomain molecule with partial homology to type IX collagen. *J Biol Chem* **264**:19772, 1989.
59. Yamagata M, Yamada KM, Yamada SS, Shinomura T, Tanaka H, Nishida Y, Obara M, Kimata K: The complete primary structure of type XII collagen shows a chimeric molecule with reiterated fibronectin type III motifs, von Willebrand factor A motifs, a domain homologous to a noncollagenous region of type IX collagen and short collagenous domains with an Arg-Gly-Asp site. *J Cell Biol* **115**:209, 1991.
60. Chu M-L, Mann K, Deutzmann R, Pribula-Conway D, Hsu-Chen CC, Bernard MP, Timpl R: Characterization of three constituent chains of collagen type VI by peptides sequences and cDNA clones. *Eur J Biochem* **168**:309, 1987.
61. Weil D, Mattei M-G, Passage E, Van Cong N'G, Pribula-Conway D, Mann K, Deutzmann R, Timpl R, Chu M-L: Cloning and chromosomal localization of human genes encoding the three chains of type VI collagen. *Am J Hum Genet* **42**:435, 1988.
62. Francomano CA, Cutting GR, McCormick MK, Chu M-L, Timpl R, Hong HK, Antonarakis SE: The COL6A1 and COL6A2 genes exist as a gene cluster and detect highly informative DNA polymorphisms in the telomeric region of human chromosome 21q. *Hum Genet* **87**:162, 1991.
63. Muragaki Y, Mattei M-G, Yamaguchi N, Olsen BR, Ninomiya Y: The complete primary structure of the human α1(VIII) chain and assignment of its gene (COL8A1) to chromosome 3. *Eur J Biochem* **197**:615, 1991.
64. Muragaki Y, Jacenko O, Apte S, Mattei M-G, Ninomiya Y, Olsen BR: The α2(VIII) collagen gene. A novel member of the short chain collagen family located on the human chromosome 1. *J Biol Chem* **266**:7721, 1991.
65. Thomas JT, Cresswell CJ, Rash B, Nicolai H, Jones T, Solomon E, Grant ME, Boot-Handford RP: The human collagen X gene. Complete primary translated sequence and chromosomal localization. *Biochem J* **280**:617, 1991.
66. Apte S, Mattei MG, Olsen BR: Cloning of human α1(X) collagen DNA and localization of the COL10A1 gene to the q21-q22 region of human chromosome 6. *FEBS Lett* **282**:393, 1991.
67. Parenta MG, Chung LC, Ryynaenen J, Woodley DT, Wynn KC, Bauer EA, Mattei MG, Chu M-L, Uitto J: Human type VII collagen: cDNA cloning and chromosomal mapping of the gene. *Proc Natl Acad Sci USA* **88**:6931, 1991.
68. Palmiter RD, Davidson JM, Gagnon J, Rowe DW, Bornstein P: NH_2-terminal sequence of the chick-proα1(I) chain synthesized in the reticulocyte lysate system. *J Biol Chem* **254**:1433, 1979.
69. Salem G, Traub W: Conformational implications of amino acid sequence regularities in collagen. *FEBS Lett* **51**:94, 1975.
70. Ramachandran GN: Structure of collagen at the molecular level, in Ramachandran GN (ed): *Treatise on Collagen*. New York, Academic, 1967, vol 2, p 103.
71. Berg RA, Prockop DJ: The thermal transition of a nonhydroxylated form of collagen. Evidence for a role for hydroxyproline in stabilizing the triple-helix of collagen. *Biochem Biophys Res Commun* **52**:115, 1973.
72. Rosenbloom J, Harsch M, Jimenez S: Hydroxyproline content determines the denaturation temperature of chick tendon collagen. *Arch Biochem Biophys* **158**:478, 1973.
73. Jimenez SA, Dehm P, Olsen BR, Prockop DJ: Intracellular collagen and protocollagen from embryonic tendon cells. *J Biol Chem* **248**:720, 1973.
74. Harwood R, Grant ME, Jackson DS: The route of secretion of procollagen. The influence of α,α'-bipyridyl, colchicine and antimycin A on the secretory process in embryonic-chick tendon and cartilage cells. *Biochem J* **156**:81, 1976.
75. Wooley DE: Mammalian collagenases, in Piez KA, Reddi AH (eds): *Extracellular Matrix Biochemistry*. New York, Elsevier, 1984, p 119.
76. Harper E: Collagenases. *Annu Rev Biochem* **49**:1063, 1980.
77. Fessler JH, Fessler LI: Biosynthesis of procollagen. *Annu Rev Biochem* **47**:129, 1978.
78. De Wet WJ, Chu M-L, Prockop DJ: The mRNAs for the proα1(I) and proα2(I) chains of type I procollagen are translated at the same rate in normal human fibroblasts and in fibroblasts from two variants of osteogenesis imperfecta with altered steady state ratios of the two mRNAs. *J Biol Chem* **258**:14385, 1983.
79. Rossi P, De Crombrugghe B: Identification of a cell-specific transcriptional enhancer in the first intron of the mouse α2 (type I) collagen gene. *Proc Natl Acad Sci USA* **84**:5590, 1987.
80. Liau G, Szapary D, Setoyama C, De Crombrugghe B: Restriction enzyme digestions identify discrete domains in the chromatin around the promoter of the mouse α2(I) collagen gene. *J Biol Chem* **261**:11362, 1986.
81. Hatamochi A, Paterson B, De Crombrugghe B: Differential binding of a CCAAT DNA binding factor to the promoters of the mouse α2(I) and α1(III) collagen genes. *J Biol Chem* **261**:11310, 1986.
82. Bornstein P, McKay J, Morishima J, Devarayalu S, Gelinas RE: Regulatory elements in the first intron contribute to transcriptional control of the human α1(I) collagen gene. *Proc Natl Acad Sci USA* **84**:5590, 1987.
83. Schmidt A, Rossi P, De Crombrugghe B: Transcriptional control of the mouse α2(I) collagen gene: Functional deletin analysis of the promoter and evidence for cell-specific expression. *Mol Cell Biol* **6**:347, 1986.
84. Bornstein P, McKay J: The first intron of the α1(I) collagen gene contains several transcriptional regulatory elements. *J Biol Chem* **263**:1603, 1988.
85. Roberts AB, Sporn MB, Assoian RK, Smith JM, Roche NS, Wakefield LM, Heine UI, Liotta LA, Falanga VA, Kehrl JH, Fauci As: Transforming growth factor type-β: Rapid induction of fibrosis and angiogenesis *in vivo* and stimulation of collagen formation *in vitro*. *Proc Natl Acad Sci USA* **83**:4167, 1986.
86. Raghow R, Postlethwaite AE, Keski-Oja J, Moses HL, Kang AH: Transforming growth factor-β increases steady state levels of type I procollagen and fibronectin messenger RNAs posttranscriptionally in cultured human dermal fibroblasts. *J Clin Invest* **79**:1285, 1987.
87. Murad S, Grove D, Lindberg KA, Reynolds G, Sivarajah A, Pinnell SR: Regulation of collagen synthesis by ascorbic acid. *Proc Natl Acad Sci USA* **78**:2879, 1981.
88. Yamada Y, Mudryj M, De Crombrugghe B: A uniquely conserved regulatory signal is found around the translation initiation site in three different collagen genes. *J Biol Chem* **258**:14914, 1983.
89. Schmidt A, Yamada Y, De Crombrugghe B: DNA sequence comparison of the regulatory signals at the 5′ end of the mouse and chick α2 type I collagen genes. *J Biol Chem* **259**:7411, 1984.
90. Bennett VC, Adams SL: Characterization of the translational control mechanism preventing synthesis of α2(I) collagen in chicken vertebral chondroblasts. *J Biol Chem* **262**:14806, 1987.
91. Paglia LM, Wilczek J, De Leon LD, Martin GR, Hörlein D, Müller P: Inhibition of procollagen cell-free synthesis by amino-terminal extension peptides. *Biochemistry* **18**:5030, 1979.
92. Horlein D, McPherson J, Goh SH, Bornstein P: Regulation of protein synthesis: Translational control by procollagen-derived fragments. *Proc Natl Acad Sci USA* **78**:6163, 1981.
93. Aycock RS, Raghow R, Stricklin GP, Seyer JM, Kang AH: Post-transcriptional inhibition of collagen and fibronectin synthesis by a synthetic homolog of a portion of the carboxyl-terminal propeptide of human type I collagen. *J Biol Chem* **261**:14355, 1986.
94. Bienkowski RS, Curran SF, Berg RA: Kinetics of intracellular degradation of newly synthesized collagen. *Biochemistry* **25**:2455, 1986.
95. Berg RA, Schwartz ML, Rome LH, Crystal RG: Lysosomal function in the degradation of defective collagen in cultured lung fibroblasts. *Biochemistry* **23**:2134, 1984.
96. Avvedimento VE, Vogeli G, Yamada Y, Maizel JV Jr, Pastan I, De Crombrugghe B: Correlation between splicing sites within an intron and their sequence complementarity with U1 RNA. *Cell* **21**:689, 1980.

97. Lichtenstein JR, Martin GR, Kohn L, Byers PH, McKusick VA: Defect in conversion of procollagen to collagen in a form of Ehlers-Danlos syndrome. *Science* **182**:298, 1973.
98. Kivirikko KI, Myllylä R: Posttranslational enzymes in the biosynthesis of collagen:Intracellular enzymes. *Methods Enzymol* **82A**:245, 1982.
99. Puistola U, Turpeenniemi-Hujanen TM, Myllylä R, Kivirikko KI: Studies on the lysyl hydroxylase reaction. II. Inhibition kinetics and the reaction mechanism. *Biochim Biophys Acta* **611**:51, 1980.
100. Risteli J, Tryggvason K, Kivirikko KI: A rapid assay for prolyl 3-hydroxylase activity. *Anal Biochem* **84**:423, 1978.
101. Kivirikko KI, Myllylä R: Biosynthesis of the collagens, in Piez KA, Reddi AH (eds). *Extracellular Matrix Biochemistry*. New York, Elsevier, 1984, p 83.
102. Olsen BR, Berg RA, Kishida Y, Prockop DJ: Collagen synthesis: Localization of prolyl hydroxylase in tendon cells detected with ferritin-labeled antibodies, *Science* **182**:825, 1973.
103. Berg RA, Kedersah NL, Guzman NA: Purification and partial characterization of the two nonidentical subunits of prolyl hydroxylase. *J Biol Chem* **254**:311, 1979.
104. Pihlajaniemi T, Helaakoski T, Tasanen K, Myllylä R, Huhtala M-L, Koivu J, Kivirikko KI: Molecular cloning of the β-subunit of human prolyl 4-hydroxylase. This subunit and protein disulphide isomerase are products of the same gene. *EMBO J* **6**:643, 1987.
105. Creighton TE, Hillson DA, Freedman RB: Catalysis by protein-disulphide isomerase of the unfolding and refolding of proteins with disulphide bonds. *J Mol Biol* **142**:43, 1980.
106. Munro S, Pelham HRB: A C-terminal signal prevents secretion of luminal ER proteins. *Cell* **48**:899, 1987.
107. Turpeenniemi-Hujanen TM, Puistola U, Kivirikko KI: Isolation of lysyl hydroxylase, an enzyme of collagen synthesis, from chick embryos as a homogenous protein. *Biochem J* **189**:247, 1980.
108. Hautala T, Byers MG, Eddy RL, Shows TB, Kivirikko KI, Myllylä R: Cloning of human lysyl hydroxylase: Complete cDNA-derived amino acid sequence and assignment of the gene (PLOD) to chromosome 1p36.3-p36.2. *Genomics* **13**:62, 1992.
109. Yeowell HN, Ha V, Walker LC, Murad S, Pinnell SR: Chracterization of a partial cDNA for lysyl hydroxylase from human skin fibroblasts; lysyl hydroxylase mRNAs are regulated differently by minoxidil derivatives and hydralazine. *J Invest Dermatol* **99**:864, 1992.
110. Myllylä R, Pihlajaniemi T, Pajunen L, Turpeenniemi-Hujanen T, Kivirikko KI: Molecular cloning of chick lysyl hydroxylase. Little homology in primary structure to the two types of subunit of prolyl 4-hydroxylase. *J Biol Chem* **266**:2805, 1991.
111. Risteli J, Tryggvason K, Kivirikko KI: Prolyl 3-hydroxylase: Partial characterization of the enzyme from rat kidney cortex. *Eur J Biochem* **73**:485, 1977.
112. Rao NV, Adams E: Partial reaction of prolyl hydroxylase $(GLY\text{-}PRO\text{-}ALA)_n$ stimulates α-ketoglutarate decarboxylation without prolyl hydroxylation. *J Biol Chem* **253**:6327, 1978.
113. Myllylä R, Kuutti-Savolainen E-R, Kivirikko KI: The role of ascorbate in the prolyl hydroxylase reaction. *Biochem Biophys Res Commun* **83**:441, 1978.
114. Peterkofsky B, Kalwinsky D, Assad R: Substance in L-929 cell extracts which replaces the ascorbate requirement for prolyl hydroxylase in a tritium release assay for reducing cofactor; correlation of its concentration with the extent of ascorbate-independent proline hydroxylation and the level of prolyl hydroxylase activity in these cells. *Arch Biochem Biophys* **199**:362, 1980.
115. Eyre DR, Paz MA, Gallop PM: Cross-linking in collagen and elastin. *Annu Rev Biochem* **53**:717, 1984.
116. Doege KJ, Fessler JH: Folding of carboxyl domain and assembly of procollagen I. *J Biol Chem* **261**:8924, 1986.
117. Koivu J: Identification of disulfide bonds in carboxy-terminal propetides of human type I procollagen. *FEBS Lett* **212**:229, 1987.
118. Bächinger HP, Bruckner P, Timpl R, Engel J: The role of *cis-trans* isomerization of peptide bonds in the coil-triple-helix conversion of collagen. *Eur J Biochem* **90**:605, 1978.
119. Bächinger HP: The influence of peptidyl-prolyl cis-trans isomerase on the *in vitro* folding of type III collagen. *J Biol Chem* **262**:17144, 1987.
120. Kivirikko KI, Myllylä R: Collagen glycosyltransferases. *Int Rev Connect Tissue Res* **8**:23, 1979.
121. Clark CC: The distribution and initial characterization of oligosaccharide units on the COOH-terminal propeptide extensions of the proα1 and proα2 chains of type I procollagen. *J Biol Chem* **254**:10798, 1979.
122. Anttinen H, Oikarinen A, Ryhanen L, Kivirikko KI: Evidence for the transfer of mannose to the extension peptides of procollagen within the cisternae of the rough endoplasmic reticulum. *FEBS Lett* **87**:222, 1978.
123. Guzman NA, Graves PN, Prockop DJ: Addition of mannose to both the amino- and carboxy-terminal propeptides of type II procollagen occurs without formation of a triple-helix. *Biochem Biophys Res Commun* **84**:691, 1978.
124. Kornfeld R, Kornfeld S: Assembly of asparagine-linked oligosaccharides. *Annu Rev Biochem* **54**:631, 1985.
125. Duksin D, Bornstein P: Impaired conversion of procollagen to collagen by fibroblasts and bone treated with tunicamycin, an inhibitor of protein glycosylation. *J Biol Chem* **252**:955, 1977.
126. Housley TJ, Rowland FN, Ledger PW, Kaplan J, Tanzer ML: Effects of tunicamycin on the biosynthesis of procollagen by human fibroblasts. *J Biol Chem* **255**:121, 1980.
127. Clark CC: Asparagine-linked glycosides. *Methods Enzymol* **82A**:346, 1982.
128. Dehm P, Prockop DJ: Time lag in the secretion of collagen by matrix-free tendon cells and inhibition of the secretory process by colchicine and vinblastine. *Biochem Biophys Acta* **264**:375, 1972.
129. Diegelmann RF, Peterkofsky B: Inhibition of collagen secretion from bone and cultured fibroblasts by microtubular disruptive drugs. *Proc Natl Acad Sci USA* **69**:892, 1972.
130. Ehrlich HP, Ross R, Bornstein P: Effects of antimicrotubular agents on the secretion of collagen. *J Cell Biol* **62**:390, 1974.
131. Fessler LI, Brosh S, Chapin S, Fessler JH: Tyrosine sulfation in precursors of collagen V. *J Biol Chem* **261**:5034, 1986.
132. Fessler LI, Chapin S, Brosh S, Fessler JH: Intracellular transport and tyrosine sulfation of procollagens V. *Eur J Biochem* **158**:511, 1986.
133. Fisher LW, Rober PG, Tuross N, Otsuka AS, Tepen DA, Esch FS, Shimasaki S, Termine JD: The M_r24,000 phosphoprotein from developing bone is the NH_2-terminal propeptide of the α1 chain of type I collagen. *J Biol Chem* **262**:13457, 1987.
134. Lapiere CM, Lenaers A, Kohn LD: Procollagen peptidase: An enzyme excising the coordination peptides of procollagen. *Proc Natl Acad Sci USA* **68**:3054, 1971.
135. Tuderman L, Prockop DJ: Procollagen N proteinase: Properties of the enzyme purified from chick embryo tendons. *Eur J Biochem* **125**:545, 1982.
136. Morris NP, Fessler LI, Fessler JH: Procollagen peptide release by procollagen peptidases and bacterial collagenase. *J Biol Chem* **254**:11024, 1979.
137. Tuderman L, Kivirikko KI, Prockop DJ: Partial purification and characterization of a neutral protease which cleaves the N-terminal propeptides from procollagen. *Biochemistry* **17**:2948, 1978.
138. Birk DE, Trelstad RL: Extracellular compartments in tendon morphogenesis: Collagen fibril, bundle, and macroaggregate formation. *J Cell Biol* **103**:231, 1986.
139. Trelstad RL: Multistep assembly of type I collagen fibrils. *Cell* **28**:197, 1982.
140. Piez KA, Trus BL: Sequence regularities and packing of collagen molecules. *J Mol Biol* **122**:419, 1978.
141. Vogel KG, Paulsson M, Heinegard D: Specific inhibition of type I and type II collagen fibrillogenesis by the small proteoglycan of tendon. *Biochem J* **223**:587, 1984.
142. Piez KA: Molecular and aggregate structures of the collagens, in Piez KA, Reddi AH (eds). *Extracellular Matrix Biochemistry*. New York, Elsevier, 1984, p 1.
143. Siegel RC: Lysyl oxidase. *Int Rev Connect Tissue Res* **83**:73, 1979.

144. Kagan HM: Lysyl oxidase, in Mecham RP (ed): *Biology of Extracellular Matrix*. Orlando, FL, Academic, 1985, vol 2, 321.
145. Cronlund AL, Kagan HM: Comparison of lysyl oxidase from bovine lung and aorta. *Connect Tissue Res* **15**:173, 1986.
146. Kuivaniemi H, Ala-Kokko L, Kivirikko KI: Secretion of lysyl oxidase by cultured human skin fibroblasts and effects of monensin, nigericin, tunicamycin and colchicine. *Biochim Biophys Acta* **883**:326, 1986.
147. Williamson PR, Moog RS, Dooley DM, Kagan HM: Evidence for pyrroloquinolinequinone as the carbonyl cofactor in lysyl oxidase by absorption and resonance Raman spectroscopy. *J Biol Chem* **261**:16302, 1986.
148. Harris ED: Copper-induced activation of aortic lysyl oxidase *in vivo*. *Proc Natl Acad Sci USA* **73**:371, 1973.
149. Hamalainen ER, Jones TA, Sheer D, Taskinen K, Pihlajaniemi T, Kivirikko KI: Molecular cloning of human lysyl oxidase and assignment of the gene to chromosome 5q23.3-31.2. *Genomics* **11**:508, 1991.
150. Mariani TJ, Trackman PC, Kagan HM, Eddy RL, Shows TB, Boyd CD, Deak SB: The complete derived amino acid sequence of human lysyl oxidase and assignment of the gene to chromosome 5 (extensive sequence homology with the murine ras recision gene). *Matrix* **12**:242, 1992.
151. Chang YS, Svinarich DM, Yang TP, Krawetz SA: The mouse lysyl oxidase gene (Lox) resides on chromosome 18. *Cytogenet Cell Genet* **63**:47, 1993.
152. McKusick VA: *Heritable Disorders of Connective Tissue*. St. Louis, Mosby, 1972.
153. Lenaers A, Ansay M, Nusgens BV, Lapiere CM: Collagen made of extended α-chains, procollagen, in genetically-defective dermatosparaxic calves. *Eur J Biochem* **23**:533, 1971.
154. Pinnell SR, Krane SM, Kenzora JE, Glimcher MJ: A heritable disorder of connective tissue: Hydroxylysine-deficient collagen disease. *N Engl J Med* **266**:1013, 1972.
155. Sykes B, Francis MJO, Smith R: Altered relation of two collagen types in osteogenesis imperfecta. *N Engl J Med* **296**:1200, 1977.
156. Holbrook KA, Byers PH: Ultrastructural characteristics of the skin in a form of the Ehlers-Danlos syndrome type IV: Storage in the rough endoplasmic reticulum. *Lab Invest* **44**:342, 1981.
157. Ogilvie D, Wordsworth P, Thompson E, Sykes B: Evidence against the structural gene encoding type II collagen (COL2A1) as the mutant locus in achondroplasia. *J Med Genet* **23**:19, 1986.
158. Wallis G, Sykes B, Byers PH, Mathew CG, Viljoen D, Beighton P: Osteogenesis imperfecta type III: Mutations in the type I collagen structural genes, COL1A1 and COL1A2, are not necessarily responsible. *J Med Genet* **30**:492, 1993.
159. Aitchison K, Oglivie D, Honeyman M, Thompson E, Sykes B: Homozygous osteogenesis imperfecta unlinked to collagen I genes. *Hum Genet* **78**:233, 1988.
160. Smith R, Francis MJO, Houghton GR: *The Brittle Bone Syndrome: Osteogenesis Imperfecta*. London, Butterworths, 1983.
161. Byers PH: Brittle bones—fragile molecules: The molecular basis of osteogenesis imperfecta. *Trends Genet* **9**:295, 1991.
162. Kuivaniemi H, Tromp G, Prockop DJ: Mutations in collagen genes in humans. *FASEB J* **5**:2029, 1991.
163. Steiner R, Byers PH: Osteogenesis imperfecta. *Annu Rev Med* **49**:310, 1992.
164. Cole WG: Etiology and pathogenesis of heritable connective tissue diseases. *J Pediatr Orthop* **13**:392, 1993.
165. Sillence DO, Senn AS, Danks DM: Genetic heterogeneity in osteogenesis imperfecta. *J Med Genet* **16**:101, 1979.
166. Seedorf KS: *Osteogenesis Imperfecta: A Study of Clinical Features and Heredity Based on 55 Danish Families Comprising 180 Affected Members*. Copenhagen, Universitetsforlaget I Arhus, 1949.
167. Wynne-Davies R, Gormley J: Clinical and genetic patterns in osteogenesis imperfecta. *Clin Orthop* **159**:26, 1981.
168. Ibsen KH: Distinct varieties of osteogenesis imperfecta. *Clin Orthop* **50**:279, 1967.
169. Sillence D: Osteogenesis imperfecta: An expanding panorama of variants. *Clin Orthop* **159**:11, 1981.
170. Paterson CR, McAllion S, Miller R: Heterogeneity of osteogenesis imperfecta type I. *J Med Genet* **20**:203, 1983.
171. Levin LS, Salinas CF, Jorgenson RJ: Classification of osteogenesis imperfecta by dental characteristics. *Lancet* **1**:332, 1978.
172. Shapiro JR, Pikus A, Weiss G, Rowe DW: Hearing and middle ear function in osteogenesis imperfecta. *JAMA* **247**:2120, 1982.
173. Quisling RW, Moore GR, Jahrsdoerfer RA, Cantrell RW: Osteogenesis imperfecta; study of 160 family members. *Arch Otolaryngol* **105**:207, 1979.
174. Pederson U: . Hearing loss in patients with osteogenesis imperfecta: A clinical and audiological study of 201 patients. *Scand Audiol* **13**:67, 1984.
175. Armstrong BW: Stapes surgery in patients with osteogenesis imperfecta. *Ann Otol Rhinol Laryngol* **93**:634, 1984.
176. Hortop J, Tsipouras P, Hanley JA, Maron BJ, Shapiro JR: Cardiovascular involvement in osteogenesis imperfecta. *Circulation* **73**:54, 1986.
177. Martin GR, Layman DL, Narayanan AS, Nigra TP, Siegel RC: Collagen synthesis by cultured human fibroblasts. *Isr J Med Sci* **7**:455, 1971.
178. Pentinnen RP, Lichtenstein JR, Martin GR, McKusick VA: Abnormal collagen metabolism in cultured cells in osteogenesis imperfecta. *Proc Natl Acad Sci USA* **72**:586, 1975.
179. Sykes B, Francis MJO, Smith R: Altered relation of two collagen types in osteogenesis imperfecta. *N Engl J Med* **296**:1200, 1977.
180. Barsh GS, David KE, Byers PH: Type I osteogenesis imperfecta: A nonfunctional allele for proα1(I) chains of type I procollagen. *Proc Natl Acad Sci USA* **79**:3838, 1982.
181. Rowe DW, Shapiro JR, Poirier M, Schlesinger S: Diminished type I collagen synthesis and reduced alpha 1(I) collagen messenger RNA in cultured fibroblasts from patients with dominantly inherited (type I) osteogenesis imperfecta. *J Clin Invest* **76**:604, 1985.
182. Genovese C, Rowe D: Analysis of cytoplasmic and nuclear messenger RNA in fibroblasts from patients with type I osteogenesis imperfecta. *Methods Enzymol* **145**:223, 1987.
183. Rowe DW, Stover ML, McKinstry M, Brufsky A, Kream B, Chipman S, Shapiro J: Molecular mechanisms (real and imagined) for osteopenic bone disease. Fourth International Conference on Osteogenesis Imperfecta, Pavia, Italy (September 9–12, 1990), Abstracts, 1990, p 57.
184. Willing MC, Pruchno CJ, Atkinson M, Byers PH: Osteogenesis imperfecta type I is commonly due to a COL1A1 null allele of type I collagen. *Am J Hum Genet* **51**:508, 1992.
185. Sykes B, Oglivie D, Wordsworth P, Anderson J, Jones N: Osteogenesis imperfecta is linked to both type I collagen structural genes. *Lancet* **2**:69, 1986.
186. Sykes B, Oglivie D, Wordsworth P, Wallis G, Mathew C, Beighton P, Nicholls A, Pope FM, Thompson E, Tsipouras P, Schwartz R, Jensson O, Arnason A, Börresen A-L, Heiberg A, Frey D, Steinmann B: Consistent linkage of dominantly inherited osteogenesis imperfecta to the type I collagen loci: COL1A1 and COL1A2. *Am J Hum Genet* **46**:293, 1990.
187. Wallis G, Beighton P, Boyd C, Mathew CG: Mutations linked to the proα2(I) collagen gene are responsible for several cases of osteogenesis imperfecta type I. *J Med Genet* **23**:411, 1986.
188. Willing MC, Cohn DH, Byers PH: Frameshift mutation near the 3′ end of the COL1A1 gene of type I collagen predicts an elongated proα1(I) chain and results in osteogenesis imperfecta type I. *J Clin Invest* **85**:282, 1990.
189. Nicholls AC, Pope FM, Craig D: An abnormal collagen α chain containing cysteine in autosomal dominant osteogenesis imperfecta. *BMJ* **288**:112, 1984.
190. Steinmann B, Nicholls A, Pope FM: Clinical variability of osteogenesis imperfecta reflecting molecular heterogeneity: Cysteine substitutions in the α1(I) collagen chain producing lethal and mild forms. *J Biol Chem* **261**:8958, 1986.
191. Cohn DH, Apone S, Eyre DR, Starman BJ, Andreassen P, Charbonneau H, Nicholls AC, Pope FM, Byers PH: Substitution of cysteine for glycine within the carboxyl-terminal telopeptide of the α1(I) chain of type I collagen produces mild osteogenesis imperfecta. *J Biol Chem* **263**:14605, 1988.

192. Nicholls AC, Oliver J, Renouf D, Pope FM: Type I collagen mutation in osteogenesis imperfecta and inherited osteoporosis. Fourth International Conference on Osteogenesis Imperfecta, Pavia, Italy (September 9–12, 1990), Abstracts, 1990, p 48.
193. Shapiro JR, Stover ML, Burn VE, McKinstry MD, Burshell AL, Chipman SD, Rowe DW: An osteopenic nonfracture syndrome with features of mild osteogenesis imperfecta with substitution of a cysteine for glycine at triple helix position 43 in the proα1(I) chain of type I collagen. *J Clin Invest* **89**:567, 1992.
194. Starman BJ, Eyre D, Charbonneau H, Harrylock M, Weis MA, Weiss L, Graham JM Jr, Byers PH: Osteogenesis imperfecta. The position of substitution for glycine by cysteine in the triple-helical domain of the proα1(I) chains of type I collagen determines the clinical phenotype. *J Clin Invest* **84**:1206, 1989.
195. Byers PH, Shapiro JR, Rowe DW, David KE, Holbrook KA: Abnormal α2-chain in type I collagen from a patient with a form of osteogenesis imperfecta. *J Clin Invest* **71**:689, 1983.
196. Crouch E, Bornstein P: Collagen synthesis by human amniotic fluid cells in culture: Characterization of a procollagen with three identical pro alpha-1(I) chains. *Biochemistry* **17**:5499, 1978.
197. Byers PH, Wenstrup RJ, Bonadio JF, Starman B, Cohn DH: Molecular basis of inherited disorders of collagen biosynthesis: Implications for prenatal diagnosis, in Gedde-Dahl T, Wuepper KD (eds): *Prenatal Diagnosis of Heritable Skin Diseases*. Basel, Karger, 1987, p 158.
198. Connor JM, Connor RA, Sweet EM, Gibson AA, Patrick WJ, McNay MB, Redford DH: Lethal neonatal chondrodysplasias in the West of Scotland 1970-1983 with a description of a thanatophoric, dysplasialike, autosomal recessive disorder, Glasgow variant. *Am J Med Genet* **22**:243, 1985.
199. Byers PH, Tsipouras P, Bonadio JF, Starman BJ, Schwartz RC: Perinatal lethal osteogenesis imperfecta (OI type II): A biochemically heterogeneous disorder usually due to new mutations in the genes for type I collagen. *Am J Hum Genet* **42**:237, 1988.
200. Shapiro JE, Phillips JA III, Byers PH, Sanders R, Holbrook KA, Levin LS, Dorst J, Barsh GS, Peterson KE, Goldstein P: Prenatal diagnosis of lethal perinatal osteogenesis imperfecta (OI type II). *J Pediatr* **100**:127, 1982.
201. Chervenak FA, Romero R, Berkowitz RL, Mahoney MJ, Tortora M, Mayden K, Hobbin JC: Antenatal sonographic findings of osteogenesis imperfecta. *Am J Obstet Gynecol* **143**:228, 1982.
202. Elejalde BR, Elejalde MM: Prenatal diagnosis of perinatally lethal osteogenesis imperfecta. *Am J Med Genet* **14**:353, 1983.
203. Sillence DO, Barlow KK, Garber AP, Hall JG, Rimoin DL: Osteogenesis imperfecta type II. Delineation of the phenotype with reference to genetic heterogeneity. *Am J Med Genet* **17**:407, 1984.
204. Young ID, Harper P: Recurrence risk in osteogenesis imperfecta congenita. *Lancet* **1**:432, 1980.
205. Young ID, Thompson EM, Hall CM, Pembrey ME: Osteogenesis imperfecta type IIA: Evidence for dominant inheritance. *J Med Genet* **24**:386, 1987.
206. Cohn DH, Starman BJ, Blumberg B, Byers PH: Recurrence of lethal osteogenesis imperfecta due to parental mosaicism for a dominant mutation in a human type I collagen gene (COL1A1). *Am J Hum Genet* **46**:591, 1990.
207. Cohn DH, Wallis GA, Edwards MJ, Starman BJ, Byers PH: Germline and somatic mosaicism in osteogenesis imperfecta. Fourth International Conference on Osteogenesis Imperfecta, Pavia, Italy (September 9–12, 1990), Abstracts, 1990, p 47.
208. Wallis GA, Starman BJ, Zinn AB, Byers PH: Variable expression of osteogenesis imperfecta in a nuclear family is explained by somatic mosaicism for a lethal point mutation in the α1(I) gene (COL1A1) of type I collagen in a parent. *Am J Hum Genet* **46**:1034, 1990.
209. Constantinou CD, Nielsen KB, Prockop DJ: A lethal variant of osteogenesis imperfecta has a single base mutation that substitutes cysteine for glycine 904 of the α1(I) chain of type I procollagen. The asymptomatic mother has an unidentified mutation producing an overmodified and unstable type I procollagen. *J Clin Invest* **83**:574, 1989.
210. Constantinou CD, Pack M, Young SB, Prockop DJ: Phenotypic heterogeneity in osteogenesis imperfecta: The mildly affected mother of a proband with a lethal variant has the same mutation substituting cysteine for α1-glycine 904 in a type I procollagen gene (COL1A1). *Am J Hum Genet* **47**:670, 1990.
211. Edwards MJ, Wenstrup RJ, Byers PH, Cohn DH: Recurrence of lethal osteogenesis imperfecta due to parental mosaicism for a mutation in the COL1A2 gene of type I collagen. The mosaic parent exhibits phenotypic features of a mild form of the disease. *Hum Mut* **1**:47, 1992.
212. Chawla S: Intrauterine osteogenesis imperfecta in four siblings. *BMJ* **5375**:99, 1964.
213. Braga S, Passarge E: Congenital osteogenesis imperfecta in three sibs. *Hum Genet* **58**:441, 1981.
214. Spranger JW, Langer LO, Wiedemann HR: *Bone Dysplasias: Atlas of Constitutional Disorders of Skeletal Development*. Philadelphia, Saunders, 1974.
215. Rimoin DL: The chondrodystrophies. *Adv Hum Genet* **5**:1, 1975.
216. Follis RH Jr: Maldevelopment of the corium in the osteogenesis imperfecta syndrome. *Bull Johns Hopkins Hosp* **93**:225, 1953.
217. Dimaio MS, Barth R, Koprivnikar KE, Sussman BL, Copel JA, Mahoney MJ, Byers PH, Cohn DH: First trimester prenatal diagnosis of osteogenesis imperfecta type II by DNA analysis and sonography. *Prenat Diagn* **13**:589, 1993.
218. Bateman JF, Mascara T, Chan D, Cole WG: Abnormal type I collagen metabolism by cultured fibroblasts in lethal perinatal osteogenesis imperfecta. *Biochem J* **217**:103, 1984.
219. Bateman JF, Chan D, Mascara T, Robers JG, Cole WG: Collagen defects in lethal perinatal osteogenesis imperfecta. *Biochem J* **240**:699, 1986.
220. Bonadio J, Byers PH: Subtle structural alterations in the chains of type I procollagen produce osteogenesis imperfecta type II. *Nature* **316**:363, 1985.
221. Byers PH, Wallis GA, Willing MC: Osteogenesis imperfecta: Translation of mutation to phenotype. *J Med Genet* **28**:433, 1991.
222. Heller RH, Winn KJ, Heller RM: The prenatal diagnosis of osteogenesis imperfecta congenita. *Am J Obstet Gynecol* **121**:572, 1975.
223. Barsh GS, Byers PH: Reduced secretion of structurally abnormal type I procollagen in a form of osteogenesis imperfecta. *Proc Natl Acad Sci USA* **78**:5142, 1981.
224. Williams CJ, Prockop DJ: Synthesis and processing of a type I procollagen containing shortened proα1(I) chains by fibroblasts from a patient with osteogenesis imperfecta. *J Biol Chem* **258**:5915, 1983.
225. Chu M-L, Williams CJ, Pepe G, Hirsch JL, Prockop DJ, Ramirez F: Internal deletion in a collagen gene in a perinatal lethal form of osteogenesis imperfecta. *Nature* **304**:78, 1983.
226. Chu M-L, Gargiulo V, Williams CJ, Ramirez F: Multiexon deletion in an osteogenesis imperfecta variant with increased type III collagen mRNA. *J Biol Chem* **260**:691, 1985.
227. Barsh GS, Roush CL, Bonadio J, Byers PH, Gelinas RE: Intron-mediated recombination may cause a deletion in an α1(I) collagen chain in a lethal form of osteogenesis imperfecta. *Proc Natl Acad Sci USA* **82**:2870, 1985.
228. Byers PH, Starman BJ, Cohn DH, Horwitz AL: A novel mutation causes a perinatal lethal form of osteogenesis imperfecta: An insertion in one α1(I) collagen allele (COL1A1). *J Biol Chem* **263**:7855, 1988.
229. Cohn DH, Pruchno CJ, Zhang X, Byers PH: Homology-mediated recombination between type I collagen gene (COL1A1) exons results in an intragenic tandem duplication and lethal osteogenesis imperfecta. *Am J Hum Genet* **47**:A110, 1990.
230. Willing MC, Cohn DH, Starman B, Holbrook KA, Greenberg CR, Byers PH: Heterozygosity for a large deletion in the α2(I) collagen gene has a dramatic effect on type I collagen secretion and produces perinatal lethal osteogenesis imperfecta. *J Biol Chem* **263**:8398, 1988.

231. Chessler SD, Byers PH: Defective folding and stable association with protein disulfide isomerase/prolyl hydroxylase of type I procollagen with a deletion in the proα2(I) chain that preserves the gly-X-Y repeat pattern. *J Biol Chem* **267**:7751, 1991.
232. Steinmann B, Rao VH, Bruckner P, Vogel A, Gitzelmann R, Byers PH: Cysteine in the triple-helical domain of one allelic product of the α1(I) gene of type I collagen produces a lethal form of osteogenesis imperfecta. *J Biol Chem* **259**:11129, 1984.
233. Cohn DH, Byers PH, Steinmann B, Gelinas RE: Lethal osteogenesis imperfecta resulting from a single nucleotide change in one human proα1(I) collagen allele. *Proc Natl Acad Sci USA* **83**:6045, 1986.
234. Valli M, Sangalli A, Rossi A, Mottes M, Forlino A, Tenni R, Pignatti PF, Cetta G: Osteogenesis imperfecta dn type-I collagen mutation. A lethal variant caused by a Gly910 to Ala substitution in the α1(I) chain. *Eur J Biochem* **211**:415, 1993.
235. Lamande SR, Dahl H-HM, Cole WG, Bateman JF: Characterization of point mutations in the collagen COL1A1 and COL1A2 genes causing lethal perinatal osteogenesis imperfecta. *J Biol Chem* **264**:15809, 1989.
236. Westerhausen A, Kishi J, Prockop DJ: Mutations that substitute serine for glycine α1-598 and glycine α1-631 in type I procollagen. The effects on unfolding of the triple-helix are position-specific, and demonstrate that the protein unfolds through a series of cooperative blocks. *J Biol Chem* **265**:13995, 1990.
237. Cohn DH, Wallis G, Zhang X, Byers PH: Serine for glycine substitutions in the α1(I) chain of type I collagen: Biological plasticity in the Gly-Pro-Hyp clamp at the carboxyl-terminal end of the triple-helical domain. *Matrix* **10**:236, 1990.
238. Wallis GA, Starman BJ, Byers PH: Clinical heterogeneity of OI explained by molecular heterogeneity and somatic mosaicism. *Am J Hum Genet* **46**:A228, 1989.
239. Pruchno CJ, Cohn DH, Wallis GA, Willing MC, Starman BJ, Zhang X, Byers PH: Osteogenesis imperfecta due to recurrent point mutations at CpG dinucleotides in the COL1A1 gene of type I collagen. *Hum Genet* **87**:33, 1991.
240. Fertala A, Westerhausen A, Morris GM, Rooney JE, Prockop DJ: Two cysteine substitutions in procollagen I: A glycine replacement near the N-terminus of α1(I) chain causes lethal osteogenesis imperfecta and a glycine replacement in the α2(I) chain markedly destabilizes the triple-helix. *Biochem J* **289**:195, 1993.
241. Steinmann B, Westerhausen A, Constantinou CD, Superti-Furga A, Prockop DJ: Substitution of cysteine for glycine α1-691 in the gene for the proα1(I) chain of type I procollagen (COL1A1) in a proband with lethal osteogenesis imperfecta. Cleavage to a thermally stable intermediate at a site COOH-terminal to the substitution. *Biochem J* **279**:747, 1991.
242. Vogel BE, Minor RR, Freund M, Prockop DJ: A point mutation in a type I procollagen gene converts glycine 748 of the α1 chain to cysteine and destabilizes the triple-helix in a lethal variant of osteogenesis imperfecta. *J Biol Chem* **262**:14737, 1987.
243. Bateman JF, Chan D, Walker ID, Rogers JG, Cole WG: Lethal perinatal osteogenesis imperfecta due to the substitution of arginine for glycine at residue 391 of the α1(I) chains of type I collagen. *J Biol Chem* **262**:7021, 1987.
244. Bateman JF, Lamande SR, Dahl H-HM, Chan D, Cole WG: Substitution of arginine for glycine 664 in the collagen α1(I) chain in lethal perinatal osteogenesis imperfecta. *J Biol Chem* **263**:11627, 1988.
245. Baker AT, Ramshaw JAM, Chan D, Cole WG, Bateman JF: Changes in collagen stability and folding in lethal perinatal osteogenesis imperfecta. *Biochem J* **261**:253, 1989.
246. Wallis GA, Starman BJ, Schwartz MF, Byers PH: Substitution of arginine for glycine at position 847 in the triple-helical domain of the α1(I) chain of type I collagen produces lethal osteogenesis imperfecta. Molecules that contain one or two abnormal chains differ in stability and secretion. *J Biol Chem* **265**:18628, 1990.
247. Zhuang J, Constantinou CD, Ganguly A, Prockop DJ: A single base mutation in type I procollagen that converts glycine α1-541 to aspartate in a lethal variant of osteogenesis imperfecta. Detection of the mutation with carbodiimide reaction. *Matrix* **10**:252, 1990.
248. Patterson E, Smiley E, Bonadio J: RNA sequence analysis of a perinatal lethal osteogenesis imperfecta mutation. *J Biol Chem* **264**:10083, 1989.
249. Westerhausen A, Constantinou CD, Prockop DJ: A mutation that substitutes valine for glycine α1-637 in a type I procollagen gene (COL1A1) and causes lethal osteogenesis imperfecta. Evidence for a cooperative block of micro-unfolding between amino acid positions 637 and 775. *Am J Hum Genet* **47**:A242, 1990.
250. Bateman JF, Hannagan M, Lamande S, Moeller I, Chan D, Cole WG: Collagen I mutations in perinatal lethal osteogenesis imperfecta. Fourth International Conference on Osteogenesis Imperfecta, Pavia, Italy (September 9–12, 1990), Abstracts, 1990, p 2.
251. Tsuneyoshi T, Constantinou CD, Mikkelson M, Prockop DJ: A substitution of arginine for glycine α2-694 in a gene for type I procollagen (COL1A2) that causes lethal osteogenesis imperfecta. Further definition of a cooperative block for micro-unfolding of the triple-helix between about residues 637 and 775. *Am J Hum Genet* **47**:A240, 1990.
252. Bonadio J, Holbrook KA, Gelinas RE, Jacob J, Byers PH: Altered triple-helical structure of type I procollagen in lethal perinatal osteogenesis imperfecta. *J Biol Chem* **260**:1734, 1985.
253. Niyibizi C, Bonadio J, Byers PH, Eyre DR: Incorporation of type I collagen molecules that contain a mutant α2(I) chain (Gly^{580}–Asp) into bone matrix in a lethal case of osteogenesis imperfecta. *J Biol Chem* **267**:23108, 1992.
254. Marini JC, Grange DK, Lewis MB: Detection of a mutation in alpha 2(I) mRNA in a proband with lethal type II osteogenesis imperfecta. *Am J Hum Genet* **45**:A205, 1989.
255. Baldwin CT, Constantinou CD, Dumars KW, Prockop DJ: A single base mutation that converts glycine 907 of the α2(I) chain of type I procollagen to aspartate in a lethal variant of osteogenesis imperfecta. The single amino acid substitution near the carboxyl terminus destabilizes the whole triple-helix. *J Biol Chem* **264**:3002, 1989.
256. Bonadio J, Ramirez F, Barr M: An intron mutation in the human α1(I) collagen gene alters the efficiency of pre-mRNA splicing and is associated with osteogenesis imperfecta type II. *J Biol Chem* **265**:2262, 1990.
257. De Wet WJ, Pihlajaniemi T, Myers J, Kelly TE, Prockop DJ: Synthesis of a shortened proα2(I) chain and decreased synthesis of proα2(I) chains in a proband with osteogenesis imperfecta. *J Biol Chem* **258**:7721, 1983.
258. De Wet W, Sippola M, Tromp G, Prockop D, Chu M-L, Ramirez F: Use of R-loop mapping for the assessment of human collagen mutations. *J Biol Chem* **261**:3857, 1986.
259. Tromp G, Prockop DJ: Single base mutation in the proα2(I) collagen gene that causes efficient splicing of RNA from exon 27 to exon 29 and synthesis of a shortened but in-frame proα2(I) chain. *Proc Natl Acad Sci USA* **85**:5254, 1988.
260. Ganguly A, Baldwin CT, Strobel D, Conway D, Horton W, Prockop DJ: Heterozygous mutation in the G+5 position of intron-33 of the pro-α2(I) gene (COL1A2) that causes aberrant RNA splicing and lethal osteogenesis imperfecta. Use of carbodiimide methods that decrease the extent of DNA sequencing necessary to define an unusual mutation. *J Biol Chem* **266**:12035, 1991.
261. Hawkins JR, Superti-Furga A, Steinmann B, Dalgleish R: A 9 base pair deletion in COL1A1 in a lethal variant of osteogenesis imperfecta. *J Biol Chem* **266**:22370, 1991.
262. Wallis GA, Kadler KE, Starman BJ, Byers PH: A tripeptide deletion in the triple-helix domain of the proα1(I) chain of type I procollagen produces lethal osteogenesis imperfecta but does not alter cleavage of the molecules by N-proteinase. *J Biol Chem* **267**:25529, 1992.
263. Bateman JF, Lamande SR, Dahl H-HM, Chan D, Mascara T, Cole WG: A frameshift mutation results in a truncated nonfunctional carboxyl-terminal proα1(I) propeptide of type I collagen in osteogenesis imperfecta. *J Biol Chem* **264**:10960, 1989.
264. Wallis GA, Starman BJ, Chessler SD, Willing MC, Byers PH: Mutations in the CB6 and carboxyl-terminal regions of COL1A1 causing lethal OI have different effects on

the stability and secretion of the type I collagen molecule. Fourth International Conference on Osteogenesis Imperfecta, Pavia, Italy (September 9–12, 1990), Abstracts, 1990, p 55.

265. Chessler SD, Wallis GA, Byers PH: Mutations in the carboxyl-terminal propeptide of the proα1(I) chain of type I collagen result in defective chain association and produce lethal osteogenesis imperfecta. *J Biol Chem* **268**:18218, 1993.
266. Follis RH Jr: Maldevelopment of the corium in the osteogenesis imperfecta syndrome. *Bull Johns Hopkins Hosp* **93**:225, 1953.
267. Thompson EM, Young ID, Hall CM, Pembrey ME: Recurrence risks and prognosis in severe sporadic osteogenesis imperfecta. *J Med Genet* **24**:390, 1987.
268. Sillence DO, Barlow KK, Cole WG, Dietrich S, Garber AP, Rimoin DL: Osteogenesis imperfecta type III: Delineation of the phenotype with reference to genetic heterogeneity. *Am J Med Genet* **23**:821, 1986.
269. Beighton P, Versfeld GA: On the paradoxically high relative prevalence of osteogenesis imperfecta type III in the Black population of South Africa. *Clin Genet* **27**:398, 1985.
270. Goldman AV, Davidson D, Pavlov H, Bullough PG: "Popcorn" calcification: A prognostic sign in osteogenesis imperfecta. *Radiology* **136**:351, 1980.
271. Sofield HA, Millar EA: Fragmentation, realignment and intramedullary rod fixation of deformities of the long bones in children: A ten year appraisal. *J Bone Joint Surg Am* **41**:1371, 1959.
272. Moorefield WG Jr, Miller GR: Aftermath of osteogenesis imperfecta: The disease in adulthood. *J Bone Joint Surg* [*Am*] **62**:113, 1980.
273. Albright JA: Systemic treatment of osteogenesis imperfecta. *Clin Orthop* **159**:88, 1981.
274. Aylsworth AS, Seed JW, Builford WB, Burns CB, Washburn DB: Prenatal diagnosis of a severe deforming type of osteogenesis imperfecta. *Am J Med Genet* **19**:707, 1984.
275. Robinson LP, Worthen NJ, Lachman RS, Adomian GE, Rimoin DL: Prenatal diagnosis of osteogenesis imperfecta type III. *Prenat Diagn* **7**:7, 1987.
276. Nicholls AC, Pope FM, Schloon H: Biochemical heterogeneity of osteogenesis imperfecta: A new variant. *Lancet* **1**:1193, 1979.
277. Nicholls AC, Osse G, Schloon HG, Lenard HG, Deak S, Myers JC, Prockop DJ, Weigel WRF, Fryer P, Pope FM: The clinical features of homozygous α2(I) collagen deficient osteogenesis imperfecta. *J Med Genet* **21**:257, 1984.
278. Deak SB, Nicholls AC, Pope FM, Prockop DJ: The molecular defect in a non-lethal variant of osteogenesis imperfecta. *J Biol Chem* **258**:15192, 1983.
279. Chu M-L, Rowe D, Nicholls AC, Pope FM, Prockop DJ: Presence of translatable mRNA for proα2(I) chains in fibroblasts from a patient with osteogenesis imperfecta whose type I collagen does not contain α1(I) chains. *Collagen Related Res* **4**:389, 1984.
280. Dickson LA, Pihlajaniemi T, Deak S, Pope FM, Nicholls A, Prockop DJ, Myers JC: Nuclease S_1 mapping of a homozygous mutation in the carboxy-propeptide coding region of the proα2(I) collagen gene in a patient with osteogenesis imperfecta. *Proc Natl Acad Sci USA* **81**:4524, 1984.
281. Pihlajaniemi T, Dickson LA, Pope FM, Korhonen VR, Nicholls A, Prockop DJ, Myers JC: Osteogenesis imperfecta: Cloning of a proα2(I) collagen gene with a frameshift mutation. *J Biol Chem* **259**:12941, 1984.
282. van der Rest M, Hayes A, Marie P, Desbarats M, Kaplan P, Glorieux FH: Lethal osteogenesis imperfecta with amniotic band lesions: Collagen studies. *Am J Med Genet* **24**:433, 1986.
283. Pack M, Constantinou C, Kalia K, Nielsen KB, Prockop DJ: Substitution of serine for α1(I)-glycine 844 in a severe variant of osteogenesis imperfecta minimally destabilizes the triple helix. The effects of glycine substitutions on thermal stability are either position or amino acid specific. *J Biol Chem* **264**:19694, 1989.
284. Cohn DH, Byers PH: Cysteine in the triple-helical domain of the α chain of type I collagen in non-lethal forms of osteogenesis imperfecta. *Hum Genet* **87**:167, 1991.
285. Wenstrup RJ, Shrago-Howe AW, Lever LW, Phillips CL, Byers PH, Cohn DH: The effects of different cysteine for glycine substitutions within α2(I) chains: Evidence of distinct structural domains within the type I collagen triple-helix. *J Biol Chem* **266**:2590, 1990.
286. Paterson CR, McAllion S, Miller R: Osteogenesis imperfecta with dominant inheritance and normal sclerae. *J Bone Joint Surg* [*Br*] **65**:35, 1983.
287. Wenstrup RJ, Willing MC, Starman BJ, Byers PH: Distinct biochemical phenotypes predict clinical severity in nonlethal variants of osteogenesis imperfecta. *Am J Hum Genet* **46**:975, 1990.
288. Tsipouras P, Schwartz RC, Goldberg JD, Berkowitz RL, Ramirez F: Prenatal prediction of osteogenesis imperfecta (OI type IV): Exclusion of inheritance using a collagen gene probe. *J Med Genet* **24**:406, 1987.
289. Tsipouras P, Myers JC, Ramirez F, Prockop DJ: Restriction fragment length polymorphisms associated with the proα2(I) gene of human type I procollagen. *J Clin Invest* **72**:1262, 1983.
290. Tsipouras P, Borresen A-L, Dickson LA, Berg K, Prockop DJ, Ramirez F: Molecular heterogeneity in the mild autosomal dominant forms of osteogenesis imperfecta. *Am J Hum Genet* **36**:1172, 1984.
291. Wenstrup RJ, Tsipouras P, Byers PH: Osteogenesis imperfecta type IV: Biochemical confirmation of genetic linkage to the proα2(I) gene of type I collagen. *J Clin Invest* **78**:1449, 1986.
292. Wenstrup RJ, Cohn DH, Cohen T, Byers PH: Arginine for glycine substitution in the triple-helical domain of the products of one α2(I) collagen allele (COL1A2) produces the osteogenesis imperfecta type IV phenotype. *J Biol Chem* **263**:7734, 1988.
293. De Vries WN, De Wet WJ: The molecular defect in an autosomal dominant form of osteogenesis imperfecta. Synthesis of type I procollagen containing cysteine in the triple-helical domain of pro-α1(I) chains. *J Biol Chem* **261**:9056, 1986.
294. Sippola M, Kaffe S, Prockop DJ: A heterozygous defect for structurally altered pro-α2 chain of type I procollagen in a mild variant of osteogenesis imperfecta. *J Biol Chem* **259**:14094, 1984.
295. Kuivaniemi H, Sabol C, Tromp G, Sippola-Thiele M, Prockop DJ: A 19-base pair deletion in the proα2(I) gene of type I procollagen that causes in-frame RNA splicing from exon 10 to exon 12 in a proband with atypical osteogenesis imperfecta and in his asymptomatic mother. *J Biol Chem* **263**:11407, 1988.
296. Minor RR, Sippola-Thiele M, McKeon J, Berger J, Prockop DJ: Defects in the processing of procollagen to collagen are demonstrable in cultured fibroblasts from patients with the Ehlers-Danlos and osteogenesis imperfecta syndromes. *J Biol Chem* **261**:10006, 1986.
297. Saraux H, Franzal J, Roy C, Aron JJ, Hayat B, Lamy M: Pseudo-gliome et fragilite osseuse hereditaire a transmission autosomal recessive. *Ann Oculist* **200**:1241, 1967.
298. Bianchine JW, Murdock JL: Juvenile osteoporosis (?) in a boy with bilateral enucleation of the eyes for pseudoglioma. *Birth Defects* **5(4)**:225, 1969.
299. Beighton P, Winship I, Behari D: The ocular form of osteogenesis imperfecta: A new autosomal recessive syndrome. *Clin Genet* **28**:69, 1985.
300. Dent CE, Friedman M: Idopathic juvenile osteoporosis. *Q J Med* **34**:177, 1965.
301. Shields ED, Bixler D, El-Kafrawy AM: A proposed classification for heritable human dentine defects with a description of a new entity. *Arch Oral Biol* **18**:543, 1973.
302. Ball SP, Cook PJL, Mars M, Buckton KE: Linkage between dentinogenesis imperfecta and Gc. *Ann Hum Genet* **46**:35, 1982.
303. Takagi Y, Veis A, Sauk JJ: Relation of mineralization defects in collagen matrices to non-collagenous protein components. Identification of a molecular defect in dentinogenesis imperfecta. *Clin Orthop* **176**:282, 1983.
304. Denholm LJ, Cole WG: Heritable bone fragility, joint laxity and dysplastic dentin in Friesian calves: A bovine syndrome of osteogenesis imperfecta. *Aust Vet J* **60**:9, 1983.
305. Fisher LW, Denholm LJ, Conn KM, Termine JD: Mineralized tissue protein profiles in the Australian form of bovine osteogenesis imperfecta. *Calcif Tissue Int* **38**:16, 1986.

306. Chipman SD, Sweet HO, McBride DJ Jr, Davisson MT, Marks SC Jr, Shuldiner AR, Wenstrup RJ, Rowe DW, Shapiro JR: Defective proα2(I) collagen synthesis in a recessive mutation in mice: A model of human osteogenesis imperfecta. *Proc Natl Acad Sci USA* **90**:1701, 1993.
307. Schnieke A, Harbers K, Jaenisch R: Embryonic lethal mutation in mice induced by retrovirus insertion into the α1(I) collagen gene. *Nature* **304**:315, 1983.
308. Harbers K, Kuehn M, Delius H, Jaenisch R: Insertion of retrovirus into the first intron of α1(I) collagen gene leads to embryonic lethal mutation in mice. *Proc Natl Acad Sci USA* **81**:1504, 1984.
309. Löhler J, Timpl R, Jaenisch R: Embryonic lethal mutation in mouse collagen I gene causes rupture of blood vessels and is associated with erythropoietic and mesenchymal cell death. *Cell* **38**:597, 1984.
310. Schnieke A, Dziadek M, Bateman J, Mascara T, Harbers K, Gelinas R, Jaenisch R: Introduction of the human proα1(I) collagen gene into proα1(I)-deficient Mov-13 mouse cells leads to formation of functional mouse-human hybrid type I collagen. *Proc Natl Acad Sci USA* **84**:764, 1987.
311. Stacey A, Bateman J, Choi T, Mascara T, Cole W, Jaenisch R: Perinatal lethal osteogenesis imperfecta in transgenic mice bearing an engineered mutant pro-α1(I) collagen gene. *Nature* **332**:131, 1988.
312. Pereira R, Khillan JS, Helminen HJ, Hume EL, Prockop DJ: Transgenic mice expressing a partially deleted gene for type I procollagen (COL1A1). A breeding line with a phenotype of spontaneous fractures and decreased bone collagen and mineral. *J Clin Invest* **91**:709, 1993.
313. Sykes B: The molecular genetics of collagen. *Bioessays* **3**:112, 1985.
314. Schnieke A, Harbers K, Jaenisch R: Embryonic lethal mutation in mice induced by retrovirus insertion into the α1(I) collagen gene. *Nature* **304**:315, 1983.
315. Bonadio J, Saunders TL, Tsai E, Goldstein SA, Morris-Wiman J, Brinkley L, Dolan DF, Altschuler RA, Hawkins JE Jr, Bateman JF, Mascara T, Jaenisch R: Transgenic mouse model of the mild dominant form of osteogenesis imperfecta. *Proc Natl Acad Sci USA* **87**:7145, 1990.
316. Holbrook KA, Byers PH: Skin is a window on heritable disorders of connective tissue. *Am J Med Genet* **34**:105, 1989.
317. Minor RR, Sippola-Thiele M, McKeon J, Berger J, Prockop DJ: Defects in the processing of procollagen to collagen are demonstrable in cultured fibroblasts from patients with the Ehlers-Danlos and osteogenesis imperfecta syndromes. *J Biol Chem* **261**:10006, 1986.
318. Dombrowski KE, Vogel BE, Prockop DJ: Mutations that alter the primary structure of type I procollagen have long-range effects on its cleavage by procollagen N-proteinase. *Biochemistry* **28**:7107, 1989.
319. Traub W, Steinmann B: Structural study of a mutant type I collagen from a patient with lethal osteogenesis imperfecta containing an intramolecular disulfide bond in the triple-helical domain. *FEBS Lett* **198**:213, 1986.
320. Beighton P: *The Ehlers-Danlos Syndrome*. London, Heinemann, 1970.
321. Byers PH, Holbrook KA: Molecular basis of clinical heterogeneity in the Ehlers-Danlos syndrome. *Ann NY Acad Sci* **460**:298, 1985.
322. Tschernogobow A: Ein fall von cutis laxa. *Jahresber Ges Med* **27**:562, 1892.
323. Ehlers E: Cutis laxa, niegung zu haemorrhagien in der haut, lockerung mehrerer artikulationen. *Derm Z* **8**:173, 1901.
324. Danlos M: Un cas de cutis laxa avec tumeurs par contusion chronique des coudes et des genoux (xanthome juvenile pseudo-diabetique de MM Hallopeau et Mace de Lepinay). *Bull Soc Franc Derm Syph* **19**:70, 1908.
325. Barabas AP: Heterogeneity of the Ehlers-Danlos syndrome: Description of three clinical types and a hypothesis to explain the basic defect. *BMJ* **2**:612, 1967.
326. Beighton P, Price A, Lord J, Dickson E: Variants of the Ehlers-Danlos syndrome. *Ann Rheum Dis* **28**:228, 1969.
327. Barabas AP: Ehlers-Danlos syndrome associated with prematurity and premature rupture of foetal membranes: Possible increase in incidence. *BMJ* **2**:682, 1966.
328. Leier CV, Call TD, Fulderson PK, Wooley CF: The spectrum of cardiac defects in the Ehlers-Danlos syndrome type I and III. *Ann Intern Med* **92**:171, 1980.
329. Sokolov BP, Prytkov AN, Tromp G, Knowlton RG, Prockop DJ: Exclusion of COL1A1, COL1A2, and COL3A1 genes as candidate genes for Ehlers-Danlos syndrome type I in one large family. *Hum Genet* **88**:125, 1991.
330. Grahame R: Physical properties of the skin in the Ehlers-Danlos syndrome, in Beighton P (ed): *The Ehlers-Danlos Syndrome*. London, Heinemann, 1970.
331. Vogel A, Holbrook KA, Steinmann B, Gitzelmann R, Byers PH: Abnormal collagen fibril structure in the gravis form (type I) of the Ehlers-Danlos syndrome. *Lab Invest* **40**:201, 1979.
332. Sevenich M, Schultz-Ehrenburg U, Organos CE: Ehlers-Danlos syndrome: A disease of fibroblasts and collagen fibrils. *Arch Dermatol Res* **267**:237, 1980.
333. Shinkai H, Hirabayashi O, Tameki A, Matsubayashi S, Seno S: Connective tissue metabolism in cultured fibroblasts of a patient with Ehlers-Danlos syndrome type I. *Arch Dermatol Res* **257**:113, 1976.
334. Sasaki T, Arai K, Ono M, Yamaguchi T, Furuta S, Nagai Y: Ehlers-Danlos syndrome. A variant characterized by the deficiency of proα2 chain of type I procollagen. *Arch Dermatol* **123**:76, 1987.
335. Sack G: Status dysvascularis; ein fall von besonderer zerreisslichkeit dev blutgefasse. *Dtsch Archiv Klin Med* **178**:663, 1936.
336. Gottron F: Familiare acrogeria. *Arch Dermatol Res* **181**:571, 1940.
337. Pope FM, Martin GR, Lichtenstein JR, Penttinen RP, Gerson G, Rowe DW, McKusick VA: Patients with Ehlers-Danlos syndrome type IV lack type III collagen. *Proc Natl Acad Sci USA* **72**:1314, 1975.
338. Pope FM, Nicholls AC, Jones PM, Wells RS, Lawrence D: EDS IV (acrogeria): New autosomal dominant and recessive types. *Proc R Soc Med* **73**:180, 1980.
339. Tsipouras P, Byers PH, Schwartz RC, Chu M-L, Weil D, Pepe G, Cassidy SB, Ramirez F: Ehlers-Danlos syndrome type IV: Cosegregation of the phenotype to a COL3A1 allele of type III procollagen. *Hum Genet* **74**:41, 1986.
340. Pope FM, Martin GR, McKusick VA: Inheritance of Ehlers-Danlos type IV syndrome. *J Med Genet* **14**:200, 1977.
341. Sulh HMB, Steinmann B, Rao VH, Dudin G, Zeid A, Slim M, Der Kaloustian VM: Ehlers-Danlos syndrome type IVD: An autosomal recessive disorder. *Clin Genet* **25**:278, 1984.
342. Rudd NL, Nimrod C, Holbrook KA, Byers PH: Pregnancy complications in type IV Ehlers-Danlos syndrome. *Lancet* **1**:50, 1983.
343. Pepin MG, Superti-Furga A, Byers PH: Natural history of Ehlers-Danlos syndrome type IV (EDS type IV): Review of 137 cases. *Am J Hum Genet* **51**:A44, 1992.
344. Imahori S, Bannerman RM, Graf CJ, Brennan JC: Ehlers-Danlos syndrome with multiple arterial lesions. *Am J Med* **47**:967, 1969.
345. Lach B, Nair SG, Russell NA, Benoit BG: Spontaneous carotid-cavernous fistula and multiple arterial dissections in type IV Ehlers-Danlos syndrome. *J Neurosurg* **66**:462, 1987.
346. Schoolman A, Kepes JJ: Bilateral spontaneous carotid-cavernous fistulae in Ehlers-Danlos syndrome. *J Neurosurg* **26**:82, 1967.
347. Fox R, Pope FM, Narcisi P, Nicholls AC, Kendall BE, Hourihan MD, Comston DAS: Spontaneous carotid cavernous fistula in Ehlers-Danlos syndrome. *J Neurol Neurosurg Psychiatry* **51**:984, 1988.
348. Halbach VV, Higashida RT, Dowd CF, Barnwell SL, Hieshima GB: Treatment of carotid-cavernous fistula in Ehlers-Danlos syndrome. *Neurosurgery* **26**:1021, 1990.
349. Pope FM, Nocholls AC: Pregancy and Ehlers-Danlos syndrome type IV. *Lancet* **1**:249, 1983.
350. Kuming BS, Joffe L: Ehlers-Danlos syndrome associated with keratoconus. *S Afr Med J* **52**:403, 1977.
351. Pope FM, Narcisi P, Nicholls AC, Liberman M, Oorthuys JWE: Clinical presentations of Ehlers-Danlos syndrome type IV. *Arch Dis Child* **63**:1016, 1988.

352. Kontusaari S, Tromp G, Kuivaniemi H, Stolle C, Pope FM, Prockop DJ: Substitution of aspartate for glycine 1018 in type III procollagen (COL3A1) causes type IV Ehlers-Danlos syndrome: The mutated allele is present in most blood leukocytes of the asymptomatic and mosaic mother. *Am J Hum Genet* **51**:497, 1992.
353. Milewicz DM, Witz AM, Smith ACM, Manchester DK, Waldstein G, Byers PH: Parental somatic and germline mosaicism for a multi-exon deletion with unusual endpoints in a type III collagen (COL3A1) allele produces Ehlers-Danlos syndrome type IV in the heterozygous offspring. *Am J Hum Genet* **53**:62, 1993.
354. Holbrook KA, Byers PH: Diseases of the extracellular matrix: Structural alterations of collagen fibrils in skin, in Uitto J, Perejda AJ (eds): *Connective Tissue Disease: Molecular Pathology of the Extracellular Matrix*. New York, Marcel Dekker, 1987, p 101.
355. Byers PH, Holbrook KA, McGillivray B, McCleod PM, Lowry RB: Clinical and ultrastructural heterogeneity of type IV Ehlers-Danlos syndrome. *Hum Genet* **47**:141, 1979.
356. Laurent R, Agache P: L'acrogeria est-elle une maladie du fibroblaste? *Dermatologica* **148**:28, 1974.
357. Byers PH, Holbrook KA, Barsh GS, Smith LT, Bornstein P: Altered secretion of type III procollagen in a form of type IV Ehlers-Danlos syndrome: Biochemical studies in cultured fibroblasts. *Lab Invest* **44**:336, 1981.
358. Aumailley M, Krieg T, Dessau W, Müller PK, Timpl R, Bricaud H: Biochemical and immunological studies of fibroblasts derived from a patient with Ehlers-Danlos syndrome type IV demonstrate reduced type III collagen synthesis. *Arch Dermatol Res* **269**:169, 1980.
359. Clark JG, Kuhn C III, Uitto J: Lung collagen in type IV Ehlers-Danlos syndrome: Ultrastructural and biochemical studies. *Am Rev Respir Dis* **122**:971, 1980.
360. Kontusaari S, Tromp G, Kuivaniemi H, Romanic AM, Prockop DJ: A mutation in the gene for type III procollagen (COL3A1) in a family with aortic aneurysms. *J Clin Invest* **86**:1465, 1990.
361. Stolle CA, Pyeritz RE, Myers JC, Prockop DJ: Synthesis of an altered type III procollagen in a patient with type IV Ehlers-Danlos syndrome. A structural change in the α1(III) chain which makes the protein more susceptible to proteinases. *J Biol Chem* **260**:1937, 1985.
362. Pyeritz RE, Stolle CA, Parfrey NA, Myers JC: Ehlers-Danlos syndrome IV due to a novel defect in type III procollagen. *Am J Med Genet* **19**:607, 1985.
363. Tromp G, Kuivaniemi H, Shikata H, Prockop DJ: A single base mutation that substitutes serine for glycine 790 of the α1(111) chain of type III procollagen exposes an arginine and causes Ehlers-Danlos syndrome IV. *J Biol Chem* **264**:1349, 1989.
364. Richards AJ, Ward PN, Narcisi P, Nicholls AC, Lloyd JC, Pope FM: A single base mutation in the gene for type-III collagen (COL3A1) converts glycine-847 to glutamic acid in a family with Ehlers-Danlos type-IV. An unaffected family member is mosaic for the mutation. *Hum Genet* **89**:414, 1992.
365. Richards AJ, Narcisi P, Lloyd JC, Johnson PH, Hopkinson DA, Pope FM: Substitution of glycine 1000, 1003 and 1006 in type III collagen all cause the acrogeric form of EDS IV, and destabilize the collagen triple-helix. *Am J Hum Genet* **51**:A105, 1992.
366. Johnson PH, Richards AJ, Pope FM, Hopkinson DA: A COL3A1 glycine 1006 to glutamic acid substitution in a patient with Ehlers-Danlos syndrome type-IV detected by denaturing gradient gel electrophoresis. *J Inherited Metab Dis* **15**:426, 1992.
367. Tromp G, Kuivaniemi H, Stolle C, Pope FM, Prockop DJ: Single base mutation in the type III procollagen gene that converts the codon for glycine 883 to aspartate in a mild variant of Ehlers-Danlos syndrome IV. *J Biol Chem* **264**:19313, 1989.
368. Richards AJ, Lloyd JC, Ward PN, De Paepe A, Narcisi PN, Pope FM: Characterisation of a glycine to valine substitution at amino acid position 910 of the triple-helical region of type III collagen in a patient with Ehlers-Danlos syndrome type IV. *J Med Genet* **28**:458, 1991.
369. Earley J, Tromp G, Kuivaniemi H, Gatalica Z, Prockop DJ: A mutation that substitutes arg for gly 136 in collagen III identified in a patient with fibromuscular dysplasia and an aortic aneurysm. Fourth International Conference on the Molecular Biology and Pathology of Matrix, 1992. (abstr. III-14)
370. Kuivaniemi H, Kontusaari S, Tromp G, Zhao M, Sabol C, Prockop DJ: Identical G^{+1} to A mutations in three different introns of the type III procollagen gene (COL3A1) produce different patterns of RNA splicing in three variants of Ehlers-Danlos syndrome IV. An explanation for exon skipping with some mutations and not others. *J Biol Chem* **265**:12067, 1990.
371. Kontusaari S, Tromp G, Kuivaniemi H, Ladda RL, Prockop DJ: Inheritance of an RNA splicing mutation (G^{+IVS20}) in the type III procollagen gene (COL3A1) in a family having aortic aneurysms and easy bruisability: Phenotypic overlap between familial arterial aneurysms and Ehlers-Danlos syndrome type IV. *Am J Hum Genet* **47**:112, 1990.
372. Anderson DW, Thakker-Varia S, Stolle CA: A G^{+1}-A change in IVS 20 of the type III procollagen gene leads of cryptic splicing of the mRNA in an EDS IV patient. Fourth International Conference on the Molecular Biology and Pathology of Matrix, 1992. (abstract III-11)
373. Lee B, Vitale E, Superti-Furga A, Steinmann B, Ramirez F: G to T transversion at position +5 of a splice donor site causes skipping of the preceding exon in the type III procollagen transcripts of a patient with Ehlers-Danlos syndrome type IV. *J Biol Chem* **266**:5256, 1992.
374. Thakker-Varia S, Anderson D, Kuivaniemi H, Tromp G, Prockop DJ, Stolle CA: An exon deletion in type III procollagen mRNA is associated with intracellular degradation of the abnormal protein in a patient with Ehlers-Danlos syndrome type IV. *Matrix* **10**:249, 1990.
375. Wu Y, Tromp G, Kuivaniemi H, Strobel D, Romanic AM, Prockop DJ: G^{+5} to T mutation in intron 37 of the type III procollagen gene (COL3A1) causes aberrant RNA splicing in a proband with the Ehlers-Danlos syndrome type IV. Fourth International Conference on the Molecular Biology and Pathology of Matrix, 1992. (abstr. III-61)
376. Cole WG, Chiodo AA, Lamande SR, Janeczko R, Ramirez F, Dahl H-HM, Chan D, Bateman JF: A base substitution at a splice site in the COL3A1 gene causes exon skipping and generates abnormal type III procollagen in a patient with Ehlers-Danlos syndrome type IV. *J Biol Chem* **265**:17070, 1990.
377. Sillence DO, Chiodo AA, Campbell PE, Cole WG: Ehlers-Danlos syndrome type IV: Phenotypic consequences of a splicing mutation in one COL3A1 allele. *J Med Genet* **28**:840, 1991.
378. Nicholls AC, De Paepe A, Narcisi P, Dalgleish R, De Keyser F, Matton M, Pope FM: Linkage of a polymorphic marker for the type III collagen gene (COL3A1) to atypical autosomal dominant Ehlers-Danlos syndrome type IV in a large Belgian pedigree. *Hum Genet* **78**:276, 1988.
379. Richards AJ, Lloyd JC, Narcisi P, Ward PN, Nicholls AC, De Paepe A, Pope FM: A 27-bp deletion from one allele of the type III collagen gene (COL3A1) in a large family with Ehlers-Danlos syndrome type IV. *Hum Genet* **88**:325, 1992.
380. Lee B, D'Alession M, Vissing H, Ramirez F, Steinmann B, Superti-Furga A: Characterization of a large deletion associated with a polymorphic block of repeated dinucleotides in the type III procollagen gene (COL3A1) of a patient with Ehlers-Danlos syndrome type IV. *Am J Hum Genet* **48**:511, 1991.
381. Vissing H, D'Alessio M, Lee B, Ramirez F, Byers PH, Steinmann B, Superti-Furga A: Multiexon deletion in the procollagen III gene is associated with mild Ehlers-Danlos syndrome type IV. *J Biol Chem* **266**:5244, 1991.
382. Superti-Furga A, Steinmann B: Impaired secretion of type III procollagen in Ehlers-Danlos syndrome type IV fibroblasts: Correction of the defect by incubation at reduced temperature and demonstration of subtle alterations in the triple-helical region of the molecule. *Biochem Biophys Res Commun* **150**:140, 1988.
383. Kuivaniemi H, Tromp G, Prockop DJ: Genetic causes of aortic aneurysms. Unlearning at least part of what the textbooks say. *J Clin Invest* **88**:1441, 1991.
384. Beighton P: X-linked recessive inheritance of the Ehlers-Danlos syndrome. *BMJ* **2**:409, 1968.

385. Beighton P, Curtis D: X-linked Ehlers-Danlos syndrome type V; the next generation. *Clin Genet* **27**:472, 1985.
386. Steinmann B, Royce PM, Superti-Furga A: The Ehlers-Danlos syndrome, in Royce PM, Steinmann B (eds): *Connective Tissue and its Heritable Disorders: Molecular, Genetic and Medical Aspects.* New York, Wiley–Liss, 1993, pp 351–407.
387. DiFerrante N, Leachman RD, Angelini D, Donnelly PW, Grancis G, Almazan A: Lysyl oxidase deficiency in Ehlers-Danlos type V. *Connect Tissue Res* **3**:49, 1975.
388. Siegel RC, Black C, Bailey AJ: Cross-linking of collagen in the X-linked Ehlers-Danlos type V. *Biochem Biophys Res Commun* **88**:281, 1979.
389. Sussman M, Lichtenstein JR, Nigra TP, Martin GR, McKusick VA: Hydroxylysine-deficient collagen in a patient with a form of the Ehlers-Danlos syndrome. *J Bone Joint Surg [Am]* **56**:1228, 1974.
390. Wenstrup RJ, Murad S, Pinnell SR: Ehlers-Danlos syndrome type VI: Clinical manifestation of collagen lysyl hydroxylase deficiency. *J Pediatr* **115**:405, 1989.
391. Steinmann B, Gitzelmann R, Vogel A, Grant ME, Harwood R, Sear CHJ: Ehlers-Danlos syndrome in two siblings with deficient lysyl hydroxylase activity in cultured skin fibroblasts but only mild hydroxylysine deficient skin. *Helv Pediatr Acta* **30**:255, 1975.
392. Elsas LJ, Miller RL, Pinnell SR: Inherited human collagen lysyl hydroxylase deficiency: Ascorbic acid response. *Pediatrics* **92**:378, 1978.
393. Dembure PP, Priest JH, Snoddy SC, Elsas LJ: Genotyping and prenatal assessment of collagen lysyl hydroxylase deficiency in a family with Ehlers-Danlos syndrome, type VI. *Am J Hum Genet* **36**:783, 1984.
394. Ihme A, Krieg T, Nerlich A, Feldmann U, Rauterberg J, Glanville RW, Edel G, Müller PK: Ehlers-Danlos syndrome type VI: Collagen type specificity of defective lysyl hydroxylation in various tissues. *J Invest Dermatol* **83**:161, 1984.
395. Ihme A, Risteli L, Krieg T, Risteli J, Feldmann U, Kuuse K, Müller PK: Biochemical characterization of variants of the Ehlers-Danlos syndrome type VI. *Eur J Clin Invest* **13**:357, 1983.
396. Krieg T, Feldmann U, Kessler W, Müller PK: Biochemical characteristics of Ehlers-Danlos syndrome type VI in a family with one affected infant. *Hum Genet* **46**:41, 1979.
397. Dembure PP, Janko AR, Priest JH, Elsas LJ: Ascorbate regulation of collagen biosynthesis in Ehlers-Danlos syndrome, type VI. *Metabolism* **36**:687, 1987.
398. McKusick VA: *Mendelian Inheritance in Man. Catlogs of Autosomal Dominant, Autosomal Recessive, and X-Linked Phenotypes*, 7th ed. Baltimore, Johns Hopkins University Press, 1986, p 949.
399. Judisch GF, Waziri M, Krachmer J: Ocular Ehlers-Danlos syndrome with normal lysyl hydroxylase activity. *Arch Ophthalmol* **94**:1489, 1976.
400. Risteli L, Risteli J, Ihme A, Krieg T, Müller PK: Preferential hydroxylation of type IV collagen by lysyl hydroxylase from Ehlers-Danlos syndrome type VI fibroblasts. *Biochem Biophys Res Commun* **96**:1778, 1980.
401. Quinn RS, Krane SM: Abnormal properties of collagen lysyl hydroxylase from skin fibroblasts of siblings with hydroxylysine-deficient collagen. *J Clin Invest* **57**:83, 1976.
402. Hyland J, Ala-Kokko L, Royce P, Steinmann B, Kivirikko KI, Myllylä R: A homozygous stop codon in the lysyl hydroxylase gene in two siblings with Ehlers-Danlos syndrome type VI. *Nat Genet* 1994.
403. Hautala T, Keikkinen J, Kivirikko KI, Myllylä R: A large duplication in the gene for lysyl hydroxylase accounts for the type VI variant of the Ehlers-Danlos syndrome in two siblings. *Genomics* **15**:399, 1993.
404. Eyre DR, Glimcher MJ: Reducible cross-links in hydroxylysine-deficient collagens of a heritable disorder of connective tissue. *Proc Natl Acad Sci USA* **69**:2594, 1972.
405. Robinow M, Duvic M, Byers PH: Unpublished observations.
406. Pope FM, Nicholls AC, Palan A, Kwee ML, De Groot WP, Hausmann R: Clinical features of an affected father and daughter with Ehlers-Danlos syndrome type VII B. *Br J Dermatol* **126**:77, 1992.
407. Fjolsted M, Helle O: A hereditary dysplasia of collagen tissues in sheep. *J Pathol* **112**:183, 1974.
408. Counts DR, Byers PH, Holbrook KA, Hegreberg GA: Dermatosparaxis in the himalayan cat: Biochemical studies of dermal collagen. *J Invest Dermatol* **74**:96, 1980.
409. Holbrook KA, Byers PH, Counts DF, Hegreberg GA: Dermatosparaxis in a himalayan cat: Ultrastructural studies of dermal collagen. J Invest Dermatol **74**:100, 1980.
410. Steinmann B, Tuderman L, Peltonen L, Martin GR, McKusick VA, Prockop DJ: Evidence for a structural mutation of procollagen type I in a patient with the Ehlers-Danlos syndrome type VII. *J Biol Chem* **255**:8887, 1980.
411. Eyre DR, Shapiro FD, Aldridge JF: Heterozygous collagen defect in a variant of the Ehlers-Danlos syndrome type VII: Evidence for a deleted amino telopeptide domain in the proα2(I) chain. *J Biol Chem* **260**:11322, 1985.
412. Cole WG, Chan D, Chambers GW, Walker ID, Bateman JF: Deletion of 24 amino acids from the proα2(I) chain of type I procollagen in a patient with the Ehlers-Danlos syndrome type VII. *J Biol Chem* **261**:5496, 1986.
413. Wirtz MK, Glanville RW, Steinmann B, Rao VH, Hollister DW: Ehlers-Danlos syndrome type VIIB. Deletion of 18 amino acids comprising the N-telopeptide region of a proα2(I) chain. *J Biol Chem* **262**:16376, 1987.
414. Weil D, Bernard M, Combata N, Wirtz MK, Hollister DW, Steinmann B, Ramirez F: Identification of a mutation that causes exon-skipping during collagen pre-mRNA splicing in an Ehlers-Danlos syndrome variant. *J Biol Chem* **263**:8561, 1988.
415. Weil D, D'Alessio M, Ramirez F, Eyre DR: Structural and functional characterization of splicing mutation in the pro-α2(I)collagen gene of an Ehlers-Danlos type VII patient. *J Biol Chem* **265**:16007, 1990.
416. Vasan NS, Kuivaniemi H, Vogel BE, Minor RR, Wootton JAM, Tromp G, Weksberg R, Prockop DJ: A mutation in the proa2(I) gene (COL1A2) for type I procollagen in Ehlers-Danlos syndrome type VII. Evidence suggesting that skipping of exon 6 in RNA splicing may be a common cause of the phenotype. *Am J Hum Genet* **48**:305, 1991.
417. Nicholls AC, Oliver J, Renouf DV, McPheat J, Palan A, Pope FM: Ehlers-Danlos syndrome type VII: A single base change that causes exon skipping in the type I collagen α2(I) chain. *Hum Genet* **87**:193, 1991.
418. Watson RB, Wallis GA, Holmes DF, Viljoen D, Byers PH, Kadler KE: Ehlers-Danlos syndrome type VIIB. Incomplete cleavage of abnormal type I procollagen by N-proteinase in vitro results in the formation of copolymers of collagen and partially cleaved pNcollagen that are near circular in cross-section. *J Biol Chem* **267**:9093, 1992.
419. D'Alessio M, Ramirez F, Blumberg BD, Wirtz MK, Rao VH, Godfrey MD, Hollister DW: Characterization of a COL1A1 splicing defect in a case of Ehlers-Danlos syndrome type VII: Further evidence of molecular homogeneity. *Am J Hum Genet* **49**:400, 1991.
420. Bateman JF, Cole WG, Pillow JJ, Ramshaw JAM: Induction of procollagen processing in fibroblast cultures by neutral polymers. *J Biol Chem* **261**:4198, 1986.
421. Cole WG, Evans R, Sillence DO: The clinical features of Ehlers-Danlos syndrome type VII due to a deletion of 24 amino acids from the pro α1(I) chain of type I procollagen. *J Med Genet* **24**:698, 1987.
422. Smith LT, Wertelecki W, Milstone LM, Petty EM, Seashore MR, Braverman IM, Jenkins TG, Byers PH: Human dermatosparaxis: A form of Ehlers-Danlos syndrome that results from failure to remove the amino-terminal propeptide of type I procollagen. *Am J Hum Genet* **51**:235, 1992.
423. Wertelecki W, Smith LT, Byers PH: Initial observations of human dermatosparaxis: Ehlers-Danlos syndrome type VIIC. *J Pediatr* **121**:558, 1992.
424. Nusgens BV, Verellen-Dumoulin C, Hermanns-Le T, De Paepe A, Nuytinck L, Pierard GE, Lapiere CM: Evidence for a relationship between Ehlers-Danlos type VIIC in humans and bovine dermatosparaxis. *Nature Genet* **1**:214, 1992.
425. Mauch C, Aumailley M, Paye M, Lapiere CM, Timple R, Krieg T: Defective attachment of dermatosparactic fibroblasts to collagens I and IV. *Exp Cell Res* **163**:294, 1986.

426. Stewart RD, Hollister DW, Rimoin DL: A new variant of the Ehlers-Danlos syndrome: An autosomal dominant disorder of fragile skin, abnormal scarring, and generalized periodontitis. *Birth Defects* **13(3B)**:85, 1977.
427. Linch DC, Acton CHC: Ehlers-Danlos syndrome presenting with juvenile destructive periodontitis. *Br Dent J* **147**:95, 1979.
428. Tiller GE, Louie JS, Rimoin DL, Cohn DH: Exclusion of linkage to the type III collagen gene (COL3A1) in a family with Ehlers-Danlos type VIII. *Pediatr Res* **29**:135A, 1991.
429. Hartsfield JK, Kousseff BG: Phenotypic overlap of Ehlers-Danlos syndrome type IV and VIII. *Am J Med Genet* **37**:465, 1990.
430. Lazoff SG, Rybak JJ, Parker BR, Luzzatti L: Skeletal dysplasia, occipital horns, diarrhea and obstructive uropathy—a new hereditary syndrome. *Birth Defects* **11(2)**:71, 1975.
431. Byers PH, Siegel RC, Holbrook KA, Narayanan AS, Bornstein P, Hall JG: X-linked cutis laxa: Defective collagen crosslink formation due to decreased lysyl oxidase activity. *N Engl J Med* **303**:61, 1980.
432. Sartoris DJ, Luzzatti L, Weaver DD, MacFarlane JD, Hollister DW, Parker BR: Type IX Ehlers-Danlos syndrome: A new variant with pathognomonic radiographic features. *Radiology* **152**:665, 1984.
433. Blackston RD, Hirschhorn K, Elsas LJ: Ehlers-Danlos syndrome (EDS), type IX: biochemical evidence for X-linkage. *Am J Hum Genet* **41**:A49, 1987.
434. Rabin JM, Hirschfield L, Badlani GH: Type IX Ehlers-Danlos syndrome: Bladder diverticula with transition cell carcinoma. *Urology* **38**:563, 1991.
435. Kuivaniemi H, Peltonen L, Palotie A, Kaitila I, Kivirikko KI: Abnormal copper metabolism and deficient lysyl oxidase activity in a heritable connective tissue disorder. *J Clin Invest* **69**:730, 1982.
436. Peltonen L, Kuivaniemi H, Palotie A, Horn N, Kaitila I, Kivirikko KI: Alterations in copper and collagen metabolism in the Menkes syndrome and a new subtype of the Ehlers-Danlos syndrome. *Biochemistry* **22**:6156, 1983.
437. Kuivaniemi H, Peltonen L, Kivirikko KI: Type IX Ehlers-Danlos syndrome and Menkes syndrome: The decrease in lysyl oxidase activity is associated with a corresponding deficiency in the enzyme protein. *Am J Hum Genet* **37**:798, 1985.
438. Vulpe C, Levinson B, Whitney S, Packman S, Gitschier J: Isolation of a candidate gene for Menkes disease and evidence that it encodes a copper-transporting ATPase. *Nature Genet* **3**:7, 1993.
439. Chelly J, Tumer Z, Tonnesen T, Petterson A, Ishikawa-Brush Y, Tommerup N, Horn N, Monaco AP: Isolation of a candidate gene for Menkes disease that encodes a potential heavy metal binding protein. *Nature Genet* **3**:14, 1993.
440. Glover TW, Mercer J, Livingston J, Hall B, Chandrasekharappa C, Begy C, Verga V: Isolation of genomic clones spanning the Xq13 translocation breakpoint in a patient with Menkes syndrome. *Am J Hum Genet* **51**:A24, 1992.
441. Levinson B, Gitschier J, Bulpe D, Whitney S, Yang S, Packman S: Are X-linked cutis laxa and Menkes disease allelic? *Nature Genet* **3**:6, 1993.
442. Arneson MA, Hammerschmidt DE, Furcht LT, King RA: A new form of Ehlers-Danlos syndrome: Fibronectin corrects defective platelet function. *JAMA* **244**:144, 1980.
443. Hegreberg GA, Padgett GA, Gorham JR, Henson JB: A connective tissue disease of dogs and mink resembling the Ehlers-Danlos syndrome of man. II. Mode of inheritance. *J Hered* **60**:249, 1969.
444. Patterson DF, Minor RR: Hereditary fragility and hyperextensibility of the skin of cats. A defect in collagen fibrillogenesis. *Lab Invest* **37**:170, 1977.
445. Counts DF: Isolation of collagen from the skins of Ehlers-Danlos syndrome-affected dogs by acetic acid extraction and pepsin digestion. *Biochim Biophys Acta* **626**:208, 1980.
446. Rowe DW, McGoodwin EB, Martin GR, Sussman MD, Grahn D, Faris B, Franzblau C: A sex linked defect in the cross-linking of collagen and elastin associated with the mottled locus in mice. *J Exp Med* **139**:180, 1974.
447. Rowe DW, McGoodwin EB, Martin GR, Grahn D: Lysyl oxidase activity in the aneurysm-prone mottled mouse. *J Biol Chem* **252**:939, 1977.
448. Hunt DM: Primary defect in copper transport underlies mottled mutants in the mouse. *Nature* **249**:852, 1974.
449. Hunt DM: A study of copper treatment and tissue copper levels in the murine congenital copper deficiency, mottled. *Life Sci* **19**:1913, 1976.
450. Port AE, Hunt DM: A study of the copper-binding proteins in liver and kidney tissue of neonatal normal and mottled mutant mice. *Biochem J* **183**:721, 1979.
451. Packman S, Chin P, O'Toole C: Cooper utilization in cultured skin fibroblasts of the mottled mouse, an animal model for Menkes' kinky hair syndrome. *J Inherited Metab Dis* **7**:168, 1984.
452. Spranger JW, Langer LO, Wiedemann HR: *Bone Dysplasias. An Atlas of Constitutional Disorders of Skeletal Development* Philadelphia, Saunders/Stuttgart, Gustav Fischer, 1974.
453. Rimoin DL: The chondrodystrophies. *Adv Hum Genet* **5**:1, 1975.
454. Sillence DO, Horton WA, Rimoin DL: Morphologic studies in the skeletal dysplasia. *Am J Pathol* **96**:813, 1979.
455. Spranger J: Radiologic nosology of bone dysplasias. *Am J Med Genet* **34**:96, 1990.
456. Horton WA, Hecht JT: The chondrodysplasias, in Royce PM, Steinmann B (eds): *Connective Tissue and its Heritable Disorders: Molecular, Genetic, and Medical Aspects*. New York, Wiley–Liss, 1993, pp 641–675.
457. Stickler GB, Belau PG, Farrell FJ, Jones JD, Pugh DG, Steinberg AG, Ward LE: Hereditary progressive arthro-ophthalmopathy. *Proc Staff Meet Mayo Clinic* **40**:433, 1965.
458. Liberfarb RM, Hirose T: The Wagner-Stickler syndrome. *Birth Defects* **18**:525, 1982.
459. Godel V, Lazar M: Wagner's vitreoretinal degeneration with generalized epiphyseal dysplasia. *Acta Ophthalmol* **60**:469, 1982.
460. Winter RM, Baraitser M, Laurence KM, Donnai D, Hall CM: The Weissenbacher-Zweymuller, Stickler, and Marshall syndromes: Further evidence for their identity. *Am J Med Genet* **16**:189, 1983.
461. Aym'e S, Preus M: The Marshall and Stickler syndromes: Objective reflection of lumping. *J Med Genet* **21**:34, 1984.
462. Francomano CA, Liberfarb R, Hirose T, Maumenee I, Streeter E, Meyers D, Pyeritz RE: The Stickler syndrome: Evidence for close linkage to the structural gene of type II collagen. *Genomics* **1**:293, 1987.
463. Knowlton RG, Weaver EJ, Struyk AF, Knoblock WH, King RA, Norris K, Shamban A, Uitto J, Jimenez SA, Prockop DJ: Genetic linkage analysis of hereditary arthro-ophthalmopathy (Stickler syndrome) and the type II procollagen gene. *Am J Hum Genet* **45**:681, 1989.
464. Priestly L, Kumar D, Sykes B: Amplification of the COL2A1 3′ variable region used for segregation analysis in a family with the Stickler syndrome. *Hum Genet* **85**:525, 1990.
465. Wilkin DJ, Cohn DH: Heteroduplex analysis can increase the informativeness of VNTR polymorphisms amplified by PCR. Application to Stickler syndrome. *Am J Hum Genet* **51**:A205, 1992.
466. Fryer AE, Upadhyaya M, Littler M, Bacon P, Watkins D, Tsipouras P, Harper PS: Exclusion of COL2A1 as a candidate gene in a family with Wagner-Stickler syndrome. *J Med Genet* **27**:91, 1990.
467. Ahmad NN, Ala-Kokko L, Knowlton RG, Jimenez SA, Weaver EJ, Maguire JI, Tasman W, Prockop DJ: Stop codon in the procollagen II gene (COL2A1) in a family with the Stickler syndrome (arthro-ophthalmopathy). *Proc Natl Acad Sci USA* **88**:6624, 1991.
468. Ahmad NN, McDonald-McGinn DM, Zackai EH, Knowlton RG, Larossa D, DiMascio J, Prockop DJ: A second mutation in the type II procollagen gene (COL2A1) causing the Stickler syndrome (arthro-ophthalmology) is also a premature termination codon. Fourth International Conference on the Molecular Biology and Pathology of Matrix. 1992. (abstr. III-10)
469. Brown DM, Nichols BE, Weingeist TA, Sheffield VC, Kimura AE, Stone EM: Procollagen II gene mutation in Stickler syndrome. *Arch Ophthalmol* **110**:1589, 1992.
470. Korkko J, Ritvaniemi P, Haataja L, Kaariainen H, Kivirikko KI, Prockop DJ, Ala-Kokko L: Mutation in

type II procollagen (COL2A1) that substitutes aspartate for glycine α1-67 and that causes cataracts and retinal detachment: Evidence for molecular heterogeneity in the Wagner syndrome and the Stickler syndrome (arthro-opthalmopathy) by denaturing gradient gel electrophoresis. *Am J Hum Genet* **53**:55, 1993.

471. Murray L, Bautista J, James PL, Rimoin DL: Type II collagen defects in the chondrodysplasias: 1. Spondyloepiphyseal dysplasias. *Am J Hum Genet* **45**:5, 1989.
472. Sher C, Ramesar R, Martell R, Learmonth I, Tsipouras P, Beighton P: Mild spondyloepiphyseal dysplasia (Namaqualand type): Genetic linkage to the type II collagen gene (COL2A1). *Am J Hum Genet* **48**:518, 1991.
473. Anderson IJ, Tsipouras P, Scher C, Ramesar RS, Martell RW, Beighton P: Spondyloepiphyseal dysplasia, mild autosomal dominant type is not due to primary defects of type II collagen. *Am J Med Genet* **37**:272, 1990.
474. Tiller GE, Rimoin DL, Murray LW, Cohn DH: Tandem duplication within a type II collagen gene (COL2A1) exon in an individual with spondyloepiphyseal dysplasia. *Proc Natl Acad Sci USA* **87**:3889, 1990.
475. Lee B, Vissing H, Ramirez F, Rogers D, Rimoin D: Identification of the molecular defect in a family with spondyloepiphyseal dysplasia. *Science* **244**:978, 1989.
476. Chan D, Cole WG: Low basal transcription of genes for tissue-specific collagen by fibroblasts and lymphoblastoid cells. Application to the characterization of a glycine 997 to serine substitution in α1(II) collagen chains of a patient with spondyloepiphyseal dysplasia. *J Biol Chem* **226**:12487, 1991.
477. Tiller GE, Weiss MA, Eyre DR, Rimoin DL, Cohn DH: An RNA splicing mutation ($G^{+5IVS20}$) in the gene for type II collagen (COL2A1) produces spondyloepiphyseal dysplasia congenita (SEDC). *Am J Hum Genet* **51**:A37, 1992.
478. Williams CJ, Considine E, Knowlton RG, Reginato AJ, Harrison DA, Buxton PG, Jimenez SA, Prockop DJ: A single base mutation in the type II procollagen gene produces an Arg—Cys mutation in one allele of the gene in a family with spondyloepiphyseal. *Am J Hum Genet* **51**:A37, 1992.
479. Whitley CB, Gorlin RJ: Achondrogenesis: New nosology with evidence of genetic heterogeneity. *Radiology* **148**:693, 1983.
480. Stanescu V, Stanescu R, Moroteaux P: Etude morphologique et biochimique du cartilage de croissance dans les osteochondrodysplasies. *Arch Fr Pediatr (suppl 3)* **34**:I, 1977.
481. Borochowitz Z, Lachman R, Adomian GE, Spear G, Jones K, Rimoin DL: Achondrogenesis type I: Delineation of further heterogeneity and identification of two distinct subgroups. *J Pediatr* **112**:23, 1988.
482. Borochowitz Z, Ornoy A, Lachman R, Rimoin DL: Achondrogenesis II-hypochondrogenesis: Variability versus heterogeneity. *Am J Med Genet* **24**:273, 1986.
483. Maroteaux P, Stanescu V, Stanescu R: The lethal chondrodysplasias. *Clin Orthop* **114**:31, 1976.
484. Eyre DR, Upton MP, Shapiro FD, Wilkinson RH, Vawter GF: Nonexpression of cartilage type II collagen in a case of Langer-Saldino achondrogenesis. *Am J Hum Genet* **39**:52, 1986.
485. Godfrey M, Keene DR, Blank E, Hori H, Sakai LY, Sherwin LA, Hollister DW: Type II achondrogenesis-hypochondrogenesis: Morphologic and immunohistopathologic studies. *Am J Hum Genet* **43**:894, 1988.
486. Horton WA, Chou JW, Machado MA: Cartilage collagen analysis in the chondrodystrophies. *Collagen Related Res* **5**:349, 1985.
487. Godfrey M, Hollister DW: Type II achondrogenesis-hypochondrogenesis: Identification of abnormal type II collagen. *Am J Hum Genet* **43**:902, 1988.
488. Horton WA, Machado MA, Ellard J, Campbell D, Bartley J, Ramirez F, Vitale E, Lee B: Characterization of a type II collagen gene (COL2A1) mutation identified in cultured chondrocytes from human hypochondrogenesis. *Proc Natl Acad Sci USA* **89**:4583, 1992.
489. Vissing H, D'Alessio M, Lee B, Ramirez F, Godfrey M, Hollister D: Glycine to serine substitution in the triple-helical domain of proαl(II) collagen results in a lethal perinatal form of short-limbed dwarfism. *J Biol Chem* **264**:18265, 1989.
490. Bogaert R, Tiller GE, Weis MA, Gruber HE, Rimoin DL, Cohn DH, Eyre DR: An amino acid substitution (Gly^{858}—Glu) in the collagen α1(II) chain produces hypochondrogenesis. *J Biol Chem* **267**:22522, 1992.
491. Alport AC: Hereditary familial congenital haemorrhagic nephritis. *BMJ* **1**:504, 1927.
492. Atkin CL, Gregory MC, Border WA: Alport syndrome, in Schrier RW, Gotschalk CW (eds): *Disease of the Kidney,* 4th ed. Boston, Little, Brown, 1988, pp 617–641.
493. Spear GS: Alport syndrome: A consideration of pathogenesis. *Clin Nephrol* **1**:336, 1973.
494. Atkin CL, Hasstedt SJ, Menlove L, Cannon L, Kirschner N, Schwartz C, Nguyen K, Skolnick M: Mapping of Alport syndrome gene to the long arm of the X chromosome. *Am J Hum Genet* **42**:249, 1988.
495. Brunner H, Schroder C, Van Bennekom C, Lambermon E, Tuerlings J, Menzel D, Olbing H, Monnens L, Wieringa B, Ropers HH: Localication of the gene for X-linked Alport's syndrome. *Kidney Int* **34**:507, 1988.
496. Flinter FA, Abbs S, Bobrow M: Localization of the gene for classic Alport syndrome. *Genomics* **4**:335, 1989.
497. Hostikka SL, Eddy RL, Byers MG, Hoeyhtyae M, Shows TB, Tryggvason K: Identification of a distinct type IV collagen α chain with restricted kidney distribution and assignment of its gene to the locus of X chromosome-linked Alport syndrome. *Proc Natl Acad Sci USA* **87**:1606, 1990.
498. Myers JC, Jone TA, Pohjolainen ER, Kadri AS, Goddard AD, Sheer D, Solomon E, Pihlajaniemi T: Molecular cloning of α5(IV) collagen and assignment of the gene to the region of the X chromosome containing the Alport syndrome locus. *Am J Hum Genet* **46**:1024, 1990.
499. Pihlajaniemi T, Pohjolainen ER, Myers JC: Complete primary structure of the triple-helical region and the carboxyl-terminal domain of a new type IV collagen chain, α5(IV). *J Biol Chem* **265**:13351, 1990.
500. Zhou J, Hostikka SL, Chow LT, Tryggvason K: Characterization of the 3′ half of the human type IV collagen α5 gene that is affected in the Alport syndrome. *Genomics* **9**:1, 1991.
501. Barker DF, Hostikka SL, Zhou J, Chow LT, Oliphant AR, Gerken SC, Gregory MC, Skolnick MH, Atkin CL, Tryggvason K: Identification of mutation in the COL4A5 collagen gene in Alport syndrome. *Science* **247**:1224, 1990.
502. Renieri A, Seri M, Myers JC, Pihlajaniemi T, Sessa A, Rizzoni G, Demarchi M: Alport syndrome caused by a 5′ deletion within the COL4A5 gene. *Hum Genet* **89**:120, 1992.
503. Knebelmann B, Deschenes G, Gros F, Hors MC, Grunfeld JP, Tryggvason K, Gubler MC, Antignac C: Substitution of arginine for glycine-325 in the collagen α5(IV) chain associated with X-linked Alport syndrome. Characterization of the mutation by direct sequencing of PCR-amplified lymphoblast cDNA fragments. *Am J Hum Genet* **51**:135, 1992.
504. Zhou J, Hertz JM, Leinonen A, Tryggvason K: Complete amino acid sequence of the human α5(IV) collagen chain and identification of a single-base mutation in exon-23 converting glycine-521 in the collagenous domain to cysteine in an Alprot syndrome patient. *J Biol Chem* **267**:12475, 1992.
505. Smeets HJM, Lemmink HH, Nelen MR, Tryggvason K, Van Oost BA, Monnens LAH, Brunner HG, Schroder CH: Mutation in the COL4A5 gene leading to different types of Alport syndrome. Fourth International Conference on the Molecular Biology and Pathology of Matrix, 1992. (abstr. III-50)
506. Antignac C, Zhou J, Sanak M, Cochat P, Roussel B, Deschenes G, Gros F, Knebelmann B, Hors-Cayla MC, Tryggvason K, Gubler M-C: Alport syndrome and diffuse esophageal leiomyomatosis: Deletions in the 5′ end of the COL4A5 collagen gene. *Kidney Int* **42**:1178, 1992.
507. Fine J-D, Bauer EA, Briggaman RA, Carter DM, Eady RAJ, Esterly NB, Holbrook KA, Hurwitz S, Johnson L, Lin A, Pearson R, Sybert VP: Revised clinical and laboratory criteria for subtypes in inherited epidermolysis bullosa. A consensus report by the subcommittee on diagnosis and classification of the National Epidermolysis Bullosa Registry. *J Am Acad Dermatol* **24**:119, 1991.
508. Coulombe PA, Hutton ME, Letai A, Hebert A, Paller AS, Fuchs E: Point mutation in human keratin 14 genes of epidermolysis bullosa simplex patients: Genetic and functional analyses. *Cell* **66**:1301, 1991.

509. Bonifas JM, Rothman A-L, Epstein E: Epidermolysis bullosa simplex: Evidence in two families for keratin gene abnormalities. *Science* **254**:1202, 1991.
510. Ryynanen M, Knowlton RG, Uitto J: Mapping of epidermolysis bullosa simplex mutation to chromosome 12. *Am J Hum Genet* **49**:978, 1991.
511. Vassar R, Coulombe PA, Degenstein L, Albers K, Fuchs E: Mutant keratin expression in transgenic mice causes marked abnormalities resembling a human genetic skin disease. *Cell* **64**:365, 1991.
512. Lane EB, Rugg EL, Navsaria H, Leigh IM, Heagerty AMH, Ishida-Yamamoto A, Eady RAJ: A mutation in the conserved helix termination peptide of keratin 5 in hereditary skin blistering. *Nature* **356**:244, 1992.
513. Savolainen E-R, Kero M, Pihlajaniemi T, Kivirikko KI: Deficiency of galactosylhydroxylysyl glucosyltransferase, an enzyme of collagen synthesis, in a family with dominant epidermolysis bullosa simplex. *N Engl J Med* **304**:197, 1981.
514. Humphries MM, Sheils D, Lawler M, Farrar GJ, McWilliam P, Kenna P, Bradley DG, Sharp EM, Gaffney EF, Young M, Uitto J, Humphries P: Epidermolysis bullosa: Evidence for linkage to genetic markers on chromosome 1 in a family with the autosomal dominant simplex form. *Genomics* 7:377, 1990.
515. Carter WG, Ryan MC, Gahr PJ: Epiligrin, a new cell adhesion ligand for integrin $\alpha3\beta1$ in epithelial basement membranes. *Cell* **65**:599, 1991.
516. Rouselle P, Lunstrum GP, Keene DR, Burgeson RE: Kalinin: An epithelium-specific basement membrane adhesion meolcule that is a component of anchoring filaments. *J Cell Biol* **114**:567, 1991.
517. Stanley JR, Tanaka T, Mueller S, Klaus-Kovtun V, Roop D: Isolation of complementary DNA for bullous pemphigoid antigen by use of patients' autoantibodies. *J Clin Invest* **82**:1864, 1988.
518. Diaz LA, Ratrie A III, Saunders WS, Futamura S, Squiquera HL, Anhalt GJ, Giudice GJ: Isolation of a human epidermal cDNA corresponding to the 180-kD autoantigen recognized by bullous pemphigoid and herpes gestationis sera. *J Clin Invest* **86**:1088, 1990.
519. Giudice G, Squiquera HL, Elias PM, Diaz LA: Identification of two collagen domains within the bullous pemphigoid autoantigen, BP180. *J Clin Invest* **87**:734, 1991.
520. Sawamura D, Li K, Chu M-L, Uitto J: Human bullous pemphigoid antigen (BPAG1): Amino acid sequence deduced from cloned cDNAs predicts biologically important peptide segments and protein domains. *J Biol Chem* **266**:17784, 1991.
521. Sawamura D, Nomura K, Sugita Y, Mattei M-G, Chu M-L, Uitto J: Genomic organization of collagenous domains and chromosomal assignment of human 180-kD bullous pemphigoid antigen (BPAG2), a novel collagen of stratified squamous epithelium. *J Biol Chem* **266**:24064, 1991.
522. Bruckner-Tuderman L: Epidermolysis bullosa, in Royce PM, Steinmann B (eds). *Connective Tissue and its Heritable Disorders: Molecular, Genetic, and Medical Aspects.* New York, Wiley–Liss, 1993, pp 507–531.
523. Palade G, Farquhar M: A special fibril of the dermis. *J Cell Biol* **27**:215, 1965.
524. Sakai LY, Keene DR, Morris NP, Burgeson RE: Type VII collagen is a major structural component of anchoring fibrils. *J Cell Biol* **103**:1577, 1986.
525. Lunstrum GP, Sakai LY, Kenne DR, Morris NP, Burgeson RE: Large complex globular domains of type VII procollagen contribute to the structure of anchoring fibrils. *J Biol Chem* **261**:9042, 1986.
526. Keene DR, Sakai Y, Lunstrum GP, Morris NP, Burgeson RE: Type VII collagen forms an extended network of anchoring fibrils. *J Cell Biol* **104**:611, 1987.
527. Ryynanen M, Ryynanen J, Sollberg S, Iozzo RV, Knowlton RG, Uitto J: Genetic linkage of type VII collagen (COL7A1) to dominant dystrophic epidermolysis bullosa in families with abnormal anchoring fibrils. *J Clin Invest* **89**:974, 1992.
528. Pearson R: Studies on the pathogenesis of epidermolysis bullosa. *J Invest Dermatol* **39**:551, 1962.
529. Briggaman RA, Wheeler CE Jr: Epidermolysys bullosa dystrophica-recessiva: A possible role of anchoring fibrils in the pathogenesis. *J Invest Dermatol* **65**:203, 1975.
530. Hashimoto I, Schnyder UW, Anton-Lamprecht I, Gedde-Dahl T Jr, Ward S: Ultrastructural studies in epidermolysis bullosa hereditaria: III. Recessive dystrophic types with dermolytic blistering (Hallopeau-Siemens types and inverse type). *Arch Dermatol Res* **256**:137, 1976.
531. Tidman MJ, Eady RAJ: Evaluation of anchoring fibrils and other components of the dermal-epidermal junction in dystrophic epidermolysis bullosa by a quantiative technique. *J Invest Dermatol* **84**:374, 1985.
532. Heagerty AHM, Kennedy AR, Leigh IM, Purkis P, Eady RAJ: Identification of an epidermal basement membrane defect in recessive forms of dystrophic epidermolysis bullosa by LH7:2 monoclonal antibody: Use in diagnosis. *Br J Dermatol* **115**:125, 1986.
533. Leigh IM, Eady RAJ, Heagerty AHM, Purkis P, Whitehead PA, Burgeson RA: Type VII collagen is a normal component of epidermal basement membrane which shows altered expression in recessive dystrophic epidermolysis bullosa. *J Invest Dermatol* **90**:639, 1988.
534. Smith LT, Sybert VP: Intra-epidermal retention of type VII collagen in a patient with recessive dystrophic epidermolysis bullosa. *J Invest Dermatol* **94**:261, 1990.
535. Hovnanian A, Duquesnoy P, Blanchet-Bardon C, Knowlton RG, Amselem S, Lathrop M, Dubertret L, Uitto J, Goossens M: Genetic linkage of recessive dystrophic epidermolysis bullosa to the type VII collagen gene. *J Clin Invest* **90**:1032, 1992.
536. Bauer EA: Recessive dystrophic epidermolysis bullosa: Evidence for an altered collagenase in fibroblast cultures. *Proc Natl Acad Sci USA* **74**:4646, 1977.
537. Stricklin PG, Welgus HG, Bauer EA: Human skin collagenase in recessive dystrophic epidermolysis bullosa. Purification of a mutant enzyme from fibroblast cultures. *J Clin Invest* **69**:1373, 1982.
538. Hovnanian A, Duquesnoy P, Amselem S, Blanchet-Bardon C, Lathrop M, Dubertret L, Goosens M: Exclusion of linkage between the collagenase gene and generalized recessive dystrophic epidermolysis bullosa phenotype. *J Clin Invest* **88**:1716, 1991.

CHAPTER 135

Marfan Syndrome and Related Disorders

Francesco Ramirez ▪ Maurice Godfrey
Brendan Lee ▪ Petros Tsipouras

1. Marfan syndrome is an autosomal dominant disorder of connective tissue characterized by manifestations in the cardiovascular, musculoskeletal, and ophthalmic systems. Well-defined diagnostic criteria differentiate Marfan syndrome from several related disorders, such as congenital contractural arachnodactyly, mitral valve prolapse syndrome, annuloaortic ectasia, and dominantly inherited ectopia lentis.

2. The basic genetic defect in Marfan syndrome was recently elucidated. A combination of experimental approaches has demonstrated that mutations in a novel extracellular matrix glycoprotein, fibrillin, are the underlying cause of this disorder. This fibrillin gene has been localized to the long arm of chromosome 15 (FBN1). Surprisingly and serendipitously, these studies revealed the existence of an additional fibrillin gene, located on chromosome 5 (FBN2) and genetically linked to congenital contractural arachnodactyly.

3. The cardinal clinical manifestations of Marfan syndrome include aortic dilatation and dissecting aneurysms, mitral valve prolapse, dolichostenomelia, arachnodactyly, and ectopia lentis. The frequency of the disorder is 1 in 10,000 individuals; 15 to 30 percent of cases are estimated to represent new mutations. The Marfan syndrome phenotype exhibits high penetrance and wide clinical variability; the diagnosis is clinical. Management must be multidisciplinary to cover all aspects of medical care, surgical intervention, and genetic counseling.

4. Among the Marfan-related conditions is congenital contractural arachnodactyly, which exhibits a marfanoid habitus but lacks ophthalmic and cardiovascular manifestations. Unlike Marfan syndrome, which is characterized by loose-jointness, the hallmark of this condition is joint contractures. Likewise, only the ocular lens is compromised in the rare, dominantly inherited form of ectopia lentis. More difficult is the diagnostic differentiation of other disorders primarily involving the cardiovascular system, such as the mitral valve prolapse syndrome and familial annuloaortic ectasia.

5. Fibrillin is a major component of the 10-nm microfibrils of extracellular matrix. The primary structure of fibrillin exhibits a multidomain organization characterized by several cysteine-rich motifs reminiscent of the epidermal growth factor module. Extracellularly, fibrillin monomers aggregate into a supramolecular structure that has a "beads on a string" profile by electron microscopy. Characterization of a variety of fibrillin mutations has emphasized the importance of the structural integrity of individual cysteine-rich repeats, as well as the requirement that the fibrillin monomer must have a certain absolute length for normal microfibril assembly.

6. In addition to Marfan syndrome, FBN1, the fibrillin locus residing on chromosome 15, has been genetically linked to dominantly inherited ectopia lentis. This result has been interpreted as suggesting that mutations in functionally distinct domains of this gene product may cause seemingly distinct clinical phenotypes. On the other hand, linkage between congenital contractural arachnodactyly and FBN2, the fibrillin locus on the chromosome 5, strongly suggests that fibrillin proteins have distinct functions in different tissues.

Marfan syndrome (MFS) has held a prominent place among the heritable disorders of connective tissue as the focus of clinical, genetic, biochemical, and molecular biologic investigations for nearly 100 years. Several aspects of MFS have stimulated the curiosity of clinicians and researchers alike. They include the wide range of pleiotropic manifestations, which in some cases overlap those of other genetic disorders; the cardiovascular complications, which are often used as paradigms of more common conditions; the great inter- and intrafamilial variability, which occasionally complicates clinical diagnosis; and, most important of all, the etiology of such a clinically heterogeneous disorder. Despite the voluminous body of work accumulated and the wealth of information available, the basic metabolic defect underlying the MFS phenotype has been elucidated only very recently by combining two distinct experimental approaches, notably the candidate gene and the positional cloning strategies.

A list of standard abbreviations is located immediately preceding the index in each volume. Additional abbreviations used in this chapter include: CCA = congenital contractural arachnodactyly; EGF-CB = epidermal growth factor—calcium-binding; EL = ectopia lentis; FBN1 and FBN2 = fibrillin loci 1 and 2; Fib 5 and Fib 15 = fibrillin protein products of FBN2 and FBN1 loci, respectively; FLP = fibrillin-like protein; MASS = mitral valve prolapse in association with aortic, skeletal, and skin manifestations; MFS = Marfan syndrome; PF-1, PF-2, etc. = pepsin-resistant fibrillin fragments; and US/LS = upper segment/lower segment.

As we are about to enter a new phase in MFS research, in which genotype/phenotype correlations will be established and the molecular pathogenesis of the disorder will be clarified, it is worthwhile to briefly recall this century-long journey.

HISTORICAL PERSPECTIVE

The history of MFS research can be broadly divided into two different phases, each characterized by a distinct scientific focus and each lasting for about five decades. The first phase could be referred to as the "phenotypic era," in that most of the investigative effort was devoted to defining the clinical manifestations and mode of inheritance of MFS. During the subsequent 50 years, the "genotypic era," the focus shifted from the bedside to the laboratory in an often frustrating attempt to identify the gene product responsible for MFS.

The *phenotypic era* began in 1896 with the publication of a case report by the French pediatrician Antoine Bernard-Jean Marfan.[1] In it, he described a 5-year-old girl, Gabrielle P., who presented with disproportionately long limbs and fingers, joint contractures of fingers and knees, and tall stature. Marfan used the term "dolichostenomelia" for this clinical presentation to emphasize the unusually long and narrow frame of the young girl. Six years later, Mery and Babonneix, in re-examining Gabrielle, added scoliosis to the previously described skeletal abnormalities and renamed the condition "hyperchondroplasia."[2] In the same year, another French clinician, Achard, coined the term "arachnodactyly" (long, spidery fingers) in describing the clinical phenotype of a seemingly identical patient.[3] In subsequent reports, displacement of the ocular lens (ectopia lentis) and mitral valve regurgitation were added to the skeletal features of the disorder.[4,5] The involvement of several mesenchymal tissues in the clinical picture of MFS, together with the demonstration of the genetic nature of the disorder, led Weve, in 1931, to propose the name of "dystrophia mesodermalis congenita, typus Marfanis."[6] Seven years later, Apert condensed Weve's designation to the current term "Marfan syndrome."[7] In 1943, one year after Marfan's death, the role of cardiovascular complications (aortic dilation and dissecting aortic aneurysms) as the major contributive factor in MFS morbidity and mortality was finally appreciated.[8,9]

Undoubtedly, the most important contribution of this era, which also signaled the beginning of the next investigative period, was a 1955 paper by McKusick.[10] In this seminal contribution, he catalogued early literature, delineated the natural history of the syndrome, proposed genetic pleiotropism as the basis of clinical variability, and firmly established the autosomal dominant mode of inheritance in MFS. In addition, McKusick used for the first time the term "heritable," as opposed to "hereditary," to emphasize the relatively high incidence of sporadic cases in MFS. He later adopted this same term in including MFS within the larger family, heritable disorders of connective tissue, described in the compilation by the same title.[11] In the 1955 article, McKusick also predicted that the complex phenotype of MFS might be ascribed to a defective component of the connective tissue, notably ". . . elastic fiber or a component intimately associated with elastic fiber."

Important historical addenda to the phenotypic period occurred in a series of articles which discriminated between MFS and disorders that shared some of the MFS stigmata while displaying distinct natural histories.[12–14] The disorders discussed in some of these papers included homocystinuria, a recessive condition of amino acid metabolism involving lens dislocation; Achard syndrome, which features arachnodactyly and joint laxity and is so named because it may have affected the patient described by Achard in 1902; and congenital contractural arachnodactyly (CCA), which shares some of the skeletal features of MFS. Indeed on reexamining the case reports on Gabrielle P., Hecht and Beals noted that she had contractures of the elbows, fingers, knees, and toes (Fig. 135-1) but neither heart nor eye malformations.[14] This clinical presentation is unique to CCA rather than MFS, in which loose-jointedness is a clinical hallmark. Accordingly, they suggested that Gabrielle P. might have been affected by the syndrome of CCA.[14]

The *genotypic era* was spurred by McKusick's prediction, and intensive research efforts immediately focused on the extracellular components of connective tissue. Initial attention was directed to the fibrillar collagens, which are the most abundant structural component of the extracellular matrix. Reports of increased urinary excretion of hydroxyproline, increased dermal collagen solubility, and decreased borohydride-resistant collagen cross-links initially supported this hypothesis.[15–17] More convincing was a paper describing a mutation in the pro-α2(I) collagen chain of an atypical MFS patient.[18] However, the mutation, later shown to be a single amino acid substitution in the triple-helical domain of α2(I) collagen,[19] was never detected in patients with the classic form of MFS. Indeed, subsequent linkage analyses using various collagen gene-specific markers convincingly excluded this protein from the etiology of MFS.[20–25] Concurrent studies focusing on defective elastin metabolism and hyaluronic acid, β-glucuronidase, and, more recently, decorin synthesis also failed to rigorously establish a causal association with MFS.[26–31] As with the collagens, these biosynthetic abnormalities probably represent a collection of secondary effects attributable to the pleiotropy of the defective MFS gene product.

In the late 1950s and early 1960s, several investigators documented the presence of elastic microfibrils in the intercellular space of several different tissues.[32] In 1986, Sakai et al.,[33] using polyclonal and monoclonal antibodies raised against microfibrils, identified a 350-kDa glycoprotein, which they named "fibrillin." The colocalization of fibrillin with microfibrils in both elastic and nonelastic tissues prompted Hollister to suggest that this macromolecule might represent a candidate gene product in MFS pathogenesis. To test this hypothesis, he performed a series of indirect immunohistofluorescence studies on the microfibrillar array of normal and MFS individuals.[34,35] Analyses on sporadic patients and ten MFS kindreds found a consistent decrease in fibrillin

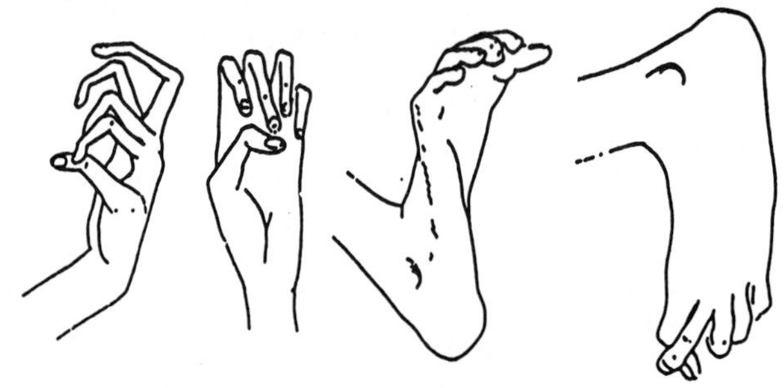

FIG. 135-1 Drawings of the original case report of Marfan[1] showing Gabrielle P.'s arachnodactyly and suggesting joint contractures.

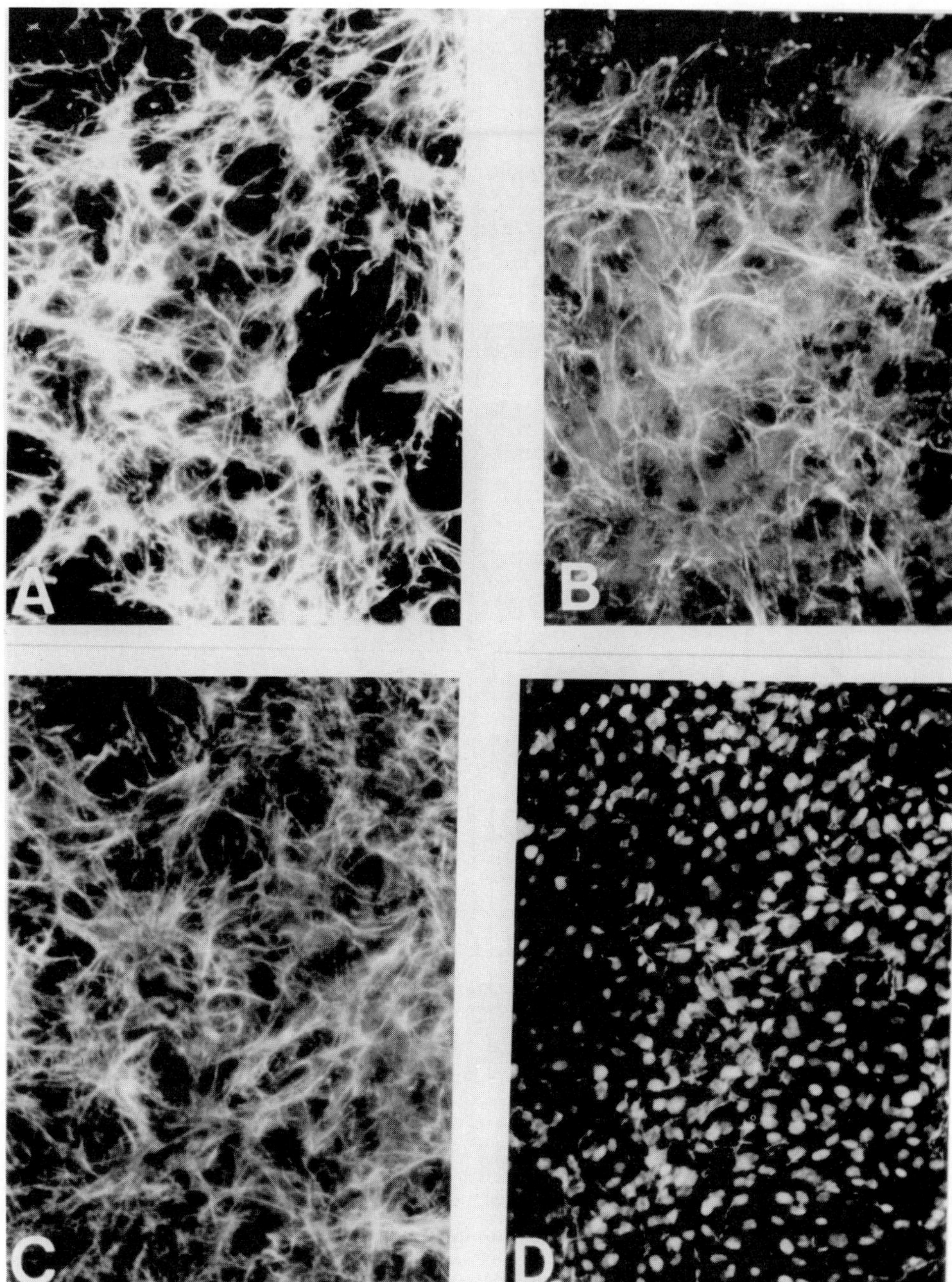

FIG. 135-2 Immunohistochemical analysis of hyperconfluent multilayers of dermal fibroblasts from *A*, a normal subject, *B*, an individual with MFS, *C*, an individual with annuloaortic ectasia, and *D*, a neonate with infantile MFS. The control and annuloaortic ectasia samples show a prominent meshwork of fibrous material, while the MFS and infantile MFS samples show a decreased amount of immunostainable fibrous meshwork. Note, however, that the morphology of the fibrils in the infantile MFS sample are different from that of MFS.

content in both skin and cultured fibroblasts of MFS patients (Fig. 135-2). These studies provided the first strong evidence of an abnormal structural aggregate in the extracellular matrix of MFS tissues. However, this work could not conclusively associate fibrillin with the MFS phenotype since the method of analysis did not discriminate between primary and secondary defects in MFS pathogenesis.

At about the same time, a consortium of investigators sought to identify the MFS gene by the positional cloning approach (see Chap. 6). This resulted in two sequential reports. The first excluded nearly 75 percent of the human genome as a possible location for the MFS gene locus.[36] The second finally mapped the MFS locus to chromosome 15q15-q23 in a linkage study of five Finnish kindreds (Fig. 135-3).[37] Shortly thereafter, studies in different ethnic groups confirmed this localization, offered specific physical order for the anonymous probes in this region, and suggested genetic locus homogeneity within MFS.[38–40] Although highly informative, this experimental approach could not elucidate the nature of the gene(s) at the MFS locus and thus independently support the immunohistologic evidence implicating fibrillin in MFS etiology.

It was at this point that two research groups concentrated on cloning the candidate fibrillin gene.[41,42] This effort resulted in the colocalization of the fibrillin gene (FBN1) and the MFS locus (Fig. 135-3),[41] and in the identification of a *de novo* fibrillin mutation in two sporadic MFS cases (Fig. 135-4).[43] Evidence was also provided for the existence of additional fibrillin genes, one of which was shown to reside on chromosome 5 (FBN2) and to be linked to the MFS-related disorder CCA.[41] Since then, additional fibrillin mutations in MFS have been reported[44–46]; another MFS-related condition (dominantly inherited ectopia lentis) has been linked to FBN1[47]; and distinct metabolic deficiencies of fibrillin have

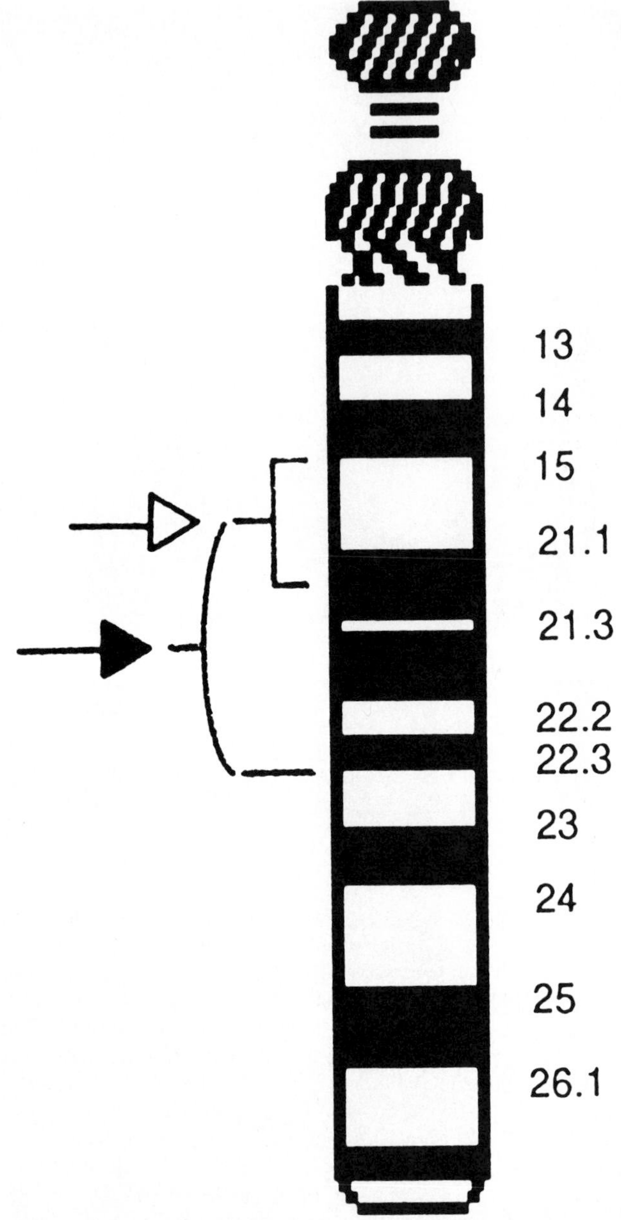

FIG. 135-3 **Idiogram of chromosome 15 showing the range of linkage with random markers[37] (curved bracket, closed arrow), and the location of fibrillin according to in situ hybridization[41] (straight bracket, open arrow).**

been demonstrated in cultured fibroblasts from MFS patients.[48]

Collectively, these studies indicate that mutations in the fibrillin gene on chromosome 15 (FBN1) are responsible for the genesis of MFS in most, if not all, cases. Moreover, they strongly suggest that mutations in fibrillin genes may cause a variety of phenotypes, broadly belonging to the clinical spectrum of MFS-related disorders.

GENETIC AND CLINICAL FEATURES OF MARFAN SYNDROME

MFS is a dominantly inherited autosomal disorder of connective tissue that occurs with an estimated frequency of approximately 1 per 10,000 individuals; 15 to 30 percent of cases represent new mutations.[49,50] Advanced paternal age may have an effect on the rate of *de novo* mutations.[51] Most infants with the severe infantile form of MFS are isolated cases, and, for some of them, the possibility of homozygosity has been raised.[52,53] MFS displays high penetrance and wide clinical variability both between and within families.

The diagnosis of MFS is clinical and relies on the presence of a combination of "major" and "minor" manifestations involving the musculoskeletal, cardiovascular, ocular, and other systems. Typical "major" manifestations are aortic root dilatation, ectopia lentis, and a characteristic habitus. In the absence of family history, the presence of a major manifestation from two of the three systems and a "minor" manifestation are needed to unequivocally establish the diagnosis of MFS in an individual. This diagnostic requirement is different in familial cases, where the presence of a major manifestation from one of the three systems and two "minor" manifestations are sufficient to establish the diagnosis.[50,54]

Musculoskeletal Manifestations

Dolichostenomelia is the characteristic skeletal abnormality observed in MFS.[49,50] Tall stature, decreased upper-to-lower segment ratio (US/LS), an arm-span that exceeds body height, dolichocephaly (disproportionately long head), and arachnodactyly of fingers and toes are some of the manifestations associated with dolichostenomelia (Fig. 135-5). The US/LS ratio is diagnostically significant, with an approximate value of 0.85 in adults with MFS compared to a segment-ratio value of 0.93 in normal Caucasians. The face is long and narrow, the palate is high-arched, and prognathism and crowding of the maxillary and mandibular teeth are frequent. Scoliosis or kyphoscoliosis, usually with onset during childhood, occurs in 30 to 60 percent of individuals with MFS. The kyphoscoliosis is particularly severe in the infantile form of MFS. Thoracic kyphosis is associated with decreased vital lung capacity and residual volume and with consequent pulmonary insufficiency.[55] Additional thoracic deformities include pectus excavatum or pectus carinatum resulting from the excessive longitudinal growth of the ribs. Pectus excavatum is a common defect seen in eight of every 1,000 live births[56]; its presence in a child makes it imperative to consider the diagnosis of MFS.

"Asthenic" habitus is frequently observed in individuals affected with MFS. This is thought to be due partly to muscular underdevelopment and to a significant decrease of subcutaneous fat. Some patients appear to have myotonic-like facies. Ligamentous laxity and generalized joint hypermobility are common in MFS (Fig. 135-6). Pes planus, genu recurvatum, and recurrent joint dislocations (especially of the hips) result from redundancy and weakness of joint capsules, ligaments, tendons, and fascia. Finally, the spinal canal is often enlarged in depth or width owing to the ectasia of the neural foramina and to sacral erosion. This feature, dural ectasia, is diagnostically suggestive when observed by computed tomography.[57,58]

Cardiovascular Manifestations

Most pediatric cardiac manifestations in MFS relate to multivalvular incompetence. In contrast, most adults with MFS exhibit manifestations primarily from the aorta.[49,50]

Although dissecting aneurysm of the aorta is the most serious and potentially fatal cardiac manifestation in MFS, it is not present at birth but develops progressively in

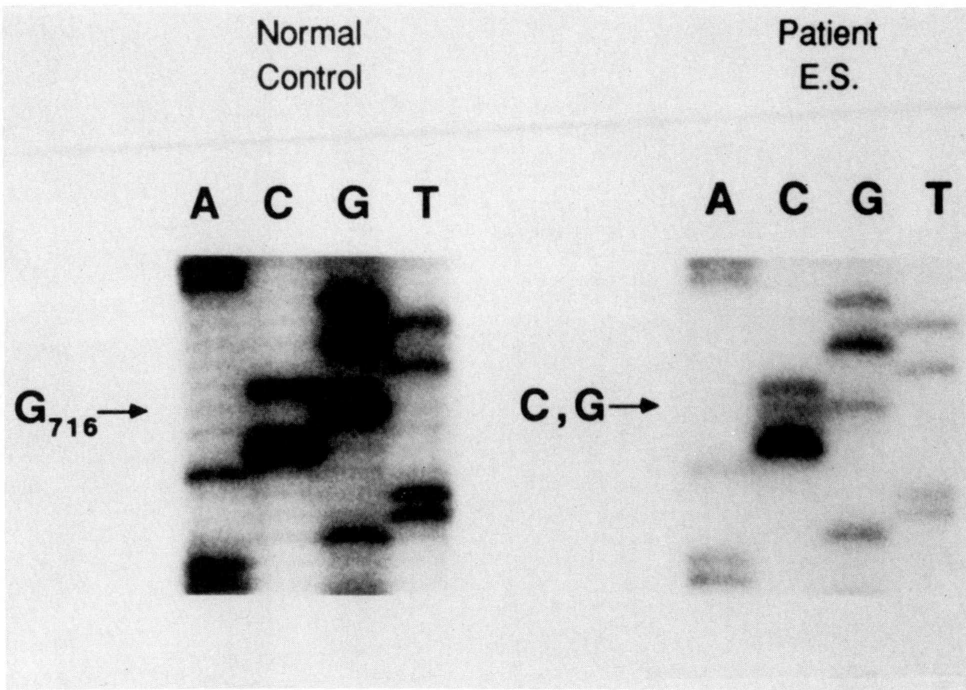

FIG. 135-4 **Identification of the first MFS mutation by direct sequencing of PCR-amplified fibrillin cDNA from a control subject and a patient showing a G-to-C transversion in one allele.** ***(From Dietz et al.[34] Used by permission.)***

postnatal life and reflects the underlying pathology of the tunica media (Fig. 135-7). Dilatation of the aorta usually precedes the development of the aneurysm and is found in approximately 50 percent of children and 70 to 80 percent of adults with MFS. The dilatation may be confined to the area around the sinuses of Valsalva or may be generalized; the latter situation is usually associated with higher morbidity.[59] Not all MFS patients develop aortic dilatation, and a small percentage of individuals with unequivocal MFS maintain a normal aortic diameter into their sixties. The dilatation can extend to the thoracic or abdominal aortic segments and, occasionally, to medium-sized arterial branches, such as the internal or external carotid arteries and even intracranial branches. Finally, enlargement of the pulmonary artery can occur in MFS, although it is much less frequent than aortic enlargement.

Aortic regurgitation is a common and usually progressive complication of MFS. It is relatively uncommon in childhood, but its frequency in adults has been estimated to be as high as 70 percent.[50] There seems to be a positive correlation between aortic root diameter and aortic regurgitation.[60] The acceleration of aortic root enlargement described in some patients with aortic regurgitation reflects the causative relationship between the two phenomena.

MFS is the leading cause of dissecting aortic aneurysms in all individuals under the age of 40. Although a dissecting aneurysm may be the first presenting manifestation in MFS, it is usually associated with underlying dilatation of the aortic root and frequently of the ascending aorta.[61] The presenting symptom is often an acute episode of severe, midline pain in the anterior chest and radiating to the back. Relatively small dissections in the ascending aorta may be asymptomatic. Most aortic dissections in MFS arise in the aortic root or proximal ascending aorta and extend distally through a variable portion of the aorta and its branches, but dissections can also begin in more distal aortic segments.[62–64]

Approximately 60 to 70 percent of MFS patients exhibit mitral valve prolapse, while tricuspid valve prolapse is observed in a much smaller fraction.[50] The mitral valve cusps and chordae tendinae may be redundant, thus resulting in mitral regurgitation.

Ocular Manifestations

Ectopia lentis (EL), usually bilateral, is a clinical hallmark of MFS. Only 50 to 80 percent of individuals with MFS have this abnormality. While the lenses are normal in shape and size, the ciliary zonules, when visualized with the slit lamp, appear redundant, attenuated, and frequently broken.[65] The lens displacement is usually upward owing to a tendency for the lower ligaments to be defective (Fig. 135-8). Iridodonesis (instability of the iris) is a reliable indicator of lens dislocation. Myopia and spontaneous retinal detachment are found in a large number of individuals affected with MFS. Spontaneous retinal detachment is also an important complication of the extirpation of the lens. While ectopia lentis is the most prevalent ocular manifestation, most of the morbidity results from secondary myopia, retinal detachment, glaucoma, and/or iritis with associated loss of vision.[65]

Other Manifestations

Spontaneous pneumothorax occurs in approximately 10 percent of individuals with MFS.[66] Apical bullae, congenital pulmonary cysts, and emphysema are some rarer pulmonary findings. Cutaneous striae distensae in the pectoral, deltoid, and lumbar areas are frequent. Inguinal, femoral, and incisional hernias occur rather often in MFS patients. Finally, the voice of individuals with MFS is sometimes high-pitched with a characteristic timbre.

Infantile Marfan Syndrome

Although MFS was first documented in infants and young children, the disorder is often difficult to recognize in early life. On the other hand, some infants present with a more severe, distinct set of clinical manifestations, which has led to the suggestion that they represent a separate entity, termed

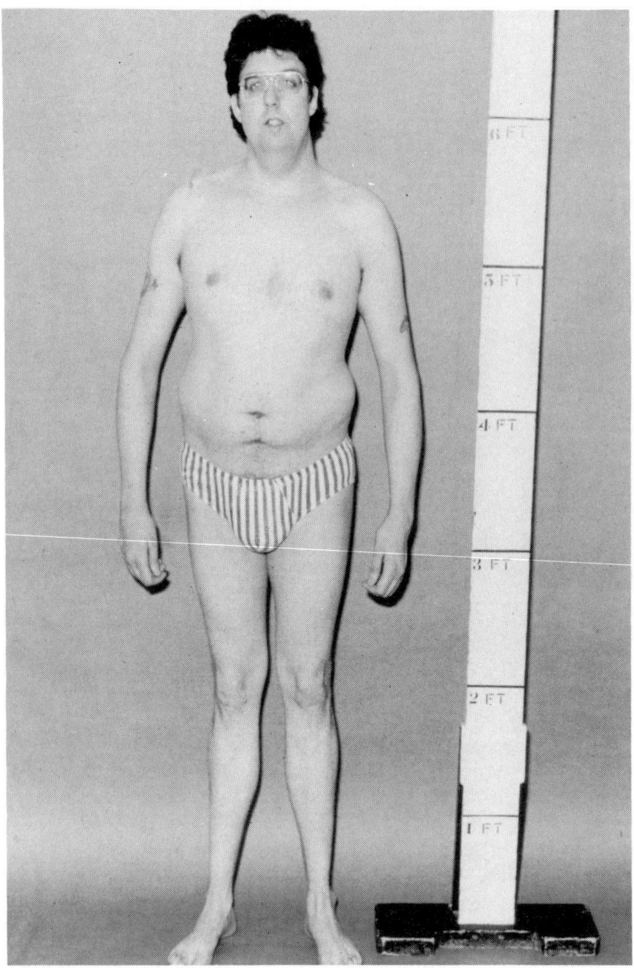

FIG. 135-5 Clinical features of MFS. Note the tall stature, excessive length of the upper and lower extremities, mild pectus excavatum, and myopia. *(Courtesy of A.H. Child, MD.)*

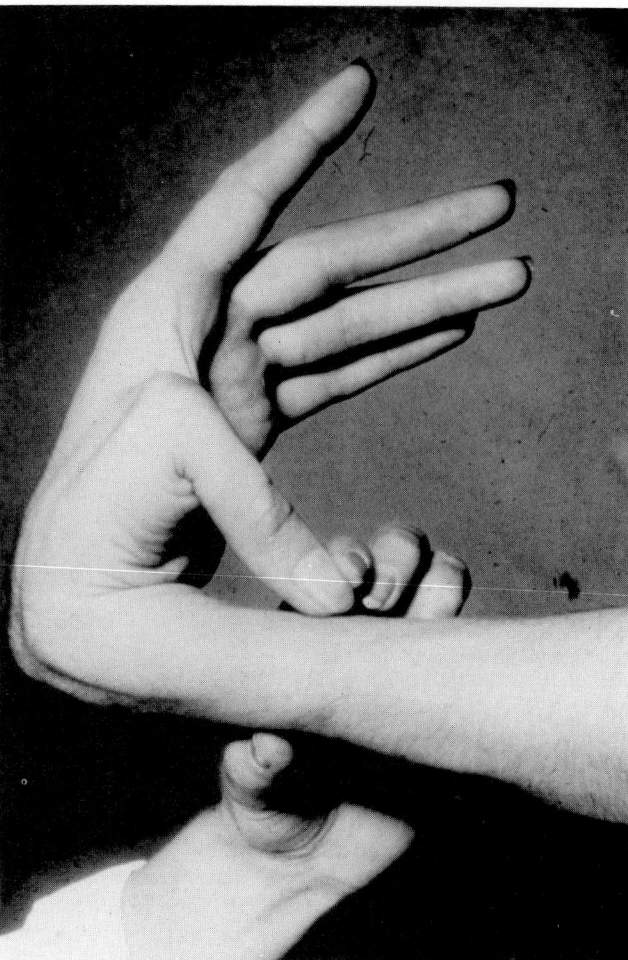

FIG. 135-6 Joint hypermobility and arachnodactyly observed in an individual affected with MFS. *(Courtesy of A.H. Child, MD.)*

infantile or neonatal MFS. The phenotypic manifestations include a characteristic elderly facial appearance due to deep-set eyes; high-arched palate; arachnodactyly; pectus deformities, flexion contractures; pes planus; multivalvular involvement; aortic root dilatation; and ectopia lentis.[67]

Management and Therapy

Individuals with MFS often require multidisciplinary management by a team of medical specialists. This setting is optimal for diagnostic confirmation or exclusion in equivocal cases. From a clinical point of view, the most serious and potentially fatal complications of the condition are associated with cardiovascular manifestations. Mortality in adult MFS patients is usually due to aortic root disease, with progressive dilatation resulting in either aortic regurgitation or dissection and rupture. The median age at death in MFS patients has been estimated to be the mid-forties, mostly as a result of cardiovascular complications.[68] Management includes a cardiologic examination schedule which depends on the severity of the cardiovascular complications. In individuals with mild clinical disease—i.e., mitral valve prolapse and minimal aortic dilatation—annual examination including an echocardiogram is sufficient. However, if aortic dilatation and regurgitation are significant, more frequent follow-up should be scheduled. In addition to echocardiography, computed tomography and magnetic resonance imaging have been used in evaluating aortic pathology in MFS. As previously stated, a direct correlation has been observed between aortic root dimension and subsequent complications of MFS.[60]

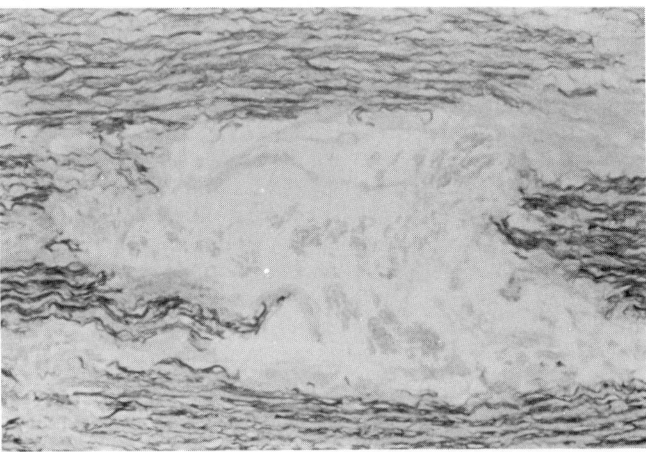

FIG. 135-7 Cystic medial necrosis, a typical histopathologic appearance of the aortic media in MFS. Note the fragmentation of the elastic fibers (stained black) and replacement by amorphous ground substance. *(Courtesy of A.H. Child, MD.)*

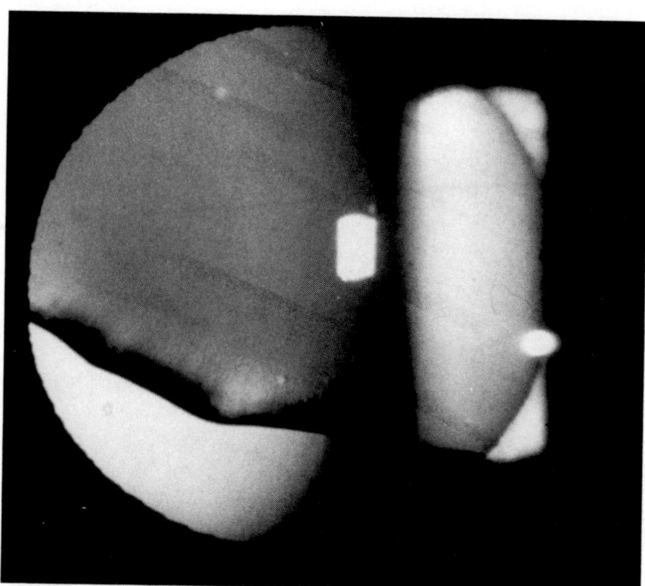

FIG. 135-8 **Ectopia lentis in MFS; note the superonasal displacement of the lens.** *(Courtesy of A.H. Child, MD.)*

Aortic regurgitation is virtually nonexistent in MFS patients whose aortic root dimension is 3.6 cm or less. In contrast, it occurs consistently in individuals who have an aortic root dimension of 6.0 cm or greater.[49,50] Patients whose aortic dilatation extends into the ascending aorta are more likely to have aortic regurgitation and, thus, are at greater short-term risk of progressive dilatation and subsequent surgery than patients whose aortic dilatation is limited to the sinuses of Valsalva.[59] Propranolol therapy is most commonly used to reduce the rate of aortic dilatation in affected children and adults.[69] However, the beneficial effects on the aorta of long-term β-blockade or negative inotropy are difficult to ascertain because they have not been studied in a rigorously controlled drug trial. It may therefore be somewhat premature to propose this treatment for all individuals with MFS.

During the past few years, improved surgical techniques for repairing the dilated or dissected aortic root and simultaneously replacing the aortic valve have greatly enhanced the survival rate of MFS patients. An elective repair, with an aortic root diameter 6 cm or less, is preferable to emergency repair. A modified Bentall procedure with a variety of composite grafts is used, with a resulting 10-year survival rate of more than 75 percent.[70,71] The occurrence of dissection prior to surgery or the presence of aneurysms in multiple aortic segments are associated with a worse postoperative prognosis and a reported 10-year survival of 56 percent.[72] While replacement of the aortic or mitral valves is a frequent procedure in MFS patients, it is often feasible in children with mitral regurgitation to reconstruct the mitral valve rather than replace it.[73]

Scoliosis is a frequent orthopedic complication in MFS. Its age of onset varies from early childhood to adolescence. Conservative treatment by bracing or surgical correction with different types of fixation and rods can be used successfully.[74,75] While pectus deformities are present in more than two-thirds of individuals with MFS, surgical correction is only warranted in cases of pulmonary compromise and not for cosmetic reasons. Since pectus abnormalities have recurred in a large number of patients in whom repair was performed at an early age, it is preferable to delay surgery until skeletal maturity is attained.[56] Pes planus and associated deformities frequently cause symptoms in the average patient and may require surgical correction. Likewise, recurrent joint dislocations and subluxations can be managed according to established orthopedic principles.

Regular ophthalmic evaluation is an important aspect of the management of individuals with MFS. Surgical removal of a dislocated lens should not be considered routinely unless correction of visual acuity is unattainable by more conventional means.[65]

Pregnancy can pose considerable risk to women affected with MFS.[76] In general, women with an aortic root diameter greater than 4 cm, valvular disease, or evidence of cardiac decompensation are at greater risk, while those with minimal cardiac findings tolerate pregnancy well.[77] Continued use of β-blockers during pregnancy remains controversial.

Although most individuals affected with MFS cope well with their condition, some require psychological counseling to help manage such a chronic and potentially debilitating condition. The National Marfan Foundation in the United States and similar lay groups in other countries provide valuable psychological and emotional support, as well as relevant information to their members and other interested individuals.

MARFAN-RELATED CONDITIONS

The establishment of an international nosology of heritable disorders of connective tissue has recently clarified the diagnostic criteria for discriminating between MFS and MFS-related conditions.[54] This distinction has prognostic value and greatly affects the clinical management and lifestyle of patients. Although the list of disorders sharing one or more stigmata with MFS is fairly long, we will briefly discuss here only those conditions which either have been linked to fibrillin loci or have been proposed as likely candidates for fibrillin mutations.[41,43,47]

Congenital Contractural Arachnodactyly

CCA is an autosomal dominant condition presenting with multiple joint contractures, arachnodactyly, dolichostenomelia, kyphoscoliosis, and abnormalities of the external ears (Figs. 135-9 to 135-11).[12,14,78,79] There are usually no cardiovascular or ocular-system manifestations, although a few isolated incidents of ectopia lentis and aortic or valvular involvement have been reported.[80]

CCA is a milder phenotype than MFS; joint contractures are most obvious in the digits and most severe in the hand, but they tend to improve with age.[78] In addition, progressive scoliosis has been observed in many patients. Although its exact incidence has not been estimated, CCA is much less common than MFS. The phenotypic distinction between these two syndromes is not always clear and, as a result, CCA has frequently been considered an allelic form of MFS. More recent studies, however, have established that CCA is genetically distinct from MFS, since the two syndromes are linked to two different fibrillin loci.[41,47]

Mitral Valve Prolapse Syndrome and Annuloaortic Ectasia

It has been proposed that the so-called MASS phenotype (mitral valve prolapse in association with aortic, skeletal, and skin manifestations), represents a phenotypic continuum

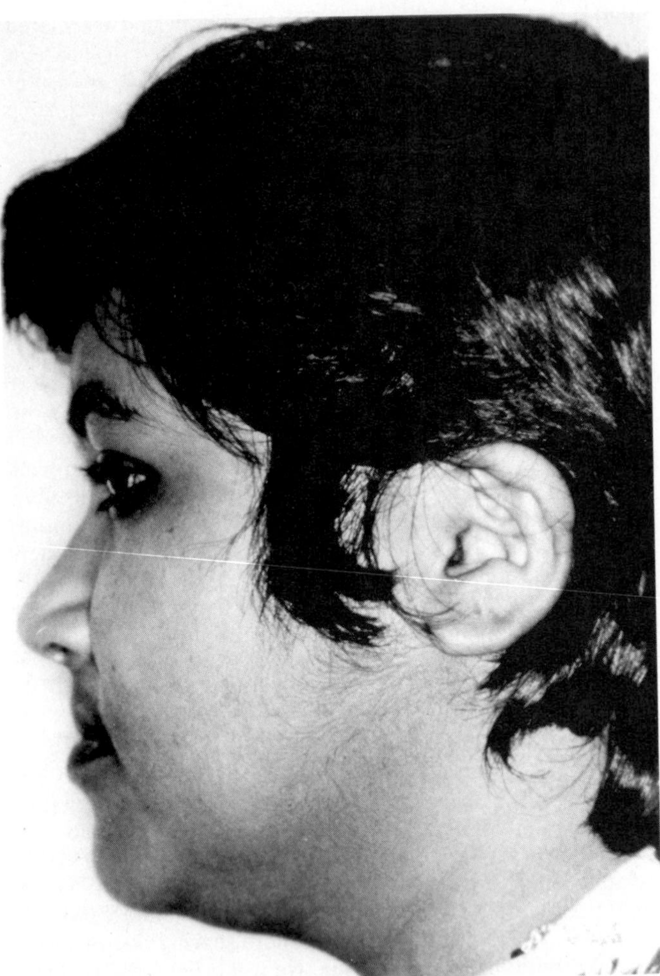

FIG. 135-9 **Characteristic "crumpled" ear in a patient with CCA.** *(From Viljoen et al.[79] Used by permission.)*

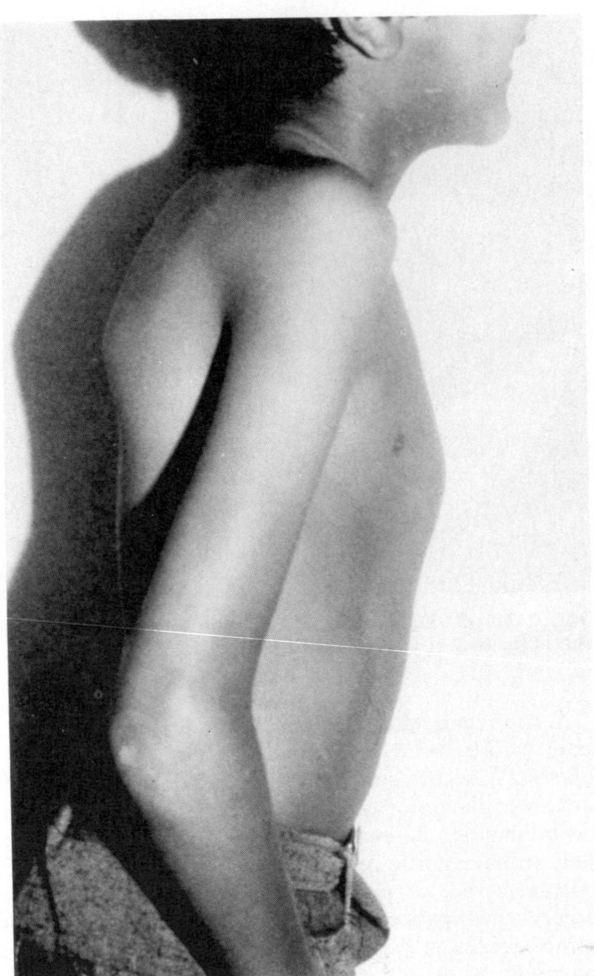

FIG. 135-10 **Contracture of the elbow in a patient with CCA.** *(From Viljoen et al.[79] Used by permission.)*

with MFS.[81] It should be noted, however, that prolapse of the mitral valve is the most common cardiac abnormality, and many individuals with mitral valve prolapse also have Marfanoid habitus.[82–84] Hence, establishment of the MASS phenotype necessitates careful clinical differentiation from MFS.

Similar diagnostic considerations apply to annuloaortic ectasia, a rare autosomal dominant disorder that exhibits isolated aortic dilatation and dissecting aortic aneurysms.[85] Patients often suffer high morbidity and mortality from sudden aneurysmal rupture in early to late adulthood. Aortic stenosis and cystic medial necrosis are common findings. Histologic studies in several patients have documented loss of elastic fibers, cystic medial changes, and deposition of polysaccharide-like materials.[86] Hitherto, only one annuloaortic ectasia family has been investigated for genetic linkage with fibrillin-specific DNA markers; it was found to be discordant with both chromosome 5 and 15 loci.[47]

Dominantly Inherited Ectopia Lentis

Dominant EL is characterized by isolated displacement of the lens behind the pupil, which results in myopia, astigmatism, and loss of vision.[87] Loss of vision usually results from marginal aberration of the lens or partial aphakia of the pupil. The cause is thought to be a weakening of specific portions of the ciliary zonule. Linkage to the fibrillin locus on chromosome 15 has been established in one three-generation EL family.[47] Dislocation of the lens sometimes coexists with a deformed and displaced pupil. Unlike isolated EL, this condition is inherited as a recessive trait.[88]

THE DEFECTIVE GENE PRODUCT IN MARFAN SYNDROME

Despite the successful identification of the MFS gene product, very little is still known about the structural/functional and metabolic features of this protein. Given such a handicap, it is almost impossible to do more than speculate about the contribution of individual mutations to the clinical spectrum of MFS. Accordingly, most of the conclusions presented here should not be accepted as definitive models; rather, they should be viewed as working hypotheses that are likely to be radically changed in both content and form by future discoveries.

The 10-nm Microfibrils

"Microfibril" is a general term originally used by Low[89] for morphologically similar matrix structures which display a diameter of less than 20 nm and lack the characteristic 67-nm banding periodicity of interstitial collagen fibers. This general term does not, however, convey the great heterogeneity

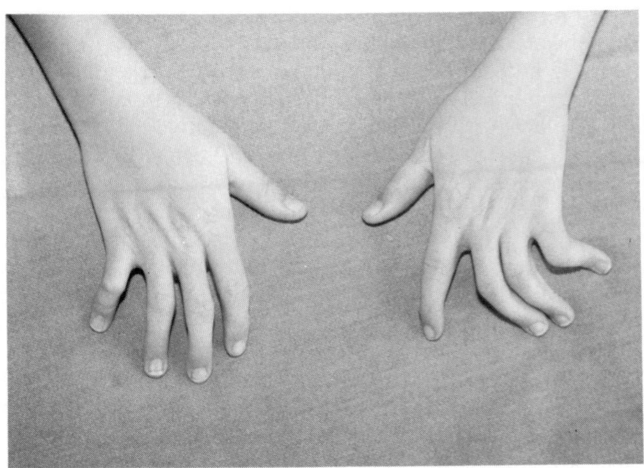

FIG. 135-11 Contractures of the fingers in a patient with CCA. *(Courtesy of D. Weaver, MD.)*

which is characteristic of microfibrils. Indeed, originally subsumed under this classification are chemically diverse matrix constituents such as thrombospondin, type VI collagen, and amyloid components, in addition to numerous as yet uncharacterized glycoproteins.[90–93]

The current definition divides the microfibrils into two separate classes according to their average diameters.[94] The largest class consists of the 10-nm microfibrils often found in association with amorphous elastin profiles and previously referred to also as "elastin-associated microfibrils."[32] Characteristically, these microfibrils are seen as "fringes" surrounding elastin cores and extending outward for a variable distance. Electron microscopy (EM) visualizes the fibers as linear bundles containing many individual, thread-like microfibrils, which are regularly beaded in longitudinal section and tubular in cross-section.[95–97] Similar fibrous profiles occur unassociated with elastin, as, for example, in the suspensory ligaments of the lens. Immunolocalization studies have identified microfibrils in periosteum, perichondrium, pleura, aorta, meninges, cartilage, tendon, muscle, and numerous other tissues.[33] Ontogenically, microfibrils are first deposited in the matrix of elastic tissues and later become invested with amorphous elastin. This is particularly true of the tunica media of the aorta, where concentric rings of microfibrils appear early in embryogenesis, prior to elastin deposition.[94]

It is believed that 10-nm microfibrils serve at least three basic functions.[94] First, they form a fibrous aggregate linking elastin to other matrix structures. For example, in skin, microfibrils are the bridge between elastin bundles and basement membranes at the dermal/epidermal junction. Second, fibrillin aggregates serve as a scaffolding on which elastin is deposited, as in the aforementioned concentric rings of elastin in the mature tunica media of the aorta. Third, they serve a structural function in tissues that do not contain elastin, such as periodontal ligament, ciliary zonule, and the mesangium of renal glomeruli.

The complete inventory of the macromolecular constituents of microfibrils is presently unknown, principally because of the highly insoluble nature of this matrix aggregate.[94] Several molecules have been shown by immunoelectron microscopy to be associated with microfibrils, although the details of these interactions remain mostly undefined. The list of the best-characterized components include the 31-kDa MAGP (microfibril-associated glycoprotein), a 34-kDa glycoprotein with amino oxidase activity, and the enzyme lysyl oxidase, in addition to fibrillin.[33,93,94,98] Overall, however, our knowledge of microfibril composition and assembly is, at best, primitive.

Structure of the Fibrillin Protein and Gene (FBN1)

The key element in the successful identification of the MFS gene was the availability of the specific antibodies that Sakai et al.[33] initially developed for characterizing microfibrillar components. These antibodies recognize three distinct pepsin-resistant fibrillin fragments, termed PF-1, PF-2 and PF-3.[99] These reagents provided the limited protein sequence necessary both for designing the oligonucleotides used in cloning the gene and for validating the cDNAs.[42] They also showed that fibrillin is an integral component of microfibrils in both elastic and nonelastic tissues and gave some insight into the structure of these matrix aggregates.[33,97,99,100]

Fibrillin is an acidic glycoprotein with an estimated molecular mass of 350 kDa under reducing conditions. Initial compositional studies showed that fibrillin has an unusually high cysteine content of 14 percent, and that one-third of the cysteines are in the free sulfhydryl form that can potentially participate in intermolecular disulfide bonds.[99,100] The existence of local intrachain disulfide bonds and interactions between fibrillin and nonfibrillin molecules via interchain disulfide bridges has been substantiated by analysis of the amino acid sequence inferred from fibrillin cDNAs.[41,42,101,102]

Superficial examination shows fibrillin to be characterized by several repeated cysteine-rich motifs. The structure of the repeats is reminiscent of the epidermal growth factor (EGF) peptide module, including the six similarly spaced cysteinyl residues.[103] Nuclear magnetic resonance has shown that this 53-amino-acid soluble peptide folds into a characteristic tertiary structure in which an N-terminal triple-stranded β sheet is stabilized by disulfide bonds involving the six cysteines. Numbering the cysteines C1 through C6, the bonds occur between C1 and C3, C2 and C4, and C5 and C6 (Fig. 135-12).[104] Variations of the EGF motif are widely distributed in a variety of macromolecules as diverse as transmembrane proteins (e.g., mammalian low-density lipoprotein receptor and the *Drosophila* homeotic gene product *Notch*), serum proteins involved in the blood coagulation cascade, and several extracellular matrix components.[103] In reference to the last group of proteins, it has been proposed that EGF-like sequences may serve as localized matrix signals for cell growth and differentiation.[105] More careful analysis shows that fibrillin appears to represent a multidomain protein consisting of at least five structurally and, plausibly, functionally distinct regions (A through E in Fig. 135-13).

The longest of the fibrillin regions, region D, spans 2240 amino acids and is arranged into 49 EGF-like repeats. This region includes peptides PF-1 and PF-2, which appear as rod-shaped structures[99] by EM rotary shadowing. The EGF-like repeats can be segregated into three separate groups on the basis of composition and sequence homology. The most common of the fibrillin EGF-like motifs (type I repeat) contains an additional consensus sequence D-D/N-N*-Y/F (where the asterisk denotes a potential hydroxylation site), which in several proteins is responsible for vitamin-K-independent high-affinity calcium binding (Fig. 135-12).[103] There is growing evidence that the EGF calcium-binding (EGF-CB) motif contributes to establishing protein–protein

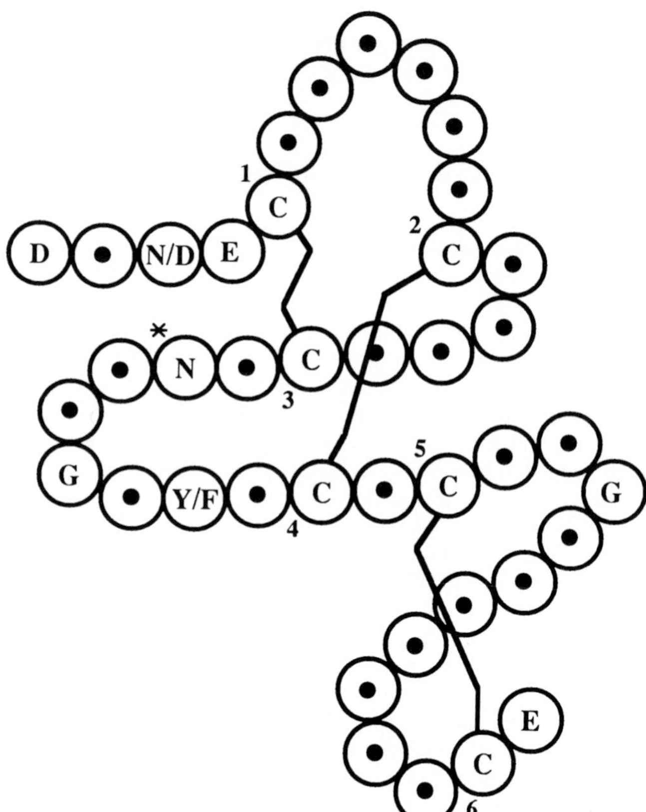

FIG. 135-12 Theoretical folding of a prototypical fibrillin EGF-CB motif modeled on the solution structure of human EGF[102] with cysteinyl residues numbered in the N-terminal to C-terminal direction.

interactions. Indeed, such a function has been demonstrated for one of the *Drosophila Notch* repeats and is implied by the presence of mutations in the EGF-CB domain of factor IX in hemophila B.[106,107]

Scattered among the numerous EGF-CD repeats are six similarly structured sequences which are analogous to the eight-cysteine module seen in transforming growth factor-β binding protein.[108] It is interesting that the eight-cysteine motif (type II repeat) is interspersed among several EGF-CB repeats in this peptide as well.[108] The cluster of three consecutive cysteines in this type II module may provide the moieties used for interchain bonds (Fig. 135-13). A similar function could also be envisioned for the last protein module of region D. This motif, present only once in fibrillin and apparently unique to it, contains eight cysteines, two of which are positioned next to each other (Fig. 135-13).

The few non-type-I modules of region D seem to demarcate clusters of EGF-CB repeats. The invariant distance between the last cysteine of one repeat and the first cysteine of the next one could lead to the formation of an additional β sheet between contiguous repeats. This configuration might in turn allow an individual cluster of multiple repeats to act as a single functional unit. Consequently, mutations that disrupt folding of one repeat would be expected to alter the conformation, and thus the function, of an entire cluster.

Several potential signals for *N*-linked glycosylation point to the substantial degree of posttranslation modification that fibrillin undergoes before being deposited in the extracellular matrix (Fig. 135-13). In addition, a putative cell-attachment site also occurs near the middle of region D (Fig. 135-13).

Contrasting with the uniformity of region D is the compositional heterogeneity of the substantially shorter region B (Fig. 135-13). This 336-amino-acid long region is made up of eight contiguous cysteine-rich sequences, three of which display clusters of two or three consecutive cysteinyl residues. Thus, compared to region D, region B has fewer cysteine-mediated interchain bonds than intrachain bonds.

The exceedingly high proline content (42 percent) of region C is consistent with an α-helical configuration (Fig. 135-13). This and the hydrophobicity of region C may allow the fibrillin molecule to bend. This could in turn favor the occurrence of interactions during the initial polymerization of the fibrillin monomers.

Flanking the aforementioned fibrillin regions are a larger basic N-terminal segment (region A), which is preceded by a signal peptide, and a lysine-rich C-terminus (region E), which contains two cysteinyl residues and three potential glycosylation sites (Fig. 135-13).

The modular arrangement of the fibrillin protein is replicated in the multicassette organization of the gene, whose coding sequence is distributed into 65 exons spanning nearly 110 kb of DNA.[101] Fifty of the 57 cysteine-rich motifs of fibrillin are encoded by single exons; in addition, 60 of the FBN1 exons begin and end with in-phase split codons. Because of this configuration, most of the genomic deletions and splicing mutations removing one or more exons from the mature transcript are expected to give rise to a shortened but in-frame fibrillin protein. Another interesting feature of the FBN1 organization is the presence of "mosaic" exons coding for the transition sequences between the major structural regions of the protein.[101]

The genomic study has also provided evidence suggesting that most of the progenitor fibrillin gene arose by multiple duplications of a type I module-coding exon.[101] It has also been postulated that various rearrangements between this ancestral unit and the one encoding a type II module gave rise to the unique peptide motifs of fibrillin.[101] Finally, preliminary results indicate that FBN2, the other fibrillin gene on chromosome 5, displays a similar configuration and thus probably originated from the same progenitor gene.[101]

Fibrillin and Microfibril Assembly

In this section we will attempt to depict a likely scenario for microfibril formation, which has been arrived at by integrating, correlating, and extrapolating from the experimental evidence described or cited in the previous two sections. More than before, the description that will emerge should be viewed as highly speculative, for it is based on indirect evidence, which is itself interpreted to fit to the proposed model.

Fibrillin is apparently synthesized in a precursor form (preprofibrillin) which, after secretion into the extracellular matrix, seems to undergo proteolytic maturation with the removal of a 30-kDa segment.[48] Once outside the cell, mature fibrillin molecules participate in the rapid formation of disulfide-bonded aggregates; first microfibrils and, later, microfibrillar bundles are built on these aggregates.[99,100] In addition, the growing microfibrils interact with and incorporate other matrix components, such as microfibril-associated glycoprotein (MAGP) and other glycoproteins or, under particular conditions, fibronectin, amyloid P, vitronectin, and thrombospondin.[90,92,94,109,110] Whether or not elastin is disulfide-bonded to microfibrils remains the subject of much speculation.[94] Regardless of the morphology of the network and its association with elastin, microfibrils appear as long,

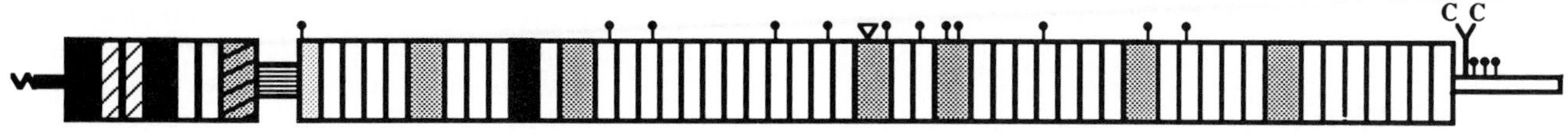

41 aa $D\,X\,{}^{N}_{D}\,E\ C\ X_6\ C\ X_4\ C\ X\,N\,X_2\,G\,X\,{}^{Y}_{F}\,X\ C\ X\ C\ X_2\,G\,X_8\ C\ X$

73 aa $D\,X\,R\,X_3\ C\,{}^{Y}_{F}\,X_8\ C\ X_{12}\,C\,C\,C\ X_{10}\ C\ E\,X\ C\ P\,X_3\,L\ C\ P\,X_{14}$

FIG. 135-13 Schematic representation of the primary structure of fibrillin. The letters above the diagram identify the five regions discussed in the text. Consensus sequences for the type I and type II modules of region D are shown below, along with their average length. The triangle on top of the type II module indicates the location of a putative cell-attachment sequence, and the black pin-heads symbolize potential glycosylation sites. Finally, the letter C identifies the two cysteines of region E.

beaded strings with EM analysis (Fig. 135-14).[95,97] The distance between beads is flexible, in that it can be stretched from 26 to 60 nm (Fig. 135-15) with the beads remaining evenly spaced.[96] In the stretched conformation, two characteristic cross-striations, suggestive of organizational sites, are noticeable in the intrabead space of the fibril (Fig. 135-15).[96] Attached to each bead are several (six to eight) fibrillin molecules.[95] The composition of the bead itself is as yet unknown.[99,100]

Antibodies raised against the N-terminal third of fibrillin (PF-3 Ab) decorate the beads,[97,99] suggesting that extracellular aggregation occurs with the establishment of disulfide bonding at this end of the molecule. The multiple interactions are probably facilitated by the proline-rich region that marks the junction of the N-terminal domain with the remainder of the fibrillin molecule and that is characterized by local folding areas and by a rod-shaped profile (Fig. 135-14). The periodicity of the arrangement is confirmed to some extent by the patterning of a second antibody that recognizes an epitope in the N-terminal half of the rod-shaped domain (PF-1 Ab).[99] Fibers subjected to immunogold labeling with either one antibody (PF-1 or PF-3) or both antibodies (PF-1 and PF-3) showed a regularly banded pattern.[100] Since both antibodies localize to the N-terminal half of fibrillin, and assuming that only one fibrillin interval stretches between each beaded structure, only a head-to-tail orientation would explain the constant periodic intervals on staining (Fig. 135-15).[100] In unstretched tissue preparations, the gold-labeled pattern on both individual microfibrils and microfibrillar bundles closely resembles the 67-nm periodicity of interstitial collagen fibers.[100]

Fibrillin Mutations in Marfan Syndrome

Characterization of fibrillin mutations in MFS has yet to reveal a pattern that would make it possible to correlate the nature of the molecular defect with the clinical severity of the resulting phenotype. This body of work nevertheless is providing indirect clues about the role of fibrillin in the assembly and maintenance of the microfibrillar meshwork. In addition, it has led to the suggestion that all MFS cases are caused by dysfunctions at the FBN1 locus.

Genetic homogeneity regarding the locus for MFS is supported by three independent lines of experimental evidence. First, fibrillin antisera were shown to stain microfibrils of MFS tissue samples consistently less than control samples.[34,35] Second, an equal proportion of cultured dermal fibroblasts from MFS patients was found to be affected by defects in fibrillin synthesis, secretion, and incorporation into the extracellular matrix.[48] Third, cosegregation between the MFS phenotype and diagnostic FBN1 markers was established in a large group of families with different clinical presentations of the disease.[47] The recent identification of three additional FBN1 polymorphisms is expected to improve substantially genetic counseling of MFS families.[11]

The variety of metabolic abnormalities identified in the biosynthesis study and the consistent reduction of epitope detection observed in the immunohistochemical work can be partly reconciled by the predominantly negative nature of the fibrillin mutations. This concept was originally proposed by Muller[112] who referred to these kind of mutations as "antagonistic mutant genes" or "antimorphs." Accordingly, the defective MFS gene product is expected to interrupt the function of the wild-type protein by interfering at many different metabolic levels, such as secretion, extracellular assembly, and association with itself and with other gene products into higher-order aggregates.

Despite its failure to define predictable genotype/phenotype correlations, molecular screening for fibrillin mutations has already yielded some new insight into the structural/functional features of this gene product.[43–46,113–117] With one

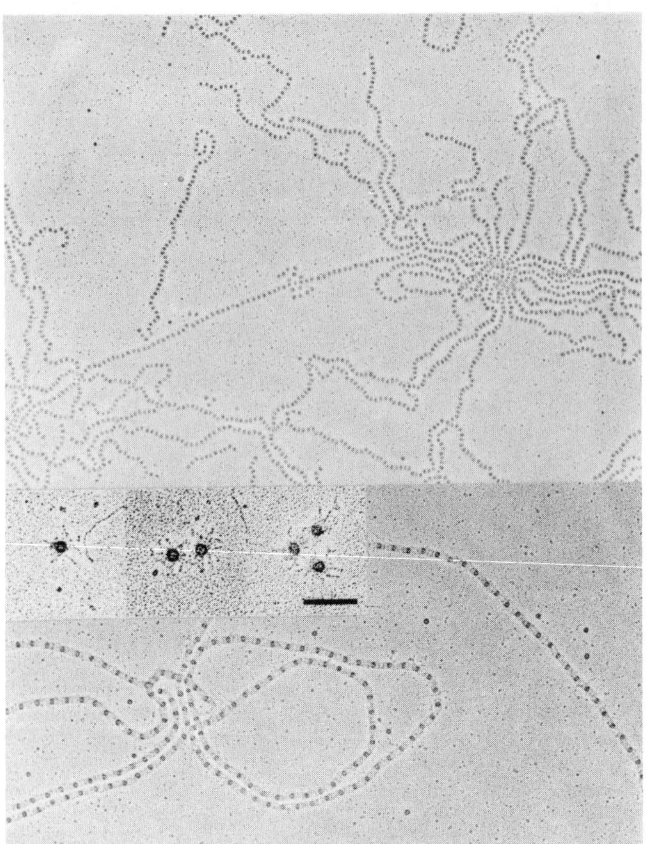

FIG. 135-14 EM images of fibrillin molecules. *Top*: rotary-shadowing EM of zonular fibrils. Note the beaded structure and the close spacing of the beads. *Bottom*: Rotary shadowing of zonular fibrils that have been stretched and fixed. Note the cross striations between the beads. *(From Ren et al.*[96] *Used by permission.) Insert*: Rotary shadowing of beaded fibrils and subunits showing filaments emerging from the surface of each bead. Bar = 100 nm. *(From Wright and Mayne.*[95] *Used by permission.)*

exception, all of the fibrillin mutations identified so far are family-specific.[43] Furthermore, most of them are single-amino-acid substitutions in different EGF-CB repeats.

Some of the substitutions affect the invariant cysteinyl residues of the EGF-CB motif. These mutations are expected to disrupt local folding of individual EGF-CB modules and, possibly, of an entire multirepeat cluster. One such mutation leads to substantial reduction and disorganized patterning of fibrillin immunostaining in cultured fibroblasts.[44] The mutation segregates in a multigeneration family that exhibits an extreme degree of variability with respect to time of disease onset, organ-system involvement, and clinical severity.

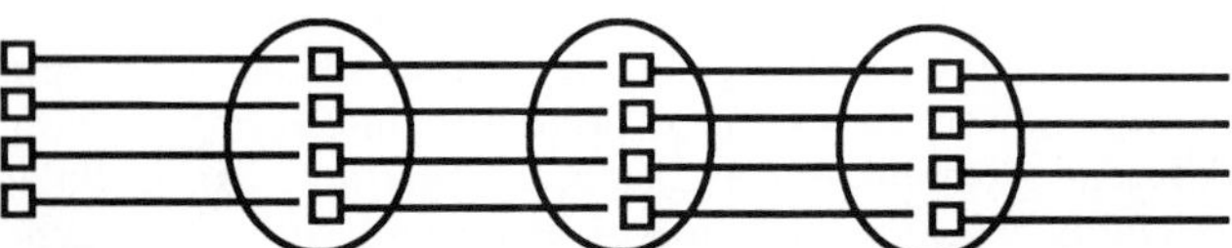

FIG. 135-15 Proposed model for the alignment of fibrillin monomers in microfibrils.[100] Squares indicate the interacting N-terminus of individual molecules, and ovals represent the beads visualized by EM. (See also Fig. 135-14.)

Similar metabolic consequences have been postulated for an arginine substitution identified in two unrelated sporadic cases with early onset and severe symptoms.[43] The mutation is located in a type I module of domain D, preceding the fourth cysteinyl residue and following the last amino acid of the calcium-binding consensus sequence.[43] Based on the structural considerations discussed above, the substitution may affect cysteine-mediated bonds by changing the secondary structure of the repeat.[43] Alternatively, the change may disrupt the calcium-binding site, thus compromising putative protein/protein interactions.[118]

More direct evidence in support of a functional role for the putative calcium-binding sequences of fibrillin has come from the characterization of three additional missense mutations.[114,115] The first was identified in the affected members of a MFS family with severe symptoms of the disease.[114] The change, asparagine to serine, is not expected to impair local folding of the repeat; rather, it eliminates the site of β-hydroxylation in the calcium-binding consensus sequence (Fig. 135-12). An isoleucine substitution in the same relative position of a different EGF-CB repeat was identified in a second family with classic MFS.[115] The third calcium-binding mutation was found in a family affected by a severe form of MFS.[115] In this case, however, the substitution affects the first residue of the calcium-binding consensus sequence, namely, the aspartic acid in the second position in the EGF-CB repeat (Fig. 135-12).

As already mentioned, most of the deletion and splicing mutations of FBN1 do not result in a truncated protein.[45,116,117] These shortened polypeptides are therefore expected to alter the phasing of, and thus the interactions among, the polymerizing fibrillin monomers. In one of these cases, the deletion causes the in-frame removal of three EGF-CB repeats of region D.[45] The shortened peptide is apparently synthesized in normal amounts, secreted efficiently, and assembled into fibrils that are structurally and functionally abnormal. The metabolic consequences of this interstitial deletion emphasize the strict length requirement of the fibrillin subunits for the assembly and function of the 10-nm microfibrils. Along these lines, a 55-year-old patient with classic manifestations of MFS was shown to be affected by a nonsense mutation resulting in the production of a truncated fibrillin peptide that lacks the last 116 residues.[45]

Another group of fibrillin mutations has focused attention on the possible contribution of quantitative defects to MFS pathogenesis.[46,115] The abnormalities are frameshift and nonsense mutations that not only produce truncated proteins but are also associated with a substantial reduction in the amount of the corresponding mature mRNA. This association is a well-documented phenomenon and is currently explained by two alternative mechanisms, the "nuclear scanning" model and the "transcriptional/translocational" model.[119,120] The latter postulates that premature termination of translation interferes with the coupled process of nuclear translocation, while the former envisions recognition of a premature stop codon in the pre-mRNA during splice-site scanning in the nuclear compartment. Regardless of the mechanism, both models predict some degradation of the abnormal transcript resulting from altered RNA nuclear transport.

The first such example in FBN1 is an early termination codon near the middle of domain D, which results in decreased synthesis (6 percent) of a truncated fibrillin molecule.[115] From a structural point of view, this finding supports the notion that the N-terminal end of the molecule plays a critical role in the polymerization of the fibrillin aggregate.

From a biosynthetic point of view, it indicates that even a relatively small amount of structurally abnormal fibrillin can give rise to a detectable phenotype. Interestingly, the clinical presentation of this MFS patient is almost undistinguishable from that of the milder MASS phenotype.[81] In contrast, a classic form of the disease was described in a different MFS patient with a similar frameshift mutation.[115] In this case, however, the defect is associated with a relatively higher level (16 percent) of mutant gene mRNA than in the previous patient.[115] Likewise, another severe case of MFS was found to exhibit 25 percent normal levels of mRNA with a splicing mutation.[46]

The apparent correlation between the amount of abnormal protein and the clinical severity is analogous to the relationship already noted in another multimeric protein system, the collagens (see Chap. 134). The 6 to 16 percent increase in the level of mutant gene expression and the concomitant transition from a milder to a more severe phenotype may, therefore, reflect a nonlinear amplification of the antimorphic effect of the mutant fibrillin pool. This amplification may in turn be dictated by one or more unknown requirements for the formation and/or maintenance of the microfibrillar meshwork. Needless to say, this and other genotype/phenotype correlations are still very premature and require more supportive evidence to be firmly established.

OTHER FIBRILLIN GENES AND MARFAN-RELATED DISORDERS

Some of the original cloning experiments identified cDNA and genomic clones harboring sequences closely resembling those of the product of the FBN1 gene.[41] This was quite unexpected, since there was no previous experimental evidence suggesting the presence of multiple fibrillin proteins. It is becoming increasingly evident, however, that the fibrillins represent a small family of structurally, functionally, and evolutionarily related proteins.

FBN2 and Congenital Contractural Arachnodactyly

The first evidence of genetic heterogeneity of fibrillin came from the original identification of Fib 5.[41] Structurally, the FBN2 gene product is highly homologous to that of Fib 5.[121] The homology extends to the total size of the protein, the length and composition of the corresponding cysteine-rich repeats, and the organization of the gene. The two proteins differ only in the composition of region C, which in Fib 5 is very rich in glycine residues.[121] This difference does not affect the postulated bending of region C, however.

The two fibrillin proteins are part of the same extracellular aggregates of elastic and nonelastic tissues.[121] In the latter, Fib 5 accumulates preferentially in elastic fiber-containing areas of the extracellular matrix.[121] This is particularly evident in the elastic cartilage of the external ear, one of the tissues that is abnormal in CCA patients.[121] Although no mutations have yet been reported, linkage between the FBN2 and CCA is based on a maximum LOD score of $Z = 6.21$ at the recombination fraction $\theta = 0.00$.[41,47]

Linkage of two distinct phenotypes, MFS and EL, to the same fibrillin locus, FBN1, suggests the differential expression of mutations in functionally distinct domains of the same molecule. On the other hand, linkage of the fibrillin loci FBN1 and FBN2 to three different clinical phenotypes, MFS, EL, and CCA, suggests these proteins have distinct functions in different tissues. In both cases, an analogy can be drawn with conditions associated with mutations in the structurally and evolutionarily related family of fibrillar collagens (see Chap. 134).

Fibrillin-Like Protein

Preliminary evidence from the bovine system indicates the existence of a third fibrillin-like transcript and protein, provisionally termed FLP.[122] FLP is structurally related to the other two fibrillins, probably undergoes alternative splicing, and colocalizes to the same elastin-associated microfibrils.[122] Moreover, the pattern of FLP gene expression is very similar to that of elastin in developing tissues.[122]

Fib 17 Gene

The last fibrillin-like candidate is a genomic clone harboring two exons potentially coding for EGF-CB repeats.[41] This locus was mapped on chromosome 17q22-q24 and called Fib 17.[41] However, emerging evidence suggests that the clone is an artifact.

ANIMAL MODELS

A more complete understanding of fibrillin pathophysiology will eventually be attained with a more comprehensive description of genotype/phenotype correlations from naturally occurring variants. In addition, the availability of suitable animal models for MFS and MFS-related disorders will greatly aid the study of fibrillin pathogenesis in these conditions. Some of these models are likely to be generated by the gene-targeting technique in mouse embryonic stem cells.[123] Aside from the transgenic model, a herd of calves affected by a disorder analogous to MFS has been reported.[124]

The animals display long thin limbs, joint laxity, ectopia lentis, and aortic dilation and aneurysm. An autopsy of a calf that died suddenly at age 16 months identified the cause of death as aortic rupture resulting in hemopericardium and cardiac tamponade. EM analysis revealed that the tunica media of the affected aorta displayed thin and irregular elastic laminae. However, there was no detectable decrease in fibrillin immunostaining of skin biopsies from affected animals compared to normal controls.[124] Subsequent immunohistochemical and biochemical analyses of cultured dermal fibroblasts and aortic smooth muscle cells have instead indicated that samples from affected calves produce and secrete a normal amount of fibrillin, but that the fibrillin is not properly assembled in the extracellular matrix.[125] Although the exact nature of the genetic defect is unknown, this animal form of MFS promises to be a suitable model for testing the efficacy of therapies designed to counteract the development of dissecting aneurysm.

ADDENDUM

The nomenclature of the fibrillin proteins has recently been changed to fibrillin-1 for Fib 15, and fibrillin-2 for Fib 5.[121] Unpublished evidence indicates that Fib 17 is a cloning artifact and excludes the existence of a profibrillin precursor molecule.[126] Finally, a mutational study[127] has recently confirmed the causal relationship between FBN1 and EL.[41,47]

ACKNOWLEDGMENTS

The authors thank Drs. Child, Dietz, Francomano, Mayne, Peltonen, Sakai, and Weaver for providing unpublished material. The continuing support of the Elster family is gratefully acknowledged, as is the help of Ms. Lingeza, Ms. Pereira, and Ms. Sozomenu in preparing this manuscript. This is article 111 from the Brookdale Center for Molecular Biology.

REFERENCES

1. Marfan AB: Un cas de déformation congenitale des quatre membres plus prononcée aux extrémités charactérisée par l'allongement des os avec un certain degré d'amincis-sement. *Bull Mem Soc Méd Hôp Paris* **13**:220, 1896.
2. Méry H, Babonneix L: Un cas de déformation congénitale des quatre membres: Hyperchondroplasie. *Bull Mem Soc Med Hop Paris* **19**:671, 1902.
3. Achard C: Arachnodactylie. *Bull Mem Soc Med Hop Paris* **19**:834,1902.
4. Boerger F: Uber zwei Fälle von Arachnodaktylie. *Z Kinderheilkd* **12**:161, 1914.
5. Piper RK, Irvine-Jones E: Arachnodactylia and its association with congenital heart disease: Report of a case and review of the literature. *Am J Dis Child* **31**:832, 1926.
6. Weve H: Veber Arachnodaktylie (Dystrophia mesodermalis congenita, typus Marfanis). *Arch Augenheilk* **104**:1, 1931.
7. Apert E: Les formes frustes du syndrome dolichosténomélique de Marfan. *Nourisson* **26**:1, 1938.
8. Etter LE, Glover LP: Arachnodactyly complicated by dislocated lens and death from rupture of dissecting aneurysm of aorta. *JAMA* **123**:88, 1943.
9. Baer RW, Taussig HB, Oppenheimer EH: Congenital aneurysmal dilatation of aorta associated with arachnodactyly. *Bull Johns Hopkins Hosp* **72**:309, 1943.
10. McKusick VA: The cardiovascular aspects of Marfan's syndrome: A heritable disorder of connective tissue. *Circulation* **11**:321, 1955.
11. McKusick VA: *Heritable Disorders of Connective Tissue*, 1st ed. St. Louis, Mosby, 1956.
12. Epstein CJ, Graham CB, Hodkin WE, Hecht F, Motulsky AG: Hereditary dysplasia of bone with kyphoscoliosis, contractures and abnormally shaped ears. *J Pediatr* **73**:379, 1968.
13. Beals RK: Homocystinuria. A report of two cases and review of the literature. *J Bone Joint Surg* **51**:1564, 1969.
14. Beals RK, Hecht F: Congenital contractural arachnodactyly: A heritable disorder of connective tissue. *J Bone Joint Surg* **53**:887, 1971.
15. Laitinen O, Uitto J, Iivanainen M, Hannuksela M, Kivirikko KI: Collagen metabolism of the skin in Marfan's syndrome. *Clin Chim Acta* **21**:321, 1968.
16. Krieg T, Müller PK: The Marfan's syndrome. In vitro study of collagen metabolism in tissue specimens of the aorta. *Exp Cell Biol* **45**:207, 1977.
17. Boucek RJ, Noble NL, Gunja-Smith Z, Butler WT: The Marfan syndrome: A deficiency in chemically stable collagen cross-links. *N Engl J Med* **305**:988, 1981.
18. Byers PH, Siegel RC, Peterson KE, Rowe DW, Holbrook KA, Smith LT, Chang Y, Fu JCC: Marfan syndrome: An abnormal $\alpha2$ chain in type I collagen. *Proc Natl Acad Sci USA* **78**:7745, 1981.
19. Phillips CL, Shrago-Howe AW, Pinnell SR, Wenstrup RJ: A substitution at a non-glycine position in the triple-helical domain of pro-α2(I) collagen chains present in an individual with a variant of the Marfan syndrome. *J Clin Invest* **86**:1723, 1990.
20. Tsipouras P, Borresen AL, Bamforth S, Harper PS, Berg K: Marfan syndrome: Exclusion of genetic linkage to the COL1A2 gene. *Clin Genet* **30**:428, 1986.
21. Dalgleish R, Hawkins JR, Keston M: Exclusion of the α2(I) and α1(III) collagen genes as the mutant loci in a Marfan syndrome family. *J Med Genet* **24**:148, 1987.
22. Ogilvie DJ, Wordsworth BP, Priestley LM, Dalgleish R, Schmidtke J, Zoll B, Sykes B: Segregation of all four major fibrillar collagen genes in the Marfan syndrome. *Am J Hum Genet* **41**:1071, 1987.
23. Francomano CA, Streeten EA, Meyers DA, Pyeritz RE: Exclusion of fibrillar procollagens as causes of Marfan syndrome. *Am J Med Genet* **29**:457, 1988.
24. Boileau C, Jondeau G, Bonaiti C, Coulon M, Delorme G, Dubourg O, Bourdarias JP, Junien C: Linkage analysis of five fibrillin collagen loci in a large French Marfan syndrome family. *J Med Genet* **27**:78, 1990.
25. Kainulainen K, Savolainen A, Palotie A, Kaitilia I, Rosenbloom J, Peltonen L: Marfan syndrome: Exclusion of genetic linkage of five genes coding for connective tissue components in the long arm of chromosome 2. *Hum Genet* **84**:233, 1990.
26. Abraham PA, Perejda AJ, Carnes WH, Uitto J: Marfan syndrome. Demonstration of abnormal elastin in aorta. *J Clin Invest* **70**:1245, 1982.
27. Royce PM, Danks DM: Normal lysyl oxidase activity in skin fibroblasts from patients with Marfan's syndrome. *IRCS Med Sci* **10**:41, 1982.
28. Appel A, Horwitz AL, Dorfman A: Cell-free synthesis of hyaluronic acid in Marfan syndrome. *J Biol Chem* **254**:12199, 1979.
29. Lamberg SI: Stimulatory effect of exogenous hyaluronic acid distinguishes cultured fibroblasts of Marfan's disease from controls. *J Invest Dermatol* **71**:391, 1978.
30. Nakashima Y: Reduced activity of serum β-glucuronidase in Marfan syndrome. *Angiology* **37**:576, 1986.
31. Pulkkinen L, Kainulainen K, Krusius T, Mäkinen P, Schollin J, Gustavsson KH, Peltonen L: Deficient expression of the gene coding for decorin in a lethal form of Marfan syndrome. *J Biol Chem* **265**:17780, 1990.
32. Cleary EG, Gibson MA: Elastin-associated microfibrils and microfibrillar proteins. *Int Rev Connect Tissue Res* **10**:97, 1983.
33. Sakai LY, Keene DR, Engvall E: Fibrillin, a new 350-kD glycoprotein, is a component of extracellular microfibrils. *J Cell Biol* **103**:2499, 1986.
34. Hollister DW, Godfrey M, Sakai LY, Pyeritz RE: Marfan syndrome: Immunohistologic abnormalities of the elastin-associated microfibrillar fiber system. *N Engl J Med* **323**:152, 1990.
35. Godfrey M, Menashe V, Weleber RG, Koler RD, Bigley RH, Lovrien E, Zonana J, Hollister DW: Cosegregation of elastin-associated microfibrillar abnormalities with the Marfan phenotype in families. *Am J Hum Genet* **46**:652, 1990.
36. Blanton SH, Sarfarazi M, Eiberg H, de Groote J, Farndon PA, Kilpatrick MW, Child AH, Pope FM, Peltonen L, Francomano CA, Boileau C, Keston M, Tsipouras P: An exclusion map of Marfan syndrome. *J Med Genet* **27**:73, 1990.
37. Kainulainen K, Pulkkinen L, Savolainen A, Kaitila I, Peltonen L: Location of chromosome 15 of the gene defect causing Marfan syndrome. *N Engl J Med* **323**:935, 1990.
38. Dietz HC, Pyeritz RE, Hall BD, Cadle RG, Hamosh A, Schwartz J, Meyers DA, Francomano CA: The Marfan syndrome locus: Confirmation of assignment to chromosome 15 and identification of tightly linked markers at 15q15-q21.3. *Genomics* **9**:355, 1991.
39. Tsipouras P, Sarfarazi M, Devi A, Weiffenbach B, Boxer M: Marfan syndrome is closely linked to a marker on 15q1.5→q2.1. *Proc Natl Acad Sci USA* **88**:4486, 1991.
40. Kainulainen K, Steinmann B, Collins F, Dietz HC, Francomano CA, Child A, Kilpatrick MW, Brock DJH, Keston M, Pyeritz RE, Peltonen L: Marfan syndrome: No evidence for heterogeneity in different populations and more precise mapping of the gene. *Am J Hum Genet* **49**:662, 1991.
41. Lee B, Godfrey M, Vitale E, Hori H, Mattei MG, Sarfarazi M, Tsipouras P, Ramirez F, Hollister DW:

Linkage of Marfan syndrome and a phenotypically related disorder to two fibrillin genes. *Nature* **353**:330, 1991.

42. Maslen CL, Corson GM, Maddox BK, Glanville RW, Sakai LY: Partial sequence of a candidate gene for the Marfan syndrome. *Nature* **352**:334, 1991.
43. Dietz HC, Cutting GR, Pyeritz RE, Maslen CL, Sakai LY, Corson GM, Puffenberger EG, Hamosh A, Nanthakumar EJ, Curristin SM, Stetten G, Meyers DA, Francomano CA: Marfan syndrome caused by a recurrent de novo missense mutation in the fibrillin gene. *Nature* **352**:337, 1991.
44. Dietz HC, Pyeritz RE, Puffenberger EG, Kendzior RJ, Corson GM, Maslen CJ, Sakai LY, Francomano CA, Cutting GR: Marfan phenotype variability in a family segregating a missense mutation in the EGF-like motif of the fibrillin gene. *J Clin Invest* **89**:1674, 1992.
45. Kainulainen K, Sakai LY, Child A, Pope MF, Puhakka L, Ryhanen L, Palotie A, Kaitila I, Peltonen L: Two unique mutations in Marfan syndrome resulting in truncated polypeptide chains of fibrillin. *Proc Natl Acad Sci USA* **88**:5917, 1992.
46. Dietz HC, Valle D, Francomano CA, Kendzior FJ, Pieritz RE, Cutting GR: The skipping of constitutive exons in vivo induced by nonsense mutation. *Science* **254**:680.
47. Tsipouras P, Del Mastro R, Sarfarazi M, Lee B, Vitale E, Child A, Godfrey M, Devereux R, Hewett D, Steinmann B, Viljoen D, Sykes BC, Kilkpatrick M, Ramirez F: Linkage of Marfan syndrome, dominant ectopia lentis and congenital contractural arachnodactyly to the fibrillin genes on chromosomes 15 and 5. *N Engl J Med* **326**:905, 1992.
48. McGookey-Milewicz D, Pyeritz RE, Crawford ES, Byers PH: Marfan syndrome: Defective synthesis, secretion and extracellular matrix formation of fibrillin by cultured dermal fibroblasts. *J Clin Invest* **89**:79, 1992.
49. Pyeritz RE, McKusick VA: The Marfan syndrome: Diagnosis and management. *N Engl J Med* **300**:772, 1979.
50. Pyeritz RE: Marfan syndrome, in Emery AEH, Rimoin DL (eds): *Principles and Practice of Medical Genetics*, 2nd ed. New York, Churchill Livingstone, 1990, p 1047.
51. Murdoch JL, Walker BA, McKusick VA: Parental age effects on the occurrence of new mutations for the Marfan syndrome. *Ann Hum Genet* **35**:331, 1972.
52. Chemke J, Nisani R, Feigl A, Garty R, Cooper M, Barash Y, Duskin D: Homozygosity for autosomal dominant Marfan syndrome. *J Med Genet* **21**:173, 1984.
53. Schollin J, Bjarke B, Gustavson KH: Probable homozygotic form of the Marfan syndrome in a newborn child. *Acta Paediatr Scand* **77**:452, 1988.
54. Beighton P, De Paepe A, Danks D, Finidori G, Gedde-Dahl T, Goodman R, Hall J, Hollister DW, Horton W, McKusick VA, Opitz JM, Pope JM, Pyeritz RE, Rimoin DL, Sillence D, Spranger JW, Thompson E, Tsipouras P, Viljoen D, Winship I, Young I: International nosology of heritable disorders of connective tissue, Berlin 1986. *Am J Med Genet* **29**:581, 1988.
55. Magid D, Pyeritz RE, Fishman EK: Musculoskeletal manifestations of the Marfan syndrome: Radiologic features. *Am J Roentgenol* **155**:99, 1990.
56. Scherer LR, Arn PH, Dressel DA, Pyeritz RM, Haller JA: Surgical management of children and young adults with Marfan syndrome and pectus excavatum. *J Pediatr Surg* **23**:1169, 1988.
57. Fishman EK, Zinreich SJ, Kumar AJ, Pyeritz RM: Sacral abnormalities in Marfan syndrome. *J Comput Assist Tomogr* **7**:851, 1983.
58. Pyeritz RE, Fishman EK, Berhardt BA, Siegelman SS: Dural ectasia is a common feature of the Marfan syndrome. *Am J Hum Genet* **43**:726, 1988.
59. Roman MJ, Devereux RB, Kramer-Fox R, Spitzer M: Aortic root dilatation in the Marfan syndrome: Patterns, familiarity, and short-term clinical courses. *J Am Coll Cardiol* **11**:74A, 1988.
60. Lima SD, Lima JAC, Pyeritz RE, Weiss JL: Relation of mitral valve prolapse to left ventricular size in Marfan's syndrome. *Am J Cardiol* **55**:739, 1985.
61. Pyeritz RE, Reider R, Fortuin NJ: Aortic complications in adult Marfan syndrome are associated with the aortic root diameter. *Clin Res* **29**:315A, 1981.
62. Crawford ES: Marfan's syndrome. Broad spectral surgical treatment of cardiovascular manifestations. *Ann Surg* **198**:487, 1983.
63. Roberts WC, Honig HS: The spectrum of cardiovascular disease in the Marfan syndrome: A clinico-morphologic study of 18 necropsy patients and comparison to 151 previously reported necropsy patients. *Am Heart J* **104**:115, 1982.
64. Larson EW, Edwards WD: Risk factors for aortic dissection: A necropsy study of 161 cases. *Am J Cardiol* **53**:849, 1984.
65. Maumenee IH: The eye in the Marfan syndrome. *Trans Am Ophthalmol Soc* **79**:684, 1981.
66. Wood JR, Bellamy D, Child AH, Citron KM: Pulmonary disease in patients with Marfan syndrome. *Thorax* **39**:780, 1984.
67. Morse RP, Rockenmacher S, Pyeritz RE, Sanders SP, Bieber FR, Lin A, MacLeod P, Hall B, Graham JM Jr: Diagnosis and management of infantile Marfan syndrome. *Pediatrics* **86**:888, 1990.
68. Murdoch JL, Walker BA, Halpern BI, Kuzma JW, McKusick VA: Life expectancy and causes of death in the Marfan syndrome. *N Engl J Med* **286**:804, 1972.
69. Pyeritz RE: Propanolol retards aortic root dilatation in the Marfan syndrome. *Circulation (Suppl. III)* **68**:365, 1983.
70. Bentall HH, DeBono AA: A technique for complete replacement of the ascending aorta. *Thorax* **23**:338, 1987.
71. Gott VL, Pyeritz RE, Magovern GJ Jr, Cameron DE, McKusick VA: Surgical treatment of aneurysms of the ascending aorta in the Marfan syndrome. *N Engl J Med* **314**:1070, 1986.
72. Crawford ES, Coselli JS: Marfan's syndrome: Combined composite valve graft replacement of the aortic root and transaortic mitral valve replacement. *Ann Thorac Surg* **45**:296, 1988.
73. Shumway SJ, Gott VL, Reitz BA: A "designer" annuloplasty ring for patients with massive mitral annular dilatation. *Ann Thorac Surg* **46**:695, 1988.
74. Birch JG, Herring JA: Spinal deformity in Marfan syndrome. *J Pediatr Orthop* **7**:546, 1987.
75. Winter RB: Thoracic lordoscoliosis in Marfan's syndrome. Report of two patients with surgical correction using rods and sublaminar wires. *Spine* **15**:233, 1990.
76. Beighton P: Pregnancy in the Marfan syndrome. *Br Med J* **285**:464, 1982.
77. Pyeritz RE: Maternal and fetal complications of pregnancy in the Marfan syndrome. *Am J Med* **71**:784, 1981.
78. Ramos-Arroyo MA, Weaver DD, Beals RK: Congenital contractural arachnodactyly. *Clin Genet* **27**:570, 1985.
79. Viljoen D, Ramesar R, Behari D: Beals syndrome: Clinical and molecular investigations in a kindred of Indian descent. *Clin Genet* **39**:181, 1991.
80. Bawle E, Quigg MH: Ectopia lentis and aortic root dilatation in congenital contractural arachnodactyly. *Am J Med Genet* **42**:19, 1992.
81. Glesby MJ, Pyeritz RE: Association of mitral valve prolapse and systemic abnormalities of connective tissue: a phenotypic continuum. *JAMA* **262**:523, 1989.
82. Salomon J, Shah PM, Heinle RA: Thoracic skeletal abnormalities in idiopathic mitral valve prolapse. *Am J Cardiol* **36**:32, 1975.
83. Devereux RB, Brown WT: Inheritance of mitral valve prolapse. *Prog Med Genet* **5**:139, 1983.
84. Cheng TO, Barlow JB: Mitral leaflet billowing and prolapse: Its prevalence around the world. *Angiology* **40**:77, 1989.
85. Nicod P, Bloor C, Godfrey M, Hollister DW, Pyeritz RE, Dittrich H, Polikar R, Peterson KL: Familial aortic dissecting aneurysms. *J Am Coll Cardiol* **13**:811, 1989.
86. Savunen T, Aho HJ: Annulo-aortic ectasia. Light and electron microscopic changes in aortic media. *Virchows Arch* **407**:279, 1985.
87. Jaureguy BM, Hall JG: Isolated congenital ectopia lentis with autosomal dominant inheritance. *Clin Genet* **15**:97, 1979.
88. Siemens HW: Veber die aetiologie der ectopia lentis et pupillae. *Graefes Arch Clin Exp Ophthalmol* **109**:359, 1920.

89. Low FN: Microfibrils: Fine filamentous components of the tissue space. *Anat Rec* **142**:131, 1962.
90. Arbeille BB, Fauvel-Lafeve FMJ, Lemesle MB, Tenza D, Legrand YJ: Thrombospondin: A component of microfibrils of various tissues. *J Histochem Cytochem* **39**:1367, 1991.
91. Gibson MA, Cleary EC: CL glycoprotein is the tissue form of type VI collagen. *J Biol Chem* **260**:11149, 1985.
92. Breathnach SM, Pepys MB, Hintner H: Tissue amyloid P component in normal human dermis is non-covalently associated with elastic fiber microfibrils. *J Invest Dermatol* **92**:53, 1989.
93. Gibson MA, Kumaratilake JS, Cleary EG: The protein components of the 12-nanometer microfibrils of elastic and nonelastic tissues. *J Biol Chem* **264**:4590, 1989.
94. Mecham RP, Heuser JE: The elastic fiber, in Hay ED (ed): *Cell Biology of the Extracellular Matrix*, 2nd ed. New York, Plenum, 1992, p 79.
95. Wright DW, Mayne R: Vitreous humor of chicken contains two fibrillar systems: An analysis of their structure. *J Ultrastruct Mol Struct Res* **100**:214, 1988.
96. Ren ZX, Brewton RG, Mayne R: An analysis by rotary shadowing of the structure of the mammalian vitreous humor and zonular apparatus. *J Struct Biol* **106**:57, 1991.
97. Keene DR, Maddox BK, Kuo HJ, Sakai LY, Glanville RW: Extraction of extendable beaded structures and their identification as fibrillin-containing extracellular matrix microfibrils. *J Histochem Cytochem* **39**:441, 1991.
98. Gibson MA, Sandberg LB, Grosso LE, Cleary EG: Complementary DNA cloning establishes microfibril-associated glycoprotein (MAPG) to be a discrete component of the elastin-associated microfibrils. *J Biol Chem* **266**:7596, 1991.
99. Maddox BK, Sakai LY, Keene DR, Glanville RW: Connective tissue microfibrils; isolation and characterization of three large pepsin-resistant domains of fibrillin. *J Biol Chem* **264**:21381, 1989.
100. Sakai LY, Keene DR, Glanville RW, Bachinger HP: Purification and partial characterization of fibrillin, a cysteine-rich structural component of connective tissue microfibrils. *J Biol Chem* **266**:14763, 1991.
101. Pereira L, D'Alessio M, Ramirez F, Lynch JR, Sykes B, Pangilinan T, Bonadio J: Genomic organization of the sequence coding for fibrillin, the defective gene product in Marfan syndrome. *Hum Mol Genet* **2**:961, 1993.
102. Corson GM, Chalberg SC, Dietz HC, Charbonneau NL, Sakai LY: Fibrillin binds calcium and is coded by cDNAs that reveal a multidomain structure and alternatively spliced exons at the 5′ end. *Genomics* **17**:476, 1993.
103. Davis CG: The many faces of epidermal growth factor repeats. *New Biol* **2**:410, 1990.
104. Cooke RM, Wilkinson AJ, Baron M, Pastore A, Tappin MJ, Campbell ID, Gregory H, Sheard B: The solution structure of human epidermal growth factor. *Nature* **327**:339, 1987.
105. Engel J: EGF-like domains in extracellular matrix proteins: Localized signals for growth and differentiation. *FEBS Lett* **251**:1, 1989.
106. Rebay I, Fleming RJ, Fehon RG, Cherbas L, Cherbas P, Artavanis-Tsakonas S: Specific EGF repeats of Notch mediate interactions with Delta and Serrate: Implications for Notch as a multifunctional receptor. *Cell* **67**:687, 1991.
107. Handford PA, Baron M, Mayhew M, Willis A, Beesley T, Brownlee GG, Campbell ID: The first EGF-like domain from human factor IX contains a high affinity calcium binding site. *EMBO J* **9**:475, 1990.
108. Kanzaki T, Olofsson A, Moren A, Wernstedt C, Hellman U, Miyazono K, Claesson-Welsh L, Heldin CH. TGF-β1 binding protein: A component of the large latent complex of TGF-β1 with multiple repeat sequences. *Cell* **61**:1051, 1990.
109. Dahlback K, Ljungquist A, Lafberg H, Dahlbäck B, Engvall E, Sakai LY: Fibrillin immunoreactive fibers constitute a unique network in the human dermis: Immunohistochemical comparison of the distribution of fibrillin, vitronectin, amyloid P component, and orcein stainable structures in normal skin and elastosis. *J Invest Dermatol* **94**:284, 1990.
110. Inoue S, Leblond CP, Rico P, Grant D: Association of fibronectin with the microfibrils of connective tissue. *Am J Anat* **186**:43, 1989.
111. Pereira L, Levran O, Ramirez F, Lynch JR, Sykes B, Pyeritz RE, Dietz HC: Diagnosis of Marfan syndrome: A molecular approach for stratification of cardiovascular risk within families. *N Engl J Med* in press, 1994.
112. Muller HJ: Further studies on the nature and causes of gene mutations, in Jones DF (ed): *Proceeding of the Sixth International Congress of Genetics*. Menasha, WI, Brooklyn Botanic Gardens, 1932, p 213.
113. Sykes B: Marfan gene dissected. *Nature Genet* **3**:99, 1993.
114. Hewett DR, Lynch JR, Smith R, Sykes B: Fibrillin mutation in the Marfan syndrome may disrupt calcium binding of the epidermal growth factor module. *Hum Mol Genet* **2**:275, 1993.
115. Dietz HC, McIntosh I, Sakai LY, Corson GM, Chalberg SC, Pyeritz RE, Francomano CA: Four novel FBN1 mutations: Significance for mutant transcript level and EGF-like domain calcium binding in the pathogenesis of Marfan syndrome. *Genomics* **17**:468, 1993.
116. Godfrey M, Vandemark N, Wang M, Velinov M, Wargowski D, Tsipouras P, Haw J, Becker J, Robertson W, Droste S, Rao VH: Prenatal diagnosis and a donor splice mutation in fibrillin in a family with Marfan syndrome. *Am J Hum Genet* **53**:472, 1993.
117. Godfrey M, Wang M, Han J, Imaizumi K, Kuroki Y: Acceptor splice site mutation in a patient with neonatal Marfan syndrome. Manuscript in preparation.
118. Handford PA, Mayhew M, Brownlee GG: Calcium binding to fibrillin? *Nature* **353**:395, 1991.
119. Urlaub G, Mitchell PJ, Ciudad CJ, Chasin LA: Nonsense mutations in the dihydrofolate reductase gene affect RNA processing. *Mol Cell Biol* **9**:2868, 1989.
120. Cheng J, Fogel-Petrovic M, Maquat LE: Translation to near the distal end of the penultimate exon is required for normal levels of spliced triosephosphate isomerase mRNA. *Mol Cell Biol* **10**:5215, 1990.
121. Zhang H, Apfelroth SD, Hu W, Davis EC, Sanguineti C, Bonadio J, Mecham RP, Ramirez F: Structure and expression of fibrillin-2, a novel microfibrillar component preferentially located in elastic matrices. *J Cell Biol* **124**:855, 1994.
122. Gibson MA, Davis E, Filiaggi M, Mecham RP: Identification and partial characterization of a new fibrillin-like protein [FLP]. *Am J Med Genet* **47**:148, 1993.
123. Capecchi MR: The new mouse genetics: Altering the genome by gene targeting. *Trends Genet* **51**:70, 1989.
124. Besser TE, Potter KA, Bryan GM, Knowlen GG: An animal model of the Marfan syndrome. *Am J Med Genet* **37**:159, 1990.
125. Potter KA, Hoffman Y, Sakai LY, Byers P, Bosser TE, Milewicz DM: Abnormal fibrillin metabolism in bovine Marfan syndrome. *Am J Pathol* **142**:803, 1993.
126. Ramirez F, Pereira L, Zhang H, Lee B: The fibrillin-Marfan syndrome connection. *Bioessays* **15**:589, 1993.
127. Kainulanen K, Karttunen L, Puhakka L, Sakai L, Peltonen L: Mutations in the fibrillin gene responsible for dominant ectopia lentis and neonatal Marfan syndrome. *Nat Genet* **6**:64, 1994.

CHAPTER 136

Hypophosphatasia

Michael P. Whyte

1. **Hypophosphatasia (McKusick 146300, 171760, 241500, 241510) is a metabolic bone disease that establishes an important (but as yet undefined) role for alkaline phosphatase (ALP) in skeletal mineralization. There is no animal model. Subnormal serum ALP activity (hypophosphatasemia) constitutes the biochemical hallmark and reflects a generalized deficiency of activity of the tissue-nonspecific (liver/bone/kidney) ALP isoenzyme (TNSALP). Activities of the three tissue-specific ALP isoenzymes in humans—intestinal, placental, and germ-cell (placental-like) ALP—are not diminished.**

2. **TNSALP is a zinc metalloglycoprotein that is catalytically active as a multimer of identical subunits. It is bound to plasma membranes by glycosylphosphatidylinositol linkage. The TNSALP gene is greater than 50 kb and has been localized to chromosome 1 (1p36.1-34). The tissue-specific ALP isoenzymes are encoded by a gene family on chromosome 2 (2q34-37). Each ALP gene has been sequenced.**

3. **Hypophosphatasia is characterized clinically by defective skeletal mineralization that manifests as rickets in infants and children and osteomalacia in adults. Clinical expressivity is, however, extremely variable. Stillbirth can occur from in utero onset in the perinatal ("lethal") form, which is apparent in newborns and associated with the most severe skeletal hypomineralization and deformity. The infantile form presents as a developmental disorder by age 6 months. It may cause craniosynostosis and nephrocalcinosis from hypercalcemia and hypercalciuria and is often fatal. Premature loss of deciduous teeth and rickets are the cardinal clinical features of childhood hypophosphatasia. Adult hypophosphatasia typically results in recurrent metatarsal stress fractures and pseudofractures in long bones and occasionally produces arthritis from calcium pyrophosphate dihydrate (CPPD) and perhaps calcium phosphate crystal deposition. Odontohypophosphatasia refers to especially mildly affected individuals who have dental, but no skeletal, manifestations. Pseudohypophosphatasia is an extremely rare variant in which serum ALP activity is normal in routine clinical assays.**

4. **Three phosphocompounds [phosphoethanolamine (PEA), PP_i, and pyridoxal 5′-phosphate (PLP)] accumulate endogenously in hypophosphatasia and are inferred to be natural substrates for TNSALP. A variety of evidence shows that PLP, a cofactor form of vitamin B_6, collects extracellularly; intracellular levels of PLP are normal. This observation explains the absence of symptoms of deficiency or toxicity of vitamin B_6 and indicates that TNSALP functions as an ectoenzyme. Extracellular accumulation of PP_i, which at low concentrations promotes calcium phosphate deposition but at high concentrations acts as an inhibitor of hydroxyapatite crystal growth, appears to account for the associated CPPD deposition and perhaps calcific periarthritis, as well as the defective mineralization of bones and teeth.**

5. **Perinatal and infantile hypophosphatasia are transmitted as autosomal recessive traits and can be due to homozygosity or compound heterozygosity for a variety of missense mutations in TNSALP gene exons. A regulatory abnormality in the biosynthesis of TNSALP may explain occasional cases. Subjects with childhood or adult hypophosphatasia can also be compound heterozygotes for TNSALP missense mutations. In some kindreds, mild forms of hypophosphatasia seem to show an autosomal dominant inheritance pattern.**

6. **There is no established medical treatment. Enzyme replacement by IV infusion of ALP from various tissue sources has generally not been of significant clinical benefit.**

7. **Prenatal diagnosis of perinatal hypophosphatasia has been successful. During the second trimester, ultrasonography, radiography, and assay of ALP activity in amniotic fluid cells have proven reliable. During the first trimester, chorionic villus samples have been used effectively for RFLP analysis as well as for quantitation of TNSALP by immunoassay and catalytic assay.**

A list of standard abbreviations is located immediately preceding the index in each volume. Additional abbreviations used in this chapter include: ALP = alkaline phosphatase; ALPL = gene mapping symbol for the TNSALP locus; CPPD = calcium pyrophosphate dihydrate; NTP-PP_i-ase = nucleoside triphosphate pyrophosphatase; PEA = phosphoethanolamine; PL = pyridoxal; PLP = pyridoxal 5′-phosphate; PTH = parathyroid hormone; TmP/GFR = tubular maximum for P_i/glomerular filtration rate; TNSALP = tissue-nonspecific (liver/bone/kidney) ALP isoenzyme.

BIOCHEMISTRY OF ALKALINE PHOSPHATASE

Alkaline phosphatase (ALP) (orthophosphoric-monoester phosphohydrolase, alkaline optimum, EC 3.1.3.1) is present in nearly all plants and animals.[1] In human beings ALPs are encoded by at least four gene loci.[2] Three isoenzymes are expressed in a tissue-specific manner—intestinal, placental, and germ-cell (placental-like) ALP. The fourth isoenzyme is ubiquitous but especially abundant in liver, bone, and kidney.[2,3] Accordingly, this "liver/bone/kidney" ALP is also called tissue-nonspecific ALP (TNSALP).[3] The distinctive physicochemical properties among the ALPs purified from liver, bone, and kidney are lost following digestion with glycosidases.[4] Thus, the various forms of TNSALP constitute a family of "secondary" isoenzymes that differ only in posttranslational modifications involving carbohydrate residues.[5]

The TNSALP gene is located near the end of the short arm of chromosome 1 (1p36.1-34)[6]; the genes for intestinal, placental, and germ-cell ALP are clustered near the tip of the long arm of chromosome 2 (2q34-37).[7] The human gene mapping symbol for the TNSALP locus is ALPL ("ALP-liver").[8] Each ALP locus has been sequenced.[9–11] The TNSALP gene is more than 50 kb and contains 12 exons, 11 of which are translated to form the 507 amino acid nascent enzyme.[2,11] The promoter region is localized within 610 nucleotides 5′ to the major transcription start site.[12] TATA and Sp1 sequences appear to be important for its function. Basal levels of TNSALP gene expression seem to reflect inherent "housekeeping" promoter activity, whereas differential gene expression in various tissues may be mediated by a posttranscriptional mechanism.[12] The tissue-specific ALP genes are much smaller primarily because of shorter introns. Amino acid profiles deduced from the human ALP cDNAs suggest positional identity of 87 percent between placental and intestinal ALP, but only 50 to 60 percent between TNSALP and the other ALP isoenzymes.[2] However, the active site of TNSALP, which is encoded by six exons, reflects base sequences that have been well conserved in ALP throughout nature.[13] TNSALP appears to be the product of the ancestral gene; the other ALP isoenzymes have arisen by a series of gene duplications.[2]

The ALPs are Zn^{2+}-metalloenzymes.[1] Catalytic activity of each isoenzyme depends on a multimeric configuration of identical monomers with molecular mass ranging from 40 to 75 kDa.[3] Each identical subunit possesses one active site and contains two Zn^{2+} molecules that stabilize its tertiary structure.[14] Catalytic activity requires Mg^{2+} as a cofactor.[1] The ALPs are generally believed to be homodimeric in the circulation.[1,3] However, ALPs may exist as homotetramers in plasma membranes.[15]

The ALP isoenzymes have broad substrate specificity and pH optimums that depend on the type and concentration of phosphocompound to be hydrolyzed.[1] Hydrolytic activity is present both for phosphoesters and for pyrophosphate.[16] Catalysis involves phosphorylation-dephosphorylation of a serine residue; dissociation of covalently linked phosphate appears to be the rate limiting step. P_i is a potent competitive inhibitor of ALP.[1,14]

Relatively little is known about the biosynthesis of ALP in higher organisms. Expression of ALP in the placenta is controlled by the fetal genome.[1] Analysis of the human ALP gene sequences indicates that each nascent polypeptide has a short signal sequence of 17 to 21 amino acids[2] and a hydrophobic domain at its C-terminus.[9–11] However, ALPs are localized primarily to the plasma membrane anchored to the polar head group of a phosphatidylinositol-glycan moiety and can be liberated by phosphatidylinositol-specific phospholipase.[15,17] The precise nature of the interaction with phosphatidylinositol may differ among the ALPs.[17]

Although lipid-free ALP is present in plasma, the mechanism of ALP release from cell surfaces is not understood. Clearance of ALP from the circulation is presumed to occur, like that of many other glycoproteins, in the liver.[18] In normal adults, most of the ALP activity in plasma reflects approximately equal amounts of TNSALP from liver and bone.[19] However, in infants and children, and particularly during the growth spurt of adolescence, blood is rich in the bone form of ALP.[1] Although some individuals (with B and O blood types and positive secretory status) increase their circulating levels of intestinal ALP after a fatty meal,[1,20] the intestinal isoenzyme usually represents just a few percent of the total serum ALP.[21] Placental ALP normally circulates only during the latter stages of pregnancy. With various malignancies, however, placental ALP or germ-cell (placental-like) ALP may be detected in the blood.[3]

PHYSIOLOGY OF SKELETAL FORMATION

The skeleton serves two important physiological functions. It acts throughout life as the framework for the body and as a reservoir for calcium, phosphate, bicarbonate, and other ions.[22,23] Skeletal development is complex and involves three processes: growth, modeling (shaping of individual bones), and remodeling (formation and resorption or "turnover" of osseous tissue).[23] Growth of the extremities occurs by endochondral bone formation until just after puberty. In the physes (growth plates) there is sequential orderly proliferation, maturation, and then degeneration of chondrocytes associated with deposition and then mineralization of extracellular matrix called "primary spongiosa."[23] Modeling occurs by resorption of selective surfaces of individual bones as they grow so that tubular structures with proper external configurations are formed. Remodeling of osseous tissue is a lifelong process and is necessary for fracture repair and is the basis for the skeleton's metabolic role.[22] Remodeling is mediated at the cell level by osteoclasts and osteoblasts that are regulated by a variety of endocrine and complex paracrine systems.[22] Osteoclasts resorb the skeleton by degrading both mineral and matrix; osteoblasts synthesize bone matrix (osteoid), which subsequently calcifies. Osteoclasts contain abundant amounts of acid phosphatase; chondrocytes and osteoblasts are rich in the bone form of TNSALP.[23]

Electron microscopic studies indicate that the earliest site of mineral deposition in the skeleton occurs within small extracellular membrane-bound structures called "matrix vesicles."[24] Matrix vesicles were first identified as buds of chondrocyte plasma membranes, but have since been found in membranous and cortical bone and in fracture callus. These vesicular structures are rich in a variety of enzymes (including TNSALP, pyrophosphatase, and ATPase) and may contain polysaccharide, phospholipid, and glycolipid among their numerous components.[25] During bone formation, spicules of hydroxyapatite are first observed within matrix vesicles. These intravesicular crystals grow and eventually rupture the membrane. Subsequently, extravesicular crystal growth continues.[24,25] Accordingly, skeletal mineralization can be described as occurring as "primary" mineralization (beginning and continuing in matrix vesicles until their disruption) and "secondary" mineralization (during which enlargement of hydroxyapatite crystals takes place in the extracellular space).[26]

Generalized impairment of skeletal mineralization in infants or children causes rickets. In adults, defective bone mineralization is manifested as osteomalacia. The important skeletal feature that distinguishes rickets from osteomalacia is the additional disturbed endochondral ossification of the growth plates.[23] Subnormal extracellular levels of calcium and/or P_i, potentially from a considerable variety of disorders (see Chaps. 100 and 124), engender nearly all forms of rickets or osteomalacia.[27] Hypophosphatasia is an interesting and instructive exception to this generalization.

PHYSIOLOGICAL ROLE OF ALKALINE PHOSPHATASE

In 1923, Robert Robison discovered that ossifying cartilage and bone from young rats and rabbits was rich in phosphatase activity. He suggested that the phosphatase conditioned skeletal mineralization by hydrolyzing some unknown phosphate ester(s) to locally increase the concentration of free P_i.[28] One year later, Robison and Soames found that this enzyme had a distinctly alkaline pH optimum.[29] Soon after its discovery, however, ALP was also noted to be abundant in tissues that do not mineralize (e.g., intestine, placenta, and a variety of fetal tissues).[1] This observation challenged a role for ALP in mineralization and suggested that it had a more universal function. Currently, the physiological roles postulated for ALP also include hydrolysis of phosphate esters to supply the nonphosphate moiety, synthesis of phosphate esters with ALP acting as a transferase, and regulation of a variety of cellular processes in which ALP acts as a phosphoprotein phosphatase.[1,30] In fact, a considerable variety of hypotheses contend for how TNSALP might function specifically in skeletal mineralization (Table 136-1).[30]

Robison's suggestion that ALP conditions skeletal mineralization by raising the concentration of P_i locally in bone tissue was challenged in part because he did not identify the enzyme's natural substrate(s). More recent studies propose that the donor source of P_i could be nucleoside phosphate that is liberated by degenerating cells.[31] An important alternative hypothesis suggests, however, that ALP functions by hydrolyzing an inhibitor of mineralization.[1,30] Indeed, the discoveries that: (1) PP_i can impair the growth of hydroxyapatite crystals,[32] (2) ALP can function as a PP_i-ase,[33] and (3) plasma levels of PP_i are increased in hypophosphatasia[34] offer a plausible candidate for this physiological inhibitor of calcification as well as an explanation for the principal clinical features of this disorder[30,35] (see below). Nevertheless, it has also been suggested that ALP might act in mineralization as: (1) a plasma membrane transport protein for P_i,[30] (2) an extracellular Ca^{2+}-binding protein that promotes calcium phosphate formation and orients its deposition into osteoid,[36] (3) a Ca^{2+}/Mg^{2+}-ATPase, or (4) a phosphoprotein phosphatase that conditions the skeletal matrix for ossification.[37]

Seventy years after its discovery, the methods used to assay ALP activity reflect our ignorance of this enzyme's physiological function(s).[1,30] In both clinical and research laboratories, ALP activity is assayed with high concentrations (m*M*) of artificial substrates (e.g., *p*-nitrophenylphosphate) at nonphysiological alkaline conditions (e.g., pH 9.2 to 10.5).[1] Understandably, however, such sensitive assays (which facilitated measurement of ALP activity in serum) were developed since they provided an extremely useful means to detect and follow the course of a variety of hepatic and skeletal disorders.[1] Nevertheless, it has been established that for certain substrates at low concentration, although the hydrolytic rate is reduced, the pH optimum of ALP is less alkaline.[1] The physiological significance of this observation has been unclear.[1,30]

In my opinion, it is characterization and study of hypophosphatasia that have best elucidated the physiological role of ALP in human beings.[30] With identification of missense mutations in the TNSALP gene in this inborn error of metabolism, there is now unequivocal evidence that TNSALP is important in mineralization of the skeleton and dentition. However, the relatively undisturbed function of other organs/tissues in hypophosphatasia poses challenging questions about the biologic significance of TNSALP elsewhere in the body.[30]

Table 136-1 Suggested Roles for ALP in Skeletal Mineralization[30]

1. Locally increase P_i levels
2. Destruction of inhibitor of hydroxyapatite crystal growth
3. Transport of P_i
4. Ca^{2+}-binding protein
5. Ca^{2+}/Mg^{2+} ATPase
6. Tyrosine-specific phosphoprotein phosphatase

HYPOPHOSPHATASIA

History

J. C. Rathbun, a Canadian pediatrician, coined the term *hypophosphatasia* in 1948 when he described an infant boy who developed and then died from severe rickets, weight loss, and seizures, yet whose ALP activity in serum, bone, and elsewhere was paradoxically subnormal.[38] Several early historical reviews mention case reports that probably referred to this entity decades earlier.[39,40] In 1953, premature loss of deciduous teeth in addition to defective skeletal mineralization was noted to be a major clinical feature.[41] About 300 patients have been described.

The metabolic basis for hypophosphatasia and the physiological role of TNSALP have been clarified by the discoveries of elevated endogenous levels of three phosphocompounds in this disorder (Fig. 136-1). In 1955, increased urinary levels of phosphoethanolamine (PEA)[42,43] provided a useful biochemical marker. In 1965 and 1971, high levels of PP_i were noted in urine[44] and in blood,[34] respectively, suggesting a mechanism for the defective mineralization of hard tissues. In 1985, elevated plasma levels of pyridoxal 5′-phosphate (PLP) were found—an observation that was consistent with an ectoenzyme function for TNSALP[45] (see below).

Clinical Features

Hypophosphatasia occurs throughout the world and apparently in all races. However, the disorder is especially prevalent in inbred Mennonite families from Manitoba, Canada, where 1 in 2500 newborns manifests severe disease and about 1 in 25 individuals is a carrier.[46] The incidence of severe forms in Toronto, Canada, has been estimated to be 1 per 100,000 live births.[40] Despite the presence of relatively high levels of TNSALP in bone, liver, kidney, and adrenal tissue (and at least some TNSALP elsewhere throughout the body) in normal subjects, the clinical consequences of hypophosphatasia involve predominantly the skeleton and dentition. However, the severity of clinical expression is remarkably variable and ranges from death in utero to merely premature loss of dentition in adult life.[40,47–50] Some individuals with characteristic biochemical abnormalities may never become symptomatic.[48,49] Although within sibships hypophosphatasia generally breeds true, variable clinical expression can occur in this setting as well.[48,49,51,52]

Since the gene defects are currently being uncovered for hypophosphatasia (see below),[13] there is promise for a precise genetic nosology in the near future. Nevertheless,

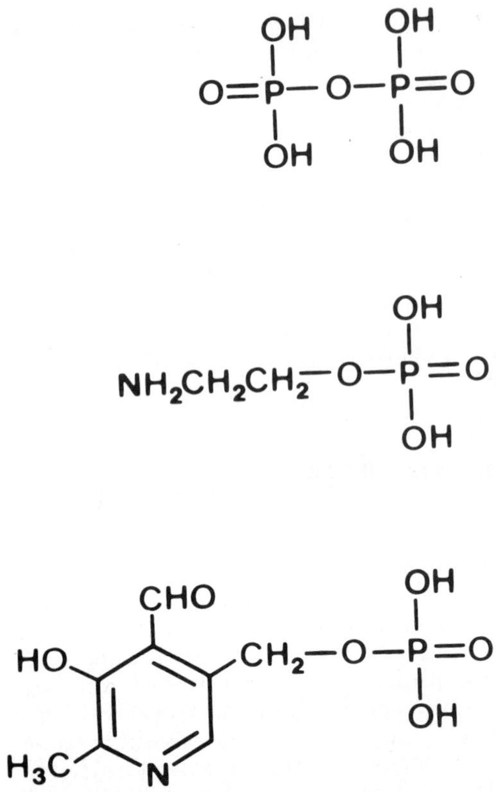

FIG. 136-1 **Natural substrates for TNSALP. Three phosphocompounds appear to be natural substrates for TNSALP, since each accumulates endogenously in hypophosphatasia: PP_i, phosphoethanolamine (PEA), and pyridoxal 5′-phosphate (PLP).**

the classification of patients for prognostication, recurrence risk estimates, and so on currently remains a clinical one. Several schemes have been proposed that attempt to deal with the remarkably variable expression.[40,47] Six clinical forms have now been identified. The age at which lesions in bone are discovered distinguishes the perinatal (lethal), infantile, childhood, and adult forms.[40,50] Subjects who have only dental manifestations are regarded as having "odontohypophosphatasia." The especially rare variant called "pseudohypophosphatasia" in all ways resembles infantile hypophosphatasia, except that serum ALP activity is not reduced (discussed below). The prognoses for these six conditions depend on the severity of the skeletal disease, which, in turn, correlates with the age at presentation. The earlier a patient becomes symptomatic, the more severe the disorder.[42] Although this clinical nosology is useful, one should bear in mind that there is variability within each clinical form and that they do not unambiguously distinguish all patients.

Perinatal (Lethal) Hypophosphatasia. Perinatal hypophosphatasia is the most severe form. It is expressed in utero and can result in stillbirth. The pregnancy may be complicated by polyhydramnios. Caput membraneceum and limbs that are shortened and deformed from profound skeletal hypomineralization are noted at birth. Unusual osteochondral spurs may protrude through the skin from the midportion of the forearms and legs.[53,54] Some affected neonates live a few days, but then suffer increasing respiratory compromise from rachitic disease of the chest and from hypoplastic lungs.[55] Clinical findings include failure to gain weight and often a high-pitched cry, irritability, periodic apnea with cyanosis and bradycardia, unexplained fever, myelophthisic anemia (perhaps from encroachment on the marrow space by excess osteoid), intracranial hemorrhage, and idiopathic seizures.[47,50]

Radiographic survey of the skeleton enables perinatal hypophosphatasia to be readily distinguished from even the most severe types of osteogenesis imperfecta and congenital dwarfism. Indeed, the radiologic changes may be considered diagnostic.[53] Nevertheless, the findings are diverse and there is marked patient-to-patient variability.[54] In some cases, the skeleton appears to be almost completely unmineralized. In others, there is marked bony undermineralization and severe rachitic changes, in which irregular extensions of growth plate cartilage and unmineralized osteoid protrude into the metaphyses from poorly ossified epiphyses. Separate diaphyseal defects may occur as well. There can be absence of ossification of individual bones. Fractures are often present. The membranous bones of the cranium may show mineralization only at their centers, so that the areas of unossified calvarium give the illusion that the sutures are widely separated, although they are functionally closed (Fig. 136-2).[53] Other unusual features include parts of or entire vertebrae that appear to be missing and spurs that protrude laterally from the midshaft of the ulnae and fibulae.[56] The teeth are poorly formed.[54]

Infantile Hypophosphatasia. Infantile hypophosphatasia presents before 6 months of age.[40] Postnatal development often seems normal until the onset of poor feeding, inadequate weight gain, and clinical features of rickets. The cranial sutures are wide. The osseous defects in the skull often constitute a "functional" craniosynostosis. True premature fusion of the cranial sutures may occur if the patient survives infancy.[53] There may be raised intracranial pressure, with bulging of the anterior fontanelle, papilledema, proptosis, mild hypertelorism, and brachycephaly. Blue sclerae have been noted.[57] A flail chest from rachitic deformity, fractures, etc. may predispose the patient to pneumonia. Hypercalcemia and hypercalciuria are common and can cause recurrent vomiting, nephrocalcinosis, and renal compromise.[40,58,59]

The radiologic features are characteristic and severe and can resemble those of the perinatal form, although they are somewhat less marked.[53] In some newly diagnosed patients, one sees a rather abrupt transition from a relatively normal-appearing diaphysis to an uncalcified metaphysis. This finding is of interest because it suggests that a metabolic change suddenly occurred.[40] Sequential radiologic studies may disclose both the persistent defective skeletal mineralization typical of rickets, and gradual demineralization of osseous tissue as well.[59] Skeletal scintigraphy can help demonstrate premature closure of cranial sutures, since these structures exhibit decreased tracer uptake, although they may appear "widened" on conventional radiography.[60]

Childhood Hypophosphatasia. Childhood hypophosphatasia is also highly variable in its clinical expression.[40,58,61] Premature loss of deciduous teeth (i.e., earlier than 5 years of age) occurs from aplasia, hypoplasia, or dysplasia of dental cementum,[62,63] with only minimal tooth root resorption. Dental radiography may show enlarged pulp chambers and root canals ("shell teeth"). The incisors are frequently lost first, but occasionally, nearly the entire dentition is disturbed. Alveolar bone attrition, especially in the anterior mandible, may occur from lack of mechanical stimulation, since defects in the cementum prevent periodontal ligaments from properly connecting the teeth to the jaw.[64]

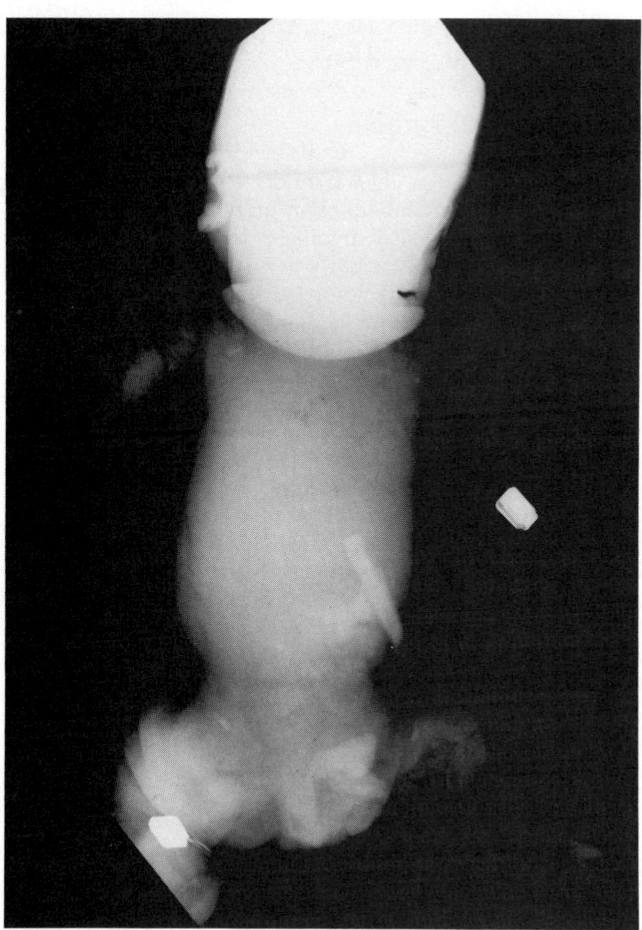

FIG. 136-2 Perinatal hypophosphatasia. Radiologic study of a stillborn with severe hypophosphatasia reveals profound skeletal hypomineralization—a finding that enables the perinatal (lethal) form to be readily distinguished from other congenital bone disorders.

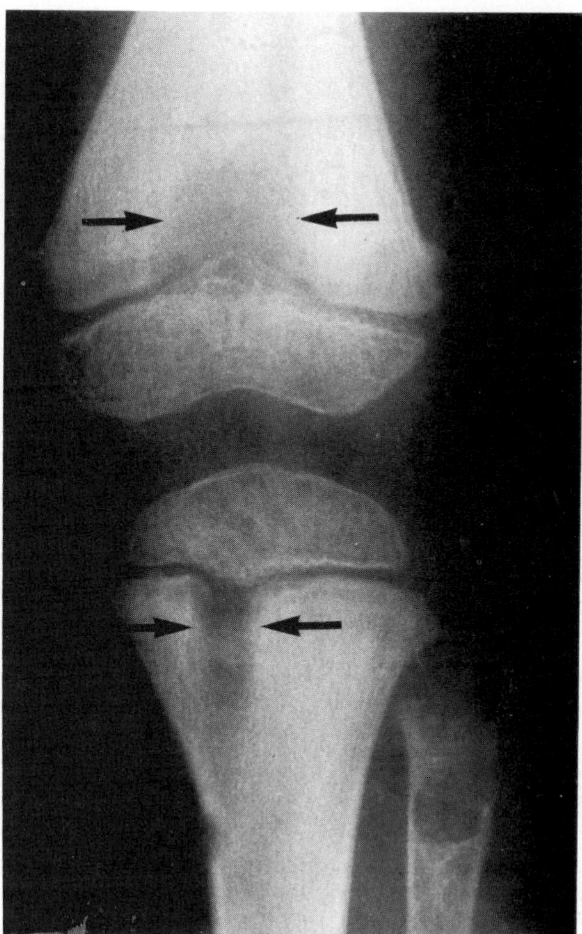

FIG. 136-3 Childhood hypophosphatasia. Posteroanterior radiograph of the knee of a 5-year-old boy with hypophosphatasia reveals growth plates that are not greatly widened, but defective endochondral bone formation is revealed by irregular radiolucencies (arrows) that project into the metaphyses. This finding is characteristic of the childhood form of hypophosphatasia.

Rickets often causes short stature, delayed walking, and a characteristic waddling gait.[40,58] Rachitic deformities include beading of the costochondral junctions; either bowed legs or knock-knees; enlargement of the wrists, knees, and ankles from flared metaphyses; and occasionally a dolichocephalic skull with frontal bossing. Patients may complain of pain and stiffness and exhibit extremity muscle weakness (especially in the proximal lower limbs) consistent with a nonprogressive myopathy.[65]

Radiography of the metaphyseal regions of long bones usually reveals characteristic focal bony defects—"tongues" of radiolucency that project from the rachitic growth plate into the metaphysis (Fig. 136-3). This feature, if present, distinguishes hypophosphatasia from other forms of rickets and metaphyseal dysplasias.[53] Epiphyseal centers of ossification may be well preserved. Functional synostosis of cranial sutures can occur in affected infants and young children despite widely "open" fontanelles and hypomineralized areas of calvarium. Later, true premature bony fusion of cranial sutures may cause raised intracranial pressure, proptosis, and brain damage. The skull may then have a "beaten-copper" appearance on radiologic study.

Adult Hypophosphatasia. Adult hypophosphatasia usually presents during middle age.[48,49] Not infrequently, however, patients recall a history of rickets and premature exfoliation of deciduous teeth that is then followed by relatively good health during adolescence and young adult life. Subsequently, osteomalacia may cause pain in the feet from recurrent, poorly healing metatarsal stress fractures and discomfort in the thighs or hips from femoral pseudofractures (Fig. 136-4). Early loss or extraction of the secondary dentition is not uncommon.[48,49,66] Calcium pyrophosphate dihydrate (CPPD) deposition, occasionally with overt attacks of arthritis (pseudogout), occurs in some patients, apparently in part from the increased endogenous levels of PP_i (see below).[49,67] Affected individuals may be troubled by degeneration of articular cartilage and pyrophosphate arthropathy. Patients appear to be predisposed to primary hyperparathyroidism (personal observation). Screening may reveal symptomatic or asymptomatic kindred members.[48,49] In some families with hypophosphatasemia there is periarticular calcium phosphate deposition that manifests clinically with "calcific periarthritis" and with ossification of ligaments (syndesmophytes) resembling spinal hyperostosis (Forrestier disease).[68,69] It has been suggested that these individuals have a mild form of hypophosphatasia.[68]

Radiologic study may show pseudofractures (Looser zones), a hallmark of defective bone mineralization. Inexplicably, they occur most often in the lateral cortexes of the proximal femora, rather than medially as in most other types of osteomalacia.[70] There may also be osteopenia,

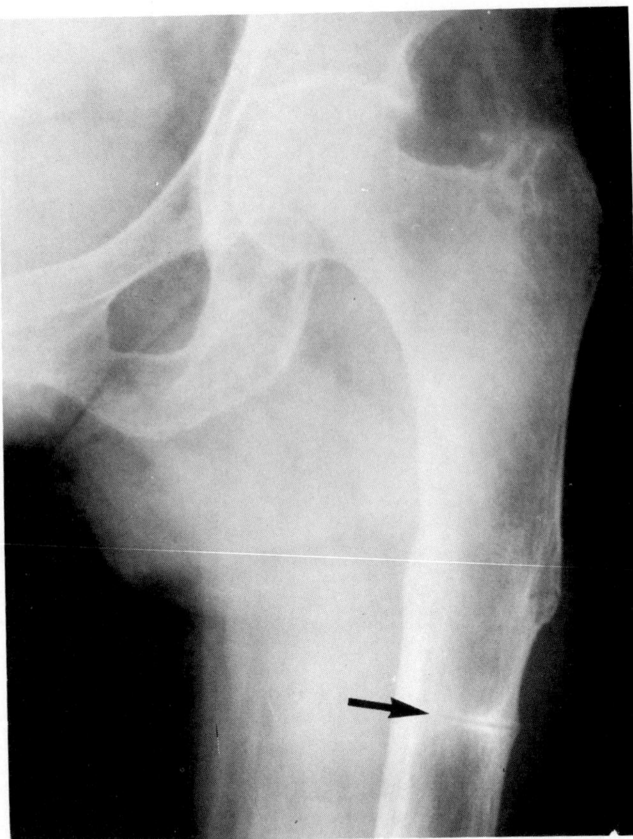

FIG. 136-4 Adult hypophosphatasia. The femur of a middle-aged woman reveals a pseudofracture (Looser zone) that has been unhealed for several years (arrow). These cortical bone defects characteristically form on the lateral aspect of the femur in adult hypophosphatasia, rather than medially as in most other forms of osteomalacia.

chondrocalcinosis, changes of pyrophosphate arthropathy, and perhaps calcific periarthritis.[49,68,69]

Odontohypophosphatasia. Odontohypophosphatasia is present when the only clinical abnormality is dental disease and radiographic studies or even bone biopsy show no sign of rickets or osteomalacia. Odontohypophosphatasia may explain some cases of "early-onset periodontitis,"[71] although hereditary leukocyte abnormalities and other factors usually account for this condition.

Pseudohypophosphatasia. Pseudohypophosphatasia is a particularly interesting but especially rare form of hypophosphatasia. It has been documented convincingly in two infants.[72,73] In this unusual hypophosphatasia variant the clinical, radiologic, and other biochemical findings are typical of subjects who have infantile hypophosphatasia, yet serum total ALP activity is consistently normal or increased.[72,73] The enzymatic defect appears to involve a mutant TNSALP that retains its catalytic activity under the artificial assay conditions of the clinical laboratory, but is inactive at physiological pH toward the natural substrates PEA, PP_i, and PLP, which then accumulate endogenously (see below).[74,75] Some reports of pseudohypophosphatasia are not very convincing[76–78] and appear to describe individuals with hypophosphatasia for whom there has been transient normalization of serum ALP activity, misinterpretation of reference ranges for serum ALP, and/or overemphasis on the significance of a raised urinary PEA level (see below).

Laboratory Diagnosis

Biochemical Findings. ***ALP Activity.*** Hypophosphatasia can be diagnosed with confidence in individuals with a typical clinical history, physical findings, and radiologic changes in whom serum ALP activity is clearly and consistently subnormal. In general, the more severe the disease the lower the serum ALP activity level appropriate for age (Fig. 136-5). Even subjects with odontohypophosphatasia can be distinguished from controls by their low serum ALP activity. In perinatal and infantile hypophosphatasia, hypophosphatasemia is present in cord blood at birth.[58,79] Indeed, in forms of rickets or osteomalacia other than hypophosphatasia, serum ALP activity is typically increased. Nevertheless, a variety of diagnostic pitfalls must be avoided. First, blood specimens must be obtained correctly.[80] Chelation of Mg^{2+} or Zn^{2+} by EDTA, etc. in collection tubes will destroy ALP activity.[1] Second, concerning the interpretation of the serum ALP level, one must recognize that it normally varies according to age and sex; for example, infants and children have considerably higher ALP levels (due to a relative

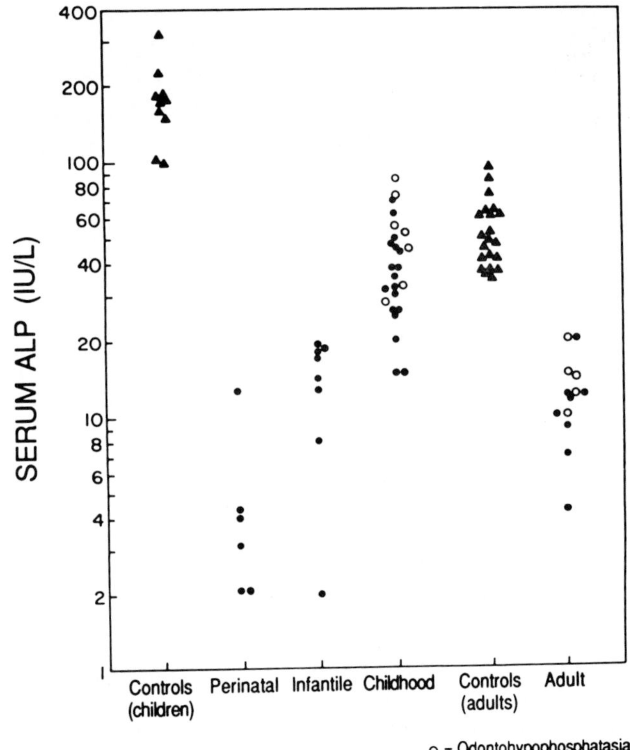

FIG. 136-5 Serum ALP activity in hypophosphatasia. ALP activity in serum in normal children and normal adults (▲) and in 52 subjects (•, ○) from 47 families with the various clinical forms of hypophosphatasia. Note the logarithmic scale. All assays were performed at the Metabolic Research Unit, Shriners Hospital for Crippled Children, St. Louis.

abundance of the bone form of TNSALP) as compared with adults. The level is especially high during the growth spurt of adolescence, which occurs earlier in girls than in boys.[1] Since the reference range for serum ALP activity provided by many clinical laboratories is only appropriate for adults, some infants or children with hypophosphatasia are mistakenly judged to have normal serum ALP activity or perhaps "pseudohypophosphatasia" if the higher pediatric reference range is not considered. Third, hypophosphatasemia may be caused by a variety of conditions (hypothyroidism, starvation, scurvy, severe anemia, celiac disease, Wilson disease, hypomagnesemia, Zn^{2+} deficiency) and drugs (glucocorticoids, chemotherapy, clofibrate, intoxication levels of vitamin D, milk-alkali syndrome), as well as exposure to radioactive heavy metals or massive transfusion of blood or plasma.[80,81] However, each of these clinical situations should be readily apparent. Especially rare cases of lethal osteogenesis imperfecta may have low serum ALP activity.[82] Finally, a few case reports of hypophosphatasia describe transient increases in serum ALP activity (probably the bone form of TNSALP) after fracture or orthopedic surgery.[48] Conditions that increase circulating activity of any form of ALP (e.g., pregnancy, liver disease) could mask the diagnosis.[58,83] Accordingly, in puzzling cases, documentation that serum ALP activity is low on more than one occasion during clinical stability seems advisable. Quantitation of ALP isoenzyme forms may also be helpful.[21]

The precise nature of the residual ALP in blood in the various clinical forms of hypophosphatasia requires further study. Leukocyte ALP activity, first noted to be absent in an adult with hypophosphatasia,[84] reflects a type of TNSALP and can be subnormal in any clinical form of the disease except perhaps pseudohypophosphatasia.[61] In serum, study of one kindred with adult hypophosphatasia using ALP isoenzyme-specific stereoinhibitors revealed that hypophosphatasemic subjects consistently showed a reduction of bone form of TNSALP and often had reduced levels of the liver form as well.[19] In a preliminary report, immunoreactive levels of both bone and liver TNSALP were found to be low in serum in all clinical forms of hypophosphatasia except pseudohypophosphatasia.[85] Furthermore, there appears to be some variation in the physicochemical and immunologic properties of the ALP in the serum of infants with severe forms of the disease.[86]

Minerals. In contrast to most types of rickets or osteomalacia, neither serum calcium nor P_i levels are low in hypophosphatasia. In fact, hypercalciuria and hypercalcemia occur frequently in infantile hypophosphatasia.[40,47,50] In childhood hypophosphatasia, severely affected patients occasionally have hypercalciuria without hypercalcemia. The pathogenesis of the calcium disturbance appears to involve defective uptake of mineral by a poorly growing skeleton. Circulating levels of the bioactive forms of vitamin D (25-hydroxyvitamin D and 1,25-dihydroxyvitamin D) and parathyroid hormone (PTH) are usually unremarkable.[87,88] Several patients have been reported to have elevated serum PTH levels,[89] but renal compromise from hypercalcemia with retention of immunoreactive fragments of the hormone may explain this finding in the severe cases. Low circulating levels of PTH, reflecting the possibility of an abnormality in the Ca^{2+}-PTH feedback system, have also been reported.[90] Subjects with the childhood and adult forms of hypophosphatasia have serum P_i levels that are above the mean value for controls, and approximately 50 percent of cases are distinctly hyperphosphatemic. Enhanced renal reclamation of P_i (increased tubular maximum for P_i/glomerular filtration rate; i.e., TmP/GFR) accounts for this finding.[91] Conversely, especially rare patients with hypophosphatasia have been reported who have hypophosphatemia from renal P_i wasting.[92,93]

Routine Biochemical Studies. Other standard laboratory tests, including serum parameters of liver or muscle function (e.g., bilirubin, aspartate aminotransferase, lactate dehydrogenase, creatine kinase, aldolase), are generally unremarkable in all forms of hypophosphatasia. Increased levels of proline in blood and urine have been reported in a few affected subjects, but the significance of this observation is not known.[94] Acid phosphatase activity in serum is generally normal,[95] but was consistently elevated in one affected woman.[96]

PEA. Documentation of increased urinary PEA levels supports a diagnosis of hypophosphatasia[97] but is not pathognomonic. Phosphoethanolaminuria has also been noted in a variety of other disorders, including several metabolic bone diseases.[98] Ideally a 24-h collection is assayed. PEA levels should always be "normalized" to creatinine content prior to interpretation. It is important for diagnosing mild cases to recognize that PEA levels are somewhat influenced by patient age, depend on diet, follow a circadian rhythm, and have been described as normal in several mildly affected individuals.[47,99] The following normal ranges have been reported: less than 15 years, 83 to 222; 15 to 30 years, 42 to 146; 31 to 41 years, 38 to 155; and over 45 years, 48 to 93 (expressed as micromoles of PEA per gram of creatinine).[98]

PLP. An increased plasma level of PLP is a sensitive and specific marker for hypophosphatasia[45,74,100] (Fig. 136-6). Even patients with odontohypophosphatasia demonstrate this biochemical feature.[45] However, to exclude false positive findings, vitamin supplements must not be taken for a week before testing.[100] In general, the more severely affected the patient, the greater the elevation in the plasma PLP level. Nevertheless, overlap occurs among the clinical types. Assay of plasma PLP levels after oral challenge with pyridoxine distinguishes patients especially well[30] and has proven helpful in identifying Canadian Mennonite carriers of severe hypophosphatasia.[101]

PP_i. Assay of PP_i in urine remains a research technique. Levels are increased in most patients, but are occasionally unremarkable in more mildly affected subjects.[35] Assay of urinary PP_i levels has been reported to be a sensitive means for carrier detection.[102]

Radiologic Findings. Radiologic studies of the skeleton are typically diagnostic in perinatal hypophosphatasia. In the other clinical forms, except odontohypophosphatasia, characteristic features are usually demonstrated (see above).

Histopathological Findings. As reviewed below, histopathological abnormalities in hypophosphatasia are observed primarily in the hard tissues. In severe cases, hypoplastic lungs have been found and extramedullary hematopoiesis is occasionally noted in the liver.[26,61]

Skeleton. In all but the mildest cases of hypophosphatasia,[48] nondecalcified sections of bone reveal evidence of defective mineralization of the skeleton.[26,61] However, features of secondary hyperparathyroidism engendered by hypocal-

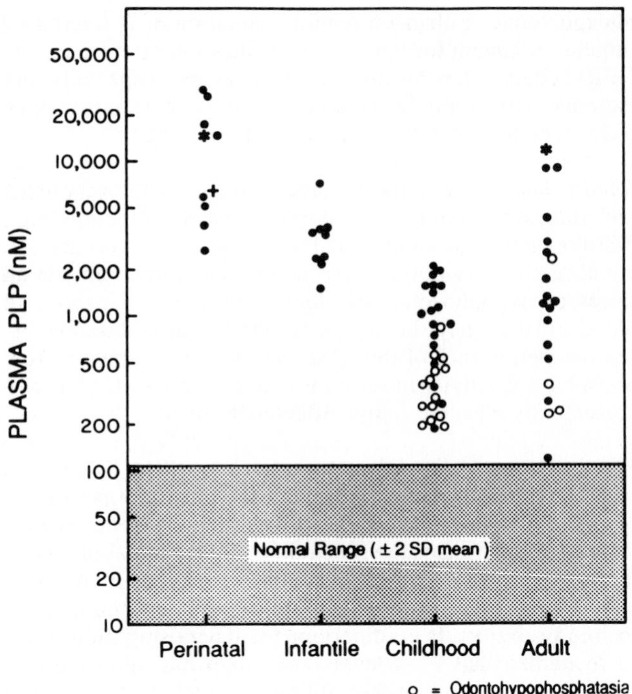

FIG. 136-6 Plasma PLP levels in hypophosphatasia. PLP levels in plasma in various clinical forms of hypophosphatasia (hatched area is the normal range for children and adults). Elevated levels have been found in all 71 affected subjects (representing 60 families). In general, the plasma PLP level reflects the disease severity. Note the logarithmic scale with some overlap among clinical forms. ***(Assays performed courtesy of Dr. Stephen P. Coburn, Fort Wayne State Developmental Center, Fort Wayne, IN.)***

cemia, as occur in many other types of rickets or osteomalacia, are generally absent.

In growth plates, characteristic rachitic changes are present. There is disruption of the normal columnar arrangement of chondrocytes, zones of provisional calcification are widened, and degenerating cartilage fails to calcify. The cellular sources of the bone form of TNSALP (chondrocytes and osteoblasts) as well as their matrix vesicles are present, but have reduced levels of TNSALP activity.[26,61]

In osseous tissue, excessive amounts of unmineralized skeletal matrix are observed because osteoid cannot calcify properly. Cranial "sutures" that are widened are not fibrous tissue, but uncalcified osteoid.[40] Woven bone, a finding that can reflect either bone repair or defective skeletal formation, may be present.[61] Impaired skeletal mineralization can be confirmed if brief courses of a tetracycline are given orally prior to bone biopsy, since fluorescence microscopy will fail to show characteristic fluorescent bands at bone surfaces where mineralization should normally occur. The magnitude of the mineralization defect generally reflects the clinical severity.[61] In lethal cases, even the bony structures of the middle ear can be poorly ossified.[103]

Unless histochemical studies of ALP activity are performed, the histopathological changes of hypophosphatasia in the skeleton cannot be distinguished from those of most other forms of rickets or osteomalacia.[61] However, the numbers and morphology of osteoblasts and osteoclasts, as well as the appearance of unmineralized osteoid, vary somewhat from case to case. The level of ALP activity in bone tissue reflects the degree of osteoid accumulation throughout the skeleton.[61] Some questionable cases reported as pseudohypophosphatasia (with normal serum ALP activity, skeletal symptoms, dental caries, elevated urinary PEA levels, and reportedly excessive amounts of osteoid in bone specimens) lack this important information from tetracycline labeling.[104]

Electron microscopy of cases of perinatal hypophosphatasia has shown normal distribution of proteoglycan granules, collagen fibers, and matrix vesicles in the extracellular space of cartilage.[26,61] However, the matrix vesicles are deficient in ALP activity and reportedly do not contain hydroxyapatite crystals. Instead, only isolated or tiny groups of crystals (calcospherites), frequently not associated with matrix vesicles, have been observed.[26,54]

Dentition. Premature loss of deciduous teeth occurs in a variety of conditions (including toxicities, metabolic errors, malignancies, and primary dental disease).[64] In hypophosphatasia, the paucity of cementum that engenders this complication is due to aplasia, hypoplasia, or dysplasia despite the presence of cells that look like cementoblasts (Fig. 136-7).[63,64,105] Cementum that is present may be afibrillar.[106] The severity of the defect varies from tooth to tooth, but generally reflects the seriousness of the skeletal disease. Incisors are usually the most notably affected. Dessicated teeth that were exfoliated years earlier may still be useful for examination. Big pulp chambers suggest retarded dentinogenesis. Dentin tubules may be enlarged though reduced in number. The excessive width of predentin, increased amounts of interglobular dentin, and impaired calcification of cementum are analogous to the excess osteoid observed in bone. The enamel is not directly affected.[63,105] The histopathological changes found in the permanent teeth appear to be similar to those in the deciduous teeth.[106]

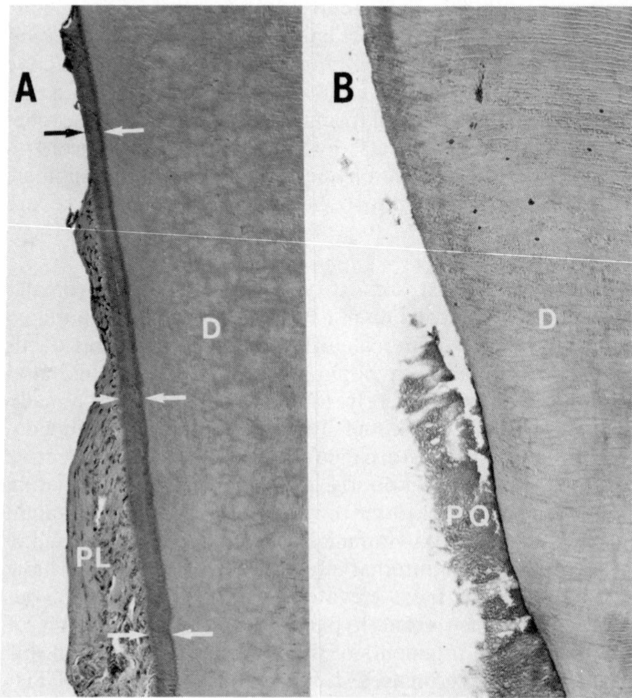

FIG. 136-7 Dental findings in hypophosphatasia. *A*. Decalcified section of part of the root of a maxillary incisor from a child with X-linked hypophosphatemic rickets is essentially normal and shows primary cementum (delineated by arrows) at the surface. *B*. In hypophosphatasia, cementum is absent. Magnification ×150. PL = periodontal ligament; PQ = plaque; D = dentin.

Biochemical and Genetic Defect. ***TNSALP Deficiency.*** Early on, autopsy studies of subjects with the perinatal and infantile forms of hypophosphatasia were important not only for clarifying the enzymatic defect for this disorder, but also for suggesting the genetic basis. Profound deficiency of ALP activity was documented in liver, bone, and kidney, but ALP activity was found not to be decreased in intestine or placenta (fetal trophoblast).[107,108] This observation was consistent with results from amino acid sequence analysis of ALP purified from various normal human tissues,[3] and indicated that the severe forms of hypophosphatasia resulted from a defect(s) that selectively diminishes the enzymatic activity of all of the secondary isoenzymes of the TNSALP family.

Investigations of the cardinal biochemical feature, hypophosphatasemia, have been consistent with, and amplify, the autopsy studies. There is deficient activity of both the liver and the bone form of TNSALP in serum.[19] Furthermore, a variety of evidence indicates that the hypophosphatasemia is not due to enhanced loss of TNSALP from the circulation.[48,109] The bone form of TNSALP (contained in plasma from patients with Paget bone disease) and purified placental ALP have essentially unremarkable circulating half-lives when given intravenously to severely affected infants in attempted enzyme-replacement therapy (see below).[59] Furthermore, coincubation experiments with mixtures of serum (as well as cell coculture and heterokaryon studies with fibroblasts from severely affected patients) do not suggest the presence of an inhibitor or absence of an activator of TNSALP.[40,48,67,110] Instead, the hypophosphatasemia of severe hypophosphatasia appears to reflect failure of especially liver and bone tissue to contribute adequate amounts of TNSALP activity into the circulation.

Autopsy studies of children or adults with hypophosphatasia have not been reported. However, general observations suggest that these clinically milder forms are also due to a defect that globally diminishes TNSALP activity within tissues. In adult hypophosphatasia, activity of both the liver and the bone forms of TNSALP can be decreased in serum.[19] Furthermore, in affected children and adults, TNSALP activity can be deficient in circulating granulocytes,[61] in bone tissue, [61] and in cultivated skin fibroblasts.[111]

Preliminary observations using a polyclonal antibody to the liver form of TNSALP indicate that tissues from severely affected subjects with hypophosphatasia can contain normal amounts of immunoreactive TNSALP.[112,113] However, a monoclonal antibody–based assay demonstrated low immunoreactive levels of the bone and liver forms of ALP in serum from patients with all clinical forms of the disease except pseudohypophosphatasia.[85] This assay measured only polymeric TNSALP.

Some ALP activity is detectable by sensitive methods in liver, bone, kidney, and skin fibroblasts in culture from infants with hypophosphatasia.[114,115] The ALP in patient fibroblasts generally has different physicochemical properties as compared with controls.[114] In one case of infantile hypophosphatasia, enzyme inhibition and isoelectric focusing studies suggested that the small amount of ALP activity detected in these organs was intestinal ALP.[108] This observation was interpreted to reflect compensatory expression of an intestinal ALP gene. Indeed, studies of homogenates of small-bowel mucosa obtained by biopsy from a family with a clinically mild childhood/adult form,[116] and at autopsy from severely affected subjects,[115] showed increased amounts of intestinal ALP. However, fibroblasts in culture from severely affected patients seem to produce low ALP activity with physicochemical properties that are primarily TNSALP-like[114] but differ from patient to patient.[86] The precise nature of the disruptive effect of TNSALP gene mutations (see below) on tissue as well as circulating TNSALP requires clarification.

Inheritance. The first evidence that hypophosphatasia was a heritable disorder came when affected sibs were reported in 1950. Early on, family studies of severely affected infants or children indicated that hypophosphatasia was transmitted as an autosomal recessive trait.[39,40,77,78,117–119] The parents of such children often demonstrated low or low-normal levels of serum ALP activity, and PEA was detectable in their urine.[39,40] Consanguinity was reported in some kindreds.

The inheritance pattern for the milder forms of hypophosphatasia has, however, remained less clear. In some reports, the childhood and adult forms of hypophosphatasia, as well as odontohypophosphatasia, have been regarded as autosomal recessive conditions.[117] Indeed, clinical expression tends to run true to form in affected sibs in all forms of the disorder, and vertical transmission of clinically apparent disease seems to be unusual.[48,49] Nevertheless, multigeneration occurrence of clinical and biochemical abnormalities has suggested that mild disease can be transmitted as an autosomal dominant trait.[48,49,120–122] Rarely, family studies are also consistent with mildly affected patients being heterozygotes for a defect that caused severe disease in their homozygous offspring.[48,122,123]

Unfortunately, it has generally been difficult to identify carriers for hypophosphatasia. It may be necessary to quantitate several biochemical parameters including urinary PP_i.[124] Pyridoxine loading followed by assay of plasma PLP levels has been shown to help in heterozygote detection among the Mennonite population in Canada.[101]

Gene Defects. Chromosomal defects have rarely been reported in hypophosphatasia. A D/D translocation was found in one adult patient, but was not present in other affected family members, and this common aberration was presumably unrelated to the disorder.[67]

Phenylketonuria has been noted in one infant with hypophosphatasemia, phosphoethanolaminuria, and generalized skeletal demineralization.[125] Morquio syndrome together with hypophosphatasia has occurred in a Canadian Hutterite kindred.[126] These patients, however, appeared to reflect the coincidental occurrence of two autosomal recessive conditions.[126]

A preliminary report of genetic complementation studies, using skin fibroblasts from individuals with perinatal or infantile hypophosphatasia, described failure to correct TNSALP activity and therefore suggested that the defect in 10 families was at the same gene locus.[110]

Some cases of hypophosphatasia may be due to a regulatory defect in the biosynthesis of TNSALP. In one boy with infantile hypophosphatasia, after a series of IV infusions of pooled normal plasma in attempted enzyme replacement therapy, a 4-month correction of hypophosphatasemia was seen due to skeletal synthesis of the bone form of TNSALP.[127] Remarkable remineralization of osseous tissue occurred during this time. This observation could not be attributed to the infused ALP, since it had a circulating half-life of just several days.[127]

Regulation of TNSALP biosynthesis may affect disease expression in other ways. Subjects with the childhood form of hypophosphatasia usually have higher serum levels of ALP activity than adult-onset cases, yet as a group overt bone disease develops earlier (see Fig. 136-5). Physiological decreases in their serum (skeletal) ALP levels during the adult years might engender clinical reexpression of the condition during adult life. However, it is noteworthy that the degree of hypophosphatasemia (relative to the serum ALP level that is normal for age) is basically similar in affected children and adults and perhaps helps to explain the "overlap" encountered in defining these two clinical forms of hypophosphatasia (see below).

Sequence analysis of the four genes for the human ALPs[2] and definition of the three-dimensional structure of *Escherichia coli* ALP by x-ray crystallography[14] have underpinned considerable recent progress in our understanding of the genetic basis for hypophosphatasia.[13,128] As summarized below, the gene defects that cause hypophosphatasia are now being revealed.

In 1987, genetic linkage of the Rh blood group to severe hypophosphatasia in six inbred Mennonite kindreds from Manitoba, Canada, provided strong supporting evidence that severe forms of the disease could result from a defect within the "candidate" TNSALP gene.[129]

In 1988, proof that hypophosphatasia can derive from a TNSALP gene abnormality came with the discovery of a missense mutation in exon 6 of the TNSALP gene in a patient with perinatal hypophosphatasia born to second cousins from Nova Scotia.[130] The patient was homozygous and both parents heterozygous for a single base transition that caused a threonine-for-alanine substitution at amino acid position 162. Site-directed mutagenesis and transfection analysis of the patient's TNSALP showed that the mutation diminished the enzyme's catalytic activity, perhaps by altering the spatial relationship of metal ligands to an important arginine residue at the catalytic pocket.[130] However, blotting studies using oligonucleotide probes failed to show this mutation in the leukocyte DNA in any of 34 additional patients who reflected all clinical forms of hypophosphatasia.[130]

In 1992, sequence analysis of the TNSALP cDNAs of four additional unrelated subjects with perinatal or infantile hypophosphatasia revealed a different missense mutation in exons of each of the eight TNSALP alleles examined.[128] Screening of leukocyte DNA from 50 unrelated patients with all clinical forms of hypophosphatasia disclosed 23 individuals who had one of these mutations but in whom the nature of the other TNSALP allele was not known. Furthermore, two sibs with typical childhood hypophosphatasia and one unrelated elderly woman with classic adult hypophosphatasia were found to be compound heterozygotes for the same two TNSALP missense mutations. This observation showed that mild forms of hypophosphatasia can indeed be transmitted as an autosomal recessive trait.[128]

In 1993, homozygosity for a tenth TNSALP missense mutation was found to account for severe hypophosphatasia with a high incidence in Canadian Mennonites,[46] presumably explained by a founder effect and inbreeding.

Thus, it has now been demonstrated that all clinical forms of hypophosphatasia, except perhaps pseudohypophosphatasia, can result from TNSALP missense mutations. Nevertheless, the precise genetic basis for most cases remains to be uncovered. Each of the ten TNSALP missense mutations identified in hypophosphatasia to date alters an amino acid residue that is conserved in all mammalian TNSALPs.[13] Indeed, several of these amino acid residues are conserved even among bacteria. The three-dimensional structure of *E. coli*[13,14] ALP suggests that some of the base substitutions would engender disturbed metal ligand binding in the mature enzyme, but how the other mutations are deleterious remains to be understood.[13]

Treatment. ***Medical.*** There is no established medical therapy for hypophosphatasia, although a variety of treatments have been studied.[40,48,89,127] Assessment of any attempted regimen is made difficult by the variable clinical course among patients. In some affected subjects there is progressive skeletal demineralization[59]; in others, there is spontaneous improvement.[131]

Traditional therapies for rickets and osteomalacia (vitamin D and mineral supplements) might best be avoided, since circulating levels of calcium, P_i, and the vitamin D metabolites are not reduced. Indeed, in infantile cases, excess vitamin D could promote intestinal absorption of calcium without enhancing skeletal formation and thus cause a predisposition to or exacerbation of hypercalcemia and hypercalciuria. However, complete restriction of vitamin D intake or exposure to sunshine should be guarded against, since superimposed vitamin D–deficiency rickets has occurred.[88] Hypercalcemia in infantile hypophosphatasia can be corrected by glucocorticoid therapy and/or restriction of dietary calcium.[58] However, progressive skeletal demineralization may follow.[59,132]

In theory, therapy with agents that could stimulate TNSALP biosynthesis or enhance its activity might be helpful for hypophosphatasia. Administration of cortisone to a few patients with severe disease was reportedly followed by periods of normalization of serum ALP activity and radiologic improvement,[40,133,134] but this has not been a consistent finding.[40] Brief treatments with zinc, magnesium, and an active fragment of PTH to stimulate ALP activity have been unsuccessful.[48,127] In other metabolic bone diseases, sodium fluoride will enhance osteoblast function and increase the activity of the bone form of TNSALP in serum.[135] However, an excessive amount of this compound can itself impair skeletal mineralization, and fluoride has not been rigorously tested in hypophosphatasia.

If extracellular accumulation of PP_i is a key pathogenetic factor in hypophosphatasia (see below), reduction in endogenous PP_i levels might enable skeletal mineralization to proceed normally.[30,35] The initial attempt to achieve this outcome by using oral P_i supplementation to promote renal PP_i excretion reportedly met with some radiologic success.[136] However, in later studies, plasma PP_i levels were found not to be changed significantly by this treatment. Indeed, increased urinary PP_i levels after P_i is administered orally may merely reflect enhanced renal PP_i synthesis.[35] This therapeutic approach has been repeated, but its efficacy has not been confirmed.[44,107]

Enzyme replacement therapy has been attempted by IV infusion of several types of ALP. The results have generally been disappointing. Serum from a patient with Paget bone disease given to one infant was associated with radiologic improvement.[137] However, subsequent trials of this therapy showed no significant clinical or radiologic benefit for four subjects affected with the infantile form.[132] IV infusions weekly of fresh normal plasma were followed by clinical and radiographic improvement in one patient.[138] Furthermore, infusions of plasma that had been frozen and then pooled were followed by well-documented correction of hypophosphatasemia and marked temporary clinical, radiographic, and histologic improvement in another subject with the infantile form (see above).[127] However, a subsequent trial of pooled plasma infusions in a different patient did not produce this response.[115] Most recently, following a brief report that suggested IV administration of ALP purified from liver improved the histologic appearance of bone and decreased urinary PEA levels in an infant with hypophosphatasia,[139] a vigorous attempt to treat infantile hypophosphatasia was conducted with IV infusion of purified placental ALP. Doses that caused hyperphosphatasemia, nevertheless, resulted in only modest decrements of plasma PLP and urinary PEA concentrations and no change in urinary PP_i levels and were not associated with clinical or radiologic improvement.[140] These cumulative observations may merely reflect the fact that tissue levels of ALP are higher than those achieved in the circulation by these treatments. Alternatively, they are consistent with a requirement for ALP to be present *in situ* to act physiologically.[140] In this regard, it should be recalled that extreme skeletal disease occurs in perinatal hypophosphatasia in which the in utero environment is clearly not protective.

Supportive. Affected infants and young children should be followed carefully for increased intracranial pressure from either "functional" or true premature cranial synostosis. As discussed, functional synostosis (that may require craniotomy) can occur despite the radiologic appearance of open fontanelles.[53]

Fractures in children do mend, although delayed healing after femoral osteotomy with casting has been reported.[141] In adult patients pseudofractures may remain stable for years, but will not heal unless they first progress to completion, or are treated orthopedically.[48] Use of intramedullary rods rather than load-sparing devices (e.g., plates) is best for the prophylactic or acute orthopedic management of femoral fractures and pseudofractures.[70] For recurrent metatarsal stress fractures, ankle-foot orthoses are useful.

Expert dental care is important for affected children and adults. Defective dentition can impair nutrition in severely affected children, and efforts to preserve teeth in position or use of complete or partial dentures may be necessary.[62,63] One study indicated that proliferation of bacteria at the tooth surface, perhaps related to deficiency of TNSALP activity in leukocytes, may contribute to loss of dentition.[106]

Symptoms from CPPD or perhaps periarticular calcium phosphate crystal deposition may respond to nonsteroidal antiinflammatory agents.[68]

Prognosis. Perinatal (lethal) hypophosphatasia is a fatal condition. Although survival may be prolonged with intensive life support, I am unaware of any case with significant longevity. Infantile hypophosphatasia can have a somewhat variable clinical course. There may be an interval of deterioration followed by improvement. However, at least 50 percent of patients die from respiratory compromise and pneumonia that follows worsening skeletal involvement of the chest.[40] The prognosis improves after infancy. Indeed, preliminary reports from Canada suggest that, in their patient population, the adult stature of patients who survive infantile hypophosphatasia may be normal (though I am aware of significant exceptions in the United States). Childhood hypophosphatasia may also spontaneously improve during adolescence,[40] but recurrence of symptoms in adulthood is possible, if not likely.[40,48,142] Adult hypophosphatasia causes chronic orthopedic problems after the onset of skeletal symptomatology.[48,49,70] Worsening osteomalacia, leading to osteopenia and fractures, seems to occur in women at menopause, but was not prevented by estrogen replacement therapy in two cases (personal observation).

Prenatal Diagnosis. Assay of total ALP activity in amniotic fluid is not helpful.[143] Indeed, at 14 to 18 weeks of gestation, most is intestinal ALP excreted from the fetus.[144] Measurement of α-fetoprotein in amniotic fluid, however, can help to differentiate anencephaly from severe hypophosphatasia.

The perinatal (lethal) form of hypophosphatasia has proven to be reliably diagnosable in utero.[79] During the first trimester, chorionic villus samples from 15 pregnancies have been asssessed successfully with a monoclonal antibody–based assay specific for TNSALP catalytic activity.[145,146] Accurate measurement of TNSALP activity requires a precisely timed and carefully prepared chorionic villus sample.[145,147] RFLP analysis, using a chorionic villus sample, has been used successfully for a Canadian Mennonite[148] and for a Japanese family.[149] During the second trimester, perinatal hypophosphatasia has been diagnosed with ultrasonography (with attention to the limbs as well as the skull),[150] radiologic study of the fetus, and assay of ALP activity in amniotic fluid cells by an experienced laboratory.[151] An ultrasound study, however, was judged to be normal at 16 to 19 weeks of gestation in three cases of the perinatal hypophosphatasia in which radiographic study at 38 weeks of gestation showed absence of a fetal skeleton.[152,153] Thus, combined use of these techniques, including serial ultrasonography, is regarded as most reliable. The utility of assaying cord blood ALP is uncertain.

Mild forms of hypophosphatasia have not been accurately diagnosed prenatally. I am aware of two children with mild disease who reportedly had normal ultrasonography in early pregnancy. Conversely, severe bowing of the lower extremities detected by ultrasound, suggestive of a potentially lethal form of skeletal dysplasia, occurred in three pregnancies in two families in whom the deformity corrected spontaneously after birth and the clinical phenotype was otherwise that of childhood hypophosphatasia.[154,155]

PHYSIOLOGICAL ROLE OF TISSUE-NONSPECIFIC ALKALINE PHOSPHATASE EXPLORED IN HYPOPHOSPHATASIA

Demonstration that missense mutations within the TNSALP gene can deactivate this enzyme and cause hypophosphatasia[130] proves that Robert Robison was correct[28,29]—that is, TNSALP functions importantly in mineralization of the skeleton (and indeed also in formation of the teeth).[30] Although the finding will require confirmation and further study (Anderson HC: personal communication), "primary mineralization" of bone appears to be disturbed in severely affected subjects, since some hydroxyapatite crystals are found in specimens of osseous tissue but not within matrix vesicles.[26] The defects in dentin and cementum in teeth appear to be analogous to those in the skeleton.[64]

Although the liver, kidneys, and adrenals are normally rich in TNSALP activity,[1] dysfunction of these organs does not appear to be a feature of hypophosphatasia (see above). It has been suggested that TNSALP deficiency might disturb the biosynthesis of the phospholipid surfactant and predispose severely affected infants to recurrent pulmonary atelectasis.[58] However, as discussed, the respiratory problems of such patients likely reflect rib cage deformities, hypoplastic lungs, etc. Although a variety of studies have suggested that TNSALP may function in cell growth and differentiation, cultivated TNSALP-deficient infantile hypophosphatasia dermal fibroblasts have been shown to grow normally.[156] Accordingly, TNSALP may have little importance except for hard tissues.[30]

Several roles for TNSALP in calcification have been proposed that could be deranged in hypophosphatasia (see Table 136-1). As reviewed below, the discovery that PEA, PLP, and PP_i accumulate endogenously, and are inferred therefore to be natural substrates for TNSALP, has been important for understanding the physiological role of TNSALP.

Phosphoethanolamine

The discovery that PEA levels are increased in urine in hypophosphatasia provided both a useful biochemical marker for this inborn error of metabolism and the first evidence from this disorder for a natural substrate for TNSALP.[42,43,97] Detailed studies of renal handling of PEA in normal subjects and in patients with hypophosphatasia showed that this phosphocompound is excreted when plasma levels are scarcely detectable; that is, there appears to be essentially no renal threshold for PEA.[97] Although its metabolic origin is unclear, PEA is thought not to be a derivative of phosphatidylethanolamine—i.e., from plasma membrane phospholipid degradation. The major source of circulating PEA has been reported to be the liver,[157] which also degrades PEA to ammonia, acetaldehyde, and P_i in a reaction that is catalyzed by *O*-phosphorylethanolamine phospholyase. Indeed, this enzyme requires PLP as a cofactor and it has been proposed that pseudohypophosphatasia might result from its deficiency.[158] In one family with adult hypophosphatasia,[19] urinary levels of PEA were found to correlate inversely with the activity in serum of the liver form of TNSALP (but not the bone) in the hypophosphatasemic adults. More recently, PEA has been found to be a constituent of the phosphatidylinositol-glycan linkage apparatus. Thus, the extracellular source of PEA could be the degradation of this anchor for cell-surface proteins.

Pyridoxal 5′-Phosphate

Discovery that plasma levels of PLP are increased in hypophosphatasia helped to clarify the physiological role of this enzyme.[45] As reviewed in Fig. 136-8, a variety of dietary forms of vitamin B_6 (including pyridoxine, pyridoxal, and pyridoxamine and their phosphorylated derivatives) are converted in the liver[159] to PLP, a cofactor form of vitamin B_6. Organ ablation studies show that the liver is the major source of PLP in the plasma. Apparently, PLP is primarily secreted from the liver into plasma coupled to albumin.[159] Some additional PLP in plasma is bound to various enzymes. Thus, only a small amount of PLP circulates freely. Like many phosphorylated compounds, however, free PLP cannot traverse plasma membranes and must first be dephosphorylated to pyridoxal (PL) before it can enter tissues. After PL crosses plasma membranes, it is rephosphorylated to PLP or converted to pyridoxamine 5′-phosphate, both of which act intracellularly as cofactors for a variety of enzymatic reactions. Ultimately, vitamin B_6 is degraded to 4-pyridoxic acid, primarily in the liver, and is then excreted into the urine.[159]

Increases in the plasma levels of PLP in hypophosphatasia suggest that TNSALP acts in the dephosphorylation of PLP.[45,100] In disorders in which serum levels of liver and bone TNSALP are increased by organ-specific increments in TNSALP activity (e.g., other skeletal and hepatic diseases), plasma PLP levels are decreased.[100,160]

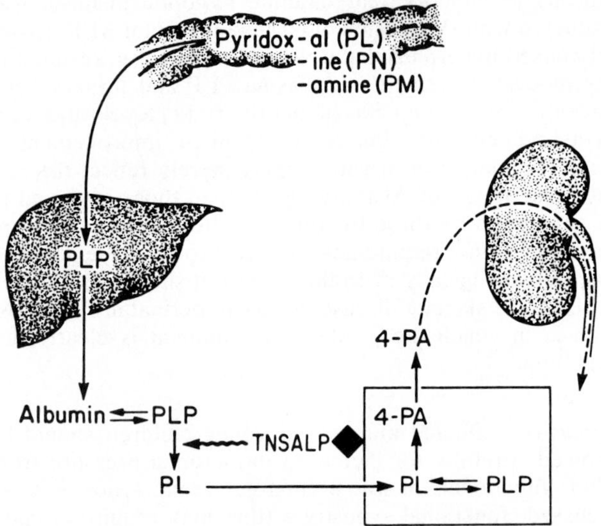

FIG. 136-8 Role of TNSALP in vitamin B_6 metabolism. The various vitameric forms of vitamin B_6 in the diet are dephosphorylated, if necessary, in the gut and then absorbed into the hepatic portal circulation. In the liver, they are each converted to PLP, which is secreted bound to albumin into the plasma. Before entering tissues, plasma PLP must be dephosphorylated to PL, which can traverse membranes. 4-Pyridoxic acid (4-PA), the major degradation product of vitamin B_6, is excreted in the urine. High plasma levels of PLP in hypophosphatasia, yet normal plasma concentrations of pyridoxal (PL), are consistent with an ectoenzyme role for TNSALP in the extracellular dephosphorylation of PLP to PL.

Since plasma membranes are impermeable to PLP, the increased levels of PLP in plasma in hypophosphatasia appear to result from failure of PLP hydrolysis extracellularly. Accordingly, plasma membrane-bound TNSALP would seem to function as an ectoenzyme.[45,100] Consonant with this hypothesis is the clinical observation that individuals with hypophosphatasia do not have symptoms of vitamin B_6 deficiency or toxicity. Dermatitis, stomatitis, peripheral neuritis, depression, or anemia—clinical hallmarks of vitamin B_6 deficiency[161]—are not present. Similarly, peripheral neuropathy, a sign of vitamin B_6 toxicity,[161] is not a feature of hypophosphatasia. Biochemical observations also indicate that intracellular levels of vitamin B_6 are normal in hypophosphatasia. Urinary concentrations of 4-pyridoxic acid were unremarkable in all of four subjects examined with the childhood form of the disease.[45] Children with hypophosphatasia respond normally during a conventional L-tryptophan loading test for vitamin B_6 deficiency (Whyte MP and Coburn SP: unpublished observation). Levels of PLP and total vitamin B_6 in homogenates of TNSALP-deficient fibroblasts obtained from subjects with infantile hypophosphatasia are the same as those from controls.[160] Finally, a study of tissues obtained at autopsy from three perinatal cases, in which plasma PLP concentrations were elevated 50 to 900 times, revealed levels of PLP, PL, and total forms of vitamin B_6 that were essentially normal.[115]

Although vitamin B_6 deficiency has been associated with renal stone disease and epilepsy, these problems in patients with hypophosphatasia appear to be explained by other factors. Nephrocalcinosis in infants with hypophosphatasia is likely due to hypercalciuria. However, the possibility of altered oxalate metabolism (a consequence of vitamin B_6 deficiency) has not been studied.[159] The epilepsy of severely affected subjects may be related to cranial deformity, hemorrhage, periodic apnea, etc. Additionally, PEA was found to be epileptogenic when given intravenously to one such infant during a study of PEA metabolism.[162] In two patients with perinatal hypophosphatasia and epilepsy, who had plasma PL levels below assay sensitivity, administration of vitamin B_6 did not correct the seizure disorder[115] (personal observation).

Since TNSALP appears to be the phosphatase that dephosphorylates PLP to PL in the extracellular space, PL in the circulation could be low in hypophosphatasia. However, subjects with hypophosphatasia usually have normal or somewhat elevated plasma PL levels.[30,45] In all forms of hypophosphatasia, there seems to be sufficient extracellular dephosphorylation of PLP to PL by some mechanism to account for the normal vitamin B_6 status.

The clinical and biochemical observations concerning vitamin B_6 status in hypophosphatasia indicate an ectoenzyme role for TNSALP.[30,100] Characterization of TNSALP as a plasma membrane-bound glycoprotein,[4] covalently linked to the polar head group of phosphatidylinositol,[15,17,163] is consistent with this conclusion. In fact, studies using cultivated dermal fibroblasts from patients with infantile hypophosphatasia[164] and human osteosarcoma cells[165] show that TNSALP is plasma membrane–associated with ectotopography and capable of dephosphorylating PLP and PEA both at natural substrate concentrations and physiological culture system pH.

Inorganic Pyrophosphate

Discovery that PP_i levels are increased in the urine[44] and plasma[34] in hypophosphatasia suggested a mechanism for the associated disorders of calcium crystal deposition and defective skeletal mineralization.[34,35]

At low concentrations, PP_i has been reported to enhance the precipitation of calcium and P_i from solution to form amorphous calcium phosphate.[35] Calcific periarthritis might then be an expected result.[68]

ALP has been shown to dissolve CPPD crystals in vitro.[16] This pyrophosphatase activity seems to be unrelated to its capacity to hydrolyze phosphoesters. Thus, CPPD deposition leading to chondrocalcinosis, pseudogout, and pyrophosphate arthropathy[49] would be explained by failure of TNSALP both to hydrolyze PP_i and to destroy CPPD crystals.[16]

At high concentrations, however, it is well established that PP_i will adsorb to amorphous calcium phosphate and prevent transformation to hydroxyapatite.[34] Additionally, adsorption of PP_i to hydroxyapatite crystals will impair their growth and dissolution.[32,35] The effect of PP_i accumulation to inhibit these processes, either within or surrounding matrix vesicles, would be expressed as rickets or osteomalacia.

Studies using cultivated TNSALP-deficient fibroblasts from perinatal and infantile hypophosphatasia patients demonstrate that generation of PP_i by these cells from ATP extracellularly is normal.[166] The level of nucleoside triphosphate pyrophosphatase (NTP-PP_i-ase) activity in such fibroblasts is unremarkable, and this enzyme therefore appears to be different from TNSALP. Clearance studies of $^{32}PP_i$ administered to adults with hypophosphatasia indicate that the endogenous accumulation of PP_i results from defective degradation rather than increased biosynthesis.[35]

Circulating Tissue-Nonspecific Alkaline Phosphatase

A variety of evidence suggests that circulating ALP is physiologically inactive.[30] Infants with hypophosphatasia who received IV infusions of plasma from patients with Paget bone disease,[132] or who were given purified placental ALP[140] (so that normal or even elevated serum ALP levels were achieved, respectively), demonstrated no clinical or radiologic improvement. Furthermore, such therapy failed to reduce substantially the urinary PEA or PP_i levels or plasma PLP concentrations.[59,140] Accordingly, deficiency of TNSALP activity in the skeleton itself appears to account for the rickets and osteomalacia of hypophosphatasia. Interestingly, Fraser and Yendt reported in 1955 that rachitic rat cartilage would calcify in serum obtained from an infant with hypophosphatasia, yet slices of the patient's costochondral junction would not mineralize in synthetic calcifying medium or in the pooled serum of healthy children.[167]

A MODEL FOR TISSUE-NONSPECIFIC ALKALINE PHOSPHATASE FUNCTION

Observations from hypophosphatasia can be formulated into an overview of how TNSALP might function physiologically (Fig. 136-9). Increased endogenous levels of PEA, PP_i, and PLP in this disorder indicate that TNSALP is catalytically active toward a variety of substrates with fairly variable chemical structure (see Fig. 136-1).

Clinical and biochemical investigations of vitamin B_6 metabolism in hypophosphatasia, supported by cell culture studies, reveal that TNSALP is an ectoenzyme. Extracellular

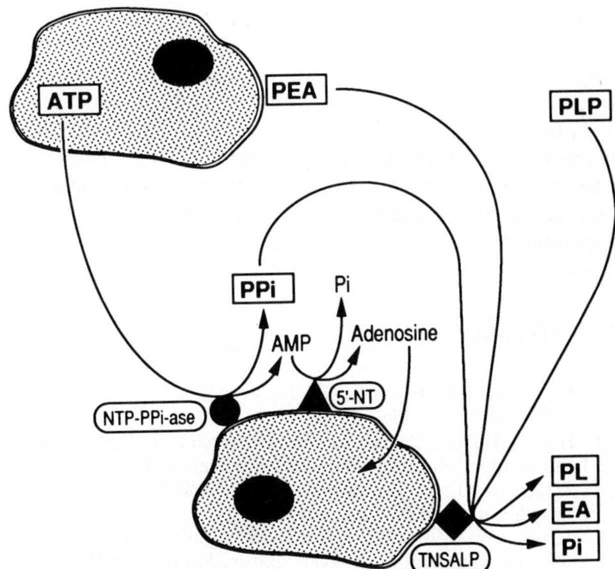

FIG. 136-9 **Metabolic basis for hypophosphatasia (hypothesis). Extracellular generation of PP_i, presumably by the action of NTP-PP_i-ase, is normal in hypophosphatasia, but extracellular degradation of PP_i, PLP, and PEA is diminished because of deficient ecto-TNSALP activity. Accumulation of PP_i extracellularly accounts for the CPPD and perhaps calcium phosphate crystal deposition as well as rickets/osteomalacia.**

accumulation of PEA, PP_i, and PLP in hypophosphatasia is a consequence of deficient ecto-TNSALP activity. The source of accumulated PEA is unclear, but it might be due to defective degradation of PEA released during the metabolism of the phosphatidylinositol moiety that anchors a variety of ectoproteins. Accumulation of membrane-impermeable PLP in plasma, but not in tissues, explains the absence of vitamin B_6 deficiency or toxicity. Generation of extracellular PP_i, perhaps from ATP, occurs normally in hypophosphatasia by the intact action of NTP-PP_i-ase. PP_i accumulation reflects instead decreased degradation by deficient ecto-TNSALP activity. Since these three phosphocompounds are normally present in extracellular fluid at nanomolar or micromolar concentrations, TNSALP acts at substrate concentrations that are much lower than those used in routine clinical assays for ALP.[165] Furthermore, it is clear that TNSALP must be active at physiological pH. Accordingly, the term *alkaline phosphatase* would appear to be a misnomer.

In hypophosphatasia, calcium phosphate crystal deposition causes calcific periarthritis and CPPD precipitation results in chondrocalcinosis and/or pyrophosphate arthropathy. Calcific periarthritis reflects the effect of PP_i at low concentrations to stimulate calcium phosphate formation. Chondrocalcinosis and pyrophosphate arthropathy occur from PP_i accumulation and failure of TNSALP to hydrolyze CPPD crystals. Rickets and osteomalacia develop in hypophosphatasia from extracellular accumulation of PP_i at sites of mineralization, since at high concentrations PP_i is an inhibitor of hydroxyapatite crystal growth. TNSALP appears to be physiologically active in tissues, but not in the circulation.

ADDENDUM

Recently, Fedde and coworkers showed by two-dimensional gel electrophoresis that fibroblasts profoundly deficient in TNSALP activity (from patients with severe forms of hypophosphatasia) appear to have unremarkable profiles of plasma membrane-associated phosphoproteins.[168] This observation suggests that TNSALP does not act as a phosphoprotein phosphatase in cell plasma membranes. ALPs are being increasingly investigated for domains in their amino acid sequences that predict binding to other proteins (including types I, II, and X collagen) and could help orient TNSALP in skeletal matrix for mineral deposition.[169]

REFERENCES

1. McComb RB, Bowers GN Jr, Posen S: *Alkaline Phosphatase.* New York, Plenum, 1979.
2. Harris H: The human alkaline phosphatases: What we know and what we don't know. *Clin Chim Acta* **186**:133, 1989.
3. Stigbrand T, Fishman WH: *Human Alkaline Phosphatases.* New York, Alan R. Liss, 1984.
4. Moss DW, Whitaker KB: Modification of alkaline phosphatases by treatment with glycosidases. *Enzyme* **34**:212, 1985.
5. Harris H: *The Principles Of Human Biochemical Genetics,* 3rd ed. Amsterdam, Elsevier/North Holland, 1980.
6. Smith M, Weiss MJ, Griffin CA, Murray JC, Buetow KH, Emanuel BS, Henthorn PS, Harris H: Regional assignment of the gene for human liver/bone/kidney alkaline phosphatase to human chromosome 1p36.1-p34. *Genomics* **2**:139, 1988.
7. Griffin CA, Smith M, Henthorn PS, Harris H, Weiss MJ, Raducha M, Emanuel BS: Human placental and intestinal alkaline phosphatase genes map to 2q34-q37. *Am J Hum Genet* **41**:1025, 1987.
8. Human gene mapping. *Cytogenet Cell Genet* **40**:1–4, 1986.
9. Berger J, Garattini E, Hua J-C, Udenfriend S: Cloning and sequencing of human intestinal alkaline phosphatase cDNA. *Proc Natl Acad Sci USA* **84**:695, 1987.
10. Henthorn PS, Raducha M, Edwards YH, Weiss MJ, Slaughter C, Lafferty MA, Harris H: Nucleotide and amino acid sequences of human intestinal alkaline phosphatase: Close homology to placental alkaline phosphatase. *Proc Natl Acad Sci USA* **84**:1234, 1987.
11. Weiss MJ, Ray K, Henthorn PS, Lamb B, Kadesch T, Harris H: Structure of the human liver/bone/kidney alkaline phosphatase gene. *Proc Natl Acad Sci USA* **263**:12002, 1988.
12. Kiledjian M, Kadesch T: Analysis of the human liver/bone/kidney alkaline phosphatase promoter in vivo and in vitro. *Nucleic Acids Res* **18**:957, 1990.
13. Henthorn PS, Whyte MP: Missense mutations of the tissue nonspecific alkaline phosphatase gene in hypophosphatasia. *Clin Chem* **38**:2501, 1992.
14. Kim EE, Wyckoff HW: Reaction mechanisms of alkaline phosphatase based on crystal structures. *J Mol Biol* **218**:449, 1991.
15. Hawrylak K, Stinson RA: Tetrameric alkaline phosphatase from human liver is converted to dimers by phosphatidylinositol phospholipase C. *FEBS Lett* **212**:289, 1987.
16. Xu Y, Cruz TF, Pritzker KP: Alkaline phosphatase dissolves calcium pyrophosphate dihydrate crystals. *J Rheumatol* **18**:1606, 1991.
17. Seetharam B, Tiruppathi C, Alpers DH: Hydrophobic interactions of brush border alkaline phosphatases: The role of phosphatidyl inositol. *Arch Biochem Biophys* **253**:189, 1987.
18. Young GP, Rose IS, Cropper S, Seetharam S, Alpers DH: Hepatic clearance of rat plasma intestinal alkaline phosphatase. *Am J Physiol* **247**:G419, 1984.
19. Millán JL, Whyte MP, Avioli LV, Fishman WH: Hypophosphatasia (adult form): Quantitation of serum alkaline phosphatase isoenzyme activity in a large kindred. *Clin Chem* **26**:840, 1980.
20. Langman MJS, Leuthold E, Robson EB, Harris J, Luffman JE, Harris H: Influence of diet on "intestinal" component of serum alkaline phosphatase in people of different ABO blood groups and secretory status. *Nature* **212**:41, 1966.
21. Mulivor RA, Boccelli D, Harris H: Quantitative analysis of alkaline phosphatases in serum and amniotic fluid: Comparison of biochemical and immunologic assays. *J Lab Clin Med* **105**:342, 1985.
22. Raisz LG, Kream BE: Regulation of bone formation. *N Engl J Med* **309**:29 & 83, 1983.
23. Williams PL, Warwick R, Dyson M, Bannister LH (eds): *Gray's Anatomy,* 37th ed. Edinburgh, Churchill Livingstone, 1989.
24. Ali SY: *Cell Mediated Calcification and Matrix Vesicles.* New York, Elsevier, 1986.
25. Anderson HC: Introduction and summary. (5th International Conference on Cell Mediated Calcification and Matrix Vesicles.) *Bone Miner* **17**:107, 1992.
26. Ornoy A, Adomian GE, Rimoin DL: Histologic and ultrastructural studies on the mineralization process in hypophosphatasia. *Am J Med Genet* **22**:743, 1985.
27. Glorieux FH (ed): *Rickets.* New York, Raven, 1991.
28. Robison R: The possible significance of hexosephosphoric esters in ossification. *Biochem J* **17**:286, 1923.
29. Robison R, Soames KM: The possible significance of hexosephosphoric esters in ossification. II. The phosphoric esterase of ossifying cartilage. *Biochem J* **18**:740, 1924.
30. Whyte MP: Alkaline phosphatase: Physiologic role explored in hypophosphatasia, in Peck WA (ed): *Bone and Mineral Research.* Amsterdam, Elsevier, 1989, vol 6, pp 175–218.
31. Majeska RJ, Wuthier RE: Studies on matrix vesicles isolated from chick epiphyseal cartilage. Association of pyrophosphatase and ATP-ase activities with alkaline phosphatase. *Biochim Biophys Acta* **391**:51, 1975.
32. Fleisch H, Russell RGG, Straumann F: Effect of pyrophosphate on hydroxyapatite and its implications in calcium homeostasis. *Nature* **212**:901, 1966.
33. Moss DW, Eaton RH, Smith JK, Whitby LG: Association

of inorganic pyrophosphatase activity with human alkaline phosphatase preparations. *Biochem J* **102**:53, 1967.

34. Russell RGG, Bisaz S, Donath A, Morgan DB, Fleisch H: Inorganic pyrophosphate in plasma in normal persons and in patients with hypophosphatasia, osteogenesis imperfecta, and other disorders of bone. *J Clin Invest* **50**:961, 1971.
35. Caswell AM, Whyte MP, Russell RGG: Hypophosphatasia and the extracellular metabolism of inorganic pyrophosphate: Clinical and laboratory aspects. *Crit Rev Clin Lab Sci* **28**:175, 1991.
36. DeBernard B, Bianco P, Bonucci E, Costantini M, Lunazzi GC, Martinuzzi P, Modricky C, Moro L, Panfili E, Pollesello P, Stagni N, Vittor F: Biochemical and immunohistochemical evidence that in cartilage an alkaline phosphatase is a Ca^{2+}-binding glycoprotein. *J Cell Biol* **103**:1615, 1986.
37. Lau KH, Farley JR, Baylink DJ: Phosphotyrosyl-specific protein phosphatase activity of a bovine skeletal acid phosphatase isoenzyme. Comparison with the phosphotyrosyl protein phosphatase activity of skeletal alkaline phosphatase. *J Biol Chem* **260**:4653, 1985.
38. Rathbun JC: Hypophosphatasia, a new developmental anomaly. *Am J Dis Child* **75**:822, 1948.
39. Currarino G, Neuhauser E, Reyersback G, Sobel E: Hypophosphatasia. *Am J Roentgenol* **78**:392, 1957.
40. Fraser D: Hypophosphatasia. *Am J Med* **22**:730, 1957.
41. Sobel EH, Clark LC, Fox RP, Robinow M: Rickets, deficiency of "alkaline" phosphatase activity and premature loss of teeth in childhood. *Pediatrics* **11**:309, 1953.
42. Fraser D, Yendt ER, Christie FHE: Metabolic abnormalities in hypophosphatasia. *Lancet* **1**:286, 1955.
43. McCance RA, Morrison AB, Dent CE: The excretion of phosphoethanolamine and hypophosphatasia. *Lancet* **1**:131, 1955.
44. Russell RGG: Excretion of inorganic pyrophosphate in hypophosphatasia. *Lancet* **2**:461, 1965.
45. Whyte MP, Mahuren JD, Vrabel LA, Coburn SP: Markedly increased circulating pyridoxal 5′-phosphate concentrations in hypophosphatasia (alkaline phosphatase acts in vitamin B_6 metabolism). *J Clin Invest* **76**:752, 1985.
46. Greenberg CR, Taylor CLD, Haworth JC, Seargeant LE, Philipps S, Triggsraine B, Chodirker BN: A homoallelic $Gly^{317} \rightarrow$ Asp mutation in ALPL causes the perinatal (lethal) form of hypophosphatasia in Canadian Mennonites. *Genomics* **17**:215, 1993.
47. Taillard F, Desbois JC, Delepine N, Gretillat F, Allaneau C, Herrault A: L'hypophosphatasie affection polymorphe de frequence peut-être sous estimee. *Med Inf (Lond)* **91**:559, 1984.
48. Whyte MP, Teitelbaum SL, Murphy WA, Bergfeld M, Avioli LV: Adult hypophosphatasia: Clinical, laboratory, and genetic investigation of a large kindred with review of the literature. *Medicine (Baltimore)* **58**:329, 1979.
49. Whyte MP, Fallon MD, Murphy WA: Adult hypophosphatasia with chondrocalcinosis and arthropathy: Variable penetrance of hypophosphatasemia in a large Oklahoma kindred. *Am J Med* **72**:631, 1982.
50. Terheggen HG, Wischermann A: Congenital hypophosphatasia. *Monatsschr Kinderheilkd* **132**:512, 1984.
51. Moore CA, Ward JC, Rivas MC, Magill HL, Whyte MP: Infantile hypophosphatasia: Autosomal recessive transmission to two related sibships. *Am J Med Genet* **36**:15, 1990.
52. Macfarlane JD, Kroon HM, van der Harten JJ: Phenotypically dissimilar hypophosphatasia in two sibships. *Am J Med Genet* **42**:117, 1992.
53. Kozlowski K, Sutcliffe J, Barylak A, Harrington G, Kemperdick H, Nolte K, Rheinwein H, Thomas PS, Uniecka W: Hypophosphatasia: Review of 24 cases. *Pediatr Radiol* **5**:103, 1976.
54. Shohat M, Rimoin DL, Gruber HE, Lachman RS: Perinatal lethal hypophosphatasia; Clinical radiologic and morphologic findings. *Pediatr Radiol* **21**:421, 1991.
55. Silver MM, Vilos GA, Milne KJ: Pulmonary hypoplasia in neonatal hypophosphatasia. *Pediatr Pathol* **8**:483, 1988.
56. Whyte MP: Spur-limbed dwarfism in hypophosphatasia (letter). *Dysmorphol Clin Genet* **2**:126, 1988.
57. Brenner RL, Smith JL, Cleveland WW, Bejar RL, Lockhart WS: Eye signs in hypophosphatasia. *Arch Ophthalmol* **81**:614, 1969.
58. Teree TM, Klein L: Hypophosphatasia: Clinical and metabolic studies. *J Pediatr* **72**:41, 1968.
59. Whyte MP, Valdes R Jr, Ryan LM, McAlister WH: Infantile hypophosphatasia: Enzyme replacement therapy by intravenous infusion of alkaline phosphatase-rich plasma from patients with Paget's bone disease. *J Pediatr* **101**:379, 1982.
60. Sty JR, Boedecker RA, Babbitt DP: Skull scintigraphy in infantile hypophosphatasia. *J Nucl Med* **20**:305, 1979.
61. Fallon MD, Teitelbaum SL, Weinstein RS, Goldfischer S, Brown DM, Whyte MP: Hypophosphatasia: Clinicopathologic comparison of the infantile, childhood, and adult forms. *Medicine (Baltimore)* **63**:12, 1984.
62. Kjellman M, Oldfelt V, Nordenram A, Olow-Nordenram M: Five cases of hypophosphatasia with dental findings. *Int J Oral Surg* **2**:152, 1973.
63. Lundgren T, Westphal O, Bolme P, Modéer T, Norén JG: Retrospective study of children with hypophosphatasia with reference to dental changes. *Scand J Dent Res* **99**:357, 1991.
64. Bixler D: Heritable disorders affecting cementum and the periodontal structure, in Stewart RE, Prescott GH (eds): *Oral Facial Genetics*. St. Louis, Mosby, 1976, p 262.
65. Seshia SS, Derbyshire G, Haworth JC, Hoogstraten J: Myopathy with hypophosphatasia. *Arch Dis Child* **65**:130, 1990.
66. Wendling D, Cassou M, Guidet M: Hypophosphatasia in adults. Apropos of 2 cases. *Rev Rhum Mal Osteoartic* **52**:43, 1985.
67. O'Duffy JD: Hypophosphatasia associated with calcium pyrophosphate dihydrate deposits in cartilage. *Arthritis Rheum* **13**:381, 1970.
68. Chuck AJ, Pattrick MG, Hamilton E, Wilson R, Doherty M: Crystal deposition in hypophosphatasia: A reappraisal. *Ann Rheum Dis* **48**:571, 1989.
69. Lassere MN, Jones JG: Recurrent calcific periarthritis, erosive osteoarthritis and hypophosphatasia: A family study. *J Rheumatol* **17**:1244, 1990.
70. Coe JD, Murphy WA, Whyte MP: Management of femoral fractures and pseudofractures in adult hypophosphatasia. *J Bone Joint Surg [Am]* **68**:981, 1986.
71. Page RC, Baab DA: New look at the etiology and pathogenesis of early onset periodontitis. *J Periodontol* **56**:748, 1985.
72. Scriver CR, Cameron D: Pseudohypophosphatasia. *N Engl J Med* **281**:604, 1969.
73. Moore CA, Wappner RS, Coburn SP, Mulivor RA, Fedde KN, Whyte MP: Pseudohypophosphatasia: Clinical, radiographic, and biochemical characterization of a second case. (abstr.) *Am J Hum Genet* **47**:A-68, 1990.
74. Cole DEC, Stinson RA, Coburn SP, Ryan LM, Whyte MP: Increased serum pyridoxal-5′-phosphate in pseudohypophosphatasia (letter). *N Engl J Med* **314**:992, 1986.
75. Fedde KN, Cole DEC, Whyte MP: Pseudohypophosphatasia: Aberrant localization and substrate specificity of alkaline phosphatase in cultured skin fibroblasts. *Am J Hum Genet* **47**:776, 1990.
76. Heaton BW, McClendon JL: Childhood pseudohypophosphatasia. Clinical and laboratory study of two cases. *Tex Dent J* **103**:4, 1986.
77. Mehes K, Klujber L, Lassu G, Kajtar P: Hypophosphatasia: Screening and family investigation in an endogamous Hungarian village. *Clin Genet* **3**:60, 1972.
78. Rubecz I, Mehes K, Klujber L, Bozzay L, Weisenbach J, Fenyvesi J: Hypophosphatasia: Screening and family investigation. *Clin Genet* **6**:155, 1974.
79. Kleinman G, Uri M, Hull S, Keene C: Perinatal ultrasound casebook. *J Perinatol* **11**:282, 1991.
80. Weinstein RS, Whyte MP: Heterogeneity of adult hypophosphatasia: Report of severe and mild cases. *Arch Intern Med* **141**:727, 1981.
81. Macfarlane JD, Sourerijn JHM, Breedveld FC: Clinical significance of a low serum alkaline phosphatase. *Neth J Med* **40**:9, 1992.
82. Royce PM, Blumberg A, Zurbrügg RP, Zimmermann A, Colombo J-P, Steinmann B: Lethal osteogenesis imperfecta: Abnormal collagen metabolism and biochemical characteristics of hypophosphatasia. *Eur J Pediatr* **147**:626, 1988.

83. Pillans PI, Berman P, Saunders SJ: Cholestatic jaundice with a normal serum alkaline phosphatase level: Another case of hypophosphatasia in an adult. *Gastroenterology* **84**:175, 1983.
84. Beisel WR, Austern KF, Rosen H, Herndon EG: Metabolic observations in adult hypophosphatasia. *Am J Med* **29**:369, 1960.
85. Whyte MP, Walkenhorst DA, Hill C, Fedde KN: Hypophosphatasemia in hypophosphatasia reflects proportionately decreased serum bone alkaline phosphatase antigen. (abstr.) *J Bone Miner Res* **5**:S-171, 1990.
86. Fedde KN, Henthorn PS, Whyte MP: Biochemical heterogeneity of alkaline phosphatase in fibroblasts from patients with the severe forms of hypophosphatasia (submitted for publication).
87. Whyte MP, Seino Y: Circulating vitamin D metabolite levels in hypophosphatasia. *J Clin Endocrinol Metab* **55**:178, 1982.
88. Opshaug O, Maurseth K, Howlid H, Aksnes L, Aarskog D: Vitamin D metabolism in hypophosphatasia. *Acta Paediatr Scand* **71**:517, 1982.
89. Wolfish NM, Heick H: Hyperparathyroidism and infantile hypophosphatasia: Effect of prednisone and vitamin D therapy. *J Pediatr* **95**:1079, 1979.
90. Taillard F, Desbois J-C, Gueris J, Delepine N, Lacour B, Gretillat F, Wyart D: Pyrophosphates inorganiques et parathormone dans l'hypophosphatasie. Etude d'une famille. *Biomed Pharmacother* **39**:236, 1985.
91. Whyte MP, Rettinger SD: Hyperphosphatemia due to enhanced renal reclamation of phosphate in hypophosphatasia (abstr. #399). *J Bone Miner Res (suppl 1)* **2**:1987.
92. Nusynowitz ML: Low serum alkaline phosphatase level; hypophosphatemia, and aching extremities (letter). *JAMA* **242**:2800, 1979.
93. Juan D, Lambert PW: Vitamin D. Metabolism and phosphorus absorption studies in a case of coexistent vitamin D resistant rickets and hypophosphatasia, in Cohn DV, Talmage RV, Matthews JL (eds): *Hormonal Control of Calcium Metabolism*. International Congress Series 511. Amsterdam, Excerpta Medica, 1981.
94. De-Vries HR, Duran M, De Bree PK, Wadman SK: A patient with hypophosphatasia and hyperprolinaemia. *Neth J Med* **21**:28, 1978.
95. Rettinger SD, Whyte MP: Normal circulating acid phosphatase activity in hypophosphatasia. *J Inherited Metab Dis* **8**:161, 1985.
96. Iqbal SJ, Taylor WH, Roberts NB, Darlow JM: Raised serum acid phosphatase activity in an adult with hypophosphatasia. *J Inherited Metab Dis* **6**:103, 1983.
97. Rasmussen K: Phosphorylethanolamine and hypophosphatasia. Studies on urinary excretion, renal handling and elimination of endogenous and exogenous phosphorylethanolamine in healthy persons, carriers, and in patients with hypophosphatasia. *Dan Med Bull (suppl II)* **15**:1, 1968.
98. Licata AA, Radfor N, Bartter FC, Bou E: The urinary excretion of phosphoethanolamine in diseases other than hypophosphatasia. *Am J Med* **64**:133, 1978.
99. Tecza S, Prandota J, Morawska Z, Rudzka M, Pankow-Prandota L: Hypophosphatasia with normal urinary phosphoethanolamine in a 22-month-old girl. *Pediatr Pol* **55**:791, 1980.
100. Coburn SP, Whyte MP: Role of phosphatases in the regulation of vitamin B_6 metabolism in hypophosphatasia and other disorders, in Leklem JE, Reynolds RD (eds): *Clinical and Physiological Applications of Vitamin B_6*. New York, Alan R. Liss, 1988, pp 65–93.
101. Chodirker BN, Coburn SP, Seargeant LE, Whyte MP, Greenberg CR: Increased plasma pyridoxal-5′-phosphate levels in carriers of infantile hypophosphatasia before and after pyridoxine loading. *J Inherited Metab Dis* **13**:891, 1990.
102. Macfarlane JD, Poorthuis BJHM, Mulivor RA, Caswell AM: Raised urinary excretion of inorganic pyrophosphate in asymptomatic members of a hypophosphatasia kindred. *Clin Chim Acta* **202**:141, 1991.
103. Nomura Y, Mori W: Hypophosphatasia: Histopathology of human temporal bones. *J Laryngol Otol* **82**:1129, 1982.
104. Manicourt D, Orloff S, Taverne-Verbanck J: Osteomalacia in hyperphosphoethanolaminuria without hypophosphatasia. *Ann Endocrinol* **40**:167, 1979.
105. Beumer J III, Trowbridge HO, Silverman S Jr, Eisenberg E: Childhood hypophosphatasia and the premature loss of teeth: A clinical and laboratory study of seven cases. *Oral Surg Oral Med Oral Pathol* **35**:631, 1973.
106. El-Labban NG, Lee KW, Rule D: Permanent teeth in hypophosphatasia: Light and electron microscopic study. *J Oral Pathol Med* **20**:352, 1991.
107. Vanneuville FJ, Leroy LG: Enzymatic diagnosis of congenital lethal hypophosphatasia in tissues, plasma, and diploid skin fibroblasts. *J Inherited Metab Dis* **4**:129, 1981.
108. Mueller HD, Stinson RA, Mohyuddin F, Milne JK: Isoenzymes of alkaline phosphatase in infantile hypophosphatasia. *J Lab Clin Med* **102**:24, 1983.
109. Gorodischer R, Davidson RG, Mosovich LL, Yaffe SJ: Hypophosphatasia: A developmental anomaly of alkaline phosphatase? *Pediatr Res* **10**:650, 1976.
110. Whyte MP, Vrabel LA: Infantile hypophosphatasia: Genetic complementation analyses with skin fibroblast heterokaryons suggest a defect(s) at a single gene locus. (abstr.) *Clin Res* **33**:332-A, 1985.
111. Whyte MP, Vrabel LA, Schwartz TD: Alkaline phosphatase deficiency in cultured skin fibroblasts from patients with hypophosphatasia: Comparison of the infantile, childhood, and adult forms. *J Clin Endocrinol Metab* **57**:831, 1983.
112. Fallon MD, Whyte MP, Weiss M, Harris H: Molecular biology of hypophosphatasia: A point mutation or small deletion in the bone/liver/kidney alkaline phosphatase gene results in an intact but functionally inactive enzyme. (abstr.) *J Bone Miner Res* **4**:S-304, 1989.
113. Goseki M, Oida S, Takagi Y, Okuyama T, Watanabe J, Sasaki S: Immunological study on hypophosphatasia. *Clin Chim Acta* **190**:263, 1990.
114. Whyte MP, Rettinger SD, Vrabel LA: Infantile hypophosphatasia: Enzymatic defect explored with alkaline phosphatase deficient patient dermal fibroblasts in culture. *Calcif Tissue Int* **40**:244, 1987.
115. Whyte MP, Mahuren JD, Fedde KN, Cole FS, McCabe ERB, Coburn SP: Perinatal hypophosphatasia: Tissue levels of vitamin B_6 are unremarkable despite markedly increased circulating concentrations of pyridoxal-5′-phosphate (evidence for an ectoenzyme role for tissue nonspecific alkaline phosphatase). *J Clin Invest* **81**:1234, 1988.
116. Danovitch SH, Baer PN, Laster L: Intestinal alkaline phosphatase activity in familial hypophosphatasia. *N Engl J Med* **278**:1253, 1968.
117. Pimstone B, Eisenberg E, Silverman S: Hypophosphatasia: Genetic and dental studies. *Ann Intern Med* **65**:722, 1966.
118. Harris B, Robson EB: A genetical study of ethanolamine phosphate excretion in hypophosphatasia. *Hum Genet* **23**:421, 1959.
119. McCance RA, Fairweather DVI, Barrett AM, Morrison AB: Genetic, clinical, biochemical and pathological features of hypophosphatasia. *Q J Med* **25**:523, 1956.
120. Eberle F, Hartenfels S, Pralle H, Kabisch A: Adult hypophosphatasia without apparent skeletal disease: "Odontohypophosphatasia" in four heterozygote members of a family. *Klin Wochenschr* **62**:371, 1984.
121. Silverman JL: Apparent dominant inheritance of hypophosphatasia. *Arch Intern Med* **110**:191, 1962.
122. Eastman JR, Bixler D: Clinical, laboratory and genetic investigations of hypophosphatasia: Support for autosomal dominant inheritance with homozygous lethality. *J Craniofac Genet Dev Biol* **3**:213, 1983.
123. Eastman J, Bixler D: Lethal and mild hypophosphatasia in half-sibs. *J Craniofac Genet Dev Biol* **2**:35, 1982.
124. Sørensen SA, Flodgaard H, Sørensen E: Serum alkaline phosphatase, serum pyrophosphatase, phosphorylethanolamine and inorganic pyrophosphate in plasma and urine: A genetic and clinical study of hypophosphatasia. *Monogr Hum Genet* **10**:66, 1978.
125. Blaskovics ME, Shaw KNF: Hypophosphatasia with phenylketonuria. *Z Kinderheilkd* **117**:265, 1974.
126. Lowry RB, Snyder FF, Wesenberg RL, Machin GA, Applegarth DA, Morgan K, Carter RJ, Toone JR, Holmes TM, Dewar RD: Morquio syndrome (MPS IVA) and hypophosphatasia in a Hutterite kindred. *Am J Med Genet* **22**:463, 1985.

127. Whyte MP, Magill HL, Fallon MD, Herrod HG: Infantile hypophosphatasia: Normalization of circulating bone alkaline phosphatase activity followed by skeletal remineralization (evidence for an intact structural gene for tissue nonspecific alkaline phosphatase). *J Pediatr* **108**:82, 1986.
128. Henthorn PS, Raducha M, Fedde KN, Lafferty MA, Whyte MP: Different missense mutations at the tissue-nonspecific alkaline phosphatase gene locus in autosomal recessively inherited forms of mild and severe hypophosphatasia. *Proc Natl Acad Sci USA* **89**:9924, 1992.
129. Chodirker BN, Evans JA, Lewis M, Coghlan G, Belcher E, Philipps S, Seargeant LE, Sus C, Greenberg CR: Infantile hypophosphatasia—linkage with the RH locus. *Genomics* **1**:280, 1987.
130. Weiss MJ, Cole DEC, Ray K, Whyte MP, Lafferty MA, Mulivor RA, Harris H: A missense mutation in the human liver/bone/kidney alkaline phosphatase gene causing a lethal form of hypophosphatasia. *Proc Natl Acad Sci USA* **85**:7666, 1988.
131. Caswell A, Russell RGG, Whyte MP: Hypophosphatasia: Pediatric forms. *J Pediatr Endocrinol* **3**:73, 1989.
132. Whyte MP, McAlister WH, Patton LS, Magill HL, Fallon MD, Lorentz WB, Herrod HG: Enzyme replacement therapy for infantile hypophosphatasia attempted by intravenous infusions of alkaline phosphatase-rich Paget plasma: Results in three additional patients. *J Pediatr* **105**: 926, 1984.
133. Scaglione PR, Lucey JF: Further observations on hypophosphatasia. *Am J Dis Child* **92**:493, 1956.
134. Fraser D, Laidlaw JC: Treatment of hypophosphatasia with cortisone, preliminary communication. *Lancet* **1**:553, 1956.
135. Riggs BL, Seeman E, Hodgson SF, Taves DR, O'Fallon WM: The effect of the fluoride/calcium regimen on vertebral fracture occurrence in postmenopausal osteoporosis: Comparison with conventional therapy. *N Engl J Med* **306**:446, 1982.
136. Bongiovanni AM, Album MM, Root AW, Hope JW, Marino J, Spencer DM: Studies on hypophosphatasia and response to high phosphate intake. *Am J Med Sci* **255**:163, 1968.
137. Macpherson RI, Kroeker M, Houston CS: Hypophosphatasia. *J Assoc Can Radiol* **23**:16, 1972.
138. Albeggiani A, Cataldo F: Infantile hypophosphatasia diagnosed at 4 months and surviving 2 years. *Helv Paediatr Acta* **37**:49, 1982.
139. Weninger M, Stinson RA, Plenk H Jr, Bock P, Pollack A: Biochemical and morphological effects of human hepatic alkaline phosphatase in a neonate with hypophosphatasia. *Acta Paediatr Scand Suppl* **360**:154, 1989.
140. Whyte MP, Habib D, Coburn SP, Tecklenburg F, Ryan L, Fedde KN, Stinson RA: Failure of hyperphosphatasemia by intravenous infusion of purified placental alkaline phosphatase (ALP) to correct severe hypophosphatasia: Evidence against a role for circulating ALP in skeletal mineralization. (abstr.) *J Bone Miner Res (suppl 1)* **7**:S155, 1992.
141. Jacobson DP, McClain EJ: Hypophosphatasia in monozygotic twins. *J Bone Joint Surg [Am]* **49**:377, 1967.
142. Weinstein RS, Whyte MP: Fifty year follow-up of hypophosphatasia (letter). *Arch Intern Med* **141**:1720, 1981.
143. Rudd NL, Miskin M, Hoar DI, Benzie R, Doran TA: Prenatal diagnosis of hypophosphatasia. *N Engl J Med* **295**:146, 1976.
144. Mulivor RA, Mennuti M, Zackai EH, Harris H: Prenatal diagnosis of hypophosphatasia: Genetic, biochemical, and clinical studies. *Am J Hum Genet* **30**:271, 1978.
145. Warren RC, McKenzie CF, Rodeck CH, Moscoso G, Brock DJH, Barron L: First trimester diagnosis of hypophosphatasia with a monoclonal antibody to liver/bone/kidney isoenzyme of alkaline phosphatase. *Lancet* **2**:856, 1985.
146. Brock DJH, Barron L: First-trimester prenatal diagnosis of hypophosphatasia: Experience with 16 cases. *Prenat Diagn* **11**:387, 1991.
147. Muller F, Oury JF, Bussière P, Lewin F, Boué J: First-trimester diagnosis of hypophosphatasia. Importance of gestational age and purity of CV samples. *Prenat Diagn* **11**:725, 1991.
148. Greenberg CR, Evans JA, McKendry-Smith S, Redekopp S, Haworth JC, Mulivor R, Chodirker BN: Infantile hypophosphatasia: Localization within chromosome region 1p36.1-34 and prenatal diagnosis using linked DNA markers. *Am J Hum Genet* **46**:286, 1990.
149. Kishi F, Matsuura S, Murano I, Akita A, Kajii T: Prenatal diagnosis of infantile hypophosphatasia. *Prenat Diagn* **11**:305, 1991.
150. Van Dongen PWJ, Hamel BCJ, Nijhuis JG, de Boer CN: Prenatal follow-up of hypophosphatasia by ultrasound: Case report. *Eur J Obstet Gynecol Reprod Biol* **34**:283, 1990.
151. Kousseff BG, Mulivor RA: Prenatal diagnosis of hypophosphatasia. *Obstet Gynecol (suppl)* **57**:9S, 1981.
152. Hausser C, Habib R, Poitras P: Hypophosphatasia: A complete absence of the fetal skeleton. *Union Med Can* **113**:978, 1984.
153. Garber AP, Sillence DO, Lachman RS, Worthen NJ, Rimoin DL, Kaback MM, Mulivor RA: Discordance between ultrasound and radiographic/biochemical findings in the prenatal diagnosis of congenital lethal hypophosphatasia. The National Foundation March of Dimes Birth Defects Conference, 1979, p 61.
154. Curry C Jr, Smith JC, O'Lague P, Wonkman LA, Golbus MS: The prenatal diagnosis of autosomal dominant hypophosphatasia. (abstr.) *Am J Hum Genet* **43**:A-230, 1988.
155. Moore CA, Curry CJR, Smith JA, Smith JC, Weaver DD, Whyte MP: In utero presentation of mild autosomal dominant hypophosphatasia. (in manuscript)
156. Whyte MP, Vrabel LA: Infantile hypophosphatasia fibroblasts grow normally in culture: Evidence against a role for constitutive alkaline phosphatase in the regulation of cell growth and differentiation. *Calcif Tissue Int* **40**:1, 1987.
157. Benke PJ, Fleshood HL, Pitat HC: Osteoporotic bone disease in the pyridoxine deficient rat. *Biochem Med* **6**:526, 1972.
158. Gron IH: Mammalian O-phosphorylethanolamine phospholyase activity and its inhibition. *Scand J Clin Lab Invest* **38**:107, 1978.
159. Dolphin D, Poulson R, Avramovic O: *Vitamin B_6 Pyridoxal Phosphate: Clinical, Biochemical, and Medical Aspects: Part B*. New York, John Wiley, 1986.
160. Whyte MP, Mahuren JD, Scott MJ, Coburn SP: Hypophosphatasia: Pyridoxal-5′-phosphate levels are markely increased in hypophosphatasemic plasma but normal in alkaline phosphatase-deficient fibroblasts (evidence for an ectoenzyme role for alkaline phosphatase in vitamin B6 metabolism). (abstr.) *J Bone Min Res* **1**:92, 1986.
161. Anderson BB, O'Brien H, Griffin GE, Mollin DL: Hydrolysis of pyridoxal 5′-phosphate in plasma in conditions with raised alkaline phosphatase. *Gut* **21**:192, 1980.
162. Takahashi T, Iwantanti A, Mizuno S, Morishita Y, Nishio H, Kodama S, Matsuo T: The relationship between phosphoethanolamine level in serum and intractable seizure on hypophosphatasia infantile form, in Cohn DV, Fugita T, Potts JT Jr, Talmage RV (eds): *Endocrine Control of Bone and Calcium Metabolism*. Amsterdam, Excerpta Medica, 1984, vol 8-B, pp 93–94.
163. Low MG, Saltiel AR: Structural and functional roles of glycosyl-phosphatidylinositol in membranes. *Science* **239**:268, 1988.
164. Fedde KN, Whyte MP: Alkaline phosphatase (tissue nonspecific isoenzyme) is a phosphoethanolamine and pyridoxal 5′-phosphate ectophosphatase: Normal and hypophosphatasia fibroblast study. *Am J Hum Genet* **47**:776, 1990.
165. Fedde KN, Lane CC, Whyte MP: Alkaline phosphatase is an ectoenzyme that acts on micromolar concentrations of natural substrates at physiologic pH in human osteosarcoma (SAOS-2) cells. *Arch Biochem Biophys* **264**:400, 1988.
166. Caswell AM, Whyte MP, Russell RGG: Normal activity of nucleoside triphosphate pyrophosphatase in alkaline phosphatase-deficient fibroblasts from patients with infantile hypophosphatasia. *J Clin Endocrinol Metab* **63**:1237, 1986.
167. Fraser D, Yendt ER: Metabolic abnormalities in hypophosphatasia. *Am J Dis Child* **90**:552, 1955.
168. Fedde KN, Michel M, Whyte MP: Evidence against a role for alkaline phosphatase in the dephosphorylation of plasma membrane proteins: hypophosphatasia fibroblast study. *J Cell Biochem* **53**:43, 1993.
169. Wu LNY, Genge BR, Wuthier RE: Evidence for specific interaction between matrix vesicle proteins and the connective tissue matrix. *Bone Miner* **17**:247, 1992.

CHAPTER 137

The Carbonic Anhydrase II Deficiency Syndrome: Osteopetrosis with Renal Tubular Acidosis and Cerebral Calcification

William S. Sly ▪ Peiyi Y. Hu

1. The carbonic anhydrase II deficiency syndrome is an autosomal recessive disorder that produces osteopetrosis, renal tubular acidosis, and cerebral calcification. Other features include mental retardation (seen in over 90 percent of reported cases), growth failure, and dental malocclusion.

2. Complications of osteopetrosis include increased susceptibility to fractures (which do, however, heal normally) and cranial nerve compression symptoms. Anemia and other hematologic manifestations of osteopetrosis are absent.

3. The renal tubular acidosis is usually a mixed type. A distal component is evident from the inability to acidify the urine, and a proximal component is evident from a lowered transport maximum for bicarbonate.

4. About 50 patients have been reported, all of whom have a quantitative deficiency of carbonic anhydrase II activity and immunoreactivity in erythrocytes. Heterozygous carriers can be identified by simple tests.

5. The carbonic anhydrase II gene is 20 kb long, contains seven exons, and maps to chromosome 8q22. Four different mutations in the structural gene have been identified by PCR amplification of genomic DNA from patients with this disorder. Two families with the His 107 → Tyr missense mutation have been notable for the relatively high frequency of skeletal fractures and absence of mental retardation. A splice junction mutation at the 5′ end of intron 2—the "Arabic mutation"—is found in most patients of Arabic descent, who account for over 75 percent of cases so far recognized. A frameshift mutation in exon 7 is the most common mutation in Hispanic patients from the Caribbean islands.

6. PCR-based diagnosis and prenatal diagnosis are available for these four mutations.

7. Symptoms of metabolic acidosis improve with treatment, but no specific treatment is available.

A list of standard abbreviations is located immediately preceding the index in each volume. Additional abbreviations used in this chapter include: CA = carbonic anhydrase; PTH = parathyroid hormone.

HISTORY

Osteopetrosis (marble bone disease) was first described in 1904 by Albers-Schonberg.[1] Subsequently, over 300 cases have been reported.[2] Among these, two principal types were distinguished. An autosomal dominant form was called the "adult, benign" form because of the relatively few symptoms and the benign course, which is compatible with a normal life span. This diagnosis is often made incidentally in adults evaluated for other complaints. At the other extreme is the clinically severe, autosomal recessive form, which has its onset in infancy and produces anemia, leukopenia, hepatomegaly, failure to thrive, cranial nerve symptoms, and early death. This form is often referred to as the "infantile," "malignant," or "lethal" form. Beighton and colleagues have pointed out the existence of clinically intermediate forms of osteopetrosis.[3] Although this genetic heterogeneity indicates that multiple genetic causes produce osteopetrosis, the common mechanism underlying all forms is thought to be failure of bone resorption.[4]

The association of renal tubular acidosis with osteopetrosis was reported independently from three different countries—France,[5] Belgium,[6] and the United States[7]—in 1972. These initial pedigrees suggested that the pattern of inheritance is autosomal recessive. The clinical course began with onset in infancy or early childhood. Though not entirely benign, it was much milder than the course of the recessive lethal form and was compatible with long survival. The hematologic abnormalities associated with the recessive lethal form of osteopetrosis were mild or absent. In 1980, Ohlsson et al.[8] reported the additional finding of cerebral calcification, documented by CT scans, in four children with osteopetrosis and renal tubular acidosis from Saudi Arabia. Calcification of the basal ganglia in the original American kindred was reported independently by Whyte et al. the same year.[9]

In an effort to explain the pleiotropic effects of the mutation underlying this disorder by a single enzyme defect, we postulated a defect in one of the three isozymes of carbonic anhydrase (CA I, CA II, CA III), which are known to be under separate genetic control in humans.[10–14] This hypothesis seemed attractive for two reasons: (1) metabolic acidosis can be produced by sulfonamide inhibitors of CA,[12] and (2) several reports had shown that CA inhibitors can block the parathyroid hormone-induced release of calcium from bone, suggesting a role for CA in bone resorption.[15–17]

The relationship of CA deficiency to cerebral calcification was less apparent, although it was known that CA II is present in brain[18] and that CA inhibitors inhibit cerebrospinal fluid production[19] and affect electrical activity of the brain.[20] A defect in the CA II isozyme seemed most likely because this is the most widely distributed of the three known soluble isozymes of CA in human tissues[10,11] and CA II is the only soluble isozyme so far identified in renal and brain tissue.[18,21,22] In addition, a genetically determined, virtually complete absence of CA I in mature erythrocytes has been found to have no clinical consequences.[23] Because both CA I and CA II are expressed in human erythrocytes, it was possible to test this hypothesis by examining these isozymes in hemolysates of peripheral blood from the family we reported previously.[8]

In 1983, Sly et al.[24] tested this hypothesis and found that the three sisters from the original American kindred with this syndrome (Fig. 137-1) lacked CA II in their erythrocytes. Their normal-appearing parents and many first-degree relatives had half-normal levels of CA II in erythrocyte lysates. These observations, coupled with the fact that CA II was the only known soluble isozyme of CA in kidney and brain, led them to propose that CA II deficiency is the primary defect in the newly recognized metabolic disorder of bone, kidney, and brain.[24]

Sly et al.[25] extended these studies to 18 additional patients in 11 unrelated families of different geographical and ethnic origins. Subsequently, Ohlsson et al.[26] reported four additional Saudi Arabian patients, including the first affected neonate, and summarized the clinical features of 21 reported patients. Cochat et al.[27] added an additional case and reviewed the clinical findings on the 30 patients reported by 1987, including a few who had not been completely described clinically. A few individual cases have been reported since, and many more have been recognized.[28–32] Whyte reviewed nearly 50 cases reported up to 1992.[32a] A deficiency of CA II has been found in erythrocyte lysates of every patient so far identified with this syndrome.

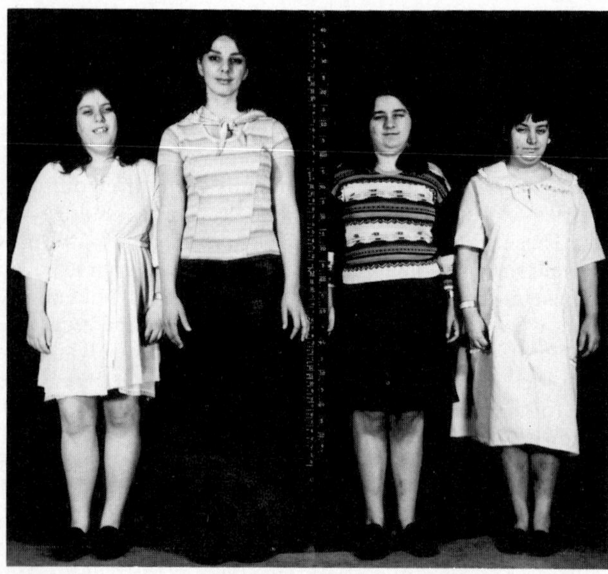

FIG. 137-1 **American family with the CA II deficiency syndrome reported by Whyte et al.[9] From left to right are patient 3, an unaffected sister, patient 2, and patient 1 (proposita). This picture was taken in 1978 when the proposita was 29. Osteopetrosis had been diagnosed at age 2 after a pathological fracture.[9] Note the short stature, unusual facial features, and squint in the three affected sisters. Patients 2 and 3 had limited vision and were considered legally blind. Vision was nearly normal in patient 1. *(From Whyte et al.[9]* Used by permission of *The American Journal of Medicine.)***

NOMENCLATURE

The syndrome of osteopetrosis with renal tubular acidosis (McKusick catalog #259730[33]) was recognized as a distinct entity in 1972.[5–7] In 1980, when Ohlsson et al.[8] pointed out that cerebral calcification was part of the syndrome, they suggested that it be referred to as "marble-brain disease," by analogy with marble-bone disease, the name given earlier to inherited forms of osteopetrosis that did not involve the brain.[2] However, since the enzymatic basis for the disorder was established,[24,25] it has been referred to as the "carbonic anhydrase II deficiency syndrome."[26,33] It has also been called the Guibaud-Vainsel syndrome after the authors of the first two full reports on the disorder.[33]

CLINICAL MANIFESTATIONS

There is considerable variability in the age of onset and the severity of clinical manifestations among the reported cases.[26,27] All have renal tubular acidosis and eventually develop osteopetrosis and cerebral calcification. Additional features include growth failure, mental retardation, and dental malocclusion. In some patients, bone fractures and other complications of osteopetrosis have dominated the clinical picture.[6,9] In others, symptoms of metabolic acidosis, including failure to thrive, developmental retardation, and growth retardation, have been more prominent.[5,8,26,27]

Osteopetrosis

The osteopetrosis results from a generalized accumulation of bone mass that is secondary to a defect in bone resorption.[4] This defect prevents the normal development of marrow cavities, the normal tubulation of long bones, and the enlargement of osseous foramina. The clinical manifestations of osteopetrosis in the CA II deficiency syndrome tend to be milder than in the recessive, lethal form of osteopetrosis. They appear later,[26,27] and they also tend to improve over time.[9,32a]

Anemia is rarely profound in patients with CA II deficiency, though two patients had sufficient anemia to be referred for bone marrow transplantation. In fact, the first reported bone marrow transplantation for osteopetrosis was done on a patient who very likely had the CA II deficiency syndrome[34] rather than the recessive lethal form of osteopetrosis, for which bone marrow transplantation has become an accepted form of therapy.[35] This patient was reported to have a favorable hematologic response, but to have been unimproved in terms of the metabolic acidosis following bone marrow transplantation.[27]

The radiologic findings in patients with CA II deficiency syndrome are not distinguishable from those in patients with other forms of osteopetrosis.[9,26,30–32a] Increased bone density (Fig. 137-2), abnormal modeling, delay or failure of normal tubulation of long bones, transverse banding of metaphyses, fractures, and a "bone-in-bone" appearance are all seen, as

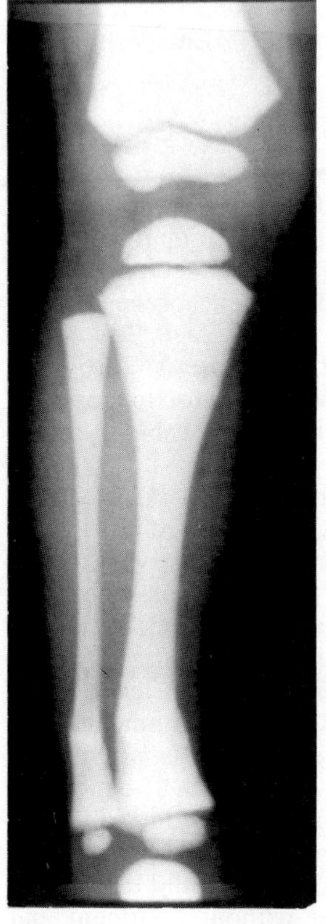

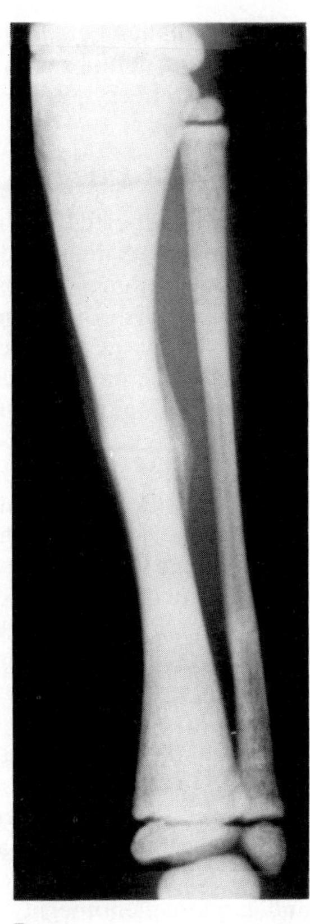

A B

FIG. 137-2 Anteroposterior radiographs of the right tibia and fibula of patient 2 at 2 years of age and of the left tibia and fibula of patient 3 at age 6. Features of osteopetrosis include diffuse osteosclerosis with absence of medullary cavities and flared metaphyses containing transverse lines. Despite the increased bone density, healing fractures are evident in both radiographs.

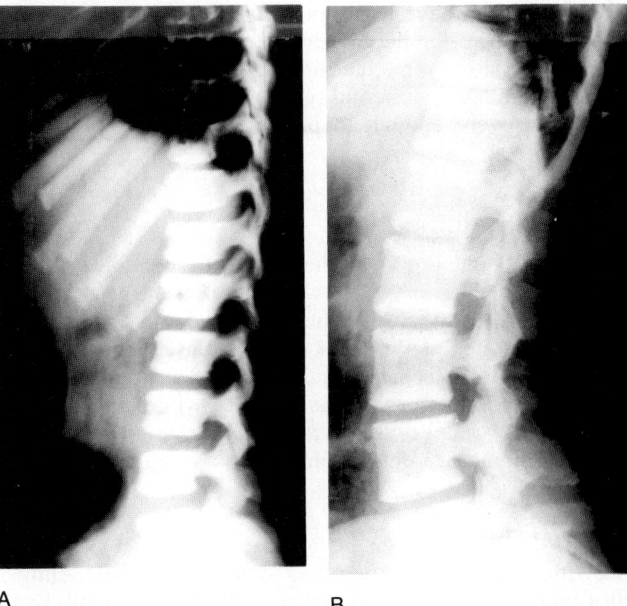

A B

FIG. 137-3 Patient 1, lumbar spine (lateral radiographs). *A*. Age 8 years. *B*. Age 25 years. Osteosclerosis diminished greatly over this interval. Persistent osteosclerosis at the vertebral end plates characterizes the "sandwich vertebrae" of osteopetrosis. *(From Whyte et al.*[9] Used by permission of *The American Journal of Medicine.)*

in other forms of osteopetrosis. However, the changes can vary with age. In the only neonate studied to date, the radiologic features were too subtle to justify the diagnosis at 23 days of age,[26] even though the hyperchloremic metabolic acidosis and alkaline urine were already prominent findings. This observation suggests that the osteopetrosis is a postpartum developmental abnormality that appears over the first year of life. The first patients reported by Guibaud[5,27] also had no osteopetrosis at age 4 months, but typical findings evolved and progressed over the first 3 years of life before stabilizing. In at least some patients followed into adulthood, the radiologic features of osteopetrosis, which were fully developed in childhood, improved substantially after puberty (Fig. 137-3). The radiographs may become nearly normal as the patients move into adulthood.[9,32a]

Bone fractures are common in childhood in many patients, with some reporting 15 to 30 fractures by midadolescence.[6,9,32a,36] After puberty, the frequency of bone fractures decreases. Fractures were the most prominent symptoms in the American patients[7] and the Belgian patient,[6] in whom mental retardation was not present (Fig. 137-2). Fractures were not seen in Guibaud's patients who were of Arabic descent.[5]

The symptoms of cranial nerve compression secondary to osteopetrosis are milder than in the recessive, lethal form of osteopetrosis. However, the cranial nerve symptoms appear in 60 percent of reported patients.[27] Optic nerve pallor is common, but frank optic nerve atrophy is less frequent. Strabismus is also common, as is hearing impairment. Facial weakness has been noted in two reports.

Renal Tubular Acidosis

Patients typically have metabolic acidosis, which varies considerably in type and severity in different pedigrees.[27] Metabolic acidosis was already present at 23 days of age in the first affected neonate.[26] Although one of the first patients reported had only proximal renal tubular acidosis, evidenced by low bicarbonate threshold, and had normal distal acidification,[5,27] most of the patients have a combination of proximal and distal renal tubular acidosis.[6,9,27,37,38] Of 21 patients in whom the renal lesion was characterized, in four the renal tubular acidosis was felt to be proximal, in six distal, and in eleven both proximal and distal.[26] Most patients had hyperchloremia, a normal anion gap, and inappropriately alkaline urine pH (>6.0). These findings are consistent with distal renal tubular acidosis. Symptomatic hypokalemia has been observed in four patients.[9,27] However, unlike other patients with distal renal tubular acidosis, these patients have neither hypercalciuria nor nephrocalcinosis. The glomerular filtration rate is not reduced, and serum creatinine and blood urea nitrogen are not elevated.

Most patients also have a reduced tubular maximum for bicarbonate. Although they usually have no bicarbonaturia when acidotic, they lose bicarbonate when plasma bicarbonate levels are raised to normal levels by loading. They do not have amino aciduria, glycosuria, or any other manifestations of the Fanconi syndrome.

Mental Retardation

The frequency and severity of mental retardation were not fully appreciated initially, because affected patients in two of the first four families recognized with this syndrome were not retarded.[6,7,9] However, over 90 percent of the patients reported to date have had significant mental retardation.[26,27] Even in the two families where intelligence was not below the normal range, some learning disabilities were observed. In most families, the mental retardation in affected patients has been severe enough to preclude education in regular schools.[26,27]

Cerebral Calcification

Cerebral calcifications, evident by CT scans, were first reported by Ohlsson.[8] They were not present at birth, but appeared some time during the first decade (in one case, by 18 months).[5,25,27] Calcifications involved the caudate nucleus, putamen, and globus pallidus, and also appeared peripherally in the periventricular and subcortical white matter (Fig. 137-4). The variability in the rate of progression of cerebral calcification in different patients has not been determined.

Growth Retardation

Growth retardation is nearly a constant finding. Almost all reported patients had short stature and many were underweight. Bone age was retarded and corresponded to height age. Genu valgum is a common finding in older patients. At least part of the growth retardation is due to the chronic metabolic acidosis. Guibaud reported acceleration of growth after correction of the acidosis,[5] but later noted that growth retardation persisted even after treatment.[27] The final height achieved by the patient who responded initially to correction of the acidosis was still nearly four standard deviations below normal.[5,27]

Dental Malocclusion

Dentition was typically delayed and dental malocclusion was a prominent finding in affected patients from several families.

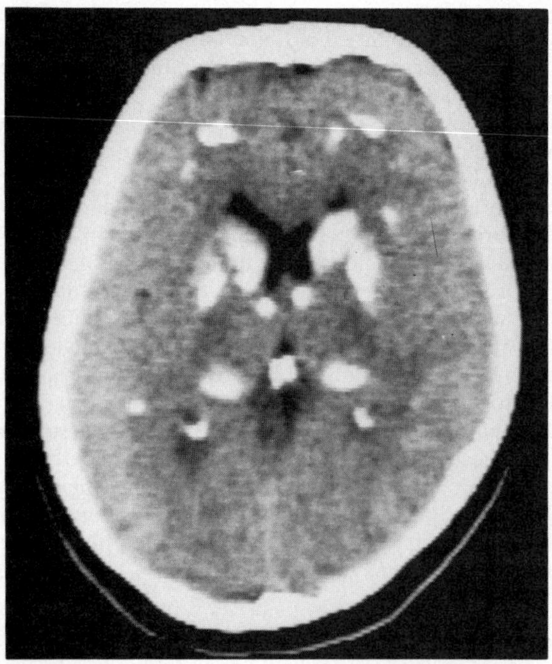

FIG. 137-4 **CT scan of the head of patient 3 at 33 years of age. Scattered dense cerebral calcifications are especially prominent in the basal ganglia.** ***(From Sly et al.***[25] **Reprinted with permission from** ***The New England Journal of Medicine,*** **vol. 313, p. 139, 1985.)**

Dental malalignment and malocclusion complicate dental hygiene, and dental caries may be severe.[9,26] Enamel hypoplasia has also been noted.[8,26]

Other Features

Ohlsson[8,26] reported a characteristic facies in the patients from Saudi Arabia, and it is present in many patients from other ethnic groups as well. These features include craniofacial disproportion with a prominent forehead and a cranial vault large relative to the size of the face. The mouth is small, and there is micrognathia. The nose is narrow but prominent. The philtrum is short, the upper lip thin, and the lower lip thick. Squint is common and contributes to the unusual facies (Fig. 137-1).

Ohlsson et al.[26] recently reported findings of restrictive lung disease in two patients. Chest films showed no signs of parenchymal lung disease, but the rib cages were very dense.

Optic atrophy has been found in patients in whom the optic foramina were of normal size.[27] The mechanism of optic atrophy in these patients is unclear.

Hematologic disorders, including anemia, leukopenia, and thrombocytopenia, which are typically prominent in the recessive malignant lethal form of osteopetrosis, are usually not seen in osteopetrotic patients with the CA II deficiency syndrome. However, anemia and hepatosplenomegaly were seen in three unrelated patients, who were even considered candidates for bone marrow transplantation until the anemia and hepatosplenomegaly improved without treatment and the more benign course became apparent.

PATHOLOGY

No autopsies have been reported on patients with the CA II deficiency syndrome. However, bone biopsy samples from the iliac crest have been analyzed and showed histologic features typical of osteopetrosis.[5,9,26] The cortical bone showed small Haversian systems widely separated from dense bone. The separation of cortical and cancellous bone was generally indistinct. Trabeculae were broad and irregular. Osteoid and normal-appearing osteoblasts were seen lining trabecular bone in several areas. On routine microscopy, osteoclast morphology was unremarkable. A minute sample of femoral cortex was obtained during open reduction of a femoral fracture. Osteoclasts were normal in appearance on light microscopy. Four osteoclasts were identified on electron microscopy, and showed a normal rim of cytoplasm adjacent to the bone surface. This "clear zone" was free of organelles. The osteoclasts appeared normal, although no "ruffled borders" were seen. In summary, the histologic findings of osteopetrosis were present, but no features appeared to distinguish the osteopetrosis of the CA II deficiency syndrome from other forms of osteopetrosis.

PATHOGENESIS

The Carbonic Anhydrase Gene Family

All three soluble isozymes of CA in humans (CA I, II, and III) are monomeric, 29-kDa zinc metalloenzymes that catalyze the reversible hydration of CO_2 (reaction I).[39]

$$CO_2 + H_2O \overset{\text{I}}{\rightleftharpoons} H_2CO_3 \overset{\text{II}}{\rightleftharpoons} H^+ + HCO_3^-$$

Reaction II involves an ionic dissociation, occurs virtually instantaneously nonenzymatically, and is not subject to enzymatic acceleration. The direction of the reaction in a given tissue or body fluid depends on the relative concentrations of CO_2, HCO_3^-, and H^+ ion (i.e., pH). There is also a distinctive membrane-bound CA in lung called CA IV,[40] which was shown to be identical to the membrane-bound CA in the brush border lining the lumen of the proximal tubules of the kidney.[41] The CA IV cDNA[42] and CA IV genomic organization[43] were recently reported. A distinct, secretory form of CA (CA VI) has been described in the saliva of the rat,[44] the human,[45] and the sheep.[46] The amino acid sequence of the ovine salivary CA was recently reported and shows 33 percent sequence identity with ovine CA II, though the residues involved in the active site were more highly conserved. A distinct CA has also been reported in mitochondria in the liver and has been designated CA V.[47]

Chromosome Localization of CA Genes

Genetic and structural evidence suggests that the CA isozymes constitute a multilocus enzyme family derived from a common ancestral gene by gene duplication.[48] CA I, II, and III are clustered at chromosome 8q22[49]; CA IV was assigned to 17q23[43]; and CA VI was assigned to chromosome 1p.[50] CA V was recently assigned to chromosome 16,[47] to which CA VIII was previously mapped.[51]

Tissue Distribution and Properties of CA Isozymes

The kinetic parameters of the different isozymes, their sensitivities to different inhibitors, and their tissue distributions differ markedly, indicating that they play different physiological roles.[52,53] The human CA II isozyme, whose turnover number for CO_2 hydration (1.3 to 1.9 $\times$ 10^6/sec) is the highest known for any enzyme,[54,55] is widely distributed. It has been identified in erythrocytes, brain, eye, kidney, cartilage, liver, lung, skeletal muscle, pancreas, gastric mucosa, and anterior pituitary body.[39,56] The other isozymes, whose activities are lower than those of CA II in the order CA II > CA IV > CA I > CA III > CA V, appear to have a more limited distribution.[47,57] CA I is found primarily in erythrocytes. CA III is found mainly in red skeletal muscle.[52,53] CA IV is expressed on the apical and basolateral surfaces of cells of the proximal tubule and thick ascending limb of the nephron[41] and on the plasma face of certain endothelial surfaces, including the pulmonary microvasculature,[58] the choriocapillaris,[59] and microcapillaries of brain,[60] heart, and skeletal muscle.[57,61] CA V is expressed in mitochondria of liver, kidney, intestine, heart, and spleen.[62]

The Biochemical Defect

In 1983, the three affected sisters reported initially by Sly et al.[7] and described in detail by Whyte et al.[9] were shown to have no detectable CA II activity in their erythrocytes.[24] CA I was present in near-normal levels. No immunoreactivity was detectable with specific antibody to CA II. The obligate heterozygote parents and several additional family members were found to have half-normal levels of CA II activity. These findings were subsequently extended to 18 similarly affected patients from 11 unrelated families of different geographic and ethnic origins.[25] Every patient with osteopetrosis and renal tubular acidosis since tested has had no detectable CA II activity.[27] Thus, there has been no exception to the finding of a quantitative defect in CA II in erythrocytes of patients with this syndrome.

Mutations in the structural gene for CA II (summarized below) have been found in most patients with CA II deficiency.[63–65,80,91] Although the complete absence of CA II activity and immunoreactivity in erythrocytes have been consistent findings in affected patients, it should be stressed that the residual activity in cells that continue to synthesize protein (such as osteoclasts in bone and cells in the proximal and distal tubules of the kidney) might be significantly higher than in erythrocytes. In fact, we suspect that some of the clinical heterogeneity in this syndrome may be explained by differences in residual CA II activity in bone and kidney in patients with different mutations in the structural gene for CA II.

Pathophysiology

The finding of a quantitative defect in CA II in these patients provided an unusual opportunity to assess the function of this enzyme and to understand its importance for bone, brain, and kidney metabolism.

Bone Metabolism. All known forms of osteopetrosis involve the failure to resorb bone.[4] Studies showing inhibition of parathyroid hormone (PTH)-induced release of CA^{2+} from bone by CA inhibitors had suggested a role for CA in bone resorption.[15–17] Also, CA had been demonstrated histochemically in chick and hen osteoclasts[66] and CA II demonstrated immunohistochemically in rat[67] and human[15] osteoclasts. The osteopetrosis seen in patients with CA II deficiency provided genetic evidence for a role of CA in bone resorption and implicated the CA II isozyme specifically.[24]

It had been suggested that CA aids the resorptive process by mediating the secretion of H^+.[16,67] We proposed that the role of CA II in acidifying the bone-resorbing component is an indirect one, analogous to its role in supporting the acidification of the lumen in the distal tubule of the kidney. It has been suggested recently that the acidification of the bone-resorbing compartment is mediated by a proton-translocating ATPase[68] that secretes protons into the lumen. This reaction would simultaneously generate an OH^- ion in the cytoplasm for each H^+ translocated to the lumen. Titration of the OH^- ions produced in the cytosol by CA II might be required to allow the proton-translocating ATPase to maintain the pH gradient (7.0 to 4.5) between the cytosol of the osteoclast and the bone-resorbing compartment. This model could explain the pharmacologic evidence that CA is required in bone resorption.[15–17] Since CA II is the only CA isozyme known to be expressed in osteoclasts,[67,68] it could also explain the osseous manifestations of CA II deficiency.

Renal Tubular Acidosis. Three things need explanation in regard to renal metabolism in these patients. First, most CA II-deficient patients have both a proximal and a distal component to the renal tubular acidosis.[26,27] Second, some patients have predominantly proximal renal tubular acidosis, while in others the distal renal tubular acidosis predominates.[26,27] Third, CA II-deficient patients have a nearly normal bicarbonaturia after ingestion or infusion of carbonic anhydrase inhibitors.[69] Some of these observations can be explained by a model in which the functions of CA II in the proximal and distal tubules are physiologically and biochemically distinct, and the major role of CA in bicarbonate reclamation is assigned not to CA II but to CA IV, the luminal CA in the brush border of the proximal tubule.[70,71] CA IV is biochemically and immunologically distinct from CA II, and appears to be normal in CA II-deficient patients,[69] based on the evidence of normal bicarbonaturia in response to infused acetazolamide. We recently showed that the affected patients in the original American family with CA II deficiency have normal CA IV levels in their urinary membranes.[71a]

We deal first with the explanation for the proximal renal tubular acidosis. There is general agreement that renal reabsorption of bicarbonate is a major factor in acid–base homeostasis. Most of the bicarbonate reclamation takes place in the proximal tubule and is blocked by inhibitors of CA. However, two distinct CA isozymes participate in bicarbonate reclamation by the proximal tubule, and they play separate roles in bicarbonate reclamation.

Bicarbonate reclamation depends on H^+ secretion, which is mediated primarily by Na^+/H^+ exchange in the proximal tubule but also by the Mg^{2+}/H^+-ATPase on the apical membrane.[72] The H^+ secreted into the lumen of the proximal tubule is titrated by the HCO_3^- in the glomerular filtrate to produce H_2CO_3, which is in contact with the membrane-bound CA IV. The luminal CA IV catalyzes the dehydration of H_2CO_3 to H_2O and CO_2.[73,74] The bicarbonaturia seen in response to infused acetazolamide in already acidotic CA II-deficient patients is attributed to inhibition of this luminal CA IV.[69]

The CO_2 produced by the CA IV-catalyzed reaction in the lumen diffuses freely into the cytosol of the proximal tubule. Here in the cytoplasm CO_2 encounters CA II, which acts to hydrate the CO_2 to produce H_2CO_3, which dissociates spontaneously to HCO_3^- and H^+. The HCO_3^- generated from CO_2 in the cytosol is transported from the cytosol to the interstitial fluid or peritubular capillary by the Na-3HCO_3 cotransporter, completing the reclamation of the filtered bicarbonate. The H^+ regenerated in the cytosol by the CA II-catalyzed reaction can be secreted in exchange for Na^+ to initiate another round of HCO_3^- reclamation.[72,74]

Thus, both the luminal CA IV and the cytosolic CA II participate in the reclamation of HCO_3^- in the proximal tubule. The fact that CA II-deficient patients do not spill HCO_3^- when acidotic suggests that CA II is not required for HCO_3^- reclamation when patients have low bicarbonate loads, i.e., when acidotic. However, they have a lowered tubular maximum for bicarbonate and lose bicarbonate when the filtered load is increased by bicarbonate infusion or ingestion, indicating that CA II is required to regenerate H^+ for bicarbonate reclamation under normal bicarbonate loads. This requirement explains the proximal component of the renal tubular acidosis in CA II-deficient patients (Fig. 137-5A).

The prominent distal component of the renal tubular acidosis in most CA II-deficient patients, evidenced by inappropriately high urine pH values when patients are

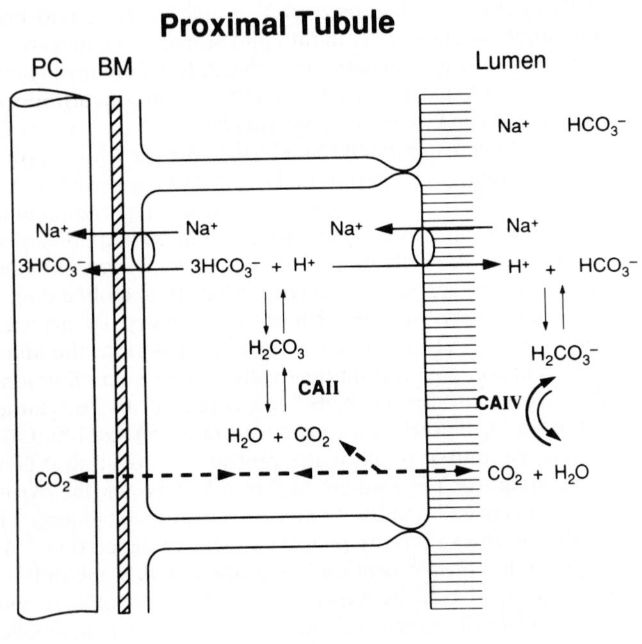

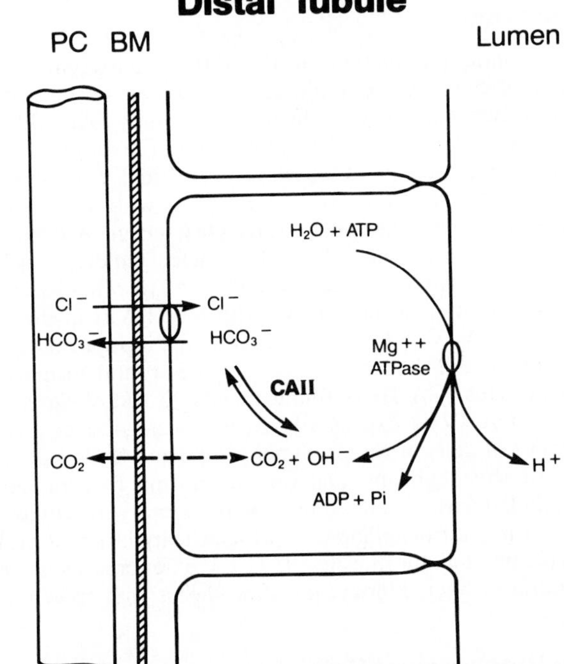

FIG. 137-5 *A*. **Proposed roles of carbonic anhydrases in bicarbonate reclamation in the proximal tubule. Na^+ and HCO_3^- enter the lumen of the proximal tubule. H^+ is secreted in exchange for Na^+, and H^+ and HCO_3^- are converted to CO_2 and H_2O in a reaction catalyzed by the luminal CA (CA IV). We propose that this enzyme functions normally in CA II-deficient patients, and its inhibition explains the positive response to acetazolamide (normal bicarbonate diuresis). CO_2 diffuses freely into the proximal tubular cell [and across the basement membrane (BM) and into the peritubular capillary (PC)] and is exposed to cytosolic CA II, which catalyzes its rehydration to form HCO_3^- and H^+. Three molecules of HCO_3^- and one of Na^+ are cotransported by the basolateral cotransporter from the contraluminal surface of the proximal tubular cell to the peritubular capillary (PC). The H^+ generated by CA II is secreted in exchange for Na^+ to initiate another cycle of HCO_3^- reabsorption. Loss of CA II-mediated regeneration of H^+ is suggested as the cause of HCO_3^- wasting in CA II-deficient patients.** *B*. **Proposed role of CA II in distal urinary acidification. The H^+ is secreted into the lumen by a proton-translocating Mg^{2+} ATPase, as in amphibians, which produces OH^- in the cytosol. CO_2 can condense with OH^- to form HCO_3^- in a CA II-catalyzed reaction, and HCO_3^- can be transported across the basement membrane and into the peritubular capillary. We suggest that failure to titrate the OH^- limits the ability to secrete H^+ and acidify the urine appropriately in CA II-deficient patients. (*From Sly et al.*[69] Used by permission of *Pediatric Research*.)**

acidotic, suggests that CA II is needed for distal acidification as well. This idea is consistent with the immunohistochemical evidence showing a much more intense reaction for CA II in the distal tubule and the intercalated cells of the collecting ducts than in the proximal tubules.[71] Why is there normally such an abundance of CA II in the distal tubules, when most of the HCO_3^- reclamation takes place in the proximal tubule? We suggested[69] that the explanation may be inferred from the analogous situation in the distal nephron and collecting system in the amphibian. In the turtle bladder, for example, the "CA-rich cells" are specialized cells that secrete H^+ and are capable of generating a steep pH gradient.[75,76] However, the acidification of the lumen is sensitive to inhibition by acetazolamide. It has been proposed that CA is needed in the amphibian nephron to titrate the OH^- produced in the cytosol by the proton-translocating Mg^{2+} ATPase. We have suggested a similar role for CA II in the distal tubule of the human kidney, i.e., catalyzing the conversion of OH^- and CO_2 to HCO_3^-.[69] Unless the OH^- is titrated by CO_2, the proton-translocating ATPase cannot generate a pH gradient and acidify the lumen. The absence of CA II for this reaction in CA II-deficient patients can explain their defect in distal tubular acidification (Fig. 137-5B).

The third point, the basis for heterogeneity in the renal lesion in CA II deficiency, still requires explanation. Why is there variation in the prominence of the proximal and distal lesions in different pedigrees? The explanation for this heterogeneity is still speculative. The different structural gene mutations producing CA II deficiency in different pedigrees may contribute to this heterogeneity in at least two ways. First, different mutations may affect the rate of enzyme turnover differently in proximal and distal tubular cells, resulting in different levels of residual enzyme activity in the two locations. Secondly, different structural gene mutations could affect the two enzymatic activities differently in the two locations. Thus, hydration of CO_2 to produce H^+ and HCO_3^- in the proximal tubule and the condensation of OH^- and CO_2 to produce HCO_3^- in the distal tubule might be differently affected by different mutations in the CA II gene. Continued delineation of the mutations in different CA II-deficient patients and studies of the enzyme produced after expression of the cloned mutant genes in prokaryotic and eukaryotic cells may allow one to test this hypothesis.

Brain Calcification and Cerebral Function. The mechanism of the cerebral calcification is unclear. CA II is primarily a glial enzyme that occurs predominantly in oligodendrocytes.[77] It is the only soluble carbonic anhydrase in brain homogenates. As much as 50 percent of the total CA II activity occurs in a membrane-bound or myelin-associated form.[78] The function of CA II in brain is not known. It is not clear whether the cerebral calcification in carbonic anhydrase II deficiency represents a direct effect of the deficiency of CA II in the brain or an indirect effect—for example, of carbonic anhydrase deficiency in erythrocytes or of chronic systemic acidosis.

While brain development and central nervous system function are not profoundly deranged in patients with this syndrome, psychomotor delay, learning disabilities, and even mental retardation are evident in most affected patients.[26,27] The mental retardation was not so obvious in the initial reports of patients with CA II deficiency syndrome, but it is now clear that over 90 percent of the reported patients have mental retardation severe enough to prevent school attendance. Whether this is a direct consequence of the CA II deficiency, or an indirect effect, is not yet clear.

Although CA II is the only soluble CA expressed in brain, CA IV is expressed on the plasma face of cerebral capillaries and is anchored to the capillary membrane by a glycosylphosphoinositol linkage.[60]

Growth Failure. Growth failure appears to result from a combination of the effect of the osteopetrosis on bone elongation and the effect of the chronic metabolic acidosis on general health. Correction of the acidosis was followed by a growth spurt in one patient,[27] but the fact that the final height achieved by this patient was still dramatically low makes it clear that the growth retardation is not due to the acidosis alone.

GENETICS

Inheritance

The CA II deficiency syndrome is inherited as an autosomal recessive trait. Affected patients are offspring of normal-appearing heterozygote carrier parents who have half-normal levels of CA II in their erythrocyte lysates. Heterozygotes have no symptoms or signs of the disorder. Males and females are affected with equal frequency and severity. Consanguinity is very common (87 percent) in parents of affected offspring.[27]

The geographical distribution of this syndrome is striking, with more than half the known cases observed in families from Kuwait, Saudi Arabia, and North Africa.[25] This probably results from both a high frequency of the carbonic anhydrase II deficiency allele in these regions and a high frequency of consanguineous marriages, particularly in the Bedouin tribes from which many of these patients originated.

Molecular Genetics

In humans, the CA I, II, and III genes (CA1, CA2, CA3) are clustered in a stretch of about 180 kb on chromosome 8q22.[48] The entire 20-kb CA II gene has been cloned and the intron/exon organization determined[63,64] (Fig. 137-6). The human CA II gene contains seven exons, as does the mouse gene, and intron/exon junctions 2 through 7 are conserved in all human CAs so far examined. The 5′ flanking region of the human CA II gene contains a TATA box and a possible CAAT box. It also contains nine potential Sp1 binding sites. Deletion analysis of the human 5′ promoter region showed a gradual but differential loss in promoter activity with loss of Sp1 binding sites.[79]

The full-length human cDNA has been expressed in both prokaryotic and eukaryotic cells. Although mRNA from CA II-deficient patients could not easily be obtained, knowledge of the genomic organization and of the intron sequences surrounding each exon has made mutational analysis on patient genomic DNA straightforward. Four mutations have been identified so far in CA II-deficient patients (Fig. 137-6). The first mutation (mutation 2 in Fig. 137-6) was identified in a Belgian patient and was a C-to-T transition in exon 3, which results in replacement of the conserved histidine at position 107 with tyrosine (His 107 → Tyr).[63] The three affected sisters in the American family in which CA II deficiency was first reported were also found to have this mutation. However, they were compound heterozygotes, having inherited the His 107 → Tyr mutation from their mother and a splice acceptor mutation in the 3′ end of intron 5 from their father.[64] Neither the Belgian patient nor the

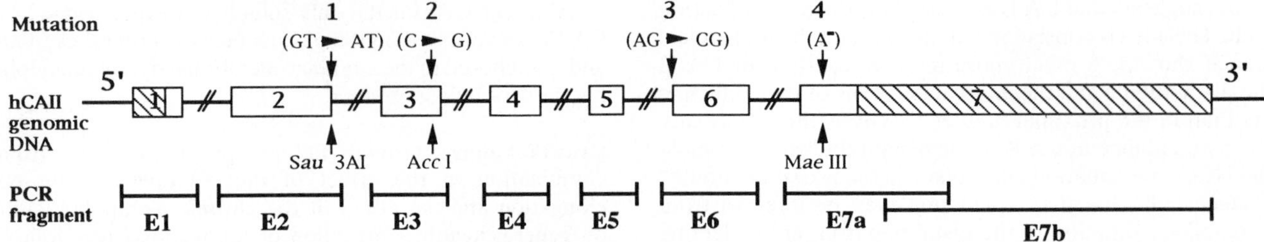

FIG. 137-6 Genomic organization, PCR fragments, and structural mutations found to date in the human CA II gene. The human CA II gene contains seven exons and six introns. Except exon 7, each exon including exon/intron boundaries can be amplified individually by PCR using intronic PCR primers. Exon 7 has 928 bp, which can be amplified in two overlapping fragments for sequencing. Similar PCR primers were described by Venta et al.[63] and Roth et al.[64] Four structural mutations have been found in the CA II gene, and are numbered here from the 5′ end. Mutation 1, which is common in Arabic patients, changes the first nucleotide of intron 2 from G to A and destroys a splice junction donor site. This change creates a new *Sau* 3AI restriction site, which can be used for diagnosis and prenatal diagnosis.[32,65] Mutation 2 is a C→G transition in exon 3, which results in replacement of the conserved histidine at position 107 with tyrosine (His 107→Tyr) and introduces a new *Acc* I restriction site. This mutation was identified in a homozygous Belgian patient[63] and also as one of two mutations in the three American sisters shown in Figure 137-1, who were compound heterozygotes, and in their mother.[64] Mutation 3 is an A-to-C transversion at the 3′ end of intron 5, which destroys a splice junction acceptor site. This mutation was the second mutation found in the American sisters, the one they inherited from their father.[64] Mutation 4 is a single-base-pair deletion in the coding region of exon 7a, which creates a new *Mae* III restriction site. This single-base deletion results in a frameshift at codon 227, which changes the next 12 amino acids and introduces a UGA stop codon 22 amino acids earlier than in the normal enzyme. This mutation was found to be common in Hispanic patients from the Caribbean islands.[80,91]

American patients were mentally retarded. Frequent skeletal fractures were the most disabling manifestation of their disease.[28] When the CA II cDNA containing the His 107 → Tyr mutation was expressed in *E. coli,* the activity of the mutant protein was drastically lower than that of the normal enzyme. However, residual activity could be easily demonstrated in cells induced at 30°C and 20°C, where a larger fraction of the expressed enzyme remained soluble (80 percent at 20°C). These experiments suggested that a small amount of residual CA II activity in patients with the His 107 → Tyr mutation may allow them to escape mental retardation.[64] The third structural gene mutation identified is a splice junction mutation at the 5′ end of intron 2, which was found in most of the patients of Arabic descent from Kuwait, Saudi Arabia, Algeria, and Tunisia.[65] More than 75 percent of the patients so far recognized have been Arabic[28] and have been severely affected. Mental retardation and metabolic acidosis were prominent in these patients, while bone fractures were less frequent.[28,65]

A novel frameshift mutation resulting from a single-base deletion in the coding region of exon 7a was found in a mildly affected Hispanic girl, who is the only patient reported so far with no renal tubular acidosis.[80,91] This single-base deletion results in a frameshift at codon 227 that changes the next 12 amino acids and introduces a UGA stop codon at codon 239. The truncated enzyme resulting from this mutation is 22 amino acids shorter than the 260 amino acids in normal CA II. When expressed in bacteria, the mutant allele produced 0.07 percent of the activity expressed by the normal allele. Unexpectedly, this mutant enzyme activity was not due to the truncated form of the mutant enzyme (27 kDa), but to a small fraction of near-normal size enzyme (29 kDa), which had about 10 percent of normal specific activity. Protein sequencing showed that the first 11 amino acids were abnormal in the 29-kDa mutant protein, as predicted by the frameshift, after which the reading frame was restored. The last 23 amino acids of the 29-kDa mutant protein were the same as in normal CA II. These results can be explained by a ribosomal −1 translational frameshift that restores the reading frame 11 codons after the original mutation and allows completion of full-length CA II. Subsequently, patients referred from seven independent Hispanic families, some having severe clinical manifestations including severe renal tubular acidosis, anemia, and hepatosplenomegaly, were found by sequencing or restriction site analysis to be homozygous for the same mutation. The basis for the wide clinical variability in these patients is unclear. However, these findings raise the possibility that individual variation in efficiency of frameshift suppression may contribute to clinical heterogeneity among patients with identical frameshift mutations.

DIAGNOSIS

Clinically, CA II deficiency should be suspected in any newborn infant with metabolic acidosis and failure to thrive, especially if the urine pH is alkaline. Osteopetrosis may not be present initially, but it usually develops over the first year of life. If osteopetrosis and renal tubular acidosis coexist, the diagnosis is virtually certain. No patient with this combination has yet been found who does not have CA II deficiency. Cerebral calcification, evident by CT scan, is usually present by the end of the first decade.

Enzymatic confirmation can be made by measuring the CA II level in erythrocyte lysates.[81,82] A relatively easy assay has been described that allows one to quantitate both CA I and CA II levels in erythrocyte lysates. This method takes advantage of the large difference in sensitivity of CA I and CA II to inhibition by sodium iodide. Normally CA I and CA II each contribute about 50 percent of the total activity, and the CA I activity is virtually completely abolished by inclusion of 8 m*M* sodium iodide in the assay. One simply measures the total activity (CA I + CA II), and also the activity seen in the presence of 8 m*M* sodium iodide (CA II). Patients with CA II deficiency have no iodide-resistant enzyme (i.e., no CA II). Obligate heterozygotes have about half-normal levels of iodide-resistant activity. Other assays have been described, including staining of individual isozymes following electrophoresis, quantitation of CA I/CA II ratios by high-pressure liquid chromatography, and immunologic identification of the isozymes on immunodiffusion with specific antisera.[24]

The identification of the structural gene mutations underlying CA II deficiency has provided simple and accurate molecular techniques for detecting these mutations, which should be useful for diagnosis, genetic counseling, and prenatal diagnosis, and also for carrier detection in certain populations. As shown in Figure 137-6, three of the four mutations in the CA II gene have introduced new restriction sites in the mutant DNA alleles. The Arabic mutation introduces an extra *Sau* 3AI site in exon 2; the His 107 → Tyr mutation creates a new *Acc* I site in exon 3; and the Hispanic mutation creates an additional *Mae* III site in exon 7a. Digestion of PCR-amplified genomic DNA fragments with the appropriate restriction enzymes followed by agarose gel electrophoresis allows one to make accurate diagnoses.[63,65,80,91] The splice-junction mutation at the 3′ end of intron 5 does not create or destroy a restriction site. In this case, dot-blot hybridization using allele-specific oligonucleotide probes proved to be useful in distinguishing patients, carriers, and normal individuals.[64]

GENETIC COUNSELING

The counseling appropriate for an autosomal recessive trait is indicated. First-degree relatives can be tested for heterozygosity. Prenatal diagnosis using the techniques described above under DNA diagnosis is now available to families where the mutation has been established. Prenatal diagnosis is not available to families in which the mutation has not yet been established. In addition, the osteopetrosis does not appear prenatally and the diagnosis cannot be made in the fetus radiologically or by ultrasound. Carbonic anhydrase levels in erythrocytes are extremely low at birth in normal infants, and it is unlikely that CA II deficiency could be diagnosed by measuring CA II activity in samples of fetal blood.

TREATMENT

No specific treatment for CA II deficiency is available. Treatment for the metabolic acidosis is recommended, at least until after adolescence.[27] It appears that the renal tubular acidosis may stabilize at a milder level after puberty. Frequent fractures require conventional orthopedic management. Bone healing is usually normal. Most patients require special education because of mental retardation. There is no specific treatment for the cranial nerve abnormalities, which may lead to impaired vision, hearing deficits, and facial nerve weakness. Attention to dental hygiene is important because of the susceptibility to caries.

In the early course of the initial American family, treatment with bicarbonate was withheld for fear that the acidosis might be compensating for the osteopetrosis and that treating the acidosis might aggravate the osteopetrosis, resulting in further loss of vision and hearing. However, prolonged treatment of several patients by Dr. Guibaud and colleagues appeared to have a beneficial effect on general health without any marked progression of the osteopetrosis and with no aggravation of cranial nerve symptoms.[27] It is not clear whether the development of cerebral calcification is influenced by correction of the acidosis.

Bone marrow transplantation is not indicated, since the hematologic manifestations that make it appropriate in the infantile, recessive lethal form of osteopetrosis[34] are usually not present in the CA II deficiency syndrome. Although the bone manifestations should theoretically improve following bone marrow transplantation, because stem cells from the donor marrow would provide CA II-containing osteoclasts, the renal insufficiency would not improve. This was actually the observation reported in the first patient treated with transplantation for osteopetrosis who, in retrospect, appears to have had CA II deficiency.[33]

We had the opportunity to replace the CA II-deficient red cells with CA II-replete blood cells following severe uterine hemorrhage in one of the patients we followed.[83] Raising the circulating erythrocyte levels of CA II to the heterozygote range by transfusion with replete erythrocytes had no effect on plasma pH or urine pH. These observations supported the proposal that the metabolic acidosis is caused by the renal CA II deficiency and is not a secondary consequence of CA II deficiency in erythrocytes.

FUTURE PROSPECTS

Delineation of the molecular defect has made prenatal diagnosis possible in many families. The PCR-based RFLP analysis may be practical for population-based screening in certain restricted populations. Perhaps the clearest example is that of the Arabic mutation, which accounts for more than 75 percent of cases reported to date. Using the PCR-based RFLP analysis, Fathallah et al. found that every affected member in 14 families in Tunisia had this mutation.[32]

Another potentially important development is the description of a mouse with CA II deficiency.[84] The mutation was produced intentionally by exposing mice that were heterozygotes for electrophoretically distinguishable CA II gene products to a powerful mutagen and screening progeny electrophoretically for loss of one of the alleles. A null mutation was found, and a breeding colony established. The affected mouse has severe acidosis but has not been found to have osteopetrosis or cerebral calcification. Although this animal model lacks some of the components of the human CA II deficiency syndrome, it is certain to be a profitable model for studying many facets of CO_2 and HCO_3^- metabolism and for studying certain experimental therapies, such as bone marrow replacement and gene therapy.

Finally, the remarkable utility of this human disease in shedding light on the physiological roles of the various carbonic anhydrases should stimulate clinical research aimed at identifying disorders caused by deficiencies of other members of the CA gene family.[56] An inherited deficiency of CA I has already been found and proved to have no clinical consequences.[56] Presumably, the latter finding reflects the facts that CA I is expressed mainly in erythrocytes and that CA II, which is expressed at normal levels in CA I-deficient patients, can more than handle the requirements for CA activity in the erythrocytes.[55] It seems likely that deficiencies of CA III, CA IV, and CA V would produce significant clinical abnormalities. Such experiments of nature probably exist, and, once they are identified, they will likely add greatly to our understanding of why we have evolved so many isozymes to catalyze a reaction as simple as the reversible hydration of CO_2.

IMPLICATIONS FOR OSTEOPOROSIS

By now, there is considerable histochemical, pharmacologic, and genetic evidence that CA II plays an important role in the generation of hydrogen ion gradients and is required for the normal functioning of osteoclasts in bone resorption.[85] Although osteopetrosis results from a defect in bone resorption, there are other metabolic disorders in which the reverse is true, and accelerated bone loss is the problem. Can one take advantage of the CA dependence of the bone resorption process to inhibit accelerated bone loss? A number of organ culture systems have been developed to study bone resorption.[55,86,87] In organ culture, Ca^{2+} release from bones was shown to be hormone responsive (parathormone and dibutyryl cyclic AMP) and sensitive to inhibition by acetazolamide and other inhibitors of CA.[87–89] Animal studies have suggested that bone loss associated with disuse can be partially prevented by CA inhibitors.[90] This observation raises hope that CA inhibitors might have a role in treating common causes of bone loss like osteoporosis. One problem, however, is that chronic administration of the currently available agents produces a systemic acidosis owing to the action of these agents on the kidney, and systemic acidosis itself can lead to calcium mobilization from bone. It has been suggested[87] that the development of effective inhibitors that might be useful in metabolic bone disease may require development of agents that act selectively on CA II in bone or that can be selectively targeted to bone-resorbing osteoclasts to avoid inhibition of CA II in kidney and other sites.

REFERENCES

1. Albers-Schonberg H: Rontgenbilder einer seltenen, Knochenerkrankung. *Muench Med Wochenschr* **51**:365, 1904.
2. Johnston CC Jr, Lavy N, Lord T, Vellios F, Merritt AD, Deiss WP Jr: Osteopetrosis: A clinical, genetic, metabolic, and morphologic study of the dominantly inherited, benign form. *Medicine (Baltimore)* **47**:149, 1968.
3. Beighton P, Hamersma H, Cremin BJ: Osteopetrosis in South Africa: The benign, lethal and intermediate forms. *S Afr Med J* **55**:659, 1979.
4. Marks SC Jr: Morphological evidence of reduced bone resorption in osteopetrotic (op) mice. *Am J Anat* **163**:157, 1982.
5. Guibaud P, Larbre F, Freycon M-T, Genoud J: Osteopetrose et acidose renale tubulaire: Deux cas de cette association dans une fratrie. *Arch Fr Pediatr* **29**:269, 1972.
6. Vainsel M, Fondu P, Cadranel S, Rocmans C, Gepts W: Osteopetrosis associated with proximal and distal tubular acidosis. *Acta Paediatr Scand* **61**:429, 1972.
7. Sly WS, Lang R, Avioli L, Haddad J, Lubowitz H, McAlister W: Recessive osteopetrosis: New clinical phenotype. *Am J Hum Genet* **24**(Suppl):34a, 1972.
8. Ohlsson A, Stark G, Sakati N: Marble brain disease: Recessive osteopetrosis, renal tubular acidosis and cerebral calcification in three Saudi Arabian families. *Dev Med Child Neurol* **22**:72, 1980.
9. Whyte MP, Murphy WA, Fallon MD, Sly WS, Teitelbaum SL, MacAlister WH, Avioli LV: Osteopetrosis, renal tubular acidosis and basal ganglia calcification in three sisters. *Am J Med* **69**:65, 1980.
10. Tashian RE: Evolution and regulation of the carbonic anhydrase isozymes, in Rattazzi MC, Scandalios JG, Whitt GS (eds): *Isozymes: Current Topics in Biological and Medical Research* **2**:21, 1977.
11. Tashian RE, Hewett-Emmett D, Goodman M: On the evolution and genetics of carbonic anhydrases I, II, and III, in Rattazzi MC, Scandalios JG, Whitt GS (eds): *Isozymes: Current Topics in Biological and Medical Research* **7**:79, 1983.
12. Maren TH: Carbonic anhydrase: Chemistry, physiology and inhibitor. *Physiol Rev* **47**:595, 1967.
13. Lindskog S, Henderson LE, Kannan KK, Liljas A, Nyman PO, Strandberg B: Carbonic anhydrase, in Boyer PD (ed): *The Enzymes*. New York, Academic, 1971, p. 587.
14. Pocker Y, Sarkanen SLL: Carbonic anhydrase: Structure, catalytic versatility, and inhibition. *Adv Enzymol* **47**:149, 1978.
15. Waite LC, Volkert WA, Kenny AD: Inhibition of bone resorption by acetazolamide in the rat. *Endocrinology* **87**:1129, 1970.
16. Waite LC: Carbonic anhydrase inhibitors, parathyroid hormone and calcium metabolism. *Endocrinology* **91**:1160, 1972.
17. Minkin C, Jennings J: Carbonic anhydrase and bone remodeling: Sulfonamide inhibition of bone resorption in organ culture. *Science* **176**:1031, 1972.
18. Kumpulainen T, Nystrom SHM: Immunohistochemical localization of carbonic anhydrase isozyme C in human brain. *Brain Res* **220**:220, 1981.
19. Vogh BP: The relation of choroid plexus carbonic anhydrase activity to cerebrospinal fluid formation: Study of three inhibitors in cat with extrapolation to man. *J Pharmacol Exp Therap* **213**:321, 1980.
20. Nair V, Bau D: Studies on the functional significance of carbonic anhydrase in central nervous system. *Brain Res* **31**:185, 1971.
21. Wistrand PJ: Human renal cytoplasmic carbonic anhydrase. Tissue levels and kinetic properties under near physiological conditions. *Acta Physiol Scand* **109**:239, 1980.
22. Dobyan DC, Bulger RE: Renal carbonic anhydrase. *Am J Physiol* **243**:F311, 1982.
23. Kendall AG, Tashian RE: Erythrocyte carbonic anhydrase I: Inherited deficiency in humans. *Science* **197**:471, 1977.
24. Sly WS, Hewett-Emmett D, Whyte MP, Yu Y-SL, Tashian RE: Carbonic anhydrase II deficiency identified as the primary defect in the autosomal recessive syndrome of osteopetrosis with renal tubular acidosis and cerebral calcification. *Proc Natl Acad Sci USA* **80**:2752, 1983.
25. Sly WS, Whyte MP, Sundaram V, Tashian RE, Hewett-Emmett D, Guibaud P, Vainsel M, Baluarte HJ, Gruskin A, Al-Mosawi M, Sakati N, Ohlsson A: Carbonic anhydrase II deficiency in 12 families with the autosomal recessive syndrome of osteopetrosis with renal tubular acidosis and cerebral calcification. *N Engl J Med* **313**:139, 1985.
26. Ohlsson A, Cumming WA, Paul A, Sly WS: Carbonic anhydrase II deficiency syndrome: Recessive osteopetrosis with renal tubular acidosis and cerebral calcification. *Pediatrics* **77**:371, 1986.
27. Cochat P, Loras-Duclaux I, Guibaud P: Deficit en anhydrase carbonique II: Osteopetrose, acidose renale tubulaire et calcifications intracraniennes. Revue de la littérature à partir de trois observations. *Pediatrie* **42**:121, 1987.
28. Strisciuglio P, Sartorio R, Pecoraro C, Lotito F, Sly WS: Variable clinical presentation of carbonic anhydrase deficiency: Evidence for heterogeneity? *Eur J Pediatr* **149**:337, 1990.
29. Bejaoui M, Kamoun A, Baraket M, Bourguiba H, Lakhoua R: Le syndrome associant: Osteopetrose, acidose tubulaire, retard mental et calcifications intracraniennes par deficit en anhydrase carbonique II. *Arch Fr Pediatr* **48**:211, 1991.
30. Schwartz GJ, Brion LP, Corey HE, Dorfman HD: Case report 668. Carbonic anhydrase II deficiency syndrome (osteopetrosis associated with renal tubular acidosis and cerebral calcification). *Skeletal Radiol* **20**:447, 1991.
31. Eddy R, Resendes M, Genant H: Case report 718. Osteopetrosis with carbonic anhydrase II deficiency. *Skeletal Radiol* **21**:135, 1992.
32. Fathallah DM, Bejaoui M, Dellagi K, Hu PY, Sly WS: A single splice junction mutation underlies the CA II deficiency syndrome in North African patients of Arab descent. *FASEB J* **7**:A813, 1993.

32a. Whyte MP: Carbonic anhydrase II deficiency. *Clin Orthopaed Rel Res* **294**:52, 1993.

33. McKusick VA: *Mendelian Inheritance in Man* 10th ed., Vol. 2. Baltimore; Johns Hopkins University Press, 1992, p. 1616.
34. Ballet JP, Griscelli C, Coutri SG, Milhaud G, Maroteaux P: Bone marrow transplantation in osteopetrosis. *Lancet* **2**:1137, 1977.
35. Coccia PF, Krivit W, Cervenka J, Clawson C, Kersey JH, Kim TH, Nesbit ME, Ramsay NK, Warkentin PI, Teitelbaum SL, Kahn AJ, Brown DM: Successful bone-marrow transplantation for infantile malignant osteopetrosis. *N Engl J Med* **302**:701, 1980.
36. Leone G: Osteopetrosis recessive con calcificazioni cerebrali: Studio di 3 sogetti adulti in due famiglie consanguine. *Radiol Med* **68**:373, 1982.

37. Baluarte J, Hiner L, Root A, Gruskin A: Osteopetrosis and renal tubular acidosis. *Pediatr Res* **7**:412, 1973.
38. Bregman H, Brown J, Rogers A, Bourke E: Osteopetrosis with combined proximal and distal tubular acidosis. *Am J Kidney Dis* **2**:357, 1982.
39. Tashian RE: Evolution and regulation of the carbonic anhydrase isozymes, in Rattazzi MC, Scandalios JG, Whitt GS (eds): *Isozymes: Current Topics in Biological and Medical Research* **2**:21, 1977.
40. Zhu XL, Sly WS: Carbonic anhydrase IV from human lung: Purification, characterization, and comparison with membrane carbonic anhydrase from human kidney. *J Biol Chem* **265**:8795, 1990.
41. Brown D, Zhu XL, Sly WS: Localization of membrane-associated carbonic anhydrase type IV in kidney epithelial cells. *Proc Natl Acad Sci USA* **87**:7457, 1990.
42. Okuyama T, Sato S, Zhu XL, Waheed A, Sly WS: Human carbonic anhydrase IV: cDNA cloning, sequence comparison, and expression in COS cell membranes. *Proc Natl Acad Sci USA* **89**:1315, 1992.
43. Okuyama T, Batanian JR, Sly WS: Genomic organization and localization of gene for human carbonic anhydrase IV to chromosome 17q. *Genomics* **16**:678, 1993.
44. Feldstein JB, Silverman DN: Purification and characterization of carbonic anhydrase from the saliva of the rat. *J Biol Chem* **259**:5447, 1984.
45. Murakami H, Sly WS: Purification and characterization of human salivary carbonic anhydrase. *J Biol Chem* **262**:1382, 1987.
46. Fernley RT, Wright RD, Coghlan JP: Complete amino acid sequence of ovine salivary carbonic anhydrase. *Biochemistry* **27**:2815, 1988.
47. Nagao Y, Platero JS, Waheed A, Sly WS: Human mitochondrial carbonic anhydrase: cDNA cloning, expression, subcellular localization, and mapping to chromosome 16. *Proc Natl Acad Sci USA* **90**:7623, 1993.
48. Tashian RE: Genetics of the mammalian carbonic anhydrases. *Adv Genet* **30**:321, 1993.
49. Nakai H, Byers MG, Venta PJ, Tashian RE, Shows TB: The gene for human carbonic anhydrase II (CA 2) is located at chromosome 8q22. *Cytogenet Cell Genet* **44**:234, 1987.
50. Southerland GR, Baker E, Fernandez KEW, Callen DF, Aldred P, Coghlan JP, Wright RE, Fernley RT: The gene for human carbonic anhydrase VI (CA VI) is on the tip of the short arm of chromosome 1. *Cytogenet Cell Genet* **50**:149, 1989.
51. Montgomery JC, Venta PJ, Eddy RL, Fukushima YS, Shows TB, Tashian RE: Characterization of the human gene for a newly discovered carbonic anhydrase, CA VII, and its localization to chromosome 16. *Genomics* **11**:835, 1991.
52. Koester MK, Pullan LM, Noltmann EA: The *p*-nitrophenyl phosphatase activity of muscle carbonic anhydrase. *Arch Biochem Biophys* **211**:632, 1981.
53. Sanyal G, Swenson ER, Pessah NI, Maren TH: The carbon dioxide hydration activity of skeletal muscle carbonic anhydrase: Inhibition by sulfonamides and anions. *Mol Pharmacol* **22**:211, 1982.
54. Sanyal G, Maren TH: Thermodynamics of carbonic anhydrase catalysis: A comparison between isozymes B and C. *J Biol Chem* **256**:608, 1981.
55. Wistrand PJ: The importance of carbonic anhydrase B and C for the unloading of CO_2 by the human erythrocyte. *Acta Physiol Scand* **113**:417, 1981.
56. Tashian RE, Hewett-Emmett D, Dodgson SJ, Forster RE, Sly WS: The value of inherited deficiencies of human carbonic anhydrase isoenzymes in understanding their cellular roles. *Ann NY Acad Sci* **429**:262, 1984.
57. Waheed A, Zhu XL, Sly WS: Membrane-associated carbonic anhydrase from rat lung. *J Biol Chem* **267**:3308, 1991.
58. Fleming RE, Crouch EC, Ruzicka CA, Sly WS: Developmentally regulated carbonic anhydrase IV gene expression in the alveolar capillary endothelium. *Pediatr Res* **33-2**:48A (abstract 275), 1993.
59. Hageman GS, Zhu XL, Waheed A, Sly WS: Localization of carbonic anhydrase IV in a specific capillary bed of the human eye. *Proc Natl Acad Sci USA* **88**:2716, 1991.
60. Ghandour MS, Langley OK, Zhu XL, Waheed A, Sly WS: Carbonic anhydrase IV on brain capillary endothelial cells: A marker associated with the blood-brain barrier. *Proc Natl Acad Sci USA* **89**:6823, 1992.
61. Waheed A, Zhu XL, Sly WS, Wetzel P, Gros G: Rat skeletal muscle membrane associated carbonic anhydrase is 39-kDA, glycosylated, GPI-anchored CA IV. *Arch Biochem Biophys* **294**:550, 1992.
62. Nagao Y, Srinivasan M, Platero JS, Svendrowski M, Waheed A, Sly WS: Mitochondrial carbonic anhydrase (CA V) in mouse and rat: cDNA cloning, expression, subcellular localization, processing, and tissue distribution. *Proc Natl Acad Sci USA*, in press, 1994.
63. Venta PJ, Welty RJ, Johnson TM, Sly WS, Tashian RE: Carbonic anhydrase II deficiency syndrome in a Belgian family is caused by a point mutation at an invariant histidine residue (107 His→Tyr): Complete structure of the normal human CA II gene. *Am J Hum Genet* **49**:1082, 1991.
64. Roth DE, Venta PJ, Tashian RE, Sly WS: Molecular basis of human carbonic anhydrase II deficiency. *Proc Natl Acad Sci USA* **89**:1804, 1992.
65. Hu PY, Roth DE, Skaggs LA, Venta PJ, Tashian RE, Guibaud P, Sly WS: A splice junction mutation in intron 2 of the carbonic anhydrase II gene of osteopetrosis patients from Arabic countries. *Hum Mutat* **1**:288, 1992.
66. Gay CV, Mueller WJ: Carbonic anhydrase and osteoclasts: Localization by labelled inhibitor autoradiography. *Science* **183**:432, 1974.
67. Väänänen HK, Parvinen E-K: High activity isoenzyme of carbonic anhydrase in rat calvaria osteoclasts: Immunohistochemical study. *Histochemistry* **78**:481, 1983.
68. Baron R, Neff L, Louvard D, Courtoy PJ: Cell-mediated extracellular acidification and bone resorption: Evidence for a low pH in resorbing lacunae and localization of a 100-kD lysosomal membrane protein at the osteoclast ruffled border. *J Cell Biol* **101**:2210, 1985.
69. Sly WS, Whyte MP, Krupin T, Sundaram V: Positive renal response to intravenous acetazolamide in patients with carbonic anhydrase II deficiency. *Pediatr Res* **19**:1033, 1985.
70. Lonnerholm G: Histochemical locations of carbonic anhydrase in mammalian tissues. *Ann NY Acad Sci* **429**:369, 1984.
71. Spicer SS, Sens MA, Tashian RE: Immunocytochemical demonstration of carbonic anhydrase in human epithelial cells. *J Histochem Cytochem* **30**:864, 1982.
71a. Sato S, Zhu XL, Sly WS: Carbonic anhydrase isozymes IV and II in urinary membranes from carbonic anhydrase II-deficient patients. *Proc Natl Acad Sci USA* **87**:6073, 1990.
72. Alpern RJ, Stone DK, Rector FC Jr: Renal acidification mechanisms, in Renner BM and Rector FC Jr (eds): *The Kidney* 4th ed. Philadephia, W.B. Saunders, 1991, p 318.
73. Lucci MS, Tinker JP, Weiner IM, DuBose TD Jr: Function of proximal tubule carbonic anhydrase defined by selective inhibition. *Am J Physiol* **F245**:443, 1983.
74. DuBose TD, Pucacco LR, Carter NW: Determination of disequilibrium pH in the rat kidney in vivo: Evidence for hydrogen secretion. *Am J Physiol* **240**:F138, 1981.
75. Schwartz JH, Rosen S, Steinmetz PR: Carbonic anhydrase function and the epithelium organization of H^+ secretion in turtle urinary bladder. *J Clin Invest* **51**:2653, 1972.
76. Gluck S, Kelly S, Al-Awqati Q: The proton-translocating ATPase responsible for urinary acidification. *J Biol Chem* **257**:9230, 1982.
77. Kumpulainen T: Immunohistochemical localization of human carbonic anhydrase isozymes. *Ann NY Acad Sci* **429**:359, 1984.
78. Lees MB, Sapirstein VS, Reiss DS, Kolodny EH: Carbonic anhydrase and 2′,3′ cyclic nucleotide 3′-phosphohydrolase activity in normal human brain and in demyelinating diseases. *Neurology (NY)* **30**:719, 1980.
79. Venta PJ, Montgomery JC, Hewett-Emmett D, Tashian RE: Comparison of the 5′ regions of human and mouse carbonic anhydrase II genes and identification of possible regulatory elements. *Biochim Biophys Acta* **826**:195, 1985.
80. Hu PY, Ernst AR, Sly WS: UGA suppression of "Hispanic mutation" for CA II deficiency syndrome suggests novel mechanism for genetic heterogeneity. *Am J Hum Genet* **51**(Suppl):A29, 1992.
81. Sundaram V, Rumbolo P, Grubb J, Strisciuglio P, Sly WS: Carbonic anhydrase deficiency: Diagnosis and carrier

detection using differential enzyme inhibition and inactivation. *Am J Hum Genet* **38**:125, 1986.
82. Conroy CW, Maren TH: The determination of osteopetrotic phenotypes by selective inactivation of red cell carbonic anhydrase isoenzymes. *Clin Chim Acta* **152**:347, 1985.
83. Whyte MP, Hamm LL, Sly WS: Transfusion of carbonic anhydrase-replete erythrocytes fails to correct the acidification defect in the syndrome of osteopetrosis, renal tubular acidosis, and cerebral calcification (carbonic anhydrase-II deficiency). *J Bone Mineral Res* **3**:385, 1988.
84. Lewis SE, Erickson RP, Barnett LB, Venta PJ, Tashian RE: *N*-ethyl-*N*-nitrosourea-induced null mutation at the mouse Car-2 locus: An animal model for human carbonic anhydrase II deficiency syndrome. *Proc Natl Acad Sci USA* **85**:1962, 1988.
85. Baron R: Molecular mechanisms of bone resorption by the osteoclast. *Anat Rec* **224**:317, 1989.
86. Bushinsky DA, Goldring JM, Coe FL: Cellular contribution to pH-mediated calcium flux in neonatal mouse calvariae. *Am J Physiol* **248**:F785, 1985.
87. Raisz LG, Simmons HA, Thompson WJ, Shepard KL, Anderson PS, Rodan GA: Effects of a potent carbonic anhydrase inhibitor on bone resorption in organ culture. *Endocrinology* **122**:1083, 1988.
88. Anderson RE, Jee WS, Woodbury DM: Stimulation of carbonic anhydrase in osteoclasts by parathyroid hormone. *Calcif Tissue Int* **37**:646, 1985.
89. Hall GE, Kenny AD: Bone resorption induced by parathyroid hormone and dibutyryl cyclic AMP: Role of carbonic anhydrase. *J Pharmacol Exp Therap* **238**:778, 1986.
90. Kenny AD: Role of carbonic anhydrase in bone: Partial inhibition of disuse atrophy of bone by parenteral acetazolamide. *Calcif Tissue Int* **37**:126, 1985.
91. Hu PY, Ernst AR, Sly WS, Venta PJ, Skaggs LA, Tashian RE: Carbonic anhydrase II deficiency: Single base deletion in exon 7 is the predominant mutation in Caribbean Hispanic patients. *Am J Hum Genet* **54**:602, 1994.

CHAPTER 138

α_1-Antitrypsin Deficiency

Diane Wilson Cox

1. Alpha$_1$-antitrypsin (α_1AT), a glycoprotein of molecular mass 52 kDa, is a major plasma serine protease inhibitor (serpin). The major physiological substrate is elastase, particularly in the lower respiratory tract.

2. The locus (PI locus) for α_1AT is on chromosome 14 at 14q32.1, close to the locus for the protease inhibitor α_1-antichymotrypsin, and in a cluster of sequence-related genes that includes corticosteroid-binding globulin and protein C inhibitor. The gene is 12.2 kb long and contains six introns. α_1AT produced in hepatocytes has a 1.4-kb mRNA transcript, while macrophages have a longer RNA transcript, beginning in exons 5′ to the first exon for hepatocyte α_1AT.

3. α_1AT shows considerable genetic variability, having more than 70 genetic variants (PI types), many of which have been sequenced. Most variants are associated with quantitatively and qualitatively normal α_1AT. Further variation can be revealed at the DNA level, where a number of restriction enzymes reveal polymorphisms.

4. The *PI*Z* allele is the most common deficiency variant. PI ZZ homozygotes have 15 to 20 percent of the normal plasma concentration of α_1AT, with a correspondingly reduced concentration in bronchoalveolar lavage fluid. The deficiency is due to lack of secretion of Z α_1AT from the hepatocyte, where inclusions are formed in the rough endoplasmic reticulum. There are several rare deficiency types, including some that show lack of secretion, and some that have no product (null or Q0).

5. Liver inclusions are formed because of a tendency for Z α_1AT to self-aggregate. This occurs because the mobile reactive center loop of one protein molecule inserts into that of another molecule instead of its own, especially at body temperature.

6. A deficiency of α_1AT results in a protease/protease inhibitor imbalance in the lung, allowing destruction of the alveolar wall. The resultant obstructive lung disease is the most prevalent clinical manifestation of α_1AT deficiency. Basal lung regions are most severely affected. In nonsmokers, onset of dyspnea occurs at a mean age of 45 to 50 years, and in smokers at about 35 years of age. Smokers show a considerably higher rate of lung destruction and have a poorer survival rate than nonsmokers with the deficiency. Smoking enhances oxidation and inactivation of α_1AT in the lung.

7. Symptoms of liver abnormalities in infancy are expressed in about 17 percent of all individuals with α_1AT deficiency. Only a few percent of all patients with the deficiency have a poor prognosis after early liver symptoms. Other familial factors may influence the prognosis.

8. α_1AT appears to be involved in regulation of the immune system, perhaps through the production of proteases by T cells. The deficiency state may contribute to diseases with an immune component. Response to inflammation is also impaired.

9. Prenatal diagnosis can be carried out using the polymerase chain reaction and then either synthetic oligonucleotide probes or digestion with restriction enzymes.

10. Avoidance of smoking is important preventative therapy. Replacement therapy with α_1AT, by infusion or aerosol, is effective at increasing protease inhibition in the pulmonary alveoli, but the clinical impact is not defined. Antioxidants could potentially delay lung and liver destruction. Lung and liver transplants offer potential therapy for end-stage destruction of these organs.

α_1-Antitrypsin (α_1AT)* plays a central role as a protease inhibitor in controlling tissue degradation. As a major protease inhibitor in human plasma, α_1AT can complex with a broad spectrum of proteases, including elastase, trypsin, chymotrypsin, thrombin, and bacterial proteases. The most important inhibitor action is that against leukocyte elastase, a protease that degrades the elastin of the alveolar walls as well as other structural proteins of a variety of tissues. Studies of the deficiency state, which began with the astute observation of an abnormal protein pattern on electrophoresis, has led us to a better understanding of the pathogenesis of pulmonary emphysema and the role of protease inhibitors in other disease states.

α_1AT, isolated by Schultze et al.[1] as α_1-3,5-glycoprotein, was later named "α_1-antitrypsin" because most of the serum trypsin inhibitory activity was associated with the α_1-globulin fraction and, particularly, with the protein they had isolated. A discussion of the early studies can be found in previous reviews.[2] α_1AT became of clinical interest when C.-B. Laurell in Malmo, Sweden, noted while examining protein

A list of standard abbreviations is located immediately preceding the index in each volume. Additional abbreviations used in this chapter include: COPD = chronic obstructive pulmonary disease; MPGN = membranoproliferative glomerulonephritis; PAS-D = periodic acid–Schiff staining after diastase treatment; PI = protease inhibitor; SGOT = serum glutamic-oxaloacetic transaminase.

*The guidelines of the PI Nomenclature Committee (see ref. 96) prefer the abbreviation α1AT for α_1-antitrypsin (not α_1AT), and the preferred style for phenotype variants is Mmalton, Pclifton, etc. (not M_{MALTON}, $P_{CLIFTON}$, etc). The reasons for the preference, among others, are ease of e-mail transmission and use in data bases. Abbreviations used in this book are both feasible for the publisher and traditional for the book.

electrophoretic patterns that a number of patients lacked an α_1-globulin band. The α_1AT component deficiency was found to occur in a number of patients with early-onset emphysema[3] and was associated with a low serum trypsin inhibitory activity. A study of this deficiency became the subject of a thesis by S. Eriksson[4] and laid the foundation for much of our basic knowledge of the clinical effects of this deficiency. The codominant nature of the trait was expressed as a partial deficiency of serum trypsin inhibitory activity in heterozygotes and as a marked deficiency in homozygotes (for a review of the early discovery, see Eriksson[5]). These findings were confirmed in many parts of the world, and the picture emerged of progressive obstructive pulmonary disease, with preferential destruction in the lung base, affecting both males and females, beginning in the second and third decades, and particularly affecting smokers.

At about the same time, Fagerhol and Braend observed electrophoretic variation in the prealbumin (Pr) region, using starch gel electrophoresis, and showed that the Pr bands were α_1AT.[6] Pi (now PI), for protease inhibitor, was chosen as the symbol for the α_1AT polymorphism, since it was already recognized that α_1AT was an effective inhibitor for other proteases in addition to trypsin.[7] The first normal variant, PI X, was recognized as a doublet in agarose gel electrophoresis.[8] The extensive polymorphism of α_1AT was recognized through a starch gel electrophoresis system developed by M.K. Fagerhol.[9] This system was not easily reproduced and has now been replaced by high-resolution isoelectric focusing in polyacrylamide gels.

Another observation of major importance came in 1969 with the observation by H. Sharp and coworkers that α_1AT deficiency was associated with liver disease in children.[10] We now know that the liver disease is not usually as devastating as first suspected.

The association between α_1AT deficiency and obstructive lung disease has led to extensive studies of the mechanisms of protease tissue destruction and of the important role of a balance between proteases and their inhibitors. Studies of α_1AT have also examined the role of protease inhibitors in immune mechanisms, nondisjunction, and recombination. The extensive genetic variation has led to population and evolution studies. The deficiency state results from abnormal plasma protein secretion from the hepatocyte, and the study of the basic defect enhances our understanding of glycoprotein secretion mechanisms. Studies at the molecular level provide possibilities for examining recombination events in and around a cluster of genes forming a protease inhibitor complex (for recent general reviews, see refs. 11–13).

For some of the other plasma protease inhibitors, such as α_2-macroglobulin and α_1-antichymotrypsin, a deficiency state has not yet been discovered, although a partial deficiency of the latter has been observed and may be associated with disease.[14] In future years, the other protease inhibitors will no doubt prove to be as complex and interesting.

STRUCTURE OF α_1-ANTITRYPSIN

Protein Structure

α_1AT is a glycoprotein consisting of a single polypeptide chain of 394 residues and a carbohydrate content of 12 percent; the resulting molecular mass is 52 kDa. Methods for purification and details of protein characterization have been reviewed.[7,15] The small size of the protein allows it to diffuse through interstitial body fluids and into tissues such as the lung. The high negative charge of α_1AT in plasma (isoelectric point 4.4 to 4.7[16,17]) may be important in preventing loss of the protein across the negatively charged glomerular membrane.[18] A somewhat larger molecule that includes a 24-residue hydrophobic signal peptide is produced in the liver and in vitro.[19] Sequencing of cDNA has confirmed the presence of the signal peptide, with an N-terminal methionine.[20,21]

α_1AT, while not crystallizable in its active form, crystallizes after proteolytic cleavage at the reactive site,[22] forming a more stable relaxed (R) form.[23] Analysis of the crystal structure indicates that the single polypeptide chain is organized into well-defined secondary structural elements: three β sheets and eight α helixes. The first 150 residues preferentially form the α helixes. α_1AT contains one cysteine residue, as indicated by both protein and DNA analysis. No disulfide bridge is present in the protein, although the thiol group can form a disulfide bond with other proteins, such as the IgA heavy chain[24] and the thiol group of immunoglobulin κ light chain, the latter being the basis for a purification method.[25] Such protein binding can also produce artifacts on isoelectric focusing, which disappear when α_1AT is exposed to a reducing agent.

Microheterogeneity

α_1AT is modified during its passage through the endoplasmic reticulum of the hepatocyte. Some of this modification is reflected in the microheterogeneity observed in acid starch gel and agarose electrophoresis and in polyacrylamide isoelectric focusing, as is typical for glycoproteins when near their isoelectric point. Eight bands were originally noted, numbered from 1 (anodal) to 8 (cathodal); bands 4 and 6 contain 40 and 35 percent, respectively, of the total α_1AT[6] and have isoelectric points of 4.52 and 4.59.[17] Much of the heterogeneity is due to differences in the type of carbohydrate side chain.[26] Three carbohydrate side chains per molecule are attached at asparagine residues 46, 83, and 247.[27] The carbohydrate chains may be biantennary or triantennary, terminating in two or three *N*-acetylneuraminic acid residues[28] (Fig. 138-1). The electrophoretic mobility of α_1AT is sequentially shifted cathodally by incubation with neuraminidase, as *N*-acetylneuraminic acid residues are removed. Isoelectric focusing after total desialylation results in one major fraction and two minor ones, the anodal fraction representing a deamidation product and the more cathodal fraction representing the asialo form of bands 7 and 8.[17] The two minor cathodal components (7 and 8) have the same carbohydrate structure as the major bands (4 and 6), but the first five amino acids (Glu-Asp-Pro-Glu-Gly) have been removed, apparently by posttranslational cleavage.[29] Alterations in the usual pattern of microheterogeneity are observed in newborns and upon estrogen administration, with an increased percentage in bands 6 and 8 relative to bands 4 and 7 (referenced in Fagerhol and Cox[7]). During inflammation or with high levels of estrogen, 80 percent of the increase in concentration of plasma α_1AT occurs in bands 2 and 4, which is explained by the replacement of biantennary by triantennary oligosaccharides.[29]

Reactive Site

Protease inhibition by α_1AT occurs by formation of a tightly bound 1:1 complex between α_1AT and the target protease, which can be one of a number of serine proteases but is

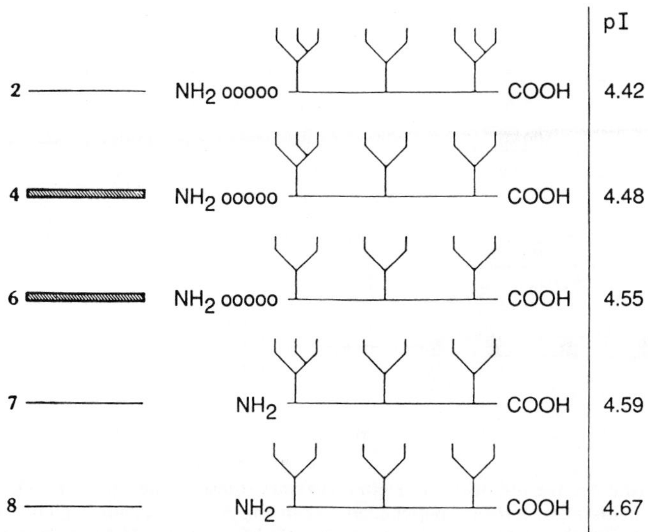

FIG. 138-1 **Distribution of biantennary and triantennary oligosaccharide chains responsible for the microheterogeneity of α_1AT. Attachments for the oligosaccharide chains are at the Asn positions 46, 83, and 247. M7 and M8 lack the first five N-terminal amino acids. The isoelectric points for each fraction are indicated. ooooo:Glu-Asp-Pro-Glu-Gly.** ***(Modified from Jeppsson et al.[29] Used by permission.)***

mainly elastase. Specificity is determined by crucial amino acids in the reactive site of α_1AT. The methionine residue at position 358 close to the C-terminus of the molecule[30] is important for functional activity (Fig. 138-2).[31] In intact inhibitor, a strand containing the methionine residue is exposed on the surface of the molecule in a loop formation, as proposed for the general mechanism for protease inhibitors.[33] This loop fits precisely the conformation of the reactive site of the target protease. The insertion of a single residue, threonine 345, into sheet A is required for activity of α_1AT. Proteolytic cleavage at the reactive site causes release of the strand and its subsequent incorporation into β sheet A,[22] a mechanism common to the serine protease superfamily.[34] The exposed position of the reactive site allows ready access for oxidation. According to this model, methionine, when oxidized to methionine sulfoxide, can no longer physically complex with elastase, and α_1AT becomes inactive.[35] The association constant for oxidized α_1AT is 1000 times lower than for native α_1AT.[36] In some situations, the release of oxygen radicals from leukocytes and the subsequent oxidation of methionine may be advantageous, for example, by allowing local tissue breakdown in areas of inflammation.[37]

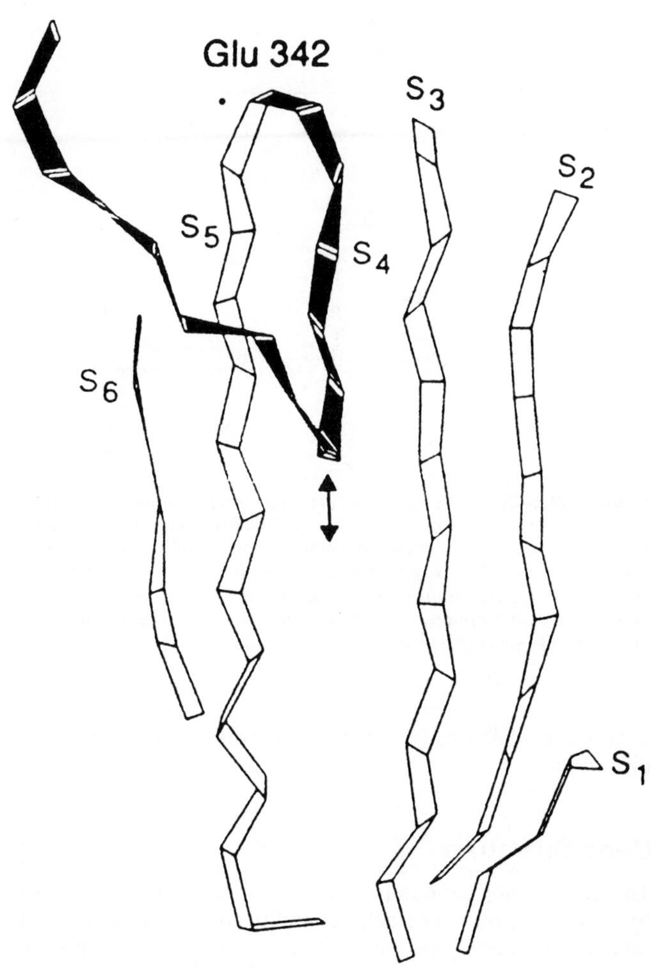

FIG. 138-2 **A diagrammatic representation of the A sheet of α_1AT. The reactive center loop (shaded) is mobile and can hinge on Glu 342 to fold back into a gap in the A sheet. Disruption of this folding by the Z mutation Glu 342→Lys allows the loop of a second PI Z molecule to insert, giving "loop-sheet polymerization."** ***(From Lomas et al.[32] Used by permission. Photograph courtesy of R.W. Carrell.)***

The reactive sites of several of the serine protease inhibitors are similar not only to each other but also to those of low-molecular-weight plant protease inhibitors. Substrate specificity is determined by the composition of the reactive site (Table 138-1). The specificity for methionine at amino acid 358 has been proved in a rare natural mutant of α_1AT, PI Pittsburgh, in which arginine is substituted for methionine 358.[359] This mutant has lost the capacity for inhibiting porcine

Table 138-1 **Reactive Centers of Selected Protease Inhibitors**

		Reactive Center*					
Inhibitor	**Substrate**	**P_1**	**P_1'**	**P_2'**	**P_3'**	**P_4'**	**P_5'**
Human α_1AT	Elastase	Met	Ser	Ile	Pro	Pro	Glu
Human α_1–antichymotrypsin	Chymotrypsin	Leu	Ser	Ala	Leu	Val	Glu
Mouse α_1AT	Elastase	Tyr	Ser	Met	Pro	Pro	Ile
Mouse contrapsin†	Trypsin	Lys	Ala	Ile	Leu	Pro	Ala
Human antithrombin III	Thrombin	Arg	Ser	Leu	Asn	Pro	Asn

*From Hill et al.[38]
†Possibly an α_1–antichymotrypsin homologue.

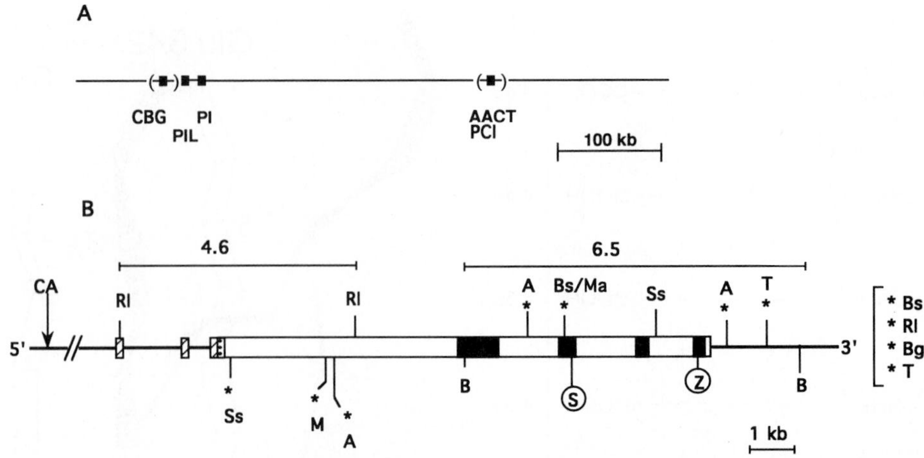

FIG. 138-3 *A.* PI and other loci in the serpin superfamily cluster on chromosome 14, as determined by pulsed field gel electrophoresis.[40] PIL = PI-like, CBG = corticosteroid-binding globulin, PCI = protein C inhibitor, AACT = α_1-antichymotrypsin. *B.* α_1AT gene and flanking regions. Coding regions are solid rectangles, introns are open rectangles, and untranslated regions are dotted rectangles. Cross-hatched regions are exons of macrophage DNA. Asterisks indicate sites of polymorphisms for the following restriction enzymes (those in the square bracket at the right indicate polymorphisms in the 3′ homologous region): A = *Ava* II; B = *Bam* HI; Bg = *Bgl* II; BS = *Bst* EII; M = *Msp* I; Ma = *Mae* III; T = *Taq* I; RI = *Eco* RI; Ss = *Sst* I; S and Z circled = sites of mutations in *PI*S* and *PI*Z*, respectively. Genomic probes, 4.6 and 6.5 kb, are indicated. The arrow marks the position of the CA repeat.

pancreatic elastase yet is a highly effective inhibitor of thrombin.

Gene Structure

The gene coding for α_1AT, 12.2 kb in length, includes a 1434 bp coding region.[20] The gene contains six introns; exons 1A through 1C, the 5′ portion of exons 2, and the 3′ portion of exon 5 are noncoding regions (Fig. 138-3). The largest intron (between exons 1C and 2), 5.3 kb in length, contains a 143-amino-acid open reading frame, an *Alu* sequence, and a pseudo-transcription-initiation region. The open reading frame does not appear to be an actual protein-coding region.

The regulatory region of the structural gene and relevant transcription factors have been well characterized (for reviews, see refs. 41 and 42). In hepatocytes, the region beginning 721 kb 5′ to the transcription start site in exon 1C is necessary for efficient expression of the α_1AT gene and for cell-specific expression.[43] In monocytes and macrophages, an initiation site 5′ to the hepatocyte initiation site is used, and a longer RNA transcript is produced.[44] This alternate form of α_1AT has a separate promoter and includes two additional exons, 1A and 1B.[45] The second of these three additional macrophage exons (1B) is optionally transcribed in macrophage α_1AT, resulting in two forms of macrophage mRNA.[45]

Homologous Proteins

DNA and protein sequencing studies have indicated homology not only between some of the protease inhibitors but also between inhibitors and other plasma proteins, as well as with chicken ovalbumin.[46] Human α_1AT and α_1-antichymotrypsin share 56 percent homology in their coding nucleotide sequences and 42 percent homology in their amino acids.[47] Human α_1AT and protein C inhibitor share 42 percent amino acid identity.[48] An unexpectedly high degree of homology has been observed between α_1AT and two noninhibitor human plasma proteins: thyroxine-binding globulin, located on the X chromosome (58 percent),[49] and corticosteroid-binding globulin, located on chromosome 14 (53 percent).[50] There is 28 percent homology between the amino acid sequences of antithrombin III and α_1AT,[51] and 27 percent between C1 inhibitor and α_1AT.[52] A similar degree of amino acid sequence homology is observed between portions of chick ovalbumin and α_1AT[46,53]; the position and number of introns is very different, however, probably indicating a relatively ancient divergence from a common ancestral gene several hundred million years ago.[53]

Localization of the Structural Gene

The PI locus that encodes α_1AT was localized to chromosome 14 by linkage studies with Gm, the system of inherited markers of the gamma immunoglobulins,[54] by analysis of protein production by somatic cell hybrids,[55,56] and by DNA analysis of somatic cell hybrids.[57] The PI locus, regionally localized to band 14q32.1,[58,59] is a member of a cluster of homologous genes with similar intron–exon structure. A region homologous to α_1AT, called PI-like (PIL locus), apparently not a functional gene, lies 8.2 kb 3′ to the α_1AT gene.[40,44,60] α_1-Antichymotrypsin,[61] the blood coagulation factor protein C inhibitor, and corticosteroid-binding globulin have been shown by pulsed field electrophoresis to lie within 280 kb of α_1AT[40] (Fig. 138-3A).

PHYSIOLOGY OF α_1-ANTITRYPSIN

Function of α_1-Antitrypsin

α_1AT inhibits a broad spectrum of serine proteases. Because of its efficiency of inhibition, broad substrate specificity, and ready access to tissue, α_1AT plays an important role in defending tissues from proteolysis. α_1AT inhibits most serine proteases tested to date, including pancreatic and neutrophil elastase, neutrophil cathepsin G, pancreatic trypsin and chymotrypsin, collagenase from skin and synovia, acrosin, kallikrein, urokinase, and renin (see refs. 7 and 36). Proteases in the clotting and fibrinolytic systems that are inhibited include plasmin, thrombin, factor XI, and Hageman factor cofactor.[7] Some of these inhibitor activities may reflect only in vitro phenomena, which have no physiological importance because of the presence in the body of other, more potent inhibitors for each specific protease.

α_1AT complex formation results in inactivation of the protease and proteolytic cleavage of the inhibitor. The rate of inactivation of α_1AT with specific proteases varies considerably, but is greatest with neutrophil elastase, for which the association constant is $6.5 \times 10^7/M$/sec, more than 10^6 times higher than that with thrombin.[36] Evidence for the important role of α_1AT as a neutrophil elastase inhibitor, reviewed previously,[62] is provided by many studies showing the effectiveness of human neutrophil elastase at inducing emphysema in experimental animals. Study of these animal models has demonstrated that the destruction of elastin fibers is of primary importance for producing the lung degradation typical of emphysema.[62] α_1AT provides approximately 90 percent of the antielastase activity in plasma. The other plasma inhibitor of elastase, α_2-macroglobulin, largely lacks access to the lower respiratory tract because of its high molecular mass (725 kDa); the small amounts of α_2-macroglobulin in the lower respiratory tract[63] may be produced locally by lung fibroblasts[64] or by macrophages.

Although a number of proteases in the clotting cascade are inhibited by α_1AT, these reactions do not appear to be of prime physiological significance, probably because of the presence of other, more effective inhibitors. Individuals with α_1AT deficiency have not been reported to have abnormalities in coagulation or fibrinolysis. However, the change of only one amino acid at the active center (in PI Pittsburgh) converts α_1AT into a potent inhibitor of thrombin and factor XI, producing a severe bleeding disorder during the acute-phase response.[65]

Since α_1AT increases during the acute-phase response and is also a trypsin inhibitor, and since trypsin inhibitors are known to have antibacterial activity, α_1AT may play some role in resistance to infection.[66,67] The association of α_1AT deficiency with a spectrum of inflammatory diseases suggests that α_1AT is important in the inflammatory response.

Function in the Immune Response

Proteases and their inhibitors have been shown, in a number of studies, to affect the immune response (reviewed by Fagerhol and Cox[7]). Trypsin and chymotrypsin act as mitogens for B lymphocytes. Trypsin, neutrophil elastase, and cathepsin G can substitute for helper T cells in B cell mitogen assays. Mouse thymocytes are triggered to synthesize DNA by neutrophils or macrophages or substances released from them. Human lymphocytes have α_1AT bound to their plasma membrane after concanavalin-A-induced blastogenic transformation.[68] Enhanced lymphocyte responsiveness to phytohemagglutinin has been observed in α_1AT-deficient individuals and decreases with the addition of highly purified α_1AT.[69] α_1AT has been reported to inhibit antibody-dependent cell-mediated cytotoxicity, T-cell-mediated cytotoxicity, and natural killer activity. α_1AT has a direct effect on adherent cells but not on proliferating T cells. There are elastase/α_1AT receptors on the surface of macrophages.[70] However, it is not clear whether α_1AT is synthesized by T lymphocytes.[71,72] This potential for increased T-helper activity and B-cell activation could lead to the exaggerated cell-mediated immunity and marked acceleration of delayed hypersensitivity responses, which have been demonstrated in vivo.[70] In addition to mitogenic activity, proteases also cleave IgG, liberating the Fc fragment, which can augment lymphocyte response.[69] The mechanism and extent of involvement of α_1AT in immune regulation still remains to be clarified.

Synthesis

α_1AT is synthesized mostly in the parenchymal cells of the liver (see Fagerhol and Cox[7]). Direct evidence is provided by the observed change of the genetic type of α_1AT to that of the donor after liver transplantation.[73,74] Cultured human fetal liver cells synthesize and secrete α_1AT; the secretion of α_1AT is suppressed by increasing concentrations of α_1AT in the medium, suggesting a feedback control mechanism.[75] Further support for feedback control comes from transgenic mice. With high production due to many gene copies, α_1AT accumulates in unaggregated form in the hepatocytes within a subset of distended cisternae of the rough endoplasmic reticulum, and secretion of murine α_1AT decreases.[76]

The production of α_1AT by monocytes[77] and alveolar macrophages[78] may be important in the regulation of local tissue injury. Transcription and translation of the α_1AT gene, followed by posttranslational processing and secretion of α_1AT in a functionally active form, has been demonstrated in human peripheral blood monocytes and in macrophages from bronchoalveoli and from breast milk.[72] Although the amount of α_1AT produced is very small, macrophage production could be important in the defense system of the lung.

In addition to showing that α_1AT is produced mainly in the liver, analysis of tissue RNA indicates that low levels are produced in the kidney, lung, and intestine.[44] In studies of transgenic mice, α_1AT production (both mRNA and protein) has been observed in chondrocytes, thymic epithelial cells and Hassall's bodies, macrophages in lymphoid tissue of the small intestine, gastric and small intestinal crypt epithelial cells, renal distal tubule brush border, and the lining of pulmonary alveoli.[44,79,80] The function and importance of α_1AT in kidney and intestine are yet to be discovered. The expression of α_1AT in the intestines is probably of some physiological importance. α_1AT is expressed in the colonic epithelial tumor cell line CACO2, a cell that differentiates into ileal-like cells. α_1AT of the hepatocyte form is produced both in this line and in jejunum.[81]

The catabolic rate of the normal type of α_1AT in plasma has been estimated at 6.7 days.[82] Removal of 20 percent and 100 percent of the sialic acid residues reduced the half-life to 4.0 and 0.8 days, respectively.[83]

Plasma Concentration

The average plasma concentration of α_1AT in healthy individuals (PI type MM) has been estimated to be 1.3 mg/ml.[17] However, concentration varies according to PI type.

The concentration of α_1AT in plasma can be measured either by functional assays or by immunochemical methods (see Cox et al.[84] for details). Functional assays, which evaluate inhibition of trypsin or elastase, can use protein substrates[85] or synthetic substrates such as alpha-*N*-benzoyl-DL-arginine-*p*-nitroanilide (BAPNA) for trypsin[86] and *N*-*tert*-butoxycarbonyl-L-alanine-*p*-nitrophenyl ester (NBA)[87] or *N*-succinyl-L-alanyl-L-alanyl-L-alanyl-L-alanine-*p*-nitroanilide (SLAPN)[88] for elastase. Appropriate immunologic methods include radial immunodiffusion,[89] electroimmuno assay,[90] and automated nephelometric methods. The results of immunologic methods frequently vary considerably between laboratories because of differences in commercial standards supplied. For this reason, many laboratories express normal values as percent of a normal pool of a large number of normal healthy individuals not pregnant or on medication, which can be assigned the value of 1.3 mg/ml.[17] Correlation between these methods is generally high, but the functional assays include a component due to α_2-macroglobulin activity. As an acute-phase protein, α_1AT can show a fourfold increase in plasma concentration during infection. A marked increase in concentration occurs in a wide range of inflammatory conditions, in response to typhoid vaccine injection, in cancer, and in liver disease (reviewed by Fagerhol and Cox[7]). Modest increases of concentration are induced by estrogen, whether during pregnancy or when administered as therapy.[91]

In addition to the inherited deficiency, low levels of α_1AT occur during the respiratory distress syndrome in newborns,[92] during severe protein-losing conditions,[4] during terminal liver failure,[93] and during the course of cystic fibrosis.[93]

GENETIC VARIATION

Genetic (PI) Variants

There are many inherited variants of α_1AT. *PI*M*, which can be further classified into subtypes, is the most common allele in all populations described to date. The *PI*S* allele reaches polymorphic frequencies in many populations, as does the *PI*Z* allele, which produces a deficiency of α_1AT.

In addition to common variants of α_1AT, more than 60 rare variants of α_1AT have been identified. The inheritance is described as codominant because expression of both alleles can be observed in the heterozygote by various electrophoretic techniques. The PI (protease inhibitor) variants, initially identified primarily by the method of acid starch gel electrophoresis developed by Fagerhol, were named in order of their mobility: F (fast), M (medium), S (slow), and Z (the most cathodal).[9] Additional variants were given alphabetic designations according to their mobility in starch. In 1974, isoelectric focusing in polyacrylamide gel was introduced for resolution of PI variants.[16,94,95] Nomenclature guidelines were established, with the position by isoelectric focusing as the criterion for designating subsequent variants.[96] Birthplace names were used to designate the more rare alleles and may be abbreviated to the first three letters of the name of the place of origin. According to the nomenclature guidelines,[96] with subsequent modification according to general guidelines for human gene nomenclature,[97] alleles at the PI locus are designated *PI*M, PI*S*, etc. Phenotypes are designated as PI MZ, PI M (or MM if confirmed in family studies). Genotype is indicated as *PI*M/PI*Z*, etc. Alleles that produce no detectable α_1AT in serum were originally designated as *PI*null*, with genotypes, –, *PI M*–, etc. According to general nomenclature guidelines, the null alleles are designated *PI*Q0*. This can be followed by a place name as for the other variants.

Earlier methods for identifying PI variants, including starch gel electrophoresis, isoelectric focusing, and agarose gel electrophoresis, have been reviewed.[7] Isoelectric focusing offers increased resolution of the variants, better reproducibility, and the possibility of typing many (up to 50) samples on a single gel. A suitable method for PI typing by isoelectric focusing has been described,[98] and many modifications have been developed. Very-narrow-range ampholytes improved the resolving power of isoelectric focusing[99] and are available commercially, as stock or in commercially prepared gels. The resolving power of isoelectric focusing has also been improved by the use of separators.[100] These methods resolved a further M subtype, M4, and other variants. As the limits of this approach were reached, immobilized pH gradients were applied to PI typing,[101] and various modifications have been described.[102,103] The use of ultrathin isoelectric focusing gels and a narrow pH gradient, e.g., 4.2 to 4.9, appears to produce resolution similar to that of immobilized gradients.[104]

Typical results using isoelectric focusing and narrow-range ampholytes for the most clinically important PI variants are shown in Figure 138-4A. The improved resolution that can be obtained with immobilized pH gradients and the additional, probably rare, M subtypes that can be differentiated are shown in Figure 138-4B. Figure 138-5 indicates the relative position by isoelectric focusing of a number of the variants and should serve as a guideline for those wishing to identify unusual variants.[96] Lists of variants, with references, have been published.[106,107]

Most PI variants are associated with normal concentrations of α_1AT. The exceptions are PI I, associated on average with 68 percent of the normal concentration of α_1AT[108]; PI S[109] and $W_{BETHESDA}$[110] at 60 percent of normal; and PI P at 30 percent of normal.[111] (A number of variants with a mobility relatively close to P have a normal concentration of α_1AT). PI S, P, and $W_{BETHESDA}$ show increased intracellular degradation. Most electrophoretic variants tested to date have normal functional capacity,[112] but the rare variant $M_{MINERALSPRINGS}$ has a modest reduction of inhibitory function. These variants have been reported to be associated with emphysema only when in combination with a true deficiency variant, and are classified here as normal variants. The types considered to be associated with high risk for disease all have less than 20 percent of the normal concentration of α_1AT; they are discussed subsequently. The normal ranges for PI types commonly found in the population are as follows, expressed as percent of a normal plasma pool ± 1 standard deviation[113] (similar to previous values[109]): M, 100 ± 23.5; MZ, 64 ±

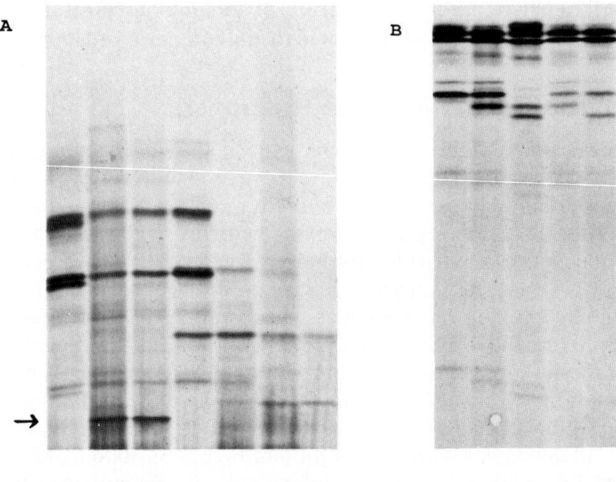

FIG. 138-4 **Selected PI variants observed in human sera using isoelectric focusing, polyacrylamide gel. Anode is at the top.** ***A.*** **Routine isoelectric focusing, as described by Cox[106] and Jeppsson and Franzen[98] but using Pharmalyte pH 4.5 to 5.5. Lane 1 = M1M2, 2 = M1Z, 3 = M1, 4 = M1S, 5 = SZ, 6 = ZZ with pronounced anodal components similar to position of S, 7 = ZZ. Dots indicate major Z bands. Lanes 2 and 3 have a cathodal component (arrow) occasionally found in patients with liver disease.** ***B.*** **Increased separation of PI M variants by hybrid PIEF, and an ultranarrow immobilized pH gradient, 4.5 to 4.75. Lane 1 = M1, 2 = M1M3, 3 = M2M3, 4 = M1M4, 5 = M1M2.** ***(From Weidinger and Cleve.[105] Used by permission.)***

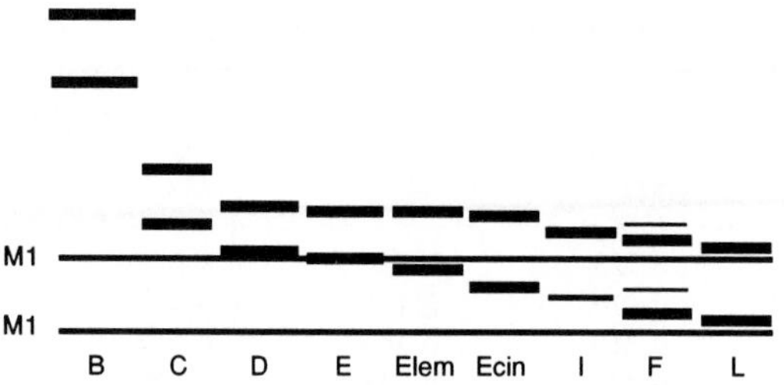

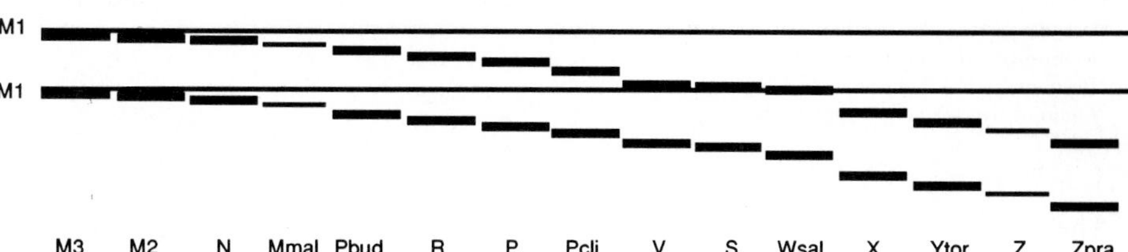

FIG. 138-5 Diagram of selected anodal (top row) and cathodal (bottom row) PI variants as revealed by isoelectric focusing in polyacrylamide gel. The positions of the two major bands of M1 are indicated by the solid lines. Anode at top. References are found in Cox et al.[96]

15.2; MS, 86 ± 20.5. Most of the quantitative variation is accounted for by PI type.[114]

Not all the variation observed electrophoretically is due to genetic differences. The cysteine in α_1AT appears able to react with a variety of other plasma components to produce artifacts, which usually disappear if plasma samples are reduced prior to isoelectric focusing.[98] Anodal variants are observed in patients with liver disease and can be mistaken for the F or E variants. A variant cathodal to Z has been described in a child with cytomegalovirus and fatty liver[115] and is also noted in other patients, mainly those with liver disease (Fig. 138-4A). Sometimes the additional bands that appear to be α_1AT are due to other proteins and are not observed when immunofixation is used. Repeat testing of patients frequently indicates the transitory nature of these unusual patterns. Family studies are a prerequisite for showing that variants are truly genetic.

Amino Acid/DNA Sequence of PI Variants

The amino acid sequence has been determined for a number of types of α_1AT, either directly or by DNA sequence analysis. The mutations identified are listed in Table 138-2. An alanine-valine substitution at amino acid position 213, noted by amino acid sequencing,[30] was further identified by DNA studies of both Z and M1.[116] The alanine substitution is found in about 34 percent of *PI*M1* alleles[116,117] and differentiates two subtypes of M1: M1(Ala213) and M1(Val213). The *PI*Z* allele has the Ala213 substitution; however, PI types M2, M3, and S all have valine at position 213.[116,117] The Z and S variant sites were confirmed by both amino acid[118–120] and DNA sequencing[20]; those for P,[121] Pittsburg,[39] $X_{CHRISTCHURCH}$,[122] and X, by amino acid sequencing only. Variants with similar electrophoretic properties do not necessarily have the same mutation.

Table 138-2 Sequenced Normal "Nondeficiency" α_1-Antitrypsin Variants

PI Type	Amino Acid No.	Exon	Ancestral Allele	Normal Amino Acid	DNA Codon	Mutant Amino Acid	DNA Codon
M1val (and Z)	213	3	M1val213	Val	GTG	—	—
M1ala	213	3	M1ala213	Ala	GCG	—	—
M3	376	5	M1val213	Glu	GAA	Asp	GAC
M2	101	2	M3	Arg	CGT	His	CAT
M4	101	2	M1val213	Arg	CGT	His	CAT
F	223	3	M1val213	Arg	CGT	Cys	TGT
$P_{SAINTALBANS}$	256 (silent)	3	M1val213	Asp	GAT	Asp	GAC
	341	5		Asp	GAC	Asn	AAC
V_{MUNICH}	2	2	M1val213	Asp	GAT	Ala	GCT
X	204	3	M1val213	Glu	GAG	Lys	(AAG)*
$X_{CHRISTCHURCH}$	363	5		Glu	GAG	Lys	(AAG)
Pittsburgh	358	5		Met	ATG	Arg	(AGG)
Reduced Plasma Concentration							
I	39	2	M1val213	Arg	CGC	Cys	TGC
S	264	3	M1val213	Glu	GAA	Val	GTA
P†	256	3	M1val213	Asp	GAT	Val	GTT
$M_{MINERALSPRINGS}$	67	2	M1ala213	Gly	GGG	Glu	GAG
$W_{BETHESDA}$	336	5	M1ala213	Ala	GCT	Thr	ACT

*Codons in parentheses are predicted as most likely from amino acid sequence.
†Identical sequence reported for *PI*Q0*$_{CARDIFF}$ and *PI*P*$_{LOWELL}$.

Table 138-3 Allele Frequencies in Selected Populations*

		PI Alleles					
Population Origin	No. Tested	M1	M2	M3	S	Z	Other
Denmark	909	0.728	0.136	0.082	0.022	0.023	0.009
Netherlands	357	0.679	0.147	0.129†	0.029	0.013	0.003
Portugal	900	0.510	0.260	0.053	0.150	0.009	0.018
U.S. (white)	904	0.724	0.137	0.095	0.023	0.014	0.007
U.S. (black)	549	0.982	—	—	0.015	0.004	—
China‡	1010	0.709	0.209	0.070	—	—	0.012
Japan	746	0.786	0.153	0.062	—	—	—

*References are listed in Cox.[125]
†Frequency of *PI*M3* plus *PI*M4*.
‡Mean of five Chinese populations.

The S variant, which is associated with a modestly reduced plasma concentration, has been shown to have slight changes in internal hydrogen bonds and salt bridge linkages, which could reduce the rate of folding and thermal stability.[123]

Population Studies

The distribution of the PI alleles has now been determined for many populations. In all populations, *PI*M* is the most common allele. The early population studies carried out by starch gel electrophoresis are summarized in refs. 2 and 124. These studies showed a low frequency of variants in Finns, Lapps, and Asians, and a high frequency of *PI*S* in Spain and Portugal. Since crossed immunoelectrophoresis was not used in the early studies, the *PI*Z* allele frequency could have been underestimated. In late studies, PI typing was carried out by acid starch gel electrophoresis with crossed immunoelectrophoresis or by isoelectric focusing. A number of the population studies, up to 1985, are summarized in refs. 7, 66, and 107.

Data from selected recent population studies, including PI M subtype frequencies, are presented in Table 138-3. This table includes only a few of the populations studied and is meant to illustrate the major population differences. The frequency of *PI*M1* is the highest in all populations studied, with *PI*M2* the next most frequent, and *PI*M3* relatively uncommon. The additional subtype allele *PI*M4* has been described in several populations at a frequency of 0.002 to 0.050.[100,126,127] In many studies, no differentiation was made between PI types M3 and M4, since these are not easily separated by isoelectric focusing. The *PI*S* allele is rare or absent in black and oriental populations, highest in Spain and Portugal, next most frequent in France, and low generally in other parts of Europe. The frequency of *PI*Z* (discussed subsequently) is highest in Scandinavian countries, and the allele is present throughout white populations, including those of the Middle East,[128] and is absent from oriental and black populations, except in those populations known to have a white admixture, as in the United States. There are two unusual exceptions to the distribution of the *PI*Z* allele. The black Somalians have been reported to have a relatively high frequency of the *PI*Z* allele.[129] However, the apparent PI ZZ types could have been caused by sample degradation and were not confirmed by family studies, or they could represent a European admixture (G. Massi, personal communication, 1987). A coastal group of New Zealand Maoris were reported to have a high frequency of the Z allele,[130] which could have been introduced by English seamen in the mid-eighteenth century.

DNA Polymorphisms

In addition to the extensive variation found in the protein by electrophoretic methods, further variation is found in the DNA sequence, as recognized by restriction enzymes, producing restriction fragment length polymorphisms (RFLP). Commonly used genomic clones[20,53] and the polymorphic sites are shown in Fig. 138-3B. Three polymorphisms have been described with probe 4.6, using the restriction enzymes *Sst* I, *Msp* I, and *Ava* II.[131] The allele frequencies are shown in Table 138-4. These polymorphisms are all in the first intron of the α_1AT gene, as shown in Fig. 138-3B, and show weaker linkage disequilibrium than expected, suggesting that this may be a region of increased recombination.[131,132] Polymorphisms are detected with probe 6.5 using the restriction enzymes *Ava* II, *Mae* III, *BstE* II, *Taq* I, and *Eco* RI (Table 138-4). *Ava* II detects polymorphisms in both the α_1AT gene and the homologous sequence and was the first enzyme to show a unique DNA haplotype for PI ZZ individuals.

When amino acid 213 is alanine, as found in Z and a portion of M1 α_1AT, a restriction site for *BstE* II[116] and *Mae* III[117,132] is not present as it is in those PI types with valine at amino acid 213. When *Mae* III is used to detect this difference, a polymorphism in the 3′ PI-like homologous region is detected in addition to the polymorphism in the α_1AT gene. The unique *Mae* III polymorphism has been found in association with all of 31 *PI*Z* alleles tested.[135] A restriction site for *BstE* II adjacent to amino acid 213 is lost in Z and in some M1 sequences,[116] but the difference in length would not be detectable using *BstE* II only. The polymorphism can be recognized using a double digest such as *BstE* II and *Bgl* II.[136] *Bgl* II also recognizes a polymorphism outside the α_1AT gene, apparently in the PI-like region,[137] producing a unique haplotype associated with *PI*Z*.[136] A *Taq* I polymorphism is located in the flanking region immediately 3′ to the α_1AT gene,[131,138,139] and an *Eco* RI polymorphism is located in the PI-like sequence.[133]

Most of the polymorphisms detected with probe 6.5 do not lie in the α_1AT gene, as determined by examining the known sequence, but instead lie in the downstream homologous sequence. The fragments appear much less intense on autoradiograms than those in the α_1AT gene. There is extensive linkage disequilibrium throughout the α_1AT gene.[132] With probe 6.5, the most useful combination

Table 138-4 Allele Frequencies for DNA Polymorphisms

Probe	Restriction Enzyme	Alleles (kb)	Allele Frequency* +	−	0	No. of Haplotypes	Heterozygosity
4.6	*Sst* I	1.8, 1.9	0.69	0.31	—	2	0.43
	Msp I	0.95, 0.98	0.47	0.53	—	2	0.49
	Ava II	0.9, 1.1	0.65	0.35	—	2	0.45
6.5	*Mae* III	2.3, 2.5	0.71	0.29	—	4	0.68
	Mae III (3′)	0.5, 0.7	0.65	0.35	—		
	Ava II (5/7)	0.48, 0.68	0.22	0.78	—	4	0.61
	Ava II (1/4)(3′)	0.72, 2.7	0.29	0.71	—		
	Taq I	1.4, 2.0	0.97	0.03	—	4	0.63
	Taq I (3′)	4.8, 6.7, 0	0.53	0.26	0.21		
	Eco RI (3′)	5.7, 8.6	0.23	0.77	—	2	0.35
(CA)n repeat		20–54 repeats				18	0.90

*+ = Presence of restriction site; − = absence of restriction site; 0 = no fragment.
NOTE: Data for 4.6 probe from Cox et al.[131] and Cox et al.[132]; data for 6.5 probe from Cox et al.[132] except *Eco* RI from Hodgson and Kalsheker[133]; (CA)n repeat from Byth and Cox.[134]

for detecting genetic variation is any enzyme that provides a polymorphism in the α_1AT gene (e.g., *Ava* II, *Mae* III, or *BstE* II) in combination with a restriction enzyme that detects a taq polymorphism in the downstream region that does not show complete equilibrium,[132] such as *Taq* I or *Bgl* II.

DNA polymorphisms and haplotypes are of particular interest for evolutionary studies. A specific DNA haplotype is associated with the *PI**Z* allele and indicates a single origin for all *PI**Z* alleles.[131] The DNA haplotype is the same irrespective of ethnic group within northern Europe and is independent of the presence or type of clinical disease.[131,135] There appears to have been an early division between M1 subtypes, since the M1A (M1A1a213) subtype, which preceded the Z allele, has the same amino acid at position 213[116,132] as found in the baboon.[51] M1(Val213) appears to have evolved into other PI subtypes such as M2, M3, and S.[12,132] Specific DNA haplotypes are associated with each of the protein variants and can be used to identify the evolutionary pathways.[132] They have also been useful for the identification of rare deficiency alleles.[140]

A highly polymorphic CA repeat has been identified 5′ to the PI locus[134] (Table 138-4, Fig. 138-3B). Additional polymorphisms, which will be useful both for linkage and for disease-association studies, have been identified in the adjacent loci for α_1-antichymotrypsin (AACT)[141] and protein C inhibitor (PC I).[142]

α_1-ANTITRYPSIN DEFICIENCY

There is no firm evidence that any of the alleles that cause a modest reduction in the plasma concentration of α_1AT (Table 138-2) are associated with disease. Even in association with the *PI**Z* allele, the risk for disease does not appear to be appreciable, and it will be presented in discussions of associated diseases. This section considers the alleles that produce a marked deficiency of α_1AT.

Deficiency Due to *PI**Z* Allele

The most common of the deficiency alleles is *PI**Z*, and most individuals with α_1AT deficiency are of PI type ZZ. As noted from population studies of PI variants, the *PI**Z* allele appears to be restricted to whites, and occurs in blacks and orientals apparently only in populations with a white admixture. The estimated frequency of the *PI**Z* allele in North American white populations is 0.0122, corresponding to a frequency of PI ZZ homozygotes of 1 in 6,700.[143,144] The frequency of *PI**Z* is higher in Scandinavia: 0.018, as calculated from 200,000 Swedish newborns in a screening program.[145]

Plasma Concentration of α_1AT

The plasma concentration of α_1AT associated with PI type ZZ is usually in the range of 12 to 18 percent of normal. In one series of 105 PI ZZ individuals, the mean plasma α_1AT concentration ($\pm$1 standard deviation) was 18 $\pm$ 5 percent of normal,[143] with a range of 9 to 27 percent in another series.[2] The plasma concentration of α_1AT in 75 PI ZZ children was similar (17 $\pm$ 3 percent)[144]; however, for children or infants with liver disease, the concentrations of α_1AT are frequently higher, and can rise to 40 percent of normal.[146]

Diagnosis

α_1AT deficiency should be considered in the differential diagnosis of patients with emphysema, jaundice in infancy, liver disease in childhood, and liver disease in adults.

Immunologic assays (radial immunodiffusion, electroimmuno assay, and nephelometry) are the most specific assays for α_1AT and should be used in clinical conditions with a relatively high probability of α_1AT deficiency. Functional assay results include a fraction of inhibitory activity due to other inhibitors, such as α_2-macroglobulin, which can prevent diagnosis of the deficiency. The α_1-globulin peak on cellulose acetate or agarose[147] electrophoresis can be used as a screening technique; it is absent or markedly reduced in most individuals with α_1AT deficiency, although not necessarily in children of PI type ZZ. Computer printouts of scans are sometimes unreliable, as the position of the baseline sometimes causes a normal concentration to be read when a visual examination of the scan clearly indicates a deficiency.

To confirm the diagnosis of α_1AT deficiency, PI typing must be carried out. The plasma concentration below which PI typing is carried out must be high enough to avoid missing affected individuals. Since patients with inflammation or liver disease, particularly children, may have a concentration of α_1AT up to about 40 percent of normal, PI typing for plasma with less than 40 percent of the normal mean concentration should detect all individuals of PI type ZZ.

Liver Inclusions

Normal α_1AT is secreted rapidly from the liver. Z-type α_1AT is retained in hepatocytes, forming intracytoplasmic inclusions, which are a characteristic sign of α_1AT deficiency.[73] Features of the inclusions have been described in detail[148] and are shown in Figure 138-6. The hepatocyte inclusions can be identified by several histochemical stains. By routine hematoxylin–eosin staining, the inclusions appear as round to oval, slightly eosinophilic, hyalin-like globules, localized predominantly in periportal hepatocytes. With periodic acid–Schiff (PAS) staining following diastase treatment (PAS-D), the inclusions are easily visualized as brilliant pink globules of various sizes. Large inclusions can be up to 15 μm in diameter. In infants with α_1AT deficiency, the inclusions may be fine and granular. Large inclusions stain brick red with Masson trichrome stain and dark purple with phosphotungstic acid–hematoxylin (PTAH) stain.

The content of these inclusions was demonstrated to be α_1AT by immunohistochemical methods.[73,149] The direct immunofluorescence method, with fluorescein- or peroxidase-labeled α_1AT antibody, is best used on frozen sections, but formalin-fixed tissue even after paraffin embedding can also be used.[150] Immunologic identification of α_1AT is useful for confirming the presence of α_1AT, particularly where other liver inclusions are present. By electron microscopy, the inclusions appear as moderately electron-dense membrane-bound masses within the membranes of the endoplasmic reticulum (ER), particularly in rough ER.[148,149]

There is considerable variability in the extent of inclusion formation. In general, the number and size of liver inclusions increases with age.[148] The presence of inclusions indicates only the presence of at least one *PI*Z* allele. In individuals heterozygous for α_1AT deficiency, PI MZ, inclusions in the liver vary considerably in amount, and they may be numerous and large in the presence of liver disease. It is not possible to differentiate heterozygotes from homozygous, deficient individuals by an examination of liver inclusions.

The occurrence of this type of liver inclusion is almost always due to the presence of a deficiency allele for α_1AT (Z or a similar type of rare deficiency allele). In a study of 1951 adult patients with suspected chronic liver disease, periportal granules were found in 30 (1.5 percent), and all but one of these carried the Z allele, mostly as MZ heterozygotes. Rare deficiency variants associated with inclusions were not sought in the remaining one, apparently PI M, individual. Of 37 granule-positive individuals, eight (22 percent) had nonhepatic cancer, a finding that can be explained by the fact that tumor necrosis factor stimulates

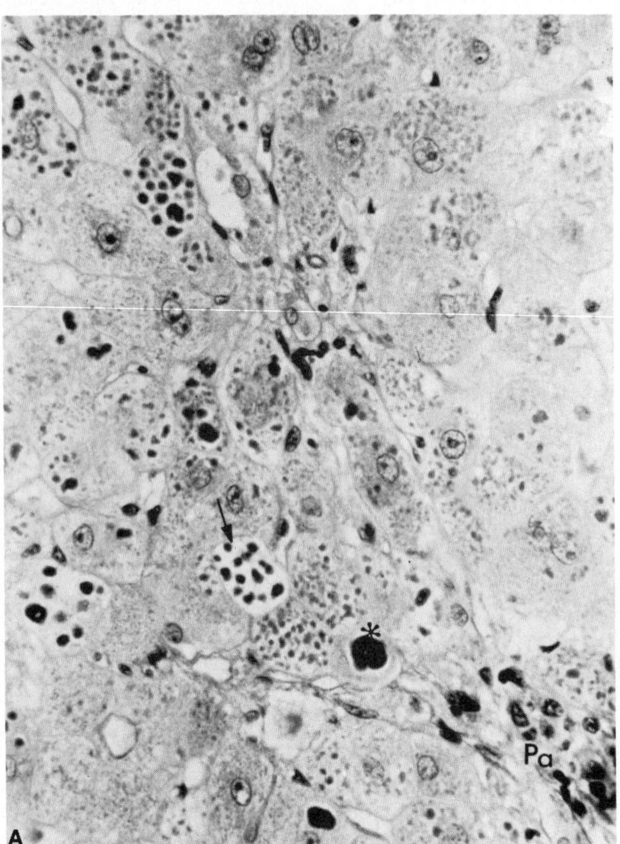

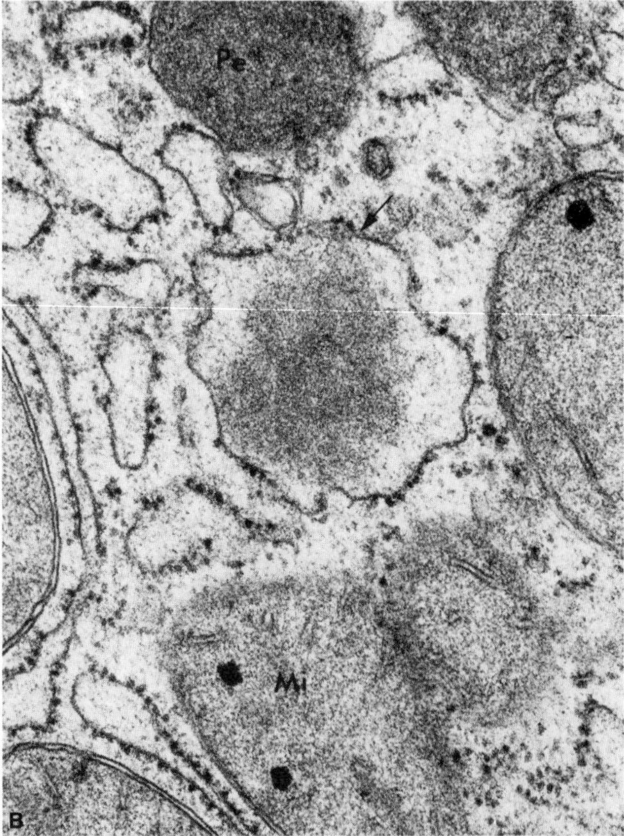

FIG. 138-6 *A*. **Appearance of hepatic inclusions with PAS-D stain. Arrow indicates multiple small inclusions of α_1AT; asterisk indicates large inclusion. Fibrosis is noted in the portal area (Pa). (PAS-D; ×800).** *B*. **Hepatic inclusion as seen with electron microscope. Arrow indicates inclusion formed from dilation of rough endoplasmic reticulum, with numerous ribosomes visible on the outer membrane. Mi = mitochondria; Pe = peroxysome. ×70,000.** ***(Photographs courtesy of E. Cutz.[148] Used by permission of Masson Publishing.)***

α_1AT production.[151] Severe systemic diseases can result in typical PAS-D-positive globules positive for α_1AT by immunofluorescence in periportal areas when the rate of α_1AT synthesis exceeds the capacity of the processing enzymes involved in secretion.[152,153] In occasional patients with alcoholic liver disease, small, scattered PAS-D globules have been observed, with no electron-microscopic confirmation of α_1AT retention.[154] Deposits of lipofuscin can produce PAS-D material that is distinctly different from α_1AT inclusions.[154]

The Basic Defect

Recent advances have increased our understanding, at the molecular level, of the basic defect leading to the plasma deficiency of α_1AT. The portion of Z α_1AT secreted into the plasma has a nearly normal specific elastase inhibitory capacity.[112] The association constants of α_1AT with neutrophil elastase are similar for M and monomer Z α_1AT[155]: $5.3 \pm 0.06 \times 10^7$ and $1.2 \pm 0.02 \times 10^7/M$/sec, respectively, for M and Z. The lower specific activity reported previously[156] could be due to the presence of aggregated and inactive α_1AT. Protease–inhibitor complexes are tight for both M and Z α_1AT. The Z α_1AT was shown to have a normal rate of synthesis[157,158] and a half-life of 5.2 days, not significantly different from that of M α_1AT.[82] These observations all suggested that the defect lies in secretion, an idea consistent with the accumulation of α_1AT in liver inclusions. PI Z individuals also show the secretion defect of α_1AT in monocytes.[159]

The inclusions in the liver do not readily dissociate,[160,161] but, when solubilized, Z α_1AT binds elastase and is functionally active as an inhibitor.[162] The Z α_1AT in the liver inclusions has an abnormal carbohydrate composition, lacking terminal *N*-acetylneuraminic acid and having a mannose-rich core that is typical of incompletely processed glycoproteins.[160–162] Incomplete processing is, however, secondary to the basic defect, since reduced secretion in comparison with M α_1AT also occurs when Z mRNA is injected into *Xenopus* oocytes.[163,164] Following up on an observation made during protein purification, Z α_1AT was noted to have a strong tendency to aggregate, even in plasma.[165] The aggregation was particularly pronounced in the presence of pH and salt concentrations typical of the hepatic intracellular fluid and was hypothesized to be the cause of the hepatic inclusions.[165] Studies of the production of M and Z α_1AT in oocytes showed that the secretion defect also occurs with nonglycosylated α_1AT,[163] indicating that the carbohydrate side chains are not involved. This result suggested that the aggregation could be explained by an examination of the three-dimensional structure of α_1AT.[125] In the Z protein, lysine replaces the glutamic acid present in normal M α_1AT at position 342.[118,119] Glutamic acid is involved in a salt bridge that is important for stabilizing the molecule and occurs at a sharp bend in the major B sheet.[22] However, when lysine 290, the other component of the 290–342 salt bridge, was altered to glutamic acid by site-directed mutagenesis, secretion of α_1AT was nearly normal after injection of mRNA into oocytes or mouse hepatoma cells.[166,167] This result indicated that alteration at the critical bend by lysine was more important than the salt bridge for normal folding.

The Glu342 residue of M α_1AT is located at a hinge region of the reactive center loop (Fig. 138-2). The reactive center loop is mobile and is able to adopt various configurations. Under mild denaturing conditions, the loop locks into the A sheet, forming a thermostable inactive protein.[168] When the temperature is elevated to 37°C, under these same conditions, the reactive center loop of one α_1AT molecule inserts into the A sheet of a second molecule. The phenomenon has been called loop–sheet polymerization,[155] but is more correctly a complex formation, or aggregation, as no chemical bonds are involved. Replacement of the hinge residue 342 in Z α_1AT apparently allows the A sheet to open, making the molecule a receptor for dimerization. This explanation is supported by the circular dichroism spectrum of Z α_1AT.[32] The extent of polymerization of Z α_1AT is temperature dependent, with acceleration at 41°C, and is also concentration dependent.[32] These facts have implications for the formation of liver inclusions. Any increase in body temperature, for example during inflammation and fever, would be expected to increase the aggregation of liver Z α_1AT. Furthermore, since α_1AT is an acute-phase protein, an increase in production, as would occur during inflammation or other stress, could also contribute to aggregation of liver Z α_1AT. M protein will also self-aggregate when the temperature is raised to 41°C and, particularly, when the concentration of α_1AT is increased.[155] This explains the occasional finding of liver inclusions in PI M individuals who are acutely ill.

Accumulation of Z α_1AT appears to proceed slowly and continuously. Stimulation of lysosomal enzymes by nonsecreted α_1AT may help to remove the abnormal Z protein.[169] Heat-shock proteins, which are produced in cells under stress, could be involved in removing the aggregated protein. Heat-shock proteins bind to secretory proteins until the assembling of the proteins is complete, and they are induced by the presence of abnormal proteins.[170] The synthesis of stress proteins has been shown to be increased in PI ZZ individuals with liver disease.[171] However, it is not clear whether such proteins induce damage or are innocent bystanders involved only in degrading the abnormal protein.

Rare Deficiency Alleles

Deficiency alleles range from those producing an amount of plasma α_1AT similar to that of the *PI*Z* allele to those that produce no detectable α_1AT by standard methods.

Alleles Expressing Detectable α_1AT. Several deficiency alleles have been reported in which the plasma concentration is detectable by standard methods and is generally in the range of about 2 to 15 percent of normal. The sites of these mutations are listed in Table 138-5. All have an electrophoretic mobility different from that of the PI Z variant.[140] PI $Z_{AUGSBURG}$ (same as PI $Z_{TUNBRIDGE\ WELLS}$) and PI $Z_{WREXHAM}$ have the Z mutation as well as another benign amino acid difference. PI M_{MALTON} is associated with PAS-positive hepatocyte inclusions identical with those found in association with PI Z,[154] and, like Z, the protein has a tendency to aggregate.[165] $M_{NICHINAN}$ has the M_{MALTON} mutation in addition to a benign alteration at residue 148.[172] S_{IIYAMA} also aggregates and forms liver inclusions.[173] Amino acid residues 52 and 53 are altered in all three variants. These mutations cause a displacement of the B helix that forms the base of the gap in the A sheet for the reactive center loop (Fig. 138-2). PI M_{DUARTE}, first reported in a 48-year-old woman with severe bullous emphysema,[174] migrates in acid starch gel and agarose similarly to PI M,[174] and the isoelectric point is similar to that of M3, as determined by isoelectric focusing.[143] PAS-D globules were present in the liver,[174] indicating that this deficient variant also has, like Z and M_{MALTON}, a defect in secretion from the liver. $M_{HEERLEN}$[175]

Table 138-5 Deficiency Alleles of α_1-Antitrypsin

Allele	Plasma Concentration (% Normal)	Amino Acid No.	Exon	Normal Codon	Normal Amino Acid	Mutant Codon	Mutation
Z	18	342	5	GAG	Glu	AAG	Lys
Z_{AUGSBURG}	<15	342	5	GAG	Glu	AAG	Lys
Z_{WREXHAM}	—	−19	—	TCG	Ser	TTG	Leu
M_{HEERLEN}	2	369	5	CCC	Pro	CTC	Leu
M_{MALTON}	12	51/52	2	TTC	Phe	—	Delete
M_{NICHINAN}	<15	52	2	TTC	Phe	—	Delete
—		148	2	GGG	Gly	AGG	Arg
M_{PROCIDA}	4	41	2	CTG	Leu	CCG	Pro
S_{IIYAMA}	—	53	2	TCC	Ser	TTC	Phe
Null							
$Q0_{\text{HONGKONG}}$	0	317/318	4	CTCTCC	Leu–Ser	CTCC	Delete, stop at amino acid 334
$Q0_{\text{BELLINGHAM}}$	0	217	3	AAG	Lys	TAG	Stop
$Q0_{\text{GRANITEFALLS}}$	0	160/161	2	TACGTG	Tyr–Val	TAGTG	Delete, stop
$Q0_{\text{MATTAWA}}$	0	353	5	TTA	Leu	TTTA	Insert, stop at amino acid 376
$Q0_{\text{ISOLA DI PROCIDA}}$	0	—	2–5	—	—	delete ex2–5	Delete 17 kb
$Q0_{\text{RIEDENBURG}}$*	0	—	2–5	—	—	delete ev2–5	Delete 15 kb
$Q0_{\text{BOLTON}}$	0	362	5	CCCG	Pro	CCG	Delete, stop at amino acid 373
$Q0_{\text{SAARBRÜCKEN}}$*	0	362	5	CCC	Pro	CCCC	Insert, stop at amino acid 376
$Q0_{\text{CARDIFF}}$	0	256	3	GAT	Asp	GTT	Val
$Q0_{\text{LUDWIGSHAFEN}}$	0	92	2	ATC	Ile	AAC	Asn
$Q0_{\text{NEWPORT}}$	0	115	2	GGC	Gly	AGC	Ser

NOTE: References are in text, in Brantley et al.[12] and in Fraizer et al.[182]
*Variant information from J.P. Faber, Ph.D. Thesis, Rheinische Friedrich-Wilhelms-Universität, Bonn, Germany (1991).

and M_{PROCIDA}[176] each have mutations involving a proline residue, which could affect stability and lead to intracellular degradation.

Individuals with rare deficiency alleles have the same risk for obstructive lung disease as PI ZZ individuals, as noted in a number of reported cases (reviewed by Cox[125]). PI MM_{MALTON} heterozygotes who smoke, like PI MZ heterozygotes, show impairment in some tests of lung function.[177] The risk for liver disease should be similar to that associated with the Z allele if liver inclusions are damaging. An adult patient has been reported with liver disease.[178] Both PI^*M_{MALTON} and PI^*M_{DUARTE} are relatively rare alleles, about 1/100th and 1/200th as frequent as the *PI*Z* allele, respectively. Their presence must be considered when no Z α_1AT can be observed in plasma from a patient with apparent α_1AT deficiency. Furthermore, these PI types will produce α_1AT inclusions in the liver, particularly in heterozygotes, in the presence of an apparently normal M phenotype. When isoelectric focusing is used, the M_{MALTON} α_1AT can be identified even in the presence of a normal M allele. M_{DUARTE} can be detected in a heterozygote with an S or Z allele but, depending on the degree of resolution with isoelectric focusing, may not be detectable in the presence of a normal M allele. Family studies should help to confirm the presence of these rare deficiency alleles. Unless their presence has been definitely excluded, these rare alleles should be considered as the most likely cause of inclusions other than *PI*Z*.

The Null (Q0) Alleles. The null alleles are associated with the most severe deficiency, producing either no α_1AT or less than 1 percent of the normal amount of plasma α_1AT. According to current nomenclature, these alleles should be designated as *PI*Q0* and homozygote phenotypes designated as PI Q0Q0. While the *PI*Z* allele has been reported only in white populations, the null alleles are widespread. In our series of 112 patients with α_1AT deficiency, we estimated the frequency of all null "alleles" to be 1.7×10^{-4}, about 1/100th the frequency of the *PI*Z* allele in a North American white population and similar to the frequency of PI^*M_{MALTON}.[143] The PI Q0 variants are listed in Table 138-5.

Clinical information on all reported null homozygotes was summarized previously.[125] Obstructive airways disease occurs as early as the second or third decade, even in nonsmokers. Data indicate that null homozygotes have more severe obstructive airways disease than individuals of PI type ZZ, whose low concentrations of α_1AT apparently provide some protection to lung tissue.[179] These individuals may particularly benefit from new methods of therapy under development. The presence of even trace amounts of α_1AT in null homozygotes may help prevent the formation of α_1AT antibodies during long-term therapy with injection of α_1AT.

There appear to be a variety of null mutants, each of which has the final result of interfering with the production of α_1AT. The most common defect is a new stop codon, although other mechanisms are reported, such as intracellular degradation ($Q0_{\text{HONGKONG}}$,[180] $Q0_{\text{MATTAWA}}$[181]), alteration of tertiary structure ($Q0_{\text{LUDWIGSHAFEN}}$[182]), and complete deletion of the α_1AT coding exons ($Q0_{\text{ISOLA DI PROCIDA}}$[183]) (for further details, see refs. 140 and 182). The use of DNA haplotypes, as described for studies of normal alleles of α_1AT, can be useful in delineating different null alleles. We have examined the DNA haplotype for six null alleles to date and have found each to have a different haplotype, probably reflecting different mutations.[184] This approach is useful for an initial identification of mutant alleles.

Selective Mechanisms for Deficiency Alleles

Since the combined frequency of *PI*Q0* alleles is about 1.7×10^{-4}, then the frequency of each allele should be considerably less. If selective advantage has allowed the frequency of the *PI*Z* allele to increase, then it is interesting that the frequency of other deficiency alleles has not similarly increased. Possible explanations are that the *PI*Z* allele has some unique selective advantage compared to other deficiency alleles, that other deficiency alleles arose much more recently than *PI*Z*, or that chance factors have been responsible for the increase in *PI*Z*.

DNA haplotypes indicate a single origin for the *PI*Z* allele with a subsequent spread of the mutation through northern Caucasian populations.[131] Increased fertility of heterozygotes has been discussed as one possible mechanism for increasing the *PI*Z* allele frequency.[7] Preferential survival of heterozygotes is another possible selection pressure, and preferential survival from tuberculosis has been suggested.[185] This is entirely speculative at present, although data suggesting that the frequency of MZ individuals is increased among older blood donors, who were adults prior to tuberculosis therapy, is of interest.[186]

OBSTRUCTIVE LUNG DISEASE

Clinical Features

Chronic obstructive pulmonary disease (COPD), specifically emphysema, is the most prevalent clinical disorder associated with α_1AT deficiency and was noted in the first patients described.[3] In a larger group of 33 patients reported by Eriksson in 1965,[4] the first symptoms of pulmonary disease were reported to occur before 40 years of age in 60 percent and before 50 years of age in 90 percent. The association with α_1AT deficiency was confirmed in many subsequent studies. The early studies, suggesting a high proportion of emphysema in patients with α_1AT deficiency, were biased by the ascertainment of patients through their illness. It is now appreciated that α_1AT-deficient patients who avoid smoking have a much later onset of clinical symptoms and may have an almost normal life span.

Surveys from several countries of groups of patients with COPD are in agreement with the initial report[3] that only 1 or 2 percent of such patients have α_1AT deficiency (earlier studies are reviewed in refs. 66 and 187). The frequency may be considerably higher: it was 18 percent of patients with emphysema in one study, in which the referral pattern favored young and more severely affected patients.[113] The male:female ratio is at least 2:1,[188,189] which may be related to smoking exposure.

Emphysema associated with α_1AT deficiency typically involves the basal more than the apical regions of the lungs. Although most patients present with emphysema, some present with symptoms of bronchial asthma or chronic bronchitis.[188,189] Thoracic radiographs show a symmetric decrease in peripheral vasculature that is most prominent in the lower lungs, but only in those patients with well-established emphysema and not in asymptomatic individuals.[190] High-resolution CT scans identify changes in patients with α_1AT deficiency which reflect changes in pulmonary structure.[191] Results of radioisotope ventilation-and-perfusion scans are usually abnormal[188] and may show slight abnormalities in asymptomatic patients.[190] Changes in lung mechanics are similar to those found in other patients with emphysema, with reduction in lung volumes and expiratory flow rates. The decreased expiratory flow rate can be attributed to loss of elastic recoil. The most sensitive parameters for detecting abnormalities in asymptomatic α_1AT-deficient patients have been reported to be closing volume, nitrogen washout volume, and lung mechanics. Clinical features of pulmonary disease were discussed extensively in an earlier edition of this text.[62]

Age of Onset and Course of Obstructive Lung Disease

The onset and severity of disease symptoms vary considerably. Nonsmokers may have normal lung function test results up to at least 30 years of age.[179] In patients identified through an affected relative, females tend to show less rapid deterioration of lung function with age[189] and better survival.[192]

True survival figures for patients with α_1AT deficiency are unknown, as it is certain that many PI ZZ individuals are never identified. Survival to the sixth and seventh decade is possible. The most extensive survival data have been obtained from Sweden and are summarized in Fig. 138-7. Mortality figures in this study differ markedly for smokers and nonsmokers. About 98 percent of nonsmoking females and 65 percent of nonsmoking males are alive at age 55, whereas only 30 percent and 18 percent of females and males, respectively, who smoke are alive at the same age.[192] However, the figures shown here are biased owing to the

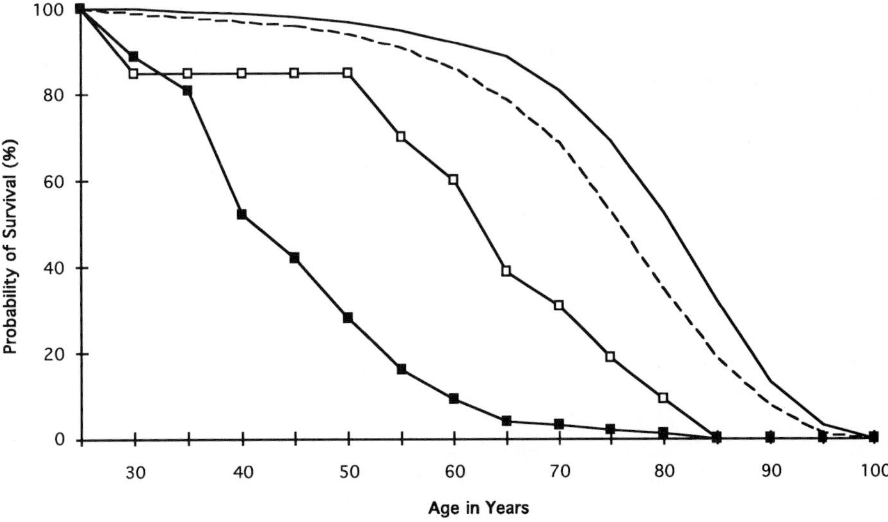

FIG. 138-7 Probability of survival to specified ages for normal females (solid line), normal males (dashed line), PI ZZ nonsmokers (open squares), PI ZZ smokers (closed squares). ***(Based on data published by Larsson.[192])***

fact that these patients were identified through hospital admissions or clinics. The prognosis, particularly in nonsmokers, is probably better than indicated by the Swedish study. A study of 54 patients with α_1AT deficiency, in which 28 of the patients were not identified through the presence of COPD or other lung problems, indicates that the risk of COPD has been overestimated.[193] Of the α_1AT-deficient patients between 30 and 60 years of age and not identified through COPD, only one in three, almost all of them smokers, had developed COPD. Nonsmokers may have a late age of onset, and α_1AT deficiency should be considered as a positive factor for emphysema in elderly nonsmokers.[194]

Smoking has a major effect on both the age of onset of pulmonary symptoms and the course of pulmonary deterioration. Onset of dyspnea appears to be rare before 40 years of age in nonsmokers.[192] In a review of patients from the literature (30 nonsmokers and 84 smokers), the mean age of onset of dyspnea was 35 years in smokers and 44 years in nonsmokers.[188] A study of 33 patients with emphysema and α_1AT deficiency in New Zealand indicated a mean age for onset of dyspnea of 32 years in smokers and 51 years in nonsmokers.[195] Lung function deteriorates continuously with time as the alveolar walls are destroyed. In a study of 65 PI ZZ Danish patients (60 percent of the group identified because of symptoms), the age to reach 50 percent of predicted FEV_1 (volume of air expired during the first second of forced vital capacity) was 17 years greater in those who had never smoked than in smokers.[196] The rate of deterioration of lung function, as measured by decline in FEV_1, showed a marked difference between six α_1AT-deficient smokers (316 ± 80 ml/year) and seven nonsmokers (80 ± 38 ml/year).[192] The rate of decline of FEV_1 for PI ZZ subjects with clinically significant pulmonary disease (17 percent of whom were smokers), as reflected by an initial FEV_1 30 to 60 percent of the normal value, was 111 ± 102 ml.[197] The subjects were tested in several U.S. cities. A comparable decline in nonsmoking control subjects is 36 ml/year.[198] Effects of smoking should be particularly detrimental in α_1AT deficiency, as in normal individuals, when begun during adolescence, as attainment of maximal lung function is prevented.[199]

Reports of emphysema in children with α_1AT deficiency are extremely rare, and emphysema in these circumstances may be due to the coexistence of other genetic abnormalities.[200] In a follow-up of 22 adolescents identified through a neonatal screening program in the U.S., all had normal pulmonary function except for two sibs known to have asthma. One subject (4 percent) was a current smoker, versus 21 percent of control subjects. In another study of 59 patients with liver disease, of whom 28 had α_1AT deficiency, PI type ZZ, patients with α_1AT deficiency tended to have higher lung volumes than healthy controls or children with extrahepatic biliary atresia.[201] Of seven patients with liver disease who responded to bronchodilator challenge, five had α_1AT deficiency, two of whom were previously diagnosed and treated for asthma. In combination, these two studies suggest that factors that predispose to liver disease may also predispose to lung disease, and indicate that children with liver disease and α_1AT deficiency should be followed closely as potential candidates for augmentation therapy if their liver disease does not lead to transplantation.

A direct measure of the presence of a peptide produced by elastase activity could be useful in identifying individuals most likely to develop severe lung disease.[202] This assay measures the amount of a specific fragment cleaved from fibrinogen, releasing a fibrinogen A-containing fragment, α1-21. The mean plasma levels were increased in PI MZ individuals, with considerable overlap, and most PI ZZ individuals had a plasma concentration above the normal upper limit. Smokers had particularly elevated levels of the peptide. Even after correction for smoking history, the plasma concentrations of peptide were four times higher in PI ZZ individuals than in PI MZ individuals, and three times higher in PI MZ individuals than in PI MM individuals. The inverse relation between peptide levels in nonsmoking PI ZZ patients and the percent of the predicted FEV_1 (FEV_1%), a measure of the extent of airways obstruction, suggests that this test might provide a useful method for identifying individuals at the greatest risk for lung destruction.

The Role of Proteases in Lung Destruction

The alveolar destruction characteristic of emphysema is generally considered to be caused by an imbalance between proteolytic enzymes, particularly elastase, and their inhibitors. Support for this concept is derived from several types of studies. Experimental studies in animals demonstrated that porcine pancreatic elastase[203] and human neutrophil elastase[204,205] produce experimental emphysema in animals. Further evidence has come from the studies of patients with α_1AT deficiency. Because of its small molecular size, α_1AT enters lung tissue and has been recovered in bronchoalveolar lavage fluid. A plasma deficiency of α_1AT is reflected by a deficiency of α_1AT in the lung.[206] The absence of adequate inhibitor allows continued destruction of lung tissue. Direct evidence for the complexing of α_1AT with elastase in the lung has been provided by the finding of elastase–α_1AT complexes in bronchial lavage fluid of normal smokers and nonsmokers, accounting for less than 1 percent of the total α_1AT in the fluid.[207]

The role of α_1AT as the major inhibitor of elastase at the epithelial lining has been demonstrated in a homozygous null individual, in whom the antineutrophil elastase capacity of lavage fluid was less than 15 percent of normal.[208] Other potential elastase inhibitors in lung tissue, such as a low-molecular-weight protease inhibitor[209,210] or locally produced α_2-macroglobulin,[64] apparently make a minor contribution.

Numerous other studies supporting the protease inhibitor imbalance hypothesis[211] and expanding on the role of neutrophils[212] have been reviewed.

Mechanisms of Exacerbation of Lung Destruction by Smoking

Mechanisms of lung destruction in normal smokers would be expected to have an even more detrimental effect in those with α_1AT deficiency. An important mechanism for the increased destruction of lung tissue in smokers appears to be oxidation, since oxidation of methionine residues interferes dramatically with complex formation of α_1AT with elastase. Since the gas phase of tobacco smoke is rich in oxidizing agents, a direct effect of smoke on α_1AT could be anticipated. In vitro, both a crude tar fraction of cigarette smoke and aqueous extracts of freshly generated cigarette smoke significantly inactivate α_1AT (reviewed by Janoff[211]).

In vivo studies assessing the effects of smoking as reflected in the serum of smokers have produced conflicting results. Although some studies have shown a decrease of elastase inhibitor activity in serum from smokers compared with nonsmokers,[88,213] other studies have not shown a difference,[214] even when carried out with careful control of timing in relation to smoking.[215] In view of the generous supply of antioxidants in plasma, a measurable effect on α_1AT in plasma would seem unlikely. A reduction of elastase inhibitor activity in lavage fluid of smokers has been reported. In a study of acute effects of smoking, there appeared to be no increase in elastaselike enzyme activity in smokers, but an increase in immunologic elastase levels indicated possible release of neutrophil elastase in the bronchoalveolar lavage fluid.[216] Slight inactivation of α_1AT was noted in lavage fluid immediately after smoking.[217] α_1AT with oxidized methionine and reduced inhibitory activity has been recovered from lungs of smokers.[218]

In addition to its oxidation effects, smoking can act on neutrophils, which are present in increased numbers in smokers. Triggered neutrophils release oxidants, which can cause local proteolytic cleavage of α_1AT by elastase.[219] Smoking causes release of elastase from neutrophils. Neutrophils are also a source of myeloperoxidase, which inactivates α_1AT.[220,221] This fact can also help account for the increased amount of proteolytically cleaved α_1AT in smokers.[222] Smoking causes impaired adherence of alveolar macrophages and promotes increased synthesis and secretion of elastase from macrophages obtained from nonsmokers (reviewed in refs. 68 and 212). Smoking acts directly on elastin by impairing its crosslinking.[223]

Other Factors Influencing the Extent of Lung Destruction

Genetic Factors. A number of population studies have indicated that respiratory symptoms show familial aggregation (reviewed by Redline et al.[224]), and genetic factors no doubt influence disease severity in α_1AT deficiency. In a study of 256 monozygotic and 158 dizygotic adult twins, a large proportion of measured variability in pulmonary function test results was accounted for by genetic influences.[224] A *Taq* I polymorphism[139] and a *Hind* III polymorphism[225] in the 3′ flanking region of the α_1AT gene have been suggested to influence predisposition to COPD. A specific *Taq* I allele has been found in approximately 20 percent of individuals with pulmonary emphysema or bronchiectasis, compared with 5 percent of a healthy control population, but is not associated with deficient α_1AT types.[139] The *Taq* I mutation is in a portion of the 3′ flanking region that carries potentially important regulatory motifs, including an AP1 binding site and a sequence similar to an enhancer region of antithrombin III.[226] These authors have thus proposed that the polymorphism either may serve as a marker for an α_1AT mutation in the PI or PI-like gene or may influence the regulation of α_1AT in the acute-phase response.

In α_1AT deficiency, the presence of emphysema in a parent or the presence of asthma appears to increase the risk for development of COPD.[193] Evidence has also been found for another major gene affecting susceptibility to COPD.[227]

A number of metabolic parameters may have a hereditary component and could alter susceptibility to lung destruction. These include number of neutrophils, extent of elastase released from neutrophils, or differences in elastase quality or quantity within neutrophils. Any increase in the protease content of neutrophils, particularly of elastase, might be expected to increase the rate of lung degradation. A number of studies have been carried out to compare neutrophil proteases in COPD patients and in individuals of PI types MZ and ZZ, all with appropriate controls (reviewed by Fagerhol and Cox[7]). No pronounced differences in neutrophil elastase concentration were found between individuals with normal lung function and those with COPD. However, the mean values were somewhat increased in patients with COPD and may indicate that some individuals have exceptionally high concentrations of neutrophil elastase. For PI MZ and ZZ individuals, there was no significant difference between those with COPD and those with normal lung function.

Detrimental effects could be produced by increased production of myeloperoxidase causing local inactivation of α_1AT, by low levels of catalase (which blocks H_2O_2 production by myeloperoxidase), by low concentrations of antioxidants, or by characteristics of lung tissue that result in susceptibility to degradation. Most of these factors have been inadequately investigated.

Antioxidant Status. Oxidation appears to play an important role in proteolytic degradation of the lung, and, therefore, antioxidants should play an important role in limiting this destruction. The damaging effects of chemical oxidants, such as those from cigarette smoke and those produced by neutrophils, could be modified by antioxidants present in lung tissue. Normal plasma and tissue components that may contribute to antioxidant activity include ascorbate, ceruloplasmin, transferrin, vitamin E, reduced glutathione (through the activity of glutathione peroxidase), NADPH reductase, methionine sulfoxide reductase, and superoxide dismutase.[228] The total antioxidant activity of plasma is somewhat less in smokers than in nonsmokers,[229,230] and individuals with a family history of lung disease may also have reduced plasma antioxidants.[229] In vitro studies of the antioxidants ascorbate, cysteine, and dapsone demonstrate that all of them can protect α_1AT from loss of inhibitory activity caused by activated neutrophils[231] but that they are not able to activate α_1AT once inactivation has occurred. The protective effects of these antioxidants are proposed to be related to their ability to scavenge the superoxide and oxidants generated by the neutrophils. In this study, it was pointed out that the concentrations of these agents that have such a protective effect are attainable in vivo. Vitamin E is particularly important as a tissue antioxidant and is believed to act predominantly on cell membranes. Animal experiments have demonstrated that vitamin E can neutralize free radicals and decrease the susceptibility of the lungs to oxidant injury (reviewed by Pacht et al.[232]). Serum levels of vitamin E and the oxidative metabolite vitamin E quinone are similar in young asymptomatic smokers and nonsmokers; however, smokers show markedly less vitamin E and vitamin E quinone in bronchoalveolar lavage fluid than nonsmokers, possibly owing to increased oxidative metabolism of vitamin E in smokers.[232] The difference was only partly corrected by vitamin E supplementation. Vitamin E was shown to have a protective role for the lung in experiments demonstrating that the killing of normal rat lung parenchymal cells by smoke or alveolar macrophages was inversely related to the vitamin E content of the parenchymal cells.[232] This study suggests that vitamin E is an important antioxidant in the lower respiratory tract and its role in therapy should be seriously considered.

Risk for Lung Disease in Heterozygotes

The extent of the risk for PI MZ heterozygotes of COPD has been controversial. Assessment of risk for these individuals is important since they constitute 2 to 5 percent of most populations. Surveys of patients with COPD have generally shown an increased frequency of individuals of PI type MZ in comparison with those of PI type M, although the difference between the two populations has varied from slight to considerable (reviewed by Cox et al.[113]). These studies usually have not distinguished smokers from nonsmokers. In studies of PI MZ subjects and appropriate PI MM control subjects, not identified because of disease, a small decrease in lung function in nonsmokers and a larger decrease in smokers was noted for parameters reflecting loss of elastic recoil.[233] The differences were not found to be significant in a multicenter study of 143 PI MZ subjects.[234] Both studies included adults of various ages, and corrections were made for age. In a study of 39 Swedish PI MZ heterozygotes identified from the general population, no significant differences were noted between PI MZ and M nonsmokers.[235] In contrast, PI MZ smokers showed a significant loss of elastic recoil, large residual volumes, and increased closing capacity, and most reported mild dyspnea on exertion. Six years later, 32 PI MZ heterozygotes and their control group were retested, and the PI MZ smokers, but not the nonsmokers, showed a significantly increased mean annual reduction in FEV_1 (75 and 40 ml/year, respectively).[236] No increased prevalence of clinical obstructive lung disease was noted in this study, although there have been numerous isolated reports in the literature of severely affected individuals of PI type MZ. The conclusions from these studies appear to be that PI MZ nonsmokers have little if any increased risk of COPD. PI MZ smokers have an increased rate of loss of lung elasticity but usually do not develop sufficient impairment to be recognized as having clinical disease. There may be certain families in which other genetic predisposing factors coexist with α_1AT heterozygosity to produce clinical disease.

An increased frequency of MZ or MS heterozygotes has been reported in association with asthma (reviewed by Fagerhol and Cox[7]). Deficiency types of α_1AT may lead to more severe lung damage for asthmatics.[7]

Individuals of PI type SZ should be more at risk than individuals of PI type MZ for developing a protease/protease inhibitor imbalance in the lungs. The risk for them of COPD must not be high, as surveys of patients with COPD have revealed few if any individuals of PI type SZ. Studies of small numbers of asymptomatic adults of PI type SZ and isolated reports of affected individuals suggest that smokers particularly may have a tendency to have impaired lung function.[237]

Although the *PI*F* allele is not associated with a decrease of α_1AT concentration, there is a suggestion that PI FM heterozygotes may be more susceptible to pulmonary function impairment, particularly when exposed to industrial pollutants.[238,239] α_1AT of the F type, which has an extra cysteine residue, appears to have an increased tendency to oxidation, as shown by its altered electrophoretic pattern after aging,[106] and this increased tendency to oxidation may make PI FM individuals susceptible to lung destruction in a polluted environment.

LIVER DISEASE

Childhood Onset

An association of α_1AT deficiency and liver disease in children was first reported by Sharp and colleagues.[10] At that time, the prognosis for liver disease with α_1AT deficiency was believed to be poor, since all of the patients identified had cirrhosis. Later studies have shown the prognosis to be more favorable. The features of α_1AT deficiency have been reviewed by Hussain et al.[240] and Povey,[241] the latter review particularly relating to neonatal liver disease.

Liver abnormalities occur in only a portion of infants of PI type ZZ. The only prospective study carried out to date is a screening of 200,000 Swedish newborns, from which 120 children of PI type ZZ (and two of PI type Z−) have been followed up.[242] Approximately 18 percent of the PI Z children developed clinically recognizable liver abnormalities: 7.3 percent had prolonged obstructive jaundice with marked evidence of liver disease, 4.1 percent had prolonged jaundice with mild liver disease, and 6.4 percent had other abnormalities suggestive of liver disease, such as hepatomegaly, splenomegaly, unexplained failure to thrive, or a stated history of prolonged jaundice without medical documentation.[242]

The most common sign of liver abnormality associated with α_1AT deficiency is the "neonatal hepatitis syndrome," characterized by conjugated hyperbilirubinemia and raised serum aminotransferases, frequently with hepatosplenomegaly. Various degrees of failure to thrive have been noted. The serum bilirubin concentration can be very high, rising to 12 to 17 mg percent (normal, less than 1).[242,243] Signs of cholestasis generally appear between 4 days and 2 months of age and can persist for a period of a few weeks to 8 months.[146,243] Cholestasis in α_1AT deficiency may be severe enough to cause acholic stools, as in extrahepatic biliary atresia. α_1AT deficiency should always be considered in a child with prolonged jaundice (conjugated hyperbilirubinemia) of unexplained origin, and PI typing should be an early diagnostic procedure. From 14 to 29 percent of infants with neonatal hepatitis have been found to have α_1AT deficiency, PI type ZZ.[146,243] While presentation as neonatal hepatitis is the most common, hepatomegaly without jaundice in infancy or childhood can be the presenting symptom. In one series of 18 children of PI type ZZ, 14 (78.6 percent) presented with the neonatal hepatitis syndrome, 3 (16.7 percent) with hepatomegaly, and 1 with hematemesis.[244]

The pathologic features of α_1AT deficiency associated with liver disease in children have been reviewed.[146] The typical PAS-D-positive inclusions, described previously, are observed in children with liver disease. They may be difficult to identify in percutaneous liver biopsy specimens from infants. Liver biopsy specimens from young, asymptomatic children usually show only very small inclusions by PAS-D staining but more extensive deposition by immunofluorescence. The amount and size of liver inclusions show no clear correlation with the severity of liver disease. Livers of older PI Z patients, particularly those in whom cirrhosis develops, contain larger amounts of α_1AT, and inclusions usually occupy 50 to 80 percent of the parenchyma. Regenerative nodules may contain focal depositions of α_1AT, while others may show no depositions.

In children who present with neonatal hepatitis, the constant histopathologic features include intrahepatic cholestasis, a varying degree of hepatocellular injury, and moderate fibrosis with inflammatory cells in portal areas. Giant-cell transformation is common. The initial liver biopsy occasionally shows marked ductular proliferation with bile plugging suggestive of biliary atresia, and the extrahepatic biliary tree may be normal[146] or may have patent but narrowed extrahepatic bile ducts.[244] Some infants have a significant decrease in the number of interlobular bile ducts. In infants who later develop cirrhosis, liver biopsy samples show moderate to heavy periportal inflammatory cell infiltrate and hepatocyte swelling with patchy necrosis but no evidence of cholestasis. In infants whose liver disease apparently resolves, the main abnormality observed on later biopsy was mild to moderate portal fibrosis with a few inflammatory cells; none of these children showed hepatocellular necrosis, cholestasis, or bile ductular changes.[146]

Once the diagnosis of α_1AT deficiency has been established, liver biopsy is usually unnecessary. Biopsy has been reported to be useful in establishing a long-term prognosis, since portal fibrosis and ductular proliferation are less common in patients with a favorable disease course. However, even patients with these liver abnormalities can have a favorable outcome.[245] Surgery has been reported to not affect the course of the disease adversely, although no supporting data were given.[246] Earlier onset and longer persistence of jaundice appear to occur in children who progress to an unfavorable outcome,[244] although this association has not been observed in all studies.[146] The level of liver enzymes such as serum alanine aminotransferase and serum glutamyl transpeptidase can be very high in PI ZZ infants,[242,243] and the degree of elevation does not appear to correlate with prognosis. γ-Glutamyl transpeptidase (γGT), found in the cell membrane in a number of tissues, is useful as a measure of the extent of bile duct damage, and elevated levels are a general feature in children with α_1AT deficiency.[247] Liver enzymes persistently elevated to more than three times the normal upper limit tend to be associated with a poor prognosis.[242,244,245,248] From birth through 8 years of age, many children who appear to be clinically well still have an elevation of liver-derived serum enzymes. The serum concentration of alanine aminotransferase was above the normal limit in 46 percent of children at 4 years of age but had decreased to 12 percent by 12 years of age[249] in the Swedish study. An elevation of enzyme levels to two or three times normal does not appear to be associated with a poor prognosis.[248] It has been suggested that measurement of urinary bile acids is useful for evaluating liver status in affected children.[250] Total bile acids remained consistently high in children whose early liver abnormalities progressed to cirrhosis.

Pathogenesis of Liver Disease

Although the structural defect leading to aggregation of Z α_1AT is known, less is known about the actual cause of liver injury. The damage could result from the presence of inclusions in the liver, from the deficiency of the inhibitor in plasma, or from both (for reviews, see refs. 251 and 252).

One hypothesis is that the α_1AT accumulated in the endoplasmic reticulum of hepatocytes directly causes the liver injury. Intracellular accumulation of α_1AT has been shown to increase lysosomal enzyme activity,[169] which could contribute to liver damage. Although the presence of stored α_1AT has not been established as the cause of fibrosis or cirrhosis, prior to cirrhosis, cell necrosis has been observed only in periportal hepatocytes with dilated endoplasmic reticulum storing α_1AT.[253] Transgenic mice expressing and storing mutant Z allele in the liver have been produced.[80,254] One study involved transgenic mouse lines in which there were multiple copies of the human α_1AT M or Z gene per mouse genome.[80] Livers from both M lines and one Z line were similar, with a few abnormal findings. However, the second Z line (12 copies) showed abundant material in the liver and areas of liver cell necrosis. It was suggested that the changes in this Z line resemble those seen in neonatal hepatitis in humans. However, as there were 12 copies of the Z allele per haploid mouse genome, this model may not be analogous to the human situation. Runting was observed in this line of mice and was later found to be strain-specific.[255] No evidence of hepatitis was found in this colony. In summary, changes were observed when 12 times the normal amount of Z protein was produced, but not with 5 times the normal amount. In another study of transgenic mice, Carlson et al.[254] studied the offspring of three lines of transgenic M mice and three lines of transgenic Z mice, the latter carrying 1, 10, and more than 10 copies of the Z gene, respectively. This study was complicated by the fact that the mice were found to carry the mouse hepatitis virus, which produced occasional necrotic and inflammatory regions in a number of mice, but the effects of the virus were shown to be no different in Z than in M transgenic mice. The degree of inflammation, necrosis, and fibrosis was assessed in each mouse. Inflammation and necrosis were significantly increased in mice with 10 or more copies of the Z gene; increase in fibrosis did not reach statistical significance in PI Z mice versus controls ($p = 0.08$). The pathology score was increased only slightly for the mice carrying one copy of the Z gene ($p < 0.028$). If the effects of the hepatitis virus can be ignored, then the conclusion from these studies is that fibrosis, necrosis, and inflammation can be produced in the liver when a sufficiently large store of inclusion granules is present. Cholestasis was not observed. The effect of an elevation in body temperature upon these mice would be of interest.[80] While there may be differences between the susceptibility of mouse and human livers, it is difficult to conclude that the storage of α_1AT alone can be responsible for the liver damage in infants and children, in whom granules are frequently scarce at the time of onset of liver damage. Additional predisposing factors may be involved. On the other hand, this exaggerated model of α_1AT retention may provide support for the inclusions themselves as the pathologic factor in adult liver disease, in which storage of the inclusion granules is pronounced.

The liver involvement could be caused by a direct injury to the hepatocytes owing to excessive uninhibited protease activity, enhanced by subsequent release of high levels of oxygen free radicals. The phagocytic cells and bacteria of the gastrointestinal tract produce large amounts of proteases, which are transported by the portal circulation to the liver. Bacterial proteases produce cell destruction in several ways, including inactivation of the complement system, direct inactivation of serum protease inhibitors,[256] and, perhaps most important, the generation of superoxide radicals leading to the formation of hydrogen peroxide (H_2O_2),[257,258] which can produce hepatic injury. This oxidant-generating system is normally kept in check by antioxidant enzymes such as superoxide dismutase, catalase, and glutathione peroxidase. These enzymes may differ in their quantities in different individuals. An imbalance in these factors might lead to the production of liver disease in some individuals with α_1AT deficiency. Newborn mammals have a very low level of superoxide dismutase, which increases dramatically just after birth.[259] This suggests that infants would be particularly susceptible to the initiation of liver damage.[260] Environmental stresses also differ between individuals. Children with impaired biliary secretion may develop deficiencies of fat-soluble vitamins. A deficiency of vitamin E in the liver could lead to excessively high oxidant levels, promoting hepatocyte membrane damage. Vitamin E therapy has been shown to improve liver function in a small number of children with cholestasis.[261] These speculations suggest further avenues for research and for potential therapy.

An autoimmune type of cellular damage could also be considered, in which abnormal α_1AT in hepatic inclusions would stimulate an immune response. As hepatocytes containing α_1AT are destroyed, the abnormal α_1AT may be released and recognized as a foreign antigen. The α_1AT in inclusions has some unique antigenic sites in comparison with normal M α_1AT, since monoclonal antibody specific for Z α_1AT has been produced.[262] Glomerular lesions found in patients with α_1AT deficiency and cirrhosis are suggestive of an autoimmune response.[263] Increased activation of complement components could account for the evidence of complement activation found in children with α_1AT deficiency and liver disease.[264]

There is probably no simple, single reason for the susceptibility of certain individuals to liver disease in infancy. The liver injury could result from a combination of inadequate protection by antioxidants against the effects of absorbed, uninhibited proteases; subsequent damage and weakening of the cell membrane by the oxidant free radicals; further destruction of the weakened cells by the presence of inclusions of α_1AT; and possibly an autoimmune effect from the eventual leakage of abnormal Z protein from the liver inclusions.

Prognosis for Childhood Liver Disease

Contrary to the initial indications of a poor prognosis in children with α_1AT deficiency and early liver symptoms, it now appears that at least two-thirds of children show recovery from their liver damage.[146] In a retrospective study from England, 20 of 82 children (24.4 percent) developed cirrhosis, 19 had persistently raised liver enzyme levels associated with clinical normality, and 23 had no evidence of liver disease.[265] The clinical presentation, course, and outcome of the disease has been reviewed in 98 patients (54 males, 55.1 percent) from 81 families in the U.S. seen over a period of 20 years.[266] This was a biased group, as many of the patients were referred because of deteriorating health or need for liver transplantation. In this group, an elevation of alanine aminotransferase (ALT) at the time of initial evaluation was associated with a poor outcome, as was a decrease in total inhibitory capacity of plasma (combination of α_1AT and α_2-macroglobulin protease inhibitory capacity). Kidney disease was found in nine females and six males (17 percent) and was usually membranoproliferative glomerulonephritis. Pulmonary symptoms developed in 18 percent, with a mean age at onset of 7 years, and usually consisting of asthma or obstructive lung disease detected in pulmonary function tests. Major infections occurred in 14 boys and 7 girls, with spontaneous bacterial peritonitis as the most common complication and *Pneumococcus* and *Escherichia coli* the most common organisms involved. The outcome tended to be poorer in females than in males. Dietary history was available for relatively few subjects, with 14 breast-fed for at least 2 months and 39 formula-fed since birth. There was no statistical difference in outcome, but the period of breast-feeding was very short. The initial indicators of poor prognosis were a serum bilirubin level that remained high, a low total inhibitory protease inhibitor capacity, and a high alanine aminotransferase level. The prognosis was slightly poorer for females than for males. At The Hospital for Sick Children, Toronto, we estimated that, at most, 37 percent of a series of PI ZZ children with liver abnormalities in the early months of life have developed chronic severe liver disease, a figure that may be biased upward because of ascertainment of more severely affected children early in the study.[146,267] Of 122 PI Z (included 2 PI Z−) α_1AT-deficient children identified from the Swedish screening program and followed up, 2 of 14 children with prolonged obstructive jaundice had died of liver cirrhosis by age 8. An additional PI ZZ child with clinical symptoms of neonatal liver disease without jaundice died of aplastic anemia at 4 years of age, with incipient liver cirrhosis at autopsy. Serum glutamic-oxaloacetic transaminase (SGOT) was elevated in 40 percent of the clinically healthy PI ZZ children. Liver cirrhosis with early death therefore occurred in only 3 of 122 PI ZZ children (2.4 percent), or in 13.6 percent of those PI Z children with clinical evidence of liver abnormalities in infancy.[268]

Factors predisposing to the development of progressive disease in the 20 to 30 percent of children who develop neonatal hepatitis have not been identified. Several studies have indicated that clinical and biochemical signs of cholestasis in PI ZZ infants occurred more frequently in males,[242,268] suggesting hormonal effects. A poorer prognosis for males has been suggested[242,268] but is not consistent in all series.[146,246,265] Hepatitis B virus infection, a suggested triggering factor for liver disease in PI ZZ infants,[269] has not been noted in other studies.[146,242,243,266] The potential effects of damage from oxygen radicals led to a study of the effects of treating heterozygotes (PI MZ) with vitamin E from infancy.[260] These infants, who were found to be at risk for subclinical hepatic involvement manifested only by an increase in liver enzymes, showed, up to 2 months of age, a decrease in abnormal liver function when treated with vitamin E supplementation. These data suggest that supplementation with vitamin E might also be useful for infants homozygous for α_1AT deficiency (PI ZZ). Vitamin E therapy has been shown also to improve liver function in children with cholestasis.[261]

Studies on the aggregation of Z proteins in the liver indicate that this process is enhanced by an increase in temperature. Therefore there is a rationale for prompt treatment of inflammatory illnesses that may lead to fever. This approach should help to prevent the production of this acute-phase reactant, which is accompanied by increased storage in the liver, which can lead to further liver damage.

The risk of liver disease progression has been reported to be reduced in infants who are breast-fed instead of bottle-fed during the first month of life.[270] Human milk has a high concentration of α_1AT, particularly in the first week of lactation, and a breast-fed infant can have an intake of 100 to 400 mg per 24 hr.[271] In the prospective Swedish study in which PI ZZ infants were identified through screening, 8 of 71 infants (11.3 percent) breast-fed for more than 1 month and 12 of 47 infants (25.5 percent) breast-fed for less than 1 month developed clinical signs of liver disease, and liver function test results were less abnormal than for the bottle-fed infants.[272] These differences were statistically significant. However, the two children who died of cirrhosis were both breast-fed for more than 1 month (T. Sveger, personal communication). An explanation for the effect of breast feeding has been proposed, according to which protease inhibitors in human milk help limit protease uptake and subsequent transport to the liver via the portal circulation.[273] Breast feeding does not offer absolute protection against the development of severe liver disease, but it may decrease the likelihood of perceptible early liver abnormality and lead to a better prognosis. Further data will be required to resolve this issue.

Unidentified genetic factors may be important in determining the prognosis in children with liver abnormalities in infancy. Sibship data from our hospital and from other series reporting a number of sibs of probands with liver disease have been reviewed.[274] In these studies, 32 families have been reported in which one or more sibs have been born to a family with a PI ZZ child with liver abnormalities. In 15 families in which a PI ZZ sib was born after a proband who had no liver disease or whose liver disease resolved, 13 percent of subsequent PI ZZ sibs developed liver disease. In 17 families in which the PI ZZ proband developed severe liver disease, 40 percent of subsequent PI ZZ sibs developed severe liver disease. Twelve families in the U.S. series had more than one child affected, and severe liver disease occurred in 21 percent of sibs.[266] The rate of occurrence of severe liver disease in a subsequent sib varies considerably between studies, with the highest risk, 67 percent, reported from Great Britain.[265] The risk of severe liver disease in a subsequent sib of a proband who had no liver disease or whose liver disease resolved may not differ significantly from that of the general population, estimated to be about 2 percent.[268] In view of the great variation between studies, further follow-up studies with larger numbers are needed, and present risk estimates must be considered as approximate. There may be a tendency for sibs to follow the same clinical disease course, but normal healthy children with no liver involvement can be born after PI ZZ children who have severe liver disease.

Therapy

In some children with cirrhosis and recurrent gastrointestinal bleeding, portacaval shunt was thought to be effective in slowing progression of the liver disease, with survival for 9 to 18 years after surgery.[245,275] The reason this procedure is proposed to be beneficial is because it diverts intestinal proteases from the liver to the systemic circulation, thus sparing the liver from further injury.[275]

The preferred surgical treatment for advanced liver disease is now liver transplantation, which, if successful, provides a cure because the α_1AT produced is that of the donor.[74] α_1AT deficiency is the heritable metabolic disease most often treated by liver transplantation. In a series of 26 patients treated with liver transplantation,[266] better results were observed when liver transplantation was performed early in the course of liver disease, and liver transplantation was recommended for those children who have a prolonged prothrombin unresponsive to vitamin K, a factor V activity of less than 65 percent, and recurrent hyperbilirubinemia. The 5-year survival of 29 children and 10 adults with α_1AT deficiency and liver disease was 72 and 60 percent, respectively.[276] Since the cause of progressive liver disease in some PI ZZ children is unknown, there is no rationale for replacement therapy with α_1AT. If the protease load from the intestine is crucial in the early weeks of life, then this is the period in which replacement therapy might be considered. The effects of therapy would be difficult to monitor, since most children recover spontaneously from their liver abnormalities.

Therapeutic recombinant DNA approaches are discussed at the end of this chapter.

Adult Onset

Cirrhosis and fibrosis of the liver were noted in Swedish adults with α_1AT deficiency.[277] In a series of 246 Swedish PI Z patients identified through hospital admissions, 12 percent were found to have liver cirrhosis.[192] Of the PI ZZ individuals over 50 years of age, 19 percent had cirrhosis, apparently without a history of neonatal hepatitis. In a series of 155 adults with α_1AT deficiency, 3.5 percent had biopsy- or autopsy-proven cirrhosis, and another had definite biochemical evidence of liver disease, providing a total figure of 5.2 percent affected with liver disease.[278] When these patients were classified by sex and age, the risks for development of liver disease for men and women, respectively, were as follows: age 20 to 40 years, 1.9 and 2.2 percent; age 41 to 50 years, 6.2 and 3.2 percent; age 51 to 60 years, 15.4 and 0 percent. These numbers should be considered approximate because of the small numbers in each class; no corresponding figures for the normal population are available. However, they indicate an appreciable risk for the development of cirrhosis, particularly in men over 50 years old. In an epidemiologic study based on autopsy cases of α_1AT deficiency in a Swedish city, a strong relation was found between α_1AT deficiency and cirrhosis, and also with primary liver cancer. These associations were statistically significant only for male patients.[279] The liver disease in adults appears to show rapid progression, and, in most patients, death has occurred within 2 years of the diagnosis of cirrhosis.[278,280] Perhaps the cirrhosis is advanced before diagnosis, and its symptoms are masked by the fatigue and dyspnea caused by pulmonary disease. Alcohol consumption does not appear to have been an important factor in the production of liver disease. In view of the appreciable risk for development of liver disease, particularly in men, avoiding significant amounts of alcohol and environmental toxins would be prudent.

Primary Liver Carcinoma

α_1AT deficiency appears to be associated with a small risk for hepatocellular carcinoma (hepatoma), with or without cirrhosis. Bile duct carcinoma has also been reported and may be a consequence of α_1AT storage in that tissue.[280] In an assessment of hepatic tissue from 14 adults of PI type Z selected through hospitalization, some of whom were also included in a later report,[281] cirrhosis of the liver was found in five and fibrosis in three, and three of these eight had hepatoma.[277] Of 246 PI Z patients over 20 years old admitted to Swedish hospitals, hepatoma was present in 3 percent,[192] which may be an underestimate, as 46 percent of the patients were less than 50 years old. A significant increase in primary liver cancer was observed in Sweden only in men with α_1AT deficiency, in comparison with population controls.[279] In a series of 140 adult Canadian patients of PI type Z, two had hepatoma; one of these had cirrhosis without lung disease and the other had lung disease without liver disease.[278] Another patient with emphysema and no evidence of cirrhosis has also been reported to have hepatoma.[282] These data suggest that primary liver carcinoma apparently can occur in α_1AT-deficient individuals without preexisting cirrhosis and may be due to the accumulation of α_1AT in the liver. α-Fetoprotein, which is usually elevated in hepatoma, is infrequently elevated in PI ZZ or MZ patients with hepatoma.[277,281]

In studies in which PI typing of patients with hepatoma has been carried out, homozygotes have not been found,[282–284] which is consistent with the rarity of α_1AT deficiency in the population and the associated small risk for developing hepatoma. α_1AT deficiency (homozygous or heterozygous) was not found in a series of 58 black South Africans with hepatoma,[285,286] but *PI*Z* is not found in black populations. Studies of pathologic tissues have yielded conflicting and unreliable results. Of 56 Danish patients with hepatoma, 23 percent were found to have PAS-D-positive globules, taken to be indicative of the presence of Z-type α_1AT, whether in the homozygous or heterozygous state.[287] Livers of 2 of 42 patients in England with hepatoma had PAS-D-positive granules, not more than expected in the normal population.[288] These studies are difficult to interpret since PI MZ individuals do not always show PAS granules in the liver, and tumor tissues can show PAS-D granules where no such granules are present in the nontumor tissue.[289]

In summary, the data suggest that α_1AT deficiency, at least in males, is associated with a small increased risk for hepatocellular carcinoma or hepatoma, usually in association with cirrhosis.

Risk for Heterozygotes

PI Type SZ Heterozygotes. A number of isolated cases of liver disease occurring in individuals of PI type SZ have been reported and have led some to conclude that these individuals are at increased risk for liver disease.[290] The reports of isolated cases in both adults and children can be explained by chance, since about 1 in 700 to 1 in 1500 of the general population is of PI type SZ. The strongest evidence for lack of risk for childhood disease comes from the Swedish screening study, which has shown a modest elevation of liver enzymes in a portion of children of PI type SZ during the early months of life but no clinical abnormalities or elevation of liver enzymes by 8 years of age.[268] Screening of 857 Swedish adults with liver disease revealed seven PI SZ individuals where one was expected, suggesting a possible increased risk for PI SZ adults.[281] Smaller studies have not confirmed this association.

PI Type MZ Heterozygotes. An increased risk for cirrhosis in PI MZ individuals has been suggested. Since 2 to 4 percent of white populations are of PI type MZ, chance associations with liver disease would be expected. In surveys, appropriate PI typing must be carried out, as it is not possible to determine the phenotype from PAS-D-positive inclusions in the liver. Individuals of PI types MZ and ZZ can both have inclusions. Furthermore, the presence of an anodal electrophoretic band migrating close to a major band of Z α_1AT can cause such patients to be misdiagnosed as being of PI type MZ (Fig. 138-4A).

In a screening study of almost 15,000 newborns in Italy, liver function tests were carried out on 101 PI MZ and 135 PI MS infants.[260] Aspartate aminotransferase (AST), alanine aminotransferase (ALT), and γ-glutamyltranspeptidase (αGT) all appeared to be similarly sensitive as indicators of liver damage. Elevation of liver enzymes as a sign of hepatic dysfunction was observed in PI MZ individuals as follows: 19 percent at 2 months, 8 percent at 5 months, and 1 percent at 12 months of age. Similarly, in 135 PI MS infants, abnormalities were observed in 15 percent at 2 months, in 7 percent at 5 months, and in none at 12 months of age. The concentration of plasma α_1AT was similar in the infants with normal and abnormal liver function tests. Uninhibited proteolytic enzymes in the liver of individuals with a partial α_1AT deficiency may allow cellular damage, perhaps through the production of highly reactive superoxide radicals.

In adults as well, a partial deficiency of α_1AT may play some role in the development of liver disease. In a study of English patients with various types of liver disease, a significant increase in PI MZ individuals was found only in patients with cirrhosis.[291] In the group with cirrhosis, PI type MZ was found in 21 percent of all patients with hepatitis Bs antigen (HBsAg*)-negative chronic active hepatitis and in 21 percent of patients with cryptogenic cirrhosis. Conflicting data have been reported from England[292]; however, the latter study may not have identified those PI MZ individuals with normal plasma levels of α_1AT. No other study has confirmed such a high risk. Among 335 patients with a variety of liver diseases, 3.3 percent were of PI type MZ, compared with 2.9 percent of normal healthy blood donors.[293] However, when examined by specific type of liver disease, PI type MZ was found in none of 53 patients with autoimmune chronic active hepatitis, in 2 of 18 patients (11.1 percent) with cryptogenic cirrhosis, in 3 of 79 patients (3.8 percent) with alcoholic liver cirrhosis, in 2 of 36 patients (5.6 percent) with primary sclerosing cholangitis, and in 1 of 26 patients (3.9 percent) with primary biliary cirrhosis. In a study in France of 159 adults with liver cirrhosis, 132 of whom had chronic alcoholism, a small and nonsignificant increase in the number of PI MZ individuals in both alcoholic and nonalcoholic groups was found.[294] In a study in Spain of 157 alcoholic patients with cirrhosis, a significant increase in individuals of PI type MZ, but not MS, was found (7 percent in cirrhotic patients, 1.7 percent in controls).[295] Of 857 Swedish patients with liver disease, 7.6 percent, rather than the expected 4.8 percent, were identified using a monoclonal antibody for detecting PI Z and were confirmed as of PI type MZ.[281] This difference, similar to those in previous studies, was significant with the larger patient group. Measurement of the concentration of serum α_1AT was not helpful in identifying adult patients with PI type MZ because of the acute-phase nature of α_1AT.[296] In this study, established liver disease was absent in 12 of 37 patients in whom α_1AT granules were detected, but the inclusions were the sole putative etiologic agent in 9.4 percent with cirrhosis of unknown etiology.

In summary, most studies suggest a small increase in risk for liver disease in individuals heterozygous for α_1AT deficiency. Environmental agents, such as viruses or alcohol, can perhaps trigger liver damage in susceptible individuals. In a study of 164 patients who were PI ZZ homozygotes and Z heterozygotes (mostly MZ), viral infections and alcohol appeared to play a prominent role in initiation of liver disease.[297]

Most studies in which PI typing rather than liver inclusions have been the basis for diagnosis indicate that PI MZ individuals are not at increased risk for hepatoma.[282–284]

OTHER DISEASE ASSOCIATIONS

A variety of disorders other than liver and lung disease have been reported to show an association with α_1AT deficiency or other variants. These disorders are generally associated with the inflammatory response and/or with hyperactivity of the immune system. The basis for hyperactivity of the immune system has been discussed above (see "Function in the Immune Response"). This increased susceptibility may be exacerbated by a decreased ability to control local inflammation. Disease associations could also be due to potential variants in adjacent genes of the serine protease inhibitor cluster; those of corticosteroid-binding protein may be particularly relevant.

Further aspects of associations with immune disorders were reviewed by Breit et al.[70]

Disorders with Immune-Response and Inflammatory Components

Kidney Disease. Membranoproliferative glomerulonephritis (MPGN) was noted in patients with α_1AT deficiency and liver disease[263,298,299] and may be a relatively frequent occurrence. Low levels of complement C3 were reported in two of these patients, and circulating immune complexes were found in the one patient tested.[299] Nephropathy was noted in 79 percent of 19 patients of PI type ZZ with chronic liver disease.[300] Seven had mesangiocapillary glomerulonephritis, and six had focal segmental mesangial proliferative glomerulonephritis, which was found at similar frequency in patients with chronic liver disease due to other causes. These authors noted that glomerular lesions might be present despite a normal urinalysis and that the type of nephropathy varies. In agreement with earlier studies by Moroz et al.,[263] the nephropathy was accompanied by granular α_1AT deposits at the subendothelial region of the glomerular basement membrane. Deposits of immunoglobulins IgG, M, and A and of complement component C3, which are frequently found in cases of MPGN, were also identified[146,298] and may represent an immune response to the abnormal circulating PI Z protein released by hepatic destruction.[263] Multiple immune complex disorders have been reported in two adults with α_1AT deficiency, obstructive lung disease, progressive glomerulonephritis, and, in addition, mild liver disease and necrotizing angiitis[301] or cutaneous vasculitis and colitis.[302] One hypothesis is that abnormal α_1AT from liver inclusions participates in the formation of an immune complex. All of the children in whom MPGN was identified had severe liver disease, suggesting that the kidney abnormality was a consequence of the liver disease. However, in a study of 246 Swedish PI Z patients, 37 (15 percent) showed signs of glomerular renal damage, indicated by constant or recurrent proteinuria or hematuria.[192] Three patients (1 percent) developed advanced renal failure. Since these patients were all identified through hospitalization, the risk of severe renal disease in PI Z patients appears to be low, although its association with liver disease in this condition may be relatively high. α_1AT deficiency is not a common cause of MPGN; among 53 patients with idiopathic MPGN, none were homozygous or heterozygous for PI Z.[299]

Panniculitis. Panniculitis is characterized by inflammation of the panniculitis adiposis, the fat layer under the dermis. The risk of panniculitis in patients with α_1AT deficiency must be relatively small, as the condition has not been identified in surveys of patients of PI type ZZ. On the other hand, a large number of cases have now been reported of severe ulcerative panniculitis associated with α_1AT deficiency. Among five patients with panniculitis, two severely affected had α_1AT deficiency.[303] Two of three sibs of a PI type ZZ individual were reported to have panniculitis.[304] In a study of 96 patients with panniculitis, 15.6 percent were found to be α_1AT deficient, as defined by the serum concentration.[305] At least 41 cases of panniculitis in association with α_1AT deficiency have now been reported. Administration of purified α_1AT was successful in the treatment of two particularly severe cases; doxycycline, a tetracycline that inhibits collagenase activity, has also been effective.[306,307]

While α_1AT is unlikely to be a cause of panniculitis, in the presence of triggering agents, among them histoplasmosis,[308] patients of PI type ZZ appear to have impaired ability to control the inflammation.

Rheumatoid Arthritis. An increased frequency of the heterozygous deficiency PI types MZ and SZ was reported in adults with rheumatoid arthritis.[309] Subsequent studies have been carried out in different populations with conflicting results. This disagreement could result from geographical differences but more likely results from differences in patient selection. In a U.S. study, no increase in the frequency of Z heterozygotes was found in a group of patients who were mostly off medication and therefore probably not severely affected.[310] No more Z heterozygotes than expected were found among patients, not selected for disease severity, in Sweden[311] or Switzerland.[312] However, in another Swedish study, in which all 200 patients had erosive rheumatoid arthritis, an increase in the frequency of Z heterozygotes was found.[313] A significant increase in the frequency of the PI MZ phenotype among patients has been shown in three British studies[314–316] and in Australia.[70] The report of an increase in the frequency of PI type MS[70] must be interpreted with caution because of marked differences in population frequencies for the *PI*S* allele. These data seem to be compatible with our conclusion that an increased frequency of Z heterozygosity occurs particularly among individuals with seropositive erosive arthritis.[317] In the Swedish study of 246 hospitalized PI Z patients, 4.4 percent had rheumatoid arthritis, and another 3 percent had a history of considerable joint pain with no confirmed diagnosis.[192] We have concluded that tissue destruction occurs more readily in the PI Z heterozygote because of inadequate α_1AT present in the joint fluid to prevent leukocyte elastase, cathepsin G, and collagenase from attacking the structural proteins of joint cartilage.[317] An increased frequency of PI FM, confirmed by family studies,[318] may be significant because of the increased sensitivity of the F variant to oxidation.[112]

A numerical but nonsignificant increase in the frequency of Z heterozygotes was found in children with juvenile rheumatoid arthritis,[317] and a study of more severely affected British children showed a significantly increased frequency of PI type MZ.[319] Juvenile arthritis consists of a number of different subgroups, and perhaps some but not all of these subgroups show increased susceptibility.

Other Disorders Associated with PI MZ or ZZ. Anterior uveitis, an immune-mediated inflammatory eye disease, has been reported to be associated with an increased frequency of Z heterozygotes,[320,321] with an increase also in the frequency of PI type MS in the latter study. The association was not confirmed in a study of 57 white American patients.[322] These discrepancies may be due to the type of patients selected. In posterior uveitis, 2 of 16 patients were of PI type MZ,[321] and further studies of these types of patients are required. Studies of PI MZ frequency in psoriasis have been contradictory.[323,324] Isolated cases of PI Z individuals with persistent cutaneous vasculitis,[325] panarteritis in association with emphysema and glomerular nephritis,[301] Hashimoto thyroiditis,[326] and severe combined immunodeficiency[327] have been reported. A slight but statistically nonsignificant increase of PI MZ from 3 to 7 percent was observed in systemic lupus erythematosis.[70] SLE occurred in 2 of 246 adult Swedish patients.[192]

The isolated reports of idiopathic hemochromatosis in PI MZ heterozygotes and in homozygotes[328,329] may be due to chance association, or hemochromatosis could promote cirrhosis when coexisting with α_1AT deficiency. In a Canadian study of 15 patients, 3 were of PI type MZ.[330] The PI Z gene, as detected by a monoclonal antibody, has not been found in either the heterozygous or homozygous state in 27 male patients with idiopathic hemochromatosis, all from the same region of Sweden.[331]

Malignancy

Studies have been carried out on a number of malignant conditions in addition to hepatoma. In a study of patients with bladder carcinoma, a significant increase in *PI*Z* frequency and decrease in *PI*M3* frequency was found in comparison with control subjects.[332] *PI*M3* frequency was also decreased in a series of lymphoma and leukemia patients. A protease–protease inhibitor imbalance could affect tumor invasiveness. A mechanism for involvement of *PI*M3* is not apparent. Because M3 is not always readily differentiated from *PI*M1*, care must be taken to avoid technical artifacts.

Other Associations

Uninhibited elastase activity could lead to arterial weakening, accounting for the increase in the frequency of PI type MZ in 47 patients with abdominal aortic aneurysm (11 percent versus 2 to 4 percent in the general population).[333] A mesenteric artery aneurysm has been described in a PI ZZ individual.[334]

An increased frequency of heterozygotes was found among parents of 21 probands with X chromosome mosaicism,[335] but the overall frequency of Z heterozygosity among patients with Down syndrome appears to be normal (reviewed by Fagerhol and Cox[7]). Proteolytic enzymes are involved in fertilization in cell division and could potentially be disturbed in the presence of inadequate protease inhibition.[336] Perhaps the same mechanisms are involved in the suggested slight increase in twinning associated with MZ[337] and MS[338] heterozygotes.

A variety of single case reports involving other disorders have been reviewed.[66]

PRENATAL DIAGNOSIS

Prenatal diagnosis was first carried out by PI typing of fetal blood obtained at fetoscopy,[339] and was accompanied by a relatively high risk to the fetus. DNA analysis is now the preferred approach, using PCR-based methods.[340] The source of fetal DNA can be amniocytes or chorion villi.

Reliable PI typing is a crucial first step in prenatal diagnosis to determine that both parents have the Z allele and that no rare deficiency or null allele is present in either parent.

Risk for an Affected Fetus

For parents of PI type MZ with no offspring, the risk of having a PI ZZ child in whom severe liver disease develops is the general population risk of 2 percent, with an overall risk (PI type undetermined) of 0.5 percent. For PI type MZ parents who have had a child with liver abnormalities, the risk for a PI ZZ child with severe liver disease is influenced by the course of liver disease in the previous child; it ranges from 13 percent of PI 22 offspring if the liver disease has resolved, to as much as 40 percent if severe liver disease persists. The basis for these risks is discussed in the section "Liver Disease" above.

Direct Mutation Detection

Synthetic oligonucleotide probes that recognize the single Z base-pair substitution can be used. This method requires that the presence of a Z allele is definitely established in both parents, as the probes will not recognize the rare deficiency mutations. Specific oligonucleotide probes have been prepared around the Z mutant site at amino acid 342 for normal M and deficiency Z DNA sequences[341] and were initially used for prenatal diagnosis on a genomic fragment cut with a specific restriction enzyme.[342] The use of the PCR offers a major improvement. The appropriate region of exon 5 can be amplified by PCR, and the Z mutation detected by using oligonucleotide probes labeled with ^{32}P[343] or with biotin.[344] A similar approach, using specific oligonucleotide probes, can also be used where one of the rare variants of α_1AT has been detected. As an alternate method for the Z mutation, a primer designed with a nucleotide substitution can create a *Taq* I site in the normal allele but not in the Z form,[345,346] an approach also used with the enzyme *Xmn* I for the S mutation.[346] A potential concern about this approach is that failure of digestion of the DNA sample for technical reasons could lead to misinterpretation of an M sample as Z. This could be overcome by incorporating another *Taq* I restriction site in the designed primer as a positive control. An advantage of the method is simplicity and lack of requirement for labeled oligonucleotide.

Restriction Site Polymorphisms

Prior to widespread use of the PCR, genomic probes from the α_1AT gene were used to identify polymorphic restriction fragments that predict the PI type of the fetus. If previous PI typing in the family has indicated the presence of a rare deficiency allele or a PI null allele for which the mutation is unknown, DNA polymorphisms can be used for prenatal diagnosis by following segregation of markers in the family. Genomic probes used for diagnosis of α_1AT deficiency lie within the gene and detect polymorphisms of both α_1AT and the α_1AT-homologous region. α_1AT deficiency is unusual, to date, in that the DNA haplotype associated with the *PI*Z* allele has been found to be specific and unique. Studies of parents and sibs are theoretically unnecessary, although in practice they are advisable because of the possibility of rare exceptions. Polymorphisms in the α_1AT region have been discussed above. When genomic probes only are used, culturing of chorionic villus cells is not required, and it is undesirable because of the possibility of maternal contamination. Two different restriction enzyme digests are advisable for verification of results. The most useful probe for prenatal diagnosis is genomic probe 6.5 (Fig. 138-3B). The restriction enzymes that have been found particularly useful for prenatal diagnosis are a combination of *BstE* II and *Bgl* II.[132] *Ava* II, the first enzyme to be applied in prenatal diagnosis, is unsatisfactory for chorionic villus DNA, apparently because of a methylation difference.[274]

POPULATION SCREENING

The screening of 200,000 Swedish infants has demonstrated that newborn screening is feasible.[145,242] In this study, a disk was punched from a dried blood sample on filter paper and eluted for a semiquantitative electroimmuno assay of both α_1AT and transferrin (as an internal standard). Infants with less than 40 percent of normal α_1AT had a blood sample drawn for PI typing. Most of the infants ascertained in this way were found to be of PI type ZZ; 28 percent of those PI typed were of PI type SZ. Although electroimmuno assay was used in this population screening, automated nephelometry could be used for the quantitation of α_1AT and transferrin. The screening program could conveniently be carried out on the same dried blood spots used for the Guthrie test for newborns for phenylketonuria. PI typing can be carried out on the dried blood samples by using silver stain following isoelectric focusing.[347]

At present, the main value of a population screening program would be to counsel the parents to encourage their affected children to avoid smoking later in life. This message must be reinforced directly with the children as they reach the teen years. Even with such reinforcement, we do not know if young adults who are then healthy will avoid smoking. Because of the known increased risk of respiratory disease in children of cigarette smokers, parents of children with α_1AT deficiency should be advised not to smoke. At 4-year follow-up of the Swedish children screened for α_1AT deficiency, 26 percent of parents had stopped smoking specifically because of their child's deficiency. However, 44 percent of mothers and 33 percent of fathers continued smoking.[248] The data are very clear, as discussed, in indicating that if smoking is avoided, the onset of obstructive pulmonary disease will be considerably delayed.

An extensive follow-up of psychological consequences of the Swedish screening program has indicated that most parents initially thought of the α_1AT deficiency as an imminent and serious threat to their child's health.[348] These negative feelings were still present in 58 percent of mothers and 44 percent of fathers when interviewed 5 to 7 years after the initial identification of α_1AT deficiency.[349] If population screening is undertaken in newborns, parents should be informed that the testing is to be undertaken and should be informed of the presence of the deficiency in their infant by an individual knowledgeable about the condition. Although specific treatment is not available for children with signs of liver disease, administration of antioxidants and encouragement of breast-feeding may help to alter the course of disease. Repeated long-term follow-up beyond the first year of life may be unnecessary for those children who show no signs of liver disturbance. Some provision must be made for later reinforcement of the need to avoid smoking, which may be difficult in families with a high degree of mobility.

While screening during the newborn period, in combination with other neonatal screening, is probably most efficient, the avoidance of smoking later in life may be more effectively accomplished by a screening program later in childhood.

TREATMENT

Preventive Therapy for Lung Destruction

The most effective therapy for the lung destruction of α_1AT deficiency is prevention, mainly through avoidance of smoking. In those individuals who begin to show relatively early signs of lung destruction, the rate of destruction may be slowed by restoring the protease–inhibitor balance in the lung through administration of suitable protease inhibitors.

In the earliest studies of α_1AT deficiency, subjects were identified mainly through pulmonary clinics, leading to the impression that most individuals with the deficiency would eventually develop emphysema. However, the outlook for those with α_1AT deficiency now appears to be more positive. In order to prevent lung destruction, the most important message for patients with the deficiency is to avoid exposure to smoke at all ages.

As previously discussed, α_1AT is known to be inactivated by oxidation. Therefore, consideration should be given to maintaining maximal antioxidant activity in lung tissue. Vitamin E status may be important in determining individual susceptibility to lung destruction. Administration of vitamin E in doses that adequately cover the daily requirements could help to protect from lung disease and is perhaps not adequately considered as a form of preventive therapy.

Augmentation Therapy

The adult human lung has a limited capacity for self-repair, and emphysema, once established, cannot be reversed. The rationale of augmentation therapy is to increase the α_1AT plasma concentration, and consequently that of the lower lung, to protective levels to delay the rate of lung deterioration or, if administered early, to prevent it. Individuals of PI type SZ have an α_1AT concentration of 22 mg/dl (35 percent of normal), which is likely to be sufficient to protect against lung destruction except in smokers. PI type MZ individuals, who appear to have an adequate level of protection against lung disease, have approximately 60 percent, or 78 mg/dl, of plasma α_1AT. The protective plasma level is therefore considered to be 80 mg/dl, or 11 μM (for reviews, see refs. 350 and 351).

Initial attempts at therapy for α_1AT deficiency focused on increasing the in vivo release of endogenous α_1AT from hepatocytes. Danazol, an isoxazole derivative of the synthetic steroid 17-ethanol testosterone, lacks major androgenic properties and was initially used because of its successful treatment of deficiency of the serum protease inhibitor C1 esterase in hereditary angioedema.[352] However, the plasma concentration of α_1AT achieved with this treatment was well below the protective level, and, furthermore, side effects were noted, including the possibility of liver damage.[353] Since increasing hepatocyte production of α_1AT also has potential for increased liver destruction owing to increased liver stores of α_1AT, this type of therapy is inappropriate.

Low-molecular-weight inhibitors, such as chloromethyl ketone peptides[354] or modified cephalosporin antibiotics,[355] have been considered for therapy. They usually disappear rapidly from the circulation, but direct administration to the lungs by aerosol may be possible. Other modes of therapy have become more promising.

All of the ways to augment lung α_1AT have application to cystic fibrosis, in which they would help combat the excessive proteolysis enhanced by the chronic inflammation associated with this disease.[351]

Guidelines for Therapy. Therapy guidelines for patients with α_1AT deficiency have been established by the American Thoracic Society[361] and by the Standards Committee, Canadian Thoracic Society.[362] The guidelines stress the importance of avoiding respiratory irritants and using maximum supportive therapy, including bronchodilators, cardiovascular conditioning, and oxygen if clinically indicated. In the U.S., augmentation therapy has been suggested for patients 18 years of age or older who show abnormal lung function test results and are believed to be capable of complying with the demanding protocol of weekly infusions. Because there is as yet no evidence from a clinical trial that aerosol or infusion therapy influences the clinical course, which costs about $25,000 per year for a 70 kg patient, the Canadian Thoracic Society has suggested that replacement therapy should not yet be standard treatment. Health care delivery systems differ from country to country and, in some (e.g., Canada), therapy would be available universally and without direct cost to the patient. This situation emphasizes the need for documentation regarding benefit of the therapy before the cost burden is added to the health-care system. Although not specifically noted in these guidelines, information is now available on the rate of decline of lung function for smokers and nonsmokers (see "Obstructive Lung Disease" above). A determination of the rate of decline of lung function in a given patient should provide a rational basis for therapy. Some patients decline very little over time, while in others, even nonsmokers, the decline is more rapid. The rate of decline would be a useful factor in deciding when this expensive augmentation therapy might be useful. Consideration might also be given to sporadic use of augmentation therapy during times of stress, such as surgery or respiratory infections. It is interesting that the guidelines do not specifically mention antioxidant therapy, which seems logically to have a place in the management of this condition.

The advantages and disadvantages of augmentation therapy must be carefully weighed in elderly persons or those with severe lung function impairment; the burden of the weekly infusions must be considered against the expectation of little real benefit in such individuals.[363]

Infusion Therapy. The current and most promising treatment for α_1AT deficiency is the administration of α_1AT purified from human plasma, by infusion at weekly or monthly intervals. Lung destruction is a chronic lifetime process; therefore, constant maintenance of an increased blood level of α_1AT would be required to prevent excessive lung destruction. Because of the variation between individuals in rate of lung decline, a properly controlled clinical study, with monitoring of decline in lung function or mortality rate, would be exceedingly difficult and costly. To show a 40 percent decrease in the decline of FEV_1 requires 500 patients and control subjects studied for a 3-year period.[356] Therefore, proof of efficacy of therapeutic products has been considered to be established if the product raises α_1AT plasma concentration to levels found in patients of PI type MZ, and if active α_1AT is found in lung wash fluids of treated patients.[357]

With weekly infusions of 60 mg/kg human α_1AT to 32 individuals with α_1AT deficiency, a consistent plasma concentration above threshold level could be maintained. A peak level greater than 40 μM of plasma α_1AT occurs shortly after infusion, with a rapid decline over the first 2 days, and a gradual decline during the remainder of the week.[358] In a further eight patients studied on weekly therapy for 30 months, no deterioration in lung function and disease was observed during the study period, where normally a decline in lung function would have been expected.[359]

Because of the inconvenience of weekly infusions of α_1AT, a regimen of monthly treatment has also been tested. In a trial of safety and pharmacologic response, 19 individuals with α_1AT deficiency were given 250 mg/kg of purified human plasma at 28-day intervals. A peak level of greater than 130 μM, greater than normal α_1AT levels and more than 10 times over threshold, was obtained, with rapid decline during the first 2 days and slower decline over the remainder of the month. The average serum level during monthly treatment was twice the threshold value. Tests of lung fluid obtained by lavage indicated that a protective level of antineutrophil elastase capacity was maintained in the lung. No significant adverse clinical reactions were observed. While the total amount of α_1AT used for monthly augmentation was the same as for weekly augmentation, the amount of time required and the administrative cost could be reduced using this approach. However, owing to the delivery of such a high protein load, infusion requires 6 to 8 h to avoid cardiovascular compromise.[360] The simultaneous combination of plasma exchange with monthly intravenous infusion permits larger amounts of α_1AT to be administered in a shorter time period (less than 2 h). However, a markedly increased amount of α_1AT is administered by this approach, with resulting plasma levels similar to those obtained with monthly treatment.

Aerosol Therapy. Since the lungs are, in most cases, the only major organ to be significantly damaged by elastase degradation, an efficient approach to therapy is to deliver α_1AT directly to the lungs. Perhaps as little as 2 percent of infused α_1AT reaches the lung during intravenous therapy.[350] Effective aerosol therapy depends on delivery of droplets of appropriate size into the lung alveoli. Studies in sheep demonstrated that aerosolized α_1AT passed through the lower respiratory tract epithelium and gained access to the interstitium of the alveolar walls.[364] These investigators also showed that aerosolized M-type α_1AT could be demonstrated in the serum of Z type individuals. Measurement of antineutrophil elastase activity in lung lavage fluid indicated that aerosol administration, 100 mg twice daily, raised the level in both lung and plasma 20-fold after 1 week, to levels within the upper range of normal and well beyond the protective threshold level.[350] There were no adverse clinical reactions. This approach would require only about 10 to 30 percent the amount of purified α_1AT used for the intravenous approach. This is an exciting potential therapy for α_1AT deficiency. If this approach continues to show effectiveness, its use, perhaps in combination with antioxidant administration, may provide an economically feasible approach to the treatment of α_1AT deficiency.

Recombinant α_1AT for Augmentation Therapy. Because of the requirements for large amounts of α_1AT and the potential risk of infection in using human blood products, large-scale synthesis of human α_1AT through recombinant DNA methodology is potentially useful. Normal human α_1AT has been produced at a high level in *Escherichia coli*[365,366] and in yeast.[21] The α_1AT from both hosts is functionally active as an elastase inhibitor, and they have similar activities for inhibiting neutrophil elastase in the presence of α_1AT-deficient plasma.[367] A modified α_1AT, resistant to oxidative inactivation, has been produced by site-directed mutagenesis, substituting valine for methionine at amino acid 385.[21,368,369] The valine form produced in yeast is as effective an inhibitor of neutrophil and pancreatic elastase as the normal methionine form, but does not inhibit cathepsin G, pancreatic trypsin, plasmin, factor Xa, or thrombin.[370] The valine form is also effective at inhibiting proteolysis of glomerular basement membrane by neutrophils.[369] This form shows effective resistance to oxidation by a variety of oxidants, including *N*-chlorosuccinimide, myeloperoxidase, activated neutrophils, and cigarette smoke, although sufficiently long exposure to these agents brings about some inactivation.[354]

The α_1AT produced in yeast and *E. coli* completely lacks carbohydrate side chains. While the functional characteristics of the synthetic α_1AT are normal, its heat stability is decreased, indicating that the carbohydrate side chains are important for normal stability.[358] Lack of side chains presents a major problem for the use of these synthetic forms, as their half-life is extremely short. The valine and methionine mutants in yeast have a half-life of 8.5 h in the rabbit, in comparison with the 2.2-day half-life of normal human α_1AT.[370] An advantage of the use of the valine form is that lower doses may be required, because of its resistance to oxidation. However, frequent administration of the synthetic α_1AT would still be necessary.

Aerosol therapy has also been tested with recombinant α_1AT.[371] Recombinant α_1AT was first administered subcutaneously to α_1AT-deficient individuals and was shown to induce no immunologic or other clinical reactions.[372] When various doses of recombinant α_1AT were administered by aerosol to 16 patients with α_1AT deficiency, the neutrophil elastase inhibitory capacity increased in the lung, and the recombinant α_1AT was detected in plasma. In spite of the short half-life of the recombinant protein, direct delivery to the lung may make it usable for treatment.

An interesting possibility for producing the large amounts of α_1AT necessary for augmentation therapy is the use of transgenic animals. The potential of this method is shown in an experiment in sheep, in which the α_1AT gene was spliced to the gene for β lactoglobin, a protein made exclusively in the milk of ruminants. When the construct was injected into sheep embryos, some of the resulting sheep were able to produce large amounts of human α_1AT[373]—as much as 35 g of human α_1AT per liter of milk. This approach, if it proves to be safe from animal pathogens, would avoid the potential risk of HIV and other human viruses that could inadvertently contaminate the product made from human blood.

Gene Therapy for α_1AT Deficiency

α_1AT deficiency has provided a useful model for testing gene therapy approaches. This approach involves altering host cells by adding a normal α_1AT gene to the host genome (for a review, see Crystal[351]). Three vector systems—plasmid, retrovirus, and replication-deficient adenovirus—have been evaluated. The general gene therapy approach of removing cells from the patient, modifying them, and reintroducing the modified cells to the patient is difficult when the product must be targeted to the lung. Plasmids are relatively inefficient in gene transfer and are sometimes linked to a ligand to target them to a particular cell type. A concern with the use of retroviral vectors is the possibility that they will target into a gene involved in tumorigenesis and lead to malignancy. Adenovirus, a virus that causes upper and lower respiratory tract infections in humans, has avidity for epithelia of the respiratory tract, and most of the retrovirus DNA remains extrachromosomal. The vector does not require host cell replication for gene expression, thus bypassing the problem of slow replication of endothelial cells.

Gene Therapy via the Lung. The α_1AT gene has been introduced, using a retroviral vector, into mouse fibroblasts, which, when transplanted into the peritoneum of nude mice, produced human α_1AT in serum and in epithelial lining fluid of the lung.[374] A recombinant adenovirus has been used to transfer human α_1AT into cultured endothelial cells.[375] Studies in rats have demonstrated that an adenovirus vector can transfer the α_1AT gene to respiratory epithelium, where it is secreted on both the air and interstitial surfaces.[376] Data from these studies have been used to suggest that gene transfer into pulmonary arteries and capillaries could provide a source of secreted α_1AT.

Gene Therapy in Hepatocytes. Another approach to gene therapy is to transfer the gene into the liver. General approaches have been reviewed.[377] Transfer of genes into hepatocytes could create a source of α_1AT, which could prevent both the liver and lung damage associated with α_1AT deficiency if circulating levels of α_1AT were sufficiently high. Primary cultures of hepatocytes infected with a recombinant adenovirus containing a human gene have been shown, in animal models, to produce human product. The Watanabe rabbit, which has heritable hyperlipidemia, was used as a model to show that allogenic hepatocytes could be transplanted into the affected rabbits to ameliorate hypercholesterolemia.[378] In this rabbit, the gene was introduced in a plasmid construct attached to an asialoglycoprotein receptor, which targets to the liver cell.

Human hepatocytes cultured in vitro have also been shown to be susceptible to retroviral infection, with expression of the transfected gene.[379] The approach of obtaining hepatocytes from an affected human, transfecting them with an adenovirus containing the defective gene, and returning the transfected cell to the affected donor into the peripheral circulation is therefore possible. This approach has been tested with α_1AT in rats and demonstrated that targeted gene expression could be achieved in the liver, although at low levels and disappearing after several weeks.[380] Deterioration of gene expression, owing in part to the instability of the targeted DNA, was found to be improved when animals were subjected to partial hepatectomy following in vivo gene transfer.[381] These investigators found that the DNA in the hepatocytes was present in stabilized plasmids, or episomes, which do not self-replicate. These episomes remain relatively stable and continue to produce α_1AT for at least 4 months, after hepatocyte regeneration is induced by partial hepatectomy.[382] The transfection of an α_1AT gene into human hepatocytes with a subsequent level, perhaps low, of production of α_1AT is technically feasible. A high level of expression would not be required to protect against the development of emphysema. However, it is not known if this approach would help to avoid liver disease, if the latter is caused by the storage of inclusions. Furthermore, there may be easier ways to protect susceptible individuals, particularly through environmental manipulation. On the other hand, as this approach develops, it may become a feasible treatment for null homozygotes. Long-term therapy with injection or gene therapy of null homozygotes needs to be approached with caution owing to the possibility of an immune reaction to replacement α_1AT protein. However, the presence of even trace amounts of endogenous α_1AT may help prevent the formation of antibodies against α_1AT.

α_1AT deficiency has provided a useful model for testing various types of gene therapy. However, at a practical level, the much simpler approaches of α_1AT infusion or delivery by aerosol, and/or antioxidant therapy may be more feasible and cost effective.

Lung Transplantation

Lung transplantation has become a feasible treatment in selected patients with end-stage lung disease. The success of lung transplantation rose markedly in the late 1980s, spearheaded by a Toronto group, with development of an omentum wrap at the site of the bronchial suture, a better understanding of potential adverse effects of corticosteroid therapy on the healing of the bronchial anastomosis, and the introduction of cyclosporin.[383] While double-lung transplantation was initially believed to be necessary for patients with chronic obstructive pulmonary disease, excellent success has now been obtained with single and bilateral sequential transplantation.[383,384] Among 66 lung transplant recipients, of whom 19 had α_1AT deficiency with emphysema, the actuarial survival at 1 year was 82 percent for the bilateral lung transplant recipients and 90 percent for the single-lung transplant recipients.[383] While the FEV_1 was significantly better after bilateral lung transplantation than after single-lung transplantation, there was little difference in exercise capacity.[383] In another group of 23 patients undergoing single-lung transplantation, of whom 5 had α_1AT deficiency, surgical procedures were slightly different and the selection criteria less stringent. In this latter study, the actuarial survival rate was 77 percent at 1 year and 73 percent at 2 years.[384] This is considered a feasible approach for patients less than 60 years of age.

ACKNOWLEDGMENTS

This chapter is dedicated to the late Andrew Sass-Kortsak, M.D., F.R.C.P. (C), my teacher, mentor, and friend, who was responsible for initiation of studies of α_1AT and provided continuous support.

I acknowledge with thanks Dr. Eve Roberts for review and helpful comments and Kristina Garrels, Dr. Barbara Byth, and Gail Billingsley for assistance in manuscript preparation.

REFERENCES

1. Schultze HE, Gollner I, Heide K, Schonenberger M, Schwick G: Zur Kenntnis der alpha globuline des menschlichen normalserums. *Z Naturforsch* **10**:463, 1955.
2. Fagerhol MK, Laurell C-B: The Pi system—inherited variants of serum α-antitrypsin, in Steinberg A, Bearn A (eds): *Medical Genetics* Vol. 7. New York, Grune and Stratton, 1970, p. 96.
3. Laurell C-B, Eriksson S: The electrophoretic α_1-globulin pattern of serum in α_1-antitrypsin deficiency. *Scand J Clin Lab Invest* **15**:132, 1963.
4. Eriksson S: Studies in α_1-antitrypsin deficiency. *Acta Med Scand [Suppl]* **432**:5, 1965.
5. Eriksson S: Discovery of α_1-antitrypsin deficiency. *Lung* **168**(Suppl):523, 1990.
6. Fagerhol MK, Laurell C-B: The polymorphism of "prealbumins" and α_1-antitrypsin in human sera. *Clin Chim Acta* **16**:199, 1967.
7. Fagerhol MK, Cox DW: The Pi polymorphism: Genetic, biochemical and clinical aspects of human α_1-antitrypsin, in Harris H, Hirschhorn K (eds): *Hum Genet* Vol. 11. New York, Plenum, 1981, p. 1.
8. Axelson U, Laurell C-B: Hereditary variants of serum α_1-antitrypsin. *Am J Hum Genet* **17**:466, 1965.
9. Fagerhol MK: Serum Pi types in Norwegians. *Acta Pathol Microbiol Scand* **70**:421, 1967.
10. Sharp HL, Bridges RA, Krivit W: Cirrhosis associated with alpha-1-antitrypsin deficiency: A previously unrecognized inherited disorder. *J Lab Clin Med* **73**:934, 1969.
11. Hutchison DC: The epidemiology of α_1-antitrypsin deficiency. *Lung* **168**(Suppl):535, 1990.
12. Brantly M, Nukiwa T, Crystal RG: Molecular basis of alpha-1-antitrypsin deficiency. *Am J Med* **84**:13, 1988.
13. Crystal RG: Alpha-1-antitrypsin deficiency, emphysema, and liver disease. Genetic basis and strategies for therapy. *J Clin Invest* **85**:1343, 1990.
14. Lindmark B, Svenonius E, Eriksson S: Heterozygous α_1-antichymotrypsin and PiZ α_1-antitrypsin deficiency. Prevalence and clinical spectrum in asthmatic children. *Allergy* **45**:197, 1990.
15. Travis J, Salvesen GS: Human plasma proteinase inhibitors. *Annu Rev Biochem* **52**:655, 1983.
16. Allen RC, Harley RA, Talamo RC: A new method for determination of alpha$_1$-antitrypsin phenotypes using isoelectric focusing on polyacrylamide gel slabs. *Am J Clin Pathol* **62**:732, 1974.
17. Jeppsson J-O, Laurell C-B, Fagerhol MK: Properties of isolated α_1-antitrypsin of Pi types M, S and Z. *Eur J Biochem* **83**:143, 1978.
18. Carrell RW, Owen MC: α_1-Antitrypsin: Structure, variation and disease. *Essays Med Biochem* **4**:83, 1978.
19. Carlson J, Stenfo J: The biosynthesis of rat α_1-antitrypsin. *J Biol Chem* **257**:12987, 1982.
20. Long GL, Chandra T, Woo, SLC, Davie EW, Kurachi K: Complete sequence of the cDNA for human α_1-antitrypsin and the gene for the S variant. *Biochemistry* **23**:4828, 1984.
21. Rosenberg S, Barr PJ, Najarian RC, Hallewell RA: Synthesis in yeast of a functional oxidation-resistant mutant of human α_1-antitrypsin. *Nature* **312**:77, 1984.
22. Loebermann H, Tokuoka R, Deisenhofer J, Huber R: Human alpha$_1$-proteinase inhibitor. Crystal structure analysis of two crystal modifications, molecular model and preliminary analysis of the implications for function. *J Mol Biol* **177**:531, 1984.
23. Carrell RW, Pemberton PA, Boswell DR: The serpins: Evolution and adaptation in a family of protease inhibitors. *Cold Spring Harbor Symp Quant Biol* **52**:527, 1987.
24. Laurell C-B, Thulin E: Complexes in human plasma between α_1-antitrypsin and IgA, and α_1-antitrypsin and fibrinogen. *Scand J Immunol* **4**:7, 1975.
25. Laurell C-B, Pierce J, Persson U, Thulin E: Purification of α_1-antitrypsin from plasma through thiol-disulfide interchange. *Eur J Biochem* **57**:107, 1975.
26. Vaughan L, Lorier MA, Carrell RW: α_1-Antitrypsin microheterogeneity: Isolation and physiological significance of isoforms. *Biochim Biophys Acta* **701**:339, 1982.
27. Carrell RW, Jeppsson J-O, Vaughan SO, Brennan SO, Owen MC, Boswell DR: Human α_1-antitrypsin: carbohydrate attachment and sequence homology. *FEBS Lett* **135**:301, 1981.
28. Chan SK, Rees DC, Li S-C, Li Y-T: Linear structure of oligosaccharide chains in α_1-protease inhibitor isolated from human plasma. *J Biol Chem* **251**:471, 1976.
29. Jeppsson J-O, Lilja H, Johansson M: Isolation and characterization of two minor fractions of α_1-antitrypsin by high-performance liquid chromatographic chromatofocusing. *J Chromatogr* **327**:173, 1985.
30. Carrell RW, Jeppsson J-O, Laurell C-B, Brennan SO, Owen MC, Vaughan L, Boswell DR: Structure and variation of human α1-antitrypsin. *Nature* **298**:329, 1982.
31. Johnson D, Travis J: Structural evidence for methionine at the reactive site of human α-1-proteinase inhibitor. *J Biol Chem* **253**:7142, 1978.
32. Lomas DA, Evans DL, Finch JT, Carrell RW: The mechanism of Z α_1-antitrypsin accumulation in the liver. *Nature* **357**:605, 1992.
33. Laskowski J, Kato I: Protein inhibitors of proteinases. *Annu Rev Biochem* **49**:593, 1980.
34. Huber R, Carrell RW: Implications of the three-dimensional structure of α_1-antitrypsin for structure and function of serpins. *Biochemistry* **28**:8951, 1989.
35. Johnson D, Travis J: The oxidative inactivation of human α-1-proteinase inhibitors. *J Biol Chem* **254**:4022, 1979.
36. Beatty K, Bieth J, Travis J: Kinetics of association of serine proteinases with native and oxidized α-1-proteinase inhibitor and α-1-antichymotrypsin. *J Biol Chem* **255**:3931, 1980.
37. Carrell RW, Owen MC: Plakalbumin, α_1-antitrypsin, antithrombin, and the mechanism of inflammatory thrombosis. *Nature* **317**:730, 1985.
38. Hill RE, Shaw PH, Boyd PA, Baumann H, Hastie ND: Plasma protease inhibitors in mouse and man: Divergence within the reactive centre regions. *Nature* **311**:175, 1984.
39. Owen MC, Brennan SO, Lewis JH, Carrell RW: Mutation of antitrypsin to antithrombin: α_1-antitrypsin-Pittsburgh (358 Met→Arg), a fatal bleeding disorder. *N Engl J Med* **309**:694, 1983.

40. Billingsley GD, Walter MA, Hammond GL, Cox DW: Physical mapping of four serpin genes: α_1-antitrypsin, α_1-antichymotrypsin, corticosteroid-binding globulin, and protein C inhibitor, within a 280-kb region on chromosome 14q32.1. *Am J Hum Genet* **52**:343, 1993.
41. Wu Y, Foreman RC: The molecular genetics of alpha 1 antitrypsin deficiency. *Bioessays* **13**:163, 1991.
42. Sifers RN, Shen RF, Woo SL: Genetic control of human alpha-1-antitrypsin. *Mol Biol Med* **6**:127, 1989.
43. Ciliberto G, Dente L, Cortese R: Cell-specific expression of a transfected human α_1-antitrypsin gene. *Cell* **4**:531, 1985.
44. Kelsey GD, Povey S, Bygrave AE, Lovell-Badge RH: Species- and tissue-specific expression of human α_1-antitrypsin in transgenic mice. *Genes Dev* **1**:161, 1987.
45. Perlino E, Cortese R, Ciliberto G: The human α_1-antitrypsin gene is transcribed from two different promoters in macrophages and hepatocytes. *EMBO J* **6**:2767, 1987.
46. Hunt LT, Dayhoff MO: A surprising new protein superfamily containing ovalbumin, anti-thrombin-III, and alpha$_1$-proteinase inhibitor. *Biochem Biophys Res Commun* **95**:864, 1980.
47. Chandra T, Stackhouse R, Kidd VJ, Robson KJH, Woo SLC: Sequence homology between human α1-antichymotrypsin, α1-antitrypsin and antithrombin III. *Biochemistry* **22**:5055, 1983.
48. Suzuki K, Deyashiki Y, Nishioka J, Kurachi K, Akira M, Yamamoto S, Hashimoto S: Characterization of a cDNA for human protein C inhibitor. *J Biol Chem* **262**:611, 1987.
49. Flink IL, Bailey TJ, Gustafson TA, Markham BE, Morkin E: Complete amino acid sequence of human thyroxine-binding globulin deduced from cloned DNA: Close homology to the serine antiproteases. *Proc Natl Acad Sci USA* **83**:7708, 1986.
50. Underhill DA, Hammond GL: Organization of the human corticosteroid binding globulin gene and analysis of its 5′-flanking region. *Genomics* **3**:1448, 1989.
51. Kurachi K, Chandra T, Friezner Degen SJ, White TT, Marchioro TL, Woo SLC, Davie EW: Cloning and sequence of cDNA coding for α_1-antitrypsin. *Proc Natl Acad Sci USA* **78**:6826, 1981.
52. Tosi M, Duponchel C, Bourgarel P, Colomb M, Meo T: Molecular cloning of human C1 inhibitor: Sequence homologies with α_1-antitrypsin and other members of the serpins super family. *Gene* **42**:265, 1986.
53. Leicht M, Long GL, Chandra T, Kurachi K, Kidd VJ, Mace M Jr, Davie EW, Woo SLC: Sequence homology and structural comparison between the chromosomal human α_1-antitrypsin and chicken ovalbumin genes. *Nature* **297**:655, 1982.
54. Gedde-Dahl T, Fagerhol MK, Cook PJL, Noades J: Autosomal linkage between the Gm and Pi loci in man. *Ann Hum Genet* **35**:393, 1972.
55. Darlington GJ, Astrin KH, Muirhead SP, Desnick RJ, Smith M: Assignment of the human alpha-1-antitrypsin gene to chromosome 14 by somatic cell hybrid analysis. *Proc Natl Acad Sci USA* **79**:870, 1982.
56. Pearson SJ, Tetri P, George DL, Francke U: Activation of human alpha$_1$-antitrypsin gene in rat hepatoma × human fetal liver cell hybrids depends on the presence of human chromosome 14. *Somatic Cell Genet* **5**:567, 1983.
57. Lai EC, Kao F-T, Law ML, Woo SLC: Assignment of the α_1-antitrypsin gene and a sequence-related gene to human chromosome 14 by molecular hybridization. *Am J Hum Genet* **35**:385, 1983.
58. Schroeder WT, Miller MF, Woo SLC, Saunders GF: Chromosomal localization of the human α_1-antitrypsin gene (PI) to 14q31-32. *Am J Hum Genet* **37**:868, 1985.
59. Purrello M, Alhadeff B, Whittington E, Buckton KE, Daniel A, Arnaud P, Rocchi M, Archidiacomo N, Filippi G, Siniscalco M: Comparison of cytologic and genetic distances between long arm subtelomeric markers of human autosome 14 suggests uneven distribution of crossing-over. *Cytogenet Cell Genet* **44**:32, 1987.
60. Hofker MH, Nelen M, Klasen EC, Nukiwa T, Curiel D, Crystal RC, Frants RR: Cloning and characterization of an α_1-antitrypsin like gene 12 kb downstream of the genuine α_1-antitrypsin gene. *Biochem Biophys Res Commun* **155**:634, 1987.
61. Sefton L, Kelsey G, Kearney P, Povey S, Wolfe J: A physical map of the human PI and AACT genes. *Genomics* **7**:382, 1990.
62. Gadek JE, Crystal RG: α_1-antitrypsin deficiency, in Stanbury JB, Wyngaarden JB, Fredrickson DS, Goldstein JL, Brown MS (eds): *Metabolic Basis of Inherited Disease* 5th ed. New York, McGraw-Hill, 1983, p 1450.
63. Gadek JE, Zimmerman RL, Fells GA, Crystal RG: Antielastases of the human alveolar structures: Assessment of the protease-antiprotease theory of emphysema. *J Clin Invest* **68**:889, 1981.
64. Brissenden JE, Cox DW: α_2-Macroglobulin production by cultured human fibroblasts. *Somatic Cell Genet* **8**:289, 1982.
65. Scott CF, Carrell RW, Glaser CB, Kueppers F, Lewis JH, Colman RW: Alpha-1-antitrypsin-Pittsburgh. A potent inhibitor of human plasma factor XIa, kallikrein and factor XII. *J Clin Invest* **77**:631, 1986.
66. Lieberman J: Alpha$_1$-antitrypsin deficiency and related disorders. *Princ Prac Med Genet* **2**:911, 1983.
67. Mirsky IA, Foley G: Antibiotic actions of trypsin inhibitors. *Proc Soc Exp Biol Med* **59**:34, 1945.
68. Lipsky JJ, Berninger RW, Hyman LR, Talamo RC: Presence of alpha-1-antitrypsin on mitogen stimulated human lymphocytes. *J Immunol* **122**:24, 1979.
69. Folds JD, Prince II, Spitznagel JK: Limited cleavage of human immunoglobulins by elastase of human neutrophil polymorphonuclear granulocytes. Possible modulator of immune complex disease. *Lab Invest* **39**:313, 1978.
70. Breit SN, Wakefield D, Robinson JP, Luckhurst E, Clark P, Penny R: The role of alpha$_1$-antitrypsin deficiency in the pathogenesis of immune disorders. *Clin Immunol Immunopathol* **35**:363, 1985.
71. Bristow CL, Lyford LK, Stevens DP, Flood PM: Elastase is a constituent product of T cells. *Biochem Biophys Res Commun* **181**:232, 1991.
72. Perlmutter DH, Cole FS, Kilbridge P, Rossing TH, Colten HR: Expression of the alpha$_1$-proteinase inhibitor gene in human monocytes and macrophages. *Proc Natl Acad Sci USA* **82**:795, 1985.
73. Sharp HL: Alpha-1-antitrypsin deficiency. *Hosp Pract* **5**:83, 1971.
74. Hood JM, Koep LJ, Peters RL, Schroter GPJ, Weil R, Redeker AG, Starzi TE: Liver transplantation for advanced liver disease with alpha-1-antitrypsin deficiency. *N Engl J Med* **302**:272, 1980.
75. Eriksson S, Alm R, Astedt B: Organ cultures of human fetal hepatocytes in the study of extra- and intracellular α_1-antitrypsin. *Biochim Biophys Acta* **542**:496, 1978.
76. Sifers RN, Rogers BB, Hawkins HK, Finegold MJ, Woo SLC: Elevated synthesis of human α1-antitrypsin hinders the secretion of murine α1-antitrypsin from hepatocytes of transgenic mice. *J Biol Chem* **264**:15696, 1989.
77. Isaacson P, Jones DB, Millward-Sadler GH, Judd MA, Payne S: Alpha-1-antitrypsin in human macrophages. *Lancet* **2**:964, 1979.
78. Cohen AB: Interrelationships between the human alveolar macrophage and alpha-1-antitrypsin. *J Clin Invest* **52**:2793, 1973.
79. Sifers RN, Carlson JA, Clift SM, Demayo FJ, Bullock DW, Woo SLC: Tissue specific expression of the human alpha-1-antitrypsin gene in transgenic mice. *Nucleic Acids Res* **15**:1459, 1987.
80. Dycaico JM, Grant SGN, Felts K, Nichols WS, Celler SA, Hager JH, Pollard AJ: Neonatal hepatitis induced by α_1-antitrypsin: A transgenic mouse model. *Science* **242**:1409, 1988.
81. Perlmutter DH, Daniels JD, Auerbach HS, De Schryver-Kecskemeti K, Winter HS, Alpers HA: The α_1-antitrypsin gene is expressed in a human intestinal epithelial cell line. *J Biol Chem* **264**:9485, 1989.
82. Laurell C-B, Nosslin B, Jeppsson J-O: Catabolic rate of α_1-antitrypsin of Pi type M and Z in man. *Clin Sci Mol Med* **52**:457, 1977.
83. Jeppsson J-O, Laurell C-B, Nosslin B, Cox DW: Catabolic rate of α_1-antitrypsin of Pi types S and Mmalton and of asialylated M protein in man. *Clin Sci Mol Med* **55**:103, 1978.
84. Cox DW, Billingsley GD, Siewertsen MA: α_1-Antitrypsin,

in Hommes FA (ed): *Techniques in Diagnostic Human Biochemical Genetics: A Laboratory Manual*. New York, Alan R. Liss, 1991, p 473.

85. Billingsley GD, Cox DW: Functional assay of α_1-antitrypsin in obstructive lung disease. *Am Rev Respir Dis* **121**:161, 1980.
86. Erlanger BF, Kokowsky N, Cohen W: The preparation and properties of two new chromogenic substrates of trypsin. *Arch Biochem* **95**:271, 1961.
87. Visser L, Blout E: The use of *p*-nitrophenyl *N-tert*-butyloxycarbonyl-L-alaninate as substrate for elastase. *Biochim Biophys Acta* **268**:257, 1972.
88. Beatty K, Robertie P, Senior RM, Travis J: Determination of oxidized alpha-1-proteinase inhibitor in serum. *J Lab Clin Med* **100**:186, 1982.
89. Mancini G, Carbonara AO, Heremans JE: Immunochemical quantitation of antigens by single radial immunodiffusion. *Immunochemistry* **2**:235, 1965.
90. Laurell C-B: Quantitative estimation of proteins by electrophoresis in agarose gel containing antibodies. *Anal Biochem* **15**:45, 1966.
91. Laurell C-B, Kullander S, Thorell J: Effect of administration of a combined estrogen-progestin contraceptive on the level of individual plasma proteins. *Scand J Clin Lab Invest* **21**:337, 1968.
92. Evans HE, Levi M, Mandl I: Serum enzyme inhibitor concentrations in the respiratory distress syndrome. *Am Rev Respir Dis* **101**:359, 1970.
93. Talamo RC: Basic and clinical aspects of the α_1-antitrypsin. *Pediatrics* **56**:91, 1975.
94. Arnaud P, Chapuis-Cellier C, Creyssel R: Polymorphisme de l'alpha-1-antitrypsin plasmatique (système Pi). Mise en évidence par électrofocalisation sur gel de polyacrylamide. *C R Soc Biol (Paris)* **168**:58, 1974.
95. Lebas J, Hayem A, Martin JP: Etude des variants génétiques de l'alpha-1-antitrypsin en immunofocalisation bidimensionelle. *C R Acad Sci (Paris)* **258**:2359, 1974.
96. Cox DW, Johnson AM, Fagerhol MK: Report of nomenclature meeting for α_1-antitrypsin. INSERM. Rouen/Bois-Guillaume-1978. *Hum Genet* **53**:429, 1980.
97. Shows TB, Alper CA, Bootsma D, Dorf M, Douglas T, Huisman T, Kit S, Klinger HP, Kozak C, Lalley PA, Lindsley D, McAlpine PJ, McDougall JK, Meerakhan P, Meisler M, Morton NE, Opitz J, Parfridge CW, Payne R, Roderick TH, Rubinstein P, Ruddle FH, Shaw M, Spranger JW, Weiss K: International system for human gene nomenclature. *Cytogenet Cell Genet* **25**:96, 1979.
98. Jeppsson J-O, Franzen B: Typing of genetic variants of α_1-antitrypsin by electrofocusing. *Clin Chem* **28**:219, 1982.
99. Charlionet R, Martin J-P, Sesboue R, Madec PJ, Lefebvre F: Synthesis of highly diversified carrier ampholytes. Evaluation of the resolving power of isoelectric focusing in the Pi system (alpha-1-antitrypsin genetic polymorphism). *J Chromatogr* **176**:89, 1979.
100. Frants RR, Noordhoek GT, Eriksson AW: Separator isoelectric focusing for identification of α1-antitrypsin (PiM) subtype. *Scand J Clin Invest* **38**:457, 1978.
101. Gorg A, Postel W, Weser J, Weidinger S, Patutschnick W, Cleve H: Isoelectric focusing in immobilized pH gradients for the determination of the genetic Pi (α_1-antitrypsin) variants. *Electrophoresis* **4**:153, 1983.
102. Pascali VL, Conte G: Improved classification of alpha-1-antitrypsin in immobilized pH gradients containing sucrose. *Electrophoresis* **6**:402, 1985.
103. Weidinger S, Cleve H: Hybrid isoelectric focusing for classification of α1-antitrypsin variants. *Prot Biol Fluids* **34**:863, 1986.
104. Budowle B, Murch RS: A high resolution, rapid procedure for α_1-antitrypsin phenotyping. *Electrophoresis* **6**:523, 1985.
105. Weidinger S, Cleve H: High resolution of alpha-1-antitrypsin PI M subtypes by isoelectric focusing with a modified immobilized pH gradient. *Electrophoresis* **5**:223, 1984.
106. Cox DW: New variants of α_1-antitrypsin: Comparison of PI typing techniques. *Am J Hum Genet* **33**:354, 1981.
107. Kamboh MI: Biochemical and genetic aspects of human serum α_1-proteinase inhibitor protein. *Disease Markers* **3**:135, 1985.
108. Arnaud P, Chapuis-Cellier C, Vittoz P, Fudenberg H: Genetic polymorphism of serum alpha-1-protease inhibitor (alpha-1-antitrypsin): Pi I, a deficient allele of the Pi system. *J Lab Clin Med* **92**:177, 1978.
109. Fagerhol MK: Quantitative studies on the inherited variants of serum α_1-antitrypsin. *Scand J Clin Lab Invest* **23**:97, 1969.
110. Holmes MD, Brantly ML, Fells GA, Crystal RG: α_1-antitrypsin Wbethesda: Molecular basis of an unusual α_1-antitrypsin deficiency variant. *Biochem Biophys Res Commun* **170**:1013, 1990.
111. Fagerhol MK, Hauge HE: The PI phenotype MP discovery of a ninth allele belonging to the system of inherited variants of serum α_1-antitrypsin. *Vox Sang* **15**:396, 1968.
112. Billingsley GD, Cox DW: Functional assessment of genetic variants of α_1-antitrypsin. *Hum Genet* **61**:118, 1982.
113. Cox DW, Hoeppner VH, Levison H: Protease inhibitors in patients with chronic obstructive pulmonary disease: The alpha$_1$-antitrypsin heterozygote controversy. *Am Rev Respir Dis* **113**:601, 1976.
114. Martin NG, Clark P, Ofulue AF, Eaves LJ, Corey LA, Nance WE: Does the PI polymorphism alone control alpha-1-antitrypsin expression? *Am J Hum Genet* **40**:267, 1987.
115. Hug G, Chuck G, Bowles B: Alpha$_1$-antitrypsin phenotype: Transient cathodal shift in serum of infant girl with urinary cytomegalovirus and fatty liver. *Pediatr Res* **16**:192, 1982.
116. Nukiwa T, Brantly M, Ogushi F, Fells G, Satoh K, Stier L, Courtney M, Crystal RG: Characterization of the M1(ala213) type of α_1-antitrypsin, a newly recognized, common "normal" α1-antitrypsin haplotype. *Biochemistry* **26**:5259, 1987.
117. Cox DW, Billingsley GD: Restriction enzyme MaeIII for prenatal diagnosis of alpha$_1$-antitrypsin deficiency. *Lancet* **2**:741, 1986.
118. Jeppsson J-O: Amino acid substitution Gly-Lys in α_1-antitrypsin Pi Z. *FEBS Lett* **65**:195, 1976.
119. Yoshida L, Lieberman J, Gaidulis L, Ewing C: Molecular abnormality of human α_1-antitrypsin variant (PiZ) associated with plasma activity deficiency. *Proc Natl Acad Sci USA* **73**:1324, 1976.
120. Owen MC, Carrell RW, Brennan SO: The abnormality of the S variant of human α_1-antitrypsin. *Biochim Biophys Acta* **453**:257, 1976.
121. Weidinger S, Jeppsson J-O: Genetic study of the deficient alpha-1-antitrypsin variant PI P. *Proc Intern Congress Human Genetics*, Berlin, 1986.
122. Brennan SO, Carrell RW: α1-Antitrypsin Christchurch, 363 Glu → Lys: Mutation at the P'5 position does not affect inhibitory activity. *Biochim Biophys Acta* **873**:13, 1986.
123. Engh R, Lobermann H, Schneider M, Wiegland G, Huber R, Laurell K-B: The S variant of human α_1-antitrypsin, structure and implications for function and metabolism. *Protein Eng* **2**:407, 1993.
124. Kellermann G, Walter H: Investigations on the population genetics of the α_1-antitrypsin polymorphism. *Humangenetik* **10**:145, 1970.
125. Cox DW: α_1-antitrypsin deficiency, in Scriver CR, Beaudet AL, Sly WS, Valle D (eds): *The Metabolic Basis of Inherited Disease* 6th ed. New York, McGraw-Hill, 1989, p 2409.
126. Constans J, Viau M, Gouaillard C: An additional PiM subtype. *Hum Genet* **55**:119, 1980.
127. Klasen ED, Bos A, Simmelink HD: Pi (α_1-antitrypsin) subtypes: Frequency of PI*M4 in several populations. *Hum Genet* **62**:139, 1982.
128. Warsy AS, El-Hazmi MAF, Sedrani SH: Alpha-1-antitrypsin phenotypes in Saudi Arabia: A study in the central province. *Ann Saudi Med* **11**:159, 1993.
129. Massi G, Vecchio FM: Alpha-1-antitrypsin phenotypes in a group of newborn infants in Somalia. *Hum Genet* **38**:265, 1977.
130. Janus EE, Sheat JM, Carrell RW: Alpha-1-antitrypsin variants in New Zealand. *NZ Med J* **82**:289, 1975.
131. Cox DW, Woo SLC, Mansfield T: DNA restriction fragments associated with alpha$_1$-antitrypsin indicate a single origin for deficiency allele PIZ. *Nature* **316**:79, 1985.
132. Cox DW, Billingsley GD, Mansfield T: DNA restriction site polymorphisms associated with the alpha$_1$-antitrypsin gene. *Am J Hum Genet* **41**:891, 1987.

133. Hodgson I, Kalsheker N: RFLP for a gene-related sequence of alpha 1-antitrypsin (AAT). *Nucleic Acids Res* **14**:6779, 1986.
134. Byth BC, Cox DW: A $(CA)_n$ repeat at the 5′ end of the α_1-antitrypsin gene. *Hum Mol Genet* **2**:1752, 1993.
135. Cox DW: DNA polymorphisms associated with α_1-antitrypsin and their clinical applications, in Mittman C, Taylor C (eds): *Pulmonary Emphysema and Proteolysis* Vol. II. New York, Academic, 1987.
136. Cox DW, Coulsen SE, Billingsley GD: Unique DNA polymorphisms associated with α_1-antitrypsin Z deficiency allele: Application to prenatal diagnosis, in Peters H (ed): *Protides of the Biological Fluids*, 1987, p 123.
137. Cox DW, Coulson SE: BglII polymorphism for the α_1-antitrypsin-related gene on chromosome 14. *Nucleic Acids Res* **15**:4701, 1987.
138. Matteson KJ, Ostrer H, Chakravarti A, Buetow KH, O'Brien WE, Beaudet AL, Phillips JA: A study of restriction fragment length polymorphisms at the human alpha-1-antitrypsin locus. *Hum Genet* **69**:263, 1985.
139. Hodgson I, Kalsheker N: DNA polymorphisms of the human α_1 antitrypsin gene in normal subjects and in patients with pulmonary emphysema. *J Med Genet* **24**:47, 1987.
140. Cox DW, Billingsley GD: Rare deficiency types of α_1-antitrypsin: Electrophoretic variation and DNA haplotypes. *Am J Hum Genet* **44**:844, 1989.
141. Byth BC, Cox DW: Two consecutive dinucleotide repeats constitute an informative marker at the α_1-antichymotrypsin locus. *Hum Mol Genet* **2**:1085, 1993.
142. Byth BC, Meijers JCM, Cox DW: A $(CA)_n$ repeat within the protein C inhibitor gene. *Hum Mol Genet* **2**:1752, 1993.
143. Cox DW, Billingsley GD, Smyth S: Rare types of α_1-antitrypsin associated with deficiency, in Allen RC, Arnaud P (eds): *Electrophoresis. Proc Third Int Conference on Electrophoresis*. New York, de Gruyter, 1981, p. 505.
144. Sveger T: Plasma protease inhibitors in α_1-antitrypsin-deficient children. *Pediatr Res* **19**:834, 1985.
145. Laurell C-B, Sveger T: Mass screening of newborn Swedish infants for α_1-antitrypsin deficiency. *Am J Hum Genet* **27**:213, 1975.
146. Moroz SP, Cutz E, Cox DW, Sass-Kortsak A: Liver disease associated with alpha$_1$-antitrypsin deficiency in childhood. *J Pediatr* **88**:19, 1976.
147. Johansson BG: Agarose gel electrophoresis. *Scand J Clin Lab Invest* **124**(Suppl):7, 1972.
148. Cutz E, Cox DW: α_1-antitrypsin deficiency: The spectrum of pathology and pathophysiology, in Rosenberg HS, Bolande RP (eds): *Pediatric Pathology*. New York, Masson, 1979, p. 1.
149. Feldmann G, Martin J-P, Sesboue R, Ropartz C, Perelman R, Nathanson M, Seringe P, Benhamou J-P: Hepatocyte ultrastructure changes in α_1-antitrypsin deficiency. *Gastroenterology* **67**:1214, 1974.
150. Huang S-N, Minassian H, More JD: Application of immunofluorescent staining on paraffin sections improved by trypsin digestion. *Lab Invest* **35**:383, 1976.
151. Darlington GJ, Wilson DR, Lachman LB: Monocyte conditioned medium, interleukin-1 and tumour necrosis factor stimulate the acute phase response in human hepatoma cells in vitro. *J Cell Biol* **103**:787, 1986.
152. Carlson J, Eriksson S, Hagerstrand I: Intra- and extracellular alpha$_1$-antitrypsin in liver disease with special reference to Pi phenotype. *J Clin Pathol* **34**:1020, 1981.
153. Bradfield JWB, Blenkinsopp WK: Alpha-1-antitrypsin globules in the liver and PiM phenotype. *J Clin Pathol* **30**:464, 1977.
154. Roberts EA, Cox DW, Medline A, Wanless IR: Occurrence of alpha-1-antitrypsin deficiency in 155 patients with alcoholic liver disease. *Am J Clin Pathol* **82**:424, 1984.
155. Lomas DA, Evans DL, Stone SR, Chang WW, Carrell RW: Effect of the Z mutation on the physical and inhibitory properties of α_1-antitrypsin. *Biochemistry* **32**:500, 1993.
156. Ogushi F, Fells GA, Hubbard RC, Straus SD, Crystal RG: Z-type α_1-antitrypsin is less competent than M1-type α_1-antitrypsin as an inhibitor of neutrophil elastase. *J Clin Invest* **80**:1366, 1987.
157. Errington DM, Bathurst IC, Janus ED, Carell RW: In vitro synthesis of M and Z forms of human α_1-antitrypsin. *FEBS Lett* **148**:83, 1982.
158. Bathurst IC, Stenflo J, Errington DM, Carrell RW: Translation and processing of normal (PiMM) and abnormal (PiZZ) human α_1-antitrypsin. *FEBS Lett* **153**:270, 1983.
159. Gross V, Vom Berg D, Kreuzkamp J, Ganter U, Bauer J, Wurtemberger G, Schulz-Huotari C, Beeser H, Gerok W: Biosynthesis and secretion of M- and Z-type α_1-proteinase inhibitor by human monocytes. Effect of inhibitors of glycosylation and of oligosaccharide processing on secretion and function. *Biol Chem Hoppe Seyler* **371**:231, 1990.
160. Eriksson S, Larsson C: Purification and partial characterization of PAS-positive inclusion bodies from the liver in alpha$_1$-Antitrypsin deficiency. *N Engl J Med* **292**:176, 1975.
161. Hercz A, Katona E, Cutz E, Wilson JR, Barton M: α_1-antitrypsin: The presence of excess mannose in the Z variant isolated from liver. *Science* **201**:1229, 1978.
162. Bathurst IC, Travis J, George PM, Carrell RW: Structural and functional characterization of the abnormal Z α_1-antitrypsin isolated from human liver. *FEBS Lett* **177**:179, 1984.
163. Foreman RC, Judah JD, Colman A: *Xenopus* oocytes can synthesize but do not secrete the Z variant of human α_1-antitrypsin. *FEBS Lett* **168**:84, 1984.
164. Errington DM, Bathurst IC, Carrell RW: Human α_1-antitrypsin expression in *Xenopus* oocytes: Secretion of the normal (PiM) and abnormal (PiZ) forms. *Eur J Biochem* **153**:361, 1985.
165. Cox DW, Billingsley GD, Callahan JW: Aggregation of plasma Z type α_1-antitrypsin suggests basic defect for the deficiency. *FEBS Lett* **205**:255, 1986.
166. Sifers RN, Hardick CP, Woo SLC: Disruption of the 290-342 salt bridge is not responsible for the secretory defect of the PiZ α_1-antitrypsin variant. *J Biol Chem* **264**:2997, 1989.
167. Foreman RC: Disruption of the Lys 290-Glu 342 salt bridge in human alpha-1-antitrypsin does not prevent its synthesis and secretion. *FEBS Lett* **216**:79, 1987.
168. Carrell RW, Evans DL, Stein PE: Mobile reactive centre of serpins and the control of thrombosis. *Nature* **353**:576, 1991.
169. Bathurst IC, Errington DM, Foreman RC, Judah JD, Carrell RW: Human Z α_1-antitrypsin accumulates intracellularly and stimulates lysosomal activity when synthesized in the *Xenopus* oocyte. *FEBS Lett* **183**:304, 1985.
170. Ananthan J, Goldberger AL, Voellmy R: Abnormal proteins serve as eukaryotic stress signals and trigger the activation of heat shock genes. *Science* **232**:522, 1986.
171. Perlmutter DH, Schlesinger MJ, Pierce JA, Punsal PI, Schwartz AL: Synthesis of stress proteins is increased in individuals with homozygous PiZZ α_1-antitrypsin deficiency and liver disease. *J Clin Invest* **84**:1555, 1989.
172. Matsunaga E, Shiokawa S, Nakamura H, Maruyama T, Tsuda K, Fukumaki U: Molecular analysis of the gene of the α_1-antitrypsin deficiency variant, Mnichinan. *Am J Hum Genet* **46**:602, 1990.
173. Seyama K, Nukiwa T, Takabe K, Takahashi H, Miyake K, Kira S: Siiyama (serine 53 (TCC) to phenylalanine 53 (TTC)). A new α_1-antitrypsin-deficient variant with mutation on a predicted conserved residue of the serpin backbone. *J Biol Chem* **266**:12627, 1991.
174. Lieberman J, Gaidulis L, Klotz SD: A new deficient variant of α_1-antitrypsin (MDuarte). Inability to detect the heterozygous state by antitrypsin phenotyping. *Am Rev Respir Dis* **113**:31, 1976.
175. Hofker MH, Nukiwa T, Van Passen HMB, Nelen M, Frants RR, Kramps JA, Klasen JC, Crystal RG: A Pro→Leu substitution in codon 369 in the α1-antitrypsin variant MHeerlen. *Hum Genet* **84**:1989.
176. Takahashi H, Nukiwa T, Satoh K, Ogushi F, Brantley M, Fells G, Stier L, Courtney M, Crystal RG: Characterization of the gene and protein of the α1-antitrypsin "deficiency" allele Mprocida. *J Biol Chem* **263**:15528, 1988.
177. Sproule BJ, Cox DW, Hsu K, Salkie ML, Herbert FA: Pulmonary function associated with the Mmalton deficient variant of alpha$_1$-antitrypsin. *Am Rev Respir Dis* **127**:237, 1983.
178. Reid CL, Wiener GJ, Cox DW, Richter JE, Geisinger KR: Diffuse hepatocellular dysplasia and carcinoma associated

with the Mmalton variant of alpha$_1$-antitrypsin. *Gastroenterology* **93:**181, 1987.

179. Cox DW, Levison H: Emphysema of early onset associated with a complete deficiency of alpha$_1$-antitrypsin (null homozygotes). *Am Rev Respir Dis* **137**:371, 1988.
180. Sifers RN, Brashears-Macatee S, Kidd VJ, Muensch H, Woo SLC: A frameshift mutation results in a truncated α_1-antitrypsin that is retained within the rough endoplasmic reticulum. *J Biol Chem* **263**:7330, 1988.
181. Curiel D, Brantly M, Curiel E, Stier L, Crystal RG: α_1-Antitrypsin deficiency caused by the α_1-antitrypsin Null$_{\text{Mattawa}}$ gene. An insertion mutation rendering the α_1-antitrypsin gene incapable of producing α_1-antitrypsin. *J Clin Invest* **83**:1144, 1989.
182. Frazier GC, Siewertsen MA, Hofker MH, Brubacher MG, Cox DW: A null deficiency allele of α_1-antitrypsin, Q0ludwigshafen, with altered tertiary structure. *J Clin Invest* **86**:1878, 1990.
183. Takahashi H, Crystal RG: α_1-Antitrypsin Null(isola di procida): an α_1-antitrypsin deficiency allele caused by deletion of all α_1-antitrypsin coding exons. *Am J Hum Genet* **47**:403, 1990.
184. Fraizer GC, Coulson SE, Cox DW: Molecular analysis of rare deficiency (PI) alleles of alpha$_1$-antitrypsin. *Am J Hum Genet* **40**(Suppl):A214, 1987.
185. Carrell RW: α_1-Antitrypsin, emphysema and smoking. *NZ Med J* **97**:327, 1984.
186. Pierce JA, Eradio B, Dew TA: Antitrypsin phenotypes in St. Louis. *J Am Med Assoc* **238**:609, 1975.
187. Morse JO: Alpha$_1$-antitrypsin deficiency. *N Engl J Med* **299**:1045, 1978.
188. Kueppers F, Black LF: α_1-antitrypsin and its deficiency. *Am Rev Respir Dis* **110**:176, 1974.
189. Tobin MJ, Cook PJL, Hutchison DCS: Alpha$_1$-antitrypsin deficiency: The clinical and physiological features of pulmonary emphysema in subjects homozygous for Pi type Z. *Br J Dis Chest* **77**:14, 1983.
190. Lieberman J, Winter B, Sastre A: Alpha$_1$-antitrypsin Pi-types in 965 COPD patients. *Chest* **89**:370, 1986.
191. Rienmuller RK, Behr J, Kalender WA, Schatzl M, Altmann I, Merin M, Beinert T: Standardized quantitative high resolution CT in lung diseases. *J Comput Assist Tomogr* **15**:742, 1991.
192. Larsson C: Natural history and life expectancy in severe alpha$_1$-antitrypsin deficiency, PiZ. *Acta Med Scand* **204**:345, 1978.
193. Silverman EK, Pierce JA, Province MA, Rao DC, Campbell EJ: Variability of pulmonary function in alpha-1-antitrypsin deficiency: Clinical correlates. *Ann Intern Med* **111**:982, 1989.
194. Jack CI, Evans CC: Three cases of alpha-1-antitrypsin deficiency in the elderly. *Postgrad Med J* **67**:840, 1991.
195. Janus ED, Phillips NT, Carrell RW: Smoking, lung function, and α_1-antitrypsin deficiency. *Lancet* **1**:152, 1985.
196. Evald T, Dirksen A, Keittelmann S, Viskum M, Kok Jensen A: Decline in pulmonary function in patients with α1-antitrypsin deficiency. *Lung* **168**(Suppl):579, 1990.
197. Buist AS, Burrows B, Eriksson S, Mittman C, Wu M: The natural history of air-flow obstruction in PiZ emphysema. *Am Rev Respir Dis* **127**:(Suppl):43, 1983.
198. Fletcher CM, Peto R, Tinker C, Speizer FE: *The Natural History of Chronic Bronchitis and Emphysema*. Oxford, Oxford University Press, 1976.
199. Tager IB, Munoz A, Rosner B, Weiss ST, Carey V, Speizer FE: Effect of cigarette smoking on the pulmonary function of children and adolescents. *Am Rev Respir Dis* **131**:752, 1985.
200. Cox DW, Talamo RC: Genetic aspects of pediatric lung disease. *Pediatr Clin North Am* **26**:467, 1979.
201. Hird MF, Greenough A, Mieli Vergani G, Mowat AP: Hyperinflation in children with liver disease due to alpha-1-antitrypsin deficiency. *Pediatr Pulmonol* **11**:212, 1991.
202. Weitz JI, Silverman EK, Thong B, Campbell EJ: Plasma levels of elastase-specific fibrinopeptides correlate with proteinase inhibitor phenotype. Evidence for increased elastase activity in subjects with homozygous and heterozygous deficiency of α_1-proteinase inhibitor. *J Clin Invest* **89**:766, 1992.
203. Kaplan PD, Kuhn CC, Pierce JA: The induction of emphysema with elastase. I. The evolution of the lesion and the influence of serum. *J Lab Clin Med* **82**:349, 1973.
204. Janoff A, Sloan B, Weinbaum G, Damiano V, Sandhaus RA, Elias J, Kimbel P: Experimental emphysema induced with purified human neutrophil elastase: Tissue localization of the instilled protease. *Am Rev Respir Dis* **115**:461, 1977.
205. Senior RM, Tegner H, Kuhn C, Ohlsson K, Starcher BC, Pierce JA: The induction of pulmonary emphysema with leukocyte elastase. *Am Rev Respir Dis* **116**:469, 1977.
206. Gadek JE, Hunninghake GW, Fells GA, Zimmerman RL, Keogh BA, Crystal RG: Evaluation of the protease-antiprotease theory of human destructive lung disease. *Bull Eur Physiopathol Respir* **16**:27, 1980.
207. Jochum M, Pelletier A, Boudier C, Pauli G, Bieth JG: The concentration of leukocyte elastase-α_1-proteinase inhibitor complex in bronchoalveolar lavage fluids from healthy human subjects. *Am Rev Respir Dis* **132**:913, 1985.
208. Wewers MD, Casolaro MA, Crystal RG: Comparison of alpha-1-antitrypsin levels and antineutrophil elastase capacity of blood and lung in a patient with the alpha-1-antitrypsin phenotype null-null before and during alpha-1-antitrypsin augmentation therapy. *Am Rev Respir Dis* **135**:539, 1987.
209. Gauthier F, Frysmark U, Ohlsson K, Bieth JG: Kinetics of the inhibition of leukocyte elastase by the bronchial inhibitor. *Biochim Biophys Acta* **700**:178, 1982.
210. Stockley RA, Morrison HM, Smith S, Tetley T: Low molecular mass bronchial proteinase inhibitor and α_1-proteinase inhibitor in sputum and bronchoalveolar lavage. *Hoppe Seylers Z Physiol Chem* **365**:587, 1984.
211. Janoff A: Elastases and emphysema. Current assessment of the protease-antiprotease hypothesis. *Am Rev Respir Dis* **132**:417, 1985.
212. Cohen AB, Rossi M: Neutrophils in normal lungs. *Am Rev Respir Dis* **127**:S3, 1983.
213. Janoff A, Carp H, Lee DK, Drew RT: Cigarette smoke inhalation decreases α_1-antitrypsin activity in rat lung. *Science* **206**:1313, 1979.
214. Stone PJ, Calorie JD, McGowan SE, Bernardo J, Snider GL, Franzblau C: Functional α_1-protease inhibitor in the lower respiratory tract of cigarette smokers is not decreased. *Science* **221**:1187, 1983.
215. Cox DW, Billingsley GD: Oxidation of plasma alpha$_1$-antitrypsin in smokers and nonsmokers and by an oxidizing agent. *Am Rev Respir Dis* **130**:594, 1984.
216. Fera T, Abboud RT, Richter A, Johal SS: Acute effect of smoking on elastaselike esterase activity and immunologic neutrophil elastase levels in bronchoalveolar lavage fluid. *Am Rev Respir Dis* **133**:568, 1986.
217. Abboud RT, Fera T, Richter A, Tabona MZ, Johal SS: Acute effect of smoking on the functional activity of alpha$_1$-protease inhibitor in bronchoalveolar lavage fluid. *Am Rev Respir Dis* **131**:79, 1985.
218. Carp H, Miller F, Hoidal JR, Janoff A: Potential mechanism of emphysema: α_1-proteinase inhibitor recovered from lungs of cigarette smokers contains oxidized methionine and has decreased elastase inhibitory capacity. *Proc Natl Acad Sci USA* **79**:2041, 1982.
219. Ossanna PJ, Test ST, Matheson NR, Regiani S, Weiss SJ: Oxidative regulation of neutrophil elastase-alpha-1-proteinase inhibitor interactions. *J Clin Invest* **77**:1939, 1986.
220. Matheson NR, Wong PS, Travis J: Enzymatic inactivation of human alpha-1-proteinase inhibitor by neutrophil myeloperoxidase. *Biochem Biophys Res Commun* **88**:402, 1979.
221. Clark RA, Stone PJ, Hag AE, Calore JD, Franzblau C: Myeloperoxidase-catalyzed inactivation of α_1-protease inhibitor by human neutrophils. *J Biol Chem* **256**:3348, 1981.
222. Stockley RA, Afford SC: Qualitative studies of lung lavage α_1-proteinase inhibitor. *Hoppe Seylers Z Physiol Chem* **365**:503, 1984.
223. Laurent P, Janoff A, Kagan HM: Cigarette smoke blocks cross-linking of elastin in vitro. *Am Rev Respir Dis* **127**:189, 1983.
224. Redline S, Tishler PV, Lewitter FI, Tager IB, Munoz A, Speizer FE: Assessment of genetic and nongenetic influences on pulmonary function. A twin study. *Am Rev Respir Dis* **135**:217, 1987.

225. Kalsheker NA, Watkins GL, Hill S, Morgan K, Stockley RA, Fick RB: Independent mutations in the flanking sequence of the alpha-1-antitrypsin gene are associated with chronic obstructive airways disease. *Dis Markers* **8**:151, 1990.
226. Morgan K, Scobie G, Kalsheker N: The characterization of a mutation of the 3′ flanking sequence of the α_1-antitrypsin gene commonly associated with chronic obstructive airway disease. *Eur J Clin Invest* **22**:134, 1992.
227. Silverman EK, Province MA, Campbell EJ, Pierce JA, Rao DC: Variability of pulmonary function in alpha-1-antitrypsin deficiency: Residual family resemblance beyond the effect of the Pi locus. *Hum Hered* **40**:340, 1990.
228. Travis J: Oxidants and antioxidants in the lung. *Am Rev Respir Dis* 127(Suppl):773, 1983. Editorial.
229. Taylor JC, Madison R, Kosinska D: Is antioxidant deficiency related to chronic obstructive pulmonary disease? *Am Rev Respir Dis* **134**:285, 1986.
230. Galdston M, Feldman JG, Levytska V, Magnusson B: Antioxidant activity of serum ceruloplasmin and transferrin available iron-binding capacity in smokers and nonsmokers. *Am Rev Respir Dis* **135**:783, 1987.
231. Theron A, Anderson R: Investigation of the protective effects of the antioxidants ascorbate, cysteine, and dapsone on the phagocyte-mediated oxidative inactivation of human alpha-1-protease inhibitor in vitro. *Am Rev Respir Dis* **132**:1049, 1985.
232. Pacht ER, Kaseki H, Mohammed JR, Cornwell DG, Davis WB: Deficiency of vitamin E in the alveolar fluid of cigarette smokers. Influence on alveolar macrophage cytotoxicity. *J Clin Invest* **77**:789, 1986.
233. Cooper DM, Hoeppner VH, Cox DW, Zamel N, Bryan AC, Levison H: Lung function in alpha$_1$-antitrypsin heterozygotes (Pi type MZ). *Am Rev Respir Dis* **110**:708, 1974.
234. Bruce RM, Cohen BH, Diamond EL, Fallat RJ, Knudson RJ, Lebowitz MD, Mittman C, Patterson CD, Tockman MS: Collaborative study to assess risk of lung disease in Pi MZ phenotype subjects. *Am Rev Respir Dis* **130**:386, 1984.
235. Larsson C, Eriksson S, Dirksen H: Smoking and intermediate alpha$_1$-antitrypsin deficiency and lung function in middle-aged men. *Br Med J* **2**:922, 1977.
236. Eriksson S, Lindell SE, Wiberg R: Effects of smoking and intermediate α_1-antitrypsin deficiency (Pi MZ) on lung function. *Eur J Respir Dis* **67**:279, 1985.
237. Larsson C, Dirksen H, Sunström G, Eriksson S: Lung function studies in asymptomatic individuals with moderately (PiSZ) and severely (PiZ) reduced levels of α_1-antitrypsin. *Scand Respir Dis* **57**:267, 1976.
238. Beckman G, Beckman L, Michaelsson O, Rudolphi N, Stjernberg N, Wiman L-G: Alpha-1-antitrypsin types and chronic obstructive lung disease in an industrial community in Northern Sweden. *Hum Hered* **30**:299, 1980.
239. Beckman G, Stjernberg NL, Eklund A: Is the Pi^F allele of α_1-antitrypsin associated with pulmonary disease? *Clin Genet* **25**:491, 1984.
240. Hussain M, Mieli Vergani G, Mowat AP: α_1-Antitrypsin deficiency and liver disease: Clinical presentation, diagnosis and treatment. *J Inherit Metab Dis* **14**:497, 1991.
241. Povey S: Genetics of α_1-antitrypsin deficiency in relation to neonatal liver disease. *Mol Biol Med* **7**:161, 1990.
242. Sveger T: Liver disease in alpha$_1$-antitrypsin deficiency detected by screening of 200,000 infants. *N Engl J Med* **294**:1316, 1976.
243. Cottrall K, Cook PJL, Mowat AP: Neonatal hepatitis syndrome and alpha-1-antitrypsin deficiency: An epidemiological study in south-east England. *Postgrad Med J* **50**:376, 1974.
244. Odievre M, Martin JP, Hadchouel M, Alagille D: Alpha$_1$-antitrypsin deficiency and liver disease in children: Phenotypes, manifestations, and prognosis. *Pediatrics* **57**:226, 1976.
245. Nebbia G, Hadchouel M, Odievre M, Alagille D: Early assessment of evolution of liver disease associated with α_1-antitrypsin deficiency in childhood. *J Pediatr* **102**:661, 1983.
246. Alagille D: α_1-Antitrypsin deficiency. *Hepatology* **4** (Suppl):11, 1984.
247. Maggiore G, Bernard O, Hadchouel M, Lemonnier A, Alagille D: Diagnostic value of serum gamma-glutamyl transpeptidase activity in liver diseases in children. *J Pediatr Gastroenterol Nutr* **12**:21, 1991.
248. Sveger T, Thelin T: Four-year-old children with alpha$_1$-antitrypsin deficiency: Clinical follow-up and parental attitudes towards neonatal screening. *Acta Paediatr Scand* **70**:171, 1981.
249. Sveger T: The natural history of liver disease in α_1-antitrypsin deficient children. *Acta Paediatr Scand* **77**:847, 1988.
250. Karlaganis G, Nemeth A, Hammarskjold B, Strandvik B, Sjovall J: Urinary excretion of bile alcohols in normal children and patients with α_1-antitrypsin deficiency during development of liver disease. *Eur J Clin Invest* **12**:399, 1982.
251. Schwarzenberg SJ, Sharp HL: Pathogenesis of α_1-antitrypsin deficiency-associated liver disease, 1990. *J Pediatr Gastroenterol Nutr* **10**:5, 1990.
252. Perlmutter DH: The cellular basis for liver injury in α_1-antitrypsin deficiency. *Hepatology* **13**:172, 1991.
253. Hultcrantz R, Mengarelli S: Ultrastructure liver pathology in patients with minimal liver disease and alpha$_1$-antitrypsin deficiency: A comparison between heteroxygous and homozygous patients. *Hepatology* **4**:937, 1984.
254. Carlson JA, Rogers BB, Sifers RN, Finegold MJ, Clift SM, Demayo FJ, Bullock DW: Accumulation of PiZ α_1-antitrypsin causes liver damage in transgenic mice. *J Clin Invest* **83**:1183, 1989.
255. Dycaico MJ, Felts K, Nichols SW, Geller SA, Sorge JA: Neonatal growth delay in alpha-1-antitrypsin disease. Influence of genetic background. *Mol Biol Med* **6**:137, 1989.
256. Maeda H, Molla A: Pathogenic potentials of bacterial proteases. *Clin Chim Acta* **185**:357, 1989.
257. Weiss SJ: Oxygen, ischemia and inflammation. *Acta Physiol Scand* **126**:9, 1986.
258. Comporti M: Lipid peroxidation and cellular damage in toxic liver injury. *Lab Invest* **53**:599, 1985.
259. Pittschieler K: Liver disease and heterozygous alpha-1-antitrypsin deficiency. *Acta Paediatr Scand* **80**:323, 1991.
260. Pittschieler K: Oxidative radicals and liver involvement of infants with alpha-1-antitrypsin deficiency. *Padiatr Padol* **26**:235, 1991.
261. Sokol RJ, Heubi JE, McGraw C, Balistreri WF: Correction of vitamin E deficiency in children with chronic cholestasis. II. Effect on gastrointestinal and hepatic function. *Hepatology* **6**:1263, 1986.
262. Wallmark A, Alm R, Eriksson S: Monoclonal antibody specific for the mutant PiZ α_1-antitrypsin and its application in an ELISA procedure for identification of PiZ gene carriers. *Proc Natl Acad Sci USA* **81**:5690, 1984.
263. Moroz SP, Cutz E, Balfe JW, Sass-Kortsak A: Membranoproliferative glomerulonephritis in childhood cirrhosis associated with alpha$_1$-antitrypsin deficiency. *Pediatrics* **57**:232, 1976.
264. Littleton ET, Bevis L, Hansen LJ, Peakman M, Mowat AP, Mieli Vergani G, Vergani D: α_1-antitrypsin deficiency, complement activation, and chronic liver disease. *J Clin Pathol* **44**:855, 1991.
265. Psacharopoulos HT, Mowat AP, Cook PJL, Carlille PA, Portmann B, Rodeck CH: Outcome of liver disease associated with alpha$_1$-antitrypsin deficiency (PiZ). *Arch Dis Child* **58**:882, 1983.
266. Ibarguen E, Gross CR, Savik SK, Sharp HL: Liver disease in alpha-1-antitrypsin deficiency: Prognostic indicators. *J Pediatr* **117**:864, 1990.
267. Cox DW: α_1-antitrypsin deficiency, in Fisher MM, Roy CC (eds): *Pediatric Liver Disease: Hepatology Research and Clinical Issues* Vol 5. New York, Plenum, 1983, p 271.
268. Sveger T: Prospective study of children with α_1-antitrypsin deficiency: Eight-year-old follow-up. *J Pediatr* **104**:91, 1984.
269. Porter CA, Mowat AP, Cook PJL, Haynes DWG, Shilkin KB, Williams R: α_1-antitrypsin deficiency and neonatal hepatitis. *Br Med J* **3**:435, 1972.
270. Udall JN, Dixon M, Newman AP, Wright JA: Liver disease in alpha$_1$-antitrypsin deficiency: A retrospective analysis of the influence of early breast- vs bottle-feeding. *JAMA* **253**:2679, 1985.
271. Davidson LA, Lonnerdal B: Fecal alpha-1-antitrypsin in breast-fed infants is derived from human milk and is not indicative of enteric protein loss. *Acta Paediatr Scand* **79**:137, 1990.

272. Sveger T: Breast-feeding, α_1-antitrypsin deficiency, and liver disease? *JAMA* **254**:3036, 1985.
273. Udall JN, Bloch KJ, Walker WA: Transport of proteases across neonatal intestine and development of liver disease in infants with α_1-antitrypsin deficiency. *Lancet* **1**:1441, 1982.
274. Cox DW, Mansfield T: Prenatal diagnosis of alpha$_1$-antitrypsin deficiency and estimates of fetal risk for disease. *J Med Genet* **24**:52, 1987.
275. Starzl TE, Porter KA, Francavilla A, Iwatsuki S: Reversal of hepatic alpha-1-antitrypsin deposition after portacaval shunt. *Lancet* **2**:424, 1983.
276. Esquivel CO, Marino IR, Fioravanti V, Vanthiel DH: Liver transplantation for metabolic disease of the liver. *Gastroenterol Clin North Am* **17**:167, 1988.
277. Berg NO, Eriksson S: Liver disease in adults with alpha$_1$-antitrypsin deficiency. *N Engl J Med* **287**:1264, 1972.
278. Cox DW, Smyth S: Risk for liver disease in adults with α_1-antitrypsin deficiency. *Am J Med* **74**:221, 1983.
279. Eriksson S, Carlson J, Velez R: Risk of cirrhosis and primary liver cancer in alpha$_1$-antitrypsin deficiency. *N Engl J Med* **314**:736, 1986.
280. Eriksson S, Hagerstrand I: Cirrhosis and malignant hepatoma in α_1-antitrypsin deficiency. *Acta Med Scand* **195**:451, 1974.
281. Carlson J, Eriksson S: Chronic 'cryptogenic' liver disease in malignant hepatoma in intermediate alpha$_1$-antitrypsin deficiency identified by a PI Z-specific monoclonal antibody. *Scand J Gastroenterol* **20**:835, 1985.
282. Schleissner IA, Cohen AH: Alpha-1-antitrypsin deficiency and hepatic carcinoma. *Am Rev Respir Dis* **111**:863, 1975.
283. Govindarajan S, Ashcavai M, Peters RL: α-1-antitrypsin phenotypes in hepatocellular carcinoma. *Hepatology* **1**:628, 1981.
284. Rabinovitz M, Gavaler JS, Kelly RH, Prieto M, Van Thiel DH: Lack of increase in heterozygous α_1-antitrypsin deficiency phenotypes among patients with hepatocellular and bile duct carcinoma. *Hepatology* **15**:407, 1992.
285. Theodoropoulos A, Fertakis A, Archimandritis A, Kapordelis C, Angelopoulos B: Alpha-1-antitrypsin phenotypes in cirrhosis and hepatoma. *Acta Gastroenterol* **23**:114, 1976.
286. Clerc M, Le Bras M, Loubiere R, Houvet D: Cancer primitif du foie: Incidence de déficit en alpha-1-antitrypsin. *Nouv Presse Med* **6**:3061, 1977.
287. Reintoft I, Hagerstrand IE: Does the Z gene variant of alpha-1-antitrypsin predispose to hepatic carcinoma? *Hum Pathol* **10**:419, 1979.
288. Kelly JK, Davies JS, Jones AW: Alpha-1-antitrypsin deficiency and hepatocellular carcinoma. *J Clin Pathol* **32**:373, 1979.
289. Palmer PE, Ucci AA, Wolfe HJ: Expression of protein markers in malignant hepatoma. Evidence for genetic and epigenetic mechanisms. *Cancer* **45**:1424, 1980.
290. Nukiwa T, Brantly M, Garver R, Paul L, Courtney M, Lecocq J-P, Crystal RG: Evaluation of "at risk" alpha-1-antitrypsin genotype SZ with synthetic oligonucleotide gene probes. *J Clin Invest* **77**:528, 1986.
291. Hodges JR, Millward-Sadler GH, Barbatis C, Wright R: Heterozygous MZ alpha1-antitrypsin deficiency in adults with chronic active hepatitis and cryptogenic cirrhosis. *N Engl J Med* **304**:557, 1981.
292. Fisher RL, Taylor L, Sherlock S: α-1-antitrypsin deficiency in liver disease: The extent of the problem. *Gastroenterology* **71**:646, 1976.
293. Bell H, Schrumpf E, Fagerhol MK: Heterozygous MZ alpha-1-antitrypsin deficiency in adults with chronic liver disease. *Scand J Gastroenterol* **25**:788, 1990.
294. Morin T, Feldmann G, Martin J-P, Rueff B, Benhamou J-P, Ropartz C: Heterozygous alpha1-antitrypsin deficiency and cirrhosis in adults, a fortuitous association. *Lancet* **1**:250, 1975.
295. Lareu MV, Alvarez-Prechous A, Pardinas C, Concheiro L, Carracedo A: Genetic markers in alcoholic liver cirrhosis. *Hum Hered* **42**:235, 1992.
296. Brind AM, Bassendine MF, Bennett MK, James OF: Alpha$_1$-antitrypsin granules in the liver—always important? *Q J Med* **76**:699, 1990.
297. Propst T, Propst A, Dietze O, Judmaier G, Braunsteiner H, Vogel W: High prevalence of viral infection in adults with homozygous and heterozygous alpha$_1$-antitrypsin deficiency and chronic liver disease. *Ann Intern Med* **117**:641, 1992.
298. Milford Ward A, Pickering JD, Shortland JR: The renal manifestations of Pi Z, in J-P Martin (ed): *L'Alpha-1-Antitrypsine et le Système Pi*. Paris, INSERM, 1975, p 131.
299. Strife CF, Hug G, Chuck G, McAdams AJ, Davis CA, Kline JJ: Membranoproliferative glomerulonephritis and α_1-antitrypsin deficiency in children. *Pediatrics* **71**:88, 1983.
300. Davis ID, Burke B, Freese D, Sharp HL, Kim Y: The pathologic spectrum of the nephropathy associated with α_1-antitrypsin deficiency. *Hum Pathol* **23**:57, 1992.
301. Miller F, Kuschner M: Alpha1-antitrypsin deficiency, emphysema, necrotizing angiitis and glomerulonephritis. *Am J Med* **46**:615, 1969.
302. Lewis M, Kallenbach J, Zaltzman M, Levy H, Lurie D, Baynes R, King P, Meyers A: Severe deficiency of alpha1-antitrypsin associated with cutaneous vasculitis, rapidly progressive glomerulonephritis, and colitis. *Am J Med* **79**:489, 1985.
303. Rubinstein HM, Jaffer AM, Kudrna JC, Lertratanakul Y, Chandrasekhar AJ, Slater D, Schmid FR: Alpha$_1$-antitrypsin deficiency with severe panniculitis. *Ann Intern Med* **86**:742, 1977.
304. Breit SN, Clark P, Robinson JP, Luckhurst E, Dawkins RL, Penny R: Familial occurrence of α_1-antitrypsin deficiency and Weber-Christian disease. *Arch Dermatol* **119**:198, 1983.
305. Smith KC, Su WP, Pittelkow MR, Winkelmann RK: Clinical and pathologic correlations in 96 patients with panniculitis, including 15 patients with deficient levels of α_1-antitrypsin. *J Am Acad Dermatol* **21**:1192, 1989.
306. Pittelkow MR, Smith KC, Su WPD: Alpha-1-antitrypsin deficiency and panniculitis: Perspectives on disease relationship and replacement therapy. *Am J Med* **84**(Suppl 6A):80, 1988.
307. Humbert P, Faivre B, Gibey R, Agache P: Use of anticollagenase properties of doxycycline in treatment of alpha$_1$-antitrypsin deficiency panniculitis. *Acta Derm Venereol (Stockh)* **71**:189, 1991.
308. Pottage JC Jr, Trenholme GM, Aronson IK, Harris AA: Panniculitis associated with histoplasmosis and alpha$_1$-antitrypsin deficiency. *Am J Med* **75**:150, 1983.
309. Cox DW, Huber O: Rheumatoid arthritis and alpha-1-antitrypsin. *Lancet* **1**:1216, 1976.
310. Collins RL, Turner RA, Johnson AM: Obstructive pulmonary disease in rheumatoid arthritis. *Arthritis Rheum* **19**:623, 1976.
311. Sjoblom KG, Wollheim FA: Alpha-1-antitrypsin phenotypes and rheumatic diseases. *Lancet* **2**:41, 1977.
312. Brackertz D, Kueppers F: Alpha-1-antitrypsin phenotypes in rheumatoid arthritis. *Lancet* **2**:934, 1977.
313. Beckman G, Beckman L, Bjelle A, Rantapaa Dahlqvist S: Alpha-1-antitrypsin types and rheumatoid arthritis. *Clin Genet* **25**:496, 1984.
314. Geddes DM, Webley M, Brewerton DA, Turton DW, Turner-Warwick M, Murphy AH, Milford Ward A: α_1-antitrypsin phenotypes in fibrosing alveolitis and rheumatoid arthritis. *Lancet* **2**:1049, 1977.
315. Buisseret PD, Pembrey ME, Lessof MH: α_1-antitrypsin phenotypes in rheumatoid arthritis and ankylosing spondylitis. *Lancet* **2**:1358, 1977.
316. Arnaud P, Galbraith RM, Faulk WP, Black C: Pi phenotypes of alpha$_1$-antitrypsin in southern England: Identification of M subtypes and implications for genetic studies. *Clin Genet* **15**:406, 1979.
317. Cox DW, Huber O: Association of severe rheumatoid arthritis with heterozygosity for α_1-antitrypsin deficiency. *Clin Genet* **17**:153, 1980.
318. Abboud RT, Chalmers A, Gofton JP, Richter AM, Enarson DA: Relationship between severity of rheumatoid arthritis and serum alpha$_1$-antitrypsin. *J Rheumatol* **18**:1490, 1992.
319. Arnaud P, Galbraith R, Faulk WP, Ansell BM: Increased frequency of the MZ phenotype of alpha-1-protease inhibitor in juvenile chronic polyarthritis. *J Clin Invest* **60**:1442, 1977.
320. Brewerton DA, Webley M, Murphy AH, Milford Ward

AM: The α_1-antitrypsin phenotype MZ in acute anterior uveitis. *Lancet* **1**:1103, 1978.
321. Wakefield D, Breit SN, Clark P, Penny R: Immunogenetic factors in inflammatory eye disease. Influence of HLA-B27 and alpha$_1$-antitrypsin phenotypes on disease expression. *Arthritis Rheum* **25**:1431, 1982.
322. Brown WT, Mamelok AE, Bearn AG: Anterior uveitis and alpha-1-antitrypsin. *Lancet* **2**:646, 1979.
323. Beckman G, Beckman L, Liden S: Association between psoriasis and the α_1-antitrypsin deficiency gene Z. *Acta Derm Venereol* **60**:163, 1980.
324. Lipkin G, Galdston M, Kueppers F: Alpha$_1$-antitrypsin deficiency genes: Contributory defect in a subset of psoriatics? *J Am Acad Dermatol* **11**:615, 1984.
325. Brandrup F, Ostergaard PA: α_1-antitrypsin deficiency associated with persistent cutaneous vasculitis. *Arch Dermatol* **114**:921, 1978.
326. Nicholls MG, Janus ED: Hashimoto's thyroiditis and homozygous alpha$_1$-antitrypsin deficiency. *Aust NZ J Med* **3**:516, 1973.
327. Gelfand EW, Cox DW, Lin MT, Dosch H-M: Severe combined immune-deficiency disease in a patient with α_1-antitrypsin deficiency. *Lancet* **2**:202, 1979.
328. Anand S, Schade R, Bendetti C, Kelley R, Rabin BS, Krause J, Starzl TE, Iwatsuki S, Van Thiel DH: Idiopathic hemochromatosis and α_1-antitrypsin deficiency: Coexistence in a family with progressive liver disease in the proband. *Hepatology* **3**:714, 1983.
329. Eriksson S, Lindmark B: A Swedish family with alpha$_1$-antitrypsin deficiency, hemochromatosis, haemoglobinopathy D and early death in liver cirrhosis. *J Hepatol* **2**:65, 1986.
330. Rabinovitz M, Gavaler JS, Kelly RH, Van Thiel DH: Association between heterozygous α_1-antitrypsin deficiency and genetic hemochromatosis. *Hepatology* **16**:145, 1992.
331. Eriksson S, Lindmark B, Olsson S: Lack of association between hemochromatosis and α_1-antitrypsin deficiency. *Acta Med Scand* **219**:291, 1986.
332. Benkmann HG, Hanssen HP, Ovenbeck R, Goedde HW: Distribution of alpha-1-antitrypsin and haptoglobin phenotypes in bladder cancer patients. *Hum Hered* **37**:290, 1987.
333. Cohen JR, Sarfati I, Ratner L, Tilson D: α_1-antitrypsin phenotypes in patients with abdominal aortic aneurysms. *J Surg Res* **49**:319, 1990.
334. Mitchell MB, McAnena OJ, Rutherford RB: Ruptured mesenteric artery aneurysm in a patient with α_1-antitrypsin deficiency: Etiologic implications. *J Vasc Surg* **17**:420, 1993.
335. Kueppers F, O'Brien P, Passarge E, Rudiger HW: Alpha$_1$-antitrypsin phenotypes in sex chromosome mosaicism. *J Med Genet* **12**:263, 1975.
336. Aarskog D, Fagerhol MK: Protease inhibitor (Pi) phenotypes in chromosome aberrations. *J Med Genet* **7**:367, 1970.
337. Lieberman J, Borhani NO, Feinleib M: α_1-antitrypsin deficiency in twins and parents-of-twins. *Clin Genet* **15**:29, 1979.
338. Clark P, Martin NG: An excess of the Pi^S allele in dizygotic twins and their mothers. *Hum Genet* **61**:171, 1982.
339. Jeppsson J-O, Franzen B, Sveger T, Cordesius E, Stromberg P, Gustabii B: Prenatal exclusion of alpha$_1$-antitrypsin deficiency in a high-risk fetus. *N Engl J Med* **300**:1441, 1979.
340. Saiki RK, Bugawan TL, Horn GT, Mullis KB, Erlich HA: Analysis of enzymatically amplified β-globin and HLA-DQα DNA with allele-specific oligonucleotide probes. *Nature* **324**:163, 1986.
341. Kidd VJ, Wallace RB, Itakura K, Woo SLC: α_1-antitrypsin deficiency detection by direct analysis of the mutation in the gene. *Nature* **304**:230, 1983.
342. Kidd VJ, Golbus MS, Wallace RB, Itakura K, Woo SLC: Prenatal diagnosis of alpha$_1$-antitrypsin deficiency by direct analysis of the mutation site in the gene. *N Engl J Med* **310**:639, 1984.
343. Bruun Petersen K, Bruun Petersen G, Dahl R, Larsen B, Kolvraa S, Koch J, Bolund L, Gregersen N: α_1-antitrypsin alleles in patients with pulmonary emphysema, detected by DNA amplification (PCR) and oligonucleotide probes. *Eur Respir J* **5**:531, 1992.
344. Gregersen N, Winter V, Petersen KB, Koch J, Kolvraa S, Rudiger N, Heinsvig E, Bolund L: Detection of point mutations in amplified single copy genes by biotin-labelled oligonucleotides: Diagnosis of variants of alpha-1-antitrypsin. *Clin Chim Acta* **182**:151, 1989.
345. Dry PJ: Rapid detection of alpha-1-antitrypsin deficiency by analysis of a PCR-induced TaqI restriction site. *Hum Genet* **87**:742, 1991.
346. Andresen BS, Knudsen I, Jensen PKA, Rasmussen K, Gregersen N: Two novel nonradioactive polymerase chain reaction-based assays of dried blood spots, genomic DNA, or whole cells for fast, reliable detection of Z and S mutations in the α_1-antitrypsin gene. *Clin Chem* **38**:2100, 1992.
347. Jeppsson J-O, Sveger T: Typing of genetic variants of α_1-antitrypsin from dried blood. *Scand J Clin Lab Invest* **44**:413, 1984.
348. Thelin T, McNeil TF, Aspegren-Jansson E, Sveger T: Psychological consequences of neonatal screening for α_1-antitrypsin deficiency. Parental reactions to the first news of their infants' deficiency. *Acta Paediatr Scand* **74**:787, 1985.
349. Thelin T, McNeil TF, Aspegren-Jansson E, Sveger T: Identifying children at high somatic risk: Parents' long-term emotional adjustment to their children's alpha$_1$-antitrypsin deficiency. *Acta Psychiatr Scand* **72**:323, 1985.
350. Hubbard RC, Crystal RG: Augmentation therapy of α_1-antitrypsin deficiency. *Eur Respir J Suppl* **9**:44s, 1990.
351. Crystal RG: Gene therapy strategies for pulmonary disease. *Am J Med* **92**:44S, 1992.
352. Gelfand JA, Sherins RJ, Alling DW, Frank MM: Treatment of hereditary angioedema with danazol: Reversal of clinical and biochemical abnormalities. *N Engl J Med* **295**:1444, 1976.
353. Wewers MD, Gadek JE, Keogh BA, Fells GA, Crystal RG: Evaluation of danazol therapy for patients with PiZZ alpha$_1$-antitrypsin deficiency. *Am Rev Respir Dis* **134**:476, 1986.
354. Powers JC, Gupton BF, Harley AD, Nishino N, Whitley RJ: Specificity of porcine pancreatic elastase, human leukocytes elastase and cathepsin-G. Inhibition with chloromethyl ketone peptides. *Biochim Biophys Acta* **485**:156, 1977.
355. Doherty JB, Ashe BM, Argenbright LW, Barker PL, Bonney RJ, Chandler GO, Dahlgren ME, Dorn CP Jr, Finke PE, Firestone RA, Fletcher D, Hagmann WK, Mumford R, O'Grady L, Maycock AL, Pisano JM, Shah SK, Thompson KR, Zimmerman M: Cephalosporin antibiotics can be modified to inhibit human leukocyte elastase. *Nature* **322**:192, 1986.
356. Burrows B: A clinical trial of efficacy of antiproteolytic therapy: Can it be done? *Am Rev Respir Dis* **127**:S42, 1983.
357. Cohen AB: The clinical usefulness of different forms of alpha-1-protease inhibitor. *Am Rev Respir Dis* **133**:349, 1986.
358. Wewers MD, Casolaro MA, Sellers SE, Swayze SC, McPhaul KM, Wittes JT, Crystal RG: Replacement therapy for alpha$_1$-antitrypsin deficiency associated with emphysema. *N Engl J Med* **316**:1055, 1987.
359. Ulmer WT, Schmidt EW, Rasche B: Long term effect on lung function of alpha1-protease inhibitor substitution therapy in COPD patients with Pi ZZ phenotype. *Eur Respir J Suppl* **9**:21s, 1990.
360. Hubbard RC, Sellers S, Czerski D, Stephens L, Crystal RG: Biochemical efficacy and safety of monthly augmentation therapy for α_1-antitrypsin deficiency. *J Am Med Assoc* **260**:1259, 1988.
361. Buist S, Burrows B, Cohen A, Crystal RG, Fallat R, Gadek J, Turino G: Guidelines for the approach to the patient with severe hereditary alpha-1-antitrypsin deficiency. Statement of the American Thoracic Society. *Am Rev Respir Dis* **140**:1494, 1989.
362. Ford GT, Abboud RT, Guenter CA: Current status of alpha-1-antitrypsin replacement therapy: Recommendations for the management of patients with severe hereditary deficiency. Ad Hoc Committee on Alpha-1-Antitrypsin Replacement Therapy of the Standards Committee, Canadian Thoracic Society. *Can Med Assoc J* **146**:841, 1992.
363. Snider GL: Pulmonary disease in alpha-1-antitrypsin deficiency. *Ann Intern Med* **111**:957, 1989.
364. Hubbard RC, Crystal RG: Strategies for aerosol therapy of alpha1-antitrypsin deficiency by the aerosol route. *Lung* **168**:565, 1990.

365. Bollen A, Herzog A, Cravador A, Herion P, Chuchana P, Vander Straten A, Loriau R, Jacobs P, Van Elsen A: Cloning and expression in *Escherichia coli* of full-length complementary DNA coding for human α_1-antitrypsin. *DNA* **2**:255, 1983.
366. Courtney M, Buchwalder A, Tessier L-H, Jaye M, Benavente A, Balland A, Kohli V, Lathe R, Tolstoshev P, Lecocq J-P: High-level production of biologically active human α_1-antitrypsin in *Escherichia coli. Proc Natl Acad Sci USA* **81**:669, 1984.
367. Straus SD, Fells GA, Wewers MD, Courtney M, Tessier L-H, Tolstoshev P, Lecocq J-P, Crystal RG: Evaluation of recombinant DNA-directed *E. coli* produced α_1-antitrypsin as an anti-neutrophil elastase for potential use as replacement therapy of α_1-antitrypsin deficiency. *Biochem Biophys Res Commun* **130**:1177, 1985.
368. Courtney M, Jallat S, Tessier L-H, Benavente A, Crystal RG, Lecocq J-P: Synthesis in *E. coli* of α_1-antitrypsin variants of therapeutic potential for emphysema and thrombosis. *Nature* **313**:149, 1985.
369. George PM, Vissers MCM, Travis J, Winterbourn CC, Carrell RW: A genetically engineered mutant of α_1-antitrypsin protects connective tissue from neutrophil damage and may be useful in lung disease. *Lancet* **2**:1426, 1984.
370. Travis J, Owen MC, George P, Carrell RW, Rosenberg S, Hallewell RA, Barr PJ: Isolation and properties of recombinant DNA produced variants of human alpha$_1$-proteinase inhibitor. *J Biol Chem* **260**:4384, 1985.
371. Hubbard RC, Brantly ML, Sellers SE, Mitchell ME, Crystal RG: Delivery of proteins for therapeutic purposes by aerosolization: Direct augmentation of anti-neutrophil elastase defenses of the lower respiratory tract in α_1-antitrypsin deficiency with an aerosol of α_1-antitrypsin. *Ann Intern Med* **111**:206, 1989.
372. Hubbard RC, McElvaney NG, Sellers SE, Healy JT, Czerski DB, Crystal RG: Recombinant DNA-produced α_1-antitrypsin administered by aerosol augments lower respiratory tract anti-neutrophil elastase defenses in individuals with α_1-antitrypsin deficiency. *J Clin Invest* **84**:1349, 1989.
373. Wright G, Carver A, Cottam D, Reeves D, Scott A, Simons JP, Wilmut I, Garner I, Coleman A: High level expression of active human α_1-antitrypsin in the milk of transgenic sheep. *Biotechnology* **9**:830, 1991.
374. Garver RI, Chytil A, Courtney M, Crystal RG: Clonal gene therapy: Transplanted mouse fibroblast clones express human α_1-antitrypsin gene in vivo. *Science* **237**:762, 1987.
375. Lemarchand P, Jaffe HA, Danel C, Cid MC, Kleinman HK, Stratford-Perricaudet LD, Perricaudet M, Pavirani A, Lecocq J-P: Adenovirus-mediated transfer of a recombinant human α_1-antitrypsin cDNA to human endothelial cells. *Proc Natl Acad Sci USA* **89**:6482, 1992.
376. Rosenfeld MA, Siegfried W, Yoshimura K, Yoneyama K, Fakayama M, Stier LE, Paakko PK, Gilardi P, Stratford-Perricaudet LD, Perricaudet M, Jallat S, Pavirani A, Lecoqc J-P, Crystal RG: Adenovirus-mediated transfer of a recombinant α_1-antitrypsin gene to the lung epithelium in vivo. *Science* **252**:431, 1991.
377. Adams RM, Soriano HE, Wang M, Darlington G, Steffen D, Ledley FD: Transduction of primary human hepatocytes with amphotropic and xenotropic retroviral vectors. *Proc Natl Acad Sci USA* **89**:8981, 1992.
378. Wilson JM, Johnston DE, Jefferson DM, Mulligan RC: Correction of the genetic defect in hepatocytes from the Watanabe heritable hyperlipidemic rabbit. *Proc Natl Acad Sci USA* **85**:4421, 1988.
379. Raper SE, Wilson JM, Grossman M: Retroviral-mediated gene transfer in human hepatocytes. *Surgery* **112**:333, 1992.
380. Jaffe HA, Danel C, Longenecker G, Metzger M, Setoguchi Y, Rosenfeld MA, Grant TW, Thorgeirsson SS, Stratford-Perricaudet LD, Perricaudet M, Pavirani A, Lecocq J-P, Crystal RG: Adenovirus-mediated in vivo gene transfer and expression in normal rat liver. *Nat Genet* **1**:372, 1992.
381. Wilson JM, Grossman M, Wu CH, Chowdhury NR, Wu GY, Chowdhury JR: Hepatocyte-directed gene transfer in vivo leads to transient improvement of hypercholesterolemia in low density lipoprotein receptor-deficient rabbits. *J Biol Chem* **267**:963, 1992.
382. Wilson JM, Grossman M, Cabrera JA, Wu CH, Wu GY: A novel mechanism for achieving transgene persistence in vivo after somatic gene transfer into hepatocytes. *J Biol Chem* **267**:11483, 1992.
383. Trulock EP, Cooper JD, Kaiser LR, Pasque MK, Ettinger NA, Dresler CM: The Washington University-Barnes Hospital experience with lung transplantation. Washington University Lung Transplantation Group. *JAMA* **266**:1943, 1991.
384. Calhoon JH, Grover FL, Gibbons WJ, Bryan CL, Levine SM, Bailey SR, Nichols L, Lum C, Trinkle JK: Single lung transplantation. Alternative indications and technique. *J Thorac Cardiovasc Surg* **101**:816, 1991.

CHAPTER 139

Amyloidosis

Merrill D. Benson

1. **Hereditary amyloidosis is characterized by the extracellular accumulation of protein fibrils having β-pleated sheet structure. Actually, hereditary amyloidosis is only one of a number of forms of amyloidosis, each characterized by the protein that is the basic subunit of the amyloid fibril. Systemic forms of hereditary amyloidosis may be associated with variant forms of transthyretin, apolipoprotein A-I, gelsolin, fibrinogen, or lysozyme. Other forms of systemic amyloidosis, which are not hereditary, include immunoglobulin (AL, primary) amyloidosis, in which the subunit protein is the variable portion of the immunoglobulin light chain; reactive (secondary) amyloidosis, in which the subunit protein is a degradation product, amyloid A (AA), of a serum acute-phase protein, serum amyloid A (SAA); and β_2-microglobulin (dialysis associated) amyloidosis, in which the subunit protein is the β_2-microglobulin protein. All forms of amyloidosis cause illness and death by physical encroachment of the deposits on normal organ structures. In autosomal dominant hereditary amyloidosis, peripheral neuropathy is the most common finding, although infiltration of vital organs such as heart, kidney, and bowel give various syndromes, which usually lead to death.**
2. **Hereditary amyloidosis is a late-onset disease with clinical symptoms beginning in most kindreds within the third to seventh decades of life. The clinical disease usually progresses over 5 to 15 years and ends with death from cardiac failure, renal failure, or malnutrition. Gene carriers in some kindreds with late-onset disease, however, have lived past age 90. Gene prevalence is not known, since there are a number of mutations in the genes for various plasma proteins, and many of the kindreds have been characterized only recently. In the United States, the prevalence of variant transthyretin genes is certainly greater than 1 in 1,000,000 and may be as high as 1 in 100,000.**
3. **The primary defect in autosomal dominant transthyretin amyloidosis results from one of a number of mutations in the gene for transthyretin, which is a single-copy sequence on chromosome 18. To date, 41 single amino acid substitutions in the transthyretin molecule that could be associated with hereditary amyloidosis have been found. In addition, two mutations each have been described in apolipoprotein A-I, gelsolin, the fibrinogen A α chain, and lysozyme, all of which are associated with systemic amyloidosis.**
4. **Direct DNA tests have been developed for many of the variant genes for transthyretin, apolipoprotein A-I, gelsolin, fibrinogen, and lysozyme. In addition, modern molecular biology techniques can provide easy detection methods for all of the demonstrated mutations. Southern blot analysis has been replaced in many cases by restriction enzyme analysis of PCR amplification products. Direct DNA sequencing based on PCR technology is used in the discovery of new mutations. DNA tests have been established for certain protein variants, and these are used for genetic counseling.**
5. **Prenatal diagnosis has been developed for at least two forms of transthyretin amyloidosis based on PCR technology.**
6. **Other forms of autosomal dominant amyloidosis that are defined by their subunit proteins include: (1) hereditary cerebral hemorrhage with amyloidosis in Iceland (cystatin C), (2) a few kindreds with Alzheimer disease or hereditary cerebral hemorrhage with amyloidosis—Dutch (amyloid beta protein or A4 protein), and (3) medullary carcinoma of the thyroid (procalcitonin).**

The term *amyloidosis* is used to describe a number of protein deposition diseases in which homogeneous protein molecules aggregate into an ordered structure to make fibrils measuring 75 to 100 Å in cross section and having indeterminate length.[1] These fibrils accumulate in extracellular spaces to form deposits which, because of their ordered structure, have the crystalline property of birefringence and, in addition, have selective affinities for certain histochemical dyes such as Congo red.

There are several types of amyloidosis, defined by the basic protein constituent of the fibrils. The most life-threatening of these disorders are systemic with involvement of major organ systems. There are, however, a number of localized forms of amyloidosis in which the amyloid deposits are restricted to a single organ. Although each type of amyloidosis is a separate disease with its own etiology and pathogenic mechanisms, all share the physicochemical properties of the amyloid fibril and cause illness in the same way. As the extracellular deposits enlarge, they displace normal tissue structures, causing disruption of cell function and ultimately cell death. The signs and symptoms of the disease depend on the strategic location and size of the fibril deposits, but the basic mechanisms and end result of their presence is the same in all types of amyloidosis. Despite this final common pathway, the etiology, pathogenesis, prognosis, and therapeutic interventions for the different forms of amyloidosis must be considered separately. To set the stage for such a discussion and prepare us for handling the rapidly accumulating data in this area, it is important to have some historical perspective.

A list of standard abbreviations is located immediately preceding the index in each volume. Additional abbreviations used in this chapter include: AA = amyloid A; AL amyloidosis = amyloid light chain amyloidosis; APP = amyloid precursor protein; FAP = familial amyloid polyneuropathy; FMF = familial Mediterranean fever; RBP = retinol binding protein; SAA = serum amyloid A; and TTR = transthyretin.

HISTORY

Although amyloidosis has undoubtedly occurred for centuries, it was not until the mid-1800s that attention was brought to the condition. Rokitansky[2] in 1842 wrote about the "lardaceous liver" found at autopsy in patients with chronic diseases, and Virchow (1854) subsequently showed that these tissues gave a unique color reaction with iodine and sulfuric acid.[3,4] Virchow coined the term *amyloid,* which means "starch-like," because of this reaction, which led him to believe that amyloid represented deposits of carbohydrates. However, in 1859, Friedreich and Kekule reported evidence that amyloid deposits were composed mainly of protein.[5] Over the next 100 years, amyloidosis associated with chronic diseases was studied histologically and epidemiologically.[6] It became obvious that some patients with amyloidosis had no predisposing illness, and that amyloidosis was occasionally seen in familial patterns. Eventually the term *primary* was applied to the sporadic form of amyloidosis and *secondary* to amyloidosis that developed in individuals with chronic inflammatory diseases such as tuberculosis, osteomyelitis, and rheumatoid arthritis. Hereditary amyloidosis was not widely recognized as such until Andrade (1952) published his finding of amyloidosis in families with polyneuropathy in northern Portugal.[7] Reviews of the literature show that, as early as the 1920s, familial occurrence of amyloidotic polyneuropathy had been described, but these cases were classified as primary.[8,9] Indeed, Ostertag in 1932 reported a family with hereditary amyloid nephropathy and subsequently published a very detailed study of this kindred in 1950, two years before Andrade's description of Portuguese families.[10] Ostertag was pathologist in the very clinic in Berlin that was named for Rudolph Virchow. So why do we revere Virchow for his description of amyloid, although he mistakenly thought it carbohydrate in character, and give little credit to Ostertag, who wrote one of the first descriptions of hereditary amyloidosis? The answer is as clear as the evolution of science in medicine. During the reign of Rudolph Virchow as the preeminent pathologist in the world, German medical science was at its pinnacle, and the accepted language of science was German. By the time of Ostertag's major publication 100 years later, American medical science had gained supremacy and with it came the installation of English as the preferred scientific language. Alas, Ostertag published in German and Andrade in English.

Characterization of amyloid remained relatively static until 1959 when Cohen and Calkins[11] and Spiro[12] showed by electron microscopy that amyloid deposits were not amorphous but contained nonbranching fibrils with diameters of 75 to 100 Å and of indeterminate length. Chemical characterization of this fibril material was hindered by its resistance to solubilization in practically all solvents. However, by 1971, Glenner et al.[13] were able to solubilize amyloid fibrils from the tissues of patients with primary amyloidosis using strong chaotropic agents, and they isolated the major subunit proteins. Amino acid sequencing revealed that these subunits were homologous to the variable segment of immunoglobulin light chains. This breakthrough in amyloid research at the chemical level was quickly followed by the demonstration that amyloid fibrils from patients with secondary amyloidosis were composed of a previously undescribed protein, which was subsequently named "amyloid A protein" (AA).[14–16] Further studies revealed that AA was derived from an acute-phase plasma protein, which was then named "serum amyloid A" (SAA).[17–23] In 1978, Costa et al. found that amyloid material from patients with hereditary amyloidosis was composed of a subunit protein which reacted with antiserum to plasma transthyretin (prealbumin).[24] The presence of transthyretin in hereditary amyloid deposits was confirmed at the structural level by 1981,[25] and since then numerous variants of this plasma protein have been found to be associated with hereditary amyloidosis.[25–30] Subsequently, various forms of other plasma proteins have been found to be associated with hereditary amyloidosis, including apolipoprotein A-I,[31] gelsolin,[32,33] and, recently, the α chain of fibrinogen.[34] In addition, advances have been made in the chemical characterization of localized forms of amyloidosis, including determination of the structure of the β-amyloid of Alzheimer plaques,[35] the prion protein of Creutzfeldt-Jakob and Gerstmann-Sträussler-Scheinker diseases,[36] and the amyloid of islets of Langerhans in type 2 diabetes mellitus.[37] This brings us to the present time where we can discuss amyloidosis at the physicochemical level and consider hypotheses on the etiology and pathogenic mechanisms of the various types.

PHYSICAL PROPERTIES OF AMYLOID FIBRILS

By light microscopy, in hematoxylin-and-eosin stained preparations, amyloid deposits of all kinds are amorphous and eosinophilic (Fig. 139-1). The deposits are extracellular and often appear to be crowding the cells aside. This phenomenon is best appreciated in peripheral nerves, where the typical nerve bundles and Schwann cell nuclei detour around large accumulations of amyloid (Fig. 139-2). In other tissues, amyloid may accumulate along cell margins. This is seen in the liver, where columns of amyloid separate the hepatic cords, and in the heart, where cross-sectional preparations show rings of amyloid around the myocardial fibers. In some tissues, large collections of amyloid may completely lack cellular elements.

While amyloid deposits of all kinds are eosinophilic, they also have unique staining properties that are useful in diagnosis. In the past, methyl violet and crystal violet, which give metachromatic reactions with amyloid, were used to stain amyloid deposits. Now Congo red has become the standard for identification of amyloid on histologic sections (Fig. 139-3).[38] In tissue sections stained with alkaline Congo red, amyloid deposits take up the dye and give a characteristic green color when viewed in the polarizing microscope. This specific marker for amyloid is due to the birefringent nature of the amyloid fibrils and to their ability to bind Congo red. Collagen is also birefringent in histologic sections, but collagen does not bind Congo red, and, therefore, the green birefringence is not seen. The fluorescent thioflavin dyes have also been used to localize amyloid but have not been universally accepted.

At the level of electron microscopy, amyloid deposits contain characteristic fibrillar structures, which are often in linear array, but lack of ordered structure is the rule (Fig. 139-4). Deep invaginations of the fibrils into the cytoplasmic membranes of reticuloendothelial cells are frequently seen and have been postulated to be the sites of amyloid formation, but controversy persists on where actual fibril formation occurs. When amyloid fibrils are physically extracted from tissue deposits, negatively stained with uranyl acetate or phosphotungstic acid, and studied by high-resolution electron microscopy, the nonbranching fibrils appear to consist of at least two and perhaps several parallel subunit filaments.[39] Helical twisting of these subunits, which measure about 25

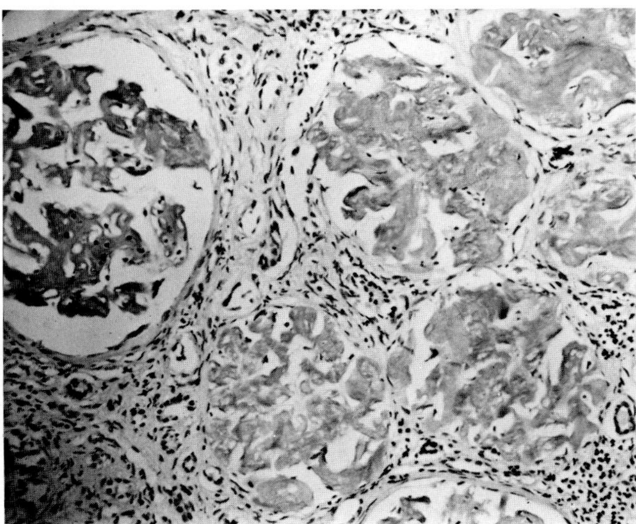

FIG. 139-1 Amyloid deposits obliterating renal glomeruli in a patient with hereditary amyloidosis. Hematoxylin and eosin stain.

to 35 Å in width, may give a beaded appearance to the fibrils. While a fair degree of structural diversity is seen from one fibril preparation to another, no ultrastructural features that distinguish immunoglobulin, AA, or transthyretin amyloid fibrils have been reported.

The substructure of amyloid fibrils has been studied by x-ray diffraction.[40,41] While amyloid fibrils basically have a crystalline structure, which gives them their birefringence, it has not been possible to solubilize and recrystallize amyloid fibrils to study the crystal lattice by x-ray diffraction. Chemical studies suggest that other substances (e.g., proteoglycans) may be involved in fibril formation, and, therefore, fibrils are a mixture of substances other than just the basic protein subunit. X-ray powder patterns, however, are consistent with β structure, and this has been the basis for developing the antiparallel β pleated sheet model of amyloid fibrils (Fig. 139-5). This is supported by x-ray crystallographic data on two of the amyloid fibril subunit proteins, immunoglobulin light chain and transthyretin. Immunoglobulin light chain domains have extensive antiparallel β configuration.[42] Similarly, the transthyretin monomer has extensive β structure, with eight polypeptide segments running in an antiparallel fashion in two planes.[43] The tertiary structure of AA protein in reactive amyloidosis is not as well understood, and structural models suggest that α helices may also be involved in intrinsic fibril formation.

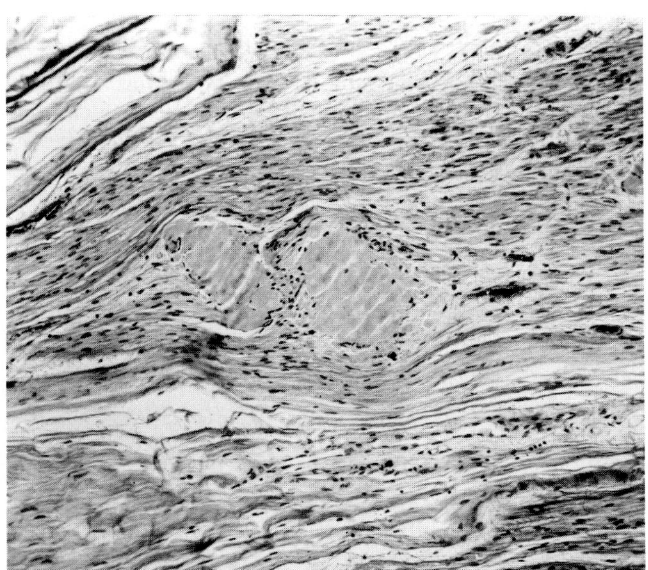

FIG. 139-2 Amyloid deposits within peripheral nerve displacing nerve fibers and supporting cells. Congo red counterstained with hematoxylin.

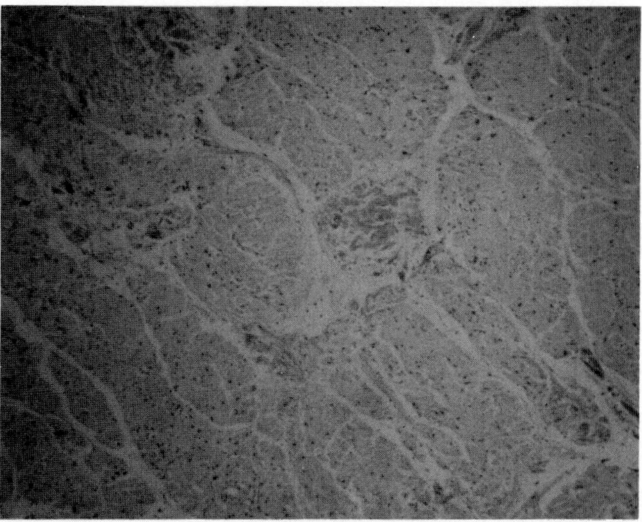

A.

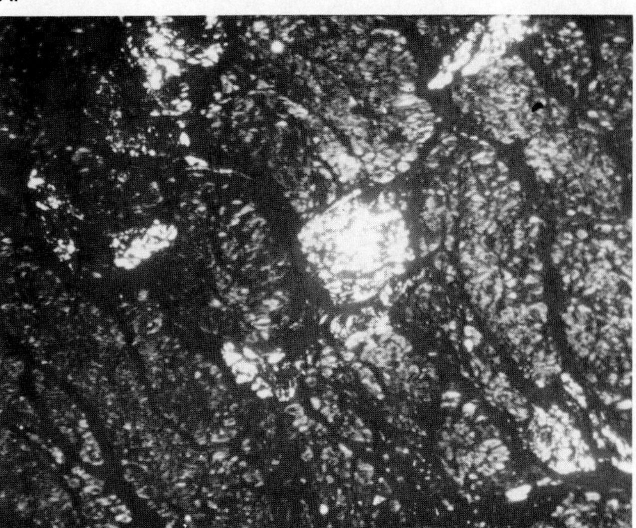

B.

FIG. 139-3 Amyloid deposits within myocardium stained with Congo red. *A*. Light microscopic view. *B*. The same section through crossed polars. Congo red-stained amyloid deposits show green birefringence. Ring structures caused by amyloid deposits around myocardial fiber bundles also become apparent in the polarizing microscope. Congo red counterstained with hematoxylin.

OVERALL CLASSIFICATION OF THE AMYLOIDOSES

Although the term *amyloid* turned out to be a misnomer, we have all become accustomed to using the term *amyloidosis* to denote the syndromes characterized by the deposition of the β pleated sheet fibrils. Amyloidosis is a more general term than such terms as *β fibrilloses* because it can accommodate

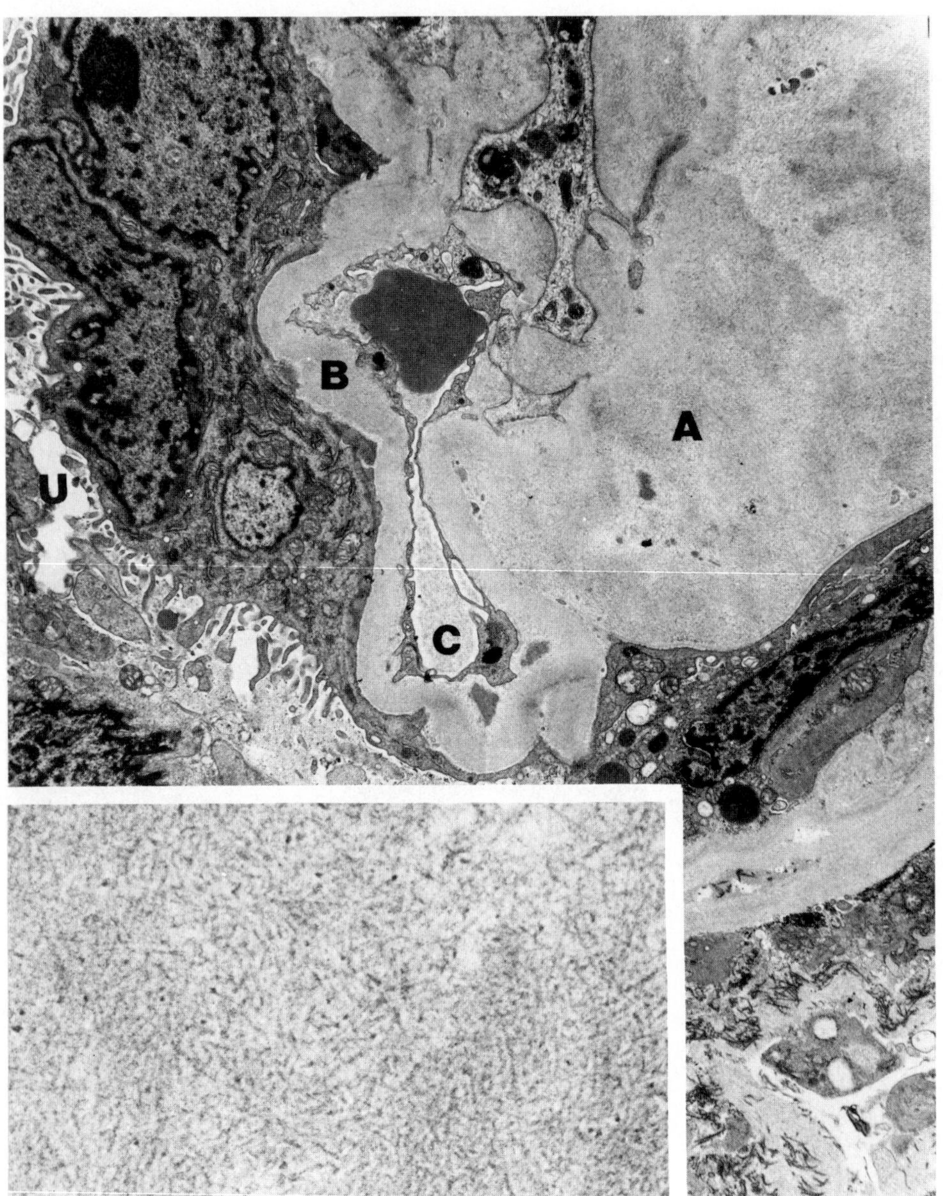

FIG. 139-4 Electron micrograph of a renal biopsy. Amyloid deposits are present throughout the basement membrane and in adjacent structures. *Inset:* higher-power micrograph showing the fibrillar structures that are characteristic of all types of amyloid deposits. A = amyloid; B = basement membrane; C = capillary loop; U = urinary space.

conditions such as immunoglobulin light chain deposition disease, a B-lymphocyte dyscrasia in which monoclonal light chain proteins (usually κ) accumulate in organs (often the kidneys) and result in death but evidently do not have the capability of forming fibrils.[44,45] This condition appears to be very closely related to immunoglobulin amyloidosis, since there have now been reports of patients who had immunoglobulin light chain deposition disease and in whom postmortem examination showed actual amyloid fibril deposits in organs other than the kidney.[46,47] Using the term *amyloidoses* to designate the entire group of protein deposition diseases, a classification has been proposed based on chemical composition of the amyloid deposits.[48] Such a classification has to be modified for clinical use, since patterns of organ involvement will continue to be important. For instance, whether an amyloidosis is systemic or localized has far-reaching significance for treatment and prognosis. Therefore, it is best to classify the systemic amyloidoses separately from the localized forms and then to use subclassifications based on chemical compositions when known.

Historically, for want of a better method, the amyloidoses were classified according to the clinical features of each syndrome. "Primary amyloidosis" was used to designate those syndromes in which there was no obvious predisposing disease. "Secondary amyloidosis" referred to those cases in which there was a predisposing chronic inflammatory disease. "Heredofamilial" or "hereditary amyloidosis" was used whenever there was a definite familial pattern. A few confusing terms were used, and these need to be mentioned because they persist in the old literature. First, patients with amyloidosis associated with multiple myeloma were frequently said to have amyloidosis "secondary" to multiple myeloma. The use of the term *secondary* in this context is unfortunate since chemical analysis now shows that myeloma-associated amyloidosis is chemically the same as primary amyloidosis. These two groups should be and are presently classified as immunoglobulin light chain amyloidosis. Further confusion has been caused by the use of the term *primary* in some of the reports of hereditary amyloidosis.

At the present time, the best classification of the amyloidoses is based on the chemical composition of the amyloid

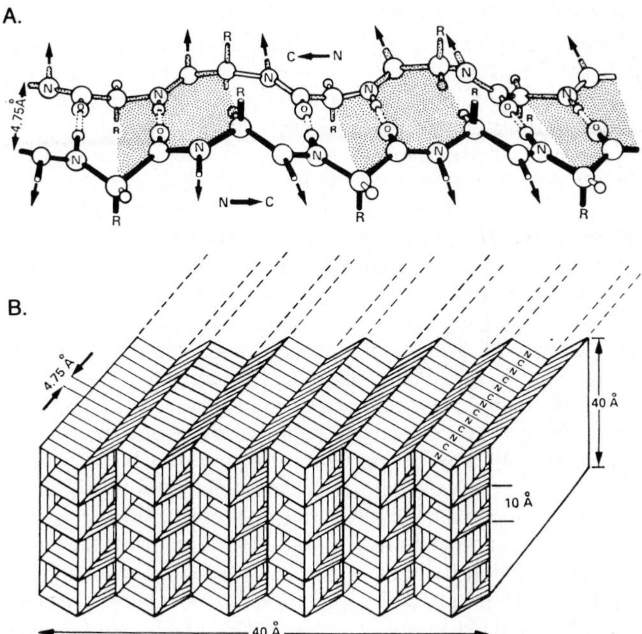

FIG. 139-5 Proposed model of antiparallel β structure. ***A.*** **The structural basis of the antiparallel β sheet. The structure is formed by a single polypeptide chain that folds back on itself. The N-terminal to C-terminal directions are as shown. The strands are held together by hydrogen bonding and have an interchain distance of approximately 4.75 Å.** ***B.*** **The proposed structure of amyloid fibrils is shown with basic dimensions of 40 × 40 Å with indefinite length. Two or more of these fibrils probably associate by twisting along the long axis to form the amyloid fibril.** ***(Modified from Sack et al.[227] Used by permission.)***

fibrils. This is of particular value in the systemic amyloidoses, where we know the chemical composition of the deposits. A word of caution is in order, however, since there may be other forms of systemic amyloidosis, particularly in the hereditary group, for which we may find as yet undescribed amyloid subunits. In the localized forms of amyloidosis, fewer subunit proteins have been characterized biochemically, so it remains necessary to classify them by a combination of factors, including organ system involvement and chemical composition, where known. It is important to realize that some hereditary amyloidoses are systemic and others are localized. In the systemic group are the autosomal dominant forms, which often show peripheral neuropathy and in which many variant forms of transthyretin have been described, as well as mutations in apolipoprotein A-I, plasma gelsolin, and fibrinogen. In addition, there is the systemic amyloidosis associated with familial Mediterranean fever, in which the pattern of inheritance is autosomal recessive.[49] Hereditary amyloid syndromes with localized deposits include medullary carcinoma of the thyroid,[50,51] familial cutaneous amyloidosis,[52,53] and those forms of Alzheimer disease in which there is a familial pattern.[54] Localized forms of amyloidosis without an apparent hereditary pattern include amyloid in the islets of Langerhans in diabetes mellitus, amyloid of the larynx and upper respiratory tract, the sporadic occurrence of amyloid tumors in the genitourinary tract, some cutaneous amyloidoses, and nonfamilial cerebral amyloid angiopathy and most Alzheimer disease.

THE SYSTEMIC AMYLOIDOSES

Three major types of systemic amyloidosis have been recognized in humans: (1) immunoglobulin (primary), (2) reactive (secondary), and (3) hereditary (Table 139-1). A fourth type, which thus far has been described only in patients with chronic renal failure, usually on hemodialysis, has deposits containing β_2-microglobulin.[55,56] While this type of amyloid deposition is predominantly restricted to bones and joints, other organ involvement has been seen.

In this chapter we are principally interested in the hereditary forms of amyloidosis, but it is important to have an understanding of the other types of human systemic amyloidosis for two reasons. First, at the clinical level, the different types of systemic amyloidosis may be very similar. They all may affect the same organ systems to varying degrees. One form of amyloidosis can be easily mistaken for another, especially in situations where a family history is not available or informative or when chronic inflammatory disease, which may predispose to reactive amyloidosis, is not readily apparent. Second, it has become increasingly evident that there is a genetic basis for both the immunoglobulin and the reactive types of amyloidosis. The monoclonal immunoglobulin light chains that are the subunit proteins of immunoglobulin amyloidosis are the products of intricate gene rearrangement mechanisms in B-lymphocyte clones. Limited structural studies of amyloid light chain proteins suggest that only certain structures are amyloidogenic (have the capability of forming amyloid fibrils). Whatever pathogenic mechanisms are involved in immunoglobulin amyloid formation, DNA rearrangements are an integral part of the process. In reactive amyloidosis, the precursor protein SAA is synthesized by the liver. Multiple genes code for this protein and, again, while structural data are limited, they suggest that certain isotypes of SAA are preferentially processed to make amyloid fibrils. While no inheritance pattern of reactive amyloidosis has been shown other than in familial Mediterranean fever and Muckle-Wells syndrome,

Table 139-1 Systemic Amyloidoses

Type	Previous Name(s)	Subunit Protein	Distinguishing Feature
Immunoglobulin (AL)	Primary Myeloma-associated	Ig light chains (kappa and lambda)	Monoclonal immunoglobulin
Reactive (AA)	Secondary	Amyloid A	Inflammatory disease
Hereditary	Familial Heredofamilial FAP	Transthyretin Apolipoprotein A-I Gelsolin Fibrinogen Lysozyme	Autosomal dominant
β_2-Microglobulin (β_2m)	Dialysis	β_2-Microglobulin	Renal dialysis

the fact that only certain SAA gene products are associated with amyloid fibrils suggests that there is a genetic basis for reactive amyloidosis as well. Therefore, we will review the clinical, pathogenic, and biochemical aspects of the two classic forms of systemic amyloidosis before we turn our attention to the hereditary amyloidoses.

Immunoglobulin Amyloidosis

Immunoglobulin amyloidosis includes all cases in which the basic building block of the amyloid fibril is immunoglobulin light chain protein. This type is referred to as "AL amyloidosis," for amyloid light chain. This group of disorders includes not only primary amyloidosis but also amyloidosis associated with multiple myeloma and other plasma cell dyscrasias, such as Waldenström macroglobulinemia and the heavy chain diseases. The unifying factor in these amyloidoses is the overproduction of monoclonal immunoglobulin protein, with the light chain of the clonal product becoming the subunit of the amyloid fibril. Recently, one case has been reported in which an incomplete immunoglobulin heavy chain protein having the approximate size of an immunoglobulin light chain has also been associated with systemic amyloidosis.[57]

Incidence. Immunoglobulin amyloidosis is the most common form of systemic amyloidosis. There are no good prevalence data, but in a large medical center there should be several patients with this disease each year.[58] Unfortunately, a fair percentage of patients with immunoglobulin amyloidosis die without the benefit of a correct diagnosis. Even when the diagnosis is made, the lack of a proven form of therapy often discourages the primary physician from referring the patient to a specialty center where that person would be entered into the published statistics. The tendency of immunoglobulin amyloidosis to affect the heart and cause heart failure or fatal arrhythmia probably adds to the number of undiagnosed cases.

Clinical Presentation. It is frequently noted that immunoglobulin amyloidosis affects the mesenchyme-derived organs such as heart, skeletal muscle, and nerve. These structures are involved much more frequently than in reactive (secondary) amyloidosis. Still, the most common presentation for immunoglobulin amyloidosis is renal involvement with nephrotic syndrome.[59] Some patients present with hepatomegaly, and a small number of patients present with clotting factor X deficiency, which may be related to amyloid infiltration of the spleen.[60] Immunoglobulin amyloidosis has been increasingly recognized in patients with cardiomyopathy and also in patients with life-threatening ventricular arrhythmias. Bowel involvement with chronic diarrhea and weight loss is common, and autonomic nervous system involvement with orthostatic hypotension and sexual impotence is also frequent. Vascular deposits in the skin may cause purpura. A small number of patients will have carpal tunnel syndrome, and some will have generalized neuropathy due to amyloid infiltration of nerves.[61] These latter cases may be confused with the hereditary syndromes.

Laboratory Findings. Laboratory test results will reflect which organ systems are infiltrated by amyloid. Electrocardiograms often show decreased voltage and evidence of anteroseptal myocardial infarction. Numerous studies have shown that no such infarction exists in these patients and that the septal Q waves and voltage abnormalities are most likely due to the amyloid deposits in the muscle. Echocardiography may show thickened ventricular walls, but good systolic function is retained. Valve thickening is much less common in this type of amyloidosis than in the hereditary syndromes. Renal amyloid usually causes proteinuria in the nephrotic range; in later stages there is increasing azotemia. Heart failure and orthostatic hypotension can frequently cause prerenal azotemia. Protein electrophoresis and immunoelectrophoresis of serum and urine will detect monoclonal immunoglobulin components in approximately 80 percent of patients with immunoglobulin amyloidosis. The bone marrow frequently has increased numbers of plasma cells which, in classic primary amyloidosis, lack malignant features but often have increased cytoplasm, which probably indicates active immunoglobulin synthesis. The percentage of plasma cells in the bone marrow is frequently in the 3 to 5 percent range but may be 20 percent or more. In patients with overt myeloma, the plasma cells will have malignant features and may constitute 50 percent or more of the bone marrow population. Recent studies using immunostaining have been particularly useful in evaluating patients with immunoglobulin amyloidosis in which circulating monoclonal proteins are not detected. The demonstration that plasma cells in a bone marrow are monoclonal supports the diagnosis of primary amyloidosis. Quantitation of Bence-Jones protein in serum or urine is not always useful in distinguishing multiple myeloma from primary amyloidosis, but it is often used as one of the parameters to diagnose multiple myeloma. If multiple myeloma is present, lytic lesions in the skull or the spine may be seen on radiographs. The clinician needs to be wary, however, since amyloid deposits in such structures as the femoral head may occasionally completely replace the bone and be misinterpreted as evidence of myeloma.

Clinical Course and Prognosis. Immunoglobulin amyloidosis is a variable disease, with the prognosis depending on which organ system is involved. Large clinical studies have shown that the median survival of patients with primary amyloidosis is 12 to 14 months,[58] although more recent studies have suggested median survival times of 20 to 24 months.[62] Survival ranges from less than 6 months for patients with serum creatinine levels greater than 4 mg/dl or with congestive heart failure to several years for patients who present with only neuropathy or carpal tunnel syndrome. All studies, however, have shown approximate 5 year survivals of 20 percent. Of the major types of systemic amyloidosis, the immunoglobulin type has the worst prognosis. The prognosis is especially grim for patients with multiple myeloma and amyloidosis, and many die within 6 months of diagnosis.

Pathogenesis. Since all immunoglobulin-type amyloid deposits are composed of monoclonal immunoglobulin light chain proteins, we know that a basic factor in the pathogenesis of this disease is the overproduction of immunoglobulin light chains by a particular B-lymphocyte clone. The factors responsible for the initiation of this process are unknown. In multiple myeloma it may be due to the malignant nature of the cell, but in most cases of classic primary amyloidosis, it would appear that normal metabolic processes are altered so that light chains are either overproduced or cannot be degraded completely. Clinical studies have suggested that certain immunoglobulin light chains are more amyloidogenic than others. For instance, more λ light chain proteins are associated with amyloid than κ proteins.[1] Since the ratio of κ to λ in the immune system is 2:1, this suggests that λ light chains are more amyloidogenic. This result may be partly due to the fact that free Bence-Jones proteins in plasma usually exist as dimers, and λ light chains have a higher association constant than κ light chains. This hypothesis is supported by the recent report of systemic amyloidosis due to a truncated heavy chain protein which, when analyzed, had essentially the same size and structure as an immunoglobulin light chain.[57] Since the domains of heavy and light chains are similar at the tertiary structure level, it would appear that the size of the immunoglobulin protein is a determining factor in fibril formation. Little is known about why certain monoclonal light chains deposit in any particular organ. Vascular organs such as kidney, liver, spleen, and heart are very prone to amyloid deposition, but bowel and nerve are also commonly involved. The light chain protein is usually processed when incorporated into fibrils, so that most amyloid subunit proteins include the entire variable segment of the light chain plus approximately the first tryptic peptide of the constant region. Since both the variable segment and the constant segment have extensive β structure, they evidently are easily incorporated into the β pleated sheet of the amyloid fibril.[42] Practically no data are available on whether the light chains are cleaved prior to incorporation into the fibril or whether incorporation occurs and then the bulk of the constant region is clipped off during the aggregation process. Occasionally, amyloid fibrils are found in which the entire light chain is incorporated into the fibril. Thus far, no *polyclonal* light chains have been found to be incorporated into fibrils, suggesting that fibril synthesis is a very selective process.

Treatment. The most frequently used treatment for immunoglobulin amyloidosis is chemotherapy with alkylating agents such as melphalan coupled with prednisone.[63] This has been a standard therapy for multiple myeloma for many years and, in selected cases, appears to be effective in immunoglobulin amyloidosis. Patients with Waldenström macroglobulinemia and amyloidosis are often treated with chlorambucil. In recent years, colchicine has been added to this regimen[64] or used alone,[65] because it has been shown that it is effective in preventing amyloid fibril formation in the murine model of amyloidosis and also in patients with familial Mediterranean fever.[66,67] It should be noted that the murine model of amyloid is of the reactive (AA) type, as is the amyloid of familial Mediterranean fever. Use of colchicine in the other forms of systemic amyloidosis is based on the hypothesis that the drug interferes with fibril formation and not with protein synthesis. At least one clinical study has suggested that the use of colchicine may be associated with prolonged survival.[65]

Numerous supportive measures have been shown to prolong the survival of patients with immunoglobulin amyloidosis. Potent diuretics can alleviate the nephrotic syndrome and congestive heart failure, and antiarrhythmia medications may prevent fatal cardiac arrhythmias. These often increase the problems of restrictive cardiomyopathy, however. Renal failure can be treated with dialysis, and some patients have received renal transplants. These transplanted organs usually develop amyloidosis if the patient lives long enough, but in selected cases survival is definitely prolonged. Bleeding diathesis from factor X deficiency has been corrected by splenectomy in a few patients.[68]

Reactive Amyloidosis

Reactive (secondary) amyloidosis is usually found in individuals with chronic inflammatory disease. Many diseases will predispose to reactive amyloidosis, but the most frequent include inflammatory arthritides, such as rheumatoid or psoriatic arthritis, granulomatous bowel disease, tuberculosis, leprosy, osteomyelitis, and suppurative infections, as may be seen in patients with quadriplegia or paraplegia. Reactive amyloidosis has also been reported in patients with cystic fibrosis, systemic lupus erythematosus, and bronchiectasis. In recent years there has been an increasing number of reports of reactive amyloidosis in intravenous drug users, presumably associated with chronic skin and other organ infection. Occasionally, reactive amyloidosis will be seen in a patient with no predisposing disease. Reactive amyloidosis occurs in a familial pattern in patients with familial Mediterranean fever. This association will be discussed in the section on hereditary amyloidosis and Muckle-Wells syndrome. The acronym classification for reactive amyloidosis is AA, which stands for amyloid A to reflect the subunit protein of the fibrils.

Incidence. Recent studies suggest that the incidence of reactive amyloidosis is decreasing. In the early part of the century, amyloidosis was common in patients with suppurative tuberculous lesions such as empyema. A lower incidence is noted in chronic cavitary disease, and now that tuberculosis is usually treated satisfactorily, it is quite uncommon to see a patient with amyloidosis associated with tuberculosis. The incidence in patients with rheumatoid arthritis was reported to be high in the past, but the figures probably reflect selection bias. Most clinicians would agree that amyloidosis is seen in less than 5 percent of patients with an inflammatory arthritis such as rheumatoid arthritis. The relatively high incidence in patients with quadriplegia or paraplegia persists despite the use of antibiotics. In certain equatorial parts of the world, leprosy is frequently associated with reactive amyloidosis.

Clinical Presentation. Reactive amyloid deposits usually involve the kidney, liver, and spleen early in the course of the disease. Many patients present with the nephrotic syndrome, and this may persist for months or years before azotemia occurs. By the time of death, major liver and spleen involvement is common. The gastrointestinal tract is commonly involved, but motility is less affected than in the immunoglobulin and hereditary amyloidoses. However, gastrointestinal bleeding, which may be life-threatening, is quite frequent, and often no definite site of bleeding can be found on clinical evaluation. Cardiac and skeletal muscle are much less commonly involved, and neuropathy has not been reported. Length of survival with reactive amyloidosis depends on how early in the course the diagnosis is made. Renal disease usually progresses slowly, and a patient may be nephrotic for 3 to 5 years before becoming significantly azotemic. Hemodialysis or peritoneal dialysis may prolong life. Amyloid infiltration in blood vessel walls, however, causes increased risk of hemorrhage, and involvement of other organs such as the liver eventually leads to death.

Pathogenesis. The precursor protein of reactive amyloid fibrils is serum amyloid A, which is synthesized mainly in the liver.[17,21,69] There is some evidence that other tissues produce SAA, but hepatic synthesis far outweighs any other origin. SAA is both an acute-phase reactant and an apolipoprotein.[70,71] The kinetics of hepatic SAA production are very similar to those for C-reactive protein, another acute-phase reactant.[21,22] Numerous studies suggest that both of these proteins are synthesized under the direction of an inducer produced by macrophages. Both interleukin 1 and interleukin 6, either alone or in concert with other factors, have been shown to stimulate hepatocytes to produce SAA by inducing the transcription of SAA genes.[72,73] In the human, there are at least four SAA genes with multiple alleles located on the short arm of chromosome 11.[74] In the mouse there are four SAA genes, and these have been localized to chromosome 7.[75–77] In the mouse, two forms of SAA (SAA1 and SAA2) are produced as acute-phase proteins by the liver. In addition, mouse serum contains another SAA isotype which does not show typical acute-phase kinetics.[78] The mouse SAA3 gene is expressed in macrophages and the product has been studied using northern blotting and electroimmunoblot analysis of serum, lipoprotein fractions, and culture medium.[79] A protein analogous to the murine SAA3 has been found in rabbit cell culture systems and the corresponding mRNA identified.[80] In the human and other primates the SAA3 gene has become a pseudogene and is not expressed.[81] Normal human serum contains another SAA (SAA4) which is normally present in higher concentration than SAA1 and 2 but which does not vary with inflammatory response.[82] In the mouse, only murine SAA2 is found in amyloid fibrils.[83] This gives support to the hypothesis that the structure of the SAA subunit protein is important in amyloid fibril formation. Human SAA has 104 amino acid residues in a single polypeptide chain.[84,85] In amyloidosis, SAA is usually processed by cleavage between residues 76 and 77, and the N-terminal 76 residues are incorporated into amyloid fibrils. Some data suggest that patients who develop reactive amyloidosis have a defect in normal degradation of SAA proteins.[86] Recent studies have shown that most of the protein in human amyloid fibrils is the SAA1 gene product, but some amyloid fibril preparations have been reported to contain up to 20 percent SAA2 protein. Reactive amyloidosis has been the most thoroughly studied because there are several animal models of this disease which lend themselves to laboratory investigations (see "Animal Models of Amyloidosis" below).

Treatment. There is no specific treatment for reactive amyloidosis. Control of the chronic inflammatory process which led to amyloidosis is a natural factor to be considered in slowing the progression of this disease. Chronic colchicine administration has been shown to prevent the occurrence of reactive amyloidosis in patients with familial Mediterranean fever, but no such finding has been reported for sporadic reactive amyloidosis.[87] Chemotherapy would seem not to be indicated since, in some animal models, cytotoxic drugs may accelerate the formation of amyloid deposits. On the other hand, suppression of chronic inflammation with antimetabolite drugs such as azathioprine and methotrexate might have a favorable effect on the overall outcome. Supportive measures are often very effective and can add significant time to survival. These include not only renal dialysis, but also the judicious use of diuretics, antibiotics, and measures to treat the primary inflammatory disease.

β_2-Microglobulin Amyloidosis

In 1980 it was reported that carpal tunnel syndrome in patients on hemodialysis for chronic renal insufficiency was associated with amyloid deposits in the soft tissues of the wrist.[88,89] While surgical decompression of the carpal tunnel resulted in relief of symptoms, these patients frequently developed diffuse arthralgias and, particularly, pain in the shoulders with decreased range of motion. Articular erosions and radiolucent cysts within juxta-articular bone of the shoulders, hips, and wrists are frequently seen and have been shown to be due to deposition of amyloid within joint capsule, synovium, subchondral bone, and articular cartilage.[90] In addition, a number of patients have presented with destructive vertebral lesions where bone is essentially replaced by amyloid.

The incidence of amyloidosis associated with chronic hemodialysis increases with increasing time on dialysis. As many as 70 percent of patients on dialysis for 10 years will have the carpal tunnel syndrome and radiolucent juxta-articular bone cysts that are typical of this syndrome. While most cases are associated with hemodialysis, the syndrome has now been observed in a number of patients treated with chronic ambulatory peritoneal dialysis, and it has also been reported in patients with chronic azotemia who have not been treated with dialysis.

In 1985, chemical analysis of amyloid deposits from dialysis patients resulted in the characterization of the fibril subunit protein as β_2-microglobulin.[91,92] β_2-Microglobulin is part of the HLA class I complex present on all nucleated cells. It is noncovalently associated with the heavy chain of the HLA complex. β_2-Microglobulin is present in the plasma in a monomeric form (11.8 kDa), and most of it is removed by glomerular filtration, after which proximal tubular reabsorption and degradation normally occur. Plasma levels are approximately 2 mg/liter but may be elevated up to sixtyfold in chronic uremia. While it was originally suspected that dialysis membranes were involved in generating high levels of β_2-microglobulin, it has now been shown that the high plasma levels can be explained by the lack of plasma clearance and degradation.[93] The current hypothesis is that decreased renal clearance of β_2-microglobulin allows markedly elevated circulating levels of the protein and subsequent amyloid formation. It is unclear why deposits tend to occur in synovium, cartilage, and juxtaarticular bone and soft tissue.

There is no specific treatment for β_2-microglobulin amyloidosis. Joint replacement has been used when destruction of the hip has occurred. Stabilizing the spine orthopedically may be necessary for destructive vertebral lesions. Some patients with this syndrome have benefited from successful renal transplantation, which presumably reestablishes normal degradation or clearance of β_2-microglobulin from the plasma. Unfortunately, many patients on chronic hemodialysis have already failed successful renal transplantation or are in an elderly group where transplantation is less indicated. Artificial means of removing β_2-microglobulin from the plasma, for instance by immunoabsorbent or other filtration techniques, are not yet clinically available.

Animal Models of Amyloidosis

Systemic amyloidosis occurs in many animal species, most often as a sporadic disease, but occasionally with hereditary aspects. The amyloid fibrils from a number of species have been analyzed and shown to contain AA proteins, which revealed the reactive nature of the disease. AA proteins have been structurally characterized for the mouse, horse, cow, dog, cat, monkey, guinea pig, hamster, mink, and Pekin duck.[69,94–100] The duck and other waterfowl are the only nonmammalian species, so far, in which AA of reactive amyloid has been characterized. In a strain of collie dogs, amyloidosis is associated with hereditary cyclic neutropenia.[101] In Abyssinian cats, amyloidosis shows a hereditary pattern.[102] Some strains of mice have spontaneous amyloid which is not of the AA type. In particular, a strain of mice showing early senescence has been shown to have amyloid fibrils composed of apolipoprotein A-II (apoA-II).[103] In this particular type of amyloidosis, an amino acid substitution (Pro5Gln) in apoA-II has been shown to be associated with the strains that develop amyloidosis. This model may be valuable in studying senescence, but, to date, human amyloidosis related to apolipoprotein A-II has not been discovered.

Reactive amyloidosis can be induced in most mammalian species. Kuczynski first showed that amyloidosis could be caused in mice by parenteral administration of sodium caseinate.[104,105] Subsequently, the murine model of induced systemic amyloidosis was used extensively as a model of the human disease. It has many features of the human disease, with major deposition of fibrils in spleen, liver, and kidney. This form of amyloid can also be produced by administration of Freund's complete adjuvant and by chronic administration of endotoxin. Studies using this model show that interleukin 1 and interleukin 6 are generated by macrophages,[72,106,107] and these cytokines induce the liver to synthesize SAA,[23] one form of which (SAA2) is incorporated into amyloid fibrils.[83] It is interesting that of all the mammalian species studied thus far, the rat does not appear to synthesize a full-length SAA and has never been shown to develop reactive amyloidosis. The murine model of casein-induced amyloidosis has been used to show that high doses of colchicine will prevent amyloid fibril formation and that discontinuing casein administration will result in some resolution of the fibril deposits.[108]

Animal models of human immunoglobulin light chain amyloidosis have not been available for study. Despite the extensive studies with myeloma proteins in mice, no strain of mice has yet been found to develop immunoglobulin amyloid deposits. The mouse is capable of processing light chain to give amyloid deposits, however, since the administration of massive doses of human amyloid-producing Bence-Jones protein into mice has been shown to result in deposition of material meeting the histologic criteria for amyloid.[109] This model has not been developed to the point where it can be used for studying human amyloid pathogenesis.

No species other than humans has been shown to have transthyretin-type amyloidosis. Transgenic mice have been created with the methionine 30 variant of transthyretin, and this model promises to be important in studying the pathogenesis of hereditary amyloidosis.[110,111] In transgenic mice with the Met-30 transthyretin gene ligated to the metallothionine promoter, amyloid deposits were noted first in intestinal mucosa at 6 months of age.[112] These increased with age along with glomerular amyloid deposits. By 24 months of age, all glomeruli had amyloid deposits, and myocardial deposits of amyloid were also reported. Amyloid deposits were not, however, detected in peripheral nerve, which is the earliest and most common site of localization in humans. Even so, this model gives a new approach to the study of pathogenesis of a hereditary disease.

HEREDITARY AMYLOIDOSIS

At present, hereditary amyloidosis is the most studied of all the various types of amyloidosis. This is a result of an intense interest in genetically determined diseases and the finding of a number of mutated plasma proteins which are associated with amyloidosis. Since the last edition of this text, the number of mutations in plasma transthyretin that are associated with systemic amyloidosis has increased from 7 to over 40. In addition, two mutations in apolipoprotein A-I, two mutations in plasma gelsolin, a mutation in cystatin C, and several mutations in the Alzheimer amyloid precursor protein (APP) have been found to be associated with amyloid fibril formation. Furthermore, recent studies suggest that a number of mutations in plasma fibrinogen may be the cause of certain types of amyloidosis. With the spread of knowledge about hereditary amyloidosis and the availability of genetic testing, it has become obvious that the hereditary amyloidoses are truly worldwide in distribution and that they affect a much larger number of families than ever previously considered.

The Transthyretin Amyloidoses

Most of the autosomal dominant amyloidoses characterized thus far are associated with variants of plasma transthyretin. So far, over 40 mutations of transthyretin have been described, and there are likely to be more. To understand the pathogenesis of these forms of amyloidosis better, it is important to review the properties of transthyretin. Transthyretin is a normal plasma protein. It was originally called "prealbumin" or "thyroxine binding prealbumin" because it migrates ahead of albumin on standard protein electrophoresis.[113] However, it has no structural relationship to albumin.[114] The name *transthyretin* (TTR) was coined because of the transport properties of the protein, which binds both thyroxine and retinol binding protein (RBP).[115] The term *transthyretin* has now gained relatively universal acceptance and is in general use. It should be noted, however, that any literature review will find many of the significant articles under the name prealbumin.

Plasma transthyretin is synthesized by the liver in a constitutive manner as a single polypeptide chain of 127 amino acid residues.[116,117] The primary structure has been known since 1974, and the secondary, tertiary, and quaternary structure has been defined by x-ray diffraction.[118] The entity circulating in plasma is a tetramer (M_r = 55,000) composed of four identical monomers[46] (Fig. 139-6). It would appear that two monomers noncovalently combine to form a stable dimer, and then two dimers associate to form the tetramer with twofold symmetry. Down the center channel of the tetramer are two binding sites for thyroxine, although binding studies suggest that these sites show negative cooperativity.[119] Transthyretin also binds RBP (M_r = 21,000), which is assumed to attach to the outside of the tetramer.[120] RBP must be saturated with retinol in order to bind to the carrier transthyretin molecule.

The transthyretin concentration in plasma normally ranges from 20 to 40 mg/dl and has been found to be significantly depressed in individuals with malnutrition. The plasma concentration also decreases at times of acute or chronic inflammation, and, therefore, transthyretin has been called a negative acute-phase protein. Plasma levels are also significantly depressed in many patients with the transthyretin amyloidoses, but the reason for this is unclear.[121–123] The single gene for transthyretin is located on human chromosome 18.[124] Most individuals with transthyretin amyloidosis have been found to be heterozygotes having one normal transthyretin allele and one variant allele. Expression of the two alleles is probably equal, but most studies have shown more of the normal gene product in the plasma than of the variant.[125,126]

Transthyretin has extensive β structure; the monomers have eight β chains arranged in an antiparallel configuration

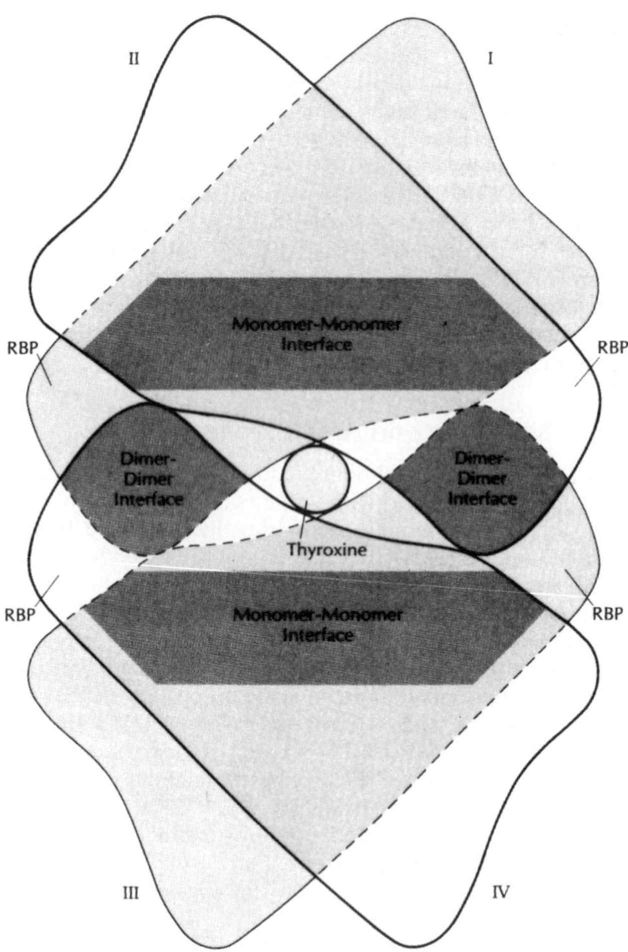

FIG. 139-6 Schematic drawing of transthyretin tetramer as viewed down the z molecular axis. Thyroxine binds in the inner channel, and RBP attaches to the outside of the molecule. *(Modified from Blake et al.[43] Used by permission.)*

in two planes (Fig. 139-7). This configuration would appear to predispose the protein toward amyloid fibril formation. Each of the amino acid substitutions that has been identified in variant transthyretins associated with hereditary amyloidosis can be hypothesized to alter the surface topography of the molecule.[127] This alteration presumably would favor aggregation and fibril formation; however, no clear unifying structural change has been noted. The identification of several transthyretin variants that do not predispose to amyloid formation has not helped to clarify this problem.[128,129]

The transthyretin cDNA sequence has been reported by a number of laboratories,[124,130,131] and the complete nucleotide sequence of the transthyretin gene in humans has been reported by two laboratories (Fig. 139-8).[132,133] The human gene has four exons (Fig. 139-9). The proximal upstream 5′ region has sequences similar to those for binding the glucocorticoid receptor.[134] However, the mouse prealbumin gene appears to have additional regulatory sequences about 2 kb upstream from the coding regions.[116] Prealbumin mRNA has been identified in choroid plexus of rats[135–137] and humans[138] and also in retina, so synthesis is not exclusively hepatic. It is unlikely that extrahepatic prealbumin synthesis plays a role in the systemic manifestations of amyloidosis, but occasional leptomeningeal involvement may be related to intracranial synthesis, and vitreous amyloid may possibly be the result of local gene expression.

Autosomal Dominant Transthyretin-Associated Amyloidosis Syndromes

Clinical Features. Most of the autosomal dominant amyloidoses have peripheral neuropathy as a major clinical manifestation. Thus, these disorders have also been called "familial amyloid polyneuropathy" (FAP). In the past, clinical classification of the syndromes has been based on whether lower-extremity neuropathy or upper-extremity neuropathy was the presenting symptom.[139] This criterion is less valid now, since the upper-extremity neuropathy, which is really a compression neuropathy from the carpal tunnel syndrome, has been seen in many of the recently described kindreds, sometimes before and sometimes after involvement of the lower extremities (Fig. 139-10).

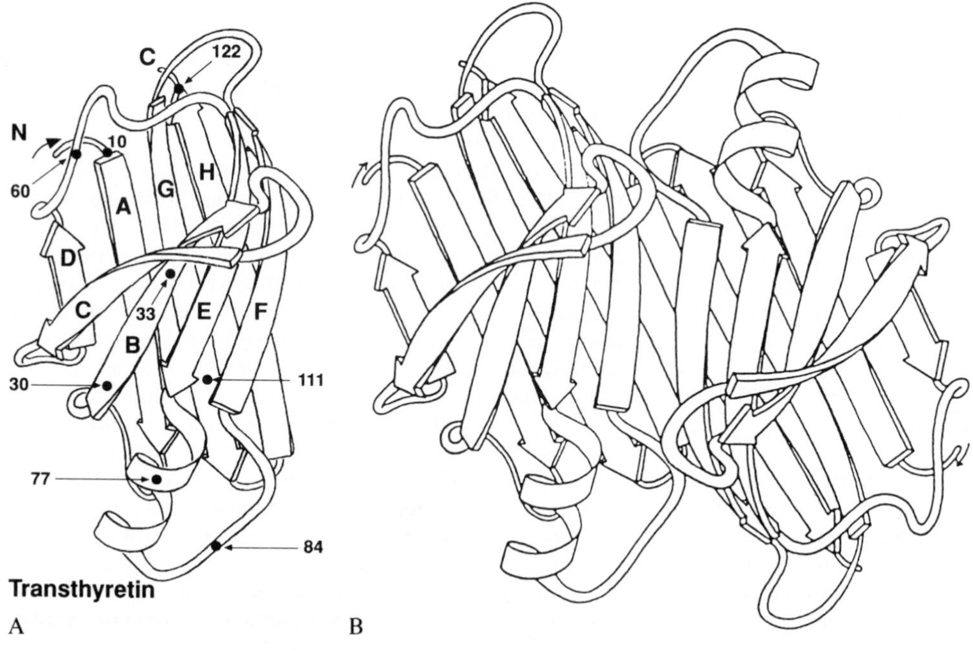

FIG. 139-7 Subunit structure of transthyretin. *A*. Antiparallel β structure of transthyretin. Eight β strands are arranged in two parallel planes. The approximate locations of eight of the mutations associated with amyloidosis are indicated. These include the mutation (Arg 10) closest to the N-terminal and the mutation (Ile 122) closest to the C-terminal. These two mutations are at the ends of the ordered β-strand structure. *B*. Two prealbumin monomers associate to form a dimer. Two dimers then associate to give the tetramer depicted in Fig. 6. *(Fig. A modified from and Fig. B from Richardson JS:* Adv Protein Chem *34:270, 1981.)*

TRANSTHYRETIN MUTATIONS

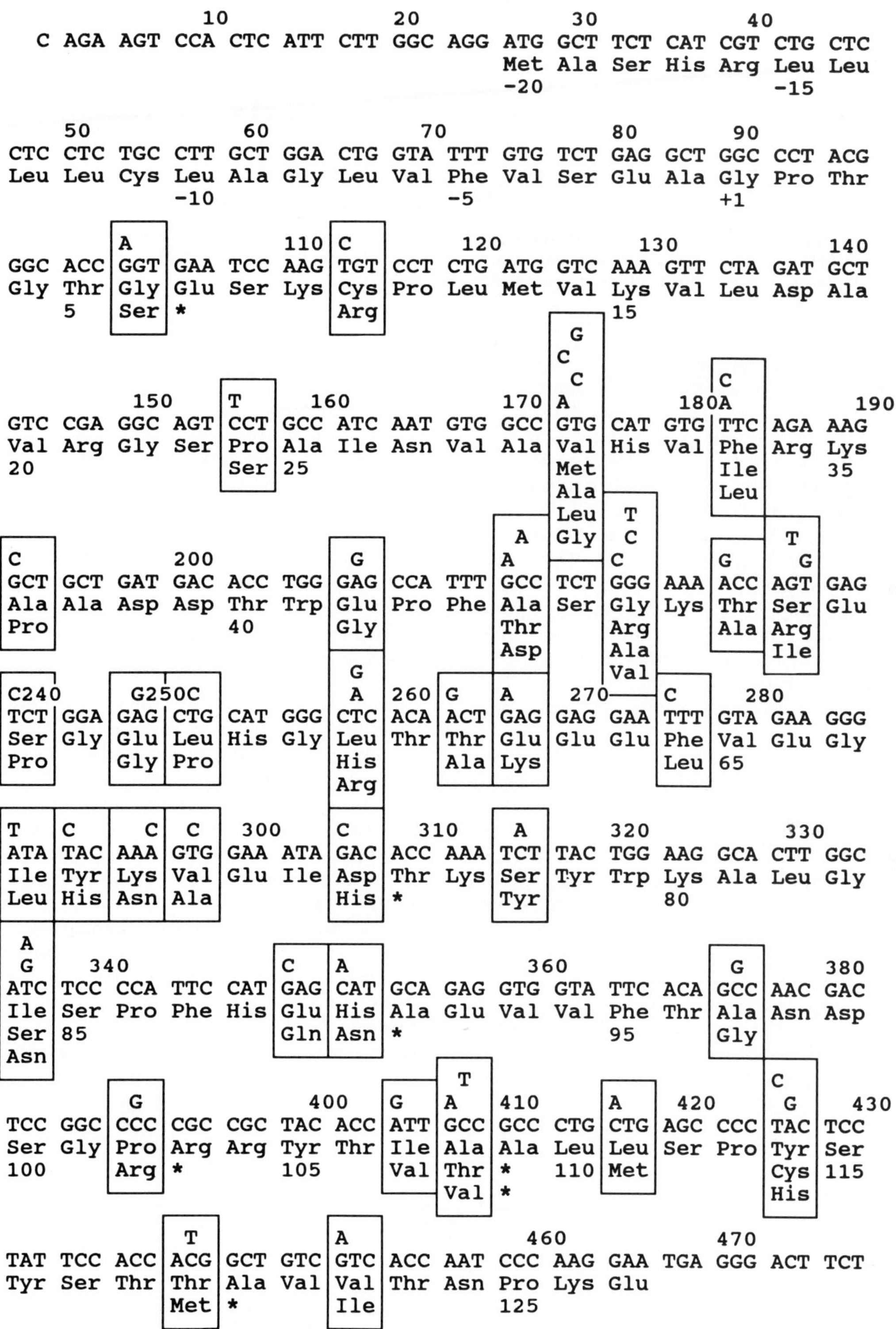

FIG. 139-8 Nucleotide sequence of transthyretin cDNA and protein amino acid sequence. All identified mutations are shown, including 40 associated with amyloidosis and 7 not associated with amyloidosis (indicated by *).

The Portuguese neuropathy (FAP type I) shows the classic and most common features of hereditary amyloidosis (Fig. 139-11). The clinical disease usually starts in the third or fourth decade, although the onset of symptoms may be delayed until old age. The disease progresses over 10 to 20 years with peripheral sensorimotor neuropathy, autonomic neuropathy, and varying degrees of systemic amyloid involvement. The neuropathy starts in the lower extremities with parasthesias and often hypesthesia, which can be debilitating. Autonomic neuropathy is an early feature, and patients may present with sexual impotence or gastrointestinal dysfunction. Sensory loss in the lower extremities follows

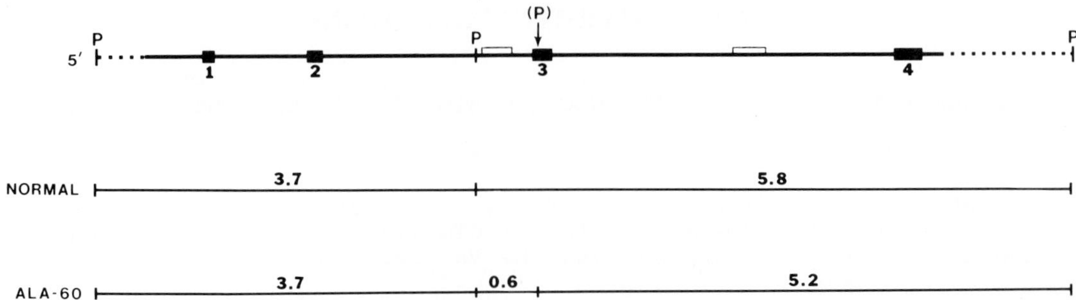

FIG. 139-9 Schematic drawing of human transthyretin gene showing four exons. Fifteen mutations associated with amyloidosis have been identified in exon 2, 19 in exon 3, and 7 in exon 4. The recognition sites for *Pvu*II are indicated (P) to show the DNA fragments generated in the Southern blot test for the Ala 60 gene (see Fig. 139-15).

a stocking distribution, and it has been noted that temperature and pain sensations are impaired earlier than proprioception. By the time sensory loss has progressed to the level of the knees, the hands usually become involved by a sensory neuropathy with a glove distribution. Motor loss develops later and frequently results in footdrop, wristdrop, and difficulty in hand function. Trophic ulcers on the lower extremities are common and, before the advent of antibiotics, were a frequent cause of infection and death. Orthostatic hypotension is common and has profound significance in patients with cardiac amyloid. Gastrointestinal symptoms are due mainly to nerve dysfunction with affected individuals having constipation alternating with diarrhea. Delayed gastric emptying may lead to distension of the organ and poor appetite. Cachexia is a frequent feature and may be a significant factor in mortality.

Visual involvement has been known to occur in the Portuguese syndrome but is much more frequently seen in Swedish kindreds and in the Indiana/Swiss amyloidosis (FAP II). Amyloid within the vitreous humor of the eye interferes with vision, but this can usually be corrected at least temporarily by surgical removal of the deposits (Fig. 139-12). The scalloped pupil deformity is another eye manifestation which has been described both in Portuguese and Swedish kindreds with FAP I, and is probably due to involvement of ciliary nerves. Autonomic neuropathy may cause urinary retention severe enough to require diversionary procedures to prevent renal damage. Hypohidrosis has also been seen.

Other clinical manifestations of hereditary amyloidosis depend on which organ systems are involved. FAP I patients (Portuguese, Swedish, Japanese) may have renal amyloid with significant protein loss and subsequent renal insufficiency. In these patients, dialysis may prolong life, but subsequent involvement of other organs is not prevented. The Indiana/Swiss kindred (FAP II), the Appalachian kindred, and several of the more recently described kindreds have severe cardiomyopathy, which is usually the cause of death. Cardiac conduction disturbances occur early and frequently require artificial pacing. The subsequent clinical picture is one of restrictive cardiomyopathy with low-output heart failure. Cardiomyopathy without peripheral neuropathy is the main feature of the amyloidosis described by Frederiksen et al. in Denmark.[140]

Chemical Classification. A number of transthyretin variants have been identified in the amyloid fibrils or plasma of patients with hereditary amyloidosis (Table 139-2). While the distribution of the amino acid substitutions gives no obvious clue to fibrillogenesis, all involve single amino acid substitutions that result from single nucleotide mutations in coding regions. The substitutions range in location from amino acid residue 10 (Cys10Arg) to residue 122 (Val122Ile) of TTR, with 15 mutations in exon 2, 19 in exon 3, and 7 in exon 4. No mutation in exon 1 (coding amino acids 1 through 3) has yet been discovered. These findings have provided a biochemical basis for classifying the transthyretin amyloidoses and have shown that, while the old classification based on the clinical syndrome and ethnic origin was basically sound, there is a great deal of overlap among the syndromes. Identification of nonsymptomatic carriers of variant transthy-

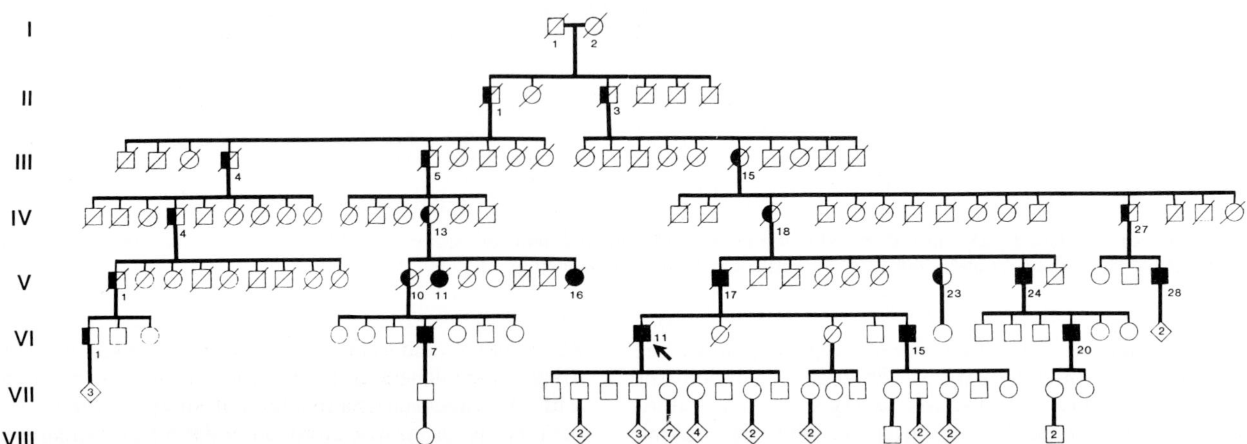

FIG. 139-10 Kindred with hereditary transthyretin amyloidosis associated with variant transthyretin showing the typical autosomal dominant pattern of inheritance. ■ = biopsy proven; ◧ = presumed affected; ◇ = multiple sibs, sex unspecified.

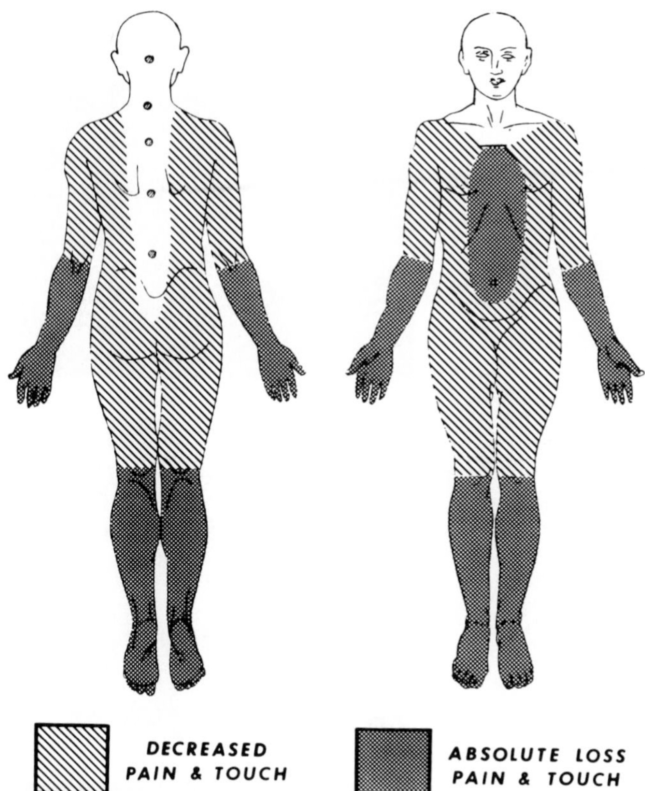

FIG. 139-11 Pattern of sensory loss in familial amyloid polyneuropathy type I.

retin genes in many of the kindreds has widened the recognized time span of clinical onset for each syndrome. The following transthyretin variants have been identified in families with hereditary amyloidosis. The clinical, geographic, and ethnic parameters that are relatively unique to each familial syndrome are emphasized to aid the clinician in recognizing and diagnosing the disease. A few additional transthyretin variants have been identified (Table 139-2), but insufficient clinical data have been reported.

Arginine 10 (C10R). This type of systemic amyloidosis presents as a peripheral neuropathy in the sixth and seventh decades of life. The only kindred that has been described is located in Pennsylvania with ancestors of Hungarian origin.[141] No evidence for the mutation in Hungary has been found to date. In three cousins who died with this syndrome and were studied in detail, severe cardiomyopathy and bowel dysfunction were the major factors leading to death between ages 64 and 70. This particular variant transthyretin has added importance for two reasons: (1) Until its description, no amyloid-associated transthyretin mutation in the N-terminal portion of the transthyretin protein proximal to position 30 had been described. (2) Arginine 10 replaces the only cysteine in the transthyretin molecule. This may be significant in terms of the possible involvement of disulfide linkage in amyloid fibrillogenesis.

Serine 24 (P24S). Transthyretin Pro24Ser was discovered in a family with relatively late-onset amyloidosis. The propositus, who was born in Kentucky, developed carpal tunnel syndrome at age 50 and severe diarrhea at age 65, and died at age 70. Three brothers died of cardiac disease, and in one, cardiac amyloidosis was proved at postmortem.

The substitution of serine for proline, the result of a $C \rightarrow T$ transition in the first position of codon 24, does not give a new restriction site, so a PCR-induced mutation restriction analysis (PCR-IMRA) (see "Detection of Gene Carriers in Hereditary Amyloidosis" below) has been used to detect the carriers of this allele.

Methionine 30 (V30M). The most common type of hereditary amyloidosis thus far reported is characterized by a substitution of methionine for valine at position 30 of the transthyretin molecule. This variant transthyretin has been found in many kindreds in Portugal and Japan, and also in American kindreds of Swedish, English, and Greek origin.[26,126,131,142–144] It has also been identified in Turkey, Majorca, Brazil, France, and England. While the largest numbers of patients and families have been identified in northern Portugal, the Met 30 gene has its highest prevalence in isolated communities in northern Sweden, where as many as 3 to 5 percent of the population may be heterozygous for the trait.[145] A number of patients homozygous for the Met 30 gene have been identified in Sweden[146] and in Turkey.[147] The onset of clinical amyloidosis and progression of the disease in these homozygous individuals does not appear to be different from that of their heterozygous kin. Clinically, most of these kindreds have been classified as FAP I with neuropathy starting in the lower extremities. Varying degrees of renal and cardiac involvement have been reported, but autonomic and gastrointestinal symptoms are present in most patients. Vitreous deposits of amyloid have been reported, as has the scalloped pupil deformity.[7] In particular, vitreous involvement appears to be much more common in the Swedish families than in the Portuguese families. Another interesting difference between Portuguese families and Swedish families with this same Met 30 mutation is the time of onset of disease. In Portugal, the mean age of onset is in the early thirties, with death often occurring by age 40. In Sweden, the mean age of onset of clinical disease is in the late fifties, and patients often live to the eighth decade. Mental functioning is generally not affected, but amyloid may be present in blood vessels of the central nervous system and in the leptomeninges.[148] There is evidence that the high prevalence and worldwide distribution of the Met 30 transthyretin mutation is in some part due to multiple mutational events. The Met 30 mutation has been found in Japan in association with three distinct haplotypes.[149] One of these haplotypes is the same as the haplotype found in Portuguese Met 30 patients and Swedish Met 30 patients, suggesting indeed that the gene has been spread from a common focus. The association of the Met 30 mutation with other haplotypes, however, suggests that separate mutation events may have occurred in Japan, and at least one Met 30 kindred of English origin in the United States does not share the Portuguese/Swedish haplotype.[150] The idea that multiple mutational events have generated the Met 30 transthyretin is supported by the fact that this position is one of the mutation hot spots in the TTR coding region, where the CpG dinucleotide sequence can be altered by deamidation of a methylated cytosine.

Alanine 30 (V30A). Substitution of alanine for valine at position 30 has been reported in association with systemic amyloidosis in one family.[151] The disease had a relatively early onset in the twenties, with death in 4 to 6 years. Clinical manifestations include autonomic neuropathy with orthostasis and gastric atony but only mild sensory neuropathy of the FAP I variety. No eye or renal involvement was clinically noted. Amyloid fibrils containing transthyretin

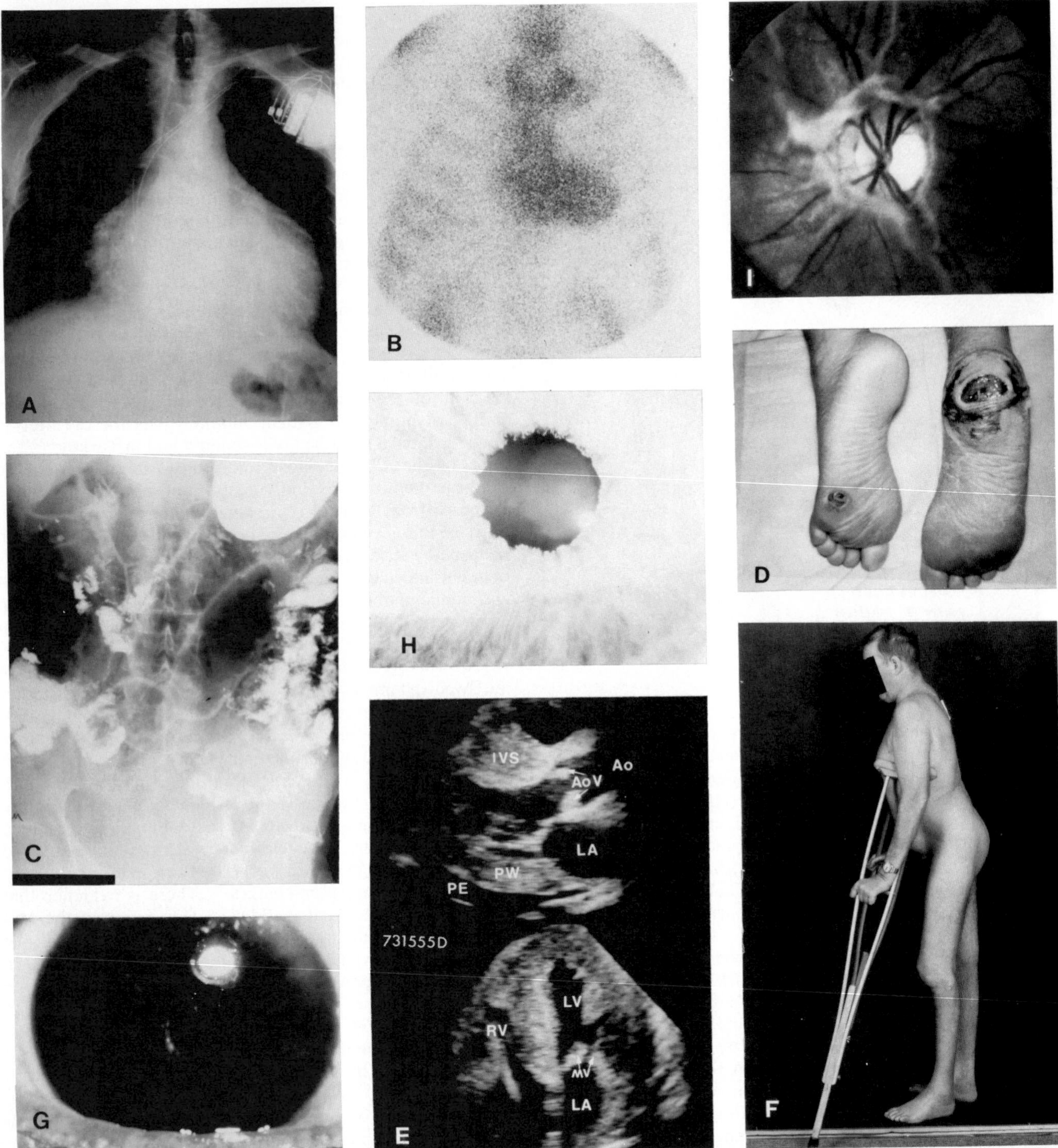

FIG. 139-12 Clinical features of the hereditary amyloidoses. *A*. Cardiomegaly in Ser 84 amyloidosis. *B*. Technetium pyrophosphate uptake in cardiac amyloidosis. *C*. Gastric distension and dilated small bowel in Ala 60 amyloidosis. *D*. Neurogenic ulcer and calcaneal osteomyelitis in Met 30 amyloidosis. *E*. Two-dimensional echocardiography in Ser 84 amyloidosis showing thickening intraventricular septum (IVS), left ventricular wall (PW), aortic (AOV), and mitral valves (MV), plus dilated left atrium (LA). *F*. Typical neuropathy of Met 30 amyloidosis. This patient has neuropathic arthropathy (Charcot knee). *G*. Lattice corneal dystrophy of Finnish amyloidosis. *H*. Scalloped pupil in Met 30 amyloidosis. *I*. Vitreous deposits in Ser 84 amyloidosis.

were isolated from the heart of one individual. The T → C mutation in the second position of codon 30 gives a new *Cfo*I restriction site in exon 2.

Leucine 30 (V30L). A third mutation at position 30 (Val30Leu) was discovered in a 53-year-old Japanese woman who presented with weight loss and diarrhea at age 51.[152,153] Sensory neuropathy was present in the lower extremities and sural nerve biopsy revealed deposits of amyloid which stained positively with anti-human transthyretin antibody. No vitreous opacities were reported, and there was no family history suggestive of FAP. The G → C transition in the third base of codon 30 results in a novel *Cfr*13I site, which can be used for identification of this mutation.

Table 139-2 Transthyretin Amyloidoses

Mutation	Clinical Name	Clinical Features*	Geographic Kindreds
Cys10Arg		Heart, eye, PN	U.S. (PA)
Pro24Ser		Heart	U.S.
Val30Met	FAP I	PN, AN, eye	Portugal, Japan, Sweden, U.S.
Val30Ala		Heart, AN	U.S.
Val30Leu		PN	Japan
Val30Gly			U.S.
Phe33Ile	Jewish	PN, eye	Israel
Phe33Leu		PN, heart	U.S.
Ala36Pro		Eye, CTS	U.S.
Glu42Gly		PN, AN, heart	Japan
Ala45Thr		Heart	U.S.
Ala45Asp		Heart, PN	U.S.
Gly47Arg		PN, AN	Japan, U.S.
Gly47Ala		Heart, AN	Italy
Gly47Val		CTS, PN, AN, heart	Sri Lanka
Thr49Ala		Heart, CTS	France, Italy
Ser50Arg		AN, PN	Japan
Ser50Ile		Heart, PN, AN	Japan
Ser52Pro		PN, AN, heart, kidney	England
Glu54Gly			
Leu55Pro		Heart, AN, eye	U.S., Taiwan
Leu58His	FAP II	CTS, heart	U.S. (MD)
Leu58Arg		CTS, AN, eye	Japan
Thr60Ala	Appalachian	Heart, CTS	U.S.
Glu61Lys		PN	Japan
Phe64Leu		PN, CTS, heart	U.S., Italy
Ile68Leu		Heart	Germany
Tyr69His		Eye	U.S.
Lys70Asn		Eye, CTS, PN	U.S.
Val71Ala		PN, eye, CTS	France, Majorca
Ser77Tyr		Kidney	U.S. (IL, TX), France
Ile84Ser	FAP II	Heart, CTS, eye	U.S. (IN), Hungary
Ile84Asn		Heart, eye	U.S.
Glu89Gln		PN, heart	Italy
Ala97Gly		Heart, PN	Japan
Ile107Val		Heart, CTS, PN	U.S.
Leu111Met	Danish	Heart	Denmark
Ser112Ile		PN, Heart	Italy
Tyr114Cys		PN, AN, eye	Japan
Tyr114His		CTS	Japan
Val122Ile	Senile cardiac	Heart	U.S.

*AN = autonomic neuropathy; CTS = carpal tunnel syndrome; eye = Vitreous deposits; PN = peripheral neuropathy.

Isoleucine 33 (F33I). This type of amyloidosis was originally called "Jewish FAP" because the only individual described with the disease was a Jewish man who was born in Poland and immigrated to Israel. The disease manifested as type I periperal neuropathy, diarrhea, and impotence. Vitreous opacities were described between ages 25 and 30.[154] Autopsy revealed amyloid in all major organs, particularly the thyroid, kidney, spleen, and nerves. The original studies of the amyloid isolated from the thyroid showed that a significant proportion of the transthyretin molecules had been cleaved between amino acid positions 48 and 49, and there was evidence for a substitution of glycine for threonine at position 49.[155] Subsequently, however, amyloid subunit protein isolated from splenic tissue showed an isoleucine substituted for phenylalanine at position 33.[156] This substitution has been verified by DNA sequence studies, which failed to show any mutation in codon 49. Incidentally, the affected individual in this kindred was found to also have the TTR mutation that gives serine at position 6, which has been described by others but not in association with amyloid formation. No other kindreds with the isoleucine 33 transthyretin amyloid have been described.

Leucine 33 (F33L). This mutation (Phe33Leu) was found in a middle-aged man of Polish and Lithuanian heritage who had lower limb neuropathy and cardiomyopathy.[157] There was no previous family history of amyloidosis, and no other kindreds have been identified. The T → C mutation at the first base of codon 33 gives a new *Dde*I site in exon 2.

Proline 36 (A36P). This mutation (Ala36Pro) has been described in two kindreds[158,159]—an American family of Greek origin and a Jewish family in which members died between ages 36 and 65. The age of onset was 28 in one individual, and the symptoms included lower limb neuropathy, autonomic neuropathy, and vitreous opacities.

Glycine 42 (E42G). One kindred with glycine substituted for glutamic acid at transthyretin position 42 has been described in Japan (Toyama Prefecture).[160] At least six members of the kindred were affected with FAP, which was manifested as lower limb neuropathy, autonomic neuropathy, cardiomyopathy, and vitreous opacities. Onset of disease was between ages 35 and 41, and major morbidity was related to restrictive cardiomyopathy. This mutation has also been found in an American Caucasian family with amyloidosis. The A → G mutation at the second position of codon 42 results in a new *Cfr*13I restriction site in exon 2.

Threonine 45 (A45T). One individual with cardiomyopathy appearing at approximately age 50 was reported to be heterozygous for a threonine substitution (Ala45Thr) at position 45 of transthyretin.[161] This individual was of Irish and Italian descent, and the family history suggested that the trait was from the Italian side of the family. Other studies of an American/Irish patient who died with restrictive cardiomyopathy showed the same mutation, but it is not known whether this single individual was a member of the previously reported kindred.

Arginine 47 (G47R). The first evidence of a de novo mutation in transthyretin is represented by the arginine-for-glycine substitution at position 47.[162] The proband of the family was a 38-year-old Japanese man who showed symptoms of autonomic neuropathy at age 29. Polyneuropathy was proved by sural nerve biopsy showing amyloid deposits that stained with anti-transthyretin. No vitreous opacities were noted. DNA studies of both parents and two siblings failed to show the mutation in codon 45, thus suggesting that the C-for-G transversion may be a de novo mutation.

Alanine 47 (G47A). A family from Italy with cardiomyopathy and peripheral neuropathy in the fifth decade of life was found to have an alanine-for-glycine substitution at position 47.[163] Although a PCR test based on mutation-induced restriction analysis to give a novel *Msp*I site has been described, no other kindred with this mutation has been found to date.

Alanine 49 (T49A). This mutation has been found in two distinct kindreds, one in France and one in Italy, both showing cardiomyopathy.[164,165] The Italian kindred was reported to have vitreous opacities, which was not a feature in the French kindred. The French kindred, first reported in 1983, showed onset of polyneuropathy and carpal tunnel syndrome between ages 35 and 40, with subsequent development of restrictive cardiomyopathy.[166] Clinical onset of disease was at a similar age in the Italian kindred, with polyneuropathy occurring in the fifth decade of life.

Arginine 50 (S50R). This mutation (Ser50Arg) was discovered in a Japanese family in which affected members presented with peripheral and autonomic neuropathy in their early forties. One man died of generalized wasting 6 years after the onset of polyneuropathy.[167] The abnormal TTR was present in serum and cardiac amyloid deposits.[168] The T → G transversion in the first position of codon 50 gives a new *Mva*I site.

Isoleucine 50 (S50I). A G → T transition in the second position of codon 50 of TTR exon 3 giving a Ser50Ile mutation was identified in a 56-year-old Japanese woman with a 7-year history of sensorimotor and autonomic neuropathy.[169] Another report of this mutation emphasized cardiomyopathy as cause of death.[170]

Proline 55 (L55P). Seven members of one kindred from West Virginia of Dutch and German descent showed early-onset, aggressive, diffuse amyloidosis which caused peripheral neuropathy, autonomic neuropathy, and vitreous opacities.[171] Death in most individuals was from restrictive cardiomyopathy, and autopsy revealed diffuse systemic amyloid deposits. The variant is due to a T → C transition in the second position of codon 55 of transthyretin, which gives a proline substitution for leucine. In the one kindred, multiple organ system involvement was noted by age 35, and all patients had died by age 38. Over four generations anticipation was suggested, with the youngest individual affected at age 19.

Histidine 58 (L58H). Mahloudji et al. originally described a number of kindreds in Maryland with this form of amyloidosis.[172] It was classified as FAP II because of onset with carpal tunnel syndrome. The disease, however, has varied manifestations, with frequent painful neuropathy and relatively slow progression. Onset may be as early as the forties, but many patients live into their seventies. Death is frequently caused by cardiomyopathy, but the syndrome is distinguished from the Indiana/Swiss (Ser 84) form of FAP II by a lack of vitreous opacities. A T → A transversion in the second position of codon 58 results in substitution of histidine for leucine.[173] The His 58 transthyretin gene has been detected in families throughout the United States.[174] It has not been reported in European kindreds, although Mahloudji et al. traced the origin of the original family to immigrants from southern Germany in the 1740s. Only one haplotype has been demonstrated in several families with this mutant transthyretin, suggesting a common origin. Recently one individual homozygous for the His 58 gene was shown to have a rapid course of generalized neuropathy with clinical presentation at age 46 and death 6 years later.[175] This is unlike the Met 30 and Ile 122 TTR variants, in which homozygous individuals do not seem to have more aggressive disease.

Arginine 58 (L58R). A single family was described in which a mother, age 62, and her son, age 39, had lower limb neuropathy, autonomic neuropathy, and carpal tunnel syndrome.[176] The mother had vitreous opacities noted at age 53, and the son developed neuropathy as early as age 36. The mutation, a T → G change in the second position of codon 58, results in a new *Bha*I restriction site.

Alanine 60 (T60A). This type of amyloidosis (also called Appalachian) was originally discovered in a large kindred from West Virginia in which the disease was traced to a couple having Irish, English, and German ancestry.[177,178] Since then, the alanine 60 transthyretin variant has been found in other U.S. families of Irish lineage, and the gene has now been reported in patients in Ireland. It is also the first mutation to be found in Australia, in a family also of Irish origin. One family of Welsh origin now in the United States has been found with this mutation. Sensorimotor neuropathy is not a prominent feature of this syndrome, although some patients have carpal tunnel syndrome. Most affected individuals have some degree of peripheral neuropathy in the lower extremities, but incapacitation is related more to bowel disease and resultant malnutrition. Sexual

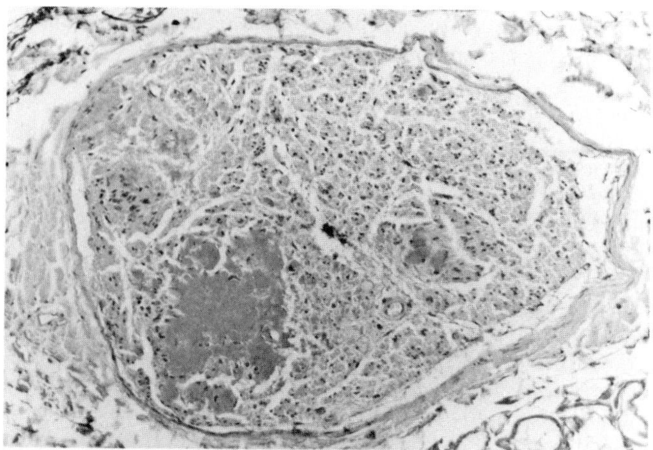

FIG. 139-13 **Section of peripheral nerve stained for transthyretin by the avidin-biotin peroxidase method. Amyloid deposits are found within the nerve structure, and the positive staining for transthyretin proves the diagnosis of hereditary amyloidosis. ×100.**

impotence is common. Many affected individuals die of cardiomyopathy, which usually starts after age 50 and may not begin until after age 60. The disease is progressive but may run a 10- to 20-year course. While most individuals have died in their sixties, some have been known to live past age 90. Postmortem examinations have shown amyloid in nerves, heart, and thyroid (Figs. 139-13 and 139-14). Significant amyloid in liver, kidney, and spleen has not been seen. The original Appalachian kindred is very large and is dispersed throughout the United States. The gene has also been detected in a large kindred in the northeastern United States.[179] The mutation (Thr60Ala) is the result of an A → G transition at the first position of codon 60 and results in a new *Pvu*II restriction site in exon 3.

Leucine 64 (F64L). This mutation (Phe64Leu) was discovered in one individual with disease beginning at age 66 as a peripheral neuropathy involving both upper and lower extremities.[180] Cardiomyopathy was present, but no eye involvement was noted. The patient was an American of Italian descent.

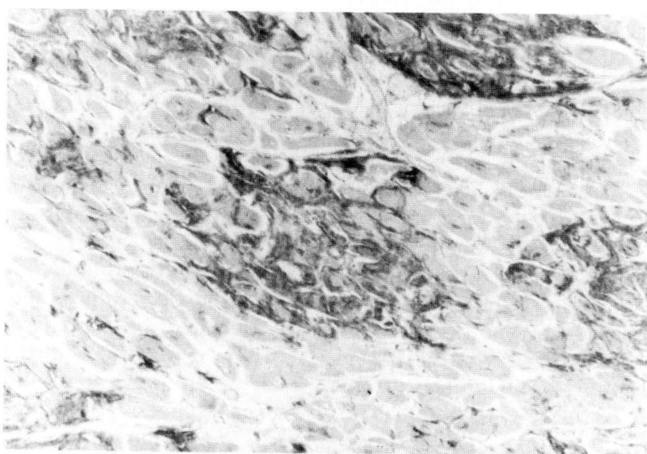

FIG. 139-14 **Section of left ventricle stained immunohistochemically using anti-transthyretin. Amyloid deposits displace myocardial fibrils and also form rings around the cardiac muscle bundles. ×100.**

Leucine 68 (I68L). A substitution of leucine for isoleucine at position 68 of transthyretin was described in a 61-year-old German individual with cardiomyopathy.[181] The mutation, an A → T transversion in the first position of codon 68, was detected in the propositus' son, who was unaffected, but not in the propositus' mother. The propositus' father died at age 56 of an accident without symptoms of amyloidosis. While polyneuropathy was suggested by complaints of dysesthesia, neurologic examination did not reveal objective pathologic findings.

Histidine 69 (Y69H). Only one family has been reported with this mutation (Tyr69His).[182] The proband noted symptoms of vitreous opacities at age 59, and amyloidosis was proved by pathologic examination of the vitrectomy specimen removed at age 62. The proband had symptoms of carpal tunnel syndrome and gastrointestinal complaints suggesting autonomic nervous system involvement. No peripheral neuropathy was noted, however. An older sibling also had vitreous opacities but died of a brain hemorrhage at age 62. The histidine-for-tyrosine substitution is the result of a T → C mutation in the first position of codon 69 of transthyretin.

Asparagine 70 (K70N). A family from New Jersey of German ancestry was found to have amyloidosis associated with a substitution of asparagine for lysine at position 70 of transthyretin.[183] This is due to an A → C mutation in the third base of codon 70. This syndrome usually presents as carpal tunnel syndrome as early as the thirties. One individual died of renal insufficiency, but nodular glomerulosclerosis characteristic of Kimmelsteil-Wilson disease was found instead of amyloid. Amyloid vitreous opacities were a common finding in this syndrome.

Alanine 71 (V71A). Val71Ala was first discovered in a family from northern France in which the proband developed carpal tunnel syndrome at age 35 and subsequently had lower limb neuropathy at age 42.[184] The proband's father had paresthesia and diarrhea starting at age 40 and subsequently developed vitreous opacities. The alanine-for-valine substitution, which is due to a C → T transition, in the second position of codon 71, has also been found in an individual in Spain.

Tyrosine 77 (S77Y). Amyloidosis associated with the tyrosine 77 transthyretin variant was originally described in a family of German extraction from Illinois.[185] The clinical syndrome shows a lower limb neuropathy and diarrhea starting about age 50. While kidney failure has been a major cause of death, cardiomyopathy has also been noted in individuals with this mutation. This transthyretin variant has now been found with the same haplotype in several families in the United States, including a large kindred in Texas.[186] A family from northern France, however, has the tyrosine 77 transthyretin with a different haplotype, suggesting a separate mutational event.[187] The mutation, a C → T transition at the second position of codon 77, gives a new *Ssp*I restriction site.

Serine 84 (I84S). Although the *Indiana/Swiss kindred* with amyloidosis was originally reported by Falls et al. in 1955,[188] Rukavina's description of the kindred in 1956 caused his name to be used in identifying the syndrome, which, because of presentation with carpal tunnel syndrome, was designated FAP II to distinguish it from the FAP I peripheral neuropathy syndrome.[189] Carpal tunnel syndrome occurs as early as the third decade of life, whereas infiltrative peripheral neuropathy tends to occur later in the course and can affect all extremities. Vitreous opacities are seen in essentially all affected individuals, and cardiomyopathy is the usual cause of death. Most patients die in their mid-fifties or sixties, although some individuals have reached age 80 with the help of artificial cardiac pacing. Sexual impotence is common in men, and bowel dysfunction with diarrhea and malabsorption is also common.[190]

The isoleucine-to-serine mutation is the result of a T → G transversion in the second position of codon 84. This gives a new *Alu*I restriction site, which can be used for DNA testing.[191] Gene carriers in this kindred, both affected and presymptomatic, have significantly reduced plasma RBP concentrations.[192] This finding suggests that the area of the molecule around residue 84 may be involved in retinol binding. The depression in the serum RBP level is such that gene carriers can usually be identified by this measurement alone. Recently a second kindred with the Ser 84 transthyretin gene has been found in Hungary; this family may be related to the original Swiss/German families.

Asparagine 84 (I84N). A second mutation in transthyretin position 84 (Ile84Asn) is due to a T → G transversion in the second position of codon 84.[193] It was reported in an individual who developed vitreous opacities at age 62. There was no family history of amyloidosis in this American family of Italian descent, although the proband's father died suddenly at age 62. Carpal tunnel syndrome developing after age 70 and mild cardiomyopathy were present in the proband.

Glutamine 89 (E89Q). The substitution of glutamine for glutamic acid at position 89 of transthyretin was discovered in a Sicilian family with carpal tunnel syndrome, cardiomyopathy, and neuropathy presenting in the fifth decade of life.[164] This is the result of a G → C transversion in the first position of codon 89.

Valine 107 (I107V). A 57-year-old man of English/German descent developed carpal tunnel syndrome at age 57 and, subsequently, generalized peripheral neuropathy at age 65.[194] Amyloid deposition was identified on muscle biopsy. There was no family history of amyloidosis. A TTR mutation, A → G in the first position of codon 107, predicts a valine-for-isoleucine substitution.

Methionine 111 (L111M). In 1962, Frederiksen et al. described a kindred in Denmark with amyloid cardiomyopathy.[195] No neuropathy was detected either at that time or on subsequent reexamination of the kindred. The clinical findings are those of restrictive cardiomyopathy. DNA sequencing showed a C → A transversion in the first position of codon 111, with the substitution of methionine for leucine.[196] A recent analysis of sera obtained at the time of the original report has detected the mutant transthyretin in all affected individuals.[197] No other kindreds have been discovered with this particular mutation, which is remarkable for its restriction of amyloid pathology to the heart.

Cysteine 114 (Y114C). Members of a kindred from Nagasaki prefecture in Japan were found to have systemic amyloidosis associated with a cysteine-for-tyrosine replacement at codon 114.[198] This is the result of an A → G change in the second position of codon 114.[199] The syndrome was manifest at age 30, with lower limb neuropathy, autonomic neuropathy, and subsequent development of vitreous opacities. Heart failure was the most common cause of death.

Isoleucine 122 (V122I). The Val122Ile mutation was discovered in an individual with cardiomyopathy but no family history of amyloidosis.[200] It was first believed to explain some cases of senile cardiac amyloidosis. It is particularly interesting because the first two individuals reported with this mutation were from separate families, and both were homozygous for isoleucine 122 transthyretin.[201,202] Subsequently other individuals have been discovered with cardiac amyloidosis who were heterozygous for the isoleucine 122 transthyretin.[203] All affected individuals so far have been elderly, presenting after age 60 with cardiomyopathy, and all have been African Americans. The mutation, a G → A transition in the first position of codon 122, has been shown to be present in approximately 2 percent of African Americans and may be the cause of heart failure in a significant portion of the elderly in this population.[204] Peripheral neuropathy has been reported but is a minor clinical manifestation of this syndrome.

Senile Systemic Amyloidosis. In addition to the characterized cases of senile cardiac amyloidosis, a number of postmortem studies have shown a high incidence of amyloid deposits in individuals dying after age 80.[205] These deposits are often in the heart, but varying degrees of systemic involvement have also been noted.[206,207]

The term *senile systemic amyloidosis* has been used for these cases as well as those previously labeled *senile cardiac amyloidosis*.[208] Immunohistochemical studies have shown that a number of these cases involve transthyretin amyloid, although some have failed to show staining with anti-transthyretin antisera.[209] DNA sequencing studies of some individuals with transthyretin cardiomyopathy without a family history of this disease failed to show mutations in the coding regions of the TTR gene.[210] This finding suggests that normal transthyretin may in some situations produce amyloid fibrils without the presence of a mutation.

Transthyretin Variants Not Associated with Amyloidosis. A number of variants of transthyretin have been reported in individuals and families without evidence of systemic amyloidosis. These have been identified either by an association with altered thyroxine binding or by an abnormal pattern on protein electrophoresis. While routine serum electrophoresis does not identify variant forms of transthyretin, both two-dimensional polyacrylamide gel electrophoresis and a system called "hybrid isoelectric focusing" have successfully discriminated several variants from normal transthyretin.[211] A variant transthyretin with serine substituted for glycine at position 6 was discovered in a family with hyperthyroxinemia.[212,213] Studies have suggested that an abnormal albumin in this kindred may cause increased thyroxine binding, giving a euthyroid state, and in vitro thyroxine binding studies on a recombinantly produced Ser 6 variant TTR failed to show increased thyroxine binding for this variant.[214] Ser 6 transthyretin may be a relatively common polymorphism since it has now been identified in unrelated individuals. Amino acid substitutions at position 109 of transthyretin have also been identified in families with euthyroid hyperthyroxinemia. Ala109Thr is the most thoroughly studied, with a fairly large kindred showing increased thyroxine binding but a euthyroid state.[215] Thyroxine binding studies of recombinant Thr 109 TTR have demonstrated increased affinity for T_4,[214] and a structural basis for this increased affinity has been demonstrated by solution of the x-ray structure at 1.7Å.[216] A valine substitution at position 109 has also been described in an individual with hyperthyroxinemia. Transthyretin Met 119 was discovered by two-dimensional polyacrylamide gel electrophoresis in a family without any evidence of hyperthyroxinemia.[129] This TTR variant may be quite common in the general population and has not yet been found to be associated with amyloid deposition. Transthyretin Met 119, like Ser 6 and Met 30, may be the result of a mutational hot spot, where deamidation of a methylated cytosine at a CG site would lead to this mutation. A transthyretin variant with histidine substituted for aspartic acid at position 74 was discovered in individuals without evidence of amyloidosis, and arginine substitution for proline at position 102 has also been described. The number of known amyloid-producing variants of transthyretin far exceeds the number of nonamyloid variants. However, no concerted effort of population screening at the DNA level has been made to discover other clinically silent variants of this protein. With such a large number of amyloid-associated variants, it would appear that the propensity for amyloid fibril formation is significantly enhanced by most pertubations in primary structure of this heavily β-structured protein.

Treatment of Transthyretin Amyloidosis. While there remains no specific treatment for autosomal dominant transthyretin amyloidosis, supportive measures can significantly prolong life. Renal dialysis may be used for patients who have severe nephropathy. The use of cardiac pacemakers has prolonged the life of many individuals in the Indiana/Swiss and also in the Appalachian and Swedish kindreds. Potent diuretics can significantly improve the quality of life of patients with restrictive cardiomyopathy, but frequently some degree of volume overload is necessary to maintain adequate cardiac filling and therefore tissue perfusion. Bowel involvement can be devastating to some individuals, and the judicious use of antibiotics to reduce intestinal flora and of agents such as metachlopramide to stimulate gastric emptying has been helpful. Vitrectomy can restore vision to some patients with vitreous opacities, although all too often this is only temporary. Patients who have had a vitrectomy for amyloidosis should be observed carefully for development of secondary glaucoma, which can be painless and can cause irreversible retinal damage. Plasmapheresis has been tried in some individuals with transthyretin amyloidosis and, while anecdotal reports suggest some improvement in quality of life, no definite therapeutic advantage has been noted. Colchicine is commonly given because of the reports of its preventing amyloid in familial Mediterranean fever. There is no definite evidence that it prevents transthyretin amyloid formation, but nevertheless it is frequently given in the hope that it might delay the onset or progression of amyloid formation, particularly in presymptomatic carriers of mutant transthyretin genes. The ability to detect carriers of variant transthyretin genes before the onset of clinical disease is a potential advantage in evaluating any future attempts at preventive therapy.

Recently several patients with transthyretin amyloidosis have received liver transplants. Since transthyretin in the general circulation is essentially completely synthesized in the liver, replacement of the organ results in rapid clearance of the variant transthyretin from the plasma.[217] Since all other liver functions were normal in these individuals, the morbidity from surgery is much less than in individuals who have liver transplants for primary liver disease. To date, definite proof of improved neurologic function has not been documented in individuals receiving liver transplants, although resolution of bowel dysfunction has been noted in several recipients.[218] While liver transplantation may represent a specific and essentially curative treatment for the systemic amyloidosis, the cost of this procedure and present-day problems with organ precurement and tissue rejection preclude its general use and acceptance.

Hereditary Amyloidosis Not Associated with Transthyretin

Apolipoprotein A-I Amyloidosis. In 1969, Van Allen et al. described a kindred from Iowa of English, Irish, and Scottish descent with autosomal-dominant amyloidosis.[219] Individuals in this kindred had prominent renal disease with nephrotic syndrome and/or renal insufficiency. Individuals in their twenties have been shown to be affected, but others have lived into their seventies. A striking incidence of peptic ulcer disease was seen in affected individuals. Lower limb neuropathy is characteristic of this syndrome, which in the past was called "FAP III," although a few reports have called it "FAP IV" (Table 139-3).

Amyloid fibrils isolated from tissues of a patient with this syndrome were found to contain a degradation product of a variant form of apolipoprotein A-I, with arginine replacing glycine at position 26.[31,220] While both normal and variant types of apolipoprotein A-I were demonstrated in the plasma of affected individuals, only the variant arginine 26 apo A-I was found in amyloid fibril deposits. A second American kindred of Italian origin has subsequently been identified

Table 139-3 Plasma Proteins (Other than Transthyretin) Associated with Autosomal Dominant Systemic Amyloidosis

Protein	Mutation	Clinical Features*	Geographic Kindreds
Apolipoprotein A-I	Gly26Arg	PN, kidney	U.S.
	Leu60Arg	Kidney	England
Gelsolin	Asp187Asn	PN, lattice corneal dystrophy	Finland, U.S., Japan
	Asp187Tyr	PN	Denmark, Czech
Cystatin C	Leu68Glu	Cerebral hemorrhage	Iceland
Fibrinogen	Arg554Leu	Kidney	Mexico
	Glu526Val	Kidney	U.S.
Lysozyme	Ile56Thr	Kidney, skin petechiae	England
	Asp67His	Kidney	England

*PN = peripheral neuropathy.

with this mutation. The Gly26Arg substitution is the result of a G → C transversion in the first position of codon 26 in exon 2.[220]

Recently a second apolipoprotein A-I mutation, Leu60-Arg, has been identified in an English family in which the propositus presented at age 24 with splenic and hepatic amyloidosis.[221] Subsequently this individual developed hypertension and thrombocytopenia. Other members of the kindred presented with renal amyloidosis but no evidence of neuropathy. Chemical analysis of amyloid fibrils revealed apo A-I degradation peptides of 88, 92, and 93 residues, whereas the original apo A-I arginine 26 mutated amyloid protein showed no peptides beyond residue 83 of apo A-I. No normal apolipoprotein A-I was found in the arginine 60 amyloid fibrils.

Gelsolin Amyloidosis. In 1969, Meretoja described familial amyloidosis with lattice corneal dystrophy, progressive corneal neuropathy, and skin changes with various internal symptoms.[222-224] The first manifestation of the disease is a dystrophic change of the cornea due to amyloid deposition. Over several decades, thickening of the skin on the forehead and back occurs, and patients may develop facial paralysis caused by cranial neuropathies. Death related to renal and cardiac amyloid has been reported. While the largest occurrence of this type of amyloidosis is in Finland, there have been reports of patients in the United States,[225-227] Denmark, and Canada. An amyloid subunit protein of 71 amino acid residues derived from plasma gelsolin was isolated from tissues of patients with this disease and shown to have an asparagine substituted for the aspartic acid at position 187.[32,33,228] This substitution is caused by a G → A transition,[229,230] which has now been demonstrated in American families[231] and in a Japanese kindred.[232] So far, haplotype analysis has not shown evidence for more than one mutational event leading to the various kindreds in Finland and Holland.[233] Individuals homozygous for the Asp187Asn variant have demonstrated early onset of severe renal amyloidosis.[234] Recently, a tyrosine-for-aspartate substitution at residue 187 has been identified in kindreds from Denmark and Czechoslovakia, with syndromes similar to the amyloidosis described by Meretoja. The same mutation, a G → T transversion at the first position of codon 187, was demonstrated for both kindreds, but they had different haplotypes, suggesting separate mutational events.[233] No other families with this mutation have been identified. At least one large kindred with lattice corneal dystrophy that is evidently not due to gelsolin deposition in the cornea has been identified.[235]

Gelsolin is a calcium-binding protein that binds to and fragments actin filaments.[236] There are two forms of gelsolin encoded by a single gene and derived through alternative splicing. A cytoplasmic gelsolin binds actin monomers and may have an important role in the reorganization of the cytoskeleton during receptor-mediated signaling.[237] Plasma gelsolin (93 kDa) also binds actin and presumably functions to clear actin from the plasma. The gelsolin gene is on chromosome 9 (9q32-q34) and spans approximately 70 kb.[238] The genomic structure has been partially determined and the gene shown to contain at least 14 exons. The higher molecular weight of plasma gelsolin is due to a 25-amino-acid extension at the N-terminal end of the protein and is the result of the alternate splicing. In the human, the plasma concentration of gelsolin is approximately 220 mg/liter. Unlike transthyretin and apolipoprotein A-I, which are synthesized mainly by the liver, plasma gelsolin is derived in large part from muscle.[239] Therefore, organ transplantation is not an option for treatment of gelsolin amyloidosis.

Fibrinogen-Associated Amyloidosis. Mutations in the fibrinogen Aα chain gene have been identified in individuals with familial autosomal dominant amyloidosis.[34] To date, two separate mutations have been found associated with amyloidosis. The disease in these families shares several features. First, it is relatively early in onset, often appearing in the patient's forties but sometimes in the twenties. Second, the principal manifestation of the amyloidosis is nephropathy, often presenting with hypertension and proteinuria. Third, there is no peripheral neuropathy. Both known mutations are in the protease-sensitive C-terminal region of fibrinogen Aα.

Fibrinogen is a major plasma protein that is involved in the final phase of blood coagulation. It is composed of two sets of three different polypeptide chains, α, β, and γ, which have molecular weights of 66,000, 52,000, and 46,500, respectively, and are the products of closely associated genes on chromosome 4.[240-242] Fibrinogen is converted to insoluble fibrin by the action of thrombin and factor VIIIa. A number of mutations in the fibrinogen Aα chain have been described in individuals with dysfibrinogenemia (Chap. 105), but none has shown an association with amyloidosis.[243] Most of these mutations have been in the N-terminal end of the fibrinogen Aα chain. The serum concentration of fibrinogen is approximately 3 mg/ml, and it functions as a moderate acute-phase reactant. A substitution of leucine for arginine at residue 554 of the fibrinogen α chain was identified in amyloid fibril subunit protein isolated from kidney tissue of a Peruvian patient who died with renal amyloidosis.[34] A sister and son also had biopsy-proven amyloidosis and died with renal failure, the sister at age 28 and the son at age 24. Genomic DNA sequencing revealed a G → T transversion at nucleotide position 4993 of the fibrinogen Aα-chain gene, corresponding to the second base of codon 554.

Another fibrinogen α-chain variant with valine substituted for glutamic acid at position 526 (A → T mutation at nucleotide 1674) was discovered in two large, unrelated American kindreds with renal amyloidosis. The disease in both kindreds had typical autosomal dominant inheritance, and there was no history of either neuropathy or coagulopathy. In at least one case, postmortem examination found amyloid deposition in the spleen but not the heart. Typical pathology in all individuals, however, is dense amyloid deposition in renal glomeruli.

Lysozyme-Associated Amyloidosis. Two mutations in human lysozyme have been reported to be associated with nonneuropathic systemic amyloidosis.[244] In one family the syndrome was characterized by a petechial skin rash from childhood and subsequent renal failure. A mutation at residue 56 of lysozyme with threonine replacing isoleucine was found by amino acid sequencing of an amyloid fibril subunit protein isolated from renal tissue. The full-length variant lysozyme molecule was present in the amyloid deposits, and no normal lysozyme was found. The isoleucine-to-threonine change is caused by a single-base T → C transition in exon 2 of the lysozyme gene. An aspartic acid-to-histidine mutation at residue 67 was found by DNA analysis of members of a second family with renal amyloidosis. This mutation is the result of a single-nucleotide change with a G → C transversion in the first base of codon 67. In both lysozyme mutations, the affected individuals were heterozygotes, consistent with an autosomal dominant form of amyloidosis.

Lysozyme is a bacteriolytic enzyme present in external secretions, polymorphonuclear leukocytes, and macrophages. Its biologic significance is not completely known, and polymorphic forms not associated with amyloidosis have not been described.

Hereditary Cerebral Hemorrhage with Amyloid (Iceland). In 1972, Gudmundsson et al. described a syndrome of premature strokes and intracranial hemorrhage in Icelandic families.[245] The syndrome usually occurred in the third or fourth decade of life and showed autosomal dominant inheritance. Neurologic symptoms varied, depending on the location and severity of hemorrhage and, while some individuals died abruptly, others suffered numerous nonfatal cerebral accidents over several years before death. Postmortem examinations showed amyloid primarily restricted to cerebral blood vessels, but subsequent studies have reported systemic deposits. Chemical analysis of this amyloid has shown a fibril subunit that is a degradation product of cystatin C (γ trace protein).[246] The amyloid subunit lacked the first 10 residues of cystatin C and, in addition, a glutamine was found at position 58 (residue 68 of intact cystatin C) instead of the normal leucine.[247] DNA analysis has shown the clinical disease segregating with the Leu68Glu substitution.[248] Individuals affected with this disease show extremely low levels of cystatin C in the cerebrospinal fluid, which provides an alternative test for detection of carriers.[249] Senile plaques containing amyloid of the type seen in Alzheimer disease are not a feature of the Icelandic amyloidosis.[250]

Cystatin C, a cysteine proteinase inhibitor, contains 120 amino acids in a single polypeptide chain. It is the product of a single-copy gene on chromosome 20. The gene, which covers approximately 7 kb, contains three exons and is expressed in many tissues, including kidney, liver, gut, pancreas, and heart.[251]

Hereditary Cerebral Hemorrhage with Amyloid (Dutch). Several families with congophilic angiopathy of the cerebral vessels resulting in intracerebral hemorrhage have been described in Holland. Affected members of these families have neither the cystatin C mutation described in hereditary cerebral hemorrhage with amyloid type I (HCHWA-I) nor low spinal fluid concentrations of cystatin C.[249] Instead, amyloid isolated from leptomeninges contains the β peptide analogous to the fibril subunit found in Alzheimer plaques and vascular deposits.[252] A glutamine substitution for glutamic acid at residue 693 of the 770-amino-acid form of β-amyloid precursor protein (β-APP) was found, and this mutation has been corroborated at the DNA level.[253] While senile dementia is not a feature of this syndrome, there have been reports of intracerebral β-amyloid deposits demonstrated by immunohistochemistry with specific antibodies. Recently, a mutation at codon 692 (Ala692Glu) of the β-APP gene, which is associated with cerebral hemorrhage, has been described.[254] Individuals in these families, which are also of Dutch origin, show an early-onset form of familial Alzheimer disease as well as cerebral hemorrhage from congophilic angiopathy.

Familial Mediterranean Fever. Familial Mediterranean fever (FMF) is the only syndrome in which systemic amyloidosis appears in a definite autosomal recessive pattern. Siegal first described FMF in 1945 and used the name *benign paroxysmal peritonitis*.[255] Other terms applied to this syndrome include *familial paroxysmal polyserositis* and *periodic fever*. Heller used the term *familial Mediterranean fever* and first noted the autosomal recessive inheritance.[256] A high percentage of patients with FMF develop systemic amyloidosis with prominent renal involvement.

FMF is seen most frequently in individuals of Mediterranean origin.[257,258] It is particularly prominent in Sephardic Jews and Armenians. The disease is characterized by periodic episodes of fever, which may be accompanied by signs of peritonitis, synovitis, pleuritis, or an erythematous rash. These attacks may occur within the first decade of life and usually persist throughout life. The clinical manifestations have wide variability, however, and some patients have only mild abdominal discomfort during attacks. Large joint effusions can be seen, but these usually resolve without residual effects.[259] The etiology of these attacks is unknown, and biopsies of either peritoneum or pleura show nothing more than evidence of mild inflammation. The attacks are self-limiting and usually resolve after two or three days. Low serum levels of C5a inhibitor in FMF patients have been reported, and this finding suggests that complement activation may be involved in pathogenesis of the syndrome.[260]

Genetic studies suggest that FMF is transmitted as a simple autosomal recessive trait, and linkage analysis has localized the FMF gene to the short arm of chromosome 16.[261] The FMF gene frequency in Sephardic Jews has been calculated as 0.22.[262,263] FMF-type illnesses have been described in other ethnic groups, however, and in some instances autosomal dominant inheritance with incomplete penetrance cannot be excluded. While systemic amyloidosis is common in patients with FMF, the relationship between the FMF and amyloidosis is not clear.[264] The development of amyloidosis does not correlate well with numbers or degrees of febrile attacks, and indeed some members of FMF kindreds have been described with amyloidosis but without the febrile attacks.[265] The incidence of amyloidosis in FMF patients of Armenian descent is much lower than in Sephardic Jews, supporting the hypothesis that FMF and amyloidosis are two separate traits with separate genetic bases.

The amyloidosis of FMF typically has a predilection for renal involvement with nephrotic syndrome followed by azotemia. Many patients die by their early twenties. Pathologically, glomerular deposits of amyloid predominate. The spleen is commonly involved, and the thyroid may be heavily infiltrated. Vascular deposits throughout the body are common but rarely lead to organ dysfunction. Treatment with either chronic hemodialysis or peritoneal dialysis has yielded fair results, and kidney transplantation has been effective.[266] Treatment with colchicine has been shown to prevent the febrile attacks in most patients and has also been associated with a lack of progression of amyloidosis.[267] This has led to treatment of all FMF patients with colchicine. In studies by Zemer et al., only patients who did not maintain this therapeutic regimen have developed progressive renal amyloidosis.[268]

The amyloid fibrils of FMF contain protein AA, and on chemical grounds this amyloidosis is the reactive type.[14,17] The serum SAA concentration usually increases during febrile attacks and returns to normal between attacks. Since SAA levels are elevated by attacks of inflammation, it would appear that the amyloidosis of FMF is indeed a reactive type not only chemically but clinically, and that at least two determining factors act in concert. Variables that may lead to the differences in expression of the amyloidosis include: (1) penetrance of the FMF genetic trait, (2) prevalence of an amyloidogenic SAA allele (on chromosome 11) in the population at risk, and (3) environmental, dietary, and metabolic factors that may modulate the expression of the SAA genes and degradation of their protein products.

Muckle-Wells Syndrome. In 1962, Muckle and Wells described a syndrome characterized by nerve deafness, fever, urticaria, malaise, and "augey" bouts (attacks of urticaria or angioedema-like symptoms).[269] Nephrotic syndrome developed by middle age, and affected individuals died of renal insufficiency. Postmortem studies showed glomerular amyloidosis plus involvement of the adrenals and spleen. Families with similar syndromes have been described, including one of Norwegian descent.[270] While the original description supports autosomal dominant inheritance, this syndrome is similar to FMF in that the amyloid has been shown to contain protein AA.[271] To date no linkage studies have been done to see if the factor for inheritance of Muckle-Wells syndrome is localized to chromosome 16, as is the FMF gene. Clinically the two syndromes seem distinct; however, given that the disease appears to be autosomal dominant in some FMF families, whereas in some Muckle-Wells families the pattern of inheritance is not clearly dominant, it may be that similar mechanisms are involved in the expression of these two conditions. There are no reports on treatment of Muckle-Wells syndrome with colchicine, but such a therapeutic trial would certainly be indicated.

Miscellaneous Hereditary Amyloidosis Syndromes. In 1932 Ostertag described a familial syndrome of renal amyloidosis.[10] More recently Weiss and Page provided an excellent pathologic description of the nephropathy in another family.[272] The main feature is renal amyloid without neuropathy and death resulting from azotemia. At autopsy the adrenals and spleen as well as the kidneys may be involved with amyloid. Possible precursor proteins associated with this type of amyloidosis include mutant forms of apolipoprotein A-I,[220,221] and the newly discovered variants of plasma fibrinogen.[34] In another family (an Ohio kindred with oculoleptomeningeal amyloidosis), patients have central nervous system complications, including dementia, seizures, strokes, abnormal gait, and vitreous deposits.[273] The Ohio family is of German origin, and postmortem examinations showed amyloid in the central nervous system, particularly in the leptomeninges and subarachnoid vessels. Traces of amyloid were found in peripheral nerves and skeletal muscles. The possible relationship to the Icelandic form of hereditary cerebral hemorrhage with amyloidosis has not been clarified, but the presence of vitreous deposits would be more consistent with a transthyretin origin for this type of amyloid.

Localized Hereditary Amyloidosis. Localized amyloidosis occurs in a number of syndromes. The first to be characterized chemically was the amyloid associated with medullary carcinoma of the thyroid. This carcinoma occurs in both sporadic and autosomal dominant patterns and is frequently associated with other endocrinopathies, including pheochromocytomas.[50,51] This syndrome has been designated "multiple endocrine adenomatosis type II" (MEA-II).[274] Chemically the amyloid is composed of peptides derived from precalcitonin and is limited to the thyroid or tumor metastases.[275]

Cutaneous amyloidosis has been reported in families and may be characterized as lichenoid changes of the skin.[276–279] Cutaneous amyloidosis appeared to be autosomal dominant in a family reported by Rajagopalan and Tay,[53] but there have also been reports of X-linked disease.[280] Familial bullous cutaneous amyloid infiltration has also been reported.

Isolated atrial amyloidosis is a localized form of amyloidosis that occurs with increasing prevalence in aging hearts[281] but is occasionally recognized in a familial pattern.[282] Small deposits of amyloid along the sarcolemma of atrial muscle cells may be observed as early as age 40, and prevalence may reach 95 percent by the ninth decade of life.[283] The hemodynamic significance of this form of amyloid is not clear, but in some families it may be associated with atrial standstill.[282]

Isolated atrial amyloid contains a 28-amino-acid residue C-terminal degradation product of atrial natriuretic peptide.[284–286] This peptide is synthesized by cardiac myocytes and may be induced as a response to congestive heart failure. This suggests that the increasing prevalence of atrial amyloidosis with age may be associated with ventricular dysfunction.[287] The familial atrial standstill syndrome, however, may show no heart failure and may be related to an unknown genetic factor.[288]

Clinically, perhaps the most important of the localized amyloidoses is Alzheimer disease, a progressive dementia characterized by accumulations of amyloid substance in the brain.[54] Amyloid deposits (plaques) in cortical tissues are associated with neurofibrillary tangles and blood vessel deposits (congophilic angiopathy), which also stain histologically as amyloid. While only 10 to 20 percent of Alzheimer disease is clearly inherited, it is a late-onset disease, and many familial cases may not be recognized.[289] The Alzheimer plaques and congophilic angiopathy deposits contain a subunit protein (amyloid β protein or β-A4 protein) having a molecular weight of approximately 4000 and from 39 to 42 amino acid residues and representing an internal fragment of the C-terminal portion of an amyloid precursor protein (APP).[35] APP is the product of a single gene on chromosome 21q and has at least three alternatively spliced transcripts, the largest encoding a protein of 770 amino acid residues.[290–292] While most cases of Alzheimer disease are sporadic, definite autosomal dominant inheritance is seen in many kindreds, and, recently, point mutations in the APP gene localized to chromosome 21 have been described that are associated with Alzheimer pathology in a small number of families. In particular, three different amino acid substitutions at codon 717 of APP have been found to be associated with Alzheimer disease,[293–295] and other amino acid substitutions in the β-amyloid peptide sequence have been shown to be associated with either cerebral hemorrhage as in hereditary cerebral hemorrhage with amyloid type D (HCHWA-D) or dementia.[253,254]

Type 2 (adult-onset) diabetes mellitus was shown to be associated with hyalinized pancreatic islets of Langerhans as early as 1900.[296] Subsequently this hyalinized material was shown to meet the criteria of amyloid and, therefore, this is a form of localized amyloidosis. Little progress was made in understanding this form of amyloidosis until it was found to be associated with age-associated diabetes in cats as well as humans and some nonhuman primates.[297] Isolation of a unique 37-amino-acid peptide, first from an insulinoma and subsequently from diabetic islets, proved that this was a new type of amyloid protein.[37,298] This peptide, which is called either "islet amyloid polypeptide" (IAPP) or "amylin,"[299] is the product of a gene on the short arm of chromosome 12.[300] It is synthesized predominantly in β cells of the pancreas and is cosecreted with insulin, although in molar amounts 100 times less. Islet amyloid polypeptide has significant (43 to 46 percent) homology with calcitonin-gene-related peptides (CGRP) 1 and 2, which are neuropeptides encoded on chromosome 11.[301]

The functions of islet amyloid polypeptide in normal physiology are not known, although various effects on insulin secretion and function have been reported. The relation of islet amyloid polypeptide to the pathogenesis of diabetes also remains to be determined. The restriction of the islet amyloid deposits to certain species (humans, apes, cats) and the association with glucose intolerance in these species suggests that it is of importance in diabetes. The idea that this form of amyloidosis represents a hereditary condition rests on its association with type 2 diabetes, which has obvious but unclear genetic features. So far, no polymorphisms in the coding regions of the islet amyloid polypeptide gene have been discovered to explain the development of this form of amyloid, but regulation of gene expression has been incompletely explored. Amyloid in the pancreatic islets of a South American rodent (*Octodon degus*) has been shown to contain insulin instead of islet amyloid polypeptide as the fibril subunit protein.[302]

Other clinically recognized types of localized amyloidosis are associated with specific syndromes. Tumoral deposits of amyloid in the urinary tract are common. To date, the chemical composition of these deposits has not been determined, but they are usually not associated with any systemic disease. Ureteral obstruction or hemorrhage from the bladder may lead to clinical recognition of these deposits.[303] Amyloid in the respiratory tract without systemic involvement has been frequently reported.[304] Again, the amyloid substance has not been chemically characterized. Amyloid deposits in senile articular cartilage may occur with or without association of calcium pyrophosphate deposition disease.[305] It is possible that these deposits are related to the β_2-microglobulin articular amyloid that is seen in chronic dialysis patients, but no studies have been reported on this topic. None of these localized tumoral amyloidoses appears to be inherited.

DETECTION OF GENE CARRIERS IN HEREDITARY AMYLOIDOSIS

Identification of carriers of genes associated with amyloidosis is important for individuals who have clinical disease and those who have not yet developed clinical evidence of amyloidosis. In the former, identification of a mutation in a gene coding for one of the amyloid-associated proteins usually allows proper diagnosis. Since the amyloidoses are heterogeneous, it is not uncommon for one syndrome to be mistaken for another. This is particularly true for distinguishing hereditary amyloidosis from the immunoglobulin type of amyloidosis. Immunoglobulin amyloidosis (AL) commonly causes cardiomyopathy with or without peripheral neuropathy, as seen in many of the transthyretin amyloidoses. Immunoglobulin amyloidosis frequently has renal involvement without neuropathy, a syndrome similar to the fibrinogen and some of the apolipoprotein A-I amyloidoses. Even the systemic manifestations of gelsolin amyloidosis may be mistaken for the AL syndrome. Since it is common to treat immunoglobulin amyloidosis with chemotherapy, it is imperative that the hereditary forms of amyloidosis be excluded from the diagnosis. Prognosis is a second major reason for distinguishing hereditary amyloid syndromes from other types of amyloidosis. The mean life span after diagnosis for individuals with AL amyloidosis is approximately 2 years. Most of the hereditary amyloidoses have a much better prognosis, with life spans of 5 to 20 years after tissue diagnosis. While the longevity with transthyretin amyloidosis may vary considerably even between families having the same mutation, disease progression is often very uniform within each kindred. Thus, attention to family histories can often lead to a more astute prognosis. For individuals in families with hereditary amyloidosis, detection of disease-associated genes is of value for genetic counseling. The autosomal dominant amyloidoses are late-onset diseases, so gene carriers usually have their children before disease onset. Gene status may be important for family planning. While the knowledge of being a carrier of a disease-producing gene may be a heavy psychological burden for an individual, those individuals who are found to be negative for the amyloid variant gene are often fortunate beneficiaries of DNA testing. In addition, for individuals in families with hereditary amyloidosis, genetic testing offers the opportunity to participate in the clinical research which, hopefully, will enhance recognition and subsequently therapeutic progress for these diseases.

Since the autosomal dominant inherited amyloidoses are associated with variant forms of plasma proteins, it is possible to detect gene carriers by isolating and analyzing the plasma protein in question. This can be done for transthyretin, gelsolin, apolipoprotein A-I, and fibrinogen with varying degrees of difficulty. A fairly small amount of plasma can be used if the test involves gel electrophoresis, as is used for variants of apolipoprotein A-I[31] or hybrid isoelectric focusing, as described for variant forms of transthyretin.[211,306] In general, these methods are not used for detecting carriers of amyloid-associated genes. One exception is the use of cyanogen bromide to cleave plasma transthyretins that have a methionine as the substituted residue.[307] This method has been used to detect the methionine 30 transthyretin, where an efficient biochemical test uses a small amount of plasma and an antibody generated against the aberrant peptide produced by cyanogen bromide cleavage at the methionine 30 residue.[308,309] Recently, cyanogen bromide cleavage of the methionine 111 transthyretin associated with the Danish type of amyloid cardiomyopathy has been used to detect the variant transthyretin in plasma samples that were stored for 30 years.[197] This test, however, is not valid for the methionine 119 transthyretin, which is not associated with amyloidosis, because the peptides generated are similar to those generated with the methionine 30 amyloid, which produces transthyretin.

DNA analysis has been used extensively for detecting variant amyloid-associated genes and presents significant advantages: (1) only small amounts of peripheral blood are required to isolate leukocyte DNA; (2) DNA can be isolated from tissues and even histologic sections of organs from individuals who have died[31,294]; (3) present-day DNA analysis techniques can be applied to amniocytes or chorionic villus samples obtained for prenatal diagnosis.[310,311]

Sasaki et al.[312] developed the first DNA test for the transthyretin methionine 30 gene using a specific restriction endonuclease and Southern blot analysis. The methionine 30 mutation creates a recognition site for *Nsi*I and *Bal*I, thus giving new hybridization bands on Southern blot analysis.[313] Similarly, the transthyretin alanine 60 variant gene can be detected using *Pvu*II since the A $\rightarrow$ G change in codon 60 creates a new *Pvu*II site (Fig. 139-15).[177] Southern blot analysis, however, usually requires the use of radioactive probes and relatively lengthy hybridization schedules followed by exposure of radiographic film. The use of Southern

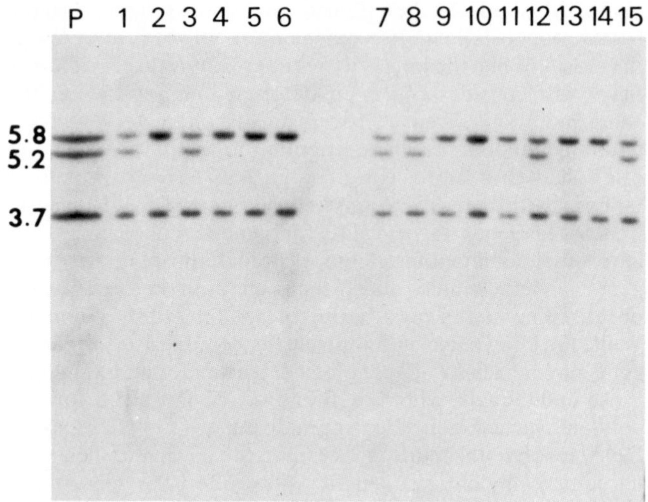

FIG. 139-15 **Southern blot analysis of members of the kindred shown in Fig. 139-10. The propositus at the left and six of his relatives have an extra 5.2-kb band which is a result of the extra *Pvu*II site in the Ala 60 gene. The transthyretin cDNA is the probe.**

blot analysis, therefore, has given way to polymerase chain reaction (PCR) technology, in which specific coding regions of the genes are amplified in vitro and then subjected to various procedures to identify base mutations.[314] There are four commonly used methods to detect mutations in PCR-amplified fragments of genomic DNA. The first, and most widely used, is PCR followed by restriction digestion (Table 139-4). Many of the disease-associated mutations in transthyretin result in new restriction endonuclease recognition sites. Therefore, digestion of PCR-amplified genomic fragments with the appropriate restriction endonuclease followed by size identification of the restriction fragments on ethidium bromide-stained agarose electrophoresis gels results in specific recognition of the mutation in question (Fig. 139-16). This method is applicable to the detection of both heterozygous and homozygous individuals and has been widely used for the methionine 30, alanine 60, tyrosine 77, and serine 84 mutations.[314] Mutations that result in loss of a restriction enzyme recognition site can also be detected by this method, but proper controls to determine the activity of the restriction endonuclease must be included in each test. In addition, since restriction endonuclease recognition sites are usually four or six bases in length, mutations in the vicinity of the disease-causing mutation will also result in lack of digestion and, therefore, spurious results. When a point mutation does not result in alteration of a restriction endonuclease recognition site, allele-specific oligonucleotides (ASO) have been used for hybridization to the variant gene sequence.[161,228] In this technique, the genomic coding sequence to be analyzed is amplified by PCR, and this product is then blotted onto nitrocellulose membrane and hybridized with a radiolabeled oligonucleotide specific for the mutation. Careful control of hybridization conditions will then differentiate between the presence of normal and variant allele products. If the proper combinations are used, homozygous and heterozygous gene products can be identified. Another method that has been used for identifying point mutations is allele-specific PCR.[31,173] In this technique, the gene segment to be analyzed is amplified using a set of oligonucleotide primers, one of which has its 3′ nucleotide complementary to the point mutation. If, under the proper conditions, amplification occurs, the variant allele is present. If no amplification occurs, the individual is assumed to lack the variant allele. This method does not identify homozygous variant individuals unless a second PCR is performed with an oligonucleotide primer that has the 3′ base complementary to the normal base at the position of the mutation. Since there are limitations to both the ASO and the allele-specific PCR techniques, a new method has been used increasingly to identify disease-associated mutations where no novel restriction endonuclease recognition site exists. In this technique, called "PCR-induced mutation restriction analysis" (PCR-IMRA)[184,315] or "PCR-induced restriction analysis" (PIRA),[316] a restriction endonuclease recognition site is created using a mutagenesis primer that induces an enzyme site when a single base mutation is created in close proximity to the disease-associated mutation (Fig. 139-17). The mutagenesis primer is usually 20 to 25 nucleotides or more long so that, when the amplification products are digested with the specific enzyme, the resulting DNA fragments can be identified on ethidium bromide-stained agarose gels. This method is capable of differentiating normal individuals from heterozygous and homozygous carriers of the variant allele. With the large number of restriction endonucleases now commercially available, it is frequently easy to plan a mutagenesis primer to create a specific endonuclease recognition site. Occasionally this method can be used to replace an enzyme site for an expensive enzyme with one for a much less expensive and/or more specific enzyme.[141,182]

These DNA tests have allowed the application of molecular biology to the practice of clinical medicine and made the latest methods of genetic counseling and treatment available to individuals with these late-onset, genetically determined diseases. DNA tests, of course, can only identify carriers of amyloid-producing genes. While they may aid in the diagnosis and subsequent treatment, they cannot change the course of the disease in affected individuals. Even more important at this time is to find some means of modifying

Table 139-4 Oligonucleotide Primers Used in Enzymatic Amplification of TTR Exons 2,3,4

Primer	Sequence*	PCR Product
E2LP1	5′-GATCCTGCAGGTTAACTTCTCACGTGTCTT-3′	215 bp containing exon 2 of transthyretin gene
E2LP2	5′-AGATCTGCAGAAGTCCTGTGGGAGGGTTCT-3′	
E3LP1	5′-GCCACTGCAGTCCTCCATGCGTAACTTAAT-3′	268 bp containing exon 3 of transthyretin gene
E3LP2	5′-ACTGCTGCAGACTGTGCATTTCCTGGAATG-3′	
E4LP1	5′-TCTGCTGCAGATGGATCTGTCTGTCTTCTC-3′	190 bp containing exon 4 of transthyretin gene
E4LP2	5′-ATGACTGCAGATCCCTCGTCCTTCAGGTCC-3′	

*The *Pst*I recognition site is underlined. The ten nucleotides at the 5′ ends (for cloning purposes) can be omitted for PCR followed by restriction analysis and for direct DNA sequencing.

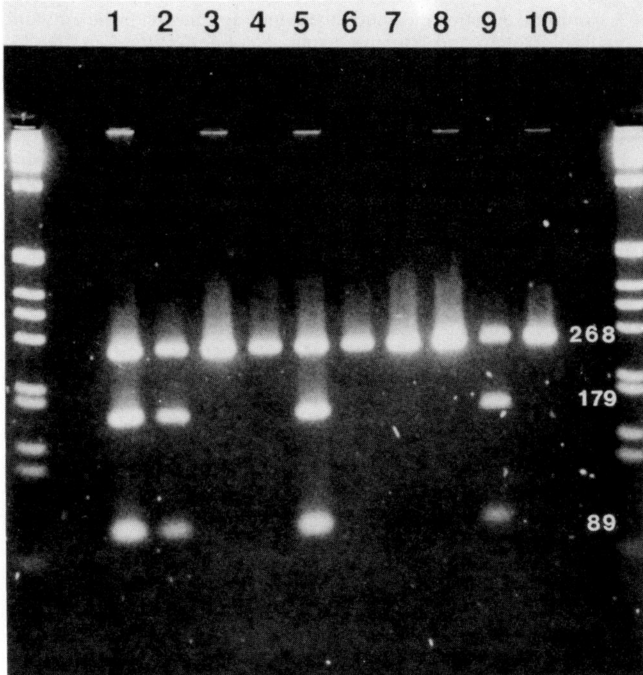

FIG. 139-16 *Pvu*II digest of the exon 3 containing amplification product for detection of the Ala 60 transthyretin gene. Lanes 3, 4, 6, 7, 8, 10: Individuals who are not carriers of the Ala 60 gene; only the normal 268-bp product is observed. Lanes 1, 2, 5, 9: Individuals who are carriers of the Ala-60 gene; the normal 268-bp product as well as 179-bp and 89-bp fragments, which result from digestion of the variant allele at the new *Pvu*II site, are observed. One kilobase ladder of molecular weight markers flanks lanes 1–10. Fragments were separated by agarose gel electrophoresis and visualized by ethidium bromide staining. Fragment sizes are indicated in base pairs.

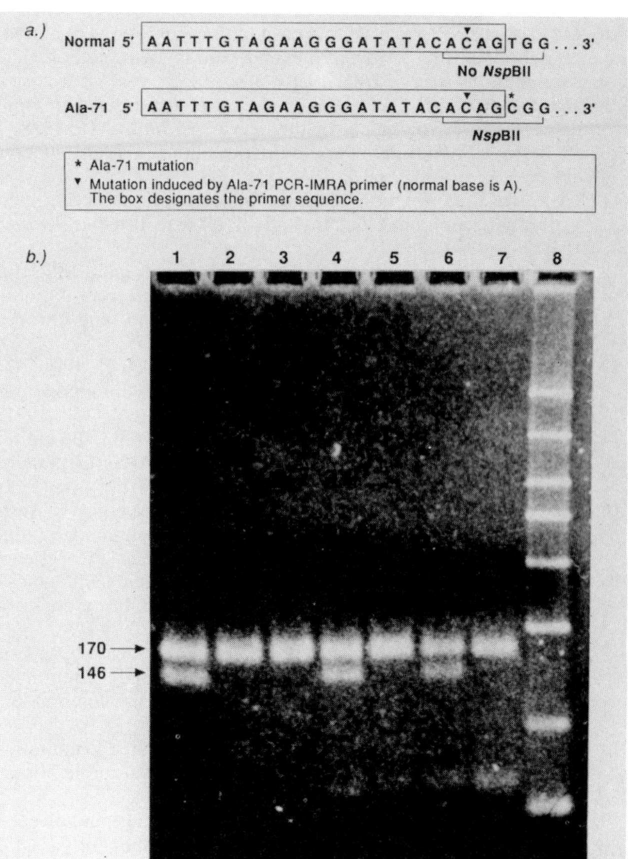

FIG. 139-17 *A*. PCR-induced mutation restriction analysis for the transthyretin Val71Ala allele. Mutation primer is shown and used in amplification reaction with E3LP2 (see Table 139-3). *B*. Ethidium bromide-stained agarose gel of *Nsp*BII-digested PCR products. Lanes 1, 4, and 6 show both the normal 170-bp and the digested variant products, indicating heterozygosity for the Ala 71 allele. Lane 8 contains size markers. PCR-IMRA = PCR-induced mutation restriction analysis.

the disease process so that fibril synthesis is decreased or stopped. Possible answers may lie in developing methods to regulate expression of specific genes or to modify the biochemical fate of their protein products.

ADDENDUM

Transthyretin Amyloidosis Syndromes

Clinical syndromes associated with a number of transthyretin variants have not been included because of insufficient data presented in the literature. This is true for the transthyretin variants Val30Gly, Ala45Asp, Gly47Val, Ser52Pro, Glu54Gly, Glu61Lys, Ala97Gly, Ser112Ile, and Tyr114His.[317-320] Although most of these mutations are listed in Table 139-2 with some of the clinical features and geographic locations of kindreds, two TTR mutations deserve mention in this Addendum. Ser112Ile has been described in one kindred in Italy in which individuals had peripheral neuropathy and cardiomyopathy. Tyr114His has been reported in patients from Japan with only the carpal tunnel syndrome. No evidence of systemic disease was noted, and therefore this particular mutation should be considered in patients with isolated carpal tunnel syndrome where tissue biopsy shows localization of transthyretin.

It has now been demonstrated that individuals in an American family with transthyretin amyloidosis have both the amyloid associated Ala42Gly and the benign His90Asn mutations.[321,322] This explains why the American family has amyloidosis, whereas other families with only the His90Asn mutation do not.

A second mutation in fibrinogen α chain associated with renal amyloidosis has been confirmed. This mutation Glu526Val of the fibrinogen α-chain gene has been detected in a number of kindreds in the United States.[323]

REFERENCES

1. Glenner GG: Amyloid deposits and amyloidosis: The B-fibrilloses. *N Engl J Med* **302:**1283 and 1333, 1980.
2. Rokitansky KF: *Handbuch der Pathologischen Anatomie*. Vienna, Braumueller and Seidel, vol 3, 1842.
3. Virchow R: Zur Cellulose-Frage. *Virchows Arch Pathol Anat* **6:**416, 1854.
4. Virchow VR: Ueber eineim Gehirn und Rueckenmark des Menschen aufgefundene Substanz mit der chemischen reaction der Cellulose. *Virchows Arch Pathol Anat* **6:**135, 1854.
5. Friedreich N, Kekule A: Zur Amyloidfrage. *Virchows Arch Pathol Anat* **16:**50, 1859.
6. Cohen AS: The constitution and genesis of amyloid. *Int Rev Exp Pathol* **4:**159, 1965.
7. Andrade C: A peculiar form of peripheral neuropathy. Familial atypical generalized amyloidosis with special involvement of the peripheral nerves. *Brain* **75:**408, 1952.

8. Debruyn RS, Stern RO: A case of the progressive hypertrophic polyneuritis of Dejerine and Sottas with pathological examination. *Brain* **52:**84, 1929.
9. Denavasquez S, Treble HA: A case of generalized amyloid disease with involvement of the nerves. *Brain* **61:**116, 1938.
10. Ostertag B: Familiere Amyloid-Erkrankung. *Z Menschl Vererbungs Konstit Lehre* **30:**105, 1950.
11. Cohen AS, Calkins E: Electron microscopic observation on a fibrous component in amyloid of diverse origins. *Nature* **183:**1202, 1959.
12. Spiro D: The structural basis of proteinuria in man. Electron microscopic studies of renal biopsy specimens from patients with lipid nephrosis, amyloidosis, and subacute and chronic glomerulonephritis. *Am J Pathol* **35:**47, 1959.
13. Glenner GG, Terry W, Harada M, Isersky C, Page D: Amyloid fibril proteins: Proof of homology with immunoglobulin light chains by sequence analysis. *Science* **172:**1150, 1971.
14. Levin M, Franklin EC, Frangione B, Pras M: The amino acid sequence of a major nonimmunoglobulin component of some amyloid fibrils. *J Clin Invest* **51:**2773, 1972.
15. Husby G, Sletten K, Michaelsen TE, Natvig JB: Antigenic and chemical characterization of non-immunoglobulin amyloid proteins. *Scand J Immunol* **1:**393, 1972.
16. Sletten K, Husby G: The complete amino acid sequence of non-immunoglobulin amyloid fibril protein AS in rheumatoid arthritis. *Eur J Biochem* **41:**117, 1974.
17. Levin M, Pras M, Franklin EC: Immunologic studies of the major non-immunoglobulin protein of amyloid I. Identification and partial characterization of a related serum component. *J Exp Med* **138:**373, 1973.
18. Husby G, Natvig JB: A serum component related to immunoglobulin amyloid protein AS, a possible precursor of the fibrils. *J Clin Invest* **53:**1054, 1974.
19. Rosenthal CJ, Franklin EC: Variation with age and disease of an amyloid A protein-related serum component. *J Clin Invest* **55:**746, 1975.
20. Linke RP, Sipe JD, Pollock PS, Ignaczak TF, Glenner GG: Isolation of a low molecular weight serum component antigenically related to an amyloid fibril protein of unknown origin. *Proc Natl Acad Sci USA* **72:**1473, 1975.
21. McAdam KPWJ, Sipe JD: Murine model for human secondary amyloidosis: Genetic variability of the acute-phase serum protein SAA response to endotoxins and casein. *J Exp Med* **144:**1121, 1976.
22. Benson MD, Scheinberg MA, Shirahama T, Cathcart ES, Skinner M: Kinetics of serum amyloid protein A in casein-induced murine amyloidosis. *J Clin Invest* **59:**412, 1977.
23. Benson MD, Kleiner E: Synthesis and secretion of serum amyloid protein A (SAA) by hepatocytes in mice treated with casein. *J Immunol* **124:**495, 1980.
24. Costa PP, Figuera AS, Bravo FR: Amyloid fibril protein related to prealbumin in familial amyloidotic polyneuropathy. *Proc Natl Acad Sci USA* **75:**4499, 1978.
25. Benson MD: Partial amino acid sequence homology between an heredofamilial amyloid protein and human plasma prealbumin. *J Clin Invest* **67:**1035, 1981.
26. Dwulet FE, Benson MD: Polymorphism of human plasma thyroxine binding prealbumin. *Biochem Biophys Res Commun* **114:**657, 1983.
27. Nakasato M, Kangawa K, Minaminoi N, Tawara S, Matsuo H, Araki S: Revised analysis of amino acid replacement in a prealbumin variant (SKO-III) associated with familial amyloidotic polyneuropathy of Jewish origin. *Biochem Biophys Res Commun* **123:**921, 1984.
28. Wallace MR, Dwulet FE, Conneally PM, Benson MD: Biochemical and molecular genetic characteristic of a new variant prealbumin associated with hereditary amyloidosis. *J Clin Invest* **78:**6, 1986.
29. Dwulet FE, Benson MD: Characterization of prealbumin variant associated with familial amyloidotic polyneuropathy type II (Indiana/Swiss). *J Clin Invest* **78:**880, 1986.
30. Benson MD: Inherited amyloidosis. *J Med Genet* **28:**73, 1991.
31. Nichols WC, Dwulet FE, Liepnieks J, Benson MD: Variant apolipoprotein AI as a major constituent of a human hereditary amyloid. *Biochem Biophys Res Commun* **156:**762, 1988.
32. Maury CPJ, Alli K, Baumann M: Finnish hereditary amyloidosis. Amino acid sequence homology between the amyloid fibril protein and human plasma gelsoline. *FEBS Lett* **260:**85, 1990.
33. Haltia M, Prelli F, Ghiso J, Kiuru S, Somer H, Palo J, Frangione B: Amyloid protein in familial amyloidosis (Finnish type) is homologous to gelsolin, an actin-binding protein. *Biochem Biophys Res Commun* **167:**927, 1990.
34. Benson MD, Liepnieks J, Uemichi T, Wheeler G, Correa R: Hereditary renal amyloidosis associated with a mutant fibrinogen α-chain. *Nat Genet* **3:**252, 1993.
35. Glenner GG, Wong CD: Alzheimer's disease: Initial report of the purification and characterization of a novel cerebrovascular amyloid protein. *Biochem Biophys Res Commun* **120:**885, 1984.
36. Tagliavini F, Prelli F, Ghiso J, Bugiani O, Serban D, Prusiner SB, Farlow MR, Ghetti B, Frangione B: Amyloid protein of Gerstmann-Sträussler-Scheinker disease (Indiana kindred) is an 11 kd fragment of prion protein with an N-terminal glycine at codon 58. *EMBO J* **10:**513, 1991.
37. Westermark P, Wernstedt C, Wilander E, Sletten K: A novel peptide in the calcitonin gene related family as an amyloid fibril protein in the endocrine pancreas. *Biochem Biophys Res Commun* **140:**827, 1986.
38. Puchtler H, Sweat F, Levine M: On the binding of Congo red by amyloid. *J Histochem Cytochem* **10:**355, 1962.
39. Shirahama T, Cohen AS: High resolution electron microscopic analysis of the amyloid fibril. *J Cell Biol* **33:**679, 1967.
40. Eanes ED, Glenner GG: X-ray diffraction studies of amyloid filaments. *J Histochem Cytochem* **16:**673, 1968.
41. Bonar L, Cohen AS, Skinner MM: Characterization of the amyloid fibrils as a cross-B protein. *Proc Soc Exp Biol Med* **131:**1373, 1969.
42. Poljak RJ, Anzel LM, Ehcn BL, Phizackerley RP, Saul F: The three-dimensional structure of the Fab′ fragment of a human myeloma immunoglobulin at 2.0 Å resolution. *Proc Natl Acad Sci USA* **71:**3440, 1974.
43. Blake CCF, Geisow MJ, Oatley SJ: Structure of prealbumin: Secondary, tertiary and quaternary interactions determined by Fourier refinement at 1.8 Å. *J Mol Biol* **121:**339, 1978.
44. Randall RE, Williamson WC Jr, Mullinax F, Tung MX, Still WJS: Manifestations of light chain deposition. *Am J Med* **60:**293, 1976.
45. Preud'homme JL, Morel-Maroger L, Brovet JC, Cerf M, Mignon F, Guglielmi P, Seligmann M: Synthesis of abnormal immunoglobulin in lymphoplasmolytic disorders with visceral light chain deposition. *Am J Med* **69:**703, 1980.
46. Hofmann-Guilaine C, Nochy D, Jacquot C, Bariety J, Camilleri JP: Association light chain deposition disease (LCDD) and amyloidosis. *Pathol Res Pract* **180:**214, 1985.
47. Jacquot C, Saint-Andre JP, Touchard G, Hochy D, De Lamartinie CD, Oriol R, Dwulet P, Bariety J: Association of systemic light-chain deposition disease and amyloidosis: A report of three patients with renal involvement. *Clin Nephrol* **24:**93, 1985.
48. WHO-IUIS Nomenclature Sub-Committee: Nomenclature of amyloid and amyloidosis. *Bull World Health Organ* **71:**105, 1993.
49. Heller H, Sohar E, Gafni J, Heller J: Amyloidosis in familial Mediterranean fever. *Arch Intern Med* **107:**539, 1961.
50. Schimke RN, Hartmann WH: Familial amyloid-producing medullary thyroid carcinoma and pheochromocytoma: Distinct genetic entity. *Ann Intern Med* **63:**1027, 1965.
51. Sipple JH: The association of pheochromocytoma with carcinoma of the thyroid gland. *Am J Med* **31:**163, 1961.
52. Sagher F, Shanon J: Amyloid cutis: Familial occurrence in three generations. *Arch Dermatol* **87:**171, 1963.
53. Rajagopalan K, Tay CH: Familial lichen amyloidosis: Report of 19 cases in 4 generations of a Chinese family in Malaysia. *Br J Dermatol* **87:**123, 1972.
54. Davies P: The genetics of Alzheimer's disease: A review and a discussion of the implications. *Neurobiol Aging* **7:**459, 1986.
55. Bardin T, Kuntz D, Zingraff J, Voisin M, Zelmar A, Lansaman J: Synovial amyloidosis in patients undergoing long-term hemodialysis. *Arthritis Rheum* **28:**1052, 1985.
56. Gejyo F, Yamada T, Odani S, Nakagawa Y, Arakawa M, Kunit-Omo T, Kataoka H, Suzuki M, Hirasawa Y, Shirahama T, Cohen AS, Schmid K: A new form of

amyloid protein associated with chronic hemodialysis was identified as B2-microglobulin. *Biochem Biophys Res Commun* **129**:701, 1985.

57. Eulitz M, Weiss DT, Solomon A: Immunoglobulin heavy-chain-associated amyloidosis. *Proc Natl Acad Sci USA* **87**:6542, 1990.
58. Kyle RA, Greipp PR: Amyloidosis (AL): Clinical and laboratory features in 229 cases. *Mayo Clin Proc* **58**:665, 1983.
59. Brandt KD, Cathcart ES, Cohen AS: A clinical analysis of the course and prognosis of 42 patients with amyloidosis. *Am J Med* 44:955, 1968.
60. Greipp PR, Kyle RA, Bowie WEJ: Factor-X deficiency in amyloidosis in a critical review. *Am J Hematol* **11**:443, 1981.
61. Benson MD, Cohen AS, Brandt KD, Cathcart ES: Neuropathy, M-components and amyloid. *Lancet* **1**:10, 1975.
62. Kyle RA, Gertz MA: Systemic amyloidosis. *Crit Rev Oncol Hematol* **10**:49, 1990.
63. Kyle RA, Wagoner RD, Holley KE: Primary systemic amyloidosis: Resolution of the nephrotic syndrome with melphalan and prednisone. *Arch Intern Med* **142**:1445, 1982.
64. Benson MD: Treatment of AL amyloidosis with melphalan, prednisone and colchicine. *Arthritis Rheum* **29**:683–687, 1986.
65. Cohen AS, Rubinow A, Anderson JJ, Skinner M, Mason JH, Libbey C, Kayne H: Survival of patients with primary (AL) amyloidosis. *Am J Med* **82**:1182, 1987.
66. Kedar (Keizman) I, Ravid M, Sohar E, Gafmi J: Colchicine inhibition of casein-induced amyloidosis in mice. *Isr J Med Sci* **10**:787, 1974.
67. Shirahama T, Cohen AS: Blockage of amyloid induction by colchicine in an animal model. *J Exp Med* **140**:1102, 1974.
68. Greipp PR, Kyle RA, Bowie EJW: Factor-X deficiency in primary amyloidosis: Resolution after splenectomy. *N Engl J Med* **301**:1050, 1979.
69. Benditt EP, Eriksen N, Hermodson MA, Ericsson LH: The major proteins of human and monkey amyloid substance: Common properties including unusual N-terminal amino acid sequences. *FEBS Lett* **19**:169, 1971.
70. Benditt EP, Eriksen N: Amyloid protein SAA is associated with high density lipoproteins from human serum. *Proc Natl Acad Sci USA* **74**:4025, 1977.
71. Benditt EP, Eriksen N, Hanson RH: Amyloid protein SAA is an apoprotein of mouse plasma high density lipoprotein. *Proc Natl Acad Sci USA* **76**:4092, 1979.
72. Sipe JD, Vogel SN, Ryan JL, McAdams KPWJ, Rosenstreich DL: Detection of a mediator derived from endotoxin-stimulated macrophages that induces the acute phase serum amyloid A response in mice. *J Exp Med* **150**:597, 1979.
73. Morrow JF, Stearman RS, Peltzman CG, Potter DA: Induction of hepatic synthesis of serum amyloid A protein and actin. *Proc Natl Acad Sci USA* **78**:4718, 1981.
74. Kluve-Beckerman B, Naylor SL, Marshal A, Gardner JC, Shows TB, Benson MD: Localization of human SAA gene(s) to chromosome 11 and detection of DNA polymorphisms. *Biochem Biophys Res Commun* **137**:1196, 1986.
75. Taylor BA, Rowe L: Genes for serum amyloid A proteins map to chromosome 7 in the mouse. *Mol Gen Genet* **195**:491, 1984.
76. Yamamoto K, Migita S: Complete primary structure of two major murine serum amyloids A proteins deduced from cDNA sequence. *Proc Natl Acad Sci USA* **82**:2915, 1985.
77. Lowell CA, Potter DA, Stearman RS, Morrow JF: Structure of the murine serum amyloid A gene family. *J Biol Chem* **261**:8442, 1986.
78. deBeer MC, Beach CM, Shedlofsky SI, deBeer FC: Identification of a novel serum amyloid A protein (SAA) in Balb/C mice. *Biochem J* **280**:45, 1991.
79. Meek RL, Eriksen N, Benditt EP: Murine serum amyloid A_3 is a high density apolipoprotein and is secreted by macrophages. *Proc Natl Acad Sci USA* **89**:7949, 1992.
80. Mitchell TI, Coon CI, Brinckerhoff CE: Serum amyloid A (SAA3) produced by rabbit synovial fibroblasts treated with phorbol esters or interleukin 1 induces synthesis of collagenase and is neutralized by specific antiserum. *J Clin Invest* **87**:1177, 1991.
81. Kluve-Beckerman B, Drumm ML, Benson MD: Nonexpression of the human serum amyloid A three (SAA3) gene. *DNA Cell Biol* **10**:651, 1991.
82. Whitehead AS, deBeer MC, Steel DM, Rits M, Lelias JM, Lane WS, deBeer FC: Identification of novel members of the serum amyloid A protein superfamily as constitutive apolipoproteins of high density lipoprotein. *J Biol Chem* **267**:3862, 1992.
83. Hoffman JS, Ericsson LH, Eriksen N, Walsh KA, Benditt EP: Murine tissue amyloid protein AA NH_2-terminal sequence identity with only one of two serum amyloid protein (ApoSAA) gene products. *J Exp Med* **159**:641, 1984.
84. Dwulet FE, Wallace DK, Benson MD: Amino acid structures of multiple forms of amyloid-related serum protein SAA from a single individual. *Biochemistry* **27**:1677, 1988.
85. Parmalee DC, Titani K, Ericsson LH, Eriksen N, Benditt EP, Walsh KA: Amino acid sequence of amyloid related apoprotein (apoSAA) from human high-density lipoproteins. *Biochemistry* **21**:3298, 1982.
86. Lavie G, Zucker-Franklin D, Franklin EC: Degradation of serum amyloid A protein by surface-associated enzymes of human blood monocytes. *J Exp Med* **148**:1020, 1978.
87. Zemer D, Pras M, Sohar E, Modan M, Cabili S, Gafni J: Colchicine in the prevention and treatment of the amyloidosis of familial Mediterranean fever. *N Engl J Med* **314**:1001, 1986.
88. Assenat H, Calemard E, Charra B, Laurent G, Terrat JC, Vanel T: Hémodialyse, syndrome du canal carpien et substance amyloïde. *Nouv Presse Med* **9**:1715, 1980.
89. Clanet M, Mansat M, Durroux R, Testut MF, Guiraud B, Rascol A, Conte J: Syndrome du canal carpien, ténosynovite amyloïde et hémodialyse périodique. *Rev Neurol (Paris)* **137**:613, 1981.
90. Bardin T, Kuntz D, Zingraff J, Voisin M-C, Zelmar A, Lansaman J: Synovial amyloidosis in patients undergoing long-term hemodialysis. *Arthritis Rheum* **28**:1052, 1985.
91. Gejyo F, Yamada T, Odani S, Nakagawa Y, Arakawa M, Kunitomo T, Kataoka H, Suzuki M, Hirasawa Y, Shirahama T, Cohen AS, Schmid K: A new form of amyloid protein associated with chronic hemodialysis was identified as β_2-microglobulin. *Biochem Biophys Res Commun* **129**:701, 1985.
92. Gorevic PD, Stone TT, Stone WJ, DiRaimondo CR, Prelli FC, Frangione B: Beta-2-microglobulin is an amyloidogenic protein in man. *J Clin Invest* **76**:2425, 1985.
93. Floege J, Bartsch A, Schulze M, Shaldon S, Koch KM, Smeby C: Clearance and synthesis rates of β_2-microglobulin in patients undergoing hemodialysis and in normal subjects. *J Lab Clin Med* **118**:153, 1991.
94. Dwulet FE, Benson MD: Primary structure of amyloid fibril protein AA in azocasein-induced amyloidosis of CBA/J mice. *J Lab Clin Med* **110**:322, 1987.
95. Westermark P, Johnson KH, Westermark GT, Sletten K, Hayden DW: Bovine amyloid protein AA: Isolation and amino acid sequence analysis. *Comp Biochem Physiol* **85B**:609, 1986.
96. Benson MD, Dwulet FE, DiBartola SP: Identification and characterization of amyloid protein AA in spontaneous canine amyloidosis. *Lab Invest* **52**:448, 1985.
97. DiBartola SP, Benson MD, Dwulet FE, Cornacoff JB: Isolation and characterization of amyloid protein AA in the Abyssinian cat. *Lab Invest* **52**:485, 1985.
98. Skinner M, Cathcart ES, Cohen AS, Benson MD: Isolation and identification by sequence analysis of experimentally induced guinea pig amyloid fibrils. *J Exp Med* **140**:871, 1974.
99. Anders RF, Nordstoga K, Natvig JB, Husby G: Amyloid-related serum protein SAA in endotoxin-induced amyloidosis of the mink. *J Exp Med* **143**:678, 1976.
100. Gorevic PD, Greenwald M, Frangione B, Pras M, Franklin EC: The amino acid sequence of duck amyloid A (AA) protein. *J Immunol* **118**:1113, 1977.
101. Machada EA, Gregory RS, Jones JB, Lange RD: The cyclic hematopoietic dog: A model for spontaneous secondary amyloidosis. *Am J Pathol* **92**:23, 1978.
102. Boyce JT, DiBartola SP, Chew DJ, Gasper PW: Familial renal amyloidosis in Abyssinian cats. *Vet Pathol* **21**:33, 1984.
103. Yonezu T, Tsunasawa S, Higuchi K, Kogishi K, Naiki H, Hanada K, Sakiyama F, Takeda T: A molecular-pathologic approach to murine senile amyloidosis. *Lab Invest* **57**:65, 1987.

104. Kuczynski MH: Neue Beitraege zur Lehre vom Amyloid. *Klin Wochenschr* **2**:727, 1923.
105. Kuczynski MH: Weitere Beitraege zur Lehre vom Amyloid 3. Mitteilung, Ueber die Rueckbildung des Amyloids. *Klin Wochenschr* **2**:2193, 1923.
106. Sipe JD, McAdams KPWJ, Uchino F: Biochemical evidence for the biphasic development of experimental amyloidosis. *Lab Invest* **38**:110, 1978.
107. Yamamoto K, Shiroo M, Migita S: Diverse gene expression for isotypes of murine serum amyloid A protein during acute phase reaction. *Science* **232**:227, 1986.
108. Shirahama T, Cohen AS: Redistribution of amyloid deposits. *Am J Pathol* **99**:539, 1980.
109. Solomon A, Weiss DT, Pepys MB: Induction in mice of human light-chain-associated amyloidosis. *Am J Pathol* **140**:629, 1992.
110. Sasaki H, Tone S, Nakazato M, Yoshioka K, Matsuo H, Kato Y, Sakaki Y: Generation of transgenic mice producing a human transthyretin variant: A possible mouse model for familial amyloidotic polyneuropathy. *Biochem Biophys Res Commun* **139**:794, 1986.
111. Wakasugi S, Inomoto T, Yi S, Naito M, Uehira M, Iwanaga T, Maeda S, Araki K, Miyazaki J, Takahashi K, Shimada K, Yamamura K: A transgenic mouse model of familial amyloidotic polyneuropathy. *Proc Jpn Acad* **63(B)**:344, 1987.
112. Yi S, Takahashi K, Naito M, Tashiro F, Wakasugi S, Maeda S, Shimada K, Yamamura K, Araki S: Systemic amyloidosis in transgenic mice carrying the human mutant transthyretin (Met30) gene. *Am J Pathol* **138**:403, 1991.
113. Branch WT Jr, Robbins J, Edelhock H: Thyroxine-binding prealbumin. *J Biol Chem* **246**:6011, 1971.
114. Robbins J: Thyroxine-binding proteins. *Prog Clin Biol Res* **5**:331, 1976.
115. NC-IUB and JCBN Newsletter, Nomenclature Committee of IUB. *J Biol Chem* **256**:12, 1981.
116. Costa RH, Lai E, Darnell JE: Transcriptional control of the mouse prealbumin (transthyretin) gene: Both promotor sequences and a distinct enhancer are cell specific. *Mol Cell Biol* **6**:4697, 1986.
117. Kanda Y, Goodman DS, Canfield RE, Morgan FJ: The amino acid sequence of human plasma prealbumin. *J Biol Chem* **249**:6796, 1974.
118. Blake CCF, Geisow MJ, Swan IDA: Structure of human plasma prealbumin at 2.5 Å resolution. *J Mol Biol* **88**:1, 1974.
119. Oatley SJ, Blaney JM, Langridge R, Kollman PA: Molecular mechanical studies of hormone-protein interactions: The interaction of T4 and T3 with prealbumin. *Biopolymers* **23**:2931, 1984.
120. Goodman DS: Retinol-binding protein, prealbumin and vitamin A transport. *Prog Clin Biol Res* **5**:313, 1976.
121. Benson MD, Dwulet FE: Prealbumin and retinol binding protein serum concentrations in the Indiana type hereditary amyloidosis. *Arthritis Rheum* **26**:1493, 1983.
122. Skinner M, Connors LH, Rubinow A, Libbey C, Sipe JD, Cohen AS: Lowered prealbumin levels in patients with familial amyloid polyneuropathy (FAP) and their non-affected but at risk relatives. *Am J Med Sci* **289**:17, 1985.
123. Westermark P, Pitkanen P, Benson L, Vahlquist A, Olofsson BO, Cornwell GG III: Serum prealbumin and retinol-binding protein in the prealbumin-related senile and familial forms of systemic amyloidosis. *Lab Invest* **52**:314, 1985.
124. Wallace MR, Naylor SL, Kluve-Beckerman B, Long GL, McDonald L, Shows TB, Benson MD: Localization of the human prealbumin gene to chromosome 18. *Biochem Biophys Res Commun* **129**:753, 1985.
125. Benson MD, Dwulet FE: Identification of carriers of a variant plasma prealbumin (transthyretin) associated with familial amyloidotic polyneuropathy type I. *J Clin Invest* **75**:71, 1985.
126. Dwulet FE, Benson MD: Primary structure of an amyloid prealbumin and its plasma precursor in a heredofamilial polyneuropathy of Swedish origin. *Proc Natl Acad Sci USA* **81**:694, 1984.
127. Hamilton JA, Steinrauf LK, Braden BC, Liepnieks J, Benson MD, Holmgren G, Sandgren O, Steen L: The X-ray crystal structure refinements of normal human transthyretin and the amyloidogenic Val-30 → Met variant to 1.7-Å resolution. *J Biol Chem* **268**:2416, 1993.
128. Moses AC, Rosen HN, Moller DE, Tsuzaki S, Haddow JE, Lawlor J, Liepnieks JJ, Nichols WC, Benson MD: A point mutation in transthyretin increases affinity for thyroxine and produces euthyroid hyperthyroxinemia. *J Clin Invest* **86**:2025, 1990.
129. Harrison HH, Gordon ED, Nichols WC, Benson MD: Biochemical and clinical characterization of prealbumin^{CHICAGO}: An apparently benign variant of serum prealbumin (transthyretin) discovered with high-resolution two-dimensional electrophoresis. *Am J Med Genet* **39**:442, 1991.
130. Mita S, Maeda S, Shimada K, Araki S: Cloning and sequence analysis of cDNA for human prealbumin. *Biochem Biophys Res Commun* **124**:558, 1984.
131. Sasaki H, Sakaki Y, Matsuo H, Goto I, Kuroiwa Y, Sahashi I, Takahashi A, Shinoda T, Isobe T, Takagi Y: Diagnosis of familial amyloidotic polyneuropathy by recombinant DNA techniques. *Biochem Biophys Res Commun* **125**:636, 1984.
132. Tsuzuki T, Mita S, Maeda S, Araki S, Shimada K: Structure of the human prealbumin gene. *J Biol Chem* **260**:12224, 1985.
133. Sasaki H, Yoshioka N, Takagi Y, Sakaki Y: Structure of the chromosomal gene for human serum prealbumin. *Gene* **37**:191, 1985.
134. Wakasugi S, Maeda S, Shimada K: Structure and expression of the mouse prealbumin gene. *J Biochem* **100**:49, 1986.
135. Soprano DR, Herber J, Soprano KJ, Schon EA, Goodman DS: Demonstration of transthyretin mRNA in the brain and other extrahepatic tissues in the rat. *J Biol Chem* **260**:11793, 1985.
136. Dickson PW, Aldred AR, Marley PD, Guo-Fen T, Howlett GJ, Schreiber G: High prealbumin and transferrin mRNA levels in the choroid plexus of rat brain. *Biochem Biophys Res Commun* **127**:890, 1985.
137. Stauder AJ, Dickson PW, Aldred AR, Schreiber G, Mendelsohn FAO, Hudson P: Synthesis of transthyretin (prealbumin) mRNA in choroid plexus epithelial cells, localized by in situ hydridization in rat brain. *J Histochem Cytochem* **34**:949, 1986.
138. Dickson PW, Schreiber G: High levels of messenger RNA for transthyretin (prealbumin) in human choroid plexus. *Neurosci Lett* **66**:311, 1986.
139. Andrade A, Araki S, Block WD, Cohen AS, Jackson CE, Kuroiwa Y, McKusick VA, Nissim J, Sohar E, Vanallen MW: Hereditary amyloidosis. *Arthritis Rheum* **13**:902, 1970.
140. Frederiksen T, Gotzsche H, Harboe N, Kiaer W, Mellemgaard K: Familial primary amyloidosis with severe amyloid heart disease. *Am J Med* **33**:328, 1962.
141. Uemichi T, Murrell JR, Zeldenrust S, Benson MD: A new mutant transthyretin (Arg 10) associated with familial amyloid polyneuropathy. *J Med Genet* **29**:888, 1992.
142. Saraiva MJM, Birken S, Costa PP, Goodman DS: Amyloid fibril protein in familial amyloidotic polyneuropathy, Portuguese type. *J Clin Invest* **74**:104, 1984.
143. Tawara S, Nakazato M, Kangawa K, Matsuo H, Araki S: Identification of amyloid prealbumin variant in familial amyloidotic polyneuropathy (Japanese type). *Biochem Biophys Res Commun* **116**:880, 1983.
144. Skinner M, Cohen AS: The prealbumin nature of the amyloid protein in familial amyloid polyneuropathy (FAP)—Swedish variety. *Biochem Biophys Res Commun* **99**:1326, 1981.
145. Holmgren G, Holmberg E, Lindstrom A, Lindstrom E, Nordenson I, Sandgren O, Steen L, Svensson B, Lundgren E, Von Gabain A: Diagnosis of familial amyloidotic polyneuropathy in Sweden by RFLP analysis. *Clin Genet* **32**:289, 1988.
146. Holmgren G, Bergström S, Drugge U, Lundgren E, Nording-Sikström C, Sandgren O, Steen L: Homozygosity for the transthyretin-Met30-gene in seven individuals with familial amyloidosis with polyneuropathy detected by restriction enzyme analysis of amplified genomic DNA sequences. *Clin Genet* **41**:39, 1992.
147. Skare J, Yazier H, Erken E, Dede H, Cohen A, Milun-

sky A, Skinner M: Homozygosity for the met30 transthyretin gene in a Turkish kindred with familial amyloidotic polyneuropathy. *Hum Genet* **86**:89, 1990.
148. Benson MD, Cohen AS: Generalized amyloid in a family of Swedish origin. A study of 426 family members in 7 generations of a new kinship with neuropathy, nephropathy and central nervous system involvement. *Ann Intern Med* **86**:419, 1977.
149. Yoshioka K, Furuya H, Sasaki H, Saraiva MJM, Costa PP, Sakaki Y: Haplotype analysis of familial amyloidotic polyneuropathy. *Hum Genet* **82**:9, 1980.
150. Kincaid JC, Wallace MR, Benson MD: Late-onset familial amyloid polyneuropathy in an American family of English origin. *Neurology* **39**:861, 1989.
151. Jones LA, Skare JC, Cohen AS, Harding JA, Milunsky A, Skinner M: Familial amyloidotic polyneuropathy: A new transthyretin position 30 mutation (alanine for valine) in a family of German descent. *Clin Genet* **41**:70, 1992.
152. Nakazato M, Ikeda S, Shiomi K, Matsukura S, Yoshida K, Shimizu H, Atsumi T, Kangawa K, Matsuo H: Identification of a novel transthyretin variant ($Val^{30} \rightarrow$ Leu) associated with familial amyloidotic polyneuropathy. *FEBS Lett* **306**:206, 1992.
153. Murakami T, Atsumi T, Maeda S, Tanase S, Ishikawa K, Mita S, Kumamoto T, Araki S, Ando M: A novel transthyretin mutation at position 30 (Leu for Val) associated with familial amyloidotic polyneuropathy. *Biochem Biophys Res Commun* **187**:397, 1992.
154. Gafni J, Fischel B, Reif R, Yaron M, Pras M: Amyloidotic polyneuropathy in a Jewish family. Evidence for the genetic heterogeneity of the lower limb familial amyloidotic neuropathies. *Q J Med* **55**:33, 1985.
155. Pras M, Prelli F, Franklin EC, Frangione B: Primary structure of an amyloid prealbumin variant in familial polyneuropathy of Jewish origin. *Proc Natl Acad Sci USA* **80**:539, 1983.
156. Nakazato M, Kangawa K, Minamino N, Tawara S, Matsuo H, Araki S: Revised analysis of amino acid replacement in a prealbumin variant (SKO-III) associated with familial amyloidotic polyneuropathy of Jewish origin. *Biochem Biophys Res Commun* **123**:921, 1984.
157. Harding J, Skare J, Skinner M: A second transthyretin mutation at position 33 (Leu/Phe) associated with familial amyloidotic polyneuropathy. *Biochim Biophys Acta* **1097**:183, 1991.
158. Jones LA, Skare JC, Harding JA, Cohen AS, Milunsky A, Skinner M: Proline at position 36: A new transthyretin mutation associated with familial amyloidotic polyneuropathy. *Am J Hum Genet* **48**:979, 1991.
159. Jacobson DR, Rosenthal CJ, Buxbaum JN: Transthyretin Pro 36 associated with familial amyloidotic polyneuropathy in an Ashkenazic Jewish kindred. *Hum Genet* **90**:158, 1992.
160. Uemichi T, Ueno S, Fujimura H, Umekage T, Yorifuji S, Matsuzawa Y, Tarui S: Familial amyloid polyneuropathy related to transthyretin Gly42 in a Japanese family. *Muscle Nerve* **15**:904, 1992.
161. Saraiva MJM, Almeida MR, Sherman W, Gawinowicz M, Costa P, Costa PP, Goodman DS: A new transthyretin mutation associated with amyloid cardiomyopathy. *Am J Hum Genet* **50**:1027, 1992.
162. Murakami T, Maeda S, Yi S, Ikegawa S, Kawashima E, Onodera S, Shimada K, Araki S: A novel transthyretin mutation associated with familial amyloidotic polyneuropathy. *Biochem Biophys Res Commun* **182**:520, 1992.
163. Ferlini A, Salvi F, Patrosso C, Fini S, Vezzoni P, Forabosco A: Gly47Ala: A new transthyretin gene mutation in hereditary amyloidosis TTR-related. *J Rheumatol* **20**:187, 1993.
164. Almeida MR, Ferlini A, Forabosco A, Gawinowicz MA, Costa PP, Salvi F, Plasmati R, Tassinari CA, Altland K, Saraiva MJ: Two transthyretin variants (TTR Ala-49 and TTR Gln-89) in two Sicilian kindreds with hereditary amyloidosis. *Hum Mutat* **1**:211, 1992.
165. Benson MD II, Julien J, Liepnieks J, Zeldenrust S, Benson MD: A transthyretin variant (alanine 49) associated with familial amyloidotic polyneuropathy in a French family. *J Med Genet* **30**:117, 1993.
166. Julien J, Vital CI, Vallat JM, Lagueny A, Ferrer X: Familial amyloid neuropathy in three families of French origin. *Rev Neurol (Paris)* **139**:259, 1983.
167. Ueno S, Uemichi T, Takahashi N, Soga F, Yorifuji S, Tarui S: Two novel variants of transthyretin identified in Japanese cases with familial amyloidotic polyneuropathy: Transthyretin (Glu^{42} to Gly) and transthyretin (Ser^{50} to Arg). *Biochem Biophys Res Commun* **169**:1117, 1990.
168. Takahashi N, Ueno S, Uemichi T, Fujimura H, Yorifuji S, Tarui S: Amyloid polyneuropathy with transthyretin Arg50 in a Japanese case from Osaka. *J Neurol Sci* **112**:58, 1992.
169. Saeki Y, Ueno S, Takahashi N, Soga F, Yanagihara T: A novel mutant (transthyretin Ile-50) related to amyloid polyneuropathy. *FEBS Lett* **308**:35, 1992.
170. Nishi H, Kimura A, Harada H, Hayashi Y, Nakamura M, Sasazuki T: Novel variant transthyretin gene (Ser^{50} to Ile) in familial cardiac amyloidosis. *Biochem Biophys Res Commun* **187**:460, 1992.
171. Jacobson DR, McFarlin DE, Kane I, Buxbaum JN: Transthyretin Pro55, a variant associated with early-onset, aggressive diffuse amyloidosis with cardiac and neurologic involvement. *Hum Genet* **89**:353, 1992.
172. Mahloudji M, Teasdall RD, Adamkiewicz JJ, Hartmann WH, Lambird PA, McKusick VA: The genetic amyloidoses. With particular reference to hereditary neuropathic amyloidosis, type II (Indiana or Rukavina type). *Medicine* **48**:1, 1969.
173. Nichols WC, Liepnieks JJ, McKusick VA, Benson MD: Direct sequencing of the gene for Maryland/German familial amyloidotic polyneuropathy type II and genotyping by allele-specific enzymatic amplification. *Genomics* **5**:535, 1989.
174. Mendell JR, Jiang X-S, Warmolts JR, Nichols WC, Benson MD: Diagnosis of Maryland/German familial amyloidotic polyneuropathy using allele-specific, enzymatically amplified genomic DNA. *Ann Neurol* **27**:553, 1990.
175. Jacobson DR, Gorevic PD, Sack GH, Malamet RL: Homozygous transthyretin His 58 associated with unusually aggressive familial amyloidotic polyneuropathy. *J Rheumatol* **20**:178, 1993.
176. Saeki Y, Ueno S, Yorifuji S, Sugiyama Y, Ide Y, Matsuzawa Y: New mutant gene (transthyretin Arg 58) in cases with hereditary polyneuropathy detected by non-isotope method of single-strand conformation polymorphism analysis. *Biochem Biophys Res Commun* **180**:380, 1991.
177. Wallace MR, Dwulet FE, Conneally PM, Benson MD: Biochemical and molecular genetic characterization of a new variant prealbumin associated with hereditary amyloidosis. *J Clin Invest* **78**:6, 1986.
178. Benson MD, Wallace MR, Tejada E, Baumann H, Page B: Hereditary amyloidosis: Description of a new American kindred with late onset cardiomyopathy. *Arthritis Rheum* **30**:195, 1987.
179. Koeppen AH, Wallace MR, Benson MD, Altland K: Familial amyloid polyneuropathy: Alanine-for-threonine substitution in the transthyretin (prealbumin) molecule. *Muscle Nerve* **13**:1065, 1990.
180. Ii S, Minnerath S, Ii K, Dyck PJ, Sommer SS: Two-tiered DNA-based diagnosis of transthyretin amyloidosis reveals two novel point mutations. *Neurology* **41**:893, 1991.
181. Almeida MR, Hesse JA, Steinmetz A, Maisch B, Altland K, Linke RP, Gawinowicz MA, Saraiva MJM: Transthyretin Leu 68 in a form of cardiac amyloidosis. *Basic Res Cardiol* **86**:567, 1991.
182. Zeldenrust SR, Skinner M, Harding J, Skare J, Benson MD: A new transthyretin variant (His-69) associated with vitreous amyloid in an FAP family. *Amyloid* **1**:17, 1994.
183. Izumoto S, Younger D, Hays AP, Martone RL, Smith RT, Herbert J: Familial amyloidotic polyneuropathy presenting with carpal tunnel syndrome and a new transthyretin mutation, asparagine 70. *Neurology* **42**:2094, 1992.
184. Benson MD II, Turpin JC, Lucotte G, Zeldenrust S, LeChevalier, Benson MD: A transthyretin variant (alanine 71) associated with familial amyloidotic polyneuropathy in a French family. *J Med Genet* **30**:120, 1993.
185. Wallace MR, Dwulet FE, Williams EC, Conneally PM, Benson MD: Identification of a new hereditary amyloid

prealbumin variant, Tyr-77, associated with autosomal dominant amyloidosis. *Am J Hum Genet* **39:**A22, 1986.

186. Libbey CA, Rubinow A, Shirahama T, Deal C, Cohen AS: Familial amyloid polyneuropathy. Demonstration of prealbumin in a kinship of German/English ancestry with onset in the seventh decade. *Am J Med* **76:**18, 1984.
187. Satier F, Nichols WC, Benson MD: Diagnosis of familial amyloidotic polyneuropathy in France. *Clin Genet* **38:**469, 1990.
188. Falls HF, Jackson JH, Carey JG, Rukavina JG, Block WD: Ocular manifestations of hereditary primary systemic amyloidosis. *Arch Ophthalmol* **54:**660, 1955.
189. Rukavina JG, Block WD, Jackson CE, Falls HF, Carey JH, Curtis AC: Primary systemic amyloidosis: A review and an experimental, genetic, and clinical study of 29 cases with particular emphasis on the familial form. *Medicine* **35:**239, 1956.
190. Dwulet FE, Benson MD: Characterization of a transthyretin (prealbumin) variant associated with familial amyloidotic polyneuropathy type II (Indiana/Swiss). *J Clin Invest* **78:**880, 1986.
191. Wallace MR, Conneally PM, Benson MD: A DNA test for Indiana/Swiss hereditary amyloidosis (FAP II). *Am J Hum Genet* **43:**182, 1988.
192. Benson MD, Dwulet FE: Prealbumin and retinol binding protein serum concentrations in the Indiana type hereditary amyloidosis. *Arthritis Rheum* **26:**1493, 1983.
193. Skinner M, Harding J, Skare I, Jones LA, Cohen AS, Milunsky A, Skare J: A new transthyretin mutation associated with amyloidotic vitreous opacities. Asparagine for isoleucine at position 84. *Ophthalmology* **99:**503, 1992.
194. Uemichi T, Gertz MA, Benson MD: Amyloid polyneuropathy in two German-American families: A new transthyretin variant (Val 107). *J Med Genet* **31**:416, 1994.
195. Frederiksen T, Gotzsche H, Harboe N, Kiaer W, Mellemgaard K: Familial primary amyloidosis with severe amyloid heart disease. *Am J Med* **33:**328, 1962.
196. Nordlie M, Sletten K, Husby G, Panløv PJ: A new prealbumin variant in familial amyloid cardiomyopathy of Danish origin. *Scand J Immunol* **27:**119, 1988.
197. Ranløv I, Alves IL, Ranløv PJ, Husby G, Costa PP, Saraiva MJM: A Danish kindred with familial amyloid cardiomyopathy revisited: Identification of a mutant transthyretin-methionine[111] variant in serum from patients and carriers. *Am J Med* **93:**3, 1992.
198. Ueno S, Fujimura H, Yorifuji S, Nakamura Y, Takahashi M, Tarui S, Yanagihara T: Familial amyloid polyneuropathy associated with the transthyretin cys114 gene in a Japanese kindred. *Brain* **115:**1275, 1992.
199. Ueno S, Uemichi T, Yorifuji S, Tarui S: A novel variant of transthyretin (Tyr[114] to Cys) deduced from the nucleotide sequences of gene fragments from familial amyloidotic polyneuropathy in Japanese sibling cases. *Biochem Biophys Res Commun* **169:**143, 1990.
200. Gorevic PD, Prelli FC, Wright J, Pras M, Frangione B: Systemic senile amyloidosis. Identification of a new prealbumin (transthyretin) variant in cardiac tissue: Immunologic and biochemical similarity to one form of familial amyloidotic polyneuropathy. *J Clin Invest* **83:**836, 1989.
201. Jacobson DR, Gorevic PD, Buxbaum JN: A homozygous transthyretin variant associated with senile systemic amyloidosis: Evidence for a late-onset disease of genetic etiology. *Am J Hum Genet* **47:**127, 1990.
202. Nichols WC, Liepnieks JJ, Snyder EL, Benson MD: Senile cardiac amyloidosis associated with homozygosity for a transthyretin variant (Ile-122). *J Lab Clin Med* **117:**175, 1991.
203. Saraiva MJM, Sherman W, Marboe C, Figueira A, Costa P, De Freitas AF, Gawinowicz MA: Cardiac amyloidosis: Report of a patient heterozygous for the transthyretin isoleucine 122 variant. *Scand J Immunol* **32:**341, 1990.
204. Jacobson DR, Reveille JD, Buxbaum JN: Frequency and genetic background of the position 122 (Val → Ile) variant transthyretin gene in the black population. *Am J Hum Genet* **49:**192, 1991.
205. Buerger L, Braunstein H: Senile cardiac amyloidosis. *Am J Med* **28:**357, 1960.
206. Pomerance A: The pathology of senile cardiac amyloidosis. *J Pathol Bacteriol* **91:**357, 1966.
207. Hodkinson HM, Pomerance A: The clinical significance of senile cardiac amyloidosis: A prospective clinico-pathological study. *Q J Med* **46:**381, 1977.
208. Pitkanen P, Westermark P, Cornwell GG: Senile systemic amyloidosis. *Am J Pathol* **117:**391, 1984.
209. Cornwell GG, Westermark P, Natvig JB, Murdoch W: Senile cardiac amyloid: Evidence that fibrils contain a protein immunologically related to prealbumin. *Immunology* **44:**447, 1981.
210. Westermark P, Sletten K, Johansson B, Cornwell GG: Fibril in senile systemic amyloidosis is derived from normal transthyretin. *Proc Natl Acad Sci USA* **87:**2843, 1990.
211. Altland K, Becher P, Banzhoff A: Paraffin oil protected high resolution hybrid isoelectric focusing for the demonstration of substitutions of neutral amino acids in denatured proteins: The case of four human transthyretin (prealbumin) variants associated with familial amyloidotic polyneuropathy. *Electrophoresis* **8:**293, 1987.
212. Lalloz MRA, Byfield PGH, Goel KM, Loudon MM, Thomson JA, Himsworth RL: Hyperthyroxinemia due to the coexistence of two raised affinity thyroxine-binding proteins (albumin and prealbumin) in one family. *J Clin Endocrinol Metab* **64:**346, 1987.
213. Fitch NJS, Akbari MT, Ramsden DB: An inherited non-amyloidogenic transthyretin variant, [Ser[6]]-TTR, with increased thyroxine-binding affinity, characterized by DNA sequencing. *J Endocrinol* **129:**309, 1991.
214. Murrell JR, Schoner RG, Liepnieks JJ, Rosen HN, Moses AC, Benson MD: Production and functional analysis of normal and variant recombinant human transthyretin proteins. *J Biol Chem* **267:**16595, 1992.
215. Moses AC, Lawlor J, Haddow J, Jackson I: Familial euthyroid hyperthyroxinemia resulting from increased thyroxine-binding prealbumin. *N Engl J Med* **306:**966, 1982.
216. Steinrauf LK, Hamilton JA, Braden BC, Murrell JR, Benson MD: X-ray crystal structure of the Ala-109 → Thr variant of human transthyretin which produces euthyroid hyperthyroxinemia. *J Biol Chem* **268:**2425, 1990.
217. Holmgren G, Steen L, Ekstedt J, Groth C-G, Ericzon B-G, Eriksson S, Andersen O, Karlberg I, Norden G, Nakazato M, Hawkins P, Richardson S, Pepys M: Biochemical effect of liver transplantation in two Swedish patients with familial amyloidotic polyneuropathy (FAP-met[30]). *Clin Genet* **40:**242, 1991.
218. Holmgren G, Ericzon B-G, Groth C-G, Steen L, Suhr O, Andersen O, Wallin BG I, Seymour A, Richardson S, Hawkins PN, Pepys MB: Clinical improvement and mayloid regression after liver transplantation in hereditary transthyretin amyloidosis. *Lancet* **341:**1113, 1993.
219. Van Allen MW, Frohlich JA, Davis JR: Inherited predisposition to generalized amyloidosis. *Neurology* **19:**10, 1969.
220. Nichols WC, Gregg RE, Brewer HB Jr, Benson MD: A mutation in apolipoprotein A-I in the Iowa type of familial amyloidotic polyneuropathy. *Genomics* **8:**318, 1990.
221. Soutar AK, Hawkins PN, Vigushin DM, Tennent GA, Booth SE, Hutton T, Nguyen O, Totty NF, Feest TG, Hsuan JJ, Pepys MB: Apolipoprotein AI mutation Arg-60 causes autosomal dominant amyloidosis. *Proc Natl Acad Sci USA* **89:**7389, 1992.
222. Meretoja J: Familial systemic paramyloidosis with lattice dystrophy of the cornea, progressive cranial neuropathy, skin changes and various internal symptoms. *Ann Clin Res* **1:**314, 1969.
223. Meretoja J: Genetic aspects of familial amyloidosis with corneal lattice dystrophy and cranial neuropathy. *Clin Genet* **4:**173, 1973.
224. Meretoja J, Teppo L: Histopathological findings of familial amyloidosis with cranial neuropathy as principal manifestation. *Acta Pathol Microbiol Immunol Scand* **79:**432, 1971.
225. Klintworth GK: Lattice corneal dystrophy. An inherited variety of amyloidosis restricted to the cornea. *Am J Pathol* **50:**371, 1967.
226. Darras BT, Adelman LS, Mora JS, Bodziner RA, Munsat TL: Familial amyloidosis with cranial neuropathy and corneal lattice dystrophy. *Neurology* **36:**432, 1986.
227. Sack GH, Dumars KW, Gummerson KS, Law A, McKu-

sick VA: Three forms of dominant amyloid neuropathy. *Johns Hopkins Med J* **149**:239, 1981.

228. Maury CPJ: Isolation and characterization of cardiac amyloid in familial amyloid poly neuropathy type IV (Finnish): Relation of the amyloid protein to variant gelsolin. *Biochim Biophys Acta* **1096**:84, 1990.
229. Maury CPJ, Kere J, Tolvanen R, de la Chapelle A: Finnish hereditary amyloidosis is caused by a single nucleotide substitution in the gelsolin gene. *FEBS Lett* **276**:75, 1990.
230. Levy E, Haltia M, Fernandez-Madrid I, Koivunen O, Ghiso J, Prelli F, Frangione B: Mutation in gelsolin gene in Finnish hereditary amyloidosis. *J Exp Med* **172**:1865, 1990.
231. de la Chapelle A, Kere J, Sack GH Jr, Tolvanen R, Maury CPJ: Familial amyloidosis, Finnish type: G654 → A mutation of the gelsolin gene in Finnish families and an unrelated American family. *Genomics* **13**:898, 1992.
232. Sunada Y, Shimizu T, Nakase H, Ohta S, Asaoka T, Amano S, Sawa M, Kagawa Y, Kanazawa I, Mannen T: Inherited amyloid polyneuropathy type IV (gelsolin variant) in a Japanese family. *Ann Neurol* **33**:57, 1993.
233. de la Chapelle A, Tolvanen R, Boysen G, Santavy J, Blecker-Wagemakers L, Maury CPJ, Kere J: Gelsolin-derived familial amyloidosis caused by asparagine or tyrosine substitution for aspartic acid at residue 187. *Nat Genet* **2**:157, 1992.
234. Maury CPJ, Kere J, Tolvanen R, de la Chapelle A: Homozygosity for the Asn187 gelsolin mutation in Finnish-type familial amyloidosis is associated with severe renal disease. *Genomics* **13**:902, 1992.
235. Wiens A, Marles S, Safneck J, Kwiatkowski DJ, Maury CPJ, Zelinski T, Phillipps S, Elkins MB, Greenberg CR: Exclusion of the gelsolin gene on 9q32-34 as the cause of familial lattice corneal dystrophy type I. *Am J Hum Genet* **51**:156, 1992.
236. Yin HL, Kwiatkowski DJ, Mole JE, Cole FS: Structure and biosynthesis of cytoplasmic and secreted variants of gelsolin. *J Biol Chem* **259**:5271, 1984.
237. Kwiatkowski DJ, Mehl R, Yin HL: Genomic organization and biosynthesis of secreted and cytoplasmic forms of gelsolin. *J Cell Biol* **106**:375, 1988.
238. Kwiatkowski DJ, Westbrook CA, Bruns GAP, Morton CC: Localization of gelsolin proximal to ABL on chromosome 9. *Am J Hum Genet* **42**:565, 1988.
239. Kwiatkowski DJ, Mehl R, Izumo S, Nadal-Ginard B, Yin HL: Muscle is the major source of plasma gelsolin. *J Biol Chem* **263**:8239, 1988.
240. Shafer JA, Higgins DL: Human fibrinogen. *CRC Crit Rev Clin Lab Sci* **26**:1, 1988.
241. Doolittle RF, Watt KWK, Cottrell BA, Strong DD, Riley M: The amino acid sequence of the α-chain of human fibrinogen. *Nature* **280**:464, 1979.
242. Rixon MW, Chan WY, Davie EW, Chung DW: Characterization of a complementary deoxyribonucleic acid coding for the α chain of human fibrinogen. *Biochemistry* **22**:3237, 1983.
243. Matsuda M, Yoshida N, Terukina S, Yamazumi K, Mackawa H: Molecular abnormalities of fibrinogen—the present status of structure elucidation, in Matsuda M, Iwanage S, Takada A, Henschen A (eds): *Fibrinogen 4: Current Basic and Clinical Aspects*. Amsterdam, Excerpta Medica, 1990, p 139.
244. Pepys MB, Hawkins PN, Booth DR, Vigushin DM, Tennent GA, Soutar AK, Totty N, Nguyen O, Blake CCF, Terry CJ, Feest TG, Zalin AM, Hsuan JJ: Human lysozyme gene mutations cause hereditary systemic amyloidosis. *Nature* **362**:553, 1993.
245. Gudmundsson G, Hallgrimsson J, Jonasson TA, Bjarnason O: Hereditary cerebral hemorrhage with amyloidosis. *Brain* **95**:387, 1972.
246. Cohen DH, Feiner H, Jensson O, Frangione B: Amyloid fibril in hereditary cerebral hemorrhage with amyloidosis (HCHWA) is related to gastroentero-pancreatic neuroendocrine protein, gamma trace. *J Exp Med* **158**:623, 1983.
247. Ghiso J, Pons-Estel B, Frangione B: Hereditary cerebral amyloid angiopathy: The amyloid fibrils contain a protein which is a variant of cystatin C, an inhibitor of lysosomal cysteine proteases. *Biochem Biophys Res Commun* **136**:548, 1986b.
248. Abrahamson M, Jonsdottir S, Olafsson I, Jensson O, Grubb A: Hereditary cystatin C amyloid angiopathy: Identification of the disease-causing mutation and specific diagnosis by polymerase chain reaction based analysis. *Hum Genet* **89**:377, 1992.
249. Jensson O, Luyendijk W, Petursdottir I, Arnason A, Gudmundsson G, Grubb A: Cystatin C values in the cerebrospinal fluid: Comparison between the Icelandic and the Dutch type of hereditary central nervous system amyloid angiopathy. *Acta Neurol Scand* **73**:313, 1986.
250. Jensson O, Thorsteinsson L, Bots GTAM, Luyendijk W, Gudmundsson G, Arnason A, Lofberg H: Immunohistochemical comparison between the Dutch and the Icelandic form of hereditary central nervous system amyloid angiopathy. *Acta Neurol Scand* **73**:312, 1986.
251. Abrahamson M, Olafsson I, Palsdottir A, Ulvsbäck M, Lundwall A, Jensson O, Grubb A: Structure and expression of the human cystatin C gene. *Biochem J* **268**:287, 1990.
252. van Duinen SG, Castano EM, Prelli F, Bots GTAM, Luyendijk W, Frangione B: Hereditary cerebral hemorrhage with amyloidosis in patients of Dutch origin is related to Alzheimer disease. *Proc Natl Acad Sci USA* **84**:5991, 1987.
253. Levy E, Carman MD, Fernandez-Madrid IJ, Power MD, Lieberburg I, van Duinen SG, Bots GTAM, Luyendijk W, Frangione B: Mutation of the Alzheimer's disease amyloid gene in hereditary cerebral hemorrhage, Dutch type. *Science* **248**:1124, 1990.
254. Hendriks L, van Duijn CM, Cras P, Druts M, van Hul W, van Harskamp F, Warren A, McInnis MG, Antonarakis SE, Martin J-J, Hofman A, van Broeckhoven C: Presenile dementia and cerebral haemorrhage linked to a mutation at codon 692 of the β-amyloid precursor protein gene. *Nat Genet* **1**:218, 1992.
255. Siegal S: Benign paroxysmal peritonitis. *Ann Intern Med* **23**:1, 1945.
256. Heller H, Sohar E, Sherf L: Familial Mediterranean fever. *Arch Intern Med* **102**:50, 1958.
257. Sohar E, Pras M, Heller J, Heller H: Genetics of familial Mediterranean fever (FMF). *Arch Intern Med* **107**:529, 1961.
258. Sohar E, Gafni J, Pras M, Heller H: Familial Mediterranean fever. *Am J Med* **43**:227, 1967.
259. Heller H, Gafni J, Michaeli D, Shahin N, Sohar E, Erlich G, Karten I, Sokoloff L: The arthritis of familial Mediterranean fever (FMF). *Arthritis Rheum* **9**:1, 1966.
260. Motzner Y, Brzozinski A: C5a inhibitor deficiency in peritoneal fluids from patients with familial Mediterranean fever. *N Engl J Med* **311**:287, 1984.
261. Pras E, Aksentijevich I, Gruberg L, Balow JE, Prosen L, Dean M, Steinberg AD, Pras M, Kastner DL: Mapping of a gene causing familial Mediterranean fever to the short arm of chromosome 16. *N Engl J Med* **326**:1509, 1992.
262. Shohat M, Bu X, Shohat T, Fischel-Ghodsian N, Magal N, Nakamura Y, Schwabe AD, Schlezinger M, Danon Y, Rotter JI: The gene for familial Mediterranean fever in both Armenians and non-Ashkenazi Jews is linked to the α-globin complex on 16p: Evidence for locus homogeneity. *Am J Hum Genet* **51**:1349, 1992.
263. Pras M, Bronshpigel N, Zemer D, Gafni J: Variable incidence of amyloidosis in familial Mediterranean fever among different ethnic groups. *Johns Hopkins Med J* **150**:22, 1982.
264. Gafni J, Ravid M, Sohar E: The role of amyloidosis in familial Mediterranean fever: A population study. *Isr J Med Sci* **4**:995, 1968.
265. Blum A, Gafni J, Sohar E, Shibolet S, Heller H: Amyloidosis as the sole manifestation of familial Mediterranean fever (FMF). *Ann Intern Med* **57**:795, 1962.
266. Benson MD, Skinner M, Cohen AS: Amyloid deposition in a renal transplant in familial Mediterranean fever. *Ann Intern Med* **87**:31, 1977.
267. Goldstain RC, Schwabe AD: Prophylactic colchicine therapy in familial Mediterranean fever: A controlled, double-blind study. *Ann Intern Med* **81**:792, 1974.
268. Zemer D, Pras M, Sohar E, Modan M, Cabili S, Gafni J: Colchicine in the prevention and treatment of the amyloidosis of familial Mediterranean fever. *N Engl J Med* **314**:1001, 1986.

269. Muckle TJ, Wells M: Urticaria, deafness and amyloidosis: A new heredofamilial syndrome. *Q J Med* **31**:235, 1962.
270. Black JT: Amyloidosis, deafness, urticaria and limb pains: A hereditary syndrome. *Ann Intern Med* **70**:989, 1969.
271. Linke RP, Heilman KL, Nathrath WBJ, Eulitz M: Identification of amyloid A protein in a sporadic Muckle-Wells syndrome. *Lab Invest* **48**:698, 1983.
272. Weiss SW, Page DL: Amyloid nephropathy of Ostertag with special reference to renal glomerular giant cells. *Am J Pathol* **72**:447, 1973.
273. Goren H, Steinberg MC, Farboody GH: Familial oculoleptomeningeal amyloidosos. *Brain* **103**:473, 1980.
274. Keiser HR, Beaven MA, Doppman J, Wells S, Buja LM: Sipple's syndrome: Medullary thyroid carcinoma, pheochromocytoma, and parathyroid disease. *Ann Intern Med* **78**:561, 1973.
275. Sletten K, Westermark P, Natvig JB: Characterization of amyloid fibril proteins from medullary carcinoma of the thyroid. *J Exp Med* **143**:993–998, 1976.
276. Eng AM, Cogan L, Gunnar RM, Blekys I: Familial generalized dyschromic amyloidosis cutis. *J Cutan Pathol* **3**:102, 1976.
277. Ozaki M: Familial Lichen Amyloidosis. *Int J Dermatol* **23**:190, 1984.
278. Newton JA, Jagjivan A, Bhogal B, McKee PH, McGibbon DH: Familial primary cutaneous amyloidosis. *Br J Dermatol* **112**:201, 1985.
279. De Pietro WP: Primary familial cutaneous amyloidosis. *Arch Dermatol* **117**:639, 1981.
280. Partington MW, Marriott PJ, Prentice RSA, Cavaglia A, Simpson NE: Familial cutaneous amyloidosis with systemic manifestations in males. *Am J Med Genet* **10**:65, 1981.
281. Cornwell GG III, Westermark P: Senile amyloidosis: A protean manifestation of the aging process. *J Clin Pathol* **33**:1146, 1980.
282. Allensworth DC, Rice GJ, Loew GW: Persistent atrial standstill in a family with myocardial disease. *Am J Med* **47**:775, 1969.
283. Steiner I: The prevalence of isolated atrial amyloid. *J Pathol* **153**:395, 1987.
284. Kaye GC, Butler MG, d'Ardenne AJ, Edmondson SJ, Camm AJ, Slavin G: Isolated atrial amyloid contains atrial natriuretic peptide: A report of six cases. *Br Heart J* **56**:317, 1960.
285. Johansson B, Wernstedt C, Westermark P: Atrial natriuretic peptide deposited as atrial amyloid fibrils. *Biochem Biphys Res Commun* **148**:1087, 1987.
286. Linke RP, Voigt C, Störkel FS, Eulitz M: N-terminal amino acid sequence analysis indicates that isolated atrial amyloid is derived from atrial natriuretic peptide. *Virchows Archiv B Cell Pathol* **55**:125, 1988.
287. Pucci A, Wharton J, Arbustini E, Grasso M, Diegoli M, Needleman P, Vigano M, Polak JM: Atrial amyloid deposits in the failing human heart display both atrial and brain natriuretic peptide-like immunoreactivity. *J Pathol* **165**:235, 1991.
288. Maeda S, Tanaka T, Hayashi T: Familial atrial standstill caused by amyloidosis. *Br Heart J* **59**:498, 1988.
289. Marotta CA, Majocha RE, Tate B: Molecular and cellular biology of Alzheimer amyloid. *J Mol Neurosci* **3**:111, 1992.
290. St George-Hyslop PH, Tanzi RE, Polinsky RJ, Haines JL, Nee L, Watkins PC, Myers RH, Feldman RG, Pollen D, Drachman D, Growdon J, Bruni A, Foncin JF, Salmon D, Frommett P, Amaducci L, Sorbi S, Piacentini S, Stewart GD, Hobbs WJ, Conneally PM, Gusella JF: The genetic defect causing familial Alzheimer's disease, maps on chromosome 21. *Science* **235**:885, 1987.
291. Tanzi RE, Gusella JF, Watkins PC, Bruns GAP, St George-Hyslop P, Van Keuren ML, Patterson D, Pagan S, Kurnit DM, Neve RL: Amyloid beta protein gene: cDNA, mRNA distribution, and genetic linkage near the Alzheimer locus. *Science* **235**:880, 1987.
292. Palmert MR, Podlinsky MB, Witker DS, Oltersdorf T, Younkin LH, Selkoe DJ, Younkin SG: The β-amyloid protein precursor of Alzheimer disease has soluble derivatives found in human brain and cerebrospinal fluid. *Proc Natl Acad Sci USA* **86**:6338, 1989.
293. Goate A, Chartier-Harlin M-C, Mullan M, Brown J, Crawford F, Fidani L, Giuffra L, Haynes A, Irving N, James L, Mant R, Newton P, Rooke K, Roques P, Talbot C, Pericak-Vance M, Roses A, Williamson R, Rossor M, Owen M, Hardy J: Segregation of a missense mutation in the amyloid precursor protein gene with familial Alzheimer's disease. *Nature* **349**:704, 1991.
294. Murrell J, Farlow M, Ghetti B, Benson MD: A mutation in the amyloid precursor protein associated with hereditary Alzheimer's disease. *Science* **254**:97, 1991.
295. Chartier-Harlin M-C, Crawford F, Houlden H, Warren A, Hughes D, Fidani L, Goate A, Rossor M, Roques P, Hardy J, Mullan M: Early-onset Alzheimer's disease caused by mutations at codon 717 of the β-amyloid precursor protein gene. *Nature* **353**:844, 1991.
296. Opie EL: On relation of chronic interstitial pancreatitis to the islands of Langerhans and to diabetes mellitus. *J Exp Med* **5**:397, 1900.
297. Yano BL, Hayden DW, Johnson KH: Feline insular amyloid: Association with diabetes mellitus. *Vet Pathol* **18**:621, 1981.
298. Westermark P, Wernstedt C, Wilander E, Hayden DW, O'Brien TD, Johnson KH: Amyloid fibrils in human insulinoma and islets of Langerhans of the diabetic cat are derived from a neuropeptide-like protein also present in normal islet cells. *Proc Natl Acad Sci USA* **84**:3881, 1987.
299. Roberts AN, Leighton B, Todd JA, Cockburn D, Schofield PN, Sutton R, Holt S, Boyd Y, Day AJ, Foot EA, Willis AC, Reid KBM, Cooper GJS: Molecular and functional characterization of amylin, a peptide associated with type 2 diabetes mellitus. *Proc Natl Acad Sci USA* **86**:9662, 1989.
300. Mosselman S, Höppener JWM, Zandberg J, van Mansveld ADM, Geurts van Kessel AHM, Lips CJM, Jansz HS: Islet amyloid polypeptide: Identification and chromosomal localization of the human gene. *FEBS Lett* **239**:227, 1988.
301. Johnson KH, O'Brien TD, Betsholtz C, Westermark P: Biology of disease. Islet amyloid polypeptide: Mechanisms of amyloidogenesis in the pancreatic islets and potential roles indiabetes mellitus. *Lab Invest* **66**:522, 1992.
302. Nishi M, Steiner DF: Cloning of complementary DNAs encoding amyloid polypeptide, insulin, and glucagon precursors froma new world rodent, the degu, *Octodon degus*. *Mol Endocrinol* **4**:1192, 1990.
303. Fujihara S, Glenner GG: Primary localized amyloidosis of the genitourinary tract: Immunohistochemical study on eleven cases. *Lab Invest* **44**:55, 1981.
304. Thompson PJ, Citron KM: Amyloid and the lower respiratory tract. *Thorax* **38**:84, 1983.
305. Athanasou NA, Sallie B: Localized deposition of amyloid in articular cartilage. *Histopathology* **20**:41, 1992.
306. Altland K, Banzhoff A: Separation by hybrid isoelectric focusing of normal human plasma transthyretin (prealbumin) and a variant with a methionine for valine substitution associated with familial amyloidotic polyneuropathy. *Electrophoresis* **7**:529, 1986.
307. Benson MD, Dwulet FE: Identification of carriers of a variant plasma prealbumin (transthyretin) associated with familial amyloidotic polyneuropathy type I. *J Clin Invest* **75**:71, 1985.
308. Nakazato M, Kurihara T, Matsukura S, Kangawa K, Matsuo H: Diagnostic radioimmunoassay for amyloidotic polyneuropathy before clinical onset. *J Clin Invest* **77**:1699, 1986.
309. Saraiva MJM, Costa PP, Goodman DS: Biochemical marker in familial amyloidotic polyneuropathy, Portuguese type. *J Clin Invest* **76**:2171, 1985.
310. Nichols WC, Padilla L-M, Benson MD: Prenatal detection of a gene for hereditary amyloidosis. *Am J Med Genet* **34**:520, 1989.
311. Morris M, Nichols WC, Benson MD: Prenatal diagnosis of hereditary amyloidosis in a Portuguese family. *Am J Med Genet* **39**:123, 1991.
312. Sasaki H, Sakaki Y, Matsuo H, Goto I, Kuroiwa Y, Sahashi I, Takahashi A, Shinoda T, Isobe T, Takagi Y: Diagnosis of familial amyloidotic polyneuropathy by recombinant DNA techniques. *Biochem Biophys Res Commun* **125**:636, 1984.

313. Mita S, Maeda S, Ide M, Tsuzuki T, Shimada K, Araki S: Familial amyloidotic polyneuropathy diagnosed by cloned human prealbumin cDNA. *Neurology* **36**:298, 1986.

314. Nichols WC, Benson MD: Hereditary amyloidosis: Detection of variant prealbumin genes by restriction enzyme analysis of amplified genomic DNA sequences. *Clin Genet* **37**:44, 1990.

315. Zeldenrust SR, Murrell J, Farlow M, Ghetti B, Roses AD, Benson MD: RFLP analysis for APP 717 mutations associated with Alzheimer's disease. *J Med Genet* **30**:476, 1993.

316. Jacobson DR: A specific test for transthyretin 122 (Val → Ile), based on PCR-primer-introduced restriction analysis (PCR-PIRA): Confirmation of the gene frequency in blacks. *Am J Hum Genet* **50**:195, 1992.

317. Shiomi K, Nakazato M, Matsukura S, Ohnishi A, Hatanaka H, Tsuji S, Murai Y, Kojima M, Kangawa K, Matsuo H: A basic transthyretin variant (GLU^{61}→LYS) causes familial amyloidotic polyneuropathy: Protein and DNA sequencing and PCR-induced mutation restriction analysis. *Biochem Biophys Res Commun* **194**:1090, 1993.

318. Yasuda T, Sobue G, Doyu M, Nakazato M, Shiomi K, Yanagi T, Mitsuma T: Familial amyloidotic polyneuropathy with late-onset and well-preserved autonomic function: A Japanese kindred with novel mutant transthyretin (Ala(97) to Gly). *J Neurol Sci* **121**:97, 1994.

319. Delucia R, Mauro A, Discapio A, Buffo A, Mortara P, Orsi L, Schiffer D: A new mutation on the transthyretin gene (Ser^{112}→Ile) causes an amyloid neuropathy with severe cardiac impairment. *Clin Neuropathol* **12**:S35, 1993.

320. Murakami T, Tachibana S, Endo Y, Kawai R, Hara M, Tanase S, Ando M: Familial carpal tunnel syndrome due to amyloidogenic transthyretin His 114 variant. *Neurology* **44**:315, 1994.

321. Skare JC, Milunsky JM, Milunsky A, Skare IB, Cohen AS, Skinner M: A new transthyretin variant from a patient with familial amyloidotic polyneuropathy has asparagine substituted for histidine at position 90. *Clin Genet* **39**:6, 1991.

322. Skinner M, Lewis WD, Jones LA, Kasirsky J, Kane K, Ju S-T, Jenkins R, Falk RH, Simms RW, Cohen AS: Liver transplantation as a treatment for familial amyloidotic polyneuropathy. *Ann Intern Med* **120**:133, 1994.

323. Uemichi T, Liepnieks JJ, Benson MD: Hereditary renal amyloidosis with a novel variant fibrinogen. *J Clin Invest* **93**:731, 1994.

Part 19

MUSCLE

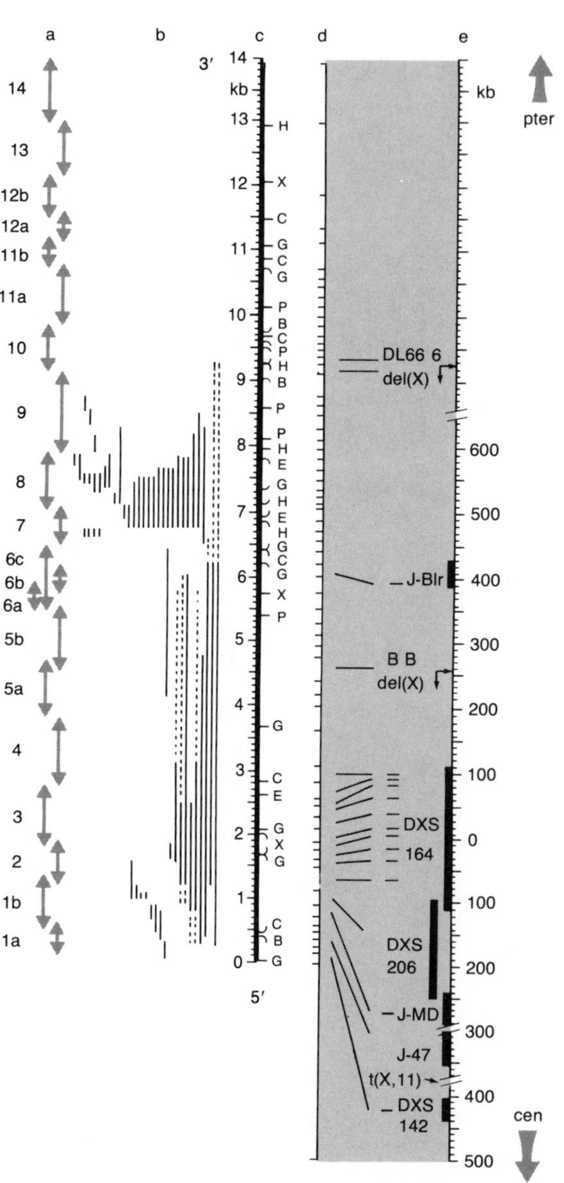

Duchenne muscular dystrophy

CHAPTER 140

The X-Linked Muscular Dystrophies

Ronald G. Worton ▪ Michael H. Brooke

1. The muscular dystrophies form a group of genetically determined, progressive, primary disorders of muscle. The various forms can be distinguished by a combination of clinical, genetic, and pathologic criteria. The forms of muscular dystrophy that follow an X-linked pattern of inheritance are the subject of this chapter. These include Duchenne and Becker muscular dystrophies (DMD and BMD) and Emery-Dreifuss muscular dystrophy (EDMD). DMD is a severe muscle-wasting disorder, resulting in early confinement to a wheelchair and often death by the age of 20. BMD is a milder form of the same disease with later onset and slower progression. EDMD is an X-linked myopathy distinct from DMD and BMD and is characterized by a specific pattern of contractures, cardiomyopathy, and slowly progressive muscle weakness in adult life.

2. The gene responsible for Duchenne and Becker muscular dystrophies (the DMD gene) maps to the short arm of the X chromosome at band Xp21. Positional cloning has resulted in the identification of the gene and its protein product, dystrophin. The DMD gene, with 79 exons spanning 2300 kb of the X chromosome, encodes a number of different mRNAs transcribed from five different promoters, with additional heterogeneity deriving from alternative splicing.

3. Dystrophin, the primary product of the DMD gene, is a high-molecular-weight (427 kDa) cytoskeletal protein that belongs to the spectrin family of proteins. In muscle it is localized at the inner surface of the sarcolemmal membrane, attached to the actin filaments of the cytoskeleton at its N-terminal end and to a complex of transmembrane proteins and glycoproteins at its C-terminal end. The complex passes through the membrane and attaches to laminin on the outer surface of the muscle cell. The biological function of dystrophin remains unknown. It may be purely mechanical—maintaining the structural integrity of the muscle membrane during contraction and relaxation, or it may have a more subtle role—providing support to the bound transmembrane complex whose function may be critical to the prevention of the disease.

4. Dystrophin is not confined to muscle. Two "brain" promoters upstream and downstream from the "muscle" promoter are responsible for two high-molecular-weight brain isoforms, each having an N-terminal end slightly different from that of muscle dystrophin. One is found in cerebral cortex and hippocampus, the other in cerebellar Purkinje cells. A dystrophin isoform is also found at the outer plexiform layer of the retina. Two lower-molecular-weight isoforms containing only the C-terminal domains of dystrophin are transcribed from promoters in introns 55 and 62. The longer form (116 kDa) is found in peripheral nerve and the shorter form (71 kDa) is expressed ubiquitously in several tissues. The function of the various isoforms remains unknown.

5. The basic defect in DMD and BMD is now clear. Boys with DMD have little or no functional dystrophin; in the milder disease BMD, dystrophin may be reduced in amount or altered in size. Approximately 60 percent of affected individuals have a deletion of one or more exons of the gene. Another 6 percent have duplications of exons, while the remaining 35 percent have a variety of subtle mutations, including point mutations, that are detectable only by detailed molecular analysis. The severe (DMD) phenotype is mainly associated with frameshifting deletions or duplications that result in truncated and nonfunctional dystrophin, whereas the milder (BMD) phenotype is associated with nonframeshifting mutations that leave the two ends of the protein intact.

6. Diagnostic evaluation of DMD and BMD patients now routinely includes analysis of dystrophin in muscle biopsies—western blot analysis to estimate quantity and molecular weight; immunolabeling of sections to determine the distribution at the muscle membrane. Diagnostic evaluation also includes Southern blot or PCR analysis of DNA to determine the nature of the mutation, since this information is of prognostic value for the patient and is a necessary prerequisite for carrier identification and prenatal diagnosis in the family.

7. Germ-line mosaicism complicates determination of carrier status, since the mother of any sporadic case might be a germ-line mosaic. The risk of having a second affected son depends on the proportion of her germ cells carrying the mutation, and the risk to the fetus of an apparent noncarrier mother may be as high as 20 percent.

8. Therapeutic approaches to DMD are in their infancy. Prednisone seems to stabilize muscle strength for up to 3 years, but the side effects are significant. Myoblast transfer therapy is controversial, but double-blind trials have shown little or no clinical improvement. Gene therapy is still at the earliest experimental stage.

9. The basic defect in EDMD is unknown and will likely await the cloning of the gene. The EDMD gene has been localized

A list of standard abbreviations is located immediately preceding the index in each volume. Additional abbreviations used in this chapter include: ARMD = autosomal recessive muscular dystrophy; BMD = Becker muscular dystrophy; CK = creatine kinase; CMD = congenital muscular dystrophy; DMD = Duchenne muscular dystrophy; EMG = electromyography; ERG = electroretinography; FCMD = Fukuyama congenital muscular dystrophy; LMD = limb-girdle muscular dystrophy; PERT = phenol-enhanced reassociation technique; SCARMD = severe childhood autosomal recessive muscular dystrophy.

to the end of the long arm of the X chromosome at band Xq28. Mapping of the gene to a region of about 2 million base pairs, near the color pigment genes, should facilitate identification of the gene and its protein product by a positional cloning strategy.

The muscular dystrophies are genetically determined diseases with progressive muscular weakness as the most prominent clinical manifestation. All display characteristic muscle degeneration on electrical, biochemical, and histologic examination, and several also show pathologic features in organ systems other than muscle. The clinical severity varies widely between the several forms of muscular dystrophy, and may even show considerable variation within a single genetic type.

As a group the muscular dystrophies rank among the most frequent of inherited diseases. The inheritance pattern may be X-linked, autosomal dominant, or autosomal recessive. The major forms of muscular dystrophy are listed according to the type of inheritance in Table 140-1. This chapter will concentrate on the X-linked muscular dystrophies. These include Duchenne and Becker muscular dystrophies (DMD and BMD), which are allelic disorders caused by mutation in the DMD gene located at band Xp21, and Emery-Dreifuss muscular dystrophy (EDMD), for which the causative gene is located at Xq28 on the long arm of the X chromosome. The autosomally inherited muscular dystrophies are described in the next chapter.

DUCHENNE AND BECKER MUSCULAR DYSTROPHIES

Duchenne muscular dystrophy (DMD) is a severe muscle-wasting disorder resulting in early confinement to a wheelchair and often death by the age of 20. Described first by Meryon[1] in 1852 and in more detail by Duchenne,[2] it was not until the mid-1950s that diagnostic criteria were developed to allow it to be clearly distinguished from other neuromuscular disorders.[3] It was not until the late 1980s that the causative gene was identified by molecular cloning and the basic defect recognized as a deficiency of the cytoskeletal protein dystrophin, the product of the DMD gene.

Becker muscular dystrophy (BMD) resembles DMD but, until recently, it was considered a separate entity because of its later onset, more benign course, and longer survival. According to traditional definitions, those confined to a wheelchair by age 12 or 13 would be classified as having DMD, and those still ambulant by age 16, as having BMD. The terms "outlier" or "intermediate phenotype" have been applied to those who become wheelchair-bound between the ages of 12 and 16. Since DMD and BMD have now been shown to result from lesions in the same X-linked gene, they represent opposite ends of the clinical spectrum of the same genetic disease. We therefore treat DMD and BMD as the same disease, and refer to the underlying gene as the "DMD gene." A comprehensive description of the disease and its pathology is contained in the recent monograph by Emery.[4]

Despite considerable research effort, including the cloning of the gene and the identification of the basic defect, the disease continues to be devastating and lethal. New approaches to treatment or cure are now under intense scrutiny, both in the research laboratory and in clinical trials. These new approaches are reviewed in a later section.

Table 140-1 **Major Forms of Human Muscular Dystrophy**

X-linked
Duchenne and Becker muscular dystrophy
Emery-Dreifuss muscular dystrophy
Autosomal recessive
Autosomal recessive childhood muscular dystrophy
Adult limb-girdle muscular dystrophy
Congential muscular dystrophy
Autosomal dominant
Myotonic dystrophy
Fascioscapulohumeral muscular dystrophy
Oculopharyngeal muscular dystrophy

Duchenne Muscular Dystrophy

Clinical Features. Boys with DMD are phenotypically unremarkable at birth and remain so for the first year or two of life. Only rarely, in families who are attuned to the illness, are symptoms noted before this stage. The first subtle indication of muscle weakness is usually noted when the child starts to walk. He is less agile than his peers and may fall frequently. At 4 to 5 years of age he will have difficulty climbing stairs and rising from a sitting position on the floor. Walking is made abnormal by a tendency to walk and balance on the ball of the foot ("toe walking"), and the ability to jump is severely compromised.

School introduces new problems, including hyperactivity and distractibility. This is complicated by an overall reduction in IQ equivalent to about 20 points, about one-fifth of patients having a significant mental handicap.[5–8]

In the untreated patient the ability to walk independently is lost at around 9 or 10 years, but aggressive use of bracing and surgery can delay this stage to about 12 years of age. Once the patient is in a wheelchair, contractures of hips and knees worsen, and severe scoliosis may develop. In the absence of treatment, scoliosis, respiratory compromise, and inanition take their toll, and death from respiratory failure may occur in the middle of the second decade. Maintenance of life to age 25 or more is now possible with the aid of a respirator.[4]

Some children have an illness that is much less progressive. Although the weakness is noticed at a young age, they decline more slowly, yet they differ from patients with classic BMD in that they lose independent ambulation before the age of 16. Members of this outlier or intermediate group are more likely to die from the complications of cardiomyopathy than from respiratory failure.

Other symptoms include muscle pain, depression, and urinary and fecal incontinence. Muscle pain in the calf or thigh may last for a day or so and then fade away. The etiology is not clear, but this type of pain is much more common in BMD, where it may be the presenting symptom. Depression, understandable in a child with a serious illness, is most noticeable at the start of school, when the patient becomes more aware of his limitations, and later when confinement in a wheelchair restricts social activity and the circle of friends. The urinary incontinence is more difficult to understand. In those with a severe disability it may be related in part to shyness in requesting assistance, but this is not the whole explanation, since incontinence is not always accompanied by such severe disability.

Signs. The earliest signs are hip weakness, an unusual rubbery feel to the muscles and tightness of the iliotibial bands and heel cords. The original name of the illness, *pseudohypertrophic muscular dystrophy*,[2] is indicative of the bulky muscles in many affected boys. Almost any muscle group may be involved, but a hypertrophic gastrocnemius is classic. The calf hypertrophy that was part of the earliest clinical descriptions of the disease is evident in Figure 140-1.

Ankle dorsiflexion to 45 degrees above horizontal is normal in a young boy, but dorsiflexion is limited to 0 to 15 degrees in an affected boy. Walking on the toes is noticeable before age 5 and is more readily observed when the child is barefoot. Strength testing at this stage is sometimes difficult, and more useful signs may be the awkward gait and Gowers

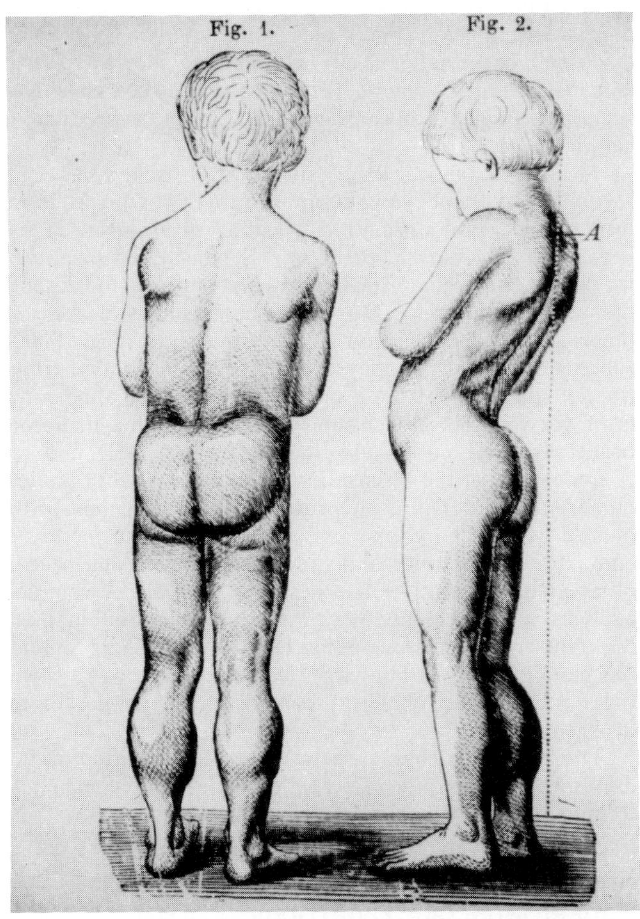

A

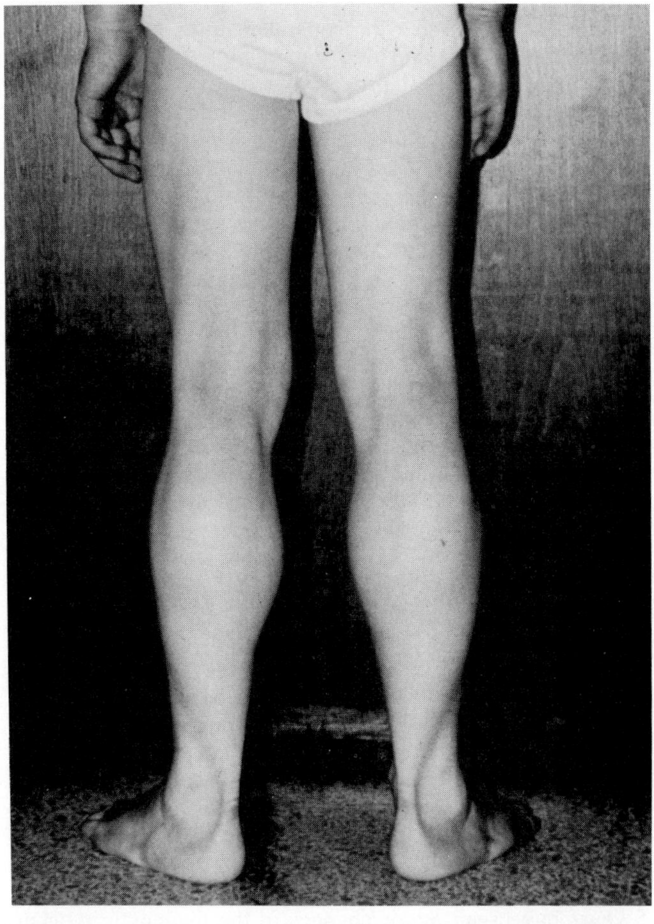

B

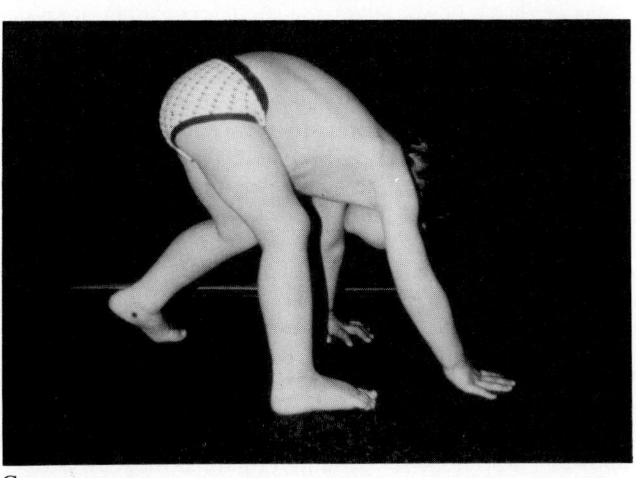

C

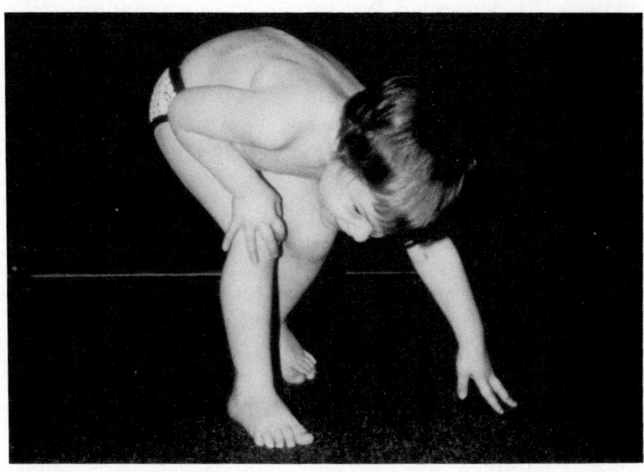

D

FIG. 140-1 **The clinical features of Duchenne muscular dystrophy. *A*. Illustration of a patient with "pseudohypertrophic muscular paralysis." *B*. Gastrocnemius hypertrophy in a patient with DMD. *C*, *D*. Young boy with DMD arising from the floor by the Gower maneuver. Initially both hands are placed on the floor for support. The hips are then raised and the weight is transferred to the thigh with the right hand and the trunk is brought upright by pushing on the thighs. *(Fig. A from Duchenne's monograph—Duchenne de Boulogne, De la paralysie musculaire pseudohypertrophique ou paralysie myosclerosique. Extrait des Archives générales de Médecine, Asselin, Pairs 1868. See also ref. 2.)***

maneuver[9] used to rise from the floor to an upright position. The waddling gait is due to weakness of the hip abductors, which allows the pelvis to tilt as the foot hits the ground. By age 6 to 8, walking is slow, usually on the toes with knees hyperextended. A compensatory lordosis, necessary to maintain balance, is part of the earliest clinical descriptions (Fig. 140-1). The Gowers maneuver, using the hands to push up from the floor, is diagrammed in Figure 140-1.

Natural History. While the general features of the disease have been well documented for individual cases, only recently has the clinical progression of a sizable cohort of affected children been recorded systematically.[10] This multicenter study included all boys whose symptoms began before 5 years of age, and therefore would include not only DMD patients but also outliers and even some who would later be classified as having BMD. The age of occurrence of a number of "milestones" was recorded, forming a database against which an individual patient could be measured. Typically, affected boys lost the ability to rise from a chair and to climb stairs by age 9 (range 7 to 13) and required a wheelchair by age 12 (range 9 to 16). For a period of about 3 years prior to the wheelchair confinement, leg braces were beneficial in maintaining a degree of ambulation.

In the teenage years, the major problems were scoliosis and reduction in forced vital capacity (FVC) of the lungs. While 25 percent of the patients maintained a relatively straight back, progressive scoliosis was common in the others. In most participating clinics, boys with curvature of >35 degrees were considered as candidates for corrective surgery. The FVC reduction and the associated risk of pneumonia were greatest in those who scored lowest in performance based on milestones. These "weak" patients, with performance ratings below the 50th percentile, generally died from respiratory failure and pneumonia, with age at death ranging from 13 to 17 years. The stronger boys, those who scored above the 50th percentile, lived a little longer (age of death 14 to 21 years), and many died of cardiac failure with respiratory function reasonably well preserved.

Diagnostic Investigations. In many medical centers, the last 5 years have seen major changes in the diagnostic workup of DMD and BMD patients. Frequently it involves DNA analysis to determine the nature of the mutation and/or protein analysis to determine the quality and quantity of dystrophin in a muscle biopsy specimen. Diagnostic testing will be discussed after the molecular genetics of DMD and BMD (see "Molecular and Diagnostic Applications for DMD and BMD" below). Prior to the development of molecular diagnostic tests, the diagnosis was confirmed primarily by measuring serum creatine kinase (CK) levels, by muscle histology, and by electromyography (EMG).

Serum CK is markedly elevated, to 50 to 100 times the upper limit of normal,[11,12] the result of leakage of the muscle isoform from the sarcoplasm into the bloodstream. While several other sarcoplasmic enzymes are elevated in the early stages of the disease, none are better than CK for diagnosis or carrier detection. Although rhabdomyolysis and hypothyroidism may also be associated with very high CK levels, these conditions can be readily differentiated on clinical grounds. In polymyositis, CK is less markedly elevated.

CK is elevated at birth in DMD and BMD, but the frequency of high CK levels in normal neonates makes it unwise to use cord blood for diagnostic evaluation. By the end of the first week the normal range is less variable, so that a high value (several thousand international units per liter) at this time is diagnostic for muscle disease. Conversely, a value in the normal range in the first few months of life provides assurance that the disease will not develop. The CK level remains high in the early stages, before the disease has become apparent clinically, and declines progressively throughout life, presumably owing to the decrease in muscle bulk.[13]

Measurement of CK is also of value for carrier detection, although in carrier females the range of values overlaps the normal range, making the test less than definitive. A thorough discussion of the value of CK testing is provided by Emery.[4] In most families, genetic testing, as described in a later section, provides a more reliable method of carrier identification.

Although a clinical diagnosis of DMD backed by a high serum CK is often beyond doubt, the gravity of the prognosis usually dictates confirmation by study of a muscle biopsy specimen. The muscle pathology is considered diagnostic for the disease even during the neonatal period in the absence of clinical symptoms.[14] Muscle histology shows evidence of muscle fiber degeneration and regeneration (Fig. 140-2). Fiber necrosis and phagocytosis may be seen, and hypercontracted opaque fibers are prominent. The overall appearance is of varying sizes of circular fibers embedded in fibrous tissue. Internal nuclei are seen often in BMD and are characteristic of the disease in the *mdx* mouse, but are less numerous in DMD muscle. Ultimately, replacement of the muscle by fat and connective tissue leads to a picture of end-stage degeneration indistinguishable from that seen in other myodegenerative diseases (Fig. 140-2B). A complete analysis of muscle histology and interpretation in many different myopathies, including DMD and BMD, is found in the monograph by Dubowitz,[14] while Engel[15] has reviewed the ultrastructural changes seen in various stages of the disease.

The EMG is characteristic, with a reduction in the duration and amplitude of action potentials and an enhanced frequency of polyphasic potentials.[16]

Becker Muscular Dystrophy

Becker and Duchenne muscular dystrophies were distinguished originally on clinical grounds. The main difference is in age of onset and rate of progression, although close questioning may reveal weakness before the age of 5 in BMD patients. The most widely accepted difference is that BMD patients remain ambulatory beyond the age of 16.

Muscle pain related to exercise is a prominent feature of BMD. Mental retardation is not part of the clinical picture. Overall, the physical picture resembles that of DMD, with a combination of axial weakness, a tendency for toe walking, and muscular hypertrophy. Laboratory studies are also similar, including elevation of CK and myopathic changes on EMG. The muscle biopsy features are somewhat different,[15] although variability in fiber size, muscle fibrosis, and necrosis as well as basophilia are still noted. Internal nuclei are much more numerous, and the distinction between type I and type II fibers, often obscured in the DMD patient, is quite clear in BMD. Fewer BMD patients require orthopedic surgery either for release of joint contractures or for scoliosis, perhaps because muscle weakness is less severe and occurs at a later time, when skeletal maturity has been reached. The natural history of BMD has not been well defined, but survival may be prolonged into the fourth decade and beyond.

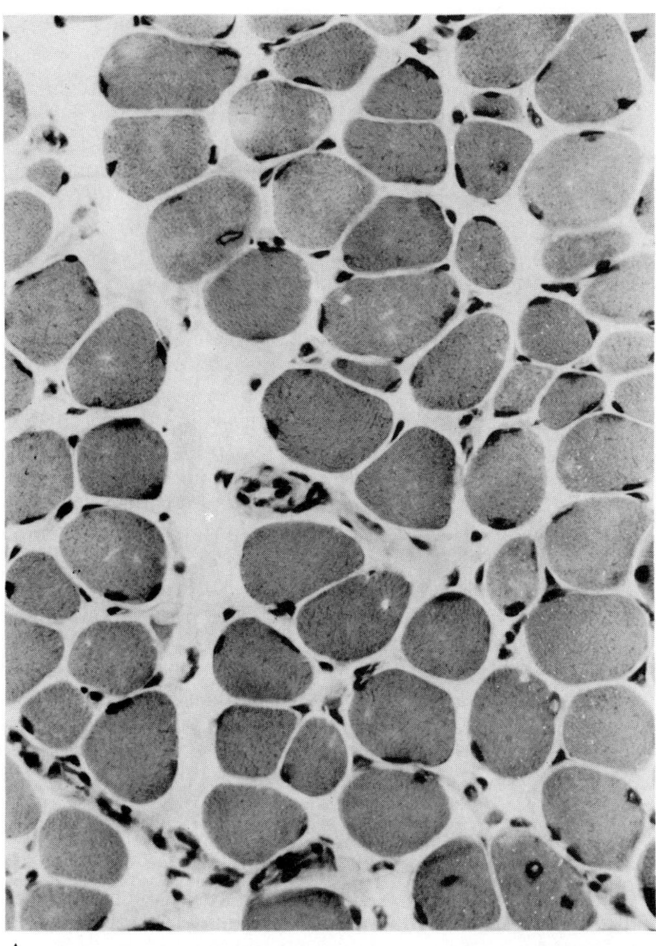

A

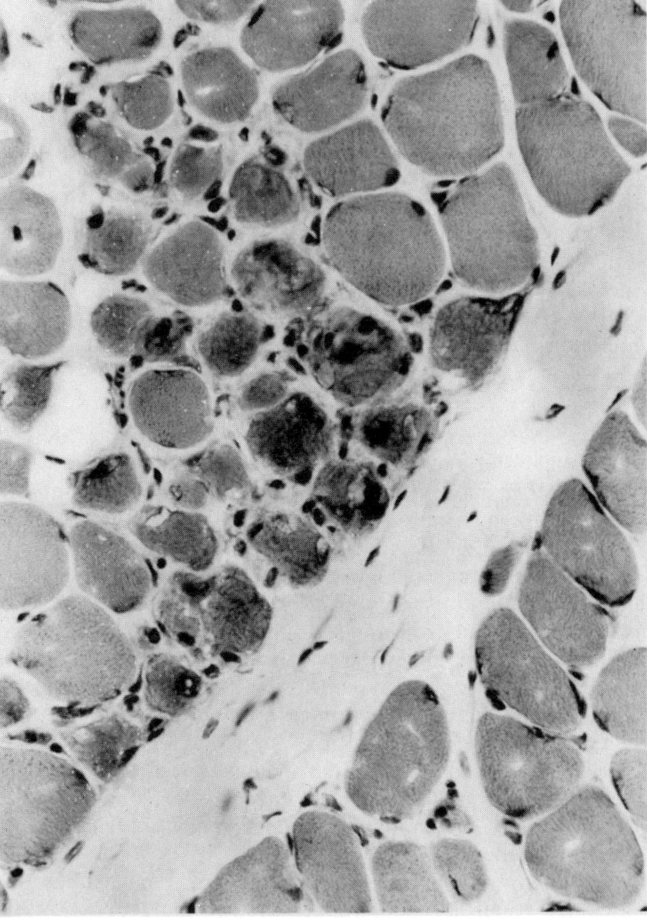

B

FIG. 140-2 **Muscle histology in Duchenne muscular dystrophy. *A*. Trichrome stain of muscle biopsy. The presence of rounded fibers of varying size embedded in a sea of connective tissue is characteristic. A group of necrotic fibers is seen toward the center of the field. *B*. A group of basophilic fibers of unknown origin, also characteristic of the muscle pathology.**

Genetics of Duchenne and Becker Muscular Dystrophy

Pattern of Inheritance. DMD and BMD display an X-linked recessive pattern of inheritance. Expression of the disease is essentially confined to males, with full expression in females found only in those with loss or inactivation of the X chromosome carrying the normal allele. The defective gene in affected males may be the result of new mutation in the germ line of the mother or may be inherited from a carrier female. The severity of the disease, and hence its classification as DMD, intermediate, or BMD, depends to a large extent on the particular mutation, as will be described in detail below.

Incidence. The incidence of DMD has been documented in numerous retrospective surveys, as well as in neonatal screening programs. Retrospective studies from Europe, North America, Australia, and Japan, summarized by Kanamori et al.[17] and by van Essen,[18] gave incidences of 14 to 29 per 100,000 male births, with little ethnic variation. In several studies corrected for ascertainment probability, the incidence was 22 to 29 per 100,000. In three neonatal screening programs in Germany,[19] Canada,[20] and Wales, the measured incidence was 48 in 176,600 (27/100,000), 5 in 18,000 (28/100,000) and 9 in 34,219 (26/100,000), respectively. Thus, a true incidence of 26 to 29 per 100,000 (approximately 1 in 3500) seems likely in most populations.

The incidence of BMD is more difficult to estimate because of the later age of onset and the phenotypic overlap with other neuromuscular diseases. Three European studies prior to 1987, summarized by Mostacciuolo et al.,[21] gave incidences of 3.3, 3.4, and 5.5 per 100,000. A recent British study[22] in which DNA and dystrophin analysis were used to confirm all cases provided a minimum incidence of 5.4/100,000. The combined incidence of DMD and BMD is therefore approximately 33/100,000, or about 1 in 3000 male births.

Mutation Rate. The mathematic analysis of mutation rate for an X-linked lethal disorder at equilibrium in the population was addressed by Haldane in 1956[23] and later by Edwards in 1986.[24] Briefly, an affected male may receive the defective gene from a heterozygous mother (carrier frequency $= h$) or by mutation in the germ line of a noncarrier mother (female mutation rate $= m$). A female heterozygote may receive the defective gene from these sources or from mutation in the germ line of her father (male mutation rate $= n$). Thus, the incidence of affected males (I) and heterozygous females (h) is given by

$$I = h/2 + m \quad (1)$$

$$h = h/2 + m + n \quad (2)$$

By rearranging terms in (2) and substituting into (1), we get

$$h = 2(m + n) \quad (3)$$

$$I = 2m + n \quad (4)$$

From (3), it is clear that the number of new mutation carriers $(m + n)$ is equal to the number of carriers who inherit their heterozygous state $(h/2)$. Thus, regardless of mutation rate, half of all carriers are the result of a new mutation and half receive the defective gene from their mothers, who are themselves subject to the same 50:50 rule.

For affected males, the proportion of cases due to new mutation is

$$c = m/I = m/(2m + n) = (m/n)/(2m/n + 1), \quad (5)$$

a value that depends on m/n, the ratio of mutation rates in the female and male. If these rates are equal, then $c = 1/3$. On the other hand, if $m >> n$, then c approaches $1/2$, and if $m << n$, then c approaches zero. Thus, c is between 0 and $1/2$, and if $m = n$, its value is $1/3$.

A priori, oogenesis and spermatogenesis are so different that equal mutation rates in males and females should not be expected. Indeed, unequal mutation rates have been found in other X-linked recessive diseases—hemophilia A and Lesch-Nyhan syndrome—in which there is a preponderance of male mutation. In contrast, direct estimation of the paternal and maternal contributions to mutations in DMD carriers[25] and estimates of the male/female mutation ratio from grandparental genotypes[26] lead to the conclusion of approximately equal mutation rates in males and females for the DMD gene.

Another way to determine if male and female mutation rates are equal is to determine whether the proportion of males who are new mutants deviates significantly from $1/3$. Several studies have attempted to estimate this quantity from recurrence data. The values, summarized by Moser to 1984,[27] ranged from 0.18 to 0.52, with most estimates falling close to the value of $1/3$. Most recently Barbujani et al.[28] evaluated segregation data from 1885 sibships from nine studies carried out in seven different countries. Assuming a segregation frequency of the defective gene of 0.5, the maximum likelihood estimate of the frequency of new mutants was 0.29, slightly but significantly lower than $1/3$. In light of recent data showing that a significant proportion of noncarrier mothers are germ-line mosaics for new mutations,[25] this value of 0.29 is an underestimate, as some new mutants would have been misclassified as familial cases. Thus, we must conclude that the proportion of new mutants is probably close to $1/3$, consistent with equal mutation rates in males and females.

Substituting $n = m$ in equation (4) gives the mutation rate as $m = 1/3 I$. The best estimate of the mutation rate for DMD is therefore one third of the incidence or approximately 10^{-4}, an order of magnitude higher than for most other genetic diseases.

The mutation rate for BMD is not quite so straightforward to calculate, since approximately 70 percent of males with BMD are capable of transmitting the gene to a carrier daughter. A higher proportion of BMD cases are therefore inherited, and the Haldane formula relating mutation rate to incidence is $m = 1/3 I(1 - f)$, where the fitness (f) is 0.7. Assuming an incidence for BMD of 5/100,000, the mutation rate is 5×10^{-6}, about 5 percent of that for DMD.

Expression in Females. The normal process of random X inactivation in females dictates that in a typical DMD carrier, the X chromosome carrying the normal DMD allele will be inactivated in approximately 50 percent of myonuclei. The amount of dystrophin in muscle of a carrier is therefore expected to be about half that in a normal male or female. Because of the random nature of X inactivation, many women are expected to have less than 50 percent functional DMD genes, and those with the most skewed X inactivation pattern may express manifestations of the disease. It is not surprising, therefore, that a mild clinical presentation is seen in about 8 percent of DMD carriers.[4]

As reviewed several years ago by Penn et al.,[29] not all females with mild muscular dystrophy are DMD carriers. In the absence of a positive family history, many such cases may be attributed to causes other than heterozygosity for mutation at the DMD gene. With the identification of dystrophin, it is now clear that those who are DMD-manifesting carriers have an abnormal amount and distribution of dystrophin in skeletal muscle and can be distinguished by immunostaining of muscle biopsies with anti-dystrophin antibodies.[30] The disease may also be expressed in Turner syndrome females who have a single X chromosome.

An extreme example of nonrandom X inactivation leading to a disease phenotype is found in monozygotic female twin carriers who are discordant for the DMD phenotype.[31–34] Recent studies have confirmed that the affected twin has preferential inactivation of the X chromosome carrying the normal DMD allele.[35–37] These cases and the lack of reports of female twins concordant for the DMD phenotype led Nance to postulate that the discordance is related to splitting of the inner cell mass shortly after X inactivation with nonrandom distribution of the cells with maternally and paternally inactivated X chromosomes.[38] He suggested that the extremely skewed X-inactivation pattern in the affected twin might be due to asymmetric splitting of the inner cell mass, with the affected twin receiving the smaller cell mass. This proposal is supported by the finding that in some twin pairs only the affected twin shows a skewed pattern, while the normal twin displays a random X-inactivation pattern.[35]

Another example of nonrandom X inactivation leading to DMD or BMD is in females with X–autosome translocations that disrupt the DMD gene. In the 22 or more cases studied to date, the translocation not only disrupts the DMD gene on one X chromosome but also causes nonrandom inactivation of the X chromosome carrying the normal allele, resulting in expression of the disease phenotype.[39] These females were instrumental in the mapping and cloning of the DMD gene and are discussed more fully in the next section.

The DMD Gene

The DMD gene was one of the first to be cloned by the positional cloning approach, in which knowledge of its position on the chromosome was the critical factor. The mapping and cloning of the gene has been reviewed extensively[40–43] and is described briefly below.

DMD Gene Localization. Three lines of evidence placed the DMD gene in band Xp21 in the middle of the X chromosome short arm—evidence from the breakpoints of translocations in affected females, linkage analysis in DMD and BMD families, and contiguous gene deletions in males with complex phenotypes (Fig. 140-3).

Translocation Mapping. The first mapping data for the DMD locus came from translocation females. From 1977 to 1981, five females were identified with X:autosome translocations.

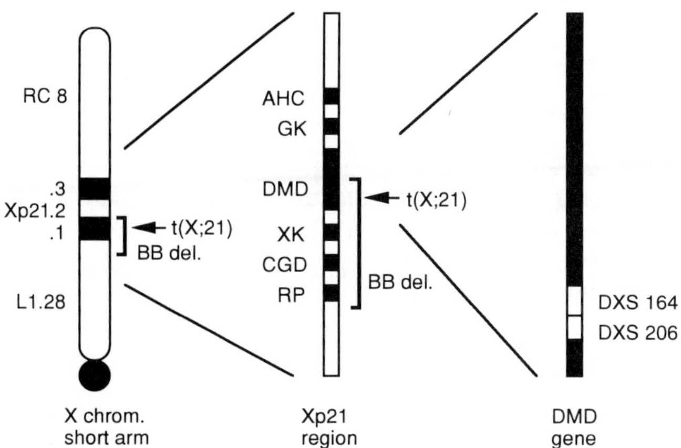

FIG. 140-3 Schematic of the short arm of the human X chromosome showing the position of genetic markers RC8 and L1.28 relative to Xp21, which is shown as three bands at high resolution (Xp21.1, Xp21.2, and Xp21.3). The expanded Xp21 region shows relative position of the genes AHC, GK, DMD, XK, CGD, and RP (see text for meaning of gene symbols). Also shown is the position of the deletion in patient BB and the t(X;21) translocation exchange point in an affected female, both of whom were instrumental in the cloning of the DMD gene. The further expansion of the DMD gene shows the position of the cloned regions DXS164 and DXS206.

In each case the exchange point in the X chromosome was in band Xp21, suggesting that a gene involved in muscular dystrophy must be located at this position in the middle of the short arm of the X chromosome.[44–48] Furthermore, in each case the normal X chromosome was the inactive one in most cells, providing an explanation for the expression of the disease in a heterozygous female.

By 1986, over 20 translocation cases were reported; they are summarized in a review by Boyd et al.[39] High-resolution banding studies revealed that the exchange points were not precisely the same in all affected females and suggested a target for disruption extending from Xp21.1 to Xp21.3, a region of perhaps 3 to 4 million base pairs.[49] This in turn suggested the possibility of a very large gene, a speculation that turned out to be correct. In one of these translocations [t(X; 21) in Figure 140-3] the DMD gene had been translocated next to a block of ribosomal RNA genes,[50] and this formed the basis for one of the successful DMD gene cloning strategies described below.

Linkage Mapping. Mutations that cause the disease in males also map to Xp21, as determined from family studies with DNA probes that detect restriction fragment length polymorphism (RFLP). By 1983 two X chromosomal probes, RC8 and L1.28, were found to detect RFLPs that segregated with the disease in Duchenne families about 80 percent of the time. This suggested a recombination frequency of about 20 percent, mapping the markers 20 cM (1 cM or centimorgan is the genetic distance corresponding to a recombination frequency of 1 percent) from the DMD gene.[51,52] Physical mapping by somatic cell hybrid analysis and *in situ* hybridization mapped RC8 to the distal third and L1.28 to the proximal third of the X chromosome short arm,[51,52] with the DMD gene between them in the middle of the short arm (Fig. 140-3).

By 1985 many additional linked markers had been identified and mapped within 10 to 20 cM of the DMD gene,[53–56] and a probe for the ornithine transcarbamylase (OTC) gene also turned out to be linked.[57] Much of the early linkage data has been summarized in several reviews.[42,43,58]

A critical discovery from the use of these new X chromosome probes was that in Becker families the markers all gave segregation results essentially similar to those for Duchenne families, providing the first indication that the genes responsible for DMD and BMD are closely linked or identical.[59,60]

Deletion Mapping. The third line of evidence came from a few boys with DMD as part of a contiguous gene deletion syndrome. One of these was a young boy, initials BB, who had DMD, retinitis pigmentosa (RP), chronic granulomatous disease (CGD), and the McLeod red-cell phenotype (XK). In 1985 high-resolution chromosome banding analysis by Francke et al.[61] demonstrated that BB had a small but cytogenetically visible deletion of part of band Xp21 (Fig. 140-3). Furthermore, Southern blot analysis with probe 754, one of the marker probes closely linked to the DMD gene, confirmed that the sequence detected by the probe was missing from BB's DNA and was not reinserted elsewhere in the genome. This established the first connection between a multidisease phenotype and a deletion of contiguous genes responsible for those diseases. DNA from BB was crucial in cloning of the DMD gene, as discussed below.

Prior to this discovery, another complex phenotype was also recognized, complex glycerol kinase deficiency, involving glycerol kinase (GK) deficiency, congenital adrenal hypoplasia (AHC) and, in some cases, Duchenne-like myopathy.[62–64] In these patients, high-resolution cytogenetic analysis and Southern blot analysis with probes closely linked to the DMD gene also confirmed the existence of deletions spanning two or more genes.[65–70]

Several later papers review the extent of the various deletions and demonstrate a gene order of AHC, GK, DMD, XK, CYBB (CGD), RP in a telomere-to-centromere direction.[71–75] Mapping of this block of contiguous genes to Xp21 provided further evidence for the location of the DMD gene and set the stage for the cloning of the gene.

DMD Gene Cloning. The unambiguous mapping of the DMD gene to band Xp21 dictated the approach to cloning the gene—cloning of genomic sequences from Xp21 followed by identification of expressed sequences from the region. This was one of the earliest attempts at positional cloning, a strategy that has already become the method of choice for cloning many disease genes. The details of the DMD gene identification have been reviewed extensively.[40–43]

Positional Cloning. The first DNA clone clearly associated with the DMD locus was isolated by Kunkel and colleagues using a competitive hybridization procedure called the phenol-enhanced reassociation technique (PERT) to enrich for DNA fragments from the region of the BB deletion.[76] Cloned fragments that mapped into the BB deletion were tested for hybridization to a panel of DNA samples from DMD patients (without visible deletions), and one clone, PERT87, failed to hybridize with DNA from 5 of 57 patients.[77] This suggested that the disease in these five boys was the result of a submicroscopic deletion that removed at least a portion of the DMD gene, including the PERT87 sequence.

The PERT87 clone was expanded by chromosome walking through the isolation of a series of overlapping DNA segments. Subclones from the cloned region (DXS164 locus; see Fig. 140-3) were sent to several laboratories around the world, which quickly confirmed the existence of PERT87 deletions in about 7 percent of DMD patients.[78] Deletions in two BMD patients confirmed the allelism of the two diseases.

Linkage analysis with RFLPs from the DXS164 locus confirmed that PERT87 polymorphisms segregated with the DMD gene in families,[79-81] but a recombination rate of 5 to 10 percent between the DXS164 locus and the disease-causing mutations in the gene was only explained later as intragenic recombination across an enormously large gene.[82]

In our own (RGW) laboratory, an alternative approach to the cloning of the DMD gene depended on a female BMD patient with a t(X;21) translocation (Fig. 140-3) in which the DMD gene had recombined with a block of ribosomal RNA genes on chromosome 21.[83] Using ribosomal gene probes, clone XJ1 was isolated from the junction of the translocation and was shown to have a portion of ribosomal gene at its telomeric end and a segment of the X chromosome at its centromeric end.[84] The region was expanded by chromosome walking from XJ1, and subclones from the region (DX206 locus; see Fig. 140-3) detected deletions in a subset of affected boys, some of them the same boys that were deleted for PERT87. Segregation studies with RFLPs from the DSX206 locus confirmed tight linkage to the DMD gene but displayed the same 5 to 10 percent recombination rate that was seen for PERT87.[85] In December 1986, a walk-step clone on the telomeric side was found to overlap Kunkel's DXS164 locus.

cDNA from the DMD Gene. To detect expressed sequences that might be derived from the DMD gene, subclones from the DXS164 and DXS206 loci were examined for the presence of conserved sequences by hybridization to DNA from multiple species in a "zoo" blot. One small DNA segment from DXS164 gave a positive signal with several species, hybridized with a 14 to 16 kb mRNA from skeletal muscle, and was used as a probe to isolate the first cDNA clone from a fetal muscle cDNA library.[86] This cDNA clone hybridized to several genomic fragments, each containing one or more exons spread over the 220-kb DXS164 locus. A similar analysis with subclones from DXS206 was initially negative (the DXS206 locus covered most of a 105-kb intron) but eventually revealed a conserved region that identified a cDNA clone overlapping the Kunkel clone and containing the first 15 exons of the DMD gene.[87]

The complete cDNA was isolated by Koenig et al.[88] in a series of overlapping cDNA clones that were sequenced and found to encode a protein of 3685 amino acids, with a predicted molecular weight of 427. The sequence and the functional protein domains it suggested, are discussed below in the section on the gene product.

The cDNA clones of this series were designated 1a, 1b, 2, 3, 4, 5a, etc. according to their approximate position along the 14-kb mRNA.[88] They were ligated into a smaller set of partial cDNA clones useful as probes to detect deletions in the genomic DNA of patients. These partial cDNAs, labeled 1-2a, 2b-3, 4-5a, 5b-7, 8, and 9-14, are shown in Figure 140-4 as bars along a schematic of the exons. Other cDNA clones shown in the figure were isolated in our own laboratory (D38, 10-69, D43 and 46-6) or Davies' laboratory[89] (Cf and Ca series). These cDNA clones, depicted in Figure 140-4, have been used in numerous laboratories to screen patients for gross chromosomal alterations by Southern blotting, as discussed in a later section.

Size of the DMD Gene. Once the full cDNA was isolated, it then became possible to use cDNA sequences as probes to identify the rest of the gene from genomic DNA of the X chromosome. The enormous size of the gene, with a few introns in excess of 100 kb, became clear from the analysis

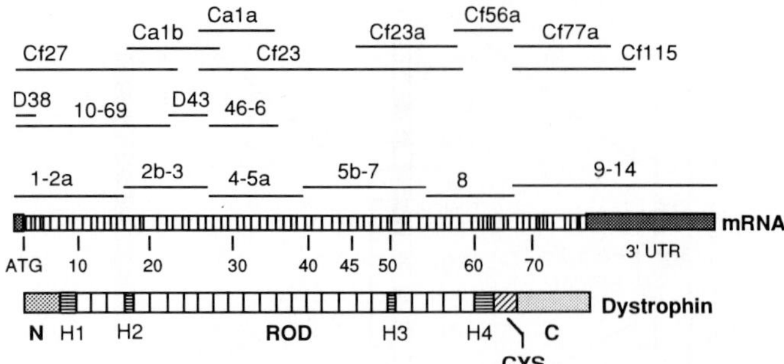

FIG. 140-4 **Schematic of the cloned cDNA fragments relative to the DMD mRNA and to the dystrophin molecule. The clone names are as described in the text. The mRNA shows the 79 exons of the gene, the ATG in exon 1, and the 3′ UTR in exon 79. The dystrophin molecule is aligned with the mRNA to show the origin of the four domains. The N, ROD, CYS, and C domains and the four hinge regions (H1 through H4) are as depicted in Figure 140-5 and as described in the text.**

of large fragments by pulsed-field gel electrophoresis.[90-92] This analysis revealed an overall size for the DMD gene of approximately 2300 kb or 1.5 percent of the X chromosome. To put this in perspective, the DMD gene is 100 times larger than an average-size gene and 1000 times larger than the b globin gene; it is half the size of the entire *Escherichia coli* genome with its estimated 5000 genes, and it is larger than any of the chromosomes of yeast.

The DMD gene appears to be about the same size in rodents and birds as in humans. The reasons for maintaining such a large gene throughout evolution are far from clear, although the possibility that other genes are contained within the introns of the DMD gene should be considered.

YAC Cloning of the DMD Gene. Recently the X chromosomal region containing the DMD gene has been cloned as a series of overlapping yeast artificial chromosome (YAC) clones,[93,94] permitting the exons of the gene to be mapped.[94] Furthermore, homologous recombination between YACs has generated a 2.4-Mb recombinant clone containing all the exons of the DMD gene except exon 60.[95] The latter appears to reside in an unstable region of the chromosome and was not contained in the original YACs. The availability of YAC clones will facilitate the determination of the overall structure of the Xp21 chromosomal region and the search for other genes within the DMD gene.

Intron–Exon Borders. Six years after the cloning of the gene, the intron–exon borders have finally been sequenced,[96-101] allowing the exons to be unambiguously numbered.[101] Table 140-2 lists the exons and presents the exon-containing fragments released by *Hin*dIII digestion, since these fragments have been extensively used in the characterization of the gene. Also presented is the 3′ border type for each exon. The border type is defined as 1, 2, or 3 depending on whether the exon ends with the first, second, or third nucleotide of a coding triplet. This border-type information is valuable in determining whether or not a deletion of an exon or group of exons causes a reading frameshift in the mRNA, as will be seen below.

Dystrophin, the Product of the DMD Gene

One important consequence of the DMD gene cloning was the identification of its protein product, given the name

Table 140-2 Exons of the DMD Gene

Exon Number	Domain	*Hin*dIII Fragment Size	3′ End of Exon: Last Nucleotide	3′ End of Exon: Border Type
1	UTR/N	3.2	239	1
2	N	3.25	301	3
3	"	4.2	394	3
4	"	8.5	472	3
5	"	3.1	565	3
6	"	8	738	2
7	"	4.6	857	1
8	N/H1	7.5	1039	3
9	H1	"	1168	3
10	H1/R1	10.5	1357	3
11	R1	"	1539	2
12	R2	3.9	1690	3
13	"	6.6	1810	3
14	R2/R3	2.7	1912	3
15	R3	"	2020	3
16	"	6	2200	3
17	H2	1.7	2376	2
18	R4	12	2500	3
19	"	3	2588	1
20	R4/R5	7.3	2830	3
21	R5	11	3011	1
22	R6	20	3157	3
23	"	"	3370	3
24	R7	"	3484	3
25	"	"	3640	3
26	R8	5.2	3811	3
27	"	"	3994	3
28	R9	1.2	4129	3
29	"	"	4279	3
30	R10	4.7	4441	3
31	"	18	4552	3
32	R11	"	4726	3
33	"	"	4882	3
34	R12	1.8	5053	3
35	"	0.45	5233	3
36	R13	1.3	5362	3
37	"	1.5	5533	3
38	R14	6	5656	3
39	"	"	5794	3
40	R15	6.2	5947	3
41	"	"	6130	3
42	R16	4.2	6325	3
43	"	11	6498	2
44	R17	4.1	6646	3
45	"	0.5	6822	2
46	R18	1.5	6970	3
47	"	10	7120	3
48	R19	1.2, 3.8	7306	3
49	"	1.6	7408	3
50	R19/H3	3.7	7517	1
51	H3/R20	3.1	7750	3
52	R20	7	7868	1
53	R20/R21	7.8, 1.0	8080	3
54	R21	8.3	8235	2
55	R22	2.3	8425	3
56	"	8.8	8598	2
57	R23	1	8755	2
58	R23/R24	6	8876	1
59	R24	"	9145	3
60	R24/H4	3.5	9292	3
61	H4	6.6	9371	1
62	"	2.8	9432	2
63	"	12	9494	1
64	"	2.4	9569	1
65	CYS	2.5	9771	2
66	"	2	9857	1
67	"	1.4	10015	3
68	C	6.6	10182	2
69	"	"	10294	3
70	"	1.5	10431	2
71	"	"	10470	2
72	"	2	10536	2
73	"	1.9	10602	2
74	"	2.4	10761	2
75	"	10	11005	3
76	"	"	11129	1
77	"	2	11222	1
78	"	3	11254	3
79	C/UTR	6.0, 7.8	13958	

dystrophin by Hoffman et al.[102] The protein is missing from muscle of boys with Duchenne muscular dystrophy, from *mdx* mice with a mutation in the equivalent mouse gene, and from dogs with canine X-linked muscular dystrophy. Its absence is clearly responsible for the disease, but how the disease pathology follows from the absence of dystrophin is far from clear. In fact, despite knowledge of the full amino acid sequence of the molecule, recognition of dystrophin as a member of the spectrin family of cytoskeletal proteins, and considerable information concerning its intracellular location in muscle and other tissues, the biological function or functions of dystrophin remain elusive. Below we summarize information concerning dystrophin's structure, its subcellular distribution in the body, its interaction with other proteins in the cell, and its various isoforms and relatives that might have different but related functions.

Structural Domains of Dystrophin. The earliest published cDNA sequence[86] led to the recognition of sequence similarity to α-actinin[103] and β-spectrin,[104] identifying dystrophin as a member of the spectrin superfamily of cytoskeletal proteins. Further sequence analysis of the complete DMD cDNA[105] predicted a protein of 3685 amino acids with a calculated molecular weight of 427 kDa and four distinct domains, three of which are characteristic of cytoskeletal proteins (Fig. 140-5).

An N-terminal domain (amino acids 14 to 240) has sequence homology to the actin-binding domain of α-actinin.

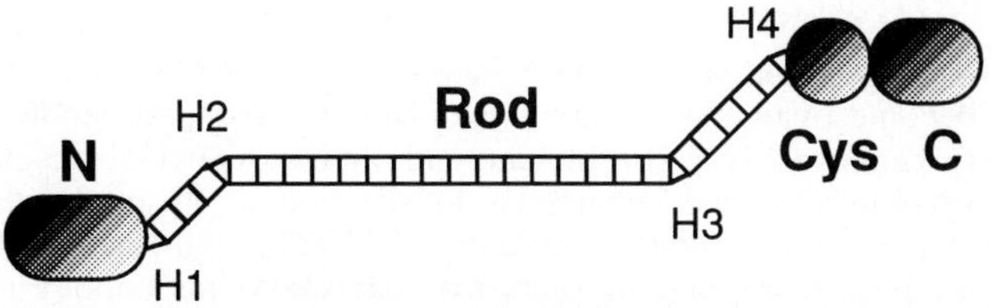

FIG. 140-5 Schematic of the dystrophin molecule. The four domains are the N-terminal domain, the spectrin-like rod domain, the cysteine-rich domain, and the C-terminal domain. The four hinge regions (H1 through H4) are thought to give flexibility to the molecule.

A large second domain (amino acids 278 to 3080) has 24 repeats of a 109-amino-acid sequence similar to the repeats found in α-actinin and spectrin. The third domain (amino acids 3080 to 3360) is cysteine-rich and also bears some homology to α-actinin. The C-terminal domain of dystrophin is different from any other previously known protein but is highly conserved in birds, rodents, and mammals, suggesting an important biologic role in the cell.[106]

The 24 triple helical segments are predicted to give the protein a rod-like character of length 125 nm[105] with four potential "hinge regions" that may give flexibility to the rod.[107] Each repeat is primarily α-helical, with two proline-rich turns that allow it to form a triple helix.[105] Rotary shadowed images of purified dystrophin from rabbit skeletal muscle[108] and from chicken gizzard smooth muscle[109] reveal dumbbell-shaped rod-like structures of length 100 to 120 nm and 175 ± 15 nm respectively. The latter study further revealed side-by-side dimers and higher-order multimeric complexes. In a third study,[110] staggered side-by-side dimers appeared to aggregate into a dumbbell-shaped tetramer 130 nm long and 5 nm wide.

Dystrophin Localization. The identification of dystrophin as the product of the DMD gene, its molecular size determination by western blot analysis, and its localization in tissue sections by light and electron microscopy (EM) depended on the generation of a number of highly specific antibodies to the dystrophin molecule.

Anti-Dystrophin Antibodies. Initial anti-dystrophin antibodies were raised in animals immunized with (1) short peptides synthesized to contain an amino acid sequence determined from the cDNA sequence,[111–114] or (2) fusion proteins synthesized by bacteria transfected with a recombinant gene containing a portion of the DMD cDNA joined to a highly expressed bacterial gene.[102,112] Now, some 5 years after the first antibodies became available, there are probably in excess of 100 different polyclonal and monoclonal antibodies available for different parts of the dystrophin molecule.[115,116]

Western Blot Analysis. Western blot analysis with anti-dystrophin antibodies identified dystrophin as a high-molecular-weight (>400 kDa) protein of skeletal and cardiac muscle with smaller amounts in smooth muscle and trace amounts in brain.[102,114] With the earliest available antisera, all directed to the N-terminal or the rod portion of the molecule, dystrophin appeared as a doublet band in extracts of skeletal and cardiac muscle. The lower band, absent from smooth muscle extracts,[102] appears to be an isoform that is missing the normal C-terminal end, as evidenced by its failure to interact with antibody D11 directed to the last 486 amino acids[107] and antibody 1461 directed to the last 17 amino acids of dystrophin.[117] Additional isoforms of much lower molecular weight are detected with a subset of antibodies, as described in a later section.

Dystrophin in Muscle. With some of the first antisera to become available, immunohistochemical and immunofluorescence analysis of human and mouse skeletal muscle sections revealed subcellular localization of the molecule at the sarcolemmal membrane[112,113,118] (Fig. 140-6A). Lack of immunostaining in sections from DMD patients (Fig. 140-6B) and *mdx* mice confirmed the specificity of the antibody reaction. Localization of dystrophin to the plasma membrane was subsequently documented for cardiac muscle and smooth muscle[113,119–122] as well as chicken gizzard smooth muscle.[123] In the heart, dystrophin is strongly expressed in the Purkinje fibers.[124]

Earlier biochemical evidence suggested that dystrophin was located primarily in the transverse tubule membranes of skeletal muscle,[125] but this idea has not been substantiated either in subsequent biochemical studies[126,127] or in additional light and electron microscopy studies.[120,128] However, dystrophin is clearly seen in both the plasma membrane and transverse tubules of cardiac muscle,[121,129] suggesting a possible functional difference between the T-tubules in cardiac and skeletal muscle.[129] Dystrophin has also been reported in the T-tubules of regenerating, but not mature, rat skeletal muscle fibers.[130]

The precise arrangement of dystrophin at the plasma membrane is not clear, but EM localization with immunogold suggests that the rod domain is 15 to 20 nm from the cytoplasmic face of the sarcolemmal membrane,[128,131,132] with the C-terminal end closer to the membrane.[133] Analysis of nearest-neighbor distances for the immunogold particles revealed a periodicity of 120 to 125 nm in both longitudinal and transverse directions.[128,131,133] Since this distance corresponds to the approximate length of dystrophin molecules, it suggests that the molecules may be associated end-to-end. A longer periodicity observed in skeletal[132] or smooth[123] muscle would also be consistent with this model. The two-dimensional nature of the pattern suggests a lattice model similar to that proposed by Koenig and Kunkel,[107] in which molecules align in antiparallel dimers in a manner analogous to α-actinin and spectrin, and then join end-to-end to form a hexagonal honeycomb array.

This simple picture of a uniform, two-dimensional lattice inside the muscle membrane is pleasing but too simplistic. Recent studies of longitudinal sections or intact teased whole fibers have clearly demonstrated that dystrophin in muscle is not uniformly distributed but occurs in a surface network with a defined relationship to the underlying contractile apparatus. Thus, colocalization of dystrophin with β-spectrin in longitudinal sections revealed a concentration of both molecules overlying the I bands, suggesting that dystrophin and spectrin, along with vinculin, might function to link the contractile apparatus to the sarcolemma.[134] A similar pattern was seen with single teased fibers, which revealed a network of dense transverse rings (costameres) overlying the Z bands, with finer longitudinal interconnections.[135] This pattern was disrupted only when blocked by the presence of a myonucleus at the membrane. Mechanical skinning of the fibers resulted in the dystrophin network peeling off with the membrane,[135] demonstrating tight membrane association. While dystrophin is clearly a part of the elaborate cytoskeletal network associated with each sarcomere, it is not required for this lattice-like organization, as the spectrin distribution is maintained in dystrophin-deficient muscle from *mdx* mice.[134]

Dystrophin at Neuromuscular and Myotendinous Junctions. Recent studies have also revealed an elevated concentration of dystrophin at the neuromuscular junction and the myotendinous junction. At the myotendinous junction, anti-dystrophin label appears to extend into the muscle away from the membrane.[120,136] While one antiserum labeled the myotendinous junction of *mdx* mice, suggesting that the enhanced reaction could be due to a cross-reacting protein,[136] antibody 6-10 of Byers et al.[120] produced no staining of the myotendinous junction in *mdx* mice, providing good evidence that the enhanced staining in normal mice was due to increased levels of dystrophin. A functional role for dystrophin in the transmission of tension from sarcomeric actin

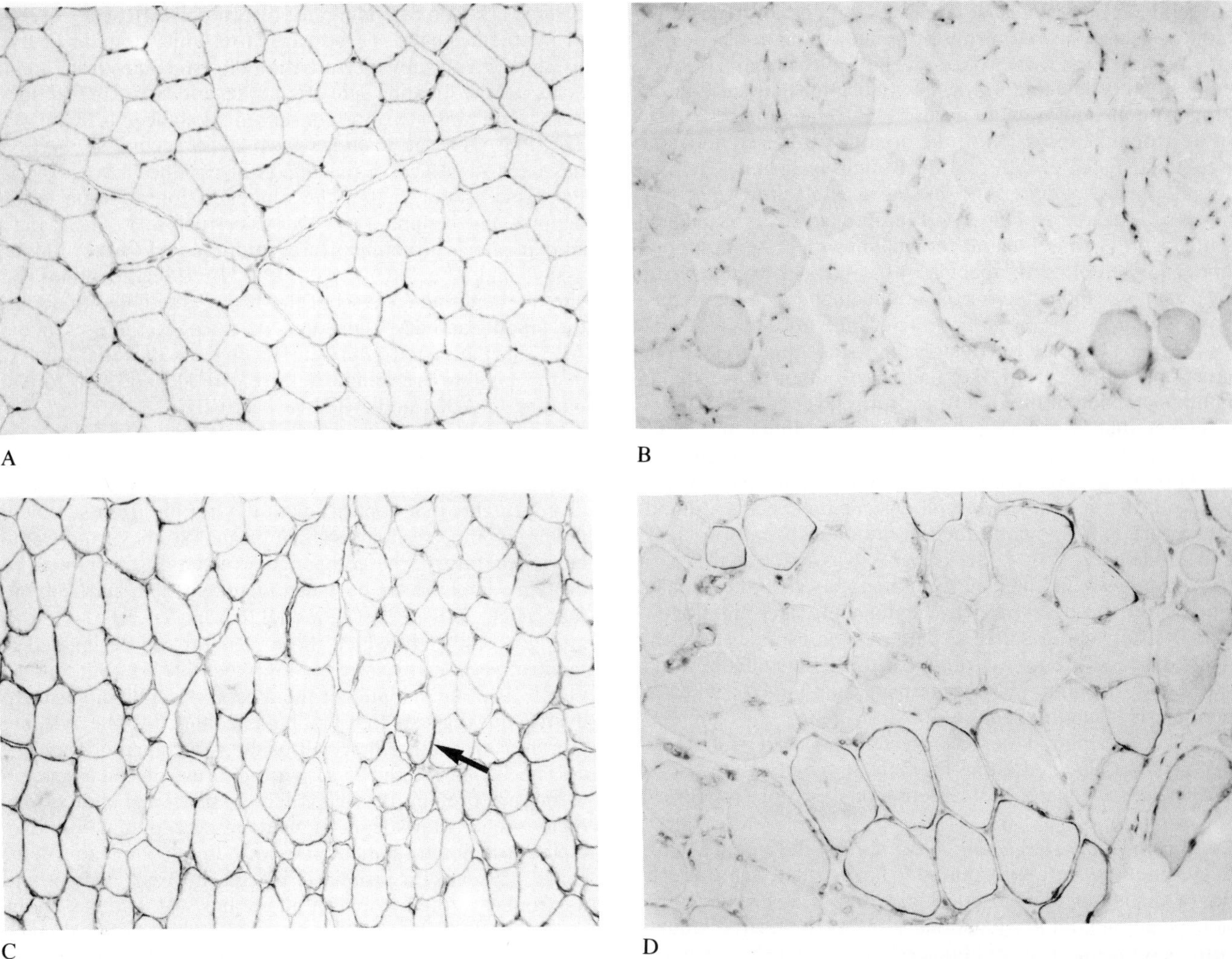

FIG. 140-6 Immunoperoxidase staining with antiserum 1461 (C-terminal anti-dystrophin antibody). *A*. Biopsy specimen from normal control muscle showing an uninterrupted sarcolemmal dystrophin immunoreactivity (×280). *B*. Biopsy from Duchenne muscular dystrophy showing complete absence of dystrophin immunoreactivity (×280) *C*. Biopsy from Becker muscular dystrophy showing variable intensity of staining with some fibers exhibiting variation of intensity within the fiber (arrow) (×280). *D*. Biopsy from outlier (intermediate phenotype) showing dystrophin-positive and -negative fibers with variable intensity (×280). *(Courtesy of Dr. Venita Jay.)*

through the membrane to the tendon is suggested by the finding of a deficiency in the attachment of actin filaments to myotendinous junctions of *mdx* mice.[137]

Initial reports of enhanced levels of dystrophin at the neuromuscular junction[138,139] failed to include dystrophin-deficient controls, so the specificity of the antibody could not be determined. Later studies with some antibodies found neuromuscular junction labeling in *mdx* controls and DMD patients,[140] indicating that the antibodies were recognizing a cross-reacting protein, probably the dystrophin-related protein discussed below. In contrast, studies with antibodies 6-10[120] and R27 (a commercial preparation of Kunkel's original anti-60kD antiserum)[141] revealed enhanced neuromuscular junction staining in normal but not *mdx* mice, providing good evidence for an elevated concentration of dystrophin at the neuromuscular junction. In these studies dystrophin appears concentrated at the postsynaptic membrane, specifically in the troughs of the synaptic folds.

Dystrophin in Electric Organs. These results are supported by the finding of dystrophin (or a highly homologous protein) at very high concentration in the electric organ of the torpedo,[142] where it is associated with the cytoplasmic surface of the postsynaptic membrane.[143-145] Electric tissue is a highly simplified, noncontractile tissue that derives embryologically from striated muscle, and the presence of dystrophin has suggested a role in the organization of the electroplate. Monoclonal antibodies against the torpedo protein react not only with the torpedo synaptic membrane but also with the synaptic and nonsynaptic membrane of normal but not dystrophic human and mouse muscle.[144,145] Cloning and sequencing of the torpedo gene has confirmed the homology of the torpedo protein with human and mouse dystrophin.[145] Anti-dystrophin antibodies also identify a membrane-associated protein in the electric organ of the skate, where localization is to both the innervated and the noninnervated surface of the electrocyte,[146] more like the situation in vertebrate muscle.

Dystrophin in the CNS and PNS. Shortly after the discovery of dystrophin, both the protein and its mRNA were detected in brain extracts. In normal mouse brain, dystrophin is most abundant in the cerebellum, where it is found in the soma and dendrites but not axons of Purkinje cells,[147,148] and in cerebral cortex, where it appears as punctate aggregates along the soma and dendrites of pyramidal neurons.[147] By *in situ* hybridization with probes specific for dystrophin mRNA, expression is detected in these two locations and also in the hippocampus and dentate gyrus.[149–151] This complex pattern of dystrophin expression in the brain is further complicated by the existence of different dystrophin isoforms generated by alternative splicing and by the use of alternative promoters, as described below. As cerebral cortex is associated with cognitive function and cerebellum with motor coordination, it is tempting to speculate that lack of dystrophin in the brain is responsible for the intellectual deficit in affected boys and/or for the tremors in older *mdx* mice.[147]

Further evidence for dystrophin localization at synaptic junctions comes from the finding of intense dystrophin immunostaining in the outer plexiform layer of the retina.[138] The fact that some but not all anti-dystrophin antibodies give retinal staining in *mdx* mice[152] suggests that there may be both dystrophin and a cross-reacting protein at this location. In a recent study with dystrophin-specific antibodies, dystrophin was confirmed in the outer plexiform layer, and its deficiency in DMD patients was correlated with a negative b-wave in the electroretinography (ERG) response, similar to that observed in congenital stationary night blindness.[153] If the abnormal ERG pattern is a direct result of the dystrophin deficiency, it provides the first evidence for a role of dystrophin in neurotransmission and provides a noninvasive functional assay for dystrophin.

In the peripheral nervous system, a short isoform of dystrophin is located along the Schwann cell membrane.[154] This is described later in the section on dystrophin isoforms.

Dystrophin in the Developing Fetus. In the developing fetus, dystrophin was initially reported to be distributed throughout the cytoplasm of skeletal muscle, with a heavier concentration at myotendinous junctions.[155] More extensive studies with several different antibodies have revealed dystrophin mRNA and the protein in developing muscle as early as 9 weeks gestation, with the level of cytoplasmic and perinuclear staining decreasing with time as the sarcolemmal localization becomes predominant by 22 to 26 weeks.[156,157] In the mouse, *in situ* hybridization detects dystrophin transcripts as early as 9 days in the heart and a little later in skeletal muscle and smooth muscle.[151] Dystrophin transcripts are also expressed in the cerebellum and forebrain from day 13.

Fetal dystrophin appears to be smaller in size than adult dystrophin, increases in amount throughout gestation, and gives a somewhat different pattern on western blot analysis with different antibodies, suggestive of developmentally regulated dystrophin isoforms.[157] These are described in more detail below in the section on isoforms.

The Actin–Dystrophin–Glycoprotein Complex. There is now substantial evidence that dystrophin is part of a complex joining the intracellular cytoskeleton to the extracellular matrix, binding cytoskeletal actin at its N-terminal end and a transmembrane glycoprotein complex at its C-terminal end.

Actin Binding. The sequence similarity of the N-terminal domain of dystrophin to the actin-binding domain of α-actinin first suggested an interaction between dystrophin and actin. Binding of dystrophin to filamentous actin (not actin of the contractile apparatus) is now well documented in several studies. Actin-binding site 1 (ABS1), located at amino acid residues 17 to 26, was identified by proton NMR spectroscopy of synthetic peptides from the N-terminal domain of dystrophin, which show perturbation of resonances from amino acids in the binding site upon the addition of F-actin.[158] ABS1 contains a highly conserved sequence, KTFT (Lys, Thr, Phe, Thr), at positions 19 to 22. A second site, ABS2, has been identified in the region of residues 128 to 156 by the same approach, but the sequence conservation is less distinct and is spread over a larger region.[159] ABS1 and a similar site in α-actinin were confirmed by direct binding assays and by cellular targeting of N-terminal peptides, but site-directed mutagenesis of the KTFT site failed to abolish the binding activity,[160] presumably owing to the presence of ABS2 in the tested peptide. The regions of actin involved in the binding are amino acids 83 to 117 and 350 to 375, binding to ABS1 and ABS2 respectively.[159]

Dystrophin–Glycoprotein Complex. At the other end of the molecule, dystrophin is bound to a complex of proteins and glycoproteins that copurify with dystrophin from sarcolemmal membrane.[161] In a series of elegant studies from Campbell's laboratory, the components of the dystrophin–glycoprotein complex have been identified and characterized from rabbit muscle.[127,162–164] The model that has emerged is shown in Figure 140-7, in which these proteins are designated by their molecular masses of 156, 59, 40, 43, 35, and 25 kDa.[162] Peptide mapping of the glycoprotein binding sites of dystrophin suggests that binding is confined to the cysteine-rich domain and the first half of the C-terminal domain.[165]

The 50, 43, 35, and 25 kDa proteins are placed as integral membrane proteins based on their possession of hydrophobic regions characteristic of transmembrane domains and on their extraction from membrane with lipid-solubilizing detergents. The 59-kDa protein is placed in direct contact with dystrophin in the cytoplasm on the basis of its cross-linking to dystrophin[166] and its lack of a hydrophobic domain. The 156-kDa protein is highly glycosylated, suggesting its placement on the exterior of the muscle cell, and it has recently been shown to bind laminin, a major component of the extracellular matrix.[163] Studies both in cultured myogenic cells[167] and in cardiac muscle[129] clearly show colocalization of dystrophin with laminin, consistent with this biochemical analysis.

Thus, dystrophin is a key element in a major glycoprotein complex that in muscle links the actin filaments of the subsarcolemmal cytoskeleton to laminin in the extracellular

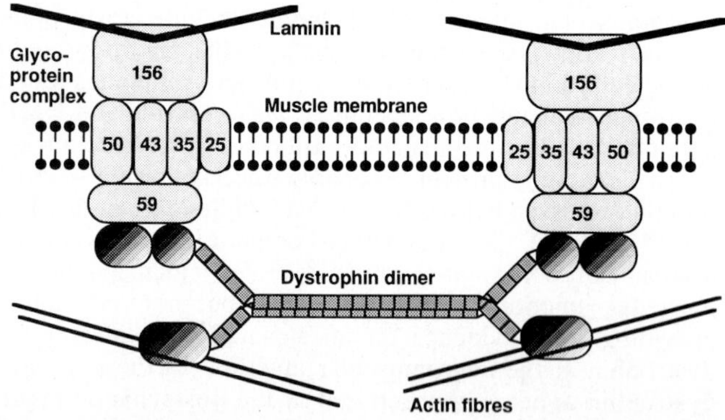

FIG. 140-7 Schematic of the actin–dystrophin–glycoprotein complex. Filamentous actin binds to dystrophin at the N-terminal end and the glycoprotein complex binds at the C-terminal end. The rationale for the model is provided in the text. ***(Adapted from Ervasti and Campbell.[162])***

matrix. The fact that dystrophin is a major component of this complex, and the fact that in the absence of dystrophin some, and perhaps all, of the associate glycoproteins are missing from the membrane, suggests that the key role of dystrophin is a structural one. Whether it forms part of a similar complex in smooth and cardiac muscle and in neurons of the brain remains to be determined. Defects in one or more of the proteins in the glycoprotein complex have been implicated in other neuromuscular disorders, as outlined in a later section.

Dystrophin Isoforms. To complicate matters further, dystrophin is not a single molecule but exists in several isoforms, generated in part by alternative splicing of the mRNA and in part by the use of alternative promoters to initiate transcription from different places in the gene.

Use of Alternative Promoters. The first promoter to be identified was that specifying the full-length skeletal muscle dystrophin. The muscle promoter is similar to other muscle-specific promoters, having MEF-1 (MyoD-binding) sites at positions −58, −535, and −583 bp, a CArG box at position −91 bp, and an MCAT consensus sequence at position −394 bp.[168] It is capable of directing transcription of a CAT (chloramphenicol acetyl transferase) reporter gene in a muscle-cell-specific and muscle-differentiation-specific manner.[168] The "core" promoter contains both positive and negative regulatory elements, and the CArG box appears to be functionally essential.[169] An enhancer sequence has also been characterized in the first intron (H. Klamut, L. Bosnoyan, R.G. Worton, and P.N. Ray, unpublished observations). In Figure 140-8 the "muscle" promoter is labeled P1.

In rat brain, mRNA from the DMD gene contains a different first exon, transcribed from a distinct promoter.[170] This result has been confirmed for the mouse[171] and human gene,[172,173] and the "brain" promoter (P2 in Fig. 140-8) has been mapped 90 kb or more upstream from the muscle-specific promoter.[173] In this brain isoform, the first 11 amino acids of the common muscle isoform are replaced with three different amino acids. Interestingly, while the "brain" promoter is highly specific to neurons, the muscle promoter is active in a wider spectrum of cell types, including striated and smooth muscle and also glial cells.[174]

By *in situ* hybridization, transcripts from P2 and to a lesser extent from P1 were found in mouse cerebral cortex and regions of the hippocampus.[150] In contrast, mRNA containing neither of these first exons was expressed in cerebellar Purkinje cells, leading to the identification of a third promoter (P3) in the middle of the 240-kb intron between the muscle-type exon 1 and exon 2.[150] In this isoform, seven amino acids encoded by the "Purkinje cell" first exon replace the first 11 amino acids of muscle-type dystrophin. This same study also identified a form of dystrophin in the dentate gyrus that was revealed by probes from the 3′ but not the 5′ end of the gene, suggesting another promoter further toward the 5′ end of the gene.

A fourth promoter had earlier been suggested by the fact that a short transcript in rat liver and other tissues was found, with probes from the 3′ but not the 5′ end of the gene.[175] Cloning and characterization of this transcript, variously described as 6.5 kb,[176,177] 4.8 kb,[178] and 4.5 kb[179] long, has revealed a unique promoter (P4 in Fig. 140-8) and first exon that maps about 8 kb upstream of exon 63. It encodes a 71-kDa protein (Dp71) that is a major product of the DMD gene in brain, liver, lung, and stomach. It is present in small amounts in cultured myogenic cells but is down-regulated during differentiation to form myotubes.[176] Dp71 contains the cysteine-rich and the C-terminal domains

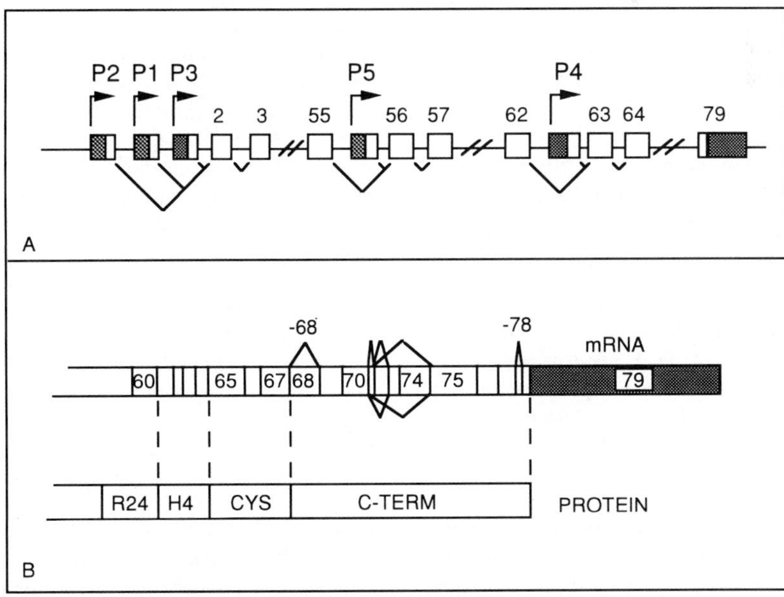

FIG. 140-8 Schematic of the dystrophin gene to illustrate the origin of dystrophin isoforms. *A*. Relative positions of the five promoters (P1 through P5). Each of the five promoters directs translation from its own first exon, and each of these has an ATG translational start site, dividing these exons into a 5′ untranslated portion (stippled) and a coding portion. The first exons at promoters P1, P2, and P3 all splice to exon 2, generating three high-molecular-weight isoforms differing only at the first few amino acids. The first exons at promoters P4 and P5 splice to exons 63 and 56, respectively, generating proteins of 71 and 116 kDa respectively. Exon 79 encodes the last several amino acids and contains a large 3′ untranslated region (stippled). *B*. Alternative splicing patterns described for the human DMD gene. Alternative splicing across exon 68 or 78 alters the reading frame of the message, thereby altering the C-terminal end of the dystrophin molecule. Alternative splicing of individual exons or combinations of exons 71 to 74 does not alter the reading frame and leaves the C-terminal end of the dystrophin molecule unchanged. The stippled area represents the untranslated portion of exon 79 when exon 78 is included in the message. This region is reduced in size in the −78 form as the C-terminal end of the protein is extended.

of dystrophin preceded by seven amino acids that are unique to this protein. The P4 promoter has features typical of a gene that is ubiquitously expressed.[179] It is possible that the 71-kDa protein is the isoform seen in the dentate gyrus by *in situ* hybridization.[150]

A fifth promoter (P5 in Fig. 140-8) has recently been recognized. Western blot analysis with antibodies against the distal part of the rod domain revealed a dystrophin isoform of 116 kDa (Dp116) uniquely expressed in peripheral nerve.[154] This isoform is encoded by a 5.2-kb message transcribed from a promoter in intron 55. The previously undetected first exon splices to muscle exon 56, resulting in a protein that begins with spectrin-like repeat 22 and includes the last 946 amino acids of dystrophin.[154]

The short isoforms encoded by the transcripts from promoters 4 and 5 lack the actin-binding domain and rod domain of dystrophin and therefore are presumed to have somewhat different functions from those of the full-length molecules derived from promoters 1, 2 and 3.

Alternative Splicing in the DMD Gene. Alternative splicing in the DMD gene was first detected by polymerase chain reaction (PCR) amplification of overlapping segments of human fetal dystrophin mRNA and sizing of the amplified fragments to detect heterogeneity in the 3′ end of the transcript.[172] Sequencing of the fragments identified six exons that were spliced out of the different products, singly or in combination, and confirmed the existence of at least three different mRNA types in skeletal muscle and brain and two in smooth muscle. With the determination of exon structure through this region of the gene,[100] it became possible to assign numbers to the alternatively spliced exons, as depicted in Figure 140-8. These same alternative splicing patterns and others have also been detected in human retina[153] as well as in embryonic and adult mouse skeletal muscle, cardiac Purkinje fibers, and brain.[124,171,180]

Removal of exon 71, 72, 71-72, 71-74, or 72-74 does not alter the reading frame of the message and results in a near-normal dystrophin missing 13, 22, 35, 97, or 110 amino acids, respectively, from the middle of the C-terminal domain. These isoforms, if functional, may have a function similar to that of full-length dystrophin, a conclusion supported by the fact that the major mRNA in chicken skeletal muscle is missing exon 72.[106] In skeletal muscle the "full-length" mRNA is the predominant form, with smaller amounts of the −71 form. In brain, retina, heart, and cardiac Purkinje fibers, a complex splicing pattern gives rise to multiple smaller transcripts. Purkinje fibers express primarily the −(71-74) form, while the −72 and −(72-74) forms are found almost exclusively in heart muscle.[180] The retina expresses the full-length form as well as the −71 and −(71-74) forms.[153]

Alternative splicing to remove exon 78 appears to be functionally and developmentally more significant. It removes 32 base pairs from the message and alters the reading frame of exon 79 such that the last 14 hydrophilic amino acids at the C-terminal end are replaced by 32 primarily hydrophobic amino acids encoded by the alternate reading frame.[180] In both mouse and human, this splicing pattern is developmentally regulated, with switching from the hydrophobic (−78) form to the hydrophilic (+78) form during fetal development.[180] An antibody directed against a synthetic peptide encoded by the alternate reading frame also detects this fetal isoform in human adult smooth muscle.[181]

Removal of exon 68 also changes the reading frame and results in loss of the entire C-terminal domain. The putative protein product therefore has three domains and is structurally similar to α-actinin and β-spectrin, perhaps an evolutionary precursor of full-size dystrophin. It is a minor splice product in all tissues examined and may have no functional significance.[180]

A cloned cDNA from the P4 promoter excluded exons 71 and 78, suggesting that these spliced products may be common to the short mRNA in nonmuscle tissues and not to the 14-kb dystrophin mRNA that is less abundant in these tissues.

Dystrophin-Related Protein (Utrophin). Detection of a dystrophin cross-reactive protein[182] in DMD patients and *mdx* mouse led to a search for a closely related protein. Cloning of cDNAs that cross-hybridize to the 3′ end of the dystrophin mRNA[183,184] identified the DMDL (DMD-like) gene on human chromosome 6 and mouse chromosome 10.[185] The gene encodes a 13-kb transcript that shows no alternative splicing at the 3′ end,[186] and the sequence of the complete cDNA shows extensive homology to dystrophin over the entire length of the molecule, suggesting derivation from a common ancestral gene.[187]

In contrast to dystrophin, skeletal muscle is not the major site of expression of dystrophin-related protein (DRP). Transcripts are detected at highest levels in placenta but occur in a broad range of fetal and adult tissues including heart, liver, intestine, kidney, and testis, some fetal tissues showing greater expression than the corresponding adult tissue.[186]

Antibodies specific to DRP reveal a protein of approximately 400 kDa, ubiquitously expressed in muscle, brain, kidney, gut, and other tissues,[184] as well as in a variety of cultured cell lines.[188] The ubiquitous expression has led to the alternate name *utrophin*.[186] In mouse skeletal muscle, utrophin levels peak during fetal life and before birth, in contrast to the pattern of expression of dystrophin.[189] The presence of the 400-kDa band in muscle of DMD and BMD males and *mdx* mice confirms that the antibodies are detecting a protein other than dystrophin.[184,190]

Immunofluorescence analysis of skeletal muscle with anti-utrophin antibodies[191,192] or with cross-reacting anti-dystrophin antibodies[193] reveals utrophin primarily at neuromuscular and myotendinous junctions of normal and *mdx* mice. With some antibodies, a weak and patchy staining is seen over the sarcolemma of normal muscle. Whether utrophin is detected at the sarcolemma as well as the neuromuscular junction appears to depend on the strength of the antibody.[194]

The presence of utrophin at the sarcolemma is greatly enhanced in the muscle of DMD patients and *mdx* mice, suggesting that a compensatory increase of utrophin occurs in response to the absence of dystrophin or to the process of regeneration.[190,195] This suggests the exciting possibility that utrophin may function in place of dystrophin in some circumstances and that upregulation of utrophin may be a potential treatment for DMD patients.

In other tissues, the distribution of utrophin is less well studied. With anti-dystrophin antibodies, cross-reacting protein has been seen at the membrane of smooth muscle in DMD boys[196] and in the pia mater of *mdx* mouse brain.[197] With utrophin-specific antibodies intense immunolabeling was seen in the pia mater, choroid plexus, and intercerebral vasculature, with minimal staining in neuronal or glial elements of brain parenchyma.[198]

Functional similarity between utrophin and dystrophin is suggested by the finding that utrophin binds to a complex of proteins and glycoproteins similar or identical to those that bind dystrophin.[199] These associated proteins colocalize with utrophin to the neuromuscular junction of skeletal muscle in DMD patients and *mdx* mice but are found throughout the sarcolemma in cardiac and small-caliber skeletal muscles of *mdx* mice.

The possible relationship of mutant utrophin to disease has been studied in both mouse and human. The human gene on chromosome 6 is a potential candidate for any of the autosomal neuromuscular disorders. RFLPs at the locus have not shown cosegregation with limb-girdle muscular dystrophy, ruling the gene out as a candidate for this disease. In mouse the gene on chromosome 10 maps in the vicinity of the *dy* locus responsible for autosomal recessive dystrophia muscularis. In *dy/dy* mice, anti-utrophin antibody detects a 400-kDa protein[186,191] that localizes at the neuromuscular junction.[191] This result suggests that mutant utrophin is not the basic defect in the *dy* mouse, although it cannot rule out a subtle mutation that destroys utrophin function without disturbing its localization in muscle.

Mutation in the DMD Gene

The first mutations to be described in the DMB gene were the deletions detected with the PERT87 and the XJ series of genomic probes, and they occurred in about 8 to 10 percent of affected boys. By Southern blot analysis with a complete set of cDNA probes or by the analysis of large fragments that cover the central portion of the gene, the frequency of detectable deletions rose to over 60 percent,[88,200,201] and duplications were detected in 6 percent of affected boys.[202] More recently a number of point mutations have been described. Translocations that disrupt the gene are the main type of mutation resulting in the expression of the disease in females.

Deletion. Deletions in the DMD gene are highly heterogeneous with respect to both size and location. The largest deletions, several thousand kilobases in size, remove neighboring genes and occur in association with a contiguous gene deletion syndrome. Smaller deletions remove from one to a few exons, and their distribution in the gene is not random (Fig. 140-9). Two deletion-rich regions are apparent in the gene, one extending over the first 20 exons and the second near the middle of the gene around exons 45 to 53.[88]

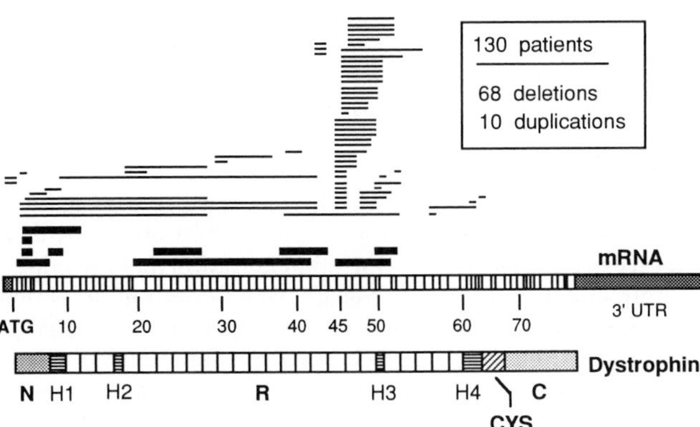

FIG. 140-9 Schematic showing the spectrum of deletions (thin bars) and duplications (thick bars) relative to the mRNA and to the dystrophin molecule. Each bar represents the extent of the deletion or duplication in a single patient. The "hot spot" for deletion around exons 45 to 52 is evident. The mRNA and dystrophin schematics are as in Figure 140-4.

Once it became possible to analyze individual mutations, it also became possible to correlate the size or location of a deletion with the phenotype of the patient. Mental capacity is one highly variable element in the DMD phenotype, with mean IQ about one standard deviation below the mean. So far there is no clear evidence of a correlation between mental functioning and the location or size of deletions, although deletion of exon 52 has been reported to be associated with an elevated risk for mental deficiency.[203]

Deletions in DMD patients are not confined to a specific region of the gene, indicating that differences in phenotype are not due to deletion of discrete domains with differing functions. Furthermore, phenotypic severity is not simply a function of deletion size, since some deletions associated with BMD are larger than, and completely encompass, deletions associated with DMD. Indeed, two BMD patients with very large deletions that remove exons 17 to 48[204] and exons 14 to 44[205] underscore this point.

Frameshift Versus Nonframeshift Deletions. The wide spectrum of severity in DMD/BMD can be largely explained as a direct consequence of the effect of the mutation on the translational reading frame of the mRNA. Deletion breakpoints are almost always in introns, so that most deletions remove a specific set of exons from the genome. If all exons began with the first nucleotide of a codon and ended with the last nucleotide of a codon, then the deletions would simply remove an integral number of codons from the message and an equal number of amino acids from the protein. Unfortunately, exon border types are variable and do not necessarily correspond to the ends of codons. In Table 140-2, exon border types are defined as 1, 2, or 3 depending on whether the exon ends with the first, second, or third nucleotide of a coding triplet.

When one or more exons are deleted from the gene, therefore, the reading frame of the mRNA may or may not be maintained. It will be maintained if the joined exon borders are of the same type, but it will be frameshifted whenever the deletion results in the joining of unlike borders. When this happens, the new reading frame specifies a completely different set of amino acids in the protein until the translation complex encounters a stop codon, at which point protein synthesis terminates. The truncated protein, missing the C-terminal end, may be nonfunctional or unstable. In contrast, a deletion that does not alter the reading frame will generate a protein that is missing those amino acids encoded by the deleted exons, but will maintain a normal amino acid sequence before and after the deleted region.

Frameshifting deletions that produce truncated dystrophin are expected to give a more severe phenotype than nonframeshifting deletions, since the latter will encode a shortened dystrophin with intact ends.[97] Several groups have evaluated their patients in relation to the frameshift model. The results, summarized in Table 140-3, indicate that most frameshift deletions are found in DMD patients, whereas most nonframeshift deletions are found in BMD patients.[96,98,206,207] Thus, the reading frame status often provides a valid prognostic indicator for the severity of the disease.

Western blot analysis has confirmed that BMD patients have significant levels of dystrophin, usually of reduced size, consistent with the model.[208] Furthermore, studies with antibodies directed to the N-terminus and the C-terminus of dystrophin show that BMD patients have dystrophin capable of reacting with both antibodies, whereas DMD patients have either no detectable dystrophin or dystrophin that is

Table 140-3 Proportion of Frameshift and In-Frame Deletions in DMD, Intermediate, and BMD Patients

Region Analyzed	DMD		Intermediate		BMD		Reference
	Frameshift	In-Frame	Frameshift	In-Frame	Frameshift	In-Frame	
Exons 1-10	11	0	8	2	6	0	Malhotra et al.[96]
Exons 1-21	5	0	2	1	0	0	Baumbach et al.[207]
Exons 44-51	20	0	2	0	1	1	Baumbach et al.[207]
Entire gene*	178	10	6	8	4	53	Koenig et al.[98]
Exons 44-51	21	0	7	1	1	8	Gillard et al.[206]
Total	235† 96%	10 4%	25† 68%	12 32%	12† 16%	62 84%	

*Excluding deletions with an end-point in a region with unknown exon border type.
†Exon 3-7 frameshift deletions were identified in 7 DMD, 10 intermediate, and 10 BMD; exon 45 frameshift deletions were identified in 9 DMD, 4 intermediate, and 2 BMD.

reduced in size and reacts with the N-terminus antibody only.[117,209,210]

As Table 140-3 indicates, there are exceptions to the reading frame rule, the most common being BMD cases with frameshifting deletions. Two examples of this type are deletions of exon 45 and exons 3 through 7, both of which are frameshifting deletions that are found in DMD, intermediate, and BMD patients. Alternative splicing of exon 44 in patients with deletion of exon 45 is apparently a common occurrence and results in a continuous reading frame, which would potentially explain the mild phenotype in some patients.[211] Alternative splicing has also been reported in a BMD patient with deletion of exons 3 through 7,[212] but this result was not confirmed in muscle biopsies of other similar patients who are nevertheless making significant amounts of dystrophin.[213] Other explanations for the production of dystrophin in these individuals include initiation of protein synthesis from an in-frame putative translational start site in exon 8 or ribosomal frameshifting in which ribosomes switch from one reading frame to another, avoiding premature termination.[214]

Deletion Mechanisms. In principle, deletion may occur by random breakage and reunion or by a specific recombination event. Recombination may involve either homologous or nonhomologous exchange and may be between chromosomes, between sister chromatids of the same chromosome, or between different regions of the same chromatid. Finally, it may occur at either meiosis or mitosis. The DMD gene is amenable to the study of some of these parameters.

The clustering of deletions around exons 45 to 53 suggests that some feature of the DNA or the chromatin structure in this region may predispose to specific breakage or recombination events. This clustering is most extreme for deletions beginning in intron 44. In a study of such deletions, however, the deletion breakpoints appear scattered throughout the 170-kb intron and not clustered at a predisposing site.[215] In contrast, the sequencing of two deletion breakpoints in this intron has identified a transposon-like element at the site of the rearrangement, suggesting predisposition to rearrangement at this site.[216] Sequencing of two other deletion junctions in this intron revealed a random breakage or nonhomologous recombination mechanism in a stretch of A-T-rich DNA, but the significance of this finding is not clear.[217] Deletions in other regions of the gene have not been examined at the nucleotide level.

There are several indications that some and perhaps many of the chromosomal rearrangements in the DMD gene occur in somatic cells or in germ-line cells prior to meiosis. This evidence, in the case of deletions, comes from families in which two or more affected boys are found to have a deletion that is not present in the blood lymphocytes of the mother. These mothers must be germ-line mosaics whose deletion arose in a diploid cell during development.[218–221] Germ-line mosaicism is reviewed in more detail in a later section.

Duplication. Duplication of one or more exons of the DMD gene can be detected in about 6 percent of patients by quantitative Southern blot analysis with cDNA probes[202] or by analysis of large gene fragments by field inversion gel electrophoresis.[90] Frameshifting duplications tend to occur more frequently in DMD patients, where they may result in a truncated protein, whereas duplications that do not shift the reading frame occur more often in BMD, and may result in a greatly enlarged dystrophin with part of the amino acid sequence repeated in the protein.[222] When examined, the mRNA is found to contain the duplicated sequence that is predicted from the genome duplication, and the protein with the duplicated set of amino acids is of the predicted size.[223]

Duplication Mechanisms. The recombination mechanisms that cause deletion can also result in duplication. In three cases a duplication has been characterized at the nucleotide level. One duplication resulted from homologous recombination between a pair of *Alu* sequences in the DMD gene, whereas two others resulted from nonhomologous recombination events.[224] In six cases where the duplication has been traced in families, the rearrangement occurred in the germ line of a maternal grandparent, in all but one the maternal grandfather.[225] Since males have a single X chromosome, the duplication must have occurred by unequal sister chromatid exchange.

Point Mutations. Mutations in the one third of patients who do not have a large deletion or duplication are difficult to identify in a 2300-kb gene. One point mutation that introduces a stop codon into the message was found in a patient previously identified with truncated dystrophin.[226] Several other mutations were found by a systematic analysis of the PCR-amplified message[227] or PCR-amplified genomic DNA.[228–232] The point mutations identified in these and other reports are tabulated in Table 140-4. Ten of these are single-base changes to a termination codon in boys with severe DMD. The affected exons are more or less evenly distributed between exons 8 and 70, with no evidence of a hot spot for mutation. One of these cases (patient 8, Table 140-4) was complicated by the fact that a two-base-pair substitution in

Table 140-4 Point Mutation in the DMD Gene

Patient Number	Nucleotide Change	Exon Affected	Effect of Change*	Reference
Mutations to Termination Codon				
1	C932T	Exon 8	Glu → term	Nigro et al.[232]
2	C2510T	Exon 19	Arg → term	Prior et al.[230]
3	G2522T	Exon 19	Glu → term	Prior et al.[230]
4	G2999T	Exon 21	Glu → term	Roberts et al.[227]
5	G3677T	Exon 26	Glu → term	Bulman et al.[226]
6	C5759T	Exon 39	Gln → term	Roberts et al.[227]
7	C7163T	Exon 48	Glu → term	Clemens et al.[229]
8	GG7609/10 → AT	Exon 51	Leu → term (s.a. in 51)	Winnard et al.[233]
9	C9152T (CpG)	Exon 60	Arg → term	Roberts et al.[227]
10	C10316T (CpG)	Exon 70	Arg → term	Roberts et al.[227]
Frameshift Deletions				
11	ΔC2568	Exon 19	fs	Prior et al.[230]
12	AG5960/1 → T	Exon 48	fs	Kilimann et al.[228]
13	ΔT10662	Exon 74	fs	Roberts et al.[227]
Frameshift Insertions				
14	T1554 → ins T	Exon 12	fs	Kilimann et al.[228]
Frameshift Splicing Alterations				
15	52-bp del. in exon 19	Exon 19 skipped	fs	Matsuo et al.[234,235]
16	5-bp del. at splice donor	Exon 44 skipped	fs	Saad et al.[231]
17	splice acceptor AG → AC	Exon 57 skipped	fs (s.a. in 57)	Roberts et al.[101]
18	splice donor GT → GA	Exon 68 skipped	fs	Roberts et al.[227]
Mutations in Animal Models of DMD				
mdx mouse	C → T	Exon 23	Glu → term	Sicinski et al.[239]
mdx (3Cv)	TG → AG, splice acceptor	Exon 66	fs, ins 14 bp of int 65	Cox et al.[241]
cxmd	splice acceptor AG → GG	Exon 6 skipped	fs	Sharp et al.[244]

*Abbreviations: fs = frameshift; ins = insertion; int = intron; s.a. = splice acceptor; term = termination.

exon 51 created both a termination codon and a new splice acceptor site.[233] This gave rise to two transcripts, a full-length transcript with the termination codon and a shorter transcript with the 3′ end of exon 50 spliced into the middle of exon 51, the latter generating a reading frameshift.

Three point mutations are classified as frameshift deletions. Two are single-base-pair deletions,[227,230] and one is a replacement of an AG dinucleotide with a single T, creating the frameshift.[228] A frameshift insertion of a T after T1554 is also listed in Table 140-2.[228]

Four of the mutations listed in Table 140-4 affect splicing. One of these, a 52-base-pair deletion from within exon 19, was originally classified as a simple frameshift deletion.[234] However, analysis of the transcript revealed that exon 19 was spliced from the message, and it has now been suggested that the aberrant splicing pattern is the result of the loss of a hairpin structure from the unspliced transcript.[235] Another is a simple 5-base-pair deletion that removes the splice donor site from intron 44, resulting in the failure of exon 44 to be included in the message.[231] The removal of either exon 19 or 44 from the message results in a reading frameshift and the introduction of a termination codon in the following exon. A third splicing mutation is a simple base substitution in the GT splice donor site of exon 68, which results in the exon being eliminated from the message, causing a shift in the reading frame.[227] The fourth mutation is more complicated and occurs in a mildly affected BMD patient. In this patient, a base substitution in the splice acceptor site of exon 57 gives rise to a message with this exon skipped. However, that is compensated by the use of a cryptic splice acceptor 18 bp 3′ to the normal one, resulting in a message with the first 18 bp of exon 57 removed. This is expected to produce a near-normal dystrophin with a six-amino-acid deletion and explains why this patient shows dystrophin staining in muscle and has a mild phenotype.

Promoter mutations have also been detected. Alterations in the muscle-specific promoter, including one deletion[173] and one point mutation,[236] lead to reduced levels of dystrophin in two mild BMD patients. A deletion of the muscle and brain promoter in a DMD patient with normal intellectual function suggests that normal brain function does not require the product from the brain promoter.[237]

Point Mutations in Animal Models of DMD. Also included in Table 140-4 are the known mutations in mouse and canine models of DMD. The original *mdx* mouse[238] has a base substitution to a termination codon in exon 23.[239] This truncates the full-size dystrophin but leaves intact the 71-kDa nonmuscle isoform. In contrast, the recently identified *mdx*^{3Cv} mouse[240] has acquired a new splice acceptor site 14 bp upstream of exon 66, which inserts 14 bp into the transcript.[241] This shifts the reading frame for both the full-length transcript and the 71-kDa nonmuscle isoform, producing a mouse that displays an abnormal breeding phenotype with reduced neonatal survival in addition to the skeletal muscle pathology that is characteristic of the original *mdx* mouse.

Canine X-linked muscular dystrophy (cxmd) is a spontaneously occurring, progressive, degenerative myopathy that is clinically and pathologically similar to human DMD.[242] The phenotype is variable despite the fact that all affected animals are descended from a single dystrophic male golden retriever, suggesting that factors other than the nature of the mutation play a role in the development of the clinical picture.[243] Many affected dogs retain some degree of ambulation, and they frequently survive to breeding age. The inheritance pattern is X-linked, and molecular studies have revealed a lack of dystrophin and reduced DMD gene transcript. The canine mutation is a single-base change in the splice site at the 3′ end of intron 6, resulting in skipping of exon 7. This alters the reading frame of exon 8, and a stop codon in the alternate reading frame results in premature termination of translation.[244]

Translocation. Translocation that disrupts the DMD gene and triggers nonrandom inactivation of the normal X chromosome is the common mutation in females with the disease.[39] Several translocation breakpoints have been mapped within the DMD gene,[245,246] and three that have been characterized at the nucleotide level involve nonhomologous recombination between the X and the autosome.[247] Without exception the translocations are *de novo* and are generated in the germ line of the father.[247,248] The fact that X–autosome translocations rarely make it through male meiosis suggests that the translocations that cause DMD/BMD are postmeiotic events occurring during spermiogenesis in the fathers of affected females.[247]

Molecular Diagnostic Applications for DMD and BMD

Now that the DMD gene has been cloned and the gene product can be visualized, the diagnosis of DMD and BMD is most readily confirmed by testing for the underlying defect directly, at the level either of the DMD gene, of the transcript from the gene, or of the protein it encodes. This is particularly useful for differentiating BMD from other muscle disorders such as limb-girdle muscular dystrophy and spinal muscular atrophy. There are now numerous reports of the use of DNA probes or anti-dystrophin antibodies for diagnosis, carrier identification, or prenatal diagnosis of DMD. It is neither possible nor helpful to review them all. Instead, a few general observations and principles will be discussed.

DNA Diagnostics. Direct analysis of the gene or its transcript is now routine in most major centers. While Southern blot analysis was the main approach initially, it has largely been replaced with PCR-based methods for routine diagnostics.

Southern Blotting. Deletions are readily visualized by Southern blot analysis with DMD cDNA probes (Fig. 140-4), and this technique has the advantage of not requiring a muscle biopsy. Generally, Southern blot analysis is performed on peripheral blood DNA digested with *Hin*dIII, as the size and order of the exon-containing fragments are best defined for this enzyme (Table 140-2). As discussed above, in many cases the effect of a given deletion on the translational reading frame can be determined from the exon/intron border types on either side of the deletion, and from this information the severity of the phenotype may be predicted. Duplications are somewhat more difficult to detect with this technology, requiring quantitative analysis to distinguish the two copies of the duplicated segment from the single copy in a normal male. Carrier identification by Southern blot analysis is also difficult, requiring quantitation to distinguish the presence of one copy of a deleted segment in a carrier from the two copies found in a normal female. The finding of a novel DNA fragment at the junction of a deletion or duplication facilitates carrier identification, since the bands generated by these fragments are readily observed in carriers without resorting to quantitative analysis.

Multiplex PCR Amplification. Southern blot analysis is now giving way to PCR as the method of choice for detecting deletions in affected boys. PCR primer pairs were initially chosen to amplify exons 4, 8, 12, 17, 19, 44, 45, 48, and 51,[249] nine exons frequently deleted in patients. The positions of the primers in the adjacent introns were chosen carefully so that each exon was amplified on a different-sized fragment in a single multiplex reaction with all nine primer pairs. The nine fragments were separated by electrophoresis and stained with ethidium bromide. In a multicenter trial of 745 patients, this simple PCR assay detected 82 percent of the deletions detectable by a full Southern blot analysis using cDNA probes.[250] Adding another nine exons to the analysis in a second multiplex reaction[251] was estimated to raise the detection efficiency to 95 percent.[250] Similar results have been obtained in single-center trials, and careful quantitation of the PCR products even makes it possible to identify duplications in affected males and deletions or duplications in carrier females.[250,252] This method does not, however, determine all the exons that are deleted and so does not allow determination of the effect on the translational reading frame.

RNA Diagnostics (RT-PCR). An alternative approach is to amplify cDNA sequences obtained by reverse transcription of mRNA. While the major site of DMD gene transcription is in the muscle, there is enough "illegitimate" transcription from the gene in blood cells to obtain diagnostic information.[253] Roberts et al.[211] have amply demonstrated the utility of RT-PCR (reverse transcript-PCR) in detecting deletions and duplications that result in altered amplified fragments. By this approach the frameshift status of the mRNA is obtained directly by sequencing the altered PCR product. While this is a powerful technology, it may be too demanding and too sophisticated for routine diagnostic use.

Dystrophin Diagnostics. Dystrophin analysis has the distinct advantage that it allows direct detection of defects in the DMD gene product, irrespective of knowledge about the underlying mutation.

Western Blotting. Western blot analysis of muscle by Hoffman et al.[254] initially suggested that Duchenne patients have no detectable dystrophin, while most Becker patients have dystrophin of abnormal size. Based on this and other studies it was suggested that patients might be classified as DMD (dystrophin <3 percent of normal), severe BMD (dystrophin 3 to 10 percent of normal), or mild BMD (dystrophin ≥ 20 percent of normal).[208] Results from other laboratories suggest that this classification is somewhat misleading. Using a highly specific monoclonal antibody and quantitative densitometry, Nicholson et al.[209] found that the abundance of dystrophin correlated well with disease severity but that the levels of dystrophin were considerably higher than those estimated by Hoffman. The majority of severe DMD patients had detectable dystrophin of altered molecular weight, with an abundance up to 25 percent of normal. In the Hoffman studies the antibodies were less sensitive and the reported dystrophin levels were based on visual estimates and not on instrument quantitation.

A more informative approach to dystrophin diagnostics is the use of antibodies against both ends of the protein.[117,210] As a general rule, DMD patients have an abnormal-sized dystrophin that is detected with N-terminal but not C-terminal antibody, consistent with a truncated molecule from a frameshift mutation. BMD patients have dystrophin that reacts with both antibodies, consistent with a mutation that maintains the translational reading frame. C-terminal antibody is therefore of value in differentiating between BMD and DMD.

Immunocytochemistry. Immunostaining of muscle sections with anti-dystrophin antibodies has the advantage of showing whether dystrophin is localized to the sarcolemma, as is assumed to be crucial for its biological function. Dystrophin staining is negative in DMD patients with the exception of rare "revertant" fibers, and has been described as "sporadic" or "diffuse" in BMD patients.[209,255] While such analysis may provide definitive diagnosis in dystrophin-negative biopsies, a "patchy" staining may be difficult to interpret, since this type of staining has been seen in other muscle disorders.

Symptomatic carriers have also been shown to have a "mosaic" or "patchy" pattern of staining, with groups of positive and negative fibers and some partially staining fibers.[209,256] Obligate carriers who do not manifest the disease may have a lower proportion of negatively stained fibers, such that reliable detection of obligate carriers by this technique may not be feasible.

Finally, dystrophin analysis has been applied to a muscle biopsy obtained in utero to determine normality in a fetus at risk for DMD.[257] Whether this will become routine procedure for prenatal diagnosis whenever DNA analysis is not informative remains to be determined.

Genetic Linkage. For the 60 to 65 percent of DMD families who have a detectable deletion, prenatal diagnosis in a subsequent pregnancy is simple and accurate. For the others, who have mutations that are not easily scored directly, linkage analysis is often the only recourse. Similarly, carrier identification remains a challenge, even in deletion families, since the deletion is difficult to score in the presence of a normal allele. Thus, linkage studies to determine the presence or absence of a mutant allele by following the inheritance of closely linked markers is a common approach to carrier identification and prenatal diagnosis.

Genetic linkage to determine carrier status began in 1983 with the first linked markers, but was limited in its use because of the high recombination rate between the DMD gene and the usable markers. With the full set of genetic markers available in 1986, carrier status could be predicted with over 98 percent accuracy for 75 percent of cases with informative markers flanking the gene, and predictive testing began in earnest. Adding intragenic markers, as these became available, improved the accuracy, but intragenic recombination still prevented accurate estimation of risk for those inheriting chromosomes that had undergone recombination.

Perhaps the most significant recent development is the identification of highly polymorphic markers within the gene and at each end of the gene. CA dinucleotide repeat polymorphisms have been described at the 5′ end,[258,259] at the 3′ end,[260,261] and in the middle of the gene.[262] Based on these markers, the recombination rate across the gene has been estimated at 11 percent.[82,259] These are now the markers of choice for linkage-based carrier identification and prenatal diagnosis. This 11 percent intragenic recombination rate is high, even for a 2.4 megabase gene, and explains the early results, which gave 5 to 10 percent recombination between the earliest intragenic probes and the mutations segregating in DMD families.

Germ-Line Mosaicism. As discussed in an earlier section, one third of DMD cases are expected to be new mutants whose mothers are noncarriers. Since 1986, however, a number of reports have documented recurrence of the same "new mutation" in multiple siblings, even when the mother has been shown not to carry the mutation in her somatic cell DNA. This is most readily explained if the mother is a mosaic for the mutation in her germ line. Similarly, male germ-line mosaicism may result in the appearance of two or more carrier daughters with the same "new mutation."

Germ-line mosaicism greatly complicates determination of carrier status, since the mother of any sporadic case might be a germ-line mosaic. Such an individual would not have an elevated CK, nor would her son's mutation, if known, be present in her own somatic cell DNA, yet the risk of having a second affected son or a carrier daughter depends on the proportion of her germ cells carrying the mutation. Based on their own patient group, Bakker et al.[218] determined the empirical recurrence risk to be 14 percent for a male fetus carrying the "at risk" haplotype (i.e., the same set of linked markers as the affected sibling). In a European collaborative study this number was 20 percent, with a 95 percent confidence interval of 10 to 31 percent.[25] Thus, all mothers of an affected boy have a significant recurrence risk even when the son's mutation is not present in their blood cell DNA, and for this reason many groups offer prenatal diagnosis to all such women.

Diagnostic Applications in Other Muscular Dystrophies

Diagnostic studies with DMD gene probes or anti-dystrophin antibodies have been applied to a number of muscular dystrophies in addition to DMD and BMD. Such analysis is particularly valuable for diseases with phenotypes that overlap that of DMD/BMD and has served to distinguish autosomal recessive limb-girdle muscular dystrophy (LMD) from BMD.[208] In two studies of patients classified as having LMD, several were found to have DMD gene mutations and/or dystrophin abnormalities characteristic of BMD; the results suggest that 30 to 40 percent of males with this diagnosis may be misclassified.[263,264] Among females classified with LMD, about 15 percent had dystrophin abnormalities and were reclassified as DMD heterozygotes.[263] Indeed, a discordant monozygotic female twin originally classified as having LMD was reclassified as a manifesting carrier of a DMD gene mutation following DMD gene analysis.[36]

Autosomal recessive muscular dystrophy (ARMD) that clinically resembles DMD can also be distinguished from the latter by DMD gene and dystrophin analysis.[265,266] Perhaps the best evidence for the existence of ARMD is the finding of brother/sister pairs with a Duchenne-like dystrophy in which the DMD gene has no apparent abnormality, dystrophin is present in the muscle, and the DMD gene alleles are different in the two affected individuals.[267-269]

In a severe childhood autosomal recessive muscular dystrophy (SCARMD) prevalent in North Africa, immunostaining for dystrophin is normal, but the 50-kDa dystrophin-associated glycoprotein is drastically diminished in the sarcolemma of all muscle fibers.[270] Whether this is due to a primary defect in the structure or expression of the gene encoding the 50-kDa protein is not yet clear.

Congenital muscular dystrophy (CMD) encompasses a heterogeneous group of disorders which present with progressive muscle wasting at birth. Fukuyama congenital muscular dystrophy (FCMD), a severe autosomal recessive form with central nervous system involvement, is endemic to Japan. While CMD muscle of the non-Fukuyama type shows normal dystrophin localization at the sarcolemma, most FCMD patients have an unusual immunostaining pattern with anti-dystrophin antibodies, and about 10 percent of patients are dystrophin-negative.[271] To explain the high frequency of dystrophin deficiency in FCMD males, it has been suggested that the FCMD gene product normally interacts with dystrophin and that the FCMD phenotype in these males is due to heterozygosity for the FCMD mutation coupled with a DMD gene mutation.[271,272] On this basis the dystrophin-associated glycoproteins are prime candidates for the defective protein in FCMD. This idea is greatly enhanced by the finding that in FCMD, immunostaining of all dystrophin-associated proteins, particularly the 43-kDa protein, is reduced.[273] The gene encoding the 43/156-kDa protein is therefore a strong candidate gene for FCMD.

Thus, a defective dystrophin–glycoprotein complex seems to be intimately linked to muscle cell degeneration in three severe neuromuscular disorders—DMD/BMD, SCARMD, and FCMD. In contrast, no abnormalities of dystrophin or its associated glycoproteins have been detected in limb-girdle, oculopharyngeal, fascioscapulohumeral, or non-Fukuyama congenital muscular dystrophies, nor in myotonic dystrophy, spinal muscular atrophy, or amyotrophic lateral sclerosis.[270]

Pathophysiology of DMD and BMD

Despite decades of intensive research into the cause of DMD, the nature of the basic defect remained elusive until the cloning of the gene allowed the identification of dystrophin as the defective protein. Even with this new knowledge, however, the biological role of dystrophin remains speculative, and our understanding of the disease remains incomplete. Certainly there are many clues from the earlier literature that should be re-examined in light of the new knowledge.

In the history of muscular dystrophy research, a number of models for the disease pathophysiology have been considered. These include (1) vascular disruption or (2) defective innervation leading to muscle degeneration; (3) increased myoplasmic Ca^{2+}, triggering activation of proteases to cause muscle breakdown; and (4) a defect in protein synthesis or degradation leading to a generalized wasting of the muscle tissue. All these ideas have suffered from inconsistent and sometimes contradictory evidence, in many cases a result of the difficulty in distinguishing the primary defect from the many secondary manifestations of the disease.

The possibility of a generalized membrane defect has had continued support. In brief, the evidence includes (1) the finding of gaps or lesions in the plasma membrane in EM studies of prenecrotic muscle tissue from affected boys, (2) the finding of greatly increased levels of certain muscle enzymes in the serum of young presymptomatic boys, suggesting leakage of macromolecules through the muscle membrane, (3) an increased level of Ca^{2+} in muscle fibers, possibly owing to increased uptake through a "leaky" membrane, (4) alterations in lectin binding to glycoproteins on the muscle cell surface, and (5) apparently altered intercellular adhesiveness of skin fibroblasts from DMD patients. These studies served to illustrate the concept of a generalized membrane defect but fell short of determining the basic defect.

An alteration in the muscle membrane is quite consistent with mutations in the gene encoding dystrophin. An attractive working model is one in which the absence of functional dystrophin results in a weakened membrane that is susceptible to contraction-induced tearing. The localized membrane lesions would be expected to give rise to segmental necrosis, followed by degeneration and then regeneration through the proliferation and differentiation of satellite cells (myoblasts) that move in to repair the damage. In the later stages of the disease, the regenerative capacity would be expected to decline as the finite proliferative potential of the satellite cells is used up and the satellite cells themselves become depleted. This view of the disease progression is consistent with the reduced growth potential of myoblasts derived from the muscle tissue of affected boys.[274]

A role for dystrophin in membrane stability and/or function is now quite clear. If the Campbell model is substantially correct, dystrophin binds to filamentous actin at its N-terminal end, and at the other end to a glycoprotein complex that traverses the membrane and connects to laminin in the basal lamina outside the membrane. It is not difficult to imagine how such a complex might protect the membrane from damage during muscle contraction and relaxation. Verification of this model will await functional analysis of the proteins that interact with dystrophin at the cell surface.

Despite the attractiveness of the proposed "structural" role for dystrophin, it is important not to become wed to any particular model. As Campbell's group have often pointed out, the biological role of dystrophin might be to maintain a particular spatial distribution of the membrane glycoprotein complex on the surface of the myofiber. The biological function of the complex is essentially unknown, and it is possible that proteins of the complex might function as an ion channel or a membrane receptor. Potentially important in this regard are the reports of alterations in Ca^{2+} channels in DMD human and *mdx* mouse muscle,[275,276] which rekindle the idea that increased cytoplasmic calcium may stimulate protease activity, resulting in proteolysis of muscle tissue. Clearly, the discovery of dystrophin may be viewed as the "end of the beginning," and the course of DMD research from here on must start from the premise that the presence of dystrophin at the muscle cell membrane is a necessary and sufficient condition to prevent the disease.

Therapeutic Options and Directions

Even before the precise function of dystrophin is learned, a number of approaches are being explored in an attempt to develop an effective therapy for Duchenne and related dystrophies. These include prednisone treatment, myoblast transfer, and gene therapy.

Prednisone Treatment. Of many drugs that have been tested for the treatment of muscular dystrophy, prednisone is the only one that has stood the test of time. Following earlier studies with limited patient numbers, a recent 6-month randomized double-blind trial comparing daily prednisone with a placebo has revealed significant improvement in several parameters relating to muscle function and total muscle mass.[277] This improvement was apparent after 1 month, peaked at about 3 months, and remained constant until 6 months. In a 3-year extension of the study (unblinded), muscle function and mass remained well above that expected for untreated natural history control subjects, with a rate of decline in strength approximately one-fifth that experienced by the natural history control subjects.[278] Side effects, including weight gain, cataracts, and cushingoid appearance, prevented maintenance of the full dosage in some boys. Recently, deflazacort, an oxazoline derivative of prednisolone, has been reported to have the beneficial effect of prednisone with less side effects,[279] and further clinical trials with this drug are currently under way in North America.

The mechanism by which steroids such as prednisone act to produce these results is unknown, although immunologic mechanisms, including suppression of cytotoxic T cells and reduced invasion of muscle by lymphocytes, may contribute to the clinical improvement.[280] It is intriguing that methylprednisolone acts to increase dystrophin gene expression in human muscle cell cultures,[281] although such stimulation would not explain the beneficial effects of steroids in DMD patients with nonfunctional dystrophin. Whatever the mechanism, prednisone must be used cautiously as a treatment for DMD. The long-term risks of prednisone act as a deterrent to its widespread use and suggest that the encouraging results should be viewed as an initial step toward identification of more satisfactory therapeutic agents.

Myoblast Transfer. With the finding that the DMD gene product is a very large cytoskeletal protein came the realization that treatment of the disease through direct replacement of the protein will be difficult, if not impossible. Therefore, introduction of a new dystrophin gene into muscle, in the hope that it will result in adequate dystrophin synthesis, appears to be an important alternative. There are potentially two routes to achieve this end—myoblast transfer and gene therapy.

Myoblast transfer was the subject of an international workshop in June of 1989. At the meeting it became clear that (1) the technical difficulties involved in the transplantation approach are considerable, perhaps even formidable, (2) animal studies are promising but fall short of answering all the questions that need to be answered, and (3) some questions can only be answered in humans. For the last of these reasons, a few groups were contemplating limited transplantation studies in patients.

Skeletal muscle is, in a sense, the ideal tissue for cell transplantation. During development, myoblasts fuse to form multinucleated fibers. Even in mature muscle, a pool of myoblasts termed "satellite cells" do not fuse but remain as single myogenic cells lying in the sarcolemma between the plasma membrane and the basal lamina. These cells are capable of fusing to one another and to the existing muscle to regenerate muscle fibers following injury or disease. In DMD, the satellite cells become depleted after several rounds of degeneration and regeneration, and the introduction of donor cells carrying an intact DMD gene and capable of fusing to the existing muscle is an attractive possibility.

Myoblast Transfer in the Mouse. The impetus for myoblast transfer came from pioneering studies in mice. Several years ago, significant functional recovery was reported following transplantation of normal myoblasts into multiple muscle groups in the *dy/dy* mouse.[282] Since the *dy* mouse has an autosomal recessive form of dystrophy, distinct from the mouse equivalent of DMD, the applicability of the results to DMD is uncertain. These results, now several years old, have never been replicated in another laboratory. It is unusual for such an important finding to remain unconfirmed or unchallenged for such a long time.

Perhaps more relevant to DMD are the studies of two groups who transplanted normal myoblasts into a single muscle of *mdx* mice and demonstrated that the donor cells fuse with the existing muscle and produce dystrophin. In these studies, dystrophin was localized to the membrane in a patchy distribution, and the amount of dystrophin on western blot analysis was as high as 30 to 40 percent of normal.[283,284] Unfortunately, *mdx* mice, despite a nearly complete absence of dystrophin, have a very mild phenotype, so it was not possible in these studies to assess the clinical impact of the procedure. No studies of myoblast transfer have been carried out in the canine model of DMD, despite the fact that dystrophin-deficient dogs have a severe muscle-wasting disease comparable to DMD in humans.

Myoblast Transfer in DMD Patients. Based on the limited studies in mouse, human myoblast transfer has begun, first with single muscle injections to determine if the introduction of myoblasts into muscle is tolerated without severe reaction and to determine if dystrophin is produced in the transplanted muscle. In a preliminary report of myoblast injection into the extensor digitorum brevis muscle of a single patient,[285] there was no clinical evidence of an adverse reaction to the injected cells. Furthermore, there was dystrophin at near-normal levels in a biopsy specimen from the injected muscle but not from the muscle on the sham-injected side, and in sections a weak dystrophin immunostaining was seen at the sarcolemmal membrane.

In another study of four patients with advanced disease who were injected with myoblasts into the tibialis anterior,[286] two were highly positive for dystrophin by western blot and immunostaining, one was weakly positive, and one had no detectable dystrophin. The best result (80 percent dystrophin-positive fibers) was brought into question by the finding of 16 percent positive fibers on the contralateral, noninjected side. To test for an effect on strength, the same four boys received myoblast transplants to their extensor carpi radialis or their biceps brachii. A dramatic 143 percent increase in wrist strength in one boy must be treated with caution, since the study was not done blind and the improvement was not sustained. The others showed little or no improvement. This study was conducted without immunosuppression, and immune rejection may play a role in the negative results even when donor and recipient are compatible for HLA classes I and II.[287]

Further results from a double-blind, placebo-controlled study of eight boys raise serious questions about the efficacy of myoblast transfer. Patients immunosuppressed with cyclosporine received myoblasts at 80 to 100 sites in the tibialis anterior on one side and placebo injections on the other.[288] One month after transplantation, the number of dystrophin-positive fibers was quite variable, and no systematic difference between the myoblast and control sides was evident. The positive fibers must be attributed to the "revertants" seen in over half of DMD patients in numerous studies. PCR analysis of posttransplant biopsies revealed mRNA from the donor DMD gene in three of the eight patients, but only after 40 cycles of PCR amplification and, according to Dr. Blau (personal communication), only when care was taken to ensure that the biopsy specimen was from the immediate vicinity of a site of injection. While some have interpreted these results as encouraging, we find them to be most discouraging and find little evidence to support further trials on children.

Very similar results have been obtained in another double-blind, placebo-controlled study of eight boys, immunosuppressed with cyclophosphamide, who received 55 injections of myoblasts into the biceps.[289] After 8 to 10 weeks one of the eight had 30 percent dystrophin-positive fibers, but this level was seen on both the myoblast-injected and the placebo-injected sides. The remaining seven patients showed only 0 to 2 percent "revertant" fibers on both sides. None of the boys had any sustained increase in muscle strength or any detectable donor mRNA after 30 cycles of PCR amplification. In fact, there was no detectable DNA from the X chromosome of the donor in any of the posttransplant biopsy specimens following 30 cycles of PCR amplification. Again, the results indicate major difficulties in the establishment of myoblast transfer as a valuable approach to the treatment of DMD.

In contrast to this bleak picture, Law's encouraging result with his first patient prompted him to proceed with "phase II" clinical trials designed to strengthen muscles of both lower limbs.[290] Twenty-one patients, immunosuppressed with cyclosporine, received five billion myoblasts, injected at 48 sites in 22 major muscles in the lower half of the body. As in the more limited studies described above, there was no evidence of adverse reaction to the myoblast injection or the cyclosporine. Functional tests using a robotic dynamometer were performed on 13 subjects at 3 months post-transplant. Of 69 muscle groups (knee extensors, knee flexors, plantar flexors) tested for isometric force generation, 43 percent showed a mean strength increase of 41 percent, 38 percent showed no change, and the remaining 19 percent showed a force reduction averaging 23 percent.

While this report impressively demonstrates that very large numbers of cells can be cultured for transplantation, and that patients are remarkably tolerant to the huge numbers of cells injected, the results are nevertheless troublesome. The major problem is that the study was conducted as a treatment and not as an experiment. First, it was not done blind and, therefore, was subject to the usual bias when both patient and observer have expectations with regard to outcome. Second, the data reported to date are short-term, and the ultimate test will not come for 3 to 5 years, by which time any real long-term benefit ought to be apparent. Third, the study did not include measurement of dystrophin or mRNA from the DMD gene, so that the biological basis for any improvement will be difficult to assess.

Of course, if the subjects all show dramatic and sustained improvement, nobody will care that dystrophin was not assessed. On the other hand, the more likely result is a variable response that is less than optimal, and any attempt to improve on the technology will suffer from a lack of critical data concerning the number of gene copies transferred, the level of expression of the donor gene, and the amount of dystrophin generated from the donor gene. Since this type of information would have required multiple biopsies, and that would have been difficult or impossible in the human subjects, we foresee a real need for detailed studies of the type described here in dogs with the disease. This is perhaps one example of a situation where detailed experimentation in animals is preferable to compromised studies in human subjects, especially when the subjects are, by necessity, children.

While all the clinical studies done to date have relied on the direct intramuscular injection of myoblasts, it is worth noting that Neumeyer et al.[291] have achieved limited success with the introduction of myogenic cells to rat muscle by an intra-arterial route. Clearly this would be the delivery route of choice should it become more efficient.

Finally, it is probably worth reminding the reader that the heart will not likely be amenable to myoblast transfer therapy since cardiac muscle is not a syncytium. It is possible that the successful correction of the basic defect in the skeletal muscle will result in a temporary improvement in the quality of life, but will put increased strain on the heart and result in the accelerated appearance of cardiomyopathy.

Gene Therapy. The alternative to donor myoblast transplantation is gene therapy. The introduction of a new gene into muscle tissue could be through direct injection of DNA into muscle tissue, or by introducing it into patient myoblasts in culture and then transplanting the transfected cells into the muscle of the patient.

Recent impetus for gene therapy came with the recognition that reporter genes such as β-galactosidase or luciferase could be expressed in muscle fibers days or even weeks after direct injection of gene constructs into mouse muscle.[292] Histologic staining revealed β-galactosidase activity in 1.5 percent of muscle fibers (10 to 30 percent within the injection area), and injected DNA persisted in the tissue for at least 30 days, although persistence is highly variable, perhaps owing to a variable rate of degradation of DNA at the site of injection.[293] The level of expression of luciferase following direct injection of plasmid DNA into monkey muscle was considerably less than in mouse, perhaps as a consequence of the thicker perimysium in these animals.[294]

For DMD, the 2400-kb size of the gene prohibits using an intact DMD gene. Several groups have constructed DMD "minigenes" consisting of a partial or full-length cDNA joined to an appropriate promoter. Both a full-length mouse[295] and a 12-kb human[296] cDNA have been constructed from smaller fragments of the gene and expressed in myogenic and nonmyogenic cells, where they determine the synthesis of a 430-kDa dystrophin that localizes at the membrane of the transfected cells. The 12-kb human minigene is missing part of the 3′ untranslated region (3′ UTR) but carries the full coding sequence. This, and a shorter 6.3-kb minigene (missing a major part of the coding sequence from the rod domain to mimic the deletion in certain mild BMD patients), when injected into muscle of *mdx* mice, produce dystrophin in about 1 percent of fibers.[297] This indicates that transfer of dystrophin minigenes to muscle by direct injection of plasmid DNA works in principle, but remains a long way from yielding a clinically significant result.

An important question not addressed in these experiments is the functionality of the shortened dystrophin encoded by the 6.3 kb minigene. To test this, Wells et al.[298] introduced this minigene driven by a constitutive MMTV promoter into transgenic *mdx* mice, and found that the gene is expressed in skeletal muscle at about one sixth the level of normal dystrophin in wild-type mice. Even at this level, however, there was a substantial correction of the muscle pathology, indicating that the minigene excodes a functional protein.[298]

An exciting recent development is the introduction of a full-length mouse cDNA controlled by a complex muscle-specific promoter into transgenic *mdx* mice, resulting in the complete correction of the muscle pathology.[299] Of equal importance to the correction of the defect was the finding that a level of dystrophin 50 times greater than normal had no toxic effect on the transgenic animal, suggesting that in developing gene therapy for humans, the level of dystrophin in the treated muscle may not have to be precisely regulated. This bodes well for gene therapy.

While plasmids may be adequate for delivering genes to transgenic mice, they may be quite inefficient at delivering genes to muscle for gene therapy. Adenovirus is a potentially more efficient vector than plasmid DNA for direct gene transfer into quiescent cells.[300] Recombinant adenovirus administered intravenously to young mice has been shown to express a β-galactosidase reporter gene from an RSV promoter in many tissues, particularly muscle and heart, over several months following injection.[301] Direct injection into muscle or use of a muscle-specific promoter would enhance the specificity for muscle. Ragot et al.[302] have recently reported positive expression from an RSV promoter of the 6.3-kb dystrophin minigene in *mdx* mouse muscle following intramuscular injection. They obtained 5 percent to 50 percent of fibers with dystrophin immunostaining at the sarcolemma, and this expression was stable for at least 3 months.

Clearly, another target organ for gene therapy is the heart. Two groups have observed expression of β-galactosidase or luciferase reporter genes following direct injection of plasmid DNA into heart muscle.[303,304] In a third study a cardiac-specific, thyroid hormone–sensitive promoter (α-myosin heavy chain promoter) was used to drive the reporter gene, whose activity in the transfected heart muscle was shown to be responsive to thyroid hormone.[305]

Altogether, these experiments demonstrate the potential for gene therapy for DMD, but much work remains to be done in animals before human gene therapy will be ready for clinical trials.

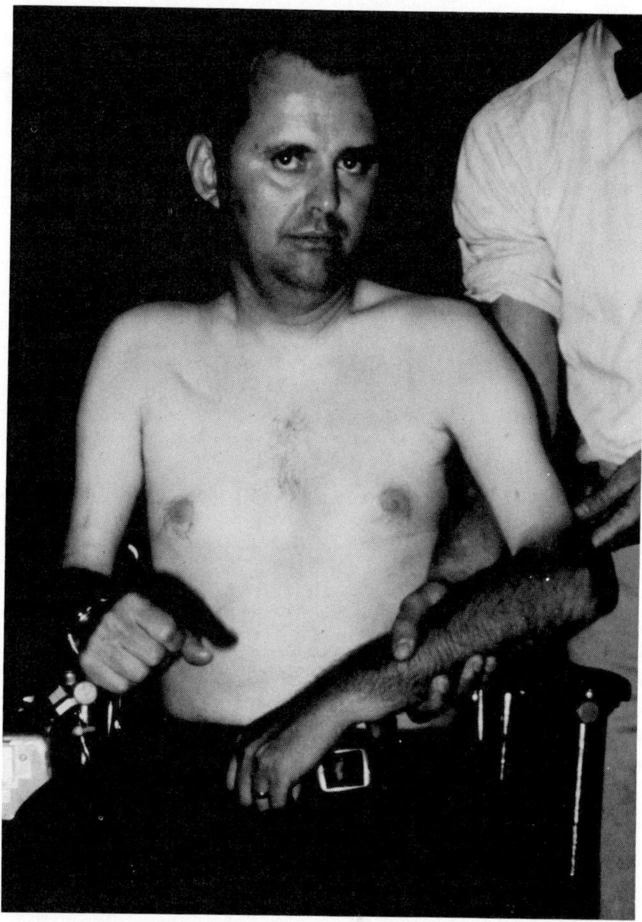

FIG. 140-10 A patient with Emery-Dreifuss muscular dystrophy. The examiner is attempting to straighten the arm, the contracture at the elbow preventing any further straightening. There is weakness of the face and wasting of the upper part of the arms.

Concluding Remarks

Our understanding of Duchenne and Becker muscular dystrophy has progressed in remarkable leaps in recent years. The identification of the DMD gene and its product, dystrophin, has given us substantial new insights into the basic defect in these diseases. Although the detailed understanding of the role of dystrophin is not yet in hand, the knowledge gained from the molecular biology approach clearly points the way to future experiments. The discovery of the responsible gene and protein has been referred to as the "end of the beginning." Let us hope that dystrophin research, coupled with studies to evaluate therapeutic approaches, will mark the beginning of the end.

EMERY-DREIFUSS MUSCULAR DYSTROPHY (EDMD)

In 1961 Dreifuss and Hogan described a kindred with relatively mild X-linked muscular dystrophy, considered then to be a benign variant of Duchenne muscular dystrophy.[306] On re-examination by Emery and Dreifuss, it was clear that there were significant differences, most notably early and widespread contractures and frequent cardiomyopathy.[307] Over the next two decades additional families were reported and the EDMD phenotype has been more clearly defined. The clinical features have been reviewed in detail by Emery.[308]

Clinical Features

The clinical features of EDMD are illustrated in Figure 140-10. In Table 140-5 the primary clinical features are compared to those in BMD, the form with which it is most likely to be confused. Onset occurs in the first decade, with the initial features including toe walking, partial flexion of the elbows, and inability to fully flex the neck and spine. Recognition of this distinct pattern of contractures of the heel cords, elbows, and neck extensors, associated with a scapulohumeroperoneal distribution of weakness, is an early clue to diagnosis. The weakness spreads to involve other muscle groups, such as those of the hip, as the disease progresses.[309]

Another consistent feature of EDMD is a cardiac conduction defect that may, unless treated, lead to sudden death. Presymptomatic detection of heart involvement by means of regular electrocardiograms and the insertion of a cardiac pacemaker at an early stage may be lifesaving.[310] Cardiac risk also appears high in some but not all female carriers.[309] The neuromuscular wasting is mild and slowly progressive, with onset during adolescence, significant disability being

Table 140-5 Emery-Dreifuss Muscular Dystrophy–Comparison of EDMD and BMD Phenotypes

Clinical Features	EDMD	BMD
Cardiac involvement	Conduction block, early, life-threatening	Cardiomyopathy, mild if present
Contractures	Early—elbows, Achilles tendon, postcervical	Late or absent except Achilles tendons
Muscle weakness	Upper limbs early, lower limbs distal	Proximal > distal hips > shoulders
Calf hypertrophy	Usually absent	Prominent early
Creatinine kinase	Moderately elevated	Greatly elevated in preclinical and early clinical stages
Inheritance	X-linked gene at Xq28	X-linked gene at Xp21

rare before adult life. Early in the course of the disease the biceps and triceps are affected most prominently. Later difficulties are due mainly to weakness of the hip and knee extensors. In the lower extremities, distal muscles seem to be affected before the proximal ones, giving a humeroperoneal distribution.[310]

Laboratory studies in EDMD have been somewhat variable and controversial. Serum CK is usually elevated 3 to 10 fold over normal levels, considerably lower than that characteristic of DMD and BMD. Disparate EMG results have been recorded showing both myopathic changes and evidence of denervation, even within the same individual.[309] Muscle biopsy changes, usually consistent with a myopathy, are also variable.[309] It would appear, therefore, that prime importance should be given to the clinical features of the disease since the disparate EMG and histologic changes are poorly understood[311,312] and may be resolved only after the underlying gene has been cloned and characterized.

Several cases classified as scapuloperoneal muscular dystrophy in early reports have since been considered by others to be EDMD.[311,312] A myopathic scapuloperoneal syndrome does appear to exist, but onset is in adult life, early contractures do not occur, and cardiac conduction defects are not consistent.[310] Other conditions with phenotypes that overlap EDMD are tabulated by Emery.[310]

Genetics of Emery-Dreifuss Muscular Dystrophy

Inheritance of EDMD is X-linked, although rare families with a similar clinical picture show autosomal dominant inheritance. In 1986 the X-linked EDMD was definitively mapped to the distal end of the long arm of the X chromosome by the demonstration of linkage to the factor VIII gene and the anonymous marker DXS15.[313-315] This agreed with the earlier finding of a family in which a "scapuloperoneal" syndrome, probably EDMD, segregated with the gene for color blindness.[316] Subsequent studies placed the EDMD gene distal to DXS15 and refined the map position of the gene with respect to several markers in the Xq28 region.[317,318]

The position of the EDMD gene in relation to Xq28 markers is diagrammed in Fig. 140-11; the order and genetic distances are based on multipoint linkage analysis of published data.[319] The EDMD gene is very close to the red-

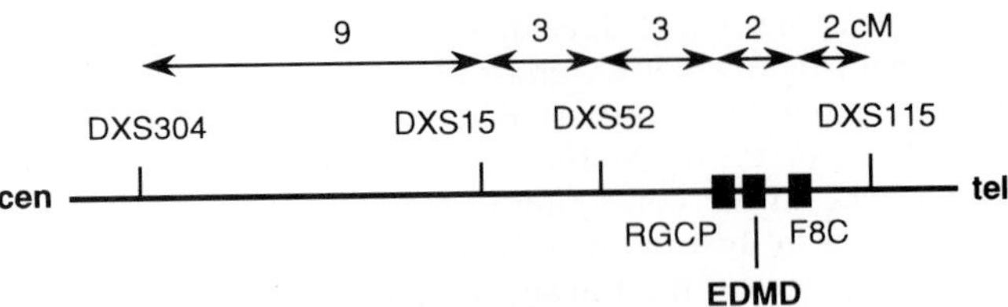

FIG. 140-11 Schematic to illustrate the position of the EDMD gene on the X chromosome in relation to genetic markers (DXS loci) and to the genes for red-green color pigment (RGCP) and factor VIII (F8C). Approximate distances are given in centimorgans.

green color pigment (RGCP) gene, about halfway between DXS15/DXS52 and factor VIII. The distance between these flanking markers is approximately 5 cM. Thus, the location of the gene has been narrowed to a region of a few million base pairs, and the gene is perhaps much closer than this to the color pigment gene cluster. Additional markers in this defined region will help to define the order of the EDMD and RGCP loci and will serve as start points for chromosomal walking to find the EDMD gene.

REFERENCES

1. Meryon E: On granular and fatty degeneration of the voluntary muscles. *Med Chir Trans* **35**:73, 1852.
2. Duchenne GBA: Recherches sur la paralysie musculaire pseudohypertrophique ou paralysie myosclerosique. *Arch Gen Med* **11**:5, 1868.
3. Walton JN, Nattrass FJ: On the classification, natural history and treatment of the myopathies. *Brain* **77**:169, 1954.
4. Emery AEH: *Duchenne Muscular Dystrophy*, 2nd ed. New York, Oxford University Press, 1993.
5. Ogasawara A: Downward shift in IQ in persons with Duchenne muscular dystrophy compared to those with spinal muscular atrophy. *Am J Ment Retard* **93**:544, 1989.
6. Glaub T, Mechler F: Intellectual function in muscular dystrophies. *Eur Arch Psychiatr Neurol Sci* **236**:379, 1987.
7. Dubowitz V: Intellectual impairment in muscular dystrophy. *Arch Dis Child* **40**:296, 1965.
8. Worden DK, Vignos PJ: Intellectual function in childhood progressive muscular dystrophy. *Pediatrics* **29**:968, 1962.
9. Gowers WR: *Pseudo-Hypertrophic Muscular Paralysis—a Clinical Lecture*, J. London and A. Churchill, 1879.
10. Brooke MH, Fenichel GM, Griggs RC, Mendell JR, Moxley R, Florence J, King WM, Pandya S, Robison J, Schierbecker J: Duchenne muscular dystrophy: Patterns of clinical progression and effects of supportive therapy. *Neurology* **39**:475, 1989.
11. Ebashi S, Toyokura Y, Momoi H, Sugita H: High creatine phosphokinase activity of sera of progressive muscular dystrophy. *J Biochem (Tokyo)* **46**:103, 1959.
12. Dreyfus JC, Schapira G, Demos J: Etude de la creatine kinase serique chez les myopathes et leurs families. *Rev Fr Etud Clin Biol* **5**:384, 1960.
13. Brooke MH, Fenichel GM, Griggs RC, Mendell JR, Moxley R, Miller JP, CIDD Group: Clinical Investigation in Duchenne muscular dystrophy. 2. Determination of the "power" of therapeutic trials based on the natural history. *Muscle Nerve* **6**:91, 1983.
14. Dubowitz V: *Muscle Biopsy—a Practical Approach* 2nd ed. London, Bailliere Tindall, 1985.
15. Engel AG: Duchenne dystrophy, in Engel AG, Banker BQ (eds): *Myology*. New York, McGraw-Hill, 1986, p 1185.
16. Daube JR: Electrodiagnosis of muscle disorders, in Engel AG, Banker BQ (eds): *Myology*. New York, McGraw-Hill, 1986, p 1195.
17. Kanamori M, Morton NE, Fujiki K, Kondo K: Genetic epidemiology of Duchenne muscular dystrophy in Japan: Classical segregation analysis. *Genet Epidemiol* **4**:425, 1987.

18. van Essen AJ, Busch HFM, te Meerman GJ, ten Kate LP: Birth and population prevalence of Duchenne muscular dystrophy in the Netherlands. *Hum Genet* **88**:258, 1992.
19. Scheuerbrandt G, Lundin A, Lovgren T, Mortier W: Screening for Duchenne muscular dystrophy: An improved screening test for creatine kinase and its application in an infant screening program. *Muscle Nerve* **9**:11, 1986.
20. Greenberg CR, Rohringer M, Jacobs HK, Averill N, Nylen E, van Ommen GJ, Wrogemann K: Gene studies in newborn males with Duchenne muscular dystrophy detected by neonatal screening. *Lancet* **2**:425, 1988.
21. Mostacciuolo ML, Lombardi A, Cambissa V, Danieli GA, Angelini C: Population data on benign and severe forms of X-linked muscular dystrophy. *Hum Genet* **75**:217, 1987.
22. Bushby KM, Thambyayah M, Gardner Medwin D: Prevalence and incidence of Becker muscular dystrophy. *Lancet* **337**:1022, 1991.
23. Haldane JBS: Mutation in the sex-linked recessive type of muscular dystrophy: A possible sex difference. *Ann Hum Genet* **20**:344, 1956.
24. Edwards JH: The population genetics of Duchenne: Natural and artificial selection in Duchenne muscular dystrophy. *J Med Genet* **23**:521, 1986.
25. van Essen AJ, Abbs S, Baiget M, Bakker E, Boileau C, van Broeckhoven C, Bushby K, Clarke A, Claustres M, Covone AE, Ferrari M, Ferlini A, Galluzzi G, Grimm T, Grubben C, Jeanpierre M, Kääriäinen H, Liechti-Gallati S, Melis MA, van Ommen G-JB, Poncin JE, Scheffer H, Schwartz M, Speer A: Parental origin and germline mosaicism of deletions and duplications of the dystrophin gene: A European study. *Hum Genet* **88**:249, 1992.
26. Muller B̄, Dechant C, Meng G, Liechti-Gallati S, Doherty RA, Hejtmancik JF, Bakker E, Read AP, Jeanpierre M, Fischbeck KH, Romeo G, Francke U, Wilichowski E, Greenberg CR, van Broeckhoven C, Junien C, Muller CR, Grimm T: Estimation of the male and female mutation rates in Duchenne muscular dystrophy (DMD). *Hum Genet* **89**:204, 1992.
27. Moser H: Duchenne muscular dystrophy: Pathogenetic aspects and genetic prevention. *Hum Genet* **66**:17, 19984.
28. Barbujani G, Russo A, Danieli GA, Spiegler AW, Borkowska J, Petrusewicz IH: Segregation analysis of 1885 DMD families: Significant departure from the expected proportion of sporadic cases. *Hum Genet* **84**:522, 1990.
29. Penn AS, Lisak RP, Rowland LP: Muscular dystrophy in young girls. *Neurology* **20**:147, 1970.
30. Minetti C, Chang HW, Medori R, Prelle A, Moggio M, Johnsen SD, Bonilla E: Dystrophin deficiency in young girls with sporadic myopathy and normal karyotype. *Neurology* **41**:1288, 1991.
31. Bonilla E, Younger DS, Chang HW, Tantravahi U, Miranda AF, Medori R, Dimauro S, Warburton D, Rowland LP: Partial dystrophin deficiency in monozygous twin carriers of the Duchenne gene discordant for clinical myopathy. *Neurology* **40**:1267, 1990.
32. Pena SD, Karpati G, Carpenter S, Fraser FC: The clinical consequences of X-chromosome inactivation: Duchenne muscular dystrophy in one of monozygotic twins. *J Neurol Sci* **79**:337, 1987.
33. Gomez MR, Engel AG, Dewald G, Peterson HA: Failure of inactivation of Duchenne dystrophy X-chromosome in one of female identical twins. *Neurology* **27**:537, 1977.
34. Chutkow JG, Hyser CL, Edwards JA, Heffner RR Jr, Czyrny JJ: Monozygotic female twin carriers discordant for the clinical manifestations of Duchenne muscular dystrophy. *Neurology* **37**:1147, 1987.
35. Lupski JR, Garcia CA, Zoghbi HY, Hoffman EP, Fenwick RG: Discordance of muscular dystrophy in monozygotic female twins: Evidence supporting asymmetric splitting of the inner cell mass in a manifesting carrier of Duchenne dystrophy. *Am J Med Genet* **40**:354, 1991.
36. Richards CS, Watkins SC, Hoffman EP, Schneider NR, Milsark IW, Katz KS, Cook JD, Kunkel LM, Cortada JM: Skewed X inactivation in a female MZ twin results in Duchenne muscular dystrophy. *Am J Hum Genet* **46**:672, 1990.
37. Burn J, Povey S, Boyd Y, Munro EA, West L, Harper K, Thomas D: Duchenne muscular dystrophy in one of monozygotic twin girls. *J Med Genet* **23**:494, 1986.
38. Nance WE: Do twin Lyons have larger spots? *Am J Hum Genet* **46**:646, 1990.
39. Boyd Y, Buckle V, Holt S, Munro E, Hunter D, Craig I: Muscular dystrophy in girls with X;autosome translocations. *J Med Genet* **23**:484, 1986.
40. Witkowski JA: The molecular genetics of Duchenne muscular dystrophy: The beginning of the end? *Trends Genet* **4**:27, 1988.
41. Monaco AP, Kunkel LM: Cloning of the Duchenne/Becker muscular dystrophy locus. *Adv Hum Genet* **17**:61, 1988.
42. Worton RG, Thompson MW: Genetics of Duchenne muscular dystrophy. *Annu Rev Genet* **22**:601, 1988.
43. Worton RG, Burghes AH: Molecular genetics of Duchenne and Becker muscular dystrophy. *Int Rev Neurobiol* **29**:1, 1988.
44. Greenstein RM, Reardon MP, Chan TS, Middleton AB, Mulivor RA, Green AE, Coriell LL: An (X; II) translocation in a girl with Duchenne muscular dystrophy. *Cytogenet Cell Genet* **27**:268, 1980.
45. Jacobs PA, Hunt PA, Mayer M, Bart RD: Duchenne muscular dystrophy (DMD) in a female with an X/autosome translocation: Further evidence that the DMD locus is at Xp21. *Am J Hum Genet* **33**:513, 1981.
46. Verellen C, Freund M, DeMeyer R, Laterre C, Scholberg B, Frederic J: Progressive muscular dystrophy of the Duchenne type in a young girl associated with an aberration of chromosome X, in Littlefield SW (ed): *Fifth International Congress of Birth Defects*; Montreal; 1977, Excerpta Medica, Amsterdam, p 42.
47. Canki N, Dutrilaux B, Tivadar I: Dystrophie musculaire de Duchenne chez une petite fille Porteuse d'une translocation t(X;3)(p(21;q13) de novo. *Ann Genet* **22**:35, 1979.
48. Lindenbaum RH, Clarke G, Patel C, Moncrieff M, Hughes JT: Muscular dystrophy in an X;1 translocation female suggest that Duchenne locus is on X-chromosome short arm. *J Med Genet* **16**:389, 1979.
49. Boyd Y, Buckle VJ: Cytogenetic heterogeneity of translocations associated with Duchenne muscular dystrophy. *Clin Genet* **29**:108, 1986.
50. Verellen-Dumoulin C, Freund M, De Meyer R, Laterre C, Frederic J, Thompson MW, Markovic VD, Worton RG: Expression of an X linked muscular dystrophy in a female due to translocation involving Xp21 and nonrandom inactivation of the normal X chromosome. *Hum Genet* **67**:115, 1984.
51. Davies KE, Pearson PL, Harper PS, Murray JM, O'Brien T: Linkage analysis of two cloned DNA sequences flanking the Duchenne muscular dystrophy locus on the short arm of the human X chromosome. *Nucleic Acids Res* **11**:2303, 1983.
52. Murray JM, Davies KE, Harper PS, Meredith L, Mueller CR, Williamson R: Linkage relationship of a cloned DNA sequence on the short arm of the X-chromosome to Duchenne muscular dystrophy. *Nature* **300**:69, 1982.
53. Hofker MH, van Ommen GJ, Bakker E, Burmeister M, Pearson PL: Development of additional RFLP probes near the locus for Duchenne muscular dystrophy by cosmid cloning of the DXS84 (754) locus. *Hum Genet* **74**:270, 1986.
54. Davies K, Speer A, Hermann F, Spiegler AWJ, McGlade S, Hofker MH, Briand P, Hanke P, Schwartz M, Steinbicker V, Szibor R, Korner H, Sommer D, Pearson PL, Coutelle CH: Human X chromosome markers and Duchenne muscular dystrophy. *Nucleic Acids Res* **13**:3419, 1985.
55. Dorkins H, Junien C, Mandel J, Wrogemann K, Moison J, Martinez M, Old J, Bundey S, Schwartz M, Carpenter N, Hill D, Lindlof M, de la Chappelle A, Pearson P, Davies K: Segregation analysis of a marker localised Xp21.2-Xp21.3 in Duchenne and Becker muscular dystrophy families. *Hum Genet* **71**:103, 1985.
56. Wilcox DE, Affara NA, Yates JR, Ferguson-Smith MA, Pearson PL: Multipoint linkage analysis of the short arm of the human X chromosome in families with X-linked muscular dystrophy. *Hum Genet* **70**:365, 1985.
57. Davies KE, Briand P, Ionasescu V, Ionasescu G, Williamson R, Brown C, Cavard C, Cathelineau L: Gene

for OTC: characterisation and linkage to Duchenne muscular dystrophy. *Nucleic Acids Res* **13**:155, 1985.

58. Shapiro F, Specht L: Orthopedic deformities in Emery-Dreifuss muscular dystrophy. *J Pediatr Orthop* **11**:336, 1991.
59. Kingston HM, Sarfarazi M, Thomas NS, Harper PS: Localisation of the Becker muscular dystrophy gene on the short arm of the X chromosome by linkage to cloned DNA sequences. *Hum Genet* **67**:6, 1984
60. Brown CS, Thomas NST, Sarfarazi M, Davies KE, Kunkel L, Pearson PL, Kingston HM, Shaw DJ, Harper PS: Genetic linkage relationships of seven DNA probes with Duchenne and Becker muscular dystrophy. *Hum Genet* **71**:62, 1985.
61. Francke U, Ochs HD, DeMartinville B, Giacalone J, Lindgren V: Minor Xp21 chromosome deletion in a male associated with expression of Duchenne muscular dystrophy, chronic granulomatous disease, retinitis pigmentosa and McLeod syndrome. *Am J Hum Genet* **37**:250, 1985.
62. Guggenheim MA, McCabe ERB, Roig M, Goodman SI, Lum GM, Bullen WW, Ringel SP: Glycerol kinase deficiency with neuromuscular, skeletal and adrenal abnormalities. *Ann Neurol* **7**:441, 1980.
63. Bartley JA, Miller DK, Hayford JT, McCabe ERB: Concordance of X-linked glycerol kinase deficiency with X-linked congenital adrenal hypoplasia. *Lancet* **2**:733, 1982.
64. Renier WO, Nabben FA, Hustinx TWJ, Veerkamp JH, Otten BJ, TerLaak HJ, ter Haar BGA, Gabreels FJM: Congenital adrenal hypoplasia, progressive muscular dystrophy and severe mental retardation, in association with glycerol kinase deficiency in male sibs. *Clin Genet* **24**:243, 1983.
65. Bartley JA, Patil S, Davenport S, Goldstein D, Pickens J: Duchenne muscular dystrophy, glycerol kinase deficiency, and adrenal insufficiency associated with Xp21 interstitial deletion. *J Pediatr* **108**:189, 1986.
66. Dunger DB, Davies KE, Pembrey M, Lake B, Pearson P, Williams D, Whitfield A, Dillon MJ: Deletion on the X chromosome detected by direct DNA analysis in one of two unrelated boys with glycerol kinase deficiency, adrenal hypoplasia, and Duchenne muscular dystrophy. *Lancet* **1**:585, 1986.
67. Wilcox DE, Cooke A, Colgan J, Boyd E, Aitken DA, Sinclair L, Glasgow L, Stephenson JB, Ferguson Smith MA: Duchenne muscular dystrophy due to familial Xp21 deletion detectable by DNA analysis and flow cytometry. *Hum Genet* **73**:175, 1986.
68. Clarke A, Roberts SH, Thomas NS, Whitfield A, Williams J, Harper PS: Duchenne muscular dystrophy with adrenal insufficiency and glycerol kinase deficiency: High resolution cytogenetic analysis with molecular, biochemical, and clinical studies. *J Med Genet* **23**:501, 1986.
69. Wieringa B, Hustinx T, Scheres J, Renier W, ter Haar B: Complex glycerol kinase deficiency syndrome explained as X chromosomal deletion. *Clin Genet* **27**:522, 1985.
70. Saito F, Goto J, Kakinuma H, Nakamura F, Murayama S, Nakano I, Tonomura A: Inherited Xp21 deletion in a boy with complex glycerol kinase deficiency syndrome. *Clin Genet* **29**:92, 1986.
71. Darras BT, Francke U: Myopathy in complex glycerol kinase deficiency patients is due to 3′ deletions of the dystrophin gene. *Am J Hum Genet* **43**:126, 1988.
72. Davies KE, Patterson MN, Kenwrick SJ, Bell MV, Sloan HR, Westman JA, Elsas LJ, Mahan J: Fine mapping of glycerol kinase deficiency and congenital adrenal hypoplasia within Xp21 on the short arm of the human X chromosome. *Am J Med Genet* **29**:557, 1988.
73. Chelly J, Marlhens F, Dutrillaux B, van Ommen GJ, Lambert M, Haioun B, Boissinot G, Fardeau M, Kaplan JC: Deletion proximal to DXS68 locus (L1 probe site) in a boy with Duchenne muscular dystrophy, glycerol kinase deficiency, and adrenal hypoplasia. *Hum Genet* **78**:222, 1988.
74. Frey D, Machler M, Seger R, Schmid W, Orkin SH: Gene deletion in a patient with chronic granulomatous disease and McLeod syndrome: Fine mapping of the Xk gene locus. *Blood* **71**:252, 1988.
75. Francke U, Harper JF, Darras BT, Cowan JM, McCabe ER, Kohlschutter A, Seltzer WK, Saito F, Goto J, Harpey JP: Congenital adrenal hypoplasia, myopathy, and glycerol kinase deficiency: Molecular genetic evidence for deletions. *Am J Hum Genet* **40**:212, 1987.
76. Kunkel LM, Monaco AP, Midlesworth W, Ochs HD, Latt SA: Specific cloning of DNA fragments absent from the DNA of a male patient with an X-chromosome deletion. *Proc Natl Acad Sci USA* **82**:4778, 1985.
77. Monaco AP, Bertelson CJ, Middlesworth W, Colletti CA, Aldridge J, Fischbeck KH, Bartlett D, Kunkel LM: Detection of deletions spanning the Duchenne muscular dystrophy locus using a tightly linked DNA segment. *Nature* **316**:842, 1985.
78. Kunkel LM, et al.: Analysis of deletions in DNA from patients with Becker and Duchenne muscular dystrophy. *Nature* **322**:73, 1986.
79. Walker A, Hart K, Cole C, Hodgson S, Johnson L, Dubowitz V, Bobrow M: Linkage studies in Duchenne and Becker muscular dystrophies. *J Med Genet* **23**:538, 1986.
80. Bertelson CJ, Bartley JA, Monaco AP, Colletti Feener C, Fischbeck K, Kunkel LM: Localisation of Xp21 meiotic exchange points in Duchenne muscular dystrophy families. *J Med Genet* **23**:531, 1986.
81. Fischbeck KH, Ritter AW, Tirschwell DL, Kunkel LM, Bertelson CJ, Monaco AP, Hejtmancik JF, Boehm C, Ionasescu V, Ionasescu R: Recombination with PERT87 (DXS164) in families with X-linked muscular dystrophy. *Lancet* **2**:104, 1986.
82. Abbs S, Roberts RG, Mathew CG, Bentley DR, Bobrow M: Accurate assessment of intragenic recombination frequency within the Duchenne muscular dystrophy gene. *Genomics* **7**:602, 1990.
83. Worton RG, Duff C, Sylvester J, Schmickel RD, Willard HF: Duchenne muscular dystrophy involving translocation of the DMD gene next to ribosomal RNA genes. *Science* **224**:1447, 1984.
84. Ray PN, Belfall B, Duff C, Logan C, Kean V, Thompson MW, Sylvester JE, Gorski JL, Schmickel RD, Worton RG: Cloning of the breakpoint of an X;21 translocation associated with Duchenne muscular dystrophy. *Nature* **318**:672, 1985.
85. Thompson MW, Ray PN, Belfall B, Duff C, Logan C, Oss I, Worton RG: Linkage analysis of polymorphisms within the DNA fragment XJ cloned from the breakpoint of an X;21 translocation associated with X linked muscular dystrophy. *J Med Genet* **23**:548, 1986.
86. Monaco AP, Neve RL, Colletti Feener C, Bertelson CJ, Kurnit DM, Kunkel LM: Isolation of candidate cDNAs for portions of the Duchenne muscular dystrophy gene. *Nature* **323**:646, 1986.
87. Burghes AH, Logan C, Hu X, Belfall B, Worton RG, Ray PN: A cDNA clone from the Duchenne/Becker muscular dystrophy gene. *Nature* **328**:434, 1987.
88. Koenig M, Hoffman EP, Bertelson CJ, Monaco AP, Feener C, Kunkel LM: Complete cloning of the Duchenne muscular dystrophy (DMD) cDNA and preliminary genomic organization of the DMD gene in normal and affected individuals. *Cells* **50**:509, 1987.
89. Cross GS, Speer A, Rosenthal A, Forrest SM, Smith TJ, Edwards Y, Flint T, Hill D, Davies KE: Deletions of fetal and adult muscle cDNA in Duchenne and Becker muscular dystrophy patients. *EMBO J* **6**:3277, 1987.
90. den Dunnen TJ, Grootscholten PM, Bakker E, Blonden LA, Ginjaar HB, Wapenaar MC, van Paassen HM, van Broeckhoven C, Pearson PL, van Ommen GJ: Topography of the Duchenne muscular dystrophy (DMD) gene: FIGE and cDNA analysis of 194 cases reveals 115 deletions and 13 duplications. *Am J Hum Genet* **45**:835, 1989.
91. Burmeister M, Monaco AP, Gillard EF, van Ommen GJ, Affara NA, Ferguson Smith MA, Kunkel LM, Lehrach H: A 10-megabase physical map of human Xp21, including the Duchenne muscular dystrophy gene. *Genomics* **2**:189, 1988.
92. van Ommen GJ, Verkerk JM, Hofker MH, Monaco AP, Kunkel LM, Ray P, Worton R, Wieringa B, Bakker E, Pearson PL: A physical map of 4 million bp around the Duchenne muscular dystrophy gene on the human X-chromosome. *Cell* **47**:499, 1986.
93. Monaco AP, Walker AP, Millwood I, Larin Z, Lehrach

H: A yeast artificial chromosome contig containing the complete Duchenne muscular dystrophy gene. *Genomics* **12**:465, 1992.

94. Coffey AJ, Roberts RG, Green ED, Cole CG, Butler R, Anand R, Giannelli F, Bentley DR: Construction of a 2.6-Mb contig in yeast artificial chromosomes spanning the human dystrophin gene using an STS-based approach. *Genomics* **12**:474, 1992.
95. den Dunnen JT: Reconstruction of the 2.4 Mb human DMD gene by homologous YAC recombination. *Hum Mol Genet* **1**:19, 1992.
96. Malhotra SB, Hart KA, Klamut HJ, Thomas NS, Bodrug SE, Burghes AH, Bobrow M, Harper PS, Thompson MW, Ray PN, Worton RG: Frame-shift deletions in patients with Duchenne and Becker muscular dystrophy. *Science* **242**:755, 1988.
97. Monaco AP, Bertelson CJ, Liechti Gallati S, Moser H, Kunkel LM: An explanation for the phenotypic differences between patients bearing partial deletions of the DMD locus. *Genomics* **2**:90, 1988.
98. Koenig M, Beggs AH, Moyer M, Scherpf S, Heindrich K, Bettecken T, Meng G, Muller CR, Lindlof M, Kaariainen H: The molecular basis for Duchenne versus Becker muscular dystrophy: Correlation of severity with type of deletion. *Am J Hum Genet* **45**:498, 1989.
99. Bebchuk KG, Bulman DE, D'Souza VN, Worton RG, Ray PN: Genomic organization of exons 22 to 25 of the dystrophin gene. *Hum Mol Genet* **2**:593, 1993.
100. Roberts RG, Coffey AJ, Bobrow M, Bentley DR: Determination of the exon structure of the distal portion of the dystrophin gene by vectorette PCR. *Genomics* **13**:942, 1992.
101. Roberts RG, Coffey AJ, Bobrow M, Bentley DR: Exon structure of the human dystrophin gene. *Genomics* **16**:536, 1993.
102. Hoffman EP, Brown RH Jr, Kunkel LM: Dystrophin: the protein product of the Duchenne muscular dystrophy locus. *Cell* **51**:919, 1987.
103. Hammonds RG: Protein sequence of DMD gene is related to actin-binding domain of alpha-actinin. *Cell* **51**:1, 1987.
104. Davison MD, Baron MD, Critchley DR, Wootton JC: Structural analysis of homologous repeated domains in alpha-actinin and spectrin. *Int J Biol Macromol* **11**:81, 1989.
105. Koenig M, Monaco AP, Kunkel LM: The complete sequence of dystrophin predicts a rod-shaped cytoskeletal protein. *Cell* **53**:219, 1988.
106. Lemaire C, Heilig R, Mandel JL: The chicken dystrophin cDNA: Striking conservation of the C-terminal coding and 3′ untranslated regions between man and chicken. *EMBO J* **7**:4157, 1988.
107. Koenig M, Kunkel LM: Detailed analysis of the repeat domain of dystrophin reveals four potential hinge segments that may confer flexibility. *J Biol Chem* **265**:4560, 1990.
108. Murayama T, Sato O, Kimura S, Shimizu T, Sawada H, Maruyama K: Molecular shape of dystrophin purified from rabbit skeletal muscle myofibrils. *Proc Jpn Acad* **66**:96, 1990.
109. Pons F, Augier N, Heilig R, Leger J, Mornet D, Leger JJ: Isolated dystrophin molecules as seen by electron microscopy. *Proc Natl Acad Sci USA* **87**:7851, 1990.
110. Sato O, Nonomura Y, Kimura S, Maruyama K: Molecular shape of dystrophin. *J Biochem (Tokyo)* **112**:631, 1992.
111. Zubrzycka Gaarn EE, Hutter OF, Karpati G, Klamut HJ, Bulman DE, Hodges RS, Worton RG, Ray PN: Dystrophin is tightly associated with the sarcolemma of mammalian skeletal muscle fibers. *Exp Cell Res* **192**:278, 1991.
112. Zubrzycka Gaarn EE, Bulman DE, Karpati G, Burghes AH, Belfall B, Klamut HJ, Talbot J, Hodges RS, Ray PN, Worton RG: The Duchenne muscular dystrophy gene product is localized in sarcolemma of human skeletal muscle. *Nature* **333**:466, 1988.
113. Arahata K, Ishiura S, Ishiguro T, Tsukahara T, Suhara Y, Eguchi C, Ishihara T, Nonaka I, Ozawa E, Sugita H: Immunostaining of skeletal and cardiac muscle surface membrane with antibody against Duchenne muscular dystrophy peptide. *Nature* **333**:861, 1988.
114. Kao L, Krstenansky J, Mendell J, Rammohan KW, Gruenstein E: Immunological identification of a high molecular weight protein as a candidate for the product of the Duchenne muscular dystrophy gene. *Proc Natl Acad Sci USA* **85**:4491, 1988.
115. Man NT, Cartwright AJ, Morris GE, Love DR, Bloomfield JF, Davies KE: Monoclonal antibodies against defined regions of the muscular dystrophy protein, dystrophin. *FEBS Lett* **262**:237, 1990.
116. Sedgwick SG, Nguyen TM, Ellis JM, Crowne H, Morris GE: Rapid mapping by transposon mutagenesis of epitopes on the muscular dystrophy protein, dystrophin. *Nucleic Acids Res* **19**:5889, 1991.
117. Bulman DE, Murphy EG, Zubrzycka Gaarn EE, Worton RG, Ray PN: Differentiation of Duchenne and Becker muscular dystrophy phenotypes with amino- and carboxy-terminal antisera specific for dystrophin. *Am J Hum Genet* **48**:295, 1991.
118. Bonilla E, Samitt CE, Miranda AF, Hays AP, Salviati G, Dimauro S, Kunkel LM, Hoffman EP, Rowland LP: Duchenne muscular dystrophy: Deficiency of dystrophin at the muscle cell surface. *Cell* **54**:447, 1988.
119. Michalak M, Zubrzycka Gaarn E: Identification of dystrophin in cardiac sarcolemmal vesicles. *Biochem Biophys Res Commun* **169**:565, 1990.
120. Byers TJ, Kunkel LM, Watkins SC: The subcellular distribution of dystrophin in mouse skeletal, cardiac, and smooth muscle. *J Cell Biol* **115**:411, 1991.
121. Yarom R, Morris GE, Froede R, Schaper J: Myocardial dystrophin immunolocalization at sarcolemma and transverse tubules. *Experientia* **48**:614, 1992.
122. Tanaka H, Ozawa E: Expression of dystrophin mRNA and the protein in the developing rat heart. *Biochem Biophys Res Commun* **172**:824, 1990.
123. Harricane MC, Augier N, Leger J, Anoal M, Cavadore C, Mornet D: Ultrastructural localization of dystrophin in chicken smooth muscle. *Cell Biol Int Rep* **15**:687, 1991.
124. Bies RD, Friedman D, Roberts R, Perryman MB, Caskey CT: Expression and localization of dystrophin in human cardiac Purkinje fibers. *Circulation* **86**:147, 1992.
125. Hoffman EP, Knudson CM, Campbell KP, Kunkel LM: Subcellular fractionation of dystrophin to the triads of skeletal muscle. *Nature* **330**:754, 1987.
126. Salviati G, Betto R, Ceoldo S, Biasia E, Bonilla E, Miranda AF, Dimauro S: Cell fractionation studies indicate that dystrophin is a protein of surface membranes of skeletal muscle. *Biochem J* **258**:837, 1989.
127. Ohlendieck K, Ervasti JM, Snook JB, Campbell KP: Dystrophin-glycoprotein complex is highly enriched in isolated skeletal muscle sarcolemma. *J Cell Biol* **112**:135, 1991.
128. Cullen MJ, Walsh J, Nicholson LV, Harris JB: Ultrastructural localization of dystrophin in human muscle by using gold immunolabelling. *Proc R Soc Lond [Biol]* **240**:197, 1990.
129. Klietsch R, Ervasti JM, Arnold W, Campbell KP, Jorgensen AO: Dystrophin-glycoprotein complex and laminin colocalize to the sarcolemma and transverse tubules of cardiac muscle. *Circ Res* **72**:349, 1993.
130. Bornemann A, Schmalbruch H: Antidystrophin stains triadic junctions in regenerating rat muscles. *Muscle Nerve* **14**:1177, 1991.
131. Watkins SC, Hoffman EP, Slayter HS, Kunkel LM: Immunoelectron microscopic localization of dystrophin in myofibres. *Nature* **333**:863, 1988.
132. Carpenter S, Karpati G, Zubrzycka Gaarn E, Bulman DE, Ray PN, Worton RG: Dystrophin is localized to the plasma membrane of human skeletal muscle fibers by electron-microscopic cytochemical study. *Muscle Nerve* **13**:376, 1990.
133. Cullen MJ, Walsh J, Nicholson LVB, Harris JB, Zubrzycka-Gaarn EE, Ray PN, Worton RG: Immunogold labelling of dystrophin in human muscle, using an antibody to the last 17 amino acids of the C-terminus. *Neuromusc Disord* **1**:113, 1991.
134. Porter GA, Dmytrenko GM, Winkelmann JC, Bloch RJ: Dystrophin colocalizes with b-spectrin in distinct subsarcolemmal domains in mammalian skeletal muscle. *J Cell Biol* **117**:997, 1992.
135. Straub V, Bittner RE, Léger JJ, Voit T: Direct visualization of the dystrophin network on skeletal muscle fiber membrane. *J Cell Biol* **119**:1183, 1992.

136. Samitt CE, Bonilla E: Immunocytochemical study of dystrophin at the myotendinous junction. *Muscle Nerve* **13**:493, 1990.
137. Tidball JG, Law DJ: Dystrophin is required for normal thin filament-membrane associations at myotendinous junctions. *Am J Pathol* **138**:17, 1991.
138. Miike T, Miyatake M, Zhao J, Yoshioka K, Uchino M: Immunohistochemical dystrophin reaction in synaptic regions. *Brain Dev* **11**:344, 1989.
139. Shimizu T, Matsumura K, Sunada Y, Mannen T: Dense immunostaining on both neuromuscular and myotendon junctions with an antidystrophin antibody. *Biomed Res* **10**:405, 1989.
140. Fardeau M, Tome FM, Collin H, Augier N, Pons F, Leger J: Presence of dystrophin-like protein at the neuromuscular junction in Duchenne muscular dystrophy and in "mdx" mutant mice. *C R Acad Sci [III]* **311**:197, 1990.
141. Huard J, Fortier L-P, Dansereau G, Labrecque C, Tremblay JP: A light and electron microscopic study of dystrophin localization at the mouse neuromuscular junction. *Synapse* **10**:83, 1992.
142. Chang HW, Bock E, Bonilla E: Dystrophin in electric organ of *Torpedo californica* homologous to that in human muscle. *J Biol Chem* **264**:20831, 1989.
143. Jasmin BJ, Cartaud A, Ludosky MA, Changeux JP, Cartaud J: Asymmetric distribution of dystrophin in developing and adult *Torpedo marmorata* electrocyte: Evidence for its association with the acetylcholine receptor-rich membrane. *Proc Natl Acad Sci USA* **87**:3938, 1990.
144. Sealock R, Butler MH, Kramarcy NR, Gao KX, Murnane AA, Douville K, Froehner SC: Localization of dystrophin relative to acetylcholine receptor domains in electric tissue and adult and cultured skeletal muscle. *J Cell Biol* **113**:1133,1991.
145. Yeadon JE, Lin H, Dyer SM, Burden SJ: Dystrophin is a component of the subsynaptic membrane. *J Cell Biol* **115**:1069, 1991.
146. Dowdall MJ, Ellis JM, Man N, Morris GE: Immunoreactivity of skate electrocytes towards monoclonal antibodies against human dystrophin and dystrophin-related (DMDL) protein. *Neurosci Lett* **138**:27, 1992.
147. Lidov HG, Byers TJ, Watkins SC, Kunkel LM: Localization of dystrophin to postsynaptic regions of central nervous system cortical neurons. *Nature* **348**:725, 1990.
148. Huard J, Tremblay JP: Localization of dystrophin in the Purkinje cells of normal mice. *Neurosci Lett* **137**:105, 1992.
149. Gorecki D, Geng Y, Thomas K, Hunt SP, Barnard EA, Barnard PJ: Expression of the dystrophin gene in mouse and rat brain. *NeuroReport* **2**:773, 1991.
150. Gorecki DC, Monaco AP, Derry JMJ, Walker AP, Barnard EA, Barnard PJ: Expression of four alternative transcripts in brain regions regulated by different promoters. *Hum Mol Genet* **1**:505, 1992.
151. Houzelstein D, Lyons GE, Chamberlain J, Buckingham ME: Localization of dystrophin gene transcripts during mouse embryogenesis. *J Cell Biol* **119**:811, 1992.
152. Miyatake M, Miike T, Zhao JE, Yoshioka K, Uchino M, Usuku G: Dystrophin: localization and presumed function. *Muscle Nerve* **14**:113, 1991.
153. Pillers DM, Bulman DE, Weleber RG, Sigesmund GA, Musarella MA, Powell PR, Murphy WH, Westall C, Panton C, Becker LE, Worton RG, Ray PN: Dystrophin expression in the human retina is required for normal function as defined by electroretinography. *Nature Genet* **4**:82, 1993.
154. Byers TJ, Lidov HGW, Kunkel LM: An alternative dystrophin transcript specific to peripheral nerve. *Nature Genet* **4**:77, 1993.
155. Wessels A, Ginjaar IB, Moorman AF, van Ommen GJ: Different localization of dystrophin in developing and adult human skeletal muscle. *Muscle Nerve* **14**:1, 1991.
156. Prelle A, Chianese L, Moggio M, Gallanti A, Sciacco M, Checcarelli N, Comi G, Scarpini E, Bonilla E, Scarlato G: Appearance and localization of dystrophin in normal human fetal muscle. *Int J Dev Neurosci* **9**:607, 1991.
157. Clerk A, Strong PN, Sewry CA: Characterisation of dystrophin during development of human skeletal muscle. *Development* **114**:395, 1992.
158. Levine BA, Moir AJG, Patchell VB, Perry SV: The interaction of actin with dystrophin. *FEBS Lett* **263**:159, 1990.
159. Levine BA, Moir AJG, Patchell VB, Perry SV: Binding sites involved in the interaction of actin with the N-terminal region of dystrophin. *FEBS Lett* **298**:44, 1992.
160. Hemmings L, Kuhlman PA, Critchley DR: Analysis of the actin-binding domain of a-actinin by mutagenesis and demonstration that dystrophin contains a functionally homologous domain. *J Cell Biol* **116**:1369, 1992.
161. Campbell KP, Kahl SD: Association of dystrophin and an integral membrane glycoprotein. *Nature* **338**:259, 1989.
162. Ervasti JM, Campbell KP: Membrane organization of the dystrophin-glycoprotein complex. *Cell* **66**:1121, 1991.
163. Ibraghimov-Beskrovnaya O, Ervasti JM, Leveille C, Slaughter CA, Sernett SW, Campbell KP: Primary structure of dystrophin-associated glycoproteins linking dystrophin to the extracellular matrix. *Nature* **355**:696, 1992.
164. Ohlendieck K, Campbell KP: Dystrophin-associated proteins are greatly reduced in skeletal muscle from mdx mice. *J Cell Biol* **115**:1685, 1991.
165. Suzuki A, Yoshida M, Yamamoto H, Ozawa E: Glycoprotein-binding site of dystrophin is confined to the cysteine-rich domain and the first half of the carboxy-terminal domain. *FEBS Lett* **308**:154, 1992.
166. Yoshida M, Ozawa E: Glycoprotein complex anchoring dystrophin to sarcolemma. *J Biochem* **108**:748, 1990.
167. Dickson G, Azad A, Morris GE, Simon H, Noursadeghi M, Walsh FS: Co-localization and molecular association of dystrophin with laminin at the surface of mouse and human myotubes. *J Cell Sci* **103**:1223, 1992.
168. Klamut HJ, Gangopadhyay SB, Worton RG, Ray PN: Molecular and functional analysis of the muscle-specific promoter region of the Duchenne muscular dystrophy gene. *Mol Cell Biol* **10**:193, 1990.
169. Gilgenkrantz H, Hugnot J-P, Lambert M, Chafey P, Kaplan J-C, Kahn A: Positive and negative regulatory DNA elements including a CCArGG box are involved in the cell type-specific expression of the human muscle dystrophin gene. *J Biol Chem* **267**:10823, 1992.
170. Nudel U, Zuk D, Einat P, Zeelon E, Levy Z, Neuman S, Yaffe D: Duchenne muscular dystrophy gene product is not identical in muscle and brain. *Nature* **337**:76, 1989.
171. Geng Y, Sicinski P, Gorecki D, Barnard PJ: Developmental and tissue-specific regulation of mouse dystrophin: The embryonic isoform in muscular dystrophy. *Neuromusc Disord* **1**:125, 1991.
172. Feener CA, Koenig M, Kunkel LM: Alternative splicing of human dystrophin mRNA generates isoforms at the carboxy terminus. *Nature* **338**:509, 1989.
173. Boyce FM, Beggs AH, Feener C, Kunkel LM: Dystrophin is transcribed in brain from a distant upstream promoter. *Proc Natl Acad Sci USA* **88**:1276, 1991.
174. Chelly J, Hamard G, Koulakoff A, Kaplan JC, Kahn A, Berwald Netter Y: Dystrophin gene transcribed from different promoters in neuronal and glial cells. *Nature* **344**:64, 1990.
175. Bar S, Barnea E, Levy Z, Neuman S, Yaffe D, Nudel U: A novel product of the Duchenne muscular dystrophy gene which greatly differs from the known isoforms in its structure and tissue distribution. *Biochem J* **272**:557, 1990.
176. Rapaport D, Lederfein D, den Dunnen JT, Grootscholten PM, van Ommen G-JB, Fuchs O, Nudel U, Yaffe D: Characterization and cell type distribution of a novel, major transcript of the Duchenne muscular dystrophy gene. *Differentiation* **49**:187, 1992.
177. Lederfein D, Levy Z, Augier N, Mornet D, Morris G, Fuchs O, Yaffe D, Nudel U: A 71-kilodalton protein is a major product of the Duchenne muscular dystrophy gene in brain and other nonmuscle tissues. *Proc Natl Acad Sci USA* **89**:5346, 1992.
178. Blake D, Love D, Tinsley J, Morris C, Turloy H, Gatter K, Dickson G, Edwards Y, Davies K: Characterization of a 4.8 kb transcript from the Duchenne muscular dystrophy locus expressed in schwannoma cells. *Hum Mol Genet* **1**:103, 1992.
179. Hugnot JP, Gilgenkrantz H, Vincent N, Chafey P, Morris GE, Monaco AP, Berwald-Netter Y, Koulakoff

A, Kaplan JC, Kahn A, Chelly J: Distal transcript of the dystrophin gene initiated from an alternative first exon and encoding a 75-kDa protein widely distributed in nonmuscle tissues. *Proc Natl Acad Sci USA* **89**:7506, 1992.

180. Bies RD, Phelps SF, Cortez MD, Roberts R, Caskey CT, Chamberlain JS: Human and murine dystrophin mRNA transcripts are differentially expressed during skeletal muscle, heart, and brain development. *Nucleic Acids Res* **20**:1725, 1992.
181. Kunkel LM, Anderson MD, Boyce FM: Dystrophin isoforms and non-deletion/duplication mutations. *Am J Hum Genet* **49**:4, 1991.
182. Hoffman EP, Beggs AH, Koenig M, Kunkel LM, Angelini C: Cross-reactive protein in Duchenne muscle. *Lancet* **2**:1211, 1989.
183. Love DR, Hill DF, Dickson G, Spurr NK, Byth BC, Marsden RF, Walsh FS, Edwards YH, Davies KE: An autosomal transcript in skeletal muscle with homology to dystrophin. *Nature* **339**:55, 1989.
184. Khurana TS, Hoffman EP, Kunkel LM: Identification of a chromosome 6-encoded dystrophin-related protein. *J Biol Chem* **265**:16717, 1990.
185. Buckle VJ, Guenet JL, Simon Chazottes D, Love DR, Davies KE: Localisation of a dystrophin-related autosomal gene to 6q24 in man, and to mouse chromosome 10 in the region of the dystrophia muscularis (dy) locus. *Hum Genet* **85**:324, 1990.
186. Love DR, Morris GE, Ellis JM, Fairbrother U, Marsden RF, Bloomfield JF, Edwards YH, Slater CP, Parry DJ, Davies KE: Tissue distribution of the dystrophin-related gene product and expression in the mdx and dy mouse. *Proc Natl Acad Sci USA* **88**:3243, 1991.
187. Tinsley JM, Blake DJ, Roche A, Fairbrother U, Riss J, Byth BC, Knight AE, Kendrick-Jones J, Suthers GK, Love DR, Edwards YH, Davies KE: Primary structure of dystrophin-related protein. *Nature* **360**:591, 1992.
188. Man NT, Thanh LT, Blake DJ, Davies KE, Morris GE: Utrophin, the autosomal homologue of dystrophin, is widely-expressed and membrane-associated in cultured cell lines. *FEBS Lett* **313**:19, 1992.
189. Koga R, Ishiura S, Takemitsu M, Kamakura K, Matsuzaki T, Arahata K, Nonaka I, Sugita H: Immunoblot analysis of dystrophin-related protein (DRP). *Biochim Biophys Acta* **1180**:257, 1993.
190. Tanaka H, Ishiguro T, Eguchi C, Saito K, Ozawa E: Expression of a dystrophin-related protein associated with the skeletal muscle cell membrane. *Histochemistry* **96**:1, 1991.
191. Ohlendieck K, Ervasti JM, Matsumura K, Kahl SD, Leveille CJ, Campbell KP: Dystrophin-related protein is localized to neuromuscular junctions of adult skeletal muscle. *Neuron* **7**:499, 1991.
192. Khurana TS, Watkins SC, Chafey P, Chelly J, Tome FMS, Fardeau M, Kaplan JC, Kunkel LM: Immunolocalization and developmental expression of dystrophin related protein in skeletal muscle. *Neuromusc Disord* **1**:185, 1991.
193. Pons F, Augier N, Leger JO, Robert A, Tome FM, Fardeau M, Voit T, Nicholson LV, Mornet D, Leger JJ: A homologue of dystrophin is expressed at the neuromuscular junctions of normal individuals and DMD patients, and of normal and mdx mice. Immunological evidence. *FEBS Lett* **282**:161, 1991.
194. Voit T, Haas K, Leger JO, Pons F, Leger JJ: Xp21 dystrophin and 6q dystrophin-related protein. Comparative immunolocalization using multiple antibodies. *Am J Pathol* **139**:969, 1991.
195. Karpati G, Carpenter S, Morris GE, Davies KE, Guerin C, Holland P: Localization and quantitation of the chromosome 6-encoded dystrophin-related protein in normal and pathological human muscle. *J Neuropathol Exp Neurol* **52**:119, 1993.
196. Augier N, Boucraut J, Léger J, Anoal M, Nicholson LVB, Voelkel MA, Léger JJ, Pellissier JF: A homologue of dystrophin is expressed at the blood vessel membrane of DMD and BMD patients: Immunological evidence. *J Neurol Sci* **107**:233, 1992.
197. Ishiura S, Arahata K, Tsukahara T, Koga R, Anraku H, Yamaguchi M, Kikuchi T, Nonaka I, Sugita H: Antibody against the C-terminal portion of dystrophin crossreacts with the 400 kDa protein in the pia mater of dystrophin-deficient mdx mouse brain. *J Biochem* **107**:510, 1990.
198. Khurana TS, Watkins SC, Kunkel LM: The subcellular distribution of chromosome 6-encoded dystrophin-related protein in the brain. *J Cell Biol* **119**:357, 1992.
199. Matsumura K, Ervasti JM, Ohlendieck K, Kahl SD, Campbell KP: Association of dystrophin-related protein with dystrophin-associated proteins in *mdx* mouse muscle. *Nature* **360**:588, 1992.
200. Forrest SM, Cross GS, Flint T, Speer A, Robson KJ, Davies KE: Further studies of gene deletions that cause Duchenne and Becker muscular dystrophies. *Genomics* **2**:109, 1988.
201. den Dunnen JT, Bakker E, Breteler EG, Pearson PL, van Ommen GJ: Direct detection of more than 50% of the Duchenne muscular dystrophy mutations by field inversion gels. *Nature* **329**:640, 1987.
202. Hu XY, Ray PN, Murphy EG, Thompson MW, Worton RG: Duplicational mutation at the Duchenne muscular dystrophy locus: its frequency, distribution, origin, and phenotype-genotype correlation. *Am J Hum Genet* **46**:682, 1990.
203. Rapaport D, Passos Bueno MR, Brandao L, Love D, Vainzof M, Zatz M: Apparent association of mental retardation and specific patterns of deletions screened with probes cf56a and cf23a in Duchenne muscular dystrophy. *Am J Med Genet* **39**:437, 1991.
204. England SB, Nicholson LV, Johnson MA, Forrest SM, Love DR, Zubrzycka Gaarn EE, Bulman DE, Harris JB, Davies KE: Very mild muscular dystrophy associated with the deletion of 46% of dystrophin. *Nature* **343**:180, 1990.
205. Love DR, Flint TJ, Genet SA, Middleton-Price HR, Davies KE: Becker muscular dystrophy patient with a large intragenic dystrophin deletion: implications for functional minigenes and gene therapy. *J Med Genet* **28**:860, 1991.
206. Gillard EF, Chamberlain JS, Murphy EG, Duff CL, Smith B, Burghes AH, Thompson MW, Sutherland J, Oss I, Bodrug SE, Ray PN, Worton RG: Molecular and phenotypic analysis of patients with deletions within the deletion-rich region of the Duchenne muscular dystrophy (DMD) gene. *Am J Hum Genet* **45**:507, 1989.
207. Baumbach LL, Chamberlain JS, Ward PA, Farwell NJ, Caskey CT: Molecular and clinical correlations of deletions leading to Duchenne and Becker muscular dystrophies. *Neurology* **39**:465, 1989.
208. Hoffman EP, Kunkel LM, Angelini C, Clarke A, Johnson M, Harris JB: Improved diagnosis of Becker muscular dystrophy by dystrophin testing. *Neurology* **39**:1011, 1989.
209. Nicholson LV, Johnson MA, Gardner Medwin D, Bhattacharya S, Harris JB: Heterogeneity of dystrophin expression in patients with Duchenne and Becker muscular dystrophy. *Acta Neuropathol* **80**:239, 1990.
210. Arahata K, Beggs AH, Honda H, Ito S, Ishiura S, Tsukahara T, Ishiguro T, Eguchi C, Orimo S, Arikawa E: Preservation of the C-terminus of dystrophin molecule in the skeletal muscle from Becker muscular dystrophy. *J Neurol Sci* **101**:148, 1991.
211. Roberts RG, Barby TF, Manners E, Bobrow M, Bentley DR: Direct detection of dystrophin gene rearrangements by analysis of dystrophin mRNA in peripheral blood lymphocytes. *Am J Hum Genet* **49**:298, 1991.
212. Chelly J, Gilgenkrantz H, Lambert M, Hamard G, Chafey P, Recan D, Katz P, de la Chapelle A, Koenig M, Ginjaar IB: Effect of dystrophin gene deletions on mRNA levels and processing in Duchenne and Becker muscular dystrophies. *Cell* **63**:1239, 1990.
213. Gangopadhyay SB, Sherratt TG, Heckmatt JZ, Dubowitz V, Miller G, Shokeir M, Ray PN, Strong PN, Worton RG: Dystrophin in frameshift deletion patients with Becker muscular dystrophy. *Am J Hum Genet* **51**:562, 1992.
214. (See ref. 96).
215. Blonden LA, Grootscholten PM, den Dunnen JT, Bakker E, Abbs S, Bobrow M, Boehm C, van Broeckhoven C, Baumbach L, Chamberlain J: 242 breakpoints in the 200-kb deletion-prone P20 region of the DMD gene are widely spread. *Genomics* **10**:631, 1991.
216. Pizzuti A, Pieretti M, Fenwick RG, Gibbs RA, Caskey

CT: A transposon-like element in the deletion-prone region of the dystrophin gene. *Genomics* **13**:594, 1992.
217. Love DR, England SB, Speer A, Marsden RF, Bloomfield JF, Roche AL, Cross GS, Mountford RC, Smith TJ, Davies KE: Sequences of junction fragments in the deletion-prone region of the dystrophin gene. *Genomics* **10**:57, 1991.
218. Bakker E, Veenema H, den Dunnen JT, van Broeckhoven C, Grootscholten PM, Bonten EJ, van Ommen GJ, Pearson PL: Germinal mosaicism increases the recurrence risk for 'new' Duchenne muscular dystrophy mutations. *J Med Genet* **26**:553, 1989.
219. Wood S, McGillivray BC: Germinal mosaicism in Duchenne muscular dystrophy. *Hum Genet* **78**:282, 1988.
220. Bakker E, van Broeckhoven C, Bonten EJ, van de Vooren MJ, Veenema H, Van Hul W, van Ommen GJ, Vandenberghe A, Pearson PL: Germline mosaicism and Duchenne muscular dystrophy mutations. *Nature* **329**:554, 1987.
221. Witkowski R: Germinal "mosaicism"—Germline mutation or chimerism? *Hum Genet* **88**:359, 1992.
222. Angelini C, Beggs AH, Hoffman EP, Fanin M, Kunkel LM: Enormous dystrophin in a patient with Becker muscular dystrophy. *Neurology* **40**:808, 1990.
223. Hu X, Bulman DE, Ray PN, Worton RG: Frame-shift duplication resulting in truncated dystrophin in a patient with Duchenne muscular dystrophy. *Hum Mutat* **1**:172, 1992.
224. Hu XY, Pay PN, Worton RG: Mechanisms of tandem duplication in the Duchenne muscular dystrophy gene include both homologous and nonhomologous intrachromosomal recombination. *EMBO J* **10**:2471, 1991.
225. Hu XY, Burghes AH, Bulman DE, Ray PN, Worton RG: Evidence for mutation by unequal sister chromatid exchange in the Duchenne muscular dystrophy gene. *Am J Hum Genet* **44**:855, 1989.
226. Bulman DE, Gangopadhyay SB, Bebchuck KG, Worton RG, Ray PN: Point mutation in the human dystrophin gene: Identification through western blot analysis. *Genomics* **10**:457, 1991.
227. Roberts RG, Bobrow M, Bentley DR: Point mutations in the dystrophin gene. *Proc Natl Acad Sci USA* **89**:2331, 1992.
228. Kilimann MW, Pizzuti A, Grompe M, Caskey CT: Point mutations and polymorphisms in the human dystrophin gene identified in genomic DNA sequences amplified by multiplex PCR. *Hum Genet* **89**:253, 1992.
229. Clemens PR, Ward PA, Caskey CT, Bulman DE, Fenwick RG: Premature chain termination mutation causing Duchenne muscular dystrophy. *Neurology* **42**:1775, 1992.
230. Prior TW, Papp AC, Snyder PJ, Burghes AHM, Sedra MS, Western LM, Bartello C, Mendell JR: Identification of two point mutations and a one base deletion in exon 19 of the dystrophin gene by heteroduplex formation. *Hum Mol Genet* **2**:311, 1993.
231. Saad, F, Vitiello L, Merlini L, Mostacciuolo M, Oliviero S, Danieli GA: A 3′ consensus splice mutation in the human dystrophin gene detected by a screening for intra-exonic deletions. *Hum Mol Genet* **1**:345, 1992.
232. Nigro V, Politano L, Nigro G, Romano SC, Molinari AM, Puca GA: Detection of a nonsense mutation in the dystrophin gene by multiple SSCP. *Hum Mol Genet* **1**:517, 1992.
233. Winnard AV, Jia-Hsu J, Gibbs RA, Mendell JR, Burghes AHM: Identification of a 2 base pair nonsense mutation causing a cryptic splice site in a DMD patient. *Hum Mol Genet* **1**:645, 1992.
234. Matsuo M, Masumura T, Nakajima T, Kitoh Y, Takumi T, Nishio H, Koga J, Nakamura H: A very small frame-shifting deletion within exon 19 of the Duchenne muscular dystrophy gene. *Biochem Biophys Res Commun* **170**:963, 1990.
235. Matsuo M, Nishio H, Kitoh Y, Francke U, Nakamura H: Partial deletion of a dystrophin gene leads to exon skipping and to loss of a intra-exon hairpin structure from the predicted mRNA precursor. *Biochem Biophys Res Commun* **182**:495, 1992.
236. Bushby KMD, Cleghorn MJ, Curtis A, Haggerty ID, Nicholson LVB, Johnson MA, Harris JB, Bhattacharya SS: Identification of a mutation in the promoter region of the dystrophin gene in a patient with atypical Becker muscular dystrophy. *Hum Genet* **88**:185, 1991.
237. den Dunnen, JT, Casula L, Makover A, Bokkev B, Yaffe D, Nudel U, van Ommen G-JB: Mapping of dystrophin brain promoter: A deletion of this region is compatible with normal intellect. *Neuromuscul Disord* **1**:327, 1991.
238. Bulfield G, Siller WG, Wight PAL, Moore KJ: X chromosome-linked muscular dystrophy (*mdx*) in the mouse. *Proc Natl Acad Sci USA* **81**:1189, 1984.
239. Sicinski P, Geng Y, Ryder Cook AS, Barnard EA, Darlison MG, Barnard PJ: The molecular basis of muscular dystrophy in the mdx mouse: a point mutation. *Science* **244**:1578, 1989.
240. Chapman VM, Miller DR, Armstrong D, Caskey CT: Recovery of induced mutations for X chromosome-linked muscular dystrophy in mice. *Proc Natl Acad Sci USA* **86**:1292, 1989.
241. Cox GA, Phelps SF, Chapman VM, Chamberlain JS: New *mdx* mutation disrupts expression of muscle and nonmuscle isoforms of dystrophin. *Nature Genet* **4**:87, 1993.
242. Valentine BA, Cooper BJ, de Lahunta A, O'Quinn R, Blue JT: Canine X-linked muscular dystrophy. An animal model of Duchenne muscular dystrophy: Clinical studies. *J Neurol Sci* **88**:69, 1988.
243. Valentine BA, Winand NJ, Pradhan D, Moise NS, de Lahunta A, Kornegay JN, Cooper BJ: Canine X-linked muscular dystrophy as an animal model of Duchenne muscular dystrophy. *Am J Med Genet* **42**:352, 1992.
244. Sharp NJH, Kornegay JN, Van Camp SD, Herbstreith MH, Secore SL, Kettle S, Hung W-Y, Constantinou CD, Dykstra MJ, Roses AD, Bartlett RJ: An error in dystrophin mRNA processing in golden retriever muscular dystrophy, an animal homologue of Duchenne muscular dystrophy. *Genomics* **13**:115, 1992.
245. Bodrug SE, Burghes AH, Ray PM, Worton RG: Mapping of four translocation breakpoints within the Duchenne muscular dystrophy gene. *Genomics* **4**:101, 1989.
246. Cockburn DJ, Munro EA, Craig IW, Boyd Y: Mapping of X chromosome translocation breakpoints in females with Duchenne muscular dystrophy with respect to exons of the dystrophin gene. *Hum Genet* **90**:407, 1992.
247. Bodrug SE, Holden JJ, Ray PN, Worton RG: Molecular analysis of X-autosome translocations in females with Duchenne muscular dystrophy. *EMBO J* **10**:3931, 1991.
248. Robinson DO, Boyd Y, Cockburn D, Collinson MN, Craig I, Jacobs PA: The parental origin of de novo X-autosome translocations in females with Duchenne muscular dystrophy revealed by M27 beta methylation analysis. *Genet Res* **56**:135, 1990.
249. Chamberlain JS, Gibbs RA, Ranier JE, Nguyen PN, Caskey CT: Deletion screening of the Duchenne muscular dystrophy locus via multiplex DNA amplification. *Nucleic Acids Res* **16**:11141, 1988.
250. Chamberlain JS, Multicenter Study Group: Diagnosis of Duchenne and Becker muscular dystrophies by polymerase chain reactions. *JAMA* **267**:2609, 1992.
251. Beggs AH, Koenig M, Boyce FM, Kunkel LM: Detection of 98% of DMD/BMD gene deletions by polymerase chain reaction. *Hum Genet* **86**:45, 1990.
252. Abbs S, Bobrow M: Analysis of quantitative PCR for the diagnosis of deletion and duplication carriers in the dystrophin gene. *J Med Genet* **29**:191, 1992.
253. Chelly J, Gilgenkrantz H, Hugnot JP, Hamard G, Lambert M, Recan D, Akli S, Cometto M, Kahn A, Kaplan JC: Illegitimate transcription. Application to the analysis of truncated transcripts of the dystrophin gene in nonmuscle cultured cells from Duchenne and Becker patients. *J Clin Invest* **88**:1161, 1991.
254. Hoffman EP, Fischbeck KH, Brown RH, Johnson M, Medori R, Loike JD, Harris JB, Waterston R, Brooke M, Specht L: Characterization of dystrophin in muscle-biopsy specimens from patients with Duchenne's or Becker's muscular dystrophy. *N Engl J Med* **318**:1363, 1988.
255. Arahata K, Hoffman EP, Kunkel LM, Ishiura S, Tsukahara T, Ishihara T, Sunohara N, Nonaka I, Ozawa E, Sugita H: Dystrophin diagnosis: Comparison of dystrophin abnormalities by immunofluorescence and immunoblot analyses. *Proc Natl Acad Sci USA* **86**:7154, 1989.

256. Arahata K, Ishihara T, Kamakura K, Tsukahara T, Ishiura S, Baba C, Matsumoto T, Nonaka I, Sugita H: Mosaic expression of dystrophin in symptomatic carriers of Duchenne's muscular dystrophy. *N Engl J Med* **320**:138, 1989.
257. Evans MI, Greb A, Kunkel LM, Sacks AJ, Johnson MP, Boehm C, Kazazian HH Jr, Hoffman EP: In utero fetal muscle biopsy for the diagnosis of Duchenne muscular dystrophy. *Am J Obstet Gynecol* **165**:728, 1991.
258. Feener CA, Boyce FM, Kunkel LM: Rapid detection of CA polymorphisms in cloned DNA: application to the 5′ region of the dystrophin gene. *Am J Hum Genet* **48**:621, 1991.
259. Oudet C, Heilig R, Hanauer A, Mandel JL: Nonradioactive assay for new microsatellite polymorphisms at the 5′ end of the dystrophin gene, and estimation of intragenic recombination. *Am J Hum Genet* **49**:311, 1991.
260. Oudet C, Heilig R, Mandel JL: An informative polymorphism detectable by polymerase chain reaction at the 3′ end of dystrophin gene. *Hum Genet* **85**:677, 1990.
261. Beggs AH, Kunkel LM: A polymorphic CACA repeat in the 3′ untranslated region of dystrophin. *Nucleic Acids Res* **18**:1931, 1990.
262. Clemens PR, Fenwick RG, Chamberlain JS, Gibbs RA, de Andrade M, Chakraborty R, Caskey CT: Carrier detection and prenatal diagnosis in Duchenne and Becker muscular dystrophy families, using dinucleotide repeat polymorphisms. *Am J Hum Genet* **49**:951, 1991.
263. Arikawa E, Hoffman EP, Kaido M, Nonaka I, Sugita H, Arahata K: The frequency of patients with dystrophin abnormalities in a limb-girdle patient population. *Neurology* **41**:1491, 1991.
264. Norman A, Thomas N, Coakley J, Harper P: Distinction of Becker from limb-girdle muscular dystrophy by means of dystrophin cDNA probes. *Lancet* **1**:466, 1989.
265. Vainzof M, Pavanello RC, Pavanello Filho I, Rapaport D, Passos Bueno MR, Zubrzycka Gaarn EE, Bulman DE, Zatz M: Screening of male patients with autosomal recessive Duchenne dystrophy through dystrophin and DNA studies. *Am J Med Genet* **39**:38, 1991.
266. Tachi N, Tachi M, Sasaki K, Nagata N, Chiba S: Dystrophin analysis in the differential diagnosis of autosomal recessive muscular dystrophy of childhood and Duchenne muscular dystrophy. *Pediatr Neurol* **6**:265, 1990.
267. Norman AM, Hughes HE, Gardner Medwin D, Nicholson LV: Dystrophin analysis in the diagnosis of muscular dystrophy. *Arch Dis Child* **64**:1501, 1989.
268. Francke U, Darras BT, Hersh JH, Berg BO, Miller RG: Brother/sister pairs affected with early-onset, progressive muscular dystrophy: Molecular studies reveal etiologic heterogeneity. *Am J Hum Genet* **45**:63, 1989.
269. McGuire SA, Fischbeck KH: Autosomal recessive Duchenne-like muscular dystrophy: Molecular and histochemical results. *Muscle Nerve* **14**:1209, 1991.
270. Matsumura K, Tomé FMS, Collin H, Azibi K, Chaouch M, Kaplan J-C, Fardeau M, Campbell KP: Deficiency of the 50K dystrophin-associated glycoprotein in severe childhood autosomal recessive muscular dystrophy. *Nature* **359**:320, 1992.
271. Arikawa E, Ishihara T, Nonaka I, Sugita H, Arahata K: Immunocytochemical analysis of dystrophin in congenital muscular dystrophy. *J Neurol Sci* **195**:79, 1991.
272. Beggs AH, Neumann PE, Arahata K, Arikawa E, Nonaka I, Anderson MS, Kunkel LM: Possible influences on the expression of X chromosome-linked dystrophin abnormalities by heterozygosity for autosomal recessive Fukuyama congenital muscular dystrophy. *Proc Natl Acad Sci USA* **89**:623, 1992.
273. Matsumura K, Nonaka I, Campbell KP: Abnormal expression of dystrophin-associated proteins in Fukuyama-type congenital muscular dystrophy. *Lancet* **341**:521, 1993.
274. Blau HM, Webster C, Pavlath GK: Defective myoblasts identified in Duchenne muscular dystrophy. *Proc Natl Acad Sci USA* **80**:4856, 1983.
275. Fong PY, Turner PR, Denetclaw WF, Steinhardt RA: Increased activity of calcium leak channels in myotubes of Duchenne human and mdx mouse origin. *Science* **250**:673, 1990.
276. Franco A Jr, Lansman JB: Calcium entry through stretch-inactivated ion channels in mdx myotubes. *Nature* **344**:670, 1990.
277. Mendell JR, Moxley RT, Griggs RC, Brooke MH, Fenichel GM, Miller JP, King W, Signore L, Pandya S, Florence J: Randomized, double-blind six-month trial of prednisone in Duchenne's muscular dystrophy. *N Engl J Med* **320**:1592, 1989.
278. Fenichel GM, Florence JM, Pestronk A, Mendell JR, Moxley RT III, Griggs RC, Brooke MH, Miller JP, Robison J, King W: Long-term benefit from prednisone therapy in Duchenne muscular dystrophy. *Neurology* **41**:1874, 1991.
279. Mesa LE, Dubrovsky AL, Corderi J, Marco P, Flores D: Steroids in Duchenne muscular dystrophy—deflazacort trial. *Neuromusc Disord* **1**:261, 1991.
280. Kissel JT, Burrow KL, Rammohan KW, Mendell JR, CIDD Study Group: Mononuclear cell analysis of muscle biopsies in prednisone-treated and untreated Duchenne muscular dystrophy. *Neurology* **41**:667, 1991.
281. Hardiman O, Sklar RM, Brown RH Jr: Methylprednisolone selectively affected dystrophin expression in human muscle cultures. *Neurology* **43**:342, 1993.
282. Law PK, Goodwin TG, Li HJ: Histoincompatible myoblast injection improves muscle structure and function of dystrophic mice. *Transplant Proc* **20**:1114, 1988.
283. Partridge TA, Morgan JE, Coulton GR, Hoffman EP, Kunkel LM: Conversion of mdx myofibres from dystrophin-negative to -positive by injection of normal myoblasts. *Nature* **337**:176, 1989.
284. Karpati G, Pouliot Y, Zubrzycka Gaarn E, Carpenter S, Ray PN, Worton RG, Holland P: Dystrophin is expressed in mdx skeletal muscle fibers after normal myoblast implantation. *Am J Pathol* **135**:27, 1989.
285. Law PK, Bertorini TE, Goodwin TG, Chen M, Fang QW, Li HJ, Kirby DS, Florendo JA, Herrod HG, Golden DS: Dystrophin production induced by myoblast transfer therapy in Duchenne muscular dystrophy. *Lancet* **336**:114, 1990.
286. Huard J, Bouchard JP, Roy R, Malouin F, Dansereau G, Labrecque C, Albert N, Richards CL, Lemieux B, Tremblay JP: Human myoblast transplantation: Preliminary results of 4 cases. *Muscle Nerve* **15**:550, 1992.
287. Huard J, Roy R, Bouchard J-P, Malouin F, Richards CL, Tremblay J-P: Human myoblast transplantation between immunohistocompatible donors and recipients produces immune reactions. *Transplant Proc* **24**:3049, 1992.
288. Gussoni E, Pavlath GK, Lanctot AM, Sharma KR, Miller RG, Steinman L, Blau HM: Normal dystrophin transcripts detected in Duchenne muscular dystrophy patients after myoblast transplantation. *Nature* **356**:435, 1992.
289. Karpati G, Ajdukovic D, Arnold D, Gledhill RB, Gittmann R, Holland P, Koch PA, Shoubridge E, Spence D, Vanasse M, Watters GV, Abrahamovicz M, Duff C, Worton RG: Myoblast transfer in Duchenne muscular dystrophy. *Ann Neurol* **34**:8, 1992.
290. Law PK, Goodwin TG, Fang Q, Duggirala V, Larkin C, Florendo JA, Kirby DS, Deering MB, Li HJ, Chen M, Yoo TJ, Cornett J, Li LM, Shirzad A, Quinley T, Holcomb RL: Feasibility, safety and efficacy of myoblast transfer therapy on Duchenne muscular dystrophy boys. *Cell Transplant* **1**:235, 1992.
291. Neumeyer AM, DiGregorio DM, Brown RH Jr: Arterial delivery of myoblasts to skeletal muscle. *Neurology* **42**:2258, 1992.
292. Wolff JA, Malone RW, Williams P, Chong W, Acsadi G, Jani A, Felgner PL: Direct gene transfer into mouse muscle in vivo. *Science* **247**:1465, 1990.
293. Wolff JA, Williams P, Acsadi G, Jiao S, Jani A, Chong W: Conditions affecting direct gene transfer into rodent muscle in vivo. *Biotech* **11**:474, 1991.
294. Jiao S, Williams P, Berg RK, Hodgeman BA, Liu L, Repetto G, Wolff JA: Direct gene transfer into nonhuman primate myofibers *in vivo*. *Hum Gene Ther* **3**:21, 1992.
295. Lee CC, Pearlman JA, Chamberlain JS, Caskey CT: Expression of recombinant dystrophin and its localization to the cell membrane. *Nature* **349**:334, 1991.

296. Dickson G, Love DR, Davies KE, Wells KE, Piper TA, Walsh FS: Human dystrophin gene transfer: Production and expression of a functional recombinant DNA-based gene. *Hum Genet* **88**:53, 1991.
297. Acsadi G, Dickson G, Love DR, Jani A, Walsh FS, Gurusinghe A, Wolff JA, Davies KE: Human dystrophin expression in mdx mice after intramuscular injection of DNA constructs. *Nature* **352**:815, 1991.
298. Wells DJ, Wells KE, Walsh FS, Davies KE, Goldspink G, Love DR, Chan-Thomas P, Dunckley MG, Piper T, Dickson G: Human dystrophin expression corrects the myopathic phenotype in mdx transgenic mice. *Hum Mol Genet* **1**:35, 1992.
299. Cox GA, Cole NM, Matsumura K, Phelps SF, Hauschka SD, Campbell KP, Faulkner JA, Chamberlain JS: Overexpression of dystrophin in transgenic mdx mice eliminates dystrophic symptoms without toxicity. *Nature* **364**:725, 1993.
300. Graham FL, Prevec L: Manipulation of adenovirus vectors. *Methods Mol Biol* **7**:109, 1991.
301. Stratford-Perricaudet LD, Makeh I, Perricaudet M, Briand P: Widespread long-term gene transfer to mouse skeletal muscles and heart. *J Clin Invest* **90**:626, 1992.
302. Ragot T, Vincent N, Chafey P, Vigne E, Gilgenkrantz H, Couton D, Cartaud J, Briand P, Kaplan J-C, Perricaudet M, Kahn A: Efficient adenovirus-mediated transfer of a human minidystrophin gene to skeletal muscle of *mdx* mice. *Nature* **361**:647, 1993.
303. Acsadi G, Jiao S, Jani A, Duke D, Williams P, Chong W, Wolff JA: Direct gene transfer and expression into rat heart in vivo. *New Biologist* **3**:71, 1991.
304. Lin H, Parmacek S, Morle G, Bolling S, Leiden JM: Expression of recombinant genes in myocardium in vivo after direct injection of DNA. *Circulation* **82**:2217, 1990.
305. Kitsis RN, Buttrick PM, McNally EM, Kaplan ML, Leinwand LA: Hormonal modulation of a gene injected into rat heart in vivo. *Proc Natl Acad Sci USA* **88**:4138, 1991.
306. Dreifuss FE, Hogan GR: Survival in X-chromosomal muscular dystrophy. *Neurology* **11**:734, 1961.
307. Emery AEH, Dreifuss FE: Unusual type of benign X-linked muscular dystrophy. *J Neurol Neurosurg Psychiatr* **29**:338, 1966.
308. Emery AE: Emery-Dreifuss syndrome. *J Med Genet* **26**:637, 1989.
309. Dickey RP, Ziter FA, Smith RA: Emery-Dreifuss muscular dystrophy. *J Pediatr* **104**:555, 1984.
310. Emery AE: X-linked muscular dystrophy with early contractures and cardiomyopathy (Emery-Dreifuss type). *Clin Genet* **32**:360, 1987.
311. Hopkins LC, Jackson JA, Elsas LJ: Emery-Dreifuss humeroperoneal muscular dystrophy: An X-linked myopathy with unusual contractures and bradycardia. *Ann Neurol* **10**:230, 1981.
312. Rowland LP, Fetell PM, Olarte M, Hays A, Singh N, Wanat FE: Emery-Dreifuss muscular dystrophy. *Ann Neurol* **5**:111, 1979.
313. Thomas NS, Williams H, Elsas LJ, Hopkins LC, Sarfarazi M, Harper PS: Localisation of the gene for Emery-Dreifuss muscular dystrophy to the distal long arm of the X chromosome. *J Med Genet* **23**:596, 1986.
314. Hodgson S, Boswinkel E, Cole C, Walker A, Dubowitz V, Granata C, Merlini L, Bobrow M: A linkage study of Emery-Dreifuss muscular dystrophy. *Hum Genet* **74**:409, 1986.
315. Yates JR, Affara NA, Jamieson DM, Ferguson Smith MA, Hausmanowa-Petrusewicz I, Zaremba J, Borkowska J, Johnston AW, Kelly K: Emery-Dreifuss muscular dystrophy: Localisation to Xq27.3–qter confirmed by linkage to the factor VIII gene. *J Med Genet* **23**:587, 1986.
316. Thomas PK, Calne DB, Elliott CF: X-linked scapuloperoneal syndrome. *J Neurol Neurosurg Psychiatr* **35**:208, 1972.
317. Romeo G, Roncuzzi L, Sangiorgi S, Giacanelli M, Liguori M, Tessarolo D, Rocchi M: Mapping of the Emery-Dreifuss gene through reconstruction of crossover points in two Italian pedigrees. *Hum Genet* **80**:59, 1988.
318. Consalez GG, Thomas NS, Stayton CL, Knight SJ, Johnson M, Hopkins LC, Harper PS, Elsas LJ, Warren ST: Assignment of Emery-Dreifuss muscular dystrophy to the distal region of Xq28: the results of a collaborative study. *Am J Hum Genet* **48**:468, 1991.
319. Yates JRW, Warner JP, Smith JA, Deymeer F, Azulay J-P, Hausmanowa-Petrusewicz I, Zaremba J, Borkowska J, Affara NA, Ferguson-Smith MA: Emery-Dreifuss muscular dystrophy: Linkage to markers in distal Xq28. *J Med Genet* **30**:108, 1993.

CHAPTER 141

Myotonic Dystrophy and Other Autosomal Muscular Dystrophies

Peter S. Harper

1. **The autosomal muscular dystrophies represent an important group of genetically determined primary disorders of muscle. Collectively they are more numerous than the X-linked muscular dystrophies, though some members of the group are extremely rare. At least eight different forms of major autosomal muscular dystrophy have been identified; heterogeneity remains to be resolved for some disorders.**
2. **Myotonic dystrophy is the most frequent autosomal muscular dystrophy. It is a multisystem disorder, involving heart, smooth muscle, central nervous system, eye, and endocrine glands as well as skeletal muscle. Unique among the progressive muscular dystrophies, it is characterized by myotonia, which results from an electrophysiological disturbance whose mechanism is likely to differ from that producing myotonia in other, nonprogressive myotonic disorders. Myotonic dystrophy has autosomal dominant inheritance, is exceptionally variable both within and between families, and shows anticipation, with earlier age at onset and more severe clinical features in successive generations. The most severe cases with congenital onset are maternally inherited.**
3. **The specific molecular defect in myotonic dystrophy has now been elucidated. The gene, which is expressed in various tissues, including heart, skeletal muscle, and brain, has been sequenced and codes for an mRNA of around 2400 bases; the derived sequence of its protein product suggests a member of the protein kinase family but is not identical with any known protein. The mutation causing myotonic dystrophy is the expansion of a CTG repeat near the 3′ end of the gene. This is present in less than 30 copies in normal individuals but in 50 copies or more in minimally affected myotonic dystrophy patients; the original premutation may have been unique, but clinically significant cases are probably replenished from a pool of healthy individuals with a high-normal repeat number. The expanded sequence in affected patients is unstable, both in meiosis and somatically, with up to 6 kb of additional DNA in severely affected individuals. The identification of this molecular defect now allows the specific diagnosis of myotonic dystrophy in relation to other neuromuscular disorders as well as accurate prenatal diagnosis and presymptomatic testing.**
4. **Facioscapulohumeral disease is a variable and relatively benign muscular dystrophy showing autosomal dominant inheritance. The gene has been located on the distal long arm of chromosome 4 but has yet to be isolated and characterized. The current closely linked markers are all proximal to the disease gene; the closest of these shows a specific alteration in a high proportion of affected patients that may reflect a subterminal deletion of DNA responsible for the disorder.**
5. **The limb-girdle muscular dystrophy group remains heterogeneous and incompletely defined. Many male patients previously thought to have an autosomal dystrophy in this group have proved to have mutations in the dystrophin gene on the X chromosome, and performing a dystrophin assay on a muscle biopsy specimen to exclude this disorder is an essential part of the diagnostic investigation of patients in this group. A rare adult autosomal dominant type has been localized to chromosome 5, while one recessive form maps to chromosome 15. The severe autosomal form of Duchenne-like childhood muscular dystrophy maps to chromosome 13q and may be caused by a defect in the 50-kDa glycoprotein associated with dystrophin.**
6. **The numerous nonprogressive forms of primary muscle disease are not covered in detail in this chapter, but important molecular advances have occurred in some of them. Two of the nonprogressive myotonias—paramyotonia congenita and adynamia (hyperkalemic periodic paralysis)—have been found to be linked to the sodium ion channel locus and are caused by mutations in this gene, while myotonia congenita is caused by defects in the chloride ion channel (ClC-1). Two other disorders, hyperpyrexic myopathy (which is likely to be heterogeneous) and central core disease, show close linkage to the ryanodine receptor gene on chromosome 19 (see Chap. 4), which, again, may be causally related in some cases.**
7. **The increasing recognition of primary molecular defects in the autosomal muscular dystrophies and allied myopathies offers possibilities for devising specific therapies for these disorders, while gene therapy may prove feasible in the future for some members of the group.**

A list of standard abbreviations is located immediately preceding the index in each volume. Additional abbreviations used in this chapter include: Clc-1 = chloride ion channel; FSHD = facioscapulohumeral muscular dystrophy.

The autosomal muscular dystrophies are responsible for a considerable proportion of chronic neuromuscular disease, particularly in adult life. Myotonic dystrophy, the most frequent member of the group and the only one so far understood in molecular terms, is the commonest adult muscular dystrophy and in its congenital form is often fatal;

Table 141-1 The Principal Autosomal Muscular Dystrophies

Disorder	Inheritance
Myotonic dystrophy	Autosomal dominant
Facioscapulohumeral muscular dystrophy	Autosomal dominant
Limb-girdle syndromes	
"Duchenne-like" autosomal dystrophy	Autosomal recessive
Autosomal recessive (Erb-type) limb-girdle dystrophy	Autosomal recessive
Benign dominant type	Autosomal dominant
Oculopharyngeal muscular dystrophy	Autosomal dominant
Distal myopathies	
Welander type	Autosomal dominant

facioscapulohumeral dystrophy, while often benign, may also be seriously disabling in some patients. Rarer members of the group may also occur at high frequency in specific populations. Table 141-1 summarizes the principal autosomal muscular dystrophies; it should be recognized that the precise classification and relationship of some of the rarer forms should be regarded as provisional.

Despite extensive research on the biochemistry, physiology, and histology of the various muscular dystrophies, no primary defect has been identified in any of the group through these approaches prior to cloning of the gene involved, nor have any less specific clues has been obtained to suggest what type of molecular defect might be responsible. Fortunately, the advent of gene mapping and positional cloning techniques, pioneered in research on the X-linked disease Duchenne muscular dystrophy, has radically altered the prospect for identifying the molecular basis of the autosomal dystrophies and has already resulted in the identification of the gene and the molecular defect in one of them, myotonic dystrophy. The Mendelian inheritance shown by all of the muscular dystrophies, with the rapid progress in construction of an overall human gene map, means that corresponding success for the other autosomal muscular dystrophies can be envisaged in the relatively near future. In the previous edition of this book, it was predicted that the focus of research would return to the nature of the protein defects as the individual genes responsible for the muscular dystrophies became more defined. This has already been strikingly born out for the X-linked muscular dystrophies (see Chap. 140); the process is now beginning for myotonic dystrophy and will undoubtedly ensue for the other forms as the genes involved are identified.

MYOTONIC DYSTROPHY

The first of the myotonic disorders to be recognized, by Thomsen in 1876,[1] was not myotonic dystrophy but the nonprogressive disease myotonia congenita; it was not until 1908 that Steinert[2] and Batten and Gibb[3] described a progressive neuromuscular disorder characterized by myotonia, thereby delineating myotonic dystrophy (dystrophia myotonica, Steinert's disease) as a specific entity. It soon became clear that myotonic dystrophy could be recognized by its specific pattern of predominant muscle involvement, especially of the face, jaw, anterior neck, and distal limb muscles, as well as by the involvement of other systems. Cataract was found to be associated as early as 1912,[4] while the regular occurrence of endocrine and central nervous system changes, as well as of smooth and cardiac muscle involvement, distinguished the condition from all other myotonic disorders, as well as from the other progressive muscular dystrophies. The early clinical studies and research on myotonic dystrophy are outlined in the author's monograph on the disorder,[5] which also gives a more detailed account of the major clinical features than is possible here. The review by Harper and Rüdel[6] discusses details of the neuromuscular aspects, in particular the physiological basis of myotonia. Table 141-2 summarizes the principal myotonic disorders; recent molecular developments in the nonprogressive myotonias are mentioned briefly in the section "Nonprogressive Myotonic Disorders" below.

Clinical Features

Myotonic dystrophy is one of the most variable disorders known, and it has presenting features that are often nonneurologic. The condition must be considered in a framework much broader than that of the other muscular dystrophies. Nevertheless, the commonest symptoms are neuromuscular, principally relating to muscle weakness and myotonia (delayed muscular relaxation; see below), the latter being most commonly interpreted as stiffness. Table 141-3 shows the most frequent presenting symptoms, while Table 141-4 gives the predominant muscle distribution. It can be seen that the muscles involved contrast strikingly with those involved in the X-linked Duchenne and Becker dystrophies, the only autosomal dystrophy with a somewhat similar pattern of muscle group involvement being facioscapulohumeral dystrophy. The mainly distal limb involvement can cause confusion with neuropathic conditions such as Charcot-Marie-

Table 141-2 The Inherited Myotonic Disorders

Disorder	Inheritance
Myotonic dystrophy	Autosomal dominant
Myotonia congenita	
Thomsen's disease	Autosomal dominant
Recessive generalized myotonia	Autosomal recessive
Paramyotonia congenita	Autosomal dominant
Periodic paralysis	
Hypokalemic	Autosomal dominant
Normo-hyperkalemic (adynamia episodica)	Autosomal dominant
Chrondrodystrophic myotonia (Schwartz-Jampel syndrome)	Autosomal recessive

Table 141-3 Presenting Symptoms in Myotonic Dystrophy*

Symptom	Percent of Patients
Muscle weakness	35
Myotonia	21
Asymptomatic (family study)	18
Mental retardation	12
Cataract	5
Neonatal problems	3
Other	5

*Data on 170 patients. From Harper.[5]

Table 141-4 Muscular Involvement in Myotonic Dystrophy

Muscles most prominently affected
Superficial facial muscles
Levator palpebrae superioris
Temporalis
Sternocleidomastoids
Distal muscles of forearm
Dorsiflexors of foot
Other muscles commonly affected
Quadriceps
Diaphragm and intercostals
Intrinsic muscles of hands and feet
Palate and pharyngeal muscles
Tongue
External ocular muscles
Muscles frequently spared
Pelvic girdle
Hamstrings
Soleus and gastrocnemius

Tooth disease, but the recognition of myotonia allows a specific clinical diagnosis of myotonic dystrophy to be made immediately. Involvement of facial and jaw muscles is almost invariable in myotonic dystrophy; ptosis can be marked, while selective weakness and wasting of sternomastoid muscles is seen in the neck. Figure 141-1 illustrates some of these features.

Myotonia can most readily be recognized by direct percussion of the muscles (in particular the thenar eminence) or by testing for rapid relaxation (especially of grip or, less commonly, eye closure). While most patients complain of stiffness in relation to their myotonia, this is frequently not mentioned unless directly inquired about. Some patients seem genuinely unaware that their myotonia is abnormal, while others may deliberately minimize their symptoms. The end result is that diagnosis is delayed in many patients, even when myotonia is obvious if actually sought.

Table 141-5 Smooth and Cardiac Muscle Involvement in Myotonic Dystrophy

Gastrointestinal tract	Widespread involvement, particularly of pharynx and esophagus
Gallbladder	Delayed emptying; high incidence of stones
Urinary bladder	Probably unaffected
Ureter	Isolated instances of dilatation
Uterus	Uncoordinated contraction in labor and in vitro
Eye	Ciliary body affected; low intraocular tension
Heart	Conduction defects, in particular heart block, atrial arrhythmias; less commonly, cardiomyopathy

The extramuscular features of myotonic dystrophy are of special importance, both in the diagnosis of relatives at risk and in terms of prognosis and management of the affected individual. Some of these can be related to smooth or cardiac muscle dysfunction (Table 141-5), while others involve entirely different systems (Table 141-6). Smooth muscle involvement may show itself in a variety of ways, but esophageal dysfunction may result in dysphagia and in bronchial aspiration causing pneumonia, while abdominal pain from colonic involvement may result in unnecessary and hazardous surgery. Among other systemic abnormalities are cataracts, characterized by highly distinctive multicolored subcortical lens opacities when viewed with the slit lamp; a variety of endocrine changes, of which testicular tubular atrophy in males is most prominent; and various degrees of central nervous system involvement, ranging from increased somnolence, apathy, and mild personality deterioration in some adults to severe mental retardation in

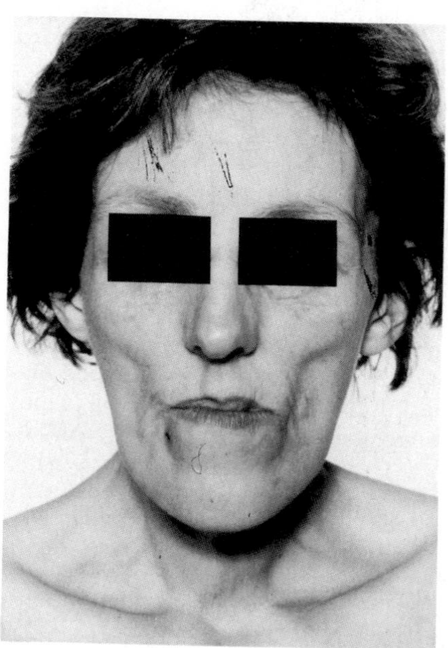

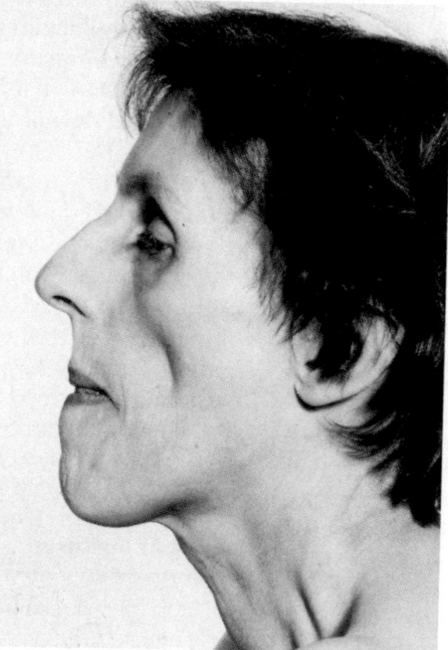

A.

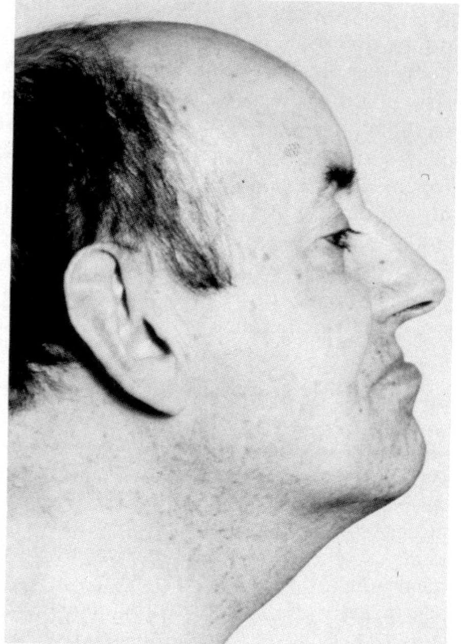

B.

FIG. 141-1 Myotonic dystrophy in adults showing *(A)* facial and jaw weakness and wasting of sternomastoid muscles and *(B)* ptosis and marked balding.

Table 141-6 Other Systems Involved in Myotonic Dystrophy

System	Symptom
Eye	Cataract, retinal degeneration, ocular hypotonia, ptosis, extraocular weakness
Endocrine	Testicular tubular atrophy; diabetes (rarely clinically significant); sometimes abnormalities of growth hormone and other pituitary functions
Brain	Severe involvement in congenital form; mild mental deterioration frequent in adults; hypersomnia
Peripheral nerves	Variable and rarely clinically significant; minor sensory loss may occur
Skeletal	Cranial hyperostosis, air sinus enlargement; jaw and palate involvement; talipes (childhood cases); scoliosis (uncommon)
Skin	Premature balding; calcifying epithelioma
Lungs	Aspiration pneumonia from esophageal and diaphragmatic involvement; hypoventilation

a proportion of congenitally affected patients. Some patients presenting with these systemic features (notably cataract) may have only minimal or occasionally no detectable muscle abnormality, even on careful investigation.

Diagnostic tests in myotonic dystrophy are summarized in Table 141-7. It should be emphasized that these are not always necessary in patients with clear-cut clinical features, while no single test apart from that for the mutation can be considered pathognomonic. However, the combined use of these tests, together with a careful clinical study of family members, will allow most diagnostic problems to be solved.[7,8] Of particular note is the ophthalmologic assessment, especially before established cataract has developed, because lens changes (as mentioned above) are characteristic, and associated retinal changes may also be found.[9]

Electromyography will confirm the presence of the myotonia and is of particular importance in distinguishing other syndromes with muscle stiffness, including various familial cramping disorders (generally electrically silent) and disorders of presynaptic origin (generally showing persistent electrical activity at rest). While the presence of myotonia will not distinguish myotonic dystrophy from other myotonic disorders such as myotonia congenita, the finding of myotonia together with "dystrophic" changes, such as diminished action potential amplitude and the presence of polyphasic potentials, in the context of a progressive neuromuscular disorder, is suggestive of myotonic dystrophy.

Further clinical investigations—such as electrocardiography, a glucose tolerance test and other endocrine studies,

Table 141-7 Diagnostic Tests Used for Myotonic Dystrophy

Test	Finding in Myotonic Dystrophy
Electromyography	Myotonic potentials
Slit-lamp examination	Multicolored lens opacities
Muscle biopsy	Internal nuclei, other specific changes
Glucose and insulin tolerance tests	Impaired glucose tolerance; hyperinsulinism
Electrocardiogram	Conduction defects; prolonged PR interval
DNA analysis	Expansion of specific unstable sequence

and gastrointestinal radiology—are all frequently helpful in management but are less definitive in the diagnosis of myotonic dystrophy. The most important clinical diagnostic aid remains awareness of the disorder and of its variable and often unexpected presentations.

Now that the specific molecular defect in myotonic dystrophy is known, DNA analysis for the expanded unstable sequence (described in detail below) is important as a diagnostic test for the disorder as well as for prediction in a family. The correlation between DNA expansion and severity may also prove helpful as an approximate guide to prognosis, while failure to find the abnormality should lead to reassessment of the diagnosis, although molecular heterogeneity of the disorder in occasional cases remains a possibility.

In the clinical management of myotonic dystrophy patients, two areas, the cardiorespiratory problems and the smooth muscle involvement, are of special importance. Cardiac arrhythmias are the main cause of death in this disorder, and they range from episodic or persistent atrial fibrillation and flutter through different degrees of heart block to sudden death.[10] Serious cardiac conduction defects may occur in patients with relatively mild physical disability, and regular electrocardiographic (EKG) monitoring should be undertaken, with more detailed cardiologic studies if abnormalities are noted.[11,12] Surgery and anesthesia pose a particular hazard, as there may be anesthetic sensitivity and postoperative respiratory muscle inadequacy as well as arrhythmia problems.[13] Surgeons and anesthetists should always be aware of the risks, while patients are advised to carry a bracelet or warning card.

Congenital Myotonic Dystrophy

Congenital myotonic dystrophy was first recognized by Vanier in 1960,[14] and it has since become clear that it is a distinctive, frequently fatal, and far from rare form of myotonic dystrophy.[15] It is seen only in offspring of women who are themselves affected with myotonic dystrophy.[16,17] These mothers are often only mildly affected but almost invariably show some neuromuscular abnormalities.[18] The relationship between the congenital and the commoner adult-onset form of the disease is still not fully understood, although molecular analysis is now providing evidence on this topic, as discussed later in the chapter.

Table 141-8 lists the main characteristics of congenital myotonic dystrophy; the features at different ages are shown in Fig. 141-2. The facial appearance is highly distinctive, largely owing to the combination of bilateral facial palsy with marked jaw weakness. The early, often intrauterine onset of muscle weakness helps to mold the facial features by creating the characteristic tented upper lip. Decreased intrauterine muscle action plays a role in many of the other features, such as the high incidence of respiratory inadequacy and pulmonary hypoplasia (caused by underdeveloped diaphragm and intercostal muscles), the occurrence of talipes and other joint contractures, the development of polyhydram-

Table 141-8 Congenital Myotonic Dystrophy: Major Clinical Features

Bilateral facial weakness	Feeding difficulties
Hypotonia	Talipes
Delayed motor development	Hydramnios in later pregnancy
Mental retardation	Reduced fetal movements
Neonatal respiratory distress	

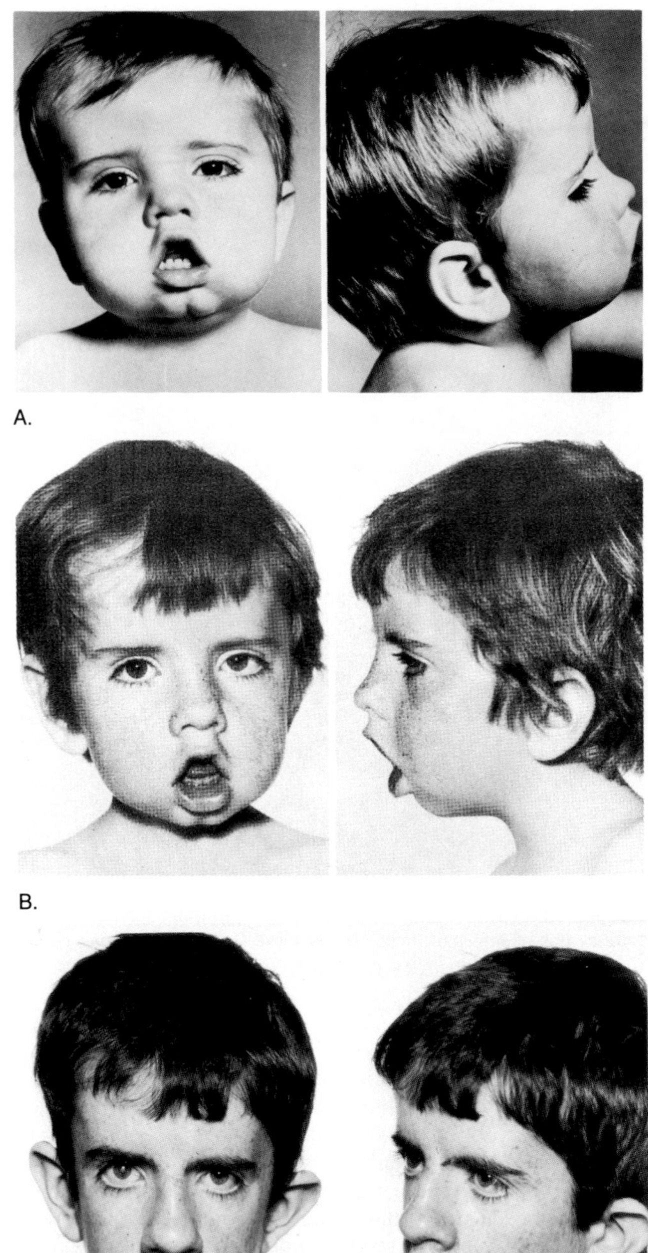

FIG. 141-2 Congenital myotonic dystrophy, showing facial features in same patient at different ages. *A*. Age 2 years. *B*. Age 6 years. *C*. Age 12 years. Note facial diplegia, tented upper lip, and open mouth caused by jaw muscle weakness.

nios (owing to lack of intrauterine swallowing), and the generally poor fetal movements. By contrast to the adult disorder, myotonia is inconspicuous or absent in affected infants, though it becomes more prominent as affected individuals reach later childhood.

The differential diagnosis of congenital myotonic dystrophy in the neonate relates not so much to other muscular dystrophies as to the broader group of congenital myopathies. These are not discussed in detail in this chapter but are listed in Table 141-9. Many patients die rapidly from respiratory

Table 141-9 Congenital Myopathies

Disorder	Inheritance
Central core disease	Autosomal dominant
Nemaline myopathy	Autosomal recessive; severe congenital form
	Autosomal dominant; milder form
Congenital myotubular (centronuclear) myopathy	X-linked recessive lethal form
	Autosomal recessive
Congenital fiber-type disproportion	Autosomal recessive; probably heterogenous
Fingerprint body myopathy	Uncertain
Multicore myopathy	Autosomal dominant?

inadequacy before the diagnosis can be made, but with the increasing success of neonatal intensive care, a higher proportion survive to be diagnosed. The relationship to adult myotonic dystrophy is important to recognize, since the discovery of a typical adult case in the family, usually the mother or another maternal relative, will confirm the diagnosis in the infant. X-linked myotubular myopathy is particularly likely to be confused with congenital myotonic dystrophy on the grounds of both clinical appearance and muscle pathology.[19] It is particularly important for all women with myotonic dystrophy who are considering child-bearing to understand the risk of the severe congenital form.

Molecular analysis, described in detail later, is proving particularly helpful in the diagnosis of congenital myotonic dystrophy, since affected individuals show a large expansion (3 to 6 kb) of the unstable DNA sequence, which should be readily recognizable. Absence of this specific abnormality would strongly suggest that another form of congenital myopathy is the cause of the problem. Detection of the molecular defect also now can be used for specific prenatal diagnosis.

Muscle Pathology

Detailed studies of muscle histology, histochemistry, and electron microscopy have given a clear picture of the changes that occur in myotonic dystrophy.[6,20] These changes are distinctive, though not totally specific. Figure 141-3 shows some of the more characteristic changes, notably increased internal nuclei, often in chains, together with ringed fibers and sarcoplasmic masses. Histochemistry shows a relative loss of type 1 fibers, while electron-microscopic changes include degeneration of microfilaments and proliferation of the sarcotubular system. More important from the viewpoint of pathogenesis are the negative ultrastructural findings, in particular absence of marked change in small blood vessels and nerve endings, showing that the muscle fiber itself is the principal site of the pathology.

Study of muscle from patients with congenital myotonic dystrophy shows several changes not present in adult patients.[21] The muscles are hypoplastic and the fibers have an immature appearance, with centrally placed nuclei and abundant satellite cells, suggesting arrested development rather than degeneration,[22] an important distinguishing feature from X-linked myotubular myopathy.[19] Histochemical studies show a peripheral area deficient in mitochondrial enzymes.[23]

Detailed reassessment of the muscle pathology will soon be possible in the light of the specific defect. As has already

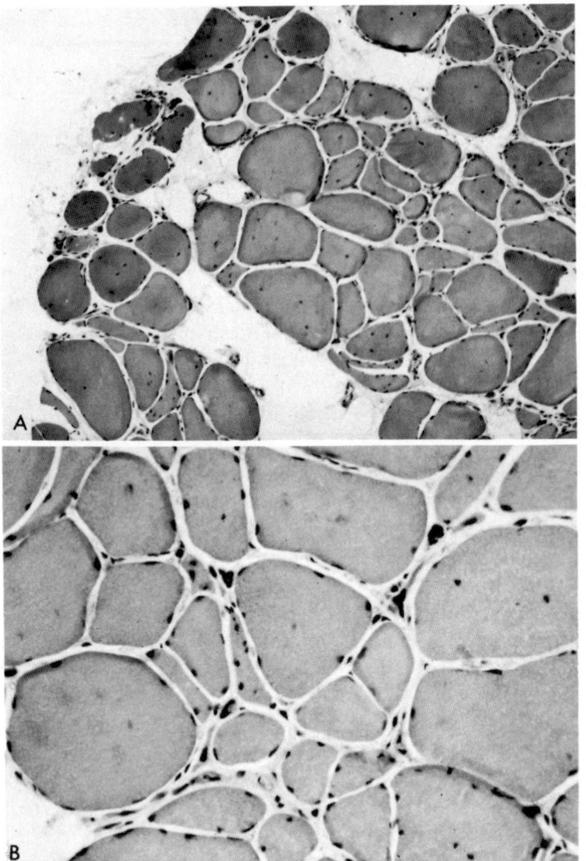

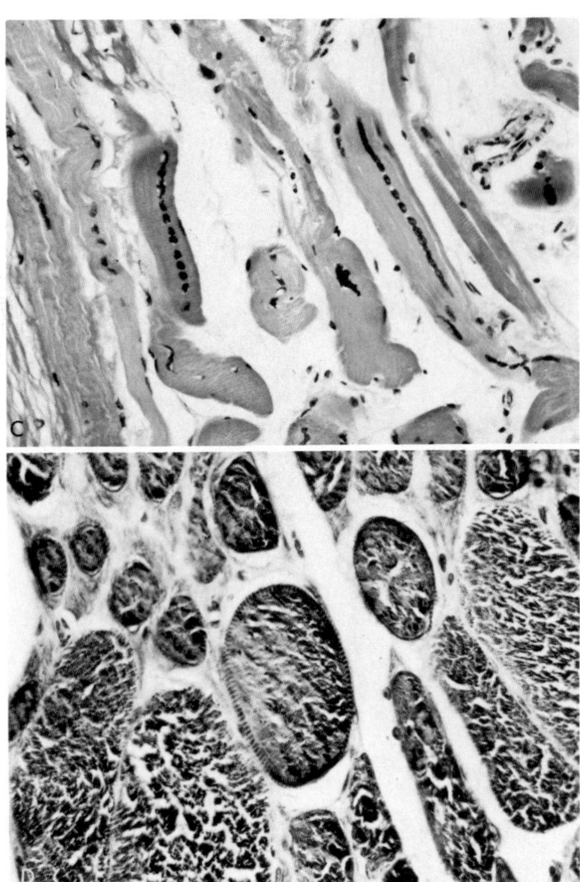

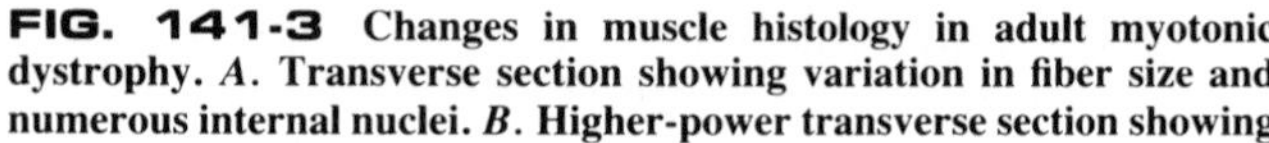

FIG. 141-3 Changes in muscle histology in adult myotonic dystrophy. *A*. Transverse section showing variation in fiber size and numerous internal nuclei. *B*. Higher-power transverse section showing atrophic fibers with clumped nuclei. *C*. Longitudinal section showing long chains of internal nuclei. *D*. Transverse section showing ringed fibers. *(From Harper.[5] Used by permission.)*

happened with Duchenne muscular dystrophy, it should be possible to study in detail the subcellular distribution of the protein (predicted to be a protein kinase) in the muscle and how this is disturbed in affected patients. Meanwhile, it is important to remember that material from a previous muscle biopsy may allow a specific diagnosis of myotonic dystrophy to be made or excluded retrospectively.

Myotonia and Disordered Physiology in Myotonic Dystrophy

The molecular basis of myotonia is considered later in relation to the nonprogressive myotonic disorders, since the great majority of the experimental work on this subject relates to those disorders in both humans and other species. Whereas there is now considerable evidence relating these types of myotonia to the dysfunction of specific muscle ion channels, notably those for sodium and chloride, the evidence for a clearly defined physiological basis for myotonia in myotonic dystrophy is much less satisfactory, with different and in some cases contradictory findings in different studies. It is likely that many of these problems will be resolved in the light of our new understanding of the molecular basis of myotonic dystrophy, but the existing evidence relating specifically to myotonic dystrophy is summarized below. A more detailed account is given by Harper and Rüdel.[6]

The initial studies of myotonic dystrophy muscle in vitro showed a reduced resting potential across the muscle cell membrane with a raised level of intracellular sodium, but a subsequent study by Lipicky[24] found the opposite, the resting potential being high and the intracellular sodium level low. A recent and more detailed study by Franke et al.[25] provides some resolution of these findings, since a reduction in resting potential was seen mainly in patients with dystrophic changes, not in those in whom myotonia was the main feature. This suggests that any change in resting membrane potential in myotonic dystrophy may be secondary to damage of muscle fibers.

Reduced chloride conductance is the principal feature of human myotonia congenita and its counterparts in the goat and mouse, a finding that led to the hypothesis, now confirmed, that a chloride channel defect is responsible for this form of myotonia. In myotonic dystrophy the results have been much less clear: Lipicky found levels varying from low to normal,[24] whereas Franke et al.,[25] using resealed muscle fiber segments, found a high level in one patient with marked myotonia and normal and low levels in others. This result clearly suggests that a chloride channel defect is not the primary mechanism. Franke et al. also showed an abnormality of sodium channel function using a patch-clamp technique.

Studies of cultured muscle have also given conflicting results in myotonic dystrophy. Merickel et al.[26] found both a reduced resting potential in cultured myotonic dystrophy fibers and a decreased after-hyperpolarization, suggesting the possibility of a primary defect in potassium conductance. These findings were not confirmed by others.[27] An interesting finding of Renaud et al.,[28] not so far confirmed, was that the potassium channel affected by the bee venom apamin was present in myotonic dystrophy fibers, in contrast to normal adult muscle and muscle in other neuromuscular disorders. While this result could relate to the immaturity of myotonic dystrophy muscle as noted by pathology studies, it could also suggest a disturbance of potassium conductance.

The results of physiological studies on myotonic dystrophy thus remain confusing, in contrast to the clear-cut results of studies on the nonprogressive myotonias, which pointed to definite and specific ion channel defects, and which led directly to the candidate gene studies that have confirmed the molecular basis of these disorders. However, in light of what we now know about the molecular basis of myotonic dystrophy, these apparently confusing findings are perhaps not so surprising. As yet we have no direct evidence on the function and spatial distribution of the myotonic dystrophy protein kinase, but it would not be surprising if an abnormality or deficiency in this protein might affect to various degrees the function of different ion channels in the muscle membrane and, thus, be responsible for the multiple and somewhat inconsistent abnormalities found so far by physiological studies. Direct experimental verification of this hypothesis will soon be possible, and it may be of considerable relevance to future therapeutic approaches in myotonic dystrophy.

Genetics of Myotonic Dystrophy

From the earliest reports, myotonic dystrophy was noted to follow an autosomal dominant pattern of inheritance, a fact confirmed by formal analysis in the studies of Bell[29] and Thomasen.[30] However, even at this early stage, unusual features were noted, such as extreme variation within a family and the phenomenon of "anticipation," discussed below. Details of the genetics of myotonic dystrophy are given in the author's monograph[5]; here those aspects most relevant to the molecular basis are noted.

Heterogeneity. No evidence has ever been found to suggest modes of inheritance other than autosomal dominant, in contrast to the situation with myotonia congenita, which has both dominant and recessive forms, nor has increased consanguinity been noted, even in areas with a particularly high incidence. Although clinical variability is extreme, the fact that this variability occurs within families has always suggested that it is not a result of genetic heterogeneity, and the possibility of genetic heterogeneity has been essentially ruled out by the fact that abundant genetic linkage data have failed to produce a single family in which the disease is not linked to chromosome 19 markers. The homogeneity of the disorder in mutational terms has now been shown, with no reported case so far resulting from a defect other than the specific unstable trinucleotide repeat.

Penetrance of the Gene. Although minimal manifestation or nonpenetrance of the gene is frequent in the "top generation" of a pedigree, skipped generations are virtually unknown, suggesting that the gene is almost fully penetrant in the adult offspring of an affected person if these individuals are examined carefully. Segregation analysis has also suggested that close to the expected 50 percent of offspring of an affected individual are affected.[8,31]

The apparent discrepancies between generations can now be explained by the expansion of the unstable DNA sequence as described later. It is clear that the proportion of clinically normal individuals carrying the mutation will vary according to their generational position within a family; the figure is likely to be low in sibships where there are congenitally affected individuals, but considerably higher in the sibs of those mildly affected; precise figures should soon emerge from molecular studies in progress.

Mutation Rate. Most older studies have agreed in finding a very low mutation rate for myotonic dystrophy,[5] but precise estimates have been hampered by the difficulty of proving that a particular case results from a new mutation, rather than having been inherited from a minimally affected parent. The recognition that an essentially harmless initial mutation precedes full disease in a family explains this situation, while the evidence from haplotype studies and linkage disequilibrium suggests that all the known cases of myotonic dystrophy from a wide geographical area, including Europe, Israel, and Japan, share a common haplotype.[32–34] Further recent molecular studies, discussed in the section "Gene Mapping" below, support the possibility that the original mutation was a unique event.

Fertility. The fertility of patients varies from essentially normal in minimally affected gene transmitters to nearly zero in patients with congenital disease, making an overall estimate difficult. A moderate reduction in fertility in both sexes has been shown in classic cases,[35] so an inescapable conclusion is that the abnormal gene must be being steadily lost from the population. This being so, it is difficult to understand why the gene persists at high frequency, even allowing for the likelihood that asymptomatic carriers of the premutation are much commoner than currently recognized. It is likely that minimal gene carriers might have some selective advantage, but that would be difficult to prove. It is also possible that the initial mutation may have become widespread before instability resulted in gene loss from clinically severe disease.

Homozygosity. The recognition of homozygosity for the myotonic dystrophy gene could have considerable importance for understanding the mode of action of the gene, but this has not been conclusively demonstrated. In one possible case,[5] where severely affected offspring were born to parents who were both affected, molecular analysis has shown that the offspring are not homozygous for the mutation. A definite homozygote for a small DNA expansion has now been documented by molecular studies,[36] and it is of interest that this individual is entirely asymptomatic.

Prevalence. The frequency of clinically obvious myotonic dystrophy in different populations varies considerably, prevalence estimates ranging from 2 to over 100 per 100,000,[5] with an average incidence around 1 in 7000 to 8000 births for most European populations.[37,38] Especially high frequencies are seen in some isolated regions that have undergone recent population expansion, notably the Saguenay region of northeastern Quebec, where all cases can be traced back to a single ancestor.[39] None of the published prevalence estimates include the asymptomatic carriers; now that molecular detection of these carriers is possible, the heterozygote and gene frequencies may prove to be considerably higher than expected on the basis of studies of clinically affected cases.

Anticipation. The progressively earlier onset of a disorder in successive generations, usually accompanied by increasing severity (Fig. 141-4), is a phenomenon that has been noted in myotonic dystrophy since the early work of Fleischer[40]

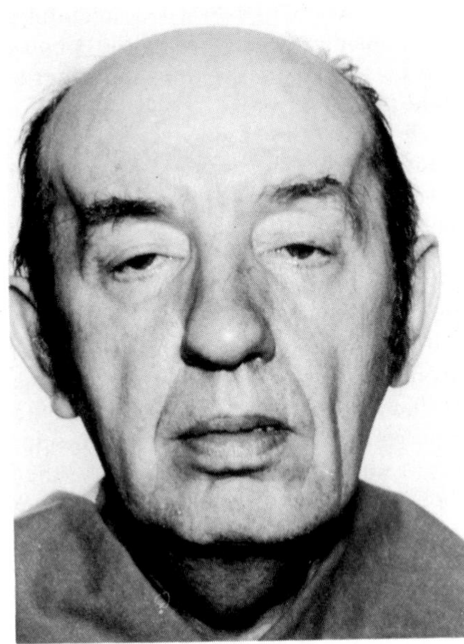

A

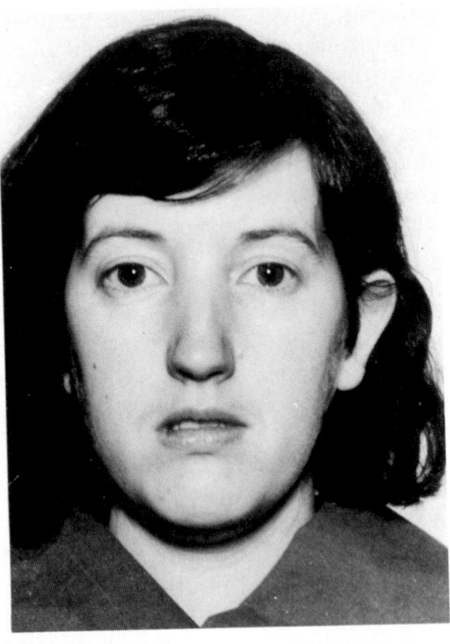

B

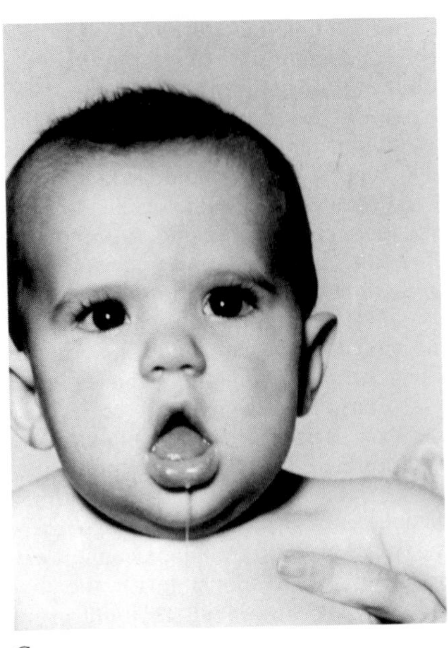

C

FIG. 141-4 Anticipation and myotonic dystrophy. Clinical features in a three-generation family, showing the increased severity in successive generations. *A*. Grandfather (age 57). Cataracts removed at age 48. Symptoms of myotonia since age 50, but no significant disability. Ptosis, facial weakness, and myotonia on examination. Myotonic dystrophy not diagnosed until birth of affected grandson. *B*. Mother (age 24). Myotonia since late teens; weakness of face and neck present on examination, together with marked myotonia. Only diagnosed after birth of affected son (right). No cataract. *C*. Son. Congenital myotonic dystrophy. Hydramnios during pregnancy; respiratory distress at birth necessitating ventilation. Subsequent improvement, but motor and mental development remains delayed. Marked facial and jaw weakness with hypotonia.

in 1918, who found that apparently separate families could be linked through individuals with cataract alone. Over the decades there has been much debate as to whether anticipation represented a real biological change in the gene and phenotype,[29,41] or whether it could be explained on the basis of ascertainment biases together with the great natural variability of the disorder.[42] The studies of Höweler[31,43] convincingly demonstrated that the phenomenon was indeed real, but its explanation only emerged with the recent identification of the myotonic dystrophy mutation and gene—the progressive expansion in the unstable DNA sequence over successive generations provides a satisfactory basis for the clinical observation of anticipation within families.

The factors that determine the expansion of the unstable sequence in myotonic dystrophy remain to be determined, as do the relative roles of meiotic and somatic instability in relation to phenotype, but it is becoming clear that unstable DNA sequences may be of general significance in producing variation in a number of genetic disorders; anticipation may be a valuable clue to the existence of this type of mutational change.[44,45]

Sex-Related Effects. Although myotonic dystrophy affects both sexes and is transmitted equally by males and females overall, there is a hidden but a very real difference relating to the congenital form of the disease discussed above. It has been recognized for many years that this form is not only clinically very different from the disease in adult life but, also, is exclusively transmitted by affected females, even though these mothers are often not severely affected themselves. Various hypotheses have been suggested for this, including a possible intrauterine effect[16,46] and the involvement of genetic imprinting,[47] but no firm evidence has yet been produced for either possibility. Molecular analysis, described later in detail, has now shown that congenital cases show a large expansion of the unstable sequence in the gene, but this does not fully explain why they should occur exclusively in the offspring of affected mothers. One aspect that is likely to be relevant is that congenitally affected children are rarely born to women without neuromuscular abnormalities,[18] suggesting that the unstable sequence does not normally progress from minimal to large expansion in a single generation.

A further sex-related effect, present but not always recognized in older studies, is an excess of males among the minimally affected "top generation,"[48] most of whom are discovered because they have more severely affected children or grandchildren. This bias may mean that there is a preferential tendency for initial DNA instability and expansion of the mutation during male meiosis.

Gene Mapping

The progress in mapping the myotonic dystrophy gene up to the year 1986 was fully reviewed in the previous edition of this text, and only work since that time is discussed in detail here. It should be emphasized, however, that the steady if unspectacular progress of this earlier work was essential for the eventual isolation of the gene, making possible the specific molecular analysis of the disorder that is described later in this chapter.

Early studies of genetic linkage, undertaken well before the advent of DNA markers, had established a firm linkage with the secretor and Lutheran blood group loci,[49,50] the C3 complement locus later being added to this linkage group. However, at that stage the chromosomal localization of these genes was unknown, and the existence of linkage offered no obvious prospect of isolating the myotonic dystrophy gene itself. This situation changed in 1982 and 1983, when the C3 gene was located by somatic cell hybrid studies to chromosome 19,[51] allowing a more focused analysis to begin. The year 1982 also saw the first use of DNA polymorphisms in the detection of genetic linkage, with the Duchenne muscular dystrophy locus linked to a DNA marker on Xp[52]; myotonic dystrophy, as an autosomal dominant disorder with a known chromosomal location, was an appropriate target for applying the new molecular techniques for gene isolation, a challenge taken up by several groups, including that of the author and his colleagues.[53,54]

That this task took 9 years should not be seen as evidence of lack of research or funding or as indicating an inappropriate strategy; rather, there were two major factors that limited the rate of advance. The first of these was the complete lack of chromosomal rearrangements that might have given a specific location and also allowed direct molecular analysis; in contrast to the case with disorders such as Duchenne muscular dystrophy[55] and neurofibromatosis,[56] the isolation of the myotonic dystrophy gene was totally the result of the positional cloning approach. At the time of the discovery it represented only the second human disease gene isolated in this way, cystic fibrosis being the first. The second relevant factor was the limitation posed by the technology available at the time of the study; were the search initiated now, success would undoubtedly come more rapidly.

The mapping and eventual isolation of the gene provides a remarkable example of how the various techniques of molecular genetics were used in succession as they became available, each making an important contribution.

The initial resources were restriction fragment length polymorphisms (RFLPs) based on libraries of genomic DNA from a variety of relatively chromosome-specific sources,[57] together with specific genes located in the relevant region.[58] Human–rodent hybrid cell lines were also valuable from an early stage and became increasingly specific,[59,60] especially when the technique of radiation mapping was evolved.[61] The introduction of pulsed field gel electrophoresis allowed a detailed physical map to be developed,[54,62] which was further refined by the use of yeast artificial chromosomes (YACs).[63] Thus, by 1989 a relatively detailed physical and genetic map of chromosome 19 was available,[62,64] but the precise location of the myotonic dystrophy gene on this framework was still far from clear. Figure 141-5 shows the chromosome 19 map at different levels of resolution in relation to myotonic dystrophy.

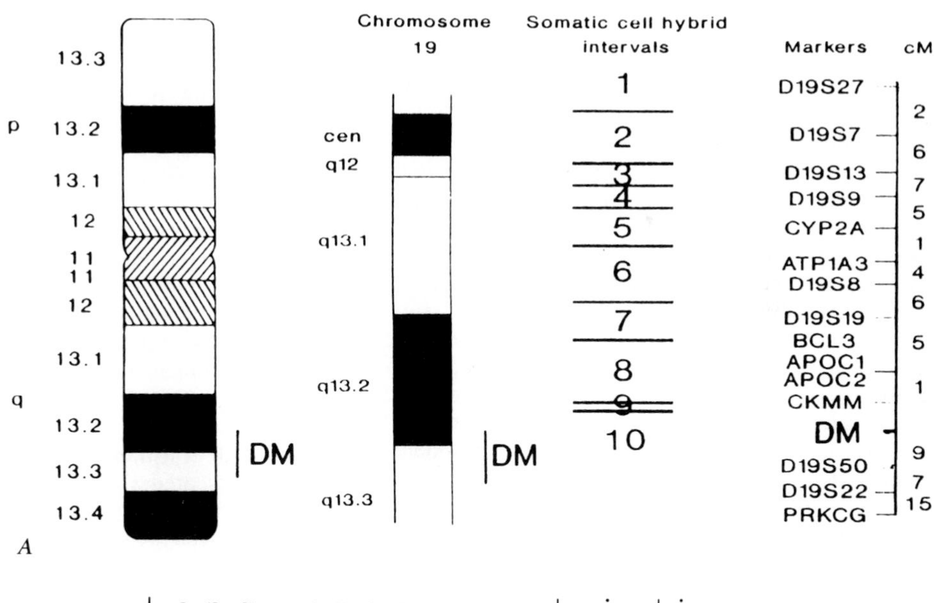

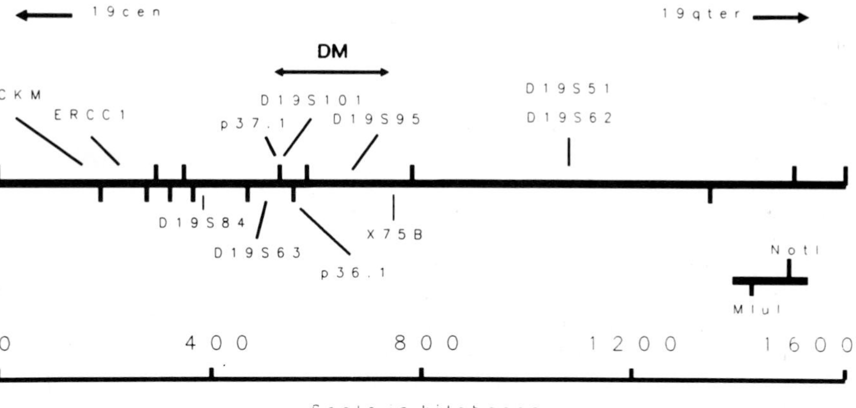

FIG. 141-5 *A*. **Mapping of the myotonic dystrophy gene locus. Diagram of chromosome 19, showing the myotonic dystrophy region of 19q in relation to principal markers.** ***B***. **Detailed long-range restriction map of the myotonic dystrophy chromosomal region.** ***(Both maps courtesy of Drs. Helen Harley and Duncan Shaw, Cardiff, Wales.)***

Although the relatively close linkage of myotonic dystrophy with the APOC2 locus had been demonstrated in 1985,[58] the exact relationship of the myotonic dystrophy gene to this and other linked markers on 19q was difficult to establish owing to the relative lack of recombination between myotonic dystrophy and these loci. The uncertainty was increased by the dependence of some of these rare events on clinical assessments of older, minimally affected patients, an area in which even experienced clinicians may be far from confident. It also became clear during this period that all the available close markers were proximal on the chromosome to myotonic dystrophy,[65] leaving a distal region of undetermined size, with the flanking markers too distant to be of much help.

One significant advance that had been achieved at this point was the exclusion of significant multilocus heterogeneity for myotonic dystrophy. Despite the analysis of many hundreds of families, no evidence of nonlinkage to chromosome 19q markers has ever been detected, a finding of practical as well as theoretical importance.

Among the closely linked markers were some that could reasonably be considered as candidate genes for the disorder. The locus for muscle-specific creatine kinase (CKM) proved to be one of the most closely linked but was excluded by the finding of recombination and the lack of specific abnormality in myotonic dystrophy patients.[66] The gene for a sodium-potassium ATPase subunit (ATP1A3) was also a relevant candidate, given the chance that a defect in ion transport was responsible for myotonia[67]; this gene was also excluded by the discovery of recombination.[68] A third gene on 19q deserving mention, though not seriously considered as a candidate, was that for the ryanodine receptor, now a likely candidate gene for some cases of hyperpyrexic myopathy (see Chap. 4). Thus, for myotonic dystrophy, the only available candidate genes proved not to be relevant, though the rapidity of their exclusion illustrates what an effective approach this can be.

At that point, the separate approach of searching for linkage disequilibrium (allelic association) became of considerable value, particularly since it does not depend on rare and easily misinterpreted recombination events. Study of the first markers to show close linkage only demonstrated linkage disequilibrium in isolated populations, such of that of Quebec,[69] known to descend from a common ancestor; more varied samples showed no such disequilibrium.[58] It was only when a new series of polymorphisms, isolated from a radiation-induced hybrid cell line,[70] was tested that striking disequilibrium was found with one of them (D10), the myotonic dystrophy gene being associated with an allele that was relatively rare in the general population.[32] This work also suggested that at least two thirds of cases from a widely scattered geographic area, including Europe, Israel, and Japan, were the result of a single mutation.

The disequilibrium data strongly suggested that the gene was located in a restricted region of around 200 kb. This region was also suggested by individual recombinants, and the combined evidence prompted a detailed molecular analysis of this entire length of DNA. By mid-1991, this region had essentially been cloned,[71] and the problem was how to identify the myotonic dystrophy gene from the considerable number of genes (estimated at 10 to 20) likely to be present in this material.

Linkage disequilibrium played a further role in focusing attention on the correct region when a sequence (D19S190; 59A) was identified that showed almost complete disequilibrium with myotonic dystrophy[33]—74 out of 75 unrelated affected individuals had the same allele, in contrast to 140 out of 232 normal individuals. Since this genomic sequence was strongly conserved, it became an important candidate for the myotonic dystrophy gene.

At that point (November, 1991), the course of the search was radically altered by the finding by two groups that a specific abnormality was present in the DNA of individuals with myotonic dystrophy. The abnormality was seen both in a cDNA sequence[72] and in the genomic sequence 59A described above.[33] Exchange of materials by the two groups showed that both probes were detecting the same change, and that the abnormality, while specific to myotonic dystrophy, appeared to vary among patients, even within the same family. It was immediately recognized that this abnormality was likely to represent expansion of an unstable DNA sequence and that the sequence was probably within the myotonic dystrophy gene itself. The findings were rapidly confirmed by a third group,[73] and the series of papers were published in *Nature* in February, 1992, thus representing the successful conclusion of almost a decade of gene mapping and positional cloning studies since the original localization of the gene to chromosome 19.

An Expanded Trinucleotide Repeat Sequence in Myotonic Dystrophy

Six months prior to the recognition of the unstable sequence in myotonic dystrophy, the molecular basis of the disorder fragile X mental retardation had been found to be the presence of an expanded and unstable sequence in this gene on the X chromosome.[74,75] Detailed analysis of the fragile X expansion showed this sequence to be a CGG repeat. Normal individuals have less than 50 copies of the repeat; clinically normal gene carriers have at least 50 copies; and clinically affected individuals have much larger expansions. The parallels with myotonic dystrophy had already been recognized at a clinical level,[5,44] and the identification of an unstable DNA sequence in the fragile X disorder made it likely that a similar trinucleotide repeat sequence was involved in myotonic dystrophy.

The Unstable DNA Sequence in Myotonic Dystrophy. As indicated above, the unstable sequence was detected independently by a genomic[33] and a cDNA clone,[72] both of which proved to identify the same specific abnormality. Figure 141-6

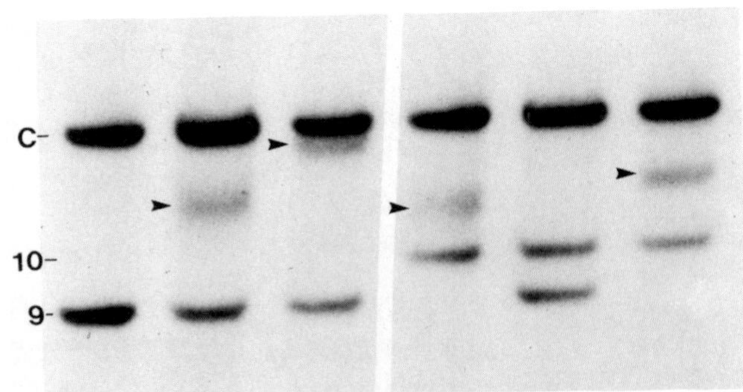

FIG. 141-6 **The unstable DNA sequence in myotonic dystrophy. *Eco*RI-digested genomic DNA probed with pBB07. All individuals have a constant band of 15kb (C). Normal individuals are either homozygous (lane 1) or heterozygous (lane 5) for bands of 9 and 10 kb. Affected individuals (lanes 2, 3, 4, 6) have one of these bands, but also show an additional larger band, whose size varies with the individual. *(Adapted from Harley et al.[33])***

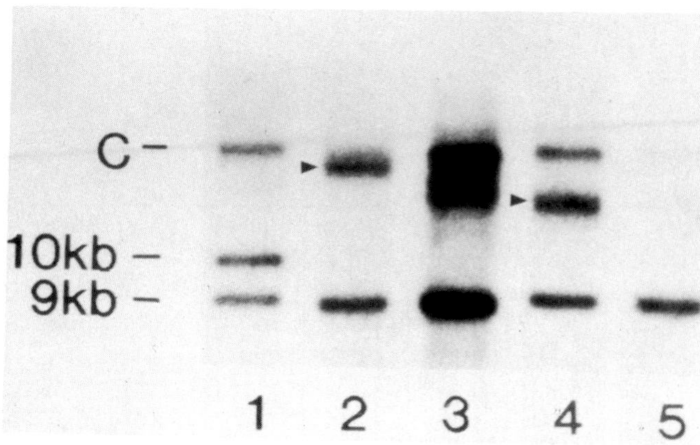

FIG. 141-7 Somatic DNA instability in myotonic dystrophy. Southern blotting with enzyme *Eco*RI (as for Fig. 141-6). Lanes 1 and 5 show blood from normal individuals. Lanes 2 through 4 are from individuals affected with myotonic dystrophy, representing the grandfather (lane 3), mother (lane 4), and son (lane 2) shown in Figure 141-4. Lane 3 illustrates the smearing of the DNA, reflecting a range of fragment sizes likely to be due to somatic instability, and making accurate estimate of band size difficult. *(Based on Harley et al.*[85]*)*

illustrates the band pattern seen for the *Eco*RI polymorphism detected by these sequences in normal and affected individuals. The normal pattern is a two-allele polymorphism with bands of 9 and 10 kb, individuals being[8] either heterozygous (lane 5) or homozygous for one or other band (lane 1). In myotonic dystrophy, one normal allele is seen, but the other (so far, invariably the 10-kb allele) is increased in size to a variable degree.

The degree of increase seen ranges from an extra 150 bp (barely visible by Southern blotting using restriction enzyme *Eco*RI and requiring the use of enzyme *Pst*I or PCR-based analysis of repeat number for accurate detection) to as much as 6 kb additional DNA, as illustrated in Figure 141-6. Most important, this variation is seen within single kindreds, notably between generations, as shown in Figures 141-7, and, particularly, 141-8. It can immediately be appreciated that the expansion of the sequence in successive generations agrees with the clinical observation of anticipation mentioned earlier[41] and discussed in detail below.

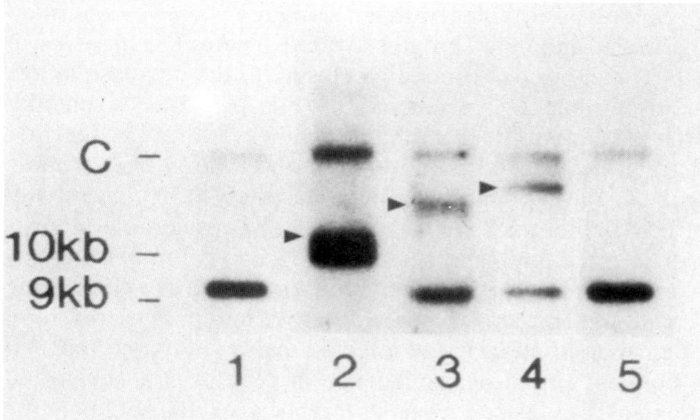

FIG. 141-8 Anticipation and unstable DNA in myotonic dystrophy. DNA samples from a three-generation family with myotonic dystrophy showing minimal DNA expansion in the mildly affected grandmother, lane 2 (CO.5 kb expansion), moderate expansion in the affected mother with adult onset, lane 3 (C2.5 kb), and large expansion in the congenitally affected son, lane 4 (C4 kb). Lanes 1 and 5 are from normal individuals. *(From Harley et al.*[85] *Used by permission.)*

The Myotonic Dystrophy Gene

While the identification of a specific unstable DNA sequence gave a clear explanation of the nature of the mutational defect in myotonic dystrophy and explained some of the genetic peculiarities associated with the disease, it did not in itself give any clue as to the nature of the gene involved. It did, however, give a way to isolate and characterize the gene, as explained in detail by Brook et al.[76]

That study used a series of clones, isolated from a radiation-reduced hybrid cell line, which spanned the region of the unstable sequence. When the minimum region containing this sequence had been defined, sequencing was undertaken to provide PCR primers that could identify the CTG repeat and the number of copies. The clone containing the normal repeat was found to show cross-species conservation and, on hybridization with cDNA libraries from various tissues, sequences were identified in heart, skeletal muscle, and brain. One of these (C28) detected a transcript of 3.0 to 3.3 kb, which was sequenced and found to correspond to a protein of at least 585 amino acids. The CTG repeat was found to be in the 3′ untranslated region of the mRNA.

Comparison of the sequence of C28 with the database of known protein sequences has shown strong homology to the cyclic-AMP dependent protein kinase group (Fig. 141-9), notably to the yeast protein kinase TKR-YKR. There is, however, no identity with any known protein, so it would appear that the normal product of the myotonic dystrophy gene is a previously unrecognized protein kinase.

Parallel to this work, a sequence corresponding to the myotonic dystrophy gene was also identified by searching for trinucleotide repeat sequences in the myotonic dystrophy region of chromosome 19,[77,78] based on the likely similarity of the mutational basis of the disorder with that of fragile X mental retardation, mentioned above. The identity of the sequence discovered in this way with the one isolated by Brook et al. is shown by both the DNA and the predicted protein structure, and the success of this independent approach suggested that other genetic disorders could be produced by unstable trinucleotide repeat sequences in the genome, and that the myotonic dystrophy and fragile X mutations may be representatives of a broader group of defects of this type. This prediction has already been fulfilled by the subsequent finding of trinucleotide repeat expansions in Huntington's disease[79] and autosomal dominant spinocerebellar ataxia,[80] as well as in the X-linked bulbospinal muscular atrophy.[81]

The Molecular Situation as of July 1993

Since the initial studies described above, which were published in the spring of 1992, numerous studies have been undertaken in many other centers, and some preliminary conclusions can now be drawn with some confidence, regarding both the mutation and the myotonic dystrophy gene itself.

The myotonic dystrophy mutation has proved to be highly specific, no normal individuals outside affected families having so far been found to show an expansion of the CTG repeat in the range shown by affected patients. The normal population shows considerable variation, with 5 repeats being the commonest value, but with up to 30 repeats being seen. There are considerable geographical differences between European,[70] Japanese,[82,83] and African[84] normal populations.

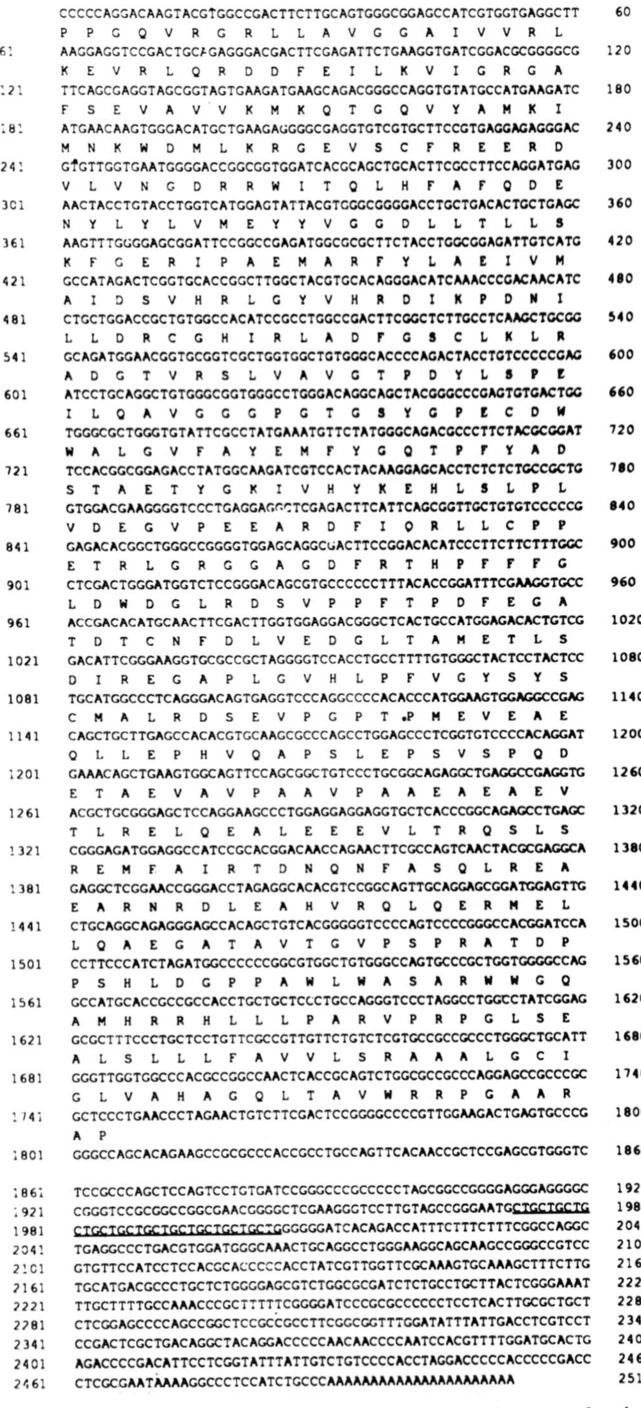

FIG. 141-9 **Sequence of the myotonic dystrophy gene, showing the location of the CTG repeat in the 3′ untranslated region of the gene. (DNA from a normal individual).** ***(From Brook et al.***[76] **Used by permission.)**

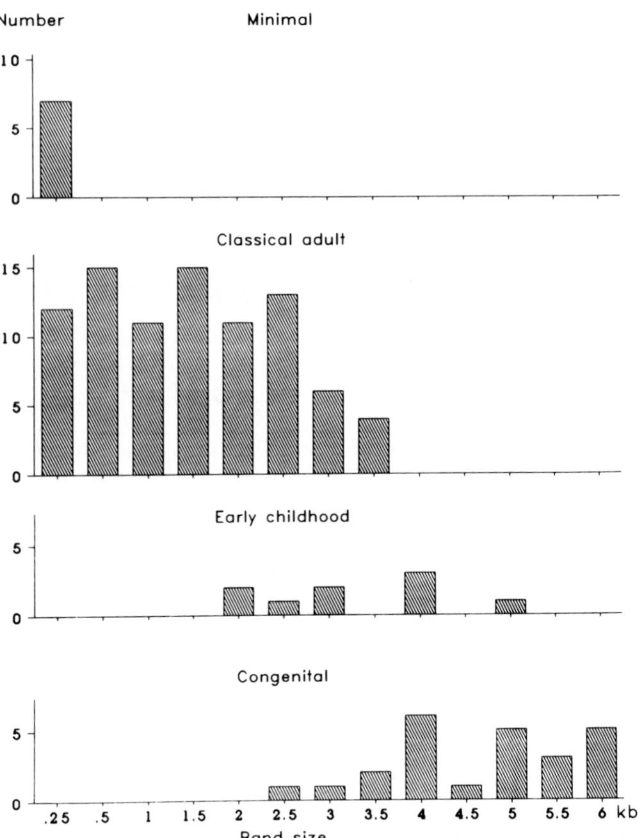

FIG. 141-10 **Size of DNA expansion in myotonic dystrophy in relation to severity of disorder.** ***Minimal:*** **Neuromuscular abnormalities absent or insignificant; cataract is the principal feature.** ***Classical adult:*** **Progressive muscle wasting with myotonia; onset in adult life.** ***Early childhood:*** **Developmental delay and other serious childhood symptoms; onset not congenital.** ***Congenital:*** **Onset of myotonic dystrophy at or before birth. DNA expansion is clearly related to these categories of severity; while individual categories show overlap, there is a distinct separation between the minimal group and those with severe childhood disease.** ***(From Harley et al.***[85] **Used by permission.)**

In myotonic dystrophy patients, several series have confirmed the initial findings of a correlation between repeat number, age at onset, and severity[85–87] (Fig. 141-10). A detailed study of minimally affected individuals and clinically normal known gene carriers in the older generations of affected families[88] has shown that these individuals have a rather narrow range of 50 to 80 repeats, while more typically affected adult-onset patients have a wide and variable repeat range of 100 to 500 copies, the number of copies not correlating closely with phenotype. Patients with congenital onset show the largest expansions[85–87] with values of 500 to 2000 copies, although there is considerable overlap with the range of noncongenital cases. Overall, there is a clear correlation of repeat number with age at onset[89,90] (Fig. 141-11).

Studies of intergenerational variation[90,91] have confirmed the initial finding of progressive expansion, the increase in repeat number corresponding closely to the decrease in age at onset in successive generations (Fig. 141-12). Congenitally affected patients in general have mothers with larger repeats, correlating well with the earlier observation that women with late onset of minimal symptoms rarely have congenitally affected children.[18] An observation of considerable interest has been the finding of a sex difference in parental transmission of the repeat[90,91]; continued expansion is seen during female transmission, while a decrease in repeat size is more often seen in offspring of affected males with large repeats, a point of practical significance in genetic counseling and prenatal diagnosis.[92,93] This difference also contributes to the maternal transmission of the congenital form.

Well over 1000 patients have now been studied by molecular analysis, and it is remarkable that no patient has so far been found to have a mutational defect other than the CTG repeat sequence expansion.[94] Most large series have encountered a few patients in whom the expansion cannot be demonstrated, but most such cases have proved to be

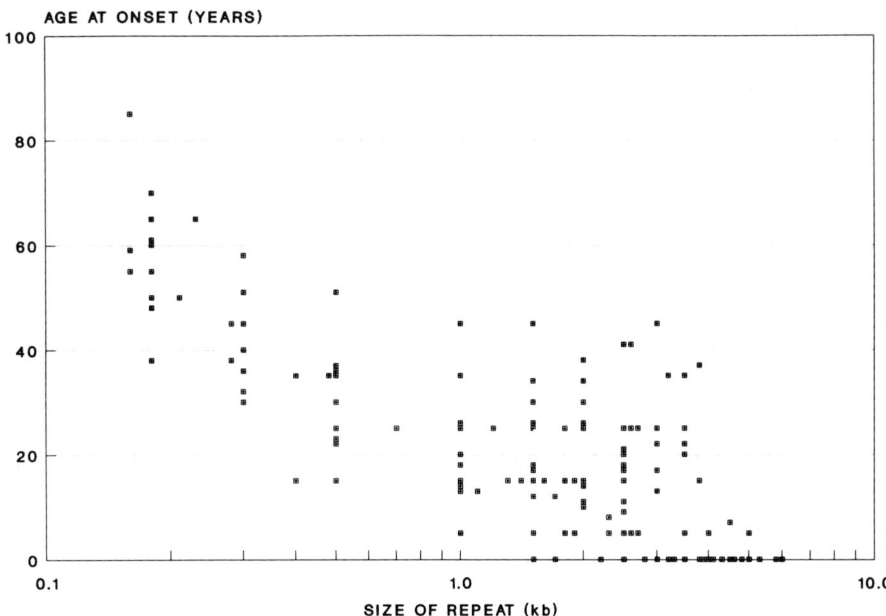

FIG. 141-11 The relationship of the age at onset of myotonic dystrophy to the size of the CTG repeat sequence. *(From Harley et al.*[90] Used by permission.)

misdiagnoses or, at the least, atypical. It thus seems likely that almost all myotonic dystrophy cases have the same mutational basis.

This homogeneity, along with the previously recognized low mutation rate in myotonic dystrophy, has reinforced the hypothesis mentioned earlier concerning the origins of the mutation.[32] Haplotype studies suggest that the original event (possibly unique and occurring many thousands of years ago) is likely to have been an expansion from an initial value of 5 copies to a "high normal" level of 20 to 30 copies,[95] with a gradual increase from this level over many generations eventually resulting in a clinically significant phenotype with apparent multiple origins. This hypothesis would suggest that those patients with minimal symptoms such as cataract only, are likely to have a repeat number that is already unstable, and that they are not the reservoir of genes that replaces those lost by reduced genetic fitness; rather, this reservoir is the pool of totally normal individuals who have repeat numbers in the high normal range. This origin, if confirmed, will have considerable implications for genetic counseling and prevention of the disorder.

Work on the mutation and its clinical correlates has been paralleled by analysis of the gene itself. The initial studies of the cDNA[76–78] have been extended to the genomic structure, which has shown 15 exons in 13 kb of genomic DNA.[96,97] As well as the kinase activity suggested by the sequence of N-terminal domain of the predicted protein, an intermediate domain suggests a filamentous structure, while the C-terminal segment should have hydrophobic properties.

The myotonic dystrophy gene is located in an extremely gene-rich region of chromosome 19, and work done on both the human gene and its mouse equivalent shows that its 5′ end is less than 500 kb from the end of another gene.[71,97] It is possible that a similar situation exists at the 3′ end of the

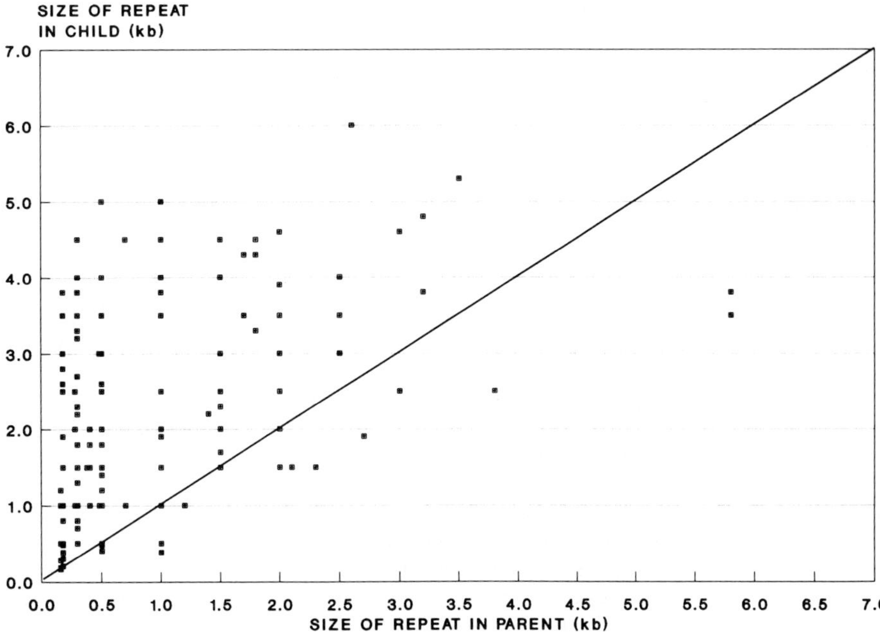

FIG. 141-12 Size of the CTG repeat in affected parent and offspring pairs, showing anticipation at the molecular level. *(From Harley et al.*[90] Used by permission.)

kinase gene, so that the clinical effects of the CTG repeat expansion could be related to disruption of the function of more than one gene.

Studies of gene expression[71] have suggested the existence of several isoforms resulting from alternative splicing in muscle, brain, and other tissues. However, the fundamental question of whether the primary defect is a deficiency or an excess of gene product is still uncertain, with one study showing a decrease of mRNA levels in muscle biopsy samples from adult patients,[98] while a second has shown increased levels.[99] Studies at the protein level likewise remain preliminary, but antibodies against various portions of the amino-acid sequence have resulted in a protein of 52 to 55 kDa being produced by more than one group,[98,100] which is likely to represent the myotonic dystrophy protein kinase.

Applied Molecular Genetics

The existence of DNA markers close to the myotonic dystrophy gene has allowed molecular predictions to be made with reasonable accuracy for the past 5 years.[101] Successively closer and more informative marker loci have been used, and several large series have been reported,[102–105] including prenatal diagnosis as well as the detection of gene carriers. In those studies that have compared the use of linked markers in gene detection with the traditional approaches of electromyography and slit-lamp examination, good agreement has been found in assigning high or low risk status for the great majority of individuals, but 8 to 10 percent of individuals classed as normal by clinical investigations proved to have a high-risk genotype in two separate studies.[103,104] Analysis of the unstable sequence is now able to confirm whether such individuals are indeed carriers of the mutation,[88,105] PCR-based analysis to determine the precise number of copies of the repeat sequence being the most definitive method. Preliminary use of this approach suggests that at least some of these clinically normal individuals do show expansion of the gene, while, conversely, some predicted as being at high risk on the basis of lens changes alone do not.[106] Thus, while direct molecular analysis has confirmed clinical and linkage predictions in most instances, mutation analysis should be undertaken in any existing cases where doubt remains, and is the approach of choice, in conjunction with clinical assessment, for new cases.

Prenatal diagnosis by specific testing for the expanded sequence has already been shown to be feasible.[85,107] In the family shown in Figure 141-13, retrospective confirmation of high- and low-risk linkage predictions was also possible in two previously studied pregnancies. An important aspect of the specific technique is the likely correlation of gene expansion with phenotype; in the family illustrated, both affected pregnancies tested using chorion biopsy samples showed expansions that were large compared with those of the affected mothers, suggesting that the children would have been severely affected. The weaker correlation of phenotype and repeat size outside congenital-onset sibships makes caution in interpretation necessary, while the observed decrease in repeat size in some male transmissions must also be taken into account. So far, no discrepancy between repeat size in chorionic villus material and that in the affected fetus has been found; however, the recent observation of a marked difference between germ-line and somatic tissues in fragile X syndrome,[108,109] with the possibility of early postconception expansion, would suggest that if preimplantation diagnosis is developed for myotonic dystrophy, it must be interpreted with great caution.

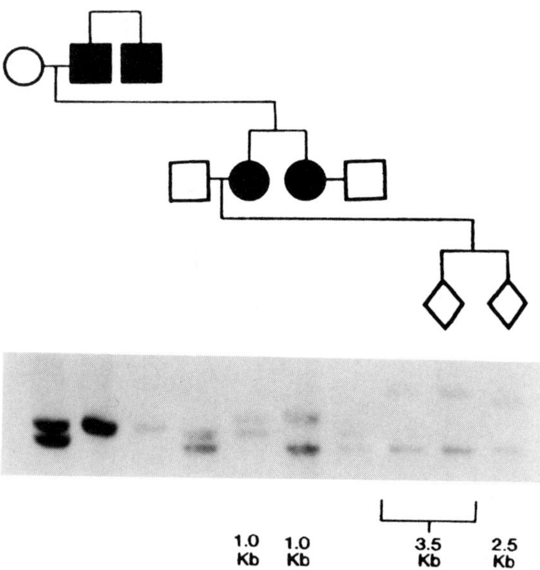

FIG. 141-13 Specific molecular prenatal diagnosis in myotonic dystrophy. Two pregnancies of an affected mother were analyzed on chorion biopsy samples, one prospectively (lanes 8 and 9), the other retrospectively on stored DNA. Both pregnancies show a large expansion, while the DNA from the affected mother and her sister (who had previously lost an infant with congenital myotonic dystrophy) shows moderate expansions. *(From Myring et al.*[107] Used by permission.)

The use of molecular analysis as a primary diagnostic tool for myotonic dystrophy, only possible since the specific defect became known, is already becoming widespread. A preliminary study of its use in patients with neuromuscular problems has shown its application in a variety of diagnostic situations, including the differential diagnosis of congenital myopathies and of puzzling cases of adult muscle disease, and the problem of distinguishing myotonic dystrophy from nonprogressive myotonic disorders.[85,110] The test may prove similarly useful in an ophthalmologic setting,[106] particularly in determining the significance of lens opacities in an otherwise healthy relative of a patient with myotonic dystrophy, or in deciding whether an isolated cataract with an appearance suggestive of myotonic dystrophy is due to a minimal mutation for this disease. However, our experience is not yet sufficient to dispense with established clinical investigations, while it also remains possible that a small proportion of myotonic dystrophy cases may result from a separate type of mutational defect. Studies on general cases of cataract do not suggest that myotonic dystrophy is a frequent cause[111] or that such cataract cases are an important pool of undetected individuals with the gene.

Previous Biochemical Studies in Myotonic Dystrophy

A large number of experimental studies of different biochemical aspects of myotonic dystrophy were undertaken before the gene and its protein were identified. As with Duchenne muscular dystrophy, most of them proved to be negative, inconclusive, or confusing, and are of little relevance now that more specific information is available. Early studies are covered in the first (1979) edition of the author's monograph.[112] One field of investigation that now merits reassessment is the series of studies by Roses, Appel, and colleagues on abnormalities in the membrane of red blood cells and muscle. These were described fully in the chapter on muscular dystrophies in the fifth edition of this text in relation to both myotonic and Duchenne muscular dystrophy,[113] but they are discussed here briefly since the finding that a protein kinase is the predicted gene product makes them again relevant. Roses and Appel's initial report[114] (now 20 years old) was of an abnormality in the phosphorylation of red blood cell membranes from myotonic dystrophy patients. The study was undertaken on the basis that the multisystem nature of myotonic dystrophy, together with the likely role of ion flow across membranes in causing myotonia, made a generalized membrane defect probable. The authors specifically suggested that a membrane-located protein kinase might be the primary defect in myotonic dystrophy, a suggestion that now indeed appears to be correct.

Subsequent work showed that muscle sarcolemmal membranes also showed decreased phosphorylation,[115] and that in both muscle and red blood cell membranes this could be located in a specific protein fraction separated by sodium dodecyl sulfate (SDS) gel electrophoresis.[116] Unfortunately, further specific characterization of the abnormality was not possible at that time, and the difficulty in obtaining consistent and repeatable results,[117,118] along with the paucity of knowledge at that period of the normal cell membrane, resulted in this work being left in an inconclusive state.[119] A contributing factor was probably the finding of similar abnormalities in Duchenne muscular dystrophy,[120] where the independent evidence for a generalized membrane defect was always much weaker.

During the subsequent 20 years our knowledge of normal cell membrane structure and function has increased immensely, as has our knowledge of the protein kinase group. Now that the myotonic dystrophy protein kinase has been isolated and is being characterized, it will be possible to study its subcellular distribution in different tissues in a much more specific way than was possible previously and to determine the precise way in which the defect in myotonic dystrophy disturbs normal membrane function.

Management and Therapy of Myotonic Dystrophy

There is currently no specific therapy that will arrest or significantly modify the progressive dystrophic changes that occur in patients with myotonic dystrophy, nor can the cardiac or other systemic abnormalities be specifically treated. It is greatly hoped that the isolation of the myotonic dystrophy gene and its protein product will alter this situation, particularly since it should now be possible to combine the physiological approaches to ion transport across the cell membrane with the more detailed information that is emerging on the nature and distribution of the myotonic dystrophy protein kinase and how its function is altered in myotonic dystrophy.

Meanwhile the lack of specific treatments makes it all the more important to use the general approaches to management that do exist and which are currently more relevant to most patients than pharmacologic treatment of their myotonia. The following aspects, discussed in more detail in the author's monograph,[7] should especially be emphasized.

1. Avoidance of hazards from anesthesia and surgery. These hazards are well described, as already mentioned, but avoidable tragedies continue to occur, sometimes in undiagnosed individuals but also in patients well known to have the disorder. All patients should be informed of the hazards, both verbally and in writing; a warning card or wrist bracelet is a useful precaution. Procedures that are not necessary should be avoided; such a statement might seem obvious and unnecessary, but the author has been surprised how often informing the surgeon and anesthetist of the risky status of their patient has led to a proposed procedure being abandoned without obvious loss of benefit. There is no reason why necessary surgery should not be undertaken, though careful preoperative assessment, avoidance of excessive anesthetic drugs, cardiac monitoring during surgery, and good postoperative respiratory care are all advisable.
2. Myotonic dystrophy patients need regular general, not just neuromuscular, assessment. Many patients seen by the author have had no continuing care of any kind, largely on the rationale that there is no specific neuromuscular therapy. Early detection of cardiac arrhythmias, impaired ventilation, or recurrent bronchial aspiration may prove life-saving, while recognition and correction of systemic features such as cataract, diabetes, and colonic problems can improve the quality of life.
3. The adaptations needed to compensate for the neuromuscular defects will depend on the patient's state. Neck weakness may be helped by a soft cervical collar; a vehicle headrest should always be used to avoid whiplash injury. Those patients with footdrop may be helped by light plastic moulded splints. A small but significant proportion will require a wheelchair at some stage, and it may need to be powered if hand and arm function is impaired.
4. Genetic counseling and the availability of appropriate molecular and other tests should be an integral part of management, even though they may be declined by some patients and relatives. The implications for the extended family must be considered by those involved in primary diagnosis, with referral to colleagues in clinical genetics where necessary.
5. Myotonia does not require specific therapy in most patients, in contrast to the nonprogressive myotonias, where myotonia may itself be quite disabling. Phenytoin, procainamide, quinine, and mexiletine are all drugs that can prove helpful, though agents with a cardiac effect should be avoided when conduction defects are present.

NONPROGRESSIVE MYOTONIC DISORDERS

This group of uncommon but important disorders cannot be considered as muscular dystrophies, but are mentioned briefly here because of the importance of distinguishing them from myotonic dystrophy and because of recent molecular advances. The value of the "candidate gene" approach is well shown by this group, providing a contrast in this respect to myotonic dystrophy. Valuable and up-to-date reviews are provided by Rüdel et al.[121] and Lehmann-Horn et al.[122]

Myotonia Congenita

Myotonia congenita exists in both autosomal dominant and autosomal recessive forms. The dominant form was first described in 1872 by Thomsen,[1] who was himself affected by the disorder; descendants with the condition are living in Denmark and Northern Germany at the present time.[123] Myotonia is the only significant feature of the disorder; it is lifelong, more generalized than is usual in myotonic dystrophy, and often more severe. Weakness may be associated with the myotonia, as may episodes of falling due to sudden generalized myotonia, often in response to being startled. Progressive muscle wasting is absent and muscles are frequently hypertrophic, with minimal changes seen on biopsy. The cardiac, ocular, and other systemic features of myotonic dystrophy are not seen.

The recessive form was first recognised by Becker[124,125] and is probably the commoner, though it lacks the multigenerational transmission that makes some pedigrees of the dominant form so conspicuous. Clinical features are similar, but more severe myotonia, a greater degree of hypertrophy, and, in some cases, appreciable weakness may be seen. The dominant and recessive forms cannot be clinically distinguished with confidence in isolated cases.

Linkage studies have clearly shown that dominant myotonia congenita is not allelic to myotonic dystrophy on chromosome 19.[126] A similar condition in goats, however, provides a well-recognized animal model, which has been used for much of the physiological work on myotonia. More recently, a mouse with nonprogressive myotonia has also been documented[127] and has been used as the basis for molecular studies that have complemented the studies of physiology.

Reduced chloride conductance has been shown to be the principal abnormality underlying myotonia in the goat model,[128,129] and most studies on human myotonia congenita agree with this conclusion.[130] Thus, a defect in the chloride ion channel seemed the most likely basis for this form of myotonia in both humans and other species.[131] That hypothesis has now been confirmed as a result of cloning of the chloride channel (ClC-1)[132] and the demonstration of mutations in its gene first in the mouse model[133] and recently in human myotonia congenita[134,135]; defects in this gene are seen in both the dominant and the recessive forms, showing that the two are allelic.

Paramyotonia and Adynamia

In paramyotonia,[122,136] the myotonia is accompanied by a prolonged specific reaction of muscle to cold, resulting in weakness and electrically silent contracture which may persist for many minutes or even hours. This cold-related abnormality distinguishes the disorder from myotonia congenita, which it otherwise resembles, being also dominantly inherited and nonprogressive. The anti-arrhythmic drug mexiletine is helpful in reducing the cold-related response; the drug tocainide was also effective[137] but has been withdrawn on account of adverse effects.[138]

In adynamia[122,139] (also known as myotonic or hyperkalemic periodic paralysis), myotonia, usually mild, is accompanied by episodes of spontaneous flaccid weakness, often generalized and lasting hours or days.[140] Following repeated severe attacks, a degree of permanent weakness may occur. A variable degree of elevation of serum potassium is seen, especially during attacks. Adynamia responds to diuretics such as acetozolamide or thiazides[141]; prophylactic use of a thiazide diuretic may be helpful in patients with frequent attacks.

The physiological and therapy-related features of these two disorders suggested that an abnormality in the skeletal muscle sodium ion channel might be responsible,[142] a hypothesis that has now been confirmed by molecular studies after the cloning of this gene.[143,144] First adynamia[145,146] and then paramyotonia[147,148] were shown to be linked to the sodium ion channel gene on chromosome 17; subsequently, specific mutations have been demonstrated in patients with each disorder, confirming that the two are allelic.[149] It should be noted that the hypokalemic form of periodic paralysis, in which myotonia does not occur, is not linked to this locus.[150]

OTHER AUTOSOMAL MUSCULAR DYSTROPHIES

As already indicated in the introduction and in Table 141-1, there are at least six other well-defined autosomal muscular dystrophies apart from myotonic dystrophy, and it is likely that considerable further heterogeneity, especially in the "limb-girdle" group, remains to be resolved. As with myotonic dystrophy, little information on the metabolic and molecular bases of these diseases has so far come from biochemical studies, so that the positional cloning approach is the one most likely to be fruitful. Indeed, results are already appearing, as summarized in Table 141-10, which

Table 141-10 Gene Mapping in Autosomal Myopathies

Disorder	Location of Gene	Comments
Myotonic dystrophy	19q	Gene isolated; no heterogeneity
Facioscapulohumeral dystrophy	4q	Heterogeneity possible in a few families
Limb girdle dystrophies		Further heterogeneity likely
Autosomal recessive	15	
Autosomal dominant	5	
Severe "Duchenne-like" "Recessive" type	13q	
Myotonia congenita (dominant and recessive)	7q	Mutations in chloride channel
Paramyotonia/hyperkalemic periodic paralysis	17	Allelic; mutations in sodium ion channel
Hyperpyrexic myopathy	19q	Defect in ryanodine receptor in some families
	7q	Possible chloride channel defect in some families
Central core disease	19q	May also be due to defect in ryanodine receptor
Nemaline myopathy (dominant)	1	Severe recessive form not yet localized

lists the current gene-mapping status for these conditions, and also includes information on other myopathies that do not fall within the remit of this chapter. It is of interest that the candidate gene approach has proved rewarding for several of the nonprogressive myopathies, such as myotonia congenita, paramyotonia, and hyperpyrexic myopathy, while none of the progressive muscular dystrophies has so far proved to be determined by a gene of previously defined function.

Facioscapulohumeral Muscular Dystrophy

Facioscapulohumeral muscular dystrophy (Landouzy-Déjerine Disease; FSHD) is a dominantly inherited disorder that is, like myotonic dystrophy, exceptionally variable. Although traditionally regarded as a benign condition, systematic family and population studies, notably those of Padberg[151] and Lunt and Harper,[152] have shown that about 20 percent of patients are severely disabled by age 40. Conversely, some individuals remain minimally affected throughout life.

Clinical Features. FSHD was first recognized as a clinical entity by Landouzy and Déjerine in 1885,[153] and has been generally accepted as a separate form of muscular dystrophy since that time. As the name of the disorder implies, facial weakness is prominent (Fig. 141-14), along with involvement of the shoulder girdle and proximal arm muscles.[154] Pelvic-girdle involvement is also seen but generally appears later and is less marked than the involvement of the shoulder girdle, in contrast to the situation in Duchenne, Becker, and other limb-girdle dystrophies, where the lower girdle is affected earlier and more severely. Lower-limb involvement in FSHD is frequently characterized by distal weakness of the peroneal muscles, resulting in footdrop, and a characteristic gait in more severe cases results from the combination of footdrop and pelvic girdle weakness.

The onset of FSHD is frequently in childhood[155,156]; facial weakness may be seen in family photographs even when the diagnosis has only been made much later. Scapular "winging" is another early sign, but a mild degree may be seen in normal, lax-jointed children. Smooth and cardiac muscle are notably unaffected, as is mental function. Some evidence of wider systemic involvement comes from the finding of associated neural hearing loss; a claim that a specific retinopathy accompanies the disorder[157] has not been confirmed.[158]

Both muscle biopsy and electromyography frequently show changes suggestive of a neurogenic basis, along with myopathic changes. These are sometimes so marked as to cause confusion with the group of spinal muscular atrophies. However, the suggestion that there is a separate spinal form of FSHD[159] has been disproved by the occurrence of such cases in typical FSHD families and by recent linkage data supporting the genetic identity of the two forms.[160]

Genetics. While autosomal dominant inheritance is not in doubt for FSHD, the variability of the disorder causes several practical difficulties in interpretation.

The penetrance of the gene is strongly age-dependent; two studies have estimated around 95 percent penetrance by age 20,[151,161] with a small number of individuals remaining undetectable even in later life; careful neurologic assessment to detect mild signs is essential in the context of genetic counseling, since around 20 percent of cases are essentially asymptomatic.

Prevalence estimates are similarly influenced by clinical variability, but a level around 5 per 100,000 has been found in several populations,[151,162] with no striking geographical variation so far noted.

Heterogeneity, as opposed to variability at the clinical level, has not been established; as mentioned above, the

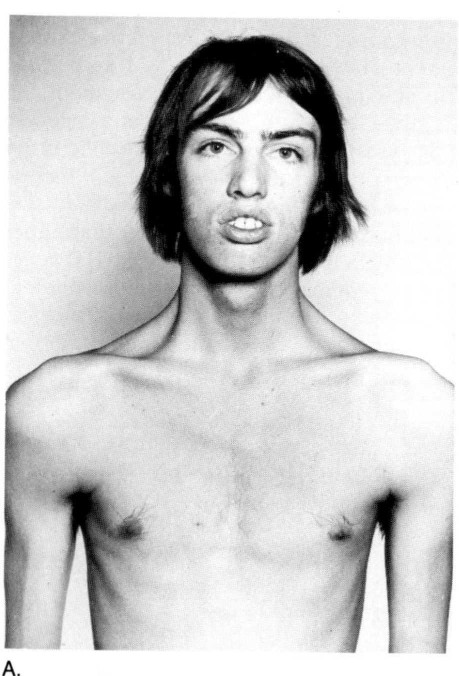

A.

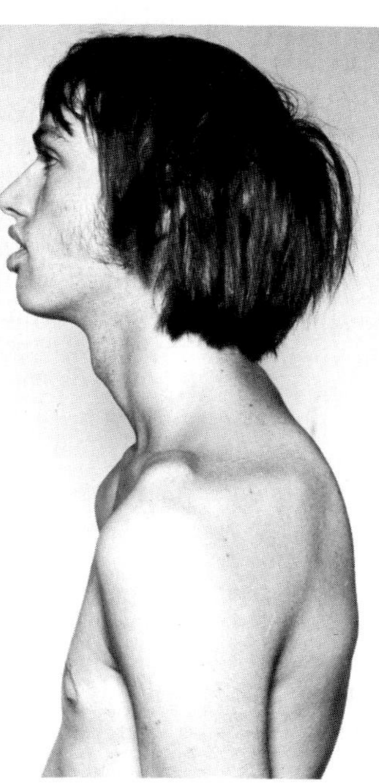

B.

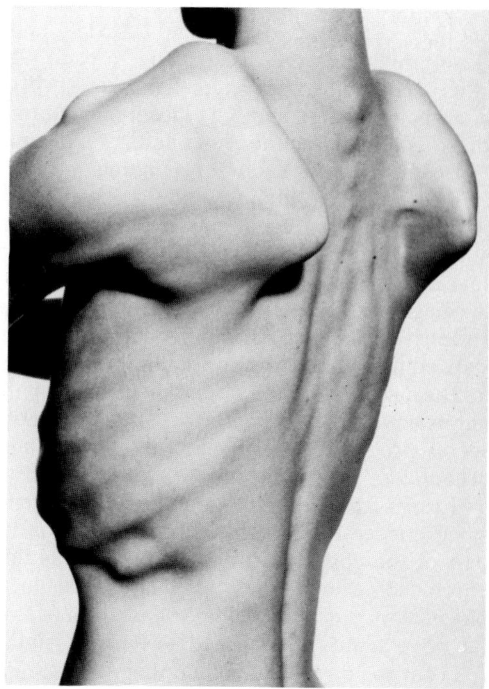

C.

FIG. 141-14 Facioscapulohumeral muscular dystrophy. *A*. Typical facial weakness and wasting of neck muscles. *B*. Another patient showing wasting and 'winging' of shoulder girdle muscles.

cases showing neuropathic changes occur within families showing more atypical features,[160] while genetic linkage data, discussed below, have so far strongly supported a single main locus.

New mutation may account for 10 to 20 percent of cases,[151] although the variability and incomplete penetrance of the disorder should give caution in accepting this as an accurate estimate. No clear sex-related effects in gene transmission, such as occur in myotonic dystrophy, are seen, nor has anticipation been noted.

Gene Mapping and Molecular Genetics. In contrast to the gene for myotonic dystrophy, the gene for FSHD has not yet (July, 1993) been identified, but we do now have an accurate chromosomal location, which makes possible the productive application of positional cloning techniques. The gene itself may well have been isolated by the time this chapter is published.

Gene-mapping studies in FSHD began with the study of Padberg et al.,[163] who used classic protein markers. Molecular genetic studies started in 1985 with the formation of an international consortium by the groups involved; this consortium rapidly provided exclusion data for most of the genome[164] and gave a strong indication of the remaining areas where the gene might be located. The assignment of FSHD to chromosome 4 in 1990 by Wijmenga et al.[165] was the first example of the power of the then newly developed microsatellite markers,[166] and it was rapidly followed by the detection of a much closer marker (D4S139) that had potential for clinical use.[160,167] The physical location was confirmed as being distal 4q,[168] previously a poorly mapped region of the genome; intensive and collaborative analysis by groups involved,[169–172] including a multipoint analysis on the pooled data set,[141] has shown that the disease locus lies distal to all marker loci detected so far, though the precise distance from the telomere remains uncertain.

Figure 141-15 indicates the provisional gene map of the relevant region; two markers (D4S139 and D4S130) are closely linked to the disease and to each other, while two others, including the original marker (D4S171), are more proximally located and only loosely linked to FSHD. Figure 141-16 shows the pattern in one large informative kindred.

Despite the lack of any flanking marker distal to the FSHD locus, the highly polymorphic nature of the linked sequences has already clarified some important aspects, notably those relating to heterogeneity. Both mild and severely affected families show linkage, as do those in which the diagnosis had been claimed to represent a spinal muscular atrophy.[160] The original pooled data set of over 50 kindreds showed no clearly unlinked families, indicating a single locus for the disorder.[172] However, at least one apparently unlinked family has since been reported,[173] so a degree of heterogeneity seems probable, though only involving a small proportion of families.

Efforts towards isolating the FSHD gene on 4q have since concentrated on the characterization of the terminal part of the chromosome, where the locus lies. Analysis of chromosome anomalies involving distal 4q is providing a physical map of this region of the chromosome, although so far no patient showing FSHD and a visible defect in the relevant region has been identified.

A recent finding of considerable importance is the recognition that a sequence derived from a human homeobox gene mapping to distal 4q[174] not only is closer to FSHD than any of the previously recognized markers but detects a specific alteration in a high proportion of affected patients.[175] Both affected and normal individuals show a high degree of polymorphism for this marker, but those affected usually show a small fragment of less than 30 kb that segregates with the disorder. In new-mutation cases, this fragment can also be shown to arise *de novo*, suggesting a specific relationship to the disease.[176] Since the sequence, like other linked markers, lies proximal to the disease gene, which is close to the telomere of the chromosome, the reduced-size fragment could reflect loss of subtelomeric DNA that either directly or indirectly affects the function of the FSHD gene. Caution is needed in the clinical application of this finding, however, since not all affected individuals show the change, while a fragment of similar size is not uncommon in normal individuals.[177]

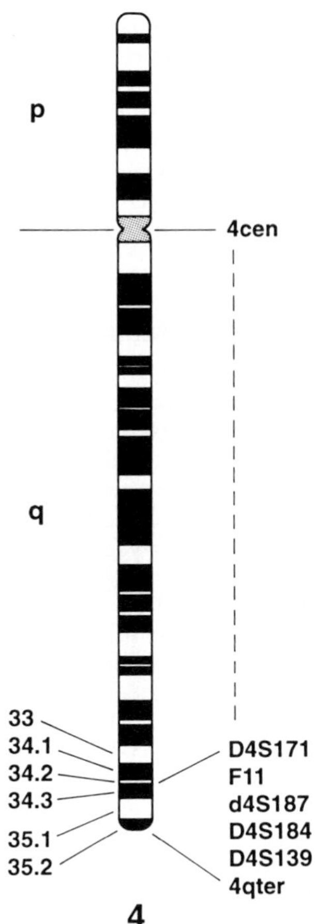

FIG. 141-15 Distal region of chromosome 4q, to show location of the facioscapulohumeral muscular dystrophy gene and adjacent genetic markers.

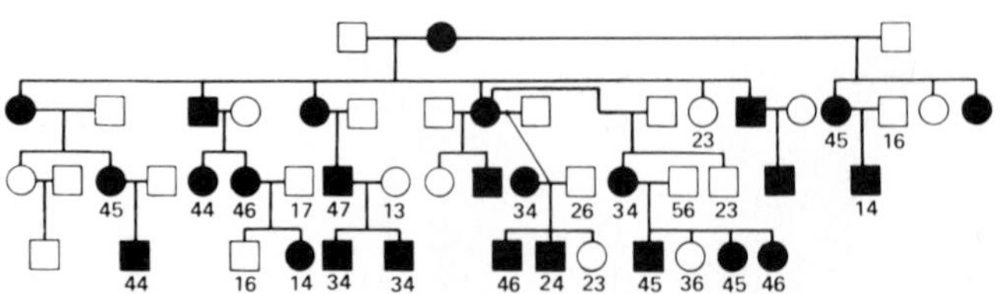

FIG. 141-16 A pedigree of facioscapulohumeral muscular dystrophy, showing coinheritance of the disorder with a closely linked multi-allelic DNA marker on chromosome 4q. All affected individuals have inherited allele 4.

The Limb-Girdle Muscular Dystrophy Group

Autosomal Recessive "Duchenne-Like" Limb-Girdle Dystrophy of Early Childhood. The rare but well-documented occurrence of a Duchenne-like disorder in chromosomally normal girls has long been recognized to imply the existence of a small subgroup that exhibit autosomal recessive inheritance.[178] While exceptionally rare in most of Europe and North America, this form appears to be more frequent in North Africa[179] and possibly in Switzerland.[180] Differences from true DMD are slight, but include lack of characteristic electrocardiographic changes and a somewhat milder course. Although this variant is too rare to significantly affect genetic counseling for DMD as a whole, it should be borne in mind when there is parental consanguinity or when multiple recombinations are observed with X-chromosome DNA markers. Most male cases are now detected when muscle dystrophin is found to be normal,[181] an indication of the importance of this analysis in clinical practice. The autosomal dystrophin-related protein (utrophin) locus on chromosome 6 (see below) has been excluded in a number of families,[182] but recently the gene present in North African families has been mapped to chromosome 13q,[183] and a specific change in muscle has been detected—the absence of the 45-kDa protein component of the dystrophin-related complex.[184] This complex constitutes a family of proteins whose structural and functional relationships are in the process of being clarified, as discussed in Chap. 140.

Late-Onset (Erb-Type) Autosomal Recessive Limb-Girdle Dystrophy. This disorder, originally described by Erb in 1884[185] has been recognized in all the major population surveys and classifications of the muscular dystrophies, but it is now considered to be only one part of a heterogeneous group.[186] Older studies probably included cases that would now be identified as being caused by chronic spinal muscular atrophy, specific metabolic myopathies such as glycogenoses, and some nongenetic causes. Incidence values of between 1 and 3 per 100,000 have been recorded, but a careful study in Scotland[187] showed a most likely maximum incidence of 0.3 per 100,000 when the excess of male cases thought probably to represent Becker muscular dystrophy was removed.

Particular care must be taken not to confuse affected females with manifesting carriers for Duchenne muscular dystrophy, the genetic risk for offspring being profoundly different. Equally important is to distinguish the isolated male case from Becker muscular dystrophy. Distinguishing points include calf hypertrophy, electrocardiographic changes, and Duchenne-like biopsy changes in Becker muscular dystrophy. The occurrence of a markedly raised creatine kinase level in the mother would also favor this diagnosis, but a good working rule is never to accept the diagnosis of "autosomal recessive limb-girdle dystrophy" unless both genetic and neuromuscular studies have been thorough and to give genetic counseling as for X-linked inheritance if there is any doubt. DNA analysis of the p21 region of the X chromosome should be undertaken in all affected males; a study of 30 isolated male cases with a limb-girdle dystrophy showed that 56 percent showed deletions in the dystrophin gene, including some cases thought on clinical grounds to be autosomal.[188] Dystrophin analysis on muscle biopsy specimens is also now an important part of clinical practice.

Unlike the severe childhood autosomal recessive form, no specific molecular defect in the adult recessive limb-girdle dystrophies has yet been found, while the small size of most affected families makes genetic linkage studies difficult. However, a large kindred from the isolated island of Reunion has shown linkage to markers on chromosome 5,[189] as have families from the Pennsylvannia Amish population[190]; other families appear to be unlinked, suggesting that further unresolved heterogeneity is present in the condition.

Autosomal Dominant Limb-Girdle Dystrophy. A few families in the limb-girdle group, usually with disease that is adult in onset and benign in clinical course, have been recognized as showing autosomal dominant inheritance,[191] and, in one large American kindred, linkage to chromosome 5q markers has been found.[192]

Autosomal Dystrophin. The detection of an autosomal homologue to dystrophin[193] represents an important advance, both in suggesting that there may be a family of such proteins and in providing an obvious candidate gene for the autosomal muscular dystrophies. This protein, called "dystrophin-related protein" and also known as "dystrophin-like protein" or "utrophin," is determined by a gene on chromosome 6[194] and has now been characterized in some detail.[194,195] It is particularly represented in smooth muscle and at neuromuscular junctions.[196,197]

The obvious candidate for a disorder that could represent a defect in this molecule is the autosomal recessive Duchenne-like dystrophy, but, as noted above, linkage has excluded this gene as the cause either of this disorder or of later-onset limb-girdle dystrophies, while so far none of the other dystrophies has shown either linkage to or any abnormality in this protein. Thus, this gene and protein remain candidates in search of a corresponding disease.

OTHER MUSCULAR DYSTROPHIES

Numerous rare and poorly defined forms of muscle disease exist which are not covered by this chapter but which are described in more extensive books on the subject, such as that of Engel.[6] A brief note is included here on forms of progressive muscular dystrophy for which gene mapping or other molecular data are likely to be obtained during the next few years. That may result from the study of individual large kindreds or from the finding of specific molecular defects in candidate genes, both approaches being actively pursued at present.

Oculopharyngeal Muscular Dystrophy

Oculopharyngeal muscular dystrophy is an autosomal dominant disorder that is generally late in onset, often appearing in the late forties or fifties, and has slow progression.[198–200] Ptosis is commonly the first clinical feature and may be visible in photographs taken many years before presentation. Limitation of eye movements is characteristic and eventually progresses to complete ocular paresis, in striking contrast to most of the other primary muscular dystrophies, in which eye movements are preserved even at a late stage. The other major problem is the involvement of pharyngeal muscles, leading to difficulty in swallowing and to aspiration of food with consequent pneumonia, the usual cause of death. More general muscle weakness is relatively mild and late.

The main differential diagnosis of oculopharyngeal dystrophy is the group of mitochondrial myopathies, which also show prominent ocular involvement, as well as a variety of central nervous system and other general problems. Since specific mutations in the mitochondrial genome, some confined to muscle, some present in all tissues, including blood, and thus heritable, have been identified in several members of this group,[201] mitochondrial DNA analysis on blood and muscle should be undertaken whenever oculopharyngeal muscular dystrophy is suspected.

In most populations, oculopharyngeal muscular dystrophy is an extremely rare disorder, but there is an unusually high frequency among French Canadians[202]; gene mapping studies in this group should provide the basis for identification of this gene in the future, but no current location has been established.

Distal Myopathies

The distal myopathies are a poorly classified group likely to contain several entities; the best delineated form is the one originally described by Welander,[203] which appears to be particularly frequent in Scandinavian countries. This dominantly inherited disorder has a variable age at onset, often late in adult life, with some individuals likely to show nonpenetrance of the gene. As the name implies, distal weakness and wasting in the hands and legs are the most prominent features, and very slow progression is usual.[203] Some more severe cases showing proximal weakness may represent homozygotes for the disorder.[204] The likelihood of genetic homogeneity in Scandinavia for this form of distal myopathy should aid gene localization.

Nonprogressive Myopathies

Even more numerous than the progressive muscular dystrophies are the nonprogressive myopathies. The various myotonic syndromes have already been mentioned briefly; Table 141-9 summarizes the group of congenital myopathies, in which onset at birth is commonly though not invariably followed by improvement and a relatively stable course in later life. Gene localization data (Table 141-10) are available for two members of this group, central core disease[205] and the dominant form of nemaline myopathy.[206] A further category not considered here is the group of metabolic myopathies, in which muscle is involved as part of a more general metabolic disorder. A final disorder deserving mention is hyperpyrexic myopathy (malignant hyperthermia), in which a subclinical myopathy predisposes a patient to potentially fatal muscle contracture with hyperpyrexia following the administration of anesthetic agents.[207] In some families, this dominantly inherited condition has been shown to be linked to chromosome 19 markers in the region of the ryanodine receptor,[208] and a specific mutation in this receptor has been detected in one case.[209] It is of interest that central core disease,[165] in which hyperpyrexia may also occur, has a similar gene location, suggesting that the two disorders may be allelic. It is also possible that some of the hyperpyrexia families not linked to chromosome 19 may prove to have chloride-channel defects, since linkage to this region of chromosome 7 has been shown for some of them.

REFERENCES

1. Thomsen J: Tonische krämpfe in willkurlich beweglichen Muskeln infolge von ererbter psychischer Disposition (Ataxia muscularis). *Arch Psychiatr Nervenkr* **6**:702, 1876.
2. Steinert H: Uber das klinische und anatomische Bild des Muskelschwundes der Myotoniker. *Dtsch Z Nervenhlk* **37**:38, 1909.
3. Batten FE, Gibb HP: Myotonia atrophica. *Brain* **32**:187, 1909.
4. Curschmann H: Uber familiare atrophische Myotonie. *Dtsch Z Nerbenhlk* **45**:161, 1912.
5. Harper PS: *Myotonic Dystrophy*. London, Saunders, 1989.
6. Harper PS, Rüdel R: Myotonic dystrophy, in Engel A (ed): *Myology*, 2d ed. New York, McGraw Hill, 1993. (In press)
7. Bundey S, Carter CO, Soothill JF: Early recognition of heterozygotes for the gene of dystrophia myotonia. *J Neurol Psychiatr* **33**:279, 1970.
8. Harper PS: Presymptomatic detection and genetic counselling in myotonic dystrophy. *Clin Genet* **4**:134, 1973.
9. Hayasaka S, Kiyosawa M, Katsumata S, Honda M, Takase S, Mizuno K: Ciliary and retinal changes in myotonic dystrophy. *Arch Ophthalmol* **102**:88, 1984.
10. Church SC: The heart in myotonica atrophica. *Arch Intern Med* **119**:176, 1967.
11. Prystowsky EN, Pritchett EL, Roses AD, Gallagher J: The natural history of conduction system disease in muscular dystrophy as determined by serial electrophysiologic studies. *Circulation* **60**:1360, 1979.
12. Forsberg H, Olofsson B-O, Erikson A, Andersson S: Cardiac involvement in congenital myotonic dystrophy. *Br Heart J* **63**:119, 1990.
13. Aldridge LM: Anaesthetic problems in myotonic dystrophy—a case report and review of the Aberdeen experience comprising 48 general anaesthetics in a further 16 patients. *Br J Anaesth* **57**:1119, 1985.
14. Vanier TM: Dystrophia myotonica in childhood. *Br Med J* **2**:1284, 1960.
15. Harper PS: Congenital myotonic dystrophy in Britain. *Arch Dis Child* **50**:505, 1975.
16. Harper PS, Dyken PR: Early onset dystrophia myotonica—Evidence supporting a maternal environmental factor. *Lancet* **2**:53, 1972.
17. Harper PS: Congenital myotonic dystrophy in Britain. II. Genetic basis. *Arch Dis Child* **50**:514, 1975.
18. Koch MC, Grimm T, Harley HG, Harper PS: Genetic risks for children of women with myotonic dystrophy. *Am J Hum Genet* **48**:1084, 1991.
19. Wallgren-Petterson C: Myotubular myopathy. Workshop report. *Neuromusc Disord* 1994. (In press.)
20. Casanova G, Jerusalem F: Myopathology of myotonic dystrophy: A morphometric study. *Acta Neuropathol* **45**:231, 1979.
21. Karpati G, Carpenter S, Watters GV, Eisen AE, Andermann F: Infantile myotonic dystrophy: Histochemical and electron microscopic features in skeletal muscle. *Neurology* **23**:1066, 1973.
22. Sarnat HB, Silbert SW: Maturational arrest of fetal muscle in neonatal myotonic dystrophy. *Arch Neurol* **33**:466, 1976.
23. Farkas E, Tomé FMS, Fardeau M, Arseniio-Nunes ML, Dreyfuss P, Diebler MF: Histochemical and ultrastructural study of muscle biopsies in 3 cases of dystrophia myotonica in the newborn child. *J Neurol Sci* **21**:273, 1974.
24. Lipicky RJ: Studies in human myotonic dystrophy, in Rowland LP (ed): *Pathogenesis of Human Muscular Dystrophy*. Amsterdam, Excerpta Medica, 1977, p 729.
25. Franke CH, Hatt H, Iaizzo PA, Lehmann-Horn F: Characteristics of Na^+ channels and Cl^- conductance in resealed muscle fibre segments from patients with myotonic dystrophy. *J Physiol (Lond)* **425**:391, 1990.
26. Merickel M, Gray R, Chauvin P, Appel S: Cultured muscle from myotonic muscular dystrophy patients: Altered membrane electrical properties. *Proc Natl Acad Sci USA* **78**:648, 1981.
27. Tahmoush AJ, Askanas V, Nelson PG, Engel WK: Electrophysiologic properties of a neurally cultured muscle from patients with myotonic muscular atrophy. *Neurology* **33**:311, 1983.
28. Renaud JF, Desnuelle C, Schmid-Antomarchi H, Hughes M, Serratrice G, Lazdunski M: Expression of apamin receptor in muscle of patients with myotonic muscular dystrophy. *Nature* **319**:678, 1986.

29. Bell J: Dystrophia myotonica and allied diseases, in Penrose LS (ed): *Treasury of Human Inheritance* Part V. Cambridge, England, Cambridge University Press, 1948.
30. Thomasen E: *Myotonia*. Aarhus, Universitetsforlaget, 1948.
31. Höweler CJ, Busch HFM, Geraedts JPM, Niermeijer MF, Staal A: Anticipation in myotonic dystrophy: Fact or fiction. *Brain* **112**:779, 1989.
32. Harley HG, Brook JD, Floyd J, Rundle SA, Crow S, Walsh KV, Thibault M-C, Harper PS, Shaw DJ: Detection of linkage disequilibrium between the myotonic dystrophy locus and a new polymorphic DNA marker. *Am J Hum Genet* **49**:68, 1991.
33. Harley HG, Brook JD, Rundle SA, Crow S, Reardon W, Buckler AJ, Harper PS, Housman DE, Shaw DJ: Expansion of an unstable DNA region and phenotypic variation in myotonic dystrophy. *Nature* **355**:545, 1992.
34. Yamagata H, Miki T, Ogihara T: Expansion of unstable DNA region in Japanese myotonic dystrophy patients. *Lancet* **339**:692, 1992.
35. Harper PS: The myotonic disorders, in Emery AEA, Rimoin DL (eds): *Principles and Practice of Medical Genetics*, 2d ed. Edinburgh, Churchill Livingstone, 1989.
36. Cobo AM, Baiget M, Lopez de Munain A, Poza JJ, Emparanza JI, Johnson K: Sex-related difference in intergenerational expansion of myotonic dystrophy gene. *Lancet* **341**:1159, 1993.
37. Pinessi L, Bergamini L, Cantello R, Di-Tizio C: Myotonia congenita and myotonic dystrophy: Descriptive epidemiological investigation in Turin, Italy (1955–1979). *Ital J Neurol Sci* **3**:207, 1982.
38. Todorov A, Jéquier M, Klein D, Morton NE: Analyse de la ségregation dans la dystrophie myotonique. *J Genet Hum* **18**:387, 1970.
39. Mathieu J, De Braekeleer M, Prévost C: Genealogical reconstruction of myotonic dystrophy in the Saguenay–Lac-Saint-Jean area. *Neurology* **40**:839, 1990.
40. Fleischer B: Uber myotonischer Dystrophie mit katarakt. *Albrecht von graefes Ztsch Ophthalmol* **96**:91, 1918.
41. Harper PS, Harley HG, Reardon W, Shaw DJ: Anticipation in myotonic dystrophy: New light on an old problem. *Am J Hum Genet* **51**:10, 1992.
42. Penrose LS: The problem of anticipation in pedigrees of dystrophia myotonica. *Ann Eugen (Lond)* **14**:125, 1948.
43. Höweler CJ: *A Clinical and Genetic Study in Myotonic Dystrophy*. University of Rotterdam, 1986, Thesis.
44. Sutherland GR, Haan EA, Kremer E, Lynch M, Pritchard M, Yu S, Richards RI: Hereditary unstable DNA: A new explanation for some old genetic questions? *Lancet* **338**:289, 1991.
45. Caskey CT, Pizzuti A, Fu Y-H, Fenwick RG, Belson DL: Triple repeat mutations in human disease. *Science* **256**:784, 1992.
46. Dyken PR, Harper PS: Congenital dystrophia myotonica. *Neurology* **23**:465, 1973.
47. Clarke A: Genetic imprinting in clinical genetics, in Monk M, Surani A (eds): *Genomic Imprinting*. Cambridge, Company of Biologists, 1990, p 131.
48. Reardon W, Newcombe N, Fenton I, Sibert J, Harper PS: The natural history of congenital myotonic dystrophy: Mortality and long term clinical aspects. *Arch Dis Child* **68**:177, 1993.
49. Renwick JH, Bundey SE, Ferguson-Smith MA, Izatt MM: Confirmation of the linkage of the loci for myotonic dystrophy and ABH secretion. *J Med Genet* **8**:407, 1971.
50. Harper PS, Rivas ML, Bias WBM, Hutchinson JR, Dyken PR, McKusick VA: Genetic linkage confirmed between the loci for myotonic dystrophy, ABH secretion and Lutheran blood group. *Am J Hum Genet* **24**:310, 1972.
51. Whitehead AS, Solomon E, Chambers S, Bodmer WF, Povey S, Fey G: Assignment of the structural gene for the third component of human complement to chromosome 19. *Proc Natl Acad Sci USA*: **79**:5021, 1982.
52. Murray JM, Davies KE, Harper PS, Meredith L, Mueller CR, Williamson R: Linkage relationship of a cloned DNA sequence on the short arm of the X chromosome to Duchenne muscular dystrophy. *Nature* **300**:69, 1982.
53. Shaw DJ, Harper PS: Myotonic dystrophy: Developments in molecular genetics. *Br Med Bull* **45**:745, 1989.
54. Wieringa B, Brunner H, Hulsebost, Stronk D, Ropers HH: Genetic and physical demarcation of the locus for dystrophia myotonica. *Adv Neurol* **48**:47, 1988.
55. Koenig M, Hoffman EP, Bertelson CJ, Monaco AP, Feener C, Kunkel LM: Complete cloning of the Duchenne muscular dystrophy (DMD) cDNA and preliminary genomic organization of the DMD gene in normal and affected individuals. *Cell* **50**:509, 1987.
56. Cawthon RM, Weiss R, Xu G, Viskochil D, Culver M, Stevens J, Robertson M, Dunn D, Gesteland R, O'Connell P, White R: A major segment of the neurofibromatosis type 1 gene: cDNA sequence, genomic structure and point mutations. *Cell* **62**:193, 1991.
57. Shaw DJ, Eiberg H: Report of the committee on the genetic constitution of chromosomes 17, 18 and 19. *Hum Gene Mapping* **9**:242, 1987.
58. Shaw DJ, Meredith AL, Sarfarazi M, Huson SM, Brook JD, Myklebost O, Harper PS: The apoliopoprotein CII gene: Sub-chromosomal localisation and linkage to the myotonic dystrophy locus. *Hum Genet* **70**:271, 1985.
59. Schonk D, Coerwinkel-Dreissen M, Van Dalen I, Oerlemans F, Smeets B, Schepens J, Hulsebos T, Cockburn D, Boyd Y, Davis M, Retting W, Shaw D, Roses A, Ropers H, Wieringa B: Definition of subchromosomal intervals around the myotonic dystrophy gene region at 19q. *Genomics* **4**:384, 1989.
60. Brook JD, Shaw DJ, Thomas NST, Meredith AL, Cowell J, Harper PS: Mapping genetic markers on human chromosome 19 using subchromosomal fragments in somatic cell hybrids. *Cytogenet Cell Genet* **41**:31, 1986.
61. Goss SJ, Harris H: A new method for mapping genes in human chromosomes. *Nature* **255**:680, 1975.
62. Smeets H, Bachinski L, Coerwinkel M, Schepens J, Hoeijmakers J, Duin M, van Grzeschik K-H, Weber CA, de Jong P, Siciliano MJ, Wieringa B: A long range restriction map of the human chromosome 19q13 region: Close physical linkage between CKMM and the ERCC1 and ECRR2 genes. *Am J Hum Genet* **46**:492, 1990.
63. Buxton J, Shelbourne P, Davies J, Jones C, Benjamin Perryman M, Ashizawa T, Butler R, Brook D, Shaw D, de Jong P, Markham A, Williamson R, Johnson K: Characterization of a YAC and cosmid contig containing markers tightly linked to the myotonic dystrophy locus on chromosome 19. *Genomics* **13**:526, 1992.
64. Shutler G, Korneluk RG, Tsilfidis C, Mahadevan M, Bailly J, Smeets H, Jansen G, Wieringa B, Lohman F, Aslanidis C, de Jong PJ: Physical mapping and cloning of the proximal segment of the myotonic dystrophy gene region. *Genomics* **13**:518, 1992.
65. Korneluk RG, MacKenzie AE, Nakamura Y, Dube I, Jacob P, Hunter AGW: A recording of human chromosome 19 long-arm DNA markers and identification of markers flanking the myotonic dystrophy locus. *Genomics* **5**:596, 1989.
66. Stallings RL, Olson E, Strauss AW, Thomspon LH, Bachinski LL, Siciliano MJ: Human creatine kinase genes on chromosomes 15 and 19, and proximity of the gene for the muscle form to the genes for apolipoprotein C2 and excision repair. *Am J Hum Genet* **43**:144, 1988.
67. Kent RB, Fallows DA, Geissler E, Glaser T, Emanuel JR, Lalley PA, Levenson R, Hoiusman DE: Genes encoding a and b subunits of Na^+, K^+-APTase are located on three different chromosomes in the mouse. *Proc Natl Acad Sci USA* **84**:5369, 1987.
68. Harley HG, Brook JD, Jackson CL, Glaser T, Walsh KV, Sarfarazi M, Kent R, Lager M, Koch M, Harper PS, Levenson R, Housman DE, Shaw DJ: Localization of a human Na^+, K^+-ATPase X subunit gene to chromosome 19q21-q13.2 and linkage to the myotonic dystrophy locus. *Genomics* **3**:380, 1988.
69. MacKenzie AE, MacLeod HL, Hunter AGW, Korneluk RG: Linkage analysis of the apolipoprotein C2 gene and myotonic dystrophy on human chromosome 19 reveals linkage disequilibrium in a French-Canadian population. *Am J Hum Genet* **44**:140, 1989.
70. Brook JD, Zemelman BV, Hadingham K, Siciliano MJ, Crow S, Harley HG, Rundle SA, Buxton J, Johnson K, Almond JW, Housman DE, Shaw DJ: Radiation-reduced

hybrids for the myotonic dystrophy locus. *Genomics* **13**:243, 1992.
71. Jansen G, de Jong PJ, Amemiya C, Aslanidis C, Shaw DJ, Harley HG, Brook JD, Fenwick R, Korneluk RG, Tsilfidis C, Shutler G, Hermens R, Wormskamp NGM, Smeets HJM, Wieringa B: Physical and genetic characterization of the distal segment of the myotonic dystrophy area on 19q. *Genomics* **13**:509, 1992.
72. Buxton J, Shelbourne P, Davies J, et al: Detection of an unstable fragment of DNA specific to individuals with myotonic dystrophy. *Nature* **335**:547, 1992.
73. Aslanidis C, Jansen G, Amemiya C, et al: Cloning of the essential myotonic dystrophy region and mapping of the putative defect. *Nature* **255**:548, 1992.
74. Oberlé I, Rousseau F, Heitz D, et al: Amazing instability of a 550bp DNA segment and abnormal methylation in fragile X syndrome. *Science* **252**:1097, 1991.
75. Yu S, Pritchard M, Kremer E, et al: Fragile X genotype characterized by an unstable region of DNA. *Science* **252**:1179, 1991.
76. Brook JD, McCurrach MR, Harley HG, et al: Molecular basis of myotonic dystrophy: Expansion of a trinucleotide (CTG) repeat at the 3′ end of a transcript encoding a protein kinase family member. *Cell* **68**:799, 1992.
77. Fu Y-H, Pizzuti A, Fenwick RG, et al: An unstable triplet repeat in a gene related to myotonic muscular dystrophy. *Science* **255**:1256, 1992.
78. Mahadevan M, Tsilfidis C, Sabourin L, et al: Myotonic dystrophy mutation: An unstable CTG repeat in the 3′ untranslated region of the gene. *Science* **255**:1253, 1992.
79. The Huntington's Disease Collaborative Research Group: A novel gene containing a trinucleotide repeat that is expanded and unstable on Huntington's disease chromosomes. *Cell* **72**:971, 1993.
80. Orr HT, Chung M, Banfi S, Kwiatkowski TJ, Servadio A, Beaudet AL, McCall AE, Duvick LA, Ranum LPW, Zoghbi HY: Expansion of an unstable trinucleotide CAG repeat in spinocerebellar ataxia type 1. *Nat Genet* **4**:221, 1993.
81. La Spada AR, Wilson EM, Lubahn DB, Harding AE, Fischbeck KH: Androgen receptor gene mutations in X-linked spinal and bulbar muscular atrophy. *Nature* **352**:77, 1992.
82. Davies J, Yamagata H, Shelbourne P, Buxton J, Ogihara R, Nokelainer P, Nakagawa M, Williamson R, Johnson K, Miki T: Comparison of the myotonic dystrophy associated CTG repeat in European and Japanese populations. *J Med Genet* **29**:766, 1992.
83. Yamagata H, Miki T, Ogihara T, Nakagawa M, Higushi I, Osame M, Shelbourne P, Davies J, Johnson K: Expansion of unstable DNA region in Japanese myotonic dystrophy patients. *Lancet* **339**:692, 1993.
84. Goldman A, Ramsay M, Jenkins T: Absence of myotonic dystrophy in Southern African Negroids is associated with a significantly lower number of CTG trinucleotide repeats. *J Med Genet* **31**:37, 1994.
85. Harley HG, Rundle SA, Reardon W, Shyring J, Crow S, Brook JD, Harper PS, Shaw DJ: Unstable DNA sequence in myotonic dystrophy. *Lancet* **339**:1125, 1992.
86. Hunter A, Tsilfidis C, Mettler G, Jacob P, Mahadevan M, Surh L, Korneluk R: The correlation of age at onset with CTG trinucleotide repeat amplification in myotonic dystrophy. *J Med Genet* **29**:774, 1992.
87. Ashizawa T, Dubel JR, Dunne PW, et al: Anticipation in myotonic dystrophy: Complex relationships between clinical findings and structure of the GCT repeat. *Neurology* **42**:1877, 1992.
88. Reardon W, Harley HG, Brook JD, Rundle SA, Crow S, Harper PS, Shaw DJ: Minimal expression of myotonic dystrophy: A clinical and molecular analysis. *J Med Genet* **29**:770, 1992.
89. Tsilfidis C, MacKenzie AE, Mettler G, Barcel J, Korneluk RG: Correlation between CTG trinucleotide repeat length and frequency of severe congenital myotonic dystrophy. *Nat Genet* **1**:192, 1992.
90. Harley HG, Rundle SA, MacMillan J, Myring J, Brook JD, Crow S, Reardon W, Fenton I, Shaw DJ, Harper PS: Size of the unstable CTG repeat sequence in relation to phenotype and parental transmission in myotonic dystrophy. *Am J Hum Genet* **52**:1164, 1993.
91. Lavedan C, Hofmann-Radvanyi H, Shelbourne P, et al: Myotonic dystrophy: Size and sex dependent dynamics of CTG meiotic instability and somatic mosaicism. *Am J Hum Genet* **52**:875, 1993.
92. Brunner HG, Jansen G, Nillesen W, Nelen MR, de Die CEM, Höweler CJ, van Oost BA, Wieringa B, Ropers H-H, Smeets HJM: Reverse mutation in myotonic dystrophy. *New Engl J Med* **238**:476, 1993.
93. Abeliovich D, Lerer I, Pashut-Lavon I, Shmueli E, Rass-Rothschild A, Frydman: Negative expansion of the myotonic dystrophy unstable sequence. *Am J Hum Genet* **52**:1175, 1993.
94. Shaw DJ, Harper PS: Workshop report: Myotonic dystrophy—advances in molecular genetics. *Neuromusc Disord* **2**:241, 1992.
95. Imbert G, Kretz C, Johnson K, Mandel J-L: Origin of the expansion mutation in myotonic dystrophy. *Nat Genet* **4**:72, 1993.
96. Mahadevan M, Amemiya C, Jansen G, Sabourin L, Baird S, Neville CE, Wormskamp N, Seegers B, Batzer M, Lamerdin J, De Jong P, Wieringa B, Korneluk R: Structure and genomic sequence of the myotonic dystrophy (DM kinase) gene. *Hum Mol Genet* **2**:299, 1993.
97. Shaw DJ, McCurrach M, Rundle SA, Harley HG, Crow SR, Sohn R, Thirion J-P, Hamshere MG, Buckler AJ, Harper PS, Housman DE, Brook JD: Genomics organisation and transcriptional units at the myotonic dystrophy locus. *Genomics* **18**:673, 1993.
98. Fu Y-H, Friedman DL, Richards S, Pearlman JA, Gibbs RA, Pizzuti A, Ashizawa T, Perryman MB, Scarlato G, Fenwick RG, Caskey CT: Decreased expression of myotonin-protein kinase messenger RNA and protein in adult form of myotonic dystrophy. *Science* **260**:235, 1993.
99. Sabourin LA, Mahedevan MS, Narang M, Lee DSC, Surh LC, Korneluk RG: Effect of the myotonic dystrophy (DM) mutation on mRNA levels of the DM gene. *Nat Genet* **4**:233, 1993.
100. Brewster BS, Jeal S, Strong PN: Identification of a protein product of the myotonic dystrophy gene using peptide specific antibodies. *Biochem Biophys Res Commun* **194**:1256, 1993.
101. Meredith AL, Huson SM, Lunt PW, Sarfarazi M, Harley HG, Brook JD, Shaw DJ, Harper PS: Application of a closely linked polymorphism of restriction fragment length to counselling and prenatal testing in families with myotonic dystrophy. *Br Med J* **293**:1353, 1986.
102. Norman AM, Floyd JL, Meredith AL, Harper PS: Presymptomatic detection and prenatal diagnosis for myotonic dystrophy by means of linked DNA markers. *J Med Genet* **26**:750, 1989.
103. Brunner HG, Smeets HJM, Nillesen W, Van Oost BA, Den Biezenbos M, van Joosten EMG, Pinickers AJLG, Hamel BCJ, Theeuwes AGM, Wieringa B, Ropers H-H: Myotonic dystrophy *Brain* **114**:2303, 1991.
104. Reardon W, Floyd JF, Myring J, Lazarou LP, Meredith AL, Harper PS: Five years experience of predictive testing for myotonic dystrophy using linked DNA markers. *Am J Med Genet* **43**:1006, 1992.
105. Brunner HG, Nillesen M, van Oost BA, Jansen G, Wieringa B, Rogers H-H, Smeets HJM: Presymptomatic diagnosis of myotonic dystrophy. *J Med Genet* **29**:780, 1992.
106. Reardon W, MacMillan JC, Myring J, Harley HG, Rundle SA, Beck L, Harper PS, Shaw DJ: Cataract and myotonic dystrophy: The role of molecular diagnosis. *Br J Ophthalmol* **77**:579, 1993.
107. Myring J, Meredith AL, Harley HG, Koch G, Norbury G, Harper PS, Shaw DJ: Specific molecular prenatal diagnosis for the CTG mutation in myotonic dystrophy. *J Med Genet* **29**:785, 1992.
108. Wöhrle D, Hennig I, Vogel W, Steinbach P: Mitototic stability of fragile X mutations in differentiated cells indicates early post-conception at trinucleotide repeat expansion. *Nat Genet* **4**:140, 1993.
109. Reyniers E, Vits L, de Boule K, Van Roy B, Van Velzen D, de Graaff E, Verkerk A, Jorens HZJ, Darby JK, Oostra B, Willems PJ: The full mutation in the FMR-

1 gene of male fragile X patients is absent in their sperm. *Nat Genet* **4**:143, 1993.

110. MacMillan JC, Myring J, Harley HG, Reardon W, Harper PS, Shaw DJ: Molecular analysis for the myotonic dystrophy mutation in neuromuscular disorders. *Neuromusc Disord* **2**:405, 1992.
111. Harley HG, Phillips MF, Shaw AM, Barnetson RA, MacMillan J, Shaw DJ, Beek L, Harper PS: No increase in the frequency of the myotonic dystrophy mutation in an unselected series of cataract patients. *J Med Genet* 1994. (In press.)
112. Harper PS: *Myotonic Dystrophy*. Philadelphia, WB Saunders, 1979.
113. Appel SH, Roses AD: The muscular dystrophies, in Stanbury JB, Wyngaarden JB, Frederickson DS (eds): *The Metabolic Basis of Inherited Disease* 5th ed. New York, McGraw-Hill, 1983, p 1260.
114. Roses AD, Appel SH: Protein kinase activity in erythrocyte ghosts of patients with myotonic muscular dystrophy. *Proc Natl Acad Sci USA* **70**:1855, 1973.
115. Roses AG, Appel SH: Muscle membrane protein kinase in myotonic muscular dystrophy. *Nature* **250**:245, 1974.
116. Appel SH, Roses AD: Membrane biochemical studies in myotonic dystrophy, in Bolis L, Hoffmann JF, Leaf A (eds): *Membranes and Disease*. New York, Raven, 1976, p 183.
117. Antoku Y, Sakai T, Tsukamoto K, Goto I, Iwashita H, Kuroiwas Y: A study on erythrocyte membrane plasmalogen in myotonic dystrophy. *J Neurochem* **44**:1667, 1985.
118. Barchi RL: Physical probes of biological membranes in studies of muscular dystrophy. *Muscle Nerve* **3**:82, 1989.
119. Lucy JA: Is there a membrane defect in muscle and other cells? *Br Med Bull* **36**:187, 1980.
120. Roses AD, Herbstreith MH, Appel SH: Membrane protein kinase alteration in Duchenne muscular dystrophy. *Nature* **254**:350, 1975.
121. Rudel R, Lehmann-Horn F, Ricker K: The non-dystrophic myotonias, in Engel AG (ed): *Myology*. New York, McGraw-Hill, 1994. (In press.)
122. Lehmann-Horn F, Engel AC, Ricker K, Rudel R: Periodic paralyses and paramyotonia congenita, in Engel AG (ed): *Myology*. New York, McGraw-Hill, 1994. (In press.)
123. Becker PE: Genetic approaches to the nosology of muscular disease: Myotonias and similar diseases. *Birth Defects* **7**:52, 1971.
124. Becker PE: Zur genetik der myotonien, in: *Progressive Muskeldystrophie, Myotonie, Myasthenia*. Berlin, Springer Verlag, 1966, p 247.
125. Becker PE: *Myotonia Congenita and Syndromes Associated with Myotonia*. Stuttgart, Thieme, 1977.
126. Koch M, Harley HG, Sarfarazi M, Zoll B, Harper PS, Bender K, Wienker T: Myotonia congenita (Thomsen's disease) excluded from the region of the myotonic dystrophy locus on chromosome 19). *Hum Genet* **82**:163, 1989.
127. Mehrke G, Brinkmeier H, Jockusch H: The myotonic mouse mutant ADR: Electrophysiology of the muscle fiber. *Muscle Nerve* **11**:440, 1988.
128. Kolb LC: Congenital myotonia in goats. *Bull Johns Hopkins Hosp* **63**:242, 1938.
129. Bryant SH: The electrophysiology of myotonia, with a review of congenital myotonia of goat, in Desmedt JE (ed): *New Developments in Electromyography and Clinical Neurophysiology*, vol 1. Basel, Karger, 1973, p 420.
130. Lipicky RJ, Bryant SH: A biophysical study of the human myotonias, in Desmedt JE (ed): *New Developments in Electromyography and Clinical Neurophysiology*, vol 1. Basel, Karger, 1973, p 451.
131. Adrian RH, Bryant SH: On the repetitive discharge in myotonic muscle fibres. *J Physiol* **240**:505, 1974.
132. Steinmeyer K, Ortland C, Jentsch T: Primary structure and functional expression of a developmentally regulated skeletal muscle chloride channel. *Nature* **354**:301, 1991.
133. Steinmeyer K, Klocke R, Ortland C, Gronomeier M, Jockusch H, Grunder S, Jentsch TJ: Inactivation of muscle chloride channel by transposon insertion in myotonic mice. *Nature* **354**:304, 1991.
134. Koch MC, Steinmeyer K, Lorenz C, Riker K, Wolf F, Otto M, Zoll B, Lehmann-Horn F, Grzeschik KH, Jentsch TJ: The skeletal muscle chloride channel in dominant and recessive human myotonia. *Science* **259**:797, 1992.
135. George AL, Crackower MA, Abdalla JA, Hudson AJ, Ebers GC: Molecular basis of Thomsen's disease (autosomal dominant myotonia congenita). *Nat Genet* **3**:305, 1992.
136. Becker PS: *Paramyotonia Congenita (Eulenberg): Fortschritte der Allgemeinen und Klinischen Humangenetik*. Stuttgart, Georg Thieme, 1970.
137. Streib EW: Paramyotonia congenita: Successful treatment with tocainide. Clinical and electrophysiological findings in seven patients. *Muscle Nerve* **10**:155, 1987.
138. Volosin K, Greenberg RM, Greenspoon AJ: Tocainide associated agranulocytosis. *Am Heart J* **109**:1392, 1985.
139. Armstrong FS: Hyperkalemic familial periodic paralysis (adynamia hyperkalaemic periodic paralysis). *Ann Intern Med* **57**(Suppl 2):455, 1962.
140. Ricker K, Camacho L, Grafe P, Lehmann-Horn F, Rudel R: Adynamia episodica hereditaria: What causes the weakness? *Muscle Nerve* **10**:883, 1989.
141. Ricker K, Bohlen R, Ronkamm R: Different effectiveness of tocainide and hydrochlorothiazide in paramyotonia congenita with hyperkalemic episodic paralysis. *Neurology* **33**:1615, 1983.
142. Cannon SC, Brown RH Jr, Corey DP: A sodium channel defect in hyperkalemic periodic paralysis: Potassium-induced failure of inactivation. *Neuron* **6**:619, 1991.
143. Trimmer JS, Coppermand SS, Tomiko SA, et al: Primary structure and functional expression of a mammalian skeletal muscle sodium channel. *Neuron* **3**:33, 1989.
144. Kallen RG, Sheng ZH, Yang J, et al: Primary structure and expression of a sodium channel characteristic of denervated and immature rat skeletal muscle. *Neuron* **4**:233, 1990.
145. Fontaine B, Khurana TS, Hoffman EP, Bruns GAP, Haines JL, Trofatter JA, Hanson MP, Rich J, MacFarlane H, Yasek DM, Romano D, Gusella JF, Brown RH: Hyperkalemic periodic paralysis and the adult muscle sodium channel alpha-subunit gene. *Science* **250**:1000, 1990.
146. Koch MC, Ricker K, Otto M, Grimm T, Hoffman EP, Rundel R, Bender K, Zoll B, Harper PS, Lehmann-Horn F: Confirmation of linkage of hyperkalemic periodic paralysis to chromosome 17. *J Med Genet* **28**:583, 1991.
147. Koch MC, Ricker K, Otto M, Grimm T, Bender K, Zoll B, Harper PS, Lehmann-Horn F, Rudel R, Hoffman EP: Linkage data suggesting allelic heterogeneity for paramyotonia congenita and hyperkalemic periodic paralysis on chromosome 17. *Hum Genet* **88**:71, 1991.
148. Ptacek LJ, George AL Jnr, Barachi RL, Griggs RC, Riggs JE, Robertson M, Leppert MF: Mutations in an S4 segment of the adult skeletal muscle sodium channel gene cause paramyotonia congenita. *Neuron* **8**:891, 1992.
149. Ptáček LJ, George AL, Griggs RC, Tarwil R, Kallen RG, Barchi RL, Robertson M, Leppert M: Identification of a mutation in the gene causing hyperkalemic periodic paralysis. *Cell* **67**:1021, 1991.
150. Fontaine B, Trofatter J, Rouleau GA, Khurana TS, Haines J, Brown R, Gusella JF: Different gene loci for hyperkalemic and hypokalemic periodic paralysis. *Neuromusc Disord* **14**:235, 1991.
151. Padberg G: *Facioscapulohumeral Disease*. University of Leiden, 1982, MD thesis.
152. Lunt PW, Harper PS: Genetic counselling in facioscapulohumeral muscular dystrophy. *J Med Genet* **28**:655, 1991.
153. Landouzy L, Déjerine J: Dé la myopathie atrophique progressive. *Res Med* **5**:253, 1885.
154. Tomé FMS, Fardeau M: Ocular myopathies, in Eagel AG, Branker BQ (eds): *Myology*. 1986, p 1327.
155. Bailey RO, Marzulo DC, Hans MB: Infantile facioscapulohumeral muscular dystrophy: New observations. *Acta Neurol Scand* **74**:512, 1986.
156. Dubowitz V: *Muscle Disorders in Childhood*. Philadelphia, Saunders, 1978.
157. Fitzsimons RB, Gurwin EB, Bird AC: Retinal vascular abnormalities in facioscapulohumeral muscular dystrophy. *Brain* **110**:631, 1987.
158. Padberg GW, Brouwer OF, de Keizer RJW, Wijmenga C: Retinal vascular disease and perception deafness in facio-

scapulohumeral muscular dystrophy. *J Neurol Sci* **98**(suppl):196, 1990.
159. Furukawa T, Toyokura Y: Chronic spinal muscular atrophy type of facioscapulohumeral dystrophy. *Arch Neurol* **17**:257, 1967.
160. Upadhyaya M, Lunt PW, Sarfarazi M, Broadhead W, Daniels J, Owen M, Harper PS: A closely linked DNA marker for facioscapulohumeral disease on chromosome 4q. *J Med Genet* **28**:665, 1991.
161. Lunt PW, Compston DAS, Harper PS: Estimation of age dependent penetrance in facioscapulohumeral muscular dystrophy by minimising ascertainment bias. *J Med Genet* **26**:755, 1989.
162. MacMillan JC, Harper PS: Single-gene neurological disorders in South Wales: An epidemiological study. *Ann Neurol* **30**:411, 1991.
163. Padberg GW, Eriksson AW, Volkers WS, deLange GG, Wintzen AR: Linkage studies in facioscapulohumeral muscular dystrophy. *Muscle Nerve* **11**:833, 1988.
164. Sarfarazi M, Upadhyaya M, Padberg G, Pericak-Vance M, Siddique T, Lucotte G, Lunt P: An exclusion map for facioscapulohumeral (Landouzy-Dejerine) disease. *J Med Genet* **26**:481, 1989.
165. Wijmenga C, Frants RR, Brouwer OF, Moerer P, Padberg GW: The facioscapulohumeral muscular dystrophy gene maps to chromosome 4. *Lancet* **2**:651, 1990.
166. Weber JL, May PE: Abundant class of human DNA polymorphisms which can be typed using the polymerase chain reaction. *Am J Hum Genet* **44**:388, 1990.
167. Upadhyaya M, Lunt PW, Sarfarazi M, Broadhead W, Farnham J, Harper PS: DNA marker applicable to presymptomatic and prenatal diagnosis of facioscapulohumeral disease. *Lancet* **2**:1320, 1990.
168. Wijmenga C, Padberg GW, Moerer P, Wiegant J, Liem L, Brower OF, Milner ECB, Frantz RR: Mapping of facioscapulohumeral muscular dystrophy gene to chromosome 4q35-qter by multipoint linkage analysis and in situ hybridisation. *Genomics* **9**:570, 1991.
169. Sarfazi M, Wijmenga C, Upadhyaya M, Weiffenbach B, Hyser C, Mathews K, Murray J, Gilbert J, Pericak-Vance M, Lunt P, Frants RR, Jacobsen S, Harper PS, Padberg GW: Regional mapping of facioscapulohumeral muscular dystrophy gene on 4q35: Combined analysis of an international consortium. *Am J Hum Genet* **51**:396, 1992.
170. Upadhyaya M, Lunt P, Sarfarazi M, Broadhead W, Franham J, Harper PS: The mapping of chromosome 4q markers in relation to facioscapulohumeral muscular dystrophy (FSHD). *Am J Hum Genet* **51**:404, 1992.
171. Weiffenbach B, Bagley RG, Falls K, Hyser C, Storvick D, Jacobsen SJ, Schultz P, Mendell JR, van Dijk KW, Milner ECB, Griggs RC: Linkage analyses of five chromosome 4 markers localizes the facioscapulohumeral muscular dystrophy (FSHD) gene to distal 4q35. *Am J Hum Genet* **51**:416, 1992.
172. Sarfarazi M, Wijmenga C, Upadhyaya M, Weiffenbach B, Hyser C, Matthews K, Murray J, Gilbert J, Pericak-Vance M, Lunt P, Frants R, Jacobsen S, Harper PS, Padberg GW: Regional mapping of facioscapulohumeral muscular dystrophy gene on 4q35: combined analysis of an international consortium. *Am J Hum Genet* **51**:396, 1992.
173. Gilbert JR, Stajich JM, Wall S, Carter SC, Qiu H, Vance JM, Stewart CS, Speer MC, Pufky J, Yamaoka LH, Rozear M, Samson F, Fardeau M, Roses AD, Pericak-Vance MA: Evidence for heterogeneity in facioscapulohumeral muscular dystrophy (FSHD) *Am J Hum Genet* **53**:401, 1993.
174. Wijmenga C, Hewitt JE, Sandkuijl LA, Clarke LN, Wright TJ, Dauwerse HG, Gruter A-M, Hofker MH, Moerer P, Williamson R, van Ommen G-J, Padberg GW, Frants RR: Chromosome 4q DNA rearrangements associated with facioscapulohumeral muscular dystrophy. *Nat Genet* **2**:26, 1992.
175. Hewitt JC, Clarke LN, Ivens A, Williamson R: Structure and sequence of the human homeobox gene HOX7. *Genomics* **11**:670, 1991.
176. Wijmenga C, Hewitt JE, Sandkuijl LA, Clarke LN, Wright TJ. *Nat Genet* **2**:26–30.
177. Upadhyaya M, Jardine P, Maynard J, Farnham J, Sarfarazi M, Wijmenga C, Hewitt JE, Frants R, Harper PS, Lunt PW: Molecular analysis of British facioscapulohumeral dystrophy families for 4q DNA rearrangements. *Hum Mol Genet* **2**:981, 1993.
178. Somer H, Voutilainen A, Kaitila I, Rapola J, Leinonen H: Duchenne-like muscular dystrophy in two sisters with normal karyotypes. Evidence for autosomal recessive inheritance. *Clin Genet* **28**:151, 1985.
179. Ben Hamida BM, Marrakchi D: Dystrophie musculaire progressive de type Duchenne en Tunisie: a propos de 13 families et 31 cas d'une forme en apparence recessive autosomique. *J Genet Hum* **28**:9, 1980.
180. Kloepfer HW, Talley C: Autosomal recessive inheritance of Duchenne-type muscular dystrophy. *Ann Hum Genet* **22**:138, 1958.
181. Vainzof M, Pavanello RCM, Pavanello-Filho I, et al: Screening of male patients with autosomal recessive Duchenne dystrophy through dystrophin and DNA studies. *Am J Hum Genet* **39**:38, 1991.
182. Azibi K, Chaouch M, Reghis A, Vinet M-C, Vignal A, Becuwe N, Beckman J, Seboun E, Nguyen S, Cometto M, Fardeau M, Tome R, Leturq F, Chafey P, Bachner L, Kaplan J-C: Linkage analysis of 19 families with autosomal recessive (Duchenne-like) muscular dystrophy from Algeria. (Abstract) *Cytogenet Cell Genet* **58**:1907, 1991.
183. Ben Othmane K, Ben Hamida M, Pericak-Vance MA, Ben Hamida C, Blel S, Carter SC, Bowcock AM, Petrukin K, Gilliam TC, Roses AD, Hentati F, Vance JM: Linkage of Tunisian autosomal recessive Duchenne-like muscular dystrophy to the pericentromeric region of chromosome 13q. *Nat Genet* **2**:315, 1994.
184. Matsumara K, Tomé FMS, Collin H, Azibi K, Chaouch M, et al: Deficiency of the 50k dystrophin-associated glycoprotein in severe childhood autosomal recessive muscular dystrophy. *Nature* **359**:320, 1992.
185. Erb W: Uber die "juvenile form" der progressiven muskelatrophie ihre Beziehungen zur sogennanten Pseudohypertrophie der Muskeln. *Dtsch Arch Klin* **34**:467, 1884.
186. Bushby K: Report on the 12th ENMC sponsored workshop—the "limb-girdle" muscular dystrophies. *Neuromusc Disord* **2**:3, 1992.
187. Yates J, Emery AEH: A population study of early onset limb-girdle muscular dystrophy. *J Med Genet* **22**:250, 1985.
188. Norman A, Thomas N, Coakley J, Harper P: Distinction of Becker from limb-girdle muscular dystrophy by means of dystrophin cDNA probes. *Lancet* **466**:8, 1989.
189. Beckman JS, Richard I, Hillaire D, Broux O, Antignac C, Bois E, Cann H, Cottingham RW Jr, Feingold N, Feingold J, et al: A gene for limb-girdle muscular dystrophy maps to chromosome 15 by linkage. *C R Acad Sci (Paris)* **312**:141, 1991.
190. Jackson CE, Stehler DA: Limb-girdle muscular dystrophy: Clinical manifestations and detection of preclinical disease. *Pediatrics* **41**:494, 1968.
191. Bethlem J, van Wijngaarden GK: Benign myopathy with autosomal dominant inheritance: A report of three pedigrees. *Neurology* **38**:5, 1976.
192. Speer MC, Yamaoka LH, Gilchrist JM, et al: Confirmation of genetic heterogeneity in limb-girdle muscular dystrophy: Linkage of an autosomal dominant form to chromosome 5q. *Am J Hum Genet* **50**:1211, 1992.
193. Love DR, Hill DF, Dickson G, et al: An autosomal transcript in skeletal muscle with homology to dystrophin. *Nature* **339**:55, 1989.
194. Voit T, Haas K, Leger JOC, Pons F, Leger JJ: Xp21 dystrophin and 6q dystrophin-related protein. Comparative immunolocalization using multiple antibodies. *Am J Pathol* **139**:969, 1991.
195. Khurana TS, Watkins SC, Chafey P: Immunolocalization and developmental expression of dystrophin related protein in skeletal muscle. *Neuromusc Disord* **1**:185, 1991.
196. Nguyen TM, Ellis JM, Love DR, Davis KE, Gatter KC, Dickson G, Morris GE: Localization of the DMDL gene-coded dystrophin-related protein using a panel of nineteen monoclonal antibodies: Presence at neuromuscular junctions, in the sarcolemma of dystrophic skeletal muscle, in vascular

and other smooth muscles, and in proliferating brain cell lines. *J Cell Biol* **115**:1695, 1991.

197. Pons F, Augier N, Leger JOC, et al: A homologue of dystrophin is expressed at the neuromuscular junctions of normal individuals and DMD patients, and of normal and mdx mice. Immunological evidence. *FEBS Lett* **282**:161, 1991.
198. Victor M, Hayes R, Adams RD: Oculopharyngeal muscular dystrophy. A familial disease of late life characterized by dysphagia and progressive ptosis of the eyelids. *N Engl J Med* **267**:1267, 1962.
199. Schotland DL, Rowland LP: Muscular dystrophy. Features of ocular myopathy, distal myopathy and myotonic dystrophy. *Arch Neurol* **10**:433, 1964.
200. Tomé FMS, Fardeau M: Ocular myopathies, in Engel AG, Banker BQ (eds): *Myology*. New York, McGraw Hill, 1986, p 1327.
201. Harding AE, Holt IJ: Mitochondrial myopathies. *Br Med Bull* **45**:760, 1989.
202. Barbeau A: Oculopharyngeal muscular dystrophy in French Canada, in Brunette JR, Barbeau A (eds): *Progress in Neuro-Ophthalmology* Vol 2. Amsterdam, Excerpta Medica ICS no 176, p 3.
203. Welander L: Myopathia distalis tarda hereditaria. *Acta Med Scand* **141**:1, 1951.
204. Udd B: Limb-girdle type muscular dystrophy in a large family with distal myopathy: Homozygous manifestation of a dominant gene? *J Med Genet* **29**:383, 1992.
205. Kausch K, Lehmann-Horn F, Grimm T, Janka M, Wieringa B, Mueller CR: Evidence of linkage of the central core disease locus to human chromosome 19q12-13.1. Human gene mapping II. *Cytogenet Cell Genet* **58**:2020, 1991.
206. Laing NG, Majda BT, Akkari PA, Layton MG, Mulley JC, Phillips H, Haan EA, White SJ, Beggs AH, Kunkel LM, Groth DM, Boundy KL, Kneebone CS, Blumbergs PC, Wilton SD, Speer MC, Kakulas BA: Assignment of nemaline myopathy (MIM 161800, NEMI) to chromosome 1. Human gene mapping II. *Cytogenet Cell Genet* **58**:1858, 1991. (abstr.)
207. Denborough MA, Ebeling P, King JO, Zapf PW: Myopathy and malignant hyperpyrexia. *Lancet* **1**:1138, 1970.
208. McCarthy TV, Healy JMS, Heffron JJA, Lehane M, Deufel T, Lehmann-Horn F, Farrall M, Johnson K: Localization of the malignant hyperthermia susceptibility locus to human chromosome 19q12-13.2. *Nature* **343**:562, 1990.
209. MacLennan DH, Duff C, Zorzato F, Fujii J, Phillips M, Korneluk RG, Frodis W, Britt A, Worton RG: Ryanodine receptor gene is a candidate for predisposition to malignant hyperthemia. *Nature* **343**:559, 1990.

CHAPTER 142

Hypertrophic Cardiomyopathy

William J. McKenna ▪ Hugh C. Watkins

1. **Hypertrophic cardiomyopathy (HCM) is a primary muscle disorder characterized clinically by myocardial hypertrophy with hyperdynamic systolic and impaired diastolic function. Typical histology reveals myocyte disorganization with myofibrillar disarray surrounding areas of increased loose connective tissue in up to 35 percent of the myocardium. HCM is usually familial with autosomal dominant inheritance; sporadic cases are uncommon.**
2. **Clinical diagnosis relies on the two-dimensional echocardiographic demonstration of unexplained left ventricular hypertrophy and is problematic when other causes (e.g., systemic hypertension, athletic training) are present, and in children in whom full expression may not occur until adolescent growth is completed.**
3. **The natural history is of a slow progression of symptoms (chest pain, dyspnea) complicated by the development of arrhythmias (atrial fibrillation, ventricular tachycardia) and sudden death. The annual mortality from sudden death is 6 percent in children and adolescents and approximately 2 percent in adults. Initial presentation with sudden death is not uncommon in the young.**
4. **Management aims to improve symptoms and prevent complications, particularly sudden death and arrhythmia-related emboli. Symptomatic treatment with β-blockers or calcium antagonists blunts the heart rate response to exertion and emotion, suppresses the hyperdynamic systolic performance, and may improve diastolic filling. Surgical removal of thickened muscle from the interventricular septum is beneficial when obstruction of the left ventricular outflow tract occurs. In adults, the finding of nonsustained ventricular tachycardia identifies the majority of those at risk of sudden death; in younger patients no such marker has yet been identified. Management for prevention of sudden death targets treatable initiating mechanisms, particularly arrhythmia and ischemia. This remains problematic in young patients.**
5. **Molecular genetic studies have revealed that up to 50 percent of familial HCM is caused by inherited mutations in the β cardiac myosin heavy chain (MHC) gene on chromosome 14 (locus designated CMH1). The mutations involved are missense mutations affecting conserved residues in the globular head or head-rod region of the myosin polypeptide.**
6. **Sporadic HCM can be caused by *de novo* mutations of the β cardiac MHC gene.**
7. **Preclinical diagnosis is possible in families in whom the disease is due to β cardiac MHC gene mutations. Different missense mutations appear to correlate with significantly different survival of affected individuals.**
8. **Two further disease loci have been identified by linkage analysis—CMH2 on chromosome 1q3 and CMH3 on chromosome 15q2. In addition, at least one more disease gene must exist. The identity of the disease genes at CMH2 and CMH3 is unknown; four contractile protein genes are candidate familial HCM genes at locus CMH2. The phenotype of familial HCM in families linked to these loci appears similar to that of families with β cardiac MHC gene mutations.**

A list of standard abbreviations is located immediately preceding the index in each volume. Additional abbreviations used in this chapter include: 2-D = two-dimensional; HCM = hypertrophic cardiomyopathy; LV = left ventricular; LVH = left ventricular hypertrophy; RNase = ribonuclease; SAM = systolic anterior motion (of the mitral valve); VO_{2max} = maximal oxygen ventilatory capacity.

HISTORICAL BACKGROUND

The clinical and morphologic features of hypertrophic cardiomyopathy (HCM) were recognized over 100 years ago in individual patients who undoubtedly had HCM.[1,2] Systematic characterization of such patients, however, was not reported until 1958, when the pathologist Donald Teare described asymmetric hypertrophy in the hearts of nine adolescents and young adults who had died suddenly.[3] Detailed clinical characterization and the recognition of the familial nature of the condition followed shortly.[4] More than 60 names have been given to the condition.[5] These reflect concepts of the disease that arise as a function of the techniques used for assessment.

In the 1960s, a left ventricular (LV) outflow tract gradient that was increased following administration of catecholamine and reduced after administration of phenylephrine was considered to be the essential feature of the condition; thus, idiopathic hypertrophic subaortic stenosis, obstructive cardiomyopathy, and muscular subaortic stenosis were early names applied to the condition.[6] In the 1970s, M-mode echocardiography became widely available. This permitted visualization of the upper anterior septum and LV posterior wall[7–10]—the thickest and thinnest myocardial segments—and thus, the asymmetric nature of the condition was reaffirmed. With the subsequent development of two-dimensional (2-D) echocardiography, the broader spectrum of the condition is now appreciated.[11–13] The majority of patients do not have LV gradients and though asymmetric septal hypertrophy is common, virtually any pattern of LV hypertrophy (LVH) may be found.[6]

DEFINITION

HCM is defined as an idiopathic heart muscle disorder characterized by a hypertrophied and nondilated left and/or right ventricle in the absence of cardiac or systemic cause.[5,14,15] This definition of unexplained myocardial hypertrophy is useful in the clinical and prognostic assessment of patients. It must be recognized, however, that such a diagnosis of exclusion often presents problems. Does the young adult with a blood pressure of 170/95 mmHg and 2.0 cm LVH have one or two diseases? Is 2.0-cm hypertrophy a physiological response in a highly trained athlete? Such diagnostic difficulties, which are not uncommon, illustrate the limitations of the current definition of HCM and underscore the need to determine the molecular basis of the condition.

DIAGNOSIS

The diagnosis of HCM is based on the demonstration of unexplained myocardial hypertrophy, which is best done using 2-D echocardiography; ideally, measurements of wall thickness should exceed 2 SD for age-, sex-, and size-matched populations. This latter consideration may be important as myocardial mass increases with both age and size. In practice, in an adult of normal size, the presence of an LV myocardial segment of 1.5 cm or greater in thickness is usually considered to be diagnostic.[11-13] Isolated right ventricular HCM is extremely rare. When the classic clinical features, including an LV outflow tract murmur, are present, or when more subtle clinical features are associated with a positive family history of the condition, echocardiography may serve only to confirm the diagnosis. More often, however, the history, physical examination, and EKG are equivocal and not diagnostic, and reliance is placed on the 2-D echocardiographic findings.

In children and adolescents, myocardial hypertrophy often develops during growth spurts.[16] Thus, a negative diagnosis made in the young must be tempered by the proviso for a subsequent reassessment. A normal EKG and 2-D echocardiogram after adolescent growth has been completed virtually excludes the diagnosis. Practical problems in diagnosis often arise in highly trained athletes and in patients with mild hypertension in whom the hypertrophic response appears greater than expected from the apparent stimulus. Highly trained athletes normally have an increase in muscle mass with an upward shift of about 3 mm in the bell-shaped curve for the distribution of LV wall thickness.[17,18] The determinants of the hypertrophic response in a patient with hypertension are seldom known. In both groups of subjects, the diagnosis of HCM is more dependent on the total clinical picture. Features that favor the diagnosis include: LVH >1.6 cm, small LV cavity dimensions, an LV outflow tract gradient, and particularly, the presence of HCM in first-degree relatives. In a middle-aged or elderly hypertensive patient with mild symmetrical LVH, it may not be clinically important whether one or two diseases are present. The diagnostic decision in the young athlete, however, could have a significant effect on his or her future career and lifestyle.

CLINICAL GENETICS

Inheritance Patterns in Familial Hypertrophic Cardiomyopathy

Early reports of HCM described single pedigrees suggesting autosomal dominant transmission of familial HCM.[19-22] Pedigree analyses based on current clinical criteria show that the majority of HCM is familial, being inherited as an autosomal dominant trait with a high degree of penetrance. Two comprehensive surveys are those of Maron et al.[23] and Greaves et al.,[24] whose findings are similar. Familial disease was identified in 56 percent and 67 percent, respectively, of the families of probands who had at least three first-degree relatives available for analysis.

Early studies basing diagnoses on clinical features and M-mode echocardiography described pedigrees consistent with autosomal recessive inheritance.[25] These accounts should be interpreted with caution because of the likelihood of diagnostic errors; there are no convincing reports of recessive transmission in families studied with 2-D echocardiography. Demonstration of previously unsuspected disease in parents or offspring has in some instances revealed that families that had appeared to show recessive inheritance were in fact carrying a dominantly expressed gene.[26]

Sporadic Hypertrophic Cardiomyopathy

Individuals with sporadic HCM show typical features of familial HCM but have no affected first-degree relatives.[27,28] In these studies, clinical features were similar in individuals with familial and apparently sporadic disease.[23] Strictly defined instances of sporadic HCM, in which both parents are available for study and are unequivocally unaffected, are not common. The family studies that estimate that up to 40 to 50 percent of HCM is sporadic include many instances in which relatives could not be studied and sporadic HCM was assumed.[23,24] The likelihood of finding familial disease increases with the number of individuals studied. No sporadic disease was found in 13 families that had six or more first-degree relatives available for study.[24] An incorrect diagnosis of sporadic disease can also result from incomplete penetrance, such that an apparently normal parent actually bears a subclinical form of the condition, but this appears to be rare. Equally, apparent sporadic disease can result from unrecognized instances of nonpaternity.

True sporadic cases may occur through etiologically distinct mechanisms. In dominant monogenic disorders, newly arising mutations in the gametes of a parent can manifest as sporadic disease in the offspring; thereafter the likelihood of transmission to the subsequent generation depends on the number of offspring. Molecular genetic analyses (see below) have demonstrated that at least some cases of sporadic HCM arise in this manner. Other mechanisms may also be involved. For example, a somatic mutation during embryogenesis that affects the heart but not the germ line might produce sporadic disease that would not be transmitted to offspring. Potentially, both environmental and genetic processes might be involved in sporadic disease. Environmental influences might perhaps act on a genetic background, conferring susceptibility; such a genetic predisposition could result from the influences of many genes.

Gene Penetrance and Phenotypic Expression

Penetrance in familial HCM is age-related, with the clinical manifestations of the disease typically developing in adolescence. Even within an adult population, penetrance may not be complete. A numerical estimate of penetrance, based on the observed incidence of disease among first-degree relatives compared with the expected incidence, is hard to obtain due to small sample size and variation in the sensitivity of diagnostic criteria. For the purposes of the genetic linkage analyses detailed below, an estimate for penetrance of $p = 0.95$ was used for family members of 16 years or older.

Mendelian inheritance in familial HCM indicates that all affected members of a given family bear an identical gene defect. However, the defect need not be the same in unrelated families with familial HCM. Either a different mutation within the same gene or a mutation in another gene could be responsible. The variable expression characteristic of familial HCM is a frequent finding in single-gene disorders and hence does not necessarily predict the presence of more than one gene. In addition, intrafamilial variation of expression is sometimes as marked as interfamilial variation.[11] Differences of expression may result from interaction with the environment and/or other genes carried by the individual or through the influence of random chance. There is evidence that at least some part of this effect is not genetic in origin, in that three pairs of monozygotic twins with HCM have been reported, each with widely differing degrees of clinical severity in the two twins.[29–31]

PATHOLOGY

Macroscopic

Although asymmetric septal hypertrophy was emphasized in Teare's original pathological report[3] and by subsequent M-mode echocardiographic studies,[7–10] it is now clear that HCM can occur in many other forms[11–13] and may involve the left, right, or both ventricles.[32,33] Hypertrophy is usually symmetric in the right ventricle,[33] but in the left ventricle it may be symmetric or asymmetric, involving the septum, free wall, posterior wall, or occasionally being isolated to the distal ventricle.[11–13,34] A patch of endocardial thickening just below the aortic valve resulting from contact with the anterior mitral leaflet is often found in patients with reduced LV dimensions, particularly that of the outflow tract.[34]

Histology

The histologic findings in HCM are distinctive and provide an almost specific morphology.[35] Within areas of affected myocardium, there is considerable interstitial fibrosis with gross disorganization of the muscle bundles resulting in a characteristic whorled pattern[36] (Fig. 142-1). The cell-to-cell orientation of muscle cells is lost (disarray) and there is disorganization of the myofibrillar architecture within a given cell.[37] Myocardial cells are wide, short, and often bizarre in shape. Foci of disorganized cells are often interspersed among areas of hypertrophied muscle cells that are otherwise normal in appearance. Although these changes are diagnostic, they are not completely specific because there is some malarrangement but no other histologic abnormality found at the junction of the septum with the anterior and posterior walls of the left ventricle in normal subjects,[38] and congenitally abnormal hearts may also show fiber disarray.[39] Although the absolute specificity of these histologic changes has been a matter of controversy, experienced pathologists agree that given the whole heart at autopsy the diagnosis is not usually difficult to make.[34,35] Occasionally, these histologic findings are found in first-degree relatives, in whom the hearts do not appear to have any macroscopic abnormality, are not hypertrophied, and do not have increased muscle mass.[40] Such families highlight a limitation of the current definition based on the demonstration of unexplained LVH, and indicate that hypertrophy is not the *sine qua non* of the condition.

PATHOPHYSIOLOGY

Myocardial disarray and hypertrophy, hyperdynamic systolic function, and impaired diastolic function account for many of the clinical features of HCM. The extent and distribution of myocardial disarray are determined post mortem; at present, they cannot be readily assessed during life. It is probable that the disorganized architecture with abnormal myofiber and myofibrillar alignment provides a substrate for electrical instability and contributes to diastolic abnormalities.[40] The precise relation of myocardial disarray with spontaneous arrhythmia and the threshold for ventricular fibrillation have not been established. The severity of myocardial hypertrophy can be readily assessed with 2-D echocardiography. It is uncertain whether the development of myocardial disarray and of myocardial hypertrophy are unrelated responses to a molecular and/or a developmental abnormality or are contingent on each other.[41] The recognition of patients who have severe LVH and minimal disarray and those who have severe disarray and minimal hypertrophy is consistent with the former hypothesis.[40]

Most patients have evidence of hyperdynamic systolic function with rapid, early, and near-complete ventricular emptying.[4,42] As LVH is usually prominent, such changes may be secondary to myocardial hypertrophy; some patients, however, have hyperdynamic systolic function with minimal

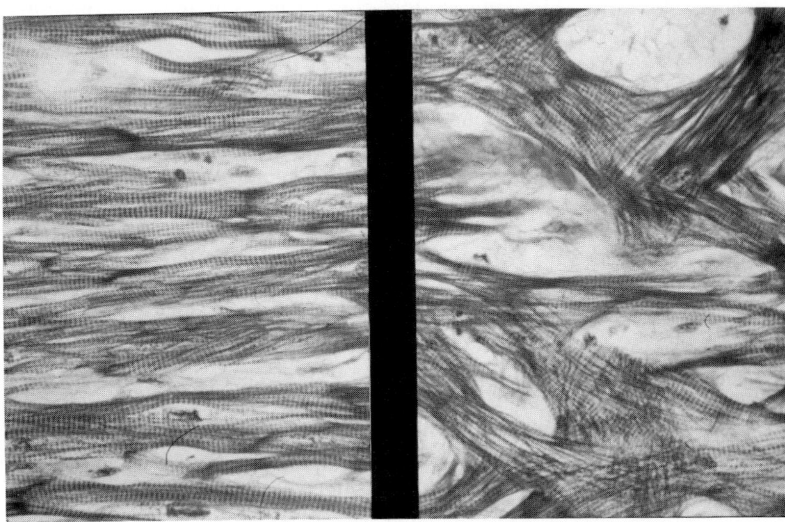

FIG. 142-1 Myofibrillar stain from a normal (left) and a 23-year-old girl with HCM who died suddenly (right) showing myocyte disorganization and myofibrillar disarray surrounding areas of increased loose connective tissue.

hypertrophy, suggesting the presence of other abnormalities, such as altered handling of calcium by the myocardium.[43–46] Approximately 30 percent of patients with hyperdynamic systolic function have recordable gradients at rest between the body and outflow tract of the left ventricle; such a gradient develops in an additional 20 to 25 percent following maneuvers that increase myocardial contractility or result in a decrease in ventricular volume with reduced afterload or venous return.[47] The mechanism and significance of such gradients have been subjects of controversy.[48,49] Many workers have claimed that the development of an LV gradient in close temporal association with the development of systolic anterior motion of the mitral valve and a fall in peak aortic velocity represents impediment or obstruction to LV emptying.[48] Another view is that gradients are generated by a dynamic left ventricle that has almost completely emptied.[49] Interpretation of the significance of an LV gradient in an individual patient requires knowledge of the relative volume ejected by the onset of the gradient.[50,51] In the majority of patients with resting LV gradients, at least 70 percent of stroke volume has already been ejected by the onset of the gradient,[51,52] and the end-systolic dimension is small. The controversy over LV gradients has dominated the interest of many investigators, to the detriment of more important issues, including the mechanism and prevention of sudden death and the molecular genetics and pathogenesis of the condition.

Diastolic abnormalities are common, although less obvious.[42,53–55] The period during which the heart is isovolumic (end systole and early diastole) is prolonged, filling is slow, and the proportion of filling volume that results from atrial systolic contraction may be increased. Occasionally, there is early rapid filling with restrictive physiology that resembles the situation in patients with constrictive pericarditis or endocardial fibrosis. It is seldom possible to identify the predominant pathophysiological mechanism of altered diastolic function because most patients have myocardial hypertrophy—evidence suggestive of ischemic as well as architectural abnormalities including myocardial disarray and fibrosis.

CLINICAL FEATURES

History

The condition is more often diagnosed in younger men and older women. Symptomatic presentation may be at any stage, with breathlessness on exertion, chest pain, syncope, or sudden death. Occasionally, HCM is found at autopsy in a stillborn infant or presents during infancy with cardiac failure that is usually fatal.[28] In children and adolescents, the diagnosis is most often made with sudden death as the initial presentation or during screening of sibs and offspring of affected family members.[56,57] Paroxysmal symptoms or mild impairment of exercise tolerance are often present, but in the absence of a murmur may not elicit a diagnostic cardiac evaluation. Approximately 50 percent of consecutive adult patient populations present with symptoms,[47] whereas in the remainder the diagnosis is made during family screening or following the incidental detection of an abnormality on physical, electrocardiographic, or echocardiographic examination.

Approximately 50 percent of patients experience dyspnea,[4,47] which is thought to be a consequence of elevated LV diastolic, left atrial, and pulmonary venous pressures resulting from impaired ventricular relaxation and filling. However, in one study, there was no relationship between an objective measurement of maximal exercise capacity and pulmonary capillary wedge pressures, indicating that, as for patients with cardiac failure, other mechanisms such as control of muscle energetics and blood flow and central perception of breathlessness may be important.[58] Approximately 50 percent of patients complain of chest pain that is exertional, atypical, or both in similar proportions of patients.[47,59] Atypical pain may have no obvious precipitant; more commonly, it follows exercise or anxiety-related tachycardia when it persists for up to several hours after the stress has been removed without enzymatic evidence of myocardial damage.[59] Speculation over the mechanism of chest pain in HCM continues; the increased metabolic demand of the greatly increased muscle mass in association with decreased diastolic perfusion of subendocardial layers, resulting from a relative increase in coronary impedance from poorly relaxing muscle and from narrowed small intramural coronary arteries, may contribute to it.[60] Approximately 15 to 25 percent of patients have experienced syncopal episodes; only in a minority are there findings suggestive of an arrhythmia or evidence of overt conduction disease.[47,61] In most patients, the mechanism cannot be determined. The surgical experience of workers in Düsseldorf is of interest. After successful myotomy/myectomy, their results have shown a greatly reduced incidence of syncope. These findings are consistent with a hemodynamically related mechanism,[61] but the view that syncope is related to an inability to increase cardiac output during exercise appears to be too simplistic. Syncopal episodes can occur at rest or during normal daily activities and can develop in patients whose cardiac output response during exercise is normal.[62] Rarely, patients present with symptoms attributable to left or right heart failure with paroxysmal nocturnal dyspnea, cough, ascites, or peripheral edema. Thus, there is a wide spectrum of clinical presentation in HCM, from severe cardiac failure in infancy to an incidental finding that may occur at any age.

PHYSICAL EXAMINATION

In the majority of patients with HCM, the physical examination is unremarkable and the detection of abnormalities depends on the elucidation of subtle physical signs. The majority of patients have a rapid upstroke arterial pulse, best felt in the carotid area, which reflects dynamic LV emptying. In children and adolescents, this pulse may be difficult to distinguish from normality, whereas in the elderly, the normal pulse transmitted by noncompliant atheromatous vessels may appear to have a rapid upstroke. The majority of patients also have a forceful LV cardiac impulse, best appreciated on full held expiration in the left lateral position. In about one-third of patients the jugular venous pulse may demonstrate a prominent "a" wave, reflecting diminished right ventricular compliance secondary to right ventricular hypertrophy. The first and second heart sounds are usually normal, and, unless patients are in atrial fibrillation, there is either a loud fourth heart sound (reflecting increased atrial systolic flow into a noncompliant ventricle) or a palpable atrial beat (reflecting forceful atrial systolic contraction that may or may not be associated with significant forward flow of blood). The most obvious physical sign in HCM is an ejection systolic murmur present only in patients (one-third) who have a resting LV-outflow-tract gradient. It is best heard at the left sternal border radiating toward the aortic and mitral areas, but not into the neck or the axilla. The intensity of outflow-tract murmurs varies with changes in ventricular volume; it can be increased by physiological and pharmacologic maneuvers that decrease afterload or venous return (amyl nitrate, standing, Valsalva) and decreased by maneuvers that increase afterload and venous return (squatting, phenylephrine). Occasionally, ejection systolic murmurs are associated at their onset with an ejection sound. The majority of patients with an LV gradient also have mild mitral regurgitation that may be difficult to distinguish by auscultation. Doppler examination reveals that mitral regurgitation usually begins just before (30 to 40 ms) the onset of the gradient and continues for the duration of systole. Radiation of the systolic murmur to the axilla is often the best auscultatory clue to the presence of coexistent mitral regurgitation. Occasionally, mitral regurgitation may be moderate to severe either alone or in association with an LV-outflow-tract gradient. A middiastolic rumble may result from increased transmitral flow in patients with severe mitral regurgitation; more commonly, it occurs in isolation, presumably reflecting inflow-tract turbulence. Early diastolic murmurs of aortic incompetence may develop following surgical myotomy/myectomy or infective endocarditis involving the aortic valve. Although such murmurs are rare in the absence of such complications, they appear to occur more commonly than would be expected by chance and may reflect traction of the noncoronary cusp of the aortic valve by the septum. An ejection systolic murmur in the pulmonary area, reflecting right-ventricular-outflow-tract obstruction, is also uncommon; when present, it is usually associated with severe biventricular hypertrophy and is more commonly seen in the young.[56,57]

INVESTIGATIONS

Cardiologic evaluation of patients with HCM is performed to confirm or make the diagnosis, to characterize the functional and morphologic features in order to guide symptomatic therapy, and to assess the risk of complications, particularly that of sudden death.

Electrocardiography

The 12-lead EKG is normal in 5 percent of symptomatic patients and in 25 percent of asymptomatic patients, particularly those who are young.[4,63] At the time of diagnosis, 10 percent of patients are in atrial fibrillation, 20 percent have left-axis deviation, and 5 percent have right bundle branch block pattern.[47,63] The majority of patients have an intraventricular conduction delay, but complete left bundle branch block pattern is rare; it may develop following surgery and as a late complication. ST-segment depression and T-wave changes are the most common abnormalities and are usually associated with voltage changes of LVH and/or deep S waves in the anterior chest leads V_1 to V_3.[63] Occasionally, giant negative T waves are seen.[64,65] Repolarization changes alone or isolated voltage criteria for LVH are unusual. Approximately 20 percent of patients have abnormal Q waves either inferiorly (2, 3, and aVF) or less commonly in leads V_1 to V_3. The distribution of the PR interval is similar to that in the normal population but occasionally a short PR interval may be associated with a slurred upstroke to the QRS complex, similar to that seen in the Wolff-Parkinson-White syndrome. At electrophysiological study, such changes are not usually associated with evidence of preexcitation, although patients with HCM and accessory pathways have been described.[66,67] P-wave abnormalities of left and/or right atrial overload are common, reflecting the difficulties faced by the atria in emptying their contents into poorly relaxing, stiff ventricles. As there are so many electrocardiographic abnormalities, there is no EKG typical of HCM; a useful rule is to consider the diagnosis whenever the EKG is bizarre, particularly in younger patients.

In adults, arrhythmias are common during 48-h ambulatory electrocardiographic monitoring.[68,69] Nonsustained ventricular tachycardia is detected in 25 to 30 percent of adults. Although this arrhythmia is invariably asymptomatic, its presence represents an approximately sevenfold increased risk of sudden death over those who do not have nonsustained ventricular tachycardia.[69–73] Established atrial fibrillation is detected in 10 to 15 percent of consecutive patient populations; a further 30 to 35 percent will have episodes of paroxysmal atrial fibrillation or supraventricular tachycardia.[68,69] Sustained supraventricular arrhythmias (>30 s) are poorly tolerated unless the ventricular response is controlled; they carry an increased risk of embolism.[74] In contrast, most children and adolescents are in sinus rhythm, and arrhythmias during ambulatory EKG monitoring are uncommon.[75] The increased incidence of supraventricular arrhythmias with age is not surprising; the development of these arrhythmias is related to increased echocardiographic left atrial dimensions and increased LV end-diastolic pressure, both of which increase with age.[68,69,76–78] The etiology of nonsustained ventricular arrhythmias is not known, but it may relate to myocyte necrosis and myocardial fibrosis that appear to be related to age. The occurrence of documented sustained ventricular tachycardia is rare.[79] The optimal duration and the method of EKG monitoring to detect asymptomatic but prognostically important ventricular arrhythmia depend on the frequency with which episodes occur. Ventricular arrhythmias have been shown to have a marked biologic variability; at initial evaluation of a patient, 5 days of EKG monitoring is necessary to ensure at least a 75 percent chance of not missing nonsustained ventricular tachycardia.[80] The recommendation of 48 h represents a pragmatic compromise that is unlikely to give rise to an important sampling error.[71,80]

Chest X-Ray Study

Chest x-ray films may be normal or show evidence of left and/or right atrial or LV enlargement; if left atrial pressure has been chronically elevated, there may be redistribution of blood flow to upper lung zones, with interstitial changes including Kerley B lines. Mitral valve annular calcification is not uncommon. Aortic valve calcification is not seen; when present, it suggests a diagnosis of aortic stenosis rather than HCM.

Two-Dimensional Echocardiography/Doppler

2-D echocardiography is used to assess the severity and distribution of myocardial hypertrophy. LVH may be symmetric or asymmetric and localized to the septum, the free wall, or most commonly, to both the septum and free wall with relative sparing of the posterior wall (Fig. 142-2). In Japan, "apical" HCM appears to be common[64,81]; in the West, hypertrophy confined to the apex is rare, although approximately 10 percent of patients have LVH that is maximal in the distal ventricle from the level of the papillary muscles down to the apex.[13,82] Approximately one-third of patients also have hypertrophy of the right ventricular free wall; the severity of right ventricular hypertrophy is strongly

Asymmetrical Hypertrophy

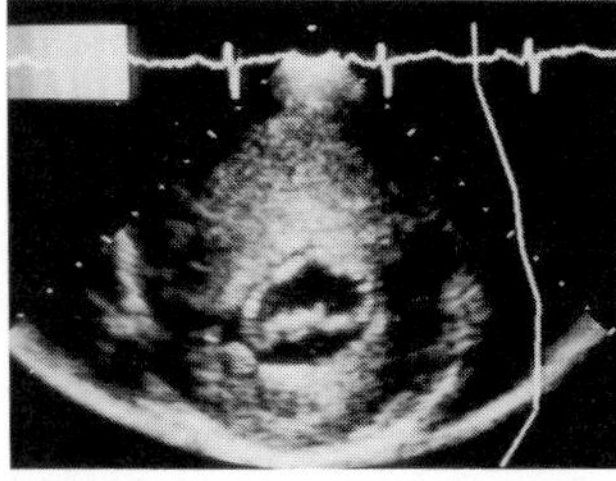

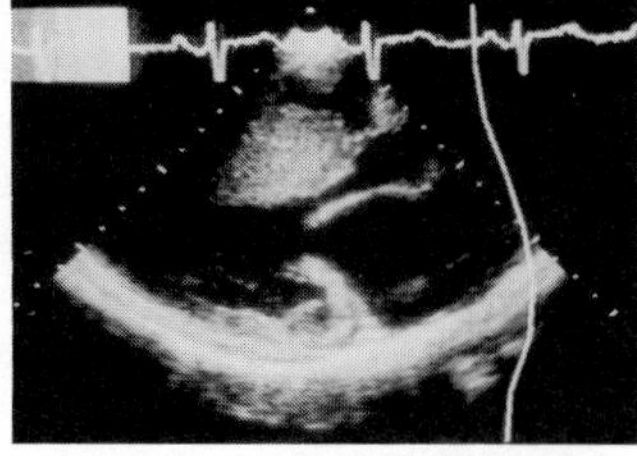

A

Symmetrical Hypertrophy

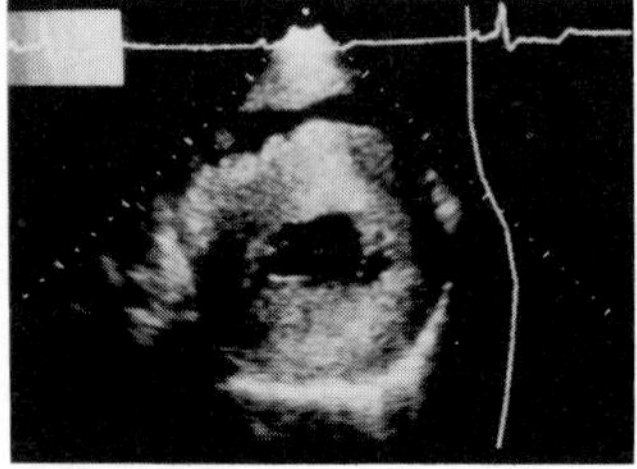

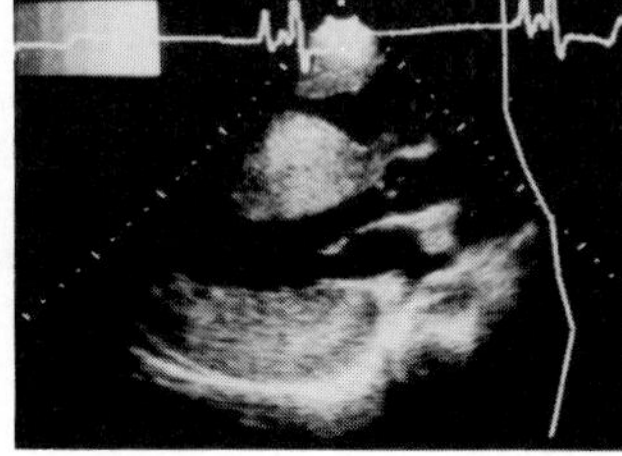

B

FIG. 142-2 2-D echocardiograms showing asymmetrical and symmetrical hypertrophy in short-axis (left) and parasternal long-axis views (right) of the left ventricle. In the view demonstrating asymmetric hypertrophy (*A*), the interventricular septum is thickened relative to the posterior wall, while the view demonstrating symmetric hypertrophy (*B*) shows concentric thickening of approximately 3.5 cm. Diastolic frames are shown with the mitral valve leaflets open.

related to the severity of LVH.[33] Typically, LV end-systolic and end-diastolic dimensions are reduced, and the left atrial dimension is increased, while indexes of systolic function, such as ejection fraction and velocity of fiber shortening, are increased. The LV outflow tract appears narrowed, particularly when there is gross upper septal hypertrophy, and right ventricular dimensions are normal. Color Doppler scanning provides a sensitive method of detecting LV-outflow-tract turbulence, and when combined with continuous-wave Doppler scanning, the peak velocity of LV blood flow can be measured and LV-outflow-tract gradients calculated by the modified Bernoulli equation[83–85]:

$$\text{pressure gradient (mmHg)} = 4V_{max^2}$$

Doppler gradients correlate well with those measured invasively. When the calculated outflow-tract gradient is >30 mmHg, systolic anterior motion of the mitral valve is usually present.[86,87] This is best demonstrated on M-mode recordings, which have the advantage of being able to time cardiac events when recorded on fast paper speed. Measurement of the time from the onset of systolic anterior motion of the mitral valve (SAM) to the onset of SAM-septal contact (x) and the duration of SAM-septal contact (y) provides another reliable noninvasive method for estimation of the pressure gradient,[88,89] where the gradient = $(y/x)25 + 25$ mmHg. Early closure or fluttering of the aortic valve leaflets and Doppler evidence of mitral regurgitation are often seen in association with SAM. Contrary to earlier reports, SAM is found in other conditions associated with LVH and hyperdynamic systolic performance.[90]

Exercise Testing

Maximal exercise testing is simple, noninvasive, and provides useful functional and possibly prognostic information. When used in association with respiratory gas analysis, it provides an objective assessment of exercise capacity that can be monitored serially. Maximal oxygen ventilatory capacity (VO_{2max}) is moderately reduced even in patients who claim their exercise tolerance is not limited.[58] Careful measurement of the blood pressure every minute or, if possible, continuously during exercise reveals that approximately one-third of patients have abnormal blood pressure response, with drops of 25 to 150 mmHg from peak recordings.[62] In the majority of patients, such changes are asymptomatic, but preliminary observations suggest that they are likely to be of prognostic significance. The mechanism of the hypotensive response during exercise in HCM is not known. The finding of an increased cardiac output with decreased systemic vascular resistance suggests it may be related to altered baroreflex control of blood flow.[62] ST-segment changes of 2 mm from base line are documented in 25 percent of patients and associated with symptoms of angina. The relation of such changes to ischemia and thallium defects requires further evaluation, and their prognostic significance has yet to be determined.[91]

Cardiac Catheterization

The combination of 2-D echocardiography and Doppler scanning has replaced cardiac catheterization of hemodynamic measurements and angiography as the method of assessing LV structure and function in patients' HCM. It is not necessary to perform cardiac catheterization for diagnosis; it is rarely indicated, unless symptoms are refractory and the direct measurement of cardiac pressures may be informative, particularly in assessing the severity of mitral regurgitation. Cardiac catheterization for the purpose of performing coronary arteriography is often necessary in patients older than 40 years of age who have significant angina or ST-segment changes during exercise. Typically, LV end-diastolic pressure, the mean left atrial pressure, and mean pulmonary capillary wedge pressure are elevated as consequences of abnormal LV diastolic filling and reduced compliance.[4] Cardiac output may be reduced, normal, or occasionally increased.[4] In approximately one-third of patients, there is a pressure gradient at rest between the body and outflow tract of the left ventricle. Such gradients are usually relatively stable but may be labile, and intraventricular pressures of up to 300 mmHg have been recorded.[92] In a small proportion of patients (<15 percent), a right ventricular infundibular gradient of >10 mmHg may be recorded.[4] Typically, right ventricular and end-diastolic and mean right atrial pressures are mildly to moderately elevated.

Left ventricular angiography reveals an abnormally shaped ventricle that typically ejects at least 75 percent of its contents in association with mild mitral regurgitation. Papillary muscles may occasionally be very prominent and obliterate the LV cavity in late systole. Usually, the left coronary arteries are large in caliber. The left anterior descending and septal perforator arteries may demonstrate phasic narrowing during systole in the absence of fixed obstructive lesions; such changes do not relate to symptoms.[93]

NATURAL HISTORY

The natural history of HCM is one of slow progression of symptoms, gradual deterioration of LV function, and a significant incidence of sudden death occurring at all ages.[94]

Data from tertiary referral centers indicate that the annual mortality from sudden death in adults is about 2.5 percent, whereas in children and adolescents it is at least 6 percent,[47,95,96] and it is even greater in those who have recurrent syncope or a family history of multiple sudden deaths from HCM[56,57,97,98] (Fig. 142-3). Although the mortality figures from nonreferral hospitals are lower, the risk of sudden death is still present.[99,100] In "low-risk" children and adolescents in whom the diagnosis of HCM was made during routine family screening or who came to medical attention because of paroxysmal symptoms or an asymptomatic murmur, the annual mortality was approximately 4 percent in two consecutive patient populations between 1960 and 1985.[75,97] Autopsy studies reveal that unsuspected HCM is the most common cause of sudden death in competitive athletes.[101,102]

Symptomatic deterioration is usually slow and associated with a gradual reduction in LV systolic performance; in the majority, the rate of deterioration is not disproportionate to other system changes with age.[76,77] Occasionally, symptomatic deterioration may be associated with progressive myocardial wall thinning, presumably reflecting myocyte necrosis and fibrosis that causes severe reduction in LV systolic performance and/or diastolic filling.[103] In such patients, end-diastolic volume increases, but even in the end stages it rarely exceeds "normal" limits; thus, such patients resemble those who have dilated cardiomyopathy mainly in the degree of impairment of systolic performance. Occasionally, patients who experience such a deterioration may present with a clinical picture resembling that of restrictive cardiomyopathy with grossly enlarged atria, signs of right heart failure, and relative preservation of left ventricular systolic performance.

Data from serial EKG revealed increased QRS voltage in 20 percent of adults, suggesting that LVH was progressive in a subset of patients.[104] However, serial echocardiographic assessment of adults has not confirmed these electrocardiographic findings.[105] The development of atrial fibrillation has long been considered to be associated with dramatic symptomatic deterioration and to indicate a poor prognosis.[92,106] One retrospective study revealed that 5-year survival in those with atrial fibrillation was similar to that of age- and sex-matched patients who remained in sinus rhythm, and symptomatic status remained stable if the ventricular response was controlled and emboli were prevented.[74] Indeed, most patients in whom atrial fibrillation develops have previously had a palpable atrial beat in the absence of a fourth heart sound, reflecting forceful atrial contraction but minimal atrial systolic contribution to filling volume.

PROGNOSIS

The major problems in the management of HCM are the identification of high-risk patients and the prevention of sudden death. In adults, the presence of nonsustained ventricular tachycardia during EKG monitoring is associated with, although probably does not cause, sudden death, and it is the best single marker of high risk, with a sensitivity of 69 percent and a specificity of 80 percent.[69–71] However, the positive predictive accuracy of ventricular tachycardia as a marker is low (22 percent), reflecting the fact that most patients with ventricular tachycardia do not die suddenly. Thus, further risk stratification of this subgroup would be helpful because a policy of aggressive therapy may include patients at relatively lower risk.[71,72] In adults, no other clinical feature is associated with or predictive of sudden death, including symptoms, LV wall thickness, filling pressures, or the presence of an LV gradient.[47,102] Children and adolescents who have experienced recurrent syncope and those who have two or more sibs with HCM who have died suddenly are clearly at increased risk.[97,98] The majority of young patients who die suddenly, however, have not experienced syncope, nor do they have a malignant family history of HCM.[75,97] The young pose problems in terms of both identification and therapy. Most are asymptomatic and many are athletic; even those at apparently low risk have an annual mortality from sudden death of 4 percent. For those with marked hypertrophy, significant gradients, arrhythmias, or adverse family history, the recommendation to abstain from competitive sports is precautionary but often

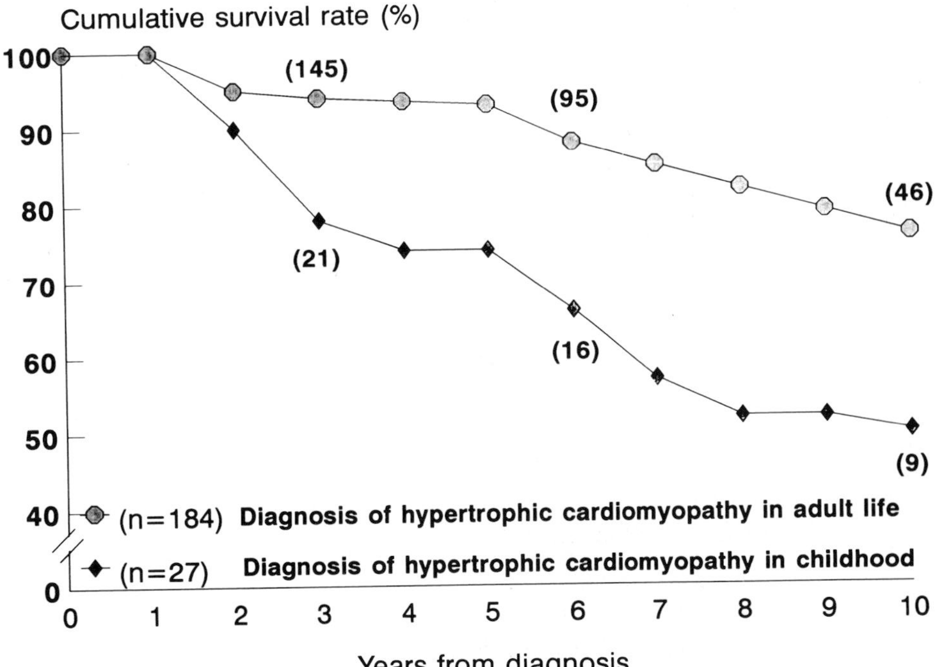

FIG. 142-3 Cumulative survival curve from the year of diagnosis for 211 medically treated patients. The probability of death = the total number of deaths for the year divided by the adjusted number at risk minus the number of deaths due to other causes. (*From McKenna et al.*[47] *Used by permission.*)

imposes a significant limitation on the lifestyle of a child, adolescent, or young adult.[107]

The ability to identify patients who are at increased risk depends on understanding the likely mechanisms of sudden death. There is evidence to suggest that hemodynamic deterioration with reduced stroke volume following a physiological tachycardia,[108] an arrhythmia,[75,109] or reduction in venous return or hypotension developing in the presence of a normal stroke volume but altered baroreflex control of peripheral blood flow are all possible initiating mechanisms.[62] The outcome (survival vs. sudden death) must be influenced by the underlying electrical stability of the myocardium, which it is reasonable to speculate is related to the extent of myocardial disarray. In adults, nonsustained ventricular tachycardia is a marker of electrical instability; in younger patients, no such marker has yet been identified.

MANAGEMENT

Symptomatic Treatment

Pharmacologic. The goal of therapy is to improve symptoms and prevent complications, especially sudden death. β-Adrenoceptor blockers, particularly propranolol, and calcium antagonists, especially verapamil, are the mainstay of pharmacologic therapy for both chest pain and dyspnea. Both propranolol and verapamil have several potentially beneficial actions, including a decrease in the determinants of myocardial oxygen consumption and thus of angina pectoris and blunting of the heart-rate response during exercise to provide increased time for filling at equivalent workloads in those with poor relaxation and slow filling. Both agents exert a negative inotropic effect, reducing hyperdynamic systolic function and LV gradients[110,111]; it is also claimed they improve diastolic filling—verapamil by improving relaxation[42,45,55,112] and propranolol by increasing compliance.[113] Such changes appear to occur in some patients receiving propranolol[113]; the effect of verapamil is more consistent and is associated with increased exercise duration in about two-thirds of patients.[42,45] Exertional chest pain usually responds to therapy with propranolol or verapamil, but when it is refractory, very high doses (propranolol, 480 mg daily; verapamil, 720 mg daily) have been beneficial.[43,114] Experience with disopyramide is limited, but in a small group of patients with reduced exercise capacity and LV-outflow-tract obstruction, LV gradients and filling pressures were reduced and symptoms of angina and dyspnea were improved.[115] Both propranolol and verapamil are usually well tolerated, and the beneficial effects outweigh the unwanted effects. None of the side effects of propranolol are serious; however, the suppressant effect of verapamil on impulse formulation and atrioventricular nodal conduction may cause problems in patients with unsuspected preexisting conduction disease, and its vasodilatory and negative inotropic effects have resulted in acute pulmonary edema and death.[116] It is not clear which patients are at particular risk for such detrimental hemodynamic effects from verapamil developing; the recommendation to avoid giving verapamil to patients who are obviously at high risk with increased filling pressures, paroxysmal nocturnal dyspnea, or orthopnea would eliminate the patients in greatest need of therapy.[116] In practice, both drugs are effective, but it is safer to use propranolol. If it is ineffective, verapamil can then be tried; in high-risk patients, verapamil should be started in the hospital. The results of preliminary studies with diltiazem are consistent with those in the extensive clinical experience with verapamil.[117] Nifedipine has also been shown to improve diastolic function by increasing compliance without significantly altering systolic performance[118]; however, the clinical experience has been disappointing and complicated by the effects of peripheral vasodilatation.[119] The potential role of β-blockers with intrinsic sympathomimetic activity in patients with impaired diastolic function has not been assessed. Dual demand pacing with short atrioventricular delay to alter the sequence of ventricular electrical activation has been advocated; selection of appropriate patients remains to be established.

Surgical. Surgery offers another major therapeutic option, with a reported experience in over 1000 patients.[94,120,121] The majority of patients operated on have had an LV-outflow-tract gradient and been refractory to medical therapy. The most common operation has been to remove a segment of the upper anterior septum (myotomy/myectomy) via a transaortic approach. Transventricular approaches have also been used but are associated with a higher incidence of late complications, particularly of cardiac failure. Despite this large experience, even in the most experienced hands, the operation carries a perioperative mortality of 5 to 10 percent.[95] Successful surgery confers symptomatic and hemodynamic (reduced LV gradient and filling pressures) improvement and is a useful therapeutic alternative for patients who are refractory to medical therapy. It is not known which patients will die and why others benefit; the optimal patient population for myotomy/myectomy has not been identified. Mitral valve replacement has also been advocated; excellent results have been achieved in patients who have had severe mitral regurgitation.[122,123] When chest pain is severe—associated with significant ST-segment changes during exercise or refractory to therapy—the performance of coronary arteriography is warranted. The results of coronary artery bypass grafting in HCM are excellent even when additional procedures are performed (myotomy/mitral valve replacement).[124] Endocarditis is a rare complication, and occurs in patients with LV-outflow-tract turbulence and/or mitral regurgitation.[125] It may involve the mitral or aortic valve and is usually associated with increased dyspnea. Antibiotic prophylaxis is important in appropriate patients.

Arrhythmia

Arrhythmias are a common complication of HCM, and supraventricular arrhythmias in particular are associated with embolic complications (Table 142-1). Once atrial fibrillation is established, treatment with anticoagulants and digoxin with or without verapamil or β-blockers is appropriate. The aim of therapy is to control the ventricular response and prevent emboli. Most patients in whom atrial fibrillation develops during EKG monitoring are unaware of changes from sinus rhythm to atrial fibrillation as long as the ventricular response is well controlled. This is consistent with the loss of a forceful atrial contraction (palpable atrial beat), which does not contribute significantly to filling volume (no fourth heart sound). In a minority, the loss of atrial systolic contribution to filling volume is important; in these patients, electrical cardioversion can be facilitated by 6 weeks of therapy with amiodarone (300 mg daily) if pharmacologic cardioversion does not occur first.[126] The role of conventional class I agents in aiding cardioversion and in the maintenance of sinus rhythm is uncertain. Sustained (>30 s) episodes of paroxysmal atrial fibrillation or supraventricular tachycardia are relatively uncommon but represent

Table 142-1 Incidence of Arrhythmia at Diagnosis in 401 Patients with HCM

	Age (Years)				
	≤15 (n = 41)	16–30 (n = 114)	31–45 (n = 103)	46–60 (n = 104)	>60 (n = 39)
Atrial fibrillation	0	0	4 (4%)	10 (10%)	2 (5%)
Supraventricular tachycardia	3 (7%)	16 (14%)	31 (30%)	30 (29%)	14 (36%)
Ventricular tachycardia	1 (2%)	19 (17%)	22 (21%)	32 (31%)	9 (23%)

a risk of hemodynamic collapse and emboli. Amiodarone in low doses (1000 to 1400 mg weekly) is effective in suppressing such episodes and also provides control of the ventricular response should breakthrough occur[126]; it is not known whether amiodarone attenuates the subsequent development of established atrial fibrillation.[107] Episodes of nonsustained ventricular tachycardia are common but are rarely symptomatic, and therapy is warranted only if prognosis can be shown to be improved (see below).

Prevention of Sudden Death

Treatment of adults is facilitated by the detection of a relatively sensitive and specific marker of increased risk, nonsustained ventricular tachycardia during electrocardiographic monitoring.[71] Subsequent investigations aim to identify likely initiating mechanism(s) amenable to treatment: paroxysmal atrial fibrillation—amiodarone; ischemia—drugs; clinical sustained ventricular arrhythmia—automatic implantable cardioverter defibrillator; supraventricular arrhythmias associated with rapid atrioventricular conduction—ablation; and obstruction—myectomy. In the majority of adults, investigations will fail to determine a likely treatable mechanism. The success of low-dose amiodarone (1000 mg/week) in preventing sudden death in patients with nonsustained ventricular tachycardia provides nonspecific but effective therapy in the remainder.[127] In the young, the higher annual mortality from sudden death in the absence of a sensitive marker of risk makes treatment problematic. As in adults, investigation is performed to identify a treatable mechanism of sudden death, but this is impractical without first being able to exclude the lower-risk patients. With plasma concentrations of amiodarone of 1.5 mg/liter or less, serious side effects are rare, although photosensitivity and sleep disturbance are common and may be troublesome.[126,128] Until practical treatment guidelines are established, young patients with HCM should undergo risk-factor characterization at specialist investigation centers.

MOLECULAR GENETIC ANALYSES

Demonstration of a Mendelian pattern of inheritance implies that familial HCM is a monogenic disorder. Associations of familial HCM with other syndromes suggested some potential genetic loci that might be involved in the etiology of familial HCM. A phenotype clinically resembling HCM has been reported in association with several familial conditions whose genetic loci have been mapped—neurofibromatosis (chromosome 17),[129,130] Friedreich ataxia (chromosome 9),[131] aniridia with catalase deficiency (chromosome 11),[132] and hereditary spherocytosis (chromosome 14).[133,134] Unexplained LVH with myocardial disarray is also seen in the Noonan syndrome, a condition of unknown genetic locus. None of these loci, however, are known to involve genes with cardiac expression that would be considered as candidates for familial HCM. It is also apparent that many of the hypertrophic phenotypes described in these syndromes show features only partly consistent with the diagnosis of familial HCM. It seems likely that these syndromes represent phenocopies with different etiologies, though perhaps sharing a final common pathway of pathological expression.

Some studies have suggested either genetic linkage of familial HCM with the major histocompatibility (HLA) locus on chromosome 6,[135,136] or association of obstructive forms of HCM with specific HLA-DR alleles.[137] Subsequent analyses have excluded linkage with the HLA locus in large pedigrees[22] and in sib-pair analyses[138] and have failed to demonstrate any disease association with HLA haplotype.[139]

Linkage Mapping of the Chromosome 14 Locus

In the absence of any apparent candidate genes or of any known cytogenetic anomaly in familial HCM, attempts to identify the underlying genetic defect depended on the use of linkage analysis. A large French Canadian family with 44 affected members was selected for study.[140] Linkage analyses were performed with DNA probes, selected randomly from a panel of probes that identify polymorphic loci spaced throughout the genome, until one was found that identified a polymorphism that cosegregated with disease. A DNA probe identifying an RFLP previously mapped to chromosome 14q11-12 (probe L436) revealed two alleles that were coinherited with the phenotypic presence or absence of familial HCM.[140] There were no recombinations. The Lod score generated for this data was +11.28 at a recombination distance of 0, indicating odds of greater than 100 billion to 1 in favor of linkage. The chromosome 14q11-12 locus for this disease has been designated CMH1.[141]

Demonstration of Genetic Heterogeneity

The mapping of the gene for familial HCM in one family provided a basis for determining whether mutations in other genes can cause this disorder independently in unrelated families. Linkage analyses with the chromosome 14q1 markers have been performed in unrelated families with familial HCM, providing evidence of further families linked to the CMH1 locus,[142,143] but also identifying others in which familial HCM is not due to mutations at this site.[142,144] Thus, these findings demonstrated the presence of genetic heterogeneity, implying the presence of one or more additional disease gene loci for familial HCM (see below).

The proportion of families showing linkage to this locus varies widely in different reports. In the original demonstration of genetic heterogeneity, two of four families were linked to the CMH1 locus.[142] Subsequent studies have been interpreted to show a range of findings—from all the families studied being linked[143] to all being unlinked.[145] In large part, these discrepancies reflect the difficulties of linkage analyses in small families. The majority of smaller families fail to generate significant Lod scores, as often some members are uninformative for any given polymorphism. In the presence of documented genetic heterogeneity it is not appropriate to sum Lod scores from unrelated families.

β Cardiac Myosin Heavy Chain Gene Mutations as a Cause of Familial Hypertrophic Cardiomyopathy

The localization of the disease locus to the chromosome 14q1 region suggested the α and β cardiac myosin heavy chain genes as candidates that might be involved in the pathogenesis of familial HCM. The two cardiac myosin heavy chain genes are tandemly arranged within 4 kb of each other, on chromosome 14 band q11.2-q13.[146,147] Myosin heavy chains constitute the major component of the thick filaments of striated muscle and exist in numerous isoforms. Of these, the α and β cardiac isoforms are the only ones expressed at high levels in the myocardium. In the adult human heart β heavy chain dimers are predominant in the ventricle and α heavy chain dimers are predominant in the atria.[148] The cardiac myosin heavy chains were therefore studied for potential involvement in familial HCM. A DNA probe, derived from the β cardiac myosin heavy chain gene, was shown to be linked without crossovers to disease status in the two families whose disease had been mapped to chromosome 14q1.[149]

During genetic linkage analysis of the CMH1 locus with the cardiac myosin heavy chain gene probe, a novel restriction fragment was identified in all affected members of one family.[150] This fragment was not seen in any of 200 other unrelated individuals. Analysis of the novel fragment revealed a hybrid gene composed of α cardiac myosin heavy chain sequence fused to β cardiac myosin heavy chain sequence, presumably caused by an unequal crossover event in meiosis.[150] Subsequent analyses revealed that each affected member of this family also carried a missense mutation in the nonrearranged β cardiac myosin heavy chain gene on the same chromosome.[151] This same missense mutation is present in an unrelated family without the hybrid gene, suggesting that the missense mutation rather than the rearrangement are responsible for the disease.[151,152] Screening of the β cardiac myosin heavy chain genes in unrelated families with familial HCM has demonstrated that missense mutations in this gene are present in up to 50 percent of families.[151]

Characteristics of Missense Mutations in the β Cardiac Myosin Heavy Chain Gene

All the missense mutations identified to date in familial HCM patients (Table 142-2) are single-nucleotide substitutions resulting in the change of a single amino acid in the globular head or head–rod junction region of the myosin heavy chain (Fig. 142-4).[151,153–158] No missense mutations have been identified in the rod region. All the mutations share certain characteristics, which supports the conclusion that they are responsible for causing the disease. First, analyses of many large families show perfect cosegregation of the presence or absence of the mutation with the disease status of adult individuals. Second, β cardiac myosin heavy chain mutations have been found only in individuals affected with familial HCM; analyses of this gene have not detected missense mutations in over 200 unrelated unaffected individuals. Third, the amino acid substitutions affect residues that have been conserved throughout vertebrate evolution, implying particular functional importance. In addition, the majority of substitutions result in a change of net charge and so are particularly likely to result in conformational changes in the polypeptide. Although the characteristics of the mutations strongly suggest that they are disease-causing, the possibility exists that they are merely polymorphisms linked to an adjacent gene, which is itself responsible for the disease. Thus, the most compelling genetic evidence has been the demonstration of the coincident appearance of *de novo* β cardiac myosin heavy chain mutations and HCM in individuals with sporadic disease[156] (also see below). When a normal copy of the β cardiac myosin heavy chain gene in an unaffected parent acquires a new mutation in an offspring in whom HCM develops, this cannot be attributed to chance association.

A single deletion mutation of the β cardiac myosin heavy chain gene has also been reported.[159] A 2.4-kb deletion was identified in a proband with familial HCM that deletes nucleotides encoding the five terminal amino acid residues and the polyadenylation signal. However, two adult offspring who inherited the deletion do not manifest familial HCM, while two sibs who do not carry the deletion have features highly suggestive of familial HCM. This suggests that the disease in this family may not be linked to the β cardiac myosin heavy chain locus and so the deletion may not be responsible for the disease. In another study, Southern blot and fluorescence *in situ* hybridization analyses did not reveal any rearrangements or deletions in 20 probands with typical familial HCM.[160]

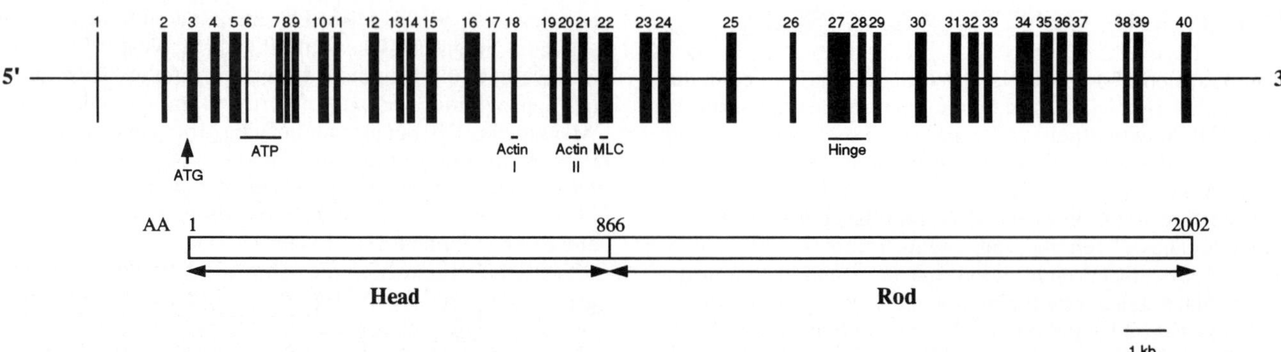

FIG. 142-4 Schematic of the normal β cardiac myosin heavy chain gene; the location of each exon is shown. Sequences that encode transcription initiation (ATG), ATPase activity (ATP), actin binding (Actin I, Actin II), myosin light chain binding (MLC), and hinge function (Hinge) are indicated. The head and rod regions of the encoded polypeptide are shown.

Table 142-2 β Cardiac Myosin Heavy Chain Missense Mutations Identified in Familial HCM

Amino Acid	Nucleotide	Exon	Charge Change	Reference
Arg_{249} → Gln	G832A	9	−1	151, 154
Arg_{403} → Gln	G1294A	13	−1	151, 154, 155, 161
Arg_{453} → Cys	C1443T	14	−1	151
Phe_{513} → Cys	T1624G	15	0	Our unpublished data
Gly_{584} → Arg	G1836C	16	+1	151
Val_{606} → Met	G1902A	16	0	151
Lys_{615} → Asn	G1931C	16	−1	157
Gly_{716} → Arg	G2232A	19	+1	Our unpublished data
Arg_{719} → Trp	C2241T	19	−1	Our unpublished data
Arg_{723} → Cys	C2253T	20	−1	156
Leu_{908} → Val	C2808G	23	0	155, 158
Glu_{924} → Lys	G2856A	23	+2	151
Glu_{949} → Lys	G2931A	23	+2	151

Myosin Mutations in Sporadic Hypertrophic Cardiomyopathy

To investigate the molecular basis of sporadic HCM, the β cardiac myosin heavy chain gene was screened in seven individuals with typical clinical features of HCM but whose parents were unaffected.[156] In two of the seven probands, missense mutations were found in the β cardiac myosin heavy chain cDNA using RNase protection assays (Arg_{723} → Cys and Glu_{924} → Lys [Fig. 142-5]). Similar analyses demonstrated that neither proband had inherited the mutation from a parent, suggesting that the mutations had arisen *de novo*. In both instances, paternity was confirmed by typing of inherited DNA polymorphisms.

It appears that, in these two examples, the mutations arose in the germ line, as they are present in both the heart and peripheral leukocytes. In addition, in one of the families the *de novo* mutation must be present in the germ cells of the affected proband because it was inherited in the next generation. Thus, *de novo* β cardiac myosin heavy chain mutations cause sporadic HCM and, in some instances, these new mutations are transmitted as familial HCM. Familial and sporadic forms of HCM are then, at least in some instances, different parts of the spectrum of a single disease process. This finding has implications for clinical treatment of individuals with sporadic HCM. Firstly, genetic counseling should take into account the potential for transmission of the disease trait to offspring. Secondly, the prognostic value of identifying a β cardiac myosin heavy chain mutation (see below) is greater in individuals for whom no family history is available as a clinical indicator of the risk of sudden death.

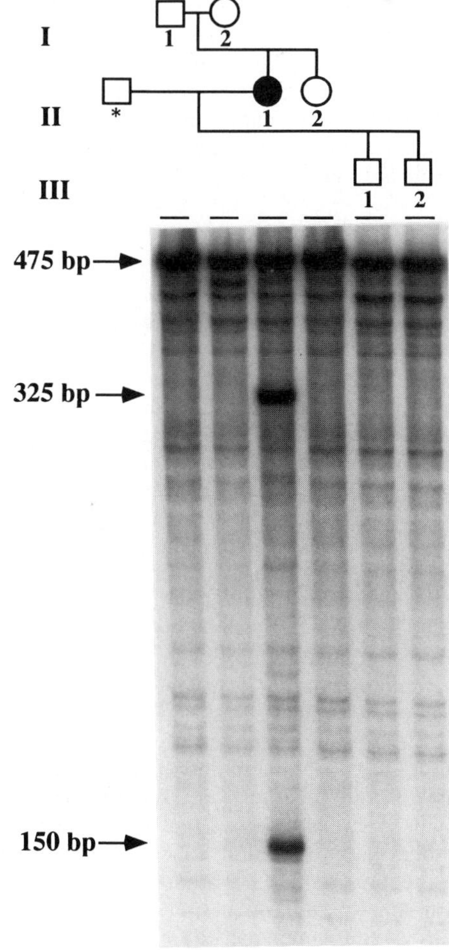

FIG. 142-5 Detection of the Arg_{723} → Cys mutation in a proband with sporadic HCM (individual II-1), as detected by RNase protection assay. The pedigree is shown in the upper panel. Squares denote males, circles females; solid symbols denote those clinically affected, open symbols those unaffected. In the lower panel is an RNase protection assay of exon 20 DNA from each individual, in positions corresponding to those of the pedigree. Cleavage due to a nucleotide mismatch is present only in affected individual II-1.

Mechanisms of Action of β Cardiac Myosin Heavy Chain Missense Mutations

To date, little direct data is available on the way in which β cardiac myosin heavy chain mutations lead to the phenotype of HCM. It is not yet possible to dissect the observed histologic and physiological abnormalities, of which many must be secondary phenomena. Mutant β cardiac myosin heavy chain mRNA has been detected by reverse transcription and PCR amplification of RNA extracted from endomyocardial biopsies of individuals affected by the $Arg_{403} \rightarrow$ Cys mutation.[161] Because of the sensitivity of the technique, this does not determine the relative levels of mutant and wild-type message. Analyses are underway to evaluate expression of mutant protein in affected individuals and to characterize the biochemical and structural properties of mutant β cardiac myosin heavy chain protein in vitro. Creation of transgenic mouse models may provide a resource for evaluating the role of disease-causing mutations and trials of therapeutic interventions.

Existing animal models may also provide insights into the role of β cardiac myosin heavy chain mutations. The mutations in HCM appear to parallel the findings in the *unc 54* myosin heavy chain gene of the nematode *Caenorhabditis elegans*. Missense mutations clustered in the globular head are associated with a dominant phenotype of body-wall paralysis.[162] The dominant expression is explained by a "poison polypeptide" mechanism, whereby structurally flawed copies of the myosin heavy chain polypeptide are incorporated at a low level into myosin filaments and then prevent normal assembly and function. In contrast, null mutations in the *C. elegans* myosin heavy chain, which cause complete disruption or failure of expression of one copy of the gene, produce a recessive phenotype. Of note, the missense mutations in the *unc 54* gene are clustered in and around the critical residues for actin binding and ATPase activity and are associated with complete loss of function. No familial HCM-causing mutations have yet been identified in these consensus sequences, perhaps indicating that such mutations are not viable.

Clinical Applications

Screening for β Cardiac Myosin Heavy Chain Gene Mutations. Clinical diagnosis of HCM is problematic in a proportion of adults and the majority of children in families with familial HCM (see above). Despite the absence of detectable myocardial hypertrophy, such individuals may be at risk of sudden death. A genetic diagnosis based on screening for myosin mutations would allow preclinical detection of the disease and might potentially be of great value. The main problem to be overcome is the extensive genetic heterogeneity in familial HCM, even within the proportion of familial HCM attributable to myosin mutations. Certain of the mutations have been identified in more than one family (e.g., $Arg_{403} \rightarrow$ Gln or $Val_{606} \rightarrow$ Met [see Table 142-2]), but others appear to be unique to a particular kindred. Even within groups of families sharing identical mutations, haplotype analysis has shown instances of independent origin of the mutations, rather than a founder effect.[163] This implies that most familial HCM-causing mutations have arisen in recent generations. Taken together with the finding of *de novo* mutations in sporadic disease (see above), this implies a relatively high new mutation rate for this gene. Thus, effective detection requires systematic screening that will detect both known and novel mutations. The β cardiac myosin heavy chain gene spans approximately 30,000 bp of genomic DNA, divided into 40 exons (see Fig. 142-5); the β cardiac myosin heavy chain mRNA contains approximately 6000 nucleotides, encoding a 2000 amino acid polypeptide. On the basis of the known mutations, screening should encompass at least the coding sequence for the head and the head–rod junction.

Fortunately, it is possible to obtain coding sequences of the β cardiac myosin heavy chain mRNA of affected individuals from peripheral blood lymphocytes, thus avoiding the need to screen individual exons of genomic DNA. This technique is based on the existence of low-level ectopic, or promiscuous, transcription of the β cardiac myosin heavy chain gene in lymphocytes, allowing amplification of the transcript by reverse transcription and nested PCR.[154] Several screening techniques have been used to analyze β cardiac myosin heavy chain DNA or cDNA sequences for point mutations. Such analyses are complicated by the presence of a normal copy of the β cardiac myosin heavy chain gene in addition to the mutated gene (affected individuals are heterozygotes). Successful techniques have included ribonuclease protection assays,[151,156] single-strand conformational polymorphism,[155] and chemical cleavage of heteroduplexes.

A group of families found not to have β cardiac myosin heavy chain gene mutations on systematic screening of cDNA by ribonuclease protection assay[151] have subsequently been studied by linkage analysis.[164] None of these families were found to be linked to the β cardiac myosin heavy chain locus, implying that no mutations were missed in this survey and suggesting that screening in this manner has a high sensitivity. As no examples were found of families that were linked to CMH1 but did not have the β cardiac myosin heavy chain gene mutations, these data also confirm that the large majority of mutations at the CMH1 locus lie in the β cardiac myosin heavy chain coding sequence, rather than in noncoding or α cardiac myosin heavy chain sequences.

Preclinical Diagnosis. While identification of β cardiac myosin heavy chain mutations remains technically demanding, genetic diagnosis in related individuals is simple once a mutation has been identified in a proband. Genetic diagnosis performed in this way provides definitive evidence of disease status in adults difficult to diagnose clinically and allows preclinical diagnosis in infants and children. The application of direct mutational analysis to preclinical diagnosis has now been shown in several kindreds.[154,155] Not surprisingly, some children and adolescents are found to carry the disease gene but do not yet manifest any detectable clinical abnormality. This provides the first opportunity to evaluate both the natural history of the disease and the efficacy of diagnostic or interventional modalities in individuals with familial HCM before established hypertrophy is present. For example, in one analysis, review of the results of noninvasive studies suggested that 12-lead EKG were more sensitive than echocardiograms as indicators of disease status in children.[154] The ultimate value of preclinical diagnosis will depend on two factors. The first is the success of therapeutic interventions in modifying the disease process or its complications. The potential for intervention may be much greater than that predicted by the clinical trials performed to date, which have involved interventions in adults with advanced morphologic features of the disease. The second is the degree to which the presence of a β cardiac myosin heavy chain mutation predicts the outcome for any individual, particularly the risk of sudden death (see below). As with any condition, preclinical screening programs within families with familial HCM will require careful evaluation of the clinical, psychosocial, and financial implications.

Prognostic Implications of Specific Myosin Mutations. The prognosis of affected individuals with familial HCM in unrelated families varies widely. A subgroup of families with an apparently higher incidence of sudden death has been qualitatively identified as having "malignant" disease,[47,98] while others have relatively benign disease.[100] Clinical indicators, particularly in the young, have been disappointing indicators of the risk of sudden death.[47,72] A family history of sudden death indicates risk,[47] but often this is unavailable or potentially misleading due to small family size. The finding of multiple different mutations within the β cardiac myosin gene provides the opportunity to determine the influence of the specific mutation on the course of the disease. If individuals from unrelated families from different backgrounds are combined for such an analysis, then differences in outcome are more likely to relate to the specific mutation that they have in common than to other genetic or environmental influences.

Such analyses have not shown clear differences among clinical parameters such as the echocardiographic features of hypertrophy,[165] but do show important differences in survival of affected individuals.[151] Kaplan-Meier analyses (Fig. 142-6) have identified some mutations associated with particularly poor prognosis (e.g., $Arg_{403} \rightarrow$ Gln and $Arg_{453} \rightarrow$ Cys), with significantly shorter survival than is seen with other mutations.[151] Two mutations have been reported to have a particularly good prognosis with near-normal survival: $Val_{606} \rightarrow$ Met[151] and $Leu_{908} \rightarrow$ Val.[155] Both these mutations differ from others in that they do not involve a net charge change and so would be predicted to cause less severe disturbance to the structure and function of the myosin polypeptide. This finding raises the possibility that conservative substitutions may in general produce less severe disease, though presumably the site as well as the charge change will determine the impact of each mutation. Of note, some of the affected members of three unrelated families with the $Val_{606} \rightarrow$ Met mutation had marked ventricular hypertrophy but still tended to survive longer than individuals with other mutations.[151] These data suggest that the specific myosin

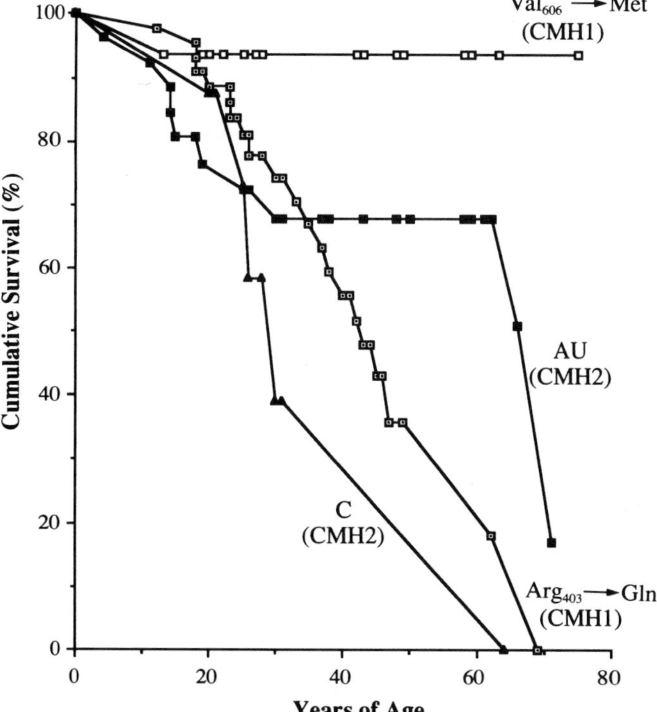

FIG. 142-6 Kaplan-Meier survival curves for affected individuals with two β cardiac MHC gene mutations ($Val_{606} \rightarrow$ Met and $Arg_{403} \rightarrow$ Gln) and for affected individuals from two families linked to CMH2 (AU and C). (*Modified from Watkins et al.,*[166] *with permission.*)

mutation is a major determinant of survival and that knowledge of the precise defect may contribute significantly to the identification of those at increased risk of sudden death.

OTHER DISEASE LOCI FOR FAMILIAL HYPERTROPHIC CARDIOMYOPATHY

Given the involvement of the β cardiac myosin heavy chain gene, other cardiac muscle contractile protein genes have been considered as candidate genes for familial HCM in families not linked to the CMH1 locus on chromosome 14. Isoforms of myosin light chain, actin, troponin, or tropomyosin interact directly or indirectly with the myosin heavy chains and might be involved in a common disease pathway. Such genes could be screened for involvement in familial HCM by either linkage analysis or direct screening for mutations. So many contractile proteins could be considered candidates, of which many are of unknown genomic location, that a more systematic approach was warranted. Two further disease loci for familial HCM have now been identified by genome-wide searches using linkage analysis.

CMH2—A Disease Locus on Chromosome 1q3

A 42-member kindred (family AU) with typical clinical and histologic features of familial HCM was studied.[166] Linkage analyses, performed with highly polymorphic short tandem repeat (STR) sequences, excluded linkage to the β cardiac myosin heavy chain gene. Thereafter, STR markers were tested systematically, being selected for their chromosomal location and predicted informativeness. Fifty-two loci were analyzed, excluding linkage to approximately 40 percent of the genome, before linkage was found to the coagulation factor XIIIB locus. The gene encoding coagulation factor XIIIB has been mapped to chromosome 1q31-q32.1 by *in situ* hybridization. Analysis of a tetranucleotide repeat polymorphism in this gene revealed four alleles in the AU pedigree, one of which was coinherited with disease status with only a single recombinant. A two-point Lod score of 6.66 was calculated at $\theta = 0$, signifying odds of 5,000,000:1 in favor of linkage to this locus, designated CMH2 (Table 142-3). Linkage analyses were performed with other markers from this region to predict the likely location of the disease gene. Multipoint linkage analyses were performed using loci of known position on the Centre d'Etude du Polymorphisme Humain (CEPH) consortium map (D1S53, F13B, and LAMB2). A peak Lod score of 8.47 was calculated for the region between loci D1S53 and F13B.

Candidate Genes at CMH2. Four genes for contractile proteins have been mapped to regions that include the CMH2 locus (Fig. 142-7, Table 142-4). The gene encoding α skeletal actin has been mapped by hybridization analysis of somatic-cell hybrids to 1p21-1qter.[167] This isoform is coexpressed with α cardiac actin in the adult ventricle; expression is

Table 142-3 Disease Loci for Familial HCM

Designation	Map Position	Disease Gene
CMH1	14q11-13	β Cardiac myosin heavy chain
CMH2	1q3	Unknown
CMH3	15q2	Unknown

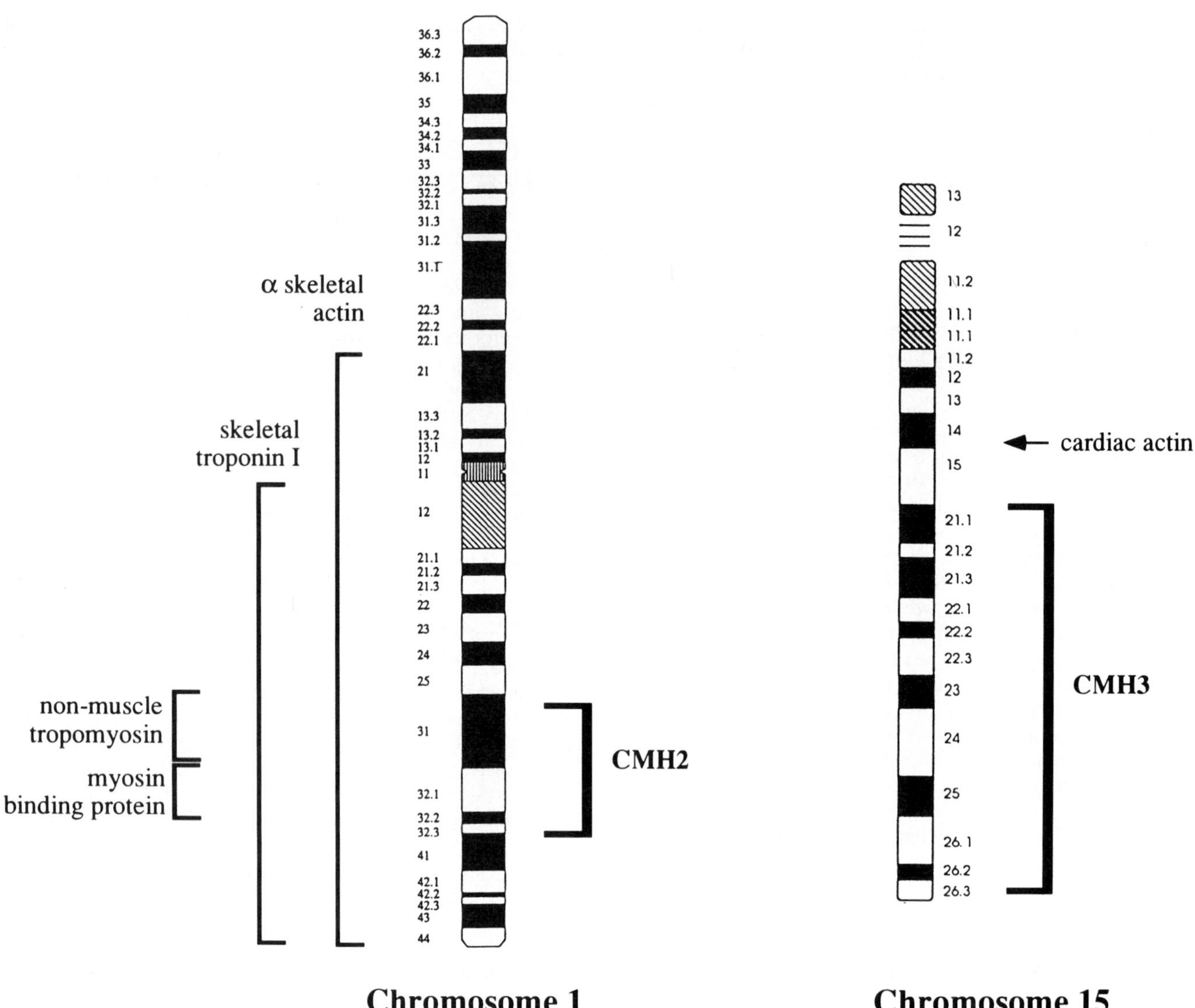

FIG. 142-7 Schematic maps of chromosomes 1 and 15 showing positions of the CMH2 and CMH3 loci (bold brackets). The published map positions of candidate contractile protein genes are indicated.

Table 142-4 Candidate Contractile Protein Genes for the CMH2 Locus

Gene	Map Position	Expression in Myocardium
α Skeletal actin	1p21-qter	Major isoform in adult, increased in hypertrophy
Nonmuscle tropomyosin	1q31	Alternatively spliced product is major cardiac isoform
Slow-twitch skeletal troponin I	1q12-qter	Expressed in embryonic and infant heart
Myosin binding protein H	1q32	Unclear

increased in models of hypertrophy, such that skeletal α actin is then the dominant isoform present in the ventricle.[168,169] The gene for nonmuscle tropomyosin has been mapped by *in situ* hybridization to 1q31.[170] By alternative splicing this gene also encodes the slow-twitch isoform of skeletal muscle α tropomyosin (skαTM.2); northern blot analysis reveals that this isoform is expressed in the adult human heart.[171] The gene for slow-twitch troponin I has been mapped to 1q12-qter[172]; although this is not the dominant troponin I isoform in the adult heart, this gene is expressed in embryonic and infant human heart.[172–174] The gene encoding the human homologue of myosin binding protein H has been mapped to 1q32.1 by *in situ* hybridization.[175] In other organisms, myosin binding protein H polypeptide has been shown to bind myosin heavy chains and has been implicated in myofibrillar assembly.[176] Northern blot analysis does not, however, demonstrate expression of this gene in human cardiac muscle.[175] Identification of polymorphisms within these candidate genes will make it possible to test for linkage to CMH2; if any is linked without recombinants, screening for mutations will be indicated.

Evidence for Further Genetic Heterogeneity

Subsequent linkage analyses in nine smaller familial HCM families not linked to the CMH1 locus demonstrated that the disease in two of these families was linked to the CMH2 locus. The two-point Lod scores in the other seven smaller families were negative. The possibility of linkage to the CMH2 locus was excluded in six by comparison of multipoint Lod scores using the HOMOG program. Thus, only 3 of 10 families whose disease is not due to β cardiac myosin heavy chain gene mutations were linked to CMH2, implying the existence of further familial HCM loci. Of the unlinked families, one, family MZ, was of sufficient size for a further genome-wide search using linkage analysis.

CMH3—A Disease Locus on Chromosome 15q2

Affected members of family MZ have a phenotype of relatively mild hypertrophy in comparison with typical familial HCM families with β cardiac myosin heavy chain gene mutations or the CMH2 locus. Penetrance is incomplete in this kindred, with some members without demonstrable hypertrophy passing the condition to offspring. Linkage analyses were performed with 120 STR polymorphisms, excluding about 50 percent of the genome, before linkage was found to an anonymous STR locus, D15S108, on chromosome 15q2.[177] Multipoint linkage analyses using flanking markers generated a peak Lod score of 4.16 at D15S108 with penetrance set at 95 percent, or 5.19 with penetrance set at 50 percent. The only known sarcomeric contractile protein gene on chromosome 15q, α cardiac actin, was excluded from the CMH3 locus by linkage analysis with an STR polymorphism within the gene (see Fig. 142-7).

Of the six available families known not to be linked to either CMH1 or CMH2, two were informative for linkage analyses with chromosome 15q2 markers. Multipoint linkage analyses showed that one of these two families was linked to CMH3 (peak Lod score 2.88), while the other was unlinked. This last unlinked family implies the existence of at least one further disease locus for familial HCM.

Characterization of Phenotype in Individuals with CMH2 and CMH3 Mutations

Allelic heterogeneity at the CMH1 locus appears to result in phenotypic differences, with correlation between a patient's life expectancy and his or her specific β myosin heavy chain missense mutation (see above). However, the overall range of life expectancies for all β myosin heavy chain missense mutations is very wide. It might be expected, then, that the disease phenotype may relate more to specific mutation than disease gene locus. Two families mapped to CMH2 (AU and C) had sufficient numbers of affected individuals for survival analysis (see Fig. 142-7). In both families, prognosis was particularly poor, with a high incidence of sudden death. Survival in families AU and C is similar to that of individuals with the more severe β myosin heavy chain mutations (e.g., $Arg_{403} \rightarrow Gln$[151]), and survival is significantly shorter in family C than for a more benign myosin mutation such as $Val_{606} \rightarrow Met$,[151] $p = 0.018$. Many further large families linked to CMH2 must be characterized before it becomes possible to dissociate whether these are the effects of locus, as opposed to allelic, heterogeneity. The family originally mapped to CMH3, MZ, had significantly less myocardial hypertrophy than other familial HCM families.[177] In contrast, affected members of the second linked family had typical hypertrophy. While these findings suggest a greater effect of allelic heterogeneity, such a conclusion must await the identification of the disease gene and mutations.

Genetic Heterogeneity—Conclusions

The clinically defined entity of HCM manifests considerable genetic heterogeneity, with at least four disease loci. Each of the three mapped loci appears to account for a minority of the total disease prevalence. Clinical application of genetic diagnosis is likely to remain complex, yet a genetic classification may offer benefits by helping to identify subgroups with a different natural history of the disease. The recent linkage assignments should ultimately lead to the identification of other genes that can be mutated to cause cardiac hypertrophy. If, as hypothesized, the disease genes encode contractile proteins, then investigation of familial HCM loci should help delineate the role of such genes in sarcomere assembly and function in normal and hypertrophied states.

ADDENDUM

A Further Disease Locus for HCM Maps to Chromosome 11p13-q13

A fourth disease locus was identified by genome-wide linkage analyses in a single large French family with typical autosomal dominant HCM,[178] mapping the disease gene in this family to a region of chromosome 11. No genes encoding cardiac contractile proteins are known to map to this region.

Identification of the Disease Genes at the CMH2 and CMH3

Candidate genes at the CMH2 and CMH3 loci have been investigated by the identification of intragenic STR markers to allow precise linkage mapping. Recombination between CMH2 and the genes encoding skeletal actin and nonmuscle tropomyosin excluded these as HCM-causing genes at CMH2. While there was no recombination between the slow-twitch troponin I gene or the myosin-binding protein H gene and CMH2, analyses of coding sequences failed to reveal abnormalities in affected individuals (our unpublished results).

Mutations in α-Tropomyosin Cause HCM Linked to the CMH3 Locus

Recent studies have mapped the murine α-tropomyosin gene to a region that is syntenic to human chromosome 15, implicating it as a candidate gene for HCM linked to the CMH3 locus. Missense mutations ($Asp_{175} \rightarrow Asn$; $Glu_{180} \rightarrow Gly$) in the α-tropomyosin gene were shown to cause HCM in the two families linked to chromosome 15q2.[179] These two missense mutations occur in exon 5, which encodes part of a putative binding domain for troponin T. These findings supported the model that HCM results from mutations in contractile protein genes and suggested other thin filament components as candidates for HCM linked to chromosome 1; in particular, cardiac troponin T was implicated.

Mutations in Cardiac Troponin T Cause HCM Linked to the CMH2 Locus

The previously unmapped gene for cardiac troponin T was mapped to chromosome 1q by hybridization to somatic cell hybrids and then shown to be tightly linked to the CMH2 locus. Mutations in this gene were demonstrated to cause HCM in affected members from three unrelated families—including family AU described above.[179] Two were missense mutations in exons 8 and 9 ($Ile_{79} \rightarrow Asn$; $Arg_{92} \rightarrow Gln$), the other a splice site mutation in intron 15 that is predicted to produce a truncated cardiac troponin T. This mutation in cardiac troponin T is analogous to that found in *D. melanogaster upheld*[2], a splice donor mutation that is functionally null. Thus, although the majority of FHC-causing mutations are missense, the splice donor mutation in cardiac troponin T may be functionally null. This would suggest that abnormal stoichiometry of sarcomeric proteins can cause cardiac hypertrophy.

The observation that defects in three contractile proteins α-tropomyosin, cardiac troponin T, and β cardiac MHC–can each cause HCM demonstrates that this condition is a disease of the sarcomere.

REFERENCES

1. Liouville H: Retrecissement cardiaque sous aortique. *Gaz Med Paris* **24:**161, 1869.
2. Hallopeau L: Retrecissement ventriculo-aortique. *Gaz Med Paris* **24:**683, 1869.
3. Teare D: Asymmetrical hypertrophy of the heart in young adults. *Br Heart J* **20:**1, 1958.
4. Braunwald E, Lambrew CT, Rockoff SD, Ross JJ Jr, Morrow AG: Idiopathic hypertrophic subaortic stenosis. I. A description of the disease based upon an analysis of 64 patients. *Circulation* **30** Suppl IV:IV-3, 1964.
5. Maron BJ, Epstein SE: Hypertrophic cardiomyopathy: A discussion of nomenclature. *Am J Cardiol* **43:**1242, 1979.
6. Criley JM, Lewis KB, White RI, Ross RS: Pressure gradients without obstruction. A new concept of "hypertrophic subaortic stenosis." *Circulation* **32:**881, 1965.
7. Abbasi AS, MacAlpin RN, Eber LM, Pearce ML: Echocardiographic diagnosis of idiopathic hypertrophic cardiomyopathy without outflow obstruction. *Circulation* **46:**897, 1972.
8. Shah PM, Gramiak R, Adelman AG, Wigle ED: Role of echocardiography in diagnostic and hemodynamic assessment of hypertrophic subaortic stenosis. *Circulation* **44:**891, 1971.
9. Tajik AJ, Giuliani ER: Echocardiographic observations in idiopathic hypertrophic subaortic stenosis. *Mayo Clin Proc* **49:**89, 1974.
10. Henry WL, Clark CE, Epstein SE: Asymmetric septal hypertrophy. Echocardiographic identification of the pathognomonic anatomic abnormality of IHSS. *Circulation* **47:**225, 1973.
11. Maron BJ, Gottdiener JS, Epstein SE: Patterns and significance of distribution of left ventricular hypertrophy in hypertrophic cardiomyopathy. A wide angle, two dimensional echocardiographic study of 125 patients. *Am J Cardiol* **48:**418, 1981.
12. Maron BJ, Gottdiener JS, Bonow RO, Epstein SE: Hypertrophic cardiomyopathy with unusual locations of left ventricular hypertrophy undetectable by M-mode echocardiography. Identification by wide-angle two-dimensional echocardiography. *Circulation* **63:**409, 1981.
13. Shapiro LM, McKenna WJ: Distribution of left ventricular hypertrophy in hypertrophic cardiomyopathy: A two-dimensional echocardiographic study. *J Am Coll Cardiol* **2:**437, 1983.
14. Report of the WHO/ISFC task force on the definition and classification of cardiomyopathies. *Br Heart J* **44:**672, 1980.
15. Goodwin JF: The frontiers of cardiomyopathy. *Br Heart J* **48:**1, 1982.
16. Maron BJ, Spirito P, Wesley Y, Arce J: Development and progression of left ventricular hypertrophy in children with hypertrophic cardiomyopathy. *N Engl J Med* **315:**610, 1986.
17. Shapiro LM, Kleinebenne A, McKenna WJ: The distribution of left ventricular hypertrophy in hypertrophic cardiomyopathy: Comparison to athletes and hypertensives. *Eur Heart J* **6:**967, 1985.
18. Pelliccia A, Maron BJ, Spataro A, Proschan MA, Spirito P: The upper limit of physiologic cardiac hypertrophy in highly trained elite athletes. *N Engl J Med* **324:**295, 1991.
19. Hollman A, Goodwin JF, Teare D, Renwick JW: A family with obstructive cardiomyopathy (asymmetrical hypertrophy). *Br Heart J* **22:**449, 1960.
20. Brent LB, Aburano A, Fisher DL, Moran TJ, Myers JD, Taylor WJ: Familial muscular subaortic stenosis, an unrecognised form of "idiopathic heart disease," with clinical and autopsy findings. *Circulation* **21:**167, 1960.
21. Pare JAP, Fraser RG, Pirozynski WJ, Shanks JA, Stubington D: Hereditary cardiovascular dysplasia: A form of familial cardiomyopathy. *Am J Med* **31:**37, 1961.
22. Haugland H, Ohm OJ, Boman H, Thorsby E: Hypertrophic cardiomyopathy in three generations of a large Norwegian family. A clinical, echocardiographic, and genetic study. *Br Heart J* **55:**168, 1986.
23. Maron BJ, Nichols PF, Pickle LW, Wesley YE, Mulvihill JJ: Patterns of inheritance in hypertrophic cardiomyopathy: Assessment by M-mode and two-dimensional echocardiography. *Am J Cardiol* **53:**1087, 1984.
24. Greaves SC, Roche AH, Neutze JM, Whitlock RM, Veale AM: Inheritance of hypertrophic cardiomyopathy: A cross sectional and M mode echocardiographic study of 50 families. *Br Heart J* **58:**259, 1987.
25. Emanuel R, Withers R, O'Brien K: Dominant and recessive modes of inheritance in idiopathic cardiomyopathy. *Lancet* **2:**1065, 1971.
26. ten Cate FJ, Hugenholtz PG, van Dorp WG, Roelandt J: Prevalence of diagnostic abnormalities in patients with genetically transmitted asymmetric septal hypertrophy. *Am J Cardiol* **43:**731, 1979.
27. Frank S, Braunwald E: Idiopathic hypertrophic subaortic stenosis. Clinical analysis of 126 patients with emphasis on the natural history. *Circulation* **37:**759, 1968.
28. Maron BJ, Tajik AJ, Ruttenberg HD, Graham TP, Atwood GF, Victorica BE, Lie JT, Roberts WC: Hypertrophic cardiomyopathy in infants: Clinical features and natural history. *Circulation* **65:**7, 1982.
29. Littler WA: Twin studies in hypertrophic cardiomyopathy. *Br Heart J* **34:**1147, 1972.
30. Reid JM, Houston AB, Lundmark E: Hypertrophic cardiomyopathy in identical twins. *Br Heart J* **62:**384, 1989.
31. Epstein ND, Lin HJ, Fananapazir L: Genetic evidence of dissociation (generational skips) of electrical from morphologic forms of hypertrophic cardiomyopathy. *Am J Cardiol* **66:**627, 1990.
32. Pomerance A, Davies MJ: Pathological features of hypertrophic obstructive cardiomyopathy (HOCM) in the elderly. *Br Heart J* **37:**305, 1975.
33. McKenna WJ, Kleinebenne A, Nihoyannopoulos P, Foale R: Echocardiographic measurement of right ventricular wall thickness in hypertrophic cardiomyopathy: Relation to clinical and prognostic features. *J Am Coll Cardiol* **11:**351, 1988.
34. Davies MJ: *Colour Atlas of Cardiovascular Pathology*. Oxford Colour Atlases of Pathology. London, Harvey Miller, 1986, p 100.
35. Davies MJ: The current status of myocardial disarray in hypertrophic cardiomyopathy. *Br Heart J* **51:**361, 1984.
36. Maron BJ, Anan TJ, Roberts WC: Quantitative analysis of the distribution of cardiac muscle cell disorganization in the left ventricular wall of patients with hypertrophic cardiomyopathy. *Circulation* **63:**882, 1981.
37. Ferrans VJ, Morrow AG, Roberts WC: Myocardial ultra-

structure in idiopathic hypertrophic subaortic stenosis. A study of operatively excised left ventricular outflow tract muscle in 14 patients. *Circulation* **45**:769, 1972.

38. Becker AE, Caruso G: Myocardial disarray. A critical review. *Br Heart J* **47**:527, 1982.
39. Bulkley BH, Weisfeldt ML, Hutchins GM: Asymmetric septal hypertrophy and myocardial fiber disarray. Features of normal, developing, and malformed hearts. *Circulation* **56**:292, 1977.
40. McKenna WJ, Stewart JT, Nihoyannopoulos P, McGinty F, Davies MJ: Hypertrophic cardiomyopathy without hypertrophy: Two families with myocardial disarray in the absence of increased myocardial mass. *Br Heart J* **63**:287, 1990.
41. Perloff JK: Pathogenesis of hypertrophic cardiomyopathy: Hypotheses and speculations. *Am Heart J* **101**:219, 1981.
42. Bonow RO, Rosing DR, Bacharach SL, Green MV, Kent KM, Lipson LC, Maron BJ, Leon MB, Epstein SE: Effects of verapamil on left ventricular systolic function and diastolic filling in patients with hypertrophic cardiomyopathy. *Circulation* **64**:787, 1981.
43. Kaltenbach M, Hopf R, Keller M: [Treatment of hypertrophic obstructive cardiomyopathy with verapamil, a calcium antagonist (author's transl).] *Dtsch Med Wochenschr* **101**:1284, 1976.
44. Goodwin JF, Krikler DM: Arrhythmia as a cause of sudden death in hypertrophic cardiomyopathy. *Lancet* **2**:937, 1976.
45. Lorell BH: Use of calcium channel blockers in hypertrophic cardiomyopathy. *Am J Med* **78**:43, 1985.
46. Pearce PC, Hawkey C, Symons C, Olsen EG: Role of calcium in the induction of cardiac hypertrophy and myofibrillar disarray. Experimental studies of a possible cause of hypertrophic cardiomyopathy. *Br Heart J* **54**:420, 1985.
47. McKenna W, Deanfield J, Faruqui A, England D, Oakley C, Goodwin J: Prognosis in hypertrophic cardiomyopathy: Role of age and clinical, electrocardiographic and hemodynamic features. *Am J Cardiol* **47**:532, 1981.
48. Wigle ED, Henderson M, Rakowski H, Wilansky S: Muscular (hypertrophic) subaortic stenosis (hypertrophic obstructive cardiomyopathy): The evidence for true obstruction to left ventricular outflow. *Postgrad Med J* **62**:531, 1986.
49. Criley JM, Siegel RJ: Obstruction is unimportant in the pathophysiology of hypertrophic cardiomyopathy. *Postgrad Med J* **62**:515, 1986.
50. Siegel RJ, Criley JM: Comparison of ventricular emptying with and without a pressure gradient in patients with hypertrophic cardiomyopathy. *Br Heart J* **53**:283, 1985.
51. Sugrue DD, McKenna WJ, Dickie S, Myers MJ, Lavender JP, Oakley CM, Goodwin JF: Relation between left ventricular gradient and relative stroke volume ejected in early and late systole in hypertrophic cardiomyopathy. Assessment with radionuclide cineangiography. *Br Heart J* **52**:602, 1984.
52. Murgo JP, Alter BR, Dorethy JF, Altobelli SA, McGranahan GMJ: Dynamics of left ventricular ejection in obstructive and nonobstructive hypertrophic cardiomyopathy. *J Clin Invest* **66**:1369, 1980.
53. Sutton MG, Tajik AJ, Gibson DG, Brown DJ, Seward JB, Guiliani ER: Echocardiographic assessment of left ventricular filling and septal and posterior wall dynamics in idiopathic hypertrophic subaortic stenosis. *Circulation* **57**:512, 1978.
54. Sanderson JE, Traill TA, Sutton MG, Brown DJ, Gibson DG, Goodwin JF: Left ventricular relaxation and filling in hypertrophic cardiomyopathy. An echocardiographic study. *Br Heart J* **40**:596, 1978.
55. Hanrath P, Mathey DG, Siegert R, Bleifeld W: Left ventricular relaxation and filling pattern in different forms of left ventricular hypertrophy: An echocardiographic study. *Am J Cardiol* **45**:15, 1980.
56. Fiddler GI, Tajik AJ, Weidman W, McGoon DC, Ritter DG, Giuliani ER: Idiopathic hypertrophic subaortic stenosis in the young. *Am J Cardiol* **42**:793, 1978.
57. Maron BJ, Henry WL, Clark CE, Redwood DR, Roberts WC, Epstein SE: Asymmetric septal hypertrophy in childhood. *Circulation* **53**:9, 1976.
58. Frenneaux MP, Porter A, Caforio AL, Odawara H, Counihan PJ, McKenna WJ: Determinants of exercise capacity in hypertrophic cardiomyopathy. *J Am Coll Cardiol* **13**:1521, 1989.
59. Cannon RO, Rosing DR, Maron BJ, Leon MB, Bonow RO, Watson RM, Epstein SE: Myocardial ischemia in patients with hypertrophic cardiomyopathy: Contribution of inadequate vasodilator reserve and elevated left ventricular filling pressures. *Circulation* **71**:234, 1985.
60. Maron BJ, Wolfson JK, Epstein SE, Roberts WC: Intramural ("small vessel") coronary artery disease in hypertrophic cardiomyopathy. *J Am Coll Cardiol* **8**:545, 1986.
61. Loogen F, Kuhn H, Gietzen F, Losse B, Schulte HD, Bircks W: Clinical course and prognosis of patients with typical and atypical hypertrophic obstructive and with hypertrophic non-obstructive cardiomyopathy. *Eur Heart J (Suppl F)* **4**:145, 1983.
62. Frenneaux MP, Counihan PJ, Caforio AL, Chikamori T, McKenna WJ: Abnormal blood pressure response during exercise in hypertrophic cardiomyopathy. *Circulation* **82**:1995, 1990.
63. Savage DD, Seides SF, Clark CE, Henry WL, Maron BJ, Robinson FC, Epstein SE: Electrocardiographic findings in patients with obstructive and nonobstructive hypertrophic cardiomyopathy. *Circulation* **58**:402, 1978.
64. Yamaguchi H, Ishimura T, Nishiyama S, Nagasaki F, Nakanishi S, Takatsu F, Nishijo T, Umeda T, Machii K: Hypertrophic nonobstructive cardiomyopathy with giant negative T waves (apical hypertrophy): Ventriculographic and echocardiographic features in 30 patients. *Am J Cardiol* **44**:401, 1979.
65. Alfonso F, Nihoyannopoulos P, Stewart J, Dickie S, Lemery R, McKenna WJ: Clinical significance of giant negative T waves in hypertrophic cardiomyopathy. *J Am Coll Cardiol* **15**:965, 1990.
66. Krikler DM, Davies MJ, Rowland E, Goodwin JF, Evans RC, Shaw DB: Sudden death in hypertrophic cardiomyopathy: Associated accessory atrioventricular pathways. *Br Heart J* **43**:245, 1980.
67. Fananapazir L, Tracy CM, Leon MB, Winkler JB, Cannon RO, Bonow RO, Maron BJ, Epstein SE: Electrophysiologic abnormalities in patients with hypertrophic cardiomyopathy. A consecutive analysis in 155 patients. *Circulation* **80**:1259, 1989.
68. Savage DD, Seides SF, Maron BJ, Myers DJ, Epstein SE: Prevalence of arrhythmias during 24-hour electrocardiographic monitoring and exercise testing in patients with obstructive and nonobstructive hypertrophic cardiomyopathy. *Circulation* **59**:866, 1979.
69. McKenna WJ, England D, Doi YL, Deanfield JE, Oakley C, Goodwin JF: Arrhythmia in hypertrophic cardiomyopathy. I: Influence on prognosis. *Br Heart J* **46**:168, 1981.
70. Maron BJ, Savage DD, Wolfson JK, Epstein SE: Prognostic significance of 24 hour ambulatory electrocardiographic monitoring in patients with hypertrophic cardiomyopathy: A prospective study. *Am J Cardiol* **48**:252, 1981.
71. McKenna WJ: Sudden death in hypertrophic cardiomyopathy: Identification of the "high risk" patient, in Brugada P, Wellens HJJ (eds): *Cardiac Arrhythmias: Where to Go From Here?* Mount Kisco, NY, Futura, 1987, p 353.
72. McKenna WJ, Camm AJ: Sudden death in hypertrophic cardiomyopathy. Assessment of patients at high risk. *Circulation* **80**:1489, 1989.
73. Maron BJ, Fananapazir L: Sudden cardiac death in hypertrophic cardiomyopathy. *Circulation* **85**:157, 1992.
74. Robinson K, Frenneaux MP, Stockins B, Karatasakis G, Poloniecki JD, McKenna WJ: Atrial fibrillation in hypertrophic cardiomyopathy: A longitudinal study. *J Am Coll Cardiol* **15**:1279, 1990.
75. McKenna WJ, Franklin RC, Nihoyannopoulos P, Robinson KC, Deanfield JE: Arrhythmia and prognosis in infants, children and adolescents with hypertrophic cardiomyopathy. *J Am Coll Cardiol* **11**:147, 1988.
76. Lewis JF, Maron BJ: Elderly patients with hypertrophic cardiomyopathy: A subset with distinctive left ventricular morphology and progressive clinical course late in life. *J Am Coll Cardiol* **13**:36, 1989.
77. Hecht GM, Panza JA, Maron BJ: Clinical course of middle-aged asymptomatic patients with hypertrophic cardiomyopathy. *Am J Cardiol* **69**:935, 1992.

78. Spirito P, Maron BJ: Relation between extent of left ventricular hypertrophy and age in hypertrophic cardiomyopathy. *J Am Coll Cardiol* **13**:820, 1989.
79. Alfonso F, Frenneaux MP, McKenna WJ: Clinical sustained uniform ventricular tachycardia in hypertrophic cardiomyopathy: Association with left ventricular apical aneurysm. *Br Heart J* **61**:178, 1989.
80. Mulrow JP, Healy MJ, McKenna WJ: Variability of ventricular arrhythmias in hypertrophic cardiomyopathy and implications for treatment. *Am J Cardiol* **58**:615, 1986.
81. Kawai C: Studies on cardiomyopathy in Japan, in Sekiguchi M, Olsen EGJ (eds): *Clinical, Pathological and Theoretical Aspects of Cardiomyopathy*. Tokyo, University of Tokyo Press, 1980, p 3.
82. Chikamori T, Doi YL, Akizawa M, Yonezawa Y, Ozawa T, McKenna WJ: Comparison of clinical, morphological, and prognostic features in hypertrophic cardiomyopathy between Japanese and western patients. *Clin Cardiol* **15**:833, 1992.
83. Maron BJ, Gottdiener JS, Arce J, Rosing DR, Wesley YE, Epstein SE: Dynamic subaortic obstruction in hypertrophic cardiomyopathy: Analysis by pulsed Doppler echocardiography. *J Am Coll Cardiol* **6**:1, 1985.
84. Yock PG, Hatle L, Popp RL: Patterns and timing of Doppler-detected intracavitary and aortic flow in hypertrophic cardiomyopathy. *J Am Coll Cardiol* **8**:1047, 1986.
85. Panza JA, Petrone RK, Fananapazir L, Maron BJ: Utility of continuous wave Doppler echocardiography in the noninvasive assessment of left ventricular outflow tract pressure gradient in patients with hypertrophic cardiomyopathy. *J Am Coll Cardiol* **19**:91, 1992.
86. Doi YL, McKenna WJ, Gehrke J, Oakley CM, Goodwin JF: M mode echocardiography in hypertrophic cardiomyopathy: Diagnostic criteria and prediction of obstruction. *Am J Cardiol* **45**:6, 1980.
87. Gilbert BW, Pollick C, Adelman AG, Wigle ED: Hypertrophic cardiomyopathy: subclassification by m mode echocardiography. *Am J Cardiol* **45**:861, 1980.
88. Pollick C, Morgan CD, Gilbert BW, Rakowski H, Wigle ED: Muscular subaortic stenosis: The temporal relationship between systolic anterior motion of the anterior mitral leaflet and the pressure gradient. *Circulation* **66**:1087, 1982.
89. Pollick C, Rakowski H, Wigle ED: Muscular subaortic stenosis: The quantitative relationship between systolic anterior motion and the pressure gradient. *Circulation* **69**:43, 1984.
90. Maron BJ, Epstein SE: Hypertrophic cardiomyopathy. Recent observations regarding the specificity of three hallmarks of the disease: Asymmetric septal hypertrophy, septal disorganization and systolic anterior motion of the anterior mitral leaflet. *Am J Cardiol* **45**:141, 1980.
91. O'Gara PT, Bonow RO, Maron BJ, Damske BA, Van Lingen A, Bacharach SL, Larson SM, Epstein SE: Myocardial perfusion abnormalities in patients with hypertrophic cardiomyopathy: Assessment with thallium-201 emission computed tomography. *Circulation* **76**:1214, 1987.
92. Wigle ED, Sasson Z, Henderson MA, Ruddy TD, Fulop J, Rakowski H, Williams WG: Hypertrophic cardiomyopathy. The importance of the site and the extent of hypertrophy. A review. *Prog Cardiovasc Dis* **28**:1, 1985.
93. Brugada P, Bar FW, de Zwaan C, Roy D, Green M, Wellens HJ: "Sawfish" systolic narrowing of the left anterior descending coronary artery: An angiographic sign of hypertrophic cardiomyopathy. *Circulation* **66**:800, 1982.
94. McKenna WJ, Goodwin JF: The natural history of hypertrophic cardiomyopathy. *Curr Probl Cardiol* **6**:1, 1981.
95. Maron BJ, Merrill WH, Freier PA, Kent KM, Epstein SE, Morrow AG: Long-term clinical course and symptomatic status of patients after operation for hypertrophic subaortic stenosis. *Circulation* **57**:1205, 1978.
96. Loogen F, Kuhn H, Krelhaus W: Natural history of hypertrophic obstructive cardiomyopathy and effect of therapy, in Kaltenbach M, Loogen F, Olsen EGJ (eds): *Cardiomyopathy and Myocardial Biopsy*. Berlin, Springer-Verlag, 1978, p 286.
97. McKenna WJ, Deanfield JE: Hypertrophic cardiomyopathy: An important cause of sudden death. *Arch Dis Child* **59**:971, 1984.
98. Maron BJ, Lipson LC, Roberts WC, Savage DD, Epstein SE: "Malignant" hypertrophic cardiomyopathy: Identification of a subgroup of families with unusually frequent premature death. *Am J Cardiol* **41**:1133, 1978.
99. Wadehra D, Gunnar RM, Scanlon PJ: Prognosis in hypertrophic cardiomyopathy with asymmetric septal hypertrophy. *Postgrad Med J* **61**:1107, 1985.
100. Spirito P, Chiarella F, Carratino L, Berisso MZ, Bellotti P, Vecchio C: Clinical course and prognosis of hypertrophic cardiomyopathy in an outpatient population. *N Engl J Med* **320**:749, 1989.
101. Maron BJ, Roberts WC, McAllister HA, Rosing DR, Epstein SE: Sudden death in young athletes. *Circulation* **62**:218, 1980.
102. Maron BJ, Roberts WC, Epstein SE: Sudden death in hypertrophic cardiomyopathy: A profile of 78 patients. *Circulation* **65**:1388, 1982.
103. Spirito P, Maron BJ, Bonow RO, Epstein SE: Occurrence and significance of progressive left ventricular wall thinning and relative cavity dilatation in hypertrophic cardiomyopathy. *Am J Cardiol* **60**:123, 1987.
104. McKenna WJ, Borggrefe M, England D, Deanfield J, Oakley CM, Goodwin JF: The natural history of left ventricular hypertrophy in hypertrophic cardiomyopathy: An electrocardiographic study. *Circulation* **66**:1233, 1982.
105. Spirito P, Maron BJ: Absence of progression of left ventricular hypertrophy in adult patients with hypertrophic cardiomyopathy. *J Am Coll Cardiol* **9**:1013, 1987.
106. Glancy DL, O'Brien KP, Gold HK, Epstein SE: Atrial fibrillation in patients with idiopathic hypertrophic subaortic stenosis. *Br Heart J* **32**:652, 1970.
107. Maron BJ, Gaffney FA, Jeresaty RM, McKenna WJ, Miller WW: Task force III: Hypertrophic cardiomyopathy, other myopericardial diseases and mitral valve prolapse. *J Am Coll Cardiol* **6**:1215, 1985.
108. McKenna W, Harris L, Deanfield J: Syncope in hypertrophic cardiomyopathy. *Br Heart J* **47**:177, 1982.
109. Stafford WJ, Trohman RG, Bilsker M, Zaman L, Castellanos A, Myerburg RJ: Cardiac arrest in an adolescent with atrial fibrillation and hypertrophic cardiomyopathy. *J Am Coll Cardiol* **7**:701, 1986.
110. Goodwin JF, Shah PM, Oakley CM, Cohen J, Yipintsoi T, Pocock W: The clinical pharmacology of hypertrophic obstructive cardiomyopathy, in Wolstenholme GEW, O'Connor M (eds): *Cardiomyopathies*. Ciba Foundation Symposium. London, J & A Churchill, 1964, p 189.
111. Rosing DR, Kent KM, Borer JS, Seides SF, Maron BJ, Epstein SE: Verapamil therapy: A new approach to the pharmacologic treatment of hypertrophic cardiomyopathy. I. Hemodynamic effects. *Circulation* **60**:1201, 1979.
112. Betocchi S, Bonow RO, Bacharach SL, Rosing DR, Maron BJ, Green MV: Isovolumic relaxation period in hypertrophic cardiomyopathy: Assessment by radionuclide angiography. *J Am Coll Cardiol* **7**:74, 1986.
113. Alvares RF, Goodwin JF: Non-invasive assessment of diastolic function in hypertrophic cardiomyopathy on and off beta adrenergic blocking drugs. *Br Heart J* **48**:204, 1982.
114. Frank MJ, Abdulla AM, Canedo MI, Saylors RE: Long-term medical management of hypertrophic obstructive cardiomyopathy. *Am J Cardiol* **42**:993, 1978.
115. Pollick C: Muscular subaortic stenosis: Hemodynamic and clinical improvement after disopyramide. *N Engl J Med* **307**:997, 1982.
116. Epstein SE, Rosing DR: Verapamil: Its potential for causing serious complications in patients with hypertrophic cardiomyopathy. *Circulation* **64**:437, 1981.
117. Suwa M, Hirota Y, Kawamura K: Improvement in left ventricular diastolic function during intravenous and oral diltiazem therapy in patients with hypertrophic cardiomyopathy: An echocardiographic study. *Am J Cardiol* **54**:1047, 1984.
118. Paulus WJ, Lorell BH, Craig WE, Wynne J, Murgo JP, Grossman W: Comparison of the effects of nitroprusside and nifedipine on diastolic properties in patients with hypertrophic cardiomyopathy: Altered left ventricular loading or improved muscle inactivation? *J Am Coll Cardiol* **2**:879, 1983.
119. Betocchi S, Cannon RO, Watson RM, Bonow RO, Ostrow HG, Epstein SE, Rosing DR: Effects of sublingual nifedipine on hemodynamics and systolic and diastolic function

in patients with hypertrophic cardiomyopathy. *Circulation* **72:**1001, 1985.

120. Kirklin JW, Barratt-Boyes BG: *Cardiac Surgery*. New York, John Wiley, 1986.
121. Seiler C, Hess OM, Schoenbeck M, Turina J, Jenni R, Turina M, Krayenbuehl HP: Long-term follow-up of medical versus surgical therapy for hypertrophic cardiomyopathy: A retrospective study. *J Am Coll Cardiol* **17:**634, 1991.
122. Cooley DA, Leachman RD, Wukasch DC: Diffuse muscular subaortic stenosis: Surgical treatment. *Am J Cardiol* **31:**1, 1973.
123. McIntosh CL, Greenberg GJ, Maron BJ, Leon MB, Cannon RO, Clark RE: Clinical and hemodynamic results after mitral valve replacement in patients with obstructive hypertrophic cardiomyopathy. *Ann Thorac Surg* **47:**236, 1989.
124. Gill CC, Duda AM, Kitazume H, Kramer JR, Loop FD: Idiopathic hypertrophic subaortic stenosis and coronary atherosclerosis. Results of coronary artery bypass alone and myectomy combined with coronary artery bypass. *J Thorac Cardiovasc Surg* **84:**856, 1982.
125. Chagnac A, Rudniki C, Loebel H, Zahavi I: Infectious endocarditis in idiopathic hypertrophic subaortic stenosis: Report of three cases and review of the literature. *Chest* **81:**346, 1982.
126. McKenna WJ, Harris L, Rowland E, Kleinebenne A, Krikler DM, Oakley CM, Goodwin JF: Amiodarone for long-term management of patients with hypertrophic cardiomyopathy. *Am J Cardiol* **54:**802, 1984.
127. McKenna WJ, Oakley CM, Krikler DM, Goodwin JF: Improved survival with amiodarone in patients with hypertrophic cardiomyopathy and ventricular tachycardia. *Br Heart J* **53:**412, 1985.
128. Harris L, McKenna WJ, Rowland E, Holt DW, Storey GC, Krikler DM: Side effects of long-term amiodarone therapy. *Circulation* **67:**45, 1983.
129. Fitzpatrick AP, Emanuel RW: Familial neurofibromatosis and hypertrophic cardiomyopathy. *Br Heart J* **60:**247, 1988.
130. Barker D, Wright E, Nguyen K, Cannon L, Fain P, Goldgar D, Bishop DT, Carey J, Baty B, Kivlin J, Willard H, Waye JS, Greig G, Leinwand L, Nakamura Y, O'Connell P, Leppert M, Lalouel J-M, White R, Skolnick M: Gene for von Recklinghausen neurofibromatosis is in the pericentromeric region of chromosome 17. *Science* **236:**1100, 1987.
131. Child JS, Perloff JK, Bach PM, Wolfe AD, Perlman S, Kark RA: Cardiac involvement in Friedreich's ataxia: A clinical study of 75 patients. *J Am Coll Cardiol* **7:**1370, 1986.
132. Gilgenkrantz S, Vigneron C, Gregoire MJ, Pernot C, Raspiller A: Association of del(11)(p15.1p12), aniridia, catalase deficiency, and cardiomyopathy. *Am J Med Genet* **13:**39, 1982.
133. Moiseyev VS, Korovina EA, Polotskaya EL, Poliyanskaya IS, Yazdovsky VV: Hypertrophic cardiomyopathy associated with hereditary spherocytosis in three generations of one family. *Lancet* **2:**853, 1987.
134. Kimberling WJ, Taylor RA, Chapman RG, Lubs HA: Linkage and gene localization of hereditary spherocytosis (HS). *Blood* **52:**859, 1978.
135. Matsumori A, Hirose K, Wakabayashi A, Kawai C, Nabeya N, Sakurami T, Tsuji K: HL-A and hypertrophic cardiomyopathy. *Am Heart J* **97:**428, 1979.
136. Kishimoto C, Kaburagi T, Takayama S, Yokoyama S, Hanyu I, Takatsu Y, Tomimoto K: Two forms of hypertrophic cardiomyopathy distinguished by inheritance of HLA haplotypes and left ventricular outflow tract obstruction. *Am Heart J* **105:**988, 1983.
137. Matsumori A, Kawai C, Wakabayashi A, Terasaki PI, Park MS, Sakurami T, Ueno Y: HLA-DRW4 antigen linkage in patients with hypertrophic obstructive cardiomyopathy. *Am Heart J* **101:**14, 1981.
138. Zezulka A, MacKintosh P, Jobson S, Lowry P, Shapiro LM: Human lymphocyte antigens in hypertrophic cardiomyopathy. *Int J Cardiol* **12:**193, 1986.
139. Gardin JM, Gottdiener JS, Radvany R, Maron BJ, Lesch M: HLA linkage vs association in hypertrophic cardiomyopathy. Evidence for the absence of an association in a heterogeneous Caucasian population. *Chest* **81:**466, 1982.
140. Jarcho JA, McKenna W, Pare JA, Solomon SD, Holcombe RF, Dickie S, Levi T, Donis Keller H, Seidman JG, Seidman CE: Mapping a gene for familial hypertrophic cardiomyopathy to chromosome 14q1. *N Engl J Med* **321:**1372, 1989.
141. Cox DW, Nakamura Y, Gedde Dahl TJ: Report of the committee on the genetic constitution of chromosome 14. *Cytogenet Cell Genet* **55:**183, 1990.
142. Solomon SD, Jarcho JA, McKenna W, Geisterfer Lowrance A, Germain R, Salerni R, Seidman JG, Seidman CE: Familial hypertrophic cardiomyopathy is a genetically heterogeneous disease. *J Clin Invest* **86:**993, 1990.
143. Hejtmancik JF, Brink PA, Towbin J, Hill R, Brink L, Tapscott T, Trakhtenbroit A, Roberts R: Localization of gene for familial hypertrophic cardiomyopathy to chromosome 14q1 in a diverse US population. *Circulation* **83:**1592, 1991.
144. Epstein ND, Fananapazir L, Lin HJ, Mulvihill J, White R, Lalouel JM, Lifton RP, Nienhuis AW, Leppert M: Evidence of genetic heterogeneity in five kindreds with familial hypertrophic cardiomyopathy. *Circulation* **85:**635, 1992.
145. Schwartz K, Beckmann J, Dufour C, Faure L, Fougerousse F, Carrier L, Hengstenberg C, Cohen D, Vosberg HP, Sacrez A, Ferrière M, Desnos M, Cambien F, Dubourg O, Komajda M: Exclusion of cardiac myosin heavy chain and actin gene involvement in hypertrophic cardiomyopathy of several French families. *Circ Res* **71:**3, 1992.
146. Saez LJ, Gianola KM, McNally EM, Feghali R, Eddy R, Shows TB, Leinwand LA: Human cardiac myosin heavy chain genes and their linkage in the genome. *Nucleic Acids Res* **15:**5443, 1987.
147. Matsuoka R, Yoshida MC, Kanda N, Kimura M, Ozasa H, Takao A: Human cardiac myosin heavy chain gene mapped within chromosome region 14q11.2----q13. *Am J Med Genet* **32:**279, 1989.
148. Nadal Ginard B, Mahdavi V: Molecular basis of cardiac performance. Plasticity of the myocardium generated through protein isoform switches. *J Clin Invest* **84:**1693, 1989.
149. Solomon SD, Geisterfer Lowrance AA, Vosberg HP, Hiller G, Jarcho JA, Morton CC, McBride WO, Mitchell AL, Bale AE, McKenna WJ, Seidman JG, Seidman CE: A locus for familial hypertrophic cardiomyopathy is closely linked to the cardiac myosin heavy chain genes, CRI-L436, and CRI-L329 on chromosome 14 at q11-q12. *Am J Hum Genet* **47:** 389, 1990.
150. Tanigawa G, Jarcho JA, Kass S, Solomon SD, Vosberg HP, Seidman JG, Seidman CE: A molecular basis for familial hypertrophic cardiomyopathy: An alpha/beta cardiac myosin heavy chain hybrid gene. *Cell* **62:**991, 1990.
151. Watkins H, Rosenzweig A, Hwang DS, Levi T, McKenna W, Seidman CE, Seidman JG: Characteristics and prognostic implications of myosin missense mutations in familial hypertrophic cardiomyopathy. *N Engl J Med* **326:**1108, 1992.
152. Watkins H, Seidman CE, MacRae C, Seidman JG, McKenna W: Progress in familial hypertrophic cardiomyopathy: Molecular genetic analyses in the original family studied by Teare. *Br Heart J* **67:**34, 1992.
153. Geisterfer Lowrance AA, Kass S, Tanigawa G, Vosberg HP, McKenna W, Seidman CE, Seidman JG: A molecular basis for familial hypertrophic cardiomyopathy: A beta cardiac myosin heavy chain gene missense mutation. *Cell* **62:**999, 1990.
154. Rosenzweig A, Watkins H, Hwang DS, Miri M, McKenna W, Traill TA, Seidman JG, Seidman CE: Preclinical diagnosis of familial hypertrophic cardiomyopathy by genetic analysis of blood lymphocytes. *N Engl J Med* **325:**1753, 1991.
155. Epstein ND, Cohn GM, Cyran F, Fananapazir L: Differences in clinical expression of hypertrophic cardiomyopathy associated with two distinct mutations in the beta-myosin heavy chain gene. A 908Leu----Val mutation and a 403Arg----Gln mutation. *Circulation* **86:**345, 1992.
156. Watkins H, Thierfelder L, Hwang DS, McKenna W, Seidman JG, Seidman CE: Sporadic hypertrophic cardiomyopathy due to de novo myosin mutations. *J Clin Invest* **90:**1666, 1992.
157. Nishi H, Kimura A, Harada H, Toshima H, Sasazuki T: Novel missense mutation in cardiac beta myosin heavy

chain gene found in a Japanese patient with hypertrophic cardiomyopathy. *Biochem Biophys Res Commun* **188:**379, 1992.

158. Al-Mahdawi S, Chamberlain S, Cleland J, Nihoyannopoulos P, Gilligan D, French J, Choudhury L, Williamson R, Oakley C: Identification of a mutation in the beta cardiac myosin heavy chain gene in a family with hypertrophic cardiomyopathy. *Br Heart J* **69:**136, 1993.
159. Marian AJ, Yu QT, Mares A Jr, Hill R, Roberts R, Perryman MB: Detection of a new mutation in the beta myosin chain gene in an individual with hypertrophic cardiomyopathy. *J Clin Invest* **90:**2156, 1992.
160. Tanigawa G, Watkins H, Jarcho JA, Morton CC, Seidman JG, Seidman CE: Absence of major deletions or rearrangements of myosin heavy chain genes in familial hypertrophic cardiomyopathy. *Circulation* **87**[Suppl IV]:11, 1993.
161. Perryman MB, Yu QT, Marian AJ, Mares AJ, Czernuszewicz G, Ifegwu J, Hill R, Roberts R: Expression of a missense mutation in the messenger RNA for beta-myosin heavy chain in myocardial tissue in hypertrophic cardiomyopathy. *J Clin Invest* **90:**271, 1992.
162. Bejsovec A, Anderson P: Functions of the myosin ATP and actin binding sites are required for C. elegans thick filament assembly. *Cell* **60:**133, 1990.
163. Watkins H, Thierfelder L, Anan R, Jarcho J, Matsumori A, McKenna WJ, Seidman JG, Seidman CE: Independent origin of identical beta cardiac myosin heavy-chain mutations in hypertrophic cardiomyopathy. *Am J Hum Genet* **53:**1180, 1993.
164. MacRae CA, Watkins HC, Jarcho JA, Thierfelder L, McKenna WJ, Seidman JG, Seidman CE: An evaluation of ribonuclease protection assays for the detection of beta-cardiac myosin heavy chain gene mutations. *Circulation* **89:**33, 1994.
165. Solomon SD, Wolff S, Watkins H, Ridker PM, Come P, Seidman CE, McKenna WJ, Lee RT: Left ventricular hypertrophy and morphology in familial hypertrophic cardiomyopathy associated with mutations of the beta-myosin heavy chain gene. *J Am Coll Cardiol* **22:**498, 1993.
166. Watkins H, MacRae C, Thierfelder L, Chou Y-H, Frenneaux M, McKenna W, Seidman JG, Seidman CE: A disease locus for familial hypertrophic cardiomyopathy maps to chromosome 1q3. *Nat Genet* **3:**333, 1993.
167. Gunning P, Ponte P, Kedes L, Eddy R, Shows T: Chromosomal location of the co-expressed human skeletal and cardiac actin genes. *Proc Natl Acad Sci USA* **81:**1813, 1984.
168. Boheler KR, Carrier L, de la Bastie D, Allen PD, Komajda M, Mercadier JJ, Schwartz K: Skeletal actin mRNA increases in the human heart during ontogenic development and is the major isoform of control and failing adult hearts. *J Clin Invest* **88:**323, 1991.
169. Bakerman PR, Stenmark KR, Fisher JH: Alpha-skeletal actin messenger RNA increases in acute right ventricular hypertrophy. *Am J Physiol* **258:**L173, 1990.
170. Radice P, Sozzi G, Miozzo M, De Benedetti V, Cariani T, Bongarzone I, Spurr NK, Pierotti MA, Della Porta G: The human tropomyosin gene involved in the generation of the TRK oncogene maps to chromosome 1q31. *Oncogene* **6:**2145, 1991.
171. Reinach FC, MacLeod AR: Tissue-specific expression of the human tropomyosin gene involved in the generation of the trk oncogene. *Nature* **322:**648, 1986.
172. Wade R, Eddy R, Shows TB, Kedes L: cDNA sequence, tissue-specific expression, and chromosomal mapping of the human slow-twitch skeletal muscle isoform of troponin I. *Genomics* **7:**346, 1990.
173. Bhavsar PK, Dhoot GK, Cumming DV, Butler Browne GS, Yacoub MH, Barton PJ: Developmental expression of troponin I isoforms in fetal human heart. *FEBS Lett* **292:**5, 1991.
174. Hunkeler NM, Kullman J, Murphy AM: Troponin I isoform expression in human heart. *Circ Res* **69:**1409, 1991.
175. Vaughan KT, Weber FE, Ried T, Ward DC, Reinach FC, Fischman DA: Human myosin-binding protein H (MyBP-H): Complete primary sequence, genomic organization and chromosomal localization. *Genomics* **16:**34, 1993.
176. Epstein HF, Fischman DA: Molecular analysis of protein assembly in muscle development. *Science* **251:**1039, 1991.
177. Thierfelder L, MacRae C, Watkins H, Tomfohrde J, Williams M, McKenna W, Bohm K, Noeske G, Schlepper M, Bowcock A, Vosberg H-P, Seidman JG, Seidman CE: A familial hypertrophic cardiomyopathy locus maps to chromosome 15q2. *Proc Natl Acad Sci USA* **90:**6270, 1993.
178. Carrier L, Hengstenberg C, Beckmann JS, Guicheney P, Dufour C, Bercovici J, Dausse E, Berebbi-Bertrand I, Wisnewsky C, Pulvenis D, Fetler L, Vignal A, Weissenbach J, Hillaire D, Feingold J, Bouhour J-B, Hagege A, Desnos M, Isnard R, Dubourg O, Komajda M, Schwartz K: Mapping of a novel gene for familial hypertrophic cardiomyopathy to chromosome 11. *Nat Genet* **4:**311, 1993.
179. Thierfelder L, Watkins H, MacRae C, Lamas R, McKenna WJ, Vosberg HP, Seidman JG, Seidman CE: α-Tropomyosin and cardiac troponin T mutations cause familial hypertrophic cardiomyopathy: A disease of the sarcomere. *Cell*, **77**:701, 1994.

Part 20

EYE

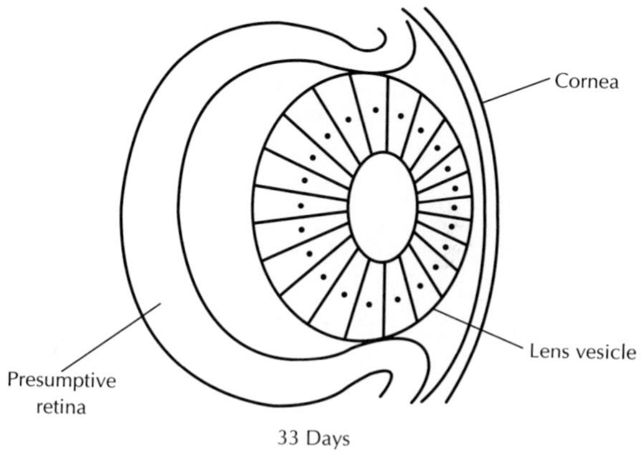

33 Days

CHAPTER 143

Color Vision and Its Genetic Defects

Arno G. Motulsky ▪ Samir S. Deeb

1. Color vision has intrigued scientists for several hundred years. Red–green color vision defects are common and were among the first recognized X-linked traits. The molecular genetics of the visual pigments mediating normal and defective color vision has been elucidated in recent years and provides the basis for a genetic understanding of normal and abnormal color vision.
2. The retina is a displaced part of the brain and includes four different photoreceptors: rods containing rhodopsin and cones containing either blue (short-wavelength), green (mid-wavelength), or red (long-wavelength) sensitive photopigments. Normal color vision is trichromatic and is subserved by these cone pigments. Rhodopsin is used in dim light, while the various cone photopigments mediate vision in bright light and color vision. The photopigments have characteristic absorption maxima with wide regions of overlap. The four human photopigments are homologous in their amino acid sequence and are members of the heptahelical transmembrane receptor family that includes olfactory receptors. The red and green pigments differ by at most 15 amino acids. Differences at three residues (180, 277, and 285) largely account for the spectral differences between these pigments.
3. The autosomal genes for rhodopsin and the blue pigment are located on chromosomes 3 and 7, respectively. The red–green pigment gene complex maps to a subterminal site on the long arm of the X chromosome (Xq28) close to the loci for adrenoleukodystrophy, glucose 6-phosphate dehydrogenase (G-6-PD), and hemophilia. The red–green gene arrays are composed of a single red pigment gene (six exons) and one or more green pigment genes (six exons) located downstream (3′) of the red gene. About 25 percent of male Caucasians have a single green gene, while the rest have two, three, or more green genes. Almost half of male Japanese and African-Americans have only a single green gene. The close homology of the red and green opsin genes (including introns) makes them prone to unequal crossing-over and accounts for the numerical polymorphism. Gene expression studies suggest that when several green pigment genes are present, only the most proximal is expressed in the retina.
4. Illegitimate recombination between the red and green pigment genes causes deletions or fusion genes and explains the genetic basis of most color vision defects. The deletion of green pigment genes leaves a single red pigment gene and is characteristically associated with deuteranopia (G^-). Affected individuals are dichromatic since they completely lack green cones. The finding of trichromatic deuteranomaly (G′) in a few individuals with this genetic makeup remains unexplained.
5. Exon 5 (which includes two of the three residues that account for the spectral difference between the red and green pigments) plays a major role in spectral tuning. The recombinational exchange of exon 5 produces hybrid pigments with large spectral shifts and corresponding effects on color vision.
6. 5′ green–red 3′ hybrid genes with or without additional green genes usually are associated with deuteranomaly—a milder type of color vision defect with a slightly red-shifted absorption maximum for the green pigment. Individuals with green–red hybrid genes who have normal color vision presumably carry the variant gene in a more downstream location of the gene array, where it is not expressed.
7. 5′ red–green 3′ fusion genes are always associated with protan abnormalities (R^- or R′). Those who have a hybrid gene only are always protanopic (R^-) and are therefore dichromats. Those who have normal green genes in addition are either protanopic (R^-) or protanomalous (R′) (milder defect with slightly green-shifted absorption maximum of the red pigment) depending on whether Ala or Ser is present at position 180 of the hybrid pigment.
8. A rare cause of red–green color vision defect (accounting for 1 in 64 color-defective males) can be a point mutation of a critical cysteine residue of the green pigment (C203R).
9. A single amino acid polymorphism (serine/alanine) at position 180 of the X-linked red pigment gene occurs in different ethnic groups. Serine occupies that position in 62 percent of Caucasians, 80 percent of African-Americans, and 84 percent of Japanese. Individuals with the serine variant with normal color vision perceive red color as a deeper red than those who have alanine at position 180, as shown by color matching. The Ser/Ala polymorphism also affects the spectral sensitivities of various hybrid genes.
10. Tritan or blue pigment abnormalities are caused by missense point mutations in the blue pigment gene and are transmitted (some with incomplete penetrance) as autosomal dominant traits.
11. The detection of color vision is often based on plate tests that require color discrimination of shapes or numbers.

A list of standard abbreviations is located immediately preceding the index in each volume. Additional abbreviations used in this chapter include: ADRP = autosomal dominant retinitis pigmentosa; BCM = blue cone monochromacy; G^- = deuteranopia; G^1 = deuteranomaly; LCR = locus control region; MYA = million years ago; R^- = protanopia; R^1 = protanomaly.

The standard test for detection of subtypes of color vision defects is quantitative anomaloscopy using color matching.

12. **Subjective color perception is most severely compromised in deuteranopes and protanopes, who cannot discriminate between green and red. More subtle abnormalities are seen in subjects with deuteranomaly and protanomaly, whose color perception for red and green is weakened but not absent. Tasks requiring practical color discrimination may be performed adequately, even by some fairly severely affected persons who test as grossly abnormal on color vision test systems.**

13. **Blue cone monochromacy is a rare disease that manifests as complete absence of red and green cone function. It can be caused by deletion of a critical regulatory gene segment upstream (5′) of the red–green gene complex which is required for expression of both the red and the green genes. Alternate causes involve point mutations of a single red–green hybrid gene that compromises function. The C203R mutation is frequently involved.**

14. **Female heterozygotes for the X-linked color vision defects are common among Caucasians (about 15 percent) and usually do not manifest color vision defects. Compound *trans*-heterozygotes for protan and deutan defects have normal color vision. Compound *trans*-heterozygotes for protanomaly/protanopia or deuteranomaly/deuteranopia, will manifest with the milder of the two defects, as expected on molecular grounds.**

15. **Deuteranomaly is the most common defect in Caucasian populations (4 to 5 percent of males). The other defects (protanopia, protanomaly, deuteranopia) have frequencies of about 1 percent each among males. The frequency of color vision defects in most other populations (e.g., Japanese and populations of African descent) is lower, ranging around 3 to 4 percent, and is largely accounted for by a lower frequency of deuteranomalous individuals. The relatively high frequency of human color vision defects is largely accounted for by unequal crossing-over between the highly homologous red and green pigment genes in this multigene complex. The high frequency of deuteranomalous individuals is unexplained. The role of selection remains undefined.**

16. **There is a high frequency (19 percent) among African-Americans of apparent green-red fusion genes that, for unknown reasons, are not expressed as color vision defects. About one-third of African-Americans have a phenotypically silent polymorphism manifesting as a shortened red pigment gene that resembles the normal (shortened) green pigment gene. This homology may predispose to more illegitimate recombination and possibly explains the higher frequency of green–red fusion genes in this population.**

Color vision as a natural phenomenon has intrigued scientists for several hundred years.[1] Severe defects in red–green color vision have been known for about 200 years,[2,3] and milder anomalies for over 100 years. Pedigrees of "color blindness" extending over several generations were reported[4] long before the rediscovery of Mendel's laws. Very early in the history of human genetics, Wilson[5], the American pioneer of fruit fly genetics, in 1911 suggested X-linked recessive inheritance as the explanation for the transmission of "color blindness." Color blindness therefore represents one of the first human traits shown to follow Mendelian inheritance. When hemophilia was later shown to be an X-linked trait, mapping of the hemophilia and color-blindness genes was undertaken by classic linkage methods in families where both genes segregated.[6] Failure of recombination between these traits suggested close linkage of their genes. Later in the 1960s, family studies also showed that the glucose 6-phosphate dehydrogenase (G-6-PD) locus is tightly linked to the red–green color vision locus.[7] More recently, the very close proximity of these three genes was demonstrated by physical mapping.[8]

Color vision has helped to establish the field of human visual psychophysics—a subfield of physiological psychology that, among other phenomena, studies the detailed perceptual characteristics of human color vision.[9] These investigations not only are interesting and important in their own right but may provide clues to other sensory phenomena in human neurobiology.

The elucidation of the molecular bases of normal and abnormal color vision pigments has revolutionized ongoing studies in this field.[10,11] Unlike elsewhere in the human central nervous system, where sophisticated gene–phenotype comparisons are not yet feasible, fundamental studies on gene structure and function can now be correlated with psychophysical observations or tests that assess the phenotype of color vision and its abnormalities quantitatively. Slight differences in red color perception among "normal" human individuals, which had been discovered earlier by psychophysical methods,[12–17] can now be related to a frequent genetic polymorphism of the red visual pigment gene caused by a single amino acid substitution.[18] It is likely that similar phenomena, i.e., minor differences in sensory perception, exist elsewhere in the human nervous system.

After the molecular biology of the photopigments underlying normal red–green and blue color vision was elucidated, various genotype–phenotype correlations in color vision defects emerged and are the topic of ongoing research in molecular biology and psychophysics.[19] While recent advances have provided a good comprehension of the biology and genetics of the visual pigments, the neurobiology of color perception involving the neural pathways of the brain is less well understood. A full understanding of color vision in all its aspects therefore requires much additional work. This chapter will be largely concerned with the biology and pathology of cone photoreceptors, their pigments, and the resulting color vision abnormalities. Ongoing work on rhodopsin and other vision-related proteins and their mutations has explained the cause of a significant proportion of cases of retinitis pigmentosa and is covered elsewhere in this book (Chap. 144).

COLOR AND COLOR VISION

The scientific study of color[20–23] started with the observation of the color spectrum by Newton over 300 years ago.[24] Sunlight or white light refracted by a glass prism could be split into a series, or rainbow, of colors. Newton suggested that any particular color was characterized by its degree of "refrangibility"—wavelength, in modern terms. Light at each angle of refraction had a characteristic color, ranging from violet for the most refracted rays through blue, green, yellow, orange, and red to the other end of the color spectrum. We know now that visible colors represent the range of electromagnetic radiation extending from about 400 nm (violet) to 700 nm (1 nm = 10^{-9} m). Under well-defined conditions, visible radiation of a particular wavelength (monochromatic light) has a characteristic color for observers with normal color vision.

Most naturally occurring colors or hues can be produced by mixtures of monochromatic light. Newton noticed this phenomenon when he observed that the human eye could not distinguish between the sensation of a mixture of red and green light and the sensation of pure yellow light having a refractive angle intermediate between those of red and green.

During the 19th century, the trichromatic theory of color perception was developed.[25–27] It was shown that lights of three different wavelengths, or primaries, mixed together were sufficient to produce light of any perceived hue and brightness. Most colors can be matched by a mixture of three primary lights. Each trio of primary lights has to include a long-wavelength, an intermediate-wavelength, and a short-wavelength light. Equal portions of these lights produce the perception of white. Color vision, therefore, was shown to be a system with only three perceptual dimensions.

The retina (see Dowling[28]) is a part of the brain that has been displaced to the eye during embryonic development, and, unlike other brain structures, can be viewed directly, for example by an ophthalmoscope. Light is absorbed by specialized retinal neurons known as photoreceptors. The resulting signals are processed to the lateral geniculate nucleus and from there to the visual cortex of the brain.

The normal human eye has several types of photoreceptors. Rods contain rhodopsin, have a maximal sensitivity at about 500 nm (the blue-green area of the spectrum), and mediate vision in dim light (scotopic vision). No color is perceived under scotopic conditions, and all colors appear grayish-white. Rods are more numerous than cones and are more common in the periphery of the retina. The photoreceptors that mediate the perception of color are the retinal cones. Historically, a variety of psychophysical approaches suggested, in conformity with the trichromatic theory, that there are three types of cones, each containing a different visual pigment. Direct proof of the existence of three color receptors came from measurements that were capable of determining the absorbance of single photoreceptor cells in the retina.[29–33] Three different but overlapping spectral sensitivity curves were obtained (Fig. 143-1). The blue or short-wavelength-sensitive pigment (peak absorption or λ_{max} of 420 nm) has only a small degree of overlap with the mid-wavelength-sensitive (green) and long-wavelength-sensitive (red) pigments, which have absorption maxima differing by only about 30 nm. Both green and red cones are active across most of the spectrum, but particularly between 450 and 650 nm.

The maximal sensitivities of long-wavelength-sensitive, mid-wavelength-sensitive, and short-wavelength-sensitive cones are at ~560, ~530, and ~420 nm, respectively. These cones are sometimes referred to as blue, green, and red cones, respectively. Although useful for characterizing the receptors and their pigments, the terms *blue*, *green*, and *red* are misnomers, since the spectrum of each pigment is spread over a considerable range and overlaps the spectra of the other pigments as well as rhodopsin (Fig. 143-1). Cones are differentiated from rods by the tapered shape of their outer segment. Each cone contains only a single type of photopigment, which is operative under well-lit (photopic) conditions.

A small area of the retina—the fovea—is centrally located on the visual axis of the eye. It is about 0.3 mm in diameter

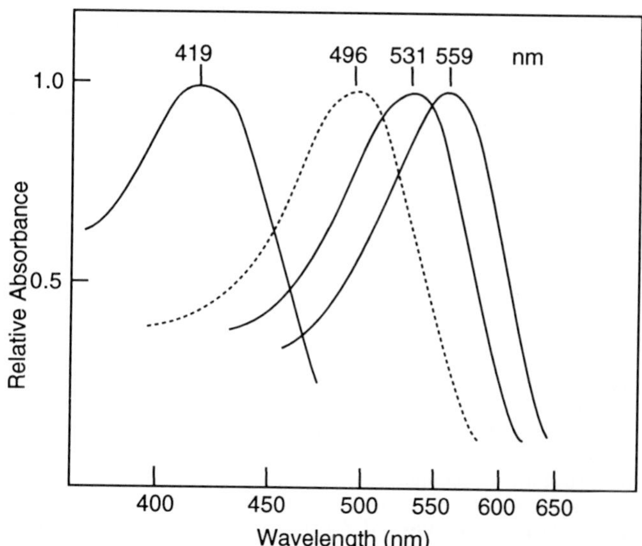

FIG. 143-1 *Absorption spectra of the four human photoreceptors.* **The dotted line is for rhodopsin and the solid lines are for the blue (λ_{max} = 419 nm), green (λ_{max} = 531 nm), and red (λ_{max} = 559 nm) cones. These curves are based on microspectrophotometric measurements of individual cones from human retinas.** *(Adapted from Dartnall et al.[31] Used by permission.)*

and contains about 10,000 cones. The central fovea has no rods and very few blue cones, and has evolved as a specialized organ of high acuity and red–green color vision.

The photoreceptors are located in the outermost layer of the retina and are overlain by a pigmented epithelial layer that absorbs strong light and prevents backscatter of light. There are about twice as many red cones as green cones in the human retina, with considerable variation between individuals.[34–38] The similarity of red and green cones (see below) precludes their direct measurement, and quantitation requires indirect psychophysical methodology. The number of blue cones can be assessed directly by immunocytochemical staining, and is 10 to 20 percent of the total number of red and green cones.[39] The various visual pigment molecules are concentrated in the outer segments of the photoreceptors, which contain about 1,000 to 2,000 transverse disks with a total of 10^9 molecules.

MOLECULAR BIOLOGY OF VISUAL PIGMENTS

The four human visual pigments—rhodopsin and the blue, red, and green pigments—are composed of a protein moiety, called opsin, which is covalently linked to the chromophore 11-*cis*-retinal via a protonated Schiff base formed between the aldehyde group of retinal and the ϵ-amino group of a highly conserved lysine residue.[40] A characteristic topographic motif of this family of photoreceptors is the heptahelical transmembrane bundle, within which the chromophore is held.[41] The transmembrane segments are believed to be largely α-helical in character.[42] The visual pigments belong to an evolutionarily related superfamily of heptahelical transmembrane receptors, which includes the adrenergic, serotonergic, dopaminergic, muscarinic, and olfactory chemoreceptors (Fig. 143-2; see Dohlman et al.[43] for a review).

In addition to the heptahelical structural motifs, members of this superfamily share many features of cellular signal

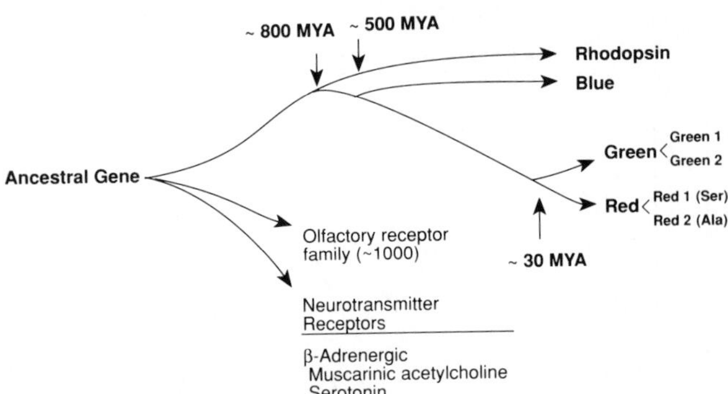

FIG. 143-2 ***Evolution of the superfamily of heptahelical G-protein-coupled receptors.*** **A chronology for the evolutionary relationships among members of the human opsin gene family. (MYA = million years ago). The terms *blue*, *green*, and *red* refer to the corresponding visual pigments. *Green 1* and *green 2* refer to the green pigment duplication (and further multiplication of the green pigment genes). *Red 1* (Ser) and *red 2* (Ala) refer to the common Ser/Ala polymorphism[18] affecting the human red pigment genes.**

transduction processes. The absorption of a single photon of light causes the retinal chromophore of photopigments to isomerize from the 11-*cis* to the all-*trans* configuration. This isomerization results in the formation of a conformationally activated intermediate of the photopigment, which triggers the signal amplification cascade.[44–46] The first step in this cascade involves activation of transducin (a G protein), which in turn activates a cyclic GMP (cGMP) phosphodiesterase. The resulting decrease in cGMP levels triggers closure of cGMP-gated membrane cation channels and hyperpolarization of the photoreceptor cell.

The four human photopigments share varying degrees of sequence homology. Figure 143-3 shows pairwise comparisons of the amino acid sequences.[10] The red and green photopigments are far more closely related to each other (96 percent amino acid sequence identity) than any other pair of pigments (40 to 45 percent identity), reflecting the more recent duplication of the ancestral red and green pigment gene (Fig. 143-2). This fact is in agreement with the observation that humans and Old World monkeys have both red and green photopigments, while New World monkeys have a single polymorphic long-wavelength photopigment.[47–49] It has been estimated that the common ancestor of the three human color-vision genes diverged from that of rhodopsin about 800 million years ago (MYA); that the ancestor of the green and red pigment genes diverged from the blue about 500 MYA; and that the red and green pigment genes diverged from each other about 30 MYA[10,50–52] (Fig. 143-2; see "Evolution" below).

Differences in amino acid residues, especially in residues at positions within the membrane bilayer that allow interaction with retinal, are likely to underlie differences in spectral characteristics among the photopigments. The absorption spectra of the blue-, red-, and green-sensitive photopigments that are involved in color vision are shown in Fig. 143-1. These spectra were determined by microspectrophotometry of individual human cone cells[31] and show absorption maxima at ~420, ~530, and ~560 nm for the blue, red, and green cone pigments, respectively. The fourth pigment, rhodopsin, which is found in the rods and mediates vision in dim light, absorbs maximally at ~495 nm. The absorption maxima of the photopigments synthesized in vitro are in good agreement with the maxima determined by microspectrophotometry.[53–55] The red and green photopigments differ in at most 15 of a total of 364 amino acid residues. The presence of a

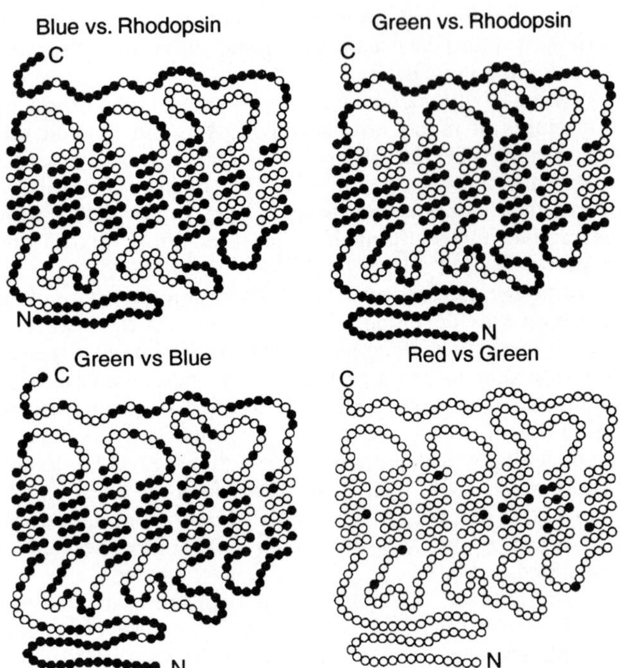

FIG. 143-3 ***Amino acid sequence identities among the human visual pigments.*** **The secondary structures of the opsins with the seven α-helical segments that span the plasma membrane are shown. The N-terminal ends (N) are exposed at the luminal surface of the disk membrane, while the C-terminal ends (C) are exposed at the cytoplasmic surface. Sequence identities are indicated by open circles and differences by filled circles. Note the remarkable identity of the red and green pigments, as contrasted with comparisons of the other pigments. *(Adapted from Nathans et al.*[10] *Used by permission.)***

hydroxyl-bearing versus a nonpolar residue constitutes the difference at 7 of these 15 positions, all lying within one turn of the helix of the location of the retinylidine group of the chromophore.[56] All other amino acid differences involve no significant changes in polarity and therefore are unlikely to influence the spectral sensitivity of the pigments.

Biochemical Basis of Spectral Tuning

Two types of evidence support the hypothesis that spectral tuning could result from the substitution of polar for nonpolar residues. One is derived from relating differences in amino acid sequence to spectral characteristics of the mid- to long-wavelength visual pigments of humans, Old World monkeys, and New World monkeys. The results indicated that the spectral tuning of these pigments depends on the presence of hydroxyl-bearing versus nonpolar residues at positions 180, 277, 285,[57] and 233.[58,59] Another line of evidence comes from experiments involving site-directed mutagenesis and expression in tissue culture cells of sequence variants of the human red photopigment. The two reconstituted red pigment variants bearing Ser or Ala at position 180 were shown to differ in wavelength of maximal absorption by 5 nm (Ser at 180 = 557 nm; Ala at 180 = 552 nm) as determined by photobleaching difference absorption spectroscopy.[60] The absorption characteristics of other pigments expressed in vitro (see below) are consistent with the earlier conclusion that differences at positions 180, 277, and 285 largely account for the spectral difference between the red and green pigments. This conclusion is further supported by in vitro spectral studies on bovine rhodopsin, which involved muta-

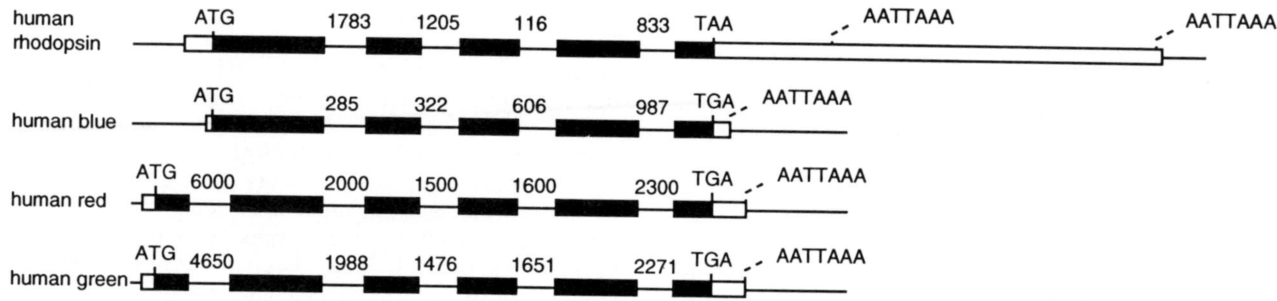

FIG. 143-4 *Comparison of the structure of the human visual pigment genes.* **Coding sequences of the genes are denoted by boxes and noncoding regions by lines (not to scale). Open boxes represent untranslated regions, and filled boxes denote coding regions. The length of introns in number of base pairs is shown. Also indicated are the initiation and termination codons and the polyadenylation signal sequences.** *(Adapted from Applebury and Hargrave.[113] Used by permission.)*

genesis of the residues equivalent to positions 180, 277, and 285 of the red and green opsins.[61]

Photopigment Genes

The recent cloning and characterization of the genes that encode the photopigment apoproteins (opsins) is largely the result of the pioneering work of Nathans and his collaborators. Based on partial amino acid sequence data, they first isolated and characterized cDNA and genomic clones of rhodopsin.[62] Using low-stringency hybridization, the bovine probe was subsequently used to isolate clones of human rhodopsin[62] and the blue, green, and red opsin genes.[10] Furthermore, cDNA probes containing coding sequences for bovine rhodopsin detected (by Southern blot hybridization) homologous sequences of other photopigment genes in DNA of a variety of vertebrate and invertebrate organisms,[63] indicating the high degree of sequence conservation among members of this family of genes.

A comparison of the intron/exon structures of some members of the photopigment gene family is given in Fig. 143-4. The rhodopsin and blue pigment genes are located on the long arms of chromosomes 3 and 7, respectively, and have remarkably similar structures, each consisting of five exons and encoding a polypeptide of 348 amino acids. On the other hand, the red and green pigment genes, which are located close to each other on the X chromosome (Xq28), are almost identical in structure. They have six instead of five exons each and encode proteins that are 364 amino acid residues long. Exon 1 of the red and green pigment genes has no homologue in the rhodopsin and blue pigment genes. The difference in length between the red and green pigment genes is caused by a 1.5-kb insertion in intron 1 of the red pigment gene. Approximately 35 percent of African-American, 2 percent of Japanese, and <1 percent of Caucasian males have a shortened red pigment gene that lacks the 1.5-kb insertion in intron 1 and is identical in size to the green pigment gene[64] (see below). The red and green pigment genes are arranged in a head-to-tail tandem array consisting of one red pigment gene 5′ to one or more green pigment genes, as determined by Southern blot hybridization, pulsed-field electrophoresis, and restriction enzyme analysis of genomic cosmid clones.[8,10,11,65] The red–green gene complex on the long arm of the X chromosome (q28) is located approximately 700 kb telomeric to the adrenoleukodystrophy gene[66] and approximately 800 to 1,000 kb centromeric from the G-6-PD and coagulation factor VIII (F8C) loci.[8] It is of interest that a recent study in families of homosexual men suggested the presence of a gene (or genes) in the Xq28 region that influences at least one subtype of male sexual orientation.[67] The exact position of this gene (or genes) within this region in not yet available.

The number of green pigment genes is polymorphic, and in addition varies in frequency distribution among males of different ethnic origin, as shown in Table 143-1.[64,68] The suggestive relationship between the frequency of green pigment genes and the frequency of hybrid genes in these three ethnic groups is intriguing (see below). Nathans et al.[11] proposed unequal recombination in the red–green pigment intergenic region (approximately 15 kb long) as a mechanism of altering the copy number of the green pigment gene (Fig. 143-5). A larger number of green opsin genes per array may lead to a higher probability of unequal recombination.

The question of whether all the green opsin genes are expressed in the retina was addressed by determining spectral luminous efficiency (which is a measure of the relative numbers of red and green cones) as a function of the number of green opsin genes in the array in a group of 26 males who had normal color vision. The results indicated that spectral luminous efficiency is not correlated with the number of

Table 143-1 **Green Pigment Gene in Different Populations with "Normal" Molecular Genotypes (Excluding Individuals with Deletions or Fusion Genes)**

		Number of Green Pigment Genes			
Population (Males)	*n*	One*	Two	Three	≥ Four
African-American	81	0.42	0.42	0.10	0.06
Japanese	97	0.48	0.31	0.15	0.05
Caucasian	113	0.22	0.51	0.19	0.08

*Proportion of single green genes: Caucasian vs. African-American, $\chi^2 = 8.79 = p < 0.01$; Caucasian vs. Japanese, $\chi^2 = 16.08 = p < 0.001$; African-American vs. Japanese, $\chi^2 = 0.74 = p > 0.3$.

SOURCE: Data from Jorgensen et al.[64]

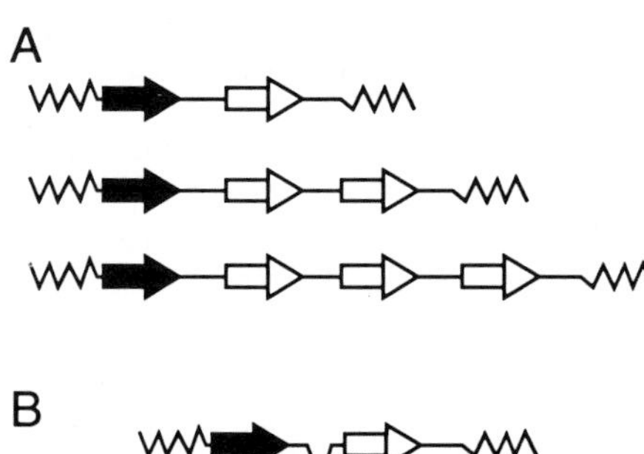

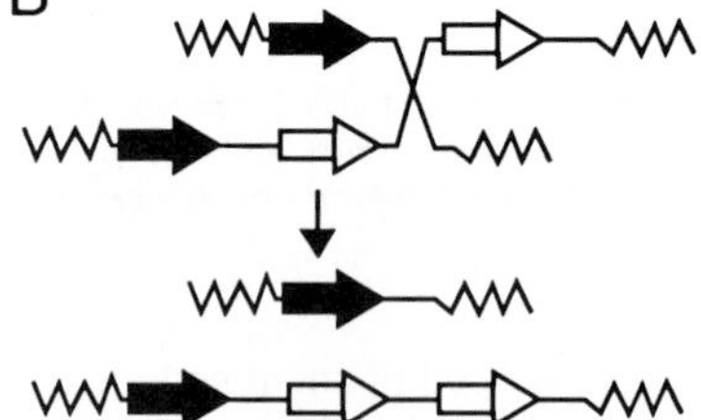

FIG. 143-5 *Polymorphism in the number of green opsin genes.* **A. Diagram of the X-linked red–green gene arrays that differ in the number of green opsin genes. Filled arrows denote red opsin genes, and open arrows denote green opsin genes. Straight lines represent intergenic regions, and wavy lines represent regions that flank the gene complex. B. Unequal recombination within intergenic regions as a mechanism of generating polymorphism in the number of green opsin genes in an array.**

green pigment gene copies in an array and support the hypothesis (see below) that only one green opsin gene is expressed in the retina (Lindsey and colleagues, unpublished observations from our group).

COLOR VISION DEFECTS

Color vision defects have been recognized for almost 200 years. The famous chemist Dalton reported his own color vision defect to the Manchester Literary and Philosophical Society in 1794.[2] Dalton reported that an "image which others call red appears to me as little more than a shade or defect of light." Orange, yellow, and green appeared to him as different shades of yellow. Color vision defects are sometimes referred to as Daltonism.

Red–green color vision defects are a group of X-linked abnormalities that are common in the male European population (8 percent).[69–71] Several types of color vision defects exist[69–71] (Table 143-2). When the color-sensitive receptors for either the long-wavelength pigment (red) or mid-wavelength pigment (green) are completely absent, color vision is dichromatic rather than trichromatic. Otherwise stated, such individuals have only two, instead of the normal three, visual pigments (i.e., green and blue or red and blue, rather than green, red, and blue). Depending on whether the long-wavelength (red) or mid-wavelength (green) pigment is absent, dichromats are classified as *deuteranopes*, persons who lack the cones with green pigment (G^-), or as *protanopes*, persons who lack cones with red visual pigment (R^-). The complete lack of the specific visual pigment in dichromats was proved first by microspectrophotometry, which failed to detect absorption of a wavelength characteristic of the red pigment in protanopes (R^-) and of the green pigment in deuteranopes (G^-).[31,32,72,73] These traits have a frequency in the Caucasian population of around 1 percent each. Molecular studies demonstrate complete absence of the green visual pigments in deuteranopes, while protanopia has been associated with red–green fusion genes that have the characteristics of normal green pigment.[11,19]

The other X-linked color-vision anomalies are associated with trichromatic color vision and are known as deuteranomaly (G′) and protanomaly (R′)[69] (Table 143-2). In these defects, all three visual pigments are present, but microspectrophotometric measurements showed a slight displacement of the green and red pigment spectral sensitivity curves in

Table 143-2 Classification of Color Vision Defects

Type	Inheritance	Frequency (Europeans)	Type of Color Vision	Symptoms
Red–green defect				
Protanopia (R-)	X-linked recessive	~1%	Dichromatic	Severe red–green color confusion
Deuteranopia (G-)		~1%	Dichromatic	Severe red–green color confusion
Protanomaly (R′)		~1%	Trichromatic	Mild red–green color confusion
Deuteranomaly (G′)		~4–5%	Trichromatic	Mild red–green color confusion
Blue–yellow defect				
Tritanopia	Autosomal dominant	1 in 500 (?) or fewer	Dichromatic*	Blue–yellow color confusion
Tritanomaly*	Autosomal dominant	?	Trichromatic*	Blue–yellow color confusion
Achromatopsias				
Complete rod monochromacy	Autosomal recessive	Very rare	Monochromatic	Onset in infancy; low visual acuity
"Atypical" rod monochromacy (with nonfunctional cone pigment)	Autosomal recessive	Very rare	Monochromatic	Pendular nystagmus, photophobia
Blue cone monochromacy	X-linked recessive	Rare	Monochromatic	No ophthalmoscopic findings
Various rare cone and cone–rod dystrophies†	Autosomal dominant autosomal recessive, X-linked recessive	Very rare	Usually monochromatic	Onset in adolescence or later; usually macular retinal pigment epithelium atrophy ("bull's eye" on ophthalmoscopy); abnormal green–red color vision

*Distinction between tritanopia and tritanomaly not fully clarified.
†See Weleber and Eisner[82] and Moore[83] for information.

deuteranomaly and protanomaly, respectively, and suggested the presence of visual pigments with altered spectral characteristics.[74–76] Deuteranomalous and protanomalous subjects thus were assumed to have variant visual pigments. Molecular studies indicated the presence of green–red fusion genes in deuteranomaly (G′)[11,19] and of red–green fusion genes in protanomaly (R′).[11,19] However, a few deuteranomalous individuals had a complete absence of green pigment genes.[19] Current molecular methodology has been unsuccessful in differentiating protanopes from protanomalous individuals, since both have red–green fusion genes (see below for details). Furthermore, green–red fusion genes are not infrequently found in persons with normal color vision,[19,64,68] but presumably are located in downstream locations where they are not expressed (see below).

There is considerable variation in the severity of the trichromatic abnormalities (protanomaly and deuteranomaly).[69,70] Some scientists have divided the various trichromatic anomalies into mild, moderate, and severe deuteranomaly or protanomaly.[77] It would be expected that a given subtype of defect generally would be expressed with a similar degree of severity in all affected male members of a family who carry the same mutation. However, intrafamilial variability of color vision defects has been occasionally observed, as in many other examples of identical mutations of a variety of human genetic diseases. Further work to relate the molecular lesion to the severity of the defect needs to be done. The frequency of deuteranomaly in Europeans ranges between 4 and 5 percent, while the frequency of protanomaly is around 1 percent (see Drummond-Borg et al.[68]).

Abnormalities affecting the blue- or short-wavelength-sensitive pigment are known as tritan defects.*[78] Differentiating tritanopia from tritanomaly is not as easy as for the green–red defects. Tritan defects are much rarer than deutan or protan abnormalities, but have been estimated to occur as frequently as one in 500 individuals.[79] Tritan individuals have problems perceiving blue color. The defect is inherited as an autosomal dominant trait, as might be expected given the location of the blue pigment gene on chromosome 7. The molecular basis of tritan abnormalities are missense mutations; three different amino acid substitutions (see below) have been observed.[80,81] Variability in expression has been noticed in several pedigrees. In fact, some individuals with the characteristic amino acid substitution did not exhibit the phenotypic color vision defect.[80]

Unlike the amino acid substitutions of rhodopsin, which often are associated with rod degeneration leading to autosomal dominant retinitis pigmentosa (Chap. 144), no other ophthalmic or clinical consequences are associated with the various deutan, protan, and tritan color vision defects. Visual acuity is unaffected. The color vision defects are expressed early in life and remain constant throughout life.

Color Vision Defects in Cone Dystrophies

Color vision defects are frequently observed in several very rare cone dystrophies (Table 143-2).[82] In achromatopsia, there may be complete absence of cone responses, causing very poor or no color discrimination, associated with a variety of eye signs or symptoms, such as low visual acuity, photophobia, and pendular nystagmus. Onset is usually in infancy. Three principal varieties[83] have been distinguished, although more complex classifications[70] have also been suggested.

1. Complete achromatopsia with rod monochromacy. There are no or very few cones, and it has been suggested that rhodopsin may be functioning in both rods and cones. This defect is autosomal recessive.
2. Atypical rod monochromacy with present but nonfunctioning cone pigments (autosomal recessive). The defect presumably occurs at a site other than the cones.
3. Blue cone monochromacy, or X-linked incomplete achromatopsia,[84] where both red and green cones are nonfunctional, while blue cone function is preserved.

Many patients with these cone dystrophies also develop electroretinographically detectable rod abnormalities that are associated with symptoms of night blindness.[83] In addition, various studies[85–92] report cone dystrophies with onset in adolescence or later, which (unlike the three achromatopsias) are associated with a characteristic ophthalmoscopic abnormality: a bull's eye appearance due to atrophy of the retinal pigment epithelium.[82] Apart from the mode of inheritance, which can be autosomal dominant, autosomal recessive, or X-linked, it has been difficult to categorize these cases. Sporadic cases in this category have also been reported, but a sporadic case could be due to autosomal recessive or X-linked inheritance, or could be a new autosomal dominant mutation.

The molecular pathology of the various cone and cone rod dystrophies requires further work. In one family[93] a 6.5-kb deletion in the red pigment gene has been detected.

Phenotypic Detection of Color Vision Defects[69,94]

Color Chart Tests. A large number of different tests have been devised for detecting color vision anomalies. Most of these have not been standardized and are not in general use. They will therefore not be discussed here. The tests discussed below are most useful for detection of genetic color vision defects.

Pseudoisochromatic plates are widely used in screening for color vision defects. The figures to be discriminated on these plates appear in shades of different chromatic quality. These tests usually use patterns of variously colored printed dots, which usually are shaped as numbers. The subject is asked to read or trace a shape or number. The charts are so designed that persons with color vision defects will miss shapes or numbers or see different shapes than persons with normal color vision. The most widely used variety are the Ishihara (Japan) charts and the American Optical H-R-R (Hardy-Rand-Ritter) polychromatic plates. Illumination should be standardized at diffused daylight during testing (100 watt blue daylight bulb or MacBeth easel lamp), since the pigments in the charts may vary in gloss, which could give clues to a color-defective person. Ordinary tungsten bulbs may allow deuteranomalous persons to read test charts correctly. Ishihara charts have had the most use. It is usually possible to distinguish between deutan and protan abnormalities on the basis of these charts, but they should not be relied on absolutely for subclassification, because severe anomalous trichromats cannot often be differentiated from dichromats.

Ishihara charts do not detect tritan defects, whereas the H-R-R charts will. When color vision abnormalities are found

*The terms *protan*, *deutan*, and *tritan* are derived from the Greek and refer to the "first," "second," and "third" variants of color defect.

on chart testing, anomaloscopy (see below) is usually done in genetic studies to confirm the type of color vision defect.

Color Arrangement Tests. The Farnsworth-Munsell 100-Hue Test[95] has been widely used to evaluate chromatic discrimination loss. In this test, the subject is asked to arrange 85 color chips in their natural order of hue. Each chip has a number on its back indicating its place in the series. The mistakes the subject makes yield a standardized score, which is recorded on a special chart. There are characteristic error patterns of protans, deutans, and tritans, but differentiating between protanomaly and protanopia is difficult.

Anomaloscopy. Anomaloscopy has been used widely and is based on color matching. Lord Rayleigh devised a simple test system to classify individuals with red–green color vision abnormalities. The observer views a pure yellow light (589 to 590 nm) on one half of a screen while the other half of the screen projects a mixture of red (650 nm) and green (545 to 550 nm) lights. The brightness or intensity of the yellow light as well as the proportion of the green and red lights are adjusted by the subject until the two fields appear identical in color and brightness. Under the color conditions of the Rayleigh match, contributions to color by the short-wavelength-sensitive (blue) pigment cones are negligible. The most frequently used instrument is the Nagel anomaloscope. The range of accepted matches of mixtures of green and red light against yellow is recorded, as is the mid-point of such matches. (See Fig. 143-9 below for typical findings for normal and various color-vision-defective persons.) Normal subjects accept matches in a narrow range. Dichromats, such as protanopic and deuteranopic subjects, will match yellow with any ratio of red and green, including red or green alone. Thus, any red/green mixture will produce a match when set to the appropriate brightness. Deuteranopes require much more yellow to match the red field than do protanopes, who need only a small amount of yellow to match the red field, which they perceive as of low intensity.

Protanomalous subjects produce match ranges that are shifted toward the red side of the mixture range, while the matches of deuteranomalous subjects are displaced toward the green. Subjects with severe deuteranomaly or severe protanomaly tend to have quite wide and characteristically displaced match ranges, while those with milder anomalous defects have narrower match ranges.

Most large-scale investigations of color vision defects start by using plate tests and employ anomaloscopy only for individuals who fail the plate test. Anomaloscopic findings in a given individual are constant and do not change. As might be expected, anomaloscopic results for different family members are usually but not always similar. The viewing angle conventionally is 2 degrees. With larger viewing angles, most protanopes are classified as protanomalous, and some deuteranopes as deuteranomalous.

Electroretinography. An objective assessment of color vision may be possible with electroretinography.[96] All other test measurements are based on the observers' subjective matching of color. In electroretinography, a corneal electrode placed on a dilated eye records the retinal response to standardized flashes of light. Because of the somewhat invasive nature of the test, no extensive experience with the various benign genetic color vision defects has been reported. However, color vision defects characterized as deutan (36 subjects) and protan (32 subjects) (with no indication of the proportion of dichromats and trichromats) could be discriminated by the log ratio of the sensitivity at short (480 nm) and long (620 nm) wavelengths.[97] Female carrier detection for protans and deutans was particularly successful for deutan carriers and less so for protan heterozygotes.[97]

Color Perception and Color Defects: Practical Implications

Color vision defects affect perception of color.[98] A large proportion of the population, therefore, lives in a different perceptual world than those with normal color vision. Normal trichromatic color vision helps to define objects in complex multicolored settings, as can be observed by comparing a colored photograph with a black and white rendering of the same scene. The color perception of color-vision-defective observers has been studied in a few individuals who, for unknown reasons, were color defective in one eye only. One otherwise healthy young woman was deuteranopic in the left eye and color-normal in the right eye (see Kalmus[69]). Her color-vision-defective eye had only three color sensations—gray, yellow, and blue—and lacked any green or red sensations. Her normal eye gave normal color vision. As shown in a film depicting the color world of this woman (MN8246—Color Vision Deficiency—Research Division Bureau Medicine and Surgery, Department of the Navy, Washington, D.C.), a room furnished entirely in gray, blue, and yellow materials had the same color appearance to her defective eye as similar objects covering the entire range of colors, including red and green. Color perception of typical deuteranopes conform to this general pattern. Protanopia appears to cause more color confusion than deuteranopia. Protanopes confuse not only red, yellow, and green, as in deuteranopia, but also deep red, dark brown, or even black, and have particular problems with red color perception. A ripe red fruit might be considered black by a protanope.

Color perception differences in anomalous trichromats are more subtle than in dichromats. Green and red are not absent but appear weakened in intensity. Deuteranomaly is considered to be the mildest anomaly. More subtle differences in color perception are seen in individuals who have either alanine (62 percent) or serine (38 percent) at position 180 of the red pigment gene. Those with 180 alanine (~62 percent) require more red in the mixture to match yellow than those who have serine at this position. Based on these findings, it is expected that about 47 percent of Caucasian women are heterozygotes for *both* the 180 alanine and the 180 serine variant, as calculated by Hardy-Weinberg statistics. Owing to X inactivation, about half of the cones will have alanine in position 180, and the other half will have serine at that site. Such women have four types of cones: blue, green, and two types of red cones, and might have tetrachromatic vision. Further tests need to be done on whether such females under certain conditions have superior color discrimination as compared with trichromats.

Color-vision-defective persons, including dichromats, can do surprisingly well in naming colors. Apparently there are enough differences in color sensation to allow them to learn to use the right terms.

It has been claimed by anecdotal evidence that color-vision-defective observers can see through colored patterns that deceive normal observers.[99] This advantage would be useful under military conditions, and could have played a role in the evolution of color vision.[100] A recent study suggests that dichromats, in fact, perform better than normal trichromats under experimental conditions in which texture was camouflaged by color.[101] No anomalous trichromats were tested in this study.

Since color vision is important for many industrial, marine, air, rail, and military occupations, color vision testing is done to screen out color-vision-defective applicants. However, when actual tasks requiring color discrimination instead of various artificial testing systems are used for testing, many color-defective persons perform adequately.[102,103] The validity of rigid color vision standards for occupational selection, therefore, has been questioned by some observers.[104] Cole[105] suggested using variable standards for the many different occupations that require color discrimination. The recommended specifications and the rigor of practical testing were based on considerations such as the probability, severity, and socioeconomic consequences of the problems that might be caused by difficulties with color discrimination.

In general, deuteranopic and protanopic dichromats perform worse on color discrimination than individuals with anomalous trichromacy. Most but not all dichromats have difficulties in selecting colored articles and materials, including foods. No studies have shown that color vision defects have been the cause of aircraft accidents.[106] On self-reporting and under conditions of confidentiality, 49 percent of dichromats reported confusing the colors of traffic lights, 33 percent found it difficult to distinguish traffic lights from street lighting, and 22 percent had difficulty detecting rear brake lights.[107] It is therefore noteworthy that rear-end collisions, particularly under conditions of poor visibility, were slightly more common among protan drivers, who have more problems with perception of red rear warning lights.[108] However, there is general agreement in most jurisdictions that nonprofessional automobile drivers with color vision defects should have no driving restrictions.

MOLECULAR GENETICS OF COLOR VISION DEFECTS

Red–Green Color Vision Defects

Nathans and his collaborators isolated and sequenced the genes that specify the three opsins responsible for normal color vision,[10] and showed how these genes are different in individuals with red–green color vision defects.[11] Based on their study of 25 red–green color-vision-deficient males, they concluded that in most cases color vision defects result from unequal recombination between the highly homologous red and green pigment genes (98 percent identity in DNA sequence of exons, introns, and 3′ flanking regions). Such events lead to deletions of the green pigment genes or to the formation of full-length hybrid genes consisting of portions of both red and green pigment genes (Fig. 143-6). With few exceptions, the deletion of green pigment genes was associated with deuteranopia (G^-R^+), 5′ green–red hybrid genes with deuteranomaly ($G'R^+$), and 5′ red–green hybrids with either protanopia (R^-G^+) or protanomaly ($R'G^+$). An interesting observation was that some males had normal green and red pigment genes in addition to the hybrids and yet tested as deutans.

Determination of the gross structure of the red and green pigment gene arrays in males was made by quantitative Southern blot analysis, taking advantage of differences in length of DNA fragments generated from the red and green opsin genes upon digestion with the restriction enzymes *Eco*RI, *Bam*HI, and *Rsa*I. Figure 143-7 shows autoradiographs of Southern blots of genomic DNA isolated from

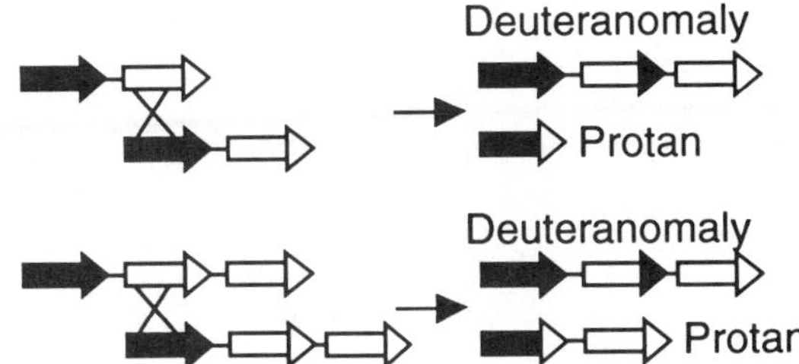

FIG. 143-6 *Generation of red/green hybrid genes.* **Unequal recombination between the highly homologous red and green opsin genes generates the 5′ red–green hybrids typically found in individuals with the protan class of color vision defects (protanopia and protanomaly) and the 5′ green–red hybrid genes found among individuals with deuteranomaly. Filled arrows denote red gene sequences and open arrows represent green opsin gene sequences.** ***(From Drummond-Borg et al.[68] Used by permission.)***

males with normal and defective color vision together with the deduced genotypes.[11]

The following important and interesting questions were raised by the above observations: Does the point of fusion in red/green hybrid genes correlate with the severity of the color vision defect? Which amino acid residues contribute significantly to the difference in absorption characteristics between the red and green opsins? Are all genes in the red–green cluster equally expressed? These questions were addressed by studying the relationship between genotype and phenotype among males who were color-vision-normal and others who had defective red–green color vision.[19] In addition to the use of quantitative Southern blot analysis to detect deletions and hybrid red–green opsin genes, amplification by the polymerase chain reaction (PCR) and single-strand conformation polymorphism (SSCP) were used to determine the approximate points of recombination in hybrid genes. Recombination between the red and green opsin genes would be expected to occur more frequently in introns than in exons, since introns are on average 10 times longer and are as homologous as exons in this gene complex.[8,10,11,65] Evidence supporting this expectation was provided by analysis of hybrid genes of 64 individuals with defective color vision (see below, and see Deeb et al.[19]). Recombinations in introns 1 and 4 could be assigned with certainty, while those in introns 2 and 3 could not be differentiated because the sequence of exon 3 does not always differ between the red and green opsin genes.[10,19,109] Recombinations in intron 1 would convert one pigment gene to the other (i.e., green to red), while those occurring in intron 5 would have no effect, since exons 1 and 6 in the red and green opsin genes have identical sequences. Recombinations in exons 2, 3, and 4 would be expected to result in hybrid genes (5′ green–red or 5′ red–green) that encode six corresponding chimeric pigments with maximal sensitivities distributed between those of the normal red and green pigments (530 to 560 nm). These six hybrid genes (three "red–green" and three "green–red") are shown in Fig. 143-8. However, since there are two common alleles of the red opsin gene, which differ in having either Ala or Ser at position 180[18] and by approximately 4 to 5 nm in absorption maxima,[60] nine instead of six common types of hybrid opsin genes would be expected to exist in the population. Merbs and Nathans[54] examined photobleaching difference spectra of in-vitro-produced red–green hybrids commonly found in the population and showed that amino acid residues in exons 2, 3, 4, and 5 that differ between the red and green pigments produce varying degrees of spectral shifts (Fig. 143-8).

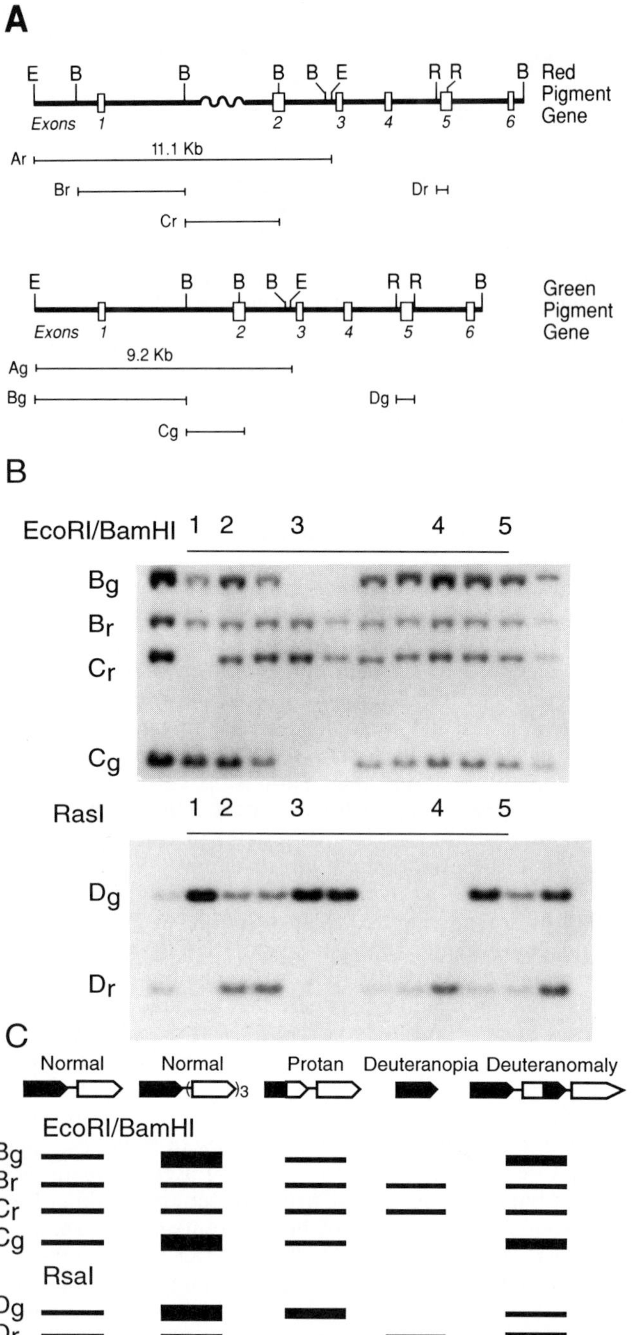

FIG. 143-7 *Southern blot analysis of the X-linked red–green gene locus. A.* **Partial restriction maps of the red and green pigment genes. E, *Eco*RI; B, *Bam*HI; R, *Rsa*I. Open boxes denote the six exons. The restriction fragments A–D used in distinguishing red-specific from green-specific sequences are shown below the genes. The A–C fragments derived from the red opsin gene (A_r, B_r, C_r) are longer than those derived from the green gene (A_g, B_g, C_g) owing to a 1.5-kb insertion in the first intron (wavy line). The absence of a *Rsa*I site in the green opsin exon 5 accounts for the larger *Rsa*I fragment of the green opsin gene (D_g).** ***B.*** **Autoradiograph of Southern blots of genomic DNA samples from males with normal and defective color vision digested with either a combination of *Eco*RI and *Bam*HI or *Rsa*I. The *Eco*RI/*Bam*HI fragments (B and C) were detected by hybridization to a 350-bp cDNA probe encompassing exon 1 and part of exon 2, whereas the D fragments were detected by a 400-bp genomic probe from the 3′ end of intron 4 of the green opsin gene.[11] Typical examples of Southern blot patterns were selected. Lane 1, an individual with protanopia who has a single red–green hybrid gene with the C and D fragments of the red gene replaced by the corresponding fragments of the green gene. Lane 2, a deuteranomalous individual who has a normal red gene and a green–red hybrid gene (see Fig. C). Lane 3, an individual with deuteranopia who has only a normal red gene (see Fig. C). Lane 4, a deuteranomalous individual with a gene array consisting of normal red and green genes as well as a green–red hybrid gene. Lane 5, individual with normal color vision who has multiple green genes. The unmarked lanes show patterns similar to those described above.** ***C.*** **Diagrammatic representation of Southern blot patterns for males with normal and defective color vision. The color vision phenotypes and the structure of the red/green gene arrays associated with the *Eco*RI/*Bam*HI and *Rsa*I Southern blot patterns are shown above the blot diagram. Filled and open arrows denote red and green gene sequences, respectively. The width of the solid lines representing restriction fragments reflects the relative quantity of DNA as quantified by densitometry. In protanomaly and protanopia (protan), the D_r fragment is missing, indicating loss of the 3′ portion of the red pigment gene, while the 5′ portion of the green gene is present. In deuteranopia, B_g, C_g, and D_g fragments are missing, indicating complete deletion of the green pigment gene. In deuteranomaly, the relative proportions of fragments is shifted, indicating the presence of green–red hybrid genes.** *(Fig. A adapted from Nathans et al.[11] Used by permission.)*

In a study of 64 red–green color-vision-defective Caucasian males, the great majority of defects were associated either with deletion of the green opsin gene or with the formation of 5′ red–green or 5′ green–red full-length hybrid genes.[19] The results, described below, were basically in agreement with those obtained in the earlier study of 25 subjects by Nathans and colleagues.[11]

Protan Subjects. Of 64 color-vision-deficient males, 23 (36 percent) were protans; their anomaloscopic Rayleigh match ranges are given in Fig. 143-9. Figure 143-10 shows the observed gene arrays, points of fusion, and class of protan defect [protanopic (P) or protanomalous (PA)] for the same subjects. The gene arrays of all protans were characterized by the presence of 5′ red–green hybrid opsin genes instead of the normal red opsin gene. In all cases, the intron of fusion was upstream of exon 5, thus indicating that exon 5 is critical in establishing the spectral characteristics of a normal red pigment. The replacement of exon 5 of the red opsin gene with that of the green opsin produced a hybrid pigment that was sufficiently green-like in its spectral properties that the subjects performed as protans. The significant role of exon 5 of the red opsin gene was somewhat predicted, since it contains two of the three amino acid residues (at positions 277 and 285) thought to be mainly responsible for the difference in spectral properties between the red and green photopigments (Fig. 143-11). The relationship between the structure of the pigment and its spectral properties as determined by electroretinography was investigated in a protanope who had a 5′ red–green hybrid gene in which the point of fusion was in intron 3.[110] The absorption spectrum of the pigment encoded by this hybrid gene (which encoded

Pigment	λ_{max} (nm)	Exons 1	2	3	4	5	6
Red (Ser)	556.7	■	■	■	■	■	■
Red (Ala)	552.4						
Green	529.7	□	□	□	□	□	□
R2G3	529.5	■	■	□	□	□	□
R3G4 (Ser)	533.3	■	■	■	□	□	□
R3G4 (Ala)	529.0						
R4G5 (Ser)	536.0	■	■	■	■	□	□
R4G5 (Ala)	531.6						
G2R3 (Ala)	549.6	□	□	■	■	■	■
G2R3 (Ser)	553.0						
G3R4	548.8	□	□	□	■	■	■
G4R5	544.8	□	□	□	□	■	■

FIG. 143-8 *Spectral characteristics of the hybrid visual pigments commonly found among individuals with defective color vision.* The right-hand column shows the exon composition of the six possible hybrid genes resulting from unequal recombination between the red and green opsin genes occurring in introns 2, 3, and 4. Filled and open boxes denote red and green gene exons, respectively. Hybrid opsins would not be formed as a result of recombinations in introns 1 and 5, since the sequences of exons 1 and 6 are identical in the two pigment genes. The normal red and green opsin genes are included for comparison. The left-hand column gives the designations for each hybrid pigment. For example, R3G4 denotes a 5′ red–green hybrid with the first three exons derived from the red gene and the last three exons from the green gene. Note that whenever exon 3 of a hybrid is derived from the red opsin gene, two forms of the hybrid are possible, depending on whether Ser or Ala is found at position 180 in exon 3. The λ_{max} or peak absorption values were determined from photobleaching difference absorption spectra of recombinant pigments expressed in tissue culture cells transfected with cDNA clones encoding the various hybrid opsins.[54] nm = nanometers.

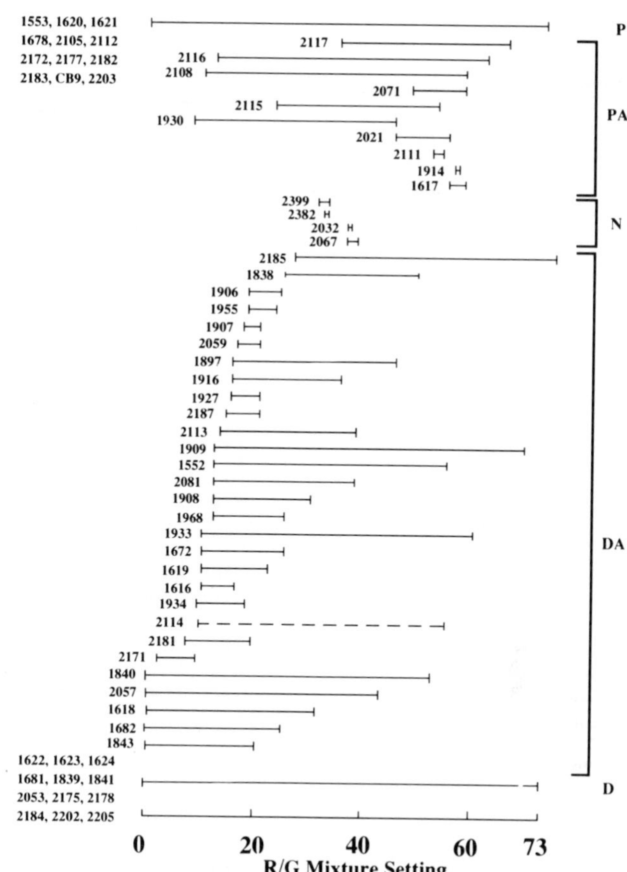

FIG. 143-9 *Anomaloscopic Rayleigh match ranges of protan, deutan, and normal male individuals.* Each horizontal line represents the range of mixtures of red and green lights that the observer could not distinguish from the standard yellow light. Identification numbers shown next to the horizontal lines refer to subjects of a large study.[19] Subject 2114 (interrupted lines) had a variable and unreliable match range. P, protanopic; PA, protanomaly; D, deuteranopia; DA, deuteranomaly; N, normal; R/G = red/green. *(From Deeb et al.[19] Used by permission.)*

Ala at position 180) was very similar to that of the green pigment, suggesting that sequence differences in exons 2 and 3 contribute little to the difference in absorption between the red and green photopigments. These results are consistent with those obtained by measuring bleaching difference spectra of in-vitro-produced types of red–green hybrid genes.[54] They showed that the exchange of exon 5 sequences resulted in a major spectral shift in λ_{max} (15 to 20 nm), whereas differences in exons 2 through 4 appeared to have smaller effects (Fig. 143-8).

Subjects who had *only* the red–green hybrid gene in their arrays tested as protanopes regardless of the point of fusion, whereas those who had one or more normal green opsin genes in addition to the hybrid gene tested as either protanopic or protanomalous. The distribution of match ranges was quite similar for subjects with fusions in either introns 2 and 3 or 4. The Ser/Ala polymorphism at position 180 in the red opsin appears to underlie the above discrepancy between genotype and phenotype. In a study of 19 protan subjects (Deeb and colleagues, unpublished observations) who had one 5′ red–green opsin gene plus one or more normal green opsin genes, protanopes and protanomalous subjects could be differentiated because (with one exception) the former had Ala and the latter had Ser at position 180 of the red portion of the hybrid gene. The presence of Ser encoded a hybrid pigment that differed by 5 nm in peak absorption from that of the normal green opsin, and this pigment was associated with protanomaly. When Ala was present at position 180 of the hybrid, there was no difference in peak absorption, and the subject was protanopic (see above and Fig. 134-12).

In addition to the above gene patterns, a rearrangement encompassing exons 2 and 3 of the red opsin gene was associated with protanopia.[93] It is noteworthy that this mutant allele cosegregated in one family with X-linked progressive cone degeneration.[93]

Deutan Subjects. The Rayleigh match ranges (Fig. 143-9) of 41 of the 64 color-vision-deficient males placed them in the deutan series. The gene arrays and estimated points of fusion for 40 of these deutans are shown in Fig. 143-13. One of the deuteranomalous subjects had a grossly normal gene array but had a point mutation in the green opsin gene (see below). All deutans had a normal red opsin gene, and all subjects (except the individual with the point mutation) had major gene rearrangements that could be detected by Southern blot analysis and/or gene-specific PCR amplification across intron 4.

Gene Deletions. Of the 41 deutans, 13 were shown to completely lack green opsin gene sequences. Of these 13 subjects, 10 were classified by anomaloscopy as deuteranopes, as expected since they have only one red opsin gene. Surpris-

Subject	Gene Array	Intron of Fusion	Phenotype
1553, 2105		2-3	P
2203		4	P
1620, 1621, 2112 2172, 2182, CB9	1-3	1	P
2177, 2183	1-3	2-3	P
1930, 2071, 2108 2116, 2117, CB8	1-3	2-3	PA
1678		4	P
1617, 1914, 2021 2111, 2115	1-3	4	PA

FIG. 143-10 ***Red/green color vision pigment gene arrays found in males with protan color vision defects.*** **Hybrid pigment genes consist of 5′ red opsin gene sequences (filled arrows) followed by green opsin gene sequences (open arrows). The subscript number 1–3 refers to the number of normal green opsin genes present (one, two, or three). The color vision phenotype, as determined by anomaloscopy, is indicated as P, protanopia; PA, protanomaly. The assignment of the intron of fusion in hybrid genes was made on the basis of results of Southern blot analysis, PCR amplification, and sequencing of exons.[19] The uncertainty in assigning the fusion point to introns 2 or 3 results from the presence of polymorphisms in exon 3, the alleles of which are shared by the red and green opsin genes. "2–3" therefore indicates fusion points in either intron 2 or 3.** ***(Subject identification numbers from Deeb et al.[19] Used by permission.)***

ingly, the remaining three tested as severely deuteranomalous trichromats. Since they have only a red opsin gene, they should be completely unable to discriminate the red and green lights from the yellow standard light in the anomaloscope, yet they can. The pattern of a single red opsin gene in a deuteranomalous subject has also been observed in a previous study.[11]

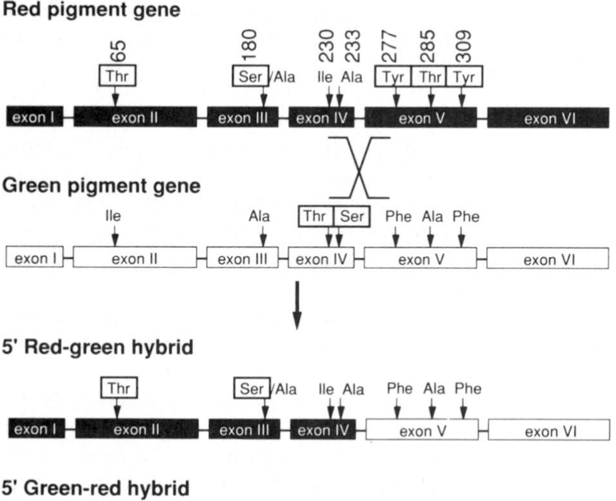

FIG. 143-11 ***The importance of exon 5 in determining spectral sensitivities of hybrid pigments.*** **The positions at which the red and green opsins differ by the presence of hydroxyl-bearing (boxed) versus nonpolar amino acid residues are shown. Recombination in intron 4 results in the exchange of three of these residues, two of which have been shown to account for the major difference in λ_{max} between the normal red and green pigments. The red–green hybrid is as observed in protan subject 2203 of Figure 143-10, and the green–red hybrid is as observed in deutan subject 1682 of Figure 143-13.** ***(From Deeb et al.[19] Used by permission.)***

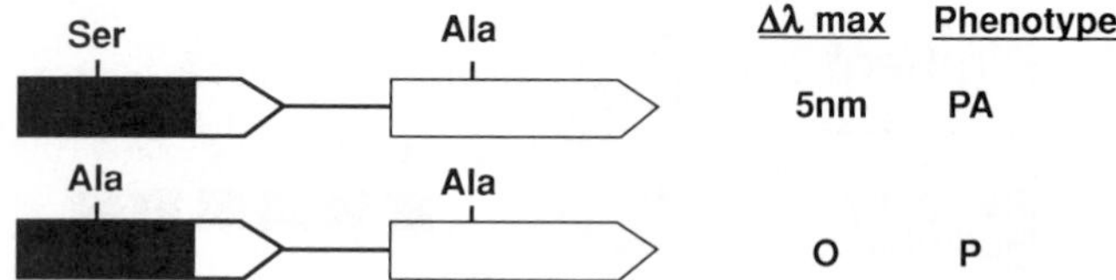

FIG. 143-12 ***The Ser/Ala polymorphism in the red opsin gene plays a role in determining protan subtypes.*** **Diagrams of X-linked gene arrays, each composed of a red–green hybrid gene (fusion in intron 4) and a normal green opsin gene. The hybrid gene with Ser at position 180 differs by 5 nm in λ_{max} from the normal green opsin. A difference in λ_{max} of this magnitude makes for protanomaly (PA), since trichromacy is preserved by this anomalous red–green pigment. In contrast, the Ala-containing hybrid has the same λ_{max} as the normal green pigment, making the carrier a protanopic (P) dichromat.**

Simple Hybrid Genes. Of the 41 deutans, 25 had gene arrays characterized by the presence of one or more full-length 5′ green–red hybrid opsin genes in addition to a normal red opsin gene (Fig. 143-13). In 18 of these subjects, one or more normal green opsin genes were found in addition to the normal red and hybrid genes. Except for two subjects who tested as deuteranopic (dichromats), these gene arrays were associated with deuteranomaly. In one of the deuteran-

Subject	Gene Array	Intron of Fusion	Phenotype
1622,1623,1839 1841, 2053, 2175 2178,2184, 2202 2205		N/A	D
1897,1933, 2185		N/A	DA
1624		1	D
1907		2-3	DA
1682, 1934, 1955 1968, 1908	1-3	4	DA
1681	2	1-3	D
1552, 1618, 1619 1843, 1916, 2057 2059, 2113, 2114 2181, 2187	1-4	1-3	DA
1616, 1672 2081, 2171	1-3	4	DA
1840, 1906	2 2	1-3	DA
1838, 1927		1-3 & 4	DA

FIG. 143-13 ***Color-vision gene arrays found in subjects with deutan color vision defects.*** **Explanations concerning the gene arrays are given in the legend to Figure 143-10. D = deuteranopia, DA = deuteranomaly. Note that 3 of 13 individuals who had only a single red opsin gene unexpectedly tested as anomalous trichromats (deuteranomalous) instead of dichromats (deuteranopic). Furthermore, individual 1681, who had normal red and green opsin genes in addition to a green–red hybrid gene, tested as a deuteranope, suggesting that the two normal green opsin genes are not expressed. Note that the hybrid genes are depicted immediately downstream of the red pigment gene by inference (see text). The methodology used cannot determine the exact position of the hybrid gene in the presence of other green genes. N/A, not applicable.** ***(From Deeb et al.[19] Used by permission.)***

opes (subject 1907), and most likely in the other (subject 1681), the points of fusion in their hybrid genes were in intron 1, causing the expected deuteranopia. The fusion points in all the other deuteranomalous subjects were located in introns 2 through 4. As seen in the protan subjects, 5′ green–red hybrid genes that resulted from a crossover in intron 4 (i.e., exchange of exons 5 and 6) encoded a pigment that was essentially red-like in absorption spectrum.

The presence of more than one hybrid gene in the array does not seem to be associated with a more severe color vision defect. Neither does the presence in arrays of normal green opsin genes in addition to normal red and hybrid genes. One explanation for these observations is that not all of the opsin genes in an array are expressed in the retina (see below).

Double Fusion Genes. Deuteranomaly in two subjects (1838 and 1927) was associated with a novel type of hybrid gene (5′ green–red–green) in which a central segment encompassing exon 4 and possibly 3 was exchanged between the red and green opsin genes, presumably owing to a double crossover or a gene conversion event. In these cases, the two hydroxyl-bearing residues at positions 230 and 233 in exon 4 of the green opsin were replaced by Ile and Ala, respectively, suggesting a role for one or both of these amino acids in determining spectral sensitivities of the photopigments. The results of Merbs and Nathans[54] support this hypothesis. They showed that amino acid differences in either exon 3 or 4 could produce a spectral shift of 4 nm (Fig. 143-8).

A Point Mutation in a Single Case of Deuteranomaly. The gene array of one of the subjects (CB 1909) with severe deuteranomaly (match range of 12 to 68) had no gross rearrangements. Examination of the coding sequences of his red and green opsin genes revealed that all of his three green opsin genes had a C-to-T transition at nucleotide 648, which translates to the substitution of Arg for Cys at position 203 (C203R).[111] Screening of 63 other color-vision-defective subjects known to have major gene rearrangements revealed another deuteranomalous individual (CB 1843) who carried the same mutation in one of his three green opsin genes. The same C203R mutation had been observed in 16 unrelated families with blue cone monochromacy.[84,112] In these cases, the mutation was in the green segments of 5′ red–green hybrid genes. These results suggest that the C203R mutant allele of the green opsin gene may be common in the general population. Indeed, the same mutation was also found in a green gene of one out of 65 male subjects with normal color vision. The Cys residue is highly conserved among all visual pigments studied so far, as well as among other seven-transmembrane-segment receptors, such as the adrenergic, muscarinic, dopaminergic, and serotonergic receptors.[43,113]

The Cys 203 residue is believed to form a disulfide bridge with another Cys at position 126, thus covalently linking the first and second extracellular loops of the opsins. Results of in vitro mutagenesis studies showed that the corresponding cysteine residues in bovine rhodopsin (residues 110 and 187) and in the hamster β-adrenergic receptor (residues 106 and 187) are essential for the function of these proteins.[114,115] Therefore, the C203R mutation is very likely to abolish function of the green-sensitive photoreceptor. Furthermore, by analogy with the mutant rhodopsin alleles associated with autosomal dominant retinitis pigmentosa,[116,117] this mutation might predispose to certain X-linked cone dystrophies as a result of accumulation of the abnormal protein. A sequence rearrangement in the red opsin gene has been found to cosegregate in one family with X-linked progressive cone degeneration.[93]

Synopsis. Based on analysis of at least 90 males with red–green color vision defects,[11,19,118] inter- and intragenic recombinations between the red and green opsin genes that result in green opsin gene deletions or shuffling of exons between the two genes account for all but the one case that was found to be due to a C203R mutation. Exon 5 plays a major role in spectral tuning, since it contains three of the seven residues that distinguish red from green opsins. Molecular analysis of the red and green opsin genes could classify subjects into either the protan or deutan series. Although certain trends were evident, the genotype at the level of coding sequence occasionally was not correlated with the color vision phenotype within the protan and deutan series. Nagel anomaloscopy may not provide a sufficiently accurate quantitative assessment of the ability of red–green color-vision-deficient subjects to discriminate color.[13] Alternatively, the severity of color vision deficiency may not be a function only of the sequence of hybrid pigments. Postreceptor neural factors[119,120] and variation in the amount of pigment synthesized or in the ratio of red to green cones[121] were proposed as explanations for variation in color discrimination. Position-dependent expression of genes of the red–green locus explains why the presence of hybrid genes and mutant green opsin genes in addition to normal red and green opsin genes does not always result in altered color vision.

Selective Expression among Multiple Green Opsin Genes—Expression of Only One Gene. The frequency of 5′ green–red hybrid genes was observed to be higher than the reported frequency of color vision defects among Caucasian and, in particular, African-American males[64,68] (see below), suggesting that such hybrid genes may not always lead to color vision defects. This was proved to be the case by showing that 4 of 129 Caucasian males with anomaloscopically determined normal color vision had a 5′ green–red hybrid gene in addition to normal red and green opsin genes.[19] In addition, a male with normal color vision was found to have the C203R mutation in one of his five green opsin genes,[111] and another (subject 1681 in Fig. 143-13), who had a green–red hybrid opsin gene in addition to normal red and green opsin genes, tested as a deuteranope, indicating that his normal green opsin genes were nonfunctional.[19]

The hypothesis that not all opsin genes in an array are expressed in the retina was advanced to explain these observations. Green opsin gene sequences in genomic DNA were compared with the corresponding mRNA sequences expressed in postmortem retinal tissues. Advantage was taken of a relatively common but silent polymorphism (A versus C at the third position of codon 283) in exon 5 of the green opsin gene.[122] The two alleles can be differentiated by PCR amplification of exon 5 followed by SSCP analysis or digestion with restriction endonuclease *Eco*O1019. Results of such a comparison in 10 male subjects who had two or more green opsin genes in their genomic DNA showed clearly that whenever the two alleles of exon 5 were present, only one was represented in expressed retinal mRNA,[122] indicating the expression of only a single green opsin gene. In addition to the expression of a single green opsin gene, retinal RNA from the same individuals contained a single red opsin-encoding mRNA sequence. In contrast, Neitz et al.[123] suggest that a large proportion of males with normal color vision have at least two expressed red pigment genes as well as at least two expressed green pigment genes. Our data[19,109,122] are most consistent with the presence of only a single red pigment gene and with the expression of only one among several green pigment genes in the retina.

The model illustrated in Fig. 143-14 was proposed[122] to explain such selective expression of one out of a set of green opsin genes in an array. In this model, a locus control region (LCR) regulates expression of the opsin genes of the array in a position-dependent manner. Thus, in red cones the LCR forms a stable transcriptionally active complex with the red opsin promoter, whereas in green cones the LCR forms a complex with the proximal green opsin promoter instead. Active complexes between the LCR and green opsin promoters located downstream of the proximal green opsin promoter are much less favored. We therefore suggest that only the most proximal green pigment gene is expressed in an array of several green pigment genes, which may include 5′ green–red hybrid pigment genes.

The concept of an LCR was first suggested for the regulatory sequences 5′ to the beta globin gene locus. The globin LCR was shown to be essential for developmental switching of expression from fetal to adult globin genes, and it was shown that the order of the genes making up this locus is important for such a transcriptional switch.[124–127] Evidence for an LCR at the red/green opsin locus has been provided by Nathans and colleagues,[84] who found that in some instances blue cone monochromacy, a disorder in which *both* red and green cone functions are absent, is associated with deletion of a regulatory sequence located 3.8 to 4.3 kb upstream of the transcription initiation site of the red opsin gene and 43 kb upstream of that of the proximal green opsin gene. They subsequently showed that a region (the LCR) between −3.1 and −3.7 kb of the red opsin gene is required for expression of a beta-galactosidase reporter gene in both long- and short-wavelength-sensitive cones in the retinas of transgenic mice.[128]

Blue Cone Monochromacy

Blue cone monochromacy (BCM), also called "Pi_1 monochromacy" or "X-linked incomplete achromatopsia,"[98] is an extremely rare disorder (prevalence less than 1 in 100,000) in which both red and green cone sensitivities are absent. The physiologic functions of both rods and blue cones are preserved. Significant linkage of BCM to the red–green pigment gene locus was established by analysis of restriction fragment length polymorphism (RFLP) alleles at the two DNA markers DXS15 and DXS52.[128] This led Nathans and colleagues[84] to analyze the red–green locus in individuals with BCM. Their studies on 38 families with BCM have uncovered two mechanisms for generating this phenotype (reviewed by Nathans et al.[112]). One, found in 14 families, involved deletions (of 587 to 55,000 bp) that included the LCR located 3.4 kb 5′ to the transcription initiation site of the red opsin gene. In some of these individuals the red and green opsin genes were unaffected, whereas in others the deletions extended into the red opsin gene. The other mechanism of generating BCM, found in 20 families, involved an unequal homologous recombination between the green and red opsin genes that reduced the gene array to only a single red gene or 5′ red–green hybrid gene. In 16 of these families, the green opsin portion of the hybrid gene had a C203R substitution, which rendered the encoded hybrid opsin nonfunctional. The same C203R mutation was found to be relatively common (2 percent) in the green opsin genes of Caucasian males.[111] Progressive central retinal dystrophy has been reported in some patients with BCM,[84] indicating that cone degeneration may result from the accumulation of an abnormally assembled photopigment, by analogy with the mutations in rhodopsin that have been found to underlie autosomal dominant retinitis pigmentosa.[116]

A. Expression in red cones

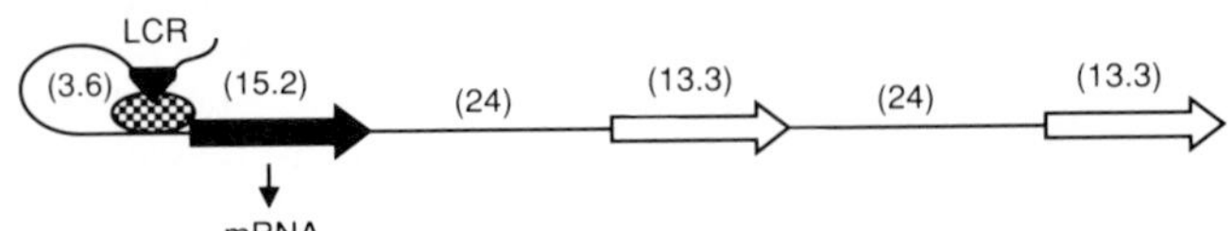

B. Expression in green cones

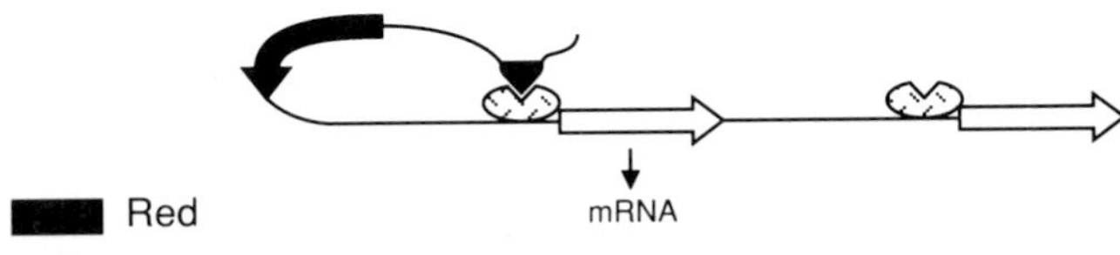

FIG. 143-14 *Model for selective expression in the X-linked red/green gene complex.* **Numbers denote length in kilobase pairs.** ***A.*** **Red cone-specific gene transcription occurs as a result of stable coupling (mediated by DNA-binding proteins) of the locus control region (LCR) to the red gene promoter.** ***B.*** **The LCR preferentially and stably couples to the proximal green opsin gene promoter and turns on its expression. Distal green opsin promoters are not activated, presumably because of the low probability of coupling to the LCR.** *(Adapted from Winderickx et al.[122] Used by permission.)*

Tritanopia

Tritanopia is a rare autosomal dominant[79] disorder characterized by selective loss of blue-sensitive photoreceptor function and greatly diminished or absent chromatic discrimination in the blue region of the spectrum. A survey in the Netherlands indicates that its frequency in the population may be as high as 1 in 500.[130] Three missense mutations in the gene encoding the blue pigment opsin, located on chromosome 7,[10] have been shown to cause tritanopia: G79R in two Japanese subjects, SZ14P in two Caucasian subjects, and P264S in three Caucasian subjects.[80,81] The three mutant alleles cosegregate with tritanopia in an autosomal dominant fashion; however, incomplete penetrance was observed in association with the G79R substitution. The mutations affect residues located in the second, fifth, and sixth transmembrane α-helical segments of the blue pigment opsin. The dominant mode of inheritance suggests that accumulation of a defective opsin within photoreceptors causes either loss of function or cell death, reminiscent of the mutations in the rhodopsin and peripherin genes that cause a subset of autosomal dominant retinitis pigmentosa (ADRP). Tritanopia has also been observed in association with some disorders of vision, such as autosomal dominant juvenile optic atrophy.[131,132]

VARIATION IN NORMAL COLOR VISION EXPLAINED BY A SINGLE AMINO ACID POLYMORPHISM

Subtle variation in color perception in the red–green region of the spectrum has been observed among individuals considered to have normal color vision. Rayleigh color match results for male subjects with normal color vision fell into two main groups[17,18,133–135] and suggested a difference of several nanometers in the red pigment absorption spectra. Females with normal color vision show a third and larger group with intermediate values of match midpoints.[17] A similar independently described Rayleigh match variability fitted transmission by X-linked inheritance in families.[16] These observations pointed to the presence of two common alleles of the red pigment gene. Assuming the occurrence of X-chromosome inactivation, females who are heterozygous for such a polymorphism would be expected to have patches of cones containing either one or the other of the pigment forms and, therefore, would show a color match distribution intermediate between those of the two homozygotes.

The subtle differences in color matching observed among individuals with normal color vision (as well as among deuteranopic dichromats who have only a red opsin gene) have been suggested to be a reflection of small variations in the absorption maxima of the red or green photopigments.[12–15,136]

Recently, a common single amino acid polymorphism (62 percent Ser, 38 percent Ala) at residue 180 of the red photopigment was discovered in the Caucasian population.[18] Fifty Caucasian males with normal color vision were used to test the hypothesis that the two major groups in the distribution of color matching could be explained by the above Ser/Ala polymorphism. The frequency distributions of Rayleigh match midpoints and of the deduced amino acid sequence of the red photopigment (Fig. 143-15) show that a higher sensitivity to red light (i.e., a requirement for less red in the mixture of red and green to match the standard yellow light) was highly correlated with the presence of Ser at position 180.[18] These males therefore have a different perception of red light than those having the alanine allele at this site. Females having both the Ala and Ser alleles would be expected to have two types of red photoreceptors owing to X-chromosome inactivation and thus might have tetrachromatic vision. This is analogous to the situation in the New World monkeys, who have only a single X-chromosome-encoded medium-long-wavelength pigment gene with several alleles, and in whom females heterozygous for two alleles of this gene achieve trichromacy, while males and homozygous females test as dichromats.[49] The frequencies of the Ser/Ala polymorphism among African-Americans were 80/20 percent and among Japanese 84/16 percent, respectively (unpublished personal observations).

The importance of the presence of Ser or Ala at position 180 in spectral tuning of photopigments had already been deduced from studies of the visual pigments of Old and New World monkeys.[57] A difference of 6 nm was observed between the peaks of maximal sensitivity (562 nm for Ser-containing and 556 nm for Ala-containing pigments, as determined by electroretinography) of the pigments of two tamarin monkeys in which the pigments differed in sequence by only Ser versus Ala at position 180. The results of Merbs and Nathans[60] for direct determination of the bleaching difference absorption spectra of human red pigments (expressed in tissue culture cells transfected with complementary DNA clones) that differed in sequence by Ser versus Ala at position 180 were thus in good agreement with the electroretinographic results in the monkeys (557 nm and 552 nm for the Ser- and Ala-containing reconstituted pigments, respectively) as well as with the human color-matching data. These results support the finding that the Ser/Ala polymorphism at position 180 of the red pigment underlies the observed variation in red–green color vision among people with normal color vision.

Other amino acid polymorphisms have been observed in both the red opsin gene (eight sites) and the green opsin gene (five sites). These polymorphisms gave rise in the general population to 15 and 18 different green and red opsins, respectively. Nine of these polymorphisms are located in exon 3. Alleles of these polymorphisms are shared between the red and green opsin genes, suggesting a history of relatively frequent gene conversion or unequal recombination, mainly localized to exon 3, during the evolution of the two lineages.[109]

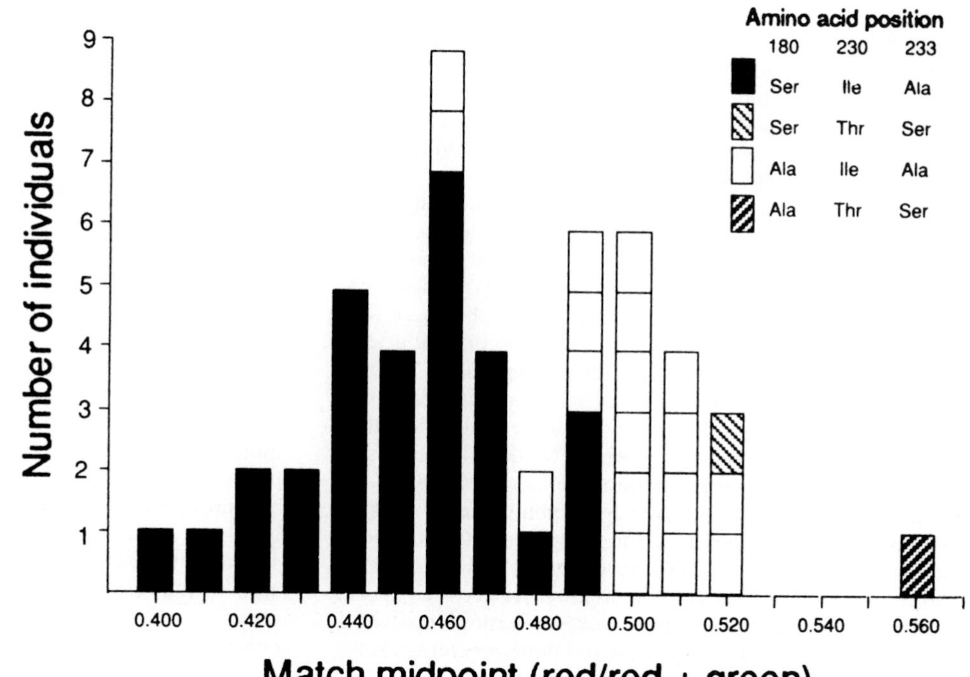

FIG. 143-15 *Correlation of the Rayleigh match midpoint (center of match range) with the presence of serine or alanine at position 180 of the red photopigment.* **The subjects (50) were Caucasian males who tested as having normal color vision. Determination of color matches was made by measuring the proportion of red in a mixture of red and green lights that was perceived to match a standard yellow light. The presence of serine at position 180 correlates with higher sensitivity to red light (i.e., less red light need be mixed with green light to match the standard yellow light). Two individuals who had Thr and Ser instead of Ile and Ala at positions 230 and 233, respectively, required more red light in the mixture in comparison to others with the same amino acid at position 180.** *(From Winderickx et al.[18] Used by permission.)*

HETEROZYGOSITY AND HOMOZYGOSITY AMONG FEMALES WITH X-LINKED COLOR VISION DEFECTS

Because of the high frequency of X-linked color vision defects among males, there will be a large number of female heterozygotes for these genes in the population. Among males, the gene frequency and trait frequency of an X-linked trait (p) are identical. Males either have (p) or lack (q) the X-linked trait under study. The expected frequency of female heterozygotes and homozygotes can be calculated by the Hardy-Weinberg law, where $2pq$ will be the number of heterozygotes and p^2 the number of abnormal homozygotes. Such homozygotes will be color-vision-defective like affected males. The number of female heterozygotes ($2pq$) for each of the color-vision defect categories is about twice the number of color-vision-defective male hemizygotes. Since the total frequency of color vision defects among male European populations is 8 percent (p), about 15 to 16 percent ($2pq$) of the female population will be heterozygotes for one or another red–green color vision defect. Most such heterozygotes (7 to 10 percent) are heterozygotes for deuteranomaly, since this abnormality is the most frequent defect.

Occasional heterozygotes who express phenotypic color vision defects may have a single X chromosome, as in Turner syndrome, or may come from the small proportion of females with extremely skewed X-inactivation who by chance have inactivated most of their X chromosomes bearing the normal allele and thus express the mutant allele.[137,138] Skewed X-inactivation appears to be more common in one member of identical female twin pairs,[139] and six pairs of heterozygote female identical twins discordant for color vision have been reported.[140–144] The expected skewed inactivation of one X chromosome has been directly demonstrated in one of these twin pairs.[139] Furthermore, two of the five Dionne identical quintuplet girls were color blind,[142] as was one of three identical Japanese female triplets.[145]

As expected by the X-inactivation hypothesis, heterozygotes are mosaics for normal and abnormal color vision in their retinas. Thus, by shining a very narrow beam of red or green light into the retinas of female heterozygotes for X-linked color vision defects, patches of defective color perception were found.[146,147] In other experiments, heterozygotes made more errors than controls when asked to identify the color of briefly presented stimuli under conditions that did not allow any eye movement.[148]

These findings are consistent with earlier data that mild abnormalities of color vision can often be detected on psychophysical testing of heterozygotes, particularly when groups of heterozygotes are compared with normal controls.[69,98] Such minor deviations have been observed with pseudoisochromatic plate reading, anomaloscopy, and tests that assessed hue and saturation discrimination.[98] The so-called Schmidt sign is the most obvious abnormality, and can be elicited by many different psychophysical techniques. It is found in protan heterozygotes. The defect consists of a reduction in the relative luminous efficiency curve compared to that in normal and affected hemizygotes.[149] Similar findings have been observed in the relative spectral luminous efficiency function of deutan heterozygotes and consisted of a lessened sensitivity at short wavelengths.[149]

Electroretinography has been successful in identifying a fairly large number of both protan and deutan heterozygotes by the ratio of sensitivity at short (480 nm) and long (620 nm) wavelengths for the rapid-off response.[97]

The molecular abnormalities in heterozygotes correspond to those observed in males with color vision defects. Current molecular methodology, which depends on Southern blots of various restriction fragments of the red and green pigment gene, does not necessarily allow molecular detection of all heterozygotes. However, when family studies are done, and affected fathers and brothers are tested by the appropriate techniques, molecular genotypes of females can be determined.[118]

Compound heterozygotes for protan and deutan defects occur. The most frequent type are females with a deuteranomaly allele on one X chromosome and an allele for one of the other color vision defects (deuteranopia, protanopia, or protanomaly) on the other. Compound heterozygotes for both deuteranomaly and deuteranopia will manifest with deuteranomaly,[69,98] as expected from the molecular findings, since a deleted green pigment gene is not expressed, whereas a visual pigment with somewhat abnormal sensitivity, such as a green–red fusion gene in deuteranomaly, will be expressed. Similarly, protanope/protanomalous heterozygotes manifest with protanomaly, demonstrating that among protans, the mild phenotype also is dominant over the more severe one, as expected from the molecular effects of the alleles.

In contrast, compound heterozygotes for both a deutan and protan defect will *not* present with color vision defects.[70,98] This finding is expected, since normal alleles for red and green pigments are present in addition to the defects in both the protan and deutan genes. Such females, therefore, are functionally heterozygotes for both the deutan and the protan genes and therefore will have normal color vision. Compound heterozygosity for protanopia/deuteranomaly and protanomaly/deuteranomaly was studied in one large family by molecular techniques; the family members with these genotypes showed no color vision abnormalities.[118]

With a population frequency among Caucasians of 1 percent each for protanopia, protanomaly, and deuteranopia and of 5 percent for deuteranomaly, the expected frequency of color-vision-defective homozygotes (q^2) is approximately 1 in 10,000 each for protanopia, protanomaly, and deuteranopia (total, 3 in 10,000) and 1 in 400 for deuteranomaly. The total frequency of color vision defects among female "homozygotes" is less than the squared number of the male frequency ($q^2 = 0.0064$), since compound heterozygotes for protan and deutan defects are phenotypically normal.

POPULATION STUDIES

The frequency of color vision defects among male populations of European origin ranges around 8 percent.[69,98] A very large number of individuals (several thousand) have been tested by anomaloscopy in many different studies. The results are very similar, in that 50 to 60 percent of the color vision defects are caused by deuteranomaly, so that 4 to 5 percent of the male population has this defect (see Drummond-Borg et al.[68]). The frequency of the other defects—protanopia, protanomaly, and deuteranopia—all range around 1 percent or slightly more. Generally, the few studies in which anomaloscopy is done on all test subjects yield a slightly higher frequency of color vision defects than the studies that rely on initial plate testing and use anomaloscopy only for subjects who test as abnormal. Because of the more complex procedures involved in anomaloscopy, studies on non-European populations, except for the Japanese, have not been done frequently. Color vision defects were found less frequently in practically all other populations than in Europeans. Among Chinese and Japanese, the frequency of all color vision defects combined together is around 4 to 6 percent,[69,150,151] while somewhat lower frequencies (4 percent or less) have been found among populations of African origin.[69,152,153] The lower frequencies among non-Europeans are largely caused by a lower frequency of deuteranomaly.[154] Deuteranopia is seen in frequencies of 1 to 2 percent in practically all populations, while protanopia is somewhat less common (0.2 to 1.2 percent). The *combined* frequency of the severe dichromatic defects in European and non-European populations everywhere varies between 1 and 3.5 percent.[155]

Molecular Population Studies

Molecular investigations of color vision genes among population groups have not been done extensively. In the first study among American males of European origin,[68] more molecular abnormalities were found than expected from the frequency of color vision anomalies. Thus, among 134 males who were not phenotypically tested, 21 (15.7 percent), showed molecular abnormalities of the red or green color vision genes; 2 (1.5 percent) had a deletion of the green pigment gene and presumably were deuteranopes; 6 (4.4 percent) had red–green fusion genes, presumably associated with protanopia or protanomaly; 9 (6.7 percent) had green–red fusion genes; and another 4 (5.2 percent) had findings suggestive of double crossovers (green–red–green). A later study of 129 American white males found 4 individuals with green–red fusion genes and *normal* color vision, as assessed by anomaloscopy.[19] The fact that green–red hybrid genes were more common than color vision defects is presumably explained by nonexpression of these hybrid genes when located in a relatively distal position in the green pigment gene array.

Red–green hybrid genes appear always to be expressed as protan defects. While the duplication of green but not red pigment genes can be explained by the fact that green pigment genes, unlike the red pigment genes, are flanked by 24 kb of almost identical intergenic DNA, which favors illegitimate recombination, the higher frequency of green–red pigment genes compared with red–green hybrids cannot be explained on this basis. The ratio of green–red and red–green hybrid genes would be expected to be 1:1, since the reciprocal product of a green–red fusion gene will be a red–green fusion gene, if the underlying mechanism is recombination (Fig. 143-6).

In a study of 102 African-American males whose phenotypic color vision was unknown, 20 (19.6 percent) were found to have green–red fusion genes.[64] A single green pigment gene deletion and no red–green fusion genes (protans) were detected in this sample. However, no less than 36 (35 percent) individuals had a polymorphism consisting of a shortened (1.5 kb) red pigment gene involving the first intron. This polymorphism, which was also seen in a small percentage of Caucasians and Japanese, had no effect on color vision—an expected effect, since the change did not involve any coding sequence. The high frequency of green–red fusion genes (19.6 percent) among African-Americans was much higher than would be expected from the frequencies of deuteranomaly observed in various population samples of African origin (1 to 2 percent). Whether the visual pigment gene pattern in Africans is such that more such green–red fusion genes are located in the second or third position of the green pigment gene complex and therefore are not expressed requires further study.

The polymorphism associated with the shortened red pigment gene may predispose to a higher frequency of unequal crossovers between the red and green pigment genes.[64] This shortened red pigment gene resembles a green pigment gene in that both the polymorphic red and the normal green pigment gene lack the 1.5-kb intervening sequence seen in the normal green pigment gene. Illegitimate pairing between these more similar shortened genes therefore may cause a higher frequency of fusion genes. Thus, 8 of 57 (14 percent) of those with the standard red pigment gene had green–red fusion genes, while 33 percent (12 of 36) of those with the polymorphic shortened red pigment gene had green–red fusion genes. The polymorphic red pigment gene was present at a similar frequency among individuals with the common polymorphisms G-6-PD A+ and A−, suggesting that there is no allelic association or linkage disequilibrium of the shortened red pigment genes and the closely linked G-6-PD locus.[64] It is therefore concluded that this red pigment gene polymorphism does not owe its existence to selection of the G-6-PD A+ and A− types (although more data on G-6-PD A− are required to be certain). Furthermore, no correlation between G-6-PD deficiency and color vision defects has been observed.[156]

A molecular study of 101 Japanese males not studied phenotypically showed three green–red (deuteranomaly) and one red–green (protan) fusion gene.[64] No green pigment gene deletions were detected. The frequency of the abnormal molecular patterns was as expected from phenotypic studies of color vision defects (4 to 5 percent). However, since the numbers are small, additional studies are needed to replicate these findings.

The distribution of the number of green genes in different polymorphisms may suggest a mechanism for a higher frequency of fusion genes in different ethnic groups. While a single green gene is only seen in 22 percent of the Caucasian population, 48 percent and 42 percent of Japanese and African-Americans have a single green gene. However, the proportions of those with two or more green genes does not differ as much (Table 143-1) in the three population groups. While these findings may explain the Japanese/Caucasian differences, the high frequency of unexpressed green–red fusion genes among African-Americans remains unexplained.

Selection in Color Vision Defects?

Since the frequency of all types of color vision defects is higher in modern Europeans than in other populations, it was hypothesized that color vision defects, regardless of type, were strongly selected against in "primitive habitats."[157–159] It was reasoned that the introduction of agriculture led to a relaxation of selection pressure and a consequent rise in the frequency of color vision defects, accounting for the current high frequencies among Europeans. The principal problem with this hypothesis is its failure to consider the different subtypes of color vision defects.[155] The frequencies of dichromats appear fairly similar in all populations (see above). Even allowing for misdiagnosis in field studies where anomaloscopic studies were not done, the detection of the more severely affected dichromats is fairly certain on plate tests, so that the finding of similar frequencies of dichromacy in all populations seems rather firm.

In view of the higher frequency of deuteranomaly in Europeans, selection might have been operative on this trait, but the nature of selection is difficult to define. Women heterozygous for deuteranomaly might be expected to be tetrachromatic, since X inactivation would render them mosaics for slightly abnormal and normal green pigment genes, in addition to having normal blue and red visual pigments. Possibly, such a tetrachromatic state in females, as well as hemizygosity for deuteranomaly, might have provided a selective advantage that has now disappeared. Why protanomalous women would not have such an advantage, however, is not clear. Cruz-Coke and Varela[160] suggested that women heterozygous for color vision defects are more fertile. However, Mollon et al. were unable to show any differences between heterozygotes and normal individuals on the basis either of the time between marriage and birth of the first child or the time between discontinuation of contraception and the beginning of pregnancy.[161] In any case, the most important reason for the relatively high frequency of the various red gene color vision defects appears to be the multigene structure of the color vision gene array, which allows relatively frequent recombination with the formation of fusion genes and deletions.

EVOLUTION

The evolution of the visual pigment genes has been elucidated.[50–52,162] An ancestral gene coded for the precursor gene of a variety of related protein molecules known as the G-protein-coupled receptors. These receptors are also known as heptahelical receptors (because they cross the membrane seven times) and include beta adrenergic receptors, serotonin receptors, the muscarinic acetylcholine receptor, and S-K receptors. The ancestral visual pigment is part of this family. Some 800 million years ago, the ancestral visual pigment diverged into the rod pigment rhodopsin and the as-yet undifferentiated cone pigment. Some 500 million years ago, a short-wavelength-sensitive (blue) pigment gene and a single middle- to long-wavelength-sensitive ("green–red") pigment gene diverged from each other (Fig. 143-2). This ancient system of short-wavelength (blue) and long-wavelength (green–red) signals probably was shared by all diurnal animals. Thirty million years ago, the green (middle-wavelength) and red (long-wavelength) system pigment genes differentiated to provide trichromatic color vision, which is shared by most humans and Old World monkeys. New World monkeys have dichromatic vision in males, but several alleles exist at their red–green locus, so that compound heterozygous females are trichromatic.[49]

The green pigment gene in all humans studied is 1.5 kb shorter than the red pigment gene. This alteration was caused by a short deletion in the first intron, presumably acquired early during evolution. The identical deletion in the red pigment gene has been observed as a polymorphic trait in one-third of African-Americans, but is much rarer in Japanese and Europeans.[64] This deletion presumably was acquired by gene conversion from the standard green pigment gene. Further differentiation in the red pigment gene occurred, in that 62 percent of Europeans carry serine at position 180 and 38 percent carry alanine, with very mild phenotypic consequences (see above). Many female heterozygotes for this polymorphism, as well as heterozygotes for the anomalous trichromacies have the genetic makeup for tetrachromacy and may therefore provide the basis for future evolution of our color vision system. However, the search for psychophysical manifestation of tetrachromacy so far has not yielded definitive results.[162]

REFERENCES

1. Gouras P: The history of colour vision, in Gouras P (ed): *Vision and Visual Dysfunctions*, vol 6, The Perception of Colour Vision. Boca Raton, CRC Press, 1992, p 1.
2. Dalton J: Extraordinary facts relating to the vision of colours, with observations. *Mem Lit Philos Soc Lond* **5**:28, 1798.
3. Emery AEH: John Dalton (1766–1844). *J Med Genet* **25**:422, 1988.
4. Horner JF: Die Erblichkeit des Daltonismus. *Amtl Ber Verwalt Med Kantons Zurich*, **108**, 1876.
5. Wilson EB: The sex chromosomes. *Arch Mikrosk Anat Enwicklungsmech* **77**:249, 1911.
6. Bell J, Haldane JBS: The linkage between the genes for colour-blindness and haemophilia in man. *Proc R Soc (Lond)* **B123**:119, 1937.
7. Porter IH, Schulze J, McKusick VA: Linkage between G6PD-deficiency and colour blindness. *Nature* **193**:503, 1962.
8. Feil R, Aubourg P, Heilig R, Mandel JL: A 195-kb cosmid walk encompassing the human Xq28 color vision pigment genes. *Genomics* **6**:367, 1990.
9. Boynton RM: *Human Color Vision*. New York, Holt, Rinehart, Winston, 1979, p 438.
10. Nathans J, Thomas D, Hogness DS: Molecular genetics of human color vision: The genes encoding blue, green and red pigments. *Science* **232**:193, 1986.
11. Nathans J, Piantanida TP, Eddy RL, Shows TB, Hogness DS: Molecular genetics of inherited variation in human color vision. *Science* **232**:203, 1986.
12. Stiles WS, Burch JM: Colour-matching investigation: Final report (1958). *Optica Acta* **6**:1, 1959.
13. Alpern M, Wake T: Cone pigments in human deutan color vision defects. *J Physiol* **266**:595, 1977.
14. Alpern M, Pugh EN Jr: Variation in the action spectrum of erythrolabe among deuteranopes. *J Physiol* **266**:613, 1977.
15. Alpern M, Moeller J: The red and green visual pigments of deuteranomalous trichromacy. *J Physiol* **266**:647, 1977.
16. Waaler GHM: Heredity of two types of colour normal vision. *Nature* **215**:406, 1967.
17. Neitz J, Jacobs GH: Polymorphism of the long-wavelength cone in normal human color vision. *Nature* **323**:623, 1986.
18. Winderickx J, Lindsey DT, Sanocki E, Teller DY, Motulsky AG, Deeb SS: Polymorphism in red photopigment underlies variation in colour matching. *Nature* **356**:431, 1992.
19. Deeb SS, Lindsey DT, Hibiya Y, Sanocki E, Winderickx J, Teller DY, Motulsky AG: Genotype-phenotype relationships in human red/green color vision defects: Molecular and psychophysical studies. *Am J Hum Genet* **51**:687, 1992.
20. Teller DY: Color vision. In Dulbecco R (ed): *Encyclopedia of Human Biology*, vol 2. San Diego, Academic Press, 1991, p 575.
21. Cornsweet TN: *Visual Perception*. New York, Academic Press, 1970.
22. Lennie P, D'Zmura M: Mechanisms of color vision. *CRC Crit Rev Neurobiol* **3**:333, 1988.
23. Mollon JD, Sharpe LT (eds): *Colour Vision: Physiology and Psychophysics*. London, Academic Press, 1983.
24. Newton I: New theory about light and colours. *Philos Trans R Soc Lond* **80**:3075, 1671/72.
25. Young T: On the theory of light and colors. *Philos Trans R Soc Lond* **92**:20, 1802.
26. Maxwell JC: On colour vision. *Proc R Inst Great Britain*, **6**:260, 1872.
27. Helmholtz HLF von: On the theory of compound colours. *Philos Mag* (Series 4) **4**:519, 1852.
28. Dowling JE: *The Retina: An Approachable Part of the Brain*. Cambridge, Harvard University Press, 1987.
29. Brown PK, Wald G: Visual pigments in single rods and cones of the human retina. *Science* **144**:45, 1964.
30. MacNichol EF, Levine JS, Mansfield RJW, Lipetz LE, Collins BA: Microspectrophotometry of visual pigments in

primate photoreceptors, in Mollon JD, Sharpe LT (eds): *Colour Vision*. London, Academic Press, 1983, p 14.

31. Dartnall HJA, Bowmaker JK, Mollon JD: Human visual pigments: Microspectrophotometric results from the eyes of seven persons. *Proc R Soc Lond* **B220**:115, 1983.
32. Rushton WAH: The Newton Lecture: The chemical basis of colour vision and colour blindness. *Nature* **206**:1087, 1965.
33. Bowmaker JK, Astell S, Hung DM, Mollon JD: Photosensitive and photostable pigments in the retinae of old world monkeys. *J Exp Biol* **55**:1, 1991.
34. Jacobs GH, Neitz J: Electrophysiological estimates of individual variation in the L/M cone ratio, in Drum B (ed): *Colour Vision Deficiencies*, vol 11. Dordrecht, Netherlands, Kluwer Academic Publishers, 1993, p 107.
35. Rushton WAH, Baker HD: Red/green sensitivity in normal vision. *Vision Res* **4**:75, 1964.
36. Vimal RLP, Pokorny J, Smith VC, Shevell SK: Foveal cone thresholds. *Vision Res* **29**:61, 1989.
37. Cicerone CM, Nerger JL: The relative numbers of long-wavelength-sensitive and middle-wavelength-sensitive cones in the human fovea centralis. *Vision Res* **19**:115, 1989.
38. Wesner MF, Pokorny J, Shevell SK, Smith VC: Foveal cone detection statistics in color normals and dichromats. *Vision Res* **31**:1021, 1991.
39. Curcio CA, Allen KA, Sloan KR, Lerea CL, Hurley JB, Klock IB, Milam AH: Distribution and morphology of human cone photoreceptors stained with anti-blue opsin. *J Comp Neurol* **312**:610, 1991.
40. Wang JH, McDowell JH, Hargrave P: Site of attachment of 11-*cis*-retinal in bovine rhodopsin. *Biochemistry* **19**:5111, 1980.
41. Caron MC, Lefkowitz RJ: Model systems for the study of seven-transmembrane-segment receptors. *Ann Rev Biochem* **60**:653, 1991.
42. Henderson R: The purple membrane from *Halobacterium holobium*. *Ann Rev Biophys Bioeng* **6**:87, 1977.
43. Dohlman G, Thorner J, Caron M, Lefkowitz R: Model systems for the study of seven-transmembrane-segment receptors. *Ann Rev Biochem* **60**:653, 1991.
44. Fung BK-K, Hurley JB, Stryer L: Flow of information in the light-triggered cyclic nucleotide cascade of vision. *Proc Natl Acad Sci USA* **78**:152, 1981.
45. Fung BK-K, Stryer L: Photolyzed rhodopsin catalyzes the exchange of GTP for bound GDP in retinal rod outer segments. *Proc Natl Acad Sci USA* **77**:2500, 1980.
46. Stryer L: Visual excitation and recovery. *J Biol Chem* **266**:1071, 1991.
47. Jacobs GH: Within-species variation in visual capacity among squirrel monkeys (*Saimiri sciureus*): Sensitivity difference. *Vision Res* **23**:239, 1983.
48. Jacobs GH: Within-species variation in visual capacity among squirrel monkeys (*Saimiri sciureus*): Color vision. *Vision Res* **24**:1267, 1984.
49. Jacobs GH, Neitz J: Inheritance of color vision in a New World monkey (*Saimiri sciureus*). *Proc Natl Acad Sci USA* **84**:2545, 1987.
50. Yokoyama S, Yokoyama R: Molecular evolution of human visual pigment genes. *Mol Biol Evol* **6**:186, 1989.
51. Mollon JD, Jordan G: Eine evolutionare Interpretation des menschlichen Farbensehen. *Die Farbe* **35/36**:139, 1988/89.
52. Bowmaker JK: The evolution of vertebrate visual pigments and photoreceptors, in Cronly-Dillon JR, Gregory RL (eds): *Vision and Visual Dysfunction*, Vol 2, *Evolution of Eye and Visual Systems*. London, Macmillan, 1991, p 63.
53. Nathans J, Weitz CJ, Agarwal N, Nir I, Papermaster DS: Production of bovine rhodopsin by mammalian cell lines expressing cloned cDNA: Spectrophotometry and subcellular localization. *Vision Res* **29**:907, 1989.
54. Merbs SL, Nathans J: Absorption spectra of the hybrid pigments responsible for anomalous trichromacy. *Science* **258**:464, 1992.
55. Oprian DD, Asenjo AB, Lee N, Pelletier SL: Design, chemical synthesis, and expression of genes for the three human color vision pigments. *Biochemistry* **30**:11367, 1991.
56. Kosower EM: Assignment of groups responsible for the "opsin shift" and light absorptions of rhodopsin and red, green, and blue iodopsins (cone pigments). *Proc Natl Acad Sci USA* **85**:1076, 1988.
57. Neitz M, Neitz J, Jacobs GH: Spectral tuning of pigments underlying red-green color vision. *Science* **252**:971, 1991.
58. Williams AJ, Hunt DM, Bowmaker JK, Mollon JD: The polymorphic pigments of the marmoset: Spectral tuning and genetic basis. *EMBO J* **11**:2039, 1992.
59. Ibbotson RE, Hunt DM, Bowmaker JK, Mollon JD: Sequence divergence and copy number of the middle- and long-wave photopigments in Old World monkeys. *Proc R Soc Lond* **B247**:145, 1992.
60. Merbs SL, Nathans J: Absorption spectra of human cone pigments. *Nature* **356**:433, 1992.
61. Chan T, Lee M, Sakmar TP: Introduction of hydroxyl-bearing amino acids causes bathochromic spectral shifts in rhodopsin. *J Biol Chem* **267**:9478, 1992.
62. Nathans J, Hogness DS: Isolation, sequence analysis, and intron-exon arrangement of the gene encoding bovine rhodopsin. *Cell* **34**:807, 1983.
63. Martin RL, Wood C, Baehr W, Applebury ML: Visual pigment homologies revealed by DNA hybridization. *Science* **232**:1266, 1986.
64. Jorgensen AL, Deeb S, Motulsky AG: Molecular genetics of X chromosome-linked color vision among populations of African and Japanese ancestry: High frequency of a shortened red pigment gene among Afro-Americans. *Proc Natl Acad Sci USA* **87**:6512, 1990.
65. Vollrath D, Nathans J, Davis RW: Tandem array of human visual pigment genes at Xq28. *Science* **240**:1669, 1988.
66. Mosser J, Douar AM, Sarde CO, Kioschis P, Feil R, Moser H, Poustka AM, Mandel JL, Aubourg P: Putative X-linked adrenoleukodystrophy gene shares unexpected homology with ABC transporters. *Nature* **361**:726, 1993.
67. Hamer DH, Hu S, Magnuson VL, Hu N, Pattatucci AML: A linkage between DNA markers on the X-chromosome and male sexual orientation. *Science* **261**:321, 1993.
68. Drummond-Borg M, Deeb S, Motulsky AG: Molecular patterns of X chromosome-linked color vision genes among 134 men of European ancestry. *Proc Natl Acad Sci USA* **86**:983, 1989.
69. Kalmus H: *Diagnosis and Genetics of Defective Colour Vision*. Oxford, Pergamon Press, 1965.
70. Piantanida T: Genetics of inherited colour vision deficiencies, in David H. Foster (ed): *Vision and Visual Dysfunction*, vol. 7, *Inherited and Acquired Colour Vision Deficiencies*. Boca Raton, CRC Press, 1991, p 88.
71. Jaeger W: Genetics of congenital colour deficiencies, in Autrum VH, Jung R, Loewenstein D, McKay M, Teuber HL (eds): *Handbook of Sensory Physiology*. Heidelberg, Springer-Verlag, 1972, p 625.
72. Rushton WAH: A foveal pigment in the deuteranope. *J Physiol (Lond)* **176**:24, 1965.
73. Mollon JD, Bowmaker JK, Dartnall HJA, Bird AC: Microspectrophotometric and psychophysical results for the same deuteranopic observer, in Verriest G (ed): *Colour Vision Deficiencies*, vol 7. The Hague, Dr W. Junk Publisher, 1984, p 303.
74. Rushton WAH, Powell DS, White KD: Pigments in anomalous trichromats. *Vision Res* **13**:2017, 1973.
75. Piantanida TP, Sperling H: Isolation of a third chromatic mechanism in the deuteranomalous observer. *Vision Res* **13**:2049, 1973.
76. Piantanida TP, Sperling HG: Isolation of a third chromatic mechanism in the protanomalous observer. *Vision Res* **13**:2033, 1973.
77. Francois J: *Heredity in Ophthalmology*. St. Louis, Mosby, 1961, p 73.
78. Wright WD: The characteristics of tritanopia. *J Opt Soc Am* **42**:509, 1952.
79. Went LN, Pronk N: The genetics of tritan disturbances. *Hum Genet* **69**:255, 1985.
80. Weitz CJ, Miyake Y, Shinzato K, Montag E, Zrenner E, Went LN, Nathans J: Human tritanopia associated with two amino acid substitutions in the blue sensitive opsin. *Am J Hum Genet* **50**:498, 1992.
81. Weitz CJ, Went L, Nathans J: Human tritanopia associated

with a third amino acid substitution in the blue-sensitive visual pigment. *Am J Hum Genet* **51**:444, 1992.

82. Weleber RG, Eisner A: Cone degeneration ("bulls eye dystrophies") and colour vision defects, in Newsome DA (ed): *Retinal Dystrophies and Degenerations*. New York, Raven Press, 1988, p 233.
83. Moore AT: Cone and cone-rod dystrophies. *J Med Genet* **29**:289, 1992.
84. Nathans J, Davenport CM, Maumenee IH, Heijtmancik JF, Litt M, Loverien E, Weleber R, Bachynski B, Zwas F, Klingman R, Fishman G: Molecular genetics of blue cone monochromacy. *Science* **245**:831, 1990.
85. Berson EL, Gouras PG, Gunkel RD: Progressive cone degeneration, dominantly inherited. *Arch Ophthalmol* **80**:77, 1968.
86. Everdingen JAM, Went LN, Keunen JEE, Oosterhuis JA: X-linked progressive cone dystrophy with specific attention to carrier detection. *J Med Genet* **29**:291, 1992.
87. Fleishman JA, O'Donnell FE: Congenital incomplete achromatopsia: Evidence for slow progression, carrier fundus findings, and possible genetic linkage with glucose-6-phosphate dehydrogenase locus. *Arch Ophthalmol* **99**:468, 1981.
88. Goodman G, Ripps H, Siegel IM: Cone dysfunction syndromes. *Arch Ophthalmol* **70**:214, 1963.
89. Hess RF, Mullen KT, Sharpe LT, Zrenner E: The photoreceptors in atypical achromatopsia. *J Physiol* **417**:123, 1989.
90. Jacobson DM, Thompson HS, Bartley JA: X-linked progressive cone dystrophy. Clinical characteristics of affected males and female carriers. *Ophthalmology* **96**:885, 1989.
91. Pearlman JT, Owen GW, Brounley DW, Sheppard JJ: Cone dystrophy with dominant inheritance. *Am J Ophthalmol* **77**:293, 1974.
92. Yagasaki Y, Jacobson SG: Cone-rod dystrophy. Phenotypic diversity by retinal function testing. *Arch Ophthalmol* **107**:701, 1989.
93. Reichel E, Bruce AM, Sandberg MA, Berson EL: An electroretinographic and molecular genetic study of X-linked cone degeneration. *Am J Ophthalmol* **108**:540, 1989.
94. Birch J, Chisholm IA, Kinnear P, Pinckers AJLG, Pokorny J, Smith VC, Verriest G: Clinical testing methods, in Pokorny J, Smith VC, Verriest G, Pinckers AJLG (eds): *Congenital and Acquired Color Vision Defects*. New York, Grune & Stratton, 1979, p 83.
95. Farnsworth D: Farnsworth-Munsell 100 hue test for the examination of color discrimination manual. Baltimore, Munsell Color Co., Inc., 1957.
96. Berson EL: Electrical phenomena in the retina, in Moses RA (ed): *Adler's Physiology of the Eye. Clinical Application*. St. Louis, Mosby, 1975, p 453.
97. Hanazaki H, Tanabe J, Kawasaki K: Electroretinographic findings in congenital red-green color deficiency, in Ohta Y (ed): *Color Vision Deficiencies*. Berkeley, Kugler & Ghedini, 1990, p 71.
98. Pokorny J, Smith VC, Verriest G: Congenital color defects, in Pokorny J, Smith VC, Verriest G, Pinckers AJLG (eds): *Congenital and Acquired Color Vision Defects*. New York, Grune and Stratton, 1979, p 183.
99. Judd DB: Color blindness and the detection of camouflage. *Science* **97**:544, 1943.
100. Adam A: A further query on color blindness and natural selection. *Soc Biol* **16**:197, 1969.
101. Morgan MJ, Adam A, Mollon JD: Dichromats detect colour camouflaged objects that are not detected by trichromats. *Proc R Soc Lond (Biol)* **248**:291, 1992.
102. Kuyk TK, Veres JG III, Lahey MA, Clark DJ: The ability of protan color defectives to perform color-dependent air traffic control tasks. *Am J Optom Physiol Opt* **63**:582, 1986.
103. Kuyk TK, Veres JG, Lahey MA, Clark DJ: Ability of deutan color defectives to perform simulated air traffic control tasks. *Am J Optom Physiol Opt* **64**:2, 1987.
104. Vingrys AJ, Cole BL: Are standards of colour vision in the transport industries justified? *Ophthalmic Physiol Opt* **8**:1257, 1988.
105. Cole B: Does defective colour vision really matter?, in Drum B (ed): *Colour Vision Deficiencies*, vol 9. Dordrecth, Netherlands, Kulwere Academic, 1993, p 67.
106. Webb N: Color-vision testing for airline pilots. *J Am Med Assoc* **258**:841, 1987.
107. Steward JM, Cole BL: What do color vision defectives say about everyday tasks? *Optometry Vision Sci* **66**:288, 1989.
108. Verriest G, Neubauer O, Marre M, Uvijls A: New investigations on the relationships between congenital colour vision defects and road traffic safety, in Verriest G (ed.): *Colour Vision Deficiencies*, vol 5. Bristol, Hilger, 1980, p 331.
109. Windericks J, Battisti L, Hibiya Y, Motulsky AG, Deeb SS: Haplotype diversity in the human red and green opsin genes: Evidence for frequent sequence exchange in exon 3. *Human Mol Genet* **2**:1413, 1993.
110. Neitz J, Neitz M, Jacobs GH: Analysis of fusion gene and encoded photopigment of colour-blind humans. *Nature* **342**:679, 1989.
111. Winderickx J, Sanocki E, Lindsey DT, Teller DY, Motulsky AG, Deeb SS: Defective colour vision associated with a missense mutation in the human green visual pigment gene. *Nat Genet* **1**:251, 1992.
112. Nathans J, Merbs SL, Sung C-H, Weitz CJ, Wang Y: Molecular genetics of human visual pigments. *Ann Rev Genet* **26**:403, 1992.
113. Applebury M, Hargrave PA: Molecular biology of the visual pigments. *Vision Res* **26**:1881, 1986.
114. Karnik SS, Sakmar TP, Chen H-B, Khorana HG: Cysteine residues 110 and 187 are essential for the formation of correct structure in bovine rhodopsin. *Proc Natl Acad Sci USA* **85**:8459, 1988.
115. Dixon RAF, Sigal IS, Candelore MR, Register RB, Scattergood W, Rands E, Strader CD: Structural features required for ligand binding to the β-adrenergic receptor. *EMBO J* **6**:3269, 1987.
116. Dryja TP, McGee TL, Hahn LB, Cowley GS, Ollson JE, Reichel E, Sandberg MA, Berson EL: Mutations within the rhodopsin gene in patients with autosomal dominant retinitis pigmentosa. *N Engl J Med* **323**:1302, 1990.
117. Inglehearn CF, Keen TJ, Bashir R, Jay M, Fizke F, Bird AC, Crombie A, Bhattacharya S: A completed screen for mutations of the rhodopsin gene in a panel of patients with autosomal dominant retinitis pigmentosa. *Hum Mol Genet* **1**:41, 1992.
118. Drummond-Borg M, Deeb S, Motulsky AG: Molecular basis of abnormal red-green color vision: A family with three types of color vision defects. *Am J Hum Genet* **43**:675, 1988.
119. Hurvich LM: Color vision deficiencies, in Jameson D, Hurvich LM (eds): *Handbook of Sensory Physiology*, vol 7. Berlin, Springer-Verlag, 1972, p 581.
120. Nagy AL, Purl KF: Color discrimination and neural coding in color vision deficients. *Vision Res* **27**:483, 1987.
121. Pokorny J, Smith VC: The functional nature of polymorphism of human color vision, in: *Frontiers of Visual Sciences: Proc 1985 Symp*. Washington, DC, National Academy Press, 1987, p 150.
122. Winderickx J, Battisti L, Motulsky AG, Deeb SS: Selective expression of the human X-linked green opsin genes. *Proc Natl Acad Sci USA* **89**:9710, 1992.
123. Neitz J, Neitz M, Jacobs GH: More than three different cone pigments among people with normal color vision. *Vision Res* **33**:117, 1993.
124. Behringer RR, Ryan TM, Palmiter RD, Brinster RL, Townes TM: Human δ to B-globin gene switching in transgenic mice. *Genes Dev* **4**:380, 1990.
125. Enver T, Raich N, Ebens AJ, Papayannopoulou T, Constantini F, Stamatoyannopoulos G: Developmental regulation of human fetal-to-adult globin gene switching in transgenic mice. *Nature* **344**:309, 1990.
126. Stamatoyannopoulos G: Human hemoglobin switching. *Science* **252**:383, 1991.
127. Hanscombe O, Whyatt D, Fraser P, Yannoutsos N, Greaves D, Dillon N, Grosveld F: Importance of globin gene order to correct developmental expression. *Genes Dev* **5**:1387, 1991.
128. Wang Y, Macke JP, Merbs SL, Zack D, Klaunberg B, Bennet J, Gearhart J, Nathans J: A locus control region adjacent to the human red and green visual pigment genes. *Neuron* **9**:429, 1992.
129. Lewis RA, Holcomb JD, Bromley WC, Wilson MC,

Roderick TH, Hejtmancik JF: Mapping X-linked ophthalmic diseases. III. Provisional assignment of the locus for blue cone monochromacy to Xq28. *Arch Ophthalmol* **105**:1055, 1987.

130. Van Heel L, Went LN, Van Norren D: Frequency of tritan disturbances in a population study. *Color Vision Defic* **5**:256, 1980.
131. Krill AE, Smith VC, Pokorny J: Further studies supporting the identity of congenital tritanopia and hereditary dominant optic atrophy. *Invest Ophthalmol* **10**:457, 1971.
132. Miyake Y, Yagasaki K, Ichikawa H: Differential diagnosis of congenital tritanopia and dominantly inherited juvenile optic atrophy. *Arch Ophthalmol* **103**:1496, 1985.
133. Eisner A, MacLeod DIA: Flicker photometric study of chromatic adaptation: Selective suppression of cone inputs by colored backgrounds. *J Opt Soc Am* **71**:705, 1981.
134. Elsner AE, Burns SA: Classes of color normal observers. *J Opt Soc Am* **4**:123, 1987.
135. Neitz J, Jacobs GH: Polymorphism in normal human color vision and its mechanism. *Vision Res* **30**:621, 1990.
136. Alpern MJ: Lack of uniformity in colour matching. *J Physiol* **288**:85, 1979.
137. Lascari AD, Hoak JC, Taylor JC: Christmas disease in a girl. *Am J Dis Child* **117**:585, 1969.
138. Ingerslev J, Schwartz M, Lamm LU, Kruse TA, Bukh A, Stenberg S: Female haemophilia A in a family with seeming extreme bidirectional lyonization tendency: Abnormal premature X-chromosome inactivation? *Clin Genet* **35**:41, 1989.
139. Jorgensen AL, Philip J, Raskind WH, Matsushita M, Christensen B, Dreyer V, Motulsky AG: Different patterns of inactivation in MZ twins discordant for red-green color-vision deficiency. *Am J Hum Genet* **51**:291, 1992.
140. Nettleship E: Some unusual pedigrees of color blindness. *Trans Ophthalmol Soc UK* **32**:309, 1912.
141. Stocks P, Karn MN: A biometric investigation of twins and their brothers and sisters. *Ann Eugenics* **5(2)**:17, 1933.
142. Walls GL: Peculiar color blindness in peculiar people. *AMA Arch Ophthalmol* **62**:41, 1959.
143. Kourlischer L, Zanen J, Meunier A: La theorie de Lyon peut-elle expliquer la desparité exceptionnellement observée de la perception colorée chez des jumelles univitellines? *Comptes-Rendus du Premier Congres International de Neuro-Ophtalmologie*. Basel, Karger, 1968, p 242.
144. Philip J, Vogelius-Anderson CH, Dreyer V, Freiesleben E, Gurtler H, Hauge M, Kissmeyer-Nielsen F, Nelson LS, Pers M, Robson EB, Svejgaard A, Sorensen B: Color vision deficiency in one of two presumably monozygotic twins with secondary amenorrhoea. *Ann Hum Genet* **33**:185, 1969.
145. Yokota A, Shin Y, Kimura J, Senos T, Seki R, Tsubota K: Congenital deuteranomaly in one of three MZ triplets, in Ohta Y (ed): *Color Vision Defects*. Tokyo, Kuguler & Ghedini, 1990.
146. Born G, Grutzner P, Hemminger H: Evidenz fur eine Mosaikstruktur der Netzhaut bei Konduktorinnen fur dichromasie. *Hum Genet* **32**:189, 1976.
147. Grutzner P, Born G, Hemminger HJ: Colored stimuli within the central visual field of carriers of dichromatism. *Mod Prob Ophthalmol* **17**:147, 1976.
148. Cohn SA, Emmerich DS, Carlson EA: Differences in the responses of heterozygous carriers of colorblindness and normal controls to briefly presented stimuli. *Vision Res* **29**:255, 1989.
149. Verriest G: Chromaticity discrimination in protan and deutan heterozygotes. *Farbe* **21**:7, 1972.
150. Ichikawa H, Akio M: Genetic studies on defective color vision in junior high school students. *Mod Prob Ophthalmol* **13**:265, 1974.
151. Nemoto H, Murao M: A genetic studies of colorblindness. *Jpn J Hum Genet* 165–173, 1961.
152. Crooks KBM: Further observations on color blindness among negroes with genealogic and geographic notes. *Hum Biol* **8**:451, 1936.
153. Adam A: Colorblindness in Africa. *Metab Pediatr Ophthalmol* **5**:181, 1981.
154. Adam A: Polymorphisms of red-green vision among populations of the tropics. *Soc Study Hum Biol Symp* **27**:245, 1986.
155. Adam A: Colorblindness in man: A call for re-examination of the selection-relaxation theory, in Ahuja YR, Neel JV (eds): *Genetic Microdifferentiation in Human and Other Animal Populations*. Dehli, India, Indian Anthropological Association, 1985 p. 181.
156. Filippi G, Rinaldi A, Palmarino R, Seravalli E, Siniscalco M: Linkage disequilibrium for two X-linked genes in Sardinia and its bearing on the statistical mapping of the human X chromosome. *Genetics* **86**:199, 1977.
157. Post RH: Population differences in red and green colour vision deficiency: Review and a query on selection relaxation. *Eugen Q* **9**:131, 1962.
158. Post RH: Possible cases of relaxed selection in civilized populations. *Humangenetik* **13**:253, 1971.
159. Neel JV, Post RH: Transitory "positive" selection for color blindness? *Eugen Q* **10**:33, 1963.
160. Cruz-Coke R, Varela A: Inheritance of alcoholism. Its association with color blindness. *Lancet* **2**:1282, 1966.
161. Mollon JD: On the origins of polymorphisms, in Committee on Vision (ed): *Frontiers of Visual Science*. Washington DC, National Academy Press, 1987.
162. Jordan G, Mollon JD: A study of women heterozygous for colour deficiencies. *Vision Res* **33**:1495, 1993.

CHAPTER 144

Retinitis Pigmentosa

Thaddeus P. Dryja

1. **Retinitis pigmentosa is the name given to a set of heritable degenerations of the retina. Patients with retinitis pigmentosa typically experience night blindness (nyctalopia) and loss of the midperipheral visual field early in the disease. As the disease progresses, a shrinking island of central vision (tunnel vision) remains. In most cases, all vision is ultimately lost during middle age. In advanced cases and sometimes even in early cases, the fundus oculi exhibits the following features: thin retinal vessels, a pale optic nerve head, and clumps of intraretinal pigment. Most forms of retinitis pigmentosa affect only the eye, although a minority of cases have other abnormalities, such as deafness in Usher's syndrome.**

2. **Measurements of the retina's electrical responses to flashes of light are the best way to distinguish the early stages of retinitis pigmentosa from nonprogressive retinal diseases such as stationary nyctalopia. These noninvasive measurements, called *electroretinograms* (ERGs), can be used to diagnose young patients with retinitis pigmentosa even before visual symptoms or funduscopic abnormalities are apparent.**

3. **Pathologic examinations of autopsy cases suggest that photoreceptors are the cells affected first. However, it is still possible that in some cases the retinal pigment epithelium could have the primary biochemical defect or that the retinal degeneration is due to a peculiar sensitivity of photoreceptors to some generalized metabolic defect.**

4. **In some families the disease is inherited as an autosomal dominant trait, in others as an autosomal recessive trait, and in still others as an X-linked trait. There is considerable nonallelic heterogeneity even within each genetic type. For example, there are at least two distinct loci implicated in X-linked retinitis pigmentosa and at least three loci known to cause dominant retinitis pigmentosa.**

5. **Mutations in the rhodopsin gene are responsible for approximately 25 percent of dominant retinitis pigmentosa cases. The dominant mutations are missense mutations or short, in-frame deletions. A null mutation (premature stop codon) has been reported in one family with autosomal recessive retinitis pigmentosa.**

6. **Mutations in the retinal degeneration slow gene (peripherin/RDS) are responsible for approximately 5 percent of cases of dominant retinitis pigmentosa without a rhodopsin mutation. Like the rhodopsin mutations causing retinitis pigmentosa, the peripherin/RDS mutations are also either missense mutations or short, in-frame deletions.**

7. **Patients with abetalipoproteinemia (Chap. 57) or Refsum's disease (Chap. 73) can exhibit the signs and symptoms of retinitis pigmentosa as the first manifestations. It is important to consider these treatable causes of retinitis pigmentosa in newly diagnosed patients. Also noteworthy in this regard is that at least some patients with a related hereditary retinal degeneration known as gyrate atrophy (Chap. 31) may benefit from specifically modifying their diet.**

8. **Except for abetalipoproteinemia and Refsum's disease, there is no therapy known to slow or stop the retinal degeneration found in retinitis pigmentosa. However, a night-vision scope can help to alleviate the symptom of night blindness in some patients.[1] Also, acetazolamide has been reported to ameliorate temporarily the cystoid macular edema that reduces central vision in some cases,[2,3] although this drug can have serious side effects.**

BACKGROUND

Retinitis pigmentosa is the name given to a set of hereditary retinal degenerations that share a number of clinical features. In fact, it has not been possible to elaborate criteria that unambiguously distinguish every patient with retinitis pigmentosa from other particular forms of retinal degeneration; thus, the phrase *retinitis pigmentosa and allied diseases* has been used to encompass related diseases such as gyrate atrophy (see Chap. 31), choroideremia (see Chap. 145), etc. This chapter will exclude discussion of the allied diseases described elsewhere in this textbook, and although this chapter centers on what is termed *"typical" retinitis pigmentosa*, it should be emphasized in the beginning that there are probably scores of hereditary retinal degenerations in humans. Some of these are designated "retinitis pigmentosa" while others have features sufficiently distinctive to warrant separate names, such as Leber's congenital amaurosis, cone-rod dystrophy, vitelliform dystrophy, Stargardt's disease, etc. Even within many of these "more-specific" diagnostic entities there is most likely considerable genetic heterogeneity, both allelic and nonallelic. Additional types of hereditary retinal dysfunction are not progressive and therefore fall outside the category of "retinal degeneration"—for example, color blindness (see Chap. 143) or stationary nyctalopia (night blindness). These diagnostic categories also display considerable genetic heterogeneity. Although they may appear to fall outside the scope of this chapter, there is evidence that some inherited, nonprogressive retinal diseases may be

A list of standard abbreviations is located immediately preceding the index in each volume. Additional abbreviations used in this chapter include: ERG = electroretinogram; RDS = retinal degeneration slow (gene).

allelic variants of retinitis pigmentosa. For instance, the locus for complete X-linked congenital stationary night blindness is closely linked to a chromosomal region also containing a locus for X-linked retinitis pigmentosa,[4] and there is speculation that these two diseases might be allelic.[5] Furthermore, missense mutations in the rhodopsin gene can be associated both with dominant retinitis pigmentosa and with a form of congenital night blindness.[6] In short, ophthalmologists have described a cornucopia of hereditary retinal diseases for which only a few have known biochemical or genetic defects.

Young patients with typical retinitis pigmentosa may have no signs or symptoms, although problems with night vision are frequently reported. As the disease progresses, an absolute scotoma in the midperipheral visual field develops.[7] This ring scotoma gradually enlarges so that in advanced cases only two islands of vision remain: a central island centered at the fixation point, and a rim of peripheral vision in the temporal field of either eye. In most cases, all vision is ultimately lost, although the age at which complete blindness occurs can vary markedly between different families and even between affected patients in the same family. The clinical symptoms and the funduscopic picture can be quite varied, however, and it is certain that a large measure of the variability in the symptoms and fundus picture is a reflection of the abundance and heterogeneity of retinal degenerations falling under the term *retinitis pigmentosa*.

Retinitis pigmentosa occurs in all races, although the incidence of the disease differs somewhat from nation to nation.[8–14] In the United States it has an prevalence of approximately 0.02 to 0.03 percent, affecting over 50,000 people.[8,9,11]

OCULAR FINDINGS

A complete ocular examination, including a dilated retinal examination and electroretinography is necessary for evaluating patients suspected of having retinitis pigmentosa or an allied disease. In most cases, central visual acuity remains good until late in retinitis pigmentosa.[7] Slit-lamp examination often reveals posterior subcapsular cataract, vitreous liquefaction, and vitreous cells. Early in the disease, the fundus can appear normal, although a subtle attenuation or thinning of the retinal vessels is usually present. As the disease progresses, the retinal vascular attenuation becomes more pronounced. The optic nerve head becomes pale. In addition, clumps of intraretinal pigment, called "bone-spicule pigmentation," appear in the midperiphery. The pattern of fundus pigmentation can vary between patients, but it is distinctively symmetrical in the two eyes.[15] A classic triad of funduscopic features is characteristic of advanced cases: retinal vascular attenuation, intraretinal pigmentation, and pallor of the optic nerve head. Cystoid macular edema is found in some cases.[16,17] Along with cataract,[18,19] it is one of the possibly treatable causes of reduced central vision.[2,3]

The ocular findings can be helpful in the genetic categorization of patients. For example, more than two diopters of myopia and astigmatism of more than one diopter are frequently found in X-linked retinitis pigmentosa.[20,21] Recording the extent of bone-spicule pigmentation in patients under the age of 20 is also of value, because if the pigmentation is not found in all four quadrants it is likely that the patient has an autosomal dominant form of retinitis pigmentosa.[20] Evaluating and interpreting these parameters will not definitively diagnose a particular genetic type of retinitis pigmentosa. Nevertheless, they can be helpful in genetic counseling, especially when dealing with an affected male with a negative or uncertain family history in whom X-linked, dominant, and recessive types of retinitis pigmentosa are all possible.

ELECTRORETINOGRAPHY

Electroretinograms (ERGs) are recordings of the retina's electrical responses to flashes of light. ERGs are generally measured noninvasively with electrodes embedded in a contact lens that rests on the cornea. One electrode rests on the cornea and the other on the inner lid; a separate, "ground" electrode is pasted to the skin of the forehead or cheek. Other arrangements of electrodes can also be used. The ERG is viewed on an oscilloscope screen with corneal voltage on the y-axis and time on the x-axis. The wave forms that are seen are due to the summation of electrical currents occurring in a variety of retinal cell types (Fig. 144-1). It is divided into components or "waves," called the a-wave, b-wave, and c-wave (for review, see Berson[22]). The a-wave, a fast, cornea-negative response, is derived from electrical currents directly generated by photoreceptors. The slower, cornea-positive b-wave has the largest amplitude. Although it is derived from fluxes of potassium ions within and surrounding Mueller cells in the inner nuclear layer,[23] it is directly dependent on functional photoreceptors, and its magnitude makes it the most convenient measure of the health of photoreceptors. The c-wave, a slow, cornea-positive response, does not customarily play a major role in the diagnosis or evaluation of patients with retinitis pigmentosa.

A flash of bright white light will stimulate both rods and cones in a dark-adapted retina to give an ERG wave form that sums the contributions of both photoreceptor types.

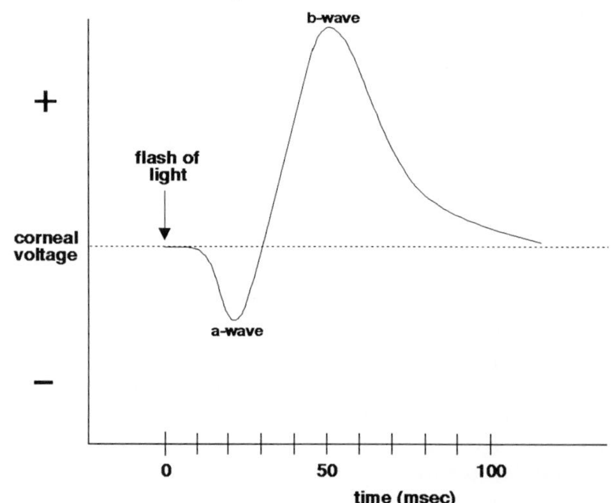

FIG. 144-1 Schematic diagram of an electroretinogram. The voltage (y-axis) is measured with an electrode embedded in a contact lens resting on the cornea (a second electrode is either in the same lens or pasted to the skin around the eye; a ground electrode is attached elsewhere on the head, e.g., to the forehead). The retina is exposed to a flash of light through a dilated pupil at time zero. The basic electrical response of the retina as an organ is a corneal-negative a-wave followed by a corneal-positive b-wave. The slow, corneal-positive c-wave is not shown on this figure. The time scale on the x-axis is approximate since the actual response times for the a- and b-waves vary according to the intensity of the light stimulus.

Conditions can be adjusted to measure rod and cone functions separately. For example, a flash of blue light, if dim enough, will stimulate the more light-sensitive rods but not the cones. In this situation, the ERG will be an indicator of rod function. Cone function can be isolated by stimulating the retina with flashes of bright white light repeated 30 times per second (30 Hz). Rods but not cones are too slow to generate respective responses to flashes of light at that frequency. In a normal individual, 30-Hz white flickering light therefore generates a 30-cycle-per-second wave form that derives exclusively from cones and indirect stimulation of Mueller cells by cones.

When evaluating a patient for a hereditary retinal degeneration, ERGs should employ full-field flashes of light (ganzfeld stimulation). ERGs should be measured after a patient's eyes have adapted to darkness for at least 30 min. With the appropriately standardized conditions, one can reliably and reproducibly measure the magnitude and timing of the ERG. Since many patients have ERG amplitudes less than 10 μV, computer averaging of signals is valuable for this purpose.[24] Such quantitation permits an objective comparison of the severity of the disease in patients. Recording the ERG at regular intervals (e.g., biannually) allows one to measure the rate of retinal degeneration,[25] making it possible to estimate the number of years of remaining vision. Also, the ERG can help in the identification of female carriers of X-linked retinitis pigmentosa, since such carriers ordinarily have subnormal responses.[26,27]

A reduction in the size (or amplitude) of the rod and/or cone responses can be observed both in patients with a progressive retinal degeneration such as retinitis pigmentosa as well as in patients with nonprogressive retinal disease such as stationary nyctalopia or self-limited or sector retinitis pigmentosa. Within a family known to have a progressive retinal degeneration, affected members over the age of 6 have a reduction in amplitude below normal for age and a delay in rod and/or cone response times (called "implicit times") even early in the disease when there may be no other symptoms or signs of the disease.[28] Patients with stationary retinal dysfunction may have reduced ERG amplitudes, but the responses, when present, will have normal timing.[29] On the other hand, a delay in the ERG responses even in the face of relatively high amplitudes signifies a progressive retinal degeneration.

RETINITIS PIGMENTOSA AS PART OF A MULTISYSTEM DISEASE

In most cases, patients with retinitis pigmentosa have no associated systemic or extraocular abnormalities. However, there are multisystem diseases in which a retinal degeneration similar to retinitis pigmentosa is a part. Although rare, the most noteworthy are diseases for which effective treatment is available to ameliorate the retinal degeneration. These are Refsum's disease and abetalipoproteinemia. Descriptions of these diseases and their underlying biochemical defects are found in Chaps. 73 and 57, respectively. It should be noted briefly that patients with abetalipoproteinemia can recover retinal function after therapy with vitamin A.[30,31] With regard to Refsum's disease, dietary modification aimed at reducing the intake of phytanic acid levels is of benefit in slowing or stopping the associated retinal degeneration.[32]

No biochemical defects are known for most other multisystem diseases in which retinitis pigmentosa is a feature, including Usher's syndrome type I (retinitis pigmentosa with vestibular ataxia and profound congenital deafness), Usher's syndrome type II (retinitis pigmentosa with partial hearing loss), and Laurence-Moon-Bardet-Biedl syndrome (retinitis pigmentosa associated with polydactyly, truncal obesity, short stature, and mental retardation). The two types of Usher's syndrome are both autosomal recessively inherited but are nonallelic (see "Genetics" below). The Lawrence-Moon-Bardet-Biedl syndrome accounts for less than 1 percent of the cases of retinitis pigmentosa and is also inherited as an autosomal recessive trait. A retinal degeneration similar to retinitis pigmentosa is also a feature of Kearns-Sayre syndrome (external ophthalmoplegia, pigmentary retinal degeneration, and cardiomyopathy). It is due to deletions of the mitochondrial genome[33–35] and is discussed in Chap. 46. The retinal degeneration found in Kearns-Sayre syndrome might be a reflection of the high metabolic demands of photoreceptors and/or the neighboring retinal pigment epithelium which makes them unusually susceptible to a relative deficiency in mitochondrial oxidative metabolism.

PATHOLOGY

There are numerous reports of pathologic examination of eyes from patients with retinitis pigmentosa.[36–45] The earliest changes are found in the photoreceptors (Fig. 144-2). Outer and inner segments are lost, followed by pyknosis and loss of the photoreceptor nuclei. In some cases rods appear to be affected earlier than cones; in others, rods and cones are equally involved. The later pathologic changes exhibited in the retina and in the other ocular tissues are presumably a consequence of the photoreceptor degeneration and are not specific to retinitis pigmentosa. Degeneration of the inner nuclear layer (bipolar, amacrine, horizontal, and Mueller cells) and even the ganglion cell layer occurs late in the disease, especially in the retinal periphery. Cataracts are very common.

There are histopathologic counterparts for each member of the funduscopic triad of retinitis pigmentosa: bone-spicule pigmentation, vascular attenuation, and pallid optic disk. The bone-spicule pigmentation is due to pigmented macrophages (thought to be metaplastic retinal pigment epithelial cells) migrating into the retina and congregating often, but not exclusively, around retinal vessels.[40] The retinal vessels may appear attenuated for two reasons. First, a reduction in the number of photoreceptors may allow the choriocapillaris to supply a larger share of the retina, thereby reducing the demands on the retinal vasculature, perhaps inducing autoregulatory reduction in blood flow. Second, a hyaline thickening of the retinal vessels has been observed in advanced cases examined pathologically. The optic disk pallor correlates with a proliferation of glial cells on the surface of the optic nerve head. This glial proliferation extends from the disk to the neighboring retina to form an epiretinal membrane.

GENETICS

Retinitis pigmentosa demonstrates allelic and nonallelic heterogeneity and can display X-linked, autosomal recessive, and autosomal dominant inheritance patterns. The proportion of cases in each genetic type varies between ethnic groups. For example, the X-linked type accounts for 14 to 16 percent of families in England,[10,13] 8 percent in the United States and Ontario, Canada,[8,9,11,14] and only 1 percent in Switzerland.[12] In the state of Maine,[9] retinitis pigmentosa was found to be

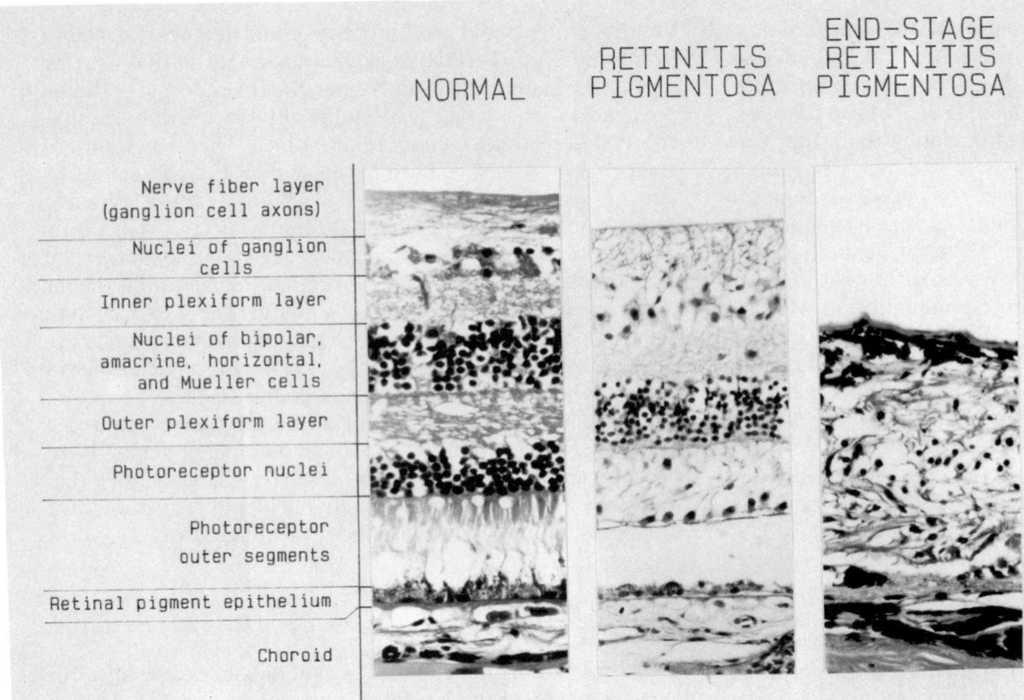

FIG. 144-2 Light micrographs of a normal human retina (left), a retina with retinitis pigmentosa (center), and a retina with end-stage retinitis pigmentosa (right). Light rays enter from the top of the figure. A light ray must pass through the nerve fiber layer, ganglion cell layer, inner plexiform layer, bipolar cell layer, outer plexiform layer, and photoreceptor nuclear layer before reaching a photoreceptor outer segment where it can interact with rod or cone opsin to initiate vision. The center panel shows histologic changes observed in eyes with early to moderately advanced retinitis pigmentosa. The photoreceptor outer segments are absent and the number of photoreceptor nuclei is reduced. The space between the remaining photoreceptor nuclei and the retinal pigment epithelium is a processing artefact. In end-stage retinitis pigmentosa, there are no recognizable cell layers. The retina is reduced in thickness and cell number. Retina with degeneration this severe would be nonfunctional.

inherited as an autosomal dominant trait in 19 percent of affected families (43 percent of cases), as an autosomal recessive trait in 19 percent of families (20 percent of cases), and as an X-linked trait in 8 percent of families (8 percent of cases). The proportions of cases differ from the proportions of families since, for example, a family with dominant retinitis pigmentosa will have on average more affected individuals than a family with recessive retinitis pigmentosa. Patients with "isolate" retinitis pigmentosa, representing 46 percent of families (23 percent of cases), are defined as those with no other affected family members (simplex cases). Most of these cases are probably autosomal recessive, although some could represent new dominant or X-linked mutations. Patients with uncertain family history (e.g., adopted) are designated "undetermined" (8 percent of families; 6 percent of cases).

Categorizing patients according to genetic type is valuable for the following reasons. One justification, of course, is to aid in genetic counseling. In this regard, it is important to note that ophthalmologic examination coupled with ERG can identify female carriers of X-linked retinitis pigmentosa.[26,27] This can be valuable for determining the mode of transmission for isolate males with retinitis pigmentosa. Second, the severity of the disease and the age at which complete blindness occurs correlates in part with the genetic type of retinitis pigmentosa. For example, patients with autosomal dominant retinitis pigmentosa often retain some useful vision after the age of 60, whereas patients with X-linked disease are usually blind by age 45 and patients with autosomal recessive disease typically retain vision until age 60. Hence, an indication of the prognosis for vision can be provided to a patient according to the genetic type of disease. Third, in the event that therapies specific for particular types of retinitis pigmentosa become available, it will be advantageous to know in advance the cohort of patients who will benefit.

Linkage analyses indicate that there are at least two separate loci on Xp that can cause X-linked retinitis pigmentosa.[46,47] One locus is in the vicinity of Xp11 and is named RP2; the other is designated RP3 and is in Xp21. It is not yet known whether there is nonallelic heterogeneity even among the families showing linkage to a particular region on Xp or whether some X-linked cases might be due to genetic defects elsewhere on the X chromosome.

With regard to autosomal dominant retinitis pigmentosa, linkage analyses point to loci on chromosomes 3q, 6p, and 8 in different pedigrees. All families linked to 3q may have defects in the rhodopsin gene (see below), although it is still possible that a second, closely linked locus is defective instead in some families.[48] Similarly, defects in the retinal degeneration slow gene (peripherin/RDS) are probably present in all families exhibiting linkage to chromosome 6p.[49,50] The gene in the pericentric region of chromosome 8 that is responsible for retinitis pigmentosa in a large American kindred remains to be identified.[51] It is possible that still other loci with dominant alleles causing retinitis pigmentosa exist.

The molecular genetics of recessive retinitis pigmentosa are the least well elucidated. A recessive, null mutation in the rhodopsin gene has been discovered in one family with recessive retinitis pigmentosa out of 126 that were screened (see below).[52] Linkage to chromosome 1q has been demonstrated in families with Usher's syndrome, type II.[53,54] No chromosomal assignment is yet known for the remainder of families, comprising the majority of recessive cases.

RHODOPSIN-RELATED RETINITIS PIGMENTOSA

Structure and Function of Rhodopsin

Rhodopsin, or rod opsin, is a member of a large family of membrane-bound, G-protein receptors.[55] It is the light-sensitive molecule in rods that initiates vision. Rhodopsin is composed of a single polypeptide, called opsin, covalently linked to 11-*cis*-retinal, a derivative of vitamin A. The retinal moiety functions as a receptor for photons of visible light.

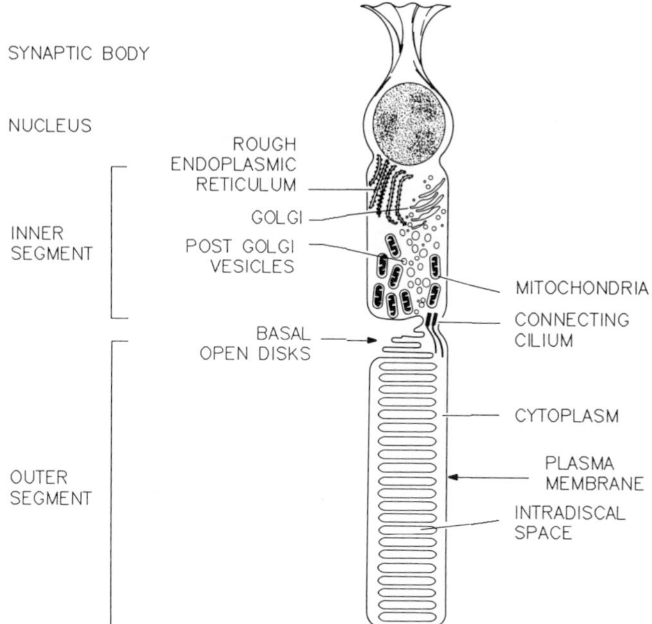

FIG. 144-3 **Schematic representation of a rod photoreceptor. The cell is oriented so that its proximal end is at the top. Disks containing rhodopsin are stacked in the outer segment. Their molecular components, including rhodopsin, are synthesized in the inner segment and transported by obscure mechanisms to the outer segment. Approximately 10 percent of the outer segment is synthesized each day, with the newly manufactured disks being the basal disks.[117,118] An equally large segment of distal outer segment is phagocytosed daily by the retinal pigment epithelium.** ***(Adapted from Fig. 6 in Berson et al.[89] Used by permission.)***

Capture of a photon changes the structure of retinal from 11-*cis* to all-*trans*. This in turn induces a conformational change in rhodopsin, which allows its interaction with a G protein called "transducin" and the initiation of the phototransduction cascade (for reviews see Stryer[56] or Hargrave and McDowell[57]).

In a rod photoreceptor, rhodopsin is concentrated in the disk membranes in the outer segment (Fig. 144-3). Disks are enclosed, flattened vesicles with membranes composed of approximately equimolar amounts of protein and lipid.[58] Rhodopsin is the most abundant disk protein, comprising over 80 percent of the membrane-bound protein in the rod outer segment.[59,60] There is a stack of approximately 1000 disks in each outer segment.[61]

According to current models, a molecule of rhodopsin traverses the disk membrane seven times (Fig. 144-4).[62] The transmembrane domains are rich in hydrophobic amino acids. They are thought to encircle the 11-*cis*-retinal moiety that is covalently linked to a lysine residue in the seventh transmembrane domain. The amino acids in the surrounding transmembrane domains form a molecular environment for 11-*cis*-retinal that tunes the peak in the absorption spectrum to 498 nm.

Dominant Rhodopsin Alleles Causing Retinitis Pigmentosa

The human gene encoding the opsin portion of rhodopsin was isolated and sequenced in 1984.[63] Later it was mapped to human chromosome 3q.[64,65] In 1989 the locus for autosomal dominant retinitis pigmentosa in a large Irish pedigree was found to be linked to an anonymous marker derived from 3q named "CRI-C17."[66] This report intensified the analysis of the rhodopsin gene in patients with dominant retinitis pigmentosa. Soon thereafter mutant alleles at this locus were identified that were specific to this disease and that cosegregated with it in affected pedigrees.[67,68] Approximately 25 percent of families with autosomal dominant retinitis pigmentosa have a defect in the rhodopsin gene, with over 30 different mutations having been reported (Table 144-1).[67–95] An examination of their distribution in the rhodopsin gene shows them to be dispersed throughout the length of the coding sequence of the gene, with the highest density near the 5′ end of exon 3 (Fig. 144-5). The reason for this cluster is still unknown; it may indicate that this is an especially mutable DNA sequence. On the other hand, it might signify a region of the encoded protein which is essential to its normal structure or function and whose alteration leads to a pathogenic molecule (see below).

The most common mutation found in North America is designated P23H (an alteration of codon 23 substituting histidine for proline). P23H is found in about 40 percent of

FIG. 144-4 **Model of rhodopsin using the single-letter amino acid code.[62,119,120] Rhodopsin comprises 348 amino acid residues, with the initial methionine in the intradiscal space. The peptide traverses the outer segment disk membrane seven times. Each circle denotes one or more amino acids that have been found to be altered by a mutation in at least one family with autosomal dominant retinitis pigmentosa. Most are missense mutations, but some are deletions (see Table 144-1). The circled lysine residue (K) in the seventh transmembrane domain is the one to which the chromophore, 11-*cis*-retinal, covalently binds; it is circled because it is replaced by a glutamic acid residue in the affected members of one family with dominant retinitis pigmentosa.[69,80] The transmembrane domains are thought to form a pocket surrounding 11-*cis*-retinal. Two asparagine-linked glycosylation sites that are present near the amino terminus in the intradiscal space are indicated.**

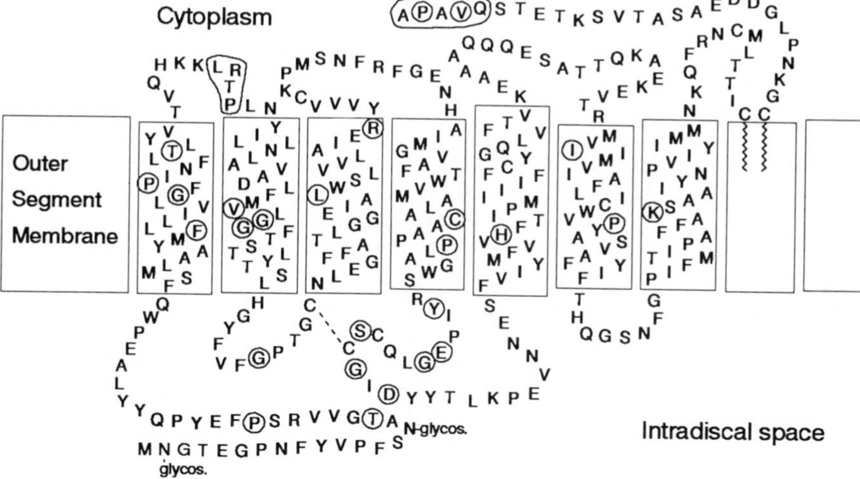

Table 144-1 Mutations Found in the Rhodopsin Gene

No.	Mutation: Protein	Mutation: DNA	Normal Sequence—Affected Base(s) Underlined	References
Mutations causing autosomal dominant retinitis pigmentosa				
1	T17M	C→T	GCG ACG GGT	71, 74, 82–86
2	P23H	C→A	AGC CCC TTC	67, 68, 71, 74, 77, 82, 84, 86–90
3	P23L	C→T	AGC CCC TTC	82
4	F45L	T→C	ATG TTT CTG	74, 84
5	G51V	G→T	CTG GGC TTC	82
6	P53R	C→G	TTC CCC ATC	80
7	T58R	C→G	CTC ACG CTC	68, 71, 74, 78, 80, 82–84, 86, 91
8	Del68–71	12 bp del	CTG CGC ACG CCT	69, 80
9	V87D	T→A	ATG GTC CTA	74, 84
10	G89D	G→A	CTA GGT GGC	74, 82, 84
11	G90D	G→A	GGT GGC TTC	6
12	G106W	G→T	TTC GGG CCC	74, 84
13	G106R	G→A	TTC GGG CCC	80
14	L125R	T→G	GCC CTG TGG	82
15	R135L	GG→TT	GAG CGG TAC	74, 83, 84
16	R135L	G→T	GAG CGG TAC	92
17	R135W	C→T	GAG CGG TAC	74, 83, 84
18	C167R	T→C	GCC TGC GCC	82
19	P171L	C→T	CCC CCA CTC	82
20	Y178C	A→G	AGG TAC ATC	72, 74, 84
21	E181K	G→A	CCC GAG GGC	82
22	G182S	G→A	GAG GGC CTG	71, 85
23	S186P	T→C	TGC TCG TGT	82
24	G188R	G→A	TGT GGA ATC	82
25	D190N	G→A	ATC GAC TAC	69, 80, 82
26	D190G	A→G	ATC GAC TAC	74, 82, 84
27	H211P	A→C	GTC CAC TTC	69, 80
28	I255Δ	3 bp del	GTC ATC ATC ATG	73, 79, 80, 93
29	P267L	C→T	GTG CCC TAC	71
30	K296E	A→G	GCC AAG AGC	69, 80
31	Q344ter	C→T	AGC CAG GTG	74, 83, 84
32	V345M	G→A	CAG GTG GCC	82, 94
33	P347R	C→G	GCC CCG GCC	70, 75
34	P347L	C→T	GCC CCG GCC	68, 74, 76, 80, 82, 84, 93, 95
35	P347S	C→T	GCC CCG GCC	68, 82
Null mutations causing rod dysfunction or recessive retinitis pigmentosa				
1	E249ter	G→T	AAG GAG GTC	52
2	5′ splice intron 4	G→T	CAG GTG CCT	52

all North American families with rhodopsin-related retinitis pigmentosa.[71,74,82] Surprisingly, this mutant allele has not been found on other continents.[96] Furthermore, P23H is in strong linkage disequilibrium with an intragenic microsatellite repeat polymorphism (see Fig. 144-5), indicating that all these families probably descend from a common ancestor who carried the P23H allele.[68,90] With few exceptions,[78,79] each of the other dominant rhodopsin mutations has been found in a single family, suggesting that this locus has a low mutation rate. The most striking exception involves codon 347, in which the mutation P347L appears to have arisen a number of times in Europe, North America, and Japan.[68,74,76,80,82] Only one instance of a new germ-line mutation has been documented, and this is also a P347L allele.[82] Still, the P347L is responsible for a minority of rhodopsin-related retinitis pigmentosa cases worldwide, probably less than 25 percent.

Characteristics of the Mutant Rhodopsins Found in Dominant Retinitis Pigmentosa

Most of the dominant rhodopsin gene defects are either missense mutations or short, in-frame deletions of a few codons. Figure 144-4 shows a schematic model of rhodopsin with the amino acids affected by dominant mutations circled. Most of the mutations involve the intradiscal or transmembrane regions of the protein, with a final cluster near the C-terminus of the molecule.

Considerable effort is currently being devoted to elucidating the pathogenic properties of these mutant opsins. So far, a number of intriguing observations of some of the mutant opsins have been reported, but no common property that might explain their pathogenicity has been discovered. Since the cytoplasmic loops of rhodopsin interact with transducin,[97] and since they are rarely affected by these mutations, one

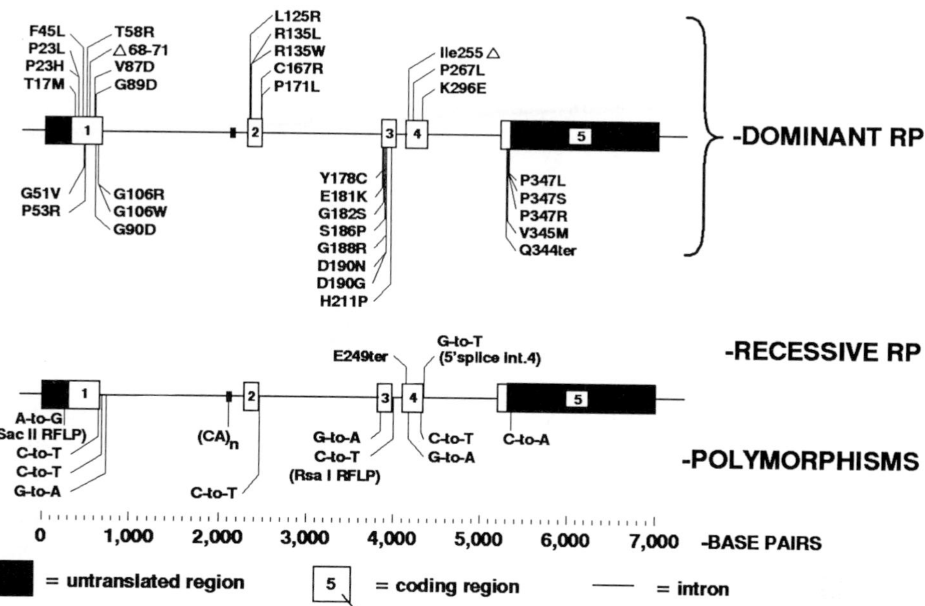

FIG. 144-5 Genomic map of the human rhodopsin locus.[63] The transcriptional unit is divided into five exons (large rectangles) and extends across approximately 7000 bp of DNA. The locations of the mutations found in dominant retinitis pigmentosa and recessive retinitis pigmentosa are indicated (see Table 144-1 for references), as are the sites of polymorphisms that have been found in the gene.[52,68,71,82,121] The small black rectangle in intron 1 denotes the site of a polymorphic CA repeat. RP = retinitis pigmentosa.

might surmise that the pathogenicity of these mutant opsins is not related to an interference with phototransduction. However, at least one mutant opsin with a defective amino acid in a transmembrane domain, K296E, constitutively activates transducin in vitro.[98] It is not yet known whether other mutant opsins share this defective function, so that it remains a possibility that constant stimulation of the phototransduction cascade might be a factor in retinal degeneration associated with a set of dominant rhodopsin mutations.

Another possible pathogenic mechanism involves probable structural defects induced by the mutations. Many of the affected amino acids in the intradiscal space, especially those near the cystine residues coupled by a disulfide bond between the second and third intradiscal loops, are in regions thought to be necessary for maintaining the three-dimensional conformation of the molecule and its ability to integrate within cellular membranes.[99] Furthermore, most of the mutations affecting amino acids in the transmembrane domains replace hydrophobic residues with charged ones. These should destabilize the transmembrane domains and distort the overall structure of the protein. Based on these observations, one might conclude that a common property of the mutant opsins is an abnormality in their conformation that interferes with their accumulation in the outer-segment disk membranes. Since rods do not ordinarily catabolize rhodopsin (instead it is phagocytosed and degraded by the adjacent retinal pigment epithelial cells), its aggregation in the inner segment could be detrimental in a manner analogous to that thought to cause hepatocyte degeneration in α_1-antitrypsin deficiency.[100,101]

In support of this hypothesis, Sung et al. reported that many of the mutant opsins expressed in vitro congregate in the ER rather than the plasma membrane.[84] However, not all of them do. The cluster of mutations near the C-terminus are among those encoding mutant opsins that localize to the plasma membrane at levels comparable to wild-type rhodopsin.[84] It is difficult to envision how the substitution of residues near the C-terminus could cause a significant alteration in the overall three-dimensional structure. Furthermore, one of the mutant opsins (P23H) that does preferentially collect in the ER in vitro can nevertheless be found within the outer segments when expressed in transgenic mice.[102] And the mutation T17M eliminates one of two asparagine-linked glycosylation sites near the N-terminus of rhodopsin, perhaps signifying that aberrant glycosylation might play a role in the toxicity of some mutant opsins. It is evident that additional work will be required to understand the pathogenic mechanisms underlying dominant rhodopsin mutations.

Clinical Findings in Rhodopsin-Related Dominant Retinitis Pigmentosa

As might be expected for defects in a rod-specific gene, rhodopsin mutations generally cause a more severe defect in rod function than cone function in young patients, as measured by ERG (Fig. 144-6).[67,68,78,83,94,103] In fact, one of the first reports of the more severe loss of rod ERG responses in some cases of autosomal dominant retinitis pigmentosa was based on a family now known to carry a rhodopsin mutation (P23H).[67,104] The decrease in rod ERG amplitudes in young patients correlates with the reduction in the amount of rhodopsin in the retina as measured by imaging fundus reflectometry.[86] Late in the disease both rods and cones are affected. Histopathology from a patient now known to have a defect in the rhodopsin gene (P23H)[89] showed no rods and a reduced number of macular cones with degenerating inner segments and absent outer segments.[37] The basis for cone degeneration in a disease due to a defect in a rod-specific gene remains unclear.

The severity of the disease appears to correlate with specific mutations. For example, it seems that T58R,[68,78,83] T17M,[85] and G182S[85] are relatively mild alleles and that K296E[69] is a relatively severe one. However, there is considerable intrafamilial variability noted in most rhodopsin-related families,[78,89,94,95] so that a rigorous analysis of visual field areas, ERG amplitudes, etc. including many affected patients with each mutation will be required to substantiate these clinical impressions. This sort of statistical

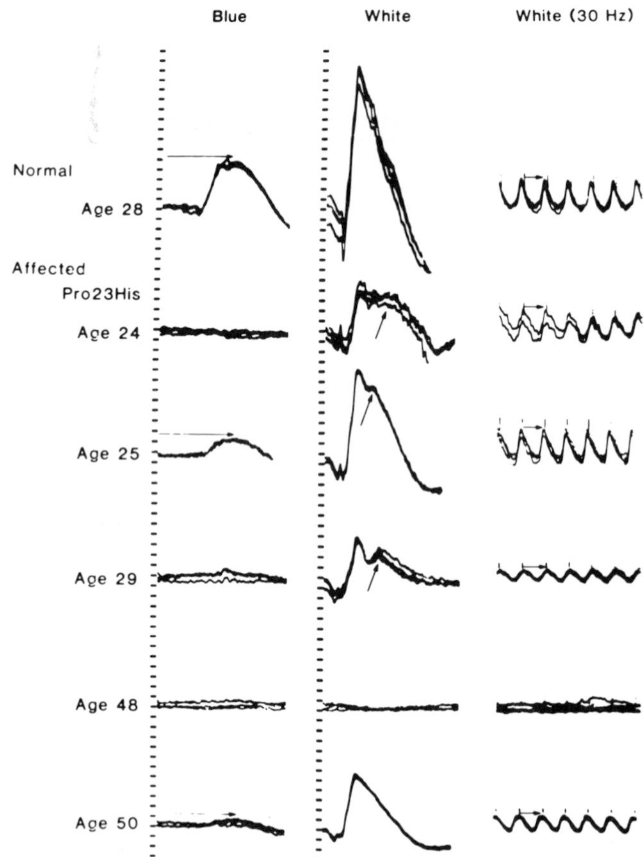

FIG. 144-6 ERGs of a normal individual (top) and five different patients with autosomal dominant retinitis pigmentosa due to a rhodopsin mutation (P23H). The tracings in the left-hand column are the responses to single flashes of blue light that is so dim that only rods are stimulated. The middle column shows the responses to bright white light flashes that stimulate both rods and cones. The right-hand column shows the responses to bright white light flashing 30 times per second; rods but not cones are able to show individual responses to light flashing at this high frequency. (In each tracing, two or three consecutive sweeps are superimposed.) Hence, going from the left to the right columns, one observes rod-isolated responses, combined rod and cone responses, and cone-isolated responses. Young patients with retinitis pigmentosa (24-, 25-, and 29-year-old patients) have dramatically reduced rod responses to dim blue light (left column) and reduced but biphasic responses to bright white light (middle column). The biphasic response is due to a delay in the response time of the rods. The arrows in the middle column point to the delayed rod-response peaks. This phenomenon is also observed in the left-hand column with the horizontal arrows that indicate rod response times. Cone responses (right column) are relatively normal in amplitude and timing (horizontal arrows) in the 24- and 25-year-old patients but reduced in amplitude and somewhat delayed in the 29-year-old patient. The 48-year-old patient with more advanced disease has markedly reduced rod and cone amplitudes. Interestingly, the 50-year-old patient (a sib of the 48-year-old) has less severe degeneration, indicated here by ERG responses which, although abnormal, are clearly detectable. The calibration symbol in the lower right corner designates 50 ms horizontally and 100 μV vertically. *(From Berson et al.[89] Used by permission.)*

analysis has been performed for two relatively common mutations—P23H and P347L. Patients with P23H have on average a larger ERG amplitude and P347L a smaller amplitude than patients with dominant retinitis pigmentosa without those mutations.[89,95] There has as yet been no prospective study of patients with rhodopsin mutations to determine if differences in severity are due to variation in the rate of progression of the retinal degeneration, to variation in the level of photoreceptor function at birth, or to a combination of the two.

Most middle-aged patients with a dominant rhodopsin mutation show intraretinal pigmentation in all four quadrants of the fundus.[89,94,95] However, some clinicians report a preferential involvement of the inferior fundus in patients with T17M,[83,85] P23H,[77,90] T58R,[83,91] G106R,[105] or G182S.[85] The basis for this preferential involvement of the inferior fundus (which corresponds to the superior visual field) is unknown, although there is speculation that it is related to phototoxic effects, with the inferior fundus being exposed to and suffering from more intense lighting overhead.[77] It certainly is not a constant finding.

After exposure to bright light, rods lose their light sensitivity and require in a normal individual 20 to 40 min of complete darkness to regain their maximal sensitivity to light. Patients with a dominant rhodopsin defect and who retain some rod function typically take a longer time to adapt to the dark. One group found that the rate of adaptation to the dark by rods and the time required for them to recover maximal sensitivity is allele-specific.[83,86] For example, patients with T58R recovered maximal sensitivity after 150 min in the dark, P23H after 3 to 6 h, and T17M after 24 h.[86]

Sieving et al. described a pedigree with an autosomal dominant form of nyctalopia associated with a missense mutation in the rhodopsin gene (G90D).[6] The family members carrying the allele had absent rod a- or b-waves irrespective of age, indicating no rod function. Most affected members with G90D had normal cone ERG. The combination of absent rod ERG and normal cone ERG is typical of stationary night blindness rather than the forms of retinitis pigmentosa that have been found to be associated with other dominant missense mutations of the rhodopsin gene. However, at least two members of the G90D pedigree, although asymptomatic, had reduced cone ERG amplitudes, and the older members had narrowed retinal vessels and some bone-spicule pigmentation in the fundus. The phenotype caused by the G90D allele may be a very mild form of retinitis pigmentosa with early, unusually severe rod impairment, although it has alternatively been termed *dominant congenital complete nyctalopia*.[6] The novelty of the phenotype suggests that the mechanism by which G90D rhodopsin disturbs rod function may be distinct from that encountered for other dominant rhodopsin alleles.

Alleles Causing Recessive Retinitis Pigmentosa and Rod Dysfunction

After screening over 100 families with recessive retinitis pigmentosa, only one was found with a mutation in the rhodopsin gene.[52] There was only one affected patient in this family, a 29-year-old female who was the offspring of a consanguineous mating. She was homozygous for a nonsense mutation (E249ter). It is possible that this mutation, like many nonsense mutations, leads to an unstable mRNA transcript and little if any translated protein.[122,123] Whatever protein is expressed by this allele would be inactive since it would have a truncated C-terminus missing the sixth and seventh transmembrane domains, including the K296 residue that is covalently linked to 11-cis-retinal. These consequences suggest that, unlike the dominant rhodopsin alleles mentioned earlier, E249ter is a "null" allele. The patient homozygous for E249ter had reduced cone function and no rod function detectable by ERG. Heterozygotes for this mutation (i.e., the parents and three sibs), or a second null mutation fortuitously found in a normal control individual without a family history of retinitis pigmentosa, showed a reduction in the amplitude of the rod responses to dim flashes of light, but normal rod responses to bright flashes of light. These findings in heterozygotes point to a subtle abnormality in rods predicted to have reduced amounts of rhodopsin. It remains to be seen whether these ERG abnormalities are specific to carriers of rhodopsin null mutations. Although the E249ter mutation is rare, it is possible that other, more prevalent null mutations of the rhodopsin gene might be the cause of other recessive retinitis pigmentosa cases.

PERIPHERIN/RETINAL DEGENERATION SLOW GENE–RELATED RETINITIS PIGMENTOSA

Structure and Function of the Peripherin/Retinal Degeneration Slow Gene

Unfortunately, two distinct proteins have been named "peripherin"; one is a neuronal intermediate filament protein[106,107] and the other is a photoreceptor protein.[108] This section will deal exclusively with photoreceptor peripherin, a glycoprotein found in the rims of outer segment disks. Two converging paths led to its isolation and identification. One was the result of studies of a spontaneously arising murine model of retinitis pigmentosa, named the *rds* strain for retinal degeneration slow.[109] Travis et al. used an mRNA subtractive hybridization technique to isolate a cDNA sequence corresponding to the wild-type allele at the murine *rds* locus.[110] The encoded protein was predicted to contain 346 amino acid residues. The mutant *rds* allele was an apparent null mutation caused by the insertion of a 10-kb, extraneous, murine sequence into the open reading frame. Concurrently and independently, Connell and Molday studied a 39-kDa protein found in the rim region of the outer segment disks (hence the name *peripherin*) that was identified on the basis of its reaction with monoclonal antibodies.[108] Monoclonal antibodies were used to isolate the corresponding bovine cDNA sequence.[111] Bovine peripherin is also composed of 346 residues and has an amino acid sequence 92.5 percent identical to the murine *rds* protein.[112] These similarities in sequence and tissue expression lead to the realization that bovine peripherin and murine RDS are cognate proteins with amino acid differences due to species variation. The protein can be designated as peripherin/RDS. More recently, the amino acid sequences of human[113] and rat[114] peripherin/RDS have been determined; they are very similar to the murine sequence (85 percent identity overall) and also have 346 residues.

Peripherin/RDS exists in outer segments as a glycosylated homodimer linked by one or more disulfide bonds.[112] It has four hydrophobic regions each thought to traverse the disk membrane, and a conserved glycosylation site in the large loop between third and fourth transmembrane domains (Fig. 144-7). Its precise structure and function remain unknown, although it is believed to play a role in maintaining the structure of the outer-segment disks.[111,115,116]

Dominant Peripherin/Retinal Degeneration Slow Alleles Causing Retinitis Pigmentosa

Two groups have encountered mutations in the peripherin/RDS gene in patients with autosomal dominant retinitis pigmentosa (Table 144-2).[49,50] Two of the reported mutations are missense, both affecting residues predicted to be in the large intradiscal loop between the third and fourth transmembrane domains (see Fig. 144-7). The other two mutations are three-base deletions that each eliminate single codons; one is in the predicted third transmembrane domain, the other is in the second intradiscal loop. It is probably too early to draw any firm conclusions regarding the nature of these mutations and the mechanism by which they lead to photoreceptor degeneration. However, it is notable that these dominant mutations are of the same class as that found for dominant mutations of the rhodopsin gene (i.e., missense mutations or short, inframe deletions). In this respect, it is likely that none of these mutations is a null allele of the sort found in the *rds* mouse. Hence, the human retinal disease that precisely corresponds to the *rds* mouse remains uncertain.

There is as yet no detailed description of the phenotype associated with dominant mutations of the peripherin/RDS gene. However, affected patients have symptoms and funduscopic features characteristic of retinitis pigmentosa and both rod and cone ERGs are affected in this disease.[49,50]

ADDENDUM

Recent work has provided evidence for chromosomal assignments and, in some cases, gene identifications for additional forms of retinitis pigmentosa and allied hereditary retinal diseases. The rate at which new loci are being implicated in this set of diseases suggests that there may be an enormous amount of nonallelic heterogeneity, perhaps involving scores of loci. Below is a brief summary that is apologetically exclusionary because of space limitations.

Linkage studies of autosomal dominant retinitis pigmentosa implicated loci within 7p and within 7q.[124,125] Each of these two chromosomal assignments was based on only one family, suggesting that they each reflect disease loci that cause small proportions of cases. The existence of a sixth dominant locus is inferred by the report of one family[126] with

Table 144-2 Mutations Found in the Peripherin/RDS Gene

No.	Mutation: Protein	Mutation: DNA	Normal Sequence—Affected Base(s) Underlined	References
Mutations causing autosomal dominant retinitis pigmentosa				
1	C118Δ	3 bp del	CTC <u>TGC</u> TGC TTT	50
2	L185P	T→C	TAC C<u>T</u>G GAC	49
3	P216L	C→T	AAT C<u>C</u>T AGC	49
4	P219Δ	3 bp del	TCG <u>CCA</u> CGG	49

AMINO ACID SEQUENCE OF PERIPHERIN/RDS
WITH RESIDUES AFFECTED IN DOMINANT RETINITIS PIGMENTOSA

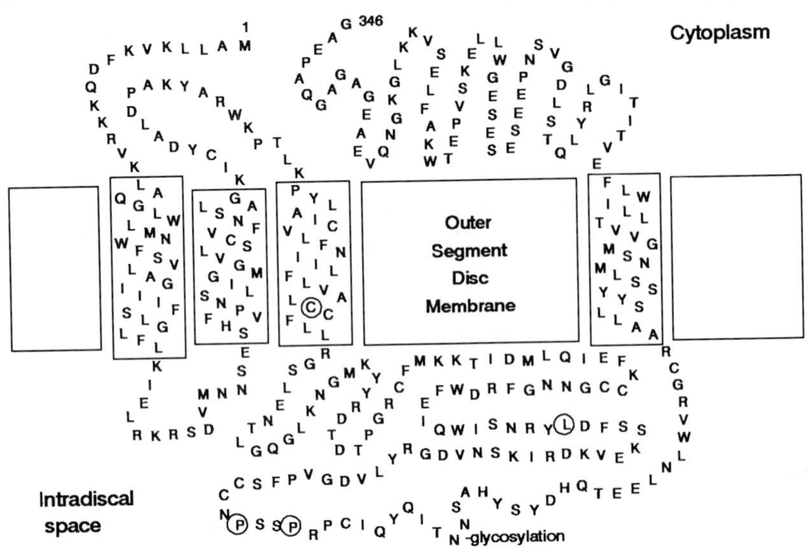

FIG. 144-7 Model of peripherin/RDS using the single-letter amino acid code.[111] Peripherin/RDS is composed of 346 amino acid residues, with the initial methionine in the cytoplasm. The peptide is thought to traverse the outer-segment disk membrane four times. Each circle denotes an amino acid that has been found to be altered by a mutation in at least one family with autosomal dominant retinitis pigmentosa. Most are missense mutations but one is a single-codon deletion (see Table 144-2). One asparagine-linked glycosylation site that is conserved in mammals is present in the second intradiscal loop.

disease not linked to any of the known chromosomal regions containing dominant retinitis pigmentosa genes [i.e., 3q (rhodopsin),[67] 6p (peripherin/RDS),[49,50] 7p, 7q, or 8[51]]. The responsible genes on 7p, 7q, and 8q remain unidentified.

A family with a form of autosomal dominant cone-rod dystrophy has disease linked to 19q.[127] Cone-rod dystrophy is a form of hereditary retinal degeneration that is distinct from retinitis pigmentosa because cones are more severely affected than rods. No gene identification has been made.

With regard to recessive retinal degenerations, mutations in the gene encoding the beta subunit of rod cGMP-phosphodiesterase have been found in a few percent of families with recessive retinitis pigmentosa.[128] In addition, linkage studies point to unidentified genes on chromosome 11p, 11q, and 14q in families with Usher's syndrome type I (retinitis pigmentosa associated with profound congenital deafness) and to 16q in one family with Bardet-Biedl syndrome (retinitis pigmentosa associated with mental retardation, polydactyly, obesity, and hypogonadism).[129–132] A set of families with autosomal recessive Stargardt's disease (a form of juvenile macular degeneration) served to implicate chromosome 1p as containing a gene responsible for that disease.[133]

Finally, Kajiwara and colleagues recently reported three families segregating a form of retinitis pigmentosa in which affected individuals were double heterozygotes for a specific peripherin/RDS allele (L185P) and null mutations in a second gene, ROM1 on 11q.[134] The ROM1 protein is closely related to peripherin/RDS and the two proteins are thought to interact noncovalently in the rim region of the photoreceptor outer segment disc membrane. Individuals heterozygous for only one of these mutations were asymptomatic. The authors suggested the term digenic retinitis pigmentosa for this phenomenon and propose that similar examples may be found in other systems in which there is intimate physical interaction of proteins encoded by different genes.

REFERENCES

1. Berson EL, Mehaffey L, Rabin AR: A night vision pocketscope for patients with retinitis pigmentosa. *Arch Ophthalmol* **91**:495, 1974.
2. Cox SN, Hay E, Bird AC: Treatment of chronic macular edema with acetazolamide. *Arch Ophthalmol* **106**:1190, 1988.
3. Fishman GA, Gilbert LD, Fiscella RG, Kimura AE, Jampol IM: Acetazolamide for treatment of chronic macular edema in retinitis pigmentosa. *Arch Ophthalmol* **107**:1445, 1989.
4. Musarella MA, Weleber RG, Murphey WH, Young RSL, Anson-Cartwright L, Mets M, Kraft SP, Polemeno R, Litt M, Worton RG: Assignment of the gene for complete X-linked congenital stationary night blindness (CSNB1) to Xp11.3. *Genomics* **5**:727, 1989.
5. Wright AF: Towards the identification of genes in X-linked retinitis pigmentosa, in Osborne NN, Chader GJ (eds): *Progress in Retinal Research*. Elmsford, Pergamon, 1990, vol 9, p. 197.
6. Sieving PA, Richards JE, Bingham EL, Naarendorp F: Dominant congenital complete nyctalopia and Gly90Asp rhodopsin mutation. *Invest Ophthalmol Vis Sci* **33(Suppl)**:1397, 1992. (Abstr.)
7. Sunga RN, Sloan LL: Pigmentary degeneration of the retina: early diagnosis and natural history. *Invest Ophthalmol Vis Sci* **6**:309, 1967.
8. Boughman JA, Conneally PM, Nance WE: Population studies of retinitis pigmentosa. *Am J Hum Genet* **32**:223, 1980.
9. Bunker CH, Berson EL, Bromley WC, Hayes RP, Roderick TH: Prevalence of retinitis pigmentosa in Maine. *Am J Ophthalmol* **97**:357, 1984.
10. Jay M: On the heredity of retinitis pigmentosa. *Br J Ophthalmol* **66**:405, 1982. (abstr.)
11. Fishman GA: Retinitis pigmentosa. Genetic percentages. *Arch Ophthalmol* **96**:822, 1978. (abstr.)
12. Ammann F, Klein D, Bohringer HR: Resultats preliminaires d'une enquête sur la fréquence et la distribution geographique des dégenerescences tapeto-retiniennes en Suisse (étude de cinq cantons). *J Genet Hum* **10**:99, 1961.
13. Bundey S, Crews SJ: A study of retinitis pigmentosa in the city of Birmingham. II. Clinical and genetic heterogeneity. *J Med Genet* **21**:421, 1984.
14. Macrae WG: Retinitis pigmentosa in Ontario—a survey. *Birth Defects* **18**:175, 1982.
15. Biro I: Symmetrical development of pigmentation as a specific feature of the fundus pattern in retinitis pigmentosa. *Am J Ophthalmol* **55**:1176, 1963.
16. Newsome DA: Retinal fluorescein leakage in retinitis pigmentosa. *Am J Ophthalmol* **101**:354, 1986.
17. Ffytche TJ: Cystoid maculopathy in retinitis pigmentosa. *Trans Ophthalmol Soc UK* **92**:265, 1992.
18. Heckenlively J: The frequency of posterior subcapsular cataract in the hereditary retinal degenerations. *Am J Ophthalmol* **93**:733, 1982.

19. Fishman GA, Anderson RJ, Lourenco P: Prevalence of posterior subcapsular lens opacities in patients with retinitis pigmentosa. *Br J Ophthalmol* **69**:263, 1985.
20. Berson EL, Rosner B, Simonoff E: Risk factors for genetic typing and detection in retinitis pigmentosa. *Am J Ophthalmol* **89**:763, 1980.
21. Fishman GA, Farber MD, Derlacki DJ: X-linked retinitis pigmentosa. Profile of clinical findings. *Arch Ophthalmol* **106**:369, 1988.
22. Berson EL: Electrical phenomena in the retina, in Hart WM (ed): *Adler's Physiology of the Eye*. St. Louis, Mosby, 1992, p 641.
23. Kline RP, Ripps H, Dowling JE: Generation of b-wave currents in the skate retina. *Proc Natl Acad Sci USA* **75**:5727, 1978.
24. Andreasson SOL, Sandberg MA, Berson EL: Narrow-band filtering for monitoring low-amplitude cone electroretinograms in retinitis pigmentosa. *Am J Ophthalmol* **105**:500, 1988.
25. Berson EL, Sandberg MA, Rosner B, Birch DG, Hanson AH: Natural course of retinitis pigmentosa over a three-year interval. *Am J Ophthalmol* **99**:240, 1985.
26. Berson EL, Rosen JB, Simonoff EA: Electroretinographic testing as an aid in detection of carriers of X-chromosome-linked retinitis pigmentosa. *Am J Ophthalmol* **87**:460, 1979.
27. Fishman GA, Weinberg AB, McMahon TT: X-linked recessive retinitis pigmentosa: Clinical characteristics of carriers. *Arch Ophthalmol* **104**:1329, 1986.
28. Berson EL: Retinitis pigmentosa and allied retinal diseases: Electrophysiologic findings. *Trans Am Acad Ophthalmol Otolaryngol* **81**:659, 1976.
29. Berson EL, Howard J: Temporal aspects of the electroretinogram in sector retinitis pigmentosa. *Arch Ophthalmol* **86**:653, 1971.
30. Gouras P, Carr RE, Gunkel RD: Retinitis pigmentosa in abetalipoproteinemia: Effect of vitamin A. *Invest Ophthalmol Vis Sci* **10**:784, 1971.
31. Sperling MA, Hiles DA, Kennerdell JS: Electroretinographic responses following vitamin A therapy in abetalipoproteinemia. *Am J Ophthalmol* **73**:342, 1972.
32. Refsum S: Heredopathia atactica polyneuritiformis. *Arch Neurol* **38**:605, 1981.
33. Zeviani M, Moraes CT, DiMauro S, Nakase H, Bonilla E, Schon EA, Rowland LP: Deletions of mitochondrial DNA in Kearns-Sayre syndrome. *Neurology* **38**:1339, 1988.
34. Lestienne P, Ponsot G: Kearns-Sayre syndrome with muscle mitochondria DNA deletion. *Lancet* **1**:885, 1988.
35. Moraes CT, DiMauro S, Zeviani M, Lombes A, Shanske S, Miranda AF, Nakase H, Bonilla E, Werneck LC, Servidei S, Nonaka I, Koga Y, Spiro AJ, Bromnell AKW, Schmidt B, Schotland DL, Zupanc M, DeVivo DC, Schon EA, Rowland LP: Mitochondrial DNA deletions in progressive external ophthalmoplegia and Kearns-Sayre syndrome. *N Engl J Med* **320**:1293, 1989.
36. Flannery JG, Farber DB, Bird AC, Bok D: Degenerative changes in a retina affected with autosomal dominant retinitis pigmentosa. *Invest Ophthalmol Vis Sci* **30**:191, 1989.
37. Kolb J, Gouras P: Electron microscopic observations of human retinitis pigmentosa, dominantly inherited. *Invest Ophthalmol Vis Sci* **13**:487, 1974.
38. Verhoeff FH: Microscopic observations in a case of retinitis pigmentosa. *Arch Ophthalmol* **5**:392, 1931.
39. Friedenwald J: Discussion of Verhoeff's observations of pathology of retinitis pigmentosa. *Arch Ophthalmol* **4**:767, 1930.
40. Cogan DG: Pathology [of retinitis pigmentosa]. *Trans Am Acad Ophthalmol Otolaryngol* **54**:629, 1950.
41. Szamier RB, Berson EL, Klein R, Meyers S: Sex-linked retinitis pigmentosa: Ultrastructure of photoreceptors and pigment epithelium. *Invest Ophthalmol Vis Sci* **18**:145, 1979.
42. Szamier RB, Berson EL: Histopathologic study of an unusual form of retinitis pigmentosa. *Invest Ophthalmol Vis Sci* **22**:559, 1982.
43. Milam AH, Jacobson SG: Photoreceptor rosettes with blue cone opsin immunoreactivity in retinitis pigmentosa. *Ophthalmology* **97**:1620, 1990.
44. Meyer KT, Heckenlively JR, Spitznas M, Foos RY: Dominant retinitis pigmentosa. A clinicopathologic correlation. *Ophthalmology* **89**:1414, 1982.
45. Gartner S, Henkind P: Pathology of retinitis pigmentosa. *Ophthalmology* **89**:1425, 1982.
46. Chen JD, Halliday F, Keith G, Sheffield L, Dickinson P, Gray R, Constable I, Denton M: Linkage heterogeneity between X-linked retinitis pigmentosa and a map of 10 RFLP loci. *Am J Hum Genet* **45**:401, 1989.
47. Ott J, Bhattacharya S, Chen JD, Denton MJ, Donald J, Dubay C, Farrar GJ, Fishman GA, Frey D, Gal A, Humphries P, Jay B, Jay M, Litt M, Machler M, Musarella M, Neugebauer M, Nussbaum RL, Terwilliger JD, Weleber RG, Wirth B, Wong F, Worton RG, Wright AF: Localizing multiple X chromosome-linked retinitis pigmentosa loci using multilocus homogeneity tests. *Proc Natl Acad Sci USA* **87**:701, 1990. (abstr.)
48. Inglehearn CF, Lester DH, Bashir R, Atif U, Keen TJ, Sertedaki A, Lindsey J, Jay M, Bird AC, Farrar GJ, Humphries P, Bhattacharya S: Recombination between rhodopsin and locus D3S47 (C17) in rhodopsin retinitis pigmentosa families. *Am J Hum Genet* **50**:590, 1992.
49. Kajiwara K, Hahn LB, Mukai S, Travis GH, Berson EL, Dryja TP: Mutations in the human retinal degeneration slow gene in autosomal dominant retinitis pigmentosa. *Nature* **354**:480, 1991.
50. Farrar GJ, Kenna P, Jordan SA, Rajendra KS, Humphries MM, Sharp EM, Sheils DM, Humphries P: A three-base-pair deletion in the peripherin-RDS gene in one form of retinitis pigmentosa. *Nature* **354**:478, 1991.
51. Blanton SH, Heckenlively JR, Cottingham AW, Friedman J, Sadler LA, Wagner M, Friedman LH, Daiger SP: Linkage mapping of autosomal dominant retinitis pigmentosa (RP1) to the pericentric region of human chromosome 8. *Genomics* **11**:857, 1991.
52. Rosenfeld PJ, Cowley GS, McGee TL, Sandberg MA, Berson EL, Dryja TP: A null mutation in the rhodopsin gene causes rod photoreceptor dysfunction and autosomal recessive retinitis pigmentosa. *Nature Genet* **1**:209, 1992.
53. Kimberling WJ, Weston MD, Moller C, Davenport SL, Shugart YY, Priluck IA, Martini A, Milan M, Smith RJ: Localization of Usher syndrome type II to chromosome 1q. *Genomics* **7**:245, 1990.
54. Lewis RA, Otterud B, Stauffer D, Lalouel JM, Leppert M: Mapping recessive ophthalmic diseases: Linkage of the locus for Usher syndrome type II to a DNA marker on chromosome 1q. *Genomics* **7**:250, 1990.
55. Applebury ML, Hargrave PA: Molecular biology of the visual pigments. *Vision Res* **12**:1881, 1986.
56. Stryer L: The molecules of visual excitation. *Sci Am* **257**:42, 1987.
57. Hargrave PA, McDowell JH: Rhodopsin and phototransduction: A model system for G protein-linked receptors. *FASEB J* **6**:2323, 1992.
58. Fliesler SJ, Anderson RE: Chemistry and metabolism of lipids in the vertebrate retina. *Prog Lipid Res* **22**:79, 1983.
59. Daemen FJM: Vertebrate rod outer segment membranes. *Biochim Biophys Acta* **300**:255, 1973.
60. Papermaster DS, Dreyer WJ: Rhodopsin content in the outer segment membranes of bovine and frog retinal rods. *Biochemistry* **13**:2438, 1974.
61. Missotten PL: Etude des batonnets de la retine humaine au microscope electronique. *Ophthalmologica* **140**:200, 1960.
62. Mirzadegan T, Liu RSH: Probing the visual pigment rhodopsin and its analogs by molecular modeling analysis and computer graphics, in Osborne NN, Chader GJ (eds): *Retinal Research*. Oxford, Pergamon, 1991, vol 11, p 57.
63. Nathans J, Hogness DS: Isolation and nucleotide sequence of the gene encoding human rhodopsin. *Proc Natl Acad Sci USA* **81**:4851, 1984.
64. Sparkes RS, Klisak I, Kaufman D, Mohandas T, Tobin AJ, McGinnis J: Assignment of the rhodopsin gene to human chromosome three, region 3q21-3q24 by in situ hybridization studies. *Curr Eye Res* **5**:797, 1986.
65. Nathans J, Piantanida TP, Eddy RL, Shows TB, Hogness DS: Molecular genetics of inherited variation in human color vision. *Science* **232**:203, 1986.
66. McWilliam P, Farrar GJ, Kenna P, Bradley DG, Humphries MM, Sharp EM, McConnell DJ, Lawler M, Sheils D, Ryan C, Stevens K, Daiger SP, Humphries P:

Autosomal dominant retinitis pigmentosa (ADRP): Localization of an ADRP gene to the long arm of chromosome 3. *Genomics* **5**:619, 1989.
67. Dryja TP, McGee TL, Reichel E, Hahn LB, Cowley GS, Yandell DW, Sandberg MA, Berson EL: A point mutation of the rhodopsin gene in one form of retinitis pigmentosa. *Nature* **343**:364, 1990.
68. Dryja TP, McGee TL, Hahn LB, Cowley GS, Olsson JE, Reichel E, Sandberg MA, Berson EL: Mutations within the rhodopsin gene in patients with autosomal dominant retinitis pigmentosa. *N Engl J Med* **323**:1302, 1990.
69. Keen TJ, Inglehearn CF, Lester DH, Bashir R, Jay M, Bird AC, Jay B, Bhattacharya SS: Autosomal dominant retinitis pigmentosa: Four new mutations in rhodopsin, one of them in the retinal attachment site. *Genomics* **11**:199, 1991.
70. Neimeyer G, Schinzel A, Gal A: Autosomal-dominant erbliche autosomal Retinopathia pigmentosa ist genetisch heterogen. *Fortschr Ophthalmol* **88**:455, 1991. (abstr.)
71. Sheffield VC, Fishman GA, Beck JS, Kimura AE, Stone EM: Identification of novel rhodopsin mutations associated with retinitis pigmentosa by GC-clamped denaturing gradient gel electrophoresis. *Am J Hum Genet* **49**:699, 1991.
72. Farrar GJ, Kenna P, Redmond R, Shiels D, McWilliam P, Humphries MM, Sharp EM, Jordan S, Kumar-Singh R, Humphries P: Autosomal dominant retinitis pigmentosa: A mutation in codon 178 of the rhodopsin gene in two families of Celtic origin. *Genomics* **11**:1170, 1991.
73. Inglehearn CF, Bashir R, Lester DH, Jay M, Bird AC, Bhattacharya SS: A 3-bp deletion in the rhodopsin gene in a family with autosomal dominant retinitis pigmentosa. *Am J Hum Genet* **48**:26, 1991.
74. Sung CH, Davenport CM, Hennessey JC, Maumenee IH, Jacobson SG, Heckenlively JR, Nowakowski R, Fishman G, Gouras P, Nathans J: Rhodopsin mutations in autosomal dominant retinitis pigmentosa. *Proc Natl Acad Sci USA* **88**:6481, 1991.
75. Gal A, Artlich A, Ludwig M, Niemeyer G, Olek K, Schwinger E, Schinzel A: Pro347Arg mutation of the rhodopsin gene in autosomal dominant retinitis pigmentosa. *Genomics* **11**:468, 1991.
76. Fujiki K, Hotta Y, Shiono T, Hayakawa M, Noro M, Sakuma T, Tamai M, Nakajima A, Kanai A: Codon 347 mutation of the rhodopsin gene in a Japanese family with autosomal dominant retinitis pigmentosa. *Am J Hum Genet (suppl)* **49**:187, 1991.
77. Heckenlively JR, Rodriguez JA, Daiger SP: Autosomal dominant sectoral retinitis pigmentosa. Two families with transversion mutation in codon 23 of rhodopsin. *Arch Ophthalmol* **109**:84, 1991.
78. Richards JE, Kuo CY, Boehnke M, Sieving PA: Rhodopsin Thr58Arg mutation in a family with autosomal dominant retinitis pigmentosa. *Ophthalmology* **98**:1797, 1991.
79. Artlich A, Horn M, Lorenz B, Bhattacharya S, Gal A: Recurrent 3-bp deletion at codon 255/256 of the rhodopsin gene in a German pedigree with autosomal dominant retinitis pigmentosa. *Am J Hum Genet* **50**:876, 1992.
80. Inglehearn CF, Keen TJ, Bashir R, Jay M, Fitzke F, Bird AC, Crombie A, Bhattacharya S: A completed screen for mutations of the rhodopsin gene in a panel of patients with autosomal dominant retinitis pigmentosa. *Hum Mol Genet* **1**:41, 1992.
81. Dryja TP: Rhodopsin and autosomal dominant retinitis pigmentosa. *Eye* **6**:1, 1992.
82. Dryja TP, Hahn LB, Cowley GS, McGee TL, Berson EL: Mutation spectrum of the rhodopsin gene among patients with autosomal dominant retinitis pigmentosa. *Proc Natl Acad Sci USA* **88**:9370, 1991.
83. Jacobson SG, Kemp CM, Sung CH, Nathans J: Retinal function and rhodopsin levels in autosomal dominant retinitis pigmentosa with rhodopsin mutations. *Am J Ophthalmol* **112**:256, 1991.
84. Sung CH, Schneider BG, Agarwal N, Papermaster DS, Nathans J: Functional heterogeneity of mutant rhodopsins responsible for autosomal dominant retinitis pigmentosa. *Proc Natl Acad Sci USA* **88**:8840, 1991.
85. Fishman GA, Stone EM, Sheffield VC, Gilbert LD, Kimura AE: Ocular findings associated with rhodopsin gene codon 17 and codon 182 transition mutations in dominant retinitis pigmentosa. *Arch Ophthalmol* **110**:54, 1992.
86. Kemp CM, Jacobson SG, Roman AJ, Sung CH, Nathans J: Abnormal rod dark adaptation in autosomal dominant retinitis pigmentosa with proline-23-histidine rhodopsin mutation. *Am J Ophthalmol* **113**:165, 1992.
87. Sorscher EJ, Huang Z: Diagnosis of genetic disease by primer-specified restriction map modification, with application to cystic fibrosis and retinitis pigmentosa. *Lancet* **337**:1115, 1991.
88. Berson EL: Ocular findings in a form of retinitis pigmentosa with a rhodopsin gene defect. *Trans Am Ophthalmol Soc* **88**:355, 1990.
89. Berson EL, Rosner B, Sandberg MA, Dryja TP: Ocular findings in patients with autosomal dominant retinitis pigmentosa and a rhodopsin gene defect (Pro23His). *Arch Ophthalmol* **109**:92, 1991.
90. Stone EM, Kimura AE, Nichols BE, Khadivi P, Fishman GA, Sheffield VC: Regional distribution of retinal degeneration in patients with the proline to histidine mutation in codon 23 of the rhodopsin gene. *Ophthalmology* **98**:1806, 1991.
91. Fishman GA, Stone EM, Gilbert LD, Kenna P, Sheffield VC: Ocular findings associated with a rhodopsin gene codon 58 transversion mutation in autosomal dominant retinitis pigmentosa. *Arch Ophthalmol* **109**:1387, 1991.
92. Andreasson S, Ehinger B, Abrahamson M, Fex G: A six-generation family with autosomal dominant retinitis pigmentosa and a rhodopsin gene mutation (arginine-135-leucine). *Ophthalmic Paediatr Genet* **13**:145, 1992.
93. Bhattacharya S, Lester D, Keen TJ, Bashir R, Lauffart B, Inglehearn CF, Jay M, Bird AC: Retinitis pigmentosa and mutations in rhodopsin. *Lancet* **337**:185, 1991.
94. Berson EL, Sandberg MA, Dryja TP: Autosomal dominant retinitis pigmentosa with rhodopsin, valine-345-methionine. *Trans Am Ophthalmol Soc* **89**:117, 1991.
95. Berson EL, Rosner B, Sandberg MA, Weigel-Difranco C, Dryja TP: Ocular findings in patients with autosomal dominant retinitis pigmentosa and rhodopsin, proline-347-leucine. *Am J Ophthalmol* **111**:614, 1991.
96. Farrar GJ, Kenna P, Redmond R, McWilliam P, Bradley DG, Humphries MM, Sharp EM, Inglehearn CF, Bashir R, Jay M, Watty A, Ludwig M, Schinzel A, Samanns C, Gal A, Bhattacharya S, Humphries P: Autosomal dominant retinitis pigmentosa: Absence of the rhodopsin proline-histidine substitution (codon 23) in pedigrees from Europe. *Am J Hum Genet* **47**:941, 1990.
97. Konig B, Arendt A, McDowell JH, Kahlert M, Hargrave PA, Hofmann KP: Three cytoplasmic loops of rhodopsin interact with transducin. *Proc Natl Acad Sci USA* **86**:6878, 1989.
98. Robinson PR, Cohen GB, Zhukovsky EA, Oprian DD: Constitutively active mutants of rhodopsin. *Neuron* **9**:719, 1992.
99. Doi T, Molday RS, Khorana HG: Role of the intradiscal domain in rhodopsin assembly and function. *Proc Natl Acad Sci USA* **87**:4991, 1990.
100. Sifers RN: Z and the insoluble answer. *Nature* **357**:541, 1992.
101. Lomas DA, Evans DL, Finch JT, Carrell RW: The mechanism of Z alpha-1 antitrypsin accumulation in the liver. *Nature* **357**:605, 1992.
102. Olsson JE, Gordon JW, Pawlyk BS, Roof D, Hayes A, Molday RS, Mukai S, Cowley GS, Berson EL, Dryja TP: Transgenic mice with a rhodopsin mutation (Pro23His): A mouse model of autosomal dominant retinitis pigmentosa. *Neuron* **9**:815, 1992.
103. Apfelstedt-Sylla E, Horn M, Kunisch M, Ruther K, Gerding H, Gal A, Zrenner E: Clinical characteristics of autosomal dominant retinitis pigmentosa (ADRP) with a deletion of 8 base pairs and shift of the reading frame in exon 5 of the rhodopsin gene. *Invest Ophthalmol Vis Sci (suppl)* **33**:1095, 1992. (abstr.)
104. Berson EL, Gouras P, Gunkel RD: Rod responses in retinitis pigmentosa, dominantly inherited. *Arch Ophthalmol* **80**:58, 1968.
105. Fishman GA, Stone EM, Gilbert LD, Sheffield VC:

Ocular findings associated with a rhodopsin gene codon 106 mutation. Glycine-to-arginine change in autosomal dominant retinitis pigmentosa. *Arch Ophthalmol* **110**:646, 1992.

106. Landon F, Lemonnier M, Benarous R, Huc C, Fiszman M, Gros F, Portier MM: Multiple mRNAs encode peripherin, a neuronal intermediate filament protein. *EMBO J* **8**:1719, 1989.
107. Thompson MA, Ziff EB: Structure of the gene encoding peripherin, an NGF-regulated neuronal-specific type III intermediate filament protein. *Neuron* **2**:1043, 1989.
108. Molday RS, Hicks D, Molday L: Peripherin. A rim-specific membrane protein of rod outer segment discs. *Invest Ophthalmol Vis Sci* **28**:50, 1987.
109. van Nie R, Ivanyi D, Demant P: A new H-2 linked mutation, rds, causing retinal degeneration in the mouse. *Tissue Antigens* **12**:106, 1978.
110. Travis GH, Brennan MB, Danielson PE, Kozak CA, Sutcliffe JG: Identification of a photoreceptor-specific mRNA encoded by the gene responsible for retinal degeneration slow (rds). *Nature* **338**:70, 1989.
111. Connell GJ, Molday RS: Molecular cloning, primary structure, and orientation of the vertebrate photoreceptor cell protein peripherin in the rod outer segment disk membrane. *Biochemistry* **29**:4691, 1990.
112. Connell G, Bascom R, Molday L, Reid D, McInnes RR, Molday RS: Photoreceptor peripherin is the normal product of the gene responsible for retinal degeneration in the rds mouse. *Proc Natl Acad Sci USA* **88**:723, 1991.
113. Travis GH, Christerson L, Danielson PE, Klisak I, Sparkes RS, Hahn LB, Dryja TP, Sutcliffe JG: The human retinal degeneration slow (RDS) gene: Chromosomal assignment and structure of the mRNA. *Genomics* **10**:733, 1991.
114. Begy C, Bridges CD: Nucleotide and predicted protein sequence of rat retinal degeneration slow (rds). *Nucleic Acids Res* **18**:3058, 1990.
115. Arikawa K, Molday LL, Molday RS, Williams DS: Localization of peripherin/rds in the disk membranes of cone and rod photoreceptors: Relationship to disk membrane morphogenesis and retinal degeneration. *J Cell Biol* **116**:659, 1992.
116. Travis GH, Sutcliffe JG, Bok D: The retinal degeneration slow (rds) gene product is a photoreceptor disc membrane-associated glycoprotein. *Neuron* **6**:61, 1991.
117. Young RW: The renewal of photoreceptor cell outer segments. *J Cell Biol* **33**:61, 1967.
118. Young RW: Visual cells and the concept of renewal. *Invest Ophthalmol Vis Sci* **15**:700, 1976.
119. Dratz EA, Hargrave PA: The structure of rhodopsin and the rod outer segment disk membrane. *Trends Biochem Sci* 1983.
120. Hargrave PA: Rhodopsin chemistry, structure and topography, in Osborne NN, Chader GJ (eds): *Progress in Retinal Research*. Elmsford, NY, Pergamon, 1982, vol 1, p 1.
121. Sheffield VC, Beck JS, Nichols B, Cousineau A, Lidral AC, Stone EM: Detection of multiallele polymorphisms within gene sequences by GC-clamped denaturing gradient gel electrophoresis. *Am J Hum Genet* **50**:567, 1992.
122. Brawerman G: mRNA decay: Finding the right targets. *Cell* **57**:9, 1989.
123. McIntosh I, Hamosh A, Dietz HC: Nonsense mutations and diminished mRNA levels. *Nat Genet* **4**:219, 1993.
124. Inglehearn CF, Carter SA, Keen TJ, Lindsey J, Stephenson AM, Bashir R, Al-Maghtheh M, Moore AT, Jay M, Bird AC, Bhattacharya SS: A new locus for autosomal dominant retinitis pigmentosa on 7p. *Nat Genet* **4**:51, 1993.
125. Jordan SA, Farrar GJ, Kenna P, Humphries MM, Sheils DM, Kumar-Singh R, Sharp EM, Soriano N, Ayuso C, Benitez J, Humphries P: Localization of an autosomal dominant retinitis pigmentosa gene to chromosome 7q. *Nat Genet* **4**:54, 1993.
126. Kumar-Singh R, Farrar GJ, Mansergh F, Kenna P, Bhattacharya S, Gal A, Humphries P: Exclusion of the involvement of all known retinitis pigmentosa loci in the disease present in a family of Irish origin provides evidence for a sixth autosomal dominant locus (RP8). *Hum Mol Genet* **2**:875, 1993.
127. Evans K, Fryer A, Inglehearn C, Duvall-Young J, Whittaker JL, Gregory CY, Butler R, Ebenezer N, Hunt DM, Bhattacharya S: Genetic linkage of cone-rod retinal dystrophy to chromosome 19q and evidence for segregation distortion. *Nat Genet* **6**:210, 1994.
128. McLaughlin ME, Sandberg MA, Berson EL, Dryja TP: Recessive mutations in the gene encoding the beta-subunit of rod phosphodiesterase in patients with retinitis pigmentosa. *Nat Genet* **4**:130, 1993.
129. Kimberling WJ, Moller CG, Davenport S, Priluck IA, Beighton PH, Greenberg J, Reardon W, Weston MD, Kenyon JB, Grunkemeyer JA, Pieke Dahl S, Overbeck LD, Blackwood DJ, Brower AM, Hoover DM, Rowland P, Smith RJH: Linkage of Usher syndrome type I gene (USH1B) to the long arm of chromosome 11. *Genomics* **14**:988, 1992.
130. Smith RJH, Lee EC, Kimberling WJ, Daiger SP, Pelias MZ, Keats BJB, Jay M, Bird A, Reardon W, Guest M, Ayyagari R, Hejtmancik JF: Localization of two genes for Usher syndrome type I to chromosome 11. *Genomics* **14**:995, 1992.
131. Kaplan J, Gerber S, Bonneau D, Rozet JM, Delrieu O. Briard ML, Dollfus H, Ghazi I, Dufier JL, Frezal J, Munnich A: A gene for Usher syndrome type I (USH1A) maps to chromosome 14q. *Genomics* **14**:979, 1992.
132. Kwitek-Black AE, Carmi R, Duyk GM, Buetow KH, Elbedour K, Parvari R, Yandava CN, Stone EM, Sheffield VC: Linkage of Bardet-Biedl syndrome to chromosome 16q and evidence for non-allelic genetic heterogeneity. *Nat Genet* **5**:392, 1993.
133. Kaplan J, Gerber S, Larget-Piet D, Rozet JM, Dollfus H, Dufier JL, Odent S, Postel-Vinay A, Janin N, Briard ML, Frezal J, Munnich A: A gene for Stargardt's disease (fundus flavimaculatus) maps to the short arm of chromosome 1. *Nat Genet* **5**:308, 1993.
134. Kajiwara K, Berson EL, Dryja TP: Digenic retinitis pigmentosa due to mutations at the unlinked peripherin/RDS and ROM1 loci. *Science* **264**:1604, 1994.

CHAPTER 145

Choroideremia

Frans P.M. Cremers ■ Hans-Hilger Ropers

1. Choroideremia (CHM) is a progressive degeneration of the retinal pigment epithelium, choroid, and retina which is inherited in an X-chromosomal recessive fashion.

2. Usually, night blindness is the first clinical sign; it may already be present in early childhood and is followed by visual loss. Typically, the central vision is not affected until late in the disease. Many patients are blind by the age of 45, but the course of the disease is very variable.

3. These symptoms are paralleled by loss of the choroidal vessels and depigmentation of the fundus which are most prominent in the midperiphery, while the macular region is conspicuously spared. In the end stage of the disorder the fundus is of scleral whiteness, choroidal vessels are absent except for possible remnants in the macular region, and retinal vessels are sometimes attenuated.

4. With an estimated incidence of 1 in 100,000, CHM is regarded as a rare disorder. Because of clinical similarities with other hereditary retinopathies, however, its frequency may have been underestimated, and by some, CHM is considered as the most frequent X-linked form of retinal degeneration.

5. Linkage studies and clinical findings in males with X-chromosomal deletions have assigned the CHM gene to Xq21, and subsequent molecular studies have led to its isolation by means of positional cloning strategies. The CHM gene encodes an mRNA of approximately 6.0 kb, of which 85 percent has been cloned as cDNA. Intragenic microdeletions, translocations, and a variety of small mutations in patients with classic CHM have established that dysfunction of this gene is the fundamental cause of choroideremia.

6. In the Western European population, roughly 14 percent of patients with CHM have deletions encompassing part of the CHM gene, but deletions have not been found elsewhere. At this writing, frameshift, stop codon, and splice site mutations have been observed in 21 percent of cases. No missense mutations have been detected yet.

7. A closely homologous and apparently functional gene, choroideremia-like (CHML) gene, has been isolated and mapped to the distal 1q region in the vicinity of the gene for Usher syndrome type 2 (USH2), another form of retinal degeneration which is associated with sensorineural deafness. The role of CHML in USH2, if any, is not yet known. Sequence comparisons involving CHML and the CHM gene of the mouse suggest that the open reading frame of the human CHM gene is larger than previously reported and may code for a protein of approximately 650 amino acids.

8. A geranylgeranyl transferase (GGT) from rat brain has been purified which specifically prenylates two ras-like GTP-binding proteins, Rab3A, found in synaptic vesicles, and Rab1A, found in the endoplasmic reticulum (ER). Tryptic digestion and sequencing revealed striking similarities between component A of this enzyme, a polypeptide of 95 kDa, and the deduced product of the murine CHM gene. Similar but weaker homologies had been detected previously between CHM and another Rab3A-binding protein from (bovine) brain—the GDP dissociation inhibitor Rab3A GDI.

9. In spite of hitherto unexplained size differences between component A of Rab GGT and the deduced CHM protein, it is likely that these proteins are identical. Thus, choroideremia may result from defective prenylation of Rab3A or a related membrane-associated small GTP-binding protein in the retina.

A list of standard abbreviations is located immediately preceding the index in each volume. Additional abbreviations used in this chapter include: AED = anhidrotic ectodermal dysplasia; CHM = choroideremia; CHML = choroideremia-like; GDI = GDP dissociation inhibitor; GGT = geranylgeranyl transferase; ORF = open reading frame; USH2 = Usher syndrome type 2.

Choroideremia (CHM) belongs to a large and heterogeneous group of genetic disorders which are characterized by progressive degeneration of the retina and the choroid. Detailed clinical, genetic and molecular studies have only just begun to shed light on the nosology, etiology, and pathogenesis of these disorders which can be inherited in an autosomal dominant, autosomal recessive, or X-linked fashion. CHM, like at least two different forms of retinitis pigmentosa, is an X-linked disorder which almost exclusively affects males. A precise clinical description of this disorder was published 120 years ago, but it took 70 years to establish its progressive nature and its mode of inheritance. Though the biochemical defect underlying this disorder is still unknown, presymptomatic diagnosis and carrier detection in families became possible in the mid-1980s, when close linkage with DNA markers was found. These studies, and subsequent molecular analyses of microdeletions encompassing the Xq21 band were instrumental for the isolation of the CHM gene on the basis of its known chromosomal location, employing "positional cloning" strategies. Sequence analysis of this gene and its protein product are beginning to provide insight into its metabolic function, and its elucidation may shed light on the basic defects underlying related disorders of the retina and choroid.

HISTORY AND CLINICAL ASPECTS

Choroideremia was first described in 1872 by Mauthner,[1] who coined this name because he thought the condition reflected the congenital absence of the choroid. Despite some earlier suggestions that CHM might be a progressive disorder,[2,3] Bedell[4] was the first to conclude, after thorough review of the literature and on the basis of own observations, that choroideremia may be defined "as a condition in which the choroid disappears . . . in a definite uniform manner." Several authors provided further evidence for progression of this disease[5–7] which was widely accepted after the description of a large Canadian family by McCulloch and McCulloch.[8] The concept of choroideremia as an X-linked disorder with full manifestation in males and minor clinical signs in female carriers was independently worked out by Waardenburg[9] and Goedbloed[10] on the basis of literature studies and their own observations. Apart from the studies of the McCullochs[8,11] and a detailed survey by Sorsby et al.,[12] several other large studies, such as those of Kurstjens,[13] Krill,[14] and Kärnä[15] have further contributed to the clinical definition of CHM.

Nightblindness is usually the first clinical sign of the disorder, and most patients report to have been nightblind since their early childhood.[4,15–17] Less frequently, nightblindness remains unnoticed before patients are 20 years old.[12,16,18,19] Occasionally, it may not be present before the midthirties[11,13] or beyond.[20]

Usually, the first signs of visual loss involve the midperiphery. Central vision is frequently preserved until the end stage of the disorder, and often there is also residual vision in the periphery. However, visual fields can vary considerably, even between the two eyes of one patient, and may appear as annular scotomas, tunnel vision, or visual fields of irregular shape. In his study of 45 patients, Kurstjens[13] observed large blind spots and reduced equatorial sensitivity, equatorial scotomas, annular scotomas, and central and peripheral temporal remnants as the most frequent findings.

Moderate myopia is more common among patients with choroideremia than in the normal population. As shown by McCulloch and McCulloch,[8] by Kurstjens,[13] and in particular by Kärnä[15] in his large and detailed study, the myopia is progressive and correlated with the course of the disease. Repeatedly, disorders of color vision have also been observed.[16,21,22] Jaeger and Grützner[23] reported on disturbances in the blue-green range of the spectrum which were correlated with the severity of the disorder. In several patients, these changes resembled protanopia while in others, deuteranopic changes were reported. Additional anomalies included punctiform and fibrillary opacities in the vitreous body.[1,8,13] Infrequently, cataract was also present, mostly of the subcapsular type.[13,24,25]

Clinical Diagnosis

According to Krill[14] the fundus changes can be divided into three stages, the first of which consists of pigmentary stippling and fine atrophy in the pigment epithelium of the posterior and equatorial parts of the fundus. These findings resemble those seen in female carriers (see below). In the first stage, there is also focal atrophy of the choroicapillary layer and atrophy of the larger choroidal vessels around the optic disk and in the equatorial area. Choroidal vascular atrophy is preceded by depigmentation of the fundus, which reflects the degeneration of the retinal pigment epithelium.

In the second stage, the atrophy of the choroid and pigment epithelium spreads from the midperiphery inward and from the disk outward. Usually, choroidal vessels of all sizes are involved, but in some cases only the choroidal capillaries are damaged. The choroidal vessels of the macula are not affected, and pigmentary mottling is no longer seen except in the far periphery. In the third stage of the disorder, atrophy of the choroidal vessels is almost complete except in the far periphery, in the macula, and sometimes near the optic disk. The fundus is yellow-whitish or greenish-white, and attenuation of the retinal vessels may occur at this stage.

The rate and degree of the atrophy varies, even within families. For example, McCulloch and McCulloch[8] described a completely white fundus in a 7-year-old patient while, on the other hand, changes were very slight in a 45-year-old patient. Not infrequently, conspicuous first-stage changes were found in boys aged between 1 and 4 years.[8,13,18,19]

Abnormal light and dark adaptation are other early signs of the disorder.[13,19,22,26–29] On dark adaptation testing, elevated rod final thresholds are observed, and usually, rod adaptation is disturbed earlier or more profoundly than cone adaptation. Changes are generally correlated with the degree of retinal degeneration.[16,25,30]

Electroretinographic signs involve both the scotopic and the photopic component. Usually, however, the degeneration follows a rod-cone pattern with reduced rod responses and normal or reduced cone responses.[13,15,31,32] Scotopic responses may even totally disappear before the photopic responses become disturbed.[13,21] At the terminal stage, the electroretinogram (ERG) is no longer recordable.[15,30] In the great majority of patients examined, the electrooculogram (EOG) was abnormal,[13,28,33] although a patient with extinguished ERG but normal EOG has been described.[34] In contrast, Krill[14] thought that abnormal ERG are mostly preceded by changes in the EOG.

Early changes in the choroidal vessels, including capillaries, can be detected by fluorescein angiography. Depending on the severity of the disorder, choroidal capillaries can be absent over large areas,[11,17,27,35] and these changes can precede ophthalmoscopic signs considerably.[14] Usually, there is macular hyperfluorescence which is due to the degeneration of the pigment epithelium.[14] In general, changes seen on fluorescein angiography are more extensive than expected from ophthalmoscopic findings.

So far, histologic examination of eyes from CHM patients has been confined to far advanced cases. Absence of the retinal pigment epithelium, the choroid, and the photoreceptor outer segments was seen with varying degrees of preservation in the macular region. McCulloch[36] reported on thickened and hyalinized choroidal vessels, but these findings were not confirmed by others. In a case studied by Grützner and Vogel,[37] proliferation of the pigment epithelium was seen, and a considerable part of the retina was substituted by glial tissue. Gliosis of the inner parts of the retina, doubling of the basal membrane of the pigment epithelium, and thickening of Bruch's membrane was observed by Ghosh and McCulloch.[38]

Choroideremia in Females

Female carriers are mostly asymptomatic. Few have minor signs of the disorder, and serious visual impairment is rare.[39,40] In contrast, the great majority of carrier females have conspicuous fundus abnormalities such as pigment changes in the periphery closely resembling the fine mottling which is characteristic of initial stages of the disease in males. As in males, fundus changes are progressive, beginning in the midperiphery and leading to degeneration of the pigment epithelium and the choroid, often including the area surrounding the optic disk. Later on, there are numerous white dots scattered throughout the retina, and with increasing age, sclerosis of the choroid is seen. While in general the severity of fundus changes in female carriers is correlated with their age, fundus changes in young heterozygotes may be far more severe than in their carrier mothers.[12,14] Variable cellular mosaicism resulting from random inactivation of one of the two X chromosomes in cells of the early female embryo[41] may be a major cause of the varying clinical manifestation of CHM in female carriers, but it is of note that in males the clinical picture and the course of the disease are also very variable. Severe manifestation of the disease in females can result from skewed X-inactivation, homozygosity, or disruption of the CHM gene by X-autosome translocations. In view of the rarity of this disorder it is not surprising that, with two possible exceptions,[42,43] homozygous females have not yet been described. In two other females with a classic CHM, X-autosome translocations have been found.[44,45] In females with reciprocal X-autosome translocations, X-chromosome inactivation is nonrandom; usually the normal X is preferentially inactivated while both translocation fragments remain active. Therefore, in line with analogous observations in Duchenne muscular dystrophy, clinical signs of CHM in the girls with *de novo* X-autosomal translocations suggested that chromosome breakage had disrupted the only active copy of the CHM gene. This has been confirmed by subsequent molecular analyses.

Other Disorders Associated with Choroideremia and Differential Diagnosis

Apart from a variety of ocular symptoms which are interpreted as direct or indirect manifestations of the fundamental defect, association of CHM with various other diseases has been reported. Sensorineural hearing loss was found in 10 of the patients studied by McCulloch and McCulloch[8] and in one of Scobee's patients.[7] One of the patients of Dachevzkaya and Polonsky[46] was mute, and Murdoch[17] described a patient with congenital hearing loss. CHM has also been described in combination with dwarfism,[47] but the absence of nightblindness in this patient and of fundus changes in the mother render the diagnosis of CHM in this case rather unlikely. Choroideremia-like symptoms have also been observed in a family with a complex, apparently X-linked disorder including anhidrotic ectodermal dysplasia (AED), skeletal abnormalities, and mental retardation[48] and in patients with choroiretinopathy and pituitary dysfunction.[49,50] The molecular relationship, if any, between these disorders and choroideremia has not yet been clarified, but in the family described by Van den Bosch,[48] a chromosomal defect spanning the CHM and AED loci has been excluded (Ropers H-H, et al.: unpublished observation). In contrast, deletions on the proximal long arm of the X chromosome have been identified as the primary defect in a variety of patients with CHM, mental retardation, deafness, and other features. As discussed below, molecular characterization of these deletions and the above-mentioned X-autosome translocations in female patients has been instrumental for fine mapping of the CHM gene and, eventually, its isolation by positional cloning.

The differential diagnosis of CHM includes gyrate atrophy (see Chap. 31) which clinically may be almost identical with CHM. Apart from characteristic circular lesions seen in the fundus of most patients with gyrate atrophy, distinguishing features are the mode of inheritance, which for gyrate atrophy is autosomal recessive, and the elevated plasma ornithine in these patients, which is due to a defect of the enzyme ornithine aminotransferase.[51,52] In early stages of the disease, CHM is sometimes indistinguishable from X-chromosomal recessive retinitis pigmentosa but in these cases, follow-up studies and examination of affected relatives will establish the diagnosis.[53] Not infrequently, autosomal dominant retinitis pigmentosa (see Chap. 144) is diagnosed in female CHM gene carriers because of similar funduscopic findings. In contrast to the situation in autosomal dominant retinitis pigmentosa, in which funduscopic changes are accompanied by alterations of the ERG and narrowed visual fields, ERG and visual fields are normal in most CHM carriers.[15,53] Other similar diseases include Bietti crystalline retinal dystrophy[54] (MIM 210370) and acquired retinal damage due to thioridazine toxicity.[55] Ocular symptoms similar to CHM have also been seen in patients with mitochondrial myopathies.[53,56]

MAPPING THE CHOROIDEREMIA GENE

Linkage Studies

As first shown by Other[57] and later confirmed by Bell and McCulloch,[58] Eriksson et al.,[59] and by Kärnä,[15] CHM is not linked to the Xg blood group on the distal short arm of the X chromosome. Likewise, linkage with X-linked color blindness could be excluded by Eriksson et al.[59] and by Kärnä,[15] thereby disproving weak evidence for cosegregation that had been reported previously.[60] Only in 1985, linkage studies with DNA markers were successful. In three informative families studied by Nussbaum et al.[61] no recombinants were detected between CHM and DXYS1, a polymorphic marker located in the Xq21 band. Measurable linkage was also detected with the DXS11 marker at Xq24-q26, whereas linkage to the HPRT gene at Xq26 could be excluded. Thus, the CHM gene was tentatively assigned to the Xq13-q24 interval. Close linkage between CHM and DXYS1 was also reported by Sankila et al.[62] in a study of three large kindreds from Northern Finland (Lod score 11.44 at zero recombination) and by Jay et al.[63] and Schwartz et al.[64,65] In a subsequent study by Nussbaum's group[66] including a total of 12 families, two recombinants were detected with the DXYS1 marker, yielding a Lod score of 10.25 at a recombination fraction of 0.02. Other recombinants were reported by MacDonald et al.[67] and by Uhlhaas et al.[68] Measurable linkage to CHM was also found for several other markers on the proximal long arm of the X chromosome, including DXS1, PGK, DXS72, DXS95, DXS3, DXYS12, and DXS17.[63–69] Multipoint linkage studies and haplotype analyses performed by Sankila et al.[70] in northeastern Finland placed the CHM gene distal to PGK1 and DXS72 but proximal to DXYS4 and DXYS12 in the vicinity of DXYS1 and DXYS5, and similar multipoint linkage analyses performed by Wright et al.[69] mapped the CHM locus between DXYS1 and DXS72 within the Xq21 band. These findings have been confirmed by linkage studies employing new markers that were generated during the molecular characterization and cloning of the relevant chromosome segment,[71–74] and by clinical and molecular analyses in patients with deletions involving part of Xq21, as discussed below.

Physical Mapping

Contiguous Gene Syndromes. The first deletion spanning part of the Xq21 band was described by Tabor et al.[75] in a male with cleft lip and palate, agenesis of the corpus callosum, and severe mental retardation. After the discovery of linkage between DXYS1 and the CHM locus[61] ophthalmologic reexamination revealed fundus changes characteristic of CHM in its early stage. The patient's mother and sister, who were both heterozygous for the deletion, were diagnosed as being carriers of CHM. Moreover, the deletion was shown to span the DXYS1 locus, thereby corroborating its linkage with CHM.[64,76,77] Since then, several other males with cytogenetically detectable Xq21 deletion have been described, and it has become apparent that their phenotypes almost invariably include CHM, congenital mixed deafness, and mental retardation. It is of note that apart from CHM, mixed deafness with or without stapes fixation, "unspecific" mental retardation and cleft lip and palate have been described as separate genetic entities segregating in families, and linkage studies have assigned these disorders to the proximal Xq.[78–81] Molecular analyses have revealed that all microscopically visible deletions span the DXYS1 locus and several other markers from Xq21.[82–88] In another patient with CHM, congenital deafness, and mental retardation that had been described previously by Ayazi,[89] a submicroscopic deletion was detected by Nussbaum and coworkers[83] by making use of two novel DNA probes. Interestingly, DXYS1 was not deleted in this patient. More precise regional mapping of the CHM locus was achieved by Cremers et al.,[90] who employed 20 anonymous probes from the Xq21 band to study five patients with CHM and Xq21 deletions. In this way, the Xq21 band could be subdivided into seven intervals, and the CHM gene as well as the DNA loci DXS95, DXS165 and DXS233 were assigned to interval 3.

Deletions Associated with Classic Choroideremia. Further refinement of the localization was achieved when Cremers et al. extended their search for deletions to patients with classic, that is, nonsyndromic CHM. With one of the probes from interval 3, p1bD5 (locus DXS165), two deletions could be found in a series of eight unrelated CHM patients (Fig. 145-1).[91] Generation of additional probes in the vicinity of the DXS165 locus by preparative field inversion gel electrophoresis, cloning of deletion endpoints, and chromosome jumping[74,85,92,93] led to the detection of eight additional deletions which ranged in size between 45 kb and approximately 5 Mb (see Fig. 145-2). While most of these deletions were overlapping, some were not; a proximal (3.5) and two distal (33.1 and LGL1101) deletions were found to be separated by at least 30 kb. This meant that the chromosome segment separating these deletions had to be part of the CHM gene, and at the same time, these observations provided a minimum estimate for its size.

X-Autosome Translocations. Molecular analyses of the breakpoints on the X chromosome in two females with balanced X-autosome translocations and choroideremia[44,45] have corroborated the results of deletion mapping. In both translocations, the breakpoints on the X chromosome were

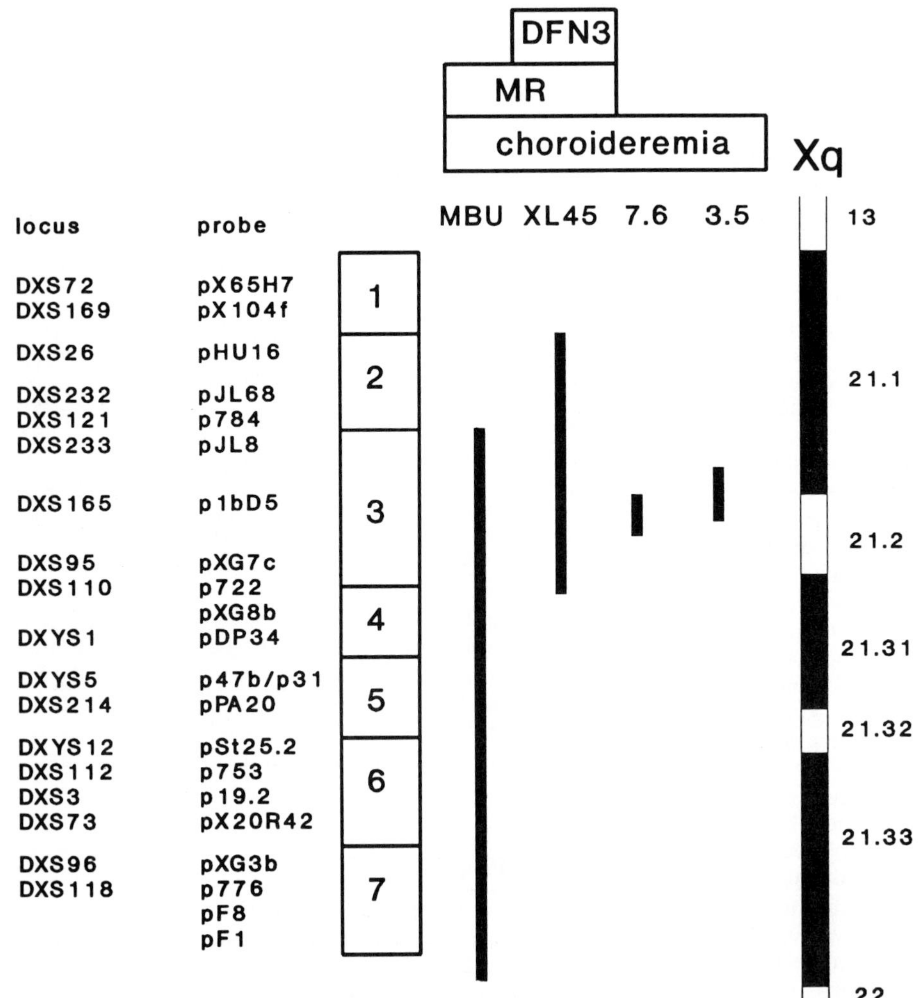

FIG. 145-1 Deletion interval map of the Xq21 region. The DNA probes used in Southern analysis are indicated at the left. Deleted chromosomal segments are indicated by vertical bars. Intervals and banding patterns are not drawn to scale.

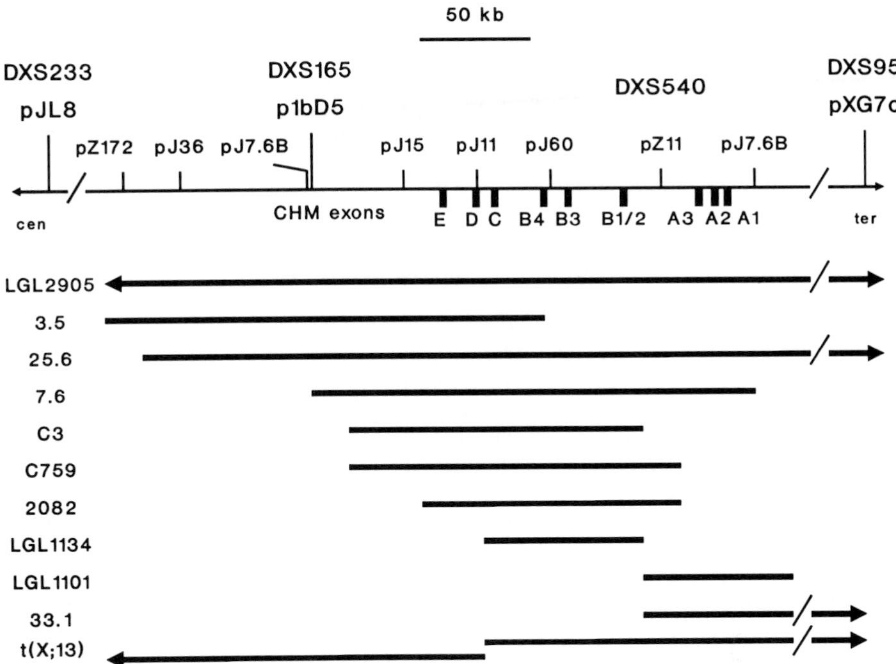

FIG. 145-2 Deletion map of the CHM locus and location of CHM exons at Xq21.2. Deleted segments are given as horizontal bars. The location of the X-chromosomal breakpoint in a female with an X;13 translocation and choroideremia is shown as a broken bar at the bottom.

situated in band Xq21.2 while the autosomal breakpoints were at 7p14 and 13p12, respectively. In addition to CHM, both females showed primary amenorrhea which is a common feature in X-autosome translocations involving the proximal Xq.[94] Cremers et al.[71] located the breakpoint of the X;13 translocation in the center of the region defined by deletion mapping as the site of the CHM gene (Fig. 145-2). These results were confirmed by Merry et al.[85,95] Evidence has indicated that the X;7 translocation breakpoint is located more distally but still within the relevant chromosome segment (Philippe C, et al.: unpublished data).

CLONING OF THE CHOROIDEREMIA GENE

Employing two clones from the critical region for CHM—pJ11 and pJ60 (see Fig. 145-2)—human genomic DNA phage clones were isolated spanning a region of 45 kb. Single- and low-copy probes were subsequently tested for evolutionary conservation by hybridization to Southern blots containing DNA from several vertebrates. Screening a human retinal cDNA library[96] with a probe that showed sequence conservation in several vertebrates, including mouse and chicken, resulted in the isolation of overlapping cDNA clones.[97] Subsequent rescreening of this and two other cDNA libraries (from fetal retina and fetal brain) with DNA probes from the 5′ and 3′ ends of the consensus cDNA enabled Cremers et al. to isolate flanking cDNA sequences, including the poly(A) tail indicative for the 3′ end of the gene (Fig. 145-3). The consensus cDNA encompasses 4.7 kb and an open reading frame (ORF) of 1257 bp corresponding to a polypeptide of 419 amino acids. Northern blotting experiments have indicated that the length of the corresponding mRNA is approximately 6.0 kb, which illustrates that the consensus cDNA is not yet complete.[95,97]

Similar findings were published by Merry et al.,[95] who independently isolated a CHM cDNA clone from a human retinal library. Their sequence is nearly identical to that published by Cremers et al. except for an inversion at the 5′ end of their sequence which is flanked by short inverted repeats. The correct orientation of this sequence could be established by Cremers et al. through comparison with the sequences of the murine CHM gene and a human autosomal homologue, CHML (see below). The open reading frames of both genes are 173 and 236 amino acids longer than the deduced product of the CHM gene. Therefore, it is likely that about one third of the CHM ORF has not yet been isolated (see Figs. 145-6 and 145-7).

Convincing evidence that this cloned cDNA is derived

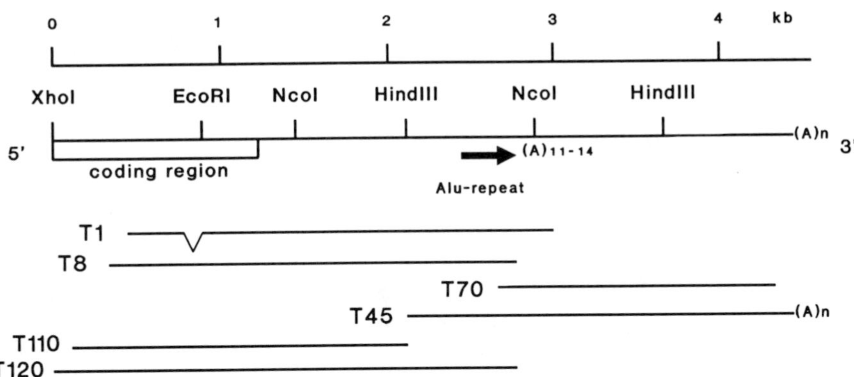

FIG. 145-3 cDNA map of the CHM gene. Schematic representation of the overlapping cDNA clones corresponding to the CHM gene with the restriction map is given at the top. The ORF encodes a polypeptide of 419 amino acids.

from the CHM gene has come from the observation that in 10 patients with deletions, and in 1 of the female patients with an X;13 translocation, the putative coding sequence was disrupted or at least partly removed (Figs. 145-2 and 145-4; unpublished data). In particular, the X-chromosomal breakpoint in the translocation patient could be mapped to an intron sequence in the middle of the ORF, between exons C and D (see Fig. 145-2). More recently, screening for point mutations in CHM patients has revealed numerous small changes in the putative CHM gene which has settled this point.[98,99]

Northern blot analyses employing RNA from several human tissues and cell lines have revealed that expression of the CHM gene is not confined to ocular tissues. With CHM cDNAs as probes, specific hybridization signals were seen in RNA from choroid and retinal pigment epithelium, retina, and different retinal cell lines but also, albeit weaker, in RNA from HeLa cells, lymphoblastoid cells, and fibroblasts (Fig. 145-5). In view of the fact that clinical signs in CHM are limited to the ocular fundus, this finding is surprising, although it is not entirely unprecedented: gyrate atrophy, a genetic eye disease with clinical similarity to CHM, is caused by the deficiency of an enzyme, ornithine aminotransferase, which is also expressed in various extraocular tissues and organs[51,52] (see also, Chap. 31). The expression of the CHM gene in fibroblasts and lymphoblastoid cells has important implications for presymptomatic diagnosis and carrier detection, as discussed below.

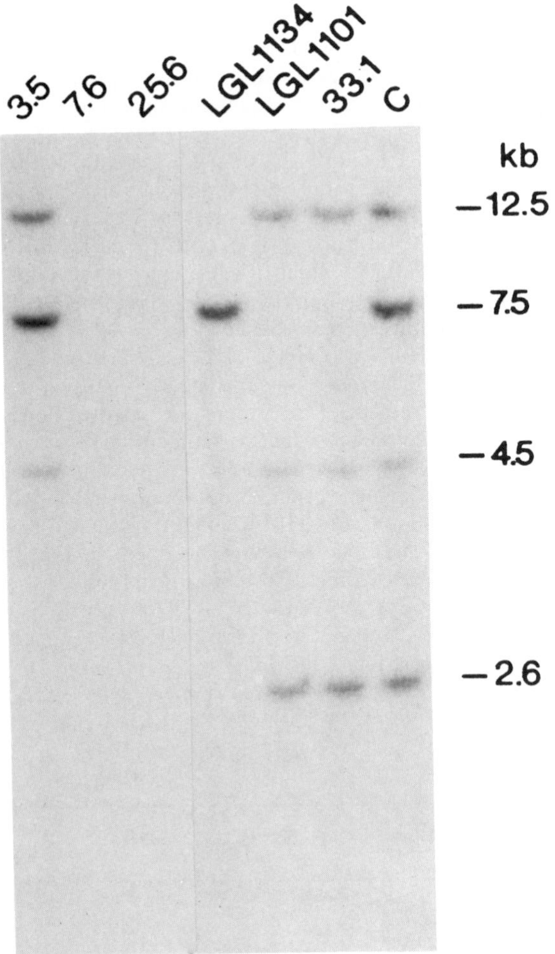

FIG. 145-4 Southern blot analysis of *Eco*RI digested DNA from several patients with classic CHM. The cDNA probe T1E0.5 encompasses exons A3, B1/2, B3, and B4 which are located on *Eco*RI fragments of 7.5, 4.5, 12.5, and 2.6 kb, respectively. *(From Cremers et al.*[97] *Used by permission of* Nature.*)*

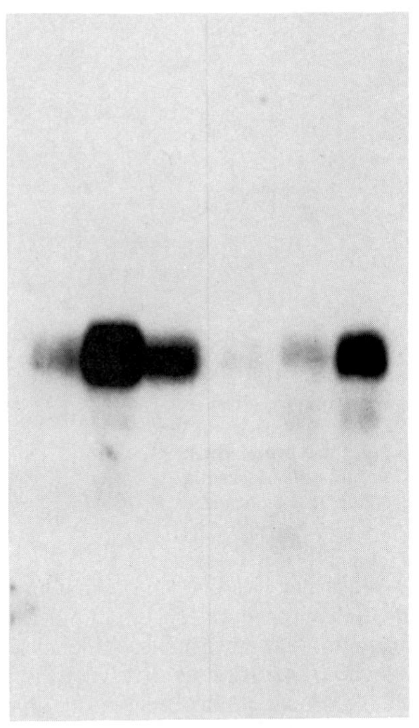

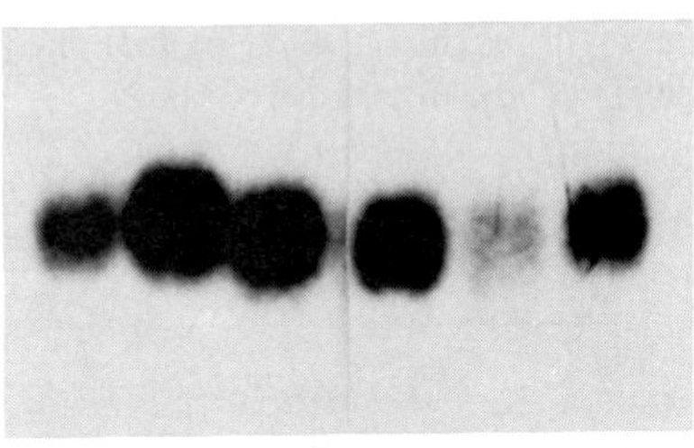

FIG. 145-5 Northern blot analysis of RNA from several human cell lines and tissues using cDNA clone T1. *A*. Blot containing RNA from HeLa, two retinal cell lines (HER RC2 and HER XC2), an Epstein-Barr-virus–immortalized lymphoblastoid cell line (LCL1154), as well as human choroid/retinal pigment epithelium (RPE) and retina screened with clone T1EN0.6 *B*. Hybridization of a hamster actin cDNA clone (pAct-1). The positions of the 18S and 28S ribosomal RNA bands are indicated. *(From Cremers et al.*[97] *Used by permission of* Nature.*)*

MUTATION SPECTRUM AND DIAGNOSTIC ASPECTS

Microdeletions

In the course of their search for deletions in patients with CHM which paved the way to the cloning of the CHM gene,

Cremers et al. examined 80 apparently unrelated patients from Germany, the Netherlands, Denmark, Finland, and other European countries. With anonymous probes from the relevant Xq21 segment, 11 deletions have been found[92] (and unpublished results), which means that in this series, approximately 14 percent of the patients carried a deletion that was detectable by Southern blotting. Against this background it is remarkable that Merry et al.[95] have not found a single functionally relevant structural rearrangement of the CHM gene in 34 American CHM patients. The marked discrepancy between these studies may be explained by founder effects resulting in a low number of different mutations in the American population. It is noteworthy in this context that even within the United States the incidence of CHM may show significant geographic differences: on the West Coast, it is considered as the most frequent form of retinal degeneration[53] while in New England, CHM seems to be much rarer than X-linked retinitis pigmentosa (Berson E, Boston: personal communication). Strong founder effects have also been detected on CHM mutation screening in Northern Finland.[99] So far, the comparison of cDNA and genomic sequences has revealed the existence of 12 exons, 9 of which have been characterized.

Single-Strand Conformation Polymorphism Analysis

For five of the CHM exons (B3 through E) which are situated at the 3′ end of the CHM gene, flanking intron sequences have been determined and were used for mutation screening (Fig. 145-6). Employing the single-strand conformation polymorphism (SSCP) technique described by Orita et al.[100] in combination with direct sequencing, Van den Hurk et al.,[98] Sankila et al.[99] and Schwartz et al. (personal communication) have detected 11 small mutations in unrelated CHM patients but none in numerous healthy controls. All mutations resulted in premature termination of the polypeptide chain, either at the site of the mutation or just downstream because of stop codons resulting from frameshifts. Five of these mutations were deletions of one or a few nucleotides, three were nucleotide substitutions, and three were splice-site mutations (see Fig. 145-6). Sankila et al.[99] were able to show that most patients in the Salla region of northern Finland carry the same mutation—an insertion into the splice donor site downstream of exon C which gives rise to aberrant splicing. By genealogical studies, this mutation could be traced back to a founder couple born 13 generations ago. Mutation screening has so far failed to detect a common defect in the CHM gene; only one mutation—a deletion of the tetranucleotide TGTT in exon C—was encountered twice. The two patients carrying this mutation, one born in Denmark and the other from southern Germany, are apparently unrelated. It is of note that in the normal CHM gene, the TGTT tetranucleotide is present in tandem, which may render this sequence particularly prone to mutation, for example, by polymerase slippage during replication. Four mutations were observed in exon B4 within a segment of only 97 bp, which may indicate that this region is a hot spot for mutations.

Until now, systematic mutation screening has been performed for 610 bp of the ORF which is thought to represent approximately one third of the protein coding sequence, as discussed above. Therefore, the percentage of mutations (11 of 45, 24 percent) detected in patients without large deletions fits the expectation, taking into account that on average, only 80 percent of the point mutations can be visualized by the SSCP technique,[101] and that mutation screening did not include the promoter region. Thus, apart from the possible clustering of mutations in exon B4, these findings suggest a relatively even distribution of mutations throughout the gene. If deletions detectable by Southern blotting are included, mutations have been detected in approximately 35 percent of patients.

So far, there is no indication for a correlation between the kind and size of the mutation and the clinical severity of the disorder, though it is possible that subtle clinical differences may be obscured by the remarkable intrafamilial variability of the disorder. On the other hand, deletions affecting the entire or part of the CHM gene and point

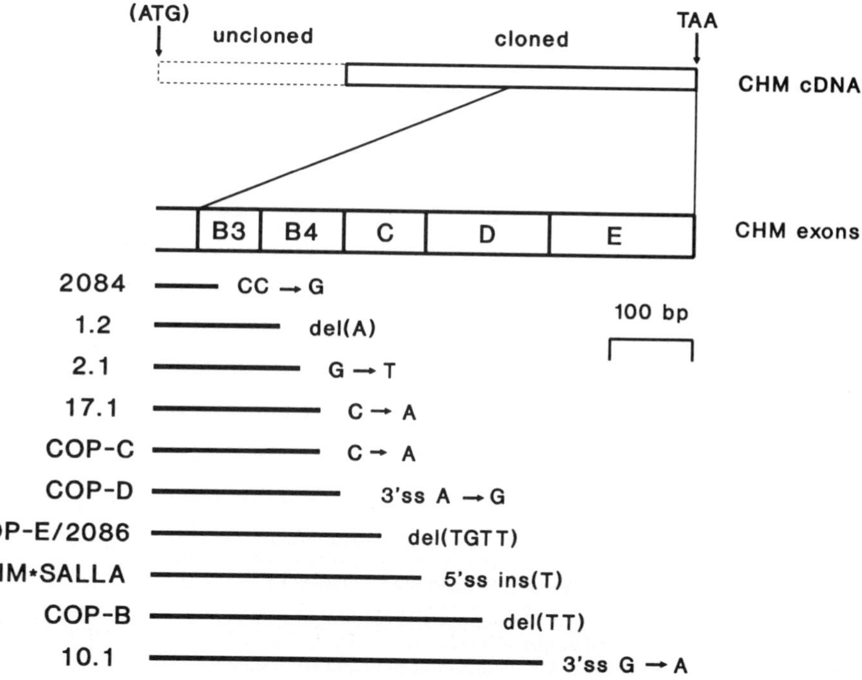

FIG. 145-6 Nonsense mutations in the CHM gene. *Upper half:* gene segment that has been investigated for small mutations by employing the SSCP technique. *Lower half:* mutations observed and length of the resulting truncated proteins.

mutations that give rise to truncated proteins are expected to abolish the function of the CHM gene. Therefore, the apparent absence of a correlation between the clinical phenotype and the genotypic changes may not be too surprising. It is striking, however, that in the 3′ part of the gene (corresponding to the C-terminal region of the protein) no missense mutations have been observed yet. This may indicate that most missense mutations in this region are functionally neutral or, alternatively, that they may give rise to an entirely different disease phenotype. It will be interesting to see whether there are missense mutations in the N-terminal portion of the protein which has not yet been studied. So far, there is no clear explanation for the conspicuous intrafamilial variability of CHM, but it is conceivable that its clinical picture and course are modulated by the CHML gene, which is structurally very similar to CHM (see below).

RNA Analyses. The CHM gene is expressed, albeit at low levels, in lymphoblasts, fibroblasts, and various other tissues (see Fig. 145-5). Expression studies in tissues of patients have indicated that a high proportion of mutations in the CHM gene can be traced in this way. Reverse transcription of RNA from lymphoblasts and subsequent amplification by means of the polymerase chain reaction enabled Merry et al.[95] to demonstrate reduced levels of CHM mRNA or its absence in 25 of 34 patients. Similarly, northern blot analyses using RNA from Epstein-Barr-virus–transformed lymphoblastoid cell lines revealed a marked reduction or absence of CHM mRNA signals in 8 of 11 patients (Cremers FPM: unpublished observations), but these analyses are complicated by the low expression level of the CHM gene in cells that are accessible for diagnostic purposes. The reverse transcriptase–PCR technique is far more sensitive than northern blotting, but here transcripts derived from CHML, an autosomal homologue of CHM, can interfere with this analysis. Because of the high sequence similarity between CHM and CHML (see below), very specific PCR primers are required to amplify CHM without contamination by CHML.

New mutations in CHM are rare, and in most cases, the disorder is familial. Therefore, closely linked markers are potentially important tools for the diagnosis of this disorder. Because of low recombination frequencies on the proximal long arm of the X chromosome, several DNA markers from Xq21 are useful for this purpose, despite their physical distance from the CHM gene, which for some is considerable. None of the markers which were originally shown to be linked to CHM mapped to the Xq21 interval carrying the CHM gene, as defined by cytogenetically visible deletions, and for some time, DXS95 was the only polymorphic marker in this segment (see Fig. 145-1). Still, with recombination frequencies between 0.04 and 0.08 (compiled by Sankila[102]), other flanking markers like DXYS1, DXYS12, DXYS3, and PGK1 can be valuable assets for diagnosis and genetic counseling. An intragenic polymorphism has been found with probe pZ11 (locus DXS540,[103]), but no highly informative variable simple sequence polymorphisms like $(CA)_n$ dinucleotide repeats have been detected yet in the vicinity of the CHM gene.

ISOLATION OF THE MURINE CHOROIDEREMIA GENE AND A HUMAN CHOROIDEREMIA-LIKE GENE ON CHROMOSOME 1

As a prerequisite for expression studies and for the generation of an animal model, Cremers et al.[104] have isolated cDNAs corresponding to the murine CHM gene, mCHM. The ORF of the murine consensus cDNA encodes 592 amino acids as compared with 419 of its human counterpart. Overlapping segments of the murine and the human CHM gene exhibit 88 percent nucleotide and amino acid sequence identity, and including conservative replacements, 97 percent of all amino acids are similar[104] (see Fig. 145-7).

An autosomal homologue of the human CHM gene was isolated by the same group in the course of experiments aiming at the cloning of the 5′ end of the CHM cDNA.

```
hCHML  MADNLPTEFDVVIIGTGLPESILAAACSRSGQRVLHIDSRSYYGGNWASFSFSGLLSWLKEYQQNNDIGEESTVVWQDLIHETEEAITLR  90
mCHM                                                                             M--EQ-L-N----L-S  16

hCHML  KKDETIQHTEAFSYASQDMEDNVEEIGALQKNPSLGVSNTFTEVLDSALPEESQLSYFNSDEMPAKHTQKSDTEISLEVTDVEESVEKEK 180
mCHM   S--K----V-V-C-----LHKD---A-------ASVM-AQA--AAEA-EAA-ATEA  AEAAEA-EAACLPTA-E--STRSC-LPA-QSQ 104

hCHML  YCGDKTCMHT   VSDKDGDKDESKST         VEDKADEPIRNRITYSQIVKEGRRFNIDLVSKLLYSQGLLIDLLIKSDVSRYV 257
mCHM   CM-PESSPQVNDAE-GEKETQS-AKS--EQSSEILPK-Q-NTET-KK--V------I----------------R----------N----A 194
hCHM                                                                         ----R----------N----A  21

hCHML  EFKNVTRILAFREGKVEQVPCSRADVFNSKELTMVEKRMLMKFLTFCLEYEQHPDEYQAFRQCSFSEYLKTKKLTPNLQHFVLHSIAMTS 347
mCHM   --------------------------------------------------V---D--G--K-YEETT-------Q-------Y---------- 284
hCHM   ----I---------T---------------Q---------------M---KY----KGYEEIT-Y-----Q-------YI-M------- 111
       ----I---------R---------------Q-------------------------------------------------------------

hCHML  ESSCTTIDGLNATKNFLQCLGRFGNTPFLFPLYGQGEIPQGFCRMCAVFGGIYCLRHKVQCFVVDKESGRCKAIIDHFGQRINAKYFIVE 437
mCHM   -TTSS-V---K---K-------Y-------------L--C----------------S---L------RK----V-Q-----IS-H-VI- 374
hCHM   -TASS-----K------H----Y-------------L--C----------------S---L------RK------Q-----ISEH-L-- 201

hCHML  DSYLSEETCSNVQYKQISRAVLITDQSILKTDLDQQTSILIVPPAEPGACAVRVTELCSSTMTCMKDTYLVHLTCSSSKTAREDLESVVK 527
mCHM   ------N---G---R----------G-V--P-S---V---T--AE-S-SF----I-----------G--------M----------R--Q 464
hCHM   ---FP-NM--R---R----------R-V----S---I---T--AE---TF----I-----------G--------T-------------Q 291

hCHML  KLFTPYTETEINEEELTKPRLLWALYFNMRDSSGISRSSYNGLPSNVYVCSGPDCGLGNEHAVKQAETLFQEIFPTEEFCPPPPNPEDII 617
mCHM   --------I-AEN-QVE---I------------D---DC--D-------------N---DN--Q---IV--K-C-N-D---A-------- 554
hCHM   ---V----M--EN-QVE---I------------D----C--D------------------DN------------C-N-D------------ 381

hCHML  FDGDDKQPEAPGTNNVVMAKLESSEESKNLESPEKHLQN 656
mCHM   L---SS-Q-VSESSVIPETNS-TPK--TV-GDS-EPSE  592
hCHM   L---SL----SESSAIPE-NS-TFK--T--GNL-ESSE  419
```

FIG. 145-7 **Alignment of the human CHML amino acid sequence with mouse CHM and human CHM sequences. Dashes indicate identical amino acids residues. The numbers at the right correspond to the amino acid residues in the respective sequences.** *(Adapted from Cremers et al.[104] Used by permission of* **Human Molecular Genetics.***)*

When a fetal brain cDNA library was probed with a murine CHM cDNA clone, four partly overlapping recombinant phages were identified whose sequence differed from those of the human CHM cDNA consensus. The consensus cDNA of this CHML gene encodes 656 amino acids. Alignment of this sequence with the human CHM consensus cDNA revealed 76 percent amino acid identity and 95 percent similarity; 80 percent of the respective nucleotide sequences are identical (Fig. 145-7). Like the CHM gene, CHML is expressed in a wide variety of tissues though generally at a lower level (Cremers FPM, et al.: unpublished observations).

Hybridization of human CHML cDNA clones to a DNA panel from 32 human rodent somatic-cell hybrids revealed that the human CHML gene resides on chromosome 1. Subsequent experiments with somatic-cell hybrids carrying defined chromosome 1 segments assigned this gene to the q42-qter segment on the distal long arm of chromosome 1[104] (and unpublished results). Linkage studies have mapped the gene for the clinically milder variant of Usher syndrome, USH2, to the same region.[105,106] Like CHM, Usher syndrome is characterized by retinal degeneration, with sensorineural deafness as an additional clinical feature and is inherited as an autosomal recessive trait. The chromosomal colocalization of the USH2 locus and the CHML gene, as well as the clinical similarity between CHM and Usher syndrome rendered the CHML gene a promising candidate for this disorder. To substantiate this hypothesis, 10 patients with USH2 were screened for point mutations in the CHML gene by making use of the SSCP technique and direct sequencing (van de Pol et al.: unpublished observations). So far, however, mutations have not been found yet.

FUNCTION OF THE CHOROIDEREMIA GENE

Initially, nucleotide and amino acid sequence comparisons had failed to detect significant homologies between the CHM gene or its deduced gene product and known genes and proteins. Therefore, Cremers et al.[97] concluded that the CHM gene had a "novel" function. Because of a so-called PEST sequence in the C-terminal portion of the gene product—a conspicuous clustering of the amino acids proline (P), glutamic acid (E), serine (S), and threonine (T) which is indicative for rapid protein turnover[107,108]—these authors speculated that the CHM gene may have a regulatory role. Shortly afterward, Fodor et al.[109] observed striking similarities between a segment of the deduced CHM gene product and a protein isolated from bovine brain which inhibits the dissociation of GDP from the Ras-like small GTP-binding protein, Rab3A.[110] These findings were confirmed by Cremers et al.,[104] who found a second region of homology between the Rab3A GDP dissociation inhibitor (GDI) and the product of the CHML gene (Fig. 145-8). To rule out the possibility that Rab3A GDI is the bovine counterpart of the human CHM or CHML genes, a bovine Rab3A GDI-cDNA was used as a probe to map the corresponding human gene on a panel of human–rodent somatic-cell hybrids. Like CHM, the Rab3A GDI gene was found to be located on the X chromosome, but subsequent analyses assigned the human GDI gene to the distal long arm of the X (Cremers FPM, et al.: unpublished observation). These results indicate that Rab3A GDI and CHM are different genes.

Seabra et al.[111] have observed striking similarities between the deduced amino acid sequence of the CHM gene product and a subunit of a geranylgeranyl transferase (GGT), Rab-GGT, from rat brain. GGT have important roles in the covalent modification of eukaryotic membrane proteins. They attach geranylgeranyl groups in thioester linkage to cysteine residues near the C-terminus.[112,113] This modification facilitates proper binding to specific membranes and is essential for the activity of the relevant proteins. As shown by Seabra et al.[114] Rab-GGT from rat brain consists of two components, A and B, of 95 and 90 kDa, respectively. Tryptic digestion and amino acid sequencing have revealed that component A is closely related, and possibly homologous, to the deduced product of the CHM gene. Rab-GGT binds specifically to two Ras-like small GTP-binding proteins one of which, Rab3A, has been implicated in the regulation of synaptic vesicle transport in brain. The similarity between component A of Rab-GGT (CHM?) and Rab3A GDI may reflect the fact that these functionally different proteins bind to the same target molecule.

At this writing, there is still no final proof for the identity of Rab-GGT component A and CHM. Unresolved questions include the molecular weight of component A, which is larger than expected from the size of the murine CHM gene product, as well as the broad expression spectrums of Rab3A and Rab-GGT which are difficult to reconcile with the retina- and choroid-specific manifestation of CHM. Wieland et al.[115,116] have detected several small GTP-binding proteins in the retina, and at least one of these seems to be involved in the visual process. It is possible that this protein is another as yet unidentified target of Rab-GGT. Given the role of Rab3A in the control of synaptic vesicle transport, it is tempting to speculate that this protein, or Rab3A itself

```
          1

bGDI      MDE    EYDVIVLGTGLTECILSGIMSVNGKKVLHMDRNPYYGGESSSIT  PLEELYKRFQL--//--RGRDWNVDLIPKFLMANGQL  87
hCHML     MADNLPTEFDVVIIGTGLPESILAAACSRSGQRVLHIDSRSYYGGNWASFSFSGLLSWLKEYQQ--//--EGRRFNIDLVSKLLYSQGLL 244
          *..    *.**...****.*.**..  * .*..***.*...****. .*..    * .  * .*          ** .*.**..*.* ..* *

bGDI      VKMLLYTEVTRYLDFKVVEGSFVYKGGKIYKVPSTETEALASNLMGMFEKRRFRKFLVFVANFDENDPKTFEGVDPQNTSMRDVYRKFDL 177
hCHML     IDLLIKSDVSRYVEFKNVTRILAFREGKVEQVPCSRADVFNSKELTMVEKRMLMKFLTFCLEYEQH PDEYQAF  RQCSFSEYLKTKKL 331
          ...*. ..*.**..** *. .....**. .**.. .....*. ..* ***...***.*  ..... *.....   .. *...  .. .*

bGDI      GQDVIDFTGHALALYRTDDYLDQPCLETINRIKLYSESLARYGKSPYLYPLYGLGELPQGFARLSAIYGGTYMLNKPVDDIIM  ENGKV 265
hCHML     TPNLQHFVLHSIAMTSESSC   TTIDGLNATKNFLQCLGRFGNTPFLFPLYGQGEIPQGFCRMCAVFGGIYCLRHKVQCFVVDKESGRC 418
          .... .*. *..*. .....   . ....* .* . ..*.*.*..*.*.**** **.**** *..*..**.* *.. *. ...  *.*.

bGDI      VGVKSE GEVARCKQLICDPSYVPDRVRKAGQ   VIRIICILSHPIKNTN DANSCQIIIPQNQVNRKSDIYVCMISYAHNVAAQGKYI 350
hCHML     KAIIDHFGQRINAKYFIVEDSYLSEETCSNVQYKQISRAVLITDQSILKTDLDQQTSILIVPPAEPG ACAVRVTELCSSTMTCMKDTYL 507
           .. .. *.  . * .* . **... . .. *   . * . * ...* .*. *.... .*.*... .   ... *   .. . ..  ...*.
```

FIG. 145-8 Comparison of part of hCHML with part of the bovine Rab3A GDI amino acid sequence.[110] Asterisks and dots below the aligned sequences indicate identical and similar positions, respectively. The regions that display the highest homology with Rab3A GDI are underlined. *(From Cremers et al.[104] Used by permission of* Human Molecular Genetics.*)*

(Seabra et al.[111]), is involved in the shedding of photoreceptor outer-segment disk and that the product of the CHM gene somehow regulates this process. This would be in keeping with the observation that the first lesions in choroideremia occur in the vicinity of the retinal pigment epithelium.

Other open questions concern the function of the CHML gene and its remarkable structural similarity to CHM. The CHML gene is nearly devoid of introns which may indicate that this gene originates from an (evolutionarily recent?) retrotransposition event. Thus, its function may not differ from that of the CHM gene, and it is possible that in patients with CHM, the course of the disease is modulated by its activity. Indeed, this may explain the conspicuous absence of symptoms in a patient with a large Xq21 deletion encompassing the entire CHM gene.[90,117] Current efforts aimed at the identification of the CHML gene in other mammals; the subcellular distribution of Rab-GGT, Rab3A, and other small GTP-binding proteins in the eye; and biochemical studies should soon shed more light on these issues. These studies should also deepen our insight into the feasibility of therapy.

ACKNOWLEDGMENTS

We thank Drs. E.M. Bleeker-Wagemakers and M. Warburg for critically reading this manuscript. Our studies were supported by the Deutsche Forschungsgemeinschaft, the British Pigmentosa Society, and the Netherlands Organization for Scientific Research (NWO). FPMC is a recipient of a career development award from the Royal Dutch Academy of Arts and Sciences.

ADDENDUM

Three recent articles have shed more light on the structure and function of the choroideremia gene and its product. By cloning and sequencing of the cDNA for component A of rat Rab geranylgeranyl transferase, Andres et al. have confirmed its identity with the human choroideremia gene product and its resemblance to Rab3A GDI.[118] In biochemical assays they also demonstrate that component A binds unprenylated Rab 1A, presents it to the catalytic component B and remains bound to the Rab molecule after the geranylgeranyl transfer reaction. Because component A escorts Rab proteins through the prenyl transfer reaction, Andres et al. have suggested renaming it Rab escort protein (REP). The apparent discrepancy between the size of the rat component A (REP-1) and the murine CHM protein could be resolved by DNA sequencing of the murine CHM gene (Cremers et al., unpublished). The murine CHM protein consists of 665 amino acids, the rat REP-1 protein is 650 amino acids long. In lymphoblastoid cells derived from patients with choroideremia, the activity of component A was markedly decreased but not completely absent,[119] in contrast with component B now renamed Rab GGT, which was normal. The deficiency of component A was more pronounced when using Rab3A instead of Rab1A as a substrate. As shown by Cremers et al.,[120] the residual activity of component A in patients lacking the choroideremia (REP-1) gene may be due to the function of the autosomal REP-2 (= CHML) gene. Rat REP-1 and human REP-2, synthesized in vitro, are approximately equivalent in facilitating the attachment of geranylgeranyl groups to different Rab proteins including Rab1A, Rab5A, and Rab6. With Rab3A and Rab3D as substrates, however, the activity of REP-2 was approximately 4 times lower than that of REP-1. Thus it appears that REP-2 can at least partially substitute for REP-1. Differential tissue distributions of these proteins, i.e., a reduced activity of REP-2 in ocular tissues, may explain why in patients with choroideremia clinical symptoms are confined to the eye.

REFERENCES

1. Mauthner H: Ein Fall von Chorioideremia. *Berl Naturw-med Ver Innsbruck* **2**:191, 1872.
2. Pöllot W: Atypische chorioretinitis pigmentosa hereditaria. *Albrecht von Graefes Arch Ophthalmol* **80**:379, 1912.
3. Usher CH: Choroideremia. (The VI Bowman lecture on a few hereditary affections). *Trans Ophthalmol Soc UK* **55**:164, 1935.
4. Bedell AJ: Choroideremia. *Arch Ophthalmol* **17**:444, 1937.
5. Schutzbach M: Über erbliche Aderhaut-Netzhaut-erkrankung. *Graefes Arch Ophthalmol* **138**:315, 1938.
6. Friedman B: Choroideremia. *Arch Ophthalmol* **23**:1285, 1940.
7. Scobee R: Choroideremia. The nature of the condition and case reports. *Am J Ophthalmol* **26**:1135, 1943.
8. McCulloch C, McCulloch RJP: A hereditary and clinical study of choroideremia. *Trans Am Acad Ophthalmol Otolaryngol* **52**:160, 1948.
9. Waardenburg PJ: Chorioideremie als Erbmerkmal. *Acta Ophthalmol (Copenh)* **20**:235, 1942.
10. Goedbloed J: Mode of inheritance in choroideremia. *Ophthalmologica* **104**:308, 1942.
11. McCulloch JC: Choroideremia: A clinical and pathologic review. *Trans Am Ophthalmol Soc* **67**:142, 1969.
12. Sorsby A, Franceschetti A, Joseph R, Davey JB: Choroideremia: Clinical and genetic aspects. *Br J Ophthalmol* **36**:547, 1952.
13. Kurstjens JH: Choroideremia and gyrate atrophy of the choroid and retina. *Doc Ophthalmol* **19**:1, 1965.
14. Krill AE: *Krill's Hereditary Retinal and Choroidal Diseases*. Hagerstown, MD, Harper & Row, 1977, vol 2 (Clinical Characteristics).
15. Kärnä J: Choroideremia: A clinical and genetic study of 84 Finnish patients and 126 female carriers. *Acta Ophthalmol Suppl (Copenh)* **176**:1, 1986.
16. François J: Choroideremia (progressive chorioretinal degeneration). *Int Ophthalmol Clin* **8**:949, 1968.
17. Murdoch JL: Choroideremia. *Birth Defects* **7(3)**:196, 1971.
18. Shapiro I, Gorlin RJ: X-linked choroidal sclerosis. A stage of choroideremia. *Minn Med* **57**:259, 1974.
19. Hammerstein W, Bischof G, Leide E: Chorioideremie im Kindesalter. *Klin Monatsbl Augenheilkd* **174**:599, 1979.
20. Magder H: Choroideremia. Report of a case. *Arch Ophthalmol* **33**:468, 1945.
21. Pameyer JK, Waardenburg PJ, Henkes HE: Choroideremia. *Br J Ophthalmol* **44**:724, 1960.
22. Rubin ML, Fishman RS, McKay RA: Choroideremia. Study of a family and literature review. *Arch Ophthalmol* **76**:563, 1966.
23. Jaeger W, Grützner P: Der Funktionsverfall bei progressiver tapeto-chorioidaler Degeneration (Chorioideremie). *Ophthalmologica* **143**:305, 1962.
24. Spear D, Stephens FE: Choroideremia, its inheritance in a family. *Trans Pacif Coast Oto-Ophthalmol Soc* **33**:215, 1952.
25. Takki K: Differential diagnosis between the primary total choroidal vascular atrophies. *Br J Ophthalmol* **58**:24, 1974.
26. Jacobson J, Stephens G: Hereditary choroidoretinal degeneration. Study of a family including electroretinography and adaptometry. *Arch Ophthalmol* **67**:321, 1962.
27. Fouanon C: La choroidérémie. Thesis. Université de Nantes, 1971.
28. Krill AE, Archer D: Classification of the choroidal atrophies. *Am J Ophthalmol* **72**:562, 1971.
29. Noble KG, Carr RE, Siegel IM: Fluorescein angiography of the hereditary choroidal dystrophies. *Br J Ophthalmol* **61**:43, 1977.

30. Sieving PA, Niffenegger JH, Berson JL: Electroretinographic findings in selected pedigrees with choroideremia. *Am J Ophthalmol* **101**:361, 1986.
31. Waardenburg PJ: Observations in choroideremia and in the female carrier of the disease. *Acta 18 Conc Ophthalmol Belge* **2**:1578, 1958.
32. Franceschetti A, François J, Babel L: *Les Héredodégénérescences Chorio-Rétiniennes*. Paris, Masson, 1963.
33. François J, De Bradendere J, Stockmans L: Choroidéremie (Dégénérescence chorio-rétinienne progressive). *Bull Soc Belge Ophtalmol* **146**:384, 1967.
34. Schmöger E, Busch I, Lukassek B: Histologischer Beitrag zur Chorioideremie. *Ophthalmologica* **166**:144, 1973.
35. Krill AE, Newell FW, Chishti MI: Fluorescein studies in diseases affecting the retinal pigment epithelium. *Am J Ophthalmol* **66**:470, 1968.
36. McCulloch JC: The pathological findings in two cases of choroideremia. *Trans Am Acad Ophthalmol Otolaryngol* **50**:565, 1950.
37. Grützner P, Vogel MH: Klinischer Verlauf und histologischer Befund bei progressiver tapeto-chorioidealer Degeneration (Chorioideremia). *Klin Monatsbl Augenheilkd* **162**:206, 1973.
38. Ghosh M, McCulloch JC: Pathological findings from two cases of choroideremia. *Can J Ophthalmol* **15**:147, 1980.
39. Fraser GRF, Friedmann AI: Choroideremia in a female. *Br Med J* **2**:732, 1968.
40. Harris GS, Miller JR: Choroideremia. Visual defects in a heterozygote. *Arch Ophthalmol* **80**:423, 1968.
41. Lyon MF: Sex chromatin and gene action in the mammalian X-chromosome. *Am J Hum Genet* **14**:135, 1962.
42. Grimsdale H: Unusual condition of choroid (congenital?). *Proc R Soc Med* **10**:29, 1917.
43. Shapira TM, Sitney JM: Choroideremia. *Am J Ophthalmol* **26**:182, 1943.
44. Kaplan J, Gilgenkrantz S, Dufier JL, Frézal J: Choroideremia and ovarian dysgenesis associated with an X;7 de novo balanced translocation. Human Gene Mapping 10: Tenth International Workshop on Human Gene Mapping. *Cytogenet Cell Genet* **51**:1022, 1989.
45. Siu VM, Gonder JR, Jung JH, Sergovich FR, Flintoff WF: Choroideremia associated with an X-autosomal translocation. *Hum Genet* **84**:459, 1990.
46. Dachevzkaya NP, Polonsky BZ: Two cases of choroideremia. *Vestn Oftalmol* **83**:89, 1970.
47. Valk LEM, Binkhorst PG: A case of familial dwarfism with choroideremia, myopia, posterior polar cataract, and zonular cataract. *Ophthalmologica* **132**:299, 1956.
48. Van den Bosch J: A new syndrome in three generations of a Dutch family. *Ophthalmologica* **137**:422, 1959.
49. Judisch GF, Lowry RB, Hanson JW, McGillivary BC: Chorioretinopathy and pituitary dysfunction. The CPD syndrome. *Arch Ophthalmol* **99**:253, 1981.
50. Menon RK, Ball WS, Sperling MA: Choroideremia and hypopituitarism: An association. *Am J Med Genet* **34**:511, 1989.
51. Trijbels JMF, Sengers RCA, Bakkeren JAJM, De Kort AFM, Deutman AF: L-ornithine-ketoacid-transferase deficiency in cultured fibroblasts of a patient with hyperornithinemia and gyrate atrophy of the choroid and retina. *Clin Chim Acta* **79**:371, 1977.
52. O'Donnel JJ, Sandman RP, Martin SR: Gyrate atrophy of the retina: Inborn error of L-ornithine: 2-oxoacid aminotransferase. *Science* **200**:200, 1978.
53. Heckenlively JR: *Retinitis Pigmentosa*. Philadelphia, Lippincott, 1988.
54. Welch RB: Bietti's tapetoretinal degeneration with marginal corneal dystrophy: Crystalline retinopathy. *Trans Am Ophthalmol Soc* **75**:164, 1977.
55. Meredith TA, Aaberg TM, Willerson WD: Progressive chorioretinopathy after receiving thioridazine. *Arch Ophthalmol* **96**:1172, 1978.
56. Herzberg NH, van Schooneveld MJ, Bleeker-Wagemakers E, Zwart R, Cremers FPM, van der Knaap MS, Bolhuis PA, de Visser M: Kearns-Sayre syndrome with a phenocopy of choroideremia instead of pigmentary retinopathy. *Neurology* **43**:218, 1993.
57. Other A: Choroideremia and the Xg blood group. *Acta Ophthalmol (Copenh)* **46**:79, 1968.
58. Bell AG, McCulloch JC: Choroideremia and the Xg locus: Another look for linkage. *Clin Genet* **2**:239, 1971.
59. Eriksson AW, Eskola MR, Forsius HR, Frants RR, Kärnä J, Sanger R: X-chromosomal intermediate choroideremia and uveal coloboma in a family: Interrelation and linkage studies. *Clin Genet* **10**:355, 1976.
60. Dreisler E, Warburg M: Xg and X-chromosome mapping, in Race RR, Sanger R (eds): *Blood Groups in Man*. Oxford, Blackwell, 1975.
61. Nussbaum RL, Lewis RA, Lesko JG, Ferrell R: Choroideremia is linked to the restriction fragment length polymorphism DXYS1 at Xq13-21. *Am J Hum Genet* **37**:473, 1985.
62. Sankila E-M, De la Chapelle A, Kärnä J, Forsius H, Frants R, Eriksson A: Choroideremia: Close linkage to DXYS1 and DXYS12 demonstrated by segregation analysis and historical-genealogical evidence. *Clin Genet* **31**:315, 1987.
63. Jay M, Wright AF, Clayton JF, Deans M, Dempster M, Bhattacharya SS, Jay B: A genetic linkage study of choroideremia. *Ophthalmic Paediatr Genet* **7**:201, 1986.
64. Schwartz M, Rosenberg T, Niebuhr E, Lundsteen C, Sardemann H, Andersen O, Yang H-M, Lamm LU: Choroideremia; further evidence for assignment of the locus to Xq13-Xq21. *Hum Genet* **74**:449, 1986.
65. Schwarz M, Rosenberg T, Page DC: Linkage analysis between choroideremia (TCD) and flanking polymorphic X chromosomal probes. *Cytogenet Cell Genet* **46**:689, 1987. (abstr.)
66. Lesko JG, Lewis RA, Nussbaum RL: Multipoint linkage analysis of loci in the proximal long arm of the human X chromosome: Application to mapping the choroideremia locus. *Am J Hum Genet* **40**:303, 1987.
67. MacDonald IM, Sandre RM, Wong P, Hunter AGW, Tenniswood MPR: Linkage relationships of X-linked choroideremia to DXYS1 and DXS3. *Hum Genet* **77**:233, 1987.
68. Uhlhaas S, Neugebauer M, van Schoonefeld M, Bleeker-Wagemakers E, Szabo P, Gal A: Multipoint linkage analysis in choroideremia. *Cytogenet Cell Genet* **46**:707, 1987. (abstr.)
69. Wright AF, Nussbaum RL, Bhattacharya SS, Jay M, Lesko JG, Evans HJ, Jay B: Linkage studies and deletion screening in choroideremia. *J Med Genet* **27**:496, 1990.
70. Sankila E-M, Lehner T, Eriksson AW, Forsius H, Kärnä J, Page D, Ott J, De la Chapelle A: Haplotype and multipoint linkage analysis in Finnish choroideremia families. *Hum Genet* **84**:66, 1989.
71. Cremers FPM, Van de Pol TJR, Wieringa B, Collins FS, Sankila E-M, Siu VM, Flintoff WF, Brunsmann F, Blonden LAJ, Ropers H-H: Chromosomal jumping from the DXS165 locus allows molecular characterization of four microdeletions and a de novo chromosome X/13 translocation associated with choroideremia. *Proc Natl Acad Sci USA* **86**:7510, 1989.
72. Merry DE, Lesko JG, Sosnoski DM, Lewis RA, Lubinsky M, Trask B, Van den Engh G, Collins FS, Nussbaum RL: Choroideremia and deafness with stapes fixation: A contiguous gene deletion syndrome in Xq21. *Am J Hum Genet* **45**:530, 1989.
73. Sankila E-M, Sistonen P, Cremers FPM, De la Chapelle A: Choroideremia: Linkage analysis with physically mapped close DNA-markers. *Hum Genet* **87**:348, 1991.
74. Van de Pol TJR, Cremers FPM, Brohet RM, Wieringa B, Ropers H-H: Derivation of clones from the choroideremia locus by preparative field inversion gel electrophoresis. *Nucleic Acids Res* **18**:725, 1990.
75. Tabor A, Andersen O, Lundsteen C, Niebuhr E, Sardemann H: Interstitial deletion in the "critical region" of the long arm of the X chromosome in a mentally retarded boy and his normal mother. *Hum Genet* **64**:196, 1983.
76. Rosenberg T, Schwartz M, Niebuhr E, Yang H-M, Sardemann H, Andersen O, Lundsteen C: Choroideremia in interstitial deletion of the X chromosome. *Ophthalmic Paediatr Genet* **7**:205, 1986.
77. Rosenberg T, Niebuhr E, Yang H-M, Parving A, Schwartz M: Choroideremia, congenital deafness and mental

retardation in a family with an X chromosomal deletion. *Ophthalmic Paediatr Genet* **8**:139, 1987.

78. Moore GE, Ivens A, Chambers J, Farrall M, Williamson R, Page DC, Bjornsson A, Arnason A, Jensson O: Linkage of an X-chromosome cleft palate gene. *Nature* **326**:91, 1987.
79. Brunner HG, Van Bennekom CA, Lambermon EMM, Oei TL, Cremers CWRJ, Wieringa B, Ropers H-H: The gene for X-linked progressive mixed deafness with perilymphatic gusher during stapes surgery (DFN3) is linked to PGK. *Hum Genet* **80**:337, 1988.
80. Wallis C, Ballo R, Wallis P, Beighton P, Goldblatt J: X-linked mixed deafness with stapes fixation in a mauritian kindred: Linkage to Xq probe pDP34. *Genomics* **3**:299, 1988.
81. Gorski SM, Adams KJ, Birch PH, Friedman JM, Goodfellow PJ: The gene responsible for X-linked cleft palate (CPX) in a British Columbia native kindred is localized between PGK1 and DXYS1. *Am J Hum Genet* **50**:1129, 1992.
82. Hodgson SV, Robertson ME, Fear CN, Goodship J, Malcolm S, Jay B, Bobrow M, Pembrey ME: Prenatal diagnosis of X-linked choroideremia with mental retardation, associated with a cytologically detectable X-chromosome deletion. *Hum Genet* **75**:286, 1987.
83. Nussbaum RL, Lesko JG, Lewis RA, Ledbetter SA, Ledbetter DH: Isolation of anonymous DNA sequences from within a submicroscopic X chromosomal deletion in a patient with choroideremia, deafness, and mental retardation. *Proc Natl Acad Sci USA* **84**:6521, 1987.
84. Schwartz M, Yang H-M, Niebuhr E, Rosenberg T, Page DC: Regional localization of polymorphic DNA loci on the proximal long arm of the X chromosome using deletions associated with choroideremia. *Hum Genet* **78**:156, 1988.
85. Merry DE, Lesko JG, Siu VM, Flintoff WF, Collins FS, Lewis RA, Nussbaum RL: DXS165 detects a translocation breakpoint in a woman with choroideremia and a de novo X;13 translocation. *Genomics* **6**:609, 1990.
86. Yang H-M, Lund T, Niebuhr E, Nørby S, Schwartz M, Shen L: A deletion panel of the long arm of the X chromosome: Subregional localization of 22 DNA probes. *Hum Genet* **85**:25, 1990.
87. Wells S, Mould S, Robins D, Robinson D, Jacobs P: Molecular and cytogenetic analysis of a familial microdeletion of Xq. *J Med Genet* **28**:163, 1991.
88. Bach I, Robinson D, Thomas N, Ropers H-H, Cremers FPM: Physical fine mapping of genes underlying X-linked deafness and non fra(X)-X-linked mental retardation at Xq21. *Hum Genet* **89**:620, 1992.
89. Ayazi S: Choroideremia, obesity and congenital deafness. *Am J Ophthalmol* **92**:63, 1981.
90. Cremers FPM, Van de Pol TJR, Diergaarde PJ, Wieringa B, Nussbaum RL, Schwarz M, Ropers H-H: Physical fine mapping of the choroideremia locus using Xq21 deletions associated with complex syndromes. *Genomics* **4**:41, 1989.
91. Cremers FPM, Brunsmann F, Van de Pol TJR, Pawlowitzki IH, Paulsen K, Wieringa B, Ropers H-H: Deletion of the DXS165 locus in patients with classical choroideremia. *Clin Genet* **32**:421, 1987.
92. Cremers FPM, Sankila E-M, Brunsmann F, Jay M, Jay B, Wright A, Pinckers AJLG, Schwartz M, Van de Pol TJR, Wieringa B, De la Chapelle A, Pawlowitzki IH, Ropers H-H: Deletions in patients with classical choroideremia vary in size from 45kb to several megabases. *Am J Hum Genet* **47**:622, 1990.
93. Cremers FPM, Brunsmann F, Berger W, Van Kerkhoff EPM, Van de Pol TJR, Wieringa B, Pawlowitzki IH, Ropers H-H: Cloning of the breakpoints of a deletion associated with choroideremia. *Hum Genet* **86**:61, 1990.
94. Teboul M, Mujica P, Chery M, Leotard B, Gilgenkrantz S: Translocations X-autosomes équilibrées et retard mental. Contribution à la cartographie des retards mentaux liés à L'X (à l'exclusion de L'X-FRA). *J Genet Hum* **37**:179, 1989.
95. Merry DE, Jänne PA, Landers JE, Lewis RA, Nussbaum RL: Isolation of a candidate gene for choroideremia. *Proc Natl Acad Sci USA* **89**:2135, 1992.
96. Nathans J, Thomas D, Hogness DS: Molecular genetics of human color vision: The genes encoding blue, green, and red pigments. *Science* **232**:193, 1986.
97. Cremers FPM, Van de Pol TJR, Kerkhoff LPM, Wieringa B, Ropers H-H: Cloning of a gene that is rearranged in patients with choroideraemia. *Nature* **347**:674, 1990.
98. Van den Hurk JAJM, Van de Pol TJR, Molloy CM, Brunsmann F, Rüther K, Zrenner E, Pinckers AJLG, Pawlowitzki IH, Bleeker-Wagemakers E, Wieringa B, Ropers H-H, Cremers FPM: Detection and characterization of point mutations in the choroideremia candidate gene by PCR-SSCP analysis and direct DNA sequencing. *Am J Hum Genet* **50**:1195, 1992.
99. Sankila E-M, Tolvanen R, Van den Hurk JAJM, Cremers FPM, De la Chapelle A: Aberrant splicing of the CHM gene is a significant cause of choroideremia. *Nature Genet* **1**:109, 1992.
100. Orita M, Iwahana H, Kanazawa H, Hayashi K, Sekiya T: Detection of polymorphisms of human DNA by gel electrophoresis as single-strand conformation polymorphisms. *Proc Natl Acad Sci USA* **86**:2766, 1989.
101. Michaud J, Brody LC, Steel G, Fontaine G, Martin LS, Valle D, Mitchell G: Strand-separating conformational polymorphism analysis: Efficacy of detection of point mutations in the human ornithine δ-aminotransferase gene. *Genomics* **13**:389, 1992.
102. Sankila E-M: Choroideremia. A genetic and molecular study. Thesis. Department of Medical Genetics, University of Helsinki, Helsinki, 1991.
103. Molloy CM, Van de Pol TJR, Brohet RM, Ropers H-H, Cremers FPM: Three RFLPs for pZ11 (DXS540) in the choroideremia gene at Xq21.2. *Nucleic Acids Res* **20**:1434, 1992.
104. Cremers FPM, Molloy CM, Van de Pol TJR, Van den Hurk JAJM, Bach I, Geurts van Kessel AHM, Ropers H-H: An autosomal homologue of the choroideremia gene colocalizes with the usher syndrome type II locus on the distal part of chromosome 1q. *Hum Mol Genet* **1**:71, 1992.
105. Kimberling WJ, Weston MD, Möller C, Davenport SLH, Shugart YY, Priluck IA, Martini A, Milani M, Smith RJ: Localization of Usher syndrome type II to chromosome 1q. *Genomics* **7**:245, 1990.
106. Lewis RA, Otterud B, Stauffer D, Lalouel J-M, Leppert M: Mapping recessive ophthalmic diseases: Linkage of the locus for Usher syndrome type II to a DNA marker on chromosome 1q. *Genomics* **7**:250, 1990.
107. Rogers S, Wells R, Rechsteiner M: Amino acids sequences common to rapidly degraded proteins: The PEST hypothesis. *Science* **234**:364, 1986.
108. Rechsteiner M, Rogers S, Rote K: Protein structure and intracellular stability. *Trends Biochem Sci* **12**:390, 1987.
109. Fodor E, Lee RT, O'Donnell JJ: Analysis of choroideraemia gene. *Nature* **351**:614, 1991.
110. Matsui Y, Kikuchi A, Araki S, Hata Y, Kondo J, Teranishi Y, Takai Y: Molecular cloning and characterization of a novel type of regulatory protein (GDI) for smg p25A, a ras p21-like GTP-binding protein. *Mol Cell Biol* **10**:4116, 1990.
111. Seabra MC, Brown MS, Slaughter CA, Südhof TC, Goldstein JL: Purification of component A of rab geranylgeranyl transferase: Apparent identity with the choroideremia gene product. *Cell* **70**:1049, 1992.
112. Rilling HC, Breunger E, Epstein WW, Crain PF: Prenylated proteins: The structure of the isoprenoid group. *Science* **247**:318, 1990.
113. Farnsworth CC, Gelb MH, Glomset JA: Identification of geranylgeranyl-modified proteins in HeLa cells. *Science* **247**:320, 1990.
114. Seabra MC, Goldstein JL, Südhof TC, Brown MS: Rab geranylgeranyl transferase: A multisubunit enzyme that prenylates GTP-binding proteins terminating in Cys-X-Cys or CysCys. *J Biol Chem* **267**:14497, 1992.
115. Wieland T, Ulibarri I, Aktories K, Gierschik P, Jakobs KH: Interaction of small G proteins with photoexcited rhodopsin. *FEBS Lett* **263**:195, 1990.
116. Wieland T, Ulibarri I, Gierschik P, Hall A, Aktories K, Jakobs KH: Interaction of recombinant rho A GTP-

binding proteins with photoexcited rhodopsin. *FEBS Lett* **274**:111, 1990.

117. Cremers FPM, Van de Pol TJR, Wieringa B, Hofker MH, Pearson PL, Pfeiffer RA, Mikkelsen M, Tabor A, Ropers H-H: Molecular analysis of male-viable deletions and duplications allows ordering of 52 DNA probes on proximal Xq. *Am J Hum Genet* **43**:452, 1988.
118. Andres DA, Seabra MC, Brown MS, Armstrong SA, Smeland TE, Cremers FPM, Goldstein JL: cDNA cloning of component A of Rab geranylgeranyl transferase and demonstration of its role as a Rab escort protein. *Cell* **73**:1091, 1993.
119. Seabra MC, Brown MS, Goldstein JL: Retinal degeneration in choroideremia: deficiency of Rab geranylgeranyl transferase. *Science* **259**:377, 1993.
120. Cremers FPM, Armstrong SA, Seabra MC, Brown MS, Goldstein JL: REP-2, a Rab escort protein encoded by the choroideremia-like gene. *J Biol Chem* **269**:2111, 1994.

CHAPTER 146

Molecular Biology and Inherited Disorders of the Eye Lens

J. F. Hejtmancik ▪ M. I. Kaiser ▪ Joram Piatigorsky

1. **Cells of the eye lens are derived from the surface ectoderm and consist of a single cell type which, as they differentiate into fiber cells, lose their protein synthetic capabilities. In addition to cytoskeletal and membrane components, lens cells contain large amounts of structural proteins called "crystallins." Because proteins in the lens nucleus cannot be replaced, they must be stable in the face of oxidative and ultraviolet insults.**

2. **Lens crystallins, which are structural proteins contributing to lens transparency, comprise more than 90 percent of the soluble protein. Lenses of most species contain α-, β-, and γ-crystallins, also called "ubiquitous crystallins." α-Crystallins are heat-shock proteins also found in a variety of nonlens tissues. The β- and γ-crystallins form a superfamily similar to microbial stress proteins.**

3. **In addition to the ubiquitous crystallins, there are also proteins called "taxon-specific crystallins," which occur at a high concentration in the lens, but are present only in selected species. Many of the taxon-specific crystallins function as enzymes in nonlens tissues, where they are expressed at low concentrations. These enzyme crystallins seem to have arisen by a process called "gene sharing," in which a single gene may acquire more than one function in several tissues.**

4. **One requirement for a protein to function as a crystallin is the ability for it to be expressed at high levels in the lens. Transcriptional regulation, which is accomplished through a complex combination of *cis-* and *trans-*regulatory elements, appears to be very important for the high expression of crystallins in the lens.**

5. **Lens transparency also requires maintenance of a reduced state to minimize oxidative damage to crystallins and other proteins over their long lifetimes. To do this, the lens uses multiple mechanisms. The glutathione redox cycle is especially important. In addition, osmotic balance is critical for lens transparency, and the lens accomplishes this by a combination of active transport by the anterior cuboidal epithelia and an extensive array of communicating channels connecting lens fiber cells.**

6. **Animal models for human cataracts have contributed a great deal to our knowledge of this disease. The Philly mouse has autosomal dominant cataracts resulting from a 12-nucleotide deletion in the βB2-crystallin mRNA. Strain 13/N guinea pigs have autosomal dominant cataracts associated with a splicing defect in ζ-crystallin, which can also function as a quinone-reductase. The eye lens obsolescence (ELO)-mouse cataract involves the γ-crystallin gene cluster. In addition, mice transgenic for diphtheria toxin, ricin, vimentin, and granulocyte–macrophage colony-stimulating factor have been used to model cataracts.**

7. **In humans, many genes appear to be able to cause cataracts. Linkage studies have implicated loci on chromosomes 1, 2, and 16. In addition, cataracts can occur as part of many inherited and chromosomal syndromes.**

The eye lens transmits and focuses light onto the retina. Containing perhaps the highest concentration of proteins found in any tissue, the lens has been intensively studied for over a century. In 1833 Sir David Brewster deduced the fine structure of the cod lens, calculating that it contained 5 million fiber cells, each 4.8 μm, using only a candle and a finely ruled steel bar.[1] Study of lens biochemistry began in 1894 when Mörner described the high concentrations of heterogeneous structural proteins now known as crystallins.[2] A cataract locus was among the first autosomal loci to be mapped.[3] Thus, the lens has served as a model system for the advancement of developmental and structural biology as well as playing an important role in inherited diseases.

BIOLOGY OF THE LENS

At birth the human lens weighs about 65 mg, increasing to about 160 mg in the first decade of life and about 250 mg by 90 years of age.[4] In the crystallin lens, the proteins may reach 60 percent of the total tissue weight.[5]

Development

The human lens can first be detected at 3 to 4 weeks of gestation, in the 4-mm embryo.[6] It is derived from surface ectoderm which begins to thicken and forms the lens placode, then invaginates toward the developing optic cup to form the lens pit. The lens pit closes, and the resulting lens vesicle is pinched off from surface ectoderm.[6] Cells along the posterior layer of the optic vesicle elongate to fill the vesicle by the seventh week of development and become primary

A list of standard abbreviations is located immediately preceding the index in each volume. Additional abbreviations used in this chapter include: ELO = eye lens obsolescence; LOCS II = lens opacity classification system; LOP = mouse lens opacity gene; MP26 = intrinsic membrane protein 26; MP70 = intrinsic membrane protein 70; NCAM2 = neural cell adhesion maleable 2; tk = thymidine kinase.

fiber cells. These will eventually become the embryonic lens nucleus (the central nonnucleated fiber cells)[6] while the remaining cells become the cuboidal anterior epithelium, some of which will divide and differentiate to become secondary fibers[7] (Fig. 146-1).

The lens is surrounded by a collagenous capsule throughout life. The basal poles of the epithelial cells face anteriorly, resting on this capsule, while those of the fiber cells face posteriorly.[7] The epithelial cells are connected by gap junctions,[8] allowing exchange of low-molecular-weight metabolites and ions but have few or no tight junctions (zonula occludens) which would seal the extracellular spaces to low-molecular-weight proteins and ions.[9,10] Ultrastructurally, anterior cuboidal epithelial cells are rich in organelles and contain large amounts of actin, myosin, vimentin, microtubules, spectrin, and α-actinin, presumably to stabilize them during accommodation.[11–13] Both the anterior epithelial cells and fiber cells contain large amounts of crystallins.

Fiber cells make up the bulk of the lens. Nucleated fiber cells form a highly ordered concentric shell around the nonnucleated central fiber cells which make up the lens nucleus. There is little extracellular space between the fiber cells, which have many interdigitations.[7,14] Adjacent fiber cells are connected by many junctional complexes, which allow for passage of metabolites between cells.[12,13] The major soluble components of fiber cells are the lens crystallins, which make up about 90 percent of the water-soluble protein, and cytoskeletal components, including actin, myosin, vimentin, α-actinin, and microtubules.[11–18]

The lens has a single cell type which follows a regular developmental pattern throughout life, resulting in the lens architecture described above with a single layer of anterior epithelial cells overlaying the fiber cells wrapped onionlike around the lens nucleus.[14] There is a germinative zone just anterior to the equator, where most mitotic division occurs. The cells then move laterally toward the equator, where the anterior epithelial cells begin to form secondary fibers. The density of organelles, including the mitochondria, Golgi bodies, and both rough and smooth ER decreases in differentiating lens fiber cells. As the cells elongate they move toward the lens nucleus, inserting anteriorly beneath the cuboidal epithelial cells and posteriorly below the posterior capsule. During this process, it seems clear that transcriptional control plays a significant role in the differential synthesis of lens crystallins (see Piatigorsky[19]). The distribution of the β-crystallins in chickens[20,21] and the β- and γ-crystallins in rats[22–24] provide examples of the spatial and temporal control of crystallin gene expression during lens development.

The lens is surrounded by a transparent basement membrane called the "lens capsule"[25] which contributes to shaping the lens during accommodation.[26,27] The major components of the lens capsule are type IV collagen, laminin, entactin, heparin sulfate proteoglycan, and fibronectin.[28,29] The capsule has a uniform parallel alignment of filaments of varying thickness.[29] The lens capsule is produced anteriorly by the cuboidal epithelium and posteriorly by the fiber cells.[25] Growth of the capsule is slower at the posterior surface, where it remains thinner. In humans, the capsule is first detectable at 5 to 6 weeks of gestation[6] and continues to thicken throughout life.[26]

Aging

The lens is susceptible to damage with aging since its cells cannot be replaced in this encapsulated tissue and its proteins cannot turn over in the nonnucleated fiber cells. Not only does this result in a decrease in function of the normal aged lens, but it also sets the stage for development of senescent cataract in individuals with additional environmental insult or genetic proclivity. As the lens ages, vacuoles and multilamellar bodies appear between fiber cells, and occasionally the fiber plasma membrane is disrupted.[30] Most of the elaborate cytoskeletal structure of the lens cells disappears with aging,[13] and by the fifth decade the ability to accommodate is essentially lost.[32,33] There is a decrease in transparency of the normal lens with aging so that the intensity of light reaching the retina is reduced by about tenfold by 80 years of age.[34]

Enzymatic activity in the lens tends to decrease with age and to be lower in the central cells of the lens nucleus than in the cortical and anterior epithelial cells.[35] As the lens ages the Na^+ and Ca^{2+} concentrations rise, reflecting an increase in lens permeability or a decrease in pumping efficiency.[36] The crystallins also show age-related changes. There is an increase in high-molecular-weight aggregates and water-insoluble protein between 10 and 50 years of age, especially in the α-crystallins, but also in the β- and γ-crystallins.[37,38] There is also partial degradation of crystallins, membranes, and enzymes. An example is the nonenzymatic cleavage of αA-crystallin between Asn 101 and Glu 102.[39] With aging, both the N- and C-terminal arms of half of the intrinsic membrane protein (MP26) molecules undergo proteolysis to form MP22.[40] The lens contains neutral proteinase, also called the "multicatalytic–proteinase complex," which preferentially degrades oxidized proteins,[41,42] leucine aminopeptidase,[43] calpains,[44] and the protease cofactor ubiquitin.[45] The activity of these proteinases is controlled by inhibitors which appear to be concentrated at the periphery of the lens.

Aging also leads to covalent modifications of crystallins and other lens proteins, including an increase in disulfide bridges, deamidation of asparagine and glutamine residues,[43] and racemization of aspartic acid residues.[46] An aspartate residue in αA-crystallin appears especially susceptible because it easily forms a succinimide intermediate.[47] This may be associated with the nonenzymatic cleavage of α-crystallin mentioned above. Phosphorylation of lens proteins also occurs.[39,48] Nonenzymatic glycosylation (glycation) occurs, especially of the ε-amino groups of lysine.[49] Through the Maillard reaction, the glycation products can result in increased pigmentation, nontryptophan fluorescence, and nondisulfide covalent crosslinks.[50] Lens proteins can also undergo carbamylation, which can induce cataract,[51] and may be the mechanism for the association of cataract with chronic diarrhea and uremia.[52] γ-Crystallins, and especially γS-crystallin, are particularly susceptible to degradation and modification in age-dependent and other cataracts, largely being degraded to low-molecular-weight peptides by increased proteolysis in the cataractous lens.[43,53–56]

Transparency

The main functions of the lens are to transmit and focus light on the retina. In fact, about 80 percent of the refraction is performed by the cornea, and the lens serves to fine tune the focusing onto the retina. The young human lens is colorless, although a gradual increase in yellow pigmentation occurs with age.[57,58] The lens transmits very little light below 390 nm, but transmits light with wavelengths up to 1200 nm efficiently. This is well above the limit of visual perception (about 720 nm). Lens transparency results from tight packing of the proteins, resulting in a constant refractive index over

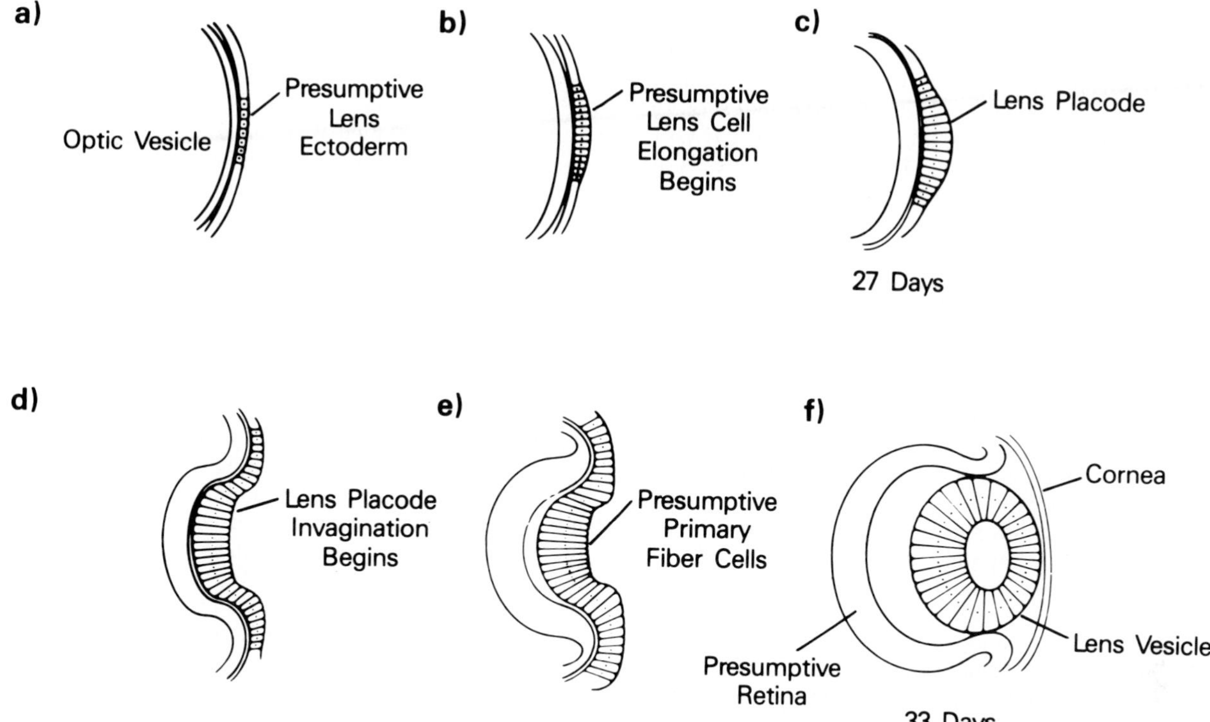

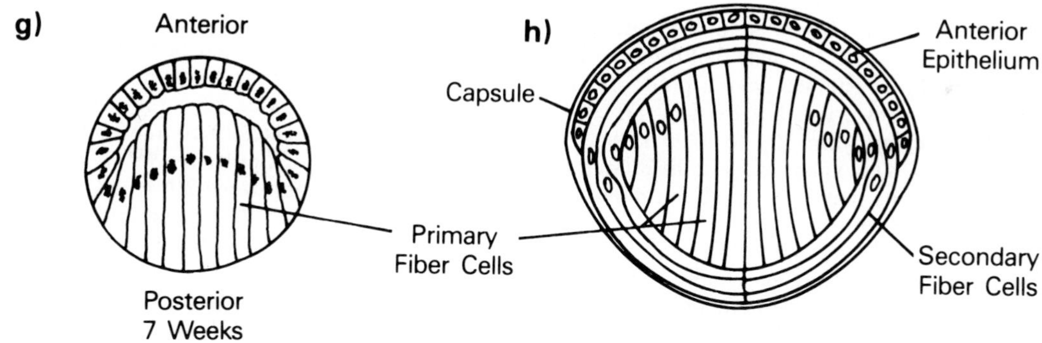

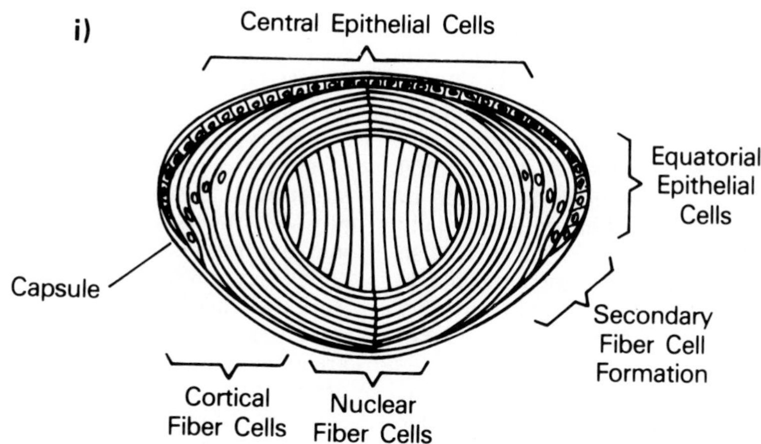

FIG. 146-1 Development and structure of the crystallin lens. Some parts of this figure are adapted from Fig. 1 of Piatigorsky,[453] indicating the conservation of developmental processes in the eye lens.

distances approximating the wavelength of light.[59,60] As the proteins are diluted to concentrations below 450 mg/ml, light scattering by lens proteins actually increases.[61,62] In addition, there is a gradual increase in the refractive index of the human lens from the cortex (1.38, 73 to 80 percent H_2O) to the nucleus (1.41, 68 percent H_2O), where there is an enrichment of tightly packed γ-crystallins.

MOLECULAR BIOLOGY OF THE LENS CRYSTALLINS

Crystallins make up more than 90 percent of the water-soluble protein, and are critical to lens function. They are most simply defined as proteins which are found in high concentration in the lens, fulfilling a structural role for transparency and refraction.[5] In 1894 Mörner first separated bovine lens proteins into three soluble and one insoluble fraction.[2] The soluble fractions represented the α-, β-, and γ-crystallins, which are found in all vertebrate lenses. In the mature human lens α-crystallin makes up 40 percent, β-crystallin 35 percent, and γ-crystallin 25 percent of total crystallin protein. The β- and γ-crystallins show sequence and tertiary structure homology, and form the βγ-superfamily (see below).

α-Crystallins

The α-crystallins are products of two similar genes, αA and αB. Human αA- and αB-crystallins have a 57 percent sequence similarity,[63–65] with αA-crystallin containing 173 and αB-crystallin 175 residues. Circular dichroism studies suggest that in solution α-crystallins have a predominantly β-sheet structure.[66] Native α-crystallins exist in the lens as globular aggregates ranging from 300 to 1200 kDa. Two models have been proposed to explain α-crystallin quaternary structure. The first suggests that the α-crystallin monomers are arranged in three concentric layers with αA-crystallin innermost and mixtures of αA- and αB-crystallins in the outer two layers.[67,68] A second model proposes that the α-crystallin aggregate behaves as a protein micelle.[69,70] The latter model seems more likely now, since it can be shown that αA and αB occupy equivalent and dynamic positions in the aggregate, with subunit exchange occurring easily.[70,71]

Both αA- and αB-crystallin have acetylated N-termini and are phosphorylated.[48] α-Crystallin is dephosphorylated by an enzyme related to calcineurin which is found in lens epithelial cells and at a low level in fiber cells.[72] It has been suggested that α-crystallin may be associated with cell membranes[73] or cytoskeletal elements.[74]

The α-crystallins are highly conserved through evolution. For example, the average rate of evolutionary change in αA-crystallin is a low 3 replacements per 100 residues per 100 million years.[75] α-Crystallins are evolutionarily related to the small heat-shock proteins of Drosophila, with especially close homology in the C-terminal half.[76] There is also similarity between α-crystallins and the egg antigen P40 from *Schistosoma mansoni*.[77] Thus, α-crystallin probably originated from the small heat-shock protein family.[5,78] Rodents[79–82] and some other mammals[82] have a second αA-crystallin protein containing an extra internal peptide as the result of alternative RNA splicing. The internal peptide (between amino acids 63 and 64 of the αA-crystallin chain) is encoded in a separate exon called the insert exon.[83] The αA^{ins} polypeptide is interchangeable with the αA and αB polypeptides in the α-crystallin aggregate.[71] Humans do not have the αA^{ins}-crystallin because the insert exon in the αA-crystallin gene is not utilized and has been inactivated by deletion of a base pair, becoming a "pseudo-exon."[84]

Studies have shown that the α-crystallins are not lens-specific. αB-crystallin is found in heart, lung, brain, skeletal muscle, kidney, and retina, although at lower levels than in the lens.[85,86] In the heart, αB-crystallin is found in aggregates of 400 to 650 kDa.[87,88] In skeletal muscle it accumulates in response stretching.[89] The brains of patients with Alexander disease accumulate αB-crystallin,[90] as do the brains of scrapie-infected hamsters.[91] αB-crystallin is also relatively abundant in fibroblasts from patients with Werner syndrome.[92] αB-crystallin is inducible by both heat[93] and osmotic shock[94] in cultured cells. αA-crystallin has been detected immunologically at low levels in many tissues and at moderate levels in spleen and thymus.[95] In the subterranean mole rat, which has nonfunctional eyes, αA-crystallin has undergone less evolutionary drift than might be expected, presumably because of a nonlens function, although its evolutionary rate is faster in the mole rat than in species which require lens transparency for vision.[96] Studies have shown that both αA- and αB-crystallin can function as molecular chaperones, and can protect both β and γ-crystallins and enzymes from thermal denaturation.[97] The chaperone function of the α-crystallins should serve to protect lens proteins from denaturing with age and probably explains their presence in nonlenticular tissues.

The structure of the duplicated αA- and αB-crystallin genes is highly conserved in all animals studied so far, except for the αA-crystallin insert exon, which is absent from some species.[5,83,98,99] There are three exons in both the αA- and αB-crystallin genes. When present, the insert exon of the αA gene is situated between exons 1 and 2.[81,83] The first exon codes for a twice repeated 30 amino acid motif, and the second and third exons contain sequences homologous to the small heat-shock proteins.[76,100] The human αA-crystallin gene maps to chromosome 21[81,101] and the αB-crystallin gene to chromosome 11.[102,103] Transcriptional activity of the αA-crystallin promoter has been extensively studied.[104] Sequences between bases −366 and +46 can initiate transcription of foreign genes introduced into transgenic mice in a lens-specific fashion,[105,106] with bases −88 to +46 being critical.[107]

γ-Crystallins

The β- and γ-crystallins are antigenically distinct, but are members of a related βγ-crystallin superfamily as determined by sequence similarities of 30 percent in aligned regions[108] and by tertiary structure.[109,110] The γ-crystallins have a molecular mass of about 21 kDa and show the highest symmetry of any crystallized protein, which may contribute to their high stability in the lens.[111,112] The first crystallin structure to be solved by high-resolution x-ray crystallography was γB-crystallin.[111,112] The 174 amino acids are arranged into four repeated segments called "Greek key" motifs. Each Greek key motif consists of an extremely stable, torqued β-pleated sheet resembling the characteristic pattern found on classical Greek pottery.[111] The first and second motifs are in the N-terminal domain and the third and fourth motifs are in the C-terminal domain of the protein (Fig. 146-2). More recently, the structure of γE-crystallin has been solved[113]; it is similar to that of γB-crystallin.

The γ-crystallins accumulate specifically in the lens fibers, and are the predominant crystallins in the lens nucleus,

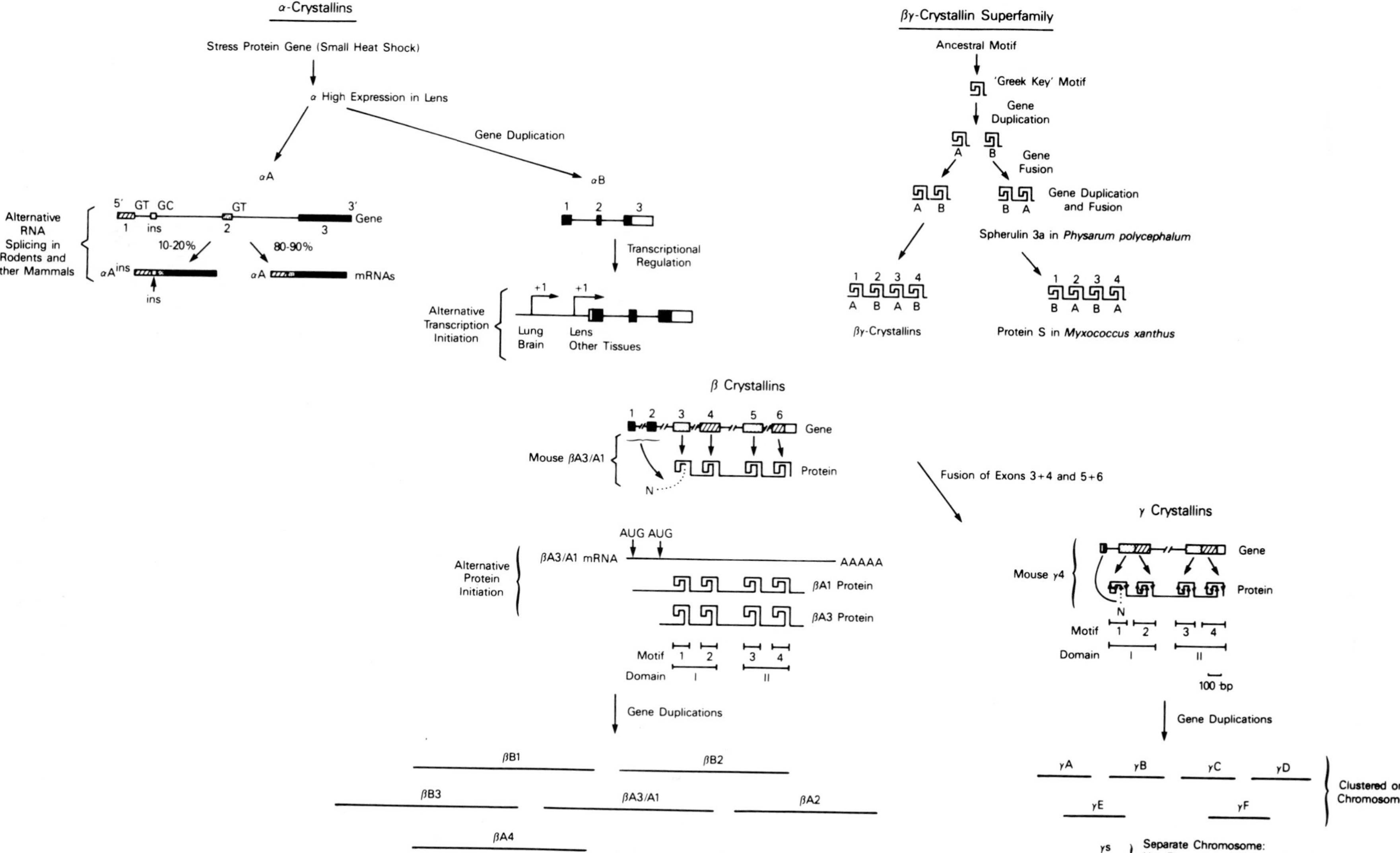

FIG. 146-2 Evolution of the ubiquitous α-, β-, and γ-crystallins and their structure. Details are described in the text. The α-crystallins are related to heat-shock proteins; the β- and γ-crystallins form a superfamily.

which maintains the highest protein concentration and is the hardest (most dehydrated) section of the lens. The γ-crystallins are abundant in almost all mammals, including humans, and species with hard lenses (such as fish and rodents) which lack the accommodative powers of the softer lenses found in birds and reptiles. Birds and reptiles, and other selected species throughout the vertebrates, use other proteins as their major crystallins in the lens nucleus (see below). Thus, γ-crystallins appear especially adapted for high-density molecular packing.[113] γ-Crystallins can be subdivided into two groups: γ^{ABC}- and γ^{DEF}-crystallins.[114,115] Proteins in the latter group have higher critical temperatures for phase separation and are largely responsible for the occurrence of the "cold cataract,"[116] a reversible opacity which occurs on cooling of the lens.

βγ-Crystallins appear distantly related to protein S, a sporulation-specific protein of the bacteria *Myxococcus xanthus,* and to spherulin 3a of the slime mold *Physarum polycephalum*.[117,118] A computer-generated model of spherulin 3a suggests that it can fold into two Greek key motifs. This would make it similar to a single domain of γ-crystallin, suggesting that evolution of the βγ superfamily originated from an ancestral gene coding for a single Greek key motif which, through successive gene duplication and fusion, gave rise to the complete βγ-crystallin structure. The order of the motifs is reversed in spherulin 3a relative to the βγ-crystallins. Protein S shows the typical fourfold repeated Greek key motifs, but as with spherulin 3a, the order of the motifs is the reverse of that in the βγ-crystallins, suggesting that divergence of these genes occurred before the initial fusion of the first two primitive motifs into a domain structure[117] (see Fig. 146-2). These microbial proteins can be induced by physiological stresses such as osmotic stress,[118] providing a functional parallel to the α-crystallins and some taxon-specific crystallins (see below).

γS-crystallin (formerly called βs), represents a link between the β- and γ-crystallins.[119–122] Many physical and chemical properties of the γS protein resemble those of β-crystallins. γS-crystallin is slightly larger than most γ-crystallins, having 177 residues including an N-terminal arm like the β-crystallins.[120] It also has a lower isoelectric point than most γ-crystallins, as do the β-crystallins. Moreover, in contrast to the N-termini of the γ-crystallins, γS has a blocked N-terminus, again like the β-crystallins. In humans, the γS-crystallin gene is on chromosome 3,[123] while all other γ-crystallin genes are clustered on chromosome 2q33-35.[124–126] Finally, γS-crystallin is expressed later in development than the other γ-crystallins, especially in the adult when expression of other γ-crystallins is low or has ceased,[127] and is expressed in birds and reptiles.[128,129] However, in contrast to the β-crystallins and like the other γ-crystallins, γS-crystallin exists in solution as a monomeric protein. It is especially important that the gene structure of γS-crystallin has three exons,[120,121] making it similar to the other γ-crystallins and distinctly different from the β-crystallins, which have six exons.[5,110]

All γ-crystallin genes have three exons (see Fig. 146-2). The first exon encodes the 5′ noncoding region and the first three amino acids, the second exon encodes the first (amino) domain consisting of the first and second Greek key motifs, and the third exon encodes the second (carboxy) domain consisting of Greek key motifs three and four.[130,131] Six functional γ-crystallin genes have been identified in rats.[110] By contrast, only three γ-crystallin polypeptides have been identified in humans, with γE and γF being pseudogenes.[132] γC- and γD-crystallins are the primary human γ-crystallins; γA is expressed at lower levels.[133,134] The promoters of the γ-crystallins appear to be lens-specific when used in combination with reporter genes (see below).[135–138]

β-Crystallins

β-Crystallins are divided into two groups, with the βA2-, βA1/A3-, and βA4-crystallins having lower isoelectric points than the βB1-, βB2-, and βB3-crystallins.[110] The lower isoelectric group is referred to as acidic and the higher isoelectric group as basic, although the isoelectric points of both are slightly above neutral. Each is encoded by a separate gene, except for the βA3 and βA1 polypeptides, which are distinguished by originating from separate AUG translation initiation codons on the same mRNA (see Fig. 146-2).[5] The β-crystallin polypeptides range in size from about 23 to 32 kDa. Globular domains of β-crystallins have about 45 to 60 percent sequence similarity with each other and about 30 percent sequence similarity with globular domains of γ-crystallins.[110,139,140] The N- and C-terminal arms are much less well conserved than the globular core, usually showing about 30 percent sequence similarity to the arms of orthologous β-crystallins.[139–141] Computer graphic analysis of sequence similarity between the β- and γ-crystallins has allowed the structure of the βB1-, βB2-, and βA3-crystallins to be predicted,[109,142–144] suggesting a highly conserved central domain structure with Greek key motifs and more divergent N- and C-terminal extensions. Basic β-crystallins have both N- and C-terminal arms, while acidic β-crystallins have only N-terminal arms. The primary structures of many β-crystallins from calves, mice, rats, chickens, frogs, and humans have been deduced from cNDA sequences.[145] βA3/A1-crystallin has more than 90 percent identity with its bovine and mouse homologues.[146] The β-crystallins may undergo posttranslational modification, including proteolytic cleavage of βB1,[147] phosphorylation of βB2 and βB3,[148,149] and glycosylation of βB1.[150]

The β-crystallins associate preferentially in a paired fashion: acidic with basic into dimers of about 50 kDa, and then in a more complex fashion into larger aggregates of 150 to 200 kDa.[151] The crystal structure of βB2-crystallin has been solved to 2.1 Å resolution.[152] This β-crystallin has an extended interchain domain. The widely separated amino and carboxy domains of one β-crystallin polypeptide are paired in an antiparallel fashion with the carboxy and amino domains of a second β-crystallin polypeptide. Thus, the tendency of the β-crystallins to dimerize appears related to the extended connecting peptide between the two domains. This connecting peptide folds back on itself in the γ-crystallins, so that the two domains of a single molecule pair with each other.[152] Higher oligomerization of β-crystallins appears to occur by association of dimers and may require at least one protein with an N-terminal extension.[147,151]

β-Crystallin genes have six exons, the first one coding for the N-terminal extension and the next four for the four Greek key motifs (see Fig. 146-2). The C-terminal arm is also encoded by the sixth exon.[110,139,144,146,153] The exons encoding the first and third motifs and second and fourth motifs show especially high homology, suggesting that an intermediate step in evolution of the βγ-crystallin superfamily might have been a two-motif structure which was then reduplicated and underwent a second fusion event to create the present βγ-crystallin core structure[154] (see Fig. 146-2). In contrast to the γ-crystallins, most β-crystallin genes are dispersed in the species examined.[110,155,156] Human βA3/A1 is on chromosome 17. However, βB2 and βB3 are linked on chromosome 22,[157] possibly representing the remnant of a primal β-crystallin gene cluster.

Taxon-Specific Crystallins

Taxon-specific crystallins are proteins which occur in the lens at a high concentration (usually 10 percent or more of the protein), but are present in only one, or more generally, a few species.[5] Many taxon-specific crystallins appear to have arisen by a process called "gene-sharing,"[158] in which a single gene product acquires an additional function without duplication, often retaining its original function in nonlens tissues.[78,159–161] When a single gene product is used for two separate functions, it becomes subject to double evolutionary selection. *Gene sharing* implies that a mutation in a regulatory sequence resulting in a change in gene expression may lead to a new function for the encoded protein before or even without gene duplication and without loss of its original function. Gene duplication and specialization of function for one of the two proteins may occur later, as appears to have happened with the δ- and α-crystallins.[161]

The occurrence of gene sharing begs the question of what criteria exist for a protein to serve as a crystallin. Amazingly, virtually all the known taxon-specific crystallins are either active metabolic enzymes or clearly related to enzymes (Table 146-1). Thus, they are generally known as enzyme crystallins. Crystallins in the lens nucleus cannot be renewed during the lifetime of the individual and so must be extremely stable. Even though many proteins can serve refractive roles as crystallins, the α- and βγ-crystallins seem to be preferred, at least in vertebrates. A comparative study of the thermal stability of crystallins in four vertebrate classes indicates that the taxon-specific crystallins tend to be more labile than the ubiquitous crystallins.[162] Interestingly, many of the crystallins are related to stress proteins or detoxification enzymes,[78,118,161] as discussed above. In addition, many of the enzyme crystallins (for example, α-enolase,/τ-crystallin, LDHB4/ϵ-crystallin, quinone reductase/ζ-crystallin, GST/S-crystallin, and Ω-crystallin) are identical to or derived from enzymes with detoxification functions, often related to oxidative stress (see Table 146-1). This suggests that crystallins might have been selected not only for their ability to satisfy the optical requirements for refraction but also for their ability to protect the transparent lens from long-term deterioration due to physiological insults throughout life. Since many proteins appear able to satisfy the requirements for optical transparency, the ability of a gene to be expressed at high levels in the lens may be a particularly important criterion for recruitment as a lens crystallin.[159]

Argininosuccinate lyase/δ-crystallin, a major enzyme-crystallin confined to bird and reptile lenses, is perhaps the most intensively studied taxon-specific crystallin.[163,164] The original argininosuccinate lyase gene has been duplicated, with one copy (δ2) continuing to code for argininosuccinate lyase and the second (δ1) evolving to code for an enzymatically inactive (or less active) but highly similar crystallin.[165–167] In other enzyme crystallins, no gene duplication has occurred, and the same gene codes for both the enzyme and refractive lens crystallin. For example, duck ϵ-crystallin is identical to lactate dehydrogenase B4 (LDHB4).[168,169] Purified duck ϵ-crystallin has a specific activity at least 70 percent of that of purified LDHB4 enzyme from the heart. LDHB4/ϵ-crystallin comprises 10 percent of duck lens protein, far beyond that needed for enzymatic activity. Several enzyme-derived crystallins have lost enzymatic activity, including cytosolic aldehyde dehydrogenase (η-crystallin in elephant shrews),[170] hydroxyacyl CoA dehydrogenase (λ-crystallin in rabbits),[171] and NADPH-dependent reductase (ρ-crystallin in frogs).[172] ζ-Crystallin in guinea pigs is structurally related to the alcohol dehydrogenases[173] but has quinone oxidoreductase activity.[174] To date, related enzymes have been identified for all taxon-specific crystallins except jellyfish J1-crystallin.[175]

Table 146-1 Enzyme Crystallins

Distribution	Crystallin	Related or Identical
Represented in all vertebrates	α	Small heat-shock proteins
		Schistosoma mansoni antigen p40
		α-Crystallins have nonlens expression
	β	*Myxococcus xanthus* protein S
	γ	*Physarum polycephalum* spherulin 3a
Some birds and reptiles	δ	Argininosuccinate lyase
	ϵ	Lactate dehydrogenase B
	ζ	Alcohol dehydrogenase and NADPH: quinone oxidoreductase
Some mammals	η	Cytoplasmic aldehyde dehydrogenase
	λ	Hydroxyacyl CoA dehydrogenases
	μ	Dehydrogenases?
Frogs	ρ	NADPH-dependent reductases
Many species	τ	α-Enolase
Cephalopods	S	Glutathione S-transferases
	ω	Aldehyde dehydrogenase
Jellyfish	J	Unknown

Crystallin Gene Regulatory Sequences

The refractive properties of the lens depend on concentrations and distributions of crystallins within the lens, which in turn depend on the precise temporal and spatial regulation of crystallin gene expression. There is a gradient of refractive index increasing from the periphery to the center of the lens which correlates with an increasing concentration and varying composition of crystallins.[60] Thus, the optical properties of the lens depend on the pattern of crystallin gene expression.

Transgenic mouse experiments using crystallin promoters and developmental studies correlating crystallin expression with their mRNAs suggest that transcriptional controls play a major role in the high and preferred expression of crystallin genes in the lens.[21–23,104,106,107,137] The great variety of regulatory sequences used by different crystallin genes is indeed surprising. Even the orthologous gene in different species may use different *cis*-elements for lens expression.[159] Detailed mutagenesis studies have shown the importance of some regulatory sequences which are confined to crystallin genes and others which are used by many genes expressed in different tissues (Fig. 146-3). Specific sequences binding lens nuclear factors have been shown to be essential for high levels of expression of mouse[105,176,177] and chicken[178,179] αA-, chicken βB1-,[180] mouse γF-,[181] and chicken δ1-crystallin[182–184] genes. Additional regulatory elements have been found in the 5′ flanking sequences of mouse γF-, rat γD-, and hamster

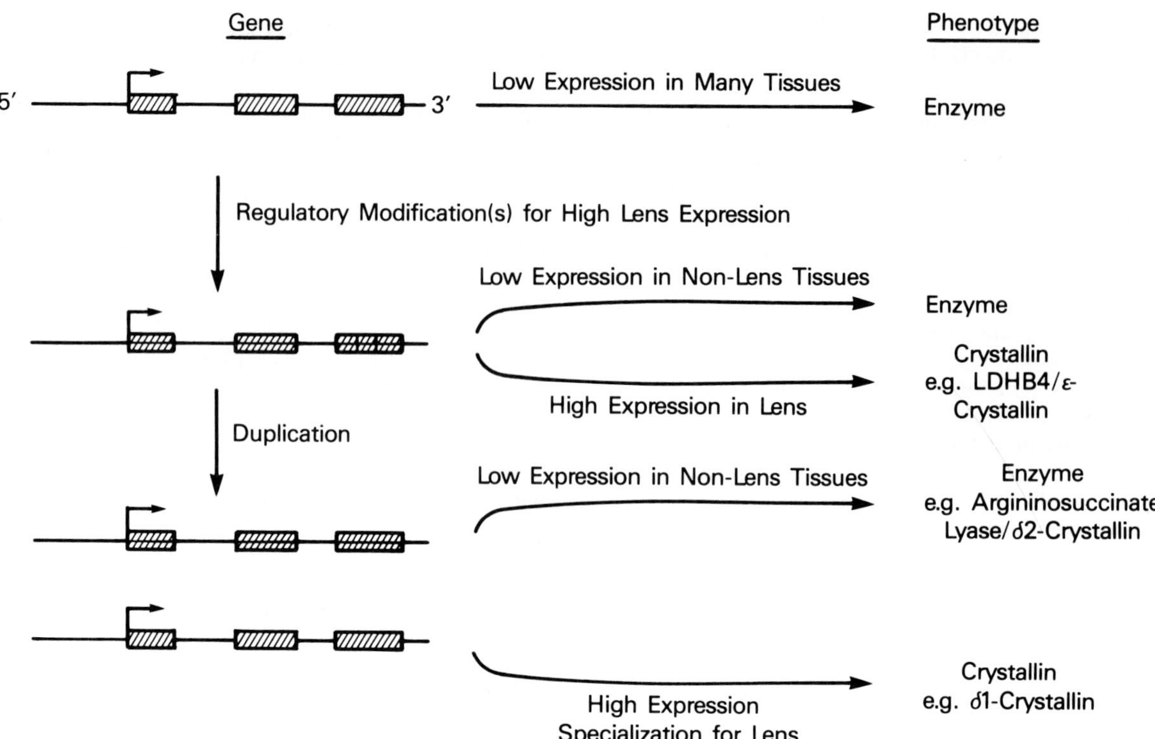

FIG. 146-3 **General evolutionary scheme for taxon-specific crystallins. High expression in the lens may occur without gene duplication or may be followed by gene duplication.**

αA-crystallin genes.[138,185,186] Methylation has also been implicated for controlling expression of chicken δ-crystallin[187] and rat γ-crystallin[188] genes. Although detailed functional studies have not yet been conducted on human crystallin genes, sequence comparisons are consistent with the idea that regulation of the αA-crystallin gene is quite similar in mice and humans.[84]

In addition to using multiple *cis*-regulatory sequences for lens expression, the present evidence suggests a corresponding diversity of *trans*-acting regulatory proteins. DNA–protein complexes generally observed in electrophoretic gel mobility shift experiments utilizing crystallin regulatory sequences form with nuclear proteins derived from many tissues,[159] suggesting that ubiquitous transcription factors play an important role in crystallin gene expression. An example is αA-CRYBP1, a cloned putative transcription factor implicated in the control of the mouse αA-crystallin gene (Fig. 146-4). The αA-CRYBP1 mRNA is found in many tissues.[177] The sequence motif to which the protein binds is present in many genes and is similar to that which binds transcription factors belonging to the NF-kB/dorsal/rel family.[189] It is possible that the αA-CRYBP1 binding protein is modified in a tissue-specific fashion, leading to a form of the protein used for preferential expression of the αA-crystallin

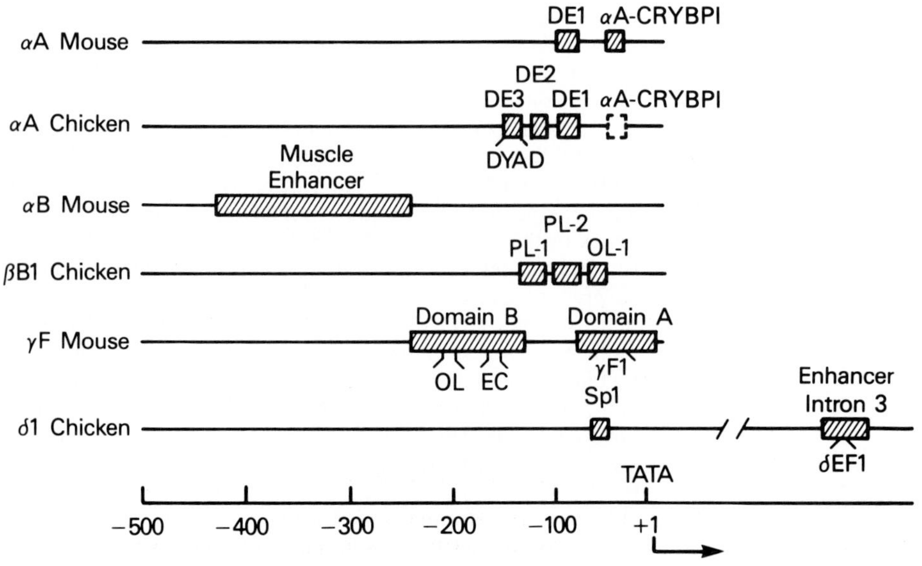

FIG. 146-4 **Summary of control elements identified in crystallin promoters. DE = distal element; αA-CRYBP1 = αA-CRYBP1 binding site; PL = polyoma enhancer-like sequence; OL = octomer-like sequence; EC = enhancer core; Sp1 = Sp1 binding site. Details are described and references given in the text. Approximate positions of *cis*-elements from transcription start sites are shown on scale below.**

gene in the lens. Quantitative aspects can also be a consideration. For example, an oligonucleotide containing a single copy of the αA-CRYBP1 gene sequence increases expression of a *Herpes simplex* thymidine kinase (tk) promoter/CAT fusion gene selectively in transfected mouse lens epithelial cells transformed with the T antigen of SV40.[190] Multiple copies of the same sequence decrease its lens-cell preference.[190] δEF1, the nuclear factor binding a key regulatory sequence in the δ1 enhancer, has been cloned and shown to contain two widely separated zinc fingers, a homeodomain, and proline- and acidic-rich domains.[183] Different complexes form with the 11-bp lens-specific regulatory sequence of the mouse γF-crystallin gene when nuclear proteins are used from fibroblasts, liver, brain, or lens.[181] The protein forming the lens complex has been called "γF-1." Further experiments are necessary in order to determine whether γF-1 or any other lens transcriptional complex involved in lens expression is due to one or more lens-specific factors, to modifications of ubiquitous factors, or to lens-specific cofactors or activators.

It is established that most (perhaps all) genes encoding proteins used as lens crystallins are expressed to some degree outside the lens. Nonlens expression has been studied most extensively in the δ-crystallin and αB-crystallin genes. As indicated above, the chicken δ1-crystallin gene is the predominant δ-crystallin gene expressed in the lens, while the linked δ2-crystallin gene is preferentially expressed in nonlens tissues.[165,191] It has been established by direct expression studies that the chicken[166] and duck[167] δ2-crystallin gene encodes active argininosuccinate lyase; no activity has been observed for the protein encoded in the chicken or duck δ1-crystallin gene. However, both chicken δ-crystallin genes have an enhancer sequence in their third intron that confers lens preference.[165,184] The molecular basis for the great excess of δ1- to δ2-crystallin expression in the lens is not yet known. Experiments with the δ1-crystallin gene have shown that its third intron also contains sequence elements responsible for directing expression to different types of nonlens cells.[182]

Multiple regulatory elements appear responsible for the nonlens expression of the αB-crystallin gene. Transcription initiates several hundred base pairs further upstream in lung, brain, and spleen than in numerous other tissues, including lens, heart, skeletal muscle, and kidney.[86,192] An enhancer conferring preference for expression in cultured muscle cells, but also affecting expression in transfected lens cells, exists between these two transcription initiation sites.[193] The broader tissue distribution of a mouse αB-crystallin minitransgene[86] than of a mouse αB promoter/CAT fusion transgene[193] in transgenic mice has suggested that 3′ regulatory elements may also exist in the αB-crystallin gene. Transfection experiments utilizing the promoter of the human αB-crystallin gene fused to the CAT reporter gene support the possible existence of 3′ regulatory elements for the αB gene.[194]

These experiments establish the complexity of expression of crystallin genes and implicate the use of multiple *cis*- and *trans*-regulatory elements. They also clearly indicate that the expression and function of crystallin genes are not limited to the lens. It follows that abnormal expression of these genes may well affect both lens and nonlens tissues; conversely, it is probable that nonlens defects involving the nonrefractive functions of crystallins or crystallin gene regulatory factors may be associated with lens abnormalities, most likely cataracts.

MEMBRANE PROTEINS, JUNCTIONS, AND THE CYTOSKELETON

Membrane Proteins

Approximately 2 percent of lens proteins are membrane-associated and have molecular masses ranging from 10 to over 250 kDa. Some are components of the cytoskeletal structure, such as *N*-cadherin, a 135-kDa intrinsic membrane protein which may be involved in cell–cell adhesion.[195] The calpactins are extrinsic membrane proteins attached to the membrane through calcium and are probably involved in membrane–cytoskeleton interactions.[12,13,196] Neural-cell adhesion molecule 2 (NCAM 2) has been implicated in cell adhesion and contributes to the appropriate arrangement of gap junctions in developing lens fiber cells.[197] Other membrane proteins are enzymes including glyceraldehyde 3-phosphate dehydrogenase and a variety of ATPases. There are also intrinsic membrane proteins specific to lens fiber cells whose function remain mysterious, for example, a 17- to 19-kDa protein.[198]

The best-studied and most abundant membrane protein of the lens is intrinsic membrane protein 26 (MP26). MP26 is a lens-specific single polypeptide with a molecular mass of 28,200 kDa (263 residues) which comprises about 50 percent of the lens membrane protein.[12,13,199] It has been suggested that MP26 may bind calmodulin.[200] Circular dichroism studies show that about half of MP26 forms an α helix. The amino acid sequence has been deduced from a cloned MP26 cDNA.[201] A model has been constructed which suggests that MP26 forms α-helical coils which traverse the membrane six times; the C- and N-termini are both on the cytoplasmic side, consistent with a possible role for MP26 as a junctional protein.[201] MP26 shows homology to nodulin-26, a major protein of the peribacteroid membrane synthesized in the roots of nitrogen-fixing plants in response to infection by the nitrogen-fixing bacteria Rhizobium.[202] In addition, MP26 shows sequence similarity with the *Escherichia coli* glycerol facilitator and a Drosophila "bib" protein (a transmembrane channel protein),[203,204] both of which appear to be involved in intercellular communication. Thus, as the crystallins, MP26 may be traced evolutionarily to other proteins with nonlens roots.

It has been determined by electron microscopic immunocytochemistry that MP26 is present in the plasma membrane and junctional complexes of lens fiber cells.[199,205–207] It was not detected in anterior lens epithelia or non-lens-cell membranes. Transfection of a human MP26 promoter/CAT fusion gene into embryonic chicken lens epithelial cells has demonstrated the ability of the MP26 gene regulatory sequences to function in lens cells.[208] MP26 can form channels permeable to ions and other small molecules in liposomes and artificial membrane systems.[209–213] MP26 may play a role in gap junctions, which are numerous in the lens. However, MP26 is more associated with thin junctions (11 to 13 nm), which may be unique to lens fibers, than with thick junctions (16 to 17 nm), which appear analogous to the gap junctions of other tissues.[205,213] MP 26 is a substrate of endogenous protein kinase,[214,215] raising the possibility that metabolic control of its structure has functional significance.

Gap Junction Proteins

The lens is avascular and must depend on its many gap junctions for nutrition and cell-to-cell communication. As stated above, the thick, 16- to 17-nm junctions may be the lens equivalent of gap junctions found in other tissues. The intrinsic membrane protein MP70 is found in these junctions.[205,216] MP70 is most prevalent in outer cortical fibers, where it undergoes age-related degradation to MP38, which remains in the functional gap junctions.[217] MP70 has sequence homology to connexins present in gap junctions of other tissues.

Cytoskeletal Proteins

Many cytoskeletal proteins found in the lens are common to other tissues, including actin, ankyrin, myosin, vimentin, spectrin, and α-actinin. It is likely that a complex network of proteins immediately below the cell membrane similar to that in erythrocytes[219] contributes to the maintenance of cell shape of differentiating fiber cells of the lens cortex. Tubulin is a component of microtubules which are lined up lengthwise in the peripheral cytoplasm in cortical fiber cells and are rare in nuclear fiber cells and epithelial cells.[220] Microtubules may contribute to the maintenance of the elongated shape of fiber cells and may be involved in the interkinetic migration of the nuclei in dividing lens epithelial cells.[18] Actin filaments are closely associated with lens-cell membranes,[221,222] and may play a role in accommodation.[14,223] Glial fibrillary acidic protein is expressed in lens anterior epithelial cells and disappears on differentiation to fiber cells.[224,225] Its role is unknown. Vimentin, which usually occurs in mesenchymally derived cells, forms the intermediate filament in lens cells.[226] It can be highly phosphorylated.[227] Vimentin expression increases approximately threefold during embryonic chicken lens development and then decreases after hatching.[228] Transfection experiments have shown that vimentin gene expression is controlled by a complex set of positive and negative *cis*-regulatory 5′ flanking sequences.[228,229]

Other cytoskeletal proteins appear to be unique to the lens.[15,16,230] One example is the beaded filament. This consists of a 709-nm backbone filament with globular protein particles,[12] and contains lens-specific proteins of 49, 95, and 115 kDa.[16,231] There are excellent reviews available of lens membrane and cytoskeletal proteins and their biochemistry.[11–13]

LENS METABOLISM

Energy Metabolism

In general, metabolic pathways of the lens are similar to those of other tissues, and detailed reviews are available.[43,232,233] However, the avascular nature of the lens, which receives the vast majority of its nutrients from the aqueous humor,[234] and the gradual loss of intracellular organelles from differentiating fiber cells place specific constraints on lens metabolism. Utilization of various metabolic pathways for energy production in the whole lens is summarized in Table 146-2. Most

Table 146-2 Lens Metabolism

Pathway	% Glucose Utilized	Additional Importance
Anaerobic glycolysis	78%	
Pentose phosphate	14%	Pentoses for NADPH
Sorbitol pathway	5%	Sugar cataract formation
Citric acid cycle	3%	Limited to epithelial cells

of the glucose metabolized in the lens is handled by anaerobic glycolysis. The citric acid cycle is active only in the anterior epithelial cells, which still contain mitochondria. This pathway produces about 20 to 30 percent of the total ATP in the lens, even though only about 3 percent of the glucose passes through this cycle.[235,236] The lens can maintain adequate ion balance, high-energy phosphate levels, and protein synthesis in the absence of oxygen, but exposure of the lens to iodoacetate, an inhibitor of 3-phosphoglyceraldehyde dehydrogenase of the Embden-Meyerhof pathway results in swelling, ionic changes, and cataracts.[237,238] Stimulation of the pentose phosphate pathway occurs when cultured lenses are exposed to oxidative stress induced by hydrogen peroxide[239–241] or hyperbaric oxygen,[242] apparently acting through an increase in hexokinase activity.

It has been suggested that aldose reductase might increase sorbitol in the lens to protect against daily diet- and disease-related changes in aqueous humor osmolality,[243] in a fashion similar to sorbitol action in the renal medulla.[244,245] The osmotic hypothesis suggests a common pathogenic mechanism in the cataracts resulting from diabetes mellitus or galactosemia. Aldose reductase reduces glucose to sorbitol and galactose (more readily) to galactitol.[246] While sorbitol is metabolized by sorbitol dehydrogenase, galactitol is not, perhaps making it a more damaging molecule. The increase in intracellular fluid in response to these polyols results in lens swelling, increased membrane permeability, electrolyte abnormalities, and metabolic dysfunction.[247–249] Although aldose reductase activity in the human lens is significantly less than that in the commonly studied rat, in vitro cultured human lenses from diabetic patients accumulate higher levels of polyols than those from nondiabetic subjects, and the accumulation is inhibited by aldose reductase inhibitors.[250] Thus, the hope that inhibition of aldose reductase might inhibit polyol accumulation, osmotic damage, and cataract in humans with abnormalities in sugar metabolism is currently being tested.

Maintenance of a Reduced State

A major threat to lens transparency lies in the accumulation of oxidative damage to the crystallins and other molecules over an individual's lifetime. Since peroxides are generated in fiber and anterior epithelial cells, the average concentration of H_2O_2 is 30 μM in the normal human eye, and it can be much higher in patients with cataracts.[251] The lens responds to this stress by accumulating reducing agents, especially glutathione, which is the most abundant low-molecular-weight thiol in aerobic organisms. There is a gradient of glutathione concentration in the lens, with the highest concentration in the anterior epithelium, next in the cortical regions, and lowest in the nucleus.[252] In the normal lens the cortical glutathione level is not age-dependent.[253] Lens glutathione presumably acts as a sulfhydryl buffer for maintaining protein thiols in a reduced state, and protecting against oxidative damage to other residues.

The lens uses both the glutathione redox cycle and catalase for the detoxification of H_2O_2.[254] Catalase is confined to peroxisomes by histochemical localization,[255] but enzymes of the glutathione redox cycle (glutathione reductase and peroxidase) are distributed throughout the cytoplasm. Although glutathione reductase is the main enzyme maintaining glutathione in reduced state in the lens,[43] the mercapturic acid pathway using glutathione S-transferase is also important in protecting the lens from oxidative damage.[256] It is interesting in this regard that the major crystallins in cephalopods are closely related to glutathione S-transferase.[164,257] The effectiveness of these reducing pathways results in only 2 to 5 percent of lens glutathione existing in the oxidized form under normal conditions.

Osmoregulation

Osmoregulation occurs by active transport, with Na^+/K^+-dependent ATPase exchanging sodium out of the lens for potassium into the lens. Most of the Na^+/K^+-dependent ATPase is in the anterior epithelium, but some is also found in the anterior cortex and fiber membranes around suture systems.[258,259] The cations are followed by passive diffusion of chloride and water.[260] Cytochemistry has indicated that Na^+/K^+-ATPase is localized to the apicolateral membranes of the anterior epithelial cells.[261,262] Because the lens capsule is slightly permeable to both sodium and potassium and most transport is by the anterior epithelium, there is a concentration gradient anterior to posterior for potassium and posterior to anterior for sodium.[263] Ca^{2+}-ATPase also occurs in the lens with the highest specific activity in the anterior epithelium but the bulk of activity is in the cortical lens fibers. This results in the lens having a lower Ca^{2+} concentration than the aqueous or vitreous humor.[264,265]

The movement of different macromolecules is controlled in various ways by the lens. The lens capsule is the first barrier for diffusion. Horseradish peroxidase (molecular weight, 40,000) can penetrate the lens capsule, whereas ferritin (molecular weight, 500,000) cannot.[9] The capsule is penetrable by low-molecular-weight crystallins but not by higher-molecular-weight α-crystallin.[266] Low-molecular-weight proteins such as horseradish peroxidase and dyes also readily penetrate the anterior epithelial layer.[8] However, passage of metabolites between the epithelial cells and fiber cells is probably through endocytotic processes rather than through the few gap junctions found connecting them.[7,9,267] The fiber cells are connected by extensive communicating channels, as shown by dye injection[10,268] and electrophysiological studies.[269,270] Sugar transport in the lens closely resembles that seen in muscle and blood cells.[271,272]

MOLECULAR BIOLOGY OF CATARACTS

Cataract, defined here as a lens opacity, can have multiple causes and is generally associated with the breakdown of the lens microarchitecture.[30,31,273] Vacuole formation will cause large fluctuations in density and hence abrupt changes in the index of refraction, resulting in light scattering. Light scattering and opacity will occur if there is a significant amount of high-molecular-weight protein aggregates in the range of 1000 Å or more.[274,275] The short-range ordered packing of the crystallins is important in this regard; crystallins must exist in a homogeneous phase. A variety of biochemical or physical insults can cause phase separation into protein-rich and protein-poor regions within the lens fibers, resulting in light scattering.[274–280] The physical basis of lens transparency is beyond the scope of this chapter and has been reviewed elsewhere.[59,274–276]

Animal Models

Since cataractogenesis is a complex process accompanied by numerous secondary changes, animal models may provide useful information for distinguishing the causes of senescent and other cataracts. The hereditary cataracts in rodents have been especially useful in this regard.

The Philly mouse displays an autosomal dominant cataract in which there is a deficiency of the βB2-crystallin polypeptide.[281,282] The βB2-crystallin cDNA has a deletion of 12 nucleotides, resulting in a four-amino-acid deletion in the encoded protein. It has been hypothesized that this causes aberrant folding of the protein and that cataract formation occurs as a result of the molecular instability of this crystallin.[283,284]

Guinea pig strain 13/N has an autosomal dominant cataract more severe in homozygotes than in heterozygotes.[285,286] A peculiarity of the guinea pig and other hystricomorphic mammals is that ζ-crystallin is a major crystallin found in the lens.[287] In the heterozygous 13/N guinea pig, levels of ζ-crystallin are reduced, and an abnormal smaller protein is present. This is due to a mutation in a splice site resulting in a loss of an entire exon during RNA processing, with consequent deletion of 34 amino acids in the protein.[288] Although it is not clear whether the molecular lesion in guinea pig strain 13/N results in a cataract by destabilizing ζ-crystallin or destroying an enzymatic activity, both the Philly mouse and guinea pig 13/N cataracts suggest that appropriate concentrations of stable crystallins are critical for maintenance of lens transparency.

A number of additional models suggest that some metabolic lesions can also cause cataracts. The Nakano mouse has autosomal recessive cataracts which show reduced synthesis of the α- and β-crystallins.[289,290] This is probably due to an increase in the Na^+:K^+ ratio occurring because of inhibition of the sodium–potassium pump.[249,291] The Fraser mouse, which displays an autosomal dominant cataract, shows preferential loss of γ-crystallins and their mRNAs.[292,293] However, the gene causing this cataract segregates independently of the γ-crystallin gene cluster.[294] It resides on chromosome 10 and has been suggested to be allelic with the mouse lens opacity gene (LOP).[295] The eye lens obsolescence (ELO) mouse cataract shows preferential reduction in γ-crystallin mRNAs.[296] The ELO locus is on chromosome 1 near the γ-crystallin gene cluster, although a recombination event has been documented between the cataract and the γ-crystallin genes.[296] In addition, many other animal cataract models have been described phenotypically but not characterized molecularly.[297–300] An interesting cataract develops in the Emory mouse after several months of life, possibly modeling senescent cataracts in humans.[301]

Transgenic Models

Transgenic mice provide an extremely powerful tool for the study of lens transparency.[104] In practice, creation of cataractous transgenic mouse lines is facilitated by the lens being readily examined for transparency, providing a rapid and efficient means to screen for phenotypic effects of transgenic insertions. Most cataracts in transgenic mice are associated with abnormalities of lens development, especially uncontrolled growth, toxic ablation of specific lens cells, or immune destruction of the lens. Lens abnormalities have been caused in transgenic mice using a variety of strategies. Expression of diphtheria toxin or ricin under the control of a lens-specific γ-crystallin or α-crystallin promoter, respectively, has caused ablations within the lens.[135,302,303] Synthesis of granulocyte–macrophage colony-stimulating factor (a leukocytic chemotactic factor) in transgenic mice resulted in inflammatory destruction of lens cells and cataract formation.[304] Transgenic mice with vimentin overexpressed in lens cells also have cataracts, probably due to developmental aberration.[305] Surprisingly, no studies have yet described creation of a cataract by transgenic alteration of lens crystallin expression or loss of osmotic or ionic homeostasis.

HUMAN CATARACTS

Definition

In the most general sense, cataract is defined as any opacity in the lens. For clinical diagnostic purposes, however, the characteristics of a cataract must be precisely defined. Opacities that are the natural result of biological aging must be distinguished from those that are secondary to pathological processes related to environmental, nutritional, or genetic factors or those that occur as a consequence of systemic disease. With aging, random fleck-like opacities in the cortex of the lens may be detected by slit-lamp biomicroscopy in normal individuals, usually beginning by the third decade of life. Age-related changes in the color and clarity of the lens also occur.[306–309] A clinically useful classification scheme must distinguish these changes of normal aging from specific pathological opacities. Rigorous clinical classification is particularly important because cataracts are an obvious and diagnostic phenotypic feature for many disorders (Table 146-3).

Table 146-3 Inherited Syndromes Associated with Cataracts

Primarily Ocular Syndromes Associated with Cataracts

Syndrome	Reference
Autosomal dominant	
Aniridia	351
Cornea guttata	352
Granular corneal dystrophy	353
Familial exudative vitreoretinopathy	354
Foveal hypoplasia	355
Hyaloideoretinal degeneration of Wagner	356
Iris pigment layer cleavage	357
Mesenchymal dysgenesis of the anterior segment	358
Microcornea	359
Microphthalmia	360
Persistent hyperplastic pupillary membrane	361
Retinitis pigmentosa	362, 363
Snowflake vitreoretinal degeneration	364
Vitreoretinochoroidopathy	365
Autosomal recessive	
Amyloid corneal dystrophy	366
Cone-rod degeneration	362
Choroideremia	362
Favre hyaloideoretinal degeneration	367
Leber congenital amaurosis type I	368
Microphthalmia and nystagmus	369
Retinitis pigmentosa	362, 363
X-linked	
Microcornea and slight microphthalmia	360
Norrie disease	370
Nystagmus	371
Retinitis pigmentosa	372

Other Genetic Syndromes Associated with Cataracts

Syndrome	Reference
Autosomal dominant	
Aberrant oral frenula and growth retardation	373
Cerebellar ataxia, deafness, and dementia	374
Chondrodysplasia punctata	375

Table 146-3 Inherited Syndromes Associated with Cataracts (*cont.*)

Other Genetic Syndromes Associated with Cataracts—Continued

Syndrome	Reference
Clouston syndrome	371
Cochleosaccular degeneration	376
Congenital lactose intolerance	377
Dwarfism with stiff joints and ocular abnormalities	378
Esophageal and vulval leiomyomatosis with nephropathy*	379
Fechtner syndrome	371
Flynn-Aird syndrome*	380
Hallermann-Streiff syndrome (new mutation)	381
Hereditary mucoepithelial dysplasia	382
Histiocytic dermatoarthritis	383
Incontinentia pigmenti (autosomal dominant new mutation)	384
Metatropic dwarfism type II (Kniest disease)	385
Kyrle disease (follicular keratosis)	386
Mitochondrial myopathy (two types)	387, 388
Marshall syndrome	389
Multiple epiphyseal dysplasia with myopia and conductive deafness*	390
Myotonic dystrophy	323
Nail-patella syndrome	391
Neurofibromatosis type II	322
Oculodentodigital syndrome	371
Optic atrophy and neurologic disorder	392
Osteopathica striata and deafness	388
Paronychia congenita syndrome	371
Progeria syndrome (autosomal dominant new mutation)	393
Schprintzen velocardiofacial syndrome	394
Sorbitol dehydrogenase	395
Split-hand and congenital nystagmus	396
Stickler syndrome	397
Trichomegaly	398
Autosomal recessive	
Absence leg deficiency*	399
Agenesis of the corpus callosum, combined immunodeficiency, and hypopigmentation*	400
Axonal encephalopathy with necrotizing myopathy and cardiomyopathy*	401
Bardet-Biedl syndrome	402
Cataract, microcephaly, failure to thrive and kyphoscoliosis (CAMFAK) syndrome	371
Cardiomyopathy	403
Cerebral cholesterinosis (cerebrotendinous xanthomatosis)	404
Cerebrooculofacioskeletal (COFS) syndrome	405
Chondrodysplasia punctata	375
Cockayne syndrome	406
Congenital ichthyosis	407
Crome syndrome*	408
Dysequilibrium syndrome	409
Galactosemia (kinase and transferase)	410
Glutathione reductase deficiency	411
Gyrate atrophy	316
Hallermann-Streiff syndrome	412
Hard-E syndrome	413
Homocysteinuria	414
Hypertrophic neuropathy*	415
Hypogonadism*	416
Osteogenesis imperfecta with microcephaly*	417
Mannosidosis	418
Majewski syndrome	419
Marinesco-Sjögren syndrome	420

Table 146-3 Inherited Syndromes Associated with Cataracts (*cont.*)

Other Genetic Syndromes Associated with Cataracts—Continued

Syndrome	Reference
Martsolf syndrome	421
Mevalonic aciduria	422
Myopathy and hypogonadism*	423
Nathalie syndrome*	424
Neu-Laxova syndrome	425
Neuraminidase deficiency	426
Neutral lipid storage disease	427
Pellagra-like syndrome*	428
Phenylketonuria	429
Polycystic kidney and congenital blindness	430
Preus oculocerebral hypopigmentation syndrome	431
Refsum syndrome	432
Roberts-SC phocomelia syndrome	433
Rothmund Thomson syndrome	434
Schwartz-Jampel syndrome	433
Short stature, mental retardation, and ocular abnormalities*	435
Smith-Lemli-Opitz syndrome	436
Tachycardia, hypertension, microphthalmos, and hyperglycinuria*	437
Toriello microcephalic primordial dwarfism*	438
Usher syndrome	439
Werner syndrome	440
Wilson disease	441
Zellweger syndrome	432
X-linked	
Albright hereditary osteodystrophy	442
Alport syndrome	443
Fabry disease	444
Glucose 6-phosphate dehydrogenase deficiency	445
Incontinentia pigmenti	446
Lenz dysplasia	447
Lowe syndrome	448
Nance-Horan syndrome	449
Pigmentary retinopathy and mental retardation	450
Renal tubular acidosis II	451
X-linked dominant chondrodysplasia punctata	452
Chromosome anomalies	
Trisomy 10q	433
Trisomy 13	433
Trisomy 18	433
18p−	433
18q−	433
Trisomy 20p	433
Trisomy 21	433
XO syndrome	433

*This syndrome has been described in a single kindred.

NOTE: Although references are given in which the cataracts found in the above syndromes are described, useful clinical summaries of most of these syndromes are found in Smith[433] or McKusick.[371] In some cases no single best source was obvious and the summary in Smith or McKusick is given as the primary reference.

Classification

Classification characteristics with diagnostic relevance include age of onset, location, size, pattern, number, shape, density, progression, and severity in terms of interfering with visual acuity or visual function.

Defined by age at onset, a congenital or infantile cataract is visible within the first year of life, a juvenile cataract occurs within the first decade of life, a presenile cataract occurs before the age of 45 years, and the so-called senile or age-related cataract, thereafter. The age of onset of a cataract does not necessarily give a clue to its etiology. Congenital cataracts may be hereditary or secondary to a noxious intrauterine event. Cataracts associated with a systemic or genetic disease may not occur until the second or third decade (e.g., cataracts associated with retinitis pigmentosa). Even age-related cataract, thought to be due to multiple insults accumulated over many years, may have a genetic component, making certain individuals more vulnerable to the environmental insults.

Classification by location is a reproducible and reliable way to identify cataracts and chart their course. There are several classification systems which have been developed based on the anatomic location of the opacity, that is, involving the nucleus, the posterior capsule, the cortex, or mixed (combinations of the former). All these systems depend on the use of slit-lamp biomicroscopy and examination through a dilated pupil. These classification systems include the LOCS II system (lens opacity classification system),[310] the Wisconsin system,[311] the Hopkins system,[312] and the Oxford system.[313] These classifications have focused primarily on acquired rather than congenital cataract. Documentation may be made either clinically by comparing the slit-lamp biomicroscopic appearance to a set of standard photographs or by direct comparison of photographs of the affected lens using slit-lamp and retroillumination photography to standard photographs (LOCS II). These techniques for the most part have been used for research studies but can be adapted to determine the presence and progression of lens opacities in a clinical setting.

In an attempt to deal with congenital cataract, Merin has proposed a system based on morphological classification. Accordingly, the cataract is classified as total (mature), polar (anterior or posterior), zonular (nuclear, lamellar, sutural), and capsular or membranous.[314]

Since lens development follows a well-documented timed sequence, the location of a lens opacity provides information about the time at which the pathological process intervened, thereby aiding in determining the etiology. Nuclear opacities from the most central region outward denote cataract formation occurring at the time of the development of that portion of the involved nucleus—embryonic (first 3 months), fetal (third to eighth month), infantile (after birth), or adult. Since the lens fibers are laid down constantly throughout life, lens opacities which develop postnatally appear in the cortex as cortical opacities or appear just beneath the posterior lens capsule as subcapsular opacities, for example, cataracts caused by topical steroid drugs and radiation. Polar opacities involve either the anterior or posterior pole of the lens and may include the posterior subcapsular lens cortex extending to the lens capsule. When both anterior and posterior poles are involved, the term *bipolar* is used. Zonular or lamellar cataracts affect the lens fibers, which are formed at the same time, resulting in a shell-like opacity at the level at which the fibers were laid down. The regions on which the lens fibers converge are referred to as the Y sutures, visible by slit-lamp biomicroscopy as an upright Y anteriorly and an inverted Y posteriorly. Theories of cataract development[315] suggest that abnormalities in lens-fiber development or maturation may lead to a predisposition to cataract development later in life. This is supported by examples in animals (the Philly mouse) and in humans (gyrate atrophy; Chap. 31).[316]

Size, pattern, shape, and density of lens opacities are determined in part by etiology, location, the ongoing process of cataractogenesis, and other, unknown, influences. Microdots and cortical flecks may be insignificant if few in number and random in location, but if the number exceeds 25 per quadrant[317,318] with a specific distribution such as the radial pattern in the Lowe carrier,[319,320] their clinical significance becomes apparent. Other examples include the cortical cataract in neurofibromatosis type 2[321,322] or the metachromasia seen in myotonic dystrophy patients.[323]

Hereditary Cataract

The frequency of hereditary cataracts in humans is not precisely known but has been estimated to be between 8.3 and 25 percent of congenital cataracts.[324,325] Hereditary cataracts include cases in which only the lens is involved, or the lens opacity may be associated with other ocular anomalies such as microphthalmia, aniridia, other anterior chamber developmental anomalies, retinal degenerations, chromosomal abnormalities, and multisystem genetic disorders such as Lowe syndrome and neurofibromatosis type 2.

Hereditary cataract may be classified by the mode of inheritance with all Mendelian inheritance patterns being described. Autosomal dominant congenital cataracts are the most frequent. Phenotypically identical cataracts have been localized to different genetic loci and may have different inheritance patterns (see below), while phenotypically variable cataracts can be found in a single large family.[326] Linkage analysis is a powerful tool to sort out the different genetic loci which can cause human cataracts. In this connection, it is interesting that a variety of different patterns of cataract occur in mouse lines transgenic for the same β-crystallin antisense construction,[327] although each transgenic line has a different integration site.

Linkage Analysis of Cataracts

Linkage analysis has been useful to identify a small number of cataractous loci and also to demonstrate the genetic heterogeneity in human hereditary cataracts. The autosomal dominant lamellar (central pulverulent) cataract (CAE) originally described by Nettleship and Ogilvie in 1906[328] was linked to the Duffy locus by Renwick and Lawler.[3] Heterogeneity in cataracts was soon proven by lack of linkage in several other families.[329–331] A Coppock-like cataract has been linked to the γ-crystallin locus in one large family with a Lod score of 7.58 and no recombinations ($\theta = 0$).[332] It is thought that this cataract might be caused by expression of a γ-crystallin gene, which is normally a pseudogene, possibly resulting in high phase separation.[134] A zonular autosomal dominant cataract initially studied by Marner has been linked to haptoglobin.[333,334] An autosomal dominant total congenital cataract has shown the possibility of linkage (Lod score of 2.1 at $\theta = 0.1$) to haptoglobin, suggesting that these loci might be allelic.[335] Phenotypically similar cataracts have also occurred in a father and son with a translocation t(3;4)p26.2.[336] These studies have established genetic heterogeneity in autosomal dominant complete cataract with loci on chromosome 1, chromosome 2, and chromosome 16, but many additional families remain which do not show linkage to these loci, and much work remains to be done.

While most studies have been of dominant cataracts, an interesting autosomal recessive congenital cataract has been associated with "i" phenotype in 17 of 18 Japanese individuals,[337] and some Caucasians.[338] Linkage analysis has been carried out on this locus in four Japanese families, giving a Lod score of 3.4 at $\theta = 0$.[339]

Cataracts also occur in association with a variety of multiple malformation syndromes listed in Table 146-3. In some cases, this association appears to be the result of truly pleiotropic effects of a single gene, while in others the cataracts appear to be secondary to pathology occurring primarily in the retina or ciliary body. As might be expected, cataracts are frequently associated with diseases resulting in marked involvement of the retina, choroid, or portions of anterior chamber structures. In addition, cataracts frequently occur with skin diseases such as epidermal dystrophies and a variety of bone and cartilage dysplasias. Inherited syndromes and diseases with which cataracts are associated are summarized in Table 146-3. Many of these diseases have been extensively studied or mapped, especially on the X chromosome.

Abnormalities of Lens Size, Shape, and Position

Coloboma of the lens, which may be associated with coloboma of the uvea (choroid, ciliary body, iris), is a congenital anomaly which may show an asymmetry of the lens with a peripheral flattening of indentation and loss of zonules usually in the six o'clock position. Associated cataractous changes are not uncommon. *Microspherophakia* refers to a small spherical lens which produces a high lenticular myopia due to the shape of the lens. Frequently these lenses can be subluxated with a displacement into the anterior chamber, resulting in a pupillary block (obstruction of the pupil by the lens) causing an acute onset of elevated intraocular pressure. Frequently these lenses become cataractous. The Weill-Marchesani syndrome is a rare example of microspherophakia, associated with short stature, brachycephaly, prognathism, and peg-shaped teeth.[340]

Lentiglobus and lenticonus are abnormalities of the shape of the lens. They usually are associated with localized axial deformities of contour of the anterior or posterior surface of the lens. Lentiglobus refers to spherical bulging of the anterior surface and lenticonus to conical changes usually of the posterior surface. Both create a central thickening and hence a high myopia. Posterior lentiglobus most frequently occurs as a unilateral condition and frequently is associated with a localized lens opacity.

Abnormal positions of the lens can occur, either with a partial dislocation, or subluxation, which may be due to weakened, stretched or broken zonules. Signs and symptoms pathognomonic of these conditions are iridodonesis (tremulous iris movement), astigmatism, and occasionally monocular diplopia. Complications include pupillary block, chorioretinal damage, or an ocular inflammatory (uveitic) response. Genetic diseases associated with subluxation of the lens include Marfan syndrome, in which the lens is usually dislocated up and outward, and homocystinuria, in which the lens is usually dislocated downward. Nonspecific dislocation can occur in the Weill-Marchesani syndrome, Ehler-Danlos syndrome, Lowe syndrome, and other rare conditions, such as sulfite oxidase deficiency and some forms of primordial dwarfism. Both Marfan syndrome and autosomal dominant ectopia lentis can be caused by a defect in the fibrillin gene on chromosome 15 (15q21.1).[341]

Evaluation

After establishing the significance of cataract by classification, case, and type, the evaluation of cataract consists of a careful assessment of its effect on the visual acuity and visual function. The first assessment in small children (0 to 3 years of age) may be done by observation-fixing, following, covering of alternative eyes to determine response (covering the eye with good vision will create a more fretful, objecting, crying child). More accurate assessment involves specialized testing by visually evoked cortical responses, preferential looking, or the forced choice method.[342,343] With older children, subjective tests, including identification of the illiterate E or the Allen cards (picture-differentiating tests) are utilized. Finally, once the alphabet is learned, conventional acuity testing by a logEDTRS or Snellen chart may be used.

Cataracts may be visualized in a variety of ways. On examination with a handlight, a cataract may present as white pupillary opacity (leukocoria). Direct ophthalmoscopy is useful with the principle that if the examiner can see the optic nerve and macula, the patient can probably see out. With either direct illumination or with retroillumination one can visualize a lens opacity silhouetted in the red reflex. Focusing on the optic nerve and macula, a hazy view of the posterior pole through a direct ophthalmoscope may indicate opacification in the visual axis and serve as an estimate of how poorly the patient may see. Nonetheless, the definitive description of a lens opacity depends on a slit-lamp biomicroscopic examination through a widely dilated pupil, allowing for direct illumination and retroillumination with appropriate magnification to visualize the lens opacity and define its clinical features. For research purposes, photographs may be used to document the features and progression of the cataract.

Differential Diagnosis and Diagnostic Tests

The differential diagnosis of a hereditary cataract includes: (1) prenatal causes which include invasion of the eye or lens by a virus or other infectious disease. Rubella directly involves the lens whereas other infectious agents result in ocular inflammation (uveitis), toxoplasmosis, mumps, measles, influenza, chickenpox, herpes simplex, herpes zoster, cytomegalovirus, and echovirus type 3. These can be screened for by TORCH titers. (2) Developmental abnormalities which include premature or dysmature patients may be associated with low birth weight, birth anoxia, or central nervous system involvement leading to seizures, cerebral palsy or hemiplegia, and retinopathy of prematurity. (3) Perinatal–postnatal problems such as hyperglycemia and hypocalcemia can cause cataracts. These are associated with the signs of diabetes and tetany, respectively, and can be screened for by serum chemistries. (4) The association with other ocular abnormalities such as anterior chamber abnormalities (e.g., Reiger syndrome or anomaly, primary hyperplastic vitreous, aniridia, retinopathies such as retinal dysplasia, Norrie disease, and microphthalmia. (5) The association with syndromes can be screened by clinical examination, chromosome analysis, and special blood and urine chemistries depending on which syndromes are suspected clinically.

Treatment

When unilateral and bilateral cataracts are thought to reduce visual acuity considerably, management should include early diagnosis with prompt evaluation to identify etiology when possible. Galactosemia is an example in which rapid diagnosis and treatment will permit recovery of the lens to a normal state of clarity.

Determination of the extent of compromise in visual acuity is important, and surgery may be required. The type of surgery, the use of intraocular lenses, and special procedures such as fitting cataract lenses and epikeratophakia are beyond the scope of this chapter, especially since the issues are controversial and the results of many procedures have yet to be adequately assessed.

Studies begun in kittens[344] and extended to nonhuman primates[345,348] show that unequal input into cortical neurons due to unilateral form deprivation results in more severe visual deficits than does bilateral deprivation. Thus, ophthalmic surgeons generally consider a unilateral dense congenital cataract to be a surgical emergency, while bilateral dense cataracts can be scheduled in a more routine fashion. Usual practice suggests that limited dense cataracts can be operated successfully in the first weeks of life, while bilateral cataracts can be operated successfully up to 3 months of age. With prompt surgery the visual prognosis is better for bilateral as compared with unilateral cases, and in less dense cataracts as compared with total opacities. When congenital cataracts are associated with other ocular abnormalities and/or systemic disease, a poorer visual outcome often results.[347–349] Lastly, it should be emphasized that communication between clinicians, therapists, and teachers is very important in the treatment of young cataract patients and their families.[350]

ADDENDUM

Since this chapter was prepared there have been a number of advances in molecular biology of the lens crystallins. It has been shown that some enzyme crystallins bind reduced nucleotides and are associated with high levels of these cofactors in the lens, which might also provide some protection from oxidative stress.[454] The α-crystallins have been shown to represent a particularly interesting case of gene sharing. Studies of these members of the family of small heat shock proteins have been considerably expanded. In addition to its chaperone ability, α-crystallin has been shown to possess autokinase activity.[455] Thus, the α-crystallins can be considered as members of the enzyme-crystallins and may be involved in metabolic pathways important for the development, maintenance or pathology of the lens and other tissues. Particularly exciting possibilities involving kinase activity for α-crystallin include a metabolic role in signal transduction or protein degradation.

Studies of transcriptional control of crystallins have progressed greatly. δEF1, the nuclear factor binding a key regulatory sequence in the δ1 enhancer, is preferentially expressed in mesoderm, nervous system and lens, and can repress the activity of the δ1-crystallin enhancer in cotransfection experiments. The negative effect of δEF1 can be counteracted by δEF2, which binds just upstream of δEF1 in the δ1 enhancer.[456] δEF2 comprises a family of proteins, with δEF2a and b predominating in the lens and δEF2c and d predominating in non-lens cells. It is believed that δEF1 and δEF2 interact in the control of δ1-crystallin gene expression. Interestingly, δEF2 also binds the promoter of the mouse γF-crystallin gene, suggesting that it may participate in the regulation of different crystallin genes in various species.[3] Another new development is the finding that the mouse γF-crystallin gene is regulated by a novel retinoic acid control element indicating that this factor might affect growth and development of the lens.[457]

In a fashion similar to the α-crystallins, both the β- and γ-crystallins have been shown to be expressed in nonlens tissue. Chicken β-crystallin mRNAs and peptides have been detected in a variety of non-lens tissues including retina, cornea, brain and kidney.[458] Four γ-crystallins were detected in nonlens tissues at various stages of *Xenopus* development.[459]

The structure-function relationships determining β-crystallin association have been further explored. Site specific mutagenesis has been used to substitute both the γ2-crystallin connecting peptide into murine βA3-crystallin and part of the βB2-crystallin connecting peptide into γ2-crystallin[460] without any effect on association in either case. Similar techniques have been used to show that although the amino terminal arm is not absolutely essential for the dimerization of βA3-crystallin, it greatly facilitates it.[461]

Finally, the mechanisms of two inherited forms of cataract, one in mice and one in humans, have been delineated. Both involve the γE-crystallin gene. In the mouse ELO cataract localized to chromosome 1, a single nucleotide deletion destroying the fourth "Greek key" motif of γE-crystallin appears to be responsible for the cataract.[462] In humans, it has been shown that the Coppock-like cataract is associated with a cluster of sequence changes located directly upstream from the human pseudogene for γE-crystallin.[463] These sequence changes result in a ten-fold increase in transcriptional activity when 1.5 kb of sequence upstream from the ψγE-crystallin gene was used to drive a CAT reporter in rat lens epithelial cells. This would turn the ψγE-crystallin transcript into a high abundance transcript, although an in-frame translation termination signal remains in the second exon. Thus, both the ELO (mouse) and Coppock-like (human) mutations would presumably result in synthesis of an improperly folded single-motif γ-crystallin which might disturb the supramolecular organization of structural proteins in the lens and cause a dominantly inherited cataract.

REFERENCES

1. Brewster D: On the anatomical and optical structure of the crystalline lens of animals, particularly that of cod. *Philos Trans R Soc* **123**:323, 1833.
2. Mörner CT: Untersuchungender protein-substanzen in den lichtbrechenden Medien des Auges. *Hoppe Seyler Z Physiol Chem* **18**:61, 1894.
3. Renwick JH, Lawler SD: Probable linkage between a congenital cataract locus and the Duffy blood group locus. *Ann Hum Genet* **27**:67, 1963.
4. Harding JJ, Rixon KC, Marriott FHC: Men have heavier lenses than women of the same age. *Exp Eye Res* **25**:651, 1977.
5. Wistow GJ, Piatigorsky J: Lens crystallins: The evolution and expression of proteins for a highly specialized tissue. *Annu Rev Biochem* **57**:479, 1988.
6. Mann I: *The Development of the Human Eye*. New York, Grune & Stratton, 1964, p 46.
7. Kuzak JR: Embryology and anatomy of the lens, in Tasman W, Jaeger EA (eds): *Duane's Clinical Ophthalmology*. Philadelphia, Lippincott, 1990, p 1.
8. Goodenough DA, Dick JSB, Lyons JE: Lens metabolic cooperation: A study of mouse lens transport and permeability visualized with freeze-substitution autoradiography and electron microscopy. *J Cell Biol* **86**:576, 1980.
9. Gorthy WC, Snavely MR, Berrong ND: Some aspects of transport and digestion in the lens of the normal young adult rat. *Exp Eye Res* **12**:112, 1971.
10. Rae JL, Stacey T: Lanthanum and procion yellow as extracellular markers in the crystalline lens of the rat. *Exp Eye Res* **28**:1, 1979.
11. Raemakers FCS, Bloemendal H: Cytoskeletal and contractile structures in lens cell differentiation, in Bloemendal H (ed): *Molecular and Cellular Biology of the Eye Lens*. New York, Wiley, 1981, p 85.
12. Benedetti L, Dunia I, Ramaekers FCS, Kibbelaar, MA: Lenticular plasma membranes and cytoskeleton, in Bloemendal H (ed): *Molecular and Cellular Biology of the Eye Lens*. New York, Wiley, 1981, p 137.
13. Alcala H, Maisel H: Biochemistry of lens plasma membranes and cytoskeleton, in Maisel H (ed): *The Ocular Lens*. New York, Marcel Dekker, 1985, p 169.
14. Rafferty NS: Lens morphology, in Maisel H (ed): *The Ocular Lens*. New York, Marcel Dekker, 1985, p. 1.
15. Ireland M, Maisel H: A family of lens fiber cell specific proteins. *Lens Eye Tox Res* **6**:623, 1989.
16. Fitzgerald PG, Gottlieb W: The Mr 115 kd fiber cell-specific protein is a component of the lens cytoskeleton. *Curr Eye Res* **8**:801, 1989.
17. Dola A, Katar M, Hussain P, Maisel H: Ankyrin of the ocular lens. *Ophthalmic Res* **22**:295, 1990.
18. Piatigorsky J: Lens cell elongation *in vitro* and microtubules. *Ann NY Acad Sci* **253**:333, 1975.
19. Piatigorsky J: Gene expression and genetic engineering in the lens. Friedenwald lecture. *Invest Ophthalmol Vis Sci* **28**:9, 1987.
20. Ostrer H, Beebe DC, Piatigorsky J: Beta-crystallin mRNAs: Differential distribution in the developing chicken lens. *Dev Biol* **86**:403, 1981.
21. Hejtmancik JF, Beebe DC, Ostrer H, Piatigorsky J: Delta- and beta-crystallin mRNA levels in the embryonic and posthatched chicken lens: Temporal and spatial changes during development. *Dev Biol* **109**:72, 1985.
22. Van Leen RW, Van Roozendaal KEP, Lubsen NH, Schoenmakers JG: Differential expression of crystallin genes during development of the rat eye lens. *Dev Biol* **120**:457, 1987.
23. Aarts HJM, Lubsen NH, Schoenmakers JGG: Crystallin gene expression during rat lens development. *Eur J Biochem* **183**:31, 1989.
24. Voorter CE, De Haard-Hoekman WA, Hermans MM, Bloemendal H, De Jong WW: Differential synthesis of crystallins in the developing rat eye lens. *Exp Eye Res* **50**:429, 1990.
25. Young RW, Ocumpaugh DE: Autoradiographic studies on the growth and development of the lens capsule in the rat. *Invest Ophthalmol Vis Sci* **5**:583, 1966.
26. Fischer RF, Pettet BE: The postnatal growth of the capsule of the human crystalline lens. *J Anat* **112**:207, 1972.
27. Koretz JF, Handelman GH: How the human eye focuses. *Sci Am* **256**:92, 1988.
28. Parmigiani C, McAvoy J: Localisation of laminin and fibronectin during rat lens morphogenesis. *Differentiation* **28**:53, 1986.
29. Cammarata PR, Cantu-Crouch D, Oakford L, Morrill A: Macromolecular organization of the bovine lens capsule. *Tissue Cell* **18**:83, 1986.
30. Vrensen G, Kappelhof J, Willikens B: Aging of the human lens. *Lens Eye Tox Res* **7**:1, 1990.
31. Kuszak JR, Deutsch TA, Brown HG: Anatomy of aged and senile cataractous lenses, in Albert D, Jacobiec F (eds): *Principles and Practice of Ophthalmology: The Harvard System*. Philadelphia, Saunders, 1994, p 82.
32. Koretz JF, Kaufman PL, Neider MW, Goeckner PA: Accommodation and presbyopia in the human eye—aging of the anterior segment. *Vision Res* **29**:1685, 1989.
33. Davson H: *Physiology of the Eye*. New York, Pergamon, 1990, p 762.
34. Sample PA, Esterson FD, Weinreb RN, Boynton RM: The aging lens: *in vivo* assessment of light absorption in 84 human eyes. *Invest Ophthalmol Vis Sci* **8**:1306, 1988.
35. Hockwin O, Ohrloff C: The eye in the elderly: Lens, in Platt D (ed): *Geriatrics*. Berlin, Springer-Verlag, 1984, p 373.
36. Sample PA, Esterson FD, Weinreb RN, Boynton RM: The aging lens: *in vivo* assessment of light absorption in 84 human eyes. *Invest Ophthalmol Vis Sci* **8**:1306, 1988.
37. Roy D, Spector A: Absence of low-molecular weight alpha-crystallin in nuclear region of old human lens. *Proc Natl Acad Sci USA* **73**:3484, 1976.
38. McFall-Ngai MJ, Ding L-L, Takemoto LJ, Horwitz J:

Spatial and temporal mapping of the age-related changes in human lens crystallins. *Exp Eye Res* **41**:745, 1985.

39. Voorter CE, De Haard-Hoekman WA, Roersma ES, Meyer HE, Bloemendal H, De Jong WW: The in vivo phosphorylation sties of bovine alpha B-crystallin. *FEBS Lett* **259**:50, 1989.
40. Horwitz J, Wong MM: Peptide mapping by limited proteolysis in sodium dodecyl sulfate of the main intrinsic polypeptides isolated from human and bovine lens plasma membranes. *Biochim Biophys Acta* **622**:134, 1980.
41. Wagner BJ, Margolis JW, Garland D, Roseman JE: Bovine lens neutral proteinase preferentially hydrolyses oxidatively modified glutamine synthetase. *Exp Eye Res* **43**:1141, 1986.
42. Wagner BJ, Margolis JW: Common epitopes of bovine lens multicatalytic-proteinase-complex subunits. *Biochem J* **257**:265, 1989.
43. Harding JJ, Crabbe MJC: The lens. Development, proteins, metabolism and cataract, in Davson H (ed): *The Eye*, 3rd ed. Orlando, FL, Academic, 1984, vol 1B, p 207.
44. David LL, Shearer TR: Purification of calpain II from rat lens and determination of endogenous substrates. *Exp Eye Res* **42**:227, 1986.
45. Jahngen JH, Lipman RD, Eisenhauer DA, Jahngen EG, Jr, Taylor A: Aging and cellular maturation cause changes in ubiquitin-eye lens protein conjugates. *Arch Biochem Biophys* **276**:32, 1990.
46. Masters PM, Bada JL, Zigler JS Jr: Aspartic acid racemisation in the human lens during ageing and in cataract formation. *Nature* **268**:71, 1977.
47. Groenen PJTA, Van Den Ijssel PR, Voorter CE, Bloemendal H, De Jong WW: Site-specific racemization in aging alpha-A-crystallin. *FEBS Lett* **269**:109, 1990.
48. Spector A, Chiesa R, Sredy J, Garner W: cAMP-dependent phosphorylation of bovine lens alpha-crystallin. *Proc Natl Acad Sci USA* **82**:4712, 1985.
49. Garlick RL, Mazer JS, Chylack LT Jr, Tung WH, Bunn HF: Nonenzymatic glycation of human lens crystallin. Effect of aging and diabetes mellitus. *J Clin Invest* **74**:1742, 1984.
50. Augusteyn RC: Distribution of flourescence in the human cataractous lens. *Ophthalmic Res* **7**:217, 1975.
51. Harding JJ: Possible causes of the unfolding of proteins in cataract and a new hypothesis to explain the high prevalence of cataract in some countries, in Regnault F, Hockwin O, Courtois Y (eds): *Aging of the Lens*. Amsterdam, Elsevier, 1980.
52. Harding JJ, Rixon KC: Carbamylation of lens proteins: A possible factor in cataractogenesis in some tropical countries. *Exp Eye Res* **31**:567, 1980.
53. Straatsma BR, Horwitz J, Takemoto LJ, Lightfoot DO, Ding LL: Clinicobiochemical correlations in aging-related human cataract. *Am J Ophthalmol* **97**:457, 1984.
54. Takemoto L, Straatsma BR, Horwitz J: Immunochemical characterization of the major low molecular weight polypeptide (10K) from human cataractous lenses. *Exp Eye Res* **48**:261, 1989.
55. Takemoto LJ, Hansen JS, Zigler JS, Horwitz J: Characterization of polypeptides from human nuclear cataracts by Western blot analysis. *Exp Eye Res* **40**:205, 1985.
56. David LL, Shearer TR: Role of proteolysis in lenses: A review. *Lens Eye Tox Res* **6**:725, 1989.
57. Ruddock KH: Light transmission through the ocular media and macular pigment and its significance for psychophysical investigating, in Jameson D, Hurvich L (eds): *Handbook of Sensory Physiology*. Berlin, Springer-Verlag, 1972, p 455.
58. Lerman S: *Radiant Energy and the Eye*. New York, Macmillan, 1980, p 131.
59. Benedek GB: Theory of transparency of the eye. *Appl Optics* **10**:459, 1971.
60. Delaye M, Tardieu A: Short-range order of crystallin proteins accounts for eye lens transparency. *Nature* **302**:415, 1983.
61. Bettelheim FA, Siew EL: Effect of changes in concentration upon lens turbidity as predicted by the random fluctuation theory. *Biophys J* **41**:29, 1983.
62. Delaye M, Gromiec A: Mutual diffusion of crystallin proteins at finite concentrations: A light scattering study. *Biopolymers* **22**:1203, 1983.
63. De Jong WW, Terwindt EC, Bloemendal H: The amino acid sequence of the A chain of human alpha-crystallin. *FEBS Lett* **58**:310, 1975.
64. Kramps JA, Deman BM, De Jong WW: The primary structure of the B_2 chain of human alpha-crystallin. *FEBS Lett* **74**:82, 1977.
65. Van Der Ouderaa FJ, De Jong WW, Hilderink A, Bloemendal H: The amino acid sequence of the alphaB_2 chain of bovine alpha-crystallin. *Eur J Biochem* **49**:157, 1974.
66. Horwitz J: Some properties of the low molecular weight alpha-crystallin from normal human lens: Comparison with bovine lens. *Exp Eye Res* **19**:49, 1974.
67. Siezen RJ, Bindels JG, Hoenders HJ: The quartenary structure of bovine alpha-crystallin. *Eur J Biochem* **111**:435, 1980.
68. Tardieu A, Laporte D, Licinio P, Krop B, Delaye M: Calf lens alpha-crystallin quarternary structure. A three-layer model. *J Mol Biol* **192**:711, 1986.
69. Augusteyn RC, Koretz JF: A possible structure for alpha-crystallin. *FEBS Lett* **222**:1, 1987.
70. Thomson JA, Augusteyn RC: On the structure of alpha-crystallin: Construction of hybrid molecules and homopolymers. *Biochem Biophys Acta* **994**:246, 1989.
71. Hendriks W, Weetink H, Voorter CE, Sanders J, Bloemendal H, De Jong WW: The alternative splicing product alpha A^{ins}-crystallin is structurally equivalent to alpha A and alpha B subunits in the rat alpha-crystallin aggregate. *Biochim Biophys Acta* **1037**:58, 1990.
72. Chiesa R, Spector A: The dephosphorylation of lens alpha-crystallin A chain. *Biochem Biophys Res Commun* **162**:1494, 1989.
73. Mulders JWM, Stokkermans J, Leunissen JAM, Benedetti EL, Bloemendal H, De Jong WW: Interaction of alpha-crystallin with lens plasma membranes: Affinity for MP26. *Eur J Biochem* **152**:721, 1985.
74. Lasser A, Balazs EA: Biochemical and fine structure studies on the water-insoluble components of the calf lens. *Exp Eye Res* **13**:292, 1972.
75. De Jong WW, Gleaves JT, Boulter D: Evolutionary changes of alpha-crystallin and the phylogeny of mammalian orders. *J Mol Evol* **10**:123, 1977.
76. Ingolia TD, Craig EA: Four small Drosophila heat shock proteins are related to each other and to mammalian alpha-crystallin. *Proc Natl Acad Sci USA* **79**:2360, 1982.
77. Nene V, Dunne DW, Johnson KS, Taylor DW, Cordingley JS: Sequence and expression of a major egg antigen from Schistosoma mansoni. Homologies to heat shock proteins and alpha-crystallins. *Mol Biochem Parasitol* **21**:179, 1986.
78. De Jong WW, Hendriks W, Mulders JW, Bloemendal H: Evolution of eye lens crystallins: The stress connection. *Trends Biochem Sci* **14**:365, 1989.
79. Cohen LH, Westerhuis LW, De Jong WW, Bloemendal H: Rat alpha-crystallin A chain with an insertion of 22 residues. *Eur J Biochem* **89**:259, 1978.
80. Cohen LH, Westerhuis LW, Smits DP, Bloemendal H: Two structurally closely related polypeptides encoded by 14-S mRNA isolated from rat lens. *Eur J Biochem* **89**:251, 1978.
81. Van Den Heuvel R, Hendriks W, Quax W, Bloemendal H: Complete structure of the hamster alpha A-crystallin gene: Reflection of an evolutionary history by means of exon shuffling. *J Mol Biol* **185**:273, 1985.
82. Hendriks W, Sanders J, De Leij L, Ramaekers F, Bloemendal H, De Jong W: Monoclonal antibodies reveal evolutionary conservation of alternative splicing of the alpha A-crystallin primary transcript. *Eur J Biochem* **174**:133, 1988.
83. King CR, Piatigorsky J: Alternative RNA splicing of the murine alpha A-crystallin gene: Protein-coding information within an intron. *Cell* **32**:707, 1983.
84. Jaworski CJ, Piatigorsky J: A pseudo-exon in the functional human alpha A-crystallin gene. *Nature* **337**:752, 1989.
85. Bhat SP, Nagineni CN: Alpha B subunit of lens-specific protein alpha-crystallin is in other ocular and non-ocular tissues. *Biochem Biophys Res Commun* **158**:319, 1989.
86. Dubin RA, Wawrousek EF, Piatigorsky J: Expression of the murine alpha B-crystallin gene is not restricted to the lens. *Mol Cell Biol* **9**:1083, 1989.

87. Bhat SP, Horwitz J, Srinivasan A, Ding L: Alpha B-crystallin exists as an independent protein in the heart and in the lens. *Eur J Biochem* **202:**775, 1991.
88. Longoni S, Lattonen S, Bullock G, Chiesi M: Cardiac alpha-crystallin. II. Intracellular localization. *Mol Cell Biochem* **97:**121, 1990.
89. Atomi Y, Yamada S, Nishida T: Early changes of alpha B-crystallin mRNA in rat skeletal muscle to mechanical tension and denervation. *Biochem Biophys Res Commun* **181:**1323, 1991.
90. Iwaki T, Kume-Iwaki A, Liem RK, Goldman JE: Alpha B-crystallin is expressed in non-lenticular tissues and accumulates in Alexander's disease brain. *Cell* **57:**71, 1989.
91. Duguid JR, Bohmont CW, Liu NG, Tourtellotte WW: Changes in brain gene expression shared by scrapie and Alzheimer disease. *Proc Natl Acad Sci USA* **86:**7260, 1989.
92. Murano S, Thweatt R, Shmookler Reis RJ, Jones RA, Moerman EJ, Goldstein S: Diverse gene sequences are overexpressed in Werner syndrome fibroblasts undergoing premature replicative senescence. *Mol Cell Biol* **11:**3905, 1991.
93. Klemenz R, Frohli E, Steiger RH, Schafer R, Aoyama A: Alpha B-crystallin is a small heat shock protein. *Proc Natl Acad Sci USA* **88:**3652, 1991.
94. Dasgupta S, Hohman TC, Carper D: Hypertonic stress induces alpha B-crystallin expression. *Exp Eye Res* **54:**461, 1992.
95. Kato K, Shinohara H, Kurobe N, Goto S, Inaguma Y, Ohshima K: Immunoreactive alpha A-crystallin in rat non-lenticular tissues detected with a sensitive immunoassay method. *Biochim Biophys Acta* **1080:**173, 1991.
96. Hendriks W, Leunissen J, Nevo E, Bloemendal H, De Jong WW: The lens protein alpha A-crystallin of the blind mole rat, Spalax ehrenbergi: Evolutionary change and functional constraints. *Proc Natl Acad Sci USA* **84:**5320, 1987.
97. Horwitz J: The function of alpha-crystallin: Proctor lecture. *Invest Ophthalmol Vis Sci* **34:**10, 1993.
98. Thompson MA, Hawkins JW, Piatigorsky J: Complete nucleotide sequence of the chicken alpha A-crystallin gene and its 5′ flanking region. *Gene* **56:**173, 1987.
99. Quax-Jeuken Y, Quax W, Van Rens G, Khan PM, Bloemendal H: Complete structure of the alpha B-crystallin gene: Conservation of the exon-intron distribution in the two nonlinked alpha-crystallin genes. *Proc Natl Acad Sci USA* **82:**5819, 1985.
100. Wistow G: Domain structure and evolution in alpha-crystallins and small heat-shock proteins. *FEBS Lett* **181:**1, 1985.
101. Hawkins JW, Van Keuren ML, Piatigorsky J, Law ML, Patterson D, Kao FT: Confirmation of assignment of the human alpha 1-crystallin gene (CRYA1) to chromosome 21 with regional localization to q22.3. *Hum Genet* **76:**375, 1987.
102. Ngo JT, Klisak I, Dubin RA, Piatigorsky J, Mohandas T, Sparkes RS, Bateman JB: Assignment of the alpha B-crystallin gene to human chromosome 11. *Genomics* **5:**665, 1989.
103. Brakenhoff RH, Guerts Van Kessel AH, Oldenburg M, Wijnen JT, Bloemendal H, Meera Kahn P, Schoenmakers JG: Human alpha B-crystallin (CRYA2) gene mapped to chromosome 11q12-q23. *Hum Genet* **85:**237, 1990.
104. Piatigorsky J, Zelenka PS: Transcriptional regulation of crystallin genes: Cis elements, trans-factors and signal transduction systems in the lens, in Wasserman PW (ed): *Advances in Developmental Biochemistry*. New York, J.A.I. 1992, p 211.
105. Chepelinsky AB, King CR, Zelenka PS, Piatigorsky J: Lens-specific expression of the chloramphenicol acetyltransferase gene promoted by 5′ flanking sequences of the murine alpha A-crystallin gene in explanted chicken lens epithelia. *Proc Natl Acad Sci USA* **82:**2334, 1985.
106. Overbeek PA, Chepelinsky AB, Khillan JS, Piatigorsky J, Westphal H: Lens-specific expression and developmental regulation of the bacterial chloramphenicol acetyltransferase gene driven by the murine alpha A-crystallin promoter in transgenic mice. *Proc Natl Acad Sci USA* **82:**7815, 1985.
107. Wawrousek EF, Chepelinsky AB, McDermott JB, Piatigorsky J: Regulation of the murine alpha A-crystallin promoter in transgenic mice. *Dev Biol* **137:**68, 1990.
108. Driessen HP, Herbrink P, Bloemendal H, De Jong WW: Primary structure of the bovine beta-crystallin Bp chain. Internal duplication and homology with gamma-crystallin. *Eur J Biochem* **121:**83, 1981.
109. Wistow G, Slingsby C, Blundell T, Driessen H, De Jong W, Bloemendal H: Eye-lens proteins: The three-dimensional structure of beta-crystallin predicted from monomeric gamma-crystallin. *FEBS Lett* **133:**9, 1981.
110. Lubsen NH, Aarts HJ, Schoenmakers JG: The evolution of lenticular proteins: The beta- and gamma-crystallin supergene family. *Prog Biophys Mol Biol* **51:**47, 1988.
111. Blundell TL, Lindley PF, Miller L, Moss DS, Slingsby C, Tickle IJ, Turnell WG, Wistow GJ: The molecular structure and stability of the eye lens: X-ray analysis of gamma-crystallin II. *Nature* **289:**771, 1981.
112. Wistow G, Turnell B, Summers L, Slingsby C, Moss D, Miller L, Linkley P, Blundell T: X-ray analysis of the eye lens protein gamma-II crystallin at 1.9 A resolution. *J Mol Biol* **170:**175, 1983.
113. White HE, Driessen HP, Slingsby C, Moss DS, Lindley PF: Packing interactions in the eye-lens. Structural analysis, internal symmetry and lattice interactions of bovine gamma IVa-crystallin. *J Mol Biol* **207:**217, 1989.
114. Siezen RJ, Wu E, Kaplan ED, Thomson JA, Benedek GB: Rat lens gamma-crystallins. Characterization of the six gene products and their spatial and temporal distribution resulting from differential synthesis. *J Mol Biol* **199:**475, 1988.
115. Broide ML, Berland CR, Pande J, Ogun OO, Benedek GB: Binary-liquid phase separation of lens protein solutions. *Proc Natl Acad Sci USA* **88:**5660, 1991.
116. Tanaka T, Benedek GB: Observation of protein diffusivity in intact human and bovine lenses with application to cataract. *Invest Ophthalmol* **14:**449, 1975.
117. Wistow G, Summers L, Blundell T: Myxococcus xanthus spore coat protein S may have a similar structure to vertebrate lens beta gamma-crystallins. *Nature* **315:**771, 1985.
118. Wistow G: Evolution of a protein superfamily: Relationships between vertebrate lens crystallins and microorganism dormancy proteins. *J Mol Evol* **30:**140, 1990.
119. Van Dam AF: Purification and composition studies of beta S-crystallin. *Exp Eye Res* **5:**255, 1966.
120. Quax-Jeuken Y, Driessen H, Leunissen J, Quax W, De Jong W, Bloemendal H: Beta S-crystallin: Structure and evolution of a distinct member of the beta gamma-superfamily. *EMBO J* **4:**2597, 1985.
121. Van Rens FLM, Raats JMH, Driessen HPC, Oldenburg M, Wijnen JT, Khan PM, De Jong WW, Bloemendal H: Structure of the bovine eye lens gamma S-crystallin gene (formerly beta S). *Gene* **78:**225, 1989.
122. Zigler JS, Russell P, Horwitz J, Reddy VN, Kinoshita JH: Further studies on low molecular weight crystallins: Relationship between the bovine $beta_s$, the human 24 kD protein and the gamma-crystallin. *Curr Eye Res* **5:**395, 1986.
123. Wijnen JT, Oldenburg M, Bloemendal H, Meera-Khan P: GS (gamma-S)-crystallin (CRYGS) assignment to chromosome 3. *Cytogenet Cell Genet* **51:**1108, 1989.
124. Willard HF, Meakin SO, Tsui LC, Breitman ML: Assignment of human gamma crystallin multigene family to chromosome 2. *Somat Cell Mol Genet* **11:**511, 1985.
125. Den Dunnen JT, Jongbloed RJE, Geurts Van Kessel AHM, Schoenmakers JGG: Human lens gamma-crystallin sequences are located in the p12-qter region of chromosome 2. *Hum Genet* **70:**217, 1985.
126. Shiloh Y, Donlon T, Bruns G, Breitman ML, Tsui LC: Assignment of the human gamma-crystallin gene cluster (CRYG) to the long arm of chromosome 2, region q33-36. *Hum Genet* **73:**17, 1986.
127. Slingsby C, Croft LR: Developmental changes in the low molecular weight proteins of the bovine lens. *Exp Eye Res* **17:**369, 1973.
128. McDevitt DS, Croft LR: On the existence of gamma-crystallin in the bird lens. *Exp Eye Res* **25:**473, 1977.
129. Van Rens GLM, De Jong WW, Bloemendal H: One member of the gamma-crystallin gene family, gamma S, is expressed in birds. *Exp Eye Res* **53:**135, 1991.
130. Moormann RJM, Den Dunnen JT, Mulleners L, Andreoli P, Bloemendal H, Schoenmakers JGG: Strict co-linearity of genetic and protein folding domains in an

intragenically duplicated rat lens gamma-crystallin gene. *J Mol Biol* **171**:353, 1983.
131. Lok S, Tsui LC, Shinohara T, Piatigorsky J, Gold R, Breitman M: Analysis of the mouse gamma-crystallin gene family: Assignment of multiple cDNAs to discrete genomic sequences and characterization of a representative gene. *Nucleic Acids Res* **12**:4517, 1984.
132. Meakin SO, Du RP, Tsui LC, Breitman ML: Gamma-crystallins of the human eye lens: Expression analysis of five members of the gene family. *Mol Cell Biol* **7**:2671, 1987.
133. Russell P, Meakin SO, Hohman TC, Tsui LC, Breitman ML: Relationship between proteins encoded by three human gamma-crystallin genes and distinct polypeptides in the eye lens. *Mol Cell Biol* **7**:3320, 1987.
134. Siezen RJ, Thomson JA, Kaplan ED, Benedek GB: Human lens gamma-crystallin: Isolation, identification, and characterization of the expressed gene products. *Proc Natl Acad Sci USA* **84**:6088, 1987.
135. Breitman ML, Clapoff S, Rossant J, Tsui LC, Glode LM, Maxwell IH, Bernstein A: Genetic ablation: Targeted expression of a toxin gene causes microphthalmia in transgenic mice. *Science* **238**:1563, 1987.
136. Lok S, Breitman ML, Chepelinsky AB, Piatigorsky J, Gold RJ, Tsui LC: Lens-specific promoter activity of a mouse gamma-crystallin gene. *Mol Cell Biol* **5**:2221, 1985.
137. Goring DR, Rossant J, Clapoff S, Breitman ML, Tsui LC: *In situ* detection of beta-galactosidase in lenses of transgenic mice with a gamma-crystallin/lacZ gene. *Science* **235**:456, 1987.
138. Lok S, Stevens W, Breitman ML, Tsui LC: Multiple regulatory elements of the murine gamma 2-crystallin promoter. *Nucleic Acids Res* **17**:3563, 1989.
139. Peterson CA, Piatigorsky J: Preferential conservation of the globular domains of the beta A3/A1-crystallin polypeptide of the chicken eye lens. *Gene* **45**:139, 1986.
140. Hejtmancik JF, Thompson MA, Wistow G, Piatigorsky J: cDNA and deduced protein sequence for the beta-B1-crystallin polypeptide of the chicken lens: Conservation of the PAPA sequence. *J Biol Chem* **261**:982, 1986.
141. Berbers GAM, Hoekman WA, Bloemendal H, De Jong WW, Kleinschmidt T, Braunitzer G: Homology between the primary structures of the major bovine beta-crystallin chains. *Eur J Biochem* **139**:476, 1984.
142. Lindley PF, Narebor ME, Summers LJ, Wistow GJ: The structure of lens proteins, in Maisel H (ed): *The Ocular Lens*. New York, Marcel Dekker, 1985, p 123.
143. Slingsby C, Driessen MPC, Mahadevan D, Bax B, Blundell TL: Evolutionary and functional relationships between the basic and acidic beta-crystallins. *Exp Eye Res* **46**:375, 1988.
144. Inana G, Piatigorsky J, Norman B, Slingsby C, Blundell T: Gene and protein structure of a beta-crystallin polypeptide in murine lens: Relationship of exons and structural motifs. *Nature* **302**:310, 1983.
145. Bloemendal H, De Jong WW: Lens proteins and their genes. *Prog Nucleic Acid Res Mol Biol* **41**:259, 1991.
146. Hogg D, Tsui LC, Gorin M, Breitman ML: Characterization of the human beta-crystallin gene Hu beta A3/A1 reveals ancestral relationships among the beta gamma-crystallin superfamily. *J Biol Chem* **261**:12420, 1986.
147. Berbers GAM, Hoekman WA, Bloemendal H, De Jong WW, Kleinschmidt T, Braunitzer G: Proline- and alanine-rich N-terminal extension of the basic bovine beta-crystallin B1 chains. *FEBS Lett* **161**:225, 1983.
148. Kleiman NJ, Chiesa R, Kolks MA, Spector A: Phosphorylation of beta-crystallin B2 (beta Bp) in the bovine lens. *J Biol Chem* **263**:14978, 1988.
149. Voorter CE, Bloemendal H, De Jong WW: In vitro and in vivo phosphorylation of chicken beta B3-crystallin. *Curr Eye Res* **8**:459, 1989.
150. Wistow G, Roquemore E, Kim HS: Anomalous behavior of beta B1-crystallin subunits from avian lenses. *Curr Eye Res* **10**:313, 1991.
151. Slingsby C, Bateman OA: Quarternary interactions in eye lens beta-crystallins: Basic and acidic subunits of beta-crystallins favor heterologous association. *Biochemistry* **29**:6592, 1990.
152. Bax B, Lapatto R, Nalini V, Driessen H, Lindley PF, Mahadevan D, Blundell TL, Slingsby C: X-ray analysis of beta B2-crystallin and evolution of oligomeric lens proteins. *Nature* **347**:776, 1990.
153. Den Dunnen JT, Moormann RJM, Lubsen NH, Schoenmakers JGG: Intron insertions and deletions in the beta/gamma-crystallin gene family: The rat beta B1 gene. *Proc Natl Acad Sci USA* **83**:2855, 1986.
154. Moormann RJM, Den Dunnen JT, Bloemendal H, Schoenmakers JGG: Extensive intragenic sequence homology in two distinct rat lens gamma-crystallin cDNAs suggests duplications of a primordial gene. *Proc Natl Acad Sci USA* **79**:6876, 1982.
155. Hogg D, Gorin MB, Heinzmann C, Zollman S, Mohandas T, Klisak I, Sparkes RS, Breitman M, Tsui LC, Horwitz J: Nucleotide sequence for the cDNA of the bovine beta B2 crystallin and assignment of the orthologous human locus to chromosome 22. *Curr Eye Res* **6**:1335, 1987.
156. Sparkes RS, Mohandas T, Heinzmann C, Gorin MB, Zollman S, Horwitz J: Assignment of a human beta-crystallin gene to 17cen-q23. *Hum Genet* **74**:133, 1986.
157. Aarts HJM, Den Dunnen JT, Lubsen NH, Schoenmakers JGG: Linkage between the beta B2 and beta B3 crystallin genes in man and rat: A remnant of an ancient beta-crystallin gene cluster. *Gene* **59**:127, 1987.
158. Piatigorsky J, O'Brien WE, Norman BL, Kalumuck K, Wistow GJ, Borras T, Nickerson JM, Wawrousek EF: Gene sharing by delta-crystallin and argininosuccinate lyase. *Proc Natl Acad Sci USA* **85**:3479, 1988.
159. Piatigorsky J: Lens crystallins: Innovation by changes in gene regulation. *J Biol Chem* **267**:4277, 1992.
160. Piatigorsky J, Wistow GJ: Enzyme/crystallins: Gene sharing as an evolutionary strategy. *Cell* **57**:197, 1989.
161. Piatigorsky J, Wistow GJ: The recruitment of crystallins: New functions precede gene duplication. *Science* **252**:1078, 1991.
162. McFall-Ngai MJ, Horwitz J: A comparative study of the thermal stability of the vertebrate eye lens: Antarctic ice fish to the desert iguana. *Exp Eye Res* **50**:703, 1990.
163. Piatigorsky J: Delta crystallins and their nucleic acids. *Mol Cell Biochem* **59**:33, 1984.
164. Wistow G, Piatigorsky J: Recruitment of enzymes as lens structural proteins. *Science* **236**:1554, 1987.
165. Thomas G, Zelenka PS, Cuthbertson RA, Norman BL, Piatigorsky J: Differential expression of the two delta-crystallin/argininosuccinate lyase genes in the lens, heart and brain of the chicken embryo. *New Biol* **2**:903, 1990.
166. Kondoh H, Araki I, Yasuda K, Matsubasa T, Mori M: Expression of the chicken 'delta 2-crystallin' gene in mouse cells: Evidence for encoding of argininosuccinate lyase. *Gene* **99**:267, 1991.
167. Barborosa P, Wistow GJ, Cialkowski M, Piatigorsky J, O'Brien WE: Expression of duck lens delta-crystallin cDNAs in yeast and bacterial hosts. *J Biol Chem* **266**:22319, 1991.
168. Wistow GJ, Mulders JWM, De Jong WW: The enzyme lactate dehydrogenase as a structural protein in avian and crocodilian lenses. *Nature* **326**:622, 1987.
169. Hendriks W, Mulders JW, Bibby MA, Slingsby C, Bloemendal H, De Jong WW: Duck lens epsilon-crystallin and lactate dehydrogenase B4 are identical: A single-copy gene product with two distinct functions. *Proc Natl Acad Sci USA* **85**:7114, 1988.
170. Wistow G, Kim H: Lens protein expression in mammals: Taxon-specificity and the recruitment of crystallins. *J Mol Evol* **32**:262, 1991.
171. Mulders JW, Hendriks W, Blankesteijn WM, Bloemendal H, De Jong WW: Lambda-crystallin, a major rabbit lens protein, is related to hydroxyacyl-coenzyme A dehydrogenases. *J Biol Chem* **263**:15462, 1988.
172. Carper D, Nishimura C, Shinohara T, Dietzschold B, Wistow G, Craft C, Kador P, Kinoshita JH: Aldose reductase and rho-crystallin belong to the same protein superfamily as aldehyde reductase. *FEBS Lett* **220**:209, 1987.
173. Borras T, Persson B, Jornvall H: Eye lens zeta-crystallin relationships to the family of "long-chain" alcohol/polyol dehydrogenases. Protein trimming and conservation of stable parts. *Biochemistry* **28**:6133, 1989.

174. Rao PV, Zigler JS Jr: Zeta-crystallin from guinea pig lens is capable of functioning catalytically as an oxidoreductase. *Arch Biochem Biophys* **284:**181, 1991.
175. Piatigorsky J, Horwitz J, Kuwabara T, Cutress CE: The cellular eye lens and crystallins of cubomedusan jellyfish. *J Comp Physiol [A]* **164:**577, 1989.
176. Chepelinsky AB, Sommer B, Piatigorsky J: Interaction between two different regulatory elements activates the murine alpha A-crystallin gene promoter in explanted lens epithelia. *Mol Cell Biol* **7:**1807, 1987.
177. Nakamura T, Donovan DM, Hamada K, Sax CM, Norman B, Flanagan JR, Ozato K, Westphal H, Piatigorsky J: Regulation of the mouse alpha A-crystallin gene: Isolation of a cDNA encoding a protein that binds to a cis sequence motif shared with the major histocompatibility complex class I gene and other genes. *Mol Cell Biol* **10:**3700, 1990.
178. Sommer B, Chepelinsky AB, Piatigorsky J: Binding of nuclear proteins to promoter elements of the mouse alpha A-crystallin gene. *J Biol Chem* **263:**15666, 1988.
179. Klement JF, Wawrousek EF, Piatigorsky J: Tissue-specific expression of the chicken alpha A-crystallin gene in cultured lens epithelia and transgenic mice. *J Biol Chem* **264:**19837, 1989.
180. Roth HJ, Das GC, Piatigorsky J: Chicken beta B1-crystallin gene expression: Presence of conserved functional polyoma enhancer-like and octomer binding-like promoter elements found in non-lens genes. *Mol Cell Biol* **11:**1488, 1991.
181. Liu QR, Tini M, Tsui LC, Breitman ML: Interaction of a lens cell transcription factor with the proximal domain of the mouse gamma F-crystallin promoter. *Mol Cell Biol* **11:**1531, 1991.
182. Goto K, Okada TS, Kondoh H: Functional cooperation of lens-specific and nonspecific elements in the delta 1-crystallin enhancer. *Mol Cell Biol* **10:**958, 1990.
183. Funahashi J, Sekido R, Murai K, Kamachi Y, Kondoh H: Delta-crystallin enhancer binding protein delta EF1 is a zinc finger-homeodomain protein implicated in postgastrulation embryogenesis. *Development* **119:**433, 1993.
184. Hayashi S, Goto K, Okada TS, Kondoh H: Lens-specific enhancer in the third intron regulates expression of the chicken delta1-crystallin gene. *Genes Dev* **1:**818, 1987.
185. Peek R, Van Der Logt P, Lubsen NH, Schoenmakers JG: Tissue- and species-specific promoter elements of rat gamma-crystallin genes. *Nucleic Acids Res* **18:**1189, 1990.
186. Yu CC-K, Tsui L-C, Breitman ML: Homologous and heterologous enhancers modulate spatial expression but not cell-type specificity of the murine gamma-crystallin promoter. *Development* **110:**131, 1990.
187. Sullivan CH, O'Farrell S, Grainger RM: Delta-crystallin gene expression and patterns of hypomethylation demonstrate two levels of regulation for the delta-crystallin genes in embryonic chick tissues. *Dev Biol* **145:**40, 1991.
188. Peek R, Niessen RW, Schoenmakers JG, Lubsen NH: DNA methylation as a regulatory mechanism in rat gamma-crystallin gene expression. *Nucleic Acids Res* **19:**77, 1991.
189. Gilmore TD: NF-kappa B, KBF1, dorsal, and related matters. *Cell* **62:**841, 1990.
190. Sax CM, Klement JF, Piatigorsky J: Species-specific lens activation of the thymidine kinase promoter by a single copy of the mouse alpha A-CRYBP1 site and loss of tissue specificity by multimerization. *Mol Cell Biol* **10:**6813, 1990.
191. Head MW, Triplett EL, Clayton RM: Independent regulation of two coexpressed delta-crystallin genes in chick lens and nonlens tissues. *Exp Cell Res* **193:**370, 1991.
192. Iwaki A, Iwaki T, Goldman JE, Liem RK: Multiple mRNAs of rat brain alpha-crystallin B chain result from alternative transcriptional initiation. *J Biol Chem* **265:**22197, 1990.
193. Gopal-Srivastava R, Piatigorsky J: The murine alphaB-crystallin/small heat shock protein enhancer: Identification of alphaBE-1, alphaBE-2, alphaBE-3, and MRF control elements. *Mol Cell Biol* **13:**7144, 1993.
194. Dubin RA, Ally AH, Chung S, Piatigorsky J: Human alpha B-crystallin gene and preferential promoter function in lens. *Genomics* **7:**594, 1990.
195. Atreya PL, Barnes J, Katar M, Alcala J, Maisel H: N-cadherin of the human lens. *Curr Eye Res* **8:**947, 1989.
196. Russell P, Zelenka P, Martensen T, Reid TW: Identification of the EDTA-extractable protein in lens as calpactin I. *Curr Eye Res* **6:**533, 1987.
197. Watanabe M, Kobayashi H, Rutishauser U, Katar M, Alcala J, Maisel H: NCAM in the differentiation of embryonic lens tissue. *Dev Biol* **135:**414, 1989.
198. Mulders JW, Voorter CE, Lamers C, De Haard-Hoekman WA, Montecucco C, Van De Ven WJ, Bloemendal H, De Jong WW: MP17, a fiber-specific intrinsic membrane protein from mammalian eye lens. *Curr Eye Res* **7:**207, 1988.
199. Fitzgerald PG, Bok D, Horwitz J: Immunocytochemical localization of the main intrinsic polypeptide (MIP) in ultrathin frozen sections of rat lens. *J Cell Biol* **97:**1491, 1983.
200. Louis CF, Hogan P, Visco L, Strasburg G: Identity of the calmodulin-binding proteins in bovine lens plasma membranes. *Exp Eye Res* **50:**495, 1990.
201. Gorin MB, Yancey SB, Cline J, Revel JP, Horwitz J: The major intrinsic protein (MIP) of the bovine lens fiber membrane: Characterization and structure based on cDNA cloning. *Cell* **39:**49, 1984.
202. Sandal NN, Marcker KA: Soybean nodulin 26 is homologous to the major intrinsic protein of the bovine lens fiber membrane. *Nucleic Acids Res* **16:**9347, 1988.
203. Baker ME, Saier MH: A common ancestor for bovine lens fiber major intrinsic protein, soybean nodulin-26 protein and E. coli glycerol facilitator. *Cell* **60:**185, 1990.
204. Rao Y, Jan LY, Jan YN: Similarity of the product of the Drosophila neurogenic gene big brain to transmembrane channel proteins. *Nature* **345:**163, 1990.
205. Zampighi GA, Gall JE, Ehring GR, Simon SA: The structural organization and protein compositions of lens fiber junctions. *J Cell Biol* **108:**2255, 1989.
206. Bok D, Dockstader J, Horwitz J: Immunocytochemical localization of the lens main intrinsic polypeptide (MIP) in communicating junctions. *J Cell Biol* **92:**213, 1982.
207. Fitzgerald PG, Bok D, Horwitz J: The distribution of the main intrinsic membrane polypeptide in ocular lens. *Curr Eye Res* **4:**1203, 1985.
208. Pisano MM, Chepelinsky AB: Genomic cloning and complete nucleotide sequence of the human gene encoding the major intrinsic protein (MIP) of the lens. *Gene* **11:**981, 1991.
209. Girsch SJ, Peracchia C: Lens cell-to-cell channel protein I. Self assembly into liposomes and permeability regulation by calmodulin. *J Membr Biol* **83:**217, 1985.
210. Gooden MM, Rintoul DA, Takehana M, Takemoto L: Major intrinsic polypeptide (MIP 26K) from lens membrane: Reconstitution into vesicles and inhibition of channel forming activity by peptide antiserum. *Biochem Biophys Res Commun* **128:**993, 1985.
211. Peracchia C, Girsch SJ: Permeability and gating of lens gap junction channels incorporated into liposomes. *Curr Eye Res* **4:**431, 1985.
212. Zampighi GA, Hall JE, Kreman M: Purified lens junctional protein forms channels in planner lipid films. *Proc Natl Acad Sci USA* **82:**8468, 1985.
213. Ehring GR, Zampighi G, Horwitz J, Bok D, Hall JE: Properties of channels reconstituted from the major intrinsic protein of lens membranes. *J Gen Physiol* **96:**631, 1990.
214. Garland D, Russell P: Phosphorylation of lens fiber cell membrane proteins. *Proc Natl Acad Sci USA* **82:**653, 1985.
215. Johnson KR, Panter SS, Johnson RG: Phosphorylation of lens membranes with a cyclic AMP-dependent protein kinase purified from the bovine lens. *Biochim Biophys Acta* **844:**367, 1985.
216. Gruijters WT, Kistler J, Bullivant S, Goodenough DA: Immunolocalization of MP70 in lens fiber 16-17-nm intercellular junctions. *J Cell Biol* **104:**565, 1987.
217. Kistler J, Schaller J, Sigrist H: MP38 contains the membrane-embedded domain of the lens fiber gap junction protein MP70. *J Biol Chem* **265:**13357, 1990.
218. Kistler J, Christie D, Bullivant S: Homologies between gap junction proteins in lens, heart and liver. *Nature* **331:**721, 1988.
219. Allen DP, Low PS, Dola A, Maisel H: Band 3 and ankyrin homologues are present in eye lens: Evidence for all major erythrocyte membrane components in same non-erythroid cell. *Biochem Biophys Res Commun* **149:**266, 1987.

220. Kuwabara T: Microtubules in the lens. *Arch Ophthalmol* **79:**189, 1968.
221. Rafferty NS, Scholz DL, Goldberg M, Lewyckyj M: Immunocytochemical evidence for an actin-myosin system in lens epithelial cells. *Exp Eye Res* **51:**591, 1990.
222. Ireland M, Lieska N, Maisel H: Lens actin: Purification and localization. *Exp Eye Res* **37:**393, 1983.
223. Kibbelaar MA, Ramaekers FC, Ringens PJ, Selten-Versteegen AM, Poels LG, Jap PH, Van Rossum AL, Feltkamp TE, Bloemendal H: Is actin in eye lens a possible factor in visual accommodation. *Nature* **285:**506, 1980.
224. Hatfield JS, Skoff RP, Maisel H, Eng L, Bigner DD: The lens epithelium contains glial fibrillary acidic protein (GFAP). *J Neuroimmunol* **8:**347, 1985.
225. Boyer S, Maunoury R, Gomes D, De Nechaud B, Hill AM, Dupouey P: Expression of glial fibrillary acidic protein and vimentin in mouse lens epithelial cells during development in vivo and during proliferation and differentiation in vitro: Comparison with the developmental appearance of GFAP in the mouse central nervous system. *J Neurosci Res* **27:**55, 1990.
226. Ramaekers FC, Osborn M, Schimid E, Weber K, Bloemendal H, Franke WW: Identification of the cytoskeletal proteins in lens-forming cells, a special epithelioid cell type. *Exp Cell Res* **127:**309, 1980.
227. Sredy J, Roy D, Spector A: Identification of two of the major phosphorylated polypeptides of the bovine lens utilizing a lens cAMP-dependent protein kinase system. *Curr Eye Res* **3:**1423, 1984.
228. Sax CM, Farrell FX, Zehner ZE, Piatigorsky J: Regulation of vimentin gene expression in the ocular lens. *Dev Biol* **139:**56, 1990.
229. Pieper FR, Slobbe RL, Ramaekers CS, Cuypers HT, Bloemendal H: Upstream regions of the hamster desmin and vimentin genes regulate expression during in vitro myogenesis. *EMBO J* **6:**3611, 1987.
230. Fitzgerald PG, Casselman J: Discrimination between the lens fiber cell 114 kd cytoskeletal protein and alpha-actinin. *Curr Eye Res* **9:**873, 1900.
231. Ireland M, Maisel H: Phosphorylation of chick lens proteins. *Curr Eye Res* **3:**961, 1984.
232. Hockwin O, Ohrloff C: Enzymes in normal, aging and cataractous lenses, in Bloemendal H (ed): *Molecular and Cellular Biology of the Eye*. New York, John Wiley, 1981, p 367.
233. Cheng H-M, Chylack LT: Lens metabolism, in Maisel H (ed): *The Ocular Lens*. New York, Marcel Dekker, 1985, p 223.
234. Reddy VN: Dynamics of transport systems in the eye. Friedenwald Lecture. *Invest Ophthalmol Vis Sci* **18:**1000, 1979.
235. Hockwin O, Blum G, Korte I, Murata T, Radetzki W, Rast F: Studies on the citric acid cycle and its portion of glucose breakdown by calf and bovine lenses in vitro. *Ophthalmic Res* **2:**143, 1971.
236. Trayhurn P, Van Heyningen R: The role of respiration in the energy metabolism of the bovine lens. *Biochem J* **129:**507, 1972.
237. Kinoshita JH, Merola LO: The utilization of pyruvate and its conversion to glutamate in calf lens. *Exp Eye Res* **1:**53, 1961.
238. Aviram A, Schalitt M, Kassem N, Groen JJ: Glucose utilization, glutathione, potassium and sodium content of isolated bovine lens. *Clin Chim Acta* **14:**442, 1966.
239. Giblin FJ, Nies DE, Reddy VN: Stimulation of the hexose monophosphate shunt in rabbit lens in response to oxidation by glutathione. *Exp Eye Res* **33:**289, 1981.
240. Giblin FJ, McCready JP, Reddan JR, Dziedzic DC, Reddy VN: Detoxification of H_2O_2 by cultured rabbit lens epithelial cells: Participation of the glutathione redox cycle. *Exp Eye Res* **40:**827, 1985.
241. Cheng HM, Aguiar E, Ford JJ, Kelleher P, Lam DM: Proton NMR spectroscopy of glucose consumption by cultured lens epithelial cells. *J Ocul Pharmacol* **2:**319, 1986.
242. Giblin FJ, Schrimscher L, Chakrapani B, Reddy VN: Exposure of rabbit lens to hyperbaric oxygen in vitro: Regional effects on GSH level. *Invest Ophthalmol Vis Sci* **29:**1312, 1988.
243. Seland JH, Chylack LT Jr: Acute glucose-derived osmotic stress in rabbit lenses. *Acta Ophthalmol (Copenh)* **64:**533, 1986.
244. Burg MB, Kador PF: Sorbitol, osmoregulation, and the complications of diabetes. *J Clin Invest* **81:**635, 1988.
245. Chylack LT Jr, Tung W, Harding R: Sorbitol production in the lens: A means of counteracting glucose-derived osmotic stress. *Ophthalmic Res* **18:**313, 1986 [erratum, *Ophthalmic Res* **19:**365, 1987].
246. Kinoshita JH: Cataracts in galactosemia: The Jonas Friedenwald Memorial Lecture. *Invest Ophthalmol* **4:**786, 1965.
247. Kador PF, Kinoshita JH: Diabetic and galactosaemic cataracts. *Ciba Found Symp* **106:**110, 1984.
248. Kinoshita JH, Fukushi S, Kador P, Merola LO: Aldose reductase in diabetic complications of the eye. *Metabolism* **28:**462, 1979.
249. Piatigorsky J: Intracellular ions, protein metabolism, and cataract formation. *Curr Top Eye Res* **3:**1, 1980.
250. Chylack LT Jr, Henriques HF, Cheng HM, Tung WH: Efficacy of Alrestatin, an aldose reductase inhibitor, in human diabetic and nondiabetic lenses. *Ophthalmology* **86:**1579, 1979.
251. Spector A, Garner WH: Hydrogen peroxide and human cataract. *Exp Eye Res* **33:**673, 1981.
252. Reddy VN: Glutathione and its function in the lens—an overview. *Exp Eye Res* **50:**771, 1990.
253. Pau H, Graf P, Sies H: Glutathione levels in human lens: Regional distribution in different forms of cataract. *Exp Eye Res* **50:**17, 1990.
254. Giblin FJ, Reddan JR, Schrimscher L, Dziedzic DC, Reddy VN: The relative roles of the glutathione redox cycle and catalase in the detoxification of H_2O_2 by cultured rabbit lens epithelial cells. *Exp Eye Res* **50:**795, 1990.
255. Mancini MA, Unaker NJ, Giblin FJ, Reddan JR: Histochemical localization of catalase in cultured lens epithelial cells. *Ophthalmic Res* **21:**369, 1989.
256. Awasthi YC, Saneto RP, Srivastava SK: Purification and properties of bovine lens glutathione S-transferase. *Exp Eye Res* **30:**29, 1980.
257. Tomarev SI, Zinovieva RD: Squid major lens polypeptides are homologous to glutathione S-transferases subunits. *Nature* **336:**86, 1988.
258. Neville MC, Paterson CA, Hamilton PM: Evidence for two sodium pumps in the crystalline lens of the rabbit eye. *Exp Eye Res* **27:**637, 1978.
259. Gorthy WC, Anderson JW: Special characteristics of polar regions of the rat lens: Morphology and phosphatase histochemistry. *Invest Ophthalmol Vis Sci* **19:**1038, 1980.
260. Kinsey VE, Reddy DVN: Studies on the crystallin lens. *Invest Ophthalmol* **4:**104, 1965.
261. Unakar NJ, Tsui JY: Sodium-potassium-dependent ATPase I. Cytochemical localization in normal and cataractous rat lenses. *Invest Ophthalmol Vis Sci* **19:**630, 1980.
262. Palva M, Palkama A: Electronmicroscopical, histochemical and biochemical findings on the Na-ATPase activity in the epithelium of the rat lens. *Exp Eye Res* **22:**229, 1976.
263. Paterson CA: Distribution and movement of ions in the ocular lens. *Doc Ophthalmol* **31:**1, 1976.
264. Hightower KR, Leverenz V, Reddy VN: Calcium transport in the lens. *Invest Ophthalmol Vis Sci* **19:**1059, 1980.
265. Borchman D, Paterson CA, Delamere NA: Ca^{+2}-ATPase activity in the rabbit and bovine lens. *Curr Eye Res* **8:**1049, 1989.
266. Francois H, Rabaey M: Permeability of the lens capsule for the lens proteins. *Arch Ophthalmol* **36:**837, 1958.
267. Brown HG, Pappas GD, Ireland ME, Kuszak JR: Ultrastructural biochemical and immunologic evidence of receptor-mediated endocytosis in the crystalline lens. *Invest Ophthalmol Vis Sci* **31:**2579, 1990.
268. Rae JL: The movement of procion dye in the crystallin lens. *Invest Ophthalmol* **13:**147, 1974.
269. Duncan G, Jacob TJC: The lens as a physicochemical system in the eye, in Davson H (ed): *The Eye*. Orlando, FL, Academic, 1984, p 159.
270. Rae JL, Mathias RT: The physiology of the lens, in Maisel H (ed): *The Ocular Lens*. New York, Marcel Dekker, 1985, p 93.

271. Kern HL, Ho CK: Localization and specificity of the transport system for sugars in the calf lens. *Exp Eye Res* **15**:751, 1973.
272. Patterson JW: A review of glucose transport in the lens. *Invest Ophthalmol* **4**:667, 1965.
273. Harding CV, Maisel H, Chylack LT: The structure of the human cataractous lens, in Maisel H (ed): *The Ocular Lens*. New York, Marcel Dekker, 1985, p 405.
274. Benedek GB, Chylack LT, Libondi T, Magnante P, Pennett M: Quantitative detection of the molecular changes associated with early cataractogenesis in the living human lens using quasielastic light scattering. *Curr Eye Res* **6**:1421, 1987.
275. Bettelheim FA: Physical basis of lens transparency, in Maisel H (ed): *The Ocular Lens*. New York, Marcel Dekker, 1985, p 265.
276. Benedek GB, Clark JI, Serrallach EU, Young CY, Mengel T, Sauke A, Bagg A, Benedek K: Light scattering and reversible cataracts in calf and human lens. *Philos Trans R Soc Lond [A]* **293**:329, 1979.
277. Clark JI, Benedek GB: Phase diagram for cell cytoplasm from the calf lens. *Biochem Biophys Res Commun* **95**:482, 1980.
278. Tanaka T, Ishimoto C, Chylack LT Jr: Phase separation of a protein-water mixture in cold cataract in the young rat lens. *Science* **197**:1010, 1977.
279. Delaye M, Clark JI, Benedek GB: Identification of scattering elements responsible for lens opacification in cold cataracts. *Biophys J* **37**:647, 1982.
280. Clark HI, Carper D: Phase separation in lens cytoplasm is genetically linked to cataract formation in the Philly mouse. *Proc Natl Acad Sci USA* **84**:122, 1987.
281. Kador PF, Fukui HN, Fukushi S, Jernigan HM Jr, Kinoshita JH: Philly mouse: A new model of hereditary cataract. *Exp Eye Res* **30**:59, 1980.
282. Carper D: Deficiency of functional messenger RNA for a developmentally regulated beta-crystallin polypeptide in a hereditary cataract. *Science* **217**:463, 1982.
283. Nakamura M, Russell P, Carper DA, Inana G, Kinoshita JH: Alteration of a developmentally regulated, heat-stable polypeptide in the lens of the Philly mouse. Implications for cataract formation. *J Biol Chem* **263**:19218, 1988.
284. Chambers C, Russell P: Deletion mutation in an eye lens beta-crystallin: An animal model for inherited cataract. *J Biol Chem* **266**:6742, 1991.
285. Amsbaugh DF, Stone SH: Autosomal dominant congenital nuclear cataracts in strain 13/N guinea pigs. *J Hered* **75**:55, 1984.
286. Huang QL, Du XY, Stone SH, Amsbaugh DF, Datiles M, Hu TS, Zigler JS Jr: Association of hereditary cataracts in strain 13/N guinea-pigs with mutation of the gene for zeta-crystallin. *Exp Eye Res* **50**:317, 1990.
287. Huang QL, Russell P, Stone SH, Zigler JS Jr: Zeta-crystallin, a novel lens protein from the guinea pig. *Curr Eye Res* **6**:725, 1987.
288. Gonzalez P, Zigler JS Jr, Borras T: A splicing-site deletion that causes defective zeta-crystallin is found in a congenital guinea-pig cataract. *Invest Ophthalmol Vis Sci* **32/4**:782, 1991. (abstr.)
289. Piatigorsky J, Fukui HN, Kinoshita JH: Differential metabolism and leakage of protein in an inherited cataract and a normal lens cultured with ouabain. *Nature* **274**:558, 1978.
290. Kobayashi S, Kasuya M, Itoi M: Changes in lens proteins induced at the early stage of cataractogenesis in cac (Nakano) mice. *Exp Eye Res* **49**:553, 1989.
291. Fukui HN, Merola LO, Kinoshita JH: A possible cataractogenic factor in the Nakano mouse lens. *Exp Eye Res* **26**:477, 1978.
292. Garber AT, Winkler C, Shinohara T, King CR, Inana G, Piatigorsky J, Gold RJ: Selective loss of a family of gene transcripts in a hereditary murine cataract. *Science* **227**:74, 1985.
293. Kuliszewski M, Rupert J, Gold R: The ontogeny of gamma-crystallin mRNAs in Cat Fraser mice. *Genet Res* **52**:45, 1988.
294. Rupert JL, Kuliszewki M, Tsui LC, Breitman ML, Gold RJ: The murine cataractogenic mutation, Cat Fraser, segregates independently of the gamma crystallin genes. *Genet Res* **51**:23, 1988.
295. Muggelton-Harris AL, Festing MFW, Hall M: A gene location for the inheritance of the cataract Fraser (CATFr) mouse congenital cataract. *Gen Res* **49**:235, 1987.
296. Quinlan P, Oda S, Breitman ML, Tsui LC: The mouse eye lens obsolescence (Elo) mutant: Studies on crystallin gene expression and linkage analysis between the mutant locus and the gamma-crystallin genes. *Genes Dev* **1**:637, 1987.
297. Graw J, Kratochvilova J, Lobke A, Reitmeir P, Schaffer E, Wulff A: Characterization of Scat (suture cataract), a dominant cataract mutation in mice. *Exp Eye Res* **49**:469, 1989.
298. Hosokawa M, Ashida Y, Tsuboyama T, Chen WH, Takeda T: Cataract in senescence accelerated mouse (SAM). 2. Development of a new strain of mouse with late-appearing cataract. *Exp Eye Res* **47**:629, 1988.
299. Graw J, Bors W, Gopinath PM, Merkle S, Michel C, Reitmeir P, Schaffer E, Summer KH, Wulff A: Characterization of Cat-2t, a radiation-induced dominant cataract mutation in mice. *Invest Ophthalmol Vis Sci* **31**:1353, 1990.
300. Zigler JS Jr: Animal models for the study of maturity-onset and hereditary cataract. *Exp Eye Res* **50**:651, 1990.
301. Kuck JF: Late onset hereditary cataract of the Emory mouse. A model for human senile cataract. *Exp Eye Res* **50**:659, 1990.
302. Kaur S, Key B, Stock J, McNeish JD, Akeson R, Potter SS: Targeted ablation of alpha-crystallin-synthesizing cells produces lens-deficient eyes in transgenic mice. *Development* **105**:613, 1989.
303. Landel CP, Zhao J, Bok D, Evans GA: Lens-specific expression of recombinant ricin induces developmental defects in the eyes of transgenic mice. *Genes Dev* **2**:1168, 1988.
304. Lang RA, Metcalf D, Cuthbertson RA, Lyons I, Stanley E, Kelso A, Kannourakis G, Williamson DJ, Klintworth GK, Gonda TJ, Dunn AR: Transgenic mice expressing a hemopoietic growth factor gene (GM-CSF) develop accumulations of macrophages, blindness, and a fatal syndrome of tissue damage. *Cell* **51**:675, 1987.
305. Capetanaki Y, Smith S, Heath JP: Overexpression of the vimentin gene in transgenic mice inhibits normal lens cell differentiation. *J Cell Biol* **109**:1653, 1989.
306. Datiles MB, Kinoshita JH: Pathogenesis of cataracts, in Tasman W, Jaeger EA (eds): *Duane's Clinical Ophthalmology*. Philadelphia, Lippincott, 1991.
307. Young R: *Age related cataract*. New York, Oxford University Press, 1991, p 119.
308. Weekers R, Delmarcelle Y, Luyckx-Bacus J, Collignon J: Morphological changes of the lens with age and cataract, in *The Human Lens—In Relation to Cataract*. Ciba Foundation 19 (new series) Amsterdam, Elsevier, 1973, p 24.
309. Weale RA: Physical changes due to age and cataract, in Duncan G (ed): *Mechanism of Cataract Formation in the Human Lens*. New York, Academic, 1981, p 47.
310. Chylack LT, Leske MC, McCarthy D, Khu T, Dashwagi T, Sperduto R: Lens opacities classification system II (LOCS II). *Arch Ophthalmol* **107**:991, 1989.
311. Klein BEK, Klein R, Linton KLP, Magli YL, Neider MW: Assessment of cataracts from photography in the Beaver Dam eye study. *Ophthalmology* **97**:1428, 1990.
312. Taylor HR, West SK: The clinical grading of lens opacities. *Aust N Z J Ophthalmol* **17**:81, 1989.
313. Sparrow J, Bron A, Brown N, Ayliff W, Hall A: The Oxford clinical cataract classification and grading system. *Int Ophthalmol* **9**:207, 1986.
314. Merin S: Congenital cataracts, in Goldberg MF (ed): *Genetic and Metabolic Eye Disease*. Boston, Little, Brown, 1974, p 337.
315. Kuszak JR: Embryology and anatomy of the lens, in Tasman W, Jaeger EA (eds): *Duane's Clinical Ophthalmology*. Philadelphia, Lippincott, 1990.
316. Kaiser-Kupfer MI, Kuwabara T, Uga S, Takki K, Valle D: Cataract in gyrate atrophy clinical and morphological studies. *Invest Ophthalmol Vis Sci* **24**:432, 1983.
317. Holmes LB, McGowan BL, Efron ML: Lowe's syndrome: A search for the carrier state. *Pediatrics* **44**:358, 1969.
318. Brown N, Gardner RJ: Lowe syndrome: Identification of the carrier state. *Birth Defects* **12**(6):579, 1976.
319. Delleman JW, Bleeker-Wapemakers EM, Vanveleen AWC: Opacities of the lens indicating carrier status in the

oculo-cerebro-renal (Lowe) syndrome. *J Pediatr Ophthalmol* **14**:205, 1976.

320. Cibis GW, Waeltermann JM, Whitcraft CT, Tripathi RC, Harris DJ: Lenticular opacities in carriers of Lowe's syndrome. *Ophthalmology* **93**:1041, 1986.
321. Pearson-Webb MA, Kaiser-Kupfer MI, Eldridge R: Eye findings in bilateral acoustic (central) neurofibromatosis: Association with presenile lens opacities and cataracts but absence of Lisch nodules. *N Engl J Med* **315**:1553, 1986.
322. Kaiser-Kupfer MI, Freidlin V, Datiles MB, Edwards PA, Sherman JL, Parry D, McCain LM, Eldridge R: The association of posterior capsular lens opacities with bilateral acoustic neuromas in patients with neurofibromatosis type 2. *Arch Ophthalmol* **107**:541, 1989.
323. Ashizawa T, Hejtmancik JF, Liu J, Perryman MB, Epstein HF, Koch DD: Diagnostic value of ophthalmologic findings in myotonic dystrophy: Comparison with risks calculated by haplotype analysis of closely linked restriction fragment length polymorphisms. *Am J Med Genet* **42**:55, 1992.
324. Francois J: Genetics of cataract. *Ophthalmologica* **184**:61, 1982.
325. Merin S, Crawford JS: The etiology of congenital cataracts. A survey of 386 cases. *Can J Ophthalmol* **6**:178, 1971.
326. Koch H-R, Wegner A: Anomalies of the lens, in Emery AEH, Rimoin DL (eds): *Principles and Practice of Medical Genetics*. New York, Churchill Livingstone, 1983, p 509.
327. Hejtmancik JF, Hope JN: Beta-crystallin structure and function: Preliminary studies. *Proc Int Soc Eye Res* **5**:72, 1988. (abstr.)
328. Nettleship E, Ogilvie FM: A peculiar form of hereditary congenital cataract. *Trans Ophthalmol Soc UK* **26**:191, 1906.
329. Hammerstein W, Scholtz W: Familiare form einer 'cataract centralis.' *Graefes Arch Klin EXP Ophthalmol* **189**:9, 1974.
330. Conneally PM, Wilson AF, Merritt AD, Helveston EM, Palmer GG, Wang LY: Confirmation of genetic heterogeneity in autosomal dominant forms of cataracts from linkage studies. *Cytogenet Cell Genet* **22**:295, 1978.
331. Barrett DJ, Sparkes RS, Gorin MB, Bhat SP, Spence MA, Marazita ML, Bateman JB: Genetic linkage analysis of autosomal dominant congenital cataracts with lens-specific DNA probes and polymorphic phenotypic markers. *Ophthalmology* **95**:538, 1988.
332. Lubsen NH, Renwick JH, Tsui LC, Breitman ML, Schoenmakers JG: A locus for a human hereditary cataract is closely linked to the gamma-crystallin gene family. *Proc Natl Acad Sci USA* **84**:489, 1987.
333. Eiberg H, Nielsen LS, Klausen J, Dahlen M, Kristensen M, Bisgaard ML, Moller N, Mohr J: Linkage between serum cholinesterase 2 (CHE2) and gamma-crystallin gene cluster (CRYG): Assignment to chromosome 2. *Clin Genet* **35**:313, 1989.
334. Marner E, Rosenberg T, Eiberg H: Autosomal dominant congenital cataract: Morphology and genetic mapping. *Acta Ophthalmol (Copenh)* **67**:151, 1989.
335. Richards J, Maumenee IH, Rowe S, Lourien EW: Congenital cataract possibly linked to haptoglobin. *Cytogenet Cell Genet* **37**:570, 1984.
336. Reese PD, Tuck-Miller CM, Maumenee IH: Autosomal dominant congenital cataract associated with chromosomal translocation [t(3;4)(p26.2;p15)]. *Arch Ophthalmol* **105**:1382, 1987.
337. Ogata H, Okubo Y, Akabane T: Phenotype i associated with congenital cataract in Japanese. *Transfusion* **19**:166, 1979.
338. MacDonald EB, Douglas R, Harden PA: A Caucasian family with the i phenotype and congenital cataracts. *Vox Sang* **44**:322, 1983.
339. Yamaguchi H, Okubo Y, Tanaka M: A note on possible close linkage between the Ii blood locus and a congenital cataract locus. *Proc Jpn Acad* **48**:625, 1972.
340. Jensen AD, Cross HE, Paton D: Ocular complications in the Weill-Marchesani syndrome. *Am J Ophthalmol* **77**:261, 1974.
341. Tsipouras P, Del Mastro R, Sarfarazi M, Lee B, Vitale E, Child AH, Godfrey M, Devereux RB, Hewett D, Steinmann B, Viljoen D, Sykes B, Kilpatrick M, Ramirez F: Genetic linkage of the Marfan syndrome, ectopia lentis, and congenital contractural arachnodactyly to the fibrillin genes on chromosomes 15 and 5. *N Engl J Med* **326**:906, 1992.
342. Dobson V, Teller DY: Visual acuity in human infants: A review and comparison of behavioral and electrophysiological studies. *Vision Res* **18**:1469, 1978.
343. Atkinson J, Braddick O: Assessment of visual acuity in infancy and early childhood. *Acta Ophthalmol Suppl (Copenh)* **157**:18, 1983.
344. Weisel TN, Hubel DH: Comparison of the effects of unilateral and bilateral eyelid closure on cortical responses in kittens. *J Neurophysiol* **28**:1029, 1965.
345. Harwerth RS, Smith EL 3D, Paul AD, Crawford ML, Von Noorden GK: Functional effects of bilateral form deprivation in monkeys. *Invest Ophthalmol Vis Sci* **32**:2311, 1991.
346. Crawford ML, Pesch TW, Von Noorden GK, Harwerth RS, Smith EL: Bilateral form deprivation in monkeys. Electrophysiologic and anatomic consequences. *Invest Ophthalmol Vis Sci* **32**:2328, 1991.
347. Nelson LB: Diagnosis and management of cataracts in infancy and childhood. *Ophthalmic Surg* **15**:688, 1984.
348. Robb RM, Mayer DL, Moore BD: Results of early treatment of unilateral congenital cataracts. *J Pediatr Ophthalmol Strabismus* **24**:178, 1987.
349. Gelbart SS, Hoyt CS, Jastrebski G, Marg E: Long-term visual results in bilateral congenital cataracts. *Am J Ophthalmol* **93**:615, 1982.
350. Burns EC, Jones RB: Long term management of congenital cataracts. *Arch Dis Child* **60**:322, 1985.
351. Elsas FJ, Maumenee IH, Kenyon KR, Yoder F: Familial aniridia with preserved ocular function. *Am J Ophthalmol* **83**:718, 1977.
352. Traboulsi EI, Weinberg RJ: Familial congenital cornea guttata with anterior polar cataracts. *Am J Ophthalmol* **108**:123, 1989.
353. Moller HU: Granular corneal dystrophy Groenouw type I: Clinical aspects and treatment. *Acta Ophthalmol (Copenh)* **68**:384, 1990.
354. Gitter KA, Rothschild H, Waltman DD, Scott B, Azar P: Dominantly inherited peripheral retinal neovascularization. *Arch Ophthalmol* **96**:1601, 1978.
355. O'Donnell FE, Pappas HR: Autosomal dominant foveal hypoplasia and presenile cataracts: A new syndrome. *Arch Ophthalmol* **100**:279, 1982.
356. Alexander RL, Shea M: Wagner's disease. *Arch Ophthalmol* **74**:310, 1965.
357. Kafer O: Dominant vererbte Spaltung des Pigmentblattes von Iris und Ciliarkoepfer mit consekutiver Microphakie, Ectopia lentis und Cataract. *Graefes Arch Klin Exp Ophthalmol* **202**:133, 1977.
358. Hittner HM, Kretzer FL, Antoszyk JH, Ferrell RE, Mehta RS: Variable expressivity of autosomal dominant anterior segment mesenchymal dysgenesis in six generations. *Am J Ophthalmol* **93**:57, 1982.
359. Friedmann MW, Wright ES: Hereditary microcornea and cataract in 5 generations. *Am J Ophthalmol* **35**:1017, 1952.
360. Capella JA, Kaufman HE, Lill FJ, Cooper G: Hereditary cataracts and microphthalmia. *Am J Ophthalmol* **56**:454, 1963.
361. Cassady JR, Light A: Familial persistent pupillary membranes. *Arch Ophthalmol* **58**:438, 1957.
362. Heckenlively J: The frequency of posterior subcapsular cataract in the hereditary retinal degenerations. *Am J Ophthalmol* **93**:733, 1982.
363. Berson EL, Rosner B, Simonoff E: Risk factors for genetic typing and detection in retinitis pigmentosa. *Am J Ophthalmol* **89**:763, 1980.
364. Hirose T, Lee KY, Schepens CL: Snowflake degeneration in hereditary vitreoretinal degeneration. *Am J Ophthalmol* **77**:143, 1974.
365. Kaufman SJ, Goldberg MF, Orth DH, Fishman GA, Tessler H, Mizuno K: Autosomal dominant vitreoretinochoroidopathy. *Arch Ophthalmol* **100**:272, 1982.
366. Stock EL, Kielar RA: Primary familial amyloidosis of the cornea. *Am J Ophthalmol* **82**:266, 1976.
367. Favre M: A propos de deux cas de degenerescence hyaloideo-retinienne. Two cases of hyaloid-retinal degeneration. *Ophthalmologica* **135**:604, 1958.

368. Alstrom CH: Heredo-retinopathia congenitalis monohybrida recessiva autosomalis: A genetical statistical study in clinical collaboration with Olof Olson. *Hereditas* **43:**1, 1957.
369. Temtamy SA, Shalash BA: Genetic heterogeneity of the syndrome: Microphthalmos with congenital cataract. *Birth Defects* **10(4):**292, 1974.
370. Warburg M: Norrie's disease: A new hereditary bilateral pseudotumour of the retina. *Arch Ophthalmol* **39:**757, 1961.
371. McKusick VA (ed.): *Mendelian Inheritance in Man,* 6th ed. Baltimore, Johns Hopkins University Press, 1992.
372. Heck AF: Presumptive X-linked intermediate transmission of retinal degenerations: Variations and coincidental occurrence with ataxia in a large family. *Arch Ophthalmol* **70:**143, 1963.
373. Wellesley D, Carman P, French N, Goldblatt J: Cataracts, aberrant oral frenula, and growth retardation: A new autosomal dominant syndrome. *Am J Med Genet* **40:**341, 1991.
374. Stromgen E, Dalby A, Dalby MA, Ranheim B: Cataracts, deafness, cerebellar ataxia, psychosis, and dementia—a new syndrome. *Acta Neurol Scand Suppl* **43:**261, 1970.
375. Spranger JW, Opitz JM, Bidder U: Heterogeneity of chondrodysplasia punctata. *Humangenetik* **11:**190, 1971.
376. Nadol JB Jr, Burgess B: Cochleosaccular degeneration of the inner ear and progressive cataracts inherited as an autosomal dominant trait. *Laryngoscope* **92:**1028, 1982.
377. Russo G, Mollica F, Mazzone D, Santonocito B: Congenital lactose intolerance of gastrogenic origin associated with cataracts. *Acta Paediatr Scand* **63:**457, 1974.
378. Moore WT, Federman DD: Familial dwarfism and stiff joints. *Arch Intern Med* **115:**398, 1965.
379. Cochat P, Guibaud P, Garcia-Torres R, Roussel B, Guarner B, Larbre F: Diffuse leiomyomatosis in Alport syndrome. *Pediatrics* **113:**339, 1988.
380. Flynn P, Aird RB: A neuroectodermal syndrome of dominant inheritance. *J Neurol Sci* **2:**161, 1965.
381. Francois J: A new syndrome: Dyscephalia with bird face and dental anomalies, nanism, hypotrichosis, cutaneous atrophy, microphthalmia, and congenital cataract. *Arch Ophthalmol* **60:**842, 1958.
382. Witkopf CJ, White JG, King RA, Dahl MV, Young WG, Dauk JJ: Hereditary mucoepithelial dysplasia: A disease apparently of desmosome and gap junction formation. *Am J Hum Genet* **31:**414, 1979.
383. Zayid I, Farraj S: Familial histiocytic dermatoarthritis: A new syndrome. *Am J Med* **54:**793, 1973.
384. Carney RG: Incontinentia pigmenti, a world statistical analysis. *Arch Dermatol* **112:**535, 1976.
385. Kniest W, Leiber B: Kniest's syndrome. *Monatsschr Kinderheilkd* **125:**970, 1977.
386. Tessler HH, Apple DJ, Goldberg MF: Ocular findings in a kindred with Kyrle disease. *Arch Ophthalmol* **90:**278, 1973.
387. Pepin B, Mikol J, Goldstein B, Aron JJ, Lebuisson DA: Familial mitochondrial myopathy with cataract. *J Neurol Sci* **45:**191, 1980.
388. Walker BA: Osteopathia striata with cataracts and deafness. *Birth Defects* **4:**295, 1969.
389. Marshall D: Ectodermal dysplasia. Report of a kindred with ocular abnormalities and hearing defect. *Am J Ophthalmol* **45:**143, 1958.
390. Beighton P, Goldberg L, Op't Hof J: Dominant inheritance of multiple epiphyseal dysplasia, myopia and deafness. *Clin Genet* **14:**173, 1978.
391. Quintanilla E, Rodrigo A, Temiño MA, Ayesa C, Olivares C: [Nail-patella syndrome with ocular involvement. Study of 5 generations.] *Actas Dermosifiliogr* **72:**415, 1981.
392. Garcin R, Delthil S, Man HX, Chimenes H: Sur une affection hérédo-familiale associant cataracte, atrophie optique, signes extra-pyramidaux et certains stigmates de la maladie de Friedreich. (Sa position nosologique par rapport au syndrome de Behr, au syndrome de Marinesco-Sjögren et à la maladie de Friedreich avec signes oculaires.) *Rev Neurol (Paris)* **104:**373, 1961.
393. Debusk FL: The Hutchinson-Gilford progeria syndrome. *J Pediatr* **80:**697, 1972.
394. Shprintzen RJ, Wang F, Goldberg R, Marion R: The expanded velo-cardio-facial syndrome (VCF): Additional features of the most common clefting syndrome. *Am J Hum Genet* **37:**A77, 1985.
395. Vaca G, Ibarra B, Bracamontes M, Garcia-Cruz D, Sanchez-Corona J, Medina C, Wunsch C, Gonzalez-Quiroga G, Cantu JF: Red blood cell sorbitol dehydrogenase deficiency in a family with cataracts. *Hum Genet* **61:**338, 1982.
396. Neugebauer H: Spalthand und fus mit familiarer besonderheit. *Z Orthop* **95:**500, 1962.
397. Seery CM, Pruett RC, Liberfarb RM, Cohen BZ: Distinctive cataract in the Stickler syndrome. *Am J Ophthalmol* **110:**143, 1990.
398. Goldstein JH, Hutt AE: Trichomegaly, cataract, and hereditary spherocytosis in two siblings. *Am J Ophthalmol* **73:**333, 1972.
399. McKusick VA, Weilbaecher RG, Gragg GW: Recessive inheritance of a congenital malformation syndrome. *JAMA* **204:**113, 1968.
400. Dionisi Vici C, Sabetta G, Gambarara M, Vigevano F, Vertini E, Boldrini R, Parisi SG, Quinti I, Aiuti F, Fiorilli M: Agenesis of the corpus callosum, combined immunodeficiency, bilateral cataract, and hypopigmentation in two brothers. *Am J Med Genet* **29:**1, 1988.
401. Lyon G, Arita F, Le Galloudec E, Vallee L, Misson J-P, Ferriere G: A disorder of axonal development, necrotizing myopathy, cardiomyopathy, and cataracts: A new familial disease. *Ann Neurol* **27:**193, 1990.
402. Riise R: Visual function in Laurence-Moon-Bardet-Biedl syndrome. *Acta Ophthalmol Suppl (Copenh)* **182:**128, 1987.
403. Sengers RCA, Ter Haar BGA, Trijbels JMF, Willems JL, Daniels O, Stadhouders AM: Congenital cataract and mitochondrial myopathy of skeletal and heart muscle associated with lactic acidosis after exercise. *J Pediatr* **86:**873, 1975.
404. Seland JH, Slagsvold JE: The ultrastructure of lens and iris in cerebrotendinous xanthomatosis. *Acta Ophthalmol* **55:**201, 1977.
405. Grizzard WS, O'Donnell JJ, Carey JC: The cerebro-oculo-facio-skeletal syndrome. *Am J Ophthalmol* **89:**293, 1980.
406. Pearce WG: Ocular and genetic features of Cockayne's syndrome. *Can J Ophthalmol* **7:**435, 1972.
407. Pinkerton OD: Cataract associated with congenital ichthyosis. *Arch Ophthalmol* **60:**393, 1958.
408. Crome L, Duckett S, Franklin AW: Congenital cataracts, renal tubular necrosis and encephalopathy in two sisters. *Arch Dis Child* **38:**505, 1963.
409. Sanner G: The dysequilibrium syndrome. A genetic study. *Neuropaediatrie* **4:**403, 1973.
410. Gitzelmann R: Hereditary galactokinase deficiency, a newly recognized cause of juvenile cataracts. *Pediatr Res* **1:**14, 1967.
411. Loos H, Roos D, Weening R, Houwerzijl J: Familial deficiency of glutathione reductase in human blood cells. *Blood* **48:**53, 1976.
412. Caspersen I, Warburg M: Hallermann-Streiff syndrome. *Acta Ophthalmol* **46:**358, 1968.
413. Pagon RA, Clarren SK, Milam DF Jr, Hendrickson AE: Autosomal recessive eye and brain anomalies: Warburg syndrome. *J Pediatr* **102:**542, 1983.
414. Spaeth GL, Barber GW: Homocystinuria—Its ocular manifestations. *J Pediatr Ophthalmol* **3:**42, 1966.
415. Gold GN, Hogenhuis LAH: Hypertrophic interstitial neuropathy and cataracts. *Neurology* **18:**526, 1968.
416. Lubinsky MS: Cataracts and testicular failure in three brothers. *Am J Med Genet* **16:**149, 1983.
417. Buyse M, Bull MJ: A syndrome of osteogenesis imperfecta, microcephaly, and cataracts. *Birth Defects* **14(6B):**95, 1978.
418. Arbisser AI, Murhree AL, Garcia CA, Howell RR: Ocular findings in mannosidosis. *Am J Ophthalmol* **82:**465, 1976.
419. Chess J, Albert DM: Ocular pathology of the Majewski syndrome. *Br J Ophthalmol* **66:**736, 1982.
420. Herva R, Von Wendt L, Von Wendt G, Saukkonen AL, Leisti J: A syndrome with juvenile cataract, cerebellar atrophy, mental retardation and myopathy. *Neuropediatrics* **18:**164, 1987.
421. Martsolf JT, Hunter AGW, Haworth JC: Severe mental retardation, cataracts, short stature and primary hypogonadism in two brothers. *Am J Med Genet* **1:**291, 1978.
422. Hoffmann G, Gibson KM, Brandt IK, Bader PI, Wappner RS, Sweetman L: Mevalonic aciduria—an inborn error of cholesterol and nonsterol isoprene biosynthesis. *N Engl J Med* **314:**1610, 1986.

423. Lundberg PO: Hereditary myopathy, oligophrenia, cataract, skeletal abnormalities and hypergonadotropic hypogonadism: A new syndrome. *Acta Genet Med Gemellol (Roma)* **23**:245, 1974.
424. Cremers CWRJ, Ter Haar BGA, Van Rens TJG: The Nathalie syndrome. A new hereditary syndrome. *Clin Genet* **8**:330, 1975.
425. Neu RL, Kajii T, Gardner LI, Nagyfy SF: A lethal syndrome of microcephaly with multiple congenital anomalies in three siblings. *Pediatrics* **47**:610, 1971.
426. Thomas PK, Abrams JD, Swallow D, Stewart G: Sialidosis type I: Cherry red spot-myoclonus syndrome with sialidase deficiency and altered electrophoretic mobility of some enzymes known to be glycoproteins. I. Clinical findings. *J Neurol Neurosurg Psychiatry* **42**:873, 1979.
427. Williams ML, Koch TK, O'Donnell JJ, Frost PH, Epstein LB, Grizzard WS, Epstein CJ: Ichthyosis and neutral lipid storage disease. *Am J Med Genet* **20**:711, 1985.
428. Salih MAM, Bender DA, McCreanor GM: Lethal familial pellagra-like skin lesion associated with neurologic and developmental impairment and the development of cataracts. *Pediatrics* **76**:787, 1985.
429. Kwashima H, Kawano M, Masaki A, Sato T: Three cases of untreated classical PKU: A report on cataracts and brain calcification. *Am J Med Genet* **29**:89, 1988.
430. Fairly KF, Leighton PW, Kincaid-Smith P: Familial visual defects associated with polycystic kidney and medullary sponge kidney. *Br Med J* **1**:1060, 1963.
431. Preus M, Fraser FC, Wigglesworth JW: An oculocerebral hypopigmentation syndrome. *J Genet Hum* **31**:323, 1983.
432. Folz SJ, Trobe JD: The peroxisome and the eye. *Surv Ophthalmol* **35**:353, 1991.
433. Jones KL: *Smith's Recognizable Patterns of Human Malformation.* 4th ed. Philadelphia, Saunders, 1988.
434. Rothmund A: Uber Cataracte in Verbindung mit einer eigenthuemlichen Hautdegeneration. *Graefes Arch Klin Exp Ophthalmol* **14**:159, 1868.
435. Mollica F, Pavone L, Antener I: Short stature, mental retardation and ocular alterations in three siblings. *Helv Paediatr Acta* **27**:463, 1972.
436. Cotlier E, Rice P: Cataracts in the Smith-Lemli-Opitz syndrome. *Am J Ophthalmol* **72**:955, 1971.
437. Adams CW, Nance WE: Persistent tachycardia, paroxysmal hypertension, and seizures: Association with hyperglycinuria, dominantly inherited microphthalmia, and cataracts. *JAMA* **202**:525, 1967.
438. Toriello HV, Horton WA, Oostendorp A, Waterman DF, Higgins JV: An apparently new syndrome of microcephalic primordial dwarfism and cataracts. *Am J Med Genet* **25**:1, 1986.
439. Hallgren B: Retinitis pigmentosa combined with congenital deafness: With vestibulo-cerebellar ataxia and mental abnormality in a proportion of cases. *Acta Psychiatr Neurol Scand Suppl* **138**:9, 1959.
440. Epstein CJ, Martin GM, Schultz AL, Motulsky AG: Werner's syndrome: A review of its symptomatology, natural history, pathologic features, genetics and relationship to the natural aging process. *Medicine (Baltimore)* **45**:177, 1966.
441. Tso MO, Fine BS, Thorpe HE: Kayser-Fleischer ring and associated cataract in Wilson's disease. *Am J Ophthalmol* **79**:479, 1975.
442. Fitch N: Albright's hereditary osteodystrophy: A review. *Am J Med Genet* **11**:11, 1982.
443. Arnott EJ, Crawford MD'A, Toghill PJ: Anterior lenticonus and Alport's syndrome. *Br J Ophthalmol* **30**:390, 1966.
444. Scher NA, Letson RD, Desnick RJ: The ocular manifestations in Fabry's disease. *Arch Ophthalmol* **97**:671, 1979.
445. Orzalesi N, Sorcinelli R, Guiso G: Increased incidence of cataracts in male subjects deficient in glucose-6-phosphate dehydrogenase. *Arch Ophthalmol* **99**:69, 1981.
446. Carney RG: Incontinentia pigmenti: A world statistical analysis. *Arch Dermatol* **112**:535, 1976.
447. Herrmann H, Opitz JM: The Lenz microphthalmia syndrome. *Birth Defects* **5(2)**:138, 1969.
448. Wadelius C, Fagerholm P, Pettersson U, Anneren G: Lowe oculocerebrorenal syndrome: DNA based linkage of the gene to X124-q26, using tightly linked flanking markers and the correlation to lens examination in carrier diagnosis. *Am J Hum Genet* **44**:241, 1989.
449. Nance WE, Warburg M, Bixler D, Helveston EM: Congenital X-linked cataract, dental anomalies and brachymetacarpalia. *Birth Defects* **10(4)**:285, 1974.
450. Mirhosseini SA, Holmes LB, Walton DS: Syndrome of pigmentary retinal degeneration, cataract, microcephaly, and severe mental retardation. *J Med Genet* **9**:193, 1972.
451. Winsnes A, Monn E, Stokke O, Feyling T: Congenital persistent proximal type real tubular acidosis in two brothers. *Acta Paediatr Scand* **68**:861, 1979.
452. Happle R: Cataracts as a marker of genetic heterogeneity in chondrodysplasia punctata. *Clin Genet* **19**:64, 1981.
453. Piatigorsky J: Lens differentiation in vertebrates: A review of cellular and molecular features. *Differentiation* **19**:134, 1981.
454. Rao CM, Zigler JS Jr: Levels of reduced pyridine nucleotides and lens photodamage. *Photochem Photobiol* **56**:523, 1992.
455. Kantorow M, Piatigorsky J: Alpha-crystallin/small heat shock protein has autokinase activity. *Proc Natl Acad Sci USA* 1994. (In Press)
456. Kamachi Y, Kondoh H: Overlapping positive and negative regulatory elements determine lens-specific activity of the delta 1-crystallin enhancer. *Mol Cell Biol* **13**:5206, 1993.
457. Tini M, Otulakowski G, Breitman ML, Tsui LC, Giguëre V: An everted repeat mediates retinoic acid induction of the gamma F-crystallin gene: evidence of a direct role for retinoids in lens development. *Genes Dev* **7**:295, 1993.
458. Head MW, Peter A, Clayton RM: Evidence for the extralenticular expression of members of the beta-crystallin gene family in the chick and a comparison with delta-crystallin during differentiation and transdifferentiation. *Differentiation* **48**:147, 1991.
459. Smolich BD, Tarkington SK, Saha MS, Grainger RM: Xenopus gamma-crystallin gene expression: evidence that the gamma-crystallin gene family is transcribed in lens and nonlens tissues. *Mol Cell Biol* **14**:1355, 1994.
460. Mayr EM, Jaenicke R, Glockshuber R: Domain interactions and connecting peptides in lens crystallins. *J Mol Biol* **235**:84, 1994.
461. Hope JN, Chen H-C, Hejtmancik JF: BetaA3/Al-crystallin association: Role of the amino terminal arm. *Prot Eng* **7**:445, 1994.
462. Cartier M, Breitman ML, Tsui LC: A frameshift mutation in the gammaE-crystallin gene of the ELO mouse. *Nat Genet* **2**:42, 1992.
463. Brakenhoff RH, Henskens HAM, van Rossum MWPC, Lubsen NH, Schoenmakers JGG: Activation of the gammaE-crystallin pseudogene in the human hereditary Coppock-like cataract. *Human Mol Genet* **3**:279, 1994.

Part 21

SKIN

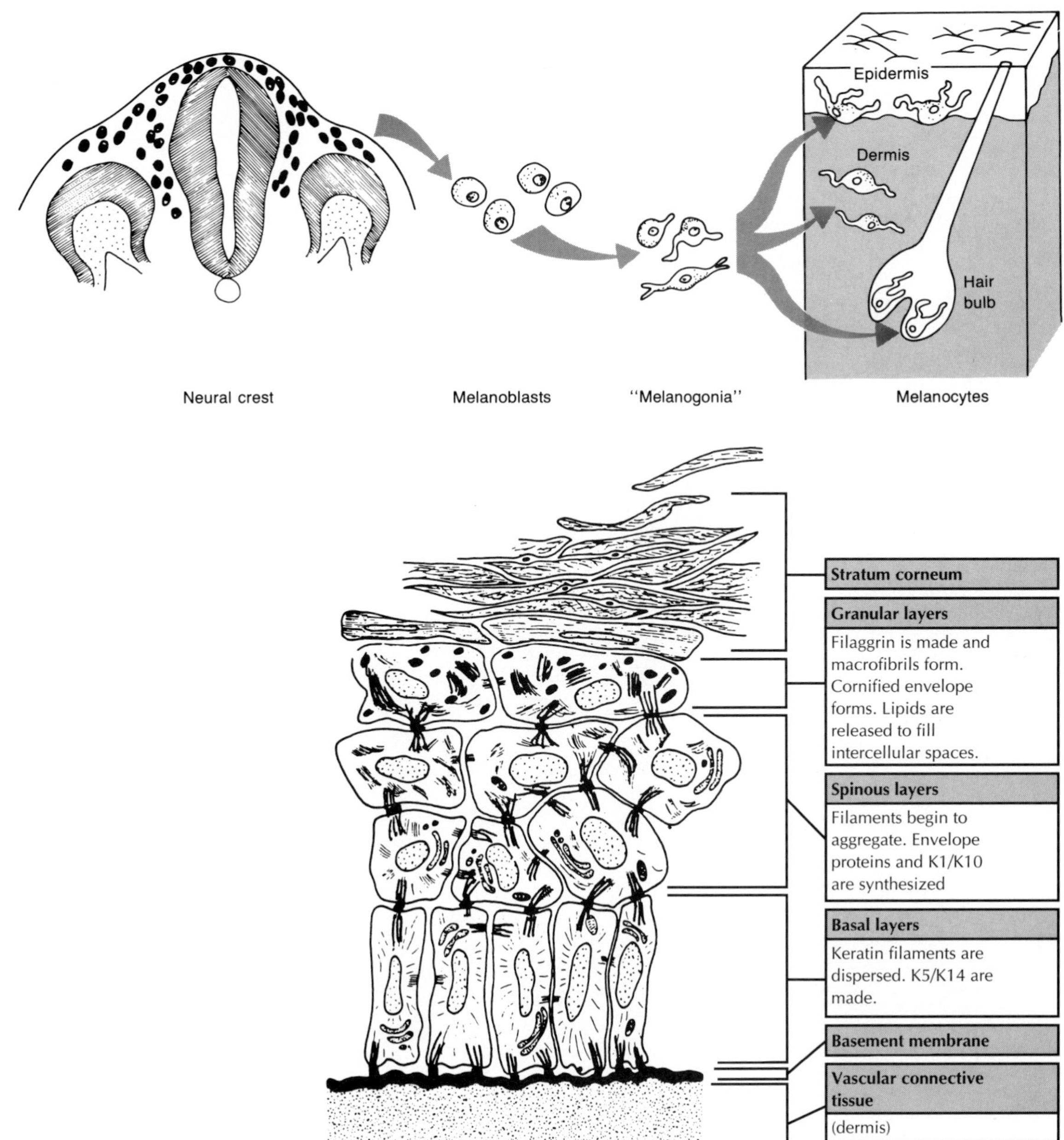

Epidermis
Dermis
Hair bulb
Neural crest
Melanoblasts
"Melanogonia"
Melanocytes
Stratum corneum
Granular layers
Filaggrin is made and macrofibrils form. Cornified envelope forms. Lipids are released to fill intercellular spaces.
Spinous layers
Filaments begin to aggregate. Envelope proteins and K1/K10 are synthesized
Basal layers
Keratin filaments are dispersed. K5/K14 are made.
Basement membrane
Vascular connective tissue
(dermis)

CHAPTER 147

Albinism

Richard A. King ▪ Vincent J. Hearing
Donnell J. Creel ▪ William S. Oetting

1. **Melanocytes represent a relatively small subpopulation of cells, yet they are exclusively responsible for producing the melanin that accounts for virtually all visible pigmentation in the skin, hair, and eyes. Normal pigmentation requires a number of critical steps during development, and a large number of genes have been shown to participate in those processes either directly or indirectly. Mutations in a number of these genes have been shown to elicit various clinical conditions of hypopigmentation, such as albinism and piebaldism.**

2. **Melanocytes in the skin interact with other types of cells either directly, as in the transfer of melanin granules to keratinocytes, or indirectly, as in the response to factors produced by other cells that influence the proliferation and/or pigmentation of melanocytes. Factors that regulate such melanocyte functions include environmental factors, such as UV light, hormones, growth factors, cytokines, and a number of other modulators present in the milieu of the skin.**

3. **Tyrosinase is the critical enzyme to melanin production by virtue of its catalytic function in the hydroxylation of tyrosine to dihydroxyphenylalanine (the rate limiting reaction in the melanin biosynthetic pathway). However, there are a number of post-tyrosinase factors and enzymes that regulate the quality and quantity of the melanins produced, and presumably their functional characteristics as well; included in that list are melanogenic inhibitors and various enzymes that can modify the sulfhydryl and carboxyl contents of the melanins.**

4. **Two distinct types of melanins can be produced in melanocytes; these are termed "eumelanin," which are black and/or brown, and "pheomelanin," which are yellow and/or red. The commitment to produce either type of melanin depends on whether sulfhydryl-containing compounds are present within the melanin granule that can interact with the nascent melanin intermediates. The chemical and physical characteristics, such as UV absorption and solubility, of the two types of melanins are significantly different, although very little is known at present about determinants affecting pheomelanogenesis.**

5. **The tyrosinase gene family currently contains three members: tyrosinase (TYR), TRP1/gp75 and TRP2/dopachrome tautomerase. The tyrosinase locus (TYR) has been mapped to chromosome 11q14-21. The gene is at least 50 kb in length and has five exons. Six polymorphic sites have been identified with TYR, and these have been used to form haplotypes for population studies. Mutations in the tyrosinase gene are responsible for tyrosinase-related oculocutaneous albinism (OCA1). The TRP1/gp75 locus has been mapped to chromosome 9p23. The role of TRP1 in pigment biosynthesis has not been conclusively determined. The dopachrome tautomerase or TRP2 gene has been isolated in mice but not in humans. The three genes have similar amino acid sequences, but their gene structures are different. The protein products of these three loci are thought to be involved in the multicomponent melanogenic complex in the melanosome.**

6. **The P gene, the human homologue of the murine "pink-eyed dilution" gene, has been mapped to chromosome 15q11.2-12. The silver/pmel 17 gene is involved in premature graying in mice. This locus is thought to be related to the proliferative state of the cells and the product of this gene is produced only in cells that are growing. The melanocyte-stimulating hormone receptor (MSH-R) and the agouti gene product regulate the production of either black/brown eumelanin or red/yellow pheomelanin through their interaction. The human KIT gene, which codes for a mast/stem cell growth factor, has been mapped to chromosome 4q11-13. Mutations in the KIT gene are responsible for piebaldism. The PAX3 gene has been mapped to chromosome 2q35-37. Mutations of the PAX3 gene are responsible for Waardenburg syndrome.**

7. **Albinism represents a group of inherited abnormalities that present with congenital hypopigmentation that can involve the skin, hair, and eyes (oculocutaneous albinism) or be limited primarily to the eyes (ocular albinism). The definition of albinism includes specific changes in the optic system, including nystagmus, reduced iris pigment, reduced retinal pigment with foveal hypoplasia, and misrouting of the optic fibers at the chiasm. These features must be present to make a diagnosis of albinism.**

8. **Oculocutaneous albinism or OCA is divided into types in which the primary defect involves the melanocyte and types in which the albinism is secondary to a primary defect that involves many cell types, including the melanocyte. Primary OCA includes OCA1 or tyrosinase-related OCA,**

A list of standard abbreviations is located immediately preceeding the index in each volume. Nonstandard abbreviations used in this chapter include: AS = Angelman syndrome; BAER = brainstem auditory evoked responses; CHS = Chediak-Higashi syndrome; DHI = dihydroxyindole; DHICA = dihydroxyindole-2-carboxylic acid; DT = DOPAchrome tautomerase; HPS = Hermansky-Pudlak syndrome; MSH = melanocyte-stimulating hormone; MSH-R = melanocyte-stimulating hormone receptor; OCA = oculocutaneous albinism; OA = ocular albinism; PDGF = platelet-derived growth factor; PWS = Prader-Willi syndrome; RPE = retinal pigmented epithelium; TRP1 = tyrosinase-related protein 1; TRP2 = tyrosinase-related protein 2; TYR = human tyrosinase locus; WS = Waardenberg syndrome.

OCA2 (or tyrosine-positive OCA), and several unclassified types, such as brown OCA. Secondary OCA includes Hermansky-Pudlak syndrome (HPS), and Chediak-Higashi syndrome (CHS). Most OCA is autosomal recessive in inheritance; rare families with autosomal dominant OCA have been incompletely reported.

9. **OCA1 is produced by mutations of the tyrosinase gene and is divided into four types according to the amount and the type of residual enzyme activity. Mutant alleles associated with no tyrosinase activity produce OCA1A or tyrosinase-negative OCA. Mutant alleles associated with some residual activity produce OCA1B (yellow OCA) and OCA1MP (minimal pigment OCA). Mutant alleles associated with unusual enzyme activity produce OCA1TS (temperature-sensitive OCA). Many mutations of the tyrosinase gene have been identified in OCA1. Most affected individuals are compound heterozygotes.**

10. **OCA2 is produced by mutations of the human P gene. The phenotype is variable but there is a distinct common phenotype in African and African-American individuals. The hypopigmentation in Prader-Willi syndrome and Angelman syndrome is also related to the P gene.**

11. **Brown OCA has been reported in African and African-American individuals, and has been recognized in the Caucasian population. Red or Rufous OCA is poorly documented and may not be a true type of albinism.**

12. **HPSyndrome is an infrequent autosomal recessive syndrome that presents with oculocutaneous albinism, a mild bleeding diathesis, and a ceroid storage disease. Platelets lack dense bodies. Pulmonary fibrosis and granulomatous colitis occur and can be severe. The responsible gene has not been identified. CHSyndrome presents with hypopigmentation associated with an increased susceptibility to bacterial infections. Cells, including the melanocyte, contain giant granules, suggesting a basic membrane defect.**

13. **Ocular albinism (OA) is divided into X-linked OA or OA1, and autosomal recessive OA. Cutaneous pigment is normal in OA1, but cutaneous and ocular melanocytes contain giant melanosomes. Heterozygous females often have pigment changes that are thought to be the result of X inactivation. Autosomal recessive OA affects both males and females. Molecular studies have suggested that many individuals with this diagnosis actually have OCA1 or OCA2.**

14. **Proper evaluation and treatment of an individual with albinism includes correct diagnosis, skin care, and ophthalmologic care.**

Melanin pigment in the cutaneous and ocular tissues represents one of the most visible markers of human variation. As a result, inherited disorders of melanin formation that present with hypopigmentation have long fascinated scientists and others interested in human biology. Albinism represents the extreme of these disorders—evidenced by reduced amounts of melanin synthesis in all parts of the involved tissue—unlike disorders such as piebaldism, in which the reduction in melanin is patchy and discrete. Albinism itself is heterogeneous, however, and can be separated clinically into types that primarily involve the eyes [ocular albinism or (OA)] and types that involve the skin and the hair as well as the eyes [oculocutaneous albinism or (OCA)].

For OCA, further separation can be made by dividing the different types into those in which the genetic abnormality alters a process that is primary to the melanocyte or the synthesis of melanin and those with a more widespread genetic abnormality that involves several different cell types including the melanocyte. The true genetic heterogeneity of the different types of OCA has been defined at the molecular level, providing insight into the pathophysiological processes of this group of disorders.

Albinism is usually recognized because of its obvious visible nature. Furthermore, because albinism is present in most animal species, it is likely that it has occurred in humans since evolutionary speciation. The earliest written records include descriptions of individuals with albinism, primarily with a total lack of visible melanin pigment.[1] Descriptions multiplied with the advent of world exploration and travel and as interest in different world ethnic groups developed. As new continents and peoples were visited, the beliefs about and toward individuals with albinism were found to vary and, in some places, to assume a mythological aura. The familial nature of albinism was recognized almost as early as albinism itself, making this one of the first genetic conditions to be recognized.[1,2]

The first scientific approach to human albinism was provided by Sir Archibald Garrod who included albinism (actually oculocutaneous albinism) as one of the four originally described inborn errors of metabolism.[387] His clear insight into the nature of this condition as an enzyme defect preceded the actual biochemical demonstration of the lack of enzyme (tyrosinase) activity by many decades. There was great confusion about the true nature of OCA in the years before and after Garrod's work, however, because of the variation in phenotype. Some affected individuals had no visible pigment, such as those described by Garrod, and were thought to have "complete" or "perfect" albinism, while others had some degree of skin, hair, and eye pigment and were (incorrectly) described as having "partial" or "incomplete" albinism. These terms persist but are inappropriate now.

This initial confusion was clarified when it was shown that there are at least two genetically different types of OCA, with one type having no visible pigment (tyrosinase-negative OCA) and the other having variable amounts of visible pigment (tyrosinase-positive OCA).[2,3] This initial distinction was made by simply incubating hairbulbs from affected individuals in tyrosine or DOPA; hairbulbs from some individuals formed pigment and those from others did not.[3–5] The hairbulb reaction tended to follow the phenotype, in that no pigment formed in hairbulbs from individuals without obvious skin, hair, or eye pigment, whereas pigment formed in hairbulbs from individuals who usually had residual melanin pigment in these tissues. The hairbulb reaction was later quantified with a precise assay, and it was shown that hairbulbs that formed no pigment had no tyrosinase activity while those that could form pigment had activity, often in amounts comparable to control values.[6]

Our understanding of OA and OCA has changed greatly in the past two decades. New types of OCA have been characterized, including Hermansky-Pudlak syndrome[7] and brown OCA.[8,9] Hypopigmentation and albinism in conditions such as Prader-Willi and Angelman syndromes have been recognized.[10–12] Most importantly, the molecular biology of normal and abnormal melanin synthesis is now being defined in many laboratories.

This chapter describes the progress in pigment biology. The basic biology of the pigment system will be described, followed by a description of the known biochemistry and molecular biology of melanin synthesis. The second half of the chapter will review the present basic and clinical knowledge of the various types of albinism.

THE MELANOCYTE AND MELANOGENIC APPARATUS

Overview

Melanocytes represent a relatively small subpopulation of the cells present in the epidermis and dermis of mammals, yet they produce the melanin that accounts for virtually all visible pigmentation.[13–19] Melanocytes are dendritic cells with two embryonic origins. Melanocytes originating in the neural crest during embryologic development subsequently migrate throughout the developing organism to three principal locations: the skin (at the epidermal–dermal border), the eyes (in the choroid and iris stroma), and the hair follicles.[20–22] Melanocytes in the retinal pigment epithelium are derived from neuroectoderm as cells originating from the outer layer of the developing optic vesicle.[23,24] Melanin is produced by melanocytes in specific subcellular organelles called "melanosomes," and can be of several types, with differing visible colors and, presumably, distinct functional properties. Melanin has several functions. It is:

1. a barrier against ionizing radiation;
2. a participant in developmental processes;
3. a cosmetic entity;
4. a potential scavenger of cytotoxic radicals and intermediates.

Normal pigmentation requires a number of critical and precise steps, including melanoblast development in the neural crest and migration of these cells to disparate parts of the body, arrest of melanoblast migration at the appropriate sites, and survival, proliferation, differentiation, and function of melanocytes in these tissues. It is little wonder that mammalian pigmentation is regulated at many different levels and is influenced, either directly or indirectly, by many genes. In the mouse for example, hundreds of different mutations have been identified that alter pigmentation at more than 65 distinct genetic loci.[25] Almost a dozen of these murine genes have been cloned. In each instance noted thus far, an analogous and highly homologous gene is also expressed by human melanocytes, which suggests that the products of these genes are important to melanocyte function. Table 147-1 presents a list of mouse pigment genes and their human homologues. The terminology found in the table will be used throughout this chapter.

Environmental Interactions

Ocular melanocytes are distributed to the choroid, iris, and retina, where they are relatively dormant in that their rates of melanogenesis are low after fetal development, and the pigment synthesized is not secreted, but remains within the melanocyte. In contrast, melanocytes that reside in the skin and hairbulbs are highly secretory. Within hairbulbs, melanocytes typically transfer melanosomes to the hair shafts, giving the hair visible color.[13,20,26] Melanocytes in the skin reside at the junction of the dermis and epidermis, and secreted melanosomes are taken up by neighboring keratinocytes (the predominant cell type in the epidermis),[18,22,27–30] as depicted in Fig. 147-1. Melanosomes in the

Table 147-1 Mouse Pigmentation Genes and Their Human Homologues

Murine Locus (symbol)	Human Locus	Protein Encoded	Function	Relevant Clinical Condition
Tissue level				
Dominant Spotting *(W)*	KIT	Tyrosine kinase receptor	KIT tyrosine kinase receptor	Piebaldism
Steel *(Sl)*		Steel factor	Ligand for KIT	Piebaldism*
Splotch *(Sp)*	PAX	Pax-3	Transcription factor*	Waardenburg syndrome
Microphthalmia *(Mi)*		Unknown	Cell/tissue development	Vitiligo*
Cellular level				
Dilute *(d)*		Myosin-related protein	Intracellular melanosome movement*	?
Pallid *(pa)* or Pearl *(pe)*		Unknown	Organellogenesis*	Hermansky-Pudlak syndrome*
Pink-eyed dilution *(p)*	P	Unknown	Tyrosine transport*	OCA2; Tyrosinase positive OCA
Extension *(e)*	MSHR	MSH receptor	Hormonal regulation	Rufous OCA*
Agouti *(a)*		171 amino acid protein	MSH receptor antagonist*	?
Beige *(be)*		Unknown	Organellogenesis	Chediak-Higashi syndrome*
Subcellular level				
Albino *(c)*	TYR	Tyrosinase	Tyrosine hydroxylase, DOPA oxidase	OCA1; Tyrosinase-related OCA
Brown *(b)*	TRP1	TRP1 (gp75)	Melanogenic catalytic function	Brown OCA*
Slaty *(slt)*	TRP2	Dopachrome tautomerase (TRP2)	Eumelanin biosynthesis	?
Silver *(si)*		gp95	Stablin* or matrix protein*	?

*Hypothetical.

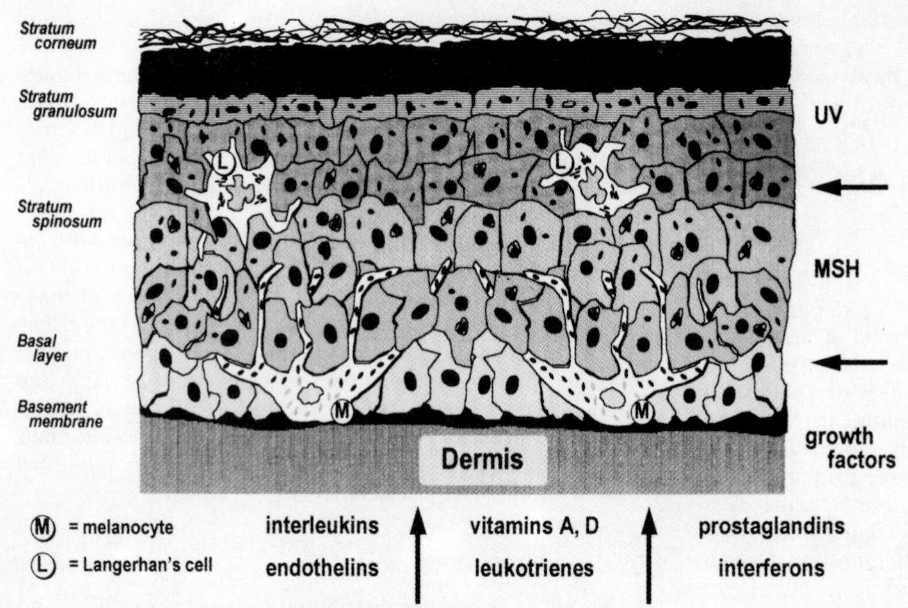

FIG. 147-1 Melanocyte functional unit. The skin is a complex system influenced by many external environmental factors. The melanocyte functional unit consists of melanocytes (M), keratinocytes, Langerhans cells (L), and other cells that produce factors regulating pigmentation, as indicated in the figure. (See text for detailed discussion.) The melanocytes reside in the basal layer with dendritic projections into the stratum spinosum of the epidermis.

keratinocytes are further processed, degraded, and redistributed either in smaller pieces and/or in larger complexes that eventually result in visible skin color.[29,31–33] The association of the melanocyte and its neighboring keratinocytes has been called the "epidermal melanin unit," but this is somewhat of a misnomer since the melanocyte interacts with many cell types in the skin. Epidermal melanocytes are highly responsive cells that continually sample their environment and modulate their levels of proliferation or melanogenesis.

Melanocytes express numerous receptors that allow interaction with other cells in their microenvironment, including keratinocytes and the immune component of the skin—the Langerhans cell.[29,30,34–37] Further, in various disease conditions, and other "abnormal" states, the skin can be infiltrated by other cell types, for example, lymphocytes or macrophages, or by foreign cells penetrating a breach in the integrity of the skin. Those types of cells can also secrete factors that bind to receptors on the melanocyte and thereby induce the melanocyte to increase or decrease its melanogenic activity. The receptors expressed on melanocytes allow these cells to respond to a wide variety of regulatory factors, including various growth factors,[36,38–45] hormones,[46–61] interferons,[55,58,62–64] interleukins,[65–67] prostaglandins,[68–73] retinoic acid,[61,74–79] and a host of other cytokines.[67,80–82] Melanocytes produce some of these factors, which then function in an autocrine manner.[83–86] In sum, the melanocyte is in a highly dynamic equilibrium with different cell types in its immediate environment, all of which participate in determining its melanocytic activity.

The Melanogenic Apparatus

The biochemical machinery to produce melanin is confined within membrane-bound organelles called "melanosomes," as shown in Fig. 147-2, perhaps for the reason that many intermediates in the melanin biosynthetic pathway are poten-

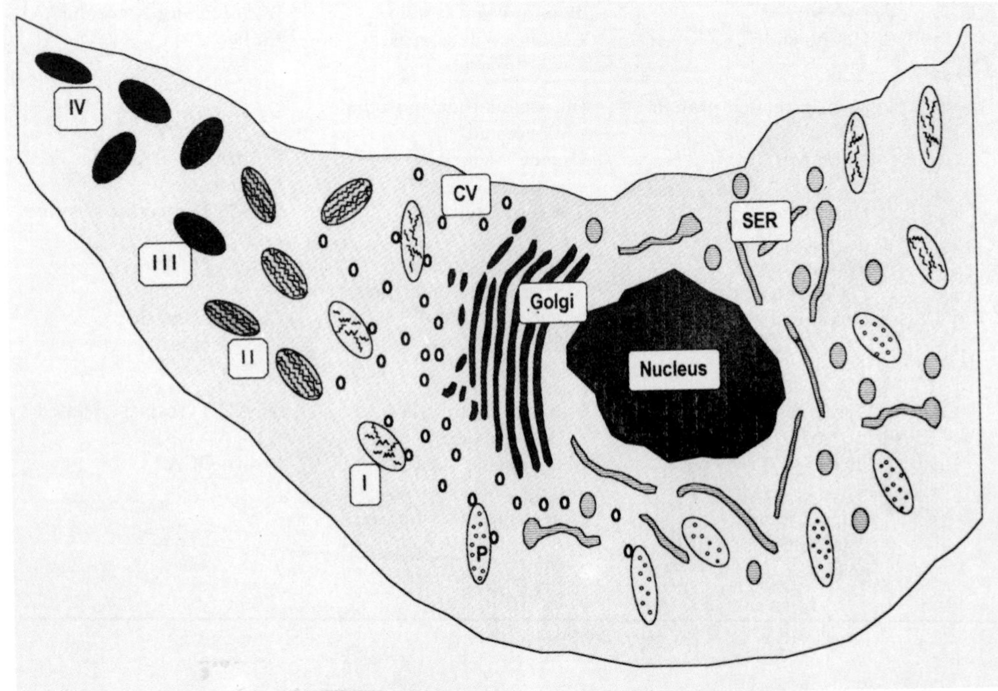

FIG. 147-2 Melanosome biogenesis. The coated vesicles (CV) contain tyrosinase and other enzymatic components. The fusion of the coated vesicles with the premelanosome (P) derived from the SER allows melanogenesis to proceed. Stages I to IV of premelanosome/melanosome development are labeled.

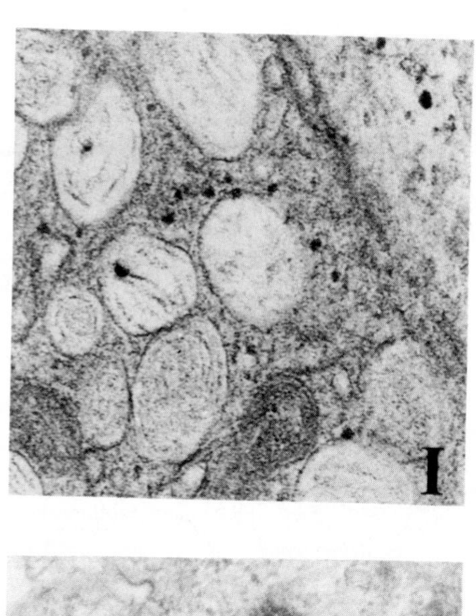

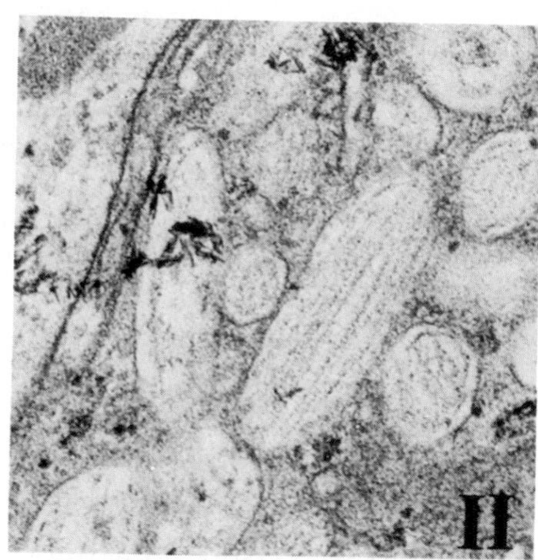

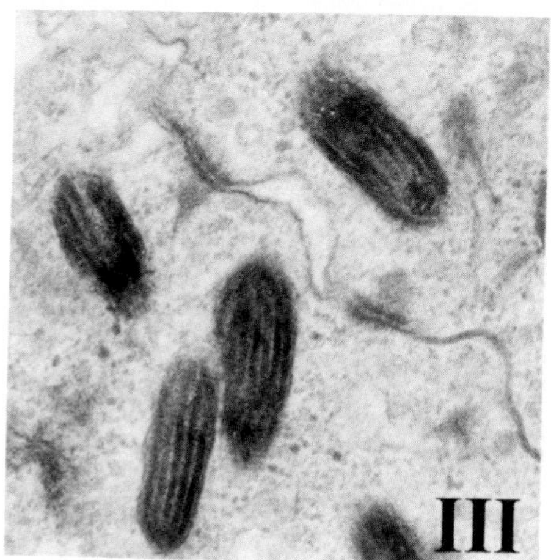

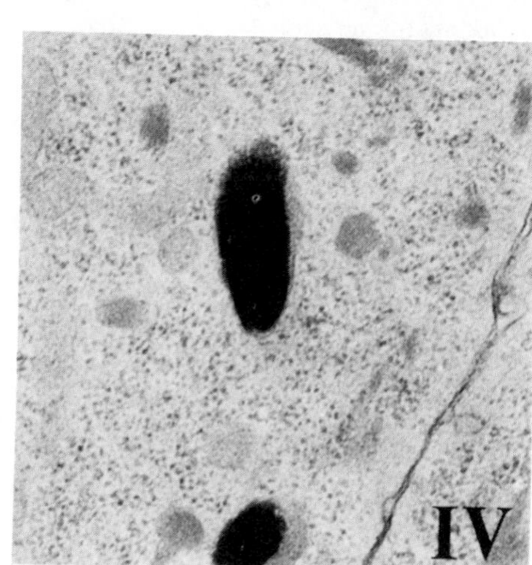

FIG. 147-3 Melanosome melanization. Ultrastructure of eumelanosome development. The maturation of melanosomes occurs in four stages: the stages I, II, and III premelanosome and stage IV fully melanized melanosome.

tially cytotoxic. The melanosome initially evolves from the SER as a cytoplasmic, membrane-bound vesicle with an amorphous interior. In this state, the organelle is referred to as a "stage I premelanosome," and does not contain any of the melanogenic enzymes required for melanin synthesis.[87–90] Tyrosinase (and probably the other melanogenic determinants) is synthesized on ribosomes, transported through the RER to the Golgi apparatus, where posttranslational processing continues.[91–98] Tyrosinase is glycosylated en route to the active face of the Golgi, secreted within coated vesicles into the cytoplasmic milieu, and then transported to the premelanosomes, where the vesicles fuse with the limiting membrane.[99–104] The melanogenic enzymes (at least those that have been characterized to date) are localized within the melanosomal membrane with their catalytic centers facing inward, and active melanogenesis begins following fusion of the coated vesicles with the melanosome. At this stage, the premelanosome has an internal matrix but contains no melanin, and is known as a "stage II premelanosome."

Tyrosinase is catalytically competent to produce pigment while in transit through the Golgi apparatus and coated vesicles, and it is unclear how melanogenesis is delayed until its arrival at the melanosome in vivo. It has been proposed that melanogenic inhibitors are responsible for preventing melanin production until incorporation within the melanosome, but this has not been satisfactorily resolved.[105–109] The mechanism involved is an important issue, since alterations in this process may result in various types of hypopigmentation conditions in which active tyrosinase is present yet no melanin is produced, such as in different types of oculocutaneous albinism. Following initiation of melanogenesis, melanin is deposited uniformly within the melanosome (stage III premelanosome), and the opacity of the organelle gradually increases until eventually all substructure is obscured, leaving only the electron-dense mature melanin granule visible (stage IV melanosome).[88,89] The different stages of melanosome development are shown in Fig. 147-3. During this process, the melanosome steadily moves away from the perinuclear region toward the periphery of the melanocyte, where it is passed to the keratinocytes and eventually degraded.

BIOCHEMISTRY AND MELANIN SYNTHESIS

Overview

The chemical reactions involved in the production of melanin from the amino acid tyrosine are relatively straightforward, and were actually described many decades ago,[110,111] but only recently has the underlying complexity of the regulatory controls involved in melanin synthesis been described. The melanin biosynthetic pathway is shown in Fig. 147-4. Several of the unusual properties of the melanin biopolymer have confounded all attempts at definitive structural analysis by conventional chemical methods, and the characterization of melanin structure is still being investigated. In addition,

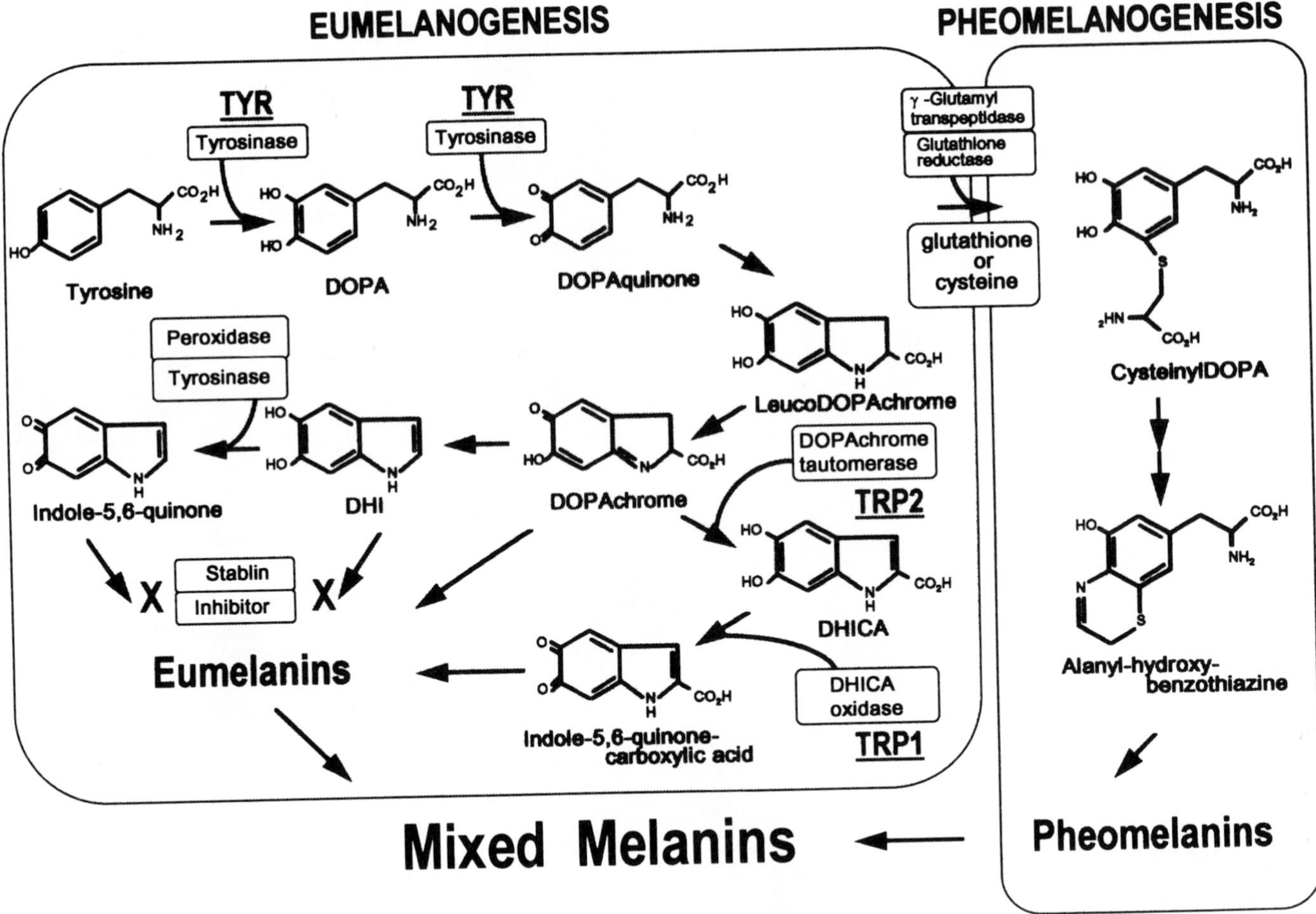

FIG. 147-4 Melanin pathway. The melanin pathway presents a summary of the known reactions and regulatory enzymes in eumelanogenesis and pheomelanogenesis.

many of the melanogenic intermediates are highly unstable, and their ability to autooxidize rapidly, forming melanin, has also hampered such analyses.

Enzymatic Components. The copper-containing enzyme tyrosinase (EC 1.14.18.1) is critical to melanin formation due to its ability to catalyze the first reaction in the biosynthetic sequence—the hydroxylation of tyrosine to DOPA. This is the most critical reaction, since the spontaneous rate of tyrosine hydroxylation is negligible, and this represents the rate limiting step in the pathway. DOPA can then spontaneously autooxidize to DOPAquinone in the absence of tyrosinase (although at slower rates than in the presence of the enzyme) and will continue through the pathway by cyclizing to form the indole rings present in leukoDOPAchrome and DOPAchrome. Without further catalytic intervention, DOPAchrome will spontaneously decarboxylate to produce 5,6-dihydroxyindole (DHI), which in turn rapidly oxidizes to indole-5,6-quinone. Early studies suggested that melanin consisted of a homogeneous polymer of indole-5,6-quinone,[112–115] but more recent evidence suggests that melanins are much more heterogeneous in nature and probably consist of mixtures of several other intermediates in the pathway.[19,116–125] Melanin synthesis will occur spontaneously in the test tube once DOPA is formed, but other constraints are put on these reactions in vivo. A number of additional factors that regulate the flow of this pathway have now been characterized, including other enzymes (i.e., DOPAchrome tautomerase),[126–137] the availability of reactive sulfhydryls (i.e., glutathione and/or cysteine),[116,118,138–145] melanogenic inhibitors,[105–109,146–151] and perhaps other regulatory factors.[152–157] The genes for several of these melanogenic factors have now been cloned, providing a glimpse of the complex mechanisms responsible for the production of different types of pigmentation. Perhaps more importantly, it is now possible to begin to understand the molecular lesions responsible for many abnormal pigmentation conditions, such as oculocutaneous albinism.

Eumelanin versus Pheomelanin Synthesis. There are two distinct types of melanins that can be produced in mammalian melanocytes: eumelanin (which is black and/or brown in color) and pheomelanin (which is red and/or yellow in color).[120,121,125,158–161] The commitment to produce either type of melanin is made following the generation of DOPAquinone. If sulfhydryl groups, typically cysteine or glutathione, are available, they will stoichiometrically react with the DOPAquinone and generate cysteinylDOPA.[141,145,162–170] There are actually three different cysteinylDOPAs that can be formed, including 2-S-, 5-S-, and 2,5-S,S-cysteinylDOPA. The cysteinylDOPAs then undergo a series of poorly understood reactions that result in the cyclization of a second ring (not of the indole type) and subsequent polymerization into a high-molecular-weight biopolymer. Pheomelanins have properties distinct from eumelanin, including a greater solubility and distinct appearance.[131,136] The pheomelanin pathway is obviously influenced by enzymes that regulate intracellular (intramelanosomal?) concentrations of available sulfhydryl groups, and it is not yet known if other enzymes are involved in the further metabolism of the cysteinyl-DOPAs and their derivatives. It seems a reasonable expectation, however, that regulatory factors similar to those of eumelanogenesis will eventually be identified for pheomelanogenesis.

In the absence of sulfhydryls, eumelanins will be produced. LeukoDOPAchrome forms and is quickly converted to DOPAchrome, which represents yet another key regulatory point in the pathway. DOPAchrome will quantitatively decarboxylate spontaneously to form DHI, although in the presence of certain divalent metal cations (e.g. Co^{2+}, Mg^{2+}, Fe^{2+}) and/or DOPAchrome tautomerase, the carboxylated intermediate 5,6-dihydroxyindole-2-carboxylic acid (DHICA) will be produced.[130,132,133,135–137,153,171] Since DHI and DHICA are not interconvertible, the carboxyl content of the melanin has essentially been determined once this step has been reached. It is not yet known if there are other enzymes that function following the production of DHI and/or DHICA (although they are expected), nor do we know the exact nature of further intermediates that may be produced subsequently. Mammalian melanins contain significant levels of carboxylated and decarboxylated intermediates,[121,172,173] although it is not known how this influences their structure and/or function.

Mutations at several gene loci in inbred mice have been identified that lead to the exclusive production of eumelanin or pheomelanin in the coat. The *brown* locus includes the wild-type *B* and the mutant *b* allele, and both are associated with eumelanin in the coat, while the *extension* locus includes the *recessive yellow* allele associated with pheomelanin in the coat.[25] In *agouti* (wild-type) mice, melanocytes produce either eumelanins or pheomelanins, resulting in hair that has alternating bands of eumelanin and pheomelanin. This occurs because all melanocytes in a single hairbulb produce one type of melanin, then switch production to the other type of melanin back and forth in regular intervals.[18,22,25,26,174–177]

The regulation of the switch to eumelanin synthesis can be induced in mice by treatment with melanocyte-stimulating hormone (MSH), and the ability to respond to this melanogenic hormone depends on the products of the *agouti* and *extension* loci.[178] The *agouti* locus in mice regulates the synthesis of eumelanin or pheomelanin by an as yet unknown mechanism[104,174–177,179,180]; however, it is known that the mechanism involves the action of MSH from exogenous sources, that is, from cells peripheral to the melanocyte.[181–183] The *agouti* gene has now been cloned,[184] and studies of the structure and function of that important gene product should be forthcoming. The MSH receptor gene has also been cloned[185] and mapped to the *extension* locus in the mouse.

In humans, MSH receptors are expressed on melanocytes, but the evidence supporting a role for MSH in human pigmentation is incomplete.[53,59] Both types of melanins can be produced in the same melanocyte in humans, and both form complexes within the same biopolymer, which is then called "mixed melanin."[97,186–189] The exact ratio of the two melanins in mixed melanins is variable, and the regulatory controls involved in determining that ratio have not yet been identified.[19] Studies currently underway on the contribution of the various intermediates (e.g., with or without sulfhydryl and/or carboxyl groups) to the structure and function of melanin should provide important insights into the understanding of the regulatory controls of this pathway and functional significance of each component.

Melanogenic Determinants of Melanin Formation

Two enzymes (tyrosinase and DOPAchrome tautomerase) and a variety of other regulating factors have been identified in the melanin synthetic pathway. Tyrosinase is absolutely essential for melanin production. DOPAchrome tautomerase and the other melanogenic factors function distal to tyrosinase to modify the type of melanin produced.

Tyrosinase. Tyrosinase is the product of the mouse *c* locus and the human TYR locus. It is a copper-dependent enzyme that is unusual in that it has three distinct catalytic functions.[6,110,111,117,123,190–194] The most critical function is the hydroxylation of tyrosine, since this is the rate limiting reaction in the melanin synthetic pathway. Tyrosinase also uses DOPA and DHI as substrates for oxidase activities (see Fig. 147-4). It has been suggested, based on kinetic data, that the various activities of tyrosinase reside at different sites on the enzyme, and biochemical evidence on the catalytic functions of various mutant human tyrosinases supports that interpretation.[195] Another distinctive characteristic of mammalian tyrosinase is its highly stereospecific requirement for DOPA as a cofactor for the initial critical hydroxylation of tyrosine, with DOPA also being the product of that reaction.[6,192,196,197] Rates of tyrosine hydroxylation in the absence of added cofactor are negligible, which raises the question of the origin of the initial DOPA cofactor, since DOPA is not a normal amino acid available within the cell. Although several suggestions have been made about the origin of the DOPA cofactor, or alternative methods of activating the enzyme, this question remains unresolved.[157,198,199]

Tyrosinase is melanocyte-specific, and studies employing various techniques to detect tyrosinase or its mRNA find that the tyrosinase gene is expressed only in melanocytes. The enzyme is synthesized as a nascent protein of approximately 60 kDa that is glycosylated en route to the melanosome to a final size of approximately 75 kDa.[54,91,92,96–98,200,201] Tyrosinase is an extremely stable protein that is highly resistant to attack by heat or by proteases, and it has an unusually long biologic half-life (~ 10 h in vivo). It has a relatively low isoelectric point (pH 4.3) and is predominantly bound to the melanosomal membrane. Many, if not all, of these physical characteristics of the enzyme are consistent with the structural features predicted by the coding sequence of the gene.

DOPAchrome Tautomerase. DOPAchrome tautomerase (DT) is the product of the mouse *slaty* locus and the human TRP2 locus.[126–137] It functions in the specific conversion of DOPAchrome to the carboxylated derivative DHICA, rather than to the decarboxylated intermediate DHI, which would be formed in its absence.[130,132,133,135–137, 153, 171] The same catalytic function can be mimicked using certain divalent metal cations, although the extent to which these function independently or by interaction with DOPAchrome tautomerase in a biologic system has not yet been determined.[135,152–154,202] The gene for this enzyme has been cloned and shows significant relationship to the tyrosinase gene.[137,203]

DOPAchrome tautomerase is expressed in melanocytes, where it localizes to the melanosomal membrane, but it is also synthesized in the developing forebrain of mice[203,204]; the reason for this is currently unknown but it has been suggested that DOPAchrome tautomerase may be required in neurons to scavenge cytotoxic byproducts of the catecholamine biosynthetic pathway. Although its route of posttranslational processing has not been as well characterized as that of tyrosinase, the similarity of their structures and glycosylation patterns suggests that their processing and delivery to the melanosome is similar.[137,205,206] The size of the nascent form of DOPAchrome tautomerase protein is close to that of tyrosinase (~65 kDa) as is its fully glycosylated size (~ 80 kDa).[137] As noted above, however, its catalytic function is quite distinct from that of tyrosinase, and, in spite of their amino acid sequence relatedness, neither enzyme has detectable levels of the other's catalytic activity. DOPAchrome tautomerase does not seem to be as biologically stable as tyrosinase, it is more labile to treatment with heat or proteases, and its activity follows a different response pattern to MSH stimulation than does that of tyrosinase.[136,207–209] Tyrosinase contains copper atoms that are required for its catalytic function, and early studies indicate that metal ions also play a role in the catalytic function of DOPAchrome tautomerase, but the metal involved may be iron rather than copper.[210]

Other Melanogenic Enzymes. Enzymes that regulate the intracellular and/or intramelanosomal concentrations of sulfhydryl compounds such as cysteine and glutathione can influence melanin synthesis by forcing the reaction toward or away from pheomelanin. Among such enzymes are glutathione reductase[138–140] and γ-glutamyl transpeptidase[166,211–214]; however, the specific role of these enzymes in melanogenesis has not yet been established. It is expected that there will be additional enzymes identified for more distal reactions in the pheomelanin pathway.

The ability of peroxidase to oxidize DHI to indole-5,6-quinone has also been documented,[155,215] and its potential role in melanogenesis is under investigation. A melanosomal specific catalase has been suggested to participate in the melanogenic process, although its potential function in the pathway is not altogether clear.[142,156]

A novel activity termed "DHICA oxidase" has been identified by several groups. This enzyme activity has been tentatively assigned to tyrosinase-related protein 1 (TRP1)—the product of the human homologue of the murine *brown* locus. Although tyrosinase can employ DHI as a substrate for its oxidase activity, it uses DHICA less efficiently, whereas TRP1 is more efficient using DHICA than DHI. In sum, the melanogenic reaction scheme is now known to be much more complex than thought just a decade ago and it seems likely that even more regulatory steps will be identified in this complex enzymatic cascade of reactions.

Melanogenic Inhibitors. Many types of natural and synthetic melanogenic inhibitors have been described.[105–109,146–151] Since the primary substrate of the melanogenic pathway, tyrosine, is a naturally occurring amino acid, many peptides and polypeptides may function as competitive inhibitors of tyrosinase if they have an exposed tyrosine or phenylalanine residue. In addition, there are other types of naturally occurring inhibitors of melanogenesis that are endogenous to melanocytes, and many laboratories are currently trying to characterize the structures and functions of those that may be biologically significant. One such inhibitor has been highly purified from amelanotic cells that have significant levels of tyrosinase, and has been partially characterized, but its exact chemical structure has not yet been defined. It is a very small molecule (~ 500 daltons) that acts as an effective competitive inhibitor of melanin production.[150,151,216] A correlation between the presence of melanogenic inhibitors and the degree of melanin pigmentation expressed in the melanocyte has been found, and it is thought that they may be critical to the regulation of tyrosinase activity in the melanocyte, particularly with respect to the rapid changes that can be induced by environmental factors, an example being the dramatic increase in melanogenesis following stimulation by MSH or by UV light. This mechanism is proposed since there are no significant differences in the transcription or translation rates of melanogenic enzymes following such stimulation, while levels of the melanogenic inhibitor decrease dramatically.[151] There is now a heightened interest in melanogenic inhibitors, since it seems probable that they are intimately related to several conditions of hypopigmentation in which normal levels of melanogenic enzyme are present, yet melanin synthesis is negligible.

Another novel melanogenic inhibitory activity that has been described is "stablin."[217,218] It apparently acts in the distal part of the eumelanin pathway by influencing the processing of DHI and DHICA to melanin in an as yet uncharacterized manner. Under biologic conditions, DHICA, and particularly DHI, are highly unstable and rapidly metabolize further to form melanin. Stablin is a high-molecular-weight, protease-sensitive, heat-stable molecule that prevents the spontaneous conversion of DHI or DHICA to melanin for relatively long periods.[218] The exact nature of this inhibition is unknown, but it seems to be associated with the expression of another pigment-related gene *(silver)*.

Further evidence for complex regulation of melanogenesis is found in studies of UV radiation. The stimulation of melanocytic differentiation (i.e., pigmentation) by MSH or UV light is not primarily dictated by increases in the translation or transcription of tyrosinase (or its mRNA).[51,54,219–222] We can now expand that concept to include the melanogenic enzyme DOPAchrome tautomerase, since levels of that enzyme's activity were increased in response to MSH, but without a concomitant increase in synthesis of the enzyme.[206–209,223] The dramatic increase in tyrosinase activity coupled with a lesser increase in DOPAchrome tautomerase activity implies that melanogenic induction leads to increased melanin formation, which would be relatively DHI-rich. Since DHI melanins are visibly darker than the DHICA melanins, this may in part explain the observed augmentation of melanocyte darkening following such stimulation.

MOLECULAR BIOLOGY OF MELANIN SYNTHESIS

Genes Involved in Melanin Synthesis

Table 147-1 lists some mouse genetic loci involved in pigmentation and their potential human homologues. The following section provides an overview of the genes that have been isolated and their role in melanogenesis as it is currently envisioned.

Tyrosinase Gene Family. Three genes, known as the *albino* or *c* locus, *brown* or *b* locus, and *slaty* or *slt* locus in mice, and the TYR, TRP1, and TRP2 genes in humans, code for proteins with very similar nucleotide and amino acid sequences. The fact that two of these were initially isolated using tyrosinase antibodies and cDNA expression libraries and that all three are recognized by tyrosinase antiserum shows that they must have common epitopes. The product of the murine *brown* locus (TRP1) has approximately 43 percent amino acid identity to tyrosinase, and the product of the murine *slaty* locus (TRP2) has a 40 percent amino acid identity to both tyrosinase and TRP1.

The Tyrosinase Gene. Tyrosinase cDNA was first isolated from a mouse melanocyte cDNA library using both mouse tyrosinase antiserum and synthetic oligonucleotides corresponding to amino acid sequences of tyrosinase determined from cyanogen bromide fragments of purified tyrosinase.[224] Subsequently, a human cDNA was isolated by screening a human melanocyte cDNA library with hamster tyrosinase antiserum.[225] The authenticity of these clones was proven by comparing the predicted amino acid sequence of the tyrosinase cDNA to the amino acid sequence of isolated mouse[224] and human tyrosinase.[226,227] The initially reported human tyrosinase cDNA lacked the initiation codon ATG, and the full-length human cDNA sequence was reported subsequently.[228]

The tyrosinase locus (TYR) in humans has been mapped to chromosome 11q14-21 using *in situ* hybridization.[229] Both the human and mouse tyrosinase gene contain five exons spanning more than 50 kb with the exons ranging in size from 819 bp for exon 1 to 148 nucleotides for exon 3.[230,231] The lengths of introns 3 and 4 are between 9 and 10 kb and the lengths of introns 1 and 2 are still unknown but thought to be much larger (20 to 50 kb).

The 5′-upstream promoter region of the human tyrosinase gene contains four transcriptional start sites with the major site −79 bp from the ATG initiation codon and minor sites at −75, −46, and −42 bp.[231,232] There are also several *cis*-regulatory elements including a putative TATA box −106 bp and CAATT box −199 bp as well as a 230-bp repeat sequence of $(GA:TC)_n$ located 713 bp upstream of the translational start site, which can assume a hinged-DNA structure that may play a role in regulation of expression.[232] This repeat sequence in humans has been found to be highly polymorphic in several different populations.[233,234] There are other *cis*-acting regulatory elements within 270 bp of the start codon, including a suppressor element and a consensus element, but the functions of these and their *trans*-acting elements have yet to be determined.[235]

Transgenic expression studies using only 270 bp of the mouse tyrosinase 5′ promoter region has shown that this region promotes both cell-type-specific expression, occurring in dermal melanocytes (neural crest in origin) and in the melanocytes of the pigmented epithelium of the retina (optic cup in origin), and faithful temporal regulation.[235,236] The critical *cis*-acting regulators appear to be between −170 and −80 bp from the translational start codon. Expression studies using a longer 5′ upstream promoter (2.5 kb) have produced mice with variation in both coat color, intensity, and in its pattern.[237–239] These pattern differences, usually observed as transverse striping, are heritable and may be due to the different integration sites of the transgene resulting in *cis*-acting positional effects,[240] or differences in the number of copies inserted into the genome. The entire mouse tyrosinase gene has been inserted into a tyrosinase deficient albino mouse using a YAC.[241,242] This transgene contained the entire coding region (80 kb) and 155 kb of the upstream sequences. The expression of this transgene in transgenic mice was found to be both position-independent and copy-number-dependent. The resulting pigmented transgenic mice were indistinguishable from wild-type. Expression studies in cell culture have shown that transfection of various plasmids containing tyrosinase cDNA and different promoter sequences into different cell types such as mouse fibroblasts (NIH 3T3 and L cells) and HeLa cells will lead to melanin synthesis in these cells.[228,243] This ability to express tyrosinase in nonmelanocytes is useful for the analysis of different tyrosinase gene mutations responsible for OCA.

The initial reported mouse tyrosinase cDNA nucleotide sequence was missing exon 3.[224,244] It is now known that tyrosinase exhibits a high percentage of transcripts that are alternatively spliced.[230,244–246] Twelve different alternatively spliced transcripts have been found in the mouse, and 41 percent of all tyroinase transcripts are alternatively spliced.[246] These alternate transcripts arise from either exon skipping, usage of alternative 5′ and/or 3′ splice sites, or retention of intron sequences.[246] There is also evidence that alternative splicing of the tyrosinase mRNA occurs in human melanoma melanocytes.[247] In many cases, the alternatively spliced tyrosinase mRNA lack important functional domains such as the copper B region and most likely these alternate mRNA, if translated, do not produce functional tyrosinase molecules. Expression studies with some of these alternative transcripts found in mice showed that they do not produce proteins with tyrosinase activity.[230,244] Alternatively spliced mRNA have been found in several different genes, including the nervous-system-specific tyrosine hydroxylase gene[248] and, of all known genes expressed in the nervous system, up to 30 percent of these genes exhibit alternative splicing.[249] It is unknown if the alternatively spliced tyrosinase mRNA encode a useful product for the melanocyte.

Six polymorphic sites have been identified with the human tyrosinase gene (Table 147-2; Figure 147-5). Two of these polymorphisms are amino acid substitutions. The Y192S

Table 147-2 Population Distribution of Polymorphisms in the Tyrosinase Gene

Polymorphism	Ethnic Group	A1	A2	A3	A4	A5	Reference
*Bgl*II RFLP	Caucasian	0.50	0.50				255
(GA) repeat	Caucasian	0.1	0.31	0.02	0.55	0.02	233
CCAATT	Caucasian	0.89*	0.11†				253
	Oriental	0.89	0.11				
Y192S	Caucasian	0.52	0.48				250
	Oriental	1.00	0				251
R402Q	Caucasian	0.85‡	0.15§				252
	Oriental	1.00	0				
*Taq*I RFLP	Caucasian	0.48	0.52				254

*A1 represents the presence of the restriction endonuclease site.
†A2 represents the absence of the restriction endonuclease site.
‡A1 represents CGA for codon 402 polymorphism.
§A2 represents CAA for codon 402 polymorphism.

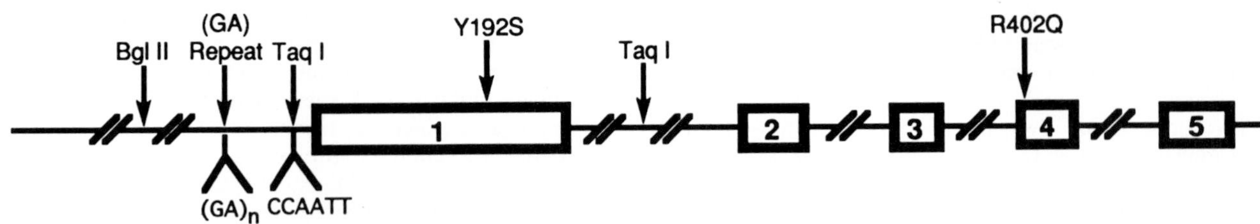

FIG. 147-5 Tyrosinase gene and polymorphisms. The tyrosinase gene (TYR) coding region is divided into five exons. There are six identified polymorphic sites in the tyrosinase gene.

polymorphism affects an *Mbo*I restriction endonuclease site and serine (TCT; presence of the *Mbo*I site) is found in all populations, whereas tyrosine (TAT; absence of the *Mbo*I site) is found only in non-Oriental populations.[250,251] The R402Q polymorphism also has one allele restricted from the Oriental population.[252] In contrast to this, both alleles of the polymorphic sites near the CCAATT box have been found in all racial groups.[253] A dinucleotide repeat sequence of $(GA{:}TC)_n$ located 713 bp upstream of the translational start site has several alleles that result from insertions or deletions of dinucleotides.[233] There are also two RFLPs, one detected with *Taq*1 and the other with *Bgl*II.[254,255] These polymorphic sites can be used to establish molecular haplotypes of the human tyrosinase gene.

There is a second tyrosinase cDNA site of hybridization located at human chromosome 11p11.2-cen, and this is called the "tyrosinase-related gene" (TYRL).[229,231,256,257] This locus consists of a truncated tyrosinase gene having only exons IV and V with the entire fourth and part of the third introns.[231,257] Sequence analysis has shown TYR and TYRL to be very similar, with 98 percent nucleotide homology for exons IV and V. Analysis of nonhuman primates has shown that gorilla DNA contains the TYRL locus while that of the chimpanzee does not, suggesting that the formation of the TYRL locus appears to have occurred relatively recently in primate evolution.[258] No transcription product of the TYRL locus is detectable in human melanocytes, and it most likely is a pseudogene.[257] The existence of a tyrosinase pseudogene presents a potential problem with PCR-based sequencing of the tyrosinase gene. Care must be taken that the amplified fragment derives from the TYR (functional) gene.

The DOPAchrome Tautomerase Gene. A second melanogenic enzyme gene to be cloned is that of DOPAchrome tautomerase (DT)—the product of the human TRP2 locus and the mouse *slaty* locus. The initial DT cDNA was isolated during an attempt to isolate the tyrosinase cDNA using rabbit antimouse tyrosinase antibody and rabbit antihamster tyrosinase antibody, and the resulting clone was first designated as 5A.[259,260] This cDNA was later termed "TRP2" and has now been identified as the coding sequence for the enzyme DOPAchrome tautomerase.[137] The cDNA was mapped to the *slaty* locus of the mouse and the only known mutant allele *(slt)* results in a reduction, but not a complete absence, of DT activity.[203] The mutant phenotype has a reduction of coat pigment from black to dark gray/brown eumelanin. Mice homozygous for the mutant *slaty* allele on a nonagouti background have a slightly diluted coat and slightly yellowish ears.[25,261] Sequencing of DNA from mice homozygous for the *slaty* mutant allele shows a mutation in one of the putative metal binding regions that results in a three- to fourfold reduction in DT activity in melanocytes.

Steel et al. have found that DT is expressed very early in developing mouse embryos (10 days postconception), while TRP1 is expressed at 11.5 days postconception and tyrosinase transcripts are seen 13.5 days postconception.[204] The DT is expressed in the developing forebrain (until 14 days postconception), suggesting that the enzyme may have more than one function. One possibility is that the enzyme may be acting as a detoxifying agent to reduce the accumulation of neural transmitters, their metabolites or other byproducts of the catecholamine pathway. DT activity may be MSH-sensitive in the adult mouse, in that some investigators have found an increase in activity in the presence of MSH,[223] while others have found no increase even when tyrosinase activity has increased.[207] The mechanism of regulation of tyrosinase appears to be different even though both reside in the same organelles.[262]

Brown/gp75 Gene. A third cDNA, isolated by using differential hybridization between mouse melanoma cells and mouse neuroblastoma cells, was initially reported as being the tyrosinase gene transcript (pMT4).[263] The eventual isolation of the true tyrosinase cDNA revealed that pMT4 was encoded by a different pigment locus. Using recombinant inbred mouse strains, this second gene was mapped to the *brown* locus (b) on chromosome 4 of the mouse and was designated as a tyrosinase-related protein or TRP, later renamed as TRP1.[259,260] The human locus is known as TRP1. There is evidence that the mouse has a truncated *brown* pseudogene but currently there is no evidence that the human genome contains a TRP1 pseudogene.[264]

Mutations at the *brown* locus produce a brown coat color rather than the wild-type black coat.[25] The common *b* allele produces wild-type levels of TRP1 mRNA but there is a cysteine-to-tyrosine substitution in codon 86 of the product.[260,265] Mice were produced that were double heterozygotes for radiation-induced mutations at the *brown* locus and were found to be fully viable and to have a complete deletion of the *brown* locus. The pigmentation of these mice was indistinguishable from the classic *b*/*b brown* mouse, showing that this latter mutation is phenotypically identical to a null phenotype.[260] The *cordovan-Harwell* allele of the *brown* locus (b^c) produces an intermediate level of pigment and is associated with very low levels of presumably normal TRP1 mRNA. The *white-based brown* allele (B^W) is dominant and appears to act by killing the melanocytes.[260] This allele has a gross rearrangement of the locus and may cause inappropriate transcription of other genes whose product is toxic to melanocytes. The *light* allele (B^{lt}) is also dominant but is the result of a point mutation thought to produce a neomorph, a mutation that confers a new function to the protein.[266] EM examination of melanocytes from 7-day-old *light* mice shows a disruption of the melanosome structure, possibly by destabilization of the melanosomal matrix. It is hypothesized that this destabilization results in the release of cytotoxic pigment intermediates that result in melanocyte death.

The human equivalent of the murine TRP1 cDNA was isolated and shares about 93 percent homology with that of the mouse.[267,268] The human cDNA codes for a polypeptide of 527 amino acids with a molecular weight of 60 kDa and has been mapped to human chromosome 9p23 using *in situ* hybridization.[269] The mature gene product is a *trans*-membrane melanosomal glycoprotein with a molecular weight of 75 kDa.

The organization of the *brown* locus is very different from that of tyrosinase locus.[264,270] In the mouse, the *brown* locus contains 8 exons and is 15 to 18 kb in length. Initial sequencing of human homologue for exons 1 and 2 has shown the human gene structure to be the same as that of the mouse.[271] The 5′ region of the *brown* gene does not contain a TATA box or a CCAAT box; however, three regulatory elements, including both positive and negative elements, have been identified in the promoter region.[264,272] One of the positive regulatory elements, a conserved 11-bp sequence (known as the M-box for melanocyte-specific sequence) binds an M-box binding factor that is found in both expressing and nonexpressing mouse cells. This sequence is also observed in the promoter region of human tyrosinase gene and may be a melanocyte-specific promoter element.[270,272] The three regulatory elements are within a region of the promoter between −44 and +107, which is the minimum promoter sequences necessary to confer cell-type specific expression.[272] This region includes the first exon that appears to act as an enhancer, increasing transient expression sixteen- to twentyfold in both melanoma cells and HeLa cells.[271] The presence of regulatory elements common to the promoter regions of the *brown* and tyrosinase genes suggests the existence of melanocyte-specific regulatory elements responsible for coordinated expression of pigment related gene products. The stimulation of pigment synthesis by environmental factors such as MSH or UV light shows that some form of coordinate control must be present to regulate the expression of these different genes. The M-box element may be one of these regulatory elements. Also like tyrosinase, the *brown* gene produces alternatively spliced transcripts.[264] The significance of this is unknown.

The TRP1 locus has been shown to encode the human melanoma autoantigenic glycoprotein 75 (gp75).[156,273] Gp75 is the most abundant glycoprotein in melanoma cell lines, but is absent in nonpigmented melanoma cell lines.[274,275] Biochemical analysis of the protein from immunoaffinity chromatography using serum antibodies against a synthetic polypeptide from the carboxy end of the TRP1 protein (PEP-1) exhibited moderate levels of tyrosinase activity (at least 20 to 30 percent of total cellular tyrosinase activity),[276,277] but protein purification using a combination of ion exchange chromatography, concanavalin A–Sepharose chromatography and immunoaffinity chromatography using a monoclonal antibody specific for the TRP1 protein, exhibited much lower tyrosinase activity (5 percent of total tyrosinase activity).[273] This discrepancy may be due to the high similarity of tyrosinase epitopes to the TRP1 protein, and the TRP1 protein immunopurified with PEP-1 may have been contaminated with tyrosinase. The TRP1 protein may have some tyrosinase (hydroxylation of tyrosine) activity but this is not thought to be the primary function of this protein.

Others have ascribed catalase activity to this protein and have given it the locus name CAS2 for the human gene, but again, this activity is thought not to be the primary catalytic function of this protein.[156,278] It has been shown that both tyrosinase and gp75 contain catalase-like activity, indicating that this activity is most likely an artifact.[208]

Interactions and Levels of Regulation

The characterization of the tyrosinase gene family (TYR, TRP1, and TRP in humans; *albino, brown,* and *slaty* in mouse) has yielded unexpected findings. The roles of the proteins encoded by those loci, and how they interact to modulate melanogenesis in mammals, has become an exciting field of study (Fig. 147-6). All three of these proteins contain a cysteine-rich domain similar to that found in proteins in the EGF family,[203] a motif that may be involved in protein–protein interaction. It has been proposed that melanin biosynthesis occurs within a complex of proteins including tyrosinase, DOPAchrome tautomerase, and gp75 as well as the melanocyte-stimulating hormone receptor (MSH-R) and lysosome-associated membrane protein-1 (Lamp-1). The potential binding domains of these proteins may play an important role in the formation and stabilization of this complex.[136,203] Furthermore, since these proteins are localized specifically in the melanosomal membrane[98,216,279] with their catalytic sites oriented inside, and all seem to function in regulating the melanogenic pathway, the possibility that these proteins interact in a melanosomal complex seems attractive. Studies have shown that tyrosinase is stabilized

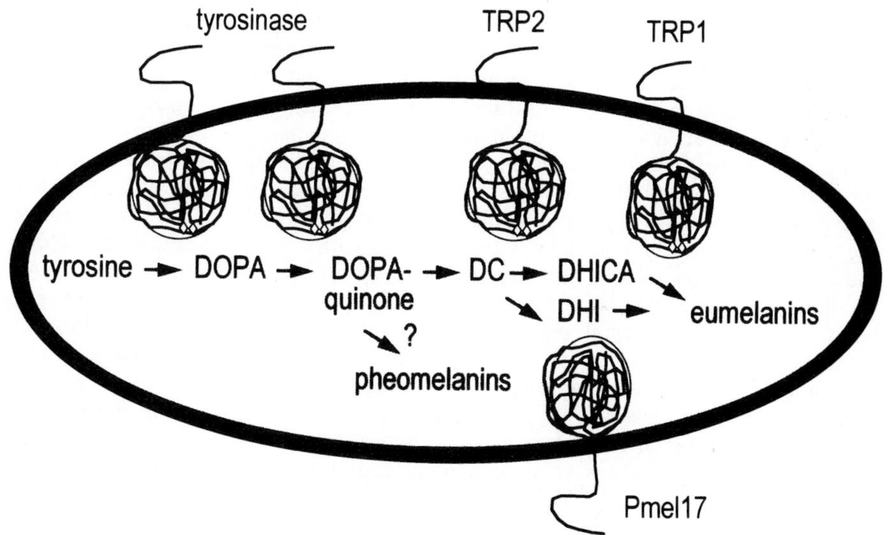

FIG. 147-6 Melanogenic complex. The biosynthesis of melanin is the result of several enzymes working as a complex within the melanosome. Tyrosinase controls the rate limiting reaction. Other enzymes and factors affect the type and quantity of melanin formed.

in the presence of TRP1 and TRP2, giving further evidence of a melanogenic complex and the melanosome matrix resulting in the correct deposition of melanin on the matrix.[208,280]

Results of the analysis of the *light* allele of the *brown* locus suggested that TRP1 interacts with melanosomal matrix proteins. It is possible that TRP1 plays a role in the interaction between the melanin biosynthesis complex and the melanosome matrix, resulting in the correct deposition of melanin on the matrix. However, the similarity between these three proteins suggests that this family of proteins is involved in melanin synthesis. These genes may have been formed from duplication of a common ancestral gene with subsequent divergence.

Other Genes Involved in Mammalian Melanogenesis

Silver/Pmel 17 Genes. A fourth cDNA isolated from human melanocytes encodes a protein called "pmel 17."[281] This cDNA, like TRP2, was co-isolated with tyrosinase using an antityrosinase antibody to screen a cDNA expression library. The pmel 17 gene maps to human chromosome 12pter-q21.[282] Its murine homology mapped near to the *silver (si)* locus in mice.[282] The *silver* phenotype is characterized by a premature graying of hair due to melanocyte loss. *Silver* melanocytes grown in culture produce pigment but have a much slower growth rate than normal melanocytes.[283] In the hair follicle, the pmel 17 protein appears to interact with the product of the *brown* locus since less pigment is produced in a silver mouse that is a *B/b* heterozygote as compared to silver mice that are homozygous for *B/B* or *b/b*.[283,284] The pmel 17 cDNA codes for a protein of 668 amino acids with a predicted molecular weight of 70.9 kDa, including a putative signal peptide. The protein has several potential glycosylation sites and a hydrophobic region at the C-terminal end, indicating that it may be membrane-bound. Studies have shown that expression of the pmel 17 protein is inducible by MSH and IBMX.[281] The pmel 17 protein has been characterized as "stablin."[217] In transfection experiments, the pmel 17 protein is associated with "indole blocking factor" or "stablin" activity, which binds and stabilizes DHICA and DHI.[218] These observations plus its abundance suggest that a possible biologic role for pmel 17 is in cellular protection from the toxic intermediates of melanin synthesis.

The pmel 17 protein has been isolated and described in several laboratories. It was isolated with a melanoma-specific antibody, HMB-50, and shown to be secreted as a 95-kDa glycoprotein in both human melanocytes and human melanomas.[285] Specifically, the protein was released by neonatal foreskin melanocytes and melanoma cell lines but not adult melanocytes. The protein was secreted in large quantities independently of the amount of pigment being produced by the cell line. It was hypothesized that the expression of pmel 17 is related to the proliferative state of the cells. This would correlate with the observation that the silver mutation affects melanocyte viability and causes premature graying. The bovine counterpart of pmel 17 has been isolated from retinal pigment epithelium using the HMB-50 antibody.[286]

Computer searches for amino acid homology between pmel 17 and other melanogenic proteins revealed similarity to the chicken melanosomal matrix protein isolated by Mochii et al.[287–290] This is a 115-kDa protein containing 762 amino acids. Immunogold EM shows that antibodies to the matrix protein recognize the matrix of the melanosome and premalanosome. Analysis of the amino acid sequence of pmel 17 and the matrix protein shows an impressive degree of similarity at the amino and carboxyl ends of the proteins. Although both have internal amino acid repeats, the sequence of these repeats differs between the two proteins. The role of pmel 17 in matrix formation and in stabilization of reaction intermediates has yet to be fully elucidated.

The Pink-Eyed Dilution Gene. Mutations at the *pink-eyed dilution* or *p* locus of the mouse alter development and produce ocular and cutaneous hypopigmentation. The hypopigmentation is associated with a reduced capacity of melanosomes to bind or store melanin. At least 16 alleles of the *p* locus have been identified.[25,291] The most severe alleles, associated with other abnormalities, were produced by radiation-induced deletions of the *p* locus and most likely affect flanking genes. Spontaneous alleles with more subtle mutations affect only pigmentation.[291] The mouse *p* locus is on chromosome 7, a region syntenic with human chromosome 15q11.2-12[292]—the region involved with Prader-Willi syndrome (PWS) and Angelman syndrome (AS).

The human homologue of the mouse *p* cDNA has been isolated from a melanoma cDNA library using the mouse *p* locus cDNA as a probe.[293] The human P locus cDNA has a high degree of homology to the mouse tyrosinase cDNA, exhibiting 84 percent amino acid identity for residues 283 to 414 of the proteins. Sequence analysis of the human P locus cDNA showed it to be the previously identified anonymous cDNA, D15S12, unequivocally mapping it to 15q11.2-13. A form of oculocutaneous albinism known as tyrosinase-positive OCA or OCA2[294] was shown to be linked to the probes D15S10 and D15S13, which also map to this region. The case for the human P locus being the OCA2 gene was strengthened by the finding of an individual with tyrosinase-positive OCA with deletions of the P locus; the entire P locus was deleted on the paternally derived chromosome 15, while the maternally derived allele was partially deleted.[295]

The 3.4-kb P locus mRNA is primarily expressed in melanocytes. The P polypeptide contains 12 transmembrane domains with several potential *N*-glycosylation sites and several potential protein kinase C phosphorylation sites.[293] Based on amino acid similarity Rinchik et al. hypothesized that the P polypeptide is a tyrosine transport protein.[295] Most likely alterations of the P locus account for the hypopigmentation found in many individuals with PWS and AS.

The Melanocyte-Stimulating Hormone Receptor (MSH-R) Gene. A number of biologic activities have been attributed to MSH, including the promotion of melanocyte differentiation and an increase in melanin biosynthesis.[296] MSH binds to the MSH-R, stimulating an increase in the amount of intracellular cAMP concentrations.[297–299] Both the mouse and human MSH-R genes have been cloned and sequenced.[185,300] The polypeptides are 76 percent similar in amino acid sequence. This receptor locus is part of a subfamily that includes the ACTH receptor and the mouse and human cannabinoid receptor having characteristics of guanine nucleotide-binding protein (G-protein)–coupled receptors.

Analysis has shown that the MSH-R maps to the extension (*e*) locus of the mouse.[301] The alleles of the *e* locus range from the most dominant allele *(E)* producing black mice to the most recessive allele *(e)* producing yellow mice.[25] This same control of eumelanin–pheomelanin synthesis is likely to be involved in hair color in humans. The *e* locus mutations do not produce albinism, but rather are responsible for variations in coat color. The *recessive yellow* allele *(e)* is the result of a frameshift mutation producing a nonfunctional receptor while the somber (E^{so-3J}) allele is the result of a point mutation that produces a hyperactive receptor that is constitutively activated.[301] Though MSH-R function is important for eumelanin synthesis in cutaneous and follicular melanocytes, retinal melanocytes produce eumelanin even in the absence of a functional MSH-R as demonstrated by the *e/e* mouse.

The Agouti Gene. The *agouti* or *a* locus in mice has been cloned and mapped to murine chromosome 2.[184] The human counterpart has not been identified. The product of this gene affects a switch from eumelanogenesis to pheomelanogenesis by its interaction with the MSH-R. More than 18 alleles have been described.[25] Some have severe pleiotropic effects, including obesity and lethality. The *agouti* wild-type *(A/A)* mouse has hair with the typical agouti banded pattern, whereas the *nonagouti (a/a)* mouse has only black hair and the lethal *yellow* A^y/a mouse has only yellow hair. Because homozygous A^y/A^y is lethal, the great variation seen with the mutant alleles on pigment has led some to hypothesize that the *a* locus is a complex locus consisting of several genes; however, the isolation of the *agouti* gene has shown that it codes for a single gene product.[184]

The *agouti* gene is 18 kb in length, contains 4 exons, and expresses a 0.8-kb transcript in cells of the hair follicle and the epidermis. The gene is not expressed in melanocytes as shown by the presence of the agouti product in W/W^v mice that lack dermal melanocytes. The gene encodes a polypeptide of 131 amino acids containing a central region rich in basic amino acids and a cysteine-rich C-terminus.[302] The product of the *agouti* locus acts as a ligand, interacting with the MSH-R. Increased expression of the agouti gene is correlated with increased production of pheomelanin pigment.[184]

Analysis of agouti mutations shows that the alleles *a*, a^t and a^{5MNU} result from insertions in the coding region. A^y transcripts are longer than normal, arising from the first exon being replaced by DNA from an unknown origin.[184] The expression of A^y is not restricted to the follicular environment, and this may be the cause of the pleiotropic effects of this allele.

Interaction Between the MSH-R, MSH and the *agouti* Locus Product. The MSH-R and MSH proteins are part of a receptor–ligand complex. The interaction of these two proteins and the product of the *agouti* locus determines if black/brown eumelanin or red/yellow pheomelanin is the predominant pigment in the melanocyte. Jackson has presented a model as to how the *agouti* protein exerts its effect on the interaction between MSH-R and MSH.[178,303] In the absence of MSH, the melanocyte produces pheomelanin. The addition of MSH results in a switch to the production of eumelanin. The *agouti* protein prevents the binding of MSH to MSH-R, reversing pigment production from eumelanin to pheomelanin. The wild-type hair of the mouse is black with yellow bands, and it is the switching on and off of the *agouti* locus that produces the yellow banding. Mutations that eliminate functional *agouti* protein or produce an MSH-R with constitutive signaling *(somber,* E^{so}*)* result in a black mouse. Conversely, mutations that eliminate the MSH-R *(extension, e)*, or result in the constitutive production of the agouti protein *(Viable yellow,* A^{v}*)* produce a yellow mouse. Mutations in the human homologue of both the MSH-R and the *agouti* loci may be partially responsible for the variation in the color and/or intensity of pigmentation in humans, including the eumelanin/pheomelanin production.

The KIT Gene. Piebaldism is an autosomal dominant genetic disorder in humans that results in patches of skin and hair that lack pigment. Melanocytes are completely absent in the white patches. The *white spotting* allele of the *dominant spotting* locus *(W)* of the mouse produces piebaldism in association with changes in hematopoiesis and gametogenesis during embryonic development and adult life.[25] The similarity of the effect of the mutant alleles of the *W* locus on pigmentation in the mouse helped lead to the isolation of the gene responsible for piebaldism in humans.

The *W* locus was shown to encode the *c-kit* proto-oncogene, a tyrosine kinase cell-surface receptor.[304,305] The human KIT gene maps to 4q11-q13, and an interstitial deletion at chromosome 4q12 was found to be associated with piebaldism,[306] suggesting that alterations in the KIT gene may result in piebaldism.[307,308] In another individual with piebaldism, a deletion of both KIT and the adjacent platelet-derived growth factor receptor gene (PDGFRTa) was found, again suggesting that mutations of the KIT gene may be responsible for human piebaldism.[309] Additionally, the murine *c-kit* gene product has been shown to be a mast/stem-cell growth factor receptor, and mutations of this gene could affect the development and/or migration of melanocytes, producing the piebald phenotype.

The human KIT cDNA and gene have been isolated and sequenced.[307,310] The gene has 21 exons, is 34 kb in length, and is similar in organization to the FMS proto-oncogene, which also maps to chromosome 4. The KIT mRNA undergoes alternative splicing.[310] Similar sequence elements in the promoters of the KIT, tyrosinase, and *brown* genes may be involved in coordinating expression of these genes.

Linkage analysis between the human KIT locus and piebaldism gave a lod score of 6.02 with no recombination, strongly suggesting that mutations in the human KIT locus are responsible for piebaldism.[308] Several different mutations have subsequently been found in the human KIT gene associated with piebaldism.[308–311] There are still unresolved differences between the phenotype of mutations in the murine *c-kit* gene and those of the KIT locus in humans. The *c-kit* locus mutations involve erythropoiesis, germ-cell development, and melanogenesis, while humans with piebaldism only appear to have alterations of melanogenesis.[312]

The ligand for the tyrosine kinase receptor encoded by the *c-kit* gene, a hematopoietic growth factor (KL) or murine stem-cell factor (SCF), is coded for by the *steel* locus, *(Sl)* of the mouse.[313–316] Mutations at the *Sl* locus prevent binding of the *c-kit* ligand to the receptor, resulting in a similar phenotype to that of the *W* locus mutations.[314,315] The *steel* mutation also affects erythropoiesis and germ-cell development, as observed with the *W* locus. The human counterpart of steel has not been cloned, but mutations in it would be expected to have a piebald phenotype.

The PAX3 Gene. Mutations of the *Splotch (Sp)* locus in mice produce areas of hypopigmentation and abnormalities in neural development, including neural-tube defects. The gene at the *Sp* locus was shown to encode a member of the *Pax* gene family, *Pax-3*, and mutations of this gene were shown to result in the *Splotch* phenotype.[321,322] The *Sp* locus maps to mouse chromosome 1 in a region syntenic to part of human chromosome 2. One form of human Waardenburg syndrome (type I, with telecanthus) also maps to this region

(2q35-37), and this co-localization was used to identify the gene for this condition.[317–320] PAX3, the human homologue to the murine *Pax-3* gene, has been isolated[323,324]; it contains three exons. Both the PAX3 and *Pax-3* proteins belong to the paired domain family of DNA binding proteins containing sequences homologous to a homeobox gene *(prd)* from *Drosophila melanogaster* associated with the *gooseberry* phenotype with disordered segmentation and segment polarity.[319,320,323] The murine protein contains three functional domains, a paired box, a conserved octapeptide, and a homeobox domain.

The *Pax-3* gene plays a role in the pattern formation in the developing neural crest of the mouse embryo. The high degree of similarity between the *Pax-3* and its human homologue PAX3 makes it likely that the latter has a similar function in the development of the human neural crest. The dominant expression of PAX3 mutations are most likely due to an inadequate amount of the functional protein.[324]

Other Pigment-Related Genes. The *dilute (d)* gene locus of the mouse has been cloned and its protein product identified as a novel myosin heavy chain.[325] Mutations at this locus produce abnormal adendritic melanocyte morphology and neurologic abnormalities. Phenotypically, *d* locus mutations produce a lightening of the coat color of the mouse, most likely resulting from the lack of melanosome distribution from the melanocyte to the keratinocytes. This is the same mechanism for reduced pigmentation caused by the *lavender (lav)* mutation in the chicken.[326] No human homologue or potential phenotype is known. Other genes that may soon be isolated include human homologues to the mouse *pearl (pe)*, *beige (bg)* and *agouti* pigment-associated loci. The *pe* gene maps to mouse chromosome 13 and has been proposed as the homologue to the human gene responsible for Hermansky-Pudlak syndrome (HPS).[327–330] The *bg* gene also maps to mouse chromosome 13 and has been proposed as a possible homologue to the human gene responsible for the Chediak-Higashi syndrome.[328,331]

ALBINISM

Definition

Albinism represents a group of inherited abnormalities with congenital hypopigmentation that is associated with a normal number and structure of melanocytes in the skin and eye.[23,332–336] A precise definition is critical for understanding the difference between true albinism and other conditions that include some type of hypopigmentation in the phenotype. A variety of terms are used to refer to genetic or acquired disorders of melanization, and the imprecise use of many of these has been confusing. For this chapter, the term *albinism* will be used to define disorders with a congenital reduction in melanin synthesis that is associated with specific ocular changes resulting from the hypopigmentation in the developing eye. The reduction in melanin synthesis can be generalized, as in OCA, or primarily localized to the eye, as in OA. The color of the hair and skin or the presence or absence of the ability to tan are no longer sufficient for definition or recognition of albinism. For example, individuals with some types of OCA can appear to have relatively normal cutaneous pigment, with tanning as a child or an adult, suggesting a diagnosis of OA; yet careful molecular analysis shows that they actually have a pigmenting type of OCA. A generalized reduction in skin pigment without ocular changes should be referred to as cutaneous hypopigmentation rather than albinism or cutaneous albinism, because there is no ocular involvement. Terms such as *partial, incomplete,* or *imperfect albinism* are not founded on genetic principles and should not be used.

The Optic System

The changes in the eye and the optic system in albinism are specific and necessary for the diagnosis or definition of albinism.[337] The abnormalities are common to all types of albinism, including OCA and OA, and are related to the reduction in melanin during development and postnatal life. In general, the ocular changes are not present in heterozygotes for autosomal recessive OCA and OA. By contrast, 80 to 90 percent of the obligate female heterozygotes for X-linked recessive OA have observable changes in ocular pigment.[338]

The characteristic changes in the eye in albinism are listed in Table 147-3. Iris melanin is normally found in the stromal melanocytes and the posterior pigment epithelium, the latter being a continuation of the ciliary body.[339] The iris has a blue color without the formation of stromal pigment, and a normal amount of melanin in the posterior surface makes the iris opaque. The reduction of melanin in the stroma and the posterior epithelial layer in albinism results in a translucent iris that transmits light through the iridial tissue on globe transillumination (Fig. 147-7).[332,340–342]

The retinal pigmented epithelium (RPE) acquires melanin early in embryogenesis and has important functions in postnatal life necessary for visual function.[343] Pigment is also present in the choroid below the retina. RPE melanin is greatly reduced or absent in albinism, making the retina transparent.[332,334,340,344–346] As a result, the choroidal blood vessels are seen below the retina on ophthalmoscopic examination (see Fig. 147-7). Despite the lack of melanin, most of the functions of the RPE are intact, and the retina is able to receive and process light. The electroretinogram is normal.[347]

Significant functional abnormalities are present, however, in the fovea, associated with a moderate to marked reduction in visual acuity.[334,344,348] The albinotic fovea is hypoplastic with a reduced or absent foveal reflex and reduced acuity that cannot be corrected to normal.[344,345,349,350] Visual acuity in albinism ranges from 20/400 to 20/40+, and is usually 20/200 to 20/100. Many individuals with albinism have myopia, hyperopia, or astigmatism, and correction of these abnormalities can often improve acuity modestly. The foveal hypoplasia does not interfere with color vision, which is normal in albinism.[351,352]

Perhaps the most striking optic system change in albinism is the abnormal decussation and misrouting of the optic fibers at the chiasm. In a mature eye that was pigmented during development, the nerve fibers of the nasal retina cross at the chiasm and terminate in the contralateral lateral

Table 147-3 Characteristic Changes in the Optic System in Albinism

Reduction in iris pigment
Reduction in retinal pigment
Foveal hypoplasia
Misrouting of the optic fibers at the chiasm
Nystagmus
Alternating strabismus

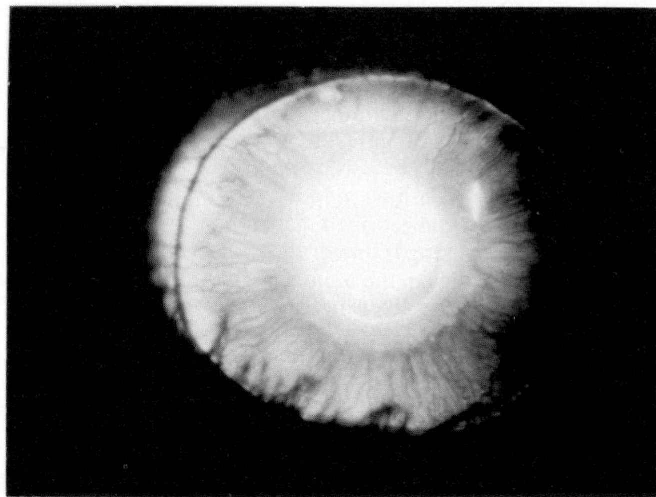

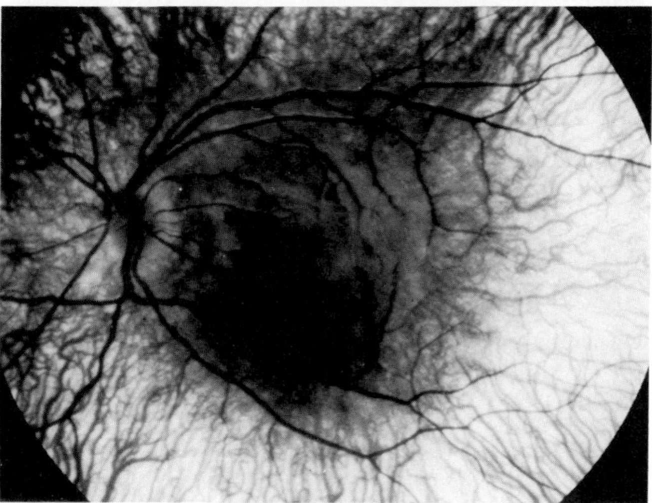

FIG. 147-7 Ocular changes in albinism. *Upper:* Translucent iris with globe transillumination. *Lower:* Fundus photograph showing lack of retinal melanin pigment and visualization of the choroidal blood vessels. There is no foveal reflex and no visual evidence of foveal development. Note that the retinal blood vessels project through the foveal area. Both photographs are from individuals with OCA.

geniculate nucleus, while the fibers of the temporal retina do not cross and terminate in the ipsilateral lateral geniculate.[337,353] In humans, the ratio of contralateral (crossed) to ipsilateral (uncrossed) fibers is in the range of 55:45. This correlates with overlapping visual fields, bilateral optic cortex input from each eye, and stereoscopic vision.[337,353] This ratio is greatly altered in albinism in humans and all other animals tested. The proportion of crossed fibers probably exceeds 90 percent in all mammals with albinism.

The abnormal decussation is due to misrouting of the temporal nerve fibers of the retina. These fibers project to the contralateral rather than to the ipsilateral geniculate, resulting in a reduction of ipsilaterally projecting fibers, as shown in Fig. 147-8.[353–357] The temporal fibers projecting to the contralateral geniculate lead to disorganization and fragmentation of the dorsal lateral geniculate[358] and to altered representation of the visual field in the geniculate and the optic cortex.[359] The effects of the changes on retinal fiber projections are a loss of stereoscopic depth perception[344] and an intermittent and alternating suppression of the vision in one eye producing an alternating strabismus.[334,344] The strabismus does not usually require surgical correction; amblyopia does not develop in most cases.[334]

The misrouting of the optic fibers at the chiasm can be detected clinically by the demonstration of an asymmetric visual evoked response.[353,354,360,361] The response to flash- or pattern-onset stimuli is recorded with right and left occipital electrodes, and the first 300 ms of the response indicates normal or abnormal decussation.[337,360] This test is often used to establish a diagnosis of albinism in children (including neonates)[362] or adults with unusual pigmentation, and the diagnosis of OCA or OA cannot be made without clinical (reduced stereoacuity) or electrophysiological (asymmetric visual evoked potential) evidence of misrouting. Congenital nystagmus due to causes other than hypopigmentation does not have an asymmetric visual evoked potential.[360,363]

Nystagmus is present in all but a few individuals with albinism. Several reports on phenotypic variation in albinism have described individuals with all of the above-mentioned features of OCA except for nystagmus.[348,364,365] The mechanism responsible for the nystagmus is not fully understood. The presence of foveal hypoplasia and reduced acuity with poor fixation may be responsible in part, but nystagmus in albinism is often present at or shortly after birth, at a time

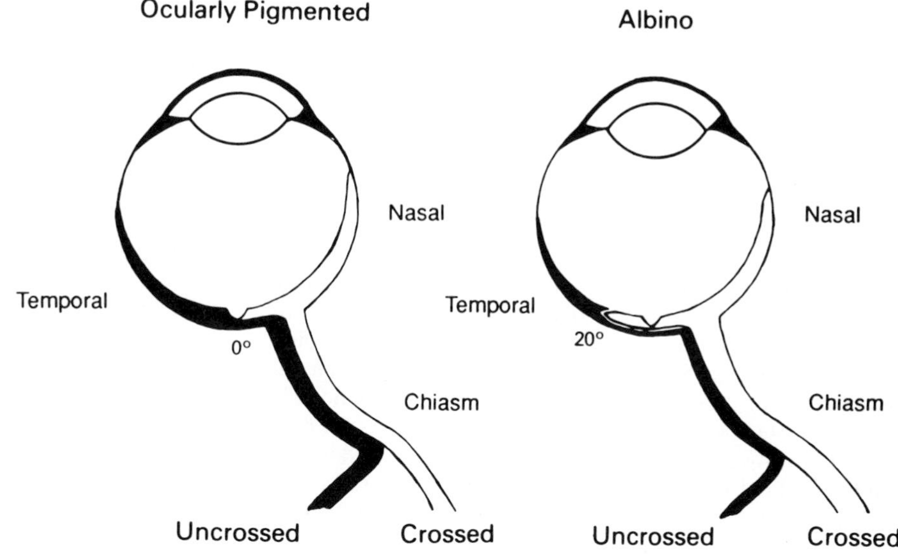

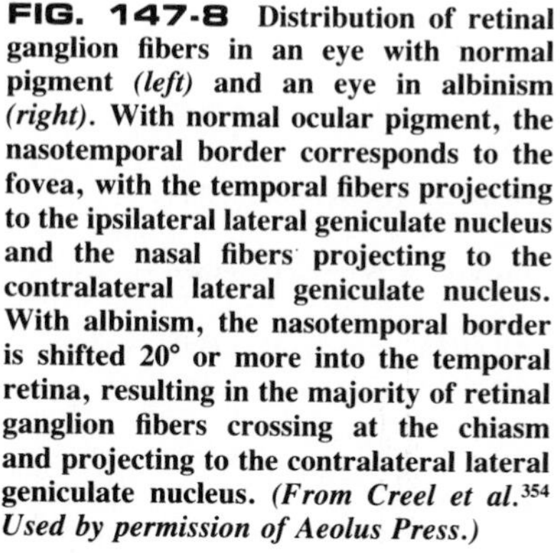

FIG. 147-8 Distribution of retinal ganglion fibers in an eye with normal pigment *(left)* and an eye in albinism *(right)*. With normal ocular pigment, the nasotemporal border corresponds to the fovea, with the temporal fibers projecting to the ipsilateral lateral geniculate nucleus and the nasal fibers projecting to the contralateral lateral geniculate nucleus. With albinism, the nasotemporal border is shifted 20° or more into the temporal retina, resulting in the majority of retinal ganglion fibers crossing at the chiasm and projecting to the contralateral lateral geniculate nucleus. *(From Creel et al.*[354] *Used by permission of Aeolus Press.)*

when the normally pigmented fovea is maturing.[334,355,366] This suggests that the lack of normal foveal function may not be critical in the development of the nystagmus.[355] Abnormal development of the ocular motor system associated with the disorganization of the lateral geniculate nucleus and its projections to the optic cortex are thought to play a more central role in the development of nystagmus in albinism.[337,355,367] Individuals with albinism often have a head posture that slows the nystagmus, with some improvement in vision.[368,369]

The pathophysiological mechanism of the misrouting of the retinal nerve fibers is unknown. The misrouting correlates with a reduction or an absence of melanin in the eye during embryogenesis, but is not a pleiotropic effect of a specific gene, since it is found in OCA and OA of all genotypes. Melanin may play a direct role in the development of the optic projections[370,371] and indirect effects of melanin topography, timing, or the presence of chemical signals in the developing optic chiasm have been suggested.[337,372–374] In humans, the optic nerve projections develop early in embryogenesis and misrouting in albinism would occur in the first trimester of a pregnancy.

The Auditory System

There are also changes in the auditory system associated with albinism. Pigmented melanocytes are found in the inner ear. In the cochlea, they are found in the stria vascularis, which provides the driving current for the hair cells—the sensory receptors in the inner ear. Although there is interspecies variation, in most species (including humans), the melanocytes are found to have an intimate relationship with the strial capillaries, and they may play a role in the microcirculation of the inner ear.[375] The number of amelanotic melanocytes, termed "intermediate cells," appears to be normal in the cochlea in individuals with albinism. The cell volume of intermediate cells is reduced in albinotic as compared with pigmented cochleas. The diminution in melanocyte volume is accompanied by both a larger volume of an adjacent cell type, the marginal cells, and a greater resting endocochlear potential in the albino inner ear.[376,377] These findings point to differences in structure and function of the cochlea in albinism that appear to be related to the presence of amelanotic melanocytes.

The absence of melanin pigment in the inner ear makes animals with albinism more susceptible to noise-induced hearing loss,[378] although in humans the only definitive demonstration related to this is evidence of prolonged temporary threshold shift following exposure to noise.[379] These occur in all humans but are greatest in individuals with little pigment.[380] Animal studies indicate that the absence of melanin pigment in the inner ear may make the albino individual more susceptible to some ototoxic drugs such as gentamicin that may be normally detoxified due to melanin pigment's ability to inactivate polycationic drugs.[376]

Individuals with albinism and animal models of albinism have abnormal brain-stem auditory evoked responses (BAER).[381,382] The abnormal components of the BAER are the potentials associated with the superior olivary complex in the brain stem. Studies of the neuronal cross-sectional area ("cell size") in the superior olive of the albino animals has shown significantly reduced cell size, on the order of 25 to 45 percent.[383–385] Whether these differences are due to dysfunction in the albino cochlea or to pleiotropic effects of the albino mutation unrelated to effects of pigmentation remains unknown.

OCULOCUTANEOUS ALBINISM

Types of Oculocutaneous Albinism

OCA is the most common inherited disorder of generalized hypopigmentation, with an estimated frequency of 1:20,000 in most populations.[1] The estimated prevalence for different albinism types in various populations is given in Table 147-4. OCA has been described in all ethnic groups and in all animal species, making it one of the most widely distributed genetic abnormalities in the animal kingdom.[386] The different types of albinism are given in Table 147-5 and the clinical features of each type of OCA are given in Table 147-6. Most types of OCA arise from a primary genetic abnormality of the melanin synthetic system, but there are several OCA types that arise from a more generalized genetic abnormality that only secondarily alters melanin synthesis. Mutations at more than 65 loci in the mouse affect hair or eye pigmentation,[25] and previous editions of this book have implied that the different types of OCA may be due to genetic alterations of many different loci. However, the molecular information now becoming available suggests that much of the variation is due to allelic rather than locus heterogeneity. This will be reviewed in detail in the discussion of each type. All types of OCA are inherited as autosomal recessive traits, except for rare families with autosomal dominant OCA, as discussed below.

OCA1: Tyrosinase-Related Oculocutaneous Albinism

One of the two most common types of albinism is tyrosinase-related OCA, which is produced by loss of function of the melanocytic tyrosinase enzyme resulting from mutations of the tyrosinase gene. Classic OCA, widely recognized in all populations and described throughout recorded history because of the total absence of melanin in the skin, hair and

Table 147-4 Estimated Prevalence of Albinism

Population	Type	Prevalence	Reference
World Survey	All types	1:10-20,000	1
United States			
Caucasian			
	All OCA	1:18,000	2
	OCA1	1:39,000	2
	OCA2	1:36,000	2
African American			
	All OCA	1:10,000	2
	OCA1	1:28,000	2
	OCA2	1:10,000	2
Amerindian			
Hopi	OCA2	1:227	439
Zuni	OCA2	1:240	435
General	OA1	1:50,000	485
Africa			
Nigeria	OCA2	1:5-15,000	431 433
	Brown OCA	1:10,000	2
Cameroon			
General	All OCA	1:35,000	432
Bamileke	All OCA	1:7,900	432
South Africa (Negro)			
	OCA2	1:3,900	438
	Red OCA	1:8,580	454

Table 147-5 Classification of Albinism

OCULOCUTANEOUS ALBINISM	OCULAR ALBINISM
Primary Defect Specific for Melanin Synthetic Pathway	OA1 (Ocular albinism, X-linked)
OCA1 (tyrosinase-related OCA)	Ocular albinism, autosomal recessive
Mutations associated with no residual enzyme activity	Ocular albinism and deafness, X-linked
OCA1A (tyrosinase-negative OCA)	
Mutations associated with residual activity	**OTHER CONDITIONS WITH ALBINISM**
OCA1B (yellow OCA)	Oculocerebral syndrome with hypopigmentation (Cross syndrome)
OCA1MP (minimal pigment OCA)	Griscelli syndrome
Mutations associated with unusual enzyme activity	
OCA1TS (temperature-sensitive OCA)	
OCA2 (tyrosinase-positive OCA) (Prader-Willi and Angelman syndromes)	
Types unclassified	
Brown OCA	
Red or rufous OCA	
Autosomal dominant OCA	
Primary Defect Not Specific for Melanin Synthetic Pathway	
Hermansky-Pudlak Syndrome	
Chediak-Higashi Syndrome	

eyes,[1,23,345,387] is the most obvious phenotype, but studies have demonstrated that a wide phenotypic variation in OCA is associated with tyrosinase gene mutations. This is predicted by the well-characterized allelic series of mutations at the *c*-locus (tyrosinase locus) in the mouse, each with a distinct phenotype.[25] In general, the different phenotypes of OCA1 are dependent on the amount or type of residual enzyme produced by the mutant alleles. The range in phenotypes extends from total absence to near normal cutaneous pigmentation, but the ocular features are always present and help identify an individual as having albinism.

An important distinguishing characteristic of OCA1 is the presence of marked hypopigmentation at birth. Most individuals affected with a type of OCA1 have white hair, milky white skin, and blue eyes at birth. The irides can be very light blue and translucent such that the whole iris appears pink or red in ambient light. During the first and second decade of life, the irides usually become a darker blue and may remain translucent or become lightly pigmented with reduced translucency. The skin remains white but may appear to have more color with time. Sun exposure produces erythema and a burn if the skin is unprotected, and a generalized tan is absent or minimal in most individuals, although occasionally an individual with OCA1 can tan well, particularly if his or her hair and eyes are pigmented. Few pigmented lesions (nevi, freckles, lentigines) develop in the skin.

The biochemical evaluation of individuals with OCA1 depends on the hairbulb incubation test to determine tyrosinase activity. Since the enzyme is localized to melanocytes, the only readily available source of enzyme is freshly plucked anagen hairbulbs.[388] Individuals with OCA1 have reduced or absent hairbulb tyrosinase activity and obligate heterozygotes generally have reduced levels of hairbulb tyrosinase activity.[388–390] Low levels are expected in OCA1A or tyrosinase-negative OCA heterozygotes, but are more variable in OCA1B or yellow OCA, in which there are differences in the amount of residual activity depending on the mutation. The reason for the marked reduction in hairbulb tyrosinase activity in heterozygotes is not entirely defined. The assay technique measures activity of soluble but not bound enzyme. Most enzyme in heterozygotes is delivered to the melanosome, where it becomes membrane-bound and active in melanin synthesis but unavailable for assay.[389]

OCA1A: Tyrosinase-Negative OCA. Individuals with tyrosinase negative OCA are unable to synthesize melanin in their skin, hair, or eyes, resulting in a characteristic phenotype. They are born with white hair and skin and blue eyes, and there is no change as they mature.[2,388,389] Melanin never develops in these tissues. The phenotype is the same in all ethnic groups and at all ages. With time, the hair may develop a darker white or a slight yellow tint but this appears to be denaturing of the hair protein related to exposure and different shampoo use. The irides are translucent and appear pink early in life and often turn a gray-blue color with time. No pigmented lesions develop in the skin, although amelanotic nevi can be present.

Hairbulb tyrosinase activity is absent in OCA1A, but the amount of inactive protein in the melanocyte has not been evaluated.[193,388,389] The ultrastructure of the hairbulb melanocyte and melanosome is normal. The melanosomes show a normal surrounding membrane and normal internal matrix formation (stages I and II premelanosomes).[87,189,391–393] No melanin forms after incubation of the hairbulb in tyrosine or DOPA.[3,5]

Table 147-6 Clinical Characteristics of Oculocutaneous Albinism

Characteristic	OCA1A (Tyrosinase-Negative)	OCA1B (Yellow)	OCA1MP (Minimal Pigment)	OCA1TS (Temperature-Sensitive)
Skin color	White, pink as baby	White	White	White
Skin tanning	Absent	Possible	Absent	Unknown
Pigmented nevi or freckles	Absent	Possible	Possible	Possible
Hair color	White throughout life	White at birth; turns yellow/blond in first few years	White at birth; slight yellow tint with time	White at birth; changes after puberty: scalp and axilla white; arm and leg pigmented
Iris color	Blue to gray; red reflex prominent	Blue to gray; some pigment may develop	Blue to gray	Blue to gray
Iris translucency	+ + + +	+ + + to + + + +	+ to + + + +	+ + + +
Retinal pigment	Absent	0 to + in adults	0	0
Nystagmus	Present throughout life	Present throughout life	Present throughout life	Present throughout life
Visual acuity	20/100 to 20/400	20/50 to 20/400	20/50 to 20/400	20/100 to 20/400
Optic tract misrouting	Present	Present	Present	Present
Hairbulb melanosomes	Stage I and II premelanosomes only	Stage I, II, and III premelanosomes	Stage I–III premelanosomes	Scalp/axilla, stage I–II; arm/leg, stage I–III premelanosomes; no stage IV melanosomes
Gene involved	Tyrosinase	Tyrosinase	Tyrosinase	Tyrosinase
Gene location	11q	11q	11q	11q

OCA1B: Yellow OCA. Yellow OCA refers to the types of OCA1 produced by mutations that result in enzyme with some residual activity rather than a total loss of activity ("leaky mutations"). The amount of residual enzyme function varies, but is sufficient to produce small to moderate amounts of iris, hair, and perhaps skin pigment. This is called "yellow OCA" because of the color of the hair, which is due to the synthesis of pheomelanin. It is believed that pheomelanin is the first melanin synthesized when DOPAquinone, the product of the initial steps of the melanin pathway, is produced in small quantities, since the affinity of DOPAquinone for sulfhydryl compounds is high and the combination of the two leads to pheomelanin.[389] Yellow OCA was first identified in the Amish of Indiana,[394] and subsequent studies identified this type of OCA in other populations. Family studies suggested the responsible gene was allelic to that of OCA1A,[395] and molecular studies eventually demonstrated tyrosinase mutations in yellow OCA.

The two distinguishing characteristics of yellow OCA are the extreme hypopigmentation at birth and the eventual development of yellow or blond hair. Affected individuals usually have white hair and skin and blue eyes at birth and appear to have OCA1A. However, hair and iris pigment develop in the first decade of life and can reach levels that are similar to those found in northern Europeans, particularly the Scandinavian populations. The hair color changes to light yellow, light blond, or golden blond first, and it can eventually turn dark blond or light brown in adolescents and adults.[394,396] The irides can develop light tan color, particularly in the inner third of the iris, and iris pigment can be present on globe transillumination, although the iris is always translucent to a degree. A small number of affected individuals have been observed to tan with sun exposure, while it is more common to burn without tanning after sun exposure. Pigmented nevi can develop with time, although most developing nevi are amelanotic. Very few freckles develop.

The variation in the phenotype of yellow OCA is broad and not completely defined. Mutations coding for enzyme with different amounts of residual activity are the primary cause of the variation, and a moderate amount of residual activity can lead to near-normal cutaneous pigmentation and the mistaken diagnosis of ocular albinism. Ethnic and family pigment patterns can also influence the phenotype, and hair color can be light red or brown in some families in whom this is the predominant pigment pattern. The frequency of yellow OCA is unknown, but molecular studies are now helping to identify an increasing number of affected individuals, suggesting that yellow OCA is not rare, and may approach the frequency of OCA1A.

Hairbulb tyrosinase activity is low or absent in individuals with yellow OCA.[389] The levels of activity in obligate heterozygotes are low but variable, most likely reflecting the differences in the genetic background of the individual and the amount of residual activity produced by the mutant allele.

Table 147-6 Clinical Characteristics of Oculocutaneous Albinism (*Continued*)

OCA2 (Tyrosinase-Positive)	Prader-Willi/ Angelman Syndromes	Type Unclassified (Brown)	Type Unclassified (Rufous or Red)	Hermansky-Pudlak Syndrome	Chediak-Higashi Syndrome
White	Normal to light; lighter than unaffected family members when hypopigmented	Light brown; identified only in African and African-American individuals	Reddish brown	Creamy white	Creamy white to slate gray
Absent	Possible	Possible	Possible	Possible	Unknown
Possible, particularly in sunexposed areas	Possible	Absent	Present	Many in sun-exposed areas; can be confluent	Possible
Usually pigmented at birth and darkens with age; Caucasian, yellow blond; African-American, yellow to dark yellow	Normal to light; blond to light brown when hypopigmented	Light to medium brown	Reddish brown to mahogany	White to blond to brown to dark brown	Blond to brown; metalic silver/gray sheen
Blue to hazel to tan	Blue to brown	Blue/gray to light brown	Hazel to reddish brown	Blue to brown	Blue to brown
+ to ++++	0 to +	++ to ++++	0 to +	++ to ++++	++ to +++
0 to ++	+ to ++++	++ to +++	+++ to +++	0 to +++	0 to +++
Present throughout life	Absent or present; may not persist throughout life	Present throughout life	Absent or present	Present throughout life	Absent or present
20/50 to 20/400	Normal or reduced	20/60 to 20/200	Normal or reduced	20/80 to 20/400	Unknown
Present	Present when hypopigmented	Present	Unknown; may be normal	Present	Absent or present
Stage II and III premelanosomes; no stage IV melanosomes	Reduced number of stage IV melanosomes when hypopigmented	Stage II and III premelanosomes; very few stage IV melanosomes.	Stage III premelanosomes and stage IV melanosomes	Stage I, II, and III premelanosomes, depending on hair color	Stage II and II premelanosomes; stage IV melanosomes; giant melanosomes
P (Pink-eyed dilution) 15q	P (Pink-eyed dilution) 15q	? TRP1 (Brown) possible 9p	Unknown	Unknown	Unknown

The architecture of hairbulb melanocytes and melanosomes from affected individuals is normal.[4,394] Stages I and II premelanosomes are present as in OCA1A, as well as some stage III partially melanized premelanosomes, but no stage IV fully melanized melanosomes are present,[189] and there is usually no increase in melanization with DOPA incubation.[4,394]

OCA1MP: Minimal Pigment OCA. Another OCA1 type that is associated with the formation of small amounts of melanin has been termed "minimal pigment OCA."[397] The originally identified individuals with this type of OCA1 had a phenotype similar to OCA1A except for the development of minimal amounts of iris pigment in the first decade of life. Biochemical evaluation suggested that this was a tyrosinase-related OCA, and molecular studies have now identified mutations of the tyrosinase gene in affected individuals.[398] It is not clear if this is truly a distinct type of OCA1. One possibility is that the expression of partially active enzyme from a mutant allele is limited to eye tissue, producing a characteristic phenotype. Supporting this is the identification of a mouse *c*-locus allele (c^{44H}) that is associated with ocular pigment formation and a phenotype known as "dark-eyed albinism."[399] A second possibility is that this is part of the spectrum of yellow OCA and not a separate type of OCA1. If this were true, then it would be hypothesized that the responsible mutant allele would encode an enzyme with less residual enzyme activity than a yellow allele. The pigment would be seen primarily in the iris because of the stable rather than deciduous nature of the pigment cells in this tissue (i.e., the pigment can accumulate without being shed with turnover of the tissue).

Affected individuals have white skin and hair and blue eyes at birth. Iris pigment is present at birth or develops in the first decade. The hair remains white or develops a very slight yellow tint. The skin remains milky white, and tanning has not been observed. To date, all individuals recognized with this type of OCA have been Caucasian, and the phenotype in other ethnic groups is unknown. The frequency is not known. "Platinum" OCA[2] most likely represents this same phenotype.

Hairbulb tyrosinase activity in affected individuals is absent.[389] The levels of activity in obligate heterozygotes are illuminating; in each identified family, one parent has had very low hairbulb tyrosinase activity, similar to that found in OCA1A or OCA1B heterozygotes, while the other parent has levels of activity that are nearly normal for hair color.[389] These results suggest that the affected individuals are genetic compounds. Parental pigmentation is normal. The architecture of hairbulb melanocytes and melanosomes from affected individuals is normal.[397] Stages I and II premelanosomes are present, but no partially melanized stage III premelanosomes or fully melanized stage IV melanosomes are present,[189] and there is no increase in melanization after DOPA incubation.

OCA1TS: Temperature-Sensitive OCA. An unusual type of OCA1 has been described.[400] The proband of the originally identified family appeared to have OCA1A through the first years of her life, with white hair and skin and blue eyes; however, her body hair color changed with puberty. The axillary hair remained white, the scalp hair remained white but developed a slight yellow tint, and arm hair turned light reddish brown, and the leg hair turned dark brown. The eyes remained blue, and the skin remained white without tan. There were three similarly affected sibs in the family and no reports of other families of this type has been published to date. OCA1TS is analogous to the Siamese cat and the Himalayan mouse.

Analysis of tyrosinase from scalp and leg hairbulbs showed that the enzyme was temperature-sensitive, losing activity above 35°C. As a result, melanin synthesis would occur in the cooler areas of the body, such as the arms and legs but not in the warmer areas. The architecture of hairbulb melanocytes and melanosomes was normal.[400] Stages I and II premelanosomes were present in the white scalp hair follicle melanocytes, and stage II premelanosomes, stage III partially melanized premelanosomes, and stage IV fully melanized melanosomes were present in the leg hair follicle melanocytes.

Molecular Pathogenesis of OCA1

Linkage analysis has shown that the tyrosinase gene is linked to OCA1,[401] and DNA sequence analysis of DNA from individuals with OCA1 has revealed many different mutant alleles, as listed in Table 147-7.[234,234,252,396,398,401–417] At present 36 mutations have been reported in the literature, including 24 missense, 4 nonsense, and 8 frameshift mutations. The majority of these mutations have been found in individuals

Table 147-7 **Mutations and Polymorphisms of the Tyrosinase Gene in Individuals with OCA1**

Mutation	Intron/Exon	Base Changes	Codon Change	Type	Population	Reference
	Promoter	AACCTT→AATCTT		Poly	All	398
	Promoter	CCAATTC→CCAATTA		Poly	All	253
P21S*	E1	CCT→TCT	Pro→Ser	IA	Caucasians	409
D42G	E1	GAC→GGC	Asp→Gly	IA	Caucasians	405
G47D	E1	GGC→GAC	Gly→Asp	IA	Caucasians and Hispanics	234, 407
C55Y	E1	TGT→TAT	Cys→Tyr	IA	Caucasians	405
R77Q	E1	CGG→CAG	Arg→Gln	IA	Japanese	415
P81L	E1	CCT→CTT	Pro→Leu	IA	Caucasians	401
C89R	E1	TGC→CGC	Cys→Arg	IA	Blacks	412
+ΔA96	E1	ATG→AATG	Term 168	IA	Caucasians	406
−ΔGA115	E1	AGA→A—	Term 167	IA	Pakastani	417
F176I	E1	TTT→ATT	Phe→Ile	IA	Caucasians	403
W178X	E1	TGG→TAG	Trp→Ter	IA	Afghans	411
−ΔG191	E1	GGA→-GA	Term 225	IA	Caucasians	406
Y192S	E1	TAT→TCT	Tyr→Ser	Poly	All except Orientals	250
A206T	E1	GCT→ACT	Ala→Thr	IA	Caucasians	405
L216M	E1	TTG→ATG	Leu→Met	IA	Hispanics	234
R217W	E1	CGG→TGG	Arg→Trp	IA	Caucasians	409
R217Q	E1	CGG→CAG	Arg→Gln	IA	Caucasians	403
W236X	E1	TGG→TAG	Trp→Ter	IA	Blacks	234
−ΔTG244	E1	TGTG→TG−	Term 244	IA	Caucasians	406
V275F	E2	GTC→TTC	Val→Phe	IB	Caucasians	396
R299H	E2	CGT→CAT	Arg→His	IA	Caucasians	409
+ΔC310	E2	CCA→CCCA	Term 317	IA	Japanese	402
N371T	E3	AAT→ACT	Asn→Thr	IA	Caucasians	407
T373K	E3	ACA→AAA	Thr→Lys	IA	Caucasians	410
Q378X	E3	CAG→TAG	Gln→Ter	IA	Caucasians	403
N382K	E3	AAC→AAA	Asn→Lys	IA	Caucasians	406
D383N	E3	GAT→AAT	Asp→Asn	IA	Caucasians	410
−ΔT388	E3	CTT→CT−	Term 484	IA	Caucasians	409
R402Q	E4	CGA→CAA	Arg→Gln	Poly	All except Orientals	252
R403S	E4	AGG→AGT	Arg→Ser	IB	Caucasians	409
P406L	E4	CCT→CTT	Pro→Leu	IB	Caucasians	396
G419R	E4	GGA→AGA	Gly→Arg	IA	Caucasians	405
R422Q	E4	CGG→CAG	Arg→Gln	ITS	Caucasians	408
−ΔCTTT438	E4	CTTT→− −	Term 484	IA	Caucasians	403
G446S	E4	GGC→AGC	Gly→Ser	IA	Caucasians	409
D448N	E4	GAC→AAC	Asp→Asn	IA	Caucasians	409
Q453X	E4	CAA→TAA	Gln→Ter	IA	Caucasians	403
+Δ489	E5	ACT→ACTT	Term 509	IA	Caucasians	414
+ΔC501	E5	CGT→CCGT	Term 509	IA	Caucasians	396

Poly = polymorphism.
*The start codon ATG (Met) is counted as codon 1. Letters represent the amino acids; numbers represent the codon.

with OCA1A or tyrosinase-negative OCA because the obvious phenotype made them the first group to study.

Mutations fall into three functional groups that help put the phenotype into perspective (see Table 147-5). The first group are mutations that are associated with no tyrosinase activity. These mutations result in OCA1A. The second group are mutations that are associated with residual tyrosinase activity, in the range of 5 to 10 percent of normal activity. These mutations in a homozygous or heterozygous dose (together with an allele yielding no tyrosinase activity) result in OCA1MP and OCA1B. The third group are mutations associated with unusual enzyme activity. The one identified mutation in this group results in OCA1TS.

The mutant alleles in OCA1A are associated with a complete lack of tyrosinase activity in cutaneous and ocular tissue. Sequence analysis has shown that many individuals with OCA1A are compound heterozygotes with different maternal and paternal alleles. Individuals have been found with all combinations of missense, nonsense and frameshift mutations. In approximately 15 percent of compound heterozygotes with one identified mutation, the mutation in the second allele has not been identified despite sequencing of the exons and flanking intronic regions. The undetected second mutation could be in a regulatory region or unsequenced intron region.

The majority of OCA1A mutations have been identified in Caucasian individuals, but mutations unique for other racial groups have been found. Two mutations have been found in Japanese individuals—a missense mutation at codon 77 (R77Q) and a single base insertion of a cytosine at codon 310 (+ΔC310), resulting in a premature termination at codon 316.[402,413,415] A missense mutation has been found in an American black (C89R), a nonsense mutation at codon 178 in an Afghan individual (W178X), and a dinucleotide deletion in a Pakistani individual (−ΔGA115).[411,412,417] Other mutations are expected as tyrosinase genes from individuals with OCA1 from different racial backgrounds is sequenced. There are two common mutations in the Caucasian OCA1A population—T373K and P81L.

Three different mutations have been found in individuals who have OCA1B or yellow OCA.[396,409] Analysis of the originally described families has shown that the affected individuals in this population are homozygous for the missense mutation P406L.[394,396] A V275F mutation has been found in OCA1B individuals who are compound heterozygotes, with P81L—a mutation that completely inactivates tyrosinase—as the second allele. The third OCA1B mutation is R403S.[409] Since the OCA1B phenotype is variable in families containing individuals homozygous for the P406L mutation as well as in individuals who are compound heterozygotes, it appears that other familial pigment genes can

Table 147-8 Alleles of Tyrosinase Locus in Humans

Allele	Name	Enzyme Activity
TYR+	Normal	100%
TYR^{A}	Tyrosinase-negative	0%
TYR^{MP}	Minimal pigment	low
TYR^{B}	Yellow	5–10%
TYR^{TS}	Temperature-sensitive	Temperature-sensitive

influence the effect of these mutations on pigmentation. Expression studies of the P406L mutation in HeLa cells showed that tyrosinase enzymatic activity was greatly reduced.[396]

The P406L mutation provides an example of the pseudogene (TYRL) interfering with the analysis of the TYR locus. The base substitution recapitulates one of the differences between the TYR and TYRL locus. In order to eliminate this problem, PCR primers that amplify only exons IV and V of the TYR gene must be used.

The individuals so far identified with OCA1TS (temperature-sensitive OCA) are compound heterozygotes[400,408] for R422Q and the P81L mutation that is common in OCA1A. Expression studies using both hairbulb tyrosinase and cells transfected with the R422Q allele showed a tyrosinase that was inactivated by temperatures above 35°C. This mutation is similar to those in the Siamese cat and Himalayan mouse, which are also temperature-sensitive.[418]

It is now possible to conceptualize a series of human TYR alleles being responsible for the different types of OCA1, as shown in Table 147-8. The TYR^{A} alleles are associated with a total loss of tyrosinase function, while the TYR^{MP} and the TYR^{B} alleles encode an enzyme with differing amounts of residual function. The TYR^{TS} alleles encode a temperature-sensitive enzyme. Given this allelic series, it can be seen that there will be a great deal of genotypic variation in OCA1, and this is demonstrated in Fig. 147-9. Many of these genotypes have been identified, as indicated in the figure.

The missense mutations in the tyrosinase gene distributed into four clusters in the protein (Fig. 147-10). Two are in the putative copper A and copper B binding regions. The third is in the N-terminal region (exon I) and the fourth is next to the copper B binding region (exon IV). It is thought that the clusters define functional domains of the tyrosinase enzyme.[403,405]

There are several mechanisms by which mutations may cause a loss of tyrosinase activity. Several mutations have been found in both the putative copper A and copper B binding region. The A206T mutation involves an alanine

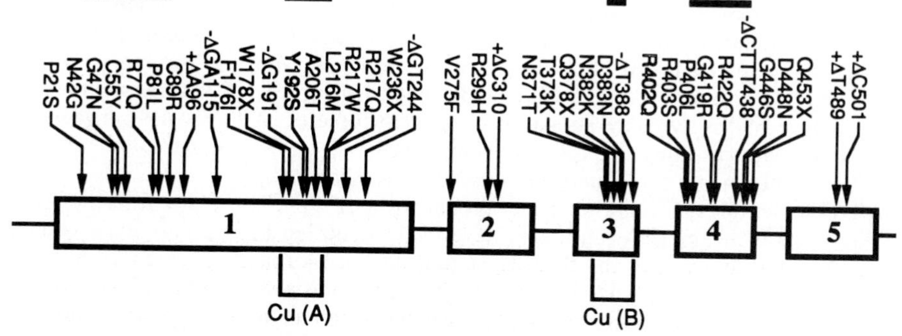

FIG. 147-9 Tyrosinase mutations. Mutations associated with OCA1 are found throughout the tyrosinase coding region. The missense mutations cluster into 4 regions (bars) thought to represent functional domains of the enzyme. Missense and nonsense mutations are indicated by codon. Frameshift mutations are indicated by +D or −D for an insertion or a deletion of one or more bases. The outlined text (Y192S, R402Q) represents nonpathological polymorphisms.

	TYR$^+$	TYR^A	TYR^{MP}	TYR^B	TYR^{TS}
TYR^{TS}	+/TS	A/TS	MP/TS	B/TS	TS/TS
TYR^B	+/B	A/B	MP/B	B/B	
TYR^{MP}	+/MP	A/MP	MP/MP		
TYR^A	+/A	A/A			
TYR$^+$	+/+				

FIG. 147-10 Potential OCA1 genotypes.

located between the proline and phenylalanine residues of a highly conserved motif (Pro-X-Phe-X-X-X-His) that is part of the copper A site. F176I in the putative copper A binding region affects the phenylalanine in a motif (Phe-X-X-X-His) that is conserved in the copper binding centers found in tyrosinase and hemocyanin.[244,419] Computer modeling of the secondary structure of the copper B binding region has shown that mutations in this area (N371T, T373K, N382K, and D383N) may alter the loop structure between the two α-helix regions responsible for correct orientation of the copper ligand and the histidine residues that bind it.[420] Missense mutations at these locations are predicted to alter the secondary structure, especially within the α-helical domains.[420] The juxtaposition of the two copper atoms is critical because of the need to form a peroxide with dioxygen, which is necessary for catalytic function. Any alteration of the histidine location would affect the copper to copper distance and most likely would render the enzyme inactive.

A second possible mechanism for loss of enzyme function is disruption of a substrate binding domain. The binding of tyrosine or DOPA must occur next to the copper atoms, and even a slight change in the chemical nature of an amino acid side chain in this region would be expected to alter enzymatic activity by reducing substrate binding. This may be the case for the cluster of missense mutations at the N-terminal of the enzyme (codons 42 to 89). One mutation in this cluster, R77Q, substitutes a neutral amino acid (glutamine) for a positively charged amino acid (arginine).[421,422] The role of arginine as an anion in the active site has been reported in over one hundred enzymes, and chemical modification of this residue results in inactivation of the enzyme. Removal of the arginine at codon 77 (and the charged group of this amino acid) may disrupt the interaction of the tyrosine substrate or DOPA cofactor at the active site resulting in an inactive enzyme.[423]

Six of the known tyrosinase missense mutations occur at CpG dinucleotides, a well-known mutational hot spot.[405,424,425] Nine different frameshift mutations have been identified in OCA1A, and analysis of the flanking sequences shows that five of these (involving codons 115, 191, 244, 310, and 438) are within repetitive sequences, suggesting the mechanism of their formation. Streisinger and others have shown that frameshift mutations occur with high frequency in regions that contain repeated base sequences.[426–429] In areas of repetitive nucleotides where L (the length of the paired but misaligned stretch of bases) is equal to or greater than 4, deletion mutations have been found to be two to four times more likely than addition mutations.[429] Of the five frameshift mutations occurring in repetitive sequences, four are deletion mutations and only one is an addition mutation. All of the identified frameshift mutations result in premature translational termination, which may reduce the stability or the processing of the protein, or result in loss of important functional domains.

The polymorphisms that have been described above in the section on the tyrosinase gene can be used to form haplotypes, and these can be used for population studies of the distribution of different mutations.[234] In one example, the missense mutation G47D has been observed in three different populations in the United States, Puerto Rico, and the Canary Islands.[234] In all instances, this mutation was associated with the same haplotype, haplotype 1, suggesting a common founder for this mutation. On the other hand, the mutation P81L found in families in the United States and the Canary Islands was on a different haplotype for each region, suggesting that there were different founders for the same mutation. Haplotype analysis is continuing in an effort to study the formation and migration of different mutations.

OCA2: Tyrosinase-Positive OCA

Overview. Individuals with albinism who have pigmented hair and eyes have long been identified, particularly in the African and African-American population, but not well characterized.[1,430–434] Terms such as *incomplete albinism, partial albinism,* or *imperfect albinism* have been used for this phenotype, but these are inappropriate and confusing. The first major insight into the separation of OCA into different types was provided by the hairbulb incubation test and tyrosinase assay.[3–5,435,436] The fact that this represented true genetic locus heterogeneity was demonstrated by the finding of normally pigmented offspring from a mating between an individual with tyrosinase-negative OCA and one with tyrosinase-positive OCA.[437] It is likely that further genetic heterogeneity exists within the broad category of OCA2 and that more precise characterizations will be possible with the identification of the responsible genes.

The general phenotypic features of OCA2 include the presence of hair pigment at birth and iris pigment at birth or early in life, and the development of localized (nevi, freckles, and lentigines) skin pigment, often in sun exposed regions of the skin.[2] The ethnic and constitutional pigment background of an affected individual are thought to have more influence on the phenotype of OCA2 than on OCA1, but further studies of individuals with OCA1B are necessary to document this point fully.[2] Most affected individuals accumulate pigment in their hair and eyes during their lifetime, and this is accentuated in individuals from darker ethnic groups. OCA2 is the most common type of OCA in the world, primarily because of its high frequency in equatorial Africa,[9,433,438] and several other smaller populations.[2,435,439]

Tyrosinase-Positive OCA. In Caucasian individuals, the amount of pigment present at birth or developing with time varies from minimal in northern European (particularly Scandinavian) to moderate in southern European and Mediterranean individuals. The hair can be very lightly pigmented at birth (having a light yellow or blond color) or more pigmented (with a definite blond, golden blond, or even red color).[333,396] The normal delayed maturation of the pigment system in many northern European individuals (i.e., very blond or towheaded as a child with later development of dark blond or brown hair) influences the phenotype early in life and can make the differentiation from OCA1 difficult. The skin is creamy white and does not tan. The iris color is blue-gray or lightly pigmented, and the degree of translucency correlates with the amount of iris pigment present. With time, pigmented nevi and lentigines may develop, and pigmented freckles are seen in exposed areas with repeated sun exposure. The hair slowly turns darker through the first two or more decades of life. Phenotypic variation between families is common, and variation within families can be seen.

The phenotype of OCA2 is distinctive in African-American and in African individuals.[1,9,430–434] The hair is yellow at birth and remains yellow through life, although the color may turn darker. Interestingly, the hair can turn lighter in older individuals, and this probably represents the normal graying with age. The skin is creamy white at birth and changes little with time. Pigmented nevi, lentigines, and freckles develop, but there is no tan. The irides are blue-gray or lightly pigmented. In the African-American population, there is some phenotypic variation within this type, particularly in the hair color, which may be brown, auburn, or red rather than yellow at birth or with time.

Hairbulb tyrosinase activity in OCA2 is normal or nearly normal when measured by a quantitative assay, and tyrosinase protein is normal when evaluated by electrophoresis.[6,388,389] The ultrastructure of the hair follicle melanocytes and melanosomes is normal.[3,5] Visible melanin forms in a freshly plucked anagen hairbulb after incubation in tyrosine or DOPA, and ultrastructural studies show that the melanin is synthesized in melanosomes as stages II and III premelanosomes are converted to stage IV melanized melanosomes.[3,5]

Prader-Willi and Angelman Syndromes. A newly recognized association with OCA2 is the hypopigmentation found with Prader-Willi syndrome (PWS) and Angelman syndrome (AS).[10–12,440] PWS is a developmental syndrome that includes neonatal hypotonia, hyperphagia and obesity, hypogonadism, small hands and feet, and mental retardation associated with characteristic behavior (see Chap. 20).[441,442] Approximately 70 percent of individuals with PWS have a deletion on the long arm of the paternal chromosome 15,[440,443,444] and most of those without a deletion of the paternal chromosome 15 have uniparental disomy for the maternal chromosome 15.[445,446]

Approximately 50 percent of individuals with PWS are hypopigmented, but most do not have the typical ocular features of albinism.[11,12,440,447] Interestingly, a number of individuals with PWS and OCA have been identified.[295] The hypopigmentation in PWS was originally described as oculocutaneous albinoidism, suggesting only cutaneous without ocular involvement,[448] but subsequent studies have now demonstrated hypopigmentation of skin, hair, and eyes, indicating that this is oculocutaneous hypopigmentation. For those without obvious OCA, hair and skin are lighter than unaffected family members, and childhood nystagmus and strabismus are common but often transient. The irides are pigmented with some translucency on globe transillumination, and retinal pigment is reduced in amount. Although foveal hypoplasia usually is not present, the fovea may not appear entirely normal.[447] Visual evoked potential studies have revealed optic tract misrouting similar to that found in albinism in some individuals with PWS and hypopigmentation.[447] This is an important observation because the presence of optic tract abnormalities implies pathological hypopigmentation during development, thus indicating that the hypopigmentation in PWS is best described as a type of albinism. The individuals with PWS and OCA have not been fully described, but the features of the albinism are typical for OCA2.

Individuals with AS are also hypopigmented, but the percentage showing this phenotypic characteristic is unknown.[10,449] AS is a complex developmental disorder that includes developmental delay and severe mental retardation, microcephaly, neonatal hypotonia, ataxic movements, and inappropriate laughter.[449–451] Those with hypopigmentation have light skin and hair and may have a history of nystagmus or strabismus.[10] Iris translucency and reduced retinal pigment may be present. No analysis of the optic tract organization is available.

Hairbulb tyrosinase activity in individuals affected with PWS or with AS is low in comparison to control values. Surprisingly, the values are low both in those with and those without hypopigmentation,[10,11] although it is somewhat higher in individuals with normal pigmentation. The ultrastructure and number of hair follicle melanocytes and melanosomes are normal.[10,11] Stages II and III premelanosomes and stage IV fully melanized melanosomes are present, but there appear to be fewer stage IV melanosomes and more stage III premelanosomes in comparison to hair follicles from normally pigmented control individuals.[10,11]

Molecular Pathogenesis of OCA2

The human homologue to the mouse pink-eyed-dilution *(p)* gene has been linked to the OCA2 phenotype.[294,295] This linkage was foreshadowed by linkage of the *p* gene to DN10, a DNA marker associated with the PWS chromosomal region.[452] This linkage made the P gene, the human homologue of the murine *p* gene, a strong candidate for OCA2. Mutations in the *p* gene of the mouse result in hypopigmentation of the coat and the eyes and many alleles have been identified.[25] Analysis with the P gene cDNA showed that this gene, which corresponds to the D15S12 marker, mapped to 15q11.2-q13, the region that is deleted in individuals with PWS and AS.[293] Linkage also was established between the classic African tyrosinase-positive OCA and markers D15S10 and D15S13, which also map to 15q11.2-q13.[294] Evidence that the P locus is synonymous with the OCA2 gene was strengthened by the finding of an individual with PWS and OCA2 who had two different deletions of the P locus—a deletion of the entire P locus on the paternally derived chromosome 15 and a partial deletion of the P locus on the maternally derived allele.[295]

More importantly, individuals with OCA2 in the Brandywine triracial isolate of Maryland (one of the original populations analyzed with OCA2) were found to be homozygous for a 2.7-Kb deletion of a single exon providing unequivocal evidence that mutations of the P gene are responsible for this type of albinism.[439a] This mutation has also been found in several unrelated African-American and African individuals showing that it is common and has an African origin. There have also been five different point mutations of the P gene associated with OCA2.[439b] These mutations include three missense mutations, one frameshift mutation, and a splice-junction mutation. The gene has been reported to be highly polymorphic, and the assignment of a base alteration as a pathogenic mutation will have to be done with care until the function of the P gene is determined and a functional assay becomes available.

The mechanism for the hypopigmentation in PWS and AS in individuals without obvious OCA has not been fully explained. The murine *p* locus is not imprinted, and it is likely that the human locus is not.[293] The deletion on the paternal chromosome 15q in PWS and the maternal chromosome 15q in AS suggests that the hypopigmentation arises from a mechanism other than gene dose effect, since heterozygotes for OCA2 are normally pigmented. Further work will be necessary after the function of the gene product of the P locus is determined.

Unclassified Types

Brown OCA. Brown OCA has been reported only in individuals in Africa or in African-American individuals, and the phenotype in Caucasian individuals has only recently been recognized.[8,9] In African and African-American individuals, the hair and skin color are light brown and the irides are gray to tan at birth. With time there is little change in skin color, but the hair may turn darker and the irides may accumulate more tan pigment. The skin is resistant to the acute effects of sun exposure and does not burn. Affected individuals are recognized as having albinism because they have all of the ocular features of albinism. The iris has punctate and radial translucency, and moderate retinal pigment is present. The skin may darken with sun exposure. Visual acuity ranges from 20/60 to 20/150. In Caucasian individuals, the phenotype would suggest tyrosinase-positive OCA. Hair color is golden blond. Skin is white. The frequency of brown OCA is unknown; in one study, approximately 29 percent of individuals with albinism in Nigeria had this type.[9]

Hairbulb tyrosinase activity has been determined in one individual with brown OCA and was normal.[8] The ultrastructural architecture of skin melanocytes was normal, but that of the melanosomes was abnormal.[8] The melanosomes were irregular and incompletely melanized in comparison with normally pigmented black skin, and large, stage IV fully melanized melanosomes typical of normal black skin were absent. Melanosomes were distributed to keratinocytes in membrane-bound packages rather than as single granules as seen in normally pigmented black skin. The architecture of hair follicle melanocytes and melanosomes was normal. Stage III partially melanized as well as stage IV fully melanized melanosomes were present.

The gene for brown OCA has not been identified. A study of cultured skin melanocytes from one child with brown OCA has shown an absence of brown protein, the product of the TRP1 gene.[453] Furthermore, the melanocyte cultures had a brown color, while those of an unaffected dizygotic twin were black. Molecular studies are in progress.

Rufous OCA. Rufous or red OCA is not well documented. Individuals with OCA who have red hair and reddish-brown pigmented skin have been reported in Africa,[1,434,454] and in New Guinea,[455,456] but clinical descriptions are incomplete, little biochemical data are available, and similar phenotypes in the U.S. population have not been reported. The cases are described in the literature as red, rufous, or xanthous albinism.[1,431,457] Individuals with red hair who have either OCA1 or OCA2 are also recognized, but the reddish-brown skin pigment is usually not present, and they should not be confused with red OCA. The phenotype in South African individuals includes red skin, ginger or reddish hair, and hazel or brown irides.[454] The ocular features were not fully consistent with the diagnosis of OCA, however, as most did not have iris translucency, nystagmus, strabismus, or foveal hypoplasia. Furthermore, a visual evoked potential study did not demonstrate misrouting of the optic fibers at the chiasm. The ultrastructural analysis of hairbulb and skin melanocytes showed eumelanosomes and pheomelanosomes in various stages of melanization, suggesting that the red color resulted from pheomelanin synthesis, as pheomelanosomes are absent in normally pigmented black skin and hairbulbs.[454] In New Guinea, the described phenotype includes reddish-brown skin, deep mahogany hair, reddish brown to brown irides with some translucency, and normal retinal pigment and foveal development.[456] Congenital nystagmus was present in this population but did not segregate specifically with the red phenotype. The true nature of red or rufous OCA must await further study. The analysis of the gene for the MSH receptor may provide important information in this regard, since this receptor is intimately involved in the pheomelanin–eumelanin switch, and mutations of this gene are responsible for red coats in several animals.[301]

Autosomal Dominant OCA. Several families have been described with autosomal dominant expression of OCA or cutaneous hypopigmentation, but characterization is incomplete and most do not fit the criteria for albinism.[458–460] In general, affected individuals have light skin that tans, light hair, and reduced iris pigment. One French family had hypopigmentation associated with skin melanocytes containing small melanosomes in three generations, suggesting a primary abnormality of melanosome structure.[459] Interestingly, one of the individuals with hypopigmentation also had PWS. The abnormal melanosomal size suggests that the hypopigmentation may not be related to the P gene on chromosome 15q, and further information on this family is not available. A second family included affected parents and children, but the grandparents were normal.[458] All the features of albinism were present in those affected, and this family is probably an example of pseudodominance. Molecular analysis of OCA1 now suggests that some families that are thought to have a dominant expression of OCA actually have mutations of the tyrosinase gene with affected individuals in several sequential generations. The third family reported does not meet the definition of albinism (i.e., no nystagmus or loss of visual acuity) and does not have OCA.[460] The final characterization of dominant OCA will await the careful evaluation of families with a clear autosomal dominant expression of OCA.

Types Of OCA in Which the Primary Defect Is Not Limited to the Melanocyte

Hermansky-Pudlak syndrome (HPS) is a complex disorder that presents with OCA, a mild bleeding diathesis, and a ceroid storage disease affecting primarily the lungs and the gut. The OCA is similar to that described in the primary OCA types described above, but obviously arises as a secondary ramification of an unknown primary defect affecting melanocytes, platelets, and possibly other tissue. HPS is inherited as an autosomal recessive trait. Hermansky and Pudlak first described this condition in two Czechoslovakian individuals in 1959[7] and it has subsequently been recognized throughout the world, with the majority of affected individuals in the Puerto Rican population.[2] HPS is not common, except in the latter population, and does not constitute a major type of OCA. The sixth edition of this book provides a detailed description.[2]

HPS is a pigmenting type of OCA in that cutaneous and ocular pigment develops in many affected individuals; however, the amount of pigment that forms is quite variable. Some affected individuals have marked cutaneous hypopigmentation similar to that of OCA1A, others have white skin and yellow or blond hair similar to OCA2, and still others have only moderate cutaneous hypopigmentation, suggesting that they may have OA rather than OCA. The variation can be seen within families as well as between families. HPS is very common in the Puerto Rican population, and affected individuals in this population have hair color that varies from white to yellow to brown.[2,344,461] Skin color is creamy white and definitely lighter than normally pigmented individuals in this population. Freckles are often present in the sun-exposed regions (face, neck, arms, and hands), often coalescing into large areas that look like normal dark skin pigment, but tanning does not occur. Pigmented nevi are common. Iris color varies from blue to brown, and all of the ocular features of albinism are present. Visual acuity ranges from 20/60 to 20/400.[344,462] The presence of OCA may not be obvious in a Puerto Rican individual with brown hair, skin pigment in exposed areas, and brown eyes unless the cutaneous pigmentation is compared to unaffected family members (who are generally darker in pigment) and unless the ocular features of albinism are recognized.

Affected individuals have been identified in other populations infrequently, and the phenotype shows the same degree of variation in pigmentation as is found in Puerto Rico.[2,333] Hair color varies from white to brown, and this correlates with the ethnic group. The skin is white and does not tan. Eye color varies from blue to pigmented.

The most severe clinical manifestations of HPS are related to the pulmonary and intestinal changes. Interstitial pulmonary fibrosis has been described in many individuals with HPS, although the actual prevalence is unknown.[463–466] The fibrosis results in moderate to severe restrictive lung disease.[465] Analysis of bronchoalveolar lavage fluid shows the presence of PDGF in homozygous affected and obligate heterozygotes, suggesting that this growth factor could be responsible for the development of the fibrosis.[465] The development of granulomatous colitis, presenting with abdominal pain and bloody diarrhea in a child or an adult, has also been described in many individuals with HPS.[467,468] The etiology of the colitis is unknown, and immunologic studies do not show an abnormality.[469] The presence of ceroid material in the epithelial cells of the gut suggests that this material may be involved in the development of the colitis, but this has not been proven.

The bleeding diathesis in HPS is related to a deficiency of storage granules in the platelets (i.e. storage pool-deficient platelets), as shown in Fig. 147-11. The storage granules or dense bodies are reduced in number or are absent, and this is associated with a deficiency of serotonin, adenine nucleotides, and calcium in the platelet.[2] As a result, platelets in HPS do not show irreversible secondary aggregation when stimulated. This deficiency produces mild hemorrhagic episodes in many affected individuals, including easy bruisability, epistaxis, hemoptysis, gingival bleeding with brushing or dental extraction, and postpartum bleeding. Occasional severe bleeding is observed, which in part may be related to normal variation in von Willebrand factor.

The basic defect in HPS is unknown. It has been hypothesized that an abnormality of a protein in the membranes of melanosomes, lysosomes, and platelet dense bodies may be involved.[327,330] HPS platelets are deficient in granulophysin, a protein found in the dense body membrane.[470] This protein has now been identified as CD63, and anti-CD63 antibodies demonstrate its deficiency in HPS platelets.[471]

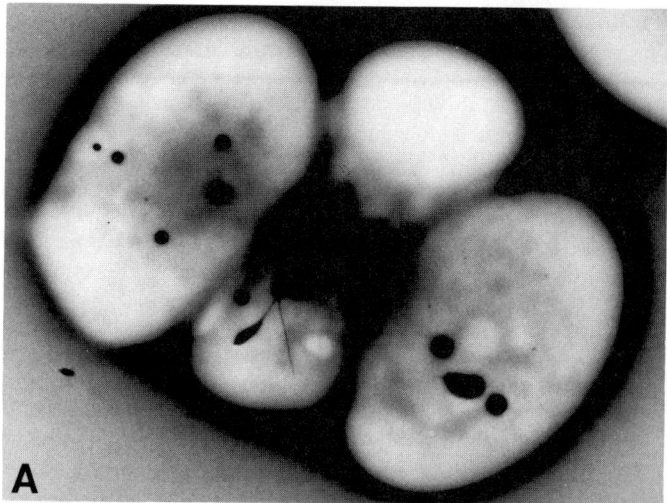

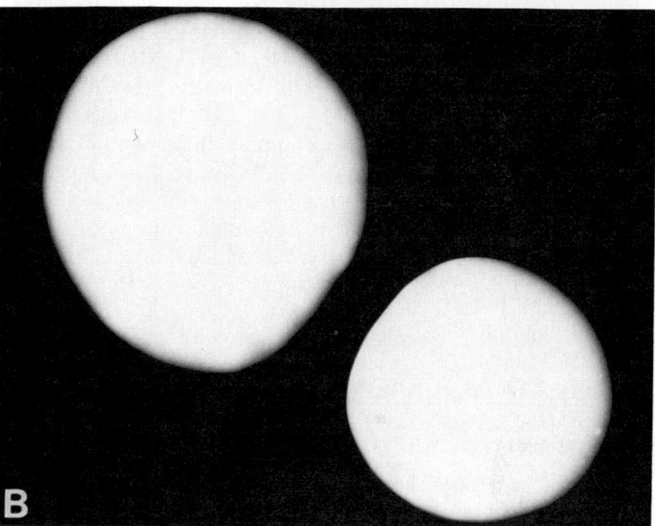

FIG. 147-11 **Platelet whole mounts. *A*. Platelets from a normal individual left in contact with a formvar-coated grid for 1 min and air-dried contain a total of 23 dense bodies. On the average, 4 to 8 dense bodies per platelet can be visualized in normal platelets by this method. *B*. Platelets from an HPS patient using the same technique contain no dense bodies. ×15,000 *(From Witkop et al.*[528] *Used by permission of the* American Journal of Hematology.)**

The mechanism for the hypopigmentation is not known. Hairbulb tyrosinase activity is present, but the level is low.[389] The ultrastructural architecture of skin and hairbulb melanocytes and melanosomes are normal.[2] There are at least 10 identified mouse loci that could be the murine counterpart of HPS because of pigment, platelet and lysosome dysfunction,[327,330] and studies are underway to identify the responsible gene.

Chediak-Higashi Syndrome (CHS). CHS is a rare autosomal recessive syndrome that consists of increased susceptibility to bacterial infections, hypopigmentation, and the presence of giant peroxidase-positive lysosomal granules in peripheral blood granulocytes.[472] As with HPS, the hypopigmentation is the result of a primary defect that affects many cell types, including the melanocyte. The skin, hair, and eye pigment is reduced or diluted in CHS, but the affected individuals often do not have obvious albinism and the hypopigmentation may be noted only when compared with other family members. Hair color is light brown to blond, and the hair has a metallic silver-gray sheen. The skin is creamy white to slate gray. Iris pigment is present and nystagmus and photophobia may be present or absent.[473] Histologic studies of the eye in CHS have shown reduced iris pigment, a marked reduction in retinal pigment granules, and infiltration of the choroid with reticuloendothelial cells.[474] Visual evoked potential studies show misrouting of the optic fibers in a pattern similar to that in individuals with OCA1 and OCA2.[475]

The primary defect in CHS is unknown. The susceptibility to bacterial infections appears to be the result of the abnormal granules in the neutrophils and other cells.[476,477] The hypopigmentation also arises from the formation of abnormal granules. Giant melanosomes form in the melanocyte and are unable to be transferred to the surrounding keratinocytes, leading to abnormal melanosome distribution and hypopigmentation. The pigment granules in the hair shaft are large and irregular in comparison with normally pigmented hair from an unaffected individual,[472,478] and this pathological change has been used to make a prenatal diagnosis of CHS.[479]

The *beige (bg)* mouse has been proposed as a model of CHS.[331] The gene for a structural protein of basement membranes known as nidogen/entactin maps to mouse chromosome 13 and is linked to the *beige* locus, suggesting that this may be involved in the pathogenesis of CHS.[480]

OCULAR ALBINISM

Overview

Albinism in which the hypopigmentation is limited to the eye is considerably less common than OCA1 or OCA2, although the true prevalence is unknown (see Table 147-4). As with OCA, there are two common types of OA and several rare variants (see Table 147-5). It is important to note that the hypopigmentation in OA is clinically limited to the eye, but changes in the cutaneous pigment system may also be present when the ultrastructure of these tissues is analyzed.

X-Linked Recessive OA (OA1)

OA1, an X-linked recessive disorder, is also known as the Nettleship-Falls type of OA.[481,482] The skin of affected Caucasian males with OA1 appears normally pigmented, while that of many African-American males may have scattered hypopigmented macules. Hair pigment is normal. The irides are blue to brown, and all of the optic changes of albinism are present.[483–485] In African-American males, iris color is often brown and there is little iris translucency.[338]

Heterozygous females can be detected clinically because of ocular pigment changes that result from X inactivation.[338] A variegated pattern of retinal pigmentation and punctate areas of iris translucency are present in approximately 80 percent of heterozygous females.[338,483,486,487] A small number of heterozygous females have ocular features of albinism, including nystagmus and reduced acuity, that are thought to be the result of nonrandom patterns of X inactivation.[488]

Melanocytes are normal in OA1, but there are changes in the melanosomes.[489] Melanocytes in the skin and hair follicles as well as those of the iris and retina contain large melanosomes—called "giant melanosomes," "macromelanosomes," or "melanin macroglobules"—along with normal melanosomes.[489–492] The giant melanosomes are also found in the tissues of obligate heterozygous females. The systemic nature of the melanosome defect in OA1 suggests that this is really a type of OCA in which the major manifestations are in the eye.

The gene for OA1 has been localized to the short arm of the X chromosome. Initial linkage studies showed OA1 linked to the Xg blood group at Xp22.32.[493,494] The OA1 gene has now been mapped more precisely to the Xp22.3-Xp22.2 region[495] and is thought to be between the markers DXS237 and DXS143,[496–499] but the gene has not been isolated, and the function of its protein product is unknown.

Autosomal Recessive Ocular Albinism

This type of OA affects males and females equally.[500] All the ocular features of the albinism are present, except that most affected individuals have some retinal pigment in the posterior pole. Skin pigment appears normal in Caucasian individuals with autosomal recessive OA. Affected African-American individuals have not been described. Most individuals reported have had light cutaneous pigment at birth with a gradual increase in skin and hair pigment with time.

The gene responsible for autosomal recessive OA has not been identified or mapped. A report of a dysmorphic child having the features of OA and an absence of giant melanosomes in association with a deletion of chromosome 6 (q13-q15) suggested that the gene for autosomal recessive OA[501] was in this region. Conversely, this may be an example of the commonly recognized pigment alterations found with many chromosomal abnormalities.[502] It is possible that OA2 is not a separate entity, and the previously described cases may actually have tyrosinase gene mutations associated with residual enzyme activity or P gene mutations that allow formation of cutaneous pigment. Individuals having tyrosinase gene mutations associated with nearly normal cutaneous pigmentation have been described.

Ocular Albinism and Deafness

Rare families have been described with ocular albinism and deafness. One large Afrikaner family with X-linked OA and late-onset sensorineural deafness segregating together was reported in 1984.[503,504] Macromelanosomes were demonstrated in skin from affected males and obligate heterozygous females, and the clinical features of albinism were similar to OA1. An additional family that contained three generations of males and females affected with congenital deafness and ocular albinism has been described, but little information on this family is available.[505]

OTHER CONDITIONS WITH ALBINISM

X-Linked Albinism and Deafness

An Israeli Jewish family of Sephardic origin has been described with albinism and deaf-mutism.[506,507] A similar syndrome has been described in the Hopi Indian population.[508] The hypopigmentation was more typical of piebaldism rather than albinism, and the ocular features of albinism were absent in affected family members. The gene for this condition has now been mapped to the long arm of the X chromosome.[509]

Oculocerebral Syndrome with Hypopigmentation (Cross Syndrome). This rare (less than 15 reported cases) syndrome presents with hypopigmentation and various neurologic changes.[510] This syndrome is often called "Cross syndrome,"[511] but the features are quite variable and may be heterogeneous in etiology. The cutaneous hypopigmentation is generalized but variable in degree, and the hair has a silver or silver-gray appearance.[512] The ocular features of albinism have not been present in all reported cases, suggesting that this is not a true type of albinism.[510]

Griscelli Syndrome. Griscelli et al. reported two unrelated individuals with hypopigmentation characterized as silver-gray hair and scattered hypopigmented areas surrounded by hyperpigmented skin.[513] Both had repeated pyogenic infections, neutropenia, and thrombocytopenia, and one died with sepsis. Melanocytes in the skin were congested with melanin granules and were surrounded by hypopigmented cells. The melanocytes had no dendrites. It was hypothesized that this condition was homologous to the *dilute (d/d)* mouse.[513]

LOCALIZED HYPOPIGMENTATION

There are a variety of conditions that present with localized hypopigmentation. The general cutaneous pigment is normal, but variably sized patches of white skin are present at birth or develop with time. The ocular features of albinism, including nystagmus, reduced retinal pigment, and misrouting of the optic fibers are absent in these conditions (i.e., they are not types of albinism), but the iris pigment may be reduced. Two conditions with congenital presentation will be discussed—piebaldism and Waardenburg syndrome.

Piebaldism

Piebaldism presents with a characteristic pattern of white forelock and multiple symmetric white or depigmented macules. This condition has been reported in the literature under a variety of names, including *partial albinism, familial white spotting, white forelock,* and *piebaldism*.[514–518] The white forelock is usually present at birth or early in life, and can be only a few strands or a large patch of white hair. The underlying skin is white. The white macules are found on the face, trunk and extremities, and the hair growing from them is white. Melanocytes are absent in the white patches of skin and the hair follicles of the white hair.[518,519] Piebaldism is inherited as an autosomal dominant trait.

Based on analogy with the murine phenotype, dominant white spotting (W), the human KIT gene, which encodes the tyrosine kinase transmembrane cellular receptor for mast/stem-cell growth factor, has been shown to be defective in piebaldism.[308–311] The protein product of the KIT gene is a 976-amino-acid peptide that is thought to homodimerize in response to ligand binding. Several mutations have been found in the KIT genes of patients with piebaldism. As was found in the mouse, these alleles of the KIT gene are associated with a spectrum of phenotypes ranging from mild to severe forms of piebaldism.[520] Three missense mutations (E583K, F584L, and G664R) are associated with severe phenotypes.[308,310] Two frameshift mutations at codon 560 (a 1-bp insertion) and 642 (a 2-bp deletion) as well as a splice site mutation at the 5′ end of intron 12 result in variable piebald phenotypes that can range from mild to severe in different members of the same family.[310] A frameshift mutation at codon 85 results in a mild phenotype.[310] This variation in the phenotypic consequences of KIT mutations may be related to subunit interactions of the dimeric KIT protein. The most severe forms are associated with missense mutations at the intracellular tyrosine kinase domain.[310] It has been suggested that the mutant protein combines with the peptide product of the normal allele producing a nonfunctional heterodimer resulting in a 75 percent reduction of functional receptors. This produces a dominant negative effect for these mutations. The frameshift mutation at codon 85 results in a truncated protein that presumably is unable to dimerize. As a consequence, all the products of the normal allele will assemble into functional receptors without interference from the abnormal protein produced by the mutant allele. The end result should be an approximately 50 percent rather than 75 percent reduction in receptor function and a milder phenotype. The two frameshift mutations and the splice site mutation associated with intermediate phenotypes would result in a 50 to 75 percent reduction in function depending on the stability of the truncated polypeptide.[310] These differing levels of stability for the product of the mutant allele may account for at least part of the variability in the phenotype for this disorder.

Waardenburg Syndrome

The combination of lateral displacement of the inner ocular canthi with a broad base of the nose, white forelock (poliosis), heterochromatic irides (different color of the two irides) hyperplasia of the medial portion of the eyebrows, and congenital sensorineural hearing loss is known as Waardenberg syndrome (WS) (see also, Chap. 155). Two types of WS are described: WS type I with lateral displacement of the inner canthi (telecanthus) and WS type II without telecanthus. Both are inherited as autosomal dominant traits. The clinical manifestations are varied and diverse, and excellent reviews are available.[521–523]

The PAX3 gene is responsible for WS type I. Analysis of PAX3 in different individuals with WS type I has revealed six different mutations that can be divided into three classes. The first class alters the paired domain of the protein. This class consists of three mutations, two missense mutations (a proline-to-leucine substitution and a glycine-to-arginine substitution) and an in-frame deletion of six amino acids (18 nucleotides).[319,320,524] Most likely the missense mutation affects the protein–DNA binding activity of the PAX3 gene like the *Pax-1* gene mutation in the mouse that causes the *undulated (un)* phenotype.[525,526] In the *Pax-1* gene, a glycine to serine missense mutation has been shown to alter the protein–DNA binding properties of this protein. The missense mutation found in the PAX3 gene is located next to one to the helixes of the paired domain structure and the 18-bp deletion mutation affects a highly conserved sequence in the paired domain. Both of these areas are important in the protein–DNA interaction for this protein. The second class of mutations does not affect the paired domain but eliminates the conserved octapeptide and homeo box domain. This class contains one mutation, a 2-bp deletion. The third class results in the elimination of all protein function. Both identified mutations are frameshift mutations resulting in a protein truncated in the paired domain.[324,524] There have been reports of heterogeneity of WS, and this may be the result of different alleles of the PAX3 gene resulting in different phenotypes.[527] The hypothesis is that the PAX gene family, and probably the PAX3 gene, encode nuclear *trans*-acting transcriptional factors that regulate several target genes. Different mutations, particularly missense mutations, may vary the DNA binding or the specificity of the DNA binding and thus produce the different phenotypes observed.

EVALUATION AND MANAGEMENT OF ALBINISM

Proper evaluation and treatment of individuals with albinism are critical to their normal growth and development and eventual adult life. It is important to note that affected individuals have only hypopigmentation and the associated ocular (and auditory) changes, and there are no changes in other functions of the brain. Specifically, mental retardation is not part of albinism, and another explanation must be considered for a child or adult with developmental delay or mental retardation. Other medical problems have been reported with different types of albinism, but most of these examples appear to be cosegregation of two conditions in a family. There are several specific areas of concern for individuals with albinism: correct diagnosis, skin care, and ophthalmologic care.

Diagnosis

The diagnosis of albinism is established when an individual with oculocutaneous or ocular hypopigmentation is found to have the ocular changes as described above. Nystagmus, reduced retinal pigment, reduced acuity, and misrouting of the optic fibers at the chiasm are present to different degrees in all patients with albinism, and the diagnosis cannot be made without these characteristic findings. Iris pigment is variable in amount in OCA and OA, and the iris translucency can vary from complete transillumination to punctate translucent areas. It is occasionally necessary to perform a visual evoked potential study to demonstrate misrouting of the optic fibers when an individual presents with moderately reduced cutaneous and retinal pigment and nystagmus. The demonstration of misrouting is the most critical diagnostic criterion; the diagnosis of albinism cannot be made without clinical or electrophysiological evidence of this abnormality. In most cases, the finding of nystagmus, alternating strabismus, foveal hypoplasia, reduced acuity, and reduced depth perception are sufficient for the diagnosis, and an evoked potential study is not necessary.

An individual with OCA can be classified as OCA1 or OCA2 by clinical, biochemical, and molecular criteria. The medical history is important. Almost all individuals with OCA1, even when they have OCA1B and form moderate amounts of hair and iris pigment as they mature, have white or nearly white hair and white skin at birth. The hairbulb incubation test and the hairbulb tyrosinase assay have been used to distinguish OCA1 from OCA2, but they are not precise, and overlap exists. Molecular analysis provides the most accurate method of diagnosis, and it should be considered if the correct diagnosis or family counseling are in question.

The diagnosis of OA1 is made when a male presents with typical features of this condition and the family history and maternal examination are consistent with this diagnosis. With no family history of OA and a normal maternal eye examination, it is necessary to demonstrate the presence of macromelanosomes in skin or hairbulbs of the affected male to make this diagnosis. EM examination of skin or hairbulb melanocytes is the preferred method for this analysis.

The diagnosis of HPS should be considered with any individual who has OCA and evidence of unusual bleeding or bruising. It is not necessary to evaluate all individuals with OCA, because HPS is not common, but the diagnosis needs to be considered in all Puerto Rican individuals with OCA. Several methods have been used to make the diagnosis of HPS,[2] and the most reliable is the demonstration of a lack of dense bodies in platelets.[528] Aspirin or aspirin-like medications must be withheld from all individuals with HPS, and should be avoided in individuals, particularly children, with OCA.

Skin Care

Individuals with albinism who have cutaneous hypopigmentation need to protect their skin from UV radiation. Physical methods, including long-sleeved shirts, long pants, and hats with a wide brim are excellent for this but often underutilized because of fashion or age. Sunscreens are very effective in protecting the skin and should be employed whenever possible. The sun protection factor or SPF rating of a sunscreen should be greater than 25 for good protection.

Some general information is helpful. The latitude is important in UV exposure, and more time in the sun can be tolerated in New Jersey than in Florida. Sand reflects UV rays, and it is possible to be burned when sitting in the shade on a beach. The greatest intensity of UV light occurs at the summer solstice, and between the hours of 10 AM and 2 PM standard time, and protection or avoidance of the sun in these periods can greatly reduce UV exposure.

Ophthalmologic Care

All individuals with albinism need regular eye care. Hyperopia, myopia, and astigmatism are common and need to be corrected to obtain the best corrected visual acuity. Correction should be reevaluated on an annual basis, starting early in life.

Most children with albinism function in a regular classroom, provided that the teacher and the school give specific attention to their special needs for vision. Braille training is rarely necessary. Teachers should be instructed to use high-contrast written materials. Copies of the teacher's board notes allow the child to read the material as it is presented to the class. Large-type books are available for many regular textbooks.

REFERENCES

1. Pearson K, Nettleship E, Usher CH: A monograph on albinism in man: Draper's company research memoirs, biometric series VI. London, Department of Applied Mathematics, Dulau, 1911, pp 1–25.
2. Witkop CJ Jr, Quevedo WC Jr, Fitzpatrick TB, King RA: Albinism, in Scriver CR, Beaudet AL, Sly WS, Valle D (eds): *The Metabolic Basis of Inherited Disease,* 6th ed. New York, McGraw-Hill, 1989, vol 2, pp 2905–2947.
3. Witkop CJ, Nance WE, Rawls RF, White JG: Autosomal recessive oculocutaneous albinism in man: Evidence for genetic heterogeneity. *Am J Hum Genet* **22**:55, 1970.
4. Witkop CJ, White JG, Nance WE, Jackson CE, Desnick S: Classification of albinism in man. *Birth Defects* **7**:13, 1971.
5. Witkop CJ, Hill CW, Desnick S, Thies JK, Thorn HL, Jenkins M, White JG: Ophthalmologic, biochemical, platelet and ultrastructural defects in the various types of oculocutaneous albinism. *J Invest Dermatol* **60**:443, 1973.
6. King RA, Olds DP, Witkop CJ: Characterization of human

hairbulb tyrosinase: Properties of normal and albino enzyme. *J Invest Dermatol* **71**:136, 1978.
7. Hermansky F, Pudlak P: Albinism associated with hemorrhagic diathesis and unusual pigmented reticular cells in the bone marrow: Report of two cases with histochemical studies. *Blood* **14**:162, 1959.
8. King RA, Lewis RA, Townsend D, Zelickson A, Olds DP, Brumbaugh JA: Brown oculocutaneous albinism. Clinical, ophthalmological, and biochemical characterization. *Ophthalmology* **92**:1496, 1985.
9. King RA, Creel DJ, Cervenka J, Okoro AN, Witkop CJ: Albinism in Nigeria with delineation of new recessive oculocutaneous type. *Clin Genet* **17**:259, 1980.
10. King RA, Wiesner GL, Townsend D, White JG: Hypopigmentation in Angelman syndrome. *Am J Med Genet* **46**:40, 1992.
11. Wiesner GL, Bendel CM, Olds DP, White JG, Arthur DC, Ball DW, King RA: Hypopigmentation in the Prader-Willi syndrome. *Am J Hum Genet* **40**:431, 1987.
12. Butler MG: Hypopigmentation: A common feature of Prader-Labhart-Willi syndrome. *Am J Hum Genet* **45**:140, 1989.
13. Montagna W, Ellis RA: *The Biology of Hair Growth*. New York, Academic, 1958, pp 1–358.
14. Montagna W, Hu F: *Advances in Biology of the Skin, The Pigmentary System*. New York, Pergammon, 1966, vol 8, pp 1–659.
15. Montagna W, Dobson RL: *Advances in Biology of the Skin*. Oxford, Pergamon, 1969, vol 9, pp 1–445.
16. Kawamura K, Fitzpatrick TB, Seiji M: *Biology of Normal and Abnormal Melanocytes*. Baltimore, University Park Press, 1971, pp 1–411.
17. Montagna W, Parakkal PF: *The Structure and Function of Skin*, 3d ed. New York, Academic, 1974, pp 1–433.
18. Quevedo WC Jr, Fitzpatrick TB, Szabo G, Jimbow K: Biology of melanocytes, in Fitzpatrick TB, Eisen AZ, Wolff K, Freedberg IM, Austen KF (eds): *Dermatology in General Medicine*, 3d ed. New York, McGraw-Hill, 1987, pp 224–251.
19. Prota G: *Melanins and Melanogenesis*. New York, Academic 1992, pp 1–290.
20. Moyer FH: Electron microscope observations on the origin, development and genetic control on melanin structure, in *The Structure of the Eye*. New York, Academic, 1967, pp 469–486.
21. Mayer TC: Enhancement of melanocyte development from piebald neural crest by a favorable tissue environment. *Dev Biol* **56**:255, 1977.
22. Quevedo WC Jr, Fleischmann RD: Developmental biology of mammalian melanocytes. *J Invest Dermatol* **75**:116, 1980.
23. Taylor WOG: Visual disabilities of oculocutaneous albinism and their alleviation. *Trans Ophthalmol Soc UK* **98**:423, 1978.
24. Ozanics V, Jakobiec FA: Prenatal development of the eye and its adnexa, in Duane TD, Jaeger EA (eds): *Biomedical Foundations of Ophthalmology*. Hagerstown, MD, Harper & Row, 1986, pp 1–86.
25. Silvers WK: *The Coat Colors of Mice. A Model for Mammalian Gene Action and Interaction*. New York, Springer-Verlag, 1979.
26. Sweet SE, Quevedo WC Jr: Role of melanocyte morphology in pigmentation of mouse hair. *Anat Rec* **162**:243, 1968.
27. Toda K, Fitzpatrick TB: Tyrosinase activity in melanosomes present within keratinocytes, in Kawamura T, Fitzpatrick TB, Seiji M (eds): *Biology of Normal and Abnormal Melanocytes*. Baltimore, University Park Press, 1971, pp 1–411.
28. Quevedo WC Jr: Genetic control of melanin metabolism within the melanin unit of mammalian epidermis. *J Invest Dermatol* **60**:407, 1973.
29. Garcia RE, Flynn E, Szabo G: Ultrastructure of melanocyte-keratinocyte interactions. *Pigment Cell Res* **4**:299, 1979.
30. Scott GA, Haake AR: Keratinocytes regulate melanocyte number in human fetal and neonatal skin equivalents. *J Invest Dermatol* **97**:776, 1991.
31. Szabo G: Racial differences in the fate of melanosomes in human epidermis. *Nature* **222**:1081, 1969.
32. Wolff K, Konrad K: Melanin pigmentation: An in vivo model for melanosome kinetics. *Science* **174**:1034, 1971.
33. Wolff K: Melanocyte:keratinocyte interactions in vivo: The fate of melanosomes. *Yale J Biol Med* **46**:384, 1973.
34. Stingl G, Wolff K: Langerhans cells and their relation to other dendritic cells and mononuclear phagocytes, in Fitzpatrick TB, Eisen AZ, Wolff K, Freedberg IM, Austen KF (eds): *Dermatology in General Medicine*, 3d ed. New York, McGraw-Hill, 1987, pp 410–426.
35. De-Luca M, D'Anna F, Bondanza S, Franzi AT, Cancedda R: Human epithelial cells induce human melanocyte growth in vitro but only skin keratinocytes regulate its proper differentiation in the absence of dermis. *J Cell Biol* **107**:1919, 1988.
36. Halaban R, Langdon R, Birchall N, Cuono C, Baird A, Scott GA, Moellmann GE, McGuire JS: Basic fibroblast growth factor from human keratinocytes is a natural mitogen for melanocytes. *J Cell Biol* **107**:1611, 1988.
37. Gordon PR, Mansur CP, Gilchrest BA: Regulation of human melanocyte growth dendricity, and melanization by keratinocyte derived factors. *J Invest Dermatol* **92**:565, 1989.
38. Eisinger M, Marko O, Ogata SI, Old LJ: Growth regulation of human melanocytes: Mitogenic factors in extracts of melanoma, astrocytoma and fibroblast cell lines. *Science* **229**:984, 1985.
39. Halaban R, Ghosh S, Baird A: bFGF is the putative natural growth factor for human melanocytes. *In Vitro Cell Dev Biol* **23**:47, 1987.
40. Ogata S, Furuhashi Y, Eisinger M: Growth stimulation of human melanocytes: Identification and characterization of melanoma-derived melanocyte growth factor (M-McGF). *Biochem Biophys Res Commun* **146**:1204, 1987.
41. Herlyn M, Mancianti ML, Jambrosic JA, Bolen JB, Koprowsky H: Regulatory factors that determine growth and phenotype of normal human melanocytes. *Exp Cell Res* **179**:322, 1988.
42. Peacocke M, Yaar M, Mansur CP, Chao MV, Gilchrest BA: Induction of nerve growth factor receptors on cultured human melanocytes. *Proc Natl Acad Sci USA* **85**:5282, 1988.
43. Rakowicz-Szulczjnska EM, Herlyn M, Koprowsky H: Nerve growth factor receptors in chromatin of melanoma cells, proliferating melanocytes and colorectal carcinoma cells in vivo. *Cancer Res* **48**:7200, 1988.
44. Pittelkow MR, Shipley GD: Serum-free culture of normal human melanocytes: Growth kinetics and growth factor requirements. *J Cell Physiol* **140**:565, 1989.
45. Abdel-Malek Z, Swope VB, Pallas J, Krug K, Nordlund JJ: Mitogenic, melanogenic, and cAMP responses of cultured neonatal human melanocytes to commonly used mitogens. *J Cell Physiol* **150**:416, 1992.
46. Wong G, Pawelek JM, Sansone M, Morowitz J: Response of mouse melanoma cells to melanocyte stimulating hormone. *Nature* **248**:351, 1974.
47. Halaban R, Lerner AB: The dual effect of melanocyte-stimulating hormone (MSH) on the growth of cultured mouse melanoma cells. *Exp Cell Res* **108**:111, 1977.
48. Hirobe T: Stimulation of dendritogenesis in epidermal melanocytes of newborn mice by melanocyte-stimulating hormone. *J Cell Sci* **33**:371, 1978.
49. Weatherhead B, Logan A: Interaction of α-melanocyte-stimulating hormone, melatonin, cyclic AMP and cyclic GMP in the control of melanogenesis in hair follicle melanocytes in vitro. *J Endocrinol* **90**:89, 1981.
50. Burchill SA, Thody AJ: Melanocyte-stimulating hormone and the regulation of tyrosinase activity in hair follicular melanocytes of the mouse. *J Endocrinol* **111**:225, 1986.
51. Fuller BB, Lunsford JB, Iman DS: α-Melanocyte stimulating hormone regulation of tyrosinase in Cloudman S91 mouse melanoma cell cultures. *J Biol Chem* **262**:4024, 1987.
52. Burchill SA, Virden R, Fuller BB, Thody AJ: Regulation of throsinase synthesis by α-melanocyte stimulating hormone in hair follicular melanocytes of the mouse. *J Endocrinol* **116**:17, 1988.
53. Ghanem G, Communale G, Libert A, Vercammen-Grandjean A, Lejeune F: Evidence for α-melanocyte stimulating hormone (α-MSH) receptors on human malignant melanoma cells. *Int J Cancer* **41**:248, 1988.
54. Jiménez M, Kameyama K, Maloy WL, Tomita Y, Hearing VJ: Mammalian tyrosinase: Biosynthesis, processing and modulation by melanocyte stimulating hormone. *Proc Natl Acad Sci USA* **85**:3830, 1988.

55. Kameyama K, Montague PM, Hearing VJ: The expression of melanocyte stimulating hormone receptors correlates with mammalian pigmentation and can be modulated by interferons. *J Cell Physiol* **137**:35, 1988.
56. McLane JA, Pawelek JM: Receptors for β-melanocyte-stimulating hormone exhibit positive cooperativity in synchronized melanoma cells. *Biochemistry* **27**:3743, 1988.
57. Ranson M, Posen S, Mason RS: Human melanocytes as a target tissue for hormones: In vitro studies with 1α-25,dihydroxyvitamin D_3, α-melanocyte stimulating hormone, and β-estradiol. *J Invest Dermatol* **91**:593, 1988.
58. Kameyama K, Tanaka S, Ishida Y, Hearing VJ: Murine α, β and γ-interferons stimulate melanogenesis by increasing the number of α-melanocyte stimulating hormone receptors on JB/MS murine melanoma cells. *J Clin Invest* **83**:213, 1989.
59. Siegrist W, Solca F, Stutz S, Siuffre L, Carrel S, Girard J, Eberle AN: Characterization of receptors for α-melanocyte stimulating hormone on human melanoma cells. *Cancer Res* **49**:6352, 1989.
60. Seechurn P, Thody AJ: The effect of ultraviolet radiation and melanocyte-stimulating hormone on tyrosinase activity in epidermal melanocytes of the mouse. *J Dermatol Sci* **1**:283, 1990.
61. Chakraborty AK, Orlow SJ, Pawelek JM: Stimulation of the receptor for melanocyte-stimulating hormone by retinoic acid. *FEBS Lett* **276**:205, 1991.
62. Fisher PB, Mufson RA, Weinstein IB: Interferon inhibits melanogenesis in B-16 mouse melanoma cells. *Biochem Biophys Res Commun* **100**:823, 1981.
63. Fisher PB, Prignoli DR, Hermo H, Weinstein IB, Pestka S: Effects of combined treatment with interferon and mezerein on melanogenesis and growth in human melanoma cells. *J Interferon Res* **5**:11, 1985.
64. Krasagakis K, Garbe C, Kruger S, Orfanos CE: Effects of interferons on cultured human melanocytes in vitro: Interferon-β but not -α or -γ inhibit proliferation and all interferons significantly modulate the cell phenotype. *J Invest Dermatol* **97**:364, 1991.
65. Birchall N, Orlow SJ, Kupper T, Pawelek JM: Interactions between ultraviolet light and interleukin-1 on MSH binding in both mouse melanoma and human squamous carcinoma cells. *Biochem Biophys Res Commun* **175**:839, 1991.
66. Swope VB, Abdel-Malek Z, Kassem LM, Nordlund JJ: Interleukins 1α and 6 and tumor necrosis factor-α are paracrine inhibitors of human melanocyte proliferation and melanogenesis. *J Invest Dermatol* **96**:180, 1991.
67. Kirnbauer R, Charvat B, Schauer E, Köck A, Urbanski A, Förster E, Neuner P, Assmann I, Luger TA, Schwarz T: Modulation of intercellular adhesion molecule-1 expression on human melanocytes and melanoma cells: Evidence for a regulatory role of IL-6, IL-7, TNBβ and UVB light. *J Invest Dermatol* **98**:320, 1992.
68. Santoro MG, Philpott GW, Jaffe BM: Inhibition of B16 melanoma growth in vivo by a synthetic analog of prostaglandin E_2. *Cancer Res* **37**:3774, 1977.
69. Bregman MD, Funk C, Fukushima M: Inhibition of human melanoma growth by prostaglandin A, D and J analogues. *Cancer Res* **46**:2740, 1986.
70. Nordlund JJ, Collins CE, Rheins LA: Prostaglandin E_2 and D_2 but not MSH stimulate the proliferation of pigment cells in the pinnal epidermis of the DBA/2 mouse. *J Invest Dermatol* **86**:433, 1986.
71. Abdel-Malek Z, Swope VB, Amornsiripanitch N, Nordlund JJ: In vitro modulation of proliferation and melanization of S91 melanoma cells by prostaglandins. *Cancer Res* **47**:3141, 1987.
72. Tomita Y, Iwamoto M, Masuda T, Tagami H: Stimulatory effect of prostaglandin E_2 on the configuration of normal human melanocytes in vitro. *J Invest Dermatol* **89**:299, 1987.
73. Abdel-Malek Z, Swope VB, Trinkle LS, Ferroni EN, Boissy RE, Nordlund JJ: Alteration of the Cloudman melanoma cell cycle by prostaglandin E_1 and E_2 determined by using a 5-bromo-2′-deoxyuridine method of DNA analysis. *J Cell Physiol* **136**:247, 1988.
74. Lotan R, Neumann G, Lotan D: Characterization of retinoic acid-induced alterations in the proliferation and differentiation of a murine and a human melanoma cell line in culture. *Ann NY Acad Sci* **359**:150, 1981.
75. Hosoi J, Abe E, Suda T, Kuraki T: Regulation of melanin synthesis of B16 mouse melanoma cells by 1α,25-dihydroxyvitamin D_3 and retinoic acid. *Cancer Res* **45**:1474, 1985.
76. Edward M, Gold JA, Mackie RM: Different susceptibilities of melanoma cells to retinoic acid-induced changes in melanotic expression. *Biochem Biophys Res Commun* **155**:773, 1988.
77. Niles RM, Loewy BP: Induction of protein kinase C in mouse melanoma cells by retinoic acid. *Cancer Res* **49**:4483, 1989.
78. Orlow SJ, Chakraborty AK, Pawelek JM: Retinoic acid is a potent inhibitor of inducible pigmentation in murine and hamster melanoma cell lines. *J Invest Dermatol* **94**:461, 1990.
79. Niles RM, Loewy BP: B16 mouse melanoma cells selected for resistance to cyclic AMP-mediated growth inhibition are cross-resistant to retinoic acid-induced growth inhibition. *J Cell Physiol* **147**:176, 1991.
80. Morelli JG, Yohn JJ, Lyons MB, Murphy RC, Norris DA: Leukotrienes C_4 and D_4 as potent mitogens of cultured human neonatal melanocytes. *J Invest Dermatol* **93**:719, 1989.
81. Zachariae COC, Thestrup-Pedersen K, Matsushima K: Expression and secretion of leukocyte chemotactic cytokines by normal human melanocytes and melanoma cells. *J Invest Dermatol* **97**:593, 1991.
82. Morelli JG, Kincannon J, Yohn JJ, Zekman T, Weston WL, Norris DA: Leukotriene C_4 and TGF-α are stimulators of human melanocyte migration in vitro. *J Invest Dermatol* **98**:290, 1992.
83. Richmond A, Lawson DH, Dixon DW, Chawla RK: Characterization of autostimulatory and transforming growth factors from human melanoma cells. *Cancer Res* **45**:6390, 1985.
84. Ellem KAO, Cullinan M, Baumann KC, Dunstan A: UVR induction of TGFα: A possible autocrine mechanism for the epidermal melanocytic response and for promotion of epidermal carcinogenesis. *Carcinogenesis* **9**:797, 1988.
85. Bogdahn U, Apfel R, Hahn M, Gerlach M, Behl C, Hoppe J, Martin R: Autocrine tumor cell growth-inhibiting activities from human malignant melanoma. *Cancer Res* **49**:5358, 1989.
86. Brocker EM, Magiera H, Herlyn M: Nerve growth factor and expression of receptors for nerve growth factor in tumors of melanocyte origin. *J Invest Dermatol* **96**:662, 1991.
87. Seiji M, Fitzpatrick TB, Birbeck MSC: The melanosome: A distinctive subcellular particle of mammalian melanocytes and the site of melanogenesis. *J Invest Dermatol* **36**:243, 1961.
88. Moyer FH: Genetic effects on melanosome fine structure and ontogeny in normal and malignent cells. *Ann NY Acad Sci* **100**:584, 1963.
89. Hearing VJ, Phillips P, Lutzner MA: The fine structure of melanogenesis in coat color mutants of the mouse. *J Ultrastruct Res* **43**:88, 1973.
90. Hirobe T: Origin of melanosome structures and cytochemical localizations of tyrosinase activity in differentiating epidermal melanocytes of newborn mouse skin. *J Exp Zool* **224**:355, 1982.
91. Hearing VJ, Nicholson JM, Montague PM, Ekel TM, Tomecki KJ: Mammalian tyrosinase: Structural and functional interrelationship of isozymes. *Biochim Biophys Acta* **522**:327, 1978.
92. Hearing VJ, Ekel TM, Montague PM: Mammalian tyrosinase: Isozymic forms of the enzyme. *Int J Biochem* **13**:99, 1981.
93. Imokawa G, Mishima Y: Isolation and biochemical characterization of tyrosinase-rich GERL and coated vesicles in melanin synthesizing cells. *Br J Dermatol* **104**:169, 1981.
94. Mishima Y, Imokawa G: Selective aberration and pigment loss in melanosomes of malignant melanoma cells in vitro by glycosylation inhibitors: Premelanosomes as glycoprotein. *J Invest Dermatol* **81**:106, 1983.
95. Imokawa G, Mishima Y: Functional analysis of tyrosinase isozymes of cultured malignant melanoma cells during the recovery period following interrupted melanogenesis induced by glycosylation inhibitors. *J Invest Dermatol* **83**:196, 1984.
96. Hearing VJ, Jiménez M: Mammalian tyrosinase: The critical regulatory control point in melanocyte pigmentation. *Int J Biochem* **19**:1141, 1987.

97. Wick MM, Hearing VJ, Rorsman H: Biochemistry of melanization, in Fitzpatrick TB, Eisen AZ, Wolff K, Freedberg IM, Austen KF (eds): *Dermatology in General Medicine,* 3d ed. New York, McGraw-Hill, 1987, pp 251–258.
98. Hearing VJ, Tsukamoto K: Enzymatic control of pigmentation in mammals. *FASEB J* **5**:2902, 1991.
99. Seiji M, Fitzpatrick TB: The reciprocal relationship between melanization and tyrosinase activity in melanosomes. *J Biochem* **49**:700, 1961.
100. Maul GG: Golgi-melanosome relationship in human melanoma in vitro. *J Ultrastruct Res* **26**:163, 1969.
101. Maul GG, Brumbaugh JA: On the possible function of coated vesicles in melanogenesis of the regenerating fowl feather. *J Cell Biol* **48**:41, 1971.
102. Tomita Y, Hariu A, Kato C, Seiji M: Transfer of tyrosinase to melanosomes in Harding-Passey mouse melanoma. *Arch Biochem Biophys* **225**:75, 1983.
103. Imokawa G: Analysis of initial melanogenesis including tyrosinase transfer and melanosome differentiation through interrupted melanization by glutathione. *J Invest Dermatol* **93**:100, 1989.
104. Granholm NH, Japs RA, Kappenman KE: Differentiation of hairbulb pigment cell melanosomes in compound agouti and albino locus mouse mutants (A^y, a, c^{2J}; C57BL/6J). *Pigment Cell Res* **3**:16, 1990.
105. Flawn PC, Wilde PF: Mechanism of action and role of a natural inhibitor of DOPA autooxidation isolated from guinea pig skin. *J Invest Dermatol* **55**:159, 1970.
106. Satoh GJZ, Mishima Y: Tyrosinase inhibitors in amelanotic and melanotic malignant melanoma. *Arch Dermatol* **140**:9, 1970.
107. Hamada T, Mishima Y: Intracellular localization of tyrosinase inhibitor in amelanotic and melanotic malignant melanoma. *Br J Dermatol* **86**:385, 1972.
108. Imokawa G, Mishima Y: Isolation and characterization of tyrosinase inhibitors and their differential actions on melanogenic subcellular compartments in amelanotic and melanotic melanomas. *Br J Dermatol* **103**:625, 1980.
109. Vijayan E, Husain I, Ramaiah A, Madan NC: Purification of human skin tyrosinase and its protein inhibitor; properties of the enzyme and the mechanism of inhibition by protein. *Arch Biochem Biophys* **217**:738, 1982.
110. Lerner AB, Fitzpatrick TB, Caukins E, Summerson WH: Mammalian tyrosinase: Preparation and properties. *J Biol Chem* **178**:185, 1949.
111. Lerner AB, Fitzpatrick TB: Biochemistry of melanin formation. *Physiol Rev* **30**:91, 1950.
112. Swan GA: Chemical structure of melanins. *Ann NY Acad Sci* **100**:1005, 1963.
113. Nicolaus RA, Piatelli M, Fattorusso E: The structure of melanins and melanogenesis. IV. On some natural melanins. *Tetrahedron* **20**:1163, 1964.
114. Hempel K: Investigation of the structure of melanin in malignant melanoma with ^{3}H- and ^{14}C-DOPA labelled at various positions, in DellaPorta G, Mühlbock O (eds): *Structure and Control of the Melanocyte*. New York, Springer-Verlag, 1966, pp 162–175.
115. Hempel K, Maennl HFK: The conversion of H^3-tyrosine to H^3-DOPA in mouse melanoma in vivo. *Biochim Biophys Acta* **124**:192, 1966.
116. Prota G, Thomson RH: Melanin pigmentation in mammals. *Endeavour* **35**:32, 1976.
117. Hearing VJ, Ekel TM: Mammalian tyrosinase: A comparison of tyrosine hydroxylation and melanin formation. *Biochem J* **157**:549, 1976.
118. Prota G: Recent advances in the chemistry of melanogenesis in mammals. *J Invest Dermatol* **75**:122, 1980.
119. Ito S, Fujita K, Takahashi H, Jimbow K: Characterization of melanogenesis in mouse and guinea pig hair by chemical analysis of melanins and of free and bound DOPA and 5-S-cysteinylDOPA. *J Invest Dermatol* **83**:12, 1984.
120. Ito S, Fujita K: Microanalysis of eumelanin and pheomelanin in hair and melanomas by chemical degradation and liquid chromatography. *Anal Biochem* **144**:527, 1985.
121. Ito S: Reexamination of the structure of eumelanin. *Biochim Biophys Acta* **883**:155, 1986.
122. Prota G: Pigment cell metabolism: Chemical and enzymatic control, in Veronesi U, Cascinelli N (eds): *Cutaneous Melanoma*. New York, Academic, 1986, pp 233–241.
123. Hearing VJ: Mammalian monophenol monooxygenase (tyrosinase): Purification, properties, and reactions catalyzed. *Methods Enzymol* **142**:154, 1987.
124. Prota G: Progress in the chemistry of melanins and related metabolites. *Med Res Rev* **8**:525, 1988.
125. Prota G: Some new aspects of eumelanin chemistry. *Prog Clin Biol Res* **256**:101, 1988.
126. Körner AM, Pawelek JM: DOPAchrome conversion: A possible control point in melanin biosynthesis. *J Invest Dermatol* **75**:192, 1980.
127. Pawelek JM, Körner AM, Bergstrom A, Bolognia J: New regulators of melanin biosynthesis and the autodestruction of melanoma cells. *Nature* **286**:617, 1980.
128. Hearing VJ, Körner AM, Pawelek JM: New regulators of melanogenesis are associated with purified tyrosinase isozymes. *J Invest Dermatol* **79**:16, 1982.
129. Barber JI, Townsend D, Olds DP, King RA: DOPAchrome oxidoreductase: A new enzyme in the pigment pathway. *J Invest Dermatol* **83**:145, 1984.
130. Leonard LJ, Townsend D, King RA: Function of DOPAchrome oxidoreductase and metal ions in DOPAchrome conversion in the eumelanin pathway. *Biochemistry* **27**:6156, 1988.
131. Aroca P, García-Borrón JC, Solano F, Lozano JA: Regulation of distal mammalian melanogenesis. I. Partial purification and characterization of a DOPAchrome converting factor: DOPAchrome tautomerase. *Biochim Biophys Acta* **1035**:266, 1990.
132. Aroca P, Solano F, García-Borrón JC, Lozano JA: A new spectrophotometric assay for DOPAchrome tautomerase. *J Biochem Biophys Methods* **21**:35, 1990.
133. Pawelek JM: DOPAchrome conversion factor functions as an isomerase. *Biochem Biophys Res Commun* **166**:1328, 1990.
134. Aroca P, Solano F, García-Borrón JC, Lozano JA: Specificity of DOPAchrome tautomerase and inhibition by carboxylated indoles. Consideration on the enzyme active site. *Biochem J* **277**:393, 1991.
135. Palumbo A, Solano F, Misuraca G, Aroca P, García-Borrón JC, Lozano JA, Prota G: Comparative action of DOPAchrome tautomerase and metal ions on the rearrangement of DOPAchrome. *Biochim Biophys Acta* **1115**:1, 1991.
136. Pawelek JM: After DOPAchrome? *Pigment Cell Res* **4**:53, 1991.
137. Tsukamoto K, Jackson IJ, Urabe K, Montague PM, Hearing VJ: A second tyrosinase-related protein, TRP2, is a melanogenic enzyme termed DOPAchrome tautomerase. *EMBO J* **11**:519, 1992.
138. Halprin KM, Ohkawara A: Glutathione and human pigmentation. *Arch Dermatol* **94**:355, 1966.
139. Prota G: Cysteine and glutathione in mammalian pigmentation, in Cavallini D, Gaull G, Zappia V (eds): *Natural Sulfur Compounds*. New York, Plenum, 1980, pp 391–398.
140. Benedetto JP, Ortonne JP, Voulot C, Khatchadourian C, Prota G, Thivolet J: Role of thiol compounds in mammalian melanin pigmentation. II. Glutathione and related enzymatic activities. *J Invest Dermatol* **79**:422, 1982.
141. Mojamdar MV, Ichihashi M, Mishima Y: Effect of DOPA loading on glutathione dependent 5-S-cysteinylDOPAgenesis in melanoma cells in vitro. *J Invest Dermatol* **78**:224, 1982.
142. Lindbladh C, Rorsman H, Rosengren E: The effect of catalase on the inactivation of tyrosinase by ascorbic acid and by cysteine or glutathione. *Acta Derm Venereol Suppl (Stockh)* **63**:209, 1983.
143. Ito S, Palumbo A, Prota G: Tyrosinase-catalyzed conjugation of DOPA with glutathione. *Experientia* **41**:960, 1985.
144. Miranda M, Dillio C, Bonfigli A, Arcadi A, Pitaro G, Dupre S, Federici G, del Boccio G: A study on the in vitro interaction between tyrosinase and glutathione-S-transferase. *Biochim Biophys Acta* **913**:386, 1987.
145. Jara JR, Aroca P, Solano F, Martínez-Liarte JH, Lozano JA: The role of sulfhydryl compounds in mammalian melanogenesis: The effect of cysteine and glutathione upon tyrosinase and the intermediates of the pathway. *Biochim Biophys Acta* **967**:296, 1988.

146. Satoh GJZ, Mishima Y: Tyrosinase inhibitor in Fortners amelanotic and melanotic malignant melanoma. *J Invest Dermatol* **48:**301, 1967.
147. Adachi K, Hu F, Kondo S: A new endogenous inhibitor for mouse melanoma cells. *Biochem Biophys Res Commun* **45:**742, 1971.
148. Menon IA, Haberman HF: Widespread occurrence of inhibitors of melanoma tyrosinase in plant and mammalian tissues. *Experientia* **27:**644, 1971.
149. Imokawa G, Mishima Y: Biochemical characterization of tyrosinase inhibitors using tyrosinase binding affinity chromatography. *Br J Dermatol* **104:**531, 1981.
150. Kameyama K, Jiménez M, Muller J, Ishida Y, Hearing VJ: Regulation of mammalian melanogenesis by tyrosinase inhibition. *Differentiation* **42:**28, 1989.
151. Kameyama K, Takemura T, Hamada Y, Sakai C, Kondoh S, Nishiyama S, Urabe K, Hearing VJ: Pigment production in murine melanoma cells is regulated by tyrosinase, tyrosinase-related protein 1 (TRP1), DOPAchrome tautomerase (TRP2) and a melanogenic inhibitor. *J Invest Dermatol* **100:**126, 1993.
152. Palumbo A, Misuraca G, d'Ischia M, Prota G: Effect of metal ions on the kinetics of tyrosine oxidation catalysed by tyrosinase. *Biochem J* **228:**647, 1985.
153. Palumbo A, d'Ischia M, Misuraca G, Prota G: Effect of metal ions on the rearrangement of DOPAchrome. *Biochim Biophys Acta* **925:**203, 1987.
154. Palumbo A, d'Ischia M, Misuraca G, Prota G, Schultz TM: Structural modifications in biosynthetic melanins induced by metal ions. *Biochim Biophys Acta* **964:**193, 1988.
155. d'Ischia M, Napolitano A, Prota G: Peroxidase as an alternative to tyrosinase in the oxidative polymerization of 5,6-dihydroxyindoles to melanin(s). *Biochim Biophys Acta* **1073:**423, 1990.
156. Halaban R, Moellmann GE: Murine and human b locus pigmentation genes encode a glycoprotein (gp75) with catalase activity. *Proc Natl Acad Sci USA* **87:**4809, 1990.
157. Palumbo A, d'Ischia M, Misuraca G, Carratu L, Prota G: Activation of mammalian tyrosinase by ferrous ions. *Biochim Biophys Acta* **1033:**256, 1990.
158. Sealy RC, Hyde JS, Felix CC, Menon IA, Prota G: Eumelanins and pheomelanins: Characterization by electron spin resonance spectroscopy. *Science* **217:**545, 1982.
159. Sato C, Ito S, Takeuchi T: Establishment of a mouse melanocyte clone which synthesizes both eumelanin and pheomelanin. *Cell Struct Funct* **10:**421, 1985.
160. Ahene AB, Chedekal MR, Koch WH, Maldonado W: Analysis and quantification of pheomelanins by radioimmunoassay. *Pigment Cell Res* **1:**326, 1988.
161. Thody AJ, Higgins EM, Wakamatsu K, Ito S, Burchill SA, Marks JM: Pheomelanin as well as eumelanin is present in human epidermis. *J Invest Dermatol* **97:**340, 1991.
162. Aubert C, Rosengren E, Rorsman H, Rouge F: Differentiation of melanocytes in culture of primary malignant melanoma indicated by 5-S-cysteinylDOPA formation. *J Natl Cancer Inst* **55:**1327, 1975.
163. Agrup C, Falck B, Rorsman H, Rosengren AM, Rosengren E: Intracellular distribution of DOPA and 5-S-cysteinyl-DOPA in Harding Passey melanoma. *Acta Derm Venereol Suppl (Stockh)* **57:**313, 1977.
164. Ito S, Novellino E, Chioccara F, Misuraca G, Prota G: Co-polymerization of DOPA and cysteinylDOPA in melanogenesis in vitro. *Experientia* **36:**822, 1980.
165. Agrup G, Hansson C, Rorsman H, Rosengren E: The effect of cysteine on oxidation of tyrosine, DOPA, and cysteinylDOPAs. *Arch Dermatol Res* **272:**103, 1982.
166. Mojamdar MV, Ichihashi M, Mishima Y: γ-Glutamyl transpeptidase, tyrosinase, and 5-S-cysteinylDOPA production in melanoma cells. *J Invest Dermatol* **81:**119, 1983.
167. Thompson A, Land EJ, Chedekal MR, Subbarao KV, Truscott TG: A pulse radiolysis investigation of the oxidation of the melanin precursors 3,4-dihydroxyphenylalanine (DOPA) and cysteinylDOPAs. *Biochim Biophys Acta* **843:**49, 1985.
168. Jiménez M, García-Cánovas F, Carcía-Carmona F, Iborra JL, Lozano JA: Kinetics and stoichiometry of cysteinylDOPA formation in the first steps of melanogenesis. *Int J Biochem* **18:**161, 1986.
169. Kato T, Ito S, Fujita K: Tyrosinase-catalyzed binding of 3,4-dihydroxyphenylalanine with proteins through the sulfhydryl group. *Biochim Biophys Acta* **881:**415, 1986.
170. Ito S, Imai Y, Jimbow K, Fujita K: Incorporation of sulfhydryl compounds into melanins in vitro. *Biochim Biophys Acta* **964:**1, 1988.
171. Körner AM, Gettins P: Synthesis in vitro of 5,6-dihydroxyindole-2-carboxylic acid by DOPAchrome conversion factor from Cloudman S91 melanoma cells. *J Invest Dermatol* **85:**229, 1985.
172. Ito S, Wakamatsu K: Melanin chemistry and melanin precursors in melanoma. *J Invest Dermatol* **92:**261S, 1989.
173. Tsukamoto K, Palumbo A, d'Ischia M, Hearing VJ, Prota G: 5,6-Dihydroxyindole-2-carboxylic acid is incorporated into mammalian melanin. *Biochem J* **286:**491, 1992.
174. Burnett JB, Holstein TJ, Quevedo WC Jr: Electrophoretic variations of tyrosinase in follicular melanocytes during the hair growth cycle in mice. *J Exp Zool* **171:**369, 1969.
175. Sakurai T, Ochiai H, Takeuchi T: Ultrastructural change of melanosomes associated with agouti pattern formation in mouse hair. *Dev Biol* **47:**466, 1975.
176. Movaghar M, Hunt DM: Tyrosinase activity and the expression of the agouti gene in the mouse. *J Exp Zool* **243:**473, 1987.
177. Movaghar M: Tyrosinase activity in the first coat of agouti and black mice. *Pigment Cell Res* **2:**401, 1989.
178. Jackson IJ: Colour-coded switches. *Nature* **362:**587, 1993.
179. Tamate HB, Hirobe T, Wakamatsu K, Ito S, Shibahara S, Ishikawa K: Levels of tyrosinase and its mRNA in coat-color mutants of C57BL/10J congenic mice: Effects of genetic substitution at the agouti, brown, albino, dilute and pink-eyed dilution loci. *J Exp Zool* **250:**304, 1989.
180. Granholm NH, Opbroek AJ, Harvison GA, Kappenman KE: Tyrosinase activity (TH, DO, PAGE-defined isozymes) and melanin production in regenerating hairbulb melanocytes of lethal yellow (A^y/a), black (a/a), agouti (A^{wJ}/A^{wJ}) and albino (a/a/c^{2J}/c^{2J}) mice (C57BL/6J). *Pigment Cell Res* **3:**233, 1990.
181. Murray M, Pawelek JM, Lamoreux ML: New regulatory factors for melanogenesis: Developmental changes in neonatal mice of various genotypes. *Dev Biol* **100:**120, 1983.
182. Lamoreux ML, Woolley C, Pendergast P: Genetic controls over activities of tyrosinase and DOPAchrome conversion factor in murine melanocytes. *Genetics* **113:**967, 1986.
183. Lamoreux ML, Pendergast P: Genetic controls over melanocyte differentiation: Interaction of agouti-locus and albino-locus genetic defects. *J Exp Zool* **243:**71, 1987.
184. Bultman SJ, Michaud EJ, Woychik RP: Molecular characterization of the mouse agouti locus. *Cell* **71:**1195, 1992.
185. Mountjoy KG, Robbins LS, Mortrud MT, Cone RD: The cloning of a family of genes that encode the melanocortin receptors. *Science* **257:**1248, 1992.
186. Carstam R, Edner C, Hansson C, Lindbladh C, Rorsman H, Rosengren E: Metabolism of 5-S-glutathionylDOPA. *Acta Derm Venereol* **126:**1, 1986.
187. Rorsman H, Pavel S: Metabolic markers and melanoma, in Cascinelli N, Santinami M, Veronesi U (eds): *Cutaneous Melanoma: Biology and Management*. Milan, Masson, 1990, pp 79–82.
188. Jimbow K, Ishida O, Ito S, Hori Y, Witkop CJ, King RA: Combined chemical and electron microscopic studies of pheomelanosomes in human red hair. *J Invest Dermatol* **81:**506, 1983.
189. Jimbow K, Oikawa O, Sugiyama S, Takeuchi T: Comparison of eumelanogenesis and pheomelanogenesis in retinal and follicular melanocytes: Role of vesiculo-globular bodies in melanosome differentiation. *J Invest Dermatol* **73:**278, 1979.
190. Körner AM, Pawelek JM: Mammalian tyrosinase catalyzes three reactions in the biosynthesis of melanin. *Science* **217:**1163, 1982.
191. Jergil B, Lindbladh C, Rorsman H, Rosengren E: DOPA oxidation and tyrosine oxygenation by human melanoma tyrosinase. *Acta Derm Venereol Suppl* **63:**468, 1983.
192. Townsend D, Guillery P, King RA: Optimized assay for mammalian tyrosinase (polyhydroxyl phenyloxidase). *Anal Biochem* **139:**345, 1984.
193. Townsend D, Olds DP, King RA: DOPA oxidase activity in human hairbulbs measured by high-performance liquid chromatography. *J Invest Dermatol* **86:**570, 1986.

194. Winder AJ, Harris H: New assays for the tyrosine hydroxylase and DOPA oxidase activities of tyrosine. *Eur J Biochem* **198**:317, 1991.
195. Tripathi RK, Hearing VJ, Urabe K, Aroca P, Spritz RA: Mutational mapping of the catalytic activities of human tyrosinase. *J Biol Chem* **267**:23707, 1992.
196. Hearing VJ, Ekel TM, Montague PM, Hearing ED, Nicholson JM: Mammalian tyrosinase: Isolation by a simple new procedure and characterization of its steric requirements for cofactor activity. *Arch Biochem Biophys* **185**:407, 1978.
197. Hearing VJ, Ekel TM, Montague PM, Nicholson JM: Mammalian tyrosinase. Stoichiometry and measurement of reaction products. *Biochim Biophys Acta* **611**:251, 1980.
198. Devi CC, Tripathi C, Ramaiah A: pH-dependent interconvertible allosteric forms of murine melanoma tyrosinase: Physiological implications. *Eur J Biochem* **166**:705, 1987.
199. Tripathi RK, Devi CC, Ramaiah A: pH-Dependent interconversion of two forms of tyrosinase in human skin. *Biochem J* **252**:481, 1988.
200. King RA, Olds DP: Electrophoretic pattern of human hairbulb tyrosinase. *J Invest Dermatol* **77**:201, 1981.
201. Tsukamoto K, Jiménez M, Hearing VJ: The nature of tyrosinase isozymes, in Mishima Y (ed): *The Pigment Cell: From the Molecular to the Clinical Level*. Copenhagen, Munksgaard, 1992, pp 84–89.
202. Palumbo A, d'Ischia M, Crescenzi O, Prota G: Isolation of a new intermediate in the oxidative conversion of 5,6-dihydroxyindole-2-carboxylic acid to melanin. *Tetrahedron Lett* **28**:467, 1987.
203. Jackson IJ, Chambers DM, Tsukamoto K, Copeland NG, Gilbert DJ, Jenkins NA, Hearing VJ: A second tyrosinase-related protein, TRP2, maps to and is mutated at the mouse slaty locus. *EMBO J* **11**:527, 1992.
204. Steel KP, Davidson DR, Jackson IJ: TRP2/DT, a new early melanoblast marker, shows that steel growth factor (c-kit ligand) is a survival factor. *Development* **115**:1111, 1992.
205. Ohkura T, Yamashita K, Mishima Y, Kobata A: Purification of hamster melanoma tyrosinases and structural studies of their asparagine linked sugar chains. *Arch Biochem Biophys* **235**:63, 1984.
206. Aroca P, Martínez-Liarte JH, Solano F, García-Borrón JC, Lozano JA: The action of glycosylases on DOPAchrome tautomerase. *Biochem J* **284**:109, 1992.
207. Martínez-Liarte JH, Solano F, García-Borrón JC, Jara JR, Lozano JA: α-MSH and other melanogenic activators mediate opposite effects on tyrosinase and DOPAchrome tautomerase in B16/F10 mouse melanoma cells. *J Invest Dermatol* **99**:435, 1992.
208. Tsukamoto K, Urabe K, Kameyama K, Hearing VJ: The tyrosinase gene family: Interactions of melanogenic proteins to regulate melanogenesis. *Proc Natl Acad Sci USA* (in preparation 1993).
209. Aroca P, Urabe K, Kabayashi T, Tsukamoto K, Hearing VJ: Melanin biosynthesis patterns following hormonal stimulation. *J Biol Chem* **268**:25650, 1993.
210. Chakraborty AK, Pawelek JM: Evidence that DOPAchrome conversion factor is a metalloenzyme. *Pigment Cell Res* **4**:132, 1991.
211. Hu F, Buxman MM: γ-Glutamyl transpeptidase in the pigment cells of rhesus eyes. *J Invest Dermatol* **76**:371, 1981.
212. Hu F: Theophylline and melanocyte-stimulating hormone effects on γ-glutamyl transpeptidase and DOPA reactions in cultured melanoma cells. *J Invest Dermatol* **79**:57, 1982.
213. Mojamdar MV, Ichihashi M, Mishima Y: Tyrosinase and γ-glutamyl transpeptidase in 5-S-cysteinylDOPAgenesis within melanotic and amelanotic membranes. *J Dermatol* **9**:73, 1982.
214. Chakraborty C, Hatta S, Ichihashi M, Hayashibe K, Mishima Y: Effects of L-glutamine on tyrosinase and τ-glutamyl transpeptidase of B-16 melanoma cells in culture. *J Dermatol* **15**:1, 1988.
215. Mondal M, Banerjee PK: Role of peroxidase in melanogenesis: Search for a control mechanism. *Int J Biochem Biophys* **18**:380, 1981.
216. Hearing VJ, Tsukamoto K, Urabe K, Kameyama K, Montague PM, Jackson IJ: Functional properties of cloned melanogenic proteins. *Pigment Cell Res* **5**:264, 1992.
217. Chakraborty AK, Park KC, Kwon BS, Hearing VJ, Pawelek JM: Stablin activity is associated with Pmel-17 gene expression. *Pigment Cell Res* **5**:84, 1992. (abstr)
218. Pawelek JM, Chakraborty AK, Pavlovich M, Osber MP, Grove K, Min K, Myerson N, Orlow SJ, Bolognia J: Stablins: Ubiquitous indole stabilizing factors. *Pigment Cell Res* **5**:91, 1992. (abstr)
219. Fuller BB, Iman DS, Lunsford JB: Comparison of tyrosinase levels in amelanotic and melanotic melanoma cell cultures by a competitive enzyme-linked immunosorbent assay and by immunotitration analysis. *J Cell Physiol* **134**:149, 1988.
220. Naeyaert JM, Eller M, Gordon PR, Park HY, Gilchrest BA: Pigment content of cultured human melanocytes does not correlate with tyrosinase message level. *Br J Dermatol* **125**:297, 1991.
221. Slominski A, Constantino R: L-tyrisone induces tyrosinase expression via a posttranslational mechanism. *Experientia* **47**:721, 1991.
222. Slominski A, Costantino R, Howe J, Moellmann GE: Molecular mechanisms governing melanogenesis in hamster melanomas: Relative abundance of tyrosinase and catalase-B (gp75). *Anticancer Res* **11**:257, 1991.
223. Barber JI, Townsend D, Olds DP, King RA: Decreased DOPAchrome oxidoreductase activity in yellow mice. *J Hered* **76**:59, 1985.
224. Yamamoto H, Takeuchi S, Kudo T, Makino K, Nakata A, Shinoda T, Takeuchi T: Cloning and sequencing of mouse tyrosinase cDNA. *Jpn J Genet* **62**:271, 1987.
225. Kwon BS, Haq AK, Pomerantz SH, Halaban R: Isolation and sequence of a cDNA locus for human tyrosinase that maps at the mouse c-albino locus. *Proc Natl Acad Sci USA* **84**:7473, 1987.
226. Wittbjer A, Dahlback B, Odh G, Rosengren AM, Rosengren E, Rorsman H: Isolation of human tyrosinase from cultured melanoma cells. *Acta Derm Venereol Suppl (Stockh)* **69**:125, 1989.
227. Wittbjer A, Odh G, Rosengren AM, Rosengren E, Rorsman H: Isolation of soluble tyrosinase from human melanoma cells. *Acta Derm Venereol Suppl (Stockh)* **70**:291, 1990.
228. Bouchard B, Fuller BB, Vijayasaradhi S, Houghton AN: Induction of pigmentation in mouse fibroblasts by expression of human tyrosinase cDNA. *J Exp Med* **169**:2029, 1989.
229. Barton DE, Kwon BS, Francke U: Human tyrosinase gene, mapped to chromosome 11 (q14→q21), defines second region of homology with mouse chromosome 7. *Genomics* **3**:17, 1988.
230. Ruppert S, Müller G, Kwon BS, Schütz G: Multiple transcripts of the mouse tyrosinase gene are generated by alternative splicing. *EMBO J* **7**:2715, 1988.
231. Giebel LB, Strunk KM, Spritz RA: Organization and nucleotide sequences of the human tyrosinase gene and a truncated tyrosinase-related segment. *Genomics* **9**:435, 1991.
232. Kikuchi H, Miura H, Yamamoto H, Takeuchi T, Dei T, Watanabe M: Characteristic sequences in the upstream of the human tyrosinase gene. *Biochim Biophys Acta* **1009**:283, 1989.
233. Morris SW, Muir W, St Clair D: Dinucleotide repeat polymorphism at the human tyrosinase gene. *Nucleic Acids Res* **19**:6968, 1991.
234. Oetting WS, Witkop CJ, Brown SA, Colomer R, Fryer JP, Bloom KE, King RA: A frequent mutation in the tyrosinase gene associated with type I-A (tyrosinase-negative) oculocutaneous albinism in Puerto Rico. *Am J Hum Genet* **52**:17, 1993.
235. Beermann F, Schmid E, Ganss R, Schütz G, Ruppert S: Molecular characterization of the mouse tyrosinase gene: Pigment cell specific expresion in transgenic mice. *Pigment Cell Res* **5**:295, 1992.
236. Kluppel M, Beermann F, Fuppert S, Schmid E, Hummler E, Schütz G: The mouse tyrosinase promoter is sufficient for expression in melanocytes and in the pigmented epithelium of the retina. *Proc Natl Acad Sci USA* **88**:3777, 1991.
237. Tanaka S, Yamamoto H, Takeuchi S, Takeuchi T: Melanization in albino mice transformed by introducing cloned mouse tyrosinase gene. *Development* **108**:223, 1990.

238. Beermann F, Ruppert S, Hummler E, Bosch FX, Müller G, Ruther U, Schütz G: Rescue of the albino phenotype by introduction of a functional tyrosinase gene into mice. *EMBO J* **9**:2819, 1990.
239. Bradl M, Larue L, Mintz B: Clonal coat color variation due to a transforming gene expressed in melanocytes of trangenic mice. *Proc Natl Acad Sci USA* **88**:6447, 1991.
240. Mintz B, Bradl M: Mosaic expression of a tyrosinase fusion gene in albino mice yields a heritable striped coat color pattern in transgenic homozygotes. *Proc Natl Acad Sci USA* **88**:9643, 1991.
241. Schedl A, Beerman F, Thies E, Montoliu L, Kelsey G, Schütz G: Transgenic mice generated by pronuclear injection of a yeast artificial chromosome. *Nucleic Acids Res* **20**:3073, 1992.
242. Schedl A, Montollu L, Kelsey G, Schütz G: A yeast artificial chromosome covering the tyrosinase gene confers copy number-dependent expression in transgenic mice. *Nature* **362**:258, 1993.
243. Winder AJ: Expression of a mouse tyrosinase cDNA in 3T3 Swiss mouse fibroblasts. *Biochem Biophys Res Commun* **178**:739, 1991.
244. Müller G, Ruppert S, Schmid E, Schütz G: Functional analysis of alternatively spliced tyrosinase gene transcripts. *EMBO J* **7**:2723, 1988.
245. Terao M, Tabe L, Garattini E, Sartori D, Studer M, Mintz B: Isolation and characterization of variant cDNAs encoding mouse tyrosinase. *Biochem Biophys Res Commun* **159**:848, 1989.
246. Porter S, Mintz B: Multiple alternatively spliced transcripts of the mouse tyrosinase-encoding gene. *Gene* **97**:277, 1991.
247. Shibahara S, Tomita Y, Tagami H, Muller RM, Cohen T: Molecular basis for the heterogeneity of human tyrosinase. *Tohoku J Exp Med* **156**:403, 1988.
248. Kobayashi K, Kaneda N, Ichinose H, Kishi F, Nakazawa A, Kurosawa Y, Fujita K, Nagatsu T: Structure of the human tyrosine hydroxylase gene: Alternative splicing from a single gene accounts for generation of four mRNA types. *J Biochem* **103**:907, 1988.
249. Sutcliffe JG, Milner RJ: Alternative mRNA splicing: The *Shaker* gene. *Trends Genet* **4**:297, 1988.
250. Giebel LB, Spritz RA: RFLP for Mbol in the human tyrosinase (TYR) gene detected by PCR. *Nucleic Acids Res* **18**:3103, 1990.
251. Johnston JD, Winder AJ, Breimer LH: An Mbol polymorphism at codon 192 of the human tyrosinase gene is present in Asians and Afrocaribbeans. *Nucleic Acids Res* **20**:1433, 1992.
252. Tripathi RK, Giebel LB, Strunk KM, Spritz RA: A polymorphism of the human tyrosinase gene is associated with temperature-sensitive enzymatic activity. *Gene Express* **1**:103, 1991.
253. Oetting WS, Roed CM, Mentink MM, King RA: PCR detection of a Taql polymorphism at the CCAATT box of the human tyrosinase (TYR) gene. *Nucleic Acids Res* **19**:5800, 1991.
254. Spritz RA, Strunk KM, Oetting WS, King RA: RFLP for Taql at the human tyrosinase locus. *Nucleic Acids Res* **16**:9890, 1988.
255. Spritz RA, Strunk KM: RFLP for BglII at the human tyrosinase (TYR) locus. *Nucleic Acids Res* **18**:3672, 1990.
256. Takeda A, Matsunaga J, Tomita Y, Tagami H, Shibahara S: Molecular analysis of the DNA segments cross-hybridize to the tyrosinase gene in patients afflicted with oculocutaneous albinism. *Tohoku J Exp Med* **159**:333, 1989.
257. Takeda A, Matsunaga J, Tomita Y, Tagami H, Shibahara S: Nucleotide sequence of the putative human tyrosinase pseudogene. *Tohoku J Exp Med* **163**:295, 1991.
258. Oetting WS, Stine OC, Townsend D, King RA: Evolution of the tyrosinase related gene (TYRL) in primates. *Pigment Cell Res* **6**:171, 1993.
259. Jackson IJ: cDNA encoding tyrosinase-related protein maps to the brown locus in mice. *Proc Natl Acad Sci USA* **85**:4392, 1988.
260. Jackson IJ, Chambers DM, Rinchik EM, Bennett DC: Characterization of TRP-1 mRNA levels in dominant and recessive mutations at the mouse brown (b) locus. *Genetics* **126**:451, 1990.
261. Green MC: Slaty (slt). *Mouse News Lett* **47**:36, 1972.
262. Aroca P, Solano F, García-Borrón JC, Salinas C, Lozano JA: Regulation of the final phase of mammalian melanogenesis. The role of DOPAchrome tautomerase and the ratio of DHICA/DHI. *Eur J Biochem* **208**:155, 1992.
263. Shibahara S, Tomita Y, Sakakura T, Nager C, Chaudhuri B, Muller R: Cloning and expression of cDNA encoding mouse tyrosinase. *Nucleic Acids Res* **14**:2413, 1986.
264. Shibahara S, Taguchi H, Muller RM, Shibata K, Cohen T, Tomita Y, Tagami H: Structural organization of the pigment cell-specific gene located at the brown locus in mouse. Its promoter activity and alternatively spliced transcript. *J Biol Chem* **266**:15895, 1991.
265. Zdarsky E, Favor J, Jackson IJ: The molecular basis of brown, an old mouse mutation, and of an induced revertant to wild-type. *Genetics* **126**:443, 1990.
266. Johnson R, Jackson IJ: Light is a dominant mouse mutation resulting in premature cell death. *Nat Genet* **1**:226, 1992.
267. Cohen T, Muller RM, Tomita Y, Shibahara S: Nucleotide sequence of the cDNA encoding human tyrosinase-related protein. *Nucleic Acids Res* **18**:2807, 1990.
268. Urquhart A: Human tyrosinase-like protein (TYRL) carboxy terminus: Closer homology with the mouse protein than previously reported. *Nucleic Acids Res* **19**:5803, 1993.
269. Murty VVVS, Bouchard B, Mathew S, Vijayasaradhi S, Houghton AN: Assignment of the Human *TYRP* (brown) locus to chromosome region 9p23 by nonradioactive *in situ* hybridization. *Genomics* **13**:227, 1992.
270. Jackson IJ, Chambers DM, Budd PS, Johnson R: The tyrosinase-related protein-1 gene has a structure and promoter sequence very different from tyrosinase. *Nucleic Acids Res* **19**:3799, 1991.
271. Shibata K, Takeda K, Tomita Y, Tagami H, Shibahara S: Downstream region of the human tyrosinase-related protein gene enhances its promoter activity. *Biochem Biophys Res Commun* **184**:568, 1992.
272. Lowings P, Yavuzer U, Goding CR: Positive and negative elements regulate a melanocyte-specific promoter. *Mol Cell Biol* **12**:3653, 1992.
273. Vijayasaradhi S, Houghton AN: Purification of an autoantigenic 75-kDa melanosomal glycoprotein. *Int J Cancer* **47**:298, 1991.
274. Tai T, Eisinger M, Ogata S, Lloyd KO: Glycoproteins as differentiation markers in human malignant melanoma and melanocytes. *Cancer Res* **43**:2773, 1983.
275. Thomson TM, Mattes MJ, Roux L, Old LJ, Lloyd KO: Pigmentation-associated glycoprotein of human melanoma and melanocytes: Definition with a mouse monoclonal anitbody. *J Invest Dermatol* **85**:169, 1985.
276. Jiménez M, Tsukamoto K, Hearing VJ: Tyrosinases from two different loci are expressed by normal and by transformed melanocytes. *J Biol Chem* **266**:1147, 1991.
277. Tsukamoto K, Urabe K, Kameyama K, Hearing VJ: Interactions of melanogenic proteins in the tyrosinase family to regulate melanogenesis. *Pigment Cell Res* **5**:97, 1992.
278. Chintamaneni CD, Ramsay M, Colman MA, Fox MF, Pickard RT, Kwon BS: Mapping the human CAS2 gene, the homologue of the mouse brown (b) locus, to human chromosome 9p22-pter. *Biochem Biophys Res Commun* **178**:227, 1991.
279. Giacomini P, Fraioli R, Cuomo M, Natali PG: Membrane compartmentalization of melanosomal gp75. *J Invest Dermatol* **98**:340, 1992.
280. Pawelek JM, Chakraborty AK, Orlow SJ: Evidence for a 'melanogenic' complex containing MSH receptors, DOPAchrome conversion factor (DCF), glycoprotein 75 (gp75), lysosome-associated membrane protein-1 (LAMP-1), tyrosinase, and tyrosinase-related protein-2 (TRP-2). *Pigment Cell Res* **4**:132, 1991.
281. Kwon BS, Halaban R, Kim GS, Usack L, Pomerantz SH, Haq AK: A melanocyte-specific complementary DNA clone whose expression is inducible by melanotropin and isobutylmethyl xanthine. *Mol Biol Med* **4**:339, 1987.
282. Kwon BS, Chintamaneni CD, Kozak CA, Copeland

NG, Gilbert DJ, Jenkins NA, Barton DE, Francke U, Kobayashi Y, Kim KK: A melanocyte-specific gene, Pmel 17, maps near the silver coat color locus on mouse chromosome 10 and is a syntenic region on human chromosome 12. *Proc Natl Acad Sci USA* **88**:9228, 1991.

283. Spanakis E, Lamina P, Bennett DC: Effects of the developmental colour mutations silver and recessive spotting on proliferation of diploid and immortal mouse melanocytes in culture. *Development* **114**:675, 1992.

284. Dunn LC, Thigpen LW: The silver mouse: A recessive color variation. *J Hered* **21**:495, 1930.

285. Vogel AM, Esclamodo RM: Identification of a secreted Mr 95,000 glycoprotein in human melanocytes and melanomas by a melanocyte specific monoclonal antibody. *Cancer Res* **48**:1286, 1988.

286. Kim RY, Wistow GJ: The cDNA RPE1 and monoclonal antibody HMB-50 define gene products preferentially expressed in retinal pigment epithelium. *Exp Eye Res* **55**:657, 1992.

287. Mochii M, Takeuchi T, Kodama R, Agata K, Eguchi G: The expression of melanosomal matrix protein in the transdifferentiation of pigmented epithelial cells into lens cells. *Cell Diff* **23**:133, 1988.

288. Mochii M, Agata K, Kobayashi H, Yamamoto TS, Eguchi G: Expression of gene coding for a melanosomal matrix protein transcriptionally regulated in the transdifferentiation of chick embryo pigmented epithelial cells. *Cell Diff* **24**:67, 1988.

289. Mochii M, Agata K, Eguchi G: Complete sequence and expression of cDNA encoding a chicken 115-kDa melanosomal matrix protein. *Pigment Cell Res* **4**:41, 1991.

290. Kwon BS: Pigmentation genes: The tyrosinase gene family and the pmel 17 gene family. *Pigment Cell Res* **100**:134S, 1993.

291. Lyon MF, King TR, Gondo Y, Gardner JM, Nakatsu Y, Eicher EM, Brilliant MH: Genetic and molecular analysis of recessive alleles at the pink-eyed dilution *(p)* locus of the mouse. *Proc Natl Acad Sci USA* **89**:6968, 1992.

292. Brilliant MH: The mouse pink-eyed dilution locus: A model for aspects of Prader-Willi syndrome, Angelman syndrome and a form of hypomelanosis of Ito. *Mammal Genome* **3**:187, 1992.

293. Gardner JM, Nakatsu Y, Gondo Y, Lee S, Lyon MF, King RA, Brilliant MH: The mouse pink-eyed dilution gene: Association with human Prader-Willi and Angelman syndromes. *Science* **257**:1121, 1992.

294. Ramsay M, Colman MA, Stevens G, Zwane E, Kromberg J, Farrah M, Jenkins T: The tyrosinase-positive oculocutaneous albinism locus maps to chromosome 15q11.2-q12. *Am J Hum Genet* **51**:879, 1992.

295. Rinchik EM, Bultman SJ, Horsthemke B, Lee ST, Strunk KM, Spritz RA, Avidano KM, John MTC, Nicholls RD: A gene for the mouse pink-eyed dilution locus and for human type II oculocutaneous albinism. *Nature* **361**:72, 1993.

296. Halaban R, Pomerantz SH, Marshall S, Lambert DT, Lerner AB: Regulation of tyrosinase in human melanocytes grown in culture. *J Cell Biol* **97**:480, 1983.

297. Tatro JB, Entwistle ML, Lester BR, Reichlin S: Melanotropin receptors of murine melanoma characterized in cultured cells and demonstrated in experimental tumors in situ. *Cancer Res* **50**:1237, 1990.

298. Pawelek JM: Evidence suggesting that a cyclic AMP-dependent protein kinase is a positive regulator of proliferation in Cloudman S91 melanoma cells. *J Cell Physiol* **98**:619, 1979.

299. Pawelek JM: Studies on the Cloudman melanoma cell line as a model for the action of MSH. *Yale J Biol Med* **58**:571, 1985.

300. Chhajlani V, Wikberg JES: Molecular cloning and expression of the human melanocyte stimulating hormone receptor cDNA. *FEBS Lett* **309**:417, 1992.

301. Robbins LS, Nadeau JH, Johnson KR, Kelly MA, Roselli-Rehfuss L, Baack E, Mountjoy KG, Cone RD: Pigmentation phenotypes of variant extension locus alleles result from point mutations that alter MSH receptor function. *Cell* **72**:827, 1993.

302. Miller MW, Duhl DMJ, Vrieling H, Cordes SP, Ollmann MM, Winkes BM, Barsh GS: Cloning of the mouse *agouti* gene predicts a secreted protein ubiquitously expressed in mice carrying the *lethal yellow* mutation. *Genes Dev* **7**:454, 1993.

303. Jackson IJ: Mouse coat colour mutations: A molecular genetic resource which spans the centuries. *Bioessays* **13**:439, 1991.

304. Geissler EN, Ryan MA, Houseman DE: The dominant-white spotting (W) locus of the mouse encodes the c-kit proto-oncogene. *Cell* **55**:185, 1988.

305. Chabot B, Stephenson DA, Chapman VM, Besmer P, Bernstein A: The proto-oncogene c-kit encoding a transmembrane tyrosine kinase receptor maps to the mouse W locus. *Nature* **335**:88, 1988.

306. Hoo JJ, Haslam RHA, van Orman C: Tentative assignment of piebald trait gene to chromosome band 4q12. *Hum Genet* **73**:230, 1986.

307. Yarden Y, Kuang W-J, Yang-Feng T, Coussens L, Munemitsu S, Dull TJ, Chen E, Schlessinger J, Francke U, Ullrich A: Human proto-oncogene *c-kit:* A new cell surface receptor tyrosine kinase for an unidentified ligand. *EMBO J* **6**:3341, 1987.

308. Giebel LB, Spritz RA: Mutation of the *KIT* (mast/stem cell growth factor receptor) protooncogene in human piebaldism. *Proc Natl Acad Sci USA* **88**:8696, 1991.

309. Fleischman RA, Saltman DL, Stastny V, Zneimer S: Deletion of the *c-kit* protooncogene in the human developmental defect piebald trait. *Proc Natl Acad Sci USA* **88**:10885, 1991.

310. Spritz RA, Giebel LB, Holmes SA: Dominant negative and loss of function mutations of the c-kit (mast/stem cell growth factor receptor) proto-oncogene in human piebaldims. *Am J Hum Genet* **50**:261, 1992.

310a. Spritz RA, Holmes SA, Ramesar R, Greenberg J, Curtis D, Beighton P: Mutations of the *KIT* (mast/stem cell growth factor receptor) proto-oncogene account for a continuous range of phenotypes in human piebaldism. *Am J Hum Genet* **51**:1058, 1992.

311. Fleischman RA: Human piebald trait resulting from a dominant negative mutant allele of the *c-kit* membrane receptor gene. *J Clin Invest* **89**:1713, 1992.

312. Spritz RA: Lack of apparent hematologic abnormalities in human patients with *c-kit* (stem cell factor receptor) gene mutations. *Blood* **79**:2497, 1992.

313. Williams DE, Eisenman J, Baird A, Rauch C, Van Ness K, March CJ, Park LS, Martin U, Mochizuki DY, Boswell HS, Burgess GS, Cosman D, Lyman SD: Identification of a ligand for the *c-kit* proto-oncogene. *Cell* **63**:167, 1990.

314. Flanagan JG, Leder P: The kit ligand: A cell surface molecule altered in steel mutant fibroblasts. *Cell* **63**:185, 1990.

315. Zsebo KM, Williams DA, Gelssler EN, Broudy VC, Martin FH, Atkins HL, Hsu RY, Burkett NC, Okino KH, Murdock DC, Jacobsen FW, Langley KE, Smith KA, Takeishi T, Cattanach BM, Galli SJ, Suggs SV: Stem cell factor is encoded at the SI locus of the mouse and is the ligand for the c-kit tyrosine kinase receptor. *Cell* **63**:213, 1990.

316. Huang E, Nocka K, Beler DR, Chu TY, Buck J, Lahm HW, Wellner D, Leder P, Besmer P: The hematopoietic growth factor KL is encoded by the SI locus and is the ligand of the c-kit receptor, the gene product of the W locus. *Cell* **63**:225, 1990.

317. Asher JH, Friedman TB: Mouse and hamster mutant as models for Waardenburg syndromes in humans. *J Med Genet* **27**:618, 1990.

318. Moase CE, Trasler DG: Splotch locus mouse mutants: Models for neural tube defects and Waardenburg syndrome type I in humans. *J Med Genet* **29**:145, 1992.

319. Tassabehji M, Read AP, Newton VE, Harris R, Balling R, Gruss P, Strachan T: Waardenburg's syndrome patients have mutations in the human homologue of the Pax-3 paired box gene. *Nature* **355**:635, 1992.

320. Baldwin CT, Hoth CF, Amos JA, daSilva EO, Milunsky A: An exonic mutation in the HuP2 paired domain gene causes Waardenburg's syndrome. *Nature* **355**:637, 1992.

321. Steel KP, Smith RJH: Normal hearing in Splotch (Sp/+), the mouse homologue of Waardengburg syndrome type 1. *Nat Genet* **2**:75, 1992.

322. Epstein DJ, Vekemans M, Gros P: Splotch (Sp2H), a mutation affecting development of the mouse neural tube, shows a deletion within the paired homeodomain of Pax-3. *Cell* **67**:767, 1991.
323. Burri M, Tromvoukis Y, Bopp D, Frigerio G, Noll M: Conservation of the paired domain in metazoans and its structure in three isolated human genes. *EMBO J* **8**:1183, 1989.
324. Morell R, Friedman TB, Moeljopawiro S, Hartono, Soewito, Asher JH Jr: A frameshift mutation in the HuP2 paired domain of the probable human homolog of murine *Pax-3* is responsible for Waardenburg syndrome type 1 in an Indonesian family. *Hum Mol Genet* **1**:243, 1992.
325. Mercer JA, Seperack PK, Strobel MC, Copeland NG, Jenkins NA: Novel myosin heavy chain encoded by murine dilute coat color locus. *Nature* **349**:709, 1991.
326. Mayerson PL, Brumbaugh JA: Lavender, a chick melanocyte mutant with defective melanosome translocation: A possible role for 10 nm filaments and microfilaments but not microtubules. *J Cell Sci* **51**:25, 1981.
327. Reddington M, Novak EK, Hurley E, Medda C, McGarry MP, Swank RT: Immature dense granules in platelets from mice with platelet storage pool disease. *Blood* **69**:1300, 1987.
328. Holcombe RF, Stephenson DA, Zweidler A, Stewart RM, Chapman VM, Seidman JG: Linkage of loci associated with two pigment mutations on mouse chromosome 13. *Genet Res* **58**:41, 1991.
329. Swank RT, Reddington M, Howlett O, Novak EK: Platelet storage pool deficiency associated with inherited abnormalities of the inner ear in the mouse pigment mutants muted and mocha. *Blood* **78**:2036, 1991.
330. Novak EK, Hui SW, Swank RT: Platelet storage pool deficiency in mouse pigment mutations associated with seven distinct genetic loci. *Blood* **63**:536, 1984.
331. Holcombe RF, Strauss W, Owen FL, Boxer LA, Warren RW, Conley ME, Ferrara J, Leavitt RY, Fauci AS, Taylor BA, Seidman JG: Relationship of the genes for Chediak-Higashi syndrome (beige) and the T-cell Receptor γ chain in mouse and man. *Genomics* **1**:287, 1987.
332. Abadi R, Pascal E: The recognition and management of albinism. *Ophthalmic Physiol Opt* **9**:3, 1989.
333. Kinnear PE, Jay B, Witkop CJ: Albinism. *Surv Ophthalmol* **30**:75, 1985.
334. King RA, Summers CG: Albinism. *Dermatol Clin* **6**:217, 1988.
335. Witkop CJ Jr: Inherited disorders of pigmentation. *Clin Dermatol* **3**:70, 1985.
336. Witkop CJ Jr, White JG, King RA: Oculocutaneous albinism, in Nyhan WL (ed): *Heritable Disorders of Amino Acid Metabolism*. New York, John Wiley, 1974, pp 177–261.
337. Creel DJ, Summers CG, King RA: Visual anomalies associated with albinism. *Ophthalmic Paediatr Genet* **11**:193, 1990.
338. Charles SJ, Moore AT, Grant JW, Yates JRW: Genetic counseling in X-linked ocular albinism. Clinical features of the carrier state. *Eye* **6**:75, 1992.
339. Rodrigues MM, Hackett J, Donohoo P: Iris, in Duane TD, Jaeger EA (eds): *Biomedical Foundations of Ophthalmology*. Hagerstown, MD, Harper & Row, 1986, chap 11, pp 1–18.
340. Krill AE: Albinism, in Krill A (ed): *Krill's Hereditary Retinal and Choroidal Diseases*. Hagerstown, MD, Harper & Row, 1977, pp 645–663.
341. Wirtschafter JD, Denslow GT, Shine IB: Quantification of iris translucency in albinism. *Arch Ophthalmol* **90**:274, 1973.
342. Donaldson DD: Transillumination of the iris, in *Transactions of the American Ophthalmological Society*. Rochester, MN, Whiting, 1975, pp 89–106.
343. Zinn KM, Benjamin-Henkind J: Retinal pigment epithelium, in Duane TD, Jaeger EA (eds): *Biomedical Foundations of Ophthalmology*. Hagerstown, MD, Harper & Row, 1986, chap 21, pp 1–20.
344. Summers CG, Knobloch WH, Witkop CJ, King RA: Hermansky-Pudlak syndrome: Ophthalmic findings. *Ophthalmology* **95**:545, 1988.
345. Usher CH: Histological examination of an adult human albino's eyeball, with a note on mesoblastic pigmentation in foetal eyes. *Biometrika* **13**:46, 1920.
346. Fulton AB, Albert DM, Craft JL: Human albinism. Light and electron microscopy study. *Arch Ophthalmol* **96**:305, 1978.
347. Wack MA, Peachey NS, Fishman GA: Electroretinographic findings in human oculocutaneous albinism. *Ophthalmology* **96**:1778, 1989.
348. Summers CG, Creel DJ, Townsend D, King RA: Variable expression of vision in sibs with albinism. *Am J Med Genet* **40**:327, 1991.
349. Abadi RV, Dickinson CM: Monochromatic fundus photography of human albinos. *Arch Ophthalmol* **101**:1706, 1983.
350. Adler JE: Histological examination of a case of albinism. *Biometrika* **7**:237, 1910.
351. Lourenco PE, Fishman GA, Anderson RJ: Color vision in albino subjects. *Doc Ophthalmol* **55**:341, 1983.
352. Pickford RW, Taylor WOG: Colour vision of two albinos. *Br J Ophthalmol* **52**:640, 1968.
353. Creel DJ, Witkop CJ, King RA: Assymetric visually evoked potentials in human albinos: Evidence for visual system anomalies. *Invest Ophthalmol* **13**:430, 1974.
354. Creel D, O'Donnell FE, Witkop CJ: Visual system anomalies in human ocular albinos. *Science* **201**:931, 1978.
355. Collewijn H, Apkarian P, Spekreijse H: The oculomotor behaviour of human albinos. *Brain* **108**:1, 1985.
356. van Dorp DB: Albinism, or the NOACH Syndrome (The book of Encoh c.v. 1-20). *Clin Genet* **31**:228, 1987.
357. Creel DJ: Inappropriate use of albino animals as models in research. *Pharmacol Biochem Behav* **12**:969, 1980.
358. Guillery RW, Okoro AN, Witkop CJ: Abnormal visual pathways in the brain of a human albino. *Brain Res* **96**:373, 1975.
359. Guillery RW: Visual pathways in albinos. *Sci Am* **230**:44, 1974.
360. Creel DJ, Spekreijse H, Reits D: Evoked potentials in albinos: Efficacy of pattern stimuli in detecting misrouted optic fibers. *Electroencephalogr Clin Neurophysiol* **52**:595, 1981.
361. Apkarian P, Eckhardt PG, van Schooneveld MJ: Detection of optic pathway misrouting in the human albino neonate. *Neuropediatrics* **22**:211, 1990.
362. Apkarian P, Eckhardt PG, van Schooneveld MJ: Detection of optic pathway misrouting in the human albino neonate. *Neuropediatrics* **22**:211, 1991.
363. Shallo-Hoffmann J, Apkarian P: Visual evoked response asymmetry only in the albino member of a family with congenital nystagmus. *Invest Ophthalmol Vis Sci* **34**:682, 1993.
364. Cheong PYY, Bateman JB, King RA: Oculocutaneous albinism: Variable expressivity of nystagmus in a sibship. *J Pediatr Ophthalmol Strabismus* **29**:185, 1992.
365. Castronuovo S, Simon JW, Kandel GL, Morier A, Wolf B, Witkop CJ, Jenkins PL: Variable expression of albinism within a single kindred. *Am J Ophthalmol* **111**:419, 1991.
366. Abramov I, Gordon J, Hendrickson A, Hainline L, Dobson V, LaBossiere E: The retina of the newborn human infant. *Science* **217**:265, 1982.
367. Hoyt CS: Nystagmus and other abnormal ocular movements in children. *Pediatr Clin North Am* **34**:1415, 1987.
368. Abadi RV, Pascal E: Visual resolution limits in human albinism. *Vision Res* **31**:1445, 1991.
369. Abadi RV, Dickinson CM, Pascal E, Papas E: Retinal image quality in albinos. A review. *Ophthalmic Paediatr Genet* **11**:171, 1990.
370. Silver J, Sapiro J: Axonal guidance during development of the optic nerve: The role of pigmented epithelia and other extrinsic factors. *J Comp Neurol* **202**:521, 1981.
371. Strongin AC, Guillery RW: The distribution of melanin in the developing optic cup and stalk and its relation to cellular degeneration. *J Neurosci* **1**:1193, 1981.
372. Colello RJ, Jeffery G: Evaluation of the influence of optic stalk melanin on the chiasmatic pathways in the developing rodent visual system. *J Comp Neurol* **305**:304, 1991.
373. Webster MJ, Shatz CJ, Silver J: Abnormal pigmentation and unusual morphogenesis of the optic stalk may be correlated with retinal axon misguidance in embryonic Siamese cats. *J Comp Neurol* **269**:592, 1988.
374. Wizenmann A, Thanos S, Boxberg YV, Bonhoeffer F: Differential reaction of crossing and non-crossing rate retinal axons on cell membrane preparations from the chiasm midline; an in vitro study. *Development* **117**:725, 1993.

375. Conlee JW, Parks TN, Schwartz IR, Creel DJ: Comparative anatomy of melanin pigment in the stria vascularis. *Acta Otolaryngol (Stockh)* **107**:45, 1989.
376. Conlee JW, Jensen RP, Parks TN, Creel DJ: Turn-specific and pigment-dependent differences in the stria vascularis of normal and gentamicin-treated albino and pigmented guinea pigs. *Hearing Res* **55**:57, 1991.
377. Conlee JW, Bennett ML: Turn-specific differences in the endocochlear potential between albino and pigmented guinea pigs. *Hear Res* **65**:141, 1993.
378. Conlee JW, Abdul-Baqi KJ, McCandless GA, Creel DJ: Effects of aging on normal hearing loss and noise-induced threshold shift in albino and pigmented guinea pigs. *Acta Otolaryngol (Stockh)* **106**:64, 1988.
379. Garber SR, Turner CW, Creel D, Witkop CJ Jr: Auditory system abnormalities in human albinos. *Ear Hear* **3**:207, 1982.
380. Barrenas M-L, Lindgren F: The influence of inner ear melanin on susceptibility to TTS in humans. *Scand Audiol* **19**:97, 1990.
381. Creel DJ, Garber SR, King RA, Witkop CJ Jr: Auditory brainstem anomalies in human albinos. *Science* **209**:1253, 1980.
382. Creel DJ, Conlee JW, Parks TN: Auditory brainstem anomalies in albino cats. I. Evoked potential studies. *Brain Res* **260**:1, 1983.
383. Conlee JW, Parks TN, Creel DJ: Reduced neuronal size and dendritic length in the medial superior olivary nucleus of albino rabbits. *Brain Res* **363**:28, 1986.
384. Conlee JW, Parks TN, Romero C, Creel DJ: Auditory brainstem anomalies in albino cats: II. Neuronal atrophy in the superior olive. *J Comp Neurol* **225**:141, 1984.
385. Baker GE, Guillery RW: Evidence for the delayed expression of a brainstem abnormality in albino ferrets. *Exp Brain Res* **74**:658, 1989.
386. Searle AG: *Comparative Genetics of Coat Colour in Mammals*. London, Logos, 1968.
387. Garrod AE: Inborn errors of metabolism, lecture II. *Lancet* **2**:73, 1908.
388. King RA, Witkop CJ: Hairbulb tyrosinase activity in oculocutaneous albinism. *Nature* **263**:69, 1976.
389. King RA, Olds DP: Hairbulb tyrosinase activity in oculocutaneous albinism: Suggestions for pathway control and block location. *Am J Med Genet* **20**:49, 1985.
390. King RA, Witkop CJ: Detection of heterozygotes for tyrosinase negative oculocutaneous albinism by hairbulb tyrosinase assay. *Am J Hum Genet* **29**:164, 1977.
391. Jimbow K, Fitzpatrick TB: Characterization of a new melanosomal structural component—the vesiculo globular body—by conventional transmission, high-voltage and scanning electron microscopy. *J Ultrastruct Res* **48**:269, 1973.
392. Fitzpatrick TB, Miyamoto M, Ishikawa K: The evolution of concepts of melanin biology. *Arch Dermatol* **96**:305, 1967.
393. Seiji M, Shimao K, Birbeck MSC, Fitzpatrick TB: Subcellular localization of melanin biosynthesis. *Ann NY Acad Sci* **100**:497, 1963.
394. Nance WE, Jackson CE, Witkop CJ: Amish albinism: A distinctive autosomal recessive phenotype. *Am J Hum Genet* **22**:579, 1970.
395. Hu F, Hanifin JM, Prescott GH, Tongue AC: Yellow mutant albinism: Cytochemical, ultrastructural, and genetic characterization suggesting multiple allelism. *Am J Hum Genet* **32**:387, 1980.
396. Giebel LB, Tripathi RK, Strunk KM, Hanifin JM, Jackson CE, King RA, Spritz RA: Tyrosinase gene mutations associated with type IB ("yellow") oculocutaneous albinism. *Am J Hum Genet* **48**:1159, 1991.
397. King RA, Wirtschafter JD, Olds DP, Brumbaugh JA: Minimal pigment: A new type of oculocutaneous albinism. *Clin Genet* **29**:42, 1986.
398. Oetting WS, King RA: Molecular basis of type 1 (tyrosinase-related) oculocutaneous albinism: Mutations and polymorphisms of the human tyrosinase gene. *Hum Mut* **2**:1, 1993.
399. Cattanach BM, Rasberry C: Dark-eyed albinism. *Mouse News Lett* **81**:64, 1988.
400. King RA, Townsend D, Oetting WS, Summers CG, Olds DP, White JG, Spritz RA: Temperature-sensitive tyrosinase associated with peripheral pigmentation in oculocutaneous albinism. *J Clin Invest* **87**:1046, 1991.
401. Giebel LB, Strunk KM, King RA, Hanifin JM, Spritz RA: A frequent tyrosinase gene mutation in classic, tyrosinase-negative (Type IA) oculocutaneous albinism. *Proc Natl Acad Sci USA* **87**:3255, 1990.
402. Tomita Y, Takeda A, Okinaga S, Tagami H, Shibahara S: Human oculocutaneous albinism caused by a single base insertion in the tyrosinase gene. *Biochem Biophys Res Commun* **164**:990, 1989.
403. Oetting WS, King RA: Molecular analysis of Type I-A (tyrosinase-negative) oculocutaneous albinism. *Hum Genet* **90**:258, 1992.
404. King RA, Oetting WS: Molecular basis of type IA (tyrosinase negative) oculocutaneous albinism. *Pigment Cell Res Suppl* **2**:19, 1992.
405. King RA, Mentink MM, Oetting WS: Non-random distribution of missense mutations within the human tyrosinase gene in Type 1 (tyrosinase-related) oculocutaneous albinism. *Mol Biol Med* **8**:19, 1991.
406. Oetting WS, Mentink MM, Summers CG, Lewis RA, White JG, King RA: Three different frameshift mutations of the tyrosinase gene in type IA oculocutaneous albinism. *Am J Hum Genet* **49**:199, 1991.
407. Oetting WS, Handoko HY, Mentink MM, Paller AS, White JG, King RA: Molecular analysis of an extended family with type IA (tyrosinase-negative) oculocutaneous albinism. *J Invest Dermatol* **97**:15, 1991.
408. Giebel LB, Tripathi RK, King RA, Spritz RA: A tyrosinase gene missense mutation in temperature-sensitive type I oculocutaneous albinism. *J Clin Invest* **87**:1119, 1991.
409. Tripathi RK, Strunk KM, Giebel LB, Weleber RG, Spritz RA: Tyrosinase gene mutations in Type I (tyrosinase-deficient) oculocutaneous albinism define two clusters of missense substitutions. *Am J Med Genet* **43**:865, 1992.
410. Spritz RA, Strunk KM, Giebel LB, King RA: Detection of mutations in the tyrosinase gene in a patient with Type IA oculocutaneous albinism. *N Engl J Med* **322**:1724, 1990.
411. Giebel LB, Musarella MA, Spritz RA: A nonsense mutation in the tyrosinase gene of Afghan patients with tyrosinase negative (type IA) oculocutaneous albinism. *J Med Genet* **28**:464, 1991.
412. Spritz RA, Strunk KM, Hsieh CL, Sekhon GS, Francke U: Homozygous tyrosinase gene mutation in an American black with tyrosinase-negative (type IA) oculocutaneous albinism. *Am J Hum Genet* **48**:318, 1991.
413. Takeda A, Tomita Y, Matsunaga J, Tagami H, Shibahara S: Molecular basis of tyrosinase-negative oculocutaneous albinism. A single base mutation in the tyrosinase gene causing arginine to glutamine substitution at position 59. *J Biol Chem* **265**:17792, 1990.
414. Chintamaneni CD, Halaban R, Kobayashi Y, Witkop CJ, Kwon BS: A single base insertion in the putative transmembrane domain of the tyrosinase gene as a cause for tyrosinase-negative oculocutaneous albinism. *Proc Natl Acad Sci USA* **88**:5272, 1991.
415. Kikuchi H, Hara S, Ishiguro S, Tamai M, Watanabe M: Detection of point mutation in the tyrosinase gene of a Japanese albino patient by a direct sequencing of amplified DNA. *Hum Genet* **85**:123, 1990.
416. Park KC, Chintamaneni CD, Halaban R, Witkop CJ, Kwon BS: Molecular analyses of a tyrosinase-negative albino family. *Am J Hum Genet* **52**:406, 1993.
417. Oetting WS, Fryer JP, King RA: A dinucleotide deletion ($-\Delta$A115) in the tyrosinase gene responsible for type I-A (tyrosinase negative) oculocutaneous albinism in a Pakistani individual. *Hum Mol Genet* **2**:1993.
418. Iljin VN, Iljin NA: Temperature effects on the color of the Siamese cat. *J Hered* **21**:309, 1930.
419. Volbeda A, Hol WG: Crystal structure of hexameric haemocyanin from Panulirus interruptus refined at 3.2 A resolution. *J Mol Biol* **209**:249, 1989.
420. Oetting WS, King RA: Analysis of mutations in the copper B binding region associated with Type I (tyrosinase-related) oculocutaneous albinism, in Takeuchi T (ed): *Molecular Biology of Pigmentation*. Copenhagen, Munksgaard, 1992, pp 274–278.
421. Shibahara S, Okinaga S, Tomita Y, Takeda A, Yamamoto H, Sato M, Takeuchi T: A point mutation in the

tyrosinase gene of BALB/c albino mouse causing the cysteine to serine substitution at position 85. *Eur J Biochem* **189**:455, 1990.

422. Shibahara S: Mutations of the tyrosinase gene in oculocutaneous albinism. *Pigment Cell Res* **5**:279, 1992.
423. Riordan JF: Arginyl residues and anion binding sites in proteins. *Mol Cell Biochem* **26**:71, 1979.
424. Abadie V, Lyonnet S, Maurin N, Berthelon M, Caillaud C, Giraud F, Mattei J-F, Rey J, Munnich A: CpG dinucleotides are mutation hot spots in phenylketonuria. *Genomics* **5**:936, 1989.
425. Cooper DN, Youssoufian H: The CpG dinucleotide and human genetic disease. *Hum Genet* **78**:151, 1988.
426. Kunkel TA: The mutational specificity of DNA polymerases-α and -γ during *in vitro* DNA synthesis. *J Biol Chem* **260**:12866, 1985.
427. Kunkel TA: Frameshift mutagenesis by eucaryotic DNA polymerases *in Vitro*. *J Biol Chem* **261**:13581, 1986.
428. Streisinger G, Okada Y, Emrich J, Newton J, Tsugita A, Terzaghi E, Inouye M: Frameshift mutations and the genetic code. *Cold Spring Harb Symp Quant Biol* **31**:77, 1966.
429. Streisinger G, Owen J: Mechanisms of spontaneous and induced frameshift mutation in bacteriophage T4. *Genetics* **109**:633, 1985.
430. McCrackin RH: Albinism. Albinism and unialbinism in twin African negroes. *Am J Dis Child* **54**:786, 1937.
431. Barnicot NA: Albinism in South-Western Nigeria. *Ann Eugenics* **17**:39, 1952.
432. Aquaron R: Oculocutaneous albinism in Cameroon: A 15-year follow-up study. *Ophthalmic Paediatr Genet* **11**:255, 1990.
433. Okoro AN: Albinism in Nigeria: A clinical and social study. *Br J Dermatol* **92**:485, 1975.
434. Stannus HS: Anomalies of pigmentation among natives of Nyasaland: A contribution to the study of albinism. *Biometrika* **9**:333, 1913.
435. Witkop CJ, Niswander JD, Bergsma DR, Workman PL, White JG: Tyrosinase positive oculocutaneous albinism among the Zuni and the Brandywine triracial isolate: Biochemical and clinical characteristics and fertility. *Am J Phys Anthropol* **36**:397, 1972.
436. Nance WE, Witkop CJ, Rawls RF: Genetic and biochemical evidence for two forms of oculocutaneous albinism in man. *Birth Defects* **7**:125, 1971.
437. Trevor-Roper PD: Marriage of two complete albinos with normally pigmented offspring. *Br J Ophthalmol* **36**:107, 1952.
438. Kromberg JGR, Jenkins T: Prevalence of albinism in the South African Negro. *S Afr Med J* **13**:383, 1982.
439. Woolf CM: Albinism among Indians in Arizona and New Mexico. *Am J Hum Genet* **17**:23, 1965.

439a. Durham-Pierre D, Gardner JM, Nakatsu Y, King RA, Francke U, Ching A, Aquaron R, Del Marmol V, Brilliant MH: African origin of a common mutation of the human P gene in African American tyrosinase positive oculocutaneous albinism (OCA2). *Nat Genet* 6, 1994.

439b. Lee S-T, Nicholls RD, Bundey S, Laxova R, Musarella M, Spritz RA: Mutations of the P gene in oculocutaneous albinism, ocular albinism, and Prader-Willi syndrome plus albinism. *New Engl J Med* **330**:529, 1994.

440. Butler MG, Meaney FJ, Palmer CG: Clinical and cytogenetic survey of 39 individuals with Prader-Labhart-Willi syndrome. *Am J Med Genet* **23**:793, 1986.
441. Cassidy SB: Prader-Willi syndrome. *Curr Prob Pediatr* **14**:5, 1984.
442. Bray GA, Dahms WT, Swerdloff RS, Fiser RH, Atkinson RL, Carrel RE: The Prader-Willi syndrome: A study of 40 patients and a review of the literature. *Medicine (Baltimore)* **62**:59, 1983.
443. Ledbetter DH, Mascarello JT, Riccardi VM, Harper VD, Airhart SD, Strobel RJ: Chromosome 15 abnormalities and the Prader-Willi syndrome: A follow-up report of 40 cases. *Am J Hum Genet* **34**:278, 1982.
444. Mutirangura A, Greenberg F, Butler MG, Malcolm S, Nicholls RD, Chakravarti A, Ledbetter DH: Multiplex PCR of three dinucleotide repeats in the Prader-Willi/Angelman critical region (15q11-q13): Molecular diagnosis and mechanism of uniparental disomy. *Hum Mol Genet* **2**:143, 1993.
445. Magenis RE, Toth-Fejel S, Allen LJ, Black M, Brown MG, Budden S, Cohen R, Friedman JM, Kalousek D, Zonana J, Lacy D, LaFranchi S, Lahr M, Macfarlane J, Williams CPS: Comparison of the 15q deletions in Prader-Willi and Angelman syndromes: Specific regions, extent of deletions, parental origin, and clinical consequences. *Am J Med Genet* **35**:333, 1990.
446. Mascari MJ, Gottlieb W, Rogan PK, Butler MG, Waller DA, Armour AL, Jeffreys AJ, Ladda RL, Nicholls RD: The frequence of uniparental disomy in Prader-Willi syndrome: Implications for molecular diagnosis. *N Engl J Med* **326**:1599, 1992.
447. Creel DJ, Bendel CM, Wiesner GL, Wirtschafter JD, Arthur DC, King RA: Abnormalities of the central visual pathways in Prader-Willi Syndrome associate with hypopigmentation. *N Engl J Med* **314**:1606, 1986.
448. Hittner HM, King RA, Riccardi VM, Ledbetter DH, Borda RP, Ferrell RE, Kretzer FL: Oculocutaneous albinoidism as a manifestation of reduced neural crest derivatives in the Prader-Willi syndrome. *Am J Ophthalmol* **94**:328, 1982.
449. Fryburg JS, Breg WR, Lindgren V: Diagnosis of Angelman syndrome in infants. *Am J Hum Genet* **38**:58, 1991.
450. Williams CA, Frias JL: The Angelman ("happy puppet") syndrome. *Am J Med Genet* **11**:453, 1982.
451. Angelman H: "Puppet" children: A report of three cases. *Dev Med Child Neurol* **7**:681, 1965.
452. Nakatsu Y, Gondo Y, Brilliant MH: The *p* locus is closely linked to the mouse homolog of a gene from the Prader-Willi chromosomal region. *Mammal Genome* **2**:69, 1992.
453. Boissy RE, Zhao H, Austin LM, Nordlund JJ, King RA: Melanocytes from an individual with brown oculocutaneous albinism lack expression of TRP-1, the product of the human homologue of the murine brown locus. *Am J Hum Genet* **53**:1993. (abstr)
454. Kromberg JG, Castle D, Zwane EM, Bothwell J, Kidson SH, Bartel P, Phillips JI, Jenkins T: Red or rufous albinism in southern Africa. *Ophthalmic Paediatr Genet* **11**:229, 1990.
455. Hornabrook RW, McDonald WI, Carroll RL: Congenital nystagmus among the red-skins of the highlands of Papua New Guinea. *Br J Ophthalmol* **64**:375, 1980.
456. Walsh RJ: A distinctive pigment of the skin in New Guinea indigenes. *Ann Hum Genet* **34**:379, 1971.
457. Loewenthal LJA: Partial albinism and nystagmus in Negroes. *Arch Dermatol Syphilol* **50**:300, 1944.
458. Bergsma DR, Kaiser-Kupfer M: A new form of albinism. *Am J Ophthalmol* **77**:837, 1974.
459. Frenk E, Calame A: [Familial oculo-cutaneous hypopigmentation of dominant transmission due to a disorder in melanocyte formation. Association of Prader-Willi syndrome with a chromosome abnormality in one of the subjects involved.] *Schweiz Med Wochenschr* **107**:1964, 1977.
460. Fitzpatrick TB, Jimbow K, Donaldson DD: Dominant oculocutaneous albinism. *Br J Dermatol (suppl 10)* **91**:23, 1974.
461. Witkop CJ, Babcock MN, Rao GHR, Gaudier F, Summers CG, Shanahan F, Harmon KR, Townsend D, Sedano HO, King RA, Cal SX, White JG: Albinism and Hermansky-Pudlak syndrome in Puerto Rico. *Bol Assoc Med P Ri* **82**:333, 1990.
462. Simon JW, Adams RJ, Calhoun JH, Shapiro SS, Ingerman CM: Ophthalmic manifestations of the Hermansky-Pudlak syndrome (oculocutaneous albinsim and hemorrhagic diathesis). *Am J Ophthalmol* **93**:71, 1982.
463. Davies BH, Tuddenham EGD: Familial pulmonary fibrosis associated with oculocutaneous albinism and platelet function defect. A new syndrome. *Q J Med* **45**:219, 1976.
464. Garay SM, Gardella JE, Fazzini EP, Goldring RM: Hermansky-Pudlak syndrome. Pulmonary manifestations of a ceroid storage disorder. *Am J Med* **66**:737, 1979.
465. Harmon KR, Witkop CJ, White JG, King RA, Peterson M, Moore D, Tashjian J, Marinelli WA, Bitterman PB: Pathogenesis of pulmonary fibrosis—PDGF precedes structural alterations in the Hermansky-Pudlak syndrome. *J Lab Clin Med* (1994 in press).
466. White DA, Smith GJW, Cooper JAD, Clickstein M, Rankin JA: Hermansky-Pudlak syndrome and interstitial lung disease: Report of a case with levage findings. *Am Rev Respir Dis* **130**:138, 1984.
467. Mahadeo R, Markowitz J, Fisher S, Daum F: Hermansky-

Pudlak syndrome with granulomatous colitis in children. *J Pediatr* **118**:904, 1991.
468. Schinella RA, Greco MA, Cobert BL, Denmark LW, Cox RP: Hermansky-Pudlak syndrome with granulomatous colitis. *Ann Intern Med* **92**:20, 1980.
469. Shanahan F, Randolph L, King R, Oseas R, Brogan M, Witkop C, Rotter J, Targan S: The Hermansky-Pudlak syndrome: An immunological assessment of 15 cases. *Am J Med* **85**:823, 1988.
470. Gerrard JM, Lint D, Sims PJ, Wiedmer T, Fugate RD, McMillan E, Robertson C, Israels SJ: Identification of a platelet dense granule membrane protein that is deficient in a patient with the Hermansky-Pudlak syndrome. *Blood* **77**:101, 1991.
471. Nishibori M, Cham B, McNicol A, Shalev A, Jain N, Gerrard JM: The protein CD63 is in platelet dense granules, is deficient in a patient with Hermansky-Pudlak syndrome, and appears identical to granulophysin. *J Clin Invest* **91**:1775, 1993.
472. Blume RS, Wolff SM: The Chediak-Higashi syndrome: Studies in four patients and a review of the literature. *Medicine (Baltimore)* **51**:247, 1972.
473. Benezra D, Mengitsu F, Cividalli G, Weizman Z, Merin S, Auerbach E: Chediak-Higashi syndrome: Ocular features. *J Pediatr Ophthalmol Strabismus* **17**:68, 1980.
474. Spencer WH, Hogan MJ: Ocular manifestations of Chediak-Higashi syndrome: Report of a case with histopathologic examination of ocular tissues. *Am J Ophthalmol* **50**:1197, 1960.
475. Creel DJ, Boxer LA, Fauci AS: Visual and auditory anomalies in Chediak-Higashi syndrome. *Electroencephalogr Clin Neurophysiol* **55**:252, 1983.
476. White JG, Clawson CC: The Chediak-Higashi syndrome: The nature of the giant neutrophil granules and their interactions with cytoplasm and foreign particulates. *Am J Pathol* **98**:151, 1980.
477. Tanaka A: Chediak-Higashi syndrome: Abnormal lysosomal enzyme levels in granulocytes of patients and family members. *Pediatr Res* **14**:901, 1980.
478. De Beer HA, Anderson R, Findlay GH: Chediak-Higashi syndrome in a black child: Clinical features, immunological studies and optics of the hair and skin. *S Afr Med J* **60**:108, 1981.
479. Durandy A, Breton-Goriust J, Guy-Grand D, Dumez C, Griscelli C: Prenatal diagnosis of syndromes associating albinism and immune deficiencies (Chediak-Higashi syndrome and variant). *Prenat Diagn* **13**:13, 1993.
480. Jenkins NA, Justice MJ, Gilbert DJ, Chu MC, Copeland NG: Nidogen-entactin *(Nid)* maps to the proximal end of mouse chromosome 13 linked to Beige *(bg)* and identifies a new region of homology between mouse and human chromosomes. *Genomics* **9**:401, 1991.
481. Nettleship E: On some hereditary diseases of the eye. *Trans Ophthalmol Soc UK* **29**:57, 1909.
482. Falls HF: Sex-linked ocular albinism displaying typical fundus changes in the female heterozygote. *Am J Ophthalmol* **34**:41, 1951.
483. Freed WJ, Adinolfi AM, Laskin JD, Geller HM: Transplantation of B16/C3 melanoma cells into the brains of rats and mice. *Brain Res* **485**:349, 1989.
484. Charles SJ, Green JS, Grant JW, Yates JRW, Moore AT: Clinical features of affected males with X-linked ocular albinism. *Br J Ophthalmol* **77**:222, 1993.
485. O'Donnell FE, Green WR: The eye in albinism, in Duane TD (ed): *Clinical Ophthalmology*. Philadelphia, Lippincott, 1989, vol 4, pp 1–23.
486. Kinoshita Y, Sato S, Takeuchi T: Cellular sialic acid level and phenotypic expression in B16 melanoma cells: Comparison of spontaneous variations and bromodeoxyuridine- and theophylline-induced changes. *Cell Struct Funct* **14**:35, 1989.
487. Smith CJ, O'Hare KB, Allen JC: Selective cytotoxicity of hydroquinone for melanocyte-derived cells is mediated by tyrosinase activity but independent of melanin content. *Pigment Cell Res* **1**:386, 1988.
488. Zuasti A, Jara JR, Ferrer C, Solano F: Occurrence of melanin granules and melanosynthesis in the kidney of Sparus auratus. *Pigment Cell Res* **2**:93, 1989.
489. O'Donnell FE, Hambrick GW, Green WR, Iliff WJ, Stone DL: X-linked ocular albinism: An oculocutaneous macromelanosomal disorder. *Arch Ophthalmol* **94**:1883, 1976.
490. Garner A, Jay BS: Macromelanosomes in X-linked ocular albinism. *Histopathology* **4**:243, 1980.
491. O'Donnell FE, Green WR, Fleischman JA, Hambrick GW: X-linked ocular albinism in blacks. *Arch Ophthalmol* **96**:1189, 1978.
492. Cortin P, Tremblay M, Lemagne JM: X-linked ocular albinism: Relative value of skin biopsy, iris transillumination and funduscopy in identifying affected males and carriers. *Can J Ophthalmol* **16**:121, 1981.
493. Fialkow PJ, Giblett ER, Motulsky AG: Measurable linkage between ocular albinism and Xg. *Am J Hum Genet* **19**:63, 1967.
494. Pearce WG, Sanger R, Race RR: Ocular albinism and Xg. *Lancet* **1**:1282, 1968.
495. Schnur RE, Nussbaum RL, Anson-Cartwright L, McDowell C, Worton RG, Musarella MA: Linkage analysis in X-linked ocular albinism. *Genomics* **9**:605, 1991.
496. Bergen AAB, Samanns C, van Dorp DB, Ferguson-Smith MA, Gal A, Bleeker-Wagemakers EM: Localization of the X-linked ocular albinism gene (OA1) between DXS278/DXS237 and DXS143/DXS16 by linkage analysis. *Ophthalmic Paediatr Genet* **11**:165, 1990.
497. Bergen AAB, Samanns C, Schuurman EJM, van Osch L, van Dorp DB, Pinckers AJLG, Bakker E, Gal A, van Ommen GJB, Bleeker-Wagemakers EM: Multipoint linkage analysis in X-linked ocular albinism of the Nettleship-Falls type. *Hum Genet* **88**:162, 1991.
498. Charles SJ, Green JS, Moore AT, Bartons DE, Yates JRW: Genetic mapping of X-linked ocular albinism: Linkage analysis in a large Newfoundland kindred. *Genomics* **16**:259, 1993.
499. Bergen AAB, Zijp P, Schuurman EJM, Bleeker-Wagemakers EM, Apkarian P, van Ommen G-JB: Refinement of the localization of the X-linked ocular albinism gene. *Genomics* **16**:272, 1993.
500. Kulkarni GA, Nathanson L: Specificity of growth inhibition of melanoma by 4-hydroxyanisole. *Pigment Cell Res* **2**:40, 1989.
501. Rose NC, Menacker SJ, Schnur RE, Jackson L, McDonald-McGinn DM, Stump T, Emanuel BS, Zackai EH: Ocular albinism in a male with del (6)(q13-q15): Candidate region for autosomal recessive ocular albinism? *Am J Med Genet* **42**:700, 1992.
502. Ohashi H, Tsukahara M, Murano I, Naritomi K, Nishioka K, Miyake S, Kajii T: Pigmentary dysplasias and chromosomal mosaicism: Report of 9 cases. *Am J Med Genet* **43**:716, 1992.
503. Beighton P, Ramesar R, Winship I, Viljoen D, Greenberg J, Young K, Curtis D, Sellars S: Hearing impairment and pigmentary disturbance. *Ann NY Acad Sci* **630**:152, 1991.
504. Winship I, Gericke G, Beighton P: X-linked inheritance of ocular albinism with late-onset sensorineural deafness. *Am J Med Genet* **19**:797, 1984.
505. Lewis RA: Ocular albinism and deafness. *Am J Hum Genet* **30**:57A, 1978.
506. Margolis E: A new hereditary syndrome—sex-linked deaf-mutism associated with total albinism. *Acta Genet* **12**:12, 1962.
507. Ziprkowski L, Krarowski A, Adam A, Costeff H, Sade J: Partial albinism and deaf mutism. *Arch Dermatol* **86**:530, 1992.
508. Woolf CM, Dolowitz DA, Aldous HE: Congenital deafness associated with piebaldness. *Arch Otolaryngol* **82**:244, 1965.
509. Shiloh Y, Litvak G, Ziv Y, Lehner T, Sandkuyl L, Hildesheimer M, Buchris V, Cremers FPM, Szabo P, White BN, Holden JJA, Ott J: Genetic mapping of X-linked albinism-deafness syndrome (ADFN) to Xq26.3-q27.1. *Am J Hum Genet* **47**:20, 1990.
510. White CP, Waldron M, Jan JE, Carter JE: Oculocerebral hypopigmentation syndrome associated with Bartter syndrome. *Am J Med Genet* **46**:592, 1993.
511. Cross HE, McKusick VA, Breen W: A new oculocerebral syndrome with hypopigmentation. *J Pediatr* **70**:398, 1967.
512. Fryns JP, Dereymaeker AM, Heremans G, Marien J, van Hauwaert J, Turner G, Hockey A, van den Berghe

H: Oculocerebral syndrome with hypopigmentation (Cross syndrome). Report of two siblings born to consanguineous parents. *Clin Genet* **34:**81, 1988.
513. Griscelli C, Durandy A, Guy-Grand D, Daguillard F, Herzog C, Prunieras M: A syndrome associating partial albinism and immunodeficiency. *Am J Med* **65:**691, 1978.
514. Jahr HM, McIntire MS: Piebaldism or familial white skin spotting (partial albinism). *Am J Dis Child* **88:**481, 1984.
515. Sundfor H: A pedigree of skin-spotting in man: 42 piebalds in a Norwegian family. *J Hered* **30:**67, 1939.
516. Comings DE, Odland GF: Partial albinism. *JAMA* **195:**111, 1966.
517. Cooke JV: Familial white skin spotting (piebaldness) ("partial albinism") with white forelock. *J Pediatr* **41:**1, 1952.
518. Ortonne J-P, Mosher DB, Fitzpatrick TB: Piebaldism, in *Vitiligo and Other Hypomelanoses of Hair and Skin.* New York, Plenum, 1983, pp 310–337.
519. Jimbow K, Fitzpatrick TB, Szabo G, Hori Y: Congenital circumscribed hypomelanosis: A characterization based on electron microscopic study of tuberous sclerosis, nevus depigmentosus and piebaldism. *J Invest Dermatol* **64:**50, 1975.
520. Reith AD, Rottapel R, Giddens E, Brady C, Forrester L, Bernstein A: W mutant mice with mild or severe developmental defects contain distinct point mutations in the kinase domain of the c-kit receptor. *Genes Dev* **4:**390, 1990.
521. Gorlin RJ, Cohen MM, Levin LS: *Syndromes of the Head and Neck,* 3d ed. New York, Oxford University Press, 1990, pp 466–469.
522. Ortonne JP: Piebaldism, Waardenburg's syndrome and related disorders: "Neural crest depigmentation syndromes." *Dermatol Clin* **6:**205, 1988.
523. da-Silva EO: Waardenburg I Syndrome: A clinical and genetic study of two large Brazilian kindreds and literature review. *Am J Med Genet* **40:**65, 1991.
524. Tassabehji M, Read AP, Newton VE, Patton M, Gruss P, Harris R, Strachan T: Mutations in the PAX3 gene causing Waardenburg syndrome type I and type 2. *Nat Genet* **3:**26, 1993.
525. Chalepakis G, Fritsch R, Fickenscher H, Deutsch U, Goulding M, Gruss P: The molecular basis of the *undulated/Pax-1* mutation. *Cell* **66:**873, 1991.
526. Hill R, van Heyningen V: Mouse mutations and human disorders are paired. *Trends Genet* **8:**119, 1992.
527. Bard LA: Heterogeneity in Waardenburg's Syndrome: Report of a family with ocular albinism. *Arch Ophthalmol* **96:**1193, 1978.
528. Witkop CJ, Krumwiede M, Sedano H, White JG: Reliability of absent platelet dense bodies as a diagnostic criterion for Hermansky-Pudlak syndrome. *Am J Hematol* **26:**305, 1987.

CHAPTER 148

Xeroderma Pigmentosum and Cockayne Syndrome

James E. Cleaver ▪ Kenneth H. Kraemer

1. **Xeroderma pigmentosum (XP) is a rare autosomal recessive disease in which patients show greater than a thousandfold increased frequency of sunlight-induced skin cancers. Two major clinical forms are seen. One form involves progressive degenerative changes of the skin and eyes. The other form also includes progressive neurologic degeneration. XP occurs at a frequency of about 1 in 1 million in the United States.**

2. **Patients with Cockayne syndrome (CS), another rare recessive disorder, have sun sensitivity, short stature, and progressive neurologic degeneration without increased frequency of skin cancer. A handful of patients have both XP and CS.**

3. **Complementation analysis has allowed a further classification of XP into at least seven groups with defective excision repair. The nonneurologic forms of XP include most patients in groups C, E, and F, plus a "variant" form with normal excision repair; the neurologic forms consist of most patients in groups A, B, D, and G. Cultured cells from patients in each group restore DNA repair processes when fused with cells from any of the other groups, suggesting that at least seven different gene products are defective. CS has similarly been classified into groups A, B, and C.**

4. **Patients in XP groups A through G are deficient in gene products required for the initial step of excision of damaged DNA. Patients in CS groups A and B are deficient in repair of actively transcribed genes.**

5. **Patients with the variant form of XP appear to be deficient in a gene product that in normal cells permits semiconservative replication past damaged sites in DNA.**

6. **Cells from different complementation groups of XP show characteristic ranges of hypersensitivity to killing and mutagenesis by ultraviolet (UV) radiation and by certain chemical carcinogens such as benz[*a*]pyrene or nitroquinoline oxide. The types of mutations observed in UV-treated DNA replicated in XP-A and XP-D cells are restricted in comparison to those in normal cells. The predominant base substitution mutation observed is the G:C-to-A:T transition.**

A list of standard abbreviations is located immediately preceding the index in each volume. Additional abbreviations used in this chapter include: AP = apurinic or apyrimidinic site; AT = ataxia-telangiectasia; CAT = chloramphenicol acetyltransferase; CNS = central nervous sytem; CS = Cockayne syndrome; SCE = sister chromatid exchange; TTD = trichothiodystrophy; XP = xeroderma pigmentosum; and XPAC = XP-A correcting (gene).

Several kinds of skin disease are caused by alterations in the normal resistance of the skin to sunlight. These occur either because of: (1) a loss in the shielding afforded by melanin, exemplified by albinism[1]; (2) the deposition of sensitizing compounds in the skin, exemplified by porphyria[2]; or (3) a decrease in the capacity of cells to repair or replicate past damage induced by sunlight, exemplified by xeroderma pigmentosum (XP).[3-5] In albinism and the porphyrias, the amount of damage caused by sunlight to the genetic material (DNA) is increased; in XP the amount of damage is unchanged, but DNA repair and DNA replication are diminished or altered[3-5] (Fig. 148-1). The major result clinically is a high incidence of sunlight-induced skin cancers[3-8] (Fig. 148-2).

An important distinction should be made between the concepts of hypersensitivity to DNA-damaging agents and of defects in repair of damaged DNA.[3] A large group of diseases are known in which cells or tissues exhibit abnormal sensitivity to one or more kinds of DNA-damaging agents.[3] In only a few of these diseases, including the various forms of XP, is the hypersensitivity caused by a defect in the repair of damaged DNA.[3-8] In other hypersensitivity diseases there may be more complex abnormalities, such as alterations in both semiconservative replication[9] and repair[10,11] in ataxia-telangiectasia after x-irradiation, and alteration in the recovery of DNA replication and defective repair of actively transcribing genes after irradiation by ultraviolet (UV) light in Cockayne syndrome (CS).[12] These are discussed in more detail below.

DNA REPAIR PATHWAYS

At least three different biochemical repair systems operate in damaged cells to safeguard DNA from permanent damage.[3,4] These are excision repair, postreplication repair, and photoreactivation (see Fig. 148-1). These systems have been found in bacteria, yeast, amphibians, fish, rodents, marsupials, and mammals. They are especially important in the skin, where they mend damage to DNA caused by the UV rays (>290 nm) present in sunlight. Some of the repair systems can also mend damage to DNA caused by chemical carcinogens.[13] These systems presumably protect internal tissues against the carcinogenic and mutagenic consequences of exposure to chemicals that damage DNA.

Excision repair is extremely versatile and can mend a large variety of UV-light, x-ray, and chemically induced forms of damage to DNA.[3,4] Excision repair may be subdivided into nucleotide excision repair and base excision repair.

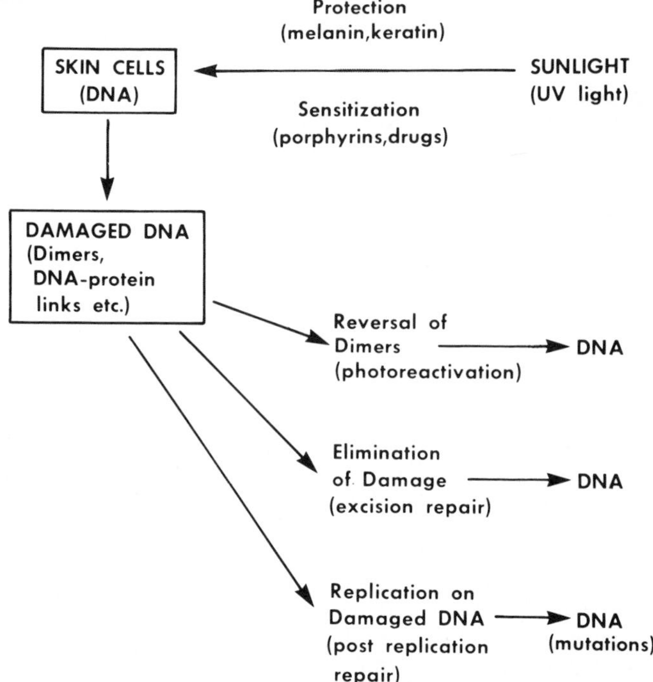

FIG. 148-1 **Schematic diagram of processes leading to damaged DNA in skin cells and three processes that repair damaged DNA. Damage to DNA of skin cells is caused by absorption of ultraviolet light; increased damage results if protection afforded by melanin is lost (e.g., albinism) or if photosensitizers are present in the skin (e.g., porphyrias). Damage is repaired by direct reversal (photoreactivation) or by excision and replacement (excision repair). Semiconservative replication of damaged templates may introduce errors (mutations) by a variety of mechanisms.**

The nucleotide excision repair system excises damaged single strands of DNA and replaces them with a new sequence of bases using as a template for base pairing the intact strand of DNA opposite the original damaged site. Excision repair is of central importance in the recovery of cells from radiation damage. It employs a wide variety of enzymes with different specificities and mechanisms for removal of damage from different regions of the genome. There appears to be specific regulation of the repair of transcribed versus nontranscribed genes, and the transcribed versus nontranscribed strand within an active gene. Base excision repair removes damaged bases, leaving the sugar-phosphate backbone of the DNA intact and creating an AP (apurinic or apyrimidinic) site which is subsequently converted to a strand break and repaired.

The second system, called "postreplication repair," is exceedingly complex and is less easily defined as a specific system for handling damage in DNA.[14] It involves multiple mechanisms by which semiconservative DNA replication can take place despite the presence of damage or incomplete excision repair in one strand of DNA.[3,4,14] *Postreplication repair* may be an operational term for a particular disturbance of DNA replication by which intact new strands of DNA can be synthesized despite the presence of unexcised damage on the parental template strands.[14]

The third repair system, photoreactivation, simply reverts the damaged DNA to the normal chemical state without removing or exchanging any material from DNA. The photoreactivation system is specific for one form of damage induced by UV light—the cyclobutane pyrimidine dimer. Photoreactivation cleaves these dimers, but the system has no ability to modify other damaged sites. Photoreactivation has been demonstrated in bacteria, yeast, fish, amphibians, and marsupials, but the existence and importance of this system in human tissue is controversial.[15–20]

At one time XP and CS were thought to be diseases involving single defects in repair systems.[3,21] However, it now appears that repair systems are more complex and interrelated or may have enzymes in common.[3,7] Both the clinical phenotype and the mechanisms of repair are varied and distinctions are unclear. Consequently, a full understanding of the biochemistry of XP and its relationship to the clinical symptoms may be more complicated than was first suspected. Because the outstanding clinical characteristic of XP is marked predisposition to skin cancers developing after exposure to sunlight, the disease involves a unique conjunction of environmental, genetic, and biochemical factors in the etiology of cancer.[3,6–8,21,22] CS, in contrast, shows a repair deficit that is not associated with cancer.[7] The elucidation of the biochemical bases of these disorders should provide clues to understanding the genetic changes involved in carcinogenesis by many physical and chemical agents.

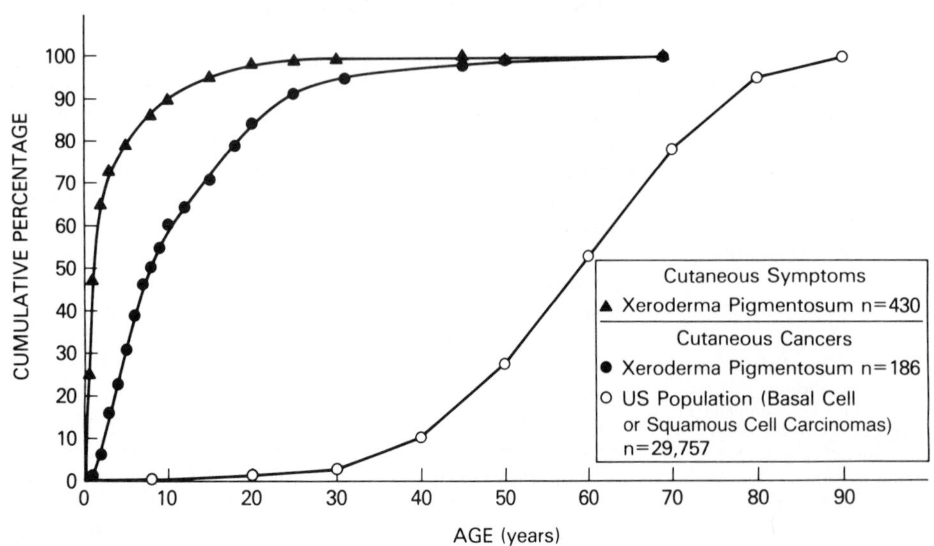

FIG. 148-2 **Age at onset of XP symptoms. Age at onset of cutaneous symptoms (generally sun sensitivity or pigmentation) was reported for 430 patients. Age at first skin cancer was reported for 186 patients and is compared with age distribution for 29,757 patients with basal-cell carcinoma or squamous-cell carcinoma in the United States general population.** ***(From Kraemer et al.[33] Used by permission.)***

CLINICAL FEATURES OF XERODERMA PIGMENTOSUM AND COCKAYNE SYNDROME

Xeroderma Pigmentosum

XP is a rare autosomal recessive disease. Affected patients (homozygotes) have sun sensitivity resulting in progressive degenerative changes of sun-exposed portions of the skin and eyes, often leading to neoplasia. Some XP patients have, in addition, progressive neurologic degeneration. Obligate heterozygotes (parents) are generally asymptomatic.

History. *Xeroderma,* or parchment skin, was the term given by Moritz Kaposi to the condition he observed in a patient in 1863 and reported in the dermatology textbook he wrote with Ferdinand von Hebra in 1874.[23] In 1882 the term *pigmentosum* was added to emphasize the striking pigmentary abnormalities. Eye involvement, including cloudiness of the cornea, was recognized by Kaposi. In 1883, Neisser reported two brothers with cutaneous xeroderma pigmentosum and neurologic degeneration beginning in the second decade.[24] DeSanctis and Cacchione in 1932 described three sibs with cutaneous XP associated with microcephaly, progressive mental deterioration, dwarfism, and immature sexual development—the DeSanctis-Cacchione syndrome.[25]

Defective DNA excision repair in UV-irradiated cultured skin fibroblasts from some XP patients was reported by Cleaver in 1968,[5] and in skin in vivo by Epstein et al.[26] The form of the disease in the first XP patient with normal excision repair described by Burk et al.[27] was subsequently named the variant form of XP[28] and was found to have an abnormality in another DNA repair system—postreplication repair.[29,30] In 1972, De Weerd-Kastelein et al.,[31] using cell-fusion techniques, demonstrated genetic heterogeneity in the DNA excision repair defect of XP.

Epidemiology. Xeroderma pigmentosum has been found in all races worldwide. The frequency is about 1 in 1 million in the United States and Europe[7] but is considerably higher in Japan (1 in 100,000)[32] and Egypt. In a literature survey of more than 800 patients[33] there were nearly equal numbers of male (54 percent) and female (46 percent) patients. Consanguinity of the patients' parents was reported in 31 percent, an elevated frequency often seen in recessive disorders. Nearly 20 percent of the patients, including a high proportion of Japanese patients, had neurologic abnormalities.[33]

Symptoms. The median age of onset of symptoms was between 1 and 2 years. In 5 percent of patients, onset of symptoms was delayed until after 14 years[33] (see Fig. 148-2). Initial symptoms included abnormal reaction to sun exposure in 19 percent (including severe sunburn with blistering and persistent erythema on minimal sun exposure) (Table 148-1). However, many patients sunburned normally. Freckling occurred by 2 years of age in most of the patients. The cutaneous abnormalities were usually strikingly limited to sun-exposed areas of the body. At an early age, the skin appears similar to that seen in farmers and sailors after many years of sun exposure: areas of increased pigment alternating with areas of decreased pigment, with atrophy and telangiectasia. A few patients who exhibit a wide spectrum of characteristic cutaneous and ocular findings have been unambiguously diagnosed as having XP, even though the erythematous response to sun exposure was normal.[34] This may be a distinctive feature of the form of XP known as variant or pigmented xerodermoid,[29,30,34,35] but this form can be diagnosed fully only by biochemical tests.[29,30]

Table 148-1 Cutaneous Manifestations of XP

Erythema and bullae (acute sun sensitivity in infancy)
Freckles
Xerosis (dryness) and scaling
Areas of hypopigmentation alternating with areas of hyperpigmentation
Telangiectasia
Atrophy
Actinic keratoses
Basal-cell and squamous-cell carcinomas
Malignant melanomas
Others (keratocanthomas, angiomas, fibromas, sarcomas)

SOURCE: From Robbins et al.[21] Used by permission.

Premalignant actinic keratoses and malignant and benign neoplasms developed.[33] The neoplasms were predominantly basal-cell or squamous-cell carcinomas (at least 45 percent of patients, many with multiple primary neoplasms) but also included melanomas (5 percent of patients), sarcomas, keratoacanthomas, and angiomas.[33] About 90 percent of the basal-cell and squamous-cell carcinomas occurred on the face, head, and neck—the sites of greatest UV exposure. The median age of onset of first skin neoplasm was 8 years, nearly 50 years younger than that in the general population of the United States (see Fig. 148-2). This represents one of the largest reductions in age of onset of neoplasia documented for any recessive human genetic disease. The frequency of basal-cell carcinomas, squamous-cell carcinomas, or melanoma of the skin was 2000 times greater than in the general population for patients under 20 years of age.[36] There was an approximate 30-year reduction in survival, with a 70 percent probability of surviving to age 40 years.[33] Many patients died of neoplasia.

Ocular abnormalities include photophobia, which may vary among patients from severe to absent; conjunctivitis of the interpalpebral (sun-exposed) area; ectropion (turning out of the lids) due to atrophy of the skin of the eyelids; exposure keratitis; and benign and malignant neoplasms of the lids, conjunctiva, and limbus (Table 148-2). The distribution of ocular damage and neoplasms corresponds closely with the sites of UV exposure. The ocular neoplasms involved the anterior portion of the eye (lids, cornea, conjunctiva) almost exclusively.[33] This portion of the eye shields the posterior eye (uveal tract, retina) from UV radiation; visible light is the only radiation that reaches the photosensitive cells of the retina. The frequency of ocular neoplasms was increased more than a thousandfold in patients under 20 years of age.[36] There was also a greater than 10,000 times increase in squamous-cell carcinoma of the tip of the tongue,[36] another sun-exposed portion of the body (Fig. 148-3).

The 18 percent of XP patients with neurologic abnormalities had a sex ratio, reported age, frequency of ocular abnormalities, and frequency of cutaneous neoplasms similar to those of patients with only skin and eye involvement.[33] The neurologic symptoms varied in age of onset and severity, but were characterized by progressive deterioration[37,38] (Table 148-3). Diminished deep tendon reflexes and sensorineural deafness were frequent early abnormalities. In some patients, progressive mental retardation became evident only in the second decade of life. Patients with the DeSanctis-Cacchione syndrome had neurologic and somatic abnormali-

Table 148-2 Ocular Abnormalities Associated with XP

Lids
- Blepharitis
- Erythema, pigmentation, keratoses
- Atrophy leading to entropion, ectropion, loss of cilia, and loss of lower lid
- Neoplasms
  - Papillomas
  - Epitheliomas of free border of lid
  - Basal-cell and squamous-cell carcinomas

Conjunctiva
- Conjunctivitis with photophobia, lacrimation, edema
- Pigmentation, telangiectasia
- Dryness
- Symblepharon
- Inflammatory nodules
- Neoplasms
  - Intraepithelial epitheliomas
  - Squamous-cell carcinomas

Cornea
- Exposure keratitis with edema, cellular invasion, vascularization
- Dryness
- Opacification
- Ulceration and scarring
- Neoplasms

Iris
- Iritis
- Synechiae
- Atrophy
- Neoplasms

SOURCE: From Robbins et al.[21] Used by permission.

ties beginning in the first years of life.[25] They had microcephaly, intellectual deterioration with loss of the ability to talk, and increasing spasticity with loss of ability to walk, leading to quadriparesis, in addition to dwarfism and immature sexual development. Among the few autopsies reported, the major finding was a primary neuronal degeneration with loss (or absence) of neurons, particularly in the cerebral cortex and cerebellum, without evidence of a storage process or inflammatory changes.[21,37–39] The severity of neurologic disease has been reported to correlate with the degree of sensitivity of cultured skin fibroblasts to UV inhibition of colony-forming ability.[40]

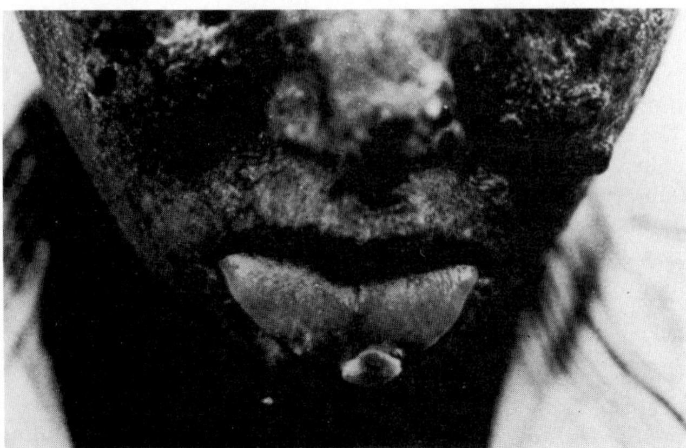

FIG. 148-3 Penduculated lingual neoplasm in patient of complementation group C (patient is described in Ref. 194). ***(Photograph kindly supplied by Dr. J German, New York Blood Center.)***

Table 148-3 Neurologic Abnormalities Associated with XP

Microcephaly

Higher cortical dysfunction
- Progressive mental deterioration
- Low intelligence
- Emotional lability
- Abnormal electroencephalogram

Basal ganglia and cerebellar involvement
- Choreoathetosis
- Ataxia

Extrapyramidal and pyramidal involvement
- Spasticity
- Extensor plantar responses
- Achilles tendon shortening

Cranial nerve involvement
- Sensorineural deafness

Lower motor neuron involvement
- Hyporeflexia or areflexia
- Neuropathic electromyogram and muscle biopsy

SOURCE: From Robbins et al.[21] Used by permission.

XP patients have a tenfold to twentyfold increase in the frequency of internal neoplasms.[36] There were reports of four patients with primary brain tumors (including two sarcomas), two with leukemia, two with lung tumors (including one patient who died at age 34 after smoking a pack of cigarettes a day for 16 years), and three with gastric carcinomas.[33,41,42] Chemical carcinogens are suspected to play a role in these neoplasms, since cultured cells from XP patients are hypersensitive to certain DNA-binding chemical carcinogens that produce damaged DNA which is normally acted on by the UV excision repair system. These include benz[*a*]pyrene derivatives (found in cigarette smoke), and tryptophan pyrolysis products (found in charred food).[43,44]

Treatment. Treatment of XP patients is a multifaceted process involving early diagnosis, genetic counseling, patient and family education, and regular monitoring of the skin.[6] The diagnosis is suspected in cases with marked sun sensitivity, photophobia, and/or early onset of freckling. Laboratory tests of UV sensitivity of fibroblasts and of excision repair confirm the diagnosis. Genetic counseling is directed toward acquainting the patients and their parents with the inherited aspects of the disease and its rarity, the increased risk in cases of familial relationship between the two parents, with the 25 percent probability that the disease will appear among subsequent offspring, and the improbability of the patient's having affected children.[22,33,45]

Patients should be shielded from sunlight by protective measures, including wearing two layers of clothing, using long hairstyles, wearing broad-brimmed hats and UV-absorbing sunglasses with side shields, and use of chemical sunscreens with sun protection factor (SPF) numbers of 15 or higher. Patients should avoid direct exposure to sunlight, especially during the peak UV hours (about 10 AM to 3 PM in the continental United States), and indirect UV reflected from snow or water. Window glass and many plastic shields for fluorescent lamps will absorb UV radiation indoors. Known chemical carcinogens such as tobacco smoke should be avoided. Patients and their families should be taught to examine their skin and to recognize and bring to medical attention any lesions suspected to be malignant. Color photographs are often useful for follow-up.

Malignant skin neoplasms are treated as in patients who do not have XP by excision, electrodesiccation and curettage, cryosurgery, or chemosurgery. XP patients have received x-ray therapy for malignant skin tumors and have had a normal response.[6] Dermabrasion or dermatome shaving has been used in patients with multiple tumors, permitting the epidermis to be repopulated by cells from the hair follicles, which are relatively shielded from sunlight.[6] Total removal of the skin of the face with grafting of skin from sun-shielded areas has been used in extreme cases. Oral retinoids have been shown to prevent new skin cancers in XP patients, but have many severe side effects.[46]

Cockayne Syndrome

CS is a very rare disorder with cutaneous, ocular, neurologic, and somatic abnormalities. Fewer than 200 cases have been recognized.[47–52] Inheritance is presumed to be autosomal recessive. Patients usually have early onset of sun sensitivity, with marked redness on minimal sun exposure. In contrast to XP, CS patients do not have severe freckling or skin cancer. CS patients have short stature, progressive neurologic degeneration, mental retardation, progressive deafness, and hyperreflexia. A pigmentary retinal degeneration often develops—a feature not seen in XP. A clinically severe form (with infantile onset, cachexia, and early death)[49] and a milder form[50,51] have been described. CS patients have microcephaly and normal pressure hydrocephalus.[53] Calcification of the basal ganglia may be visible on CT scan.[54] Pathologically, there is a primary demyelination in CS while there is primary neuronal degeneration in XP.[38]

Laboratory studies show cultured CS cells to have a similar hypersensitivity to killing by UV as is found with XP.[55–59] CS differs from XP in that the usual assays of DNA excision repair in the total genomic DNA are normal. Venema et al.[60] have demonstrated that while repair of total genomic DNA is normal, the increased rate of repair of active genes usually seen in repair-proficient cells is absent in CS cells. Confirmatory studies using a plasmid vector also showed reduced expression of a UV-damaged transcriptionally active gene in CS cells.[61] This defect is reflected in delayed recovery of DNA and RNA synthesis following UV radiation,[12,62–64] which has provided the basis for prenatal diagnosis.[65] The assay was also used to assess genetic heterogeneity[63,64] and demonstrated three complementation groups.[64] Complementation groups A and B consist of patients with CS, while complementation group C consists of a patient (XP11BE) who has both XP and CS in XP complementation group B. One patient was reported with a cytogenetic abnormality on chromosome 10.[50] This region includes the location of a rodent repair gene ERCC 6.

Xeroderma Pigmentosum–Cockayne Syndrome Complex

Five patients have been identified with clinical features of both XP and CS[7,21] (see Table 148-6). These patients had the cutaneous pigmentary and neoplastic features of XP with the dwarfism, mental retardation, increased reflexes, and retinal degeneration typical of CS. Complementation studies have revealed that these patients have different excision repair defects; they are the members of complementation groups B,[4] D,[21] and G.

Trichothiodystrophy

Patients with trichothiodystrophy (TTD), an autosomal recessive disorder, have sulphur-deficient brittle hair, short stature, mental retardation, and ichthyosis (fish-scale-like skin).[66–74] Some patients are also sun sensitive. TTD is not associated with cancer.

Fibroblasts from TTD patients with sun sensitivity have been found to have similar abnormalities to patients with XP.[75–77] The cells are hypersensitive to killing by UV radiation and have reduced unscheduled DNA synthesis. Fusion studies revealed them to be in XP group D (see Table 148-6). Fibroblasts from TTD patients without sun sensitivity had normal UV survival and normal unscheduled DNA synthesis.[74,76]

PRODUCTION OF CELLULAR DAMAGE BY SUNLIGHT

Sunlight is the major environmental agent that precipitates the clinical symptoms of XP; it does so by damaging cutaneous cells. Understanding the biochemical defects in XP requires knowledge of the way the damaging wavelengths in sunlight are absorbed by macromolecules and the nature of the damage that is produced.

The wavelengths of sunlight reaching the surface of the earth extend into the near-UV region, the shortest detectable being about 290 nm. Shorter-wavelength UV (present in solar radiation in space) is blocked from reaching the ground by ozone and other components of the atmosphere. This lower limit slightly overlaps the upper region of the absorption spectra of nucleic acids and proteins. Energy in this region of overlap is absorbed by macromolecules in the skin, producing harmful effects that include erythema, burns, and actinic carcinogenesis.[78–80] Comparisons between direct sunlight and short-wavelength UV light (254 nm) indicate that sunlight in the midwestern United States is equivalent in germicidal activity to about 0.1 to 0.2 J per square meter of surface per minute [J/m^2-min] of 254-nm UV light.[81,82] Since normal human cells in culture have a D_{37}* of only about 3 to 5 J/m^2 of radiation at 254 nm, the direct exposure of human proliferating cells to sunlight can result in significant amounts of cell killing.

Radiation at the UV end of the sun's spectrum produces its biologic effects through absorption of quanta in molecules that have unsaturated chemical bonds, such as aromatic amino acids in proteins and purine and pyrimidine components of DNA and RNA. The action spectra for production of DNA damage (pyrimidine photoproducts),[84] cell killing,[85,86] production of aberrant chromosomes,[87] and induction of unscheduled DNA repair synthesis (i.e., DNA synthesis not associated with the normal cell cycle)[88] are all similar, exhibiting maximum efficiency in wavelengths from 260 to 280 nm. Although there is negligible energy in this region of the sun's spectrum, there is sufficient overlap of the shortest end of the sun's spectrum with the longer-wavelength side of the absorption spectrum of DNA for significant photochemical reaction to occur. Short-wavelength UV is absorbed by the outer, nondividing layers of skin cells. An action

*The D_{37} is the dose required to reduce survival to 0.37 from the initial value of 1.0, and in target theory corresponds to the dose required to produce an average of one lethal hit on the sensitive target of an irradiated organism when the survival curve is exponential.[83]

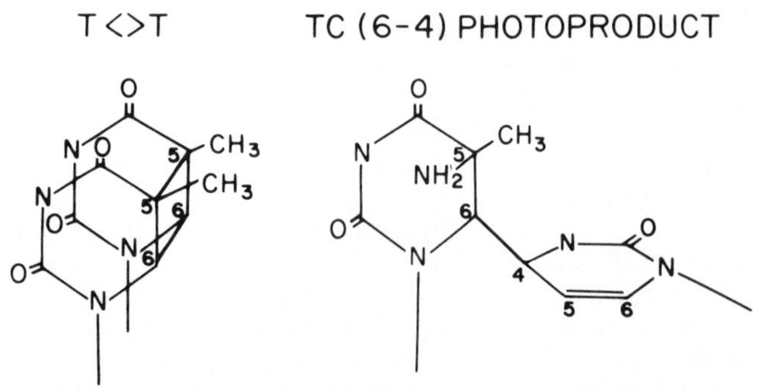

T<>T TC (6-4) PHOTOPRODUCT

FIG. 148-4 **Cyclobutane pyrimidine dimer (type I, meso) and [6-4] pyrimidine–pyrimidone products formed by UV light in DNA. *Left.* Cyclobutane dimer between adjacent thymines on the same strand of DNA with 5-5 and 6-6 bonds produced by irradiation. *Right.* [6-4] Photoproduct between adjacent thymine and cytosine on same strand of DNA. Structures shown are schematic. In DNA, the structures consist of pyrimidine bases stacked one above the other with considerable distortion of the phosphodiester backbone of DNA. *(Illustration provided by D. E. Brash.)***

spectrum of production of DNA damage in human skin shows a peak at about 302 nm.[89]

Two kinds of pyrimidine photoproducts are formed in DNA by absorption of UV light. The more frequent is the cyclobutane pyrimidine dimer (Fig. 148-4). This is formed between adjacent pyrimidines in the same strand of DNA by the formation of two new bonds between the 5 positions and between the 6 positions on the pyrimidine rings. At least four possible isomers (forms I to IV)[90] can be formed by irradiating frozen solutions of pyrimidines; the form I (meso) dimer corresponds to the one formed in DNA and can be isolated from sunlight and UV-irradiated cells and skin.[82,91,92] An alternative dipyrimidine photoproduct is the [6-4] pyrimidine–pyrimidone product mainly consisting of 5′TC or 5′CC (see Fig. 148-4), which is formed at lower rates than the cyclobutane dimer but is also important biologically. Various estimates suggest that the [6-4] photoproduct is formed at 10 to 50 percent of the frequency of cyclobutane dimers by low doses of 254-nm light, but there is a strong influence of local base sequences on photoproduct yields.[93] At some 5′TC sites the frequency of 6-4 photoproducts is nearly equal to that of the 5′TC cyclobutane dimer.[93,94] This lesion has been shown to be important in production of mutations in bacteria[93] and has been associated with mutagenic sites in shuttle vector plasmids replicated in XP cells, although structural features of chromatin strongly affect mutant yields.[94] Numerous biologic effects, such as cell killing, production of chromosome aberrations, mutagenesis, and carcinogenesis, can be attributed to these photoproducts in DNA.[84–88,91,95] Other photoproducts have biologic effects in some circumstances. These include the unstable cytosine hydrate, purine photoproducts, and, at relatively high doses, locally denatured regions, DNA-protein crosslinks, and single-strand breaks.[95]

CELLULAR CHARACTERISTICS OF XERODERMA PIGMENTOSUM AND COCKAYNE SYNDROME

Chromosomal Features

Cultured cells from most XP and CS patients have a normal karyotype. One CS case has been identified with a chromosomal deletion on chromosome 10[50] which has led to the identification of a CS-B gene. Distinctive karyotypic changes characteristic for some diseases with a high cancer incidence, such as Down syndrome, ataxia-telangiectasia, Fanconi anemia, and Bloom syndrome,[22] are not seen in XP patients, although karyotypic changes have occasionally been reported in XP cells.

Spontaneous and induced sister chromatid exchanges (SCE) can be visualized in human fibroblasts by a combination of growth in bromodeoxyuridine and staining with a photochemical reaction plus Giemsa[96,97] (Fig. 148-5). XP cells show a normal frequency of spontaneous SCE[98] but a greater than normal frequency after exposure to UV light and most chemical carcinogens (see Fig. 148-4).[99,100] Similarly, XP cells show more chromosome aberrations than normal cells after exposure to UV light and chemical carcinogens.[101,102]

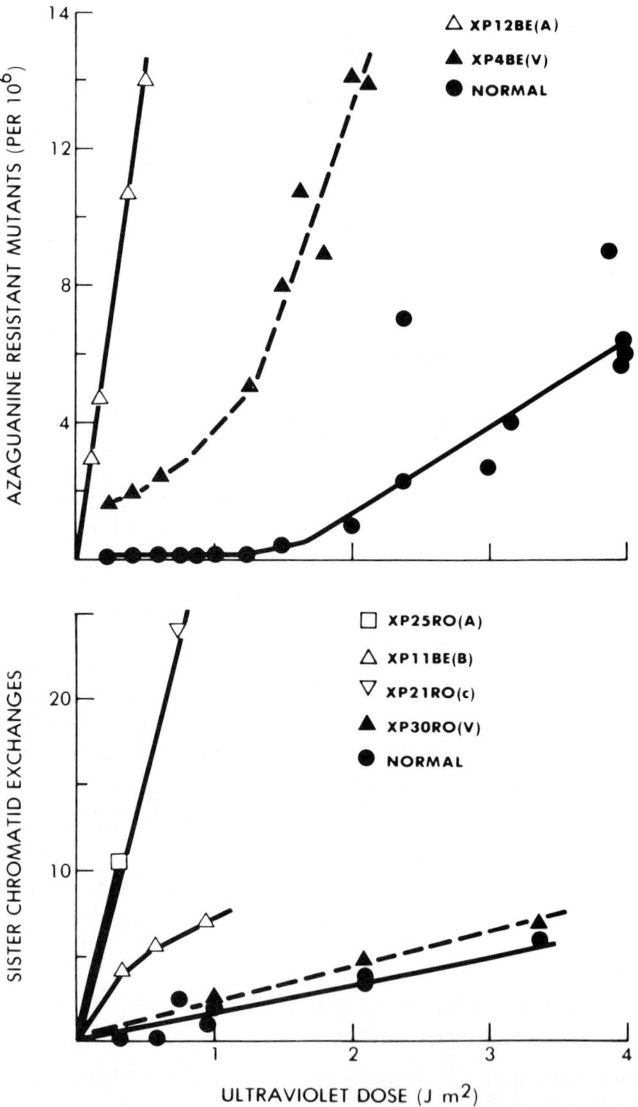

FIG. 148-5 **Relative frequencies of UV-induced mutations to 8-azaguanine (20 μ*M*) resistance or of SCE in normal (●), excision-defective XP (△, ▽, □), and XP variant (▲) cells as a function of ultraviolet dose. *Top.* Mutation frequencies. *(Redrawn from Maher et al.*[123,124] *Used by permission). Bottom.* SCE frequencies. *(Redrawn from De Weerd-Kastelein et al.*[100] *Used by permission.)***

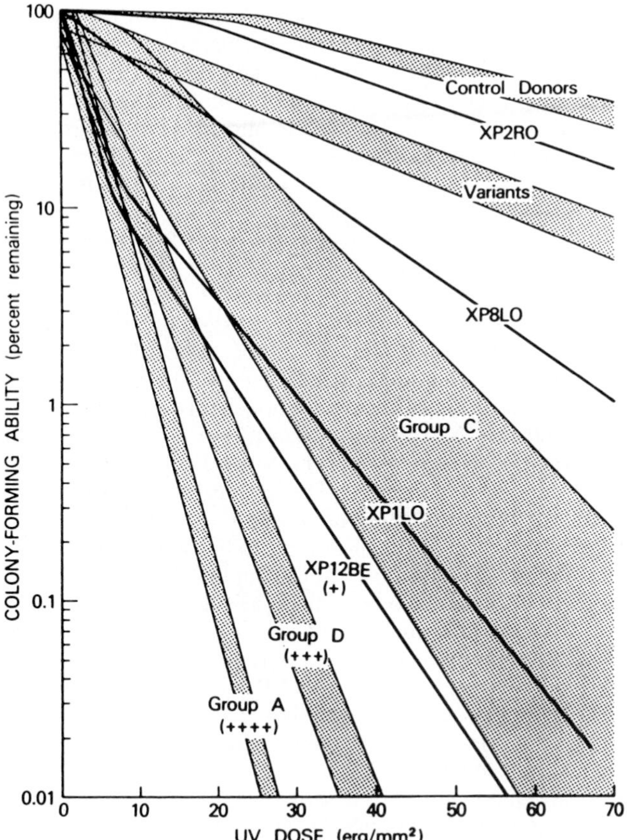

FIG. 148-6 **UV (254 nm) inactivation curve for fibroblasts from normal and various XP patients. Each complementation group (A to E, variant) is represented either by a range encompassing data from several patients in that group or as a single line for data from a single patient (i.e., the exceptional group A patients with little neurologic involvement—XP1LO, XP8LO, XP12BE—and group E, XP2RO). The severity of neurologic abnormalities is indicated by: + + + + = numerous clinical manifestations by age 7; + + + = numerous clinical manifestations between ages 7 and 12; + = areflexia and abnormal electroencephalogram at age 10.** ***(From Andrews et al.[40] Used by permission.)***

Sensitivity of Colony Formation to DNA Damage

The number of cells in culture that can grow into colonies after UV irradiation can be used as an in vitro measurement of sensitivity. Fibroblast cultures from patients who exhibit neurologic abnormalities are generally the most sensitive (Figs. 148-6 and 148-7).[40] The colony-forming ability of cells from subjects with most forms of XP and CS are much more sensitive than that of normal cells to UV radiation and some chemicals; the sensitivity increase corresponds to a dose-modifying factor between 3 and 10.[40,103–109] XP cells are also more sensitive to 4-nitroquinoline-1-oxide, benz[*a*]anthracene, and a variety of aromatic amides, but are normal in response to *N*-methyl-*N*′-nitro-*N*-nitrosoguanidine.[105–109]

Fibroblasts from some variant XP patients without neurologic complications do not exhibit a great increase in UV sensitivity (e.g., XP7TA and XP30RO).[27,28,40]

Host-Cell Reactivation

The ability of UV-damaged viruses to undergo DNA repair and replication in infected cells depends on the genetic constitution of the cells. This is because most viruses depend on cellular enzymes for their repair and reproduction. The degree of dependence is greater for the smaller viruses [e.g., Simian virus 40 (SV40)] than for the larger ones (e.g., herpes simplex, cytomegalovirus).[110–119] UV treatment of a virus suspension before it is used to infect host cells damages the viral DNA and inactivates a certain fraction of the viruses. The fraction inactivated depends on the ability of the host cell to repair the damaged DNA in the infecting virus. The extent of this "host-cell reactivation" by various cell types often parallels the cells' ability to survive UV damage. Host-cell reactivation is therefore an important assay of the functional capacity of the DNA repair system. The survival of various UV-damaged viruses, including vaccinia,[110,111] herpes simplex virus,[111,112] adenovirus,[113,114] SV40,[115] and Epstein-Barr virus (EBV)[116,117] is less in XP cells than in normal cells. All of these are DNA viruses that replicate in the cell nucleus.

The D_{37} of irradiated viruses grown in XP complementation group A cells is about 20 times less than in normal cell strains for adenovirus[113,114] and about 3 times less for herpes virus.[111,112] The D_{37} for adenovirus in XP cells corresponds to the production of about one pyrimidine dimer per viral genome. Irradiated adenoviruses grown in XP variant cells show reductions in survival of a factor of only about 2, as compared with those grown in normal cells.[118] This may be the only assay that consistently demonstrates an abnormality in every form of XP. UV-damaged adenovirus grown in fused, complementing XP-A and XP-D cells shows normal survival,[119] indicating that fusion results in complementation of the functional activity of DNA repair in vivo.

Host-cell reactivation has been used to measure effects of the cellular repair system in the absence of replication, using UV-damaged nonreplicating expression vector plasmids.[120,121] The plasmids contain a bacterial enzyme, chloramphenicol acetyltransferase (CAT), in a construction that

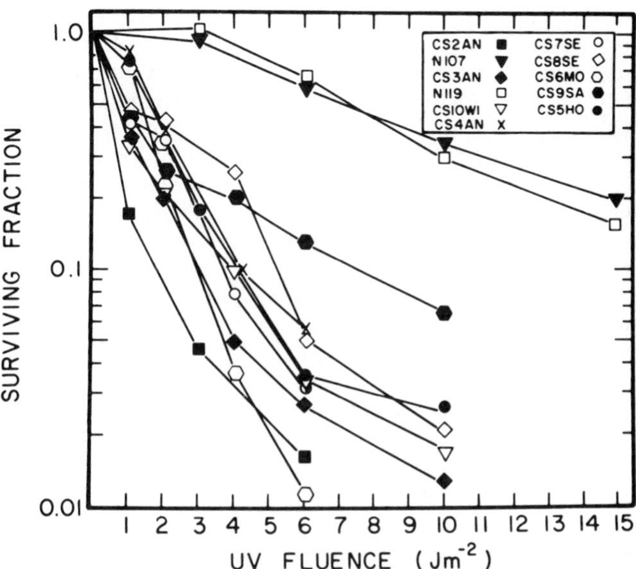

FIG. 148-7 **UV (254 nm) sensitivity as measured by colony-forming ability in diploid skin fibroblast strains derived from nine unrelated Cockayne syndrome patients and two normal donors. The UV flux was 1 J/m²/s as determined by the Black-Ray UV meter, model J-225. Plating efficiencies of fibroblasts varied between 10 and 50 percent. All points are the result of 5 to 10 replicate plates.** ***(From Wade and Chu.[57] Used by permission.)***

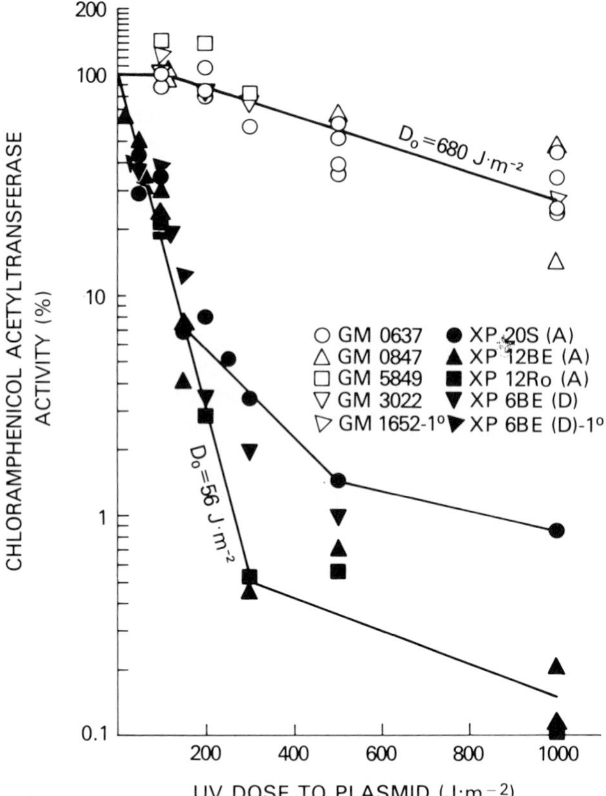

FIG. 148-8 **Transient expression of CAT gene in SV40-transformed xeroderma pigmentosum, ataxia-telangiectasia (GM 5849), retinoblastoma (GM 3022), Lesch-Nyhan (GM 0847), and normal human cells (GM 0637) and primary human skin fibroblasts (GM 1652-1°) transfected with UV-treated pSV2catSVgpt DNA. Cell types and designations are indicated in the figure.** ***(Reproduced from Protic-Sabljic and Kraemer.***[120] ***Used by permission.)***

permits expression of this novel activity on transfection into mammalian cells. Expression of transfected CAT activity following UV damage is much less in XP group A and D cells than in normal cells (Fig. 148-8). The unrepaired DNA damage appears to block transcription efficiently. In fact, with the XP-A and XP-D cells, about one cyclobutane pyrimidine dimer in the CAT gene results in its inactivation. Removal of 99 percent of the cyclobutane dimers by treatment of UV-damaged plasmid with photolyase prior to transfection did not completely restore CAT expression to normal levels. This implies that nondimer photoproducts also are poorly repaired by these XP cells.[121] Similar studies have been performed on cells from patients with CS.[61] Like XP, expression of UV-damaged CAT gene was lower in the CS than in the normal cells, but unlike XP, removal of the cyclobutane dimers did completely restore CAT expression to normal levels. This result suggests that CS cells have defective repair of cyclobutane dimers but normal repair of other DNA photoproducts.

Induction of Mutations by Ultraviolet Light

A small proportion of the cells that recover from irradiation carry mutations in the form of base-pair changes or deletions in the DNA. These are thought to arise from faulty replication of DNA that contains damaged bases. Some mutations can be detected through the cells' gain of drug resistance—that is, by growing cells in drugs that are lethal analogues of normal metabolites (e.g., 8-azaguanine or 6-thioguanine as analogues of purines) and observing the growth of mutant cells that have acquired resistance. One locus that has been studied extensively is the defective gene in the Lesch-Nyhan syndrome.[122] The key step in this pathway consists of an enzyme (HPRT) that attaches a phosphoribosyl group to 8-azaguanine or 6-thioguanine so that it can be incorporated into DNA. Resistant mutants produced by irradiation can survive high concentrations of these analogues because HPRT activity has been lost. Other gene loci amenable to study are those that regulate resistance to toxic chemicals such as ouabain or diphtheria toxin.

The frequency with which cells resistant to 6-thioguanine, ouabain, diphtheria toxin, or other toxic chemicals are produced by irradiation with UV light or artificial sunlight, or by exposure to chemical carcinogens, is greater in all XP cells, including XP variants, than in normal cells[123–127] (see Fig. 148-5). This implies that the genetic defects in XP cells confer increased mutability. The similar responses of all the XP cells in this mutagenesis assay contrast with the variability in their responses in the UV-light toxicity assay (see Figs. 148-5 and 148-6). This observation implies that the hypersensitive XP cells (later to be defined as the excision-defective groups A through G) have lost a system that normally repairs UV-induced damage in such a way as to avoid the errors that lead to mutations. In the XP variant, the damage is repaired in such a way as to allow cell survival. However, the repair system has lost fidelity and so produces a high frequency of mutations.

A newly developed host-cell reactivation assay using a replicating plasmid has been used to measure UV-induced base substitution mutagenesis in XP and normal cells.[94,128,129] This "shuttle vector" plasmid, pZ189, contains SV40 sequences that permit replication in some mammalian cells, plasmid sequences facilitating replication in bacteria, and a 150-bp marker gene (a bacterial suppressor tRNA) that serves as the target for mutations. The UV-damaged plasmid is transfected into the XP or normal cells where DNA repair, replication, and mutation occur. The replicated plasmids are harvested and then used to transform an indicator strain of *Escherichia coli* containing a suppressible (amber) mutation in the β-galactosidase gene. Plasmid survival and mutations are reflected in the number and color of bacterial colonies obtained by plating the bacteria on selective agar plates containing ampicillin and an indicator dye (X-gal), which is metabolized by β-galactosidase. Mutations that inactivate the suppressor tRNA function will result in white or light-blue colonies, while an active marker gene gives blue colonies. The mutant plasmids are purified, and the DNA sequence is determined.

The mutational spectrum found with pZ189 replicated in XP-A, XP-D, XP-F, and XP variant cells was restricted in comparison with that found in the normal cells[128,130–132] (Table 148-4). There were significantly fewer plasmids with tandem or multiple base substitution mutations or with single or tandem transversion mutations. With all cell lines, the predominant base substitution mutation was the G:C-to-A:T transition. Thus, with these human cells, the major UV photoproduct, the TT cyclobutane dimer, is not the major premutagenic lesion. This finding is consistent with observations made in bacteria more than 20 years ago, and more recently explained by the "A" rule: a tendency of polymerases to insert adenines opposite noninstructional lesions.[93,128] Thus, insertion of A opposite TT dimers results in the correct pairing, while insertion of A opposite a C involved in photoproducts results in G:C-to-A:T transitions. The G:C-to-A:T mutations common to the XP and normal cells may

Table 148-4 **Mutations Observed in UV-Treated Shuttle Vector pZ189 Replicated in Xeroderma Pigmentosum or Repair-Proficient Cells**

	Number (%) of Plasmids with Base Changes*							
	XP-A		XP-C	XP-D	XP-F	Variant	Normal	
	XP12BE	XP20S	XP4PA	XP6BE	XP2YO	GM2359	GM637	WI38
Independent plasmids sequenced[†]	61 (100)	61 (100)	67 (100)	69 (100)	72 (100)	53 (100)	89 (100)	91 (100)
Point mutations								
Single base substitutions	47[‡] (77)	46[§] (75)	48 (72)	59 (86)	51 (71)	41 (77)	48 (54)	53 (58)
Tandem base substitutions[¶]	12 (20)	8 (13)	11 (17)	4[‖] (6)	11 (15)	3 (6)	16 (18)	15 (16)
Multiple base substitutions[**]	1[‡] (2)	7 (11)	8 (12)	6[‡] (9)	8[‖] (11)	8 (15)	24 (27)	20 (22)
Base insertions and deletions								
Single base insertion	0	0	0	0	2 (3)	0	2 (2)	1 (1)
Single or tandem base deletion	1	0	0	1 (2)	0	0	3 (2)	2 (2)
Types of Single or Tandem Mutations and Number (%) of Changes								
Transitions	67[‡] (94)	52[‡] (84)	54 (75)	59 (88)	56[‖] (77)	34 (53)	61 (75)	52 (62)
G:C to A:T	66[‡] (93)	49[‡] (79)	51[‖] (71)	57 (85)	53[§] (73)	29 (45)	59 (73)	47 (56)
A:T to G:C	1 (1)	3 (5)	3 (4)	2 (3)	3 (4)	5 (8)	2 (2)	5 (6)
Transversions	4[‡] (6)	10[‡] (16)	18 (25)	8 (12)	17[‖] (23)	30 (47)	20 (25)	32 (38)
G:C to T:A	0[‡]	4[§] (6)	11 (15)	5 (7)	6[§] (8)	14 (22)	8 (10)	18 (21)
G:C to C:G	1 (1)	5 (8)	2[‖] (3)	1 (1)	6 (8)	3 (5)	5 (6)	9 (11)
A:T to T:A	3 (4)	0[‖]	4 (6)	0[‖]	5 (7)	9 (14)	6 (8)	3 (4)
A:T to C:G	0	1 (2)	1 (1)	2 (3)	0	4 (6)	1 (1)	2 (2)
Total mutations	71 (100)	62 (100)	72 (100)	67 (100)	73 (100)	64 (100)	81 (100)	84 (100)

*50 to 1000 J/m^2 to plasmid with xeroderma pigmentosum, 100 to 5000 J/m^2 to plasmid with normal. UV-treated plasmid replicated in the xeroderma pigmentosum cells had lower survival and higher mutation frequency than plasmid replicated in the repair proficient cells (see text for details).
†From separate transfections or different mutations in the same transfection, including all experiments.
‡$p<0.01$ versus normal.
§$p<0.02$ versus normal.
¶Two base substitutions 0 to 2 bases apart, or 3 adjacent base substitutions.
‖$p<0.05$ versus normal.
**At least two base substitutions more than 3 bases apart.
SOURCES: XP12BE and GM637—Bredberg et al.[128]; XP20S, XP2YO, and WI38—Yagi et al.[130]; XP6BE—Seetharam et al.[131]; XP variant—Wang et al.[132]; XP4PA—Yagi et al.[285]

be particularly important in somatic mutagenesis by UV radiation.

Both cyclobutane dimers (mainly 5′TC and 5′CC) and nondimer photoproducts, such as the [6-4] pyrimidine–pyrimidone photoproduct, have been shown to be mutagenic in monkey[129] and XP[128] cells by use of UV-exposed shuttle vector plasmids treated with photoreactivating enzyme prior to transfection.

BIOCHEMICAL CHARACTERISTICS OF XERODERMA PIGMENTOSUM

Excision Repair Pathways

The first studies of cultured fibroblasts from patients with the common and the neurologic forms of XP[5,133] showed that both classes of patients are defective to varying degrees in their ability to perform excision repair of damaged DNA. This is normally accomplished by several different repair enzyme systems with different mechanisms and efficiencies for removing various kinds of damaged DNA bases.[3,4,134] The sites of damage and rates of repair are influenced by the organization of DNA in the nucleus, which consists of histone particles around which 200 bp of DNA are wrapped to form each structural unit, or nucleosome[135–138] (Fig. 148-9).

Two major pathways of excision repair—the nucleotide and base excision repair pathways—operate on different kinds of damage in DNA.[3,4,134] The nucleotide pathway removes pyrimidine dimers and large chemical adducts to DNA (e.g., benz[*a*]anthracene adducts, methoxypsoralen monoadducts, acetoxyacetylaminofluorene adducts) and replaces the damaged site with a newly synthesized polynucleotide patch approximately 12 to 13 bases long in prokaryotes[139,141] but about 30 bases long in human cells.[140,141] The base excision pathway removes DNA bases that have undergone relatively small degrees of modification, such as alkylation or deamination, by a glycosylase and an apurinic endonuclease and replaces them with a patch that may be smaller than in nucleotide repair.[139,141] A further type of repair has been found in human cells that is specific for damage in the form of O^6-alkylguanine produced by alkylating agents. Some human tumor-cell strains are defective in this repair,[142] which operates by direct removal of the alkyl group itself with its transfer to the protein.[139,141,142]

Detailed analysis of the enzymes responsible for the first step in removal of pyrimidine dimers in various bacteria—the UV endonucleases—has demonstrated two distinct mechanisms. UV endonucleases from *Micrococcus luteus* and T4 phage-infected *E. coli* catalyze a glycosyl cleavage of the thymine deoxyribose bond on the 5′-thymine of the dimer.[143,144] This mechanism does not occur in *E. coli* itself, however, where a true endonucleolytic cleavage occurs on either side of the damage to release a 12- or 13-base oligonucleotide.[145] The mechanism that occurs in human

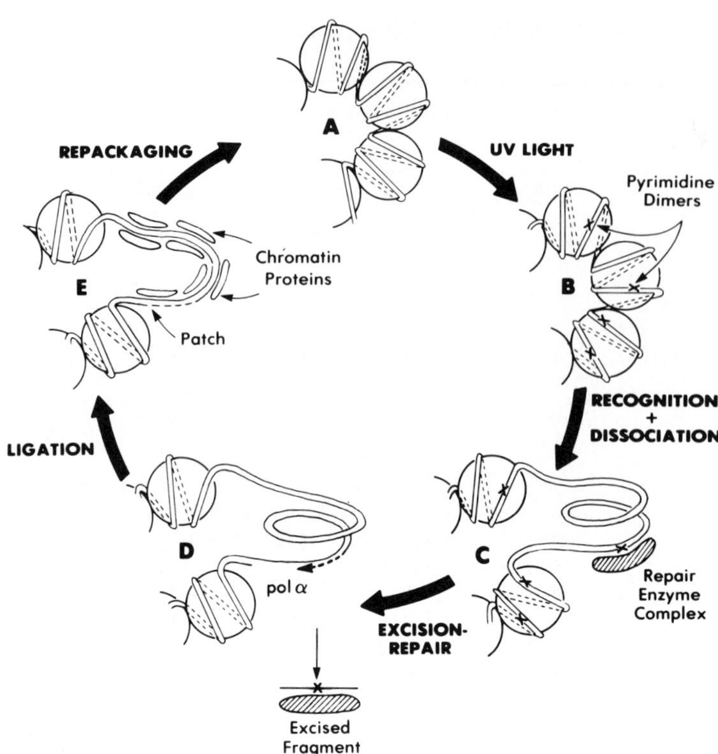

FIG. 148-9 **Heuristic scheme for excision repair of damaged sites on DNA in mammalian chromatin. The first step involves mechanisms that recognize damage and dissociate nucleoproteins to make the DNA accessible to repair enzymes. This is followed by sequential incision by a DNA polymerase, sealing of the patch by a polynucleotide ligase, and final reassembly and repackaging of nucleoprotein.** ***(Reproduced from Cleaver and Kraemer.[3] Used by permission.)***

cells is currently unknown, but may be similar to that in *E. coli* (Fig. 148-10).

The polymerization step of excision repair of UV damage is catalyzed predominantly by DNA polymerase alpha[146] or delta,[147] although polymerase beta may also be involved.[148]

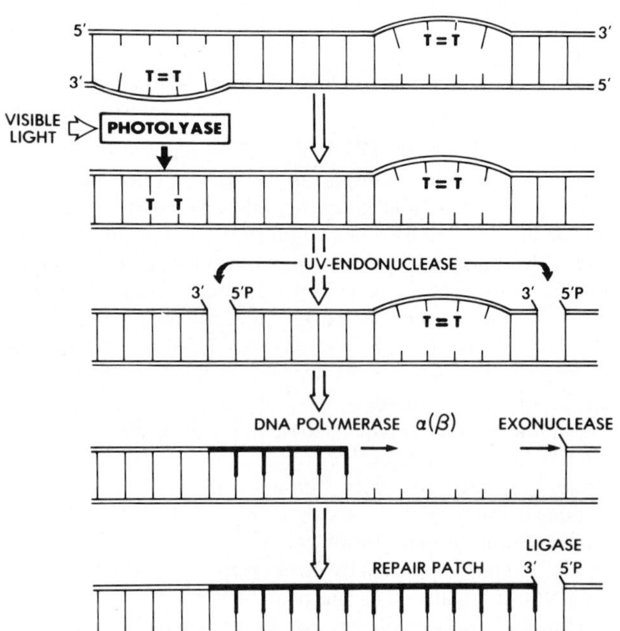

FIG. 148-10 **Biochemical steps for excision repair of pyrimidine dimers (nucleotide excision repair) in DNA prokaryotes showing biochemical details of events represented schematically in Fig. 148-9. The initial step of nucleotide excision occurs when a UV-specific endonuclease makes an incision on the 5′ and 3′ sides. Excision and subsequent polymerization releases a small oligonucleotide containing the dimer.**

The final step of repair is the sealing of the 5′, 3′ gap, a reaction catalyzed by polynucleotide ligase. Excision repair presumably requires a temporary relaxation of nucleosomal structure so that repaired regions are more accessible to exogenous nucleases (see Fig. 148-9).[134–138] Repair is strongly influenced by the transcriptional state of DNA[149,150]; actively transcribed genes are repaired more rapidly than untranscribed genes or the genome overall, and within transcribed regions the transcribed strand is repaired more rapidly than the untranscribed strand (Fig. 148-11). A role has also been demonstrated for single-strand DNA binding protein in excision repair.[151]

The process by which new bases are inserted into DNA during repair has been given various names according to the methods used for study, and a full description of methods is available elsewhere.[4,152] Autoradiographic methods of detection gave rise to the term *unscheduled synthesis*.[153] Cesium chloride isopyknic gradient methods led to the term *repair replication*,[154] which is also used in the bromouracil photolysis method.[155] The term *radiation-stimulated [^{3}H]thymidine incorporation*[27] describes an increase in total radioactivity incorporated into DNA by excision repair in cells in which normal DNA synthesis is naturally low (e.g., lymphocytes, plateau-phase tissue cultures), or is depressed by inhibitors of semiconservative DNA synthesis such as hydroxyurea. These various terms all describe the same biochemical process and are essentially equivalent. The different methods are chosen according to the cells or tissues under study. A conclusion derived from the use of each of the methods is that the patches that replace excised dimers are relatively large—10 to 50 bases long[4,5,13,140,141,155,156]—and contain both purines and pyrimidines.[13]

The continuous excision of dimers (Fig. 148-12) and insertion of the bases (see Figs. 148-9 to 148-11) is associated with a very low net frequency of DNA strand breaks.[4,157–164] This suggests that during excision repair a dynamic balance is established between strand breakage and rejoining. The actual number of sites involved in excision repair at any

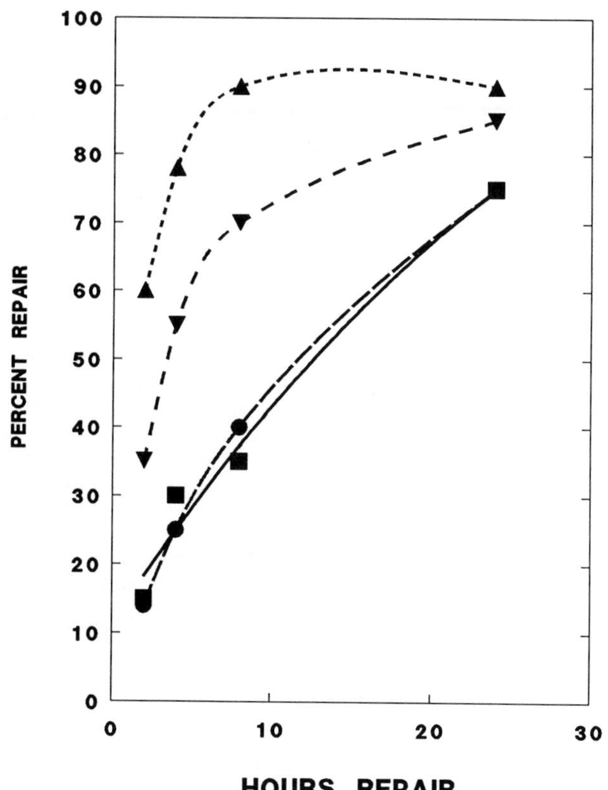

FIG. 148-11 **Preferential DNA repair. This plot shows the time course of repair following UV damage in normal human repair-proficient and Cockayne syndrome cells. There is more rapid repair in the actively transcribing c-*myc* (▲) and *dhfr* (▼) genes in the normal repair-proficient cells, in comparison with repair in the overall genome or in noncoding sequences (●). With the cells from a Cockayne syndrome patient the rate of repair was the same in the active *dhfr* gene as in the overall genome (■).** ***(Redrawn from Bohr.[150] Used by permission.)***

instant is small, no more than about 1 in 2×10^8 daltons of DNA. Only about 1 percent of the dimers produced in DNA by a dose of 10 J/m^2 is undergoing excision at any instant. The excision rate must therefore be dictated by the enzymes involved in the early steps of repair, not the number of substrates. The enzyme system must also move from site to site repairing different sites according to a set of endogenous priorities, such as the relative importance of the damaged regions or their transcriptional state.[149,150]

DEFECTIVE REPAIR IN XERODERMA PIGMENTOSUM

Cells from patients with XP excise pyrimidine dimers and carry out repair replication at rates that are between 0 and 90 percent of normal[165,166] (see Figs. 148-9 and 148-11). Cells from affected sibs usually carry out these processes at similar rates. XP cell lines that do not excise a detectable number of dimers also have low levels of repair replication, and those that excise at only a slightly reduced level also show only slightly reduced rates of repair replication. The reductions are similar in all tissues thus far investigated, including skin in vivo,[26] isolated epidermal cells, conjunctival cells, vascular smooth muscle cells, peripheral lymphocytes,[27] fibroblasts,[5] liver-cell cultures,[167] and tumor cells.[6] Patients with the XP variant exhibit normal levels of both dimer excision and repair replication.[27–30]

Repair of Damage from Chemical Mutagens and Carcinogens in Xeroderma Pigmentosum

Most chemical mutagens and carcinogens damage many cellular components, but the damage they cause to DNA is the most serious. XP cells show differential sensitivity to different agents. In response to damage from some mutagens and carcinogens, XP cells perform the same amounts of excision repair and have the same sensitivity to killing as do normal cells.[13,106,168,169] However, in response to damage from other carcinogens, XP cells perform less excision repair and have greater sensitivity than normal cells.[13,105–109,170–173] Since XP cells also respond normally to x-ray-induced damage, but not to UV-induced damage, the chemicals to which XP cells respond normally can be considered "x-ray-like" and those to which XP cells are sensitive, "UV-like"[13] (Table 148-5). The patch sizes synthesized in response to damage from x-ray-like chemicals may be smaller than those synthesized in response to UV-like chemicals.[4,172,173] The impaired response of XP cells to various carcinogens and mutagens appears to depend on the type of damage to DNA and the extent to which repair of the damage requires enzymes that are deficient in XP cells.

GENETICS

Genetic Heterogeneity in Xeroderma Pigmentosum and Cockayne Syndrome

Genetic heterogeneity in XP and CS patients whose cells are defective in excision repair is suggested by the different residual activities of dimer excision (see Fig. 148-12) and repair replication (Fig. 148-13; Table 148-6) and by the different clinical patterns. In addition to these quantitative differences are genetic differences between patients that can be analyzed by somatic-cell hybridization. Cells from different patients can be hybridized in culture using inactivated Sendai virus or polyethylene glycol as cell-fusing agents (Fig. 148-14). Cell fusion produces multinucleated cells with nuclei from each patient (heterokaryons). Heterokaryons from some combination of patients exhibit complementation and increased repair, whereas other combinations remain repair-deficient.[6,21,31,174–178] Complementation has been assayed by increased repair, survival, or recovery of RNA synthesis. If complementation occurs, it is an indication that the cell types contain defects in different genes and each supplies what the other is lacking.

Numerous studies in which cells from many patients were hybridized in pairs have demonstrated seven excision-repair-deficient complementation groups[6,21,31,174–178] (see Table 148-6 and Fig. 148-12). These groups represent different gene loci and distinctive excision deficiencies (see Table 148-6). This implies that the initial step of repair, which once appeared to be the action of a single UV endonuclease, actually requires the cooperative function of many interacting gene products. The three major groups include A (63 patients, 27 percent), C (60 patients, 25 percent), and variant (54 patients, 23 percent). The next most frequent is group D (35 patients, 15 percent). The remaining groups are represented by only one or two families.

The characteristic cellular phenotype of CS is indicated by a failure of RNA and DNA synthesis to recover to normal levels after moderate doses of UV light (5 to 10 J/m^2). This failure of recovery has been used in cell-fusion studies to permit identification of two CS complementation groups—A and B—and a third that coincides with XP group B.[12,62,64]

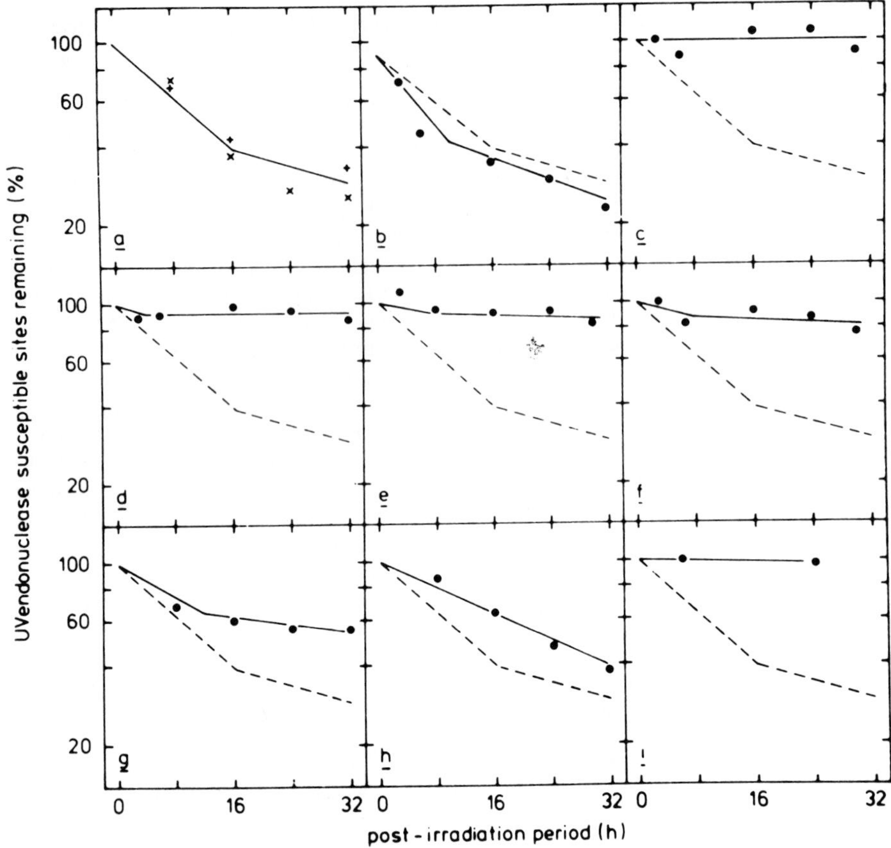

FIG. 148-12 Time course of disappearance of UV endonuclease-susceptible sites (pyrimidine dimers) from the DNA of normal human cells and cells from each complementation group of XP after radiation at 254 nm. After specified periods of post-UV incubation, cell samples were assayed to determine the number of dimers remaining in the extracted DNA. The percentages shown for the incubated samples are relative to those found for the parallel nonincubated ones and normalized to 100 percent for the number of dimers present immediately after irradiation. Panel *a*, two normal cell lines. The other panels give data for one patient from each XP group; *b*, XP variant; *c*, group A; *d*, group B; *e*, group C; *f*, group D; *g*, group E; *h*, group F; *i*, group G. The dashed lines indicate the mean response of normal cells. *(Reproduced from Zelle and Lohman.[166] Used by permission.)*

The question of assignment to a CS group for patients who display CS and XP signs clinically, but who also fall into XP groups D and G, is currently unresolved. This is because a failure to recover RNA and DNA synthesis can also be caused by the deficient repair of XP. For this reason, cellular definition of CS in the presence of concomitant XP defects in DNA excision repair is difficult. Therefore, whether the groups that coincide with XP groups D and G are distinct from CS A and B or represent a complex consequence of a single excision repair defect itself has not yet been clarified. Distributions for CS are not available since only a small number of patients have been classified, but more CS group A patients are known than group B.[64]

Patients with Combined Xeroderma Pigmentosum and Cockayne Syndrome Symptoms

The presence of several patients in XP groups B, D, and G who also show symptoms of CS is particularly difficult to explain (see Table 148-6).[179] Since groups B and D each appear to correspond to mutations in a single gene, and the in vitro phenotype of UV sensitivity is almost completely correctable by the appropriate gene, it is unlikely that these complex mixed phenotypes represent mutations in more than one gene. A provisional explanation could be based on the model in which excision repair is mediated by multiple interacting gene products[180] involving DNA binding proteins, protein–protein associations, and secondary modification by phosphorylation. If there are primary sets of XP and CS gene products, but some of these are required to interact with each other, symptoms of both diseases could develop if mutations involve the regions of XP or CS proteins that are involved in specific, mutual interactions.

Interspecies Comparison in DNA Repair

Human and rodent cells have similar mechanisms for UV repair and contain homologous repair genes, but there are certain notable differences. In particular, rodent cells are similar to human cells in excision of [6-4] photoproducts,

Table 148-5 Classification of Carcinogens and Mutagens on the Basis of the Total Amount of DNA Repair in XP Cells

Agents Causing Damage That Is Repaired Defectively in XP Cells	Agents Causing Damage That Is Repaired Normally in XP Cells
UV light	X-rays
Methoxypsoralen adduct	Bromouracil photoproducts
4-Nitroquinoline-1-oxide	Dimethyl sulfate
Bromobenz[*a*]anthracene	Methyl methanesulfonate
Benz[*a*]anthracene epoxide	*N*-methyl-*N*′-nitro-*N*-nitrosoguanidine
1-Nitropyridine-1-oxide	Methylnitrosourea
Acetylaminofluorene	ICR 170
Aromatic amides	
Benz[*a*]pyrene	

NOTE: The measurements of repair are biased toward those lesions in DNA that predominate and that are repaired more rapidly with larger patches. Therefore, quantitatively minor lesions, such as those from 4-nitroquinoline-1-oxide that are normally repaired or from 4-nitroquinoline-1-oxide that are normally repaired, will not be resolved in measurements of the total amount of repair. For references to specific chemicals, see text.

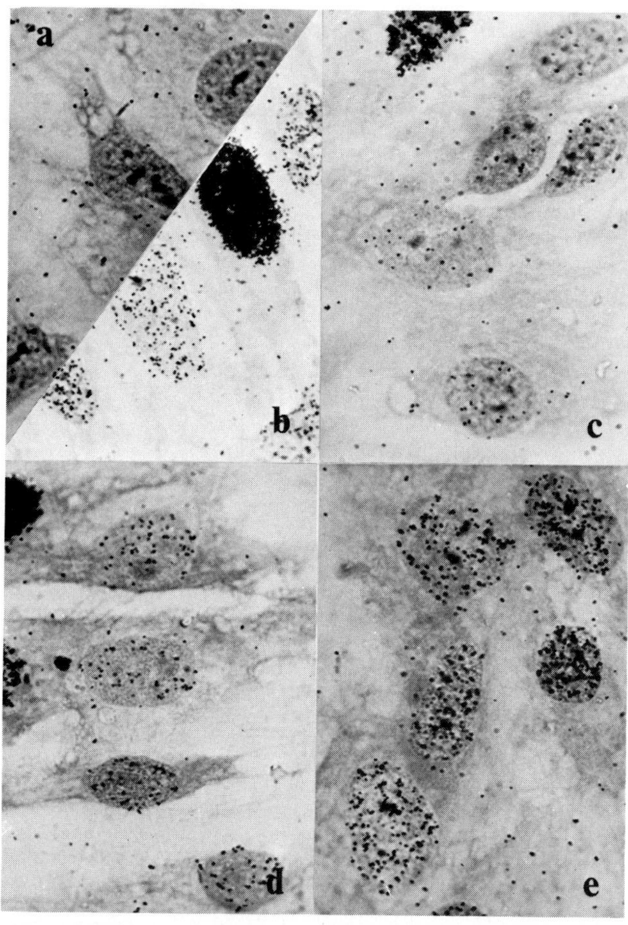

FIG. 148-13 **Autoradiographs of normal and XP cells irradiated with 30 J/m² of UV light and labeled for 3 h with [³H]thymidine (10 μCi/ml, 21.9 Ci/mmol). *A*. Normal (JEC) cells, nonirradiated. *B*. Normal (JEC) cells, irradiated. *C*. Repair-deficient XP23SF cells, irradiated. *D*. Partially repair-deficient XP20SF cells, irradiated. *E*. XP variants, irradiated. *(From J. E. Cleaver, unpublished data, 1975.)***

but are relatively poor at excision of cyclobutane dimers. Rodent cells appear to excise dimers mainly from actively transcribed genes; human cells have additional capacity for excising dimers from the nontranscribed regions of their genome.[149,150]

UV-sensitive mutant cell lines have been isolated from Chinese hamster ovary (CHO) cells[181] and mouse cells,[182] and both species demonstrate multiple complementation groups. About 12 UV-sensitive groups have thus far been identified in rodent cell lines, and their genes are denoted as ERCC (excision repair cross complementing). These mutants are also sensitive to varying degrees to mitomycin C, an alkylating agent that crosslinks DNA. This property is exhibited strongly by human cell lines from patients with Fanconi anemia but less so from patients with XP.[183]

The gene for CHO complementation group 1 (ERCC1) has been cloned and corresponds to a human gene of 15 kb on human chromosome 19q13.2-13.3 coding for a 297 amino acid protein.[184–187] This gene does not correct any XP cell lines, but mutations are lethal in transgenic mice.[185] Two other genes (ERCC2 and ERCC3) have been found to correspond to XP groups D and B, respectively. The ERCC6 gene corresponds to CS group B.

Genetic studies of yeast have found at least 24 genes to be involved in UV sensitivity (called RAD1 through RAD24).[187] Ten genes in the RAD3 epistasis group are involved in excision repair of DNA damage induced by UV radiation (RAD1, RAD2, RAD3, RAD4, RAD10, RAD7, RAD23, RAD14, RAD16, and MMS19). RAD3, a DNA helicase, has homologies to rodent ERCC2 gene, RAD10 is similar to ERCC1,[188] RAD2 corresponds to ERCC5, and RAD14 is homologous to the XPAC gene.[189]

Cloning Studies in Xeroderma Pigmentosum and Cockayne Syndrome

Isolation and cloning of the genes involved in UV-sensitivity disorders has been an extremely long and difficult project.

Table 148-6 **Level of Unscheduled DNA Synthesis (UDS), Clinical Features, XP Patient Frequency and Location, and Chromosome Site in the XP Complementation Groups**

Complementation Group	UDS (% of Normal)	Clinical Features		XP Patients		
		Skin Cancer	Neuro Abnl*	Number Reported	Location†	Chromosome Site
A	<2%	Yes	Severe	63	Japan, Europe, United States, Egypt	9q34.1
B‡	3–7%	Yes	XP-CS§	3	United States, Europe	2q21
C	10–20%	Yes	None	60	Europe, United States, Egypt, Japan	3p25.1
D‡	25–50%	Yes	Moderate	28	Europe, United States, Japan	19q13.2
D‡	25–50%	Yes	XP-CS	1	France	19q13.2
D‡	25–50%	No	TTD¶	6	United States, Europe	19q13.2
E	40–50%	Yes	None	6	Europe, Japan	?
F	10–20%	Yes	None	11	Japan, Europe	16p13
G	<2%, 25%	Yes	Variable	3	Europe, Japan	13q32–33
G	<2%, 25%	No	XP-CS	2?	United States, Europe	13q32–33
Variant	100%	Yes	None	54	Japan, Europe, United States, Egypt	?

*Neurologic abnormalities classified as severe, moderate, or none.
†Location of XP patients listed by relative frequency of country or area of origin of patients.
‡These genes code for products that are components of transcription factor TFIIH, which may also contain other DNA repair genes.
§Xeroderma pigmentosum–Cockayne syndrome complex. See text for details.
¶Trichothiodystrophy. See text for details.

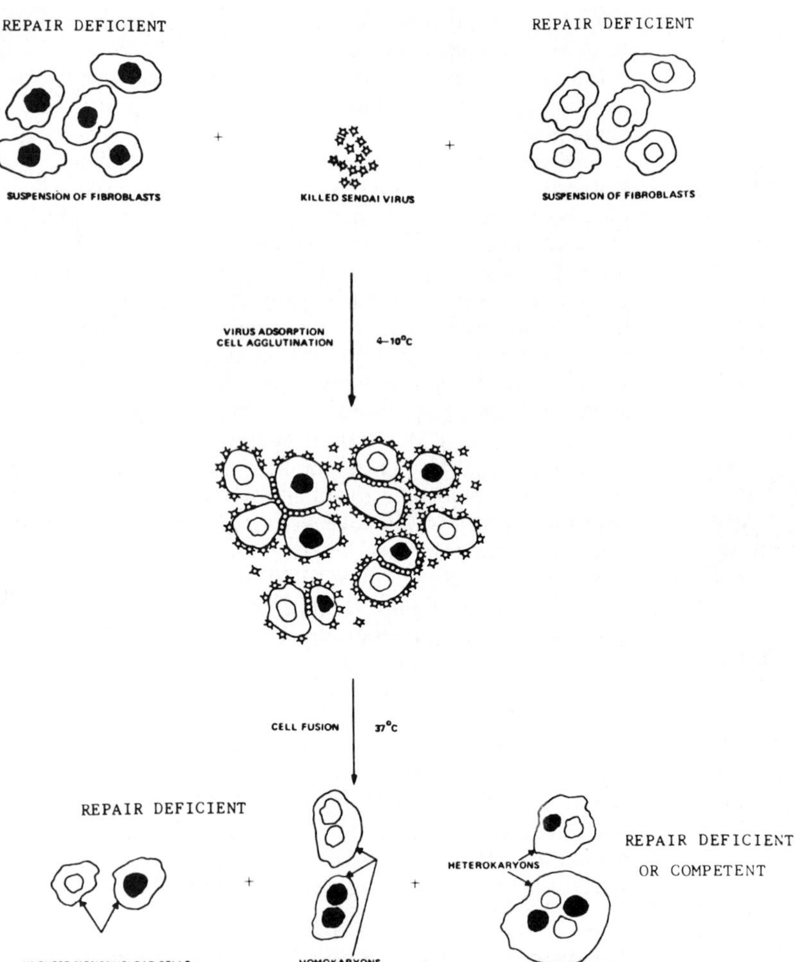

FIG. 148-14 Schematic representation of cell fusion under the influence of inactivated Sendai virus as it is employed to detect complementation between different genetic defects. Fibroblasts from two XP patients who are both repair-deficient (denoted by dark and light nuclei) are allowed to agglutinate in the cold and fuse at 37°C to form multinucleate cells. Multinucleate cells with nuclei from the same cell line (homokaryons) will exhibit a repair defect similar to that of the original mononuclear cells. Multinucleate cells with nuclei from each cell line (heterokaryons) will be either repair-deficient or repair-competent, depending on whether the repair defects in the original cell lines are in the same or different complementation groups. One complementation group will usually comprise XP patients with defects in a single gene that codes for an enzyme, an enzyme subunit, or a single polypeptide.

This is mainly because human cell lines proved to be refractory to the incorporation of large quantities of exogenous DNA in comparison to rodent cell lines and few chromosome markers have been available in families sufficiently large to permit chromosome walking. The approach available, therefore, was functional complementation of UV sensitivity by exogenous DNA. This has been a slow and difficult route. Eventual success has been considerably facilitated by the use of the ERCC series of UV-sensitive Chinese hamster cell mutants.

Table 148-7 Cloned Human NER Genes

Gene*	Phenotype*	Chromosome Location	Yeast Homolog	Function
ERCC1	Lethal in a mouse model	19q13.2	RAD10	Component of nuclease complex (with ERCC4)
ERCC2/XPD	XP-D	19q13.2	RAD3	Transcription factor BTF2/TFIIH†
ERCC3/XPB	XP-B	2q21	RAD25	Transcription factor BTF2/TFIIH†
ERCC4	XP-F	16p13	RAD1	Component of nuclease complex (with ERCC1)
ERCC5	XP-G	13q32–33	RAD2	Nuclease
ERCC6	CS-B	10q21.1	ERCC6^{cer}	Transcription coupling factor
XPA	XP-A	9q34.1	RAD14	Damage recognition
XPC	XP-C	3p25.1‡	RAD4	Repair genome overall
XPE	XP-E	?	?	Damage recognition
HHR23A		19p13.2‡	RAD23	
HHR23B		3p25.1‡	RAD23	Complex with XP-C protein

*The nomenclature ERCC is based on Chinese hamster cell mutants; XP, CS nomenclature is based on complementation between human fibroblasts. A proposed simplification under consideration is that when a gene is proved to carry mutations in affected patients, the disease nomenclature listed under phenotype above supplants previous uses.

†The following proteins are associated with BTF2/TFIIH complex and may play a role in NER: TTD-A, TTD-B, p62 (TFB1), p44 (SSL1), p41, and p34.

‡P.J. van der Spek, J.H.J. Hoeijmakers, and A. Hagemeijer, personal communication.

The first UV repair gene to be cloned was that for complementation group 1 in CHO cells, subsequently known as ERCC1.[175] This small gene has not proved to correspond to any known human disorder and may therefore constitute an essential gene. It contains sequences homologous to RAD10 in yeast and UVRA and UVRC in bacteria, but its functional significance has yet to be elucidated.[186] Other genes cloned by this route include ERCC2, 3, 5, and 6. Of these, ERCC2 has been found to correspond to XP group D and ERCC3 to XP group B.

The cloning of complementation group A for XP was achieved, however, by direct transfer of mouse genomic DNA into XP group A cells, and searching for complementation of the UV sensitivity. This led to the successful cloning of the XP-A gene by Tanaka et al.[190] The identities of XP-A, XP-B, and XP-D genes have been confirmed by direct and specific complementation of several cell lines within each group by the cDNA in question, and in some cases the identification of specific mutations in the gene in individual XP patients. Identification of CS group B was facilitated by the identification of a patient in whom a chromosome deletion occurred at the site that has been mapped for ERCC6, the CHO gene with putative helicase function.

Most recently, functional complementation has been considerably facilitated by the development of EBV-based vectors that can transfect functional cDNA libraries into competent cells. The complementing gene is then easy to recover because the complementing sequence is retained in an episomal-based vector. Therefore, the remaining genes that have not yet been cloned are highly likely to be found within the next few years. At that point a complete analysis of the genetic regulation and the gene products involved in XP and CS should be possible, and detailed understanding of the regulation of DNA repair at genomic and subgenomic levels should become possible.

Characteristics of Complementation Groups

Group A. Group A usually corresponds to the most severe clinical form of XP, in which there are both skin symptoms and central nervous system (CNS) disorders. Many patients exhibit disorders from birth or early in life and correspond to the clinical category of the DeSanctis-Cacchione syndrome with progressive neurologic degeneration.[25,33,191–194]

There are exceptions to these general characteristics of group A cells. One British patient without CNS disorders, XP8LO, exhibited about 30 percent of normal excision repair and higher survival after UV than other group A cells.[195] Cells from one 35-year-old Egyptian male (XP13CA) had a low level of unscheduled synthesis typical of most group A cells, but the patient was neurologically normal, had normal stature, and was fertile[194] (Fig. 148-15). Two other group A patients, XP12BE and XP1LO, also show minimal neurologic abnormalities, and the cells have higher survival after UV irradiation than the majority in group A.[21,40] In one Italian family, group A sibs exhibited different clinical symptoms; only one had disorders of the CNS.[196] In cell cultures, it appeared that the sib with no CNS disorder had, on average, higher repair due to a subpopulation of cells, with normal repair mixed with typical group A cells. Therefore, although group A patients usually have the associated neurologic abnormalities of the DeSanctis-Cacchione syndrome, several are known who are neurologically normal or who have less severe neurologic abnormalities.

Excision repair is very low (<2 percent of normal) in these cells and they are about 10 times more sensitive than normal to killing by UV radiation or other carcinogens (see Fig. 148-6). They are also about four times more sensitive to methyl methanesulfonate[197] and have slightly reduced levels of apurinic endonuclease.[198]

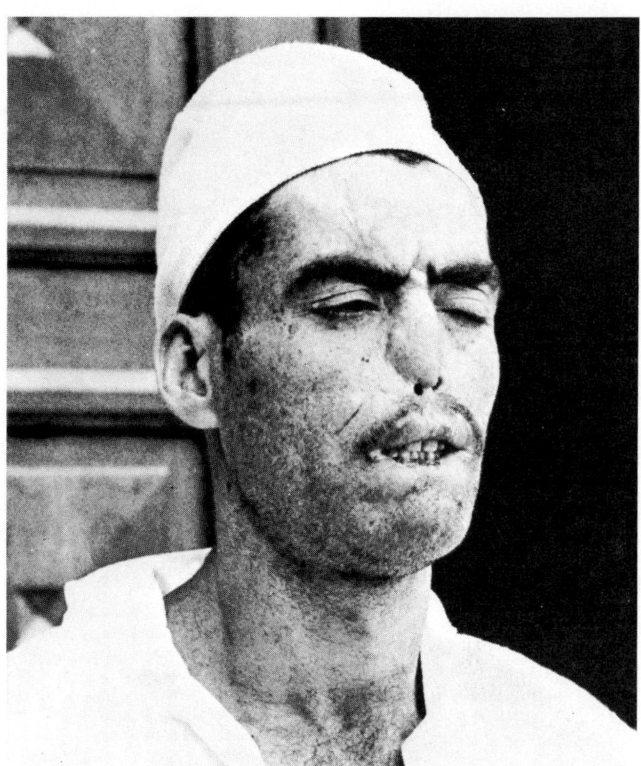

FIG. 148-15 Exceptional group A patient (XP13CA) from complementation group A exhibiting skin abnormalities, including the consequences of invasive skin carcinoma of the nose, but with normal neurologic status, unlike most group A patients. ***(Photograph kindly supplied by Dr. J. German, New York Blood Center.)***

The cloned gene for this complementation group, known as XPAC (XP-A correcting), consists of a cDNA of about 0.8 kb that codes for a DNA binding protein of 273 amino acids containing a Zn finger motif.[190] The 25-kb gene has six exons and is located on chromosome 9q34. This gene is homologous to the RAD14 gene of yeast.[189] The predicted molecular weight of the gene product is 31 kDa. Direct analysis of the XPAC protein identified multiple species between 38 and 42 kDa.[199,200] The protein's binding affinity for UV-damaged DNA is about 103 times greater than for undamaged DNA,[199] and the protein appears to be present in excess. Exon 1 of the XPAC gene is not essential for DNA repair activity, but exons 2 to 6 are required.[190] The gene product may be mainly responsible for repair of [6-4] photoproducts.[201]

More is known about the molecular details of Japanese XPAC gene mutations.[190,202,283,284] The majority of Japanese cases result from one of three classes of mutations: a G-to-C transversion at the 3′ splice acceptor site of intron 3, a nonsense mutation in exon 3, and a nonsense mutation in exon 6. The frequency of these mutant alleles is about 85 percent:4 percent:13 percent in Japanese XP-A patients. Different mutations are found in U.S. and European XP-A patients. The mild case XP8LO contains a missense mutation in exon 6.

Group B. There are only two reported families (Fig. 148-16) in group B—one U.S. patient (XP11BE) and two European

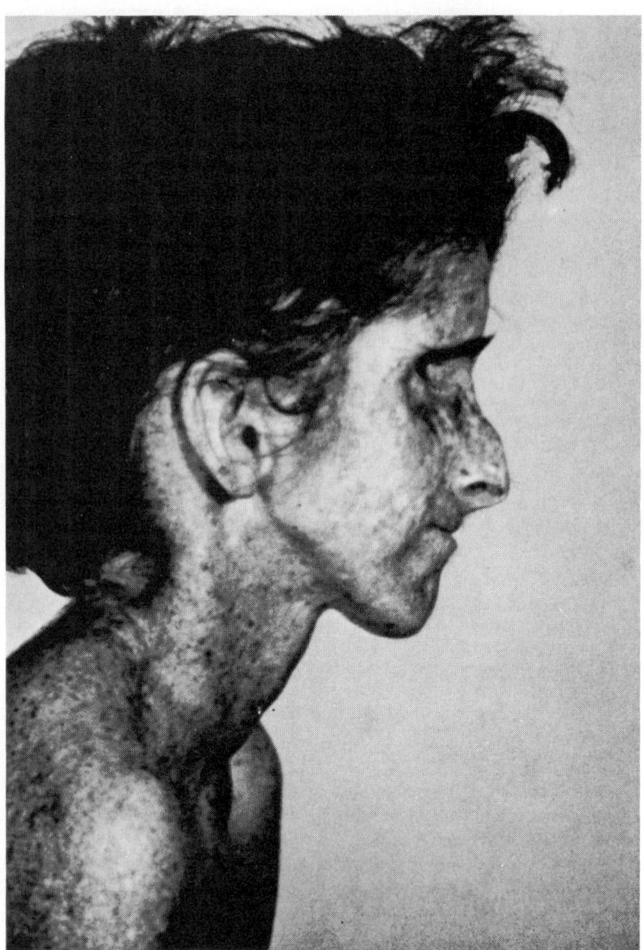

FIG. 148-16 XP patient (XP11BE) from complementation group B exhibiting skin, ocular, and neurologic characteristics that have been ascribed to both XP and Cockayne syndrome. ***(From Kraemer.[282] Used by permission.)***

brothers—all of whom have symptoms of both XP and Cockayne syndrome.[21] The patient XP11BE died of acute hypertension at age 33. She had reduced stature, deafness, mental retardation, immature sexual development, premature senility, absence of subcutaneous fat, and optic nerve and retinal pigment degeneration characteristic of Cockayne syndrome. She exhibited acute sun sensitivity, ocular changes, and multiple cutaneous malignancy at age 18, all typical of XP. The European patients were identified at about age 40; they had no tumors. The conjunction of two extremely rare disorders in individual patients is statistically unlikely, so this constellation of symptoms may instead be regarded as characteristic of this group. Cells in this group have low levels of excision repair and are very sensitive to killing by UV light.

The gene for this group (XPBC) was cloned indirectly by first cloning the gene correcting the hamster group ERCC3, which was then found to correspond to XP group B.[203,204] This gene is located on chromosome 2q21, is 45 kb in size with at least 14 exons, and encodes a protein of 782 amino acids. The deduced amino acid sequence resembles that of a DNA binding helicase in yeast. In one allele of XP11BE, who was severely affected, a C-to-A transversion in the splice acceptor sequence resulted in a 4-bp insertion and an inactivating frameshift close to the C-terminus of the protein.[203] In the newly identified European family, consisting of less severely affected patients, there is a point mutation close to the N-terminus.[205]

Group C. Group C is one of the largest groups (see Fig. 148-3) and is often referred to as the common or classic form of XP. The patients usually show only skin disorders. These vary considerably in severity, depending on the climate. Tumors of the tip of the tongue have been observed in several patients[32,186] (see Fig. 148-3). Cells have low but heterogeneous levels of excision repair (10 to 20 percent of normal) and are less sensitive to killing by UV light and chemical carcinogens than cells from groups A and D.[21,40,107] One characteristic of repair unique to this group is that it is clustered rather than random, due to a loss in the capacity to repair transcriptionally inactive regions.[206–209]

One exceptional patient (XP1M1) exhibited symptoms of XP, systemic lupus erythematosus, microcephaly, and a marginal degree of mental retardation.[210] Cells from this patient had typical DNA repair levels but were the most UV-sensitive of any in group C.[40] Two reported instances of CNS tumors in XP patients—XP106LO[211] and Hawaiian patient XP15BE[212]—are in this group.

The XPCC gene has been cloned, but no detailed information is yet available.[213,214]

Group D. Patients in XP complementation group D resemble those in group A in exhibiting both skin and CNS disorders, although the latter usually develop later in life than in patients in group A.[193,211] This group shows considerable clinical heterogeneity. Some patients have been reported in both the United States and Europe with TTD, a disorder with sulfur deficiency of the hair and mental retardation.[75,76] Some other cases, notably a patient originally classified as group H but now reclassified as group D,[215–218] have additional symptoms of CS. Group D is consequently a complex group involving diverse clinical syndromes.[179] Representatives of this group have been reported more frequently in Britain than elsewhere, but their distribution is not as restricted as that of groups B, F, and G. Excision repair is low (10 to 20 percent), as in group C cells, but functionally poorer. Some evidence suggests that the amount of unscheduled DNA synthesis is higher than expected from the low amount of dimer excision observed in these cells due perhaps to better repair of [6-4] photoproducts (see Table 148-6).[219] Cells are almost as sensitive to cell killing as are group A cells.[21,40] Cells in this group were claimed in one study to have reduced levels of apurinic endonuclease,[220] but this was not confirmed in another study.[221]

The gene for this group (XPDC) was cloned indirectly by first cloning the gene correcting the hamster group ERCC2, which was then found to correspond to XP group D.[222–225] This gene is located on chromosome 19q13.2-13.3, is 19 kb in size, and encodes a protein of 760 amino acids, with sequence motifs that resemble a DNA helicase. In one patient an amino acid change from Leu to Val in position 461 has been identified.[224]

Group E. Patients in the rare group E exhibit mild degrees of skin symptoms and are neurologically normal.[21] The level of excision repair is high (more than 50 percent of normal), and the level relative to normal cells increases with increasing UV dose. The cells are only slightly more sensitive than normal to UV damage. Patients have been reported from Europe and Japan.[226–228]

Deficiencies in a DNA binding protein have been reported for patients from two unrelated families in this group, but the general significance of this is unknown.[229] Cells from other XP-E patients have normal levels of this protein.[230]

Group F. Most representatives of group F have been described in Japan (XP230S, XP107TO, XP2YO, and XP3YO).[177,231,232] The patients had acute sun sensitivity in infancy but relatively mild symptoms with late onset of skin cancer despite a substantially reduced level of repair. Excision repair was 10 to 15 percent of normal but increased to 60 percent with incubation. The cells appear to be more defective in repair of damage that occurs at rapid rates and at early times after irradiation such as [6-4] photoproducts.[219] The cells showed an intermediate sensitivity to killing by UV light and a high degree of excision of pyrimidine dimers. There was a marked enhancement of UV survival when cells were held in a density-inhibited condition for 1 to 4 days after irradiation.[232] The gene may be located on chromosome 15.[233]

Group G. Two representatives of group G have been described in England (XP3BR, XP2B1)[178,234] and one in Japan (XP31KO),[235] and two patients with XP-G and CS have also been identified.[179] The European patients had mental retardation, microcephaly, and sun sensitivity, but no neoplasms. The cells had extremely low levels of dimer excision and unscheduled synthesis and were as sensitive as groups A and D to killing by UV light. XP3BR is unusual in having a slightly increased sensitivity to killing by x-rays.[178,234] There is heterogeneity within this group: the Japanese patient was 37 years old with no neurologic abnormalities, a normal skin phototest reaction, and a basal-cell carcinoma.[235] Unscheduled DNA synthesis of XP31KO was 25 percent, a level much higher than in the other group G cells.

XP Variant. Patients in the variant group (Fig. 148-17) have mild to severe skin symptoms and usually have normal CNS functions. The variant form is found worldwide and is a frequently occurring and distinct group, even though it cannot often be clinically discriminated without cell culture studies. Originally defined as a clinically recognized XP without any biochemical defect in excision repair,[27,28] it was also described earlier under the clinical designation *pigmented xerodermoid*.[29,35,236] With careful clinical investigation, some patients in this group may be recognized by relatively mild symptoms and the absence of an enhanced erythematous response,[34] but this is insufficient for unambiguous diagnosis, and other XP variant patients may have severe clinical symptoms.[21]

The high level of mutagenesis[126,132,237] involving reduced insertion of adenine bases opposite dimers[132] with near-normal levels of cell survival after UV irradiation[40] could be interpreted as indicating that the inherited disorder has made XP variant cells error-prone. The outstanding feature of this form of XP is that after UV irradiation, replication forks appear to stop or to be interrupted during semiconservative replication at every site of DNA damage. This radiation effect on replication is exaggerated by growth in 1 m*M* caffeine,[14,29,30,238,239] which stimulates many new replication forks,[14,29] and survival is concomitantly diminished. These observations can be explained if it is assumed that normal cells and cells from XP groups A through G have gene product(s) that normally facilitate replication without interruption at damaged sites and that XP variant cells have lost one or more of these gene product(s).[29,30] This is correlated with a reduced rate of recovery of DNA replication after UV irradiation.[238]

Whether the variant group is homogeneous or has multiple subgroups is not known, but the clinical heterogeneity is suggestive.[27-30,34,35,236] The pigmented xerodermoid family of Jung et al.,[35,236] although biochemically identical to other XP variants, is unusual because no clinical symptoms were evident until after the age of 40, and patients lived into their eighties. These mild symptoms contrast with other variant families from comparable environments in whom the disease is quite severe.[21,29] One attempt at studying complementation between cells from different XP variant patients indicated a single XP variant group.[240]

Xeroderma Pigmentosum Heterozygotes

The XP gene defects appear to have a significant effect on clinical symptoms and DNA repair only when present in both alleles. Clinical and laboratory investigations of XP heterozygotes have failed to uncover consistent clinical or

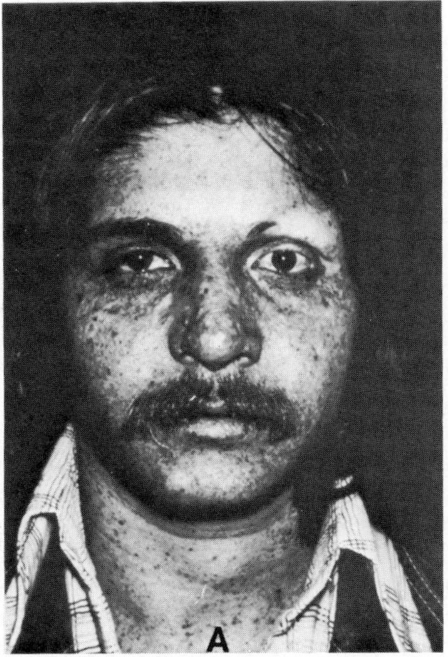

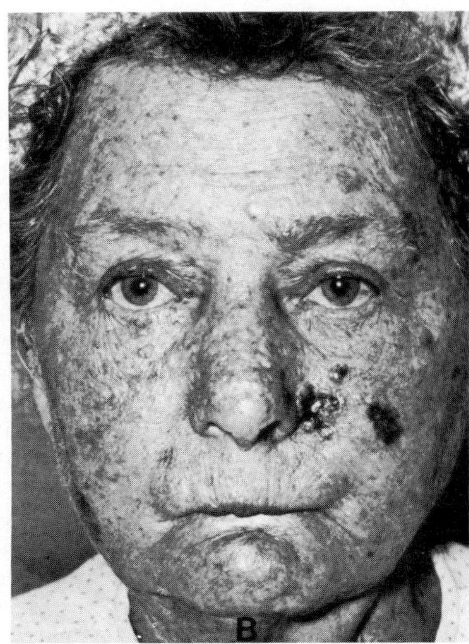

FIG. 148-17 **XP variants (*A*, XP115LO; *B*, XP5MA) exhibiting skin symptoms characteristic of XP and normal neurologic status. *(Photographs kindly provided by Drs. H. Hoffmann and E. G. Jung [A] and Dr. F. Giannelli [B].)***

cellular abnormalities.[25,26,28,194] In a study of XP cases in the United States,[241] the majority of XP heterozygotes were asymptomatic, although a few families in one geographical location had nonmelanoma skin cancers. In Egypt no skin abnormalities were seen in nearly 100 heterozygotes, despite the intense sunlight and the severe skin abnormalities seen in homozygotes.[194,242]

Studies of DNA repair in cell cultures from heterozygotes also fail to detect any consistent DNA repair defects, although slight reductions in repair have been reported in occasional studies at high UV doses.[243,244] In one study, fusion of heterozygote with homozygote cells produced multinucleated cells, each of which contained many repair-deficient nuclei and one heterozygous XP nucleus.[243] Slight reductions in repair were then evident in comparison with normal cells.[243] Also, a slightly lower rate of dimer excision from DNA of heterozygotes as compared with normal cells has been observed at high UV doses.[244] An increased level of chromosome rearrangements has been reported for XP heterozygotes.[245] An assay of sensitivity of XP lymphocytes to recovery of chromosome breaks and gaps following x-ray exposure revealed a slow recovery rate in XP homozygotes.[246] The XP heterozygotes had a rate intermediate between the XP homozygotes and normal.[246] Identification of the defective gene in Japanese patients with XP complementation group A has enabled detection of XP-A heterozygotes by molecular biologic techniques.[190]

Measurements of host-cell reactivation of irradiated adenovirus[113] or herpes virus[247] did not show any differences between normal hosts and XP heterozygotes. However, measurements of the rate of production of viral antigen from irradiated adenovirus did show lower rates in heterozygotes.[248] A plasmid host-cell reactivation assay measuring CAT activity following transfection of UV-treated plasmid into peripheral blood lymphocytes has been field tested (see Fig. 148-8 for comparison).[249] There was a broad range of reactivity with the normal population and obligate XP heterozygotes showed activity at the low portion of this range.

PRENATAL DIAGNOSIS OF XERODERMA PIGMENTOSUM

Once the main biochemical features of XP were delineated, the assays were adapted for use in prenatal diagnosis. Cell suspensions can be obtained from amniotic fluid by transabdominal puncture during the second half of the first trimester of pregnancy and used to grow fibroblasts in tissue culture representative of the fetus. Fibroblasts from normal fetuses have normal capacities for excision repair,[103] whereas those from XP fetuses are expected to be defective. It is possible to identify a family at risk for the XP genotype when one homozygous child has already appeared in the family. Prenatal diagnosis was first achieved in such a family by Ramsay et al.[250]

Speed is paramount in tests for DNA repair in amniocentesis specimens. One of the main purposes is to provide a family with reliable information on which to base a decision whether to interrupt pregnancy within the period allowed by law. Autoradiographic analysis of DNA repair and many other assays for excision repair deficiency or postreplication repair deficiency can be completed in a few days. The longest delay is due to the time required for fibroblast cultures to develop from amniocentesis cell suspensions (about 1 week or longer). Autoradiographic analysis can be done on smaller cultures and is technically easier than most other assays. In the first successful prenatal diagnosis of XP,[250] fibroblast cultures were ready to assay for unscheduled synthesis 6 days after amniocentesis, and autoradiography was completed in 3 days. In families in whom the defective gene has been identified (e.g., Japanese XP-A patients), molecular biologic techniques such as PCR of DNA obtained from trophoblast or amniotic fluid cells should be useful for rapid prenatal diagnosis at an early stage of pregnancy.

One potential problem in all amniocentesis tests is that of an error in diagnosis because of contamination of a sample with unrepresentative cells (e.g., nonviable or maternal cells). Usually, the presence of nonviable cells can be excluded because they will be lost from cultures during the first days of growth. The probability of contamination with maternal cells is low (on the order of 0.5 percent or less) and can be excluded for male fetuses by observing sex chromatin in interphase or karyotypic analysis. The risk of false diagnosis should be less than 1 in 500.

OTHER HYPERSENSITIVITY DISEASES

XP is only one of a large number of human disorders in which cells (fibroblasts, lymphocytes, etc.) are more sensitive than normal (i.e., hypersensitive) to DNA-damaging agents.[3] Only for XP, however, is there a clear correlation between the hypersensitivity to UV light, the biochemical defect in DNA repair, and the etiology of the disease. In several of the hypersensitive diseases, abnormalities have been found in DNA replication rather than repair. Other diseases in which there is only about twice as much sensitivity as normal appear more difficult to attribute to specific defects in repair or replication of DNA; secondary or more subtle defects may be involved.

Ataxia-telangiectasia (AT) is a disorder associated with neurologic symptoms, vascular telangiectasia, and frequent development of lymphoreticular malignancy.[9–11,251–256] AT patients have clinical hypersensitivity to therapeutic doses of x-radiation (e.g., as used in treatment of lymphoma), and cultured cells show increased sensitivity to killing by ionizing radiation. This disorder involves a complex spectrum of defects in repair of lesions in DNA caused by ionizing radiation[9,10,251,253,254] or chemical agents.[252] In addition, DNA replication is resistant to inhibition by x-rays.[9–11] A small fraction of x-ray-induced chromosomal breaks appears to remain unrejoined in AT cells in comparison with normal cells.[254] AT involves four complementation groups, A, C, D, and VI, which all appear clustered in the chromosomal region 11q22[255]; the gene for group D has been cloned.[256]

Fanconi anemia is a disease involving a deficiency in bone development and bone marrow function. Although cells are markedly hypersensitive to DNA–DNA crosslinking agents,[183] the biochemical defect is poorly understood and results have thus far been quite variable.[183,257–259] A gene for Fanconi anemia has been located on chromosome 20q.[260]

Patients with Bloom syndrome have high spontaneous frequencies of lymphatic and other malignancies, high baseline levels of sister chromatid exchanges,[261] and a high frequency of somatic-cell mutation.[262,263] Neither consistent hypersensitivity, other than that involving SCE,[264] nor any defect in DNA repair has been demonstrated in Bloom syndrome.[265] DNA ligase I was reported to have reduced activity and increased heat sensitivity in cells from patients with this syndrome,[266,267] but no mutations are found in ligase I. Instead, a patient with an immunodeficient disease classified as 46BR has been found to be homozygous for mutations in DNA ligase I.[268]

Several patients have been described with cellular characteristics typical of CS cells, but quite varied and atypical clinical symptoms, and named simply as a UV sensitive syndrome, UV^S.[269,270]

Patients with basal-cell nevus syndrome (Gorlin syndrome), an autosomal dominant disease, have multiple cutaneous basal-cell carcinomas, cysts of the jaw bone, calcification of the membranes covering the brain (falx), and skeletal abnormalities such as bifid ribs.[271] They have an increased frequency of internal neoplasms such as medulloblastoma of the brain. Patients have clinical radiosensitivity manifested by myriad cutaneous basal-cell carcinomas in portions of the skin receiving radiation therapy as treatment for brain tumors or skin cancers. This x-ray hypersensitivity was not found with cultured cells,[272] but there is one report of hypersensitivity of fibroblasts to UV-B radiation[273] and of increased sensitivity to transformation by oncogenes.[274] The underlying cellular defect is unknown. A gene for basal-cell nevus syndrome has been located on chromosome 9q.[275–277]

DNA REPAIR AND CARCINOGENESIS IN XERODERMA PIGMENTOSUM

One theory of carcinogenesis[278] invokes an accumulation of genetic damage as part of the underlying mechanism. Environmental mutagens are postulated to damage some critical region(s) of the genome of somatic cells.[279,280] If the damage is not repaired before DNA replication occurs, then that region becomes the site of a somatic mutation or chromosomal rearrangements and amplifications. If these changes occur in genes involved in growth control, then they might become early events in carcinogenesis. Incomplete, inefficient, or inaccurate repair in some hereditary diseases should therefore be correlated with increased carcinogenesis. Carcinogenesis induced by radiation or chemicals in normal individuals would then be due to the normal amount of inaccuracy present in repair, or perhaps to inhibition of repair by the damaging agents themselves, or to replication of a damaged region before repair was complete. XP would be an example of increased damage remaining in DNA during replication, with a resultant accumulation of mutations.

Carcinogenesis often appears to proceed by a multistep process, the first step being an initiation event and the later steps, which can often occur much later, being promotional events. One theory of carcinogenesis would correlate initiation with the induction of somatic mutations, and promotion with an alteration in the expression of the mutations (e.g., by induction of aneuploidy, which produces haploid cells that can express recessive mutations generated by the initiating carcinogenic event).

Substantial evidence from microorganisms and mammalian cells supports a theory in which initiating events in carcinogenesis are akin to mutagenic events caused by damage to DNA. Generally, there is a high correlation between the mutagenic activity of a chemical and its carcinogenic activity.[279,280] In XP there is a correlation between high levels of carcinogenesis and susceptibility to UV-induced mutagenesis[3,8,21,123–132] in all forms of the disease, both excision-repair-defective and variant, although UV-induced rearrangements of DNA in the form of SCE are elevated only in excision defective XP. In support of this idea, examination of the p53 tumor suppressor gene in sunlight-induced human cutaneous squamous-cell carcinomas identified a high proportion of mutations that are typical of those expected from UV-induced dipyrimidine photoproducts.[281]

These kinds of results suggest that the various cellular factors studied experimentally, such as DNA damage, repair, mutation, and transformation, are but a few of the complex mechanisms involved in carcinogenesis. Further elucidation of details of the biochemical, cellular, and clinical characteristics of XP should provide a better understanding of one kind of carcinogenesis, but might have implications for carcinogenesis in general.

ACKNOWLEDGMENTS

This work was supported by the Office of Health and Environmental Research, U.S. Department of Energy, contract no. DE-AC03-76-SF01012, and by the National Cancer Institute.

ADDENDUM

D. Bootsma ▪ K.H. Kraemer ▪ J.E. Cleaver

Links Between DNA Repair and Transcription

A coupling of nucleotide excision repair (NER) with transcription was first recognized through the increased repair of DNA lesions in the transcribed strand of active genes.[149,150] Venema et al.[60] demonstrated a defect in this pathway in cells of CS patients, and the defective gene in the CS complementation group B, ERCC6, was cloned by Troelstra et al.[286] This gene likely encodes one of the transcription repair coupling factors and is the first human gene cloned that is specifically involved in transcription-coupled repair.

A different association of DNA repair and transcription was disclosed by Schaeffer et al.[287] These investigators characterized a multisubunit factor involved in the initiation of transcription of most of our genes (the RNA polymerase II-mediated basal transcription process). The p89 subunit of the BTF2/TFIIH transcription complex appeared to be identical to the ERCC3 protein, earlier characterized by Weeda et al.[203] as a protein involved in NER and defective in XP complementation group B. ERCC3 in the context of the multiprotein BTF2/TFIIH complex exerts a DNA unwinding function in NER and in basal transcription.[288,289] This reveals a dual involvement of the protein in two intrinsically distinct types of DNA transactions: transcription and repair. It is most likely that the function of the complex in both processes is the catalysis of a similar biochemical step in the context of an otherwise different process. One possibility is that the helicase activity of ERCC3 in BTF2/TFIIH[289] is required for translocation of the RNA polymerase or the NER damage-recognition complex along the DNA template. This suggests that the BTF2/TFIIH complex may be a separate DNA translocation carrier that can be coupled to the transcription as well as to the NER machinery. Alternatively, or in addition, it is possible that local denaturation is an obligatory step in loading the RNA polymerase onto the strand to be transcribed. In the NER reaction such a step may be needed to assemble the scanning complex onto the DNA or to induce a specific DNA conformation around a lesion so that the incision complex is properly positioned to perform a dual incision.

DNA Repair and DNA Transcription Syndromes

Recently, experiments with microneedle injection and an in vitro repair assay have revealed that the highly purified BTF2/TFIIH complex contains at least three NER proteins, all associated with distinct human NER syndromes.[290] An intriguing observation is that all three proteins fall into a specific subclass of NER disorders that display the exceptional combination of XP and CS (XPB/ERCC3 and XPD/ERCC2) or the peculiar PIBIDS syndrome (XPD/ERCC2) and one newly identified, very rare PIBIDS complementation group, TTD-A.[291] These findings support the notion that the entire BTF2/TFIIH complex is recruited for repair purposes. Because the ERCC2, ERCC3, and TTD-A proteins also participate directly in transcription, it is plausible that at least some of the unusual symptoms associated with the corresponding disorders are related to this other function of the complex. This sheds new light on the clinical features of XP, XP/CS, and PIBIDS that were difficult to rationalize on the sole basis of an NER defect.[292] These include the neurological abnormalities associated with neurodysmyelination, which could be due to poor expression of one of the myelin genes; the brittle hair symptoms, which could be related to low expression of a cysteine-rich matrix protein; and the severe growth defect involving dwarfism, microcephaly, and immature sexual development. It seems likely that these findings reveal a novel type of syndrome caused by a subtle defect in general transcription that also may occur in the absence of a repair deficiency, such as in the form of TTD without photosensitivity.[290] In this "transcription syndrome," BTF2/TFIIH plays a crucial role.

Cloned Human NER Genes

At least five and perhaps all seven XP excision repair genes have now, as of early 1994, been isolated and their chromosome locations identified (Tables 148-6, 148-7).

The XP-C correcting gene cloned by Legerski and Peterson[214] was found to act in a complex with one of the human homologs of the yeast RAD23 NER protein, HHR23B.[293] This is the first protein complex isolated that is uniquely involved in the repair pathway that acts on the whole genome. In addition, a second human homolog of RAD23 (HHR23A) has been cloned.[293] Its function in NER is at present unknown. It will be of interest to find out whether this gene and the closely related HHR23B gene are implicated in any of the remaining XP, CS, and TTD complementation groups.

Two XP-E families are known in which patients are deficient in an abundant UV-damage DNA binding protein of 120 kDa, which appears to be complexed with a 41-kDa protein,[294] but XP-E patients from other families appear to have normal amounts of this protein. Recently, Keeney et al.[294] demonstrated correction of the XP-E repair defect, in the cell lines that lack it, by microinjection of the purified protein. The gene encoding the large subunit has been cloned by Takao and coworkers,[295] but evidence that it contains mutations causing the defect or that it is definitely the XP-E gene product is still lacking.

The XP-F factor was found to be part of a complex that also includes ERCC1, ERCC4, and ERCC11.[296,297] At present, it is unknown whether XP-F is identical to either ERCC4 or ERCC11. The ERCC4 gene was cloned by Thompson and collaborators (L. Thompson, personal communication). This complex is thought to be involved in the incision stage of the NER reaction. An additional association between the XP-A and ERCC1 gene products has recently been reported.[298]

The XP-G correcting gene has been isolated[299] and found to be equivalent to ERCC5.[300] Its function has yet to be resolved. There are indications, based on parallels with the ERCC5 yeast homolog, RAD2, that this protein may be a single-stranded endonuclease.[301] In conclusion, in 1992 and 1993, considerable progress was been made in cloning and characterizing DNA repair genes and proteins. This has resulted in new insights into the molecular bases of the clinical features of the NER syndromes and into a new class of human genetic diseases, the transcription syndromes.[290,292]

REFERENCES

1. Witkop CJ Jr, Quevedo WC Jr, Fitzpatrick TB, King RA: Albinism, in Scriver CR, Beaudet AL, Sly WS, Valle D (eds): *The Metabolic Basis of Inherited Disease,* 6th ed. New York, McGraw-Hill, 1989, vol 2, p 2905.
2. Kappas A, Sassa S, Galbraith RA, Nordmann Y: The porphyrias, in Scriver CR, Beaudet AL, Sly WS, Valle D (eds): *The Metabolic Basis of Inherited Disease,* 6th ed. New York, McGraw-Hill, 1989, vol 2, p 1305.
3. Cleaver JE, Kraemer KH: Xeroderma pigmentosum, in Scriver CR, Beaudet AL, Sly WS, Valle D (eds): *The Metabolic Basis of Inherited Disease,* 6th ed. New York, McGraw-Hill, 1989, vol 2, p 2949.
4. Cleaver JE: Repair processes for photochemical damage in mammalian cells, in Lett JT, Adler H, Zelle M (eds): *Advances in Radiation Biology,* New York, Academic, 1974, vol 4, p 1.
5. Cleaver JE: Defective repair replication of DNA in xeroderma pigmentosum. *Nature* **218:**652, 1968.
6. Kraemer KH, Slor H: Xeroderma pigmentosum. *Clin Dermatol* **3:**33, 1985.
7. Kraemer KH: Heritable diseases with increased sensitivity to cellular injury, in Fitzpatrick TB, Eisen AZ, Wolff K, Freedberg IM, Austen KF (eds): *Dermatology in General Medicine,* 4th ed. New York, McGraw-Hill. 1993, p. 1974.
8. Cleaver JE: DNA damage and repair in light-sensitive human skin disease. *J Invest Dermatol* **54:**181, 1970.
9. Painter RB, Young B: Radiosensitivity in ataxia telangiectasia: A new explanation. *Proc Natl Acad Sci USA* **77:**7315, 1980.
10. Paterson MC, Smith BP, Lohman PHM, Anderson AK, Fishman L: Defective excision repair of gamma-ray-damaged DNA in human (ataxia-telangiectasia) fibroblasts. *Nature* **260:**444, 1976.
11. Taylor AMR, Harnden DG, Arlett CF, Harcourt SA, Lehmann AR, Stevens S, Bridges BA: Ataxia telangiectasia: A human mutation with abnormal radiation sensitivity. *Nature* **258:**427, 1975.
12. Lehmann AR, Kirk-Bell S, Mayne L: Abnormal kinetics of DNA synthesis in ultraviolet light irradiated cells from patients with Cockayne's syndrome. *Cancer Res* **3:**4237, 1979.
13. Cleaver JE: DNA repair with purines and pyrimidines in radiation- and carcinogen-damaged normal and xeroderma pigmentosum human cells. *Cancer Res* **33:**362, 1973.
14. Park SD, Cleaver JE: Postreplication repair: Questions of its definition and possible alteration in xeroderma pigmentosum cell strains. *Proc Natl Acad Sci USA* **76:**3927, 1979.
15. Cleaver JE: Photoreactivation: A radiation repair mechanism absent from mammalian cells. *Biochem Biophys Res Commun* **24:**569, 1966.
16. Sutherland BM: Photoreactivating enzyme from human leukocytes. *Nature* **248:**109, 1974.
17. Sutherland BM, Rice M, Wagner EK: Xeroderma pigmentosum cells contain low levels of photoreactivating enzyme. *Proc Natl Acad Sci USA* **72:**103, 1975.
18. Sutherland JC, Sutherland BM: Human photoreactivating enzyme. Action spectrum and safelight conditions. *Biophys J* **15:**435, 1975.
19. Mortelmans K, Cleaver JE, Friedberg EC, Paterson MC, Smith BP, Thomas GH: Photoreactivation of thymine

dimers in UV-irradiated human cells: Unique dependence on culture conditions. *Mutat Res* **44**:433, 1977.
20. Sutherland BM, Harber LC, Kochevar IE: Pyrimidine dimer formation and repair in human skin. *Cancer Res* **40**:3181, 1980.
21. Robbins JH, Kraemer KH, Lutzner MA, Festoff BW, Coon HG: Xeroderma pigmentosum. An inherited disease with sun sensitivity, multiple cutaneous neoplasms, and abnormal DNA repair. *Ann Intern Med* **80**:221, 1974.
22. McKusick VA: Mendelian inheritance in man, in *Catalogs of Autosomal Dominant, Autosomal Recessive, and X-Linked Phenotypes*, 3rd ed. Baltimore, Johns Hopkins, 1971, p 294.
23. von Hebra F, Kaposi M: *On Diseases of the Skin, Including the Exanthemata*. Tay W, trans. London, New Sydenham Society, 1874, vol 3, p 252.
24. Neisser A: Ueber das 'Xeroderma pigmentosum' (Kaposi) Lioderma essentailis cum melanosi et telangiectasia. *Viertel Dermatol Syphil* 47, 1883.
25. DeSanctis C, Cacchione A: L'idiozia xerodermica. *Riv Sper Freniatr* **56**:269, 1932.
26. Epstein JH, Fukuyama K, Reed WB, Epstein WL: Defect in DNA synthesis in skin of patients with xeroderma pigmentosum demonstrated in vivo. *Science* **168**:1477, 1970.
27. Burk PG, Lutzner MA, Clarke DD, Robbins JH: Ultraviolet-stimulated thymidine incorporation in xeroderma pigmentosum lymphocytes. *J Lab Clin Med* **77**:759, 1971.
28. Cleaver JE: Xeroderma pigmentosum: Variants with normal DNA repair and normal sensitivity to ultraviolet light. *J Invest Dermatol* **58**:124, 1972.
29. Cleaver JE, Arutyunyan RM, Sarkisian T, Kaufmann WK, Greene AE, Coriell L: Similar defects in DNA repair and replication in the pigmented xerodermoid and the xeroderma pigmentosum variants. *Carcinogenesis* **1**:647, 1980.
30. Lehmann AR, Kirk-Bell S, Arlett CF, Paterson MC, Lohman PHM, De Weerd-Kastelein EA, Bootsma D: Xeroderma pigmentosum cells with normal levels of excision repair have a defect in DNA synthesis after UV-irradiation. *Proc Natl Acad Sci USA* **72**:219, 1975.
31. De Weerd-Kastelein EA, Kleijzer W, Bootsma D: Genetic heterogeneity of xeroderma pigmentosum demonstrated by somatic cell hybridization. *Nature New Biol* **238**:80, 1972.
32. Takebe H, Nishigori C, Satoh Y: Genetics and skin cancer of xeroderma pigmentosum in Japan. *Jpn J Cancer Res (Gann)* **78**:1135, 1987.
33. Kraemer KH, Lee MM, Scotto J: Xeroderma pigmentosum: Cutaneous, ocular and neurologic abnormalities in 830 published cases. *Arch Dermatol* **123**:241, 1987.
34. Ramsay CA, Giannelli F: The erythemal action spectrum and deoxyribonucleic acid repair synthesis in xeroderma pigmentosum. *Br J Dermatol* **92**:49, 1975.
35. Jung EG: New form of molecular defect in xeroderma pigmentosum. *Nature* **228**:361, 1970.
36. Kraemer KH, Lee MM, Scotto J: DNA repair protects against cutaneous and internal neoplasia: Evidence from xeroderma pigmentosum. *Carcinogenesis* **5**:511, 1984.
37. Mimaki T, Itoh N, Abe J, Tagawa T, Sato K, Yabuuchi H, Takebe H: Neurological manifestations of xeroderma pigmentosum. *Ann Neurol* **20**:70, 1986.
38. Robbins JH, Brumack RA, Mendiones M, Barrett SF, Carl JR, Cho S, Denckla MB, Ganges MB, Gerber LH, Guthrie RA, Meer J, Moshell AN, Polinsky RJ, Ravin PD, Sonies BC, Tarone RE: Neurological disease in xeroderma pigmentosum: Documentation of a late onset type of the juvenile onset form. *Brain* **114**:1335, 1991.
39. Roytta M, Anttinen A: Xeroderma pigmentosum with neurological abnormalities. A clinical and neuropathological study. *Acta Neurol Scand* **73**:191, 1986.
40. Andrews AD, Barrett SF, Robbins JH: Xeroderma pigmentosum neurological abnormalities correlate with colony-forming ability after ultraviolet radiation. *Proc Natl Acad Sci USA* **75**:1984, 1978.
41. Puig L, Marti R, Matias-Guiu X, Lecha M, Guix M: Gastric adenocarcinoma in a patient with xeroderma pigmentosum. *Br J Dermatol* **113**:632, 1985.
42. Takebe H, Tatsumi K, Satoh Y: DNA repair and its possible involvement in the origin of multiple cancer. *Jpn J Clin Oncol (suppl 1)* **15**:299, 1985.
43. Okui T, Fujiwara Y: Defective repair of tryptophan pyrolysate (Trp P-1 and Trp P-2) and aflatoxin B1 damage in xeroderma pigmentosum cells. *J Radiat Res (Tokyo)* **24**:356, 1983.
44. Protic-Sabljic M, Whyte DB, Kraemer KH: Hypersensitivity of xeroderma pigmentosum cells to dietary carcinogens. *Mutat Res* **145**:89, 1985.
45. Lynch HT, Anderson DE, Smith JL, Howell JB, Krush AJ: Xeroderma pigmentosum, malignant melanoma and congenital ichthyosis. *Arch Dermatol* **96**:625, 1967.
46. Kraemer KH, Digiovanna JJ, Moshell AN, Tarone RE, Peck GL: Prevention of skin cancer with oral 13-cisretinoic acid in xeroderma pigmentosum. *N Engl J Med* **318**:1633, 1988.
47. Cantani A, Bamonte G, Bellioni P, Tucci-Bamonte M, Ceccoli D, Tacconi ML: Rare syndromes. I. Cockayne syndrome: A review of 129 cases so far reported in the literature. *Riv Eur Sci Med Farmacol* **9**:9, 1987.
48. Nance MA, Berry SA: Cockayne syndrome: Review of 140 cases. *Am J Med Genet* **42**:68, 1992.
49. Jaeken J, Klocker H, Schwaiger H, Bellmann R, Hirsch-Kauffmann M, Schweiger M: Clinical and biochemical studies in three patients with severe early infantile Cockayne syndrome. *Hum Genet* **83**:339, 1989.
50. Fryns JP, Bulcke J, Verdu P, Carton H, Kleczkowska A, van den Berghe H: Apparent late-onset Cockayne syndrome and interstitial deletion of the long arm of chromosome 10 (del(10)(q11.23q21.2)). *Am J Med Genet* **40**:343, 1991.
51. Kennedy RM, Rowe VD, Kepes JJ: Cockayne syndrome: An atypical case. *Neurology* **30**:1268, 1980.
52. Norris PG, Arlett CF, Cole J, Lehmann AR, Hawk JL: Abnormal erythemal response and elevated T lymphocyte HPRT mutant frequency in Cockayne's syndrome. *Br J Dermatol* **124**:453, 1991.
53. Brumback RA, Yoder FW, Andrews AD, Peck GL, Robbins JH: Normal pressure hydrocephalus: Recognition and relationship to neurological abnormalities in Cockayne's syndrome. *Arch Neurol* **35**:337, 1978.
54. Riggs W, Seibert J: Cockayne's syndrome: Roentgen findings. *Am J Roentgenol* **116**:623, 1972.
55. Schmickel RD, Chu EHY, Trosko JE, Chang CC: Cockayne syndrome: A cellular sensitivity to ultraviolet light. *Pediatrics* **60**:135, 1977.
56. Andrews AD, Barrett SF, Yoder FW, Robbins JH: Cockayne's syndrome fibroblasts have increased sensitivity to ultraviolet light but normal rates of unscheduled DNA synthesis. *J Invest Dermatol* **70**:237, 1978.
57. Wade MH, Chu EHY: Effects of DNA damaging agents on cultured fibroblasts derived from patients with Cockayne's syndrome. *Mutat Res* **59**:49, 1979.
58. Marshall RR, Arlett CF, Harcourt SA, Broughton BA: Increased sensitivity of cell strains from Cockayne's syndrome to sister chromatid exchange induction and cell killing by UV light. *Mutat Res* **69**:107, 1980.
59. Chang WS, Tarone RE, Andrews AD, Whang-Peng JS, Robbins JH: Ultraviolet light-induced sister chromatid exchanges in xeroderma pigmentosum and in Cockayne syndrome lymphocyte cell lines. *Cancer Res* **38**:1601, 1978.
60. Venema J, Mullenders LH, Natarajan AT, Van Zeeland AA, Mayne LV: The genetic defect in Cockayne syndrome is associated with a defect in repair of UV-induced DNA damage in transcriptionally active DNA. *Proc Natl Acad Sci USA* **87**:4707, 1990.
61. Barrett SF, Robbins JH, Tarone RE, Kraemer KH: Defective repair of cyclobutane pyrimidine dimers with normal repair of other DNA photoproducts in a transcriptionally active gene transfected into Cockayne syndrome cells. *Mutat Res* **255**:281, 1991.
62. Cleaver JE: Normal reconstruction of DNA supercoiling and chromatin structure in Cockayne syndrome cells during repair of damage from ultraviolet light. *Am J Hum Genet* **34**:566, 1982.
63. Tanaka K, Kawai K, Kumahara Y, Ikenaga M, Okada Y: Genetic complementation groups in Cockayne syndrome. *Somat Cell Genet* **7**:445, 1981.
64. Lehmann AR: Three complementation groups in Cockayne syndrome. *Mutat Res* **106**:347, 1982.
65. Lehmann AR, Francis AJ, Giannelli F: Prenatal diagnosis of Cockayne's syndrome. *Lancet* **1**:486, 1985.

66. Price VH, Odom RB, Ward WH, Jones FT: Trichothiodystrophy. *Arch Dermatol* **116:**1375, 1980.
67. Przedborski S, Ferster A, Goldman S, Wolter R, Song M, Tonnesen T, Pollitt RJ, Vamos E: Trichothiodystrophy, mental retardation, short stature, ataxia, and gonadal dysfunction in three Moroccan siblings. *Am J Med Genet* **35:**566, 1990.
68. Itin PH, Pittelkow MR: Trichothiodystrophy: Review of sulfur-deficient brittle hair syndromes and association with the ectodermal dysplasias. *J Am Acad Dermatol* **22:**705, 1990.
69. Tay CH: Ichthyosiform erythroderma, hair shaft abnormalities, and mental and growth retardation: A new recessive disorder. *Arch Dermatol* **104:**4, 1971.
70. Nuzzo F, Zei G, Stefanini M, Colognola R, Santachiara AS, Lagomarsini P, Marinoni S, Salvanesdic L: Search for consanguinity within and among families of patients with trichothiodystrophy associated with xeroderma pigmentosum. *J Med Genet* **27:**21, 1990.
71. Jackson CE, Weiss L, Watson JHL: "Brittle" hair with short stature, intellectual impairment, and decreased fertility: An autosomal recessive syndrome in an Amish kindred. *Pediatrics* **54:**201, 1974.
72. Howell RR, Arbisser AI, Parsons DS, Scott CI, Fraustadt U, Collie WR, Marshall RN, Ibarra OC: The Sabinas brittle hair syndrome. *Am J Hum Genet* **33:**957, 1981.
73. Pollitt RJ, Stonier PD: Proteins of normal hair and of cystine-deficient hair from mentally retarded siblings. *Biochem J* **122:**433, 1971.
74. Broughton BC, Lehmann AR, Harcourt SA, Arlett CF, Sarasin A, Kleijer WJ, Beemer FA, Naim R, Mitchell DL: Relationship between pyrimidine dimers, 6-4 photoproducts, repair synthesis and cell survival: Studies using cells from patients with trichothiodystrophy. *Mutat Res* **235:**33, 1990.
75. Stefanini M, Lagomarsini P, Arlett CF, Marinoni S, Borrone C, Crovato F, Trevisan G, Cordone G, Nuzzo F: Xeroderma pigmentosum (complementation group D) mutation is present in patients affected by trichothiodystrophy with photosensitivity. *Hum Genet* **74:**107, 1986.
76. Lehmann AR, Arlett CF, Broughton BC, Harcourt SA, Steingrimsdottir H, Stefanini M, Taylor AMR, Natarajan AT, Green S, King MD, Mackie RM, Stephenson JBP, Tolmie JL: Trichothiodystrophy, a human DNA repair disorder with heterogeneity in the cellular response to ultraviolet light. *Cancer Res* **48:**6090, 1988.
77. Rebora A, Crovato F: PIBI(D)S syndrome: Trichothiodystrophy with xeroderma pigmentosum (group D) mutation. *J Am Acad Dermatol* **16:**940, 1987.
78. Setlow RB: The wavelengths in sunlight effective in producing skin cancer: A theoretical analysis. *Proc Natl Acad Sci USA* **71:**3363, 1974.
79. Epstein JH: Ultraviolet carcinogenesis. *Photophysiology* **5:**235, 1970.
80. Blum HF: *Carcinogenesis by Ultraviolet Light*. Princeton, NJ, Princeton University Press, 1959.
81. Harm W: Use of an *E. coli* uvr- rec- mutant for monitoring the germicidal activity of sunlight. *Radiat Res* **39:**517, 1969. (abstr.)
82. Trosko JE, Krause D, Isoun M: Sunlight-induced pyrimidine dimers in human cells in vitro. *Nature* **228:**358, 1970.
83. Zimmer KG: *Studies on Quantitative Radiation Biology*. Griffith HD, trans. New York, Hafner, 1961.
84. Rothman RH, Setlow RB: An action spectrum for cell killing and pyrimidine dimer formation in Chinese hamster V-79 cells. *Photochem Photobiol* **29:**57, 1979.
85. Todd P, Coohill TP, Mahoney JA: Responses of cultured Chinese hamster cells to ultraviolet light of different wavelengths. *Radiat Res* **35:**390, 1968.
86. Kantor GJ, Sutherland JC, Setlow RB: Action spectra for killing nondividing normal human and xeroderma pigmentosum cells. *Photochem Photobiol* **31:**459, 1980.
87. Chu EHY: Effects of ultraviolet radiation on mammalian cells. I. Induction of chromosome aberrations. *Mutat Res* **2:**75, 1965.
88. Ichihashi M, Ramsay CA: The action spectrum and dose response studies of unscheduled DNA synthesis in normal human fibroblasts. *Photochem Photobiol* **23:**103, 1975.
89. Freeman SE, Hacham H, Gange RW, Maytum DJ, Sutherland JC, Sutherland BM: Wavelength dependence of pyrimidine dimer formation in DNA of human skin irradiated in situ with ultraviolet light. *Proc Natl Acad Sci USA* **86:**5605, 1989.
90. Smith KC: An isomer of the cyclobutane-type thymine dimer produced in the presence of adenine. *Biochem Biophys Res Commun* **25:**426, 1966.
91. Pathak MA, Kramer DM, Gungerich U: Formation of thymine dimers in mammalian skin by ultraviolet radiation in vivo. *Photochem Photobiol* **15:**177, 1972.
92. Setlow RB: Cyclobutane-type pyrimidine dimers in polynucleotides. *Science* **153:**379, 1966.
93. Brash DE, Haseltine WA: UV-induced mutation hotspots occur at DNA damage hotspots. *Nature* **298:**189, 1982.
94. Brash DE, Seetharam S, Kraemer KH, Seidman MM, Bredberg A: Photoproduct frequency is not the major determinant of ultraviolet mutation hotspots or coldspots in human cells. *Proc Natl Acad Sci USA* **84:**3782, 1987.
95. Smith KC, Hanawalt PC: *Molecular Photobiology: Inactivation and Recovery*. New York, Academic, 1969.
96. Kato H: Spontaneous sister chromatid exchanges detected by a BUdR-labeling method. *Nature* **251:**70, 1974.
97. Perry P, Wolff S: New Giemsa method for the differential staining of sister chromatids. *Nature* **251:**156, 1974.
98. Wolff S, Bodycote J, Thomas GH, Cleaver JE: Sister chromatid exchange in xeroderma pigmentosum cells that are defective in DNA excision repair or post-replication repair. *Genetics* **81:**349, 1975.
99. Wolff S, Rodin B, Cleaver JE: Sister chromatid exchanges induced by mutagenic carcinogens in normal and xeroderma pigmentosum cells. *Nature* **265:**347, 1977.
100. De Weerd-Kastelein EA, Keijzer W, Rainaldi G, Bootsma D: Induction of sister chromatid exchanges in xeroderma pigmentosum cells after exposure to ultraviolet light. *Mutat Res* **45:**253, 1977.
101. Parrington JM, Delhanty JDA, Baden HP: Unscheduled DNA synthesis, UV-induced chromosome aberrations and SV40 transformation in cultured cells from xeroderma pigmentosum. *Ann Hum Genet* **35:**149, 1971.
102. Sasaki MS: DNA repair capacity and susceptibility to chromosome breakage in xeroderma pigmentosum cells. *Mutat Res* **20:**41, 1973.
103. Cleaver JE: DNA repair and radiation sensitivity in human (xeroderma pigmentosum) cells. *Int J Radiat Biol* **18:**557, 1970.
104. Goldstein S: The role of DNA repair in aging and cultured fibroblasts from xeroderma pigmentosum and normals. *Proc Soc Exp Biol Med* **137:**730, 1971.
105. Takebe H, Furuyama JI, Miki Y, Kondo S: High sensitivity of xeroderma pigmentosum cells to the carcinogen 4-nitroquinoline-1-oxide. *Mutat Res* **15:**98, 1972.
106. Stich HF, San RHC, Kawazoe Y: Increased sensitivity of xeroderma pigmentosum cells to some chemical carcinogens and mutagens. *Mutat Res* **17:**127, 1973.
107. Hoffman ME, Menighini R: Action of hydrogen peroxide on human fibroblasts in culture. *Photochem Photobiol* **30:**151, 1979.
108. Stich HF, San RHC: DNA repair synthesis and survival of repair deficient human cells exposed to the K-region epoxide of benz(a)anthracene. *Proc Soc Exp Biol Med* **142:**155, 1973.
109. Maher VM, Birch N, Otto JR, McCormick JJ: Cytotoxicity of carcinogenic aromatic amides in normal and xeroderma pigmentosum fibroblasts with different DNA repair capabilities. *J Natl Cancer Inst* **54:**1287, 1975.
110. Zavadova Z: Host-cell repair of vaccinia virus and of double stranded RNA of encephalomyocarditis virus. *Nature New Biol* **233:**123, 1971.
111. Lytle CD, Aaronson SA, Harvey E: Host-cell reactivation in mammalian cells. II. Survival by herpes simplex virus and vaccinia virus in normal human and xeroderma pigmentosum cells. *Int J Radiat Biol* **22:**159, 1972.
112. Rabson AS, Tyrrell SA, Legallais FY: Growth of ultraviolet-damaged herpes virus in xeroderma pigmentosum cells. *Proc Soc Exp Biol Med* **132:**802, 1969.
113. Day RS III: Studies on repair of adenovirus 2 by human fibroblasts using normal, xeroderma pigmentosum, and xero-

derma pigmentosum heterozygous strains. *Cancer Res* **34:**1965, 1974.
114. Day RS III: Cellular reactivation of ultraviolet-irradiated human adenovirus 2 in normal and xeroderma pigmentosum fibroblasts. *Photochem Photobiol* **19:**9, 1974.
115. Aaronson SA, Lytle CD: Decreased host-cell reactivation of irradiated SV40 virus in xeroderma pigmentosum. *Nature* **228:**359, 1970.
116. Henderson EE: Host cell reactivation of Epstein-Barr virus in normal and repair defective leukocytes. *Cancer Res* **38:**3256, 1978.
117. Henderson EE, Long WK: Host cell reactivation of UV- and X-ray damaged herpes simplex virus by Epstein-Barr (EBV)-transformed lymphoblastoid cells. *Virology* **115:**237, 1981.
118. Day RS III: Xeroderma pigmentosum variants have decreased repair of UV-damaged DNA. *Nature* **253:**748, 1975.
119. Day RS III, Kraemer KH, Robbins JH: Complementing xeroderma pigmentosum fibroblasts restore biological activity to UV damaged DNA. *Mutat Res* **28:**251, 1975.
120. Protic-Sabljic M, Kraemer KH: One pyrimidine dimer inactivates expression of a transfected gene in xeroderma pigmentosum cells. *Proc Natl Acad Sci USA* **82:**6622, 1985.
121. Protic-Sabljic M, Kraemer KH: Reduced repair of non-dimer photoproducts in a gene transfected into xeroderma pigmentosum cells. *Photochem Photobiol* **43:**509, 1986.
122. Kelley WN, Wyngaarden JB: The Lesch-Nyhan syndrome, in Stanbury JB, Wyngaarden JB, Fredrickson DS, Goldstein JL, Brown MS (eds): *The Metabolic Basis of Inherited Disease*, 5th ed. New York, McGraw-Hill, 1983, p 1115.
123. Maher VM, Ouelette LM, Curren RD, McCormick JJ: Frequency of ultraviolet light-induced mutations is higher in xeroderma pigmentosum variant cells. *Nature* **261:**593, 1976.
124. Maher VM, Dorney DJ, Mendrala AL, Konze-Thomas B, McCormick JJ: DNA excision-repair processes in human cells can eliminate the cytotoxic and mutagenic consequences of ultraviolet irradiation. *Mutat Res* **62:**311, 1979.
125. Glover TW, Chang CC, Trosko JE, Li SS: Ultraviolet light induction of diphtheria toxin-resistant mutants of normal and xeroderma pigmentosum human fibroblasts. *Proc Natl Acad Sci USA* **76:**3982, 1979.
126. Patton JD, Rowan LA, Mendrala AL, Howell JN, Maher VM, McCormick JJ: Xeroderma pigmentosum fibroblasts including cells from XP variants are abnormally sensitive to the mutagenic and cytotoxic action of broad spectrum simulated sunlight. *Photochem Photobiol* **39:**37, 1984.
127. Deluca JG, Kaden DA, Komives EA, Thilly WG: Mutation of xeroderma pigmentosum lymphoblasts by far-ultraviolet light. *Mutat Res* **128:**47, 1984.
128. Bredberg A, Kraemer KH, Seidman M: Restricted ultraviolet mutational spectrum in a shuttle vector propagated in xeroderma pigmentosum cells. *Proc Natl Acad Sci USA* **83:**8273, 1986.
129. Protic-Sabljic M, Tuteja N, Munson PJ, Hauser J, Kraemer KH, Dixon K: UV light-induced cyclobutane dimers are mutagenic in mammalian cells. *Mol Cell Biol* **6:**3349, 1986.
130. Yagi T, Tatsumi-Miyajima J, Sato M, Kraemer KH, Takebe H: Analysis of point mutations in a UV-irradiated shuttle vector plasmid propagated in cells from Japanese xeroderma pigmentosum patients in complementation groups A and F. *Cancer Res* **51:**3177, 1991.
131. Seetharam S, Protic-Sabljic M, Seidman MM, Kraemer KH: Abnormal ultraviolet mutagenic spectrum in DNA replicated in cultured fibroblasts from a patient with the skin cancer-prone disease, xeroderma pigmentosum. *J Clin Invest* **80:**1613, 1987.
132. Wang YC, Maher VM, McCormick JJ: Xeroderma pigmentosum variant cells are less likely than normal cells to incorporate dAMP opposite photoproducts during replication of UV-irradiated plasmids. *Proc Natl Acad Sci USA* **88:**7810, 1991.
133. Cleaver JE: Xeroderma pigmentosum: A human disease in which an initial stage of DNA repair is defective. *Proc Natl Acad Sci USA* **63:**428, 1969.
134. Cleaver JE: DNA repair and its coupling to DNA replication in eukaryotic cells. *Biochim Biophys Acta* **516:**489, 1978.
135. McGhee JD, Felsenfeld G: Nucleosome structure. *Ann Res Biochem* **49:**115, 1980.
136. Bodell WJ: Nonuniform distribution of DNA repair in chromatin after treatment with methylmethane sulfonate. *Nucleic Acids Res* **4:**2619, 1977.
137. Cleaver JE: Nucleosome structure controls rates of excision repair in DNA of human cells. *Nature* **270:**451, 1977.
138. Smerdon MJ, Tlsty TD, Lieberman MW: Distribution of ultraviolet-induced DNA repair synthesis in nuclease sensitive and resistant regions of human chromatin. *Biochemistry* **17:**2377, 1978.
139. Sancar A, Sancar GB: DNA repair enzymes. *Annu Rev Biochem* **57:**29, 1988.
140. Cleaver JE, Jen J, Charles WC, Mitchell DL: Cyclobutane dimers and (6-4) photoproducts are mended with the same patch sizes. *Photochem Photobiol* **54:**393, 1991.
141. Hanawalt PC, Cooper PK, Ganesan AK, Smith CA: DNA repair in bacteria and mammalian cells. *Annu Rev Biochem* **48:**783, 1979.
142. Day RS III, Ziolkowski CH, Scudiero DA, Meyer A, Mattern MR: Human tumor cell strains defective in the repair of alkylation damage. *Carcinogenesis* **1:**21, 1980.
143. Haseltine WA, Gordon LK, Lindan CP, Grafstrom RH, Shaper NL, Grossman L: Cleavage of pyrimidine dimers in specific DNA sequences by a pyrimidine dimer DNA glycosylase of *M. luteus*. *Nature* **285:**634, 1980.
144. Demple B, Linn S: DNA N-glycosylases and UV repair. *Nature* **287:**203, 1980.
145. Sancar A, Rupp WD: A novel repair enzyme: UVRABC excision nuclease of *Escherichia coli* cuts a DNA strand on both sides of the damaged region. *Cell* **33:**249, 1983.
146. Hubscher U, Kuenzle CC, Spadari S: Functional roles of DNA polymerases beta and alpha. *Proc Natl Acad Sci USA* **76:**2316, 1979.
147. Dresler SL, Frattini MG: DNA replication and UV-induced DNA repair synthesis in human fibroblasts are much less sensitive than DNA polymerase alpha to inhibition of butylphenyl-deoxyguanosine triphosphate. *Nucleic Acids Res* **14:**7093, 1986.
148. Ciarrocchi G, Jose JG, Linn S: Further characterization of a cell-free system for measuring replicative and repair DNA synthesis with cultured human fibroblasts and evidence for the involvement of DNA polymerase alpha in DNA repair. *Nucleic Acids Res* **7:**1205, 1979.
149. Terleth C, van de Putte P, Brouwer J: New insights in DNA repair: Preferential repair of transcriptionally active DNA. *Mutagenesis* **6:**103, 1991.
150. Bohr VA: Gene specific DNA repair. *Carcinogenesis* **12:**1983, 1991.
151. Coverley D, Kenny MK, Munn M, Rupp WD, Lane DP, Wood RD: Requirement for the replication protein SSB in human DNA excision repair. *Nature* **349:**538, 1991.
152. Cleaver JE: Methods for studying repair of DNA damaged by physical and chemical carcinogens, in Busch H (ed): *Methods in Cancer Research*. New York, Academic, 1975, vol 2, p 123.
153. Djordjevic B, Tolmach LJ: Responses of synchronous population of HeLa cells to ultraviolet irradiation at selected stages of the generation cycle. *Radiat Res* **32:**327, 1967.
154. Pettijohn D, Hanawalt PC: Evidence for repair-replication of ultraviolet damaged DNA in bacteria. *J Mol Biol* **9:**395, 1964.
155. Regan JD, Setlow RB, Ley RD: Normal and defective repair of damaged DNA in human cells: A sensitive assay utilizing the photolysis of bromodeoxyuridine. *Proc Natl Acad Sci USA* **68:**708, 1971.
156. Edenberg H, Hanawalt PC: Size of repair patches in the DNA of ultraviolet-irradiated HeLa cells. *Biochim Biophys Acta* **272:**361, 1972.
157. Setlow RB, Regan JD, German J, Carrier WL: Evidence that xeroderma pigmentosum cells do not perform the first step in the repair of ultraviolet damage to their DNA. *Proc Natl Acad Sci USA* **64:**1035, 1969.
158. Cleaver JE: Sedimentation of DNA from human fibroblasts irradiated with ultraviolet light: Possible detection of excision breaks in normal and repair-deficient xeroderma pigmentosum cells. *Radiat Res* **57:**207, 1974.

159. Cleaver JE, Thomas GH, Trosko JE, Lett JT: Excision repair (dimer excision, strand breakage and repair replication) in primary cultures of eukaryotic (bovine) cells. *Exp Cell Res* **74:**67, 1972.
160. Kleijzer WJ, Hoeksema JL, Sluyter ML, Bootsma D: Effects of inhibitors on repair of DNA in normal human and xeroderma pigmentosum cells after exposure to X rays and ultraviolet irradiation. *Mutat Res* **17:**385, 1973.
161. Ben-Hur E, Ben-Ishai R: DNA repair in ultraviolet light irradiated HeLa cells and its reversible inhibition by hydroxyurea. *Photochem Photobiol* **13:**337, 1971.
162. Fornace AJ Jr, Kohn KW, Kann HE Jr: DNA single-stranded breaks during repair of UV damage in human fibroblasts and abnormalities of repair in xeroderma pigmentosum. *Proc Natl Acad Sci USA* **73:**39, 1976.
163. Dingman CW, Kakunaga T: DNA strand breaking and rejoining in response to ultraviolet light in normal human and xeroderma pigmentosum cells. *Int J Radiat Biol* **30:**55, 1976.
164. Dunn WC, Regan JD: Inhibition of DNA excision repair in human cells by arabinofuranosyl cytosine: Effects on normal and xeroderma pigmentosum cells. *Mol Pharmacol* **15:**367, 1976.
165. Bootsma D, Mulder MP, Pot F, Cohen JA: Different inherited levels of DNA repair replication in xeroderma pigmentosum cell strains after exposure to ultraviolet irradiation. *Mutat Res* **9:**507, 1970.
166. Zelle B, Lohman PHM: Repair of UV-endonuclease-susceptible sites in the 7 complementation groups of xeroderma pigmentosum A through G. *Mutat Res* **62:**363, 1979.
167. Dupuy JM, Lafforet D, Rachman F: Xeroderma pigmentosum with liver involvement. *Helv Paediatr Acta* **29:**213, 1975.
168. Cleaver JE: Repair of alkylation damage in ultraviolet sensitive (xeroderma pigmentosum) human cells. *Mutat Res* **12:**453, 1971.
169. Kleijer WJ, Lohman PHM, Mulder MP, Bootsma D: Repair of X-ray damage in DNA of cultivated cells from patients having xeroderma pigmentosum. *Mutat Res* **9:**517, 1970.
170. Setlow RB, Regan JD: Defective repair of N-acetoxy-2-acetylaminofluorene-induced lesions in the DNA of xeroderma pigmentosum cells. *Biochem Biophys Res Commun* **16:**1019, 1972.
171. Stich HF, San RHC, Miller JA, Miller EC: Various levels of DNA repair synthesis in xeroderma pigmentosum cells exposed to the carcinogens N-hydroxy and N-acetoxy-2-acetylaminofluorene. *Nature New Biol* **238:**9, 1972.
172. Regan JD, Setlow RB: Two forms of repair in the DNA of human cells damaged by chemical carcinogens and mutagens. *Cancer Res* **34:**3318, 1974.
173. Painter RB, Young BR: Repair replication in mammalian cells after X-irradiation. *Mutat Res* **14:**225, 1972.
174. Kraemer KH, Coon HG, Petinga RA, Barrett SF, Rash AE, Robbins JH: Genetic heterogeneity in xeroderma pigmentosum. Complementation groups and their relationship to DNA repair rates. *Proc Natl Acad Sci USA* **72:**59, 1975.
175. De Weerd-Kastelein EA, Keijzer W, Bootsma D: A third complementation group in xeroderma pigmentosum. *Mutat Res* **22:**87, 1974.
176. Kraemer KH, De Weerd-Kastelein EA, Robbins JH, Keijzer W, Barrett SF, Petinga RA, Bootsma D: Five complementation groups in xeroderma pigmentosum. *Mutat Res* **33:**327, 1975.
177. Arase S, Kozuka T, Tanaka K, Ikenaga M, Takebe H: A sixth complementation group in xeroderma pigmentosum. *Mutat Res* **59:**143, 1979.
178. Keijzer W, Jaspers NGJ, Abrahams PJ, Taylor AMR, Arlett CF, Zelle B, Takebe H, Kanmont PDS, Bootsma D: A seventh complementation group in excision deficient xeroderma pigmentosum. *Mutat Res* **62:**183, 1979.
179. Wood RD: DNA repair. Seven genes for three diseases. *Nature* **350:**190, 1991.
180. Van Houten B: Nucleotide excision repair in *Escherichia coli. Microbiol Rev* **54:**18, 1990.
181. Thompson LH, Busch DB, Brookman K, Mooney CL, Glaser DA: Genetic diversity of UV-sensitive DNA repair mutants of Chinese hamster ovary cells. *Proc Natl Acad Sci USA* **78:**3734, 1981.
182. Hori TA, Shiomi T, Sato K: Human chromosome 13 compensates a DNA repair defect in UV sensitive cells by mouse-human cell hybridization. *Proc Natl Acad Sci USA* **80:**5655, 1983.
183. Fujiwara Y, Tatsumi M, Sasaki MS: Cross-link repair in human cells and its possible defect in Fanconi's anemia cells. *J Mol Biol* **113:**635, 1977.
184. Thompson LH, Mooney CL, Burkhart-Schultz K, Carrano AV, Siciliano MJ: Correction of a nucleotide-excision repair mutation by human chromosome 19 in hamster-human hybrid cells. *Somat Cell Genet* **11:**87, 1985.
185. McWhir J, Selfridge J, Harrison DJ, Squires S, Melton DW: Mice with DNA repair gene (ERCC-1) deficiency have elevated levels of p53, liver nuclear abnormalities and die before weaning. *Nat Genet* **5:**217, 1993.
186. Van Duin M, De Wit J, Odijk H, Westerveld A, Yasui A, Koken MHM, Hoeijmakers JHJ, Bootsma D: Molecular characterization of the human excision repair gene ERCC1: cDNA cloning and amino acid homology with the yeast DNA repair gene RAD10. *Cell* **44:**913, 1986.
187. Prakash S, Sung P, Prakash L: Structure and function of RAD3, RAD6, and other DNA repair genes of *Saccharomyces cerevisiae,* in Strauss PR, Wilson SH (eds): *The Eukaryotic Nucleus, Molecular Biochemistry and Macromolecular Assemblies.* Caldwell, NJ, Telford, 1990, vol 1, p 275.
188. Prakash L, Prakash S: Excision repair genes of *Saccharomyces cerevisiae. Ann Ist Super Sanita* **25:**99, 1989.
189. Bankmann M, Prakash L, Prakash S: Yeast RAD14 and human xeroderma pigmentosum group A DNA-repair genes encode homologous proteins. *Nature* **355:**555, 1992.
190. Tanaka K, Miura N, Satokata I, Miyamoto I, Yoshida MC, Satoh Y, Kondo S, Yasui A, Okayama H, Okada Y: Analysis of a human DNA excision repair gene involved in group A xeroderma pigmentosum and containing a zinc-finger domain. *Nature* **348:**73, 1990.
191. Reed WB, May SB, Nickel WR: Xeroderma pigmentosum with neurological complications: The DeSanctis Cacchione syndrome. *Arch Dermatol* **91:**224, 1965.
192. Reed WB, Landing B, Sugarman G, Cleaver JE, Melnyk J: Xeroderma pigmentosum. Clinical and laboratory investigation of its defect. *JAMA* **207:**2073, 1969.
193. Thrush DC, Holti G, Bradley WG, Campbell MI, Walton JN: Neurological manifestations of xeroderma pigmentosum in two siblings. *J Neurol Sci* **22:**91, 1974.
194. Cleaver JE, Zelle B, Hashem N, German J: Xeroderma pigmentosum in Egypt. II. Epidemiology, clinical symptoms and molecular biology. *J Invest Dermatol* **77:**96, 1981.
195. De Weerd-Kastelein EA, Keijzer W, Sabour M, Parkington JM, Bootsma D: A xeroderma pigmentosum patient having a high residual activity of unscheduled DNA synthesis after UV is assigned to complementation group A. *Mutat Res* **37:**307, 1976.
196. Stefanini M, Kleijer W, Dalpra L, Elli R, Porro MN, Nicoletti B, Nuzzo F: Differences in the levels of UV repair and in clinical symptoms in two sibs affected by xeroderma pigmentosum. *Hum Genet* **634:**1, 1980.
197. Thillmann HW, Witte J: Correlation of the colony-forming abilities of xeroderma pigmentosum fibroblasts with repair-specific DNA incision reactions catalyzed by cell-free extracts. *Arch Toxicol* **44:**197, 1980.
198. Kuhnlein U, Penhoet EE, Linn S: An altered apurinic endonuclease activity in group A and group D xeroderma pigmentosum fibroblasts. *Proc Natl Acad Sci USA* **73:**1169, 1976.
199. Robins P, Jones JJ, Biggerstaff M, Lindahl T, Wood RD: Complementation of DNA repair in xeroderma pigmentosum group A cell extracts by a protein with affinity for damaged DNA. *EMBO J* **10:**3913, 1991.
200. Miura N, Miyamoto I, Asahina H, Satokata I, Tanaka K, Okada Y: Identification and characterization of the XPAC protein, the gene product of the human XPAC (xeroderma pigmentosum group A complementing) gene. *J Biol Chem* **266:**19786, 1991.
201. Ishizaki K, Matsunaga T, Kato M, Nikaido O, Ikenaga M: Repair of thymine dimers and (6-4) photoproducts in group A xeroderma pigmentosum cell lines harboring a transferred normal chromosome 9. *Photochem Photobiol* **56:**365, 1992.

202. Satokata I, Tanaka K, Miura N, Miyamoto I, Satoh Y, Kondo S, Okada Y: Characterization of a splicing mutation in group A xeroderma pigmentosum. *Proc Natl Acad Sci USA* **87:**9908, 1990.
203. Weeda G, Bootsma D, Van Ham RCA, Vermeulen W, Van Der Eb AJ, Hoeijmakers JHJ: A presumed DNA helicase encoded by ERCC-3 is involved in the human repair disorder xeroderma pigmentosum and Cockayne's syndrome. *Cell* **62:**777, 1990.
204. Weeda G, Ma L, Van Ham RCA, Van Der Eb AJ, Hoeijmakers JHJ: Structure and expression of the human XPBC/ERCC-3 gene involved in DNA repair disorders xeroderma pigmentosum and Cockayne's syndrome. *Nucleic Acids Res* **19:**6301, 1991.
205. Troelstra C, Koken M, Weeda G, Van Der Spek P, Van Den Berg J, Hoeijmakers JHJ, Bootsma D: Molecular analysis of the genes involved in mammalian DNA repair, in Proceedings of the American Association for Cancer Research Special Conference on Cellular Responses to Environmental DNA Damage, Banff, Canada, December 1–6, 1991.
206. Mansbridge JN, Hanawalt PC: Domain-limited repair of DNA in ultraviolet irradiated fibroblasts from xeroderma pigmentosum complementation group C, in Friedberg EC, Bridges BR (eds): *Cellular Responses to DNA Damage*. New York, Alan R. Liss, 1983, p 195.
207. Karentz D, Cleaver JE: Excision repair in xeroderma pigmentosum group C but not group D is clustered in a small fraction of the total genome. *Mutat Res* **165:**165, 1986.
208. Cleaver JE: DNA repair in human xeroderma pigmentosum group C cells involves a different distribution of damaged sites in confluent and growing cells. *Nucleic Acids Res* **14:**8155, 1986.
209. Venema J, Van Hoffen A, Natarajan AT, Van Zeeland AA, Mullenders LHF: The residual repair capacity of xeroderma pigmentosum complementation group C fibroblasts is highly specific for transcriptionally active DNA. *Nucleic Acids Res* **18:**443, 1990.
210. Hananian J, Cleaver JE: Xeroderma pigmentosum exhibiting neurological disorders and systemic lupus erythematosus. *Clin Genet* **17:**39, 1980.
211. Pawsey SA, Magnus IA, Ramsay CA, Benson PF, Giannelli F: Clinical, genetic and DNA repair studies on a consecutive series of patients with xeroderma pigmentosum. *Q J Med* **48:**179, 1979.
212. Goldstein N, Hay-Roe V: Prevention of skin cancer with a PABA in alcohol sunscreen in xeroderma pigmentosum. *Cutis* **15:**61, 1975.
213. Legerski RJ, Brown DB, Peterson CA, Robberson DL: Transient complementation of xeroderma pigmentosum cells by microinjection of poly(A)$^+$ RNA. *Proc Natl Acad Sci USA* **81:**5676, 1984.
214. Legerski R, Peterson C: Expression cloning of a human DNA repair gene involved in xeroderma pigmentosum group C. [Published erratum appears in *Nature* **360:**610, 1992.] *Nature* **359:**70, 1992.
215. Robbins JH, Moshell AN, Lutzner MA, Ganges MB, Dupuy JM: A new patient with both xeroderma pigmentosum and Cockayne syndrome is in a new complementation group. *J Invest Dermatol* **80:**331A, 1983.
216. Dupuy JM, Moshell AN, Lutzner MA, Robbins JH: A new patient with both xeroderma pigmentosum and Cockayne syndrome is not in complementation group B. *J Invest Dermatol* **78:**356, 1982.
217. Johnson RT, Elliot GC, Squires S, Joysey VC: Lack of complementation between xeroderma pigmentosum complementation groups D and H. *Hum Genet* **81:**203, 1989.
218. Vermeulen W, Stefanini M, Giliani S, Hoeijmakers JHJ, Bootsma D: Xeroderma pigmentosum group H falls into complementation group D. *Mutat Res* **255:**201, 1991.
219. Galloway AM, Liuzzi M, Chan JR, Paterson MC: Processing of UV-induced DNA damage in cultured human fibroblasts, in Proceedings of the American Association for Cancer Research Special Conference on Cellular Responses to Environmental DNA Damage, Banff, Canada, December 1–6, 1991.
220. Kuhnleun U, Lel B, Penhoet E, Linn E: Xeroderma pigmentosum fibroblasts of the group D lack an apurinic DNA endonuclease species with a low apparent Km. *Nucleic Acids Res* **5:**951, 1978.
221. Moses RE, Beaudet AL: Apurinic endonuclease activities in repair-deficient human cell lines. *Nucleic Acids Res* **5:**463, 1978.
222. Weber CA, Salazar EP, Stewart SA, Thompson LH: Molecular cloning and biological characterization of a human gene ERCC2 that corrects the nucleotide excision repair defect in CHOUV5 cells. *Mol Cell Biol* **8:**1137, 1988.
223. Weber CA, Salazar EP, Stewart SA, Thompson LH: ERCC2: cDNA cloning and molecular characterization of a human nucleotide excision repair gene with high homology to yeast RAD3. *EMBO J* **9:**1437, 1990.
224. Weber CA, Thompson LH, Salazar EP: Characterization of ERCC2 and its correction of xeroderma pigmentosum group D, in Proceedings of the American Association for Cancer Research Special Conference on Cellular Responses to Enviromental DNA Damage, Banff, Canada, December 1–6, 1991.
225. Flejter W, McDaniel LD, Johns D, Friedberg EC, Schultz RA: Correction of xeroderma pigmentosum complementation group D mutant cell phenotypes by chromosome and gene transfer: Involvement of the human ERCC2 DNA repair gene. *Proc Natl Acad Sci USA* **89:**261, 1992.
226. Fischer E, Schnyder UW, Jung EG: Report of three sisters with XP-E, a rare xeroderma pigmentosum complementation group. *Photodermatology* **1:**232, 1984.
227. Kawada A, Satoh Y, Fujiwara Y: Xeroderma pigmentosum complementation group E: A case report. *Photodermatology* **3:**233, 1986.
228. Fujiwara Y, Uehara Y, Ichihashi M, Yamamoto Y, Nishioka K: Assignment of 2 patients with xeroderma pigmentosum to complementation group E. *Mutat Res* **145:**55, 1985.
229. Chu G, Chang E: Xeroderma pigmentosum group I cells lack a nuclear factor that binds to damaged DNA. *Science* **242:**564, 1988.
230. Keeney S, Wein H, Linn S: Biochemical heterogeneity in xeroderma pigmentosum complementation group E. *Mutat Res* **273:**49, 1992.
231. Fujiwara Y, Uehara Y, Ichihashi M, Nishioka K: Xeroderma pigmentosum complementation group F: More assignments and repair characteristics. *Photochem Photobiol* **41:**629, 1985.
232. Nishigori C, Fujiwara H, Uyeno K, Kawaguchi T, Takebe H: Xeroderma pigmentosum patients belonging to complementation group F and efficient liquid-holding recovery of ultraviolet damage. *Photodermatol Photoimmunol Photomed* **8:**146, 1991.
233. Saxon PJ, Schultz RA, Stanbridge EJ, Friedberg EC: Human chromosome 15 confers partial complementation of phenotypes to xeroderma pigmentosum group F cells. *Am J Hum Genet* **44:**474, 1989.
234. Arlett CF, Harcourt SA, Lehmann AR, Stevens S, Ferguson-Smith MA, Mosley WN: Studies on a new case of xeroderma pigmentosum (XP3BR) from complementation group G with a cellular sensitivity to ionizing radiation. *Carcinogenesis* **1:**745, 1980.
235. Ichihashi M, Fujiwara Y, Uehara Y, Matsumoto A: A mild form of xeroderma pigmentosum assigned to complementation group G and its repair heterogeneity. *J Invest Dermatol* **85:**284, 1985.
236. Hofmann H, Jung EG, Schnyder UW: Pigmented xerodermoid: First report of a family. *Bull Cancer* **65:**347, 1978.
237. Myhr BC, Turnbull D, Dipaolo JA: Ultraviolet mutagenesis of normal and xeroderma pigmentosum variant fibroblasts. *Mutat Res* **62:**341, 1979.
238. Cleaver JE, Thomas GH, Park SD: Xeroderma pigmentosum variants have a slow recovery of DNA synthesis after irradiation with ultraviolet light. *Biochim Biophys Acta* **564:**122, 1979.
239. Cleaver JE, Carter DM: Xeroderma pigmentosum variants: Influence of temperature on DNA repair. *J Invest Dermatol* **60:**29, 1973.
240. Jaspers NGJ, Jansen VD, Kuilen G, Bootsma D: Complementation analysis of xeroderma pigmentosum variants. *Exp Cell Res* **136:**81, 1981.

241. Swift M, Chase C: Cancer in families with xeroderma pigmentosum. *J Natl Cancer Inst* **62:**1415, 1979.
242. Hashem N, Bootsma D, Keijzer W, Greene AE, Coriell L, Thomas GH, Cleaver JE: Clinical characteristics, DNA repair, and complementation groups in xeroderma pigmentosum patients from Egypt. *Cancer Res* **40:**13, 1980.
243. Giannelli F, Pawsey SA: DNA repair synthesis in human heterokaryons. II. A test for heterozygosity in xeroderma pigmentosum and some insight into the structure of the defective enzyme. *J Cell Sci* **15:**163, 1974.
244. Ritter MA: Reduced DNA repair in xeroderma pigmentosum (XP) heterozygotes, in *Sixth International Congress of Radiation Research*. Tokyo, Japan, Toppan, 1979, p 264.
245. Casati A, Stefanini M, Giorgi R, Ghetti P, Nuzzo F: Chromosome rearrangements in normal fibroblasts from xeroderma pigmentosum homozygotes and heterozygotes. *Cancer Genet Cytogenet* **51:**89, 1991.
246. Parshad R, Sanford KK, Kraemer KH, Jones GM, Tarone RE: Carrier detection in xeroderma pigmentosum. *J Clin Invest* **85:**135, 1990.
247. Selsky CA, Greer S: Host-cell reactivation of ultraviolet irradiated and chemically treated herpes simplex virus I by xeroderma pigmentosum, xeroderma pigmentosum heterozygotes and normal skin fibroblasts. *Mutat Res* **50:**395, 1978.
248. Rainbow AJ: Reduced capacity to repair irradiated adenovirus in fibroblasts from xeroderma pigmentosum heterozygotes. *Cancer Res* **40:**3945, 1980.
249. Athas W, Hedayati M, Matanoski G, Farmer E, Grossman L: Development and field-test validation of an assay for DNA repair in circulating human lymphocytes. *Cancer Res* **51:**5786, 1991.
250. Ramsay CA, Coltart TM, Blumt S, Pawsey SA, Giannelli F: Prenatal diagnosis of xeroderma pigmentosum. Report of the first successful case. *Lancet* **2:**1109, 1974.
251. Paterson MC, Anderson AK, Smith BP, Smith PJ: Enhanced radiosensitivity of cultured fibroblasts from ataxia telangiectasia heterozygotes manifested by defective colony-forming ability and reduced DNA repair replication after hypoxic gamma-irradiation. *Cancer Res* **39:**3725, 1979.
252. Scudiero DA: Decreased DNA repair synthesized defective colony forming ability of ataxia telangiectasia fibroblast cell strains treated with N-methyl-N′-nitro-N-nitrosoguanidine. *Cancer Res* **40:**984, 1980.
253. Smith PJ, Paterson MC: Defective DNA repair and increased lethality in ataxia telangiectasia cells following gamma-ray irradiation. *Nature* **287:**745, 1980.
254. Cornforth MN, Bedford JS: On the nature of the defect in cells from individuals with ataxia telangiectasia. *Science* **227:**1589, 1985.
255. Gatti RA, Berkel I, Boder E, Braedt G, Charmley P, Concannon P, Ersoy F, Foroud T, Jaspers NGJ, Lange K, Lathrop GM, Leppert M, Nakamura Y, O'Connell P, Paterson M, Salser W, Sanal O, Silver J, Sparkes RS, Susi E, Weeks DE, Wei S, White R, Yoder F: Localization of an ataxia-telangiectasia gene to chromosome 11q22.23. *Nature* **336:**577, 1988.
256. Kapp LN, Painter RB, Yu L-C, Van Loon N, Richard CW, James MR, Cox DR, Murnane JP: Cloning of a candidate gene for ataxia-telangiectasia group D. *Am J Hum Genet* **51:**45, 1992.
257. Fornace AJ, Little JB, Weichselbaum RR: DNA repair in a Fanconi's anemia fibroblast cell strain. *Biochim Biophys Acta* **561:**99, 1979.
258. Kaye J, Smith CA, Hanawalt PC: DNA repair in human cells containing photoadducts of 8-methoxypsoralen or angelicin. *Cancer Res* **40:**696, 1980.
259. Poon PK, O'Brien RL, Parker JW: Defective DNA repair in Fanconi's anemia. *Nature* **250:**223, 1974.
260. Mann WR, Venkatraj VS, Allen RG, Liu Q, Olsen DA: Fanconi anemia: Evidence for linkage heterogeneity on chromosome 20q. *Genomics* **9:**329, 1991.
261. Chaganti RSK, Schonberg S, German J: A manyfold increase in sister chromatid exchanges in Bloom's syndrome lymphocytes. *Proc Natl Acad Sci USA* **71:**4508, 1974.
262. Vijayalaxmi EHJ, Ray JH, German J: Bloom's syndrome: Evidence for an increased mutation frequency in vivo. *Science* **221:**851, 1983.
263. Langlois RG, Bigbee WL, Jensen RH, German J: Evidence for increased in vivo mutation and somatic recombination in Bloom's syndrome. *Proc Natl Acad Sci USA* **86:**670, 1989.
264. Krepinsky AB, Rainbow AJ, Heddle JA: Studies on the ultraviolet light sensitivity of Bloom's syndrome fibroblasts. *Mutat Res* **69:**357, 1980.
265. Remsen JF: Repair of damage by N-acetoxy-2-acetylaminofluorene in Bloom's syndrome. *Mutat Res* **72:**151, 1980.
266. Willis AE, Lindahl T: DNA ligase I deficiency in Bloom's syndrome. *Nature* **325:**357, 1987.
267. Chan JYH, Becker FF, German J, Ray JH: Altered DNA ligase I activity in Bloom's syndrome cells. *Nature* **325:**357, 1987.
268. Barnes DE, Tomkinson AE, Kodama K, Lindahl T: DNA ligase defect in Bloom's syndrome. *Am J Hum Genet (suppl)* **49:**61, 1991.
269. Fujiwara Y, Ichihashi M, Kano Y, Goto K, Shimizu K: A new human photosensitive subject with a defect in the recovery of DNA synthesis after ultraviolet-light irradiation. *J Invest Dermatol* **77:**256, 1981.
270. Greenhaw G, Hebert A, Duke-Woodside ME, Butler IJ, Hecht JT, Cleaver JE, Thomas GH, Horton WA: Xeroderma pigmentosum and Cockayne syndrome: Overlapping clinical and biochemical phenotypes. *Am J Hum Genet* **50:**277, 1992.
271. Gorlin RJ: Nevoid basal-cell carcinoma syndrome. *Medicine (Baltimore)* **66:**98, 1987.
272. Little JB, Nichols WW, Troilo P, Nagasawa H, Strong LC: Radiation sensitivity of cell strains from families with genetic disorders predisposing to radiation-induced cancer. *Cancer Res* **49:**4705, 1989.
273. Applegate LA, Goldberg LH, Ley RD, Ananthaswamy HN: Hypersensitivity of skin fibroblasts from basal cell nevus syndrome patients to killing by ultraviolet B but not by ultraviolet C radiation. *Cancer Res* **50:**637, 1990.
274. Shimada T, Dowjat WK, Gindhart TD, Lerman MI, Colburn NH: Lifespan extension of basal cell nevus syndrome fibroblasts by transfection with mouse pro or v-myc genes. *Int J Cancer* **39:**649, 1987.
275. Farndon PA, Del Mastro RG, Evans DGR, Kilpatrick MW: Location of gene for Gorlin syndrome. *Lancet* **339:**581, 1992.
276. Reis A, Kuster W, Linss G, Gebel E, Hamm H, Fuhrmann W, Wolff G, Groth W, Gustafson G, Kuklik M: Localisation of gene for naevoid basal-cell carcinoma syndrome. *Lancet* **339:**617, 1992.
277. Gailani MR, Bale SJ, Leffell DJ, DiGiovanna JJ, Peck GL, Poliak S, Drum MA, Pastakia B, McBride OW, Kase R, Greene M, Mulvihill JJ, Bale AE: Developmental defects in Gorlin syndrome related to a putative tumor suppressor gene on chromosome 9. *Cell* **69:**111, 1992.
278. Burnet M: Cancer—A biological approach. I. The processes of control. *Br Med J* 799, 1957.
279. Ames BN: The detection of chemical mutagens with enteric bacteria, in Hollander A (ed): *Chemical Mutagens, Principles and Methods for Their Detection*. New York, Plenum, 1971, vol 1, p 267.
280. Ames BN: Dietary carcinogens and anticarcinogens, oxygen radicals and degenerative diseases. *Science* **221:**1256, 1983.
281. Brash DE, Rudolph JA, Simon JA, Lin A, McKenna GJ, Baden HP, Halperin AJ, Ponten J: A role for sunlight in skin cancer: UV-induced p53 mutations in squamous cell carcinoma. *Proc Natl Acad Sci USA* **88:**10124, 1991.
282. Kraemer KH: Xeroderma pigmentosum, in Demis DJ, Dobson RL, McGuire J (eds): *Clinical Dermatology 4*. Philadelphia, Harper & Row, 1980, unit 19-7, p 1.
283. Satokata I, Tanaka K, Miura N, Narita M, Mimaki T, Satoh Y, Kondo S, Okada Y: Three nonsense mutations responsible for group A xeroderma pigmentosum. *Mutat Res* **273:**193, 1992.
284. Satokata I, Tanaka K, Yuba S, Okada Y: Identification of splicing mutations of the last nucleotides of exons, a nonsense mutation, and a missense mutation of the XPAC gene as causes of group A xeroderma pigmentosum. *Mutat Res* **273:**203, 1992.
285. Yagi T, Sato M, Tatsumi-Miajima J, Takebe H: UV-induced base substitution mutations in a shuttle vector plasmid

propagated in group C xeroderma pigmentosum cells. *Mutat Res* **273:**213, 1992.

286. Troelstra C, van Gool A, de Wit J, Vermeulen W, Bootsma D, Hoeijmakers JHJ: *ERCC6*, a member of a subfamily of putative helicases, is involved in Cockayne's syndrome and preferential repair of active genes. *Cell* **71:**939, 1992.
287. Schaeffer L, Roy R, Humbert S, Moncollin V, Vermeulen W, Hoeijmakers JHJ, Chambon P, Egly J-M: DNA repair helicase: a component of BTF2 (TFIIH) basic transcription factor. *Science* **260:**58, 1993.
288. van Vuuren AJ, Vermeulen W, Ma L, Weeda G, Appeldoorn E, Jaspers NGL, van der Eb AJ, Bootsma D, Hoeijmakers JHJ, Humbert S, Schaeffer L, Egly J-M: Correction of xeroderma pigmentosum repair defect by basal transcription factor BTF2 (TFIIH). *EMBO J* **13:**645, 1994.
289. Schaeffer L, Moncollin V, Roy R, Staub A, Mezzina M, Sarasin A, Weeda G, Hoeijmakers JHJ, Egly J-M: The ERCC2/DNA repair protein is associated with the class II BTF2/TFIIH transcription factor. *EMBO J* **13:**2388, 1994.
290. Vermeulen W, van Vuuren AJ, Chipoulet M, Schaeffer L, Appeldoorn E, Weeda G, Jaspers NGJ, Priestley A, Arlett CF, Lehmann AR, Bootsma D, Egly J-M, Hoeijmakers JHJ: Three excision repair proteins associated with transcription factor BTF2 (TFIIH). Evidence for the existence of a transcription syndrome. (Submitted for publication.)
291. Stefanini M, Vermeulen W, Weeda G, Giliani S, Nardo T, Mezzina M, Sarasin A, Harper JI, Arlett CF, Hoeijmakers JHJ, Lehmann AR: A new nucleotide-excision-repair gene associated with the disorder trichothiodystrophy. *Am J Hum Genet* **53:**817, 1993.
292. Bootsma D, Hoeijmakers JHJ: DNA repair, engagement with transcription. *Nature* **363:**114, 1993.
293. Masutani C, Sugasawa K, Yanagisawa J, Sonoyama T, Ui M, Enomoto T, Takio K, Tanaka K, van der Spek PJ, Bootsma D, Hoeijmakers JHJ, Hanaoka F: Purification and cloning of a nucleotide excision repair complex involving the xeroderma pigmentosum group C protein and a human homolog of yeast RAD23. *EMBO J* **13:**1831, 1994.
294. Keeney S, Eker APM, Brody T, Vermeulen W, Bootsma D, Hoeijmakers JHJ, Linn S: Correction of the DNA repair defect in xeroderma pigmentosum group E by injection of a DNA damage binding protein. *Proc Natl Acad Sci USA* **91:**4053, 1994.
295. Takao M, Abramic M, Moos M Jr, Otrin VR, Wootton JC, McLenigan M, Levine AS, Protic M: A 127 kDa component of a UV-damaged DNA-binding complex, which is defective in some xeroderma pigmentosum group E patients, is homologous to a slime mold protein. *Nucl Acids Res* **21:**4111, 1993.
296. van Vuuren AJ, Appeldoorn E, Odijk H, Yasui A, Jaspers NGJ, Bootsma D, Hoeijmakers JHJ: Evidence for a repair enzyme complex involving ERCC1 and complementing activities of ERCC4, ERCC11 and xeroderma pigmentosum group F. *EMBO J* **12:**3693, 1993.
297. Biggerstaff M, Szymkowski DE, Wood RD: Co-correction of the ERCC1, ERCC4 and xeroderma pigmentosum group F DNA repair defects *in vitro*. *EMBO J* **12:**3685, 1993.
298. Li L, Elledge SJ, Peterson CA, Bales ES, Legerski RJ: Specific association between the human DNA repair proteins XPA and ERCC1. *Proc Natl Acad Sci USA* **91:**5012, 1994.
299. Scherly D, Nouspikel T, Corlet J, Ucla C, Bairoch A, Clarkson SG: Complementation of the DNA repair defect in xeroderma pigmentosum group G cells by a human cDNA related to yeast *RAD2*. *Nature* **363:**182, 1993.
300. O'Donovan A, Wood RD: Identical defects in DNA repair in xeroderma pigmentosum group G and rodent ERCC group 5. *Nature* **363:**185, 1993.
301. Habraken Y, Sung P, Prakash L, Prakash S: Yeast excision repair gene RAD2 encodes a single-stranded DNA endonuclease. *Nature* **366:**365, 1993.

CHAPTER 149

Genetic Skin Disorders of Keratin

Elaine Fuchs

1. **Keratins belong to the supergene family of >40 intermediate filament (IF) proteins, which assemble into 10 nm cytoskeletal filaments in all eukaryotic cells. Approximately 30 keratins of two distinct types are coexpressed as pairs in epithelial cells, at various stages of differentiation and development. In the epidermis, keratins (K) 5 and 14 are the major structural proteins of basal cells. As keratinocytes commit to differentiate terminally, they switch off expression of this pair and switch on expression of K1 and K10, which constitute ~85 percent of total protein in the fully differentiated squame.**
2. **More than 5000 type I and II keratin subunits comprise each 10-nm filament. Filaments are composed of ~4 intertwined protofibrils (4.5 nm), which in turn are composed of ~2 protofilaments (2 to 3 nm). Protofilaments can accommodate linear chains of tetramers, which for keratins, are composed of coiled-coil heterodimers arranged in antiparallel fashion. In vitro, 10-nm filament assembly relies only on type I and II keratins, and does not require auxiliary proteins or factors. In vivo, keratin filaments interact with both the nuclear envelope and desmosomes, generating an extensive cytoplasmic network imparting mechanical strength to the keratinocyte.**
3. **Genetic engineering has enabled construction of a series of keratin and other IF mutants, many of which act in a dominant negative fashion to perturb IF network formation in transfected cells and alter 10-nm filament assembly in vitro. A number of amino acid residues essential for proper 10-nm filament assembly have been identified.**
4. **Transgenic mice expressing dominant negative mutant human K14 genes show clinical and biochemical features of human epidermolysis bullosa simplex (EBS), an autosomal dominant blistering skin disease typified by alterations in basal keratin networks and basal-cell cytolysis upon mild mechanical trauma. Severity in phenotype correlates with the degree to which 10-nm filament assembly is perturbed. Human families with any of the three major subtypes of EBS have genetic defects that map to either chromosome 12 or chromosome 17, near or at locations where the respective K5 and K14 genes reside. Point mutations in K5 or K14 genes have been found in >10 distinct instances of Dowling-Meara EBS, four instances of Koebner EBS, and in six families with Weber-Cockayne EBS. These mutations are functionally responsible for EBS. Nine of the Dowling-Meara EBS instances involve C or H mutations at arginine residue 125 of K14, suggesting that CpG methylation and deamination play a role in the mutagenesis.**
5. **Transgenic mice expressing mutant human K10 genes have morphologic and biochemical features of human epidermolytic hyperkeratosis (EH), a blistering skin disease typified by alterations in keratin networks and cell cytolysis in terminally differentiating cells. Point mutations in K1 or K10 genes have been found in 19 distinct instances of EH. These mutations appear to be functionally responsible for EH. Six incidences involve Cys or His mutations at arginine residue 156 of K10, suggesting that CpG methylation and deamination play a role in the mutagenesis. Interestingly, arginine 156 of K10 is equivalent to residue 125 of K14, indicating that mutations in the same highly conserved residue of two differentially expressed keratin genes account for a significant number of EH and EBS mutations thus far identified.**
6. **Studies involving genetic disorders of keratin are relatively new, but the field has opened up exciting new prospects for elucidating the genetic bases of other human diseases that are typified by alterations in IF networks and cell degeneration. It seems likely that many of these diseases will either involve IF gene defects or defects in proteins or organelles that associate with 10-nm filaments. Finally, studies revealing the genetic basis of EBS illustrate well the power of combining classic genetic approaches with "reverse" approaches (involving cell biology and transgenic mouse technology) in understanding the genetic bases of human diseases.**

A list of standard abbreviations is located immediately preceding the index in each volume. Additional abbreviations used in this chapter include: EBS = epidermolysis bullosa simplex; EH = epidermolytic hyperkeratosis; IF = intermediate filament; K = keratin.

THE EPIDERMIS: PROGRAMS OF TERMINAL DIFFERENTIATION AND DIFFERENTIAL KERATIN EXPRESSION

The epidermis and its appendages provide the protective interface between various traumas of the environment and the body.[1] The epidermis manifests its protective role by building a three-dimensional network of interconnected keratinocytes, each containing an extensive cytoskeleton of specialized 10-nm keratin filaments, encased by a membranous envelope of highly cross-linked proteins. How the epidermis produces its armor is considerably simpler than the program of differentiation carried out by its appendages. In the epidermis, the innermost, basal, layer has the capacity for DNA synthesis and mitosis. As cells commit to differentiate terminally, they begin their journey to the skin surface. In transit, they undergo a series of morphologic and biochemical changes culminating in the production of dead, flattened, enucleated squames, which are sloughed from the surface and continually replaced by inner cells differentiating outward.

The process of epidermal growth and differentiation is illustrated in Fig. 149-1. Mitotically active basal cells adhere to the basement membrane and underlying dermis via specialized, calcium-activated adhesion plaques, called "hemidesmosomes."[2,3] Hemidesmosomes contain unique anchoring proteins, including the α6β4 integrin heterodimer and several proteins identified by autoimmune antibodies from serums of patients with bullous pemphigoid. Basal cells interact laterally and suprabasally with their neighbors through calcium-activated membranous plaques, called "desmosomes."[2,3] Despite their ultrastructural similarity to hemidesmosomes, desmosomes are composed of distinct proteins, including desmoplakins, desmoglein, and desmocollins.

Intracellularly, hemidesmosomes and desmosomes connect with the cytoskeletal network of keratin filaments. As in basal cells of all stratified squamous epithelia, basal epidermal cells display a keratin network composed of the type II keratin K5 (58 kDa) and the type I keratin K14 (50 kDa)[4-7] (see following section and Table 149-1 for taxonomy of keratins discussed in this chapter). These keratins constitute ~15 to 25 percent of basal-cell protein. As basal epidermal cells differentiate, they down-regulate expression of K5/K14 and induce expression of a new set of differentiation-specific keratins.[4,5,7] For most body regions, the type II keratins K1 (67 kDa) and K2 (65 kDa) and the type I keratins K10 (56.5 kDa) and K11 (56 kDa) are expressed.[4,7] Some evidence suggests that K10 and K11 arise from polymorphisms, rather than gene multiplicity,[8,9] although this has not been unequivocally resolved. In palmar and plantar skin, an additional type I keratin, K9 (63 kDa) is expressed suprabasally.[4,5,10]

Even though terminally differentiating cells are postmitotic, they are nevertheless metabolically active, and the differentiation-associated changes in keratin expression are regulated transcriptionally.[11] In the inner spinous layers, keratins are a mixture of residual K5/K14 and newly synthesized differentiation-specific keratins. As spinous cells continue their path to the skin surface, they devote most of their protein-synthesizing machinery to manufacturing keratins. Keratins are highly stable in filament form, and K1 and K10 eventually constitute >85 percent of the total protein of a fully differentiated squame. Although the functional significance of the keratin switch has not yet been unequivocally resolved, K1/K10 filaments aggregate to form tonofibrillar bundles, which are thicker than tonofilament bundles in basal cells (for review, see Montagna and Lobitz[12]). This process also takes place in vitro, and appears to depend on the pair(s) of keratins.[13] The increase in filament bundling may enhance the ability of keratins to be among the sole survivors of the terminal differentiation process.

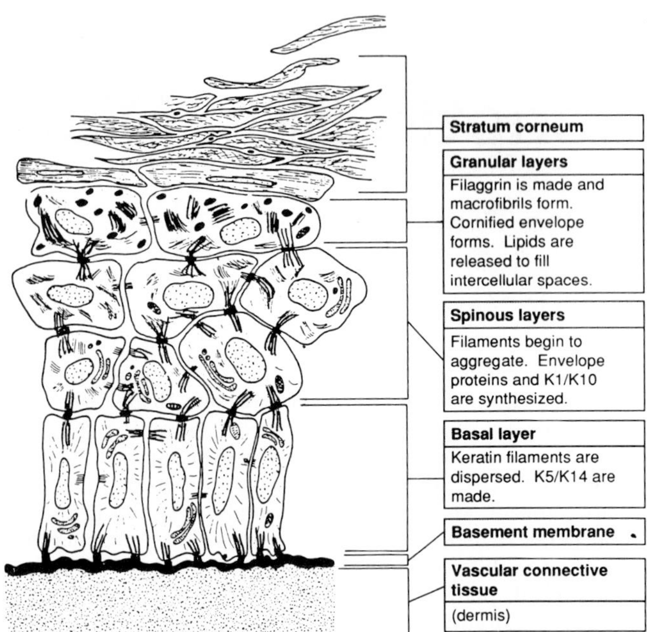

FIG. 149.1 Epidermal differentiation. Schematic outlining the basic features of terminal differentiation in epidermis. Outermost layer of cells is skin surface. (*From Fuchs E, Albers K, Kopan R: Terminal differentiation in cultured human epidermal cells.* Adv Cell Culture *6:1, 1988. Used by permission of Academic Press.*)

As spinous cells reach the granular layer, they undergo a final tailoring in protein synthesis, producing filaggrin, a histidine-rich, basic protein that may be involved in bundling tonofibrils into large macrofibrillar cables.[14] This process may impart to keratin filaments their final protection against the destructive phase that soon ensues.

Several other changes occur in the later stages of differentiation. Membrane-coating granules, made earlier, fuse with the plasma membrane and release lipids into intercellular spaces of granular and stratum corneum cells (for review, see Schurer et al.[15]). In addition, glutamine- and lysine-rich proteins are deposited on the inner surface of the plasma membrane.[16] Some of these proteins, such as involucrin, are made early during differentiation (see refs. 16 and 17 and references therein). Others, such as loricrin, are synthesized later.[18] As each differentiating cell becomes permeable during the destructive phase, a calcium influx activates epidermal transglutaminase, which then catalyzes formation of ε-(γ-glutamyl) lysine isopeptide bonds. The envelope proteins

Table 149-1 Properties and Distribution of Intermediate Filament Proteins

IF Protein	Subtype	Mass (kDa)	Approx. No.	Tissue Distribution
Keratin	I	40–63	15 (K9–K20; Ha1–Ha4)	Epithelia
Keratin	II	53–67	15 (K1–K8; Hb1–Hb4)	Epithelia
Vimentin	III	57	1	Mesenchymal cells
Desmin	III	53–54	1	Myogenic cells
Glial fibrillary acidic protein	III	50	1	Glial cells and astrocytes
Peripherin, α-internexin	III	57	1	Peripheral neurons
Neurofilament proteins	IV	62–210	3	Neurons of central and peripheral nerves
Lamin proteins	V	60–70	3	All cell types
Nestin	VI	240	1	Neuronal stem cells

are thereby cross-linked into a cage to contain the keratin macrofibrils (for review, see Greenberg et al.[19]). As lytic enzymes are released, all vestiges of metabolic activity terminate, and the resulting flattened squames are merely cellular skeletons, chock full of keratin macrofibrils. The stratum corneum, composed of squames sealed together by lipids, is an impermeable fortress, keeping microorganisms out and essential bodily fluids in.

In development, progenitor cells for the epidermis are embryonic basal cells.[12] They are the first cells to express epidermal markers, synthesizing very low levels of K14 and K5 (see refs. 20 and 21 and references therein). If embryonic basal cells do not come into contact with specialized mesenchymal cells, called "dermal papilla cells," they elevate K5/K14 expression concomitant with a commitment to an epidermal cell fate. In rodents, this occurs shortly before birth, whereas in humans, this occurs after the first trimester in utero. Upon differentiation, K1 and K10, and presumably other differentiation-specific markers, appear in the stratified layers. This pattern of keratin expression is then maintained in the adult.

Terminal differentiation continues throughout life. It takes approximately 2 to 4 weeks for an epidermal cell to leave the basal layer and reach and be sloughed from the skin surface. Thus, the adult epidermis is rejuvenated every few weeks.

THE KERATINS

Protein and 10-nm Filament Structure

The keratins constitute a group of ~30 related proteins (40 to 67 kDa) that are differentially expressed in epithelia at various stages of differentiation and development.[5] Keratins are only one group of a number of proteins with a remarkable capacity to self-assemble into 10-nm cytoskeletal or nuclear matrix fibers. This group has been called the intermediate filament (IF) supergene family (for reviews, see refs. 22 to 25). Based on amino acid sequence, IF proteins (40 to 240 kDa) have been subdivided into distinct types, of which keratins constitute type I and type II (see Table 149-1). Members within a type share 50 to 99 percent sequence identity, whereas members of different types share 25 to 35 percent identity. The typifying feature of IF polypeptides is a central α-helical rod domain, which can be subdivided into four smaller regions, referred to as 1A, 1B, 2A, and 2B. Within these helixes, sequences have heptad repeats of hydrophobic residues. Separating the helixes are short linker regions that interrupt the heptad repeat and helix continuity. In cytoskeletal IF proteins, the central domain encompasses 310 amino acids, whereas for the nuclear lamins, this length is increased by an insertion of 42 amino acids (6 heptads). Homology between different IF proteins is particularly high at the start of helix 1A and at the end of helix 2B. Flanking the rod domain are nonhelical amino (head) and carboxy (tail) domains that are variable in size and in sequence among all IF proteins, even within a single type. This variability in end domains accounts for much of the wide variability in size of IF proteins, despite their otherwise similar secondary structure. A comparison of selected IF protein sequences is shown in Fig. 149-2. Most notably, sequences are given for the four major human epidermal keratins.[26–31]

The sequences of IF proteins are compatible with the subunit structures that these proteins form. While the roles of the linker sequences that segment the rod remain to be elucidated, the unique α-helical, heptad repeat structure of the rod generates a surface stripe of hydrophobicity, enabling two IF proteins to intertwine in a coiled-coil fashion, aligned in parallel and in register (reviewed in refs. 22 to 25). These dimers are likely to be further stabilized by periodic ionic interactions. While most IF proteins can form homodimers, keratins form obligatory heterodimers, composed of type I and type II proteins.[32–34]

Tetramers form readily in vivo and in vitro, and all IF dimers appear to align in an antiparallel fashion, forming an apolar structure (for review, see Fuchs and Weber[24]). The most stable tetramer configuration seems to be a partially staggered arrangement of dimers, overlapping at their amino ends of the rod (see refs. 32, 35, and 36 and references therein). However, dimers aligned in exact register have also been observed, and there is some evidence that both configurations may play a role in filament assembly at least in vitro (see refs. 32, 36, and 37 and references therein).

Figure 149-3 illustrates a model of the structure of an IF. The mechanisms leading to higher-ordered packing of IF subunits are complex. Scanning transmission EM has revealed that ~32 polypeptides contribute to the overall width of the 10-nm filament, although some polymorphism in mass-per-unit width has been described (for review, see Aebi et al.[23]). Each filament is subdivided into ~4 intertwined protofibrils (4.5 nm), which in turn are composed of ~2 protofilaments (2 to 3 nm). Protofilaments can thus accommodate linear chains of tetramers aligned in a head-to-tail fashion. The precise arrangement of subunits in IF has been difficult to assess, because many of the lateral and end-to-end interactions occur under similar conditions. However, it has been proposed that dimers are in a staggered array within the protofilament and that the unstaggered alignment occurs at a higher level of lateral alignment.[37] In vitro, in the absence of auxiliary proteins or factors, assembly of ~8000 IF proteins can take place to form a single IF of 10 to 20 μm in length.

Mutagenesis Studies I: Importance of the Rod Domain in 10-nm Filament Structure

In the mid-1980s, investigators began to assess the sequences required for IF formation. Initially, mutant IF cDNAs were expressed in transfected cultured cells, and perturbations in IF networks were examined using indirect double immunofluorescence. Later, wild-type and mutant IF proteins were expressed in bacteria, purified by anion exchange chromatography, and assayed by in vitro IF assembly. Relevant to the epidermis, many of these experiments were conducted using the human keratins K5 and K14.[32,38–41] Additional studies were conducted on simple epithelial keratins[42–45] and other IF proteins (see refs. 46 to 50 and references therein).

Given the appreciable degree of sequence conservation among all IF rod domains, the universal importance of this segment in 10-nm filament structure is not surprising. From secondary structure analyses alone, it is clear that the rod domain is involved in formation of the coiled-coil dimer.[25,28] The ability of different IF proteins to recognize their respective partners in dimer and tetramer formation is also imparted by sequences in the rod. Removing a portion of the rod from an IF protein does not necessarily prevent it from forming dimers and tetramers,[40] but such deletions do interfere with filament formation in vivo and in vitro.[38–49] In many cases, these mutants interfere with filament elongation.[40]

The individual roles of amino acids within the rod have been explored through point mutagenesis studies. Even

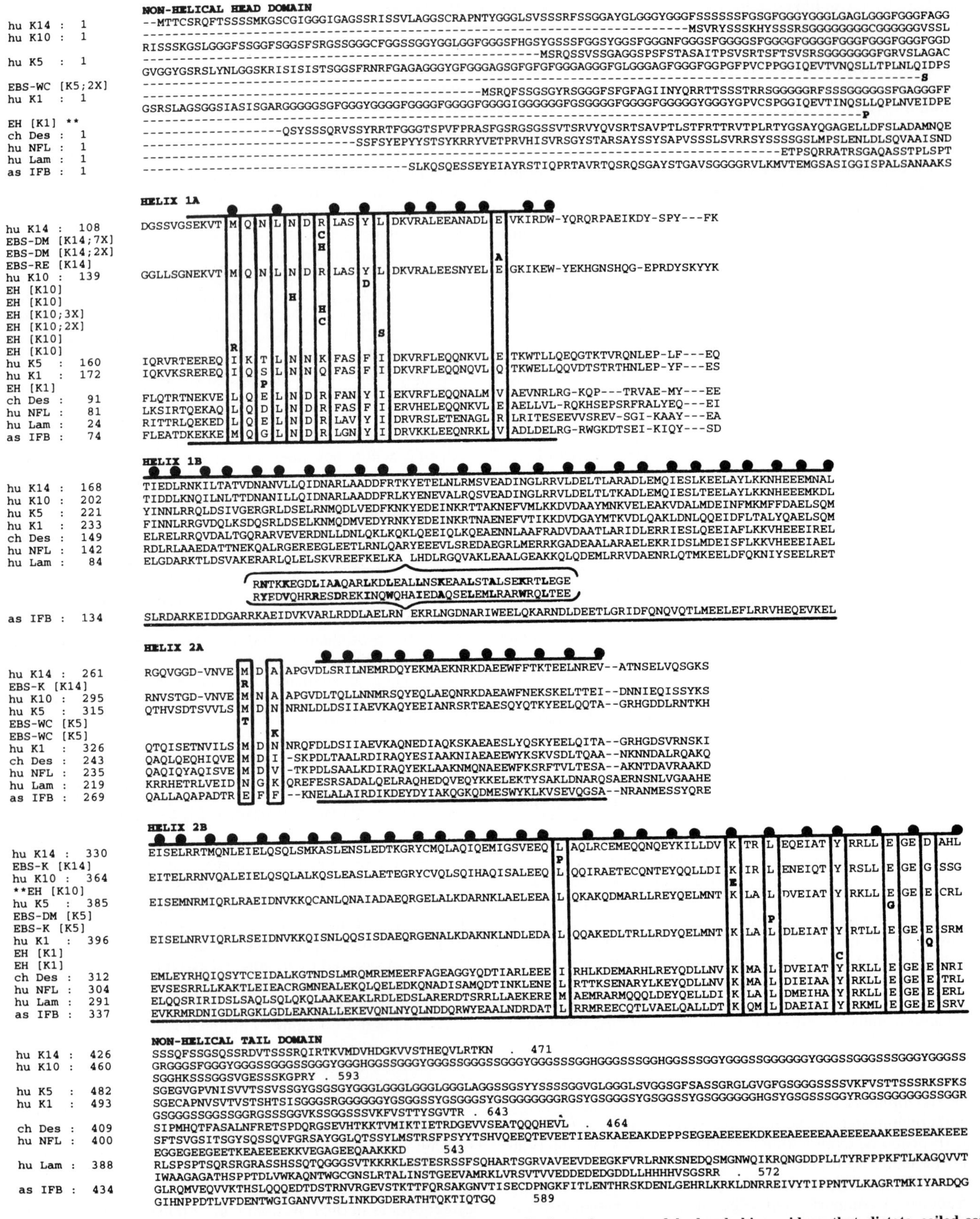

FIG. 149-2 Sequence comparisons of keratins and other IF proteins. Shown are amino acid sequences of the human epidermal keratins, K14,[26,28] K10,[30,31] K5,[27] and K1,[29] and other IF proteins, including human vimentin, human neurofilament protein L, human lamin C, and the invertebrate IF-B protein isolated from *Ascaris lumbricoides* (for sequences, see Albers and Fuchs[22]). Bars indicate positions of α-helical domains. Dots above the helical domains indicate the heptad repeat of hydrophobic residues that dictate coiled-coil formation. These residues are shown in bold for the additional helix 1B sequences of the lamin and invertebrate IF proteins. The boxed areas are residues where K5 or K14 point mutations have been found in patients with epidermolysis bullosa simplex, or where K1 or K10 point mutations have been found in patients with epidermolytic hyperkeratosis. **denotes mild case of EH.

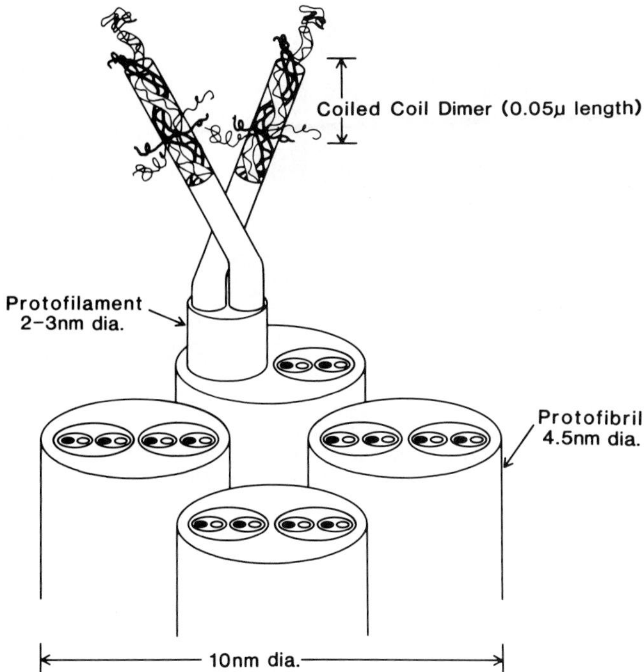

FIG. 149-3 **Model of 10-nm filament assembly. Model depicting inner structure of a keratin filament, revealing the heterodimeric nature of the coiled-coil, and the higher-ordered series of intertwining of protofilaments and protofibrils to yield the 10 nm-structure.** *(From Fuchs E, Tyner AL, Giudice GJ, Marchuk D, RayChaudhury A, Rosenberg M: The human keratin genes and their differential expression.* **Curr Topics Dev Biol** *22:5, 1987. Used by permission of Academic Press.)*

conservative amino acid substitutions in the highly conserved ends of the rod domain can be deleterious to filament formation both in vivo[41,44,46] and in vitro.[41,43] In contrast, even helix-disrupting residues such as proline can sometimes be tolerated within the central portion of the rod, without gross perturbations to 10-nm filament structure.[41]

Mutagenesis Studies II: Importance of Head and Tail Domains in 10-nm Filament Assembly

The highly divergent nonhelical head and tail domains of IF seem specifically tailored to suit particular 10-nm filament networks in different tissues. Given the obligatory heteropolymeric nature of keratin IF, this adds even more to the diversity of head and tail sequences and contributes to differences between the functions of these domains in keratin filaments versus other IF. In this regard, experiments focusing on IF end domains are often applicable only to a single IF subgroup, or in some instances to a single IF protein.

For keratins, the major findings obtained with tailless, headless and tailless/headless epidermal proteins are consistent with results from similar filament assembly studies conducted with simple epithelial proteins. One general role that seems to be shared among the tail domains of keratins is to stabilize protein–protein interactions between IF subunits.[42,45,51] Thus, while tailless keratins can assemble into 10-nm structures, they often do so only under conditions that provide additional stabilization, such as elevated ionic strength. Moreover, the absence of a tail domain is less deleterious to stabilization when only one of the two keratin types in the filament is tailless.[42,51] Similar results have been obtained for type III and type IV IF proteins missing at least a part of their tail domain (e.g., see refs. 48, 49, and 52).

The role of the keratin head domain seems to be more complex. A headless K14 can assemble into filaments, at least in the presence of wild-type K5.[39,40] In contrast, even in the presence of wild-type K14, K5 requires at least a portion of its head to assemble into 10-nm filaments.[51] Although the precise function of the K5 head domain remains to be elucidated, it may play some role in the spacial alignment of subunits during IF assembly.[51] Whether the head domains of other type II keratins play a similar role is unresolved.[42,44]

The head and tail domains of nonkeratin IF proteins seem to impart a greater dynamic instability to 10-nm filament networks than is typical of keratins.[47–50,52] Specific sites have been identified in type III IF nonhelical domains that may interact with the rod, perhaps regulating the assembly process.[53,54] In addition, head and tail domains of type III and type V IF proteins contain specific phosphorylation sites, which appear to play a role either in cdc2 kinase–mediated reorganization of IF during mitosis or in other models of filament dynamics (for review, see Erikson et al.[55]). It is interesting that keratins do not have the sequences that target the types III and V proteins for cell cycle–mediated phosphorylation and disassembly. Moreover, in epidermal cells, a keratin network persists throughout the cell cycle. This said, it is nevertheless possible that the stability of keratin filament networks in vivo might be influenced by phosphorylation.

The functions of head and tail domains are likely to extend beyond mere 10-nm filament structure. It is known that at least a portion of these ends protrude along the surface of IF,[56] thereby coating IF with different sequences. Thus, it seems likely that end domains are involved in intracellular interactions between IF and other organelles or structures, including the nucleus and plasma membrane.[57] A compelling study regarding tail function comes from a report by Bader et al.,[44] revealing that tailless K8/K19 filaments concentrate in the nucleus of transfected fibroblast cultures. Thus, it seems likely that some protein(s) or other factor(s) interacts with tail domains to maintain cytoplasmic localization of the keratin filament network. For the epidermal keratins, it seems likely that head and/or tail domains will be involved in the well-known associations between IF and desmosomes, hemidesmosomes, and filaggrin. More studies will be necessary to elucidate the precise biochemical natures of these interactions and to assess how differential expression of keratins might contribute to the diversity of interactions between IF and other proteins.

Keratin Gene Structure and Chromosomal Organization

Many keratin genes have now been sequenced, and they have similar structures.[22] Most human type I keratin genes reside on chromosome 17,[58–61] and most human type II keratin genes are on chromosome 12.[60–63] Most importantly, the functional genes for the epidermal keratins K14 and K10 reside at 17q12 → q21,[58,60] and many other skin type I genes are clustered in this same region.[58,60,62] Similarly, the genes for the type II epidermal keratins K5 and K1 are clustered at the q11 → q14 locus of chromosome 12.[60,62,63]

Studies have localized epidermal type I keratin genes to murine chromosome 11, at a homologous syntenic region of human chromosome 17, and the epidermal type II keratin genes to murine chromosome 15, at a homologous syntenic region of human chromosome 12.[64] The murine homologues of the type I human keratin genes map in close proximity to three dominant mutations, *Re*, *Bsk*, and Re^{den}, known to cause abnormal hair and epidermal development (see Nadeau et al.[64] and references therein). Moreover, additional mutations affecting the development of epidermis and its appendages map to the equivalent segment of mouse chromosome 15. It is not yet known whether keratin gene mutations are the cause of these skin diseases, nor is it known whether there are human counterparts to the diseases. However, given the findings with epidermolysis bullosa simplex and epidermolytic hyperkeratosis (see below), this is clearly an interesting avenue for future research.

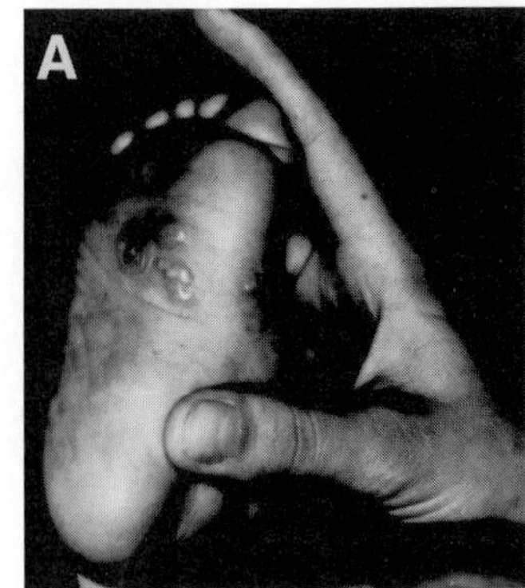

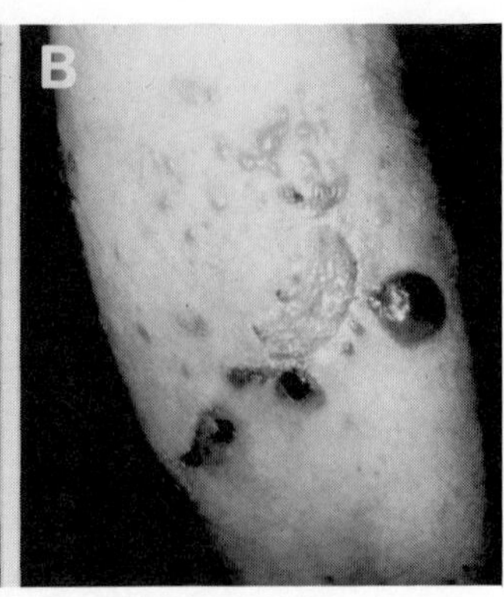

FIG. 149-4 Clinical features of epidermolysis bullosa simplex. *A*. Weber-Cockayne EBS: note plantar blisters. *B*. Dowling-Meara EBS: note dermatitis herpetiformis-like clustering of blisters on leg. (*Courtesy of Dr. Amy S. Paller, Northwestern University.*)

INHERITED DISORDERS OF KERATIN

Epidermolysis Bullosa Simplex

Classification. Epidermolysis bullosa simplex (EBS) is a group of rare genetic skin diseases affecting 1:50,000 population. It is typified by intraepidermal blistering due to cell degeneration within the basal layer.[65] In most cases, the diseases are autosomal dominant, although a recessive phenotype has been reported.[66–69] Clinical manifestations are often present at birth, with blistering associated with mild physical trauma. Blisters heal, often without scarring. Hyperpigmentation at areas of previous blisters has also been reported (see Fischer and Gedde-Dahl[70] and references therein). Additional curious features of the disease are that clinical manifestations improve with age and that the severity of blistering decreases during periods of fever (severe forms), but increases during warmer weather (milder forms).

EBS has been subdivided into three major and several minor subtypes (Table 149-2).[71,72] Weber-Cockayne is the mildest form of the disease. Blisters are usually confined to palmar and plantar regions of the body, and not surprisingly, the onset of the disease is often most apparent when a child begins to walk (Fig. 149-4*A*).[73] As judged by ultrastructural analysis, basal-cell cytolysis is evident, albeit sparse, over whole body trunk regions. Cytolysis occurs in a defined zone, beneath the nucleus and above the hemidesmosomes (Fig. 149-5*A* and 149-5*B*).[74] Keratin filaments often appear nearly normal, and as in all EBS subtypes, suprabasal layers are unperturbed, indicating a normal differentiation process.[74]

In EBS Koebner, blistering is more generalized than in Weber-Cockayne.[75] However, as in all forms of EBS, cytolysis is typically most extensive in areas susceptible to mechanical trauma, and this includes palmar and plantar epidermis. Noncutaneous involvement is rare in EBS Koebner, and when it occurs, it is usually the nails that become loosened when subjected to physical stress. Oral blistering has been reported.

Dowling-Meara is the most severe form of EBS (see Fig. 149-4*B*).[71,75–77] This disease is apparent at birth, and the incidence of neonatal death can be appreciable. Blistering

Table 149-2 Clinical Features of the Major Subtypes of EBS

	EBS Subtype		
	Weber-Cockayne	Koebner	Dowling-Meara
Mode of inheritance	AD	AD	AD
Onset	Infancy to childhood	Birth to infancy	Birth
Distribution	Primarily palmoplantar	Generalized	Generalized
Cutaneous anomalies			
Blisters	+	+ + +	+ + + + +
Scarring	Very rare	Rare	Rare
Pigmentation	OK	+/−*	+/−
Nail dystrophy	+/−	+/−	+ + +
Mechanical fragility	+	+ +	+ + +
Oral cavity anomalies			
Erosions	+†	+†	+ +
Scarring	−	−	−
Dental anodontia/ hypodontia	−	−	+
Other extracutaneous involvement	−	−	Corneal, esophageal
Growth	OK	Retarded (+)‡	Retarded (+ +)‡

AD = Autosomal dominant.
*Rare, except as postinflammatory hyperpigmentation in darkly pigmented races.
†Seen in a substantial minority, primarily during early infancy.
‡No eventual growth retardation, but growth may be slow during infancy.

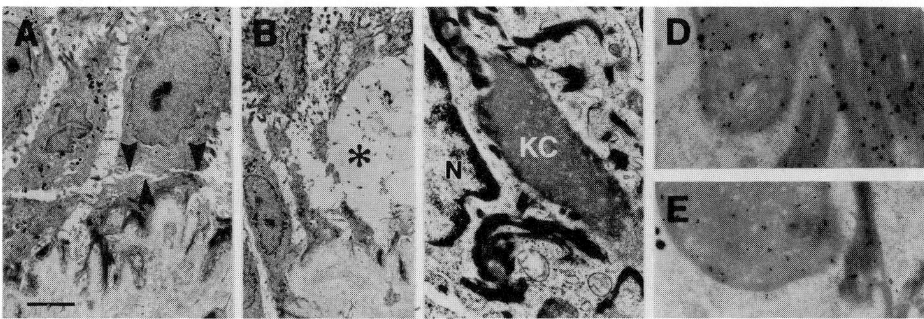

FIG. 149-5 Ultrastructural appearance of keratin in basal epidermal cells of EBS patients. *A*. Basal layer of skin from Weber-Cockayne patient, depicting split in basal cells beneath nucleus and above hemidesmosomes (arrowheads). *B*. Basal cell from same patient as in (*A*), this time exhibiting signs of cytolysis.* *C*. Tonofilament clumping (*KC*), in basal cell of skin from Dowling-Meara patient. *D* and *E*. Immunogold labeling of tonofilament clumps with specific antibodies against the basal epidermal keratins 14 (*D*) or 5 (*E*). N = nucleus. Bar in *A* represents 4 μm for *A*, 5 μm for *B*, 0.8 μm for *C*, and 0.4 μm for *D* and *E*. (Courtesy of Drs. Q.-C. Yu and P.A. Coulombe, University of Chicago). (See also, refs. 78, 85, and 86).

is extensive, and can occur over the entire body trunk and proximal extremities, often in herpetiform clusters.[75] In severe cases, denuding of skin can also occur. Plaquelike hyperkeratoses with extensive lamellar exfoliation also occur, particularly on the hands and feet.[78] Nail dystrophy, loss and regrowth, oral mucosal blistering, and tooth destruction are relatively frequent. In addition, other stratified squamous epithelia, such as cornea, can also be affected, albeit to a lesser extent.[67,75,78–82] In very rare cases, esophageal involvement can occur (Pearson R: personal communication).

The major ultrastructural feature of Dowling-Meara that distinguishes it from other EBS subtypes is the appearance of clumps or aggregates of tonofilaments within the basal-cell cytoplasm (see Fig. 149-5*C*).[71,78,84] In some cases, these aggregates are so amorphous that it is not clear whether keratins are in filamentous form. In other cases, the filamentous nature of the keratins is evident. EBS tonofilament clumps are recognized by antibodies against K14 or K5, indicating that the aggregates are composed of these keratins (see Fig. 149-5*D* and 149-5*E*).[85,86] As in other EBS subtypes, the organization of hemidesmosomes and desmosomes, and the program of terminal differentiation, appear normal. In the dermal connective tissue, inflammatory cells are typically present.

A few forms of EBS do not fit into the three classic subtypes. Like other EBS subtypes, EBS Ogna exhibits blistering due to cytolysis in the basal layer. However, in this subtype, small traumatic blood blebs have been observed on the distal extremities, elicited by short-acting trauma and serous seasonal blistering of the hands and feet, and occasionally elsewhere.[79] The relation of EBS Ogna to other subtypes is unknown, although genetic linkage to the glutamic pyruvic transaminase locus on chromosome 8q has been reported.[87,88] In addition to EBS Ogna, there are some reported cases of autosomal recessive EBS associated with appreciable extracutaneous disease, including anemia, neuromuscular disease, growth retardation, and infant mortality.[69] The extent to which these cases are genetically related to EBS is unknown.

Epidermolysis Bullosa Simplex: Studies Leading to the Genetic Basis of the Disease. The pioneering electron microscopy studies of Dr. Ingrun Anton-Lamprecht provided the first insights that EBS might be a keratin disorder.[74,78,83,84] In careful ultrastructural studies of skin biopsies of Dowling-Meara EBS patients, tonofilament clumping seemed to occur at the beginning of the pathogenetic process. Since clumping of tonofilaments preceded blister formation and cytolysis, it was argued that EBS was likely to arise from structural defects in keratin.[84]

In the 1980s, the implications of these elegant EM studies received little attention in the literature, as most studies focused on an interesting earlier theory by Pearson[89] that cytolytic enzymes might be responsible for the blistering in EBS. Indeed, many of the biochemical reports published during that decade seemed consistent with this hypothesis. In one study, deficient levels of galactosylhydroxylysyl glucosyltransferase, an enzyme of collagen synthesis, were found in affected members of one EBS family.[90] In another set of studies, there was controversy about whether skin fibroblast cultures from patients with Koebner EBS did[91] or did not[92] exhibit decreased levels of gelatinase. In one report, blister fluid from a patient with EBS was able to induce intraepidermal blistering in the basal layer of a normal skin explant culture, and follow-up studies suggested that the active factor in the blister fluid was a neutral protease (see Takamori et al.[93] and references therein). Finally, in another study, it was discovered that clinically uninvolved skin from patients with EBS had an abnormal staining pattern with peanut agglutinin, indicating that one or more glycosylated cell membrane components may be present in reduced amounts in EBS skin.[94] In contrast, immunofluorescence staining patterns obtained with antibodies against various epidermal keratins appeared normal,[94,95] providing seemingly additional support against the notion that EBS was a structural defect in keratin.

In the 1990s, attention again turned to the possibility that EBS may have as its genetic basis defects in keratin. Kitajima et al.[96] demonstrated that keratinocytes cultured from patients with EBS Dowling-Meara have a perturbed keratin network, similar to that of keratinocytes transfected with mutant K14 genes.[38,39] Then, using a reverse genetic approach, Vassar et al.[85] introduced a mutant human keratin 14 gene into the germ line of transgenic mice. The encoded truncated K14 protein had previously been shown to perturb keratin filament network formation severely in both keratinocytes in culture[38] and in vitro assembly.[40] In mice, the human keratin gene was appropriately expressed in the basal layer of the epidermis and other stratified squamous epithelia (see Vassar et al.[85] and references therein). Mice expressing the truncated human K14 gene, but not the wild-type human K14 gene, exhibited nearly all of the phenotypic, morphologic, and biochemical traits characteristic of EBS Dowling-

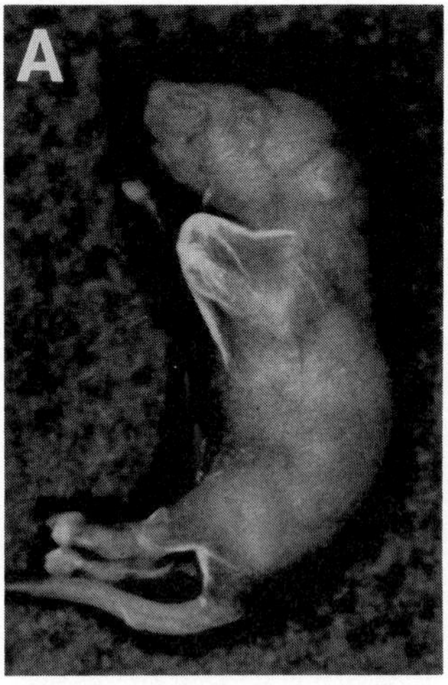

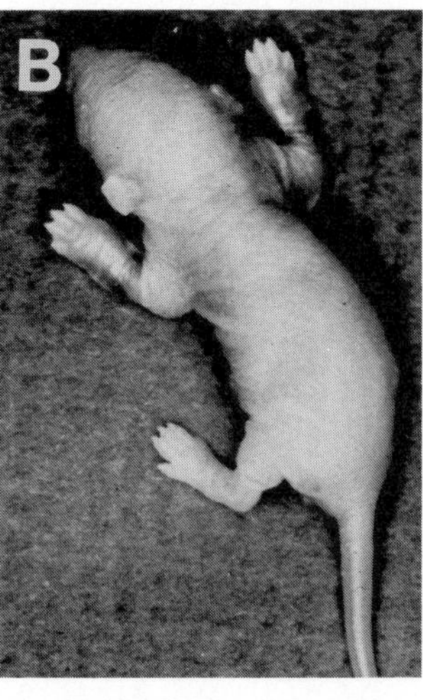

FIG. 149-6 **Transgenic mice expressing mutant human K14 genes. *A*. Mouse expressing mutant K14 at levels causing severe disruption of 10-nm filament assembly.[85] Note blistering over whole body. *B*. Mouse expressing mutant K14 at levels causing mild perturbations in 10-nm filament assembly. Note blistering of front paws. (*From Coulombe et al.*[97] *Used by permission.*)**

Meara, including total body trunk blistering (Fig. 149-6*A*), basal-cell cytolysis, and tonofilament clumping in the basal-cell cytoplasm, with an otherwise normal program of terminal differentiation.[85] These mice also had oral blistering and a high rate of neonatal death.

When transgenic mice were engineered that either expressed low levels of keratin mutants that severely disrupted keratin filament assembly, or high levels of mutants that mildly disrupted keratin filament assembly, they had a phenotype more similar to Weber-Cockayne EBS, with blistering predominantly over their front paws (Fig. 149-6*B*).[97] As in Weber-Cockayne and Koebner EBS, the epidermis of these mice still showed basal-cell cytolysis, but in this case tonofilament clumping was not observed.[97] Thus, multiple mutations in a single gene, namely K14, could give rise to phenotypes characteristic of most if not all of the major EBS subtypes, thereby suggesting a possible genetic relation among EBS subtypes. Collectively, the transgenic mouse studies provided compelling evidence that (1) structural defects in K14 and K5 genes could generate an EBS phenotype, and (2) the degree to which a specific K14 or K5 mutant perturbed 10-nm filament assembly correlated with the corresponding severity of the EBS phenotype.

The Genetic Basis of Human Epidermolysis Bullosa Simplex: Mapping to Chromosomes 17 and 12, and Point Mutations in the Genes Encoding Keratins 14 and 5. While transgenic mouse studies suggested that EBS might be a disease of K14 or K5 gene mutations, initial chromosomal mapping did not support this notion.[87,88,98,99] However, two of these studies applied to Ogna EBS, a form of EBS that may be genetically distinct from the other forms,[87,88] and the lod scores from the other early studies left chromosomal assignments questionable. More recent studies using improved markers showed that the genetic defect of several Koebner and Weber-Cockayne families mapped to human chromosomes 17 or 12,[100–104] at locations corresponding to the loci for epidermal types I and II keratin gene clusters, respectively.[58,60,62,63]

Unequivocal evidence that human EBS can arise from genetic defects in K14 and K5 came from sequencing the corresponding genes from normal and EBS patients, and from conducting a functional analysis of the defects. In the first studies, two patients with spontaneous cases of Dowling-Meara EBS were found to have single point mutations in amino acid 125 of K14, giving rise to R125C and R125H mutations,[105] and affected members of a family with Koebner EBS had Leu → Pro mutations at amino acid 384 of K14.[100] In the following year, affected members of a family with Dowling-Meara EBS were shown to have an E475G mutation in K5.[106] The mildest form, Weber-Cockayne (W-C) EBS has also been shown to be a disorder of K5 or K14.[102,103,168] Additional mutations have also been reported for D-M EBS and for Koebner EBS.[104,107–110,169] Finally, a rare case of recessive EBS has also been shown to have a point mutation in the K14 gene.[111] The locations of these mutations are indicated in Fig. 149-2.

In several cases, functional evidence was provided to demonstrate that the keratin point mutations are in fact responsible for generating the EBS phenotypes.[103,105,112] Mutations were genetically engineered into an epitope-tagged, but otherwise wild-type, human K14 or K5 cDNA. When expressed in transfected human epidermal cells, the EBS mutant keratins caused perturbations in the filament networks (Fig. 149–7A) similar to those detected in cells cultured from the patients (Fig. 149-7*B*). In addition, bacteria expressing K14 and K4 EBS mutants had perturbed filament assembly with their wild-type counterparts in vitro, in a fashion similar to the altered filaments formed with keratins

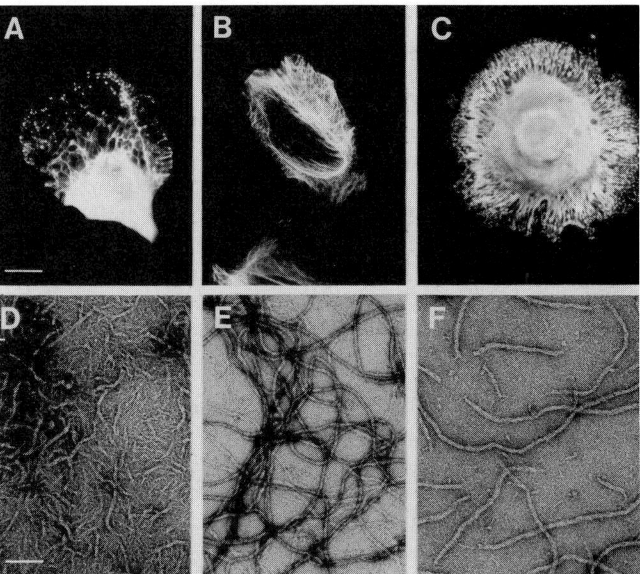

FIG. 149-7 **Comparison of the effects of a genetically engineered and natural Dowling-Meara EBS mutation in keratinocytes and in 10-nm filament assembly. *A*. Human keratinocytes transfected with a genetically engineered, mutant K14 gene, harboring the 125 (Arg → Cys) mutation. *B*. Keratinocytes transfected with a tagged, but otherwise wild-type, K14 gene. *C*. Keratinocytes from a patient with Dowling-Meara EBS, containing the 125 (Arg → Cys) mutation. Keratin networks were examined using antibodies specific for the transgene (*A* and *B*) or human K14 (*C*). Note collapsed keratin networks and punctate peripheral staining in *A* and *C*, but not in *B*. *D*. The genetically engineered 125 (Arg → Cys) K14 was expressed in bacteria, purified, and used in a filament reconstitution assay with wild-type K5. *E*. Filament reconstitution of wild-type K14 and K5. *F*. Filaments assembled from keratins isolated from keratinocytes of a patient with Dowling-Meara EBS containing the K14 (Arg → Cys) mutation. Bar represents 10 μm in *A* to *C* and 50 nm in *D* to *F*. (*From Coulombe et al.*[105] *Used by permission.*)**

isolated from the EBS patients (Fig. 149-7*D*, compare with 149-7*F*). Overall, there was a good correlation between the severity of the EBS disease, the location of the EBS point mutation with respect to keratin structure, and the degree to which a particular mutation perturbed filament assembly.[112]

While the relation between structural defects in keratin filaments and EBS seems clear, it is nevertheless possible that some cases of EBS arise from mutations in genes encoding proteins that are not keratins, but that interact with the keratin filament network in cells. Based on the number of EBS cases solved thus far, it is expected that if genetic heterogeneity exists in EBS, the numbers of such cases relative to K14 and K5 defects would be predicted to be small.

Combining Cell Biology and Epidermolysis Bullosa Simplex Biology. Now that the genetic basis for at least some cases of EBS is known, what additional information about EBS can we learn from the myriad molecular studies already conducted on K14 and K5? For one thing, we can predict where additional EBS mutations are likely to be found. Indeed, just as the severity of EBS in mice correlated with the severity with which a mutant perturbed 10-nm filament assembly,[85,97] the locations of K14 and K5 point mutations in Dowling-Meara EBS correlated with amino acids known to be critical for keratin filament assembly in vitro.[41,43,50] All Dowling-Meara patients thus far analyzed have mutations either in the amino end of helix 1A or the carboxy end of helix 2B.[105,106,108,109] While the precise importance of these small sequence motifs remains to be elucidated, it is interesting that these sequences come into close proximity, and may even overlap, in aligning linear arrays of tetramers within each protofilament.[35–37] In addition, these regions are also predicted to come into close contact with each other at higher-order levels.[36,37] These multiple modes of interactions required for both elongation and lateral packing of subunits most likely account for the high degree of evolutionary conservation of these sequences and for their critical importance to IF structure.

In contrast to the Dowling-Meara EBS mutations, the Koebner mutations reside in less conserved α-helical segments of the rod domain.[100,104,110,169] Interestingly, two of these Koebner EBS mutations are prolines. A priori, while a proline in the coiled-coil segment of the rod might be expected to perturb IF structure dramatically, in fact, proline residues can be accommodated at a number of central positions within the K14 (and presumably K5) rod domain, with only a rather subtle effect on filament assembly.[41] Finally, it is intriguing that in all six Weber-Cockayne EBS cases studied thus far, mutations reside outside the α-helical segments.[102,103,168] Affected members of two families have the same mutation, I161:S, in the nonhelical head domain of K5.[102] Not only is this region critical for filament assembly,[51] but it is also a region regulated by phosphorylation in the lamins and type III IF proteins.[50,55] It remains to be determined whether this site is phosphorylated in these Weber-Cockayne EBS patients, and if so, whether the phosphorylation might contribute to filament destabilization. A major finding to come out of combined molecular and clinical studies is that even subtle perturbations to IF structure in vitro can cause EBS in vivo. Continued mapping of mutations in these mild EBS cases should afford additional insights into amino acids that are critical for more subtle features of IF structure.

Given that the pattern of mutations found in EBS patients correlates well with in vitro mutagenesis studies, it seems likely that as additional EBS mutations are mapped, the pattern will continue. Thus, we might expect to find more Dowling-Meara EBS mutations in conserved residues within the rod ends, with less severe EBS cases mapping to regions of K5 and K14 that do not have as severe an effect on filament assembly. This said, there is an added element to consider that is exemplified by the propensity of mutations at R125 of K14 in D-M EBS. While the equivalent of K14's residue 125 is arginine or lysine in 50 of 51 published IF protein sequences,[105] and therefore is highly conserved, it was nevertheless curious to find this residue as the source of 9 of the 10 published D-M mutations, when many other residues in K5 and K14 are as highly conserved. A likely explanation is that this site is a hot spot for mutagenesis.[105,109] Indeed, both the R125C and the R125H mutations occur as a result of a C → T transition at a CpG dinucleotide on either the coding strand (R125C) or the noncoding strand (R125H). It is well known that eukaryotic methyltransferases can act at CpG sequences, and if a 5-methyl cytosine is subsequently deaminated, this can lead to C → T transitions at CpG residues. This natural method of hotspot mutagenesis can play a major role in human genetic diseases,[113] as it appears to be doing in EBS.

In addition to enabling predictions about the possible locations of future EBS mutations, the cell biology has provided an understanding of many previously unexplained aspects of human EBS. The autosomal dominance arises because mutant keratins are able to recognize their obligatory heterotypic partners and act in a dominant negative fashion to perturb keratin network formation. The disease is manifested predominantly in the basal layer of the epidermis because K14 and K5 are expressed only in basal cells. If cells can escape lysis, then they recover when they commit to differentiate terminally, because they down-regulate K5/K14 expression and induce K1/K10 expression. In severe cases of EBS, clinical manifestations can occur in other stratified squamous epithelia, including nail, oral mucosa, cornea, and esophagus, because these cells also express K5 and K14, albeit to a lesser extent in other tissues than in epidermis. Precisely why extracutaneous involvement is manifested most strikingly in the more severe EBS cases is presently unknown.

A major question concerns why EBS cells are prone to cytolysis. A number of findings point to the hypothesis that without a proper keratin network, cells become fragile and prone to breakage on mechanical stress. Particularly in Dowling-Meara, cytolytic blisters form in areas of basal cells that are deprived of tonofilaments.[71,78,83,86] In the initial phases of blistering, these areas are often in a d fined zone—beneath the nucleus and above the hemidesmosomes.[74] Transgenic animals expressing a mutant that mildly affects filament assembly have cells that lyse in this defined zone of fragility.[97] These cells do not exhibit tonofilament clumping, although they do show some disorganization in the tonofilament network. If the function of keratin filaments is to impart mechanical integrity to the cell, then when the network is perturbed, the zone between the nucleus and hemidesmosomes (i.e., the longest portion of the cytoplasm) might be expected to be fragile and prone to rupture on physical stress.

Another finding supporting this notion is that both in mice and humans, with the exception of very severe cases, EBS blisters generally heal without scarring. In mice, it was shown that during the wound-healing process, basal cells flatten, reduce their level of K5 and K14 synthesis, and do not lyse.[97] In addition, when EBS keratinocytes are allowed to flatten out on the surface of a cell culture dish, they are no longer as susceptible to lysis as they are when in tissue.[97,105] Collectively, these results support the notion that lysis is a mechanical trauma–dependent phenomenon, one likely to occur from a direct compromise to mechanical integrity, and that mechanical stress may be greater when cells are cuboidal or columnar than when cells are flattened. If enzymatic aberrancies occur secondarily in EBS as a consequence of tonofilament disorganization and subsequent blister formation,[90,91,93–95] these changes are not likely to be essential to the initial rupture process.

Another interesting feature of EBS is that the phenotypic aspects of Dowling-Meara and Koebner EBS improve with age. What accounts for this difference? It is likely that mechanical stress on basal cells is greatest during development. In neonatal skin, the papillary tips and rete pegs anchoring the epidermis to the dermis are much smaller. In addition, the epidermis is undergoing rapid expansion, and the underlying support structures for the epidermis are not fully formed. Maturation is thus likely to improve the mechanical strength of the skin in general, and this may lessen basal-cell fragility. Additionally, it may be that the internal mechanical strength of a basal cell might increase during development, perhaps as a consequence of as yet unidentified biochemical changes in the cytoskeleton and/or the plasma membrane.

Paradoxical questions are Why does Dowling-Meara EBS improve with fever? and Why does Koebner EBS get worse during summer months? At the moment, we can only speculate. In this regard, however, it seems plausible that heat could cause temperature-sensitive changes in the mechanical integrity of a cell, particularly if membrane fluidity plays a role in this process. Furthermore, it is known that induction of heat-shock proteins can induce alterations in keratin filament networks, at least in simple epithelial cells.[114] Finally, the stability of the keratin network or its interaction(s) with other cellular components could change in a temperature-dependent fashion. As additional studies are conducted, the extent to which these factors play a role in the clinical features of EBS should become more apparent.

Diagnosis and Therapy of Epidermolysis Bullosa Simplex. Methods for diagnosis of EBS are quite good, and a preliminary diagnosis can often be made through a routine patient examination. Blistering at birth or in early childhood, lesions on mild physical trauma, and healing without scarring are signs that a patient may have EBS. However, ultrastructural analysis of a skin biopsy from a lesion is essential for accurate diagnosis, since the hallmarks of EBS, namely intraepidermal cytolysis of the basal-cell layer without perturbations in the suprabasal layers, can often be missed by clinical or light microscopic examinations.

Certain broad distinctions between the mildest and most severe EBS subtypes can sometimes be made by visual analysis. The mildest form of EBS, Weber-Cockayne, is largely restricted to palmar and plantar areas, although some minor blistering can occur elsewhere. In contrast, the Koebner and Dowling-Meara subtypes exhibit more generalized blistering over body trunk areas, including palmar and plantar blistering. Dowling-Meara EBS is often more severe than Koebner EBS and is frequently typified by dermatitis herpetiformis-like (clustered) lesions and cutaneous and oral cavity anomalies (see Table 149-2). However, according to a recently agreed on classification,[72] the most distinctive feature of the Dowling-Meara form is the unique tonofilament clumping in the cytoplasm of basal cells, readily assessed only by ultrastructural analysis. Since cases with severe blistering and no tonofilament clumping can occur (Paller AS, Fuchs E: unpublished results; see also, ref. 83), accurate distinction between Dowling-Meara and Koebner EBS subtypes is reliant on ultrastructural analysis.

As additional genetic data are accumulated, it may be possible to develop DNA screening methods for the diagnosis of EBS. It is already apparent that Dowling-Meara mutations tend to be clustered at the ends of the K5 and K14 rods, and it should be possible to develop DNA probes capable of rapidly identifying most Dowling-Meara basal keratin mutations. Alternatively, immunologic tools could be developed to distinguish the wild-type from the mutant sequences at the ends of the α-helical rod domains. In this regard, an antibody is already available that can distinguish mutant from wild-type sequences at the C-terminus of the IF rod end.[106] Once the location of an EBS mutation has been identified in an affected parent, DNA probes could then be used to diagnose the disease from genomic DNA isolated from chorionic villus samples. This would be a distinct improvement over currently employed methods of EM of fetal skin biopsies (for reviews, see refs. 115 to 117). Finally, as in vitro methods are developed to distinguish normal and mutant embryos, it may be possible in the future to eliminate the disease in future offspring of an EBS family.

The clinical treatment of children with Dowling-Meara EBS represents the most difficult challenge to physicians and others caring for individuals with this disease. The primary objectives are to provide affected babies with the greatest protection against physical trauma and bacterial infections during their first few years of life. In the most severe cases, this generally means application of topical antibiotics to guard against infection, protecting affected areas with bandages, and continual care. Since blistering is exacerbated by heat, a cool environment is also important, particularly for Koebner EBS. In most cases, blistering improves with age, even in the most severe cases. Therapeutic methods have been largely ineffective.[118]

Now that the relation between keratin mutations and EBS has been established, what are the prospects for future improved therapeutic methods? It is too early to say. However, one curious finding from transgenic mouse studies suggests that EBS may be a disease amenable to gene therapy. In mosaic transgenic mice, in which the mutant human keratin gene integrated into the mouse's chromosomal DNA after the first cell division of the embryo, only a fraction of the transgenic animal's epidermal cells contained the mutant gene, while the remainder were wild-type.[85] Interestingly, within a relatively short period, these animals recovered and appeared healthy. Subsequent analysis of the skin revealed no evidence of mutant keratin transgene expression (Vassar R, Fuchs E: unpublished data). While an unequivocal molecular understanding of these results must await more extensive studies, it seems likely that given the tremendous selection pressure against autolysing EBS cells, the healthy wild-type cells rapidly replaced basal layer vacancies left by cytolysed EBS cells. If true, then it may be possible to develop the technology to engineer out or replace the mutant keratin gene from cells cultured from an EBS patient and then use skin grafting to replenish badly affected areas with these now-healthy cultured keratinocytes. The technology to culture human epidermal cells from patients is already well established. This technology has been adapted for severely burned individuals, in which sheets of keratinocytes cultured from a patient's skin are grafted back onto the same patient.[119] Thus, the rate limiting step for gene therapy in EBS will be to develop the technology for rapidly engineering out a defective keratin gene from the cultured keratinocytes. This could be helpful in extremely severe incidences of EBS, in which the disease can be life-threatening. Whether this will be possible or feasible should be answered within the next decade.

Genetic Disorders of Suprabasal Keratins

There are a number of autosomal dominant skin diseases that involve disorganization of tonofilaments in the suprabasal layers of the epidermis. Some of these, such as Hailey-Hailey disease and Darier disease, exhibit anomalies in desmosomes or other structures as well as aberrancies in tonofilament organization.[120,121] Other diseases, however, exhibit suprabasal alterations in tonofilament organization that are extraordinarily similar to the basal-cell-layer aberrancies that occur in EBS. Given the switch in keratin expression that takes place as epidermal cells commit to differentiate terminally, diseases involving suprabasal keratin abnormalities are prime candidates for having defects in the genes encoding the terminal differentiation-specific keratins.

Epidermolytic Hyperkeratosis. ***Complexity and Characteristics of Epidermolytic Hyperkeratosis.*** Epidermolytic hyperkeratosis (EH), previously called "bullous congenital ichthyosiform erythroderma," is a rare form of ichthyosis.[122,123] Like EBS, it is an autosomal dominant disease, with clinical manifestations usually present at birth (Fig. 149-8). The histopathology of EH is typified by (1) a normal, but hyperproliferative, basal epidermal layer, (2) tonofilament clumping and perinuclear shells of tonofilament aggregates in suprabasal cells, (3) vacuolization and cytolysis in suprabasal layers, beginning in the lower spinous layers and increasing during terminal differentiation, (4) a markedly thickened granular layer and stratum corneum, and (5) keratohyalin granules of irregular shape and size.[84,123,124] These features are also typical of several other autosomal dominant diseases, including (1) ichthyosis hystrix Curth-Macklin,[125–127] (2) epidermolytic palmoplantar keratoderma,[128–130] (3) epidermolytic leukoplakia,[131] and (4) ichthyosis bullosa of Siemens.[132,133] The distinctions between bullous congenital ichthyosiform erythroderma (EH) and epidermolytic palmoplantar keratoderma of the Voerner type are somewhat similar to the distinctions between generalized EBS and Weber-Cockayne EBS. EH is typified by verrucous thickening with a predisposition to suprabasal blistering. This occurs over entire body trunk regions, with the flexural regions being the most affected. In contrast, epidermolytic palmoplantar keratoderma is typified by hyperkeratotic palms and soles, also accompanied by painful fissuring. While epidermolytic hyperkeratosis is not associated with all cases of keratoderma, there are a number of cases referred to as "epidermolytic palmoplantar keratoderma," in which features of epidermolytic hyperkeratosis are seen.

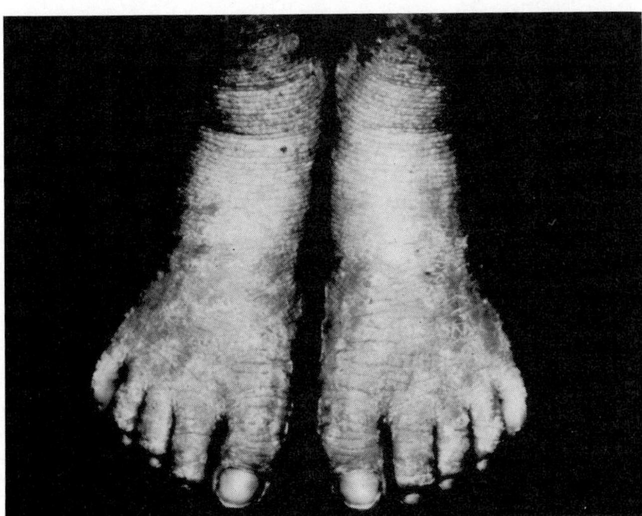

FIG. 149-8 Clinical features of EH (bullous congenital ichthyosiform erythroderma). Note verrucous thickening of ankle skin, around flexural area. (*Courtesy of Dr. Amy S. Paller, Northwestern University.*)

The disinctions between bullous congenital ichthyosiform erythroderma and some EH-related diseases are even more subtle. Ichthyosis hystrix Curth-Macklin may have morphologic features resembling EH, but with a distinctly different appearance of tonofilament organization yielding concentric perinuclear shells and no tonofilament clumping.[84,125,134] However, perinuclear shells of tonofilaments have also been seen in the suprabasal layers of skin from patients with EH[83,84,124,126] (and Paller AS, Pearson R, Fuchs E: unpublished observations). Similarly, ichthyosis bullosa of Siemens has been distinguished by the presence of cytolysis only in the very superficial layers of the epidermis, by lichenification and superficially denuded areas ("mauserung").[133] However, initiation of cytolysis in EH can vary, ranging from the first suprabasal layer to nearly the granular layer (Yu QC, Paller AS, Pearson R, Fuchs E: unpublished observations; see also, ref. 83). Given the significant parallels in the histopathologies of these three diseases, the extent to which they might be genetically distinct is still not clear.

Genetic Basis for Epidermolytic Hyperkeratosis. A clue to the genetic basis for EH stems from the striking similarity between tonofilament clumping in suprabasal cells of EH skin and in basal cells of EBS skin. This parallel was first noted by Anton-Lamprecht.[84] Since clumping of tonofilaments in EH preceded blister formation, it was argued that EH was likely to be a genetic defect involving keratin.[126] That EH is a genetic disorder of keratin became increasingly likely, given the transgenic studies of Fuchs et al.[135] When expressed in transgenic mice, a truncated human K10 gene gave rise to the pathobiologic and biochemical characteristics of EH. Although mouse skin is thinner than human skin, vacuolization and cytolysis were still seen in the upper spinous and granular layers of transgenic mouse skin in a fashion nearly indistinguishable from that of human EH skin (Fig. 149-9). Similarly, tonofilament clumping was seen in the first suprabasal layer, and this increased as cells progressed through terminal differentiation (Fig. 149-10*A* to 149-10*C*). Perinuclear shells of keratin aggregates surrounded some nuclei, and seemingly binucleate cells were seen (Fig. 149-10*D* to 149-10*G*).

The parallel between mutant keratin expression, perinuclear filament shells, and nuclear distortion was intriguing. Early reports on human EH also described binucleate suprabasal cells,[124] particularly in ichthyosis hystrix Curth-Macklin,[84] and the existence of a nucleolus in each of the two nuclei has been suggested as verification that the EH cells were truly binucleate.[124] However, normal uninuclear keratinocytes can have double nucleoli; therefore, this is not a reliable measure. Since the two nuclear masses are sometimes of unequal size and shape, since they occur in both EBS basal cells and in EH suprabasal cells, and since

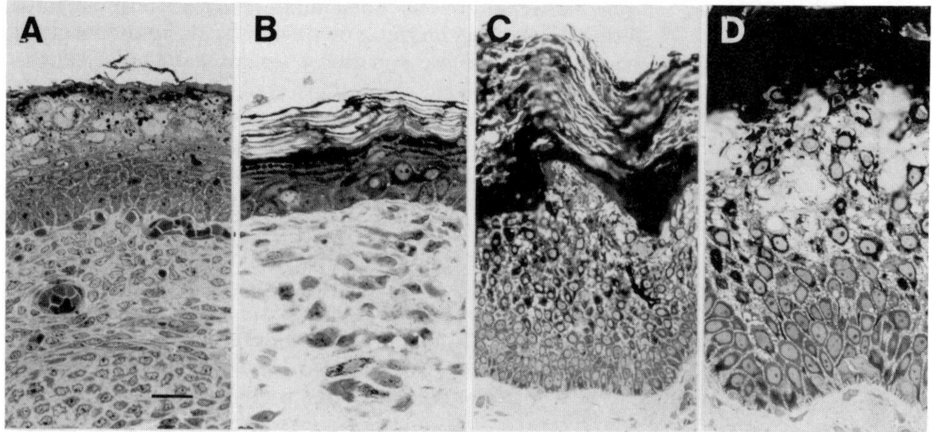

FIG. 149-9 Morphologic appearance of EH skin from transgenic mouse expressing a mutant K10 gene and from human patient with EH. Semithin sections (0.75 μ) of skin from: *A*. Transgenic mouse expressing a truncated human K10 gene. *B*. Normal control mouse. *C* and *D*. Human patient with EH. Bar in *A* represents 50 μ for *A* and *D*, 33μ for *B*, and 86μ for *C*. (*See also, Fuchs et al.*[135])

in mice these two diseases arise from defective keratin genes, it seems equally possible that a novel function of keratin filaments may be to provide a supportive scaffold to the nucleus and perhaps to other cytoplasmic organelles.[109] When this scaffold is perturbed, the shape and/or structural integrity of the organelles might be compromised. An alternative interpretation is that formation of perinuclear keratin shells alters the ability of a cell to divide, either in the basal layer (EBS), or at the point at which it exits the basal layer (EH).[135] Future experiments should provide additional insights into this question.

The transgenic mouse data provided strong evidence that a genetic basis for human EH resides in defective keratin networks within differentiating epidermal cells. The data also demonstrated that aberrant suprabasal keratin networks can affect filaggrin-containing keratohyalin granules and granular-cell shape, perhaps explaining why some researchers had suggested that EH may be a filaggrin defect.[136] However, the timing of K1/K10, rather than filaggrin, synthesis more closely paralleled the appearance of aberrations in the differentiation process. Coupled with the generation of an EH phenotype in K10 mutant mice, it seemed more likely that EH involves primarily perturbations in suprabasal keratin networks, and secondarily, perturbations in keratohyalin granules. This was subsequently confirmed by analysis of the K1 and K10 genes in EH patients.

In 1992, point mutations were found in the K10 and K1 genes of six distinct cases of human EH (see Fig. 149-2).[137–139] Chromosomal linkage analyses have also been provided to confirm that EH is indeed a keratin disorder.[140–142] Interestingly, in two unrelated families[137] and in one spontaneous case,[139] affected EH members had identical mutations, namely an R156H mutation in K10 gene. This was not a polymorphic variation, since in more than 200 wild-type alleles, the encoded residue was arginine.[137] Remarkably, the R156H K10 point mutation was in the exact same highly conserved arginine residue as the mutations in K14 (R125C and R125H) previously reported for EBS. This represents the first mutation in a highly conserved residue of two differentially expressed, but related, genes giving rise to two distinct genetic diseases. As in EBS, the high frequency of mutation of this arginine in EH appears to be due to a

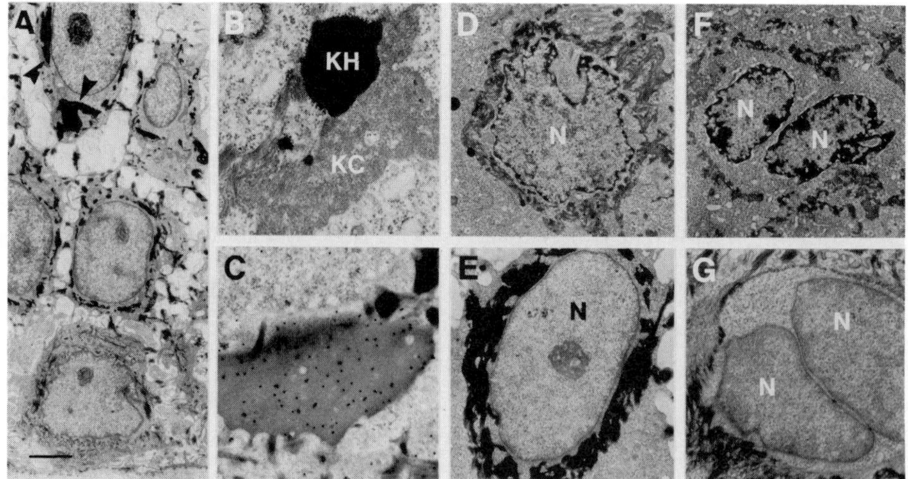

FIG. 149-10 Ultrastructural appearance of epidermal cells of an EH transgenic mouse and a patient with EH. *A*. Epidermis of EH patient, with normal basal-cell and tonofilament clumping (arrowheads) in spinous cells. *B* and *C*. Granular layer cell of epidermis from transgenic EH mouse (*B*) or EH patient (*C*). Note cell degeneration. Note also tonofilament clumping (KC) and association of clumps with keratohyalin granules (KH). (*C*) is immunogold labeled with antibodies against K1, showing that the clumps are composed of suprabasal keratins. *D* and *E*. Perinuclear shell of keratin aggregates in suprabasal cell of epidermis from transgenic EH mouse (*D*) or human EH (*E*). N = nucleus. *F* and *G*. Seemingly binucleate suprabasal cell of epidermis from transgenic EH mouse (*F*) or human EH (*G*). Bar represents 3.3 μm for *A*, 1 μm for *B* and *E* to *G*, 0.4 μm for *C*, and 2 μm for *D* (Courtesy of Dr. Q.-C. Yu, University of Chicago.) (*See also, Fuchs et al.*[135])

combination of the special importance of this residue in 10-nm filament structure and the naturally high frequency of C → T transitions due to CpG methylation and deamination in the human genome.[137]

Of the other three EH mutations reported in 1992, two are in residues located in the highly conserved ends of the keratin rod domain.[139] Only one mutation occurred outside the rod ends, and interestingly, this mutation was L160P in the nonhelical head domain of K1 in a mild EH case.[138] This region of type II keratins may be important in 10-nm filament assembly.[51,102,143]

Several additional reports of K1 or K10 mutations in EH have recently appeared.[144–146] While the number of EH incidences analyzed is still small, like EBS, there appears to be a correlation between the severity of the disease and the location of point mutations within the keratin polypeptides.[138,146] Finally, a new consideration for EH not relevant for EBS is that in palmar/plantar skin, there is a unique keratin, K9, expressed suprabasally.[4,10] Thus, it might be predicted that some cases of epidermolytic palmoplantar keratoderma will arise from K9 mutations. Intriguingly, the genetic defect in a family with epidermolytic palmoplantar keratoderma has been mapped to chromosome 17.[147]

Future Studies: Insights into Additional Genetic Disorders of Keratin and Other Intermediate Filament Proteins through a Knowledge of Intermediate Filament Function

Perhaps more than any other tissue, the epidermis and its appendages have evolved to utilize cytoplasmic intermediate filaments as their major structural components. Epidermal keratins form some of the most stable protein–protein interactions known in nature,[32,148] and this may enable the keratin filaments to be among the few survivors of the terminal differentiation process.

Given the self-destructing environment of a terminally differentiating keratinocyte, survival is certainly an important feature of keratins. Furthermore, the correlations of keratin defects with skin diseases involving intraepidermal cytolysis demonstrates convincingly that keratin networks play a vital role in the mechanical integrity of an epidermal cell.[149] This notion is also supported by rheologic studies, which showed that wild-type intermediate filaments harden and resist breakage under stresses with which other cytoskeletal networks will rupture.[150] Coupled with findings demonstrating that mutations in both the K5/K14 and the K1/K10 pairs can lead to cell fragility and degeneration, it seems likely that the ability to impart mechanical strength may extend to other keratins in particular, and to other IF proteins in general.[149] In this regard, transgenic studies on hair keratin genes revealed that alterations in the normal architecture of keratin tonofibrils in the hair can compromise mechanical integrity.[151] Thus, when overexpressed in cortical hair cells of transgenic mice, a type II hair keratin caused abnormalities in keratin IF organization, presumably because the resulting imbalance in the ratio of type I and type II keratins interfered with normal IF organization.[151] This led to brittleness, and caused hair breakage.[149]

Are there genetic diseases involving hair keratin defects? At present, the answer to this question is unknown. However, given the nature of 10-nm filament assembly, if such diseases exist, they might be expected to be autosomal dominant. In addition, given the previous studies with K5/K14 and K1/K10 gene defects, coupled with the transgenic studies described above, hair brittleness and follicle-cell fragility would be expected to be a consequence of putative hair keratin defects. Several possible candidate diseases share these features (for review, see refs. 1, 152, and 153). These include congenital hypotrichosis and monilethrix. In some cases, abnormalities in two-dimensional gel patterns and amino acid compositions of hair keratins from patients with these diseases have been reported (see, e.g., ref. 152). However, given the complexity of Ha/Hb keratins, high-sulfur keratins (IF-associated proteins), and high glycine and tyrosine keratins (IF-associated proteins),[153–157] coupled with the complexity of differentiation programs within hair, it may be a far greater challenge to dissect out the genetic bases for these diseases than the challenge in understanding the genetic disorders of epidermal keratins.

At present, it is not known whether hair IF keratin genes are linked to epidermal IF genes. However, it has been shown that high-sulfur keratin genes expressed in hair cuticles are clustered on human chromosome 11 at 11q13 and 11q15.[158] If high glycine and tyrosine genes are also at a chromosomal locus distinct from that of the other keratin genes, then some valuable insights into sorting out the potential complexity may be gained by classic chromosomal mapping of families with these hair defects. As these and transgenic mouse studies are conducted, it seems likely that at least some of the genetic defects involving hair structure and fragility will arise from mutations in keratins. In this regard and as noted previously, it is interesting that several autosomal dominant mouse mutants, *Re*, *Bsk*, and *Re*^{den}, map in close proximity to the type I epidermal keratin genes (see Nadeau et al.[64] and references therein). Rex mice have curly whiskers and bent hair shafts, and denuded mutant mice and bare-skin mice undergo hair loss after completion of the first hair cycle.

CONCLUSION

This chapter has focused on skin disorders of keratin. The reader is referred elsewhere for recent studies on nonkeratin genetic skin diseases, in particular, other forms of epidermolysis bullosa, which are due to defects in other structural proteins such as collagen VII (see Chap. 134), laminins, and integrins.[159–163] More closely related disorders to EBS and EH are likely to be as yet unidentified non–skin disorders that have as their origin defects in one of the other 40 to 50 members of the human intermediate filament gene superfamily. Indeed, an intriguing feature of the IF family is its complexity in expression patterns. Virtually all cells in the human body express not only nuclear lamin IF, but in addition, at least one cytoskeletal IF protein. As originally hypothesized by Lazarides in 1980,[164] IF play a vital role as mechanical integrators of cytoplasmic space, in addition to having more specialized functions. Some of those disorders may include certain types of motor neuron diseases, which could arise from neurofilament anomalies,[165,166] and a fraction of cardiomyopathies, which could arise from desmin defects.[167] As additional studies are conducted on human diseases involving IF aberrations and cell fragility, it seems likely that as in skin diseases, some of these diseases will arise from genetic defects in one of the myriad of IF genes.

ACKNOWLEDGMENTS

I thank Dr. Pierre A. Coulombe (Johns Hopkins University Medical School) and Dr. Q.-C. Yu (Howard Hughes Medical

Institute, University of Chicago) for providing electron micrographs and Dr. Amy S. Paller (Northwestern Medical School) for providing clinical photographs. I also thank Dr. Ingrun Anton-Lamprecht (Institut fur Ultrastrukturforschung der Haut, Hautklinik der Ruprecht-Karls-Universitaet, Heidelberg, Germany), Dr. Amy S. Paller, and Dr. Pierre Coulombe for their careful reading of this manuscript, and for their valuable comments. Finally, I would like to express my sincere gratitude to the members of my laboratory, past and present, who have so enthusiastically devoted their time and scientific expertise to enhancing our understanding of keratin structure and function and its relation to human skin diseases.

ADDENDUM

In early 1994, two groups reported that epidermolytic palmoplantar keratoderma cosegregates with keratin 9 mutations,[169,170] thereby establishing that this disease is also a keratin disorder.

REFERENCES

1. Fitzpatrick TB, Eisen AZ, Wolff K, Freedberg IM, Austen KF (eds): *Dermatology in General Medicine*, 3rd ed. New York, McGraw-Hill, 1987, vol 1.
2. Jones JC, Green KJ: Intermediate filament-plasma membrane interactions. *Curr Opin Cell Biol* **3**:127, 1991.
3. Schwarz MA, Owaribe K, Kartenbeck J, Franke WW: Desmosomes and hemidesmosomes: Constitutive molecular components. *Annu Rev Cell Biol* **6**:461, 1990.
4. Fuchs E, Green H: Changes in keratin gene expression during terminal differentiation of the keratinocyte. *Cell* **19**:1033, 1980.
5. Moll R, Franke W, Schiller D, Geiger B, Krepler R: The catalog of human cytokeratins: Patterns of expression in normal epithelia, tumors and cultured cells. *Cell* **31**:11, 1982.
6. Nelson W, Sun TT: The 50- and 58-kdalton keratin classes as molecular markers for stratified squamous epithelia: Cell culture studies. *J Cell Biol* **97**:244, 1983.
7. Roop DR, Huitfeldt H, Kilkenny A, Yuspa SH: Regulated expression of differentiation—associated keratins in cultured epidermal cells detected by monospecific antibodies to unique peptides of mouse epidermal keratins. *Differentiation* **35**:143, 1987.
8. Mischke D, Wild G: Polymorphic keratins in human epidermis. *J Invest Dermatol* **88**:191, 1987.
9. Korge BP, Gan SQ, McBride OW, Mischke D, Steinert PM: Extensive size polymorphism of the human keratin 10 chain resides in the C-terminal V2 subdomain due to variable numbers and sizes of glycine loops. *Proc Natl Acad Sci USA* **89**:910, 1992.
10. Knapp AC, Franke WW, Heid H, Hatzfeld M, Jorcano JL, Moll R: Cytokeratin No. 9, an epidermal type I keratin characteristic of a special program of keratinocyte differentiation displaying body site specificity. *J Cell Biol* **103**:657, 1986.
11. Stellmach V, Leask A, Fuchs E: Retinoid-mediated transcriptional regulation of keratin genes in human epidermal and squamous cell carcinoma cells. *Proc Natl Acad Sci USA* **88**:4582, 1991.
12. Montagna W, Lobitz WC (eds): *The Epidermis*. New York, Academic, 1964.
13. Eichner R, Sun TT, Aebi U: The role of keratin subfamilies and keratin pairs in the formation of human epidermal intermediate filaments. *J Cell Biol* **102**:1767, 1986.
14. Dale BA, Holbrook KA, Steinert PM: Assembly of stratum corneum basic protein and keratin filaments in macrofibrils. *Nature* **276**:729, 1978.
15. Schurer NY, Plewig G, Elias PM: Stratum corneum lipid function. *Dermatologica* **183**:77, 1991.
16. Rice RH, Green H: Presence in human epidermal cells of a soluble protein precursor of the cross-linked envelope: Activation of the cross-linking by calcium ions. *Cell* **18**:681, 1979.
17. Simon M, Green H: Enzymatic cross-linking of involucrin and other proteins by keratinocyte particulates in vitro. *Cell* **40**:677, 1985.
18. Mehrel T, Hohl D, Rothnagel JA, Longley MA, Bundman D, Cheng C, Lichti U, Bisher ME, Steven AC, Steinert PM: Identification of a major keratinocyte cell envelope protein, loricrin. *Cell* **61**:1103, 1990.
19. Greenberg CS, Birckbichler PJ, Rice RH: Transglutaminases: Multifunctional cross-linking enzymes that stabilize tissues. *FASEB J* **5**:3071, 1991.
20. Dale BA, Holbrook KA, Kimball JR, Hoff M, Sun TT: Expression of epidermal keratins and filaggrin during human fetal skin development. *J Cell Biol* **101**:1257, 1985.
21. Kopan R, Fuchs E: A new look into an old problem: Keratins as tools to investigate determination, morphogenesis, and differentiation in skin. *Genes Dev* **3**:1, 1989.
22. Albers K, Fuchs E: The molecular biology of intermediate filament proteins. *Int Rev Cytol* **134**:243, 1992.
23. Aebi U, Haner M, Troncoso J, Eichner R, Engel A: Unifying principles in intermediate filament (IF) structure and assembly. *Protoplasma* **145**:73, 1988.
24. Fuchs E, Weber K: Intermediate filaments: Structure, dynamics, function and disease. *Ann Rev Biochem* **63**:345, 1994.
25. Conway JF, Parry DAD: Intermediate filament structure: 3. Analysis of sequence homologies. *Int J Biol Macromol* **10**:79, 1988.
26. Marchuk D, McCrohon S, Fuchs E: Remarkable conservation of structure among intermediate filament genes. *Cell* **39**:491, 1984.
27. Lersch R, Stellmach V, Stocks C, Giudice G, Fuchs E: Isolation, sequence, and expression of a human keratin K5 gene: Transcriptional regulation of keratins and insights into pairwise control. *Mol Cell Biol* **9**:3685, 1989.
28. Hanukoglu I, Fuchs E: The cDNA sequence of a type II cytoskeletal keratin reveals constant and variable structural domains among keratins. *Cell* **33**:915, 1983.
29. Johnson L, Idler W, Zhou XM, Roop D, Steinert P: Structure of a gene for the human epidermal 67-kda keratin. *Proc Natl Acad Sci USA* **82**:1896, 1985.
30. Rieger M, Franke WW: Identification of an orthologous mammalian cytokeratin gene. High degree of intron sequence conservation during evolution of human cytokeratin 10. *J Mol Biol* **204**:841, 1988.
31. Zhou XM, Idler WW, Steven AC, Roop DR, Steinert PM: The complete sequence of the human intermediate filament chain keratin 10. Subdomainal divisions and model for folding of end domain sequences. *J Biol Chem* **263**:15584, 1988.
32. Coulombe P, Fuchs E: Elucidating the early stages of keratin filament assembly. *J Cell Biol* **111**:153, 1990.
33. Hatzfeld M, Weber K: The coiled coil of in vitro assembled keratin filaments is a heterodimer of type I and II keratins: Use of site-specific mutagenesis and recombinant protein expression. *J Cell Biol* **110**:1199, 1990.
34. Steinert PM: The two-chain coiled-coil molecular of native epidermal keratin intermediate filaments is a type I-type II heterodimer. *J Biol Chem* **265**:8766, 1990.
35. Geisler N, Schunemann J, Weber K: Chemical cross-linking indicates a staggered and antiparallel protofilament of desmin intermediate filaments and characterizes one higher-level complex between protofilaments. *Eur J Biochem* **206**:841, 1992.
36. Steinert PM, Marekov LN, Fraser RDB, Parry DAD: Keratin intermediate filament structure: Crosslinking studies yield quantitative information on molecular dimensions and mechanisms of assembly. *J Mol Biol* **230**:436, 1993.
37. Heins S, Wong PC, Muller S, Goldie K, Cleveland DW, Aebi U: The rod domain of NF-L determines neurofilament architecture, whereas the end domains specify filament assembly properties. *J Cell Biol* **123**:1517, 1993.
38. Albers K, Fuchs E: The expression of mutant epidermal keratin cDNAs transfected in simple epithelial and squamous cell carcinoma lines. *J Cell Biol* **105**:791, 1987.
39. Albers K, Fuchs E: Expression of mutant keratin cDNAs

in epithelial cells reveals possible mechanisms for initiation and assembly of intermediate filaments. *J Cell Biol* **108**:1477, 1989.

40. Coulombe P, Chan YM, Albers K, Fuchs E: Deletions in epidermal keratins that lead to alterations in filament organization and assembly: In vivo and in vitro studies. *J Cell Biol* **111**:3049, 1990.
41. Letai A, Coulombe P, Fuchs E: Do the ends justify the mean? Proline mutations at the ends of the keratin coiled-coil rod segment are more disruptive than internal mutations. *J Cell Biol* **116**:1181, 1992.
42. Lu X, Lane EB: Retrovirus-mediated transgenic keratin expression in cultured fibroblasts: Specific domain functions in keratin stabilization and filament formation. *Cell* **62**:681, 1990.
43. Hatzfeld M, Weber K: Modulation of keratin intermediate filament assembly by single amino acid exchanges in the consensus sequence at the C-terminal end of the rod domain. *J Cell Sci* **99**:351, 1991.
44. Bader BL, Magin TM, Freundenmann M, Stumpp S, Franke WW: Intermediate filaments formed de novo from tailless cytokeratins in the cytoplasm and in the nucleus. *J Cell Biol* **115**:1293, 1991.
45. Hatzfeld M, Weber K: Tailless keratins assemble into regular intermediate filaments in vitro. *J Cell Sci* **97**:317, 1990.
46. Loewinger L, McKeon F: Mutations in the nuclear lamin proteins resulting in their aberrant assembly in the cytoplasm. *EMBO J* **7**:2301, 1988.
47. Raats JMH, Pieper FR, Vree Egberts WTM, Verrij KN, Ramaekers FCS, Bloemendal H: Assembly of amino terminally deleted desmin in vimentin-free cells. *J Cell Biol* **111**:1971, 1990.
48. Gill SR, Wong PC, Cleveland DW: Assembly properties of dominant and recessive mutations in the small mouse neurofilament (NF-L) subunit. *J Cell Biol* **111**:2005, 1990.
49. Wong PC, Cleveland DW: Characterization of dominant and recessive assembly defective mutations in mouse neurofilament NF-M. *J Cell Biol* **111**:1987, 1990.
50. Heald R, McKeon F: Mutations of phosphorylation sites in lamin A that prevent nuclear lamina disassembly in mitosis. *Cell* **61**:579, 1990.
51. Wilson AK, Coulombe PA, Fuchs E: The role of K5 and K14 head, tail and R/KLLEGE domains in keratin filament assembly in vitro. *J Cell Biol* **119**:401, 1992.
52. Kaufmann E, Weber K, Geisler N: Intermediate filament forming ability of desmin derivatives lacking either the amino-terminal 67 or the carboxy-terminal 27 residues. *J Mol Biol* **185**:733, 1985.
53. Birkenberger L, Ip W: Properties of the desmin tail domain: Studies using synthetic peptides and antipeptides antibodies. *J Cell Biol* **111**:2063, 1990.
54. Kouklis PD, Papamarcaki T, Merdes A, Georgatos SD: A potential role for the COOH-terminal domain in the lateral packing of type III intermediate filaments. *J Cell Biol* **114**:773, 1991.
55. Eriksson JE, Opal P, Goldman RD: Intermediate filament dynamics. *Curr Opin Cell Biol* **4**:99, 1992.
56. Steinert PM, Rice DRR, Trus ACS: Complete amino acid sequence of a mouse epidermal keratin subunit and implications for the structure of intermediate filaments. *Nature* **302**:794, 1983.
57. Georgatos SD, Blobel G: Two distinct attachment sites for vimentin along the plasma membrane and the nuclear envelope in avian erythrocytes: A basis for a vectorial assembly of intermediate filaments. *J Cell Biol* **105**:105, 1987.
58. Rosenberg M, RayChaudhury A, Shows TB, LeBeau MM, Fuchs E: A group of type I keratin genes on human chromosome 17: Characterization and expression. *Mol Cell Biol* **8**:722, 1988.
59. Bader BJ, Jahn L, Franke WW: Low level expression of cytokeratins 8, 18, and 19 in vascular smooth muscle cells of human umbilical cord and in cultured cells derived therefrom, with an analysis of the chromosomal locus containing the cytokeratin 19 gene. *Eur J Cell Biol* **47**:300, 1988.
60. Lessin SR, Huebner K, Isobe M, Croce CM, Steinert PM: Chromosomal mapping of human keratin genes: Evidence of non-linkage. *J Invest Dermatol* **91**:572, 1988.
61. Romano V, Bosco P, Rocchi M, Costa G, Leube RE, Franke WW, Romeo G: Chromosomal assignments of human type I and type II cytokeratin genes to different chromosomes. *Cytogenet Cell Genet* **48**:148, 1988.
62. Popescu NC, Bowden PE, DiPaolo JA: Two type II keratin genes are localized on human chromosome 12. *Hum Genet* **82**:109, 1989.
63. Rosenberg M, Fuchs E, Le Beau MM, Eddy R, Shows TB: Three epidermal and one epithelial keratin gene map to human chromosome 12. *Cell Cytogenet* **57**:33, 1991.
64. Nadeau JH, Berger FG, Cox DR, Crosby JL, Davisson MT, Ferrara D, Fuchs E, Hart C, Hunihan L, Lalley PA, Langley SH, Martin GR, Nichols L, Phillips SJ, Roderick TH, Roop DR, Ruddle FH, Skow LC, Compton JG: A family of type I keratin genes and the homeobox-2 gene complex are closely linked to the rex locus on mouse chromosome 11. *Genomics* **5**:454, 1989.
65. Pearson RW, Spargo B: Electron microscope studies of dermal-epidermal separation in human skin. *J Invest Dermatol* **36**:213, 1961.
66. Salih MAM, Lake BD, Hag MAEL, Atherton DJ: Lethal epidermolytic epidermolysis bullosa: A new autosomal recessive type of epidermolysis bullosa. *Br J Dermatol* **113**:135, 1985.
67. Neilsen PB, Sjolund E: Epidermolysis bullosa simplex localisata associated with anodontia, hair and nail disorders: A new syndrome. *Acta Derm Venereol (Stockh)* **65**:526, 1985.
68. Niemi KM, Sommer H, Kero M, Kanerva L, Haltia M: Epidermolysis bullosa simplex associated with muscular dystrophy with recessive inheritance. *Arch Dermatol* **124**:551, 1988.
69. Fine JD, Stenn J, Johnson L, Wright R, Bock HGO, Horiguchi Y: Autosomal recessive epidermolysis bullosa simplex. *Arch Dermatol* **125**:931, 1989.
70. Fischer T, Gedde-Dahl T: Epidermolysis bullosa simplex and mottled pigmentation: A new dominant syndrome. *Clin Genet* **15**:228, 1979.
71. Gedde-Dahl T, Anton-Lamprecht I: *Principles and Practice in Medical Genetics: Epidermolysis Bullosa*. New York, Churchill Livingstone, 1981.
72. Fine JD, Bauer EA, Briggaman RA, Carter DM, Eady RAJ, Esterly NB, Holbrook KA, Hurwitz S, Johnson L, Lin A, Pearson R, Sybert VP: Revised clinical and laboratory criteria for subtypes of inherited epidermolysis bullosa. *J Am Acad Dermatol* **24**:119, 1991.
73. Cockayne EA: Recurrent bullous eruption of the feet. *Br J Dermatol* **55**:358, 1938.
74. Haneke E, Anton-Lamprecht I: Ultrastructure of blister formation in epidermolysis bullosa hereditaria: V. Epidermolysis bullosa simplex localista type Weber-Cockayne. *J Invest Dermatol* **78**:219, 1982.
75. Gedde-Dahl T: *Paediatrische Dermatologie: Classification of epidermolysis bullosa*. New York, Schattauer Verlag, 1978.
76. Dowling GB, Meara RH: Epidermolysis bullosa resembling juvenile dermatitis herpetiformis. *Br J Dermatol* **66**:139, 1954.
77. Gedde-Dahl T: Sixteen types of epidermolysis bullosa. On the clinical discrimination, therapy and prenatal diagnosis. *Acta Derm Venereol (Stockh)* **95**:74, 1981.
78. Anton-Lamprecht I, Schnyder UW: Epidermolysis bullosa herpetiformis Dowling-Meara: Report of a case and pathogenesis. *Dermatologica* **164**:221, 1982.
79. Gedde-Dahl T: Phenotype-genotype correlations in epidermolysis bullosa. *Birth Defects* **7**:107, 1971.
80. Granek H, Baden HP: Corneal involvement in epidermolysis bullosa simplex. *Arch Ophthalmol* **98**:469, 1980.
81. Buchbinder LH, Lucky AW, Ballard E, Stanley JR, Stolar E, Tabas M, Bauer EA, Paller AS: Severe infantile epidermolysis bullosa simplex. Dowling-Meara type. *Arch Dermatol* **122**:190, 1986.
82. Hacham-Zadeh S, Rappersberger K, Livshin R, Konrad K: Epidermolysis bullosa herpetiformis Dowling-Meara in a large family. *J Am Acad Dermatol* **18**:702, 1988.
83. Anton-Lamprecht I: In Papadimitriou JF, Henderson DW, Spagnolo DV (eds): *Diagnostic Ultrastructure of Non-neoplastic Diseases*. Edinburgh, Churchill Livingstone, 1992, pp 459–550.

84. Anton-Lamprecht I: Genetically induced abnormalities of epidermal differentiation and ultrastructure in ichthyoses and epidermolysis: Pathogenesis, heterogeneity, fetal manifestation, and prenatal diagnosis. *J Invest Dermatol* **81**:149s, 1983.
85. Vassar R, Coulombe PA, Degenstein L, Albers K, Fuchs E: Mutant keratin expression in transgenic mice causes marked abnormalities resembling a human genetic skin disease. *Cell* **64**:365, 1991.
86. Ishida-Yamamoto A, McGrath JA, Chapman SJ, Leigh IM, Lane EB, Eady RAJ: Epidermolysis bullosa simplex (Dowling-Meara type) is a genetic disease characterized by an abnormal keratin-filament network involving keratins K5 and K14. *J Invest Dermatol* **97**:959, 1991.
87. Olaisen B, Gedde-Dahl T: GPT-epidermolysis bullosa simplex (EBS Ogna) linkage in man. *Hum Hered* **23**:189, 1973.
88. Gedde-Dahl T, Olaisen B, Aarum G, Brevik K, Bye R: Linkage relations of chromosome 16 marker PGP to GPT: EBS1 and unassigned markers. *Cytogenet Cell Genet* **37**:474, 1984.
89. Pearson RW: *Dermatology in General Medicine: The Mechanobullous Disease* (*Epidermolysis bullosa*), 1st ed. New York, McGraw-Hill, 1971.
90. Savolainen ER, Kero M, Pihlajaniemi T, Kivirikko KI: Deficiency of galactosylhydroxylysyl glucosyltransferase, an enzyme of collagen synthesis, in a family with dominant epidermolysis bullosa simplex. *N Engl J Med* **304**:197, 1981.
91. Sanchez G, Seltzer JL, Eisen AZ, Stapler P, Bauer EA: Generalized dominant epidermolysis bullosa simplex: Decreased activity of a gelatinolytic protease in cultured fibroblasts as a phenotypic marker. *J Invest Dermatol* **83**:576, 1983.
92. Winberg JO, Real D, Gedde-Dahl T: Gelatinase expression in generalized epidermolysis bullosa simplex fibroblasts. *J Invest Dermatol* **87**:326, 1986.
93. Takamori K, Ikeda S, Naito K, Ogawa H: Proteases are responsible for blister formation in recessive dystrophic epidermolysis bullosa and epidermolysis bullosa simplex. *Br J Dermatol* **112**:533, 1985.
94. Fine JD, Griffith RD: A specific defect in glycosylation of epidermal cell membranes: Definition in skin from patients with epidermolysis bullosa simplex. *Arch Dermatol* **121**:1292, 1985.
95. Tidman MJ, Eady RA, Leigh IM, MacDonald DM: Keratin expression in epidermolysis bullosa simplex (Dowling-Meara). *Acta Derm Venereol* (*Stockh*) **68**:15, 1988.
96. Kitajima Y, Inoue S, Yaoita H: Abnormal organization of keratin intermediate filaments in cultured keratinocytes of epidermolysis bullosa simplex. *Arch Dermatol Res* **281**:5, 1989.
97. Coulombe PA, Hutton ME, Vassar R, Fuchs E: A function for keratins and a common thread among different types of epidermolysis bullosa simplex diseases. *J Cell Biol* **115**:1661, 1991.
98. Mulley JC, Nicholls CM, Propert DN, Turner T, Sutherland GR: Genetic linkage analysis of epidermolysis bullosa simplex, Koebner type. *Am J Med Genet* **19**:573, 1984.
99. Humphries MM, Sheils D, Lawler M, Farrar GJ, McWilliam P, Kenna P, Bradley DG, Sharp EM, Gaffney EF, Young M, Uitto J, Humphries P: Epidermolysis bullosa: Evidence for linkage to genetic markers on chromosome 1 in a family with the autosomal dominant simplex form. *Genomics* **7**:377, 1990.
100. Bonifas JM, Rothman AL, Epstein EH: Epidermolysis bullosa simplex: Evidence in two families for keratin gene abnormalities. *Science* **254**:1202, 1991.
101. Ryynanen M, Knowlton RG, Uitto J: Mapping of epidermolysis bullosa simplex mutation to chromosome 12. *AM J Hum Genet* **49**:978, 1991.
102. Chan YM, Yu QC, Fine JD, Fuchs E: The genetic basis of Weber-Cockayne epidermolysis bullosa simplex. *Proc Natl Acad Sci USA* **90**:7414, 1993.
103. Chan YM, Yu QC, Christiano A, Uitto J, Fuchs E: Mutations in the non-helical linker segment L1-2 of keratin 5 in patients with Weber-Cockayne Epidermolysis Bullosa Simplex. *J Cell Sci* **107**, 1994 (in press).
104. McKenna KE, Hughes AE, Bingham EA, Nevin NC: Linkage of epidermolysis bullosa simplex to keratin gene loci. *J Med Genet* **29**:568, 1992.
105. Coulombe PA, Hutton ME, Letai A, Hebert A, Paller AS, Fuchs E: Point mutations in human keratin 14 genes of epidermolysis bullosa simplex patients: Genetic and functional analyses. *Cell* **66**:1301, 1991.
106. Lane EB, Rugg EL, Navsaria H, Leigh IM, Heagerty AHM, Ishida-Yamamoto A, Eady RAJ: A mutation in the conserved helix termination peptide of keratin 5 in hereditary skin blistering. *Nature* **356**:244, 1992.
107. Dong W, Ryynanen M, Uitto J: Identification of a leucine-to-proline mutation in the keratin 5 gene in a family with the generalized Koebner type of epidermolysis bullosa simplex (EBS). *Hum Mutat* **2**:94, 1993.
108. Stephens K, Sybert VP, Wijsman EM, Ehrlich P, Spencer A: A keratin 14 mutational hot spot for epidermolysis bullosa simplex, Dowling-Meara: Implications for diagnosis. *J Invest Dermatol* **101**:240, 1993.
109. Fuchs E, Coulombe PA: Of mice and men: Genetic skin diseases of keratin. *Cell* **69**:899, 1992.
110. Humphries MM, Sheils DM, Farrar GJ, Kumar-Singh R, Kenna PF, Mansergh FC, Jordan SA, Young M, Humphries P: A mutation (Met → Arg) in the type I keratin (K14) gene responsible for autosomal dominant epidermolysis bullosa simplex. *Hum Mutat* **2**:37, 1993.
111. Hovnanian A, Pollack E, Hilal L, Rochat A, Prost C, Barrandon Y, Goossens M: A missense mutation in the rod domain of keratin 14 associated with epidermolysis bullosa simplex. *Nat Genet* **3**:327, 1993.
112. Letai A, Coulombe PA, McCormick MB, Yu QC, Hutton E, Fuchs E: Disease severity correlates with position of keratin point mutations in patients with epidermolysis bullosa simplex. *Proc Natl Acad Sci USA* **90**:3197, 1993.
113. Cooper DN, Youssoufian H: The CpG dinucleotide and human genetic disease. *Hum Genet* **78**:151, 1988.
114. Shyy TT, Asch BB, Asch HL: Concurrent collapse of keratin filaments, aggregation of organelles, and inhibition of protein synthesis during the heat shock response in mammary epithelial cells. *J Cell Biol* **108**:997, 1989.
115. Anton-Lamprecht I: Prenatal diagnosis of genetic disorders of the skin by means of electron microscopy. *Hum Genet* **59**:392, 1981.
116. Eady RA: Fetoscopy and fetal skin biopsy for prenatal diagnosis of genetic skin disorders. *Semin Dermatol* **7**:2, 1988.
117. Sybert VP, Holbrook KA, Levy M: Prenatal diagnosis of severe dermatologic diseases. *Adv Dermatol* **7**:179, 1992.
118. Fine JD, Johnson LB, Wright JT: Inherited blistering diseases of the skin. *Pediatrician* **18**:175, 1991.
119. Green H: Cultured cells for the treatment of disease. *Sci Am* **265**:96, 1991.
120. Burge SM, Garrod DR: An immunohistological study of desmosomes in Darier's disease and Hailey-Hailey disease. *Br J Dermatol* **124**:242, 1991.
121. Ishibashi Y, Kajiwara Y, Andoh I, Inoue Y, Kukita A: The nature and pathogenesis of dyskeratosis in Hailey-Hailey's disease and Darier's disease. *J Dermatol* **11**:335, 1984.
122. Frost P, Van Scott EJ: Ichthyosiform dermatoses: Classification based on anatomic and biometric observations. *Arch Dermatol* **94**:113, 1966.
123. Ackerman AB: Histopathologic concept of epidermolytic hyperkeratosis. *Arch Dermatol* **102**:253, 1970.
124. Wilgram GF, Caulfield JB: An electron microscopic study of epidermolytic hyperkeratosis. *Arch Dermatol* **94**:127, 1966.
125. Anton-Lamprecht I, Curth HO, Schnyder UW: Ultrastructure of inborn errors of keratinization. II. Ichthyosis hystrix type Curth-Macklin. *Arch Dermatol Res* **246**:77, 1973.
126. Anton-Lamprecht I, Schnyder UW: Ultrastructure of inborn errors of keratinization. *Arch Derm Forsch* **250**:207, 1974.
127. Curth HO, Macklin MT: The genetic basis of various types of ichthyosis in a family group. *Am J Hum Genet* **6**:371, 1954.
128. Voerner H: Zur Kenntris des Keratoma hereditarium palmare et plantare. *Arch Dermatol Syphilol* **56**:3, 1901.
129. Fritsch P, Hoenigsmann H, Jaschke E: Epidermolytic hereditary palmoplantar keratoderma. *Br J Dermatol* **99**:561, 1978.
130. Klaus S, Weinstein GD, Frost P: Localized epidermolytic hyperkeratosis. *Arch Dermatol* **101**:272, 1970.

131. Kolde G, Vakilzadeh F: An ultrastructural study of epidermolytic leukoplakia. *Arch Dermatol Res* **275**:86, 1983.
132. Siemens HW: The as yet undescribed regular dominant form of bullous congenital ichthyosiform erythroderma. *Hautarzt* **21**:252, 1970.
133. Traupe H, Kolde G, Hamm H, Happle R: Ichthyosis bullosa of Siemens: A unique type of epidermolytic hyperkeratosis. *J Am Acad Dermatol* **14**:1000, 1986.
134. Ollendorff-Curth H, Allen FH, Schnyder UW, Anton-Lamprecht I: Follow-up of a family group suffering from ichthyosis hystrix type Curth-Macklin. *Hum Genet* **17**:37, 1972.
135. Fuchs E, Esteves RA, Coulombe PA: Transgenic mice expressing a mutant keratin 10 gene reveal the likely genetic basis for Epidermolytic Hyperkeratosis. *Proc Natl Acad Sci USA* **89**:6906, 1992.
136. Holbrook KA, Dale BA, Sybert VP, Sagebiel RW: Epidermolytic hyperkeratosis: Ultrastructure and biochemistry of skin and amniotic fluid cells from two affected fetuses and a newborn infant. *J Invest Dermatol* **80**:222, 1983.
137. Cheng J, Syder AJ, Yu QC, Letai A, Paller AS, Fuchs E: The genetic basis of epidermolytic hyperkeratosis: A disorder of differentiation-specific epidermal keratin genes. *Cell* **70**:811, 1992.
138. Chipev CC, Korge BP, Markova N, Bale SJ, DiGiovanna JJ, Compton JG, Steinert PM: A leucine→proline mutation in the H1 subdomain of keratin 1 causes epidermolytic hyperkeratosis. *Cell* **70**:821, 1992.
139. Rothnagel JA, Dominey AM, Dempsey LD, Longley MA, Greenhalgh DA, Gagne TA, Huber M, Frenk E, Hohl D, Roop DR: Mutations in the rod domains of keratins 1 and 10 in epidermolytic hyperkeratosis. *Science* **257**:1128, 1992.
140. Compton JG, DeGiovanna JJ, Santucci SK, Kearns KS, Amos CI, Abangan DL, Korge BP, McBride OW, Steinert PM, Bale SJ: Linkage of epidermolytic hyperkeratosis to the type II keratin gene cluster on chromosome 12q. *Nat Genet* **1**:301, 1992.
141. Bonifas JM, Bare JW, Chen MA, Lee MK, Slater CA, Goldsmith LA, Epstein EH Jr: Linkage of the epidermolytic hyperkeratosis phenotype and the region of the type II keratin gene cluster on chromosome 12. *J Invest Dermatol* **99**:524, 1992.
142. Pulkkinen L, Christiano AM, Knowlton RG, Uitto J: Epidermolytic hyperkeratosis (bullous congenital ichthyosiform erythroderma): Genetic linkage to chromosome 12q in the region of the type II keratin gene cluster. *J Clin Invest* **91**:357, 1993.
143. Steinert PM, Parry DAD: The conserved H1 domain of the type II keratin 1 chain plans an essential role in the alignment of nearest neighbor molecules in mouse and human keratin 1/keratin 10 intermediate filaments at the two- to four-molecular level of structure. *J Biol Chem* **268**:2878, 1993.
144. Chipev CC, Yang J-M, Di Giovanna JJ, Steinert PM, Marekov L, Compton JG, Bale SJ: Preferential sites in keratin 10 that are mutated in epidermolytic hyperkeratosis. *Am J Hum Genet* **54**:179, 1994.
145. McLean WHI, Eady RAJ, Dopping-Hepenstal PJC, McMillan JR, Leigh IM, Navsaria HA, Higgins C, Harper JI, Paige DG, Morley SM, Lane EB: Mutations in the rod 1A domain of keratins 1 and 10 in Bullous Congenital Ichthyosiform Erythroderma (BCIE). *J Invest Dermatol* **102**:24, 1994.
146. Syder AJ, Yr QC, Paller AS, Giudice GJ, Dale B, Sybert VJ, Pearson R, Fuchs E: Genetic mutations in the K1 and K10 genes of patients with epidermolytic hyperkeratosis: Correlation between location and disease severity. *J Clin Invest* **93**, 1994 (in press).
147. Reis A, Kuster W, Eckardt R, Sperling K: Mapping of a gene for epidermolytic palmoplantar keratoderma to the region of the acidic keratin gene cluster at 17q12-q21. *Hum Genet* **90**:113, 1992.
148. Franke WW, Schiller DL, Hatzfeld M, Winter S: Protein complexes of intermediate-sized filaments: Melting of cytokeratin complexes in urea reveals different polypeptide separation characteristics. *Proc Natl Acad Sci USA* **80**:7113, 1983.
149. Fuchs E: Threads between useful and useless. *Curr Biol* **1**:284, 1991.
150. Janmey PA, Euteneuer U, Traub P, Schliwa M: Viscoelastic properties of vimentin compared with other filamentous biopolymer networks. *J Cell Biol* **113**:155, 1991.
151. Powell BC, Rogers GE: Cyclic hair-loss and regrowth in transgenic mice overexpressing an intermediate filament gene. *EMBO J* **9**:1485, 1990.
152. Baden HP, Hooker PA: Advances in genetics in dermatology. *Adv Hum Genet* **12**:89, 1982.
153. Marshall RC, Gillespie JM: Variations in the proteins of wool and hair, in Rogers GE, Marshall RC, Reis PJ, Ward KA (eds): *The Biology of Wool and Hair*. London, Chapman & Hall, 1989, pp 117–125.
154. Gillespie JM, Marshall RC: Effect of mutation on the proteins of wool and hair, in Rogers GE, Marshall RC, Reis PJ, Ward KA (eds): *The Biology of Wool and Hair*. London, Chapman & Hall, 1989, pp 257–274.
155. Lynch MH, O'Guin WM, Hardy C, Mak L, Sun TT: Acidic and basic hair/nail ("hard") keratins: Their colocalization in upper cortical and cuticle cells of the human hair follicle and their relationship to "soft" keratins. *J Cell Biol* **103**:2593, 1986.
156. Heid HW, Werner E, Franke WW: The complement of native alpha-keratin polypeptides of hair-forming cells: A subset of eight polypeptides that differ from epithelial cytokeratins. *Differentiation* **32**:101, 1986.
157. Powell BC, Nesci A, Rogers GE: Regulation of keratin gene expression in hair follicle differentiation. *Ann NY Acad Sci* **642**:1, 1991.
158. MacKinnon PJ, Powell BC, Roger GE, Baker EG, MacKinnon RN, Hyland VJ, Callen DF, Sutherland GR: An ultrahigh-sulphur keratin gene of the human hair cuticle is located at 11q13 and cross-hybridizes with sequences at 11q15. *Mamm Genet* **1**:53, 1991.
159. Burgeson RE: Type VII collagen, anchoring fibrils, and epidermolysis bullosa. *J Invest Dermatol* **101**:252, 1993.
160. Epstein EH: Molecular genetics of epidermolysis bullosa. *Science* **256**:799, 1992.
161. Christiano AM, Greenspan DS, Hoffman GG, Zhang X, Tamai Y, Lin AN, Dietz HC, Hovnanian A, Uitto J: A missense mutation in type VII collagen in two affected siblings with recessive dystrophic epidermolysis bullosa. *Nat Genet* **1**:62, 1993.
162. Ryynanen M, Ryynanen J, Sollberg S, Iozzo RV, Knowlton RG, Uitto J: Genetic linkage of type VII collagen (COL7A1) to dominant dystrophic epidermolysis bullosa in families with abnormal anchoring fibrils. *J Clin Invest* **89**:974, 1992.
163. Marinkovich MP, Verrando P, Keene DR, Meneguzzi G, Lunstrum GP, Ortonne JP, Burgeson RE: Basement membrane proteins kalinin and nicein are structurally and immunologically identical. *Lab Invest* **69**:295, 1993.
164. Lazarides E: Intermediate filaments as mechanical integrators of cellular space. *Nature* **283**:249, 1980.
165. Xu Z, Cork LC, Griffin JW, Cleveland DW: Increased expression of neurofilament subunit NFL produces morphological alterations that resemble the pathology of human motor neuron disease. *Cell* **73**:23, 1993.
166. Cote F, Collard JF, Julien JP: Progressive neuronopathy in transgenic mice expressing the human neurofilament heavy gene: a mouse model of amyotrophic lateral sclerosis. *Cell* **73**:35, 1993.
167. Pellissier JF, Pouget J, Charpin C, Figarella D: Myopathy associated with desmin type intermediate filaments: an immunoelectron microscopic study. *J Neurol Sci* **89**:49, 1989.
168. Rugg EL, Morley SM, Smith FJD, Boxer M, Tidman MJ, Navsaria H, Leigh IM, and Lane EB: Missing links: Weber-Cockayne keratin mutations implicate the L12 linker domain in effective cytoskeleton function. *Nat Genet* **5**:294, 1993.
169. Torchard D, Blanchet-Bardon C, Serova O, Langbein L, Narod S, Janin N, Goguel AF, Bernheim A, Franke WW, Lenoir GM, and Feunteun J: Epidermolytic palmoplantar keratoderma cosegregates with a keratin 9 mutation in a pedigree with breast and ovarian cancer. *Nat Genet* **6**:106, 1994.
170. Reis A, Hennies HC, Langbein L, Digweed M, and Mischke D: Keratin 9 gene mutations in Epidermolytic Palmoplantar Keratoderma (EPPK). *Nat Genet* **6**:174, 1994.

Part 22

INTESTINE

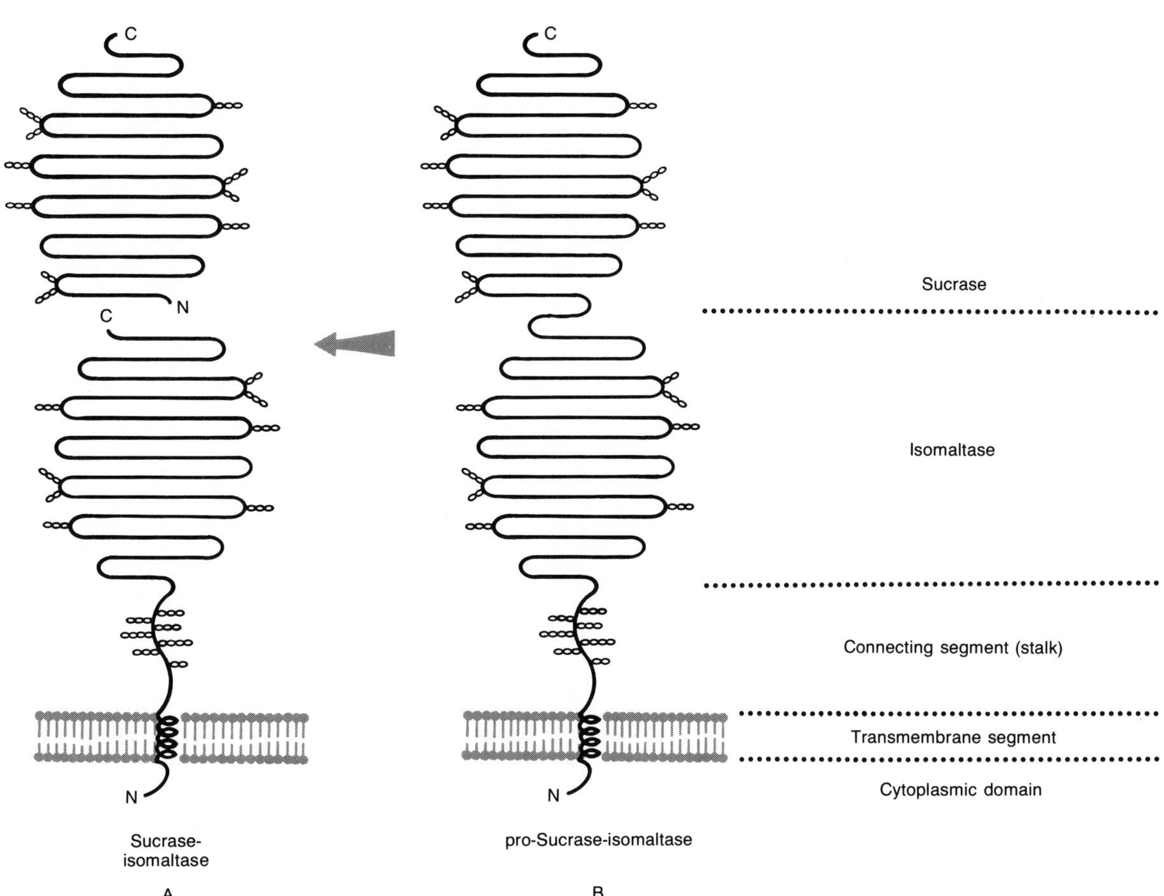

CHAPTER 150

The Genetic Polymorphism of Intestinal Lactase Activity in Adult Humans

Gebhard Flatz

1. The utilization of lactose for human nutrition requires the hydrolysis of this disaccharide in the intestinal tract. This is achieved by the enzyme lactase, a β-galactosidase located in the brush border of small-intestinal epithelial cells. Lactase activity is high during infancy, when milk is the main nutrient. As in most other mammals, lactase activity normally declines in a majority of humans after the weaning phase and remains low throughout life (phenotype: lactase restriction). In other healthy humans, lactase activity persists at a level not much lower than in infants (phenotype: lactase persistence). Subjects with lactase restriction have a low lactose digestion capacity (low LDC); those with lactase persistence can hydrolyze large amounts of lactose (high LDC). The adult lactase phenotypes can be diagnosed through small-intestinal biopsy or lactose-tolerance tests.

2. Family studies, measurement of relative lactase activity, and a study of lactose digestion in twins prove that the lactase phenotypes are genetically determined. The observed segregation is satisfactorily explained by a Mendelian system of two autosomal alleles (or groups of alleles), the globally more frequent lactase restriction gene(s)—*LAC*R*—and the lactase persistence gene(s)—*LAC*P*. Multiple allelism at the lactase locus is possible but not definitely proved. *LAC*P* allele(s) are dominant over the recessive *LAC*R* allele(s), which means that only subjects homozygous for the restriction allele(s) have the phenotype low LDC.

3. The structural locus for intestinal lactase is located on chromosome 2. Molecular studies have so far not revealed a difference in the DNA sequence of the gene between subjects with lactase persistence and repression. Studies of the expression of lactase activity in animals and in humans suggest that there may be various (pretranslational and posttranslational) causes of the low enzyme activity in lactase restriction, but this requires further clarification.

4. The distribution of the lactase phenotypes in human populations is highly variable. In most tropical and subtropical countries and in all East Asian populations, lactase restriction is predominant. According to the Hardy-Weinberg rule, the frequency of *LAC*P* alleles is higher than that of *LAC*R* in populations with less than 25 percent lactase restriction. In the Old World, there are only two human population groups in which the lactase persistence gene predominates: northwestern Europeans and milk-dependent nomads of the Afro-Arabian desert zone. Natural selection in favor of the lactase persistence gene due to improved utilization of animal milk in the nutrition of older children and adults with high LDC is the most likely cause of the unusual lactase phenotype distribution in Europeans and Afro-Arabian nomads.

5. In self-chosen nutritional conditions, the disease potential of lactase restriction is low. In countries where animal milk is part of the usual diet, most people seem to adjust milk consumption to their individual lactose tolerance threshold. The role of lactase restriction in the causation of recurrent abdominal pain in children, irritable bowel syndrome in adults, and osteoporosis in postmenopausal women and the role of lactase persistence in promoting coronary heart disease and premature cataract are controversial.

A list of standard abbreviations is located immediately preceding the index in each volume. Additional abbreviation used in this chapter is: LDC = lactose digestion capacity.

A difference in lactase activity between suckling and adult animals has been known since 1895, when Röhmann and Lappe[1] showed that cows and adult dogs have a much lower small-intestinal lactose digestion capacity than calves and puppies. The developmental rule derived from this observation was not applied to humans for a long time, probably because medical research was most active in countries where the majority of the population retain high small-intestinal lactase activity throughout life. Constitutionally low lactase activity in healthy adult humans was discovered independently by two groups of researchers in 1963.[2,3] The term *lactase deficiency* for this type of enzymatic variation is not preferred by me because it seems inappropriate to speak of a trait that is present in the majority of adult humans as a pathological or abnormal condition. It is important to realize that both high and low lactase activity in healthy adult humans are normal phenotypes and should be seen on the same level as similar genetically determined variations, for example, the human blood groups. This is increasingly supported by current nomenclature.[4] The biochemical, physiological, and nutritional implications of genetically determined "lactase deficiency" have been treated in Chap. 151. The main objective of this chapter is to stress the formal and population genetic aspects of lactase variability in adults.

Only 3 years after the discovery of constitutionally low lactase activity in healthy adult humans,[2,3] the idea that the variability of lactase activity represents a genetic polymorphism was clearly expressed by Bayless and Rosensweig.[5] According to Ford,[6] "genetic polymorphism is a type of variation in which individuals with sharply distinct qualities co-exist as normal members of a population" and is defined as "the occurrence together in the same habitat of two or more discontinuous forms, or 'phases,' of a species in such proportions that the rarest of them cannot be maintained merely by recurrent mutation." Therefore, the prerequisites for designating an observed variability as genetic polymorphism are the demonstration that the phases of a trait in the population are distinct, that is, that the expression of the traits is discontinuous; that the variable expression of the trait is genetically determined; and that the rarest of the phases has a frequency of more than approximately 1 percent (thus precluding recurrent mutation as the cause of the variability). It will be shown that these three characteristics of a genetic polymorphism apply to the variability of lactase activity in healthy adult humans.

LOW AND HIGH ADULT LACTASE ACTIVITY AS PHYSIOLOGICAL TRAITS

When lactase activity is determined in biopsies of morphologically normal small intestine, a bimodal distribution is obtained in most human populations. In Central and Northern Europeans and their overseas descendants, the average lactase activity is not much lower than that of normal infants of the same population. Some individuals, however, exhibit a distinctly low lactase activity. Depending on the conditions of analysis, the two modes of lactase activity may be separated or overlapping. The fact that any of no less than three reference parameters—wet weight of the biopsy specimen, protein concentration, or DNA content of the homogenate—are recommended in disaccharidase activity determinations, attests to the difficulties in defining a reliable base for the calculation of intestinal enzyme activities. The overlapping of low and high lactase activities is probably caused in part by variations of the reference parameters. In contrast to activities of a single enzyme, the ratios of disaccharidase activities are fairly constant in a given individual, and maltase:lactase or sucrase:lactase ratios are superior to simple lactase activities in resolving two distinct groups of adults with high and low lactase activity (Fig. 150-1).[7] It is convenient to designate these two groups of differing lactase activity as physiological lactase phenotypes.

That these two groups are biologically different is proved by the result of lactose-tolerance tests. Subjects with high lactase activity can completely digest the usual test dose of 50 g lactose. They have a significant rise in blood glucose concentration within 15 to 45 min following lactose administration, and since no undigested lactose reaches the colon, they lack colonic hydrogen formation and hydrogen excretion in the breath. In contrast, the lactose digestion capacity of subjects in the group with low lactase activity is usually overtaxed by a single dose of 50 g lactose. There is no increase or only a small increase in blood glucose concentration; lactose reaching the colon is fermented by colonic bacteria; the hydrogen produced in this process is partially excreted in the expired air; and the osmotic effects of undigested lactose, the acidification of the colonic contents by short-chain fatty acids, and the formation of copious amounts of gas cause symptoms of lactose intolerance, such as nausea, meteorism, flatulence, borborygmi, and diarrhea. Comparative studies have shown that the lactose-tolerance test with breath hydrogen determination and the lactose–ethanol test with blood galactose determination reliably separate the two phenotypic groups of adults with high and low lactase activity[8,9]

Phylogenetically, low lactase activity in adult mammals is normal.[10] In all lactose-producing mammals, a characteristic developmental pattern of lactase activity has been observed. Lactase activity is high in the newborn and suckling period, declines regularly after the species-specific weaning phase, and remains low in adolescent and adult animals. The concept that humans are an exception to this rule is no longer tenable. Worldwide studies have shown that the majority of adult humans belong to the phenotypic group with low lactase activity and low lactose digestion capacity. In analogy to the ontogenetic development in other mammals, mature human newborns and normal human infants have high lactase activity. In subjects in whom physiological low adult lactase activity develops, the decrease occurs during childhood. The decline of lactase activity begins between 2 and 3 years and is usually complete by the age of 5 to 10 years.[11–13] Rare exceptions to this developmental pattern with a conversion from high to low lactase activity during adolescence have been observed in Finland.[14] In other healthy subjects this decline of lactase activity does not take place; lactase activity and lactose digestion capacity remain high throughout life. There is ample evidence of the independence of these developmental patterns and the resulting phenotypes from nutritional factors, such as the amount of milk in the diet.[15–17] The usual terms for the two distinct lactase phenotypes fail to recognize that the difference between them is not a matter of lactose absorption but rather one of lactose digestion. Therefore, the terms high lactose digestion capacity (high LDC) and low lactose digestion capacity (low LDC) seem more appropriate.

GENETIC DETERMINATION OF THE LACTASE PHENOTYPES

A genetic basis of the two physiological adult lactase phenotypes was suspected soon after the discovery of low lactase activity ("lactase deficiency") as a common trait among healthy adult humans.[18] Different genetic models were proposed, but experimental evidence of a simple mode of inheritance of the lactase phenotypes was lacking. Sahi[19] summarized earlier segregation studies and showed that insufficient numbers and/or unreliable methods—for example, the lactose tolerance test with blood gluose determination (which gives particularly poor results in children)[20]—precluded proof of Mendelian inheritance of the two adult lactase phenotypes. It was not until 1973 that the classic methods of segregation analysis and reliable methods of lactase phenotype diagnosis were applied in a family study.[21]

This work was facilitated by the relatively high frequency of low lactase activity among Finns, but also by the fact that the Finnish study group was first to apply a reliable diagnostic procedure—the lactose–ethanol tolerance test with blood galactose determination[22,23]—to a sufficiently large number of informative families. They proved convincingly that healthy adult subjects with low lactase activity are homozygous for a recessive autosomal allele causing the physiological postweaning decline of lactase activity, whereas subjects with high adult lactase activity are either

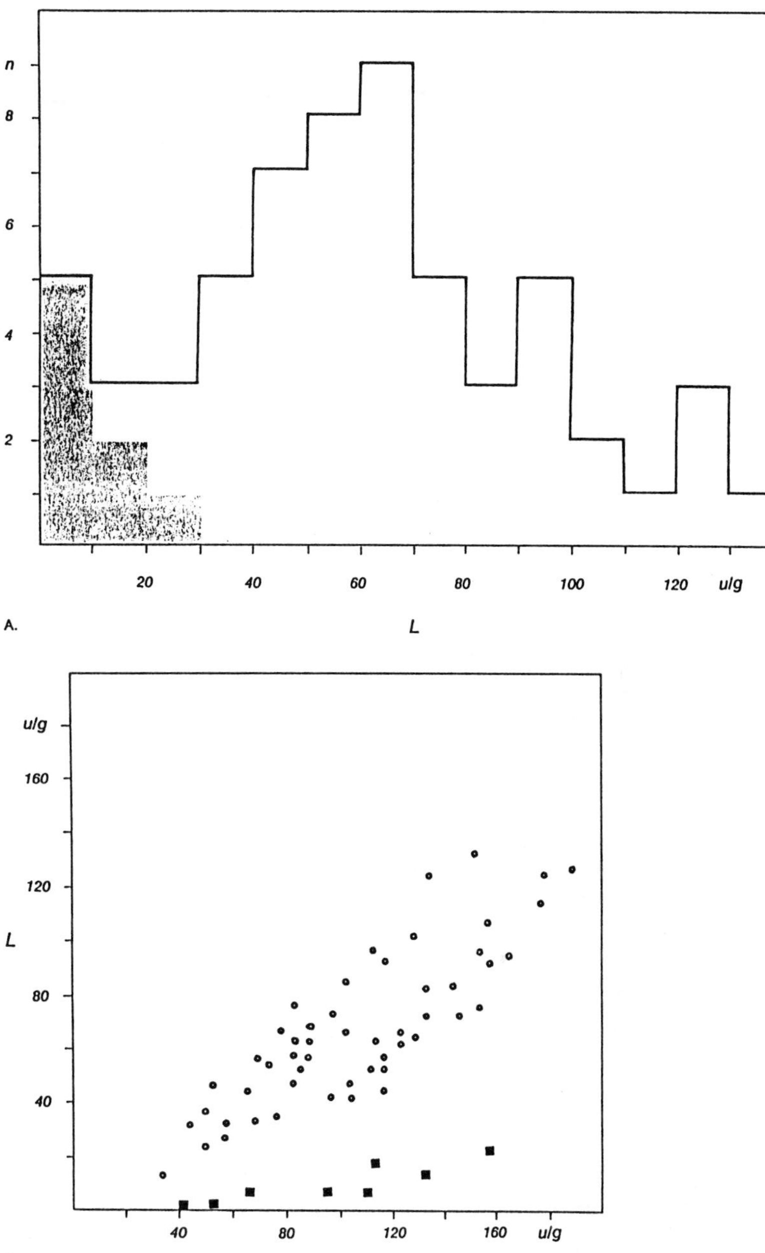

FIG. 150-1 *A*. **Lactase activity (*L*, in units/g protein in intestinal biopsy homogenates) and *B*. lactase:sucrase activity ratios (L:S) in 60 healthy male adult Germans (age 20 to 53 years). Shading (in *A*) and squares (in *B*) represent subjects with low lactose digestion capacity (LDC); the remaining subjects (clear in *A* and circles in *B*) have high LDC. The lactase phenotype diagnosis was determined by two independent lactose tolerance tests. *n* = number of subjects.**

heterozygous or homozygous for a dominant allele preventing the normal decline of lactase activity.

The results of this study were soon confirmed by independent segregation analyses in different populations.[24,25] The postweaning decrease in lactase activity can thus be described as a regular genetic switch and a developmental program that is characteristic of almost all species of mammals. At present, the molecular mechanisms of this ontogenetic switch (restriction of lactase activity during childhood) and its failure (persistence of lactase activity throughout life) are unknown. Since the physicochemical, immunologic, and kinetic properties of lactase in infants and adults—and in individuals with lactase restriction and those with lactase persistence—are identical (see Chap. 151), it is clear that the difference between the physiological adult lactase phenotypes is regulatory and not structural. In this respect, lactase restriction differs fundamentally from enzyme deficiencies due to gene deletions or structural mutations. At the present state of knowledge, it seems advisable to use a system of neutral descriptive terms and to avoid expressions implying definite genetic mechanisms, such as *lactase r pression*. The suggested nomenclature for the physiological adult lactase phenotypes and the underlying genotypes is listed in Table 150-1. *LAC*R* is a designation for the allele(s) causing *lactase restriction* in childhood and *LAC*P* for the allele(s) determining *lactase persistence*.

Although the genetic etiology of low and high adult lactase activity and their Mendelian segregation is now generally recognized, it is rarely appreciated that additional independent evidence for the formal genetic model of the two alleles (or group of alleles) *LAC*R* and *LAC*P* has accumulated. The first type of evidence concerns the relationship between lactase phenotype and genotype. If there is a correlation between lactase gene dosage and lactase activity, a trimodal distribution of lactase activity would be expected in populations possessing both lactase alleles. Such a trimodality has not been convincingly demonstrated using conventional lactase activity determination. Only disaccharidase

Table 150-1 Relation between Enzymatic and Digestive Adult Lactase Phenotypes and Genotypes

Enzymatic Phenotype	Digestive Phenotype	Genotype
Lactase restriction	Low LDC	*LAC*R/LAC*R*
Lactase persistence	High LDC	*LAC*R/LAC*P*
		*LAC*P/LAC*P*

The designations *LAC*P* and *LAC*R* may represent groups of alleles with similar physiological action.

activity ratios determined with optimized methods have uncovered a trimodal distribution of sucrase:lactase or maltase:lactase activity ratios compatible with Hardy-Weinberg expectations of the distribution of the three genotypes *LAC*R/LAC*R*, *LAC*R/LAC*P*, and *LAC*P/LAC*P*.[26,27] Additional proof of monogenic inheritance of the lactase phenotypes was obtained in a study of lactose digestion in twins, using two independent methods of assessing LDC. Concordance of the lactase phenotypes among monozygous twins was complete, and the distribution of dizygous twins pairs concordant for low LDC, discordant pairs, and pairs concordant for high LDC corresponded with Hardy-Weinberg expectations.[9]

In view of occasional doubts concerning the simple genetic etiology of the lactase phenotypes, it is important to note that their diagnosis requires the administration of unphysiological doses of lactose. Therefore, low LDC and lactase restriction are not synonymous with lactose intolerance. Many healthy subjects with low lactase activity experience no symptoms or only minimal symptoms with ordinary amounts of milk or other lactose-containing foods. Many genetic and nutritional factors influence lactose tolerance in a single individual.[28] Therefore, it is expected that familial aggregation, but not Mendelian segregation, will be found in family studies if lactose tolerance is ascertained by personal nutritional history and the lactase phenotype is not determined using biochemical methods.[29]

MOLECULAR STUDIES OF THE LACTASE PHENOTYPES

Only a brief review of molecular studies pertinent to the formal and population genetic problems is given here (see Chap. 151 for a more complete coverage). The lactase structural locus has been localized to chromosome 2.[30] No differences in the nucleotide sequence were observed between subjects with high and low lactase activity.[31] Evidence for transcriptional and posttranscriptional mechanisms of the maturational decline in lactase activity has been obtained in animal and human studies.[32–35] Histochemically, subjects with lactase restriction showed either no lactase or a patchy distribution of lactase-specific staining enterocytes,[36] a finding that suggested different mechanisms. Studies in rats[37] and in humans[38,39] have suggested that the regulation of lactase activity is mainly determined at the transcriptional level.

It would be surprising if a genetic switch common to almost all mammals is caused by different mechanisms, but if this is proved, studies of the regulation of lactase activity in animals may not be relevant for the mechanism in humans. In analogy with the perinatal switch of globin production multiple allelism seems more likely in the evolutionarily younger trait of lactase persistence and may explain the observed differences in the age of onset of low LDC.

DISTRIBUTION OF THE LACTASE PHENOTYPES IN HUMAN POPULATIONS: THE LACTASE POLYMORPHISM

The data on the distribution of the lactase phenotype in the world population are not as reliable as those of other monogenic traits. This is due mainly to the difficulties in performing lactose tolerance tests (in comparison with serologic or electrophoretic studies on single blood samples) and to the inadequacy of the methods of lactose testing in earlier studies. Even if specific enzymatic methods for the glucose assay are used, the lactose-tolerance test based solely on blood glucose determination is unreliable and liable to overestimate the number of subjects with high LDC.[8,9,20] Despite these limitations, the available data of lactose tests in about 24,000 subjects permit a sufficiently precise description of the distribution of the lactase phenotypes in the world population. Detailed summaries of the lactase phenotype distribution have already been published.[40,41]

As is evident from the distribution data summarized in Table 150-2, lactase restriction is predominant and often the ubiquitous lactase phenotype in the native populations of Australia and Oceania, East and Southeast Asia, tropical Africa, and the Americas. The opposite distribution, predominance of the lactase persistence alelle, is found in two separate groups of populations: (1) Central and Northern Europeans (the Scandinavian countries, Germany, Austria, Switzerland, northern France, Belgium, the Netherlands, Britain and Ireland), and (2) nomadic, milk-dependent populations in the arid zones of North Africa and Arabia (Tuareg, Fulbe, Kabbabish, Beja, and Bedouin people). In these populations the lactase persistance allele *LAC*P* is more frequent than *LAC*R*. According to the Hardy-Weinberg rule, this means that less than 25 percent of the population have low LDC. Contrary to common opinion, lactase persistence is obviously not predominant in all European populations. The two regions of high prevalence of lactase persistence are separated by a wide peri-Mediterranean belt inhabited by peoples with predominant lactase restriction. This includes the littoral of North Africa, the Near East, Turkey, the Balkans, Italy and southern France—areas where the frequency of low LDC is between 45 and 95 percent. In the eastern part of Central Europe (Hungary, Poland), 30 to 40 percent of the people have low LDC, and there may be a continuous west-east gradient extending from this region to the Far East, where 76 percent of the Kasakhs of northwestern China, 88 percent of Mongols in China, and 95 to 100 percent of southern Chinese have low lactase activity. Lactase restriction is also predominant in Southeast Asia and in South Asia (Iran, Afghanistan, Pakistan, India, and Sri Lanka). As expected, intermediate frequencies of the lactase phenotypes are found in populations originating from recent mixing of peoples with high and low frequencies of low LDC. In some of these, for example, American Indians[51] and Eskimos,[52] the frequency of lactase persistence is correlated with the number of European ancestors. Figure 150-2 shows the distribution of the lactase phenotypes in the Old World, the region where lactase polymorphism evolved.

Table 150-2 Distribution of the Adult Lactase Phenotypes in Human Populations

Population or Country	Subgroup	No. of Subjects	High LDC	Low LDC	Percent Low LDC
Finland	Finns	449	371	78	17
	Lapps	521	305	216	41
	Swedes	91	84	7	8
Sweden	Swedes	400	396	4	1
Denmark	Danes	761	743	18	3
Britain	British	96	90	6	6
Ireland	Irish	50	48	2	4
Netherlands	Dutch	14	14	0	0
Germany	Germans	1872	1596	276	15
France	North	73	56	17	23
	South	82	47	35	43
	West[42]	102	78	24	24
Spain	Spaniards	265	225	40	15
Switzerland	Swiss	64	54	10	16
Austria	Austrians	528	422	106	20
Italy	North	565	301	264	47
	South	128	41	78	68
	Sicily	100	29	71	71
Yugoslavia	Slovenia	153	99	54	35
	South	51	25	26	51
Hungary	Hungarians	707	446	61	37
Czechoslovakia	Czechs	217	189	28	13
Poland	Poles	296	187	109	37
Estonia	See refs. 41 and 43	720	515	205	28
Russia	Leningrad	248	210	38	15
Greece	Greeks	972	452	520	53
Cyprus	Greeks	67	19	48	72
Gypsies	Europe	253	83	170	67
Turkey	Turks	470	135	335	71
Morocco	Maghrebi	55	12	43	78
Egypt		584	157	427	73
Sudan	Arabs	387	179	208	54
	Nomads	364	294	70	19
	South	366	92	274	75
Ethiopia		58	6	52	90
Somalia		244	58	186	76
Kenya	Bantu	71	19	52	73
Uganda, Rwanda	Bantu	114	14	100	88
	Hima, Tussi	70	65	5	7
	mixed	75	38	37	49
Central Africa	Bantu	112	6	106	95
South Africa	Bantu	57	3	54	95
	Bushmen	65	3	62	95
	Mixed	152	26	126	83
Gabun	See ref. 44	20	8	12	60
Nigeria	Ibo, Yoruba	113	12	101	89
	Hausa	48	9	39	81
	Fulani (Fulbe)	9	7	2	22
Niger	Tuareg	118	103	15	13
Senegal	Agriculture	131	85	46	35
	Peuhl (Fulbe)	29	29	0	0
Israel	Israeli	272	92	180	66
	Arabs	67	13	54	80
Jordan	Agriculture	204	43	161	79
	Bedouins	162	123	39	24
Saudi Arabia	Bedouins	22	17	5	23
	Other Arabs	18	8	10	56
Lebanon		225	48	177	79
Syria		75	7	68	91
Arabs	Mixed groups	30	5	25	83
Iran	Iranians	40	7	33	83
Afghanistan	Afghans	270	47	223	83
Pakistan		467	195	272	58

(*Continues*)

Table 150-2 Distribution of the Adult Lactase Phenotypes in Human Populations *(Continued)*

Population or Country	Subgroup	No. of Subjects	High LDC	Low LDC	Percent Low LDC
India	North	264	194	70	27
	Central	125	46	79	63
	South	60	20	40	67
	Nagaland[45]	29	8	21	72
Indians	Overseas	87	22	65	75
Sri Lanka	Singhalese	200	55	145	73
Thailand	Thai	428	8	420	98
Vietnam	Vietnamese in United States	31	0	31	100
China	Han North	641	49	592	93
	Han South	405	17	388	96
	Mongols	198	24	174	88
	Kasakhs	195	46	149	76
	Uygurs	202	37	165	82
	Hui	177	24	153	86
	Koreans	198	12	186	94
	Hakka	202	22	180	89
	Bai/Zhuang	359	27	332	93
	Taiwan	71	0	71	100
Chinese overseas	See refs. 41 and 46	220	28	192	87
Japan	Japanese	66	10	56	85
Indonesia	Java	53	5	48	91
Papua-N. Guinea	Tribals	123	12	111	90
Fidji	Fidjians	12	0	12	100
Australia	Whites	133	127	6	5
	Aborigenes	145	48	97	67
Greenland	Eskimo	119	18	101	85
	Mixed	108	67	41	38
Canada	Whites	16	15	1	6
	Indians	30	11	19	63
United States	Alaska	36	6	30	83
	Indians	221	11	210	95
	Whites	1101	887	214	19
	Blacks	390	138	252	65
	Mexicans	305	147	158	52
	Puerto Rico[47]	50	23	27	54
Mexico	Mexicans	401	69	332	83
Guatemala	See ref. 47	20	7	13	65
Colombia	Mestizos	45	30	15	33
	Chami Indian	24	0	24	100
Peru	Mestizos	94	26	68	72
Bolivia	Aymara	31	7	24	77
Chile	See ref. 49	195	51	136	70
Brazil[41,50]	White	85	37	48	56
	Not white	49	9	40	82
	Japanese	20	0	20	100

For entries without reference see Tables IV, V and Addenda in ref. 41

The distinctness of the two lactase phenotypes, their proved genetic determination, and the highly variable distribution in human populations leave no doubt that the variability of intestinal lactase activity in healthy adults represents a genetic polymorphism. It is also clear that lactase restriction in childhood or adolescence occurs in the majority of humans. Postweaning lactase restriction conforms to the developmental pattern in most of the mammalian species. Lactase persistence is the "unusual" or even "abnormal" condition, and its high prevalence in some populations requires explanation.[53] Therefore, the rationale in calling genetically determined low lactase activity in healthy adults "lactase deficiency" is to be questioned. Are individuals lacking the Rhesus blood group factor D "Rhesus-factor deficient"? Would one designate blood group O as "combined sphingolipid *H-N*-acetylgalactosamyl-galactosyl transferase deficiency"?

EXPLANATIONS FOR THE VARIABLE DISTRIBUTION OF THE LACTASE PHENOTYPES IN HUMAN POPULATIONS

High frequencies of adult lactase persistence are found only in populations with a tradition of substantial production and consumption of animal milk. It is generally assumed that the lactase persistence gene has reached high frequencies by

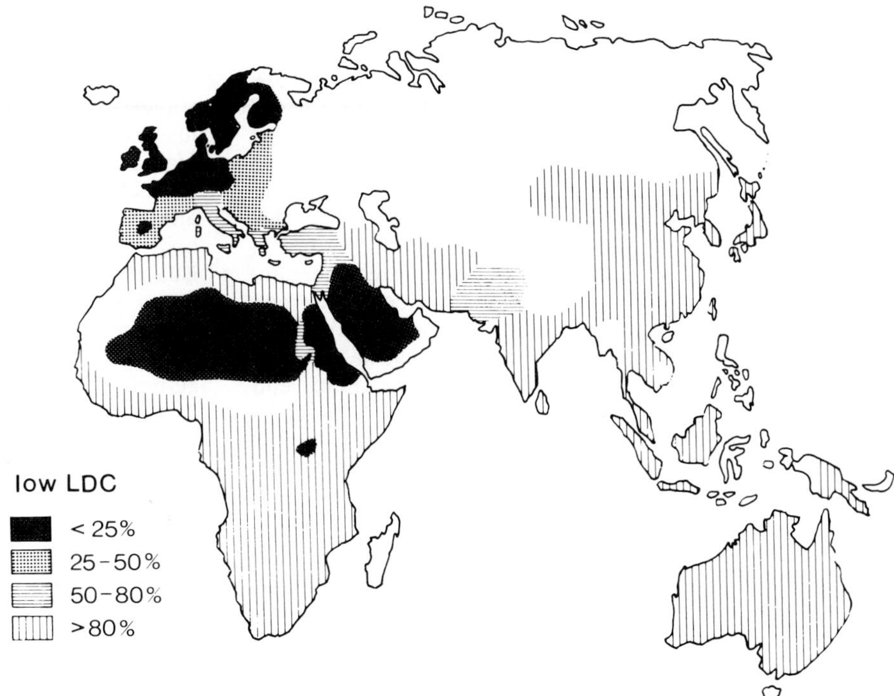

FIG. 150-2 **Distribution of the lactase phenotypes [shown as percent of population with low lactase digestion capacity (see key)] in the native populations of the Old World. Blank areas = insufficient data.**

natural selection in pastoralist populations that developed dairying during the Neolithic period. On the individual level, however, people adjust their dietary intake of milk and milk products consciously or unconsciously to their individual lactose tolerance threshold. Even in populations with generally high milk intake, subjects with low LDC rarely experience severe symptoms of lactose intolerance. This observation may also be relevant on the population level, and the question must be raised whether people adopted dairying and milk consumption because the majority among them were lactase-persistent. Most writers addressing this problem assume a selective advantage of subjects with high LDC, but an opposite, neutralistic hypothesis has been advanced. On the basis of the observation that the lactase persistence gene seems to be present in variable frequencies in most human populations, Nei and Saitou[54] reason that this gene originated before the separation of the major human races—that is, long before the domestication of milking animals. Populations in which the lactase persistence gene attained high frequencies by chance (genetic drift) are presumed to have been able to utilize the benefit of animal milk in adult nutrition. Subsequent selection in favor of the lactase persistence gene is held possible but not essential for the present distribution of the lactase phenotypes.

The validity of this hypothesis must be questioned for two reasons: (1) as mentioned before, the usual field tests for lactose digestion tend to overestimate the frequency of lactase persistence, and lactase restriction may be ubiquitous in many populations for which frequencies of low LDC in excess of 95 percent have been reported; and (2) there is evidence for migration of nomadic pastoralist peoples with a presumably high frequency of lactase persistence to economically more promising agricultural areas with absent or low milk production.[55,56] If these factors are taken into consideration, natural selection in favor of the lactase persistence gene(s) is a more likely cause of the high prevalence of lactase persistence in Afro-Arabian nomads and in the populations of Central and Northern Europe. Johnson, Kretchmer, and Simoons[57] have aptly described the appropriate environmental conditions: "Such selective advantage would only develop among peoples, whether farmers or pastoralists, who had a plentiful milk supply, who did not process their milk into products that were low in lactose and for whom milk provided essential nutrients that could not be readily obtained in the other foods available." This statement is the salient argument of the "culture historical hypothesis," first advanced by Simoons in 1970.[58] Such environmental conditions, conveniently described as "milk dependence," are present in the arid desert areas of North Africa and Arabia,[55] and therefore the culture historical hypothesis plausibly explains the high frequency of lactase persistence among all examined nomadic populations of this area.

Assuming nutritional milk dependence as a selective factor in populations other than nomadic pastoralists raises difficulties. In most agricultural populations of the Old World except tropical Africa and East Asia, animal milk is used in moderate amounts in the nutrition of older children and adults. The frequency of low LDC in milk-using populations of the Mediterranean area and the Near East varies between 50 and 100 percent, and there is no correlation between present and traditional milk use on the one hand, and the frequency of lactase persistence, on the other. Moderate milk consumption does not seem to result in selection in favor of lactase persistence, and the adaptation of milk by fermentation is a procedure permitting innocuous consumption of relatively large amounts of milk products by subjects with low LDC. The variable lactase phenotype distribution in agricultural populations in the Mediterranean area and in Southwest Asia is more likely due to migrations of pastoralist populations with presumably high frequencies of *LAC*P* than to differences in selective pressure in favor of lactase persistence.[59]

The application of the culture historical hypothesis to European populations is even more problematic. The frequency of *LAC*P* does not correspond to the known genetic gradient caused by the migratory settlement of Europe from the Near East in the postglacial period.[60] On the contrary, the highest frequency of $LAC^{*}P$ is found in southern Scandinavia, an area where agriculture and dairying were introduced late, probably not more than 4000 years ago.[61] This means that the period available for selection in favor of $LAC^{*}P$ was only about half as long as that in the Afro-Arabian arid zone. It seems likely, therefore, that European lactase persistence developed independently of that in nomadic pastoralists and may be due to a different mutation. This view is strengthened by the fact that Northern European populations are and were characterized by a mixed economy of farming and dairying that is not conducive to milk dependence. To explain the relatively rapid establishment of high frequencies of a lactase persistence allele in Northern Europe in the absence of milk dependence, Flatz and Rotthauwe advanced the "calcium absorption hypothesis."[62] This is based on the observation that lactose increases the absorption of calcium in subjects with high LDC in the absence of monosaccharides,[63,64] and on the assumption that rickets and osteomalacia were potent selective factors in the conditions of low solar irradiation that are characteristic of Northwestern Europe.[65,66] Notwithstanding the difficulties in obtaining experimental evidence for the calcium absorption hypothesis, the wide geographical distance between the two population groups with predominance of $LAC^{*}P$ suggests an independent origin of the lactase persistence gene in these groups and legitimates the proposition of differing selective mechanisms in the two areas. Refined molecular studies may tell us whether Afro-Arabian and European lactase persistence have a common or a separate mutational origin.

NUTRITIONAL AND MEDICAL IMPLICATIONS

The majority of humans with genetically determined low LDC live in countries where animal milk is not used in the normal diet. Consequently, lactose intolerance is not likely to occur. Even in milk-consuming societies, lactose intolerance is not a frequent medical problem, because individuals with lactase restriction seem to adjust milk intake to their individual tolerance level. This is exemplified by the observation that the diet manuals in 58 percent of 323 American hospitals did not contain instructions with respect to lactose intolerance.[67] Lactose intolerance is most likely to develop when people with low LDC change their dietary habits—for example, following the move from a country with low milk consumption to an area where milk use is high, or when nutrients with high lactose concentration, such as powdered milk, are distributed during relief programs in communities where the majority of people have low LDC. In these cases, the pharmacologic action of lactose in subjects with lactase restriction should be kept in mind. Personal communications from several professionals from Southern European or tropical countries indicate that a glass of cold milk is a convenient and inexpensive laxative in subjects with low lactase activity.

Several associations between the adult lactase phenotypes and diseases have been reported, but the evidence is controversial. A role of low LDC in recurrent abdominal pain in children[68-70] and in irritable bowel syndrome in adults[71-77] has been claimed, but there are other reports that do not support this association.[78-83] Only a few of these studies are satisfactory with respect to matching in ethnicity between the patient and control groups, which seems mandatory in view of the great variation in the distribution of the lactase phenotypes. The possible placebo effect of milk withdrawal must also be taken into consideration.[84] Lactase persistence is not devoid of possible disease associations. There is some evidence for a role of milk consumption by lactase-persistent subjects in the causation of hyperlipidemia,[85] coronary heart disease,[86] and cataract.[87] A study in Italy demonstrated a high frequency of premature cataract in milk-consuming subjects with high LDC,[88] but similar surveys in Sweden and Mexico were negative.[89,90] Since the cataracts observed in genetic disorders of galactose metabolism are attributed to galactitol, physiological differences in galactose metabolism and milk consumption may play a role in the development of cataracts. One study revealed a high risk of cataract formation in subjects with high lactose intake and low activities of galactokinase.[91]

An even more controversial subject is the role of lactase restriction in presenile osteoporosis. It is not possible to discuss this aspect of the association between lactase phenotypes and disease fully in the context of this chapter. Several reports describe a significantly higher frequency of lactase restriction in osteoporotic women in comparison with control groups,[92-95] and a reduction of calcium availability by milk avoidance and by reduced absorption is claimed to be a causative factor. However, there are doubts[96] that a high calcium intake can prevent osteoporosis, and the recommendations for daily adult calcium intake vary considerably.[97-99] No ill effects have been observed following prolonged restriction of calcium intake to less than 200 mg/day,[100] an amount easily supplied by a milk-free diet. Furthermore, in contrast to osteomalacia, osteoporosis is not primarily due to calcium deficiency. It is rather a defect of bone matrix formation that is influenced by several other factors, such as physical activity, exposure to sunshine, hormonal status, and vitamin and protein nutrition. At present, one can hardly say more about the role of lactase restriction in osteoporosis of the elderly than that it may be a contributory factor in milk-consuming societies where a large part of the daily protein and calcium requirement is covered by milk and milk products.

REFERENCES

1. Röhmann F, Lappe J: Über die Lactase des Dünndarms. *Ber Dtsch Chem Ges* **28:**2506, 1895.
2. Auricchio S, Rubino A, Semenza G, Landolt M, Prader A: Isolated intestinal lactase deficiency in the adult. *Lancet* **2:**324, 1963.
3. Dahlqvist A, Hammond B, Crane RK, Dunphy JV, Littman A: Intestinal lactase deficiency and lactose intolerance in adults: Preliminary report. *Gastroenterology* **45:**488, 1963.
4. McKusick V: *Mendelian Inheritance in Man, Catalogs of Autosomal Dominant, Autosomal Recessive, and X-linked Phenotypes,* 9th ed. Baltimore, Johns Hopkins University Press, 1990.
5. Bayless TM, Rosensweig NS: A racial difference in the incidence of lactase deficiency. A survey of milk intolerance and lactase deficiency in healthy adult males. *JAMA* **197:**968, 1966.
6. Ford EB: *Genetic Polymorphism.* London, Faber & Faber, 1965.
7. Newcomer AD, McGill DB: Distribution of disaccharidase activity in the small bowel of normal and lactase-deficient subjects. *Gastroenterology* **51:**481, 1966.
8. Newcomer AD, McGill DB, Thomas PJ, Hofmann AF: Prospective comparison of indirect methods for detecting lactase deficiency. *N Engl J Med* **293:**1232, 1975.
9. Metneki J, Czeizel A, Flatz SD, Flatz G: A study of lactose absorption capacity in twins. *Hum Genet* **67:**296, 1984.

10. Blaxter KL: Lactation and the growth of the young, in Kow SK, Cowie AS (eds): *Milk: The Mammary Gland and Its Secretion*. New York, Academic, 1961, p 329.
11. Simoons FJ: Age of onset of lactose malabsorption. *Pediatrics* **66**:646, 1980.
12. Thomas S, Walker-Smith JA, Senewiratne B, Hjelm M: Age dependency of the lactase persistence and lactase restriction phenotypes among children in Sri Lanka and Britain. *J Trop Pediatr* **36**:80, 1990.
13. Wittenberg DF, Moosa A: Lactose maldigestion—age specific prevalence in black and Indian children. *S Afr Med J* **78**:470, 1990.
14. Sahi T, Launiala K, Laitinen H: Hypolactasia in a fixed cohort of young Finnish adults, a follow-up study. *Scand J Gastroenterol* **18**:865, 1983.
15. Flatz G, Rotthauwe HW: Evidence against nutritional adaption of tolerance to lactose. *Hum Genet* **13**:118, 1971.
16. Knudsen KB, Welsh MD, Kronenberg RS, Vanderveen JE, Heidelbauch ND: Effect of a nonlactose diet on human intestinal disaccharidase activity. *Am J Dig Dis* **13**:593, 1968.
17. Lebenthal E, Sunshine P, Kretchmer N: Effect of prolonged nursing on the activity of intestinal lactase. *Gastroenterology* **64**:1136, 1973.
18. Cuatrecasas PD, Lockwood H, Caldwell J: Lactase deficiency in the adult: A common occurrence. *Lancet* **1**:14, 1965.
19. Sahi T: The inheritance of selective adult-type lactose malabsorption. *Scand J Gastroenterol Suppl* **30**:1, 1974.
20. Krasilnikoff PA, Gudmand-Hoyer E, Moltke HH: Diagnostic value of disaccharidase tolerance in children. *Acta Paediatr Scand* **64**:693, 1975.
21. Sahi T, Isokoski M, Jussila J, Launiala K, Pyörälä K: Recessive inheritance of adult-type lactose malabsorption. *Lancet* **2**:823, 1973.
22. Fischer W, Zapf J: Zur erworbenen Laktoseintoleranz. *Klin Wochenschr* **43**:1243, 1965.
23. Isokoski M, Jussila J, Sarna S: A simple screening method for lactose malabsorption. *Gastroenterology* **62**:28, 1972.
24. Lisker R, Gonzales B, Daltabuit M: Recessive inheritance of the adult type of intestinal lactase deficiency. *Am J Hum Genet* **227**:662, 1975.
25. Ransome-Kuti O, Kretchmer N, Johnson JD, Gribble JT: A genetic study of lactose digestion in Nigerian families. *Gastroenterology* **68**:431, 1975.
26. Ho MW, Povey S, Swallow D: Lactase polymorphism in adult British natives: Estimating allele frequencies by enzyme assays in autopsy samples. *Am J Hum Genet* **34**:650, 1982.
27. Flatz G: Gene dosage effect on lactase activity demonstrated in vivo. *Am J Hum Genet* **36**:306, 1984.
28. Flatz G, Rotthauwe HW: The human lactase polymorphism: Physiology and genetics of lactose absorption and malabsorption. *Prog Med Genet* **2**:205, 1977.
29. Johnson RC, Schwitters SY, Cole RE, Ahern FM, Au K: A family study of lactose intolerance. *Behav Genet* **11**:369, 1981.
30. Kruse TA, Bolund L, Grzeschik KH, Ropers HH, Sjöström H, Noren O, Mantei N, Semenza G: The human lactase-phlorizin hydrolase gene is located on chromosome 2. *FEBS Lett* **240**:123, 1988.
31. Boll W, Wagner P, Mantei N: Structure of the chromosomal gene and cDNAs coding for lactase-phlorizin hydrolase in humans with adult-type hypolactasia or persistence of lactase. *Am J Hum Genet* **48**:889, 1991.
32. Freund JN, Duluc I, Raul F: Discrepancy between the intestinal lactase enzymatic activity and mRNA accumulation in sucklings and adults. Effect of starvation and thyroxine treatment. *FEBS Lett* **248**:39, 1989.
33. Sebastio G, Hunziker W, Ballabio A, Auricchio S, Semenza G: On the primary site of control of the spontaneous development of small-intestinal sucrase-isomaltase after birth. *FEBS Lett* **208**:460, 1986.
34. Witte J, Lloyd M, Lorenzson V, Korsmo H, Olsen W: The biosynthesic basis of adult lactase deficiency. *J Clin Invest* **86**:1338, 1990.
35. Sterchi EE, Lentze MJ, Naim HY: Molecular aspects of disaccharidase deficiencies. *Baillieres Clin Gastroenterol* **4**:79, 1990.
36. Maiuri L, Raia V, Potter J, Swallow D, Ho MW, Fiocca R, Finzi G, Cornaggia M, Capella C, Quaroni A, Auricchio S: Mosaic pattern of lactase expression by villous enterocytes in human adult-type hypolactasia. *Gastroenterology* **100**:359, 1991.
37. Büller HA, Kothe MJ, Goldman DA, Grubman SA, Sasak WV, Matsudaira PT, Montgomery RK, Grand RJ: Coordinate expression of lactase-phlorizin hydrolase mRNA and enzyme levels in rat intestine during development. *J Biol Chem* **265**:6978, 1990.
38. Escher JC, De Koning ND, Van Engen CGJ, Arora S, Büller HA, Montgomery RK, Grand RJ: Molecular basis of lactase levels in adult humans. *J Clin Invest* **89**:480, 1992.
39. Lloyd M, Mevissen G, Fischer M, Olsen W, Goodspeed D, Genini M, Boll W, Semenza G, Mantei N: Regulation of intestinal lactase activity in adult hypolactasia. *J Clin Invest* **89**:524, 1992.
40. Simoons FJ: The geographic hypothesis and lactose malabsorption: A weighing of the evidence. *Am J Dig Dis* **23**:963, 1978.
41. Flatz G: Genetics of lactose digestion in humans. *Adv Hum Genet* **16**:1, 1987.
42. Cloarec D, Gouilloud S, Bornet F, Bruley des Varannes S, Bizais Y, Galmiche JP: Déficit en lactase et symptomes d'intolérance au lactose dans une population adulte saine originaire de l'ouest de la France. *Gastroenterol Clin Biol* **15**:588, 1991.
43. Lember M, Tamm A: Lactose absorption and milk drinking habits in Estonians with myocardial infarction. *Br Med J* **296**:95, 1988.
44. Gendrel D, Dupont C, Richard-Lenoble D, Gendrel C, Nardou M, Choussain M: Milk lactose malabsorption in Gabon measured by the breath hydrogen test. *J Pediatr Gastroenterol Nutr* **8**:545, 1989.
45. Kar P, Tandon RK: Lactose intolerance in Nagaland. *Indian J Med Res* **82**:254, 1985.
46. Yap I, Berris B, Kang JY, Math M, Chu M, Miller D, Pollard A: Lactase deficiency in Singapore-born and Canadian-born Chinese. *Dig Dis Sci* **34**:1085, 1989.
47. Goldman B, Corcino JJ: Adult lactose malabsorption in Puerto Rico. *Ann Clin Lab Sci* **6**:352, 1976.
48. Solomons NW, Garcia-Ibanez R, Viteri FE: Hydrogen breath test of lactose absorption in adults: The application of physiological doses and whole cow's milk sources. *Am J Clin Nutr* **33**:545, 1980.
49. Lacassie Y, Weinberg R, Monckeberg F: Poor predictability of lactose malabsorption from clinical symptoms for children populations. *Am J Clin Nutr* **31**:799, 1978.
50. Troncon LED, Collares EF, Oliveira RB, Padovan N, Meneghelli UG: Lactose malabsorption in adult patients of the Hospital das Clinicas de Ribeirao Preto. *Arqu Gastr* **18**:106, 1981.
51. Newcomer AD, Thomas PJ, McGill DB, Hofmann AF: Lactase deficiency: A common genetic trait of the American Indian. *Gastroenterology* **72**:234, 1977.
52. Gudmand-Hoyer E, McNair A, Jarnum S, Broersma L, McNair J: Laktosemalabsorption i Vestgronland. *Ugeskr Laeger* **135**:169, 1973.
53. Dahlqvist A: The basic aspects of the chemical background of lactase deficiency. *Postgrad Med J* **53**:57, 1977.
54. Nei M, Saitou N: Genetic relationship of human populations and ethnic differences in relation to drugs and food, in Kalow W, Goedde HW, Agarwal DP (eds): *Ethnic Differences in Reactions to Drugs and Other Xenobiotics*. New York, Alan R. Liss, 1986, p 21.
55. Bayoumi RAL, Flatz SD, Kühnau W, Flatz G: Beja and Nilotes: Nomadic pastoralist groups in the Sudan with opposite distributions of the adult lactase phenotypes. *Am J Phys Anthropol* **58**:173, 1982.
56. Hijazi SS, Abulaban A, Ammarin Z, Flatz G: Distribution of adult lactase phenotypes in Bedouins and in urban and agricultural populations of Jordan. *Trop Geogr Med* **35**:157, 1983.
57. Johnson JD, Kretchmer N, Simoons FJ: Lactose malabsorption: Its biology and history. *Adv Pediatr* **21**:197, 1974.
58. Simoons FJ: Primary adult lactose intolerance and the milking

habit: A problem in biological and cultural interrelations, II. A culture historical hypothesis. *Am J Dig Dis* **15:**695, 1970.

59. Flatz G: Laktase-Phänotypen in seßhaften und nomadischen Bevölkerungsgruppen des Nahen Ostens. *Homo* **35:**173, 1984.
60. Piazza A, Menozzi P, Cavalli-Sforza LL: The HLA-A,B gene frequencies in the world: Migration or selection? *Hum Immunol* **4:**297, 1980.
61. Ammermann AJ, Cavalli-Sforza LL: Measuring the rate of spread of early farming in Europe. *Man* **6:**674, 1971.
62. Flatz G, Rotthauwe HW: Lactose nutrition and natural selection. *Lancet* **2:**76, 1973.
63. Cochet B, Jung A, Griessen M, Bartholdi P, Schaller P, Donath A: Effects of lactose on intestinal calcium absorption in normal and lactase deficient subjects. *Gastroenterology* **84:**935, 1983.
64. Birlouez-Aragon I: Effect of lactose hydrolysis on calcium absorption during duodenal milk perfusion. *Reprod Nutr Dev* **28:**1465, 1988.
65. Jonxis JHP: Some investigations on rickets. *J Pediatr* **59:**607, 1961.
66. Loomis WF: Skin-pigment regulation of vitamin-D biosynthesis in man. *Science* **157:**501, 1967.
67. Welsh JD: Diet therapy in adult lactose malabsorption: Present practices. *Am J Clin Nutr* **31:**592, 1978.
68. Bayless TM, Huang SS: Recurrent abdominal pain due to milk and lactose intolerance in school-aged children. *Pediatrics* **47:**1029, 1971.
69. Barr RG, Levine MD, Watkins JB: Recurrent abdominal pain of childhood due to lactose intolerance: A prospective study. *N Engl J Med* **300:**1449, 1979.
70. Liebman WM: Recurrent abdominal pain in children: Lactose and sucrose intolerance. *Pediatrics* **64:**43, 1979.
71. McMichael HB, Webb J, Dawson AM: Lactase deficiency in adults: A cause of 'functional' diarrhoea. *Lancet* **1:**717, 1965.
72. Weser E, Rubin W, Ross L, Sleizenger MH: Lactase deficiency in patients with the 'irritable-colon syndrome.' *N Engl J Med* **273:**1070, 1965.
73. McDonaugh TJ: Lactose intolerance: A newly recognized cause of gastrointestinal symptoms seen in the practice of occupational medicine. *J Occup Med* **11:**57, 1969.
74. Fung WP, Kho KM: The importance of milk intolerance in patients presenting with chronic (nervous) diarrhoea. *Aust N Z J Med* **1:**374, 1971.
75. Pena AS, Truelove SC: Hypolactasia and the irritable colon syndrome. *Scand J Gastroenterol* **7:**433, 1972.
76. Gudmand-Hoyer E, Riis P, Wulff HR: The significance of lactose malabsorption in the irritable colon syndrome. *Scand J Gastroenterol* **8:**273, 1973.
77. Porro GB, Petrillo M, Parente F, Sangaletti O, Della Vedova G: Recurrent abdominal pain and lactose intolerance. *Br Med J* **283:**501, 1981.
78. Newcomer AD, McGill DB: Irritable bowel syndrome: Role of lactase deficiency. *Mayo Clin Proc* **58:**339, 1983.
79. Blumenthal I, Kelleher J, Littlewood JM: Recurrent abdominal pain and lactose intolerance in childhood. *Br Med J* **282:**2013, 1980.
80. Christensen MF: Prevalence of lactose malabsorption in children with recurrent abdominal pain. *Pediatrics* **65:**681, 1980.
81. Lebenthal E, Rossi TM, Nord KS, Branski D: Recurrent abdominal pain and lactose malabsorption in children. *Pediatrics* **67:**828, 1981.
82. Dearlove J, Dearlove B, Pearl K, Primavesi R: Dietary lactose and the child with abdominal pain. *Br Med J* **286:**1936, 1983.
83. Wald A, Chandra R, Fisher SE: Lactose malabsorption in recurrent abdominal pain of childhood. *J Pediatr* **100:**65, 1982.
84. MacLean WC: Lactose intolerance. *N Engl J Med* **302:**177, 1980.
85. Sahi T, Jussila J, Penttilä I, Sarna S, Isokoski M: Serum lipids and proteins in lactose malabsorption. *Am J Clin Nutr* **30:**476, 1977.
86. Segall JJ: Hypothesis. Is lactose a dietary risk factor for ischaemic heart disease? *Int J Epidemiol* **9:**271, 1980.
87. Simoons FJ: A geographic approach to senile cataracts. Possible links with milk consumption, lactase activity and galactose metabolism. *Dig Dis Sci* **27:**257, 1982.
88. Rinaldi E, Albini L, Costagliola C, Derosa G, Auricchio G, Devizia B, Aurichio S: High frequency of lactose absorbers among adults with idiopathic senile and presenile cataract in a population with a high prevalence of primary adult lactose malabsorption. *Lancet* **1:**355, 1984.
89. Bengtson B, Steen B, Dahlqvist A, Jägerstad M: Does lactose intake induce cataract in man? *Lancet* **1:**1293, 1984.
90. Lisker RL, Cervantes G, Perez-Briceno R, Alva G: Lack of relationship between lactose absorption and senile cataracts. *Ann Ophthalmol* **20:**436, 1988.
91. Jacques PF, Phillips J, Hartz SC, Chylack LT: Lactose intake, galactose metabolism and senile cataract. *Nutr Res* **10:**255, 1990.
92. Birge SJ, Keutmann HT, Cuatrecasas P, Whedon GD: Osteoporosis, intestinal lactase deficiency and low dietary calcium intake. *N Engl J Med* **276:**445, 1967.
93. Newcomer AD, Hodgson SF, McGill DB, Thomas PJ: Lactase deficiency: Prevalence in osteoporosis. *Ann Intern Med* **89:**218, 1978.
94. Velebit L, Cochet B, Courvoisier B: Incidence de l'intolerance au lactose dans l'osteoporose post-menopausique. *Schweiz Med Wochenschr* **108:**2061, 1978.
95. Kocian J, Vulterinova M, Beijblova O, Skala I: Influence of lactose intolerance on the bones of patients after partial gastrectomy. *Digestion* **8:**324, 1973.
96. Alhava EM, Jussila J, Karjalainen P, Vuojolahti P: Lactose malabsorption and bone mineral content. *Acta Med Scand* **201:**281, 1977.
97. Food and Nutrition Board: *Recommended Dietary Allowances*. Washington, DC: National Academy of Sciences, 1968, p 233.
98. Walker ARP: The human requirement of calcium: Should low intake be supplemented? *Am J Clin Nutr* **25:**518, 1972.
99. Passmore R, Nicol BM, Rac MN: *Handbook on Human Nutritional Requirements*. Geneva, World Health Organization, 1974, p 453.
100. Hegstedt DM, Moscosco I, Collazos C: A study of the minimum calcium requirement of adult men. *J Nutr* **48:**181, 1952.

CHAPTER 151

Small-Intestinal Disaccharidases*

Giorgio Semenza ▪ Salvatore Auricchio

1. **The brush-border membrane of the human small intestine is endowed with a total of seven glycosidases, which give rise to free monosaccharides by splitting dietary disaccharides and oligosaccharides that arise in the intestinal lumen from the α amylolysis of starch. The four "maltases" occur as two heterodimers (i.e., the glucoamylase complex and the sucrase–isomaltase complex); the β-glycosidase complex, which is composed of a single type of polypeptide, has two catalytic sites (lactase and glycosylceramidase). Trehalase is composed of a single type of subunit(s) (Table 151-1). These glycosidases are "stalked" intrinsic proteins of the membrane; the "body" of the protein mass, including the catalytic sites, protrudes toward the small-intestinal lumen.**
2. **The glycosidases (with the possible exception of trehalase, the synthesis of which is still little known) are synthesized as large polypeptide chains, each of which has an apparent molecular weight in the range 200,000 to 250,000. These "pro" forms are each split into the final forms either extracellularly (as are the α-glucosidase complexes) or intracellularly (the β-glycosidase complex; see Table 151-2). Since the two catalytic domains in each of these complexes belong to a single translational unit, they are subjected to the same biologic control mechanism(s).**
3. **Mammals other than humans are equipped at birth with the β-glycosidase and the glucoamylase complexes. Sucrase–isomaltase and trehalase develop at the time of weaning, when the β-glucosidase complex begins to decline, eventually reaching a level as low as 5 to 10 percent of that at birth. In contrast, in human beings the brush-border disaccharidases develop before birth, beginning prior to the tenth week of gestation, with a developmental "burst" (particularly in the β-glycosidase complex) a few weeks before birth. The level of the β-glycosidase complex—in effect, the level of lactase activity—remains high throughout adulthood in most white people and a few other races.**
4. **The primary site of control in the spontaneous physiological development of sucrase–isomaltase is in all likelihood at the level of transcription. Dietary and hormonal factors also control the levels of disaccharidase activities.**
5. **Both secondary and primary (genetic) disaccharidase deficiencies are known, which may lead to malabsorption and intolerance of the corresponding disaccharide(s), but not of the constituent monosaccharides. Diagnosis depends on determination of enzyme activities through small-intestinal biopsies and/or on oral tolerance test with the corresponding disaccharides; among the latter, the breath hydrogen test is particularly reliable.**
6. **All genetic defects of intestinal disaccharidases are monofactorial, autosomal, and recessive. The most common of them (indeed, perhaps the most common of all genetic disturbances in humans, affecting one-third to one-half of the human race) is adult hypolactasia; in this condition intestinal lactase declines in childhood or shortly thereafter (as it does in mammals other than human beings) to 10 percent or less of the level at birth.**
7. **Sucrase–isomaltase deficiency is much rarer and is genetically heterogeneous. Congenital lactase deficiency and trehalase deficiency are extremely rare, and virtually nothing is known about their molecular basis.**

A list of standard abbreviations appears immediately preceding the index in each volume.

LUMINAL HYDROLYSIS OF STARCH

In the average Western diet, starch provides approximately 50 percent of absorbable carbohydrates, but disaccharides (mainly sucrose and lactose) are also important nutrients. In addition, small amounts of free fructose, of the disaccharide trehalose (which is hydrolyzed into two molecules of glucose), and of nonabsorbable carbohydrates including dietary fiber, stachyose, and raffinose are ingested.[1–3]

Starch is a mixture of two types of polysaccharides, amylose and amylopectin. Amylose has a linear structure and is made up of 1-4-α-linked glucose units. Amylopectin has a branched structure: the majority of the glucose residues are connected by 1,4-α-glucosidic bonds (the linear chains); the branch points are made by 1,6-α-glucosidic linkages. In the digestive tract, starch is eventually hydrolyzed to yield free glucose by the cumulative action of both the salivary and pancreatic α-amylases, the latter being present in solution in the intestinal lumen (but also adsorbed at the surface of the brush-border membrane), and of the α-glucosidases of the intestinal mucosa.

The hydrolysis in vitro of amylose by salivary or pancreatic α-amylase starts as a random hydrolysis of the internal 1,4 bonds. As it proceeds, it becomes more and more selective, as a result of the greater resistance to enzymatic attack of the last and next-to-last 1,4-α-glucopyranosyl bonds at the nonreducing end of the small linear 1,4-α-glucans and of the 1,4-α bond adjacent to the reducing end.[4–10] The final (limit) products resulting from amylose hydrolysis in vitro are maltose and maltotriose[11]; those from amylopectin are

*In this chapter we will use the term *disaccharidases* to refer to the enzymes in Tables 151-1 and 151-2. The term will be used even in cases in which the substrates of interest are oligosaccharides or glycosides other than disaccharides.

Table 151-1 Major Intestinal Disaccharidases

Enzyme or Complex	Representative Data on Substrate Specificities
Glucoamylase complex (EC 3.2.1.20; the "heat-stable" maltases): glucoamylase-(maltase)-1 + glucoamylase-(maltase)-2	See Fig. 151-2. In detail, the two catalytic sites have similar but probably not quite identical substrate specificities.[36,41] They split 1,4-α-glucopyranosidic bonds from the nonreducing ends of amylose, amylopectin, glycogen, and straight-chain 1,4-α-glucopyranosyl oligomers, including maltose.[40,42] Minor 1,6-α-glucopyranosidase activity.[39,42–44]
Sucrase–isomaltase complex (the "heat-labile" maltases): sucrase–(maltase) (EC 3.2.1.48) + isomaltase–(maltase) (EC 3.2.1.10)	See Fig. 151-2. In addition, both subunits split maltose (see, for example, refs. 43, 44, and 56), maltotriose,[46] maltitol (Semenza G, Balthazar AK: unpublished), α-*F*-glucopyranoside,[47] and (less well) aryl-α-glucopyranosides.[48] In addition, the sucrase subunit splits sucrose and turanose[49]; the isomaltase subunit splits the 1,6-α-glucopyranosyl bonds in isomaltose, isomaltulose (palatinose), and panose and in a number of branched limit α-dextrins.[38,43–45,50,51]
Trehalase (EC 3.2.1.28)	α,α′-Trehalose and 6,6′-dideoxy-α-α′-trehalose[52]; α- and β-*F*-glucopyranoside (tested on renal trehalase)[53]
β-Glycosidase complex: lactase (EC 3.2.1.23) + glycosylceramidase (EC 3.2.1.45–46; also called phlorizin hydrolase, EC 3.2.1.62)	A number of β-glycosides: α- and β-lactose, 3-(β-D-galactosido)-D-glucose, 6-(βD-galactosido)-D-glucose, aryl-β-galactopyranosides, aryl-β-glucopyranosides, methyl-β-galactopyranoside.[54,55] The "lactase" site preferentially splits β-glycosides with hydrophilic aglycons (typically lactose, but also cellobiose,[56–59] cellotriose, and cellotetrose, and also, but much less, cellulose[59]), whereas the "glycosylceramidase" site preferentially splits β-glycosides with a large, hydrophobic aglycon (typically, galactosyl- and glycosyl-β-ceramides,[58] phlorizin,[60] and other aryl-β-glycosides.[55,61]

glucose (in small amounts), maltose, maltotriose, and branched dextrins (Fig. 151-1).[12–16]

In humans older than 1 year, the α-amylase activity of duodenal juice after a test meal is very high; the intestinal hydrolysis of starch in vivo is thus very rapid. The amylopectin of a test meal consisting of more than 5000 glucose units is digested at the end of the duodenum into oligosaccharides composed of an average of three glucose units.[17] The major components of this carbohydrate mixture are maltose, maltotriose, and branched dextrins with both 1,4-α and one or more 1,6-α branching links. (Isomaltose is not produced in the digestion of starch by α-amylase.[17]) Maltose, maltotriose, and at least some of these branched dextrins must be considered limit products of the α amylolysis in vivo, which are further hydrolyzed into free glucose by brush-border α-glucosidases; see "Intestinal (Membrane Surface) Hydrolysis of Oligosaccharides" below.

Although the intraluminal hydrolysis of free starch does proceed rapidly in vivo, the starch in most staple foods (wheat, corn, oats, potatoes) may escape *complete* digestion and absorption in the small intestine, and thus some may reach the colon.[18,19] From the amount of hydrogen excreted in the breath[20] (see "Diagnosis of Disaccharidase Deficiency, Carbohydrate Malabsorption, and Carbohydrate Intolerance" below) after an oral load of 100 g of flours from different sources, the proportion of starch not absorbed by the healthy small bowel was estimated to be 5 to 20 percent.[18,19] These values were then confirmed by measuring directly the ileal recovery of carbohydrates after ingestion of starch.[21,22] The type of starch and the protein content of

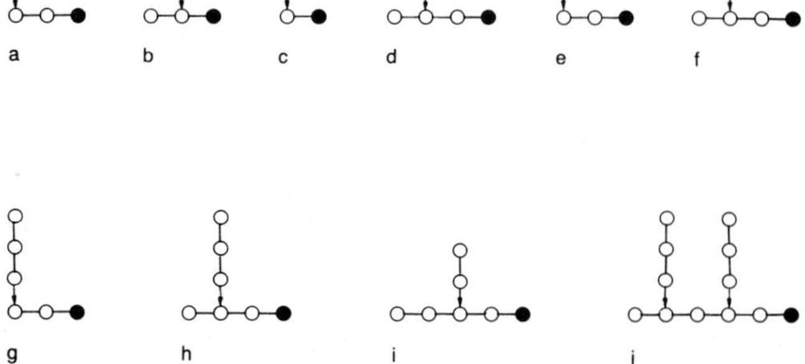

FIG. 151-1 Branched limit dextrins from the α amylolysis of amylopectin in vitro. ○ = nonreducing glucose unit; ● = reducing glucose unit; — = 1,4-α-glucopyranosidic bond; → = 1,6-α-glucopyranosidic bond. (*From Auricchio et al.*[452] *Used by permission.*)

Table 151-2 Molecular Weights of the Small-Intestinal Disaccharidases and of Their Precursors*

Enzyme	Species	M_r (thousands) of the Primary Translation Product, Nonglycosylated Form†	Brush-Border Form (in parentheses, the M_r (thousands) of Proteolytically Cleaved Mature Forms)	References
Glucoamylase complex	Pig	200	~245 (125, 135)	97, 116
(maltases-glucoamylases)	Human	~230	~335	82d
Sucrase–isomaltase complex	Rabbit	210.139	~275 (120,140)‡	76,80,84,89,124
	Human	209.074	~235 (145,150)	82a, 117
	Rat		~240 (140,160)	82c
	Pig	225	~265 (140,150)	115,116
Trehalase	Rabbit	65.516	~66	141
β-Glycosidase complex	Rabbit	215.629	121.221§	99
(Lactase–phlorizin	Human	216.393	120.068§	99,102,103,107,117
hydrolase; lactase–			262 (156)⁺	446,447
glycosylceramidase)	Rat	217.266	225 (130)⁺	82b, 101,104,205
	Pig	210	245 (160)	101

*During their migration from the ER membrane through the Golgi stacks to the brush-border membrane, these membrane proteins are N-glycosylated first (to high-mannose, endo-H sensitive forms), trimmed and eventually complex-glycosylated (see text). The glycosylated forms naturally have larger molecular weights than the nonglycosylated forms. Trehalase exchanges its transient C-terminal hydrophobic peptide sequence for the final phosphoinositol anchor in the ER. Pre-pro-lactase-phlorizin hydrolase is subjected to extensive proteolytic processing (see text).

†The M_r values are either estimates from SDS-PAGE or have been deduced from the cDNA. In the latter case, the M_r values of the primary translation products have been calculated from the initiation methionine to the stop codon, i.e., they include the cleavable, or noncleavable, signal, and, in the case of trehalase, the transient hydrophobic anchoring sequence that is exchanged in the ER for a phosphoinositol anchor.

‡The smaller subunit is sucrase, the larger one is isomaltase and carries the hydrophobic anchor not far the N-terminus.[79,85] Sucrase stems from the C-terminal and isomaltase from the N-terminal portion of pro-sucrase-isomaltase.[83]

§Calculated from the cDNA and from the position of the secondary N-terminus.

⁺The differences in apparent molecular sizes (by SDS-PAGE) between human and rat lactase–phlorizin hydrolases are real,[82c] and are probably due to different extents of glycosylation.

the flours appear to be important, because starch from all-purpose wheat flour and from potato is absorbed by the small intestine less completely than that from rice flour or low-gluten wheat flour.[18,19] With other foods, such as legumes or rices rich in amyloses,[23] the percentage of carbohydrates reaching the colon may be even higher. It has been calculated that a substantial amount of dietary starch, perhaps as much as 40 g/day, may reach the colon.[21]

The diarrhea that would otherwise ensue from the delivery of such large quantities of carbohydrates to the large intestine is prevented by the action of the colonic flora. Inadequately absorbed carbohydrates are in fact salvaged through fermentation to gases (hydrogen, methane, and carbon dioxide) and to acetic, propionic, and butyric acids; these acids are readily absorbed from and/or metabolized in the colon. This organ, therefore, makes an important contribution to the absorption of carbohydrates escaping small-intestinal digestion,[24] so that, as a rule, sugars are absent from the stool. As a matter of fact, after the first year of life children are able to absorb, almost completely, 170 g/m² of body surface of cooked wheat or potato starch, administered in biscuits and macaroni.[25] The human colon is able to metabolize anaerobically up to 50 g of unprocessed wheat starch without changing the stool content of volatile fatty acids and lactic acid or its bacterial mass.[26,27]

DIGESTION OF STARCH AND GLUCOSE POLYMERS IN HUMAN INFANTS

α-Amylase activity in the duodenal lumen does not reach normal adult levels until well after birth.[17] There is practically no α-amylase activity in the duodenal fluid of premature and term infants at birth.[28] After the first month of life, amylase activity can be increased on stimulation by pancreozymin and secretin and in response to ingested starch.[29] As a consequence of the low levels of α-amylase activity in duodenal juice, in most infants younger than 6 months of age the duodenal hydrolysis of amylopectin is incomplete, with large amounts of dextrin composed of more than 30 glucose units and, in comparison with older infants, less maltose and more maltotetrose in the luminal fluid; maltotetrose accounts for only 1 to 3 percent of total carbohydrates in the duodenal juice by the end of the first year of life.[17]

This does not mean that young infants may not absorb even sizable quantities of starch and glucose polymers almost completely.[25,30–32] One-month-old infants may tolerate up to 100 g/m² of rice starch per day, whereas larger quantities cause fermentative diarrhea.[25] However, healthy young infants do not absorb glucose polymers longer than 43 glucose units as completely as short-chain glucose polymers (e.g., 3 to 8 glucose units).[33] The capability of young infants to digest limited amounts of starches and glucose polymers in spite of low levels of pancreatic α-amylase may depend on various factors. First of all, the low levels of salivary[34] and of pancreatic α-amylase activity in duodenal juice may still be sufficient if the quantities of starch or glucose polymers are small. Furthermore, the glucoamylase of the small-intestinal mucosa probably plays an important role in digestion of dextrins and glucose polymers during the first few months of life, even if this enzyme is best suited for the hydrolysis of oligomers smaller than 10 glucose residues.[35,36] Finally, at this age also the colonic flora undoubtedly plays a significant role in salvaging unabsorbed starch and glucose polymers.[31]

INTESTINAL (MEMBRANE SURFACE) HYDROLYSIS OF OLIGOSACCHARIDES

The elaborate structure of the brush border greatly expands the surface area of the apical plasma membrane (to some 200 m² in a normal adult man!), making it better suited to carry out the final steps in digestion and to absorb the resulting products. The tight packing of microvilli, however, also results in thick, unstirred layers, to which mucus also contributes. The limiting factor in membrane digestion in vivo is often the diffusion of the substrate from the lumen to the membrane surface. It seems very appropriate, therefore, that large molecules such as starch and glycogen are first split by enzymes present in solution in the lumen (through "cavital digestion") and that their smaller, partial degradation products diffuse onto the brush-border membrane to be split further ("membrane digestion"[37]).

Table 151-1 reports the essentials of the substrate specificities of brush-border glycosidases (more can be found in the original literature cited). Considering only the digestion of the oligosaccharides and disaccharides commonly occurring as such in the diet, or arising during the digestion of starch and glycogen, the β-glycosidase complex accounts for all the lactase activity; trehalase for all the trehalase activity; the sucrase–isomaltase complex for all the sucrase activity, for almost all or all of the isomaltase (1,6-α-oligosaccharidase) activity, and for about 80 percent of the maltase activity; and the maltase–glucoamylase complex for a few percent (if any) of the isomaltase activity, for about 20 percent of the maltase activity, and for all the glucoamylase activity.*

Hence, the limit dextrins arising from the α amylolysis of starch in the lumen are completely split to free glucose by the combined action of the glucoamylase and the sucrase–isomaltase complexes (Fig. 151-2).[38–40] The linear 1,4-α-glucans are split, with different V_{max} and K_m values, by the four maltases listed in Table 151-2. The 1,6-α-branched dextrins are split almost exclusively by the isomaltase subunit of the sucrase–isomaltase complex. It should be noted that these branched dextrins can be as much as 25 percent of the original starch.

In adult human small intestine, lactase–glycosylceramidase and sucrase–isomaltase activities are highest in the jejunum and lower at the proximal and distal ends. In contrast, glucoamylase activity increases along the small intestine and reaches maximal values in the ileum, or distal end.[62,63] Similar distribution patterns have been demonstrated in the intestine of the human newborn.[64,65]

The capacity for digestion of most oligosaccharides of α-glucose exceeds the capacity for absorption of the component monosaccharides. The anatomic structure of the brush-border region provides a diffusion barrier to the movement of monosaccharides (liberated by the disaccharidases) back from the outer surface of the brush-border membrane into the intestinal lumen. It thus favors the absorption of monosaccharides originating from the disaccharides.[66–70] In spite of this, some of the monosaccharides liberated do appear in the intestinal lumen[71,72]; i.e., for most oligosaccharides, hydrolysis is not rate limiting. However, the glucose itself inhibits intestinal maltases somewhat.[73]

In contrast to the hydrolysis of other oligosaccharides, that of lactose is the rate limiting step for the absorption of this sugar.[74] Even in apparently normal individuals, mucosal lactase activity is the lowest of all disaccharidase activities. (Indeed, the capacity of this enzyme can be exceeded easily, which results in the presence of unsplit lactose in the lumen.) The monosaccharides arising from the hydrolysis of lactose never appear in significant amounts at the luminal side of the brush border, indicating that the transport system or systems for its component monosaccharides, glucose, and galactose, are capable of completely absorbing the hydrolysis products presented to them.[75]

*Pancreatic α-amylase and brush-border glucoamylase hydrolyze only 1,4-α-glucopyranosidic bonds, as they occur, for example, in starch and other 1,4-α glucans. They differ, however, in several respects. α-Amylase prefers long chains, and does not split maltose; glucoamylase prefers short chains and does split maltose. The end products of the action of α-amylase on linear chains are maltose and maltotriose, whereas the end product of glucoamylase is glucose only. (It is set free progressively from the nonreducing ends.) Finally, different compounds are known that activate or inhibit either α-amylase or glucoamylase without affecting the other; they allow the quantitative determination of either enzyme in the presence of the other (see, for example, refs. 46 and 57).

MEMBRANE ANCHORING AND BIOSYNTHESIS OF DISACCHARIDASES

The mode of anchoring and the biosynthesis of brush-border glycosidases have been the object of some reviews,[76–78a] to which the reader is referred for details. See also, Table 151-2.

The Sucrase–Isomaltase, Maltase–Glucoamylase, and β-Glycosidase (Lactase–Phlorizin Hydrolase) Complexes*

The α-glucosidase complexes are heterodimers, each composed of two similar but not identical subunits; each subunit consists of a single glycosylated polypeptide chain with an apparent molecular weight in the 120,000 to 160,000 range (see Table 151-2). The sucrase–isomaltase[79,80] and the glucoamylase[81,82] complexes are anchored to the membrane via one subunit only. The anchoring segment in the transmembranal subunit is located not far from the N-terminus of the subunit.

The positioning of the sucrase–isomaltase complex is now known in a fair amount of detail (reviewed in refs. 76–78); (see Fig. 151-3*A*). The N-terminus of the isomaltase subunit is located at the *cytosolic* side of the membrane[80]; a number of positive charges occur in the first four amino acid residues; an extremely hydrophobic stretch of approximately 20 residues[80,83] crosses the membrane once[80] in a helical configuration[84]; and most of the protein mass of isomaltase, including the C-terminus, protrudes to the outer, luminal side of the membrane. The sucrase subunit has a peripheral positioning[85], interacting with the membrane fabric solely via isomaltase[79]; the only hydrophobic segment present in the whole complex is the one that occurs at the N-terminal region of the isomaltase subunit[80] and accounts for approximately 1 percent of the total protein mass.

In the glucoamylase complex, also, the "anchor" is confined to one subunit only[81,82]; it is located not far from the N-terminal region of that subunit.[86]

Both the sucrase–isomaltase[87] and the glucoamylase[86]

*The β-glycosidase activity associated with lactase was initially described as phlorizin hydrolase (β-glucosidase).[60] It was later recognized[58] that the "natural" substrates of β-glycosidase are β-glucosyl and β-galactosyl ceramides. These substrates, however, are costly and are so little soluble in water that they are impractical in routine determinations. In this chapter we will refer interchangeably to this β-glycosidase activity as *phlorizin hydrolase* activity or *glycosylceramidase activity.*

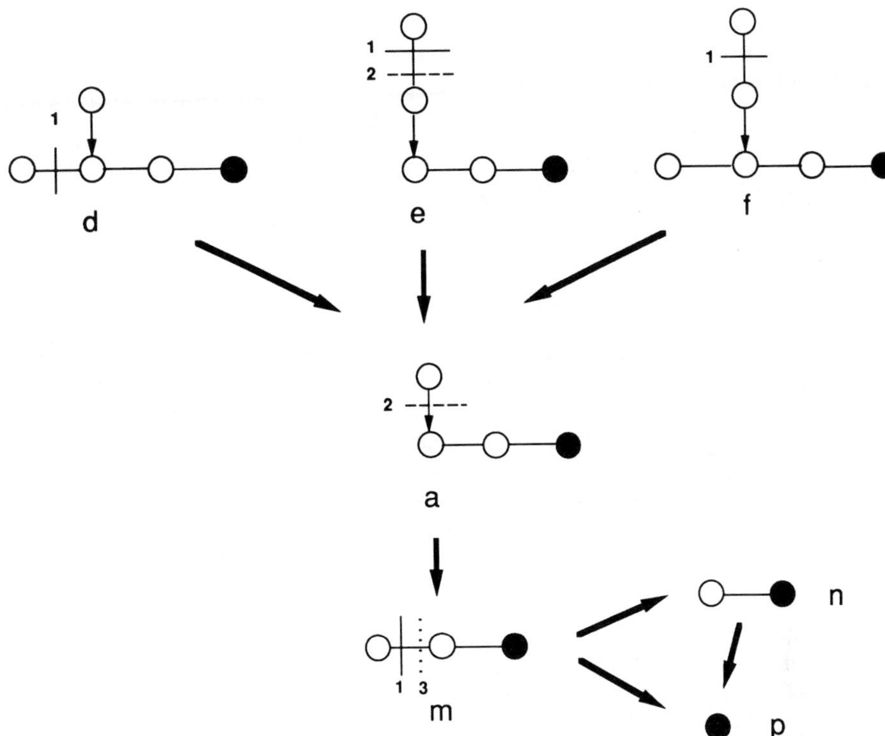

FIG. 151-2 Hydrolysis by glucoamylases by the sucrase-isomaltase of the shortest limit dextrins resulting from exhaustive digestion of starch by α-amylase. ○ = nonreducing glucopyranose unit; ● = reducing glucopyranose unit; ——— = 1,4-α-glucopyranosidic bond; → = 1,6-α-glucopyranosidic bond. *d* = 6-α-D-glucopyranosyl-maltotetraose; *e* = 6-α-D-maltopyranosyl-maltotriose; *f* = 6-α-D-maltopyranosyl-maltotetraose; *a* = 6-α-D-glucopyranosyl-maltotriose; *m* = maltotriose; *n* = maltose; *p* = D-glucose; 1 ——— = bond hydrolzyed by a glucoamylase; 2 - - - - = bond hydrolyzed by isomaltase; 3 · · · · = bond hydrolyzed by sucrase.

Hence glucoamylases hydrolyze the pentasaccharides *d* and *e* and hexasaccharide *f* to the tetrasaccharide *a*. The further degradation of *a* (6-α-D-glucopyranosyl-maltotriose) to maltotriose *(m)*, maltose *(n)* and eventually to glucose *(p)* is accomplished mainly by the sucrase-isomaltase complex. *(Data from Auricchio.*[453]*)*

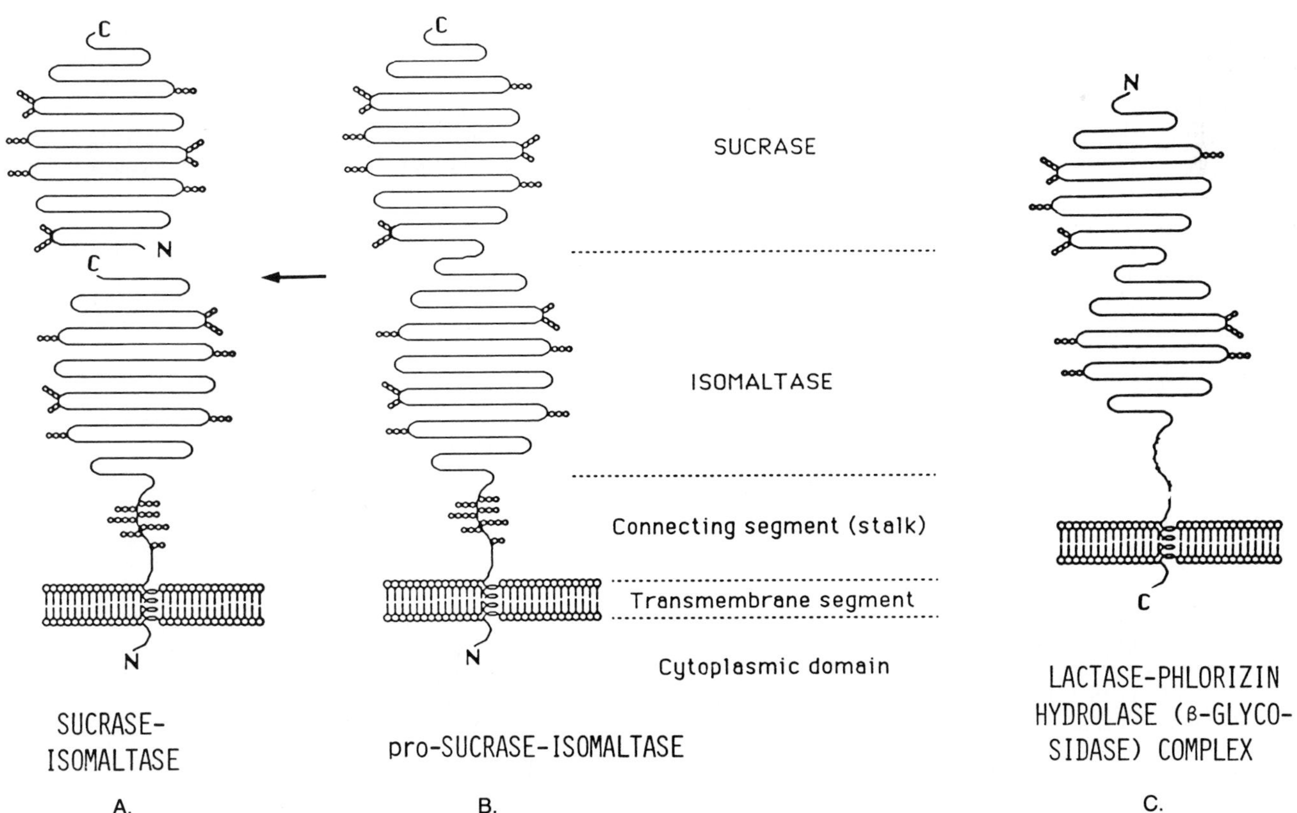

FIG. 151-3 Positioning of sucrase–isomaltase (*A*) and of pro-sucrase–isomaltase (*B*) in the small-intestinal brush-border membrane. The (unspecified) interactions within and between the sucrase and isomaltase domains (or subunits) are not indicated. ○○○ = sugar chains. (*From Semenza.*[77] *Used by permission.*) (*C*) Positioning of the lactase–phlorizin hydrolase (β-glycosidase) complex. Note the opposite direction of the polypeptide chain spanning the brush-border membrane, and also that this "complex" is composed of a *single* polypeptide chain, with the two catalytic activities associated with different domains. (*Adapted from Mantei et al.*[99]) The domain more remote from the membrane is lactase; the other, closer to it is phlorizin hydrolase.[85]

complexes dimerize further, thus forming homo-hetero-tetramers of the type $(\alpha, \beta)_2$ in the brush-border membrane.

The major lines in the biosynthesis of these heterodimers have been established in some detail for sucrase–isomaltase, but again, they seem to hold true for the other α-glucosidase complex as well.

As discussed in later sections, sucrase and isomaltase activities develop simultaneously, respond identically to hormonal and dietary stimuli, and in most cases are equally affected by genetic defects. Their identical or closely related biologic control mechanism(s), *plus* a very close similarity in the functional (and, where known, structural) properties of the two subunits,[88-90] *plus* the mode of membrane insertion of sucrase—isomaltase (in Fig. 151-3*A*, notice the peripheral positioning of sucrase and the anchoring of isomaltase via the N-terminal region) prompted one of us to formulate the "one polypeptide chain, two active sites" precursor hypothesis,[91-93] as follows: (1) An ancestral gene existed, coding for a one–polypeptide chain, one–active site enzyme that split both maltose and isomaltose (a simple isomaltase). (2) The gene was partially duplicated, resulting in a gene coding for a long single polypeptide chain with two identical active sites (a double isomaltase). (3) Point mutation(s) and/or deletion(s) changed one of these active sites from an isomaltase–maltase into a sucrase–maltase. Thereby, a long polypeptide chain was formed, carrying two similar, but not identical, active sites (the pro-sucrase–isomaltase). (4) Posttranslational modification of this single long polypeptide chain by pancreatic proteases leads to the two subunits that make up the final sucrase–isomaltase complex. The subunits remain associated with one another via interactions formed during the folding of the original single-chain pro-sucrase–isomaltase.

When sucrase–isomaltase is synthesized unexposed to pancreatic juice—whether in vivo or in vitro, whether produced in cultivated tissue or cells or translated in a cell-free system—it is always in the form of a 260,000-dalton single-chain polypeptide, i.e., of pro-sucrase–isomaltase.[76,77] Furthermore, the total sequencing of the 1827 amino acid residues of this pro-sucrase–isomaltase (by cDNA cloning and sequencing[80]) has revealed a 41 percent identity between the isomaltase and sucrase portions, with another 40 percent of nonidentical but conservative changes, 28 percent of which result from single-base mutations of the codons. This has brought final evidence, therefore, for the partial gene duplication postulated by the "one polypeptide chain, two active sites" mechanism. Finally, the characteristics and mode of membrane insertion of fowl (pro-) sucrase–isomaltase, which are very similar to those of the mammalian enzyme, strongly suggest that the mutation of double isomaltase into pro-sucrase–isomaltase took place prior to the separation of mammals from reptiles and birds, that is, more than 350 million years ago.[82]

This phylogenetic pedigree of sucrase–isomaltase has been enriched by two more observations. The membrane-spanning domains of (1) pro-sucrase–isomaltase, maltase–glucoamylase, and endopeptidase 24.11[94] (all three are brush-border enzymes) and (2) the asialoglycoprotein receptors (proteins of the basolateral membrane)[95] show significant homology to one another and have apparently evolved from an exon unrelated to those of the glucosidase portions. Furthermore, lysosomal α-glucosidase (the enzyme whose absence leads to glycogenosis type II, Pompe's disease) is reported to have a highly significant homology with brush-border sucrase and isomaltase.[96] The lysosomal enzyme lacks both the stalk and the N-terminal hydrophobic anchor of pro-sucrase–isomaltase and is synthesized with an N-terminal *cleavable* signal. Lysosomal α-glucosidase is thus likely to have evolved from the same ancestral gene as brush-border isomaltase before it acquired the hydrophobic anchor and the stalk portion. These mammalian α-glucosidases are homologous to a yeast glucoamylase.[82a]

The maltase-glucoamylase complex also is synthesized as a single polypeptide chain of 220 kDa or more,[82d,97] which is split (but not always completely) extracellularly by pancreatic proteases into the "final" unequal subunits.

The individual steps in biosynthesis and membrane insertion of these polypeptides are less well understood. It is clear, however, that pro-sucrase–isomaltase, and presumably the maltase–glucoamylase complex also, are synthesized *without* a cleavable signal, that is, that the hydrophobic stretch at the N-terminal region of isomaltase has a dual function: that of the signal ("leading sequence") during biosynthesis and insertion into the membrane of the ER, and that of the anchor in the final protein (Fig. 151-4). This was demonstrated by the pro-sucrase–isomaltase cDNA sequence, which showed no signal prior to the N-terminus of the final polypeptide.[80] Also, the N-terminal sequence of the primary translation product (in vitro, in a cell-free system, without microsomal membranes) corresponded exactly to that of "mature" pro-sucrase-isomaltase.[98]

The complete primary structure of the β-glycosidase complex (lactase–phlorizin hydrolase) and of its pre-pro form has been established.[99] It shows no homology with the sucrase–isomaltase complex or, in fact, with any other vertebrate glycosidase (homology with bacterial β-glucosidases has been reported[100]). The long pre-pro-lactase–phlorizin hydrolase (1927 amino acid residues for the human enzyme; 1926 for the rabbit homologue) comprises five domains: (1) a putative cleaved signal of 19 amino acids; (2) a large "pro" portion of 847 amino acids (in the rabbit), or 849 amino acids (in humans), none of which appears in the mature brush-border lactase–phlorizin hydrolase; (3) the mature enzyme, which contains both catalytic sites in a single polypeptide chain, lactase being distal and phlorizin hydrolase being proximal to the brush-border membrane[85];

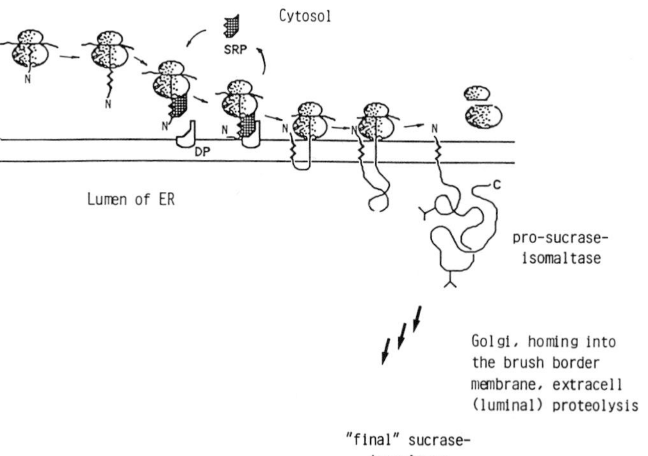

FIG. 151-4 Suggested minimum mechanism for the synthesis and membrane assembly of pro-sucrase–isomaltase. The highly hydrophobic stretch between positions 12 and 31 is suggested to play a dual role of (uncleaved) signal during biosynthesis and of membrane anchor in the final pro-sucrase–isomaltase. SRP = signal recognition particle; DP = docking protein. The sugar chains in pro-sucrase–isomaltase are shown as branches. (*From Semenza.*[77] *Used by permission.*)

(4) a membrane-spanning hydrophobic segment near the C-terminus, which serves as the membrane anchor; and (5) a short hydrophilic segment at the C-terminus, which must be cytosolic. The positioning of "final" lactase–phlorizin hydrolase in the brush-border membrane is shown in Fig. 151-3*C*.

Whereas pro-sucrase–isomaltase shows a twofold internal homology, pro-lactase–phlorizin hydrolase shows a fourfold internal homology (which indicates that partial gene duplications have occurred twice)—two of the homologous regions occur in the "pro" portion and two in mature lactase–phlorizin hydrolase. Pre-pro-lactase–phlorizin hydrolase, therefore, in addition to not showing any homology with α-glucosidases, differs from them in several respects. The degree of internal homology is different; its mode of anchoring in the brush-border membrane is different; and its mode of biosynthesis is also different in part, since it is endowed with a cleavable, rather than an uncleavable, signal.[100a]

The proteolytic processing of pre-pro-lactase to lactase differs in several respects from that of pro-sucrase–isomaltase to sucrase–isomaltase. In the ER, signal peptidase in all likelihood splits off the leading ("pre") sequence of pre-pro-lactase–phlorizin hydrolase after position 19, thereby yielding pro-lactase–phlorizin hydrolase. This is, as we will discuss below, "high-mannose" glycosylated (~200 kDa) and then "complex" glycosylated (~220 kDa). Splitting of these glycosylated forms of pro-lactase takes place in one or two steps (i.e., with the possible formation of intermediate 180- to 190-kDa polypeptides). The N-terminus of "final" lactase–phlorizin hydrolase is formed by the action of a (presumably) monobasic processing protease, splitting the Arg-Ala bond at position 866–867 (in rabbit) or position 868–869 (in humans)[101–106], or the Arg-Val bond at position 869–870 (in the rat).[82b]

These proteolytic events, which eventually lead to final lactase–phlorizin hydrolase, take place intracellularly,[101–105] most probably past the trans-Golgi network,[106a] although it is quite possible that some unsplit pro-lactase–phlorizin hydrolase escapes this processing (at least in the rat) and is cleaved by luminal proteases.[106b] Some pro-lactase–phlorizin hydrolase appears in the basolateral membrane (at least in vitro in transfected MDCK cells); its proteolytic processing into "final" lactase–phlorizin hydrolase is *not* a prerequisite for correct sorting.[106c]

The destiny and role, if any, of the pro-sequence and of fragments thereof (i.e., of nearly 850 amino acid residues in pre-pro-lactase–phlorizin hydrolase) are still unclear. Since this sequence lacks hydrophobic stretches of any length,[99] it is unlikely to be targeted to a membrane. It may be secreted into the intestinal lumen or into the intracellular space, or targeted to some intracellular compartment, or rapidly degraded. Most probably this pro-sequence does not have glycosidase activity. Indirect evidence has shown that it does not split either lactose or phlorizin (pro-lactase and "final" lactase have identical specific activities for these substrates[107]) and that it has no configuration-retaining glycosidase activity.[85] The pro-sequence is needed for the protein to reach the plasma membrane, perhaps by playing the role of an intramolecular chaperone.[106d]

From the ER membrane the pro-disaccharidases proceed to the brush-border membrane; en route they are *N*-glycosylated, trimmed, complex-glycosylated, and *O*-glycosylated by processes that have been well established for other glycoproteins of the plasma membranes. Pro-sucrase–isomaltase, and perhaps other disaccharidases also, occur in two high-mannose forms,[108] which can be distinguished immunologically. Fructose induces a block in the expression of sucrase–isomaltase and of other brush-border glycoproteins, probably via abnormal high-mannose glycosylation followed by rapid proteolytic degradation within the ER.[109] Proper folding, which in turn requires proper glycosylation and oligomerization (for an important review, see ref. 110), is needed for the synthesized protein to proceed past the ER (see refs. 111 and 112 and the references therein). Pro-lactase–phlorizin hydrolase, however, seems to move out of the ER as a monomer.[112a] In the *trans*-Golgi network pro-sucrase–isomaltase, pro-glucoamylase, aminopeptidases N and A, and a few other microvillar proteins are tyrosine-sulfated.[113,114] This process had been reported previously for secretory, but never for membrane proteins. Its possible biologic significance is still unclear.

The in vivo turnover of both sucrase–isomaltase and lactase–phlorizin hydrolase has recently been determined in adult rats.[100a] Interestingly, the mean residence time in the brush-border membrane is as short as 5.8 h for sucrase and 7.8 h for lactase. The fractional synthesis rates were more than 400 percent per day for sucrase and more than 300 percent per day for lactase.

In tissue cultures and in Caco-2 cells, movement of the glycosidases from the ER through the Golgi membranes takes 60 to 90 minutes (refs. 115 to 117 and others), which is much longer than for peptidases. This asynchronous transport to the cell surface is likely to be due to differential transit through the Golgi apparatus.[112,118,119] Pro-sucrase–isomaltase seems to be transferred to the brush-border membrane directly from the *trans*-Golgi complex, apparently without passing transiently through the basolateral membrane[120–123] (see, however, ref. 124). But pro-lactase–phlorizin hydrolase and processed lactase–phlorizin hydrolase (at least in transfected MDCK cells) appear in the basolateral membrane.[106c] This may indicate that (some?) pro-lactase–phlorizin hydrolase passes transiently through the basolateral membrane before reaching the brush border. In in vitro cultures, microvillar proteins are arrested in their high-mannose form by lowering the temperature to 20°C (e.g., ref. 125). Some sucrase–isomaltase reaches the lysosomes,[126] either via the brush-border membrane, or directly.[126b] The sugar moieties of these glycoproteins may have some effect on their enzymatic activities (and, when they have some effect, it is still unclear whether the effect is direct or indirect [e.g., via effects on stability]). "Mature" human lactase–phlorizin hydrolase, both *N*- and *O*-glycosylated, is reported to have a fourfold higher lactase activity than the solely *N*-glycosylated form[126a]; on the other hand, the high-mannose form of human pro-lactase–phlorizin hydrolas has the same specific activities as mature lactase that has undergone, in addition to proteolytic processing, complex glycosylation.[107] Pig pro-sucrase–isomaltase also is about twice as active in the fully glycosylated as in the high-mannose form.[127]

The sugar chains are often responsible for the blood group specificity of these enzymes.[128] They are likely to be responsible, also, for the high-affinity binding of *C. difficile* toxin A to sucrase–isomaltase.[129] Electrophoretic microheterogeneity may be related to the extent of sialylation (e.g., refs. 130 to 132).

Sucrase–isomaltase, glucoamylases, and lactase–phlorizin hydrolase are all configuration-retaining glycosidases. The reader interested in their catalytic mechanism is referred to the reviews in refs. 90 and 133; see also, ref. 48.

The genes for sucrase–isomaltase and for lactase–phlorizin hydrolase have been assigned to different human chromosomes, the former to chromosome 3q25-26 (refs. 134 and

135) and the latter to chromosome 2q21 (refs. 136, 137, and 137a).

The human chromosomal lactase–phlorizin hydrolase gene is approximately 50 kb long and has 17 introns. All exons and their intron borders as well as 1 kb of 5′-flanking region, have been sequenced.[138] In the rabbit (but not so in the rat or in humans) three chromosomal lactase–phlorizin hydrolase genes exist; they are expressed differently along the small intestine.[138a]

Trehalase

Trehalase is unique among intestinal brush-border glycosidases in several respects. It is a very minor component, accounting for about 0.1 percent of the intrinsic protein,[139] but has a far larger turnover number; as a result, trehalase and sucrase activities are at comparable levels in the brush-border membrane. Trehalase occurs either as a monomer or as a homooligomer.[139,140] Its apparent molecular size is approximately 75 kDa (refs. 139 and 140), or 65 kDa (from its 578 amino acid residues, including the cleavable leading sequence and the transient hydrophobic C-terminal anchor, as deduced from the cDNA of rabbit intestinal pretrehalase[141]). Trehalase is thus considerably smaller than the other brush-border glycosidases (see Table 151-2). Among the glysosidases, it alone is anchored to the membrane via phosphatidylinositol.[141,142]

The amino acid sequence of rabbit intestinal trehalase is known.[141] It has no homology with any other known glycosidase, except for *Escherichia coli* trehalase[143] (38 percent identical residues). Like other phosphatidylinositol-anchored proteins, its primary translation product begins with a cleavable signal sequence (19 to 22 amino acids long) and ends with a hydrophobic stretch located not far from the (cytosolic) C-terminal segment. This hydrophobic stretch is exchanged for the final phosphatidylinositol anchor while still in the ER. Other than this, very little is known about trehalase biosynthesis; also, the exact location of the junction between the polypeptide chain and the phosphatidylinositol anchor, or the exact structure of the latter, are not known. Trehalase can be expressed in *Xenopus laevis* oocytes, where it appears at the membrane surface, again anchored via phosphatidylinositol.[141]

The catalytic mechanism of trehalase is little known; it leads to inversion of the configuration at C1, liberating the "α-glucosyl" moiety as β-glucopyranose (ref. 53 and Wacker H, Semenza G, 1991: unpublished observations). Therefore, in this respect also trehalase differs from all other brush-border glycosidases. The trehalase gene is located on human chromosome 11 (Kruse T, et al., 1992: unpublished observations).

DEVELOPMENT AND REGULATION OF THE DISACCHARIDASES

In Mammals Other than Humans

At birth the small-intestinal brush-border membrane of most mammals is endowed with lactase–phlorizin hydrolase and the glucoamylase complex only. The other α-glucosidases develop during extrauterine life—in the rat (see e.g., ref. 144) and the rabbit (ref. 145) from days 15 to 18 and approximately days 25 to 30, respectively, that is, during weaning. At the same time, lactase (ref. 146 and a great many others) and phlorizin hydrolase[147] activities begin to decline. Their levels in adulthood are eventually approximately 10 percent of those at birth. Initiation of the postnatal ontogenic events in the rat gastrointestinal tract is probably determined by the genetic program,[148,149] while the terminal phase of intestinal development seems to be influenced by environmental factors such as nutrients and hormones.[150–152]

Enterocytes arising in the crypts acquire the ability to digest and absorb during subsequent migration along the intestinal villi. Interestingly, columnar cells may display a nonhomogeneous pattern of differentiation along the villus, as indicated by the variable expression of the lactase protein in adult animals.[153] The basic program describing this differentiation is carried within the enterocyte, but the signal(s) to differentiate depends on the interactions taking place between crypts, enterocytes, and underlying fibroblasts.[154,155] On weaning the suckling rat, an enzymatically active sucrase–isomaltase first appears in crypt cells and then progresses gradually to uniform distribution along the villus.[156–158]*

The primary site of control in spontaneous development of brush-border disaccharidases is most probably at the level of transcription, because in rats and rabbits the enzyme activities appear concordantly with the cognate mRNAs (sucrase–isomaltase, at weaning,[160,161] Fig. 151-5; lactase, in fetal life[162]). Also, studies along the crypt–villus axis (in rats) agree with the site of control of sucrase–isomaltase biosynthesis being at the level of transcription,[163,164] as the bulk of sucrase–isomaltase mRNA is located at the crypt–villus junction and proximal villus.

The expression of α-glucosidase activities responds to hormonal administration—cortisonelike steroids,[165–168] thyroxine,[166] insulin,[169] and epidermal growth factor[170]—which can induce their appearance (in rats, rabbits, and mice) if administered approximately 1 week before the time of their spontaneous development. Glucocorticosteroid-induced precocious development of rat intestinal epithelium and increased turnover rate (see below) may be mediated, at least in part, through alterations in the synthesis of extracellular matrix proteins by differential regulation of their gene expression.[171] The response of sucrase–isomaltase mRNA to hydrocortisone administration parallels that of enzyme activity,[172,173] as does that of trehalase in RNA (J. Riby and N. Kretchmer; G. Galand, personal communications.) The glucocorticoid receptor occurs at high concentrations in the small intestine during the suckling period and decreases thereafter[173a]; after weaning, hydrocortisone fails to elicit an increase of sucrase activity.[173b] This does not necessarily mean, though, that the physiological trigger of development of sucrase during weaning is a glucocorticosteroid, because an antagonist of these hormones for their receptor does not prevent the normal development of sucrase.[173c] The reader will find a discussion of this complicated topic and of the equally complicated dietary regulation of disaccharidases in other reviews.[151,174–177a]

*This pro-sucrase–isomaltase should not be confused with the enzymatically inactive protein cross-reacting with sucrase–isomaltase that has been obtained in homogeneous or highly purified form from the intestine of baby rats[159] or rabbits.[145] The kind and amount of information on these cross-reacting proteins is somewhat different for the two species, but perhaps what is known for one species complements what is known for the other. The protein from rabbit intestine appears at about the sixth day of life, reaches a maximum at about the eightieth day, and decreases thereafter, still remaining detectable in adult life, particularly at the apical pole of crypt cells. It has a somewhat larger molecular weight ($S_{20,w}$ = 9.8 S) than sucrase–isomaltase ($S_{20,w}$ = 9.2 S). The cross-reacting proteins from the rat are, unlike sucrase–isomaltase, periodic acid–Schiff-negative. These proteins may derive from endocytosed, partially degraded sucrase–isomaltase or from incompletely or nonglycosylated (pro-)sucrase–isomaltase, or they may have another origin.

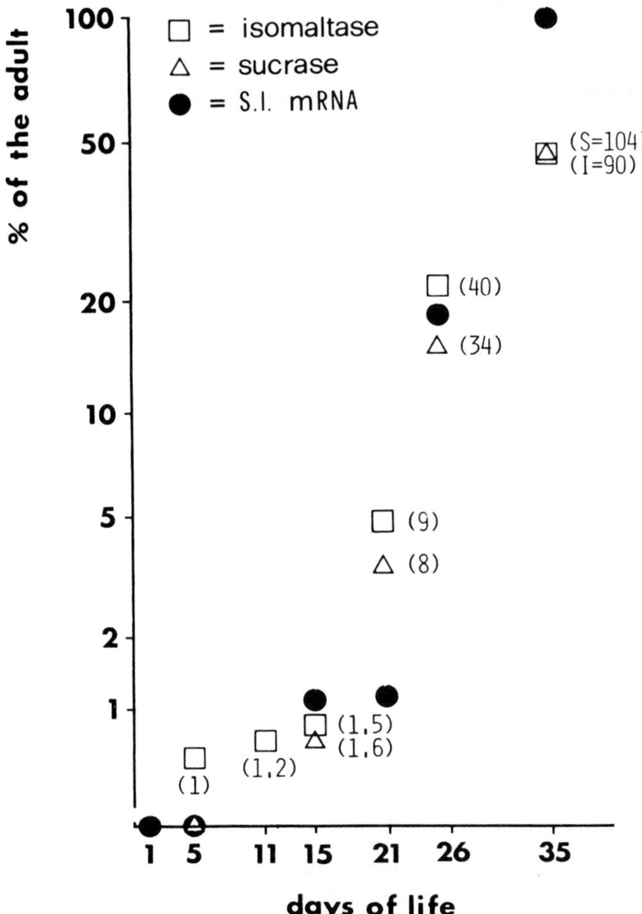

FIG. 151-5 **Development of sucrase and isomaltase activities and of sucrase–isomaltase mRNA in baby rabbits. Sucrase (△) and isomaltase (□) activities and the mRNA levels (●) are expressed as percentages of adult values. In parentheses are the sucrase and isomaltase activities at the different ages, as units per gram of protein.** ***(From Sebastio et al.*[160] *Used by permission.)***

At weaning, intestinal lactase–phlorizin hydrolase declines to very low levels in most mammals other than man. The mechanism(s) of this decline is not fully understood, and is under intensive investigation in several laboratories.

What factor triggers this decline? Since weaning is accompanied by the progressive removal of lactose from the diet, it was suggested 30 years ago that dietary lactose may be necessary to "sustain" the presence of high levels of lactase in enterocytes. However, the large amount of work (carried out in a number of species, under a number of experimental conditions, and testing a variety of β-glycosides) has produced comparatively disappointing results—administering even large amounts of lactose could achieve only a moderate delay in the onset and a less steep decline of lactase activity.[57,176–182] Dietary lactose, therefore, does not seem to have more than a marginal effect.

A similar statement can probably be made about the effects of hormones on the decline of lactase at weaning; glucocorticosteroids increase lactase activity only little (ref. 183 and literature quoted therein), which is in keeping with the observation that the consensus sequence for the glucocorticosteroid-receptor binding was not found in 1000 bp upstream in the human lactase gene.[138] Thyroxine, at pharmacologic dose levels,[183–189] does produce a decline in lactase, particularly if it follows cortisone administration.[183]

Parallel to the decline of lactase activity at the time of weaning, the life span of the enterocyte also decreases.[152,190–194] Indeed, the correlation between the decline of lactase and shortened life span of enterocytes is reported to be so close[192,193] that the former has been suggested to derive from the latter. Accurate cytokinetic measurements by another group[195] have also led to the conclusion that accelerated cell migration can contribute to the decline of lactase, at least during a part of the weaning time. But pathological conditions have also been identified in the experimental animal, under which crypt-cell hyperplasia correlates with an increase of intestinal lactase.[196,197]

In suckling rats and rabbits, lactase protein and activity can be visualized along the whole length of the small intestine and in all enterocytes along the villus: contrary to this, in adult animals, some populations of enterocytes in the proximal and distal segments of the small intestine do not express lactase, whereas other, neighboring ones do. This patchy expression of lactase (which, incidentally, is not observed for sucrase, for example) undoubtedly contributes to the low average lactase in these intestinal segments.[201]

The levels of lactase–phlorizin hydrolase mRNA are reduced in the small intestine of the adult mammal, but they are still present in very substantial amounts, particularly in the middle and proximal part of the intestine. That is, lactase activity is reduced in adulthood to far lower levels than its cognate mRNA. This has been shown for rats[162,185,198,199] (save for a single report[200]), rabbit,[162] mouse,[199] and pig.[185] In the sheep lactase and lactase mRNA decline in a parallel fashion[199]; however, this observation may well be worth a more quantitative evaluation, because the decline of the Na, glucose cotransporter, which occurs at the same time, is accompanied by a fairly small decline in its cognate mRNA.[199a,b]

Shortly before birth, lactase appears also in the colon, and declines thereafter. In the colon the levels of the enzyme and those of the mRNA parallel one another.[202,203]

In vivo studies on the rate of biosynthesis and processing of lactase using pulse and chase of methionine, in preweaning and postweaning rats[193,204,205] have indicated that its velocity of synthesis does not significantly change at weaning. (Although previous authors[194] reported that [again in rats in vivo, but referring their incorporation rates to total tissue protein], lactase biosynthesis does decrease at weaning.) In vitro cultures of small intestine from adult rabbits synthesize less lactase precursor than cultures from suckling rabbits.[205a]

In an important paper, Troelsen et al.[206] have identified a nuclear factor in pig enterocytes that binds to a sequence of the lactase gene promoter located close to the TATA box. This factor is present in high amounts in pig enterocytes with high lactase activity, but in low amounts in enterocytes of adult animals with low lactase activity.

Additional reasons may blur the reported observations further. Relatively little attention has been paid, for example, to individual variability, which we find remarkable, even among animals with similar pedigrees. Also, prior to ref. 198, little attention was paid to the fact that the lactase/lactase–mRNA ratios change along the intestine, and that the pattern of these ratios is modulated by the diet during weaning.[198a] The former observation was expanded in the experiment of Fig. 151-6 on rabbit small intestine[206b]: the rates of in vitro biosynthesis correlated well with the lactase–mRNA levels (Fig. 151-6G) but the lactase/lactase–mRNA ratios were much smaller in the proximal third of the intestine, than in more distal segments (Fig. 151-6C). (Similar observations were made for sucrase, right panels in Fig.

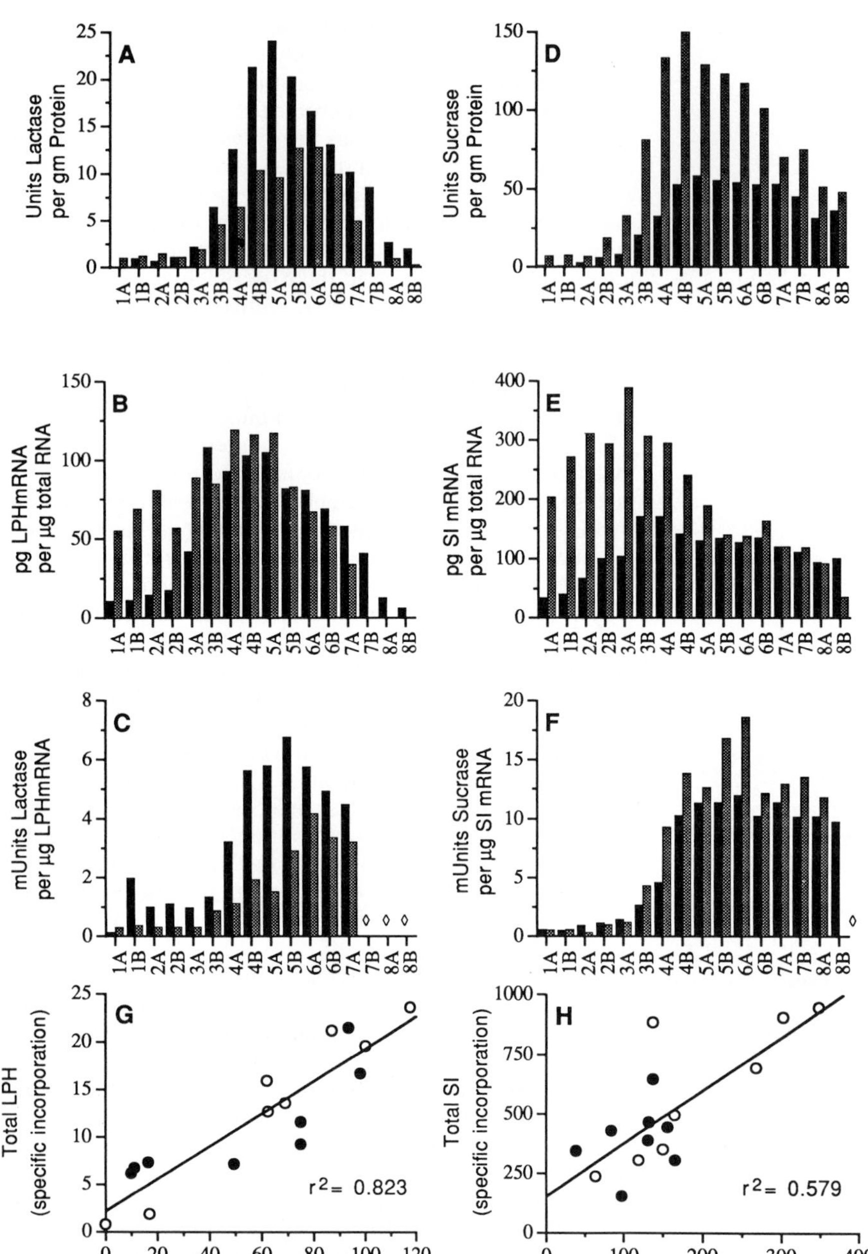

FIG. 151-6 Lactase–phlorizin hydrolase (LPH; A,B,C,G) and sucrase–isomaltase (SI; D, E, F, H) along the small intestine of rabbits. A and D, lactase and sucrase enzymatic activities, respectively. B and E, their cognate mRNAs. C and F, ratios between the enzymatic activities and the cognate mRNAs. G and H, correlation between the in vitro biosynthesis of LPH (G) and SI (H) and the respective mRNA levels. The enzymatic and mRNA levels were determined in 16 segments from the pylorus to the ileal–coecal valve; the rates of biosynthesis were in 8 samples in between. Black bars and black dots, 36-day-old rabbit; shaded bars and open circles, 3.5-year-old rabbit. Diamonds: these ratios (not reported) were too inaccurate, due to the small magnitudes involved. (*Reproduced by permission from Keller et al.*[206b])

151-6). It is quite possible, therefore, that pancreatic proteases may act locally as a "posttranslational" factor degrading in part intestinal brush-border enzymes; they are probably the reason why lactase, for example, is often absent from the tip of the villi.[201] But the role of pancreatic proteases is certainly not essential in the decline of lactase at weaning (ref. 206c, and references therein). A very accurate study by Duluc et al.[206f] clearly shows that the lactase gene (in suckling rats) is transcribed actively in distal duodenum, jejunum, and proximal ileum, but much less so in proximal duodenum, and nearly not at all in distal ileum. After weaning, neither mRNA nor lactase were detected in distal ileum, while mosaicism appeared in duodenum.

The decisive factors deciding the decline of lactase must reside primarily in the small intestine itself (and/or in the animal's hormonal setup), because isografts of fetal or newborn mouse[206d] or rat[206e] small intestine do show this decline, albeit with some delay, as compared with the controls (and develop sucrase at the same time as the controls).

Therefore, it may well be that the origin of the decline of intestinal lactase at weaning has multiple causes and may differ in different species. Indeed, as it has been pointed out by Mantei,[206a] past the weaning age, mammals as a rule do not come across lactose in their diets. No special advantage arises from persistent intestinal lactase, and no major disadvantage from its disappearance. Chance may decide the mechanism by which a given species loses intestinal lactase, and the mechanism—transcriptional, translational, posttranslational—may well be different in different species or even ethnic groups, or even individual cells in the same villus.

As will be mentioned below, brush-border glycoproteins are richer in terminal sialic acid residues before than after weaning. It would be conceivable, therefore, that, for example, postweaning lactase–phlorizin hydrolase, which is poorer in or even devoid of sialic acid residues, would be more prone to be degraded by intracellular (processing?) proteases. It seems, however, that the switch in glycosylation does not exactly correlate with the decline of lactase.[207]

In Humans

The developmental pattern of disaccharidases is different in humans from that in other mammals. In humans, both α- and β-glycosidase activities develop during fetal life. The newborn is therefore able to digest not only lactose, but also α-glucosides; thus, with due precautions, a newborn can be precociously weaned. This contrasts with other mammalian species, which survive after birth on mother's milk only.

Intestinal lactase activity is detectable in human fetal intestine by the 8th week of gestation. Mucosal enzyme activity rises gradually between the 8th and 34th weeks of gestation and more rapidly shortly before birth, so that lactase activity in term neonates is two to four times higher than that in infants 2 to 11 months of age (Fig. 151-7*A*).[65,208–212] Within the first week of life, enterally fed preterm infants show a rapid postnatal rise in lactase activity.[65,213] Most premature infants do not experience lactose intolerance. Although the absorption of this disaccharide in the small bowel is incomplete in both preterm and term infants, adequate colonic salvage of malabsorbed carbohydrates is achieved by colonic flora.[214–220] In human fetuses, the biosynthesis of lactase is most probably controlled by the level of their mRNA.[221]

α-Glucosidase activities appear between the 8th and 10th weeks of gestation. Thereafter, they remain at levels comparable to those in adulthood, and increase greatly at term (Fig. 151-7*A*).[208,209] The primary site of control is likely to be again at the level of transcription, since the appearance of sucrase–isomaltase mRNA parallels that of the enzymatic activities (Fig. 151-7*B, C*).[172] Likewise, the expression of the sucrase–isomaltase gene along the crypt–villus axis is regulated by the level of its mRNA.[221a] In two important papers, Traber's group have identified the promoter of the sucrase–isomaltase gene, three nuclear protein binding sites within this promoter, each acting as a positive regulatory element for transcription; and the proximal and distal elements regulating intestine-specific transcription.[221b,221c]

Established cell lines derived from human colonic cancer show an "enterocytelike" differentiation similar to that which occurs in fetal colon. Glucose is a powerful negative modulator of the biosynthesis of sucrase–isomaltase in these cells.[222–224]

Glycosylation of Disaccharidases and Development

Before weaning, the sugar moieties of brush-border disaccharidases are rich in sialic acid residues; after weaning they are nearly or totally devoid of them and rich in fucosyl residues.[131,207,225–228] This change in composition of the sugar moieties corresponds to changes in the levels of two sugar transferases: sialyltransferase is high before and low after weaning; fucosyltransferase is the opposite.[229,230]

The increase of fucosyltransferase at the time of weaning, as in other organs, is probably under transcriptional control,[230a] but the process in the small intestine seems to be more complex, involving an inhibitor of this enzyme,[230b] which declines in rat small intestine between the 18th and the 23rd days of extrauterine life.[231,231a]

Treatment of rats with hydrocortisone during the suckling period (but not after weaning) leads to a precocious increase of fucosyltransferase activity. However, administration of an antagonist of glucocorticosteroids to suckling rats does not prevent the normal increase of fucosyltransferase activity at weaning.[231b,231c] This response of fucosyltransferase activity to hormone is thus reminiscent of the response of sucrase mentioned above.

Dietary manipulations at weaning can modulate the levels of small-intestinal transglycosidase activities and hence the composition of the glycosyl moieties of these glycoproteins.[230] For an important review, see ref. 231c.

CHANGES OF DISACCHARIDASES IN ACQUIRED DISEASES

Several factors such as dietary components, hormones, and endoluminal enzymes may alter the activity of brush-border oligosaccharidases by varying the rates of their synthesis, their degradation, or both, and may also lead to a change in their covalent structure. The turnover of disaccharidases is much faster than cell turnover. In fact, rather than being simply synthesized once and for all by an intestinal cell, a particular membrane protein is turned over repeatedly during the cell's life cycle: whereas the life of rat intestinal villus is about 36 h, that of sucrase can vary from 2.5 to 14 h, depending on the experimental conditions.[232,233] Turnover of brush-border proteins is also heterogeneous. Large-molecular-weight proteins, including disaccharidases, have a more rapid turnover than lower-molecular-weight proteins.[234,235] The sucrase and the isomaltase parts of the sucrase–isomaltase complex appear to be degraded at different rates (see below), and the carbohydrate moiety may be selectively removed at least in part, whereas the protein core remains attached to the membrane.[236] Altered degradation rate is an important mechanism controlling levels of brush-border enzymes in various pathological and physiological conditions.

In the following, we briefly discuss some representative conditions in which changes of disaccharidase activities are brought about by a variety of mechanisms.

Diabetes

Diabetes, either in humans or in experimental animals, is accompanied by an increase in activity of membrane transport systems (for a review, see ref. 237) and in hydrolytic enzyme activities including those of disaccharidases; the enhanced sucrase in diabetic animals reflects a selective increase in sucrase–isomaltase *protein,* which is due (mainly) to a decreased rate of degradation,[233] perhaps related to altered glycosylation of intestinal microvillus[238] and of the sucrase–isomaltase itself.[239] The turnover of brush-border proteins as a whole and of the enterocyte is either normal or increased. In congenital diabetic BioBreed rats, but not in streptozocin-induced diabetic rats, changes in the glycosylation of sucrase–isomaltase have been observed.

The increased disaccharidase activity in diabetic rats appears to be the result of insulin deficiency: it is independent of intraluminal factors, such as food intake or pancreatobiliary secretions.[240] (For a review, see ref. 176.)

Exocrine Pancreatic Insufficiency

In addition to processing some "pro" forms to the final heterodimers (see the earlier section on biosynthesis of

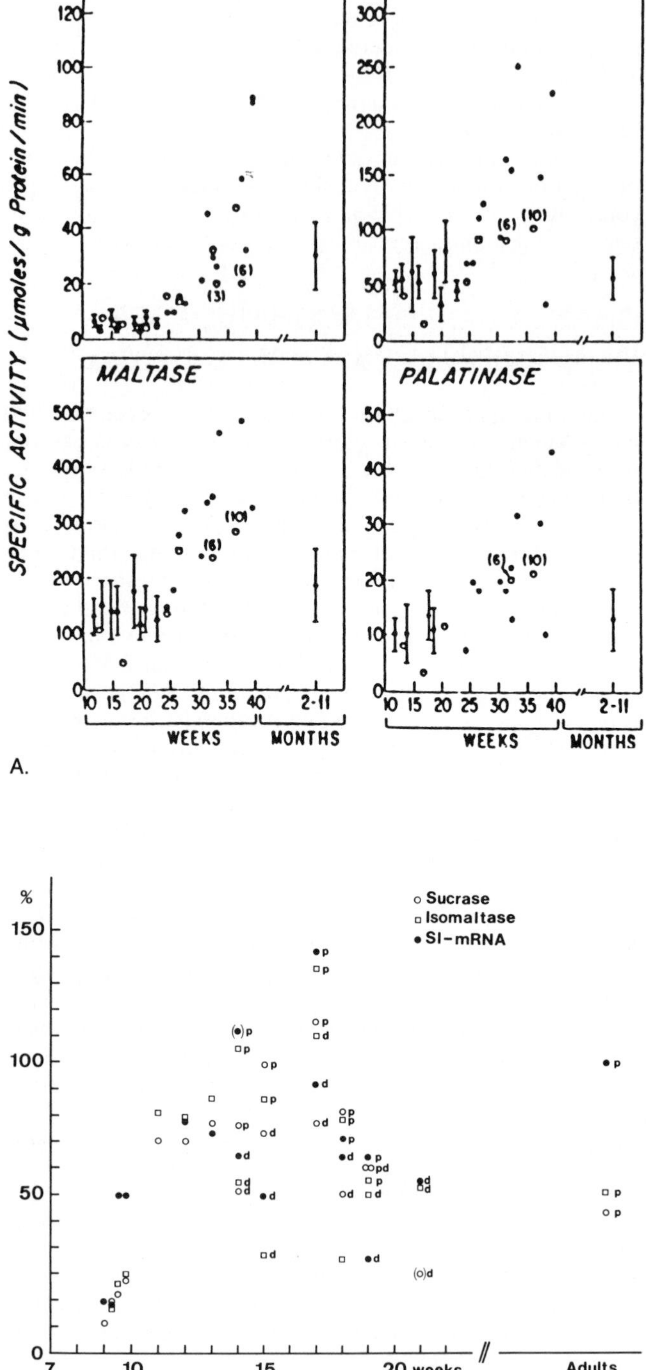

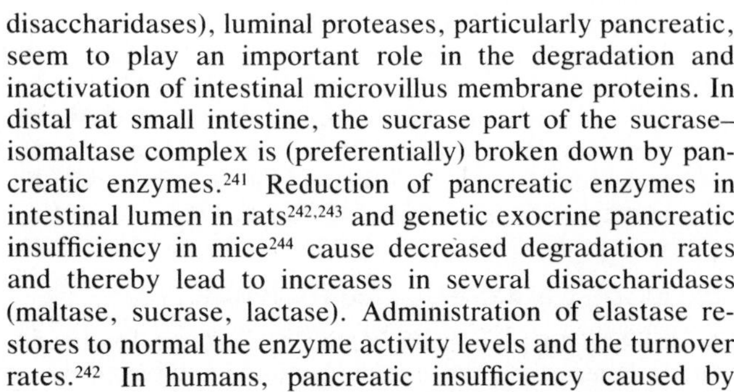

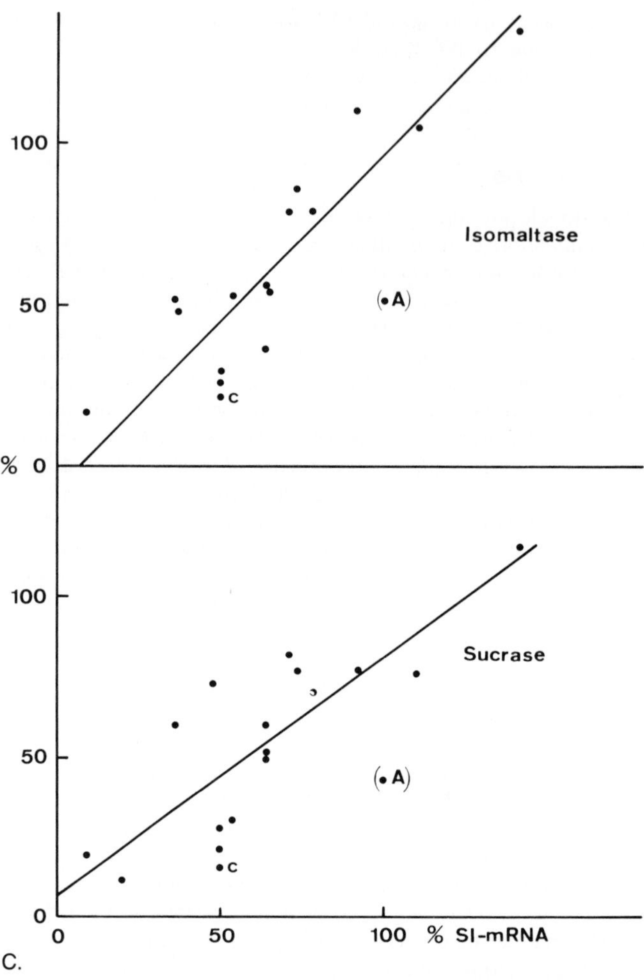

FIG. 151-7 *A.* Development of disaccharidase activities in human fetal jejunum. Values in parentheses are numbers of observations. For infants 2 to 11 months of age, n = 25. Where possible, data are means ±SD (bars). *(From Mobassaleh et al.*[212] *Original data from refs. 208, 210, and 211. Used by permission.) B.* Simultaneous appearance of sucrase (◯) and isomaltase (□) activities and of sucrase–isomaltase mRNA (SI-mRNA, ●). Enzymatic activities are expressed as a percentage of the values at 15 to 18 weeks of gestation; the mRNA levels as a percentage of adult levels in proximal small intestine. p = samples from proximal half of small intestines; d = samples from distal half. Samples without either p or d were from total intestine. *(From Sebastio et al.*[172] *Used by permission.) C.* Correlation between isomaltase activity (top panel), isomaltase activity (bottom panel), and SI-mRNA in the samples of Fig. 151-6*B*. c = sample of colon (18 weeks old; A = sample from proximal part of small intestine from a healthy adult. The correlation coefficients r (0.889 for isomaltase; 0.812 for sucrase) and the lines were calculated utilizing all points with the exception of A. The slopes of the lines are not different from 1, and their intercepts are not different from the origin. *(From Sebastio et al.*[172] *Used by permission.)*

disaccharidases), luminal proteases, particularly pancreatic, seem to play an important role in the degradation and inactivation of intestinal microvillus membrane proteins. In distal rat small intestine, the sucrase part of the sucrase–isomaltase complex is (preferentially) broken down by pancreatic enzymes.[241] Reduction of pancreatic enzymes in intestinal lumen in rats[242,243] and genetic exocrine pancreatic insufficiency in mice[244] cause decreased degradation rates and thereby lead to increases in several disaccharidases (maltase, sucrase, lactase). Administration of elastase restores to normal the enzyme activity levels and the turnover rates.[242] In humans, pancreatic insufficiency caused by chronic pancreatitis or by cystic fibrosis also leads to increased levels of sucrase and maltase, which are also ascribed to a decrease in degradation of these enzymes. Oral administration of pancreatic proteases in patients causes a decrease in sucrase, maltase, and lactase activities.[245]

Secondary Generalized Glycosidase Deficiency

In a number of intestinal diseases with various degrees of mucosal atrophy of the small intestine, there is a generalized decrease in glycosidase activity of varying severity. In atrophic intestinal mucosa from proximal small intestine of children with active celiac disease or cow's milk protein intolerance[246] or of patients with infectious diarrheas (particularly those accompanied by malnutrition and/or small-intestinal lesion[247]), glycosidase activities are significantly reduced as compared with those of normal controls. In all these conditions, lactase is usually the first glycosidase affected, is the one to reach the lowest level, and is the last to recover. Glucoamylase activity is only slightly reduced.[248–252] Various mechanisms may underlie this decrease in disaccharidase activity: atrophy of small-intestinal mucosa, with reduced surface; reduced microvillus surface area[253]; presence on the villi of immature enterocytes with low levels of digestive enzymes[254]; altered cell kinetics; or increased degradation of proteins of the brush-border membrane by luminal enzymes of bacterial origin, either proteases or deglycosylating enzymes, with partially deglycosylated disaccharidases then becoming more susceptible to luminal proteolysis.[255] The last mechanism could be the cause of decreased disaccharidase activity in contaminated small-bowel syndrome[256] or in giardiasis.[257]

DIAGNOSIS OF DISACCHARIDASE DEFICIENCY, CARBOHYDRATE MALABSORPTION, AND CARBOHYDRATE INTOLERANCE

Disaccharidase Deficiency

Disaccharidase activity is usually measured in homogenates of small-intestinal biopsies obtained only from the proximal small intestine and therefore gives little information on the ability of the total bowel mucosa to hydrolyze disaccharide.*

Assay of disaccharidases in biopsies involves use of D-glucose-oxidase[258,259] or D-glucose-dehydrogenase[260] to measure glucose released from the substrate. Lactase activity should be assayed in the presence of *p*-chloromercurybenzoate, so that only the relevant brush-border enzyme is measured.[261] Alternatively, brush-border lactase can be selectively determined by using cellobiose as the substrate,[262] since cellobiose is not hydrolyzed by the other β-galactosidases present in the cell homogenate. For the assay of glucoamylase with glycogen or high-molecular-weight soluble starch as the substrate, it is necessary to inactivate the pancreatic α-amylase adsorbed on the small-intestinal mucosa; with maltose as the substrate, the sucrase–isomaltase complex must first be heat-inactivated.[43,263,264] Appropriate inhibitors can also be used.[46,57]

Disaccharidases may also be measured by quantitative immunoelectrophoresis of proteins from individual small-intestinal biopsies using specific antiserums.[265]

Enzymatic activity is usually expressed either in units per gram of wet mucosa or in units per gram of protein (1 g wet weight of mucosa contains approximately 100 mg protein). There are no advantages in one way of expressing the results over another. (For a discussion on this point, see also ref. 237.)

Most investigators agree satisfactorily on the mean values and the SDs of normal α-glucosidase activities (e.g., refs. 258, 259, and 266–268). Normal enzymatic values are usually defined as those of histologically normal small-intestinal mucosa.[269–271] Disaccharidase "deficiency" is defined as the reduction of an enzyme activity to levels lower than the normal mean by at least 2 SD.[268,271]

Most studies carried out in the past investigated disaccharidase activities present in *jejunal* mucosa removed from near the ligament of Treitz using such instruments as the Crosby capsule. Over recent years jejunal biopsy has been replaced more and more by *endoscopic duodenal* biopsy. The disaccharidase activities—and particularly lactase activities—show a rising gradient in the distal direction (Fig. 151-8), which contributes to the individual spread of "normal" disaccharidase activities.[272] Only a few studies have attempted to determine the reference ranges for *duodenal* disaccharidases. In one such study mean lactase activity was about 40 percent lower in duodenum than in jejunum, and the individual variability was quite large.[273]

Important pieces of information still missing are whether the proximal–distal enzyme distribution reported in the classical study of Newcomer and McGill[272] holds true for disaccharide *absorbers* other than Caucasians and how it changes within age. In the absence of this information one should not classify a patient as "lactose malabsorber" solely on the basis of enzyme determinations in endoscopic duodenal biopsies without carrying out oral load tests (see below), which alone provide an estimate of the total digestive capacity of the patient beyond the ligament of Treitz.

In congenital sucrase–isomaltase deficiency, sucrase activity is absent or nearly so, isomaltase activity is either absent or heavily reduced, and maltase activity is severely reduced (see "Molecular Defects" below).[274]

In heterozygotes for congenital sucrase–isomaltase deficiency, sucrase and isomaltase levels are intermediate between those of affected patients and normal controls,[274,275] and the sucrase:lactase ratio is abnormal (the normal value for the ratio having been determined for subjects with persistent high lactase activity in adult life).[276] Heterozygotes are best identified by comparing the activity of the relevant enzyme with a weighted average of other enzymatic activities in their own brush-border membrane.[277]

In normal humans, lactase activity varies widely according to age and ethnic group (see Chap. 150). It is conventional to regard levels of lactase activity less than 8 units per gram of protein or 0.7 unit per gram wet weight as diagnostic of primary adult hypolactasia.[278–280]

Carbohydrate Malabsorption

Sugar malabsorption is the failure to digest and absorb carbohydrates adequately, with or without signs of clinical intolerance. *Intolerance* and *malabsorption* should thus not be used as synonyms.

The oral absorption tests used routinely in humans are based either on the extent of the blood glucose increase following oral administration of the sugar,* on the appearance of gases (mainly hydrogen) in the expired air, or on the presence in feces of the malabsorbed carbohydrates and/or of their fermentation products created by the colonic flora.

*One source of error, often not recognized, is the circadian rhythm in disaccharidase activities. Activity may vary by a factor of 2 between minimum and maximum (for a review, see ref. 176).

*Mention should also be made of the oral tolerance test with 3-*O*-methyllactose. This substituted disaccharide is split by small-intestinal lactase to yield galactose and 3-*O*-methylglucose. The latter is absorbed in the small intestine (but not in the colon), and is not metabolized to any significant extent. Hence, the appearance of 3-*O*-methylglucose in urine following oral administration of 3-*O*-methyllactose is an indirect measure of total small-intestinal lactase activity.[281]

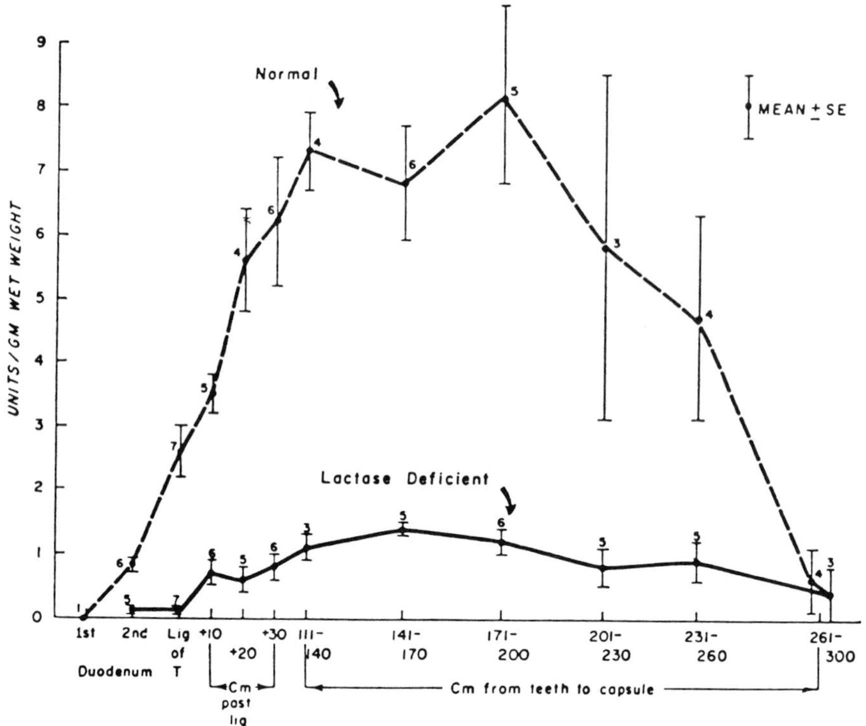

FIG. 151-8 Distribution of lactase activity in the small bowel of seven normal and seven hypolactasic adults. (*From Newcomer and McGill.*[272] *Used by permission.*)

The first two tests measure the capacity of the small bowel to digest and absorb a carbohydrate load; the third one includes information on the efficiency of colonic mechanisms to compensate for small-bowel failure.

The amount of sugar administered in oral tolerance tests is usually much larger than that present in a physiologically balanced diet.

Blood samples are obtained at chosen times after ingestion of the load (2 g of sugar per kilogram of body weight; maximum, 50 g). After sucrose and lactose are administered, a peak rise in serum glucose of less than 20 to 25 mg/dl (during the first 90 min) is diagnostic of sugar malabsorption.[259,278,282] The rise in blood glucose following administration of the disaccharide is best compared with that observed after administration of the component monosaccharides.[259,278]

Whereas this oral load test is reliable in adults, it is not so reliable in children, for whom both false positive and false negative results are reported with either lactose or sucrose in 20 to 30 percent of cases.[283] It is imperative that the child have no diarrhea at the time of the test.

The extent of rise in blood glucose following oral administration of a sugar provides no information, however, as to whether the sugar has been absorbed *completely* or not. Incomplete absorption can be deduced only by measuring parameters directly related to the carbohydrates reaching the colon, such as the increase in breath hydrogen after ingesting a sugar load.

The breath hydrogen test is the most reliable and also the least invasive procedure for measuring carbohydrate malabsorption, even in children.[284–287] A peak rise in breath hydrogen greater than 20 parts per million (10, according to Kneepkens et al.[288]) over the fasting base-line value after ingestion of a carbohydrate load or a carbohydrate-containing meal indicates sugar malabsorption. When the test meal consists of solids, breath hydrogen collection should be continued for 8 h in recognition of the delayed orocecal transit of solids as compared with liquids.[289] No antibiotic should be given before or during the test. False negative hydrogen breath tests due to the inability of colonic bacterial flora to produce hydrogen from unabsorbed carbohydrates amount to 2 to 9 percent.[290–293] Excretion of hydrogen in breath after a test meal may be quantitated by comparing it with hydrogen excretion after a dose of lactulose, which is not split by lactase[18,19] and can thus be used as a reference for totally nonabsorbable sugar. This method has been validated in vivo in humans.[26] The lactose breath hydrogen test gives the best discrimination between lactose absorbers and malabsorbers.[267,280]

Acetate is another product of the bacterial colonic fermentation of unabsorbed carbohydrate. Venous blood acetate in the nonfasting state can be quantitatively related to carbohydrate breakdown in the colon, although the concentration of acetate in blood may vary with different types of malabsorbed carbohydrates. Breath hydrogen and blood acetate correlate with one another.[24]

When the colon fails to compensate fully for the carbohydrate malabsorption in the small intestine, the sugars themselves and the products of their bacterial breakdown (such as lactic acid or volatile fatty acids) appear in a liquid stool. Detection of reducing substances in feces using copper sulfate tablets (Clinitest)[294] is useful as a screening test for lactose malabsorption in infants after a milk-containing meal or after administration of an oral lactose load but is relatively unreliable in newborns[295] and adults.[296]

Malabsorbed carbohydrates can be also detected in feces by chromatographic methods,[297] or by measuring fecal excretion of ^{13}C-enriched sugars.[32,33]

A new test for assessment of lactose absorption is based on the measurement of urinary galactose after ingestion of 50 g of lactose in adults. The ratio between urinary galactose and urinary creatinine completely separates lactose absorbers from lactose malabsorbers.[298]

Carbohydrate Intolerance

Sugar intolerance refers to abdominal symptoms that result from sugar malabsorption, such as flatulence, borborygmi, abdominal distension, pain, and diarrhea. Final confirmation of the role of disaccharide intolerance in producing these symptoms in an individual patient requires resolution of symptoms following elimination from the diet of the foods containing the offending disaccharide.

Clinical intolerance of lactose may correlate poorly with the levels of intestinal lactase activity[299] or with the results of oral tolerance tests[300] or of the breath hydrogen test (see the next section[301,302]).

PATHOGENESIS OF CARBOHYDRATE INTOLERANCE

General

Whether sugar malabsorption produces symptoms[18,26,303–305] depends not only on the intestinal digestive and absorptive capacity, but also on factors such as the quantity of the ingested sugar, the rate of gastric emptying, the response of the small intestine to the osmotic load, the metabolic activity of colonic bacteria, and the absorptive capacities of the colon, mainly for water and short-chain fatty acids.[306] We will discuss some of these factors, one at a time.

Gastric emptying is delayed and duodenal-ileal transit is accelerated by the insufficient digestion of the sugar itself: The unabsorbed carbohydrate, when present in the distal small intestine, inhibits gastric emptying by an ill-defined mechanism; at the same time, it stimulates duodenal-ileal transit, because of the decreased water and sodium absorption.[27,307–311] (The delayed gastric emptying thus partially compensates for the effects of the high sugar levels in the intestine.[283])

As a consequence, the reduced digestion per se, the delayed gastric emptying, and the accelerated duodenal-ileal transit all concur in reducing monosaccharide absorption.[27,312] The ensuing flattened blood glucose profile elicits, in turn, little or no increase in the plasma levels of insulin, C peptide, and gastric inhibitory polypeptide.

Accelerated duodenal-ileal transit may entail the malabsorption of unrelated nutrients, such as starch or fat.[313–315] Furthermore, ileal flow rates may exceed the critical values above which the right colon propels fluid onward.[316–318]

The colonic bacterial flora salvages some of the dietary carbohydrate not digested and absorbed by the small bowel,[20] and in so doing limits both colonic wastage and diarrhea. In normal adults it has been calculated that the colon may salvage up to 20 to 25 g of lactose (or lactulose) and up to 50 g of starch.[26,319,320] Adaptation of the colonic flora to a particular dietary carbohydrate may further increase this salvaging capacity.[321–323] Diarrhea ensues either when this capacity is exceeded because the amount of unsplit carbohydrates is excessive, or when it is reduced for one reason or another. The latter mechanism has been suggested as the cause of lactose intolerance in milk-fed infants treated with antibiotics.[324]

Individual differences in intestinal microflora are a reason for variation in severity of abdominal symptoms in lactose malabsorption. The fecal concentrations and the relative contributions of isobutyric and isovaleric acids in fecal short-chain fatty acids of lactose-tolerant lactose malabsorbers is significantly higher than those of the intolerant ones. This is probably due to larger colonization of the small bowel of lactose-tolerant malabsorbers with anaerobes such as the Bacteroides species. The fermentation of unabsorbed lactose by bacteria colonizing the small intestine may act as a complementary protective mechanism reducing the osmotic load of the sugar, and avoiding the development of diarrhea.[325]

In Sucrase–Isomaltase Deficiency

The intolerance of sugars in congenital sucrase–isomaltase deficiency deserves a special comment. The clinical symptoms are mainly those of intolerance of ingested sucrose—abdominal distension and osmotic-fermentative diarrhea with liquid feces containing sucrose and glucose (see, for example, ref. 297). This correlates well with the lack of sucrase activity in this disease.

The situation with respect to 1,6-α-glucopyranosides is more complex. The oral tolerance of substrates of isomaltase (e.g., palatinose, i.e., 1,6-α-glucopyranosylfructose; and 1,6-α-glucose oligomers) may be as poor as that of sucrose[326]; that of dextrins, amylopectin, or starch may also be reduced.[326] When present in the diet, the latter glucans may nevertheless elicit diarrhea to a much milder degree than sucrose, particularly during the first year of life.[282,297,326] The milder symptoms are due to the low content of 1,6-α-glucosyl bonds in these glucans (as compared with the oligosaccharides used in the oral tolerance tests just mentioned); to the reduced, but not necessarily absent, 1,6-α-glucosidase (isomaltase) activity (see "Molecular Defects"); to the salvaging role of colonic flora; and to a sufficient residual capacity to hydrolyze 1,4-α-glucopyranosidic bonds.

The last point must be discussed further. The hydrolysis of amylopectin and of starch by α-amylase(s) is, as a rule, normal in these patients (but see below).[327] The capacity to hydrolyze completely the 1,4-α-glucans arising from α-amylolysis is severely reduced in patients with sucrase–isomaltase deficiency, yet the level is still sufficient to ensure adequate digestion. This level is mainly due to the glucoamylase complex (see Table 151-1), which is generally unaffected (but see refs. 328 to 330: in some cases of sucrase–isomaltase deficiency, glucoamylase also is affected, which can lead to reduced starch tolerance); also, the maltase activity of the "residual, altered isomaltase" present in some patients with sucrase–isomaltase deficiency (see under "Molecular Defects" below) may contribute an adequate digestion of 1,4-α-glucopyranosidic bonds.

Finally, as mentioned in the above section "Digestion of Starch and Glucose Polymers in Human Infants," in *normal* infants younger than 6 months of age the α-amylolytic digestion of starch in the lumen is either nil (during the first month of life) or incomplete. Infants of this age, if affected by sucrase–isomaltase deficiency, therefore show a very poor tolerance to starch.[299,327]

TYPES OF HEREDITARY CARBOHYDRATE INTOLERANCE

Primary Adult-type Hypolactasia

Primary adult-type hypolactasia is the most common form of genetically determined disaccharidase deficiency (see also Chap. 150). Isolated low lactase activity in adults was first described in Europe[331] and the United States[332] in individuals from populations that typically have persistent high lactase activity in adult life. The latter phenotype was considered "normal" until it was realized that, in the majority of the world's human populations, intestinal lactase declines during childhood and adolescence to about 5 to 10 percent of the level at birth,[333] as it does in most mammals after weaning.

Subjects with primary adult hypolactasia have no feeding problems during infancy, since the enzyme deficiency is not present at birth. The "postweaning" decline in intestinal lactase activity may start at different ages in the different ethnic groups: by age 3 years in blacks and Mexicans, later in North European and American white groups.[276,280,334–337] In the Finnish population, hypolactasia manifests itself between 10 and 20 years of age.[338] Evidence of sugar malabsorption by oral tolerance test or breath hydrogen test suggests increasing prevalence of malabsorption with age in these populations, with a substantial percentage of individuals demonstrating abnormal responses to the tests only as teenagers.[339–342] Intolerance to consumption of 250 ml of milk is rare in preadolescents.

Clinical and Nutritional Consequences of Hypolactasia. Shortly after drinking milk, lactose malabsorbers usually suffer from borborygmi and abdominal symptoms such as meteorism, abdominal fullness, loose stools or diarrhea, and abdominal pain.[303,343–346] The clinical effects of lactose ingestion are related to dose, with a wide variation in response among individuals.[335,344,347] The relationship of symptoms to milk ingestion may even go unrecognized by some patients. The conventional lactose load used in the tolerance test, 50 g, will produce symptoms in 70 to 90 percent of malabsorbers, whereas 10 to 15 g of lactose or half a pint of milk will produce abdominal symptoms in only 30 to 60 percent.[304,347,348]

Lactose intolerance due to lactase deficiency should be considered as the possible cause of gastrointestinal complaints in a number of patients with "idiopathic" diarrhea, irritable bowel syndrome, or recurrent abdominal pain, particularly in children[288] and in gastrectomized adults. A coincident lactose intolerance may modify the pattern of clinical presentation of gastrointestinal or other disease, and a period on a lactose-free diet may often be of diagnostic value in patients with abdominal complaints.[349]

Intolerance to lactose may also have nutritional consequences. Most lactose malabsorbers drink less milk than do lactose-tolerant individuals[304,350]; this behavior may decrease the intake of calcium. An increased incidence of intestinal lactase deficiency has been reported in subjects with osteoporosis,[351,352] which has been attributed to the avoidance of dairy products because of symptoms induced by lactose malabsorption and/or to a deleterious effect of lactose malabsorption on calcium absorption.[353–357] The presence of moderate amounts of lactose in the diet of lactose malabsorbers is reported to favor intestinal calcium absorption.[358,359]

It is not clear whether consumption of moderate quantities of milk may be dangerous to lactose malabsorbers. It certainly induces loss of calories and nutrients in feces; but this may become a problem only if the overall intake is only marginally adequate.[360,361] It is probably inadvisable to encourage the consumption of lactose-rich food, for example, fresh milk, in populations with a high frequency of lactose malabsorbers, since in these very populations the caloric and nutritional intake is often deficient.[361,362]

There is also no answer to the opposite question—whether a lactose-rich diet in adult life may entail some danger in subjects with persistent *high* lactase activity. Oral administration of D-galactose is, of course, known to produce cataracts in rats and other species (the lenses of which have a quite high aldose-reductase activity, as compared with humans[363]); in galactosemic patients dietary galactose is responsible for the cataract. It seems most likely that the main mechanism leading to galactose-induced cataract involves accumulation of the sparingly water-soluble galactitol in the lenses, although other mechanisms cannot be ruled out—for example, nonenzymatic glycosylation of proteins (to which galactose is more prone than glucose), followed by Amadori rearrangement and eventual formation of cross-links, etc. The suggestion has thus been put forward that persistence of high lactase activity into adulthood, and hence larger intake of lactose, may favor the formation of *senile* cataract. A high incidence of senile cataract has been noted in populations who consume large quantities of milk and lactose-rich milk products and who have, in addition, a high frequency of persistent lactase into adulthood.[364] A high frequency of lactose absorbers was found among adults with idiopathic, diabetic, and senile and presenile cataracts, as compared with controls, in a population with a high prevalence of primary adult-type hypolactasia[365,366]; in another study[367] high milk intake correlated with cortical cataracts. (For reviews, see refs. 368 and 369.) These observations indicate, therefore, that adults able to absorb galactose from a lactose-rich diet are more prone to having cataract. If this is so, however, nothing can be said at the moment about the possible mechanism(s) involved: attempts at detecting galactitol in lenses with senile or diabetic cataracts of subjects with adult-type hypolactasia have failed.[370]

Finally, in two population studies[371,372] significant positive correlations have been noted between the incidence of ovarian cancer, per capita milk consumption, and lactase persistence (and, in one study, low red-cell galactose-1-phosphate uridyltransferase). Lactose consumption may be a dietary risk factor, and low transferase a genetic risk factor for ovarian cancer.

Diagnosis. The diagnosis of lactose intolerance relies first of all on objective measurements of the clinical effects of the withdrawal and reintroduction of lactose. If the symptoms are due solely to lactose intolerance, response to a lactose-poor diet is excellent. Partial resolution of symptoms may suggest a coincidental problem of lactose malabsorption with another disorder, most often irritable bowel syndrome.[349] When gastrointestinal symptoms occur after ingestion of cow's milk, they need not be due to late-onset lactase deficiency. They may relate to a secondary lactase deficiency resulting from some gastrointestinal disease, to malabsorption of the monosaccharides deriving from the intestinal hydrolysis of lactose (glucose and galactose), to an allergic reaction to cow's milk protein,[373,374] or to some other cause.

Thus, the diagnosis of lactose malabsorption and lactase deficiency should be secured by appropriate tests (i.e., an oral tolerance test, a breath hydrogen test, and/or an assay of lactase in a jejunal biopsy specimen); see the section on diagnosis of malabsorption and intolerance, above.

Genetics and the Geographic Hypothesis. Lactase activity in human jejunum after infancy is genetically determined (see Chap. 150). The two adult human lactase phenotypes (either high or low activity) are attributable to different alleles at one autosomal locus. The effect of the allele responsible for the persistence of lactase after childhood is dominant to that of the allele causing decline of lactase activity.[333,376] Accordingly, lactase deficiency of adulthood (called *low* *lactase digestion capacity* by Flatz in Chap. 150) is the recessive phenotype. By calculating the lactase:maltase or lactase:sucrase ratio[376,377] in small-intestinal biopsies, a trimodal distribution was found, indicating a homozygous lactase-deficient phenotype, and heterozygous or homozygous lactase-persistent phenotypes (see Chap. 150 and refs. 362, 375, and 378 to 381).

Simoons has pointed out the striking similarity between the geographic areas of persistent high lactase activity and the traditional areas of milking. According to this *geographic hypothesis*,[333] humans in the Paleolithic period, like other land mammals, underwent a normal decline in intestinal lactase activity after weaning. With the appearance of milkable domesticated animals, a mutated human being with persistent high lactase activity would have a significant selective advantage, probably because of facilitated access to calories and nutrients, particularly calcium,[382] provided by milk. That advantage would occur within groups, especially pastoral and semipastoral ones, living under marginal nutritional conditions and consuming substantial amounts of lactose-rich dairy products. This hypothesis suggests, therefore, that the genetic change causing persistent high lactase activity may have taken place under the influence of the spread of agriculture, when humans, during the last few thousand years, ceased being food collectors (hunter-gatherers) and became food producers, thanks to the domestication of plants and animals.[383]

Therapy. In most cases it is sufficient to avoid foods rich in lactose (fresh milk, powdered milk, and milk puddings), whereas foods containing small amounts of lactose are usually well tolerated. Some individuals with hypolactasia can drink small amounts of milk without symptoms.

Lactose malabsorbers do not have symptoms when they ingest appreciable quantities of lactose in yogurt, since the lactase of the yogurt microorganism itself markedly contributes to the digestion of the disaccharide in vivo.[384–387] Furthermore, the calcium in the yogurt is absorbed normally by lactose malabsorbers; thus, yogurt is an excellent source of dietary calcium for them.[388]

Pretreatment of milk with β-galactosidase makes it well tolerated. In some countries milk previously percolated through immobilized β-galactosidase, and thus made poor in lactose, is available to the general public. The addition of microbial β-galactosidase directly to milk at mealtime also represents an effective enzyme replacement therapy.[389]

Congenital Lactase Deficiency

Congenital lactase deficiency is a very rare disease.[390–393] It is relatively more frequent in Finland, where 16 cases have been described.[394] Not more than 40 cases have been reported altogether.

A severe diarrhea starts during the first hours or days of life, with dehydration, malnutrition, and large amounts of lactose in the feces. On a lactose-free diet, children show good growth and psychomotor development. The disease appears in sibs and seems to have an autosomal recessive inheritance mode.[394] On a lactose-free diet, jejunal biopsies are morphologically normal; lactase activity is the only one affected. Lactase was originally thought to be totally absent in this disease,[395,396] even when a very sensitive assay method was used,[397] but most probably lactase is present, albeit at trace levels,[394,398] much lower than in adult hypolactasia.

Congenital lactase deficiency should not be confused with severe infantile lactose intolerance, first described by Durand[399]; in the latter disease the infant is critically ill, suffering from vomiting and failure to thrive on a lactose-containing diet, with lactosuria, aminoaciduria, and acidosis.[400–403] Cataract may also be present.[400,401,403] This disorder is not a mucosal enzyme deficiency, because substantial evidence exists that jejunal lactase activity is normal. It is probably due to an abnormal permeability of the gastric mucosa.[402]

Congenital Sucrase–Isomaltase Deficiency

Hereditary sucrose malabsorption was first described by Weijers et al.[404] in 1960. Shortly thereafter it was realized that in this condition isomaltose malabsorption is also present,[297,326,405] because of an absence of or severe reduction in not only sucrase but also isomaltase activity.[274,406–408] The disease occurs in families and is inherited as an autosomal recessive trait.[275,408]

Symptoms appear when sucrose or starch dextrins are added to the diet. Breast-fed infants or infants fed formulas containing only lactose remain well. The clinical manifestations are watery, osmotic-fermentative diarrhea, which may lead to dehydration and malnutrition, and even to occasional vomiting and milk steatorrhea. Failure to thrive and other symptoms are severe in the young child, but there is a tendency toward spontaneous improvement of symptoms with age; starch tolerance improves after the first years of life.[409] Symptoms, if they persist into adult life, may be limited to some increase in frequency of bowel movement and to minor abdominal distension, although episodes of diarrhea associated with high sucrose intake may still occur. In spite of this spontaneous favorable evolution, it is important that this condition be recognized as early as possible, so that the normal development of the child can be secured by removal of sucrose from the diet.[410]

The diagnosis can be missed in children with chronic diarrhea,[410,411] particularly in older children with a mild clinical presentation and normal growth and development.[412] In adults, the disease is a possible cause of refractory diarrhea or gastrointestinal complaints.[413] Many adults with this disorder have symptoms dating back to childhood, but occasionally the symptoms may appear as late as the time of puberty.[305,414–417]

Hereditary sucrase–isomaltase deficiency is probably rare in most human populations; only some 200 cases were reported up to 1984.[418] Welsh et al. found a 2 percent frequency of heterozygotes in a large series of small-intestinal biopsies from white American subjects.[276] The disease is more common among Greenland and Canadian Inuit and in Canadian Amerindians, the reported incidence of homozygotes varys between 4 and 10 percent.[376,377,419] It is not known whether the high frequency of the disease in these populations is the result of the high degree of inbreeding or whether this mutation produced an unidentified biologic advantage in populations that do not traditionally eat foods containing sucrose. Such an advantage might be related to some role of sucrase–isomaltase other than its digestive function. In the rabbit, the sucrase–isomaltase complex may serve as an intestinal receptor for an enteropathogenic *Escherichia coli*[420] and (along with other membrane glycoproteins) as a high-affinity receptor of *Clostridium difficile* toxin A.[290]

The diagnosis is based on the demonstration that osmotic-fermentative diarrhea, with increased fecal excretion of lactic acid, is elicited by sucrose and starch dextrins in the diet. A sucrose-tolerance test will produce a flat blood glucose curve and will result in acid watery diarrhea and presence of sucrose in the feces, whereas the absorption of a mixture of glucose and fructose will be normal. The sucrose hydrogen breath test consistently demonstrates excessive H_2 excretion in the breath.[286,421,422] The final diagnosis is based on the demonstration of deficiencies of α-glucosidase enzymes typical of the disease.

Treatment in the first years of life consists of the elimination of sucrose, glucose polymers, and starch from the diet. Symptoms subside within a few days. Restriction of starch intake is usually unnecessary after 2 to 3 years of age, although excessive amounts should be avoided.

Trehalase Deficiency

Trehalose is a disaccharide that occurs mainly in insects and in mushrooms.[423] Isolated trehalase malabsorption has been reported in an elderly woman[424] and in a family.[425] In the latter case, a 24-year-old man presented with diarrhea and vomiting after ingestion of a large amount of *edible* mushrooms. Peroral biopsies of the patient and of his father showed lack of trehalase activity: both subjects presented trehalose malabsorption on oral tolerance test with the disaccharide. Trehalase deficiency appears to be an autosomal recessive phenotype.[425]

Trehalase deficiency is likely to go undetected, since ingestion of large quantities of foods containing trehalose is not common; therefore its real frequency is unknown. Studies on disaccharidase activities in intestinal biopsies suggest that this defect in adult white Americans is rare,[276] whereas it is very frequent (10 to 15 percent) in Greenland Inuit.[418,426]

MOLECULAR DEFECTS

Congenital Sucrase–Isomaltase Deficiency

In the complex chain of events coding for the expression and hormonal regulation of a polypeptide chain of nearly 2000 amino acid residues, its membrane insertion, its glycosylation, its homing to the brush-border membrane, and so on (see the section on disaccharidase biosynthesis and anchoring, above), many steps can conceivably be affected by mutations. The result may be a lack of sucrase–isomaltase, or the appearance of an abnormal sucrase–isomaltase. Indeed, it was realized fairly early that sucrose–isomaltose malabsorption is a heterogeneous condition: whereas all patients lack sucrase, some have only traces of isomaltase activity while others have reduced but still conspicuous isomaltase activity.[274,329,398,427–430] The reports on the molecular defects in cases of sucrose–isomaltose malabsorption differ widely; they certainly agree with the concept that this condition has molecular genetic heterogeneity. But it is unfortunate that most of the papers dealing with this infrequent condition have investigated only a few patients (mostly belonging to a single pedigree) and have considered only a few properties. What follows is a list of reported and/or potential molecular defects.

1. Absence of sucrase–isomaltase activity and of immunologically cross-reacting material in total homogenates of jejunal biopsies was reported by Gray's group.[428] These conditions could be the consequence of mutations in the sucrase–isomaltase gene, in its promoter, or in a regulatory gene.

2. Absence of sucrase–isomaltase activity and of the corresponding protein band in SDS-PAGE of brush-border *membranes* was reported by Crane's group[431] and by others.[427,429,430] This finding would be compatible with the finding in item 1 above and also with a defective homing mechanism of pro-sucrase–isomaltase into the brush border.

3. Defective homing of pro-sucrase–isomaltase en route to the brush-border membrane,[112,432–434] (for a review, see ref. 435): various phenotypes could be identified by the combined use of electrophoresis, monoclonal antibodies, and electron microscopy. In one, the sucrase–isomaltase protein accumulated probably in the ER as a high-mannose precursor; in another, the intracellular transport was apparently blocked in the Golgi apparatus, and sucrase–isomaltase displayed an "immature" conformation[112]; in a third, a catalytically altered enzyme was transported to the cell surface; in a fourth, pro-sucrase–isomaltase did not undergo normal glycosylation in the Golgi apparatus and was mistargeted to the basolateral membrane[436]; in a fifth, high-mannose pro-sucrase–isomaltase was slowly and incompletely complex-glycosylated and cleaved intracellularly, with an isomaltaselike subunit being transferred to the brush-border membrane.[436] In some patients with defective homing, the high-mannose form is reported to be more easily degraded.[434] In most of these phenotypes, the block along the route was shown in in vitro pulse-chase experiments using peroral biopsies.

4. Absence of the sucrase and isomaltase bands in SDS-PAGE of the brush-border membranes and presence of abnormal band(s) have been reported. In one case a high-molecular-weight single-chain isomaltase was found that cross-reacted with anti-sucrase–isomaltase antiserums.[437] Is it a "back-mutated" protease-resistant double isomaltase? (See the section on disaccharide biosynthesis, above, for the "one polypeptide chain, two active sites" hypothesis.) Is it a mutated pro-sucrase–isomaltase with enzymatically inactive sucrase portion and with resistance to proteolytic processing?

5. Absence of the sucrase subunit and presence of a low-activity isomaltase subunit has been reported.[429,430] This finding may be related to that in item 3, above, or if this isomaltase is located in the brush-border membrane, it may indicate a mutated isomaltase subunit with (evidently) lower enzymatic activity and impaired capacity to interact normally with sucrase. It may be due, also, to a stop in the expression of the pro-sucrase–isomaltase polypeptide chain somewhere near the end of the isomaltase portion, which prevents synthesis of the sucrase portion (and hence of the sucrase subunit).

6. Presence of an immunologically cross-reacting, enzymatically inactive protein was reported by Dubs et al.[438] in patients with nonzero isomaltase activity.

7. Reduction in the amount[329,427,429,430] and/or change in the sedimentation properties[328] of the maltase–glucoamylase complex, present in some cases of sucrose–isomaltose malabsorption, may indicate that the biologic regulation of mechanisms of the two α-glucosidase heterodimeric complexes are related.

8. A possible regulatory gene controlling the expression of sucrase–isomaltase and its response to diet has been demonstrated in mice,[439] which may indicate that mutations in the regulatory gene are potentially responsible for (human) sucrose–isomaltose malabsorption: the sucrase and isomaltase activities in the brush-border membranes can indeed be equally and severely reduced.[440]

The regulatory gene demonstrated in mice does not influence either maltase–glucoamylase or trehalase.

Primary Adult-type Hypolactasia

The β-glycosidase complex present in the small intestine of subjects affected with primary adult-type hypolactasia seems to be indistinguishable from that present in lactose digesters: it has the same electrophoretic mobility,[277,441] the same immunologic properties,[441,442] and the same specific lactase[441,442] and phlorizin hydrolase activities[443] (although individual enterocytes may have inactive, or inactivated, lactase; see below). Sequence analysis (at the mRNA level) has shown that subjects with hypolactasia and persistence of lactase can code for identical pre-pro-lactase enzymes.[138]

The molecular defect(s) leading to the adult-type human hypolactasia cannot, at the time of this writing, be ascribed to a single cause. As in the case of the decline of lactase at weaning in the experimental animal, various, sometimes contradictory observations have been reported; thus, different molecular mechanisms have been suggested. Some contradictions may well eventually turn out to be apparent only. For example, different sites of control may be operative in different regions of the small intestine. If this is so, it may well be misleading to derive conclusions from samples obtained from the duodenum alone (the only segment of small intestine accessible to peroral duodenal endoscopy), even more so because in the duodenum the oral–aboral gradient of lactase is the steepest and its variability the largest.[272] Also, the proximal–distal gradient of lactase activity in lactose absorbers need not be identical with that of Fig. 151-8 in all ethnic or age groups (as discussed under "Diagnosis" above). Hence, studies carried out on endoscopic duodenal biopsies alone[444] are subject to question.

On the other hand, genetic variability may well be real, that is, the molecular mechanism operating in different pedigrees may well be different, depending on the ethnic group, and perhaps other factors. (See "Development and Regulation of the Disaccharidases" above). Keeping these limitations in mind, we will try to summarize below the present state of knowledge. (See also, ref. 444a.)

At the cellular level, the proximal small intestine of hypolactasic subjects is characterized by the existence of two types of populations of enterocytes—one expressing and the other not expressing lactase.[445] This is undoubtedly (one of) the mechanism(s) that can lead to the hypolactasia in the proximal small intestine of some adult humans. In fact, it agrees with the biochemical findings that the proximal small intestines of hypolactasic adults often synthesize lactase at reduced rates: reduced synthesis is observed in in vitro surviving cultures of peroral biopsies.[446–448] Also, markedly reduced mRNA levels are found in endoscopic duodenal biopsies[444,449] and in several (but not all; see below) surgical biopsies from proximal jejunum.[162,449a]

On the other hand, in the jejunal specimen of many Neapolitan adults we have studied[162] and also of North American subjects[450] some decrease of the level of lactase mRNA was found, but far less conspicuous than that of the lactase activity. Indeed, in a few subjects the levels of mRNA were comparable to those of adults with persistent high lactase activity, suggesting a posttranscriptional control of lactase in the intestinal tissue of these subjects with adult-type hypolactasia.

Delayed maturation of lactase[446,448] associated with the accumulation of immunoreactive material in the Golgi region on immunoelectromicroscopy[446] has been observed in some hypolactasic adults.[446] Furthermore, in the intestinal tissue of one subject, lactase biosynthesis was characterized by normal synthesis of high-molecular-weight precursors, followed by reduced conversion of these precursors to mature enzyme.[447] Finally, the proximal small intestine of a few hypolactasic adult Neapolitans was found to be able to synthesize high amounts of precursor forms and of mature lactase.[448,449a]

Summing up, both pretranslational and posttranslational factors seem to produce the decline of lactase in adult-type hypolactasia. Among the former ones are those leading to decreased levels of lactase mRNA—often, however, to levels quite as high as compared to the very low steady-state levels of the enzyme. Among the posttranslational factors, defective processing (and perhaps homing) of the lactase precursor and degradation of lactase have been reported. The posttranslational factors in particular make adult hypolactasia so very heterogeneous; the lactase mRNA levels in some hypolactasics[162,448–450b] may even be higher than those of some lactase persistents. Furthermore, the enterocyte of the proximal small intestinal villi from hypolactasic individuals show a conspicuously complicated patchy pattern[450a,b]: enterocytes with neither lactase mRNA nor lactase protein (probably as a consequence of reduced transcription or increased degradation of lactase mRNA); enterocytes with lactase mRNA, but without lactase protein in the brush borders (probably due to degradation of the lactase protein by luminal or cellular proteases, or to failure of the lactase protein to reach the microvillus membrane); enterocytes with lactase protein devoid of lactase activity (probably due to inactivation of the enzyme), and finally, enterocytes with lactase mRNA protein and activity (i.e., "persistent" enterocytes in an otherwise hypolactasic small intestine).

There is therefore no doubt that multiple mechanisms are responsible for the loss of lactase in adult mammals. The tenfold reduction in the steady-state levels of lactase activity may result from the combined, indeed multiplicative effects of such factors—increased cell kinetics, decreased transcription, and also, posttranslational degradation of the synthesized protein. Different factors act in the same individual, indeed in the very same villus, and some may be more prominent in some individuals than in others.

In the intestine of the suckling, on the contrary, high levels of lactase mRNA, the commitment of all enterocytes emerging from the crypts to produce lactase, the low enterocyte turnover, and the low intraluminal pancreatic (and bacterial) proteolysis favor high expression of lactase activity. *Persistence* of high lactase activity in the adult mutated man is most probably primarily due to increased biosynthesis of lactase; while a variety of factors lead to the *decline* of lactase activity, a single constant factor in *lactase persistence* is the high rate of its synthesis.[449a] Indeed, when it became advantageous to some human populations to keep having intestinal lactase activity in adulthood (see Simoons' "geographical hypothesis" mentioned above[333]), it was probably biologically "simpler" acting on a single biological event (i.e., increasing the rate of lactase biosynthesis via increased transcription), rather than acting on the host of factors causing lactase decline. (See also above, "Development and Regulation of the Disaccharidases, in Mammals Other than Humans"). The concept that lactase decline may be due to various factors, even acting in the very same individual, whereas lactase persistence is due to a single overriding factor (i.e., increased transcription) simplifies, therefore, our present understanding of these phenomena by focussing on persistence rather on the decline of the enzyme.

Congenital Lactase Deficiency

In a Finnish subject with this condition, the coding region of the lactase–phlorizin hydrolase gene has been sequenced[451] and found to be identical with that reported in lactase persistence,[99] save for minor allelic differences.

REFERENCES

1. McMichael HB: Disorders of carbohydrate digestion and absorption. *Clin Endocrinol Metab* **5**:627, 1976.
2. Gray GM: Carbohydrate absorption and malabsorption, in Johnson LR (ed): *Gastrointestinal Disease*. New York, Raven, 1981, p 1063.
3. Gitzelmann R, Auricchio S: The handling of soya α-galactosides by a normal and a galactosemic child. *Pediatrics* **36**:231, 1965.
4. Pazur JH, French D, Knapp DW: Mechanism of salivary amylase action. *Proc Iowa Acad Sci* **57**:203, 1950.
5. Pazur JH: The hydrolysis of amylotriose and amylotetraose by salivary amylase. *J Biol Chem* **205**:75, 1953.
6. Pazur JH, Budovich T: Hydrolysis of amylotriose by cristalline salivary amylase. *Science* **121**:702, 1955.
7. Pazur JH: Radioisotopes and enzymatic transformation of oligosaccharides. *Abstr 134th Am Chem Soc Meeting* 6D. New York, 1958.
8. Nordin PH: Action pattern of salivary amylase. Thesis. Iowa State College, 1953.
9. Bird R, Hopkins RH: The action of some α-amylases on amylose. *Biochem J* **56**:86, 1954.
10. Walker GJ, Whelan WJ: The action patterns of alfa-amylases. *Starke* **12**:358, 1960.
11. Whelan WJ, Roberts PJP: The mechanism of carbohydrase action. Part II, Alfa-amylolysis of linear substrate. *J Chem Soc* 1928, 1953.
12. Whelan WJ: The action patterns of α-amylases. *Starke* **12**:358, 1960.
13. Roberts PJP, Whelan WJ: The mechanism of carbohydrase action. 5. Action of human salivary α-amylase on amylopectin and glycogen. *Biochem J* **76**:246, 1960.
14. Bines J, Whelan WJ: The mechanism of carbohydrase action. 6. Structure of a salivary α-amylase limit dextrin from amylopectin. *Biochem J* **76**:253, 1960.
15. Heller J, Schramm M: α-Amylase limit dextrins of high molecular weight obtained from glycogen. *Biochim Biophys Acta* **81**:96, 1964.
16. Nordin PH, French D: I-Phenyl-flavazole derivates of starch dextrins. *J Am Chem Soc* **80**:1445, 1958.
17. Auricchio S, Della Pietra D, Vegnente A: Studies on intestinal digestion of starch in man. II. Intestinal hydrolysis of amylopectin in infants and children. *Pediatrics* **39**:853, 1967.
18. Anderson IH, Levine AS, Levitt MD: Incomplete absorption of the carbohydrate in all-purpose wheat flour. *N Engl J Med* **304**:891, 1981.
19. Levine AS, Levitt MD: Malabsorption of starch moiety of oats, corn, and potatoes. *Gastroenterology* **80**:1209, 1981.
20. Bond JH, Levitt MD: Use of pulmonary hydrogen (H2) measurements to quantitate carbohydrate absorption. Study of partially gastrectomized patients. *J Clin Invest* **51**:1219, 1972.
21. Stephen AM, Haddad AC, Phillips SF: Passage of carbohydrate into the colon. *Gastroenterology* **85**:589, 1983.
22. Chapman RW, Sillery JK, Graham MM, Saunders DR: Absorption of starch by healthy ileostomates: Effect of transit time and carbohydrate load. *Am J Clin Nutr* **41**:1244, 1985.
23. Goddard MS, Young G, Marcus R: The effect of amylose content on insulin and glucose responses to ingested rice. *Am J Clin Nutr* **39**:388, 1984.
24. Pomare EW, Branch WJ, Cunnings JH: Carbohydrate fermentation in the human colon and its relation to acetate concentration in venous blood. *J Clin Invest* **75**:1448, 1985.
25. De Vizia B, Ciccimarra F, De Cicco N, Auricchio S: Digestibility of starches in infants and children. *J Pediatr* **86**:50, 1975.
26. Flourie B, Florent C, Jouany JP, Thivend P, Etanchaud F, Rambaud JC: Colonic metabolism of wheat starch in healthy humans. *Gastroenterology* **90**:111, 1986.
27. Layer P, Zinsmeister AR, Di Magno E: Effects of decreasing intraluminal amylase activity on starch digestion and postprandial gastrointestinal function in humans. *Gastroenterology* **91**:41, 1986.
28. Lebenthal E, Lee PC: Development of functional response in human exocrine pancreas. *Pediatrics* **66**:556, 1980.
29. Zoppi G, Andreotti G, Pajno-Ferrara F, Njai DM, Gaburro D: Exocrine pancreas function in premature and fullterm neonates. *Pediatr Res* **6**:880, 1972.
30. Senterre J: Net absorption of starch in low birth weight infants. *Acta Paediatr Scand* **69**:653, 1980.
31. Shulman RJ, Wong WW, Irving CS, Nichols BL, Klein PD: Utilization of dietary cereal by young infants. *J Pediatr* **103**:23, 1983.
32. Klein PD, Klein ER: Application of stable isotopes to pediatric nutrition and gastroenterology: Measurement of nutrient absorption and digestion using 13C. *J Pediatr Gastroenterol Nutr* **4**:19, 1985.
33. Shulman RJ, Kerzner B, Sloan HR, Boutton TW, Wong WW, Nichols BL, Klein PD: Absorption and oxidation of glucose polymers of different lengths in young infants. *Pediatr Res* **20**:740, 1986.
34. Murray RD, Kerzner B, Sloan HR, McClung J, Gilbert M, Ailabouni A: The contribution of salivary amylase to glucose polymers hydrolysis in premature infants. *Pediatr Res* **20**:186, 1986.
35. Kerzner B, Sloan HR, McClung HJ, Ailabouni A: The jejunal absorption of glucose oligomers in the absence of pancreatic enzymes. *Pediatr Res* **15**:250, 1981.
36. Kelly JJ, Alpers DH: Properties of human intestinal glucoamylase. *Biochem Biophys Acta* **315**:113, 1981.
37. Ugolev AM: Membrane (contact) digestion. *Physiol Rev* **45**:555, 1965.
38. Gray GM, Lally BC, Conklin KA: Action of intestinal sucrase-isomaltase and its free monomers on an α-limit dextrin. *J Biol Chem* **254**:6038, 1979.
39. Taravel FR, Datema R, Woloszczuk W, Marshall JJ, Whelan WJ: Purification and characterization of a pig intestinal α-limit dextrinase. *Eur J Biochem* **130**:147, 1983.
40. Rodriguez IR, Taravel FR, Whelan WJ: Characterization and function of pig intestinal sucrase isomaltase and its separate subunits. *Eur J Biochem* **143**:575, 1984.
41. Sjöström H, Norén O, Danielsen EM, Skovbjerg H: Structure of microvillar enzymes in different phases of their life cycles, in Porter R, Collins G (eds): *Brush Border Membranes*. Ciba Foundation Symposium 95. London, Pitman, 1983, p 95.
42. Sφrensen SH, Norén O, Sjöström H, Danielsen EM: Amphiphilic pig intestinal microvillus maltase/glucoamylase. Structure and specificity. *Eur J Biochem* **126**:559, 1982.
43. Dahlqvist A: Specificity of the human intestinal disaccharidases and implications for hereditary disaccharide intolerance. *J Clin Invest* **41**:463, 1962.
44. Auricchio S, Semenza G, Rubino A: Multiplicity of human intestinal disaccharidases. II. Characterization of the individual maltases. *Biochim Biophys Acta* **96**:498, 1965.
45. Kolínská J, Semenza G: Studies on intestinal sucrase and on intestinal sugar transport. V. Isolation and properties of sucrase-isomaltase from rabbit small intestine. *Biochim Biophys Acta* **146**:181, 1967.
46. Messer M, Kerry KR: Intestinal digestion of maltotriose in man. *Biochim Biophys Acta* **132**:432, 1967.
47. Barnett JEG, Jarvis WTS, Munday KA: Enzymic hydrolysis of the carbon-fluorine bond of a α-D-glucosyl fluoride by rat intestinal mucosa. *Biochem J* **103**:699, 1967.
48. Cogoli A, Semenza G: A probable oxocarbonium ion in the reaction mechanism of small intestinal sucrase and isomaltase. *J Biol Chem* **250**:7802, 1975.
49. Dahlqvist A: Characterization of hog intestinal invertase as a glucosidoinvertase. III. Specificity of purified invertase. *Acta Chem Scand* **14**:63, 1960.
50. Larner J, McNickle CM: Gastrointestinal digestion of starch. I. The action of oligo-1,6-glucosidase on branched saccharides. *J Biol Chem* **215**:723, 1955.

51. Seiji M: Studies on digestion of starch by α-limit-dextrinase. *J Biochem* **40:**519, 1953.
52. Labat-Robert J, Baumann FC, Bar-Guilloux E, Robic D: Comparative specificities of trehalases from various species. *Comp Biochem Physiol [B]* **61:**111, 1978.
53. Hehre EJ, Sawai T, Brewer CF, Nakano M, Kanda T: Trehalase: Stereocomplementarity hydrolytic and glucosyl transfer reactions with α- and β-D-glucosyl fluoride. *Biochemistry* **21:**3090, 1982.
54. Wallenfels K, Fischer J: Untersuchungen über milchzuckerspaltende Enzyme. X. Die Laktase des Kälberdarms. *Z Physiol Chem* **321:**223, 1960.
55. Kraml J, Kolínská J, Elledérová H, Hiršová D: β-Glucosidase (phlorizin hydrolase) activity of the lactase fraction isolated from the small intestinal mucosa of infant rat and the relationship between β-glucosidases and β-galactosidases. *Biochim Biophys Acta* **258:**520, 1972.
56. Semenza G, Auricchio S, Rubino A: Multiplicity of human intestinal disaccharidases. 1. Chromatographic separation of maltases and of two lactases. *Biochim Biophys Acta* **96:**487, 1965.
57. Schlegel-Haueter S, Hore P, Kerry KR, Semenza G: The preparation of lactase and glucoamylase of rat small intestine. *Biochim Biophys Acta* **258:**506, 1971.
58. Leese HJ, Semenza G: On the identity between the small-intestinal enzymes phlorizin-hydrolase and glycosylceramidase. *J Biol Chem* **248:**8170, 1973.
59. Skovbjerg H, Norén O, Sjöström H, Danielsen EM, Enevoldsen BS: Further characterization of intestinal lactase-phlorizin hydrolase. *Biochim Biophys Acta* **707:**89, 1982.
60. Malathi P, Crane RK: Phlorizin hydrolase: A β-glucosidase of hamster intestinal brush border membrane. *Biochim Biophys Acta* **173:**245, 1969.
61. Colombo V, Lorenz-Meyer H, Semenza G: Small-intestinal phlorizin hydrolase: The β-glycosidase complex. *Biochim Biophys Acta* **327:**412, 1973.
62. Skovbjerg H: Immunoelectrophoretic studies on human small intestinal brush border proteins. The longitudinal distribution of peptidases and disaccharidases. *Clin Chim Acta* **112:**205, 1981.
63. Triadou N, Bataille J, Schmitz J: Longitudinal study of the human intestinal brush border membrane proteins. Distribution of the main disaccharidases and peptidases. *Gastroenterology* **85:**1326, 1983.
64. Raul F, Lacroix B, Aprahamian M: Longitudinal distribution of brush border hydrolases and morphological maturation in the intestine of the preterm infant. *Early Hum Dev* **13:**225, 1986.
65. Auricchio S, Rubino A, Mürset G: Intestinal glycosidase activities in the human embryo, fetus and newborn. *Pediatrics* **35:**944, 1965.
66. Miller D, Crane RK: The digestive function of the epithelium of the small intestine. 1. An intracellular locus of disaccharide and sugar phosphate ester hydrolysis. *Biochim Biophys Acta* **52:**281, 1961.
67. Parson DS, Pritchard JS: Hydrolysis of disaccharides during absorption by the perfused small intestine of amphibia. *Nature* **208:**1097, 1965.
68. Hamilton JD, McMichael HB: Role of microvillous in the absorption of disaccharides. *Lancet* **2:**154, 1968.
69. Malathi P, Ramaswamy K, Caspary WF, Crane RK: Studies on the transport of glucose from disaccharides by hamster small intestine in vitro. 1. Evidence for a disaccharidase-related transport system. *Biochim Biophys Acta* **307:**613, 1973.
70. Ramaswamy K, Malathi P, Caspary WF, Crane RK: Studies on the transport of glucose from disaccharides by hamster small intestine in vitro. II: Characteristic of the disaccharidase-related transport system. *Biochim Biophys Acta* **345:**39, 1974.
71. Gray GM, Ingelfinger FJ: Intestinal absorption of sucrose in man: The site of hydrolysis and absorption. *J Clin Invest* **44:**390, 1965.
72. McMichael HB, Webb J, Dowson AM: The absorption of maltose and lactose in man. *Clin Sci* **33:**135, 1967.
73. Alpers DH, Cote MN: Inhibition of lactose hydrolysis by dietary sugars. *Am J Physiol* **221:**865, 1971.
74. Dawson DJ, Lobley RW, Burrows PC, Miller W, Holmes R: Lactose digestion by human jejunal biopsies: The relationship between hydrolysis and absorption. *Gut* **27:**521, 1986.
75. Gray GM, Santiago N: Disaccharide absorption in normal and diseased human intestine. *Gastroenterology* **51:**489, 1966.
76. Wacker H, Jaussi R, Sonderegger O, Dokow M, Ghersa P, Hauri HP, Christen PH, Semenza G: Cell-free synthesis of the one-chain precursor of a major intrinsic protein complex of the small-intestinal brush border membrane (pro-sucrase-isomaltase). *FEBS Lett* **136:**329, 1981.
77. Semenza G: Anchoring and biosynthesis of stalked brush border membrane proteins: Glycosidases and peptidases of enterocytes and renal tubuli. *Annu Rev Cell Biol* **2:**255, 1986.
78. Spiess M, Hunziker W, Lodish HF, Semenza G: Molecular cell biology of brush border hydrolases: Sucrase isomaltase and γ-glutamyl transpeptidase, in Kenny AJ, Turner AJ (eds): *Ectoenzymes*. Amsterdam, Elsevier, 1987, p 87.
78a. Semenza G: The insertion of stalked proteins of the brush border membranes: The state of the art in 1988. *Biochem Int* **18:**15, 1989.
79. Brunner J, Hauser H, Braun H, Wilson KJ, Wacker H, O'Neill B, Semenza G: The mode of association of the enzyme complex sucrase-isomaltase with the intestinal brush border membrane. *J Biol Chem* **254:**1821, 1979.
80. Hunziker W, Spiess M, Semenza G, Lodish H: The sucrase-isomaltase complex: Primary structure, membrane orientation and evolution of a stalked intrinsic brush border protein. *Cell* **46:**227, 1986.
81. Lee L, Forstner G: Hydrophobic binding domains of rat intestinal maltase-glucoamylase. *Biochem Cell Biol* **64:**782, 1986.
82. Hu C, Spiess M, Semenza G: The mode of anchoring and precursor forms of sucrase-isomaltase and maltase-glucoamylase in chicken intestinal brush border membrane. Phylogenetic implications. *Biochim Biophys Acta* **896:**275, 1987.
82a. Chantret I, Lacasa M, Chevalier G, Ruf J, Islam I, Mantei N, Edwards Y, Swallow D, Rousset M: Sequence of the complete cDNA and the 5′ structure of the human sucrase isomaltase gene: Homology with a yeast glucoamylase. *Biochem J* **285:**915, 1992.
82b. Duluc I, Boukamel R, Mantei N, Semenza G, Raul F, Freund J-N: Sequence of the precursor of intestinal lactase-phlorizin hydrolase from fetal rat. *Gene* **103:**275, 1991.
82c. Montgomery RK, Sybicki MA, Forcier AG, Grand RJ: Rat intestinal microvillus membrane sucrase-isomaltase is a single high molecular weight protein and fully active enzyme in the absence of luminal factors. *Biochim Biophys Acta* **661:**346, 1981.
82d. Naim HY, Sterchi EE, Lentze MJ: Structure, biosynthesis, and glycosylation of human small intestinal maltase-glucoamylase. *J Biol Chem* **263:**19709, 1988.
82e. Castillo RO, Kwong LK, Reisenauer AM, Tsuboi KK: Human intestinal lactase-phlorizin hydrolase: Isolation and preparation of a specific antiserum. *Biochem Biophys Res Commun* **164:**94, 1989.
83. Sjöström H, Norén O, Christiansen L, Wacker H, Spiess M, Bigler-Meier B, Rickli EE, Semenza G: N-terminal sequences of pig intestinal sucrase-isomaltase and pro-sucrase-isomaltase. Implications for the biosynthesis and membrane insertion of pro-sucrase-isomaltase. *FEBS Lett* **148:**321, 1982.
84. Spiess M, Brunner J, Semenza G: Hydrophobic labeling, isolation and partial characterization of the NH_2-terminal membranous segment of sucrase-isomaltase complex. *J Biol Chem* **257:**2370, 1982.
85. Wacker H, Keller P, Falchetto R, Legler G, Semenza G: Location of the two catalytic sites in intestinal lactase-phlorizin hydrolase: Comparison with sucrase-isomaltase and with other glycosidases. The membrane anchor of lactase-phlorizin hydrolase. *J Biol Chem* **267:**18744, 1992.
86. Norén O, Sjöström H, Cowell G, Tranum-Jensen J, Hansen OC, Welinder KG: Pig intestinal microvillar maltase-glucoamylase. Structure and membrane insertion. *J Biol Chem* **261:**12306, 1986.
87. Cowell GM, Sjöström H, Norén O, Tranum-Jensen J: Topology and quaternary structure of pro-sucrase-isomaltase

and final forms of sucrase isomaltase. *Biochem J* **237:**455, 1986.

88. Semenza G: Intestinal oligo- and disaccharides, in Randle PJ, Steiner DF (eds): *Carbohydrate Metabolism and Its Disorders.* London, Academic, 1981, p 425.
89. Hauser H, Semenza G: Sucrase-isomaltase: A stalked intrinsic protein of the brush border membrane. *Crit Rev Biochem* **14:**319, 1983.
90. Semenza G: Glycosidases, in Kenny AJ, Turner AJ (eds): *Ectoenzymes.* Amsterdam, Elsevier, 1987, p 265.
91. Semenza G: The sucrase-isomaltase complex, a large dimeric amphipathic protein from the small intestinal brush border membrane: Emerging structure-function relationships, in Ahlberg P, Sundelöf LO (eds): *Structure and Dynamics of Chemistry. Symposium 500th Jubilee Univ Uppsala, Sweden, Stockholm* Almquist and Wiksell, 1977, p 226.
92. Semenza G: Mode of insertion of the sucrase-isomaltase complex in the intestinal brush border membrane: Implications for the biosynthesis of this stalked intrinsic membrane protein, in Elliot K, Whelan WJ (eds): *Development of Mammalian Absorptive Processes.* Ciba Foundation Symposium. Amsterdam, Excerpta Medica, 1979, vol 70, p 133.
93. Semenza G: The mode of anchoring of sucrase-isomaltase to the small-intestinal brush border membrane and its biosynthetic implications, in Rapoport S, Schewe T (eds): *Proc 12th FEBS Meeting, Dresden.* Oxford, Pergamon, 1978, vol 53, p 21.
94. Fulcher IS, Pappin JC, Kenny AJ: The N-terminal amino acid sequence of pig kidney endopeptidase 24.11 shows homology with pro-sucrase-isomaltase. *Biochem J* **240:**305, 1986.
95. Spiess M, Mantei N, Semenza G: Unpublished observations 1989.
96. Hoefsloot LH, Hoogeveen-Westerveld M, Kroos MA, Van Beeumen J, Reuser AJJ, Oostra BA: Primary structure and processing of lysosomal α-glucosidase; homology with the intestinal sucrase-isomaltase complex. *EMBO J* **7:**1697, 1988.
97. Danielsen EM, Sjöström H, Norén O: Biosynthesis of microvillar proteins. Pulse-chase labeling studies on maltase-glucoamylase, aminopeptidase A and dipeptidyl peptidase IV. *Biochem J* **210:**389, 1983.
98. Ghersa P, Huber P, Semenza G, Wacker H: Cell-free synthesis, membrane integration and glycosylation of pro-sucrase-isomaltase. *J Biol Chem* **261:**7969, 1986.
99. Mantei N, Villa M, Enzler T, Wacker H, Boll W, James P, Hunziker H, Semenza G: Complete primary structure of human and rabbit lactase-phlorizin hydrolase: Implications for biosynthesis, membrane anchoring and evolution of the enzyme. *EMBO J* **7:**2705, 1988.
100. Gräbnitz F, Seiss M, Rücknagel KP, Staudenbauer WL: Structure of the β-glucosidase gene *bglA* of *Clostridium thermocellum. Eur J Biochem* **200:**301, 1991.
100a. Dudley MA, Hachey DL, Quaroni A, Hutchens TW, Nichols BL, Rosenberger J, Perkinson JS, Cook G, Reeds PJ: In vivo sucrase-isomaltase and lactase-phlorizin hydrolase turnover in fed adult rat. *J Biol Chem* **268:**13609, 1993.
101. Danielsen EM, Skovbjerg H, Norén O, Sjöström H: Biosynthesis of intestinal microvillar proteins. Intracellular processing of lactase-phlorizin hydrolase. *Biochem Biophys Res Commun* **122:**82, 1984.
102. Skovbjerg H, Danielsen EM, Norén O, Sjöström H: Evidence for biosynthesis of lactase-phlorizin hydrolase as a single-chain high-molecular weight precursor. *Biochim Biophys Acta* **789:**247, 1984.
103. Naim HY, Sterchi EE, Lentze MJ: Biosynthesis and maturation of lactase-phlorizin hydrolase in the human small intestinal epithelial cells. *Biochem J* **241:**427, 1987.
104. Büller HA, Montgomery RK, Sasak WV, Grand RJ: Biosynthesis, glycosylation and intracellular transport of intestinal lactase-phlorizin hydrolase in rat. *J Biol Chem* **262:**17206, 1987.
105. Witte J, Lloyd M, Lorenzsonn V, Korsmo H, Olsen WA: The biosynthetic basis of adult lactase deficiency. *J Clin Invest* **86:**1338, 1990.
106. Rossi M, Maiuri L, Russomanno C, Auricchio S: In vitro biosynthesis of lactase in preweaning and adult rabbit. *FEBS Lett* **313:**260, 1992.
106a. Lottaz D, Oberholzer T, Bähler P, Semenza G, Sterchi EE: Maturation of human lactase-phlorizin hydrolase. Proteolytic cleavage of precursor occurs after passage through the Golgi complex. *FEBS Lett* **313:**270, 1992.
106b. Yeh KY, Yeh M, Pan PC, Holt PR: Posttranslational cleavage of rat intestinal lactase occurs at the luminal side of the brush border membrane. *Gastroenterology* **101:**312, 1991.
106c. Grünberg J, Luginbühl U, Sterchi EE: Proteolytic processing of human intestinal lactase-phlorizin hydrolase precursor is not a prerequisite for correct sorting in Madin Darby canine kidney (MDCK) cells. *FEBS Lett* **314:**224, 1992.
106d. Oberholzer T, Mantei N, Semenza G: The pro sequence of lactase-phlorizin hydrolase is required for the enzyme to reach the plasma membrane. An intramolecular chaperone? *FEBS Lett* **333:**127, 1993.
107. Naim HY, Lacely SW, Sambrook JF, Gething M-JH: Expression of a full-length cDNA coding for human intestinal lactase-phlorizin hydrolase reveals an uncleaved, enzymatically active and transport-competent protein. *J Biol Chem* **266:**12313, 1991.
108. Beaulieu JF, Nichols B, Quaroni A: Post-translational regulation of sucrase-isomaltase expression in intestinal crypt and villus cells. *J Biol Chem* **264:**20000, 1989.
109. Danielsen EM: Perturbation of intestinal microvillar enzyme biosynthesis by amino acid analogues. *J Biol Chem* **264:**13726, 1989.
110. Hurtley SM, Helenius A: Protein oligomerization in the endoplasmic reticulum. *Annu Rev Cell Biol* **5:**277, 1989.
111. Danielsen EM: Folding of intestinal brush border enzymes. Evidence that high mannose glycosylation is an essential early event. *Biochemistry* **31:**2266, 1992.
112. Matter K, Hauri HP: Intracellular transport and conformational maturation of intestinal brush border hydrolases. *Biochemistry* **30:**1916, 1991.
112a. Danielsen EM: Biosynthesis of intestinal microvillar proteins. Dimerization of aminopeptidase N and lactase-phlorizin hydrolase. *Biochemistry* **29:**305, 1990.
113. Danielsen EM: Tyrosine sulfation, a post-translational modification of microvillar enzymes in the small intestinal enterocyte. *EMBO J* **6:**2891, 1987.
114. Danielsen EM: Tyrosine sulfation is not required for microvillar expression of intestinal aminopeptidase N. *Biochem J* **254:**219, 1988.
115. Danielsen EM: Biosynthesis of intestinal microvillar proteins. Pulse-chase labeling studies on aminopeptidase N and sucrase-isomaltase. *Biochem J* **204:**639, 1982.
116. Danielsen EM, Cowell GM, Norén O, Sjöström H: Biosynthesis of microvillar proteins. *Biochem J* **221:**1, 1984.
117. Hauri HP, Sterchi EE, Bienz D, Fransen JAM, Marxer A: Expression and intracellular transport of microvillus membrane hydrolases in human intestinal epithelial cells. *J Cell Biol* **101:**838, 1985.
118. Danielsen EM, Cowell GM: Biosynthesis of intestinal microvillar proteins. The intracellular transport of aminopeptidase N and sucrase-isomaltase occurs at different rates pre-Golgi but at the same rate post-Golgi. *FEBS Lett* **190:**69, 1985.
119. Stieger B, Matter K, Baur B, Höchli M, Hauri HP: Dissection of the asynchronous transport of intestinal microvillar hydrolases to the cell surface. *J Cell Biol* **106:**1853, 1988.
120. Danielsen EM, Cowell GM: Biosynthesis of intestinal microvillar proteins. Evidence for an intracellular sorting taking place in, or shortly after, exit from the Golgi complex. *Eur J Biochem* **152:**493, 1985.
121. Hansen G, Dabelsteen E, Sjöström H, Norén O: Immunomicroscopic localization of aminopeptidase N in the pig enterocyte. Implication for the route of intracellular transport. *Eur J Cell Biol* **43:**53, 1987.
122. Matter K, Brauchbar M, Bucher K, Hauri HP: Sorting of endogenous plasma membrane proteins occurs from two sites in cultured human intestinal epithelial cells (Caco-2). *Cell* **60:**429, 1990.
123. LeBivic A, Quaroni A, Nichols B, Rodriguez-Boulan E: Biogenetic pathways of plasma membrane proteins in Caco-2, a human intestinal epithelian cell line. *J Cell Biol* **111:**1351, 1990.
124. Hauri HP, Quaroni A, Isselbacher K: Biogenesis of intestinal plasma membrane: Posttranslational route and cleav-

age of sucrase-isomaltase. *Proc Natl Acad Sci USA* **76:**5183, 1979.

125. Danielsen EM, Hansen GH, Cowell GM: Biosynthesis of intestinal microvillar proteins. Low temperature arrests both processing and intracellular transport. *Eur J Cell Biol* **49:**123, 1989.
126. Fransen JAM, Ginsel LA, Hauri HP, Sterchi EE, Blok J: Immunoelectromicroscopical localization of a microvillus membrane disaccharidase in the human small-intestinal epithelium with monoclonal antibodies. *Eur J Cell Biol* **38:**6, 1985.

126a. Naim HY, Lentze MJ: Impact of O-glycosylation on the function of human intestinal lactase-phlorizin hydrolase. *J Biol Chem* **267:**25494, 1992.

126b. Matter K, Stieger B, Klumperman J, Ginsel L, Hauri HP: Endocytosis, recycling, and lysosomal delivery of brush border hydrolases in cultured human intestinal epithelial cells (Caco-2), *J Biol Chem* **265:**3503, 1990.

127. Sjöström H, Norén O, Danielsen EM: The enzymatic activity of "high mannose" glycosylated forms of intestinal microvillar hydrolases. *J Pediatr Gastroenterol Nutr* **4:**980, 1985.
128. Kelly JJ, Alpers DH: Blood group antigenicity of purified human intestinal disaccharidases. *J Biol Chem* **248:**8216, 1973.
129. Pothoulakis C, Gao N, Cladaras C, Offner G, LaMont JT: *C. difficile* toxin A binds to rabbit ileal sucrase-isomaltase. *Gastroenterology* 1994. (In Press) (abstr)
130. Cousineau J, Green JR: Isolation and characterization of the proximal and distal forms of lactase-phlorizin-hydrolase from the small intestine of the suckling rat. *Biochim Biophys Acta* **615:**147, 1980.
131. Kraml J, Kolínská J, Kadlecová L, Zákostelecká M, Lojda Z: Analytical isoelectric focusing of rat intestinal brush border enzymes: Postnatal changes and effect of neuraminidase in vitro. *FEBS Lett* **151:**193, 1983.
132. Kraml J, Kolínská J, Kadlecová L, Zákostelecká M, Lojda Z: Effect of hydrocortisone on the desialylation of intestinal brush border enzymes of the rat during postnatal development. *FEBS Lett* **172:**25, 1984.
133. Semenza G: The minimum catalytic mechanism of intestinal sucrase and isomaltase. *Indian J Biochem Biophys* **28:**331, 1991.
134. Green F, Edwards Y, Hauri HP, Povey S, Ho WM, Pinto M, Swallow D: Isolation of a cDNA probe for a human jejunum brush-border hydrolase, sucrase-isomaltase, and assignment of the gene locus to chromosome 3. *Gene* **57:**101, 1987.
135. West LF, Davis MB, Green FR, Lindenbaum RH, Swallow D: Regional assignment of the gene coding for human sucrase-isomaltase (SI) to chromosome 3q25-26. *Ann Hum Genet* **52:**57, 1988.
136. Kruse TA, Bolund L, Grzeschik KH, Ropers HH, Sjöström H, Norén O, Mantei N, Semenza G: The human lactase-phlorizin hydrolase gene is located on chromosome 2. *FEBS Lett* **240:**123, 1988.
137. Kruse TA, Bolund L, Byskov A, Sjöström H, Norén O, Mantei N, Semenza G: Mapping of the human lactase-phlorizin hydrolase gene to chromosome 2. *Cytogenet Cell Genet* **51:**1026, 1989.

137a. Harvey CB, Fox MF, Jeggo PA, Mantei N, Povey S, Swallow DM: Regional localization of the lactase-phlorizin hydrolase gene, LCT, to chromosome 2q21. *Ann Hum Genet* **57:**179, 1993.

138. Boll W, Wagner P, Mantei N: Structure of the chromosomal gene and cDNAs coding for lactase-phlorizin hydrolase in humans with adult-type hypolactasia or persistence of lactase. *Am J Hum Genet* **48:**889, 1991.

138a. Villa M, Brunschwiler D, Gächter T, Boll W, Semenza G, Mantein N: Region-specific expression of multiple lactase-phlorizin hydrolase genes in intestine of rabbit. *FEBS Lett* **336:**70, 1993.

139. Galand G: Purification and characterization of kidney and intestinal brush-border membrane trehalases from the rabbit. *Biochim Biophys Acta* **789:**10, 1984.
140. Yokota K, Nishi Y, Takesue Y: Purification and characterization of amphiphilic trehalase from rabbit small intestine. *Biochim Biophys Acta* **881:**405, 1986.
141. Ruf J, Wacker H, James P, Maffia M, Seiler P, Galand G, von Kieckenbush A, Semenza G, Mantei N: Rabbit small intestinal trehalase. Purification, cDNA cloning, expression, and verification of glycosylphosphatidylinositol anchoring. *J Biol Chem* **265:**15034, 1990.
142. Takesue Y, Yokota K, Nishi Y, Taguchi R, Ikesawa H: Solubilization of trehalase from rabbit renal and intestinal brush-border membranes by a phosphoinositol-specific phospholipase C. *FEBS Lett* **201:**5, 1986.
143. Gutierrez C, Ardourel M, Bremer E, Middendorf A, Boos W, Ehmann U: Analysis and DNA sequence of the osmoregulated *treA* gene encoding the periplasmic trehalase of *Escherichia coli* K12. *Mol Gen Genet* **217:**347, 1989.
144. Rubino A, Zimbalatti F, Auricchio S: Intestinal disaccharidase activities in adult and suckling rats. *Biochim Biophys Acta* **92:**305, 1964.
145. Dubs R, Gitzelman R, Steinmann B, Lindenmann J: Catalytically inactive sucrase antigen of rabbit small intestine: The enzyme precursor. *Helv Paediatr Acta* **30:**89, 1975.
146. Doell RG, Kretchmer N: Studies of small intestine during development. I. Distribution and activity of β-galactosidase. *Biochim Biophys Acta* **62:**353, 1962.
147. Colombo V, Lorenz-Meyer H, Semenza G: Small-intestinal phlorizin hydrolase: The "β-glycosidase complex." *Biochim Biophys Acta* **327:**412, 1973.
148. Lee PC, Lebenthal E: Early weaning and precocious development of small intestine in rats: Genetic, dietary or hormonal control. *Pediatr Res* **17:**645, 1983.
149. Yeh KJ, Holt PR: Ontogenic timing mechanism initiates the expression of rat intestinal sucrase activity. *Gastroenterology* **90:**520, 1986.
150. Henning SJ: Postnatal development: Coordination of feeding, digestion and metabolism. *Am J Physiol* **241:**G199, 1981.
151. Henning SJ: Ontogeny of enzymes in the small intestine. *Annu Rev Physiol* **47:**231, 1985.
152. Klein RM, McKenzie JC: The role of cell renewal in the ontogeny of the intestine. I. Cell proliferation patterns in adult, fetal and neonatal intestine. *J Pediatr Gastroenterol Nutr* **2:**204, 1983.
153. Maiuri L, Garipoli V, Norén O, Dabelsteen E, Swallow D, Auricchio S: Mosaic pattern of expression of lactase protein and mRNA by villus enterocytes in adult rabbit. *Gastroenterology* **100:**A227, 1991.
154. Kedinger M, Simon PM, Grenier JF, Haffen K: Role of epithelial mesenchymal interactions in the ontogenesis of intestinal brush border enzymes. *Dev Biol* **86:**339, 1981.
155. Haffen K, Lacroix B, Kedinger M, Simon-Assmann PM: Inductive properties of fibroblastic cell cultures derived from rat intestinal mucosa on epithelial differentiation. *Differentiation* **23:**226, 1983.
156. Simon PM, Kedinger M, Raul F, Grenier JF, Haffen K: Developmental pattern of rat intestinal brush border enzymic proteins along the villous-crypt axis. *Biochem J* **178:**407, 1979.
157. Boyle JT, Kokonos M, Koldovský O: Developmental profile of jejunal lactase and sucrase activity along the villous-crypt in the rat. *Pediatr Res* **16:**157A, 1982.
158. Lund EK, Smith MW: Rat jejunal disaccharidase activity increases biphasically during early development. *J Physiol (Lond)* **391:**487, 1987.
159. Kolínská J, Kraml J, Zákostelecká M, Lojda Z: Low molecular weight antigens of sucrase-isomaltase in the intestinal mucosa of suckling rats. *Mol Physiol* **5:**133, 1984.
160. Sebastio G, Hunziker W, Ballabio A, Auricchio S, Semenza G: On the primary site of control in the spontaneous development of small intestinal sucrase isomaltase after birth. *FEBS Lett* **208:**460, 1986.
161. Leeper LL, Henning SJ: Development and tissue distribution of sucrase-isomaltase mRNA in rats. *Am J Physiol* **258:**652, 1990.
162. Sebastio G, Villa M, Sartorio R, Guazzetta V, Poggi V, Auricchio S, Boll W, Mantei N, Semenza G: Control of lactase in human adult-type hypolactasia and in weaning rabbits and rats. *Am J Hum Genet* **45:**489, 1989.
163. Traber PG: Regulation of sucrase-isomaltase gene expression along the crypt-villus axis of rat small intestine. *Biochem Biophys Res Commun* **173:**765, 1990.
164. Lorenzsonn V, Lloyd M, Olsen WA: Transcription of mRNA for sucrase-isomaltase peaks before the protein on the

crypt-villus axis of rat small intestine. *J Cell Biol* **109:**124a, 1989.

165. Doell RG, Kretchmer N: Intestinal invertase: Precocious development of activity after injection of hydrocortisone. *Science* **143:**42, 1964.
166. Malo CH, Ménard D: Hormonal control of intestinal glucoamylase activity in suckling and adult mice. *Comp Biochem Physiol [B]* **65:**169, 1980.
167. Kedinger M, Simon PM, Raul F, Grenier JF, Haffen K: The effect of dexamethasone on the development of rat intestinal brush border enzymes in organ culture. *Dev Biol* **74:**9, 1980.
168. Beaulieu JF, Calvert R: Influences of dexamethasone on the maturation of fetal mouse intestinal mucosa in organ culture. *Comp Biochem Physiol [A]* **82:**91, 1985.
169. Ménard D, Malo CH, Calvert R: Insulin accelerates the development of intestinal brush border hydrolytic activities of suckling mice. *Dev Biol* **85:**150, 1981.
170. Malo CH, Ménard D: Influence of epidermal growth factor on the development of suckling mouse intestinal mucosa. *Gastroenterology* **83:**28, 1982.
171. Walsh MJ, Leleiko NS, Sterling KM: Glucocorticoid-induced development of the rat small intestine is associated with differential regulation of intestinal and basement membrane collagen in RNA synthesis. *Gastroenterology* **90:**1683(A), 1986.
172. Sebastio G, Hunziker W, O'Neill B, Malo C, Ménard D, Auricchio S, Semenza G: The biosynthesis of intestinal sucrase-isomaltase in human embryo is most likely controlled at the level of transcription. *Biochem Biophys Res Commun* **149:**830, 1987.
173. Sebastio G, Hunziker W, Ballabio A, Maiuri S, Auricchio S, Semenza G: On the primary site of control in spontaneous and glucocorticoid-triggered precocious development of small-intestinal sucrase-isomaltase complex. *Pediatr Res* **22:**99, 1987. (abstr.)

173a. Henning SJ, Ballard PL, Kretchmer N: A study on the cytoplasmic receptors for glucocorticoid in intestine of pre- and postweaning rats. *J Biol Chem* **250:**2073, 1975.

173b. Henning SJ, Leeper LL: Coordinate loss of glucocorticoid responsiveness by intestinal enzymes during postnatal development. *Am J Physiol* **242:**G89, 1982.

173c. Galand G: Effect of an antiglucocorticoid (RU-38486) on hydrocortisone induction of maltase-glucoamylase, sucrase-isomaltase and trehalase in brush border membranes of suckling rats. *Experientia* **44:**516, 1988.

174. Kedinger M, Haffen K, Simon-Assman P: Control mechanisms in the ontogenesis of villus cells, in Desnuelle P, Sjöström H, Norén O (eds): *Molecular and Cellular Biology of Digestion*. Amsterdam, Elsevier, 1986, p 323.
175. Moog F: Perinatal development of the enzymes of the brush border membrane, in Lebenthal E (ed): *Textbook of Gastroenterology and Nutrition*. New York, Raven, 1981, p 139.
176. Koldovský O: Developmental, dietary and hormonal control of intestinal disaccharidases in mammals (including man), in Randle PJ, Steiner DF, Whelan WJ (eds): *Carbohydrate Metabolism and Its Disorders*. London, Academic, 1981, vol 3, p 418.
177. Enck P, Whitehead WE: Lactase deficiency and lactose malabsorption. A review. *Z Gastroenterol* **24:**125, 1986.

177a. Galand G: Brush border membrane sucrase-isomaltase, maltase-glucoamylase and trehalase in mammals. Comparative development, effects of glucocorticoids, molecular mechanisms, and phylogenetic implications. *Comp Biochem Physiol [B]* **94:**1, 1989.

178. Leichter J: Effect of dietary lactose on intestinal lactase activity in young rats. *J Nutr* **103:**392, 1973.
179. Ferguson A, Gerskowitch VP, Russell RI: Pre- and postweaning disaccharidase patterns in isografts of fetal mouse intestine. *Gastroenterology* **64:**292, 1973.
180. Bolin TD, McKern A, Davis AE: The effect of diet on lactase activity in the rat. *Gastroenterology* **60:**432, 1971.
181. Bolin TD, Pirola RC, Davis AE: Adaptation of intestinal lactase in the rat. *Gastroenterology* **57:**406, 1969.
182. Montgomery RK, Sybicki MA, Grand RJ: Autonomous biochemical and morphological differentiation in the fetal rat intestine transplanted at 17 and 20 days of gestation. *Dev Biol* **87:**76, 1981.
183. Yeh KY, Yeh M, Holt PR: Intestinal lactase expression and epithelial cell transit in hormone-treated suckling rats. *Am J Physiol* **260:**G379, 1991.
184. Nsi-Emvo E, Launay JF, Raul F: Is adult-type hypolactasia in the intestine of mammals related to changes in the intracellular processing of lactase? *Cell Mol Biol* **33:**335, 1987.
185. Freund JN, Duluc I, Raul F: Discrepancy between the intestinal lactase enzymatic activity and the mRNA accumulation in suckling and adults. Effect of starvation and thyroxine treatment. *FEBS Lett* **248:**39, 1989.

185a. Freund JN, Duluc I, Foltzer-Jourdainne C, Gosse F, Raul F: Specific expression of lactase in the jejunum and colon during postnatal development and hormone treatments in the rat. *Biochem J* **268:**99, 1990.

186. Moog F: The functional differentiation of the small intestine. II. The differentiation of alkaline phosphomonoesterases in the duodenum of the mouse. *J Exp Zool* **118:**187, 1951.
187. Moog F: The functional differentiation of the small intestine. III. The influence of the pituitary-adrenal system on the differentiation of phosphatase in the duodenum of the suckling mouse. *J Exp Zool* **124:**329, 1953.
188. Yeh K, Moog F: Intestinal lactase activity in the suckling rat: Influence of hypophysectomy and thyroidectomy. *Science* **183:**77, 1974.
189. Malo CH, Ménard D: Opposite effects of one and three injections of cortisone or thyroxine on intestinal lactase activity in suckling mice. *Experiéntia* **35:**493, 1979.
190. Buts JP, De Meyer R: Postnatal proximodistal development of the small bowel mucosal mass in growing rats. *Biol Neonate* **40:**62, 1981.
191. Buts JP, De Meyer R: Intestinal development in the suckling rat: Effects of weaning, diet composition and glucocorticoids on thymidine kinase activity and DNA synthesis. *Pediatr Res* **18:**145, 1984.
192. Tsuboi KK, Kwong LK, Neu J, Sunshine P: A proposed mechanism of normal intestinal lactase decline in the postweaned mammal. *Biochim Biophys Res Commun* **101:**645, 1981.
193. Tsuboi KK, Kwong LK, D'Harlingue AE, Stevenson DK, Kerner JA, Sunshine P: The nature of maturational decline of intestinal lactase activity. *Biochim Biophys Acta* **840:**69, 1985.
194. Jonas MM, Montgomery RK, Grand RJ: Intestinal lactase synthesis during postnatal development in the rat. *Pediatr Res* **19:**956, 1985.
195. Smith MW, James PS: Cellular origin of lactase decline in postweaning rats. *Biochim Biophys Acta* **905:**503, 1987.
196. Smith MW, Lloyd S: Intestinal infection with *Nematospiroides dubius* selectively increases lactase expression in mouse jejunal enterocytes. *Clin Sci* **77:**139, 1989.
197. Smith MW, Lloyd S, James PS: Testing the hypothesis that crypt cell hyperplasia inhibits lactase expression by mouse jejunal enterocytes. *Q J Exp Physiol* **73:**777, 1988.
198. Freund JN, Duluc I, Raul F: Lactase expression is controlled differently in the jejunum and ileum during development in rats. *Gastroenterology* **100:**388, 1991.

198a. Duluc I, Galluser M, Raul F, Freund J-F: Dietary control of the lactase mRNA distribution along the rat small intestine. *Am J Physiol* **262:**G954, 1992.

199. Lacey SW, Naim HY, Magness RR, Gething MJ, Sambrook JF: Lactase-phlorizin hydrolase activity, protein, and mRNA are coordinately regulated in the sheep. *Gastroenterology* **100:**A223, 1991.

199a. Lescale-Matys L, Dyer J, Scott D, Freeman TC, Wright EM, Shirazi-Beechey SP: Regulation of ovine intestinal Na^+/glucose co-transporter (SGLT1) is dissociated from mRNA abundance. *Biochem J* **291:**435, 1993.

199b. Freeman TC, Wood IS, Sirinath-singhij DJS, Beechey RB, Dyer J, Shirazi-Beechey SP: The expression of the NA^+/glucose cotransporter (SGLT1) gene in lamb small intestine during postnatal development. *Biochim Biophys Acta* **1146:**203, 1993.

200. Büller HA, Kothe MJC, Goldman DA, Grubman SA, Sasak WV, Madsudaira PT, Montgomery RK, Grand RJ: Coordinate expression of lactase-phlorizin hydrolase mRNA and enzyme levels in rat intestine during development. *J Biol Chem* **265:**6978, 1990.

201. Maiuri L, Rossi M, Raia V, Swallow D, Quaroni A, Auricchio S: Patchy expression of lactase protein in adult rabbit and rat intestine. *Gastroenterology* **103:**1739, 1992.
202. Foltzer-Jourdainne C, Kedinger M, Raul F: Perinatal expression of brush-border hydrolases in rat colon: Hormonal and tissue regulations. *Am J Physiol* **257:**G496, 1989.
203. Freund JN, Duluc I, Foltzer-Jourdainne C, Gosse F, Raul F: Specific expression of lactase in the jejunum and colon during postnatal development and hormone treatments in the rat. *Biochem J* **268:**99, 1990.
204. Quan R, Santiago NA, Tsuboi KT, Gray GM: Intestinal lactase. Shift in intracellular processing to altered, inactive species in the adult rat. *J Biol Chem* **265:**15882, 1990.
205. Castillo RO, Reisenauer AM, Kwong LK, Tsuboi KT, Quan R, Gray GM: Intestinal lactase in the neonatal rat. Maturational changes in intracellular processing and brush-border degradation. *J Biol Chem* **256:**15889, 1990.
205a. Rossi M, Maiuri L, Salvati VM, Russomanno C, Capparelli R, Auricchio S: In vitro biosynthesis of lactase in suckling and adult rabbits. Regulatory mechanisms involved in the decline of the lactase activity. *FEBS Lett* **329:**106, 1993.
206. Troelsen JK, Olsen J, Norén O, Sjöström H: A novel intestinal trans-factor (NF-LPH1) interacts with the lactase-phlorizin hydrolase promoter and co-varies with the enzymatic activity. *J Biol Chem* **267:**20407, 1992.
206a. Mantei N: Afterthought: How did the decline of lactase in adults evolve? in Auricchio S, Semenza G (eds): *Milk in Human Nutrition and Adult-type Hypolactasia*. Dyn Nutr Res. Basel, Karger, vol 3, 1993, p 208.
206b. Keller P, Zwicker E, Mantei N, Semenza G: The levels of lactase and of sucrase-isomaltase along the rabbit small intestine are regulated both at the mRNA level and post-translationally. *FEBS Lett* **313:**265, 1992.
206c. Keller P, Poirée JC, Giudicelli G, Semenza G: Do pancreatic proteases play a role in the processing of pro lactase and/or in the post-weaning decline of lactase? submitted, 1994.
206d. Ferguson A, Gerskowich VP, Russel RI: Pre- and post-weaning disaccharidase patterns in isografts of fetal mouse intestine. *Gastroenterology* **64:**292, 1973.
206e. Yeh KY, Holt PR: Ontogenic timing mechanism initiates the expression of rat intestinal sucrase activity. *Gastroenterology* **90:**520, 1986.
206f. Duluc I, Jost B, Freund JF: Multiple levels of control of the stage- and region-specific expression of rat intestinal lactase. *J Cell Biol* **123:**1577, 1993.
207. Büller HA, Rings EHHM, Pajkrt D, Montgomery RK, Grand RJ: Glycosylation of lactase-phlorizin hydrolase in rat small intestine during development. *Gastroenterology* **98:**667, 1990.
208. Antonovicz I, Chang SK, Grand RJ: Development and distribution of lysosomal enzymes and disaccharidases in human fetal intestine. *Gastroenterology* **67:**51, 1974.
209. Antonovicz I, Lebenthal E: Development pattern of small intestinal enterokinase and disaccharidase activity in the human fetus. *Gastroenterology* **72:**1299, 1977.
210. Dahlqvist A, Lindberg T: Fetal development of the small intestinal disaccharidase and alkaline phosphatase activities in the human. *Biol Neonate* **9:**24, 1965.
211. Jiřšová V, Koldovský O, Heringová, Uher J, Jodl J: Development of invertase activity in the intestines of human fetuses, appearance of jejunoileal differences. *Biol Neonate* **13:**143, 1968.
212. Mobassaleh M, Montgomery RK, Biller JA, Grand RJ: Development of carbohydrate absorption in the fetus and neonate. *Pediatrics (suppl)* **75:**160, 1985.
213. Mayne A, Hughes CA, Sule D, Brown GA, McNeish AS: Development of intestinal disaccharidases in preterm infants. *Lancet* **2:**622, 1983.
214. MacLean WC Jr, Fink BB: Lactose malabsorption by premature infants: Magnitude and clinical significance. *J Pediatr* **97:**383 1980.
215. MacLean WC, Fink BB, Schoeller DA, Wong W, Klein PD: Lactose assimilation by full-term infants: Relations of (13C) and H2 breath test with fecal (13C) excretion. *Pediatr Res* **17:**629, 1983.
216. Schoeller DA, Kelin PD, MacLean WC, Watkins JB, VanSanten E: Fecal 13C analysis for the detection and quantitation of intestinal malabsorption. Limits of detection to disorders of intestinal cholylglycine metabolism. *J Lab Clin Med* **97:**439, 1981.
217. Lifshitz CH, O'Brian Smith E, Garza C: Delayed complete functional lactase sufficiency in breast-fed infants. *J Pediatr Gastroenterol Nutr* **2:**478, 1983.
218. Chiles C, Watkins JB, Barr RG, Tsaj PY, Goldman DA: Lactose utilization in the newborn: Role of colonic flora. *Pediatr Res* **13:**365, 1979.
219. Bond JH, Currier BE, Buchwald H, Levitt MD: Colonic conservation of malabsorbed carbohydrate. *Gastroenterology* **78:**444, 1980.
220. Murray RD, Boutton TW, Klein PD, Gilbert M, Paule CL, MacLean WC: Comparative absorption of [^{13}C]glucose and [^{13}C]lactose by premature infants. *Am J Clin Nutr* **51:**59, 1990.
221. Villa M, Ménard D, Semenza G, Mantei N: The expression of lactase enzymatic activity and mRNA in human fetal jejunum: Effect of organ culture and of treatment with hydrocortisone. *FEBS Lett* **301:**202, 1992.
221a. Traber PG, Yu L, Wu GD, Judge TA: Sucrase-isomaltase gene expression along the crypt-villus axis of human small intestine is regulated at the level of mRNA abundance. *Am J Physiol* **262:**G123, 1992.
221b. Traber PG, Wu GD, Wang W: Novel DNA-binding proteins regulate intestine-specific transcription of the sucrase-isomaltase gene. *Mol Cell Biol* **12:**3614, 1992.
221c. Wu GD, Wang W, Traber PG: Isolation and characterization of the human sucrase-isomaltase gene and demonstration of intestine-specific transcriptional elements. *J Biol Chem* **267:**7863, 1992.
222. Trugnan G, Rousset M, Chantret I, Barbat A, Zweibaum A: The posttranslational processing of sucrase-isomaltase in HT-29 cells is a function of their state of enterocytic differentiation. *J Cell Biol* **104:**1199, 1987.
223. Zweibaum A, Pinto M, Chevalier G, Dussaulx E, Triadou N, Lacroix B, Haffen K, Rousset M: Enterocytic differentiation of a subpopulation of the human colon tumor cell line HT-29 selected for growth in sugar-free medium and its inhibition by glucose. *J Cell Biol* **100:**118, 1985.
223a. Chantret I, Trugnan G, Dussaulx E, Zweibaum A, Rousset M: Monensin inhibits the expression of sucrase-isomaltase in Caco-2 cells at the mRNA level. *FEBS Lett* **235:**125, 1988.
224. Rousset M, Chantret I, Darmoul D, Trugnan G, Sapin C, Green F, Swallow D, Zweibaum A: Reversible forskolin-induced impairment of sucrase-isomaltase mRNA levels, biosynthesis, and transport to the brush border membrane in Caco-2 cells. *J Cell Physiol* **141:**627, 1989.
225. Auricchio S: "Fetal" forms of brush border enzymes in the intestine and meconium. *J Pediatr Gastroenterol Nutr (suppl)* **2:**164, 1983.
226. Auricchio S, Caporale C, Santamaria F, Skovbjerg H: Fetal forms of oligoaminopeptidase, dipeptidylaminopeptidase IV and sucrase in human intestine and meconium. *J Pediatr Gastroenterol Nutr* **3:**28, 1984.
227. Triadou N, Zweibaum A: Maturation of su .rase-isomaltase complex in human fetal small and large intestine during gestation. *Pediatr Res* **19:**136, 1985.
228. Kraml J, Kolínská J: Sialylated forms of intestinal brush-border enzymes. Lecture presented at the 14th International Congress of Biochemistry, Prague, 1988. (abstract no. TU:C18-3)
229. Chu SW, Walker WA: Developmental changes in the activities of sialyl- and fucosyltransferases in rat small intestine. *Biochim Biophys Acta* **883:**496, 1986.
230. Biol MC, Pintori S, Mathian B, Louisot P: Dietary regulation of intestinal glycosyl-transferase activities: Relation between developmental changes and weaning in rats. *J Nutr* **121:**114, 1991.
230a. Paulson JC, Colley KJ: Glycosyltransferases. *J Biol Chem* **264:**17615, 1989.
230b. Martin A, Ruggiero-Lopez D, Biol MC, Louisot P: Evidence for the presence of an endogenous cytosolic protein inhibitor of intestinal fucosyltransferase activities. *Biochem Biophys Res Commun* **166:**1024, 1990.
231. Ruggiero-Lopez D, Biol MC, Louisot P, Martin A:

Participation of an endogenous inhibitor of fucosyltransferase activities in the developmental regulation of intestinal fucosylation process. *Biochem J* **279**:801, 1991.

231a. Ruggiero-Lopez D, Martin A, Louisot P: Caractérisation et évolution post-natale d'un inhibiteur protéique endogène des fucosyl-transférases intestinales. *Gastroenterol Clin Biol* **15**:939, 1991.

231b. Biol MC, Lenoir D, Hugueny I, Louisot P: Hormonal regulation of glycosylation process in rat small intestine: Responsiveness of fucosyl-transferase activity to hydrocortisone during the suckling period, unresponsiveness after weaning. *Biochim Biophys Acta* **1133**:206, 1992.

231c. Biol MC, Martin A, Louisot P: Nutritional and developmental regulation of glycosylation processes in digestive organs. *Biochimie* **74**:13, 1992.

232. James WPT, Alpers DH, Gerber JE, Isselbacher KJ: The turnover of disaccharidases and brush border proteins in rat intestine. *Biochim Biophys Acta* **230**:194, 1971.

233. Olsen WA, Korsmo H: The intestinal brush border membrane in diabetes. Studies of sucrase-isomaltase metabolism in rats with streptozotocin diabetes. *J Clin Invest* **60**:181, 1977.

234. Alpers DH: The relation of size to the relative rates of degradation of intestinal brush border proteins. *J Clin Invest* **51**:2621, 1972.

235. Forstner G, Galand G: The influence of hydrocortisone on the synthesis and turnover of microvillus membrane glycoproteins in suckling rat intestine. *Can J Biochem* **54**:224, 1976.

236. Ahnen DJ, Santiago NA, Yoshioka C, Gray GM: Intestinal sucrase-α-dextrinase: Differential degradation of its protein and carbohydrate components in vivo. *Gastroenterology* **82**:1006, 1982.

237. Karasov WH, Diamond JM: Adaptive regulation of sugar and amino acid transport by vertebrate intestine. *Am J Physiol* **245**:G443, 1983.

238. Jacobs LR: Alterations in labeling of cell-surface glycoproteins from normal and diabetic rat intestinal microvillus membranes. *Biochim Biophys Acta* **649**:155, 1981.

239. Najjar S, Hampp LT, Rabkin R, Gray GM: Sucrase-α-dextrinase in diabetic BioBreed rats: Reversible alteration of subunit structure. *Am J Physiol* **260**:G275, 1991.

240. Schedl HP, Al-Jurf AS, Wilson DH: Elevated intestinal disaccharidase activity in the streptozotocin diabetic rat is independent of enteral feeding. *Gastroenterology* **82**:1171, 1982.

241. Goda T, Koldovský O: Evidence of degradation process of sucrase-isomaltase in jejunum of adult rats. *Biochem J* **229**:751, 1985.

242. Alpers DH, Tedesco FJ: The possible role of pancreatic proteases in the turnover of the intestinal brush border proteins. *Biochim Biophys Acta* **401**:28, 1975.

243. Riby JE, Kretchmer N: Participation of pancreatic enzymes in the degradation of intestinal sucrase-isomaltase. *J Pediatr Gastroenterol Nutr* **4**:971, 1985.

244. Kwong WKL, Seetharam B, Alpers DH: Effect of exocrine pancreatic insufficiency on small intestine in the mouse. *Gastroenterology* **74**:1277, 1978.

245. Seetharam B, Perrillo R, Alpers DH: Effect of pancreatic proteases on intestinal lactase activity. *Gastroenterology* **79**:827, 1980.

246. Smith MW, Phillips AD, Walker-Smith JA: Selective inhibition of brush border hydrolase development in coeliac disease and cow's milk protein intolerance. *Pediatr Res* **20**:693, 1986. (abstr.)

247. Lifshitz F: Perspectives of carbohydrate intolerance in infants with diarrhea, in Lifshitz F (ed): *Carbohydrate Intolerance in Infancy*. New York, Marcel Dekker, 1982, p 3.

248. Shmerling DH, Auricchio S, Rubino A, Hadorn B, Prader A: Der sekundäre Mangel an intestinalen Disaccharidaseakvität bei der Coeliakie. Quantitative Bestimmung der Enzymaktivität und klinische Beurteilung. *Helv Paediatr Acta* **19**:507, 1964.

249. Lebenthal E, Lee P: Possible alternative pathway for starch digestion in infants and mucosal glucamylase activity in small intestinal atrophy. *Pediatr Res* **29**:504, 1980.

250. Gray GM, William MW Jr, Eugene H: Persistent deficiency of intestinal lactase in apparently cured tropical sprue. *Gastroenterology* **54**:552, 1968.

251. Romer H, Urbach R, Gomez MA, Lopez A, Perozo-Ruggeri G, Vegas ME: Moderate and severe protein energy malnutrition in childhood: Effects of jejunal mucosae morphology and disaccharidase activities. *J Pediatr Gastroenterol Nutr* **2**:459, 1983.

252. Greene HL, McCabe DR, Merenstein GB: Protracted diarrhea and malnutrition in infancy: Changes in intestinal morphology and disaccharidase activities during treatment with total intravenous nutrition or oral elemental diets. *J Pediatr* **87**:695, 1975.

253. Phillips AD, Avigad S, Sacks J, Rice SJ, France NE, Walker-Smith SA: Microvillous surface area in secondary disaccharidase deficiency. *Gut* **21**:44, 1980.

254. Boyle JT, Celano R, Koldovský O: Demonstration of a difference in expression of maximal lactase and sucrase activity along the villus in the adult rat jejunum. *Gastroenterology* **79**:503, 1980.

255. Alpers DH, Seetharam B: Pathophysiology of diseases involving intestinal brush border proteins. *N Engl J Med* **296**:1047, 1977.

256. Sherman P, Wesley A, Forstner G: Sequential disaccharidase loss in rat intestinal blind loops: Impact of malnutrition. *Am J Physiol* **248**:626, 1985.

257. Welsh JD, Poley JR, Hensley J, Bathia M: Intestinal disaccharidase and alkaline phosphatase activity in Giardiasis. *J Pediatr Gastroenterol Nutr* **3**:37, 1984.

258. Dahlqvist A: Method for assay of intestinal disaccharidases. *Anal Biochem* **7**:18, 1964.

259. Auricchio S, Rubino A, Tosi R, Semenza G, Landolt M, Kistler HJ, Prader A: Disaccharidase activities in human intestinal mucosa. *Enzymol Biol Clin* **3**:193, 1963.

260. Banauch D, Brummer W, Ebeling W, Metz H, Rindfrey M, Land H: Eine Glucose-Dehydrogenase für die Glucose-Bestimmung in Körperflüssigkeiten. *Z Klin Chem Klin Biochem* **13**:101, 1975.

261. Asp NG, Dahlqvist A: Human small-intestinal β-galactosidases specific assay of three different enzymes. *Anal Biochem* **47**:527, 1972.

262. Tsuboi KK, Schwarz SM, Burrill PH, Kwong LK, Sunshine P: Sugar hydrolases of the infant rat intestine and their arrangement on the brush border membrane. *Biochim Biophys Acta* **554**:234, 1979.

263. Eggermont E: The hydrolysis of the naturally occurring alpha-glucosides by the human intestinal mucosa. *Eur J Biochem* **9**:483, 1969.

264. Auricchio S, Ciccimarra F, Starace E, Vegnente A, Giliberti P, Provenzale L: Glucamylase activity of human intestinal mucosa. *Rend Gastroenterol* **3**:1, 1971.

265. Skovbjerg H, Sjöström A, Norén O, Gudmand-Høyer E: Immunoelectrophoretic studies on human small intestinal brush border proteins. A quantitative study from single, small intestinal biopsies. *Clin Chim Acta* **92**:315, 1979.

266. Lebenthal E, Antonowicz I, Shwachman H: Correlation of lactase activity, lactose tolerance and milk consumption in different age groups. *Am Clin Nutr* **28**:595, 1975.

267. Newcomer AD, McGill DB, Thomas PM, Hofmann AF: Prospective comparison of indirect methods for detecting lactase deficiency. *N Engl J Med* **293**:1232, 1975.

268. Eggermont E, Carchon H, Eeckels R: Centile values of small intestinal mucosal enzymatic activities in Caucasian children. *Pediatr Res* **15**:1205A, 1981.

269. Niessen KH, Schmidt K, Bruggmann G: Disaccharidasen der Dünndarmschleimhaut bei Säuglingen und Kindern. *Z Gastroenterol* **13**:565, 1975.

270. McMichael WB, Webb J, Dawson AM: Jejunal disaccharidases and some observations on the cause of lactase deficiency. *Br Med J* **2**:1037, 1966.

271. Calvin RT, Klish WJ, Nichols BL: Disaccharidase activities, jejunal morphology, and carbohydrate tolerance in children with chronic diarrhea. *J Pediatr Gastroenterol Nutr* **4**:949, 1985.

272. Newcomer AD, McGill DB: Distribution of disaccharidase activity in the small bowel of normal and lactase-deficient subjects. *Gastroenterology* **51**:481, 1966.

273. Langman JM, Rowland R: Activity of duodenal disaccharidases in relation to normal and abnormal mucosal morphology. *J Clin Pathol* **43**:537, 1990.

274. Auricchio S, Rubino A, Prader A, Rey J, Jos J, Frézal J, Davidson M: Intestinal glycosidase activities in congenital malabsorption of disaccharides. *J Pediatr* **66**:555, 1965.
275. Kerry KR, Townley RRW: Genetic aspects of intestinal sucrase-isomaltase deficiency. *Aust Pediatr J* **1**:223, 1965.
276. Welsh JD, Poley JR, Bhatia M, Stevenson DE: Intestinal disaccharidase activities in relation to age, race, and mucosal damage. *Gastroenterology* **75**:855, 1978.
277. Crane RK, Ménard D, Preiser H, Cerda J: The molecular basis of brush border membrane disease, in Bolis L, Hoffman JF, Leaf A (eds): *Membranes and Disease*. New York, Raven, 1976, p 229.
278. Haemmerli UP, Kistler HJ, Ammann R, Marthaler T, Semenza G, Auricchio S, Prader A: Acquired milk intolerance in the adult caused by lactose malabsorption due to a selective deficiency of intestinal lactase activity. *Am J Med* **38**:7, 1965.
279. Newcomer AD, McGill DB: Disaccharidase activity in the small intestine: Prevalence of lactase deficiency in 100 healthy subjects. *Gastroenterology* **53**:881, 1967.
280. Forget P, Lambet J, Grandfils C, Dandrifosse G, Genbelle F: Lactase insufficiency revisited. *J Pediatr Gastroenterol Nutr* **4**:868, 1985.
281. Martinez-Pardo M, Montes PG, Martin-Lomas M, Sols A: Intestinal lactase evaluation in vivo with 3-methyllactose. *FEBS Lett* **98**:99, 1979.
282. Weijers HA, Van De Kamer JH, Dicke WK, Ijsseling J: Diarrhoea caused by deficiency of sugar-splitting enzymes. I. *Acta Paediatr* **50**:55, 1961.
283. Krasilnikoff PA, Gudmann-Høyer E, Moltke HH: Diagnostic value of disaccharide tolerance tests to children. *Acta Paediatr Scand* **64**:693, 1975.
284. Fernandes J, Vos CE, Douwes AC, Slotema E, Degenhart HJ: Respiratory hydrogen excretion as a parameter for lactose malabsorption in children. *Am J Clin Nutr* **31**:597, 1978.
285. Maffei HVL, Metz G, Bampoe V, Shiner M, Herman S, Brook CGD: Lactose intolerance, detected by breath hydrogen test in infants and children with chronic diarrhoea. *Arch Dis Child* **52**:766, 1977.
286. Perman JA, Barr RG, Watkins JB: Sucrose malabsorption in children: Non-invasive diagnosis by interval breath hydrogen determination. *J Pediatr* **93**:17, 1978.
287. Robb TA, Davidson GP: Advances in breath hydrogen quantitation in paediatrics: Sample collection and normalization to constant oxygen and nitrogen levels. *Clin Chim Acta* **111**:281, 1981.
288. Kneepkens CMF, Bijleveld CMA, Vonk RJ, Fernandes J: The daytime breath hydrogen profile in children with abdominal symptoms and diarrhoea. *Acta Paediatr Scand* **75**:632, 1986.
289. Kerlin P, Phillips SF: Differential transit of liquids and solid residue through the ileum of man. *Am J Physiol* **245**:G38, 1983.
290. Douwes AC, Schaap C, Van Der Kei Van Moorsel JM: Hydrogen breath test in schoolchildren. *Arch Dis Child* **60**:333, 1985.
291. Levitt MD, Donaldson RM: Use of respiratory hydrogen to detect carbohydrate malabsorption. *J Lab Clin Med* **75**:937, 1970.
292. Bjorneklett A, Jenssen E: Relationship between hydrogen (H_2) and methane (CH_4) in man. *Scand J Gastroenterol* **17**:985, 1982.
293. Gardiner AJ, Tarlow MJ, Symonds J, Hutchinson GJP, Shuterland JT: Failure of the hydrogen breath test to detect primary sugar malabsorption. *Arch Dis Child* **56**:368, 1981.
294. Kerry KR, Anderson CM: A ward test for sugar in faeces. *Lancet* **1**:981, 1964.
295. Davidson AGF, Mullinger M: Reducing substances in neonatal stool detected by Clinitest. *Pediatrics* **46**:632, 1970.
296. McMichael HB, Webb J, Dawson AM: Lactase deficiency in adult: A cause of functional diarrhoea. *Lancet* **1**:717, 1965.
297. Auricchio S, Prader A, Mürset G, Witt G: Saccharoseintoleranz: Durchfall infolge hereditären Mangels an intestinaler Saccharaseaktivität. *Helv Paediatr Acta* **16**:483, 1961.
298. Grant JD, Bezerra JA, Thompson SH, Lemen RJ, Koldovský O, Udall JN: Assessment of lactose absorption by measurement of urinary galactose. *Gastroenterology* **97**:895, 1989.
299. Harrison M, Walker-Smith JA: Reinvestigation of lactose intolerant children: Lack of correlation between continuing lactose intolerance and small intestinal morphology, disaccharidase activity and lactose tolerance tests. *Gut* **18**:48, 1977.
300. Dawson DJ, Newcomer AD, McGill DB: Lactose tolerance tests in adults with normal lactase activity. *Gastroenterology* **50**:340, 1966.
301. Davidson GP, Robb TA: Value of breath hydrogen analysis in management of diarrheal illness in childhood: Comparison with duodenal biopsy. *J Pediatr Gastroenterol Nutr* **4**:381, 1985.
302. Lifshitz CH, Bautista A, Gapalachrishna GS, Stuff J, Garza C: Absorption and tolerance of lactose in infants recovering from diarrhea. *J Pediatr Gastroenterol Nutr* **4**:942, 1985.
303. Welsh JD: Isolated lactase deficiency in humans: Reports on 100 patients. *Medicine (Baltimore)* **49**:257, 1970.
304. Bayless TM, Rothfeld B, Massa C, Wise L, Paige D, Bedine MS: Lactose and milk intolerance: Clinical implications. *N Engl J Med* **292**:1156, 1975.
305. Ringrose RE, Preiser H, Welsh JD: Sucrase-isomaltase (Palatinase) deficiency diagnosed during adulthood. *Dig Dis Sci* **25**:384, 1980.
306. Ravich WJ, Bayless TM: Carbohydrate absorption and malabsorption. *Clin Gastroenterol* **12**:335, 1983.
307. Launiala K: The effect of unabsorbed sucrose and mannitol on small intestinal flow rate and mean transit time. *Scand J Gastroenterol* **3**:665, 1968.
308. Launiala K: The effect of unabsorbed sucrose- or mannitol-induced accelerated transit on absorption in the human small intestine. *Scand J Gastroenterol* **4**:25, 1969.
309. Goda T, Bustamante S, Edmond J, Grimes J, Koldovský O: Precocious increase of sucrase activity by carbohydrates in the small intestine of suckling rats. II. Role of digestibility of sugars, osmolality, and stomach evacuation in producing diarrhea. *J Pediatr Gastroenterol Nutr* **4**:634, 1985.
310. Caspary WF, Kalish H: Effect of alpha-glucosedehydrolase inhibition on intestinal absorption of sucrose, water, and sodium in man. *Gut* **20**:750, 1979.
311. Azpiroz F, Malagelada JR: Luminal nutrients in the proximal and distal small intestine elicit gastric relaxation. *Dig Dis Sci* **29**:564, 1984.
312. Jenkins DFA, Taylor RH, Goff WD: Scope and specificity of acarbose in slowing carbohydrate absorption in man. *Diabetes* **31**:951, 1981.
313. Holgate AM, Read NW: Relationship between small bowel transit time and absorption of a solid meal. *Dig Dis Sci* **28**:812, 1983.
314. Chapman RW, Graham MM: Absorption of starch by healthy ileostomatoses: Effect of transit time and of carbohydrate load. *Am J Clin Nutr* **41**:1244, 1985.
315. Auricchio S, Ciccimarra F, De Vizia B: *Starch Malabsorption*. XIII International Congress of Pediatrics, Vienna, Aug. 29–Sept. 4, 1971, p 139.
316. Chauve A, Devroede G, Bastin E: Intraluminal pressures during perfusion of the human colon in situ. *Gastroenterology* **70**:336, 1976.
317. Debongnie JC, Philips FS: Capacity of the human colon to absorb fluid. *Gastroenterology* **74**:698, 1978.
318. Palma R, Vidon N, Bernier JJ: Maximal capacity for fluid absorption in human bowel. *Dig Dis Sci* **26**:929, 1981.
319. Newcomer AD, McGill DB, Thomas PM, Hoffman AF: Tolerance to lactose among lactase deficient American Indians. *Gastroenterology* **74**:44, 1978.
320. Saunders DR, Wiggins HS: Conservation of mannitol, lactulose and raffinose by the human colon. *Am J Physiol* **241**:G387, 1981.
321. Argenzio RA, Southworth M: Sites of organic acid production and absorption in gastrointestinal tract of the pig. *Am J Physiol* **228**:454, 1975.
322. Orskov ER, Frase C, Mason WC, Mann SO: Influence of starch digestion in the large intestine of sheep on caecal fermentation, caecal microflora and faecal nitrogen excretion. *Br J Nutr* **24**:671, 1970.
323. Florent CH, Flourie B, Leblond A, Rautureau M,

Bernier JJ, Rambaud JC: Influence of chronic lactulose ingestion on the colonic metabolism of lactulose in man (an in vivo study). *J Clin Invest* **75**:608, 1985.

324. Bhatia J, Prihoda AR, Richardson CJ: Parenteral antibiotics and carbohydrate intolerance in term neonates. *Am J Dis Child* **149**:111, 1986.
325. Siigur U, Tamm A, Tammur R: The fecal SCFAs and lactose tolerance in lactose malabsorbers. *Eur J Gastroenterol* **3**:321, 1991.
326. Auricchio S, Dahlqvist A, Mürset G, Prader A: Isomaltose intolerance causing decreased ability to utilize dietary starch. *J Pediatr* **62**:165, 1963.
327. Auricchio S, Ciccimarra F, Moauro L, Rey F, Jos J, Rey J: Intraluminal and mucosal starch digestion in congenital deficiency of intestinal sucrase and isomaltase activities. *Pediatr Res* **6**:832, 1972.
328. Eggermont E, Hers HG: The sedimentation properties of the intestinal alpha-glucosidases of normal human subjects and of patients with sucrose intolerance. *Eur J Biochem* **9**:488, 1969.
329. Hadorn B, Green JR, Sterchi EE, Hauri HP: Biochemical mechanism in congential enzyme deficiencies of the small intestine. *Clin Gastroenterol* **10**:671, 1981.
330. Skovbjerg H, Krasilnikoff PA: Maltase-glucoamylase and residual isomaltase in sucrose intolerant patients. *J Pediatr Gastroenterol Nutr* **5**:365, 1986.
331. Auricchio S, Rubino A, Landolt M, Semenza G, Prader A: Isolated intestinal lactase deficiency in the adult. *Lancet* **2**:324, 1963.
332. Dahlqvist A, Hammond JD, Crane RK, Dunphy JV, Littman A: Intestinal lactase deficiency and lactose intolerance in adults: Preliminary report. *Gastroenterology* **45**:488, 1963.
333. Simoons FJ: The geographic hypothesis and lactose malabsorption. A weighing of the evidence. *Dig Dis* **23**:963, 1980.
334. Cook GC: Lactase activity in newborn and infant Baganda. *Br Med J* **1**:527, 1967.
335. Keusch GT, Troncale FJ, Miller LH, Promadhat V, Anderson PR: Acquired lactose malabsorption in Thai children. *Pediatrics* **43**:540, 1969.
336. Sahi T, Isokoski M, Jussila J, Launiala K: Lactose malabsorption in Finnish children of school age. *Acta Paediatr Scand* **61**:11, 1972.
337. Sahi T, Launiala K: Manifestation and occurrence of selective adult-type lactose malabsorption in Finnish teenagers. *Am J Dig Dis* **23**:699, 1978.
338. Sahi T, Launiala K, Laitinen H: Hypolactasia in a fixed cohort of young Finnish adults: A follow-up study. *Scand J Gastroenterol* **18**:865, 1983.
339. Paige DM: Lactose malabsorption in children: Prevalence, symptoms, and nutritional considerations, in Paige DM, Bayless TM (eds): *Lactose Digestion: Clinical and Nutrition Implications*. Baltimore, Johns Hopkins University Press, 1981, p 151.
340. Newcomer AD, Thomas PT, McGill D, Hofmann AF: Lactase deficiency: A common genetic trait of the American Indian. *Gastroenterology* **72**:234, 1977.
341. Caskey DA, Payne-Bose D, Welsh JD, Gearhart HI, Nance RD, Morrison RD: Effect of age on lactose malabsorption in Oklahoma native Americans as determined by breath hydrogen analysis. *Am J Dig Dis* **22**:113, 1977.
342. Roggero P, Offredi ML, Mosca F, Perazzani M, Mangiaterra B, Ghislanzoni P, Marenghi L, Careddu P: Lactose absorption and malabsorption in healthy Italian children: Do the quantity of malabsorbed sugar and the small bowel transit time play roles in symptoms production? *J Pediatr Gastroenterol Nutr* **4**:82, 1985.
343. Jussila J, Launiala K, Gorbatow O: Lactase deficiency and a lactose-free diet in patients with "unspecific abdominal complaints." *Acta Med Scand* **186**:217, 1969.
344. Gudmand-Høyer E, Dahlqvist A, Jarnum S: The clinical significance of lactose malabsorption. *Am J Gastroenterol* **53**:460, 1970.
345. Mitchell KJ, Bayless TM, Huang SS, Paige DM, Goodgame RW, Rothfeld B: Intolerance of a glass of milk in healthy teenagers. *Gastroenterology* **64**:773, 1973.
346. Sahi T: Dietary lactose and aetiology of human small intestinal hypolactasia. *Gut* **19**:1074, 1978.
347. Bedine MS, Bayless TM: Intolerance of small amount of lactose by individuals with low lactase levels. *Gastroenterology* **65**:735, 1973.
348. Jones DW, Latham MC, Kosikowski FW, Woodward G: Symptom response to lactose-reduced milk in lactose-intolerant adults. *Am J Clin Nutr* **29**:633, 1976.
349. Ferguson A: Diagnosis and treatment of lactose intolerance. *Br Med J* **283**:1423, 1981.
350. Fowkes FGR, Ferguson A: Prevalence of self-diagnosed irritable bowel syndrome and cows' milk intolerance in white and non white doctors. *Scott Med J* **26**:41, 1980.
351. Birge SJ Jr, Keutmann HT, Cuatrecasas P, Wheaton GD: Osteoporosis, intestinal lactase deficiency and low dietary calcium intake. *N Engl J Med* **276**:445, 1967.
352. Newcomer AD, Hodgson SF, McGill DB, Thomas BJ: Lactase deficiency prevalence in osteoporosis. *Ann Intern Med* **89**:218, 1978.
353. Condon JR, Nassim JR, Millard JC, Hilbe A, Stainthorpe EM: Calcium and phosphorus metabolism in relation to lactose tolerance. *Lancet* **1**:1027, 1970.
354. Kocian J, Skala I, Bakos K: Calcium absorption from milk and lactose free milk in healthy subjects and patients with lactose intolerance. *Digestion* **9**:317, 1973.
355. Editorial: Lactase deficiency in osteoporosis. *Lancet* **1**:86, 1979.
356. Editorial: Lactose malabsorption and lactose intolerance. *Lancet* **2**:831, 1979.
357. Cochet BA, Jung M, Griessen P, Schaller P, Donath A: Effects of lactose on intestinal calcium absorption in normal and lactase-deficient subjects. *Gastroenterology* **84**:935, 1983.
358. Tremaine WJ, Newcomer AD, Riggs CB, McGill DB: Calcium absorption from milk in lactase-deficient and lactase-sufficient adults. *Dig Dis Sci* **31**:376, 1986.
359. Griessen M, Cochet B, Infante F, Jung A, Bartholdi P, Donath A, Loizeau E, Courvoisier B: Calcium absorption from milk in lactase-deficient subjects. *Am J Clin Nutr* **49**:377, 1989.
360. Sahi T, Jussila J, Penttila IM, Sarna S, Isokoski M: Serum lipids and protein in lactose malabsorption. *Am J Clin Nutr* **30**:476, 1977.
361. Simoons FJ, Johnsson JB, Kretchmer N: Perspective on milk-drinking and malabsorption of lactose. *Pediatrics* **59**:98, 1977.
362. Flatz G, Rotthauwe HW: The human lactase polymorphism: Physiology and genetics of lactose absorption and malabsorption. *Prog Med Genet* **2**:205, 1977.
363. Pottinger PK: A study of the three enzymes acting on glucose in the lens of different species. *Biochem J* **104**:663, 1967.
364. Simoons FJ: A geographic approach to senile cataracts: Possible links with milk consumption, lactase activity and galactose metabolism. *Dig Dis Sci* **27**:257, 1982.
365. Rinaldi E, Albini L, Costagliola C, De Rosa G, Auricchio G, De Vizia B, Auricchio S: High frequency of lactose absorbers among adults with idiopathic senile and presenile cataract in a population with a high prevalence of primary adult lactose malabsorption. *Lancet* **1**:357, 1984.
366. Auricchio S, Costagliola C, De Rosa G, De Vizia B, Rinaldi E, Simonelli F: High frequency of lactose absorbers among adults with idiopathic and diabetic cataract in a population with high prevalence of primary adult-type hypolactasia. *Gastroenterology* **96**:A18, 1989.
367. Bhatnagar R, Sharma YR, Vajpayee RB, Madan M, Chhabra VU, Ram N, Mukesh K, Azad RV, Sharma R: Does milk have a cataractogenic effect? Weighing of clinical evidence. *Dig Dis Sci* **34**:1745, 1989.
368. Birlouet-Aragon I, Stevenin L, Rouzier C, Brivet M: Consommation de lactose et activité lactasique: Deux facteurs de risque de la cataracte sénile et diabétique. *Age Nutr* **1**:74, 1990.
369. Couet C, Jan P, Debrey G: Lactose and cataract in humans: A review. *J Am Coll Nutr* **10**:79, 1991.
370. Wacker H, Soldati L, Simonelli F, Richter C, Gazzaniga A, Auricchio S, Semenza G: Senile cataractic lenses do not accumulate galactitol in either lactose tolerant or intolerant subjects. *Clin Chim Acta* **220**:12901, 1993.

371. Cramer DW: Lactase persistence and milk consumption as determinants of ovarian cancer risk. *Am J Epidemiol* **130:**904, 1989.
372. Cramer DW, Harlow BL, Willett WC, Welch WR, Bell DA, Scully RE, Ng WG, Knapp RC: Galactose consumption and metabolism in relation to the risk of ovarian cancer. *Lancet* **2:**66, 1989.
373. Jackson W: Clinical manifestations, in Jackson W (ed): *Proceedings of the First Food Allergy Workshop*. Oxford, Medical Education Service, 1980, p 41.
374. Lessoff MH, Wraith DG, Merrett TG, Merrett J, Buisseret PD: Food allergy and intolerance in 100 patients—Local and systemic effects. *Q J Med* **49:**259, 1980.
375. Sahi T: The inheritance of selective adult-type lactose malabsorption. *Scand J Gastroenterol Suppl* **30:**1, 1974.
376. Ellestead-Sayed JJ, Haworth JC, Hildes JA: Disaccharide consumption and malabsorption in Canadian Indians. *Am J Clin Nutr* **30:**698, 1977.
377. Ellestead-Sayed JJ, Haworth JC, Hildes JA: Disaccharide malabsorption and dietary patterns in two Canadian Eskimo communities. *Am J Clin Nutr* **31:**1473, 1978.
378. Rosenzweig NS, Huang SS, Bayless TM: Transmission of lactose intolerance. *Lancet* **2:**777, 1967.
379. Ho MW, Poley S, Swallow D: Lactase polymorphism in adult British natives: Estimating allele frequencies by enzyme assays in autopsy samples. *Am J Hum Genet* **34:**650, 1982.
380. Flatz G: Gene-dosage effect of intestinal lactase activity demonstrated in vivo. *Am J Hum Genet* **36:**306, 1984.
381. Kretchmer N: Memorial lecture: Lactose and lactase—A historical perspective. *Gastroenterology* **61:**805, 1971.
382. Flatz G, Rotthauwe HW: Lactose nutrition and natural selection. *Lancet* **2:**76, 1973.
383. Simoons FJ: Celiac disease as a geographic problem, in Walcker DN, Kretchmer N (eds): *Food, Nutrition and Evolution*. Paris, Masson, 1981, p 179.
384. Kolars JC, Levitt MD, Aouji M, Savaiano DA: Yoghurt—An autodigesting source of lactose. *N Engl J Med* **310:**1, 1984.
385. Lerebours E, Djitoyap Ndam CN, Lavoine A, Hellot MF, Antoine JM, Colin R: Yogurt and fermented-then-pasteurized milk: Effects of short-term and long-term ingestion on lactose absorption and mucosal lactase activity in lactase-deficient subjects. *Am J Clin Nutr* **49:**823, 1989.
386. Onwulata CI, Rao DR, Vankineni P: Relative efficiency of yogurt, sweet acidophilus milk, hydrolyzed-lactose milk, and a commercial lactase tablet in alleviating lactose maldigestion. *Am J Clin Nutr* **49:**1233, 1989.
387. Marteau P, Flourie B, Pochart P, Chastang C, Desjeux JF, Rambaud JC: Effect of the microbial lactase (EC 3.2.1.23) activity in yoghurt on the intestinal absorption of lactose: An in vivo study in lactase-deficient humans. *Br J Nutr* **64:**71, 1990.
388. Smith TM, Kolars JC, Savaiano DA: Absorption of calcium from milk and yoghurt. *Am J Clin Nutr* **42:**1197, 1985.
389. Rosado JL, Solomons NW, Lisker R, Bourges H, Anrubio G, Garcia A, Perez-Briceno R, Aizupuru E: Enzyme replacement therapy for primary adult lactase deficiency. Effective reduction of lactose malabsorption and milk intolerance by direct addition of beta-galactosidase to milk at mealtime. *Gastroenterology* **87:**1072, 1984.
390. Holzel A, Schwarz V, Sutcliffe KW: Defective lactose absorption causing malnutrition in infancy. *Lancet* **1:**1126, 1959.
391. Lifshitz F: Congenital lactase deficiency. *J Pediatr* **69:**229, 1966.
392. Launiala K, Kuitunen P, Visakorpi J: Disaccharidases and histology of duodenal mucosa in congenital lactose malabsorption. *Acta Paediatr Scand* **55:**257, 1966.
393. Levin B, Abraham JM, Burgess EA, Wallis PG: Congenital lactose malabsorption. *Arch Dis Child* **45:**173, 1975.
394. Savilathi E, Launiala K, Kuitunen P: Congenital lactase deficiency: A clinical study on 16 patients. *Arch Dis Child* **58:**246, 1983.
395. Asp NG, Dahlqvist A: Intestinal β-galactosidases in adult low lactase activity and in congenital lactase deficiency. *Enzyme* **18:**84, 1974.
396. Asp NG, Dahlqvist A, Kuiunen P, Launiala K, Visakorpi JK: Complete deficiency of brush border lactase in congenital lactose malabsorption. *Lancet* **2:**329, 1973.
397. Dahlqvist A, Asp NG: Accurate assay of low intestinal lactase activity with a fluorimetric method. *Anal Biochem* **44:**654, 1971.
398. Freiburghaus AU, Schmitz J, Schindler M, Rotthauwe HW, Kuitunen P, Launiala K, Hadorn B: Protein patterns of brush border fragments in congenital lactose malabsorption and in specific hypolactasia of the adult. *N Engl J Med* **294:**1030, 1976.
399. Durand P: Lattosuria idiopatica in una paziente con diarrea cronica ed acidosi. *Minerva Pediatr* **1:**706, 1958.
400. Russo G, Molica F, Mazzone D, Santonocito B: Congenital lactose intolerance of gastrogen origin associated with cataracts. *Acta Paediatr Scand* **63:**457, 1974.
401. Hirashima Y, Shinozuka S, Ieiri T, Matsuda I, Ono Y, Murata T: Lactose intolerance associated with cataracts. *Eur J Pediatr* **130:**41, 1979.
402. Berg NO, Dahlqvist A, Lindberg T: A boy with severe infantile gastrogen lactose intolerance and acquired lactase deficiency. *Acta Paediatr Scand* **68:**751, 1979.
403. Hoskova A, Sabacky J, Mrskos A, Pospisil R: Severe lactose intolerance with lactosuria and vomiting. *Arch Dis Child* **55:**304, 1980.
404. Weijers HA, Van De Kamer JH, Mosel DAA, Dick WK: Diarrhoea caused by deficiency of sugar splitting enzymes. *Lancet* **2:**296, 1960.
405. Prader A, Auricchio S, Mürset G: Durchfall infolge hereditären Mangels an intestinaler Saccharaseaktivität (Saccharoseintoleranz). *Schweiz Med Wochenschr* **91:**465, 1961.
406. Anderson CM, Messer M, Townley RRW, Freeman M, Robinson RJ: Intestinal isomaltase deficiency in patients with hereditary sucrose and starch intolerance. *Lancet* **2:**556, 1962.
407. Anderson CM, Messer M, Townley RRW, Freeman M: Intestinal sucrase and isomaltase deficiency in two siblings. *Pediatrics* **31:**1003, 1963.
408. Burgess EA, Levin B, Mahalanabis D, Tonge RE: Hereditary sucrose intolerance. Levels of sucrase activity in jejunal mucosa. *Arch Dis Child* **39:**431, 1964.
409. Prader A, Auricchio S: Defects of intestinal disaccharide absorption. *Annu Rev Med* **13:**345, 1965.
410. Gudmand-Høyer E, Krasilnikoff PA: The effect of sucrose malabsorption on the growth pattern in children. *Scand J Gastroenterol* **12:**103, 1977.
411. Ament ME, Perera DR, Esther LJ: Sucrase-isomaltase deficiency, a frequently misdiagnosed disease. *J Pediatr* **83:**721, 1973.
412. Antonovicz I, Lloyd JD, Khaw KT, Shwachman H: Congenital sucrase isomaltase deficiency. Observation over a period of 6 years. *Pediatrics* **49:**847, 1972.
413. Sonntag WM, Brill ML, Troyer WE, Welsh JD, Semenza G, Prader A: Sucrose-isomaltose malabsorption in an adult female. *Gastroenterology* **47:**18, 1964.
414. Neale G, Clark M, Levin B: Intestinal sucrase deficiency presenting as sucrose intolerance in adult life. *Br Med J* **2:**1223, 1965.
415. Starnes CW, Welsh JD: Intestinal sucrase-isomaltase deficiency and renal calculi. *N Engl J Med* **202:**1023, 1970.
416. Jansen W, Que CS, Veeger W: Primary combined saccharase and isomaltase deficiency. *Arch Intern Med* **116:**1125, 1972.
417. Cooper BT, Scott J, Hopkins J, Peters TJ: Adult onset sucrase-isomaltase deficiency with secondary disaccharidase deficiency resulting from severe dietary carbohydrate restriction. *Dig Dis Sci* **28:**473, 1983.
418. Gudmand-Høyer E, Krasilnikoff PA, Skovbjerg H: Sucrose-isomaltose malabsorption, in Draper H (ed): *Advances in Nutritional Research*. New York, Plenum, 1984, vol 6, p 233.
419. Gudmand-Høyer E: Sucrose malabsorption in children: A report of thirty-one Greenlanders. *J Pediatr Gastroenterol Nutr* **4:**873, 1985.
420. Cheney CP, Boedeker EC: Evidence that the sucrase/isomaltase complex may serve as an intestinal receptor for an enteropathogenic "Escherichia coli." *Gastroenterology* **82:**1032, 1982.

421. Metz G, Jenkins DJA, Newman A, Blendis LM: Breath hydrogen in hyposucrasia. *Lancet* **1**:119, 1976.
422. Douwes AC, Fernandes J, Jongbloed AA: Diagnostic value of sucrose tolerance test in children evaluated by breath hydrogen measurement. *Acta Paediatr Scand* **69**:79, 1980.
423. Birch JB: Trehalose. *Adv Carbohydr Chem* **18**:201, 1963.
424. Bergoz R: Trehalose malabsorption causing intolerance to mushrooms. *Gastroenterology* **5**:909, 1971.
425. Madzarovová-Nohejilová J: Trehalase deficiency in a family. *Gastroenterology* **65**:130, 1973.
426. McNair A, Gudmand-Høyer E, Jarnum S, Orrild L: Sucrose malabsorption in Greenland. *Br Med J* **2**:19, 1972.
427. Schmitz J, Bresson JL, Triadou N, Bataille J, Rey J: Analyse en electrophorèse sur gel de polyacrylamide des protéines de la membrane microvillositaire et d'une fraction cytoplasmique dans 8 cas d'intolérance congénitale au saccharose. *Gastroenterol Clin Biol* **4**:251, 1980.
428. Gray GM, Conklin KA, Townley RRW: Sucrase-isomaltase deficiency. Absence of an inactive enzyme variant. *N Engl J Med* **294**:750, 1976.
429. Skovbjerg H, Krasilnikoff PA: Maltase-glucoamylase and residual isomaltase in sucrose intolerant patients. *J Pediatr Gastroenterol Nutr* **3**:365, 1986.
430. Skovbjerg H, Krasilnikoff PA: Immunoelectrophoretic studies on human small intestinal brush border protein. The residual isomaltase in sucrose intolerant patients. *Pediatr Res* **15**:214, 1981.
431. Preiser H, Ménard D, Crane RK, Cerda JJ: Deletion of enzyme protein from brush border membrane in sucrase-isomaltase deficiency. *Biochim Biophys Acta* **363**:279, 1974.
432. Naim HY, Roth J, Sterchi EE, Lentze M, Milla P, Schmitz J, Hauri HP: Sucrase-isomaltase deficiency in humans. Different mutations disrupt intracellular transport, processing and function of an intestinal brush border enzyme. *J Clin Invest* **82**:667, 1988.
433. Naim HY, Sterchi EE, Hauri HP, Schmitz J, Lentze MJ: Defective posttranslational processing of sucrase-isomaltase (SI) in congenital sucrase-isomaltase deficiency. Presented at the XIX Annual Meeting of the European Society for Paediatric Gastroenterology and Nutrition (ESPAGN) Edinburgh, June 25–27, 1986. (abstr. 26)
434. Lloyd ML, Olsen WA: A study of the molecular pathology of sucrase-isomaltase deficiency. A defect in the intracellular processing of the enzyme. *N Engl J Med* **316**:438, 1987.
435. Sterchi EE, Lentze MJ, Naim HY: Molecular aspects of disaccharidase deficiencies. *Baillieres Clin Gastroenterol* **4**:79, 1990.
436. Fransen JAM, Hauri HP, Ginsel LA, Naim HY: Naturally occurring mutations in intestinal sucrase-isomaltase provide evidence for the existence of an intracellular sorting signal in the isomaltose subunit. *J Cell Biol* **115**:45, 1991.
437. Freiburghaus AU, Dubs R, Hadorn B, Gaze H, Hauri HO, Gitzelmann R: The brush border membrane in hereditary sucrase-isomaltase deficiency: Abnormal protein pattern and presence of immunoreactive enzyme. *Eur J Clin Invest* **7**:455, 1977.
438. Dubs R, Steinmann B, Gitzelmann R: Demonstration of an inactive enzyme antigen in sucrase-isomaltase deficiency. *Helv Paediatr Acta* **28**:187, 1973.
439. James PS, Smith MW, Butcher GW, Brown D, Lund EK: Evidence for a possible regulatory gene (Suc-1) controlling sucrase expression in mouse intestine. *Biochem Genet* **24**:169, 1986.
440. Cooper BT, Candy DCA, Harries JT, Peters TJ: Subcellular fractionation studies of the intestinal mucosa in congenital sucrase-isomaltase deficiency. *Clin Sci Mol Med* **57**:181, 1979.
441. Skovbjerg H, Gudmand-Høyer E, Fenger HJ: Immunoelectrophoretic studies on human small intestinal brush border proteins. The amount of lactase protein in adult-free hypolactasia. *Gut* **21**:360, 1980.
442. Potter J, Ho M-W, Bolton H, Eurth AJ, Swallow DM, Griffith B: Human lactase and the molecular basis of lactase persistence. *Biochem Genet* **23**:432, 1985.
443. Lorenz-Meyer H, Blum AL, Haemmerli HP, Semenza G: A second enzyme defect in acquired lactase deficiency. Lack of small-intestinal phlorizin-hydrolase. *Eur J Clin Invest* **2**:326, 1972.
444. Escher JC, de Koning ND, van Engen CGJ, Arora S, Büller H, Montgomery RK, Grand RJ: Molecular basis of lactase levels in adult humans. *J Clin Invest* **89**:480, 1992.
444a. Auricchio S, Semenza G (eds): *Milk in Human Nutrition and Adult-type Hypolactasia*. Dyn Nutr Res Basel, Karger, 1993, vol 3.
445. Maiuri L, Raia V, Potter J, Swallow D, Ho MW, Fiocca R, Finzi G, Cornaggia M, Capella C, Quaroni A, Auricchio S: Mosaic pattern of lactase expression by villous enterocytes in human small adult-type hypolactasia. *Gastroenterology* **100**:359, 1991.
446. Sterchi EE, Mills RP, Fransen JAM, Hauri HP, Lentze MJ, Naim HI, Ginsel L, Bond J: Biogenesis of intestinal lactase-phlorizin hydrolase in adults with lactase intolerance. *J Clin Invest* **86**:1329, 1990.
447. Witte J, Lloyd M, Lorenzsonn V, Korsmo H, Olsen W: The biosynthetic basis of adult lactase deficiency. *J Clin Invest* **86**:1338, 1990.
448. Rossi M, Maiuri L, Fusco MI, Danielsen EM, Auricchio S: The human adult-type hypolactasia is a heterogeneous condition *in vitro* biosynthetic studies, in Aurricchio S, Semenza G (eds): *Milk in Human Nutrition and Adult-type Hypolactasia*. Dyn Nutr Res Basel, Karger, vol 3. 1993, p. 174
449. Lloyd M, Mevissen, Fischer M, Olsen W, Goodspeed D, Genini M, Boll W, Semenza G, Mantei N: Regulation of intestinal lactase in adult hypolactasia. *J Clin Invest* **89**:524, 1992. (See also *Gastroenterology* **100**:A226, 1991.)
449a. Rossi M, Maiuri L, Fusco MI, Salvati VM, Fuccio A, Auricchio S, Mantei N, Semenza G: Lactase decline and lactase persistence in human adults. Submitted, 1994.
450. Musy P, Kastern W, Cerda J, Neu J: Maturational decline of lactase-phlorizin hydrolase is not due to decreased mRNA synthesis. *Pediatr Res* **29**:109A, 1991.
450a. Mairui L, Rossi M, Raia V, Paparo F, Garipoli V, Auricchio S: Surface staining on the villus of lactase protein and lactase activity in adult-type hypolactasia. *Gastroenterology* **105**:708, 1993.
450b. Maiuri L, Rossi M, Raia V, Garipoli V, Hughes LA, Swallow D, Norén O, Sjöström H, Auricchio S: The cellular basis of adult-type hypolactasia. *Gastroenterology* 1994. (In Press)
451. Poggi V, Savilhati E, Sebastio G, Mantei N, Boll W, Congia H, Santantonio AA, Muro V, Auricchio S: Primary sequence of coding region of lactase-phlorizin hydrolase gene in congenital human lactase deficiency. *J Pediatr Gastroenterol Nutr*. **13**:A17, 1991.
452. Auricchio S, Ciccimarra F, Della Pietra D, Vegnente A: Intestinal hydrolysis of starch. *Mod Probl Pediatr* **11**:23, 1968.
453. Auricchio S: Brush border enzymes, in Anderson CM, Burke V, Gracey M (eds): *Paediatric Gastroenterology*, 2d ed. Australia, Blackwell, 1986, chap 5, part III, p 185.

Part 23

NEUROGENETICS

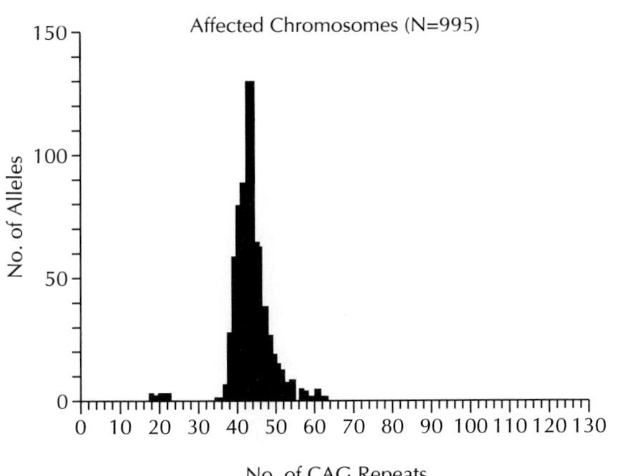

Control Chromosomes (N=600)

No. of Alleles

No. of CAG Repeats

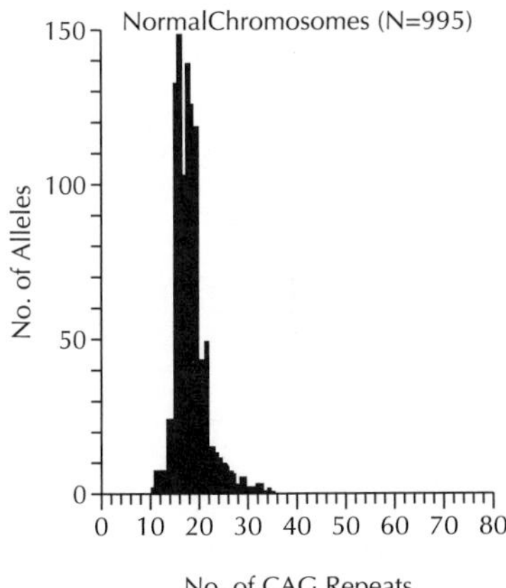

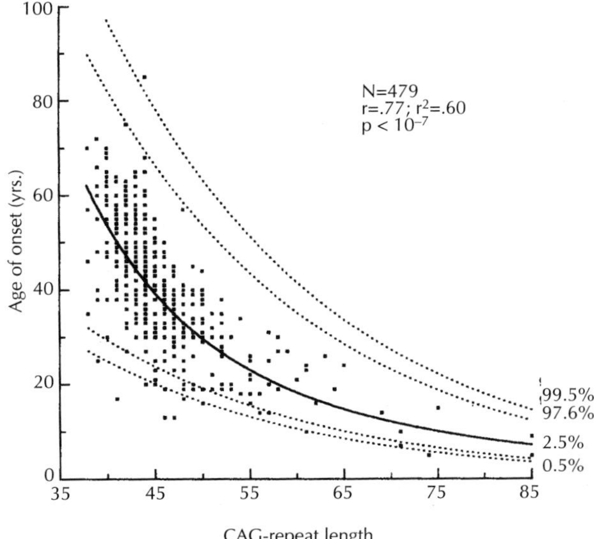

Huntington disease and CAG repeats

CHAPTER 152

Huntington Disease

Michael R. Hayden ▪ Berry Kremer

1. **Huntington disease (HD) is a slowly progressive autosomal dominant neurodegenerative disease with complete penetrance. Onset is usually in adult life, with a mean age at onset of around 40 years. However, onsets before age 20 or after age 60 have been described. The disease progresses inexorably, with death occurring approximately 18 years from onset. Prevalence is between 3 and 7 per 100,000 in populations of Western European descent, but HD has been described in populations of many different ancestries.**
2. **The neuropathological hallmark of the disease is neuronal loss and gliosis in the caudate nucleus and the putamen (the striatum), with resultant atrophy. Medium-sized striatal neurons that contain GABA and enkephalin or GABA and substance P as their neurotransmitters, are selectively depleted. Other, neurochemically distinct, striatal neuronal populations are spared, such as large aspiny acetylcholinesterase-containing neurons or NADPH-diaphorase neurons with somatostatin and neuropeptide Y. Apart from the striatum, the whole brain undergoes generalized atrophy. No specific pathological changes have been found outside the central nervous system.**
3. **Clinical manifestations consist of gradually evolving involuntary movements, progressive dementia, and psychiatric disturbances, especially mood disorder and personality changes. Chorea is the most prominent abnormality, but parkinsonism, dystonia, and involuntary motor impairment may all be present. Minor motor abnormalities, including clumsiness, hyperreflexia, and eye movement disturbances, often appear as early manifestations of HD. Patients with onset before age 20 frequently have prominent bradykinesia, rigidity, epilepsy, severe dementia, and a shorter duration of illness. In contrast, cognitive decline is often less severe in patients with onset after age 60.**
4. **The diagnosis is based on the clinical presentation. The demonstration of caudate nucleus atrophy on CT or MRI scan will confirm the diagnosis. Caudate hypometabolism, as detected by positron emission tomography using ^{18}fluorodeoxyglucose, is already present at the earliest phase of the illness, when caudate nucleus atrophy is still invisible.**
5. **A novel gene containing a CAG trinucleotide repeat that is expanded on HD chromosomes has been identified. This highly polymorphic CAG repeat located in the 5′ end of the gene has been shown to range between 10 and 30 copies on normal chromosomes, while it is expanded to a range of 36 to 121 on HD chromosomes. The vast majority of patients with the clinical diagnosis of HD have expansion of the CAG repeat. Sequence analysis has not revealed any obvious homology, and no further understanding of the pathogenesis of HD is currently forthcoming. Age of onset shows a highly significant association with the length of the CAG repeat.**
6. **The biochemical defect underlying HD is unknown. The most consistent hypothesis for the striatal neuronal death postulates a neurotoxic effect of glutamate or other neuroexcitatory substances. There is no known treatment to retard disease progression. Neuroleptic medication is able to alleviate choreic movements to some extent, but side effects may be severe. Antidepressant therapy may be helpful in the early stages to alleviate the mood disorder.**

A list of standard abbreviations is located immediately preceding the index in each volume. Additional abbreviations used in this chapter include: AChE = acetylcholinesterase; AD = Alzheimer disease; AMPA = α-amino-3-hydroxy-5-methylisoxazole-4-propionic acid; EAA = excitatory amino acids; Enk = enkephalin; GFAP = glial fibrillary acidic protein; GP = globus pallidus; GPi/e = globus pallidus, pars interna/externa; HD = Huntington disease; IA = intermediate allele; NMDA = *N*-methyl-D-aspartate; PET = positron emission tomography; SNr = substantia nigra, pars reticulata; STN = subthalamic nucleus.

HISTORICAL BACKGROUND

How did this disease get its name? At the age of 21, only a year after graduating from Columbia University as a doctor, George Huntington presented his paper on chorea to the Meigs and Mason Academy of Medicine in Middleport, Ohio (Fig. 152-1). The text of the lecture appeared in the *Medical and Surgical Reporter* on April 13, 1872.[1] After a general discussion on the subject of childhood chorea, he provided in approximately 1200 words a comprehensive description of hereditary chorea. Sir William Osler, professor of medicine at Johns Hopkins University in Baltimore remarked that "there are few instances in the history of medicine in which a disease has been more graphically or more briefly described."[2] This account of the disorder was abstracted into German,[3] with the result that Huntington's name very quickly became attached to the disease in different parts of the world, including Germany,[4] France,[5] Italy,[6] and England.[7]

Both his father and grandfather were medical doctors and Huntington reported in 1910[8] that his grandfather had observed patients with inherited chorea when he had moved to East Hampton, NY, in 1797. George Huntington was only 8 years old when he first saw patients with this disorder while riding with his father on his professional rounds in East Hampton. Approximately 13 years later, he wrote out the original draft on chorea, with his father's penciled revisions still visible in the margins of the original manuscript.[9] The eventual delineation of the disorder was therefore the outcome of the cooperation between three generations of doctors in the Huntington family. Extracts from Huntington's original and only major contribution to medical literature,

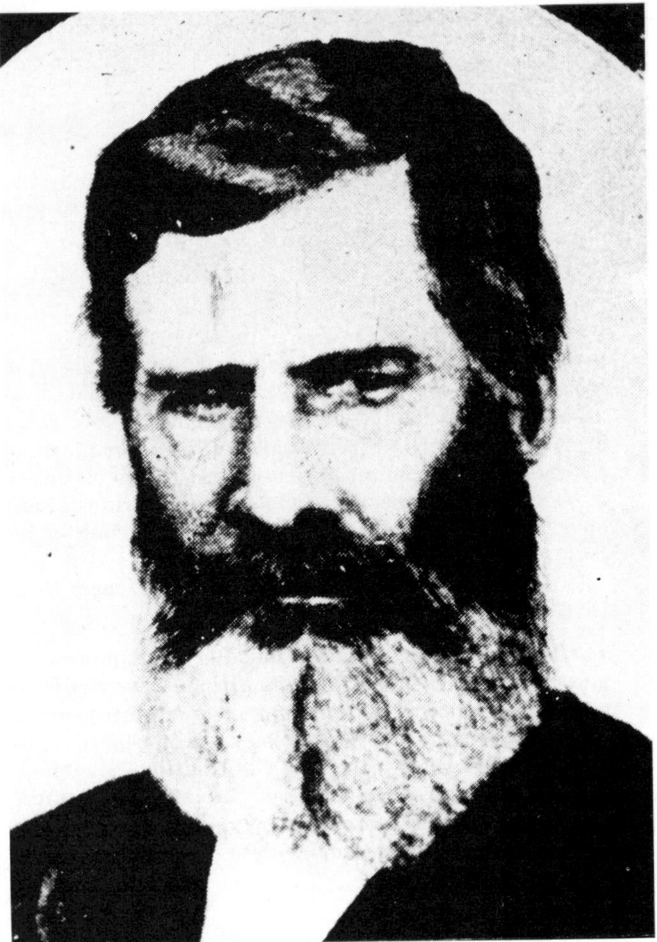

FIG. 152-1 Photograph of George Huntington.

which encompassed the core features of this disease, are cited here.

> The hereditary chorea as I shall call it is confined to certain and fortunately few families and has been transmitted to them as an heirloom from generations way back in the dim past. It is spoken of by those in whose veins the seeds of the disease are known to exist with a kind of horror and not at all alluded to except through dire necessity with it being mentioned as "that disorder." It is attended generally by all the symptoms of common chorea only in an aggravated degree, hardly ever manifesting itself until adult or middle life and then coming on gradually but surely, increasing by degrees and often occupying years in its development until the hapless sufferer is but a quivering wreck of his former self. . . . There are three marked peculiarities in this disease; 1) its hereditary nature, 2) a tendency to insanity and suicide, and 3) its manifesting itself as a grave disease only in adult life.
>
> 1. Of its hereditary nature. When either or both the parents have shown manifestations of the disease, and more especially when these manifestations have been of a serious nature, one or more of the offspring almost invariably suffer from the disease if they live to adult age. But if by any chance these children go through life without it, the thread is broken and the grandchildren and great grandchildren of the original sufferers may rest assured that they are free of the disease. . . .
>
> 2. The tendency to insanity and sometimes that form of insanity which leads to suicide is marked. I know of several instances of suicide in people suffering from this form of chorea, or who belonged to families in which the disease existed. . . .
>
> 3. Its third peculiarity is its coming on at least as a grave disease only in adult life. I do not know of a single case that has shown any marked signs of chorea before the age of thirty or forty years while those who pass the fortieth year without symptoms of the disease are seldom attacked. . . . I've never known a recovery even an amelioration of symptoms in this form of chorea; when once it begins it clings to the bitter end. No treatment seems to be of any avail and indeed nowadays, its end is so well known to the sufferer and his friends that medical advice is seldom sought. It seems at least to be one of the incurables.[1]

EPIDEMIOLOGY

Prevalence

Many different epidemiologic surveys have been presented from different parts of the world, including northwestern Europe, the United Kingdom, Scandinavia, North America, Australia, Japan, and South Africa. While recorded rates differ, there is general agreement that the frequency of HD in populations of Western European descent is between 3 and 7 affected individuals per 100,000 population. However, a few areas show particularly high or low prevalence rates.

Areas of Low Prevalence. HD appears to be particularly uncommon in Japan[10] and among African blacks.[11] The frequency of HD in Japan has been estimated at between 0.1 and 0.38 per 100,000, which is just below the frequency in Finland of 0.5 per 100,000.[12] This frequency is between 10 and 20 times less common than seen in most Western countries (Table 152-1). Extensive studies in South Africa revealed that the disease is approximately 40 times less frequent in African blacks than in South African Whites. Earlier studies from the United States[13,14] also showed that this disorder was approximately three times less frequent in American blacks than in American whites. However, a more detailed study by Folstein et al.[15] revealed that a prevalence in blacks was quite similar to that seen in whites in the state of Maryland. In this study, multiple sources for ascertainment were used. The studies by Reed et al.[13] and Wright et al.[16] in South Carolina were based on very small numbers of patients and therefore might reflect bias in ascertainment.

Table 152-1 Areas of Low Prevalence of Huntington's Disease*

Location	Author(s)	Rate (per 100,000)	No. of Patients	Population Size
Japan	Kishimoto	0.38	13	3,916,922
Finland	Palo	0.5	26	±4,900,000
African blacks	Hayden	0.06	11	16,640,314

*Adapted from Hayden.[25]

Table 152-2 Areas of High Prevalence of Huntington Disease*

Location	Author(s)	Rate (per 100,000)	No. of Patients	Population Size
North Sweden	Sjögren	144	18	±12,500
Tasmania, Australia	Brothers	174	105	60,344
	Pridmore	12.1	54	±447,000
Moray Firth, Scotland	Lyon	560	5	896
Lake Maracaibo, Zulia, Venezuela	Avila-Giron	±700	28	±4,000
Mauritius (Caucasian)	Hayden	46	16	±132,000

*Adapted from Hayden.[25]

However, the low prevalence of HD in Japan and Finland and in South African blacks clearly are not the result of underestimates but represent real racial differences.

The explanation for the geographic variation in frequency is related to the ethnic origins of these particular populations and the origins of HD in that country. Most genealogical studies have indicated that migration from northwestern Europe was a primary factor responsible for the spread for the gene for HD around the world. A low prevalence of the disorder would be expected in populations who have their origins outside Europe. However, there is mounting evidence from studies of DNA haplotypes linked to the HD gene (see "Molecular Genetics" below) that HD is not due to a single mutation but might be caused by multiple mutations. The low prevalence of the disorder in these populations might reflect a more recent introduction of the gene for HD in that population.

Areas of Higher Prevalence. The prevalence of HD exceeds 15 per 100,000 in five areas listed in Table 152-2. An important factor to be considered when assessing prevalence in a particular region is the total size of the surveyed population. In a small population, the presence of a few affected individuals will raise the disease prevalence.

This is obvious in the study in the Moray Firth area of Scotland, where a total of 5 affected individuals resulted in calculated prevalence of 560 per 100,000 because the total of inhabitants in this region was less than 1000. Similarly, an artificially high prevalence was found in Mauritius.[17]

The highest frequency of HD in the world in a larger population occurs in Venezuela at the edge of Lake Maracaibo.[18,19] The gene was introduced into an isolated community sometime in the early nineteenth century. The gene frequency has rapidly increased as a result of the aggregation of affected persons in this relatively isolated area.

This population has offered a unique research opportunity for investigation of the natural history of this disorder as well as the understanding of the clinical features of the homozygous form of HD.[20] The identification of this large family with HD served to confirm the suspected linkage to G8, which was the initial discovery of linkage for the gene for HD to a polymorphic genetic marker on 4p. In addition, this family has continued to serve as a reference pedigree for gene mapping studies.

The high frequency of HD in Tasmania[21] relative to other regions also reflects the introduction of the gene by a single ancestor from Somerset, England, who after being widowed for the second time left her village with her 13 children and migrated to Australia. By 1964 there were 120 affected persons in five generations in Tasmania. A study by Pridmore[21] revealed that this family was still the major factor in the higher prevalence for HD in Tasmania.

Areas of Unknown Prevalence. While there have been numerous studies on the epidemiology of HD in most Western countries, which have indicated that this disease may be ubiquitous, there are regions for which information is extremely scanty. These include the Middle East and most of Asia. There have been at least 20 families who appear to be well documented in China but the prevalence remains unknown. There is also no information concerning the frequency of HD in the Arab population, and it is uncertain whether this reflects a low frequency or underreporting.

Mortality Data

Mortality data are a poor indication of the frequency of the illness primarily due to underreporting. This has been particularly exacerbated since January 1, 1979, when HD was classified under the International Statistical Classification of Diseases (ISC) as the rubric 333.4, of which the 333 root is often the only one completed. Under the latter code are included many other diseases that occur with greater frequency than HD. Therefore, ISC data are of less value when trying to assess the number of deaths due to HD.

Detailed comparison of death rates due to HD for different countries have revealed that the similar results for northwestern Europe and for U.S. whites range between 1 and 2.27 deaths per 1 million population per year.[22] Careful analysis of mortality data for HD between 1968 and 1974 in the United States[23] revealed major variations in rates, with the highest being reported from South Dakota, Wyoming, and New Hampshire. North Dakota, Alaska, and Hawaii had no deaths coded for HD. These differences might again reflect biases of ascertainment, with a small number of deaths in very small populations. High mortality rates in the states of California, Oregon, and Washington might reflect a true increase in prevalence in that part of the country.

NATURAL HISTORY

Age at Onset

A broad definition of age of onset is the first time any neurologic or psychiatric symptoms appear that represent a permanent change from the normal state. However, with this interpretation the estimation of the age of onset may be most difficult. Doctors seldom witness the earlier signs and symptoms of HD, and assessment of these early and insidious changes often depends on the patient themselves or their family. In some families, denial of early HD is commonplace with acknowledgment of the presence of the disorder only in a more advanced form while in others any restlessness or clumsiness is ascribed to onset of the illness. In either situation age of onset is commonly miscalculated.

International Comparisons. Different studies have revealed marked variation in ages of onset. Before biologic significance can be attached to these comparisons, methodologic issues need to be assessed. Clearly, different criteria for age at onset explain part of this variation, for example, onset of psychiatric symptoms or chorea as the defining event. Another major problem is the truncated interval of observation, which may artificially lower the age of onset as this may contain no information from asymptomatic heterozygotes who have not yet manifested signs of the disorder at the time of the study.[24] Different methods of ascertainment or true geographic factors currently not understood may also confound this variable.

The age at which signs of symptoms for HD occur has a normal distribution, with a mean of around 40 and an SD of approximately 10 years.[25,26] The earliest age of onset has been approximately 2 years, and patients with onset of the disorder in their 70s and even early 80s have been noted.

To correct the problem of truncated intervals of observation, Wendt et al.[27] restricted their analysis to cohorts born 60 years prior to the time of data analysis and reported a mean age of onset of 43.97, which is higher than other studies. When Newcombe's study[24] was limited to persons born before 1909, the mean age of onset was 48.4 years. A successive decrease in the mean age of onset occurred as one got closer to the current time of analysis. Similarly, in the study of Adams et al.[26] the mean age of onset in the total sample of 611 patients was 38.6 years. However, restriction of the analysis to persons born in 1920 resulted in a mean age at onset of 43.7 years.

Therefore, the mean age of onset in most of the studies[25,28] may have been underestimated as a result of the effect of the truncated intervals of observation. The corrected studies consistently show that the mean age of onset is between 43 and 48 years of age.

Zone of Onset

HD does not have a specific single presenting sign or symptom. In the earliest phases, there is an insidious and slow deterioration of intellectual functions as well as mild personality change. A most comprehensive way of assessing the signs and symptoms of HD is to follow a cohort for an extended period. The longitudinal study of the kindred in Venezuela[29] has clearly demonstrated that patients pass through a zone of onset that represents a transitional state from the normal presymptomatic phase to the time at which the diagnosis can be clearly made on neurologic examination. This zone of onset during which the diagnosis of HD cannot be made unequivocally is frequently witnessed by changes in caudate metabolic rates of glucose as seen on positron emission tomography.[30,31]

Age at Death

While the age of death is a specific point, a survey of the mean ages of death in a population would be subject to the same biases of ascertainment as seen with age of onset—for example, the assessment of a recent cohort would not include those who are longer survivors.

The mean age of death in different studies varies from a low of 51.4[32] to a high of 62.9 years.[33] In all instances, studies with lower ages of death have had lower ages of onset, suggesting that this does not reflect variation in duration of the disease. The mean age of death in Tasmania is the oldest reported for any geographical region and is consistent with the finding of mean age at onset of 48.3 years in that region. The largest study of HD mortality and causes of death reported is based on the national data made available through the U.S. National Center of Health Statistics for all causes of death reported on death certificates.[22] In this study of 3058 persons, the mean age of death was 56.5 years. The leading causes of death in persons with HD were pneumonia (33 percent) and heart disease (24 percent).[34,35] Suicide represented only 1 to 3 percent of deaths but is likely to be underreported. If one assumes death due to suicide in all cases in which accidental poisonings and violence were reported, this would account for approximately 8 percent of deaths. Pneumonia occurs five times more commonly in HD than in controls and is likely to be secondary to the significant dysphagia that results in choking and aspiration pneumonia.

Duration of Huntington Disease

The duration of HD is estimated by subtracting the age at onset from age of death. In contrast to the considerable differences in the age at onset and age of death in different studies, there are no significant variations in duration of disease, which is around 15 years, with no differences between the sexes.[25] Survival with HD has not significantly changed over the past 50 years, which reflects the failure of medical therapy to delay disease progression. Even though the mean duration in many different studies has been constant, there are marked individual variations, extending up to as much as 40 years from time of onset on rare occasions.[27] It would appear that in some families, HD follows a milder course with longer survival. Factors associated with longer survival in families are unknown.

NEUROPATHOLOGICAL AND NEUROCHEMICAL ALTERATIONS

Striatal Changes. Since the descriptions of Anglade,[36] Jelgersma,[37] and Alzheimer,[38] atrophy of the caudate nucleus and the putamen (the neostriatum), has been considered the most characteristic pathological feature of the disease.[39] Yet, the severity of neostriatal abnormalities is highly variable. In a series of 163 clinically diagnosed cases, 13 lacked macroscopically visible atrophy, while in 18 cases the caudate was extremely shrunken and the putamen markedly atrophic[40] (Fig. 152-2). This variability is reported in all large series[41–44] and is documented in numerous case reports.[39–45]

Microscopically, the neostriatal atrophy is characterized by neuronal loss and gliosis[39,40] (Fig. 152-3), which again may be highly variable. Full appreciation of neuronal loss, however, can only be obtained by cell counting. In these instances, even in the absence of caudate abnormalities macroscopically, regional loss of up to 40 percent of the normal neurons may be found.[46] Medium- and small-sized neurons, which are the most abundant class in human striatum[47] disappear, while larger neurons appear relatively preserved.[39,42,48,49] The remaining neurons often show irregu-

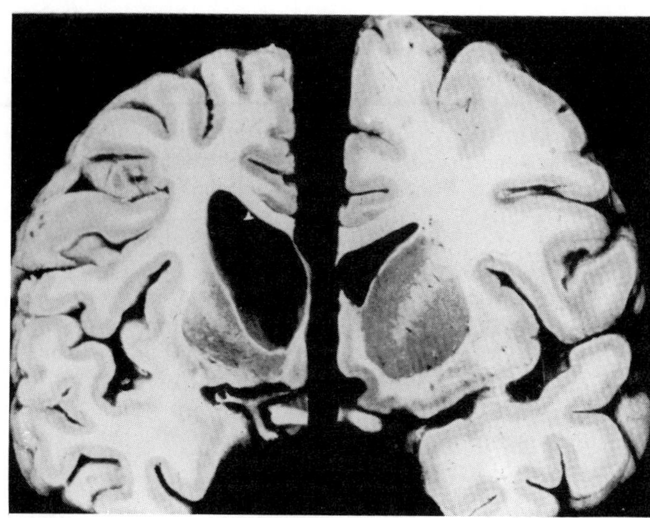

FIG. 152-2 Coronal brain sections. Severe striatal atrophy in the brain of a patient with HD *(left)*, compared to a control *(right)* *(From Hayden[25] Used by permission.)*

lar loss and pallor of the cytoplasm, some shrinkage, and pyknosis of the nucleus.[42]

Ultrastructural (EM) studies of caudate neurons may reveal abnormalities in the nucleus and nucleolus, the ER, ribosomes, the Golgi apparatus, mitochondria, and lysosomes.[50] In affected cells both degenerative and regenerative changes can be observed. In Golgi stains of medium-sized spiny neurons, abnormal dendritic branching, elongation and abnormal recurvations of distal dendrites, and alterations in spine densities were visualized.[51,52] Intense immunohistochemical labeling of abnormally shaped neurites by both nonphosphorylated and phosphorylated antineurofilament antibodies,[53] displacement of calbindin (D28k) immunostaining toward the distal dendrites,[52] and increased expression of neural cell adhesion molecule immunoreactivity in the HD neostriatum[53] may all be additional manifestations of these changes. As proliferation of dendrites occurs more frequently in the moderately affected cases, with loss of dendrites in the severely affected, it has been suggested that neuritic growth may actually precede neuronal loss.[52]

Gliosis particularly manifest by astrocytosis may be prominent. In the HD neostriatum, an increased density of fibrillary astrocytes is found.[40,44] These astrocytes express glial fibrillary acidic protein (GFAP), have nuclei that appear larger and more vesicular than normal,[42,54] and possess an increased number of bundles of glial filaments in astrocytic processes on EM examination[55] (Fig. 152-4). Fibrillary astrocytosis is often easier to appreciate than mild neuronal loss.[40] It is currently unknown whether the increased density in astrocytes, as well as oligodendrocytes, represents a truly increased total number,[46] or in reality obscures a normal or even decreased number of cells,[49,57] compacted in a smaller volume of shrunken tissue.

No specific cellular markers characteristic of HD have been found. Accumulation of lipofuscin in remaining neurons and astrocytes[39,42,50,54] is evident, as is an increased neostriatal iron content,[43,54,58] probably stored in siderophages in the perivascular spaces.[42] Corpora amylacea[54] that may even occur in synaptic terminals,[59] and an increased proportion of neurons with nuclear membrane indentations[60,61] have all been noted to accompany the neostriatal neuronal loss and gliosis. None of these phenomena, however, is specific to HD.

Although the neostriatum is the most severely and obviously affected structure in the brains of HD patients, it is not uniformly atrophied. The caudate seems more affected than the putamen.[40,44] The nucleus accumbens is least affected.[40,42,62] Within the caudate, a gradient of atrophic changes can be discerned. The tail is more affected than the body, and the head displays the least changes. The mediodorsal parts of the caudate are initially more affected than the ventrolateral parts, but ultimately the whole caudate becomes diffusely atrophic.[40] Within the putamen a similar gradient exists with the posterior putamen being most affected and the anterior ventral putamen least involved.[62]

The earliest and most extensively affected neurons are the medium-sized spiny neurons that express GABA and enkephalin (Enk) or GABA and substance P as their neurotransmitter.[63] Their cell bodies are located in the striatal matrix and they project to the external part of the globus pallidus (GPe; GABA/Enk), or to the internal part of the globus pallidus (GPi) and the substantia nigra, pars reticulata (SNr; GABA/substance P)[64,65] (see Fig. 152-9). Their disappearance explains the previously found reductions in tissue

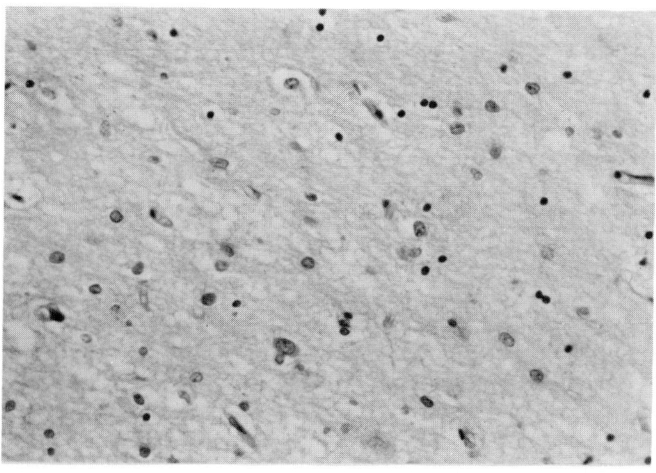

A

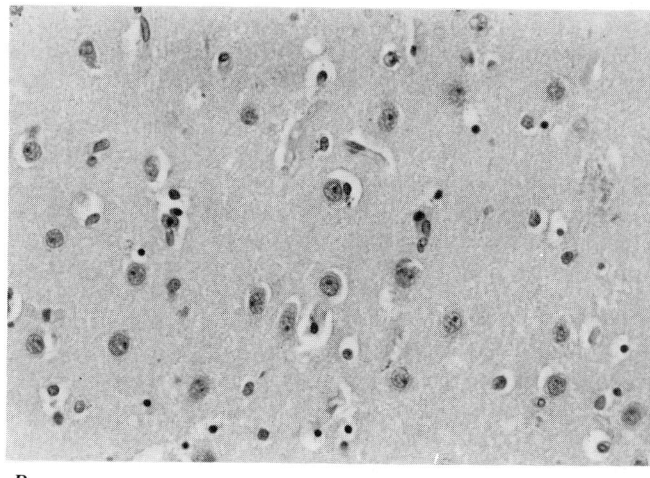

B

FIG. 152-3 Microscopic view, showing severe neuronal loss, increased density of glial cells, and rarefaction of the neuropil in the striatum of a patient with HD *(A)*, as compared with a control *(B)* *(From Kremer et al.[337] Used by permission.)*

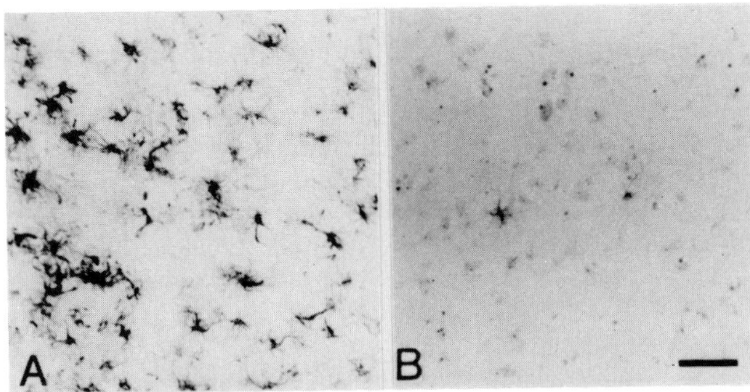

FIG. 152-4 **Immunohistochemistry for glial fibrillary acidic protein (GFAP), showing densely staining fibrillary astrocytes in the caudate of an HD patient *(A)* but not in a control *(B)* *(From Kremer et al.*[337] *Used by permission.)***

or cerebrospinal fluid GABA content.[65a] The GABA/Enk projection to GPe may be more severely affected than the GABA/substance P projection to GPi.[66] The substance P projection to SN pars compacta, originating from striosomes,[64] appears to be involved in the disease process only in the later stages.[66–68] A decreased number of fibers immunoreactive for Enk and substance P in GPe and SNr, respectively, was already observable in the brain of an asymptomatic individual at high risk for having inherited the HD gene.[268,269]

Medium-sized and large neurons containing the enzyme NADPH-diaphorase (recently identified as a nitric oxide synthase)[69] remain intact.[70] These neurons contain somatostatin and neuropeptide Y as their neurotransmitter and are localized in the striatal matrix,[71,72] probably serving as interneurons. Another relatively spared group are large aspiny acetylcholinesterase (AChE)-containing and locally arborizing interneurons,[73] which seem not to be localized in any particular compartment.[74] Again, it should be appreciated that the absence of studies applying formal morphometric methods precludes the assessment of whether these "resistant" neurons do not die at all, or only die less rapidly than their vulnerable counterparts.

The globus pallidus (GP) may show a general volume reduction as large as the neostriatum.[49,75] Part of this reduction is due to the loss of striatopallidal fibers.[44,66] Demyelinization of remaining fibers, with astrocytosis and crowding of oligodendrocytes, is common. The large neurons in the GPe appear shrunken and laden with lipofuscin, while GPi neurons seem affected only in severe cases.[39]

Changes in Extrastriatal Structures. The selective nature of neuronal loss may be demonstrated by the patterns of cell loss within the neostriatum. However, other regions of the brain are also affected. Macroscopically, the whole brain often appears atrophic, with narrowed gyri, widened sulci, and a reduction of brain weight, sometimes by as much as 400 g.[39,44,75]

Cortical atrophy with changes in neocortical architecture have been frequently reported.[36–39,41,45] Morphometric analysis of 30 HD brains revealed up to 30 percent reduction of mean cortical area and a reduction to 16 percent of cortical ribbon thickness associated with increasing severity of the neostriatal changes.[75] The normal layered architecture is preserved, but alterations occur in layers III, V, and VI,[39,42,44,77,77a] with layer IV possibly also involved.[39,42,78] Ganglion cells in these layers appear shrunken, basophilic, and abnormally shaped,[41,42,45] with ultrastructural changes similar to the striatum.[50,79] The major class of neurons affected are the large pyramidal projection neurons[77] that express nonphosphorylated neurofilament epitopes.[80] Loss of their extensive cortical dendritic arborizations may explain part of the general decrease in cortical thickness and volume. Neuropeptide Y–containing cortical interneurons, in contrast, are spared,[80] as are the large Betz cells in the precentral gyrus that give rise to descending corticobulbar and corticospinal connections.[44,45]

Gliosis in the cortex is less conspicuous.[44,81] However, on counting, both astrocyte and oligodendroctyte densities were found to be significantly increased in all layers in the prefrontal cortex.[77] Astrocytic changes were visible on EM, with lipofuscin accumulation and prominent bundles of glial filaments in astrocytic processes as the most characteristic changes.[79]

In mildly affected cases, the cortical changes are patchy, while in severe cases they are spread throughout the cortex.[41] The changes may be most marked in the neocortical frontal areas,[45] with the parietal and temporal lobes sometimes equally affected.[42] Changes in the occipital lobe vary from mild to severe.[42,45,57] Hippocampal changes are usually less pronounced than in the neocortex.[42] A relatively recent finding is the severe cell loss in the entorhinal cortex.[82]

Cortical changes in HD do not differ qualitatively from that seen in senile and other atrophies.[42,63] In some instances, senile plaques and neurofibrillary tangles may be found in neocortical and limbic areas of the brains of elderly HD patients.[44,83–85] The patchy nature of the cortical changes in less severely affected cases may lead to underrepresentation due to sampling errors. What is certain, however, is that at least one neuronal population, the large projection neurons, is predictably affected. As this population makes up a much smaller part of the cortex than the medium-sized spiny neurons in the neostriatum, the apparent atrophy in the cortex is less impressive.

The diminution in size of the subcortical white matter and the reduced size of the corpus callosum supports the described loss of cortical projection neurons.[42,75]

The amygdala, although reduced in cross-sectional area,[75] is microscopically well preserved, with only a few instances of slight astrocytosis and some neuronal atrophy.[42]

The thalamus, similar to most structures, may be reduced in proportion to the rest of the brain.[49,75] The density of small neurons in the ventrobasal complex is considerably reduced (50 percent), while the large neurons persist normally.[76] Astrocytosis in defined thalamic nuclei may be present.[39,42,44]

The subthalamic nucleus, which receives significant projections from the cerebral cortex and from the GPe, projects to the GPe, GPi, neostriatum, and substantia nigra[86] and may be significantly reduced (by 23 percent) in volume, but not in absolute number of nerve cells.[49]

In contrast to variable changes in other extrastriatal structures, the hypothalamic lateral nucleus is severely atrophied.[87,88] Morphometric analysis has revealed a consistent reduction (by 90 percent) of the normal neuronal content of about 60,000; in some cases less than 2000 neurons remained.[89,90] Accompanied by gliosis, the atrophic process seems similar to that in the neostriatum.[89]

Brain-stem nuclei, including the substantia nigra, pars compacta, and the neurons of the ventral tegmental mesencephalic area (with dopamine as a neurotransmitter), the locus ceruleus (noradrenaline), the raphe nuclei (serotonin), the tuberomammillary nucleus (histamine), and the large cholinergic basal forebrain neurons of the substantia innominata, including the basal nucleus of Meynert, are generally intact.[44,59,89–93] However, in severely demented patients there may be neuronal loss in the locus ceruleus,[94] while cell loss in the substantia nigra is absent or only mild.[39,42,44]

Gross cerebellar atrophy is rare[95] but some cerebellar changes are well established[39,42] and are especially prominent in early-onset cases.[96,97] But even in adult cases, the density of cortical Purkinje cells may often be decreased, on average, to half the value of age-matched controls.[98] This decrease bears no obvious relation to the general brain atrophy.[98] The dentate nucleus is often depleted,[39,42] but the fastigial nucleus is usually normal.[44]

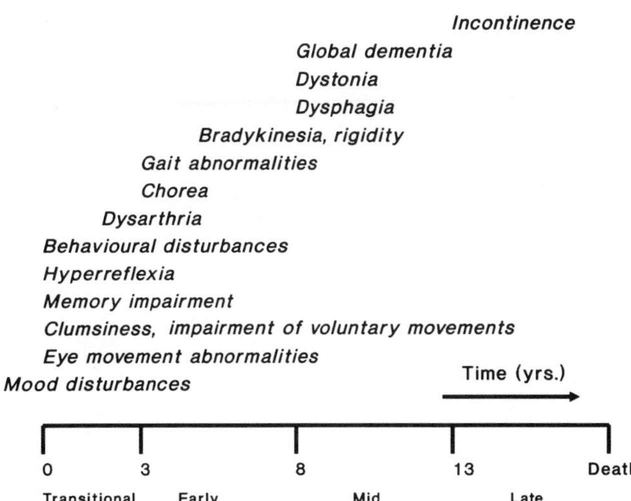

FIG. 152-5 **Clinical phases and associated signs and symptoms in the natural history of Huntington disease** *(From Kremer et al.[337] Used by permission.)*

CLINICAL MANIFESTATIONS AND DIAGNOSIS

Diagnosis of Huntington Disease

Traditionally a definite diagnosis of HD was made in the presence of (1) a positive family history, consistent with autosomal dominant inheritance; (2) progressive motor disability involving both involuntary and voluntary movement; and (3) mental disturbances including cognitive decline, affective disturbances, and/or changes in personality.

The diagnosis of HD is made primarily on clinical examination. Demonstration of atrophy of the caudate nucleus and the putamen by CT or MRI provide additional support. Positron emission tomography (PET) may reveal a decrease in the uptake and metabolism of glucose in the caudate nucleus before structural tissue loss becomes evident. A finding of CAG expansion in the HD range in a symptomatic patient is further support for the diagnosis of HD.[356]

Despite the clinical criteria, misdiagnosis still occurs fairly frequently. In a community-based survey in the state of Maryland, 11 percent of 212 patients who met their diagnostic criteria had previously received another (false) diagnosis, while 15 percent could not be confirmed to have HD on closer examination.[99] In an older unselected autopsy series, 7 percent of the cases clinically diagnosed as having HD had some other neurologic condition.[100] DNA approaches are likely to reduce the frequency of misdiagnoses.

Early Signs of Huntington Disease: Transitional Phase

The clear appearance of extrapyramidal signs such as chorea, hypokinesia, rigidity, or dystonia, marks a phase in the disease progression, not the beginning of disease. In recent years the longitudinal study of a large cohort of at-risk people in Venezuela,[19,29] follow-up of individuals in predictive testing programs, and the application of PET scanning to individuals without overt chorea have provided valuable information on the earliest clinical manifestations of the disease. Most individuals will initially display minor motor abnormalities. These include general restlessness, abnormalities of eye movements or optokinetic nystagmus, hyperreflexia, impairments of finger tapping or rapid alternating hand movements, and excessive and inappropriate movements of the fingers, hands, or toes during emotional stress,[19,29,99] as well as mild dysarthria. Minor motor abnormalities usually precede the obvious signs of extrapyramidal dysfunction by at least 3 years.[29,99] Persons with a completely normal neurologic examination have a 3 percent chance of being diagnosed within the next 3 years.[19,29]

The clinical onset of HD is gradual, with patients passing from an asymptomatic period through a transitional phase during which diagnosis is still difficult, to a stage when overt signs and symptoms allow a definitive diagnosis to be made (Fig. 152-5). The proportion of people initially at risk and displaying minor motor abnormalities who later turn out not to have HD is unknown. These changes most likely are early signs of HD, but may also be due to anxiety, the recent use of alcohol or drugs, or other neurologic illnesses.

Extrapyramidal Motor Signs

Chorea. Chorea is the major motor sign of the disease, hence the old name "Huntington chorea." These involuntary movements are continuously present during waking hours, cannot be voluntarily suppressed by the patient, and worsen during stress. Although the pattern of the movements may differ between affected patients, they occur in individual patients in a stereotypic manner. Choreic movements of the face are common and present as pouting of the lips, irregular grimacing, twitching of the cheeks, and alternate lifting of the eyebrows and frowning (Fig. 152-6). The neck is often involved, causing forward or backward bending of the head or rotation. Choreic movements of the trunk moves the body in different directions. Breathing may become irregular. In the limbs, there is frequent flexion and extension of the fingers. The legs may be alternately crossed and uncrossed and the toes flexed and extended. Chorea is a feature of HD in over 90 percent of patients, increasing during the first phase (about 10 years) of the patients' illness. With advancing duration, features of bradykinesia, rigidity, and dystonia become more evident.[19,25,101] Chorea is seen less frequently in patients with juvenile onset[25] and may rarely be absent in adult-onset cases.[102]

Bradykinesia and Rigidity. Bradykinesia and rigidity, best known as the core features of Parkinson disease, are infrequent in the early phases of adult-onset Huntington disease. However, they gradually appear until they often dominate the final stages of the illness, in which the patient will become severely rigid and grossly akinetic.[19,39] Early in the illness, bradykinesia alone may contribute to an impairment

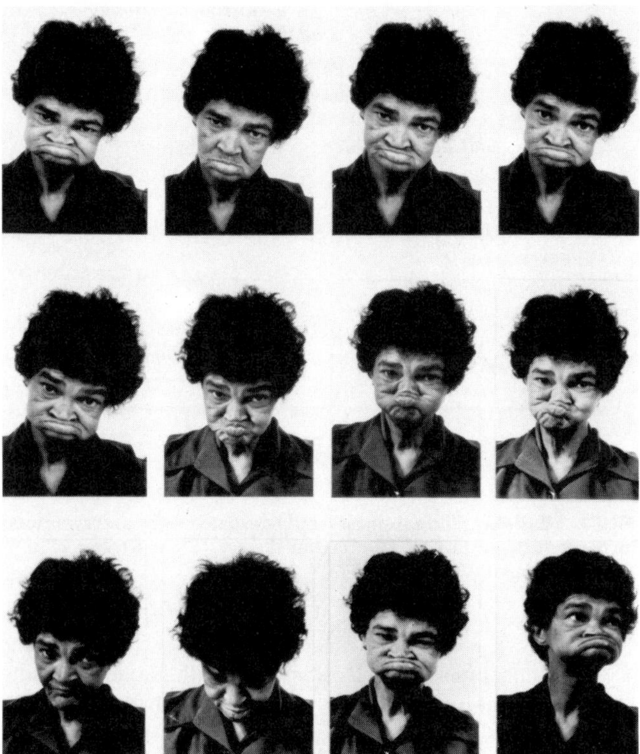

FIG. 152-6 Orofacial dyskinesia in a patient with Huntington's disease. ***(From Hayden.[25] Used by permission.)***

in voluntary motor performance.[103] In both juvenile and adult rigid cases a coarse resting tremor, distinct from a parkinsonian tremor, may complement the clinical picture.[102,104] The use of neuroleptic drugs, intended to suppress choreic movements, may aggravate the existing bradykinesia and rigidity.

Dystonia. Dystonia, characterized by slow abnormal movements and abnormal posturing, is infrequent in the early symptomatic period but worsens and becomes a prominent feature in the later stages of the illness.[19,104]

Other Motor Abnormalities

Oculomotor Dysfunction. Oculomotor disturbances, apart from being among the earliest signs in the transitional phase, are present in the vast majority of affected patients.[99,105] Slowing of saccades may be seen in up to 75 percent of symptomatic individuals,[105,106] especially in early-onset cases,[107] more particularly affecting the vertical rather than horizontal movements. Abnormalities in saccadic movements, including impaired pursuit with saccadic intrusions, impairment of gaze fixation due to distractability, slowing of optokinetic nystagmus, and inability to suppress blinking during saccades, are also evident.[29,99,106–108] Conjugate gaze disturbances may be prominent in rigid cases.[105]

Voluntary Motor Dysfunction. A nonspecific, but early sign is impairment of voluntary motor function.[103,109] Patients and their family describe clumsiness in common daily activities. Clear abnormalities of rapid alternating movements may already be observed in the transitional phase. Disturbances in motor speed, fine motor control, and gait correlate with disease progression and appear to be better measures of duration of illness than chorea.[101] Clumsiness may increase with deterioration of functional capacity.[19]

Reflexes. Hyperactive reflexes occur early in up to 90 percent of patients, while clonus and extensor plantar responses occur late and are less frequent.[19,25] Again, these latter phenomena are predominant in juvenile and advanced adult cases.[19] Frontal release reflexes like snouting, sucking, or grasping typically accompany significant cognitive decline.

Gait. Gait disturbances ultimately result in severe disability.[25,39] Subtle changes in gait may be observed early in the illness, including difficulty with tandem walking, sudden stopping on command, and turning.[110] With more advanced disease, walking difficulties are more pronounced. As a consequence, patients experience frequent falls, with significant associated morbidity, and often ultimate confinement to a wheelchair. Gait disturbances exist at least partially independently from chorea, as neuroleptic treatment that suppresses choreic movements does not improve the gait disturbance.[110]

Speech. Most patients display speech abnormalities,[25] which are present early in the illness.[19,111,112] Initially mild disturbance of clarity appears, which is aggravated by changes in rate and rhythm of speech as the disease progresses.

Dysphagia. Disturbances in swallowing generally occur late with progression of the illness. Initially, this may primarily affect intake of fluids but later will also affect intake of solids. Choking with aspiration secondary to dysphagia is a common cause of morbidity.

Cognitive Disturbances

Subcortical Dementia. A global decline in cognitive capabilities is ultimately present in all HD patients.[39] While global measurements of cognitive function may still be preserved,[113–116] a typical pattern of decline becomes apparent very early in the disease, including slowness of thought, altered personality, affective changes, and impaired ability to integrate new knowledge. The designation *subcortical dementia* evokes anatomical correlations, but its main value is to stress the difference from the pattern of dementia occurring in Alzheimer, Pick, or Creutzfeldt-Jakob disease. In these, aphasia, alexia, agnosia and apraxia are prominent, while they are rare in HD.[117,118]

Memory. Memory impairment is common early in the disease and is often one of the patient's presenting symptoms.[113] Visuospatial memory is particularly affected, involving visual retention,[116] while verbal memory remains fairly well preserved until late.[116,119] For example, patients have difficulty reproducing geometric designs but may remember facts, words, or stories.

Retrieval of information is impaired[120,121] but verbal cues, priming, and sufficient time may lead to partial or correct recall.[114,120–123] Recall of recent and remote events is equally impaired.[114,124] Learning and acquisition of new motor skills (procedural memory) is also affected.[125–127] In contrast to other amnestic syndromes, orientation in both time and place remains intact until late in the illness.[128]

Attention and Concentration. Attention and concentration are affected early,[116] resulting in easy distractability by interfering stimuli. The difficulty in performing sustained simple motor tasks such as gazing laterally, sticking out the tongue, or tightly closing the eyelids may be a manifestation of this distractability rather than motor disturbance. Problems with organizing, sequencing, and planning; inability to coordinate and initiate complex actions; and inability to maintain a mental set or organize cognitive strategies constitute other early impairments.[113,114,129] These functions have been traditionally ascribed to circuitry in which the frontal lobe plays an important role.

Language and Related Functions. Although speech production and fluency may be severely reduced, the dementia of HD is nonaphasic.[113] Dysarthria, slowness, and lack of initiative interfere significantly with fluency and spontaneous speech,[130] but semantic and syntactic structure, word finding, and speech comprehension remain intact until the final stages of the disease.[102,111] Difficulties in writing and recognition of objects have been ascribed to defective nonlinguistic modalities, such as visuoperceptual analysis, attention and concentration, and overall cognition.[111,113,130,131] In contrast, simple naming of daily objects, as tested in the Mini Mental State Examination, may remain intact until the latest stages of the disease.[128]

Expression and perception of the musical, tonal, rhythmic, nonlinguistic aspects of language (prosody), which is a function of nondominant hemisphere structures, (analogous to those mediating language in the dominant hemisphere) seem to be impaired in affected HD patients.[132]

Visuospatial Functions. Specialized neuropsychological tests reveal impaired visuospatial abilities, particularly in later stages of disease.[113] However, patients are oriented to time and place, able to dress themselves, and have no obvious spatial neglect until late in the illness. Clearly, in comparison with Alzheimer disease, visuospatial functions are relatively preserved in HD.[102] Similarly, a patient's insight into his or her deteriorating cognitive abilities, which is absent in Alzheimer disease, remains intact.

Psychiatric Disturbances

Although psychiatric disturbances are as characteristic for the disease as motor and cognitive abnormalities, these appear less consistently and are not necessarily related to the severity of chorea or dementia.[113,133]

Mood and Affect. Changes in mood and affect are common, ranging from anxiety and ill-defined irritability to prolonged periods of depression.[102,134] Suicide is more common in patients than in the affected population and may be a significant cause of death of patients in their earlier stages.[135] Manic or hypomanic episodes also occur with increased frequency. Approximately 10 percent of patients have transient episodes of increased activity, pressured speech, uncharacteristic cheerfulness, and transient return of sexual interest after a long period of libido loss and impotence.[102] Affective syndromes may precede the first signs of motor impairment by many years[102] and do not usually manifest for the first time late in the illness.[136]

Behavioral Disturbances. Apathy, aggressive behavior, sexual disinhibition, and alcohol abuse are other symptoms seen in HD patients.[134] They may be either a manifestation of the progressive cognitive decline or, alternatively, manifestations of the mood disturbances, especially if they are reversible and related to the premorbid personality.[137]

Delusions and Hallucinations. Delusions are common, occurring in more than 50 percent of the patients with advanced disease.[134] They may be seen in depressive or manic episodes, or they may be isolated and are frequently paranoid in nature. In contrast, hallucinations are less common.[25]

Other Abnormalities

Weight Loss. Striking emaciation is one of the features of advanced HD.[39] Clinical follow-up[138] and anthropometric studies[139,141] with dietary assessment[140] show that the vast majority of HD patients lose weight in the course of the disease. This weight loss may occur in conjunction with adequate dietary intake[138,140] or even increased carbohydrate intake.[139] Intriguingly, a relationship has been found between weight at initial examination and rate of progress of the disease.[56]

Sleep. Sleep may be disturbed in advanced disease, with frequent nocturnal sleeplessness and reversal of the day–night pattern of sleep.[142] In early disease, sleep is essentially normal.[142–144] Choreic movements disappear during sleep.

Incontinence. Approximately 20 percent of all patients are incontinent of urine and feces in the terminal phases of the illness, while in early symptomatic persons, incontinence rarely occurs.[25] In incontinent patients with frequency, urgency, and nocturia, detrusor hyperreflexia without sphincter dyssynergia is apparent. Choretic contractions have been electromyographically recorded from perineal musculature in affected patients.[145]

Problems in Anesthesia. It has been suggested that patients are abnormally sensitive to barbiturate anesthesia and may exhibit prolonged apnea,[146–148] but these reports have been disputed.[149–151] The weight loss and poor general condition of these patients may make them susceptible to adverse effects of anesthesia.

Assessment of Functional Decline. Questionnaires have been developed that rate disability in terms of how the patient functions in daily life.[152,153] An example is shown in Table 152-3. Simple to score, the results of these disability rating scales correlate strongly with various clinical parameters of disease progression.[19,29]

Chorea, unless very severe, does not appear to constitute a major impairment to normal function. Neuroleptic drugs that suppress choreic movements do not improve the functional ratings.[154] Furthermore, during the late stages, a diminished severity of choretic movements without improvement of function is apparent. These findings caution against use of neuroleptic medication in the later stages of illness.

Early- and Late-Onset Disease

Juvenile Cases. Approximately 10 percent of all patients with HD have onset before age 20. The youngest patient described had onset at age 2.[25]

In contrast to adult cases, bradykinesia and rigidity are conspicuous from early on, dominating the neurologic findings in about 50 percent of the cases.[25,39,155–157] Chorea is present in almost all cases but is often of short duration and is superseded by rigidity.[25] Frequent falls, dysarthria, clumsiness, hyperreflexia, and oculomotor disturbances are frequent in children with HD and occur early. Although

Table 152-3 Functional Designation of Patients with Huntington Disease*

Stage	Engagement in Occupation	Score	Capacity to Handle Financial Affairs	Score	Capacity to Manage Domestic Responsibility	Score	Capacity to Perform Activities of Daily Living	Score	Care Can be Provided at	Score
1	Usual level	3	Full	3	Full	2	Full	3	Home	2
2	Lower level	2	Requires slight help	2	Full	2	Full	3	Home	2
3	Marginal	1	Requires major help	1	Impaired	1	Mildly impaired	2	Home	2
4	Unable	0	Unable	0	Unable	0	Moderately impaired	1	Home or extended-care facility	1
5	Unable	0	Unable	0	Unable	0	Severely impaired	0	Total-care facility only	0

*From Shoulson and Fahn.[152] Adapted from Hayden.[25]

difficult to assess in HD,[158] cerebellar dysfunction is more prominent than in adult patients.[19,25]

Mental deterioration is first manifested by declining school performance. Over the years severe progressive dementia develops.

Epileptic seizures, occurring in adult HD patients with a frequency similar to that in the general adult population (1 percent),[25] are more common in early-onset cases with an estimated 30 to 50 percent of the juvenile patients affected.[25,96,157] Partial or generalized, tonic–clonic, or absence seizures may all appear. Seizures should be differentiated from myoclonic jerks, which also rarely occur in adult cases.[159] The epilepsy of juvenile HD patients is often difficult to control.

Late-Onset Disease. In contrast, the manifestations in late-onset disease are less severe. Approximately 25 percent of all patients will display first signs and symptoms after age 50, and in these patients the disease will follow slower progression than usual.[153] Chorea is the presenting motor disorder, and gait disturbances and dysphagia are common though not severe. Cognitive impairment, although invariably present, may be less debilitating than in younger patients.[153] Older onset is associated with a slower disease progression, as measured by functional disability.[153]

Differential Diagnosis

Noninherited Chorea. Many different conditions are associated with chorea,[160] but most are rare and can easily be excluded in a patient with suspected HD. The most common cause of isolated chorea to be considered is tardive dyskinesia associated with the use of neuroleptics. Many different medications may induce chorea, including medication-induced dyskinesias in Parkinson disease (L-dopa), anticonvulsant drugs (especially in children), noradrenergic stimulant drugs (cocaine, amphetamine, aminophylline), digoxin intoxication, and oral contraceptives. Other causes of chorea, including thyrotoxicosis, cerebrovascular disease of arteriolosclerotic or vasculitic origin such as bilateral lacunar infarcts of the striatum, cerebral lupus erythematosus, and polycythemia can easily be excluded based on the family history, associated findings, and course of the illness.

Inherited Chorea. Neuroacanthocytosis (McKusick no. 100500) is inherited as an autosomal dominant trait. However, the occurrence of muscle wasting, absent lower limb tendon reflexes, clinical and electrophysiological signs of motor neuropathy, epilepsy, orolingual dystonia, self-mutilation, and only mild dementia aid in the differentiation from HD. Laboratory findings are typical acanthocytes in a thick wet blood smear, and an elevated serum creatine kinase level.[161]

Benign hereditary chorea (McKusick no. 118700 for the common autosomal dominant form; 215450 for a rare possibly recessive form) is usually nonprogressive without dementia. However in rare instances the phenotype may be more severe. The absence of linkage between markers on 4p16 and benign hereditary chorea would indicate a different genetic etiology in most instances. However, these patients with a more severe phenotype could still represent allelic variants of HD.

Hereditary cerebellar ataxias should be distinguishable from HD because of prominent cerebellar and long tract signs. Dentato-rubro-pallido-luysian atrophy (McKusick no. 125370) (DRPLA) may closely resemble HD, and sometimes neuropathology may provide the only distinction.[162] However, the disease seems to be extremely rare in patients of non-Japanese descent. Familial paroxysmal kinesiogenic (McKusick no. 128200) or dystonic choreoathetosis (McKusick no. 118800) is not associated with dementia, and the attacks of involuntary movements are easily suppressed by antiepileptic drugs.[163] Mitochondrial myoencephalopathies may occasionally present with an extrapyramidal syndrome.[164] Wilson's disease (McKusick no. 277900) should also be considered as this has significant therapeutic implications.

Chorea and Dementia. Creutzfeldt-Jakob disease, which may be familial and be inherited as an autosomal dominant trait in some families (McKusick no. 123400) progresses much more rapidly than HD. The major involuntary movements are myoclonus. In elder patients in whom dementia is insidious, Alzheimer disease (AD) deserves consideration, as it sometimes presents with myoclonus. Abnormalities typical for AD may be found in the brains of elder HD patients (see section on neuropathology). The rare coincidence of AD and HD might occasionally be expected based on the frequency of both in the population.

Chorea and Psychiatric Disturbances. If affective disturbances or psychosis dominate the initial syndrome, a carefully taken family history and a neurologic examination may lead to a correct diagnosis. Chorea in these patients may be wrongly considered tardive dyskinesia.

Juvenile Huntington Disease. The diagnosis of HD in children should present no problems if the details of the clinical phenotype are recognized and the family is known, but it may be extremely difficult in isolated cases. The complex tics of Tourette syndrome (McKusick no. 137580) should be well distinguishable from the motor disorder in HD. Hallervorden-Spatz syndrome (McKusick no. 234200) is very rare,[165] as are a large number of various metabolic diseases. Lesch-Nyhan syndrome (McKusick no. 308000) can be diagnosed by its laboratory findings.

Diagnosis of Huntington Disease without a Positive Family History. (See "Genetics" below.) Although the combination of progressive chorea and cognitive dysfunction in a patient with a positive family history establishes the diagnosis of HD, a special clinical challenge is posed by those in whom the family history is lacking. The most obvious causes may be nonpaternity, adoption, nonrecognition of the existence of the disorder in family members, or early death or late onset in the affected parent. Furthermore new mutations may be accounting for a larger proportion of such patients than previously recognized.[354]

Is it possible to make a diagnosis in the absence of a family history? In these cases the constellation of characteristic signs and symptoms, a progressive course of the illness over time, and the demonstration of caudate atrophy (CT, MRI), or caudate hypometabolism of glucose by PET, in the absence of any other demonstrable cause, make the diagnosis of HD highly likely. Furthermore, assessment for expansion of the CAG repeat in such instances will be absolutely critical to confirm that the patient has the genetic changes consistent with the diagnosis of HD (see "Genetics" below).

Laboratory Investigations

CT and MRI. CT and MRI scanning can demonstrate caudate atrophy in affected patients, but appreciable atrophy usually appears after the appearance of chorea.[170] Measurements of the area of the head of the caudate nucleus,[171] or standardized measurements such as the ratio of the distance of the caudate heads and the inner tables of the skull,[172] or the ratio of the bicaudate diameter and distances between the frontal heads[173] will achieve up to 90 percent discrimination between patients with established disease and controls. A number of other conditions may also be associated with caudate atrophy, such as normal aging, multiple infarcts, obstructive hydrocephalus, and neuroacanthocytosis.[161,174] A CT or MRI scan is also useful in the detection of basal ganglia calcifications. Obviously, a scan showing caudate atrophy supports a diagnosis, but a normal scan does not exclude the diagnosis.

MRI. MRI is similar to CT scanning in accuracy and diagnostic value. However in advanced cases, it may reveal widespread cortical and subcortical atrophy more clearly.[175] In addition, it allows volumetric measurements.

PET. PET using [^{18}F]deoxyglucose demonstrates decreased glucose metabolism in the caudate nucleus that appears normal on CT or MRI scan in affected persons and some persons at risk.[30,31,176–178] This later finding has not been replicated in all studies.[179] PET scanning may be a sensitive method to detect early HD-related changes, particularly during the transitional clinical phase when a definitive diagnosis cannot yet be made (Fig. 152-7). However, the finding of caudate hypometabolism lacks specificity. Significantly decreased caudate glucose metabolism has been demonstrated in neuroacanthocytosis, dentato-rubro-pallido-luysian atrophy,[180] and Wilson's disease,[181] while chorea due to systemic lupus erythematosus[182] seems associated with normal glucose metabolism. Both abnormal[183] and normal results[184] have been found in patients with benign hereditary chorea. It has been claimed that single-photon emission CT may yield equivalent results, but the method has not yet been sufficiently validated.[185–188]

Electrophysiology. Electromyography and the recording of sensory action potentials may be helpful in the differentiation of HD from neuroacanthocytosis.[161] Asymmetry, absence, or delayed onset of the long-latency responses of the stretch reflex[103,189–192] are electrophysiological correlates of chorea and may precede overt choreic movements. Peak latencies of somatosensory or auditory evoked potentials may be increased or normal.[193–199] Motor evoked potentials elicited by magnetic stimulation of the cortex were normal.[190] While these results provide insights into the physiology of the motor and cognitive disorder in HD, they are nonspecific and too insensitive to be used for diagnostic purposes.

DNA Testing. Approximately 99 percent of all patients (995 of 1007 affected persons in one series) with the clinical phenotype of HD have expansion of the CAG repeat.[358] Therefore, in patients with signs and symptoms suggestive

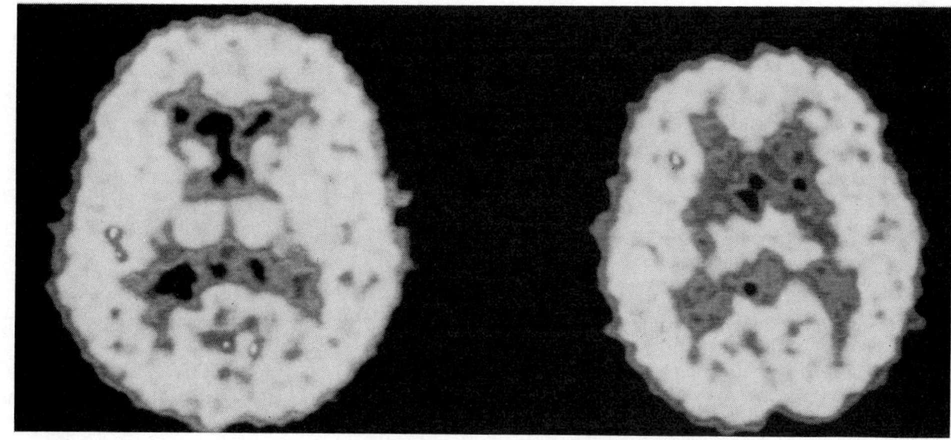

FIG. 152-7 **Positron emission tomography scan using [^{18}F]deoxyglucose, showing marked hypometabolism in the caudate nucleus and the putamen in a patient *(right)* as compared to a control subject *(left)*. The basal ganglia were of normal size on a CT scan *(From Kremer et al.*[337] *Used by permission.)***

of HD, DNA assessment will be the single most helpful test to confirm that the patient has the molecular changes associated with HD.

GENETICS

HD is inherited as an autosomal dominant trait. This implies that the gene is transmitted by parents of either sex to children of either sex. Each child of an affected parent has an even chance of inheriting the gene. All heterozygotes for Huntington disease show signs of symptoms if they live long enough. There are no described instances of incomplete penetrance for this disorder.[15,28]

Homozygosity for Huntington Disease

Offspring of two parents affected with HD are rare, and only a few occurrences have been well documented. Discovery of markers linked to the HD gene has allowed assessment of possible homozygotes.

One such family has been described within the population of HD in the state of Zulia in Venezuela. Avila-Giron[18] had noted that within this community up to 30 percent of the patients had two parents affected with the same illness. In one family, 4 of the 14 sibs were shown by DNA segregation analysis to be homozygous for the DNA haplotype with which the HD gene was segregating.[20] Interestingly, there were no clinical features that would distinguish these persons from heterozygotes for this illness. The suggestion that the homozygous form of HD has no increasing severity of clinical phenotype as compared with the heterozygote was supported by a separate study from Myers et al.,[200] who again showed that offspring who are likely to be homozygous for the HD gene have no features that distinguish them from affected heterozygotes within that family.

Therefore the homozygous form for HD may be different to other autosomal dominant inherited disorders such as familial hypercholesterolemia or hereditary hemoragic telangictasia where homozygotes have a much more severe manifestation of the illness.

This suggests that the underlying biochemical defect in HD is not likely to be due to a deficiency of a particular gene product, because this would be expected to result in a more severe phenotype when present in two copies. A better explanation would be a defect that confers a gain of a new function or a gene producing an abnormal gene product.

Genetic Heterogeneity

Prior to the discovery of linkage of markers on 4p16.3 to HD, arguments in favor of heterogeneity centered around the greater variation of clinical presentation of affected individuals between different families as compared with that observed within kindreds.[201] However, varying clinical phenotypes could equally be due to specific and different mutations within the same gene. The most comprehensive assessment showed that data were most consistent with a single locus underlying HD.[202]

Mapping of the Huntington Disease Defect to 4p16.3

Only 3 years after RFLPs had been recognized as powerful tools for mapping gene loci,[223] HD was shown to be linked to polymorphisms detected by the DNA marker G8 (D4S10)[224] (Fig. 152-8). Subsequently, G8 was mapped to distal 4p16.[225–228] Refined mapping using a panel of somatic-cell hybrid lines with various deletions in distal 4p16 placed the D4S10 locus within the proximal region of the most distal subband 4p16.3.[229] Additional polymorphic markers that were also shown to be in strong linkage with HD were identified.[230] Multipoint linkage analysis of two proximal markers (Raf2 and D4S62) and D4S10 and HD, in combination with informative crossovers within the D4S10 locus,[231]

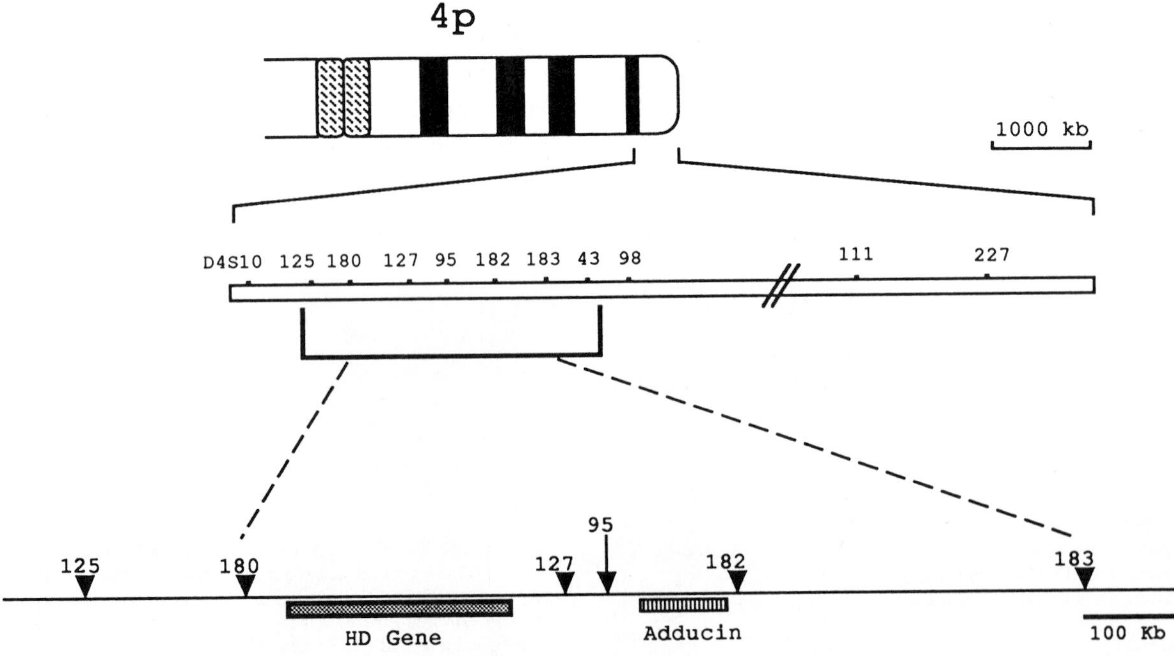

FIG. 152-8 Localization of the HD gene on the tip of the short arm of chromosome 4. Linked markers are indicated (e.g., D4S10, 95), as is the localization of the adducin gene.

unambiguously localized the HD gene to a 6-mb region between D4S10 and the telomere[232] (see Fig. 152-8).

Refined Localization of the Huntington Disease Locus between D4S10 and the Telomere

In the absence of any cytogenetically detectable abnormalities involving the most distal subband 4p16.3, two approaches have been taken to refine the location of the HD gene. First, the analysis of informative crossover events in HD pedigrees,[203,204] and second, the assessment of linkage disequilibrium of DNA markers spanning the entire 6-mb region with the disease (see Fig. 152-8). These studies have initiated an extensive search for new polymorphic DNA markers from the HD region distal to D4S10[230,233–241] and have also facilitated the construction of detailed genetic[237] and physical[242,243] maps of the 4p16.3 region (see Fig. 152-8).

Region between D4S10 and D4S168

Analysis of different recombinant HD chromosomes localized the HD defect to a region distal to a crossover between DNA markers D4S125 and D4S180[243] and proximal to a crossover between D4S168 and D4S113/D4S114[245,247] (see Fig. 152-8). Additional support for this region was provided by linkage disequilibrium data that have consistently demonstrated significant nonrandom allelic association between HD and alleles at D4S95[246,247,249–252] and D4S127. Allele association had also been detected initially at D4S98[246,247,250] but this was no longer significant in one larger sample.[249]

The entire region between D4S10 and D4S168 was then cloned using YAC[254,255] and cosmid technology facilitating the identification of numerous genes.

Cloning of the Huntington Disease Gene

Several genes were identified from 4p16.3 using classic approaches of detection of multiple CpG islands and associated phylogenetically conserved sequences.[336–338] Other genes, such as the human *N*-methyl-D-aspartate (NMDA) receptor gene, which has been implicated as a candidate for HD based on its potential function, were excluded by mapping to other chromosomes.[339]

The development of new approaches to identify genes in relatively large regions of the genome facilitated progress. Exon amplification, which exploits the presence of splice and donor sites in DNA and uses these to generate exons after transfection into cultured cells, represented the technique of choice for the HD Collaborative Research Group.[340] Another approach was to develop a transcriptional map of the HD region using a modification of a direct DNA selection strategy derived from immobilized cosmids and YAC. Numerous genes were rapidly identified, including the a-adducin gene,[342,343] which was shown in all likelihood to be excluded as the cause for HD at least in a few patients.[342]

The region extending around D4S95 and D4S127 proved to be gene-rich, as many genes were quickly located. Apart from a-adducin, a novel member of the family of G protein–coupled receptor genes was found,[343] as well as another gene located between D4S95 and the 3′ end of a-adducin (cD510), which has no obvious homology to known sequences.[344] A total of approximately 58 cDNA clones encoding at least nine different transcription units were obtained from this region using cDNA selection strategies.[345]

A novel gene containing a trinucleotide repeat (CAG) that is expanded on HD chromosomes has been described.[346] This highly polymorphic CAG repeat, located in the 5′ region of the Huntington gene, has been shown to range from 10 to 30 copies on normal chromosomes, while it is expanded beyond 35 repeats in HD. The largest expansion found to date was 121 trinucleotides.

Two mRNA species were observed to originate from this single gene and accounted for by 3′ differential polyadenylation leading to transcripts of different sizes.[347] Currently there are no obvious homologies for this gene, and detailed sequence analysis has provided no clues as to the pathogenesis of this illness.

Relationship between Trinucleotide (CAG) Repeat Length and Clinical Features of Huntington Disease

A significant correlation between the number of CAG repeats and the age of onset of HD was demonstrated, with earlier age of onset associated with longer repeat lengths.[348–351] This association was present irrespective of the mode of clinical presentation at time of onset. The number of trinucleotide repeats in the upper allele accounted for about 50 percent of the variation in the age of onset (Fig. 152-9).[348] However, repeat length is not indicative of any other particular clinical phenotype, as there is no independent association between any particular clinical feature of the illness and the number of repeats.

Curves for age of onset in offspring have been constructed previously that gave estimations of the age of onset in offspring based on the age of onset in the parent.[208] In counseling programs, persons at risk have been informed that there is in general an aggregation of age of onset among sibs, with less correlation of the age of onset between parent

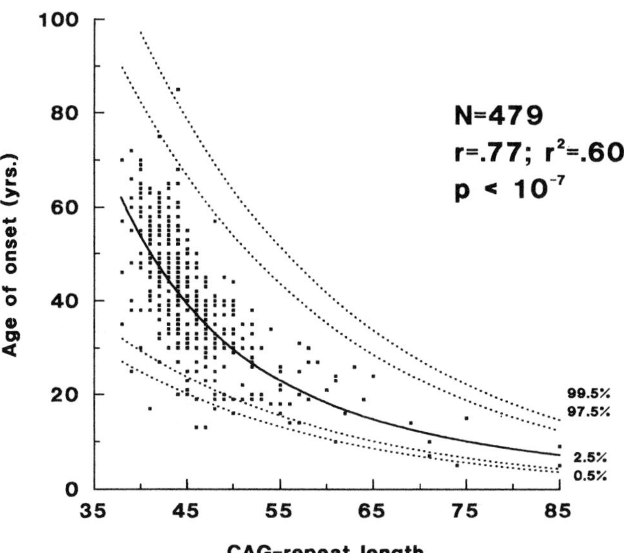

FIG. 152-9 Plot depicting the relation between age of onset of HD and CAG trinucleotide repeat length in the HD gene. Repeat lengths over 85 are omitted for scaling purposes. The regression line (derived from log-transformed onset data and back-transformed to the original ages) in black. The 95 percent and 99 percent confidence intervals for prediction of onset age from CAG repeat length are indicated as interrupted lines.

and child. Specific estimates of age of onset with appropriate confidence limits were developed based on the relationship between repeat length and age at onset. However, because of the broad confidence limits around the predicted age at onset, this will help in counseling only a small proportion of patients, particularly those with large expansions (Fig. 152-9).[348]

Molecular Analysis of New Mutations

New mutations causing HD have been proposed to be exceedingly rare, with the mutation rate estimated as the lowest for any human genetic disease.[28,353] This may reflect that proof of a new mutation in HD is difficult, as prior criteria for identification of a new mutation have stipulated that parents of the sporadic case must have lived beyond the expected age of onset of HD without any manifestations of the disease, paternity of the sporadic case must be confirmed, and the disease should be transmitted to the offspring of the sporadic case.[166]

The CAG repeat length in 21 sporadic cases of HD and their families has been assessed in order to learn more about the molecular events underlying new mutations for HD. In 18 of these families the sporadic HD patient had an upper allele that was in the size range seen in patients with this disorder. In all eight families for whom DNA was available from parents ($n = 6$) or there were a sufficient number of sibs to reconstruct genotypes in the parents ($n = 2$), one parental allele was found to be significantly greater than that seen in the general population (>30), but below the range seen in patients with HD [an intermediate allele (IA)].[354] Similar findings were also seen in a related study.[357]

The sex of origin of the premutation was determined by examining DNA from parents. In 7 of 7 families, a preferential origin of the new mutation from the paternally derived allele ($p = 0.0078$) was demonstrated. This would suggest that the paternal allele in the premutation range is more likely to undergo significant expansion to a repeat length in the range seen in patients affected with HD.

Patients with suspected HD on clinical criteria without a positive family history are not rare and initially represented 11 percent of a cohort that was biased toward ascertainment of familial cases.[354] The finding that 18 of 21 sporadic cases of HD had CAG expansion suggested in most instances that the diagnosis of HD can be made correctly in the absence of a positive family history. However, it is apparent from this study that new mutations for HD are not rare, and it is likely that the mutation rate for this disorder has been underestimated.

These findings have significant genetic implications for family members of sporadic cases, in particular for sibs and second-degree relatives of such affected persons. In the past, there was no appreciation that the unaffected sibs of a sporadic case for HD might indeed have an increased risk of manifesting with HD in the future since they may also inherit an expanded HD allele. Similarly, children of unaffected male sibs with an IA are also at increased risk of having children with HD. This latter risk would depend on whether the premutation allele undergoes expansion during transmission through the male germ line. Female sibs who carry the premutation allele, however, may have a lower probability of passing on an expanded allele resulting in HD in their offspring. Thus, the risk for the children of females carrying the premutations for HD would be considerably lower than that seen in the offspring of males.

Molecular Analysis of Juvenile Huntington Disease

Juvenile HD shows remarkable features with respect to the sex of the transmitting parent. While the sex incidence for juvenile HD is equal, approximately 80 percent of juvenile patients inherit the defective gene from their father.[28] For children who have onset up to 10 years of age (childhood onset), approximately 90 percent inherit the gene from their father, while approximately 75 percent of persons with adolescent onset (11 to 20 years) have paternal descent.[25]

Different factors have been proposed to account for this finding. Maternal protective factors mediated through mitochondria or other cytoplasmic influences are compatible with the results of some studies that have shown a greater correlation for age of onset for mother–child than for father–child pairs.[205–207] Imprinting[210,211] and, more recently, selective amplification of repeat sequences within the genome have been suggested as mechanisms to explain the paternal transmission effect.[353]

Similar to adults, there is a highly significant correlation between length of the CAG trinucleotide repeat in the HD gene and age of onset for persons with juvenile HD.[355] Children with earliest onset have the highest number of repeats. In fact, the juvenile patients present the end of a continuum of the curve that describes the relation between age at onset and CAG size.

The predominance of paternal descent in juvenile HD is not in accordance with classic Mendelian genetics and until now has remained a statistical fact with no adequate biologic explanation. However, it has been shown that the size of the CAG repeat may expand, and that CAG repeat is most unstable, leading to amplification, when transmitted through the male germ line.

There was a remarkable aggregation of juvenile-onset HD within families.[209] This has previously been observed within juvenile sibs and led to the development of algorithms for prediction of age of onset in a sib of a child with juvenile HD.[208,209] The presence of juvenile HD in multiple sibs associated with repeat expansion is evidence against an additional single mutation occurring in the germ line of the transmitting parent accounting for this phenomenon. Furthermore, in some kindreds, the aggregation of juvenile onset is also seen beyond the nuclear family.[355] The observation that affected relatives of probands with juvenile HD either had early onset themselves or were more likely to have children with juvenile HD suggests that there might be a familial factor present in these families rendering them more likely to have children with juvenile HD. This finding can also be taken into account when counseling first- or second-degree relatives of probands with juvenile HD by informing them of this familial effect.

Therefore a strong biologic correlate for juvenile HD is the size of the CAG repeat, which is primarily influenced by the sex of the affected parent (Fig. 152-10).[355] However, the mechanism conferring sex-specific effects on the likelihood of amplification and the familial predisposing effect leading to juvenile HD remain to be determined.

Genetic Counseling

The geneticist and genetic counselor commonly encounter a healthy person at risk for HD who wants to know his or her risk for having inherited the illness. In this particular instance, it is most important to estimate the risk, taking

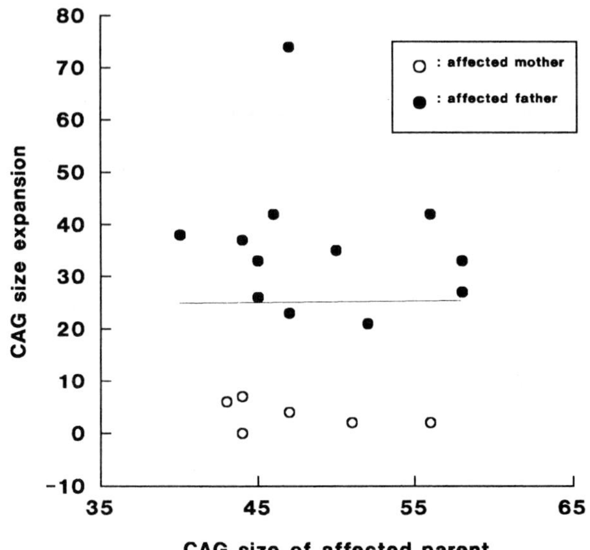

FIG. 152-10 Plot depicting the expansion (patient's minus parental CAG repeat size) in 18 juvenile-onset HD patients as compared with the allele size of their affected parent. Note the striking effect of the parental sex and the absence of an effect of parental CAG size on subsequent expansion in the child, as illustrated by the straight regression line.

into account the subject's age. For a person in early adult life who has an affected parent, the risk is very close to 50 percent. However, by the time the person is beyond the age of 60 the risk will have decreased considerably. The risk for a healthy subject of 50 percent prior risk of carrying the HD gene at different ages is shown in Table 152-4 and is based on the life-table analysis of data from South Wales.[212]

Familial aggregation of age of onset can also be taken into account in assessing the risk for an asymptomatic individual who has a parent affected with HD. This has been thoroughly investigated for sibs of persons with juvenile HD.[209] Therefore, both familial aggregation of age of onset as well as age of the person at risk for HD should be taken into account when deriving risks for asymptomatic individuals for having inherited the HD gene. In addition, as noted, estimates of repeat length may also be helpful in instances when repeat length is greatly expanded (>55 repeats).

Predictive Testing

Predictive testing for HD has been offered in different parts of the world for several years. Prior to the introduction of these programs research protocols were developed to evaluate the psychological impact of receiving either an increased or decreased risk result.[213–216] There was major concern that an increased risk result would precipitate catastrophic reactions such as emotional breakdown or suicide.

Short-term follow-up of participants in the Canadian Predictive Testing Program has revealed that predictive testing for HD may maintain or even improve the psychological well-being of individuals at risk.[217] Most individuals who receive a decreased-risk result have shown marked improvement in psychological health, while the individuals

Table 152-4 Risk for a Healthy Subject at 50 Percent Prior Risk of HD Carrying the HD Gene at Different Ages*

Age (yr)	Risk (%)	Age (yr)	Risk (%)
20.0	49.6	47.5	34.8
22.5	49.3	50.0	31.5
25.0	49.0	52.5	27.8
27.5	48.4	55.0	24.8
30.0	47.6	57.5	22.1
32.5	46.6	60.0	18.7
35.0	45.5	62.5	15.2
37.5	44.2	65.0	12.8
40.0	42.5	67.5	10.8
42.5	40.3	70.0	6.2
45.0	37.8	72.5	4.6

*Adapted from Harper and Newcombe.[212]

who have received an increased-risk result have not responded to predictive testing in the negative manner feared when predictive testing programs for HD were first developed.[217] Despite the fact that both groups as a whole responded well to predictive testing programs, several individuals did have difficulties in adjusting to their new status. For those who received an increased-risk result, there has been a new focus on physical symptoms, with requests for physical examination and the need for continued support and reassurance that DNA testing is not synonymous with diagnosis of illness.[217] Though it was expected that some individuals might have difficulty coping with an increased-risk result, a similar frequency of problems was not expected among those receiving a decreased-risk result.[218] About 10 percent of the decreased-risk group have had serious difficulties adapting to their new status. The major hurdle for these individuals appears to be the realization that they are facing an unplanned future.

The demand for predictive testing has been lower than expected in studies conducted prior to the advent of predictive testing.[214,219,220] In addition, prenatal testing for HD is not a frequently chosen option.[221] Only 7 of 38 persons who became pregnant while part of a predictive testing program chose to participate in prenatal testing. The most frequently cited reason for declining prenatal testing was the hope for the development of a cure in time for their children.[222]

Cloning of the gene for HD will have impact on the demand for attitudes of individuals at risk toward both predictive and prenatal testing. The demand for predictive testing is likely to increase as the cloning of the gene is likely to herald new hope for treatment. However, the possibility of effective therapy for HD is likely to reduce the demand for prenatal testing further since termination of a pregnancy for a curable or potentially treatable adult-onset illness is likely to be even less acceptable. This would be similar to the very low demand for prenatal testing for other late-onset autosomal dominant disorders such as polycystic kidney disease, for which there are some effective therapies that might retard progression of the illness. The medium- and long-term effects of predictive testing for HD are not known, and there is a continued need for longitudinal investment to examine the psychological and social effects of testing and to collect data that best predict responses to change in risk status.

PATHOPHYSIOLOGY OF HUNTINGTON DISEASE

Clinicopathological Correlations

Striatal atrophy has long been postulated to be responsible for the occurrence of choreic movements in HD. However, only recently have the distinct features of the disease been more definitely related to the particular pattern of pathological changes.

Significant correlations have been found between the severity of caudate atrophy as seen on CT and impairment of daily activities, various neuropsychological test scores, total neurologic impairment, and eye-movement abnormalities.[74,129,256,257] Both the absence[129] and presence[256] of a relationship between voluntary motor impairment and chorea score on the one hand and caudate atrophy on the other have been reported. PET scanning has also provided new insights. Chorea, voluntary motor abnormalities, and slowing of saccades have been shown to correlate more closely with putaminal glucose metabolism than with caudate metabolism. In contrast, memory abnormalities (as measured by the Wechsler Memory Scale) were found significantly associated with caudate but not with putaminal hypometabolism.[258]

These findings are consistent with the current notion, derived from both neuroanatomical[259] and neurophysiological[260] data that the caudate nucleus is predominantly involved in cognitive and complex associative processing, while the putamen is involved in sensorimotor processing.[260,261]

Lesions of the striatum generally fail to produce chorea in experimental animals.[260] However, lesions of the subthalamic nucleus (STN), accidental in humans or experimental in monkeys, produce severe choreic movements (called "hemiballismus") in the contralateral side of the body. It is therefore possible that dysfunction (not atrophy) of the STN is the primary pathophysiological condition contributing to chorea in HD. This dysfunction then would be caused by a tonically exaggerated inhibition of the nucleus by GABA-ergic projections originating from the external part of the globus pallidus. The inhibitory activity of these pallidal neurons themselves is normally inhibited by the GABA-Enk-containing medium-sized spiny projection neurons of the striatum[262,263] (Fig. 152-11).

Striatal GABA-Enk projections to the external globus pallidus degenerate earlier than striatal GABA-substance P projections to the internal globus pallidus[66,67] (see Fig. 152-9). While the initial degeneration of the former may cause chorea, the later disappearance of the projections to the internal global pallidus may be responsible for the gradually increasing bradykinesia.[67] Thus, the feature that discriminates rigid from choreic cases seems to be the extent of involvement of the striatal GABA-substance P projections to the internal globus pallidus. In rigid cases, they degenerate together with GABA-Enk projections, while in choreic cases they are relatively spared.[67]

Delayed initiation and other abnormalities of saccades may result from overinhibition of neurons in the tectum mesencephali. This overinhibition is caused by the action of GABA-ergic afferent neurons from the SNr, that are normally inhibited by striatal GABA-substance P-containing projections.[262] This class of neurons seems to degenerate earlier than the GABA-substance P neurons to the internal globus pallidus, and may be affected as early as the GABA-Enk projections to the external pallidum,[66,265,266] explaining the occurrence of saccadic abnormalities already in the transitional period.

Role of Dopamine

Alterations in dopaminergic neurotransmission in the degenerating neostriatum have been implicated in the appearance

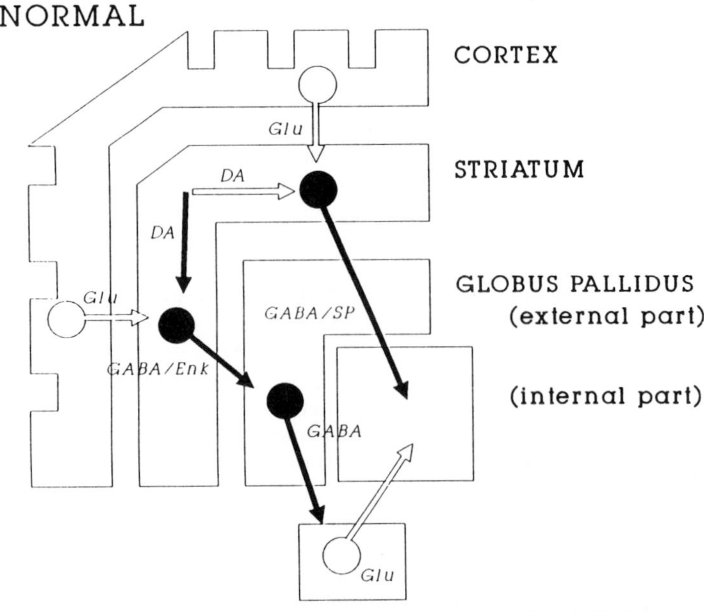

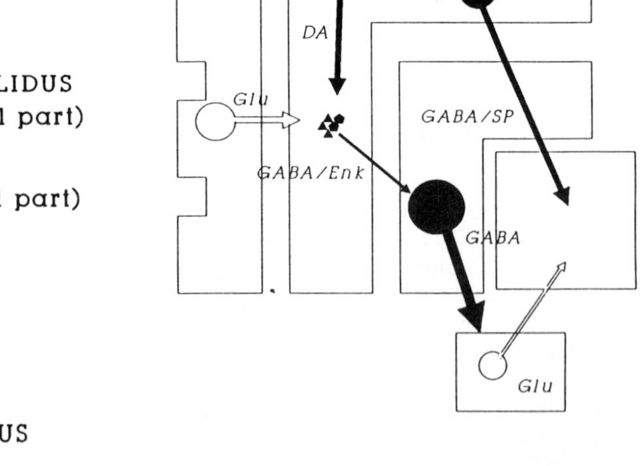

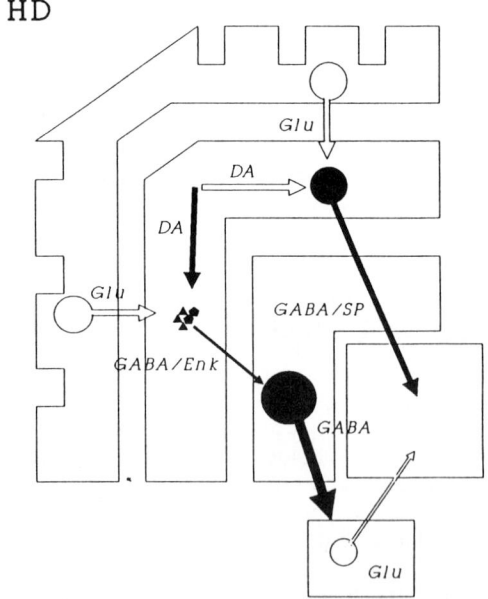

FIG. 152-11 Schematic representation of neuronal connections in the basal ganglia in a normal person *(left)* and a person with HD *(right)*. Inhibitory neurons and their connections are in black, excitatory neurons in white. Dopamine probably exerts both excitatory and inhibitory effects. The GABA-Enk neurons projecting from the striatum are first affected in HD. As a result, inhibitory GABA neurons in the external part of the globus pallidus become hyperactive, depressing the activity of glutamatergic neurons in the subthalamic nucleus. Glu = glutamate; DA = dopamine; Enk = enkephalin; SP = substance P.

of choreic movements. Arguments in support of this are the contrast between the hyperkinesia in HD and the hypokinesia in Parkinson disease (the classic dopamine-deficient basal ganglia disorder); the normal or increased dopamine concentrations in the neostriatum of HD patients[267]; the provocation of choreic movements by dopamine-enhancing drugs in patients with advanced Parkinson disease or tardive dyskinesia; the exacerbation of choreic movements in HD patients receiving dopamine agonists[268]; and the observed suppression of involuntary movements of HD patients by neuroleptic drugs (i.e., dopamine-receptor blocking agents).

Dopamine is thought to inhibit striatal GABA-Enk neurons and may stimulate GABA-substance P neurons.[269] This may explain the partial success of neuroleptic treatment of chorea, as the dopamine-induced suppression of remaining GABA-Enk neurons will be diminished.

Although a PET study of patients with juvenile-onset HD suggested deficient nigrostriatal dopaminergic neurotransmission,[270] striatal dopamine concentrations, and cerebrospinal fluid homovanillic acid (a dopamine metabolite) levels in rigid cases were similar to those in choreic cases.[267,271] Tyrosine hydroxylase immunoreactive neurons in the substantia nigra are preserved.[67] Thus, unlike Parkinson disease, parkinsonism in HD is not clearly caused by a deficient nigrostriatal system.

Cognitive Changes and the Role of Cortical Dysfunction

The pattern of neuropsychological impairment partly resembles that seen in patients with unequivocal frontal lobe disease. Currently, the most important argument in favor of a cortical contribution to cognitive dysfunction is the reduced cortical metabolism as visualized by PET scanning. This begins in frontal and inferior parietal areas, but gradually involves all cortical regions.[272] Whether this phenomenon is caused by local structural damage or by functional disturbance due to the interruption of cortico-striato-pallido-thalamo-cortical loops is unknown.

Why Do Neurons Die in Huntington Disease? The Excitotoxic Hypothesis

The excitotoxic hypothesis of neuronal loss in Huntington disease proposes that endogenously produced excitatory amino acids (EAA), or closely related substances, physiologically involved in neurotransmission, damage and kill neurons that are chronically exposed to their effects.[273] Neurons affected are those that possess receptors for EAA neurotransmitters, including the NMDA, the α-amino-3-hydroxy-5-methylisoxazole-4-propionic acid (AMPA), and the kainate receptor.

The potential pathogenic role of excitotoxic mechanisms in the HD neostriatum is supported by different observations. Injections of kainic acid, a glutamate analogue, in the rat striatum destroyed almost all neurons, while glial cells and afferents remained intact.[274,275] The NMDA agonists quinolinic acid, L-homocysteic acid, and NMDA itself, produce striatal damage that closely mimic the structural and neurochemical changes of HD.[276] EAA receptors are abundant in the striatum, and NMDA, AMPA, and kainate binding are significantly decreased in HD patients.[277] In a presymptomatic individual carrying the HD gene, NMDA receptor binding was already found to be decreased.[265] In primates with striatal excitotoxin lesions, levodopa may result in dyskinesias.[278,279] The hypothalamic lateral tuberal nucleus, prominently involved in HD, has NMDA and AMPA receptors as well.[280] All these findings support the hypothesis of EAA-mediated, and particularly NMDA-mediated, cell death in HD.

Yet, several problems currently hamper the excitotoxic hypothesis in HD. Excitotoxic mechanisms clearly play a role in acute exposure to excitotoxins.[281] It is more difficult, however, to assess their role experimentally in chronic disease. Some of the early experiments with quinolinic acid injections could not be reproduced, although this controversy has apparently been resolved in favor of the hypothesis.[282] The excitotoxin itself has not been identified. Most importantly, the presence of EAA receptors alone provides insufficient explanation for neuronal death in HD. Many apparently unaffected neuronal populations elsewhere in the brain do contain EAA receptors (e.g., in the hippocampus, the amygdala, the cerebellum, or the frontal cortex).[283,284] Even if careful morphometrics would show some neuronal loss in these areas, the extent of the damage does not resemble that in the striatum. Apparently, other factors must be operative that either protect EAA receptor–bearing neurons against the effects of the HD gene or render striatal and some other neuronal populations, like the lateral tuberal nucleus, especially vulnerable.[267] These factors could be the nature of their afferents; abnormal metabolism of regional EAA-like substances; different EAA receptor subtypes; abnormal mitochondrial energy metabolism in postsynaptic cells; or deficiencies in intracellular calcium-clearing mechanisms[264,282] (Fig. 152-12). The theory of EAA-mediated neuronal loss in HD supports drug trials aimed at protecting the remaining neurons from the deleterious effects of excitatory amino acids. The discovery of the CAG repeat associated with HD has not yet provided any additional insights to the pathogenesis of HD.

MANAGEMENT

Drug therapy for the management of HD is still limited to symptomatic treatment. Choreic movements can be partially suppressed by neuroleptics, while hypokinesia and rigidity may be ameliorated by antiparkinsonian agents. Psychiatric disturbances may react well to psychotropic drugs. Cognitive impairment is not amenable to drug treatment. Successful symptomatic treatment, however, does not lead to a significant improvement of functional capacity. Therefore, an important part of management is to help the patient and the family cope with the disease. Effective therapy to retard disease progression has not yet been achieved, although recent pathophysiological insights suggest novel approaches.

Nonpharmacologic Management

It should be stressed that the contribution of nonpharmacologic approaches to the general well-being of HD patients is more important than medication. For patients still living in the community, the close attention of family and friends, the family doctor, the social worker, or a public health nurse will be increasingly required. While there are obvious declines in functional capacity, patients with HD can in many instances remain in partial employment and fulfill domestic responsibilities until far into the illness. Premature withdrawal from these activities may further exacerbate the feelings of inadequacy and loss of power associated with the illness.

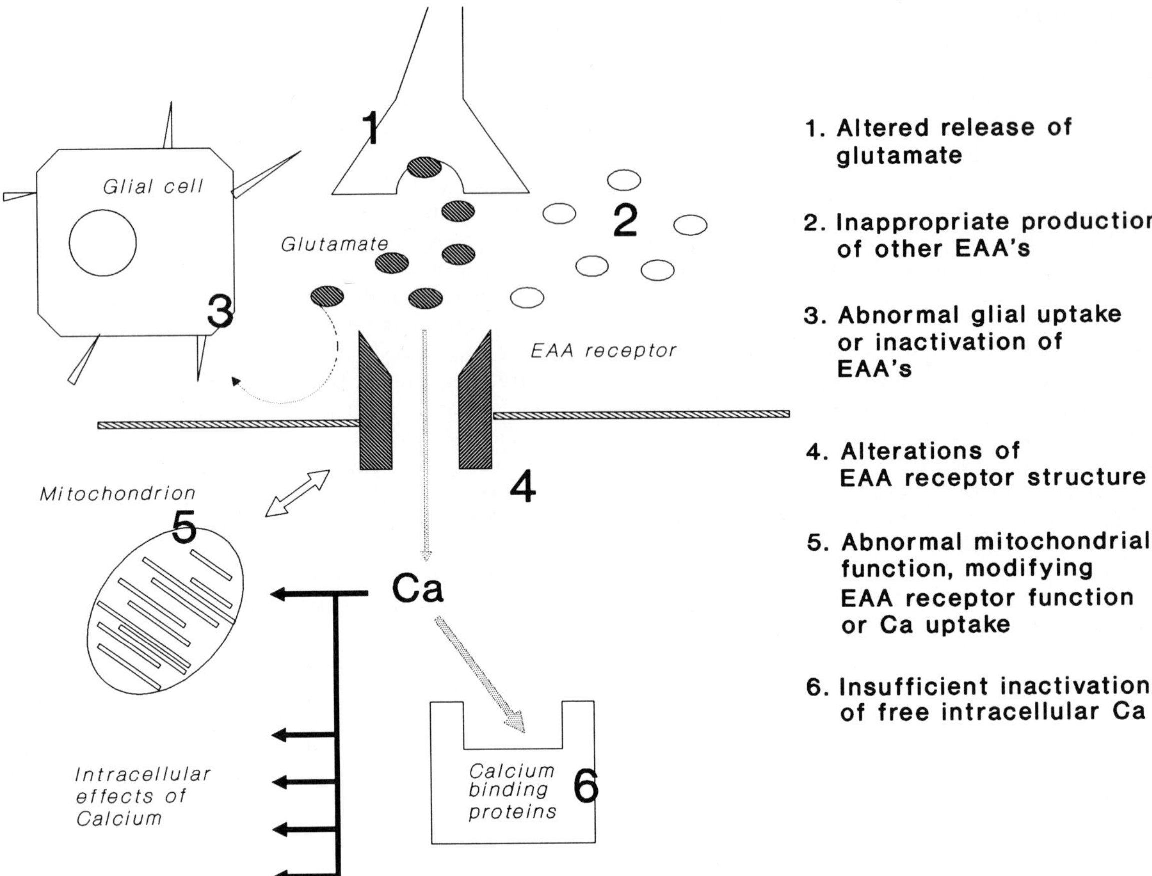

FIG. 152-12 Some suggested mechanisms of excitatory amino acid neurotoxicity *(From Kremer et al.[337] Used by permission.)*

Physical therapy is generally useful for patients. Initially, it should be directed at maintaining activity, but in the final stages, the prevention of painful contractures will be most important. Speech therapy can help the patient in communication and may improve swallowing. An occupational therapist can provide valuable advice regarding domestic adaptations such as toilet and bathing facilities. If gait problems are prominent, a wheelchair will be required. Walking canes are often of limited value. Because of frequent weight loss, nutrition requires close attention, and a high-calorie, high-protein diet may be required. Extensive nursing care plans have been described.[25,285]

Attention should also be paid to the well-being of family members. Apart from possibly being at risk for HD, they also suffer from their daily burden of providing adequate care for the patient. Intermittent, temporary relief from this burden through respite care may encourage them to continue. A crisis at home is the most common reason for forced institutionalization of HD patients.

Many of these options will depend on the society in which the patient lives. The advice, help, and expertise of the national lay societies, therefore, is indispensable in accumulating knowledge about the specific problems and opportunities for people with HD in their country.

Pharmacotherapy of Chorea

The most widely used drugs to suppress choretic movements are dopamine-receptor blocking neuroleptics such as phenothiazines or butyrophenones. The phenothiazine compound perphenazine was recommended in the United States as the first choice for this purpose in the past.[286] Haloperidol in low doses,[287] pimozide, or substituted benzamides such as sulpiride[288] or tiapride[289,290] are suitable alternatives. Tetrabenazine, a synthetic benzochinozoline, with the reserpine-like property of depleting presynaptic monoamines, may be even more effective.[291–294] This drug however, is not registered in many countries. The ultimate choice of neuroleptic will depend to a large extent on the individual clinician's experience with these drugs. Depot neuroleptics to suppress chorea should be avoided.

Drugs are only partially successful in suppressing chorea. Moreover, although they suppress involuntary movements, they do not improve the patient's functional capacity[154,288,295] or fine motor performance.[101] Side effects may be prominent and confer additional disability on the patient. Drowsiness, a dry mouth, blurred vision, constipation, or difficulties on micturition are well-known parasympatholytic effects of these drugs. Tetrabenazine, although in general remarkably well tolerated,[296] may cause depression. All neuroleptics may aggravate parkinsonian signs. Acute dystonia[297] or rigidity[298] and akathesia may occur early during treatment. Obviously, these side effects are difficult to discriminate from the extrapyramidal movement disorder of HD, causing considerable diagnostic uncertainty in some instances.

Neuroleptic drug treatment does not improve swallowing, speaking, or walking difficulties, and may in fact aggravate these through its parasympatholytic and parkinsonian effects.[110,299] In juvenile patients, neuroleptics may complicate the treatment of epilepsy. The neuroleptic malignant syndrome has been described in an HD patient receiving dopamine-depleting agents.[300]

Therefore, drug treatment of chorea should be undertaken only in those with severe movements. A crucial question prior to implementation of drug therapy is whether the movements are causing significant concern to the patient. A low initial dose, gradual increments, and frequent reassessment are required. Determining when the maximal effect is obtained is difficult but can be monitored clinically. When a certain dose is exceeded, no further suppression of chorea will occur.[287] Side effects may even further limit reaching maximal effect. The use of standardized assessments, such as the quantified neurologic examination,[101,119] chorea score,[301] functional capacity scale,[152] or videotaping, may be helpful in objectively monitoring drug efficacy. A proposed list of drugs useful in HD is given in Table 152-5.

Apart from neuroleptics, many other drugs have been proposed to ameliorate dyskinesia, but their effects have been observed in a few patients only, and in most cases these effects have not been substantiated by formal trials. These drugs include low-dose bromocriptine[302,303]; apomorphine[304,305]; transdihydrolisuride[306]; benzodiazepines[307]; isoniazid[308–310]; baclofen[311,312]; lithium[313]; and corticosteroids.[314]

Theoretical considerations concerning the pathophysiology of chorea have led to additional drugs being tested, but none of these has been shown to be effective. This category includes drugs intended to stimulate GABA-ergic transmission, such as sodium valproate,[315,316] muscimol,[317] gamma-acetylenic GABA,[318] gamma-vinyl GABA,[319] progabide,[320] and various other substances.[25] Cysteamine, a putative somatostatin-depleting agent, was equally ineffective.[321] Anticholinergic drugs used in Parkinson disease, aggravate choreic movements in HD. The cholinergic agents choline[322] and 2-dimethylaminoethanol (Deanol)[323] are ineffective, while arecoline, another acetylcholine-agonist, paradoxically has exacerbated choreic movements.[324]

Stereotactic surgery, in the past sometimes advocated to control chorea, is not a treatment modality to be considered. Surgical implantation of human fetal tissue in the striatum in an attempt to connect the biochemical balance, as assessed in primates, may offer new hopes for future treatment.[325]

Pharmacotherapy of Hypokinesia and Rigidity

Levodopa and anticholinergics may ameliorate rigidity and bradykinesia.[25,299] They will, however, exacerbate chorea. Their effect on overall functional capacity has not been evaluated. Their greatest use is for predominantly rigid cases of early onset. In the individual patient, the contribution of neuroleptic medication to hypokinesia and rigidity should be assessed before starting antiparkinsonian agents.

Table 152-5 Drugs That May Be Useful in the Treatment of HD

Compound	Recommended Daily Dose for: Chorea	Psychosis	Depression
Neuroleptics			
Perphenazine	2–8 mg	2–16 mg	
Sulpiride	300–1200 mg	300–2000 mg	
Tiapride	300–1200 mg	—	
Haloperidol	2–10 mg	2–16 mg	
Pimozide	2–8 mg	2–16 mg	
Tetrabenazine	25–100 mg	—	*
Antidepressants			
Amitryptiline			25–100 mg
Imipramine			25–200 mg
Fluoxetine			20–80 mg
Amoxepine			30–90 mg

*Stop when depression occurs.

Pharmacotherapy of Psychiatric Disturbances

Depression may contribute to early disability,[154] and suicide occurs with increased frequency.[135] Antidepressant therapy is warranted whenever symptoms of depression become recognizable. This class of drugs is still frequently underused in the management of HD. Antidepressants fail to delay the progressive deterioration of functional capacity,[154] but they may provide valuable and important temporary symptomatic relief. Conventional tricyclic antidepressants, like amitryptiline or imipramine have proven to be useful.[326] In general, insufficient experience with the modern noradrenergic (mianserin) or serotoninergic (fluvoxamin, fluoxetin) antidepressants exists, but there are no reasons to exclude them from use. It should be borne in mind that the effects of antidepressant treatment may become apparent only after 3 weeks. The experience with MAO-inhibitors in HD patients is limited, but they may be effective when classic antidepressants have failed.[327] Electroconvulsive therapy may have a role as the final treatment of intractable depression.[326]

Benzodiazepines will be the first choice in anxious or irritable patients. Neuroleptics may be helpful for the aggressive patient. Propranolol has been used to treat aggressive behavior in patients with organic brain disease, including HD,[328,329] but paradoxical reactions (i.e., increased aggressive behavior) to these agents have been reported.[329,330] The usefulness of lithium for mood disorders or aggression in HD patients has not yet been formally established. The need for monitoring, careful dosing, and repeated blood sampling may make it less suitable for HD patients.[326] A new drug to treat mania is carbamazepine but its effects in HD are unknown.[136] Sexual disinhibition may also respond well to low doses of neuroleptics.

In patients with hallucinations or delusions, the classic neuroleptic drugs (see above) are probably as efficacious as in non-HD patients. The dosages required will be higher than used to treat chorea. Tetrabenazine is not indicated in this condition. Depot neuroleptics should be avoided as the ability to respond immediately to the advent of side effects is limited. Clozapine, in line with its current status, may be effective in otherwise intractable psychoses, but requires extra precautions.[331]

Antiepileptic Drugs

Epilepsy in juvenile HD patients requires similar drugs as in other forms of convulsive disorders, such as carbamazepine, dilantin, or valproic acid. Seizures are often difficult to control. Blood levels have to be regularly monitored, as it may be difficult to discern toxic side effects. Moreover, long-term weight loss will tend to increase blood concentrations. Standard values for optimal therapeutic concentrations can be applied.

Retarding Disease Progression

The excitotoxic hypothesis is currently an accepted model for neurodegeneration in HD (see "Pathophysiology" above). This concept has stimulated attempts to block the neurotoxic effects of glutamate or other excitotoxic amino acids. Thus far, the only reported trial used baclofen to retard disease progression, as this drug inhibits corticostriatal glutamate release and displayed some protective effects against kainic acid in animal models of HD. Follow-up of 60 patients for at least 30 months in a double-blind placebo-controlled study failed to show any effect of the drug.[312] Attempts to influence excitatory amino acid transmission, however, remain attractive.

REFERENCES

1. Huntington G: On chorea. *Med Surg Rep* **26**:317, 1872.
2. Osler W: *On Chorea and Choreiform Affections*. Philadelphia, Blakiston, 1894.
3. Kussmaul A, Nothnagel CWH: *Virchow-Hirsch's Yahrbuch für 1872*. New York, 1872, p 175.
4. Huber A: Chorea hereditaria der Erwachsenen (Huntington's chorea). *Virchows Arch [A]* **108**:267, 1887.
5. Klippel M, Ducellier F: Un cas de chorée héréditaire de l'adulte (maladie de Huntington). *Encephale* **8**:716, 1888.
6. Seppili G: Corea ereditaria (Corea d'Huntington—corea cronica progressiva). *Riv Sper Freniat* **13**:453, 1888.
7. Suckling CW: Hereditary chorea (Huntington's disease). *Br Med J* **2**:1039, 1889.
8. Huntington G: Recollections of Huntington's chorea as I saw it as East Hampton, Long Island, during my boyhood. NY Neurological Society, Dec 1909. *J Nerv Ment Dis* **37**:255, 1910.
9. De Jong RN: The history of Huntington's chorea in the United States of America, in Barbeau A, Chase TN, Paulson GW (eds): *Advances in Neurology*. New York, Raven, 1973, vol 1, p 19.
10. Kishimoto K, Nakamura M, Sotokawa Y: Population genetics study—Huntington's chorea in Japan. *Ann Rep Res Inst Environ Med* **9**:195, 1957.
11. Hayden MR, MacGregor JM, Beighton PH: The prevalence of Huntington's chorea in South Africa. *S Afr Med J* **58**:193, 1980.
12. Palo J, Somer H, Ikonen E, Karila L, Peltonen L: Low prevalence of Huntington's disease in Finland (letter). *Lancet* **2**:805, 1987.
13. Reed TE, Chandler JH, Hughes EM, Davidson RT: Huntington's chorea in Michigan. I. Demography and genetics. *Am J Hum Genet* **10**:201, 1958.
14. Kurtzke JF, Anderson VE, Beebe GW, Elston RC, Higgins I, Hogg J, Kurland L, Muenter M, Myrianthopoulos N, Reed TE, Schoenberg B, Schull WJ, Li CC: Report of workgroup on epidemiology, biostatistics and population genetics, in *Commission for the Control of Huntington's Disease and its Consequences*. DHEW publication (NIH) 718-1503, Washington, DC, Government Printing Office, 1977, vol 3, p 133.
15. Folstein SE, Chase GA, Wahl WE, McDonnell AM, Folstein MF: Huntington disease in Maryland: Clinical aspects of racial variation. *Am J Hum Genet* **41**:168, 1987.
16. Wright HH, Still CN, Abramson RK: Huntington's disease in black kindreds in South Carolina. *Arch Neurol* **38**:412, 1981.
17. Hayden MR: Huntington's Chorea in South Africa. PhD Thesis. Cape Town, South Africa, University of Cape Town, 1979.
18. Avila-Giron R: Medical and social aspects of Huntington's chorea in the State of Zulia, Venezuela, in Barbeau A, Chase TN, Paulson GW (eds): *Advances in Neurology*. New York, Raven, 1973, vol 1, p 261.
19. Young AB, Shoulson I, Penney JB, Starosta-Rubinstein S, Gomez F, Travers H, Ramos-Arroyo MA, Snodgrass SR, Bonilla E, Moreno H: Huntington's disease in Venezuela: Neurologic features and functional decline. *Neurology* **36**:244, 1986.
20. Wexler NS, Young AB, Tanzi RE, Travers H, Starosta-Rubinstein S, Penney JB, Snodgrass SR, Shoulson I, Gomez F, Ramos Arroyo MA: Homozygotes for Huntington's disease. *Nature* **326**:194, 1987.
21. Pridmore SA: The prevalence of Huntington's disease in Tasmania. *Med J Aust* **153**:133, 1990.
22. Lanska DJ, Lavine L, Lanska MJ, Schoenberg BS: Huntington's disease mortality in the United States. *Neurology* **38**:769, 1988.
23. Hogg JE, Massey EW, Schoenberg BS: Mortality from Huntington's disease in the United States. *Adv Neurol* **23**:27, 1979.
24. Newcombe RG: A life table for onset of Huntington's chorea. *Ann Hum Genet* **45**:375, 1981.
25. Hayden MR: *Huntington's Chorea*. Berlin, Springer-Verlag, 1981.
26. Adams P, Falek A, Arnold J: Huntington disease in Georgia: Age at onset. *Am J Hum Genet* **43**:695, 1988.
27. Wendt GG, Landzettel I, Unterreiner I: Erkrankungsalter bei der Huntingtonschen Chorea. *Acta Genet (Basel)* **9**:18, 1959.
28. Harper PS: *Major Problems in Neurology, Huntington Disease*, 22d ed. Philadelphia, Saunders, 1991.
29. Penney JB Jr, Young AB, Shoulson I, Starosta-Rubenstein S, Snodgrass SR, Sanchez-Ramos J, Ramos-Arroyo M, Gomez F, Penchaszadeh G, Alvir J: Huntington's disease in Venezuela: 7 years of follow-up on symptomatic and asymptomatic individuals. *Mov Disord* **5**:93, 1990.
30. Hayden MR, Hewitt J, Stoessl AJ, Clark C, Ammann W, Martin WR: The combined use of positron emission tomography and DNA polymorphisms for preclinical detection of Huntington's disease. *Neurology* **37**:1441, 1987.
31. Grafton ST, Mazziotta JC, Pahl JJ, St. George-Hyslop P, Haines JL, Gusella J, Hoffman JM, Baxter LR, Phelps ME: A comparison of neurological, metabolic, structural, and genetic evaluations in persons at risk for Huntington's disease. *Ann Neurol* **28**:614, 1990.
32. Brothers CRD: Huntington's chorea in Victoria and Tasmania. *J Neurol Sci* **1**:405, 1964.
33. Pridmore SA: Age of death and duration in Huntington's disease in Tasmania. *Med J Aust* **153**:137, 1990.
34. Lanska DJ, Lanska MJ, Lavine L, Schoenberg BS: Conditions associated with Huntington's disease at death. A case-control study. *Arch Neurol* **45**:878, 1988.
35. Haines JL, Conneally PM: Causes of death in Huntington disease as reported on death certificates. *Genet Epidemiol* **3**:417, 1986.
36. Anglade M: Une autopsie de chorée de Huntington. *Gaz Hebd Sci Med Bordeaux* **27**:89, 1906.
37. Jelgersma G: Die anatomische Veränderungen bei Paralysis agitans und chronischer Chorea. *Verh Ges Dtsch Naturf Artz* **2**:383, 1908.
38. Alzheimer A: Über die anatomische Gründlage der Huntington' schen Chorea und der choreatischen Bewegungen überhaupt. *Neurol Zentralbl* **30**:891, 1911.
39. Bruyn GW: Huntington's chorea. Historical, clinical and laboratory synopsis, in Vinken PJ, Bruyn GW (eds): *Diseases of the Basal Ganglia. Handbook of Clinical Neurology*. Amsterdam, North Holland, 1968, vol 6, p 298.
40. Vonsattel JP, Myers RH, Stevens TJ, Ferrante RJ, Bird ED, Richardson EP Jr: Neuropathological classification of Huntington's disease. *J Neuropathol Exp Neurol* **44**:559, 1985.
41. Dunlap CB: Pathologic changes in Huntington's chorea with special reference to the corpus striatum. *Arch Neurol Psychiatry (Chicago)* **18**:867, 1927.
42. McCaughey WTE: The pathologic spectrum of Huntington's chorea. *J Nerv Ment Dis* **133**:91, 1961.
43. Earle KM: Pathology and experimental models of Huntington's chorea, in Barbeau A, Chase TM, Paulson GW (eds): *Huntington's Chorea 1872–1972. Advances in Neurology, vol 1*. New York, Raven, 1973, p 341.
44. Forno LS, Jose C: Huntington's chorea: A pathological study, in Barbeau A, Chase TN, Paulson GW (eds): *Huntington's Chorea 1872–1972. Advances in Neurology*. New York, Raven, 1973, vol 1, p 453.
45. Stone TT, Falstein EI: Pathology of Huntington's chorea. *J Nerv Ment Dis* **88**:602, 1938.
46. Myers RH, Vonsattel JP, Paskevich PA, Kiely DK, Stevens TJ, Cupples LA, Richardson EP Jr, Bird ED: Decreased neuronal and increased oligodendroglial densities

in Huntington's disease caudate nucleus. *J Neuropathol Exp Neurol* **50:**729, 1991.
47. Graveland GA, Williams RS, DiFiglia M: A golgi study of the human neostriatum: Neurons and afferent fibers. *J Comp Neurol* **234:**317, 1985.
48. Dom R, Baro F, Brucher JM: A cytometric study of the putamen in different types of Huntington's chorea, in Barbeau A, Chase TN, Paulson GW (eds): *Huntington's Chorea 1872–1972. Advances in Neurology*. New York, Raven, 1973, vol 1, p 369.
49. Lange H, Thorner G, Hopf A, Schroder KF: Morphometric studies of the neuropathological changes in choreatic diseases. *J Neurol Sci* **28:**401, 1976.
50. Roizin L, Stellar S, Liu JC: Neuronal nuclear-cytoplasmic changes in Huntington's chorea: Electron microscope investigations, in Chase TN, Wexler NS, Barbeau A (eds): *Huntington's disease. Advances in Neurology*. New York, Raven, 1979, p 95.
51. Graveland GA, Williams RS, DiFiglia M: Evidence for degenerative and regenerative changes in neostriatal spiny neurons in Huntington's disease. *Science* **227:**770, 1985.
52. Ferrante RJ, Kowall NW, Richardson EP Jr: Proliferative and degenerative changes in striatal spiny neurons in Huntington's disease: A combined study using the section-Golgi method and calbindin D28k immunocytochemistry. *J Neurosci* **11:**3877, 1991.
53. Nihei K, Kowall NW: Neurofilament and neural cell adhesion molecule immunocytochemistry of Huntington's disease striatum. *Ann Neurol* **31:**59, 1992.
54. Klintworth GK: Huntington's chorea—morphologic contributions of a century, in Barbeau A, Chase TN, Paulson GW (eds): *Huntington's Chorea 1872–1972. Advances in Neurology*. New York, Raven, 1973, vol 1, p 353.
55. Forno LS, Norville RL: Ultrastructure of the neostriatum in Huntington's disease, in Chase TN, Wexler NS, Barbeau A (eds): *Huntington's Disease. Advances in Neurology*. New York, Raven, 1979, p 123.
56. Myers RH, Sax DS, Koroshetz WJ, Mastromauro C, Cupples LA, Kiely DK, Pettengill FK, Bird ED: Factors associated with slow progression in Huntington's disease. *Arch Neurol* **48:**800, 1991.
57. Lange HW: Quantitative changes of telencephalon, diencephalon, and mesencephalon in Huntington's chorea, postencephalitic, and idiopathic parkinsonism. *Verh Anat Ges* **75:**923, 1981.
58. Dexter DT, Carayon A, Javoy-Agid F, Agid Y, Wells FR, Daniel SE, Lees AJ, Jenner P, Marsden CD: Alterations in the levels of iron, ferritin and other trace metals in Parkinson's disease and other neurodegenerative diseases affecting the basal ganglia. *Brain* **114:**1953, 1991.
59. Averback P: Lesions of the nucleus ansae peduncularis in neuropsychiatric disease. *Arch Neurol* **38:**230, 1981.
60. Roos RA, Bots GT: Nuclear membrane indentations in Huntington's chorea. *J Neurol Sci* **61:**37, 1983.
61. Roos RA, Bots GT, Hermans J: Quantitative analysis of morphological features in Huntington's disease. *Acta Neurol Scand* **73:**131, 1986.
62. Roos RA, Pruyt JF, de Vries J, Bots GT: Neuronal distribution in the putamen in Huntington's disease. *J Neurol Neurosurg Psychiatry* **48:**422, 1985.
63. Kowall NW, Ferrante RJ, Martin JB: Patterns of cell loss in Huntington's disease. *Trends Neurosci* **10:**24, 1987.
64. Graybiel AM: Neurotransmitters and neuromodulators in the basal ganglia. *Trends Neurosci* **13:**244, 1990.
65. Smith AD, Bolam JP: The neural network of the basal ganglia as revealed by the study of synaptic connections of identified neurons. *Trends Neurosci* **13:**259, 1990.
65a. Perry TL, Hansen S, Kloster M: Huntington's chorea. Deficiency of gamma-aminobutyric acid in brain. *N Engl J Med* **288:**337, 1973.
66. Reiner A, Albin RL, Anderson KD, D'Amato CJ, Penney JB, Young AB: Differential loss of striatal projection neurons in Huntington disease. *Proc Natl Acad Sci USA* **85:**5733, 1988.
67. Albin RL, Reiner A, Anderson KD, Penney JB, Young AB: Striatal and nigral neuron subpopulations in rigid Huntington's disease: Implications for the functional anatomy of chorea and rigidity-akinesia. *Ann Neurol* **27:**357, 1990.
68. Albin RL, Qin Y, Young AB, Penney JB, Chesselet MF: Preproenkephalin messenger RNA-containing neurons in striatum of patients with symptomatic and presymptomatic Huntington's disease: An in situ hybridization study. *Ann Neurol* **30:**542, 1991.
69. Hope BT, Michael GJ, Knigge KM, Vincent SR: Neuronal NADPH-diaphorase is a nitric oxide synthase. *Proc Natl Acad Sci USA* **88:**2811, 1991.
70. Ferrante RJ, Kowall NW, Beal MF, Richardson EP Jr, Bird ED, Martin JB: Selective sparing of a class of striatal neurons in Huntington's disease. *Science* **230:**561, 1985.
71. Dawbarn D, De Quidt ME, Emson PC: Survival of basal ganglia neuropeptide Y-somatostatin neurons in Huntington's disease. *Brain Res* **340:**251, 1985.
72. Ferrante RJ, Kowall NW, Beal MF, Martin JB, Bird ED, Richardson EP Jr: Morphologic and histochemical characteristics of a spared subset of striatal neurons in Huntington's disease. *J Neuropathol Exp Neurol* **46:**12, 1987.
73. Ferrante RJ, Beal MF, Kowall NW, Richardson EP Jr, Martin JB: Sparing of acetylcholinesterase-containing striatal neurons in Huntington's disease. *Brain Res* **411:**162, 1987.
74. Young AB, Penney JB: Striatal inhomogeneities and basal ganglia function. *Mov Disord* **1:**3, 1986.
75. De la Monte SM, Vonsattel JP, Richardson EP Jr: Morphometric demonstration of atrophic changes in the cerebral cortex, white matter, and neostriatum in Huntington's disease. *J Neuropathol Exp Neurol* **47:**516, 1988.
76. Dom R, Malfroid M, Baro F: Neuropathology of Huntington's chorea. Studies of the ventrobasal complex of the thalamus. *Neurology* **26:**64, 1976.
77. Sotrel A, Paskevich PA, Kiely DK, Bird ED, Williams RS, Myers RH: Morphometric analysis of the prefrontal cortex in Huntington's disease. *Neurology* **41:**1117, 1991.
77a. Hedreen JC, Peyser CE, Folstein SE, Ross CA: Neuronal loss in layers V and VI of cerebral cortex in Huntington's disease. *Neurosci Lett* **133:**257, 1991.
78. Savvopoulos S, Golaz J, Bouras C, Constantinidis J, Tissot R: [Huntington chorea. Anatomoclinical and genetic study of 17 cases.] *Encephale* **16:**251, 1990.
79. Tellez-Nagel I, Johnson AB, Terry RD: Studies on brain biopsies of patients with Huntington's chorea. *J Neuropathol Exp Neurol* **33:**308, 1974.
80. Cudkowicz M, Kowall NW: Degeneration of pyramidal projection neurons in Huntington's disease cortex. *Ann Neurol* **27:**200, 1990.
81. Zalneraitis EL, Landis DMD, Richardson EP, Selkoe DJ: A comparison of astrocytic structure in cerebral cortex and striatum in Huntington disease. *Neurology (suppl 1)* **31:**151, 1981. (abstr)
82. Braak H, Braak E: Allocortical involvement in Huntington's disease. *Neuropathol Appl Neurobiol* **18:**539, 1992.
83. McIntosh GC, Jameson HD, Markesbery WR: Huntington disease associated with Alzheimer disease. *Ann Neurol* **3:**545, 1978.
84. Reyes MG, Gibbons S: Dementia of the Alzheimer's type and Huntington's disease. *Neurology* **35:**273, 1985.
85. Bruyn GW, Roos RA: Senile plaques in Huntington's disease: A preliminary report. *Clin Neurol Neurosurg* **92:**329, 1990.
86. Parent A: Extrinsic connections of the basal ganglia. *Trends Neurosci* **13:**254, 1990.
87. Wahren W: Anatomy of the hypothalamus, in Schaltenbrand G, Bailey P (eds): *Introduction to Sterotaxis with an Atlas of the Human Brain*. Stuttgart, Thieme, 1959, p 119.
88. Wahren M, Trzepacz PT: Zur pathoklise des Nucleus Tuberis lateralis. *Prog Brain Res* **5:**161, 1964.
89. Kremer HP, Roos RA, Dingjan G, Marani E, Bots GT: Atrophy of the hypothalamic lateral tuberal nucleus in Huntington's disease. *J Neuropathol Exp Neurol* **49:**371, 1990.
90. Kremer HP, Roos RA, Dingjan GM, Bots GT, Bruyn GW, Hofman MA: The hypothalamic lateral tuberal nucleus and the characteristics of neuronal loss in Huntington's disease. *Neurosci Lett* **132:**101, 1991.
91. Tagliavini F, Pilleri G: Basal nucleus of Meynert. A neuropathological study in Alzheimer's disease, simple senile dementia, Pick's disease and Huntington's chorea. *J Neurol Sci* **62:**243, 1983.

92. Clark AW, Parhad IM, Folstein SE, Whitehouse PJ, Hedreen JC, Price DL, Chase GA: The nucleus basalis in Huntington's disease. *Neurology* **33**:1262, 1983.
93. Mann DM: Subcortical afferent projection systems in Huntington's chorea. *Acta Neuropathol (Berl)* **78**:551, 1989.
94. Zweig RM, Ross CA, Hedreen JC, Peyser C, Cardillo JE, Folstein SE, Price DL: Locus coeruleus involvement in Huntington's disease. *Arch Neurol* **49**:152, 1992.
95. Rodda RA: Cerebellar atrophy in Huntington's disease. *J Neurol Sci* **50**:147, 1981.
96. Jervis GA: Huntington's chorea in childhood. *Arch Neurol* **9**:244, 1963.
97. Byers RK, Gilles FH, Fung C: Huntington's disease in children. Neuropathologic study of four cases. *Neurology* **23**:561, 1973.
98. Jeste DV, Barban L, Parisi J: Reduced Purkinje cell density in Huntington's disease. *Exp Neurol* **85**:78, 1984.
99. Folstein SE, Leigh RJ, Parhad IM, Folstein MF: The diagnosis of Huntington's disease. *Neurology* **36**:1279, 1986.
100. Bird ED: The brain in Huntington's chorea. *Psychol Med* **8**:357, 1978.
101. Folstein SE, Jensen B, Leigh RJ, Folstein MF: The measurement of abnormal movement: Methods developed for Huntington's disease. *Neurobehav Toxicol Teratol* **5**:605, 1983.
102. Folstein SE: *Huntington's Disease. A Disorder of Families.* Baltimore, Johns Hopkins University Press, 1989.
103. Thompson PD, Berardelli A, Rothwell JC, Day BL, Dick JP, Benecke R, Marsden CD: The coexistence of bradykinesia and chorea in Huntington's disease and its implications for theories of basal ganglia control of movement. *Brain* **111**:223, 1988.
104. Bittenbender JB, Quadfasel FA: Rigid and akinetic forms of Huntington's chorea. *Arch Neurol* **7**:275, 1962.
105. Beenen N, Büttner U, Lange HW: The diagnostic value of eye movement recordings in patients with Huntington's disease and their offspring. *Electroencephalogr Clin Neurophysiol* **63**:119, 1986.
106. Oepen G, Clarenbach P, Thoden U: Disturbance of eye movements in Huntington's chorea. *Arch Psychiatrie Nervenkr* **229**:205, 1981.
107. Lasker AG, Zee DS, Hain TC, Folstein SE, Singer HS: Saccades in Huntington's disease: Slowing and dysmetria. *Neurology* **38**:427, 1988.
108. Tian JR, Zee DS, Lasker AG, Folstein SE: Saccades in Huntington's disease: Predictive tracking and interaction between release of fixation and initiation of saccades. *Neurology* **41**:875, 1991.
109. Hefter H, Hömberg V, Lange HW, Freund HJ: Impairment of rapid movement in Huntington's disease. *Brain* **110**:585, 1987.
110. Koller WC, Trimble J: The gait abnormality of Huntington's disease. *Neurology* **35**:1450, 1985.
111. Podoll K, Caspary P, Lange HW, Noth J: Language functions in Huntington's disease. *Brain* **111**:1475, 1988.
112. Coleman R, Anderson D, Lovrien E: Oral motor dysfunction in individuals at risk of Huntington disease. *Am J Med Genet* **37**:36, 1990.
113. Caine ED, Fisher JM: Dementia in Huntington's disease, in Vinken PJ, Bruyn GW, Klawans HL, Frederiks JAM (eds): *Handbook of Clinical Neurology,* vol 46, rev series 2, *Neurobehavioural Disorders.* Amsterdam, Elsevier, 1985, p 305.
114. Brandt J, Butters N: The neuropsychology of Huntington's disease. *Trends Neurosci* **9**:118, 1986.
115. Jason GW, Pajurkova EM, Suchowersky O, Hewitt J, Hilbert C, Reed J, Hayden MR: Presymptomatic neuropsychological impairment in Huntington's disease. *Arch Neurol* **45**:769, 1988.
116. Pillon B, Dubois B, Ploska A, Agid Y: Severity and specificity of cognitive impairment in Alzheimer's, Huntington's, and Parkinson's diseases and progressive supranuclear palsy. *Neurology* **41**:634, 1991.
117. Albert ML, Feldman RG, Willis AL: The subcortical dementia of progressive supranuclear palsy. *J Neurol Neurosurg Psychiatry* **37**:121, 1974.
118. Cummings JL, Benson DF: Subcortical dementia. Review of an emerging concept. *Arch Neurol* **41**:874, 1984.
119. Folstein SE: *Huntington's Disease. A Disorder of Families.* Appendix 1. The documentation of clinical features of Huntington's disease: Clinical assessment instruments. Baltimore, Johns Hopkins University Press, 1989, p 189.
120. Wilson RS, Como PG, Garron DC, Klawans HL, Barr A, Klawans D: Memory failure in Huntington's disease. *J Clin Exp Neuropsychol* **9**:147, 1987.
121. Massman PJ, Delis DC, Butters N, Levin BE, Salmon DP: Are all subcortical dementias alike? Verbal learning and memory in Parkinson's and Huntington's disease patients. *J Clin Exp Neuropsychol* **12**:729, 1990.
122. Scholz OB, Berlemann C: Memory performance in Huntington's disease. *Int J Neurosci* **35**:155, 1987.
123. Randolph C: Implicit, explicit, and semantic memory functions in Alzheimer's disease and Huntington's disease. *J Clin Exp Neuropsychol* **13**:479, 1991.
124. Beatty WW, Salmon DP, Butters N, Heindel WC, Granholm EL: Retrograde amnesia in patients with Alzheimer's disease or Huntington's disease. *Neurobiol Aging* **9**:181, 1988.
125. Heindel WC, Butters N, Salmon DP: Impaired learning of a motor skill in patients with Huntington's disease. *Behav Neurosci* **102**:141, 1988.
126. Heindel WC, Salmon DP, Butters N: The biasing of weight judgments in Alzheimer's and Huntington's disease: A priming or programming phenomenon. *J Clin Exp Neuropsychol* **13**:189, 1991.
127. Knopman D, Nissen MJ: Procedural learning is impaired in Huntington's disease: Evidence from the serial reaction time task. *Neuropsychologia* **29**:245, 1991.
128. Brandt J, Folstein SE, Folstein MF: Differential cognitive impairment in Alzheimer's disease and Huntington's disease. *Ann Neurol* **23**:555, 1988.
129. Starkstein SE, Brandt J, Folstein S, Strauss M, Berthier ML, Pearlson GD, Wong D, McDonnell A, Folstein M: Neuropsychological and neuroradiological correlates in Huntington's disease. *J Neurol Neurosurg Psychiatry* **51**:1259, 1988.
130. Wallesch CW, Fehrenbach RA: On the neurolinguistic nature of language abnormalities in Huntington's disease. *J Neurol Neurosurg Psychiatry* **51**:367, 1988.
131. Hodges JR, Salmon DP, Butters N: The nature of the naming deficit in Alzheimer's and Huntington's disease. *Brain* **114**:1547, 1991.
132. Speedie LJ, Brake N, Folstein SE, Bowers D, Heilman KM: Comprehension of prosody in Huntington's disease. *J Neurol Neurosurg Psychiatry* **53**:607, 1990.
133. Caine ED, Shoulson I: Psychiatric syndromes in Huntington's disease. *Am J Psychiatry* **140**:728, 1983.
134. Morris M, Tyler A: Management and therapy, in Harper PS (ed): *Huntington's Disease.* London, Saunders, 1991, p 205.
135. Farrer LA: Suicide and attempted suicide in Huntington disease: Implications for preclinical testing of persons at risk. *Am J Med Genet* **24**:305, 1986.
136. Folstein SE: The psychopathology of Huntington's disease. *Res Publ Assoc Res Nerv Ment Dis* **69**:181, 1991.
137. Burns A, Folstein S, Brandt J, Folstein M: Clinical assessment of irritability, aggression, and apathy in Huntington and Alzheimer disease. *J Nerv Ment Dis* **178**:20, 1990.
138. Sanberg PR, Fibiger HC, Mark RF: Body weight and dietary factors in Huntington's disease patients compared with matched controls. *Med J Aust* **1**:407, 1981.
139. Farrer LA, Yu PL: Anthropometric discrimination among affected, at-risk, and not-at-risk individuals in families with Huntington disease. *Am J Med Genet* **21**:307, 1985.
140. Morales LM, Estévez J, Suárez H, Villalobos R, Chacín de Bonilla L, Bonilla E: Nutritional evaluation of Huntington disease patients. *Am J Clin Nutr* **50**:145, 1989.
141. Oepen H: Über 217 Korpersektionsbefunde bei der Huntingtonscher Krankheit. *Beitr Pathl Anat Alg Path* **128**:12, 1963.
142. Hansotia P, Wall R, Berendes J: Sleep disturbances and severity of Huntington's disease. *Neurology* **35**:1672, 1985.
143. Bollen EL, Den Heijer JC, Ponsioen C, Kramer C, van der Velde EA, Van Dijk JG, Roos RA, Kamphuisen HA, Buruma OJ: Respiration during sleep in Huntington's chorea. *J Neurol Sci* **84**:63, 1988.
144. Emser W, Brenner M, Stober T, Schimrigk K: Changes

in nocturnal sleep in Huntington's and Parkinson's disease. *J Neurol* **235:**177, 1988.
145. Wheeler JS, Sax DS, Krane RJ, Siroky MB: Vesicourethral function in Huntington's chorea. *Br J Urol* **57:**63, 1985.
146. Davies DD: Abnormal response to anaesthesia in a case of Huntington's chorea. *Br J Anaesth* **38:**490, 1966.
147. Gualandi W, Bonfanti G: [A case of prolonged apnea in Huntington's chorea.] *Acta Anaesthesiol Suppl 19* **6:**235, 1968.
148. Blanloeil Y, Bigot A, Dixneuf B: Anaesthesia in Huntington's chorea (letter). *Anaesthesia* **37:**695, 1982.
149. Farina J, Rauscher LA: Anaesthesia and Huntington's chorea. A report of two cases. *Br J Anaesth* **49:**1167, 1977.
150. Browne MG, Cross R: Huntington's chorea (letter). *Br J Anaesth* **53:**1367, 1981.
151. Browne MG: Anaesthesia in Huntington's chorea. *Anaesthesia* **38:**65, 1982.
152. Shoulson I, Fahn S: Huntington disease: Clinical care and evaluation (editorial). *Neurology* **29:**1, 1979.
153. Myers RH, Sax DS, Schoenfeld M, Bird ED, Wolf PA, Vonsattel JP, White RF, Martin JB: Late onset of Huntington's disease. *J Neurol Neurosurg Psychiatry* **48:**530, 1985.
154. Shoulson I: Huntington disease: Functional capacities in patients treated with neuroleptic and antidepressant drugs. *Neurology* **31:**1333, 1981.
155. Markham CH, Knox JW: Observations on Huntington's chorea in childhood. *J Pediatr* **67:**46, 1965.
156. Oliver J, Dewhurst K: Childhood and adolescent forms of Huntington's disease. *J Neurol Neurosurg Psychiatry* **32:**455, 1969.
157. Osborne JP, Munson P, Burman D: Huntington's chorea. Report of 3 cases and review of the literature. *Arch Dis Child* **57:**99, 1982.
158. Paulson GW: Diagnosis of Huntington's disease, in Chase TN, Wexler NS, Barbeau A (eds): *Huntington's Disease. Advances in Neurology*. New York, Raven, 1979, vol 23, p 177.
159. Vogel CM, Drury I, Terry LC, Young AB: Myoclonus in adult Huntington's disease. *Ann Neurol* **29:**213, 1991.
160. Padberg G, Bruyn GW: Chorea—differential diagnosis, in Vinken PJ, Bruyn GW, Klawans HL (eds): *Handbook of Clinical Neurology 5(49). Extrapyramidal Disorders*. Amsterdam, Elsevier, 1986, p 549.
161. Hardie RJ, Pullon HWH, Harding AE, Owen JS, Pires M, Daniels GL, Imai Y, Misra VP, King RHM, Jacobs JM, Tippett P, Duchen LW, Thomas PK, Marsden CD: Neuroacanthocytosis. A clinical, haematologic and pathological study of 19 cases. *Brain* **114:**12, 1991.
162. Iiuzuka R, Hirayama K, Maehara K: Dentato-rubro-pallido-luysian atrophy: A clinico-pathological study. *J Neurol Neurosurg Psychiatry* **47:**1288, 1984.
163. Buruma OJS, Roos RAC: Paroxysmal choreoathetosis, in Vinken PJ, Bruyn GW, Klawans HL (eds): *Handbook of Clinical Neurology, vol 5(49). Extrapyramidal Disorders*. Amsterdam, Elsevier, 1986, p 349.
164. Truong DD, Harding AE, Scaravilli F, Smith SJM, Morgan-Hughes JA, Marsden CD: Movement disorders in mitochondrial myopathies: A study of nine cases with two autopsy studies. *Mov Disord* **5:**109, 1990.
165. Swaiman KF: Hallervorden-Spatz and brain iron metabolism. *Arch Neurol* **48:**1285, 1991.
166. Stevens D, Parsonage M: Mutation in Huntington's chorea. *J Neurol Neurosurg Psychiatry* **32:**140, 1969.
167. Wolff G, Deuschl G, Wienker TF, Hummel K, Bender K, Lücking CH, Schumacher M, Hammer J, Oepen G: New mutation to Huntington's disease. *J Med Genet* **26:**18, 1989.
168. Quarrell OW, Tyler A, Cole G, Harper PS: The problem of isolated cases of Huntington's disease in South Wales 1974–1984. *Clin Genet* **30:**433, 1986.
169. Bateman D, Boughey AM, Scaravilli F, Marsden CD, Harding AE: A follow-up of isolated cases of suspected Huntington's disease. *Ann Neurol* **31:**293, 1992.
170. Terrence CF, Delaney JF, Alberts MC: Computed tomography for Huntington's disease. *Neuroradiology* **13:**173, 1977.
171. Wardlaw JM, Sellar RJ, Abernethy LF: Measurement of caudate nucleus area—a more accurate measurement for Huntington's disease? *Neuroradiology* **33:**316, 1991.
172. Starkstein SE, Folstein SE, Brandt J, Pearlson GD, McDonnell A, Folstein M: Brain atrophy in Huntington's disease. A CT-scan study. *Neuroradiology* **31:**156, 1989.
173. Clark C, Hayden M, Hollenberg S, Li D, Stoessl AJ: Controlling for cerebral atrophy in positron emission tomography data. *J Cereb Blood Flow Metab* **7:**510, 1987.
174. Serra S, Xerra A, Scribano E, Meduri M, Di Perri R: Computerized tomography in amyotrophic choreoacanthocytosis. *Neuroradiology* **29:**480, 1987.
175. Simmons JT, Pastakia B, Chase TN, Shults CW: Magnetic resonance imaging in Huntington disease. *AJNR* **7:**25, 1986.
176. Kuhl DE, Phelps ME, Markham CH, Metter EJ, Riege WH, Winter J: Cerebral metabolism and atrophy in Huntington's disease determined by 18FDG and computed tomographic scan. *Ann Neurol* **12:**425, 1982.
177. Hayden MR, Martin WR, Stoessl AJ, Clark C, Hollenberg S, Adam MJ, Ammann W, Harrop R, Rogers J, Ruth T: Positron emission tomography in the early diagnosis of Huntington's disease. *Neurology* **36:**888, 1986.
178. Mazziotta JC, Phelps ME, Pahl JJ, Huang SC, Baxter LR, Riege WH, Hoffman JM, Kuhl DE, Lanto AB, Wapenski JA: Reduced cerebral glucose metabolism in asymptomatic subjects at risk for Huntington's disease. *N Engl J Med* **316:**357, 1987.
179. Young AB, Penney JB, Starosta-Rubinstein S, Markel D, Berent S, Rothley J, Betley A, Hichwa R: Normal caudate glucose metabolism in persons at risk for Huntington's disease. *Arch Neurol* **44:**254, 1987.
180. Hosokawa S, Ichiya Y, Kuwabara Y, Ayabe Z, Mitsuo K, Goto I, Kato M: Positron emission tomography in cases of chorea with different underlying diseases. *J Neurol Neurosurg Psychiatry* **50:**1284, 1987.
181. Hawkins RA, Mazziotta JC, Phelps ME: Wilson's disease studies with FDG and positron emission tomography. *Neurology* **37:**1707, 1987.
182. Lang AE, Garnett ES: Positron emission tomography in cases of chorea with different underlying diseases (letter). *J Neurol Neurosurg Psychiatry* **51:**1010, 1988.
183. Suchowersky O, Hayden MR, Martin WR, Stoessl AJ, Hildebrand AM, Pate BD: Cerebral metabolism of glucose in benign hereditary chorea. *Mov Disord* **1:**33, 1986.
184. Kuwert T, Lange HW, Langen KJ, Herzog H, Hefter H, Aulich A, Feinendegen LE: Normal striatal glucose consumption in two patients with benign hereditary chorea as measured by positron emission tomography. *J Neurol* **237:**80, 1990.
185. Reid IC, Besson JA, Best PV, Sharp PF, Gemmell HG, Smith FW: Imaging of cerebral blood flow markers in Huntington's disease using single photon emission computed tomography. *J Neurol Neurosurg Psychiatry* **51:**1264, 1988.
186. Nagel JS, Johnson KA, Ichise M, English RJ, Walshe TM, Morris JH, Holman BL: Decreased iodine-123 IMP caudate nucleus uptake in patients with Huntington's disease. *Clin Nucl Med* **13:**486, 1988.
187. Smith FW, Gemmell HG, Sharp PF, Besson JA: Technetium-99m HMPAO imaging in patients with basal ganglia disease. *Br J Radiol* **61:**914, 1988.
188. Botsch H, Oepen G, Deuschl G, Wolff G: [SPECT studies with 99mTc-HMPAO in Huntington's chorea patients.] *ROFO* **147:**666, 1987.
189. Noth J, Podoll K, Friedemann HH: Long-loop reflexes in small hand muscles studied in normal subjects and in patients with Huntington's disease. *Brain* **108:**65, 1985.
190. Eisen A, Bohlega S, Bloch M, Hayden M: Silent periods, long-latency reflexes and cortical MEPs in Huntington's disease and at-risk relatives. *Electroencephalogr Clin Neurophysiol* **74:**444, 1989.
191. Leblhuber F, Windhager E, Reisecker F, Rittmannsberger H: Long latency EMG responses in early diagnosis of Huntington's chorea. *Eur Arch Psychiatry Clin Neurosci* **241:**113, 1991.
192. Huttunen J, Hömberg V: EMG responses in leg muscles to postural perturbations in Huntington's disease. *J Neurol Neurosurg Psychiatry* **53:**55, 1990.

193. Abbruzzese G, Dall' Agata D, Morena M, Reni L, Favale E: Abnormalities of parietal and prerolandic somatosensory evoked potentials in Huntington's disease. *Electroencephalogr Clin Neurophysiol* **77**:340, 1990.
194. Ehle AL, Stewart RM, Lellelid NA, Leventhal NA: Evoked potentials in Huntington's disease. A comparative and longitudinal study. *Arch Neurol* **41**:379, 1984.
195. Noth J, Engel L, Friedemann HH, Lange HW: Evoked potentials in patients with Huntington's disease and their offspring. I. Somatosensory evoked potentials. *Electroencephalogr Clin Neurophysiol* **59**:134, 1984.
196. Filipovic S, Kostic VS, Sternic N, Marinkovic Z, Ocic G: Auditory event-related potentials in different types of dementia. *Eur Neurol* **30**:189, 1990.
197. Josiassen RC, Curry LM, Mancall EL, Shagass C, Roemer RA: Relationship between evoked potential and neuropsychological findings in persons "at risk" for Huntington's disease. *J Clin Exp Neuropsychol* **8**:21, 1986.
198. Hennerici M, Hömberg V, Lange HW: Evoked potentials in patients with Huntington's disease and their offspring. II. Visual evoked potentials. *Electroencephalogr Clin Neurophysiol* **62**:167, 1985.
199. Bollen E, Arts RJ, Roos RA, van der Velde EA, Buruma OJ: Brainstem reflexes and brainstem auditory evoked responses in Huntington's chorea. *J Neurol Neurosurg Psychiatry* **49**:313, 1986.
200. Myers RH, Leavitt J, Farrer LA, Jagadeesh J, McFarlane H, Mastromauro CA, Mark RJ, Gusella JF: Homozygote for Huntington disease. *Am J Hum Genet* **45**:615, 1989.
201. Wallace DC, Hall AC: Evidence of genetic heterogeneity in Huntington's chorea. *J Neurol Neurosurg Psychiatry* **33**:789, 1972.
202. Conneally PM, Haines JL, Tanzi RE, Wexler NS, Penchaszadeh GK, Harper PS, Folstein SE, Cassiman JJ, Myers RH, Young AB: Huntington disease: No evidence for locus heterogeneity. *Genomics* **5**:304, 1989.
203. Robbins C, Theilmann J, Youngman S, Haines J, Altherr MJ, Harper PS, Payne C, Junker A, Wasmuth J, Hayden MR: Evidence from family studies that the gene causing Huntington disease is telomeric to D4S95 and D4S90. *Am J Hum Genet* **44**:422, 1989.
204. Pritchard C, Zhu N, Zuo J, Bell L, Pericak-Vance MA, Vance JM, Roses AD, Milatovitch A, Franke U, Cox DR, Myers RM: Recombination of 4p.16 DNA markers in an unusual family with Huntington disease. *Am J Hum Genet* **50**:1218, 1992.
205. Boehnke M, Conneally PM, Lange K: Two models for a maternal factor in the inheritance of Huntington disease. *Am J Hum Genet* **35**:845, 1983.
206. Bird ED, Caro AJ, Pilling JB: A sex related factor in the inheritance of Huntington's chorea. *Ann Hum Genet* **37**:255, 1974.
207. Ridley RM, Frith CD, Crow TJ, Conneally PM: Anticipation in Huntington's disease is inherited through the male line but may originate in the female. *J Med Genet* **25**:589, 1988.
208. Farrer LA, Conneally PM: A genetic model for age at onset in Huntington disease. *Am J Hum Genet* **37**:350, 1985.
209. Hayden MR, Soles JA, Ward RH: Age of onset in siblings of persons with juvenile Huntington disease. *Clin Genet* **28**:100, 1985.
210. Reik W: Genomic imprinting: A possible mechanism for the parental origin effect in Huntington's chorea. *J Med Genet* **25**:805, 1988.
211. Ridley RM, Frith CD, Farrer LA, Conneally PM: Patterns of inheritance of the symptoms of Huntington's disease suggestive of an effect of genomic imprinting. *J Med Genet* **28**:224, 1991.
212. Harper PS, Newcombe RG: Age at onset and life table risks in genetic counselling for Huntington's disease. *J Med Genet* **29**:239, 1992.
213. Skraastad MI, Verwest A, Bakker E, Vegter-van der Vlis M, van Leeuwen-Cornelisse I, Roos RA, Pearson PL, van Ommen GJ: Presymptomatic, prenatal, and exclusion testing for Huntington disease using seven closely lined DNA markers. *Am J Med Genet* **39**:217, 1991.
214. Craufurd D, Dodge A, Kerzin-Storrar L, Harris R: Uptake of presymptomatic predictive testing for Huntington's disease. *Lancet* **2**:603, 1989.
215. Brandt J, Quaid KA, Folstein SE, Garber P, Maestri NE, Abbott MH, Slavney PR, Franz ML, Kasch L, Kazazian HH Jr: Presymptomatic diagnosis of delayed-onset disease with linked DNA markers. The experience in Huntington's disease. *JAMA* **261**:3108, 1989.
216. Wiggins S, Whyte P, Huggins M, Adam S, Theilmann J, Bloch M, Sheps SB, Schechter MT, Hayden MR: The psychological consequences of predictive testing for Huntington disease. *N Engl J Med* **327**:1401, 1992.
217. Bloch M, Adam S, Wiggins S, Huggins M, Hayden MR: Predictive testing for Huntington disease in Canada: The experience of those receiving an increased risk. *Am J Med Genet* **42**:499, 1992.
218. Huggins M, Bloch M, Wiggins S, Adam S, Suchowersky O, Trew M, Klimek M-L, Greenberg C, Eleff M, Thompson LP, Knight J, MacLeod P, Girard K, Theilmann J, Hedrick A, Hayden MR: Predictive testing for Huntington disease in Canada: Adverse effects and unexpected results in those receiving a decreased risk. *Am J Med Genet* **42**:508, 1992.
219. Meissen GJ, Berchek RL: Intended use of predictive testing by those at risk for Huntington disease. *Am J Med Genet* **26**:283, 1987.
220. Mastromauro C, Myers RH, Berkman B: Attitudes toward presymptomatic testing in Huntington disease. *Am J Med Genet* **26**:271, 1987.
221. Tyler A, Quarrell OW, Lazarou LP, Meredith AL, Harper PS: Exclusion testing in pregnancy for Huntington's disease. *J Med Genet* **27**:488, 1990.
222. Adam S, Wiggins S, Whyte P, Bloch M, Shokeir MHK, Soltan H, Meschino W, Summers A, Suchowersky O, Welch JP, Huggins M, Theilmann J, Hayden MR: Five year study of prenatal testing for Huntington disease: Demand, attitudes and psychological assessment. *J Med Genet* **30**:549, 1993.
223. Botstein D, White RL, Skolnick M, Davis RW: Construction of a genetic linkage map in man using restriction fragment length polymorphisms. *Am J Hum Genet* **32**:314, 1980.
224. Gusella JF, Wexler NS, Conneally PM, Naylor SL, Anderson MA, Tanzi RE, Watkins PC, Ottina K, Wallace MR, Sakaguchi AY: A polymorphic DNA marker genetically linked to Huntington's disease. *Nature* **306**:234, 1983.
225. Landegent JE, Jansen in de Wal N, Fisser-Groen YM, Bakker E, van der Ploeg M, Pearson PL: Fine mapping of the Huntington disease linked D4S10 locus by non-radioactive in situ hybridization. *Hum Genet* **73**:354, 1986.
226. Magenis RE, Gusella J, Weliky K, Olson S, Haight G, Toth-Fejel S, Sheehy R: Huntington disease-linked restriction fragment length polymorphism localized within band p16.1 of chromosome 4 by in situ hybridization. *Am J Hum Genet* **39**:383, 1986.
227. Wang HS, Greenberg CR, Hewitt J, Kalousek D, Hayden MR: Subregional assignment of the linked marker G8 (D4S10) for Huntington disease to chromosome 4p16.1-16.3. *Am J Hum Genet* **39**:392, 1986.
228. Zabel BU, Naylor SL, Sakaguchi AY, Gusella JF: Mapping of the DNA locus D4S10 and the linked Huntington's disease gene to 4p16----p15. *Cytogenet Cell Genet* **42**:187, 1986.
229. MacDonald ME, Anderson MA, Gilliam TC, Tranejaerg L, Carpenter NJ, Magenis E, Hayden MR, Healey ST, Bonner TI, Gusella JF: A somatic cell hybrid panel for localizing DNA segments near the Huntington's disease gene. *Genomics* **1**:29, 1987.
230. Wasmuth JJ, Hewitt J, Smith B, Allard D, Haines JL, Skarecky D, Partlow E, Hayden MR: A highly polymorphic locus very tightly linked to the Huntington's disease gene. *Nature* **332**:734, 1988.
231. Skraastad MI, Bakker E, de Lange LF, Vegter-van der Vlis M, Klein-Breteler EG, van Ommen GJ, Pearson PL: Mapping of recombinants near the Huntington disease locus by using G8 (D4S10) and newly isolated markers in the D4S10 region. *Am J Hum Genet* **44**:560, 1989.
232. Gilliam TC, Tanzi RE, Haines JL, Bonner TI, Faryniarz

AG, Hobbs WJ, MacDonald ME, Cheng SV, Folstein SE, Conneally PM: Localization of the Huntington's disease gene to a small segment of chromosome 4 flanked by D4S10 and the telomere. *Cell* **50**:565, 1987.

233. Pohl TM, Zimmer M, MacDonald ME, Smith B, Bucan M, Poustka A, Volinia S, Searle S, Zehetner G, Wasmuth JJ: Construction of a NotI linking library and isolation of new markers close to the Huntington's disease gene. *Nucleic Acids Res* **16**:9185, 1988.
234. Richards JE, Gilliam TC, Cole JL, Drumm ML, Wasmuth JJ, Gusella JF, Collins FS: Chromosome jumping from D4S10 (G8) toward the Huntington disease gene. *Proc Natl Acad Sci USA* **85**:6437, 1988.
235. Smith B, Skarecky D, Bengtsson U, Magenis RE, Carpenter N, Wasmuth JJ: Isolation of DNA markers in the direction of the Huntington disease gene from the G8 locus. *Am J Hum Genet* **42**:335, 1988.
236. Whaley WL, Michiels F, MacDonald ME, Romano D, Zimmer M, Smith B, Leavitt J, Bucan M, Haines JL, Gilliam TC: Mapping of D4S98/S114/S113 confines the Huntington's defect to a reduced physical region at the telomere of chromosome 4. *Nucleic Acids Res* **16**:11769, 1988.
237. MacDonald ME, Haines JL, Zimmer M, Cheng SV, Youngman S, Whaley WL, Wexler N, Bucan M, Allitto BA, Smith B: Recombination events suggest potential sites for the Huntington's disease gene. *Neuron* **3**:183, 1989.
238. Pritchard CA, Casher D, Uglum E, Cox DR, Myers RM: Isolation and field-inversion gel electrophoresis analysis of DNA markers located close to the Huntington disease gene. *Genomics* **4**:408, 1989.
239. Youngman S, Sarfarazi M, Bucan M, MacDonald M, Smith B, Zimmer M, Gilliam C, Frischauf AM, Wasmuth JJ, Gusella JF: A new DNA marker (D4S90) is located terminally on the short arm of chromosome 4, close to the Huntington disease gene. *Genomics* **5**:802, 1989.
240. Lin CS, Altherr M, Bates G, Whaley WL, Read AP, Harris R, Lehrach H, Wasmuth JJ, Gusella JF, MacDonald ME: New DNA markers in the Huntington's disease gene candidate region. *Somat Cell Mol Genet* **17**:481, 1991.
241. Weber B, Hedrick A, Andrew S, Riess O, Collins C, Kowbel D, Hayden MR: Isolation and characterization of new highly polymorphic DNA markers from the Huntington disease region. *Am J Hum Genet* **50**:382, 1992.
242. Bucan M, Zimmer M, Whaley WL, Poustka A, Youngman S, Allitto BA, Ormondroyd E, Smith B, Pohl TM, MacDonald M: Physical maps of 4p16.3, the area expected to contain the Huntington disease mutation. *Genomics* **6**:1, 1990.
243. Bates GP, MacDonald ME, Baxendale S, Youngman S, Lin C, Whaley WL, Wasmuth JJ, Gusella JF, Lehrach H: Defined physical limits of the Huntington disease gene candidate region. *Am J Hum Genet* **49**:7, 1991.
244. Allitto BA, MacDonald ME, Bucan M, Richards J, Romano D, Whaley WL, Falcone B, Ianazzi J, Wexler NS, Wasmuth JJ: Increased recombination adjacent to the Huntington disease-linked D4S10 marker. *Genomics* **9**:104, 1991.
245. Whaley WL, Bates GP, Novelletto A, Sedlacek Z, Cheng S, Romano D, Ormondroyd E, Allitto B, Lin C, Youngman S: Mapping of cosmid clones in Huntington's disease region of chromosome 4. *Somat Cell Mol Genet* **17**:83, 1991.
246. Theilmann J, Kanani S, Shiang R, Robbins C, Quarrell O, Huggins M, Hedrick A, Weber B, Collins C, Wasmuth JJ: Non-random association between alleles detected at D4S95 and D4S98 and the Huntington's disease gene. *J Med Genet* **26**:676, 1989.
247. Snell RG, Lazarou LP, Youngman S, Quarrell OW, Wasmuth JJ, Shaw DJ, Harper PS: Linkage disequilibrium in Huntington's disease: An improved localisation for the gene. *J Med Genet* **26**:673, 1989.
248. Andrew S, Theilmann J, Hedrick A, Mah D, Weber B, Hayden MR: Nonrandom association between Huntington disease and two loci separated by about 3 Mb on 4p16.3. *Genomics* **13**:301, 1992.
249. Adam S, Theilmann J, Buetow K, Hedrick A, Collins C, Weber B, Huggins M, Hayden M: Linkage disequilibrium and modification of risk for Huntington disease. *Am J Hum Genet* **48**:595, 1991.
250. Barron L, Curtis A, Shrimpton AE, Holloway S, May H, Snell RG, Brock DJ: Linkage disequilibrium and recombination make a telomeric site for the Huntington's disease gene unlikely. *J Med Genet* **28**:520, 1991.
251. Novelletto A, Mandich P, Bellone E, Malaspina P, Vivona G, Ajmar F, Frontali M: Non-random association between DNA markers and Huntington disease locus in the Italian population. *Am J Med Genet* **40**:374, 1991.
252. MacDonald ME, Lin C, Srinidhi L, Bates G, Altherr M, Whaley WL, Lehrach H, Wasmuth J, Gusella JF: Complex patterns of linkage disequilibrium in the Huntington disease region. *Am J Hum Genet* **49**:723, 1991.
253. MacDonald ME, Novelletto A, Lin C: The Huntington's disease candidate region exhibits many different haplotypes. *Nat Genet* **1**:99, 1992.
254. Bates GP, Valdes J, Hummerish J: Characterization of a yeast artificial chromosome contig spanning the Huntington's disease gene candidate region. *Nat Genet* **1**:180, 1992.
255. Zuo J, Robbins C, Taillon-Miller P, Cox DR, Myers RM: Cloning of the Huntington disease region in yeast artificial chromosomes. *Hum Mol Genet* **1**:149, 1992.
256. Young AB, Penney JB, Starosta-Rubinstein S, Markel DS, Berent S, Giordani B, Ehrenkaufer R, Jewett D, Hichwa R: PET scan investigations of Huntington's disease: Cerebral metabolic correlates of neurological features and functional decline. *Ann Neurol* **20**:296, 1986.
257. Bamford KA, Caine ED, Kido DK, Plassche WM, Shoulson I: Clinical-pathologic correlation in Huntington's disease: A neuropsychological and computed tomography study. *Neurology* **39**:796, 1989.
258. Berent S, Giordani B, Lehtinen S, Markel D, Penney JB, Buchtel HA, Starosta-Rubinstein S, Hichwa R, Young AB: Positron emission tomographic scan investigations of Huntington's disease: Cerebral metabolic correlates of cognitive function. *Ann Neurol* **23**:541, 1988.
259. Parent A: *Comparative Neurobiology of the Basal Ganglia.* New York, John Wiley, 1986.
260. DeLong MR, Georgopoulos AP: Motor functions of the basal ganglia, in Brooks VB (ed): *Handbook of Physiology: The Nervous System II.* Washington, DC, American Physiology Society, 1981, p 1017.
261. Alexander GE, Crutcher MD: Functional architecture of basal ganglia circuits. Neural substrates of parallel processing. *Trends Neurosci* **13**:266, 1990.
262. Albin RL, Young AB, Penney JB: The functional anatomy of basal ganglia disorders. *Trends Neurosci* **12**:366, 1989.
263. DeLong MR: Primate models of movement disorders of the basal ganglia. *Trends Neurosci* **13**:281, 1990.
264. Albin RL, Greenamyre JT: Alternative excitotoxic hypothesis. *Neurology* **42**:733, 1992.
265. Albin RL, Young AB, Penney JB, Handelin B, Balfour R, Anderson KD, Markel DS, Tourtellotte WW, Reiner A: Abnormalities of striatal projection neurons and N-methyl-D-aspartate receptors in presymptomatic Huntington's disease. *N Engl J Med* **322**:1293, 1990.
266. Albin RL, Reiner A, Anderson KD, Dure LS, Handelin B, Balfour R, Whetsell WO, Penney JB, Young AB: Preferential loss of striato-external pallidal projection neurons in presymptomatic Huntington's disease. *Ann Neurol* **31**:425, 1992.
267. Spokes EG: Neurochemical alterations in Huntington's chorea: A study of post-mortem brain tissue. *Brain* **103**:179, 1980.
268. Klawans HL, Paulson GW, Ringel SP, Barbeau A: Use of L-Dopa in the detection of presymptomatic Huntington's chorea. *N Engl J Med* **286**:1332, 1972.
269. Gerfen CR: The neostriatal mosaic: Multiple levels of compartmental organization. *Trends Neurosci* **15**:133, 1992.
270. Stoessl AJ, Martin WR, Hayden MR, Adam MJ, Ruth TJ, Rajput A, Pate BD, Calne DB: Dopamine in Huntington disease—studies using positron emission tomography. *Neurology* **36**:310, 1986. (abstr)
271. Kurlan R, Goldblatt D, Zaczek R, Jeffries K, Irvine C, Coyle J, Shoulson I: Cerebrospinal fluid homovanillic acid and parkinsonism in Huntington's disease. *Ann Neurol* **24**:282, 1988.

272. Martin WR, Clark C, Ammann W, Stoessl AJ, Shtybel W, Hayden MR: Cortical glucose metabolism in Huntington's disease. *Neurology* **42**:223, 1992.
273. DiFiglia M: Excitotoxic injury of the neostriatum: A model for Huntington's disease. *Trends Neurosci* **13**:286, 1990.
274. Coyle JT, Schwartz R: Lesion of striatal neurones with kainic acid provides a model for Huntington's chorea. *Nature* **263**:244, 1976.
275. McGeer EG, McGeer PL: Duplication of biochemical changes of Huntington's chorea by intrastriatal injections of glutamic and kainic acids. *Nature* **263**:517, 1976.
276. Beal MF, Ferrante RJ, Swartz KJ, Kowall NW: Chronic quinolinic acid lesions in rats closely resemble Huntington's disease. *J Neurosci* **11**:1649, 1991.
277. Dure LS, Young AB, Penney JB: Excitatory amino acid binding sites in the caudate nucleus and frontal cortex of Huntington's disease. *Ann Neurol* **30**:785, 1991.
278. Kanazawa I, Tanaka Y, Cho F: Choreic movements induced by unilateral kainate lesions of the striatum and L-dopa administration in monkey. *Neurosci Lett* **71**:241, 1985.
279. Hantraye P, Riche D, Maziere M, Isacson O: A primate model of Huntington's disease: Behavioral and anatomical studies of unilateral excitotoxic lesions of the caudate-putamen in the baboon. *Exp Neurol* **108**:91, 1990.
280. Kremer B, Tallaksen-Greene SJ, Albin RL: AMPA and NMDA binding sites in the hypothalamic lateral tuberal nucleus: Implications for Huntington's disease. *Neurology* **43**:1593, 1993.
281. Choi DW, Rothman SM: The role of glutamate neurotoxicity in hypoxic-ischemic neuronal death. *Annu Rev Neurosci* **13**:171, 1990.
282. Beal MF: Does impairment of energy metabolism result in excitotoxic neuronal death in neurodegenerative illnesses? *Ann Neurol* **31**:119, 1992.
283. Cotman CW, Monaghan DT, Ottersen OP, Storm-Mathisen J: Anatomical organization of excitatory amino acid receptors and their pathways. *Trends Neurosci* **7**:273, 1987.
284. Young AB, Cha J-HJ, Makowiec RL, Albin RL, Penney JB: The anatomy of non-N-methyl-D-aspartate excitatory amino acid binding sites in mammalian brain, in Meldrum BS, Moroni F, Simon RP, Woods JH (eds): *Excitatory Amino Acids*. New York, Raven, 1991, p 55.
285. Drapo PJ: Huntington's disease: The nursing process. *J Adv Nurs* **6**:377, 1981.
286. Shoulson I, Caine E, Fahn S, Kobayashi R, Kokmen E, Sax D, Weingartner H, Wexler NS: Clinical care of the patient and family with Huntington's disease, in *Commission for the Control of Huntington's Disease and its Consequences*. Bethesda, Md, Department of Health, Education and Welfare, National Institutes of Health, 1977, vol 11, p 421.
287. Barr AN, Fischer JH, Koller WC, Spunt AL, Singhal A: Serum haloperidol concentration and choreiform movements in Huntington's disease. *Neurology* **38**:84, 1988.
288. Quinn N, Marsden CD: A double blind trial of sulpiride in Huntington's disease and tardive dyskinesia. *J Neurol Neurosurg Psychiatry* **47**:844, 1984.
289. Deroover J, Baro F, Bourguignon RP, Smets P: Tiapride versus placebo: A double-blind comparative study in the management of Huntington's chorea. *Curr Med Res Opin* **9**:329, 1984.
290. Roos RA, Buruma OJ, Bruyn GW, Kemp B, van der Velde EA: Tiapride in the treatment of Huntington's chorea. *Acta Neurol Scand* **65**:45, 1982.
291. Swash M, Roberts AH, Zakko H, Heathfield KW: Treatment of involuntary movement disorders with tetrabenazine. *J Neurol Neurosurg Psychiatry* **35**:186, 1972.
292. McLellan DL, Chalmers RJ, Johnson RH: A double-blind trial of tetrabenazine, thiopropazate, and placebo in patients with chorea. *Lancet* **1**:104, 1974.
293. Asher SW, Aminoff MJ: Tetrabenazine and movement disorders. *Neurology* **31**:1051, 1981.
294. Jankovic J, Orman J: Tetrabenazine therapy of dystonia, chorea, tics, and other dyskinesias. *Neurology* **38**:391, 1988.
295. Girotti F, Carella F, Scigliano G, Grassi MP, Soliveri P, Giovannini P, Parati E, Caraceni T: Effect of neuroleptic treatment on involuntary movements and motor performances in Huntington's disease. *J Neurol Neurosurg Psychiatry* **47**:848, 1984.
296. Mikkelsen BO: Tolerance of tetrabenazine during long-term treatment. *Acta Neurol Scand* **68**:57, 1983.
297. Schott K, Ried S, Stevens I, Dichgans J: Neuroleptically induced dystonia in Huntington's disease: A case report. *Eur Neurol* **29**:39, 1989.
298. Moss JH, Stewart DE: Iatrogenic parkinsonism in Huntington's chorea. *Can J Psychiatry* **31**:865, 1986.
299. Shoulson I: Care of patients and families with Huntington's disease, in Marsden CD, Fahn S (eds): *Movement Disorders*. London, Butterworths, 1982, p 277.
300. Burke RE, Fahn S, Mayeux R, Weinberg H, Louis K, Willner JH: Neuroleptic malignant syndrome caused by dopamine-depleting drugs in a patient with Huntington disease. *Neurology* **31**:1022, 1981.
301. Marsden CD, Quinn N: Appendix 6, in Lader MH, Richens A (eds): *Methods in Clinical Pharmacology—Central Nervous System*. London, Macmillan, 1981.
302. Frattola L, Albiazzati MG, Spano PF, Trabucchi M: Treatment of Huntington's chorea with bromocriptine. *Acta Neurol Scand* **56**:37, 1977.
303. Kartzinel R, Perlow MD, Carter AC, Chase TN, et al: Metabolic studies with bromocriptine in patients with idiopathic parkinsonism and Huntington's chorea. *Trans Am Neurol Assoc* **101**:53, 1976.
304. Tolosa ES, Sparber SB: Apomorphine in Huntington's chorea: Clinical observations and theoretical considerations. *Life Sci* **15**:1371, 1974.
305. Corsini GU, Onali P, Masala C, Cianchetti C, Mangoni A, Gessa G: Apomorphine hydrochloride-induced improvement in Huntington's chorea: Stimulation of dopamine receptor. *Arch Neurol* **35**:27, 1978.
306. Bassi S, Albizzati MG, Corsini GU, Frattola L, Piolti R, Suchy I, Trabucchi M: Therapeutic experience with transdihydrolisuride in Huntington's disease. *Neurology* **36**:984, 1986.
307. Peiris JB, Boralessa H, Lionel ND: Clonazepam in the treatment of choreiform activity. *Med J Aust* **1**:225, 1976.
308. Perry TL, Wright JM, Hansen S, MacLeod PM: Isoniazid therapy for Huntington's disease, in Chase TN, Wexler NS, Barbeau A (eds): *Huntington's Disease. Advances in Neurology*. New York, Raven, 1979, vol 23, p 785.
309. Neophytides AN, Lieberman A, Foo SH, Walker R: Treatment of Huntington's disease with isoniazid and pyridoxine. *Neurology* **30**:383, 1980.
310. McLean DR: Failure of isoniazid therapy in Huntington disease. *Neurology* **32**:1189, 1982.
311. Paulson GW: Lioresal in Huntington's disease. *Dis Nerv Syst* **37**:465, 1976.
312. Shoulson I, Odoroff C, Oakes D, Behr J, Goldblatt D, Caine E, Kennedy J, Miller C, Bamford K, Rubin A: A controlled clinical trial of baclofen as protective therapy in early Huntington's disease. *Ann Neurol* **25**:252, 1989.
313. Schou M: Lithium in the treatment of other psychiatric and nonpsychiatric disorders. *Arch Gen Psychiatry* **36**:856, 1979.
314. Brown WT, Sanberg PR, McGeer PL: Corticosteroids and chorea (letter). *Arch Neurol* **36**:452, 1979.
315. Pearce I, Heathfield KW, Pearce MJ: Valproate sodium in Huntington chorea. *Arch Neurol* **34**:308, 1977.
316. Symington GR, Leonard DP, Shannon PJ, Vajda FJ: Sodium valproate in Huntington's disease. *Am J Psychiatry* **135**:352, 1978.
317. Shoulson I, Goldblatt D, Charlton M, Joynt RJ: Huntington's disease: Treatment with muscimol, a GABA-mimetic drug. *Ann Neurol* **4**:279, 1978.
318. Tell G, Böhlen P, Schechter PJ, Koch-Weser J, Agid Y, Bonnet AM, Coquillat G, Chazot G, Fischer C: Treatment of Huntington disease with gamma-acetylenic GABA an irreversible inhibitor of GABA-transaminase: Increased CSF GABA and homocarnosine without clinical amelioration. *Neurology* **31**:207, 1981.
319. Scigliano G, Giovannini P, Girotti F, Grassi MP, Caraceni T, Schechter PJ: Gamma-vinyl GABA treatment of Huntington's disease. *Neurology* **34**:94, 1984.

320. Mondrup K, Dupont E, Braendgaard H: Progabide in the treatment of hyperkinetic extrapyramidal movement disorders. *Acta Neurol Scand* **72**:341, 1985.
321. Schults C, Steardo L, Barone P, Mohr E, Juncos J, Seratti C, Fedio P, Tamminga CA, Chase TN: Huntington's disease: Effect of cysteamine, a somatostatin-depleting agent. *Neurology* **36**:1099, 1986.
322. Aquilonius SM, Eckernas SA: Choline therapy in Huntington chorea. *Neurology* **27**:887, 1977.
323. Caraceni TA, Girotti F, Celano I, Parati E, Balboni L: 2-dimethylaminoethanol (Deanol) in Huntington's chorea. *J Neurol Neurosurg Psychiatry* **41**:1114, 1978.
324. Nutt JG, Rosin A, Chase TN: Treatment of Huntington disease with a cholinergic agonist. *Neurology* **28**:1061, 1978.
325. Hantraye P, Riche D, Mazière M, Isacson O: Intrastriatal transplantation of cross-species fetal striatal cells reduces abnormal movements in a primate model of Huntington disease. *Proc Natl Acad Sci USA* **89**:4187, 1992.
326. Folstein S, Folstein M: Diagnosis and treatment of Huntington's disease. *Compr Ther* **7**:60, 1981.
327. Ford MF: Treatment of depression in Huntington's disease with monoamine oxidase inhibitors. *Br J Psychiatry* **149**:654, 1986.
328. Greendyke RM, Schuster DB, Wooton JA: Propranolol in the treatment of assaultive patients with organic brain disease. *J Clin Psychopharmacol* **4**:282, 1984.
329. Stewart JT: Paradoxical aggressive effect of propranolol in a patient with Huntington's disease (letter). *J Clin Psychiatry* **48**:385, 1987.
330. von Hafften AH, Jensen CF: Paradoxical response to pindolol treatment for aggression in a patient with Huntington's disease (letter). *J Clin Psychiatry* **50**:230, 1989.
331. Sajatovic M, Verbanac P, Ramirez LF, Meltzer HY: Clozapine treatment of psychiatric symptoms resistant to neuroleptic treatment in patients with Huntington's chorea. *Neurology* **41**:156, 1991.
332. Sjögren T: Vererbungsmedizinische Untersuchungen über Huntingtons chorea in einer schwedischen Bauernpopulation. *Vererb Konstit Lehre* **19**:131, 1936.
333. Brothers CRD: The history and incidence of Huntington's chorea in Tasmania. *Proc R Coll Physicians* **4**:48, 1949.
334. Lyon RL: Huntington's chorea in the Moray Firth area. *Br Med J* **1**:1301, 1962.
335. Kremer B, Weber B, Hayden MR: New insights into the clinical features, pathogenesis and molecular genetics of Huntington disease. *Brain Pathol* **2**:321, 1992.
336. Thompson LM, Plummer S, Schailing M, Altherr M, Gusella JF, Housman DE, Wasmuth JJ: A gene encoding a fibroblast growth receptor isolated from the Huntington disease gene region of human chromosome 4. *Genomics* **11**:1133, 1991.
337. Collins C, Schappert K, Hayden MR: The genomic organization of a novel regulatory myosin light chain gene (MYL5) that maps to chromosome 4p.16.3 and shows different patterns of expression between primates. *Hum Mol Genet* **9**:727, 1992.
338. Weber B, Collins C, Kowbel D, Riess O, Hayden MR: Identification of multiple CpG islands and associated conserved sequences in a candidate region for the Huntington disease gene. *Genomics* **11**:1113, 1991.
339. Collins C, Duff C, Montal M, Duncan A, Norremolle A, Michaelis E, Worton R, Hayden MR: Mapping of the human NMDA receptor subunit (NMDARI) and the proposed NMDA receptor glutamate-binding subunit (NMDARAI) to chromosomes 0134.3 and chromosome 8 respectively. *Genomics* **17**:237, 1993.
340. Buckler AJ, Chang DD, Graw SL, Brook JD, Haber DA, Sharp PA, Housman DE: Exon amplification: A strategy to isolate mammalian genes based on RNA splicing. *Proc Natl Acad Sci USA* **88**:4005, 1991.
341. Taylor SAM, Snell RG, Buckler A, Ambrose C, Duyao M, Church D, Lin CS, Altherr M, Bates GP, Groot N, Barnes G, Shaw DJ, Lehrach H, Wasmuth JJ, Harper PS, Housman DE, MacDonald ME, Gusella JF: Cloning of the α-adducin gene from the Huntington's disease candidate region of chromosome 4 by exon amplification. *Nat Genet* **2**:223, 1992.
342. Goldberg YP, Lin B-Y, Andrew SE, Nasir J, Graham R, Glaves ML, Hutchinson GB, Theilmann J, Ginzinger DG, Schappert K, Clarke LA, Rommens JM, Hayden MR: Cloning and mapping of the α-adducin gene close to D4S95 and assessment of its relationship to Huntington disease. *Hum Mol Genet* **9**:669, 1992.
343. Ambrose C, James M, Barnes G, Lin C, Bates G, Altherr M, Duyao M, Groot N, Church D, Wasmuth JJ, Lehrach H, Housman D, Buckler A, Gudella JF, MacDonald ME: A novel G protein-coupled receptor kinase cloned from 4p16.3. *Hum Mol Genet* **1**:697, 1992.
344. Goldberg YP, Rommens JM, Andrew SE, Hutchinson GB, Lin B-Y, Theilmann J, Graham R, Glaves ML, Starr E, McDonald H, Nasir J, Schappert K, Kalchman MA, Clarke LA, Hayden MR: Identification of an Alu transposition event in close proximity to a strong candidate gene for Huntington disease. *Nature* **362**:370, 1993.
345. Rommens JM, Lin B-Y, Hutchinson GB, Andrew SE, Goldberg YP, Glaves ML, Graham R, Lai V, McArthur J, Nasir J, Theilmann J, McDonald H, Kalchman M, Clarke LA, Schappert K, Hayden MR: A transcription map of the region containing the Huntington disease gene. *Hum Mol Genet* **2**:901, 1993.
346. The Huntington's Disease Collaborative Research Group: A novel gene containing a trinucleotide repeat that is expanded and unstable on Huntington's disease chromosomes. *Cell* **72**:971, 1993.
347. Lin B-Y, Rommens JM, Graham RK, Kalchman MA, McDonald H, Nasir J, Delaney A, Goldberg YP, Hayden MR: Differential 3′ polyadenylation of the Huntington disease gene results in two mRNA species with variable tissue expression. *Hum Mol Genet* **2**:1541, 1993.
348. Andrew SE, Goldberg YP, Kremer B, Telenius H, Theilmann J, Adam S, Starr E, Squitieri F, Lin B, Kalchman MA, Graham RK, Hayden MR: The relationship between trinucleotide repeat length (CAG) and clinical features of Huntington disease. *Nat Genet* **4**:398, 1993.
349. Norremolle A, Riess O, Epplen JT, Fenger K, Hasholt L, Sorenson SA: Trinucleotide repeat elongation in the Huntington gene in Huntington disease patients from 71 Danish families. *Hum Mol Genet* **2**:1475, 1993.
350. Snell RG, MacMillan JC, Cheadle JP, Fenton I, Lazarou LP, Davies P, MacDonald ME, Gusella JF, Harper PS, Shaw DJ: Relationship between trinucleotide repeat expansion and phenotypic variation in Huntington's disease. *Nat Genet* **4**:393, 1993.
351. Duyao M, Ambrose C, Myers R, Novelletto A, Persichetti F, Frontali M, Folstein S, Ross C, Franz M, Abbott M, Gray J, Conneally P, Young A, Penney J, Hollingsworth Z, Shoulson I, Lazzarini A, Falek A, Koroshetz W, Sax D, Bird E, Vonsattel J, Bonilla E, Alvir J, Bickham Conde J, Cha J-H, Dure I, Gomez F, Ramos M, Sanchez-Ramos J, Snodgrass S, de Young M, Wexler N, Moscowitz C, Penchaszadeh G, MacFarlane H, Anderson M, Jenkins B, Srinidhi J, Barnes G, Gusella J, MacDonald M: Trinucleotide repeat length instability and age of onset in Huntington's disease. *Nat Genet* **4**:387, 1993.
352. Stevens DL: The heterozygote frequency for Huntington's chorea, in Barbeau A, Chase TN, Paulson GW (eds): *Huntington's Chorea: 1872–1972*. New York, Raven, 1973, pp 191–198.
353. Vogel F, Motuksky AG: *Human Genetics*, 2d ed. New York, Springer-Verlag, 1986.
354. Goldberg YP, Kremer B, Andew SE, Theilmann J, Graham RK, Squitieri F, Telenius H, Adam S, Sajoo A, Starr E, Heiberg A, Wolff G, Hayden MR: Molecular analysis of new mutations causing Huntington disease: Identification of a premutation and sex of origin effects. *Nat Genet* **5**:174, 1993.
355. Telenius H, Kremer HPH, Theilmann J, Andrew SE, Almquist E, Anvret M, Greenberg C, Greenberg J, Lucotte G, Squitieri FS, Starr E, Goldberg YP, Hayden MR: Molecular analysis of juvenile Huntington disease: The major influence of paternal descent on $(CAG)_n$ repeat length. *Hum Mol Genet* **2**:1535, 1993.

356. Kremer B, Goldberg P, Andrew SE, Squitieri F, Theilmann J, Telenius H, Zeisler J, Lin B, Adam S, Benjamin C, Hayden MR, and the International Huntington Disease Research Group: Worldwide distribution of the Huntington disease mutation: The sensitivity and specificity of CAG repeat length assessment. *N Engl J Med* (in press)

357. Myers RH, MacDonald ME, Koroshetz WJ, Duyao MP, Ambrose CM, Taylor SAM, Barnes G, Srinidhi J, Lin CS, Whaley WL, Lazzarini AM, Schwartz M, Wolff G, Bird ED, Vonsattel J-PG, & Gusella JF: De novo expansion of a $(CAG)_n$ repeat in sporadic Huntington's disease. *Nat Genet* **5(2):**168, 1993.

CHAPTER 153

Prion Diseases

Stanley B. Prusiner

1. **Many advances in our knowledge of the transmissible pathogens causing scrapie and other transmissible neurodegenerative diseases over the past decade support the hypothesis that these pathogens are novel and different from both viroids and viruses. After convincing evidence was obtained showing that scrapie infectivity depends on a protein component, the term "prion" was introduced to distinguish these infectious pathogens from others including viroids and viruses.**

2. **Enriching fractions from Syrian hamster (SHa) brain for scrapie prion infectivity led to the discovery of the prion protein (PrP). Determination of the N-terminal sequence of the protease-resistant core of PrP permitted retrieval of molecular clones encoding PrP from cDNA libraries. The finding of PrP mRNA in uninfected tissues led to discovery of the normal PrP isoform, denoted PrP^{C}, while the abnormal PrP isoform is designated PrP^{Sc}. Immunoaffinity chromatography with monoclonal antibodies to PrP 27-30 demonstrated copurification of PrP^{Sc} and scrapie infectivity. The prion diseases include scrapie of sheep, transmissible mink encephalopathy (TME), chronic wasting disease (CWD) of mule deer and elk, bovine spongiform encephalopathy (BSE) of cattle, feline spongiform encephalopathy (FSE), exotic ungulate encephalopathy, as well as kuru, Creutzfeldt-Jakob disease (CJD), Gerstmann-Sträussler-Scheinker syndrome (GSS) and fatal familial insomnia of humans.**

3. **Transgenic (Tg) mice expressing both SHa and mouse (Mo) PrP genes were used to probe the molecular basis of the species barrier and the mechanism of scrapie prion replication. Four Tg lines expressing SHa PrP exhibited distinct incubation times ranging from 48 to 277 days after SHa prion inoculation, which were inversely correlated with the steady state levels of SHaPrP mRNA and $SHaPrP^{C}$. Bioassays of brain extracts from two scrapie-infected Tg lines showed that the prion inoculum dictates which prions are synthesized *de novo,* even though the cells express both PrP genes. Tg mice inoculated with SHa prions had $\sim10^9$ median infective dose (ID_{50}) units of SHa prions per gram of brain, while <10 units of Mo prions were found. Conversely, Tg mice inoculated with Mo prions had $\sim10^6$ ID_{50} units of Mo prions and <10 units of SHa prions. These results argue that the species barrier for scrapie prions resides in the primary structure of PrP and formation of infectious prions is initiated by a species-specific interaction between PrP^{Sc} in the inoculum and homologous PrP^{C}. Studies on Syrian, Armenian, and Chinese hamsters suggest that the domain of the PrP molecule between codons 100 and 120 controls both the length of the incubation time and the deposition of PrP in amyloid plaques.**

4. **Ataxic GSS in families shows genetic linkage to a mutation in the PrP gene leading to the substitution of Leu for Pro at codon 102. Discovery of a point mutation in the PrP gene from humans with GSS and familial CJD established that prion diseases are unique among human illnesses—they are both genetic and infectious. Tg mice expressing MoPrP with the GSS point mutation have spontaneous neurologic dysfunction, spongiform degeneration, and astrocytic gliosis. Inoculation of brain extracts prepared from these Tg(GSSMoPrP) mice into Syrian hamsters and Tg mice expressing PrP transgenes has produced neurodegeneration in recipient animals after prolonged incubation times. If convincing data on serial passage of prions from the inoculated recipients can be obtained, then these results will argue that prions are devoid of foreign nucleic acid. The foregoing investigations have revised thinking about sporadic CJD, suggesting that it may arise from a somatic mutation.**

5. **Pulse-chase radiolabeling experiments of scrapie-infected cultures of mouse neuroblastoma cells indicate that protease-resistant PrP^{Sc} is synthesized during the chase period with $t_{1/2}$ ~1 to 3 h from a protease-sensitive precursor, consistent with the conclusion that PrP^{C} and PrP^{Sc} differ due to a posttranslational event. The acquisition of PrP protease resistance in scrapie-infected cultured cells was found to be independent of Asn-linked glycosylation. Neither tunicamycin nor mutation of Asn-linked glycosylation sites prevented PrP^{Sc} formation. PrP^{C} is bound to external surface of cells by a glycoinositol-phospholipid anchor. In**

A list of standard abbreviations is located immediately preceding the index in each volume. Additional abbreviations used in this chapter include: AD = Alzheimer's disease; AH = amphipathic helix (domain); BSE = bovine spongiform encephalopathy; CJD = Creutzfeldt-Jakob disease; CSF = cerebrospinal fluid; CWD = chronic wasting disease; FSE = feline spongiform encephalopathy; GPI = glycosyl-phosphaditylinositol; GSS = Gerstmann-Sträussler-Scheinker syndrome; HGH = human growth hormone; Mo = mouse; NFT = neurofibrillary tangle; ORF = open reading frame; *Pid-1* = gene in mice on chromosome 17 that controls Creutzfeldt-Jakob disease and probably scrapie incubation times; Prn = prion gene complex formed by *Prn-i* and *Prn-p*; *Prn-i* = gene in mice on chromosome 2 controlling experimental scrapie and Creutzfeldt-Jakob disease incubation times; PRNP = PrP gene in humans located on chromosome 20; PrP = prion protein; PrP 27-30 = limited digestion of PrP^{Sc} with proteinase K generates PrP 27-30; PrP^{C} = cellular isoform of the prion protein; PrP^{Sc} = scrapie isoform of the prion protein; SAF = scrapie-associated fibril; SHa = Syrian hamster; *Sinc* = gene in mice controlling experimental scrapie incubation times (this genetic locus is probably the same as *Prn-i*); STE = stop transfer effector (domain); Tg = transgenic; TM = transmembrane (domain); TME = transmissible mink encephalopathy.

contrast, PrP^{Sc} accumulates within cytoplasmic vesicles of cultured cells.

6. **Attempts to demonstrate a scrapie-specific nucleic acid within highly purified preparations of prions have been unrewarding to date.[1] These observations are in accord with the preliminary findings noted above that brain extracts prepared from Tg(GSSMoPrP) mice with spontaneous neurodegeneration transmit central nervous system disease to inoculated recipients and with many unsuccessful attempts to inactivate prion infectivity by procedures that specifically hydrolyze or modify nucleic acids.[2] Although it seems likely that transmissible prions are composed only of PrP^{Sc} molecules, a hypothetical second component such as a small polynucleotide remains a formal possibility.**
7. **Studies on the structure of PrP^{Sc} and PrP^{C} have been unsuccessful in defining a posttranslational chemical modification that distinguishes one PrP isoform from the other. These findings suggest that the difference between PrP^{Sc} and PrP^{C} may be conformational. Distinct prion isolates or "strains" produce different patterns of PrP^{Sc} accumulation. The molecular mechanism responsible for these different isolates of prions remains to be established. Whether distinct prion isolates result from multiple conformers of PrP^{Sc} or they arise from differences in Asn-linked oligosaccharides is unknown. The study of prion diseases seems to be emerging as a unique area of investigation at the interface of such disciplines as genetics, cell biology, and virology.**

The prion diseases are a group of neurodegenerative diseases of animals and humans.[1,2] They are transmissible under some circumstances, but unlike other transmissible disorders, the prion diseases can also be caused by mutations in the prion protein (PrP), which is encoded by a chromosomal gene. Six diseases of animals and four of humans are caused by prions (Table 153-1). Scrapie of sheep and goats is the prototypic prion disease. Transmissible mink encepalopathy (TME), chronic wasting disease (CWD), bovine spongiform encephalopathy (BSE), feline spongiform encephalopathy (FSE), and exotic ungulate encephalopathy are all thought to occur after the consumption of prion-infected foodstuffs. Similarly, kuru of the Papua New Guinea Fore people is thought to have resulted from the consumption of brains from dying relatives during ritualistic cannibalism.[3,4] Creutzfeldt-Jakob disease (CJD) occurs primarily as a sporadic disorder,[5] but iatrogenic CJD is thought to result from the accidental inoculation of patients with prions.[6,7] Familial CJD, Gerstmann-Sträussler-Scheinker syndrome (GSS), and fatal familial insomnia are all dominantly inherited prion diseases that have been shown to be caused by mutations in the PrP gene.[8–11]

From studies of a once obscure disease of sheep, a new area of biologic research is beginning to emerge. For many decades, scrapie was considered an enigmatic disorder of sheep and goats, the etiology of which was unknown. By 1938, experimental transfer of scrapie from one sheep to another began to argue for an infectious etiology.[12] Meanwhile, observations that the genetic backgrounds of flocks profoundly influence their susceptibility to scrapie raised the possibility that scrapie might be an inherited disorder.[13] These opposing views sparked many controversial encounters[14,15] and foreshadowed a series of equally bitter arguments about the possible structure of the transmissible scrapie agent.[16]

A decade has passed since the term "prion" was introduced[17] and the prion protein discovered.[18,19] Prions are defined as small proteinaceous infectious particles that resist inactivation by procedures that modify nucleic acids.[17] Although the notion of prions was initially met with considerable skepticism, the steady accumulation of experimental data over the past 10 years has created a rather convincing argument that prions are unique among all infectious pathogens.[2,17] While the human prion diseases once presented a rather confusing picture, the finding that prion diseases may be both inherited and transmissible has begun to bring some clarity. The situation with the natural prion diseases of animals remains more problematic. Progress in understanding the human prion diseases has its roots in their transmission to animals[20] and the discovery of the prion protein[18,19] followed by the molecular cloning of the PrP gene.[21–23]

As molecular biologic and genetic analyses of both the human and animal prion diseases have advanced, the biochemistry of the prion protein has continued to pose both methodologic and conceptual problems. For example, transmissible prions are composed largely, if not entirely, of an abnormal isoform of cellular PrP designated PrP^{Sc}.[2,24] Although PrP^{Sc} is synthesized from cellular PrP (PrP^{C}) by a posttranslational process,[25–28] the precise nature of this protein transformation remains unknown. Whether the conversion of PrP^{C} to PrP^{Sc} involves an as yet unidentified chemical modification, perhaps labile under the conditions of analysis or only involves a conformational change[29] remains to be established. Furthermore, the function of PrP^{C} is unknown, but PrP^{C} molecules appear to be unnecessary, since mice homologous for disruption of the PrP gene develop normally and are healthy for more than 24 months.[30] These results argue that scrapie and the other prion diseases do not result from an inhibition of PrP^{C} function due to PrP^{Sc} but rather the accumulation of PrP^{Sc} interferes with some as yet undefined cellular process.

INFECTIOUS, SPORADIC, AND GENETIC FORMS OF PRION DISEASES

The three human prion diseases (kuru, CJD, and GSS) are likely to be variants of the same disorder, and they share many features. By analogy with studies on experimental scrapie, it seems likely that all three of these human diseases will require the appearance of an abnormal isoform of the prion protein. The prion protein is encoded by a single-copy gene in rodents and probably in humans.[22,25,31]

The human prion diseases illustrate three manifestations of central nervous system degeneration—infectious, sporadic, and inherited forms. The three human prion diseases have been transmitted to experimental animals.[5,32,33] Kuru is thought to have been spread exclusively through the slow infectious mechanism by ritualistic cannibalism.[3,4]

While a few CJD cases can be attributed to inoculation with prions—for example, human growth hormone (HGH), cornea transplantation, and cerebral electrode implantation—most are sporadic despite considerable effort to implicate scrapie-infected sheep as an exogenous source of prions.[34–36] Although sporadic CJD could be explained by prions being ubiquitous in our food chain with their efficiency of infection being very low, there is no evidence to support this hypothesis. Of note, infection by the oral route is 10^9 times less efficient than intracerebral inoculation in hamsters.[37] Whether CJD can arise endogenously without

Table 153-1 Prion Diseases*

Disease	Natural Host
Scrapie	Sheep and goats
Transmissible mink encephalopathy (TME)	Mink
Chronic wasting disease (CWD)	Mule deer and elk
Bovine spongiform encephalopathy (BSE)†	Cattle
Feline spongiform encephalopathy (FSE)	Cats
Exotic ungulate encephalopathy	Nyala and greater kudu
Kuru	Humans—Papua New Guinea Fore people
Creutzfeldt-Jakob disease (CJD)	Humans
Gerstmann-Sträussler-Scheinker syndrome (GSS)	Humans
Fatal familial insomnia	Humans

*Alternative terminologies include slow virus infections, subacute transmissible spongiform encephalopathies, and unconventional slow virus diseases.[4]
†BSE is frequently called "mad cow disease."

any exogenous prion source remains to be established but somatic mutation of the PrP gene seems a much more likely mechanism, as discussed below.[2,38]

About 10 to 15 percent of cases of CJD and virtually all of GSS are inherited. These diseases as well as fatal familial insomnia are caused by germ-line mutations in the PrP gene. Twelve mutations of the PrP gene have been genetically linked to the development of the human prion diseases. Although some investigators argue that PrP^C is a receptor for the putative scrapie "virus" and mutations in PrP^C render people more susceptible to this ubiquitous "virus," there is no evidence to support such a hypothesis.

TERMINOLOGY

The term *prion* is used to denote the small proteinaceous infectious particles that resist inactivation by procedures that modify nucleic acids (Table 153-2). Prions cause scrapie and other related transmissible neurodegenerative diseases of animals and humans (see Table 153-1). Prions are composed largely, if not entirely, of a protein designated as the scrapie isoform of the prion protein, or PrP^{Sc}. A posttranslational process, as yet undefined, generates PrP^{Sc} from the normal, cellular isoform of the prion protein designated PrP^C. A major feature that distinguishes prions from viruses is the finding that both PrP isoforms are encoded by a chromosomal gene. In humans the PrP gene is designated PRNP and is located on the short arm of chromosome 20. The McKusick catalogue number is 176640.[39] In mice, the PrP gene is designated *Prn-p* and is located on chromosome 2. PrP^{Sc} is readily distinguished from PrP^C by its different biochemical and biophysical properties. Limited proteolysis of PrP^{Sc} produces a smaller protease-resistant molecule of ~131 amino acids designated PrP 27-30; under the same conditions, PrP^C is completely hydrolyzed. In the presence of detergent, PrP 27-30 polymerizes into amyloid rods. These prion amyloid rods formed by limited proteolysis and detergent extraction are indistinguishable from the filaments that aggregate to form PrP amyloid plaques in the central nervous system. Both the rods and the PrP amyloid filaments found in brain tissue exhibit similar ultrastructural morphology and green-gold birefringence after staining with Congo red dye. To differentiate the amyloid plaques found in the prion diseases from those found in aged brains, Alzheimer's disease (AD) and Down syndrome, it is suggested that the former be labeled "PrP plaques" and the latter be called "β plaques."[40]

The term *scrapie-associated fibrils* (SAF) continues to be used by some investigators as a synonym for the prion rods, even though the ultrastructure of these polymers was used to differentiate them from amyloids.[41]

Four diseases of humans are caused by prions or mutations in the PrP gene: kuru, CJD, GSS, and FFI (see Table 153-1). While kuru is confined to the mountainous Fore region of Papua New Guinea, the other three diseases are found worldwide. To distinguish between these three disorders is increasingly difficult, with the recognition that familial CJD, GSS, and fatal familial insomnia are autosomal dominant diseases caused by mutations in the PRNP gene. Initially, we thought that a specific PrP mutation was very frequently associated with a particular clinical and neuropathological presentation.[8] While that is often the case, an increasing number of exceptions are beginning to accumulate. In a single family with a particular PrP mutation, different clinical and neuropathological manifestations of the same

Table 153-2 Glossary of Prion Terminology

Pid-1	Gene in mice on chromosome 17 controlling CJD and probably scrapie incubation times.
Prion	Small proteinaceous infectious particle that resists inactivation by procedures that modify nucleic acids. Prions are composed largely, if not entirely of PrP^{Sc} molecules; they cause scrapie of animals and related neurodegenerative diseases of humans such as CJD. *Scrapie agent* is a synonym.
Prion rod	An aggregate of prions composed largely, if not entirely, of PrP 27-30 molecules. Created by detergent extraction and limited proteolysis of PrP^{Sc}. Morphologically and histochemically indistinguishable from many amyloids.
Prn-i	Gene in mice on chromosome 2 controlling experimental scrapie and CJD incubation times. *Prn-i* and *Prn-p* form the prion gene complex (*Prn*).
Prn-p	PrP gene in mice located on chromosome 2.
PRNP	PrP gene in humans located on chromosome 20.
PrP 27-30	Digestion of PrP^{Sc} with proteinase K generates PrP 27-30 by hydrolysis of the N-terminal ~67 amino acids.
PrP amyloid plaque	Amyloid plaque composed of PrP in the brain of an animal or human with a prion disease.
PrP^C	Cellular isoform of the prion protein.
PrP^{Sc}	Scrapie isoform of the prion protein. This protein is the only identifiable macromolecule in purified preparations of scrapie prions.
Sinc	Gene in mice controlling experimental scrapie incubation times. This genetic locus is probably the same as *Prn-i*.

genetic disease can be seen.[42] These different constellations of central nervous system symptoms, signs, and neuropathological lesions would seem to render the old system of classification obsolete since the precise chemical cause is now known. Instead, it has been suggested that these disorders be labeled "prion diseases," followed by the mutation. For example, most patients with a PrP mutation at codon 102 present primarily with ataxia and have PrP amyloid plaques; these patients are generally labeled GSS but a few within these families present with a dementing disorder characteristic of CJD. Would it not be most expeditious to give these patients the diagnosis of prion disease codon 102?

The proposal for a new terminology delineated above is likely to be adopted over the next decade since it is based on the molecular lesion and not on phenotypic features described in clinical or pathological terms. Yet, in the interest of clarity, some aspects of current terminology are retained in this manuscript.

BIOASSAYS OF PRION INFECTIVITY

The experimental transmission of scrapie from sheep[43] to mice[44] gave investigators a more convenient laboratory model, which yielded considerable information on the nature of the unusual infectious pathogen that causes scrapie.[45–51] Yet progress was slow because quantitation of infectivity in a single sample required holding 60 mice for 1 year before accurate scoring could be accomplished.[44] The availability of a more rapid and economical bioassay for the scrapie agent in Syrian golden hamsters accelerated purification of the infectious particles.[52,53]

Bioassays for transmission of the human prion diseases to experimental animals was initially confined to apes and monkeys. The incubation periods were quite prolonged (Table 153-3), making experimental studies difficult. Subsequently, CJD and GSS were transmitted to laboratory rodents with incubation times comparable to those observed in experimental scrapie.[54,55]

Table 153-3 Incubation Periods and Durations of Illness in Creutzfeldt-Jakob Disease and Kuru (Months)

	Incubation Period		Duration of Illness	
Host	CJD	Kuru	CJD	Kuru
Natural				
Humans	18–360	60–360	1–55	3–12
Experimental				
Apes	11–71	10–82	1–6	1–15
Monkeys	4–73	8–92	1–27	1–23
Sheep				
Goats	36–48	39		2–6
Ferrets		18–71		
Mink		45		
Domestic cats	19–30	2–6		
Guinea pigs	7–16	1		
Hamsters	5–18			
Mice	3–20	1–2		

*Data compiled from refs 3, 54, 55, 256, 455–458, and Hadlow WJ: unpublished observations.
SOURCE: From Prusiner et al.[459]

HYPOTHESES ON THE NATURE OF THE SCRAPIE AGENT

The literature on scrapie contains a fascinating record of all the structural hypotheses proposed to explain the physicochemical structure of the infectious particles (Table 153-4). Among the earliest hypotheses was the notion that scrapie was a disease of muscle caused by the parasite Sarcosporidia.[56,57] With the successful transmission of scrapie to animals, the hypothesis that scrapie is caused by a "filterable" virus became popular.[12,58] A few investigators continue to persist with the belief that scrapie is caused by a virus, despite much evidence to the contrary. With the findings of Tikvah Alper and her colleagues that scrapie infectivity resists inactivation by UV and ionizing radiation,[45,46] a myriad of hypotheses on the chemical nature of the scrapie agent emerged. Among the hypothetical structures proposed were a small DNA virus,[59] a replicating protein,[49,51,60,61] replicating abnormal polysaccharide with membranes,[48,62] a DNA subvirus controlled by a transmissible linkage substance,[63,64] and a provirus consisting of recessive genes generating RNA particles.[14,65] Based on the resistance of scrapie infectivity to inactivation by UV and ionizing radiation,[45,46] it was proposed that the scrapie agent might be a naked nucleic acid similar to plant viroids.[66] Subsequent studies showed that suggestion to be incorrect.[67] The term "unconventional virus" was proposed, but no structural details were ever given with respect to how these unconventional virions differ from the conventional virus particles.[4] Some investigators have suggested that this term obscured the ignorance that continued to shroud the infectious scrapie agent[16]; in retrospect, that view was correct. Other suggestions included: aggregated conventional virus with unusual properties,[68] replicating polysaccharide,[69] nucleoprotein complex,[70] nucleic acid surrounded by a polysaccharide coat,[71–73] spiroplasma-like organism,[74,75] multicomponent system with one component quite small,[76,77] membrane-bound DNA,[78] virino (viroid-like DNA complexed with host proteins), filamentous

Table 153-4 Hypotheses on the Nature of the Scrapie Agent*

Sarcosporidia-like parasite
"Filterable" virus
Small DNA virus
Replicating protein
Replicating abnormal polysaccharide with membranes
DNA subvirus controlled by a transmissible linkage substance
Provirus consisting of recessive genes generating RNA particles
Naked nucleic acid similar to plant viroids
Unconventional virus
Aggregated conventional virus with unusual properties
Replicating polysaccharide
Nucleoprotein complex
Nucleic acid surrounded by a polysaccharide coat
Spiroplasma-like organism
Multicomponent system with one component quite small
Membrane-bound DNA
Virino (viroid-like DNA complexed with host proteins)
Filamentous animal virus (SAF)
Aluminum–silicate amyloid complex
Computer virus

*References cited in text.

animal virus (SAF),[79] aluminum–silicate amyloid complex, and a computer virus.[80]

PURIFICATION OF SCRAPIE INFECTIVITY

Many investigators attempted to purify the scrapie agent for several decades, but with relatively little success. The slow, cumbersome, and tedious bioassays in sheep and later mice greatly limited the number of samples that could be analyzed. Since the ease of purifying any biologically active macromolecule is directly related to the rapidity of the assays, it is not surprising that little progress was made with sheep and goats, where only very limited numbers of samples could be analyzed and incubation times exceeding 18 months were required.[16,81–83] Experimental transmission of scrapie to mice allowed many more samples to be analyzed, but 1 year was required to complete the measurement of scrapie infectivity by end-point titration using 60 animals to evaluate one sample.[44]

The transmission of scrapie to Syrian hamsters by an inoculum previously passaged in rats produced disease in about 70 days.[84] These shorter incubation times coupled with the development of standard curves relating the length of the incubation time to the size of the inoculated dose permitted much more rapid quantitation of specimens.[52,53] This methodologic advance made possible the development of protocols for the significant enrichment of scrapie infectivity.[19,85,86]

DEVELOPMENT OF THE PRION CONCEPT

With partially purified fractions of scrapie agent from hamster brain, it became possible to demonstrate that procedures that modify or hydrolyze proteins produce a diminution in scrapie infectivity.[17,87] At the same time, tests done in search of a scrapie-specific nucleic acid were unable to demonstrate any dependence of infectivity on a polynucleotide,[17] in agreement with earlier studies reporting the extreme resistance of infectivity to UV irradiation at 254 nm.[46]

Based on these observations, it seemed likely that the infectious pathogen capable of transmitting scrapie was neither a virus nor a viroid. For this reason, the term *prion* was introduced to embolden the concept that the scrapie agent was likely to be unique in its molecular structure.[17] Indeed, considerable evidence has accumulated over the past decade to support this hypothesis.[2,88] Furthermore, the replication of prions and their mode of pathogenesis also appear to be unique and without precedent.

DISCOVERY OF THE PRION PROTEIN

Once it was established that scrapie prion infectivity depended on protein,[87] the search for a scrapie-specific protein intensified. While the insolubility of scrapie infectivity made purification problematic, we took advantage of this property, along with its relative resistance to degradation by proteases, to extend the degree of purification. Radioiodination of partially purified fractions revealed a protein unique to preparations from scrapie-infected brains.[18,19] This protein was later named prion protein (PrP) with an apparent, M_r of 27 to 30 (PrP 27-30).[89]

Subsequent studies showed that PrP 27-30 is derived from a larger protein of M_r 33 to 35 designated PrP^{Sc}.[22,90] At the same time, it was found that the brains of normal and scrapie-infected hamsters express similar levels of PrP mRNA and a protease-sensitive prion protein designated PrP^C.[22] PrP^C or a subset of PrP molecules are the substrate for PrP^{Sc}. Many lines of evidence argue that PrP^{SC} is an essential component of the infectious prion particle (Table 153-5). To date, all attempts to find a second prion component have been unsuccessful.

The function of PrP^C is unknown, although it has been suggested that a PrP-like molecule from chickens may have acetylcholine receptor–inducing activity.[91] Furthermore, PrP^C does not seem to be essential, at least in young mice, since disruption of the PrP gene has not caused any detectable abnormalities in the nervous, musculoskeletal or lymphoreticular systems at 9 months of age.[30] Perhaps, the absence of PrP^C will result in abnormalities later in life, as is the case for the p53 tumor-suppressor protein—young animals lacking p53 are normal, but as they age neoplasms develop.[92]

Table 153-5 Evidence that PrP^{SC} is a Major and Necessary Component of the Infectious Prion

1. Copurification of PrP 27-30 and scrapie infectivity by biochemical methods. Concentration of PrP 27-30 is proportional to prion titer.[18,19,89,460–462]
2. Kinetics of proteolytic digestions of PrP 27-30 and infectivity are similar.[18,19,89]
3. Copurification of PrP^{Sc} and infectivity by immunoaffinity chromatography. α-PrP antiserum neutralization of infectivity.[24,99]
4. PrP^{Sc} detected only in clones of cultured cells producing infectivity.[168,170,172]
5. PrP amyloid plaques are specific for prion diseases of animals and humans.[40,110,112,113] Deposition of PrP amyloid is controlled, at least in part, by the PrP sequence.[156]
6. Correlation between PrP^{Sc} (or PrP^{CJD}) in brain tissue and prion diseases in animals and humans.[93,262,263]
7. Genetic linkage between mouse PrP gene and scrapie incubation times.[184–187] PrP gene of mice with long incubation times encodes amino acid substitutions at codons 108 and 189, as compared to mice with short or intermediate incubation times.[134]
8. Syrian hamster PrP transgene and PrP^{Sc} in the inoculum govern the "species barrier," scrapie incubation times, neuropathology, and prion synthesis in mice.[156,428]
9. Genetic linkage between human PrP gene mutation at codon 102 and development of GSS.[42] Association between codon 200 point mutation or codon 53 insertion of six additional octarepeats and familial CJD.[9,375–377,379, 393]
10. Mice expressing mouse PrP transgenes with the point mutation of GSS have spontaneous neurologic dysfunction, spongiform brain degeneration, and astrocytic gliosis.[259]

SOURCE: From Prusiner.[463]

PRION PROTEIN AMYLOID

The discovery of PrP 27-30 in fractions enriched for scrapie infectivity was accompanied by the identification of rod-shaped particles.[19,85] In fractions containing human CJD

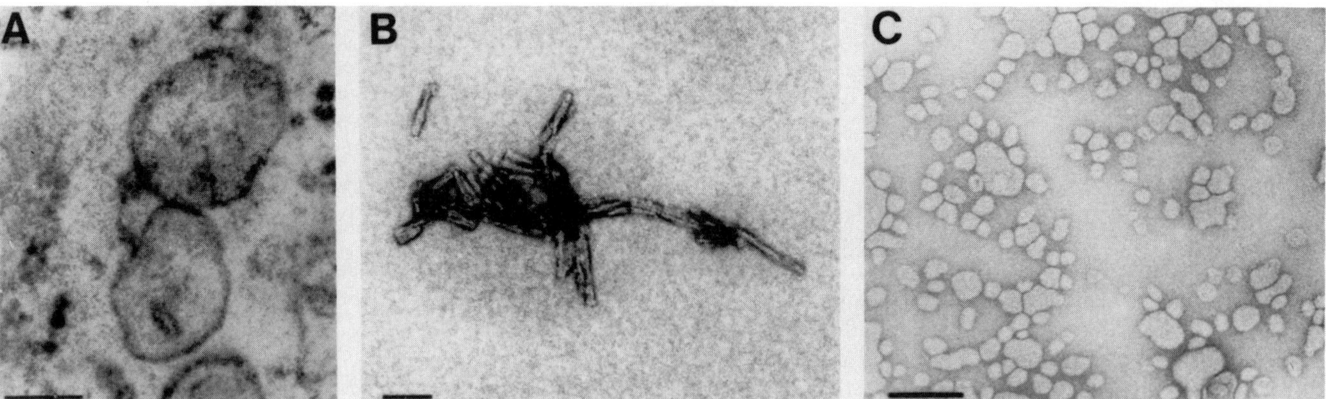

FIG. 153-1 Multiple forms of scrapie prions isolated from infected Syrian hamster brains. *A*. Microsomal membranes containing prions. *B*. Purified prion rods are generated by limited proteolysis and detergent extraction of membranes isolated from scrapie infected brain. *C*. Prion liposomes generated by sonication of rods isolated by sucrose gradient sedimentation with phosphatidylcholine. All three forms contain high levels of prion infectivity ($>10^7$ ID_{50} units/ml). Bars are 100 nm. *(Adapted from refs. 98 and 264.)*

prion proteins, rod-shaped particles were also found by electron microscopy after negative staining.[93] Most of the particles were of uniform diameter of ~11 nm; their mean lengths were ~165 nm, but they varied from 25 to 550 nm. The rods exhibited a smooth surface and appeared almost ribbon-like; infrequently, the rods were twisted. Many of the prion rods resemble purified amyloids both ultrastructurally and histochemically (Fig. 153-1)[85] as well as filamentous structures described earlier in thin sections of kuru, CJD, and scrapie-infected brain.[94–96]

The formation of prion rods requires limited proteolysis in the presence of detergent (see Fig. 153-1).[97] Thus, the prion rods in fractions enriched for scrapie infectivity are largely, if not entirely, artifacts of the purification protocol. Solubilization of PrP 27-30 into liposomes with retention of infectivity[98] demonstrated that large PrP polymers are not required for infectivity and permitted the immunoaffinity copurification of PrP^{Sc} and infectivity.[24,99]

Some investigators believe that SAF are synonymous with the prion rods and are composed of PrP even though these fibrils can be distinguished ultrastructurally and tinctorially from amyloid polymers.[41,79,86,100–105] These helically wound fibrils have a distinctive ultrastructural morphology and have been found in CJD and scrapie extracts.[41,106] The regularly twisted structure of the SAF has been used to distinguish them from amyloid,[41,106,107] and it has been suggested that they are the first example of filamentous animal viruses.[107,108] While the fibrils are presumed by some investigators to be composed of prion proteins,[86] these structures as originally described are found in neither purified preparations of prions nor infected tissues.[83,85,103,109–111]

Prion Protein Amyloid Plaques

The description of prion rods as a form of amyloid was followed by the demonstration that amyloid plaques in prion diseases contain PrP (Fig. 153-2), as determined by immunoreactivity[40,110,112,113] and eventually amino acid sequencing.[114,115]

The PrP amyloid plaques of CJD, kuru, and natural[5,20,116] and experimental scrapie are similar morphologically.[117] They consist of discrete eosinophilic glassy-appearing masses often having radiating amyloid fibrils at their periphery (see Fig. 153-2). Because this appearance of the plaques was first described in kuru, investigators sometimes refer to these types of plaques in CJD and scrapie as "kuru" plaques. The term "kuru" plaque has created considerable confusion. The PrP amyloid plaques of GSS are numerous and diffuse; they are often surrounded by smaller satellite plaques. Most of these plaques are found in the cerebellum, but they can also be found throughout the cerebral cortex, thalamus, and brain stem. Amyloid deposits also develop in and around small blood vessels in the central nervous system (see Fig. 153-2).

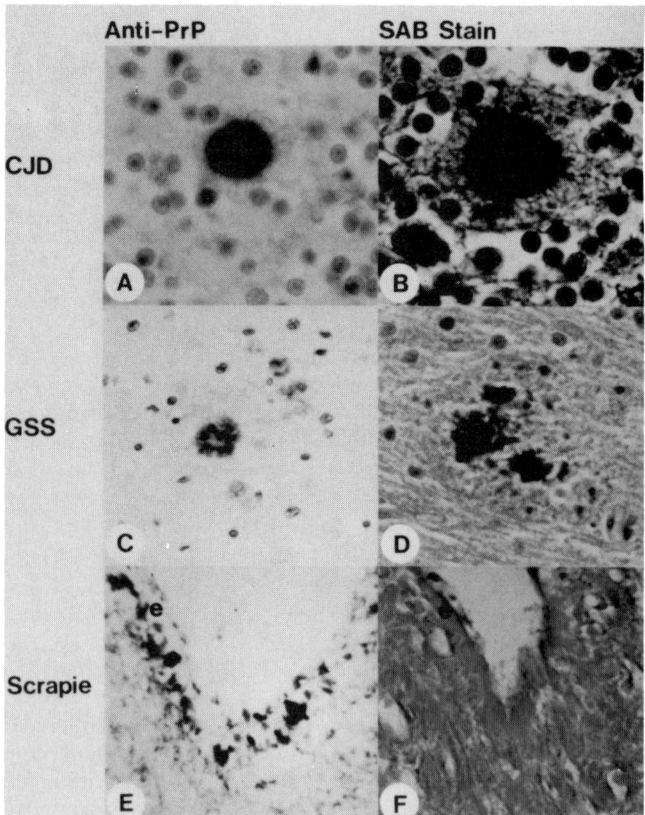

FIG. 153-2 Amyloid plaques in CJD (*A*, *B*), GSS (*C*, *D*), and scrapie (*E*, *F*), histochemically stained by the sulfated alcian blue (SAB) procedure and by peroxidase immunohistochemistry using PrP-specific antibodies. In scrapie, plaques are located beneath the ependyma. *(From Snow et al.*[123] *Used by permission.)*

PrP amyloid plaques have been found in the cerebellar cortex in natural sheep scrapie.[116] The plaques that develop in mice following intracerebral inoculation of scrapie prions were distributed among nerve-cell bodies in the hippocampus (dentate gyrus), thalamus, hypothalamus, cerebral cortex, granular-cell layer of the cerebellum, and medulla.[118,119] They were also located in the corpus callosum and along the intracerebral inoculation tract.

In studies by my colleagues and I of the hamster scrapie model, every terminally ill animal has had cerebral amyloid plaques.[110,112,120,121] The plaques were primarily subependymal, subpial, and perivascular; some were found in the cerebral neuropil and corpus callosum, but not in the cerebellum. Filaments that form the amyloid plaques stain with antiserums specific for the prion protein.[110] The anatomic distribution of the plaques may result in part from pathways of interstitial fluid flow. Based on the behavior of macromolecules injected into the brain, it has been postulated that there is a net bulk flow of fluid that presumably originates from the capillary–astrocyte complex and that flows toward the ependyma and pia by way of perivascular spaces.[122] Therefore, the following sequence of events might occur: (1) In the prion diseases, it is conceivable that PrP^{Sc} synthesized in neurons is released into the central nervous system extracellular space as a result of overproduction and focal nerve-cell membrane necrosis. (2) PrP^{Sc} is then carried to perivascular, subependymal, and subpial regions, where it polymerizes into insoluble amyloid filaments during limited proteolysis.[97] (3) The PrP amyloid filaments coalesce into amyloid plaques as a result of increased local concentration, the presence of sulfated glycosaminoglycans,[123,124] and/or the action of local cells such as macrophages.

PrP amyloid accumulates extracellularly like other amyloid deposits.[125–128] Although macrophages are not a characteristic feature of scrapie, a few are seen by electron microscopy in the vicinity of amyloid deposits in scrapie and are generally believed to play an important role in the formation of amyloid plaques.[125,127,129]

The senile amyloid plaques of AD do not react with PrP antiserums. This is in agreement with amino acid sequencing studies of the βA4 peptide, which is thought to be a major component of amyloid plaques in AD and Down syndrome[130,131]; the amino acid sequence of the AD amyloid protein exhibits no significant homology with PrP.

PRION PROTEIN GENE STRUCTURE AND ORGANIZATION

The entire open reading frame (ORF) of all known mammalian and avian PrP genes is contained within a single exon (Fig. 153-3).[25,42,132–134] This feature of the PrP gene eliminates the possibility that PrP^{Sc} arises from alternative RNA splicing[25,134,135]; however, mechanisms such as RNA editing and protein splicing remain a possibility.[136,137] The two exons of the Syrian hamster (SHa) PrP gene are separated by a 10-kb intron: exon 1 encodes a portion of the 5′ untranslated leader sequence, while exon 2 encodes the ORF and 3′ untranslated region.[25] The mouse (Mo) PrP gene is comprised of three exons, with exon 3 analogous to exon 2 of the hamster.[135] The promoters of both the SHa and Mo PrP genes contain copies of G-C–rich repeats 3 and 2, respectively, but are devoid of TATA boxes. These G-C nonamers represent a motif that may function as a canonical binding site for the transcription factor Sp1.[138]

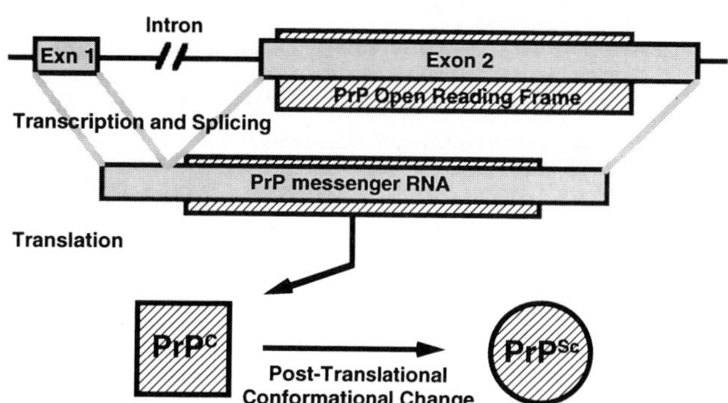

FIG. 153-3 Structure and organization of the chromosomal prion protein gene. In all mammals examined, the entire ORF is contained within a single exon. The 5′ untranslated region of the PrP mRNA is derived from either one or two additional exons [25,132] (and Westaway D, et al: unpublished data). Only one PrP mRNA has been detected. PrP^{Sc} is thought to be derived from PrP^C by a posttranslational process.[25–28,169] The amino acid sequence of PrP^{Sc} is identical to that predicted from the translated sequence of the DNA encoding the PrP gene,[25,29] and no unique posttranslational chemical modifications have been identified that might distinguish PrP^{Sc} from PrP^C. Thus, it seems likely that PrP^C undergoes a conformational change as it is converted to PrP^{Sc}.

Four regions of the mammalian PrP gene ORF are highly conserved when the translated amino acid sequences are compared (Fig. 153-4*A*)[22,23,25,139–143] (and Scott M, et al.: unpublished data). The Mo PrP sequence is ~30 percent homologous with chicken PrP.[91,133,144] Twenty-three of 24 amino acids encoded by Mo *Prn-p^a* correspond to codons 104 to 127 and are identical to those found in avian PrP. Within the N-terminal conserved regions of mammalian PrP, five Gly:Pro-rich octarepeats and two hexarepeats (Fig. 153-5) have been found, while chicken PrP has eight hexarepeats.

Mapping PrP genes to the short arm of human chromosome 20 and the homologous region of Mo chromosome 2

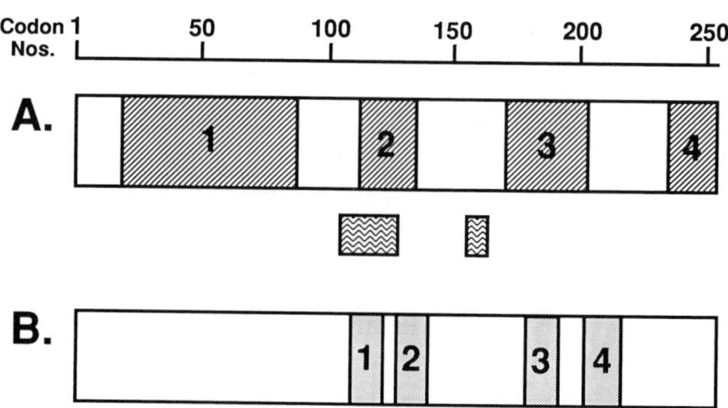

FIG. 153-4 Genetic map of PrP ORF and regions predicted to be α-helixes. Codon numbers are indicated at the top of the figure. *A*. Four regions among mammalian PrP molecules (hatched);[22,23,25,139–143,476] homologous regions of the chicken PrP (wave).[133,144] *B*. By comparing the amino acid sequences of 11 mammalian and one avian PrP, structural analyses predicted 4 α-helical regions, denoted H1 to H4. H1 corresponds to SHa PrP codons 109 to 122, H2 to codons 129 to 140, H3 to codons 178 to 191, and H4 to codons 202 to 218. The amino acid sequences of these peptides are given in Fig. 153-5. Peptides corresponding to these regions of the SHa PrP were synthesized and contrary to predictions, H1, H3, and H4 spontaneously formed amyloids as shown by electron microscopy and Congo red staining. By infrared spectroscopy, these amyloid peptides were found to exhibit a secondary structure comprised largely of β-sheets.

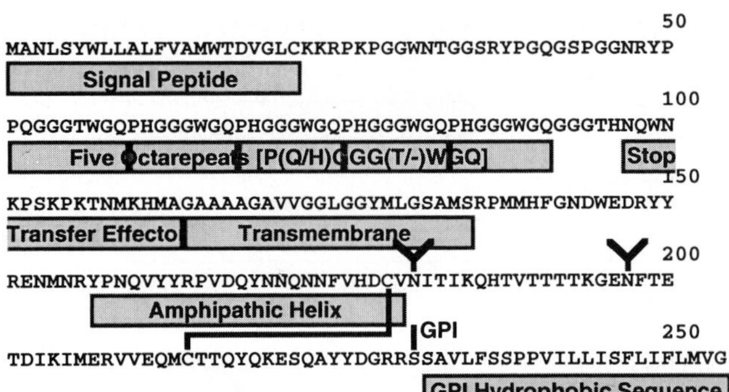

FIG. 153-5 Amino acid sequence and structural features of the SHaPrP. Codon numbers are indicated above the sequence. NH_2-terminal signal peptide of 22 amino acids is removed during biosynthesis.[22,25,460–462] The NH_2-terminal region contains five Gly-Pro-rich octarepeats and two hexarepeats; between codons 96 and 112 a domain controlling PrP topology is designated as the stop-transfer effector[176,177]; codons 113 to 135 encode a transmembrane α-helix; codons 157 to 177 encode an amphipathic helix,[176–180] and codons 232 to 254 encode a hydrophobic signal sequence that is removed when a glycosyl-phosphalidylinositol (GPI) anchor is added.[163,165] Both PrP isoforms contain a disulfide (S—S) bond between Cys 179 and Cys 214[461]; asparagine-linked glycosylation (Y) occurs at residues 181 and 197,[158–162] and a GPI anchor is attached to Ser 231.[165] The molecule denoted PrP 27-30 is derived from PrP^{Sc} by limited proteolysis that removes the NH_2-terminal 67 amino acids and leaves a protease-resistant core of 141 amino acids.[22,25]

argues for the existence of PrP genes prior to the speciation of mammals.[31,145–147] Hybridization studies demonstrated <0.002 PrP gene sequence per ID_{50} unit in purified prion fractions, indicating that a gene encoding PrP^{Sc} is not a component of the infectious prion particle.[22] This is a major feature that distinguishes prions from viruses, including retroviruses that carry cellular oncogenes, and from satellite viruses that derive their coat proteins from other viruses previously infecting plant cells.

EXPRESSION OF THE PRION PROTEIN GENE

Although PrP mRNA is constitutively expressed in the brains of adult animals,[22,23] it is highly regulated during development. In the septum, levels of PrP mRNA and choline acetyltransferase were found to increase in parallel during development.[148] In other brain regions, PrP gene expression occurred at an earlier age. *In situ* hybridization studies show that the highest levels of PrP mRNA are found in neurons.[149] In both adult and embryonic rodent organs, PrP gene expression is highest in neuronal cells but significant levels of expression have been recorded in other tissues.[22,149–151]

PrP^C expression in brain was defined by standard immunohistochemistry[121] and by histoblotting (Fig. 153-6).[152] Immunostaining of PrP^C in the SHa brain was most intense in the stratum radiatum and stratum oriens of the CA1 region of the hippocampus and was virtually absent from the granule-cell layer of the dentate gyrus and the pyramidal cell layer throughout Ammon's horn. PrP^{Sc} staining was minimal in these regions, which were intensely stained for PrP^C. A similar relationship between PrP^C and PrP^{Sc} was found in the amygdala. In contrast, PrP^{Sc} accumulated in the medial habenular nucleus, the medial septal nuclei, and the diagonal band of Broca; these areas were virtually devoid of PrP^C.

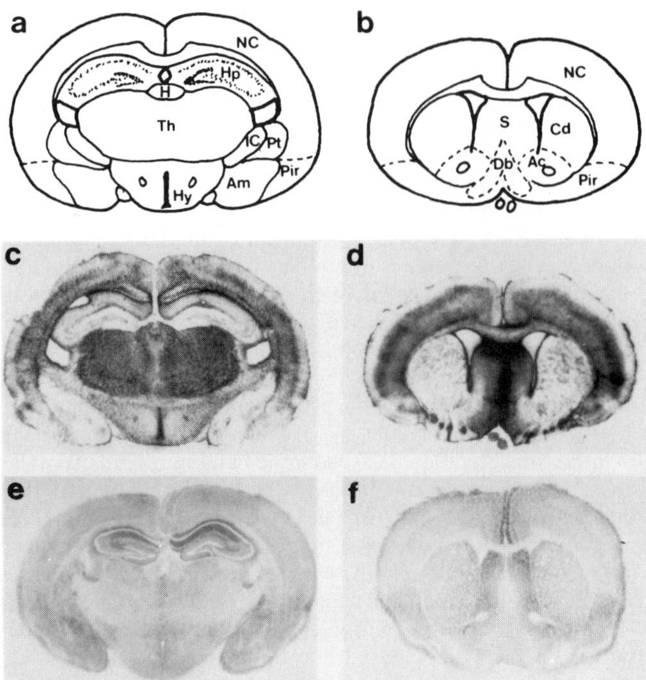

FIG. 153-6 Histoblots of Syrian hamster brain immunostained for PrP^C or PrP^{Sc}. Coronal sections through the hippocampus-thalamus (*a, c,* and *e*) and the septum-caudate (*b, d,* and *f*). Brain sections of a Syrian hamster clinically ill after inoculation with Sc237 prions (*c* and *d*) and an uninfected, control animal (*e* and *f*). Immunostaining for PrP^{Sc} shown in panels *c* and *d*: for PrP^C in *e* and *f*. Ac-nucleus accumbens; Am-amygdala; Cd-caudate nucleus; Db-diagonal band of Broca; H-habenula; Hp-hippocampus; Hy-hypothalmus; IC-internal capsule; NC-neocortex. *(From Taraboulos et al.[152] Used by permission.)*

In white matter, bundles of myelinated axons contained PrP^{Sc} but were devoid of PrP^C. These findings suggest that prions are transported along axons, in agreement with an earlier finding that scrapie infectivity was found to migrate in a pattern consistent with retrograde transport.[153–155] While the rate of PrP^{Sc} synthesis appears to be a function of the level of PrP^C expression in transgenic (Tg) mice, the level to which PrP^{Sc} accumulates appears to be independent of PrP^C concentration.[156]

SYNTHESIS OF PRION PROTEIN ISOFORMS

Metabolic labeling studies of scrapie-infected cultured cells have shown that PrP^C is synthesized and degraded rapidly, while PrP^{Sc} is synthesized slowly by an as yet undefined posttranslational process (Table 153-6).[26–28,157] These observations are consistent with earlier findings showing that PrP^{Sc} accumulates in the brains of scrapie-infected animals, while PrP mRNA levels remain unchanged.[22] Furthermore, the structure and organization of the PrP gene made it likely that PrP^{Sc} is formed during a posttranslational event.[25]

Both PrP isoforms appear to transit through the Golgi apparatus, where their Asn-linked oligosaccharides are modified and sialylated.[158–162] PrP^C is presumably transported within secretory vesicles to the external cell surface, where it is anchored by a glycosyl phosphaditylinositol (GPI) moiety (see Fig. 153-5).[163–167] In contrast, PrP^{Sc} accumulates primarily within cells, where it is deposited in cytoplasmic vesicles, many of which appear to be secondary lysosomes.[28,168–172]

Table 153-6 Properties of Cellular and Scrapie PrP Isoforms

Property	PrP^{C}	PrP^{Sc}
Concentration in normal SHa brain[156]	~1 to 5 μg/g	
Concentration in scrapie-infected SHa brain[156]	~1 to 5 μg/g	~5 to 10 μg/g
Presence in purified prions[18,19,21,85,89]	—	+*
Protease resistance[18,19,21,22,25,85,89]	—	+†
Presence in amyloid rods[40,85,110,112,113]	—	+‡
Subcellular localization in cultured cells[163–168, 170, 172]	?	vesicles
PIPLC§ release from membranes[163–167]	+	–
Synthesis ($t_{1/2}$)¶[26,157]	<0.1 h	~1 to 3 h¶
Degradation ($t_{1/2}$)[26,157]	~5 h	>>24 h

*Copurification of PrP^{Sc} and prion infectivity demonstrated by two protocols: (1) detergent extraction followed by sedimentation and protease digestion and (2) PrP 27-30 monoclonal antibody affinity chromatography.
†Limited proteinase K digestion of SHaPrP^{Sc} produces PrP 27-30.
‡After limited proteolysis of PrP^{Sc} (PrP 27-30 is produced) and detergent extraction, amyloid rods form; except for length, the rods are indistinguishable from amyloid filaments forming plaques.
§PIPLC = phosphatidylinositol-specific phospholipase C.
¶PrP^{Sc} *de novo* synthesis is a posttranslational process.
SOURCE: Adapted from Prusiner.[463]

PrP^{Sc} is also thought to accumulate within neuronal lysosomes of mice with scrapie.[173]

Several experimental results argue that PrP molecules destined to become PrP^{Sc} exit to the cell surface, as does PrP^{C},[163] prior to their conversion into PrP^{Sc} (Fig. 153-7).[27,28,169] Interestingly, the GPI anchors of both PrP^{C} and PrP^{Sc}, which presumably feature in directing the subcellular trafficking of these molecules, are sialylated (Fig. 153-8).[174] It is unknown whether sialylation of the GPI anchor participates in some aspect of PrP^{Sc} formation.

Although most of the difference in mass of PrP 27-30 predicted from the amino acid sequence and that observed after posttranslational modification is due to complex-type oligosaccharides, these sugar chains are not required for the synthesis of protease-resistant PrP in scrapie-infected cultured cells based on experiments with the Asn-linked glycosylation inhibitor tunicamycin and on site-directed mutagenesis studies.[175] Whether unglycosylated PrP^{Sc} is associated with scrapie prion infectivity remains to be established, but experiments with Tg mice may resolve this issue.

Cell-free translation studies have demonstrated two forms of PrP—a transmembrane form that spans the bilayer twice at the transmembrane (TM) and amphipathic helix (AH) domains and a secretory form (see Fig. 153-5)[176–180] The stop transfer effector (STE) domain controls the topogenesis of PrP. That PrP contains both a TM domain and a GPI anchor poses a topologic conundrum. It seems likely that membrane-dependent events feature in the synthesis of PrP^{Sc} especially since brefeldin A, which selectively destroys the Golgi stacks,[181,182] prevents PrP^{Sc} synthesis in scrapie-infected cultured cells.[169] For many years, the association of scrapie infectivity with membrane fractions has been appreci-

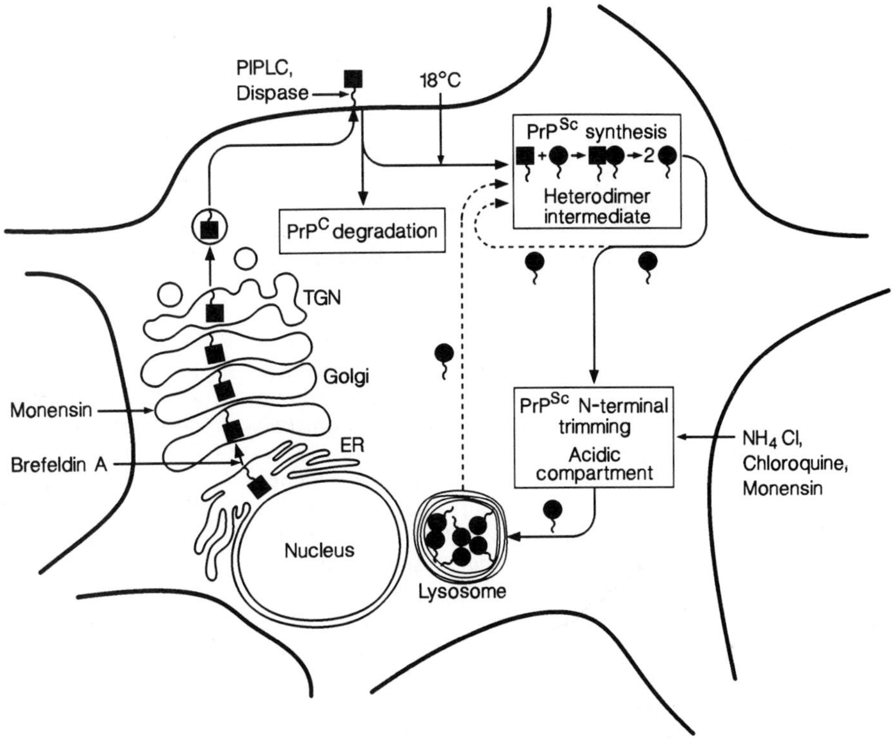

FIG. 153-7 Subcellular localization of PrP^{C} and PrP^{Sc} in cultured cells. Synthesis of PrP^{C} occurs in the ER; subsequently, PrP^{C} is transported through the Golgi, where its complex type Asn-linked oligosaccharides are modified and sialylated. Presumably, the GPI anchor of PrP^{C} also acquires sialic acid in the Golgi compartment. PrP^{C} is bound to the external surface of cells by its GPI anchor; PrP^{C} can be released from cells by phosphoinositol phospholipase C-catalyzed hydrolysis of the anchor. PrP^{Sc} synthesis occurs after reentry of PrP^{C} into the cell through caveolae or endosomes. The precise subcellular location(s) at which PrP^{C} is converted into PrP^{Sc} is unknown. ***(From Taraboulos et al.[169] Used by permission.)***

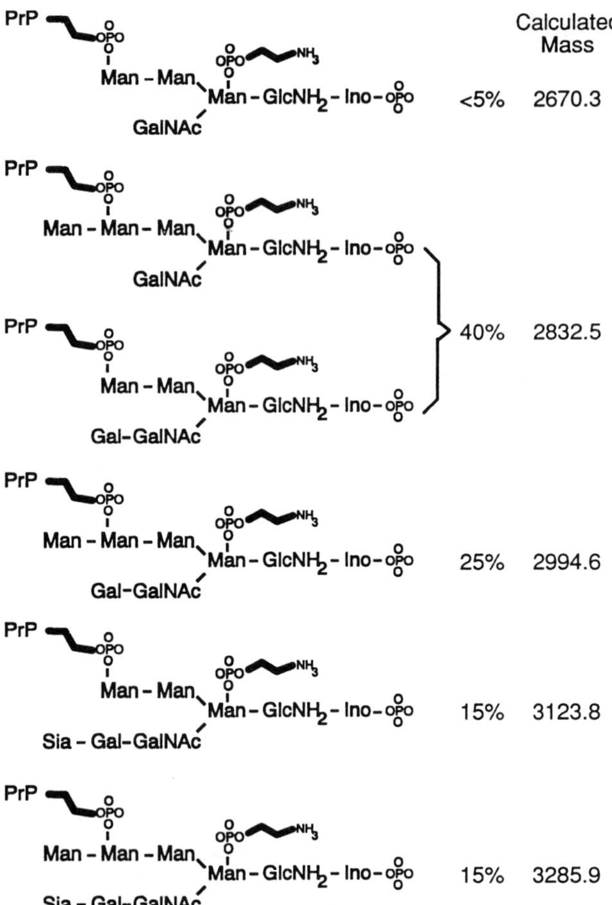

FIG. 153-8 **Glycoinositol phospholipid anchors of the PrP. The proposed GPI anchor structures were determined for SHaPrP^{Sc} by mass spectrometry.[174] The percentages indicate an estimate of the approximate relative abundance of each glycoform. The calculated masses are based on the average molecular weight of each element in the GPI and include the mass of the C-terminal PrP (K12) peptide, which accounts for 1312.5 mass of the total.** ***(From Stahl et al.[174] Used by permission.)***

ated[48–50]; indeed, hydrophobic interactions are thought to account for many of the physical properties displayed by infectious prion particles.[53,98,183]

GENETIC LINKAGE OF PRION PROTEIN WITH SCRAPIE INCUBATION TIMES

Studies of PrP genes (*Prn-p*) in mice with short and long incubation times demonstrated genetic linkage between a *Prn-p* RFLP and a gene modulating incubation times (*Prn-i*).[184] Other investigators have confirmed the genetic linkage, and one group has shown that the incubation time gene (*Sinc*) is also linked to PrP.[185–187] *Sinc* was first described by Dickinson and colleagues over 20 years ago[188]; whether the genes for PrP, *Prn-i,* and *Sinc* are all congruent remains to be established. The PrP sequences of NZW (*Prn-p^a*) and I/Ln (*Prn-p^b*) mice with short and long scrapie incubation times, respectively, differ at codons 108 (L → F) and 189 (T → V).[134] While these amino acid substitutions argue for the congruency of *Prn-p* and *Prn-i,* experiments with *Prn-p^a* mice expressing *Prn-p^b* transgenes demonstrated a paradoxical shortening of incubation times[135] instead of a prolongation, as predicted from (*Prn-p^a* × *Prn-p^b*) F1 mice, which exhibit long incubation times that are dominant.[184–188] Whether this paradoxical shortening of scrapie incubation times in Tg(*Prn-p^b*) mice results from high levels of PrP^C-B expression remains to be established.[135]

Loci other than *Prn-i* that modify scrapie incubation times in mice have been identified, including the gene on chromosome 17 that influences CJD and probably scrapie incubation times (*Pid-i*).

PRION DISEASES OF ANIMALS

Scrapie of Sheep and Goats

Even though scrapie was recognized as a distinct disorder of sheep with respect to its clinical manifestations, as early as 1738, the disease remained enigmatic, even with respect to its pathology, for more than two centuries. Some veterinarians thought that scrapie was a disease of muscle caused by parasites, while others thought that it was a dystrophic process. An investigation into the etiology of scrapie followed the vaccination of sheep for looping ill virus with formalin-treated extracts of ovine lymphoid tissue unknowingly contaminated with scrapie prions.[43] Two years later, more than 1500 sheep had contracted scrapie from this vaccine.

While the transmissibility of scrapie became well established, the spread of scrapie within and among flocks of sheep remained puzzling. Parry argued that host genes were responsible for the development of scrapie in sheep. He was convinced that natural scrapie is a genetic disease that could be eradicated by proper breeding protocols.[14,190] He considered its transmission by inoculation of importance primarily for laboratory studies and communicable infection of little consequence in nature. Other investigators viewed natural scrapie as an infectious disease and argued that host genetics only modulates susceptibility to an endemic infectious agent.[15] The incubation time gene for experimental scrapie in Cheviot sheep, called *"Sip"* is said to be linked to a PrP gene RFLP,[191] a situation perhaps analogous to *Prn-i* and *Sinc* in mice. However, the null-hypothesis of nonlinkage has yet to be tested, and this is important, especially in view of earlier studies that argue that susceptibility of sheep to scrapie is governed by a recessive gene.[14,190] In Suffolk sheep, a polymorphism in the PrP ORF was found at codon 171 (Q → R)[141,142] (and Westaway D, et al.: unpublished data); whether it or other amino acid variants segregate with a *Sip* phenotype in Cheviot sheep is unknown.[192,193]

Bovine Spongiform Encephalopathy

Since 1986, more than 130,000 cattle have died of BSE in Great Britain.[194–198] Neither the cause of BSE, often referred to as "mad cow disease," nor methods of controlling the spread of this disorder are known. Many investigators contend that BSE resulted from the feeding of meat and bone meal prepared from rendered sheep offal. The diminished use of hydrocarbon extraction in the rendering of sheep offal has been suggested as the reason that scrapie prions survived the rendering process. Since 1988, the practice of using dietary protein supplements for domestic animals derived from rendered sheep or cattle offal has been forbidden in the United Kingdom. Curiously, almost half of the BSE cases have occurred in herds in which only a single affected animal has been found; several cases of BSE in a single herd are infrequent.[194–196] Whether the distribution of BSE cases within herds will change as the epidemic progresses and whether BSE will disappear with the cessation of feeding rendered meat and bone meal are uncertain.

Of particular importance to the BSE epidemic is the transmission of BSE to the nonhuman primate marmoset after a prolonged incubation period (see ref. 468).The potential parallels with kuru of humans, confined to the Fore region of Papua New Guinea[4,32] are worthy of consideration. Once the most common cause of death among women and children, kuru has almost disappeared with the cessation of ritualistic cannibalism.[199] These findings argue that kuru was transmitted orally as proposed for BSE among cattle. Of note are cases of kuru that have occurred in people exposed to prions more than three decades ago. Whether BSE poses any risk to humans is unknown.

Besides BSE, four other animal diseases appear to have arisen from the oral consumption of prions. It has been suggested that an outbreak of TME in 1985 arose from feeding the colony with meat from a sporadic case of BSE.[200] The source of prions in CWD is unclear.[201,202] The prion-contaminated meat and bone meal thought to be the cause of BSE are also hypothesized to be the cause of FSE and exotic ungulate encephalopathy. FSE has been found in almost 30 domestic cats in Great Britain as well as in a puma and a cheetah. Three cases of FSE in domestic cats have been transmitted to laboratory mice, and PrP^{Sc} has been identified in their brains by immunoblotting (see ref. 469). Spongiform encephalopathies have been found in the brains of five exotic ungulates in British zoos; brain extracts prepared from a nyala and a greater kudu have transmitted disease to mice (see refs. 470, 471).

CREUTZFELDT-JAKOB DISEASE

The discovery of human prion diseases came from the recognition that the neuropathology of a cerebellar disorder of Papua New Guinea natives was similar to that of scrapie. Spongiform degeneration in kuru prompted Hadlow to suggest that transmission studies in apes be performed.[203] The success of those studies[32] was followed by the transmission of CJD to apes[33] based on the earlier recognition that the neuropathological changes in kuru were similar to those found in CJD.[204] In 1920, Creutzfeldt reported the case of a 23-year-old woman who died of a neurodegenerative disease,[205] and the following year Jakob reported five cases.[206–208] Ironically, some investigators doubt that Creutzfeldt described the disease that now bears his name.[209]

Three forms of CJD are now recognized—infectious, sporadic, and inherited. The only documented cases of the infectious form of CJD are iatrogenic. The great majority of CJD cases are sporadic, while 10 to 15 percent of cases are familial and inherited as an autosomal dominant trait with variable penetrance.[20,210,211]

Epidemiology of Creutzfeldt-Jakob Disease

CJD is found throughout the world, and the incidence of sporadic CJD is approximately one case per million population.[212] Although many geographical clusters of CJD have been reported,[212–215] each has been shown to segregate with a PRNP gene mutation that results in a nonconservative substitution. To date attempts to identify a common exposure to some etiologic agent have been unsuccessful both for the sporadic and familial cases. Some families have multiple cases of both CJD and AD.[20] The relationship, if any, between CJD and AD remains to be established.[21]

Epidemiologic studies have failed to implicate the ingestion of scrapie-infected sheep or goat meat in the pathogenesis of CJD in humans. But speculation about this potential route of inoculation continues.[34,212,216–219] On the other hand, it is assumed that the transmission of kuru among Papua New Guinea tribesmen occurred after the consumption of kuru-infected brain during ritualistic cannibalism.[4] Studies with SHa provided convincing evidence that the oral route of inoculation, although extremely inefficient, can with regularity be a source of prion infection.[37]

General Clinical Features

Nonspecific prodromal symptoms occur in about a third of CJD patients, and may include fatigue, sleep disturbance, weight loss, headache, general malaise, and ill-defined pain.[220] The majority of CJD patients present with deficits in higher cortical function.[220–228] These deficits virtually always progress to a state of profound dementia characterized by memory loss, impaired judgment and a decline in virtually all aspects of intellectual function.[229] A minority of patients present with either visual impairment or cerebellar gait and coordination deficits. Frequently, the cerebellar deficits are rapidly followed by progressive dementia.[230,231] Visual problems often begin with blurred vision and diminished acuity, rapidly followed by dementia.

Generally, patients with CJD are between 50 and 65 years of age; however, patients as young as 17 and as old as 83 have been recorded.[220,225,227,232]

Other symptoms and signs include extrapyramidal dysfunction manifested as rigidity, mask-like facies, or choreoathetoid movements; pyramidal signs (usually mild); seizures (usually major motor); and, less commonly, hypesthesia; supranuclear gaze palsy; optic atrophy; and vegetative signs such as changes in weight, temperature, sweating, or menstruation.[220,233] One study indicates that lower motor neuron disease in association with a progressive dementing syndrome is not transmissible to apes and monkeys.[234] Based on these findings, the authors argue that the term "amyotrophic Creutzfeldt-Jakob disease" is not a useful label.

Myoclonus in Creutzfeldt-Jakob Disease

Most patients (~90 percent) with CJD exhibit myoclonus appearing at various times throughout the illness.[220,224,227] Unlike other involuntary movements, myoclonus persists during sleep. Startle myoclonus elicited by loud sounds or bright lights is frequent. It is important to stress that myoclonus is neither specific nor confined to CJD. Dementia with myoclonus can also be due to AD,[235] as well as cryptococcal encephalitis[236] or Unverricht-Lundborg disease.

Electroencephalogram in Creutzfeldt-Jakob Disease

The EEG is often useful in the diagnosis of CJD. During the early phase of CJD, the EEG is usually normal or shows only scattered theta activity. In most advanced cases, repetitive, high-voltage triphasic and polyphasic sharp discharges are seen. The presence of these sterotyped periodic bursts of <200 msec in duration occurring every 1 to 2 sec makes the diagnosis of CJD very likely.[229,237–242] These discharges are frequently but not always symmetrical; there may be a one-sided predominance in amplitude. As CJD progresses, normal background rhythms become fragmentary and slower. The appearance of these periodic electrical; complexes during the clinical course of CJD is variable, and in many cases their presence is transient.

Clinical Course

In documented cases of accidental transmission of CJD to human subjects, an incubation period of 1.5 to 2.0 years preceded the development of clinical disease.[243,244] In other cases, incubation periods of up to 30 years have been suggested. Most patients with CJD live only 6 to 12 months after the onset of clinical signs and symptoms,[220,227,232] but some live for up to 5 years.[245]

Clinical Diagnosis of Creutzfeldt-Jakob Disease

The constellation of dementia, myoclonus, and periodic electrical bursts in an afebrile 60-year-old patient is generally diagnosed as CJD. Clinical abnormalities in CJD are confined to the central nervous system. Fever, elevated sedimentation rate, leukocytosis in blood, or a pleocytosis in cerebrospinal fluid (CSF) should alert the physician to another etiology to explain the patient's central nervous system dysfunction.

Differential Diagnosis

Many conditions may mimic CJD superficially. AD is occasionally accompanied by myoclonus,[235] but is usually distinguished by its protracted course and lack of motor and visual dysfunction.

Intracranial vasculitides may produce nearly all of the symptoms and signs associated with CJD, sometimes without systemic abnormalities. Myoclonus is exceptional with cerebral vasculitis, but focal seizures may confuse the picture; furthermore, myoclonus is often absent in the early stages of CJD. Stepwise change in deficits, prominent headache, abnormal CSF, and focal tomographic or angiographic abnormalities all favor vasculitis.

Neurosyphilis may present with dementia and myoclonus relatively rapidly,[246] but is easily distinguished from CJD by CSF findings, as is crytopococcal meningoencephalitis.[236] Diffuse intracranial tumor may occasionally be confused with CJD. In rare cases of central nervous system neoplasia in which the CT is normal and there are no signs of increased intracranial pressure, CSF protein is usually elevated. Kufs disease and myoclonic epilepsy with Lafora bodies may be responsible for dementia, myoclonus, and ataxia, but the less acute courses and prominent seizures distinguish them from CJD.[247]

A number of diseases that may simulate CJD are easily discriminated by noting the clinical setting in which they occur. These include anoxic encephalopathy, subacute sclerosing panencephalitis, progressive rubella panencephalitis, herpes simplex encephalitis (in immunoincompetent hosts), dialysis dementia, uremia, and portosystemic shunt encephalopathy.[246,248,249]

When CJD begins atypically, it may for a short time resemble other disorders, such as Parkinson disease, progressive supranuclear palsy, or progressive multifocal leukoencephalopathy. However, this resemblance usually fades early in the course of CJD.[220,250]

The AIDS (acquired immunodeficiency syndrome) dementia complex may occasionally imitate CJD in onset, early course, physical signs, CT findings, and lack of abnormalities on routine CSF studies.[249,251] The few such patients without manifestations of systemic immunodeficiency (<10 percent) should be asked about risk factors and should be tested for serum antibodies to human immunodeficiency virus (HIV) determined. Additionally, more specific CSF tests are likely to be abnormal—in one study, CSF oligoclonal bands were present in six of nine patients, and intra-blood–brain barrier synthesis of IgG specific for HIV was elevated in eight of nine.[252]

Ancillary Tests

With the exception of brain biopsy, there are no specific tests for CJD. EEG is the most helpful. CT may be normal or show cortical atrophy; to date, MRI studies have not been more helpful.[233] Positron emission tomography shows a loss of normal metabolic landmarks, which is thought by some investigators to be of differential significance[233] but by others to be indistinguishable from the pattern produced by AD.[253] CSF is nearly always normal, but may show a minimal protein elevation.[220] Two-dimensional gel electrophoresis of CSF proteins from CJD patients has been reported to identify two abnormal proteins of 26 and 29 kDa, but these proteins were also found in the CSF of patients with herpes simplex virus encephalitis.[254] The lack of specificity found with this test argues that these proteins are released into the CSF as result of injury to the central nervous system.

Brain Biopsy

If the constellation of pathological changes frequently found in CJD are seen in a brain biopsy, the diagnosis is reasonably secure. However, the enthusiasm for brain biopsies in patients with suspected CJD is quite low for two reasons: first, there is no specific effective treatment for CJD, and second, decontamination of surgical instruments requires special protocols, described below.

Transmission to Animals

CJD has been transmitted to a variety of laboratory animals (see Table 153-3). Over 250 cases of CJD have been transmitted to apes and monkeys[255] (and Gajdusek DC, Gibbs, CJ, Jr: personal communication). Many fewer cases have been transmitted to goats, marmosets, cats, and laboratory rodents. Most cases of CJD cannot be transmitted to nonprimates.[256] The chemical basis for these differences among isolates is unknown. Nearly 80 percent of all Japanese CJD cases were found to be transmissible to rats and mice.[257] With the discovery of PrP gene mutations, Tateishi and colleagues have reanalyzed their data and now report that while most cases of sporadic CJD are transmissible to rodents, only ~50 percent of inherited cases are transmissible.[258] These findings raise the possibility that mutant PrP^C molecules may cause central nervous system dysfunction without prior conversion to PrP^{Sc}. A similar situation may attend with Tg mice expressing the codon 102 GSS mutation, since central nervous system dysfunction develops with little or no PrP^{Sc}.[259]

Prolonged incubation times ranging from 4 months to more than 4 years have been recorded for CJD in experimental animals. Like CJD patients, a progressive central nervous system disorder develops in the infected animals, leads to death in a comparatively short time. With a few exceptions, the neuropathological changes in animals are similar to those described here for humans.

Immunologic Studies

The rapid and reliable diagnosis of CJD post mortem can be accomplished during antiserums to PrP.[93,260–262] Initially, partial purification of 1 to 2g of infected brain tissue using detergent extractions, differential centrifugation, and enzyme digestions was required to detect PrP^{Sc} in 14 cases of CJD analyzed by immunoblots.[261] Antibodies raised against SHa PrP 27-30, were found to react with protease-resistant PrP in the partially purified fractions prepared from human CJD brain. Six of the CJD cases had been previously transmitted to mice, and all of these demonstrated the presence of CJD prion proteins. Brains from control patients with anoxic encephalopathy or AD did not contain these protease-resistant, immunoreactive prion proteins. Two new procedures have been developed for diagnostic evaluations of CJD; one protocol uses a dot blot, in which the sample is first digested with proteinase K and then denatured with GdHCI.[262] The other protocol is designated histoblotting and utilizes the same limited proteolysis followed by GdHCI denaturation to enhance PrP^{Sc} antigenicity.[152] These procedures have, for the most part, replaced transmission studies using apes and monkeys.

In one study, 100 percent of the CJD cases (14 of 14) examined were found to have PrP immunoreactive proteins that were proteinase K–resistant.[261] In another report, 17 of 24 CJD cases (71 percent) showed PrP immunoreactive proteins by immunoblotting with PrP 27-30 antiserums.[263] All 24 of those cases had been previously transmitted to apes and monkeys. Since considerable data indicate that the scrapie isoform of the prion protein (by analogy the CJD isoform) is required for infectivity,[99,264] we would expect that all cases of authentic, noninherited CJD will contain the protease-resistant isoforms of the human prion protein.

In support of the argument that all cases of CJD should have demonstrable CJD prion proteins is my experience with the immunostaining of CJD amyloid plaques. In 16 of 17 CJD cases with amyloid plaques (94 percent), my colleagues and I have found PrP immunoreactive plaques.[40,113,265] Since all cases of CJD do not have readily identifiable amyloid plaques, immunostaining of tissue sections fixed in formaldehyde and embedded in paraffin is useful only when positive. The use of other fixatives such as McLean's appears to be superior to formaldehyde in preserving PrP antigenicity.[121]

Care of Creutzfeldt-Jakob Disease Patients

It is important to stress that CJD is neither a contagious nor a communicable disease, but it is transmissible. While the risk of accidental inoculation by aerosols is very small, procedures producing aerosols should be performed in certified biosafety cabinets. Biosafety level 2 practices, containment equipment, and facilities are recommended.[266]

The primary problem in caring for patients with CJD is the inadvertent infection of health care workers by needle and stab wounds, while the possible transmission of contagion through the air has never been documented. Accidental parenteral inoculation especially with neural tissues and including formalin-fixed specimens is potentially very hazardous.[267–270] EEG and electromyographic needles should not be reused after procedures have been performed on CJD patients.

There is no rational, scientific reason for surgeons or nurses to resist performing biopsies on demented patients when this operation is warranted medically. Likewise, there is no reason for pathologists or morgue dieners to resist performing autopsies on patients whose clinical diagnosis was CJD. Progress in the diagnosis, care, and treatment of CJD patients requires the dedicated efforts of physicians, nurses, and other health care workers. The standard microbiologic practices outlined here, along with specific recommendations for decontamination seem to be adequate precautions for the care of CJD patients and the handling of infected specimens.

Decontamination of Creutzfeldt-Jakob Disease Prions

The scrapie prion is extremely resistant to common inactivation procedures.[4,17,43,46,271] Similar structural features for CJD prions in human brain have been described.[93]

Procedures for decontamination of CJD-infected materials have been defined.[4,82,271–276] While there is general agreement about the extreme resistance of prions to inactivation, there is some disagreement about the optimal conditions for sterilization. Little is known about the resistance of the human CJD prion to inactivation; most of our knowledge comes from animal models of experimental CJD and scrapie. The most widely studied murine CJD model uses an isolate from a Japanese patient with CJD.[55] Whether this murine CJD prion accurately reflects the properties of human CJD prions from other racial backgrounds remains to be established. It is noteworthy that human CJD prions from British and American patients can rarely be transmitted to mice,[256] while most cases from Japanese patients are readily transmitted.[257]

Although some investigators recommend treating CJD-contaminated materials once with 1 *N* NaOH at room temperature,[219,276] I believe this procedure may be inadequate for sterilization. Autoclaving at 132°C for 5 h or treatment with 2 *N* NaOH for several hours is recommended for sterilization of prions.[82] The term "sterilization" implies complete destruction of prions; any residual infectivity can be hazardous.

The greatest possible contamination of hospital equipment will most likely occur in the neurosurgical operating room.[277] Sterilization of surgical instruments by 2 *N* NaOH or autoclaving at 132°C seems mandatory, especially if the cranium has been opened. By analogy to experimental scrapie, the human CJD brain probably has higher titers of prions than any other organ.[278] Furthermore, the intracerebral route of inoculation of scrapie prions in hamsters is approximately 10^9 times more efficient than oral ingestion.[37] These data emphasize the extreme danger of introducing small numbers of prions into the central nervous system tissue during neurosurgical procedures.

It has been argued that subclinical cases of CJD will harbor high titers of the infectious prions, but these will not be manifest until some time after the surgery is completed, when a neurologic disorder develops. Though this is particularly disconcerting, the rarity of CJD clearly indicates that very few, if any, patients contract CJD as a result of neurosurgical procedures.

Therapeutic Intervention

There is no known effective therapy for treating or preventing CJD. There are no well-documented cases of patients with CJD showing recovery either spontaneously or after therapy, with one possible exception.[54]

Treatment with amantadine has been unsuccessful.[279–281] HPA-23 is an inhibitor of viral glycoprotein synthesis and when given to scrapie-infected animals around the time of inoculation, but not later, it profoundly extends the length of the incubation period.[282] The effects in human CJD are uncertain.[220] DEAE dextran and cortisone have also extended the incubation period in experimental scrapie.[283,284] Interferon has been used in experimental scrapie of rodents, but the incubation times were unaltered.[285–287] Although amphotericin has been used to prolong scrapie incubation periods in rodents,[288–290] it is not effective in treating patients with CJD.[291]

Although antibodies have been raised against the scrapie prion protein and these cross-react with prion proteins in CJD human brains,[93] passive immunization or even vaccination would seem to be of little value. CJD and scrapie both progress in the absence of any immune response to the offending prions; however, neutralization of scrapie prion infectivity was accomplished when the infectious particles were dispersed into detergent–lipid–protein complexes.[292]

IATROGENIC CREUTZFELDT-JAKOB DISEASE

Accidental transmission of CJD to humans appears to have occurred with corneal transplantation,[243] contaminated EEG electrode implantation,[244] and surgical operations using contaminated instruments or apparatus (Table 153-7).[212,277,293,294] Corneas unknowingly removed from donors with CJD have been transplanted to apparently healthy recipients in whom CJD developed after prolonged incubation periods; corneas of animals have significant levels of prions,[295] making this scenario seem quite probable. The same improperly decontaminated EEG electrodes that caused CJD in two young patients with intractable epilepsy were found to cause CJD in a chimpanzee 18 months after their experimental implantation.[296]

Surgical procedures may have resulted in accidental inoculation of patients with prions during their operations,[4,277,297] presumably because some instrument or apparatus in the operating theater became contaminated when a CJD patient underwent surgery. Although the epidemiology of these studies is highly suggestive, no proof for such episodes exists.

Table 153-7 Infectious Prion Diseases of Humans*

Diseases	No. of Cases
Kuru (1957–1982)	
Adult females	1739
Adult males	248
Children and adolescents	597
Total	2584
Iatrogenic Creutzfeldt-Jakob disease	
Depth electrodes	2
Corneal transplants	3
Human pituitary growth hormone	40
Human pituitary gonadotropin	3
Dura mater grafts	8
Neurosurgical procedures	4
Total	60

*References cited in text.

Since 1988, eight cases of CJD developing after implantation of dura mater grafts have been recorded.[297–303] All the grafts were thought to have been acquired from a single manufacturer, whose preparative procedures were inadequate to inactivate human prions.[297] One case of CJD occurred after repair of an eardrum perforation with a pericardium graft.[304]

Human Growth Hormone Therapy

The possibility of transmission of CJD from contaminated HGH preparations derived from human pituitaries has been raised by the occurrence of fatal cerebellar disorders with dementia in more than 40 patients ranging in age from 10 to 41 years (see Table 153-7).[7,297,305,306] One case of spontaneous CJD in a 20-year-old woman has been reported,[6,305,307] but CJD in patients under 40 years of age is very rare. These patients received injections of HGH every 2 to 4 days for 4 to 12 years.[6,308–316] Interestingly, most of the patients presented with cerebellar syndromes that progressed over periods varying from 6 to 18 months. Some patients became demented during the terminal phase of their illnesses. The clinical courses of some patients with dementia occurring late resemble kuru more than ataxic CJD in some respects.[317] Assuming CJD developed in these patients from injections of prion-contaminated HGH preparations, the possible incubation periods range from 4 to 30 years.[297] Incubation periods of two to three decades have been suggested to explain some cases of kuru.[317–319] Many patients received several common lots of HGH at various times during their prolonged therapies, but no single lot was administered to all the American patients. An aliquot of one lot of HGH has been reported to transmit central nervous system disease to a chimpanzee after a prolonged incubation period.[320] The number of lots of the HGH that might have been contaminated with prions is unknown.

Although CJD is a rare disease, with an incidence of approximately one per million population,[212] it is reasonable to assume that CJD occurs with a proportional frequency among people who have died. About 1 percent of the population dies each year and most CJD patients die within 1 year of symptoms developing. Thus, we estimate that one per 10^4 dead people had CJD. Since 10,000 human pituitaries were typically processed in a single HGH preparation, the possibility of hormone preparations contaminated with CJD prions is not remote. The concentration of CJD prions within infected human pituitaries is unknown; however, it is interesting that widespread degenerative changes have been observed in both the hypothalamus and pituitary of sheep with scrapie.[116] The forebrains from scrapie-infected mice have been added to human pituitary suspensions to determine if prions and HGH copurify.[321] Bioassays in mice suggest that prions and HGH do not copurify with currently used protocols.[322] Although these results seem reassuring, especially for patients treated with HGH over much of the last decade, the relatively low titers of the murine scrapie prions used in these studies may not have provided an adequate test.[305] The extremely small size and charge heterogeneity exhibited by scrapie[45,85,158,183,323] and presumably CJD prions[93,324] may complicate procedures designed to separate pituitary hormones from these slow infectious pathogens. Even though additional investigations argue for the efficacy of inactivating prions in HGH fractions prepared from human pituitaries using 6 *M* urea,[325] it seems doubtful that such protocols will be used for purifying HGH now that recombinant HGH is available.

Three cases of CJD have occurred in women receiving human pituitary gonadotropin.[326]

KURU

For many decades kuru devastated the lives of the Fore Highlanders of Papua New Guinea.[4] The high incidence of the disease among women left a society of motherless children raised by their fathers (see Table 153-7). It was unusual in the Fore region to see an elderly woman. With the cessation of traditional warfare, older men are now found. Many of these older men have had a succession of wives, each dying of kuru, leaving several children. Because contamination during ritualistic cannibalism appears to have been the mode of spread of kuru among the Fore people, and since cannibalism had ceased by 1960 in the Fore region, the patients in whom kuru now develops presumably were exposed to the kuru agent more than three decades ago.[3,4] In many cases, histories from patients and their families of the episode in which they cannibalized the remains of a near relative who had died of kuru have been obtained, presumably providing the source of infection. That the kuru prions could remain apparently quiescent in these patients for periods of two decades and then manifest themselves in the form of a fatal neurologic disease is supported by incubation periods of over 7.5 years in some monkeys inoculated with the kuru agent.[327]

Clinical Features

In one report describing 15 patients with kuru seen in 1978 and 1980, 13 of these received detailed neurologic examinations.[317] Ten of the 15 patients were women, and all were adults. The mean age of all the patients was 40.2 years, and their ages ranged from 29 to 60. The mean age of the 10 women was 43.2 years, and of the 5 men, 34.2. Five men and four women were under 40; all those over 40 were female. The youngest patient, a male, was 29 years old. All but three of the patients lived in the South Fore, the others in the North Fore. The duration of clinical disease ranged from 5 to 22 months (onset was dated from difficulty with walking).

All 15 patients related a history of joint pain preceding onset difficulty walking by several months. Eleven of the 15 also reported diffuse headache as a prodomal symptom. The diagnosis of kuru was first made by the patients themselves on recognizing that they were having difficulty walking. The rugged, mountainous terrain, which is frequently muddy from tropical rains, provided an ample test for assessing their balance on a daily basis.

Eleven of the 15 patients showed no signs of dementia at the time of examination, while 4 were disoriented and confused and had loss of memory. The latter individuals exhibited speech and frontal lobe release signs consisting of suck, snout, bite, and both hand and foot grasps. Three of the demented patients required a stick to maintain their balance while standing, and one was unable to stand. With advanced kuru, truncal ataxia and tremor were so severe that the stick had to be implanted into earth, and patients with advanced disease were unable to walk without the assistance of another person. In all patients still able to walk with the assistance of a stick or an assistant, marked truncal ataxia was evident.

All the patients exhibited an apprehensive facial expression, which remained unchanged for as long as 30 minutes. It could be interrupted, however, by laughter with other members of the village. All patients were able to smile when requested to do so. Examination of the cranial nerves revealed no abnormalities except for ataxic movements of the eyes during tests of conjugate gaze. Optokinetic nystagmus was diminished or absent bilaterally in most kuru patients even at an early stage of the disease.

There was no evidence of muscle wasting or diminished strength, though one patient had course fasciculations intermittently in the triceps, quadriceps, and gastrocnemius muscles. No fasciculations of the tongue were observed.

Of the 13 patients who had neurologic examinations, 4 showed increased resistance to passive movements, while an additional 7 exhibited mild rigidity with demonstrable cogwheeling. The initial clinical descriptions of kuru emphasized this aspect of the disease as well as the cerebellar dysfunction.[328,329] No patient was hypotonic. Nine of the 15 patients exhibited choreiform movements. All 15 had normal strength. In 8 of 13 patients, hyperactive deep tendon reflexes were demonstrable but confined to the lower extremities. Seven patients had ankle clonus. Two showed unilateral extensor plantar responses, while two others exhibited bilateral responses. In one case, a unilateral extensor plantar response was accompanied by normal deep tendon reflexes. In five patients in whom clonus at the ankles was readily elicited, no extensor plantar response was seen.

On sensory examination, responses to pinprick, temperature, touch, and vibration were normal. Cortical sensory testing failed to reveal deficits.

Marked ataxia of the upper and lower extremities was pronounced in all patients, and all exhibited a prominent intention tremor. Marked difficulties with all tests for coordination were observed. Rapid alternating movements were of uneven amplitude and rhythm.

Uniformity of Clinical Signs

The uniform clinical presentation of kuru is remarkable.[329–334] The prodomal symptoms and onset of the disease were similar in all the patients investigated in one study.[317] Even the time between the prodomal symptoms of headache and joint pain and the onset of difficulty walking was always 6 to 12 weeks. In most cases the disease progressed to death within 12 months, and all patients were dead within 2 years of onset. The average duration of illness for the 15 patients was 16 months.[317] Invariably, signs of cerebellar dysfunction dominated the clinical picture. All patients remained ambulatory with the aid of a stick for more than half of the clinical phase of their illness. These clinical characteristics were similar to those reported for adult patients at the peak of the kuru epidemic.[329–334]

There has been debate about dementia in kuru.[329–334] Findings of memory loss and disorientation accompanied by primitive reflexes such as snout, bite, suck, rooting, and hand grasps leave no doubt that patients become demented at an advanced stage of the disease.[317] The same patients also exhibited considerable muscle paratonia or gegenhalten.

The uniformity of presentation and clinical course in kuru contrasts with that of CJD, in which a wide spectrum of clinical manifestations is found.[223,224] While most CJD patients exhibit dementia, myoclonus, and pyramidal tract dysfunction at an early stage of the clinical illness, 10 to 20 percent present with an ataxic illness.[231,335] However, the dementia appears at an earlier clinical stage in ataxic CJD than in kuru. During the ambulatory phase of disease, no patients with kuru were found to be as severely demented as are most patients with CJD.

Incubation Periods That Exceed Three Decades

Kuru has not developed in any individual born in the South Fore after 1959. It has progressively disappeared, first among children and thereafter among adolescents. The number of deaths of adult females has decreased steadily, and adult male deaths have remained almost invariant. No one born in a village since cannibalism ceased has had kuru.[3,199] Each year the youngest new patients are older than those of the previous year.

Of several hundred kuru orphans born since 1957 to mothers who died of kuru, none has shown signs of the disease. Thus, the many children with kuru seen in the 1950s were not infected prenatally, perinatally, or neonatally by their mothers. There is no evidence for transmission in utero or by human milk. The regular disappearance of kuru is inconsistent with the existence of any natural reservoirs for kuru besides humans. Indeed, there is no evidence for animal or insect reservoirs.

While patients currently afflicted with kuru exhibit greatly prolonged incubation periods, children with kuru who were observed 20 years ago provide some information on the minimum incubation period. The youngest patient with kuru was 4 years old at the onset of the disease and died at age 5. It is not known at what age young children were infected. Accidental transmission of CJD to humans has required only 18 months after intracerebral or intraoptic inoculation.[243,244] An incubation period of 18 months has also been found in chimpanzees inoculated intracerebrally with the kuru agent.

Transmission by Cannibalism

Considerable evidence implicates ritualistic cannibalism as the mode of transmission for kuru among the Fore and neighboring tribes.[4] Oral transmission of kuru to monkeys has been documented.[327] Proposed transmission routes through laceration of the skin and rubbing of the eyes remains to be established.[4] These routes were suggested when early experiments on oral transmission to apes and monkeys failed. The experimental results from oral transmission of scrapie to hamsters suggests that insufficient doses of the kuru agent or prion were used in those protocols.[37]

Origin of Kuru

It has been suggested that kuru began at the turn of the century as a spontaneous case of CJD that was propagated by ritualistic cannibalism.[3,4] Whether the Fore people and their immediate neighbors provide an especially permissive genetic background on which kuru prions multiply remains to be established. Sequencing of the ORF of the PrP gene from three kuru patients failed to reveal any mutations.[336] Noteworthy is a case of CJD outside the kuru region in Papua New Guinea.

Transmission to Animals

Kuru has been regularly transmitted after intracerebral inoculation to apes and monkeys.[4,32] Occasional cases have been transmitted to cats but not to rodents.[256] The prolonged incubation periods in experimental animals are similar to those observed with CJD and GSS (see Table 153-3). Oral transmission of kuru to apes and monkeys has been difficult,[4] but studies have demonstrated transmission to monkeys.[327] Presumably, the difficulties in transmitting human kuru prions to apes and monkeys orally are due to the inefficiency of this route[37] and the crossing of a species barrier.

Immunologic Studies

Using PrP antiserum, protease-resistant immunoreactive proteins have been demonstrated in the brain extracts of one of two patients (50 percent) dying of kuru.[260] Presumably, these two patients are included in a larger series, in which three of four kuru patients (75 percent were found to have the abnormal isoforms of the prion protein.[263]

GERSTMANN-STRÄUSSLER-SCHEINKER SYNDROME

GSS, also known as Sträussler's disease and Gerstmann-Sträussler syndrome, was first described by Gerstmann and coworkers in 1936.[337] This syndrome originally referred to a familial condition, but sporadic cases resembling GSS clinically and pathologically have been reported and are now generally included under the same rubric.[20,338] The different clinical presentations of GSS suggested that it may be a heterogeneous disorder, and it was defined as a "spinocerebellar ataxia with dementia and plaque-like deposits."[339]

Molecular genetic investigations of GSS have defined four syndromes each with a different PRNP gene point mutation (Table 153-8). The ataxic form of GSS is caused by a point mutation at codon 102,[42] while a telencephalic form is caused by a mutation at codon 117.[340,341] A form of GSS in which ataxia is often accompanied by Parkinsonism and dementia is genetically linked to a PRNP mutation at codon 198.[342,343] In the codon 198 form of GSS and another caused by a mutation at codon 217, PrP amyloid plaques are found surrounded by numerous neurofibrillary tangles (NFT).[343]

Epidemiology

GSS is rare[20,338,344–347]; it comprises less than 2 percent of nearly 1000 cases of CJD or CJD-related diseases.[20] Assuming that the incidence of CJD is less than one per million, a

Table 153-8 Four Forms of Human Inherited Prion Disease with Amyloid Plaques*

PrP Mutation†	Predominant Clinical Presentation	Neuropathology
P102L	Ataxia	PrP plaques
A117V	Dementia and pseudobulbar signs	PrP plaques
F198S	Ataxia, Parkinsonism and dementia	PrP plaques and NFT‡
Q217R	Dementia	PrP plaques and NFT

*These disorders have generally been labeled GSS because of the amyloid plaques. References are cited in text.
†Point mutations are designated by the wild-type amino acid preceding the codon number, and the mutant residue follows.
‡NFT = neurofibrillary tangles.

rough estimate of the incidence of GSS is less than two per hundred million. This estimate may underrepresent GSS, since GSS frequently resembles other chronic degenerative diseases such as spinocerebellar degeneration, olivopontocerebellar degeneration, and multiple sclerosis.[20]

All reported cases of GSS have originated in the northern hemisphere—in Europe, Canada, the United States, and Japan.[20,338,344–347] Cases from the southern hemisphere may be recognized in the future.

Clinical Features

The diversity of clinical manifestations in GSS, even within the same pedigree, is well documented; however, patients typically complain of difficulty walking and unsteadiness, sometimes accompanied by leg pains or paresthesias in the early stages of the disease. On examination, cerebellar ataxia, dysarthria, ocular dysmetria, hyporeflexia or areflexia in the lower extremities with extensor plantar responses, and mild wasting or weakness in the lower extremities may be found. Hyporeflexia or areflexia in the lower extremities may be helpful in distinguishing GSS from dominantly inherited olivopontocerebellar degenerations. Sensory disturbances, usually impairment of vibratory and proprioceptive sensations, are occasionally detected on examination. Later in the course, mental deterioration may occur; sometimes it is quite mild or is difficult to assess because of severe dysarthria. Dysphagia frequently develops and contributes to inanition in the late stages of disease. Deafness, blindness, gaze palsies, and extrapyramidal rigidity have been reported in several cases. Convulsions may occur but are rare. Myoclonus seldom occurs; when it does occur, it may be confined to the lower extremities.

The majority of patients present with symptoms in the fourth to sixth decades. The average age of onset is 43 years old and ranges from 24 to 66. Symptoms may initially be relapsing; thus, GSS can be mistaken for multiple sclerosis. Eventually, inexorable progression of symptoms leads to death. The duration of illness ranges from 1 to 11 years, with a mean of 5 years. The mean age at death is 48 years. The age of onset may vary as much as three decades within a single pedigree.[346]

Clinically, GSS is thought to be distinguished from CJD by the prominence of ataxia in the former and the prominence of dementia with myoclonus in the latter. Yet, paradoxically, the clinical manifestations of both GSS and CJD may occur in different members of the same family. In one such family, the characteristic amyloid plaques of GSS were found in all afflicted members, including one member who died with a rapidly progressive dementia and myoclonus clinically consistent with CJD.[20,210] This patient's father and sister had both been afflicted with slowly progressive ataxia and little or no accompanying dementia, as is characteristic for GSS. Such a pedigree raises the question of whether CJD and GSS are distinct entities and perhaps demonstrates how a single allele can be variably expressed against different genetic backgrounds.

GSS and kuru are different in duration of clinical illness (up to 5 years in GSS vs. 1 to 2 years in kuru), morphology of amyloid plaques (multicentric in GSS vs. unincentric in kuru), and mode of transmission (vertical in GSS vs. horizontal in kuru). However, the symptomatology and distribution of neuropathological lesions in GSS and kuru are strikingly similar, thus also calling into question whether they are separate diseases.

Genetics and Diagnostic Evaluation

Most cases of GSS are familial,[20] exhibiting an autosomal dominant pattern with nearly complete penetrance. The premortem diagnosis of GSS is secure if a nonconservative mutation of the PrP gene is found.[8] Prior to the discovery of PrP gene mutations causing GSS, the diagnosis of GSS was rarely made prior to autopsy. Biopsy of the cerebellum was occasionally diagnostic when PrP amyloid plaques were found. Serologic and CSF examinations are normal. CT of the brain sometimes reveals cerebellar and brainstem atrophy. The EEG is normal or shows nonspecific, diffuse changes. Periodic complexes have not been reported in GSS except in cases in which clinical manifestations resembled CJD. Electromyography may reveal denervation potentials in lumbosacral myotomes. Sensory and motor nerve conduction velocities are normal.

Transmission to Animals

In 1978, Tateishi and coworkers produced experimental spongiform encephalopathy in mice and rats using brain tissue from a patient with a chronic spongiform encephalopathy and kuru plaques.[55,348] Although this case was not thought to be familial at the time, its clinicopathological features resembled GSS, and subsequently Masters et al. suggested that this case be classified as GSS.[20] In 1981, transmission of GSS to monkeys using brain tissue from a patient with familial disease was reported.[20] Subsequently, brain tissue from another afflicted member of the same family was used to transmit disease to marmosets.[349] No diagnostic conclusions can yet be made from such transmission studies because transmissibility of GSS appears to be variable, even within a single pedigree.[20,349]

Immunologic Studies

Using PrP antiserum, protease-resistant immunoreactive proteins have been demonstrated in the brain extracts of two of four patients (50 percent with GSS).[260] Presumably, these two patients are included in a second report, in which three of four GSS patients (75 percent) were stated to have the abnormal isoforms of the prion protein.[263] Partially purified, the protease-resistant PrP from the brain of one patient dying of GSS were found to be PrP-immunoreactive on Western immunoblots.[261] Subsequent studies with larger numbers of GSS patients have documented the PrP immunoreactivity of amyloid plaques and the presence of PrP^{Sc}.[350,351] A dot blot procedure for detection of PrP^{Sc} in brain homogenates provides a rapid and reliable method for the diagnosis of GSS, provided multiple regions of the brain are sampled.[262] Isolation of amyloid plaques from the brains of GSS patients and subsequent purification of a major 11-kDa protein have shown by protein sequencing that this protein is a proteolytic fragment of PrP extending from 58 to 150.[114]

NEUROPATHOLOGY OF THE HUMAN PRION DISEASES

The triad of microscopic features that characterize the prion diseases consists of (1) spongiform degeneration of neurons, (2) severe astrocytic gliosis, which often appears to be out of proportion to the degree of nerve cell loss, and (3) amyloid plaque formation (see Fig. 153-2).[5,20,33,116,118,352,353]

Spongiform degeneration consists of intracellular vacuoles that focally dilate neuronal processes, giving the gray matter a microvacuolated appearance on light microscopy. Ultrastructurally, the vacuoles display splitting of the unit cell membrane with the formation of blister-like membrane expansions and multiple septae.[354] In addition, the abnormal single-component membranes are focally thickened and necrotic. These neuronal membrane alterations as primary targets of the disease, strongly correlate with the PrP being an integral membrane sialoglycoprotein,[17,19,89,90,158,179] which, during the course of the disease, accumulates in neuronal cell membranes.

Neuropathology of CJD

Frequently, the brains of patients with CJD show no recognizable abnormalities on gross examination. In patients surviving several years, variable degrees of cerebral atrophy are likely to result in brain weights as low as 850 g.

The pathological hallmarks of CJD at the light microscopic level are spongiform degeneration and astrogliosis. The lack of an inflammatory response in CJD and other prion diseases is an important pathological feature of these degenerative disorders. Generally, the spongiform changes occur in the cerebral cortex, putamen, caudate nucleus, thalamus, and molecular layer of the cerebellum.[355–357] Spongiform degeneration is characterized by many 1 to 5 μm vacuoles in the neuropil between nerve-cell bodies.[212] On electron microscopy the vacuoles appear to be swollen neuronal processes and seem to be surrounded by a membrane.[356,358] Frequently, many membrane fragments can be seen within them. In some brains with CJD, we have seen no recognizable spongiform degeneration. Generally, the white matter is devoid of lesions, but several cases of CJD in Japan have exhibited well-documented vacuolar changes.[359] In natural scrapie of sheep, vacuolization is very limited,[360] while experimental scrapie of rodents is accompanied by widespread vacuolar changes, In TME, generally there is widespread vacuolation, but infected Aleutian mink fail to show vacuolar changes.[361] Thus, vacuolation, while a common feature of prion diseases, does not seem to be an obligatory change.

Astrogliosis is a more constant feature, though nonspecific, of prion diseases. Widespread proliferation of fibrous astrocytes is found throughout the gray matter of brains infected with CJD prions. Astrocytic processes filled with glial filaments form extensive networks. Whether prions possess some glial growth or maturation activity remains to be established. Alternatively, changes in neuronal function may provoke this attendant gliosis.

Amyloid plaques have been found in 5 to 10 percent of CJD. Purified CJD prions from humans and animals exhibit the ultrastructural and histochemical characteristics of amyloid.[85,93] In first passage from some human Japanese CJD cases, amyloid plaques have been found in mouse brains.[362] These plaques stain with antiserums raised against scrapie hamster PrP 27-30 protein.[40,113,265,363]

The majority of cases of kuru show plaques that are presumably comprised of amyloid within their cores.[204,357] The kuru plaques differ from senile plaques in that senile plaques have a collection of amorphous material, presumably degenerating dendrites, around their amyloid core. The kuru plaques do not possess such a large halo. Both kuru and senile plaques have been reported in CJD, but they are not a constant feature of the disease.[364,365] Kuru plaques do seem to be a constant feature of GSS.[20,366]

Neuropathology of GSS

The neuropathological diagnosis of GSS is based on the presence of characteristic amyloid plaque deposition, degeneration of white matter tracts, and neuronal loss throughout the brain, variably accompanied by spongiform changes and gliosis. The distribution and extent of these neuropathological changes differs widely between patients, even within one pedigree.

The amyloid plaques of GSS are distinct from those seen in kuru, AD, or scrapie. GSS plaques consist of a central dense core of amyloid surrounded by smaller globules of amyloid. Ultrastructurally, they consist of a radiating fibrillar network of amyloid fibrils with scant or no neuritic degeneration. The plaques can be distributed throughout the brain but are most frequently found in the cerebellum. They are often located adjacent to blood vessels. Congophilic angiopathy has been noted in some cases of GSS. In addition to the multicentric plaques of GSS, unicentric kuru plaques may also be seen.[20]

In numerous cases of GSS, there are PrP-immunoreactive proteins within the amyloid plaques.[113,120,265] Thus, like CJD and kuru, the amyloid plaques of GSS specifically stain with antiserums raised against PrP 27-30 that was isolated from scrapie-infected hamster brains. PrP immunostaining of formalin-fixed brain embedded in paraffin blocks as well as dot blot immunostaining of PrP^{Sc} in brain homogenates can be used to establish the diagnosis of GSS.[113,262]

The pattern of white matter degeneration resembles that of other systems degenerations, such as hereditary spinocerebellar degeneration (Friedreich's), cerebellar degeneration (Marie), and dentatorubral degeneration (Ramsay Hunt). The principal tracts involved include the dorsal and ventral spinocerebellar tracts, the posterior columns, the superior, middle, and inferior cerebellar peduncles, and the corticospinal tracts.

Neuronal loss occurs in scattered areas throughout the brain and spinal cord. The nuclei and regions that may be affected include Clarke's column, anterior horn cells, vestibular and cochlear nuclei, dentate nuclei, Purkinje and granule cells in the cerebellum, pontine nuclei, inferior olive, thalamus, substantia nigra, striatum, globus pallidus, subthalamic nucleus, and all layers of the cerebral cortex and hippocampus.

The presence of spongiform changes can vary even within a given pedigree.[20] Transmission of GSS to experimental animals was achieved only in cases with severe spongiform changes[20] until Tateishi and coworkers demonstrated transmission to rodents from a case of GSS with minimal spongiform changes.[117]

Prior to the availability of immunocytochemical analyses for PrP, some cases of GSS were incorrectly diagnosed as familial AD, since histochemistry showed NFT and amyloid plaques of the Alzheimer type.[347,367] While NFT confined to the hippocampus may be incidental, the distribution of NFT throughout the cerebral cortex along with plaques suggests AD or the simultaneous occurrence of AD with GSS.[347] Subsequent immunostaining studies have shown that the amyloid plaques in some of these cases are composed of prion proteins and do not bind antibodies raised to the β-amyloid peptide.[368–371] Molecular genetic investigations elucidated the point mutations of the PrP gene point mutations in each of these prion disorders.

Neuropathology of Kuru

The neuropathological changes in kuru are much like those described for CJD and GSS. Spongiform changes, astrogliosis, and amyloid or "kuru" plaques are the pathological hallmarks of kuru. Most, but not all, cases of kuru exhibit amyloid plaques.[204] These plaques have been found to contain prion proteins by immunostaining.[265]

MOLECULAR GENETICS OF INHERITED HUMAN PRION DISEASES

Human Prion Protein Gene Mutations

In humans, genes were first thought to play a role in CJD with the recognition that ~10 percent of cases are familial.[4,5] Like sheep scrapie, the relative contributions of genetic and infectious etiologies in the human prion diseases remained puzzling. The discovery of the PrP gene raised the possibility that mutation might feature in the hereditary human prion diseases. A point mutation at codon 102 (P → L) was shown to be linked genetically to development of GSS with a Lod score exceeding 3 (Fig. 153-9).[42] This mutation may be due to the deamination of a methylated CpG in a germ-line PrP gene resulting in the substitution of a T for C. The codon 102 mutation has been found in 10 different families in nine different countries, including the original GSS family (Table 153-9).[340,372–374]

An insert of 144 bp at codon 53 containing six octarepeats has been described in patients with CJD from four families all residing in southern England (see Fig. 153-9).[9,375–381] This mutation must have arisen through a complex series of events, because the human PrP gene contains only five octarepeats, indicating that a single recombination event could not have created the insert. Genealogic investigations have shown that all four families are related, arguing for a single founder born more than two centuries ago.[378] The Lod score for this extended pedigree exceeds 11. Studies from several laboratories have demonstrated that two, four, five, six, seven, eight, or nine octarepeats in addition to the normal five have been found in individuals with inherited CJD,[9,375–377,382–384] whereas, deletion of one octarepeat has been identified without the neurologic disease[385,386] (see ref. 472).

For many years the unusually high incidence of CJD among Israeli Jews of Libyan origin was thought to be due to the consumption of lightly cooked sheep brain or eyeballs.[211,217,387–390] Studies have shown that some Libyan and Tunisian Jews in families with CJD have a PrP gene point mutation at codon 200, resulting in a E → K substitution.[391–393] One patient was homozygous for the mutation (Fig. 153-10), but her clinical presentation was similar to that of heterozygotes,[393] arguing that familial prion diseases are true autosomal dominant disorders, like Huntington's disease.[394] The codon 200 mutation has also been found in Slovaks originating from Orava in North Central Czechoslovakia,[391] in a cluster of familial cases in Chile,[395] and in a large German family living in the United States.[396] Some investigators have argued that the codon 200 mutation originated in a Sephardic Jew whose descendants migrated

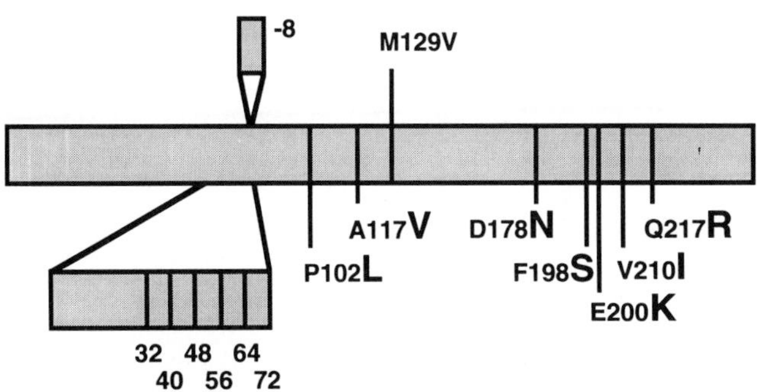

FIG. 153-9 Human prion protein gene (PRNP). The ORF is denoted by the large gray rectangle. Human PRNP wild-type polymorphisms are shown above the rectangle, while mutations that segregate with the inherited prion diseases are depicted below. The wild-type human PrP gene contains five octarepeats [P(Q/H)GGG (G/−)WGQ] from codons 51 to 91.[140] Deletion of a single octarepeat at codon 81 to 82 is not associated with prion disease[132,385,386]; whether this deletion alters the phenotypic characteristics of a prion disease is unknown. There are common polymorphisms at codons 117 (Ala → Ala) and 129 (Met → Val); homozygosity for Met or Val at codon 129 appears to increase susceptibility to sporadic CJD.[411] Octarepeat inserts of 32, 40, 48, 56, 64, and 72 amino acids at codon 67, 75, or 83 are designated by small rectangle below the ORF. These inserts segregate with familial CJD, and significant genetic linkage has been demonstrated when sufficient specimens from family members are available[9,336,375–378,382] (see also ref. 472). Point mutations are designated by the wild-type amino acid preceding the codon number, and the mutant residue follows. These point mutations segregate with the inherited prion diseases, and significant genetic linkage has been demonstrated when sufficient specimens from family members are available. Mutations at codons 102 (Pro → Leu), 117 (Ala → Val), 198 (Phe → Ser), and 217 (Gln → Arg) are found in patients with GSS.[8,42,336,340,341,351,372,391,464,465] Point mutations at codons 178 (Asp → Asn), 200 (Glu → Lys), and 210 (Val → Iso) are found in patients with familial CJD.[392,393,398,466,467] Point mutations at codons 198 (Phe → Ser) and 217 (Gln → Arg) are found in patients with GSS who have PrP amyloid plaques and neurofibrillary tangles.[342,343] The single-letter codes for amino acids are as follows: A = Ala; D = Asp; E = Glu; F = Phe; I = Iso; K = Lys; L = Leu; M = Met; N = Asn; P = Pro; Q = Gln, R = Arg; S = Ser; T = Thr; V = Val.

from Spain and Portugal at the time of the inquisition.[395] It is more likely that the codon 200 mutation has arisen independently multiple times by the deamidation of a methylated CpG as described above the codon 102 mutation.[42,393] In support of this hypothesis are historical records of Libyan and Tunisian Jews, indicating that they are descended from Jews living on the island of Jerba, where Jews first settled around 500 B.C. and not from Sephardim.[397]

Many families with CJD have been found to have point mutations at codon 178.[398–402] In these patients, as well as those with the codon 200 mutation, PrP amyloid plaques are rare; the neuropathological changes generally consist of widespread spongiform degeneration. A new prion disease that presents with insomnia has been described in three Italian families with the codon 178 mutation.[403] The neuropathology in these patients with fatal familial insomnia is restricted to selected nuclei of the thalamus. It is unclear whether all patients with the codon 178 mutation or only a subset present with sleep disturbances. It has been proposed that the allele with the codon 178 mutation encodes a Met at position 129 in fatal familial insomnia while a Val is encoded at position 129 in familial CJD.[404] The discovery that fatal familial insomnia is an inherited prion disease clearly widens the clinical spectrum of these disorders and

Table 153-9 Geographic Distribution of Patients with Inherited Prion Diseases*

PrP Mutation†	Prion Disease	Countries of Residence
P102L	Ataxic GSS	United States, United Kingdom, Japan, Germany, Italy, Canada, Austria, Israel, France
A117V	Dementing GSS	France, United States
D178N	Familial CJD	Finland, France, Italy, United States, (Hungary and Holland)‡
F198S	GSS with NFTs	United States
E200K	Familial CJD	Poland, Czechoslovakia, Italy, France, Greece, Japan, Chile, Israel, (Libya and Tunisia)‡
V210I	Familial CJD	France
Q217R	GSS with NFT	United States (Sweden)
Inserts	Familial CJD	United Kingdom, Japan, France, United States

*References cited in text and Fig. 153-9 legend.
†Point mutations are designated by the wild-type amino acid preceding the codon number, and the mutant residue follows.
‡Parentheses signify countries of origin.

raises the possibility that many other degenerative diseases of unknown etiology may be caused by prions.[403,405]

Other point mutations at codons 117, 198, and 217 also segregate with inherited prion diseases.[340,341,343,384,406] Patients with a dementing or telencephalic form of GSS have a mutation at codon 117. These patients as well as some in other families were once thought to have familial AD, but are now known to have prion diseases on the basis of PrP immunostaining of amyloid plaques and PrP gene mutations.[368,370,407,408] Patients with the codon 198 mutation have numerous NFT that stain with antibodies to τ and have amyloid plaques[368,370,407,408] that are composed largely of a PrP fragment extending from residues 58 to 150.[114] A genetic linkage study of this family produced a Lod score exceeding 6.[342] The neuropathology of two patients of Swedish ancestry with the codon 217 mutation[371] was similar to that of patients with the codon 198 mutation.

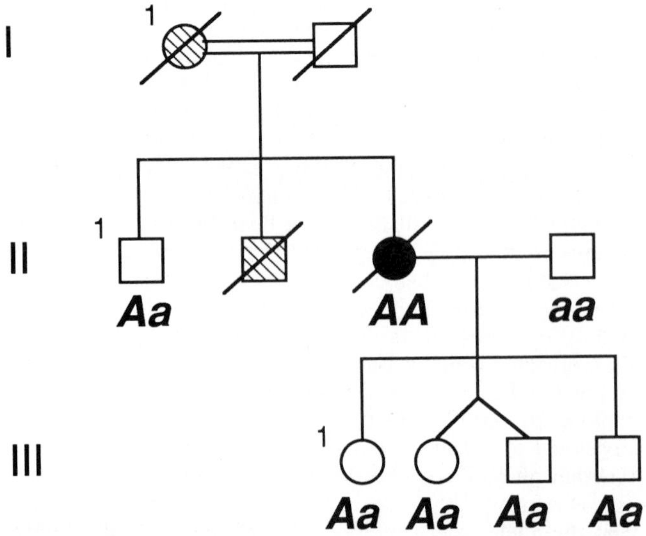

FIG. 153-10 Pedigree of a Libyan Jewish family with CJD. In this family, the ages of the subjects with the *A* haplotype who were at risk for disease were 25 years in subject II-1, 8 in subject III-1, 10 in subjects III-2 and III-3, and 12 in subject III-4. Subject II-3 died at age 42; she was homozygous for the PrP gene condon 200 lysine mutation, and all four of her children had the *A* haplotype. *(Adapted from Hsiao et al.,[393] by permission.)*

Human Prion Protein Gene Polymorphisms

At PrP codon 129, an amino acid (Met/Val) polymorphism (see Fig. 153-9) has been identified.[409] Patients with CJD following treatment with human pituitary growth hormone[7,306] or gonadotropin have a significant preponderance of the Val allele[410] as compared with the general population (Table 153-10). Sporadic CJD patients were found to be homozygous for the Met or Val allele at codon 129 but were rarely heterozygous.[411] This finding was interpreted[411,412] as consistent with the hypothesis that PrP^{C}/PrP^{Sc} heterodimers feature in the replication of prions.[2,156]

ATTEMPTS TO DEMONSTRATE *DE NOVO* SYNTHESIS OF PRIONS IN TRANSGENIC MICE EXPRESSING GERSTMANN-STRÄUSSLER-SCHEINKER MUTANT MOUSE PRION PROTEIN

When the codon 102 point mutation was introduced into MoPrP in Tg mice, spontaneous central nervous system

Table 153-10 PrP Gene Codon 129 Polymorphism in Patients with Iatrogenic, Sporadic, and Atypical CJD

	Number with Polymorphism			
Polymorphism	Iatrogenic	Sporadic	Atypical	General Population
Met/Met	1	16	11	54
Met/Val	2	1	4	39
Val/Val	4	5	6	13

NOTE: Data compiled from refs. 409 to 411.

degeneration occurred, characterized by clinical signs indistinguishable from experimental murine scrapie and neuropathology consisting of widespread spongiform morphology and astrocytic gliosis.[259] By inference, these results suggest that PrP mutations cause GSS and familial CJD. It is unclear whether low levels of protease-resistant PrP in the brains of Tg mice with the GSS mutation are PrP^{Sc} or residual PrP^{C}. Undetectable or low levels of PrP^{Sc} in the brains of these Tg mice are consistent with the results of transmission experiments that suggest low titers of infectious prions. Brain extracts transmit central nervous system degeneration to inoculated recipients, and the *de novo* synthesis of prions has been demonstrated by serial passage from Tg(GSSMoPrP) mice in which spontaneous neurodegeneration developed.[413] If these observations can be supported by additional studies with similar results and the possibility of contamination eliminated, then it can be argued that prions are devoid of foreign nucleic acid, in accord with many studies that use other experimental approaches.[1,67,292,414–422]

One view of the PrP gene mutations has been that they render individuals susceptible to a common "virus."[104,423,424] In this scenario, the putative scrapie virus is thought to persist within a worldwide reservoir of humans, animals, or insects without causing detectable illness. Yet 1 in 10^6 individuals have sporadic CJD and die from a lethal "infection," while ~100 percent of people with PrP point mutations or inserts appear eventually to have neurologic dysfunction. That germ-line mutations found in the PrP genes of patients and at-risk individuals are the cause of familial prion diseases is supported by experiments with Tg(GSSMoPrP) mice as described above.[8,413,425] The Tg mouse studies also argue that sporadic CJD might arise from the spontaneous conversion of PrP^{C} to PrP^{CJD} due to either a somatic mutation of the PrP gene or rare event involving modification of wild-type PrP^{C}.[2]

SPECIES BARRIERS IN THE TRANSMISSION OF PRION DISEASES

Passage of prions between species is a stochastic process characterized by prolonged incubation times.[51,426,427] Prions synthesized *de novo* reflect the sequence of the host PrP gene and not that of the PrP^{Sc} molecules in the inoculum.[261] On subsequent passage in the homologous host, the incubation time shortens to that recorded for all subsequent passages, and it becomes a nonstochastic process. The species-barrier concept is of practical importance in assessing the risk of CJD in humans after they have consumed scrapie-infected lamb or BSE beef.

To test the hypothesis that differences in PrP gene sequences might be responsible for the species barrier, Tg mice expressing SHaPrP were constructed.[156,428] The PrP genes of SHa and mice encode proteins differing at 16 positions. Incubation times in four lines of Tg(SHaPrP) mice inoculated with Mo prions were prolonged as compared with those observed for non-Tg, control mice (Fig. 153-11*A*). Inoculation of Tg(SHaPrP) mice with SHa prions demonstrated abrogation of the species barrier, resulting in abbreviated incubation times due to a nonstochastic process (Fig. 153-11*B*).[156,428] The length of the incubation time after inoculation with SHa prions was inversely proportional to the level of $SHaPrP^{C}$ in the brains of Tg(SHaPrP) mice (Fig. 153-11*B* and 153-11*C*).[156] $SHaPrP^{Sc}$ levels in the brains of clinically ill mice were similar in all four Tg(SHaPrP) lines inoculated with SHa prions (Fig. 153-11*D*). Bioassays of brain extracts from clinically ill Tg(SHaPrP) mice inoculated with Mo prions revealed that only Mo prions but no SHa prions were produced (Fig. 153-11*E*). Conversely, inoculation of Tg(SHaPrP) mice with SHa prions led to only the synthesis of SHa prions (Fig. 153-11*F*). Thus, the *de novo* synthesis of prions is species-specific and reflects the genetic origin of the inoculated prions. Similarly, the neuropathology of Tg(SHaPrP) mice is determined by the genetic origin of prion inoculum. Mo prions injected into Tg(SHaPrP) mice produced a neuropathology characteristic of mice with scrapie. A moderate degree of vacuolation in both the gray and white matter was found, while amyloid plaques were rarely detected (Fig. 153-11*G*) (Table 153-11). Inoculation of Tg(SHaPrP) mice with SHa prions produced intense vacuolation of the gray matter, sparing of the white matter and numerous SHaPrP amyloid plaques characteristic of SHa with scrapie (Fig. 153-11*H*)

These investigations indicate that PrP transgenes modulate virtually all phases of scrapie, including: replication of prions, incubation times, synthesis of PrP^{Sc}, species barrier, and neuropathological changes.

ABLATION OF THE PRION PROTEIN GENE

Ablation of the PrP gene in Tg ($Prn\text{-}p^{0/0}$) mice has, unexpectedly, not affected the development of these animals.[30] In fact, they are healthy at almost 2 years of age. $Prn\text{-}p^{0/0}$ mice are resistant to prions and do not propagate scrapie infectivity;[429] mice heterozygous ($Prn\text{-}p^{0/+}$) for ablation of the PrP gene had prolonged incubation times when inoculated with mouse prions (see ref. 473). This finding is in accord with studies on Tg(SHaPrP) mice, in which increased SHaPrP expression was accompanied by diminished incubation times.[156] Furthermore, since the absence of PrP^{C} expression does not provoke disease, we can conclude that scrapie and other prion diseases are a consequence of PrP^{Sc} accumulation rather than an inhibition of PrP^{C} function. To date, the function of PrP^{C} remains unknown.

PRION DIVERSITY

There is good evidence for multiple "strains" or distinct isolates of prions as defined by specific incubation times, distribution of vacuolar lesions, and patterns of PrP^{Sc} accumulation.[188,430–432] The mechanism by which isolate-specific information is carried by prions remains enigmatic; indeed, explaining the molecular basis of prion diversity seems to be a formidable challenge. For many years some investigators argued that scrapie is caused by a virus-like particle that contains a scrapie-specific nucleic acid that encodes the information expressed by each isolate.[433] To date, no such polynucleotide has been identified by a wide variety of techniques, including measurements of the nucleic acids in purified preparations. An alternative hypothesis has been suggested that PrP^{Sc} alone is capable of transmitting disease, but the characteristics of PrP^{Sc} might be modified by a cellular RNA.[88] This accessory cellular RNA is postulated to induce its own synthesis on transmission from one host to another.

Two additional hypotheses not involving a nucleic acid have been offered to explain distinct prion isolates: a nonnucleic acid second component might create prion diversity or posttranslational modification of PrP^{Sc} might be responsible

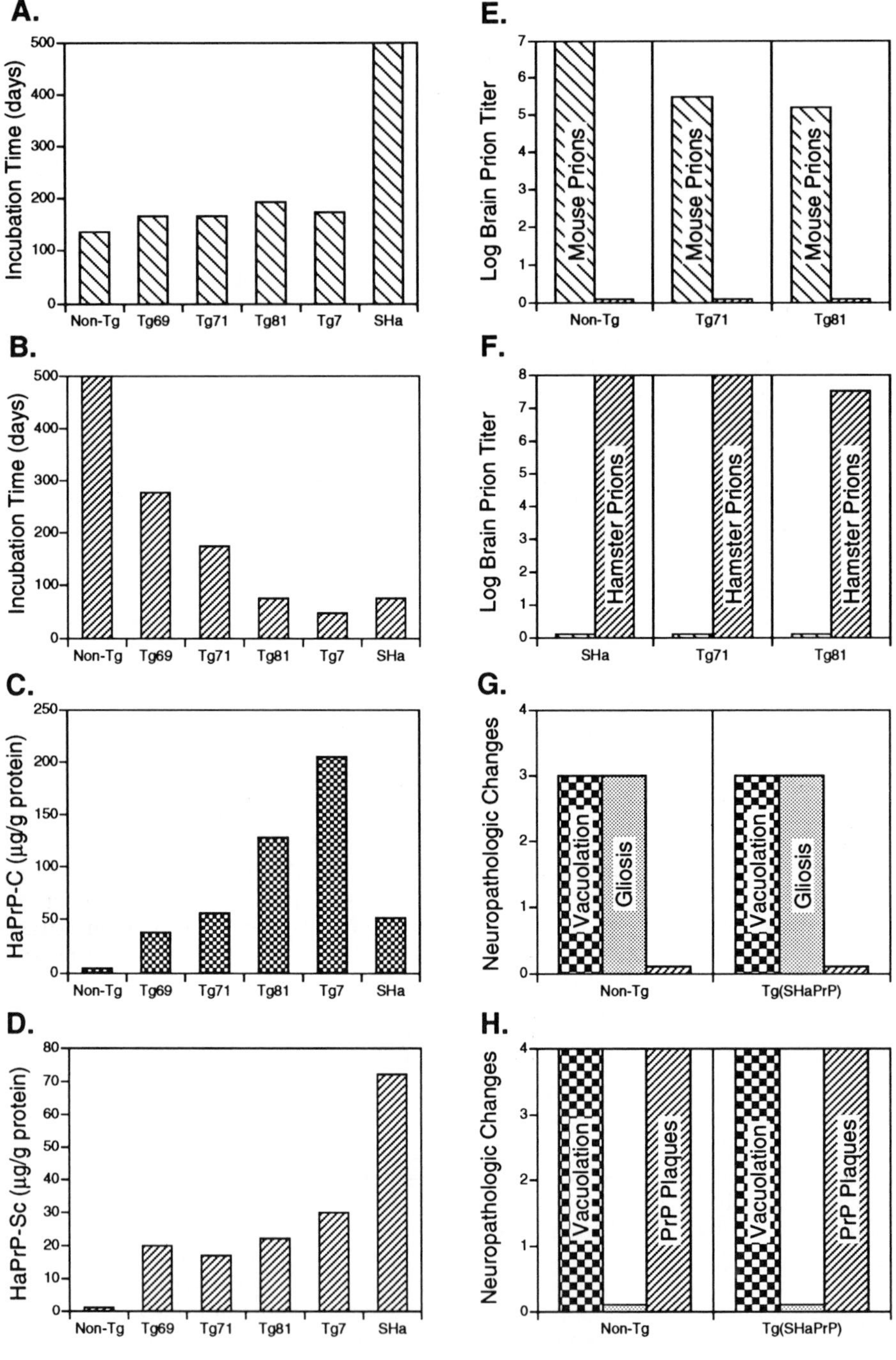

FIG. 153-11 Tg mice expressing SHa prion protein exhibit species-specific scrapie incubation times, infectious prion synthesis, and neuropathology.[156] *A.* Scrapie incubation times in non-Tg mice and four lines of Tg mice expressing SHaPrP and H inoculated intracerebrally with $\sim 10^6$ ID$_{50}$ units of Chandler Mo prions serially passaged in Swiss mice. The four lines of Tg mice have different numbers of transgene copies: Tg69 and 71 mice have two to four copies of the SHaPrP transgene, whereas Tg81 have 30 to 50 and Tg7 mice have >60. Incubation times are numbers of days from inoculation to onset of neurologic dysfunction. *B.* Scrapie incubation times in mice and hamsters inoculated with $\sim 10^7$ ID$_{50}$ units of Sc237 prions serially passaged in Syrian hamsters and as described in *A. C.* Brain SHaPrP^{C} in Tg mice and hamsters. SHaPrP^{C} levels were quantitated by ELISA. *D.* Brain SHaPrP^{Sc} in Tg mice and hamsters. Animals were killed after exhibiting clinical signs of scrapie. SHa-PrP^{Sc} levels were determined by immunoassay. *E.* Prion titers in brains of clinically ill animals after inoculation with Mo prions. Brain extracts from non-Tg, Tg71, and Tg81 mice were bioassayed for prions in mice (left) and hamsters (right). *F.* Prion titers in brains of clinically ill animals after inoculation with SHa prions. Brain extracts from SHa as well as Tg71 and Tg81 mice were bioassayed for prions in mice (left) and hamsters (right). *G.* Neuropathology in non-Tg mice and Tg(SHaPrP) mice with clinical signs of scrapie after inoculation with Mo prions. Vacuolation in gray (left) and white matter (center) and PrP amyloid plaques (right). Vacuolation score: 0 = none; 1 = rare; 2 = modest; 3 = moderate; 4 = intense. *H.* Neuropathology in SHa and Tg mice inoculated with SHa prions. Degree of vacuolation and frequency of PrP amyloid plaques as described in *G.* *(Adapted from Prusiner,[2] by permission.)*

for the different properties of distinct prion isolates.[2] Whether the PrP^{Sc} modification is chemical or conformational alone remains to be established, but no candidate chemical modifications have been identified. Structural studies of the GPI anchors of two SHa isolates have failed to reveal any differences; interestingly, about 40 percent of the anchor glycans have sialic acid residues (see Fig. 153-8).[174] A portion of the PrP^{C} GPI anchors also have sialic acid residues; PrP is the first protein found to have sialic acid residues attached to GPI anchors.

Although the structures of Asn-linked carbohydrates have been analyzed for PrP^{Sc} of one isolate,[161] no data are available for PrP^{Sc} of other isolates or PrP^{C}. The great diversity of glycosylation makes them candidates for isolate-specific information, but there is no precedent for Asn-linked glycosylates instructing the synthesis of more of the same. In some studies, it has been found that distinct isolates produce different, reproducible patterns of PrP^{Sc} accumulation.[432] These findings have given rise to the hypothesis that PrP^{Sc} synthesis occurs in particular sets of cells for a given distinct prion isolate. Whether different Asn-linked carbohydrates function to target PrP^{Sc} of a distinct isolate to a particular set of cells, where similarly Asn-linked glycosylates will be coupled to PrP^{C} prior to its conversion to PrP^{Sc}, remains to be established. Even though this hypothesis is attractive, it must be noted that PrP^{Sc} synthesis in scrapie-infected cells occurs in the presence of tunicamycin, which inhibits Asn-linked glycosylation, and with PrP molecules mutated at the Asn-linked glycosylation consensus sites.[168] Whether SHa scrapie prions can be synthesized in Tg mice expressing

Table 153-11 Species-Specific Prion Inoculums Determine the Distribution of Spongiform Change and Deposition of PrP Amyloid Plaques in Tg Mice

	SHa Prions					Mo Prions			
		Spongiform Change*		PrP Plaques†			Spongiform Change*		PrP Plaques†
Animal	n‡	Gray	White	Frequency	Diameter§	n‡	Gray	White	Frequency
Non-Tg		N.D.		N.D.		10	+	+	–
Tg 69	6	+	–	Numerous	6.5±3.1 (389)	2	+	+	–
Tg 71	5	+	–	Numerous	8.1±3.6 (345)	2	+	+	–
Tg 81	7	+	–	Numerous	8.3±3.0 (439)	3	+	+	Few
Tg 7	3	+¶	–	Numerous	14.0±8.3 (19)	4	+	+	–
SHa	3	+	–	Numerous	5.7±2.7 (247)		ND		ND

*Spongiform change evaluated in hippocampus, thalamus, cerebral cortex, and brain stem for gray matter and the deep cerebellum for white matter.
+ = present; – = not found; N.D. = not determined.
†Plaques in the subcallosal region were stained with SHaPrP mAb 13A5, anti-PrP rabbit antiserum R073, and trichrome stain.
‡n = number of brains examined.
§Mean diameter of PrP plaques given in microns ± SE, with the number of observations in parentheses.
¶Focal: confirmed to the dorsal nucleus of the raphe.
SOURCE: From Prusiner.[463]

SHaPrP with mutated Asn-linked glycosylation consensus sites and the properties exhibited by distinct isolates is currently under investigation. Of note, two different isolates from mink dying of TME exhibit different sensitivities of PrP^{Sc} to proteolytic digestion, supporting the suggestion that isolate-specific information might be carried by PrP^{Sc}.[200,434,435]

PRION REPLICATION

The mechanism by which prions multiply is unknown. Although the search for a scrapie-specific nucleic acid continues to be unrewarding, some investigators steadfastly cling to the notion that this putative polynucleotide drives prion replication. If prions are found to contain a scrapie-specific nucleic acid, then such a molecule would be expected to direct scrapie agent replication using a strategy similar to that employed by viruses (Fig. 153-12*A*). In the absence of any chemical or physical evidence for a scrapie-specific polynucleotide,[1,67,292,414–422,436–443] it seems reasonable to consider some alternative mechanisms that might feature in prion biosynthesis. The multiplication of prion infectivity is an exponential process in which the posttranslational conversion of PrP^{C} or a precursor to PrP^{Sc} appears to be obligatory.[26] As illustrated in Fig. 153-12*B*, PrP^{Sc} molecules combine with two heterodimers, which are subsequently transformed into two homodimers. In the next cycle, four PrP^{Sc} molecules combine with four PrP^{C} molecules, giving rise to four homodimers that dissociate to combine with eight PrP^{C} molecules, creating an exponential process. Studies with Tg(SHaPrP) mice argue that prion synthesis involves "replication," not merely "amplification."[156] Assuming prion biosynthesis simply involves amplification of posttranslationally altered PrP molecules, we might expect Tg(SHaPrP) mice to produce both SHa and Mo prions after inoculation with either prion since these mice produce both SHa and Mo PrP^{C}. Yet, Tg(SHaPrP) mice synthesize only prions present in the inoculum (Fig. 153-11*E* and 153-11*F*). These results argue that the incoming prion and PrP^{Sc} interact with the homologous PrP^{C} substrate to replicate more of the same prions (Fig. 153-12*C*).

Additional evidence in support of the proposed model for prion replication comes from Tg(Mo/SHaPrP) mice expressing chimeric Mo/SHaPrP^{C} (see ref. 474). The chimeric Mo/SHaPrP gene was constructed by substituting the SHaPrP sequence for Mo PrP from codon 94 to 188; within this domain, there are five amino acid substitutions that distinguish Mo from SHaPrP. When inoculated with either Mo or SHa prions, these Tg(Mo/SHaPrP) mice have scrapie after ~140 days. The chimeric Tg mice produce Mo/SHaPrP^{Sc} and Mo/SHa prions and inoculation with SHa prions and probably Mo prions as well. Evidence for chimeric Mo/SHa prions comes from the development of scrapie in Tg(Mo/SHaPrP) mice ~70 days after inoculation with brain extracts from Tg(Mo/SHaPrP) mice containing the chimeric prions.

In the absence of any candidate posttranslational chemical modifications[29] that differentiate PrP^{C} from PrP^{Sc}, we are forced to consider the possibility that conformation distinguishes these isoforms. By comparing the amino acid sequences of 11 mammalian and one avian PrP, structural analyses predicted 4 α-helical regions (see Fig. 153-4*B*)[444] (and Gabriel J-M, Cohen F, Fletterick, RA, Prusiner SB: unpublished data). Peptides corresponding to these regions of the SHaPrP were synthesized, and contrary to predictions, three of the four spontaneously formed amyloids as shown by electron microscopy and Congo red staining.[445] By infrared spectroscopy, these amyloid peptides were found to exhibit a secondary structure comprised largely of β-sheets. The first of the predicted helixes is the 14-residue peptide corresponding to codons 109 to 122; this peptide and the overlapping 15-residue sequence 113 to 127 both form amyloid. The most highly amyloidogenic peptide is the sequence AGAAAAGA corresponding to PrP codons 113 to 120. This peptide is in a region of PrP that is conserved across all known species (see Fig. 153-4*A*). Two other predicted α-helixes corresponding to codons 178 to 191 and 202 to 218 form amyloids and exhibit considerable β-sheet structure when synthesized as peptides. These findings suggest the possibility that the conversion of PrP^{C} to PrP^{Sc} involves the transition of one or more putative PrP α-helixes into β-sheets. Infrared spectroscopy of PrP 27-30 showed a high β-sheet content,[446] which decreased when PrP 27-30 was denatured, and scrapie infectivity diminished concomitantly.[447]

These structural investigations of synthetic PrP peptides and the correlations between PrP 27-30 secondary structure and scrapie infectivity offer a structural model for the

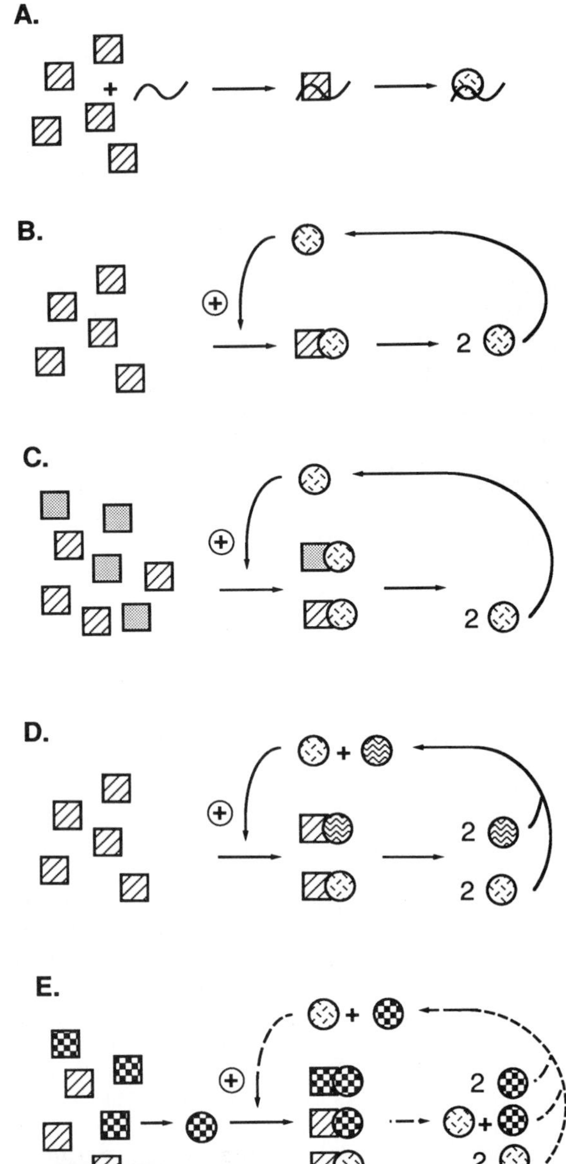

FIG. 153-12 Some possible mechanisms of prion replication. *A*. Two-component prion model. Prions contain a putative, as yet unidentified, nucleic acid or another second component (solid, thick wavy line) that binds to PrP^{C} (squares) and stimulates conversion of PrP^{C} or a precursor to PrP^{Sc} (circle). *B*. One-component prion model—prions devoid of nucleic acid. PrP^{Sc} binds to PrP^{C}-forming heterodimers that function as replication intermediates in the synthesis of PrP^{Sc}. Repeated cycles of this process result in an exponential increase in PrP^{Sc}. *C*. Prion synthesis in Tg mice.[156] SHaPrP^{Sc} (broken, cross-hatched circles) binds to SHaPrP^{C} (diagonally striped squares), leading to the synthesis of PrP^{Sc}. Binding to MoPrP^{C} (stippled squares) does not produce PrP^{Sc}. Species barrier for scrapie between mice and hamsters represented by MoPrP^{C}-SHaPrP^{Sc} heterodimer. *D*. Scrapie isolates or strains in hamsters or mice. Multiple PrP^{Sc} conformers (cross-hatched and wavy patterns in circles) bind to PrP^{C} and constrain the conformational changes that PrP^{C} undergoes during its conversion into PrP^{Sc}. *E*. Inherited prion diseases in humans and Tg mice. Mutant PrP^{C} molecules (checkered pattern in squares) might initiate the conversion of PrP^{C} to PrP^{Sc} (or PrP^{CJD}). If infectious prions are produced (dashed lines), then they stimulate the synthesis of more PrP^{CJD} in humans and PrP^{Sc} in experimental animals. Alternatively, prion infectivity is not generated, but neurologic dysfunction, spongiform degeneration, astrocytic gliosis, and possibly PrP amyloid plaques develop.[4,5,8,42,336,340,341,351,372,391,393,413,464–466] *(From Prusiner.[2] Used by permission.)*

conversion of PrP^{C} to PrP^{Sc} as well as the replication of infectious prion particles involving a transition from α-helixes to β-sheets in PrP (see ref. 475). Whether any of the synthetic PrP peptides described here can induce brain degeneration, PrP^{Sc} formation, or prion infectivity is currently being investigated. If additional data can be obtained to support the hypothesis set forth here, then it may be useful to examine other degenerative diseases with respect to proteins undergoing similar structural changes.

The diversity of scrapie prions[433,448–450] poses an interesting conundrum. The finding that the pattern of PrP^{Sc} accumulation in the central nervous system is characteristic for a particular strain offers a mechanism for the propagation of distinct prion isolates.[432] In this model, a different set of cells would propagate each isolate. Whether the isolates are targeted to specific sets of cells by the Asn-linked oligosaccharides of PrP^{Sc} remains to be established. It is noteworthy that PrP^{Sc} synthesis can occur in the absence of Asn-linked glycosylaton in scrapie-infected cultured cells[175]; further studies are needed to determine the molecular basis of the cellular trophism exhibited by prions. Alternatively, explaining the problem of multiple distinct prion isolates might be accommodated by multiple PrP^{Sc} conformers that act as templates for the folding of PrP^{Sc} molecules synthesized *de novo* during prion "replication" (see Fig. 153-12*D*). Although both these proposals are rather unorthodox, they are consistent with observations generated from Tg(SHaPrP)Mo studies contending that PrP^{Sc} in the inoculum binds to homologous PrP^{C} or a precursor to form a heterodimeric intermediate in the replication process.[156] Whether "foldases," "chaperonins," or other types of molecules feature in the conversion of the PrP^{C}/PrP^{Sc} heterodimer to two molecules of PrP^{Sc} is unknown. The molecular weight of a PrP^{Sc} homodimer is consistent with the ionizing radiation target size of 55±9 kDa as determined for infectious prion particles independent of their polymeric form.[451]

In humans carrying point mutations or inserts in their PrP genes, mutant PrP^{C} molecules might spontaneously convert into PrP^{Sc} (see Fig. 153-12*E*). While the initial stochastic event may be inefficient, once it happens the process becomes autocatalytic. The proposed mechanism is consistent with individuals harboring germ-line mutations in whom central nervous system dysfunction does not develop for decades and with studies on Tg(GSSMoPrP) mice in which central nervous system degeneration spontaneously develops.[259] Whether all GSS and familial CJD cases contain infectious prions or some represent inborn errors of PrP metabolism in which neither PrP^{Sc} nor prion infectivity accumulates is unknown. If the latter is found, then presumably, mutant PrP^{C} molecules alone can produce central nervous system degeneration.

Some investigators have suggested that scrapie agent multiplication proceeds through a crystallization process involving PrP amyloid formation.[80,452,453] Against this hypothesis is the absence or rarity of amyloid plaques in many prion diseases, as well as the inability to identify any amyloid-like polymers in cultured cells chronically synthesizing prions.[97,156] Purified infectious preparations isolated from scrapie-infected hamster brains exist as amorphous aggregates; only if PrP^{Sc} is exposed to detergents and limited proteolysis does it then polymerize into prion rods exhibiting the ultrastructural and tinctorial features of amyloid.[97] Furthermore, dispersion of prion rods into detergent–lipid–protein complexes results in a tenfold to one-hundredfold increase in scrapie titer and no rods could be identified in these fractions on electron microscopy.[98]

AN OVERVIEW OF PRION STRUCTURE AND REPLICATION

Although many experimental studies reviewed above argue persuasively that prions are devoid of nucleic acid, the complete structure of the prion particle remains to be established. Whether the enigma of prion diversity will eventually be shown to depend on an as yet undetected scrapie-specific nucleic acid or it arises through an unorthodox mechanism such as Asn-linked glycosylation of PrP^{Sc} is uncertain.

Consider the remote possibility that prions do contain an as yet undetected polynucleotide; then presumably, prion replication would involve a virus-like strategy. The putative scrapie-specific nucleic acid would act as a template for its own synthesis using cellular polymerases. By an as yet undefined mechanism, the putative scrapie-specific nucleic acid would stimulate the conversion of PrP^{C} to PrP^{Sc}. While this putative scrapie-specific nucleic acid would provide a plausible explanation for prion diversity, it would require that this nucleotide sequence be able to discriminate between SHaPrP and MoPrP in Tg(SHaPrP) mice. In addition, the putative scrapie-specific nucleic acid would have to be ubiquitous in order to explain how sporadic CJD occurs with an incidence of 1 in 10^6 population[232,454] all over the planet, while in virtually all people who carry PrP gene mutations prion disease develops.

A more likely scenario is that prions do not contain a scrapie-specific nucleic acid; rather, they are composed entirely of PrP^{Sc} molecules. If this is the case, then the species barrier for prion transmission, the results with Tg(SHaPrP) mice, and infectious prions in the brains of patients with inherited prion diseases can be more readily explained. If prions are composed entirely of PrP^{Sc}, then replication must involve the interaction of nascent PrP^{C} or a precursor with PrP^{Sc}.[2,156] Although there is no physical data at this time demonstrating the existence of PrP^{C}/PrP^{Sc} heterodimers, it is difficult to explain the results obtained with Tg(SHaPrP) mice in studies of prion replication. Moreover, other studies have shown that patients homologous for the Met/Val polymorphism at codon 129 are predisposed to sporadic CJD, while those with heterozygous alleles at codon 129 are relatively protected.[411] These findings have been interpreted as being consistent with the hypothesis that prion replication is most efficient when the primary structures of PrP^{C} and PrP^{Sc} are the same. As noted above, although the PrP^{Sc} model is consistent with all of the experimental data, it continues to be problematic with respect to explaining the molecular basis of multiple distinct scrapie prion isolates or "stains."

The formal possibility remains that prions contain a second component that is not a nucleic acid. A small polypeptide, a polysaccharide, a lipid-glycan, or a phospholipid–sterol complex are all possibilities, but there is no evidence at this time for any of these molecules to be prion components.

CONCLUSIONS AND PROSPECTS

The study of prions has taken several unexpected directions over the past few years. The discovery that prion diseases in humans are uniquely both genetic and infectious has greatly strengthened and extended the prion concept. To date, 12 different mutations in the human PrP gene all resulting in nonconservative substitutions have been found to be either linked genetically to or to segregate with the inherited prion diseases. Yet, the transmissible prion particle is composed largely, if not entirely, of an abnormal isoform of the prion protein designated PrP^{Sc}.[2] These findings argue that prion diseases should be considered pseudoinfections, since the particles transmitting disease appear to be devoid of a foreign nucleic acid and thus differ from all known microorganisms as well as viruses and viroids. Because much information, especially about scrapie of rodents, has been derived using experimental protocols adapted from virology, we continue to use terms such as *infection, incubation period, transmissibility,* and *end-point titration* in studies of prion diseases.

Although relatively little is known about the replication of prions, Tg mice expressing foreign or mutant PrP genes now permit virtually all facets of prion diseases to be studied and have created a framework for future investigations. Furthermore, the structure and organization of the PrP gene suggested that PrP^{Sc} is derived from PrP^{C} or a precursor by a posttranslational process. Studies with scrapie-infected cultured cells have provided much evidence that the conversion of PrP^{C} to PrP^{Sc} is a posttranslational process that probably occurs in the endocytic pathway. The molecular basis of the PrP^{Sc} synthetic process remains to be elucidated, but extensive protein chemical studies suggest that this process is likely to involve a conformational change.

It seems likely that the principles learned from the study of prion diseases will be applicable to elucidating the causes of more common neurodegenerative diseases. Such disorders include AD, amyotrophic lateral sclerosis, and Parkinson disease. Since people at risk for inherited prion diseases can now be identified decades before neurologic dysfunction is evident, the development of an effective therapy is imperative. If PrP^{C} can be diminished in humans without deleterious effects, as is the case for Prn-$p^{0/0}$ mice,[30] then reducing the level of PrP mRNA with antisense oligonucleotides might prove an effective therapeutic maneuver in delaying the onset of central nervous system symptoms and signs.

The study of prion biology and diseases seems to be a new and emerging area of biomedical investigation. While prion biology has its roots in virology, neurology, and neuropathology, its relationships to the disciplines of molecular and cell biology as well as protein chemistry have become evident only recently. Certainly, the possibility that learning how prions multiply and cause disease will open up new vistas in biochemistry and genetics seems likely.

ACKNOWLEDGMENTS

I thank M. Baldwin, D. Borchelt, G. Carlson, F. Cohen, C. Cooper, S. DeArmond, R. Fletterick, D. Foster, M. Gasset, R. Gabizon, D. Groth, L. Hood, K. Hsiao, V. Lingappa, W. Mobley, D. Riesner, M. Scott, A. Serban, N. Stahl, A. Taraboulos, M. Torchia, and D. Westaway for their help in these studies. Special thanks to L. Gallagher who assembled this manuscript. This work was supported by grants from the National Institutes of Health (NS14069, AG08967, AG02132, and NS22786) and the American Health Assistance Foundation, as well as by gifts from Sherman Fairchild Foundation,

Bernard Osher Foundation, and National Medical Enterprises.

REFERENCES

1. Meyer N, Rosenbaum V, Schmidt B, Gilles K, Mirenda C, Groth D, Prusiner SB, Riesner D: Search for a putative scrapie genome in purified prion fractions reveals a paucity of nucleic acids. *J Gen Virol* **72**:37, 1991.
2. Prusiner SB: Molecular biology of prion diseases. *Science* **252**:1515, 1991.
3. Alpers MP: Epidemiology and ecology of kuru, in Prusiner SB, Hadlow WJ (eds): *Slow Transmissible Diseases of the Nervous System*. New York, Academic, 1979, vol. 1, pp 67–90.
4. Gajdusek DC: Unconventional viruses and the origin and disappearance of kuru. *Science* **197**:943, 1977.
5. Masters CL, Gajdusek DC, Gibbs CJ Jr: The familial occurrence of Creutzfeldt-Jakob disease and Alzheimer's disease. *Brain* **104**:535, 1981.
6. Gibbs CJ Jr, Joy A, Heffner R, Franko M, Miyazaki M, Asher DM, Parisi JE, Brown PW, Gajdusek DC: Clinical and pathological features and laboratory confirmation of Creutzfeldt-Jakob disease in a recipient of pituitary-derived human growth hormone. *N Engl J Med* **313**:734, 1985.
7. Fradkin JE, Schoenberger LB, Mills JL, Gunn WJ, Piper JM, Wysowski DK, Thomson R, Durako S, Brown P: Creutzfeldt-Jakob disease in pituitary growth hormone recipients in the United States. *JAMA* **265**:880, 1991.
8. Hsiao K, Prusiner SB: Inherited human prion diseases. *Neurology* **40**:1820, 1990.
9. Collinge J, Harding AE, Owen F, Poulter M, Lofthouse R, Boughey AM, Shah T, Crow TJ: Diagnosis of Gerstmann-Sträussler syndrome in familial dementia with prion protein gene analysis. *Lancet* **2**:15, 1989.
10. Brown P, Goldfarb LG, Gajdusek DC: The new biology of spongiform encephalopathy: Infectious amyloidoses with a genetic twist. *Lancet* **337**:1019, 1991.
11. Medori R, Tritschler H-J, LeBlanc A, Villare F, Manetto V, Chen HY, Xue R, Leal S, Montagna P, Cortelli P, Tinuper P, Avoni P, Mochi M, Baruzzi A, Hauw JJ, Ott J, Lugaresi E, Autilio-Gambetti L, Gambetti P: Fatal familial insomnia, a prion disease with a mutation at codon 178 of the prion protein gene. *N Engl J Med* **326**:444, 1992.
12. Cuillé J, Chelle PL: Experimental transmission of trembling to the goat. *C R Seances Acad Sci* **208**:1058, 1939.
13. Gordon WS: Variation in susceptibility of sheep to scrapie and genetic implications, *Report of Scrapie Seminar, ARS 91-53*. Washington, DC, Department of Agriculture, 1966, pp 53–67.
14. Parry HB: Scrapie: A transmissible and hereditary disease of sheep. *Hereditary* **17**:75, 1962.
15. Dickinson AG, Young GB, Stamp JT, Renwick CC: An analysis of natural scrapie in Suffolk sheep. *Heredity (Edinburgh)* **20**:485, 1965.
16. Pattison IH: Fifty years with scrapie: A personal reminiscence. *Vet Rec* **123**:661, 1988.
17. Prusiner SB: Novel proteinaceous infectious particles cause scrapie. *Science* **216**:136, 1982.
18. Bolton DC, McKinley MP, Prusiner SB: Identification of a protein that purifies with the scrapie prion. *Science* **218**:1309, 1982.
19. Prusiner SB, Bolton DC, Groth DF, Bowman KA, Cochran SP, McKinley MP: Further purification and characterization of scrapie prions. *Biochemistry* **21**:6942, 1982.
20. Masters CL, Gajdusek DC, Gibbs CJ Jr: Creutzfeldt-Jakob disease virus isolations from the Gerstmann-Sträussler syndrome. *Brain* **104**:559, 1981.
21. Prusiner SB, Groth DF, Bolton DC, Kent SB, Hood LE: Purification and structural studies of a major scrapie prion protein. *Cell* **38**:127, 1984.
22. Oesch B, Westaway D, Wälchli M, McKinley MP, Kent SBH, Aebersold R, Barry RA, Tempst P, Teplow DB, Hood LE, Prusiner SB, Weissmann C: A cellular gene encodes scrapie PrP 27-30 protein. *Cell* **40**:735, 1985.
23. Chesebro B, Race R, Wehrly K, Nishio J, Bloom M, Lechner D, Bergstrom S, Robbins K, Mayer L, Keith JM, Garon C, Haase A: Identification of scrapie prion protein-specific mRNA in scrapie-infected and uninfected brain. *Nature* **315**:331, 1985.
24. Gabizon R, Prusiner SB: Prion liposomes. *Biochem J* **266**:1, 1990.
25. Basler K, Oesch B, Scott M, Westaway D: Wälchli M, Groth DF, McKinley MP, Prusiner SB, Weissmann C: Scrapie and cellular PrP isoforms are encoded by the same chromosomal gene. *Cell* **46**:417, 1986.
26. Borchelt DR, Scott M, Taraboulos A, Stahl N, Prusiner SB: Scrapie and cellular prion proteins differ in their kinetics of synthesis and topology in cultured cells. *J Cell Biol* **110**:743, 1990.
27. Caughey B, Raymond GJ: The scrapie-associated form of PrP is made from a cell surface precursor that is both protease- and phospholipase-sensitive. *J Biol Chem* **226**:18217, 1991.
28. Borchelt DR, Taraboulos A, Prusiner SB: Evidence for synthesis of scrapie prion proteins in the endocytic pathway. *J Biol Chem* **267**:6188, 1992.
29. Stahl N, Baldwin MA, Teplow DB, Hood L, Gibson BW, Burlingame AL, Prusiner SB: Structural analysis of the scrapie prion protein using mass spectrometry and amino acid sequencing. *Biochemistry* **32**:1991, 1993.
30. Büeler H, Fischer M, Lang Y, Blüthmann H, Lipp H-L, DeArmond SJ, Prusiner SB, Aguet M, Weissmann C: The neuronal cell surface protein PrP is not essential for normal development and behavior of the mouse. *Nature* **356**:577, 1992.
31. Sparkes RS, Simon M, Cohn VH, Fournier REK, Lem J, Klisak I, Heinzmann C, Blatt C, Lucero M, Mohandas T, DeArmond SJ, Westaway D, Prusiner SB, Weiner LP: Assignment of the human and mouse prion protein genes to homologous chromosomes. *Proc Natl Acad Sci USA* **83**:7358, 1986.
32. Gajdusek DC, Gibbs CJ Jr, Alpers M: Experimental transmission of a kuru-like syndrome to chimpanzees. *Nature* **209**:794, 1966.
33. Gibbs CJ Jr, Gajdusek DC, Asher DC, Alpers MP, Beck E, Daniel PM, Matthews WB: Creutzfeldt-Jakob disease (spongiform encephalopathy): Transmission to the chimpanzee. *Science* **161**:388, 1968.
34. Brown P: An epidemiologic critique of Creutzfeldt-Jakob disease. *Epidemiol Rev* **2**:113, 1980.
35. Cousens SN, Harries-Jones R, Knight R, Will RG, Smith PG, Matthews WB: Geographical distribution of cases of Creutzfeldt-Jakob disease in England and Wales 1970–84. *J Neurol Neurosurg Psychiatry* **53**:459, 1990.
36. Harries-Jones R, Knight R, Will RG, Cousens S, Smith PG, Matthews WB: Creutzfeldt-Jakob disease in England and Wales, 1980–1984: A case-control study of potential risk factors. *J Neurol Neurosurg Psychiatry* **51**:1113, 1988.
37. Prusiner SB, Cochran SP, Alpers MP: Transmission of scrapie in hamsters. *J Infect Dis* **152**:971, 1985.
38. Prusiner SB: Scrapie prions. *Annu Rev Microbiol* **43**:345, 1989.
39. McKusick VA (ed): *Mendelian Inheritance in Man—Catalogs of Autosomal Dominant, Autosomal Recessive, and X-Linked Phenotypes*, 10th ed. Baltimore, Johns Hopkins University Press, vol 1, 1992.
40. Roberts GW, Lofthouse R, Allsop D, Landon M, Kidd M, Prusiner SB, Crow TJ: CNS amyloid proteins in neurodegenerative diseases. *Neurology* **38**:1534, 1988.
41. Merz PA, Somerville RA, Wisniewski HM, Iqbal K: Abnormal fibrils from scrapie-infected brain. *Acta Neuropathol (Berl)* **54**:63, 1981.
42. Hsiao K, Baker HF, Crow TJ, Poulter M, Owen F, Terwilliger JD, Westaway D, Ott J, Prusiner SB: Linkage of a prion protein missense variant to Gerstmann-Sträussler syndrome. *Nature* **338**:342, 1989.
43. Gordon WS: Advances in veterinary research. *Vet Res* **58**:516, 1946.
44. Chandler RL: Encephalopathy in mice produced by inoculation with scrapie brain material. *Lancet* **1**:1378, 1961.
45. Alper T, Haig DA, Clarke MC: The exceptionally small

size of the scrapie agent. *Biochem Biophys Res Commun* **22**:278, 1966.
46. Alper T, Cramp WA, Haig DA, Clarke MC: Does the agent of scrapie replicate without nucleic acid? *Nature* **214**:764, 1967.
47. Alper T, Haig DA, Clarke MC: The scrapie agent: Evidence against its dependence for replication on intrinsic nucleic acid. *J Gen Virol* **41**:503, 1978.
48. Gibbons RA, Hunter GD: Nature of the scrapie agent. *Nature* **215**:1041, 1967.
49. Griffith JS: Self-replication and scrapie. *Nature* **215**:1043, 1967.
50. Millson G, Hunter GD, Kimberlin RH: An experimental examination of the scrapie agent in cell membrane mixtures. II. The association of scrapie infectivity with membrane fractions. *J Comp Pathol* **81**:255, 1971.
51. Pattison IH, Jones KM: The possible nature of the transmissible agent of scrapie. *Vet Rec* **80**:1, 1967.
52. Prusiner SB, Cochran SP, Groth DF, Downey DE, Bowman KA, Martinez HM: Measurement of the scrapie agent using an incubation time interval assay. *Ann Neurol* **11**:353, 1982.
53. Prusiner SB, Groth DF, Cochran SP, Masiarz FR, McKinley MP, Martinez HM: Molecular properties, partial purification, and assay by incubation period measurements of the hamster scrapie agent. *Biochemistry* **19**:4883, 1980.
54. Manuelidis E, Kim J, Angelo J, Manuelidis L: Serial propagation of Creutzfeldt-Jakob disease in guinea pigs. *Proc Natl Acad Sci USA* **73**:223, 1971.
55. Tateishi J, Ohta M, Koga M, Sato Y, Kuroiwa Y: Transmission of chronic spongiform encephalopathy with kuru plaques from humans to small rodents. *Ann Neurol* **5**:581, 1979.
56. M'Gowan JP: *Investigation into the Disease of Sheep Called "Scrapie."* Edinburgh, William Blackwood, 1914, p 114.
57. M'Fadyean J: Scrapie. *J Comp Pathol* **31**:102, 1918.
58. Wilson DR, Anderson RD, Smith W: Studies in scrapie. *J Comp Pathol* **60**:267, 1950.
59. Kimberlin RH, Hunter GD: DNA synthesis in scrapie-affected mouse brain. *J Gen Virol* **1**:115, 1967.
60. Lewin P: Scrapie: An infective peptide? *Lancet* **1**:748, 1972.
61. Lewin P: Infectious peptides in slow virus infections: A hypothesis. *Can Med Assoc J* **124**:1436, 1981.
62. Hunter GD, Kimberlin RH, Gibbons RA: Scrapie: A modified membrane hypothesis. *J Theor Biol* **20**:355, 1968.
63. Adams DH, Field EJ: The infective process in scrapie. *Lancet* **2**:714, 1968.
64. Adams DH: The nature of the scrapie agent: A review of recent progress. *Pathol Biol* **18**:559, 1970.
65. Parry HB: Scrapie—natural and experimental, in Whitty CWM, Hughes JT, MacCallum FO (eds): *Virus Diseases and the Nervous System*. Oxford, Blackwell, 1969, pp 99–105.
66. Diener TO: Is the scrapie agent a viroid? *Nature* **235**:218, 1972.
67. Diener TO, McKinley MP, Prusiner SB: Viroids and prions. *Proc Natl Acad Sci USA* **79**:5220, 1982.
68. Rohwer RG, Gajdusek DC: Scrapie—virus or viroid, the case for a virus. in, Boese A (ed): *Search for the Cause of Multiple Sclerosis and Other Chronic Diseases of the Central Nervous System*. Weinheim, Verlag Chemie, 1980, pp 333–355.
69. Field EJ: The significance of astroglial hypertrophy in scrapie, kuru, multiple sclerosis and old age together with a note on the possible nature of the scrapie agent. *Dtsch Z Nervenheilkd* **192**:265, 1967.
70. Latarjet R, Muel B, Haig DA, Clarke MC, Alper T: Inactivation of the scrapie agent by near monochromatic ultraviolet light. *Nature* **227**:1341, 1970.
71. Adams DH, Caspary EA: Nature of the scrapie virus. *Br Med J* **3**:173, 1967.
72. Narang HK: Ruthenium red and lanthanum nitrate a possible tracer and negative stain for scrapie "particles"? *Acta Neuropathol (Berl)* **29**:37, 1974.
73. Siakotos AN, Raveed D, Longa G: The discovery of a particle unique to brain and spleen subcellular fractions from scrapie-infected mice. *J Gen Virol* **43**:417, 1979.
74. Bastin FO: Spiroplasma-like inclusions in Creutzfeldt-Jakob disease. *Arch Pathol Lab Med* **103**:665, 1979.
75. Humphrey-Smith I, Chastel C, Le Goff F: Spiroplasmas and spongiform encephalopathies. *Med J Aust* **156**:142, 1992.
76. Hunter GD, Kimberlin RH, Collis S, Millson GC: Viral and non-viral properties of the scrapie agent. *Ann Clin Res* **5**:262, 1973.
77. Somerville RA, Millson GC, Hunter GD: Changes in a protein-nucleic acid complex from synaptic plasma membrane of scrapie-infected mouse brain. *Biochem Soc Trans* **4**:1112, 1976.
78. Marsh RF, Malone TG, Semancik JS, Lancaster WD, Hanson RP: Evidence for an essential DNA component in the scrapie agent. *Nature* **275**:146, 1978.
79. Merz PA, Rohwer RG, Kascsak R, Wisniewski HM, Somerville RA, Gibbs CJ Jr, Gajdusek DC: Infection-specific particle from the unconventional slow virus diseases. *Science* **225**:437, 1984.
80. Gajdusek DC: Transmissible and non-transmissible amyloidoses: Autocatalytic post-translational conversion of host precursor proteins to β-pleated sheet configurations. *J Neuroimmunol* **20**:95, 1988.
81. Hunter GD: Scrapie: A prototype slow infection. *J Infect Dis* **125**:427, 1972.
82. Prusiner SB, McKinley MP, Bolton DC, Bowman KA, Groth DF, Cochran SP, Hennessey EM, Braunfeld MB, Baringer JR, Chatigny MA: Prions: Methods for assay, purification and characterization, in Maramorosch K, Koprowski H (eds): *Methods in Virology*. New York, Academic, 1984, pp 293–345.
83. Prusiner SB: Molecular structure, biology and genetics of prions. *Adv Virus Res* **35**:83, 1988.
84. Marsh RF, Kimberlin RH: Comparison of scrapie and transmissible mink encephalopathy in hamsters. II. Clinical signs, pathology and pathogenesis. *J Infect Dis* **131**:104, 1975.
85. Prusiner SB, McKinley MP, Bowman KA, Bolton DC, Bendheim PE, Groth DF, Glenner GG: Scrapie prions aggregate to form anyloid-like birefringent rods. *Cell* **35**:349, 1983.
86. Diringer H, Gelderblom H, Hilmert H, Ozel M, Edelbluth C, Kimberlin RH: Scrapie infectivity, fibrils and low molecular weight protein. *Nature* **306**:476, 1983.
87. Prusiner SB, McKinley MP, Groth DF, Bowman KA, Mock NI, Cochran SP, Masiarz FR: Scrapie agent contains a hydrophobic protein. *Proc Natl Acad Sci USA* **78**:6675, 1981.
88. Weissmann C: A "unified theory" of prion propagation. *Nature* **352**:679, 1991.
89. McKinley MP, Bolton DC, Prusiner SB: A protease-resistant protein is a structural component of the scrapie prion. *Cell* **35**:57, 1983.
90. Meyer RK, McKinley MP, Bowman KA, Braunfeld MB, Barry RA, Prusiner SB: Separation and properties of cellular and scrapie prion proteins. *Proc Natl Acad Sci USA* **83**:2310, 1986.
91. Harris DA, Falls DL, Johnson FA, Fischbach GD: A prion-like protein from chicken brain copurifies with an acetylcholine receptor-inducing activity. *Proc Natl Acad Sci USA* **88**:7664, 1991.
92. Donehower LA, Harvey M, Slagle BL, McArthur MJ, Montgomery CAJ, Butel JA, Bradley A: Mice deficient for p53 are developmentally normal but susceptible to spontaneous tumours. *Nature* **356**:215, 1992.
93. Bockman JM, Kingsbury DT, McKinley MP, Bendheim PE, Prusiner SB: Creutzfeldt-Jakob disease prion proteins in human brains. *N Engl J Med* **312**:73, 1985.
94. Field EJ, Matthews JD, Raine CS: Electron microscopic observations on the cerebellar cortex in kuru. *J Neurol Sci* **8**:209, 1969.
95. Vernon ML, Horta-Barbosa L, Fuccillo DA, Sever JL, Baringer JR, Birnbaum G: Virus-like particles and nucleoprotein-type filaments in brain tissue from two patients with Creutzfeldt-Jakob disease. *Lancet* **1**:964, 1970.
96. Narang HK: An electron microscopic study of the scrapie mouse and rat: Further observations on virus-like particles with ruthenium red and lanthanum nitrate as a possible trace and engative stain. *Neurobiology* **4**:349, 1974.
97. McKinley MP, Meyer R, Kenaga L, Rahbar F, Cotter

R, Serban A, Prusiner SB: Scrapie prion rod formation *in vitro* requires both detergent extraction and limited proteolysis. *J Virol* **65**:1440, 1991.
98. Gabizon R, McKinley MP, Prusiner SB: Purified prion proteins and scrapie infectivity copartition into liposomes. *Proc Natl Acad Sci USA* **84**:4017, 1987.
99. Gabizon R, McKinley MP, Groth DF, Prusiner SB: Immunoaffinity purification and neutralization of scrapie prion infectivity. *Proc Natl Acad Sci USA* **85**:6617, 1988.
100. Merz PA, Wisniewski HM, Somerville RA, Bobin SA, Masters CL, Iqbal K: Ultrastructural morphology of amyloid fibrils from neuritic and amyloid plaques. *Acta Neuropathol (Berl)* **60**:113, 1983.
101. Merz PA, Kascsak RJ, Rubenstein R, Carp RI, Wisniewski HM: Antisera to scrapie-associated fibril protein and prion protein decorate scrapie-associated fibrils. *J Virol* **61**:42, 1987.
102. Somerville RA, Ritchie LA, Gibson PH: Structural and biochemical evidence that scrapie-associated fibrils assemble in vivo. *J Gen Virol* **70**:25, 1989.
103. Diener TO: PrP and the nature of the scrapie agent. *Cell* **49**:719, 1987.
104. Kimberlin RH: Scrapie and possible relationships with viroids. *Semin Virol* **1**:153, 1990.
105. Liberski PP, Brown P, Xiao S-Y, Gajdusek DC: The ultrastructural diversity of scrapie-associated fibrils isolated from experimental scrapie and Creutzfeldt-Jakob disease. *J Comp Pathol* **105**:377, 1991.
106. Merz PA, Somerville RA, Wisniewski HM, Manuelidis L, Manuelidis EE: Scrapie-associated fibrils in Creutzfeldt-Jakob disease. *Nature* **306**:474, 1983.
107. Merz PA, Kascsak R, Rubenstein R, Carp RI, Wisniewski HM: Variations in SAF from different scrapie agents, in Tateishi J (ed): *Proceedings of Workshop on Slow Transmissible Diseases*. Tokyo, Japanese Ministry of Health and Welfare, 1984, pp 137–145.
108. Rohwer RG: Scrapie-associated fibrils. *Lancet* **2**:36, 1984.
109. Prusiner SB: Prions and neurodegenerative diseases. *N Engl J Med* **317**:1571, 1987.
110. DeArmond SJ, McKinley MP, Barry RA, Braunfeld MB, McColloch JR, Prusiner SB: Identification of prion amyloid filaments in scrapie-infected brain. *Cell* **41**:221, 1985.
111. McKinley MP, Prusiner SB: Scrapie prions, amyloid plaques, and a possible link with Alzheimer's disease, in Altman HJ (ed): *Alzheimer's Disease: Problems, Prospects and Perspectives*. New York, Plenum, 1987, pp 75–86.
112. Bendheim PE, Barry RA, DeArmond SJ, Stites DP, Prusiner SB: Antibodies to a scrapie prion protein. *Nature* **310**:418, 1984.
113. Kitamoto T, Tateishi J, Tashima I, Takeshita I, Barry RA, DeArmond SJ, Prusiner SB: Amyloid plaques in Creutzfeldt-Jakob disease stain with prion protein antibodies. *Ann Neurol* **20**:204, 1986.
114. Tagliavini F, Prelli F, Ghisto J, Bugiani O, Serban D, Prusiner SB, Farlow MR, Ghetti B, Frangione B: Amyloid protein of Gerstmann-Sträussler-Scheinker disease (Indiana kindred) is an 11-kd fragment of prion protein with an N-terminal glycine at codon 58. *EMBO J* **10**:513, 1991.
115. Kitamoto T, Yamaguchi K, Doh-ura K, Tateishi J: A prion protein missense variant is integrated in kuru plaque cores in patients with Gerstmann-Sträussler syndrome. *Neurology* **41**:306, 1991.
116. Beck E, Daniel PM, Parry HB: Degeneration of the cerebellar and hypothalamo-neurohypophysial systems in sheep with scrapie; and its relationship to human system degenerations. *Brain* **87**:153, 1964.
117. Tateishi J, Sato Y, Nagara H, Boellaard JW: Experimental transmission of human subacute spongiform encephalopathy to small rodents. IV. Positive transmission from a typical case of Gerstmann-Sträussler-Scheinker's disease. *Acta Neuropathol (Berl)* **64**:85, 1984.
118. Bruce ME, Fraser H: Amyloid plaques in the brains of mice infected with scrapie: Morphological variation and staining properties. *Neuropathol Appl Neurobiol* **1**:189, 1975.
119. Wisniewski HM, Bruce ME, Fraser H: Infectious etiology of neuritic (senile) plaques in mice. *Science* **190**:1108, 1975.
120. DeArmond SJ, Kretzschmar HA, McKinley MP, Prusiner SB: Molecular pathology of prion diseases, in Prusiner SB, McKinley MP (eds): *Prions—Novel Infectious Pathogens Causing Scrapie and Creutzfeldt-Jakob Disease*. Orlando, FL, Academic, 1987, pp 387–414.
121. DeArmond SJ, Mobley WC, DeMott DL, Barry RA, Beckstead JH, Prusiner SB: Changes in the localization of brain prion proteins during scrapie infection. *Neurology* **37**:1271, 1987.
122. Cserr HF, Cooper DN, Milhorat TH: Flow of cerebral interstitial fluid as indicated by the removal of extracellular markers from rat caudate nucleus. *Exp Eye Res (suppl)* **25**:461, 1977.
123. Snow AD, Kisilevsky R, Willmer J, Prusiner SB, DeArmond SJ: Sulfated glycosaminoglycans in amyloid plaques of prion diseases. *Acta Neuropathol (Berl)* **77**:337, 1989.
124. Snow AD, Wight TN, Nochlin D, Koike Y, Kimata K, DeArmond SJ, Prusiner SB: Immunolocalization of heparan-sulfate proteoglycans to the prion protein amyloid plaques of Gerstmann-Sträussler syndrome, Creutzfeldt-Jakob disease and scrapie. *Lab Invest* **63**:601, 1990.
125. Terry RD, Gonatas NK, Weiss M: Ultrastructural studies in Alzheimer's presenile dementia. *Am J Pathol* **44**:269, 1964.
126. Wisniewski H, Johnson AB, Raine CS, Terry RD: Senile plaques and cerebral amyloidosis in aged dogs. *Lab Invest* **23**:287, 1970.
127. Glenner GG: Current knowledge of amyloid deposits as applied to senile plaques and Congophilic angiopathy, in Katzman R, Terry RD, Bick KL, (eds): *Alzheimer's Disease: Senile Dementia and Related Disorders*. New York, Raven, 1978, pp 493–501.
128. Cohen AS, Shirahama T, Skinner M: Electron microscopy of amyloid, in Harris (ed): *Electron Microscopy of Proteins*. New York, Academic, 1982, vol 3, pp 165–206.
129. Gueft B, Kikkawa Y, Hirschl S: An electron-microscopic study of amyloidosis from different species, in Mandema E, Ruinen L, Scholten JH, Cohen AS (eds): *Amyloidosis*. Amsterdam, Excerpta Medica, 1968, pp 172–183.
130. Glenner GG, Wong CW: Alzheimer's disease and Down's syndrome: Sharing of a unique cerebrovascular amyloid fibril protein. *Biochem Biophys Res Commun* **122**:1131, 1984.
131. Masters CL, Simms G, Weinman NA, Multhaup G, McDonald BL, Beyreuther K: Amyloid plaque core protein in Alzheimer disease and Down syndrome. *Proc Natl Acad Sci USA* **82**:4245, 1985.
132. Puckett C, Concannon P, Casey C, Hood L: Genomic structure of the human prion protein gene. *Am J Hum Genet* **49**:320, 1991.
133. Gabriel J-M, Oesch B, Kretzschmar H, Scott M, Prusiner SB: Molecular cloning of a candidate chicken prion protein. *Proc Natl Acad Sci USA* **89**:9097, 1992.
134. Westaway D, Goodman PA, Mirenda CA, McKinley MP, Carlson GA, Prusiner SB: Distinct prion proteins in short and long scrapie incubation period mice. *Cell* **51**:651, 1987.
135. Westaway D, Mirenda CA, Foster D, Zebarjadian Y, Scott M, Torchia M, Yang S-L, Serban H, DeArmond SJ, Ebeling C, Prusiner SB, Carlson GA: Paradoxical shortening of scrapie incubation times by expression of prion protein transgenes derived from long incubation period mice. *Neuron* **7**:59, 1991.
136. Blum B, Bakalara N, Simpson L: A model for RNA editing in kinetoplastid mitochondria: "Guide" RNA molecules transcribed from maxicircle DNA provide edited information. *Cell* **60**:189, 1990.
137. Kane PM, Yamashiro CT, Wolczyk DF, Neff N, Goebl M, Stevens TH: Protein splicing converts the yeast TFP1 gene product to the 69-kD subunit of the vacuolar H+-adenosine triphosphatase. *Science* **250**:651, 1990.
138. McKnight S, Tijan R: Transcriptional selectivity of viral genes in mammalian cells. *Cell* **46**:795, 1986.
139. Locht C, Chesebro B, Race R, Keith JM: Molecular cloning and complete sequence of prion protein cDNA from mouse brain infected with the scrapie agent. *Proc Natl Acad Sci USA* **83**:6372, 1986.
140. Kretzschmar HA, Stowring LE, Westaway D, Stubblebine WH, Prusiner SB, DeArmond SJ: Molecular cloning of a humam prion protein cDNA. *DNA* **5**:315, 1986.

141. Goldman W, Hunter N, Foster JD, Salbaum JM, Beyreuther K, Hope J: Two alleles of a neural protein gene linked to scrapie in sheep. *Proc Natl Acad Sci USA* **87**:2476, 1990.
142. Goldman W, Hunter N, Manson J, Hope J: The PrP gene of the sheep, a natural host of scrapie. VIIIth International Congress of Virology, Berlin, Aug. 26–31, 1990, p 284. (abstr.)
143. Lowenstein DH, Butler DA, Westaway D, McKinley MP, DeArmond SJ, Prusiner SB: Three hamster species with different scrapie incubation times and neuropathological features encode distinct prion proteins. *Mol Cell Biol* **10**:1153, 1990.
144. Falls DL, Harris DA, Johnson FA, Morgan MM, Corfas G, Fischbach GD: 42 kD ARIA: A protein that may regulate the accumulation of acetylcholine receptors at developing chick neuromuscular junctions. *Cold Spring Harb Symp Quant Biol* **55**:397, 1990.
145. Liao Y-C, Lebo RV, Clawson GA, Smuckler EA: Human prion protein cDNA: Molecular cloning, chromosomal mapping, and biological implication. *Science* **233**:364, 1986.
146. Robakis NK, Devine-Gage EA, Kascsak RJ, Brown WT, Krawczun C, Silverman WP: Localization of a human gene homologous to the PrP gene on the p arm of chromosome 20 and detection of PrP-related antigens in normal human brain. *Biochem Biophys Res Commun* **140**:758, 1986.
147. McKusick VA (ed): *Mendelian Inheritance in Man—Catalogs of Autosomal Dominant, Autosomal Recessive, and X-Linked Phenotypes,* 10th ed. Baltimore, Johns Hopkins University Press, 1992, vol 1, p ccxlv.
148. Mobley WC, Neve RL, Prusiner SB, McKinley MP: Nerve growth factor increases mRNA levels for the prion protein and the beta-amyloid protein precursor in developing hamster brain. *Proc Natl Acad Sci USA* **85**:9811, 1988.
149. Kretzschmar HA, Prusiner SB, Stowring LE, DeArmond SJ: Scrapie prion proteins are synthesized in neurons. *Am J Pathol* **122**:1, 1986.
150. Manson J, West JD, Thomas V, McBride P, Kaufman MH, Hope J.: The prion protein gene: A role in mouse embryogenesis? *Development* **115**:117, 1992.
151. Bendheim PE, Brown HR, Rudelli RD, Scala LJ, Goller NL, Wen GY, Kascsak RJ, Cashman NR, Bolton DC: Nearly ubiquitous tissue distribution of the scrapie agent precursor protein. *Neurology* **42**:149, 1992.
152. Tarboulos A, Jendroska K, Serban D, Yang S-L, DeArmond SJ, Prusiner SB: Regional mapping of prion proteins in brains. *Proc Natl Acad Sci USA* **89**:7620, 1992.
153. Jendroska K, Heinzel FP, Torchia M, Stowring L, Kretzschmar HA, Kon A, Stern A, Prusiner SB, DeArmond SJ: Proteinase-resistant prion protein accumulation in Syrian hamster brain correlates with regional pathology and scrapie infectivity. *Neurology* **41**:1482, 1991.
154. Kimberlin RH, Field HJ, Walker CA: Pathogenesis of mouse scrapie: Evidence for spread of infection from central to peripheral nervous system. *J Gen Virol* **64**:713, 1983.
155. Fraser H, Dickinson AG: Targeting of scrapie lesions and spread of agent via the retino-tectal projection. *Brain Res* **346**:32, 1985.
156. Prusiner SB, Scott M, Foster D, Pan K-M, Groth D, Mirenda C, Torchia M, Yang S-L, Serban D, Carlson GA, Hoppe PC, Westaway D, DeArmond SJ: Transgenetic studies implicate interactions between homologous PrP isoforms in scrapie prion replication. *Cell* **63**:673, 1990.
157. Caughey B, Race RE, Ernst D, Buchmeier MJ, Chesebro B: Prion protein biosynthesis in scrapie-infected and uninfected neuroblastoma cells. *J Virol* **63**:175, 1989.
158. Bolton DC, Mayer RK, Prusiner SB: Scrapie PrP 27-30 is a sialoglycoprotein. *J Virol* **53**:596, 1985.
159. Manuelidis L, Valley S, Manuelidis EE: Specific proteins associated with Creutzfeldt-Jakob disease and scrapie share antigenic and carbohydrate determinants. *Proc Natl Acad Sci USA* **82**:4263, 1985.
160. Haraguchi T, Fisher S, Olofsson S, Endo T, Groth D, Tarantino A, Borchelt DR, Teplow D, Hood L, Burlingame A, Lycke E, Kobata A, Prusiner SB: Asparagine-lined glycosylation of the scrapie and cellular prion proteins. *Arch Biochem Biophys* **274**:1, 1989.
161. Endo T, Groth D, Prusiner SB, Kobata A: Diversity of oligosaccharide structures linked to asparagines of the scrapie prion protein. *Biochemistry* **28**:8380, 1989.
162. Rogers M, Taraboulos A, Scott M, Groth D, Prusiner SB: Intracellular accumulation of the cellular prion protein after mutagenesis of its Asn-linked glycosylation sites. *Glycobiology* **1**:101, 1990.
163. Stahl N, Borchelt DR, Hsiao K, Prusiner SB: Scrapie prion protein contains a phosphatidylinositol glycolipid. *Cell* **51**:229, 1987.
164. Stahl N, Borchelt DR, Prusiner SB: Differential release of cellular and scrapie prion proteins from cellular membranes by phosphatidylinositol-specific phospholipase C. *Biochemistry* **29**:5405, 1990.
165. Stahl N, Baldwin MA, Burlingame AL, Prusiner SB: Identification of glycoinositol phospholipid-linked and truncated forms of the scrapie prion protein. *Biochemistry* **29**:8879, 1990.
166. Baldwin MA, Stahl N, Reinders LG, Gibson BW, Prusiner SB, Burlingame AL: Permethylation and tandem mass spectrometry of oligosaccharides having free hexosamine: Analysis of the glycoinositol phospholipid anchor glycan from the scrapie prion protein. *Anal Biochem* **191**:174, 1990.
167. Safar J, Ceroni M, Piccardo P, Liberski PP, Miyazaki M, Gajdusek DC, Gibbs CJ Jr: Subcellular distribution and physicochemical properties of scrapie associated precursor protein and relationship with scrapie agent. *Neurology* **40**:503, 1990.
168. Taraboulos A, Serban D, Prusiner SB: Scrapie prion proteins accumulate in the cytoplasm of persistently-infected cultured cells. *J Cell Biol* **110**:2117, 1990.
169. Taraboulos A, Raeber AJ, Borchelt DR, Serban D, Prusiner SB: Synthesis and trafficking of prion proteins in cultured cells. *Mol Biol Cell* **3**:851, 1992.
170. McKinley MP, Taraboulos A, Kenaga L, Serban D, Stieber A, DeArmond SJ, Prusiner SB, Gonatas N: Ultrastructural localization of scrapie prion proteins in cytoplasmic vesicles of infected cultured cells. *Lab Invest* **65**:622, 1991.
171. Caughey B, Raymond GJ, Ernst D, Race RE: N-terminal truncation of the scrapie-associated form of PrP by lysosomal protease(s): Implications regarding the site of conversion of PrP to the protease-resistant state. *J Virol* **65**:6597, 1991.
172. Butler DA, Scott MRD, Bockman JM, Borchelt DR, Taraboulos A, Hsiao KK, Kingsbury DT, Prusiner SB: Scrapie-infected murine neuroblastoma cells produce protease-resistant prion proteins. *J Virol* **62**:1558, 1988.
173. Laszlo L, Lowe J, Self T, Kenward N, Landon M, McBride T, Farquhar C, McConnell I, Brown J, Hope J, Mayer RJ: Lysosomes as key organelles in the pathogenesis of prion encephalopathies. *J Pathol* **166**:333, 1992.
174. Stahl N, Baldwin MA, Hecker R, Pan K-M, Burlingame AL, Prusiner SB: Glycosylinositol phospholipid anchors of the scrapie and cellular prion proteins contain sialic acid. *Biochemistry* **31**:5043, 1992.
175. Taraboulos A, Rogers M, Borchelt DR, McKinley MP, Scott M, Serban D, Prusiner SB: Acquisition of protease resistance by prion proteins in scrapie-infected cells does not require asparagine-linked glycosylation. *Proc Natl Acad Sci USA* **87**:8262, 1990.
176. Yost CS, Lopez CD, Prusiner SB, Meyers RM, Lingappa VR: A nonhydrophobic extracytoplasmic determinant of stop transfer in the prion protein. *Nature* **343**:669, 1990.
177. Lopez CD, Yost CS, Prusiner SB, Myers RM, Lingappa VR: Unusual topogenic sequence directs prion protein biogenesis. *Science* **248**:226, 1990.
178. Hay B, Prusiner SB, Lingappa VR: Evidence for a secretory form of the cellular prion protein. *Biochemistry* **26**:8110, 1987.
179. Hay B, Barry RA, Lieberburg I, Prusiner SB, Lingappa VR: Biogenesis and transmembrane orientation of the cellular isoform of the scrapie prion protein. *Mol Cell Biol* **7**:914, 1987.
180. Bazan JF, Fletterick RJ, McKinley MP, Prusiner SB: Predicted secondary structure and membrane topology of the scrapie prion protein. *Protein Eng* **1**:125, 1987.
181. Doms RW, Russ G, Yewdell JW: Brefeldin A redistributes resident and itinerant Golgi proteins to the endoplasmic reticulum. *J Cell Biol* **109**:61, 1989.

182. Lippincott-Schwartz J, Yuan LC, Bonifacino JS, Klausner RD: Rapid redistribution of Golgi proteins into the ER in cells treated with Brefeldin A: Evidence for membrane cycling from the Golgi to ER. *Cell* **56**:801, 1989.
183. Prusiner SB, Hadlow WJ, Garfin DE, Cochran SP, Baringer JR, Race RE, Eklund CM: Partial purification and evidence for multiple molecular forms of the scrapie agent. *Biochemistry* **17**:4993, 1978.
184. Carlson GA, Kingsbury DT, Goodman PA, Coleman S, Marshall ST, DeArmond SJ, Westaway D, Prusiner SB: Linkage of prion protein and scrapie incubation time genes. *Cell* **46**:503, 1986.
185. Hunter N, Hope J, McConnell I, Dickinson AG: Linkage of the scrapie-associated fibril protein (PrP) gene and Sinc using congenic mice and restriction fragment length polymorphism analysis. *J Gen Virol* **68**:2711, 1987.
186. Race RE, Graham K, Ernst D, Caughey B, Chesebro B: Analysis of linkage between scrapie incubation period and the prion protein gene in mice. *J Gen Virol* **71**:493, 1990.
187. Carlson GA, Goodman PA, Lovett M, Taylor BA, Marshall ST, Peterson-Torchia M, Westaway D, Prusiner SB: Genetics and polymorphism of the mouse prion gene complex: The control of scrapie incubation time. *Mol Cell Biol* **8**:5528, 1988.
188. Dickinson AG, Meikle VMH, Fraser H: Identification of a gene which controls the incubation period of some strains of scrapie agent in mice. *J Comp Pathol* **78**:293, 1968.
189. Kingsbury DT, Kasper KC, Stites DP, Watson JD, Hogan RN, Prusiner SB: Genetic control of scrapie and Creutzfeldt-Jakob disease in mice. *J Immunol* **131**:491, 1983.
190. Parry HB: *Scrapie Disease in Sheep*. New York, Academic, 1983, p 192.
191. Hunter N, Foster JD, Dickinson AG, Hope J: Linkage of the genes for the scrapie-associated fibril protein (PrP) to the Sip gene in Cheviot sheep. *Vet Rec* **124**:364, 1989.
192. Hunter N, Foster JD, Benson G, Hope J: Restriction fragment length polymorphisms of the scrapie-associated fibril protein (PrP) gene and their association with susceptibility to natural scrapie in British sheep. *J Gen Virol* **72**:1287, 1991.
193. Goldmann W, Hunter N, Benson G, Foster JD, Hope J: Different scrapie-associated fibril proteins (PrP) are encoded by lines of sheep selected for different alleles of the *Sip* gene. *J Gen Virol* **72**:2411, 1991.
194. Wilesmith JW, Wells GAH, Cranwell MP, Ryan JBM: Bovine spongiform encephalopathy: Epidemiological studies. *Vet Rec* **123**:638, 1988.
195. Wilesmith J, Wells GAH: Bovine spongiform encephalopathy. *Curr Top Microbiol Immunol* **172**:21, 1991.
196. Dealler SF, Lacey RW: Transmissible spongiform encephalopathies: The threat of BSE to man. *Food Microbiol* **7**:253, 1990.
197. Wilesmith JW, Ryan JBM, Hueston WD, Hoinville LJ: Bovine spongiform encephalopathy: Epidemiological features 1985 to 1990. *Vet Rec* **130**:90, 1992.
198. Wilesmith JW, Hoinville LJ, Ryan JBM, Sayers AR: Bovine spongiform encephalopathy: Aspects of the clinical picture and analyses of possible changes 1986-1990. *Vet Rec* **130**:197, 1992.
199. Alpers M: Epidemiology and clinical aspects of kuru, in Prusiner SB, McKinley MP (eds): *Prions—Novel Infectious Pathogens Causing Scrapie and Creutzfeldt-Jakob Disease*. Orlando, FL, Academic, 1987, pp 451–465.
200. Marsh RF, Bessen RA, Lehmann S, Hartsough GR: Epidemiological and experimental studies on a new incident of transmissible mink encephalopathy. *J Gen Virol* **72**:589, 1991.
201. Williams ES, Young S: Chronic wasting disease of captive mule deer: A spongiform encephalopathy. *J Wildl Dis* **16**:89, 1980.
202. Williams ES, Young S: Spongiform encephalopathy of Rocky Mountain Elk. *J Wildl Dis* **18**:465, 1982.
203. Hadlow WJ: Scrapie and kuru. *Lancet* **2**:289, 1959.
204. Klatzo I, Gajdusek DC, Zigas V: Pathology of kuru. *Lab Invest* **8**:799, 1959.
205. Creutzfeldt HG: Über eine eigenartige herdförmige Erkrankung des Zentralnervensystems. *Z Gesamte Neurol Psychiatrie* **57**:1, 1920.
206. Jakob A: Über eine der multiplen Sklerose klinisch nahestehende Erkrankung des Zentralnervensystems (spastische Pseudosklerose) mit bemerkenswertem anatomischem Befunde. Mitteilung eines vierten Falles. *Med Klin* **17**:372, 1921.
207. Jakob A: Über eigenartige Erkrankungen des Zentralnervensystems mit bemerkenswertem anatomischen Befunde (spastische Pseudosklerose-Encephalomyelopathie mit disseminierten Degenerationsherden). *Z Gesamte Neurol Psychiatrie* **64**:147, 1921.
208. Jakob A: Über eigenartige Erkrankungen des Zentralnervensystems mit bemerkenswertem anatomischen Befunde (spastische Pseudoscklerose-Encephalomyelopathie mit disseminierten Degenerationscherden). Preliminary communication. *Dtsch Z Nervenheilk* **70**:132, 1921.
209. Richardson EPJ: Myoclonic dementia—Introduction, in Rottenberg DA, Hochberg FH (eds): *Neurological Classics in Modern Translation*. New York, Hafner, 1977, 95–96.
210. Rosenthal NP, Keesey J, Crandall B, Brown WJ: Familial neurological disease associated with spongiform encephalopathy. *Arch Neurol* **33**:252, 1976.
211. Neugut RH, Neugut AI, Kahana E, Stein Z, Alter M: Creutzfeldt-Jakob disease: Familial clustering among Libyan-born Israelis. *Neurology* **29**:225, 1979.
212. Masters CL, Richardson EP Jr: Subacute spongiform encephalopathy Creutzfeldt-Jakob disease—the nature and progression of spongiform change. *Brain* **101**:333, 1978.
213. Goldberg H, Alter M, Kahana E: The Libyan Jewish focus of Creutzfeldt-Jakob disease: A search for the mode of natural transmission, in Prusiner SB, Hadlow WJ (eds): *Slow Transmissible Diseases of the Nervous System*. New York, Academic, 1979, vol 1, pp 195–211.
214. Malmgren R, Kurland L, Mokri B, Kurtzke J: The epidemiology of Creutzfeldt-Jakob disease, in Prusiner SB, Hadlow WJ (eds): *Slow Transmissible Diseases of the Nervous System*. New York, Academic, 1979, vol 1, pp 93–112.
215. Mayer V, Mitrova E, Orolin D: Creutzfeldt-Jakob disease in Czechoslovakia and a working concept of its surveillance, in Prusiner SB, Hadlow WJ (eds): *Slow Transmissible Diseases of the Nervous System*. New York, Academic, 1979, vol 1, pp 287–303.
216. Bobowick AR, Brody JA, Matthews MR, Roos R, Gajdusek DC: Creutzfeldt-Jakob disease: A case-control study. *Am J Epidemiol* **98**:381, 1973.
217. Alter M, Kahana E: Creutzfeldt-Jakob disease among Libyan Jews in Israel. *Science* **192**:428, 1976.
218. LoRusso F, Neri G, Figa-Talamanca L: Creutzfeldt-Jakob disease and sheep brain—a report from central and southern Italy. *Ital J Neurol Sci* **3**:171, 1980.
219. Rosenberg RN, White LL III, Brown P, Gajdusek DC, Volpe JJ, Posner J, Dyck PJ: Precautions in handling tissues, fluids, and other contaminated materials from patients with documented or suspected Creutzfeldt-Jakob disease. *Ann Neurol* **19**:75, 1986.
220. Cathala F, Baron H: Clinical aspects of Creutzfeldt-Jakob disease, in Prusiner SB, McKinley MP (eds): *Prions—Novel Infectious Pathogens Causing Scrapie and Creutzfeldt-Jakob Disease*. Orlando, FL, Academic, 1987, pp. 467–509.
221. Siedler H, Malamud N: Creutzfeldt-Jakob's disease. Clinicopathologic report of 15 cases and review of the literature (with special reference to a related disorder designated as subacute spongiform encephalopathy). *J Neuropathol Exp Neurol* **22**:381, 1963.
222. May WW: Creutzfeldt-Jakob disease. 1. Survey of the literature and clinical diagnosis. *Acta Neurol Scand* **44**:1, 1968.
223. Kirschbaum WR: Jakob-Creutzfeldt Disease. New York, Elsevier, 1968, p 251.
224. Roos R, Gajdusek DC, Gibbs CJ Jr: The clinical characteristics of transmissible Creutzfeldt-Jakob disease. *Brain* **96**:1, 1973.
225. Brown P, Cathala F, Sadowsky D, Gajdusek DC: Creutzfeldt-Jakob disease in France. II. Clinical characteristics of 124 verified cases during the decade 1968-1977. *Ann Neurol* **6**:430, 1979.
226. Lechi A, Tadeschi F, Mancia D, Pietrini V, Tagliavini F, Terzano MG, Trabattoni G: Creutzfeldt-Jakob disease: Clinical, EEG and neuropathologic findings in a cluster of eleven patients. *Ital J Neurol Sci* **1**:47, 1983.

227. Will RG, Matthews WB: A retrospective study of Creutzfeldt-Jakob disease in England and Wales 1970-79. I. Clinical features. *J Neurol Neurosurg Psychiatry* **47:**134, 1984.
228. Mizutani T, Shiraki H: *Clinicopathological Aspects of Creutzfeldt-Jakob Disease*. Amsterdam, Elsevier, 1985, p 325.
229. Nevin S, McMenemy WH, Behrman S, Jones DP: Subacute spongiform encephalopathy—a subacute form of encephalopathy attributable to vascular dysfunction (spongiform cerebral atrophy). *Brain* **83:**519, 1960.
230. Brownell B, Oppenheimer DR: An ataxic form of subacute presenile polioencephalopathy (Creutzfeldt-Jakob disease). *J Neurol Neurosurg Psychiatry* **28:**350, 1965.
231. Gomori AJ, Partnow MJ, Horoupian DS, Hirano A: The ataxic form of Creutzfeldt-Jakob disease. *Arch Neurol* **29:**318, 1973.
232. Masters CL, Harris JO, Gajdusek DC, Gibbs CJ Jr, Bernouilli C, Asher DM: Creutzfeldt-Jakob disease: Patterns of worldwide occurrence and the significance of familial and sporadic clustering. *Ann Neurol* **5:**177, 1978.
233. Benson DF: Neuroimaging and dementia. *Neurol Clin* **4:**341, 1986.
234. Salazar AM, Masters CL, Gajdusek DC, Gibbs CJ Jr: Syndromes of amyotrophic lateral sclerosis and dementia: Relation to transmissible Creutzfeldt-Jakob disease. *Ann Neurol* **14:**17, 1983.
235. Watson CP: Clinical similarity of Alzheimer and Creutzfeldt-Jakob disease. *Ann Neurol* **6:**368, 1979.
236. Steiner I, Polacheck I, Melamed E: Dementia and myoclonus in a case of cryptococcal encephalitis. *Arch Neurol* **41:**216, 1984.
237. Burger LJ, Rowan AJ, Goldensohn ES: Creutzfeldt-Jakob disease. An electroencephalographic study. *Arch Neurol* **26:**428, 1972.
238. Lee RG, Blair RDG: Evolution of EEG and visual evoked response changes in Jakob-Creutzfeldt disease. *Electroencephalogr Clin Neurophysiol* **35:**133, 1973.
239. Chiafalo N, Fuentes AN, Galvez S: Serial EEG findings in 27 cases of Creutzfeldt-Jakob disease. *Arch Neurol* **37:**143, 1980.
240. Au WJ, Gabor AJ, Vijayan N, Markand ON: Periodic lateralized epileptiform complexes (PLEDs) in Creutzfeldt-Jakob disease. *Neurology* **30:**611, 1980.
241. Kuroiwa Y, Celesia GG: Clinical significance of periodic EEG patterns. *Arch Neurol* **37:**15, 1980.
242. Traub RD, Pedley TA: Virus-induced electrotonic coupling: Hypothesis on the mechanism of periodic EEG discharges in Creutzfeldt-Jakob disease. *Ann Neurol* **10:**405, 1981.
243. Duffy P, Wolf J, Collins G, Devoe A, Streeten B, Cowen D: Possible person to person transmission of Creutzfeldt-Jakob disease. *N Engl J Med* **290:**692, 1974.
244. Bernouilli C, Siegfried J, Baumgartner G, Regli F, Rabinowicz T, Gajdusek DC, Gibbs CJ Jr: Danger of accidental person to person transmission of Creutzfeldt-Jakob disease by surgery. *Lancet* **1:**478, 1977.
245. Brown P, Rodgers-Johnson P, Cathala F, Gibbs CJ Jr, Gajdusek DC: Creutzfeldt-Jakob disease of long duration: Clinicopathological characteristics, transmissibility, and differential diagnosis. *Ann Neurol* **16:**295, 1984.
246. Castleman B, Richardson EPJ: *Neurologic Clinicopathologic Conferences of the Massachusetts General Hospital*. London, Churchill, 1968.
247. Austin J, Sakai M: Disorder of glycogen and related molecules in the nervous system, in Vinken PJ, Bruyn GW (eds): *Handbook of Clinical Neurology*. New York, Elsevier, 1976, vol 27, pp 169–219.
248. Raskin NH, Bredesen D, Ehrenfeld WK, Kerlan R: Periodic confusion caused by congenital extrahepatic portacaval shunt. *Neurology* **34:**666, 1984.
249. Levy RM, Bredesen DE, Rosenblum ML: Neurological manifestations of the acquired immunodeficiency syndrome (AIDS): Experience at UCSF and review of the literature. *J Neurosurg* **62:**475, 1985.
250. Bertoni JM, Label LS, Sackelleres JC, Hicks SP: Supranuclear gaze palsy in familial Creutzfeldt-Jakob disease. *Arch Neurol* **40:**618, 1983.
251. Snider WD, Simpson DM, Nielsen S, Gold JW, Metroka CE, Posner JB: Neurological complications of acquired immune deficiency syndromes: Analysis of 50 patients. *Ann Neurol* **14:**403, 1983.
252. Resnick L, DiMarzo-Veronese F, Schupbach J, Tourtellotte WW, Ho DD, Muller F, Shapshak P, Vogt M, Groopman JE, Markham PD, Gallo RC: Intra-blood-brain-barrier synthesis of HTLV-III-specific IgG in patients with neurologic symptoms associated with AIDS or AIDS-related complex. *N Engl J Med* **313:**1498, 1985.
253. Friedland RP, Prusiner SB, Jagust WJ, Budinger TF, Davis RL: Bitemporal hypometabolism in Creutzfeldt-Jakob disease measured by positron emission tomography with [^{18}F]-2-fluorodeoxyglucose. *J Comput Assist Tomogr* **8:**978, 1984.
254. Harrington MG, Merril CR, Asher DM, Gajdusek DC: Abnormal proteins in the cerebrospinal fluid of patients with Creutzfeldt-Jakob disease. *N Engl J Med* **315:**279, 1986.
255. Brown P, Cathala F, Castaigne P, Gajdusek DC: Creutzfeldt-Jakob disease: Clinical analysis of a consecutive series of 230 neuropathologically verified cases. *Ann Neurol* **20:**597, 1986.
256. Gibbs CJ Jr, Gajdusek DC, Amyx H: Strain variation in the viruses of Creutzfeldt-Jakob disease and kuru, in Prusiner SB, Hadlow WJ (eds): *Slow Transmissible Diseases of the Nervous System*. New York, Academic, 1979, vol 2, pp 87–110.
257. Tateishi J, Sato Y, Ohta M: Creutzfeldt-Jakob disease in humans and laboratory animals, in Zimmerman HM (ed): *Progress in Neuropathology*. New York, Raven, 1983, vol 5, pp 195–221.
258. Tateishi J, Doh-ura K, Kitamoto T, Tranchant C, Steinmetz G, Warter JM, Boellaard JW: Prion protein gene analysis and transmission studies of Creutzfeldt-Jakob disease, in Prusiner SB, Collinge J, Powell J, Anderton B (eds): *Prion Diseases of Humans and Animals*. London, Ellis Horwood, 1992, pp 129–134.
259. Hsiao KK, Scott M, Foster D, Groth DF, DeArmond SJ, Prusiner SB: Spontaneous neurodegeneration in transgenic mice with mutant prion protein of Gerstmann-Sträussler syndrome. *Science* **250:**1587, 1990.
260. Brown P, Coker-Vann M, Gajdusek DC: Immunological study of patients with Creutzfeldt-Jakob disease and other chronic neurological disorders: Western blot recognition of infection-specific proteins by scrapie virus antibody, in Bignami A, Bolis CL, Gajdusek DC (eds): *Molecular Mechanisms of Pathogenesis of Central Nervous System Disorders*. Geneva, Foundation for the Study of the Nervous System, 1986, pp 107–109.
261. Bockman JM, Prusiner SB, Tateishi J, Kingsbury DT: Immunoblotting of Creutzfeldt-Jakob disease prion proteins: Host species-specific epitopes. *Ann Neurol* **21:**589, 1987.
262. Serban D, Taraboulos A, DeArmond SJ, Prusiner SB: Rapid detection of Creutzfeldt-Jakob disease and scrapie prion proteins. *Neurology* **40:**110, 1990.
263. Brown P, Coker-Vann M, Pomeroy K, Franko M, Asher DM, Gibbs CJ Jr, Gajdusek DC: Diagnosis of Creutzfeldt-Jakob disease by Western blot identification of marker protein in human brain tissue. *N Engl J Med* **314:**547, 1986.
264. Prusiner SB: Prions causing degenerative neurological diseases. *Annu Rev Med* **38:**381, 1987.
265. Roberts GW, Lofthouse R, Brown R, Crow TJ, Barry RA, Prusiner SB: Prion-protein immunoreactivity in human transmissible dementias. *N Engl J Med* **315:**1231, 1986.
266. Richardson JH, Barkley WE (eds): *Biosafety in Microbiological and Biomedical Laboratories, US Department of Health and Human Services, Public Health Service, Centers for Disease Control and National Institutes of Health*. Washington, DC, Government Printing Office, 1988.
267. Miller DC: Creutzfeldt-Jakob disease in histopathology technicians. *N Engl J Med* **318:**853, 1988.
268. Sitwell L, Lach B, Atack E, Atack D, Izukawa D: Creutzfeldt-Jakob disease in histopathology technicians. *N Engl J Med* **318:**854, 1988.
269. Gorman DG, Benson DF, Vogel DG, Vinters HV: Creutzfeldt-Jakob disease in a pathologist. *Neurology* **42:**463, 1992.
270. Schoene WC, Masters CL, Gibbs CJ Jr, Gajdusek DC, Tyler HR, Moore FD, Dammin GJ: Transmissible spongiform encephalopathy (Creutzfeldt-Jakob disease). *Arch Neurol* **38:**473, 1981.

271. Chatigny MA, Prusiner SB: Biohazards of investigations on the transmissible spongiform encephalopathies. *Rev Infect Dis* **2:**713, 1980.
272. Kimberlin RH, Walker CA, Millson GC, Taylor DM, Robertson PA, Tomlinson AH, Dickinson AG: Disinfection studies with two strains of mouse-passaged scrapie agent. *J Neurol Sci* **59:**355, 1983.
273. Walker AS, Inderlied CB, Kingsbury DT: Conditions for the chemical and physical inactivation of the K. Fu. strain of the agent of Creutzfeldt-Jakob disease. *Am J Public Health* **73:**661, 1983.
274. Brown P, Gibbs CJ Jr, Amyx HL, Kingsbury DT, Rohwer RG, Sulima MP, Gajdusek DC: Chemical disinfection of Creutzfeldt-Jakob disease virus. *N Engl J Med* **306:**1279, 1982.
275. Brown P, Rohwer RG, Green EM, Gajdusek DC: Effect of chemicals, heat, and histopathologic processing on high-infectivity hamster-adapted scrapie virus. *J Infect Dis* **145:**683, 1982.
276. Brown P, Rohwer RG, Gajdusek DC: Sodium hydroxide decontamination of Creutzfeldt-Jakob disease virus. *N Engl J Med* **310:**727, 1984.
277. Will RG, Matthews WB: Evidence for case-to-case transmission of Creutzfeldt-Jakob disease. *J Neurol Neurosurg Psychiatry* **45:**235, 1982.
278. Eklund CM, Kennedy RC, Hadlow WJ: Pathogenesis of scrapie virus infection in the mouse. *J Infect Dis* **117:**15, 1967.
279. Braham J: Creutzfeldt-Jakob disease: Treatment by amantadine. *Br Med J* **4:**212, 1971.
280. Herishanu Y: Antiviral drugs in Jakob-Creutzfeldt disease. *J Am Geriatr Soc* **21:**229, 1973.
281. Terzano MG, Montanari E, Calzetti S, Mancia D, Lechi A: The effect of amantadine on arousal and EEG patterns in Creutzfeldt-Jakob disease. *Arch Neurol* **40:**555, 1983.
282. Kimberlin RH, Walker CA: The antiviral compound HPA-23 can prevent scrapie when administered at the time of infection. *Arch Virol* **78:**9, 1983.
283. Dickinson AG, Fraser H, Outram GW: Scrapie incubation time can exceed natural lifespan. *Nature* **256:**732, 1975.
284. Ehlers B, Diringer H. Dextran sulphate 500 delays and prevents mouse scrapie by impairment of agent replication in spleen. *J Gen Virol* **65:**1325, 1984.
285. Katz M, Koprowski H: Failure to demonstrate a relationship between scrapie and production of interferon in mice. *Nature* **219:**639, 1968.
286. Field EJ, Joyce G, Keith A: Failure of interferon to modify scrapie in the mouse. *J Gen Virol* **5:**149, 1969.
287. Worthington M: Interferon system in mice infected with the scrapie agent. *Infect Immun* **6:**643, 1972.
288. Pocchiari M, Salvatore M, Ladogana A, Ingrosso L, Xi YG, Cibati M, Masullo C: Experimental drug treatment of scrapie: A pathogenetic basis for rationale therapeutics. *Eur J Epidemiol* **7:**556, 1991.
289. Casaccia P, Ladogana A, Xi YG, Ingrosso L, Pocchiari M, Silvestrini MC, Cittadini A: Measurement of the concentration of amphotericin B in brain tissue of scrapie-infected hamsters with a simple and sensitive method. *Antimicrob Agents Chemother* **35:**1486, 1991.
290. Xi YG, Ingrosso L, Ladogana A, Masullo C, Pocchiari M: Amphotericin B treatment dissociates *in vivo* replication of the scrapie agent from PrP accumulation. *Nature* **356:**598, 1992.
291. Masullo C, Macchi G, Xi YG, Pocchiari M: Failure to ameliorate Creutzfeldt-Jakob disease with amphotericin B therapy. *J Infect Dis* **165:**784, 1992.
292. Gabizon R, McKinley MP, Groth DF, Kenaga L, Prusiner SB: Properties of scrapie prion liposomes. *J Biol Chem* **263:**4950, 1988.
293. Kondo K, Kuroina Y: A case control study of Creutzfeldt-Jakob disease: Association with physical injuries. *Ann Neurol* **11:**377, 1981.
294. Davanipour Z, Goodman L, Alter M, Sobel E, Asher D, Gajdusek DC: Possible modes of transmission of Creutzfeldt-Jakob disease. *N Engl J Med* **311:**1582, 1984.
295. Buyukmihci N, Rorvik M, Marsh RF: Replication of the scrapie agent in ocular neural tissues. *Proc Natl Acad Sci USA* **77:**1169, 1980.
296. Bernouilli CC, Masters CL, Gajdusek DC, Gibbs CJ Jr, Harris JO: Early clinical features of Creutzfeldt-Jakob disease (subacute spongiform encephalopathy), in Prusiner SB, Hadlow WJ (eds): *Slow Transmissible Diseases of the Nervous System*. New York, Academic, 1979, vol 1, pp 229–251.
297. Brown P, Preece MA, Will RG: "Friendly fire" in medicine: Hormones, homografts, and Creutzfeldt-Jakob disease. *Lancet* **340:**24, 1992.
298. Otto D: Creutzfeldt-Jacob disease associated with cadaveric dura. *J Neurosurg* **67:**149, 1987.
299. Thadani V, Penar PL, Partington J, Kalb R, Janssen R, Schonberger LB, Rabkin CS, Prichard JW: Creutzfeldt-Jakob disease probably acquired from a cadaveric dura mater graft. Case report. *J Neurosurg* **69:**766, 1988.
300. Nisbet TJ, MacDonaldson I, Bishara SN: Creutzfeldt-Jakob disease in a second patient who received a cadaveric dura mater graft. *JAMA* **261:**1118, 1989.
301. Masullo C, Pocchiari M, Macchi G, Alema G, Piazza G, Panzera MA: Transmission of Creutzfeldt-Jakob disease by dural cadaveric graft. *J Neurosurg* **71:**954, 1989.
302. Willison HJ, Gale AN, McLaughlin JE: Creutzfeldt-Jakob disease following cadaveric dura mater graft. *J Neurol Neurosurg Psychiatry* **54:**940, 1991.
303. Miyashita K, Inuzuka T, Kondo H, Saito Y, Fujita N, Matsubara N, Tanaka R, Hinokuma K, Ikuta F, Miyatake T: Creutzfeldt-Jakob disease in a patient with a cadaveric dural graft. *Neurology* **41:**940, 1991.
304. Tange RA, Troost D, Limburg M: Progressive fatal dementia (Creutzfeldt-Jakob disease) in a patient who received homograft tissue for tympanic membrane closure. *Eur Arch Otorhinolaryngol* **247:**199, 1989.
305. Brown P: Virus sterility for human growth hormone. *Lancet* **2:**729, 1985.
306. Buchanan CR, Preece MA, Milner RDG: Mortality, neoplasia and Creutzfeldt-Jakob disease in patients treated with pituitary growth hormone in the United Kingdom. *Br Med J* **302:**824, 1991.
307. Packer RJ, Cornblath DR, Gonatas NK, Bruno LA, Asbury AK: Creutzfeldt-Jakob disease in a 20-year-old woman. *Neurology* **30:**492, 1980.
308. Koch TK, Berg BO, DeArmond SJ, Gravina RF: Creutzfeldt-Jakob disease in a young adult with idiopathic hypopituitarism. Possible relation to the administration of cadaveric human growth hormone. *N Engl J Med* **313:**731, 1985.
309. Powell-Jackson J, Weller RO, Kennedy P, Preece MA, Whitcombe EM, Newsome-Davis J: Creutzfeldt-Jakob disease after administration of human growth hormone. *Lancet* **2:**244, 1985.
310. Titner R, Brown P, Hedley-Whyte ET, Rappaport EB, Piccardo CP, Gajdusek DC: Neuropathologic verification of Creutzfeldt-Jakob disease in the exhumed American recipient of human pituitary growth hormone: Epidemiologic and pathogenetic implications. *Neurology* **36:**932, 1986.
311. Croxson M, Brown P, Synek B, Harrington MG, Frith R, Clover G, Wilson J, Gajdusek DC: A new case of Creutzfeldt-Jakob disease associated with human growth hormone therapy in New Zealand. *Neurology* **38:**1128, 1988.
312. New MI, Brown P, Temeck JW, Owens C, Hedley-Whyte ET, Richardson EP: Preclinical Creutzfeldt-Jakob disease discovered at autopsy in a human growth hormone recipient. *Neurology* **38:**1133, 1988.
313. Marzewski DJ, Towfighi J, Harrington MG, Merril CR, Brown P: Creutzfeldt-Jakob disease following pituitary-derived human growth hormone therapy: A new American case. *Neurology* **38:**1131, 1988.
314. Anderson JR, Allen CMC, Weller RO: Creutzfeldt-Jakob disease following human pituitary-derived growth hormone administration. *Br Neuropatholog Soc Proc* **16:**543, 1990.
315. Billette de Villemeur T, Beauvais P, Gourmelon M, Richardet JM: Creutzfeldt-Jakob disease in children treated with growth hormone. *Lancet* **337:**864, 1991.
316. Macario ME, Vaisman M, Buescu A, Neto VM, Araujo HMM, Chagas C: Pituitary growth hormone and Creutzfeldt-Jakob disease. *Br Med J* **302:**1149, 1991.
317. Prusiner SB, Gajdusek DC, Alpers MP: Kuru with incubation periods exceeding two decades. *Ann Neurol* **12:**1, 1982.
318. Gajdusek DC, Gibbs CJ Jr, Asher DM, Brown P, Diwan

A, Hoffman P, Nemo G, Rohwer R, White L: Precautions in medical care of and in handling materials from patients with transmissible virus dementia (CJD). *N Engl J Med* **297**:1253, 1977.

319. Klitzman RL, Alpers MP, Gajdusek DC: The natural incubation period of kuru and the episodes of transmission in three clusters of patients. *Neuroepidemiology* **3**:3, 1984.
320. Gibbs CJ Jr, Asher DM, Brown PW, Fradkin JE, Gajdusek DC: Creutzfeldt-Jakob disease infectivity of growth hormone derived from human pituitary glands. *N Engl J Med* **328**:358, 1993.
321. Lumley Jones R, Benker G, Salacinski PR, Lloyd TJ, Lowry PJ: Large-scale preparation of highly purified pyrogen-free human growth hormone for clinical use. *Br J Endocrinol* **82**:77, 1979.
322. Taylor DM, Dickinson AG, Fraser H, Robertson PA, Salacinski PR, Lowry PJ: Preparation of growth hormone free from contamination with unconventional slow viruses. *Lancet* **2**:260, 1985.
323. Prusiner SB, Groth DF, Cochran SP, McKinley MP, Masiarz FR: Gel electrophoresis and glass permeation chromatography of the hamster scrapie agent after enzymatic digestion and detergent extraction. *Biochemistry* **19**:4892, 1980.
324. Bendheim PE, Bockman JM, McKinley MP, Kingsbury DT, Prusiner SB: Scrapie and Creutzfeldt-Jakob disease prion proteins share physical properties and antigenic determinants. *Proc Natl Acad Sci USA* **82**:997, 1985.
325. Pocchiari M, Peano S, Conz A, Eshkol A, Maillard F, Brown P, Gibbs CJJ, Xi YG, Tenham-Fisher E, Macchi G: Combination ultrafiltration and 6 *M* urea treatment of human growth hormone effectively minimizes risk from potential Creutzfeldt-Jakob disease virus contamination. *Horm Res* **35**:161, 1991.
326. Cochius JI, Mack K, Burns RJ, Alderman CP, Blumbergs PC: Creutzfeldt-Jakob disease in a recipient of human pituitary-derived gonadotrophin. *Aust N Z J Med* **20**:592, 1990.
327. Gibbs CJ Jr, Amyx HL, Bacote A, Masters CL, Gajdusek DC: Oral transmission of kuru, Creutzfeldt-Jakob disease and scrapie to nonhuman primates. *J Infect Dis* **142**:205, 1980.
328. Zigas V, Gajdusek DC: Kuru: Clinical study of a new syndrome resembling paralysis agitans in natives of the Eastern Highlands of Australian New Guinea. *Med J Aust* **2**:745, 1957.
329. Gajdusek DC, Zigas V: Clinical, pathological and epidemiological study of an acute progressive degenerative disease of the central nervous system among natives of the eastern highlands of New Guinea. *Am J Med* **26**:442, 1959.
330. Gajdusek DC, Zigas V: Degenerative disease of the central nervous system in New Guinea—The endemic occurrence of "kuru" in the native population. *N Engl J Med* **257**:974, 1957.
331. Simpson DA, Lander H, Robson HN: Observations on kuru. II. Clinical features. *Aust Ann Med* **8**:8, 1959.
332. Alpers M: Kuru: A clinical study, in *Mimeographed Manuscript, Reissued.* Bethesda, DHEW, NIH, NINCDS, 1964, pp 1–38.
333. Hornabrook RW: Kuru—a subacute cerebellar degeneration: The natural history and clinical features. *Brain* **91**:53, 1968.
334. Hornabrook RW: Kuru and clinical neurology, in Prusiner SB, Hadlow WJ (eds): *Slow Transmissible Diseases of the Nervous System.* New York, Academic, 1979, vol 1, pp 37–66.
335. Zarranz JJ, Rivera-Pomar JM, Salisachs P: Kuru plaques in the brain of two cases with Creutzfeldt-Jakob disease. *J Neurol Sci* **43**:291, 1979.
336. Goldfarb LG, Brown P, Goldgaber D, Asher DM, Rubenstein R, Brown WT, Piccardo P, Kascsak RJ, Boellaard JW, Gajdusek DC: Creutzfeldt-Jakob disease and kuru patients lack a mutation consistently found in the Gerstmann-Sträussler-Scheinker syndrome. *Exp Neurol* **108**:247, 1990.
337. Gerstmann J, Sträussler E, Scheinker I: Über eine eigenartige hereditär-familiäre erkrankung des zentralnervensystems zugleich ein beitrag zur frage des vorzeitigen lokalen alterns. *Z Neurol* **154**:736, 1936.
338. Kuzuhara S, Kanazawa I, Sasaki H, Nakanishi T, Shimamura K: Gerstmann-Sträussler-Scheinker's disease. *Ann Neurol* **14**:216, 1983.
339. Seitelberger F: Sträussler's disease. *Acta Neuropathol Suppl (Berl)* **7**:341, 1981.
340. Doh-ura K, Tateishi J, Sasaki H, Kitamoto T, Sakaki Y: Pro→Leu change at position 102 of prion protein is the most common but not the sole mutation related to Gerstmann-Sträussler syndrome. *Biochem Biophys Res Commun* **163**:974, 1989.
341. Hsiao KK, Cass C, Schellenberg GD, Bird T, Devine-Gage E, Wisniewski H, Prusiner SB: A prion protein variant in a family with the telencephalic form of Gerstmann-Sträussler-Scheinker syndrome. *Neurology* **41**:681, 1991.
342. Dlouhy SR, Hsiao K, Farlow MR, Foroud T, Conneally PM, Johnson P, Prusiner SB, Hodes ME, Ghetti B: Linkage of the Indiana kindred of Gerstmann-Sträussler-Scheinker disease to the prion protein gene. *Nature Genet* **1**:64, 1992.
343. Hsiao K, Dloughy S, Ghetti B, Farlow M, Cass C, Da Costa M, Conneally M, Hodes ME, Prusiner SB: Mutant prion proteins in Gerstmann-Sträussler-Scheinker disease with neurofibrillary tangles. *Nature Genet* **1**:68, 1992.
344. Dolman CL, Daly LL: Spino-cerebello-cerebral degeneration with amyloid plaques (Gerstmann, Sträussler, Scheinker syndrome). *Can J Neurol Sci* **9**:439, 1982.
345. Peiffer J: Gerstmann-Sträussler disease, atypical multiple sclerosis and carcinomas in a family of sheepbreeders. *Acta Neuropathol (Berl)* **56**:87, 1982.
346. Hudson AJ, Farrell MA, Kalnins R, Kaufmann JCE: Gerstmann-Sträussler-Scheinker disease with coincidental familial onset. *Ann Neurol* **14**:670, 1983.
347. Azzarelli B, Muller J, Ghetti B, Dyken M, Conneally PM: Cerebellar plaques in familial Alzheimer's disease (Gerstmann-Sträussler-Scheinker variant?). *Acta Neuropathol (Berl)* **65**:235, 1985.
348. Tateishi J, Koga M, Sato Y, Mori R: Properties of the transmissible agent derived from chronic spongiform encephalopathy. *Ann Neurol* **7**:390, 1980.
349. Baker HF, Ridley RM, Crow TJ: Experimental transmission of an autosomal dominant spongiform encephalopathy: Does the infectious agent originate in the human genome? *Br Med J* **291**:299, 1985.
350. Tateishi J, Kitamoto T, Hashiguchi H, Shii H: Gerstmann-Sträussler-Scheinker disease: Immunohistological and experimental studies. *Ann Neurol* **24**:35, 1988.
351. Tateishi J, Kitamoto T, Doh-ura K, Sakaki Y, Steinmetz G, Tranchant C, Warter JM, Heldt N: Immunochemical, molecular genetic, and transmission studies on a case of Gerstmann-Sträussler-Scheinker syndrome. *Neurology* **40**:1578, 1990.
352. Wisniewski HM, Moretz RC, Lossinsky AS: Evidence for induction of localized amyloid deposits and neuritic plaques by an infectious agent. *Ann Neurol* **10**:517, 1981.
353. Tateishi J, Nagara H, Hikita K, Sato Y: Amyloid plaques in the brains of mice with Creutzfeldt-Jakob disease. *Ann Neurol* **15**:278, 1984.
354. Chou SM, Payne WN, Gibbs CJ Jr, Gajdusek DC: Transmission and scanning electron microscopy of spongiform change in Creutzfeldt-Jakob disease. *Brain* **103**:885, 1980.
355. Blackwood W, McMenemy WH, Meyer A, Norman RM, Russell DS (eds): *Greenfield's Neuropathology,* 2nd ed. London, Edward Arnold, 1971, pp 558–567.
356. Lampert PW, Gajdusek DC, Gibbs CJ Jr: Subacute spongiform virus encephalopathies. Scrapie, kuru and Creutzfeldt-Jakob disease: A review. *Am J Pathol* **68**:626, 1972.
357. Beck E, Daniel PM: Kuru and Creutzfeldt-Jakob disease; neuropathological lesions and their significance, in Prusiner SB, Hadlow WJ (eds): *Slow Transmissible Diseases of the Nervous System.* New York, Academic, 1979, vol 1, pp 253–270.
358. Beck E, Daniel PM, Davey AJ, Gajdusek DC, Gibbs CJ Jr: The pathogenesis of transmissible spongiform encephalopathy—an ultrastructural study. *Brain* **105**:755, 1982.
359. Tateishi J, Doi H, Sato Y, Suetsugu M, Ishii K, Kuroiwa Y: Experimental transmission of human subacute spongiform encephalopathy to small rodents. III. Further transmission from three patients and distribution patterns of lesions in mice. *Acta Neuropathol (Berl)* **53**:161, 1981.
360. Zlotnik I: The pathology of scrapie: A comparative study of lesions in the brain of sheep and goats. *Acta Neuropathol Suppl (Berl)* **1**:61, 1962.

361. Marsh RF, Sipe JC, Morse SS, Hanson RP: Transmissible mink encephalopathy: Reduced spongiform degeneration in aged mink of the Chediak-Higashi genotype. *Lab Invest* **34:**381, 1976.
362. Tateishi J, Hikita K, Nagara H, Sato Y, Koga M: Transmission of Creutzfeldt-Jakob disease and production of amyloid plaques in rodents. Sixth International Congress of Virology. Sendai, Japan, Sept. 1–7, 1984, p 76.
363. Kitamoto T, Tateishi J, Sato Y: Immunohistochemical verification of senile and kuru plaques in Creutzfeldt-Jakob disease and the allied disease. *Ann Neurol* **24:**537, 1988.
364. Chou SM, Martin JD: Kuru-plaques in a case of Creutzfeldt-Jakob disease. *Acta Neuropathol (Berl)* **17:**150, 1971.
365. Yagishita S: Creutzfeldt-Jakob disease with kuru-like plaques in Japan. *Acta Pathol Jpn* **31:**923, 1981.
366. Seitelberger F: Spinocerebellar ataxia with dementia and plaque-like deposits (Sträussler's disease), in Vinken PJ, Bruyn GW (eds): *Handbook of Clinical Neurology*. Amsterdam, North-Holland, 1981, vol 42, pp 182–183.
367. Heston LL, Lowther DLW, Leventhal CM: Alzheimer's disease: A family study. *Arch Neurol* **15:**255, 1966.
368. Ghetti B, Tagliavini F, Masters CL, Beyreuther K, Giaccone G, Verga L, Farlo MR, Conneally PM, Dlouhy SR, Azzarelli B, Bugiani O: Gerstmann-Sträussler-Scheinker disease. II. Neurofibrillary tangles and plaques with PrP-amyloid coexist in an affected family. *Neurology* **39:**1453, 1989.
369. Sumi SM, Nochlin D, Bird TD: Familial presenile dementia with neurofibrillary tangles but without senile (neuritic) plaques: Is this familial Alzheimer's disease? *Neurology (suppl 1)* **38:**266, 1988.
370. Nochlin D, Sumi SM, Bird TD, Snow AD, Leventhal CM, Beyreuther K, Masters CL: Familial dementia with PrP-positive amyloid plaques: A variant of Gerstmann-Sträussler syndrome. *Neurology* **39:**910, 1989.
371. Ikeda S, Yanagisawa N, Allsop D, Glenner GG: A variant of Gerstmann-Sträussler-Scheinker disease with β-protein epitopes and dystrophic neurites in the peripheral regions of PrP—immunoreactive amyloid plaques, in Natvig JB, Forre O, Husby G, Husebekk A, Skogen B, Sletten K, Westermark P (eds): *Amyloid and Amyloidosis 1990*. Dordrecht, The Netherlands, Kluwer, 1991, pp 737–740.
372. Goldgaber D, Goldfarb LG, Brown P, Asher DM, Brown WT, Lin S, Teener JW, Feinstone SM, Rubenstein R, Kascsak RJ, Boellaard JW, Gajdusek DC: Mutations in familial Creutzfeldt-Jakob disease and Gerstmann-Sträussler-Scheinker's syndrome. *Exp Neurol* **106:**204, 1989.
373. Kretzschmar HA, Honold G, Seitelberger F, Feucht M, Wessely P, Mehraein P, Budka H: Prion protein mutation in family first reported by Gerstmann, Sträussler, and Scheinker (letter). *Lancet* **337:**1160, 1991.
374. Kretzschmar HA, Kufer P, Riethmuller G, DeArmond SJ, Prusiner SB, Schiffer D: Prion protein mutation at codon 102 in an Italian family with Gerstmann-Sträussler-Scheinker syndrome. *Neurology* **42:**809, 1991.
375. Owen F, Poulter M, Lofthouse R, Collinge J, Crow TJ, Risby D, Baker HF, Ridley RM, Hsiao K, Prusiner SB: Insertion in prion protein gene in familial Creutzfeldt-Jakob disease. *Lancet* **1:**51, 1989.
376. Owen F, Poulter M, Shah T, Collinge J, Lofthouse R, Baker H, Ridley R, McVey J Crow T: An in-frame insertion in the prion protein gene in familial Creutzfeldt-Jakob disease. *Mol Brain Res* **7:**273, 1990.
377. Collinge J, Owen F, Poulter H, Leach M, Crow T, Rosser M, Hardy J, Mullan H, Janota I, Lantos P: Prion dementia without characteristic pathology. *Lancet* **336:**7, 1990.
378. Crow TJ, Collinge J, Ridley RM, Baker HF, Lofthouse R, Owen F, Harding AE: Mutations in the prion gene in human transmissible dementia. Seminar on Molecular Approaches to Research in Spongiform Encephalopathies in Man, Medical Research Council, London 1990. (abstr.)
379. Owen F, Poulter M, Collinge J, Leach M, Shah T, Lofthouse R, Chen YF, Crow TJ, Harding AE, Hardy J: Insertions in the prion protein gene in atypical dementias. *Exp Neurol* **112:**240, 1991.
380. Poulter M, Baker HF, Frith CD, Leach M, Lofthouse R, Ridley RM, Shah T, Owen F, Collinge J, Brown G, Hardy J, Mullan MJ, Harding AE, Bennett C, Doshi R, Crow TJ: Inherited prion disease with 144 base pair gene insertion. 1. Geneological and molecular studies. *Brain* **115:**675, 1992.
381. Collinge J, Brown J, Hardy J, Mullan M, Rossor MN, Baker H, Crow TJ, Lofthouse R, Poulter M, Ridley R, Owen F, Bennett C, Dunn G, Harding AE, Quinn N, Doshi B, Roberts GW, Honavar M, Janota I, Lantos PL: Inherited prion disease with 144 base pair gene insertion. 2. Clinical and pathological features. *Brain* **115:**687, 1992.
382. Goldfarb LG, Brown P, McCombie WR, Goldgaber D, Swergold GD, Wills PR, Cervenakova L, Baron H, Gibbs CJJ, Gajdusek DC: Transmissible familial Creutzfeldt-Jakob disease associated with five, seven, and eight extra octapeptide coding repeats in the *PRNP* gene. *Proc Natl Acad Sci USA* **88:**10926, 1991.
383. Owen F, Poulter M, Collinge J, Leach M, Lofthouse R, Crow TJ, Harding AE: A dementing illness associated with a novel insertion in the prion protein gene. *Mol Brain Res* **13:**155, 1992.
384. Brown P: The clinico-pathological features of transmissible human spongiform encephalopathy, with a discussion of recognized risk factors and preventive strategies, in *International Meeting on Transmissible Spongiform Encephalopathies, Impact on Animal and Human Health, Heidelberg, Germany, June 23–24, 1992*. Heidelberg, Germany, International Association of Biological Standardization, 1992. (abstr.)
385. Laplanche J-L, Chatelain J, Launay J-M, Gazengel C, Vidaud M: Deletion in prion protein gene in a Moroccan family. *Nucleic Acids Res* **18:**6745, 1990.
386. Vnencak-Jones CL, Phillips JA: Identification of heterogeneous PrP gene deletions in controls by detection of allele-specific heteroduplexes (DASH). *Am J Hum Genet* **50:**871, 1992.
387. Kahana E, Milton A, Braham J, Sofer D: Creutzfeldt-Jakob disease: Focus among Libyan Jews in Israel. *Science* **183:**90, 1974.
388. Herzberg L, Herzberg BN, Gibbs CJ Jr, Sullivan W, Amyx H, Gajdusek DC: Creutzfeldt-Jakob disease: Hypothesis for high incidence in Libyan Jews in Israel. *Science* **186:**848, 1974.
389. Zilber N, Kahana E, Abraham MPH: The Libyan Creutzfeldt-Jakob disease focus in Israel: An epidemiologic evaluation. *Neurology* **41:**1385, 1991.
390. Kahana E, Zilber N, Abraham M: Do Creutzfeldt-Jakob disease patients of Jewish Libyan origin have unique clinical features? *Neurology* **41:**1390, 1991.
391. Goldfarb LG, Mitrova E, Brown P, Toh BH, Gajdusek DC: Mutation in codon 200 of scrapie amyloid protein gene in two clusters of Creutzfeldt-Jakob disease in Slovakia. *Lancet* **336:**514, 1990.
392. Gabizon R, Meiner Z, Cass C, Kahana E, Kahana I, Avrahami D, Abramsky O, Scarlato G, Prusiner SB, Hsiao KK: Prion protein gene mutation in Libyan Jews with Creutzfeldt-Jakob disease. *Neurology* **41:**160, 1991. (abstr.)
393. Hsiao K, Meiner Z, Kahana E, Cass C, Kahana I, Avrahami D, Scarlato G, Abramsky O, Prusiner SB, Gabizon R: Mutation of the prion protein in Libyan Jews with Creutzfeldt-Jakob disease. *N Engl J Med* **324:**1091, 1991.
394. Wexler NS, Young AB, Tanzi RE, Travers H, Starosta-Rubinstein S, Penney JB, Snodgrass SR, Shoulson I, Gomez F, Ramos Arroyo MA, Penchaszadeh GK, Moreno H, Gibbons K, Faryniarz A, Hobbs W, Anderson MA, Bonilla E, Conneally PM, Gusella JF: Homozygotes for Huntington's disease. *Nature* **326:**194, 1987.
395. Goldfarb LG, Brown P, Mitrova E, Cervenakova L, Goldin L, Korczyn AD, Chapman J, Galvez S, Cartier L, Rubenstein R, Gajdusek DC: Creutzfeldt-Jacob disease associated with the PRNP codon 200^{Lys} mutation: An analysis of 45 families. *Eur J Epidemiol* **7:**477, 1991.
396. Bertoni JM, Brown P, Goldfarb L, Gajdusek D, Omaha NE: Familial Creutzfeldt-Jakob disease with the PRNP codon 200^{lys} mutation and supranuclear palsy but without myoclonus or periodic EEG complexes. *Neurology (suppl 3)* **42:**350, 1992. (abstr.)
397. Udovitch AL, Valensi L: *The Last Arab Jews: The Communities of Jerba, Tunisia*. London, Harwood, 1984, p 178.

398. Goldfarb LG, Haltia M, Brown P, Nieto A, Kovanen J, McCombie WR, Trapp S, Gajdusek DC: New mutation in scrapie amyloid precursor gene (at codon 178) in Finnish Creutzfeldt-Jakob kindred. *Lancet* **337**:425, 1991.
399. Goldfarb LG, Brown P, Haltia M, Cathala F, McCombie WR, Kovanen J, Cervenakova L, Goldin L, Nieto A, Godec MS, Asher DM, Gajdusek DC: Creutzfeldt-Jakob disease cosegregates with the codon 178^{Asn} *PRNP* mutation in families of European origin. *Ann Neurol* **31**:274, 1992.
400. Brown P, Goldfarb LG, Kovanen J, Haltia M, Cathala F, Sulima M, Gibbs CJJ, Gajdusek DC: Phenotypic characteristics of familial Creutzfeldt-Jakob disease associated with the codon 178^{Asn} *PRNP* mutation. *Ann Neurol* **31**:282, 1992.
401. Haltia M, Kovanen J, Goldfarb LG, Brown P, Gajdusek DC: Familial Creutzfeldt-Jakob disease in Finland: Epidemiological, clinical, pathological and molecular genetic studies. *Eur J Epidemiol* **7**:494, 1991.
402. Fink JK, Warren JT Jr, Drury I, Murman D, Peacock BA: Allele-specific sequencing confirms novel prion gene polymorphism in Creutzfeldt-Jakob disease. *Neurology* **41**:1647, 1991.
403. Medori R, Montagna P, Tritschler HJ, LeBlanc A, Cortelli P, Tinuper P, Lugaresi E, Gambetti P: Fatal familial insomnia: A second kindred with mutation of prion protein gene at codon 178. *Neurology* **42**:669, 1992.
404. Goldfarb LG, Petersen RB, Tabaton M, Brown P, LeBlanc AC, Montagna P, Cortelli P, Julien J, Vital C, Pendelbury WW, Haltia M, Wills PR, Hauw JJ, McKeever PE, Monari L, Schrank B, Swergold GD, Autilio-Gambetti L, Gajdusek DC, Lugaresi E, Gambetti P: Fatal familial insomnia and familial Creutzfeldt-Jakob disease: Disease phenotype determined by a DNA polymorphism. *Science* **258**:806, 1992.
405. Johnson RT: Prion disease. *N Engl J Med* **326**:486, 1992.
406. Tranchant C, Doh-ura K, Warter JM, Steinmetz G, Chevalier Y, Hanauer A, Kitamoto T, Tateishi J: Gerstmann-Sträussler-Scheinker disease in an Alsatian family: Clinical and genetic studies. *J Neurol Neurosurg Psychiatry* **55**:185, 1992.
407. Farlow MR, Yee RD, Dlouhy SR, Conneally PM, Azzarelli B, Ghetti B: Gerstmann-Sträussler-Scheinker disease. I. Extending the clinical spectrum. *Neurology* **39**:1446, 1989.
408. Giaccone G, Tagliavini F, Verga L, Frangione B, Farlow MR, Bugiani O, Ghetti B: Neurofibrillary tangles of the Indiana kindred of Gerstmann-Sträussler-Scheinker disease share antigenic determinants with those of Alzheimer disease. *Brain Res* **530**:325, 1990.
409. Owen F, Poulter M, Collinge J, Crow TJ: Codon 129 changes in the prion protein gene in Caucasians. *Am J Hum Genet* **46**:1215, 1990.
410. Collinge J, Palmer MS, Dryden AJ: Genetic predisposition to iatrogenic Creutzfeldt-Jakob disease. *Lancet* **337**:1441, 1991.
411. Palmer MS, Dryden AJ, Hughes JT, Collinge J: Homozygous prion protein genotype predisposes to sporadic Creutzfeldt-Jakob disease. *Nature* **352**:340, 1991.
412. Hardy J: Prion dimers—a deadly duo. *Trends Neurosci* **14**:423, 1991.
413. Hsiao KK, Groth D, Scott M, Yang S-L, Serban A, Rapp D, Foster D, Torchia M, DeArmond SJ, Prusiner SB: Neurologic disease of transgenic mice which express GSS mutant prion protein is transmissible to inoculated recipient animals, in Prion Diseases of Humans and Animals Symposium, London, Sept 2–4, 1991. (abstr.)
414. McKinley MP, Masiarz FR, Isaacs ST, Hearst JE, Prusiner SB: Resistance of the scrapie agent to inactivation by psoralens. *Photochem Photobiol* **37**:539, 1983.
415. Bellinger-Kawahara C, Cleaver JE, Diener TO, Prusiner SB: Purified scrapie prions resist inactivation by UV irradiation. *J Virol* **61**:159, 1987.
416. Bellinger-Kawahara C, Diener TO, McKinley MP, Groth DF, Smith DR, Prusiner SB: Purified scrapie prions resist inactivation by procedures that hydrolyze, modify, or shear nucleic acids. *Virology* **160**:271, 1987.
417. Weitgrefe S, Zupancic M, Haase A, Chesebro B, Race R, Frey W II, Rustan T, Friedman RL: Cloning of a gene whose expression is increased in scrapie and in senile plaques. *Science* **230**:1177, 1985.
418. Diedrich J, Weitgrefe S, Zupancic M, Staskus K, Retzel E, Haase AT, Race R: The molecular pathogenesis of astrogliosis in scrapie and Alzheimer's disease. *Microb Pathog* **2**:435, 1987.
419. Duguid JR, Rohwer RG, Seed B: Isolation of cDNAs of scrapie-modulated RNAs by subtractive hybridization of a cDNA library. *Proc Natl Acad Sci USA* **85**:5738, 1988.
420. Oesch B, Groth DF, Prusiner SB, Weissmann C: Search for a scrapie-specific nucleic acid: A progress report, in Bock G, Marsh J (eds): *Novel Infectious Agents and the Central Nervous System*. Ciba Foundation Symposium 135. Chichester, England, John Wiley, 1988, pp 209–223.
421. Neary K, Caughey B, Ernst D, Race RE, Chesebro B: Protease sensitivity and nuclease resistance of the scrapie agent propagated in vitro in neuroblastoma-cells. *J Virol* **65**:1031, 1991.
422. Kellings K, Meyer N, Mirenda C, Prusiner SB, Riesner D: Further analysis of nucleic acids in purified scrapie prion preparations by improved return refocussing gel electrophoresis (RRGE). *J Gen Virol* **73**:1025, 1992.
423. Aiken JM, Marsh RF: The search for scrapie agent nucleic acid. *Microbiol Rev* **54**:242, 1990.
424. Chesebro B: PrP and the scrapie agent. *Nature* **356**:560, 1992.
425. Weissmann C: Spongiform encephalopathies—the prion's progress. *Nature* **349**:569, 1991.
426. Pattison IH: Experiments with scrapie with special reference to the nature of the agent and pathology of the disease, in Gajdusek DC, Gibbs CJ Jr, Alpers MP (eds): *Slow, Latent and Temperate Virus Infections*. NINDB Monograph 2. Washington, DC, Government Printing Offices, 1965, pp 249–257.
427. Pattison IH: The relative susceptibility of sheep, goats and mice to two types of the goat scrapie agent. *Res Vet Sci* **7**:207, 1966.
428. Scott M, Foster D, Mirenda C, Serban D, Coufal F, Wälchli M, Torchia M, Groth D, Carlson G, DeArmond SJ, Westaway D, Prusiner SB: Transgenic mice expressing hamster prion protein produce species-specific scrapie infectivity and amyloid plaques. *Cell* **59**:847, 1989.
429. Büeler H, Aguzzi A, Sailer A, Greiner R, Autenried P, Aguet M, Weissmann C: Mice devoid of PrP are resistant to scrapie. *Cell* **73**:1339, 1993.
430. Fraser H, Dickinson AG: Scrapie in mice. Agent-strain differences in the distribution and intensity of grey matter vacuolation. *J Comp Pathol* **83**:29, 1973.
431. Bruce ME, McBride PA, Farquhar CF: Precise targeting of the pathology of the sialoglycoprotein, PrP, and vacuolar degeneration in mouse scrapie. *Neurosci Lett* **102**:1, 1989.
432. Hecker R, Taraboulos A, Scott M, Pan K-M, Torchia M, Jendroska K, DeArmond SJ, Prusiner SB: Replication of distinct prion isolates is region specific in brains of transgenic mice and hamsters. *Genes Dev* **6**:1213, 1992.
433. Bruce ME, Dickinson AG: Biological evidence that the scrapie agent has an independent genome. *J Gen Virol* **68**:79, 1987.
434. Bessen RA, Marsh RF: Biochemical and physical properties of the prion protein from two strains of the transmissible mink encephalopathy agent. *J Virol* **66**:2096, 1992.
435. Bessen RA, Marsh RF: Identification of two biologically distinct strains of transmissible mink encephalopathy in hamsters. *J Gen Virol* **73**:329, 1992.
436. Braig H, Diringer H: Scrapie: Concept of a virus-induced amyloidosis of the brain. *EMBO J* **4**:2309, 1985.
437. Sklaviadis TK, Manuelidis L, Manuelidis EE: Physical properties of the Creutzfeldt-Jakob disease agent. *J Virol* **63**:1212, 1989.
438. Sklaviadis T, Akowitz A, Manuelidis EE, Manuelidis L: Nuclease treatment results in high specific purification of Creutzfeldt-Jakob disease infectivity with a density characteristic of nucleic acid-protein complexes. *Arch Virol* **112**:215, 1990.
439. Aiken JM, Williamson JL, Marsh RF: Evidence of mitochondrial involvement in scrapie infection. *J Virol* **63**:1686, 1989.
440. Aiken JM, Williamson JL, Borchardt LM, Marsh RF: Presence of mitochondrial D-loop DNA in scrapie-infected

brain preparations enriched for the prion protein. *J Virol* **64**:3265, 1990.

441. Akowitz A, Sklaviadis T, Manuelidis EE, Manuelidis L: Nuclease-resistant polyadenylated RNAs of significant size are detected by PCR in highly purified Creutzfeldt-Jakob disease preparations. *Microb Pathog* **9**:33, 1990.
442. Murdoch GH, Sklaviadis T, Manuelidis EE, Manuelidis L: Protential retroviral RNAs in Creutzfeldt-Jakob disease. *J Virol* **64**:1477, 1990.
443. Manuelidis L, Manuelidis EE: Creutzfeldt-Jakob disease and dementias. *Microb Pathog* **7**:157, 1989.
444. Cohen FE, Abarbanel RM, Kuntz ID, Fletterick RJ: Turn prediction in proteins using a pattern-matching approach. *Biochemistry* **25**:266, 1986.
445. Gasset M, Baldwin MA, Lloyd D, Gabriel J-M, Holtzman DM, Cohen F, Fletterick R, Prusiner SB: Predicted α-helical regions of the prion protein when synthesized as peptides form amyloid. *Proc Natl Acad Sci USA* **89**:10940, 1992.
446. Caughey BW, Dong A, Bhat KS, Ernst D, Hayes SF, Caughey WS: Secondary structure analysis of the scrapie-associated protein PrP 27-30 in water by infrared spectroscopy. *Biochemistry* **30**:7672, 1991.
447. Gasset M, Baldwin MA, Fletterick RJ, Prusiner SB: Perturbation of the secondary structure of the scrapie prion protein under conditions associated with changes in infectivity. *Proc Natl Acad Sci USA* **90**:1, 1993.
448. Dickinson AG, Fraser H: An assessment of the genetics of scrapie in sheep and mice, in Prusiner SB, Hadlow WJ (eds): *Slow Transmissible Diseases of the Nervous System.* New York, Academic, 1979, vol 1, pp 367–386.
449. Kimberlin RH, Cole S, Walker CA: Temporary and permanent modifications to a single strain of mouse scrapie on transmission to rats and hamsters. *J Gen Virol* **68**:1875, 1987.
450. Dickinson AG, Outram GW: Genetic aspects of unconventional virus infections: The basis of the virino hypothesis, in Bock G, Marsh J (eds): *Novel Infectious Agents and the Central Nervous System.* Ciba Foundation Symposium 135. Chichester, England, John Wiley, 1988, pp 63–83.
451. Bellinger-Kawahara CG, Kempner E, Groth DF, Gabizon R, Prusiner SB: Scrapie prion liposomes and rods exhibit target sizes of 55,000 Da. *Virology* **164**:537, 1988.
452. Gajdusek DC: Subacute spongiform encephalopathies: Transmissible cerebral amyloidoses caused by unconventional viruses, in Fields BN, Knipe DM, Chanock RM, Hirsch MS, Melnick JL, Monath TP, Roizman B (eds): *Virology*, 2nd ed. New York, Raven, 1990, pp 2289–2324.
453. Gajdusek DC, Gibbs CJ Jr: Brain amyloidoses-precursor proteins and the amyloids of transmissible and nontransmissible dementias: Scrapie-kuru-CJD viruses as infectious polypeptides or amyloid enhancing vactor, in Goldstein A (ed): *Biomedical Advances in Aging.* New York, Plenum, 1990, pp 3–24.
454. Brown P, Cathala F, Raubertas RF, Gajdusek DC, Castaigne P: The epidemiology of Creutzfeldt-Jakob disease: Conclusion of 15-year investigation in France and review of the world literature. *Neurology* **37**:895, 1987.
455. Gibbs CJ Jr, Gajdusek DC: Experimental subacute spongiform virus encephalopathies in primates and other laboratory animals. *Science* **182**:67, 1973.
456. Manuelidis E, Gorgacz EJ, Manuelidis L: Interspecies transmission of Creutzfeldt-Jakob disease to Syrian hamsters with reference to clinical syndromes and strains of agent. *Proc Natl Acad Sci USA* **75**:3422, 1978.
457. Masters CL, Gajdusek DC, Gibbs CJ Jr, Bernouilli C, Asher DM: Familial Creutzfeldt-Jakob disease and other familial dementias: An inquiry into possible models of virus-induced familial diseases in, Prusiner SB, Hadlow WJ (eds): *Slow Transmissible Diseases of the Nervous System.* New York, Academic, 1979, vol 1, pp 143–194.
458. Hadlow WJ, Kennedy RC, Race RE, Eklund CM: Virologic and neurohistologic findings in dairy goats affected with natural scrapie. *Vet Pathol* **17**:187, 1980.
459. Prusiner SB, Hsiao KK, Bredesen DE, DeArmond SJ: Prion disease, in Vinken PJ, Bruyn GW, Klawans HL (eds): *Handbook of Clinical Neurology.* vol 12(56): Viral Disease, Amsterdam, Elsevier, 1989, pp 543–580.
460. Hope J, Morton LJD, Farquhar CF, Multhaup G, Beyreuther K, Kimberlin RH: The major polypeptide of scrapie-associated fibrils (SAF) has the same size, charge distribution and N-terminal protein sequence as predicted for the normal brain protein (PrP). *EMBO J* **5**:2591, 1986.
461. Turk E, Teplow DB, Hood LE, Prusiner SB: Purification and properties of the cellular and scrapie hamster prion proteins. *Eur J Biochem* **176**:21, 1988.
462. Safar J, Wang W, Padgett MP, Ceroni M, Piccardo P, Zopf D, Gajdusek DC, Gibbs CJ Jr: Molecular mass, biochemical composition, and physicochemical behavior of the infectious form of the scrapie precursor protein monomer. *Proc Natl Acad Sci USA* **87**:6373, 1990.
463. Prusiner SB: Molecular biology and genetics of neurodegenerative diseases caused by prions. *Adv Virus Res* **41**:241, 1992.
464. Goldfarb L, Brown P, Goldgaber D, Garruto R, Yanaghiara R, Asher D, Gajdusek DC: Identical mutation in unrelated patients with Creutzfeldt-Jakob disease. *Lancet* **336**:174, 1990.
465. Hsiao KK, Doh-ura K, Kitamoto T, Tateishi J, Prusiner SB: A prion protein amino acid substitution in ataxic Gerstmann-Sträussler syndrome. *Ann Neurol* **26**:137, 1989.
466. Goldfarb L, Korczyn A, Brown P, Chapman J, Gajdusek DC: Mutation in codon 200 of scrapie amyloid precursor gene linked to Creutzfeldt-Jakob disease in Sephardic Jews of Libyan and non-Libyan origin. *Lancet* **336**:637, 1990.
467. Ripoll L, Laplanche J-L, Salzmann M, Jouvet A, Planques B, Dussaucy M, Chatelain J, Beaudry P, Launay J-M: A new point mutation in the prion protein gene at codon 210 in Creutzfeldt-Jakob disease. *Neurology* **43**:1934, 1993.
468. Baker HF, Ridley RM, Wells GAH: Experimental transmission of BSE and scrapie to the common marmoset. *Vet Rec* **132**:403, 1993.
469. Pearson GR, Wyatt JM, Gruffydd-Jones TJ, Hope J, Chong A, Higgins RJ, Scott AC, Wells GA: Feline spongiform encephalopathy: Fibril and PrP studies. *Vet Rec* **131**:307, 1992.
470. Cunningham AA, Wells GAH, Scott AC, Kirkwood JK, Barnett JEF: Transmissible spongiform encephalopathy in greater kudu (*Tragelaphus strepsiceros*). *Vet Rec* **132**:68, 1993.
471. Kirkwood JK, Cunningham AA, Wells GAH, Wilesmith JW, Barnett JEF: Spongiform encephalopathy in a herd of greater kudu (*Tragelaphus strepsiceros*): epidemiological observations. *Vet Rec* **133**:360, 1993.
472. Palmer MS, Mahal SP, Campbell TA, Hill AF, Sidle KC, Leplanche JL, Collinge J: Deletions in the prion protein gene are not associated with CJD. *Hum Molec Genet* **2**:541, 1993.
473. Prusiner SB, Groth D, Serban A, Koehler R, Foster D, Torchia M, Burton D, Yang SL, DeArmond SJ: Ablation of the prion protein (PrP) gene in mice prevents scrapie and facilitates production of anti-PrP antibodies. *Proc Natl Acad Sci USA* **90**:10608, 1993.
474. Scott M, Groth D, Foster D, Torchia M, Yang SL, DeArmond SJ, Prusiner SB: Propagation of prions with artificial properties in transgenic mice expressing chimeric PrP genes. *Cell* **73**:979, 1993.
475. Pan K-M, Baldwin M, Nguyen J, Gasset M, Serban A, Groth D, Mehlhorn I, Huang Z, Fletterick RJ, Cohen FE, Prusiner SB: Conversion of α-helices into β-sheets features in the formation of the scrapie prion proteins. *Proc Natl Acad Sci USA* **90**:10962, 1993.
476. Prusiner SB, Füzi M, Scott M, Serban D, Serban H, Taraboulos A, Gabriel J-M, Wells GA, Wilesmith JW, Bradley R, DeArmond SJ, Kristensson K: Immunologic and molecular biological studies of prion proteins in bovine spongiform encephalopathy. *J. Infect Dis* **167**:602, 1993.

Part 24

SIGNIFICANT DEVELOPMENTS IN PROGRESS

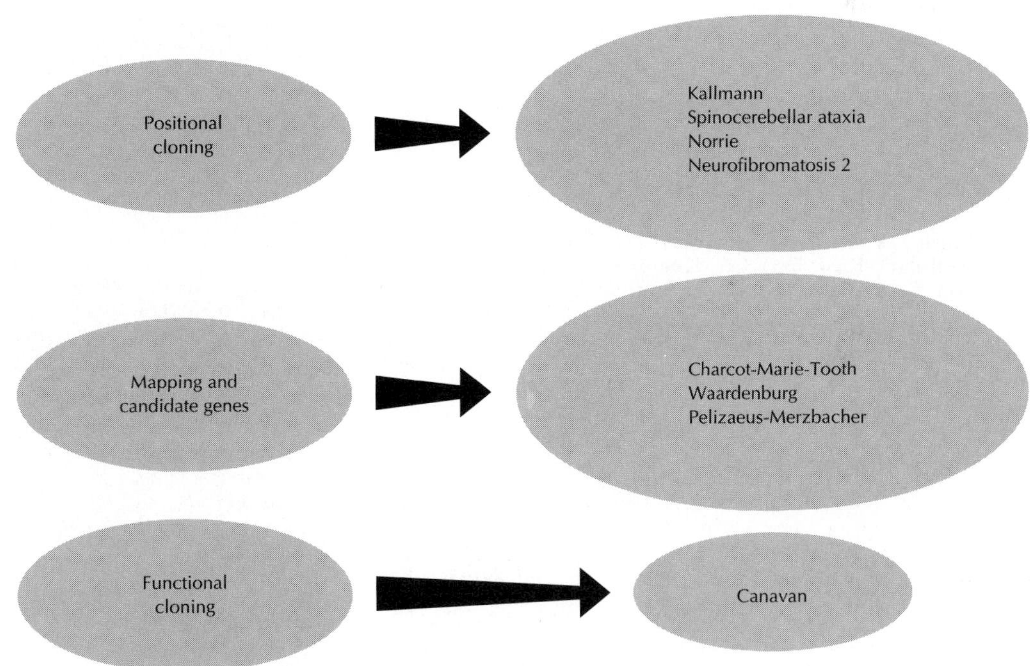

CHAPTER 154A

Kallmann Syndrome

Andrea Ballabio ▪ Huda Y. Zoghbi

1. **Kallmann syndrome is an inherited disorder characterized by the association of hypogonadotropic hypogonadism, due to gonadotropin-releasing hormone (GnRH) deficiency, with inability to smell (anosmia). These symptoms are the result of a defect in migration and targeting of two specific neuronal subpopulations, the GnRH producing neurons and the olfactory neurons.**
2. **Autosomal dominant, autosomal recessive, and X-linked recessive inheritance patterns have been described in Kallmann syndrome, indicating the presence of genetic heterogeneity. Deletion mapping and positional cloning efforts in the distal short arm of the X chromosome (Xp22.3) led to the isolation of the gene involved in the X-linked type of Kallmann syndrome (KAL). Patients with Kallmann syndrome carrying deletions in the Xp22.3 region may have contiguous gene syndromes and, therefore, may display the phenotype of several X-linked disorders associated with Kallmann syndrome.**
3. **In addition to deletions, several point mutations in the KAL gene have been identified in patients with isolated Kallmann syndrome.**
4. **The KAL gene encodes a protein that shares significant similarities with neural-cell adhesion molecules as well as with other molecules involved in neuronal migration and axonal pathfinding.**
5. **The characterization of KAL spatiotemporal expression pattern in chick embryos has provided important clues to the understanding of Kallmann syndrome pathogenesis.**
6. **Within the olfactory system, the gene is expressed by the mitral cells of the olfactory bulb, which represent the target of the olfactory axons.**
7. **It appears likely that the primary defect in Kallmann syndrome is an abnormality of olfactory system development affecting axonal targeting and/or synaptogenesis.**

CLINICAL FEATURES, DIAGNOSIS, AND THERAPY

In 1856, Maestre de San Juan observed the association of hypogonadism with olfactory system abnormalities.[1] Later de Morsier described, under the term "olfactogenital dysplasia," a series of patients with hypogonadism and anosmia who had various abnormalities of the olfactory system associated with multiple malformations.[2,3] The inherited nature of this condition was first identified by Kallmann in 1944.[4] Subsequently, the term Kallmann syndrome (KS) has come to designate an inherited disorder characterized by the association of hypogonadotropic hypogonadism and anosmia.

The hypogonadism in KS is due to a reduced secretion of gonadotropin-releasing hormone (GnRH) by the hypothalamus.[5] The degree of GnRH deficiency in KS patients is variable, ranging from complete deficiency, in which both follicle-stimulating hormone (FSH) and luteinizing hormone (LH) levels are low and there is no evidence of sexual maturation, to partial deficiency, in which FSH secretion predominates, allowing a certain degree of germinal-cell maturation in the testis but resulting in incomplete sexual development.[6] Typical patients with KS have a eunuchoid habitus. Gynecomastia, micropenis, and cryptorchidism have been reported in some cases.[7]

The other cardinal feature of patients with KS is the presence of nonselective anosmia or hyposmia. Therefore, a precise determination of the olfactory threshold in patients with hypogonadotropic hypogonadism is of fundamental importance in confirming the diagnosis of KS.

The complete spectrum of clinical features associated with KS is shown in Table 154A-1. Additional features found in several patients with KS include synkinesia (mirror movements), pes cavus, high arched palate, and unilateral renal agenesis.[8–11] Hardelin et al. demonstrated that these features represent pleiotropic effects of point mutations in the X-linked KS gene.[12,13] Synkinesia is thought to arise from the lack of the fibers that typically cross within the corpus callosum and inhibit the contralateral uncrossed pyramidal tract.[14] When asked to perform unilateral intentional movements, patients with synkinesia move muscles of the contralateral side together with the primary movement. Danek et al. measured movement-related cortical potentials in families with X-linked KS and demonstrated a complete correlation between the presence of the KS phenotype and bilaterality of evoked motor responses.[15] Additional neurologic symptoms described in some patients with KS include eye-movement abnormalities, cerebellar ataxia, gaze-evoked horizontal nystagmus,[10,11] sensorineural deafness,[9] spatial-attention abnormalities,[16] spastic paraplegia,[17] and mental retardation.[8] Moreover, somatic defects such as cleft lip and palate and congenital heart defects have been described.[9,11,18]

Occasional patients with KS also manifest features of other distinct X-linked diseases such as ichthyosis, chondrodysplasia punctata, mental retardation, short stature, and ocular albinism. This combination of disorders results from

A list of standard abbreviations is located immediately preceding the index in each volume. Additional abbreviations used in this chapter include: FN = fibronectin; FSH = follicle-stimulating hormone; GnRH = gonadotropin-releasing hormone; KAL or *KAL* = Kallmann syndrome protein or gene symbol, respectively; KAL-X = Kallmann gene on the X chromosome; KAL-Y = Kallmann pseudogene on the Y chromosome; KAL_c = chicken Kallmann gene or protein; KS = Kallmann syndrome; LH = luteinizing hormone; NCAM = neural-cell adhesion molecule.

Table 154A-1 Clinical Features Associated with Kallmann Syndrome

Cardinal features found in most patients with Kallmann syndrome
Hypogonadotropic hypogonadism
Anosmia
Pleiotropic effects of mutations in the KAL gene
Synkinesia (mirror movements)
Unilateral renal agenesis
High arched palate
Pes cavus
Rare features observed in a few cases
Eye-movement abnormalities
Cerebellar ataxia
Gaze-evoked horizontal nystagmus
Sensorineural deafness
Spatial-attention abnormalities
Spastic paraplegia
Mental retardation
Cleft lip and palate
Features found in patients with Xp22.3 deletions (contiguous gene syndrome)
Ichthyosis
Mental retardation
Chondrodysplasia punctata
Short stature
Ocular albinism

deletions of the distal short arm of the human X chromosome, leading to a contiguous gene syndrome (see Chap. 20).[19]

Patients with KS usually present at puberty with a delay in the appearance of secondary sex characteristics. Laboratory tests reveal low serum concentrations of FSH and LH[6] and very low levels of testosterone in males or of estradiol in females. Differentiation between KS and delayed puberty requires a complete family history and a thorough assessment of olfactory function, which can be tested by the method proposed by Henkin and Bartter[20] or by the Smell Identification Test.[21] Sporadic cases of KS may be difficult to differentiate from idiopathic hypogonadotropic hypogonadism because of the variability in expression of anosmia in KS.[22] Hypogonadotropic hypogonadism can also be due to central nervous system tumors, histiocytosis, radiation therapy, idiopathic hypopituitary dwarfism, Prader-Willi syndrome, Laurence-Moon-Biedl syndrome, chronic diseases, malnutrition, anorexia nervosa, or hypothyroidism. All of these disorders are easily distinguishable from KS.[6]

Treatment for KS is directed toward restoration of normal gonadal steroid levels to allow sexual maturation and induce fertility. The exogenous administration of testosterone is usually effective in inducing virilization. Achieving fertility, however, requires administration of gonadotropins or GnRH. Controversy exists regarding the effectiveness of gonadotropin versus GnRH replacement therapy in hypogonadotropic males, as reviewed elsewhere.[23] Combined gonadotropin replacement by administration of human chorionic gonadotropin (hCG) and human menopausal gonadotropin (hMG) appears to be the most common treatment for hypogonadotropic hypogonadism. Comparable results have been obtained with either subcutaneous or intramuscular administration. Subcutaneous applications, however, seem to be preferred because they are less painful and can be done by the patient.[24] Response to gonadotropin therapy varies considerably among individuals.[24] Although pulsatile subcutaneous administration of GnRH is the most physiological treatment,[25] the need for a programmable infusion pump makes this therapy difficult to carry out and often decreases compliance. Hormonal replacement therapy, either by gonadotropins or GnRH, is required over many months, since shorter treatments usually fail to induce normal sexual development and spermatogenesis. The patient's compliance and his desire for fertility play a fundamental role in achieving successful treatment.

HISTOPATHOLOGY

The presence of anatomical defects of the olfactory system in patients with hypogonadism and anosmia was first described by Maestre de San Juan.[1] More recent anatomical studies of patients with KS revealed the absence or hypoplasia of olfactory bulbs and tracts.[26–28] In addition, biopsies of nasal mucosa from a patient with KS revealed immature olfactory neurons and degenerating axons in the olfactory epithelium.[29]

The first clue to the pathogenesis of KS came from the observation of a developmental relationship between GnRH-secreting neurons and the olfactory system. Two independent studies performed in mice demonstrated that GnRH-secreting neurons share a common origin and migration pathway with olfactory axons during development (Fig. 154A-1).[30,31] Immunohistochemistry and mRNA *in situ* hybridization studies were performed in mouse embryos using anti-GnRH antibodies and a GnRH probe, respectively. These studies demonstrated that GnRH neurons originate in the olfactory placode, a discrete thickening of the head ectoderm that goes on to form the olfactory epithelium. During development, GnRH neurons migrate along the olfactory, terminalis, and vomeronasal nerves, traverse both the cribriform plate and the meninges, enter the forebrain, and eventually reach their final destination in the hypothalamus.[30,31] It was evident from these data that interactions between the olfactory axons and the bulb were of essential importance for GnRH neuronal

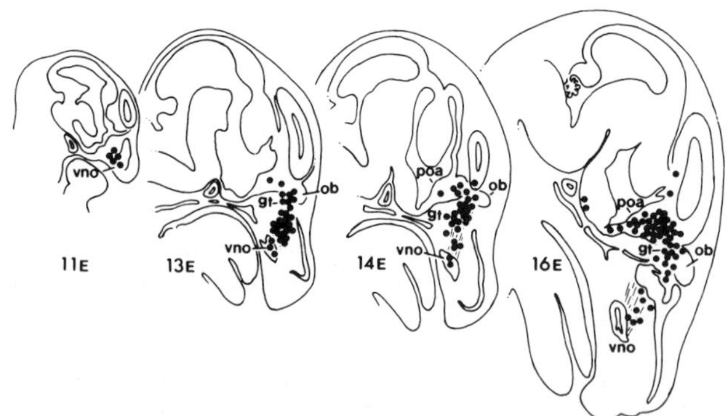

FIG. 154A-1 Migratory route of GnRH-immunoreactive neurons from derivatives of the medial olfactory placode to the forebrain is shown in microprojection drawings in the sagittal plane of 6-μm sections through the whole heads of fetal mice on embryonic (E) days 11, 13, 14, and 16. The black dots represent GnRH-immunoreactive neurons. On day 11, GnRH-immunoreactive cells are seen in the anlage of the vomeronasal organ and medial wall of the olfactory placode. On day 13, most of the GnRH cells are seen on the nasal septum, with the nervus terminalis and the vomeronasal nerves, and on day 14, most of these cells are in the ganglion terminale and in the central roots of the nervus terminalis. The 16-day-old fetal brain had most GnRH neurons arching through the forebrain into the hypothalamus and preoptic areas. gt = ganglion terminale; ob = olfactory bulb; poa = preoptic area; vno = vomeronasal organ. ***(From Schwanzel-Fukuda M, Pfaff D.[30] Used by permission of* Nature.*)***

migration. Therefore, the hypothesis was formulated that KS was due to a defect in a molecule involved in the migration of olfactory axons.[30]

The concept that migration of GnRH neurons depends on contact between olfactory axons and the olfactory bulb was substantiated by data obtained from the study of a 19-week-old human fetus with X-linked KS.[27] In this fetus, olfactory axons developed normally and started their migration toward the forebrain but arrested prematurely within the meninges, between the cribriform plate and the forebrain, ending in a tangle of nerve fibers and connective tissue. Immunohistochemical analysis, using human anti-GnRH antibodies, revealed that the majority of GnRH neurons were located at the dorsal surface of the cribriform plate, in the region where olfactory, terminalis, and vomeronasal nerves ended their migration. A similar analysis, performed in three age-matched normal fetuses, showed that all GnRH neurons had reached their final destination in the hypothalamus. This study supported the hypothesis (as did previous investigations) that the contact between olfactory axons and the olfactory bulb was an essential factor in GnRH neuronal migration.[27]

MRI studies have been performed in patients with KS.[32-36] This method provides accurate in vivo imaging of the neuroanatomical defect and appears, therefore, to be a very useful diagnostic tool.[36] Using MRI, aplasia or hypoplasia of olfactory sulci and of olfactory bulbs and tracts can be detected in all KS patients examined. Interestingly, one of these studies[34] demonstrated by MRI the presence of an abnormal mass of heterotopic soft tissue located between the upper nasal vault and the forebrain. This mass might represent the radiologic correlate of the dysplastic tangle of nerve fibers that Schwanzel-Fukuda et al. observed in a KS fetus.[27]

GENETICS

The incidence of KS has been estimated to be 1:10,000 in males and 1:50,000 in females.[37] Therefore, KS is the most common type of isolated gonadotropin deficiency. Autosomal dominant, autosomal recessive, and X-linked recessive inheritance patterns have been described, indicating the presence of genetic heterogeneity.[9,38] The five- to sixfold excess of male over female patients suggests that the X-linked form is the most frequent. Penetrance is not always complete in KS, and identical twins discordant for KS have been described.[39] Expressivity is also variable in KS, with both interfamilial and intrafamilial variability of the phenotype described by several groups.[9,38,40]

To date there are no genetic mapping data on the autosomally inherited forms of KS, although four patients with KS carrying chromosomal rearrangements have been identified: a balanced translocation involving chromosome breaks at 7q22 and 12q24,[41] an extra metacentric chromosome of unknown origin,[42] a balanced complex rearrangement involving chromosome breaks at 3q13, 9q13q21, and 12q15,[43] and a balanced translocation involving chromosomes 1 and 10 (Schinzel A: personal communication). These translocations may be causally associated with KS and, therefore, may pinpoint map locations of autosomal genes involved in KS.

Early reports can be found in which features of KS were described as part of complex X-linked syndromes.[10,44-49] A constant clinical feature in these cases was the presence of X-linked ichthyosis, a dermatologic condition characterized by dark scaly skin due to steroid sulfatase deficiency (see Chap. 96). Although most of these patients had both hypogonadotropic hypogonadism and anosmia, a diagnosis of KS was not made, perhaps due to the complexity of the observed phenotype. In some of these patients a translocation involving the distal short arm of the X chromosome (Xp22.3) and the long arm of the Y chromosome (Yq11) was detected.[47,48]

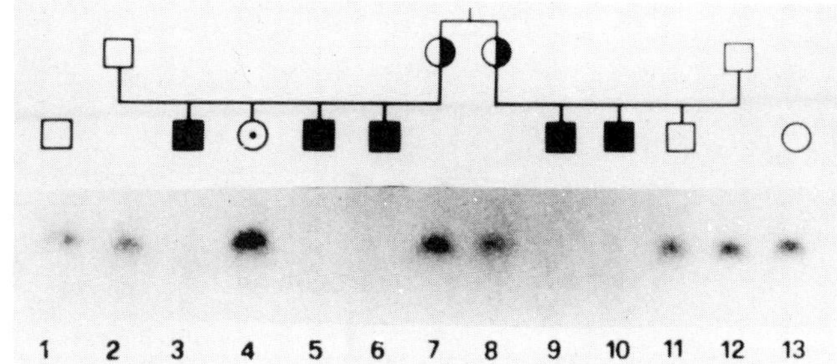

FIG. 154A-2 **Autoradiograph of a Southern blot and pedigree of a family with X-linked ichthyosis associated with Kallmann syndrome. The pedigree is mounted so that each lane is below the symbol identifying the individual whose DNA was run in that lane. The first and last lane contain male and female controls, respectively. The probe used was a steroid sulfatase cDNA clone.[51] A deletion of the steroid sulfatase gene is evident in the lanes corresponding to all affected individuals from this family.** *(From Ballabio et al.[52] Used by permission of* **Human Genetics.***)*

In 1986, the study of a family in which several affected males had hypogonadotropic hypogonadism, anosmia, and ichthyosis led to the hypothesis that these males were affected by a contiguous gene syndrome, in which a codeletion of adjacent KS and steroid sulfatase genes on the X chromosome resulted in simultaneous expression of KS and ichthyosis (see Fig. 20-9).[50] This led to the first tentative chromosomal assignment of the X-linked KS gene to the region of the steroid sulfatase gene in Xp22.3.[50] In keeping with this hypothesis, a deletion of the steroid sulfatase gene was subsequently demonstrated in the DNA of these patients by Southern blot analysis using a steroid sulfatase cDNA probe (Fig. 154A-2), which was previously isolated by the immunoscreening of a cDNA expression library.[51,52] The map assignment of the X-linked KS gene (KAL) to the Xp22.3 region was confirmed by linkage analysis in families with isolated KS.[53]

THE X-LINKED KALLMANN SYNDROME GENE (KAL)

Molecular characterization of patients with contiguous gene syndromes carrying deletions and translocations involving the Xp22.3 region permitted the construction of a deletion map of this region and the assignment of KAL to a specific interval within this map.[54] A candidate KAL gene was isolated from this interval by two independent groups using a positional cloning strategy.[55,56] Evidence that this gene was the KAL gene came from the molecular analysis of two brothers with KS carrying a small (3 kb) intragenic deletion, removing the C-terminal region of the predicted protein product (Fig. 154A-3).[57]

The KAL gene is expressed by both the active and the inactive X chromosomes[55]; it has a closely related nonfunctional homologue on the long arm of the Y chromosome (Yq11.2),[58,59] and it is highly conserved in many distantly related species except mice and hamsters.[60] All these features are not unique to KAL, since they are shared

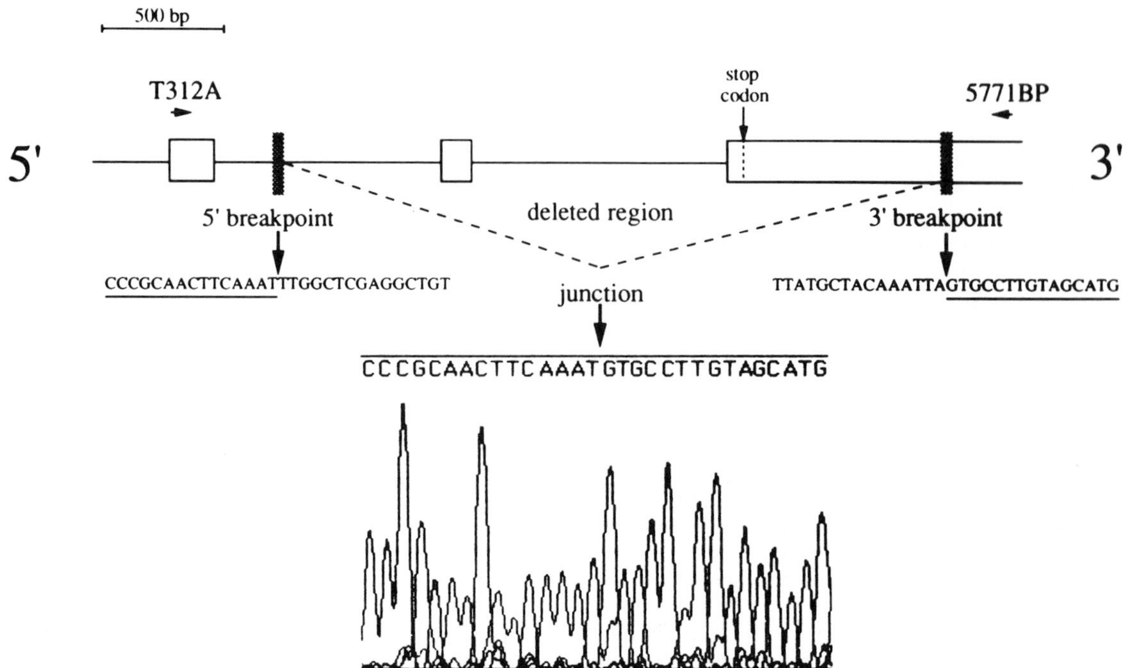

FIG. 154A-3 Schematic representation of the 3′ end of the KAL gene and of the genomic region involved in a deletion detected in a family with X-linked Kallmann syndrome.[57] The sizes of the exons (*open rectangles*) and of the introns (*solid lines*) were derived by both sequencing and restriction mapping. The position of the stop codon at the end of KAL open reading frame is indicated. The 5′ and 3′ boundaries of the deleted region are indicated by hatched bars. The positions of two oligonucleotide primers (T312A and 5771BP) used for PCR amplification of the patient's DNA are indicated at the top. The sequences of 5′ and the 3′ deletion breakpoints in normal DNA are shown under each position. The nucleotides retained in the DNA of patients 1 and 2 are underlined. The sequence chromatogram of the junction fragment is shown at the bottom. The arrows indicate the breakpoints. *(From Bick et al.[57] Used by permission of* New England Journal of Medicine.*)*

by most of the genes localized in Xp22.3 and may be the result of recent evolutionary changes undergone by the X chromosome.[58]

The KAL cDNA sequence analysis has provided insights into the pathogenesis of KS. The gene encodes a 680 amino acid protein that shares homologies with several molecules involved in neural development. These homologies are summarized in Table 154A-2. The N-terminal part of the protein contains a cysteine-rich domain, referred to as a "four-disulfide core" domain, which is found in a number of proteins such as protease inhibitors and neurophysins.[61] This finding is intriguing since proteases (e.g., plasminogen activator–like proteases) regulate adhesion of axons to specific components of the extracellular matrix, thus facilitating their elongation. Protease inhibitors may, therefore, modulate this interaction.[62–64]

The C-terminal two-thirds of KAL protein contains regions of significant similarity with the fibronectin (FN) type III repeat, first detected in fibronectin and also found in several neural-cell adhesion molecules[65] and in receptor-linked protein kinases and phosphatases.[66] Many of these molecules containing FN type III repeats have been implicated in neuronal migration and axonal growth and guidance.[67–70] The specific function of FN type III repeats in these molecules is not known.

KAL protein is clearly different from the other molecules containing the FN type III repeat since only part of this repeat sequence is present in KAL while all the other molecules contain the entire sequence (often repeated several times).[67] Furthermore, the association of a "four-disulfide core" domain with FN type III repeats seems to be unique to KAL. Features of the KAL protein, such as the presence of a leader peptide and the absence of transmembrane domains or of sequences indicative of a phosphoinositol linkage to the membrane, suggest that it may be secreted as an extracellular matrix protein. However, experimental evidence needs to be obtained for localization of the KAL protein in vivo.

MOLECULAR BASIS OF X-LINKED KALLMANN SYNDROME

A study of over 70 unrelated cases of isolated KS showed evidence of a deletion in KAL in only one family. While in some of the sporadic cases this likely reflects the fact that KS is genetically heterogeneous, deletions appear to be infrequent in X-linked KS.[57]

Mutation detection strategies have relied on a detailed characterization of the KAL gene structure. The KAL gene contains 14 exons spanning approximately 210 kb on Xp22.3.[58,59] The KAL homologue on the Y chromosome (KAL-Y) shares a very high degree of similarity with KAL but lacks exons 3, 8, and 9 and contains several stop and frameshift mutations (Fig. 154A-4). This high degree of X-Y sequence similarity is present also in intronic regions and is not limited to KAL but is shared also by a large genomic region in which both the steroid sulfatase and KAL genes are located. In one patient with KS it was demonstrated that abnormal pairing and exchange between the X and Y copies of KAL resulted in an X/Y translocation, which created a nonfunctional KAL X/Y fusion gene.[71]

The presence of a nonfunctional KAL homologue on the Y chromosome hampered mutation scanning strategies, since

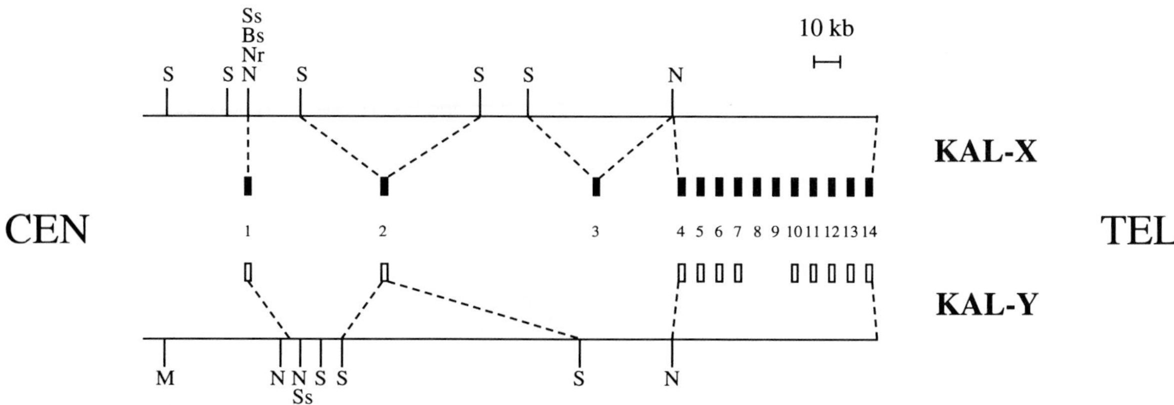

FIG. 154A-4 Genomic structure of KAL-X and KAL-Y.[58] The long-range restriction maps of the regions spanning KAL-X and KAL-Y were determined by PFGE on the YAC contigs. Restriction sites are as follows: Bs = *Bss*HII; M = *Mlu*I; N = *Not*I; Nr = *Nru*I; S = *Sal*I; Ss = *Sst*I. Each exon of KAL-X and KAL-Y was localized within these maps by Southern blot analysis. Exons from KAL-X and KAL-Y are indicated as solid and open boxes, respectively. Dashed lines indicate the restriction fragment to which each exon has been localized. Exons 3, 8, and 9 are missing from KAL-Y. *(From Incerti et al.[58] Used by permission of* Nature Genetics.*)*

most of them rely on the amplification of patients' genomic DNA. Therefore, primers and PCR conditions were carefully designed to minimize cross-amplification of Y-derived sequences[59] (and Meitinger T, et al.: personal communication). The results of mutation detection studies are summarized in Table 154A-3[12,13] (and Meitinger T, et al.: personal communication). A high degree of heterogeneity of mutations was found, with an identical mutation found only in two individuals. Several stop codon mutations were identified, probably representing null alleles and resulting in a complete loss of function of KAL protein. In some patients, missense and splice site mutations were identified in regions of putative functional importance (based on sequence homology data).[12] Some of the patients in whom point mutations were identified displayed, in addition to KS, mirror movements, pes cavus, high arched palate, and unilateral renal aplasia. This finding indicates that these additional features probably represent pleiotropic effects of KAL gene defects (see Table 154A-1) and suggests that KAL plays a role in various developmental systems.[12,13]

Based on these data, molecular diagnosis can now be offered to families with X-linked KS in which a specific mutation has been identified. In families in which the mutation has not yet been identified, male individuals can be tested for deletions by Southern blotting, using KAL cDNA as a probe before proceeding to sequence-based mutation detection. Patients with KS displaying complex phenotypes should undergo chromosome analysis, and their DNA should be tested with KAL and other Xp22.3 markers in order to detect a contiguous gene syndrome (see Chap. 20). There

Table 154A-2 Molecules Sharing Homology with KAL

4-Disulfide Core Domain	Fibronectin Type III Repeat
Protease inhibitors	Neural-cell adhesion molecules
Whey acidic protein	Axonal glycoprotein TAG-1
Elafin	Neural-cell adhesion molecule L1
Antileukoproteinase I	Neural-cell surface F3
ATPase inhibitor	Contactin
Neurophysin	Integrin β4 subunit
Chelonianin	Protein kinases
WDNM (cDNA from nonmetastatic mammary adenocarcinoma)	Twitchin
Na/K = ATPase inhibitor	Myosin-light-chain kinase
	ROS proto-oncogene tyrosine kinase
	Insulin receptor–related receptor eck
	Tyrosine phosphatases
	Leukocyte antigen-related protein
	Protein-tyrosine-phosphatase delta
	Protein-tyrosine-phosphatase DLAR (Drosophila leukocyte common antigen related)
	Protein-tyrosine-phosphatase DPTP (Drosophila protein tyrosine phosphatase)
	Others
	Fibronectin
	Adenylate cyclase
	C protein

Bibliography is available in references 55,56, and 79.

Table 154A-3 Mutations in the KAL Gene

Patient	Nucleotide Substitution	Amino Acid Change	Exon
1*	G → A	Trp 237 → Stop	5
2*†	C → T	Arg 257 → Stop	6
3*	G → A	Trp 258 → Stop	6
4†	G → A	Trp 258 → Stop	6
5*	C → T	Gln 421 → Stop	9
6*	C → T	Arg 423 → Stop	9
7†	C → T	Arg 262 → Stop	6
8*	T → A	Asn 267 → Lys	6
9†	A → G	Val 534 → Ile	11
10*	1 bp deletion (C)	Frameshift at 277	6
11*	1 bp insertion (A)	Frameshift at 339	7
12†	2 bp insertion (AG)	Frameshift at 433	9
13*	G → A	Splice mutation (acceptor site)	Intron 12

*Mutations reported by Hardelin et al.[12,13]
†T. Meitinger et al., personal communication.

has been one report of prenatal diagnosis of KS in a fetus with an Xp22.3 contiguous gene syndrome.[28]

KAL EXPRESSION STUDIES AND A PATHOGENETIC MODEL OF KALLMANN SYNDROME

The characterization of the KAL spatiotemporal expression pattern has provided important clues to the understanding of the molecular pathogenesis of Kallmann syndrome. KAL mRNA was detected at very low levels by RT-PCR analysis in some human adult tissues, including brain, muscle, kidney, liver, and intestine.[55,56] The chicken homologue of KAL (KAL_c) was isolated in order to study the developmental expression pattern of this gene.[60,72] The entire coding region of KAL_c was sequenced and compared to its human homologue.[60] The predicted protein product of KAL_c shows 77 percent amino acid identity with the human protein (84 percent when conservative substitutions are included); this value increases to over 90 percent in regions spanning the putative functional domains.[60]

RNA *in situ* hybridization studies were performed in chick embryos using KAL_c as a probe (Fig. 154A-5).[60,72] Neither the olfactory epithelium nor the meningeal tissue through which the olfactory axons migrate expresses the gene at any developmental stage. Within the olfactory system, KAL_c expression was first detected in the presumptive bulb region at day 7 of chick embryonal development. As the olfactory bulb acquires its characteristic structure, KAL_c expression increases and persists in adult chickens. In the bulb, the gene is expressed by the mitral cells, which are the secondary sensory neurons forming synapses with the olfactory axons. Up-regulation of transcription is seen when the first synaptic contacts between the olfactory axons and mitral cells are established.

Prominent expression was also found in the Purkinje cells of the cerebellum.[60,72] This pattern of expression could be related to the occurrence of cerebellar symptoms in KS patients. Multiple additional sites of KAL_c expression were detected, both within and outside the nervous system. In the brain, KAL_c mRNA was detected in the oculomotor nucleus primordium, ectostriatum, trigeminal motor nucleus, and choroid plexus. Other tissues expressing KAL_c include the developing limb buds, mesonephros and metanephros, facial mesenchyme, and retina.[60,72,73] Table 154A-4 shows a

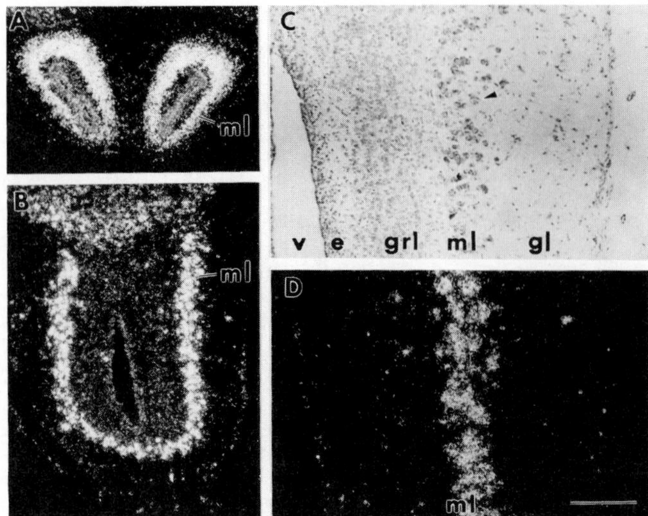

FIG. 154A-5 Expression of the chicken Kallmann syndrome gene (KAL_c) during the development of the olfactory system.[60] *A*. Transverse section through both olfactory bulbs of a $7\frac{1}{2}$ day-old chick embryo. *In situ* hybridization reveals high levels of KALc expression in the mitral cell layer. *B*. Transverse section through the olfactory bulb of a newly hatched chicken (21 days). *C*. Neighboring section of panel *B* stained with thionin. *D*. Enlarged view of panel *B*. The KAL_c-positive area in the olfactory bulb corresponds to the mitral-cell layer. *e* = ependymal layer; *gl* = glomerular layer; *grl* = granule-cell layer; *ml* = mitral-cell layer; *v* = lateral ventricle. Scale bar is equal to 100 μm for panels *C* and *D* and to 250 μM for panels *A* and *B*. *(From Rugarli et al.[60] Used by permission of* Nature Genetics.*)*

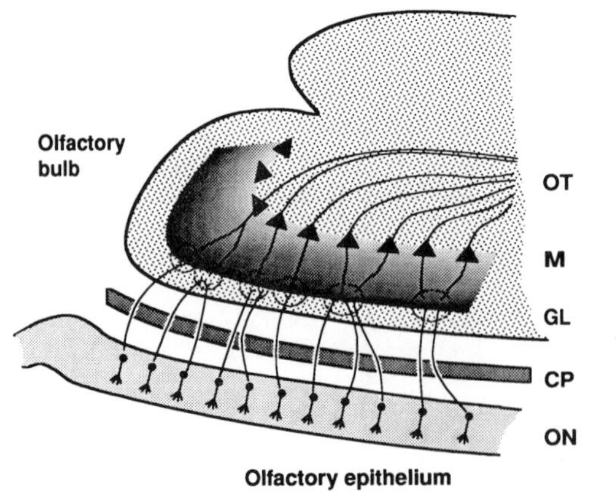

NORMAL

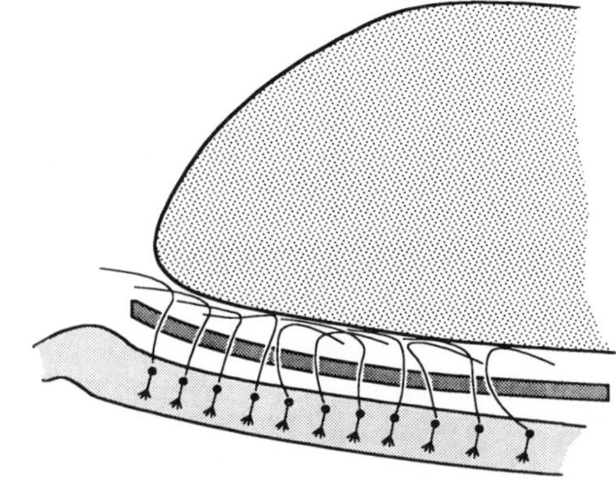

KALLMANN SYNDROME

FIG. 154A-6 Model for KAL function and KS pathogenesis. In normal individual axons of olfactory neurons (ON) traverse the cribriform plate (CP) to reach the olfactory bulb. Within the glomerular layer of the bulb (GL), they make synapses with dendrites of mitral cells (M), whose axons will form the olfactory tracts (OT). A tentative model is proposed in which the KAL protein (*shaded area*) is secreted by the mitral cells and is required in the glomerular layer for the establishment/maintenance of proper interactions with olfactory axons. In KS, KAL protein is absent; therefore, olfactory axons cannot interact properly with their target, ending their migration between the cribriform plate and the forebrain. The migration defect of GnRH neurons in KS would be a secondary effect caused by lack of contact between olfactory nerves and forebrain, resulting in the absence of a "migration route." *From Rugarli and Ballabio.[77] Used by permission of* JAMA.*)*

Table 154A-4 Tentative Correlation Between KAL Expression Pattern and Kallmann Syndrome Phenotype

Expression Pattern		Clinical Features
Olfactory bulb (mitral cells)	↔	Anosmia
Cerebellum (Purkinje cells)	↔	Cerebellar dysfunction
Oculomotor nucleus	↔	Eye-movement defects
Mesonephros/metanephros	↔	Unilateral renal aplasia
Facial mesenchyme	↔	Cleft palate

tentative correlation between some of the sites of KAL_c expression and KS symptoms. Although in some cases there is a clear relationship between the site of KAL expression and a symptom observed in KS, sometimes this correlation cannot be made. In these cases, the possibility of a different pattern of expression in human and chick, and of compensatory mechanisms preventing the appearance of a phenotype, should be considered.

KS was the first neuronal migration defect in vertebrates for which the gene has been identified. Two more examples of genes involved in human neuronal migration defects are the L1-CAM gene in X-linked hydrocephalus[74,75] and the lissencephaly/Miller-Dieker gene.[76] It is an intriguing observation that both X-linked hydrocephalus and X-linked KS are due to mutations in genes containing FN type III domains.

A tentative pathogenic model for KS is depicted in Fig. 154A-6. According to this model, the primary defect in KS is an abnormality of olfactory system development that affects axonal targeting and/or synaptogenesis, rather than neuronal migration directly. KAL protein may be a substrate adhesion molecule of the extracellular matrix mediating interactions between dendrites of mitral cells in the olfactory bulb and incoming olfactory axons. Since these interactions are essential for olfactory bulb morphogenesis, the absence of KAL prevents the bulb from acquiring its normal structure. The migration defect of GnRH neurons in KS would, therefore, be a secondary effect caused by lack of the "migration route" for GnRH neuronal migration that is normally provided by the contact between olfactory nerves and forebrain.[73,77] It is likely that several different molecules are involved in the establishment of proper interactions between olfactory axons and the olfactory bulb and in the migration process of GnRH neurons. For example, immunohistochemical data suggest that the neural-cell adhesion molecule NCAM has a role in the formation of a scaffold of cells and axons that link the olfactory epithelium with the forebrain.[78] The genes involved in the autosomal types of Kallmann syndrome may encode additional factors participating in this fascinating developmental system.

ACKNOWLEDGMENTS

We thank Drs. E. Rugarli, B. Lutz, and G. Eichele for helpful comments and for providing us with Fig. 154A-5.

REFERENCES

1. Maestre de San Juan A: Teratologia: Falta total de los nervios olfactorios con anosmian en un individuo en quien existia un atrofia congentia de los testiculos y miembro viril. *El Siglo Med* **3**:211, 1856.
2. de Morsier G: Etudes sur les dysraphies cranio-encephaliques. 1. Agenesie des lobes olfactifs (telencephaloschizis lateral) et des commissures calleuse et anterieure (telencephaloschizis median). La dysplasie olfacto-genitale. *Schweiz Arch Neurol Neurochir Psychiatr* **74**:309, 1954.
3. de Morsier G: Median cranioencephalic dysraphias and olfactogenital dysplasia. *World Neurol* **3**:485, 1962.
4. Kallmann F, Schoenfeld WA, Barrera SE: The genetic aspects of primary eunuchoidism. *Am J Ment Defic* **48**:203, 1944.
5. Naftolin F, Harris GW, Bobrow M: Effect of purified luteinizing hormone releasing factor on normal and hypogonadotropic anosmic men. *Nature* **232**:496, 1971.
6. Griffin JE, Wilson JD: Disorders of the testes and the male reproductive tract, in Wilson JD, Foster DW (eds): *Williams Textbook of Endocrinology,* 8th ed. Philadelphia, Saunders, 1992, p 822.
7. Turner RC, Bobrow LG, MacKinnon PCB, Bonnar J, Hockaday TDR, Ellis JD: Cryptorchidism in a family with Kallmann's syndrome. *Proc R Soc Med* **67**:33, 1974.
8. Wegenke JD, Uehling DT, Wear JB Jr, Gordon ES, Bargman JG, Deacon JSR, Herrmann JPR, Opitz JM: Familial Kallmann syndrome with unilateral renal aplasia. *Clin Genet* **7**:368, 1976.
9. White BJ, Rogol AD, Brown SK, Lieblich JM, Rosen WS: The syndrome of anosmia with hypogonadotropic hypogonadism: A genetic study of 18 new families and a review. *Am J Med Genet* **15**:417, 1983.
10. Sunohara N, Sakuragawa N, Satoyoshi E, Tanae A, Shapiro LJ: A new syndrome of anosmia, ichthyosis, hypogonadism and various neurological manifestations with deficiency of steroid sulfatase and arylsulfatase C. *Ann Neurol* **19**:174, 1986.
11. Schwankhaus JD, Currie J, Jaffe MJ, Rose SR, Sherins RJ: Neurologic findings in men with isolated hypogonadotropic hypogonadism. *Neurology* **39**:223, 1989.
12. Hardelin J-P, Levilliers J, del Castillo I, Cohen-Salmon M, Legouis R, Blanchard S, Compain S, Bouloux P, Kirk J, Moraine C, Chaussain J-L, Weissenbach J, Petit C: X chromosome-linked Kallmann syndrome: Stop mutations validate the candidate gene. *Proc Natl Acad Sci USA* **89**:8190, 1992.
13. Hardelin J-P, Levilliers J, Blanchard S, Carel J-C, Leutenegger M, Pinard-Bertelletto J-P, Bouloux P, Petit C: Heterogeneity in the mutations responsible for X chromosome-linked Kallmann syndrome. *Hum Mol Genet* **2**:373, 1993.
14. Nass R: Mirror movement asymmetries in congenital hemiparesis: The inhibition hypothesis revisited. *Neurology* **35**:1059, 1985.
15. Danek A, Heye B, Schroedter R: Cortically evoked motor responses in patients with Xp22.3-linked Kallmann's syndrome and in female gene carriers. *Ann Neurol* **31**:299, 1992.
16. Kertzman C, Robinson DL, Sherins RJ, Schwankhaus JD, McClurkin JW: Abnormalities in visual spacial attention in men with mirror movements associated with isolated hypogonadotropic hypogonadism. *Neurology* **40**:1057, 1990.
17. Tuck RR, O'Neill BP, Gharib H, Mulder DW: Familial spastic paraplegia with Kallmann's syndrome. *J Neurol Neurosurg Psychiatry* **46**:671, 1983.
18. Cortez AB, Galindo A, Arensman FW, Van Dop C: Congenital heart disease associated with sporadic Kallmann syndrome. *Am J Med Genet* **46**:551, 1993.
19. Ballabio A, Andria G: Deletions and translocations involving the distal short arm of the human X chromosome: Review and hypotheses. *Hum Mol Genet* **1**:221, 1992.
20. Henkin RI, Bartter FC: Studies on olfactory thresholds in normal man and in patients with adrenal cortical insufficiency: The role of adrenal cortical steroids and of serum sodium concentration. *J Clin Invest* **45**:1631, 1966.
21. *The Smell Identification Test Administration Manual.* Haddonfield, NJ, Sensonics, 1983.
22. Spratt DI, Carr DB, Merriam GR, Scully RE, Rao PN, Crowley WF Jr: The spectrum of abnormal patterns of gonadotropin-releasing hormone secretion in men and idiopathic hypogonadotropic hypogonadism: Clinical and laboratory correlations. *J Clin Endocrinol Metab* **64**:283, 1987.
23. Giusti M, Cavagnaro P: Update on pulsatile luteinizing hormone-releasing hormone therapy in males with idiopathic hypogonadotropic hypogonadism and delayed puberty. *J Endocrinol Invest* **14**:419, 1991.

24. Saal W, Happ J, Cordes U, Baum RP, Schmidt M: Subcutaneous gonadotropin therapy in male patients with hypogonadotropic hypogonadism. *Fertil Steril* **56**:319, 1991.
25. Hurley DM, Clarke IJ, Shelton R, Burger HG: Subcutaneous administration of gonadotropin-releasing hormone: Absorption kinetics and gonadotropin responses. *J Clin Endocrinol Metab* **65**:46, 1987.
26. Males JL, Townsend JL, Schneider RA: Hypogonadotropic hypogonadism with anosmia—Kallmann's syndrome. *Arch Intern Med* **131**:501, 1973.
27. Schwanzel-Fukuda M, Bick D, Pfaff DW: Luteinizing hormone-releasing hormone (LHRH)-expressing cells do not migrate normally in an inherited hypogonadal (Kallmann) syndrome. *Mol Brain Res* **6**:311, 1989.
28. Bick DP, Schorderet DF, Price PA, Campbell L, Huff RW, Shapiro LJ, Moore CM: Prenatal diagnosis and investigation of a fetus with chondrodysplasia punctata, ichthyosis, and Kallmann syndrome due to an Xp deletion.*Prenat Diagn* **12**:19, 1992.
29. Schwob JE, Leopold DA, Mieleszko-Szumowsi KE, Emko P: Histopathology of olfactory mucosa in Kallmann's syndrome. *Ann Otol Rhinol Laryngol* **102**:117, 1993.
30. Schwanzel-Fukuda M, Pfaff DW: Origin of luteinizing hormone-releasing hormone neurons. *Nature* **338**:161, 1989.
31. Wray S, Grant P, Gainer H: Evidence that cells expressing luteinizing hormone-releasing hormone mRNA in the mouse are derived from progenitor cells in the olfactory placode. *Proc Natl Acad Sci USA* **86**:8132, 1989.
32. Klingmüller D, Dewes W, Krahe T, Brecht G, Schweikert H-U: Magnetic resonance imaging of the brain in patients with anosmia and hypothalamic hypogonadism (Kallmann's syndrome). *J Clin Endocrinol Metab* **65**:581, 1987.
33. Knorr JR, Ragland RL, Brown RS, Gelber N: Kallmann's syndrome: MR findings. *Am J Neuroradiol* **14**:845, 1993.
34. Truwit CL, Barkovich AJ, Grumbach MM, Martini JJ: MR imaging of Kallmann syndrome, a genetic disorder of neuronal migration affecting the olfactory and genital systems. *Am J Neuroradiol* **14**:827, 1993.
35. Yousem DM, Turner WJD, Li C, Snyder PJ, Doty RL: Kallmann's syndrome: MR evaluation of olfactory system. *Am J Neuroradiol* **14**:839, 1993.
36. Bick DP, Ballabio A: Bringing Kallmann syndrome into focus. *Am J Neuroradiol* **14**:852, 1993.
37. Jones J, Kemman E: Olfacto-genital dysplasia in the female. *Obstet Gynecol Annu* **5**:443, 1976.
38. Hermanussen M, Sippell WG: Heterogeneity of Kallmann's syndrome. *Clin Genet* **28**:106, 1985.
39. Hipkin LJ, Casson IF, Davis JC: Identical twins discordant for Kallmann's syndrome. *J Med Genet* **27**:198, 1990.
40. Parenti G, Carrozzo R, Ghezzi M, Di Maio S, Ballabio A, Andria G: Molecular studies on the clinical heterogeneity in a family with X-linked ichthyosis and Kallmann syndrome. *Am J Hum Genet (suppl)* **49**:155, 1991.
41. Best LG, Wasdahl WA, Larson LM, Sturlaugson J: Chromosome abnormality in Kallmann syndrome. *Am J Med Genet* **35**:306, 1990.
42. Ventruto V, Cali A, Farina L, Festa B, Ricciardi I, Sebastio L: A case of hypogonadotrophic hypogonadism with anosmia (Kallmann's syndrome) in a male, with familial incidence of a small metacentric chromosome (47, XY, mat?+). *J Med Genet* **13**:71, 1976.
43. Casamassima AC, Wilmot PL, Vibert BK, Shapiro LR: Kallmann syndrome associated with complex chromosome rearrangement. *Am J Med Genet* **45**:539, 1993.
44. Lynch HT, Ozer F, McNutt CW, Johnson JE, Jampolsky NA: Secondary male hypogonadism and congenital ichthyosis: Association of two rare genetic diseases. *Am J Hum Genet* **12**:440, 1960.
45. Perrin JCS, Idemoto JY, Sotos JF, Maurer WF, Steinberg AG: X-linked syndrome of congenital ichthyosis, hypogonadism, mental retardation and anosmia. *Birth Defects* **12**:267, 1976.
46. Abe K, Matsuda I, Matsuura N, Murayama T, Uzuki K, Endo M, Miyakoshi M, Okuno A: X-linked ichthyosis, bilateral cryptorchidism, hypogenitalism and mental retardation in two siblings. *Clin Genet* **9**:341, 1976.
47. Tiepolo L, Zuffardi O, Fraccaro M, di Natale D, Gargantini L, Muller CR, Ropers H-H: Assignment by deletion mapping of the steroid sulfatase X-linked ichthyosis locus to Xp22.3. *Hum Genet* **54**:205, 1980.
48. Metaxotou C, Ikkos D, Panagiotopoulou P, Alevizaki M, Mavrou A, Tsenghi C, Matsaniotis N: A familial X/Y translocation in a boy with ichthyosis, hypogonadism and mental retardation. *Clin Genet* **24**:380, 1983.
49. Andria G, Ballabio A, Parenti G, Di Maio S, Piccirillo A: Steroid sulphatase deficiency is present in patients with the syndrome "Ichthyosis and male hypogonadism" and with "Rud syndrome." *J Inherit Metab Dis* **7**:159, 1984.
50. Ballabio A, Parenti G, Tippett P, Mondello C, Di Maio S, Tenore A, Andria G: X-linked ichthyosis due to steroid sulphatase deficiency associated with Kallmann syndrome (hypogonadotropic hypogonadism and anosmia): Linkage relationships with Xg and cloned DNA sequences from the distal short arm of the X chromosome. *Hum Genet* **72**:237, 1986.
51. Ballabio A, Parenti G, Carrozzo R, Sebastio G, Andria G, Buckle V, Fraser N, Boyd Y, Craig I, Rocchi M, Romeo G, Jobsis AC, Persico MG: Isolation and characterization of a steroid sulphatase cDNA clone: Genomic deletions in patients with X-linked ichthyosis. *Proc Natl Acad Sci USA* **13**:4519, 1987.
52. Ballabio A, Sebastio G, Carrozzo R, Parenti G, Piccirillo A, Persico MG, Andria G: Deletions of the steroid sulphatase gene in "classical" X-linked ichthyosis and in X-linked ichthyosis associated with Kallmann syndrome. *Hum Genet* **77**:338, 1987.
53. Meitinger T, Heye B, Petit C, Levilliers J, Golla A, Moraine C, Dallapiccola B, Sippell WG, Murken J, Ballabio A: Definitive localization of X-linked Kallman syndrome (hypogonadotropic hypogonadism and anosmia) to Xp22.3: Close linkage to the hypervariable repeat sequence CRI-S232. *Am J Hum Genet* **47**:664, 1990.
54. Ballabio A, Bardoni B, Carrozzo R, Andria G, Bick D, Campbell L, Hamel B, Ferguson-Smith MA, Gimelli G, Fraccaro M, Maraschio P, Zuffardi O, Guioli S, Camerino G: Contiguous gene syndromes due to deletions in the distal short arm of the human X chromosome. *Proc Natl Acad Sci USA* **86**:10001, 1989.
55. Franco B, Guioli S, Pragliola A, Incerti B, Bardoni B, Tonlorenzi R, Carrozzo R, Maestrini E, Pieretti M, Taillon-Miller P, Brown CJ, Willard HF, Lawrence C, Persico MG, Camerino G, Ballabio A: A gene deleted in Kallmann's syndrome shares homology with neural cell adhesion and axonal path-finding molecules. *Nature* **353**:529, 1991.
56. Legouis R, Hardelin J-P, Levilliers J, Claverie J-M, Compain S, Wunderle V, Millasseau P, Le Paslier D, Cohen D, Caterina D, Bougueleret L, Delemarre-Van de Waal H, Lutfalla G, Weissenbach J, Petit C: The candidate gene for the X-linked Kallmann syndrome encodes a protein related to adhesion molecules. *Cell* **67**:423, 1991.
57. Bick D, Franco B, Sherins RJ, Heye B, Pike L, Crawford J, Maddalena A, Incerti B, Pragliola A, Meitinger T, Ballabio A: Intragenic deletion of the *KALIG-1* gene in Kallmann's syndrome. *N Engl J Med* **326**:1752, 1992.
58. Incerti B, Guioli S, Pragliola A, Zanaria E, Borsani G, Tonlorenzi R, Bardoni B, Franco B, Wheeler D, Ballabio A, Camerino G: Kallmann syndrome gene on the X and Y chromosomes: Implications for evolutionary divergence of human sex chromosomes. *Nature Genet* **2**:311, 1992.
59. del Castillo I, Cohen-Salmon M, Blanchard S, Lutfalla G, Petit C: Structure of the X-linked Kallmann syndrome gene and its homologous pseudogene on the Y chromosome. *Nat Genet* **2**:305, 1992.
60. Rugarli EI, Lutz B, Kuratani SC, Wawersik S, Borsani G, Ballabio A, Eichele G: Expression pattern of the Kallmann syndrome gene in the olfactory system suggests a role in neuronal targeting. *Nat Genet* **4**:19, 1993.
61. Drenth J, Low BM, Richardson JS, Wright CS: The toxin-agglutinin fold. *J Biol Chem* **255**:2652, 1980.
62. McGuire PG, Seeds NW: Degradation of underlying extracellular matrix by sensory neurons during neurite outgrowth. *Neuron* **4**:633, 1990.
63. Monard D: Cell-derived proteases and protease inhibitors as regulators of neurite outgrowth. *Trends Neurosci* **11**:541, 1988.

64. Letourneau PC, Condic ML, Snow DM: Extracellular matrix and neurite outgrowth. *Curr Opin Genet Dev* **2**:625, 1992.
65. Lander AD: Understanding the molecules of neural cell contacts: Emerging patterns of structure and function. *Trends Neurosci* **12**:189, 1989.
66. Fischer EH, Charbonneau H, Tonks NK: Protein tyrosine phosphatases: A diverse family of intracellular and transmembrane enzymes. *Science* **253**:401, 1991.
67. Dodd J, Jessell TM: Axon guidance and the patterning of neuronal projections in vertebrates. *Science* **242**:692, 1988.
68. Reichardt LF, Tomaselli KJ: Extracellular matrix molecules and their receptors: Functions in neural development. *Annu Rev Neurosci* **14**:531, 1991.
69. Chiquet M, Wehrle-Haller B, Koch M: Tenascin (cytotactin): An extracellular matrix protein involved in morphogenesis of the nervous system. *Semin Neurosci* **3**:341, 1991.
70. Hynes RO, Lander AD: Contact and adhesive specificities in the associations, migrations, and targeting of cells and axons. *Cell* **68**:303, 1992.
71. Guioli S, Incerti B, Zanaria E, Bardoni B, Franco B, Taylor K, Ballabio A, Camerino G: Kallmann syndrome due to a translocation resulting in an X/Y fusion gene. *Nat Genet* **1**:337, 1992.
72. Legouis R, Ayer-Le Lievre C, Leibovici M, Lapointe F, Petit C: Expression of the KAL gene in multiple neuronal sites during chicken development. *Proc Natl Acad Sci USA* **90**:2461, 1993.
73. Lutz B, Rugarli EI, Eichele G, Ballabio A: X-linked Kallmann syndrome: A neuronal targeting defect in the olfactory system? *FEBS Lett* **325**:128, 1993.
74. Rosenthal A, Jouet M, Kenwrick S: Aberrant splicing of neural cell adhesion molecule L1 mRNA in a family with X-linked hydrocephalus. *Nat Genet* **2**:107, 1992.
75. Van Camp G, Vits L, Coucke P, Lyonnet S, Schrander-Stumpel C, Darby J, Holden J, Munnich A, Willems PJ: A duplication in the *L1CAM* gene associated with X-linked hydrocephalus. *Nat Genet* **4**:421, 1993.
76. Reiner O, Carrozzo R, Shen Y, Wehnert M, Faustinella F, Dobyns WB, Caskey CT, Ledbetter DH: Isolation of a Miller-Dieker lissencephaly gene containing G protein β-subunit-like repeats. *Nature* **364**:717, 1993.
77. Rugarli EI, Ballabio A: Kallmann syndrome: From genetics to neurobiology. *JAMA* **270**:2713, 1993.
78. Schwanzel-Fukuda M, Abraham S, Crossin KL, Edelman GM, Pfaff DW: Immunocytochemical demonstration of neural cell adhesion molecule (NCAM) along the migration route of luteinizing hormone-releasing hormone (LHRH) neurons in mice. *J Comp Neurol* **321**:1, 1992.
79. Ballabio A, Camerino G: A gene for the human neuronal migration defect Kallmann syndrome. *Curr Opin Genet Dev* **2**:417, 1992.

CHAPTER **154B**

Spinocerebellar Ataxia Type 1

Huda Y. Zoghbi ▪ Andrea Ballabio

1. **Spinocerebellar ataxia type 1 (SCA1) is an autosomal dominant disorder characterized by progressive ataxia, dysarthria, amyotrophy, and bulbar dysfunction. The onset of symptoms is typically in the third or fourth decade, although juvenile-onset cases with more rapid progression of the disease have been reported in the most recent generations of some families, suggesting the presence of anticipation.**

2. **Linkage studies localized the SCA1 gene to the short arm of human chromosome 6 (6p). A combination of detailed genetic and physical mapping studies assigned the gene to a critical region on 6p spanning 1.2 Mb of DNA. Since anticipation has been observed in other neurologic disorders shown to be caused by the expansion of trinucleotide repeats, the candidate region for SCA1 was searched for such repeats. This led to the identification of an expressed, highly polymorphic trinucleotide repeat that was found to be expanded and unstable in SCA1 individuals. Normal alleles range in size from 19 to 36 repeats, while SCA1 alleles contain from 42 to 81 repeats. A direct correlation between the size of the expanded repeat and the age of onset of SCA1 was demonstrated, with larger alleles occurring in juvenile cases.**

3. **Sequence analysis of the CAG repeat revealed an interrupted repeat configuration in 98 percent of the unexpanded alleles, whereas 100 percent of the expanded alleles revealed an uninterrupted $(CAG)_n$ configuration. Analysis of the SCA1 CAG repeat can be used for the identification of SCA1 families and for genetic counseling.**

4. **The SCA1 transcript is approximately 10 kb and has a wide tissue expression pattern. The SCA1 gene encodes an 816 amino acid protein, ataxin-1, with no detectable sequence homology to previously identified molecules. The CAG repeat resides within the coding region at amino acid 196.**

5. **Given that the mutational mechanism in four late-onset neurodegenerative disorders (spinobulbar muscular atrophy, Huntington disease, SCA1, and dentatorubral and pallidoluysian atrophy) involves the expansion of a polyglutamine tract, it is possible that the pathogenetic mechanism is similar in all these disorders and possibly in other late-onset neurodegenerative disorders.**

A list of standard abbreviations is located immediately preceding the index in each volume. Additional abbreviations used in this chapter include: DM = gene symbol for myotonic dystrophy; DRPLA = dentatorubral and pallidoluysian atrophy; FRAXA = gene for common form of fragile X syndrome; GDH = glutamate dehydrogenase; HD = Huntington disease; SBMA = spinobulbar muscular atrophy; SCA = spinocerebellar ataxia, including SCA1, SCA2, etc.

CLINICAL FEATURES, DIFFERENTIAL DIAGNOSIS, AND BIOCHEMICAL STUDIES

The inherited spinocerebellar ataxias (SCA) are a heterogeneous group of neurologic disorders characterized by variable degrees of degeneration of the cerebellum, spinal tracts, and brain stem.[1,2] The first report of an inherited ataxia was that by Friedreich in 1863.[3] In 1893, Marie[4] reported a hereditary ataxia distinct from that described by Friedreich. This clinical entity, then referred to as "Marie's ataxia" was characterized by late onset of symptoms, increased deep tendon reflexes, and an autosomal dominant pattern of inheritance. Holmes indicated that the cases described by Marie were clinically and pathologically heterogenous.[5] Since then several studies attempting to classify the dominantly inherited SCA have been published (for review see Harding[6] and Zoghbi[7]). Most of these classifications were based on clinical and pathological findings that rendered them unsatisfactory given the interfamilial and intrafamilial variability of clinicopathological findings. Indeed there were instances in which patients from the same kindred were classified into two or more distinct types of SCA.[8] This demonstrated the pitfalls of classifying the SCA based on limited clinical and pathological findings and emphasized the need to adopt a classification scheme that relies on the mapping and identification of the relevant SCA genes.

The first subtype of SCA to be identified based on genetic mapping data was SCA type 1 (SCA1), which maps to the short arm of chromosome 6 (see below). Identification of families with SCA1 permitted analysis and documentation of the clinical features seen in this subtype of hereditary ataxia.

In retrospect, the first clinical description of a kindred later shown to have SCA1 was the one published by Gray and Oliver in 1941.[9] The authors documented an autosomal dominant mode of inheritance and provided a detailed clinical description of the disorder. In 1950, J. W. Schut reported the results of detailed clinical studies on the same kindred.[10] He differentiated between four clinical forms of the disease on the basis of the degree of incoordination and the activity of the deep tendon reflexes. In a more recent report, L.J. Schut[11] reported his findings after a 25-year follow-up of over 25 affected members from the same family, which is now referred to as the Minnesota (MN-SCA1) kindred. Many of the patients were examined prior to the onset of symptoms and were followed for the duration of illness until death. Over the past 20 years detailed clinical descriptions of several SCA1 kindreds have been published.[12–17] From reviewing the reported clinical features the following observations can be made: extensive interfamilial and intrafamilial variability occurs, and all affected individuals from all the reported families suffered from ataxia, dysarthria, and eventually bulbar dysfunction.

In the early stages of the disease, patients with SCA1 report slight gait and limb incoordination, slurred speech, and deteriorating handwriting. In the family described by Schut[11] a cough, which seems to represent a throat-clearing attempt, often precedes the onset of the disease. Neurologic findings in the early stages include gait ataxia, dysarthria, hypermetric saccades, and nystagmus. As the disease progresses, hyperreflexia may be detected, the ataxia worsens, and other cerebellar signs such as dysmetria, dysdiadochokinesis, hypotonia, and the rebound phenomenon become apparent. Optic nerve atrophy and variable degrees of ophthalmoparesis may be detected in some patients. Amyotrophy, decreased or absent deep tendon reflexes, and loss of proprioception or vibration sense may occur in the middle or late stages of the disease. Mild cognitive dysfunction, manifested as emotional lability, decreased attention and abstractional abilities, and reduction in recent and remote memory, has been documented in some members of SCA1 families.[18] The degree of cognitive impairment correlated with the severity of disease but did not interfere with daily functions. Extrapyramidal signs, including dystonic posturing and choreiform movements, have been observed in the later stages of the disease in some individuals. In the final stage of the disease, brain-stem involvement results in facial weakness and bulbar signs, including tongue atrophy and fasciculations, severe dysarthria, and dysphagia. Frequent choking spells develop, as well as loss of the ability to cough effectively; the patients eventually die from aspiration and pneumonia. A summary of the clinical features is provided in Table 154B-1. The typical age of onset for SCA1 is in the third or fourth decade, but early onset in the first decade has been documented in two large families from Texas and Minnesota, referred to as the TX-SCA1 and MN-SCA1 kindreds, respectively.[10,14] An increase in the severity of the phenotype in later generations, a phenomenon known as "anticipation," has been observed in at least two large SCA1 kindreds.[10,14] The disease typically progresses over 10 to 15 years, but a more rapidly progressive course has been described in juvenile-onset cases.[14]

The clinical features observed in SCA1 families are not unique to this type of ataxia and have been observed in patients known to have a genetically distinct form of SCA such as type 2 spinocerebellar ataxia (SCA2), which maps to chromosome 12q23-q24,[19] or Machado-Joseph disease (MJD), which maps to chromosome 14q24.3-q32[20] (Table 154B-2). Furthermore, these clinical features are observed in several dominantly inherited SCA families that do not map to any of the three known loci on 6p, 12q, or 14q.[21,21a]

Table 154B-1 Clinical Features of SCA1

Established disease
- Ataxia
- Dysarthria
- Nystagmus and restricted gaze
- Hyperreflexia
- Vibration and proprioceptive loss

Advanced disease
- Severe ataxia and dysarthria
- Gaze palsy
- Amyotrophy and areflexia
- Vibration and proprioceptive loss
- Dysphagia, tongue atrophy, and fasciculations
- Dystonia and choreiform movements

Table 154B-2 Genetic Classification of Dominantly Inherited Ataxias

Type	Chromosome
SCA1	6p22–p23
SCA2	12q23–q24.1
MJD	14q24.3–q31
SCA3	?

Biochemical studies aimed at detecting a metabolic defect in SCA1 have not identified any specific abnormality. Such studies included measurement of glutamate dehydrogenase (GDH) activity in leukocytes, muscle, and brain[22–25] and measurements of amino acids and neurotransmitters in postmortem brains of SCA patients, including some with SCA1.[26–28] Although reductions of GDH activity have been observed in recessively and dominantly inherited SCA,[23,24] normal brain GDH activity has been reported in four patients with SCA1.[25] This, combined with additional studies of GDH activity in patients with other neurodegenerative disorders, has led to the conclusion that reduced GDH activity is not a specific finding, nor is it involved in the pathogenesis of SCA1 or other types of hereditary ataxia.[29,30] Decreased levels of aspartate, glutamate, and GABA in the cerebellar cortex and dentate nucleus have been observed in postmortem brains from SCA1 patients.[27,28] However, given that similar reductions were documented in other types of SCA, it is likely that these changes are secondary to the neuronal loss seen in this group of disorders. Lastly, reductions in the activities of choline acetyltransferase and acetylcholine esterase have been demonstrated in postmortem brains of SCA1 patients[31,32] and were similar to those observed in brains of patients with Alzheimer disease. The significance of this finding is unknown.

Given that the pathophysiology and biochemistry underlying the SCA1 symptomatology is not yet understood, there is no effective treatment for the cerebellar tremor or ataxia. Several trials using precursors of serotonin or acetylcholine, anticholinergic drugs, or GABA receptor agonists did not demonstrate therapeutic efficacy of any of these drugs.[33] Accordingly, the only treatment available to SCA1 patients is supportive physical therapy aimed at reducing spasticity.

NEUROIMAGING AND NEUROPATHOLOGICAL STUDIES

Neuroimaging studies have been carried out on some members of known SCA1 kindreds.[11,16] Both CT and MRI scans revealed atrophy of the brachia pontis and anterior lobe of the cerebellum and enlargement of the fourth ventricle. In advanced disease, severe atrophy of the pons, enlargement of the third ventricle, and mild cerebral atrophy were noted. Such findings are similar to those observed in other dominantly inherited ataxias and hence are not helpful in establishing a diagnosis.

Detailed postmortem examination has been carried out on some members of five different SCA1 kindreds. Schut and Haymaker[34] reported their findings on five cases from the MN-SCA1 kindred. They showed that the disease affects many areas within the nervous system. The cerebellum was reduced in size, with definite loss of Purkinje cells and dentate nucleus neurons. Severe neuronal degeneration in the inferior olive and cranial nerve nuclei IX, X, and XII was noted in all cases. Demyelination was found in the restiform body and brachium conjunctivum, dorsal and ventral spinocerebellar tracts, and to a lesser degree in the posterior columns; variable degeneration of the anterior horn cells in the spinal cord also occurred. Similar but variable findings have been reported in studies of other SCA1 families.[12,13,35] Spadaro et al.[16] examined the brain and the spinal cord from a 32-year-old female who died 12 years after the onset of SCA1. Their findings were similar to those previously reported, but in addition severe neuronal loss in cranial nerve nuclei III and IV and severe demyelination of the posterior columns were noted, in addition to the typical demyelination of the spinocerebellar tracts.

D. Amstrong (unpublished data, Baylor College of Medicine) performed detailed neuropathological examination on the brain from the youngest known genetically proven SCA1 patient. This patient, a member of the TX-SCA1 kindred, became symptomatic at 4 years of age and died at 10 years of age after a rapidly progressive course. Gross examination revealed mild to moderate cerebellar atrophy and a normal-appearing cerebral cortex and basal ganglia. Microscopic examination of the cerebellum was remarkable for focal loss of Purkinje cells and internal granular cells. Eosinophilic spheres ("torpedoes") were identified in the internal granular layer and some were related to Purkinje-cell bodies (Fig. 154B-1). Gliosis and neuronal loss were noted in the fastigial nucleus of the cerebellum and in the nuclei for cranial nerves III, X, and XII. The most dramatic change was in the inferior olive, where there were almost no neurons and there was severe gliosis. Other findings included mild gliosis in the anterior horn cells of the spinal cord, mild demyelination of the spinocerebellar tracts, and marked demyelination of the dorsal columns.

Based on the above studies, it is clear that there is both interfamilial and intrafamilial variability with respect to the involvement of certain cranial nerve nuclei and the degree of demyelination in the dorsal columns. It is interesting that the most dramatic findings in the above-described patient with juvenile-onset SCA1 involved the inferior olive, cranial nerves, and dorsal columns. This is consistent with her rapidly deteriorating clinical picture, which was dominated by bulbar dysfunction, severe deep sensation loss, and minimal ataxia.

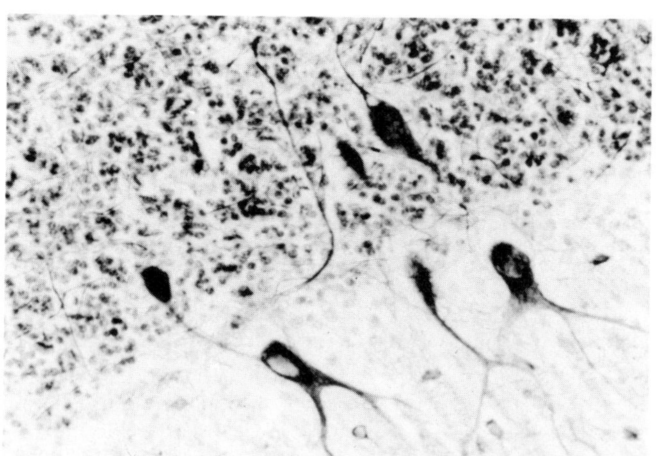

FIG. 154B-1 **Section of the cerebellum stained with Seivier Munger preparation from the brain of a 10-year-old SCA1 patient who died after 6 years of symptoms. Three Purkinje cells are in a state of degeneration, with their axons showing "torpedos" in the internal granular cell layer.** ***(Courtesy of Dr. D. Armstrong, Baylor College of Medicine.)***

GENETIC AND PHYSICAL MAPPING OF THE SCA1 LOCUS

In 1974, Yakura and colleagues suggested that an ataxia gene locus might map to the short arm of chromosome 6 based on an association of a particular HLA haplotype with disease in a sibship of five individuals with a dominantly inherited SCA.[36] In 1977, Jackson and coworkers[37] performed HLA typing and linkage analysis on 19 members from the SCA kindred previously described by Currier et al.[12] Their analysis confirmed the presence of an SCA locus near the HLA loci on chromosome 6.[37] Since then, more than 22 studies on linkage between SCA and HLA have been reported; six of these studies provided evidence for linkage to HLA in the evaluated kindreds.[13,14,17,38–40] These studies confirmed that at least one type of SCA maps to chromosome 6; the disease locus for this type was designated SCA1 in 1985.[41]

In 1990, Litt and Luty identified D6S89, a highly polymorphic DNA marker of the dinucleotide repeat type, and showed that it mapped telomeric to the HLA loci on 6p.[42] Two genetic studies demonstrated that the SCA1 gene maps telomeric to HLA and is very closely linked to D6S89.[43,44] Subsequent to these studies, Keats et al.[15] demonstrated very close linkage between SCA1 and D6S89 in a family in whom linkage to HLA or coagulation factor XIIIA (F13A) could not be detected. This emphasized the need to replace HLA typing by D6S89 genotyping for the identification of SCA1 families. Linkage analysis using D6S89 and approximately 120 affected individuals from nine SCA1 kindreds revealed a single recombinational event between SCA1 and D6S89.[45] These results identified D6S89 as one flanking marker that is extremely close to SCA1 (at a genetic distance $\leq$1 cM). New DNA markers were identified in 6p22-p23, YAC clones were isolated, and a large set of overlapping YAC, spanning approximately 2.5 Mb was developed.[46] To determine the minimal critical region for the SCA1 gene within this contig, five highly informative DNA markers of the dinucleotide repeat type were developed.[45,47,48] Genotypic analysis at these markers revealed that the AM10GA marker was very closely linked to SCA1 at a peak Lod score of 42.1 and 0 recombination fraction. These data, combined with the genotypic data at the remaining four markers (D6S109, SB1, LR40, and D6S202), indicated that SCA1 maps centromeric to D6S89. A single recombination event between D6S274 (a marker that maps centromeric to D6S89) and SCA1 identified this marker as the closest flanking marker at the centromeric end.[46] Long-range restriction analysis of the critical SCA1 region (identified as the region between D6S274 at the centromeric and D6S89 at the telomeric end) determined the size of the region to be 1.2 Mb.[46] This region was represented in a minimum of four overlapping YAC clones, which were subsequently cloned into cosmids. The isolation of the critical SCA1 region in overlapping YAC and cosmids allowed the eventual cloning of the SCA1 gene, as will be described below.

EXPANSION OF A TRINUCLEOTIDE REPEAT IN SCA1

Over the 2 years preceding the identification of the SCA1 gene, four human diseases were shown to result from a novel mutational mechanism involving expansion of unstable trinucleotide repeat sequences. These disorders include the fragile X syndrome (FRAXA), myotonic dystrophy (DM), Huntington disease (HD), and spinobulbar muscular atrophy (SBMA)[49–59] (see Chaps. 19, 141, 152 and 95, respectively). Three of these disorders—FRAXA, DM, and HD—display anticipation, as has been observed in SCA1. This led to the hypothesis that the amplification of an unstable trinucleotide repeat could be the underlying mechanism for the genetic defect in SCA1. To test this hypothesis, cosmid clones from the candidate SCA1 region were screened for the presence of trinucleotide repeat sequences. A CAG repeat was detected on a 3.36-kb *Eco*RI fragment derived from a set of 22 overlapping cosmids[60] that map between D6S288 and AM10GA (two DNA markers that reveal no recombination with SCA1).[46]

To test the genetic stability of this CAG repeat in SCA1, the 3.36-kb *Eco*RI fragment was hybridized to *Bst*NI- or *Taq*I-digested DNA from individuals with juvenile-onset disease. Expanded fragments were noted in all SCA1 individuals but in none of the unaffected individuals. All SCA1 individuals had a fragment in the normal size range in addition to the expanded allele. Sequence analysis of a 500-bp $(CAG)_n$-containing subclone of the 3.36-kb *Eco*RI fragment revealed the following repeat configuration: $(CAG)_{12}$ CAT CAG CAT $(CAG)_{15}$.[60] Using oligonucleotide primers that flank the CAG repeat, radioactively labeled PCR products were analyzed from normal and SCA1 individuals. Normal individuals displayed 15 alleles ranging from 19 to 36 repeat units (Table 154B-3), whereas individuals with SCA1 had two alleles—one within the size range seen in normal individuals and one within a range of 42 to 81 repeat units (Table 154B-3 and Fig. 154B-2). This repeat was highly polymorphic with a heterozygosity rate of 84 percent. The number of repeat units on SCA1 chromosomes was inversely correlated with the age of onset (Fig. 154B-3). A linear correlation coefficient of −0.845 was obtained, indicating that 71.4 percent of the variability in the age of onset can be accounted for by the number of CAG repeat units. Further analysis of the SCA1 CAG repeat in nine previously documented SCA1 kindreds revealed an expanded allele in the 42 to 81 range in all affected individuals, and confirmed the inverse correlation between repeat number and age of onset (linear correlation coefficient of −0.801 based on 111

Table 154B-3 Comparison of the Number of CAG Repeat Units on Normal and SCA1 Chromosomes

Number of Repeats	Normal Chromosomes Number	Normal Chromosomes Frequency	SCA1 Chromosomes Number	SCA1 Chromosomes Frequency
≥61	0	0	5	0.053
58–60	0	0	4	0.042
55–57	0	0	14	0.149
52–54	0	0	23	0.245
49–51	0	0	23	0.245
46–48	0	0	14	0.149
43–45	0	0	9	0.096
40–42	0	0	2	0.021
37–39	0	0	0	0
34–36	8	0.042	0	0
31–33	37	0.193	0	0
28–30	117	0.609	0	0
25–27	26	0.135	0	0
≤24	4	0.021	0	0
Total	192	1.00	94	1.00

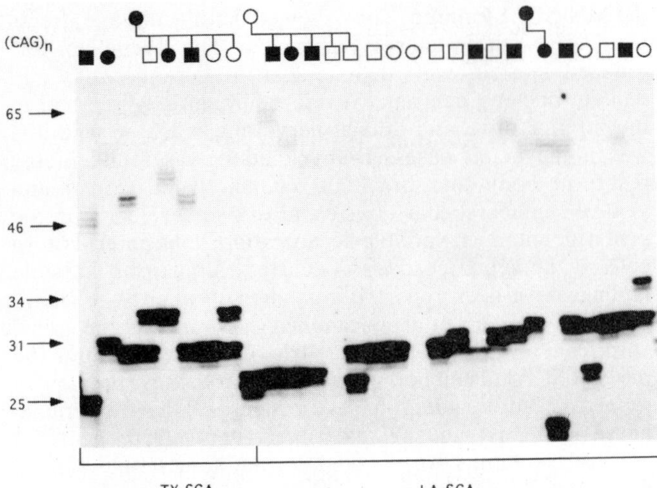

FIG. 154B-2 Analysis of the PCR-amplified products containing the trinucleotide repeat from normal SCA1 members of the TX- and LA-SCA1 kindreds. The sizes of the CAG repeats are ≤34 for the normal alleles and ≥46 for the expanded alleles on this autoradiograph.

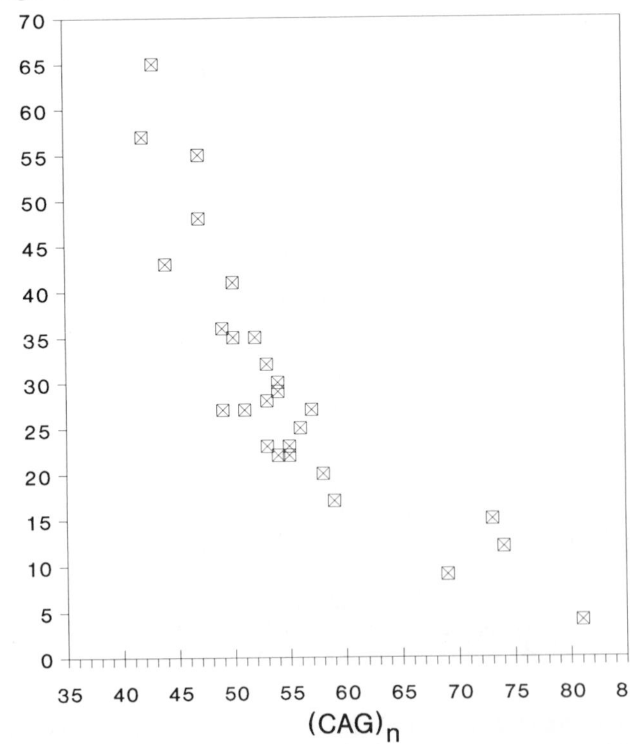

FIG. 154B-3 Scatter plot for the age of onset of SCA1 in years versus the number of CAG repeat units demonstrates the inverse correlation between the age of onset and the number of repeats. *(From Orr et al.[60] Used by permission of* Nature Genetics.*)*

SCA1 individuals[21a]). Analysis of the SCA1 CAG repeat in 42 families with dominantly inherited ataxia, not proven to be SCA1 because of the limited kindred size, identified three families (7 percent) with the expansion. These data suggest that analysis of the trinucleotide repeat at the SCA1 locus should allow rapid identification of SCA1 families in which the mutational mechanism involves a trinucleotide repeat expansion. It is not yet known if other mutations in the SCA1 gene will result in the same phenotype.

The intergenerational variation in the number of CAG repeats was examined in five SCA1 kindreds by studying 28 maternal- and 16 paternal-offspring pairs.[61] Increases and decreases in the number of repeats were found in both maternal and paternal transmissions of the SCA1 alleles. However, a significant difference in the type or size of variation was noted in maternal versus paternal transmissions (Fig. 154B-4). Sixty-nine percent of the maternal transmissions had no change or a decrease in the number of CAG repeats with an average change of −0.4 repeat; whereas 63 percent of the paternal transmissions had an increase in the number of CAG repeats with an average of +3.3 repeats.[61] The difference in intergenerational change between maternal and paternal transmissions is statistically significant ($p < 0.005$) and is similar to the variations observed in HD.[62,63]

The configuration of the CAG repeat on normal and SCA1 chromosomes was examined by sequence analysis and a combination of PCR and restriction analysis using *Sfa*NI, which cleaves GCATC$(N)_5$, allowing the identification of CAG repeats with a CAT interruption. Sequence analysis of the CAG repeat from 46 normal chromosomes revealed an interrupted repeat configuration in 43/46. The three chromosomes, which had a contiguous CAG repeat configuration, had the shortest normal alleles observed (one with 19 and two with 21 CAG repeats). Restriction analysis of the PCR products from 80 additional normal chromosomes revealed that all were cleaved with *Sfa*NI, indicating the presence of at least one CAT interruption. Thus, 98 percent of normal chromosomes had an interrupted repeat configuration. In contrast, the CAG repeats on SCA1 chromosomes were contiguous on all 30 alleles examined (13 by sequence and 17 by restriction analysis). These expanded SCA1 alleles were from seven unrelated SCA1 families who displayed at least four different haplotypes at D6S288 and D6S274 (markers within the SCA1 gene), indicating that the contiguous CAG repeat on SCA1 chromosomes is not the result of a single founder chromosome.[61] These data raise the possibility that the CAT interruptions that normally break the CAG repeat tracts into two smaller units may stabilize an allele with repeat number of 21 or more. Loss of the interruption then renders such alleles unstable. The configuration of the CAG repeat in the TATA-binding protein is analogous to the SCA1 repeat. Analysis of the CAG repeat tracts in the TATA-binding protein revealed that among 2003 chromosomes examined, the repeat tracts were interrupted by CAACAGCAA, with the exception of one very short allele that had 17 contiguous CAG repeats. Gostout et al.[64] proposed that contiguous repeats arise from cryptic or interrupted repeats and that the interruption functions to stabilize the repeat possibly by suppressing polymerase stuttering. The data for the SCA1 locus support the hypothesis that loss of the CAT interruption renders the CAG repeat unstable on SCA1 chromosomes.[61]

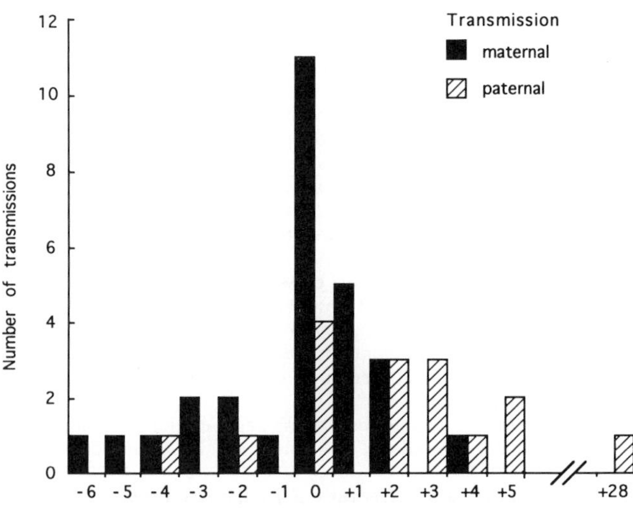

FIG. 154B-4 Intergenerational variation of CAG repeat number in maternal (*solid bars*) and paternal (*hatched*) transmissions. Repeat variation is shown as a decrease (−) or an increase (+) of repeat units. (*From Chung et al.*[61] *Used by permission of* Nature Genetics.)

THE SCA1 GENE PRODUCT

The CAG repeat at the SCA1 locus was documented to lie within a gene by RT-PCR and northern analysis. RT-PCR using primers immediately flanking the repeat as well as primers adjacent to the repeat confirmed that the CAG repeat is present in mRNA from lymphoblasts and cerebellar tissue (Orr HT, Zoghbi HY: unpublished data). Northern blot analysis using human poly(A)+ RNA from various tissues and cDNA clones containing and flanking the repeat sequence identified a 10.66-kb transcript that is expressed in brain, skeletal muscle, placenta, kidney, lung, and heart (Fig. 154B-5).

Sequence analysis of several independent and overlapping cDNA clones spanning approximately 10 kb of the SCA1 transcript identified a coding region of 2448 bp encoding 816 amino acids. The SCA1 protein, termed "ataxin-1," appears to represent a novel protein that does not share any homology with previously identified proteins. It does not have a prominent hydrophobic domain and hence may be soluble. One large internal exon of 2079 bp encodes the first 660 amino acids, and the remaining 156 amino acids are encoded by the last exon. There are seven exons in the 5′ untranslated region (spanning 935 bp of the cDNA). The 3′ untranslated region contains 7277 bp.[85] The features of ataxin-1 are summarized in Table 154B-4. Mammalian genes with either large internal exons or a large 5′ untranslated region are not commonly described. Examples of such genes include the human acidic fibroblast growth factor and human c-*fgr* proto-oncogene, which have four and seven 5′ untranslated exons, respectively.[65,66] Human genes with large internal exons include coagulation factors V and VIII and apolipoprotein

Table 154B-4 Features of Ataxin-1

Coding region of 816 amino acids
Transcript is 10.66 kb
5′ untranslated region includes 7 exons and is 935 bp
3′ untranslated region is 7277 bp
$(CAG)_n$ is within coding region at amino acid 196

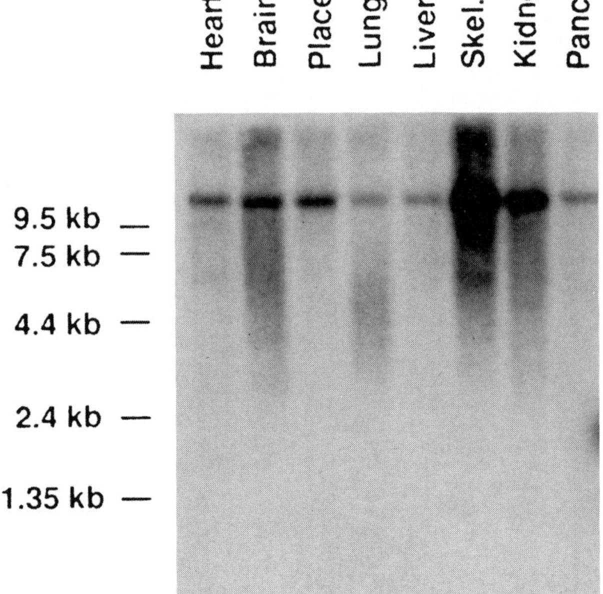

FIG. 154B-5 Expression analysis of the SCA1 gene using a multiple-tissue northern blot. Approximately 2 μg of human poly(A)+ RNA is in each lane. Using a 3-kb cDNA from the 3′ untranslated region of the SCA1 gene, an approximately 11-kb transcript is detected in all tissues. The same size transcript was detected using cDNA clones containing the CAG repeat or 5′ to the repeat (data not shown).

B, which have exons measuring 2820, 3106, and 7572 bp, respectively.[67,68]

TENTATIVE PATHOGENETIC MODEL

The role of the expanded polyglutamine tract in the pathogenesis of SCA1 has not yet been elucidated. An attractive hypothesis is that SCA1, HD, and SBMA involve gain-of-function mutations related to the polyglutamine tract in a regulatory protein.[60] A fourth dominantly inherited neurodegenerative disorder, dentatorubral pallidoluysian atrophy (DRPLA), has been shown to be due to an expanded polyglutamine tract in a novel gene.[69,70] DRPLA, like HD and SCA1, displays anticipation with propenderance of male transmission in juvenile cases. As evident from Table 155B-5, disorders caused by an expansion of trinucleotide repeats can be divided into two broad categories, neurodegenerative and other (so far neurologic but with no evidence of neurodegeneration). The common features among the neurodegenerative disorders include late-onset selective neuronal loss (motor neurons in SBMA, striatal neurons in HD, and Purkinje cells in SCA1), a polyglutamine tract in the protein, wide tissue expressivity of the mutated genes, and most likely a gain-of-function pathogenetic mechanism given that deletions of the androgen receptor gene[71,72] and disruption of the HD gene by a translocation (MacDonald M: personal communication) do not result in SBMA or HD, respectively.

Polyglutamine tracts are present in a number of transcription factors and in Drosophila proteins involved in neural development and developmental stage-specific transcription factors.[73–79] Proposed functional roles for the polyglutamine

Table 154B-5 Trinucleotide Repeat Expansions and Human Diseases

Disorder	Inheritance	Nucleotide	Coding
Neurodegenerative Disorders			
SBMA	XL	CAG	Gln
HD	AD	CAG	Gln
SCA1	AD	CAG	Gln
DRPLA	AD	CAG	Gln
Other Disorders			
FRAXA	XL	CGG	5′ UT
DM	AD	CTG	3′ UT
Fragile XE	AD	CGG	?

XL = X-linked; AD = autosomal dominant; UT = untranslated.

tracts include transcriptional activation as in the case of transcription factor Sp1[80] or a spacer between two different functional domains of a protein. The expansion of the polyglutamine tracts in four neurodegenerative disorders suggests that a common mechanism is involved in producing the phenotype. It is conceivable that the protein with an expanded polyglutamine tract retains its normal function totally or partially (as in the case of the androgen receptor in SBMA), but the gain of function represents an aberrant regulatory interference with a biologically unrelated gene.[60,81] The neurodegenerative phenotype could then be explained by the dysfunction of the aberrant target gene, which remains to be identified. This model would explain the gain-of-function phenotype and the exquisite cellular and tissue specificity seen in these neurodegenerative disorders.

The identification of a polyglutamine tract expansion in four neurodegenerative disorders with anticipation suggests that the same mechanism may be involved in the many other disorders displaying these features. Such disorders include SCA2,[19,82] MJD,[20,83] and other dominantly inherited SCA; and might include bipolar affective disorders, schizophrenia, and autism.[81,84]

REFERENCES

1. Greenfield JG: *The Spino-cerebellar Degenerations*. Springfield, IL, Charles C Thomas, 1954.
2. Koeppen AH, Barron KD: The neuropathology of olivopontocerebellar atrophy, in Duvoisin RC, Plaitakis A (eds): *The Olivopontocerebellar Atrophies*. New York, Raven, 1984, p 13.
3. Friedreich N: Ueber degenerative Atrophie der spinalen Hinterstrange. *Virchows Arch Pathol Anat* **26**:433, 1863.
4. Marie P: Sur l'hérédoataxie cérébelleuse. *Semin Med (Paris)* **13**:444, 1893.
5. Holmes G: An attempt to classify cerebellar disease with a note on Marie's hereditary cerebellar ataxia. *Brain* **30**:545, 1907.
6. Harding AE: The clinical features and classification of the late onset autosomal dominant cerebellar ataxias: A study of eleven families, including descendants of the "Drew family of Walworth." *Brain* **105**:1, 1982.
7. Zoghbi HY: The spinocerebellar degenerations, in Appel SH (ed): *Current Neurology*. St. Louis, Mosby–Year Book, 1991, p 121.
8. Konigsmark BW, Weiner LP: The olivopontocerebellar atrophies: A review. *Medicine (Baltimore)* **49**:227, 1970.
9. Gray RC, Oliver CP: Marie's hereditary cerebellar ataxia (Olivopontocerebellar atrophy). *Minn Med* **24**:327, 1941.
10. Schut JW: Hereditary ataxia: Clinical study through six generations. *Arch Neurol Psychiatr* **63**:535, 1950.
11. Schut LJ: Schut family ataxia, in de Jong JMBV (ed): *Handbook of Clinical Neurology*. Amesterdam, Elsevier, 1991, vol-

ume 16 (Hereditary Neuropathies and Spinocerebellar Atrophies), p 481.

12. Currier RD, Glover G, Jackson JF, Tipton AC: Spinocerebellar ataxia: Study of a large kindred. *Neurology* **22:**1040, 1972.
13. Nino HE, Noreen HJ, Dubey DP: A family with hereditary ataxia: HLA typing. *Neurology* **30:**12, 1980.
14. Zoghbi HY, Pollack MS, Lyons LA, Ferell RE, Daiger SP, Beaudet AL: Spinocerebellar ataxia: Variable age of onset and linkage to human leukocyte antigen in a large kindred. *Ann Neurol* **23:**580, 1988.
15. Keats BJB, Pollack MS, McCall A, Wilensky MA, Ward LJ, Lu M, Zoghbi HY: Localization of the gene for spinocerebellar ataxia to the short arm of chromosome 6 in a kindred for which close linkage to HLA is excluded. *Am J Hum Genet* **49:**972, 1991.
16. Spadaro M, Giunti P, Lulli P, Frontali M, Jodice C, Cappellacci S, Morellini M, Persichetti F, Trabace S, Anastasi R, Morocutti C: HLA-linked spinocerebellar ataxia: A clinical and genetic study of large Italian kindreds. *Acta Neurol Scand* **85:**257, 1992.
17. Bryer A, Martell RW, du Toif ED, Beighton P: Adult onset spinocerebellar ataxia linked to HLA in a South African kindred of mixed ancestry. *Tissue Antigens* **40:**111, 1992.
18. Kish SJ, Schut L, Simmons J, Gilbert J, Change L, Rebbetoy M: Brain acetocholinesterase activity is markedly reduced in dominantly-inherited olivopontocerebellar atrophy. *J Neurol Neurosurg Psychiatr* **51:**544, 1988.
19. Gispert S, Twells R, Orozco G, Brice A, Weber J, Heredero L, Scheufler K, Riley B, Allotey R, Nothers C, Hillerman R, Lunkes A, Khati C, Stevanin G, Hernandez A, Magarino C, Klockgether T, Durr A, Chneiweiss H, Enczmann J, Farrall M, Beckmann J, Mullan M, Wernet P, Agid Y, Freund H-J, Williamson R, Auburger G, Chamberlain S: Chromosomal assignment of the second locus for autosomal dominant cerebellar atxia (SCA2) to chromosome 12q23-24.1. *Nature Genet* **4:**295, 1993.
20. Takiyama Y, Nishizawa M, Tanaka H, Kawashima S, Sakamoto H, Karube Y, Shimazaki H, Soutome M, Endo K, Ohta S, Kagawa Y, Kanazawa I, Mizuno Y, Yoshida M, Yuasa T, Horikawa Y, Oyanagi K, Nagai H, Kondo T, Inuzuka T, Onodera O, Tsuji S: The gene for Machado-Joseph disease maps to human chromosome 14q. *Nat Genet* **4:**300, 1993.
21. Stevanin G, Chneiweiss H, Le Guern E, Ravise N, Durr A, Penet C, Agid Y, Brice A: Genetic heterogeneity of autosomal dominant cerebellar ataxia type I: Evidence for the existence of a third locus. *Hum Mol Genet* **2:**1483, 1993.

21a. Ranum LPW, Chung M-Y, Banfi S, Bryer A, Schut LJ, Ramesar R, Duvick LA, McCall AE, Subramony SH, Goldfarb L, Gomez C, Sandkuijl LA, Orr HT, Zoghbi HY: Molecular and clinical correlations in spinocerebellar ataxia type 1 (SCA1): Evidence for familial effects on the age of onset. *Am J Hum Genet* **55:**244, 1994.

22. Plaitakis A, Nicklas WJ, Desnick RJ: Glutamate dehydrogenase deficiency in three patients with spinocerebellar syndrome. *Ann Nuerol* **7:**297, 1980.
23. Plaitakis A, Berl S, Yahr MD: Neurological disorders with deficiency of glutamate dehydrogenase. *Ann Neurol* **15:**144, 1984.
24. Finocchiaro G, Taroni F, Di Donato S: Glutamate dehydrogenase in olivopontocerebellar atrophies: Leukocytes, fibroblasts, and muscle mitochondria. *Neurology* **36:**550, 1986.
25. Grossman A, Rosenberg RN, Warmoth L: Glutamate and malate dehydrogenase activities in Joseph's disease and olivopontocerebellar atrophy. *Neurology* **37:**106, 1987.
26. Perry TL, Currier RD, Hansen S, MacLean J: Aspartate-taurine imbalance in dominantly inherited olivopontocerebellar atrophy. *Neurology* **27:**257, 1977.
27. Perry TL, Kish SJ, Hansen S, Currier RD: Neurotransmitter amino acids in dominantly inherited cerebellar disorders. *Neurology* **31:**257, 1981.
28. Perry TL: Four biochemically different types of dominantly inherited olivopontocerebellar atrophy, in Duvoisin RC, Plaitakis A (eds): *The Olivopontocerebellar Atrophies.* New York, Raven, 1984, p 205.
29. Auby D, Saggu HK, Jenner P, Quinn NP, Harding AE, Marsden CD: Leukocyte dehydrogenase activity in patients with degenerative neurological disorders. *J Neurol Neurosurg Psychiatr* **8:**635, 1988.
30. Rosenberg RN, Banner C: Normal cerebellar glutamate dehydrogenase protein in spinocerebellar degeneration. *J Neurol Neurosurg Psychiatr* **52:**666, 1989.
31. Kish SJ, Currier RD, Schut L, Perry TL, Morito CL: Brain choline acetyltransferase reduction in dominantly inherited olivopontocerebellar atrophy. *Ann Neurol* **22:**272, 1987.
32. Kish GJ, El-Awar M, Schut L, Leach L, Oscar-Berman M, Freedman M: Cognitive deficits in olivopontocerebellar atrophy: Implications for the cholinergic hypothesis of Alzheimer's dementia. *Ann Neurol* **24:**200, 1988.
33. Oertel WH: Neurotransmitters in the cerebellum: Scientific aspects and clinical relevance, in Harding AE, Deufel T (eds): *Advances in Neurology.* New York, Raven, 1993, volume 61 (Inherited Ataxias), p 33.
34. Schut JW, Haymaker W: Hereditary ataxia. A pathologic study of five cases of common ancestry. *J Neuropathol Clin Neurol* **1:**183, 1951.
35. Bebin EM, Bebin J, Currier RD, Smith EE, Perry TL: Morphometric studies in dominant olivopontocerebellar atrophy. *Arch Neurol* **47:**188, 1990.
36. Yakura H, Wakisaka A, Fujimoto S, Itakura K: Hereditary ataxia and HLA genotypes. *N Engl J Med* **291:**154, 1974.
37. Jackson JF, Currier RD, Terasaki PI, Morton NE: Spinocerebellar ataxia and HLA linkage: Risk prediction by HLA typing. *N Engl J Med* **296:**1138, 1977.
38. Haines JL, Schut LJ, Weitkamp LR: Spinocerebellar ataxia in large kindred: Age at onset, reproduction, and genetic linkage studies. *Neurology* **34:**1542, 1984.
39. Sasaki H, Wakisaka A, Katoh T, Yoshida MC, Hamada T, Shima K, Matsuura T: Linkage study of dominantly inherited olivo-ponto-cerebellar atrophy (OPCA) and Holmes' ataxia. *Jpn J Hum Genet* **33:**423, 1988.
40. Frontali M, Jodice C. Lulli P, Spadaro M, Cappellacci S, Giunti P, Malaspina P, Morellini M, Morocutti C, Novelletto A, Persichetti F, Trabace S, Anastasi R, Terrenato L: Spinocerebellar ataxia (SCA1) in two large Italian kindreds: Evidence in favour of a locus position distal to Glo1 and the HLA cluster. *Ann Hum Genet* **55:**7, 1991.
41. Lamm LU, Olaisen B: Report on the committee on the genetic constitution of chromosome 5 and 6. *Cytogenet Cell Genet* **40:**128, 1985.
42. Litt M, Luty JA: A TG microsatellite VNTR detected by PCR is located on 6p (HGM10 No. D6S89). *Nucleic Acids Res* **18:**4301, 1990.
43. Zoghbi HY, Jodice C, Sandkuijl LA, Kwiatkowski TJ Jr, McCall AE, Huntoon SA, Lulli P, Spadaro M, Litt M, Cann HM, Frontali M, Terrenato L: The gene for autosomal dominant spinocerebellar ataxia (SCA1) maps telomeric to HLA complex and is closely linked to the D6S89 locus in three large kindreds. *Am J Hum Genet* **49:**23, 1991.
44. Ranum LPW, Duvick LA, Rich SS, Schut LJ, Litt M, Orr HT: Localization of the autosomal dominant, HLA-linked spinocerebellar ataxia (SCA1) locus in two kindreds within an 8cM subregion of chromosome 6p. *Am J Hum Genet* **49:**31, 1991.
45. Kwiatkowski TJ Jr, Orr HT, Banfi S, McCall AE, Jodice C, Persichetti F, Novelletto A, LeBorgne-Demarquoy F, Duvick LA, Frontali M, Subramony SH, Beaudet AL, Terrenato L, Zoghbi HY, Ranum LPW: The gene for autosomal dominant spinocerebellar ataxia (SCA1) maps centromeric to D6S89 and shows no recombination, in nine large kindreds, with a dinucleotide repeat at the AM10 locus. *Am J Hum Genet* **53:**391, 1993.
46. Banfi S, Chung M-Y, Kwiatkowski TJ Jr, Ranum LPW, McCall AE, Chinault AC, Orr HT, Zoghbi HY: Mapping and cloning of the critical region for the spinocerebellar ataxia type 1 gene in a yeast artificial chromosome contig spanning 1.2Mb. *Genomics* **18:**355, 1993.
47. Ranum LPW, Chung MY, Duvick LA, Zoghbi HY, Orr HT: Dinucleotide repeat polymorphism at the D6S109 locus. *Nucleic Acids Res* **19:**1171, 1991.
48. Le Borgne-Demarquoy F, Kwiatkowski TJ Jr, Zoghbi HY: Two dinucleotide repeat polymorphisms at the D6S202 locus. *Nucleic Acids Res* **19:**6060, 1991.
49. Kremer EJ, Pritchard M, Lynch M, Yu S, Holman K,

Baker E, Warren ST, Schlessinger D, Sutherland GR, Richards RI: Mapping of DNA instability at the fragile X to a trinucleotide repeat sequence p(CCG)n. *Science* **252**:1711, 1991.

50. Verkerk AJMH, Pieretti M, Sutcliffe JS, Fu Y-H, Kuhl DPA, Puzutti A, Reiner O, Richards S, Victoria MF, Zhang R, Eussen BE, van Ommen G-JB, Blonden LAJ, Riggins GJ, Chastain JL, Kunst CB, Galjaard H, Caskey CT, Nelson DL, Oostra BA, Warren ST: Identification of a gene (FMR-1) containing a CGG repeat coincident with a breakpoint cluster region exhibiting length variation in fragile X syndrome. *Cell* **65**:905, 1991.
51. Fu Y-H, Kuhl DPA, Pizutti A, Pieretti M, Sutcliffe JS, Richards S, Verkerk AJMH, Holden JJA, Fenwick Jr RG, Warren ST, Oostra BA, Nelson DL, Caskey CT: Variation of the CGG repeat at the fragile X site results in genetic instability: Resolution of the Sherman paradox. *Cell* **67**:1047, 1991.
52. Fu Y-H, Pizutti A, Fenwick RG, King JJ, Rajnarayan S, Dunne PW, Dubel J, Nasser GA, Ashizawa T, De Jong P, Wieringa B, Korneluk R, Perryman MB, Epstein HF, Caskey CT: An unstable triplet repeat in a gene related to myotonic muscular dystrophy. *Science* **255**:1256, 1992.
53. Brook JD, McCurrach ME, Harley HG, Buckler AJ, Church D, Aburatani H, Hunter K, Stanton VP, Thirion J-P, Hudson T, Sohn R, Zemelman B, Snell RG, Rundle SA, Crow S, Davies J, Shelbourne P, Buxton J, Jones C, Juvonen V, Johnson K, Harper PS, Shaw DJ, Houseman DE: Molecular basis of myotonic dystrophy: Expansion of a trinucleotide (CTG) repeat at the 3′ end of a transcript encoding a protein kinase family member. *Cell* **68**:799, 1992.
54. Buxton J, Shelbourne P, Davies J, Jones C, Van Tongeren T, Aslanidis C, de Jong P, Jansen G, Anvret M, Riley B, Williamson R, Johnson K: Detection of an unstable fragment of DNA specific to individuals with myotonic dystrophy. *Nature* **355**:547, 1992.
55. Harley HG, Brook JD, Rundle SA, Crow S, Reardon W, Buckler AJ, Harper PS, Housman DE: Expansion of an unstable DNA region and phenotypic variation in myotonic dystrophy. *Nature* **355**:545, 1992.
56. Mahadevan M, Tsilfidis C, Sabourin L, Shutler G, Amemiya C, Jansen G, Neville C, Narang M, Barcelo J, O'Hoy K, Leblond S, Earle-MacDonald J, De Jong PJ, Wieringa B, Korneluk RG: Myotonic dystrophy mutation: An unstable CTG repeat in the 3′ untranslated region of the gene. *Science* **255**:1253, 1992.
57. The Huntington's Disease Collaborative Research Group: A novel gene containing a trinucleotide repeat that is expanded and unstable on Huntington's disease chromosomes. *Cell* **72**:971, 1993.
58. Bruner HG, Jansen G, Nillesen W, Nelen MR, de Die CEM, Howeller CJ, van Oost BA, Wieringa B, Ropers H-H, Smeets HJM: Reverse mutation in myotonic dystrophy. *N Engl J Med* **328**:476, 1993.
59. LaSpada AR, Wilson EM, Lubahn DB, Harding AE, Fishbeck H: Androgen receptor gene mutations in X-linked spinal and bulbar muscular atrophy. *Nature* **352**:77, 1991.
60. Orr H, Chung M-y, Banfi S, Kwiatkowski TJ Jr, Servadio A, Beaudet AL, McCall AE, Duvick LA, Ranum LPW, Zoghbi HY: Expansion of an unstable trinucleotide (CAG) repeat in spinocerebellar ataxia type 1. *Nat Genet* **4**:221, 1993.
61. Chung M-Y, Ranum PW, Duvick L, Servadio A, Zoghbi HY, Orr HT: Analysis of the CAG repeat expansion in spinocerebellar ataxia type I: Evidence for a possible mechanism predisposing to instability. *Nat Genet* **5**:254, 1993.
62. Duyao M, Ambrose C, Myers R, Novelletto A, Persichetti F, Frontali M, Folstein S, Ross C, Franz M, Abbott M, Gray J, Conneally P, Young A, Penney J, Hollingsworth Z, Shoulson I, Lazzarini A, Falek A, Koroshetz W, Sax D, Bird E, Vonsattel J, Bonilla E, Alvir J, Bickham Conde J, Cha J-H, Dure L, Gomez F, Ramos M, Sanchez-Ramos J, Snodgrass S, de Young M, Eexler N, Moscowitz C, Penchaszadeh G, MacFarlene H, Anderson M, Jenkins B, Srinidhi J, Barnes G, Gusella J, MacDonald M: Trinucleotide repeat length and age of onset in Huntington's disease. *Nat Genet* **4**:387, 1993.
63. Snell RG, MacMillan JC, Cheadle JP, Fenton I, Lazarou LP, Davies P, MacDonald ME, Gusella JF, Harper PS, Shaw DJ: Relationship between trinucleotide repeat expansion and phenotypic variation in Huntington's disease. *Nat Genet* **4**:393, 1993.
64. Gostout B, Liu Q, Sommer SS: "Cryptic" repeating triplets of purines and pyrimidines (cRRY(i)) are frequent and polymorphic: Analysis of coding cRR(i) in the proopiomelanocortin (POMC) and TATA-binding protein (TBP) genes. *Am J Hum Genet* **52**:1182, 1993.
65. Myers RL, Payson RA, Chotani MA, Deaven LL, Chiu IM: Gene structure and differential expression of acidic fibroblast growth factor mRNA: Identification and distribution of four different transcripts. *Oncogene* **8**:341, 1993.
66. Link DC, Gutkind SJ, Robbins KC, Ley TJ: Characterization of the 5′ region of the human c-fgr and identification of the major myelomonocytic c-fgr promoter. *Oncogene* **7**:877, 1992.
67. Cripe LD, Moore KD, Kane WH: Structure of the gene for human coagulation factor V. *Biochemistry* **31**:3777, 1992.
68. Ludwig EH, Blackhart BD, Pierotti VR, Caiati L, Fortier C, Knott T, Scott J, Mahley RW, Levy-Wilson B, McCarthy BJ: DNA sequence of the human apolipoprotein B gene. *DNA* **6**:363, 1987.
69. Nagafuchi S, Yanagisawa H, Sato K, Shirayama T, Ohsaki E, Bundo M, Takedo T, Tadokoro K, Kondo I, Maruyama N, Tanaka Y, Kikushima H, Umino K, Kurosawa H, Furukawa T, Nihei K, Inoue T, Sano A, Komure O, Yoshizawa T, Kanazawa I, Yamada M: Expansion of an unstable CAG trinucleotide on chromosome 12p in dentatorubral and pallidoluysian atrophy. *Nat Genet* **6**:14, 1993.
70. Koide R, Ikeuchi T, Onodera O, Tanaka H, Igarashi S, Endo K, Takashashi H, Kondo R, Ishikawa A, Hayashi T, Saito M, Tomoda A, Miike T, Naito H, Ikuta F, Tsuji S: Unstable expansion of CAG repeat in hereditary dentatorubral-pallidoluysian atrophy (DRPLA). *Nat Genet* **6**:9, 1993.
71. Quigley CA, Friedman KJ, Johnson A, Lafreniere RG, Silverman LM, Lubahn DB, Brown TR, Wilson EM, Willard HF, French FS: Complete deletion of the androgen receptor gene: Definition of the null phenotype of the androgen insensitivity syndrome and determination of carrier status. *J Clin Endocrinol Metab* **74**:927, 1992.
72. Trifiro M, Gottlieb B, Pinsky L, Kaufman M, Prior L, Belsham DD, Wrogemann K, Brown CJ, Willard HF, Trapman J, Brinkmann AO, Chang C, Liao S, Sergovich F, Jung J: The 56/58 kDa androgen-binding protein in male genital skin fibroblasts with a deleted androgen receptor gene. *Mol Cell Endocrinol* **75**:37, 1991.
73. Wharton KA, Johansen KM, Xu T, Artavanis-Tsakonas S: Nucleotide sequence from the neurogenic locus Notch implies a gene product that shares homology with proteins containing EGF-like repeats. *Cell* **43**:567, 1985.
74. Duboule D, Maenlin M, Galliot B, Mohier E: DNA sequences homologous to the drosophila *opa* repeat are present in murine mRNAs that are differentially expressed in fetus and adult tissues. *Mol Cell Biol* **7**:2003, 1987.
75. Kadonaga JT, Courey A, Ladika J, Tjian R: Distinct regions of Sp1 modulate DNA binding and transcriptional activation. *Science* **242**:1566, 1988.
76. Courey AJ, Tijan R: Analysis of Sp1 in vivo reveals multiple transcriptional domains, including a novel glutamine-rich activation motif. *Cell* **55**:887, 1988.
77. Kao CC, Liebrman PM, Schmidt MC, Zhou Q, Pei R, Berk AJ: Cloning of a transcriptionally active TATA binding factor. *Science* **248**:1648, 1990.
78. Vaessin H, Ellsworth G, Wolff E, Bier E, Jan LY, Jan YN: *Prospero* is expressed in neuronal precursors and encodes a nuclear protein that is involved in the control of axonal outgrowth in drosophila. *Cell* **67**:941, 1991.
79. Bellen HJ, Kooyer S, D'Evelyn D, Pearlman J: The *Drosophila* couch potato protein is expressed in nuclei of peripheral neuronal precursors and shows homology to RNA-binding proteins. *Genes Dev* **6**:2125, 1992.
80. Courey AJ, Holtzman DA, Jackson SP, Tjian R: Synergis-

tic activation by the glutamine-rich domains of human transcription factor Sp1. *Cell* **59:**827, 1989.

81. Ross CA, McInnis MG, Margolis RL, Li S-H: Genes with triplet repeats: Candidate mediators of neuropsychiatric disorders. *Trends Neurosci* **16:**254, 1993.
82. Orozco G, Estrada R, Perry TL, Araña J, Fernandez R, Gonzalez-Quevedo A, Galarraga J, Hansen S: Dominantly inherited olivopontocerebellar atrophy from eastern Cuba. Clinical, neuropathological, and biochemical findings. *J Neurol Sci* **93:**37, 1989.
83. Coutinho P, Andrade C: Autosomal dominant system degeneration in Portuguese families of the Azores Islands: A new genetic disorder involving cerebellar, pyramidal, extrapyramidal, and spinal cord motor functions. *Neurology* **28:**703, 1978.
84. Mandel J-L: Questions of expansion. *Nat Genet* **4:**8, 1993.
85. Banfi S, Servadio A, Chung M-y, Kwiatkowski Jr TJ, McCall AE, Duvick LA, Shen Y, Roth EJ, Orr HT, Zoghbi HY: Identification and characterization of the gene causing type 1 spinocerebellar ataxia. *Nat Genet* **7:**513, 1994.

CHAPTER 154C

Charcot-Marie-Tooth Disease and Hereditary Neuropathy with Liability to Pressure Palsies

Andrea Ballabio ▪ Huda Y. Zoghbi

1. **Distal muscle weakness and atrophy, mild sensory impairment, and segmental demyelination are the hallmarks of inherited disorders of the peripheral nerves. Charcot-Marie-Tooth (CMT) disease represents a heterogeneous group of peripheral neuropathies characterized by a late-onset, slowly progressive phenotype that in some patients is associated with decreased nerve conduction velocity.**

2. **Hereditary neuropathy with liability to pressure palsies (HNPP) is characterized by periodic sensory-motor findings and in some cases by palsies following minor compression or trauma of the peripheral nerve.**

3. **Molecular analysis has permitted the identification of several genetic loci involved in distinct types of peripheral neuropathies. The majority of patients with CMT type 1A (CMT1A) have a submicroscopic duplication involving the short arm of chromosome 17 (17p11.2).**

4. **Patients with HNPP have a deletion that involves the same region and appears to represent the reciprocal product of an unequal crossing over underlying the CMT1A duplication. Point mutations have been identified in the gene encoding the peripheral myelin protein 22 (*PMP22*) in patients with CMT1A. It appears likely that both CMT1A and HNPP are due to mutations affecting gene dosage for *PMP22*.**

5. **Mutations in a gene encoding another peripheral myelin protein, myelin protein zero (P_0), have been found in patients with CMT type 1B.**

CLINICAL, ELECTROPHYSIOLOGICAL, AND PATHOLOGICAL FINDINGS

Charcot-Marie-Tooth (CMT) disease, also known as "peroneal muscular atrophy," is characterized by a progressive muscular atrophy with initial involvement of feet and legs.[1,2] Symptoms start in the first or second decade of life. Muscle weakness is usually detected as an abnormality of gait (typically steppage or equine gait) or clumsiness in running. Cramps are frequently reported. Physical examination often reveals foot deformities, including pes cavus or equinovarus, and an "inverted champagne bottle" appearance of lower limbs. Deep tendon reflexes are usually absent. Sensory symptoms are very mild, and they are reported by the patients as diminished sensation over the feet. This results in calluses, and less often ulcers, which develop over pressure points. Later in life, patients may experience weakness of intrinsic hand muscle, which may lead to a "claw hand" appearance. Both interfamilial and intrafamilial variability of phenotypic expression has been described in CMT.[3,4]

Electrophysiology represents an important diagnostic tool for CMT disease. On the basis of the electrophysiological data, CMT patients can be divided into two major categories: CMT type 1 disease (CMT1) patients showing decreased motor-nerve conduction velocity (MCV) and CMT2 patients with normal MCV. The conduction velocities of peroneal and ulnar nerves in the patients are, on average, less than half the values of normal individuals. There is a general agreement that 38 m/sec is considered to be the threshold MCV value for defining CMT1.[3,4] However, some patients with values slightly above 38 m/sec have been described in families with CMT1. Therefore, it has been recommended that mean values of MCV of all affected members in the kindred be used for CMT1 diagnosis.[4] Although not practical for screening purposes, sensory-nerve conduction velocity (SNCV) measurements are also abnormal in CMT1, and it has been suggested that they may provide a better discrimination between CMT1 and CMT2.[3] Little information is available on the age at which MCV abnormalities first appear; patients with CMT1 have normal MCV at birth, and they clearly show MCV abnormalities by 4 to 5 years of age. There is no correlation between the degree of MCV abnormalities and the severity of the phenotype.[3,4]

The pathology findings in CMT patients have been extensively described. These include spinal cord and peripheral nerve abnormalities. Demyelination and gliosis, often associated with enlargement of the peripheral nerves, are the most frequent findings. Onion bulb structures, consisting of circumferentially directed Schwann cells and their processes, can be observed at internodes under phase and electron microscopy.[3,5]

Since there is no pharmacologic treatment available for CMT, the therapy is symptomatic. Patients are advised to

A list of standard abbreviations is located immediately preceding the index in each volume. Additional abbreviations used in this chapter include: CMT = Charcot-Marie-Tooth disease, including CMT1, CMT2, etc.; HNPP = hereditary neuropathy with liability to pressure palsies; MCV = motor-nerve conduction velocity; p_0 = myelin protein zero; *PMP22* = peripheral myelin protein 22; SNCV = sensory-nerve conduction velocity.

maintain normal body weight, to have good foot care, and to enroll in physical fitness programs. More severely affected individuals should undergo proper physical therapy.[3,4]

Hereditary neuropathy with liability to pressure palsies (HNPP), also termed "familial recurrent polyneuropathy" or "tomaculous neuropathy," has been considered a distinct entity from CMT on the basis of different clinical presentation and of a different histopathological and electrophysiological pattern. The clinical features of HNPP, usually appearing during adolescence, are recurrent attacks of numbness, muscular weakness, and atrophy. In some cases, these are associated with palsies triggered by compression or trauma.[6,7] Segmental demyelination and thickenings of the myelin sheath (tomaculous or "sausage-like" structures) are typical pathological findings in HNPP.[8,9] Patients with HNPP frequently have carpal tunnel syndrome and other entrapment neuropathies. Electrophysiology is usually normal; therefore it is not helpful in HNPP, but it may reveal a reduction of nerve-conduction velocity or a conduction block in a few cases.[10]

GENETICS

Inheritance Pattern and Chromosomal Assignment

As a group, CMT disease is the most common peripheral neuropathy, having an estimated prevalence of 1:2500 individuals.[11] However, it is now clear from electrophysiological and genetic studies, that the term *CMT* generally refers to phenotypically similar conditions caused by mutations at distinct genetic loci. The concept that mutations at different genetic loci can have the same phenotypic consequences and that, conversely, different mutations at the same locus can cause different phenotypes, finds full representation in CMT. The first clear indication of genetic heterogeneity came from the observation of families in which the CMT phenotype appeared to segregate in a Mendelian fashion, with autosomal dominant transmission most commonly observed,[3,4] but other patterns also seen. A summary of the genetic classification of CMT disorders and the associated electrophysiological features is shown in Table 154C-1.

A major aid in the classification of disorders collectively referred to as "CMT disease" has come from linkage studies in CMT pedigrees (see Table 154C-1). CMT1 has been assigned to two defined genetic loci, one on chromosome 17 for CMT1A[12] and another on chromosome 1 for CMT1B.[13] A third undefined locus for CMT1 (CMT1C) can be inferred from the analysis of some CMT1 families in whom the disease locus does not segregate with markers on either chromosome 17 or chromosome 1.[14,15] CMT1A has been shown to be tightly linked to several DNA markers assigned

Table 154C-1 **Genetic Classification of CMT Disease and Correlation with Neurophysiological Data**

	Decreased MCV	Chromosomal Assignment	Protein (Gene Symbol)
CMT1A	Yes	17p11.2–p12	PMP22 (*PMP22*)
CMT1B	Yes	1q21.2–q23	P_0 (*MPZ*)
CMT1C	Yes	—	—
CMT2A	No	1p35–p36	—
CMTX	Yes	Xq13–q21	Connexin 32 (*GJβ1*)

to the 17p11.2-p12 region, as reviewed elsewhere.[4] Linkage data originally obtained with the Duffy blood group, and subsequently with the FcδRII receptor gene, have assigned CMT1B to the 1q21.2-q23 region.[13,16] Both CMT1A and CMT1B are typically inherited with an autosomal dominant pattern; however, there is evidence that recessive point mutation at the CMT1A locus may also cause CMT1.[17] Multipoint linkage analysis revealed linkage of CMT2 to markers located in the distal short arm of chromosome 1 (1p35-p36) in three families, establishing a map location for at least one form of autosomal dominant CMT2 (CMT2A).[18]

CMT1 families with X-linked dominant (CMTX1) and with X-linked recessive (CMTX2) inheritance patterns have been reported as reviewed elsewhere.[3,4] In some cases it was difficult to distinguish unequivocally between autosomal and X-linked dominant patterns. It is not clear whether CMTX1 and CMTX2 represent two distinct loci or if they are the results of mutations with a different effect on the penetrance of the phenotype in heterozygous females. In some families with X-linked CMT1, significant linkage has been reported with X chromosome markers located in the Xq13-q21 region.[19–27] A locus for X-linked CMT has also been assigned to the Xp22 region; however, it is questionable whether the phenotype described in this family can be considered a form of CMT disease or a completely different entity.[24]

A DNA Duplication in Charcot-Marie-Tooth Disease Type 1A

In 1991, two research groups simultaneously reported on the identification of a large submicroscopic duplication of the 17p11.2-p12 region in patients with CMT1A.[28,29] This conclusion was supported by multiple experimental observations. First, using a polymorphic DNA marker mapping to 17p11.2 (D17S122), both groups detected the simultaneous presence of three copies. Similar results were obtained using a highly polymorphic short tandem repeat at the D17S122 locus, which also detected three alleles in the majority of the patients.[28] The duplication invariably segregated with the disease within the families, and it was later found to be completely concordant with the neurophysiological diagnosis of CMT1A.[30] Second, a duplication junction fragment, also segregating in a Mendelian fashion with CMT1A, was identified by long-range restriction mapping, using PFGE.[28] Third, when D17S122 was used as a probe in fluorescence *in situ* hybridization (FISH) analysis, three positive signals were observed on chromosomes from patients with CMT1A, two from the duplicated 17 and one from the normal 17.[28] Together these data demonstrated the presence of a duplication in patients with CMT1A. Furthermore, the identification of a homozygous duplication in a severely affected case with CMT1A,[28] and of a *de novo* duplication associated with new onset of the disease in another CMT1A family,[29] provided evidence that the duplication is the disease-causing mutation.

The identification of a DNA duplication in patients with CMT1A raised several important questions, including the frequency, similarity, stability, and size of the duplication among CMT1A patients. Molecular studies have been performed in many CMT1A families of different ethnic origins.[28,29,31–33] These studies have shown that the DNA duplication is the most common defect in CMT1 and is seen in approximately 70 percent of the patients,[34] that the duplication is stably transmitted through both meiosis and mitosis,[35] and that there is a high frequency of *de novo* duplication events.[29,34,36]

The region of chromosome 17 spanning the duplication (17p11.2-p12) has been characterized in detail in normal and duplicated chromosomes. Physical mapping of this region, using PFGE, has provided evidence that the CMT1A duplication monomer measures approximately 1.5 Mb.[37–40] The entire duplicated region was isolated in overlapping YAC clones.[37,41] All patients carrying the CMT1A duplication, regardless of their ethnic origin or their haplotype, have the same PFGE junction fragment, suggesting a common DNA rearrangement mechanism in CMT1A.[28,34,38] A low copy number repeat was identified at the duplication junction. Two copies of this repeat were found in normal chromosomes 17, while three copies were detected in CMT1A duplication chromosomes, suggesting that the duplication arises from unequal crossing over at the repeat site.[37]

A DNA Deletion in Hereditary Neuropathy with Liability to Pressure Palsies

If the mechanism underlying the CMT1A duplication is indeed an unequal crossing over, one would expect to observe chromosomes carrying the reciprocal product of this event, which would be characterized by a deletion of the same region involved in the duplication. Deletions resulting from abnormal recombination at repeat sites have already been described for other diseases.[42,43]

Evidence for the presence of such a reciprocal event was presented by Chance et al., who found an interstitial deletion in three unrelated kindreds with HNPP.[44] The deletion measured approximately 1.5 Mb and included all the markers that were found to be duplicated in CMT1A. Supporting data were obtained by genetic analysis using polymorphic DNA markers and by FISH analysis. The deletion breakpoints appeared to map exactly to the same intervals to which the CMT1A duplication breakpoints were assigned.[17] As in the case of the CMT1A duplication, the deletion cosegregated completely with the HNPP phenotype within the families analyzed.[44]

Mutations in the Peripheral Myelin Protein 22 and P-Myelin Protein Zero Genes in Patients with Charcot-Marie-Tooth Disease Type 1

Two allelic mutations resulting in a hypomyelinating neuropathy (*trembler* and *trembler-J*) have been identified in mice.[45,46] The *trembler* locus has been assigned to a region of mouse chromosome 11 that is syntenic to the human 17p11.2 region.[47] The similarity between the neuropathological and electrophysiological features of *trembler* and CMT1A, and the syntenic map location of the two loci, led to the suggestion that *trembler* is a mouse model for CMT1A.

Suter et al. demonstrated that the *trembler* and *trembler-J* mice carry mutations in a gene, termed "*PMP22*" (peripheral myelin protein 22), which encodes a 22-kDa peripheral myelin protein and is localized to mouse chromosome 11.[48,49] *PMP22* is highly expressed in the peripheral nervous system and in the spinal cord. The product of the *PMP22* gene is a 160 amino acid glycosylated polypeptide, displaying four putative transmembrane domains that have been highly conserved throughout evolution. Analysis of the *PMP22* gene in the *Trembler* mice revealed a G-to-A transition in *Trembler,* resulting in glycine to aspartic acid substitution (G150D) in the fourth putative transmembrane domain, and a T-to-C transition in *Trembler-J,* resulting in a leucine to proline substitution (L16P) in the putative first transmembrane domain.[48,49]

An important next step was to test if the human homologue was localized in the 17p11.2 region and if it was included in the CMT1A duplication. Four independent research groups simultaneously reported direct evidence that *PMP22* is localized within the CMT1A duplication and proposed that an increased dosage of this gene is responsible for the CMT1A phenotype.[39,50–52] The evidence was based on PFGE, FISH, and dosage analyses. One of these groups cloned and characterized the human *PMP22* gene and found a high degree of similarity between the human and mouse genes in both sequence and expression patterns.[50]

Subsequently, CMT1 patients showing no evidence of duplication were tested for point mutations in the *PMP22* gene. Valentijn et al. identified a mutation identical to the *Trembler-J* mouse mutation on one allele of the PMP-22 gene.[53] The mutation was found to segregate with the CMT1A phenotype within this large family. This finding strongly implicated *PMP22* as the major gene contributing to the CMT1A phenotype. Subsequently, a large study performed on 32 unrelated CMT1 patients who did not have the duplication identified an additional point mutation, causing a cysteine to serine substitution in the second putative transmembrane domain. This mutation was detected in three patients from this family and was found to arise *de novo* simultaneously with the CMT1 phenotype.[54]

The gene encoding another peripheral myelin protein, myelin protein zero (P_0), an adhesion glycoprotein of the immunoglobulin superfamily, was assigned to human chromosome 1q22-1q23,[55] which is the same chromosomal region to which CMT1B was previously assigned.[13] This prompted two research groups to test for mutations in this gene in patients affected by CMT1B.[56,57] Mutations in the extracellular domain of the P_0 gene (Lys 96, Asp 90 and Ser 34) were identified in three families with CMT1B.[56–58] Four different mutations in the extracellular domain of the mature P_0 protein, involving Lys 67,[56] Asp 61,[58] Ile 1,[58] and deletion of Ser 34[57] have been identified in CMT1B patients.

During the preparation of this chapter mutations in the gene encoding *Connexin,* a gap-junction protein, were detected in patients with CMTX (Fischbeck K, et al.: personal communication).

Molecular Pathogenesis of Charcot-Marie-Tooth Disease Type 1A and Hereditary Neuropathy with Liability to Pressure Palsies

A summary of genotype/phenotype correlation data for CMT and HNPP peripheral neuropathies is shown in Fig. 154C-1, as adapted from Suter and Patel[59] Duplications and deletions involving the same chromosomal region have been found in patients with CMT1A and HNPP, respectively. This suggests that these two disorders, like other genetic disorders (see "Contiguous Gene Syndromes Result from Dosage Imbalance" in Chap. 20), are sensitive to dosage imbalance of a gene(s) located in this region.[60,61] The identification of four patients with 17p trisomy, displaying the CMT1A phenotype, reinforces this hypothesis.[62–65]

The *PMP22* point mutations found in CMT1A patients clearly identify *PMP22* as the major gene involved in CMT1A and, most likely, also in HNPP. The observation that both duplications and point mutations of the same gene can give rise to a dominantly inherited condition is intriguing. It seems reasonable to speculate that *PMP22* point mutations represent gain-of-function mutations. Conversely, HNPP

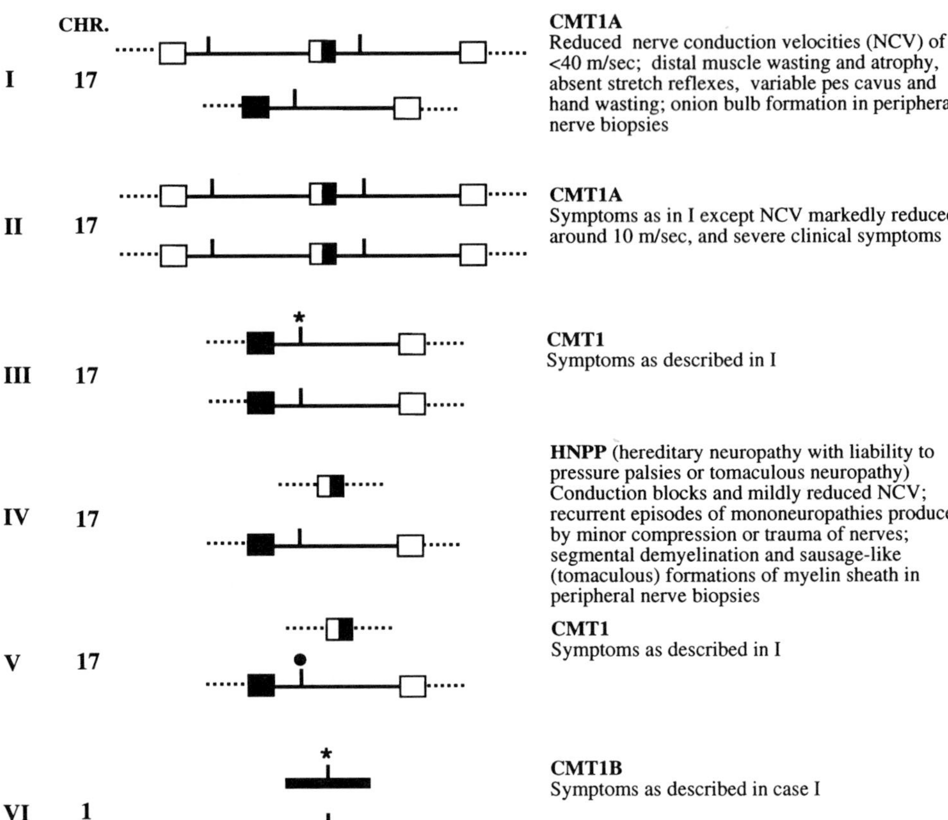
GENOTYPE
PHENOTYPE
CHR.
I 17
CMT1A
Reduced nerve conduction velocities (NCV) of <40 m/sec; distal muscle wasting and atrophy, absent stretch reflexes, variable pes cavus and hand wasting; onion bulb formation in peripheral nerve biopsies
II 17
CMT1A
Symptoms as in I except NCV markedly reduced to around 10 m/sec, and severe clinical symptoms
III 17
*
CMT1
Symptoms as described in I
IV 17
HNPP (hereditary neuropathy with liability to pressure palsies or tomaculous neuropathy)
Conduction blocks and mildly reduced NCV; recurrent episodes of mononeuropathies produced by minor compression or trauma of nerves; segmental demyelination and sausage-like (tomaculous) formations of myelin sheath in peripheral nerve biopsies
V 17
CMT1
Symptoms as described in I
VI 1
*
CMT1B
Symptoms as described in case I

FIG. 154C-1 Genotype/phenotype correlation of inherited peripheral neuropathies. The gross arrangement of sequence in the relevant region on the indicated chromosome (CHR) is depicted schematically under "GENOTYPE." Filled and open rectangular boxes represent CMT1A-REP sequences that flank the 1.5-Mb region duplicated in the 17p11.2-p12 region of the majority of CMT1A patients, which have been postulated to mediate the unequal exchange resulting in the duplication and deletion seen for example in genotypes I and IV, respectively. The horizontal solid lines on chromosome 17 represent the duplication interval, while the dotted lines represent the sequence outside the duplication/deletion interval. The vertical line represents the PMP22 gene on chromosome 17 and P_0 gene on chromosome 1. The asterisk and filled circles denote the presence of a dominant and a recessive mutation in the candidate genes, respectively. Genotype I has been seen in the majority of CMT1 patients, II in one patient, III in two families, IV in four families, V in one patient, and VI in four families. (*From Suter and Patel*[59] *Used by permission of* Human Mutation.)

would be due to loss of function of the *PMP22* gene, although this remains to be proved.

Two complex families with CMT1A have been described. The first is a family in which a duplication, including the *PMP22* gene, was observed to segregate independently from the disease phenotype. Four individuals from this family showed a mild CMT1A phenotype, but they did not have the duplication.[66] The duplication found in the other affected members of the family seems to be smaller than the previously described CMT1A duplication. The possibility exists that two different forms of CMT are present in this family, although duplication and nonduplication patients appear to have the same haplotype. A search for point mutations by single-strand conformational polymorphisms (SSCP) in the nonduplication cases gave negative results.[66]

The second family includes one individual with CMT1 and her three sons.[17] A deletion similar to the one reported in HNPP patients was detected in the mother and in two of the children. The mother had classic CMT1 and the two sons had HNPP. In addition to the deletion, the mother carried a point mutation in the *PMP22* gene on the other chromosome, causing a methionine to threonine amino acid substitution (M118T) at the end of the third putative transmembrane domain. The same point mutation was detected in the third son, who had a normal phenotype. Thus, in this family, the deletion/M118T genotype was associated with a classic CMT1 phenotype, the deletion/normal genotype with an HNPP phenotype, and the M118T/normal genotype with a normal phenotype.[17]

Since the physiological role of the *PMP22* protein is not known, it is difficult to envision the biologic steps leading from the *PMP22* gene rearrangements or mutations to the CMT1A phenotype. It has been proposed that the *PMP22* protein could function as a pore or channel protein.[49] According to this hypothesis, mutations may change the structure of the *PMP22* protein, thereby altering the macromolecular stoichiometry.[54]

Molecular Diagnosis

The finding of a duplication in the majority (>65 percent) of patients with CMT1 greatly facilitates diagnosis. Presymptomatic and prenatal diagnosis can be offered to families with CMT1A. Molecular diagnosis can now be performed also in sporadic CMT1 cases to differentiate between CMT1A and other types of CMT1. As previously mentioned, the duplication can be identified by the following methods:

1. RFLP analysis by Southern blotting
2. PCR analysis using short tandem repeats (STR)
3. PFGE analysis
4. FISH analysis.

A large study on 75 unrelated patients diagnosed clinically with CMT compared the efficiency of the various methods.[34] The conclusions of this study were that RFLP analysis was the most efficient method in most cases, while the identification of a specific duplication junction fragment by PFGE analysis was the most definitive. It is, therefore, suggested that RFLP analysis should be performed first and that PFGE analysis may be used in uninformative cases, and as an independent molecular method to confirm the RFLP results. FISH is probably the best method to detect the HNPP deletion.[44]

ACKNOWLEDGMENTS

We thank Drs. P. Patel and J. Lupski for helpful comments.

REFERENCES

1. Charcot JM, Marie P: Sur une forme particulière d'atrophie musculaire progressive souvent familiale debutante par les pieds et les jambes et atteignante plus tard les mains. *Rev Med* **6**:97, 1886.
2. Tooth HH: *The Peroneal Type of Progressive Muscular Atrophy*. London, H. K. Lewis, 1886.
3. Dyck PJ, Chance P, Lebo R, Carney JA: Hereditary motor and sensory neuropathies, in Dyck PJ (ed): *Peripheral Neuropathy,* 3rd ed. Philadelphia, Saunders, 1992, p 1094.
4. Lupski JR, Garcia CA, Parry GJ, Patel PI: Charcot-Marie-Tooth polyneuropathy syndrome: Clinical, electrophysiologic, and genetic aspects, in Appel S (ed): *Current Neurology*. St. Louis, Mosby–Year Book, 1991, p 1.
5. Lupski JR, Garcia CA: Molecular genetics and neuropathology of Charcot-Marie-Tooth disease type 1A. *Brain Pathol* **2**:337, 1992.
6. Earl CJ, Fullerton PM, Wakefield GS, Schutta HS: Hereditary neuropathy, with liability to pressure palsies. *Q J Med* **33**:481, 1964.
7. Staal A, De Weerdt CJ, Went LN: Hereditary compression syndrome of peripheral nerves. *Neurology* **15**:1008, 1965.
8. Madrid R, Bradley WG: The pathology of neuropathies with focal thickening of the myelin sheath (tomaculous neuropathy): Studies on the formation of the abnormal myelin sheath. *J Neurol Sci* **25**:415, 1975.
9. Debruyne J, Dehaene I, Martin JJ: Hereditary pressure-sensitive neuropathy. *J Neurol Sci* **47**:385, 1980.
10. Dyck PJ, Oviatt KF, Lambert EH: Intensive evaluation of unclassified neuropathies yields improved diagnosis. *Ann Neurol* **10**:222, 1981.
11. Skre H: Genetic and clinical aspects of Charcot-Marie-Tooth's disease. *Clin Genet* **6**:98, 1974.
12. Vance JM, Nicholson GA, Yamaoka LH, Stajich J, Stewart CS, Speer MC, Hung WY, Roses AD, Barker D, Pericak-Vance MA: Linkage of Charcot-Marie-Tooth neuropathy type 1a to chromosome 17. *Exp Neurol* **104**:186, 1989.
13. Bird TD, Ott J, Gilbert ER: Evidence for linkage of Charcot-Marie-Tooth disease neuropathy to the Duffy locus on chromosome number 1. *Am J Hum Genet* **34**:388, 1982.
14. Chance PF, Bird TD, O'Connell P, Leppert M, Lipe H, Lalouel J-M: Linkage and heterogeneity in type 1 Charcot-Marie-Tooth disease (hereditary motor and sensory neuropathy I). *Am J Hum Genet* **47**:915, 1990.
15. Chance PF, Matsunami N, Lensch MW, Smith BS, Bird TD: Analysis of the DNA duplication 17p11.2 in Charcot-Marie-Tooth neuropathy type 1 (HMSN1) pedigrees: Additional evidence for a third autosomal *CMT1* locus. *Neurology* **42**:2037, 1992.
16. Lebo RV, Chance PF, Dyck PJ, Redila-Flores MT, Lynch ED, Golbus MS, Bird TD, King MC, Anderson LA, Hall J, Wiegant J, Jiang Z, Dazin PF, Punnett HH, Schonberg SA, Moore K, Shull MM, Gendler S, Hurko O, Lovelace RE, Latov N, Trofatter J, Conneally PM: Chromosome 1 Charcot-Marie-Tooth syndrome (HMSN1B) locus in FcyRII gene region. *Hum Genet* **88**:1, 1991.
17. Roa BB, Garcia CA, Pentao L, Killian JM, Trask BJ, Suter U, Snipes GJ, Ortiz-Lopez R, Shooter EM, Patel PI, Lupski JR: Evidence for a recessive *PMP22* point mutation in Charcot-Marie-Tooth disease type 1A. *Nat Genet* **5**:189, 1993.
18. Othmane KB, Middleton LT, Loprest LJ, Wilkinson KM, Lennon F, Rozear MP, Stajich JM, Gaskell PC, Roses AD, Pericak-Vance MA, Vance JM: Localization of a gene (CMT2A) for autosomal dominant Charcot-Marie-Tooth disease Type 2 to chromosome 1p and evidence of genetic heterogeneity. *Genomics* **17**:370, 1993.
19. Gal A, Mücke J, Theile H, Wieacker PF, Ropers H-H, Wienker TF: X-linked dominant Charcot-Marie-Tooth disease: Suggestion of linkage with a cloned DNA sequence from the proximal Xq. *Hum Genet* **70**:38, 1985.
20. Fischbeck KH, ar-Rushdi N, Rozear M, Pericak-Vance M, Fryns JP: X-linked neuropathy: Gene localization with DNA probes. *Am J Hum Genet* **37**:A153, 1985.
21. Goonewardena P, Welihinda J, Anvret M, Gyftodimou J, Haegermark A, Iselius L, Lindsten J, Pettersson U: A linkage study of the locus for X-linked Charcot-Marie-Tooth disease. *Clin Genet* **33**:435, 1988.
22. Haites N, Fairweather N, Clark C, Kelly KF, Simpson S, Johnston AW: Linkage in a family with X-linked Charcot-Marie-Tooth disease. *Clin Genet* **35**:399, 1989.
23. Mostacciuolo ML, Muller E, Fardin P, Micaglio GF, Bardoni B, Guioli S, Camerino G, Danieli GA: X-linked Charcot-Marie-Tooth disease. *Hum Genet* **87**:23, 1991.
24. Ionasescu VV, Trofatter J, Haines JL, Summers AM, Ionasescu R, Searby C: Heterogeneity in X-linked recessive Charcot-Marie-Tooth neuropathy. *Am J Hum Genet* **48**:1075, 1991.
25. Ionasescu VV, Trofatter J, Haines JL, Ionasescu R, Searby C: Mapping of the gene for X-linked dominant Charcot-Marie-Tooth neuropathy. *Neurology* **42**:903, 1992.
26. Ionasescu VV, Trofatter J, Haines JL, Summers AM, Ionasescu R, Searby C: X-linked recessive Charcot-Marie-Tooth neuropathy: Clinical and genetic study. *Muscle Nerve* **15**:368, 1992.
27. Bergoffen J, Trofatter J, Pericak-Vance MA, Haines JL, Chance PF, Fischbeck KH: Linkage localization of X-linked Charcot-Marie-Tooth disease. *Am J Hum Genet* **52**:312, 1993.
28. Lupski JR, Montes de Oca-Luna R, Slaugenhaupt S, Pentao L, Guzzetta V, Trask BJ, Saucedo-Cardenas O, Barker DF, Killian JM, Garcia CA, Chakravarti A, Patel PI: DNA duplication associated with Charcot-Marie-Tooth disease type 1A. *Cell* **66**:219, 1991.
29. Raeymaekers P, Timmerman V, Nelis E, de Jonghe P, Hoogendijk JE, Baas F, Barker DF, Martin JJ, de Visser M, Bolhuis PA, van Broeckhoven C, HMSN Collaborative Research Group: Duplication in chromosome 17p11.2 in Charcot-Marie-Tooth neuropathy type 1a (CMT 1a). *Neuromus Disord* **1**:93, 1991.
30. Kaku DA, Parry GJ, Malamut R, Lupski JR, Garcia CA: Nerve conduction studies in Charcot-Marie-Tooth polyneuropathy associated with a segmental duplication of chromosome 17. *Neurology* **43**:1806, 1993.
31. Brice A, Ravisé N, Stevanin G, Gugenheim M, Bouche P, Penet C, Agid Y, French CMT Research Group: Duplication within chromosome 17p11.2 in 12 families of French ancestry with Charcot-Marie-Tooth disease type 1a. *J Med Genet* **29**:807, 1992.
32. Hallam PJ, Harding AE, Berciano J, Barker DF, Malcolm S: Duplication of part of chromosome 17 is commonly associated with hereditary motor and sensory neuropathy type 1 (Charcot-Marie-Tooth disease type 1). *Ann Neurol* **31**:570, 1992.
33. Bellone E, Mandich P, Mancardi GL, Schenone A, Uccelli A, Abbruzzese M, Sghirlanzoni A, Pareyson D, Ajmar F: Charcot-Marie-Tooth (CMT) la duplication at 17p11.2 in Italian families. *J Med Genet* **29**:492, 1992.
34. Wise CA, Garcia CA, Davis SN, Zhang H, Pentao L, Patel PI, Lupski JR: Molecular analyses of unrelated Charcot-Marie-Tooth (CMT) disease patients suggest a high frequency of the CMT1A duplication. *Am J Hum Genet* **53**:853, 1993.
35. Lupski JR, Pentao L, Williams LL, Patel PI: Stable inheritance of the CMT1A DNA duplication in two patients with CMT1 and NF1. *Am J Med Genet* **45**:92, 1993.
36. Hoogendijk JE, Hensels GW, Gabreëls-Festen AAWM, Gabreëls FJM, Janssen EAM, de Johnghe P, Martin J-J, van Broeckhoven C, Valentijn LJ, Baas F, de Visser M, Bolhuis PA: *De-novo* mutation in hereditary motor and sensory neuropathy type 1. *Lancet* **339**:1081, 1992.
37. Pentao L, Wise CA, Chinault AC, Patel PI, Lupski JR:

Charcot-Marie-Tooth type 1A duplication appears to arise from recombination at repeat sequences flanking the 1.5 Mb monomer unit. *Nat Genet* **2**:292, 1992.

38. Raeymaekers P, Timmerman V, Nelis E, van Hul W, de Jonghe P, Martin J-J, van Broeckhoven C, HMSN Collaborative Research Group: Estimation of the size of the chromosome 17p11.2 duplication in Charcot-Marie-Tooth neuropathy type 1a (CMT1a). *J Med Genet* **29**:5, 1992.
39. Valentijn LJ, Bolhuis PA, Zorn I, Hoogendijk JE, van den Bosch N, Hensels GW, Stanton VP Jr, Housman DE, Fischbeck KH, Ross DA, Nicholson GA, Meershoek EJ, Dauwerse HG, van Ommen GJB, Baas F: The peripheral myelin gene *PMP-22/GAS-3* is duplicated in Charcot-Marie-Tooth disease type 1A. *Nat Genet* **1**:166, 1992.
40. Hoogendijk JE, Hensels GW, Zorn I, Valentijn L, Janssen EAM, de Visser M, Barker DF, de Visser BWO, Baas F, Bolhuis PA: The duplication in Charcot-Marie-Tooth disease Type 1a spans at least 1100 kb on chromosome 17p11.2. *Hum Genet* **88**:215, 1991.
41. Nieuwenhuijsen BW, Chen KL, Chinault AC, Wang S, Valmiki VH, Meershoek EJ, van Ommen GJB, Fischbeck KH: A yeast artificial chromosome contig spanning the Charcot-Marie-Tooth disease type 1A duplication region. *Hum Mol Genet* **1**:605, 1992.
42. Yen PH, Li X-M, Tsai SP, Johnson C, Mohandas T, Shapiro LJ: Frequent deletions of the human X chromosome distal short arm result from recombination between low copy repetitive elements. *Cell* **61**:603, 1990.
43. Ballabio A, Bardoni B, Guioli S, Basler E, Camerino G: Two families of low-copy-number repeats are interspersed on Xp22.3: Implications for the high frequency of deletions in this region. *Genomics* **8**:263, 1990.
44. Chance PF, Alderson MK, Leppig KA, Lensch MW, Matsunami N, Smith B, Swanson PD, Odelberg SJ, Disteche CM, Bird TD: DNA deletion associated with hereditary neuropathy with liability to pressure palsies. *Cell* **72**:143, 1993.
45. Falconer DS: Two new mutants, "Trembler" and "reeler," with neurological action in the house mouse (Mus. Musculus L). *J Genet* **50**:192, 1951.
46. Henry EW, Cowen JS, Sidman RL: Comparison of Trembler and Trembler-J mouse phenotypes: Varying severity of peripheral hypomyelination. *J Neuropathol Exp Neurol* **42**:688, 1983.
47. Davisson MT: X-linked genetic homologies between mouse and man. *Genomics* **1**:213, 1987.
48. Suter U, Welcher AA, Ozcelik T, Snipes GJ, Kosaras B, Francke U, Billings-Gagliardi S, Sidman RL, Shooter EM: The *Trembler* mouse carries a point mutation in a myelin gene. *Nature* **356**:241, 1992.
49. Suter U, Moskow JJ, Welcher AA, Snipes GJ, Kosaras B, Sidman RL, Buchberg AM, Shooter EM: A leucine-to-proline mutation in the putative first transmembrane domain of the 22-kDa peripheral myelin protein in the *Tembler-J* mouse. *Proc Natl Acad Sci USA* **89**:4382, 1992.
50. Patel PI, Roa BB, Welcher AA, Schoener-Scott R, Trask BJ, Pentao L, Snipes GJ, Garcia CA, Francke U, Shooter EM, Lupski JR, Suter U: The gene for the peripheral myelin protein PMP-22 is a candidate for Charcot-Marie-Tooth disease type 1A. *Nat Genet* **1**:159, 1992.
51. Timmerman V, Nelis E, van Hul W, Nieuwenhuijsen BW, Chen KL, Wang S, Ben Othman K, Cullen B, Leach RJ, Hanemann CO, de Jonghe P, Raeymaekers P, van Ommen G-JB, Martin J-J, Müller HW, Vance JM, Fischbeck KH, van Broeckhoven C: The peripheral myelin protein gene *PMP-22* is contained within the Charcot-Marie-Tooth disease type 1A duplication. *Nat Genet* **1**:171, 1992.
52. Matsunami N, Smith B, Ballard L, Lensch MW, Robertson M, Albertsen H, Hanemann CO, Müller HW, Bird TD, White R, Chance PF: Peripheral myelin protein-22 gene maps in the duplication in chromosome 17p11.2 associated with Charcot-Marie-Tooth 1A. *Nat Genet* **1**:176, 1992.
53. Valentijn LJ, Baas F, Wolterman RA, Hoogendijk JE, van den Bosch NHA, Zorn I, Gabreëls-Festen AAWM, de Visser M, Bolhuis PA: Identical point mutations of *PMP-22* in *Trembler-J* mouse and Charcot-Marie-Tooth disease type 1A. *Nat Genet* **2**:288, 1992.
54. Roa BB, Garcia CA, Suter U, Kulpa DA, Wise CA, Mueller J, Welcher AA, Snipes GJ, Shooter EM, Patel PI, Lupski JR: Charcot-Marie-Tooth disease type 1A association with a spontaneous point mutation in the *PMP22* gene. *N Engl J Med* **329**:96, 1993.
55. Hayasaka K, Himoro M, Wang Y, Takata M, Minoshima S, Shimizu N, Miura M, Uyemura K, Takada G: Structure and chromosomal localization of the gene encoding the human myelin protein zero (MPZ). *Genomics* **17**:755, 1993.
56. Hayasaka K, Himoro M, Sato W, Takada G, Uyemura K, Shimizu N, Bird TD, Conneally PM, Chance PF: Charcot-Marie-Tooth neuropathy type 1B is associated with mutations of the myelin P_0 gene. *Nat Genet* **5**:31, 1993.
57. Kulkens T, Bolhuis PA, Wolterman RA, Kemp S, te Nijenhuis S, Valentijn LJ, Hensels GW, Jennekens FGI, de Visser M, Hoogendijk JE, Baas F: Deletion of the serine 34 codon from the major peripheral myelin protein P_0 gene in Charcot-Marie-Tooth disease type 1B. *Nat Genet* **5**:35, 1993.
58. Hayasaka K, Takada G, Ionasescu VV: Mutation of the myelin Po gene in Charcot-Marie-Tooth neuropathy type 1B. *Hum Mol Genet* **2**:1369, 1993.
59. Suter U, Patel PI: Genetic basis of inherited peripheral neuropathies. *Hum Mut* **3**:95, 1994.
60. Lupski JR: An inherited DNA rearrangement and gene dosage effect are responsible for the most common autosomal dominant peripheral neuropathy: Charcot-Marie-Tooth disease type 1A. *Clin Res* **40**:645, 1992.
61. Patel PI: Charcot-Marie-Tooth disease type 1A: Mutational mechanisms and candidate gene. *Curr Opin Genet Dev* **3**:438, 1993.
62. Lupski JR, Wise CA, Kuwano A, Pentao L, Parke JT, Glaze DG, Ledbetter DH, Greenberg F, Patel PI: Gene dosage is a mechanism for Charcot-Marie-Tooth disease type 1A. *Nat Genet* **1**:29, 1992.
63. Roa BB, Garcia CA, Wise CA, Anderson K, Greenberg F, Patel PI, Lupski JR: Gene dosage as a mechanism for a common autosomal dominant peripheral neuropathy: Charcot-Marie-Tooth disease type 1A, in Epstein CJ (ed): *Phenotypic Mapping of Down Syndrome and Other Aneuploid Conditions*. New York, Wiley–Liss, 1993, p 187.
64. Chance PF, Bird TD, Matsunami N, Lensch MW, Brothman AR, Feldman GM: Trisomy 17p associated with Charcot-Marie-Tooth neuropathy type 1A phenotype: Evidence for gene dosage as a mechanism in CMT1A. *Neurology* **42**:2295, 1992.
65. Upadhyaya M, Roberts SH, Farnham J, MacMillan JC, Clarke A, Heath JP, Hodges ICG, Harper PS: Charcot-Marie-Tooth disease type 1A (CMT1A) associated with a maternal duplication of chromosome 17p11.2-12. *Hum Genet* **91**:392, 1993.
66. Ionasescu VV, Ionasescu R, Searby C, Barker DF: Charcot-Marie-Tooth neuropathy type 1A with both duplication and non-duplication. *Hum Mol Genet* **2**:405, 1993.

CHAPTER 154D

Waardenburg Syndrome

Huda Y. Zoghbi ■ Andrea Ballabio

1. **Waardenburg syndrome (WS) is the most common form of inherited congenital deafness. It is inherited in an autosomal dominant pattern with variable penetrance. Based on clinical classification at least three distinct types have been identified, of which WS type I (WS-I) is the most common.**

2. **WS-I is characterized by depigmentation of the hair and skin, heterochromia irides, dystopia canthorum, congenital deafness, a broad nasal root, and confluent eye brows. The absence of dystopia canthorum has been the distinguishing feature of WS-II, and upper-limb abnormalities are characteristic of WS-III.**

3. **The identification of a paracentric inversion of chromosome 2 in a WS-I patient and linkage studies allowed the mapping of the WS-I gene to human chromosome 2q37. Genetic heterogeneity for WS-I was demonstrated based on the finding that only 45 percent of WS-I families show linkage to chromosome 2q.**

4. **The *splotch* (*Sp*) mouse mutant, a well-characterized mutant with neural-tube defects and neural-crest migration abnormalities in homozygous animals, maps to the proximal portion of mouse chromosome 1 which is syntenic with human 2q37. *Sp* heterozygotes have pigmentary disturbances involving the feet, tail, and abdomen.**

5. ***Sp* was proposed as a model for WS-I based on the phenotypic similarity between WS and *Sp*, the mapping of both disorders to syntenic chromosomal regions, and the implication of neural-crest-derived cells in both disorders.**

6. **The mapping of a paired-box gene *Pax-3* to the proximal portion of mouse chromosome 1 led to the discovery that *Pax-3* is mutated in several *Sp* allele variants. Mutations in the human homologue *PAX3* were subsequently identified in several patients with WS-I, one family with possible WS-II, and another with WS-III. The PAX proteins are a family of transcription factors active in developmental regulation; the pattern of expression of *PAX3* is consistent with the phenotypic abnormalities in *Sp* and WS. It is hypothesized that these phenotypes result from the differential expression of genes regulated by *PAX3*.**

A list of standard abbreviations is located immediately preceding the index in each volume. Additional abbreviations used in this chapter include: e5 = a conserved regulatory sequence first described in the *even-skipped* gene of Drosophila; PAX, *PAX*, or *Pax* = paired box protein, human gene, or mouse gene respectively; *Sey* = *small-eye* mouse locus; *Sp* = *splotch*, including Sp^4 Sp^d, etc. alleles; WS = Waardenburg syndrome, including WS-I, WS-II, etc.

CLINICAL FEATURES AND CLASSIFICATION

In August of 1947 David Klein presented the case of a 10-year-old deaf and mute child at a meeting of the Swiss Society of Genetics. The child had partial depigmentation of the hair and skin, slate-blue irides, and musculoskeletal abnormalities of the upper limbs. A full case report about this patient was published by Klein in 1950.[1] In December of 1947 Petrus Waardenburg presented the case of a deaf and mute 72-year-old man and subsequently published a case report in 1948.[2] In 1951, Waardenburg published a full account of the syndrome,[6] describing it as an autosomal dominant disorder characterized by the following features:

1. Depigmentation of the eyes, hair, and skin
2. Dystopia canthorum (increase in the distance between the inner angles of the eyelids)
3. Congenital deafness
4. Broad nasal root
5. Synophrys (confluent eyebrows).

This disorder, now known as Waardenburg syndrome (WS), is also called "Klein-Waardenburg syndrome," although the latter term is generally used for a particular subtype of WS distinguished by the presence of limb malformations, as will be described below.

More than 1500 cases of WS, representing all ethnic groups, have been reported.[3] In 1971, Arias raised the issue of possible heterogeneity in WS and suggested that the disorder can be divided into three distinct types: type I with dystopia canthorum, type II without dystopia canthorum, and type III ("pseudo-Waardenburg" syndrome) without dystopia canthorum but with unilateral ptosis.[4] Hageman and Delleman[5] reviewed 1285 patients from the literature and 34 patients from families in the Netherlands. They concluded that there are two distinct types that can be distinguished clinically: type I with dystopia canthorum and type II without dystopia canthorum. Both types are inherited in an autosomal dominant fashion. Today the classification of WS includes type I and type II; the "Waardenburg-Klein" variant; and two other possible variants, "pseudo-Waardenburg" and "Waardenburg-Shah" syndrome.

Waardenburg syndrome type 1 (WS-I) is responsible for 0.5 to 3 percent of congenital deafness based on several published studies.[6–12] The frequency of the syndrome has been estimated between 1:32,400 and 1:42,000.[6,10,11] The syndrome is inherited with an autosomal dominant pattern with variability in penetrance. The most frequent cutaneous pigmentary abnormality is a white forelock; the skin beneath the forelock is usually depigmented. Premature graying, occurring as early as the teens, can involve the scalp, eyebrows, ciliary body of the eye, and body hair.[13] Patches of depigmentation on the face, neck, anterior chest, abdomen, and limbs are also a common feature. The patches of depigmentation are similar to those observed in piebaldism. Hyperpigmented macules may occur on depigmented or normal skin. Partial or total heterochromia irides is found in more than 20 percent of the reported cases.[13] Unilateral depigmentation of the irides typically gives rise to irides of different colors, one usually being slate-blue. Bilateral involvement results in pale-blue eyes. In addition, confluent eyebrows and broadened nasal root are two fairly common facial features.

Sensorineural deafness occurs in 9 to 37.5 percent of the patients.[5,6,13] The deafness may be unilateral or bilateral, moderate or severe. Auditory brain-stem responses typically demonstrate sensorineural deafness without any particular distinguishing features unique to this syndrome. Histopathological study of the inner ear from one patient with WS revealed absence of the organ of Corti, atrophy of the spinal ganglion and nerve, and absence of melanocytes.[13] Numerous anomalies have been reported in WS type I. These include cleft lip and palate, Hirschsprung disease, facial asymmetry, facial palsy, hypoplasia of the middle ear ossicles, iris coloboma, genitourinary abnormalities, and neural-tube defects, as reviewed elsewhere.[3,14]

Histopathological findings in WS include absent or reduced number of melanocytes in depigmented skin. Abnormal migration of neural crest cells has been suggested by Kaplan and de Chadérevian.[15] Histologic analysis of the temporal bones from two cases of WS revealed atrophy of the vestibular neuroepithelia and stria vascularis of the inner ear.[16]

Waardenburg syndrome type II (WS-II) is also an autosomal dominant disorder; its clinical features are similar to those described in type I. The major feature that led several investigators to distinguish this type from WS type I is the absence of dystopia canthorum. In the review by Hageman and Delleman[5] the authors commented on the higher incidence of bilateral deafness in type II (50 percent) as compared with type I (25 percent).

A few patients with the characteristic features of WS type I and upper limb defects have been described. This association is referred to as WS type III or Klein-Waardenburg syndrome. These patients typically have the pigmentary and craniofacial features of WS-I in combination with a myoosteoarticular defect of the upper limbs and pectoral region. Musculoskeletal hypoplasia, rigidity of joints, axillary webs, and camptodactyly were observed in the patient reported by Klein as well as in other reported cases.[17,18] An autosomal dominant inheritance pattern for this syndrome was suggested by Klein.[19]

In 1981 Shah et al.[20] described a syndrome that they considered a variant of WS in spite of an autosomal recessive inheritance pattern. This is a rare, potentially fatal disorder in which affected individuals have depigmentation of the hair, eye, and skin associated with Hirschsprung disease of the long segment type. Several families with parental consanguinity, multiple affected sibs, and normal parents have been reported with this variant, termed "Waardenburg-Shah syndrome," supporting the hypothesis for an autosomal recessive inheritance.[20–22]

The pseudo-Waardenburg syndrome is a rare variant characterized by congenital unilateral ptosis of the eyelid, heterochromia irides, congenital deafness, light hair with scattered white hairs, dystopia canthorum, and a broad nasal root.[4]

MAPPING OF THE WS-I LOCUS

The first hint on the mapping of the WS-I gene came from the finding of a paracentric inversion of chromosome 2 in a 20-month-old boy with this disorder.[23] This boy had heterochromia irides, hypopigmentary and hyperpigmentary abnormalities of the skin, and sensorineural deafness. Chromosome analysis demonstrated a *de novo* paracentric inversion of chromosome 2 [inv(2)(q35q37.3)]. This finding suggested that the WS-I gene might be located at one of the breakpoints of the chromosomal inversion: either at 2q35 or at 2q37.3. Foy and colleagues performed genetic studies using a number of genetic markers on five multigeneration kindreds with WS type I.[24] These studies allowed them to exclude the WS type I locus from approximately 23 percent of the human genome. Based on the finding of the *de novo* inversion of 2q35-q37,[23] a probe derived from the placental alkaline phosphatase (ALPP) locus, which maps to 2q37, was used for additional linkage analyses. Linkage was demonstrated between the WS-I locus and ALPP with a peak Lod score of 4.76 at a recombination fraction of 0.023. This finding permitted the assignment of WS-I to 2q37, the region containing the distal breakpoint of the inversion.

Asher et al.[25] confirmed the previous genetic mapping data by demonstrating tight linkage with ALPP and fibronectin 1 (FN1) in a large four-generation kindred. In the first report of the WS consortium, Farrer et al.[26] described the results of genetic studies on 41 WS-I and three WS-II families. These studies were aimed at refining the location of WS locus and at evaluating the extent of genetic heterogeneity. The data from the study confirmed that WS-I is responsible for the disorder in approximately 45 percent of all the families they studied. Among the WS-II families, the disease was unlinked to 2q in the two families which were informative.

SPLOTCH, A MOUSE MODEL FOR WAARDENBURG SYNDROME TYPE I

The mouse mutant *splotch* (*Sp*) arose spontaneously on a C57BL inbred background,[27] and since then, several other mutants, either spontaneous as in the case of *Sp*-delayed (Sp^d),[28] or radiation-induced as in the cases of *Sp*-retarded (Sp^r), Sp^{1H}, Sp^{2H}, and Sp^{4H}, which map to the proximal portion of mouse chromosome 1, have been shown to be allelic to *Sp*. These mutants are classified as semidominant lethal and serve as mouse models for neural-tube defects and deficiencies in neural-crest cell derivates. Most *Sp*, Sp^{1H}, and Sp^{2H} homozygotes have meningoceles, spina bifida, or malformed inner ears, and over half have exencephaly.[29,30] Defects in structures derived from neural-crest cells, such as spinal ganglia, Schwann cells, and neural-crest-derived heart tissue have also been observed in *Sp* mutants and their variants. All these mutants die in utero at approximately 14 to 16 days of gestation.[29,31] Sp^{4H} homozygotes die prenatally, but the approximate time of death is unknown. Sp^d is the least severe allele; spina bifida develops in homozygotes, who survive until birth,[28] while Sp^r homozygotes are presumed to die before implantation. The Sp^r mutation involves a cytogenetically detectable deletion of chromosome 1 band C4.[32]

All heterozygous *Sp* mutants and their allelic variants have a similar phenotype characterized by white spotting of the abdomen, feet, and tail tip. Sp^r heterozygotes display growth retardation in addition to the white patches. Based on the phenotypic similarity between *Sp* and WS (pigmentary abnormalities), the implication of neural-crest-derived cell in both disorders, and the mapping of both disorders to a syntenic chromosomal region in mice and humans, it was suggested that WS-I is the human homologue of the mouse *Splotch* mutant.[24,33] It is interesting to note that *Sp* heterozygotes, unlike WS patients, have normal hearing and do not have any sign of abnormal morphogenesis of the inner ear.[34]

THE *Pax-3* GENE

The paired box is a DNA-binding domain that is highly conserved throughout evolution.[35,36] Eight different genes containing this domain have been identified to date in several species and compose the PAX multigene family.[37,38] Table 154D-1 lists the chromosomal localizations of the PAX genes in humans and mice and the phenotypes associated with various deletions and point mutations in some of these genes. As shown in the table, one of these genes, *Pax-3,* was mapped to the proximal portion of mouse chromosome 1, which is the same chromosomal region where *Sp* is located.[39] This led to the hypothesis that the *Splotch* mouse mutant was due to a mutation in the *Pax-3* gene. This hypothesis was strengthened by the study of the spatial and temporal expression of *Pax-3,* which revealed expression in neural-crest cell derivatives just before neural-tube closure. Furthermore, linkage analysis of *Pax-3* and *Splotch* showed no recombination between these two loci in two independent studies involving large panels of backcross mice.[40,41]

To understand the molecular basis of the genetic defect in *Sp* mutants the *Pax-3* gene was analyzed in these mutants. *Sp*, Sp^r, and Sp^{2H} mutants were tested for alterations in the *Pax-3* gene. *Pax-3* was found to be completely deleted on the mutant chromosome in heterozygous $Sp^{r/+}$ mice. A 32-bp deletion within the paired box of the *Pax-3* gene was detected in Sp^{2H}/Sp^{2H} embryos.[31] The deletion interrupts the reading frame and creates a termination codon downstream of Ala 237 that results in a truncated protein lacking the C-terminal half. No gross rearrangements were detected in the *Pax-3* gene of *Sp*/*Sp* embryos. To identify the putative mutation in the *Pax-3* gene in *Sp*/*Sp* mice, mRNA from mutant and wild-type mice was analyzed by PCR amplification, resulting in the identification of novel fragments in the mutant mice. Cloning and sequencing of cDNA and genomic DNA from *Pax-3* from *Sp*/*Sp* mutants identified a sequence variation in intron 3 involving five nucleotides including an A→T transversion at the invariant 3′ AG splice acceptor site of intron 3. This mutation impairs the splicing of intron 3 and results in four aberrantly spliced mRNA transcripts that encode for presumably, nonfunctional *Pax-3* proteins.[42] Several additional mutations of the *Pax-3* gene have been identified in different *Splotch* alleles.[41,43] A summary of the mutations/deletions identified to date in *Sp* mice and their allelic variants is presented in Table 154D-2.

MOLECUALR BASIS OF WAARDENBURG SYNDROME

Several human genes homologous to mouse and *Drosophila melanogaster* PAX genes have been identified (see Table 154D-1).[39,44,45] Given the overlap between the phenotypes of WS-I and *Splotch* and the syntenic map positions of these two disorders, the human homologue of the *Pax-3* gene, termed "HuP2," was tested for mutations in families with WS-I.[46,47] Tassabehji et al. identified a deletion of six amino acids in the paired domain,[46] and Baldwin et al. identified a C-to-T substitution in exon 2, resulting in the alteration of proline to leucine at a position within the paired domain, which is invariant in PAX proteins.[47] Of interest is the fact that the Brazilian family studied by Baldwin et al. had a high incidence of hearing loss (78 percent) as compared with

Table 154D-1 PAX3 Mutations in Mice and Humans

Phenotype	Nucleotide(s) Substitution/Deletion	Amino Acid Change	Domain	Reference
Sp^r	Complete deletion of *Pax-3*			31, 41
Sp^{1H}, Sp^{2H}	32 bp deletion	Deletion Ala 237 → Thr 248	Homeobox domain presumed to result in a truncated protein	31, 43
Sp	AG → TG	Splice acceptor site mutation at the intron 3–exon 4 boundary		31, 41
Sp^{4H}	Complete deletion of *Pax-3*			41
Sp^d	GGA → CGA	GLy 42 → Arg	Paired domain	43
WS-I	18-bp deletion	Met 29 → Ile 34	Paired domain	46
WS-I	CCG → CTG	Pro 50 → Leu	Paired domain	47
WS-I	14-bp deletion	Arg 56 or Tyr 57 → Thr 60	Paired domain stop codon in exon 3	48
WS-I	Single base deletion	Frameshift	Paired domain stop condon in exon 3	49
WS-I	2-bp deletion	Frameshift	Octapeptide motif premature termination in exon 5	49
WS-II	GGC → GCC	Gly 48 → Ala	Paired domain	49
WS-I	Complete deletion of *PAX3*			49, 51
WS-I	CGC → CTC	Arg 56 → Leu	Paired domain	45
WS-III	AAC → CAC	Asn 47 → His	Paired domain	45
WS-III	Complete deletion of *PAX3*			52

Table 154D-2 Paired-Box-Containing Genes, Chromosomal Localization, and Associated Phenotypes in Humans and Mice

Gene	Human Map Position	Human Syndromes	Mouse Map Position	Mouse Mutants
Pax-1, PAX1 (HuP48)	20		2 (distal)	*Undulated*
Pax-2, PAX2	10q11.2–qter		19	
Pax-3, PAX3 (HuP2)	2	Waardenburg type 1	1	*Splotch*
Pax-4, PAX4	7q22–qter		6	
Pax-5, PAX5	9p		4	
Pax-6, PAX6	11	Aniridia	2 (central)	*Small-eye*
Pax-7, PAX7 (HuP1)	1p36		4	
Pax-8, PAX8	2		2 (proximal)	

the typical incidence (20 percent) in WS-I families. It is possible that the proline-to-leucine mutation within the paired domain in this family has an important effect on ear development and hearing.

Many additional mutations in the HuP2 gene were identified in patients with WS-I. These included deletions[48] and point mutations most of which involve the paired box domain.[45,49] Tsukamoto et al.[50] cloned and characterized the inversion breakpoint in the patient with WS-I and the paracenteric inversion (2q35-37.3) and demonstrated that HuP2 was disrupted by the inversion event.

Mutations in the *PAX3* gene (previously referred to as HuP2) have also been identified in one family with possible WS-II and another with WS-III. Both mutations were in the highly conserved paired domain.[45,49] Interstitial deletions of distal 2q encompassing the *PAX3* gene have been described in patients with WS-I[49,51] and in one patient with WS-III.[52] These data suggest that, although WS-I, WS-II, and WS-III are in general distinct clinical entities, a subset of families with these phenotypes share a common molecular mechanism. The observation that genetic linkage to chromosome 2q37 is demonstrated in 45 to 70 percent of WS-I families suggests that at least one other locus is involved in the WS-I phenotype.[26,53] It is intriguing that sizable deletions involving the *PAX3* gene have been also observed in patients with other congenital anomalies but without the features of WS.[54,55] Pasteris et al. suggested that the severe developmental anomalies typically associated with the larger deletions in chromosome 2q might obscure or interfere with the development of the WS phenotype.[52]

TENTATIVE PATHOGENETIC MODEL FOR *SPLOTCH* AND WS-I

Comparison of the murine and human PAX3 with other known paired proteins reveals three conserved domains within the PAX3 protein, the paired domain, the octapeptide motif, and the homeodomain. As is apparent from Table 154D-2, all the mutations described to date affect the paired box, except for one case in which the highly conserved octapeptide motif was involved. Paired domain–containing genes have been shown to be transcription factors involved in developmental regulation.[56–58] Although biologically relevant target genes have not yet been discovered, sequences that serve as DNA binding sites and allow transactivation of downstream reporter genes have been identified. The e5 sequence in the *Drosophila even-skipped* promoter represents a target for the *Drosophila* paired gene.[59] The e5 sequence consists of two overlapping recognition elements, one that is recognized by the paired domain and the other by the homeodomain. Goulding et al.[60] demonstrated that the PAX3 protein is able to bind in vitro to e5 and that both the paired domain and the homeodomain of PAX3 are involved in the DNA binding.

Mutations in *PAX3* in WS-I and *Pax-3* in *Splotch* mice either alter highly conserved amino acids within the paired domain and subsequently alter binding to the e5 sequence, as it has been demonstrated for the 18-bp deletion,[46] or change the structure of the PAX3 protein to result in a truncated protein that lacks either the homeodomain or both the octapeptide motif and the homeodomain. The pattern of expression of PAX3 is consistent with the phenotypic abnormalities seen in WS-I and *Splotch*. PAX3 is expressed in the primordial cells involved in the dorsal-ventral organization of the neural tube prior to neural-tube differentiation. Also expression of *PAX3* has been shown in a subpopulation of craniofacial neural-crest cells. Given that the cell type thought to be affected in WS-I and *Splotch* is of neural-crest origin, it is speculated that differential expression of *PAX3* controlled genes may lead to these phenotypes.[61] The expression of *PAX3* on days 10 and 11 in the undifferentiated mesenchyme of the forelimb and hindlimb[60] may be relevant to the limb abnormalities in WS-III patients.

To date three mouse mutants have been identified in the eight-member PAX family of genes. These are: *undulated*, which is caused by a mutation in *Pax-1*[58]; *Splotch*, which is caused by mutations in *Pax-3*, and *Small-eye* (*Sey*) caused by mutations in *Pax-6*.[62] Mutations in the human homologue, *PAX-6*, have been shown to cause aniridia in humans.[63,64] At this time it is not clear whether the *Pax-3* mutations result in neural-tube defects via loss of function or gain of function. However, given that different mutations in the mouse *Pax-3* gene produce the same phenotype in both spontaneous (*Sp*) and radiation-induced (Sp^{1H} and Sp^{2H}) mouse mutants and that deletion and point mutations in the human *PAX3* result in a similar phenotype, it is speculated that these are loss-of-function mutations.[42] This implies that gene dosage may be critical for PAX genes and that the activity provided by one allele is already below a critical threshold, which will subsequently result in the altered phenotypes.

REFERENCES

1. Klein D: Albinisme partiel (leucisme) avec surdi-mutite, blepharophimosis et dysplasie myo-osteo-articulaire. *Helv Paediatr Acta* **5**:38, 1950.
2. Waardenburg P: Dystopia punctorum lacrimalium, blepharophimosis en partiele iris atrophie bij een doofstomme. *Ned Tijdschr Geneeskd* **92**:3463, 1948.
3. da-Silva EO: Waardenburg I Syndrome: A clinical and genetic

study of two large Brazilian kindreds, and literature review. *Am J Med Genet* **40**:65, 1991.

4. Arias S: Genetic heterogeneity in the Waardenburg syndrome. *Birth Defects* **7**:87, 1971.
5. Hageman MJ, Delleman JW: Heterogeneity in Waardenburg Syndrome. *Am J Hum Genet* **29**:468, 1977.
6. Waardenburg PJ: A new syndrome combining developmental anomalies of the eyelids, eyebrows, and nose root with pigmentary defects of the iris and head hair and with congenital deafness. *Am J Hum Genet* **3**:195, 1951.
7. DiGeorge AM, Olmsted RW, Harley RD: Waardenburg's syndrome. *J Pediatr* **57**:649, 1960.
8. Partington MW: Waardenburg's syndrome and heterochromia iridium in a deaf school population. *Can Med Assoc J* **90**:1008, 1964.
9. Reed WB, Stone VM, Boder E, Ziprkowski L: Pigmentary disorders in association with congenital deafness. *Arch Dermatol* **95**:176, 1967.
10. Hanta Y, Azumi M: Waardenburg syndrome in Japan. *Jpn J Hum Genet* **11**:94, 1967.
11. Hageman MJ: Waardenburg's syndrome in Kenyan Africans. *Trop Geogr Med* **30**:45, 1978.
12. Sellars S, Beighton P: The Waardenburg syndrome in deaf children in Southern Africa. *S Afr Med J* **63**:725, 1983.
13. Ortonne J-P: Piebaldism, Waardenburg's syndrome, and related disorders. "Neural crest depigmentation syndromes?" *Dermatol Clin* **6**:205, 1988.
14. Kromberg JGR, Krause A: Waardenburg syndrome and spina bifida. *Am J Med Genet* **45**:536, 1993.
15. Kaplan P, de Chadérevian JP: Piebaldism-Waardenburg syndrome: Histopathologic evidence for a neural crest syndrome. *Am J Med Genet* **31**:679, 1988.
16. Rarey KE, Davis LE: Inner ear anomalies in Waardenburg's syndrome associated with Hirschsprung's disease. *Int J Pediatr Otorhinolaryngol* **8**:181, 1984.
17. Marx P, Bertrand J: Un cas de syndrome Waardenburg-Klein. *Bull Mem Soc Fr Ophthalmol* **68**:444, 1968.
18. Goodman RM, Lewithal I, Soloman A: Upper limb involvement in the Klein-Waardenburg syndrome. *Am J Med Genet* **11**:425, 1982.
19. Klein D: Historical background and evidence for dominant inheritance of the Klein-Waardenburg syndrome (type III). *Am J Med Genet* **14**:231, 1983.
20. Shah KN, Dalal SJ, Desai MP, Sheth PN, Joshi NC, Ambani LM: White forlock, pigmentary disorders of iridis, and long segment Hirschsprung disease. Possible variant of Waardenburg syndrome. *J Pediatr* **99**:432, 1981.
21. Farndon PA, Bianchi A: Waardenburg's syndrome associated with total aganglionosis. *Arch Dis Child* **58**:932, 1983.
22. Kulkarni ML, Kurian M, Guruprasad G, Panchaksariah MS: Genetic heterogeneity in Waardenburg's syndrome. *J Med Genet* **26**:411, 1989.
23. Ishikiriyama S, Tonoki H, Shibuya Y, Chin S, Harada N, Abe K, Niikawa N: Waardenburg syndrome type I in a child with de novo inversion (2) (q35q37.3). *Am J Med Genet* **33**:505, 1989.
24. Foy C, Newton V, Wellesley D, Harris R, Read AP: Assignment of the locus for Waardenburg syndrome type I to human chromosome 2q37 and possible homology to the Splotch mouse. *Am J Hum Genet* **46**:1017, 1990.
25. Asher JJR, Morell R, Friedman TB: Confirmation of the location of a Waardenburg syndrome type I mutation on human chromosome 2q. Tight linkage to FN1 and ALPP. *Ann NY Acad Sci* **630**:295, 1991.
26. Farrer LA, Grundfast KM, Amos J, Arnos KS, Asher JH, Beighton P, Diehl SR, Fex J, Foy C, Friedman TB, Greenberg J, Hoth C, Marazita M, Milunsky A, Morell R, Nance W, Newton V, Ramesar R, San Augustin TB, Skare J, Stevens CA, Wagner RGJ, Wilcox ER, Winship I, Read AP: Waardenburg Syndrome (WS) Type I is caused by defects at multiple loci, one of which is near ALPP on chromosome 2: First report of the WS consortium. *Am J Hum Genet* **50**:902, 1992.
27. Russell WL: Splotch, a new mutation in the house mouse *Mus musculus*. *Genetics* **32**:107, 1947.
28. Dickie MM: New splotch alleles in the mouse. *J Hered* **5**:97, 1964.
29. Auerbach R: Analysis of the development effects of a lethal mutation in the house mouse. *J Exp Zool* **127**:305, 1954.
30. Beechey CV, Searle AG: Mutations at the *Sp* locus. *Mouse News Lett* **75**:28, 1986.
31. Epstein DJ, Vekemans M, Gros P: *splotch* (Sp^{2H}), a mutation affecting development of the mouse neural tube, shows a deletion within the paired homeodomain of *Pax-3*. *Cell* **67**:767, 1991.
32. Evans EP, Burtenshaw MD, Beechey CV, Searle AG: A splotch locus deletion visible by Giemsa banding. *Mouse News Lett* **81**:66, 1988.
33. Asher JHJ, Friedman TB: Mouse and hamster mutants as models for Waardenburg syndromes in humans. *J Med Genet* **27**:618, 1990.
34. Steel KP, Smith RJH: Normal hearing in *Splotch* (*Sp*/+), the mouse homologue of Waardenburg syndrome type 1. *Nat Genet* **2**:75, 1992.
35. Bopp D, Burri M, Baumgartner S, Frigerio G, Noll M: Conservation of a large protein domain in the segmentation gene *paired* and in functionally related genes of Drosophila. *Cell* **47**:1033, 1986.
36. Gruss P, Walther C: Pax in development—Minireview. *Cell* **69**:719, 1992.
37. Kessel M, Gruss P: Murine developmental control genes. *Science* **249**:374, 1990.
38. Scott MP, Tamkun JW, Hartzell GW III: The structure and function of the homeodomain. *Biochim Biophys Acta* **989**:25, 1989.
39. Walther C, Guenet J-L, Simon D, Deutsch U, Jostes B, Goulding MD, Plachov D, Balling R, Gruss P: Pax: A murine multigene family of paired box-containing genes. *Genomics* **11**:424, 1991.
40. Mancino F, Vekemans M, Trasler DG, Gros P: Segregation analysis reveals tight genetic linkage between the spontaneously arising neural tube defect gene splotch (Sp) and Pax-3 in an intraspecific mouse backcross. *Cell* **67**:767, 1991.
41. Goulding M, Sterrer S, Fleming J, Balling R, Nadeau J, Moore KJ, Brown SDM, Steel KP, Gruss P: Analysis of the *Pax-3* gene in the mouse mutant *Splotch*. *Genomics* **17**:355, 1993.
42. Epstein DJ, Vogan KJ, Trasler DG, Gros P: A mutation within intron 3 of the Pax-3 gene produces aberrantly spliced mRNA transcripts in the splotch (*Sp*) mouse mutant. *Proc Natl Acad Sci USA* **90**:532, 1993.
43. Vogan KJ, Epstein DJ, Trasler DG, Gros P: The *Splotch-Delayed* (*Spd*) mouse mutant carries a point mutation within the paired box of the *Pax-3* gene. *Genomics* **17**:364, 1993.
44. Burri M, Tromvoukis Y, Bopp D, Frigerio G, Noll M: Conservation of the paired domain in metazoans and its structure in three isolated human genes. *EMBO J* **8**:1183, 1989.
45. Hoth CF, Milunsky A, Lipsky N, Sheffer R, Clarren SK, Baldwin CT: Mutations in the paired domain of the human PAX3 gene cause Klein-Waardenburg Syndrome (WS-III) as well as Waardenburg Syndrome Type I (WS-I). *Am J Hum Genet* **52**:455, 1993.
46. Tassabehji M, Read AP, Newton VE, Harris R, Balling R, Gruss P, Strachan T: Waardenburg's syndrome patients have mutations in the human homologue of the *Pax-3* paired box gene. *Nature* **355**:635, 1992.
47. Baldwin CT, Hoth CF, Amos JA, da-Silva EO, Milunsky A: An exonic mutation in the *HuP2* paired domain gene causes Waardenburg's syndrome. *Nature* **355**:637, 1992.
48. Morell R, Friedman TB, Moeljopawiro S, Hartono, Soewito, Asher JHJ: A frameshift mutation in the HuP2 paired domain of the probable human homolog of murine *Pax-3* is responsible for Waardenburg syndrome type 1 in an Indonesian family. *Hum Mol Genet* **1**:243, 1992.
49. Tassabehji M, Read AP, Newton VE, Patton M, Gruss P, Harris R, Strachan T: Mutations in the *Pax3* gene causing Waardenburg syndrome type 1 and type 2. *Nat Genet* **3**:26, 1993.
50. Tsukamoto K, Tohma T, Ohta T, Yamakawa K, Fukushima Y, Nakamura Y, Niikawa N: Cloning and characterization of the inversion breakpoint at chromosome 2q35 in a patient with Waardenburg syndrome type 1. *Hum Mol Genet* **1**:315, 1992.
51. Kirkpatrick SJ, Kent CM, Laxova R, Sekhon GS: Waar-

denburg syndrome type I in a child with deletion (2) (q35q36.2). *Am J Med Genet* **44**:699, 1992.

52. Pasteris NG, Trask BJ, Sheldon S, Gorski JL: Discordant phenotype of two overlapping deletions involving the PAX3 gene in chromosome 2q35. *Hum Mol Genet* **2**:953, 1993.
53. Reynolds JE, Landa B, Duke B, Arnos KS, Stevens C, Israel J, Marazita M, Bodurtha J, MacLean C, Meyer J, Nance WE, Diehl SR: Molecular genetic studies of Waardenburg syndrome (WS1). *Am J Hum Genet* **51**:A200, 1992.
54. Palmer CG, Heerema N, Bull M: Deletions in chromosome 2 and fragile sites. *Am J Med Genet* **36**:214, 1990.
55. Barr FG, Galili N, Holick J, Biegel JA, Rovera G, Emanuel BS: Rearrangement of the PAX3 paired box gene in the pediatric solid tumour alveolar rhabdomyosarcoma. *Nat Genet* **3**:1993.
56. Treisman J, Gonczy P, Vashishtha M, Harris E, Desplan C: A single amino acid can determine the DNA binding specificity of homeodomain proteins. *Cell* **59**:553, 1989.
57. Treisman J, Harris E, Desplan C: The paired box encodes a second DNA-binding domain in the paired homeo domain protein. *Genes Dev* **5**:594, 1991.
58. Chalepakis G, Fritsch R, Fickenscher H, Deutsch U, Goulding M, Gruss P: The molecular basis of the *undulated/Pax-1* mutation. *Cell* **66**:873, 1991.
59. Hoey T, Levine M: Divergent homeo box proteins recognize similar DNA sequences in *Drosophila*. *Nature* **332**:858, 1988.
60. Goulding MD, Chalepakis G, Deutsch U, Erselius JR, Gruss P: Pax-3, a novel murine DNA binding protein expressed during early neurogenesis. *EMBO J* **10**:1135, 1991.
61. Pierpont JW, Erickson RP: Invited editorial: Facts on *PAX*. *Am J Hum Genet* **52**:451, 1993.
62. Hill RE: Mouse small eye results from mutations in a paired-like homeobox-containing gene. *Nature* **354**:522, 1991.
63. Ton CC, Hirvonen H, Miwa H, Weil MM, Monaghan P, Jordan T, van Heyningen V, Hastie ND, Meijers-Heijboer H, Drechsler M, Royer-Pokora B, Collins F, Swaroop A, Strong LC, Saunders GF: Positional cloning and characterization of a paired box- and homeobox-containing gene from the Aniridia region. *Cell* **67**:1059, 1991.
64. Glases T, Walton DS, Maas RL: Genomic structure, evolutionary conservation and aniridia mutations in the human *PAX6* gene. *Nat Genet* **2**:232, 1992.

CHAPTER 154E

Pelizaeus-Merzbacher Disease

Huda Y. Zoghbi ▪ Andrea Ballabio

1. **Pelizaeus-Merzbacher disease (PMD) is an X-linked leukodystrophy characterized by nystagmus, ataxia, choreoathetosis, spasticity, and mental deterioration. Typically, PMD has an onset in early childhood but earlier onset in the first 3 months of life is noted in the more severe connatal form.**
2. **Neuropathological findings in PMD include diffuse symmetrical demyelination in the central nervous system, loss of oligodendrocytes, and gliosis. The demyelination is detected as low signal intensity of the white matter on T_1-weighted MRI.**
3. ***Jimpy (jp),* a mouse mutant with an X-linked demyelinating disorder characterized by seizures, tremors, and motor paralysis has been proposed as an animal model for PMD. With the cloning of the human and murine genes for proteolipid protein (PLP), it became evident that PLP mutations underlie PMD and *jp*.**
4. **Human PLP consists of 276 amino acids with five hydrophobic domains and is extremely conserved between different species. A defect in RNA splicing of PLP was shown to be the basis of the *jimpy* phenotype, and an amino acid substitution at position 242 was shown to be the cause of myelin-synthesis-deficient *jimpy* (jp^{msd}), which is allelic to *jp*.**
5. **Several mutations as well as complete deletion of the *PLP* gene have been demonstrated in both the connatal and childhood-onset forms of PMD. Mutations in the *PLP* gene have also been identified in dysmyelination disorders in rats and dogs.**

HISTORY AND CLASSIFICATION

In 1885 Pelizaeus described a family with an X-linked demyelinating disorder that extended over a number of generations,[1] and in 1910 Merzbacher examined a brain from an affected individual from the same kindred.[2] Hence, the eponym *Pelizaeus-Merzbacher* was originally used to denote the disease entity observed in this particular family. In describing the clinical features of the disease, Merzbacher wrote that this disorder "starts early in infancy but progresses slowly, following a very chronic course. It is characterized by speech disturbances, bradylalia, foolish grimacing, ataxia, intention tremor, athetosis, choreiform movements, spasticity, and mental deterioration." In 1927 Bostroem reported a family suffering from the same disease,[3] which was subsequently confirmed histologically by Wicke.[4] Since then a number of families and individual cases have been reported as having Pelizaeus-Merzbacher disease (PMD), based on the similarity of their clinical and neuropathological features to those reported by Pelizaeus and Merzbacher. Seitelberger classified the disease as a leukodystrophy based on progressive myelin degeneration in the brain.[5] Among the cases described by Seitelberger, three brothers had clinical features very similar to those observed in the family studied by Pelizaeus and Merzbacher, but they differed in that they had a very early onset of disease in the neonatal period or early infancy, death in the first decade of life, and complete demyelination of the central nervous system. Based on these observations and on the finding of families who have adult onset of the disease,[6] Norman[7] proposed in 1961 a classification that distinguishes three types: the completely demyelinating "congenital Seitelberger type"; the "classical Pelizaeus-Merzbacher type"; and the adult form of Pelizaeus-Merzbacher disease.

In 1970 Seitelberger proposed a classification based on clinical findings (particularly age of onset and age of death), pattern of demyelination, pattern of inheritance, and neurochemical findings.[8] Based on this classification six types were identified: type I, the classic Pelizaeus-Merzbacher disease; type II, the connatal Seitelberger type; type III, the transitional type between I and II; type IV, the adult type; type V, which includes cases with patchy myelination; and type VI, a demyelinating variant of the Cockayne syndrome.

The major criticism of the classification proposed by Seitelberger is that it includes entities that are not inherited in an X-linked pattern and are thus different genotypically from those originally described by Pelizaeus and Merzbacher. This is particularly true for type IV, which is inherited in an autosomal dominant pattern[9] and type VI (Cockayne syndrome) which is an autosomal recessive disorder probably caused by defects in DNA repair.[10–12] Accordingly, the discussion in this chapter will focus on the X-linked form of PMD. In X-linked PMD, the phenotype is quite consistent within a family.

CLINICAL FEATURES

Typically, Pelizaeus-Merzbacher has an onset in infancy or early childhood. The classic clinical features in affected males include eye rolling; nystagmus, which can be vertical, horizontal, or rotary; intermittent nodding; side-to-side tremor of the head; and poor head control. The infants are usually floppy early on and have significant psychomotor

A list of standard abbreviations is located immediately preceding the index in each volume. Additional abbreviations used in this chapter include: DM-20 = a shortened (~20 kDa) isoform of proteolipid protein; MBP = myelin basic protein; PLP = proteolipid protein; PMD = Pelizaeus-Merzbacher disease.

delay; speech typically does not develop, and patients are unable to walk.[2,8,13–17] Choreoathetosis is a common clinical finding and, like the head tremor, it disappears during sleep. As the child matures, nystagmus disappears and cerebellar ataxia, spastic quadriparesis, and bowel and bladder dysfunction become apparent.[8,13,14] The disease often progresses to cause death in late adolescence or young adulthood, although there are patients who survived until the sixth decade.[1,13]

Onset of the disease in the first 3 months of life has been reported by several investigators and referred to as the common connatal form.[8,14,18,19] Laryngeal stridor due to a floppy larynx has been observed in these patients,[14,19] and they typically have a more severe course and die in infancy or childhood.

NEUROIMAGING AND NEUROPATHOLOGY

The diagnosis of Pelizaeus-Merzbacher disease is usually made on the basis of histopathological findings in the brain. The first report on the neuropathological findings was by Merzbacher in 1910, who found diffuse symmetrical white-matter atrophy that originated at the ventricular surface and spread peripherally. The myelin sheaths were severely affected with little islands of sparing, and the cerebellum and brain stem were found to be reduced in size. Additional neuropathological studies[8] confirmed the earlier findings reported by Merzbacher. Typically, the brain was shrunken, particularly in the cerebellum and brain stem, and the white matter was atrophic and sclerotic. Lack of oligodendrocytes was apparent, and astrocytes were normal to increased, suggestive of gliosis. Discontinuous parts of preserved myelin islets were detected in the demyelinated areas; these were frequently found perivascularly as zones of preserved myelin along stretches of blood vessels, hence giving rise to the characteristic "tigroid" appearance (Fig. 154E-1).

Demyelination of the gray matter was also noted, indicating involvement of the myelinated fibers in that area. The neuropathological findings in the connatal form are similar to those in the typical cases except that demyelination is more extensive, involving all parts of the brain so that not a single myelinated fiber can be found.[8] The myelin is replaced by fibrillary gliosis, the number of oligodendrocytes is reduced, and the number of reactive astrocytes is increased.

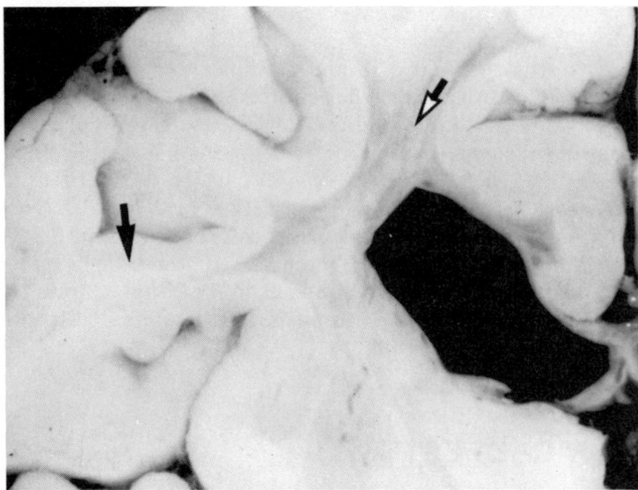

FIG. 154E-1 Left cerebral hemisphere from a 10-year-old boy with PMD-I. The section is at the level of the body of the caudate. The lateral ventricle is enlarged and most of the white matter is abnormal except for the U fibers (*open arrowhead*), which preserve their normal white myelin. The remainder of the white matter shows a patchy loss of myelin surrounding streaks of preserved white myelin creating the so-called tigroid appearance (*closed arrowhead*). (*Courtesy of Drs. C. M. Shaw and T. D. Bird.*)

Over the past two decades neuroimaging studies have been carried out on patients with PMD in an attempt to identify such patients at an early stage. CT is usually normal in the early stages of the disease and nonspecific in the late stages, showing abnormalities such as diffuse atrophy. MRI proved to be superior to CT in the evaluation of white matter abnormalities in the central nervous system. Caro et al.[20] studied six patients with classic PMD to determine if MRI would be useful in the case of a tentative early diagnosis. The MRI showed reversal of white-matter signal intensity on T_1- and T_2-weighted images. There was symmetrical and homogenous low signal intensity in the T_1-weighted images with small scattered areas of normal signal. These islets of normal-appearing white matter are reminiscent of the "tigroid" images observed on histopathology. The amount of white matter was decreased and the corpus callosum was thin. In contrast, CT images revealed cerebral and cerebellar atrophy without any evidence of white-matter abnormality. André et al.[21] performed MRI on a 3-month-old infant with clinical features compatible with connatal PMD and found total inversion of signals between white and gray matter on T_1- and T_2-weighted images. Signal inversion abnormalities have also been documented in older children with PMD.[18,22–24] The consistent finding of symmetrical and homogeneous inversion of the myelin signal on MRI images in PMD suggests that this is a useful test in the early stages of the disease.

GENETICS AND MOLECULAR BIOLOGY OF PELIZAEUS-MERZBACHER DISEASE

The myelin sheath in the central nervous system is an extension of the plasma membrane of the oligodendrocyte, which enwraps axons and permits fast saltatory conduction of nerve impulses. It is composed of 75 percent lipids and a number of specific proteins, 70 to 80 percent of which are the membrane proteins myelin basic protein (MBP) and myelin proteolipid protein (PLP), also known as lipophilin.[25] Another proteolipid, DM-20, a shortened (~20 kDa) isoform of PLP, is found in lesser amounts in the myelin sheath. Both PLP and DM-20 are hydrophobic integral membrane proteins and account for approximately half of the protein content of myelin in the adult central nervous system.[25,26]

Genetic analysis of the role of PLP in the nervous system became possible when the bovine cDNA for PLP was cloned and characterized.[27] Using the bovine cDNA, Willard and Riordan[28] mapped the PLP gene to the human X chromosome in the Xq13-q22 region. Using a somatic-cell hybrid that retained the mouse X chromosome in a Chinese hamster background, the same authors demonstrated that the murine PLP gene is also on the X chromosome.

In 1964 Sidman et al. described *jimpy (jp),* a mouse with an X-linked recessive mutation.[29] Hemizygous males, carrying the *jimpy* mutation, had generalized seizures, tremors, and weak hind limbs by weaning age. Complete paralysis of hind limbs later developed, and these animals typically died by 30 days after the onset of seizures. Brains of *jimpy* mice, examined at 12 to 39 days of age, revealed far less myelin than littermate controls. Based on the clinical and neuropathological findings, the authors suggested that *jimpy* is an animal model for human inherited leukodystrophies.

Eicher and Hoppe described the *jimpy* myelin synthesis deficient (jp^{msd}) mutant mouse, which is allelic to *jimpy*, and like *jimpy* was found to be lacking mature oligodendrocytes and was depleted for a number of myelin constituents, including PLP.[30] The syntenic mapping of *jp* and jp^{msd} in the mouse and PLP in humans suggested that *jp* and jp^{msd} are caused by mutations of the murine *Plp*. Willard and Riordan[28] also suggested that a mutation in the human *PLP* gene might underline PMD given the clinical and neuropathological similarities between PMD and *jp*.

Protein sequence studies on bovine and human *PLP* revealed a 276 amino acid polypeptide with five hydrophobic domains.[31–33] With the cloning of the rat[34–36] and bovine[27] cDNAs for PLP, molecular characterization of this gene in various species became feasible.

The first evidence that the PLP gene is mutated in *jimpy* mice was provided in 1986, when Dautigny and colleagues[34] performed S1 nuclease protection experiments using a probe corresponding to the 5′ end of rat PLP mRNA, and poly(A)$^+$ brain RNA from *jimpy* and normal wild-type mice. These studies revealed a protected fragment of 800 nucleotides in wild-type mice, whereas protection extended over approximately 630 nucleotides for *jimpy* mice, indicating an apparent loss of protection over a region of 160 nucleotides in *jimpy* mRNA. No differences were detected between the *jimpy* and wild-type S1 profiles when using a 3′ noncoding PLP fragment.

In 1986, the human cDNA for PLP was isolated by Fahim and Riordan[37] and the molecular organization of the human gene encoding PLP was determined by Diehl et al.[38] Human PLP consists of 276 amino acids encoded by a single gene that is about 17 kb and spans seven exons and six introns.[38]

Hudson et al.[39] isolated genomic and cDNA clones for both human and mouse cDNA clones and reported the sequence of the murine *Plp* cDNA. PLP was found to be highly conserved among mice,[39] rat,[34,35] cow,[27] and humans[38] at the amino acid and nucleotide level. PLP was identical in rats, humans, and mice and displayed two conservative amino acid differences from the bovine protein.[27,39] One distinction among the *PLP* genes in different species is the use of alternative polyadenylation sites. All species used the major site at about 3000 bases, but a different secondary site at position 2290 in mice and 1480 in rats was found.[39] The DM-20 isoform of PLP is missing an internal domain of 32 amino acids (positions 119 to 150) and is postulated to represent an alternatively spliced form of PLP.[40]

Using the human cDNA for PLP, Fahim and Riordan[37] demonstrated a five- to tenfold decrease in *PLP* mRNA in *jimpy* mice as compared with controls. Analysis of *PLP* and DM-20 transcripts in *jimpy* mice revealed a partial deletion of 74 nucleotides in both isoforms as determined by ribonuclease protection analysis.[39] Detailed restriction enzyme analysis of wild-type and *jimpy* mouse DNA did not reveal any differences. The fact that the 5′ and 3′ borders of the deleted region coincided with the boundaries of the fifth exon in the gene suggested that a mutation within the donor or acceptor splice sites of the *jimpy Plp* gene resulted in the shortened transcript, which explains the lack of evidence for deletion on genomic DNA analysis. Analysis of the *jimpy* mutant mRNA and gene by Nave and colleagues provided further evidence for a primary defect in RNA splicing and identified the single base mutation (AG→GG) causing aberrant splicing of exon V.[41,42] Gencic et al.[43] analyzed the exons of the *Plp* gene in myelin-synthesis-deficient mice ($jimpy^{msd}$), which are allelic to *jimpy*, and found a C → T transition in exon VI that resulted in the substitution of valine for alanine at position 242.

In 1989 the first mutation in the human *PLP* gene was identified in a patient with PMD.[44] A single base change (T → C) in exon IV resulted in the substitution of an arginine residue for tryptophan at amino acid 162 (W162R). Such substitution introduced a charged amino acid in one of the hydrophobic domains, which is usually devoid of charged amino acids. If the hydrophobic, α-helical domains of PLP are critical for correct folding of the protein and compaction of the myelin sheath, the introduction of a charged arginine residue into one of these domains may perturb the function of the protein. Additional mutations in the gene encoding PLP have been identified in several patients with PMD[15,19,26,45–50] (summarized in Table 154E-1). Mutations in this gene have also been identified in dysmyelination disorders in other species such as the myelin-deficient rat.[46] In addition to

Table 154E-1 Proteolipid Protein Mutations in Human and Animal Models

Species	Phenotype	Nucleotide(s) Substitution/Deletion	Amino Acid Change	Exon	Reference
Human	PMD-I	TGC → CGG	Tryp 162 → Arg	IV	44
	PMD-II	CCT → TCT	Pro 215 → Ser	V	15
	PMD-I	CCC → CTC	Pro 14 → Leu	II	45
	PMD-I	ACC → ATC	Thr 155 → Ile	IV	48, 49
	PMD-I	GTT → TTT	Val 218 → Phe	V	26
	PMD-I	Complete deletion of PLP gene			16
	PMD-I	GAT → CAT	Asp 202 → His	IV	54
	PMD-I	GGA → AGA	Gly 73 → Arg	III	54
	PMD-II	ACC → CCC	Thr 181 → Pro	IV	19
	PMD-II	CTT → CCT	Leu 223 → Pro	V	19
	PMD-II	GGC → TGC	Gly 220 → Cys	V	50
Mouse	*jimpy*	AG → GG	splicing site	V	42
	$jimpy^{msd}$	GCG → GTG	Ala 242 → Val	VI	43
	rumpshaker	ATT → ACT	Ile 186 → Thr	IV	53
Rat	md	ACT → CCT	Thr 74 → Pro	III	46
Dog	shaking	CAT → CCT	His 36 → Pro	II	47

PMD-I = classic type; PMD-II = connatal type.

single base mutations, complete deletion of the *PLP* gene has been documented in a kindred with typical PMD.[16] Altogether these findings have provided additional evidence that defects in PLP are the cause of PMD. An interstitial duplication of Xq21-q22 (spanning the region where *PLP* maps) has been identified in a male patient with hypotonia, motor and developmental delay, and PMD.[51] This finding raises the possibility that dosage is critical for PLP, and a demyelinating phenotype may result from either an increase or decrease in the levels of the gene product. All the mutations listed in Table 154E-1 have been carefully analyzed to exclude the possibility that they represent polymorphisms. The facts that the PLP amino acid sequence is extremely conserved between different species (one amino acid difference among rat, mouse, dog, and human sequences) and that several different amino acid substitutions result in severe dysmyelinating disorders suggest that variation in this protein is not tolerated and that multiple functional sites may exist within this molecule. Hypotheses about which regions of the molecule are critical for the function of the protein relied on the topological models of the arrangement of PLP in the membrane in view of the absence of a three-dimensional structure of PLP. Several such models have been proposed and are reviewed by Popot et al.[52] One of these models suggests that PLP and its isoform DM-20 form four membrane-spanning α-helixes designated A through D (Fig. 154E-2).[52] According to this model interactions with molecules in the cytosol would involve the N-terminus, the C-terminus, or the central extramembrane loop. Two intraluminal–extracellular loops allow interaction with extracellular molecules. DM-20 lacks approximately half of the intracellular loop. This model helps explain the deleterious effect of all the nucleotide substitutions observed in PLP. These mutations, which occur either in the hydrophobic transmembrane helices or in the intraluminal loop, may result in marked change of the helix geometry or side-chain structure, which may interfere with proper folding or stability of PLP, as well as with the interactions with other molecules in the extracellular matrix.[26,52]

The signature of all of the above PLP mutations is dysmyelination and loss of oligodendrocytes. The PLP mutant *rumpshaker (rsh)* in mice is characterized by hypomyelination but unlike *jimpy* and PMD, it is not associated with a lack of oligodendrocytes. An isoleucine-to-threonine substitution at residue 186 in a transmembrane domain was found in this mutant.[53] This finding suggested that changes of PLP structure can cause severe hypomyelination not associated with degeneration of oligodendrocytes. Furthermore, the inability to assemble myelin is not the underlying cause of oligodendrocytes loss, as *rsh* mutants are definitively myelin-deficient.[53] The *rsh* mutation may interfere with different aspects of PLP function, and it is possible that PLP plays a specific role in glial-cell development in addition to its role in myelin assembly.

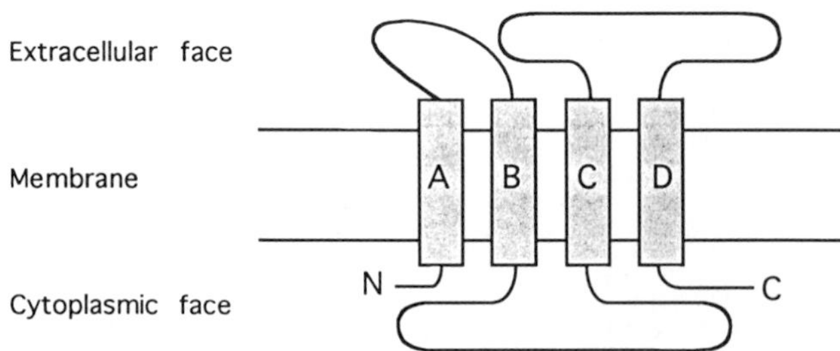

FIG. 154E-2 Schematic diagram of the four-helix model of proteolipid protein. (***Modified from Pham-Dinh et al.***[26])

Detailed genotype/phenotype analyses have not been carried out in humans to determine if specific PLP mutations result in a more or less severe PMD. It is important to note that all the mutations identified to date have been in patients with the classic PMD type, with the exception of three that were found in the connatal form (see Table 154E-1). Although the latter type is classified as such because it occurs within the first 3 months of life, the finding of PLP mutations in both the classic and connatal forms suggests that such mutations generate a continuum of phenotypes in the same X-linked disorder. As none of the patients with any of the other types proposed by Seitelberger[8] have been found to have mutations in the *PLP* gene, and some clearly have an unrelated disorder (type VI is Cockayne syndrome), it is best to restrict the term *Pelizaeus-Merzbacher disease* to patients with X-linked inheritance of the classic or connatal form of the disease. Several patients with an X-linked leukodystrophy and a phenotype compatible with PMD have had detailed characterization of the PLP gene, and no mutations were detected, suggesting that PLP mutations may not account for all X-linked PMD-like phenotypes.[44,54] Given the heterogeneity of the mutations at the PLP locus, it is clear that rapid molecular diagnostic evaluation of PMD patients, in search of a defect in the PLP gene, is not straightforward, nor is it widely available at present. Molecular diagnosis will be an option for families in whom a mutation in the PLP gene has already been identified. For families for whom molecular data are not available, the diagnosis can be made based on clinical findings, pattern of inheritance, neuroimaging, and histopathological studies when available.

REFERENCES

1. Pelizaeus F: Uber eine eigentumliche Form spastischer Lahmung mit Zerebralerscheinungen auf hereditarer Grundlage (multiple Sklerose). *Arch Psychiatr Nervenkr* **16**:698, 1885.
2. Merzbacher L: Eine eigenartige familiare Erkrankungsform (Aplasia axialis extracorticalis congenita). *Z Gesamte Neurol Psychaitr* **3**:1, 1910.
3. Bostroem A: uber die Pelizaeus-Merzbachersche Krankheit. *Dtsch Z Nervenheilkd* **100**:63, 1927.
4. Wicke R: Ein Beitrag zur Frage der familiaren diffusen Sklerosen einschlieslich der Pelizaeus-Merzbacherschen Krankheit und ihrer Beziehung zur amaurotischen Idiotie. *Z Gesamte Neurol Psychiatr* **162**:741, 1938.
5. Seitelberger F: Die Pelizaeus-Merzbachersche Krankheit, Klinisch-anatomische Untersuchungen zum Prolbem ihrer Stellung unter den diffusen Sklerosen. *Wien Z Nervenheilkd* **9**:228, 1954.
6. Lowenberg K, Hill TS: Diffuse sclerosis with preserved myelin islands. *Arch Neurol Psychiatry (Chic)* **29**:1232, 1933.
7. Norman RM: Lipid diseases of the brain, in Williams D (ed): *Modern Trends in Neurology*. London, Butterworths, 1962, p 173.
8. Seitelberger F: Pelizaeus-Merzbacher disease, in Vinken PJ, Bruyn GW (eds): *Handbook of Clinical Neurology. Leucodystrophies and Poliodystrophies*. Amsterdam, North Holland, 1970, p 150.
9. Zerbin-Rudin E, Peiffer J: Ein genetischer Beitrag zur Frage der Spatform der Pelizaeus-Merzbacherschen Krankheit. *Hum Genet* **1**:107, 1964.
10. Robbins JH, Kraemer KH, Lutzner MA, Pestoff BW, Coon HG: Xeroderma pigmentosum: An inherited disease with sun sensitivity, multiple cutaneous neoplasms and abnormal DNA repair. *Ann Intern Med* **80**:221, 1974.
11. Otsuka F, Robbins JH: The Cockayne syndrome—An inher-

ited multisystem disorder with cutaneous photosensitivity and defective repair of DNA. *Am J Dermatopathol* **4**:387, 1985.
12. Vermeulen W, Jaeken J, Jaspers NGJ, Bootsma D, Hoeijmakers JHJ: Xeroderma pigmentosum complementation group G associated with Cockayne Syndrome. *Am J Hum Genet* **53**:185, 1993.
13. Tyler HR: Pelizaeus-Merzbacher disease: A clinical study. *Arch Neurol Psychiatry* **80**:162, 1958.
14. Renier WO, Gabreels FJM, Hustinx TWJ, Jaspar HHJ, Geelen JAG, Van Haelst UJG, Lommen EJP, Ter Haar BGA: Connatal Pelizaeus-Merzbacher disease with congenital stridor in two maternal cousins. *Acta Neuropathol (Berl)* **54**:11, 1981.
15. Gencic S, Abuelo D, Ambler M, Hudson LD: Pelizaeus-Merzbacher disease: An X-linked neurologic disorder of myelin metabolism with a novel mutation in the gene encoding proteolipid protein. *Am J Hum Genet* **45**:435, 1989.
16. Raskind WH, Williams CA, Hudson LD, Bird TD: Complete deletion of the proteolipid protein gene (PLP) in a family with X-linked Pelizaeus-Merzbacher disease. *Am J Hum Genet* **49**:1355, 1991.
17. Johnson VP, Carpenter NJ, Kelts KA: Pelizaeus-Merzbacher disease: Clinical and DNA-linkage study of an extended family. *Am J Med Genet* **41**:355, 1991.
18. Haenggeli CA, Engel E, Pizzolato GP: Connatal Pelizaeus-Merzbacher disease. *Dev Med Child Neurol* **31**:803, 1989.
19. Strautnieks S, Rutland P, Winter RM, Baraitser M, Malcolm S: Pelizaeus-Merzbacher disease: Detection of mutations Thr181 → Pro and Leu223 → Pro in the proteolipid protein gene, and prenatal diagnosis. *Am J Hum Genet* **51**:871, 1992.
20. Caro PA, Marks HG: Magnetic resonance imaging and computed tomography in Pelizaeus-Merzbacher disease. *Magn Reson Imaging* **8**:791, 1990.
21. André M, Monin P, Moret C, Braun M, Picard L: Pelizaeus-Merzbacher disease. Contribution of magnetic resonance imaging to an early diagnosis. *J Neuroradiol* **17**:216, 1990.
22. Journel H, Roussey M, Gandon Y, Allaire C, Carsin M, La Marec B: Magnetic resonance imaging in Pelizaeus-Merzbacher disease. *Neuroradiology* **29**:403, 1987.
23. Penner MW, Gebarski SS, Allen RS: MR imaging of Pelizaeus-Merzbacher disease. *J Comput Assist Tomogr* **11**:591, 1987.
24. Jasek F, Chateil JL, Fontan D, Diard F, Desforges J: La maladie de Pelizaeus-Merzbacher: Contribution diagnostique de l'IRM. *Arch Fr Pediatr* **47**:265, 1990.
25. Lees MB, Brostoff SW: Proteins of myelin, in Morell P (ed): *Myelin*, 2d ed. New York, Plenum, 1984, p 197.
26. Pham-Dinh D, Popot JL, Boespflug-Tanguy O, Landrieu P, Deleuze JF, Boue J, Jolles P, Dautigny A: Pelizaeus-Merzbacher disease: A valine to phenylalanine point mutation in a putative extracellular loop of myelin proteolipid. *Proc Natl Acad Sci USA* **88**:7562, 1991.
27. Naismith AL, Hoffman-Chudzik E, Tsui L-C, Riordan JR: Study of the expression of myelin proteolipid protein (lipophilin) using a cloned complimentary DNA. *Nucleic Acids Res* **13**:7413, 1985.
28. Willard HF, Riordan JR: Assignment of the gene for myelin proteolipid protein to the X chromosome: Implications for X-linked myelin disorders. *Science* **230**:940, 1985.
29. Sidman RL, Dickie MM, Appel SH: Mutant mice (quaking and jimpy) with deficient myelination in the central nervous system. *Science* **144**:309, 1964.
30. Eicher EM, Hoppe PC: Use of chimeras to transmit lethal genes in the mouse and to demonstrate allelism of the two X-linked male lethal genes jp and msd. *J Exp Zool* **183**:118, 1973.
31. Stoffel W, Schroder W, Hillen H, Deutzmann R: Analysis of the primary structure of the strongly hydrophobic brain myelin proteolipid apoprotein (lipophilin). Isolation and amino acid sequence determination of proteolytic fragments. *Hoppe Seyler Z Physiol Chem* **363**:1117, 1982.
32. Stoffel W, Hillen H, Schroder W, Deutzmann R: The primary structure of bovine myelin lipophilin (proteolipid apoprotein). *Hoppe Seyler Z Physiol Chem* **364**:1455, 1983.
33. Stoffel W, Hillen H, Giersiefen H: Structure and molecular arrangement of proteolipid protein of central nervous system myelin. *Proc Natl Acad Sci USA* **81**:5012, 1984.
34. Dautigny A, Alliel PM, d'Auriol L, Pham-Dinh D, Nussbaum JL, Galibert F, Jolles P: Molecular cloning and nucleotide sequence of a cDNA clone coding for rat brain myelin proteolipid. *FEBS Lett* **188**:33, 1985.
35. Milner RJ, Lai C, Nave K-A, Lenoir D, Ogata J, Sutcliffe JG: Nucleotide sequences of two mRNAs for rat brain myelin proteolipid protein. *Cell* **2**:931, 1985.
36. Schaich M, Budzinski R-M, Stoffel W: Cloned proteolipid protein and myelin basic protein cDNA. Transcription of the two genes during myelination. *Biol Chem Hoppe Seyler* **367**:825, 1986.
37. Fahim S, Riordan JR: Lipophilin (PLP) gene in X-linked myelin disorders. *J Neurosci Res* **16**:303, 1986.
38. Diehl HJ, Schaich M, Budzinski RM, Stoffel W: Individual exons encode the integral membrane domains of human myelin proteolipid protein. *Proc Natl Acad Sci USA* **83**:9807, 1986.
39. Hudson LD, Berndt J, Puckett C, Kozak CA, Lazzarini RA: Aberrant splicing of proteolipid protein mRNA in the dysmyelinating jimpy mouse. *Proc Natl Acad Sci USA* **84**:1454, 1987.
40. Nave KA, Lai C, Bloom FE, Milner RJ: Splice site selection in the proteolipid protein (PLP) gene transcript and primary structure of the DM-20 protein of central nervous system myelin. *Proc Natl Acad Sci USA* **84**:5665, 1987.
41. Nave KA, Lai C, Bloom FE, Milner RJ: Jimpy mutant mouse: A 74-base deletion in the mRNA for myelin proteolipid protein and evidence for a primary defect in RNA splicing. *Proc Natl Acad Sci USA* **83**:9264, 1986.
42. Nave KA, Bloom FE, Milner RJ: A single nucleotide difference in the gene for myelin proteolipid protein defines the jimpy mutation in mouse. *J Neurochem* **49**:5665, 1987.
43. Gencic S, Hudson LD: Conservative amino acid substitution in the myelin proteolipid protein of *jimpy*^{msd} mice. *J Neurosci* **10**:117, 1990.
44. Hudson LD, Puckett C, Berndt J, Chan J, Gencic S: Mutation of the proteolipid protein gene PLP in a human X chromosome-linked myelin disorder. *Proc Natl Acad Sci USA* **86**:8128, 1989.
45. Trofatter JA, Dlouhy SR, DeMyer W, Conneally PM, Hodes ME: Pelizaeus-Merzbacher disease: Tight linkage to proteolipid protein gene exon variant. *Proc Natl Acad Sci USA* **86**:9427, 1989.
46. Boison D, Stoffel W: Myelin-deficient rat: A point mutation in exon III (A → C, Thr75 → Pro) of the myelin proteolipid protein causes dysmyelination and oligodendrocyte death. *EMBO J* **8**:3295, 1989.
47. Nadon NL, Duncan ID, Hudson LD: A point mutation in the proteolipid protein gene of the 'shaking pup' interrupts oligodendrocyte development. *Development* **110**:529, 1990.
48. Weimbs T, Dick T, Stoffel W, Boltshauer E: A point mutation at the X-chromosomal proteolipid protein locus in Pelizaeus-Merzbacher disease leads to disruption of myelinogenesis. *Biol Chem Hoppe Seyler* **371**:1175, 1990.
49. Pratt VM, Trofatter JA, Schinzel A, Dlouhy SR, Conneally PM, Hodes ME: A new mutation in the proteolipid protein (PLP) gene in a German family with Pelizaeus-Merzbacher disease. *Am J Med Genet* **38**:136, 1991.
50. Iwaki A, Muramoto T, Iwaki T, Furumi H, Dario-deLeon ML, Tateishi J, Fukumaki Y: A missense mutation in the proteolipid protein gene responsible for Pelizaeus-Merzbacher disease in a Japanese family. *Hum Mol Genet* **2**:19, 1993.
51. Cremers FPM, Pfeiffer RA, van de Pol TJR, Hofker MH, Kruse TA, Wieringa B, Ropers HH: An interstitial duplication of the X chromosome in a male allows physical fine mapping of probes from the Xq13-q22 region. *Hum Genet* **77**:23, 1987.
52. Popot J-L, Pham-Dinh D, Dautigny A: Major myelin proteolipid: The 4-α-helix topology. *J Membr Biol* **120**:233, 1991.
53. Schneider A, Montague P, Griffiths I, Fanarraga M, Kennedy P, Brophy P, Nave KA: Uncoupling of hyomyelination and glial cell death by a mutation in the proteolipid protein gene. *Nature* **358**:758, 1992.
54. Doll R, Natowicz MR, Schiffmann R, Smith FI: Molecular diagnostics for myelin proteolipid protein gene mutations in Pelizaeus-Merzbacher disease. *Am J Hum Genet* **51**:161, 1992.

CHAPTER **154F**

Norrie Disease

Andrea Ballabio ▪ Huda Y. Zoghbi

1. **Norrie disease is a rare, X-linked form of congenital blindness characterized by severe, bilateral abnormalities of eye development. These abnormalities include the presence of a tumorlike retrolental mass, termed "*pseudoglioma*," which is composed of layered and highly vascularized collagenous tissue, probably resulting from an early arrest of embryonic retinal development.**
2. **Approximately one-third of patients with Norrie disease have sensorineural hearing loss, which usually appears in early or middle childhood and maintains a progressive course to complete deafness.**
3. **Linkage analysis and the identification of submicroscopic deletions in families with Norrie disease led to the mapping assignment of the Norrie gene to the Xp11.3 region and opened the way to the subsequent positional cloning of this gene. Mutation detection in patients with Norrie disease identified several deletion, nonsense, frameshift, splice site, and missense mutations in this gene. A mutation in the Norrie gene was also identified in a family with X-linked exudative vitreoretinopathy, indicating that the two diseases are allelic.**
4. **The Norrie gene encodes a protein sharing sequence and structural similarities with proteins containing a cysteine knot C-terminal domain. These proteins include mucins, von Willebrand factor, transforming growth factor (TGFβ), the slit protein in Drosophila, and a family of growth regulators, including the connective-tissue growth factor (CTGF). The protein product of the Norrie gene may represent a growth factor primarily involved in normal eye development.**

CLINICAL, GENETIC, AND HISTOPATHOLOGICAL FEATURES

Norrie disease (ND) [McKusick (MIM no. 31060)], first described by Norrie in 1927,[1] is a rare inherited form of congenital blindness. In most patients the phenotype is evident at birth and is characterized by severe, bilateral abnormalities of eye development. These abnormalities include the presence of a tumorlike retrolental mass, retinal detachment, iris atrophy and synechiae, corneal and vitreous opacities, and glaucoma (Fig. 154F-1).[2,3] The detached retina often can be detected as leukokoria (white pupil reflex). Most patients are blind at birth or by the end of the second month of life, but some preserve light perception in the first few years. Phthisis bulbi (severe shrunken atrophy of the optic globe) usually develops by the end of the first decade.[2–4]

In some patients eye abnormalities are associated with defects involving other organs and tissues. Approximately one-third of ND patients have sensorineural hearing loss, which usually appears in early or middle childhood and follows a progressive course to complete deafness.[5] Mental retardation and psychotic behavior are also common findings in ND patients. Goodyear et al. pointed out that blindness by itself can cause developmental stasis or regression, particularly when the developmental climate is suboptimal.[4] There is, however, no doubt about the causal relationship between ND and mental retardation, given the number of patients with mental retardation described who had received adequate care and in whom a point mutation in the ND gene was found.

ND is transmitted as a fully penetrant, X-linked trait. Heterozygous females typically do not show any signs of the disease, however, in a few instances they may be symptomatic.[6] Expressivity of the phenotype is variable, even within the same family, and particularly with respect to deafness and mental retardation. Dysmorphic features,

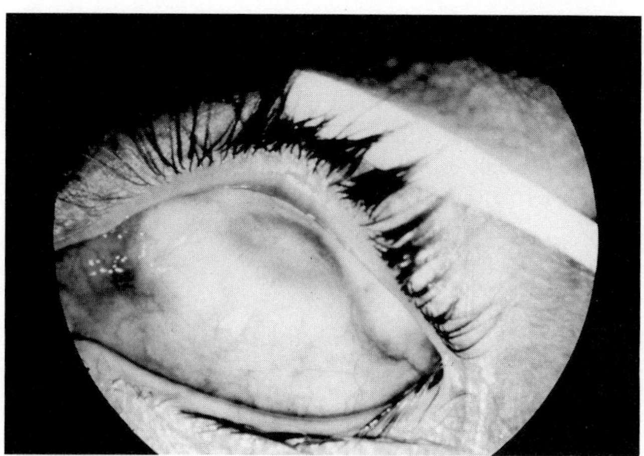

FIG. 154F-1 **Eye findings in a patient with Norrie disease. Severe enophthalmus due to atrophic changes and subtotal corneal clouding with moderate vascularization are evident. Deeper ocular structures are not visible. A previous ultrasound examination had revealed the presence of highly reflective structures between the lens and the posterior wall of the globe. A point mutation in the ND gene (R74C) was subsequently demonstrated in the patient and in both his mother and maternal grandmother (see below).** ***(Courtesy of Dr. Brigit Lorentz.)***

A list of standard abbreviations in located immediately preceding the index in each volume. Additional abbreviations used in this chapter include: MAOA = monamine oxidase A; MAOB = monamine oxidase B; ND = Norrie disease; TGFβ = transforming growth factor β; XLFEVR = X-linked familial exudative vitreoretinopathy.

including a typical "Norrie facies," microcephaly, cryptorchidism, growth retardation, and limb anomalies have been reported in some patients with ND. These patients had large deletions probably involving other flanking genes in addition to the Norrie gene and resulting in a contiguous gene syndrome.[4]

There is no pharmacologic treatment available for ND. Symptomatic therapy includes enucleation and replacement with an artificial eye and the use of hearing aids.[3]

The histopathological hallmark of ND is the presence of a yellowish-white, tumorlike, retrolental mass called a "pseudoglioma."[3] This mass is composed of layered collagenous tissue that is highly vascularized. Histopathological examination of the retina, performed after vitrectomy, reveals signs of an early arrest of embryonic retinal development.[7] This arrest results in the persistence of a hyaloidal vascular system, which is the source of the retrolental mass formation. Other histopathological changes typically observed in the eyes of ND patients include disruption of the inner and outer neuroblastic layers and absence of ganglion cells. It has been suggested that the arrest of retinal development in ND may occur as early as 7 weeks of gestation.[7]

The pseudoglioma usually represents the diagnostic clue for ND. However, other ocular conditions should be considered in the differential diagnosis, including retinoblastoma, fibrolental dysplasia, and persistent hyperplastic primary vitreous.[8] The presence of an X-linked inheritance pattern represents another important diagnostic clue. However, X-linked familial exudative vitreoretinopathy (XLFEVR), like ND, is also characterized by a severe retinopathy and by the presence of fibrovascular mass lesions.[9] The degree of differentiation of the retina and of other eye structures in patients with XLFEVR and with ND suggests that the developmental defect causing XLFEVR occurs much later in gestation (29 to 40 weeks) than that causing ND.[9] Linkage studies and mutation analysis suggest that XLFEVR and ND are in fact allelic.[9,10]

POSITIONAL CLONING OF THE NORRIE DISEASE GENE

The ND locus was first mapped to the Xp11.3 region by linkage analysis.[11,12] An anonymous polymorphic DNA marker, L1.28 (DXS7), was found in tight linkage with the disease locus, with no recombination events observed in six kindreds with ND.[12] Following the mapping assignment of the ND gene, de la Chapelle et al. identified a family in whom a submicroscopic interstitial deletion spanning the DXS7 locus was found to cosegregate with the ND phenotype.[13] Subsequently, several additional patients with ND carrying deletions or other types of chromosomal rearrangements were identified.[14–17]

Molecular characterization of these deletion cases greatly facilitated physical mapping of the ND locus region. Deletions were found to span several markers, including, in some patients, the genes for monoamine oxidases A and B (MAOA and MAOB), which had been assigned to the same chromosomal region.[18,19] For some time, therefore, MAOA and MAOB were considered candidate genes for ND. Sims et al. definitively excluded these genes as etiologic factors in ND on the basis of normal MAOA and MAOB activities in ND patients.[20]

A specific genomic region spanning the ND gene (the ND "critical region") was identified by both deletion and genetic mapping (Fig. 154F-2). By searching for evolutionarily conserved sequences and screening of cDNA libraries using cosmid and PFGE fragments as probes, two independent groups simultaneously reported the isolation of the same gene from the ND critical region.[21,22] This gene was found to be highly conserved throughout evolution and to be expressed in retina, choroid, and fetal brain,[21] indicating that it was a strong candidate for being the ND gene.

MOLECULAR BASIS OF NORRIE DISEASE

The availability of a candidate gene for ND provided the opportunity for mutation detection in ND patients. The structure of the ND gene was elucidated in order to design an effective mutation detection strategy for analysis of genomic DNA from ND patients.[23] The gene contains three exons and spans approximately 27 kb. Four pairs of oligonucleotide primers were used for the amplification of exonic regions of DNA from patients.[23] Table 154F-1 is a summary of the mutations that have been identified in 22 unrelated Norrie patients tested by either single-strand conformation polymorphism (SSCP) or by direct sequencing. Several deletion, nonsense, frameshift, and splice site mutations were identified, most of which probably represent functionally null

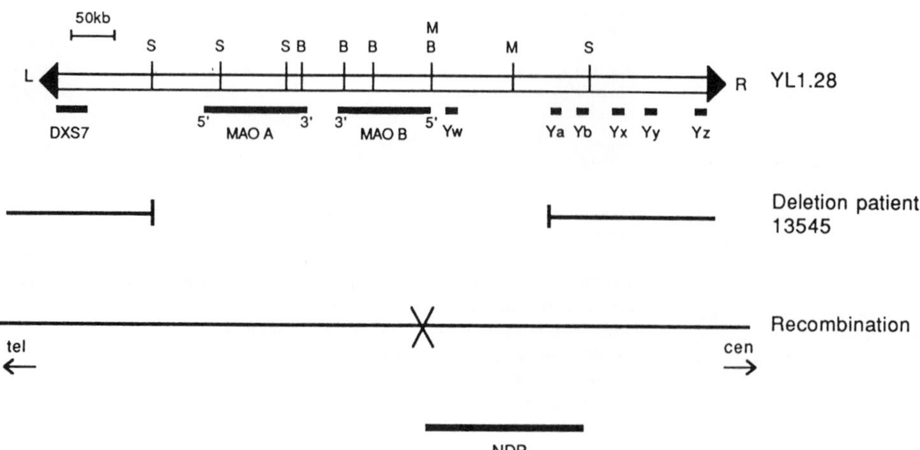

FIG. 154F-2 Physical map of the Norrie gene (NDP) region. Restriction map of YL1.28 indicating locations of MAOA, MAOB, DXS7, and various phage subclones (Ya to Yz) used in mapping the end points of the deletion patient 13545. The most distal position for a single recombination event reported,[27] which orients MAOB and NDP with respect to the centromere, is designated by a cross. Left and right ends of the YAC are designated by L and R, respectively. Restriction enzyme sites are as follows: M = *MluI*, S = *SstI*, and B = *BssHII*. The lower solid bar represents the 160-kb region identified as important in the etiology of NDP. *(From Chen et al.[22] Used by permission of* Nature Genetics.*)*

alleles. In the remaining patients missense mutations at highly conserved amino acid residues were found.[23-25] As shown in Table 154F-1, there was no correlation between the type of mutation found and the severity or complexity of the phenotype. Therefore, the presence of deafness and mental retardation in ND represents a pleiotropic effect of mutations in the ND gene and is probably influenced by other genetic, environmental, and stochastic factors.[25] The high degree of heterogeneity of the detected mutations is in keeping with a high proportion of new mutations usually observed in X-linked disorders affecting male reproductive fitness. The small size of the coding region in the ND gene will permit molecular diagnosis by direct amplification and sequencing.

Norrie Disease Gene Mutations in X-Linked Exudative Vitreoretinopathy

The phenotypic similarity and coincident map locations of ND and XLFEVR led to the hypothesis that these two disorders were allelic.[9] Therefore, mutations in the ND gene were searched for in patients with XLFEVR. A missense mutation, causing a neutral amino acid substitution in a highly conserved region of the ND gene, was detected in all affected individuals from a family with XLFEVR. This suggests that mutations in the ND gene can also cause XLFEVR, which is most likely allelic to ND.[10]

The Norrie Disease Gene Product

The ND gene encodes a 133 amino acid polypeptide that shows a high proportion of basic amino acids and cysteine residues and no sites for glycosylation. The presence of a signal peptide at the N-terminal region suggests that the protein is secreted. No significant homologies with other previously identified proteins were reported in the original studies describing the ND gene.[21,22] Subsequently, a more detailed analysis revealed homologies with a C-terminal domain common to a group of proteins including mucins.[23]

Meitinger et al. thoroughly analyzed sequence homologies and performed three-dimensional modeling of the ND protein.[26] The results of these studies are shown in Fig. 154F-3. A high degree of conservation in the number and spacing of cysteine residues was found between the ND protein and a number of other proteins containing a cysteine-knot C-terminal domain. These include mucins, von Willebrand factor, transforming growth factor (TGFβ), the slit protein in Drosophila, and a family of growth regulators including the connective-tissue growth factor (CTGF). Secondary structure prediction and three-dimensional modeling revealed a remarkable structural similarity between ND protein and TGFβ, supported by comparison of disulfide patterns, all-atom model building, and conservation mapping. This structural similarity suggests that the ND protein, like TGFβ, is also subject to dimerization.[26]

From these data it can be postulated that the ND protein

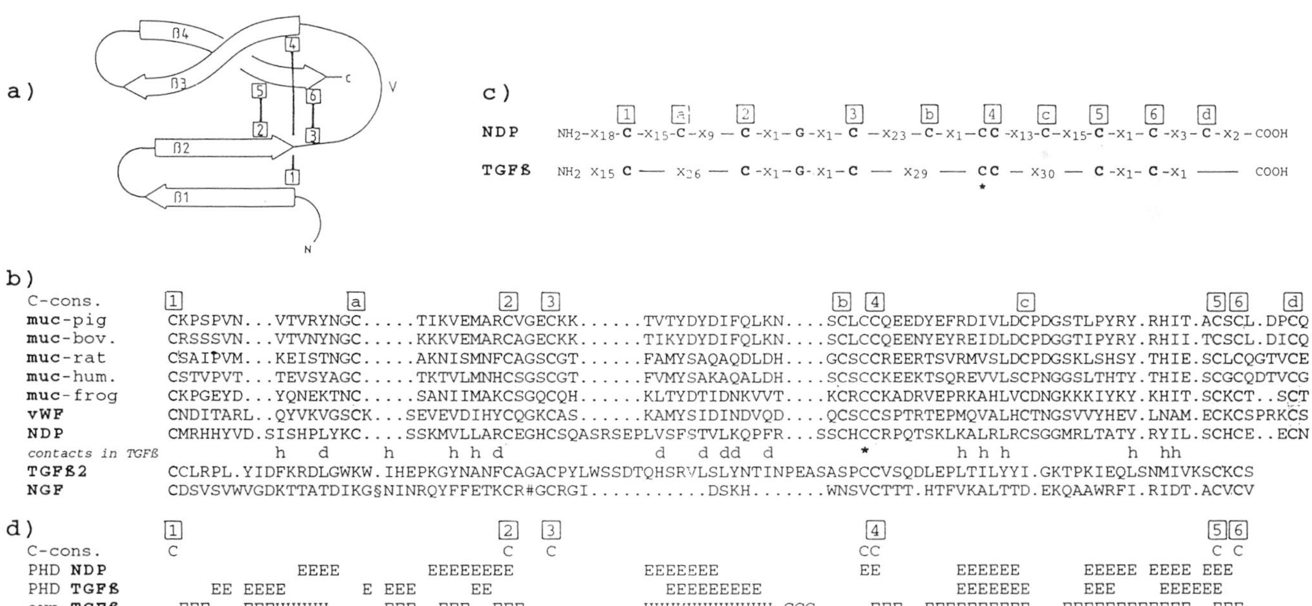

FIG. 154F-3 **Cysteine residues, sequence alignment, and secondary structure prediction of transforming growth factor β (TGFβ) and Norrie disease protein (NDP).** ***A.*** **Schematic representation of a TGFβ-like monomer, modified from refs. 2 and 8. β Strands are drawn as arrows (β1 to β4). Cysteine-knot–forming residues are numbered 1 to 6; disulfide bridges are indicated. The loop between β strands 2 and 3 shows *variable lengths* (V) and crystal structure in TGF, nerve growth factor (NGF), and PDGF.** ***B.*** **Multiple alignment of NDP and related C-terminal cysteine-rich domains (CT domains) with TGFβ and NGF. All sequences are aligned to match the cysteine residues numbered 1 to 6 and lettered a to d. Insertions/deletions are indicated by dots. The cysteine forming an intermolecular disulfide bridge in TGFβ is marked by an asterisk. Dimer contacts (d) and hydrophobic core contacts (h) in TGFβ are consistent with corresponding positions in the CT domains. Two inserts in the NGF sequence have been deleted (§ = KEVTVLAEV; # = ASNPVES). Abbreviations are muc = mucin and vWD = von Willebrand factor.** ***C.*** **Alignment of cysteine and glycine residues in TGFβ with those in NDP. The number of amino acids (X_n) between conserved cystein residues (C) is given. Cysteines involved in the cysteine knot are numbered 1 to 6. The additional cysteines conserved in the CT domain are lettered a to d. An asterisk indicates the cysteine residue involved in dimerization.** ***D.*** **Comparison between observed β strands and helices in TGFβ and predicted second structures of TGFβ and NDP (exp = crystal structure; PHD = prediction from sequence family; E = β strand, H = nα-helix, G = 3_{10}-helix, space = loop). NDP is predicted to consist predominantly of β sheets, with strand placements roughly in agreement with those experimentally observed in TGFβ. The central predicted β strand (sequence LVSFSTV in NDP) actually is a helix in TGFβ, involved in dimerization, and is likely to be present in NDP; the incorrect prediction of this strand is probably due to the hydrophobic residues at the surface involved in the dimer contacts.** ***(From Meitinger T, et al.[26] Used by permission of*** **Nature Genetics.*)***

Table 154F-1 Mutations in the Norrie Gene

Patient	Mutation	Mutation Type	Reference
1 (12316)	del ex2	Deletion	22
2 (3883)	del ex2	Deletion	22
3 (2844)	del (ex2)	Deletion	21
4 (200)	del (ex2u3)	Deletion	21
5 (1609)	del (ex1)	Deletion	21
6 (P.Ru.)	delG706	Frameshift	24
7 (9500)	delT813	Frameshift	24
8 (1443)	insATCC443	Frameshift	24
9 (204)	S29X (nt502C→G)	Stop	23
10 (1650)	Y44C (nt547A→G)	Missense	23
11 (2248)	590 + 1G→?	Splice	24
12 (2843)	S57X (nt586C→G)	Stop	24
13 (167)	V60Q (nt595T→A)	Missense	23
14 (2942)	L61F (nt597C→T)	Missense	24
15 (3710)	R74C (nt636C→T)	Missense	24
16 (1245)	S75C (nt640C→G)	Missense	24
17 (1127)	R90P (nt685G→C)	Missense	24
18 (Cyp)	C96Y (nt703G→A)	Missense	23,24
19 (G)	C110X (nt746C→A)	Stop	24
20 (A.La.)	C110X (nt746C→A)	Stop	24
21 (FEVR1)	L124F (nt788C→T)	Missense	10
22 (III-1)	C69S (nt614G→C)	Missense	6

is a member of a family of growth factors containing a cysteine knot C-terminal domain. The ND protein may be a growth factor particularly important for normal development of the retina. Loss of function of this protein in ND patients would result in the phenotypic consequences of ND, which are localized primarily to the eye. The lower frequency of symptoms affecting other organs, such as the ear and the central nervous system, may be related to the development of compensating pathways. Unfortunately, because of the nature of the defect in ND, which involves early stages of embryonal development, it is difficult to envision a therapeutic approach to cure this disease. Nevertheless, a more complete knowledge of the ND protein and its function may lead to the discovery of fundamental biologic processes involved in eye development. Genetic counseling, carrier detection, and prenatal diagnosis are possible using linkage and mutation analysis.

ACKNOWLEDGMENTS

We thank Drs. T. Meitinger and I. Craig for helpful comments and for providing us with some of the figures and tables.

REFERENCES

1. Norrie G: Causes of blindness in children. *Acta Ophthalmol (Copenh)* **5**:357, 1927.
2. Warburg M: Norrie's disease: A new hereditary bilateral pseudotumor of the retina. *Acta Ophthalmol (Copenh)* **39**: 757, 1961.
3. Warburg M: Norrie's disease: A congenital progressive oculo-acoustico-cerebral degeneration. *Acta Ophthalmol Suppl (Copenh)* **89**:1, 1966.
4. Goodyear HM, Sonksen PM, McConachie H: Norrie's disease: A prospective study of development. *Arch Dis Child* **64**:1587, 1989.
5. Parving A, Warburg M: Audiological findings in Norrie's disease. *Audiology* **16**:124, 1977.
6. Chen Z-Y, Battinelli EM, Woodruff G, Young I, Breakefield XO, Craig IW: Characterization of a mutation within the NDP gene in a family with a manifesting female carrier. *Hum Mol Genet* **2**:1727, 1993.
7. Barlow Enyedi L, de Juan E Jr, Gaitan A: Ultrastructural study of Norrie's disease. *Am J Ophthalmol* **111**:439, 1991.
8. LaRussa F, Wesson MD: Norrie's disease vs. PHPV: One family's dilemma. *J Am Optom Assoc* **63**:404, 1992.
9. Fullwood P, Jones J, Bundey S, Dudgeon J, Fielder AR, Kilpatrick MW: X linked exudative vitreoretinopathy: Clinical features and genetic linkage analysis. *Br J Ophthalmol* **77**:168, 1993.
10. Chen Z-Y, Battinelli EM, Fielder A, Bundey S, Sims K, Breakfield XO, Craig IW: A mutation in the Norrie disease gene (NDP) associated with X-linked familial exudative vitreoretinopathy. *Nat Genet* **5**:180, 1993.
11. Gal A, Stolzenberger C, Wienker T, Wieacker P, Ropers H-H, Friedrich U, Bleeker-Wagemakers L, Pearson P, Warburg M: Norrie's disease: Close linkage with genetic markers from the proximal short arm of the X chromosome. *Clin Genet* **27**:282, 1985.
12. Bleeker-Wagemakers LM, Friedrich U, Wienker TF, Warburg M, Ropers H-H: Close linkage between Norrie disease, a cloned DNA sequence from the proximal short arm, and the centromere of the X chromosome. *Hum Genet* **71**:211, 1985.
13. de la Chapelle A, Sankila E-M, Lindlof M, Aula P, Norio R: Norrie disease caused by a gene deletion allowing carrier detection and prenatal diagnosis. *Clin Genet* **28**:317, 1985.
14. Zhu D, Antonarakis SE, Schmeckpeper BJ, Diergaarde PJ, Greb AE, Maumenee IH: Microdeletion in the X-chromosome and prenatal diagnosis in a family with Norrie disease. *Am J Med Genet* **33**:485, 1989.
15. Diergaarde PJ, Wieringa B, Bleeker-Wagemakers EM, Sims KB, Breakefield XO, Ropers H-H: Physical fine-mapping of a deletion spanning the Norrie gene. *Hum Genet* **84**:22, 1989.
16. Pettenati MJ, Rao PN, Weaver RG Jr, Thomas IT, McMahan MR: Inversion (X)(p11.4q22) associated with Norrie disease in a four generation family. *Am J Med Genet* **45**:577, 1993.
17. Donnai D, Mountford RC, Read AP: Norrie disease resulting from a gene deletion; clinical features and DNA studies. *J Med Genet* **25**:73, 1988.
18. Sims KB, de la Chapelle A, Norio R, Sankila EM, Hsu Y-PP, Reinhart WB, Corey TJ, Ozelius L, Powell JF, Bruns G, Gusella JG, Murphy DL, Breakefield XO: Monoamine oxidase deficiency in males with an X chromosome deletion. *Neuron* **2**:1069, 1989.
19. Lan NC, Heinzmann C, Gal A, Klisak I, Orth U, Lai E, Grimsby J, Sparkes RS, Mohandas T, Shih JC: Human monoamine oxidase A and B genes map to Xp11.23 and are deleted in a patient with Norrie disease. *Genomics* **4**:552, 1989.
20. Sims KB, Ozelius L, Corey T, Rinehart WB, Liberfarb R, Haines J, Chen WJ, Norio F, Sankila E, de la Chapella A, Murphy DL, Gusella J, Breakefield XO: Norrie disease gene is distinct from the monoamine oxidase genes. *Am J Hum Genet* **45**:424, 1989.
21. Berger W, Meindl A, van de Pol TJR, Cremers FPM, Ropers H-H, Döerner C, Monaco A, Bergen AAb, Lebo R, Warburg M, Zergollern L, Lorenz B, Gal A, Bleeker-Wagemakers EM, Meitinger T: Isolation of a candidate gene for Norrie disease by positional cloning. *Nat Genet* **1**:199, 1992.
22. Chen Z-Y, Hendriks RW, Jobling MA, Powell JF, Breakefield XO, Sims KB, Craig IW: Isolation and characterization of a candidate gene for Norrie disease. *Nat Genet* **1**:204, 1992.
23. Meindl A, Berger W, Meitinger T, van de Pol D, Achatz H, Dörner C, Haasemann M, Hellebrand H, Gal A, Cremers F, Ropers H-H: Norrie disease is caused by mutations in an extracellular protein resembling C-terminal globular domains of mucins. *Nat Genet* **2**:139, 1992.
24. Berger W, van de Pol D, Warburg M, Gal A, Bleeker-Wagemakers L, de Silva H, Meindl A, Meitinger T, Cremers F, Ropers H-H: Mutations in the candidate gene for Norrie disease. *Hum Mol Genet* **1**:461, 1992.

25. Meitinger T, Meindl A, Berger W, Ropers HH: The Norrie disease gene: Positional cloning, mutation analysis and protein homologies, in Hollyfield JG, LaVail M, Anderson RE (eds): *Retinal Degeneration: Clinical and Laboratory Applications*. New York, Plenum, 1993, p 135.
26. Meitinger T, Meindl A, Bork P, Rost B, Sander C, Haasemann M, Murken J: Norrie disease protein (NDP) predicted to be a cysteine knot growth factor. *Nat Genet* **5**:376, 1993.
27. Sims KB, Lebo RV, Benson G, Shalish C, Schuback D, Chen ZY, Bruns G, Craig IW, Golbus MS, Breakefield XO: The Norrie disease gene maps to a 150 kb region on chromosome Xp11.3. *Hum Mol Genet* **1**:83, 1992.

CHAPTER **154G**

Neurofibromatosis 2

Huda Y. Zoghbi ▪ Andrea Ballabio

1. **Neurofibromatosis type 2 (NF2) is an autosomal dominant disorder characterized by bilateral Schwann-cell tumors of the vestibular branch of the eighth cranial nerve, vestibular schwannomas, in 95 percent of gene carriers. Additional findings include subcapsular cataracts, occasional café au lait spots, and meningiomas or ependymomas. The diagnosis is usually made on the basis of family history, hearing loss, or associated brain-stem findings secondary to the mass effect of vestibular schwannomas. Gadolinium-enhanced MRI is the most definitive test to confirm the presence of a vestibular schwannoma.**
2. **The NF2 gene was mapped to human chromosome 22q12 first, based on the loss of the heterozygosity for chromosome 22 markers in tumor samples from NF2 patients, and subsequently by linkage analysis in families with NF2. The NF2 gene was isolated by positional cloning and was found to share high sequence homology with the cytoskeleton-associated proteins moesin, ezrin, radixin, and erythrocyte protein 4.1. This family of proteins is proposed to act as a link between the cytoskeleton and the cell membrane.**
3. **NF2 gene deletions as well as single base substitutions resulting in a truncated protein have been identified in several patients. Loss of heterozygosity for chromosome 22 alleles was detected in NF2-related tumors such as schwannomas and meningiomas. The absence of a normal NF2 allele in these tumors and the homology detected with cytoskeleton-associated proteins support the hypothesis that NF2 may represent a novel class of tumor-suppressor genes.**

CLINICAL FEATURES, DIFFERENTIAL DIAGNOSIS, AND THERAPY

In 1822, Wishart described a case of bilateral acoustic neuromas that he presumed to be a form of neurofibromatosis (NF)[1] which was previously described by von Recklinghausen.[2] In 1902, Henneberg and Koch recognized a clinically distinct form of NF, which they referred to as "central" neurofibromatosis, and emphasized the lack of skin alterations and the presence of acoustic neuromas.[3] In 1915, Bassoe and Nuzum described a patient with bilateral cerebellopontine angle tumors and multiple central neurofibromas.[4] In 1930, Gardner and Frazier[5] reported a family with 38 members who had acoustic neuromas transmitted in an autosomal dominant fashion. In 1937, Worster-Drought et al.[6] proposed a classification of NF and suggested three forms—"peripheral", "central," and combined. Later, Riccardi proposed eight provisional categories based on clinical findings in a large cohort of patients.[7] Several family studies subsequently indicated that the form of NF characterized by bilateral cerebellopontine angle tumors is a distinct disorder most likely caused by a single mutant gene.[8–10] Currently, *neurofibromatosis* is used to describe two distinct autosomal dominant diseases that primarily involve tumors of the nervous system.[10,11] NF1, or von Recklinghausen NF, is one of the most common single gene disorders affecting the nervous system with an incidence of 1:3000 to 1:4000 (see Chap. 14). It is characterized by multiple brown skin macules (café au lait spots), iris hamartomas (Lisch modules), and multiple cutaneous neurofibromas. Although patients with NF1 are predisposed to optic gliomas and spinal and peripheral nerve neurofibromas, cerebellopontine angle tumors are virtually nonexistent in these patients.[12,13] NF1 is caused by defects in a gene mapping to chromosome 17,[14–16] whose product (neurofibromin) is presumed to be involved in modulating a signal transduction pathway.[17–21] NF1 is extensively described in Chap. 14. NF2, which occurs with an incidence of 1:40,000,[22] is mainly characterized by bilateral vestibular schwannomas (Fig. 154G-1).

The term *vestibular schwannoma* will be used throughout this chapter, as it has replaced the term *acoustic neuroma* based on the consensus statement from the National Institutes of Health Consensus Development Conference on Acoustic Neuroma.[23] The term *vestibular schwannoma* was

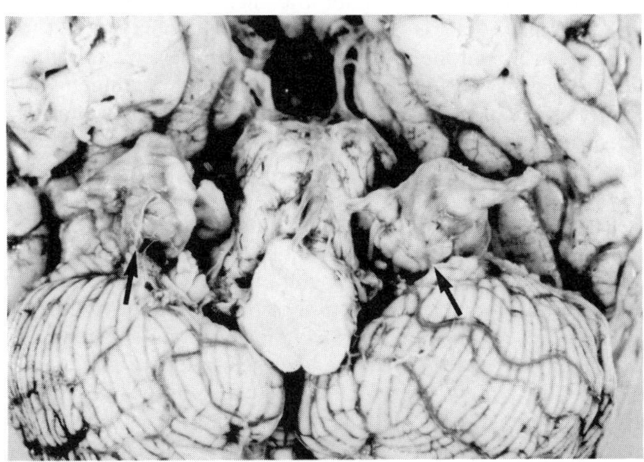

FIG. 154G-1 **View of the base of the brain showing the transected medulla in the midline. Shwannomas of the eighth cranial nerve are seen on each side (*arrows*) in the cerebellopontine angles. *(Courtesy of Dr. D. Armstrong.)***

A list of standard abbreviations is located immediately preceding the index in each volume. Additional abbreviations used in this chapter include: BAER = brain-stem auditory evoked responses; NF = neurofibromatosis, including NF, NF1, and NF2.

adopted because the tumors are composed of Schwann cells and involve the vestibular rather than the acoustic branch of the eighth cranial nerve. Symptoms of vestibular schwannomas are usually caused by pressure from the tumors and most often develop during the second or third decade. The first symptom in NF2 is typically hearing loss, which is generally unilateral but may be symmetric. A frequently reported symptom is distorted sound perception when using the telephone.[10] The hearing loss is usually progressive; however, approximately 10 percent of patients report sudden hearing loss. Other, less commonly reported symptoms, include ringing or roaring in one or both ears, with or without dizziness or unsteadiness.

Other findings related to compression by the tumor mass on neighboring structures may include facial weakness, sensory changes, ataxia, headache, or diplopia.[10] Juvenile lens opacities or subcapsular cataracts are estimated to occur in half of NF2 patients and may precede the onset of other symptoms, allowing early identification of affected individuals. NF2 patients may have café au lait spots and skin neurofibromas but typically these are much less common in NF2 than in NF1. Tumors of the brain, spinal cord, and peripheral nerve are commonly seen in NF2. Schwann-cell tumors are the most common, but tumors of meningeal and glial origin may also be found in the same patient.[10] Penetrance is high in FN2, such that individuals carrying a mutant allele have a 95 percent chance of bilateral vestibular schwannomas developing.[8,24]

The diagnosis of NF2 should be suspected in the following instances: in the parent, sib, or child of a person with NF2; in a person with an apparent unilateral vestibular schwannoma and onset of symptoms before 30 years of age (because sporadic vestibular schwannomas present later in life); in a child with meningeal or Schwann-cell tumor; in an individual of any age with multiple nervous system tumors of unknown etiology; and in a person with a few café au lait spots, one or more neurofibromas, no Lisch nodules, and a negative family history for NF1.[10] Such individuals require detailed evaluation, including careful skin and eye examination, audiologic evaluation, and neuroimaging of the head if indicated. Brain-stem auditory evoked responses (BAER) are ideal for the evaluation of audiologic dysfunction. The sensitivity of the BAER test is 94 percent, and the specificity is greater than 85 percent for the diagnosis of vestibular schwannoma.[23] MRI is considered the most definitive test to confirm or rule out the presence of a vestibular schwannoma. When MRI is performed with gadolinium enhancement, using thin-slice scans in the axial plane, vestibular tumors measuring a few millimeters in diameter can be detected. Early diagnosis of vestibular schwannomas is critical for successful treatment.

The ideal treatment for symptomatic patients is the total excision of the tumor with minimal morbidity and mortality. Other management options include observation, subtotal removal, and radiation. Selection of the treatment option is typically based on the clinical findings, patients' age, and size and growth rate of the tumor. Surgery is clearly indicated in a young patient with evidence of tumor growth or a progressive neurologic deficit. On the other hand, long-term observation is appropriate for the elderly patient without severe neurologic deficits or evidence of tumor growth and for patients with imperfect but stable and useful hearing and no evidence of tumor progression.[10] The use of gadolinium-enhanced MRI has resulted in the identification of patients with very small, relatively asymptomatic vestibular schwannomas. Given that the natural history for these patients is still not known, conservative management may be more appropriate.

MOLECULAR GENETIC AND BIOLOGIC STUDIES

The mapping of the NF2 gene was accomplished first by identifying a candidate region of the genome because of loss of heterozygosity for chromosome 22 markers in tumor samples, and the localization was subsequently confirmed by linkage analysis in families with NF2. Vestibular schwannomas are found relatively frequently in the general population as unilateral, sporadic tumors. This situation, coupled with familial bilateral occurrence of these tumors in NF2, was reminiscent of the clinical presentation of retinoblastoma and Wilms tumor. Hence, it was hypothesized that the same model of tumorigenesis in retinoblastoma and Wilms tumor applies to NF2.[25] This model, first proposed by Knudson,[26] invoked a single locus that normally suppresses tumor formation; two mutations causing loss of function of both alleles at this locus must occur for a sporadic tumor to develop. As this requires two rare events within a single cell, a single unilateral tumor is typically observed. In familial cases, a constitutional mutation predisposing to tumor formation is inherited in an autosomal dominant pattern, and a single somatic mutation affecting the normal homologue will lead to more frequent formation of tumors resulting in bilateral tumors (see Chap. 11).

To test this hypothesis, Seizinger et al.[25] looked for loss of heterozygosity for DNA markers in tumor DNA as compared with leukocyte DNA extracted from patients with unilateral sporadic vestibular schwannomas. Because loss of chromosome 22 had been previously detected in meningiomas (tumors also typically seen in NF2 patients), the initial effort focused on chromosome 22 markers. Loss of heterozygosity for chromosome 22 markers was found in tumors from 44 percent of the patients with sporadic unilateral vestibular schwannoma and in the tumor of one patient with NF2. Subsequently, several studies of sporadic and NF2 tumors confirmed loss of alleles on chromosome 22 and provided further support for the hypothesis that a recessive tumor-suppressor gene involved in NF2 was located on chromosome 22.[27–35]

Proof that the NF2 gene maps to the same chromosomal region frequently found to be deleted in vestibular schwannomas came from a genetic study of one kindred with NF2 in whom linkage between the disease and two chromosome 22 markers was demonstrated.[36] Additional linkage studies confirmed the assignment of the NF2 gene to chromosome 22q12 and suggested that NF2 is genetically homogeneous.[30,35,37,38]

The genetic mapping of the NF2 gene to a well-delineated region on chromosome 22q12 was the first step toward the isolation of this gene by positional cloning. The NF2 gene was isolated independently by two research groups.[39,40] The first group used DNA markers from the candidate NF2 region and PFGE to look for deletions in the DNA of NF2 patients. An altered fragment was detected in the DNA of one patient using a probe derived from the neurofilament heavy chain gene (NEFH). Chromosome walking toward the deletion was initiated from neurofilament locus using cosmid clones, and the size of the deletion was delineated to be approximately 35 to 45 kb. Exon trapping was subsequently used to isolate sequences at, or flanking, the deleted region. In another study, Rouleau et al.[40] identified the candidate NF2 region to be between the markers D22S212 and D22S32. They cloned this region, which spans approximately one Mb, in YAC and cosmids. Using single-copy probes from cosmids in the candidate region, they subsequently analyzed, by PFGE, DNA from 42 unrelated NF2 patients in search of deletions or other alterations. Two deletions were identified, and a candidate region of 40 kb was delineated following detailed analysis of these deletions. Cosmid clones mapping to this 40-kb region were screened for the presence of hypomethylated CpG sequences and for phylogenetic conservation. These efforts resulted in the identification of a gene termed "merlin" by Trofatter et al.[39] and "schwannomin" (SCH) by Rouleau et al.[40] The gene shares high sequence homology with the cytoskeleton-associated proteins, moesin, ezrin, radixin, and erythrocyte protein 4.1 (Fig. 154G-2). The open reading frame for the predicted NF2 protein contains 587 to 595 amino acids.

Northern analysis using total and poly(A)$^+$ RNA from a variety of human tissues (tumor cells, heart, brain, lung, muscle, kidney, pancreas, and liver) indicated that the gene is widely expressed and revealed two major hybridizing RNA species of 7 and 2.6 kb, and one less intensely hybridizing RNA of 4.4 kb. Whether these larger RNA species have a longer 3′ untranslated region or arise by alternative splicing was not determined. Two nonoverlapping germ-line deletions in the NF2 gene, removing 112 amino acids from the N-terminus in one case and 78 amino acids

```
                    1                                                                                                     100
Human Moesin                  .PKT..VR..TMDAE. EF.......GK.LFD.V..T.GLRE.WFFGLQY...K....WLK..KKV...DV.KE.P..F.F.AKFYPE...
Mouse Radixin                 .PK...VR..TMDAE. EF.......GK.LFD.V..T.GLRE.WFFGLQY...K....WLK..KKV...DV.KE.P..F.F.AKF.PE...
Human Ezrin                   .PK...VR..TMDAE. EF.......GK.LFD.V..T.GLRE.W.FGL.Y...K....WLK.DKKV....V.KE.P..F.F.AKFYPE...
Human Merlin        MSFSSLKRKQPKTFTVRIVTMDAEM EFNCEMKWKGKDLFDLVCRTLGLRETWFFGLQY TIKDTVAWLKMDKKVLDHDVSKEEPVTFHFLAKFYPENAE
Ech.mult. tegument     .LKR...KT..VR..T..... EF.......G.DLFD.V.RT.GLRE.W.FG.QY.........L..DKK....D........F.F..KFYPEN.E
Human eryth. 4.1                 ........D....E...E...KG.DL...VC..L.L.E...FGL.........WL...K.....  ....P..F.F..KFYP....

                    101                                                                                                   200
Human Moesin        EEL.Q.ITQ.LFFLQVK..IL...IYCPPE..VLLASYAVQ.KYGD....VHK.G.LA...LLP.RV..........WEERI..W..EHRG..R..A..E
Mouse Radixin       EEL.QEITQ.LFFLQVK..IL...IYCPPE..VLLASYAVQAKYGDY....HK.G.LA...LLP.RV......T.E.WEERI..W..EHRG..R....ME
Human Ezrin         EEL.Q.ITQ.LFFLQVK..IL...IYCPPE..VLL.SYAVQAK.GDY...VHK.G.L..E.L.P.RV......T...WE.RI..W.AEHRG...D.A..E
Human Merlin        EELVQEITQHLFFLQVKKQILDEKIYCPPEASVLLASYAVQAKYGDYDPSVHKRGFLAQEELLPKRVINLYQMTPEMWEERITAWYAEHRGRARDEAEME
Ech.mult. tegument  EEL.Q..T...F.LQVK..I...KIYCP....VLLASYA..AKYG.YDP...... L....L....  ..Y..T.E.W.ERI.A.Y..H....R..A...
Human eryth. 4.1     .L...IT.....LQ....I......C......LL.SY..Q...GDYDP..H.........L.P.....          .EE.........R......A..E

                    201                                                                                                   300
Human Moesin        YLKIAQDLEMYGVNYF.I.NKKG.EL.LGVDALGL.IY....RLTPKI.FPW.EIRNIS..DK.F.IK    P.DKK...F.F....LR.NK.IL.LC.G
Mouse Radixin       YLKIAQDLEMYGVNYF.I.NKKGTEL.LGVDALGL.IY.....LTPKI.FPW.EIRNIS..DK.F.IK    P.DKK...F.F....LR.NK.IL.LC.G
Human Ezrin         YLKIAQDLEMYG.NYF.I.NKKGT.L.LGVDALGL.IY.....LTPKI.FPW.EIRNIS..DK.F.IK    P.DKK...F.F....LR.NK.ILQLC.G
Human Merlin        YLKIAQDLEMYGVNYFAIRNKKGTELLLGVDALGLHIYDPENRLTPKISFPWNEIRNISYSDKEFTIK    PLDKKIDVFKFNSSKLRVNKLILQLCIG
Ech.mult. tegument  YL.IAQDLEMYGV..F.I.NKKGT.L.LGVDALGL.IY.P.N.L.PKI.FPW.EIRN.S..DK.F.IK    P.DK....F.F...K...NK.IL.LC.G
Human eryth. 4.1    .L..A..L.MYGV.........G....LGV...GL..Y....R...    FPW.....ISY....F.IK.............F.....R..K.....C..

                    301                                                                                                   400
Human Moesin        NH.L.MRRRK.D..EVQQMKAQAREEK..KQMER..L..EK..RE.AE......ER.......RL.Q..E....A...L......A..L.....
Mouse Radixin       NH.L.MRRRK.D..EVQQMKAQARE....KQ.ER..L..EK..RE.AE......ER.......RL.Q..E....A...L......A..L....Q
Human Ezrin         NH.L.MRRRK.D..EVQQMKAQAREEK..KQ.ERQ.L..EK..RE..ER......R.......RL....E....A...L......A..L.E...
Human Merlin        NHDLFMRRRKADSLEVQQMKAQAREEKARKQMERQRLAREKQMREEAERTRDELER        RLLQMKEEATMANEALMRSEETADLLAEKAQ
Ech.mult. tegument  NH.L.MRRRK.DS.EVQQMK.QA.EE...K..ERQRL..E...R.E.E    ..L...................A........E...LL.....
Human eryth. 4.1    .H..F R....D........A............     A...Q......R.....ER.......R.L........A...........A......A.......

                    401                                                                                                   500
Human Moesin              ....EA..LA....EAE.........................E.................EA....Q..Q...E........L......
Mouse Radixin             ...EEA..L......AE.....I...A...............E.........E.......EA.........A.E.....K..L.........P.
Human Ezrin               ...EEA..L......A..........A...............E.........E...R...E.........EA.......K..L.........P.
Human Merlin              ITEEEAKLLAQKAAEAEQEMQRIKATAIRTEEEKRLMEQKVLEAEVLALKMAEESERRAKEADQLKQDLQEAREAERRAKQKL   LEIATKPT
Ech.mult. tegument           ....L..............K.......EE.........E.................E..Q        A....RR...K
Human eryth. 4.1    ...................................KR...............M.E.......E.........E......................T

                    501                                                                                                   600
Human Moesin         P....................   S.DL.... M....  .E.E.....EK....Q..L..L..E.........   .TA.D..H.EN. R.G..K..T
Mouse Radixin       .PP..P...............   S..L.... .....  .E.E.V....K......QL..L..E.........   .T..D.LH.EN. ..G..K..T
Human Ezrin         .P...P...................S..L.... .....  .E.......EK....Q.QL..L..E.........   .T..DI.HNEN. R.G..K..T
Human Merlin        YPPMNPIPAPLPPDIPSFNLIGDSLSFDFKDTD MKRLSMEIEKEKVEYMEKSKHLQEQLNELKTEIEALKLKER   ETALDILHNENSDRGGSSKHNT
Ech.mult. tegument       ..........S............K... ........E...V....K...LQ..L..LK.E.........   ....D..H..N. R.G..K..T
Human eryth. 4.1    ..P...........................D...................E......E.....K..I.......R.......DI.H.............

                    601                 623
Human Moesin        .........K.R...FE..*
Mouse Radixin       .........K.....FE..*
Human Ezrin         .........K.R...FE.L*
Human Merlin        IKKLTLQSAKSRVAFFEEL*
Ech.mult. tegument  ..........RV..FE..*
Human eryth. 4.1    ....  ...K..V....E....*
```

FIG. 154G-2 Comparison of the amino acid sequence identities between the NF2 gene product (merlin) and other merlin-related proteins. Dots indicate nonidentical amino acids, and empty spaces represent gaps introduced by the program. *(From Trofatter et al.[39] Used by permission of* Cell.*)*

from the C-terminus in the other, were detected in unrelated NF2 families. Alterations resulting from 4-bp and 1-bp deletions in meningiomas from two unrelated NF2 patients were also demonstrated.[39]

In search of point mutations in NF2 patients, Rouleau et al.[40] performed denaturing gradient-gel electrophoresis on the amplified exons of the NF2 gene from 90 unrelated NF2 patients. Fifteen variants were identified and sequenced; 14 of the 15 mutations identified were predicted to result in a truncated protein. One variant caused a nonconservative leucine-to-proline substitution.[40] Mutations were also detected in two schwannomas and two meningiomas from non-NF2 patients, and in two schwannomas from NF2 patients. Loss of heterozygosity for the chromosome 22 allele in three of the non-NF2 tumors, and the loss of a normal NF2 allele in one and a germ-line mutation in the other tumors from NF2 patients, support the hypothesis that the NF2 gene is a tumor-suppressor gene that is inactivated by two hits.[40]

The NF2 gene product (merlin/schwannomin) is a novel member of a family of proteins proposed to act as a link between the cytoskeleton and the cell membrane.[41,42] All members of this family (moesin, ezrin, radixin, protein 4.1, and talin) have a large N-terminal domain (~200 amino acids), a large α-helix domain, and a small highly charged C-terminal domain. Erythrocyte protein 4.1, which is one of the best-studied members of this family, maintains membrane stability and cell shape in the erythrocyte by linking the integral membrane glycoproteins to the spectrin–actin complex of the cytoskeleton (see Chap. 115 for discussion of genetic defects in protein 4.1).[43,44]

The protein encoded by the NF2 gene has an N-terminal domain that is closely related to moesin, ezrin, and radixin (approximately 63 percent identity for the first 342 amino acids). It also possesses a long α-helical domain of which the first third overlaps with the region of highest homology to moesin, ezrin, and radixin.[39] The C-terminal region of the protein is also homologous to other members of the family. These structural similarities suggest that the NF2 protein, like other members of this family of proteins, may act as a link between the cytoskeleton and cell membrane and hence may represent a novel class of tumor-suppressor genes. The implications of cloning the NF2 gene are both biologic and clinical. Investigating the mechanism by which a protein presumed to link the cell membrane with the cytoskeleton disrupts cell growth and causes tumor formation will be crucial for exploring how this class of tumor-suppressor genes functions. From a clinical perspective, members of NF2 families in whom the mutation has been identified can now be directly tested for mutations of this gene and can be spared repeated medical evaluations. For the remaining families, mutation detection strategies must be employed for molecular diagnosis.

REFERENCES

1. Cushing H: *Tumors of the Nervus Acusticus*. Philadelphia, Saunders, 1917.
2. von Recklinghausen F: *Ueber die multiplen Fibrome der Haut und ihre Beziehung zu den multiplen Neuromen*. Berlin, Hirschwald, 1882.
3. Henneberg R, Koch M: Ueber "centrale" Neurofibromatose und die Geschwulste des Kleinhirnbruckenwinkels (Acusticusneurome). *Arch Psychiatrie* **36:**251, 1902.
4. Bassoe P, Nuzum F: Report of a case of central and peripheral neurofibromatosis. *J Nerv Ment Dis* **42:**785, 1915.
5. Gardner WJ, Frazier CH: Bilateral acoustic neurofibromas: A clinical study and field survey of a family of five generations with bilateral deafness in thirty-eight members. *Arch Neurol Psychiatry* **23:**266, 1930.
6. Worster-Drought C, Carnegie Dickson WE, McMenemey WH: Multiple meningeal and perineural tumours with analogous changes in the glia and ependyma (neurofibroblastomatosis): With report of two cases. *Brain* **60:**85, 1937.
7. Riccardi VM: Neurofibromatosis: Clinical heterogeneity. *Curr Probl Cancer* **7:**1, 1982.
8. Young DF, Eldridge R, Nager GT, Deland FH, McNew J: Hereditary bilateral acoustic neuroma (central neurofibromatosis). *Birth Defects* **7:**73, 1971.
9. Kanter WR, Eldridge R, Fabricant R, Allen JC, Koerber T: Central neurofibromatosis with bilateral acoustic neuroma: Genetic, clinical and biochemical distinctions from peripheral neurofibromatosis. *Neurology* **30:**851, 1980.
10. Martuza RL, Eldridge R: Neurofibromatosis 2 (bilateral acoustic neurofibromatosis). *N Engl J Med* **318:**684, 1988.
11. Mulvihill JJ, Parry DM, Sherman JL, Pikus A, Kaiser-Kupfer MI, Eldridge R: NIH conference. Neurofibromatosis 1 (Recklinghausen disease) and neurofibromatosis 2 (bilateral acoustic neurofibromatosis). An update. *Ann Intern Med* **113:**39, 1990.
12. Riccardi VM: von Recklinghausen neurofibromatosis. *N Engl J Med* **305:**1617, 1981.
13. Riccardi VM, Eichner JE: *Neurofibromatosis: Phenotype, Natural History, and Pathogenesis*. Baltimore, Johns Hopkins University Press, 1986.
14. Viskochil D, Buchberg AM, Xu G, Cawthon RM, Stevens J, Wolff RK, Culver M, Carey JC, Copeland NG, Jenkins NA, White R, O'Connell P: Deletions and a translocation interrupt a cloned gene at the neurofibromatosis type 1 locus. *Cell* **62:**187, 1990.
15. Cawthon RM, Weiss R, Xu G, Viskochil D, Culver M, Stevens J, Robertson M, Dunn D, Gesteland R, O'Connell P, White R: A major segment of the neurofibromatosis type 1 gene: cDNA sequence, genomic structure, and point mutations. *Cell* **62:**193, 1990.
16. Wallace MR, Marchuk DA, Anderson LB, Letcher R, Odeh HM, Saulino AM, Fountain JW, Brereton A, Nicholson J, Mitchell AL, Brownstein BH, Collins FS: Type 1 neurofibromatosis gene: Identification of a larger transcript disrupted in three NF1 patients. *Science* **249:**181, 1990.
17. Ballester R, Marchuk D, Boguski M, Saulino A, Letcher R, Wigler M, Collins F: The *NF1* locus encodes a protein functionally related to mammalian GAP and yeast *IRA* proteins. *Cell* **63:**851, 1990.
18. Buchberg AM, Cleveland LS, Jenkins NA, Copeland NG: Sequence homology shared by neurofibromatosis type-1 gene and IRA-1 and IRA-2 negative regulators of the RAS cyclic AMP pathway. *Nature* **347:**291, 1990.
19. Xu G, O'Connell P, Viskochil D, Cawthon R, Robertson M, Culver M, Dunn D, Stevens J, Gesteland R, White R, Weiss R: The neurofibromatosis type 1 gene encodes a protein related to GAP. *Cell* **62:**599, 1990.
20. DeClue JE, Papageorge AG, Fletcher JA, Diehl SR, Ratner N, Vass WC, Lowy DR: Abnormal regulation of mammalian $p21^{ras}$ contributes to malignant tumor growth in von Recklinghausen (type 1) neurofibromatosis. *Cell* **69:**265, 1992.
21. Basu TN, Gutmann DH, Fletcher JA, Glover TW, Collins FS, Downward J: Aberrant regulation of *ras* protein in malignant tumour cell from type 1 neurofibromatosis patients. *Nature* **356:**713, 1992.
22. Evans DGR, Huson SM, Donnai D, Neary W, Blair V, Teare D, Newton V, Strachan T, Ramsden R, Harris R: A genetic study of type 2 neurofibromatosis in the United Kingdom. I. Prevalence, mutation rate, fitness and confirmation of maternal transmission effect on severity. *J Med Genet* **29:**841, 1992.
23. Eldridge R, Parry DM: Summary: Vestibular schwannoma (acoustic neuroma). Consensus Development Conference. *Neurosurgery* **30:**961, 1992.
24. Eldridge R: Central neurofibromatosis with bilateral acoustic neuroma. *Adv Neurol* **29:**57, 1981.
25. Seizinger BR, Martuza RL, Gusella JF: Loss of genes on chromosome 22 in tumorigenesis of human acoustic neuroma. *Nature* **322:**644, 1986.

26. Knudson AG: Mutation and cancer: A statistical study. *Proc Natl Acad Sci USA* **68**:820, 1971.
27. Seizinger BR, Rouleau GA, Ozelius LJ, Lane AH, St. George-Hyslop P, Gusella JF: Common pathogenetic mechanism for three tumor types in bilateral acoustic neurofibromatosis. *Science* **236**:317, 1987.
28. Seizinger BR, de La Monte S, Atkins L, Gusella JF, Martuza RL: Molecular genetic approach to human meningioma: Loss of genes on chromosome 22. *Proc Natl Acad Sci USA* **84**:5419, 1987.
29. Couturier J, Delattre O, Kujas M, Philippon J, Peter M, Rouleau G, Aurias A, Thomas G: Assessment of chromosome 22 anomalies in neurinomas by combined karyotype and RFLP analyses. *Cancer Genet Cytogenet* **45**:55, 1990.
30. Rouleau GA, Seizinger BR, Wertelecki W, Haines JL, Superneau DW, Martuza RL, Gusella JF: Flanking markers bracket the neurofibromatosis type 2 (*NF2*) gene on chromosome 22. *Am J Hum Genet* **46**:323, 1990.
31. Fiedler W, Claussen U, Ludecke HJ, Senger G, Horsthemke B, Geurts Van Kessel A, Goertzen W, Fashold R: New markers for the neurofibromatosis-2 region generated by microdissection of chromosome 22. *Genomics* **10**:786, 1991.
32. Fontaine B, Hanson MP, VonSattel JO, Martuza RL, Gusella JF: Loss of chromosome 22 alleles in human sporadic spinal schwannomas. *Ann Neurol* **29**:183, 1991.
33. Fontaine B, Sanson M, Delattre O, Menon AG, Rouleau GA, Seizinger BR, Jewell AF, Hanson MP, Aurias A, Martuza RL, Gusella JF, Thomas G: Parental origin of chromosome 22 loss in sporadic and NF2 neuromas. *Genomics* **10**:280, 1991.
34. Bijlsma EK, Brouwer-Mladin R, Bosch DA, Westerveld A, Hulsebos TJ: Molecular characterization of chromosome 22 deletions in schwannomas. *Genes Chrom Cancer* **5**:201, 1992.
35. Wolff RK, Frazer KA, Jackler RK, Lanser MJ, Pitts LH, Cox DR: Analysis of chromosome 22 deletions in neurofibromatosis type 2-related tumors. *Am J Hum Genet* **51**:478, 1992.
36. Rouleau GA, Wertelecki W, Haines JL, Hobbs WJ, Trofatter JA, Seizinger BR, Martuza RL, Superneau DW, Conneally PM, Gusella JF: Genetic linkage of bilateral acoustic neurofibromatosis to a DNA marker on chromosome 22. *Nature* **329**:246, 1987.
37. Wertelecki W, Rouleau GA, Superneau DW, Forehand LW, Williams JP, Haines JL, Gusella JF: Neurofibromatosis 2: Clinical and DNA linkage studies of a large kindred. *N Engl J Med* **319**:278, 1988.
38. Narod SA, Parry DM, Parbossingh J, Lenoir GM, Rutledge M, Fisher G, Eldridge R, Martuza RL, Frontali M, Haines J, Gusella JF, Rouleau GA: Neurofibromatosis type 2 appears to be a genetically homogeneous disease. *Am J Hum Genet* **51**:486, 1992.
39. Trofatter JA, MacCollin MM, Rutter JL, Murrell JR, Duyao MP, Parry DM, Eldridge R, Kley N, Menon AG, Pulaski K, Haase VH, Ambrose CM, Munroe D, Bove C, Haines JL, Martuza RL, MacDonald ME, Seizinger BR, Short MP, Buckler AJ, Gusella JF: A novel moesin-, ezrin, radixin-like gene is a candidate for the neurofibromatosis 2 tumor suppressor. *Cell* **72**:791, 1993.
40. Rouleau GA, Merel P, Lutchman M, Sanson M, Zucman J, Marineau C, Hoang-Xuan K, Demczuk S, Desmaze C, Plougastel B, Pulst S, Lenoir G, Bijlsma E, Fashold R, Dumanski J, de Jong P, Parry D, Eldridge R, Aurias A, Delattre O, Thomas G: Alteration in a new gene encoding a putative membrane-organizing protein causes neurofibromatosis type 2. *Nature* **363**:515, 1993.
41. Luna EJ, Hitt AL: Cytoskeleton-plasma membrane interactions. *Science* **258**:955, 1992.
42. Sato N, Funayama N, Nagafuchi A, Yonemura S, Tsukita S, Tsukita S: A gene family consisting of ezrin, radixin and moesin. Its specific localization at actin filament/plasma membrane association sites. *J Cell Sci* **103**:131, 1992.
43. Leto TL, Marchesi VT: A structural model of human erythrocyte protein 4.1. *J Biol Chem* **259**:4603, 1984.
44. Conboy J, Kan YW, Shohet SB, Mohandas N: Molecular cloning of protein 4.1, a major structural element of the human erythrocyte membrane skeleton. *Proc Natl Acad Sci USA* **83**:9512, 1986.

CHAPTER **154H**

Aspartoacylase Deficiency (Canavan Disease)

Arthur L. Beaudet

HISTORICAL

The disorder now identified as aspartoacylase deficiency is equivalent to the condition variously called spongy degeneration of the brain, spongy degeneration of the central nervous system in infancy, or spongy degeneration of infancy, and many publications have used the eponymic designation, Canavan disease. The first definition of this condition as a distinct clinical entity is properly credited to van Bogaert and Bertrand in 1949.[1,2] In retrospect, the first clinical description is attributed to Globus and Strauss in 1928.[3] In 1931 Canavan described an infant with prominent enlargement of the head and cerebral and cerebellar spongy degeneration under the designation "Schilder's encephalitis periaxialis diffusa".[4] Eiselsberg is credited with the recognition of the familial nature of the disorder in 1937,[5] but like Jervis,[6,7] she described the condition as Krabbe disease. The reports of von Bogaert and Bertrand[1,2] were comprehensive and described the essential pathologic and clinical features as well as the predilection for the occurrence of the disorder in Ashkenazic infants. In a more detailed review of the historical literature,[8] Banker et al. pointed out that the Canavan eponym is hardly justified, since her report was not the first clinical description, did not recognize the familial or ethnic aspect to the disorder, and did not recognize spongy degeneration as the unique pathologic feature; the designation *aspartoacylase deficiency* may be most appropriate at this time, but the eponym is widely used.

Unraveling of the biochemical basis of infantile spongy degeneration began with the description of urinary excretion of *N*-acetylaspartic acid (NAA) by Kvittingen et al.,[9] but aspartoacylase was reported to be normal in cultured fibroblasts; presumably the failure to demonstrate the enzyme deficiency was due to the choice of conditions for enzyme analysis. In 1987 Hagenfeldt et al. reported *N*-acetylaspartic aciduria and identified aspartoacylase deficiency,[10] but neither of these biochemical reports recognized the association with infantile spongy degeneration. Matalon et al.,[11,12] and Divry et al.[13,14] are credited with the recognition that aspartoacylase deficiency correlated with infantile spongy degeneration (Canavan disease). Kaul et al. went on to isolate a cDNA clone for human aspartoacylase and identified the common mutation in Jewish patients.[15]

A list of standard abbreviations is located immediately preceding the index in each volume. Additional abbreviations used in this chapter include: NAA = *N*-acetylaspartic acid; NAAG = *N*-acetyl-aspartyl-glutamate.

CLINICAL FEATURES

In addition to the landmark descriptions of von Bogaert and Bertrand,[1,2] Banker and colleagues and others have provided excellent reviews of the clinical and pathologic features of infantile spongy degeneration.[8,16,17] Ungar and Goodman reviewed cases of infantile spongy degeneration in Israel from 1965 to 1980.[18] Although infants are virtually always normal in the first month of life, they demonstrate poor head control, seizures, and abnormal muscle tone beginning in the second to fourth month, and all those with the classic phenotype are clearly neurologically abnormal before six months of age (Table 154H-1). Some skills such as grasping, visual attentiveness, and smiling may be acquired and subsequently lost. Increase in head circumference is uniformly present by six months of age and may be associated with delayed closure of the anterior fontanelle. This correlates with a substantial increase in brain weight at necropsy, which is most conspicuous if death occurs before three years of age. Brain weight is closer to the normal range thereafter (Fig. 154H-1).[19] Motor activity is consistently abnormal with diminished muscle tone and decreased motor activity early in life and spasticity at later times, although this transition may occur as early as five weeks of age or as late as three years of age.[8] Increased deep tendon reflexes and the presence of Babinski signs are common, and the patients progress to extreme hypertonicity with pseudobulbar palsy and decerebrate or decorticate posturing. Tonic extensor

Table 154H-1 Clinical Features of Aspartoacylase Deficiency

Normal first month of life
Poor head control and hypotonia at 2–4 months
Generalized seizures
Opisthotonic posturing
Loss of very early milestones
Increased head circumference
Leukodystrophy on MRI or CT
Hypotonia progresses to spasticity
Decerebrate or decorticate posturing late

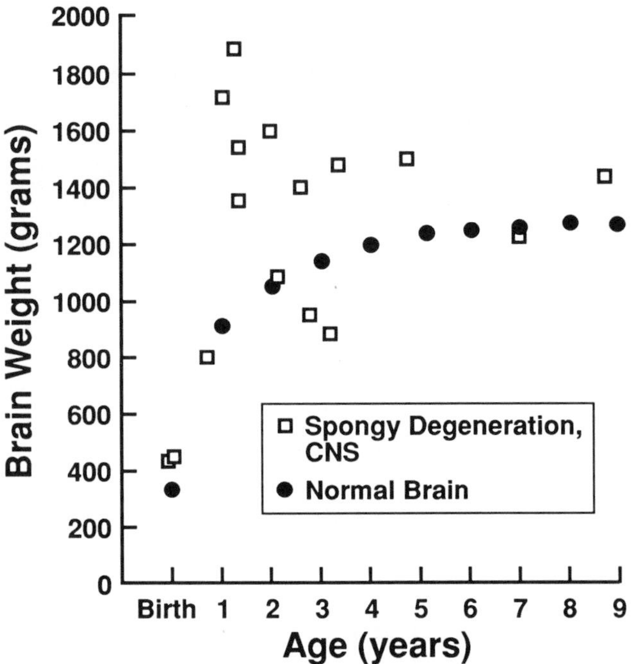

FIG. 154H-1 Brain weights in infantile spongy degeneration compared to normal mean values. (From Adachi and Aronson,[19] by permission of Pergamon Press.)

spasms are common with exaggerated opisthotonic posturing in response to stimuli. Seizures, usually generalized tonic and clonic type, occur in about half of patients; dysphagia, optic atrophy, and nystagmus are reported in a significant but lesser fraction.[18] There has been a suggestion that the phenotype may include a mild hypopigmentation,[16,18] but this finding is of uncertain significance.

Occasional patients may have a somewhat later age of onset,[20] and prolonged survival can occur in some cases.[21] Suggestions that there might be a juvenile form of disease[22–25] require further study to determine if there are milder mutations or other modifying factors which might account for such a phenotype. Cholelithiasis has been reported in one case,[26] but this association may not be significant. Based on necropsy data,[19] it would appear that the majority of deaths are relatively evenly distributed over the first three years of life with some patients surviving substantially longer.

Depending on the clinical presentation, differential diagnoses might include disorders where biochemical studies should clarify the diagnosis as for G_{M1} gangliosidosis or Krabbe disease. The increased head circumference can raise the possibility of Sotos syndrome, but the neurological progression should distinguish this disorder. Although megalencephaly also occurs in Alexander disease, the pathological findings are distinct. Other disorders with familial megalencephaly and leukodystrophy with unknown biochemical defect are reported.[27] At this time, biochemical analysis for aspartoacylase deficiency or the associated *N*-acetylaspartic aciduria can be readily utilized to provide a definitive diagnosis.

Cerbral Imaging

There are numerous reports of CT and MRI studies of the brain in aspartoacylase deficiency.[28–37] The most consistent findings are diffuse symmetrical abnormalities of white matter which are sometimes quite nonuniform. The white matter disease can be seen using CT and also using ultrasound.[35] Many investigators have used proton magnetic resonance spectroscopy to quantitate the levels of NAA in the brain in vivo. Most have reported increased amounts of this compound in the brain relative to other metabolites such as choline and creatinine,[28,30–32] although some reports emphasize normal levels of NAA with reduced levels of these other metabolites.[32,33] Although changes in white matter are not always present,[34] MRI studies usually show symmetrical diffuse low signal intensity on T1-weighted images and high signal intensity on T2-weighted images (Fig. 154H-2).

GENETICS AND INCIDENCE

Infantile spongy degeneration due to aspartoacylase deficiency is an autosomal recessive disorder (McKusick MIM# 271900). A review of cases reported from 1928 to 1977 appeared in 1979 and identified 83 cases in 48 families which were felt to meet the appropriate clinical and pathologic criteria for a diagnosis of infantile spongy degeneration.[16]

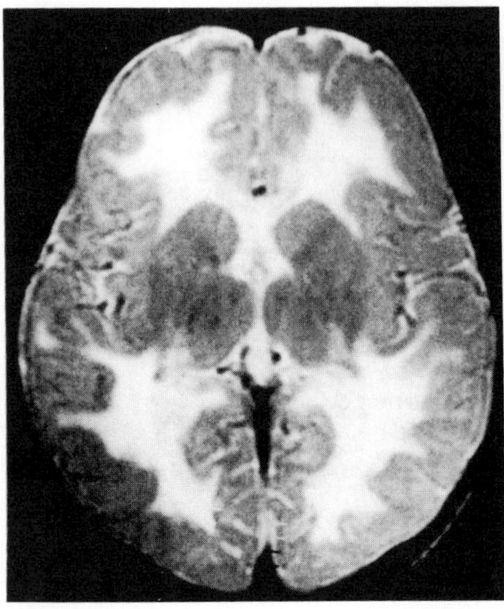
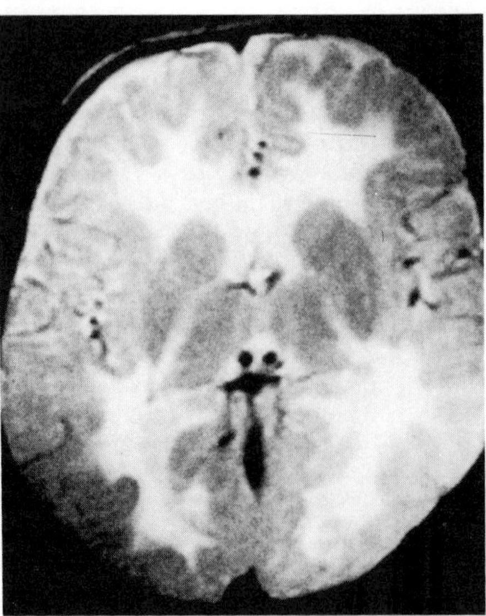

FIG. 154H-2 MRI of the brain showing severe white matter changes. *Left:* MRI (2300/80) in a 2 year old girl showing severe changes in the subcortical white matter. *Right:* MRI (2000/80) in a 12 month old boy also showing severe changes in the subcortical white matter. (From Brismar,[29] by permission of *AJNR American Journal of Neuroradiology*.)

Consanguinity was found in 23 percent of 48 families in one study[16] being slightly more frequent in the non-Jewish families than in the Jewish families. Although there was a suggestion of a statistically significant difference in male:female ratio,[16] there was no difference when the Jewish and non-Jewish cases were conmbined, and this is unlikely to be of significance. Of the 42 families with known ethnic origin, 28 were Jewish (mostly Ashkenazic) with multiple other ethnic groups represented including German, Swiss, Austrian, Irish, Italian, French Canadian, Ojibway Indian, and Iranian (see Banker and Victor[16] for bibliography). Of eleven families identified in Israel, seven were Ashkenazic with the others being Iraqi, Yemenite, or Spanish Moroccan.[18] There is some evidence that the ancestors of Ashkenazic patients originated from eastern Poland, Lithuania, and western Ukraine,[8] but some may have come from more scattered regions in Europe.[18] Although the disease is definitely relatively rare and occurs preferentially in the Ashkenazic population, one group reported diagnosing 145 patients biochemically by 1993[15] suggesting that the disorder may be somewhat more common than has been appreciated. In more recent years, there have been numerous reports of patients documented biochemically by the presence of *N*-acetylaspartic aciduria and/or aspartoacylase deficiency[13,20,21,26,29,31,33,34,38–45] including at least 24 patients from Saudi Arabia.[46]

PATHOLOGY

Histopathology of the brain provided the primary diagnostic criterion for infantile spongy degeneration from the time of the classic delineation of van Bogaert and Bertrand in 1949 until the biochemical delineation of the disorder in the late 1980s, and detailed descriptions are available.[1,2,8,16,19] At autopsy, the white matter is characteristically soft and gelatinous. The spongy or vacuolization change (Fig. 154H-3) is seen in the lower layers of the gray matter and in the subcortical white matter with the more central white matter tending to be relatively or entirely spared. There is extensive loss of myelin, maintenance or slight increase in numbers of oligodendroglia, and a prominent increase in protoplasmic astrocytes. It was postulated by van Bogaert and Bertrand that these changes might represent a form of chronic edema. Interestingly in the context of the newer biochemical knowledge, Wolman had suggested in 1958[47] that catabolites of low molecular value might contribute to edema formation, although he proposed that these might be breakdown products of myelin.

Extensive ultrastructural studies have been performed by Adachi and colleagues.[19,22,48] At the electron microscopic level, vacuoles are demonstrated to be within the swollen cytoplasm and processes of protoplasmic astrocytes in the cortex, and the vacuolated appearance of the white matter is primarily related to swelling of the protoplasmic astrocytes. The membrane bound vacuoles in the cytoplasm appear to arise from the smooth portion of the endoplasmic reticulum. In the subcortical white matter, vacuoles are also found between split lamellae of the myelin spirals. The split occurs between the major dense lines of myelin. Vacuoles are thought to communicate through ruptured membranes into widened extracellular spaces. Mitochondria in astrocytes showed elongations and contain distended and distorted cristae. Biochemically, there is marked loss of proteolipid protein and total lipids in the white matter,[49,50] but these changes are thought to be nonspecific.

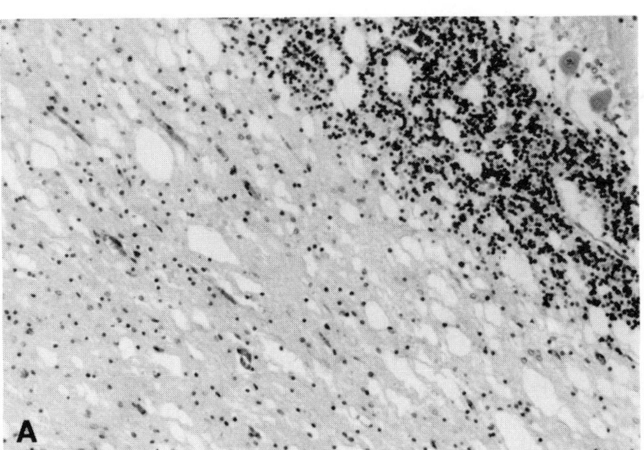

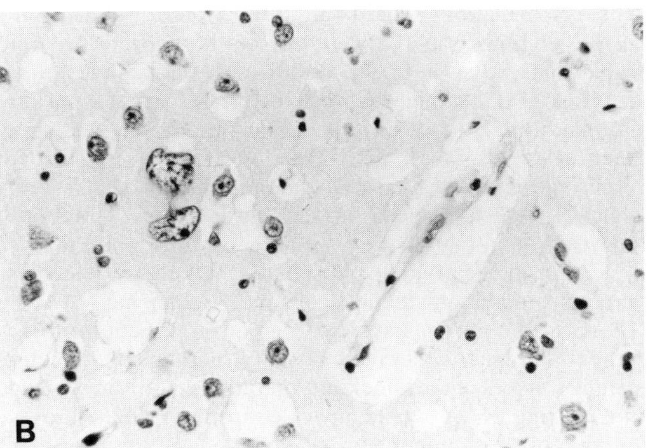

FIG. 154H-3 **Histopathology showing spongy degeneration. Panel A: Cerebellar folia showing spongy degeneration. The vacuoles tend to be oriented parallel to the fibers, and are concentrated in the sub-Purkinje cell layer, and in the white matter adjacent to the internal granular cell layer. (H&Ex40). Panel B: White matter showing Alzheimer type II astrocytes. The nuclei are enlarged, altered in shape and have a well defined nuclear membrane. (H&Ex100) (Courtesy of Dawna Armstrong, M.D. and Hannes Vogel, M.D.)**

BIOCHEMISTRY

N-acetyl-L-aspartic acid (NAA) is a compound of particular interest because it is found only in the nervous system, because the concentration of free NAA is enormous, and because its function is almost totally enigmatic. NAA was discovered in 1956,[51] and a review of the literature published in 1989[37] provides an extensive bibliography regarding topics such as regional distribution and quantitation within the brain, species differences, changes induced by exogenous substances and treatments, synthesis, breakdown, and possible functions. The concentration of NAA is second only to glutamate in total concentration of free amino acids in mammals. The fact that concentrations of NAA can be studied in vivo using proton magnetic resonance spectroscopy should prove to be an important tool for understanding the clinical signifance of this compound.

NAA is synthesized from acetyl-CoA and L-aspartic acid by an enzyme termed acetyl-CoA-L-aspartate *N*-acetyltransferase (EC 2.3.1.2) (Fig. 154H-4).[37,52–54] The enzyme is not in the supernatant of cellular extracts and is thought to be located in a subcellular organelle, perhaps mitochondria,[55] and its distribution within the nervous system has been

acetyl-CoA-L-aspartate *N*-acetyltransferase
(EC 2.3.1.2)

acetyl-CoA + L-aspartate → acetylaspartate + CoA-SH

aspartoacylase
(*N*-acyl-L-aspartate amidohydrolase; EC 3.5.1.15)

acetylaspartate → L-aspartate + acetate

FIG. 154H-4 Pathways for synthesis and degradation of *N*-acetylaspartic acid.

suggested to be similar to that of *N*-acetyl-aspartyl-glutamate (NAAG),[56] suggesting that NAA may act as a precursor for NAAG. The function of NAAG is also unclear, although there is some evidence for action on receptors of Purkinje cells.[57] Speculations regarding the function of NAA include the possibilities that the acetyl group is incorporated into brain lipids, that it might stabilize the concentration of acetyl-CoA, that it might serve as a storage form of aspartate, and that it might serve as a precursor for NAAG. NAA may function as a cofactor in conversion of lignoceric acid to cerebronic acid.[58] NAA is found in the synaptosomal fraction while NAAG is present in the mitochondrial fraction.[59] NAAG, but not NAA, serves as a cofactor for the urea cycle enzyme, carbamyl phosphate synthetase. There are numerous immunohistochemical studies localizing NAA and NAAG in the nervous system,[60–62] but the function of each compound remains relatively obscure. Perhaps the development of mice with knockout mutations for the enzyme synthesizing NAA would provide further insight into the function of this compound.

Aspartoacylase was first described as a form of amino acid acylase.[63] Subsequently amino acid acylase II was found to hydrolyze NAA preferentially[64] and was designated aspartoacylase (*N*-acyl-L-aspartate amidohydrolase; EC 3.5.1.15). The enzyme hydrolyzes NAA to acetic acid and aspartic acid (Fig. 154H-4). Aspartoacylase was purfied from bovine brain and found to be a 55-kDa monomer with highest abundance in white matter.[65] The enzyme is variously reported to be cytosolic or membrane associated and is solubilized by detergent,[65,66] but the cDNA sequence does not suggest the existence of a leader peptide.[15]

The pathogenesis of the phenotype in aspartoacylase deficiency is unclear. Since there are many alternative sources for acetate and aspartate in the brain, it would seem unlikely that deficiency of the products of the reaction is important. Increased concentrations of NAA in tissues and fluids would suggest the possibility that NAA or related metabolites might have toxic effects. There is no explanation for the fact that patients are asymptomatic for the first month of life and then rapidly develop symptoms, although enzymatic and metabolite abnormalities are present prenatally. Concentrations of NAA are reported to increase sixfold from birth to 20 days of age in rats,[67] but findings in humans regarding changes in concentration after birth are inconclusive.[37]

MOLECULAR GENETICS

Matalon and colleagues purified bovine aspartoacylase to obtain partial amino acid sequence which was then used to construct primers to isolate a bovine cDNA clone.[68] The bovine cDNA was then used to isolate a human cDNA of 1,435 bp with 158 bp of 5′ untranslated and 316 bp of 3′ untranslated sequence.[15] The human cDNA predicts a 313 amino acid protein that is 92 percent identical to the bovine sequence. The predicted molecular mass of 36 kDa contrasts with the biochemical determination of 58 kDa for the bovine enzyme, but there are five potential phosphorylation sites and one potential *N*-glycosylation site in the human sequence. Northern blot analysis revealed transcripts of 1.44 and 5.4 kb with intensity greatest in skeletal muscle followed by kidney and brain. Expression of the human cDNA sequence in bacteria resulted in modest levels of aspartoacylase activity. The gene for aspartoacylase (gene symbol = *ASPA*) was found to be comprised of six exons spread over 29 kb of genomic DNA,[69] and the human gene was mapped to chromosome 17p13-pter.

In the initial cloning report,[15] a single nucleotide change was found in patients with aminoacylase deficiency changing Glu at codon 285 to Ala (E285A). This mutation was found in 85 percent of 34 mutant chromosomes tested.[15] Additional mutations have been identified (Table 154H-2) including mutation of Tyr at codon 231 to nonsense (Y231X), Ala at codon 305 to Glu (A305E), and a splicing mutation in intron 2 (433-2A→G).[70] Analysis of 88 disease chromosomes from Ashkenazic Jewish patients identified the mutation in all but one with E285A, Y231X, and 433-2A→G representing 83, 15 and 1 percent of the chromosomes respectively.[70] Analysis of 40 disease chromosomes from non-Jewish families of European descent identified the A305E mutation in 24 and the E285A mutation in one with unknown mutations of 15 chromosomes.

Table 154H-2 Aspartoacylase Mutations

Nucleotide Change	Protein Coding	Ethnicity
854A→C	E285A	Ashkenazic
693C→A	Y231X	Ashkenazic
914C→A	A305E	European, non-Jewish
433-2A→G	Splicing	One Ashkenazic

DIAGNOSIS AND TREATMENT

It should be possible to suspect the diagnosis of aspartoacylase deficiency based on clinical features and cranial imaging studies. Ashkenazic ancestry is present in a substantial fraction of cases. If the disorder is suspected, a diagnosis can be confirmed by the demonstration of increased amounts of NAA in the urine using gas chromatography/mass spectroscopy (GC/MS)[71,72] and/or by enzyme analysis of cultured fibroblasts,[11,73]; enzyme analysis of leukocytes is not reported. The mass spectra for derivitized metabolites of NAA have been published, and accurate quantitation of levels in urine, plasma, and cerebrospinal fluid have been reported using stable isotope dilution methods.[71,72] Normal ranges of NAA in urine were reported as 6.6 to 35.4 or 12.7 ± 7.8μmol/mmol of creatinine in two studies with affected values typically being more than 20 fold above the upper limits of normal. Activity of aspartoacylase is readily detected in cultured skin fibroblasts with values being profoundly reduced in affected patients.[71,72] Enzyme activity has been measured spectrophotometrically as aspartic acid produced using absorbance at 340 nm to quantitate conversion of NADH to NAD in the presence of malate dehydrogenase and aspartate aminotransferase.[10,11] A sensitive radiometric assay utilizes ion exchange chromatography to quantitate the production of [^{3}H]acetate from[^{3}H]NAA.[73] Since the first two cases of *N*-acetylaspartic aciduria were reported without recognizing the association with infantile spongy degeneration, it seems likely that some infants will continue to be diagnosed on the basis of urinary organic acid analysis in patients with neurological symptoms where the diagnosis of infantile spongy degeneration is not specifically being considered. For this reason, laboratories performing urinary organic acid analysis should be alert to the conditions necessary for extraction and detection of NAA and to the significance of this compound in the urine. Mutation analysis will also permit diagnosis in the majority of Jewish patients and in a significant fraction of non-Jewish patients, but biochemical studies should remain the primary basis for diagnosis or ruling out the condition.

PRENATAL DIAGNOSIS

Prenatal diagnosis has been attempted primarily utilizing quantitation of NAA in amniotic fluid and measuring aspartoacylase activity in cultured amniotic fluid cells or chorionic villus samples. Early reports[46,74] have been supplanted by subsequent more extensive experience. Prenatal diagnosis using stable isotope dilution to quantitate NAA in the amniotic fluid found values within the normal range in a fetus later born and found to be healthy,[71] and retrospective analysis of amniotic fluid revealed elevation of NAA in two affected pregnancies.[75] In one report, 19 pregnancies at 1 in 4 risk were analyzed using enzyme assay on cultured CVS and amniocytes as well as measurement of NAA in amniotic fluid,[76] and 16 pregnancies were predicted to be normal and three were predicted to be affected. With expansion of this series, the same group found that 4 of 24 fetuses predicted to be normal were born affected.[68] One study of 17 pregnancies[77] compared quantitation of amniotic fluid NAA in four laboratories; 8 of 17 pregnancies were predicted to be affected, and biochemical or clinical data were available in 6 of these 8 to indicate a correct diagnosis. One case yielded ambiguous data, and one false negative result occurred. Enzyme analysis of cultured amniotic fluid cells in the same study[77] concluded that activity was too low to be of value. It has been emphasized that isotope dilution methods are more reliable for quantitation of NAA and that normal values in amniotic fluid increase during gestation.[75]

Overall, the data suggest that there are modest elevations of NAA in amniotic fluid during the second trimester, but these increases are minimal by comparison to the findings in postnatal urine. Although prenatal diagnosis by measurement of amniotic fluid NAA is accurate in the majority of cases, the separation of values in affected and unaffected pregnancies is marginal, and numerous diagnostic errors have occurred. Use of isotope dilution methods and appropriate gestational controls should provide improved reliability. Levels of aspartoacylase activity in cultured CVS and cultured amniocytes are very low by comparison to cultured skin fibroblasts, and are not reliable for prenatal diagnosis. Given these problems, diagnosis by DNA analysis would now be far preferable and can be used in addition to measurement of NAA in amniotic fluid. DNA diagnosis should be straightforward in cases where the mutations can be identified in the index case or parents and could be performed using linkage analysis if DNA was available from the index case and if polymorphisms can be identified within the gene.

Treatment

There is no known treatment for aspartoacylase deficiency at the present time. It would be of interest to know if inhibitors of the enzyme which synthesizes NAA could be developed and perhaps tested for safety and efficacy in animal models.

ANIMAL MODELS

Spongy degeneration of white matter has been reported in silver foxes,[78] Hereford calves,[79] an Egyptian Mau kitten, a Silkie terrier puppy, a Samoyed puppy, and Labrador retrievers (see Hagen and Bjerkå[76] for bibliography). In cases where adequate samples are available, it would be of interest to know if any of these animal models are associated with aspartoacylase deficiency, but not data have been reported to date. The literature implies that additional affected animals can be bred in the case of the silver foxes[78] and Hereford calves.[79] Obviously it would be possible to prepare a mouse model using gene targeting methodology.

REFERENCES

1. van Bogaert L, Bertrand I: Sur une idiotie familiale avec dégénérescence spongieuse de nevraxe. *Acta Neurol Belg* **49:**572, 1949.
2. van Bogaert L, Bertrand I: *Spongy Degeneration of the Brain in Infancy*. Amsterdam, North Holland Publishing Co., 1967, p. 3.
3. Globus JH, Strauss I: Progressive degenerative subcortical encephalopathy (Schilder's disease). *Arch Neurol Psychiat* **20:**1190, 1928.
4. Canavan MM: Schilder's encephalitis periaxialis diffusa. *Arch Neurol Psychiat* **25:**299, 1931.
5. Eiselsberg F: Über frühkindliche familiäre diffuse Hirnsklerose. *Z Kinderheilk* **58:**702, 1937.
6. Jervis GA: Early infantile acute diffuse sclerosis of the brain (Krabbe's type). *Am J Dis Child* **64:**1055, 1942.
7. Jervis GA: Early infantile acute diffuse sclerosis of brain (Krabbe's disease) *Mod Probl Pediatr* **1:**781, 1954.
8. Banker BQ, Robertson JT, Victor M: Spongy degeneration of the central nervous system in infancy. *Neurology* **14:**981, 1964.
9. Kvittingen EA, Guldal G, Børsting S, Skalpe IO, Stokke O, Jellum E: *N*-acetylaspartic aciduria in a child with a progressive cerebral atrophy. *Clin Chim Acta* **158:**217, 1986.
10. Hagenfeldt L, Bollgren I, Venizelos N: *N*-acetylaspartic aciduria due to aspartoacylase deficiency—a new aetiology of childhood leukodystrophy. *J Inherit Metab Dis* **10:**135, 1987.
11. Matalon R, Michals K, Sebesta D, Deanching M, Gashkoff P, Casanova J: Aspartoacylase deficiency and *N*-acetylaspartic aciduria in patients with Canavan disease. *Am J Med Genet* **29:**463, 1988.
12. Matalon R: Reply to Drs. Divry and Mathieu. *Am J Med Genet* **32:**551, 1989.
13. Divry P, Vianey-Liaud C, Gay C, Macabeo V, Rapin F, Echenne B: *N*-acetylaspartic aciduria: report of three new cases in children with a neurological syndrome associating macrocephaly and leukodystrophy. *J Inherit Metab Dis* **11:**307, 1988.
14. Divry P, Mathieu M: Aspartoacylase deficiency and *N*-acetylaspartic aciduria in patients with Canavan disease. *Am J Med Genet* **32:**550, 1989.
15. Kaul R, Gao GP, Balamurugan K, Matalon R: Cloning of the human aspartoacylase cDNA and a common missense mutation in Canavan disease. *Nat Genet* **5:**118, 1993.
16. Banker BQ, Victor M: Spongy degeneration of infancy, in Goodman RM, Motulsky AG (eds): *Genetic Diseases Among Ashkenazi Jews*. New York, Raven Press, 1979, p 201.

17. Buchanan DS, Davis RL: Spongy degeneration of the nervous system. *Neurology* **15**:207, 1965.
18. Ungar M, Goodman RM: Spongy degeneration of the brain in Israel: A retrospective study. *Clin Genet* **23**:23, 1983.
19. Adachi M, Aronson SM: Studies on spongy degeneration of the central nervous system (van Bogaert-Bertrand type), in Aronson SM, Volk BW (eds): *Inborn Disorders of Sphingolipid Metabolism*. Oxford, Pergamon Press, 1967, p 129.
20. von Moers A, Sperner J, Michael T, Scheffner D, Schutgens RHB: Variable course of Canavan disease in two boys with early infantile aspartoacylase deficiency. *Dev Med Child Neurol* **33**:824, 1991.
21. Zelnik N, Luder AS, Elpeleg ON, Gross-Tsur V, Amir N, Hemli JA, Fattal A, Harel S: Protracted clinical course for patients with Canavan disease. *Dev Med Child Neurol* **35**:355, 1993.
22. Adachi M, Volk BW: Protracted form of spongy degeneration of the central nervous system (van Bogaert and Bertrand type). *Neurology* **18**:1084, 1968.
23. Brucher JM, Dom R, Robin A: Degenerescence spongieuse juvenile du système nerve central. Ses rapports avec la maladie d'Hallervorden-Spatz et let dystrophies neuroaxonales. *Rev Neurol* **119**:425, 1968.
24. Jellinger K, Seitelberger F: Juvenile form of spongy degeneration of the CNS. *Acta Neuropathol* **13**:276, 1969.
25. Goodhue WW, Couch RD, Nakimi H: Spongy degeneration of the CNS. An instance of the rare juvenile form. *Arch Neurol* **36**:481, 1979.
26. Bakon M, Strauss S, Shental I, Elpeleg ON: Cholelithiasis in Canavan disease. *J Ultrasound Med* **12**:363, 1993.
27. Harbord MG, Harden A, Harding B, Brett EM, Baraitser M: Megalencephaly with dysmyelination, spasticity, ataxia, seizures and distinctive neurophysiological findings in two siblings. *Neuropediatrics* **21**:164, 1990.
28. Grodd W, Krägeloh-Mann I, Petersen D, Trefz FK, Harzer K: In vivo assessment of *N*-acetylaspartate in brain in spongy degeneration (Canavan's disease) by proton spectroscopy. *Lancet* **336**:437, 1990.
29. Brismar J, Brismar G, Gascon G, Ozand P: Canavan disease: CT and MR imaging of the brain. *AJNR Am J Neuroradiol* **11**:805, 1990.
30. Marks HG, Caro PA, Wang ZY, Detre JA, Bogdan AR, Gusnard DA, Zimmerman RA: Use of computed tomography, magnetic resonance imaging, and localized ^{1}H magnetic resonance spectroscopy in Canavan's disease: A case report. *Ann Neurol* **30**:106, 1991.
31. Austin SJ, Connelly A, Gadian DG, Benton JS, Brett EM: Localized ^{1}H NMR spectroscopy in Canavan's disease: A report of two cases. *Magn Reson Med* **19**:439, 1991.
32. Grodd W, Krägeloh-Mann I, Klose U, Sauter R: Metabolic and destructive brain disorders in children: Findings with localized proton MR spectroscopy. *Radiology* **181**:173, 1991.
33. Barker PB, Bryan RN, Kumar AJ, Naidu S: Proton NMR spectroscopy of Canavan's disease. *Neuropediatrics* **23**:263, 1992.
34. Toft PB, Geiss-Holtorff R, Rolland MO, Pryds O, Müller-Forell W, Christensen E, Lehnert W, Lou HC, Ott D, Hennig J, Henriksen O: Magnetic resonance imaging in juvenile Canavan disease. *Eur J Pediatr* **152**:750, 1993.
35. Bührer C, Bassir C, von Moers A, Sperner J, Michael T, Scheffner D, Kaufmann HJ: Cranial ultrasound findings in aspartoacylase deficiency (Canavan disease). *Pediatr Radio* **23**:395, 1993.
36. McAdams HP, Geyer CA, Done SL, Deigh D, Mitchell M, Ghaed VN: CT and MR imaging of Canavan disease. *AJNR Am J Neuroradiol* **11**:397, 1990.
37. Birken DL, Oldendorf WH: *N*-acetyl-L-aspartic acid: A literature review of a compound prominent in ^{1}H-NMR spectroscopic studies of brain. *Neurosci Biobehav Reb* **13**:23, 1989.
38. Elpeleg ON, Amir N, Barash V, Glick B, Gross-Tsur V, Shachar E, Shapira Y, Tzelnik N: Canavan disease and *N*-acetylaspartic aciduria. *Neuropediatrics* **20**:238, 1989.
39. Ozand PT, Gascon GG, Dhalla M: Aspartoacylase deficiency and Canavan disease in Saudi Arabia. *Am J Med Genet* **35**:266, 1990.
40. Yalaz K, Topçu M, Topaloğlu H, Gürçay Ö, Özcan OE, Önol B, Renda Y: N-acetylaspartic aciduria in Canavan disease: Another proof in two infants. *Neuropediatrics* **21**:140, 1990.
41. Michelakakis H, Giouroukos S, Divry P, Katsarou E, Rolland MO, Skardoutsou A: Canavan disease: Findings in four new cases. *J Inherit Metab Dis* **14**:267, 1991.
42. de Coo IFM, Gabreëls FJM, Renier WO, DePont JJHHM, van Haelst UJGM, Veerkamp JH, Trijbels JMF, Jaspar HHJ, Renkawek K: Canavan disease: Neuromorphological and biochemical analysis of a brain biopsy specimen. *Clin Neuropathol* 10:73, 1991.
43. Ozand PT, Devlo EB, Gascon GG: Neurometabolic diseases at a national referral center: Five years experience at the King Faisal Specialist Hospital and Research Centre. *J Child Neurol Suppl* **7**:S4, 1992.
44. Bartalini G, Margollicci M, Balestri P, Farnetani MA, Cioni M, Fois A: Biochemical diagnosis of Canavan disease. *Child Nerv Syst* **8**:468, 1992.
45. Matalon R, Kaul R, Casanova J, Michals K, Johnson A, Rapin I, Gashkoff P, Deanching M: Aspartoacylase deficiency: The enzyme defect in Canavan disease. *J Inherit Metab Dis Suppl* **12**:329, 1989.
46. Ozand PT, Gascon GG, Al Aqeel A, Nester MJ, Feryal RR, Gleispach H, Cook JD, Al Odaib A, Leis HJ: Prenatal detection of Canavan disease. *Lancet* **337**:735, 1991.
47. Wolman M: The spongy type of diffuse sclerosis. *Brain* **81**:243, 1958.
48. Adachi M, Torii J, Schneck L, Volk BW: Electron microscopic and enzyme histochemical studies of the cerebellum in spongy degeneration (van Bogaert and Bertrand type). *Acta Neuropathol (Berl)* **20**:22, 1972.
49. Lees MB, Folch-Pi J: A study of some human brains with pathological changes, in Folch-Pi J (ed): *Chemical Pathology of the Nervous System*. Oxford, Pergamon Press, 1961, p 75.
50. Kamoshita S, Rapin I, Suzuki K, Suzuki K: Spongy degeneration of the brain. *Neurology (Minneap)* **19**:975, 1968.
51. Tallan HH, Moore S, Stein WH: *N*-acetyl-L-aspartic acid in brain. *J Biol Chem* **219**:257, 1956.
52. Knizley Jr, H.: The enzymatic synthesis of *N*-acetyl-L-aspartic acid by a water-insoluble preparation of a cat brain acetone powder. *J Biol Chem* **242**:4619, 1967.
53. Goldstein FB: Biosynthesis of *N*-acetyl-L-aspartic acid. *J Biol Chem* **234**:2702, 1959.
54. Goldstein FB: The enzymatic synthesis of *N*-acetyl-L-aspartic acid by subcellular preparations of rat brain. *J Biol Chem* **244**:4257, 1969.
55. Patel TB, Clark JB: Synthesis of *N*-acetyl-L-aspartate by rat brain mitochondria and its involvement in mitochondrial/cytosolic carbon transport. *Biochem J* **184**:539, 1979.
56. Truckenmiller ME, Namboodiri MAA, Brownstein MJ, Neale JH: *N*-acetylation of L-aspartate in the nervous system: Differential distribution of a specific enzyme. *J Neurochem* **45**:1658, 1985.
57. Sekiguchi M, Okamoto K, Sakai Y: Excitatory action of *N*-acetylaspartylglutamate on Purkinje cells in guinea pig cerebellar slices: an intrasomatic study. *Brain Res* **423**:23, 1987.
58. Shigematsu H, Okamura N, Shimeno H, Kishimoto Y, Kan L-s, Fenselau C: Purification and characterization of the heat-stable factors essential for the conversion of lignoceric acid to cerebronic acid and glutamic acid: Identification of *N*-acetyl-L-aspartic acid. *J Neurochem* **40**:814, 1983.
59. Reichelt KL, Fonnum F: Subcellular localization of *N*-acetyl-aspartyl-glutamate, *N*-acetyl-glutamate and glutahione in brain. *J Neurochem* **16**:1409, 1969.
60. Moffett JR, Namboodiri MAA, Cangro CB, Neale JH: Immunohistochemical localization of *N*-acetylaspartate in rat brain. *NeuroReport* **2**:131, 1991.
61. Moffett JR, Namboodiri MAA, Neale JH: Enchanced carbodiimide fixation for immunohistochemistry: Application to the comparative distributions of *N*-acetylaspartylglutamate and *N*-acetylaspartate immunoreactivities in rat brain. *J Histochem Cytochem* **41**:559, 1993.
62. Ory-Lavollée L, Blakely RD, Coyle JT: Neurochemical and immunocytochemical studies on the distribution of *N*-acetyl-aspartylglutamate and *N*-acetyl-aspartate in rat spinal cord and some peripheral nervous tissues. *J Neurochem* **48**:895, 1987.

63. Birnbaum SM: Aminoacylase: Amino acid acylases I and II from hog kidney. *Methods Enzymol* **2:**115, 1955.
64. Birnbaum SM, Levintow L, Kingsley RB, Greenstein JP: Specificity of amino acid acylases. *J Biol Chem* **194:**455, 1952.
65. Kaul R, Casanova J, Johnson AB, Tang P, Matalon R: Purification, characterization, and localization of aspartoacylase from bovine brain. *J Neurochem* **56:**129, 1991.
66. Goldstein FB: Amidohydrolases of brain; enzymatic hydrolysis of *N*-acetyl-L-aspartate and other *N*-acetyl-L-amino acids. *J Neurochem* **26:**45, 1976.
67. Tallan HH: Studies on the distribution of *N*-acetyl-L-aspartic acid in brain. J Biol Chem **224:**41, 1957.
68. Matalon R, Kaul R, Michals K: Canavan disease: Biochemical and molecular studies. *J Inherit Metab Dis* **16:**744, 1993.
69. Kaul R, Balamurugan K, Gao GP, Matalon R: Canavan disease: Genomic organization and localization of human *ASPA* to 17p13-ter and conservation of the *ASPA* gene during evolution. *Genomics* **21:**364, 1994.
70. Kaul R, Gao GP, Aloya M, Balamurugan K, Petrosky A, Michals K, Matalon R: Canavan disease: Mutations among Jewish and non-Jewish patients. *Am J Hum Genet* **55:**34, 1994.
71. Jakobs C, ten Brink HJ, Langelaar SA, Zee T, Stellaard F, Macek M, Sršňová K, Sršeň Š, Kleijer WJ: Stable isotope dilution analysis of *N*-acetylaspartic acid in CSF, blood, urine and amniotic fluid: Accurate postnatal diagnosis and the potential for prenatal diagnosis of Canavan disease. *J Inherit Metab Dis* **14:**653, 1991.
72. Kelley RI, Stamas JN: Quantification of *N*-acetyl-L-aspartic acid in urine by isotope dilution gas chromatography-mass spectrometry. *J Inherit Metab Dis* **15:**97, 1992.
73. Barash V, Flhor D, Morag B, Boneh A, Elpeleg ON, Gilon C: A radiometric assay for aspartoacylase activity in human fibroblasts: Application for the diagnosis of Canavan's disease. *Clin Chim Acta* **201:**175, 1991.
74. Jakobs C, ten Brink HJ, Divry P, Rolland MO: Prenatal diagnosis of Canavan disease. *Eur J Pediatr* **151:**620, 1992.
75. Kelley RI: Prenatal detection of Canavan disease by measurement of *N*-acetyl-L-asparate in amniotic fluid. *J Inherit Metab Dis* **16:**918, 1993.
76. Matalon R, Michals K, Gashkoff P, Kaul R: Prenatal diagnosis of Canavan disease. *J Inherit Metab Dis* **15:**392, 1992.
77. Bennett MJ, Gibson KM, Sherwood WG, Divry P, Rolland MO, Elpeleg ON, Rinaldo P, Jakobs C: Reliable prenatal diagnosis of Canavan disease (aspartoacylase deficiency): Comparison of enzymatic and metabolite analysis. *J Inherit Metab Dis* **16:**831, 1993.
78. Hagen G, Bjerkås I: Spongy degeneration of white matter in the central nervous system of silver foxes (*Vulpes vulpes*). *Vet Pathol* **27:**187, 1990.
79. Duffel SJ: Neuraxial oedema of Hereford calves with and without hypomyelinogenesis. *Vet Rec* **118:**95, 1986.

STANDARD ABBREVIATIONS

Abbreviation	Name
ACTH	corticotropin (adrenocorticotropin, adrenocorticotropic hormone)
ADA	adenosine deaminase
AdoMet	s-adenosylmethionine
Ag	antigen
AIDS	acquired immunodeficiency syndrome
ALT	alanine aminotransferase
AMP, ADP, and ATP*	adenosine 5′-mono-, di-, and triphosphates
apo A-I	apolipoprotein A-I
apo A-II	apolipoprotein A-II
apo A-III	apolipoprotein A-III
apo B	apolipoprotein B
apo C-I	apolipoprotein C-I
apo C-II	apolipoprotein C-II
apo C-III	apolipoprotein C-III
apo D	apolipoprotein D
apo E	apolipoprotein E
APRT	adenine phosphoribosyltransferase
ASO	allele specific oligonucleotide
AST	aspartate aminotransferase
ATPase	adenosine triphosphate
α_1AT	α_1-antitrypsin
cAMP, cGMP, etc.	cyclic AMP (adenosine 3′: 5′-monophosphate), etc.
cDNA	complementary DNA
CHO cells	Chinese hamster ovary cells
CoA (or CoASH)	coenzyme A
CoASAc	acetyl coenzyme A
cM	centimorgan
Cm-cellulose	O-(carboxymethyl)cellulose
CMP, CDP, and CTP*	cytidine 5′-mono-, di-, and triphosphates
COS cells	CV-I origin, SV40; cells widely used for transfection studies
CPK	creatine phosphokinase
CRM	cross-reacting material
CT	computerized tomography
CVS	chorionic villus sampling
DEAE-cellulose	O-(diethylaminoethyl)cellulose
DNA	deoxyribonucleic acid
DNase	deoxyribonuclease
DOPA	3,4-dihydroxyphenylalanine
DPN, DPN^+, $DPNH^+$	diphosphopyridine nucleotide and its oxidized and reduced forms
dTMP, dTDP, and dTTP*	thymidine 5′-mono-, di-, and triphosphates
DTT	dithiothreitol
EBV	Epstein-Barr virus
EDTA	ethylenediaminetetraacetate
EEG	electroencephalogram
EGF	epidermal growth factor
EGTA	[ethylenebis(oxyethylenenitrilo)] tetraacetic acid
EKG	electrocardiogram
ELISA	enzyme-linked immunosorbent assay
EM	electron microscopy or microscopic
ER	endoplasmic reticulum
FAD and $FADH_2$	flavin-adenine dinucleotide and its fully reduced form
FISH	fluorescence in situ hybridization
FITC	fluorescein isothiocyanate
FMN	riboflavin 5′-phosphate
G, G_i, G_s	guanine nucleotide binding protein, inhibitory form, stimulatory form
G-6-PD	glucose 6-phosphate dehydrogenase
GABA	γ-aminobutyric acid
GC	gas chromotography
GC/MS	gas chromotography/mass spectroscopy
GERL	golgi endoplasmic reticulum-like
GFR	glomerular filtration rate
GMP, GDP, and GTP*	guanosine 5′-mono-, di-, and triphosphates
GSH and GSSG	glutathione and its oxidized form
Hb, HbCO, HbO_2	hemoglobin, carbon monoxide hemoglobin, oxyhemoglobin
HDL	high density lipoprotein
HEPES	4-(2-hydroxyethyl)-1-piperazine ethanesulfonic acid
Hep G2	hepatocellular carcinoma human cell line
HIV	human immunodeficiency virus
HLA	human leukocyte antigens
HMG-CoA	3-hydroxy-3-methylglutaryl-coenzyme A
HPLC	high performance (or pressure) liquid chromotography
HPRT	hypoxanthine-guanine phosphoribosyltransferase
Ig	immunoglobulin
IgA	gamma A immunoglobulin
IgG	gamma G immunoglobulin
IgM	gamma M immunoglobulin
IL	interleukin, including IL-1, IL-2, etc.
IMP, IDP, and ITP*	inosine 5′-mono-, di, and triphosphates
LDH	lactate dehydrogenase
LDL	low density lipoproteins
lod	logarithm of the odds
MCH	mean corpuscular hemoglobin
MCHC	mean corpuscular hemoglobin concentration
MCV	mean corpuscular volume
MHC	histocompatibility complex
MPS	mucopolysaccharide or mucopolysaccharidosis
MRI	magnetic resonance imaging
mRNA	messenger RNA
MS	mass spectrometry
mtDNA, mtRNA	mitochondrial DNA, RNA
NAD, NAD^+, and $NADH^+$	nicotinamide adenine dinucleotide and its oxidized and reduced forms
NADP, $NADP^+$, and $NADPH^+$	nicotinamide adenine dinucleotide phosphate and its oxidized and reduced forms
NMN	nicotinamide mononucleotide
NMR	nuclear magnetic resonance
p	probability
P_i	inorganic phosphate
PAS	periodic acid Schiff
PCR	polymerase chain reaction
PEG	polyethylene glycol
PFGE	pulsed-field gel electrophoresis
PKU	phenylketonuria
PP_i	inorganic pyrophosphate
PP-ribose-P	phosphoribosylpyrophosphate
RER	rough endoplasmic reticulum
RFLP	restriction fragment length polymorphism
rRNA	ribosomal RNA
RNase	ribonuclease
RT-PCR	reverse transcription-polymerase chain reaction
SD	standard deviation
SDS	sodium dodecyl sulfate

(*Continues*)

STANDARD ABBREVIATIONS (*Cont.*)

Abbreviation	Name	Abbreviation	Name
SDS-PAGE	sodium dodecyl sulfate polyacrylamide gel electrophoresis	TPN, TPN^+, TPNH†	triphosphopyridine nucleotide and its oxidized and reduced forms
SE	standard error	Tris	tris(hydroxymethyl)aminomethane
SEM	standard error of mean	tRNA	transfer RNA
SER	smooth endoplasmic reticulum	UDP-Gal	uridine diphosphogalactose
SSCP	single strand conformational polymorphism	UDP-Glc	uridine diphosphoglucose
STR	short tandem repeat	UMP, UDP, and UTP*	uridine 5′-mono-, di-, and triphosphates
SV40	Simian virus 40	UV	ultraviolet light
T_3	triiodothyronine	VLDL	very low density lipoprotein
T_4	thyroxine	VNTR	variable number tandem repeat
TMP, TDP, and TTP*	ribosylthymine 5′-mono-, di-, and triphosphates	YAC	yeast artificial chromosome

*The d prefix may be used to represent the corresponding deoxyribonucleoside phosphates, e.g. dADP.
†Note that DPN = NAD and TPN = NADP.

AMINO ACID SYMBOLS

Name	Symbols		Name	Symbols	
alanine	Ala	A	leucine	Leu	L
arginine	Arg	R	lysine	Lys	K
asparagine	Asn	N	methionine	Met	M
aspartic acid	Asp	D	phenylalanine	Phe	F
cysteine	Cys	C	proline	Pro	P
glutamic acid	Glu	E	serine	Ser	S
glutamine	Gln	Q	threonine	Thr	T
glycine	Gly	G	tryptophan	Trp	W
histidine	His	H	tyrosine	Tyr	Y
isoleucine	Ile	I	valine	Val	V

CARBOHYDRATE SYMBOLS

Name	Symbols	Name	Symbols
fructose	Fru	N-acetylgalactosamine	GalNAc
fucose	Fuc	N-acetylglucosamine	GlcNAc
galactose	Gal	N-acetylneuraminic acid	NeuAc
glucosamine	GlcN	ribose	Rib
glucose	Glc	sialic acid	Sia
glucuronic acid	GlcA	xylose	Xyl
mannose	Man		

INDEX

Three-volume set code

ISBN 0-07-909826-6

P/N 060729-X Volume I
P/N 060730-3 Volume II
P/N 060731-1 Volume III

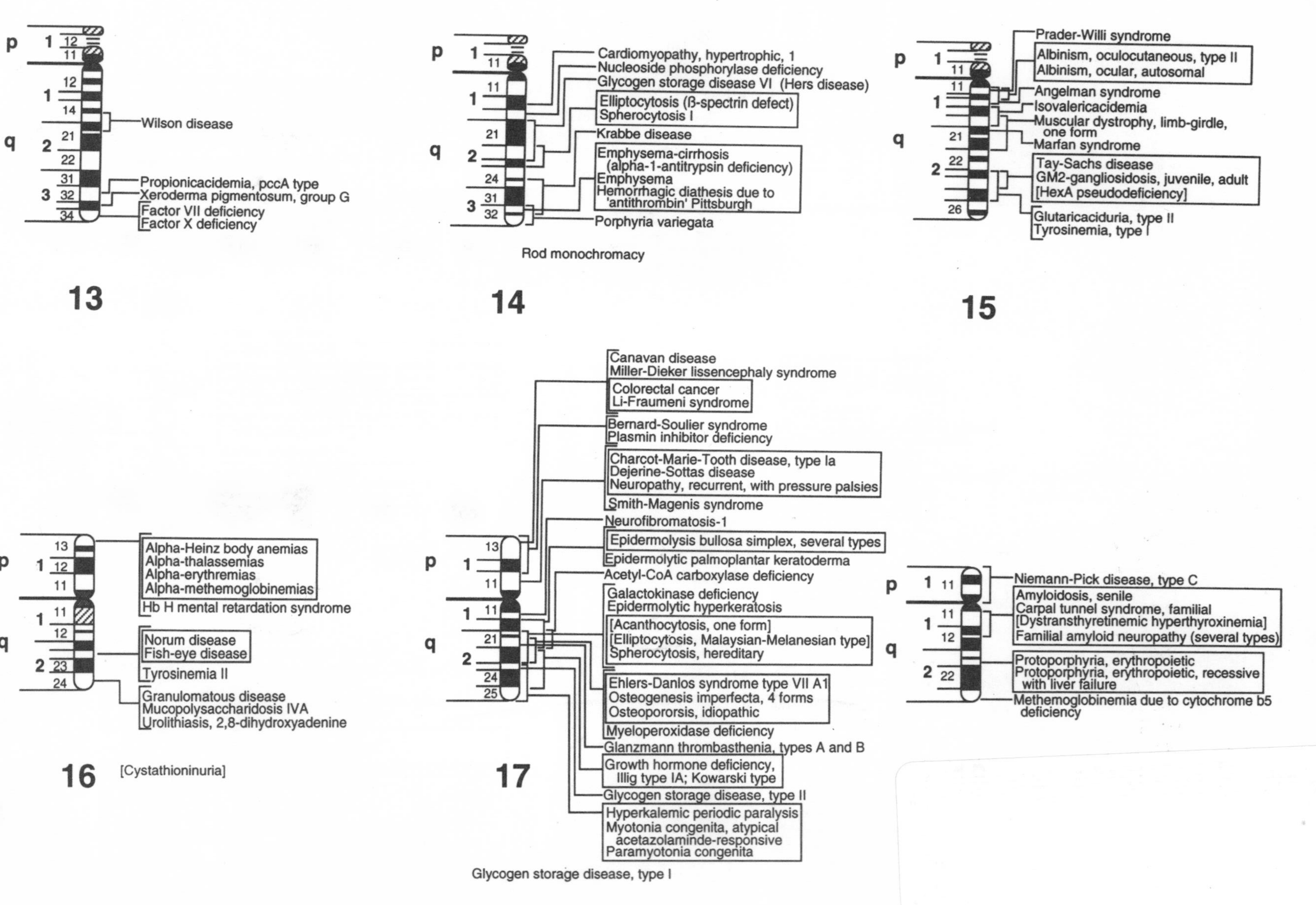

13
Wilson disease
Propionicacidemia, pccA type
Xeroderma pigmentosum, group G
Factor VII deficiency
Factor X deficiency
14
Cardiomyopathy, hypertrophic, 1
Nucleoside phosphorylase deficiency
Glycogen storage disease VI (Hers disease)
Elliptocytosis (ß-spectrin defect)
Spherocytosis I
Krabbe disease
Emphysema-cirrhosis (alpha-1-antitrypsin deficiency)
Emphysema
Hemorrhagic diathesis due to 'antithrombin' Pittsburgh
Porphyria variegata
Rod monochromacy
15
Prader-Willi syndrome
Albinism, oculocutaneous, type II
Albinism, ocular, autosomal
Angelman syndrome
Isovalericacidemia
Muscular dystrophy, limb-girdle, one form
Marfan syndrome
Tay-Sachs disease
GM2-gangliosidosis, juvenile, adult
[HexA pseudodeficiency]
Glutaricaciduria, type II
Tyrosinemia, type I
16
Alpha-Heinz body anemias
Alpha-thalassemias
Alpha-erythremias
Alpha-methemoglobinemias
Hb H mental retardation syndrome
Norum disease
Fish-eye disease
Tyrosinemia II
Granulomatous disease
Mucopolysaccharidosis IVA
Urolithiasis, 2,8-dihydroxyadenine
[Cystathioninuria]
17
Canavan disease
Miller-Dieker lissencephaly syndrome
Colorectal cancer
Li-Fraumeni syndrome
Bernard-Soulier syndrome
Plasmin inhibitor deficiency
Charcot-Marie-Tooth disease, type Ia
Dejerine-Sottas disease
Neuropathy, recurrent, with pressure palsies
Smith-Magenis syndrome
Neurofibromatosis-1
Epidermolysis bullosa simplex, several types
Epidermolytic palmoplantar keratoderma
Acetyl-CoA carboxylase deficiency
Galactokinase deficiency
Epidermolytic hyperkeratosis
[Acanthocytosis, one form]
[Elliptocytosis, Malaysian-Melanesian type]
Spherocytosis, hereditary
Ehlers-Danlos syndrome type VII A1
Osteogenesis imperfecta, 4 forms
Osteopororsis, idiopathic
Myeloperoxidase deficiency
Glanzmann thrombasthenia, types A and B
Growth hormone deficiency, Illig type IA; Kowarski type
Glycogen storage disease, type II
Hyperkalemic periodic paralysis
Myotonia congenita, atypical acetazolaminde-responsive
Paramyotonia congenita
Glycogen storage disease, type I
18
Niemann-Pick disease, type C
Amyloidosis, senile
Carpal tunnel syndrome, familial
[Dystransthyretinemic hyperthyroxinemia]
Familial amyloid neuropathy (several types)
Protoporphyria, erythropoietic
Protoporphyria, erythropoietic, recessive with liver failure
Methemoglobinemia due to cytochrome b5 deficiency

(*Continued*)

suggested also by linkage studies[185–187]) could produce similar phenotypes (see Fig. 134–6).

Diagnosis, Treatment, and Prenatal Diagnosis. The diagnosis of OI type I is first suspected clinically, usually because of the presence of a dominant family history, the observation of blue sclerae in the patient, and bone fractures, and is confirmed by measuring the production of type I procollagen by dermal fibroblasts in culture. Ordinarily, about 85 percent of the collagen synthesized by these cells is type I procollagen and most of the remainder is type III procollagen; cells from patients with OI type I synthesize about half the normal amount of type I procollagen but a normal amount of other proteins. In rare families (see above), other types of mutations may be found. Diagnosis is particularly important in the newly affected infant for whom there is no family history because it can facilitate genetic counseling and help to reassure the family about prognosis. It can also remove the concern of child abuse in some families, and it may be important for families to have a letter from the child's physician stating the diagnosis.

There are currently no treatments for OI type I that reliably and predictably decrease the frequency of bone fracture or increase bone density. From a theoretical point of view, agents that increase the production of type I collagen have therapeutic potential but none has yet been proved effective in controlled tests.

Prenatal identification of affected fetuses can be provided by any of several methods that identify the mutant allele including segregation studies with an appropriate family structure, identification of the nonexpressed allele in mRNA from the fetus, or by recognition of fracture or bowing of long bones by ultrasound. Allele segregation studies would provide diagnosis at 11 to 12 weeks of gestation if chorionic villus samples were used. Analysis of the amount of type I procollagen synthesized by cells cultured from chorionic villus samples taken at 9 to 10 weeks of gestation could provide a means to detect affected fetuses early in gestation. However, our experience has been that the amount of type I procollagen synthesized by cultured chorionic villus cells varies with time in culture so that the ability to identify alterations in the proportions of different molecules made by the cells may be compromised. Because of this experience, we have been reluctant to use cultured chorionic villus cells, even with age-in-culture and gestational-age–matched controls, for diagnostic studies based on protein analysis alone. Amniotic fluid cells are not useful in establishing the diagnosis at the protein level because the major population of cells that grows out does not synthesize normal type I procollagen.[196,197]

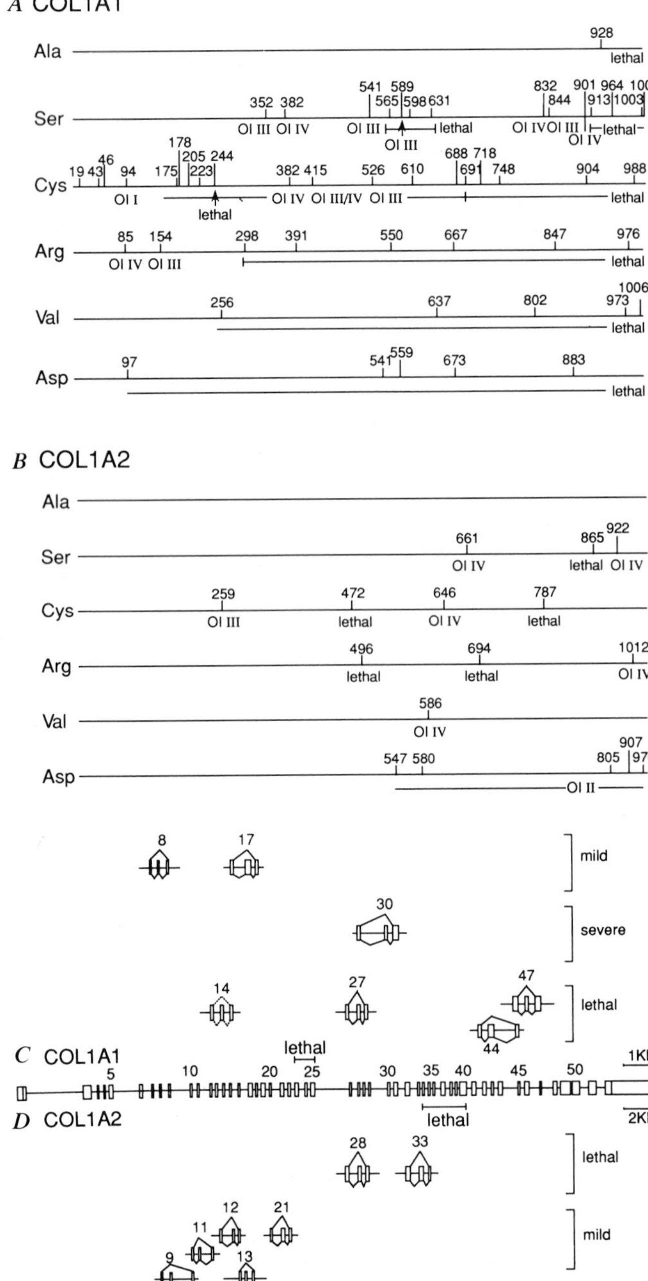

FIG. 134-6 Summary of known mutations that result in OI. Point mutations (*A* and *B*) are shown along horizontal lines representing the triple-helical domain of the proα1(I) (*A*) and proα2(I) (*B*) chains. The amino acid at the left indicates the substituting residue and the number indicates the position of the glycine within the triple helix that is substituted. The phenotype is indicated below the line. Exon skipping mutations and genomic deletions in the COL1A1 and COL1A2 genes that result in OI (*C* and *D*).

Osteogenesis Imperfecta Type II (Perinatal Lethal)

Genetics and Natural History. OI type II, the perinatal lethal form of OI, affects between 1 in 20,000 and 1 in 60,000 infants.[198] Prematurity and low birth weight are common. Affected infants have a characteristic facial appearance with dark sclerae, beaked nose, and extremely soft calvarium. The extremities are short, the legs are bowed, and the hips are usually in a flexed and abducted (frog-leg) position; the thoracic cavity is generally very small. The radiologic picture is characteristic but exhibits some heterogeneity[199] (Fig. 134-7). All infants have markedly telescoped femurs, bowed tibias, and virtual absence of calvarial mineralization. The ribs are generally beaded, although they may be broad throughout; frank fractures are rare in the newborn period and the vertebral bodies may be flattened. Death usually results from respiratory failure and frequently occurs during the first few hours following birth. More than 60 percent of infants with OI type II die during the first day, 80 percent die within the first month, and survival beyond a year must be rare.[199] With the increasing use of routine early gestational ultrasound, first affected infants in families are being detected during the second trimester of pregnancy.[200–202]